D0204247

Maternal-Child Nursing Care

Optimizing Outcomes for Mothers, Children, & Families

MATERNAL-CHILD NURSING CARE

with The Women's Health Companion

SECOND EDITION

LOOK FOR THESE ICONS.

They identify the themes you'll follow throughout your text.

  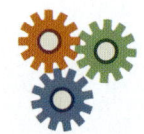   

HOLISTIC CARE   **VALIDATING PRACTICE**   **TOOLS OF CARE**   **CRITICAL THINKING**

PREVIEW WHAT YOU'LL LEARN

Learning Targets introduce you to the major concepts and important information in each chapter.

PICO(T) Questions (**p**opulation • **i**ntervention or **i**ssue • **c**omparison of interest • **o**utcome • **t**imeframe) emphasize the importance of evidence-based practice and how it relates to the content in the chapter.

---

chapter
20

Caring for the Developing Child

"**It** is when we include caring and love in our science, we discover our caring-healing professions and disciplines are much more than a detached scientific endeavor, but a life-giving and life-receiving endeavor for humanity."

—Watson, 2005 p. 3

LEARNING TARGETS   *At the completion of this chapter, the student will be able to:*

- Describe the principles inherent in the developmental process.
- Identify and explain the theories of growth and development.
- Discuss the components for each developmental stage.
- Address anticipatory guidance for each developmental stage.
- Develop a developmental care plan for the child and family.

PICO(T) Questions

The intent of evidence-based practice (EBP) is to provide nursing care that integrates the best available evidence. An initial step in EBP is to write a PICO(T) question that effectively guides the research. A PICO(T) question is an acronym that stands for population (P), intervention or issue (I), comparison of interest (C), outcome (O), and timeframe (T). Depending on the question, all or some of the question components are used in the research process. Use these

PICO(T) questions to spark your thinking as you read the chapter.

1. Does (I) being raised in a single-parent household (O) impact behavioral development (P) in toddlers?

2. Do (P) preschool-age children without siblings who attend group day care (I) develop physical skills (O) at the same rate on average as (C) preschool children with siblings who do not attend group day care?

PREPARE FOR THE REAL WORLD OF NURSING PRACTICE.

"What to say" — *When asked about sexual activity during pregnancy*

Couples have many questions regarding sexual activity during pregnancy. These questions relate to the safety of sexual intercourse, potential complications, when to stop having intercourse, and sexual positions that facilitate comfort. It is important for the health-care provider to address sexual activity early in the pregnancy in an honest, open manner and to encourage the couple to communicate with each other. The nurse can address the couple's concerns with the following statements:

"What to Say" develops your communication skills through examples and helpful hints.

Optimizing Outcomes show you how to establish the course of action that achieves the best possible outcomes for your patient.

 Optimizing Outcomes— **Teaching patients to avoid bone meal supplements**

Bone meal, sometimes used as a calcium source, should be avoided during pregnancy. This supplement is frequently contaminated with lead, a toxin that readily crosses the placenta and can result in high levels in the fetus.

Evidence-Based Practice

O'Connor, P. J., Poudevigne, M. S., Cress, M. E., Motl, R. W., & Clapp, J. F. (2011). Safety and efficacy of supervised strength training adopted in pregnancy. *Journal of Physical Activity and Health 8*, 309–320.

Previous studies have found that physical inactivity predisposes to reduced fitness and increased fetal and maternal risks during pregnancy. Maternal fitness and several aspects of fetal and maternal health have previously been found to improve through the use of low- to moderate-intensity exercise during pregnancy. The purpose of this study was to describe the progression of supervised, low- to moderate-intensity strength training program implemented among a sample of pregnant women. A further purpose was to explore the incidence of associated musculoskeletal injuries, lumbar endurance, blood pressure changes, and the occurrence of problematic symptoms, (e.g., swelling in hands or feet; headache or visual disturbance; chest, pelvic, or abdominal pain; irregular heartbeats or dizziness; and unexpected vaginal bleeding or leaking).

The sample was composed of 32 healthy pregnant women who were primarily recruited through midwives and obstetricians. The participants were between 21 and 25 weeks of gestation and their ages ranged from 18 to 38 years of age. They were at low risk for any pregnancy-related complications and free from back pain or a history of back pain. Women who reported use of regular strength training and those who reported uncontrolled psychiatric conditions and orthopedic or cardiovascular limitations were excluded.

Prior to initiating the exercise program, experienced trainers taught and supervised participants on the use of strength training and specific types of exercises. The participants were then expected to implement strength training twice a week for a 12-week period. Data recorded included blood pressure, extension endurance exercise test, and report of symptoms or musculoskeletal injuries. Participants were instructed to complete a warm-up that included 5 minutes of walking on a treadmill. Following the warm-up, participants performed six resistance exercises: dual leg extension, dual leg press, dual arm lat pull, dual leg curl, lumbar extensions, and a transverse abdominis muscle (abdominal) exercise. Using the Universal Gym and Cybex Eagle for the first five exercises, the number of sets and repetitions were constant throughout the

training at a low to moderate velocity with scheduled rest periods between exercises. Participants were instructed to rate exercise intensity using a rated perceived exertion (RPE) scale. A rating of 13 represented moderate intensity, 11 represented fairly light, and ratings of 10 or less represented low intensity. External load was progressively increased based on RPE responses to each exercise. Participants usually performed the abdominal exercise from a standing position and were asked to draw in their abdominal muscles as if trying to reach the spine. Repetitions were held at 8 throughout the training. Five minutes after completing the training, the blood pressures were measured, and participants were asked about potential problematic symptoms and back pain.

The researchers stated that no musculoskeletal injuries were reported for women at risk for low back pain. No chest palpitations or chest pains were reported. Symptoms were reported 13 times and included dizziness (8/13) and abdominal/pelvic pain (4/13). One person reported a headache. Most symptoms were reported within the first 3 weeks of the study. The percentage of increase in the external load across the 12 weeks was found to be statistically significant and reported as follows: leg presses (36%), leg curl (39%), lat pull down (39%), lumbar extension (41%), and leg extensions (56%). The researchers reported that exercises were performed at a low to moderate perceived intensity with a mean RPE of 10.5 to 12.9, which did not change significantly throughout the 12-week period. A 14% increase in lumbar endurance was reported. No significant changes in blood pressure were reported during and at the conclusion of the 12-week training. The researchers concluded that use of supervised, low- to moderate-intensity strength training during pregnancy is safe and efficacious.

1. "How is this information useful to clinical nursing practice?"
2. "Based on these findings, what are implications for further research?"

See Suggested Responses for Evidence-Based Practice on Davis*Plus*.

Evidence-Based Practice Boxes and Questions highlight current research and encourage you to think about how you can incorporate evidence-based findings into your practice.

Focus on Safety highlights important protective measures to keep mothers and children out of harm's way.

Review Questions

Multiple Choice

1. The pediatric nurse assesses the toddler's fine motor skills by observing which task?
   A. Buttoning a shirt
   B. Writing with a pencil
   C. Holding a spoon to eat
   D. Using the pincer grasp

2. According to Piaget, an infant uses his or her senses to learn and explore the environment. Which action is the most appropriate for the nurse to implement to determine object permanence?
   A. Playing the game of peek-a-boo
   B. Encouraging the infant to shake a rattle
   C. Pushing a button on an overhead mobile
   D. Placing the child in a stroller and going for a walk

NCLEX-Style Review Questions at the end of each chapter help you identify your areas of strength/weakness and prepare you for course tests and national licensure examination.

Nursing Care Plans provide the in-depth information you need to plan and care for patients with commonly encountered normal and pathological conditions.

Nursing Diagnoses, based on the information you obtain during your nursing assessment, form the basis for your selection of the nursing interventions that will address the problem.

Nursing Care Plan Delayed Growth and Development

Nursing Diagnosis: Delayed growth and development, related to chronic illness

Measurable Short-term Outcome: Child will maintain current weight and participate in age-appropriate activities, as possible.

Measurable Long-term Outcome: Child will reach age-appropriate growth and developmental milestones.

NOC Outcomes:
   Growth (0110) Normal increase in bone size and body weight during growth years
   Child Development: Middle Childhood (0108) Milestones of physical, cognitive, and psychosocial progression from 6 through 11 years of age (specify other age groups as appropriate)
   Play Participation (0116) Use of activities by a child from 1 year through 11 years of age to promote enjoyment, entertainment, and development

NIC Interventions:
   Nutrition Management (1100)
   Developmental Enhancement: Child (8274)
   Normalization Promotion (7200)
   Activity Therapy (4310)

Nursing Interventions:

1. Build a trusting, supportive relationship with child and caregivers by taking time, actively listening to concerns, and offering information and encouragement.
   RATIONALE: A trusting relationship facilitates implementation of developmental interventions.

2. Monitor child's height and weight (specify frequency) and record on a continuous flow sheet.
   RATIONALE: A flow sheet provides a continuous record of the child's growth over time.

CONCEPT MAP

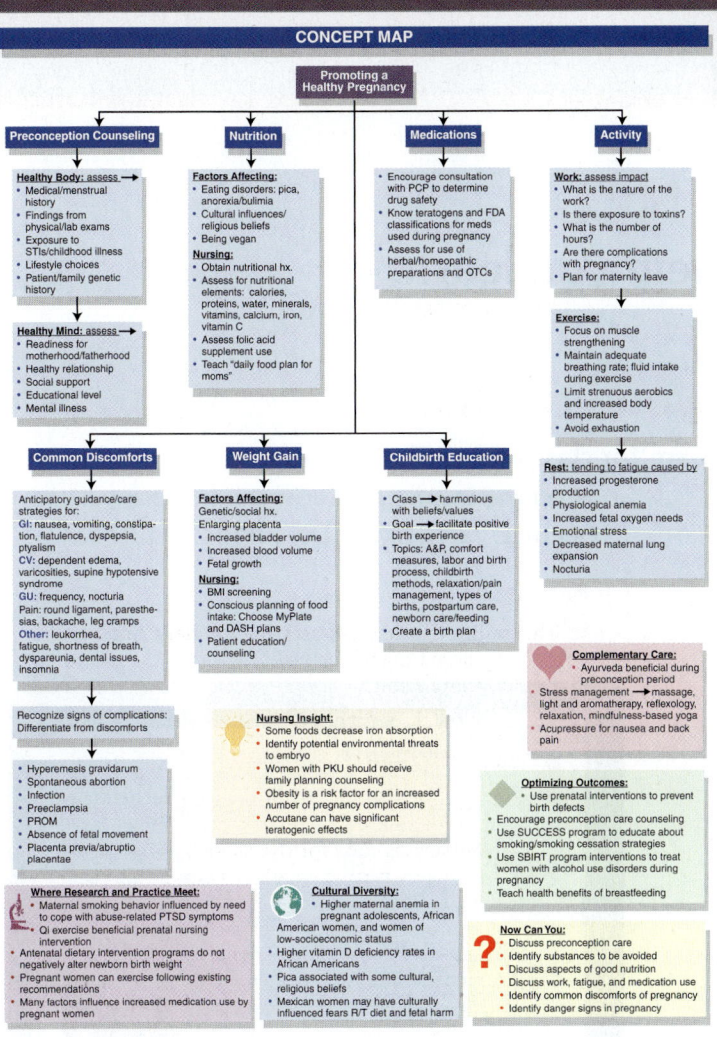

Promoting a Healthy Pregnancy

Preconception Counseling

Healthy Body: assess →
- Medical/menstrual history
- Findings from physical/lab exams
- Exposure to STIs/childhood illness
- Lifestyle choices
- Patient/family genetic history

Healthy Mind: assess →
- Readiness for motherhood/fatherhood
- Healthy relationship
- Social support
- Educational level
- Mental illness

Nutrition

Factors Affecting:
- Eating disorders: pica, anorexia/bulimia
- Cultural influences/religious beliefs
- Being vegan

Nursing:
- Obtain nutritional hx.
- Assess for nutritional elements: calories, proteins, water, minerals, vitamins, calcium, iron, vitamin C
- Assess folic acid supplement use
- Teach "daily food plan for moms"

Medications
- Encourage consultation with PCP to determine drug safety
- Know teratogens and FDA classifications for meds used during pregnancy
- Assess for use of herbal/homeopathic preparations and OTCs

Activity

Work: assess impact
- What is the nature of the work?
- Is there exposure to toxins?
- What is the number of hours?
- Are there complications with pregnancy?
- Plan for maternity leave

Exercise:
- Focus on muscle strengthening
- Maintain adequate breathing rate; fluid intake during exercise
- Limit strenuous aerobics and increased body temperature
- Avoid exhaustion

Rest: tending to fatigue caused by
- Increased progesterone production
- Physiological anemia
- Increased fetal oxygen needs
- Emotional stress
- Decreased maternal lung expansion
- Nocturia

Common Discomforts

Anticipatory guidance/care strategies for:
GI: nausea, vomiting, constipation, flatulence, dyspepsia, ptyalism
CV: dependent edema, varicosities, supine hypotensive syndrome
GU: frequency, nocturia
Pain: round ligament, paresthesias, backache, leg cramps
Other: leukorrhea, fatigue, shortness of breath, dyspareunia, dental issues, insomnia

Recognize signs of complications: Differentiate from discomforts
- Hyperemesis gravidarum
- Spontaneous abortion
- Infection
- Preeclampsia
- PROM
- Absence of fetal movement
- Placenta previa/abruptio placentae

Weight Gain

Factors Affecting:
Genetic/social hx.
Enlarging placenta
- Increased bladder volume
- Increased blood volume
- Fetal growth

Nursing:
- BMI screening
- Conscious planning of food intake: Choose MyPlate and DASH plans
- Patient education/counseling

Childbirth Education
- Class → harmonious with beliefs/values
- Goal → facilitate positive birth experience
- Topics: A&P, comfort measures, labor and birth process, childbirth methods, relaxation/pain management, types of births, postpartum care, newborn care/feeding
- Create a birth plan

Complementary Care:
- Ayurveda beneficial during preconception period
- Stress management → massage, light and aromatherapy, reflexology, relaxation, mindfulness-based yoga
- Acupressure for nausea and back pain

Nursing Insight:
- Some foods decrease iron absorption
- Identify potential environmental threats to embryo
- Women with PKU should receive family planning counseling
- Obesity is a risk factor for an increased number of pregnancy complications
- Accutane can have significant teratogenic effects

Optimizing Outcomes:
- Use prenatal interventions to prevent birth defects
- Encourage preconception care counseling
- Use SUCCESS program to educate about smoking/smoking cessation strategies
- Use SBIRT program interventions to treat women with alcohol use disorders during pregnancy
- Teach health benefits of breastfeeding

Where Research and Practice Meet:
- Maternal smoking behavior influenced by need to cope with abuse-related PTSD symptoms
- Qi exercise beneficial prenatal nursing intervention
- Antenatal dietary intervention programs do not negatively alter newborn birth weight
- Pregnant women can exercise following existing recommendations
- Many factors influence increased medication use by pregnant women

Cultural Diversity:
- Higher maternal anemia in pregnant adolescents, African American women, and women of low-socioeconomic status
- Higher vitamin D deficiency rates in African Americans
- Pica associated with some cultural, religious beliefs
- Mexican women may have culturally influenced fears R/T diet and fetal harm

Now Can You:
- Discuss preconception care
- Identify substances to be avoided
- Discuss aspects of good nutrition
- Discuss work, fatigue, and medication use
- Identify common discomforts of pregnancy
- Identify danger signs in pregnancy

Concept Maps visually summarize the relationships among the most important concepts. Use them to review the chapter content and better understand how to apply it in practice.

Procedure Boxes provide step-by-step instructions (and rationales) for performing common procedures.

Purpose

To maintain optimum nutrition using a feeding tube that is passed through the mouth or nares and into the stomach

Equipment
- Oro- or nasogastric tube
- Tap water or a water-soluble lubricant
- Syringe
- pH indicator paper

Steps

1. Wash hands and don gloves.

2. Determine tube length required by measuring from the nose to the earlobe and to the midway point between the end of the xiphoid process and the umbilicus (Fig. 21-19).

   RATIONALE: *Proper measurement determines the distance that the catheter is inserted.*

3. Note the measurement by finding the manufacturer's black mark on the proximal end of the tube near the nares.

4. Lubricate the tube with tap water or a water-soluble lubricant. Follow manufacturer guidelines.

   RATIONALE: *Lubrication eases catheter insertion.*

5. Using the dominant hand, gently direct the tube toward the back of the throat or, if using the nose, toward the occiput.

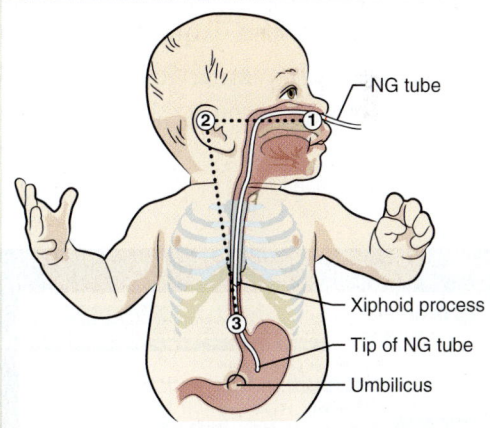

NG tube
Xiphoid process
Tip of NG tube
Umbilicus

Figure 21-19 Nasogastric tube insertion measurement.

Nursing Insight— *When teaching about iron supplements*

Nurses can teach patients about substances known to decrease the absorption of iron. Women should be taught to avoid consuming bran, tea, coffee, milk, oxylates (found in Swiss chard and spinach), and egg yolk at the same time as they take the iron supplement. Also, iron is best absorbed when taken between meals with a beverage other than tea, coffee, or milk.

Nursing Insight boxes show you how experienced nurses use their five senses to gain a deeper understanding of the clinical situation or the patient's condition.

BUILD YOUR CONFIDENCE.
Don't miss all of the ways we help you learn.

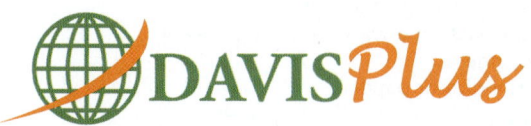

Beyond the text...
Prepare for class and clinical success.
The *Plus* Code on the inside front cover unlocks a wealth of learning resources. **Visit www.DavisPlus.com today!**

Your Davis*Plus* Resources are waiting for you.

- Davis Digital Version—Your complete text online. Quickly search for the content you need. Add notes, highlights, and bookmarks.

- Online Study Guide—Chapter Resources
  - Question Bank
  - Interactive Exercises
  - Nursing Care Plans
  - Bonus Nursing Care Plans
  - Clinical Pathways
  - Case Studies with CT questions
  - Answers to Chapter Review Questions
  - Suggested Answers to Case Studies in Text

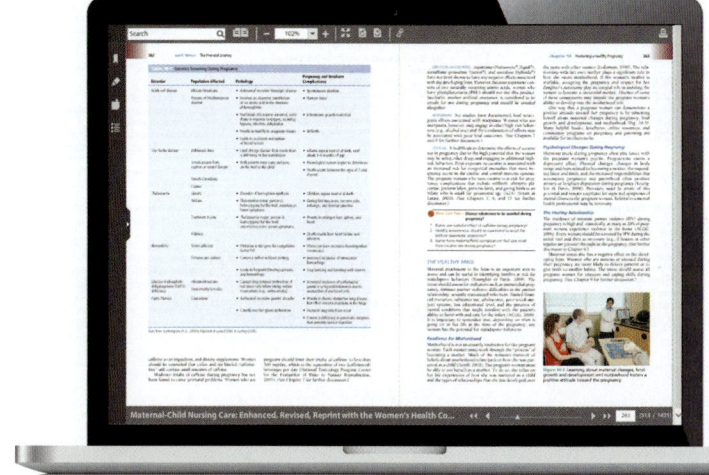

- Test Bank
- Interactive Exercises
- Interactive Clinical Scenarios
- Animations
- Audio Library of Maternal and Pediatric Sounds
- Concept Maps and Concept Map Generator
- Family Teaching Guides
- Additional Family Teaching Guides
- Glossary (PDF)
- Audio Glossary
- Podcast Library
- Dosage Calculation Module

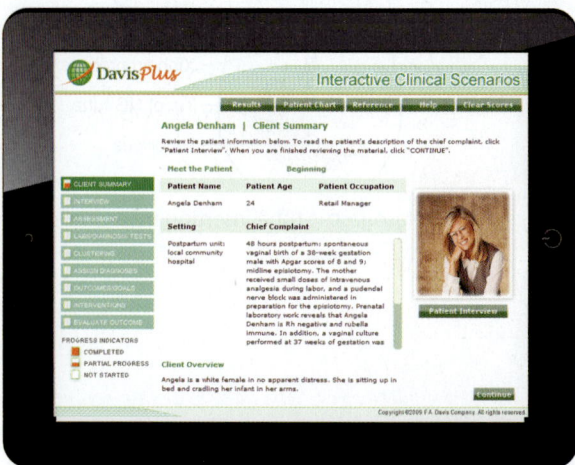

Visit Davis*Plus*.com today!

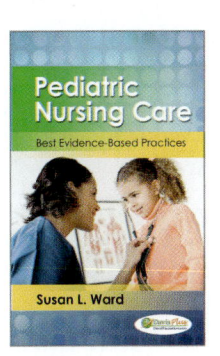 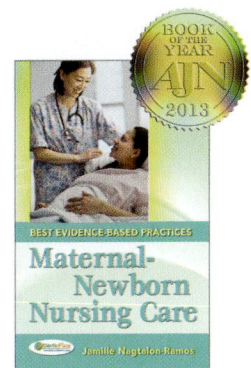
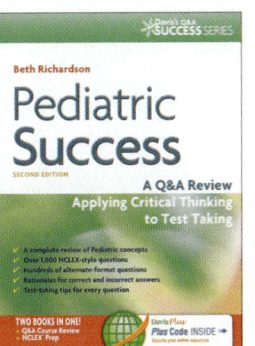 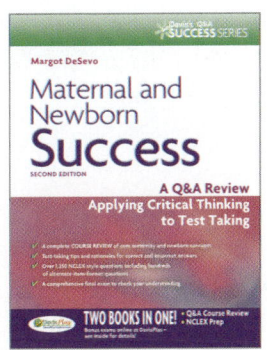
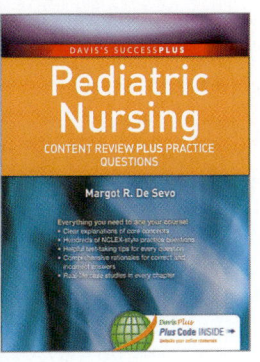
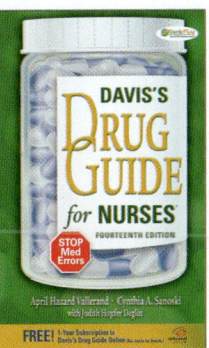 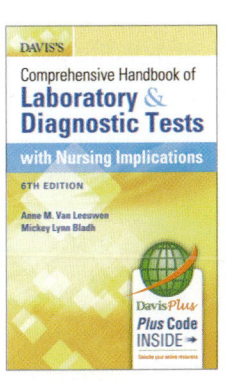
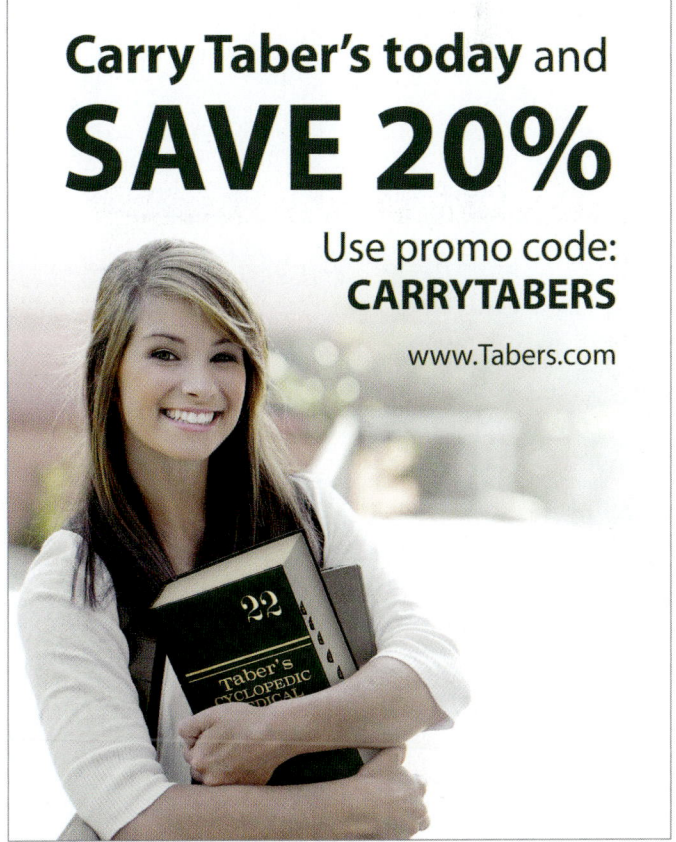

Maternal-Child Nursing Care

Optimizing Outcomes for Mothers, Children, & Families

SECOND EDITION

Susan L. Ward, PhD, RN

Professor of Nursing and Director of Nursing, Special Programs
Nebraska Methodist College
Omaha, Nebraska

Shelton M. Hisley, PhD, RNC, WHNP-BC

Assistant Professor of Nursing (Retired)
University of North Carolina at Wilmington
Wilmington, North Carolina

Amy Mitchell Kennedy, MSN, RN, Associate Editor

Adjunct Faculty, AAS Registered Nursing Program
ECPI University: School of Health Science
Newport News, VA

F.A. Davis Company • Philadelphia

F.A. Davis Company
1915 Arch Street
Philadelphia, PA 19103
www.fadavis.com

Printed in the United States of America

Last digit indicates print number: 10 9 8 7 6 5 4

Publisher, Nursing: Lisa Houck
Developmental Editor: Beth LoGiudice
Content Development Manager: Darlene Pedersen
Content Project Manager: Christina L. Snyder
Manager of Art and Design: Carolyn O'Brien

As new scientific information becomes available through basic and clinical research, recommended treatments and drug therapies undergo changes. The author(s) and publisher have done everything possible to make this book accurate, up to date, and in accord with accepted standards at the time of publication. The author(s), editors, and publisher are not responsible for errors or omissions or for consequences from application of the book, and make no warranty, expressed or implied, in regard to the contents of the book. Any practice described in this book should be applied by the reader in accordance with professional standards of care used in regard to the unique circumstances that may apply in each situation. The reader is advised always to check product information (package inserts) for changes and new information regarding dose and contraindications before administering any drug. Caution is especially urged when using new or infrequently ordered drugs.

Library of Congress Cataloging-in-Publication Data

Ward, Susan L., author.
 Maternal-child nursing care : optimizing outcomes for mothers, children, and families / Susan L. Ward, Shelton M. Hisley, Amy Mitchell Kennedy.—Second edition.
     p. ; cm.
 Includes bibliographical references and index.
 ISBN 978-0-8036-3665-1—ISBN 0-8036-3665-2
 I. Hisley, Shelton M., author. II. Kennedy, Amy Mitchell, author. III. Title.
 [DNLM: 1. Maternal-Child Nursing--methods. 2. Cultural Diversity. 3. Evidence-Based Nursing—methods. 4. Holistic Nursing—methods. WY 157.3]
 RG951
 618.2'0231—dc23
                                2014037091

The successful development of this second edition could not have become a reality without the enthusiasm and creative support of family and friends, who offered encouragement and fueled our commitment to the project with their patience, understanding, humor, opinions, and love. Our contributors' and reviewers' collective expertise provided ongoing guidance and direction in chapter development and content. To all of these wonderful, caring, and talented people, it is our honor and privilege to dedicate this book.

Susan L. Ward
Shelton M. Hisley

Preface

Maternal-Child Nursing Care: Optimizing Outcomes for Mothers, Children, and Families springs from our passionate commitment to providing the best nursing care possible to mothers and children and our desire to inspire others to make that same commitment. In this all-inclusive source, we provide students with current, comprehensive information about maternal-child nursing in creative, dynamic ways and in a concise, easy-to-use format. Building on theoretical foundations in basic nursing care, communication skills, and principles of health promotion, the text challenges students to optimize outcomes for their patients using critical thinking as they care for pregnant women and children in the hospital and community environments. We focus on aesthetics, cultural sensitivity, and a caring approach. This textbook also serves as an excellent resource for practicing nurses who work with women, children, and families in a variety of settings. We believe that combining essential information about the two specialties into a single textbook supports good educational practice while being economically advantageous.

Philosophy

The primary intent of this textbook is to identify the myriad options for holistic, evidence-based practice in maternal and child nursing care based on a philosophy of physiological and developmental normalcy and stressing safety and optimization of outcomes for mother and child. In addition to comprehensive coverage of maternal and child nursing care in traditional settings, we present essential elements for providing cost-effective, high-quality, innovative nursing care in community settings. Discussion of health-care delivery in community settings is crucial in contemporary nursing education and reflects today's trend for women, families, and children to obtain health care in the diverse settings in which they live, grow, play, work, or go to school.

This book is built on a framework that views the delivery of nursing care as a continuum spanning the traditional hospital inpatient environment to the community setting. Students are presented with information essential to providing appropriate, culturally informed nursing care to women, families, and children. A variety of creative learning aids are used to assist students in subject mastery and prompt the delivery of care that appropriately addresses contemporary needs while incorporating innovative approaches that integrate provider–patient partnerships and alliances with coalitions that serve women, families, and children across the lifespan.

Because the traditional hospital experience constitutes an important component of nursing education, content on hospital-based nursing care for women, families, and children examines acute, traumatic, chronic, and terminal conditions. Likewise, content that addresses community-based nursing care for women, families, and children explores strategies and resources for the provision of appropriate care in many different outpatient settings. With this text, students learn that community-based care can take place in a variety of ways at any time and in any place. It is our hope that the users of this textbook will acquire the essential knowledge for professional nursing practice in the specialties of maternal and child nursing and that they will gain insights about providing nursing care in a myriad of settings and with diverse populations.

Organization

Each chapter opens with a culturally or spiritually oriented story, literary piece, caring element, or quotation that creatively expresses various dimensions of aesthetics in nursing. Because contemporary nursing is a dynamic profession with a rich past, present, and future, we emphasize and promote the importance of innovative, state-of-the-art technology balanced with compassionate, humanistic care. "Learning Targets" offer a guided approach to chapter content and provide a gauge for assessing outcomes. "Growth and Development" offers additional information about how children grow and develop, based on various physiological and psychological conditions.

Chapter introductions provide a preview of content and assist students in identifying essential information and major concepts. Key words appear in boldface print accompanied by brief definitions in the text and are available grouped in the glossary for easy, quick reference on the electronic study guide. Color illustrations and photos provide visual cues to enhance understanding. These features facilitate students' learning and promote an understanding of the relationship between classroom or textbook information and the delivery of nursing care in the clinical setting.

A short review of anatomy, physiology, and pathophysiology is provided at the beginning of applicable chapters and interspersed where appropriate to foster understanding of new applications of concepts previously learned. Eye-catching display boxes draw students' attention to essential information about medications, critical nursing actions, nursing procedures, related research studies, assessment tools, diagnostic modalities, safety issues, therapeutic communication strategies, and family teaching guidelines.

Each chapter concludes with a concept map that visually summarizes the relationships among the most important concepts presented. This map reinforces students' learning, mastery of information, and also assists students in critical analysis. The concept map is a useful tool for confirming that students have identified the essential chapter elements and for applying classroom information to the clinical setting.

A number of strategies designed to prompt and enhance critical thinking weave through the text. Case studies, nursing care plans, NCLEX-style review questions, and exercises in clinical decision making assist students in mastering content and in integrating new information. These creative learning activities help students to assimilate and internalize information as they build on previously learned nursing knowledge and prepare to apply newly introduced concepts in various maternal-child clinical practice areas.

Themes and Key Features

The overarching theme of this comprehensive maternal-child resource focuses on how to provide contemporary nursing care to women, families, and children in the traditional hospital setting as well as in the community. In service to that goal are the broad themes of holistic care, critical thinking, validating practice, and tools for care. We use the following key features throughout the chapters to creatively illustrate and emphasize information essential for the delivery of safe, effective nursing care to diverse populations across care settings, thus ensuring an educational experience rich with critical thinking activities and clinical application opportunities.

HOLISTIC CARE

- Each chapter begins with a culturally or spiritually oriented story, literary piece, caring element, or quotation that creatively expresses aesthetics in nursing.
- "Nursing Insight" boxes show students how experienced nurses use their five senses to gain a deeper understanding about the clinical situation or the patient's condition.
- "Collaboration in Caring" provides guidelines for working with other health-care professionals to care for patients and families in inpatient and in community-based environments.
- "Cultural Diversity" emphasizes cultural sensitivity in both the hospital and community settings.
- "What to Say" helps students develop and enhance their communication skills by providing verbatim examples or helpful hints.
- Nursing Care Plans incorporating NANDA, NOC, and NIC terminology relate classroom and textbook knowledge to clinical practice, while evidence-based rationales for interventions show how research supports practice.
- "Complementary Care" shows students the wide range of complementary options available for integration with conventional approaches to provide safe, timely, and compassionate care.
- "Across Care Settings" fosters students' responsiveness to trends in health care by understanding holistic health care in acute care and community-based settings in which children and families live, grow, play, work, or go to school. Sensitivity to diverse patient populations is also included.
- "Family Teaching Guidelines" help students teach families essential components about caring for themselves and their children and are offered both in English (in the text and on the Electronic Study Guide) and Spanish (on the Electronic Study Guide).
- "Focus on Safety" helps students learn important protective measures to keep mothers and children out of harm's way.

CRITICAL THINKING

- "Learning Targets" offer a guided approach to chapter content and provide a gauge for assessing outcomes.
- "Key Words" appear in boldface type accompanied by brief definitions. Key words are also stored in the glossary for easy, quick reference on the electronic study guide and Davis*Plus*.
- "Case Studies" facilitate students' practice in the assimilation of content from various chapters into actual patient situations. As students work through the various case studies, they are challenged to apply critical thinking and practice clinical decision making.
- "Global Health Case Studies" facilitate students' practice in the assimilation of content from various cultural and geographic areas into actual patient situations.
- "Nursing Diagnoses" foster the development of new nursing knowledge by which diagnoses are developed based on information obtained during a nursing assessment. A standardized statement about the health of a patient for the purpose of providing nursing care is created. The nursing diagnosis portrays the patient's response to his or her condition so the nurse can address the problems independently.
- "Clinical Alerts" help students recognize emergent or critical situations and relate classroom or textbook information as they deliver safe, effective nursing care in the hospital and community-based environments.
- "Pediatric Math Worksheet" challenges students with realistic math problems; using dimensional analysis helps them to solve the problems.
- "Critical Nursing Actions" prompt students to assimilate and internalize information as they prepare to apply important concepts in the clinical area.
- "NCLEX-Style Review Questions" located at the end of each chapter prompt and enhance critical thinking and help to prepare students for licensure examination. An extensive NCLEX-style test bank is also available online for faculty use.
- "Concept Maps" visually summarize the relationships among the most important concepts presented in every chapter. Students can use the concept maps to review chapter content, enhance critical thinking, and to more readily grasp the application of classroom information in the clinical setting.

VALIDATING PRACTICE

- "PICO(T) Questions" foster students' understanding of evidence-based practice.
- "Where Research and Practice Meet" focuses on investigative initiatives that may impact practice in the future while underscoring the value of clinical inquiry in ensuring positive outcomes for patients and their families.
- "Optimizing Outcomes" enhance critical thinking skills for clinical application and help establish the best possible outcomes and how to obtain them.
- "Legal Alerts" introduce new nurses to important legal issues that impact the clinical environment and shows them, guides them, assists them, and helps them recognize how to critically analyze potentially litigious situations.

- "Now Can You?" prepares students to assimilate and internalize information presented throughout the chapter and serves as a mini check to ensure mastery of material before proceeding to the next section.
- "What to Say" gives students information and examples of statements to assist them in their care of mothers and children.
- "Evidence-Based Practice" highlights current relevant research and encourages students to incorporate evidence-based findings into their everyday practice.
- "Concept Methodology" assists students in focusing their learning on key building blocks as they develop a deeper understanding of the plethora of complex health information needed today by the practicing nurse.
- "Summary Points" bring together the information students should be most careful to comprehend from the chapter.
- "Appendices" provide in-depth information that helps students identify specific aspects of care.
- References provide current citations that validate practice and support the chapter content.

TOOLS FOR CARE

- "A & P Review" of chapter-specific anatomy, physiology, and pathophysiology fosters understanding of new applications of previously learned concepts.
- "Labs" boxes present crucial information about laboratory testing and its relationship to the patient's overall health status.
- "Procedures" provide step-by-step instructions for performing common procedures in maternal-child nursing and the rationales for why things are done a particular way. Each procedure includes an example of documentation to emphasize the critical nature of proper, accurate documentation.
- "Medication Boxes" present crucial information about commonly prescribed medications and help students in their care of mothers, children, and families.
- "Assessment Tools" facilitate understanding of clinical evaluation and help students make the connection between classroom or textbook knowledge and the clinical setting.
- "Diagnostic Tools" present crucial information about common diagnostic measures and their relationship to various disease entities.
- "Family Teaching Guidelines" provide relevant information that families need as they move through illness to recovery or acceptance of chronic or terminal illness.
- "Growth and Development" present additional information about how children grow and develop and is specifically related to physiological or psychosocial information in each chapter.

Teaching Ancillaries and Other Related Products

INSTRUCTOR'S GUIDE

The "Course Syllabus" includes a proposed class schedule for a traditional 15-week semester and for an accelerated 8-week semester along with reading assignments and testing content. The syllabi provide a guide for using the text in the most efficient way.

"Teaching Plans" provide a user-friendly lesson plan for each chapter, whether teaching in separate or combined courses. The lesson plans integrate teaching tips, PowerPoint presentations, and suggested students' assignments.

"Tips for Teaching a Combined Maternal-Child Course" offer suggestions about how to effectively teach these two specialties in one course.

Faculty Case Studies

The case studies provided to the instructor are more extensive and detailed than those provided in the text or on the Electronic Study Guide so they can be used for testing as well as for post-conference discussions. Answers to the faculty case studies are provided to promote and enhance critical thinking skills and facilitate the application of theoretical concepts into the clinical setting.

Concept Maps

Concept maps are constructed to underscore the relationships between the essential concepts in each chapter. These pieces prompt critical thinking and may be used as a guide for students assigned to create additional maps about other important theoretical elements.

Electronic Test Bank

A collection of NCLEX-style questions and rationales enables students to identify areas of strength and weakness and prepare for course tests and for the national licensure examination.

PowerPoint Presentations

A collection of slides that form the basis for lecture for each chapter is provided; these can be modified to meet the instructor's specific needs.

Media Ancillary

Electronic files of images from the text may be used in the classroom; audio selections of heart sounds are also included.

ELECTRONIC STUDY GUIDE

A free electronic study guide is included with the text. This resource, intended to assist and enhance students' learning, offers creative ways to supplement and reinforce the textbook information. It contains the following:

Interactive Exercises

A creative and fun way to supplement and reinforce learning with

- Hangman
- Quiz Show
- Critical Thinking
- Drag and Drop Bucket
- Fill-in-the-Blank Clue

Student Case Studies

Thirty-one relevant case studies from selected chapters facilitate students' practice in the assimilation of content from various chapters into actual patient situations.

Expanded Nursing Care Plans

All care plans from the textbook are provided and are printable. There are also 12 expanded care plans that are not included in the text (6—Maternity care; 6—Pediatric care). These are intended to provide in-depth information and guidance for planning and providing care to maternity and pediatric patients with commonly encountered normal and pathological conditions.

Family Teaching Guidelines

English and Spanish versions of the Family Teaching Guidelines from the text, as well as additional ones unique to the electronic study guide can be personalized and printed and used in actual patient care situations.

NCLEX-Style Review Questions

A collection of NCLEX-style questions and rationales can help students identify areas of strength and weakness and prepare for course tests and for the national licensure examination.

Sound Collection

Heart sounds depicting various normal and abnormal heart sounds are included to help students recognize when there is a problem.

Davis*Plus*

Davis*Plus* contains Internet links related to specific content areas presented throughout the book, links to useful Web sites, links to the F.A. Davis Web site, and product page; and bonus material, including interactive exercises for pediatric dosage calculations including dimensional analysis.

Second Edition Contributors

Sharon Bator, RN, MSN, PNP, CPE, PhD
Assistant Professor of Nursing
Southern University School of Nursing
Baton Rouge, Louisiana
Chapter 31

Meg Blair, PhD, RN
Professor of Nursing
Nebraska Methodist College
Omaha, Nebraska
End of Chapter Questions, NCLEX Testbank

Diane M. Bligh, MS, RN
Associate Professor, Nursing
Front Range Community College
Westminster, Colorado
Chapter Concept Maps

Michelle Lynn Burke, MSN, ARNP, CPN, CPON
Clinical Specialist
Department of Hematology Oncology
Miami Children's Hospital
Miami, Florida
Chapter 32

Cassandra Frost RN, MSN
Assistant Professor
Nebraska Methodist College
Omaha, Nebraska
Chapter 35, Growth and Development for Chapters 19–35, Pediatric Main Work Sheet, Transplant Content Consultant, Ancillaries

Elizabeth Gephart, DNP, APRN, PNP-BC
Assistant Professor
School of Nursing
Millikin University
Decatur, Illinois
Pediatric Content Consultant

Maryann Godshall, PhD, RN, CCRN, CPN, CNE
Assistant Clinical Professor
Drexel University
Philadelphia, Pennsylvania
Chapters 33, 34

Ann Harms, RN, EdD
Assistant Professor
Creighton University College of Nursing—Mary Lanning Campus
Hastings, Nebraska
Chapter 22

Corlis Hayden, MSN, RN
Assistant Professor
Nebraska Methodist College
Omaha, Nebraska
Chapter 22

Mary Helming, PhD, APRN, FNP-BC, AHN-BC
Professor of Nursing, FNP Track Coordinator, and Acting Director of Graduate Nursing
Quinnipiac University
Hamden, Connecticut
Chapters 25, 31

Shelton M. Hisley, PhD, RNC, WHNP-BC
Assistant Professor of Nursing (Retired)
University of North Carolina at Wilmington
Wilmington, North Carolina
Chapters 1–18

Lin Hughes, PhD, RN
Professor of Nursing and Dean of Nursing
Nebraska Methodist College
Omaha, Nebraska
Concept Methodology

Nellie Johnson, MSN, RN, CCRN
Assistant Professor
Nebraska Methodist College
Omaha, Nebraska
Chapter 35

Cyn Kildare MSN, APRN, FNP-C
Family Nurse Practitioner
Advanced Health
Chantilly, Virginia
Chapter 30

Marla Kniewel RN, EdD
Associate Professor of Nursing
Nebraska Methodist College Omaha, Nebraska
Concept Methodology for Web

Nancy Kramer EdD, CPNP, ARNP, CNE
Professor and Vice Chancellor of Academic Affairs
Allen College
Waterloo, Iowa
Chapters 23, 24, 27, Evidence-Based Practice Feature

Karla Luxner, DNP, RNC
Assistant Professor of Nursing
Millikin University
Decatur, Illinois
Nursing Care Plans and Expanded Nursing Care Plans

Judy M. Marshall, RN, NP
Family Nurse Practitioner
Children's Memorial Hospital
Chicago, Illinois
Chapter 26, Cardiac Figures for Chapter 26, 27

Tina Martin RN, PhD, FNP-BC
Professor of Nursing
Assistant Professor of Neurology
Director of Accelerated BSN Program
School of Nursing, University of Mississippi Medical
    Center
Jackson, Mississippi
    Chapter 28

Deborah Naccarini, DNP, RN, CNE
Assistant Professor of Nursing
Notre Dame of Maryland University
Baltimore, MD
    Chapters 20, 21, and SBAR Appendix on Davis*Plus*

Margaret (Peggy) O'Connor, MSN, BSN, RN
Assistant Clinical Professor
Lawrence Memorial/Regis College Nursing Program
Medford, Massachusetts
    Chapters 29, 30, and Burn Consultant

Ruth Wittmann-Price, DNSc, RN, CNE, Perinatal CNS
Professor and Chair, Nursing
Francis Marion University
Florence, South Carolina
    Chapter 19

Deborah Salani, DNP, ARNP, CPON
Assistant Professor of Clinical
University of Miami
Miami, Florida
    Chapter 32

Lorin Schumacher, BA
English Teacher
Our Lady of Mt Carmel
Essex, Maryland
    *Grammatical Editing for Chapters 19–35, PowerPoints
    and Teaching Plans for Chapters 19–35*

First Edition Contributors

Sharon Akes-Caves, RN, MS, MSN
Corporate Nursing Education Program and Interim ADN
  Program Director
Pima Medical Institute
Mesa, Arizona
  Chapter 1

Jan Andrews, RNC, PhD, WHNP
Professor and Associate Dean of Nursing and Health
  Sciences
Macon State College
Macon, Georgia
  Chapter 6

Kimberly Attwood, PhD(c), MSN, CRNP, APRN, BC, NP-C
Assistant Professor of Nursing
DeSales University
Center Valley, Pennsylvania
  Chapter 15

Bridget Bailey, RN, MSN
Associate Professor
Iowa Lakes Community College
Emmetsburg, Iowa
  Chapter 22

Deborah Bambini, PhD, WHNP-BC, CNE
Assistant Professor
Grand Valley State University
Grand Rapids, Michigan
  Clinical Pocket Companion

Sharon Bator, RN, MSN, PNP, CPE, PhD Student
Assistant Professor of Nursing
Southern University School of Nursing
Baton Rouge, Louisiana
  Chapter 32

Diane M. Bligh, MS, RN
Associate Professor, Nursing
Front Range Community College
Westminster, Colorado
  Chapter Concept Maps

Michelle Lynn Burke, MSN, ARNP, CPN, CPON
Clinical Specialist
Department of Hematology Oncology
Miami Children's Hospital
Miami, Florida
  Chapter 33

Irma Bustamante-Gavino, PhD, RN
Associate Professor
The Aga Khan University School of Nursing
Karachi, 74800, Pakistan
  Chapter 24

Marsha Cannon, MSN, RN
Associate Professor
University of West Alabama
Livingston, Alabama
  Chapter 29

Patricia M. Connors, RNC, MS, WHNP
Perinatal Clinical Nurse Specialist
Massachusetts General Hospital
Boston, Massachusetts
  Chapter 11

Sherrill Anne Conroy, D Phil, Med, BN, RN
Assistant Professor
University of Alberta
Edmonton, Alberta, Canada
  Chapter 21

Wendy A. Darby, PhD, CRNP
Associate Professor, Family Nurse Practitioner
University of North Alabama
Florence, Alabama
  Case Studies for Pediatric Chapters in Ancillaries

Michele D'Arcy-Evans, CNM, PhD
Professor
Lewis-Clark State College
Lewiston, Idaho
  Chapter 9

Jacqueline Maria Dias, RN, RM, MEd
Assistant Professor
The Aga Khan University School of Nursing
Karachi, 74800, Pakistan
  Chapter 24

Elizabeth Fahrenholtz, APRN, MSN
Assistant Professor
Creighton University
Hastings, Nebraska
  Chapter 5

Brian G. Fonnesbeck, RN, BSN, MN
Associate Professor
Lewis Clark State College
Lewiston, Idaho
  Chapter 3

Marcia L. Gasper, EdD, RNC
Associate Professor of Nursing
East Stroudsburg University
East Stroudsburg, Pennsylvania
  Interactive Exercises

Maryann Godshall, MSN, CPN
Assistant Professor of Nursing
DeSales University
Center Valley, Pennsylvania
Chapters 34, 35

Jacqueline L. Gonzalez, ARNP, MSN, FAAN, CNAA-BC
Senior Vice President/ Chief Nursing Officer
Miami Children's Hospital
Miami, Florida
Chapter 22

Linda Nicholson Grinstead, PhD, RN, CPN, CNE
Professor
Grand Valley State University
Grand Rapids, Michigan
Clinical Pocket Companion

Ann M. Harms, RN, MSN, CS
Assistant Professor
Creighton University School of Nursing
Hastings-Mary Lanning Campus
Hastings, Nebraska
Chapters 20, 23

Dawn Hawthorne, MSN, RN, CCRN, IBCLC
Family Educator and Lactation Consultant
Joe DiMaggio Children's Hospital at Memorial Hospital
Hollywood, Florida
Chapter 15

Mary A. Helming, PhD, APRN, FNP-BC, AHN-BC
Professor of Nursing and FNP Track Coordinator
Quinnipiac University
Hamden, Connecticut
Chapter 32

Shelton M. Hisley, PhD, RNC, WHNP-BC
Assistant Professor of Nursing (Retired)
University of North Carolina at Wilmington
Wilmington, North Carolina
Chapter 18

Jodi L. Jenson, RN, MSN
Assistant Professor
Nebraska Methodist College
Omaha, Nebraska
PowerPoints for Pediatric Chapters

Helen W. Jones, RN, APN, C., PhD
Chairperson of Health Science Education
Raritan Valley Community College
Somerville, New Jersey
PowerPoints for Maternity Chapters

Marcia Jones, RN, ND
Assistant Professor of Nursing
Bronx Community College
Bronx, New York
*Case Studies and Family Teaching Guidelines for
   Maternity Chapters in Ancillaries*

Esperanza Villanueva Joyce, EdD, CNS, RN
CHSS Associate Dean for Nursing Education and Director
   of Nursing
New Mexico State University School of Nursing
Las Cruces, New Mexico
Spanish Translations of Family Teaching Guidelines

Kathy Jo Bertelsen Keever, RNC, CNM, MS
Associate Professor of Nursing
Women's Health
Anne Arundel Community College
Arnold, Maryland
Chapter 8

Patricia A. Kiladis, MS, RN
Director of Undergraduate Nursing Program
Northeastern University
Boston, Massachusetts
Chapter 14

Cynthia Kildare, RN, MSN, APRN-BC
Assistant Professor
Bryan LGH College of Health Sciences
Lincoln, Nebraska
Chapter 31

Nancy Kramer, EdD, CPNP, CNE, ARNP
Associate Dean, Head of the Division of Nursing,
   Professor
Allen College
Waterloo, Iowa
*Chapter 25, Evidence-Based Practice Features, and
   Family Teaching Guidelines for Ancillaries*

Marilee LeBon, BA
Developmental Editor/Writer
Mountaintop, Pennsylvania
NCLEX-Style Questions for Pediatrics

Karla Luxner, DNP, RNC
Assistant Professor of Nursing
Millikin University
Decatur, Illinois
Nursing Care Plans

Judy M. Marshall, RN, NP
Family Nurse Practitioner
Children's Memorial Hospital
Chicago, Illinois
Chapter 27

Betsy B. McCune, MSN, RNC
OB Clinical Nurse Specialist
Borgess Medical Center
Kalamazoo, Michigan
Chapter 16

Karen McQueen, RN, MA(N), PhD
Assistant Professor
Lakehead University School of Nursing
Thunder Bay, Ontario, Canada
Chapter 12

Deborah Naccarini, DNP, RN, CNE
Assistant Professor Nursing
Notre Dame of Maryland University
Baltimore, Maryland
Chapter 21

Margaret A. O'Connor, RN, MS
Assistant Clinical Professor
Lawrence Memorial/Regis College Nursing Program
Medford, Massachusetts
Chapter 30

Nicole K. Olshanski, MSN, RN
Instructor of Nursing
University of Pittsburgh School of Nursing
Pittsburgh, Pennsylvania
Chapter 13

Helen Papas-Kavalis, RNC, MA Nursing
Bronx Community College
Bronx, New York
NCLEX-Style Questions as Review Questions in Pediatric Chapters

Karen Joy Poole, RN, BScN, ME, MA
Director and Associate Professor
Lakehead University
Thunder Bay, Ontario, Canada
Chapter 12

Karen L. Pulcher, MSN, BSN, ARNP, BC
Assistant Professor of Nursing
University of Central Missouri
Lee's Summit, Missouri
Chapter 29

Fatima Ramos-Marcuse, PhD, APRN, BC
Adjunct Assistant Professor and Psychotherapist
University of Maryland School of Nursing
Baltimore, Maryland 21201
Chapter 23

Nancy Redfern-Vance, PhD, MN, CNM
Associate Professor
Valdosta State University
Valdosta, Georgia
Chapter 2

Sarah Roland
Associate Degree Nursing Instructor
Central Carolina Technical College
Sumter, South Carolina
Teaching Plans for Pediatric Chapters

Maria A. Rosen, RN, PNP, PhD
Program Director
Becker College
Worcester, Massachusetts
Chapter 21

Melodie Rowbotham, PhD, RN
Assistant Professor
Southern Illinois University School of Nursing
Edwardsville, Illinois
Teaching Plans for Maternity Chapters

Deborah Salani, ARNP, MSN, CPON
Director of the Emergency Department
Miami Children's Hospital
Miami, Florida
Chapter 33

Jacoline Sommer, RN, RM, BScN
Senior Instructor
The Aga Khan University School of Nursing
Karachi, 74800, Pakistan
Chapter 24

Deborah Stiffler, PhD, RN, CNM
Assistant Professor
Coordinator, Women's Health Nurse Practitioner Major
Indiana University School of Nursing
Indianapolis, Indiana
Chapter 10

Angela S. Taylor, PhD, RN, BC
Director of Nursing Program and Associate Professor
Department of Nursing, School of Health Sciences and Human Performance
Lynchburg College
Lynchburg, Virginia
Chapters 4, 10

Dawn Michele Teeple, RN, BSN, MS, CCE
Assistant Professor
Anne Arundel Community College
Baltimore, Maryland
Chapter 17

Joan Nalani Thompson, NNP, MSN, RNC
Assistant Professor
University of Hawaii at Hilo
Hilo, Hawaii
Chapter 7

Wendy Thomson, EdD(c), MSN, BSBA, RN, IBCLC
Assistant Professor and Technology Coordinator
Nursing Department
Nova Southeastern University
Fort Lauderdale, Florida
Chapter 15

Kelly Tobar, RN, EdD
Associate Professor
California State University Sacramento
Sacramento, California
Chapter 26

Chandra Vig, BSN
Curriculum Developer
Bow Valley College
Calgary, Alberta, Canada
Chapter 20

Susan L. Ward, PhD, RN
Professor of Nursing
Nebraska Methodist College
Omaha, Nebraska
Chapter 18

Nancy Watts, RN, MN, PNC (C)
Clinical Nurse Specialist
London Health Sciences Centre
London, Ontario, Canada
  *Maternity NCLEX-Style Questions for Text, Electronic
    Study Guide and Instructors' Materials*

Ruth A. Wittmann-Price, DNSc, RN, CNE
Assistant Professor
Drexel University
Philadelphia, Pennsylvania
  Chapter 19

Roseann Mary Zahara-Such, APRN, BC, MSN, CCNS
Assistant Clinical Professor of Nursing
Purdue University
Hammond, Indiana
  Chapter 28

Kelly K. Zinn, MSN, RN
Assistant Professor
Nebraska Methodist College
Omaha, Nebraska
  Coordinator for All Ancillary Components

Second Edition Reviewers

Civita Allard, RN, MS
Associate Professor of Nursing
Utica College
Utica, New York

Marilyn A. Beard, MSN, RNC
Clinical Instructor of Nursing
Clayton State University
Morrow, Georgia

Carol Caico, PhD, CS, NP
Assistant Professor of Nursing and NP
New York Institute of Technology
Old Westbury, New York

Vicki Caraway, RN, MSN, CNE
Nursing Instructor/Associate Degree
Nursing Program Coordinator
Mayland Community College
Spruce Pine, North Carolina

Valerie Cline, RNC-OB, MSN
Nursing Faculty
Clark College
Vancouver, Washington

Gloria Haile Coats, RN, MSN, FNP
Professor of Nursing
Modesto Junior College
Modesto, California

Leslie Collins, RN, MS
Instructor of Nursing
Northwestern Oklahoma State
University
Alva, Oklahoma

Amy Mitchell Corbitt, MSN, RN
Adjunct Faculty
ECPI University, RN Program
Newport News, Virginia

Allan Joseph V. Cresencia, MSN, CPN, RN
Assistant Professor
West Coast University, College of
Nursing
North Hollywood, California

Jenny Cronkhite, RN, MSN, Med
Nursing Faculty
State College of Florida
Bradenton, Florida

Joanne Denz, RN, BSN, MSN, PNP
Instructor
TriCounty Technical College
Pendleton, South Carolina

Debbie Diamond, MSN, RN-BC
Nursing Faculty
Nova Southeastern University,
Baptist Health South Florida
Miami, Florida

Teresa Diekmann, RNC, BSN, MSN
Nursing Instructor
Illinois Eastern Community Colleges
Mt. Carmel, Illinois

Cathleen Dowe, MSN, RN
Adjunct Nursing Faculty
Jefferson Community College
Watertown, New York

Karen A. Eberle, MSN, RNC-OB, CNE
Associate Professor
St. Luke's College, Department of
Nursing Education
Sioux City, Iowa

Deepika Goyal, RN, FNP-C, PhD
Associate Professor
San Jose State University, The Valley
Foundation School of Nursing
San Jose, California

Maria Grandinetti, MS, RN, PhD (c)
Assistant Professor of Nursing
Wilkes University
Wilkes-Barre, Pennsylvania

Karen M. Bennett Gural, RN, MS
RN Faculty
Crouse Hospital College of Nursing
Syracuse, New York

Lola A. Hardy, RN, MS
Assistant Professor
Corning Community College, Nurse
Education Program
Corning, New York

Judith Ingrasin, MS, RN
Assistant Professor of Nursing
Kansas City Kansas Community
College
Kansas City, Kansas

Jodi L. Jenson-Bassett, MSN, RN
Assistant Professor of Nursing
Nebraska Methodist College
Omaha, Nebraska

Laura M. Karnitschnig, MN, RN, CPNP
Assistant Clinical Professor
Northern Arizona University, School
of Nursing
Flagstaff, Arizona

Barbara L. Lange, PhD, RN
Executive Director
University of Arkansas - Fort Smith
Fort Smith, Arkansas

Sister Corinne Lemmer, PhD, RN
Professor of Nursing
Mount Marty College
Yankton, South Dakota

Brenda Lennon, MS, RN, BC
Course Chair of Pediatrics/OB/
Newborn/Women's Health
Albany Memorial School of Nursing,
AD Program
Albany, New York

Robyn C. Leo, MS, RN
Associate Professor
Worcester State University
Worcester, Massachusetts

Beverly Witt Lester, RN, MSN
Associate Professor of Nursing
Southwest Virginia Community
College
Cedar Bluff, Virginia

Amy Lippert, MSN, RN
Lecturer of Nursing
Mount Mercy University
Cedar Rapids, Iowa

Rebecca Loth Luetke, BA, BSN, MSN, RN
Professor of Nursing
Colorado Mountain College
Glenwood Springs, Colorado

Cherie L. McCann, MSN, RN-BC, CPN
Instructor
Armstrong Atlantic State University
Savannah, Georgia

Andrea McCrink, EdD, WHNP-BC, RN
Assistant Professor of Nursing
Adelphi University
Garden City, New York

Paula McNichols, MSN, BSN, RNC, RN
Resident Faculty/Lead Faculty
Mohave Community College
Kingman, Arizona

Randy Miller, MSN, BS, RN-BC, CNE
Professor of Nursing
Seminole State College of Florida
Altamonte Springs, Florida

Tracy A. Moshier, MSN, RN, CCE
Nursing Instructor
Lake Superior College
Duluth, Minnesota

Patricia Novak, MSN
Nursing Professor
Phoenix College
Phoenix, Arizona

Noreen Nutting, RN, BSN, MAIS
Associate Professor
Northern Virginia Community
    College
Springfield, Virginia

Margery Orr, DNS, RN
Nursing Education Specialist
Becker College
Worcester, Massachusetts

Alissa Parrish, RN, MSN
Assistant Professor
The University of Tennessee at
    Martin
Martin, Tennessee

Valerie N. Rakes, MSN, RN
Assistant Professor
Cabarrus College of Health Sciences
Concord, North Carolina

Laura Rodriguez, DNP, MSN, RN, CNS
Clinical Assistant Professor
University of Texas – El Paso
El Paso, Texas

Cynthia D. Rothenberger, MSN, RN, ACNS, BC
Assistant Professor of Nursing
Alvernia University
Reading, Pennsylvania

Kerry Rusk, MN, BScN, RN
Faculty Lecturer
University of Alberta
Edmonton, Alberta
Canada

Nancy I. Simpson, MSN, RN-BC, CNE
Associate Professor
University of New England
Portland, Maine

Kathy Snider, MSN, MA, BSN
Instructor of Nursing
West Texas A&M University
Canyon, Texas

Kristy Strother, RD
Adjunct Instructor
Butler Community College
Lawrence, Kansas

Marcy Tanner-Garrett, MSN, RN, CNE
RN to BSN Coordinator/Instructor
Southwestern Oklahoma State
    University
Weatherford, Oklahoma

Pat Durham Taylor, RN, PhD
Faculty
Truckee Meadows Community
    College
Reno, Nevada

Rhonda K. Tower-Siddens, MSN, RN
Associate Professor of Associate
    Degree Nursing and Clinical
    Coordinator of Nursing Programs
McLennan Community College
Waco, Texas

Laura Vanyo, MSN, RNC-OB
College Assistant Professor
New Mexico State University
Las Cruces, New Mexico

Max Veltman, RN, PhD (c), CPNP-PC
Associate Professor
Boise State University
Boise, Idaho

Deb Williams, MSN, RNC, CNE
Maternal Child Nursing Instructor
Northwest College
Powell, Wyoming

Sue Willms, RN, MSN
Director of Nursing
Iowa Western Community College
Council Bluffs, Iowa

Michele Woodbeck, MS, RN
Professor of Nursing
Hudson Valley Community College
Troy, New York

Hollace (Holly) Yowler, MSN, RN, CNE
Professor of Nursing
Ivy Tech Community College
Madison, Indiana

Phyllis Zimmerman MSN, BGS, RN
Director of Continuing Education,
    Professional Development
Nebraska Methodist College
Omaha, Nebraska
Chapter PICOT Questions

First Edition Reviewers

Randee L. Masciola, RN, MS, CNP
Clinical Instructor and Women's
    Health Nurse Practitioner
Ohio State University
Columbus, Ohio

Kathleen Matta, MSN, CNS, IBCLC
Visiting Faculty
University of New Mexico
Albuquerque, New Mexico

Sheila Matye, MSN, RNC
Adjunct Assistant Professor
Montana State University
Great Falls, Montana

Trilla Mays, RN, MSN
Nursing Instructor
Midlands Technical College
Columbia, South Carolina

Barbara McClaskey, PhD, MN, RNC, ARNP
Professor, Department of Nursing
Pittsburg State University
Pittsburg, Kansas

Michelle Michitsch, RN, MS, CPNP-PC
Adjunct Nursing Professor
Borough of Manhattan Community
    College
New York, New York

Nancy Miller, MSN, RNC, CCM
Nursing Professor
Keiser University
Fort Lauderdale, Florida

Georgia Moore, PhD, MSNed, RN-BC
Consultant/ Online educator
Louisville, Kentucky

Julie Moore, RNC, MSN, MPH, WHNP
Associate Professor of Nursing
Hawaii Community College
Hilo, Hawaii

Cindy Morgan, CNM
Instructor
University of Tennessee at
    Chattanooga
Chattanooga, Tennessee

Deborah Naccarini, DNP, RN, CNE
Assistant Professor
Notre Dame of Maryland University
Baltimore, Maryland

Debbie Ocedek, RN, BSN, MSN
Professor of Nursing
Mott Community College
Flint, Michigan

Donna Paulsen, RN, MSN
Nursing faculty
North Carolina Agricultural and
    Technical State University
Greensboro, North Carolina

Melissa A. Popovich, RN, MSN
Clinical Faculty
Ohio State College of Nursing
Columbus, Ohio

Karen L. Pulcher, ARNP/CPNP, MSN, RN
Assistant Professor in Nursing
University of Central Missouri
North Kansas City, Missouri

Jacquelyn Reid, MSN, EdD, CNM, CNE
Associate Professor
Indiana University Southeast
New Albany, Indiana

Jean Rodgers, RN, BSN, MN
Nursing Faculty
Hesston College
Hesston, Kansas

Kathryn Rudd, RNC, MSN, MSN
Clinical Educator
MetroHealth Medical Center
Cleveland, Ohio

Christine L. Sayre, MSN, RN
Auxiliary Faculty
Ohio State University
Columbus, Ohio

Gwenneth C. Simmonds, PhDc, CNM, MSN, RN
Clinical Instructor
Ohio State University
Columbus, Ohio

Lisa H. Simmons, RN, MSN
Instructor and Coordinator Child
    Health Nursing
University of South Carolina Aiken
North Augusta, South Carolina

Cordia A. Starling, BSN, MS, EdD
Division Chair of Nursing
Dalton State University
Dalton, Georgia

Nora F. Steele, DNS, RNC, PNP
Professor
Charity/Delgado Community College
New Orleans, Louisiana

Suzan Stewart, RN, BS
Lab Coordinator
Community College of Denver
Denver, Colorado

Deborah Terrell, RN, MSN, APN, DNSc
Associate Professor
Harry S. Truman College
Chicago, Illinois

Barbara Tewell, RNC, BSN
Perinatal Staff Nurse
Naval Medical Center
San Diego, California

Donna J. Gryctz Thomas, RN, BSN, MSN
Assistant Professor of Nursing
Kent State University
New Philadelphia, Ohio

Joan Thompson, NNP, MSN, RNC
Assistant Professor
University of Hawaii at Hilo
Hilo, Hawaii

Pat Twedt, RN, MS, Med, MS
Associate Professor of Nursing
Dakota Wesleyan University
Mitchell, South Dakota

Becky C. Vicknair, RNBS, APRN, MSN, PNP
Pediatric Instructor
Delgado/Charity School of Nursing
New Orleans, Louisiana

Sherry Warner, RN
Nursing Instructor
Fulton-Montgomery Community
    College
Johnstown, New York

Maribeth Wilson, MSN, MSPH
Nursing Faculty
Keiser University
Tallahassee, Florida

Jennifer J. Woods, RN, MSN
Instructor
Delgado/Charity School of Nursing
New Orleans, Louisiana

Acknowledgments

It has taken a village of professionals to bring this project to fruition, and we thank the editors and production staff of the F.A. Davis Company for their expertise and guidance, especially:

- Lisa Houck, Publisher, Nursing
- Amy Mitchell Kennedy, Associate Editor
- Beth LoGiudice, Special Projects Editor
- Christina L. Snyder, Content Project Manager
- Darlene Pedersen, Director of Content Development

We are indebted to the following for helping us shoot and collect the photographs used in the text:

Billings Photography, Omaha Nebraska

Children's Hospital and Medical Center, Omaha, Nebraska

Methodist Health System, Women's Hospital, Omaha, Nebraska

Nebraska Methodist College, Omaha, Nebraska

Betsy Toole Media Production Services, St. Luke's Hospital & Health Network, Bethlehem, Pennsylvania

Miami Children's Hospital, The Mary Ann Knight International Institute of Pediatrics, Founded as Variety Children's Hospital, Miami, Florida

Chandra Vig, Ann Harms, and Susan Ward's nursing students, family members, and friends

Many thanks to the following people who helped us supply sketches for the professional illustrator to create many of the line drawings in the text for the first and second editions: John C. Hisley, MD, William Ward, BFA, MAT, and Matthew T. Blaszko.

Second Edition Dedicated Participants

Many colleagues and friends assisted the chapter contributors through mentoring, editing, and offering content expertise. A special thank you goes to the following individuals:

Tem Adair, BS
Tim Connor, MSW
Kathleen Clark, RN, BSN
Alissa Dornink, MLS
Heather D. Henrichs, BS, DC
Steve Hess, MS, RDMS
Tim Landolt, RN, MSN, MSHP
Sonya Maddox, BSG
Jose Villegas, MD, MSHP

First Edition Dedicated Participants

Many colleagues and friends assisted the chapter contributors through mentoring, editing, and offering content expertise. A special thank you goes to the following individuals:

Tem Adair, BS
Rita Atwell MS, CRNP
Joanna E. Cain, BSN, RN
Kathy Cassandra RN, MS
Megan Connelly MSN, APRN, CCRN, CPNP-AC
Carolyn Gilmore, BSN
Christine A. Hamilton, DHSc, RRT, AE-C
Patricia Harris MS, CRNP-PMH
Sue Hinds RN, MSN, CPN
Nancy Koster, MS, APN
Melissa Lanza RN, MS, APRN-BC
Kerry Lazewski, MS, PNP
Casey O'Brien, BSN
Barbara Paliughi, RN, BSN
Ellen Reyerson, MS, NP
Judith Rocchiccioli, PhD, RN,
Sherrie Rodgers, MS, PNP
Cathy Webb, RN, MA
Joyce Weisshar, MS, CNS
Renee Zubay Fife, RN, MSN

Contents in Brief

Detailed Table of Contents

chapter 4

Caring for Women, Families, and Children Across the Life Span   81

unit two
The Process of Human Reproduction   129

chapter 5

Reproductive Anatomy and Physiology   131

chapter 6

Human Sexuality and Fertility   155

chapter 10

Promoting a Healthy Pregnancy   293

chapter 11

Caring for the Woman Experiencing Complications During Pregnancy   335

unit four
The Birth Experience   409

chapter 12
The Process of Labor and Birth   *411*

chapter 13

Promoting Patient Comfort During Labor and Birth   471

chapter 14

Caring for the Woman Experiencing Complications During Labor and Birth   503

unit five
Care of the New Family   551

chapter 15

Caring for the Postpartal Woman and Her Family   553

chapter 16

Caring for the Woman Experiencing Complications During the Postpartal Period   604

chapter 17

Physiological Transition of the Newborn   638

chapter 18

Caring for the Normal Newborn   662

chapter 19

Caring for the Newborn at Risk   707

unit six
Caring for the Child and Family   753

chapter 20
Caring for the Developing Child   755

chapter 21
Caring for the Child in the Hospital, the Community, and Across Care Settings   786

chapter 25

Caring for the Child With an Immunological or Infectious Condition   969

chapter 26

Caring for the Child With a Cardiovascular Condition   1017

chapter 27

Caring for the Child With an Endocrinological or Metabolic Condition   1059

chapter 28

Caring for the Child With a Neurological or Sensory Condition   1112

chapter 29

Caring for the Child With a Musculoskeletal Condition   1160

chapter 30

Caring for the Child With an Integumentary Condition   1203

chapter 34
Caring for the Child With a Chronic Condition or the Dying Child   1386

chapter 35
Caring for the Critically Ill Child   1411

Special Features

Global Health/Case Studies

Clinical Alerts

Collaboration in Caring

Complementary Care

Critical Nursing Actions

Cultural Diversity

Diagnostic Tools

Family Teaching Guidelines

Focus on Safety

Labs

Legal Alerts

Medications

Now Can You

Nursing Care Plan

Nursing Diagnoses

Nursing Insight

Optimizing Outcomes

Procedures

What to Say

Where Research and Practice Meet

one
two
three
four
five
six
seven

Foundations
in Maternal, Family,
and Child Care

Traditional and Community Nursing Care for Women, Families, and Children

 As a Family-Centered Nurse

Learn of the essence of family-centered nursing,
while you walk with a worried family
until you wear side-by-side paths in the carpet;
Suffer the emotions of a troubled family
When they soar in their hope for healing and recovery;
Stay through the darkest hour of a mother, father, sister or brother,
as they silently cry for a member's pain;
Experience the failure, disappointment and challenges
presented with each health care encounter;
Never cease to be amazed at the resilience
of a family's strength, spirit and protective value.

—S. Caves

LEARNING TARGETS *At the completion of this chapter, the student will be able to:*

◆ Explore the impacts of ethnocentrism, ethnopluralism, paternalism, the medical model, and consumerism on nursing.

◆ Compare the roles of nurses, families, and patients in various health-care settings.

◆ Discuss theories of caring and holism as they apply to the nursing care of women, families, and children.

◆ Clarify nursing responsibilities using NANDA, NIC, and NOC taxonomy related to diagnosis, management, and outcome evaluation of family-centered medical and nursing problems.

◆ Summarize the importance of cultural humility in fulfilling the role of nurse teacher.

◆ Discuss how responsibility and professional accountability are enhanced by evidence-based knowledge.

PICO(T) Questions

The intent of evidence-based practice (EBP) is to provide nursing care that integrates the best available evidence. An initial step in EBP is to write a PICO(T) question that effectively guides the research. A PICO(T) question is an acronym that stands for population (P), intervention or issue (I), comparison of interest (C), outcome (O), and timeframe (T). Depending on the question, all or some of the question components are used in the research process.

Use these PICO(T) questions to spark your thinking as you read the chapter.

1. How do (P) nurses with 1 year of experience (O) view the importance of (I) incorporating the art of nursing in their practice (C) compared with nurses with 10 years of experience?

2. How do (P) patients who use (I) CAM (complementary and alternative health care/medicine) methods along with traditional treatment (O) rate their level of overall health (C) compared with those who do not use CAM methods?

Evidence-Based Practice

Rappaport, D. I., Ketterer, T. A., Nilforoshan, V., & Sharif, I. (2012). Family-centered rounds: Views of family, nurses, trainees, and attending physicians. *Clinical Pediatrics, 51*(3), 260–266.

The purpose of this study was to examine the impact of family-centered rounds (FCR) on the general pediatric inpatient population. According to the literature, bedside rounds typically include only the physician. Family-centered rounds include the physician and the multidisciplinary team and seek family involvement. Family-centered rounds are advocated by the American Academy of Pediatrics and recommended as a standard for practice. According to the literature, families are eager to participate, the practice may lead to earlier hospital discharge, and nursing staff are positive and supportive of the strategy.

The study, which compared the impact of FCR versus non-FCR, examined associations with the following outcomes: "longer duration of rounds," "higher family satisfaction," "staff perception of more difficulty managing rounds and less teaching," and "increased nurse and family participation during rounds with increased nurse satisfaction." Inpatient teams included attending physicians, senior residents, interns, and medical students. The teams, generally responsible for seeing an average of 10 patients during the rounds, also included the bedside nurse, unit nurse manager, pharmacist, dietician, and social worker and/or interpreter as needed. The decision regarding which professionals were included in rounding teams was based on the physician's preference, though FCR were encouraged. Rounds were traditionally made regardless of whether the family members participated.

The study, conducted over a 12-week period, used an observation tool completed once a week by a research assistant for each team's rounds. The research assistant used a stopwatch to record start and stop times, and total time included teaching activities with the residents and students, even though they may have occurred after leaving the patient's room. Time was also measured between the end of one round and the beginning of the next, and this component was referred to as "transition time." Surveys developed to measure family and staff satisfaction with the rounds included the "Family Survey" (11 questions with a 5-point Likert scale) completed by the parent or guardian and the "Staff Satisfaction Survey" (7 questions with a 5-point Likert scale) completed by physicians, residents, interns, medical students, and nurses. Surveys were coded to include the following three categories: no family present, family present but no nurse present, and both family and nurse present.

Study participants for this study included 295 patients and 257 staff members, and data were collected on 35 nonconsecutive days. A family member was present for 117 patients (40%), and a nurse was present for 172 patients (58%). Both family and nurse were present for 76 patients (26%). The rounds averaged 9.2 minutes with a range from 1 to 28 minutes. Interestingly, rounding time was significantly shorter when family members were present. The Family Survey was returned by 46% (137) of the family members, and of these, 85% agreed or strongly agreed with each item on the survey (indicative of satisfaction with the rounds). The Staff Satisfaction Survey was completed by 78 medical students, 60 interns, 59 nurses, 31 residents, and 29 attending physicians. Overall, the staff agreed or strongly agreed that "it was easy to manage the length of rounds," "family contributions were helpful," "families participated in decision making," and the staff disagreed that "patients and family concerns took too much time." Moreover, the staff generally agreed that on the days that more families were present, the amount of time spent on patient rounds was more easily managed. Staff respondents reported being comfortable when discussing patient cases with family members present.

The researchers concluded that the satisfaction level for families experiencing FCR versus non-FCR was essentially equal, although those experiencing FCR had a better understanding of the various roles of the team members. Furthermore, there was no significant variation in family satisfaction whether or not a nurse was present, although the nurses' level of satisfaction was improved when families were present for patient rounds. Consistent with previous studies were findings regarding medical students' expressions of concern over being questioned by the attending physician in front of the family.

1. How is this information useful to clinical nursing practice?

2. Based on these findings, what are implications for further research?

See Suggested Responses for Evidence-Based Practice on Davis*Plus.*

Introduction

Most nurses and students have personal understandings of what it means to be a nurse caring for women, families, and children—the field of family and child nursing. They may have even developed a broad range of strategies, knowledge, values, and competencies to use when caring for women, families, and children. Nurses conversely may approach family and child nursing no differently than they would if providing care for any other patient. Realizing how the nurse, the patient, other health-care providers, and outside forces of influence have framed

family and child nursing through the last century provides the nurse with insights into the level and outcome of care historically and currently received and given to families and children.

There is a fairly consistent view of how family and child patients are defined, from one of three family and children perspectives: an individual affected by some health event; the family unit involved in that event; and the whole of supporting mind-body-spirit, culture, and community affected by the experience (Rowe Kaakinen, Padgett Coehlo, Steele, Tabacco, & Harmon Hanson, 2014). Nurses and families are being challenged by ever-increasing numbers of health-care and societal changes to adapt and expand these perspectives on family and child health.

The traditional hospital that served as the center of care for families and children has been replaced by a myriad of community-based settings. With this change in setting, often the thrust of power has shifted from the traditional nursing and medical models to one of family-centered decision making.

Becoming a part of this care experience—engaging in the patient's lived experience throughout its entirety instead of functioning as a part of the process by doing "for" the patient—is one of the emerging roles for the family and child nurse. Using this engaging transpersonal approach to understanding the experience of the patient's entire mind-body-and-soul during times of health threats may offer one of the most fulfilling roles for the nurse, and one of the first experiences of empowered caring for the patient. This return to the development of a therapeutic nurse–patient relationship through communication and the artistry of nursing provides the nurse the opportunity to experience the ultimate caring component of nursing for which the profession is known.

This chapter begins with a historical overview of nursing, family and child health care, and the influences that have shaped and driven some of the changes toward a more contemporary approach to family and child nursing. It discusses the many professional roles of the family and child nurse, how they have changed over time, and where the future will take them, irrespective of the type of care setting. The focus of the chapter is on the art of caring and its centrality to the family and child nurse experience.

Traditional Nursing Care

Taking a look at the traditional role of nursing in the care of families and children helps identify the significance of both positive and unfavorable changes that have occurred during the past century and framed current standards of care.

HISTORICAL PERSPECTIVE

Physicians, the general public, and the nursing profession historically viewed health as the absence of disease and the presence of optimal functioning. Illness was seen as pathological and something of which the health-care provider worked to rid, heal, or cure the patient. This curative approach commonly was referred to as the **medical model**. It often entailed a paternalistic, one-way channel of communication between the powerfully dominant and more knowledgeable health-care provider and the submissive and uneducated patient or family. The power base for all decisions rested with the medical or, infrequently, the nurse provider who together often took an objective, detached biomedical approach (Gordon & Nelson, 2005).

Over the previous quarter century, a number of influences have affected how family and child health and nursing care are now defined in the 21st century (Fig. 1-1). The infusion of multiple cultures and beliefs about health-care systems, along with exponential growth in scientific and technological capabilities, have been major forces in shaping the structure and delivery of nursing care. In addition,

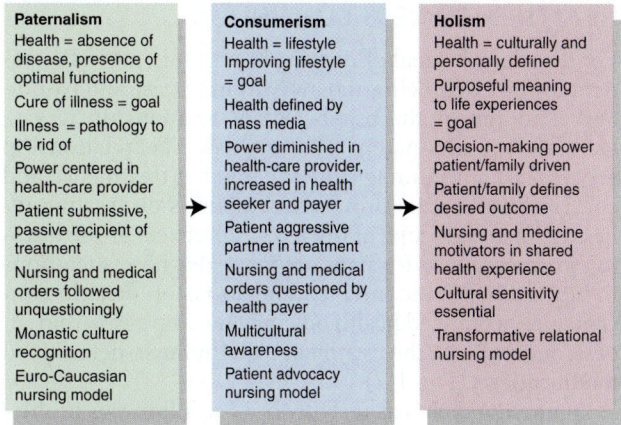

Figure 1-1 Evolution of family and child health nursing model.

increased consumer access to health-related information via the Internet, mass media, and other sources that may or may not be accurate, the unprecedented rise in health-care costs, and increasing imposition of cumbersome regulations have also contributed to change.

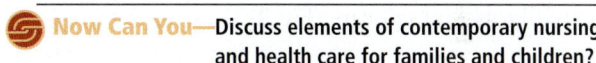

Now Can You—Discuss elements of contemporary nursing and health care for families and children?

1. Identify a major force that accounts for the present-day shift toward family-centered decision making in health matters?
2. Describe a nursing approach that fosters empowered caring for the patient?
3. Name four factors that have shaped contemporary family and child health and nursing care?

The growth of **ethnopluralism** (diverse cultures) impacts health-care systems and providers daily. Often each culture comes with its own beliefs, values, and practices about health and illness. The United States Department of Commerce, Bureau of the Census projects that within the next 10 to 12 years only one-half of the U.S. population will be of Euro-Caucasian descent, although the medical model formed and that continues to be supported is based on this group (U.S. Census Bureau, 2011). The population of other ethnicities and cultures will double and triple in that time, rapidly making up the other half of the U.S. population and bringing to the forefront their beliefs, values, and health practices.

During the past century the values, beliefs, and practices of the predominantly Euro-Caucasian male health-care provider system drove health-care decisions, interactions, and treatments based on the belief that these were unquestioningly in everyone's best interest and by far superior to all others: a belief referred to as **ethnocentrism** (Leininger & McFarland, 2006).

In a culture changing as rapidly as is that of the United States today, ethnocentrism can critically compromise effective health care. One of the predominant problems with a health-care system founded on ethnocentrism, paternalism, and the medical model is the system's closed-mindedness and prejudice toward other solutions and viewpoints of health. It is this viewpoint that often alienates people in need of health care and deters them from seeking or accepting help.

HEALTH–WELLNESS CONTINUUM

For decades, the goal of nursing has been to move the patient toward well-being and away from disease and pathology. The aim of the nurse–patient relationship was to facilitate the attainment of that goal. The relationship process had a beginning (illness), middle (treatment), and end (wellness). This prominent emphasis on treating illness defined the scope of the nurse's practice, or the **nursing process:** assess for signs of illness, diagnose alterations in health, determine interventions to restore health, conceptualize a targeted health outcome moving away from illness, and evaluate the treatment plan for nurse-determined modifications (Fig. 1-2).

In nursing there has recently been a shift in this health–wellness continuum and process. The emphasis is changing from a linear beginning-to-end, illness-to-wellness process. No longer is the predominant nursing perspective to return the patient from illness (beginning) to a prior disease-free state (end) but toward a shared experience of transcending or controlling the health threat and changing it into one of purposeful meaning (Wilson, 2007). The nurse–patient relationship now is a circular or spiral process formed to motivate the patient or family toward promotion, maintenance, and restoration of health; health potential; prevention of illness; and self-care (Fig. 1-3).

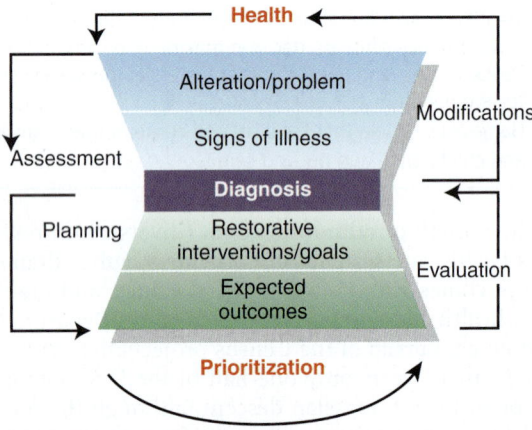

Figure 1-2 Traditional nursing process.

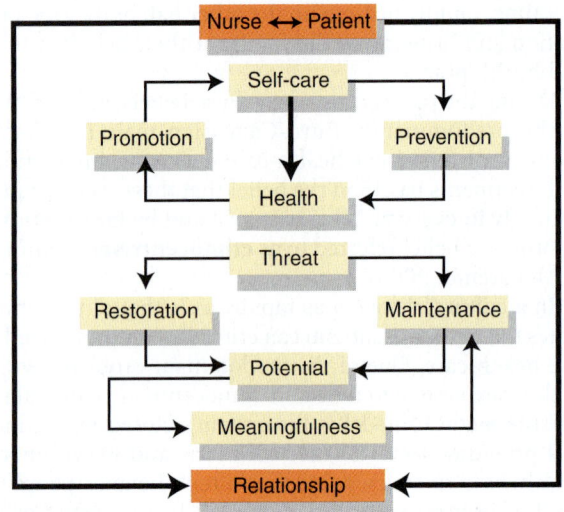

Figure 1-3 Health promotion nursing process.

Cultural Diversity: Perceptions of Desired Health and Health Outcomes

Based on personal beliefs, values, and practices, an ever-increasing culturally diverse population has many differing definitions of health and the outcomes desired during health-seeking encounters.

Through health promotion, the nurse helps the woman, child, or family understand health risk factors and adopt lifestyle changes that foster health maintenance, prevent health threats through early detection and recognition, and explore options for health restoration.

Across Care Settings: Health protection for families

With increasing international travel comes also the transport of illness vectors previously unknown in certain locales. Providing information about ways to protect children and families from these new sources of illness and injury through the use of individual instruction, educational videos, and use of the mass media can help the family maintain confidence in their ability to protect themselves from new threats.

This form of nursing entails a shared connectedness between patient and nurse. The goal is to experience the illness or health threat in the same way the patient perceives it. The nurse moves with the patient beyond the illness through the patient's own inner healing process to a patient-defined state of coping, harmony, wholeness **(holism),** and unity with the illness and healing outcome and hope, purpose, meaning **(spirituality),** and health potential beyond the illness toward healing. The power base for this healing and future health decisions rests in the patient's belief in her or his health potential.

The approach of the nurse provider is to form a caring relationship through listening, understanding, experiencing, presencing, facilitating, valuing, and using nursing aesthetics. **Nursing aesthetics,** or the art of nursing, is the low-tech, high-touch artistry of caring that strengthens the patient's confidence in her or his ability to manage the healing process, make change, or master the threatening health event (Stichler & Weiss, 2001). It is the way the nurse and patient help each other find meaning in the experience. It is a transformative, spiral process with a beginning (a threat), middle (relational building of trust and connection), and future (experiencing new possibilities for health change and outcomes) (Sanford, 2000).

Now Can You—Discuss aspects of health promotion and nursing aesthetics?

1. Describe present-day trends in nursing focus related to the health–wellness continuum?
2. Identify the elements of a health promotion nursing process?
3. Define "nursing aesthetics" and the role it plays in realizing health potential?

Some nursing interventions that fall under this art of aesthetics include imagery, music therapy, and touch. Guiding the family or child's imagination **(guided imagery)** to visualize repeatedly a positive outcome has been demonstrated to enhance healthy outcomes. Music has been shown to improve mood, reduce fatigue and agitation, and increase spirituality among patients (Ko, 2010). Music therapy helps bond the mind–body–spirit components of health and is especially successful with children. Touch and speech patterns of the nurse have descriptively been shown to soothe, calm, and encourage patients toward the health outcome of their choosing. One only needs to watch a caregiver stroke, rock, and sing to a sick child to know that this form of the nursing art works.

 ### Across Care Settings: Teaching simple strategies for stress relief

Most have heard of the beneficial effects of slow, deep, deliberate abdominal breathing patterns on the stress, anxiety, and pain associated with labor and birth. Nurses can teach these simple techniques to patients who anticipate stress, anxiety, or pain in any care setting.

 ### Cultural Diversity: Use of Imagery, Chanting, and Afterlife Encounters

One often thinks of imagery as a collection of nurse-initiated instructions given to the patient. To the woman undergoing treatment for cancer, the nurse may suggest, "Imagine all of the cancer cells flowing up through your body, gathering all of the bad cells with them, and finally bursting into an explosion of color and sparkles like an explosion of fireworks from your body. Out into the atmosphere they go, floating higher and higher as they disintegrate into outer space." But, have nurses considered the healing power connected with objects used by some non-European non-Caucasian cultures? For example, the healing feather used by Native Americans, the "seeing" of spirits practiced in Asian cultures, the casting of spells performed in the Caribbean Island culture, and the prayer beads used in Middle Eastern cultures. Spiritual treatments are an integral part of health promotion and healing for Native Americans, whose healing ceremonies rely heavily on a combination of traditional and Christian religious symbols, icons, and ritualistic objects (Koithan & Farrell, 2010). The healing effects of music and speech patterns have also been well documented. But do health professionals consider of equal value the healing value of chanting by the Native American or the wails of sorrow of the Central and Eastern European culture? One's awareness of various cultural practices is important. Even more important to their healing powers is the nurse's sensitivity and incorporation of such practices into a shared perspective of healing with the patient and family.

While the family or child relates stories of a lived experience, maintaining en-face eye contact, symbolically enfolding them through proximity, and staying focused solely on them acknowledges their worthiness. Imaginatively being in the patient's experience, reflectively sharing that experience through the use of body language, and avoiding demonstrations of disappointment and frustration gives the nurse a shared point of reference from which to help the family and child create meaning out of a threatening health experience (Fig. 1-4).

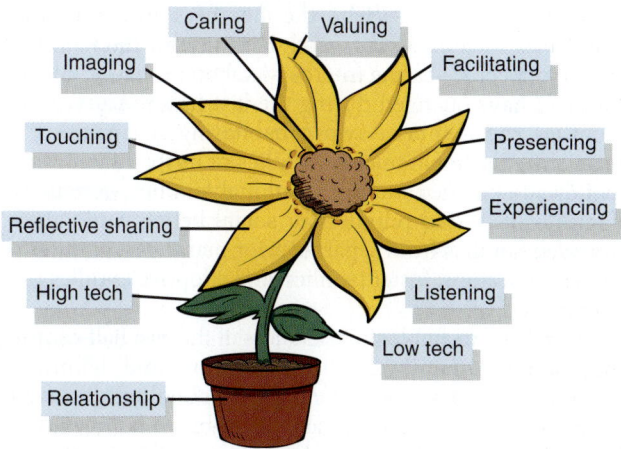

Figure 1-4 Nursing aesthetics that strengthen confidence in mastering a health threat.

CHANGING DEMANDS AND DEMOGRAPHICS

This nursing approach of **engaging transpersonal care** has evolved from the simple nursing basics of providing treatment-driven, high-technology-centered care. It is an opportunity for the family–child nurse to use the nursing process in a new way. The nurse assesses the patient and family's confidence to address and manage the health threat, diagnoses the health alteration from the patient's viewpoint, conceptualizes the outcome as the patient and family envision it, and supports the patient in his or her chosen changes directed at restoring health or transcending the threat. Finally, the nurse evaluates the ongoing maintenance of health as it is lived by the patient and family.

Over the last half-century, public trust in health-care providers has continually declined. Some surveys have noted that the public trusts health-care providers only slightly more than they do the Internal Revenue Service and the tobacco industry (Fottler, Ford & Heaton, 2010). According to data from the National Coalition on Health Care (2011), much of this is likely because of health-care providers' minimal awareness of consumer preferences and desire for personal control. Starting in the 1960s, health-care seekers became increasingly critical of health-care providers.

Family–child nursing responded to this call for consumer advocacy (consumerism) by supporting the consumer demand for a shift in the thrust of decision-making power. Other strategies included advocating for the provision of health care in facilities outside the standard hospital setting (accessibility) and by providing family-centered approaches to care that emphasized health promotion and education. During the next half-century, other societal changes occurred that continued to alter health-care delivery.

 ### Across Care Settings: Family-centered care

The need for family members to feel significant and competent to care for their loved ones is universal and should not be affected by the setting in which care is provided. Being friendly, encouraging family participation, and modeling of care are techniques that accomplish this goal in any setting.

Family structures (who the members are), functions (the roles members play), and definition of the family (a group of people sharing interpersonal bonds, tasks, and activities) have changed during the last half-century. Dyad families can comprise two cohabitating companions or spouses; traditional nuclear families of husband, wife, and children; extended multigenerational families; communal families of shared religious or social beliefs and values; blended families from separate prior marriages; families of same-sex unions; foster families; and adoptive families (see Chapter 3).

Social and technological advances of the past half-century have changed family structure, function, and definition. With the increasing acceptance and technologically available birth control options made available to families since the 1970s, family size has also changed. The sexual revolution of the 1960s resulted in an increase in the number of single-parent families. The feminist movement of the 1970s sent ever-growing numbers of mothers outside the home into a second work environment. As the workforce increased, industries flourished, cities grew, and families became more mobile in search of better lives for themselves, often leaving behind the extended multigenerational family they had learned to depend on.

In the family's search for a better life, family health consciousness increased, as did usage of health-care services and costs. The changes had implications for the way nursing delivered care and families sought it. Smaller families, single-parent families, families dispersed in search of better lives, and dual-income families meant fewer support persons present during family illnesses and crises. As a result, the role of the nurse inevitably changed from a focus on carrying out medical orders to a fuller scope of providing family support services.

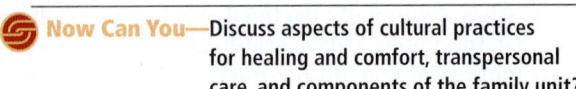

Now Can You—Discuss aspects of cultural practices for healing and comfort, transpersonal care, and components of the family unit?

1. Explain why nurses should develop awareness and understanding of cultural practices intended to foster comfort and promote healing?
2. Discuss a nursing approach that incorporates engaging transpersonal care?
3. Differentiate among family, family structures, and family functions?

PROFESSIONAL NURSING ROLES: HISTORICAL CONTEXT

Since the time of Florence Nightingale, nurses have played a role that involved clinical interventions, patient and family education, empathetic support, development of therapeutic relationships, and unique opportunities to make a difference in the lives of families during illness. Nursing's domain in the earlier times consisted of being a provider of care and a teacher. As a provider of care, the nurse would change elements of the patient's environment through hygienic measures, nourishment, and comfort to enable the best opportunity for recovery. As a teacher, the nurse would prepare the patient for procedures, surgery, and the uncertainties of hospitalization.

Even in the 1860s, nurses saw their patient responsibilities not only for the individual for whom they ministered but also for the living conditions of the individual's family. The most frequent cause of illness and death during these years was infectious diseases. The nursing emphasis on sanitation, nutrition, and family education played a key role in the decline in deaths well into the 1950s when antibiotic drugs and scientific treatments became widely available.

Until the late 20th century, nurses continued to be seen as passive, deferential, and compliant advocates to paternalistic physicians. Within the prevailing health-care system of the time, nurses practiced from the male-dominated, ethnocentric, patriarchal medical model of the professional nurse. In 1963, however, the nursing process began to change that.

DEVELOPMENT OF THE NURSING PROCESS

The **nursing process** was developed as a framework of systematic problem solving and actions to be used by nurses in identifying, preventing, or treating the individual health needs of patients. The nursing process was problem oriented, goal directed, and involved critical thinking and decision making. Clear differentiations were made between nursing and medical diagnoses, interventions, and outcomes. Ten years later, the North American Nursing Diagnosis Association (NANDA) developed a list of standardized nursing diagnoses used by the nurse through individualized patient care plans to express to other caregivers the findings of the nurse's assessment, diagnosis, and plans of action (Johnson, Moorhead, Bulechek, Butcher, Maas, & Swanson, 2012). An example of the use of the NANDA-I Diagnosis to formulate a nursing care plan for a child with culturally different verbal communication is presented in Box 1-1.

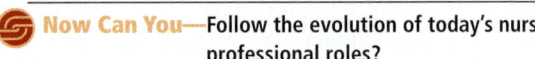

Now Can You—Follow the evolution of today's nursing professional roles?

1. Explain the central focus of the nurse as a provider of care and teacher before the 1950s?
2. Describe how the introduction of the nursing process as a systematic framework changed the nurse's professional role?

Contemporary Nursing Care

As families became more prosperous in the late 20th century, they also became more conscious of health promotion and advanced health technology. They demanded more knowledge about how to stay healthy, prevent common illnesses, and use technology to detect and treat early signs of health alterations. With this increased demand on the health-care system came increasing costs. In response to increased health-care costs, health-care systems and third-party payers focused on monitoring, controlling, and curtailing expenditures. As the costs for health care rose, the resultant changes impacted family and child health and nursing's professional role.

Hospitals and third-party payers responded to increasing costs in a number of ways that included managed care

Box 1-1 Use of NANDA-I Diagnosis to Formulate a Nursing Care Plan
Care Plan for the Patient With Culturally Different Verbal Communication

Patient and Family Data: Extended three-generational family comes to the health-care provider with a complaint of weakness and loss of appetite in a 3-year-old family member. The family has arrived from a Middle Eastern country within the previous 2 weeks; they do not speak English and converse among themselves loudly and with much gesturing.

NANDA Nursing Diagnosis: Impaired Verbal Communication related to patient-care provider cultural and language difference

Measurable Short-Term Goal: The family will have an opportunity through appropriate interpretation resources to share and interpret information regarding the well-being of the child.

Measurable Long-Term Goal: The family will express concerns, needs, wants, ideas, questions, and understanding about immediate and long-term home care of the child.

NOC Outcome:
Communication (0902): Reception, interpretation, and expression of spoken, written, and nonverbal messages

NIC Interventions:
Active Listening (4920)
Culture Brokerage (7330)

Nursing Interventions:

1. Assist the family and patient to establish means of communication via a professional interpreter.

2. Assess contributing cultural and language factors that may impede simple communication between the family and care providers.

   RATIONALE: A shared understanding of culture and language is necessary for communication to take place.

3. Evaluate the nature and extent and level of impairment differences that the family and care provider have related to the patient's health problem.

   RATIONALE: Misunderstandings of intent and content are heightened with increased levels of communication disparity.

4. Establish a therapeutic relationship by appearing relaxed, allowing extra time, and listening carefully.

   RATIONALE: Communication is enhanced when intent of trust and understanding is established.

5. Assist the family and patient to establish means of communication via an interpreter.

   RATIONALE: Law mandates that interpretation services be made available for accurate and precise basic understanding of medical terminology and care provided.

6. Validate the meaning of nonverbal and verbal communication.

   RATIONALE: Words and gestures can easily be misinterpreted and affect the delivery and reception of important concepts.

Documentation Focus:

1. Assessment of pertinent patient physical, psychological, and cultural concerns

2. Description and meaning of nonverbal cues as related by interpreter

3. Type of interpreter services used

4. Teaching and explanations communicated

5. Level of outcome (NOC) completion/accomplishment

6. Discharge needs, referrals, and stated family/patient understanding

NIC (Nursing Interventions Classification); NOC (Nursing Outcomes Classification).
Source: Adapted from Doenges, M. E., Moorhouse, M. F., & Murr, A. C. (2014). *Nursing care plans: Guidelines for individualizing client care across the life span* (9th ed.). Philadelphia, PA: F.A. Davis.

systems and the development of alternative settings for health-care delivery. In addition, greater emphasis was placed on patient and family accountability and responsibility for their own health promotion and disease prevention. This approach shifted the thrust of decision-making power to the consumer. Other measures included a redefining of nursing functions, workloads, and methods for care delivery.

CURRENT HEALTH-CARE SETTINGS

Cost containment, tightened reimbursement for services, and advanced technology have become important determinants of the current settings in which health care is received. Patients are being discharged earlier from acute care hospitals. Care is being provided in the home by family members using highly technical equipment. Many conditions that previously required acute care hospital stays are now being treated in ambulatory settings and the community-based health-care service sector is almost limitless. Hospitals, homes, and community service centers have become interdependent providers in the ever-expanding health-care arena.

Regional and specialized acute care hospitals for women, families, and children have undergone a multitude of changes since their inception in the late 1950s. Liberalized family, sibling, and children visiting; 24-hour family partnering with caregivers; policies and procedures based on theories of child and family growth and development; and a heightened level of acuity in these acute care settings have had both beneficial and challenging effects on nurses, families, and children. A strong knowledge base in the care of families and children, highly developed critical thinking skills, expertise with advanced technology, and dedication to evidence-based practice are stringent requirements for nurses caring for families and children in all settings.

When referred to these modern, highly technologically advanced facilities, family members are often separated by great distances from children and other support persons. Emotions of separation, anxiety, abandonment, fear, and guilt compound already tenuous physical conditions. The accessibility to follow-up care in these comprehensive settings is frequently made difficult by time, distance, and coordination of return visits to multiple providers of segmented and specialized care.

Even with the heightened acuity of patients in acute and tertiary care hospitals, the length of stay in the settings continues to decrease. With these decreasing hospital stays, alternative settings were created for what once was considered "inpatient care."

At the other end of the health provider environment from the specialized tertiary and acute care hospitals are the acute care 24-hour observation unit, freestanding short stay, and urgent care centers. The facilities are less costly than acute care settings, in part because they minimize the high cost of advanced technology in specialized hospitals. These settings present their own challenges for the nurse, family, and patient. Assessment, risk identification, counseling, and teaching must all be accomplished in a crucially compressed time. The nurse in these settings may be responsible for direction of unlicensed assistive personnel (UAP, also known as nursing assistive personnel [NAP]) who may not have the highly developed expertise needed to recognize subtle physiological changes in a patient's condition before discharge. Follow-up procedures that once were performed and monitored by nurses in the acute care setting now must be taught to the patient and family as they prepare for a rapid return to their home (Association of Women's Health, Obstetric and Neonatal Nurses [AWHONN], 2009).

 Collaboration in Caring—*Preparing the family for community-based care*

The nurse can prepare the patient and family for care outside the acute setting by:

- Discussing the feasibility of using specialized equipment in the home
- Encouraging the patient and family to investigate health insurance coverage for home care
- Suggesting the parents of a young patient contact school officials before a child returns after an illness
- Evaluating the family's transportation needs for follow-up care
- Discerning when an interaction in the acute care setting is conducive to teaching and learning

Since the early 1990s, there has been a dramatic increase in home- and community-based nursing care. Home- and community-based nursing care is provided in settings such as adult and child day-care centers, public and private schools, churches and religious body parishes, penal systems, health- and disease-related camps, foster homes and homeless shelters, physicians' offices, public health systems, and nurse-managed care centers (Fig. 1-5). Nurses in these settings often experience different degrees of professional independence and accountability, yet still need to possess expert skills as providers of clinical interventions, health history interviewers, culturally competent teachers, coordinators of extended care services, managers of allied health colleagues, supporters of family functionality, and advocates for family-centered care.

 Now Can You—Recognize the changes created by family-centered care for professional nursing in acute care settings?

1. List at least four characteristics of acute care hospitalization that have changed since the introduction of family-centered care?
2. Identify at least five community-based care settings in which the nurse may practice family-centered care?
3. Compare and contrast the role of the professional nurse in acute and specialized care hospitals and alternative care settings?

FAMILY-CENTERED CARE

Acute care providers have made strides toward keeping family members informed of hospital procedures and

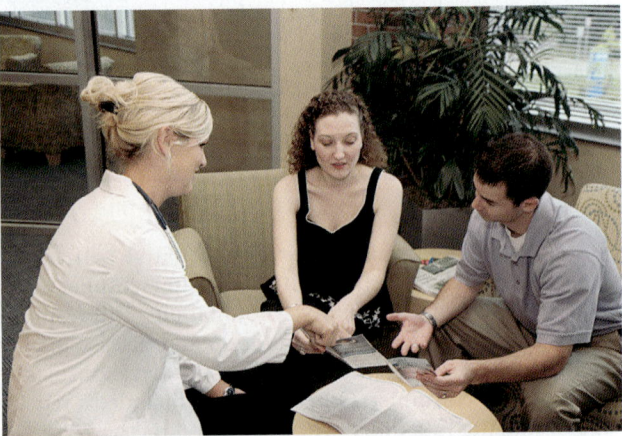

Figure 1-5 The nurse is instrumental in providing family-centered care in the community setting.

processes affecting their loved ones and the patient outcomes expected. Acute care settings still, however, are major sources of family disruption during times of stress and illness. Placing family relationships, their coping mechanisms, values, priorities, and perceptions at the center of a patient's health-care needs is the essence of **family-centered care (FCC).**

Family-centered care requires sensitivity to the beliefs, values, and customs of each family member and those of their supporting culture or community. The role of the family-centered nurse is to facilitate and assist the family in making informed choices toward the outcome the patient and family desire. Family-centered care necessitates that the nurse relinquish an authoritarian role that tells the family what is best for them while the nurse does things to and for them. The nurse becomes a human just like all other members of the family, each with their special abilities to support the patient. The center of power shifts from the one with the most clinical knowledge to the whole of the group's knowledge.

This is a large shift for the nurse educated under traditional Euro-Caucasian theories of nursing care. The global nature of health care as a multiethnic (ethnopluralitic), multicultural composite of health-seeking people requires an ever-growing sensitivity on the part of the nurse. Culture encompasses gender, faith, sexual orientation, profession, tastes, age, socioeconomic status, disability, ethnicity, and race (American College of Obstetricians and Gynecologists [ACOG], 2011). Cultural skill, which involves collecting cultural data and conducting a culturally relevant physical examination, requires effectiveness in cultural communication. Culturally sensitive communication is open, respectful, nonjudgmental, and reflective of the nurse's willingness to learn (Campinha-Bacote, 2002; Dean, 2010; Lewallen, 2011; Zander, 2007).

Consideration of the family's cultural influences allows the nurse to take a more in-depth approach to health assessment and outcome-directed interventions. For example, the proximity and quality of the family's support systems; religious and spiritual beliefs; customs and traditions, especially as they relate to health, illness, and healing; micro-living environment of the home; and macro-living environment of the neighborhood all must be incorporated into the plan of care. Other elements to be considered include financial resources, including willingness to ask for and accept additional resources; significant historical events, especially crises, losses, and new beginnings; and the members' communication patterns and verbal abilities, coping strategies, and problem-solving techniques.

One format used for assessing the health of a family is the community health map. With this tool, the nurse assesses the family structure, function, and support networks. The map provides a diagram of significant data and helps the nurse focus on the family as it interacts with the social systems within and around them (Falk-Rafael, 2005) (Fig. 1-6). Actively including the family members in the development of the community health map provides the nurse insights into the family's health experience and fosters the nurse–family alliance. The nurse should remember that the focus is on family health, past successes, and current strengths, not on family problems.

Learning, recognizing, and comprehending that these cultural factors are what shape a family's perception of their health and health-related events is known in nursing as **cultural awareness.** The nurse does not need to seek congruency between these factors, values, traditions, and beliefs and his or her own. The nurse does, however, need to recognize that how the patient and family comprehend and respond to a particular health event is shaped by these factors, values, and beliefs.

Structural Family Assessment
- Number males/females
- Marriage status
- Number/order children
- Family members loss/death
- Significant contacts and strength of relationship (work, church, medical, school, friends, extended family, clubs/organizational participation)
- Ethnicity
- Religion
- Socioeconomic status/environment
- Culture
- Health problems
- Living difficulties

Developmental Family Assessment
- Parent's family of origin
- Emotional reactions to changes
- Spiritual beliefs
- Recent life changes
- Degree of family stability
- Recent or expected shifts in family structure/relationships
- Affectional bonds
- Feelings about family roles
- Child care–work–relaxation balance
- Alone time balance
- Hopes for future
- View of extended family
- Previous health crises
- Method of coping with crises

Functional Family Assessment
- Socioeconomic systems in place
- Physical problems and strengths of patient
- Family strengths and weaknesses in shared caregiving
- Who identifies and problem solves what issues
- Parental discipline habits
- Perceptions of health, control over health, strengths, and weaknesses
- Health priorities (individual and shared)
- Health values (individual and shared)
- Cultural values (individual and shared)
- Spiritual values (individual and shared)
- Goals for a fulfilling life
- Permeability of family boundaries—who is allowed into inner circle and for what function
- Willingness to accept help
- Communication styles, patterns
- Use of power, by whom, when
- Emotional closeness

Figure 1-6 Community health map.

Nursing Insight—*Appreciating the related concepts of cultural sensitivity, cultural competence, and cultural humility*

In clinical settings, *cultural sensitivity* is a way of approaching individuals who hold health beliefs that are different from those of the provider, while *cultural competence* focuses on the ability of nurses to interact effectively with people of different cultures. Cultural competency implies that one can function with a thorough knowledge of the mores and beliefs of another culture. By contrast, *cultural humility* acknowledges that it is impossible to be adequately knowledgeable about cultures other than one's own, and there is no objective of mastering another culture. Instead, cultural humility is a lifelong continual process of self-reflection and self-critique that overtly addresses power inequities between providers and patients. To this end, the attainment of cultural humility is not a goal, but an active, dynamic process and an ongoing way of being in the world and being in relationships with others and self (Foster, 2009; Levi, 2009; Miller, 2009).

Cultural competence is the ability to understand and effectively respond to the needs of individuals and families from different cultural backgrounds (Jirwe, Gerrish, & Emami, 2006; Spector, 2012). To use cultural competence as a nursing assessment tool, the nurse must be open and receptive to gaining awareness and respect of these cultural influences. Nursing interventions that are based on a solid knowledge of these values and practices have been demonstrated to achieve much higher levels of successful outcomes for families and patients. Listening to the cultural voices and experiences of family and patients affirms their value and is critically important to unifying the nurse–patient relationship as it motivates the patient toward positive health-promoting activities.

 Across Care Settings: Ensuring cultural sensitivity and reliable information

In all care settings, nurses should use the services of professionals who can interpret word meanings correctly. Relying on family members often results in literal translation of words and omission of information—problems that create confusion and misunderstanding. In settings where professional interpreters are not available, the use of services such as an international thesaurus, or handheld personal information devices, can be useful alternatives.

Delivering nursing care that is sensitive to and understands cultural differences, whether in knowledge, values, beliefs, or role expectations, should help the nurse evolve into a culturally sensitive professional who makes assessments and plans interventions from a holistic framework. Framing one's nursing assessment, intervention, outcome expectation, and evaluation with a holistic perspective gives the nurse a better assurance that no significant physiological, psychological, cultural, spiritual, or social component is excluded.

 Cultural Diversity: Cultural Prescriptions and Proscriptions for Women and Children

Cultural prescriptions are folk beliefs, practices, and values of a group that tell women and children what they should do—what their respective roles should be.

Cultural proscriptions are folk beliefs, practices, and values of a group that tell women and children what they should not do—what is "not" incorporated in their respective roles. When assessing cultural prescriptions and proscriptions, it is helpful to consider elements such as clothing, exercise, sexual participation, disciplinary efforts, dietary habits, family roles and relationships, verbal and nonverbal communication, cleanliness, illness remedies, and displays of emotion.

In some cultures, women and children do not have the permission, the decision-making power, or the means to access the American health-care system. Legal barriers, language differences that restrict access to medical care, and lack of diversity in the health-care workforce are some of the obstacles that may prevent immigrant minorities from accessing care. In addition to the barrier(s) that culture may place on accessibility of modern health care for women and children, in many situations, health-care providers are not available in the areas where culturally bound groups reside. The real or perceived lack of accessibility, affordability, and availability of health-care services to growing numbers of individuals leaves the provision of health-care delivery to the family, especially in multicultural societies. In these situations, nurses must help family members identify needs, strengths, resources, coping mechanisms, and desired outcomes. The functions of the nurse and family are intertwined and require collaborative planning, delegation, coordination, and provision of care.

COMBINING MODERN TECHNOLOGY WITH THE CARING TOUCH

In settings where modern health care may not be accessible, affordable, and available or is culturally restricted, **complementary and alternative health care/medicine (CAM)** methods often are used. Complementary therapy is nontraditional medical treatment that is used together with conventional medical treatment; an alternative therapy is used to address health concerns in place of conventional medical treatment (National Center for Complementary & Alternative Medicine [NCCAM], 2011). The focus of these low-tech high-touch noninvasive, nonintrusive, nontraditional interventions is the support of the family and child's whole mind, body, energy, environment, and spiritual healing. The nurse approaches this healing methodology from a holistic philosophy of caring, aimed toward a goal of patient-centered autonomy and a patient-defined sense of well-being.

 Cultural Diversity: Ethnicity and Use of CAM

African Americans and Hispanics are more likely to use CAM based on recommendations from friends and family while non-Hispanic whites look to multiple information CAM sources such as social networks, media, and the Internet. The particular type of CAM used frequently relates to cultural patterns within a family. For example, there is greater use of acupuncture, green tea, and soy products among Asian Americans, whereas Hispanics are more likely to use a greater number of herbal products (Campesino & Koithan, 2010).

In 1998 an Advanced Practice Nurse established a "Nurses' Tool Box" of CAM nursing interventions found to be effective in establishing patient and family autonomy—relieving various illness symptoms, controlling pain, improving immune function, decreasing anxiety and depression, improving circulation, excreting toxins, and enhancing healing (Ward, 2002). CAM interventions range from guided imagery; aromatherapy; imagining; creating art and writing; prayer, chanting, meditation, and channeling; therapeutic touch, stroking, and cuddling; acupressure, tai chi, magnetic forces, and massage; music, singing, tonal vibrations, and various water therapies; to storytelling, joking, and humor (Fig. 1-7).

 ### Complementary Care: *Natural Healing With Functional Medicine*

Functional medicine focuses on restoring balance to a dysfunctional system by investigating and correcting underlying imbalances. The philosophy behind functional medicine grew out of naturopathy, which centers on supporting the body's ability to heal itself through dietary and lifestyle changes in combination with complementary and alternative medicine therapies. Functional medicine views each patient as a system of interconnecting unique genetic, psychosocial, and pathophysiological elements whose interactions with the environment influence health (Provencher, 2010).

Approximately 38 million U.S. adults use herbal and dietary supplements, and it is estimated that Americans spent more than 5.03 billion dollars on herbs and other botanical supplements in 2009 (Anastasi, Chang, & Capili, 2011;

Cavaliere, Rea, Lynch, & Blumenthal, 2010). This statistic reflects the increasing level of consumer interest and demand for low-tech medical and nursing interventions and self-directed healing. Certain CAM methods (e.g., acupuncture, natural products [herbs], qigong and t'ai chi) are used mostly by individuals with higher educations and incomes (Darby, 2009; NCCAM, 2008). The nurse must be aware that not all CAM interventions are noninvasive, nonintrusive, or free from side effects and negative consequences. It is important to remember that CAM may involve the use of nutritional and herbal supplements, diet adjustments and fasting, chiropractic and body manipulation, and the use of drugs that have not been fully tested for safety and efficacy. Today, much confusion about CAM remains in both the consumer and health provider sectors (Box 1-2).

 ### Collaboration in Caring—*Supporting the family that uses CAM*

The nurse can provide support to the patient or family that uses CAM by:

- Investigating what they think caused a health event and how they have been able to avoid it in the past
- Encouraging them to seek all approaches of healing that are evidence-based, including both traditional and alternative medicine
- Respecting the participation of a family-chosen folk healer
- Acknowledging the patient's/family's religious and spiritual beliefs
- Reflecting on and understanding personal beliefs and recognizing when they may conflict with those of the patient
- Avoiding judgment

The family-centered nurse has a responsibility to advocate for the patient and family who choose to use CAM; to assess for and educate about the implications, contraindications, and benefits of CAM to the family and patient; and to promote health practices that have been proven safe and effective in restoring well-being, whether via conventional treatments or CAM. The nurse must recognize that health can be achieved through various means, both high-tech and high-touch, and that individual well-being is most optimally accomplished when care is directed by concerns

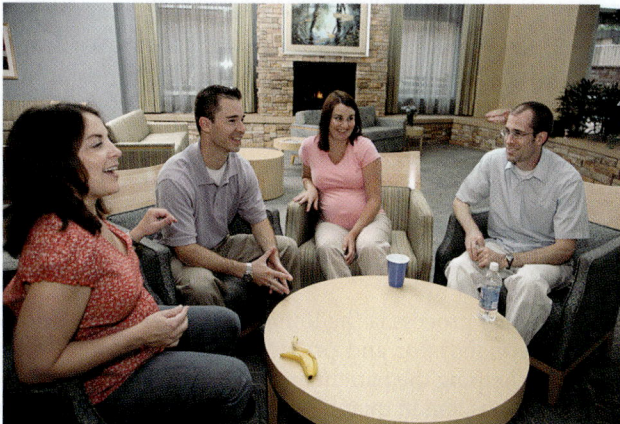

Figure 1-7 Storytelling, joking, and humor are therapeutic complementary and alternative medicine interventions.

Box 1-2 Confusion About CAM Through the Ages

A HISTORY OF MEDICINE
(Author unknown)

2000 B.C.	"Here, eat this root."
1000 A.D.	"That root is heathen. Say this prayer."
1850 A.D.	"That prayer is superstitious. Drink this potion."
1940 A.D.	"That potion is snake oil. Swallow this pill."
1985 A.D.	"That pill is ineffective. Take this antibiotic."
2000 A.D.	"That antibiotic doesn't work anymore. Here, eat this root."

Source: Helms, J. E. (2006). Complementary and alternative therapies: A new frontier for nursing education? *Journal of Nursing Education, 45*(3), 117.

expressed, interventions chosen, and outcomes defined by the patient. It is easy to understand why the nurse–patient relationship and a focus on the patient as a whole being (mind, body, energy, environment, and spirit) are key to the success of CAM healing.

Also key to a healthy outcome when using CAM therapy, as with all nursing interventions, is the responsibility to encourage evidence-based decision making. Patients must have an understanding of the most up-to-date information available, and nurses are central to helping patients understand evidence. This method of **evidence-based practice** is built on the premise that interventions need to be questioned, examined, and confirmed or refuted in their ability to support healthy outcomes. The nurse using evidence-based practice searches computer databases and current literature for reports that evaluate the safety, quality, and credibility of particular interventions. These searches produce reports from rigorous research studies, textbook and journal readings, stated expert opinions, and best practices resulting from quality improvement activities. Evidence-based practice has the potential to improve clinical outcomes and quality of care. It is the nurse's responsibility to use the best evidence available and to make decisions accordingly, especially when working with practices such as CAM that are viewed by many as mythical, magical, and nontraditional (Harrington, 2012; Stevens, 2013).

Another source of evidence-based guidelines available to the nurse is the standards of care/practice developed by nursing professional organizations such as the American Nurses Association (ANA); Society of Pediatric Nurses (SPN); National Association of Neonatal Nurses (NANN); National Association of Pediatric Nurse Associates and Practitioners (NAPNAP); and Association of Women's Health, Obstetric and Neonatal Nurses. These published guidelines promote consistency and quality in nursing care and outcomes. Because of the time it takes to search and retrieve evidence-based knowledge, these guidelines provide the nurse a reliable source of high-quality interventions on which to base practice. As health-care professionals, nurses must guide patients to the best possible evidence and explain it to them in a way that they can understand it and use it.

teaches the patient and family by helping them gain knowledge and skills about the health risk affecting them and of behaviors that can assist in accomplishing the health outcome they desire. There is a sharing of knowledge, and through that knowledge, a gathering of strength that can be directed toward the health condition.

The nurse, patient, and family combine their strengths, through collaboration, to describe the health issue, what it means in their lives, and what interventions and decisions are possible and preferable. This collaboration results from, and becomes an act of, mutual respect for each other's values, abilities, expectations, and experiences with the health event and life (Sanford, 2000). Collaboration with the patient and family about health education needs pulls the nurse away from the traditional "banking" concept of patient teaching and learning in which facts, skills, and knowledge are offered by the nurse and deposited for storage in the patient's vault (Freire as cited in Sanford, 2000, p. 6).

Collaboration requires two-way dialogue and sharing between the patient and nurse of both personal and health-related problems and solutions. Each participant is an equal possessor of knowledge and shares the power of determining what is to be learned. Each has a desire to learn more from and about the other. Participants become personally engaged and share a deeper level of understanding of each other, the health risk as each perceives it, and the available and chosen interventions to explore in collaboration.

The nurse still holds responsibility as the provider of care to implement the chosen interventions or to accept accountability for their delivery. Even though family-centered care encourages patient and family involvement in therapy delivery, it is still expected that the nurse will be actively involved and skilled in the provision of health assessment, treatment, care, and follow-up evaluation. The nurse plays a vital role in collaborative care across a range of settings, especially in the follow-up evaluation and ongoing treatment. It is the nurse's task to collaborate with the discharge planner, child's teacher, physician, physical or speech therapist, dietitian, and community services worker to develop with the family the best plan of care for the desired long-range health outcome.

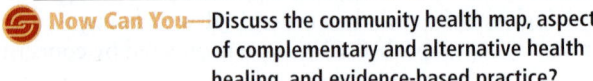 **Now Can You**—Discuss the community health map, aspects of complementary and alternative health healing, and evidence-based practice?

1. Discuss the value of a community health map as a nursing assessment tool?
2. Identify at least five ways that nurses can offer support for the patient/family who uses CAM?
3. Explain what is meant by evidence-based practice?

Now Can You—Describe the role of the nurse as a teacher, collaborator, and provider?

1. Explain how the nurse functions in the role of patient/family teacher?
2. Discuss aspects of therapeutic nurse–patient collaboration?
3. Describe the need for accountability on the part of the nurse as a provider of care?

PROFESSIONAL NURSING ROLES: TEACHER, COLLABORATOR, AND PROVIDER

Ever since Florence Nightingale's time, helping patients and families gain understanding into their health practices has been integral to the profession of nursing (Nightingale, 1859). The role of the nurse as patient and family teacher has been sustained over the years as a foundation of the profession and continues to be reinforced through professional standards of care/practice. The professional nurse

THE NURSING PROCESS IN CONTEMPORARY CARE

The nursing process is the foundation for the professional role as collaborator and provider of care and guides the nurse in helping the patient and family choose appropriate interventions and in quantifying and evaluating the chosen outcome goal. By using the NANDA International **Nursing Outcomes Classification (NOC)** and **Nursing Interventions Classification (NIC)**, the nurse is able to evaluate more clearly associations between interventions and outcomes (Johnson et al., 2012). Using these standards also helps nursing students and novice professionals develop the intellectually and technically complex competencies required to link assessment cues accurately with outcomes and interventions (Smith & Craft-Rosenberg, 2010).

Nursing interventions are more than the actions nurses take to help patients and families toward their desired outcome. One NIC may entail up to 30 actions or activities the nurse and family selectively choose from to individualize the intervention to the specific health condition as it is perceived at that moment (Johnson et al., 2012). The NIC also involves the evidence-based practices and critical thinking processes the nurse undertakes when judging for appropriateness and feasibility of activities chosen to reach resolution of the health problem and achieve desired outcomes.

Nursing interventions must be appropriate for both the selected nursing outcomes and diagnoses. They require comprehensive, preliminary assessment of patient and family strengths and health concerns; acceptability to the patient and family of the chosen interventions; and the nurse's and family's capabilities to fulfill or coordinate the chosen health outcomes with other health-care providers, both professional and familial.

Before nursing interventions are selected, appropriate, feasible, and family-agreed-on outcomes must be clearly identified. The chosen NOCs help the nurse identify, prioritize, and differentiate the critical from the sometimes exhaustive list of other relevant interventions and actions. Just as nursing interventions are more than the sum of outcome-directed actions, outcomes are more than the ultimate end goal of the health state. Outcomes are dynamic and demand frequent measurement of the responsiveness of the chosen interventions. Outcomes should be evaluated for continuing meaningfulness, both physiologically and personally; for direction and purpose, whether health restoration, maintenance, promotion, or threat prevention; and for consistency with the culturally lived experience of the patient and family.

The Caring Art and Science of Nursing

Just as a family's culture is their centering foundation in times of health and illness, caring is the centering foundation of nursing. "Caring transcends language, customs, and cultural differences . . . it is universal" (Watson as cited in Rexroth & Davidhizar, 2003, p. 298). It "defines the characteristics and parameters of practice" (Falk-Rafael, 2005, p. 38). The Accreditation Commission for Education in Nursing (ACEN), formerly known as the National League for Nursing Accrediting Commission (NLNAC), supports caring as a vital core value of nursing (ACEN, 2013). Caring often leads to new outcomes and new ways of being and experiencing life for a patient and family (Watson, 2011).

"Many circumstances in contemporary society have made caring more difficult now than in the past" (Rosalynn Carter as cited in Cluff & Binstock, 2003, p. 15). Advanced technology, the rapid pace of health care, and a focus on the legal ramifications of one's professional actions have placed great demands on the time and support a nurse can offer a patient and family. Understanding the many dimensions of caring

one brings to, and gets from, the patient encounter is essential to the nurse's ability to recognize the pain, suffering, and vulnerability that patients experience.

THEORIES THAT FRAME CARING AS THE CORE OF NURSING

Florence Nightingale's model of nursing encouraged a focus on the spiritual, physical/environmental, emotional, mental, and social needs of the patient and is known as a holistic view of the patient (Nightingale, 1859). She described the base of nursing activities as observation; experience; knowledge of sanitation, nutrition, caring, and compassion; and the focus of nursing as the patient rather than the illness. Nightingale viewed all people as equal in their abilities to attain health. In addition to her emphasis on improving the patient's environment, she encouraged the use of imagination and retelling of pleasant life events as appropriate healing interventions to help restore the patient to the best possible condition so that natural healing could occur (Nightingale, 1859).

Watson and Leininger are two modern-day theorists known for their inclusion of caring as a core of nursing. The commonalities between these two theorists are especially important in understanding how to incorporate caring as a recognized nursing intervention with a measurable outcome.

In her *Theory of Human Caring*, **Jean Watson** contends that caring as a nurse demands that attention be given not only to the body but also to the soul and spiritual dimension of the patient and family. She defines the soul as the ideal self of an individual and notes that the individual is constantly striving to achieve that ideal self by creating harmony among the body, mind, and spirit—between the ideal self (referred to as "I") and the current self as living the experience (referred to as "me"). The state of health is related to the congruence between I and me and the effect that the differences in I and me is having on the body, mind, and spirit (Watson, 2005). As Watson and Woodward (2010) explain, "a caring occasion occurs whenever the nurse and client come together in a human-to-human transaction" (p. 358). The caring moment involves an action and choice by both the nurse and the other individual and presents them with an opportunity to decide how to be in the moment (Theroux, 2011).

By participating in transpersonal therapeutic relational nurse–patient communication in which each participant gives and gains equally and learns to identify with the other, the nurse and patient demonstrate mutual caring, recognize the other as more than an object, and move the patient toward a desired state. This caring by the nurse begins with the feelings elicited and responses demonstrated toward the patient's condition, allowing or encouraging the patient to also release feelings and thoughts about the condition and self. The focus of the encounters, referred to by Watson as caring occasions, is on "caring, healing and wholeness, rather than on disease, illness and pathology" (Watson, 2005).

The goals of the nurse–patient transpersonal therapeutic relational communication are to find meaning and develop a wholeness in the body–mind–spirit; assist the patient in transcending beyond the current health state toward his or her ideal; give meaning to the patient's being; and "release some of the disharmony, the blocked energy that interferes with the natural healing processes; thus the nurse helps another through this process to access the healer within, in the fullest sense Nightingale's view of nursing" (Watson, 2011, p. 108).

Madeleine Leininger also believes that caring is the core value of nursing. "Caring is essential for curing, but curing is not essential for caring" (Leininger as cited in Jeffreys, 2010, p. 37). Her *Theory of Transcultural Care Diversity and Universality* sees caring and culture as embedded within each other. You cannot have one without the other.

Caring necessitates understanding of the patient's cultural beliefs, values, methods of providing or showing caring, causes of illness and how it is viewed, and how wellness is achieved. This level of understanding only comes through a trusting relationship. Developing that trusting relationship is an ongoing process. When the nurse takes the time to clarify the patient's health beliefs and practices, reflect on one's own health values and actions, and validate through an unprejudiced and unbiased eye (avoiding judgment of what seems logical, sensible, or reasonable) the strengths and weaknesses of each, a caring relationship is established.

 Now Can You—Compare and contrast the caring base of nursing as described by Nightingale, Watson, and Leininger?

1. Describe Nightingale's focus of nursing?
2. List three of Watson's goals for a caring, therapeutic nurse–patient relational communication?
3. Discuss Leininger's advice for a nurse who wishes to develop a caring nurse–patient relationship?

ESSENTIAL CHARACTERISTICS OF CARING

Trust, built through an interactional relationship in which the nurse is cognizant of both personal and the patient's feelings and meaning of the health experience, is an essential characteristic of caring. It can involve such concrete actions as listening and observing for cues as to what the health event means to the patient and what the patient views as her needs, how they should be met, and what the desired outcome should be. It is the aesthetic engagement, or art, of nursing that is defined as caring (see Fig. 1-4).

Caring provides a sense of empowerment (some believe caring is the opposite of power), capability, inner peace, and self-determination. It requires an understanding of one's own beliefs, prejudices, and values so that those of the patient can be addressed with respect and dignity (Davis, 2005; Rhodes, Morris, & Lazenby, 2011).

A study of patients in an intensive care unit (Rosenthal as cited in Rexroth & Davidhizar, 2003, p. 301) helped divide caring characteristics into instrumental behaviors of caring and expressive behaviors of caring, or technical and nontechnical components. It is important to know that nursing behavior that is considered caring first depends on clinical competence and technical expertise. "Without knowledge, caring is just a matter of good intentions" (Mayeroff as cited in Falk-Rafael, 1998, p. 41). It was found that where the patient perceived himself to be on the health-wellness continuum, or how critically ill, played a big role in the value he placed on the instrumental versus expressive caring behavior of the nurse (Mayeroff as cited in Falk-Rafael, 1998, p. 41) (Fig. 1-8).

 Collaboration in Caring—*Enhancing family and patient coping*

The nurse caring for a patient in an intensive care unit can facilitate coping by:

- Encouraging family presence, interaction, and touching
- Encouraging the family to adhere to home/daily routines as much as possible
- Including the family in the plan of care, offering choices when possible
- Encouraging discussion of family fears and anxieties
- Offering to contact a spiritual leader or healer
- Encouraging the family to place familiar and comforting articles nearby

In a study that explored patients' perceptions of caring, expressive behaviors such as smiling, gentleness in touch, praising the patient for her efforts, and making the patient feel important were consistently classified as central expressions of caring (Davis, 2005). Communication was identified as another essential element. Communication with the patient and family that they mattered to the nurse personally; about the patient's hopefulness for the future and awareness of a higher source of healing; and

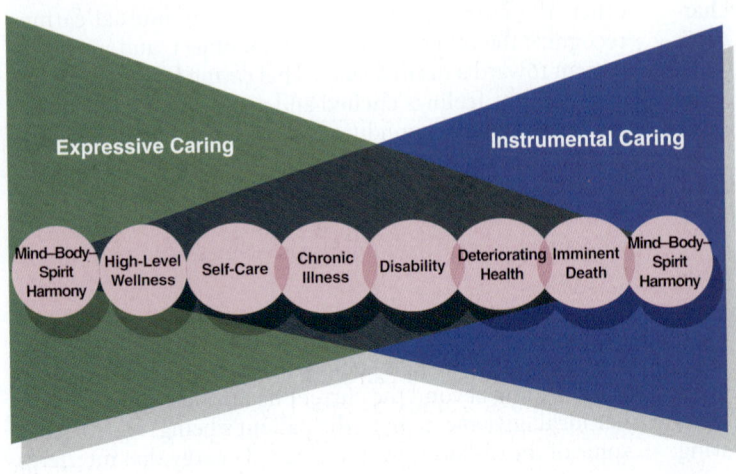

Figure 1-8 Health–illness continuum and the patient's need for caring behaviors.

with the physician that things were going well or not going well as defined mutually by the patient and caregiver were all recognized as supportive, caring ways of conveying concern, interest, and compassion (Cluff & Binstock, 2003).

In addition to instrumental and expressive characteristics of caring, a spiritual component was reported by patients. Spiritual caring, however, did not necessarily equate with attention to one's religion, rituals, or beliefs. Rather, **spirituality** addressed the meaning of life, including the present as being experienced, the past, and the future. It entailed learning about a patient's and one's own perceived weaknesses, vulnerabilities, and mortality and where the power lies to transcend or accept them (Kelly, 2004). Again, many of the same expressive characteristics were found when describing nurses who addressed spiritual caring (touching, listening, respecting, trusting, and humor). It is important to note that more than 80% of the patients questioned about caring stated they did not expect the nurse to address their spiritual needs, although they would have liked it (Davis, 2005).

Helms (2009) suggests that the simple act of touch, such as placing a hand on the shoulder or holding hands, is capable of creating a spiritual, person-to-person connection. Another way that nurses can help to create a spiritual connection with their patients is by teaching them self-care measures such as centering meditation using a holy word, the relaxation response, or deep breathing. **Therapeutic presence** has been defined as a spirit-to-spirit connection using mind, body, spirit, and emotion (Geller & Greenberg, 2011). Offering presence constitutes perhaps the simplest spiritual gift of all, as it is the gift of self (Helms, 2009).

Tolstoy said that "the essence of caring is the need to have one's position grasped" (Cluff & Binstock, 2003, p. 47). Caring's "unifying essence, however, is concern for and responsiveness to the needs and worth of the person receiving it. . . . How often do I turn my focus from my performance to the needs of the patient?" (Cluff & Binstock, 2003, p. 1).

 Now Can You—Define the essential characteristics of caring?

1. List three nursing actions designed to build trust?
2. Discuss the importance of instrumental, expressive, and spiritual behaviors of caring?
3. Identify three ways that communication is translated into caring behavior?

PROFESSIONAL NURSING ROLES: CARE PROVIDER, THINKER, AND ADVOCATE

Provider of Care

As a provider of care, the nurse expertly includes caring behaviors that address all the physical, psychosocial, and spiritual needs of the patient and family. Through careful assessment of all three categories of needs, diagnosis of the patient's response to the health event, planning of interventions that promote the patient's strengths and follow-up, and evaluation of the patient's transition and potential for a new health state, the nurse can accomplish the most effective, efficient, and desirable outcome.

 Nursing Insight—*Public trust in nurses*

In 2012, for the 12th year, nurses were voted the most trusted profession in America in Gallup's annual survey that ranks professions based on their honesty and ethical standards. Eighty-four percent of Americans rated nurses' honesty and ethical standards as "very high" or "high." Since the profession's first appearance in the poll in 1999, nurses have received the highest ranking each year except in 2011, when firefighters ranked first.

One of the major responsibilities of the nurse as a provider of care is to stay current and competent in the operation of technical procedures and monitoring equipment. This professional responsibility requires knowledge of not only how to perform the procedures and operate the equipment but also an understanding of why the procedure and equipment are necessary.

It means the nurse is not only responsible for safely executing the procedure but also accountable for recognizing and interpreting the data gathered during the procedure and from the equipment read-outs. This level of responsibility and accountability evolves from an ongoing development of critical, analytical thinking on the part of the nurse.

Critical Thinker

Critical thinking is the "precise, disciplined thinking that promotes accuracy and depth of data collection and seeks to clearly identify the problems, issues, and risks at hand" (Alfaro-LeFevre, 2011, p. 87). Much of what it entails comes from experience, knowledge seeking, practiced hands-on work, and contextual discernment. Much of critical thinking is also built on inner personal skills, including the ability and willingness to self-reflect on values and beliefs, open-mindedness to diverse and unique perspectives, persistence in seeking the most reasonable answer, comfort and confidence with calculated risk-taking, and devotion to listening with a passion for true comprehension and understanding (Alfaro-LeFevre, 2011). The overriding purpose of critical thinking always is to make the best clinical judgment possible.

 Now Can You—Describe why critical thinking is key to the successful clinical practice of nursing?

1. Define critical thinking?
2. Name four avenues for developing successful analytical critical thinking?
3. Discuss the personal skills that help build critical thinking analysis?

Effective Communicator

Good listening and communication skills are essential to the nurse, especially when providing care for children and families. Often the nurse receives key information through subtle tones of voice and snippets of dialogue with a child or parent. Listening carefully allows the nurse to evaluate the level of language development of a child and to effectively use words that can be understood. It also offers the nurse an opportunity to view how the family communicates with each member, often delineating the family roles and structure. Listening to communication patterns can clue the nurse to components of the patient's value system and cultural approaches. For example, some cultures consider it rude to offer an immediate response when asked a question. Silence signifies that the receiver values the question and the person and is giving it serious consideration. Some cultures communicate through storytelling, "Remember when Aunt Margie was in the hospital and. . . ." The nurse can use this insight to help tailor much of the interactions that will take place during the health event encounter. Listening to the family communicate can provide insight into the most favorable method of interacting.

The nurse often has the potential to role model for the child, and even the parent, effective ways of verbally expressing ideas, thoughts, and feelings. One way of role modeling appropriate expressive language is by the use of reflective listening and rephrasing. A parent who tells a 3-year-old, "Now be a good boy and stop crying. Big boys don't cry," might benefit from the nurse rephrasing the statement for her by saying, "Mommy knows your head hurts, and it's all right to cry. You did such a good job helping the nurse see how warm your body was."

Tone and quality of voice sometimes communicate more than the actual words themselves. This is especially true with infants and toddlers. All audible sounds convey meaning, even when the tone is incongruent with the word. Caution should be taken when using a stern tone to express endearments like, "Get over here so I can put some love on you." The young child is more likely to hear the stern tone of the voice than he or she is to hear the loving words. Touch, eye contact, and body language are also key components of communication the nurse must recognize as having the potential for enhancing or impeding a healthy outcome.

Cultural Diversity: Patterning Effective Communication Styles

Most of us have seen the way an infant responds to the pace of our speech. Talk slowly, and the infant's body movements become slower to match the pace of the spoken words. Talk very quickly, and the infant becomes very active with her movements. To communicate effectively with various cultures, nurses need to become aware of the pacing of their speech. The pacing of the spoken word for people from the southern United States is often slow and drawn out, commonly called a "Southern drawl," while the spoken word of the person from New York City is often rapid and clipped, commonly called "rapid-fire chatter." Responding to a Southerner with rapid-fire answers, or to a New Yorker with slow, drawn out responses, may be perceived as rude. Listening to the speech pattern of the patient can allow the nurse to match that pattern when communicating with her.

Listening, touching, establishing eye contact, patterning, and paying attention to body language are all essential components of effective communication. The vital distinguishing factors of therapeutic communication, however, are that it is purposeful, goal driven, and focused on the outcome. Therapeutic communication should most often start with an introduction of the nurse, by name and role. This helps differentiate the purpose of therapeutic communication from that of social interaction. Maintaining focus of the communication on the outcome desired (i.e., meeting the patient's needs) helps not only in the nurse's time management but also in identifying data that are important from that which may be interesting but not necessary for a healthy outcome.

Optimizing Outcomes—Conveying empathy to enhance communication

Empathy is the process through which one attempts to project oneself into the life of another and imagine a situation from the other individual's point of view. Empathy plays an important role in caring for and healing the whole patient, especially in the field of reproductive medicine, where events often take place at critical stages of the development of individuals and families. To provide empathetic care, one must develop an appreciation of each patient's story and an understanding of the differences among individual patients and their unique situations (American College of Obstetricians and Gynecologists [ACOG], 2011).

Teacher

The nurse's professional role as a teacher relies heavily on effective therapeutic communication. To meet the patient's desired health outcome, in addition to caring and competent nursing care, the patient needs information and education. Teaching what to expect regarding a procedure, surgery, or hospitalization; how to prevent complications, injuries, or illnesses; preparation toward discharge and continuing self-care efforts; guidance in nutrition, safety, and general wellness behaviors; and identification and avoidance of high-risk behaviors are all professional obligations of the nurse. With patient encounters sometimes controlled by the clock, opportunities for effective teaching must be expertly recognized, planned, and executed.

Using multiple communication approaches can facilitate the nurse's health education encounter with the patient and family. Because children are introduced to television, animated computer games, and interactive learning early in their development, simply talking to them may not achieve the effect the nurse desires. Just as health assessment is a key role for the nurse when providing care, so is learning assessment. Finding out the desired educational outcome of the patient, her preferred learning style, and the most effective methods of delivery are fundamental to the nurse's role as a health teacher.

It is especially important to allow additional time for questions and answers. Most have experienced a precocious 3-year-old child's persistent and repeated use of the word "Why?" and the adolescent's ongoing "Yeah, but what if?" The nurse must feel comfortable in permitting the child all the time necessary to have these questions answered, no matter how seemingly insignificant. Not only does it provide an avenue for teaching and learning, but it also demonstrates to the child and parent that the child is important to the nurse. Taking the time to exhaust all the questions helps establish and enhance therapeutic nurse–patient communication. Keep answers and explanations simple until asked for more elaboration.

Optimizing Outcomes—Identifying patient expected learning outcomes

Best Outcome: The nurse establishes the targeted learning outcome by talking and negotiating with the patient and family about what is most important. For example, an 8-year-old child learning how to control his asthma may be more interested in the mechanics of the use of the inhaler, while a 13-year-old might want to know how long he can wait to use his inhaler when he first experiences difficulty breathing (wanting to avoid at all costs the appearance of being different from the other children). Finding out what the child or adult wants to learn increases the success of changed behavior through new knowledge—always the underlying goal of teaching.

Mutually establishing the patient desired learning outcome is important to the success of the teaching encounter. Discussion of outcomes is futile if the patient is not ready to learn. Assessing readiness to learn is critical to the outcome of teaching. If there are basic needs yet unmet, such as physical hunger, safety, or pain; psychological anxiety, fear, or guilt; and spiritual rituals, fears, and traditions; then learning is likely to be less effective. After ensuring that basic needs are met, the nurse can then assess for the patient's readiness to learn while taking into consideration the language development; current level of knowledge and experience with the topic; growth and development stage of life and capabilities; psychomotor, cognitive, and emotional skills; cultural rituals, beliefs, and values; and the learning environment.

In addition to setting mutually understood learning outcomes and assessing the readiness of the learner, there are some other key principles the nurse needs to be cognizant of when performing health teaching. Praise and positive feedback foster feelings of competence and motivation to learn more. The nurse is the ultimate role model for health teaching. Actions are remembered and patterned much more easily and create a more lasting effect than words. It is important to remember that along with the topic that the child, his family, and the nurse have chosen, growth and development learning tasks are also under way, so the teaching should be planned as not to overwhelm the child. Topics should be taught in a manner that moves from the simple to the complex, with the recognition that follow-up teaching may need to be delivered in another setting at a later date.

Collaborator

The nurse plays a key role as a collaborator and coordinator of health teaching, especially when it must occur and be reinforced across multiple care settings and with multiple caregivers. Continuity of care involves not only addressing the continuing physical, emotional, and spiritual needs of the patient, but also the learning needs. Planning, implementing, and evaluating a teaching plan should involve members of multiple health disciplines: dietitians, community health nurses, social workers, home health aides, discharge planners, respiratory therapists, criminal justice workers, schoolteachers, pharmacists, physical therapists, ministers, respite providers, physicians, clinical nurse specialists, nurse practitioners, and family supporters.

Optimizing Outcomes—With nurse bedside reporting

"Nurse Bedside Reporting" is an innovative communication model that allows patients and family members to participate in the daily report conversation between nurses and other health-care providers concerning the patient's treatment. Traditionally, daily reports took place in secluded conference rooms or other private areas far away from patients and their families who rarely had an opportunity to participate. Nurse Bedside Reporting, which may occur when patients are transferred to other units or during a change of staff, provides a safe method to hand off patient care, fosters patient/family involvement in the plan of care, returns nurses to patient care needs more quickly, and promotes patient safety, understanding, and satisfaction with their hospital experience (Laws & Amato, 2010).

In today's managed care health environment in which patients are being pushed farther and farther away from the acute care setting, it is unreasonable to expect the patient's learning needs to be assessed, met, and adequately evaluated all during the brief initial nurse–patient encounter. Coordinating and collaborating about the learning needs of the patient with health-care providers present during the provision of continuing care beyond the initial encounter are critical to a successful outcome.

Now Can You—Discuss three professional nursing roles that rely heavily on therapeutic communication?

1. Explain why listening skills are important to the nurse's role as provider of care?
2. Discuss five areas of readiness to learn that the nurse must assess before teaching begins?
3. Clarify the professional nursing role of collaborator as it relates to patient teaching and learning?

Advocate

When coordinating care for the patient who is receiving services from multiple providers, the nurse may be called on to speak on the patient's behalf. As the number of providers increases, the potential for patient confusion and disillusionment also increases. Making certain that the patient's wishes, needs, plans, decisions, resources, and expected outcomes are recognized and guiding the provision of care is a vital role for the nurse. In this role as advocate, the nurse can promote patient- and family-centered care while ensuring that the patient's and family's vision of health and healing remain the ultimate goal.

As an advocate for the patient and family, however, the nurse must take caution to avoid influencing the care from a personal values perspective rather than from that of the patient and family. Self-reflection of one's own values, beliefs, perceptions, and moral standards can help the nurse minimize the imposition of health-related decisions driven by personal values rather than the values of the patient and family. Advocacy should always provide the patient more control, power, and self-determination of the outcome of the health experience (Falk-Rafael, 2005). There should be clear agreement concerning when the patient wants, or needs, the nurse to speak for him. A well-established transpersonal relationship can foster this level of understanding and agreement.

Advocating for patients through group organizations (political, social, and professional; local, statewide, national, and international) can also have an important impact on health care. Finding solutions to broad-based health problems and disparities among groups of people, such as children, women, and the poor, can be accomplished through nurses' political and social advocacy on their behalf.

The percentage of children living in poverty has remained between 17% and 20% for the past two decades. Economic security has been identified as a key indicator of well-being and health. Poverty affects the child's and family's ability to access health care, educational opportunities, housing, transportation, health prevention measures, adequate nutrition, and continuity of care (Forum on Child and Family Statistics [FCFS], 2011).

Impoverished children are at higher risk for a number of health threats including obesity, violence, asthma, lead poisoning, teen pregnancy, and mental disorders. Nurses have the ability, opportunity, and ethical responsibility to advocate for this group of vulnerable individuals. Nurses can use their image, knowledge, and numbers to advocate for change in these and other health disparities that exist between the economically secure and the impoverished (McCrink, 2010).

Collaboration in Caring—*Helping impoverished families*

The nurse can be instrumental in helping impoverished families by:

- Providing the telephone number/contact information for federal food stamps; reduced-fee community health clinics and dental and mental health programs; Women, Infants and Children Special Supplemental Food Programs (WIC); State Children's Health Insurance Program (SCHIP); State Medicaid: HeadStart; and Lion's Eyeglass Services
- Helping the patient investigate reduced-fee pharmaceutical options
- Connecting the family with Big Brother and Sister programs for family respite

EVIDENCE-BASED RESEARCH, PRACTICE, AND GUIDELINES

Evidence-based research requires the practitioner to possess a strong foundation in research methodology and in the pathological or physiological process being investigated and critically analyze the findings (Edmunds, 2010). The link between poverty as a risk factor and the health outcomes of obesity, violence, asthma, lead poisoning, teen pregnancy, and mental disorders has been demonstrated through epidemiological, controlled quantitative and qualitative studies, and nursing research (FCFS, 2011). Nurses and others interested in improving the health of these vulnerable groups have taken research findings and developed evidence-based practices (EBPs) that promote, prevent, and protect health behaviors in vulnerable populations.

This scientific literature helps nurses not only stay current in their technical clinical abilities, but also in their choice of the most effective interventions. Professional organizations such as Association of Women's Health, Obstetric and Neonatal Nurses (AWHONN), Society of Pediatric Nurses (SPN), American Nurses Association (ANA), National Association of Pediatric Nurse Associates and Practitioners (NAPNAP), and National Association of Neonatal Nurses (NANN) have developed evidence-based clinical practice guidelines for the safest, most consistent, and effective provision of family-centered nursing care. Not only are these evidence-based practice guidelines beneficial to the individual nurse's practice, but they can also be used by the nurse to advocate for change in the ritualistic, unverified, rules-oriented, and opinion-laced traditions (i.e., accustomed practice) of institutional nursing. With an ever-increasing level of patient knowledge and health-seeking sophistication, the demand for higher level nursing knowledge quickly becomes evident (Catalano, 2012; Jolivet, 2011).

Evidence-based guidelines are available for a number of interventions including newborn bathing, use of adhesives on premature newborns, positioning and snuggling of premature newborns, childhood asthma management, HIV/AIDS treatment, childhood cancer treatments, hypertension management, pregnancy weight gain, play therapy, and family-centered care (National Guideline Clearinghouse, 2013). The nurse must be diligent in seeking out these evidence-based guidelines so that excellence in practice can always be achieved, measured, and held up for scrutiny. However, as one nurse researcher (Schultz, 2005) cautions, nurses must be careful to remember that evidence-based practice is not "best practice" until it combines the investigational guidelines and scientifically sound interventions with clinical expertise and the patient's values and preferences.

Accessing a wide variety of evidence-based information is important when evaluating the quality of data to be used in one's nursing practice (Box 1-3). Examples of three sources of peer-reviewed, critically evaluated research summaries and reports available to the nurse for use in assessing research studies are The Cochrane Database of Systematic Reviews Library, the Agency for Healthcare Research and Quality (AHRQ), and MEDLINE.

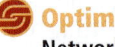

Optimizing Outcomes—The Cochrane Nursing Care Network

The Cochrane Collaboration, an international nonprofit and independent organization, has recently registered a new nursing entity. The Cochrane Nursing Care Network (CNCN) is one of 16 Fields and Networks within the Cochrane Collaboration. The purpose of a Field or Network is to support the conduct, dissemination, and utilization of systematic reviews relevant to the field. Membership of the Network is open to nurses, formal and informal care providers, other health-care professionals, researchers, and others involved in the delivery of nursing care.

Questioning nursing practice, collecting relevant evidence to support or change practice, and evaluating the best data for the desired patient outcome help provide the best care. As more responsibility and accountability for practice and patient outcome are shifted to the individual nurse, the role of the nurse will continue to change. Advancing nurses' accountability for the quality of care provided also advances autonomy of practice.

The advanced practice registered nurse (APRN) enjoys the highest level of autonomy because of additional education, occasionally through certification (alone) but most often through a master's level of postsecondary education. There are four advanced practice nursing roles: clinical nurse specialist (CNS), certified registered nurse anesthetist (CRNA), certified nurse midwife (CNM), and certified nurse practitioner (CNP) and six populations of practice focus: family/individual across the life span, adult gerontology, pediatrics, neonatal, women's health/gender-related, and psychiatric/mental health. Regardless of the chosen specialty area, nurse practitioners are first registered nurses who embrace a *nursing* paradigm (Apgold, 2011; Lowe, 2010).

 ### *Across Care Settings:* Practice possibilities for advanced practice nursing

The Advanced Practice Registered Nurse can practice in all types of health-care settings: nurse-owned and -run clinics, nursing homes, rehabilitation centers, hospitals, physician offices, sports health centers, surgical centers, student health centers, birthing centers, private outpatient practice, community health centers, primary and secondary schools, research centers, private consultation, academia, military fields, and state and federal legislature.

APRNs make independent clinical judgments and provide primary care to individuals and groups of patients. Of the 3,063,163 licensed registered nurses living and working in the United States in 2008, 158,348 (8.2%) were prepared for advanced practice in various roles (Ford & Pronsati, 2010; Health Resources and Services Administration [HRSA], 2010).

The clinical nurse specialist has more autonomy and authority than a direct care nurse. This leadership role encompasses direct patient and family care and staff education, along with multidisciplinary collaboration and an opportunity for influencing patient outcomes (Wetzel & Kalman, 2012). The CRNA's focus centers on a patient's anesthesia needs before, during, and after surgery or childbirth. CNMs work in hospitals, birthing centers, and private practices and are prepared to manage independently the care of women at low risk for complications

throughout the childbearing year. They also provide healthy newborn care, along with family planning and other gynecological services (AWHONN, 2010). The role of the nurse practitioner encompasses decision-making skills; clinical judgment and knowledge; and the ability to care for not only physical health, but also mental, emotional, and spiritual health—and this holistic aspect of patient care is one for which nurses are most often known (Bartol, 2011; Chichester, 2011).

In 2004, the American Association of Colleges of Nursing (AACN) published a position statement on the Practice Doctorate in Nursing (doctor of nursing practice, or DNP), which called for doctoral preparation to provide leadership in light of today's "growing complexity of health care, burgeoning growth in scientific knowledge, and increasing sophistication of technology" (American Association of Colleges of Nursing [AACN], 2004, p. 7). The practice-focused doctoral programs are designed to prepare experts in specialized advanced nursing practice. The nurse practitioner (NP) with a DNP degree possesses improved skills in information technology and interprofessional collaboration and mentoring (American Nurses Association [ANA], 2010; Emanuele, 2011; O'Dell, 2011; Smith, 2010), and currently there is a push from academia to require a DNP for NPs by the year 2015 (Ford, 2010; Wysocki, 2010). The AACN has defined research-focused doctoral programs (i.e., PhD programs) as those that prepare nurse scientists and scholars with curricula focused on scientific content and research methodology (Vincent, Johnson, Velasquez, & Rigney, 2010). The PhD graduate "develops the science, stewards the profession, educates the next generation of nurses, defines its uniqueness and maintains its professional integrity" (AACN, 2004 p. 2).

 ### Optimizing Outcomes—Advancing nursing education for the future

According to a new report ("Future of Nursing: Leading Change, Advancing Health") released by the Institute of Medicine (2011), nurses' roles, responsibilities, and education should change significantly to meet the increased demand for health care that will be created by health-care reform and to advance needed improvements in the United States' increasingly complex health system. Nurses must collaborate with other health-care professionals and assume leadership roles, both in the clinical context and in the arenas of public policy, nonprofits, and the private sector, in redesigning health care in this country. Nurses should be viewed as valued decision makers in considering ways to implement health reform because of their unique perspective and because they are highly trusted and relied on by health-care consumers. Strategies to ensure that members of the profession are well prepared for the challenges ahead include residency training for nursing, increasing the percentage of nurses who attain a bachelor's degree to 80% by 2020, doubling the number who pursue doctorates, and ensuring that all nurses engage in lifelong learning. Additional information on the report is available at http://www.iom.edu/nursing (Committee on the Robert Wood Johnson Foundation Initiative on the Future of Nursing, 2011; Hassmiller, 2011; Hellwig, 2011, 2012; Lowe, 2011; Ridgway, 2011; Scott, 2011).

The University of Pennsylvania conducted a 1-year study (Kennedy, 2004) to evaluate the effect of APRN versus traditional hospital-based care on death, re-hospitalization, complications, and cost for elderly patients with congestive heart failure health problems. There was a 13.7% lower death and re-hospitalization rate, an average of 110 days longer period of time without complications, and a savings of $4,845.00 for patients cared for by APRNs. Although not statistically linked, it was hypothesized that the difference resulted from the holistic mind–body–soul perspective taken by the APRNs in their approach to patient care; the more patient-friendly atmosphere of a primary, non-acute care setting; and a focus on health prevention, promotion, and protection.

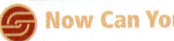 **Now Can You**—Discuss evidence-based practice and contrast the focus of the advanced practice nurse with that of the professional registered nurse?

1. Describe the difference(s) between "best practice" and "evidence-based practice"?
2. Explain six key elements to look for when evaluating the quality of evidence-based data found in journals or on Web sites?
3. Compare and contrast the licensed Registered Nurse and the Advanced Practice Nurse's role and preparation?

THE NURSING PROCESS AND EVIDENCE-BASED CARE

Evidence-based practice constantly questions the status quo and focuses on the outcome rather than the process of treatment. It helps to take the nursing process to the next level, from treating illness to predicting and preventing health problems, complications, and risks (Alfaro-LeFevre, 2011). A nurse using the traditional nursing process of assess, diagnose, plan, implement, and evaluate most likely uses some form of a body systems approach to data collection, focused primarily on medical systems health problems. A nurse practicing from an evidence-based focus assesses for health risk factors; patient and family strengths and self-worth; learning needs; family role and relationship patterns; values, cultural beliefs, and spiritual health; and patient perception of or response to the risk or problem, in addition to the medical body systems assessment (Alfaro-LeFevre, 2011).

The evidence-based nurse diagnoses not only health problems but is also able to predict potential problems based on knowledge of prior research. That evidence-based knowledge includes awareness of signs, symptoms, and related health factors of potential problems as well as a grounded understanding of their etiology. The use of a concept map, clinical pathway, or care map can aid the nurse in this awareness of relationships. The maps also help in prioritizing diagnoses.

The concept map is a five-step process, just as the traditional nursing process is. It is built on the nursing process and is especially helpful in the analysis of relationships of data to the health problem and the development of critical thinking.

Although there are different ways to create a concept map, a format that is often used parallels the steps in the traditional nursing process. First, assessment data are gathered. In Step 2 of the map, the nurse analyzes the data to determine the patient's key medical and nursing problems. The medical diagnosis occupies the center of the map. The nursing diagnoses are those problems or responses the medical diagnosis has caused for the patient.

When creating a concept map, one begins by drawing a skeleton diagram with the medical diagnosis placed in the center and the nursing diagnoses, patient responses, or general impressions of health threats surrounding the medical diagnosis (Fig. 1-9). At this point in the map development, potential problems are yet to be addressed. The initial focus is on problems that are currently major issues in maintaining wellness.

After the initial diagram is constructed, depicting what is believed to be the key problems, it is then time to investigate the medical diagnosis and gain knowledge of the treatment options. A review of assessment and evidence-based information on the following patient areas guide the nurse in the next step of the map:

- Growth and development tasks
- Past medical history
- Current laboratory values
- Medication taken and likely to be ordered
- Allergies
- Pain rating
- Diet and fluid intake, needs, and preferences
- Recent elimination patterns
- Usual activity rituals and current limitations

Step 2 in developing the concept map is to categorize the assessment data gathered under one or more of the identified patient problem areas (Fig. 1-10). Then the nurse describes the essential ongoing assessment data that signify improvement or deterioration in the health status of the primary medical diagnosis (Fig. 1-11). Step 3 of the map involves analyzing the relationships among the data and prioritizing the patient responses that led to the nursing diagnoses. The problem or diagnosis with the most supporting data is usually the most important (Fig. 1-12).

Step 4 of the concept map requires the nurse, along with the patient and family, to develop the beneficial goals and outcomes they hope to attain. This step corresponds to the planning phase of the nursing process. The outcomes are

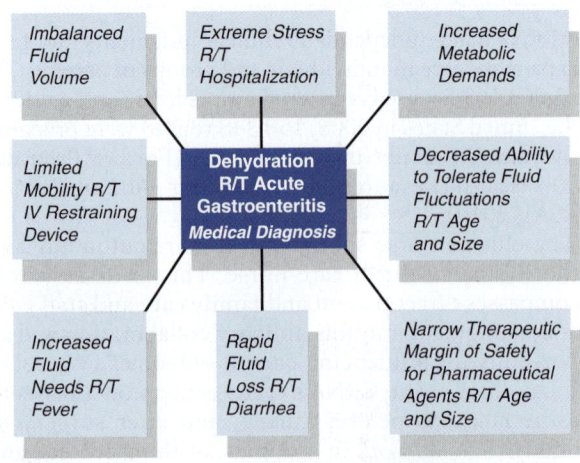

Figure 1-9 Concept map construction begins with gathering and analyzing assessment data.

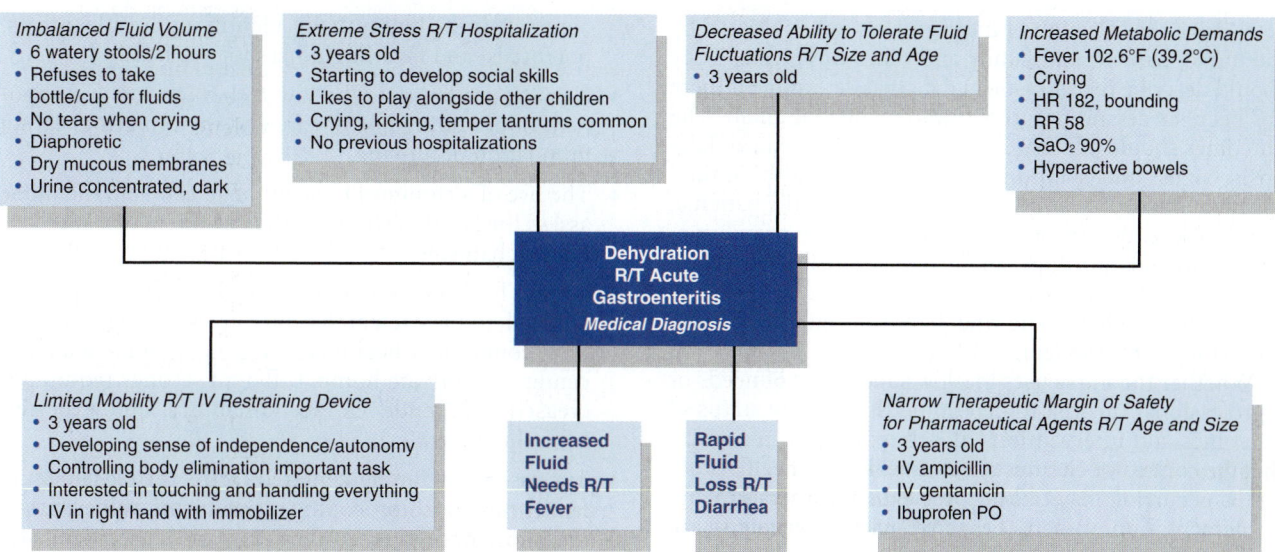

Figure 1-10 Categorizing the assessment data.

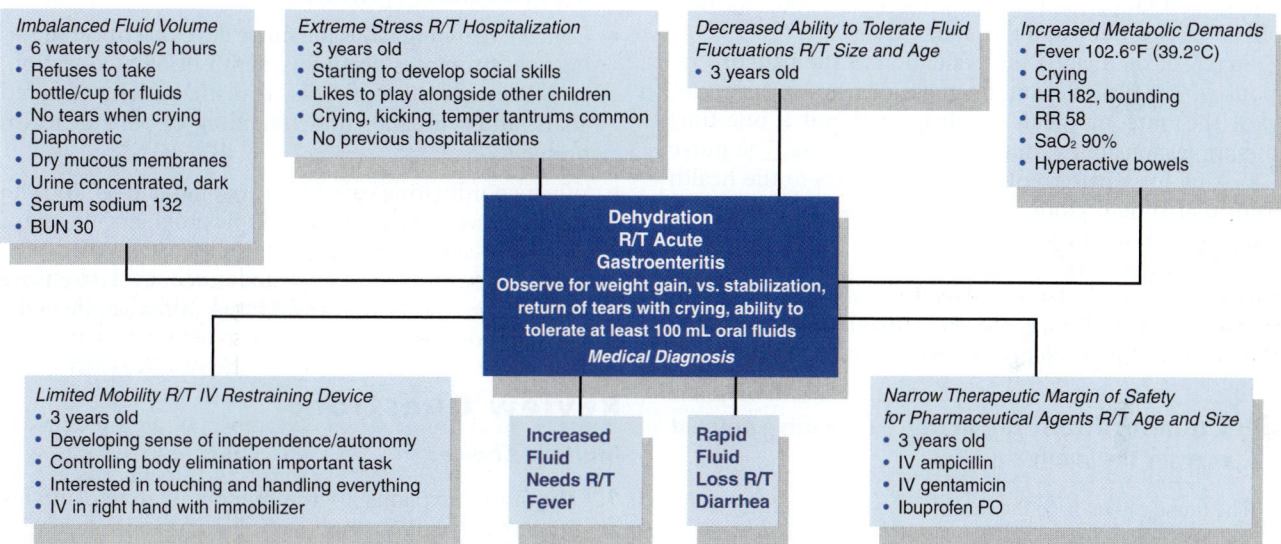

Figure 1-11 Identifying essential assessment data to evaluate the health status.

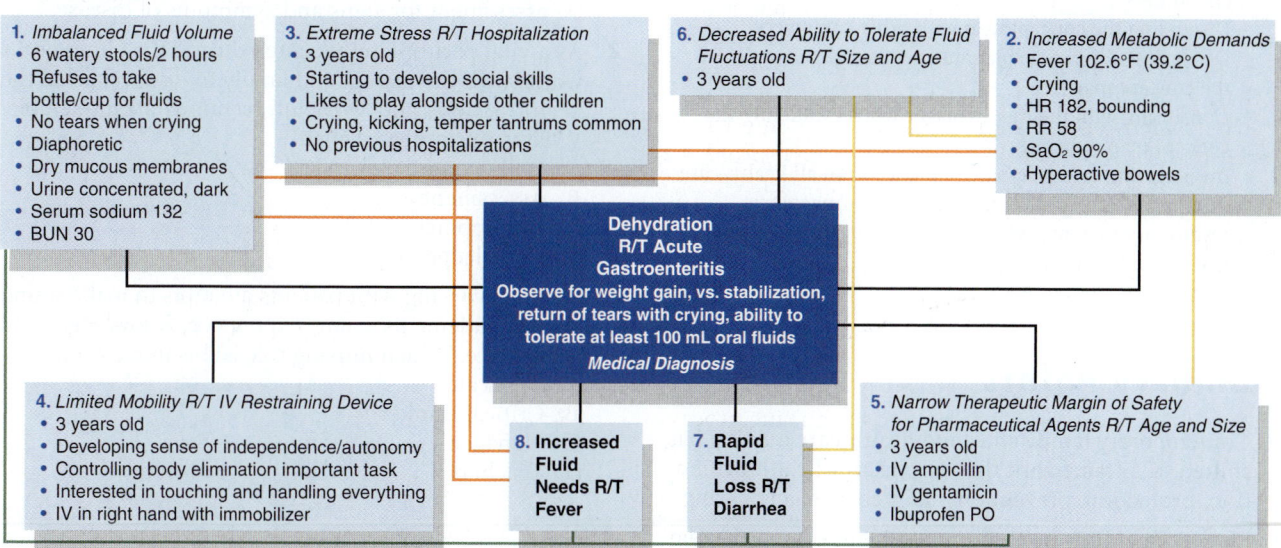

Figure 1-12 Analyzing relationships and prioritizing patient responses.

what drive the selection of interventions to be initiated by the nurse, patient, and family and other caregivers. They should describe the assessment data that determine if there has been successful progress toward achieving them. The outcomes should address clinical health (the medical diagnosis, signs, and symptoms), functional health (mind–spirit–emotions), quality of life (as defined by the patient), health risk reduction, health protection, health promotion, therapeutic relationships, and personal satisfaction. "Simply put, determining expected outcomes requires you to reverse the problem (state what happens when the person doesn't have the problem)" (Alfaro-LeFevre, 2011, p. 267).

Whether the nurse uses Maslow's hierarchy of needs or a professional theorist to determine the priority status of outcomes and interventions, it is important to recognize that the context or circumstances in which the health problem is occurring plays a key role in the prioritization and implementation. When the above-mentioned steps are completed, it becomes much easier to choose interventions that are achievable within the time and environmental constraints of the health event; build on the strengths of the patient and family; and increase the likelihood that they will be carried out by all those providing care.

Step 5 of the map is the evaluation of the patient's response to the health event, interventions, and progress toward the outcome goals. Evaluation is not a one-time nursing responsibility, but an ongoing process. The nurse is looking for a pattern of patient responses to the health event that should guide ongoing reassessment, planning, and provision of safe and effective care. Concept mapping helps the nurse develop disciplined, critical thinking that promotes accuracy, depth of data collection, early identification of risks, realistic goals, and a broader understanding of patient health problems (Alfaro-LeFevre, 2011).

 Collaboration in Caring—*Promoting optimal care for the family*

The nurse can manage the care of the family best by:

- Establishing therapeutic communication with the patient and family
- Developing relationship-centered, patient-focused encounters
- Discussing the concept map with other caregivers
- Designating discharge planning needs and personnel in the concept map
- Consulting with the case manager when evaluating the concept map outcomes
- Investigating evidence-based practice from all health-care disciplines (e.g., medicine, nursing, pharmacology, respiratory therapy, primary school education, criminal justice, and social sciences)

Summary Points

- Contemporary family and child health-care nursing has shifted to a framework that emphasizes health promotion, protection, prevention, maintenance, and caring.

- Modern family-centered nursing applies a circular or spiral process that builds a nurse–patient–family

connectedness by mutually identifying health threats, potentials, and meaningfulness for the family.

- Nursing aesthetics is the low-tech, high-touch component of providing health care and the centering, caring foundation of nursing.

- The use of a community health map can help the nurse assess the family's support systems, strengths, and coping mechanisms.

- Today, health care may be provided in the acute care hospital, tertiary research center, freestanding short stay unit, community health center, school, nurse-managed center, and private home. Different settings require increased independence, accountability, and expertise from the nurse.

- The essence of family-centered care is the placement of family relationships, coping mechanisms, values, priorities, and perceptions at the center of the health event.

- A holistic view of the patient and family includes the spiritual, physical, emotional, mental, social, and cultural indicators of patient health.

- Concept mapping helps the nurse develop critical thinking that promotes accuracy, depth of data collection, early identification of risks, realistic patient-centered goals, and a broader understanding of patient health problems.

- When coordinating care for the patient and family who are receiving services from multiple providers, the nurse must advocate for the patient's wishes, needs, plans, decisions, resources, and expected outcomes and ensure that they are recognized and are the guiding force in the provision of care.

Review Questions

Multiple Choice

1. The nurse explains to the student that the nursing process currently being taught has an emphasis on
   A. health promotion.
   B. disease and illness.
   C. linear progression of an illness.
   D. assessment for signs and symptoms of disease.

2. As a vital part of family-centered care, the clinic nurse works with the patient and family to discover what the health issue is and what interventions are preferable. What is this process called?
   A. Collaboration
   B. Assessment
   C. Development
   D. Knowledge

3. A nurse working with patients attempts to make sound clinical judgments using experience, knowledge, and persistence. Which nursing role is this nurse using?
   A. Advocate
   B. Critical thinker
   C. Manager
   D. Teacher

4. A community-based nurse is worried that many individuals from a refugee population do not seek health care routinely or appropriately. Which action by the nurse would best address this situation?
A. Assess local factors that encourage ethnocentrism in the health-care system.
B. Design an educational seminar on appropriate use of health-care resources.
C. Investigate whether community agency hours are convenient for the population.
D. Provide transportation and translation services for the refugee community.

5. The nursing instructor explains to students that a major development in the evolution of the nursing role was the creation of what aspect of contemporary nursing care?
A. Paternalism
B. Role of advocate
C. The nursing process
D. Watson's theory of caring

6. A nurse has taken a job in an alternative care setting after working in a hospital for many years. What important concept does this nurse need to understand to be successful in the new job?
A. Because the patients are less ill, the nurse has more time for interaction.
B. Because of lower costs of providing care, only the poorest patients are in this setting.
C. Risk identification and teaching cannot be accomplished in this setting.
D. Teaching patients involves covering the most crucial information first.

7. The nurse practicing with children and families is aware that family-centered care (FCC) is a major component of working with this population. Which idea is most important to this concept?
A. Decreasing the disruption illness causes to families
B. Including cultural and spiritual beliefs into care
C. Increased paternalism on the part of physicians
D. Making health care more affordable to more people

8. Which asset is most important for a nurse to practice in a culturally competent way?
A. Being able to conduct a detailed cultural assessment of all patients
B. Educating the patient on the Euro-Caucasian view of health care
C. Having a thorough understanding of patient's different cultures
D. Willingness to consider health and illness from the patient's point of view

9. A patient wishes to use a complementary and alternative medicine practice. Which action by the nurse is most appropriate?
A. Encouraging the patient to use tested Western medical treatments
B. Helping the patient find approaches that are evidence-based
C. Supporting CAM because there are usually no side effects
D. Teaching the patient that modern medical practices are safer

10. Which nursing theorist focused on nurse–patient encounters described as "caring occasions"?
A. Clara Barton
B. Florence Nightingale
C. Jean Watson
D. Madeleine Leininger

See Answers to End of Chapter Review Questions on Davis*Plus*.

REFERENCES

Accreditation Commission for Education in Nursing. (2013). *Accreditation Manual*. Retrieved 9-26-13 from http://acenursing.org/

Alfaro-LeFevre, R. (2011). *Critical thinking and clinical judgment: A practical approach* (5th ed.). St. Louis, MO: Elsevier Health Sciences.

American Association of Colleges of Nursing. (2004). *AACN position statement on the practice doctorate in nursing*. Retrieved 9-26-13 from http://www.aacn.nche.edu/publications/position/DNPpositionstatement.pdf

American College of Obstetricians and Gynecologists. (2011). Committee Opinion No. 480: Empathy in women's health care. *Obstetrics & Gynecology, 117*(3), 756–761.

American Nurses Association (ANA). (2010).The Doctor of Nursing Practice: Advancing the nursing profession. *Position Statement 2010*. Retrieved from http://www.nursingworld.org/drpractice.aspx

Anastasi, J. K., Chang, M., & Capili, B. (2011). Herbal supplements: Talking with your patients. *The Journal for Nurse Practitioners, 7*(1), 29–35.

Apgold, S. (2011). Support for distinguishing between NPs and PAs. *The Journal for Nurse Practitioners, 7*(2), 131.

Association of Women's Health, Obstetric and Neonatal Nurses (AWHONN). (2009). AWHONN Position Statement: The role of unlicensed assistive personnel (nursing assistive personnel) in the care of women and newborns. *Nursing for Women's Health, 13*(6), 526–528.

Association of Women's Health, Obstetric and Neonatal Nurses (AWHONN). (2010). AWHONN Position Statement: Midwifery. *Journal of Obstetric, Gynecologic, & Neonatal Nursing, 39*(6), 734–737.

Bartol, T. (2011). It's time to collaborate. *The American Journal for Nurse Practitioners, 15*(1/2), 36–37.

Campinha-Bacote, J. (2002). The process of cultural competence in the delivery of healthcare services: A model of care. *Journal of Transcultural Nursing, 13*(3), 181–184. doi:10.1177/10459602013003003

Campesino, M., & Koithan, M. (2010). Complementary therapy use among racial/ethnic groups. *The Journal for Nurse Practitioners, 6*(8), 647–648.

Catalano, J. T. (2012). *Nursing now! Today's issues, tomorrow's trends* (6th ed.). Philadelphia, PA: F.A. Davis.

Cavaliere, C., Rea, P., Lynch, M. E., & Blumenthal, M. (2010). Herbal supplement sales rise in all channels in 2009. *Herbalgram, 86*(4), 62–65.

Chichester, M. (2011). Lifelong Learning, Part 2. *Nursing for Women's Health, 15*(2), 171–175.

Cluff, L. E., & Binstock, R. H. (2003). *The lost art of caring: A challenge to health professionals, families, communities, and society*. Baltimore: The Johns Hopkins University Press.

Committee on the Robert Wood Johnson Foundation Initiative on the Future of Nursing at the Institute of Medicine. (2011). *The future of nursing: Leading change, advancing health*. Washington, DC: National Academies Press.

Darby, S. B. (2009). Traditional Chinese medicine: A complement to conventional. *Nursing for Women's Health, 13*(3), 199–206.

Davis, L. A. (2005). A phenomenological study of patient expectations concerning nursing care. *Holistic Nursing Practice, 19*(3), 126–133.

Dean, R. A. K. (2010). Cultural competence: Nursing in a multicultural society. *Nursing for Women's Health, 14*(1), 52–60.

Doenges, M. E., Moorhouse, M. F., & Murr, A. C. (2014). *Nursing care plans: Guidelines for individualizing client care across the life span* (9th ed.). Philadelphia, PA: F.A. Davis.

Edmunds, M. W. (2010). Increasing the quality of evidence-based publication. *The Journal for Nurse Practitioners, 6*(7), 494.

Emanuele, D. M. (2011). Support for the DNP as a degree. *The Journal for Nurse Practitioners, 7*(8), 645.

Falk-Rafael, A. (2005). Advancing nursing theory through theory-guided practice: The emergence of a critical caring perspective. *Advances in Nursing Science, 28*(1), 38–49.

Ford, J. (2010). Common ground: Understanding NPs & PAs. *Advance for NPs & PAs, 11*(1), 25–26.

Ford, J., & Pronsati, M. (2010). Front & Center – News for NPs & PAs. *Advance for NPs & PAs, 1*(4), 10.

Forum on Child and Family Statistics (FCFS). (2011). America's children: Key national indicators of well-being. Retrieved from http://www.childstats.gov

Foster, J. (2009). Cultural humility and the importance of long-term relationships in international partnerships. *Journal of Obstetric, Gynecologic, and Neonatal Nursing, 38*(1), 100–107.

Fottler, M. D., Ford, R. C., & Heaton, C. P. (2010). *Achieving service excellence, strategies for healthcare* (2nd ed.). Chicago, IL: Health Administration Press.

Freire, P. (1997). Pedagogy of the oppressed. Cited in Sanford, R. C. (2000). Caring through relation and dialogue: A nursing perspective for patient education (healing and caring). *Advances in Nursing Science, 22*(3), 1–15.

Geller, S. M., & Greenberg, L. S. (2011). *Therapeutic presence: A mindful approach to effective therapy*. Washington, DC: American Psychological Association.

Gordon, S., & Nelson, S. (2005). An end to angels. *American Journal of Nursing, 105*(5), 62–69.

Harrington, C. C. (2012). Why evidence-based practice matters. *Advance for NPs & PAs, 3*(4), 14.

Hassmiller, S. B. (2011). The national perspective on the future of nursing: Where are we going? *North Carolina Medical Journal, 72*(4), 324–326.

Health Resources & Services Administration (HRSA). (2010). The registered nurse population: Findings from the 2008 National Sample Survey of Registered Nurses. Washington, DC: U.S. Department of Health and Human Services.

Hellwig, J. P. (2011). The future of nursing. *Nursing for Women's Health, 15*(1), 75–76.

Hellwig, J. P. (2012). Charting nursing's future. *Nursing for Women's Health, 16*(1), 80.

Helms, J. E. (2006). Complementary and alternative therapies: A new frontier for nursing education? *Journal of Nursing Education, 45*(3), 117.

Helms, M. A. (2009). Integrating spirituality into nurse practitioner practice: The importance of finding the time. *The Journal for Nurse Practitioners, 5*(8), 598–605.

Jeffreys, M. R. (2010). *Teaching cultural competence in nursing and health care* (2nd ed.). New York, NY: Springer Publishing Company.

Jirwe, M., Gerrish, K., & Emami, A. (2006). The theoretical framework of cultural competence. *The Journal of Multicultural Nursing & Health, 12*(3), 240–250.

Johnson, M., Moorhead, S., Bulechek, G., Butcher, H., Maas, M., & Swanson, E. (2012). *NOC and NIC linkages to NANDA-I and clinical conditions: Supporting critical reasoning and quality care* (3rd ed.). St. Maryland Heights, MO: Elsevier Mosby.

Jolivet, R. (2011). Current resources for evidence-based practice, September/October 2010. *Journal of Midwifery and Women's Health, 55*(5), 469–471.

Kelly, J. (2004). Spirituality as a coping mechanism. *Dimensions in Critical Care Nursing, 23*(4), 162–168.

Kennedy, M. (2004). APNs: Improved outcomes at lower costs. *American Journal of Nursing, 104*(9), 19.

Ko, J. Y. (2010). Music therapy in palliative care. *The Clinical Advisor, 13*(9), 112.

Koithan, M., & Farrell, C. (2010). Indigenous Native American healing traditions. *The Journal for Nurse Practitioners, 6*(6), 477–478.

Laws, D., & Amato, S. (2010). Incorporating bedside reporting into change-of-shift report. *Rehabilitation Nursing, 35*(2), 70–74.

Leininger, M., & McFarland, M. R. (2006). *Culture care diversity and universality: A worldwide nursing theory* (2nd ed.). Burlington, MA: Jones & Bartlett.

Levi, A. (2009). The ethics of nursing student international clinical experiences. *Journal of Obstetric, Gynecologic, and Neonatal Nursing, 38*(1), 94–99.

Lewallen, L. P. (2011). The importance of culture in childbearing. *Journal of Obstetric, Gynecologic, and Neonatal Nursing, 40*(1), 4–8.

Lowe, N. K. (2010). The landscape of advanced practice nursing. *Journal of Obstetric, Gynecologic, and Neonatal Nursing, 39*(4), 359–360.

Lowe, N. K. (2011). The future of nursing. *Journal of Obstetric, Gynecologic, and Neonatal Nursing, 30*(3), 253–254.

Mayeroff, M. (1971). *On caring*. New York: Harper Perennial. Cited in Falk-Rafael, A. R. (1998). Nurses who run with the wolves: The power and caring dialectic revisited. *Advances in Nursing Science, 21*(1), 29–42.

McCrink, A. (2010). Ethical nursing practice: Why it should concern us all. *Nursing for Women's Health, 14*(6), 443–446.

Miller, S. (2009). Cultural humility is the first step in becoming global care providers. *Journal of Obstetric, Gynecologic, and Neonatal Nursing, 38*(1), 92–93.

National Center for Complementary & Alternative Medicine. (2008). *The Use of Complementary and Alternative Medicine in the United States.* Retrieved 9-16-11 from http://nccam.nih.gov/news/camstats/2007/camsurvey_fs1.htm

National Center for Complementary & Alternative Medicine. (2011). *What Is Complementary and Alternative Medicine?* Retrieved 9-16-11 from http://nccam.nih.gov/health/whatiscam/

National Coalition on Health Care. (2011). Curbing costs and improving care. The path to an affordable health care future. Retrieved 9-21-14 from http://www.nchcbeta.org/wp-content/uploads/2012/05/NCHC-Plan-for-Health-and-Fiscal-Policy.pdf

National Guideline Clearinghouse. (2013). Guidelines by topic. Retrieved from http://www.guideline.gov/browse/by-topic.aspx

Nightingale, F. (1859). *Notes on nursing*. Philadelphia, PA: Lippincott Williams & Wilkins.

O'Dell, D. G. (2011). Support for the DNP as a role. *The Journal for Nurse Practitioners, 7*(8), 645.

Provencher, G. (2010). Restoring balance: An introduction to functional medicine. *Advance for Nurse Practitioners 18*(5), 33–39.

Rexroth, R., & Davidhizar, R. (2003). Caring: Utilizing the Watson theory to transcend culture. *The Health Care Manager, 22*(4), 295–304.

Rhodes, M. K., Morris, A. H., & Lazenby, R. B. (2011). Nursing at its best: Competent and caring. *The Online Journal of Issues in Nursing, 16*(2), 1–11. doi:10.3912/OJIN.Vol16No.02PPT01

Ridgway, C. (2011). Assessing the future of health care through the future of nursing. *Clinician Reviews/Convenient Care, 14*(1), 13–15.

Rowe Kaakinen, J., Padgett Coehlo, D., Steele, R., Tabacco, A., & Harmon Hanson, S. M. (2014). *Family health care nursing: Theory, practice, and research* (5th ed.). Philadelphia, PA: F.A. Davis.

Sanford, R. C. (2000). Caring through relation and dialogue: A nursing perspective for patient education (healing and caring). *Advances in Nursing Science, 22*(3), 1–15.

Schultz, A. (2005). Clinical scholars at the bedside: An EBP mentorship model for today. *Online Journal of Excellence in Nursing Knowledge, 2.* Retrieved from http://www.nursingknowledge.org/

Scott, E. S. (2011). Educational preparation to strengthen nursing leadership. *North Carolina Medical journal, 72*(4), 296–299.

Smith, K. J., & Craft-Rosenberg, M. (2010). Using NANDA, NIC, and NOC in an undergraduate nursing practicum. *Nurse Educator, 35*(4), 162–166.

Smith, M. A. (2010). Making a difference: DNP can pave the way. *Advance for Nurse Practitioners, 18*(5), 65.

Spector, R. E. (2012). *Cultural diversity in health and illness* (8th ed.). Upper Saddle River, NJ: Pearson Prentice Hall.

Stevens, K. (2013). The impact of evidence-based practice in nursing and the next big ideas. *The Online Journal of Issues in Nursing, 18*(2), 1–8. doi:10.3912/IJIN.Vol18No02Man04

Stichler, J. F., & Weiss, M. E. (2001). Through the eye of the beholder: Multiple perspectives on quality in women's health care. *Journal of Nursing Care Quality, 15*(3), 59–74.

Theroux, R. (2011). Not just another annual exam: Thoughts on the nurse-patient relationship. *Nursing for Women's Health, 15*(3), 195–198.

U.S. Census Bureau. (2011). The 2012 Statistical Abstract: The national data book. Retrieved from http://www.census.gov/compendia/statab

Vincent, D., Johnson, C., Velasquez, D., & Rigney, T. (2010). DNP-Prepared nurses as practitioner-researchers: Closing the gap between research and practice. *The American Journal for Nurse Practitioners, 14*(11/12), 28–34.

Ward, S. L. (2002). Ask the expert: Balancing high-tech nursing with holistic healing. *Journal for Specialists in Pediatric Nursing, 7*(2), 81–84.

Watson, J. (2005). Theory of human caring. Retrieved from http://watsoncaringscience.org/images/features/library/THEORY%20OF%20HUMAN%20CARING_Website.pdf

Watson, J. (2011). *Human Caring Science. A theory of nursing* (2nd ed.). Sudbury, MA: Jones & Bartlett.

Watson, J., & Woodward, T. (2010). Jean Watson's theory of human caring. In M. Parker & M. Smith (Eds.), *Nursing theories & nursing practice* (3rd ed., pp. 351–369). Philadelphia, PA: F.A. Davis.

Wetzel, C., & Kalman, M. (2012). Critical care clinical nurse specialist: Is this the role for you? *Dimensions of Critical Care Nursing, 29*(1), 29–32. doi:10.1097/DCC.0b013e3181be4ae2

Wilson, Deborah W. (2007). From their own voices. *Journal of Transcultural Nursing, 18* (2), 142–149.

Wysocki, S. (2010). How will the Doctor of Nursing Practice program impact women's health? *The Female Patient, 35*(5), 47–48.

Zander, P. (2007). Cultural competence: Analyzing the construct. *Journal of Theory Construction and Testing, 11*(2), 50–54.

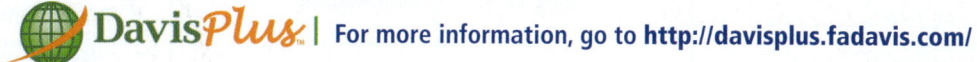 **For more information, go to http://davisplus.fadavis.com/**

CONCEPT MAP

Nursing Care: Women, Families, and Children

Traditional Nursing Care

Contemporary Nursing Care

Caring: The Centering Foundation of Nursing

Historic Nursing Approach:
- Health = absence of disease
- Medical model
  - Rid, heal, cure
  - Paternalistic
- Submissive patient
- Ethnocentrism
- Treatment-driven care

Theories of Caring:
- Nightingale
- Leininger
- Watson

Characteristics:
- Establish trust
- Recognize patient feelings/perception of illness
- Expressive behavior ➝ touch, smile, praise
- Communication
- Technical skill/knowledgeable
- Spiritual awareness/connection

Family-Centered Care:
- Sensitivity to culture, beliefs/values of family and community
- Use of culturally sensitive communication
- Collaborative versus authoritarian role
- Recognize knowledge of family group
- In-depth assessment of family ➝ use of Community Health Map

Forces of Change:
- Consumerism
- Change in family structure/accessibility
- Increase in health consciousness
- Social/technical advances
- Increased patient/family accountability
- Ethnopluralism

A New Nursing View:
- Transcend/control health threat
- Motivate patient/family toward health promotion, prevention, maintenance and self-care
- Shared connectedness
- Patient-defined wholeness
- Engaged, transpersonal care
- Power base for healing within patient

Nursing Roles:
- Provider
  - Use up-to-date, evidence-based interventions
  - Form a caring relationship
  - Implement the art of nursing aesthetics ➝ imagery, music therapy, art
  - Use concept map for plan of care
- Collaborator across care settings
- Implement nursing process using NIC/NOC
- Critical/analytical thinker
- Communicator
- Patient advocate
  - Support decision-making power
  - Increase access to health care
  - Emphasize education
  - Increase family-centered approaches
- Patient/family teacher

Home- and Community-Based Care:
- Independent practice
- Expert skill in:
  - Health history
  - Cultural competence
  - Coordinating extended care
- Manage other health-care workers
- Advocate for family-centered care
- Advocate for patients using CAM

24-Hour Observation/Urgent Care:
- Manage time to:
  - Assess, ID those at risk, counsel, teach
  - Direct unlicensed personnel
  - Teach follow-up procedures to family

Collaboration in Caring:
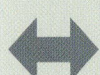
- Prepare the family for community-based care
- Support CAM use; respect family healer; reflect on personal beliefs
- Enhance family/patient coping
- Help impoverished families

Nursing Insight:
- Define cultural sensitivity, competency, and humility.

Specialized Acute Care:
- Strong knowledge base ➝ care of the family/child
- Critical thinking
  - Technological expertise
  - Evidence-based

Across Care Settings:
- Teach families who travel about protection against illness vectors
- Encourage family participation in care across all settings
- Use professional translator when possible
- Identify role of APRN and utilize in all settings

Cultural Diversity:

- Health-care beliefs and desired outcomes vary among cultures
- Use of imagery/music ➝ based on cultural definition of said therapies
- Include cultural prescriptions/proscriptions
- Match pace of speech to the patient's speech pattern
- Type of CAM used is R/T cultural pattern in family

Optimizing Outcomes:
- Communication is enhanced by empathy
- Search Cochrane Nursing Care Network for EBP
- Establish learning outcomes by negotiating with family

Now Can You:
?
- Identify a major force that accounts for the present-day shift toward family-centered decision making in health matters
- Define present-day trends in nursing focus related to the health–wellness continuum
- Discuss a nursing approach that incorporates engaging transpersonal care
- Explain what is meant by evidence-based practice
- Identify how the nursing process has changed the professional role of the nurse
- Identify the essential characteristics of caring

Contemporary Issues in Women's, Families', and Children's Health Care

 In these days of investigation and statistics, where results are described with microscopic exactness and tabulated with mathematical accuracy, we seem to think figures will do instead of facts, and calculation instead of action. We remember the policeman who watched his burglar enter the house and waited to make quite sure whether he was going to commit robbery with violence or without, before interfering with his operations. So as we read such an account as this we seem to be watching, not robbery, but murder going on, and to be waiting for the rates of mortality to go up before we interfere; we wait to see how many of the children playing round the houses shall be stricken down. We wait to see whether the filth will really trickle into the well, and whether the foul water really will poison the family, and how many will die of it. And then, when enough have died, we think it time to spend some money and some trouble to stop the murders going further, and we enter the results of our "masterly inactivity" neatly in tables; but we do not analyse and tabulate the saddened lives of those who remain, and the desolate homes in our "sanitary districts."

—Florence Nightingale,
writing on rural hygiene

LEARNING TARGETS *At the completion of this chapter, the student will be able to:*

- ◆ Describe a multilevel approach for prevention and intervention in addressing contemporary health-care issues.
- ◆ Explain social, political, economic, and cultural trends that affect the health status of women, children, and families.
- ◆ Evaluate current gaps in health-care delivery systems that impact women's, children's, and families' health.
- ◆ Discuss examples of major barriers to accessing health care in the United States.
- ◆ Apply four bioethics principles to analyze ethical issues in maternal–child and family health.
- ◆ Describe vulnerable populations in the United States and the nurse's role in advocating for neglected and stigmatized persons.

PICO(T) Questions

The intent of evidence-based practice (EBP) is to provide nursing care that integrates the best available evidence. An initial step in EBP is to write a PICO(T) question that effectively guides the research. A PICO(T) question is an acronym that stands for population (P), intervention or issue (I), comparison of interest (C), outcome (O), and timeframe (T). Depending on the question, all or some of the question components are used in the research process. Use these

PICO(T) questions to spark your thinking as you read the chapter.

1. Does (I) prepregnancy counseling related to the effects of tobacco and/or alcohol use during pregnancy lead to a (O) decrease in the number of (P) babies born with birth defects?

2. Do (P) students in schools with a (I) school nurse nutritional education program have a (O) lower incidence of obesity (C) than students in schools without a program?

Evidence-Based Practice

Lewin, L., & Graham, G. (2012). Interpersonal violence: Secondary analysis of the keep your children/yourself safe and secure (KySS) data. *Journal of Pediatric Health Care, 26*(2), 102–108.

The purpose of this study was to perform a secondary analysis of data from the original Keep Your Children/Yourself Safe and Secure (KySS) survey originally used in a descriptive study conducted by the National Association of Pediatric Nurses Practitioners (NAPNAP) in 2002. The present study purported to examine parent-child agreement on items related to interpersonal violence. The researchers wished to determine if there were any differences between parents and their children in attitude, knowledge, and frequency of worries about interpersonal violence as well as the frequency of worries.

The original study participants included 621 children/adolescents and 603 parents, which provided 563 dyads examined in the current study. Dyad was defined as a parent-child combination (e.g., mother/son or father/daughter). To be included, each dyad was required to have responded to every interpersonal violence item in the original study. In the current study, the mean age of the children was 14 years, 65.1% self-identified as Caucasian and over one-half (62.4%) were female. The parents' ages ranged from 18 to 60+ years. Nearly 84% were ages 31 to 50. Of these, 85.9 were female, 64.4% were married, and 71.8% identified themselves as Caucasian.

Data analysis focused on examining the strength of the agreement or differences between parent and child responses to select items. The study included 10 items related to interpersonal violence attitudes/knowledge and five items related to frequency of worry about neglect, sexual abuse, physical abuse, school violence, and the parent-child relations. Findings indicated that the single mother/son dyad shared less agreement than did any other dyad combinations. The 10- to 12-year-old age group disagreed with the parent more than any other age group in their responses to items related to interpersonal violence. Of the 563 dyads, 68 shared no differences on interpersonal violence items, 122 disagreed on only one item, 138 disagreed on two items, 86 disagreed on three items, and 149 disagreed on four or more items.

Based on their findings, the researchers proposed that parents and providers may not always be aware of how their understanding of interpersonal violence differs from that of children and adolescents. They suggested that an enhanced comprehension of the differences in understanding between parents and children may better prepare parents and providers to address education and preventive efforts. Interestingly, the item showing the least agreement between parents and children on attitude/knowledge was the one that stated, "children who are sexually abused are more likely to abuse their children when they are parents." The item that demonstrated the greatest agreement between parents and children concerned worry about physical abuse/neglect.

1. How is this information useful to clinical nursing practice?

2. Based on these findings, what are implications for further research?

See Suggested Responses for Evidence-Based Practice on Davis*Plus*.

Introduction

This chapter examines contemporary trends in women's, children's, and families' health care from a holistic, action-oriented perspective. Emphasis is on the professional nurse's role as change agent using the intervention wheel model and the national *Healthy People* initiative as guides for improvement. Biostatistical data are used to assess the current status of women, children, and family health, highlighting health inequities, vulnerable populations, and gaps in health-care access and delivery. Societal trends and issues are examined from political, social, economic, and cultural perspectives, illustrating how these important dimensions become determinants of health. An overview of legal, ethical, and social justice is presented, with the nurse as a key player in transforming and maintaining a more effective health-care system in the future.

Framework: The Public Health Intervention Model

Nurses have always been tenacious in their responsiveness to the rapidly changing health and societal landscape and are well situated to address contemporary family health issues. This is an era of unprecedented change in health care.

Some of these fast-paced trends include rapid technological advances, escalating health-care costs, managed care, demands for increased accountability for public agencies, and terrorism threats. Modern nurses maintain a readiness to address new and resurfacing health-related issues, illnesses, or disaster management responsibilities. Nurses frequently serve as catalysts to help coordinate societal, community, and individual efforts to help achieve health and wellness goals.

It is useful to have a framework when thinking critically about the complex topics encountered in family health. The Intervention Wheel, formerly known as Minnesota's "public health intervention model," is particularly well suited for examining health issues with an action-oriented, holistic lens. The lens used to view the intervention model is population-based, meaning that epidemiology of the population's health status as a whole is assessed (Keller, Strohschein, Schaffer, & Lia-Hoagberg, 2004b) (Fig. 2-1).

The model is an inclusive framework and was developed, refined, and extensively critiqued by more than 200 nurses throughout the country (Keller et al., 2004a). It encompasses three levels at which interventions can be initiated, from the micro-level of the individual to the macro-level environment. Interventions are targeted toward individuals/families, communities, and larger institutional and societal systems. Thus, broad determinants of health such as environment, employment, insurance, class, race, social support,

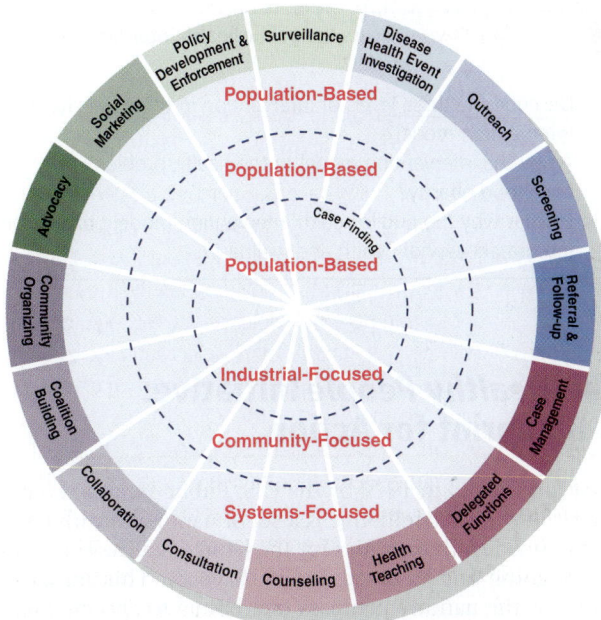

Figure 2-1 The Public Health Intervention Model.

access to health services, genetic endowment, and personal histories can be integrated, making health-care interventions more comprehensive and effective.

In short, the public health intervention model is population-based, defines levels of practice, and has a comprehensive prevention focus. There are 17 categories of intervention tactics outlined in the model: social marketing, advocacy, policy development, surveillance, disease investigation, outreach, screening, case finding, referral, case management, delegated functions, health teaching, counseling, consultation, collaboration, coalition building, and community organizing (Keller et al., 2004b).

HOW THE INTERVENTION WHEEL WORKS

The issue of childhood obesity provides a good example for demonstrating how the Minnesota public health intervention model can be used to confront a contemporary health problem. Approaches that are currently being used to address the problem of childhood obesity range from those at the micro-level to the macro-level spheres of practice.

Childhood obesity has traditionally been framed as an issue of personal or parental responsibility. Viewing childhood obesity as merely a personal responsibility excuses society's responsibility and limits shared solutions. Nurses need to broaden their scope to examine health processes more globally. For example, nurses need to ensure that social, political, and structural conditions are addressed so that it is possible for people to achieve health.

There are many interesting and promising strategies for addressing childhood obesity. Some urban areas are proactively collaborating to redesign their communities. One intervention is to build community sidewalks, establishing a more inviting environment for children to bicycle or walk to school. Communities have formed coalitions that advocate for neighborhood safety, so that walking, biking, and running can be safe. Some have looked at the strategic geographical proximity of fast food restaurants to schools and have brought those observations to public consciousness.

Fast food restaurants are clustered three to four times more often within walking distances of schools (Davis & Carpenter, 2009). This deliberate geographical placement exposes America's children to poor quality food that is frequently inadequate for health promotion.

Other strategies are targeted at schools, such as altering choices in school vending machines and cafeterias to include healthy alternatives to junk food. Some schools have already done so on their own. Others are advocating interventions at the state and federal levels, such as bringing back physical education courses in schools where they have been eliminated (Lockwood, 2011).

In 2011, 29% of U.S. public high school students surveyed had participated in at least 60 minutes per day of physical activity on all 7 days before the survey, and only 31% attended physical education class daily (Centers for Disease Control and Prevention [CDC], 2011a). Some schools collaborate with community health programs, screen for body mass index (BMI), and refer overweight children for early intervention and follow-up. Several schools have implemented the *Planet Health* program, developed by The Harvard School of Public Health. The *Planet Health* curriculum is intertwined with existing lessons already being taught in middle schools, such as science, math, and English. Students who participated in the pilot *Planet Health* interdisciplinary studies increased their fruit and vegetable intake, decreased their television viewing time, and lowered their BMI (CDC, 2012).

Television presents another avenue for targeting obesity in children. It is used more as an electronic babysitter than ever before. The American Academy of Pediatrics recommends that children under 2 years of age not watch any TV and that those older than 2 watch no more than 1 to 2 hours a day of quality programming. Yet, two-thirds of infants and toddlers watch a screen an average of 2 hours a day. Television has evolved as a tool to help parents manage busy schedules, provide an ever-changing distraction, and facilitate family routines such as eating, relaxing, and falling asleep (KidsHealth.org, 2013). Television viewing contributes to childhood obesity because it fosters physical inactivity and exposes children to a bombardment of junk food advertising (Fig. 2-2).

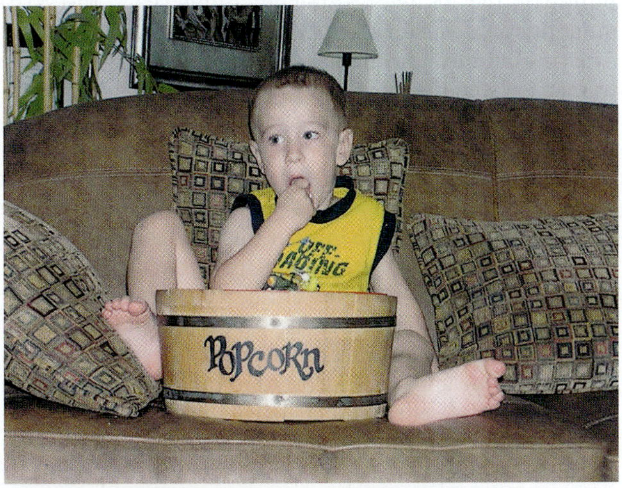

Figure 2-2 Typical American child fixed on the television set while snacking on popcorn.

The American Psychological Association has a task force that researches television advertising that is specifically aimed at children. The task force has learned that children younger than the age of 8 do not yet have the experience and knowledge to critically evaluate advertising messages, and they tend to accept advertising as factual. American children view an average of 40,000 television ads per year (Kunkel, 2007). Many messages are aimed at marketing unhealthy foods to children and are aired strategically at times when children are most likely to watch. One study demonstrated an average of 11 food commercials per hour during children's Saturday morning cartoons. Therefore, an average child is exposed to approximately one food commercial every 5 minutes. Advertising strategies for snacks, sugared cereals, soft drinks, and fast food contribute to the epidemic of childhood obesity, and the task force is urging policymakers to better protect young children from this exposure (Kunkel, 2007; Dembek, Harris, & Schwartz, 2013).

There are initiatives at the federal level to address the childhood obesity problem as well. For example, the U.S. Food and Drug Administration (FDA) recommends strengthening food labeling in grocery stores and in restaurants. In some cases, consultation with restaurants is resulting in healthier portion sizes and the offering of lower fat options. The Centers for Disease Control and Prevention (CDC) is using a multicultural social marketing technique to spread the word nationally about exercise benefits to children.

In 2010, the U.S. Preventive Services Task Force (USPSTF) published recommendations that clinicians screen children ages 6 and older, and when appropriate, refer them to intensive counseling and behavioral interventions to promote improvements in weight. The Task Force found new and existing evidence that comprehensive, moderate-to high-intensity programs that include dietary changes, physical activity, behavioral counseling, and parent involvement (for younger children) were effective in producing improvements in weight (USPSTF, 2010). Recognizing the fact that more than two-thirds of adults and one-third of children nationwide are overweight or obese, the U.S. Department of Agriculture (USDA) recently released "Dietary Guidelines for Americans, 2015" that builds on the 23 key recommendations (from the 2010 guidelines) most important to improving public health. The tips fall into four main categories: balancing calories to manage weight, foods and food components to reduce, foods and nutrients to increase, and building healthy eating patterns (USDA, 2013).

The public health intervention model gives an integrated view because it includes both the local and the more global system realms. The use of this model guides health professionals toward enhancing the capacity of all segments of society to move toward health and wellness. For nurses, it is becoming increasingly clear that the traditional approach to "caring" must be broadened beyond the individual patient and instead become oriented toward the public's health to effect real change in health outcomes. Intervention programs must be multitiered and oriented toward the broader social context because this is where most patients are located.

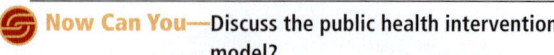 **Now Can You**—Discuss the public health intervention model?

1. Describe the three levels of intervention in the public health intervention model?
2. Apply the intervention model to the health problem of childhood obesity?
3. Discuss why the public health intervention model provides an integrated view of health and wellness?

The *Healthy People* Initiative: A Blueprint for Action

First formulated in 1979 by the U.S. Public Health Service, the *Healthy People* initiative is a set of national health goals that define health priorities for the United States. The goals are ongoing and updated every 10 years. This initiative serves as the nation's compass that points to specific focus areas that will guide progress toward the ultimate goal of optimal health for all Americans. The *Healthy People* blueprint for action is coordinated by the Office of Disease Prevention and Health Promotion in the U.S. Department of Health and Human Services. Prominent health scientists, both inside and outside government, use population-based studies to create this blueprint for national health goals. *Healthy People 2020* can be accessed at www.healthypeople.gov.

Healthy People 2020 includes four overarching health outcome goals that overlie all others:

- To attain high-quality, longer lives free of preventable disease, disability, injury, and premature death
- To achieve health equity, eliminate disparities, and improve the health of all groups
- To create social and physical environments that promote good health for all
- To promote quality of life, healthy development, and health behaviors across all life stages

Healthy People 2020 contains approximately 1,200 objectives in 42 topic areas designed to serve as the current framework for improving the health of all people in the United States. Objectives in the latest initiative include an emphasis on the importance of social and physical environments on health. Leading health indicators include several prevention factors such as physical activity, control of overweight and obesity, abstention from tobacco use and substance abuse, and responsible sexual behavior. Other leading indicators include mental health, prevention of injury and violence, environmental quality, immunization, and access to health care (Koh, 2010; Levi & Quang Dau, 2011).

Ideally, the best method to address health priorities is through the early prevention of health problems. There are three levels of prevention. The most desirable level is **primary prevention,** which encompasses health promotion as well as activities specifically meant to prevent disease from occurring. **Secondary prevention** refers to early identification and prompt treatment of a health problem before it has an opportunity to spread or become more serious. Finally, **tertiary prevention** is intended to restore health to the highest functioning state possible. These three levels of prevention may be applied to a child's day-care setting. Primary prevention would involve teaching children and workers proper hand hygiene to prevent illness. Secondary prevention would encompass screening and isolating children who develop signs and symptoms of infection to prevent its spread. Tertiary prevention would involve strategies such as keeping the child at home, administering fluids, encouraging rest, and administering antibiotics if indicated, until the child is once again restored to health. This focus on prevention has the potential to make an enormous difference in family health status.

Current health indicators demonstrate that Americans today are healthier than they have ever been, with a steady upward trend to an average life expectancy of 77.9 years. Dreaded diseases that struck terror in families 100 years ago such as plague, polio, tetanus, and whooping cough (pertussis) are under control even though new health problems continually threaten to surface. Although heart disease remains the leading cause of death in the United States, rates have plummeted in recent years, most likely because of the present emphasis on healthy lifestyles and the availability of cholesterol-lowering medications.

However, there is no room for complacency regarding the present state of the nation's health. Despite some positive trends, the United States lags behind other industrialized countries. The World Health Organization ranks the United States as 37th in health system status, even though health spending per capita in the United States exceeds that of all other countries. Remarkably, health spending consumes one-seventh of the United States' gross national budget.

Despite large health-care expenditures, health care and other resources are unevenly distributed in the United States. Persistent health disparities remain disturbing. An African American baby, for example, is more than twice as likely to be low birth weight and two and one-half times more likely to die during the first year of life than a European American baby. Sudden infant death syndrome (SIDS) is more than two times higher in American Indian and Alaska native babies than in European American babies (U.S. Department of Health and Human Services, 2013). Additional information about health disparities can be accessed at the Centers for Disease Control's Web site, http://www.cdc.gov/.

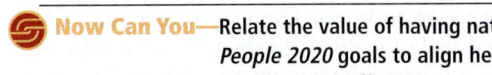 **Now Can You**—Relate the value of having national *Healthy People 2020* goals to align health-care improvement efforts?

1. Discuss the four overarching goals of *Healthy People 2020*?
2. Define the three levels of prevention and give an example of each?
3. Describe prevention measures that have made a difference in reducing heart disease, the leading cause of death in the United States?

Overview of Selected Societal Trends

What is meant by the term "health"? Is health merely the absence of illness? If nurses are to effect improvements in national health status, a more comprehensive definition of health is needed. A holistic definition would include more than the physical body and instead extend into the interconnected mental, social, and spiritual realms. Health would encompass energy levels, balance, and resiliency. The World Health Organization defines health as a state of complete physical, mental, and social well-being and not merely the absence of disease or infirmity. Purnell (2012) expands this definition by describing health as a state of wellness that includes physical, mental, and spiritual states and is defined by individuals within their ethnocultural group.

Health as a concept may be self-defined, but to examine a population's health, one is limited to using health status indicators that can be directly measured. The health of a nation is measured by collecting statistical data and making inferences. **Epidemiology** is the statistical analysis of the distribution and determinants of disease in populations over time. **Mortality** (death) and **morbidity** (illness) rates are examined for trends. For example, epidemiological studies of heart disease reveal how many people develop heart disease, what type of heart disease they have, and what factors are associated with heart disease, such as smoking, obesity, diet, hyperlipidemia, working hazards, family dynamics, and other environmental factors. Mortality rates provide information about where nursing efforts should be focused. Morbidity rates identify populations where the illness occurs most frequently.

There have been many achievements that translate to measurable improvements in health status indicators. Yet the nation still has a long way to go. A report published in the academic journal *Health Affairs* (Muennig & Glied, 2010) states that the United States has dropped to 49th place in the world in overall life expectancy, lagging behind countries with half the national income per capita and with a fraction of the expenditure on medical care. Certain national health problems, including acquired human immunodeficiency virus (AIDS), drug abuse, family violence, and homelessness, continue to signal special cause for concern. More than 3 million people will experience homelessness in a given year, and families with children compose 33% of the homeless population. In addition, in 2010, more than 17 million U.S. households were "food insecure" (Coleman-Jensen, Nord, Andrews, & Carlson, 2011).

To understand better the myriad of issues that impact the nation's health, it is helpful to consider some of the major trends that exert an influence on health status. These include the aging population, ethnic diversity, health-care disparities, childbirth trends, and patterns of physical fitness.

Now Can You—Discuss why analysis of statistical health data in the United States is useful?

1. Define the term epidemiology and describe how analysis of epidemiological data may guide public health interventions?
2. Discuss why mortality/morbidity biostatistics about disease and illness are useful?
3. Describe three health problems in the United States today that are of particular concern?

AGING POPULATION WITH MORE CHRONIC ILLNESSES

The population of persons ages 65 and older (one in eight in the United States) is growing steadily. This trend is attributed to the present increase in life expectancy and is expected to continue as the baby boom generation ages. It is predicted that by 2030, one in five persons will be elderly (U.S. Census Bureau, 2011a). With the increased length of life comes more chronic illnesses, such as strokes, diabetes, arthritis, and Alzheimer's disease. Management of chronic illnesses presents a major challenge to health-care systems that is expected to continue well into the years ahead.

INCREASED RACIAL AND ETHNIC DIVERSITY

The composition of the U.S. population is rapidly changing, and racial and ethnic diversity (difference) is greater than ever before. The historically designated U.S. minority populations can be classified as Hispanic, Black/African American, Asian, and Native American. White Americans (non-Hispanic/Latino and Hispanic/Latino) constitute the racial majority and share 72% of the total U.S. population according to the 2010 U.S. Census. Hispanic and Latino Americans constitute 15% of the population and make up the largest minority. African Americans are the largest racial minority and amount to approximately 13% of the population, while the White, non-Hispanic or Latino population makes up 63% of the nation's total (U.S. Census Bureau, 2011b). As the population becomes more diverse, delivering culturally competent care becomes crucial for nurses. The delivery of health care within a culturally appropriate framework will help patients to feel better satisfied with their care and empower nurses to contribute more actively to the healing process.

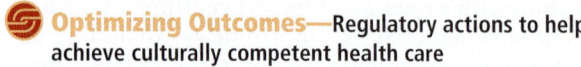

Optimizing Outcomes—Regulatory actions to help achieve culturally competent health care

The growing diversity of the nation has prompted health-care regulators to institute requirements related to the provision of culturally competent care. To successfully implement these requirements, health-care providers must use population-based data (e.g., census figures, voter registration data, school enrollment profiles) to accommodate the patient's cultural, religious, spiritual, and personal values; beliefs and preferences in the care; and treatment and services rendered (Ardoin & Wilson, 2010).

Everyone, regardless of his or her professional status, is interested in the concept of racial and ethnic diversity. However, a most important point to remember is that racial and ethnic categories (Hispanic, Black/African American, Asian, European American, and Native American) are constructed by social systems (i.e., people) and their differences are based on visible physical characteristics. In scientific terms, these differences are phenotypic genetic expressions. There is no known biological basis for what society calls "race." Scientists have noted that there is more diversity within each of these artificial categories than there is between them. Migration, intermarriage, and genetic modifications have served to form one race: the human race. Despite the fact that "race" cannot be supported by scientists as a biological concept, as a social concept (i.e., how persons see one another and label one another) it is still very real.

DISPARITIES IN HEALTH CARE

Health disparities can be viewed as the extra burden carried by certain racial, ethnic, gender, and age groups for different health problems. Statistics indicate that the risk of death for women of color, for example, is nearly four times higher than it is for Caucasian women. More than half of 45- to 64-year-old African American women have hypertension, an incidence that is twice the rate for European Americans. Although Hispanic and African American women have a lower incidence of breast cancer than European Americans, they experience greater mortality from this disease. For reasons that include gender bias and difficulty establishing a correct diagnosis, a woman who presents to the hospital with symptoms of a heart problem is less likely than a man to receive a heart catheterization or to be given certain heart medications. The same scenario applies to Hispanics and African Americans of both genders (National Conference of State Legislatures, 2013).

Optimizing Outcomes—Advancing advocacy for women at the national level

The mission of the Office on Women's Health (OWH) of the U.S. Department of Health and Human Services is to protect and advance the health of women through policy, science, and outreach and to advocate for the participation of women in clinical trials and for sex, gender, and subpopulation analyses. Examples of OWH initiatives include the "Use Medicines Wisely" campaign to promote safe medicine use, the Pink Ribbon Sunday campaign to educate African American and Hispanic women about the early detection of breast cancer through mammography, and the Menopause Hormone Therapy campaign to educate women about the risks and benefits of hormone therapy (Office on Women's Health, 2013).

Access to health care is disproportionate among different population groups. The status of one's health insurance remains the greatest factor that determines access. Insurance status is also the largest predictor of the quality of the health care that one receives. The Commonwealth Fund (2011) reported that during 2010, one of three women ages 19 to 64 was without health insurance, and 48% of working women reported that, because of the associated cost, they did not fill a prescription or obtain a recommended test or follow-up (The Commonwealth Fund, 2011; Ruhl, 2012). Yet insurance status alone cannot explain racial and ethnic disparities. Disparities exist even when clinical factors, such as comorbidities, age, stage of disease presentation, and severity of disease, are taken into account (Clingerman & Fowles, 2010; Isaacs & Colby, 2012).

Racism can be defined as the assumption that one's "race" is superior to others', resulting in unfair and harmful treatment. Racism can include attitudes and behaviors, it can be overt or covert, and it can exist at the individual and the institutional levels. Many other factors, such as the role of discrimination and stereotyping in health-care settings, must also be considered when health disparities are analyzed. Nurses have long considered themselves to be "caring professionals." However, nurses are not immune from societal beliefs and values that result in discrimination and stereotyping of different populations. Nurses must continually remain vigilant for signs of these attitudes in themselves, and in turn, develop an awareness of how they influence their nursing practice. To heighten awareness of these issues, the Institute of Medicine published *Unequal Treatment: Confronting Racial and Ethnic Disparities in Health Care* in 2002. This compilation of studies clearly demonstrated that racism does indeed exist in medicine—and nursing is no exception.

 Optimizing Outcomes—The National Institutes of Health initiative to reduce health disparities

The National Institutes of Health (NIH) has launched a multidisciplinary network of scientists to explore new approaches to understanding the origins of health disparities. With the use of cutting edge conceptual and computational models, the network's goal is to identify important areas where interventions or policy changes could have the greatest impact in eliminating health disparities. NIH will be the first network to apply systems science approaches to the study of health inequities and has plans to produce ongoing reports and publications on the collaborative work of network members (Hellwig, 2010).

Nurses are perfectly situated to partner with representatives of the disparities populations for whom they wish to advocate or seek to better serve. Such partnerships allow nurses and other professionals to gain a deeper understanding of the context of disparities and to work collaboratively with representatives of disparities populations. Taking these actions empowers nurses to help promote social justice for individuals traditionally marginalized by various health disparities (Logsdon & Davis, 2010; Walker & Chesnut, 2010).

Now Can You—Discuss health inequities and limited access to health care?

1. Identify both the age and racial/ethnic diversity trend of the U.S. population and discuss what that means in terms of nursing and health-care provision?
2. Describe the greatest factor that limits access to health care?
3. Explain the roles that discrimination, stereotypes, and racism play in perpetuating health inequities?

CHILDBIRTH TRENDS

Today, many women are choosing to delay childbirth, and this trend is believed to be a result of the desire to complete education and to securely establish careers, relationships, and finances. In 1970, the average age for a woman to have her first baby was 23.4 years; in 2001, the average age had risen to 27.6 years. Births to women ages 35 and older grew 64% between 1990 and 2008, increasing in all major race and ethnic groups (Livingston & Cohn, 2010). The birth rate for women aged 35 to 39 was 47.2 births per 1,000 women in 2011, and the birth rate for women aged 40 to 44 was 10.3 births per 1,000 women—the highest rate in more than four decades (Martin, Hamilton, Ventura, Osterman,

& Mathews, 2013). Because fertility decreases with age, some couples may miss the opportunity to have children altogether. Other related trends in society include children leaving home later and forming unions such as marriage at an older age.

In addition, more women are electing to give birth by cesarean section even when there is no medical reason for doing so. Patient-choice cesarean births in 2001 accounted for 1.87% of births. However, data from a recent (2011) review of over 32,000 births at a major academic hospital between 2003 and 2009 revealed that maternal request for cesarean delivery was the most rapidly increasing category (27% per year) (Barber, Lundsberg, Belanger, Pettker, Funai, & Illuzzi, 2011). Much controversy continues to surround this trend because a cesarean birth is major abdominal surgery with all of the accompanying risks and potentially negative outcomes for women, newborns, and their families (Campbell, 2011; Ehrenthal, Jiang, & Strobino, 2010).

PATTERNS OF PHYSICAL FITNESS

Physical inactivity and its consequences are becoming a significant health problem for families in the United States. According to the Centers for Disease Control (CDC), children and adolescents should engage in at least 1 hour of physical activity every day (CDC, 2011b). To maintain and promote adult health, the American Heart Association advocates a lifestyle that centers on weight control, increased physical activity, alcohol moderation, sodium restriction, and the regular consumption of fresh fruits, vegetables, and low-fat dairy products (American Heart Association [AHA], 2013).

Obesity has made a steady climb upward. In 2000, the World Health Organization (WHO) labeled obesity as the most blatantly visible, but most neglected, public health problem worldwide (WHO, 2013). In this country, more than half of all Americans are overweight or obese (Ogden & Carroll, 2010). It makes sense that increasing physical activity and reducing obesity are underscored in the *Healthy People* initiative as a primary means for reaching the nation's major health outcome goal: increasing the quality and years of healthy life.

THE INTERSECTION OF RACE, CLASS, AND HEALTH

While great strides have been made in family health, the progress achieved is not universal. The gap is widening between persons in lower and upper socioeconomic classes. "Upper class" in this context refers to those who live in contented neighborhoods, have a quality education, and bring home adequate wages. Persons from the lower classes, many of whom are African American, Hispanic, or Native American, live shorter and less healthy lives. According to researchers at the University of New Hampshire, between 2009 and 2010, 1 million more children in America joined the ranks of those living in poverty, bringing the total to an estimated 15.7 million poor children in 2010 (University of New Hampshire, 2011).

It is important for nurses to work toward eliminating discrimination and racism, but if they are to make a difference in rates of illness and premature death, it is also important to work toward improving socioeconomic opportunities for all Americans (Isaacs & Colby, 2012). All too often, life and health choices are limited by socioeconomic status. The vision of the "American dream" and the ideology of "personal choice" obscure the fact that there are enormous constraints and limited choices that accompany poverty. A hungry and desperate person loses the capacity to choose.

 Now Can You—Identify certain population trends that relate to health?

1. Discuss U.S. fertility trends and trends toward surgical birth and what it means for women's health?
2. Discuss the trend toward inactivity in the United States and describe what consequences might be seen in the future health-care status of Americans as a result?
3. Describe the role poverty plays in increasing health-care disparities?

The Current Health Status of the Nation

INFANTS AND YOUNG CHILDREN

The plummeting rates of infant mortality in the past century allowed health-care professionals to move forward beyond infant survival and focus on prevention and early intervention with children's health. Ideally, health prevention strategies targeting children's health would begin as early as preconception. It has been learned, for example, that folic acid supplementation helps to prevent certain birth defects. A fetus' exposure to harm could potentially be prevented if a woman were counseled *before* pregnancy about the harmful effects of alcohol, tobacco, toxoplasma, and other **teratogens** (substances that adversely affect normal cellular development in the embryo/fetus). The fetal neurological system, especially the brain, is extremely vulnerable to even small amounts of potentially toxic substances.

Early intervention is especially important when it comes to growth and developmental delays. There is a well-established link between developmental delays and learning difficulties. Once children reach school age, interventions are less likely to be effective if they have already begun to fail academically or socially. Today, a number of infant and child development screening tools have been developed and refined. Unfortunately, however, close to one-third of developmental or behavioral disorders are not detected until children begin to attend school (Marks, Glascoe, & Macias, 2011).

The leading causes of death by age groups are revealing and offer clues about how to prioritize nursing interventions. Sudden Infant Death Syndrome (SIDS) is the leading cause of death among infants between the ages of 1 and 12 months. Accidents, or unintentional injuries, constitute the leading cause of death in children older than 1 year of age, which suggests that more community education and effort are needed to address child safety hazards. Although the incidence varies by age group, congenital malformations and malignant neoplasms shift between the second and fourth place for the leading cause of death in children (CDC, 2013).

Violence also takes a harsh toll on America's children. Homicidal assaults are the third leading cause of death of children in the 1- to 4-year-old age group, and also in the 15- to 19-year-old age group. Suicide is the third leading cause of death in teenagers and young adults, ages 15 to 24; it is the sixth leading cause of death among children ages 5 to 14. Family violence, child maltreatment, and violence in schools such as bullying are also issues of great concern (CDC, 2011a; U.S. Department of Health and Human Services, 2012).

Anthropologists such as Sanday (2007) note that in American culture, "inter-personal violence has become a national pastime" (p. 2). The most watched television shows of 2005, *Law and Order* and *CSI*, were routinely based on violent acts. It is estimated that the average child will witness 9,000 media murders by the time he or she finishes elementary school (Kunkel, 2007). Findings from a 2008 study of over 800 youth concluded that violent media exposure is associated with involvement in violent behavior (Boxer, Huesmann, Bushman, O'Brien, & Moceri, 2009).

Violent video games are a more recent trend, and research is still sparse regarding their effects on children. A study by Anderson and Dill (2000) suggests that they may be even more harmful because they are interactive and the aggressor is the one glorified and with whom the player identifies.

There are other potentially preventable children's health issues. Lead exposure provides another example where early intervention and teaching can have a positive impact on children's health. Exposure to lead can occur from contact with lead-based paint in older homes; contaminated soil; a parent's occupation; certain vinyl mini-blinds; various folk remedies; living close to major highways; and from contact with imported pottery, jewelry, or cosmetics. The American Academy of Pediatrics (AAP) (2005) recommends that all children between the ages of 1 and 2 years receive testing for lead exposure, because 25% of homes presently occupied by children younger than the age of 6 have known lead contamination. Lead exposure has been linked to a number of medical and developmental problems, including anemia, seizures, and mental retardation.

A trend not well understood is the alarming increase in childhood asthma, a condition that constitutes the most common cause of time missed from school. Asthma and allergies account for the loss of an estimated 2 million school days per year. In fact, the number one reason for pediatric emergency room visits because of chronic illness is for asthma-related problems.

Other trends in children's health status include a significant rise in the diagnoses of attention-deficit/hyperactivity disorder (ADHD) and developmental delays caused by autism. Children with ADHD are typically fidgety, act without thinking, and have difficulty focusing. ADHD now affects 4% to 8% of all school-age children (CDC, 2010). Autism is the third most common type of developmental delay in the United States. An autistic child presents as a solitary child and notably lacks social responsiveness to others. Autism affects language, which is absent, abnormal, or delayed. Autistic children may demonstrate a strong resistance to change and show an abnormal attachment to objects. The prevalence of this disorder is difficult to gauge because autism is not an easily accepted diagnosis. However, it is estimated that it affects approximately 6 out of every 1,000 children (National Institute of Neurological Disorders and Stroke, 2013).

One way to visualize children's health is to view it as an obstacle course. The fortunate child is one who was desired and planned for before conception and who has parents with a good genetic profile, adequate resources, and who harbor no chronic illnesses. The fortunate child's mother would have healthy eating habits; maintain her ideal body weight; access early and regular prenatal care; and abstain from the use of alcohol, tobacco, and other harmful substances. The child who does well through fetal life must then encounter birth and avoid major complications such as prematurity or aspiration pneumonia.

Following birth, the child must encounter the hurdles of the first year of life to avoid becoming an infant mortality statistic. She has to dodge SIDS and shaken baby syndrome and needs to be taken to health-care providers for the hectic schedule of immunizations needed to prevent major childhood diseases. She must be fed and stimulated enough to grow physically, psychologically, socially, and emotionally. The child whose mother breastfeeds her gains an added bonus of immunities.

As the child matures, there are more obstacles to confront. The child who attends day care faces a significantly higher risk of infections. The tendency toward obesity and all the tempting fast food commercials on television offer additional stumbling blocks. She has to dodge all kinds of accidents that cause unintentional injury, tackle each developmental milestone, and land solidly in the "normal" grid of childhood growth charts. Ideally, she will not develop asthma, autism, or ADHD. She will hope to avoid the stumbling blocks of sexual abuse or coping with poverty and poor housing in unsafe neighborhoods. While parents work, the child's day-care environment may be laden with communicable childhood illnesses to be avoided. School-age children need to dodge being one of the 50% who are bullied (American Academy of Adolescent & Child Psychiatry, 2011). The obstacle course continues to pose challenges throughout childhood, and when adolescence arrives, the child again faces new foothills and crags.

ADOLESCENTS

Adolescents represent a population group with a set of issues uniquely their own. With regard to health care, adolescents are most often at risk for falling through the cracks. The adolescent must confront issues of self-esteem along with demands to meet a cultural ideal, while at the same time deal with pressure to conform to gain peer acceptance. The adolescent may have to cope with changes in appearance such as acne and awkwardness. Reproductive issues also arise. Girls must bridge the experience of menses, while boys encounter embarrassing erections and emissions. Issues such as sexuality, teen pregnancy, and sexually transmitted infections may pose further stumbling blocks. Alcohol, tobacco, and drug use as well as bullies, gangs, and school violence may force more hurdles in the envisioned obstacle course for the child to seek a full and healthy life.

One way nurses can make a difference is by learning and teaching others how to listen to children respectfully and value their experiences. Nursing can be called a "narrative profession" because patients present first and foremost with their narratives of symptoms and illness. Children do so as well, but it takes patience to really listen.

 Nursing Insight—*Listening to our youngest patients*

Children tell us that we do not respect their expertise. The child who lives with an illness day by day holds the greatest insight into what it is to experience that illness. They come to know what the illness feels like, what treatments are necessary, what works, and what does not work. They often develop quite sophisticated knowledge about their medications and treatment. The difficulty is that we do not give this knowledge and experience the same value as that held by the adults around them. Children also tell us that we do not give them uninterrupted time to tell their story their way. Children, with their varying cognitive and communication abilities, need time to explain their illness experience and time to respond to our questioning. Sometimes, through adult eyes, their way of telling us seems long and convoluted, and we therefore cannot resist the temptation of jumping in or interpreting what we think they are trying to say. Long storytelling does not fit well in the busy world of practice (Dickinson, 2006).

Two of the priority goals for children in the *Healthy People* initiative address childhood vaccinations. One goal is to achieve and maintain effective vaccination coverage levels for universally recommended vaccines to 90% of children from 19 to 35 months of age and increase routine vaccination coverage for adolescents. The second goal is to reduce vaccine-preventable diseases as follows: (a) measles, mumps, and rubella to zero cases and (b) pertussis in children younger than 7 years to no more than 2,000 cases per year (USDHHS, 2014).

 Now Can You—Describe nursing actions that can serve to improve the current status of children's health in the United States?

1. Describe two benefits of preconceptual health guidance and early intervention?
2. Discuss major causes of child mortality and describe nursing interventions that can make a difference?
3. Compare and contrast communication strategies for children with those of adults?

FAMILIES

Today's world is full of complex, overlapping conditions and trends that influence the health of American families. Families are often the core unit where health habits are first formed. One of nursing's most important roles is to foster the health capacity of families, whether those families are blood-related or are families of choice.

Families do not exist in a vacuum but are situated within communities and regions that often have unique social and physical characteristics. Surrounding environmental hazards affect family health. Natural disasters such as earthquakes, hurricanes, tornadoes, floods, and fires have favorite regional targets. Such disasters cause more damage when they strike high-population areas. Communities with high poverty rates are more likely to have older, run-down homes with more asthma-producing sources, such as mold, lead, and pests. Poorer neighborhoods are more likely to be closer to highways and regional waste sites.

Access to health insurance is an enormous factor that affects the health status of families in what is considered the richest country in the world. There is an ever increasing number of uninsured and underinsured citizens in the United States. More than 49 million Americans were uninsured at last count in 2010 (U.S. Census Bureau, 2011b). One concerning trend is the erosion of employer-provided insurance. Today's employees are no longer guaranteed health insurance coverage through their jobs. According to the U.S. Census Bureau (2011c), the percentage of people covered by employment-based health insurance decreased to 55.3% in 2010 from 56.1% in 2009.

A 2009 study conducted by Himmelstein and colleagues at Harvard University found that illness and medical bills constitute the leading cause of personal bankruptcy and affect approximately 2 million Americans each year (Himmelstein, Thorne, Warren, & Woolhandler, 2009). It has been estimated that in 2013, 1 in 5 Americans will experience difficulty paying medical bills, and 3 in 5 personal bankruptcies will be caused by medical bills (LaMontagne, 2013). Those with health insurance coverage frequently have gaps in coverage that can lead to missed appointments or the inability to fill a needed prescription. Health-care problems among children extend beyond the millions who are uninsured, because for each of those children is another who misses a doctor's appointment or filled prescription as a result of coverage gaps in their parents' plans. Researchers suggest there are many more children in the nation receiving inadequate health care than are reflected in the uninsured figures. Persons without health insurance have limited access to health care and are left vulnerable to the effects of illness, both physical and financial. One of the more ambitious goals of *Healthy People 2020* is to increase to 100% the proportion of persons with health insurance.

WOMEN

The leading cause of death for women in the United States in 2006 was heart disease, which accounted for 25.8% of all female deaths. Cancer represented the second leading cause at 22.0%, followed by cerebral vascular disease (stroke) as third, which accounted for 6.7% (CDC, 2011d).

There is plenty of room for improvement in health behaviors that are precursors to heart disease. According to the 2011 CDC's Behavioral Risk Factor Surveillance System (BRFSS), two-thirds of women in the 25- to 65-year-old age group do not get the recommended 30 minutes of daily physical activity. One in five adult women smoke tobacco. With regard to nutrition, 72% of women do not get the recommended five or more servings of vegetables and fruits per day. There are also deficiencies in calcium and folic acid intake, nutrients important to women's health. Folic acid is a B vitamin that is linked to prevention of certain birth defects. Calcium is important to bone health. Lack of calcium contributes to osteoporosis, which makes a person susceptible to fractures, which can lead to disability and death (CDC, 2011d).

Perinatal Health

Maternal and newborn morbidity and mortality place huge burdens on families, communities, and societies as a whole. The United States currently ranks 42nd in the world in the infant mortality rate, and over the past three decades, there has been no decline in the number of pregnancy-associated deaths. According to the CDC (2010), 2 to 3 women in the United States die from pregnancy complications each day. Studies show that at least one-half of pregnancy-related deaths could be prevented. One reason for the recent escalation in high-risk pregnancies is related to pregnancies that occur in women with preexisting chronic conditions. Complications before childbirth account for more than 2 million hospital days of care and more than $1 billion spent each year in this country. In actuality, this number would be even higher if it also included complications that occur during and after childbirth (CDC, 2011e).

Four million women give birth each year in the United States. Interestingly, in this day where there are more contraceptive methods than ever before, at least one-half of all pregnancies are unintended or mistimed. Another *Healthy People 2020* goal is to improve pregnancy planning and spacing and to prevent unintended pregnancies. Currently, there are some positive trends in perinatal health. For example, women are starting their prenatal care earlier. In the latest CDC Behavioral Risk data (2011d), 83.9% of women initiated prenatal care during the first trimester. Smoking during pregnancy decreased from 20% in 1989 to less than 11% in 2003. Also, today, there is more published information about proper nutrition, folic acid, and healthy lifestyles than ever before (Speidel & Grossman, 2011).

There is evidence that contemporary health-care systems are more cognizant of women's needs. Children maneuvering giant balloons as they eagerly bounce down the postpartum hall en route to visit their mothers and newborn siblings is a welcome and familiar sight. There is more understanding in research circles about the differences in the health-care needs of women and men. Women are being empowered more in health-care settings, enabling them, in turn, to make better health-care decisions for their families.

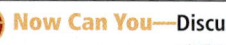 **Now Can You**—Discuss elements of the current health status of American families and women?

1. Discuss how recent national trends have affected families' access to health insurance?
2. Identify the three leading causes of death in women in the United States?
3. Help develop a statewide model to improve pregnancy outcomes and reduce maternal mortality?

Politics, Socioeconomics, and Culture: Contemporary Influences and Trends

To facilitate understanding of present-day health-care issues, it is helpful to consider political, socioeconomic, and cultural influences and trends. Family health issues are shaped, in part, by other elements as well. These elements include historical factors, family features, and biological and ecological influences. All of these factors intermingle and intersect with personal life experiences to constitute a health issue.

❀ *Nursing Insight—Global health challenges and the millennium development goals*

The rapid growth of world population from 2.6 billion in 1950 to almost 7 billion in 2011, coupled with dramatically increased consumption of natural resources, contributes to global food insecurity, climate change, and economic instability. In 2000, world leaders committed their nations to a new global partnership to reduce extreme poverty, hunger, illiteracy, maternal mortality, and disease through the Millennium Development Goals. The eight goals, with targeted achievement by 2015, form a blueprint agreed on by various countries and leading development institutions (Callister & Edwards, 2010; Gilliam, 2009; Mattson, 2010; Speidel & Grossman, 2011; Tyer-Viola & Cesario, 2010). Today's global health problems include HIV infection leading to AIDS, other infectious diseases, sexual and reproductive health, maternal and child health, chronic diseases, climate change, nutrition and food security, and health systems strengthening. Efforts to find and implement solutions for these varied and complex health concerns will require the effective mobilization of science, technology, and interdisciplinary research. To meet these challenges, nurses and other health-care professionals must collaborate with other disciplines in designing and participating in ongoing research, providing evidence-based interventions, and pooling resources to find effective solutions to the myriad global health problems (Callister & Edwards, 2010; Campbell & Moran, 2010; Edwards, 2011; Hawley, Fouche, Cates, Jr., & Bentley, 2010; McKee, Jr., & Cohen, 2010).

POLITICAL INFLUENCES AND TRENDS

Health policy decisions always involve choices, and whenever there are choices to be made, values and the potential for values conflicts are involved. One of the most polarizing political debates in modern times concerns the issue of abortion. Throughout the years since the passage of *Roe vs. Wade*, "abortion has kept its grip on the American imagination . . . dividing the body politic on issues of control of women's bodies, rights to privacy, fetal viability, and broader concerns over the moral shape of our country . . ." (Ginsburg, 1998, p. ix).

How and where a nation spends money has a major influence on the overall health of the population. National economic policies often dictate who has access to health care and who will be able to obtain medications. Policies related to social income programs such as Social Security and welfare assistance significantly affect the health of populations. Transportation issues and housing policies are critical as well. Education policies, such as the removal of physical education requirements from schools, have far-reaching and long-lasting effects on the health of children.

HEALTH-CARE DELIVERY

Changes in health-care delivery are omnipresent. The current health-care delivery system is less a system than it is a collection of entities. Health care today is corporate and thus is more market driven than based on the common good or the actual needs of populations. Care is increasingly centralized into major medical centers. Small hospitals are closing because of an inability to remain solvent.

Managed care is the rule rather than the exception and is expanding as more and more health-care providers and institutions are pressured into joining networks for health-care delivery. Many of the provider networks operate on capitation, in which they negotiate and are paid a set amount to provide complete health care for a certain number of clients.

Quality of health care and consumer satisfaction are the drivers of health care, just as in the retail industries. National databases regarding quality of care and specific conditions are only now beginning to be organized. Although a dearth of information is available on the quality of health care in the United States, this is changing as the focus on accountability in government and institutions moves to the forefront. The trend toward increased media attention concerning health-care errors represents a vivid example of a growing demand for accountability. Workplace satisfaction and nursing shortages are issues that need to be addressed as well.

PUBLIC POLICIES AND PROGRAMS

There are several public policies and programs that make a difference in women's, children's, and families' health. One highly influential program is the Women, Infants, and Children (WIC) program. WIC targets pregnant women, infants, and children, age 5 or younger, who are nutritionally at risk and provides supplemental nutritious foods and nutrition counseling and education. WIC serves low-income families and any pregnant woman who has particular nutrition challenges such as diabetes or anemia. Forty-five percent of infants born in the United States participate in the WIC program. Another nutrition program, The National School Lunch/Breakfast program, provides free or reduced-price meals to children from low-income families.

Medicaid, legislated through Title XIX of the Social Security Act, is a major publicly funded program that helps to boost the health status of women, children, and families. Funding for Medicaid is shared between federal and state governing bodies. Medicaid offers medical assistance after specific sets of complex eligibility criteria have been met. The Medicaid program is the largest safety net source of funding for health-care services for the poorest populations in the United States.

The Newborn and Mothers Health Protection Act was passed in 1996. This legislation ensures that mothers and their newborn infants can remain in the hospital for at least 48 hours after a vaginal birth or 96 hours following a cesarean birth. Another influential source of legislation for families is the Family and Medical Leave Act (FMLA) of 1993. This law permits American workers to take up to 12 weeks of unpaid leave per year from their jobs for recovery from serious illness or to provide care for a sick family member.

Signed into law in 2010, the Affordable Care Act (ACA) takes significant steps forward in the areas of health promotion, prevention, and primary care. In addition to policies designed to extend health-care benefits to more than 30 million previously uninsured Americans, the ACA contains a host of provisions aimed at lowering overall health-care costs and improving quality of care at the same time. Under the ACA, health plans must now cover preventive services such as flu shots, childhood and adult vaccinations, and screening tests without charging a co-payment or deductible. An expanded package of women's preventive health services enacted in 2011 provided coverage for all FDA-approved contraceptive methods and devices, including sterilization procedures. The ACA better enables physicians and patients to work together as a team to promote health rather than to simply treat illness. Registered nurses will continue to play an important role in ensuring the delivery of quality health care. The ACA provides expanded access to primary care, increases the reimbursement for primary care services, and expands payments for graduate medical education for primary care (ACOG, 2012; Buppert, 2011; Kohlenberg, 2011; Ricketts, 2011; Ruhl, 2012; Seligson, 2010; Shore & Griggs, 2010; Slywotzky & Main, 2011).

SELECTED SOCIOECONOMIC INFLUENCES AND TRENDS

The most egregious effects of inequality in the United States are seen on the streets of the inner cities among persons with little hope for the future. The more subtle but far-reaching effects are seen in workers with insecure jobs. These are persons who rightly fear that major illness would result in personal catastrophe. According to the U.S. Census Bureau (2011c), between 2008 and 2009, the poverty rate increased for children under age 18 and adults aged 18 to 64 (U.S. Census Bureau, 2011c).

In addition, there are the elderly who must expend nearly all of their resources before they can accept public funding for needed long-term care. For the elderly, the cost of medications can add up at the same rapid rate as do the chronic health conditions associated with the aging process. There are also those who may be classified in a low- or a high-income group; may be young or may be elderly; and may be living in a busy metropolis, in suburbia, or in a lonesome rural area and yet are maintaining lives that offer little opportunity for control or meaningful social participation. Certainly these inequalities are, in part, inequalities in income. However, more than an inequality of income is at issue. In a fundamental sense, these inequalities are reflective of a society that works well for those at the top and far less well for everyone else.

THE INCREASING RATE OF POVERTY

Most persons consider items like adequate food, housing, clothing, heat, electricity, telephone service, and essential health care as necessities rather than luxuries. This is not true for everyone. Overall, 12.7% of Americans were living in poverty in the United States in 2004. The number has risen each year since 2000 (U.S. Census Bureau, 2011a). Economic changes, racial inequality, suburban movement, man-made and natural disasters, and industrialization all contribute to poverty circumstances.

THE FEMINIZATION OF POVERTY

Women are the most impoverished demographic group in American society. In 2005, 56% of persons older than age 18 living in poverty were women. In 2013, more than one in seven women lived in poverty. The poverty rate among women was 14.5 %; for men, the poverty rate was 11%. Single mothers with their children constitute 82% of the poverty population. More than 60% of U.S. women

with children younger than the age of 2 now work outside the home (National Women's Law Center, 2014; U.S. Census Bureau, 2011a).

The poverty rate for children has historically been higher than the overall poverty rate, and the poverty rate for persons living in households headed by single women is significantly higher than the overall poverty rate. For example, in 2000, one-fifth of all U.S. children were living in poverty. Between 2000 and 2003, the number and percentage of single mothers living in poverty increased while the percentage of single mothers with jobs fell. At the same time, poverty among children rose, and the number of children living below half of the poverty line (about $732 a month in 2010 for a single mother with two children) has increased by nearly 1 million. These structural features of U.S. society have contributed to what has been coined as the "feminization of poverty" (National Poverty Center, 2013).

Single mothers face oppressive barriers to achieve "economic self-sufficiency," now legislatively prescribed for them, commonly referred to as "welfare to work." The essence of the new legislation, entitled Temporary Assistance for Needy Families (TANF), is that work now becomes compulsory and lifetime limits are imposed. TANF replaces the former public assistance program that was known as Aid to Families with Dependent Children (AFDC). There is a maximum period that a person is allowed to receive public assistance at one time and a lifetime limit. The mandates apply to pregnant women and women with infants older than the age of 3 months.

THE WAGE GAP

Gender inequity persists, and the ratio of full-time working women's weekly earnings to those of men was 77 cents to the men's dollar in 2011. Proportionately, more families are being supported by women today than ever before, and women constitute over half of the 39 million Americans living in poverty today. According to the U.S. Census Bureau, there are twice as many female head of households (with no males present) living in poverty than male head of households (with no females present). Furthermore, men continue to earn more money than women, even for the same type of work (U.S. Census Bureau, 2011c).

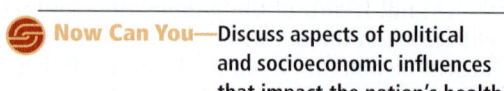

Now Can You—Discuss aspects of political and socioeconomic influences that impact the nation's health?

1. Identify and discuss three socioeconomic trends that have a negative impact on the health of persons living in the United States?
2. Describe two public programs intended to improve the health of American women, children, and families?
3. Describe what is meant by the phrase "the feminization of poverty"?

COMMUNICATIONS AND THE DIGITAL DIVIDE

One of the factors promoting patient empowerment is the ready access to health-care information over the Internet. Fox (2011), reporting on health and electronic media, found that 59% of the U.S. adult population seeks health information online, most often searching for specific symptoms and treatments. Approximately 44% of Internet users look online for information about doctors or other health-care professionals, and one-third seek information related to health insurance, Medicare, or Medicaid. Interestingly, 17% of cell phone users have used their phone to look up health or medical information.

In modern society, however, there exists what has been termed the "digital divide." Families with discretionary income and with some formal education are more likely to access health information and educational resources from the worldwide Web. Those with less income, in particular those from racial and ethnic minority backgrounds, are less likely to have access to electronic materials. In addition, there is what is called the "gray gap," referring to seniors who do not use Internet technology. Approximately 82% of American households reported ready access to the Internet in 2010. In families with incomes of $75,000, 95% of children have a computer at home. Yet over 30% of Americans claim they have never used the Internet or e-mail. Again, the "digital divide" separates and discriminates against the poor or elderly who do not have access to computers or who have not learned computer skills (U.S. Census Bureau, 2011d).

VULNERABLE POPULATIONS

As a society, it behooves Americans to focus on a shared vision and goals, such as those afforded to us by the *Healthy People* initiative. To do so, it is important to consider the vulnerable populations in the United States. As Aday (2001) notes, "as members of human families and communities, we are all potentially vulnerable" (p. 53). Vulnerability encompasses threats to physical and psychological health, as well as vulnerable social circumstances and stages within the life course.

HOMELESS PERSONS. Homelessness is rising among all populations but most noticeably for families. There is an increase in families at the extreme poverty level (about $11,500 for a family of four in 2011). Income levels such as this are woefully inadequate to maintain a household. The increase in homelessness has resulted in more and more entire families who regularly visit homeless shelters and soup kitchens across the country. In New York City, 78% of the shelter population comprises children and their parents (Coalition for the Homeless, 2013). The random collection of community shelters and free food kitchens that have proliferated throughout the United States during the past several years have had a difficult time keeping up with needs. It has not helped that recent policy changes have resulted in the elimination of several programs that previously served as safety nets for health-care and housing subsidies. Persons displaced as a result of wars and disasters have also added to the number of those desperately seeking assistance.

For homeless persons and families, health is a momentous challenge. The poverty, stigma, poor nutrition, and increased susceptibility to violence and mental illness all take their toll. Access to health care is a problem because of lack of transportation and finances, so that hospital emergency rooms are often the only option for medical attention. It is difficult to obtain accurate numbers on the homeless population, but the Coalition for the Homeless estimates that currently there are about 2 million homeless persons in the United States, with 9,864 homeless families in New York City alone (Coalition for the Homeless, 2013).

 Nursing Insight—*Putting homelessness into proper perspective*

To enhance understanding of the magnitude of the problem of homelessness in the United States, it is useful to consider the following statistics. These figures relate to families with children who slept in Department of Homeless Services (DHS) city shelters in New York City during a single night in the fall of 2011:

- 8,338 families
- 16,121 children
- 11,245 adults
- Average daily shelter census—families with children: 8,338
- Average daily shelter census—adult families: 1,337
- Average daily shelter census—total number of individuals: 38,655 (New York City Department of Homeless Services, 2013).

UNDOCUMENTED IMMIGRANTS AND REFUGEES. Undocumented persons (foreign nationals residing in the United States without legal immigration status) who enter the United States illegally to work constitute another highly vulnerable population. Many are drawn to the United States for economic reasons or to escape political conflicts. Undocumented persons are willing to work in what are considered the lowest paid and least desirable occupations in the United States. They generally have no job security, health-care access, or decent housing. Most face language barriers as well. Without financial resources, hospital and health clinic doors are generally closed to them.

PERSONS RESIDING IN RURAL AREAS. Persons living in rural neighborhoods are less likely to have access to quality health care. Primary care providers are increasingly reluctant to locate in rural areas. Many small, rural hospitals have been forced to close because of centralization of intensive care services. In 2009, the American College of Obstetricians and Gynecologists (ACOG) published a position paper urging OB/GYN doctors to help increase rural women's health-care access. The summary statement discusses how lack of access to adequate women's health care puts rural women in the United States at greatly increased risk of poor health outcomes and suggests ways in which physicians can help to improve the situation (ACOG, 2009).

PERSONS WITH LIMITED HEALTH LITERACY. According to the Institute of Medicine (2004), health literacy is defined as the degree to which individuals have the capacity to obtain, process, and understand basic health information and services needed to make appropriate health decisions and to use such information and services in ways that are health enhancing. Adults with limited health literacy are at increased risk of hospitalization, encounter more barriers to receiving necessary health-care services, and are less likely to understand medical advice that can affect their disease progression. An important target area in the

Healthy People 2020 national initiative identifies objectives to improve health communication with goals related to health literacy and cultural competency. In today's health-care climate, patients are expected to be articulate and accurate about their conditions and symptoms, have access to and use a computer and the Internet, and possess sophisticated decision-making skills. Often individuals with the greatest health-care needs have limited skills to synthesize and interpret health information. Patients with specific educational or linguistic challenges may also have limited health literacy. Nurses can use several strategies to help to address the needs of those with low health literacy, such as obtaining training in improving communication with patients; asking open-ended questions; checking for comprehension by asking patients to restate health information; using plain, culturally sensitive language; using professional interpreters and informing patients of their right to receive bilingual services and language assistive services in their preferred language; and by developing health information appropriately tailored for the intended users (ACOG, 2011a, 2011b; Harrington, 2012; Lee, 2011; McLeod-Sordjan, 2011; Moore, 2012; Warner & Washington, 2011).

ABUSED AND NEGLECTED CHILDREN. The National Child Abuse and Neglect Data System (NCANDS) is the federal reporting system that analyzes data on child abuse that are collected on an annual basis. In 2011, NCANDS reported that the information obtained in the 2009 count included over 3 million cases of reported child abuse. Child abuse can take many forms. The most common is child neglect, which can mean withholding food, clothing, shelter, love, supervision, or medical attention. Physical and child sexual abuse are other types, and it is not uncommon for all three forms of abuse and neglect to overlap. According to the American Academy of Pediatrics, study estimates predict that 1 out of 4 girls and 1 out of 6 boys will be inappropriately touched sexually by the time they turn 18 (Child Welfare Information Gateway, 2011; The National Center for Victims of Crime, 2011).

NCANDS reports that three children die of child abuse in the home each day. Fewer than 1% of children are abused by strangers. Children are most commonly abused by someone they know. In 79% of cases, the perpetrator is a parent. Child abuse can set up a perpetuating cycle of suffering and more violence later in life, potentially reaching into future generations (Child Welfare Information Gateway, 2011).

Nurses have a legal obligation to report any observed known or suspected child abuse to child protective services. Thus, it is critical for nurses to learn to assess the signs and symptoms of child abuse (see Chapter 22).

VICTIMS OF VIOLENCE AGAINST WOMEN.

Sexual Violence. Historical beliefs and attitudes toward women continue to influence women's lives and health. In the past, women were viewed as physically and psychologically inferior to men. They were denied rights and privileges routinely granted to men, such as owning property and voting.

Sexual violence haunts the lives of all women, both with its frequency and its impact. In 2010, the Centers for Disease Control and Prevention published a summary report with findings from a national survey (National Intimate Partner and Sexual Violence Survey [NISVS]) intended to provide baseline data that will be used to track intimate partner violence, sexual violence, and stalking trends (Black et al., 2011). Some have called the United States a "rape-prone" society (Buchwald, Fletcher, & Roth, 2005; Sanday, 2007). Sexual violence is linked with deleterious long-term psychological, social, and physical effects such as substance abuse, major depression, gynecological disorders, and others. Unwanted sexual attention also devalues women and takes a toll on their health. Lewd sexual comments, cat calls, whistling, and intrusive looks are demeaning actions that negatively affect women's health (Alpert, 2010).

Female Genital Cutting/Mutilation/Circumcision. Female genital cutting (FGC) (also known as female genital mutilation or circumcision) is a commonly performed practice worldwide that affects approximately 3 million girls each year. According to the World Health Organization (WHO), female genital mutilation is any procedure that intentionally alters or injures female genital organs for non-health-related reasons (WHO, 2010). Rooted in cultural values, beliefs, and social patterns, genital cutting is considered a rite of passage and confers on females a right to belong to, participate in, and own property in that culture. While female genital cutting can be performed at any time from birth to adulthood, most girls undergo the procedure between ages 4 and 8 years. Complications resulting from genital cutting may be acute (e.g., hemorrhage, shock, and death) or long-term (e.g., painful menses and urination, fear of first intercourse, dyspareunia, physical scarring, mental trauma, and anxiety). Efforts to eradicate FGC have been in place since the 1950s. Today, the practice is widely perceived as a violation of human rights, and multiple governments throughout the world are now enforcing legislation against FGC and initiating educational programs to teach citizens about the immediate and long-reaching harmful effects of the practice (Ibe & Johnson-Agabakwu, 2011; Sandy, 2011).

Intimate Partner Violence. It is difficult to obtain accurate numbers about intimate partner violence because of varying definitions and widespread under-reporting. The National Intimate Partner and Sexual Violence Survey: 2010 Summary Report (Black et al., 2011) revealed that nearly 1 in 5 women (18.3%) and 1 in 71 men (1.4%) in the United States have been raped at some time in their lives. More than half (51.1%) of female victims of rape reported being raped by an intimate partner and 40.8% by an acquaintance at some point in their lifetime. Furthermore, most female and male victims of rape, physical violence, and/or stalking by an intimate partner experienced some form of intimate partner violence for the first time before reaching 25 years of age (Black et al., 2011).

Research suggests that nurses in clinical settings are still reluctant to question patients about intimate partner violence (Kang, Gottlieb, Raker, Aneja, & Boardman, 2010). Nurses need to routinely ask the violence screening questions and offer to help abused patients develop a safety plan. It is important for nurses to know that the most dangerous times for abused women are during pregnancy and when a woman tries to leave her partner.

Human Trafficking. Human trafficking, or "trafficking in persons," an egregious violation of human rights, is the enslavement of individuals for profit. It is both a global and a domestic problem that affects nearly 1 million people worldwide and approximately 20,000 persons in the United States each year (U.S. Department of State, 2011). Often used in the sex trade or in forced labor servitude, women and children are the most frequent victims of this modern-day form of slavery. The majority of victims are domestically trafficked, meaning persons of the same nationality force them into labor for another's profit within their own countries (McClain & Garrity, 2011). Human trafficking also crosses international borders. Adult victims, commonly uneducated and jobless, are promised gainful employment as nannies, maids, dancers, models, and agricultural/factory workers in the United States. Once here, traffickers use methods such as threats, physical force, rape, torture, and starvation to coerce them into prostitution, pornography, and involuntary servitude. The health risks for victims of human trafficking are substantial and include torture, rape, exposure to sexually transmitted diseases, hazardous work environments, poor nutrition, and drug and alcohol addiction (ACOG, 2011c; Hodge & Lietz, 2007). Nurses working in any setting must be aware of this problem and remain alert for clues that may point to trafficking victimization (e.g., poor health status; inability or reluctance to discuss self/injury/work/living arrangements; lack of any official identification papers; malnourishment and signs of physical abuse/depression/posttraumatic stress disorder; and obvious fearfulness of the "sponsor"). Indicators of possible forced labor of a child include situations in which the child appears to be in the custody of a non-family member who has the child perform work that financially benefits someone outside the child's family and does not offer the child the option of leaving (ACOG, 2011c; U.S. Department of State, 2011).

GAY/LESBIAN/TRANSGENDERED INDIVIDUALS. Studies repeatedly demonstrate that access to sensitive health care for gay, lesbian, and gender-transitioning patients is extremely limited. Stigma and prejudice continue to prevail in attitudes toward those living an "other than heterosexual" lifestyle (see Chapter 6 for further discussion about specific health issues among this population).

Optimizing Outcomes—Health care for transgender individuals

In late 2011, the American College of Obstetricians and Gynecologists (ACOG) released a Committee Opinion calling for increased awareness of barriers to health care (e.g., lack of insurance coverage for mental health services, cross-sex hormone therapy, and gender affirmation surgery) faced by transgender individuals. ACOG urged health-care providers to foster nondiscriminatory practices and policies to increase identification of transgender individuals and to facilitate quality health care in all clinical settings (ACOG, 2011d).

INCARCERATED WOMEN. An invisible population of marginalized women exists within the hidden pockets of the richest country in the world. One hears very little about incarcerated women, yet they currently inhabit U.S. jails and prisons in ever-increasing numbers, with a sixfold increase during the past 20 years. The growth rate of women prisoners has now overtaken the growth rate of male prisoners, and at present, women constitute 10% of the total inmate population. In this country, which has the highest incarceration rate in the world, there are approximately 1 million women behind bars (U.S. Department of Justice, 2011), and the majority of female inmates are between 24 and 35 years of age (Sarteschi & Vaughn, 2010).

As a population, incarcerated women are not healthy. They tend to have a myriad of health problems, particularly illnesses that stem from the stresses of poverty, physical and sexual abuse, addiction, and motherhood. Imprisoned women frequently do not have access to the benefits of health education. Mental health issues abound in this vulnerable population as well (Harner & Burgess, 2011).

Pregnancies among incarcerated women are frequently unplanned and high risk. Complications arising from lack of prenatal care, poor nutrition, intimate partner violence, chronic diseases, infectious diseases, mental illness, and drug and alcohol abuse are not uncommon. According to ACOG (2011e), every woman of childbearing age should be assessed for pregnancy risk upon entry into a prison or a jail and tested for pregnancy as appropriate to enable the provision of adequate perinatal care and abortion services. Incarcerated women who wish to continue their pregnancies should have ready access to regularly scheduled obstetric care and access to unscheduled or emergency obstetric visits on a 24-hour basis (ACOG, 2011e; Clarke & Adashi, 2011).

Optimizing Outcomes—Advocating for discontinuing the practice of shackling incarcerated pregnant women

In late 2011, the Association of Women's Health, Obstetric and Neonatal Nurses (AWHONN) released a position statement to address the practice of shackling incarcerated pregnant women. According to the organization, shackling a pregnant woman should only take place if prison officials reasonably believe that a particular individual may attempt to harm herself or others or presents a legitimate flight risk. Underscoring the need for the continued safety of registered nurses and other health-care personnel, AWHONN acknowledges the benefit of adequate correctional staff to monitor incarcerated women during routine prenatal examinations, labor and delivery, and the postpartum recovery period but emphasizes that shackles should not be used as a substitute for adequate correctional staff monitoring (AWHONN, 2011a).

More than 70% of incarcerated women are mothers. This is an issue that greatly impacts the health of families. Approximately 1.3 million minor children have no mother to care for them on a daily basis. Inevitably, children are affected by the abrupt changes commonly associated with incarceration of a parent. They may experience a sudden change in caretaking arrangements, social stigma, the potential for abandonment, and the loss of family support and financial resources.

The Girl Scouts of America organization has developed a unique program for girls who are separated from their mothers because of incarceration. Called "Girl Scouts Beyond Bars," this program is similar to regular scouting programs and has the same goals of self-esteem building and incremental accomplishments. It includes prison visitation between mothers and daughters and especially targets social risks for which these young women are more vulnerable. The program also attempts to help incarcerated women hone their parenting skills. Forensic psychiatric nurses play an important consulting role in this national program, now operational in 13 states.

A nurse who is able to deliver culturally competent care to incarcerated populations quickly becomes cognizant of the challenges and the importance of raising standards and improving the present system. Clinicians in correctional facilities have a unique opportunity to help ensure that incarcerated women leave jails and prisons in better physical and mental health than when they arrived (Harner & Burgess, 2011). Work performed with this vulnerable population is significant far beyond the prison walls. Nearly 95% of prisoners will eventually be released into communities where they will likely face poverty, stigma, unemployment, and deficiencies in health care.

PERSONS WHO ARE SUBSTANCE ABUSERS. Substance abuse is a major health issue for families. Unfortunately, children are often the ones who suffer the most. Children in families with substance use problems are likely to be abused and neglected. These same children are also more likely to become substance users themselves. See Chapters 11 and 23 for further information.

 Now Can You—Identify vulnerable populations of women, children, and families that exist in the United States today?

1. Identify and describe four vulnerable populations in the United States?
2. Describe the population group at present experiencing the largest rise in homelessness?
3. Explain why undocumented immigrants are considered a vulnerable population?

PERSONAL AND CULTURAL INFLUENCES AND TRENDS

In today's world, nursing students are likely to use their mobile phones to contact their friends via text message. The population relies on mass media for news, information, and entertainment, and the electronic gaming industry is thriving. In addition to an abundance of online resources, many professional organizations offer individuals free tablet apps for various health-related topics. For example, AWHONN's consumer magazine "Healthy Mom & Baby" is now available as an iPad application that includes special features such as videos, click-to-reveal articles, quizzes, and online-only content.

 Across Care Settings: Text4Baby

It is estimated that 90% of U.S. women have a mobile phone, and texting is especially prevalent among women of childbearing age and among minority populations, who face higher infant mortality rates (Pew Internet & American Life Project, 2010). Text4baby is a free service that provides ongoing vital health information to pregnant women and new mothers via text messages. Developed by a multifaceted public-private partnership, the service may be implemented as a component of prenatal education during the initial obstetric visit. Topics covered in the Text4baby messages include nutrition, seasonal flu prevention and treatment, mental health, risks of tobacco use, oral health, immunization schedules, breastfeeding, and safe infant sleeping practices (Jordan, Ray, Johnson, & Evans, 2011).

---

 legal alert—Use social networking sites responsibly

It is reported that 60 million professionals regularly use online sites to exchange information, ideas, and opportunities (Walker, 2011). Professionals in health care may use social networking to share information for business and marketing endeavors or to learn through communication with colleagues. For nurses, sharing patient care experiences with colleagues can serve as a powerful learning tool that encourages reflection, enhances empathy, and deepens understanding. However, for these kinds of communications, a private site for professional purposes only should be considered. Nurses must always be mindful of maintaining patient confidentiality, an important component of the Health Insurance Portability and Accountability Act (HIPAA) and long held standard in health care (Balestra, 2011; Kirby, 2011; Madden & Zickuhr, 2011; Walker, 2011).

Other cultural changes include an increase in language barriers and cultural differences within the U.S. population. There is also a cultural component to many health issues. For example, the dramatic rise in eating disorders demonstrates how present-day popular culture can strongly influence health. Media images of so-called "perfection" flood the media, yet these images rarely represent healthy role models.

SELF-CARE AND PATIENT INVOLVEMENT

Autonomy and social participation have important influences on health status. Trends that present themselves in the health-care arena include a focus on more consumer involvement and self-care tactics. Today there is an abundance of self-help groups, many of which are modeled along the lines of Alcoholics Anonymous, with varying purposes.

 Where Research and Practice Meet: Patients and Social Media

Although Americans readily use e-mail as a mode of correspondence, they do not like the idea of using social media (e.g., Twitter and Facebook) to consult with their doctors. A national telephone survey determined that more than 5 of every 6 of the 843 respondents said that if given the opportunity, they would not use social media for communicating with their doctors. Nearly 75% said they would not take advantage of chat or instant messaging if offered by their doctor, and 54% would not use a private online forum. However, 52% of respondents said they would be willing to confer with their doctor via e-mail (57% of women, 47% of men), and 72% would use a nurse helpline (82% of women and 61% of men) (Capstrat Public Policy Polling, 2011). This information is helpful to nurses who may wish to routinely ask patients about their preferred method of contact and provide information about practice resources such as a nurse helpline.

For example, there are groups for tobacco dependency, "co-dependency" (CODA), drug addictions (Narcotics Anonymous), eating disorders (Overeater's Anonymous), and for families of addicts (Al-Anon and Alateen). In addition, there are self-help groups for nearly every medical ailment or illness imaginable. Some communities offer peer visitation programs whereby a person with the same illness or condition shares personal experiences with the newly diagnosed patient to help him or her understand what to expect in the days ahead.

In many situations, increased patient autonomy has resulted in more of a partnership model for the nurse. The nurse's role becomes increasingly one of facilitator and "cultural broker" to help the patient negotiate mutually acceptable plans of care. In obstetrics, it has meant that traditional childbirth practices of the past are increasingly challenged to become more personalized and family-centered. In pediatrics, it has meant that parents are encouraged to remain in their everyday roles as the primary support persons for their children.

The trend toward early discharge from hospitals has resulted in sicker patients in hospitals. Early discharge trends have also led to the blossoming of home health organizations. It is estimated that within the next few years, 70% of nursing care will be administered in the home setting. Literature has indicated that community-based care will be essential to nursing in the 21st century.

COMPLEMENTARY AND ALTERNATIVE THERAPIES

As noted in Chapter 1, there is a growing trend toward the use of complementary and alternative medicine (CAM) therapies. The majority of persons in the United States now use some sort of CAM therapy, but many are reluctant to disclose that information to traditional medical personnel. There is sometimes the perception that nurses and physicians, because most are trained using the biomedical model, may not approve of the use of CAM. It is important for health-care providers to have a working knowledge of CAM and try to integrate the two types of medicine. In this way, the patient obtains the benefit of each. Integrating CAM with conventional health care is called "integrative health care." Ideally, the nurse can thread integrative health care with the practice of conventional maternal child nursing for the maximum benefit of the patient.

One common lay perspective that is difficult to counter is the belief that because something is marketed as "natural," it means that it is harmless or without side effects. There have been publicized incidences of children being given unsafe treatments that resulted in harm or death. Mantle (2005) notes that the Children's Act of 1989 states the "interests of the child are paramount. This includes the child's physical welfare and anything relevant to this, including nutrition and access to appropriate medical care" (p. 24).

Complementary Care: *Blogging As Therapy*

Some health programs recommend "blogging" to facilitate healing when faced with serious diseases. Patients write daily about their experiences in diary format on the Internet. Blogs are a recording of personal experience, a participatory form of self-expression. Blogs help the creativity of individuals to surface and can be comforting during health crises. Blogs bypass editors and publishers and can be produced at the person's own pace. A strong sense of community can grow from blogging for health, and it is free of charge for those with computers and Internet access.

Now Can You—Discuss personal and cultural trends that may impact an individual's health status?

1. Discuss some of the effects of self-care and autonomy on a person's health status?
2. Explain what is meant by the term "integrative health care"?
3. Discuss why blogging may be viewed as a complementary care method?

Health Care for the Nation

Recent years have brought an exponential growth of information and knowledge in all areas, especially in the field of health care. It is estimated that the total amount of information doubles every 6 years. Knowledge becomes obsolete at a rapid pace. Learning how to access current and accurate knowledge is critical for all health-care providers. The implementation of community-based programs that are responsive to population needs for health promotion, education, and screening is an important nursing strategy to help meet many of the national goals of the *Healthy People 2020* initiative.

Across Care Settings: Serving the public through faith community nursing

Faith community nursing, sometimes known as parish nursing, congregational nursing, or church nursing, is a phenomenon born from the marriage of nursing to the healing ministry of churches and religion. Faith community nursing is a practice specialty that focuses on the intentional care of the spirit, promotion of an integrative model of health, and the prevention and minimization of illness within the context of a higher power. The faith community nurse embraces a holistic approach that recognizes the spiritual domain as an essential component of health. Practitioners of faith community nursing consider the spiritual, physical, psychological, and social aspects of an individual to create a sense of harmony with self, others, the environment, and a higher power (American Nurses Association [ANA] and the Health Ministries Association, 2012).

There is also a growing trend toward the use of "high-tech" medical care. Remarkable advances in technology have fostered the development of new strategies for delivering health services across care settings. The United States is a world leader in its investment in biomedical technology (the application of technology to the solution of medical problems) and owns 85% of the intellectual property associated with biotechnology (SelectUSA, 2013). Telemedicine/home telecare provide one example of an innovative approach that has become increasingly available during the past decade.

DELIVERY SYSTEMS

Telemedicine

Telemedicine, whereby specialists can be remotely based and still assess and counsel patients, is another growing trend in health-care delivery systems. Digital photos can be sent by the Internet from the patient's location to the specialist, at substantial cost savings. For example, in sexual assault crisis centers, a nurse practitioner can capture a colposcopy image and have ready access to a consultant through telecommunications technology. Wireless technology has progressed to the point where remote telemetry is possible. Wireless sensors are capable of detecting changes in blood pressure or respiratory rate and sending alerts. It is possible to monitor medication adherence, and when a pill is missed an alert can be sent to the patient's pharmacist or provider. Webcams can be used to assess patients who have disabilities or live in remote areas. As the aging population increasingly grows, so do chronic health disabilities. Because the majority of health-care providers remain concentrated in metropolitan areas, this type of technology may help bridge the gap in health-care access, especially for those in remote or rural locations.

Telemedicine technology can be used for access to medical interpreters, desperately needed in many areas with multiethnic populations. It can also be used for home surveillance of elderly persons. Eighty percent of elderly persons who need help with their activities of daily living are cared for by family members, most of whom work. It is now possible to turn on a webcam at work to "look in" on a grandparent who is at home alone. In some areas, pediatric remote home monitoring services are offered to reach underserved children who have asthma. School-based telemedicine programs have been found to decrease emergency department visits and diabetes- and asthma-related hospitalizations (Kattlove, 2009). Telepsychiatry, a service that allows for patient psychiatric services, consultation with other clinical professionals, and mobilization of crisis teams, has made a significant impact on the delivery of mental health services, particularly to individuals with limited access (Saeed, Diamond, & Bloch, 2011).

Optimizing Outcomes—Using modern media technology to promote health

Today's new media methods can provide an alternative presentation method and communication link for health promotion and chronic-disease management. Cell phone and text-messaging interventions have been shown to improve medication adherence; appointment attendance; asthma symptoms; and, in diabetic patients, HbA1C levels (Ito & Brown, 2011; Thomas, Stephens, & Blanchard, 2010). In some states, Planned Parenthood offers a text message–based medication reminder (Pill Pixy) to remind patients to take their birth control pills, and in California, SEXINFO is a text-messaging system that provides sexual health information and referrals (Levine, McCright, Dobkin, Woodruff, & Klausner, 2008). Various online programs for disease-specific self-management are beneficial in educating and empowering individuals by providing a combination of health information, online peer support, decision support, and cognitive behavioral therapy (Facchiano & Snyder, 2011). In Minnesota, an online convenient care model (Zipnosis) was recently founded by a nurse practitioner. Staffed by nurse practitioners and physician assistants, Zipnosis is a Web site that provides for treatment of a small set of simple conditions such as upper respiratory conditions, bladder infections, acne, and smoking cessation. Once logged on to the Web site, patients read over their HIPAA notice, pay a small fee, and complete a questionnaire. Within an hour, a Zipnosis clinician sends a response that could result in support and recommendations for over-the-counter medications, a prescription, or a referral to a primary care provider. Since the company's launch in 2009, clinicians with Zipnosis have provided more than 2,300 visits (Ford, 2011).

CHALLENGES FOR NURSES IN CONTEMPORARY SOCIETY

An Ethical Framework for Professional Practice

Nurses study ethics and are taught about the American Nurses Association (ANA) Code of Ethics for Nurses (ANA, 2001). They learn that they must be of good moral character and must act for the benefit of the public. According to the Code, a nurse has the freedom to express an informed personal opinion while upholding professional and moral boundaries (Philipsen & Soeken, 2011). Throughout their careers, nurses are intimately drawn into daily encounters with other humans and as a result often face difficult legal and ethical concerns. The Patient's Bill of Rights, informed consent, confidentiality, pain relief, and end of life care are examples of ethical concerns.

There are four basic principles that are commonly used to help solve ethical dilemmas. Those principles are beneficence, nonmaleficence, respect for autonomy, and justice or fairness. **Beneficence** means acting for the patient's benefit. **Nonmaleficence** is known best by the saying that is credited to Hippocrates, "First, do no harm" or "*Primum non nocere*" in Latin. **Respect for autonomy** means that patients have a right to make decisions about themselves and the right to have the information that is needed to make certain decisions. **Justice** or **fairness** means that all patients should be treated equally. Discrimination should not occur based on social or economic status or type of illness.

The problem is that it is not unusual for those principles to be in conflict. Consider, for example, the Jehovah's Witness mother who refuses to accept blood, even if it means the death of herself or her child. Beneficence and respect for autonomy are clearly in conflict. Jonsen, Siegler, and Winslade (2010) suggest that beyond the four principles, ethics must consider contextual data to be more useful in the complex medical world that nurses work in today. These authors developed a clinical pocket guide to help clinicians analyze case circumstances in context (Table 2-1).

Collaboration in Caring—*Providing a nursing perspective for resolving ethical dilemmas*

Many health-care settings have bioethics committees who confront the more difficult ethical problems, and some individual health systems such as the Veterans Health Administration have established a mandate requiring ethical consultation committees. Nurses are often asked to sit on these types of interdisciplinary committees that usually include clergy, attorneys, social workers, physicians, and ethics consultants (Sego, 2011).

Table 2-1 Ethics Guide for Clinical Practice

Medical Indications	Patient Preferences
THE PRINCIPLES OF BENEFICENCE AND NONMALEFICENCE	THE PRINCIPLE OF RESPECT FOR AUTONOMY
1. What is the patient's medical problem? history? diagnosis? prognosis? 2. Is the problem acute? chronic? critical? emergent? reversible? 3. What are the goals of treatment? 4. What are the probabilities of success? 5. What are the plans in case of therapeutic failure? 6. In sum, how can this patient be benefited by medical and nursing care and how can harm be avoided?	1. Is the patient mentally capable and legally competent? Is there evidence of incapacity? 2. If competent, what is the patient stating about preferences for treatment? 3. Has the patient been informed of benefits and risks, understood this information, and given consent? 4. If incapacitated, who is the appropriate surrogate? Is the surrogate using appropriate standards for decision making? 5. Has the patient expressed prior preferences (e.g., advance directives?) 6. Is the patient unwilling or unable to cooperate with medical treatment? If so, why? 7. In sum, is the patient's right to choose being respected to the extent possible in ethics and law?
Quality of Life	**Contextual Features**
THE PRINCIPLES OF BENEFICENCE AND NONMALEFICENCE AND RESPECT FOR AUTONOMY	THE PRINCIPLES OF LOYALTY AND FAIRNESS
1. What are the prospects, with or without treatment, for a return to normal life? 2. What physical, mental, and social deficits is the patient likely to experience if treatment succeeds? 3. Are there biases that might prejudice the provider's evaluation of the patient's quality of life? 4. Is the patient's present or future condition such that his or her continued life might be judged undesirable? 5. Is there any plan and rationale to forgo treatment? 6. Are there plans for comfort and palliative care?	1. Are there family issues that might influence treatment decisions? 2. Are there provider (physicians and nurses) issues that might influence treatment decisions? 3. Are there financial and economic factors? 4. Are there religious or cultural factors? 5. Are there limits on confidentiality? 6. Are there problems of allocation of resources? 7. How does the law affect treatment decisions? 8. Is clinical research or teaching involved? 9. Is there any conflict of interest on the part of the providers or the institution?

Source: Jonsen, A. R., Siegler, M., & Winslade, W. J. (2010). *Clinical ethics: A practical approach to ethical decisions in clinical medicine* (7th ed.). New York, NY: McGraw-Hill.

IMPLICATIONS OF THE HEALTH INSURANCE PORTABILITY AND ACCOUNTABILITY ACT (HIPAA). The Health Insurance Portability and Accountability Act (HIPAA) is a law that was passed in 1996. It has several components, including procedural mandates (Title II) designed to protect the privacy of an individual's health information. The portability component (Title I) ensures that a person moving from one health plan to another will be able to continue his or her insurance coverage. Expanded federal sanctions attached to health-care fraud are also included in the HIPAA law (U.S. Department of Health and Human Services, 2013). The American Recovery and Reinvestment Act of 2009, which includes the Health Information Technology for Economic and Clinical Health Act (HITECH), also has provisions to address health information technology for economic and clinical health. It is aimed at enhancing health care while promoting electronic health records (EHRs) and electronic transactions (Murray, Calhoun, & Philipsen, 2011).

When passed, HIPAA resulted in a flurry of health-care system–wide modifications. Many office settings were required to reorganize their sign-in procedures. Others had to rebuild patient interviewing spaces, install expensive computer safeguarding mechanisms, supply units with paper shredders, and extend continuous training to employees. With this law, patients clearly have the right to protected health information (PHI). The consequences for breaking a HIPAA law can be both civil and criminal charges. Substantial fines and imprisonment can be imposed if a patient's health information is knowingly disclosed.

Because nurses frequently have ready access to confidential patient data, extreme vigilance is required. Addresses, telephone numbers, occupations, and e-mail addresses need to be protected, along with the patient's medical history, diagnosis, and condition. Nurses must be particularly cautious with conversations that take place in public places such as elevators and lunchrooms. Communication needs to be limited to only those who *need* to know the specific information to provide care for the patient.

THE HUMAN GENOME PROJECT. The Human Genome Project (HGP) was a 13-year project completed by the U.S. Department of Energy and the National Institutes of Health. In 2003, the project produced the first draft of a map that identified the estimated 20,000 to 25,000 genes in human DNA. More than 3 billion sequences of human DNA base pairs were revealed. The base pairs are the chemical building blocks (A, T, C, and G) that are contained in the long, twisted chains that make up the DNA of the 23 pairs of human chromosomes. It is the DNA that provides the gene with detailed instructions about how to manage all the processes within the human body. In May 2006, HGP researchers filled in gaps from the first draft and completed the DNA sequence for the last of the 23 human chromosomes. Dr. Francis Collins, the director of the NIH, predicts that within the next 5 years it will be financially feasible to sequence every person's genome (Darr, 2010). Once that occurs, the era of personalized genomics and individualized risk assessment will be ushered in. Presently, scientists around the globe are moving in that direction with various projects including the haplotype map (HapMap) (a global catalog of common genetic variants) and genome-wide association studies (GWAS) (Seibert, 2010).

Knowledge gained from these projects offers great potential in health care. It also brings to the surface some difficult ethical issues. For example, who will control genetic information? Commercialization has already begun in the areas of genetic testing and exploration of the promise of gene therapy, including more targeted medications. Yet social consequences have not been fully resolved. If sophisticated genetic testing is available, how will privacy be maintained? What will be the psychological impact of having genetic information, especially if it is thought to be predictive of a genetically related illness or condition? Could the information potentially jeopardize insurance coverage for an entire family? Technologies developed for more sophisticated fetal testing will invariably lead to more controversy regarding reproductive rights. The ethical, legal, and social issues associated with the HGP were built in as part of the scientific study, and many have called the project the "world's largest bioethics program."

The American Nurses Association (ANA) (2007) proactively produced a thoughtful position statement supporting the use of stem cell research in preparation for future ethics challenges. In their statement, the ANA recognizes that stem cell research will significantly impact health and the quality of life as research and therapeutic processes use adult, fetal, and embryonic stem cells to "explore the possibilities of growing new organs and tissues to replace those that are damaged or diseased" (p. 4). The ANA supports nursing education in matters related to stem cell research and therapies and encourages nurses as individuals and as a professional community ". . . to maintain awareness of the practice outcomes translated from stem cell research and respond appropriately" (p. 4).

 Nursing Insight—Professional responsibilities and genetics research

The possibility of using cloning techniques to create human embryos and possibly human beings raises profound ethical, social, and health concerns. It is crucial that nurses understand the science of cloning techniques and appreciate the implications of related developments in germ line gene therapy and stem cell research.

 Now Can You—Discuss aspects of an ethical framework for nursing practice?

1. Describe the four basic principles involved in resolving ethical dilemmas?
2. Define HIPAA and give two examples of a breach of this legislation?
3. Discuss implications of the HGP for professional nursing practice?

CURRENT TRENDS IN CLINICAL PRACTICE

Innovative approaches in health-care delivery systems coupled with technological advances in patient management have prompted the emergence of new trends in nursing. Increased complexities in modern-day patient care are evident. Programmable electronic pumps that deliver specific rates of fluid and medications have replaced tedious bedside calculations of IV drips. "Paperless" (computerized) charting has become the norm, replacing the alternating black and red inked pens that separated night shift from the day. Use of the electronic medical record (EMR—a digital version of the paper charts in the clinician's office) and the electronic health record (EHR—an expanded health record that includes the standard clinical data collected in the provider's office but focuses on the total health of the patient) is thought to enhance provider adherence to evidence-based practice guidelines, streamline patient encounter documentation, help generate medication and problem lists, and reduce health-care errors. The clinician uses systems that have interactive alerts integrated into the EHR (Conrad & Schneider, 2011; Murray, Calhoun, & Philipsen, 2011; Peace, 2011; Schram, 2010). Also gone are the large vats of medications that once lined the shelves of medicine rooms. Today, medications are dispensed in individually dosed packages stored in locked robotic machines that require computerized entry.

 Optimizing Outcomes—Health information technology to enhance health-care delivery in the perinatal setting

The Association of Women's Health, Obstetric and Neonatal Nurses (AWHONN) published a Position Statement in 2011 in support of standard data collection across the perinatal setting, regardless of the format of the patient's record (electronic or paper). Recognizing the need for interoperability and archiving in data collection systems, AWHONN advocates for hospital- and institution-wide health information technology (HIT) systems to incorporate specialty-specific data (e.g., neonatal intensive care unit and obstetric outpatient records) into patient records. To accomplish this goal, AWHONN advocates for nursing involvement both in the selection, design, and implementation of the HIT systems and in providing continuous feedback while using the systems at the patient's bedside (AWHONN, 2011b). To work effectively with HIT, nurses must possess basic computer skills, typically defined as the ability to use office software, communicate electronically, and conduct Internet searches (Peace, 2011).

The aging of the population has created a shift in focus from acute to chronic care. Nurses in every specialty area are challenged to manage a rapidly expanding evidence base to guide their clinical practice. The global community, evident in patient populations, has underscored the need for collaboration and the use of "interdisciplinary" models to manage care.

Nurses are involved in cutting-edge approaches to health-care delivery to patients in a variety of settings. Nursing resources and expertise have helped to develop cost-effective, innovative programs. For example, children with asthma can be monitored in their own homes for blood pressure, pulse rate, temperature, blood oxygenation, and breathing rate. The results, quickly relayed to a secure server, are sent to health centers where nurses can assess and manage the patient who remains comfortable in the home environment.

 Nursing Insight—*Differentiating among the terms "telehealth," "telemedicine," and "telenursing"*

Telehealth is the removal of time and distance barriers for the delivery of health-care services or related health-care activities. *Telemedicine* is the use of telecommunication technologies and computers to provide medical and health-care information and services to patients at another site, and *telenursing* is the use of telemedicine technology to deliver nursing care and conduct nursing practice. The terms "telehealth" and "telemedicine" are often used interchangeably and are sometimes encompassed within the term "telenursing" (Hebda & Czar, 2013; Schlachta-Fairchild, 2008; Schlachta-Fairchild, Varghese, Deickman, & Castelli, 2010).

Some professional organizations have promoted the "medical home" concept. Medical homes are reimbursed not only on a fee-for-service basis but they also receive a monthly fee for the oversight function. With this model, one provider oversees and coordinates each individual's care, attending to preventive measures and screening as well as episodic and chronic illness. The Medicaid Pregnancy Medical Home initiative, for example, is designed to bring clinical improvement to pregnant women and their newborn children (Buppert, 2011; Gray, 2011; Schram, 2010).

The concept of the group health-care visit provides another example of an innovative care delivery model. Developed in response to patients' and practitioners' dissatisfaction with the traditional model of health care, the group health-care model seeks to maximize the outpatient health-care experience through provision of care to multiple patients simultaneously during one extended appointment. With this care delivery design, the group setting enables patients and practitioners to spend increased time together to cultivate trusting and productive relationships while benefiting from the power of peer support. Group care may be used with a variety of patient populations, for example, to deliver maternal–child services (e.g., prenatal care and well-baby visits) and to address needs for persons with chronic conditions (e.g., diabetes, polycystic ovary syndrome, and osteoporosis) (Moore & Caldwell, 2011; Sikon & Bronson, 2010; Thacker, Maxwell, Saporito, & Bronson, 2010).

In the area of maternal health care, a perinatal nursing service may be prescribed for women at risk for preterm labor. The service provides daily contact with a perinatal nurse and the use of an electronic device for conducting home monitoring to detect uterine contractions. Telecare is also used to monitor wound healing in medical-surgical patients. An inexpensive digital camera attached to a computer allows specialists to view the various stages of wound healing, make clinical assessments, and provide patient consultation.

The Patient Provider Telehealth Network (PPTN) in North Carolina offers an example of a patient/primary care provider model that has proven to be cost efficient and improve access to care. Providers determine the need for, nature of, and frequency of health education and monitoring and set patient-specific critical indicators and parameters. Telehealth registered nurses customize the technology software and visit the patient's home to install the telehealth equipment, educate the patient about its use, and validate the patient's competency with its use. Patients perform daily self-monitoring as ordered (e.g., blood pressure, pulse, body weight, blood sugar level, and oxygen saturation) and transmit the data to a secure server accessed by the registered nurses, who assess, educate, and contact the patient and/or physician as needed. Every 2 weeks, the data are compiled and transferred into the patient's EMR (Schwartz & Britton, 2011).

The use of telemedicine has great potential for reducing the need for hospital admissions and frequent office visits. Some nurses resist home telecare, fearful that "high-touch" care is being replaced by "high-tech" care. However, home telecare, when creatively and appropriately used, can serve to administer personalized patient care and communication, result in better outcomes, and increase patient satisfaction. The increased application of technology ensures that nurses' caring presence in the virtual world will continue to expand. Despite the movement into "high technology," nurses must remain cognizant of the need to provide "human-centered," holistic care. Holism is a philosophy of care that is built on a framework that values the human relationship and focuses on meeting the physical, emotional, spiritual, and social needs of the person.

To practice holistic nursing is to blend technology with healing while providing care that encompasses the interrelated relationships between the patient, the patient's family and other support persons, the provider(s), and the community.

NANDA-I Nursing Diagnoses for Holistic Nursing

NANDA-I Classification of Nursing Diagnoses, Nursing Interventions Classification (NIC), and Nursing Outcomes Classification (NOC) were described in Chapter 1 as classification systems used to name nursing interventions. Examples of how holistic nursing and complementary therapies fit nicely into nursing taxonomies for documenting care are presented in Table 2-2.

 Nursing Insight—*A holistic approach to care*

The practice of holistic nursing encompasses approaches and interventions that address the needs of the whole person: mind, body, and spirit. Florence Nightingale recognized the value of caring for the whole person and encouraged the use of touch, light, aromatics, empathetic listening, music, quiet reflection, and other methods to empower the individual's ability to draw on inner strengths to promote healing (American Holistic Nurses Association, 2013).

Table 2-2 Selected Nursing Diagnoses and Nursing Interventions: Possible Pairings of Nursing Concerns and Complementary/Alternative Interventions

Impaired Comfort	Acupressure, therapeutic touch	To decrease perceived pain
Disturbed Sleep Pattern	Massage	To promote relaxation, rest
Social Isolation	Pet therapy	To provide affection
Impaired Coping	Humor	To facilitate appreciation of that which is funny, to relieve tensions
Hopelessness	Hope instillation	To promote a positive sense of the future
Spiritual Distress	Spiritual support	To facilitate a sense of inner peace
Spiritual Well-Being	Spiritual growth facilitation	To support growth/reflection/reexamination of values
Anxiety or Fear	Guided imagery, relaxation therapy, biofeedback, calming techniques	To reduce sense of anxiety
Impaired Communication	Art therapy	To facilitate expression

Source: Frisch, N. (May 31, 2001). Nursing as a context for alternative/complementary modalities. *Online Journal of Issues in Nursing, 6*(2), Manuscript 2. Available online: http://www.nursingworld.org/MainMenuCategories/ANAMarketplace/ANAPeriodicals/OJIN/TableofContents/Volume62001/No2May01/AlternativeComplementaryModalities.html

 Now Can You—Discuss current trends in clinical nursing practice?

1. Provide two examples of ways that home telecare can improve patient outcomes?
2. Explain how nurses can provide sensitive, personalized care that enhances the "high-tech" methods used?
3. Describe what is meant by holistic care?

CONTEMPORARY ISSUES AND NURSING ROLES

The scope and complexity of current health problems continue to present formidable challenges for nurses. There is no room for complacency in nursing's future. Nurses will inevitably need to struggle to keep up with the exponential growth of information, evidence-based knowledge, and technological advances. Nurses are likely to deal with ethics questions that have never been faced before. The growth and diversity of the population will require more cultural sensitivity than ever before. The continual threat of chronic diseases demands creative, holistic approaches. Infectious disease threats will continue to challenge health-care resources at the national and international levels. Terrible natural and man-made disasters will tax the nation's systems to their fullest extent. All citizens will feel the effects of HIV/AIDS as the disease trends toward women and children.

Nurses must extend their caring work beyond individual patients and families to communities, sociopolitical systems, and national and global health arenas if they are to have a significant impact on health promotion. Major disparities in health outcomes between families and children from racial and ethnic backgrounds and those of European American backgrounds must be confronted. Nurses have serious work to do to empower the many Americans who are without adequate health-care coverage and access to services.

Broad-based efforts are needed to work through societal, economic, and cultural issues. Nursing's passion for evidence-based solutions must continue and remain focused on conditions that determine the health of individuals and populations. The *Healthy People 2020* national initiative is a step in the right direction. States, communities, and national organizations have rallied behind the priorities, goals, and objectives set in the *Healthy People* initiative and have used it to guide their own health planning efforts.

A caring, holistic nurse is one who endeavors to develop and apply critical thinking skills to bring about changes, not only to bedside nursing of the individual, but to social justice issues that are determinants of health. Nurses have continually been ranked as the top professionals in the public trust in Gallup's annual Honesty and Ethics Poll since they were added to the list in 1999. The only exception occurred in the year after the World Trade Center attacks, when firefighters were ranked number one. As a profession, nursing's challenge is to step up and claim that popular power with the public and use it to be a dynamic force in transforming family and community health systems.

Summary Points

- There is much work to be done, and health-care challenges can best be faced by using multitiered, holistic approaches such as those articulated in the Intervention Wheel model.

- *Healthy People 2020*'s visionary blueprint prioritizes national goals for health so that health promotion efforts can be focused and aligned.

- A priority goal of *Healthy People 2020* centers on resolving health inequities in the United States.

- An overview of societal trends reveals where present and future health problems are arising and where efforts should be concentrated.

◆ Technological trends such as the Internet, telemedicine, and genetics research highly influence health issues.

◆ Cultural trends must be used to guide the designing of effective, culturally acceptable health interventions and programs.

◆ Nurses need to be vigilant and confront the negative effects of racism and prejudice in all health-care settings.

◆ Nurses need to be familiar with health policy and programs of assistance so that patients can be referred to needed resources whenever possible.

◆ There are numerous vulnerable populations in the United States and the "common good" ethic needs to be rediscovered.

◆ The nurse of the future will face unprecedented ethical challenges that can be analyzed using a systematic framework like the one described by Jonsen and colleagues.

Review Questions

Multiple Choice

1. A clinic nurse is providing information to a parent whose 5-year-old child has been diagnosed with rubella. The nurse counsels the parent on rest, acetaminophen (Tylenol), and increased fluids. What type of intervention is this?
   A. Primary prevention
   B. Secondary prevention
   C. Tertiary prevention
   D. Mandatory health care

2. The clinic nurse is aware that which of the following is a specific health concern for African American women between 45 and 65 years of age?
   A. Stroke
   B. Breast cancer
   C. Hypertension
   D. Motor vehicle collisions

3. The clinic nurse works with many ethical principles, including nonmaleficence. What does this ethical principle mean?
   A. First do no harm
   B. Acting on the patient's behalf
   C. Patients have a right to information
   D. Patients should be treated equally

4. Which of the following is a primary goal of the *Healthy People* initiative?
   A. Helping people attain longer lives free of disease or disability
   B. Improving the insurance industry's responsiveness
   C. Increasing the average American's life span
   D. Promoting evidence-based acute care for episodic illnesses

5. The community-based nurse works with all populations and age groups. What concept is important regarding diverse populations?
   A. Different races have no true biological basis and are social creations.
   B. Disparities in health care are rapidly disappearing in America.
   C. Many social networks exist to support minority health-care needs.
   D. Providing culturally competent care is not a regulatory requirement.

6. What current trend has a major negative impact on the health of individuals and families living in rural areas?
   A. An increase in telemedicine
   B. Impact of Affordable Care Act
   C. Loss of rural hospitals
   D. Increased use of home health care

7. A nurse working with an impoverished, inner city population is concerned with the community's low health literacy level and lack of empowerment in their own health. Which action by the nurse would best address this problem?
   A. Encourage adults to ask questions of their health-care providers.
   B. Have events at the local library where computer skills are taught.
   C. Promote the distribution of health pamphlets at grocery stores.
   D. Teach healthy lifestyle habits to increase control over one's health.

8. A nurse is teaching a patient who has low health literacy to manage a chronic health condition. Which action by the nurse is best?
   A. Ask the patient to restate the information in his or her own words.
   B. Assess learning by asking a series of simple, yes or no questions.
   C. Determine if the patient is able to synthesize the information.
   D. Give pamphlets that have detailed information in large type.

9. A nurse believes that all patients should be treated equally. What ethical principle does this relate to?
   A. Autonomy
   B. Beneficence
   C. Justice
   D. Nonmaleficence

10. A nurse working with incarcerated women knows that what information about this population is true?
   A. Incarcerated women rarely are pregnant.
   B. Mental health issues are not common in imprisoned women.
   C. The majority of women in prison are mothers.
   D. Women are a declining part of the prison population.

See Answers to End of Chapter Review Questions on Davis*Plus*.

REFERENCES

Aday, L. A. (2001). *At risk in America: The health and health care needs of vulnerable populations in the United States* (2nd ed.). San Francisco, CA: John Wiley & Sons, Inc.

Alpert, E. J. (2010). *Intimate partner violence: The clinician's guide to identification, assessment, intervention, and prevention.* (5th ed.). Waltham, MA: Massachusetts Medical Society.

American Academy of Child & Adolescent Psychiatry. (2011). Bullying. Publication #80; March 2011. Retrieved from http://www.aacap.org/cs/root/facts_for_families/bullying

American Academy of Pediatrics. (2005). Lead exposure in children: Prevention, detection, and management. *Pediatrics, 116*(4), 1036–1046. doi:10.1542/peds.2005-1947

American College of Obstetricians and Gynecologists (ACOG). (2009). Committee Opinion Number 429: Health disparities for rural women. *Obstetrics & Gynecology, 113*(3), 762–765.

American College of Obstetricians and Gynecologists (ACOG). (2011a). Committee Opinion Number 491: Health literacy. *American Journal of Obstetrics & Gynecology, 117*(5), 1250–1252.

American College of Obstetricians and Gynecologists (ACOG). (2011b). Committee Opinion Number 490: Partnering with patients to improve safety. *American Journal of Obstetrics & Gynecology, 117*(5), 1247–1249.

American College of Obstetricians and Gynecologists (ACOG). (2011c). Committee Opinion Number 507: Human trafficking. *American Journal of Obstetrics & Gynecology, 118*(3), 767–770.

American College of Obstetricians and Gynecologists (ACOG). (2011d). Committee Opinion Number 512: Health care for transgender individuals. *American Journal of Obstetrics & Gynecology, 118*(6), 1454–1458.

American College of Obstetricians and Gynecologists (ACOG). (2011e). Committee Opinion Number 511: Health care for pregnant and postpartum incarcerated women and adolescent females. *American Journal of Obstetrics & Gynecology, 118*(5), 1198–1202.

American College of Obstetricians and Gynecologists (ACOG). (2012). Committee Opinion Number 516: Health care systems for underserved women. *American Journal of Obstetrics & Gynecology, 119*(1), 206–209.

American Heart Association (AHA). (2013). *Heart disease & stroke statistics: 2013 update.* Retrieved from http://www.heart.org/HEARTORG/General/Heart-and-Stroke-Association-Statistics_UCM_319064_SubHomePage.jsp

American Holistic Nurses Association (AHNA). (2013). *American Holistic Nurses Association: About us.* Retrieved from http://www.ahna.org/About-Us/Mission-Statement

American Nurses Association. (2001). *Code of ethics for nurses.* Retrieved from http://www.nursingworld.org/MainMenuCategories/EthicsStandards/CodeofEthicsforNurses/Code-of-Ethics.pdf

American Nurses Association (ANA). (2007). *Position Statement on Stem Cell Research.* Retrieved from http://www.nursingworld.org/MainMenu-Categories/Policy-Advocacy/Positions-and-Resolutions/ANAPosition-Statements/Position-Statements-Alphabetically/StemCellResearch.txt

American Nurses Association (ANA) and the Health Ministries Association. (2012). *Faith Community Nursing: Scope and Standards of Practice* (2nd ed.). Silver Spring, MD: ANA.

Anderson, C. A., & Dill, K. E. (2000). Video games and aggressive thoughts, feelings, and behavior in the laboratory and in life. *Journal of Personality and Social Psychology, 78*(4), 772–790.

Ardoin, K. B., & Wilson, K. B. (2010). Cultural diversity: What role does it play in patient safety? *Nursing for Women's Health, 14*(4), 322–326.

Association of Women's Health, Obstetric and Neonatal Nurses (AWHONN). (2011a). Position Statement: Shackling incarcerated pregnant women. *Journal of Obstetric, Gynecologic & Neonatal Nursing, 40*(12), 549–550. doi:10.1111/j.1552-6909.2011.01300.x

Association of Women's Health, Obstetric and Neonatal Nurses (AWHONN). (2011b). Position Statement: Health information technology for the perinatal setting. *Journal of Obstetric, Gynecologic & Neonatal Nursing, 40*(3), 383–385.

Balestra, M. (2011). Nurse practitioners & social media: Unprofessional behavior can impact your license. *The Journal for Nurse Practitioners, 7*(9), 715.

Barber, E. L., Lundsberg, L. S., Belanger, K., Pettker, C. M., Funai, E. F., & Illuzzi, J. L. (2011). Indications contributing to the increasing cesarean delivery rate. *Obstetrics & Gynecology, 118*(1), 29–36.

Black, M. C., Basile, K. C., Breiding, M. J., Smith, S. G., Walters, M. L., Merrick, M. T., . . . Stevens, M. R. (2011). *The National Intimate Partner and Sexual Violence Survey (NISVS): 2010 Summary Report.* Atlanta, GA: National Center for Injury Prevention and Control, Centers for Disease Control and Prevention.

Boxer, P., Huesman, L. R., Bushman, B. J., O'Brien, M., & Moceri, D. (2009). The role of violent media preference in cumulative developmental risk for violence and general aggression. *Journal of Youth and Adolescence, 38*(3), 417–428.

Buchwald, E., Fletcher, P., & Roth, M. (Eds.). (2005). *Transforming a rape culture* (2nd ed.). Minneapolis, MN: Milkweed Editions.

Buppert, C. (2011). Where do nurse practitioners stand with health care? *The Journal for Nurse Practitioners, 7*(8), 687–688.

Callister, L. C., & Edwards, J. E. (2010). Achieving Millennium Development Goal 5, the improvement of maternal health. *Journal of Obstetric, Gynecologic & Neonatal Nursing, 39*(5), 590–599. doi:10.1111/j.1552-6909.2010.01161.x

Campbell, C. (2011). Elective cesarean delivery: Trends, evidence and implications for women, newborns and nurses. *Nursing for Women's Health, 15*(4), 310–319.

Campbell, D., & Moran, B. (2010). Sustaining the vision for Millennium Development Goal 6, to halt and reverse the spread of HIV/AIDS and other infections. *Journal of Obstetric, Gynecologic & Neonatal Nursing, 39*(5), 600–605.

Capstrat Public Policy Polling. (2011). *Millennials do not favor social media for personal healthcare communication.* Retrieved from https://www.capstrat.com/posts/millennials-do-not-favor-social-media-personal-healthcare-communication/

Centers for Disease Control and Prevention (CDC). (2010). Attention-Deficit Hyperactivity Disorder (AD/HD). Retrieved from http://www.cdc.gov/ncbddd/adhd/data.html

Centers for Disease Control and Prevention (CDC). (2011a). Youth risk behavior surveillance-United States, 2011. *MMWR 2012; 61*(SS-4).

Centers for Disease Control and Prevention (CDC). (2011b). Physical activity for everyone. Retrieved from http://www.cdc.gov/physicalactivity/everyone/guidelines/children.html

Centers for Disease Control and Prevention (CDC). (2011d). Behavioral Risk Factor Surveillance System Survey Data. Atlanta, Georgia: U.S. Department of Health and Human Services, Centers for Disease Control and Prevention, 2011.

Centers for Disease Control and Prevention (CDC). (2011e). National vital statistics reports, Vol. 58, No. 17. Retrieved from http://www.cdc.gov/nchs/data/nvsr/nvsr58/nvsr58_17.pdf

Centers for Disease Control and Prevention (CDC). (2012). Planet health for obesity reduction in school children—readily accepted and cost-effective. Retrieved from http://www.cdc.gov/prc/prevention-strategies/planet-health-obesity-reduction-school-children.htm

Centers for Disease Control and Prevention (CDC). (2013). Sudden unexpected infant death and sudden infant death syndrome. Retrieved from http://www.cdc.gov/sids/

Child Welfare Information Gateway. (2011). *Child abuse and neglect fatalities 2009: Statistics and interventions.* Washington, DC: U.S. Department of Health and Human Services, Children's Bureau.

Clarke, J., & Adashi, E. (2011). Perinatal care for incarcerated patients: A 25-year-old woman pregnant in jail. *Journal of the American Medical Association, 305*(9), 923–929.

Clingerman, E., & Fowles, E. (2010). Foundations for social justice-based actions in maternal/infant nursing. *Journal of Obstetric, Gynecologic & Neonatal Nursing, 39*(3), 320–327.

Coalition for the Homeless. (2013). *Basic facts about homelessness.* Retrieved from http://www.coalitionforthehomeless.org/pages/basic-facts

Coleman-Jensen, A., Nord, M., Andrews, M., & Carlson, S. (2011). Household food insecurity in the United States in 2010. Economic Research Report-125, U.S. Dept. of Agriculture, Economic Resource Service, September 2011, 1–37.

Conrad, D., & Schneider, J. S. (2011). Enhancing the visibility of NP practice in electronic health records. *The Journal for Nurse Practitioners, 7*(12), 832–838.

Darr, A. S. (2010). Vision of a personal genomics future. *Nature, 643*(21), 298–299.

Davis, B., & Carpenter, C. (2009). Proximity of fast-food restaurants to schools and adolescent obesity. *American Journal of Public Health, 99*(3), 505–510.

Dembek, C. R., Harris, J. L., & Schwartz, M. B. (2013). Rudd Report: Where children and adolescents view food and beverage ads on TV: Exposure by channel and program. Retrieved from http://www.yaleruddcenter.org/resources/upload/docs/what/reports/Rudd_Report_TV_Ad_Exposure_Channel_Program_2013.pdf

Dickinson, A. R. (2006, May). 'We are just kids': Children within healthcare relationships. *Contemporary Nurse, 21*(2), 24–28.

Edwards, J. E. (2011). Why global health matters. *Nursing for Women's Health, 15*(5), 419–421.

Ehrenthal, D. B., Jiang, X., & Strobino, D. M. (2010). Labor induction and the risk of a cesarean delivery among nulliparous women at term. *Obstetrics & Gynecology, 116*(1), 35–42.

Facchiano, L., & Snyder, C. H. (2011). Challenges surrounding provider/client electronic-mail communication. *The Journal for Nurse Practitioners, 7*(4), 309–315.

Ford, J. (2011). Online healthcare: A new wave in convenience. *Advance for NPs & PAs, 2*(4), 17.

Fox, S. (2011). Health, digital divide. Pew Internet & American Life Project. Retrieved from http://www.pewinternet.org/Reports/2011/Health-Topics/Summary-of-Findings/Symptoms-and-treatments.aspx

Gilliam, M. L. (2009). The Millennium Development Goals and providers of women's health care. *Obstetrics & Gynecology, 114*(2), 209–210.

Ginsburg, F. D. (1998). *Contested lives: The abortion debate in an American community.* Berkeley, CA: University of California Press.

Gray, C. L. (2011). The Pregnancy Medical Home: Use of the power of the Medicaid program to improve standard of care across North Carolina. *North Carolina Medical Journal, 72*(3), 232–234.

Harner, H., & Burgess, A. W. (2011). Using a trauma-informed framework to care for incarcerated women. *Journal of Obstetric, Gynecologic & Neonatal Nursing, 40*(4), 469–476.

Harrington, C. C. (2012). The power of culture and language in patient care. *Advance for NPs & PAs, 3*(1), 17–18.

Hawley, L., Fouche, N., Cates Jr., W., & Bentley, M. E. (2010). Understanding the relevance of global health to North Carolina. *North Carolina Medical Journal, 71*(5), 429–433.

Hebda, T., & Czar, P. (2013). *Handbook of informatics for nurses and health care professionals.* (5th ed.). Upper Saddle River, NJ: Prentice Hall.

Hellwig, J. P. (2010). Reducing health disparities. *Nursing for Women's Health, 14*(6), 512–514.

Himmelstein, D. U., Thorne, D., Warren, E., & Woolhandler, S. (2009). Medical bankruptcy in the United States, 2007: Results of a national study. *The American Journal of Medicine, 122*(9), 741–746.

Hodge, D. R., & Lietz, C. A. (2007). The international sexual trafficking of women and children: A review of the literature. *Journal of Women & Social Work, 22*(2), 163–174.

Ibe, C., & Johnson-Agabakwu, C. (2011). Female genital cutting: Addressing the issues of culture and ethics. *The Female Patient, 36*(8), 28–31.

Institute of Medicine (U.S.). (2004). Health literacy: A prescription to end confusion. Washington, DC: National Academies Press.

Isaacs, S. L., & Colby, D. C. (Eds.). (2012). *To improve health and health care: Volume XV.* Hoboken, NJ: Jossey-Bass.

Ito, K. E., & Brown, J. D. (2010). To friend or not to friend: Using new media for adolescent health promotion. *North Carolina Medical Journal, 71*(4), 367–372.

Jonsen, A. R., Siegler, M., & Winslade, W. J. (2010). *Clinical ethics: A practical approach to ethical decisions in clinical medicine* (7th ed.). New York, NY: McGraw-Hill.

Jordan, E. T., Ray, E. M., Johnson, P., & Evans, W. D. (2011). Text4Baby: Using text messaging to improve maternal and newborn health. *Nursing for Women's Health, 15*(3), 208–212.

Kang, J. A., Gottlieb, A. S., Raker, C. A., Aneja, S. S., & Boardman, L. A. (2010). Interpersonal violence screening for ambulatory gynecology patients. *Obstetrics & Gynecology, 115*(6), 1159–1166.

Kattlove, J. (2009). *School-Based Telehealth: An Innovative Approach to Meet the Health Care Needs of California's Children.* Santa Monica, CA: The Children's Partnership.

Keller, L. O., Strohschein, S., Schaffer, M. A., & Lia-Hoagberg, B. (2004a). Population-based public health interventions: Innovations in practice, teaching, and management, part II. *Public Health Nursing, 21*(5), 469–487.

Keller, L. O., Strohschein, S., Schaffer, M. A., & Lia-Hoagberg, B. (2004b). Population-based public health interventions: Practice-based and evidence supported, part I. *Public Health Nursing, 21*(5), 453–468.

KidsHealth.org (2013). How TV affects your child. Retrieved from http://kidshealth.org/parent/positive/family/tv_affects_child.html

Kirby, S. G. (2011). Practicing medicine in the Facebook age: Maintaining professionalism online. *The Forum – NC Medical Board, 15*(Summer), 6–8.

Koh, H. K. (2010). A 2020 vision for Healthy People. *New England Journal of Medicine, 362*(18), 1653–1656.

Kohlenberg, E. (2011). Contribution of nursing education programs to the implementation of the Affordable Care Act in North Carolina. *North Carolina Medical Journal, 72*(4), 289–292.

Kunkel, D. (2007). The effects of media violence on children. Testimony before the U.S. Senate Committee on Commerce, Science, and Transportation. Washington, DC. (Remarks begin at 41:10).

LaMontagne, C. (2013). *NerdWallet health finds medical bankruptcy accounts for majority of personal bankruptcies.* Retrieved from http://www.nerdwallet.com/blog/health/2013/06/19/nerdwallet-health-study-estimates-56-million-americans-65-struggle-medical-bills-2013/

Lee, B. H. (2011). Get your patient an interpreter. *The Clinical Advisor, 14*(3), 142.

Levi, A., & Quang Dau, K. (2011). Meeting the national health goal to reduce unintended pregnancy. *Journal of Obstetric, Gynecologic & Neonatal Nursing, 40*(6), 775–781.

Levine, D., McCright, J., Dobkin, L., Woodruff, A. J., & Klausner, J. D. (2008). SEXINFO: A sexual health text messaging service for San Francisco youth. *American Journal of Public Health, 98*(3), 393–395.

Livingston, G., & Cohn, D. (2010). The new demography of American motherhood. *Pew Research Center Publications.* Retrieved from http://www.pewsocialtrends.org/2010/05/06/the-new-demography-of-american-motherhood/

Lockwood, C. J. (2011). The changing face of maternal mortality. *Contemporary OB/GYN, 56*(3), 8–11.

Logsdon, M. C., & Davis, D. W. (2010). Social justice as a wider lens of support for childbearing women. *Journal of Obstetric, Gynecologic & Neonatal Nursing, 39*(3), 339–348.

Madden, M., & Zickuhr, K. (2011). *Report: Social networking.* PEW Internet & American Life Project. Washington, DC.

Mantle, F. (2005). Complementary medicine and children. *Primary Health Care, 15*(8), 23–25.

Marks, K. P., Glascoe, F. P., & Macias, M. M. (2011). Enhancing the algorithm for developmental-behavioral surveillance and screening in children 0 to 5 years. *Clinical Pediatrics, 7*(9), 853–868.

Martin, J. A., Hamilton, B. E., Ventura, S. J., Osterman, M. J., & Mathews, T. J. (2013). National Vital Statistics Reports: *Births: Final data for 2011.* Retrieved from http://www.cdc.gov/nchs/data/nvsr/nvsr62/nvsr62_01.pdf

Mattson, S. (2010). Millennium Development Goals and global women's and infants' health. *Journal of Obstetric, Gynecologic & Neonatal Nursing, 39*(5), 573–579.

McClain, N. M., & Garrity, S. E. (2011). Sex trafficking and the exploitation of adolescents. *Journal of Obstetric, Gynecologic & Neonatal Nursing, 40*(2), 243–252.

McKee, K. T., Jr., & Cohen, O. (2010). Advancing the global public health agenda with commercial clinicl research infrastructure. *North Carolina Medical Journal, 71*(5), 474–476.

McLeod-Sordjan, R. (2011). Assessing functional health literacy among Hispanic elders with chronic disease. *The Journal for Nurse Practitioners, 7*(10), 839–846.

Moore, A., & Caldwell, J. (2011). The importance of collaboration in treating chronic disease: A focus on PCOS and group medical visits. *Women's Health Care: A Practical Journal for Nurse Practitioners, 10*(9), 10–18.

Moore, V. (2012). Assessing health literacy. *The Journal for Nurse Practitioners, 8*(3), 243–244.

Muennig, P. A., & Glied, S. A. (2010). What changes in survival rates tell us about U.S. health care. *Health Affairs, 29*(11), 11–16. doi:10.1377/hlthaff.2010.0073

Murray, T. L., Calhoun, M., & Philipsen, N. C. (2011). Privacy, confidentiality, HIPAA, and HITECH: Implications for the health care practitioner. *The Journal for Nurse Practitioners, 7*(9), 747–752.

National Conference of State Legislatures (2013). *Disparities in health.* Retrieved from http://www.ncsl.org/issues-research/health/health-disparities-overview.aspx

National Institute of Neurological Disorders and Stroke. (2013). Autism Fact Sheet. Retrieved from http://www.ninds.nih.gov/disorders/autism/detail_autism.htm

National Poverty Center. (2013). *Poverty in the United States.* Retrieved from http://www.npc.umich.edu/poverty/

National Women's Law Center. (2014). *NWLC analysis of 2013 census poverty data.* Retrieved from http://www.nwlc.org/nwlc-analysis-2013-census-poverty-data

New York City Department of Homeless Services. (2013). *Daily DHS shelter census.* Retrieved from http://www.nyc.gov/html/dhs/html/home/home.shtml

Office on Women's Health, U.S. Department of Health and Human Services. (2013). *Government in Action.* Retrieved from http://www.womenshealth.gov/about-us/government-in-action/index.html

Ogden, C. L., & Carroll, M. D. (2010). Prevalence of overweight, obesity, and extreme obesity among adults: United States, Trends 1961–1962 Through 2007–2008. Retrieved from http://www.cdc.gov/NCHS/data/hestat/obesity_adult_07_08/obesity_adult_07_08.pdf

Peace, J. (2011). Nurses and health information technology: Working with and around computers. *North Carolina Medical Journal, 72*(4), 317–320.

Pew Internet & American Life Project. (2010). *Cell phones and American adults.* Retrieved from http://www.pewinternet.org/files/old-media//Files/Reports/2010/PIP_Mobile_Access_2010.pdf

Philipsen, N. C., & Soeken, D. (2011). Preparing to blow the whistle: A survival guide for nurses. *The Journal for Nurse Practitioners, 7*(9), 740–746.

Purnell, L. D. (2012). *Transcultural health care: A culturally competent approach* (4th ed.). Philadelphia, PA: F.A. Davis.

Ricketts, T. C., III. (2011). New models of health care payment and delivery. *North Carolina Medical Journal, 72*(3), 197–200.

Ruhl, C. (2012). Contraception is health promotion. *Nursing for Women's Health, 16*(1), 73–77. doi:10.1111/j.1751-486X.2012.01703.x

Saeed, S. A., Diamond, J., & Bloch, R. M. (2011). Use of telepsychiatry to improve care for people with mental illness in rural North Carolina. (2011). *North Carolina Medical Journal, 72*(3), 219–222.

Sanday, P. R. (2007). *Fraternity gang rape: Sex, brotherhood, and privilege on campus.* (2nd ed.). New York, NY: NYU Press.

Sandy, H. P. (2011). Female genital cutting: An overview. *The American Journal for Nurse Practitioners, 15*(1/2), 53–60.

Sarteschi, C. M., & Vaughn, M. G. (2010). Double jeopardy: A review of women offenders; mental health and substance abuse characteristics. *Victims and Offenders, 5*(2), 161–182.

Schlachta-Fairchild, L. (2008). *International competencies for telenursing.* Geneva, Switzerland: International Council of Nurses.

Schlachta-Fairchild, L., Varghese, S. B., Deickman, A., & Castelli, D. (2010). Telehealth and telenursing are live: APN policy and practice implications. *The Journal for Nurse Practitioners, 6*(2), 98–106.

Schram, A. P. (2010). Medical home and the nurse practitioner: A policy analysis. *The Journal for Nurse Practitioners, 6*(2), 132–139.

Schwartz, K. A., & Britton, B. (2011). Use of telehealth to improve chronic disease management. *North Carolina Medical Journal, 72*(3), 216–218.

Sego, S. (2011). Navigating ethics in a health-care setting. *The Clinical Advisor, 15*(6), 72–77.

Seibert, D. C. (2010). Genetics and disease prevention: Complementary or contradictory? *The Journal for Nurse Practitioners, 6*(7), 507–518.

SelectUSA. (2013). *The health and medical technology industry in the United States.* Retrieved from http://selectusa.commerce.gov/industry-snapshots/health-and-medical-technology-industry-united-states

Seligson, R. W. (2010). Putting patients at the forefront of good health care reform. *North Carolina Medical Journal, 71*(5), 424–427.

Shore, S., & Griggs, G. K. (2010). Health care reform: A perspective from primary care. *North Carolina Medical Journal, 71*(5), 421–423.

Sikon, A., & Bronson, D. L. (2010). Shared medical appointments: Challenges and opportunities. *Annals of Internal Medicine, 152*(11), 745–646. doi:10.7326/000e-4819-152-11-201006010-00012

Slywotzky, A., & Main, T. (2011). The quiet health-care revolution. *The Atlantic, 308*(4), 92–98.

Speidel, J. J., & Grossman, R. A. (2011). Addressing global health, economic, and environmental problems through family planning. *Obstetrics & Gynecology, 117*(6), 1394–1398.

Thacker, H. L., Maxwell, R., Saporito, J., & Bronson, D. (2010). Shared medical appointments: Facilitating interdisciplinary care for midlife women. *Journal of Women's Health, 14*(9), 867–870.

The Commonwealth Fund. (2011). Women without health insurance. Retrieved from http://www.commonwealthfund.org/Search.aspx?search=women+without+health+insurance&filefilter=1

The National Center for Victims of Crime. (2011). Child Sexual Abuse. Retrieved from http://www.victimsofcrime.org/media/reporting-on-child-sexual-abuse/child-sexual-abuse-statistics

Thomas, T. L., Stephens, D. P., & Blanchard, B. (2010). Hip hop, health, and Human Papilloma Virus (HPV): Using wireless technology to increase HPV vaccination uptake. *The Journal for Nurse Practitioners, 6*(6), 464–470.

Tyer-Viola, L. A., & Cesario, S. K. (2010). Addressing poverty, education, and gender equality to improve the health of women worldwide. *Journal of Obstetric, Gynecologic & Neonatal Nursing, 39*(5), 580–589.

University of New Hampshire. (2011, September 23). One million more U.S. children living in poverty since 2009, new census data shows. Retrieved from http://www.sciencedaily.com/releases/2011/09/110922152631.htm

U.S. Census Bureau. (2011a). 2010 Census demographic profiles. Retrieved from http://www.census.gov/2010census/data/

U.S. Census Bureau. (2011b). Highlights: 2010. Retrieved from http://www.census.gov/hhes/www/hlthins/data/incpovhlth/2010/highlights.html

U.S. Census Bureau. (2011c). Income, poverty and health insurance coverage in the United States: 2010. Retrieved from http://www.census.gov/prod/2011pubs/p60-239.pdf

U.S. Census Bureau. (2011d). Household Internet usage in and outside of the home by selected characteristics: 2010. Retrieved from https://www.census.gov/compendia/statab/2012/tables/12s1155.pdf

U.S. Department of Agriculture (USDA). (2013). Dietary guidelines for Americans, 2015. Retrieved from http://www.health.gov/dietaryguidelines/2015.asp

U.S. Department of Health and Human Services. Centers for Medicare & Medicaid Services. (2013). *HIPAA–General Information Overview.* Retrieved from http://www.hhs.gov/ocr/privacy/

U.S. Department of Health and Human Services, Health Resources and Services Administration, Maternal and Child Health Bureau. (2012). *Child Health USA 2011.* Rockville, MD: U.S. Department of Health and Human Services.

U.S. Department of Health and Human Services. Office of Minority Health. (2013). *Infant mortality and American Indians/Alaska Natives.* Retrieved from http://minorityhealth.hhs.gov/templates/content.aspx?ID=3038

U.S. Department of Health and Human Services. (2014). *Healthy People 2020: Improving the health of Americans.* Retrieved from http://www.healthypeople.gov/2020/topicsobjectives2020/default.aspx

U.S. Department of Justice. National Criminal Justice Reference Service. (2011). Women & girls in the criminal justice system–facts and figures. Retrieved from https://www.ncjrs.gov/spotlight/wgcjs/facts.html

U.S. Department of State. (2011). *Trafficking in Persons Report 2011.* Retrieved from http://www.state.gov/g/tip/rls/tiprpt/2011/

U.S. Preventive Services Task Force (USPSTF). (2010). Screening for obesity in children and adolescents. Retrieved from http://www.uspreventiveservicestaskforce.org/uspstf/uspschobes.htm

Walker, C. (2011). Online social networking: Think before you post! *Nursing Bulletin, 7*(1), 12–14.

Walker, L. O., & Chesnut, L. W. (2010). Identifying health disparities and social inequities affecting childbearing women and infants. *Journal of Obstetric, Gynecologic & Neonatal Nursing, 39*(3), 328–338.

Warner, W. A., & Washington, G. (2011). The role of effective communication in reducing health care disparities. *The Journal for Nurse Practitioners, 7*(7), 612–614.

World Health Organization (WHO). (2010). Female genital mutilation. Retrieved from http://www.who.int/mediacentre/factsheets/fs241/en/

World Health Organization (WHO). (2013). Overweight and obesity. Retrieved from http://www.who.int/gho/ncd/risk_factors/overweight/en/index.html

CONCEPT MAP

Societal Health Trends ←→ **Contemporary Issues in Women's, Families', and Children's Health Care** ←→ **Factors/Trends Influencing Health Issues**

- U.S.: 49th in life expectancy
- National health problems of social concern:
  - AIDS; homelessness: drug abuse; domestic violence
- Increased need for chronic illness management in the aged
- Increasing need for delivering culturally competent health care
- Disparities in HC: access; treatment; role discrimination
- Childbirth trends: increased maternal age at birth; more elective C-sections
- Physical inactivity/obesity
- "Class" gap = shorter, less healthy lives for "lower" class due to limited choices

Politics:
- 2010 Affordable Care Act
- How and where $$$ is spent
- How health care is delivered
- Public programs/policies (e.g., WIC, Medicaid)

Socioeconomics:
- Poverty rates: women most impoverished
- Male–female wage-gap
- Internet digital divide and gray gap: have/have not
- Increasing vulnerable populations (e.g., homeless, gay/lesbian, transgender, incarcerated women)

Personal/Cultural Trends:
- Increased use of technology
- Cultural/language barriers
- Degree of patient autonomy/self-care
- Trend toward early discharges
- Increased use of CAM therapies

Current Health Status/ Health Issues

Infants/Children:
- Infant mortality rate falling
- Leading causes of death:
  - SIDS; accidents/violence; malignant neoplasms; homicidal assaults; suicide
- Health issues/trends
  - Obesity/type II diabetes
  - Lead exposure
  - Asthma
  - Rise in ADHD/autism
  - Self-image issues
  - Sexuality/pregnancy
  - Substance abuse
- Health affected by status of parents' insurance

Families:
- Environmental hazards
- Natural disasters
- Poverty-related concerns → asthma and waste sources
- Increased rates of uninsured/ under-insured

Nursing Insight:
- Critical to listen to young patients' illness stories
- Develop awareness of relevant statistics
- Understand implications of genetic research
- Holistic nursing = addressing needs of mind/body/spirit
- Millennium Development Goals to address global health issues

Women:
- Causes of death: heart disease, cancer, stroke
- Nutritional deficits
- Lack of exercise
- Increased smoking
- Chronic diseases lead to high-risk pregnancies and pregnancy related deaths
- 1/2 of all pregnancies unintended/unwanted
- Trends:
  - Seeking earlier prenatal care
  - Smoking during pregnancy decreasing
  - Women more empowered r/t health-care decisions

Intervention Wheel ←— Guided by — **Professional Nursing Role: Change Agent** — Guided by → **Healthy People Initiative**

- Assesses epidemiology of population's health
- Uses broad determinants of health
- Encompasses three intervention "levels" and 17 intervention categories
- Comprehensive focus on prevention

- Know how to access current/accurate knowledge
- Implement community-based programs for screening/ prevention/education
- Be aware of alternative HC delivery systems and nursing role
- Develop an ethical framework for practice

- U.S. Dept. HHS
- Blueprint for national health goals
- Framework to improve health
- 42 topic areas
- 1200 objectives

Collaboration in Caring:
- Bioethical committees

Complementary Care:
- Blogging to facilitate healing; promote sense of community

Optimizing Outcomes:
- Use population-based data to provide culturally competent care
- Use Office of Women's Health initiatives
- AWHONN initiative to incorporate specialty-specific data into EMR

Now Can You:
- Discuss the Intervention Wheel and Healthy People 2020 goals
- Identify population trends that relate to health, including identifying vulnerable populations
- Describe nursing actions that improve U.S. children's health
- Discuss influences that impact the nation's health

Across Care Settings:
- Faith community nurse serving the church community
- Text4Baby: health care information for pregnant and new moms

The Evolving Family

 Question of Family

What is a family but a collection of beings
    dwelling together?
But it is more than that.
One person might see a refuge from the
    storms of society. . . .
Another, a prison to prevent help from the
    outside world.
It can be both and more.
We draw our first breath in the presence of
    our family and hopefully . . .
we are held in family's arms when we sigh
    our last.

We learn all that is good in its caring
    boundaries or keep secrets of terror
    locked in its heart.
The difference between knowing love and
    trust and learning never to love or trust is
    in what passes between members of the
    family and what is passed on through
    members to their families.
What have you learned from your family?
What will you pass to your family?

      —Brian Fonnesbeck, 2006

LEARNING TARGETS *At the completion of this chapter, the student will be able to:*

◆ Identify different structures of the modern American family.

◆ Describe theoretical concepts that apply to the family.

◆ Assess the family using selected family assessment tools during an interview.

◆ Apply specific family nursing diagnoses and interventions to the family.

◆ Compare various family cultural characteristics that may impact nursing care.

◆ Expand patient care to include and involve the family in every nursing setting.

PICO(T) Questions

The intent of evidence-based practice (EBP) is to provide nursing care that integrates the best available evidence. An initial step in EBP is to write a PICO(T) question that effectively guides the research. A PICO(T) question is an acronym that stands for population (P), intervention or issue (I), comparison of interest (C), outcome (O), and timeframe (T). Depending on the question, all or some of the question components are used in the research process. Use these

PICO(T) questions to spark your thinking as you read the chapter.

1. Do (P) single-parent households view (I) preventative health strategies as being as (O) important as (C) traditional families view them?

2. Does a (I) bereavement program provide (O) positive support to (P) families as they cope with the death of a loved one?

Evidence-Based Practice

Respler-Herman, M., Mowder, B. A., Yasik, A. E., & Shamah, R. (2012). Parenting beliefs, parental stress, and social support relationships. *Journal of Child & Family Studies, 21,* 190–198.

The purpose of this study was to explore the relationship between parenting beliefs, parental stress, and social support. Previous research has explored the effects of parenting styles on children's growth and development and ways that parenting beliefs impact parenting behaviors. Six dimensions of parenting have been described: bonding, discipline, education, general welfare and protection, responsivity, and sensitivity. Other studies support the likelihood that social support constitutes a significant factor in reducing parental stress and exerts a cumulative influence on parenting.

Participants in this study included 87 upper middle-class parents of preschool and elementary students from a small, private school. Of this group, 97.7% were identified as the "parent," 1.1% was identified as a "stepparent," and 1.1% was classified as "other." All participants were married, the majority (74.7%) was female, and the parents' ages ranged from 20 to 60+ years. The majority (92%) of the participants were self-identified as Caucasian. Parents of more than one child were asked to select only one child about whom they would be referring when responding to the questionnaire. The children's genders included 44 females and 42 males; the mean age of all children was 6.8 years. The mean number of children in each family was 2.6, and 3.4% of the children were identified as having special needs.

Participants were asked to complete several questionnaires. The Parent Behavior Importance Questionnaire-Revised (PBIQ-R), which included the domains of bonding, discipline, education, general welfare and protection, responsivity, sensitivity, and negativity, was used to evaluate parent beliefs about the importance of various parenting behaviors. The participants also completed the Parenting Stress Index-Short Form (PSI-SF), a tool that measures parenting stress (i.e., Parental Distress, Parent-Child Dysfunction Interaction, and Difficult Child). A third questionnaire, the Multidimensional Scale of Perceived Social Support (MSPSS), measured participants' perceptions of social support from family, friends, and significant other(s).

Descriptive statistics were used to analyze the data. The researchers concluded that lower total parenting stress scores (indicative of less stress) were related to more positive beliefs about the importance of parenting behaviors. More stress was related to less positive beliefs about parenting behaviors. Also, participants who attached a high level of importance with bonding, education, general welfare and protection, responsivity, and sensitivity on the PBIQ-R were more likely to demonstrate low total parenting stress scores on the PSI-SF. High total parenting stress scores on the PSI-SF were associated with high scores on the negativity subscale of the PBIQ-R. High levels of importance associated with responsivity and general welfare and protection were significantly associated with high total social support scores on the MSPSS. Interestingly, the relationship between parental stress and parenting ideas did not appear to be influenced by social support. The investigators concluded that their study extended prior research exploring the relationship of stress and social support on parenting.

1. How is this information useful to clinical nursing practice?
2. Based on these findings, what are implications for further research?

See Suggested Responses for Evidence-Based Practice on Davis*Plus.*

Introduction

This chapter addresses the assessment of families and highlights interventions for families encountered in a variety of nursing settings. Viewed through the lens of the media, actual and perceived changes that have taken place in the American family since the 1940s are explored. Modern-day family structures and challenges are described, and various theories from psychology, sociology, and nursing are presented to provide a reference point for family assessments and interventions. A nursing diagnosis is presented and described in detail to illustrate the possible goals, interventions, and evaluation criteria that could be used with a family that is experiencing problems with daily functioning.

Concepts such as developmental and group stages of the family, communication, roles and relationships, and special need families are presented to assist with the planning and implementation of family-centered care. Cultural characteristics and comparisons of American family orientation with families from various ethnic backgrounds provide the nurse with a starting point for the delivery of culturally sensitive care for American and international families.

The Evolving Family

VIEWING THE FAMILY IN A NURSING CONTEXT

A nurse hears in report, ". . . that family is starting to get to me. They have a million questions and want to be involved in any decisions that are made related to the patient." Another nurse asks, "Why is this patient still a full-code status? Someone needs to clue the family in on what the actual prognosis is. They are grasping at straws!" Another's comments are, "I had to ask the boyfriend to leave again . . . the family does not want him around their daughter any more."

The preceding statements reflect an often-prevailing narrow point of view related to families and their involvement in nursing care. The literature describes the ideal nursing approach as one that views the entire family as the recipient of care, rather than only the individual patient (Rowe Kaakinen, Padgett Coehlo, Steele, Tabacco, & Harmon Hanson, 2014). In most practice settings, under the best circumstances, the family is seen as contextual background for the patient, and, under the worst, the family represents a pesky interference or additional stressor in the patient's hospitalization and treatment. Nurses should lead the team of health professionals who welcome and embrace the involvement of families in every care setting. In most situations, the family represents a rich source of information and support for the patient. An important role for nursing involves tailoring each plan of care to include the family in interventions that will assist the patient's reintegration back into the family unit following discharge.

THE *HEALTHY PEOPLE* NATIONAL INITIATIVE

The family is the starting point for societal changes needed to ensure the health of families in the future. The national initiative *Healthy People 2020* outlines objectives and indicators that provide the basis for interventions, education, and policy on improving health in this decade. All of the indicators encompassed in this important national health initiative have an impact on the family, such as physical activity, overweight and obesity, tobacco use, substance abuse, responsible sexual behavior, mental health, injury and violence, environmental quality, immunization, and access to health care. Target areas concerning social policy and access to health care for families are underscored in the charge to ". . . reduce the proportion of families that experience difficulties or delays in obtaining health care or do not receive needed care for one or more family members" (U.S. Department of Health and Human Services [USDHHS], 2011).

Families Today

The family is widely defined by many different sources reflective of the social, biological, and legal domains. Various definitions describe members who compose the family, their interdependence, and methods of interaction. A **family** consists of two or more members who self-identify as a "family" and interact and depend on one another socially, emotionally, and financially. Most often, family structure involves either the **family of origin** (the family that reared the individual) or the **family of choice** (the family adopted through marriage or cohabitation). A single person belongs to a family of origin but may choose not to become a member of a family of choice. A single individual cannot constitute a family. Instead, most definitions of family include a prerequisite of at least one other person who is self-defined as being a part of the family (Rowe Kaakinen et al., 2014; Wright & Leahey, 2012).

 Nursing Insight—*Differentiating among various family configurations*

In contemporary society, the traditional **nuclear family**, which consists of a male partner, female partner, and their children, actually represents only a small number of families. Other family members, termed **extended family**, may also live in the same household. There are many variations of family and household structures. For example, the **married-blended family**, formed as a result of death or divorce, consists of unrelated family members who join together to form a new household. A **single-parent family** includes an unmarried biological or adoptive parent. A **commune** is a group of men, women, and children. **Cohabitation**, or domestic partnership, describes an unmarried man and woman who share a household; a **homosexual family** (lesbian and gay) consists of same-sex partners who live together with or without children, and a **no-parent family** is one in which children live independently in foster or kinship care, such as living with a grandparent or aunt (Rowe Kaakinen et al., 2014).

 ### Cultural Diversity: Patterns of Family Structure

Patterns of family structure tend to be culturally influenced. For example, Hispanic children are more than twice as likely as African American children to live in cohabiting-parent families, and they are approximately four times as likely as Caucasian children to live in this type of family configuration (U.S. Census Bureau, 2012).

THE CHANGING FAMILY AS REFLECTED IN THE MEDIA

Family changes and adaptations from the Cro-Magnon era to the present day have been well researched and documented, but it is useful to examine the more recent changes that have taken place over the past 20 to 40 years. During this time, family structure and roles have changed rapidly and at present seem to be in a state of flux. As American families transition and evolve, television and theater often provide useful insights into the predominant family themes of the time.

For example, in the 1950s and 1960s, a nuclear family was presented with little emphasis on the extended family. Programs such as *Ozzie and Harriet*, *Leave It to Beaver*, *The Dick Van Dyke Show*, and *Father Knows Best* portrayed the typical family as one that included the mother and father along with one to three children. Family roles typically portrayed a father-dominated household and a homemaker mother who would occasionally flex her decision-making authority when the father's advice did not work. Issues were generally simple and resolvable with an occasional foray into societal issues such as racism or mental health. When problems such as alcoholism were presented, they tended to be in the context of an outsider who temporarily touched the family and then left. Rarely was there depiction of a serious internal family mental health problem. Instead, scenarios involved events such as girlfriend–boyfriend situational crises or friend-related peer pressure. Occasional variations in family structure were offered in weekly programs such as *Bonanza*, *Family Affair*, and *My Three Sons* that portrayed households run by males who received assistance from a housekeeper or relative.

Programming during the 1960s and early 1970s reflected a growing trend toward themes that included blended families with shows such as *The Brady Bunch*. These weekly programs tended to present upper-income families with housekeepers and stay-at-home mothers who deferred major decisions to the father. Widowhood, as opposed to divorce, usually constituted the reason for remarrying, and this situation neatly sidestepped the unpleasantness of a broken home resulting from divorce.

Family issues continued to relate primarily to difficulties associated with school and dating. Major breakthroughs were achieved with *All in the Family*, *The Jeffersons*, *What's Happening*, and other sitcoms in the 1970s that dealt with the turbulent issues of civil rights and sex equality and changing views on race and gender.

During this time, there were also shows that began to present selected variations of family. For example, *The Mary Tyler Moore Show* centered on a career woman whose close work relationships served as a central component of family. *Gilligan's Island* presented family-like associations that dealt with work or survival issues as a team and shared support and platonic love and loyalty that would have normally been received from a family. The 1990s to 2000s version of this theme was expanded in *Friends* and *Seinfeld*, programs that introduced the idea that people could remain single longer without the expectation that a family was defined by marriage and procreation. This trend is again reflected in more recent programs such as *Grey's Anatomy*, in which unrelated individuals form a family with "ties" that sometimes are actually stronger than those with their biological relatives who may not always "be there" for them.

Television programs during the 1980s and 1990s also began to address variations in social class and politics with shows such as *Family Ties*, which explored social issues such as premarital sex, dealing with the death of friends, and Alzheimer's disease. Interestingly, the episodes did not always present a clean resolution of an issue but instead focused on the importance of family closeness and support in dealing with the problem within the context of battling political views. *The Cosby Show* depicted an African American upper middle-class family in which both parents were white-collar professionals.

The 1990s brought increased awareness of the challenges facing families dealing with poverty, alcoholism, and abuse within their own ranks rather than as a problem that occurred only outside the family. *Grace Under Fire* presented a single head of household who was a recovering alcoholic. *Roseanne* revolved around a matriarchal family structure in a lower economic setting in which both parents had to work to make ends meet. One particular episode in this series dealt with how to write a check in a way that delayed cashing (and subsequently, "bouncing") it, to allow extra time for sufficient funds to be deposited into the account.

Television sitcoms in the new millennium continue to reflect trends consistent with societal changes. Family structures such as the binuclear arrangement (two intact nuclear families sharing a home) and the divorced family living with a brother and sharing responsibility for rearing a son (*Two and a Half Men*) are examples of alternate family themes that have emerged in recent times. Programs such as these may be preparing the way for shows that depict same-sex unions with or without children.

Also reflective of contemporary society is the trend of sitcoms that feature extended family members such as the live-in father in *King of Queens* and the very intrusive parents in *Everybody Loves Raymond*. The success of the movie *My Big Fat Greek Wedding* opened the door for depicting ethnic families that were keeping their own values and beliefs separate from those of the prevailing culture. *Modern Family* focuses on a nuclear family, a blended family (older man, younger woman and two sons), and a gay couple with an adopted girl of Asian descent. Over the years, Hispanic, Jewish, Asian, and other ethnic groups have revealed their differences in humorous but culturally sensitive ways. The media, however, generally provides only a superficial representation of the varied and complex challenges faced by the modern-day family.

 Collaboration in Caring—*Five functions of the family*

1. Physical Needs: Meets the primary basic needs such as food, water, clothing, and shelter
2. Economic Needs: Access to enough financial resources to adequately meet the family's needs and wishes
3. Reproductive Needs: Ways that add new life to the family unit and maintain a healthy sexual relationship between parents
4. Affective and Coping Needs: Strategies to deal with everyday stresses of life and encourage a nurturing environment
5. Socialization Needs: Processes whereby families acquire the skills, knowledge, attitudes, and values necessary for performing their social roles

STRESSORS ON FAMILIES TODAY

Health Care

Today's families face varied and complex challenges. Baby boomers are aging and entering retirement. This shift in the contemporary workforce leaves openings and shortages in critical areas such as education and health care and at the same time adds increased demands on a health-care system already burdened with an aging population. For many, insurance coverage changes and often becomes more expensive as retirees transition from employment insurance to retirement insurance options such as Medicare and Social Security. In many instances, families have no options for insurance because of part-time work or unemployment.

Mental Illness

Other problems that arise from both internal and external causes also impact families. According to the Centers for Disease Control and Prevention (CDC) (2011), approximately 25% of U.S. adults have a mental illness. Affected families not only face dealing with a potentially chronic illness that continues to be stigmatized by society, but they also must grapple with paying for treatment of a diagnosis that is largely exempt from insurance coverage. Challenges that come from external forces outside the family system include environmental assaults such as catastrophic weather, forest fires, and earthquakes. An entire region of families continues to be affected by problems that follow in the aftermath of hurricanes, fires, and floods.

 Nursing Insight—*Recognizing the relationship between family stressors and poor health outcomes*

Families may have multiple stressors that increase their vulnerability to poor health outcomes. Problems such as substance abuse, mental illness, domestic violence, and limited access to medical care because of unemployment, loss of medical insurance, or inadequate insurance coverage can affect families across all strata of society.

Societal Pressures

The family also faces societal pressures. The incidence of violent crimes has decreased in major urban areas, but suicide among children and adolescents continues to represent an important societal issue. The number of families currently affected by AIDS is increasing at a startling rate. Women and children, a vulnerable population because of barriers associated with access to health care, constitute the fastest growing segment of the population to contract HIV. Public education is in a state of crisis as demands increase on teachers who are confronted with diminishing resources.

These and many other issues continue to challenge families. Meanwhile, family structure and roles are undergoing changes that frequently increase the potential for further family problems. Present trends show a diminishing number of nuclear family households. The traditional family structure is being replaced by one that includes a single head of household, most frequently a divorced or abandoned mother. The number of unmarried mothers continues to increase. Statistics reflect the current trend: The percentage of children living with both parents decreased from 85% in 1970 to 67% in 2008. A divorced or single woman is usually the head of household in those families, although recently there has been an increase in single male head of household families from 1% to 4% (Child Trends DataBank, 2011). In other situations, the head of household is homosexual or sharing a home with a same-sex partner.

These trends reflect increasing opportunities for alternative forms of parenthood within contemporary American society. The nontraditional parenting arrangements result from more liberal social mores and the technological and medical advances that now offer the possibility of parenthood to single men and women. Same-sex partnerships/marriages and their effects on the family raise political, social, and religious issues that have increasingly found their way into present-day discussions. While the far-reaching impact of same-sex relationships on family structure and function continues to be investigated, areas that frequently must be addressed concern child custody, legal consent, power of attorney, and confidentiality (Rosenfeld, 2010). The following case study provides an example of some of the issues and questions that may need to be addressed by the family and the patient's care providers.

66What to say 99 —*Effective tools for families*

Covey (2006) discusses effective tools that may enhance family performance. The nurse can communicate these principles to families that may promote healthy family functioning.

- Be proactive: Become an agent of change in the family.
- Begin with the end in mind: Develop a family mission statement.
- Put first things first: Make the family a priority in a turbulent world.
- Think "win–win": Move from me to we.
- Seek first to understand then be understood: Solve family problems through empathetic communication.
- Synergize: Build family unity through celebrating differences.
- Sharpen the saw: Renew family spirit through traditions.

 Global Health Case Study An Australian Family With Same-Sex Partners

Sienna, a 37-year old comatose Australian woman, is dying of ovarian cancer. She is on life support in the hospital. The family, which includes ex-husband, William, and two children—Lucas, age 12 and Olivia, age 14—has gathered in the visitors' lounge. Lily, Sienna's life partner, is also present in the lounge. The family is discussing whether to extend Sienna's present level of care or to begin to wean her from life support. Although Sienna has a living will, there is concern and conflict among the family members and Lily regarding how and when the will should be honored. William questions the appropriateness of Lily's being in attendance for the discussion.

critical thinking questions

1. What would the nurse need to know to help the family problem-solve in this situation?

2. What resources are available to the family and the nursing staff to help clarify these issues?

◆ See Suggested Answers to Global Health Case Studies on Davis*Plus*.

The **skip generation**, an arrangement in which the grandparents rear grandchildren with or without the parents' help, describes another present-day variation in family structure. In the United States today, approximately 5.8 million children are living in grandparents' homes, and more than 2.5 million grandparents assume primary responsibility for these children (American Association of Retired Persons, 2013).

 Now Can You—**Discuss contemporary family changes and stressors?**

1. Define family and identify five family categories?
2. Identify three changes in family structure that have been highlighted in the media?
3. Identify five stressors faced by the American family today?

Family Theories and Models

Development of a specialized body of knowledge provides the foundation for a profession. While nursing theories and models are essential in defining nursing and nursing practice, theories from other disciplines are important in providing insights into other dimensions of health and human behavior. For example, family theory, which draws from a number of related disciplines (Rowe Kaakinen et al., 2014), helps to guide assessment and intervention within a holistic framework that views the entire family as client. The following discussion presents several theoretical models representing a cross section of useful concepts to assist in the nursing assessment and to facilitate a creative application to various family interactions.

FAMILY SYSTEMS THEORY

A systems approach to understanding the family centers on the recognition that changes that occur in one member affect the entire family. The family systems theory, which views persons as "open systems," has a central theme: "The sum of the parts is greater than the whole" (Rowe Kaakinen et al., 2014). According to this theory, the family shares a unique identity that is far more complex than that of its collective members. The family is dynamic, constantly adjusting to information that filters in from the surrounding environment and from within the family.

Nursing Insight—*Clinical application of the family systems theory*

When working with families, the nurse uses the family systems theory to "view the family as a unit and focus on observing the interaction among family members rather than studying family members individually" (Wright & Leahey, 2012).

The following situation helps to illustrate application of the family systems theory: An addicted member receives help for the addiction and then returns to the family system. The changes in the recovering family member have a significant impact on how the entire family acts and reacts. A new system of communication is established. In the new system, the family members communicate assertively and supportively with each other and no longer adhere to the former framework of denial that a problem exists and secret keeping. The nurse working with the family recognizes that teaching and referrals to appropriate community resources are most likely needed to facilitate the family's healthy adjustment to the changes.

Boundaries

Another concept inherent in family systems theory concerns boundaries. Each system contains a boundary that affects how the outside world is allowed to interact with the family members. Stated another way, boundaries identify the family's control of how the family system interacts with the outside world. A family whose children obtain food and shelter by begging from the neighbors demonstrates a problem with boundaries that are too permeable. Permeability refers to the degree that information and interchange are allowed to flow between systems. An ideal system is one that is semipermeable. In a semipermeable system, the boundaries are secure enough to keep the family intact but still allow for free interchange with the outside world. In this situation, the family system readily interacts with outside systems. A healthy family has a semipermeable boundary that allows and encourages interaction with outside agencies such as work, school, religious organization, and friends.

A closed boundary serves to keep family secrets inside and therapeutic interventions outside. Closed boundaries often occur in families with issues of addiction or abuse. Families of alcoholics soon learn not to disclose information about their problems to outsiders. Conversely, a family that is so lacking in structure that it allows an uninterrupted free flow of information/intervention to and from outsiders can be said to have an open boundary or no boundary at all. For example, an open boundary exists with a family whose children are so neglected that they rely on friends or neighbors to feed them.

Nursing Insight—*Recognizing the childbearing family's boundary permeability*

The extent to which the **suprasystem** (the broad system that surrounds the family unit, such as the cultural community) influences the childbearing family's participation in activities such as childbirth education, prenatal care, and infant care is dependent on the family's boundary permeability.

Subsystems

Family systems are further divided into subsystems. A family of four may constitute the "main" system. The mother and father represent a subsystem that has a permanent or temporary relationship that is a part of, yet separate from, the main family system. Children often form alliances with other siblings or with one parent. A subsystem can develop when a sibling marries or cohabits with another individual who is temporarily or permanently accepted into the family. Subsystems are necessary parts of family functioning, especially in health crisis situations when families must make decisions for sick or disabled members or when new dependent members join the family. For example, the birth of a baby introduces a new member who becomes part of the family system but is also a subsystem with the mother or father or other family caregiver(s).

Cultural Diversity: *Boundaries and Receptivity to Information*

Families that have recently immigrated to this country may be receptive to health information only from extended family members or from persons within their cultural community.

Balance and Homeostasis

The family system continually strives to return to balance or achieve homeostasis after a crisis. When a family member is sick or injured, or when an emergency arises that requires a reorganization of the family (e.g., an evacuation during a storm), the family quickly attempts to return to former routines and rules as a way of reestablishing homeostasis. At certain times the family is unable to return to former normalcy and instead must adjust or form adaptive behaviors. For example, the family may learn to work with a wheelchair and other adaptive devices when a member suffers a stroke or spinal cord injury. Over time, adaptations become the norm for the family.

Maladaptive behaviors are an alternate adaptation that involves the use of unhealthy or abnormal behaviors to adapt to a family crisis. Enabling and codependency are common maladaptive behaviors that are often adopted by an addictive family (Townsend, 2010). Enabling involves making excuses or obtaining substances for the addictive family member. Codependency is a maladaptive behavior in which the non-addicted family member joins the addicted member in the use of alcohol or other substances as a way of interacting or communicating.

FAMILY DEVELOPMENTAL STAGES AND THEORY

Developmental theory (Friedman, Bowden, & Jones, 2003; Rowe Kaakinen et al., 2014) has at its core the idea that every life moves through developmental stages with tasks that need to be accomplished before moving on to the next stage. Duvall identifies eight family stages: beginning, childbearing, preschool children, school-age, teenagers, launching, middle-aged, and retirement (Friedman et al., 2003). Each stage is accompanied by specific tasks that are performed to assist with the physical and emotional development of the family members in that particular stage.

When working with families, the nurse should identify what stage(s) the family is in and assess how well the needs for that particular stage are being met. Learning, attachment, and grieving represent specific tasks that are affected by the developmental stage. Teaching needs and nursing interventions are structured and implemented according to the developmental stages of the family and its members. Although the stages follow one another in a linear progression, some families may simultaneously be in more than one stage or they may revert to previous stages (Wilkinson & Treas, 2011).

Beginning Families

Beginning families are those that have just been formed through marriage or that self-identify as family, as in the case of common-law unions. The beginning family identifies shared goals that may include career paths, homebuilding, and planning for children. Creating shared time together to build the relationship constitutes a central developmental task for all families, and this special together time traditionally is initiated during the honeymoon period. Combined households and property are common features of all families. One of the limitations of Duvall's theory concerns its application with the childless family. If the family has no children, many of the developmental stages are not applicable until the couple reaches middle age and beyond. If the family does have a child, the family developmental stage parallels the age of the child. When more than one child is present, the family is usually in more than one developmental stage.

Childbearing Stage

The childbearing developmental stage begins with conception. Early tasks during this stage include seeking prenatal care and planning for space for the child. If there are other children already in the home, the family begins to prepare and socialize the other children into a sibling role. Ideally, the family involves the children in decision making related to preparation for the expected baby. For example, siblings can help to choose paint colors for the baby's room or offer advice regarding toys or clothes to select for the baby. When the baby is born, the family must adapt its routines to include the various tasks associated with feeding and caring for the baby. Family teaching needs may include dealing with sleep pattern disturbances related to feeding and changing diapers through the night. Along with strategies for successfully coping with these adjustments, the nurse can offer support and reassurance. The nurse assesses the family's readiness and openness to learn and receive help and, according to specific needs, may provide additional information concerning nutrition, the importance of well-baby visits, car seats, immunization schedules, and infant crib monitors.

 Optimizing Outcomes—Applying developmental theory when caring for the childbearing family

An understanding of the normal phases of the life cycle helps the nurse to provide anticipatory guidance for the childbearing family. Strategies to bolster the young child's sense of security when a newborn is brought home may divert a potential family crisis.

Preschool Stage

The preschool developmental stage includes toddlerhood and attending kindergarten. During this stage, the child has learned to walk and actively explore her world, which encompasses siblings and other family members and friends. At this time, families need information about the prevention of injuries and interventions for accidents that usually result from the child's increased motor abilities coupled with less-developed judgment and coordination. The nurse should be alert for signs of abuse or neglect during this stage. Points of contact that allow the nurse to assess developmental progress occur during well-child checks, immunization appointments, and office or hospital visits for the child or other family members.

School-Age and Adolescent/Teenage Stages

The school-age and adolescent/teenage developmental stages provide the optimal opportunity for teaching about drugs, sex, and health promotion. Personal values are shaped and clarified, and ethical development occurs during this time. Surveys have shown that nurses are included among the top 10 trusted people sought by school-aged children to discuss issues important to them.

Launching, Middle-Age, and Retirement Stages

The launching, middle-age, and retirement developmental stages bring the family full-circle back to the early issues of self and couple-building with less emphasis on children (if successfully launched) and more involvement in community and hobby-related interests. The young adult who is not successfully launched from the childhood home presents a complication of incomplete launching. This situation may represent a temporary arrangement necessary for continuing education, or it may provide a convenient and economical "non-action" by the son or daughter until ties with others have been established. The nurse's role in this situation is to assess whether the living arrangement creates a problem (e.g., anger, frustration, and delay in meeting goals) for either the parents or the child. Interventions may include strategies to improve communication between the parents and the child and/or community referrals for assistance with goal setting and vocational training.

STRUCTURAL–FUNCTIONAL THEORY

Structural–functional theory focuses on the functioning of the family and the roles assumed by each family member to promote family function. Necessary roles include provider, housekeeper, child caregiver, socializer, sexual partner, therapist, recreational organizer, and kinship member. Although a family member often assumes more than one role, some roles may be exclusive to only one identified member. This arrangement takes on added significance concerning the family's ability to move forward when a member is unable to fulfill his or her exclusive role (Friedman et al., 2003; Rowe Kaakinen et al., 2014; Wright & Leahey, 2012). According to structural–functional theory, if any of the roles are not managed by one or more members of the family, problems such as disorganization, deficits in hygiene, isolation, and other negative situations will emerge that may require a nurse's intervention to help the family return to balance (Rowe Kaakinen et al., 2014).

Provider Role

The provider role is the money-earner or the resource gatherer. One or more family members pay the bills and distribute resources to other family members for clothing, food, and recreation. If the provider is sick or hospitalized, the family identifies an alternate provider to temporarily meet that need or identifies other resources such as savings, insurance, or public assistance to pay bills.

Housekeeper

During recent years, the housekeeper role has evolved from the traditional stay-at-home mother as increasing numbers of women are engaged in full-time employment outside the home. Housekeeping involves not only the physical cleaning and maintenance of the family environment but also the organization of family duties to maintain a stable, healthy living situation for the family.

Child-Caregiver

The child-caregiver role is assumed by the person (usually the mother) who is designated as the primary care provider for the children. This role is performed by a designated member such as the mother, father, grandmother, or uncle, depending on the family structure. Someone (e.g., child care facility or babysitter) is responsible to ensure that the children are supervised and cared for even when the primary child-caregiver is away from home.

Socializer and Recreational Organizer

The socializer and recreational organizer roles may not be as consciously directed as the previous roles, but they encompass how the family interacts with others. Initially, the parents or guardians may arrange interactions for the children through family and friend gatherings, trips, and activities. Eventually, most members begin to organize their own social events through personal friendship choices and preferred activities outside the home. Socialization is taught by the family and may be a role that is shared equally among family members unless a problem occurs. Family trips, holidays, and birthdays are important events that teach family patterns that children will later use to help them develop their own family's social and recreational roles.

Sexual Partner

The sexual partner role should exist between the parental units. Variations exist in different family structures. In every structure, children should have education and role modeling on how to interact in socially and sexually appropriate ways. Healthy family interactions constitute the first defense against abuse and violence.

Therapist

The therapist role is assumed when one family member expresses concern for another's health or emotional well-being. For example, concern about the husband's blood pressure prompts the wife to make him an appointment with his health-care practitioner. The therapist role can also involve active listening and other expressions of caring as family members help one another through a loss or a crisis.

Kinship

The family member who organizes family reunions, corresponds with friends, sends birthday and holiday greetings, and reminds children to write thank-you notes assumes the kinship role. The wife most often assumes this role and is charged with the responsibility of remembering important dates for her spouse's family as well as for her own.

Optimizing Outcomes—Applying the structural–functional theory

Structural–functional theories view the family as a social system and focus on outcomes, not process. Nurses can use structural–functional theory to assess how well the family functions internally among family members and externally with outside systems.

COMMUNICATION THEORY

Communication theory asserts that emotional problems result from the way people interact with each other in the context of the family (Rowe Kaakinen et al., 2014). Healthy families have clear rules such as "we don't interrupt each other when speaking" or "we don't yell at each other." Communication is clear and congruent and nonverbal cues match what is being said. Unhealthy families give mixed or double-binding messages, which are statements accompanied by nonverbal expressions that are inconsistent and incongruent with the verbal message. Healthy families communicate love and support clearly and often. Verbal communication is matched by nonverbal communication (such as hugs, voice tone, and eye-contact) that supports the intended message. Families check with each other to make sure the intended meaning is understood. For example, a parent explains; "I am setting a curfew because I care about you and want you to be safe. Does that make sense to you?" The parent then encourages discussion to ensure clarity and understanding of the purpose of curfew.

Nursing Insight—*Family communication patterns*

Patterns of family communication reveal much about family functioning. In addition to providing information about "who is saying what and to whom," they also convey information about the structure and functions of family relationships in relation to the power base, decision-making processes, affection, trust, and coalitions. Dysfunctional communication inhibits healthy nurturing and diminishes personal feelings of self-esteem and self-worth.

The nurse or family therapist assesses a repeating negative pattern such as excessive drinking to determine if it has been replaced instead by an assertive yet supportive and positive communication. For example, a wife complains to the nurse that her husband drinks more whenever they have an argument about their children. The husband notes that his wife complains to him about the children whenever he tries to relax by drinking. The nurse educates the family that interventions regarding either the arguing or the drinking could help to break the pattern of negative communication and refers them to a support group or a counselor to learn new patterns.

GROUP THEORY

Group theory can be applied to the family as a group. Norms (rules of conduct), roles, goals, and power structure are inherent family concepts along with the division of household chores, expectations of completed homework, and curfew enforcement. According to group theory, stages of groups (forming, storming, norming, performing, and adjourning/terminating) explain expected behaviors that occur in any given stage (Clark, 2008; Johnson & Johnson, 2012).

Forming describes the beginning phase of the group. In families, the forming stage usually occurs through marriage or cohabitation. *Storming*, the next stage, is the disordered time of confusion or chaos when two or more distinct personalities discover their differences. Norming describes how groups (or families) adjust to individual members by applying rules and procedures that the members agree to obey. *Performing* is the ideal stage in which the group (i.e., the family) accomplishes their goals and produces results. In the family, desirable results would include good citizenship, education and health of its members, and active contribution to society. *Adjourning/terminating* represents the final stage in a group when it has accomplished its goals and disbands to possibly form a different group. Families experience this stage when members die, divorce, or leave the family to begin their own families.

Because families represent long-term relationships anchored in the performing stage of meeting goals and taking care of one another, the stages tend to be more stable than with groups. Forming occurs when a child is brought into the family by birth or by adoption. Storming describes the emotional clashes that occur during times of transition (e.g., an adolescent testing the rules) or crisis (e.g., adjusting to a move or job change). Norming generally occurs when parental rules are imposed. For example, family norming may involve teaching the children to talk more softly inside the house than when playing in the yard. Performing occurs as each family member performs specific duties to accomplish the daily tasks of life. Adjourning or termination may follow a death in the family, or it can also follow the launching of a high school graduate into college. The healthy family adjusts for the loss and resets roles and norms to fit the new family structure.

BOWEN FAMILY SYSTEMS THEORY

Bowen family systems theory is a human behavior theory that views the family as an emotional unit and uses systems thinking to describe the complex interactions within the family unit (The Bowen Center for the Study of the Family,

2013). The theory is useful when identifying family problems or challenges that are rooted in family processes such as communication, connecting between members, and teaching values (Rowe Kaakinen et al., 2014). The nuclear family emotional system describes the pattern of adaptive/maladaptive emotional expression that exists as a theme in the family. According to this theory, one family could be characterized as stoic or cold in their interactions with others, while another is described as emotional and highly reactive to situations and circumstances.

According to family systems theory, differentiation of self is demonstrated when a family member breaks away from the learned emotional system and instead expresses emotions that differ from the learned family pattern. For example, a father whose family of origin is nondemonstrative of love and caring may openly hug and kiss his spouse and children and verbally express his love for them. In an emotional cutoff, a family member has separated from the original family pattern in a dramatic and sometimes permanent way. This may occur when a family member who was reared in a dysfunctional family chooses not to perpetuate the learned pattern of alcoholism or abuse.

Family systems theory also views birth order as a predictor of certain patterns of behavior that may be desirable or conflicting, depending on the birth order of the chosen mate. A firstborn child with behaviors related to high responsibility and control may clash with a spouse who is also a firstborn. The "baby of the family" (youngest sibling) may seek out a spouse who was a firstborn to serve as a caretaker.

With the family systems approach, most interactions take place in the form of a duo or dyad. Triangulation occurs when the dyad diverts attention away from its own conflict by focusing on a third person such as the child, teacher of the problem child, or police officer who comes into a domestic disturbance. Police, nurses, and counselors have often taken the displaced anger of a couple they are trying to help and have instead unwittingly become the third part of a triangle.

The multigenerational transmission process describes how one learns or transmits family emotional systems across generations. Watching grandparents express affection teaches patterns to grandchildren who will model similar behaviors to their children (unless self-differentiation or an emotional cutoff changes the pattern). Family projection process is how and what children are taught. Societal regression describes patterns of the family projection process that exist in cultures as part of a dominant theme. For example, in the United States, independence and individuality are recognized as desirable qualities and thus are replicated throughout family culture. This is in contrast with some Asian cultures that value interdependence and the importance of being a part of a group.

NURSING THEORIES

Nursing theories define the family–nurse relationship in various ways. Nightingale viewed family as a support system for the primary patient. King described interactions that result in a shared or mutual transaction (similar to the nursing care plan). Roy placed family in the context of the adaptive system of the client. Neuman viewed families as systems and subsystems. According to this framework, the family can become the self-care agent of a patient who is unable to meet her own needs. Rogers described the family as an open system that interacts through the exchange of matter and energy (George, 2010).

Many nursing theorists and practitioners blend theories, which then become "integrated" nursing theories. Friedman et al. (2003) merged concepts from general systems theory and structural functional theory to form an assessment model. Rowe and colleagues (2009) used the family assessment intervention model with the Family Systems Stressor-Strength Inventory to apply Neuman's theory in a quantitative measurement tool for assessing families. The Calgary Family Assessment Model (Wright & Leahey, 2012) draws on postmodernism, systems theory, cybernetics, communication theory, change theory, and biology of cognition to form a multidimensional assessment model for family nursing care.

The theories described in this chapter have been selected for their clarity and applicability to a variety of family structures and situations. Many theories from nursing and related disciplines have utility in a range of family settings and can be successfully applied to guide and direct nursing care. Familiarization with a variety of theories allows for selection of the theory or theories that best fits the family nursing assessment and interventions. Nursing is both an art and a science. The science component involves the research of concepts and development of theories to describe phenomena. The art of nursing is the application of theory or theories to a specific family interaction.

 Now Can You—Discuss family theory for nursing practice?

1. Identify at least four types of theories used in family nursing?
2. Name three components of Bowen Family Systems Theory?
3. Discuss a theory that describes stages experienced by the family during the life span of the children?

Family Assessment

Theories are useful for helping to explain and categorize behaviors of individuals and families. The next logical step, applying theory to the assessment of families, provides information from which to base interventions to either improve or correct the family's health. The nurse is sensitive to family needs and is in a unique position to interact with the family during the assessment process.

THE NURSING ROLE IN FAMILY ASSESSMENT

It is difficult to fit modern American families into any particular mold. Variations in size, structure, and parenting style, along with religious, cultural, and socioeconomic orientation all affect how the family deals with economic, educational, social, and health-care issues. To guide the delivery of appropriate care to the family unit, it is helpful to examine the nurse's role in assessment and intervention and explore some of the major factors that influence family structure. During the assessment interview, the nurse addresses important concepts including family size and structure; parenting style; and religious, cultural, and socioeconomic orientation.

Family Size and Structure

Family size has generally decreased since the founding of the country when large families ensured more workers for the family business. As recently as one generation ago, families consisting of more than six members were more reflective of the norm than today's families that average two and a half children. Birth rates have declined in Caucasian families while remaining the same in some ethnic cultures. It has been predicted that by the year 2020, the "minority" family will represent 51% of the total American population.

Family structure is becoming increasingly different from the traditional two-parent, two-child nuclear family portrayed during the 1950s. Single-parent (mother or father head of household), binuclear (two families living together), skip-generation (grandparents rearing grandchildren), and extended family (grandparents or other relatives living with the nuclear family) are all represented in the American family of today.

Parenting Style

Parenting style is the manner in which knowledge and values first observed and ingrained during one's own upbringing and other observed experiences are then used in rearing one's own children. Parenting style includes discipline, communication, and distribution of power. Some families tend to view corporal punishment (usually in the form of spanking) as the normal approach to discipline; others favor disciplinary measures that include times-out, positive reinforcement, and other nonphysical methods. Three distinct styles of parenting have been identified:

- **Authoritarian** or **dictatorial**: Enforces absolute rule; parents enforce rules and strict expectations of each family member; children have little say in decision making, and punishment follows any deviation from the established rules; punishment is not necessarily corporal but often includes withdrawal of approval; children from this style of parenting tend to be shy, sensitive, conforming, submissive, loyal, and honest.
- **Laissez-faire** or **permissive**: Allows the children control over their environment and subsequent behavior with less input from the parents; few rules to follow; children are able to make their own decisions; punishment is inconsistent when used; children from this family tend to be disrespectful, aggressive, and disobedient, possibly growing up to be irresponsible members of the community.
- **Authoritative** or **democratic**: Parents have a combination of characteristics from both the authoritarian and laissez-faire parenting styles; parents find a common ground between enforcing rules and allowing some freedom for their children to participate in decisions; parents are firm, set realistic standards, and punishment centers on assisting the child develop an inner consciousness about behavior; produces children who are assertive, self-reliant, and highly interactive with high self-esteem (Hockenberry, 2012). Although each type of parenting style has benefits and drawbacks, authoritative parenting tends to meet the child's needs better than the other styles.

The nurse recognizes that disciplining children is an important concept for parents to understand. Discipline is training the child to meet a pattern of behavior with the intention of instilling good moral judgment, achieving competence and maintaining self-control, promoting self-direction, and learning to respect others. Consistency with rule setting is a key concept that parents must understand. A reliable and steady discipline approach by parents reinforces to the child that their misbehavior will be corrected. Often, redirecting the child away from the behavior to alternative activity can be an effective way to discipline. With older children, reasoning or explaining to the child why the behavior is unacceptable may also be useful. The nurse can help parents understand that positive and effective child-rearing practices can be straightforward and firm without being negative or abusive.

During the family parenting-style assessment, the nurse observes for indicators of neglect or physical abuse but otherwise supports consistent and predictable consequences and rewards appropriate to the age of the child. Parents should be given information about disciplining consistently and without anger. When indicated, parents can be referred to parenting courses or support groups.

Religious, Cultural, and Socioeconomic Orientation

Religious orientation has varying effects on families. The majority of Americans claim some affiliation with a church or spiritual group, but according to a 2012 Gallup report, fewer than 60% actually attend a spiritual institution on a regular basis (Newport, 2012). Values that tend to be rooted in religious beliefs include practices concerning the observation of holidays and beliefs toward abortion, birth control, marriage, and advance directives (legal documentation that directs that "no heroic" measures be taken to extend life).

Religion also influences attitudes toward alternate lifestyle choices such as homosexuality and sexual abstinence and other moral choices such as euthanasia or suicide. Religious beliefs can provide comfort and a sense of peace to believers in times of sickness or grieving. Religion-based movements such as the "Promise-Keepers" and the "Million Man March" were created, in part, as a positive force to encourage men to become more responsible fathers and husbands.

The nurse assesses the family's religious or spiritual affiliation, and when indicated, assists in contacting the appropriate spiritual advisor or clergy member. Hospitals provide clergy and chaplain services for a variety of needs and occasions. The nurse avoids imposing personal beliefs and values on the family but instead helps them obtain the resources necessary to help them to regain balance in crisis situations.

Cultural orientation includes family communication styles, structure of family, health beliefs, and power distribution. The nurse assesses family cultural affiliation and avoids generalities or stereotypes by validating all cultural information with the family.

🌼 *Cultural Diversity: When Assessing Families*

It is important for the nurse to be aware of cultural variations that may exist in family structure and communication styles. Many cultures emphasize the extended family to a much greater extent than the American nuclear family. Often, grandparents as well as aunts, uncles, and cousins may be considered a part of the primary family. In some Native American tribes, a sister or aunt or grandparent may be the primary caretaker of the family, and this individual needs to be included in health planning and teaching. Certain cultures give preference to the matriarch, while others are more male-dominated. In some Hispanic cultures, the adult son makes health-care decisions for the family. Nonverbal forms of communication can vary widely across cultures. There may be differences in eye contact, the practice of formal and informal touch, the level and tone of voice, and how respect is shown. A nod by individuals in some Pacific Rim countries may be an indicator of respect but does not necessarily convey an understanding of the nursing instructions given. Although a translator who is a family member may be comforting to the family, this situation is not reflective of best practice methods, especially for informed consent purposes. Instead, a non-family, professional translator should be used (Spector, 2012; Wilkinson & Treas, 2011).

Socioeconomic status impacts the family's ability to access and pay for health care and other services. The nurse assists with referrals to social workers or other community experts to secure resources appropriate to the family's needs. Available resources include state and government supplemental programs, insurance sources, loans and grants, and church or community programs that aid families through catastrophic losses such as fire or health crises.

Historically recognized as important advocates for the family, nurses lead efforts to change or adjust laws and legislation to assist and empower families in areas such as child care, elder care, work leave for births or care of sick family members, tax breaks for dependents including elderly members, assistance with health-care costs, and public service education for health-care choices. Legislation concerning helmets, seat belts, and child safety seats illustrates several government interventions designed to foster and enhance the well-being of families and individuals. Policies concerning stem-cell research, same-sex marriage, property laws, pro-choice rights, and minimum wages are but a few examples of the government's far-reaching impact on the family.

TOOLS TO FACILITATE THE FAMILY ASSESSMENT

Qualitative and Quantitative Surveys

For most hospital settings, assessment of the family is limited to gathering a history, usually during admission, related to the patient's illness. However, in a family nursing approach that encompasses care of the entire family, more thorough formats for family assessment are used. Friedman et al. (2003), Rowe Kaakinen et al. (2014), Wright and Leahey (2012), and others have developed family nursing assessment forms to provide either a qualitative or a quantitative view of the family. A variety of assessment tools are available and those frequently used include surveys, genograms, ecomaps, and strengths and problems lists.

Qualitative tools assess the description and depth of family experiences. **Quantitative** tools measure the frequency with which behaviors or situations exist. Most survey tools emphasize either the qualitative or quantitative dimensions of family but usually contain elements of both. Friedman et al. (2003) have developed both a long form and a short form to qualitatively assess the roles and structure of the family and its members. Rowe Kaakinen et al. (2014) utilize the Family Systems Stressors-Strength Inventory, an instrument that elicits a numbered ranking of each family member's perception of the severity of stressors in selected categories. Wright and Leahey (2012) use the Calgary Family Assessment Model (CFAM) and combine this tool with the Calgary Family Intervention Model (CFIM) to provide a complete assessment and treatment map.

Before implementation of the selected assessment tool, agreements and sometimes written consents are obtained that relate to the confidentiality of the information sought, how it will be used, and what treatment options and referrals may be recommended. Before the assessment, it is important for the family to understand that the nurse is legally bound to mandatory reporting obligations in cases of abuse or violence and also that member safety remains a priority above all other interventions. Following these disclosures, or "ground rules," the family may choose to end the therapeutic relationship with the nurse before any information is shared.

Genogram and Ecomap

Family assessment usually begins with a simple diagram (of the family history) in the form of a **genogram** (Fig. 3-1). A genogram is a set of symbols that is used to illustrate the present family structure and compare generations within the same family. The genogram may be used to highlight generational influences of behaviors, illnesses, vocational information, or any other pertinent information that provides a larger picture of patterns that exert influence on the family's current situation. Dates of births, divorces, deaths, stillbirths, and other pertinent elements of family information are represented. A key to guide interpretation of the various symbols is included on the form. Depending on the situation, the nurse either assists the family in drawing the genogram or instructs them in producing a genogram that will be reviewed during the next assessment visit. To make the information more meaningful to the assessor, the genogram should include at least three family generations.

The nurse also helps the family create an ecomap. An ecomap is a tool that displays the various outside systems used by the family. An ecomap illustrates the relationship between the family as a whole system and the various systems with which the family most often interacts, including school, job, church, and other institutions (Fig. 3-2).

To create a family ecomap, the nurse inquires about schools, health-care agencies, employment, church, and other outside systems with which the family has routine interaction. Families may have closed boundaries with some systems and maintain open boundaries with others. For example, the parents may conduct home schooling yet contract with the public schools to provide their children with opportunities for extracurricular involvement. During the family assessment, the nurse looks for balance and self-regulation in the family system.

Strengths and Problems Lists

Early in the assessment process, the nurse asks the family to list their strengths (strengths list). The strengths list gives the family an opportunity to express the positive characteristics, or attributes, of their family as a whole and strengths that each member brings to the constellation. The family also creates a problems list, which identifies the difficult or negative characteristics. The family and the nurse collaboratively create both lists. The nurse can provide input based on observations related to the family's strengths and weaknesses but should not take over this process. In the therapeutic situation, the family must assume ownership of all identified strengths and problems so that they can participate fully during the assessment and treatment phases of the nursing intervention. The nurse

helps the family focus on major issues or problems that will form the starting point of intervention.

Next, the family makes a commitment with the nurse and appropriate referral agencies to participate in the mutually agreed on interventions. Depending on the situation, the family may be assisted in completion of the assessment tools, or the tools may be given to each member to complete and return at a later date. Usually, more tools are completed when the family is assisted with this task in the nurse's presence.

The nurse compiles and summarizes the information provided and discusses the results with the family. The initial assessment, which utilizes the selected assessment tools and surveys, is frequently completed within an hour and is then followed by daily or weekly conferences, depending on the setting and the time available. The follow-up conference provides an opportunity to review the assessment information and to identify progress made

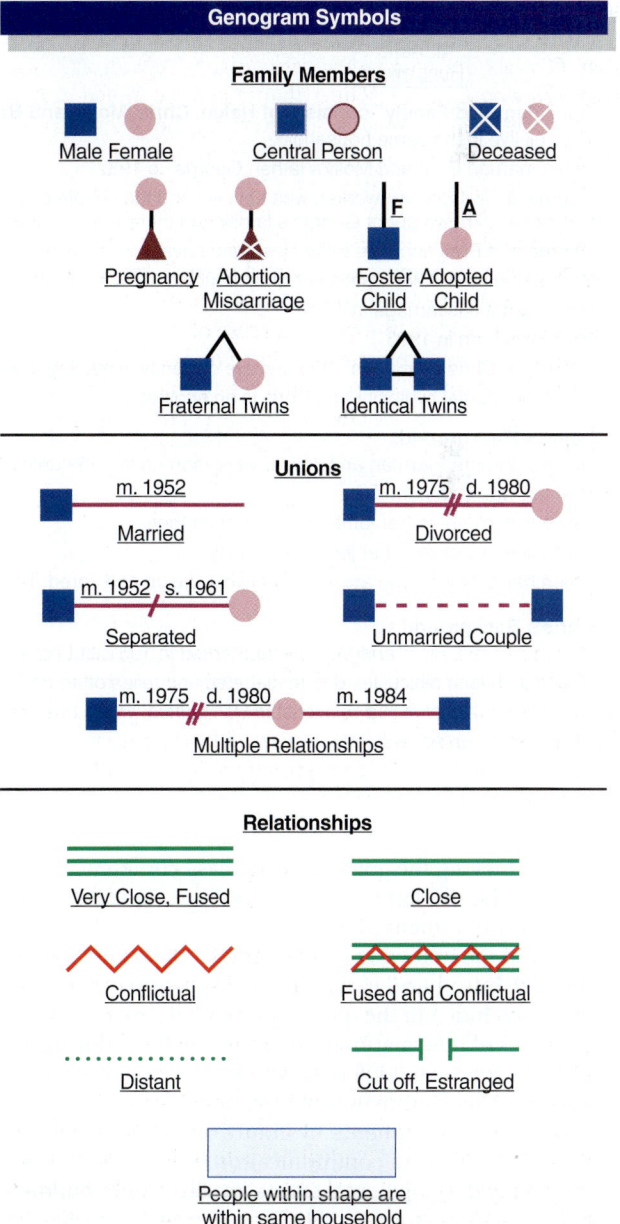

Figure 3-1 Example of a genogram template.

(continued)

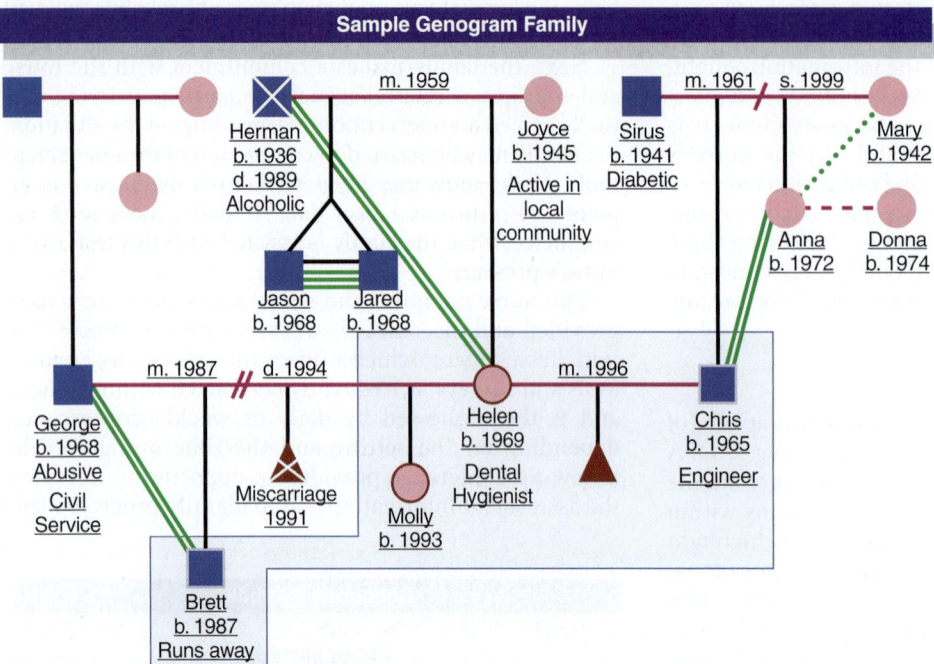

Sample Genogram Family

Our "Identified Family" consists of Helen, Chris, Molly, and Brett.
They all live in the same household.
Helen married Brett and Molly's father, George, in 1987.
George, a Civil Service worker, was abusive and the couple divorced in 1994.
Not much is known about George's family and there is little contact with Helen.
George and Brett continue to be close and have weekly visits.
Brett was born in 1987 and is currently troubled, running away often to his father George's house.
Helen had a miscarriage in 1991.
Molly was born in 1993.
Helen and Chris married in 1996 and are currently expecting their first child together.
Helen is a dental hygienist and Chris is an engineer.

Helen's Background:
Helen's parents, Herman and Joyce, were married in 1959 until Herman's death in 1989.
Herman was an alcoholic.
Helen was closer to her father than to her mother.
Joyce is very active in her local community.
Helen has brothers who are identical twins, Jason and Jared. They are very close.

Chris's Background:
Chris's parents, Sirus and Mary, were married in 1961, but have been separated since 1999.
Sirus has health difficulties due to diabetes and relies often on Chris to help him.
Chris' sister, Anna, is in a relationship with Donna, which has distanced her from their mother, Mary.
Chris is close to Anna.

Figure 3-1 (continued)

toward achieving the goals. During these conferences, the nurse and family agree on priority issues and begin to formulate a treatment plan.

Many of the following components of the family assessment were introduced earlier in the discussion of theories. They are included in the discussion that follows to demonstrate types of information that can be obtained during assessments conducted via observation, direct questioning, or through the administration of various assessment tools and surveys. Components of family assessment include but are not limited to communication, roles and relationships, family developmental stages, rituals, family-building activities, triangulation, and other concepts from selected theories.

COMPONENTS OF THE FAMILY ASSESSMENT

Assessment of Communication Patterns

Communication is how the family exchanges information, values, and emotional connection. The nurse assesses the type, frequency, and direction of communication among the family members. For example, the nurse seeks answers to questions such as, "What is the nature of the interpersonal messages—supportive or attacking?" "What emotional content is expressed?" "Who is sending and receiving the messages?" and "Are there any patterns of dominance or powerlessness?" In some situations, one family member may dominate the responses to the assessment. The nurse assesses whether the entire family agrees

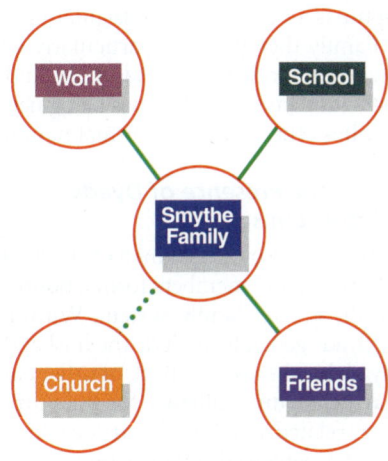

Key to Ecomap

Circles represent systems that interact with Smythe Family

Dotted line indicates strained relationship

Figure 3-2 Example of an ecomap.

with the information presented or if one member's point of view is ignored or suppressed. A family with addiction issues may present information cautiously and censure members who give information that indicates a problem.

The nurse looks for themes of emotional connectedness or isolation among the family members. There may also be clues that indicate the presence of family violence or neglect. In their interactions, the healthy family conveys a sense of connection and an appreciation of the family unit and of its individual members. The healthy family is open with problem identification and exploring coping patterns. There may also be clues that indicate the presence of family violence or neglect. Conversely, the unhealthy family tends to control or hide information or block access (of information) from other family members. The nurse should always conduct follow-up interviews with family members who were absent or not accessible during the initial interview.

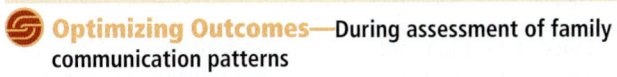

Optimizing Outcomes—**During assessment of family communication patterns**

During the family interview, the nurse should be cautious not to rely solely on information provided by family members. Often, dysfunctional communication patterns are suppressed as members attempt to present themselves most favorably. It is important to observe verbal and nonverbal communication with and *among* family members.

Assessment of Roles and Relationships

Roles and relationships are the job descriptions and connections of the individual family members. One or more family members assumes the responsibility of earning or obtaining money and resources, paying bills, providing meals, cleaning the living space, transporting family members, choosing entertainment and recreation activities, and promoting health and emotional security. The

nurse assesses (through observation and/or application of assessment tools/surveys) for the delegation of tasks that meet the family needs on a daily basis. Certain roles clearly fall in the domain of specific family members, such as the parent who pays the bills. Other roles may be more fluid, like the mother or older sister with a driver's license who take turns transporting the younger child to soccer practice. Relationships are usually clearly delineated: father, mother, brother, and sister. Relationships may also be self-declared or assigned. Examples of these types of relationships include brothers or cousins who are best friends or an oldest sibling who becomes the "boss" of younger siblings while the parents are away. Some roles and relationships are blended together: the mother who is also the nurturer; the father who is also the enforcer of rules. Roles and relationships should have an observable outcome on the family home/household.

 Nursing Insight—*Family roles, cultural influences, and maternity care*

When working with the childbearing family, nurses need to be aware that social class and cultural norms frequently affect the roles of various family members. The male's likelihood to participate in the childbearing experience, for example, is culturally influenced. Traditional Mexican and Arab families may view pregnancy and birth as events that are strictly "female affairs."

The nurse assesses the effectiveness of family roles by observing the condition of the house and living conditions (by conducting a home visit, if possible, or by obtaining the information during the interview), the clothing and personal hygiene of the family members. The nurse gathers other information to determine if family members are carrying out individual role assignments. There is much variation on how different family members meet their role requirements. For example, a single mother may need to seek public assistance to fulfill the provider role and obtain essential resources for her family. This process involves contacting various agencies, completing lengthy forms, waiting in lines, and engaging in other activities that can sometimes take as much time as working at a job to meet the family's needs. Fulfilling roles also encompasses the completion of tasks appropriate to each member's and the family's stage of development.

Assessment of the Family Developmental Stage

The Family Developmental Stage (Friedman et al., 2003; Rowe Kaakinen et al., 2014; Wright & Leahey, 2012) is the time in the family's life span that is focused on a particular age of a child or a specific family situation. This stage is assessed by means of the interview, the application of tools and surveys, and during observation of the family. At any given time, most families exist in simultaneous stages. They may be launching a high school graduate off to work or college and still have an infant (their child or grandchild) in the home. The family must accomplish a specific set of tasks for each stage. An infant requires feeding, changing, napping, and nurturing throughout the day. The high school graduate most likely needs assistance and support whether planning for college or making career choices. An extended living situation at home may be needed while a family member is in transition. The nurse assesses (by the observation of the presence or absence of resources and material goods such as clothing, food, and furniture appropriate to the family stage) that the family is successfully meeting the tasks for each stage or that they are obtaining appropriate assistance from outside resources (e.g., a student loan) to help meet their needs.

Assessment of Family Rituals

Family rituals consist of routines or activities that the family performs and teaches its members as a part of continuity and stability. Rituals encompass meal and bedtime routines, greeting and dismissing behaviors (a kiss goodbye or good night or a hello or a good-morning shout across the room), and observation of celebrations or terminations (birthdays or funerals). The nurse assesses (through observation and direct inquiry, or as guided by the assessment survey) for family member agreement on how important days are observed or if they are acknowledged at all. For example, birthday celebrations may be elaborate, informal, or summarily dismissed. Holiday presents may be opened before or during the holiday or not exchanged at all. Families may always or never share meals together.

 Nursing Insight—*Family-building activities, rules, mottos, and beliefs*

Family-building activities are an extension of rituals that center on recreation and leisure, such as family trips and vacations. Although a best friend may be invited to participate in some family events, a healthy family generally designates special "together time" that isn't open to non-family members. Family rules, mottos, and beliefs are the ways the family views itself and describes itself to others. "We always finish what we start" or "We stick together through thick and thin" are oft-used sayings that a family may identify with, whether or not they are consistent in holding to those beliefs. As a component of the assessment, the nurse can ask for three or four sayings or beliefs that the family feels are important in maintaining their family system. The nurse then asks for examples of responses to situations that illustrate or confirm this belief.

Assessment for Triangulation

Triangulation, assessed through family observation, occurs when two family members focus on or team up against a third family member to compensate for friction between the two members (Bowen, 1978; Rowe Kaakinen et al., 2014). Triangulation balances the family in a manner similar to how a furniture builder adds a third leg to balance a two-legged stool. The family reaches out or even attacks a third member or outside person as a way to decrease tension between two members and to obtain balance. For example, rather than blame one another for the child's asthma symptoms, the parents instead focus on seeking outside medical help for the condition. This scenario illustrates a positive use of triangulation.

Conversely, tobacco-using parents who focus on their child's asthma symptoms while ignoring their own tobacco addiction (and the unhealthy environment that accompanies it) illustrate a potentially negative triangulation. Two brothers who team up against the policeman called to break up their drunken dispute is an example of triangulating with an outside source. Family therapists are particularly vulnerable to triangulation when working with families, and they must learn to recognize when triangulation is being negatively used and teach families other strategies for maintaining stability.

Assessment for the Presence of Dyads and Other Subsystems

A dyad (Bowen, 1978; Rowe Kaakinen et al., 2014) is a structure in which two family members form a bond to become a subsystem of the greater family system. Within a family of four, existing dyads generally include the husband–wife dyad, father–son dyad, brother–sister dyad, or other combinations. The dyad may be a natural alliance for the purposes of intimacy or play or related activities. Dyads may form as siblings team up against a perceived unfair parental rule. The nurse observes for the presence of dyads and notes whether they are self-identified and whether a positive or negative impact on the family is known or acknowledged.

❝**What to say**❞—*Specific questions to ask during the family assessment*

To elicit family identifying data, the nurse may ask:

"Who in your family lives in your home?"

"What other family members live elsewhere?"

"What are the sources of income or other resources for your family?"

Questions to determine the family's developmental stage can include:

"What are the ages of the children in the family?"

"What jobs or tasks take up the most time in providing care for the children?"

Environmental data include information about the neighborhood of residence and local resources such as stores, schools, hospitals, and entertainment centers. Other questions are intended to elicit information concerning family structure ("Who makes decisions?"), function ("How are emotion and affection shown?"), and health care ("What health appointments are made and by whom?") (Friedman et al., 2003).

Once all pertinent information has been obtained and documented, the nurse elicits the family's assistance in prioritizing the most pressing and problematic issues. These issues are then addressed in the family treatment plan that forms the basis for all family-centered interventions. Depending on the specific situation, nursing interventions for families most often include referrals, education, and counseling.

 Optimizing Outcomes—With nursing interventions for families

Referrals may be made to support groups (e.g., Alcoholics Anonymous, Al-Anon, Gamblers Anonymous), physicians, social services, and mental health agencies. Education may center on the use of prescribed medications and therapies, nutrition, and family health promotion. When indicated, licensed professional counselors, nurse practitioners, psychologists, and family therapists provide in-depth family counseling.

Family-Centered Care

After the assessment process has been completed, the nurse selects all applicable nursing diagnoses and formulates the family care plan. The family's assistance is elicited to ensure that they are in agreement with the identified diagnoses. The nurse guides the family in writing mutually agreed-on goals that they will work on together. Diagnoses may be psychosocial, physiological, or both, and they may be focused on the individual or on the family (Box 3-1).

In the following discussion, the nursing diagnosis "Altered Family Processes" is presented and described in detail to illustrate the possible goals, interventions, and evaluation criteria that could be appropriate for families experiencing problems in their day-to-day functioning.

NURSING DIAGNOSIS: ALTERED FAMILY PROCESSES

This nursing diagnosis describes a family that experiences problems in their everyday functioning. Problems often center on communication issues or difficulties with member role fulfillment. In these situations, the family is in need of education and/or intervention to help them return to normal daily functioning. As an example, a family with an infant may not be communicating about sharing the new roles brought about by the baby's arrival. The mother feels resentful that the father is not helping more; the father senses the resentment but doesn't recognize what is wrong. The nurse identifies clues to tension in the relationship during well-baby checkups or perhaps even prior to discharge from the hospital.

GOAL: RETAIN/MAINTAIN OPEN LINES OF COMMUNICATION. The family will discuss feelings openly and nonjudgmentally with each other using "I feel" statements (Clark, 2008) and avoiding defensive communication techniques (Johnson & Johnson, 2012). All members will negotiate what it is they would want for the other member to understand about their feelings and needs.

GOAL: ADAPT TO CHANGES IN FAMILY PROCESS/SITUATION BY SHARING RESPONSIBILITIES. To meet this goal, various family roles need to be adjusted. For example, having an older sister help babysit the infant to give the mother more time for rest represents a family adaptation necessitated by a change in the home situation. After the birth of a baby, the father may need to take family leave so that he can share in child care. In another family, the mother-in-law may be asked to assume a more active role in assisting with newborn or child care.

GOAL: RESPECT THE INDIVIDUALITY OF EACH MEMBER'S ACTIONS. The family may need to allow a member to isolate from an event until he or she is able to handle the situation with the rest of the family. For example, it is developmentally appropriate for a teenager to want to continue with contact from friends while the family is experiencing a situational crisis.

GOAL: PARTICIPATE IN THE CARE OF INDIVIDUALS. The family needs to prioritize care for its sick or disabled members over lesser psychosocial needs such as having friends over for the school-aged children. All needs should be addressed eventually, but safety and physiological needs should be addressed first.

GOAL: SEEK/ACCEPT RESOURCES AS NEEDED. As a system, the family opens its boundaries to appropriate outside sources (e.g., the pediatrician, internist, and social worker or community health department) as needed to help provide appropriate health care for its members. Families with issues such as domestic violence often have difficulty trusting another system because of the fear of legal intervention. The family may have difficulty accepting help if they do not perceive or acknowledge the problem. The nurse may use a number of interventions to help the family obtain their goals under this nursing diagnosis.

The following are examples of applicable nursing interventions.

INTERVENTION: IDENTIFY FAMILY DYSFUNCTION AND THE FAMILY'S AWARENESS OF THE PROBLEM(S). As part of an ongoing collaborative process with the family, the nurse adds entries to the problems list as needed to keep the list current and applicable. The problems list is then reviewed during each nursing visit. For example, the nurse may recognize that the family does not use proper car safety seats for the younger children. Throughout the collaborative process, as problems are identified by a family member, the nurse assesses other members' understanding and willingness to participate in the proposed solutions.

Box 3-1 Examples of Family Nursing Diagnoses

Any NANDA diagnosis may be appropriate for describing an individual family member's health status. A family diagnosis is intended to describe the health status of the family as a whole. Examples of family diagnoses include the following:

Caregiver Role Strain (actual and risk for)
Dysfunctional Family Processes: Alcoholism
Family Coping: Compromised
Family Coping: Disabled
Impaired Parenting (actual and risk for)
Ineffective Family Therapeutic Regimen Management
Readiness for Enhanced Family Coping
Readiness for Enhanced Parenting
Risk for Parent-Infant-Child Attachment
Social Isolation
Spiritual Distress

NOC outcomes specifically for families as units are included in the NOC domain "Family Health." This category includes the following classes: Family Caregiver Status, Family Member Health Status, Family Well-Being and Parenting. Outcomes from other domains may also apply. *NIC interventions* for families as units are included in the NIC domain "Family." This category includes the following classes: Childbearing Care, Childrearing Care, and Life-Span Care.

Sources: Carpenito (2012); Wilkinson & Treas (2011).

INTERVENTION: GUIDE THE FAMILY THROUGH MEDICAL ADMISSIONS/ INTERVENTIONS. The nurse acts as the liaison with family member hospitalizations and other referrals. In this role, the nurse provides information about medical procedures, coordinates care with various community resources, and helps to clarify medical explanations to the family when one of the members receives medical assistance.

INTERVENTION: ASSESS THE IMPACT OF IDENTIFIED PROBLEMS ON THE STABILITY AND FUNCTIONING OF THE FAMILY. The nurse identifies roles or functions that are neglected by the family and helps the family adjust as they struggle to meet the health needs of members.

INTERVENTION: LISTEN ATTENTIVELY TO ALL MEMBERS. The nurse helps the family to identify the meaning of the dysfunction and assists the family in improving communication among its members.

INTERVENTION: SCHEDULE FAMILY CONFERENCES. Family conferences give all members an opportunity to express themselves and share in the family situation. This strategy is particularly important in an emergency hospitalization when the family members are not all initially involved in the decision making concerning treatments received. For example, a sister who arrives late from out of town may not initially understand the decision to withhold treatment in respect to advance directives.

INTERVENTION: IDENTIFY, REFER, AND INFORM THE FAMILY OF AVAILABLE RESOURCES. After hospitalization of a family member, the nurse may identify a social worker to assist with discharge plans and payment issues. In another situation, the nurse may serve as an advocate to help the family receive rehabilitative care for a member with a head injury.

INTERVENTION: DISCUSS ROLE CHANGES AND THEIR IMPACT ON FAMILY MEMBERS. A family situation may involve a sister caring for a parent with Alzheimer's disease who needs support and respite care to meet her own needs and those of her children. The nurse has the objectivity to identify the sister's needs and facilitate her communication of these needs to other family members.

Periodically, the nurse and family assess the extent to which the goals have been accomplished and the effectiveness of the nursing interventions. Adjustments in goals and interventions are made when necessary.

Evaluation

Expected outcomes may include the following:

- Effective communication takes place among family members in an assertive and nonthreatening manner that allows members' needs to be expressed and met.
- Family tasks and roles are appropriately distributed so that students attend school and employed members go to work, medical appointments are made and kept, and food and shelter are adequately provided.

Many other nursing diagnoses are applicable for the family experiencing health or social problems. For example, Family Coping: Potential for Growth is particularly useful for the family that is not experiencing health or social crisis but can still benefit from nursing education for improvement in selected areas.

Now Can You—Apply family nursing diagnoses to a family?

1. Identify two family nursing diagnoses that may be applied to a variety of situations?
2. List three goals for each nursing diagnosis identified?
3. List three nursing interventions for each nursing diagnosis identified?

Families With Special Needs

Sometimes families are in special need of nursing intervention because of situational or developmental crises that go beyond the family's internal resources. Situational crises include environmental disasters such as floods, hurricanes, or fires. The loss of a home, job, family member, or close friend are all unexpected and unplanned-for events that initially send the family into a state of chaos and often require outside help for the process of reorganization. Developmental crises occur as part of expected growth events that can take place during any developmental stage of the family or its individual members. Toddlerhood and adolescence are examples of two developmental stages that often disrupt family balance if no preparations were made in anticipation of the changing needs of the child and young teen.

Whether related to developmental stages or situational changes, certain events often require some level of intervention to help restore the family's balance and function, such as hospitalization, chronic mental illness, developmental disorders, substance abuse, sexual or physical abuse, posttraumatic stress disorder, chronic illness, and loss of a family member.

HOSPITALIZATION

The hospitalization of a family member often triggers a crisis that requires assistance and interventions from various outside sources. The scope of the family's needs is related to their resources, level of adaptability, and prior experience. In most situations, intervention includes treatment and education provided by the physician, care and additional education provided by the nurse, and discharge planning with community support arranged by designated hospital staff. Depending on the circumstance, the chaplain, social worker, community health nurse, and rehabilitation professional may all be members of the health-care team that assists in the transition from the hospital to the home or community facility. At times, the nurse is responsible for identifying and coordinating these resources to facilitate the patient's and family's transition and may initiate various other interventions.

CHRONIC MENTAL ILLNESS

A family with a member who has a chronic mental illness such as schizophrenia or bipolar disorder is a lifelong partner with the mental health system. This partnership can be therapeutic or antagonistic, depending on the resources available, the family's history in using these resources, and the amount of continuity that exists between the professionals and the families as they work together. The nurse's role is that of mediator/facilitator between the family system and the mental health system.

Establishing a diagnosis serves as the beginning point in helping the family to proceed with care for their family member. This task can be accomplished with the assistance of outpatient experts such as psychiatrists, social workers, psychologists, and advanced practice nursing specialists. Diagnostic work-ups are usually conducted as a team approach and most often involve an initial hospitalization for patient stabilization and medication. The family should be educated about prescribed medications, their side effects and planned treatments, and provided with information about financial resources such as Medicaid, Social Security, vocational rehabilitation, and other resources. The family is also in need of information and guidance concerning voluntary and involuntary commitment, guardianship, and other legal issues that often emerge as the illness progresses.

In many cases, problems with treatment are related to noncompliance or taking medications improperly (e.g., skipping doses or combining them with other substances). Sometimes the family assumes responsibility for the administration of medications for the family member. Another issue that often arises concerns an inability to pay for the medication. The nurse assists the family and/or family member in securing financial resources.

An important problem that should be addressed with families that have a mentally disabled member concerns social isolation. Social isolation is a situation that occurs when the ill family member is afraid or does not have the energy to participate in activities without continued prompting and encouragement by the family. Another potential problem involves nutritional deficit because of paranoia about harmful substances in the food or changes in eating habits related to depression. Certain medications are associated with weight gain, a problem that can lead to other health issues. Mental illness can also affect sleeping and rest patterns, and this problem is often associated with bipolar disease.

Special attention must be paid to the patient's suicidal potential and risk for harm to others. The nurse teaches the family to be especially vigilant when the patient is recovering from an immobilizing depression, an especially vulnerable time associated with newfound energy to carry out a plan. The person suffering from depression, bipolar disorder, or schizophrenia is also at risk when the normal impulse control becomes affected by influences such as drug or alcohol abuse or the rapid cycling associated with bipolar disorder. An important nursing role involves teaching the family techniques to assess for deficits, strategies for intervention, and recognizing when to call for assistance. Extended family should be recruited to help prevent caregiver strain by being available to help with the family member or offer respite care. Caregiver strain occurs when the main caregiver becomes overwhelmed and feels "under helped" in regard to the tasks concerned with the care of the family member. In this situation, mounting bitterness and withdrawal from other family members may cause caregivers to push away any potential helpers. Respite care occurs when someone else assumes the care of the sick family member to give the caregiver time off to rest.

Case Study The Family of a Young Adult With Schizophrenia

Ricky, age 24, was diagnosed with schizophrenia at the age of 16. His symptoms include paranoia, auditory hallucinations (hearing voices), and social isolation. He has been hospitalized several times over the years but his symptoms are currently stable on a newer antipsychotic medication. The family is willing for him to be discharged from the state hospital where he had been receiving treatment and come back home to live with them.

critical thinking questions

1. What information would the family require to be able to properly care for Ricky at home?

2. What are some of the resources the nurse should provide to help Ricky and his family cope with his illness?

◆ See Suggested Answers to Case Studies on Davis*Plus*.

SUBSTANCE ABUSE

Substance abuse negatively affects the family system. Family functions frequently become reorganized to sustain and cover up the addiction. If a parent is the substance abuser, parental roles are shifted to the other parent or to a child to provide meals, wash clothes, get the children to school, and call in sick for the affected parent. This process, termed enabling, is necessary for the addicted member to appear to be functioning normally. Sometimes another member of the family is so closely enmeshed with the affected member's addiction that he or she becomes codependent (Townsend, 2010). Although the codependent member may not be abusing substances with the addict, he or she is equally impaired through the continued cooperation in the addiction.

Often the remaining family members assume roles that help the addiction to continue. One child, usually the oldest, takes on the learned role of responsible child. This responsible child, who is either self-selected or is family assigned by default, takes over for the mother if she is drinking with the alcoholic partner or engaging in other enabling behaviors that make her unavailable to the family and makes sure the younger children are being cared for. The responsible child makes lunches, gets the siblings off to school and extracurricular activities, and may even help with paying the bills. The hero is another role that may evolve in children of families with an impaired member. The child in a hero role serves as the family standard-bearer, ready to proclaim that the family cannot really be impaired if it produced such a star. The hero is academically successful and excels in sports and other extracurricular activities.

Two additional roles that may be found in the substance- or alcohol-impaired family are the scapegoat and the lost child. The scapegoat is the opposite of the hero. The scapegoat fails at school and social activities and may have run-ins with the law for vandalism, shoplifting, or fighting at school. The family presents the scapegoat to the world with the message, "Look at what we have to endure! No wonder we have a difficult life!" The hero and the scapegoat are actually diversions for what is really happening to the family because of substance abuse. The lost child is a symptom of a family that is too chaotic to meet the needs of the child or notice the child at all. The lost child keeps a low profile at home and school and does not usually fail but also does not particularly stand out in anything, either.

Along with the family roles are family rules that are implicitly followed by all members, such as, "Don't talk and don't feel." Family members know not to discuss family problems with outsiders such as teachers, nurses, or even friends. Secrets are the hallmark of addictive families both for social and legal reasons. Family members also learn not to feel the disappointment or anger or sadness that the addiction causes them. Parents do not make it to the children's games or teacher conferences, or even to major events such as graduation. The children deny that the parent's lack of involvement impacts their feelings. If changes do not take place in these types of family systems, there is a great likelihood that the children will be socially and personally impaired, and a high percentage turns to substance abuse themselves (Townsend, 2010).

The nurse and the family with substance abuse/alcohol abuse must assess the amount, type, and length of time the addiction has been a part of the family. If the main substance abuser is actively engaged in treatment, the family should be referred to therapy or support groups such as Al-Anon that can help them to identify and change their own behaviors, wants, and needs apart from those of the alcoholic. If treatment is not obtained for the affected member, the nurse should refer family members to organizations such as Alcoholics Anonymous or to legal agencies that can identify options for getting the member into treatment or strategies for keeping the family safe from the member.

 Case Study The Family Members of an Alcoholic

A 9-year-old boy has been sent home from school several times for fighting. The father has a history of scrapes with the law related to public drunkenness and bar fights. The mother tells the school nurse that the father has been laid off at work and has a lot of issues on his mind to work through. She further states that the boy has been nothing but trouble and is an embarrassment to the family, unlike his sister, who is a junior high cheerleader and "straight A" student.

critical thinking questions

1. What roles are being played in this family?

2. What is the purpose of these roles?

3. What interventions would the nurse bring to this family?

◆ See Suggested Answers to Case Studies on Davis*Plus*.

SEXUAL OR PHYSICAL ABUSE

Sexual or physical abuse in the family is similar to substance abuse in how it affects the family system. In general, this problem can exist only in a family system that keeps secrets and creates specific roles that allow its continuance. When an incestuous father/child sexual relationship occurs, the mother or marital partner has taken on the role of either ignoring or covering up the abuse. In some situations, the mother feels threatened and acts as a sexual competitor (against the daughter) for the husband's affection.

In many cases, one person is singled out for the physical or sexual abuse. Other family members have a relatively normal relationship with the abuser and with one other. If the abused member is removed from the family, there may be a transfer of the behavior to another member.

In all situations, the nurse is legally obligated to report the abuse to the proper investigating agency. However, the nurse is not responsible for investigating or intervening with the family once the report has been made. When unsure, the nurse can verify suspicions of abuse with other treatment team members, but once the suspicions are confirmed, either the nurse, nursing supervisor, or treatment team leader is mandated to report the abuse. The nurse then makes a therapeutic alliance with the family unit (probably without the abuser) to help return them to normal roles and relationships. The nurse must remain vigilant for signs of continued abuse or violence with the remaining members or with the primary abuser if he (or she) is returned to the family.

? **Case Study** Family Elder Abuse

The nurse is conducting a home visit with an 85-year-old mother who is being cared for by her adult daughter. The daughter exhibits an attitude of detachment toward her mother. A general assessment of the elderly patient is remarkable for strong body odor, stained clothes, and an overall disheveled appearance. The mother is alert but hesitant to talk with the nurse and evasive with her answers. The daughter appears to be impatient and explains that she needs to go to the market.

critical thinking questions

1. What other assessment information would be needed to verify whether the patient was being neglected?

2. What steps should be taken if abuse or neglect is suspected?

◆ See Suggested Answers to Case Studies on Davis*Plus*.

POSTTRAUMATIC STRESS DISORDER

Posttraumatic stress disorder (PTSD) is an anxiety disorder that results from experiencing a catastrophic event such as rape, battering, accident, mugging, or war. The survivor or survivors of the traumatic event may experience nightmares and flashbacks (vivid re-experiencing of events while awake) and frequently develop a detached view of life. Involved families "lose" an active participant in their lives while the family member with PTSD vacillates between apathy and extreme vigilance and overprotectiveness. The affected family member may also turn to substance abuse in an attempt to dull the memories associated with the event (Lorth, 2011).

An entire family may experience PTSD after a shared event such as surviving a flood or tornado that destroyed everything and left them homeless. Often, symptoms do not appear for days or weeks following the event. The delay may result from the initial gestures of support provided by the family and the community. The nurse assesses for symptoms of PTSD during the interview, with questions focused on sleep disturbances or flashbacks of the traumatic event and the individual's inability to participate fully in the family's life. When identified, the family member(s) is referred for appropriate intervention. Alternately, the nurse may elicit the assistance of an expert trained in Critical Incident Stress Debriefing or who has experience with other proven techniques for treating survivors. Support groups are usually therapeutic in helping both the victim and the family ease the affected member back into their world.

CHRONIC PHYSICAL ILLNESS

Asthma, diabetes, and Crohn's disease are often viewed as medical conditions that are affected by psychological factors (Kneisl & Trigoboff, 2012) because of the strong emotionality involved. Although emotions do not cause these illnesses, they may exacerbate the symptoms by decreasing the family member's compliance with the treatment or by increasing the anxiety related to the symptoms. Families need to be educated about various aspects of daily care for members who experience chronic illness. For example, the nurse may teach about monitoring the diabetic family member's blood glucose analysis or self-administration of insulin or how to assist the asthmatic with inhalation therapy.

In some situations, a teenager may not fully accept his illness and choose not to take prescribed medications. This behavior often stems from a need to prove to self or others that he does not truly need the medications or treatment. An older adult living in the home may not fully understand the temporal demands associated with a medication schedule and may require additional teaching and close monitoring, especially if the medications have recently been changed. The nurse helps the family transition from dependence on the health-care worker to family member independence, although, depending on the circumstances, some supervision by the family may always be necessary. The family benefits through an ongoing partnership with a provider or clinic that enables them to receive progress reports, treatment updates, and needed medications. The nurse facilitates family empowerment by helping them to get the information necessary to provide continued support and treatment of their family member. To learn more about caring for the family with chronic physical illness, see Chapter 34.

DEATH OF A FAMILY MEMBER

The nurse is often the first point of contact when a family member has died in the hospital, or at home, if home nursing was involved in the member's care. The particular developmental stage affects the way in which each family member grieves. While the length of time that elapses between the stages of grief and the manifestations of grief vary, all family members grieve in some manner. Stages of grieving have been described by a number of theorists; several are presented in Table 3-1. The nurse provides time and space (family visiting room, chapel, or the patient's room) for the family to gather. The nurse also inquires about the family's preferences concerning participation in preparation activities before the arrival of the mortuary representatives. Some cultures and religions wish to ritually bathe and dress the body.

The family must also decide which members should be involved in the various tasks, and this decision is affected by the age or developmental level of the child or adult. For example, a developmentally challenged adult may need the same approach as a younger child. In most situations, viewing the deceased (after equipment such as tubes and drainage bags have been removed) helps family members of all ages accept that death has occurred. They can then begin the grieving process.

The nurse participates in the accepting/searching for answers stage that often occurs early during grieving by providing answers regarding the illness or procedures or treatments that were involved. As appropriate, the nurse may seek assistance from the physician, other members of the health-care team, or from other resources. The family's minister or hospital chaplain may be asked to offer spiritual support, provide counseling, and address concerns. The nurse may wish to participate in prayer led by the family's clergy or hospital chaplaincy. Providing a presence and remaining with the family as long as possible are often the best nursing approaches for the family that has experienced a loss. The nurse may also have an opportunity to advise family friends that a critical time for them to be available to the family is around the third or fourth week after the funeral, when the family is left to deal with the full impact of the loss (Wilkinson & Treas, 2011).

(?) Case Study The Family of a Diabetic Teen

Shelley is a 15-year-old with type 1 diabetes mellitus who presents periodically to the emergency department with a blood sugar level of greater than 300 mg/dL. The family states she has been snacking on foods not on her diet, is sporadic with her blood sugar testing, and inconsistent in the management of her sliding scale method of insulin administration. The nurse's conversation with Shelley reveals that Shelley is resentful of her illness and angry that she has to do things that "The other girls do not have to do."

critical thinking questions

1. In view of Shelley's developmental stage, what information should the nurse give to Shelley and her family regarding diabetes?

2. How would the information be presented differently if Shelley were 6 years old?

◆ See Suggested Answers to Case Studies on Davis*Plus*.

 Across Care Settings: **Family care in inpatient, outpatient, and hospice settings**

In hospital inpatient units, families should be oriented to visiting hours, waiting rooms, meals, and overnight accommodations. Nurses reinforce patient admission data such as advance directives and organ donation policies and encourage an open discussion between the patient and family to prevent confusion regarding who would act as the patient's agent to make decisions in the event of incapacity or death. Families often need assistance with medical information, billing information, and admission and discharge information. In pediatric units, families should be alerted to policies concerning staying with their sick child, and assistance should be offered in making arrangements for the care of other children. In long-term inpatient settings, families rely on visits, telephone calls, mail, and e-mail to stay in touch with members. In outpatient units, nurses can educate the family about strategies to enhance patient

Table 3-1 The Grieving Process as Described by Various Theorists

Kübler-Ross' Stages of Grieving	Rodebaugh's Stages of Grieving	Harvey's Phases of Grieving	Epperson's Phases of Grieving	Rando's Reactions of Bereaved Parents
Denial (shock and disbelief)	Reeling (stunned disbelief)	Shock, Outcry, and Denial (external response to loss)	High Anxiety (physical response to emotional upheaval)	Avoidance (confusion and dazed state, avoidance of reality of loss)
Anger (toward God, relatives, the health-care system)	Feelings (emotionally experiencing the loss)	Intrusion of thoughts, distractions, and obsessive reviewing of the loss (internal response, isolation)	Denial (protective psychological reaction)	Confrontation (intense emotions, anger, sadness, feeling the loss)
Bargaining (trying to attain more time, delaying acceptance of the loss)	Dealing (taking care of details, taking care of others)	Confiding in others to emote and cognitively restructure (integration of internal thoughts and external actions to move on)	Anger (directed inwardly, toward another family member, or toward others)	Reestablishment (intensity declines, and the parents resume their lives)
Depression (feelings of sadness, regret, fear, and uncertainty indicate the griever has begun to accept the situation)				
Acceptance (readiness to move forward with newfound meaning or purpose in one's own life)	Healing (recovering and reentering life)		Remorse (feelings of guilt and sorrow)	
			Grief (overwhelming sadness)	
			Reconciliation (adaptation to existing circumstances)	

recovery, reinforce discharge instructions, and provide written information about follow-up visits.

In home health and hospice settings, the nurse assists the family in reaching a comfortable balance between direct involvement in the family member's care and respite time for family-building activities with other members. Demystifying medical procedures such as medication administration, catheterization, and tube feeding empowers the family to decide what they can do and how and when to seek assistance from the nurse and other care staff.

 Now Can You—Identify and plan care for special problems and issues faced by the American family?

1. List eight special problems that may be experienced by families?
2. Identify various nursing roles and interventions appropriate for these families?
3. Describe the nurse's role when abuse is suspected?

Family Cultural Characteristics

An understanding of the prevailing concepts of acculturation, assimilation identity, time, connectedness, communication, and social class facilitates the nursing assessment and guides the application of interventions within different cultural frameworks. To enhance understanding of the concepts, it is

helpful to examine characteristics of the "typical" American family. General comparisons with selected cultural groups provide the nurse with a starting point for understanding and interacting with families in a culturally appropriate way.

ACCULTURATION AND ASSIMILATION

The American family exhibits many variations owing to its unique blending with other cultures. The rich cultural heritage that has evolved from the mixing of various ethnic groups that compose the American family constitutes the hallmark of this relatively new culture. **Acculturation** describes the changes in one's cultural pattern to match those of the host society (Spector, 2012). The changes occur within one group or among several groups when individuals from different cultures come into contact with one another. Certain characteristics of the primary culture may be retained, while other practices of the dominant cultural society are adopted. For example, culturally influenced customs and traditions such as food choice and preparation, language patterns, and health practices are usually retained for long periods of time. **Assimilation** is the process in which the family loses its unique cultural identity and identifies instead with the prevailing or dominant culture (Spector, 2012).

IDENTITY

The identity (how the family views itself) of the American family is related to whether the family aligns itself with a particular ethnic group (e.g., Italian American and Irish American) or instead only sees itself as "American." Identifying with a particular ethnic group usually involves adopting that group's world view or approach to life. Anglo-Americans, for example, view themselves as independent individuals often separate from families (Friedman et al., 2003). Other cultures (e.g., Hispanic, Asian, and Pacific Islander) consider individuals in the context of family members and place less of an emphasis on who they are as individuals (Wilkinson & Treas, 2011).

The American family may influence a member's choice of occupation but usually to a lesser degree than that found in some cultures. For example, in earlier times, the English names of "Butcher" and "Baker" reflected a family occupation and set of expectations. In general, an American child is free to choose a career based on personal preferences and talents that have been developed in outside systems such as school, church, or extracurricular activities rather than one exclusively imposed by the family.

Time orientation is a concept that refers to whether the family views itself to be strongly connected to previous generations. The American family tends to be focused on the present and future much more so than many cultures. This current-future time orientation may be related to the relative newness of America as a country, as compared with an ancient civilization such as China. In the American family, the individual is expected to be punctual and conform to deadlines at school and work. Making future plans by saving money or pursuing higher education is also valued. Many industrialized countries share a present and future time orientation, while other countries value a slower pace with greater emphasis on the connection to the past in terms of ancestors and traditional beliefs (Friedman et al., 2003; Townsend, 2010).

CONNECTEDNESS

Connectedness is a concept that emphasizes who the family identifies with and relates to as family members. Some American families and many other cultures highly value and place great importance on the inclusion of grandparents, aunts, uncles, and cousins in their family circle. That level of extended connectedness may also include the community, especially if other members of the same ethnic group live in the neighborhood. In some American families, members spend more time commuting to outside interests than engaging in neighborhood and home-based family activities.

COMMUNICATION PATTERNS

Patterns of communication vary according to ethnic group. Cultural customs often guide selection of the family member who will be designated as the primary historian in a health-care interview. American families tend to be more fluid and open in designating which member speaks to outsiders, although legal contracts most often favor the parents. Other cultures (e.g., Hispanic families from Mexico) may be more patriarchal (male dominant) or matriarchal (female dominant), and the caregiver role may rely heavily on a grandparent or aunt rather than the parents. The designated caregiver is usually the communicator in the health-care setting. When planning interventions, it is important to consider the cultural role of the family member who makes the primary decisions (Wilkinson & Treas, 2011).

 Nursing Insight—*Culture, communication, and emotional expression*

Culture is the essence of what defines us as people. Gaining an understanding of culture gives insights into family patterns of human interaction as well as expressions of emotion (Munoz & Luckmann, 2005).

The American family member is more likely to speak on her own behalf in public situations such as in schools and health-care settings and is encouraged (within legal limits) to do so. Language other than American English often contains built-in formal and informal variations of words intended to convey respect to parents and elders, who frequently serve as spokespersons in settings such as hospitals and physicians' offices.

SOCIOECONOMIC CLASS

Social class refers to occupation and economic status. In America, status is related to social and economic variables, and mobility between the different classes is more fluid than in some countries. Religious and political influences significantly influence how the family interacts and responds to outside systems such as schools and community health programs. For example, some religious groups advocate home, rather than public schooling; political and religious orientation often shapes family beliefs about abortion or birth control. Other values are influenced by the prevailing societal view. For example, the contemporary American family tends to value its members according to the individual's line of work and educational achievements rather than the family's identity (Rowe Kaakinen et al., 2014).

HOLISTIC NURSING ENCOMPASSES A CULTURALLY SENSITIVE FAMILY APPROACH

Family assessment is integral to the delivery of competent, appropriate, holistic care. For most nurses, developing a knowledge base that is sensitive to the cultural variations of structure and function in the American family presents a personal challenge. Awareness of personal perceptions and values that may negatively impact therapeutic interactions with families is a professional responsibility. Nurses at every level of preparation and throughout their professional careers must engage in an ongoing process of developing and refining attitudes and behaviors that will promote culturally competent care (Taylor, 2005). The professional nurse grows in cultural competence by seeking more knowledge through review of literature and evidence-based practice, attendance at cultural seminars, and exposure to other cultures in a variety of settings. The more we learn about other cultures, the more we learn about ourselves as nurses and as human beings.

 Now Can You—Recognize cultural differences that may impact the nursing assessment and interventions with the family?

1. Identify "typical" characteristics of the American family related to time and goal orientation?
2. Explain how culture influences the family's degree of connectedness and patterns of communication in the health-care setting?

3. Describe adjustments the nurse may make to heighten cultural awareness and enhance a culturally appropriate family assessment and intervention?

Summary Points

◆ The competent nurse views the family as a focus of care, not as an inconvenient intrusion into the nursing routine.

◆ While family structure has undergone dramatic changes over the past 60 years, the importance of family has not diminished.

◆ Family theories and models give the nurse a reference point from which to analyze the information obtained from a family assessment.

◆ The nursing process is applicable and appropriate to guide nursing interventions with the family.

◆ The family nurse possesses an understanding of the norms related to roles, relationships, developmental stages, and family functioning and uses this information to guide the family assessment and plan appropriate interventions.

◆ The nurse recognizes special needs that affect family functioning and applies strategies to assist the family in the fulfillment of healthy roles and relationships.

◆ Culture is the context by which family behavior is understood.

◆ Working with families in the home and in community health-care settings is a challenging and rewarding aspect of nursing.

Review Questions

Multiple Choice

1. A nurse is taking a history from a woman and her common-law husband. What is the best description of this type of family?
A. Family
B. Family of origin
C. Family of choice
D. Extended family

2. An obstetric nurse understands and works within the systems theory of family interaction. This nurse is aware that an integral part of the nursing role is to facilitate the development of a bond between the
A. new subsystem of mother/infant and the father.
B. subsystem of mother/father and the new infant.
C. subsystem of mother/father/infant and extended family.
D. new subsystem of mother/infant and significant others.

3. The pediatric nurse understands and works within the developmental theory of families. According to this theory, which information would be most important to provide to families with preschool children?
A. Injury prevention and immunizations
B. Sibling rivalry
C. Sleep-wake patterns
D. Couple-building and family adjustment

4. The clinic nurse is providing assistance to a family who lost their son in a motorcycle collision. Future planning would include counseling the family that one of the most critical times in the grieving process usually takes place in the
A. first two weeks.
B. third to fourth week.
C. fifth to sixth week.
D. eighth to tenth week.

5. A nurse is working with a family whose members appear cold and distant toward each other. None of the family members seems able to manage stress. Which familial role has not been met by this family?
A. Affective and coping needs
B. Economic needs
C. Physical needs
D. Socialization needs

6. A nurse is planning interventions to assist a family that has had a death in the immediate family group. The nurse is helping other family members to take on some of the roles left by the deceased person. Under which family theory is this nurse working?
A. Communication Theory
B. Family Developmental Stages and Theory
C. Family Systems Theory
D. Structural-Functional Theory

7. A nurse is planning to assess a family using a standardized tool. Before beginning the assessment, which action by the nurse is most important?
A. Ensure the family that the nurse will maintain strict confidentiality of all data.
B. Inform the family that all assessments will be shared with the health-care team.
C. Instruct the family on the various types of tools available for use.
D. Obtain agreements over the confidentiality of the information obtained.

8. A nurse has assessed a family that has difficulty with communication and blurring of roles, affecting daily function. Which nursing diagnosis best fits this situation?
A. Altered Family Processes
B. Caregiver Role Strain
C. Readiness for Enhanced Coping
D. Situational Family Dysfunction

9. A patient admitted to the hospital is from a culture with which the nurse is unfamiliar. The patient has limited English skills. The patient needs surgery but will not consent until her oldest son arrives. Which action by the nurse is best?
A. Describe all the complications that can occur if the operation is delayed.
B. Make the patient as comfortable as possible while waiting for the son.
C. Teach the patient about the value of autonomy in American health care.
D. Using an interpreter, attempt to convince the patient to consent.

10. A nurse is working with a patient who became critically ill and was admitted emergently. The patient's large family is coming to the hospital from several different states over several different days. Which of the following would be the best intervention to promote family cohesion and function?

A. Arrange for visitation by the hospital or family clergy member.

B. Ask the family to appoint a single spokesperson who will get all information.

C. Create a visitation schedule so that the nurses are not overwhelmed by the family.

D. Schedule a family conference when all family members have arrived.

See Answers to End of Chapter Review Questions on Davis*Plus*.

REFERENCES

American Association of Retired Persons (AARP). (2013). Grandfacts: State fact sheets for grandparents and other relatives raising children. Retrieved from http://www.aarp.org/relationships/friends-family/grandfacts-sheets/

Bowen, M. (1978). A classic! *Family therapy in clinical practice*. New York, NY: Jason Aronson.

Carpenito, L. (2012). *Handbook of nursing diagnosis* (14th ed.). Philadelphia, PA: Lippincott Williams & Wilkins.

Centers for Disease Control and Prevention (CDC). (2011). U.S. adult mental illness surveillance report. Retrieved from http://www.cdc.gov/Features/MentalHealthSurveillance/

Child Trends DataBank. (2011). Family structure and living arrangements. Retrieved from http://www.childtrendsdatabank.org/?q=node/231

Clark, C. (2008). *Group Leadership Skills for Nurses and Health Professionals*. (5th ed.). New York, NY: Springer Publishing Company.

Covey, S. R. (2006). *The 7 habits of highly effective families*. New Delhi, India: B. Jain Publishers.

Friedman, M. R., Bowden, V. R., & Jones, E. (2003). *Family Nursing: Research, theory and practice* (5th ed.). Upper Saddle River, NJ: Prentice-Hall.

George, J. B. (2010). *Nursing theories: The base for professional nursing practice* (6th ed.). Upper Saddle River, NJ: Prentice-Hall.

Hockenberry, M. (2012). Family influences on child health promotion. In M. J. Hockenberry & D. Wilson, *Wong's Essentials of Pediatric Nursing* (9th ed., pp. 23-41). St. Louis, MO: C.V. Mosby.

Johnson, D., & Johnson, F. (2012). *Joining together: Group theory and group skills* (11th ed.). Upper Saddle River, NJ: Pearson Publishing.

Kneisl, C., & Trigoboff, E. (2012). *Contemporary psychiatric-mental health nursing* (3rd ed.). Upper Saddle River, NJ: Pearson Prentice Hall.

Lorth, P. (2011). Understanding PTSD in Cambodian survivors: Implications for primary care. *The American Journal for Nurse Practitioners, 15*(7/8), 10–17.

Munoz, C., & Luckmann, J. (2005). *Transcultural communication in nursing* (2nd ed.). Clinton Park, NY: Thompson Delmar Learning.

Newport, F. (2012). Gallup: Mississippi is most religious U.S. State. Retrieved from http://www.gallup.com/poll/153479/Mississippi-Religious-State.aspx?ref=more

Rosenfeld, M. J. (2010). Nontraditional families and childhood progress through school. *Demography, 47*(3), 755–775.

Rowe Kaakinen, J., Padgett Coehlo, D., Steele, R., Tabacco, A., & Harmon Hanson, S. M. (2014). *Family health care nursing: Theory, practice, and research* (5th ed.). Philadelphia, PA: F.A. Davis.

Spector, R. E. (2012). *Cultural diversity in health and illness* (8th ed.). Upper Saddle River, NJ: Prentice Hall.

Taylor, R. (2005). Addressing barriers to cultural competence. *Journal for Nurses in Staff Development, 21*(4), 135–142.

The Bowen Center for the Study of the Family. (2013). *Bowen Theory*. Retrieved from http://www.thebowencenter.org/pages/theory.html

Townsend, M. (2010). *Essentials of psychiatric mental health nursing: Concepts of care in evidence-based practice* (5th ed.). Philadelphia, PA: F.A. Davis.

U.S. Census Bureau. (2012). Households and families: 2010 Census. Retrieved from http://www.census.gov/prod/cen2010/briefs/c2010br-14.pdf

U.S. Department of Health and Human Services (USDHHS). (2011). *Healthy People 2020*. Retrieved from http://www.healthypeople.gov/2020/topicsobjectives2020/default.aspx.

Wilkinson, J. M., & Treas, L. S. (2011). *Fundamentals of nursing: Theory, concepts & applications* (2nd ed.). Philadelphia, PA: F.A. Davis.

Wilson, D., Hockenberry-Eaton, M., Winkelstein, M. L., & Schwartz, M. (2001). *Wong's essentials of pediatric nursing*. St. Louis, MO: C.V. Mosby.

Wright, L., & Leahey, M. (2012). *Nurses and families* (6th ed.). Philadelphia, PA: F.A. Davis.

CONCEPT MAP

The Evolving Family

Family Theories/Models:
Guide Holistic Nursing Care
- Family systems theory
- Developmental theory: family stages
- Structural-functional theory
- Communication theory
- Group theory
- Bowen's Family Systems theory
- Nursing theories: Florence Nightingale; King, Roy; Neuman; Friedman; Hansen: Calgary Family model

Family Stressors:
- Health-care access
- Insurance/lack of
- Homelessness
- Catastrophic events
- Societal pressures:
  - Crime, suicide, AIDS
- Changing family structure
- "Skip" generation responsibilities

Family with Special Needs:
- In situational crises
  - Disasters, losses
- Developmental crises
  - e.g., adolescence
- Hospitalization
- Chronic mental illness
- Substance abuse
- Physical/sexual abuse
- PTSD
- Chronic physical illness
- Death of a member

Family Cultural Characteristics:
- Acculturation and assimilation
- Identity
- Time orientation
- Connectedness
- Communication
- Social class

Guides Nursing Assessment and Interventions

Nursing Insight
Family Configurations:

No-parent

Cohabitation/domestic partnership

Commune

Married blended

Single parent

Married parent

Homosexual

Nuclear and Extended

Family
Patient

Family of origin

- Two or more members
- Self-identify as family
- Interact/depend on each other: socially, emotionally, financially

Cultural Diversity:
- Pattern of family structure influenced by culture
- Recent immigrants may only be receptive to info from person in their cultural community
- Styles of communication vary by culture

Family of choice

Nursing Assessment of Families;
Concepts; Components; Factors
that Influence Structure
- Family size/structure: roles and relationships
- Parenting styles
- Communication styles/patterns
- Religious orientation/beliefs/affiliation
- Ethnicity/culture
- Socioeconomic status
- Developmental stage of the family
- Family rituals/rules/mottos/beliefs
- Family-building activities
- Family dyads/subsystems
- Triangulation within the family

Assessment Tools: Family Assessment
- Discuss legalities and ground rules prior to using
- Family Systems Stressors-Strengths Inventory
- Calgary Family Assessment Model
- Genogram and Ecomap

Potential Nursing Interventions: Family-Centered Care
Dx: Altered Family Processes
- Identify family dysfunction/family's awareness
- Guide family through medical admissions/interventions
- Assess impact of problems on family stability/functioning
- Listen attentively to all members
- Schedule family conferences
- Identify resources and refer
- Discuss role changes and impact on family members
Evaluation: Outcomes may include effective family communication patterns; appropriate distribution of family tasks and roles

Now Can You:
- Discuss contemporary family changes/stressors
- Discuss family theory for nursing practice
- Apply family nursing diagnoses to a family
- Identify families with special needs/distinct cultures

chapter

4

Caring for Women, Families, and Children Across the Life Span

 The secret of health for both mind and body is not to mourn for the past, not to worry about the future, or not to anticipate troubles, but to live the present moment wisely and earnestly.

—The Buddha

LEARNING TARGETS *At the completion of this chapter, the student will be able to:*

◆ Determine appropriate timing for health screening examinations based on national recommendations.

◆ Discuss health promotion and disease prevention strategies related to infants and children, including nutrition, dental care, safety, activity, immunizations, and sexuality.

◆ Discuss health promotion and disease prevention strategies related to adolescents, including nutrition, dental care, safety, health promotion screening, sexual behavior, and menstrual disorders.

◆ Discuss health promotion and disease prevention strategies related to young adults, including safety, health promotion screening, and gynecological disorders.

◆ Discuss health promotion and disease prevention strategies related to middle-aged adults, including health promotion screening, perimenopause, menopause, and gynecological disorders.

◆ Discuss health promotion and disease prevention strategies related to older adults, including health promotion screening, gynecological disorders, prostate cancer, and mental and emotional health.

PICO(T) Questions

The intent of evidence-based practice (EBP) is to provide nursing care that integrates the best available evidence. An initial step in EBP is to write a PICO(T) question that effectively guides the research. A PICO(T) question is an acronym that stands for population (P), intervention or issue (I), comparison of interest (C), outcome (O), and time-frame (T). Depending on the question, all or some of the question components are used in the research process. Use

these PICO(T) questions to spark your thinking as you read the chapter.

1. Does it make a difference in (O) the ability for (P) infants to (I) learn to self soothe if they are (C) breastfed versus bottle-fed?

2. Is there a (O) greater impact on the rate of sexually transmitted infections (STIs) in (P) high school students after (I) an educational program if presented to (C) a coed group versus a same-sex group?

Evidence-Based Practice

Cassidy, B., & Schlenk, E. A. (2012). Uptake of the human papillomavirus vaccine: A review of the literature and report of a quality assurance project. *Journal of Pediatric Health Care, 26*(2), 92–101.

The purpose of this descriptive study was to review predictors of knowledge about human papillomavirus (HPV) as found in previous studies and to compare previously collected HPV vaccine dose completion data. Earlier research has supported the notions that higher levels of education, Caucasian race, personal experience with cervical cancer, knowledge of the risks associated with acquiring HPV, and having been educated about HPV and the HPV vaccine were associated with increased knowledge levels and higher rates of vaccine completion. Concerns related to receiving the vaccine were noted to include the cost of the medication, the young age of the girls, a fear of adverse reactions to the vaccine, and a fear of promoting early sexual activity. Research has also reported higher HPV prevalence rates among non-Hispanic Black women.

The convenience sample was composed of 195 patients in a private, urban, pediatric practice well-child clinic who were scheduled for well-child or episodic visits. One hundred fifty-three of the participants were between the ages of 12 and 17; 42 participants were between the ages of 18 and 21.

Data were collected through computer query and chart review. Of the 195 participants, a total of 189 received the HPV vaccine according to the following schedule: 72% (n=110) of the younger group and 79% (n=33) of the older group during a scheduled well-child visit, and 24% (n=46) scheduled for an episodic visit. Of the girls who received the initial HPV vaccine dose, 63.5% (n=120/189) completed the full three-dose series and 66.7% (n=80/120) did so within 12 months.

The researchers found that, in this study, HPV vaccine rates were higher than those reported by the Centers for Disease Control and Prevention (CDC). The CDC reported the HPV vaccine rate in 2007 to be 25.1% in girls ages 13 to 17 years of age. This rate increased modestly to 37.2% in 2008. The researchers indicated that the three-dose completion rate of 66.7%, although only moderate, compares with a 17.9% rate reported by the CDC. While predictors of knowledge were not formally measured in this study, the researchers concluded from a review of previous studies that race, level of education, costs, experience with cancer, and knowledge of risks were all factors associated with vaccine completion rates.

1. How is this information useful to clinical nursing practice?

2. Based on these findings, what are implications for further research?

See Suggested Responses for Evidence-Based Practice on Davis*Plus*.

Introduction

This chapter focuses on health promotion and disease prevention across the life span. Health promotion refers to the advancement of health to the highest degree possible for an individual. Disease prevention focuses on the implementation of strategies to reduce the incidence of disease or the development of comorbid illnesses in individuals with existing diseases. Health promotion has become a focus of health care since the advent of managed care. *Healthy People 2000* identified areas of priority for people of all ages regarding health promotion, which have been updated in *Healthy People 2020* and include physical activity, control of overweight and obesity, responsible sexual behavior, and immunization (U.S. Department of Health and Human Services [USDHHS], 2011).

Health assessment and health promotion screening are perhaps the most important aspects related to promotion of health and prevention of disease. For women, this includes breast cancer screening and pelvic examinations on a recommended basis. For men, it is important to encourage screening for testicular and prostate cancer. Colorectal cancer screening should be routinely performed on all adults.

Nurses are perfectly situated to provide anticipatory guidance in areas of health promotion, thereby making accurate information available to family members. With all of the health information currently available in popular magazines, television programming, advertisements, and the Internet, patients do not always have the backgrounds to separate accurate information and practices from propaganda. A solid foundation in anatomy, physiology, sociology, and psychology, along with knowledge of current health promotion research, enables nurses to provide accurate patient information in the areas of nutrition, physical activity, stress management, and safer sexual practices.

Nurses assume many roles when caring for families. Theory-driven knowledge, experiential understanding, and evidence-based clinical practice are essential tools that enable nurses to teach patients at a variety of age and developmental levels. In the areas of infant and child health, major health promotion concerns include nutrition, safety, activity and play, and immunizations.

Adolescents can be considered to be relatively healthy individuals. As such, health promotion for this age group is often ignored. Because peer relationships constitute an important component of adolescent development, peer pressure can precipitate high-risk behaviors that may lead to health complications and the early initiation of chronic illnesses. Nurses play a vital role in the education of adolescents in health-care settings and in the community. A holistic approach is tremendously beneficial with this patient population. Teaching healthy practices regarding nutrition, safety, health screening, and safe sexual practices and sexual health can provide avenues for improvement in health practices that can last a lifetime.

During young adulthood, there continue to be health concerns related to nutrition and safety. However, the primary focus of health promotion for this population shifts to reproductive concerns, because this is the time when many patients are engaging in more mature relationships, marriage, and childbearing. For women, gynecological disorders including infertility may be diagnosed, requiring additional education for maintaining health and preventing complications.

Health screening is essential for patients in middle adulthood. For this age group, health promotion screening includes mammography, colonoscopy, cholesterol and lipid screening, and osteoporosis screening. While gynecological disorders are still a major health concern for women, reproductive health begins to concentrate on the period preceding menopause, known as perimenopause, with interest targeted on the physiological and psychological changes that occur, the hormone therapy debate, and the use of complementary and alternative therapies for symptom relief.

Older adults experience physical and psychological changes caused by the aging process. These changes shift health promotion concerns for older adults, including concerns related to sexual functioning, exercise and activity, and cognitive functioning. Gynecological topics that nurses should address for women include menopause, osteoporosis, cancer, and pelvic floor dysfunction.

Health Promotion Screening

Health screening is essential for all family members. Recommendations for examinations, laboratory, and diagnostic tests have been developed by diverse professional and community agencies. Guidelines for addressing high-priority services through preventive screening delivery have been developed and are presented in Table 4-1.

Table 4-1 Preventive Services Delivery Schedule: High-Priority Services			
Service	**19–39 Years**	**40–64 Years**	**65+ Years**
Aspirin Prophylaxis	Discuss with women ages 55–79 years, men over age 40, and younger individuals at increased risk for coronary heart disease. The benefits of stroke prevention must outweigh the harm of gastrointestinal bleeding.		
Breast Cancer Screening	Periodic mammogram for high-risk groups (women who have had breast cancer or who have a first-degree relative or multiple other relatives who have a history of premenopausal breast or breast and ovarian cancers; Clinical breast exam every 1–3 years ages 20–39 (ACOG, 2011e)	Mammogram every year beginning at age 40; clinical breast exam every year (ACOG, 2011e)	Annual mammogram, clinical breast exam every year (ACOG, 2011e)
Cervical Cytology Screening	First Pap test at age 21; then every 2 years Age 30 or older: Option 1: Screen every 3 years after 3 consecutive negative test results with no history of cervical intraepithelial neoplasia (CIN) 2 or 3, immunosuppression, HIV infection, or diethylstilbestrol (DES) exposure in utero; or Option 2: Screen every 3 years after negative human papillomavirus DNA test and negative cervical cytology (ACOG, 2010a)	Pap test every 3 years after 3 consecutive negative results if no history of cervical intraepithelial neoplasia (CIN) 2 or 3, immunosuppression, HIV infection, or diethylstilbestrol (DES) exposure in utero, or every 3 years after negative human papillomavirus DNA test and negative cervical cytology (ACOG, 2011a)	Consider discontinuing Pap test at age 65 years or 70 years if patient has had 3 or more normal results in a row, no abnormal results in 10 years, no history of cervical cancer, no history of diethylstilbestrol (DES) exposure in utero, is HIV negative, is not immunosuppressed; if cervical cytology has been discontinued, annual review of risk factors to evaluate need for reinitiation of screening. If cervical cytology is needed: may screen every 3 years after 3 consecutive negative test results if no history of cervical intraepithelial neoplasia (CIN) 2 or 3, immunosuppression, HIV infection, or diethylstilbestrol (DES) exposure in utero or every 3 years after negative human papillomavirus DNA test and negative cervical cytology (ACOG, 2011a)
Bone Mineral Density Screening			In the absence of new risk factors, screen no more frequently than every 2 years
Chlamydia and Gonorrhea Screening	All sexually active females, including asymptomatic women aged 25 years and younger; for patients ages 13–18 years, urine-based sexually transmitted disease screening is an efficient means for accomplishing such screening without a speculum examination (ACOG, 2011a)		
Colorectal Cancer Screening	Patients ages 13–18 years: only those with a family history of familial adenomatous polyposis or 8 years after the start of pancolitis. Patients ages 19–49 years: only high-risk groups (colorectal cancer or adenomatous		Beginning at age 50 years: colonoscopy (preferred method) every 10 years for all persons. Other methods include: (a) fecal occult blood testing or fecal immunochemical test, annual patient-collected (fecal occult

(continued)

Table 4-1   Preventive Services Delivery Schedule: High-Priority Services (continued)

Service	19–39 Years	40–64 Years	65+ Years
Colorectal Cancer Screening (continued)	polyps in first-degree relative younger than age 60 years or in two or more first-degree relatives of any ages; family history of familial adenomatous polyposis or hereditary nonpolyposis colon cancer; history of colorectal cancer, adenomatous polyps, inflammatory bowel disease, chronic ulcerative colitis, or Crohn's disease) (ACOG, 2011e)		blood testing and fecal immunochemical testing require 2 or 3 samples of stool collected by the patient at home and returned for analysis). A single stool sample obtained by digital rectal examination is not adequate for the detection of colorectal cancer); (b) flexible sigmoidoscopy every 5 years; (c) double contrast barium enema every 5 years; (d) computed tomography colonography every 5 years; and (e) stool DNA (ACOG, 2011e).
Hypertension Screening	Blood pressure screening every 2 years if less than 120/80 mm Hg; annual blood pressure screening if 120–139/80–90 mm Hg		
Thyroid Screening		Thyroid-stimulating hormone testing (every 5 years beginning at age 50 years)	
Fasting Glucose Testing		Every 3 years after age 45 years	
IMMUNIZATIONS:			
Influenza Vaccine	Ages 19–65+ years: Annually between October and March Use trivalent inactivated influenza vaccine for women who are pregnant or who plan to become pregnant during flu season; vaccination may be given at any time during pregnancy.		
Pneumococcal Vaccine	Immunize individuals at high risk with pneumococcal polysaccharide vaccine (PPSV23); wait at least one year and then immunize with pneumococcal conjugate vaccine (PCV13)		At age 65 immunize with PCV13 first, followed by PPSV23 6 to 12 months later.
Hepatitis A Vaccine	One series (2 doses) for those not previously immunized		
Hepatitis B Vaccine	One series (3 doses) for those not previously immunized		
Human Papillomavirus Vaccine	One series (3 doses) for those ages 9–26 years and not previously immunized		
Meningococcal Conjugate Vaccine	Before entry into high school for those not previously immunized		
Diphtheria and Reduced Tetanus Toxoids and Acellular Pertussis Vaccine	Substitute one-time dose of Tdap for Td booster; then boost with Td every 10 years		
Varicella Vaccine	One series (2 doses) for those without evidence of immunity (contraindicated if pregnant, immunocompromised, or HIV+)		
Herpes Zoster	Single dose in adults aged 60 years or older		
Fasting Glucose Testing	Every 3 years at age 45 years		
Problem Drinking Screening	Screen for problem drinking among all adults and provide brief counseling		
Tobacco Cessation Counseling	Assess all adults for tobacco use and provide ongoing cessation services for those who smoke or are at risk for smoking relapse		
Total Cholesterol and HDL Cholesterol Screening		Fasting fractionated lipid screening for men older than age 35 and for women older than age 45 every 5 years (ACOG, 2011a); USPSTF recommends that women at any age be screened only if other risk factors for cardiovascular disease are present.	
Vision Screening		Asymptomatic elderly adults	

Sources: American College of Obstetricians and Gynecologists [ACOG] (2010a, 2011a, 2011e); Centers for Disease Control and Prevention, 2013f, 2013g, 2014; Institute for Clinical Systems Improvement [ICSI] (2013); U.S. Preventive Services Task Force (2011a)

HEALTH SCREENING SCHEDULE

The health maintenance examination (HME) (Michigan Quality Improvement Consortium, 2011a, 2011b) is one of the primary components of health promotion screening. Screening should begin in adolescence and should cover a diversity of health promotion topics (Box 4-1). According to these guidelines, adolescents and young adults 18 to 49 years of age should have one HME every 1 to 5 years according to their risk status, and adults 50 to 65+ years of age should have one HME every 1 to 3 years based on their risk status.

Infant and Child Health

Health promotion and anticipatory guidance are particularly important in infant and child health. Parents need to have an understanding of nutritional needs, including selection of healthy snacks. Proper dental care is also important in maintaining a child's health. Because infants and children are developing cognitively and physically during this time, there are specific considerations that must be given to safety needs. Immunizations provide protection from and prevention of disease, and selection of appropriate toys encourages developmental play that meets safety requirements and facilitates development of social roles. Sexual development and sexual education promote healthy sexual behavior in later years.

NUTRITIONAL GUIDANCE

Infant Feeding

The first decision that parents make regarding infant nutrition is the decision to breastfeed or bottle-feed their newborn. Although the composition of infant formula is similar to that of breast milk, and many babies thrive on proprietary formula, breast milk is still considered to be the best option for optimal health promotion and disease prevention in the newborn. One of the primary benefits of breastfeeding is the decreased incidence of bacterial and viral infections as a result of passive immunity, acquired via the transfer of maternal antibodies. According to the U.S. Department of Health and Human Services (USDHHS), Office on Women's Health (2010), breastfed infants are less likely to develop allergies, gastrointestinal tract diseases, respiratory tract diseases, ear infections, and childhood obesity. They also have fewer systemic bacterial infections, urinary tract infections, and bacterial and viral infections of the respiratory tract.

Because an infant's immune system does not become fully mature until 2 years of age, the maternal transfer of antibodies and immune factors enhances development of the immune system and facilitates the neonate's immune system response. The longer an infant is breastfed, the stronger the protection against infection and the earlier the maturation of the infant's immune system. In addition, some studies have indicated that breastfed infants experience lower rates of diabetes, lymphoma, leukemia, Hodgkin's disease, and sudden infant death syndrome (SIDS) (American Academy of Pediatrics [AAP], 2012; DHHS, Office on Women's Health, 2010).

Human breast milk contains more carbohydrates, less protein, and less casein than cow's milk or infant formulas. This difference in chemical composition facilitates digestion of breast milk and enables the infant to more readily use the nutrients provided. At 1 year of age, breastfed infants are leaner than their formula-fed counterparts. In addition, breastfed infants tend to gain less weight during childhood, a factor that may lead to reduced overweight and obesity in later life.

While breastfeeding and breast milk are associated with many benefits, commercially prepared formula, based on cow's milk, also provides the essential nutrients for infant growth and development. Soy-based formulas are available for infants who have an intolerance to formulas based on cow's milk. Sucrose and corn syrup, the carbohydrates in soy formulas, tend to be more easily digested than lactose, the carbohydrate in cow's milk–based formula. However, cow's milk formulas provide a better source of protein than the soy formulas. Hydrolyzed-protein formulas are also available for infants with intolerance to cow's milk–based formula. Because the protein has already been broken down, the likelihood of an allergic response is diminished.

Whole milk should be introduced into the infant's diet at 1 year of age. By this time, the infant's digestive system has developed enough to provide the enzymes necessary for appropriate absorption and use. The use of whole milk is important in ensuring that the child receives enough fat and calories to meet nutritional and developmental needs (Table 4-2).

Table 4-2 Infant Feeding Patterns	
Birth–1 month	Breast every 2–3 hours Bottle every 3–4 hours 2–3 oz per feeding
2–4 months	Breast or bottle every 3–4 hours 3–4 oz per feeding
4–6 months	Breast or bottle 4–6 times per day 4–5 oz per feeding
6–8 months	Iron-fortified rice cereal Breast or bottle 4 times per day 6–8 oz per feeding
8–10 months	Finger foods Chopped or mashed foods Sippy cup with formula, breast milk, juice, or water Breast or bottle 4 times per day 6–8 oz per feeding
10–12 months	Self-feeds with fingers and spoon Most table foods are allowed Breast or bottle 4 times per day 6–8 oz per feeding

Cultural Diversity: Infant Feeding

Culture plays an important role in infant feeding. For many immigrants and members of ethnic minorities, the traditions of their homeland, the consumption of traditional foods, and maintaining traditional food preparations provide comfort in an environment that is new and unknown and is a way of sustaining cultural identity. Some cultural practices include breastfeeding on demand and early introduction of solid foods, whereas others feel that exposure of the breast is indecent—a view that may decrease the mother's comfort with breastfeeding. It is imperative for nurses to recognize biases that the Western view of health and nutrition is the only appropriate method to feeding an infant. Nurses need to evaluate the effect of the cultural practices objectively and intervene only if the mother or baby is at risk for harm.

Introduction of Solid Foods

As a child moves from infancy to toddlerhood, parents should introduce solid foods into the diet, including finger foods. The foods that should be introduced are based on the developmental stage and nutritional need. Solid food should not be introduced until the infant is at least 4 months of age because the digestive tract is still developing until this point. In addition, solid food should not be put in an infant's bottle. Instead, the child needs to learn that food is to be eaten and taken from a spoon.

Between 4 and 6 months of age, infants begin to exhibit signs of readiness for the introduction of solid foods. These signs include the ability to hold up the head, sit in a high chair, and move the tongue around the mouth without pushing food out of the mouth (as the extrusion reflex disappears). In addition, the infant should be teething, gaining weight (should be doubled from the birth weight), and remain hungry after 8 to 10 breastfeedings or after consuming 40 ounces of formula per day. The first solid food offered to the infant should consist of an iron-fortified rice cereal prepared by mixing 1 teaspoon of cereal with 4 to 5 teaspoons of breast milk or formula. Over the following weeks, the cereal mixture consistency should be thickened and the amount gradually increased to 1 tablespoon of cereal per day. New cereals, such as those containing oats and barley, may be added, but parents should wait at least 1 week before adding each new food to identify signs of potential allergy.

Between the ages of 6 and 8 months, the infant's cereal intake should increase to 3 to 9 tablespoons per serving, given two to three times per day. In addition, parents should introduce pureed or strained fruits, such as bananas, pears, apples, and peaches, into the diet, beginning with 1 teaspoon and increasing to one-fourth to one-half cup in two to three feedings. At 1-week intervals, pureed or strained vegetables such as carrots, squash, sweet potatoes, avocado, green beans, and peas should also be introduced in the same form as the fruit.

Finger foods can be introduced once the infant reaches 8 to 12 months of age. Signs of readiness for finger foods include the ability to pick up objects with the thumb and forefinger (known as development of the pincer grasp), the ability to transfer items from one hand to the other, and the tendency to put everything into the mouth. Examples of appropriate finger foods include small pieces of lightly toasted bagels, small pieces of ripe bananas, well-cooked spiral pasta, teething crackers, and low-sugar "O"-shaped cereal. During this age, mixed cereals may also be introduced, along with small amounts of yogurt and cottage cheese, small amounts of protein (e.g., egg yolk, pureed meats and poultry, and mashed beans with soft skins), and apple and pear juice. Citrus juices should not be introduced, because the digestive system has not developed enough to process the nutrients.

From 1 year to 18 months of age, the toddler should begin to use a spoon and eat some of the same foods (mashed or chopped into bite-size pieces) as the older family members. Whole milk, eggs, full-fat yogurt and cottage cheese, and citrus juices can be introduced at this time. New vegetables, such as broccoli and cauliflower, can also be introduced.

New foods are then introduced over the next 18 months as the infant begins to feed himself more and make his own choices. Fruit, cut up into bite-size pieces, and diced vegetables may be added to the diet. As the toddler develops his own taste, combination foods such as macaroni and cheese and spaghetti may also be introduced.

Family Teaching Guidelines...
Introducing Solid Foods to Infants

The baby is ready for the introduction of solid foods at approximately 6 months of age. To help determine if the baby is ready for solid foods, look for developmental cues such as the ability to sit well with support and the decrease or disappearance of the extrusion reflex. The baby may watch very intently as you eat and may seem hungry between bottles or breastfeeding.

- Iron-fortified rice cereal is recommended as baby's first solid food for a couple of reasons. Rice is the least allergenic of the grains, and the iron helps the rapidly growing baby replenish the iron needed for motor and mental function. When introducing the rice cereal to the baby, you can mix it with formula, breast milk, or boiled and cooled water until it is very soupy. As the baby becomes accustomed to solid foods, the consistency of the cereal can be gradually adjusted to create a less soupy texture.

- When the baby is eating about 4 tablespoons of cereal twice a day, introduce vegetables and fruits. It is recommended to start with vegetables and then expose the baby to the sweet taste of fruits, because babies are typically more accepting of the sweet tastes.

- Introduce one food at a time, wait 3 to 5 days between new foods so you will be able to identify any reactions to particular foods.

- Introduce food before formula or breastfeeding when the infant is hungry and follow each solid food meal with breast milk or formula.

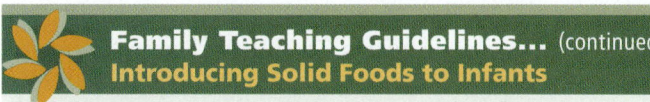

Family Teaching Guidelines... (continued)
Introducing Solid Foods to Infants

SEEKING ADDITIONAL HELP:

◆ If the infant is not growing or gaining weight or if he or she is unable to suck or swallow or shows any signs of an allergic reaction, it is important to promptly seek help from the primary health-care provider, nearby clinic, or emergency room.

ESSENTIAL INFORMATION:

◆ Keep salt, sugar, and additives to a minimum or avoid them altogether. If you make your baby's food, do not add salt or sugar.

◆ **Never** put food in bottles or mix food with formula because it can cause choking.
◆ Offer only small bites of food to prevent choking and pay close attention to your baby when feeding.

_____

Source: Data from American Academy of Pediatrics. (2012). Policy statement: Breastfeeding and the use of human milk. *Pediatrics, 129*(3), 827–841.

 Now Can You—Discuss infant and child nutrition?

1. Discuss the benefits of breastfeeding when compared with bottle feeding?
2. Describe the recommended process for introducing solid foods into an infant's diet?
3. Identify at least four safe, nutritious finger foods for infants and toddlers?

Childhood Nutrition

Once the child reaches 3 years of age, parents should be introduced to the MyPlate for Kids (U.S. Department of Agriculture, 2011). As with the MyPlate developed for adults, the servings per day are calculated based on weight and activity. Specific suggestions are included, such as limiting the intake of juice, ensuring that all juices are 100% natural, and incorporating whole grains to make up half of the daily grain intake. The MyPlate for Kids campaign offers various materials (e.g., interactive computer game, coloring page, and worksheet) and a double-sided poster specifically designed for children aged 6 to 11.

Snacks for children are often the most difficult aspect of planning meals. Parents need to be taught that snacks should be nutritious, and that any food item that is appropriate for a meal is appropriate for a snack. Children typically need to eat every 3 to 4 hours to maintain energy needs. Thus, parents must consider portion sizes when providing snacks for their children. Nutritious snacks include grain products, fruit and vegetable juices, fresh fruits and vegetables, dried fruit, nuts, and seeds (Box 4-2).

DENTAL CARE

Teething typically begins between 4 and 7 months of age. The first teeth to erupt are usually the bottom central incisors followed by the upper central and lateral incisors. The next to erupt are the bottom lateral incisors followed by the first molars. An infant may have any range from no teeth to eight or more teeth by her first birthday. Most children will have all 20 of their primary teeth by their third birthday.

Signs of teething include increased drooling, irritability, desire to chew on objects, crying episodes, and disrupted sleeping and eating patterns. Caregivers can be encouraged to give teething infants a cool wet washcloth, teething rings that have been cooled in the refrigerator, or a clean finger rubbed on the gums to help ease the discomfort.

The American Dental Association (ADA) recommends that a dentist examine a child within 6 months of the eruption of the first tooth and no later than the first birthday. Daily dental care can begin even before the first tooth emerges. Gums can be gently wiped with a damp washcloth or gauze, and when the first tooth emerges, a soft toothbrush and water can be used. To prevent enamel fluorosis (cosmetic defects such as faint, white streaks that can appear on tooth enamel during their development), fluoridated toothpaste should not be used until age two (ADA, 2013).

SLEEP AND REST

Newborns sleep approximately 15 to 20 hours per day in 2- to 3-hour increments. By 3 months of age, infants sleep approximately 15 hours in a 24-hour period. At 6 months, the infant may have two naps of 2 hours each during the day and sleep 9 to 14 hours per night. From 9 months to 1 year, the length of naps may decrease slightly, with nighttime sleep remaining in the 9- to 14-hour range.

Box 4-2 Snacks for Children

- Grain products.
- Bread products: Yeast breads and quick breads, made from whole wheat, rye, oatmeal, mixed grains, and bran; rye crisps; whole-grain crackers. Serve with crackers and cheese, peanut butter, or milk.
- Cereals: Dry cereals with less than 5 grams of sugar. Serve with milk. Add dried fruits.
- Popcorn: Top with grated cheese instead of butter and salt.
- Cookies: Use whole-wheat flour for baking. Try oatmeal or peanut butter cookies. Serve with milk.
- Beverages: Fruit juices and vegetable juices. Serve milk with breads, cereals, and cookies. Blend fruit with milk in a blender.
- Vegetables: Cut up raw vegetables. Serve with peanut butter, cheese, or milk. Include broccoli, carrots, celery, green beans, zucchini, and others.
- Fresh fruit: Serve with peanut butter, yogurt, or milk. Include apples, bananas, grapes, melons, oranges, and peaches.
- Nuts and seeds: Include almonds, cashews, and peanuts.

Infants are not born knowing how to put themselves to sleep. To help the infant learn to fall asleep on his own, caregivers can put the infant to bed drowsy but awake, rather than breastfeeding or rocking the infant to sleep. By training the infant to fall asleep independently, if he wakens in the night, he is more likely to self-soothe back to sleep.

Dr. T. Berry Brazelton describes six states of behavior in the newborn: quiet sleep, active sleep, drowsiness, quiet alert, active awake, and crying. These states include body activity, eye movements, facial movements, breathing patterns, and response to external and internal stimuli. The nurse can provide anticipatory guidance by educating caregivers about how to recognize these states in the newborn. Often caregivers think the infant is waking, when the infant is actually in a period of active sleep, and if left for a few minutes, he will settle back into a quiet sleep state.

In 1992, the American Academy of Pediatrics (AAP) recommended that infants be placed on their backs to sleep to reduce the risk of sudden infant death syndrome (SIDS). According to the Centers for Disease Control and Prevention (CDC) (2013a), overall SIDS rates have declined up to 50% in recent years. Premature infants and infants with certain illnesses may be required to sleep in a prone or side-lying position. In 2011, the AAP updated its policy on how to prevent SIDS, adding three important measures to the existing recommendations: Breastfeeding is recommended and is associated with a reduced risk of SIDS; infants should receive all recommended vaccinations, because evidence suggests that immunization reduces the risk of SIDS by 50%; and bumper pads, associated with a potential risk of suffocation, strangulation, or entrapment, should not be used in cribs (AAP, 2011a).

Toddlers and preschoolers require the same amount of sleep per day as do infants. Toddlers and preschoolers sleep approximately 14 hours in a 24-hour period, 11 of those hours at night. One 1.5- to 3-hour afternoon nap provides the additional needed rest. Bedtime resistance is likely to appear in this developmental stage. The nurse can provide anticipatory guidance by recommending sleep strategies for caregivers to implement with toddlers.

School-age children require about 10 to 12 hours of sleep per night. Depending on activity level, some children may require a little more or a little less. The nurse can educate the caregiver to assess the child's mood, temperament, and energy levels throughout the day to determine if the amount of sleep is sufficient.

SAFETY

Infants and children are at particular risk for accidents and injuries as a result of their cognitive and physical development during these years. Parents need to be taught how to prevent injuries and accidents and how to prepare for risk-taking behaviors that may arise in late childhood.

Injury Prevention

One of the best methods for prevention of injury to infants and children is for parents to prepare and keep their homes safe. This process, ideally begun before the infant is brought home from the hospital, should be reevaluated and modified as the child moves through each developmental stage. Smoke and carbon monoxide detectors should be installed throughout the home. Medications and chemicals should be moved to a high shelf, placed in a sealed area, or

---

Family Teaching Guidelines...
Preventing Plagiocephaly

◆ Infant skulls are soft and flexible during the first year of life to allow the skull to enlarge to accommodate the growing brain. During this time, the infant's skull can become misshapen or deformed by external pressure. This condition is rarely life threatening but can cause permanent facial and skull deformities, or in severe cases, the child's vision can be affected.

◆ Constant pressure on one area of the infant's head can flatten or reshape it. The Back to Sleep campaign initiated by the American Academy of Pediatrics has had the unintended effect of increasing the incidence of plagiocephaly. Proper positioning during sleep and waking periods spent in car seats and baby chairs often require the infant to spend considerable time on his or her back.

◆ Place the baby on the stomach to play for several times each day. When the baby is very young, placing a rolled towel or blanket under his arms for support helps the infant to be more comfortable. This intervention removes pressure from the skull and facilitates the development of strong neck and arm muscles needed for sitting and crawling.

◆ Alternating the direction the baby faces in the bassinet or crib during sleep times is also helpful. If the baby's crib is positioned against a wall, alternating the end of the bed where the baby's head is placed allows her to look out toward the room rather than at the less stimulating wall.

SEEKING ADDITIONAL HELP:

◆ If you notice a flattened area on the baby's skull that does not seem to be improving with positioning changes, you should talk with the physician. The baby may need to be fitted with a customized helmet that is worn for 23 hours a day. This helmet is designed to prevent the baby's head from assuming one position and allows the skull to expand into the flattened area.

ESSENTIAL INFORMATION:

◆ The baby may also be placed on his side while he is awake. The mother can lie on her side, face the baby, and both parties can entertain each other with toys and facial expressions. It is a wonderful way to bond with the baby. Newborn babies love to look at their parents' faces, so this is a very enjoyable activity for them.

Source: Data from American Academy of Pediatrics (2011b).

stored in a cupboard equipped with child safety locks. A fire extinguisher should be readily available on every floor in the home and an additional unit placed in the kitchen. A fire escape route should be planned.

An appropriate car seat should be obtained in anticipation of bringing the new infant home from the hospital. Proper use of a car seat, which has been shown to reduce the chance of death by 71% for infants, and by 54% for toddlers ages 1 to 4, includes placing the unit in a backward-facing direction in the backseat (AAP, 2013a; CDC, 2013b).

When the infant is brought home from the hospital, new areas of concern must be considered. Crib safety is one of these. Parents should be cautioned about buying older (made prior to 1989) models of cribs because they do not meet current safety standards. The distance between the slats of the crib railings should be less than 2 ⅜ inches to prevent head entrapment and potential strangulation. There should be no sharp edges, and the crib mattress should fit snugly with the end panels extending below the mattress to prevent suffocation. Bumper pads should not be used to pad the crib. There is currently no evidence that these products prevent injuries, and they create a potential risk of suffocation, strangulation, or entrapment. The furniture paint should be nontoxic, and all furniture in the infant's nursery should be positioned to avoid windows, curtains, blinds, lamps, electrical cords, outlets, and appliances.

With regard to infant feeding and safety, teach parents to warm bottles slowly, never to use a microwave oven to heat breast milk or formula (heats unevenly), and never prop a bottle in the infant's mouth because this practice creates a choking hazard. Remind parents to keep all hot liquids and foods away from the baby and to place them well away from the edges of tables and countertops. If a pacifier is used, one with shields large enough to prevent placement of the entire pacifier in the mouth should be selected, and the pacifier should be frequently inspected for breakage or cracks. To reduce choking hazards, never place the pacifier on a cord around the infant's neck or attached to the infant's clothes with a clip or cord.

At 3 months of age, infants begin to roll over from stomach to back and to turn toward loud sounds. These activities can pose a safety hazard related to the changing tables used for changing diapers. Teach parents to keep one hand on the infant at all times and never to leave the infant alone on the table. Powders, oils, and lotions should be used cautiously to prevent inhalation poisoning or illness if swallowed. To prevent aspiration, powders should never be shaken close to the infant's face. Current recommendations for powder use include having the parents first place the powder in their hands and then rub it onto the infant (AAP, 2013b).

Because serious falls and injuries can occur with the use of high chairs, playpens, strollers, and swings, these items should be used only under supervision of an adult. Playpens should not be used in place of cribs to prevent injury from suffocation that can occur while the infant is asleep. The use of walkers is not recommended, because serious brain injury, fractures, and concussions have resulted from accidents that involve the walker tipping over or falling down a staircase. Also, the development of gross motor skills may be hindered with walker use because babies who use them learn to walk on the tips of the toes.

Play time and bath time are associated with potential hazards as well. Risks of accidental choking and suffocation are significant for children younger than the age of 6 months who tend to place small objects in their mouths as their cognitive and fine motor skills are developing. Parents must ensure that crib gyms and mobiles are placed at an appropriate height, toys and stuffed animals have no removable parts or sharp edges, and pull toys do not have long cords. Bath safety includes ensuring that the water temperature is below 120°F. Teach parents to test the water temperature before placing the child in the bath and to use bath mats or towels to prevent slipping. During the bath, the parent should keep both hands positioned securely on the infant while using one hand to constantly hold the infant and the other hand to wash the infant.

By 14 months of age, the child has developed the skills necessary for walking; the majority of children walk well by this time. Once the child begins to crawl, creep, and walk, additional environmental safety hazards are present. Kitchen and bathroom cabinets should be equipped with firm latches or locks to prevent injury from medications, poisonous chemicals, and sharp implements. Stove guards should be placed over knobs and burners to prevent accidental injury from burns. Remind parents to turn all pot handles away from the front of the stove and to install locks or latches on appliance doors to prevent entrapment and suffocation.

Stairs and windows present safety hazards related to falls. Safety gates at the tops and bottoms of staircases should be used at all times; accordion gates are not recommended. Railings on steps, decks, and balconies should be covered with netting to prevent children from getting trapped between the posts or falling. Safety guards can be placed on windows to prevent them from opening more than 4 inches; however, these should not be used on windows designated for fire escape. Furniture should not be placed near windows because children can climb on the furniture and fall through the windows. Poisoning accidents can occur through the ingestion of harmful plants or peeling paint chips, particularly in homes built before 1978 that contain lead-based paint.

Now Can You—Discuss strategies to ensure infant and toddler safety?

1. Describe methods for ensuring crib safety?
2. Identify ways to promote bath safety?
3. Discuss strategies for making stairways and window areas safe?

By 24 months of age, cognitive skills have developed that allow the toddler to begin logical reasoning. During this time, play activities pose the greatest risk of injury. While playing indoors, children should always be supervised, and the kitchen and bathroom should be off limits. Refrigerators and freezers should be locked, and closets, attics, and basements should be sealed to prevent accidental injuries. Outside safety includes having a fenced-in yard with a locked gate and ensuring that all playground equipment is installed securely. A soft surface should be placed under playground areas to provide cushioning for falls. All yard equipment should be safely stored away from children.

Water safety is also important. Swimming in pools, lakes, and rivers should take place only under adult supervision, and children should not be allowed to dive or jump into water less than 12 feet in depth. Chemicals used in pools and hot tubs are poisonous and should be kept out of the reach of children. If possible, a separate fence should be placed around the pool, equipped with a safety alarm system to alert parents when children are near the water.

Risk-Taking Behaviors

Children engage in risk-taking behaviors as a normal progression through cognitive development. Risk-taking enables children to develop skills and self-confidence and to understand their strengths and limitations. Through risk-taking behavior, children learn boundaries and develop an awareness of the outside world.

TESTING LIMITS. Risk-taking actually begins in infancy, as infants explore their worlds, place objects in their mouths, and learn to identify parental facial expressions and gestures. Once the child begins to walk, limit-testing heightens through activities such as climbing, reaching, and balancing. Parents who allow the child's exploration send a message that when performed in appropriate situations, a certain degree of risk-taking is necessary for development. Conversely, parents who do not allow exploration convey the message that experimentation is undesirable and should not be done. Close to age 2, when the child enters the developmental stage of *autonomy versus shame and doubt*, risk-taking may present itself in the form of saying "no" to parents (Erikson, 1959).

Preschoolers may engage in risk-taking behaviors as a result of their physical development. As gross motor skills develop, their physical abilities exceed their ability to logically reason the danger associated with their activities. Parents need to monitor their children's activities, while allowing them to maintain a sense of control. In so doing, the parent helps the child to develop the confidence needed to try something new or difficult in the future and facilitates the child's successful mastery of the developmental task associated with *initiative versus guilt*.

School-age children's risk-taking behavior, as opposed to the preschoolers' behavior, is more closely related to cognitive rather than physical development. At this time, the child has moved into the stage of *industry versus inferiority* and is developing a sense of self-esteem. Risk-taking allows the school-age child to experience heightened feelings of self-worth following success and to learn to evaluate mistakes and develop alternative strategies for the future when they meet with failure. See Chapter 20 for more information on developmental stages.

PLAY

Play enables children to explore their world, express their thoughts and feelings, and meet and solve problems. The foundation for play begins immediately after birth. The infant reflexively grasps objects or moves extremities and through this discovers enjoyment of the sounds, tastes, textures, and smells. These discoveries gradually lead the infant to perform such activities purposefully. Playing with an infant begins with engaging

all of the senses. Infants enjoy looking at faces, black-and-white objects, hearing voices, and sucking on hands in the reflexive play stage. It is important for caregivers to play with their babies because much of an infant's learning occurs through play. For the first few months, the caregiver must play with the baby during quiet alert periods. This is the best learning time for a young infant. As the baby grows and abilities and mobility increase, the infant plays for longer periods and becomes adept at expressing feelings. Signs of boredom or lack of interest become more obvious, at which point the caregiver can switch to a new game.

As physical coordination and sensory ability increase rapidly, the infant is able to examine objects more closely. By looking, touching, and placing objects in the mouth, the infant discovers different textures, tastes, and colors. As the infant develops, he learns cause and effect. For example, when an infant shakes the rattle, it makes a pleasant sound. This recognition of cause and effect encourages the infant to repeat activities to achieve the desired result.

As the infant approaches the 1-year mark, the play environment increases dramatically as the infant learns to crawl and walk. In addition, the ability to communicate increases steadily as the infant reaches 12 months. At this time, the infant can point to objects, voice frustrations at having toys taken away, and use body language and sounds in an attempt to express emotions. Play in childhood is based on cognitive as well as physical development. While there are five types of developmental play in which older children can participate, children must progress from the lower levels to the higher levels. To meet the developmental needs of each stage of play as the child grows and matures, specific activities, toys, and games should be introduced (Table 4-3).

- Solitary play (type 1): The child plays alone, without regard for those around him.
- Onlooker play (type 2): The child observes the other children around him as he plays alone; may alter own play activities based on what he sees the others doing or may be content to continue in his play while simply talking with the other children; play activities are different (e.g., one child may be bouncing a ball while another is playing with jacks).
- Parallel play (type 3): Children play with the same materials and items, but they do not yet play together.
- Associative play (type 4): The peer group is developed to the extent that children play together but in a loosely organized manner.
- Cooperative play (type 5): Children assume designated roles in the games, have goals for the games, and rely on one another for the game to continue and progress.

 Now Can You—Provide developmentally appropriate play activities for school-age children?

1. Identify the five types of play?
2. Describe the developmental tasks associated with each type of play?
3. Identify play activities that are appropriate for each type of play?

Table 4-3 Play Activities for Children

Developmental Age	Type of Play	Purpose of Play	Activities/Toys
Infant	Solitary Play—The infant plays alone, without regard for those around him/her.	Stimulates sensorimotor development with simple imitative games	• Blocks • Books • Teething toys or rattles • Push or pull toys • Musical toys or toys that make sounds and/or have bright lights • Finger/Hand games (e.g., pat-a-cake, peek-a-boo, itsy-bitsy spider) • Balls • Soft toys • Songs/Music • Tummy toys • Mobiles
Toddler	Onlooker Play—Children observe other children play but don't participate. Parallel Play—Children play with the same materials and items, but they do not yet play together.	Helps children make the transition from solitary play to associative play by stimulating sensorimotor and psychosocial development	• Push or pull toys • Musical toys or toys that make sounds and/or have bright lights • Ride-on toys • Balls • Soft toys • Songs/Music • Dolls or stuffed animals • Outside toys (e.g., shovel and bucket, ride-on toys, small swim pools) • Books • Video movies • Imitative toys (e.g., broom for sweeping or dishes for playing house) • Matching games • Simple puzzles • Blowing bubbles • Bean-bag toss • Catching fireflies • Interactive games (e.g., ring-around-the-rosie, London Bridge is falling down, duck-duck-goose, hide and seek) • Coloring or drawing
Preschooler	Associative Play—The peer group is developed to the extent that children play together, in a loosely organized manner.	Helps children learn how to share and play in small groups and helps them to learn simple games with rules, concepts of language, and social rules	• Imitative games (e.g., house, fire or police person) • Simple arts and crafts • Simple board games (e.g., Memory, Chutes and Ladders, Candy land, Checkers) • Interactive games (e.g., Ring-around-the-rosie, London Bridge is falling down, duck-duck-goose, hide and seek) • Alphabet or know your colors games • Coloring, drawing, • Simple computerized games
School-age	Cooperative Play—Children assume designated roles in games, have goals for games, and rely on one another for the game to continue and progress.	Teaches children how to bargain, cooperate, and compromise to develop logical reasoning, which increases social skills	• Music • Books • Arts and crafts • Bikes, skates, roller-blades, scooters, skateboarding • Team sports (e.g., baseball, soccer, gymnastics, swimming, basketball, volleyball) • Group games (e.g., dodge-ball, tag, hide and seek) • Imitative games (e.g., school, doctor, business person) • Board games • Card games • Computerized games • Video movies and games • Puzzles

(continued)

Table 4-3 Play Activities for Children (continued)

Developmental Age	Type of Play	Purpose of Play	Activities/Toys
School-age (continued)			• Crossword or word search puzzles • Organizations (e.g., girls' or boys' clubs, after-school clubs, faith community activities, sponsored events)
Adolescent	Cooperative Play—Children assume designated roles in the games, have goals for the games, and rely on one another for the play to continue and progress.	Teaches children how to bargain, cooperate, and compromise to develop logical reasoning, which increases social skills	• Team sports (e.g., baseball, basketball, cross-country, gymnastics, running, soccer, swimming, track & field, volleyball) • Video games • Computer games • Board games • Card games • Art • Concerts/Music • "Hanging out" • Social events (e.g., dances, clubs, friends' houses) • Organizations (e.g., girls' or boys' clubs, after-school and/or faith community activities, sponsored events)

Updated by Jodi Jenson-Bassett RN, MSN

IMMUNIZATIONS

Immunizations are the child's first and best defense against several diseases that can be fatal or cause serious disability. Because the child's immune system is immature, the administration of vaccines enables the child to develop antibodies against specific potential organisms. The CDC (2013f, 2013g) has developed recommended schedules to enable health-care practitioners and parents to ensure that early and appropriately timed immunization is in place; immunization schedules are available for persons aged 0 through 18 years and for adults aged 19 years and older (Figs. 4-1 and 4-2).

SEXUALITY

It is never too early to begin sexual education with children. Correct information enhances appropriate decision making regarding sexual behavior in the later years. The infant is aware of the differences in touch in certain parts of the body and is capable of deriving comfort and pleasure from touch. Male babies have erections, and female babies experience vaginal lubrication. Infants can experience orgasm as early as 4 or 5 months of age. Sexuality at these young ages is an expression of exploration and comfort.

As early as 18 months of age, toddlers begin to explore their bodies and express concerns and questions about their bodies. Parents should teach their children the proper names for sex organs and allow masturbation, in a private manner, as children begin normal body exploration. By age 4, children can be taught that males and females have different sexual organs. While sexual exploration with other children is normal developmentally, the parents should set limits and discourage it if seen. During the preschool years, the question of where babies come from usually arises. It is best if parents are direct and honest and provide a simple and straightforward answer that babies come from inside the mother. School-age children, who tend to associate and play more with children of their same gender, are still attempting to learn the difference between the sexes. At this time, parents must continue to provide truthful, direct information and encourage questions to prevent their children from receiving incorrect information from friends.

During the years between ages 8 and 11, children begin to focus on their own development and contrast it with that of their friends. Reassurance from parents decreases anxiety and helps children to realize that they are in the normal range of development. At this time, parents should begin to educate their children about the names and functions of the male and female sexual organs, puberty, the menstrual cycle, sexual intercourse, pregnancy, pregnancy prevention, same-sex relationships, masturbation, and the spread of sexually transmitted infections. They should also encourage dialogue about personal expectations and values regarding sexual activity.

Adolescent Health

Adolescents are in a vulnerable life stage because they are between the states of childhood and adulthood and are experiencing significant physical and emotional growth. A number of developmental tasks are associated with this period (Box 4-3). The most important changes that occur between the ages of 11 and 18 are sexual developmental changes. The influx of sexual hormones, combined with the growth of primary and secondary sexual characteristics and the focus on peer relationships, place adolescents at increased risk of injury and disease. During this developmental period, special attention needs to be placed on

Figure 1. Recommended immunization schedule for persons aged 0 through 18 years – United States, 2014.
(FOR THOSE WHO FALL BEHIND OR START LATE, SEE THE CATCH-UP SCHEDULE [FIGURE 2]).
These recommendations must be read with the footnotes that follow. For those who fall behind or start late, provide catch-up vaccination at the earliest opportunity as indicated by the green bars in Figure 1. To determine minimum intervals between doses, see the catch-up schedule (Figure 2). School entry and adolescent vaccine age groups are in bold.

Vaccine	Birth	1 mo	2 mos	4 mos	6 mos	9 mos	12 mos	15 mos	18 mos	19–23 mos	2-3 yrs	4-6 yrs	7-10 yrs	11-12 yrs	13–15 yrs	16–18 yrs
Hepatitis B[1] (HepB)	1st dose	◄──── 2nd dose ────►			◄──────────────── 3rd dose ────────────────►											
Rotavirus[2] (RV) RV1 (2-dose series); RV5 (3-dose series)			1st dose	2nd dose	See footnote 2											
Diphtheria, tetanus, & acellular pertussis[3] (DTaP: <7 yrs)			1st dose	2nd dose	3rd dose		◄──── 4th dose ────►					5th dose				
Tetanus, diphtheria, & acellular pertussis[4] (Tdap: ≥7 yrs)														(Tdap)		
Haemophilus influenzae type b[5] (Hib)			1st dose	2nd dose	See footnote 5		◄── 3rd or 4th dose, See footnote 5 ──►									
Pneumococcal conjugate[6] (PCV13)			1st dose	2nd dose	3rd dose		◄── 4th dose ──►									
Pneumococcal polysaccharide[6] (PPSV23)																
Inactivated poliovirus[7] (IPV) (<18 yrs)			1st dose	2nd dose	◄──────────── 3rd dose ────────────►							4th dose				
Influenza[8] (IIV; LAIV) 2 doses for some: See footnote 8					◄──────── Annual vaccination (IIV only) ────────►					◄──────── Annual vaccination (IIV or LAIV) ────────►						
Measles, mumps, rubella[9] (MMR)							◄──── 1st dose ────►					2nd dose				
Varicella[10] (VAR)							◄──── 1st dose ────►					2nd dose				
Hepatitis A[11] (HepA)							◄──── 2-dose series, See footnote 11 ────►									
Human papillomavirus[12] (HPV2: females only; HPV4: males and females)														(3-dose series)		
Meningococcal[13] (Hib-MenCY ≥ 6 weeks; MenACWY-D ≥9 mos; MenACWY-CRM ≥ 2 mos)					◄──────────────── See footnote 13 ────────────────►									1st dose		Booster

	Range of recommended ages for all children		Range of recommended ages for catch-up immunization		Range of recommended ages for certain high-risk groups		Range of recommended ages during which catch-up is encouraged and for certain high-risk groups		Not routinely recommended

This schedule includes recommendations in effect as of January 1, 2014. Any dose not administered at the recommended age should be administered at a subsequent visit, when indicated and feasible. The use of a combination vaccine generally is preferred over separate injections of its equivalent component vaccines. Vaccination providers should consult the relevant Advisory Committee on Immunization Practices (ACIP) statement for detailed recommendations, available online at http://www.cdc.gov/vaccines/hcp/acip-recs/index.html. Clinically significant adverse events that follow vaccination should be reported to the Vaccine Adverse Event Reporting System (VAERS) online (http://www.vaers.hhs.gov) or by telephone (800-822-7967). Suspected cases of vaccine-preventable diseases should be reported to the state or local health department. Additional information, including precautions and contraindications for vaccination, is available from CDC online (http://www.cdc.gov/vaccines/recs/vac-admin/contraindications.htm) or by telephone (800-CDC-INFO [800-232-4636]).

This schedule is approved by the Advisory Committee on Immunization Practices (http://www.cdc.gov/vaccines/acip), the American Academy of Pediatrics (http://www.aap.org), the American Academy of Family Physicians (http://www.aafp.org), and the American College of Obstetricians and Gynecologists (http://www.acog.org).

NOTE: The above recommendations must be read along with the footnotes of this schedule.

Figure 4-1 Recommended immunization schedule for persons aged 0 through 18 years (CDC, 2013f).

nutrition, safety, sexual health promotion, and prevention of illness (Krowchuk, 2010).

NUTRITION

Diet and nutrition are especially important for facilitating optimal growth and development during adolescence. Adequate nutritional intake is essential to accommodate the growth spurt that occurs during this time. Adolescents gain approximately 25% of their adult height and 50% of their adult weight throughout this time period. In addition to the nutritional needs to promote growth and development, adolescents are tasked with developing a positive body image and a personal identity. When conflicts exist, adolescents are at increased risk for eating disorders, which can lead to overweight, underweight, hypertension, and diabetes mellitus.

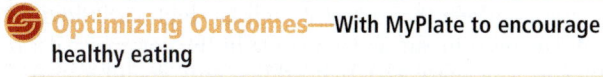

Optimizing Outcomes—With MyPlate to encourage healthy eating

The Dietary Guidelines for Americans are developed and released jointly by the U.S. Department of Agriculture and the U.S. Department of Health and Human Services every

5 years to ensure the public receives the most current, scientifically sound nutrition advice available. Recently, the Food Pyramid was replaced with a plate icon ("MyPlate") designed to help Americans understand what a balanced meal should look like (Fig. 4-3). Simply stated, MyPlate offers suggestions on how to build a healthy plate. Included with the plate are recommendations ("10 Tips to a Great Plate"), which are based on the Dietary Guidelines. A Web site (http://www.ChooseMyPlate.gov) is available for more information on building a healthy plate and diet.

Obesity in Adolescence

During adolescence, it is common for the appetite to increase. In addition, adipose cells develop rapidly, leading to an increased potential for adipose tissue development and overweight. This growth is dependent on both nutritional and environmental factors. It is essential to balance the energy intake and output in the adipose cells to prevent the growth of larger adipose cells, which can lead to obesity.

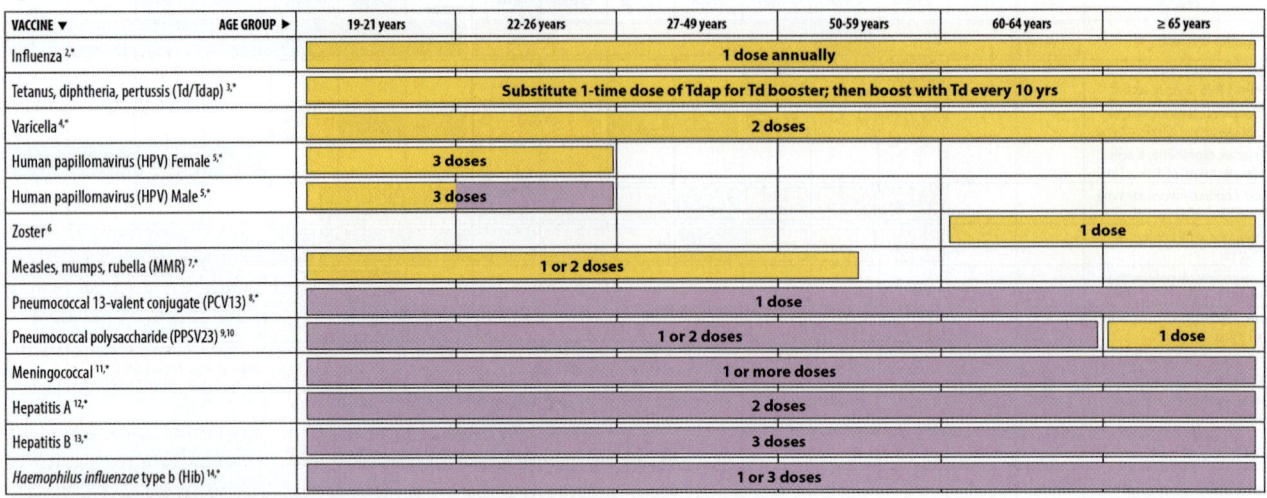

Recommended Adult Immunization Schedule—United States - 2014

Note: These recommendations must be read with the footnotes that follow
containing number of doses, intervals between doses, and other important information.

Figure 1. Recommended adult immunization schedule, by vaccine and age group[1]

VACCINE ▼ AGE GROUP ►	19-21 years	22-26 years	27-49 years	50-59 years	60-64 years	≥ 65 years
Influenza [2,*]	1 dose annually					
Tetanus, diphtheria, pertussis (Td/Tdap) [3,*]	Substitute 1-time dose of Tdap for Td booster; then boost with Td every 10 yrs					
Varicella [4,*]	2 doses					
Human papillomavirus (HPV) Female [5,*]	3 doses					
Human papillomavirus (HPV) Male [5,*]	3 doses					
Zoster [6]					1 dose	
Measles, mumps, rubella (MMR) [7,*]	1 or 2 doses					
Pneumococcal 13-valent conjugate (PCV13) [8,*]	1 dose					
Pneumococcal polysaccharide (PPSV23) [9,10]	1 or 2 doses					1 dose
Meningococcal [11,*]	1 or more doses					
Hepatitis A [12,*]	2 doses					
Hepatitis B [13,*]	3 doses					
Haemophilus influenzae type b (Hib) [14,*]	1 or 3 doses					

*Covered by the Vaccine Injury Compensation Program

	For all persons in this category who meet the age requirements and who lack documentation of vaccination or have no evidence of previous infection; zoster vaccine recommended regardless of prior episode of zoster	Report all clinically significant postvaccination reactions to the Vaccine Adverse Event Reporting System (VAERS). Reporting forms and instructions on filing a VAERS report are available at www.vaers.hhs.gov or by telephone, 800-822-7967.

Information on how to file a Vaccine Injury Compensation Program claim is available at www.hrsa.gov/vaccinecompensation or by telephone, 800-338-2382. To file a claim for vaccine injury, contact the U.S. Court of Federal Claims, 717 Madison Place, N.W., Washington, D.C. 20005; telephone, 202-357-6400. |

Additional information about the vaccines in this schedule, extent of available data, and contraindications for vaccination is also available at www.cdc.gov/vaccines or from the CDC-INFO Contact Center at 800-CDC-INFO (800-232-4636) in English and Spanish, 8:00 a.m. - 8:00 p.m. Eastern Time, Monday - Friday, excluding holidays.

Recommended if some other risk factor is present (e.g., on the basis of medical, occupational, lifestyle, or other indication)

Use of trade names and commercial sources is for identification only and does not imply endorsement by the U.S. Department of Health and Human Services.

No recommendation

The recommendations in this schedule were approved by the Centers for Disease Control and Prevention's (CDC) Advisory Committee on Immunization Practices (ACIP), the American Academy of Family Physicians (AAFP), the American College of Physicians (ACP), American College of Obstetricians and Gynecologists (ACOG) and American College of Nurse-Midwives (ACNM).

Figure 4-2 Recommended immunization schedule for adults aged 19 years and older (CDC, 2013g. Available at http://www.cdc.gov/mmwr/preview/mmwrhtml/su6201a3.htm)

Box 4-3 Developmental Tasks of Adolescence

- Formal Operational Thought: Piaget's Theory of Cognitive Development indicates that adolescents' thought becomes more abstract. They develop the ability to logically reason, generating hypotheses and potential consequences of action.

- Learning Identity: Erikson's Theory of Psychosocial Development suggests that the adolescent experiments with different roles in an attempt to identify the role with which he or she is most comfortable. The adolescent, through achievement, becomes more confident in his abilities and gradually develops a set of ideals with which he can identify. As the adolescent experiments with different societal roles, peer influences play an increasingly important role in development.

- Sexual Identity: Freud's Theory of Psychosexual Development proposes that, as adolescents enter puberty, instinctual impulses create stress and uncertainty. As the adolescent develops a sense of sexuality, the stress is decreased, and balance is restored, allowing the adolescent to engage in healthy sexual relationships.

 ### Where Research and Practice Meet:
Overweight, Obesity, and Adolescent Risk-Taking Behavior

Overweight is defined as a body mass index (BMI) between the 85th and 94th percentiles for age and sex, while *obesity* is defined as a BMI at or above the 95th percentile for age and sex (Ogden, Carroll, Curtin, Lamb, & Flegal, 2010). A recent (2011) study was conducted by a team of nurse researchers (Polfuss, Liebhart, & Greenley) to examine the possibility of a relationship between overweight/obesity and risk-taking behaviors in adolescents. The investigators concluded that overweight/obesity status appears to be a predictor of certain adolescent health-related risk-taking behaviors such as smoking tobacco, chewing tobacco, and neglecting to wear a seat belt. Also, the belief that one is loved and supported by one's family members appeared to have a general protective role with respect to health-related risk-taking behaviors. Nurses can use this information to guide the development and implementation of appropriate patient education materials for adolescents and their parents.

The effects of heredity and environment should be considered as contributing factors in adolescent obesity. A child born to two obese parents has a 75% chance of being obese. A child born to parents where only one is obese has a 25% chance of being obese. However, the influence of heredity must be considered in the context of the adolescent's environment. Psychological, social, and health factors collectively shape the adolescent's environment and its impact on nutritional health.

PSYCHOLOGICAL FACTORS. Perhaps the factor that has the greatest psychological effect on body image and nutritional health is the media. Television and advertising both encourage and condone the eating of high-fat, high-carbohydrate foods, using thin, attractive people in the commercials. In addition, the mere fact that adolescents spend approximately 3 to 4 hours each day watching television adds to the problem of obesity because television viewing is a sedentary activity.

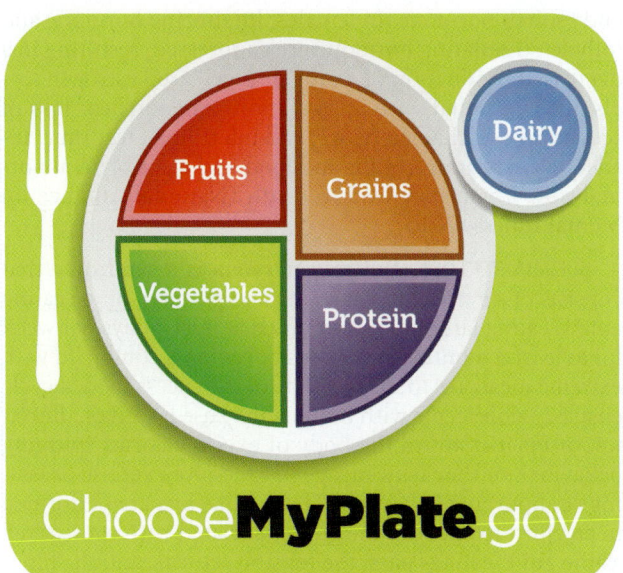

Figure 4-3 MyPlate (*Source:* www.choosemyplate.gov; U.S. Department of Agriculture, 2011).

The impact of the media on the developing adolescent's body image is crucial. Body image is affected by physical characteristics, body-related experiences, social response to appearance, and social value placed on body characteristics. Each of these factors has an effect on personality development and is influenced by individual responses. Many times, these factors combine to create a focus on excessive dieting and scale-weighing behaviors. In addition, there is a relationship between impaired body image in adolescents and depression.

SOCIAL FACTORS. Social factors such as the influence of family and peers interact with the psychological factors that impact adolescent obesity. In many families, eating and mealtime behaviors are instituted at an early age. Little time may be spent on meal preparation, and time spent with family members while eating may be nonexistent. As the dual-income family has become the norm in modern society, fast food and eating "on the go" has also become the norm. Eating patterns that lead to adolescent obesity may include the regular consumption of high-calorie, low-nutrient-dense foods, a lack of understanding about nutrition, a lack of structure and sociability in eating patterns, a tendency to eat late in the evening, binge eating when hungry or bored, and the habit of eating rapidly.

Adolescence is also a time when peer relationships become extremely important in the development of a personal identity. Adolescents frequently congregate and socialize in areas where food is consumed, such as fast food restaurants, pizza parlors, and at parties. For many, eating becomes a social event in and of itself. In these settings, peer pressure may influence the healthy eaters to consume high-fat, high-caloric food to fit in with the majority. Over time, many adolescents become conditioned to eat poorly and to elude structure in their eating behaviors.

One's level of physical activity is associated with weight, and a sedentary lifestyle constitutes a significant factor in obesity. When overweight adolescents are not with their peers, they are often engaging in sedentary activities, such as watching television, using the computer, talking on the telephone, and text messaging. Without energy expenditure, the excess in calorie consumption increases the number of adipose cells and leads to further weight gain.

MEDICAL FACTORS. The psychological and social factors may predispose to an increased risk for disease related to overeating and obesity. Depression is one of the most common disorders associated with adolescent obesity. While attempting to fit into the peer group by engaging in unhealthy eating behaviors, adolescents are meanwhile being bombarded with media images of thin, attractive individuals overeating and societal messages that obesity is unattractive and shameful. There is an unspoken viewpoint that obese individuals are overindulgent and lack self-control. These influences negatively impact the adolescent's body image and self-esteem, and create a risk for depression, feelings of social isolation, rejection, failure, and thoughts of suicide.

Obesity in adolescence leads to medical problems, including cardiovascular disease, type 2 diabetes mellitus, kidney disease, gallbladder disease, liver disease, and orthopedic problems. Hypercholesterolemia and hyperlipidemia increase the workload on the heart, resulting in hypertension. These disorders, when combined with hyperinsulinemia, result in insulin resistance syndrome. Insulin resistance is highly associated with the development of type 2 diabetes mellitus, long thought to be an adult disease. Over the past 10 years, however, there has been an increased incidence of type 2 diabetes mellitus developing in childhood and adolescence (Polotsky, 2010).

For the adolescent female, insulin resistance and obesity may affect reproductive and gynecological health. Insulin resistance causes an increase in circulating insulin and stimulates an increase in the production of androgens. Increased androgens, combined with the increased levels of circulating insulin, have been reported to trigger polycystic ovarian syndrome (PCOS) (Polotsky, 2010). PCOS is associated with anovulation and is manifested by dysmenorrhea, hirsutism, and acne. Insufficient progesterone production results in infertility and an increased risk of endometrial cancer (American College of Obstetricians and Gynecologists [ACOG], 2011c).

❝**What to say**❞—*When talking with an adolescent about losing weight*

Discussions about weight loss can be a sensitive issue for many overweight patients. During adolescence, body weight has a dramatic effect on the development of self-image and self-esteem and can be an even more sensitive issue for discussion. An important strategy in discussions about weight and weight loss with adolescents is to begin the conversation with expressions of respect that are sensitive to cultural differences related to food choices and eating patterns. Regardless of whether the patient is ready to begin a weight control program, she may still benefit from talking openly about healthy eating and exercise. To open the conversation, the nurse can begin with a simple question to determine if the patient is willing to talk about the issue:

"Cindy, can we talk about your weight? What are your thoughts about your weight right now?"

To determine the degree of readiness to engage in weight control, additional questions can be asked:

"What are your goals concerning your weight?"

"What kind of help would you like from me regarding your weight?"

Nurses should avoid the use of words that may make patients feel uncomfortable, such as "obese," "obesity," "fat," and "excess fat."

Eating Disorders

In addition to overweight and obesity associated with overeating, other eating disorders such as anorexia nervosa and bulimia nervosa may develop during adolescence. These two eating disorders adversely affect nutrition and the overall health status and impact growth and development. The underlying issue associated with eating disorders concerns the improper use of food: eating too little, eating too much, or eating too much and purging in an attempt to rid the body of excessive calories.

Eating disorders are rooted in issues related to body image development. The core of the problem involves a distortion in body image and a delay in achieving progress toward a healthy, adult body image. In essence, adolescents with severe eating disorders are struggling with another developmental task, that of autonomy. They tend to have an unrealistic view of themselves and depend on social opinions and judgments, as evidenced by their preoccupation with food, dieting, and exercise patterns.

ANOREXIA NERVOSA. **Anorexia nervosa** is a chronic eating disorder that stems from a distorted body image. This condition develops as a result of obesity or a perception of obesity that creates an obsession with weight loss and a denial of hunger. The fear of gaining weight, combined with a low self-esteem, creates a life-threatening disorder that can, if not properly treated, lead to serious medical complications and death. Individuals with anorexia nervosa undertake strict and severe diets and engage in rigorous excessive exercise to maintain an unrealistic body weight. Psychological traits associated with anorexia nervosa include perfectionism, obsessive–compulsive behavior, social isolation, a focus on high achievement without satisfaction, and depression (Carr & Kaplan, 2010; Williams, 2012).

 Nursing Insight—*The female athlete triad eating disorder*

The female athlete triad is a syndrome consisting of three interrelated components: disordered eating, amenorrhea, and osteoporosis. The condition is most common in sports that emphasize leanness or low body weight, such as gymnastics, long-distance running, diving, swimming, ballet dancing, and figure skating. The triad is a serious illness with lifelong health consequences and can potentially be fatal (The Nemours Foundation, 2013).

Because of a pervasive malnutrition that affects all organ systems, symptoms include weakness, dizziness, excessive weight loss, intolerance to cold, bradycardia, hypotension, bone loss with consequent fractures, constipation from dehydration, and the development of lanugo. The continued restriction of calories suppresses the hypothalamic–pituitary–adrenal axis and results in decreased production of cortisol and growth hormone. In females, luteinizing hormone and follicle-stimulating hormone are suppressed, resulting in a decreased production of estrogen. Decreased estrogen levels are associated with anovulation, amenorrhea, loss of secondary sex characteristics, and infertility. Over time, inadequate nutrition results in blood and electrolyte abnormalities, which may lead to death (National Alliance on Mental Illness, 2013).

BULIMIA NERVOSA. **Bulimia nervosa** is a syndrome that consists of a cycle of binge eating and purging. Binge eating entails eating large amounts of food at least 2 days per week for at least 3 months. When this behavior is combined with extreme measures to rid the body of the excess food, a cycle ensues. Adolescents with bulimia may use laxatives, diuretics, or emetics to rid the body of excess calories (purging behavior), or they may engage in excessive exercise or fasting (nonpurging behavior). These behaviors are performed in an effort to alleviate the guilt associated with overeating; as the guilt feelings pass, the tension returns, and the binging behavior begins once again.

Adolescents with bulimia nervosa typically maintain a normal weight, although psychological factors associated with bulimia include poor impulse control, low self-esteem, depression, and anxiety disorder. In addition, comorbid behaviors such as alcohol and substance abuse, unprotected sexual activity, self-mutilation, and suicide attempts may be present. Similar to anorexia, bulimia is an eating disorder that is usually associated with some degree of depression.

Physically, the adolescent with bulimia nervosa may present with symptoms related to forced excessive vomiting: cracked and damaged lips, tooth damage, callused fingers and hands, and broken blood vessels in the face. Symptoms that may not be physically noticeable include throat irritation, esophageal inflammation, and parotitis from vomiting, as well as rectal bleeding from overuse of laxatives. While life-threatening conditions are less common in adolescents with bulimia than in adolescents with anorexia, they may still be at risk for dehydration, electrolyte imbalances, ruptures in the gastrointestinal tract, kidney disease, and cardiac arrhythmias.

 Nursing Insight—*Diabulimia for weight loss*

Among persons with type 1 diabetes, diabulimia—skipping or shortchanging insulin doses—is sometimes practiced to achieve weight loss. Diabulimia tends to begin in adolescence and is more likely to occur in women than in men. The administration of inadequate amounts of insulin for the carbohydrates consumed during a meal may result in hyperglycemia, glycosuria, and polyuria with resultant short-term reduction in weight from fluid loss. Over time, this dangerous eating pattern can progress to diabetic ketoacidosis. Nurses can help to prevent this type of disordered eating in diabetic patients by reinforcing a healthy body image and by teaching about the importance of healthy eating, regular exercise, and adherence to the prescribed treatment plan. Emphasis should be placed on eating and diabetes in relation to good health, not in relation to weight (Murdoff, 2011).

DENTAL CARE

For adolescents, twice yearly dental visits for checkups and cleaning are required. It is common for adolescents to have dental work performed to correct tooth malformations.

Obvious dental correction can create body image problems, particularly if wearing braces or a headgear is required. Education regarding the proper care of teeth with dental appliances must be received at the dentist's office and reinforced by caregivers at home.

SLEEP AND REST

Adolescents are commonly chronically sleep deprived as activities, schoolwork, and after-school jobs keep them up later at night. Often the adolescent sleeps extensively on weekends to make up for the deficiency during the week, but this is generally more detrimental because the body has difficulty adapting to irregular sleeping patterns. Sleep deprivation can impair memory and inhibit creativity, making it difficult for sleep-deprived adolescents to learn.

The nurse can encourage caregivers and adolescents to keep evening activities to a manageable level that allows for some quiet time before bed and an appropriate bedtime. Involving the adolescent in the decision-making process regarding which activities to reduce or eliminate will help the teen comply with the limits set. In addition, if the adolescent adheres to a similar bedtime and wake time on the weekends as during the week, excessive fatigue can be controlled.

SAFETY

Because adolescents are still developing formal thought operations, they may not have the cognitive abilities to make appropriate decisions regarding safety. Their decisions are likely to result in accidents and injuries and risk-taking behaviors for which adults may not be at risk. However, the accidents and injuries most common in adolescents differ from those in infancy and childhood. In addition, adolescents must be taught information related to safe sexual practices, substance use and abuse, violence, and suicide prevention.

Accidents and Injuries

The three leading causes of death in adolescents are motor vehicle accidents, homicide, and suicide, respectively. The risk for motor vehicle accidents is greater among adolescents than for any other age group, with 3,023 young persons between the ages of 13 and 19 dying from injuries related to crashes in 2011 (Insurance Institute for Highway Safety, 2013). For male adolescents, the risk is two times higher than that of female adolescents. Risk factors for these statistics include the inability to assess hazardous situations while driving, speeding, driving under the influence of drugs or alcohol, and a low compliance with seat belt use.

In relation to homicides, approximately one-third of all homicides in the United States occur among adolescents. Individual factors related to this level of violence in adolescence include a history of abuse and the observation of violent acts at home. Certain familial characteristics have also been linked to adolescent homicide: distant, passive, or absent fathers; dominant, overprotective, and sexually inappropriate mothers; violence between family members; turmoil in the home setting; and feelings of distrust among the children in the home. Health-care providers need to be aware of protective factors that have been identified in order to provide health-care teaching to adolescents and empower them with strategies to reduce their risk. Education, spiritual support, improved economic conditions, conflict resolution skills, and reduced use of drugs and alcohol are areas of education focus and patient advocacy that can be addressed by health-care providers. Finally, because access to guns impacts the adolescent homicide rate, implementation of gun safety classes is another appropriate area for intervention.

Suicide is the third leading cause of death in adolescents, and as such, needs to be understood and addressed by health-care providers. As a result of their developing personality and peer and family pressures, adolescents may become easily overwhelmed and anxious and look to suicide as an answer to their distress. Although female adolescents are more likely to engage in suicide attempts, males are more likely to complete them and account for approximately 85% of all suicides, while females account for 15%. Adolescent Native Americans and Alaskan Natives have the highest rates of suicide; African Americans, Hispanics, and Asians have the lowest rates of suicide (National Institute of Mental Health [NIMH], 2010; Varghese & Gray, 2011).

Common symptoms of suicidal ideation that can be addressed by health-care providers include the following: reports of crying frequently, fatigue and insomnia, feelings of isolation, and changes in body weight. Adolescents may exhibit additional symptoms, such as behavior problems, violence, sexual promiscuity, a drop in academic performance, and school absence. Nurses who are aware of any of these symptoms should ask if the adolescent has plans to commit suicide, the means to commit suicide, and if there have been any previous attempts at suicide. Adolescents who are determined to be at low risk for suicide should be referred to a mental health professional; those determined to be at high risk for suicide should be immediately evaluated by a mental health professional (Shropshire & Thornton, 2011; Varghese & Gray, 2011; Williams, Daley, & Iennaco, 2010).

Risk-Taking Behaviors

As in childhood, it is normal for adolescents to engage in risk-taking behavior. Taking healthy risks provides an avenue for discovering and developing one's own identity. Parents need to be taught that they can facilitate healthy risk-taking through talking with their adolescent openly and honestly and helping their child to understand the consequences of healthy versus unhealthy risk-taking behaviors. Ongoing dialogue provides an opportunity to explore alternative actions, and sharing a personal history of past risk-taking behaviors conveys the message that making mistakes is not a fatal act.

Health-care providers and parents can assist adolescents in finding alternative behaviors to provide outlets for identity development through providing them with challenges that create risk while promoting healthy decision making (Box 4-4).

Injury Prevention

Unhealthy risk-taking often leads to injuries for adolescents, and the most common injuries are related to motor vehicles, bicycles, firearms, and water. Nurses and parents can provide valuable teaching to adolescents and empower them to take necessary precautions to avoid injury. One of

---

Box 4-4 **Healthy Risk Alternatives for Adolescents**

PHYSICAL ACTIVITIES
- Team sports
- Horseback riding
- Camping
- Rock climbing (with supervision)
- White water rafting (with supervision)

CREATIVE ACTIVITIES
- Joining a band
- Acting in a play
- Photography
- Dance
- Producing a video

DEVELOPING RELATIONSHIPS
- Talking openly about sex and relationships
- Volunteering in the community
- Participating in a student exchange program

LEARNING RESPONSIBILITY
- Getting a part-time job
- Tutoring

---

the most important ways in which parents can affect adolescent safety is to set a good example and be a positive role model.

DRIVING SAFELY. Because motor vehicle accidents occur so commonly and cause such significant injury, there needs to be a strong focus on injury prevention for this activity. Recommendations for parents to ensure safe driving include establishing limits, such as the number of passengers and restriction to daytime driving, enforcing penalties for unsafe driving practices, adult supervision of adolescents while driving, ensuring mechanical safety, and mandating the use of seat belts.

BICYCLE SAFETY. Another common area of injury in adolescence, and one that is not often discussed includes activities that involve bicycles, in-line skating, and skateboarding. Head injuries related to these activities are quite common in this age group. Approximately 50% of young adolescents hospitalized for a bicycle-related injury have some degree of brain injury. Behaviors that cause the majority of the injuries include riding into a street without yielding or stopping, swerving into traffic, and riding against the flow of traffic.

Consistent use of a helmet is one of the best preventive strategies. It is essential that the helmet fit properly—it should not move around when the straps are fastened—and the straps should remain fastened when in use. When worn and used correctly, helmets can reduce the risk of a head injury by 85% and the risk of brain damage by 88%. All helmets should meet the standards established by the American National Standards Institute, the American Society for Testing and Materials, and the United States Consumer Product Safety Commission.

FIREARM SAFETY. Curiosity and impulse control remain important factors in firearm-related injuries and deaths among adolescents. Parents should consider the risks associated with storing a firearm in the home. In this age group, ready access to a firearm is the most frequent cause of the experimentation. If parents choose to keep a firearm in the home for protection or for hunting, it should be safely stored in a locked cabinet and all ammunition placed in a separate, locked location. A firearm safety class should be mandatory for adolescents who engage in the sport of hunting with parents or peers.

WATER SAFETY. Adolescents, who are in the process of developing formal operational thought, have an increased risk of drowning when swimming because of an overestimation of ability and skill, a lack of awareness of water depth and currents, and the use of alcohol and drugs. Safety measures include insisting that adolescents do not swim alone and teaching them never to dive into shallow water, above-ground pools, or the shallow end of an inground pool. In addition, adolescents riding in a boat should be required to wear personal flotation devices that are securely fastened. Parents and health-care providers should routinely incorporate safety education into discussions with adolescents.

Now Can You—Provide safety education to adolescents?

1. Identify the three leading causes of death in adolescents?
2. Discuss methods for improving driving safety?
3. Identify the best method of preventing injury related to bicycle riding?
4. Describe methods to facilitate firearm safety?

REPRODUCTIVE HEALTH SAFETY. Safety with regard to reproductive health can be positively impacted through proper, sensitive, and honest education on topics related to sexual activity. While the majority of parents indicate that they believe education on issues of sexual health should be taught in the family, most also agree that they do not feel prepared to do so alone. Many schools have subsequently incorporated education on sexuality into curricula in an effort to facilitate transfer of factual information.

Developmentally, adolescence is characterized by attempts to develop a personal identity, which includes sexual and gender identity. Young people are bombarded with sexual images from music, television, advertisements, and movies on a daily basis. Providing adolescents with correct information on issues of sexuality helps to empower them to make healthy decisions regarding their own sexual behavior. Whether taught by parents, health-care providers, or classroom educators, educational content should include human development, reproductive anatomy and physiology, relationships, personal coping skills and decision making, sexual behavior, contraceptive use, condom use, sexual health, and gender role development (Fantasia & Fontenot, 2011; Fantasia, Fontenot, Harris, Hurd, & Chui, 2011).

It is also important that the information provided is appropriate to the age and sexual experience of the adolescent. For those who have not engaged in sexual intercourse, an approach that focuses on abstinence as the only absolute way to avoid pregnancy and sexually transmitted infections may be appropriate. Education that focuses on the avoidance of unprotected sex by the use of a condom with every sexual encounter may be an appropriate approach for adolescents who have begun to have sexual intercourse. Life-building skills that are necessary for adolescents, and which may facilitate appropriate decision making, include negotiation skills, values clarification, goal setting, and interpersonal communication (Harris, 2011).

SUBSTANCE ABUSE. Experimentation and risk-taking behavior as a means of self-discovery and identity development are common during adolescence. Often this experimentation involves the use of drugs and alcohol. The reasons that adolescents give for trying drugs and alcohol include: to satisfy curiosity, to achieve a feeling of well-being while under the influence, to reduce stress, and to fit in with peers. Adolescents who are at an increased risk for developing dependency are those with low self-esteem, a family history of substance abuse, depression, and those who do not feel accepted by their peers.

Alcohol and marijuana are the most common drugs used by adolescents. On average, alcohol use begins at age 12 and marijuana use at age 14. Adolescent substance use is associated with school failure, an increased risk for accidents, violence, suicide, and unplanned and unsafe sexual activity (Substance Abuse and Mental Health Services Administration [SAMHSA], 2012).

Nursing Insight—*Hazards of psychoactive "bath salts"*

Marketed under compelling names such as "White Rush," "Ocean Snow," and "Red Dove," psychoactive bath salts (PABS) are not intended for bathing at all. Instead, these highly toxic designer drugs contain powerful stimulants that are inhaled, injected, instilled per rectum, or taken by mouth. PABS are said to have the worst characteristics of lysergic acid diethylamide (LSD), phencyclidine (PCP), ecstasy, cocaine, and methamphetamine. Adverse effects include liver failure, tachycardia, seizures, hyperthermia, rhabdomyolysis, panic attacks, and violent behavior. Available for about $20 at convenience stores, gas stations, and on the Internet, the drugs are often taken with other substances such as marijuana, opiates, cocaine, and amphetamines and in combination or alone have been fatal. Recently, the U.S. Drug Enforcement Administration (DEA) issued an order to temporarily classify the stimulants used in PABS (similar in effect to illegal drugs but dissimilar in structure) as Schedule I controlled substances (Benzie, Hekman, Cameron, Wade, Miller, Smolinske, et al., 2011; Jordan & Harrison, 2013; Ross, Watson, & Goldberger, 2011; Rutecki, 2011).

There are many warning signs to alert parents to adolescent substance abuse. Physical signs include fatigue, red and glazed eyes, chronic cough, and health complaints. Emotional signs include personality changes, sudden mood swings, irritability, poor judgment and decision making, depression, and lack of interest in things that were of previous interest. As the substance abuse continues, adolescents may demonstrate a negative attitude, withdraw from the family or from previous friends, and become increasingly argumentative and secretive. Academic performance often drops and school officials report problems with truancy and discipline.

Parents need to be informed about the types of drugs that adolescents may use and the possible adverse consequences associated with each. Early and ongoing parent-adolescent education, open communication, appropriate role modeling, and the early recognition of developing problems are the best strategies for prompt identification and interventions for substance use.

VIOLENCE AND ABUSE. Negative consequences are also seen in the rising degree of violence and abuse in the adolescent population. In 2006, there were 29 violent crimes at school per 1,000 students. This included rape, both sexual and aggravated assault, and robbery. It is estimated that over 32% of all middle school students encounter some type of bullying, either as the bully, as a victim of the bully, as a victim of cyber bullying, or both (CDC, 2013c).

Violence is a learned behavior. Adolescents learn to solve problems through violence by watching parents, teachers, and others in the community and in the media and by role modeling their behavior. To engage in problem-solving behavior without violence, adolescents need to be taught how to assess the conflict, see the other person's point of view, and then redefine the conflict so that they and the others involved can negotiate to a decision without violence.

Parents need to allow the adolescent to develop social relationships outside the family to mature and define their identity. At the same time, they need to continue to set limits to adolescent behavior, maintain open and honest communication on problem-solving, and allow the adolescent to evaluate options to conflict resolution in passive, yet assertive ways.

Successful conflict resolution strategies enable the adolescent to remain calm in a potentially violent situation and to understand that the aggressor is attempting to resolve the conflict in ways that are understood by him. If communication and respect are not facilitating conflict resolution, the adolescent should be taught to remove himself from the potentially dangerous situation (Sutherland, 2011).

Cultural Diversity: *Exploring Differences in Ethnicity and Race in Adolescent Violence*

- African Americans, Native Americans, and Hispanics are more likely to be victims or the persons responsible for fatal violence than Asians or Caucasians.
- These differences are more pronounced in adolescent aggression resulting in homicide than adolescent aggression not resulting in homicide.
- Homicide rates were consistently higher for Non-Hispanic African Americans than for all other race/ethnicity groups from 1994 to 2010. Homicide rates for Non-Hispanic African Americans declined from 60.6 per 100,000 population in 1994 to 28.8 per 100,000 in 2010.
- African Americans, Native Americans, and Hispanics are arrested more often for acts of interpersonal violence than Asians or Caucasians.
- Hispanic adolescent males are more likely to be victims of homicide than African Americans or Caucasians.
- African Americans account for the majority of all adolescents known to have committed murder.

Sources: CDC, 2013d; Center for the Study and Prevention of Violence, 2010.

Adolescents are particularly vulnerable to violence and abuse in dating relationships as well. Parents should be encouraged to discuss these issues openly before dating begins to prevent this type of abuse from occurring. Dating provides an opportunity to develop healthy love relationships that are built on mutual respect and trust. Similar to abusive situations, relationships can become coercive and escalate to physical abuse at a later time. Indicators of a coercive relationship include:

- Telling a partner what to wear
- Telling a partner where she is allowed to go
- Telling a partner who she can be friends with or talk to
- Making a partner do something she does not want to do
- Destroying the partner's personal property
- Threatening to hurt oneself if the partner breaks up with him
- Repeatedly contacting the partner after a breakup

Indications of abuse, which may be directed toward the male or female partner, can include rude and swearing talk, forcing sexual activity against the partner's will, humiliating one's partner in front of other people, and hitting or hurting one's partner in any way. If parents are aware of any of these behaviors, it is their responsibility to intervene, even to the point of legal action. Through interaction and communication, parents can have a lasting effect on helping their adolescent to develop future healthy relationships with others (Fontenot & Fantasia, 2011; Hanson, 2010; Kang, Gottlieb, Raker, Aneja, & Boardman, 2010).

TATTOOING AND BODY PIERCING. Tattooing and body piercing are examples of adolescent risk-taking behavior (Rutecki, 2010; Ziegler, 2011) and are associated with other high-risk activities, including smoking, alcohol use, use of smokeless tobacco, and riding in a vehicle driven by another individual who has been drinking. Health risks associated with tattooing and body piercing may be infectious or noninfectious.

Infectious health risks include viral, bacterial, and fungal diseases, most commonly infections caused by viruses and bacteria. The most common infections associated with tattooing and body piercing include hepatitis, HIV, and human papillomavirus (HPV). Bacterial infections may be caused by *Staphylococcus*, *Streptococcus*, *Pseudomonas*, *Clostridium*, and *Mycobacterium* (Ziegler, 2011). These organisms have the potential to cause lifelong infection with adverse effects on various body systems or the progression to other diseases, such as cancer and tuberculosis. Allergic or hypersensitivity reactions are the most common noninfectious responses to tattooing and body piercing. Although these reactions may be transient, they can lead to the development of more serious lesions that require surgical intervention.

HEALTH PROMOTION

Although the majority of adolescents have not yet become sexually active, it is important that health-care providers promote activities to prevent health problems from developing as they mature. Adolescents should be taught about skin cancer, the hazards associated with indoor/outdoor tanning, and the importance of consistent sunscreen use. They should also be taught about breast self-awareness (being aware of how the breasts normally look and feel), how to perform breast self-examination (BSE) early in their development, and how to engage in activities to promote

optimal bone health. Once adolescents become sexually active, they should be encouraged to have regular gynecological examinations.

Prevention of Skin Cancer

Each year more than 2 million U.S. residents are diagnosed with skin cancer. At current rates, 1 in 5 Americans will develop skin cancer in their lifetime. Approximately 75% of skin cancer deaths result from melanoma, and the incidence of melanoma has been rising for at least 30 years, particularly among young, white women (ACS, 2011a; Zoller, 2011).

Although melanoma is the least common form of skin cancer, it is more likely to metastasize than other skin cancers and thus is considered to be more dangerous. Originating in the melanocyte cells, common sites for this skin cancer type are the trunk (men) and the legs (women), but melanoma can appear anywhere on the body, including the face, neck, eyes, mouth, and vagina. Darker skinned individuals who develop melanoma often have cancer under their nails (Hutchinson's sign), on the palms of the hands, and on the soles of the feet (ACS, 2011a; Zoller, 2011).

Most skin cancers are basal cell carcinomas (BCC) or squamous cell carcinomas (SCC). Originating in the epidermal basal cell layer, BCC commonly develops in sun-exposed areas such as the head and the neck. Although it tends to grow slowly, if left untreated, BCC can invade tissue or bone close to the original lesion. Interestingly, approximately 50% of individuals who are diagnosed and treated for BCC experience a recurrence within 5 years. Also appearing on sun-exposed areas (e.g., ears, lips, face, neck, and backs of the hands), SCC tends to be more invasive than BCC. Areas of likely metastasis include the fatty tissues beneath the skin and the lymph nodes (ACS, 2011a; Zoller, 2011).

Although most individuals are aware that exposure to ultraviolet (UV) radiation is the leading risk factor for skin cancer, teens and young women continue to use tanning beds or intentionally sun bathe outdoors to enhance their skin tone. Results of a survey conducted in 2011 by the American Academy of Dermatology (AAD) revealed that women ages 18 to 22 were almost twice as likely to have used indoor tanning (40%) compared with the 14 to 17 age group (22%). Caucasian girls and women, primarily aged 16 to 29 years, account for nearly 70% of tanning salon patrons. A separate study (Mosher & Danoff-Burg, 2010) suggests that some individuals may develop an addiction to indoor tanning because of the production of endorphins via exposure to UV light. Although spray tans are considered a safe alternative to UV exposure from the sun and indoor tanning beds, 85% of survey respondents indicated that they never received a spray tan in the past year (AAD, 2011).

Despite claims by the tanning industry to the contrary, indoor tanning is so dangerous that the U.S. Department of Health and Human Services and the World Health Organization's International Agency of Research on Cancer panel have declared UV radiation from the sun and artificial light sources (such as tanning beds and sun lamps) as a known carcinogen. Studies show indoor tanning increases a person's risk of melanoma by 75%, and presently, melanoma is increasing faster in females 15 to 29 years old than in males of the same age group (AAD, 2011).

⊜ Optimizing Outcomes—Counseling to prevent skin cancer

In late 2011, the U.S. Preventive Services Task Force (USPSTF) updated its recommendations regarding behavioral counseling to prevent skin cancer. Stating that the goal of behavioral counseling is to increase sun-protective behaviors shown to be effective in reducing UV radiation from the sun and from indoor tanning, the USPSTF made the following recommendation: To reduce the risk for and prevent incidence of skin cancer, the USPSTF recommends counseling children, adolescents, and young adults aged 10 to 24 years who have fair skin about minimizing their exposure to UV radiation. The task force concluded that current evidence is insufficient to determine the balance of benefits and harms of counseling adults older than age 24 years about minimizing their risks to prevent skin cancer (USPSTF, 2011a).

Adolescents and young women should be educated about the hazards of intentional sun exposure and encouraged to take measures to prevent skin cancer. Nurses can teach them to avoid sun exposure between the hours of 11 a.m. and 3 p.m. and to generously apply sunscreen (sun protection factor [SPF] 15 or higher) to all sun-exposed areas, with reapplication after swimming or heavy perspiration. During periods of sun exposure, patients should understand that tightly woven fabrics provide better UV protection than loosely woven clothing and that FDA-certified protective eyewear should be worn. Nurses can encourage them to consider tanning alternatives such as sunless tanning lotions and sprays. Also, patients should be made aware that certain medications (e.g., doxycycline) cause photosensitivity and thus increase skin cancer risk (AAD, 2011; ACS, 2011a; Zoller, 2011).

❋ Cultural Diversity: Skin Color and Skin Cancer Risk

Individuals with lighter skin and eyes and those with freckles and blond or red hair tend to burn more easily and thus are at a greater risk for skin cancer. Although people of color may be less likely than Caucasians to develop melanoma, those who do develop this deadliest form of skin cancer are more likely than Caucasians to die from it. The 5-year survival rate for African Americans with melanoma is 59% compared with 85% for Caucasians. Although skin cancer constitutes only 1% to 2% of all cancers in African Americans, patients in this population are more likely to be diagnosed later with advanced cases (Skin Cancer Foundation, 2011).

Prevention of Osteoporosis

Osteoporosis has been described as a "pediatric disease with geriatric consequences" (Chesnut, 1989). While adolescents are not at high risk for the development of this condition, which is characterized by loss of bone mass throughout the skeleton, it is essential that steps be taken at this early age to decrease the risk later in life. Strategies that are appropriate for adolescents include maintaining an adequate intake of calcium and vitamin D and engaging in regular exercise. Adolescents are at an increased risk for unhealthy eating behaviors that result in a calcium intake that falls far short of the amount needed for bone strengthening. Thus, nutritional intake during the adolescent years becomes even more important. In addition, adequate amounts of vitamin D are necessary to facilitate the absorption of calcium. Regular exercise helps the adolescent to achieve peak bone density levels. Weight-bearing exercises, including walking, dancing, certain sports, and hiking, are the best activities for young people to develop strong muscles and bones (Nelson, 2010).

⊜ Optimizing Outcomes—With vitamin D for lifelong skeletal health

Vitamin D, an important steroid hormone that controls calcium and phosphorus homeostasis and the development and preservation of bone integrity, is essential to women's health. According to the Office of Dietary Supplements, both breastfed infants and nonbreastfed/weaned infants require 400 IU/d, with the latter also consuming 1,000 mL/d of fortified milk. Children and adults are likewise advised to receive 600 IU/d of vitamin D in fortified milk or as a supplement. The general recommendation for healthy adults under the age of 71 is 600 IU/d, and healthy people over the age of 71 should have 800 IU/d. Individuals who have very little sun exposure, dark skin, osteoporosis, problems absorbing dietary fat, or who are taking medicines that interfere with vitamin D absorption may need more (Emeis, 2011; Hoffman, 2010; Office of Dietary Supplements, 2011).

Gynecological Examinations

Another aspect of developing health practices that continues into later years is the initiation of gynecological examinations during adolescence. It is important for parents and adolescents to understand that the first visit may not necessarily include an internal pelvic examination and collection of specimens.

The first visit, which should occur between the ages of 13 and 15, should be used as an introduction to reproductive health care. The health-care provider should discuss issues of sexuality with the adolescent to help prepare her for making appropriate decisions. Information and reassurance can be provided regarding normal development, and education on sexually transmitted infections and sexual behavior can empower the adolescent for informed sexual decision making. It is essential that nurses take measures to ensure the adolescent's right to confidential health-care services and promote policies in health-care settings to ensure this right (ACOG, 2010a,b; Association of Women's Health, Obstetric and Neonatal Nurses (AWHONN), 2010a; Braverman & Breech, 2010).

The first pelvic examination should be performed at age 21 or 3 years after the initiation of sexual activity, whichever comes first. Other reasons for pelvic examination include unexplained pain in the lower abdomen or pelvic region; vaginal discharge that causes itching, burning, or has an odor; delayed menstruation; prolonged menstruation lasting more than 10 days; dysmenorrhea; and missed periods.

PELVIC EXAMINATION. The frequency of pelvic examinations varies based on age. Females should have pelvic examinations once they become sexually active. Women ages

21 to 40 should undergo a pelvic examination at least every 3 years or annually if high risk. "High risk" includes those with abnormal findings on previous examinations, the presence of a sexually transmitted infection, sexual activity before age 18, multiple sexual partners, or abnormal spotting or bleeding. After the age of 40, pelvic examinations should be performed every 1 to 3 years, based on personal risk factors and history (Institute for Clinical Systems Improvement, 2013).

The nurse assists the patient with relaxation techniques before the pelvic examination, performed in a lithotomy position, is initiated. Anxiety is common, especially in women with a history of sexual abuse or assault. Deep breathing, a helpful relaxation strategy, is easy to perform. The patient is encouraged to take slow, deep breaths, in through the nose and out through the mouth. She should be observed for signs of hyperventilation and instructed to slow down her breathing if necessary. Visual imagery is another useful relaxation technique. Many health-care providers place engaging pictures on the ceiling for the recumbent patient to view. Some women relax with conversation. Others prefer to quietly concentrate on deep breathing and visualization. It is important to ask the patient if she prefers to talk during the examination.

EXTERNAL INSPECTION. The skin, including the labia majora, is inspected for color, bruising, erythema, lesions, and hair distribution (Fig. 4-4). Using a gloved hand, the examiner gently spreads the labia to assess the external genital structures (Fig. 4-5). The clitoris, labia minora, urethral opening, and vaginal opening are inspected for inflammation, lesions, and lumps. Bartholin's glands, which secrete fluid for lubrication, are palpated using the index finger and thumb and are assessed for edema, pain, and discharge. The vaginal orifice is opened slightly, and the patient is asked to squeeze the vaginal muscles. This technique allows the examiner to inspect for cystocele, rectocele, uterine prolapse, and incontinence.

VULVAR SELF-EXAMINATION. Nurses can play a vital role in the early detection and treatment of vulvar and vaginal cancer by teaching patients about monthly self-examination.

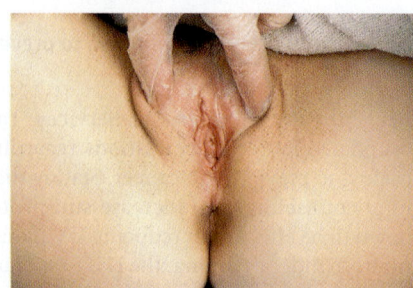

Figure 4-5 Using the fingers to separate the labia to assess the external genital structures.

Routine self-examination frequently allows for the early identification and evaluation of abnormalities.

INTERNAL INSPECTION. The examiner uses a speculum for the internal inspection (Fig. 4-6). The speculum should be warmed or maintained at room temperature and moistened with a small amount of water or lubricating gel, which has been shown to be associated with decreased patient pain during vaginal speculum insertion (Hill & Lamvu, 2012). Depending on the situation, specimens may be collected for cervical cancer screening (Papanicolaou test), gonorrhea, chlamydia, trichomoniasis, bacterial vaginosis, candidiasis, group B *Streptococcus*, and herpes simplex virus. The specimens for cervical cancer screening must be obtained first to avoid cell damage during the collection of additional specimens. Common sexually transmitted infections (STIs), symptoms, and methods of diagnosis are presented in Table 4-4. (See Chapters 9, 11, and 19 for further discussion.)

Once the speculum is inserted, the blades are opened fully to allow complete visualization of the cervix and cervical os (Fig. 4-7). The cervix should be pink, smooth, and absent of lesions or lacerations. It should be midline with no lateral displacement. The cervical os is rounded in nulliparous women and slit-shaped in multiparous women. Secretions in the cervical area may appear thin and watery or thick and stringy, depending on the day of the menstrual cycle. The secretions should be clear to opaque and have no foul odor. Around the time of ovulation, the cervical secretions are more profuse, slippery, and stretchy to facilitate sperm transport through the cervical mucus. Once the specimens have been collected, the speculum is slowly removed and the vaginal vault is inspected for color and the presence of inflammation, edema, bleeding, and discharge. (See Chapter 9 for further discussion.)

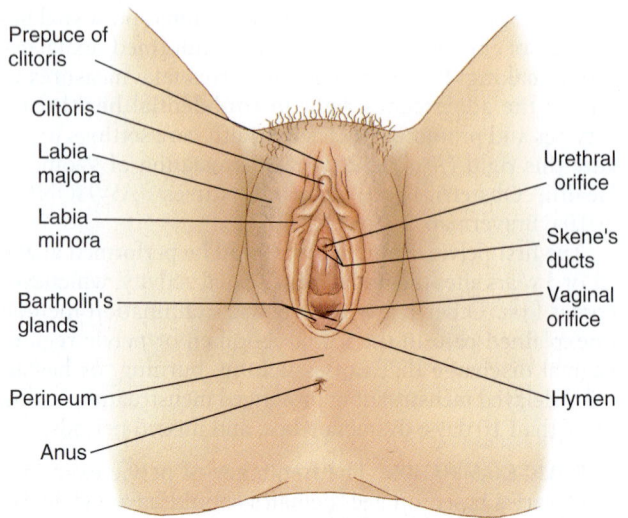

Figure 4-4 Female external genitalia.

Prepuce of clitoris
Clitoris
Labia majora
Labia minora
Bartholin's glands
Perineum
Anus
Urethral orifice
Skene's ducts
Vaginal orifice
Hymen

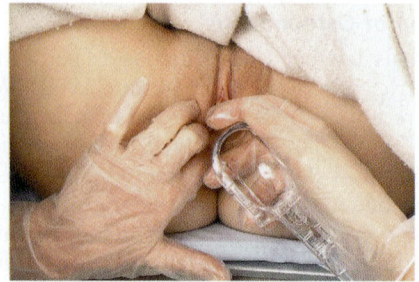

Figure 4-6 Inserting the speculum.

Table 4-4 Summary of Common Sexually Transmitted Infections

Infection	Symptoms (May Be Asymptomatic)	Detection
Gonorrhea	Purulent vaginal discharge Dyspareunia Abdominal pain Dysuria	Endocervical culture Urine test
Chlamydia	Mucopurulent discharge Postcoital bleeding Dyspareunia Abdominal pain Dysuria	Endocervical culture Urine test
Trichomoniasis	Frothy malodorous vaginal discharge Dyspareunia Vaginal itching/irritation Dysuria	Saline wet mount of vaginal discharge viewed under microscope
Hepatitis B	Fatigue Nausea/anorexia Dark urine Clay-colored stool Jaundice/abdominal pain	Serological testing With acute infection: Test — Result HbsAg — Positive Anti-Hbc — Positive IgM anti-Hbc — Positive Anti-Hbs — Negative
Human papillomavirus (HPV)	Visible wart-like growths in genital area associated with subtypes including 6, 11, 16, 18, 42, 44, and others	Pap test report Physical examination Colposcopy/biopsy
Syphilis	**Primary** Chancre (painless raised ulcer) **Secondary** Skin rash, lymphadenopathy **Tertiary** Cardiac, ophthalmic, auditory involvement	**Serological Testing** Nontreponemal test (RPR, VDRL) • Reported quantitatively (titers) Fourfold decrease in titers indicates treatment success • False-positive possible • Treponemal test (FTA-ABS) • Specific for syphilis • Reported as positive or negative
HIV	Fever Malaise Lymphadenopathy Skin rash Rapid weight loss Night sweats	Screening Enzyme-linked immunosorbent assay (ELISA): Positive screen must be confirmed by more specific test (e.g., Western blot or immunofluorescence assay [IFA])
Herpes simplex virus (HSV)	Painful, recurrent vesicular lesions Fever, malaise Enlarged lymph nodes	Viral culture

Note: Please visit the CDC Web site (http://www.cdc.gov) for current information regarding STI treatment guidelines.
Source: Holloway, B. W., & Moredich, C. (2011). *OB/GYN Peds Notes: Nurse's clinical pocket guide.* Philadelphia, PA: F.A. Davis.

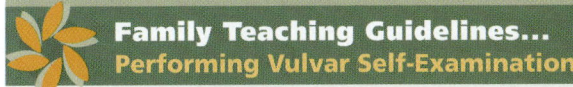

Family Teaching Guidelines...
Performing Vulvar Self-Examination

To prepare for vulvar self-examination, the woman places a flashlight and mirror within easy reach. She washes her hands, removes clothing from the waist down, and sits comfortably on the floor or bed, with a pillow support behind her back. The following steps should then be performed:

1. While bending her knees, she leans backward and allows her knees to fall slightly apart to expose the genital area. The mirror and flashlight should be positioned for optimal visualization.

2. External inspection of the genital area includes visualizing the labia, the clitoris, the urethral meatus, the vaginal opening, and the anal opening.

3. Using her fingers, the woman should gently spread the labia and inspect the vaginal vault. The vaginal walls should be pink and contain small folds or ridges, called rugae.

4. The vaginal discharge should be evaluated at this time as well. Normal vaginal discharge is clear to cloudy and white, with a slightly acidic odor; it may be thick or thin,

(continued)

depending on the timing of the examination with regard to the menstrual cycle.

5. Findings that need to be reported to the health-care provider include the presence of sores or growths on the labia or vaginal walls, an unpleasant odor to the vaginal discharge, and tissue redness. Sores, redness, abnormal

growths, malodorous or excessive vaginal discharge, and itching may indicate irritation or infection.

Source: Vulval Pain Society. (2012). *How to do vulval self-examination*. Retrieved from http://vulvalpainsociety.org/index.php?page=self-examination

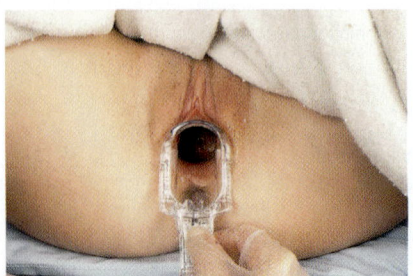

Figure 4-7 Opening the speculum.

PAPANICOLAOU TEST. The Papanicolaou test (Pap test) is the microscopic examination of cells taken from the cervical area by various techniques. It is the most reliable method used to screen the patient for preinvasive cervical cancer. The American College of Obstetricians and Gynecologists (ACOG) and the U.S. Preventive Services Task Force (USPSTF) recommend the first Pap test at age 21 years regardless of sexual history. Cervical cytology screening is recommended every 2 years for women aged 21 to 29 years, with either conventional or liquid-based cytology. After age 30 and three consecutive negative Pap tests, screening may be performed every 3 years, in consultation with the health-care provider. Women ages 65 to 70 who have had three or more negative cytology test results in a row and no abnormal test results in the past 10 years may choose to stop Pap screening. Women in high-risk categories should continue to have more frequent Pap tests, according to standard guidelines and their care provider's recommendations (ACOG, 2010a, 2010b, 2012; Burkman, 2010; Carter & Downs, 2011; USPSTF, 2012).

The Papanicolaou test should not be performed if the woman is menstruating or has an infection. The best time to collect the specimen is at mid-cycle to ensure the absence of menstrual blood, which may distort results. The nurse should confirm that the woman has not had intercourse or douched within the 24 hours preceding the test. Using a spatula or an endocervical sampling device, cells are scraped from the cervical os and from around the cervical opening. With one cytological preparatory technique, the sample is smeared onto a slide, sprayed immediately with a fixative solution, and allowed to dry. With another method (e.g., ThinPrep Pap Test or BD SurePath Pap Test), the specimen is placed directly into a prepared vial of preservative. Regardless of the method used, the sample is labeled and sent to a laboratory for cytological examination (Afify & Howell, 2010).

BIMANUAL PALPATION. The examiner lubricates the first and second (gloved) fingers with water-soluble lubricant. The vaginal canal is palpated for the presence of tenderness, lesions, and nodules (Fig. 4-8). The cervix is palpated for position, consistency, contour, and mobility. It should be soft and movable without tenderness. The uterus is palpated to determine if it is in a midposition or retroverted or anteverted (Fig. 4-9). It should be soft, movable, and nontender. The uterine fundus (upper area above the openings of the fallopian tubes) should be rounded. The examiner then palpates the adnexa to assess for masses or tenderness. The ovaries may or may not be palpable. If palpable, they should be mobile, smooth, and firm. Ovarian palpation may cause some slight discomfort (Fig. 4-10). Structures on each side of the uterus are palpated. As the examiner's fingers are removed, the patient is asked to tighten her vaginal muscles to facilitate assessment of pubococcygeal muscle strength. This component of the examination provides an opportune time to teach about pelvic floor (Kegel) exercises. (See Chapter 9 for further discussion.)

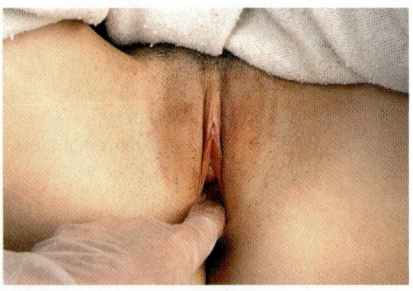

Figure 4-8 The vaginal canal is palpated for the presence of tenderness, lesions, and nodules.

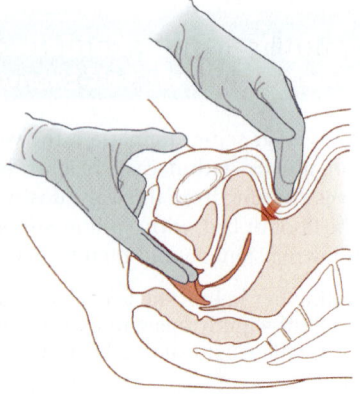

Figure 4-9 Palpating the uterus.

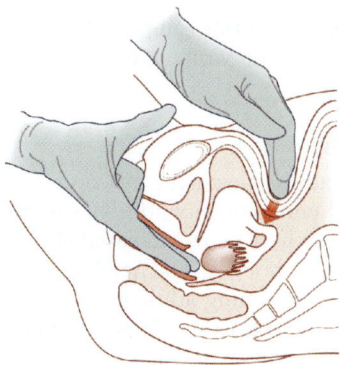

Figure 4-10 Palpating the ovaries.

RECTOVAGINAL PALPATION. The examiner changes gloves before this component of the examination. Following application of a water-based lubricant, the examiner inserts the index finger into the vagina and the middle finger into the rectum. To facilitate insertion and assessment of muscle strength, the patient is asked to bear down during the insertion. The procedures of the bimanual palpation are repeated, allowing the examiner to palpate the rectovaginal wall, the posterior side of the uterus, and the area behind the adnexa. Palpation should reveal no tenderness or the presence of fissures or masses along the rectovaginal wall. The uterus and adnexa should be nontender, soft, movable, and absent of masses (Figs. 4-11, 4-12, and 4-13).

Now Can You—Discuss the pelvic examination process?

1. Discuss patient preparation for the procedure?
2. Identify the structures that are examined during the external assessment?
3. Identify the specimens collected during the internal inspection and explain their importance?
4. List the structures that are evaluated during the bimanual palpation?

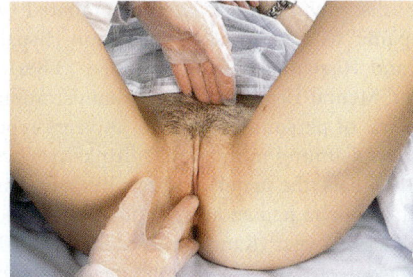

Figure 4-11 Inserting fingers for the rectovaginal exam.

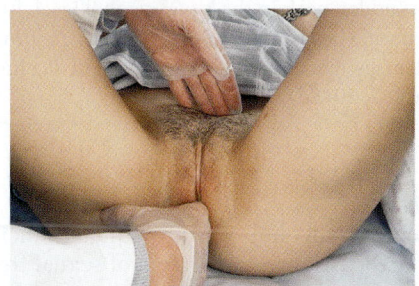

Figure 4-12 Performing the rectovaginal exam.

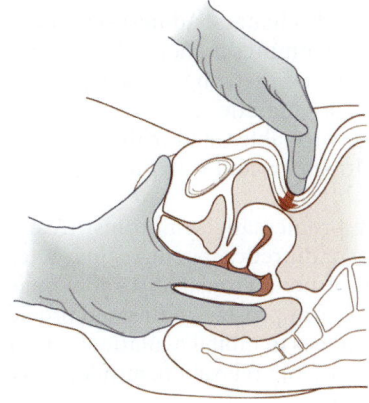

Figure 4-13 Proper position of the hands.

MENSTRUAL DISORDERS

Various menstrual disorders may occur during adolescence. The most common conditions are menstrual cramps, **dysmenorrhea** (painful menstruation that interferes with daily activities), and premenstrual syndrome (PMS). Painful cramping in the uterus during menstruation occurs from myometrial contractions induced by prostaglandins during the second phase of the menstrual cycle. **Prostaglandins** are chemical mediators that cause pain as part of the inflammatory response; during menstruation, the cramps are frequently accompanied by back pain and headache. Peaking levels of prostaglandins cause the symptoms to begin a day or two before the beginning of menstrual flow and continue until about the second or third day of menstrual flow.

Dysmenorrhea is painful menstruation that affects a woman's ability to perform daily activities for 2 or more days each month. Health-care teaching for females experiencing dysmenorrhea should be holistic in nature and include relaxation and breathing techniques, the use of heat to reduce uterine contractions and increase blood flow to the uterine tissues, exercise or rest, and the use of nonsteroidal anti-inflammatory drugs to inhibit the synthesis of prostaglandin. For some women, dysmenorrhea is symptomatic of other conditions, including pelvic inflammatory disease and endometriosis. Severe pain and dysmenorrhea that disrupts a woman's life should be evaluated by a health-care provider (Gilliam, 2010; Woo & McEneaney, 2010).

PMS is another commonly occurring disorder associated with menstruation that affects adolescents. Approximately 85% of all females experience some degree of symptoms related to PMS. Symptoms range from irritability and mood changes to fluid retention, heart palpitations, and visual disturbances. While the most common cause of PMS is the normal fluctuation of estrogen and progesterone during the menstrual cycle, other factors may be associated with PMS symptoms as well. For example, some PMS symptoms may result from the following: an imbalance in the levels of estrogen and progesterone, **hyperprolactinemia** (an excessive secretion of prolactin, the hormone responsible for stimulation of breast development), alterations in carbohydrate metabolism and hypoglycemia, and an excessive production of aldosterone resulting in sodium and water retention.

Recommendations for reducing the severity of the symptoms associated with PMS include the incorporation of simple lifestyle changes. Adolescents should be encouraged to have 60 minutes or more of physical activity daily, eat a well-balanced diet, and get adequate sleep and rest. Dietary changes include increasing the daily intake of whole grains, vegetables, and fruits, while decreasing the intake of salt, sugar, and caffeine (CDC, 2013e; Raines, 2010).

For more problematic symptoms, treatment may include the use of diuretics to reduce fluid retention, the administration of nonsteroidal anti-inflammatory drugs to inhibit synthesis of prostaglandins and provide pain relief, oral contraceptives to inhibit ovulation, central nervous depressants to promote relaxation, antidepressants, and vitamin supplements.

Young Adulthood Health

Formal operational thought is completed as individuals move from adolescence into young adulthood (ages 19 to 34). The developmental stage during this time period is *intimacy versus isolation*. The individual no longer views the family as the primary source of identity, and developmental tasks center on making a personal commitment to another individual as a partner or spouse. With the increased independence associated with young adulthood and the concomitant increase in age, new challenges to health promotion and disease prevention arise. During young adulthood there is a focus on safety, sexual health, reproductive health promotion that includes breast awareness (with monthly practice of self-examination if desired) and yearly clinical breast examinations, and awareness of potential gynecological disorders common to this age group.

NUTRITION

In 2011, the U.S. Department of Health and Human Services released an updated *Dietary Guidelines for Americans 2010*. These new nutritional recommendations are evidence-based and designed to promote health and reduce the risk of chronic diseases through improved nutrition (e.g., there are 23 recommendations on healthy eating) and physical activity. The longstanding food pyramid has been replaced with a plate divided into four unequal quadrants of vegetables, grains, fruits, and protein with a circle (representing the top view of a glass) off to the side for dairy (see Fig. 4-3).

The two larger quadrants of the ChooseMyPlate graphic stress an increased consumption of vegetables and whole grains. Essentially, adults are encouraged to eat less food and avoid oversized portions. Approximately one-half of the plate should be filled with fruits and vegetables, one-half of the grains consumed should consist of whole grains, and foods with lower sodium content should be selected. Also, adults should drink water instead of sugary drinks and switch to fat free or low fat milk (Sulak, 2011).

SAFETY

As young adults attempt to engage in dating relationships, the safety risks associated with substance use, sexual practices, and intimate partner violence become more evident. It is during this time, when young adults are developing relationships with members of the opposite or same sex in

intimate ways, that nurses can provide education and counseling and empower women to care for themselves in healthy ways.

Substance Use

Once young adults reach the age of 21, they can legally purchase and consume alcoholic beverages. This "rite of passage" places them at an increased risk for problems associated with alcohol use. The newly gained independence that comes as the young adult moves out of the parent's home, combined with the social acceptance of drinking during this time, may coincide to place the young adult in situations where excessive and binge drinking can be common and frequent. Although formal operational thought has been developed by this age, the brain continues to mature during young adulthood. Heavy or binge drinking during this time of brain development and independent decision making may cause serious health risks as well as risks to social growth.

In addition to alcohol consumption, young adults continue to be at risk for the use of illicit drugs. Peak use, similar to that of alcohol, occurs during the early 20s, declines in the late 20s, and tends to come to an end around age 30. The most reliable theory related to illicit substance use focuses on role development during young adulthood, specifically with regard to role normalization and role compatibility. As young adults take on more adult roles associated with employment, marriage, and parenting, the use of illicit drugs may decrease as performance is altered or the person is unable to meet role expectations. Similarly, when the adult roles are seen as being incompatible with illicit drug use and non-normative behavior, substance use declines.

Cultural Diversity: At-Risk Drinking and Alcohol Dependence Among Women

According to national surveys, American Indian and Alaska Native women (13.7%) were the most likely race to have an alcohol use disorder. This may be compared with white non-Hispanic women (5.6%), black non-Hispanic women (3.5%), and Hispanic or Latino women (3.8%) (Substance Abuse and Mental Health Services Administration, 2012). In 2009, 25.6% of persons aged 18 to 24 years reported binge drinking (consuming more than 3 drinks per occasion). Of those individuals, the majority were white non-Hispanic, college graduates who had an average household income greater than $50,000 per year (Kanny, Liu, & Brewer, 2011). Among women aged 18 to 34 years who binge drink, approximately one-third report drinking eight or more drinks per occasion (Naimi, Nelson, & Brewer, 2010). Binge drinking, which causes a sudden peak in the blood alcohol level, frequently results in unsafe behavior and the risk of more reproductive and organ damage than sustained high levels of alcohol consumption (ACOG, 2011d).

Sexual Health

While increased alcohol consumption and illicit drug use are associated with greater degrees of sexual freedom and loss of sexual inhibition, young adults are faced with sexual decision making regardless of substance use. Both males and females tend to have their sexual peak, with regard to interest, desire, ability, and performance in the mid- to late 20s, with sexual interest and ability beginning to decrease during the 30s. This is particularly true of males, because testosterone production and ejaculation decline later in young adulthood.

With regard to safe sex practices during young adulthood, it is essential for nurses to educate women regarding the anatomy and physiology of their bodies in an effort to facilitate an understanding of the heightened risk of susceptibility to sexually transmitted infections. Physiological factors that predispose women to increased susceptibility include an increased genital mucosal surface area, retention of semen in the vagina for several hours following intercourse, and the pH of the vagina. During menstruation, women are more vulnerable to infection as the pH of the vagina becomes more alkaline, thereby becoming more hospitable to viral and bacterial transmission and growth.

During young adulthood, abstinence remains the only safe method for protection against sexually transmitted infections. However, as young adults begin to experiment with sexual activity, nurses must continue to educate them on the proper use of condoms, including the use of a water-based lubricant to prevent tears in the mucosa, use of a barrier during oral sex, and protection and cleaning of sexual toys that may be used. While some nurses may find these topics difficult to approach and discuss openly, it is only through open communication that young adults are likely to incorporate safe practices into their development and experimentation.

HEALTH PROMOTION

Health practices, both positive and negative, that were initiated during adolescence will likely continue into young adulthood. During this time, dietary and exercise behaviors are more likely to either protect from or increase the risk of developing obesity, hypertension, type 2 diabetes mellitus, and cardiovascular disease. Specifically, the chronic illnesses that are more likely to emerge during young adulthood include cancer, cardiovascular disease, type 2 diabetes mellitus, and autoimmune diseases such as lupus erythematosus and multiple sclerosis.

For women, stress-related disorders become more apparent during this time. Stress can trigger behaviors such as overindulgence in comfort foods, alcohol abuse, and the use of marijuana and other drugs to reduce tension. It is encouraging that women in young adulthood are more likely to experiment with alternative therapies to relieve stress. Herbal methods, homeopathic remedies, spiritual approaches, music and dance, and art therapy may be used. Nurses need to understand and support these positive, alternative methods for stress reduction to promote a holistic approach to health and wellness.

🌸 Complementary Care: *Anxiety and Depression*

Herbal remedies for anxiety and depression include the use of kava kava, passionflower, valerian root, gotu kola, and St. John's wort. While these herbs are believed to reduce anxiety, stress, and muscle tension, the nurse should provide education on the potential side effects of these substances, which include gastrointestinal discomforts, nausea, and dizziness.

TESTICULAR CANCER SCREENING. Although considered rare, testicular cancer is the most common cancer found in young men 20 to 34 years of age. It is the second most common cancer in men 35 to 39 years of age, and the third most common cancer in men between the ages of 15 and 19. Risk factors for testicular cancer include a positive family history and a personal history of undescended testes; congenital gonadal dysgenesis; and Klinefelter's syndrome, a sex-linked genetic disorder. Interestingly, the majority of testicular tumors are discovered during self-examination. The National Cancer Institute (2012) does not recommend routine screening, other than clinical palpation, for testicular cancer because treatment is effective at each state of diagnosis. However, all males should be taught to palpate the testes for abnormal lumps, hardness, thicknesses, and masses on a regular basis.

GYNECOLOGICAL DISORDERS. Along with specific medical problems, certain gynecological disorders are more common during young adulthood as well. Endometriosis, cervical cancer, breast cancer, and urinary tract infections are more likely to occur during this time. Also, because young adulthood marks the time when most women try to begin a family, problems associated with infertility may be discovered at this time as well (Ruhl, 2011).

ENDOMETRIOSIS. Endometriosis, a benign disorder of the reproductive tract, is characterized by the presence and growth of endometrial tissue outside the uterus. Women ages 30 to 40 are most likely to develop endometriosis. Endometrial tissue may implant on the fallopian tubes, ovaries, and the tissues surrounding and lining the pelvis. The endometrial tissue responds to hormonal influences during the secretory and proliferative stages of the menstrual cycle, where it grows and thickens, in a similar fashion to the endometrial tissue lining the uterus. However, during the ischemic and menstrual phases of the cycle, the misplaced endometrial tissue breaks down and bleeds into the surrounding tissue, causing inflammation. The blood

Family Teaching Guidelines…
Testicular Self-Examination

The best time to perform a testicular self-examination is during or immediately following a hot shower or bath because the scrotum is more relaxed at this time. The following steps should be performed, examining one testicle at a time:

1. Examine the testicles. One should be slightly larger than the other, usually the right testicle.
2. Feel for lumps and bumps along the front and sides.
3. Using both hands, place your thumbs over the top of the testicle and your index fingers and middle fingers underneath the testicle. Gently roll the testicle, using slight pressure, between your fingers (Fig. 4-14).
4. The epididymis, which carries the sperm, can be felt at the top of the back part of each testicle. It should feel soft and ropelike and be slightly tender to pressure. This is a normal finding.
5. Notify your doctor if you notice any swelling, lumps, pain, or changes in color or size of either testicle.

Source: The Nemours Foundation (2012). *How to perform a testicular self-examination*. Retrieved from http://www.kidshealth.org/teen/sexual_health/guys/tse.html

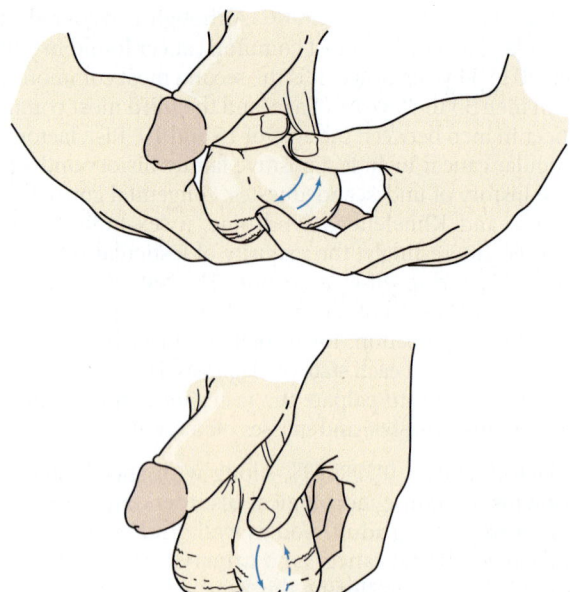

Figure 4-14 Testicular self-examination.

becomes trapped in the surrounding tissues causing the development of blood-containing cysts. Recurring inflammation in the areas outside the uterus eventually result in scarring, fibrosis, and the development of adhesions, scar tissue that binds the organs together causing increased abdominal pain and a risk of infertility.

Abdominal pain of varying intensity is the most common symptom associated with endometriosis. However, the degree of pain associated with endometriosis is not a reliable indicator of the extent of the disorder. Other symptoms may include pain during ovulation (**mittelschmerz**), heavy bleeding during menstruation, and episodes of diarrhea and constipation, which may be mistaken for irritable bowel syndrome. Women may also experience dyspareunia or pain during defecation.

Although the etiology of endometriosis is unknown, the most commonly held theory is "retrograde menstruation." During menstruation, endometrial tissue is refluxed through the fallopian tubes and out into the peritoneal cavity where it implants on the ovaries and surrounding organs. While 90% of all women experience retrograde menstruation, only about 5% to 10% develop endometriosis, indicating a possible difference in immune function, genetic predisposition, or environmental influence (ACOG, 2010c; Appelbaum & Nentin, 2010).

The diagnosis of endometriosis may be made by pelvic examination, although it is often impossible to palpate small areas of localized endometrial tissue. A vaginal ultrasound may be performed to provide imaging of the displaced endometrial tissue or cyst. The physician may also perform a laparoscopy to visualize the abdominal organs and locate sites of abnormally located endometrial tissue. Laparoscopy provides information concerning the location, size, extent of disease, and the presence of scars and adhesions and allows for biopsy of the lesions.

Medical management includes pain control, the use of hormonal therapy to shrink the abnormal tissue, and at times, surgery to remove the abnormal tissue. The pain associated with tissue inflammation may be managed with nonsteroidal anti-inflammatory drugs, such as ibuprofen, to inhibit the synthesis of prostaglandin and reduce the inflammation. If conservative treatment is not helpful, supplemental hormonal therapy may be introduced, with the goal of stabilizing the release of estrogen and progesterone to decrease tissue swelling and bleeding.

When pregnancy is not an immediate goal, oral contraceptives with a low estrogen to progestin ratio may be used to inhibit the production of hormones and suppress ovulation. Gonadotropin-releasing hormone (Gn-RH) agonists and antagonists, such as leuprolide (Lupron) or nafarelin (Synarel), suppress the secretion of pituitary gonadotropins, decrease the release of follicle-stimulating hormone (FSH) and luteinizing hormone (LH), and diminish ovarian function. Danazol (Danocrine), another medication that suppresses the release of FSH and LH, may be used. However, the side effects of acne and facial hair growth make danazol a less commonly prescribed medication. Medroxyprogesterone (Depo-Provera) is an injectable medication used to reduce the growth of the endometrial tissue, but its undesired side effects include weight gain and depression. Other pharmacological modalities utilize aromatase inhibitors, including anastrozole (Arimidex), exemestane (Aromasin), and letrozole (Femara), chemicals that block the conversion of androgens to estrogen and suppress the production of estrogen from the abnormal endometrial tissue, thereby decreasing tissue growth.

When pharmacological approaches are not successful, or when pregnancy is desired, the endometrial tissue growths, scar tissue, and adhesions can be removed surgically through laparoscopy. When endometriosis is severe, however, radical surgery that includes removal of the uterus, fallopian tubes, and ovaries (bilateral salpingo-oophorectomy) may be indicated.

CERVICAL CANCER. Cervical cancer develops gradually as cells change their growth pattern. Precancerous cellular changes, called **cervical intraepithelial neoplasia** or **dysplasia,** may eventually become cancerous. There are two types of cervical cancer: squamous cell carcinoma and adenocarcinoma. Approximately 80% to 90% of all cervical cancers are squamous cell carcinomas that cover the surface of the cervix.

 Nursing Insight—Understanding the Bethesda System terminology for interpretation of cervical cytology findings

The Bethesda System is the classification for abnormal cervical cytology and histology that is most commonly used today. First developed in 1988 under sponsorship of the National Institutes of Health (NIH), the updated 2001 Bethesda System terminology is used to describe the categories of epithelial cell abnormalities, including atypical squamous cells (ASC), low-grade or high-grade squamous intraepithelial lesions (LSIL or HSIL), and glandular cell abnormalities, including atypical glandular cells (AGC) and adenocarcinoma in situ (AIS) (ACOG, 2008; Frey & Gupta, 2011).

While not all cervical epithelial and glandular cell abnormalities develop into carcinoma, screening and appropriate treatment significantly reduce the chances that carcinoma will develop. This fact lends credence to the recommendation that screening through Papanicolaou testing be performed on all young adults. Furthermore, 50% of all women diagnosed with cervical cancer are diagnosed during the ages of young adulthood.

The primary risk factor for cervical cancer is human papillomavirus (HPV) infection. There is a strong correlation between infection with the high-risk types of HPV and the development of cervical cancer. Seventy percent of cervical cancers are caused by HPV-16 or HPV-18. Other types of HPV are associated with the development of **papillomas,** which are benign growths found primarily in the genital and anal regions.

A vaccine (Gardasil) against HPV types 6, 11, 16, and 18 became available in 2006. The quadrivalent recombinant (non-live virus) vaccine is recommended for females ages 9 to 26 years. The CDC Advisory Committee on Immunization Practices also recommends routine quadrivalent HPV vaccination for boys aged 11 or 12 years and for others up to age 21 years who haven't already received the vaccine. The quadrivalent HPV vaccine reduces the likelihood of acquiring genital warts; ideally the vaccine should be administered before potential exposure to HPV through sexual contact. Vaccination consists of three intramuscular injections given over 6 months, with the second dose to be given 2 months after the first dose and the third dose given 6 months after the first dose. If the HPV vaccine schedule is interrupted, the vaccine series does not need to be restarted. In late 2014, the FDA approved a 9-valent recombinant HPV vaccine (Gardasil 9) that also covers HPV types 31, 33, 45, 52, and 58. These latter five are responsible for roughly one in five cases of cervical cancer. Gardasil 9, also administered as three intramuscular injections given over 6 months, is approved for use in females ages 9 through 26 and in males ages 9 through 15. Another immunogen, Cervarix, is a bivalent vaccine that protects against HPV 16 and 18. Approved by the FDA in 2009, Cervarix also consists of three intramuscular injections given over 6 months; the second dose is given 1 month after the first dose, and the third dose is given 6 months after the first dose (American Society for Colposcopy and Cervical Pathology [ASCCP], 2013; CDC, 2011). It is important for nurses to remind patients receiving the vaccines to return for each dose and to continue to have routine cervical cancer screenings (AWHONN, 2010b).

Following identification of abnormal cervical cytology screening results, **colposcopy** (use of a stereoscopic binocular microscope to examine the cervix under magnification) is usually performed. An acetic acid solution applied to the cervix enhances visualization of the epithelium and helps to identify areas for biopsy. Cervical biopsies are then obtained and pathologically examined for the presence and extent of cancer. Several outpatient biopsy methods are available. The endocervical curettage (ECC) is an effective diagnostic method in about 90% of cases. The **cone biopsy** involves removal of a cone- or cylinder-shaped sample of tissue. **Loop electrosurgical excision procedure** (LEEP) is a newer method for cervical biopsy and the removal of abnormal cells. With this procedure, an electrically charged wire loop is inserted through a speculum, and a thin layer of cells is removed from the cervix. The LEEP technique provides excision and cautery with minimal tissue damage. Patients should be instructed that vaginal drainage is normal and expected following the procedure and may last up to 3 weeks. The patient should refrain from using tampons or having sexual intercourse for the following 4 weeks to minimize the risk of infection. Nonsteroidal anti-inflammatory medications may be taken to reduce the mild cramping that may occur following the procedure.

Following the biopsy, further and more extensive treatment may be required if the cancer has spread to other areas of the cervix or beyond the cervix. The three primary methods of cervical cancer treatment include surgery, radiation, and chemotherapy. It is not uncommon for a combination of two treatment methods to be used.

 Global Health Case Study African American Adult With an Abnormal Pap Test Result

Vanessa, a 32-year-old African American woman, visits the women's health clinic in a small, rural community. She requests a gynecological examination and states this is her first exam in 3 years. Vanessa has recently married and engages in normal sexual activity with her husband. Her medical history is positive for asthma, and she takes one Singulair 10 mg tablet at bedtime and Flovent two puffs twice daily. Following an abnormal Pap test result, Vanessa is scheduled for a colposcopy. She is frightened and asks about the procedure.

critical thinking questions

1. What information can you provide Vanessa about colposcopy?

2. Vanessa asks how she should prepare for the scheduled colposcopy.

◆ See Suggested Answers to Global Health Case Studies on Davis*Plus*.

URINARY TRACT INFECTIONS. Urinary tract infections (UTIs) can be very serious in young adults and may lead to major problems if not diagnosed or treated. Infections of the urinary tract are the second most common type of infection in adults, and young adults are more susceptible, in most instances, as a result of increased sexual activity during this time. Women tend to be more vulnerable than men because the short urethral length and the proximity of the urethral meatus to the anus allow for the easy ascension of bacteria. However, urinary tract infections in men can be more serious than in women. The majority of UTIs are caused by the microorganism *Escherichia coli* (*E coli*), which is normally found in the colon. Once introduced into the urethra, the bacteria colonize, causing urethritis. As the bacteria multiply and migrate into the bladder, cystitis develops. Left untreated, the infection can spread up the ureters and into the kidneys, causing pyelonephritis.

Symptoms of urinary tract infections include burning, urinary frequency, urgency during urination, and a strong sensation of the need to void followed by passage of only a small amount of urine. Women often report a sensation of fullness noted above the symphysis pubis; in men, infection triggers a sensation of rectal fullness. Other clinical manifestations of infection include fever, general malaise and fatigue, elevated white blood cell count, and chills. The urine may appear cloudy because of the presence of white blood cells.

Medical management centers on the use of antibiotics. Trimethoprim/sulfamethoxazole (Bactrim, Septra) are the medications most commonly prescribed. Depending on the strain of bacteria and results from culture and sensitivity testing, other agents such as amoxicillin (Amoxil, Trimox) and ampicillin (Omnipen) may be used. Nitrofurantoin (Macrodantin) or ciprofloxacin (Cipro) may be prescribed for more complicated infections.

Patient education should focus on the prevention of urinary tract infections. Everyone should drink adequate water each day and urinate when the urge is felt. Following urination and defecation, women should wipe from front to back to prevent bacteria from entering the urethra from the colon and be encouraged to take showers instead of tub baths. Bath oils, perfume, and bubble baths should be avoided if tub baths are taken. Feminine hygiene sprays and scented douches should be avoided to prevent irritation, and cotton underwear should be worn to decrease perineal moistness and warmth that can enhance the growth of bacteria.

Middle Adulthood Health

As the young adult matures into middle age, which includes ages 40 to 64, there is a decrease in the risk for some health problems and an increased risk for others. It is during this age group that mammography screenings should begin, along with colonoscopies, cholesterol and lipid screening, and osteoporosis screening. Most women begin to experience symptoms of perimenopause during middle age and need to make decisions on managing these symptoms. Certain gynecological disorders become more common during middle age, including fibroid tumors, ovarian cysts, ovarian cancer, and endometrial cancer.

HEALTH PROMOTION SCREENING

Health promotion screenings can be of great benefit to people in middle age because there are a variety of diseases that become more prevalent during this time. Breast cancer is the second leading cause of cancer death in U.S. women, and the chance of a woman developing invasive breast cancer at some point during her lifetime is a little less than 1 in 8. In women between the ages of 40 and 55, breast cancer is the leading cause of death (American Cancer Society, 2011f).

The promotion of breast health encompasses several areas, including breast self-awareness (women's awareness of the normal appearance and feel of their breasts), cancer screening, optimal nutrition, and physical activity. It is important for nurses to educate women throughout the life span about strategies for promoting breast health. Nurses who work with women must be able to educate them about normal breast anatomy, breast cancer risk factors, and the benefits, limitations, and risks of breast screening techniques (AWHONN, 2010d). Personal awareness of the normal appearance and feel of the breasts constitutes an essential first step in promoting and maintaining breast health (Box 4-5).

⑤ Optimizing Outcomes—Teaching about fibrocystic breast changes

When teaching women about breast self-awareness, nurses can include information about **fibrocystic changes**, palpable thickening in the breasts often associated with pain and tenderness that fluctuates with the menstrual cycle. Fibrocystic changes are common, benign, and tend to appear during the second and third decades of life. First-line treatment for the condition, which may be related to an imbalance in estrogen and progesterone, centers on patient education and reassurance. Other interventions focus on relief of symptoms and may include analgesics, topical and oral nonsteroidal anti-inflammatory drugs (e.g., ibuprofen), the use of gamma-linolenic acid (the active ingredient of evening primrose oil), the use of a supportive bra, a reduction in saturated dietary fat, and the application of heat to the breasts (Chase, Wells, & Eley, 2011; Pearlman & Griffin, 2010).

Breast self-awareness, which may include breast self-examination, along with clinical breast exams and **mammography** (x-ray filming of the breasts) can assist in early

---

Box 4-5 Knowing and Understanding Your Breasts

- As you age, your breasts experience loss of milk glands and shrinkage of collagen. This causes an increase in the fat tissue and loosening of the breast tissue. Instead of getting larger with the increase in fat tissue, however, the breast tissue begins to sag, causing the breasts to drop.
- Breast tissue weighs less than most people think: an A-cup weighs 1/4 lb, a B-cup weighs 1/2 lb, a C-cup weighs 3/4 lb, and a D-cup weighs about 1 lb.
- The skin covering the breasts stretches as you grow, causing the skin to become thinner than the skin on other parts of the body.
- It is not uncommon for women to have some degree of hair surrounding their nipples. The darker the skin, the more hair there is likely to be.
- A woman's nipples may be different sizes and may be located in slightly different locations on each breast. This may cause the nipples to point in different directions, which is considered a normal finding.
- Fluctuating hormone levels during the monthly cycle cause changes in breast tissue. Following menstruation, when hormone levels are at their lowest, the breast tissue is smooth and nontender. As estrogen levels increase mid-cycle, breasts may become more sensitive. Also, just before menstruation, when progesterone is elevated, the breasts become swollen and tender, with palpable nodules.

- The health-care provider should perform clinical breast examinations 1 week following menstruation, when the breast tissue is nontender and smooth.
- Breast implants still pose health risks, including deflation, leakage, and wrinkling. In addition, capsular contraction can occur, causing the scar tissue surrounding the implant to tighten and the breast to become hard.
- The area between the breasts has several oil and sweat glands, creating an atmosphere conducive to the growth of bacteria.
- Sleeping on your side, with a pillow to support your breasts, provides the best position for maintaining breast shape and contour over time.
- Regular exercise can strengthen the pectoral muscles, reducing sagging over time and creating a natural lift.
- It is not uncommon to have a third nipple, stemming from breast buds that form during early fetal development. These extra nipples, however, rarely contain milk glands.
- Pregnancy darkens the color of the nipple, which is an enhancement for the breastfeeding baby. This darker color does not disappear after pregnancy.
- The left breast is usually larger than the right breast.
- Breasts do not reach their full size until the early 20s.

detection and early treatment. The initiation and frequency of mammography depends on the woman's age and risk factors. Magnetic resonance imaging (MRI) appears to be more sensitive in detecting tumors in women with an inherited susceptibility to breast cancer, and recent findings suggest that this diagnostic method can detect cancer in the contralateral breast that was missed by mammography in women with recently diagnosed breast cancer (ACOG, 2011e; Griffin & Pearlman, 2010).

While breast cancer is more common in women, colon cancer is the fourth most common cancer in both men and women. In addition, risk for heart disease related to elevated cholesterol and lipids increases in both genders during middle age. Osteoporosis, which may also occur in men, becomes more common and debilitating in women in the latter years of middle age, as they move from perimenopause into menopause.

 ### Cultural Diversity: Gender, Race, Ethnicity, and Breast Cancer

Breast cancer is approximately 100 times less common among men than among women, and a male's lifetime risk of developing breast cancer is about 1 in 1,000. At one time it was believed that the prognosis for men with breast cancer was worse than that for women, but recent evidence now indicates that men and women with the same stage of breast cancer have a similar outlook for survival. Overall, white women are slightly more likely to develop breast cancer than are African American women, but African American women are more likely to die from this cancer because of late diagnosis. In women under 45 years of age, breast cancer is more common in African American women. Asian, Hispanic, and Native American women have a lower risk of developing and dying from breast cancer (ACS, 2011b, 2011c).

Breast Self-Examination

Familiarization with one's breasts facilitates the early detection of problems and allows for prompt evaluation. Presently, there is an evolution away from teaching breast self-examination (BSE) toward the newer concept of breast self-awareness. Nurses should encourage breast self-awareness (which may include BSE) and the prompt reporting of any breast changes. Women who wish to perform self-examination as a component of breast self-awareness should be instructed in the appropriate technique, although emphasis is not on examination techniques. BSE provides one way for women to learn how their breasts normally feel. Routinely performing BSE is an approach that focuses on the importance of self-awareness and helps women to notice changes in breast tissue (Allen, Van Groningen, Barksdale, & McCarthy, 2010; ACS, 2011d; ACOG, 2011e; Griffin & Pearlman, 2010).

Clinical Breast Examination

All women should have a clinical breast examination performed at recommended intervals by a skilled health-care practitioner. The clinical breast exam should be performed every 1 to 3 years for women aged 20 to 39 and every year for women aged 40 and over (ACOG, 2011e; ACS, 2011e; National Comprehensive Cancer Network, 2011).

Mammography

A mammography examination is used to aid in the early diagnosis of breast cancer. The examination, which requires exposure to small doses of ionizing radiation, allows for identification of small breast tissue abnormalities that may require further investigation. In recent times, two enhancements have been made to traditional mammography: digital mammography and computer-aided detection (CAD). Digital mammography, also called full-field digital mammography (FFDM), converts the x-rays to electrical signals, similar to those found in digital cameras. These signals produce images that can be viewed on a computer screen or printed on special film. The images are stored for future comparison. This latest technology may be enhanced with the use of a computer-aided detection system that highlights areas of increased density, masses, and calcifications. Recent data indicate that overall, digital mammography demonstrates a slightly higher detection rate than film mammography, particularly for women aged 60 years or younger (ACOG, 2011e).

 ### Optimizing Outcomes—Breast cancer screening guidelines

In 2009, the U.S. Preventive Services Task Force issued revised breast cancer screening recommendations for the general population. Based on evidence review, the updated guidelines recommend against routine mammography screening for women before age 50 years, suggest that screening end at age 74 years, and recommend changing the screening interval from 1 year to 2 years. Several professional organizations have voiced their objections to the new recommendations. The American Cancer Society, the American College of Radiology, and several other expert groups recommend that clinicians and patients continue to follow the earlier guidelines; the American College of Obstetricians and Gynecologists now recommends that women undergo a screening mammography once a year beginning at age 40 years (ACOG, 2011e; ACS, 2011e; Burkman, 2010; Stern, 2010; USPSTF, 2011a).

Lifestyle Choices and Breast Health

Lifestyle choices, including moderate alcohol consumption, weight maintenance, and avoidance of smoking, can affect breast health as well. Alcohol consumption is known to be associated with an increased risk of breast cancer. The American Cancer Society (2011b) recommends limiting alcohol intake to one drink per day. The risk of breast cancer is increased 1.5 times in women who consume two to five drinks per day.

Routine exercise, which helps to maintain a healthy weight, is associated with a decreased risk of breast cancer. Maintenance of a healthy weight is recommended for optimum breast health. Obesity is associated with an increased risk of breast cancer, particularly in postmenopausal women. Following menopause, estrogen is produced in the fat cells. In combination with dietary fat, estrogen significantly increases the likelihood of breast cancer development. Smoking is associated with an increased risk of breast cancer, lung cancer, and heart disease in women (ACOG, 2011b; AWHONN, 2010c; Gies, 2011).

BREAST CANCER. While the majority of lumps found in the breast and axillary tissue are not cancerous, discovery of a mass remains the most common sign of breast cancer. Other signs of breast cancer include a clear or bloody discharge from the nipple, retraction or indentation of the nipple, dimpling of the breast tissue, and change in the size or contour of the breast. While the exact etiology of breast cancer remains unclear, there are factors that place a woman at greater risk for developing breast cancer (Box 4-6).

 Now Can You—Discuss ways to enhance breast health?

1. Teach a patient about breast self-awareness?
2. Discuss recommendations regarding clinical breast examination and mammography?
3. Discuss risk factors associated with breast cancer?
4. Identify lifestyle choices that decrease the risk of developing breast cancer?

 Family Teaching Guidelines...
Breast Self-Examination (ACS, 2011d)

1. Lie down on your back and place your right arm behind your head. Remember, this step is done while lying down. In this position, the breast tissue spreads evenly over your chest wall and is as thin as possible. This makes it much easier to feel all of the breast tissue.

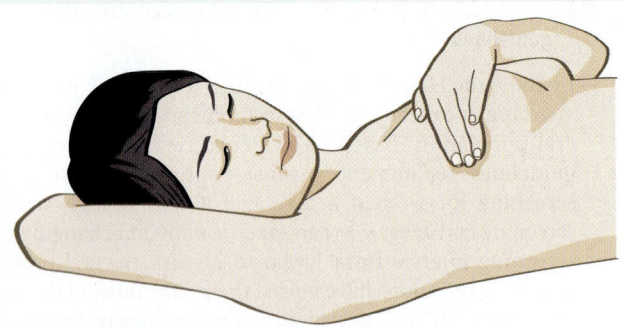

2. Use the pads of your three middle fingers on the left hand to feel for lumps in the right breast. Use overlapping dime-sized circular motions of the finger pads to feel all of the breast tissue.

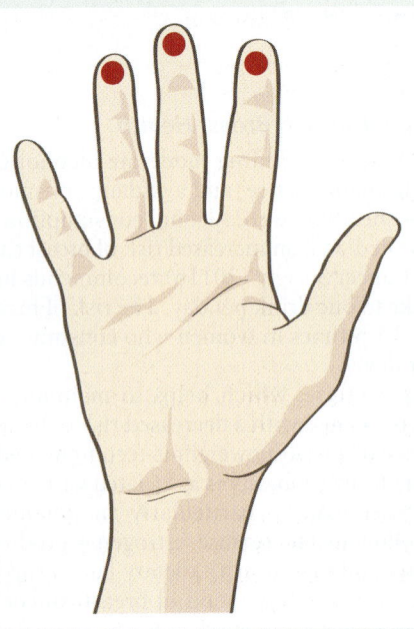

3. When feeling the breast tissue, you will use three different levels of pressure. Light pressure is needed to feel the tissue closest to the skin. Medium pressure allows you to feel a little deeper, and firm pressure allows you to feel the tissue closest to your chest and ribs. Remember, it is normal to feel a firm ridge in the lower curve of each breast. If you feel anything else out of the ordinary, be sure to tell your health-care practitioner. It is important to use each pressure level to feel all of the breast tissue before you move on to the next spot.

4. Move around the breast in an up and down pattern, starting at an imaginary line drawn straight down your side from the underarm and moving across the breast to the middle of the chest bone (sternum, breastbone). Make sure that you check the entire breast area going down until you feel only your ribs and then up to the neck or collarbone (clavicle). Using the up and down, or vertical, pattern is probably the most effective way to examine the entire breast without missing any breast tissue.

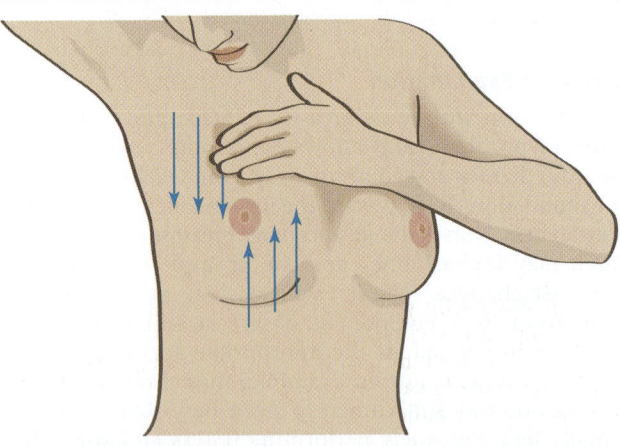

5. Repeat step 4 on your left breast, putting your left arm behind your head and using the finger pads of your right hand to do the exam.

6. Stand before a mirror, place your hands on your hips, and press down firmly. In the mirror, look at your breasts for any changes of size, shape, contour, or dimpling or redness or scaliness of the nipple or breast skin. (Pressing down on your hips contracts the muscles of the chest wall and enhances any breast changes).

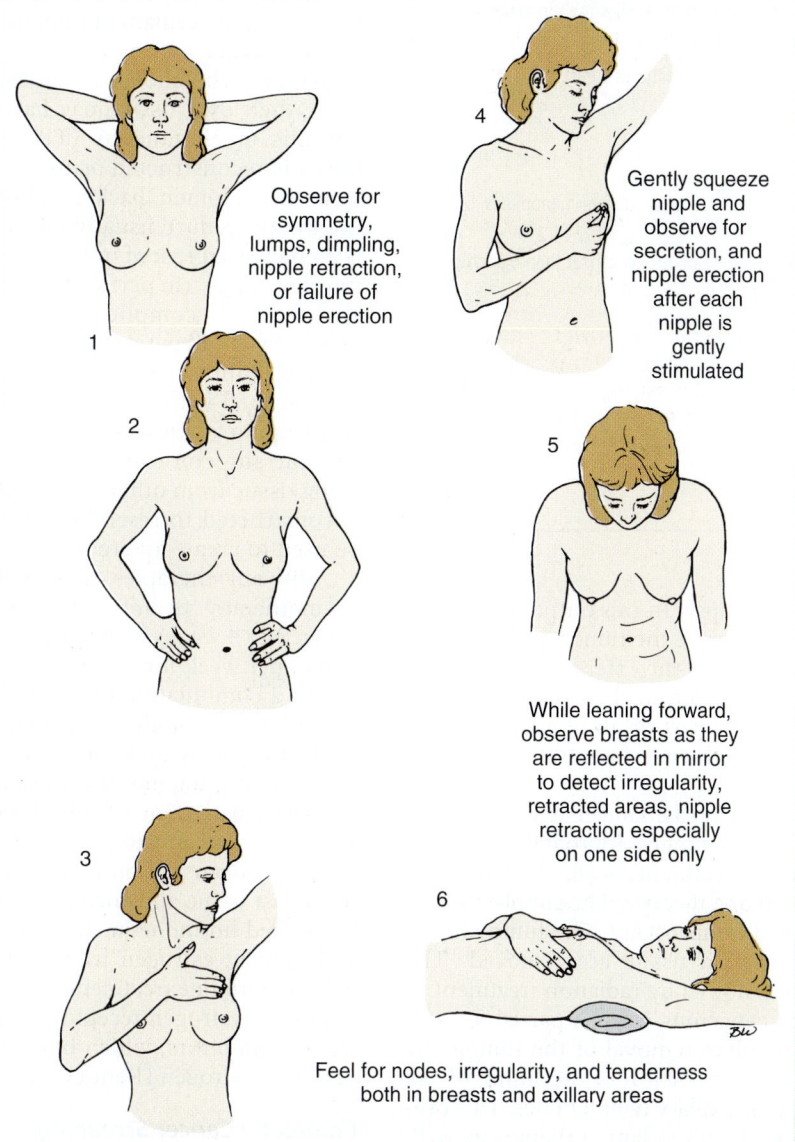

1 Observe for symmetry, lumps, dimpling, nipple retraction, or failure of nipple erection

4 Gently squeeze nipple and observe for secretion, and nipple erection after each nipple is gently stimulated

5 While leaning forward, observe breasts as they are reflected in mirror to detect irregularity, retracted areas, nipple retraction especially on one side only

6 Feel for nodes, irregularity, and tenderness both in breasts and axillary areas

7. Sit or stand with your arm only slightly raised so that you can easily feel the underarm area. Do this on each side, feeling for lumps or thickened areas. (Raising the arm straight up causes a tightening of the tissue and makes it more difficult to examine).

⚬ Optimizing Outcomes—Screening for breast cancer

Best outcome: Breast-self awareness (may include BSE), clinical breast examinations, and routine mammography allow health-care practitioners to detect potentially cancerous tumors at the earliest stage possible. This multipronged screening approach facilitates early diagnosis and early treatment, providing the best outcome possible (National Comprehensive Cancer Network, 2011).

When BSE, clinical breast examination, mammography, and MRI detect possible cancerous tumors in the breast or axillae, a biopsy procedure is performed to determine if cancer is indeed present. One type of biopsy procedure is the fine-needle aspiration, which is the simplest method. A thin, hollow needle is used to withdraw cells for histological analysis. Core needle biopsy may be performed to withdraw multiple (e.g., up to 15) tissue samples. This procedure is used when tissues, instead of cells, are necessary for diagnosis. A stereotactic biopsy removes more

---

Box 4-6 Risk Factors Associated With Breast Cancer

- Defects in breast cancer gene 1 (*BRCA1*) or breast cancer gene 2 (*BRCA2*)
- Gender: 100 times more likely to occur in females than in males
- Age: Increasing age, with 50% appearing by age 50
- Personal history of breast cancer in at least one breast
- Family history of breast cancer
- Exposure to radiation
- Excess weight
- Exposure to estrogen: early onset of menarche, late menopause, or use of hormonal therapy
- Race: Caucasians more likely to develop breast cancer than Hispanics or African Americans
- Smoking
- Exposure to carcinogens
- Excessive use of alcohol
- Diagnosis of precancerous breast changes
- Increased breast density revealed on mammography

Source: American Cancer Society (2011b).

---

tissue than a core needle biopsy. In this outpatient procedure, MRI may be used to locate the tumor, plot its coordinates, and precisely aim the stereotactic biopsy instrument into the tumor. Surgical, or open, biopsy, which involves removal of a part or all of a breast lump for microscopic analysis, is the most accurate method of breast biopsy.

Medical management of breast cancer is complicated and may require a multi-treatment approach, including surgery and adjunctive treatment, such as radiation, chemotherapy, and hormone therapy. The simplest surgical treatment option is a lumpectomy: The lump and an area of surrounding normal tissue are removed. The lumpectomy is usually followed by radiation treatment to remove any remaining cancerous cells. A partial, or segmental, mastectomy involves removal of the tumor, the surrounding breast tissue, a portion of the lining of the chest wall, and some of the axillary lymph nodes. This procedure is usually followed with radiation therapy as well. A simple mastectomy involves the removal of all of the breast tissue along with the area surrounding the nipple and areola. Radiation, chemotherapy, or hormone therapy may follow this surgical procedure. In a modified radical mastectomy, the entire breast and several axillary lymph nodes are removed, leaving the chest wall intact. While this procedure makes breast reconstruction easier for the patient, complications including lymphadenopathy and paresthesia are more likely to occur (ACS, 2011e).

Many women choose to undergo breast reconstruction after a mastectomy. This surgical option, performed by a plastic surgeon, is a personal decision that requires considerable individualized counseling and education. Because the reconstruction can be performed at the same time as the mastectomy, it is important to consider the options early. Breast reconstruction methods include use of a synthetic breast implant or reconstruction using one's own tissue. Synthetic implants typically are composed of a silicone shell filled with a saline solution. A tissue expander may be needed to cover the implant. To accomplish tissue expansion, an empty implant shell is placed under the skin and muscles and gradually filled with the saline solution over several months. Once the skin is stretched sufficiently, the expander is removed and replaced with a permanent implant. Recovery usually takes several weeks.

Women who choose to undergo breast reconstruction using their own tissue may have a transverse rectus abdominis myocutaneous (TRAM) flap procedure. The breast is reconstructed using fat and muscle tissue taken from the abdomen, back, and buttocks. Recovery following the procedure usually takes 6 to 8 weeks, and there is an increased risk of infection and tissue necrosis. Deep inferior epigastric perforator (DIEP) reconstruction is a slightly less complicated surgical procedure. This method is similar to the TRAM flap procedure, but the abdominal muscles are left intact. The DIEP procedure is associated with fewer complications and less postoperative pain. Following reconstruction of the breast tissue, the surgeon can reconstruct the nipple and areola using tissue from other areas of the body. A small mound is constructed to resemble a nipple, and tattooing may be used to create an areola.

Adjuvant therapies may include radiation therapy, chemotherapy, or hormone therapy. Radiation is usually begun 3 to 4 weeks after surgery, and treatments are given 5 days per week for 5 to 6 weeks. Chemotherapy that includes a combination of two or more drugs may also be prescribed. Chemotherapeutics may be administered orally or intravenously and usually require four to eight treatments over 3 to 6 months. Hormone therapy is most commonly used to treat advanced metastatic cancer or as an adjuvant treatment to prevent recurrence of cancer. Normally, estrogen and progesterone bind to receptor sites in the breast tissue and encourage growth of cancerous cells. Prescribed hormone medications bind to the sites instead and prevent estrogen from reaching them. Medications used in hormone treatment include tamoxifen (Nolvadex), a selective estrogen receptor modulator (SERM), and aromatase inhibitors, which block the conversion of androgens into estrogen (Kentley, 2011).

Colorectal Cancer Screening

Colorectal cancer (CRC), which occurs in the large intestine and rectum, is the third leading cause of cancer death in the United States. The primary goal of CRC screening is to reduce mortality through the reduction of advanced disease. Although several CRC screening options are available (Box 4-7), colonoscopy is considered the best method for identifying possible colon and rectal cancer. Because more than 90% of colon and rectal cancers are diagnosed after the age of 50, recommendations suggest having a colonoscopy at this age. Individuals who have a family history of colorectal cancer, colon polyps, or other cancer should have colonoscopies in their 40s, and younger patients with actual symptoms such as rectal bleeding, blood in the stool, or vague abdominal pain should be evaluated by colonoscopy. The U.S. Preventive Services Task Force does not recommend routine CRC screening for persons age 75 to 85 and recommends against screening for persons age 85 years or older (ACOG, 2011e; USPSTF, 2011a).

Box 4-7 Other Screening Tests for Colorectal Cancer

- Fecal testing (encompasses 3 types: fecal occult blood test and fecal immunochemical [detect blood in the stool] and DNA fecal markers [screens for 21 genetic mutations associated with colorectal cancer])
- Flexible sigmoidoscopy (detects adenomatous polyps and cancer inside the descending colon)
- Virtual or computed tomography (CT) colonography (an x-ray of the colon; detects adenomatous polyps and cancer although small lesions and polyps may be missed)
- Lower colon double-contrast barium enema (x-ray films are taken of the colon and rectum)

Sources: ACOG (2011f); USPSTF (2011a).

Box 4-8 Lipid Screening Results

GUIDELINES FOR INTERPRETING LIPID SCREENING RESULTS

Total Cholesterol

Below 200 mg/dL:	Desirable
240 mg/dL and above:	High, increased risk of cardiac disease

LDL Cholesterol

Below 100 mg/dL:	Desirable; target goal for those with cardiac disease or multiple risk factors
100–129 mg/dL:	Elevated; target goal for those with two or more risk factors
130–160 mg/dL:	Borderline high; target goal for those with zero to one risk factor
Above 160 mg/dL:	Significantly elevated

HDL Cholesterol

Below 40 mg/dL:	Adds a risk factor for cardiac disease
60 mg/dL and above:	Desirable

Triglycerides

Below 150 mg/dL:	Desirable
200 mg/dL and above:	High

Source: Veterans Health Administration, Department of Defense (2011). *VHA/DoD clinical practice guideline for the management of dyslipidemia in primary care.* Washington, DC: Author.

A colonoscopy is an examination that involves insertion of a colonoscope (a long, flexible scope) into the colon to the ileocecal valve. Removal of polyps or abnormal tissue is performed as necessary. Preparation for the procedure usually includes a clear liquid diet for 1 to 3 days before the examination and administration of a laxative or enema on the evening prior to the procedure. Patients who take anticoagulants, nonsteroidal anti-inflammatory drugs, or oral antidiabetic agents are instructed when to withhold their medications in preparation for the procedure.

Colonoscopy is performed under conscious sedation. The patient is placed on the left side and given an analgesic and a sedative. Once the patient is relaxed and the colonoscope is inserted into the rectum, the patient is asked to change positions several times to enhance visualization of the colon. Abnormal growths or tissue are removed for laboratory analysis. The procedure usually takes about 30 to 60 minutes and the patient may experience mild cramping and slight bleeding afterwards.

Cholesterol and Lipid Screening

Cholesterol is essential for cell membranes, synthesis of bile acids, and synthesis of steroid hormones. Included in the cholesterol are chylomicrons, very low density lipids (VLDLs), low-density lipids (LDLs), and high-density lipids (HDLs). **Chylomicrons** are lipoproteins that are present shortly after eating, then disappear within a couple of hours following a meal. HDLs are considered to exert a positive influence on prevention of heart disease: They carry cholesterol to the liver for excretion in the bile. Conversely, LDLs carry cholesterol into the bloodstream. Comparison of results with normal values provides the nurse with information to evaluate cardiac disease risk and provide patient education on healthy eating behaviors (Box 4-8).

THE CLIMACTERIC, MENOPAUSE, PERIMENOPAUSE, AND POSTMENOPAUSE

The **climacteric** is a transitional time in a woman's life marked by declining ovarian function and decreased hormone production. The climacteric begins at the onset of ovarian decline and ends with the cessation of postmenopausal symptoms. **Menopause** (a term derived from Latin *mensis* for month and Greek *pausis*, meaning to cease) refers to the last menstrual period and can be dated with certainty only 1 year after menstruation ceases. The average age at menopause in the United States is 51.4 years; the normal age at menopause ranges from 35 to 60 years.

Perimenopause is the period of time preceding menopause, usually between 2 and 8 years before menopause. The age at onset of perimenopause ranges from 39 to 51 years (Speroff & Fritz, 2010). Although perimenopause may last as few as 2 or as many as 10 years, on average it lasts 4 years. During this time of transition, levels of estrogen and progesterone increase and decrease at uneven intervals, causing the menstrual cycle to become longer, shorter, and eventually absent. Ovulation is sporadic. Symptoms of perimenopause, including irregular menses, hot flashes, vaginal dryness, dyspareunia, and mood changes, are associated with the fluctuation and decline in hormone levels.

During **postmenopause** (the time after menopause) estrogen is produced solely by the adrenal glands, and the ovaries are no longer involved in estrogen production.

While there is no specific treatment for perimenopause, use of oral contraceptives may help to regulate menstrual periods and alleviate hot flashes and vaginal dryness. **Hormone therapy** (HT), provided as estrogen only or a combination of estrogen and progestin, may be a consideration for the short-term treatment of moderate to severe vasomotor symptoms (e.g., hot flashes and night sweats). Estrogen-only HT increases the risk of endometrial cancer; HT is not recommended for women with a history of endometrial cancer. Estrogen–progestin therapy increases the risk of venous thromboembolism (VTE), especially in women with a history of VTE or factor V Leiden (a hypercoagulability disorder), and breast cancer (when taken longer than 3 to 5 years). In a recent position statement, The North American Menopause Society (NAMS) suggests that estrogen therapy (for women who have had hysterectomies) or the combination of estrogen and progesterone therapy offers the greatest benefit and smallest risk to women who are within 10 years of menopause. The lowest effective estrogen dose should be provided for the shortest duration necessary because risks increase with increasing age, time since menopause, and duration of use (NAMS, 2010a; Shifren & Schiff, 2010). (See Chapter 5 for further discussion.)

 legal alert—Provide patients with accurate information on menopause hormone therapy

In 2002, the National Heart, Lung and Blood Institute of the National Institutes of Health halted a major landmark study, called the Women's Health Initiative. The study was intended to evaluate the risks and benefits of **menopausal hormonal therapy.** The study was immediately stopped when results indicated an increased risk of invasive breast cancer and a lack of overall benefit for the relief of menopausal symptoms with the use of estrogen and progestin, known as hormonal replacement therapy (HRT) (Writing Group for the Women's Health Initiative Investigators, 2002). The findings also indicated an increased risk of heart attack, stroke, and blood clots; a reduced risk of colorectal cancer; fewer fractures; and no improvement in cognitive function.

The study component designed to investigate the use of **estrogen-only replacement therapy** (ERT) was allowed to continue. The findings from this branch of the study revealed no difference in the risk for heart attack or colorectal cancer, an increased risk of stroke and blood clots, an uncertain effect on breast cancer risk, and a reduced risk of fractures (The Women's Health Initiative Steering Committee, 2004).

Given the findings of this 15-year study, nurses should focus perimenopausal counseling on:

- Strategies for health promotion: recommendations for Pap tests and screening mammography, blood pressure monitoring, immunization updates, screening for blood lipids, thyroid function, diabetes, bone loss, and colorectal cancer
- Healthy lifestyle changes: smoking cessation, consuming a variety of foods low in saturated fat and cholesterol, limiting salt and alcohol intake, maintaining a healthy weight, and being physically active
- Prevention of osteoporosis: consuming foods rich in vitamin D and calcium, obtaining moderate exposure to sunlight, engaging in weight-bearing exercises; smoking cessation; and limiting alcohol intake
- Treatment of menopausal symptoms with complementary and alternative medicine approaches (e.g., stress management, guided imagery, massage therapy, yoga, acupuncture, dietary supplements, and exercise)
- Education about various hormone therapy options and nonhormonal prescription medications (including contraindications and side effects) for severe vasomotor symptoms

 Complementary Care: *Managing the Symptoms of Menopause*

Dietary supplements and herbal therapies have long provided women with alternative treatments to alleviate some of the symptoms associated with menopause. These biologically based therapies include soy, vitamins, probiotics, and herbs such as black cohosh. However, research evidence does not support the ideas that they are efficacious in minimizing menopausal symptoms (NAMS, 2011).

Complementary therapies that are currently being studied for their benefit in diminishing menopausal symptoms include:

- Mind–body medicine (e.g., hypnosis, dance, meditation, music, and yoga)
- Energy medicine (e.g., putative energy fields and veritable energy [electromagnetic] fields)
- Manipulative and body-based therapy (e.g., Chiropractic, osteopathy, and massage)
- Traditional Chinese medicine (e.g., acupuncture, herbal medicine, and qi gong)

While there is no current evidence to support their effectiveness in minimizing the symptoms of menopause, these complementary methods are considered to be much safer than herbal and vitamin therapies.

 Nursing Insight—Framing menopause as a celebration of midlife

Once considered by many to be a sign of "old age," menopause has come to be viewed as a natural passage in a maturing woman's life. Through education and support, nurses can help empower women to embrace menopause and midlife as a liberating time that brings freedom from the worry of an unplanned pregnancy; an end to childrearing responsibilities; and an opportunity to focus on hobbies, career, interpersonal relationships, and self-discovery.

GYNECOLOGICAL DISORDERS

During middle age, there is an increased incidence of certain gynecological disorders because of hormonal and environmental influences. Leiomyomas are present in about 20% of women during this age period. Ovarian cysts, which may occur at any age, are most common during the childbearing years up to the time of menopause. Endometrial cancer is the most common malignancy of the reproductive system. Ovarian cancer, which accounts for about 3% of all cancers in women, is the most common cause of death of all of the reproductive cancers because of its rapid growth and nonspecific symptomatology. Endometrial cancer is slow-growing, and when detected at a localized stage, the survival rate is much greater than with ovarian cancer (ACS, 2011f).

Leiomyomas

Leiomyomas, or uterine fibroid tumors, are benign growths that arise from the smooth muscle in the uterus. They occur most often after age 50 and are more common in African American women and in women who have never been pregnant. While the exact cause is unknown, their growth is dependent on estrogen. Leiomyomas begin as small masses of tissue that spread into and throughout the myometrium. They rarely become malignant and shrink after menopause when levels of the ovarian hormones have declined.

Leiomyomas are often asymptomatic and may not be detected until there is evidence of infertility. Symptoms, if present, may include a sensation of fullness or pressure in the lower abdomen, increased pain and cramping with menstrual periods, abdominal distention, urinary frequency, or heavy menses. Uterine tumors may be identified during a pelvic examination through palpation of the uterus. A transvaginal ultrasound may be performed to confirm the diagnosis. If cancer is suspected, a laparoscopy may be indicated.

Medical management may include the use of nonsteroidal anti-inflammatory drugs for dysmenorrhea. Oral contraceptives may be prescribed to control heavy periods and decrease tumor growth. Leuprolide (Lupron), a medication that suppresses the production of estrogen and progesterone, may be used to shrink leiomyomas although patients may complain of menopausal symptoms such as vaginal dryness, hot flashes, and mood changes.

If the fibroid tumors are growing inside the uterus, a hysteroscopic uterine **ablation** (vaporization of tissue) may be performed under local or general anesthesia. In this procedure, a hysteroscope, a small camera, and surgical instruments are inserted through the vagina and into the uterus. After the procedure, scarring and adhesions that interfere with fertility may form in the uterine cavity. **Uterine artery embolization,** a procedure performed by an interventional radiologist, involves the injection of polyvinyl alcohol pellets into selected blood vessels to block the blood supply to the fibroid and cause shrinkage and resolution of symptoms. Women who undergo this procedure should be advised that data are lacking about the long-term effects on fertility and future pregnancies. **Myomectomy** (removal of the fibroid tumor) is an alternative surgical treatment that may be performed for women who wish to preserve their fertility. Myomectomy can be done through an abdominal incision or through a laparoscopic or vaginal (hysteroscopic) approach. Although symptoms of menorrhagia and pelvic pressure are relieved, this procedure is associated with a risk of recurrence (ACOG, 2008).

Ovarian Cysts

Ovarian cysts are benign fluid-filled sacs that develop on the ovaries and cause pain and, at times, bleeding. A follicular cyst is the most common growth that occurs on the ovary. It develops during the first half of the menstrual cycle (the follicular phase). This type of ovarian cyst, termed a "functional" or "simple" cyst, forms when ovulation does not occur. Instead, the developing dominant follicle continues to grow and evolves into a large, fluid-filled cyst that contains a high concentration of estrogen. The follicular cyst can also form from one of the smaller follicles that failed to regress after another ovarian follicle gained dominance. Follicular cysts usually produce no symptoms and disappear spontaneously within a few months. However, approximately one-fourth of women with follicular cysts report symptoms such as pain or the sensation of a heavy, achy feeling in the pelvis. Rupture of a persistent follicular cyst causes severe pelvic pain.

A corpus luteum cyst occurs after ovulation. Under normal circumstances, if fertilization does not occur, the corpus luteum shrinks and disappears. When the corpus luteum persists, it can become filled with fluid or blood and remain on the ovary. Symptoms associated with a corpus luteum cyst include abdominal pain, ovarian tenderness, and delayed or irregular menses. If bleeding occurs within the cyst, it is known as a hemorrhagic cyst. Rupture can cause an intraperitoneal hemorrhage. Corpus luteum cysts typically resolve spontaneously within one or two menstrual cycles.

A dermoid cyst is a germ cell tumor that usually affects women at an earlier age. This type of ovarian cyst may grow to 6 inches in diameter and can contain fat, teeth, bone, hair, and cartilage. Dermoid cysts can develop bilaterally and may cause lower abdominal pain or complications related to torsion. Surgical removal is the usual treatment.

Endometrioid cysts result from the growth of endometrial tissue in the ovaries. They are often filled with dark blood and may cause chronic pelvic pain. Treatment involves removal to prevent rupture and the development of a hemoperitoneum.

Ovarian Cancer

Cancer of the ovary is the ninth most common cancer among women, excluding non-melanoma skin cancers. It ranks fifth in cancer deaths among women and accounts for more deaths than any other cancer of the female reproductive system. A woman's risk of getting ovarian cancer during her lifetime is about 1 in 71 (ACS, 2011f). While the cause is unknown, there are identified risk factors, including nulliparity, pregnancy later in life, obesity (body mass index of at least 30), presence of *BRCA1* and *BRCA2* genes, a personal history of breast cancer, and a family history of breast, ovarian, or colorectal cancer. Associative causes include the use of fertility medications, exposure to asbestos, genital exposure to talcum powder, a high-fat diet, and childhood mumps infection. Older women are at increased risk as compared with younger women. About half of the women who are diagnosed with ovarian cancer are over the age of 63, and it is more common in Caucasian women than in African American women. Pregnancy, oral contraceptive use, tubal ligation, and hysterectomy provide some protection against ovarian cancer, and the use of postmenopausal estrogen may increase the risk (ACS, 2011f).

Symptoms are usually vague and nonspecific and include pelvic fullness, lower abdominal pain, weight gain, irregular menstrual cycles, back pain, abdominal distention and increased abdominal girth (related to ovarian enlargement or ascites), urinary urgency, urinary frequency, indigestion, lack of appetite, feeling full after eating only a little bit, and bloating. Because ovarian cancer is a rapidly growing neoplasm, the diagnosis is usually not made until the cancer has metastasized, giving rise to the nickname for ovarian cancer as "the silent killer."

The diagnosis is made via transvaginal ultrasonography, serum CA-125 antigen (a tumor-associated antigen) testing, or laparotomy. The preferred treatment for ovarian cancer is surgical removal and usually requires a hysterectomy with bilateral salpingo-oophorectomy. After surgery, chemotherapy, sometimes combined with immunotherapy, is used to treat any remaining cancer. Radiation therapy may be used as a palliative measure although it is not typically used as a treatment option for ovarian cancer.

Older Adulthood Health

As individuals move into the later stages of life, physiological and psychological changes alter their health and increase their risk of disease. During these years, health promotion and disease prevention are imperative to maintain quality of life and encourage empowerment in managing health and daily activities. Health-care management focuses on gynecological health and mental and emotional health.

HEALTH PROMOTION

Health promotion is complex and challenging in older adults because they are experiencing changes in sexual functioning, exercise and activity, cognition, and function. Many considerations must be incorporated into patient education during older age.

Sexual Functioning

Intimacy and sexual activity during the later years remain important in fulfilling relationships that can positively affect one's physical and emotional health. However, physical and psychological changes that occur in the body can affect intimacy as one ages. Testosterone, the hormone that regulates the sex drive, does not decrease significantly as one ages. Instead, other changes exert a more immediate impact on intimacy and sexual functioning.

For women, the most significant change is the decrease in estrogen that accompanies menopause. Low levels of estrogen are associated with decreased vaginal lubrication and a slowed response to sexual stimulation. In addition, the vaginal tissue loses elasticity, resulting in increased dryness and dyspareunia. Prolonged foreplay and use of a water-soluble lubricant or an estrogen cream that can be applied directly to the vagina can facilitate lubrication and help in maintaining elasticity.

For men, it may take longer to achieve an erection. Once achieved, the erection may not be as firm or last as long as in previous years. To help with this problem, the health-care provider can make recommendations including medications, a penile vacuum pump, or vascular surgery.

For both genders, changes in physical appearance can adversely affect one's emotional ability to develop an intimate relationship with another. The presence of gray hair, wrinkles, and increased body fat may cause the older adult to feel less attractive and experience a reduced libido. Talking to one's partner about these feelings and emotions can stimulate intimacy and help the couple connect on a more comfortable level with one other.

For those who are single, it is imperative that health providers address sexually transmitted infections and safe sex practices. About 20% of all adults with HIV infection are older adults, and the risk increases for women because of the increased dryness and loss of elasticity of the vaginal mucosa. Barriers should be used for sexual intercourse as well as for oral sex for all sexually active adults.

Exercise and Activity

Maintaining exercise and activity during the later years can improve an adult's strength, balance, flexibility, and endurance, which can combine for healthier living and increased independence. Strength exercises build muscles, increase metabolism, and help with maintaining healthy body weight and blood sugar levels. Exercises that can be performed safely by older adults to help in strength building include arm raises, bicep curls, triceps extensions, and knee flexion. Balance exercises help adults to build leg muscles, which can help to prevent falls. Included in the balance exercises are side leg raises, hip flexion, and hip

extension. Stretching exercises improve movement and allow one to be more physically active during the later years. Included in the stretching exercises are triceps stretches and double hip rotations. Endurance exercises include cardiovascular exercises that increase the heart rate and respiratory rate and help to build up endurance gradually. The activities can include any activity that builds cardiovascular health in this way, from walking to jogging to swimming and biking. Older adults who have not engaged in endurance exercises should begin slowly, with only about 5 minutes of activity per day.

Cognitive Functioning

While cognition includes memory and knowledge, there are other factors incorporated into cognitive ability. Cognition is a combination of acquiring knowledge, perceiving events that surround us, using language, making decisions, using judgment, and executing motor skills. As cognitive changes occur because of the aging process, older adults begin to notice changes in memory and the ability to execute normal daily functions.

Most of the decline seen in cognitive functioning because of the aging process is irreversible. However, there are some factors that can slow the decline. Stress management and coping strategies can lessen depression and increase concentration and memory. Medical management of physical illnesses can control renal disease, liver disease, endocrine disorders, and electrolyte imbalances that can contribute to diminishing cognitive functioning. Good nutritional intake, including folate, riboflavin, and thiamine can improve cognition. Finally, moderation or elimination of alcohol use can reduce cognitive impairment.

A simple cognitive assessment that can be performed on all adults includes the use of clock drawing, box copying, and narrative writing to describe a pictured scene. These activities allow the health-care provider to gather information regarding cognitive function in a relatively quick fashion. The Mini-Mental State Examination (MMSE) can be performed to provide a better gauge of cognitive difficulty. The specific components in the MMSE are time orientation, place orientation, registration of three words, serial 7's as a test of attention and calculation, recall of three words, naming, repetition, comprehension, reading, writing, and drawing (National Institutes of Health, 2011). A newer cognitive test, the "Sweet 16," includes 16 measurements for testing a person's temporal/spatial orientation, registration, sustained attention, and short-term memory. The "Sweet 16" can be administered in 3 minutes, requires no pen, paper, or special forms, and has the ability to accurately characterize mental status without being influenced by the individual's education level or other socio-demographic factors. Other cognitive screening tools include the Computerized Self-Test (CST) and the Self-Administered Gerocognitive Examination (SAGE), both of which were created as early-screening tools for persons with mild thinking and memory impairments (Fong, Jones, Rudolph, Yang, Tommet, Habtemariam, et al., 2011).

Functional Ability

Functional ability may also decrease with aging, especially if the older adult has any disability or does not engage in physical activity and exercise. When assessing functional ability, it is important to consider how a person manages her day-to-day activities, the impact of any disease on the daily activities, and the overall quality of life being experienced by the individual. To gain this information, the health-care provider should perform a functional assessment.

The functional assessment needs to incorporate physical, social, psychological, demographic, financial, and legal issues. Questions asked should be designed to provide answers regarding self-concept and self-esteem, occupation, activity and exercise, sleep and rest, nutrition and elimination, interpersonal relationships and resources, coping and stress management, and environmental hazards (Bonnel, 2011).

 ### *Across Care Settings:* Optimizing senior health

Older adults should be encouraged to become more involved in activities that can improve health, endurance, and the enjoyment of life. Whether the individual is at home, in the workplace, in the community, or residing in a senior living environment, regular activity needs to be promoted. Physical activities may include walking, exercise classes, strength training, or swimming. In addition, cognitive functioning can be improved through conversation, puzzles, board games, and card games. Many communities have organizations that provide activities to promote healthy living for seniors, and nurses can play an integral role in encouraging and providing information on available resources.

Immunizations

Recommended immunizations for the older adult focus on disease prevention related to highly communicable illnesses. An influenza vaccination should be administered annually to prevent infection from influenza, and this is particularly important in older adults with chronic respiratory and cardiac diseases. The pneumococcal vaccine, which provides protection against pneumococcal pneumonia, should be administered to all adults around the age of 65. Individuals at higher risk for infection and complications related to infection are those who reside in assisted living or long-term care facilities and older adults with chronic respiratory, cardiac, renal, and hepatic disease.

COMMON HEALTH PROBLEMS IN OLDER WOMEN

Health problems that frequently develop in women during older age include osteoporosis, endometrial cancer, and pelvic floor dysfunction. Medical management of each of these disorders can prolong life and in many cases provide for a healthier ability to engage in daily activities.

Osteoporosis

As individuals age, there is a progressive decrease in bone density. **Osteoporosis** is a generalized, metabolic disease characterized by decreased bone mass and an increased incidence of bone fractures. Although osteoporosis occurs primarily in older women, it can also occur in older men, in persons with decreased levels of calcium and phosphorus, and in conjunction with increased corticosteroid release or administration. The most common problem associated with osteoporosis is the increased risk of bone

---

Box 4-9 **Risk Factors for Developing Osteoporosis**

Risk factors for developing osteoporosis include:

- Age, because of decreased estrogen following menopause
- Slender build and small frame
- Low body weight (150 lb <70 kg])
- Shortened exposure to estrogen, through late menarche or early menopause
- Family history of osteoporosis
- Smoking
- Decreased physical activity or sedentary lifestyle
- Excessive caffeine or alcohol use
- Low calcium and vitamin D intake
- Southeast Asian and Caucasian ethnicity
- Use of corticosteroids, commonly used to treat chronic respiratory disorders and arthritis

---

fracture, primarily in the spine, hip, or wrist. While normal changes in bone density occur with aging, there are a number of risk factors that are associated with the development of osteoporosis (Box 4-9).

SCREENING. Screening for osteoporosis through measurement of bone density should begin for all women at age 65 and initiated earlier for women younger than 65 whose clinical risk factors place them at a fracture risk similar to a 65-year-old woman (USPSTF, 2011b).

A variety of tests are available for osteoporosis screening. Dual-energy x-ray absorptiometry (DEXA), measured at the femoral head of the hip, spine, and wrist, is the best indicator of an increased risk for hip fracture, although measurements at different areas can be used to determine the presence and degree of osteoporosis. Peripheral sites can also be used for screening purposes, through quantitative ultrasonography, radiographic absorptiometry, single-energy x-ray absorptiometry, peripheral dual-energy x-ray absorptiometry, and peripheral quantitative computed tomography (NAMS, 2010b).

Medical management of osteoporosis is usually pharmacological and focuses on the goals of preventing increased bone density loss and, if possible, increasing bone density over time. Bisphosphonates, the most common group of medications used, inhibit osteoclast activity, preserve bone mass, and increase bone density. The most common bisphosphonates are alendronate (Fosamax), ibandronate (Boniva), and risedronate (Actonel), which can be taken on a weekly or monthly basis. Denosumab (Prolia) has a different mechanism of action than the bisphosphonates. This agent inhibits a soluble protein needed for the formation of osteoclasts and is responsible for bone resorption. It is administered subcutaneously every 6 months. Raloxifene (Evista), formerly known as a selective estrogen-receptor modulator (SERM), is used for both prevention and treatment of osteoporosis in postmenopausal women. This medication, indicated for the reduction in risk of invasive breast cancer in postmenopausal women with osteoporosis, increases the risk of deep vein thrombosis, and it also increases the frequency of night sweats and hot flashes (NAMS, 2010b; Wilton, 2011).

Prevention is the best strategy for reducing the risk of fractures associated with osteoporosis. Health-promoting activities that facilitate prevention include adequate amounts of calcium and vitamin D, moderate exposure to sunlight, strength training exercises, endurance exercises, consuming a diet that is composed primarily of plant-based, unprocessed whole foods, cessation of smoking, and the avoidance of excess caffeine and alcohol.

⑨ Optimizing Outcomes—Potential nursing diagnoses for women with osteoporosis

Nursing diagnoses for women with osteoporosis may focus on potential or real problems such as trauma, pain, or impaired mobility:

Risk for Trauma (related to loss of bone density/integrity; increasing risk of fracture with minimal or no stress)

Acute/Chronic Pain (related to vertebral compression on spinal nerves/muscles/ligaments, spontaneous fractures, possibly evidenced by verbal reports, guarding/distraction behaviors, self-focus, and changes in sleep pattern)

Impaired Physical Mobility (related to pain and musculoskeletal impairment, possibly evidenced by limited range of motion, reluctance to attempt movement/expressed fear of reinjury, and imposed restrictions/limitations) (Venes, 2013)

Pelvic Floor Dysfunction

The pelvic muscles atrophy after menopause, becoming weak and unable to adequately support the pelvic structures and organs. As the pelvic organs shift position, they begin to press against the vagina, resulting in prolapse, usually of the vagina or bladder. The most common cause of pelvic muscle weakness results from damage to the muscles during vaginal birth, particularly if the baby was large or if the labor was difficult. Other factors related to weakening of the pelvic floor include obesity, chronic cough, chronic constipation, and strenuous exercise. A prolapse can result in pain during intercourse and urinary incontinence. In severe cases, the vagina may prolapse and protrude through the vaginal orifice.

Different types of prolapse can occur, depending on the muscles and organs that are affected. A **cystocele** results when the bladder herniates into the vagina. Symptoms include difficulty in voiding, incontinence, and dyspareunia. A **rectocele** occurs when the muscles behind the vagina are damaged, allowing the rectum to press into the vagina. When the muscle damage occurs in a higher location in the colon, it is referred to as an **enterocele.** Symptoms associated with both of these types of prolapse include constipation, difficulty in completing a bowel movement, and dyspareunia. Uterine and vaginal vault prolapses occur when the uterus and cervix press downward, resulting in a sensation of pressure in the abdomen and vagina, dyspareunia, and back pain.

Exercise can strengthen the muscles; however, muscle damage cannot be reversed. Surgery is the primary treatment for pelvic prolapse; the timing of the surgery depends on the woman's symptoms and their effect on her daily activities.

Some symptoms can be medically managed until surgery is appropriate. Many treatment options are available for urinary incontinence, especially if it is not accompanied by a cystocele. Exercises to strengthen the pelvic muscles, including Kegel exercises, can be beneficial in decreasing the incidence of urinary incontinence (see Chapter 10 for more information). Vaginal cones, which may also be vaginal weights, can be used to strengthen the vaginal muscles as well. These tampon-shaped cones are inserted into the vagina, beginning with the lightest weight. Once inserted, the patient should contract the pelvic muscles in an effort to keep the cone in place for minutes. As the muscles strengthen, the patient then transitions, one at a time, to the next heaviest cone. It is helpful to use the cone while doing the pelvic floor exercises as well. As the pelvic muscles strengthen, patients can use the cones while engaging in exercise.

Electrical stimulation during Kegel exercises stimulates and contracts the pelvic muscles in a manner similar to the Kegels. This approach, conducted in the health-care practitioner's office, may be helpful for women who have difficulty contracting the pelvic muscles voluntarily. With an electrode attached to the skin, biofeedback machines measure the electrical signals elicited when the pelvic muscles and urinary sphincter are contracted. With biofeedback through the visual cues from the graph shown on the monitor, patients can learn to control these muscles voluntarily.

Some women choose to use a **pessary,** which is a device inserted into the vagina to support the prolapsed bladder or uterus. This device must be fitted by a health-care practitioner and needs to be removed and cleaned regularly with soap and water to reduce the risk of infection.

Pharmacological management of incontinence is aimed at relaxing the involuntary contractions that occur in the bladder. For overactive bladder, common medications include tolterodine (Detrol), oxybutynin (Ditropan), and imipramine (Tofranil). Common side effects associated with these medications include dry mouth, nausea, dizziness, drowsiness, and constipation. For **urinary stress incontinence** (USI), in which there is an involuntary loss of urine during sneezing, coughing, or laughing, the goal of treatment is to increase muscle tone in the urinary sphincter. Postmenopausal women may choose to use estrogen replacement therapy following careful consideration of the risks and benefits. For weak or underactive bladder problems, bethanechol (Urecholine) is the usual medication of choice.

Surgical interventions include laparoscopic or abdominal procedures to support the bladder and urethra in the correct anatomical position or methods to tighten the sphincter muscles. In one type of procedure, the surgeon sutures the vaginal wall to the tissue near the pubic bone. Another involves the creation of a sling using synthetic material or tissue taken from the abdomen or from beneath the thigh. The sling is then positioned beneath the urethra to provide support and prevent urine leakage. A newer procedure uses a mesh-like tape, called tension free transvaginal tape (TVT), which is surgically inserted through the vagina and positioned to support the neck of the urethra and the bladder. This procedure is performed under local anesthesia and intravenous sedation. A final procedure involves injections of collagen or silicone into the lining of the urethra. The injected substance increases the bulk of the surrounding tissues, allowing the urethra to close tightly and prevent leakage of urine. This technique usually requires two to three injections before symptom improvement is noticed.

Following either type of surgical repair, the patient should not engage in exercise for 2 weeks and avoid lifting objects weighing more than 10 pounds for 3 months after the surgery. At that time, exercises to protect and strengthen the pelvic muscles are initiated.

Endometrial Cancer

Endometrial cancer occurs most often in women between the ages of 50 and 69 and is the most common malignancy of the reproductive system. Endometrial cancer is slow growing, and most women are symptomatic in the early stages, factors that lead to early diagnosis, and frequently, successful treatment. For postmenopausal women, the cardinal symptom is vaginal bleeding; perimenopausal women may have heavy or prolonged menstruation or spotting or bleeding between menses. Other symptoms for all women with endometrial cancer include pelvic pain, dyspareunia, and/or weight loss.

An increased estrogen level, which stimulates growth of the endometrium during the menstrual cycle, is the most common cause of endometrial cancer. However, several additional risk factors have been identified: early age of menarche (before the age of 12); late menopause (after age 55); nulliparity or low parity; irregular ovulation, which may result from obesity or polycystic ovarian syndrome; a high-fat diet, which increases the levels of circulating estrogen; diabetes (a condition closely related to obesity and a high-fat dietary intake); estrogen-only replacement therapy; ovarian tumors that produce estrogen; age greater than 40 years; ovarian granulosa-theca cell tumors; therapy with tamoxifen (an anti-estrogen medication used in the prevention and treatment of breast cancer); Caucasian race; and hereditary nonpolyposis colorectal cancer (HNPCC), a specific type caused by a gene that inhibits DNA repair.

The diagnosis is made by histological examination. Most often, tissue is obtained by endometrial biopsy, an outpatient procedure performed using local anesthesia. A suction-type curette is used to remove the tissue for laboratory analysis. Fractional curettage, a surgical procedure that involves a scraping of the endocervix and the endometrium to obtain tissue for histological evaluation, may also be performed. Other diagnostic tests include hysteroscopy (examination of the uterus through an endoscope) and transvaginal ultrasound. If endometrial cancer is present, staging, which may include chest radiography, abdominal CT scan, MRI, cystoscopy, proctoscopy, liver function tests, renal function tests, bone scans, and serum testing for the presence of cancer antigen 125 (CA 125, released by some endometrial and ovarian cancers), is done to determine the extent of metastasis.

Total abdominal hysterectomy (surgical removal of the uterus) is the most common treatment for endometrial cancer. In most cases, a bilateral salpingo-oophorectomy is also performed, along with removal of local lymph nodes. Following the surgery, radiation therapy, chemotherapy, or hormone therapy may be prescribed, depending on the clinical findings. When diagnosed and treated early, survival rates are greater than 90%.

PROSTATE CANCER SCREENING

Other than skin cancers, prostate cancer is the most common neoplasm diagnosed in men. The highest prevalence occurs among African American men, and the lowest rate occurs among Asians and American Indian/Alaskan Native men. Other risk factors include a positive family history, having had a vasectomy, consuming a diet high in fats and red meats and low in fruits and vegetables, environmental exposure to carcinogens, hormonal influences, especially elevated levels of androgens, and advancing age. Benign hypertrophy of the prostate (BPH) is associated with prostate cancer. However, there is no evidence that a causative link exists. While BPH does not usually cause symptoms in men before the age of 40, more than 50% of men in their 60s and 90% of men in their 80s have some symptoms of BPH, such as urinary frequency, hesitancy, urgency, nocturia, and weak urinary stream.

Screening for prostate cancer is a controversial issue in health care today. The U.S. Preventive Services Task Force has determined that there is insufficient evidence to recommend for or against routine screening for prostate cancer (USPSTF, 2011a). Most professional medical organizations recommend that men over the age of 50 or men with a strong family history of prostate cancer discuss screening with their health-care practitioners. The available options include digital rectal examination (DRE), blood tests to assess levels of prostate specific antigen (PSA), or assessment of the gland with ultrasonography. To perform a DRE, the examiner inserts a gloved and lubricated finger into the rectum and carefully palpates the prostate gland. The examination is considered normal when palpation reveals a prostate that is smooth, absent of nodules, and of normal size and shape. A symmetrically firm, soft, and enlarged prostate by DRE is indicative of BPH.

When prostate cancer is suggested by screening methods, biopsies are required to confirm the diagnosis. Biopsies are usually performed using guided imagery via transrectal ultrasound. During the procedure, an ultrasound probe is inserted into the rectum and ultrasonographic pictures are transmitted for viewing. This procedure allows the health-care practitioner to determine the size and shape of the prostate and location of abnormal growths. A fine needle is then inserted into the gland and several samples of prostate tissue are removed for pathological examination. Further studies may include MRIs, CTs, and bone scans to determine if the disease has spread. While there is no curative treatment for metastatic disease, several options are available for the treatment of localized prostate cancer. These include watchful waiting/expectant therapy, radical prostatectomy, three-dimensional external beam radiation (with or without hormone therapy), brachytherapy (the use of implants of radioactive materials), and cryosurgery (the use of extremely cold probes to destroy neoplastic tissue).

Preparation for Prostate Biopsy

Patients are provided with the necessary information for biopsy preparation at least 2 weeks before the procedure. Although men who have a history of cardiac valvular disease must receive antibiotic prophylaxis before the procedure, many physicians prescribe prophylactic antibiotic therapy for all patients prior to the procedure to decrease the incidence of postprocedure infection. Patients who are taking coagulation-modifier agents or anti-inflammatory agents are instructed to discontinue the use of these medications 7 to 10 days before the procedure, and blood tests, including prothrombin time (PT) and international normalized ratio (INR), are performed before the procedure on the day of the biopsy to determine if bleeding times are normal. The patient is also instructed to administer an enema for bowel cleansing the day before the scheduled procedure.

After the procedure, the patient is instructed to refrain from taking coagulation-modifier agents and anti-inflammatory agents for 3 days and to drink plenty of water. A sitz bath or warm soak is recommended for rectal tenderness. Antibiotics are prescribed for all postprocedure patients to prevent infection.

MENTAL AND EMOTIONAL HEALTH

Some older adults may experience declines in health and cognitive ability, which can lead to behavioral and emotional problems and physical complaints. Signs of altered mental and emotional health may begin with subtle changes in personality or with dramatic alterations that require immediate intervention from a health-care professional. Symptoms that require immediate intervention include hallucinations, paranoia, incoherent thinking or language, extreme lack of motivation or flat affect, and expression of suicidal thoughts or actions. Less serious symptoms that also require intervention include changes in sleeping or eating patterns, loss of interest in activities, neglect of grooming and personal hygiene, changes in sexual habits, and refusal to take prescribed medications.

Treatment for alterations in mental and emotional health requires a collaborative approach. Psychologists and neurologists may be involved in initial testing and diagnosis, while psychiatrists and nurses become an integral part of the treatment and management team. Pharmacists are an important part of the team because they have specialized knowledge in drugs and drug interactions. Psychologists provide psychotherapy treatment and counseling for the patient and the family. Social workers are essential in coordinating care with regard to medical care, benefits, and housing. Occupational therapists are experts that evaluate and restructure a person's physical environment as well as provide mental activities to enhance independent functioning. Community health nurses visit the home to assess the patient and family and to gauge understanding and acceptance of the treatment plan.

 Collaboration in Caring—*Culturally sensitive community approaches to enhanced health care for older citizens*

Organizations, groups, and health-care facilities recognize the importance of culturally sensitive approaches to meet the health needs of older citizens. Information gained from these collaborative endeavors benefits diverse communities by generating new knowledge and understanding and by providing insights for further investigation. Examples of successful projects include the following:

- The National Asian Pacific Center on Aging (NAPCA) organized community forums to share assessment results with participants. Three translators were available throughout the forums. Working groups were then developed to implement interventions to meet the identified needs.

- An advisory committee was used to evaluate the methodology and language used for a breast cancer study in Vietnamese women conducted by the University of California at San Francisco. Vietnamese women were hired to conduct the interventions in the study to improve accuracy of the results.

- The American Society on Aging conducted a study to determine the drinking habits of elders in the Chinese community. The written survey was translated into Chinese and included alcoholic beverages specific to that culture, including plum wine. The researchers were able to acquire more accurate results by using culturally appropriate content (American Society on Aging, 2012).

Advancing age raises issues related to death and dying for most individuals. As they age, individuals may lose a spouse, family member, or close friend, which can significantly alter their living situation and their emotional health. As with persons of any age, the patient needs to be encouraged to grieve. However, it is essential for the nurse to be sensitive to the specific issues that frequently arise following the loss of the loved one: fear about living arrangements, preoccupation with one's own death, agitation and an inability to perform daily activities, and an overwhelming sadness or withdrawal. Counseling, support groups, and antidepressant medications are often beneficial for individuals who are experiencing difficulty with coping.

Another issue related to emotional and mental health concerns the older person's ability to remain connected to other people. Declines in health, physical mobility, and cognitive function may contribute to problems of isolation for the older adult. Family members should be encouraged to maintain frequent contact and engage the elderly in a variety of social activities to keep their loved ones involved in life and socially connected. Many community health agencies or elder day-care facilities offer programs with supervised stimulation for adults experiencing difficulty in these areas. Respite care, which allows family members an opportunity for time away from the caregiving situation, may also be beneficial.

Summary Points

- Health promotion screening can provide early detection and treatment of health disorders, including skin and reproductive cancers, hyperlipidemia, osteoporosis, and gynecological disorders.

- Nurses play a key role in collaborative care for all patients, at each stage of the life span, from infancy to older age.

- A holistic approach to health promotion includes focusing on nutrition, dental care, safety, injury prevention, screening for early diagnosis and treatment, and other strategies to facilitate healthy development.

- Cultural and ethnic differences must be taken into consideration when providing anticipatory guidance and health promotion education to patients.

Review Questions

Multiple Choice

1. The outpatient clinic nurse correctly makes a recommendation that a 65-year-old man schedule a health maintenance examination every
A. year.
B. 2 years.
C. 3 years.
D. 5 years.

2. The pediatric nurse is teaching the mother of a 1-year-old child about nutrition. Which milk selection is most appropriate to introduce to the child at this point?
A. Whole milk
B. 1% milk
C. 2% milk
D. Skim milk

3. The clinic nurse teaches new parents that the most normal time for children to ask about "where babies come from" is approximately
A. 2 to 3 years of age.
B. 3 to 5 years of age.
C. 5 to 7 years of age.
D. 7 to 9 years of age.

4. The clinic nurse is assessing a child's risk for obesity. Both the child's parents have a body mass index (BMI) of 32. What risk of obesity does this give the patient?
A. 25%
B. 50%
C. 75%
D. 90%

5. The clinic nurse is teaching a new mother the signs of feeding readiness she may see in her child. Which of the following is the most important sign of readiness for solid food?
A. Absence of the extrusion reflex
B. Appropriate weight gain
C. Development of the pincer grasp
D. Reaching 4 months of age

6. The father of a 9-month-old infant asks about appropriate finger foods for the child. Which of the following should the nurse suggest?
A. Well-cooked hot dogs cut into small pieces
B. Pastas cooked al dente (firm)
C. Small pieces of ripe banana
D. Tiny bites of whole wheat cereal

7. The clinic nurse is educating the parents of an adolescent about risk-taking behaviors. Which factor most increases the likelihood of the teen's engaging in risky behavior?
A. The effect of media and advertising on teens
B. The fact that teens are chronically sleep deprived
C. The importance placed on peer relationships
D. The need to find boundaries and explore the world

8. A nurse is working with a teen group. One of the participants is thin but "always on a diet" and claims to never be hungry. Which eating disorder does the nurse suspect?
A. Anorexia nervosa
B. Bulimia nervosa
C. Diabulimia
D. Pica

9. A nurse sees a teen in the adolescent health clinic. The teen has damaged teeth, a hoarse voice, and seems to be mildly dehydrated. Which action by the nurse is best?
A. Ask about eating habits.
B. Assess for strep throat.
C. Refer the teen to a dentist.
D. Start an intravenous line.

10. A nurse is working with a teen after-school group. Which of the following is the best primary prevention measure the nurse can implement to reduce the risk of death from preventable cancer?
A. Conduct screening clinics for cervical and skin cancers.
B. Create a family genogram to assess the risk of cancer.
C. Encourage the teens to get 30 minutes of exercise daily.
D. Teach the adolescents about the dangers of sun exposure.

See Answers to End of Chapter Review Questions on Davis*Plus*.

REFERENCES

Afify, A., & Howell, L. P. (2010). Cervical cancer screening: Effective clinician and laboratory partnership. *The Female Patient, 35*(8), 27–30.

Allen, T. L., Van Groningen, B. J., Barksdale, D. J., & McCarthy, R. (2010). The breast self-examination controversy: What providers and patients should know. *The Journal for Nurse Practitioners, 6*(6), 444–451.

American Academy of Dermatology (AAD). (2011). Indoor tanning: Teen and young adult women. Retrieved from http://www.aad.org/media-resources/stats-and-facts/prevention-and-care/indoor-tanning

American Academy of Pediatrics (AAP). (2011a). Policy statement: SIDS and other sleep-related infant deaths: Expansion of recommendations for a safe infant sleeping environment. *Pediatrics, 128*(11), 1030–1039. doi:10.1542/peds.2011-2284

American Academy of Pediatrics (AAP). (2011b). Clinical report: Prevention and management of positional skull deformities in infants. *Pediatrics, 128*(6), 1236–1241. doi:10.1542/peds.2011–2220

American Academy of Pediatrics (AAP). (2012). Policy statement: Breastfeeding and the use of human milk. *Pediatrics, 129*(3), 827–841. doi:10.1542/peds.2011-3552

American Academy of Pediatrics (AAP). (2013a). Car seats: Information for families 2013. Retrieved from http://www.healthychildren.org/English/safety-prevention/on-the-go/pages/Car-Safety-Seats-Information-for-Families.aspx

American Academy of Pediatrics (AAP). (2013b). Safety & prevention: Make baby's room safe. Retrieved from http://www.healthychildren.org/English/safety-prevention/at-home/pages/Make-Babys-Room-Safe.aspx

American Cancer Society (ACS). (2011a). Skin cancer prevention and early detection. Retrieved from http://www.cancer.org/cancer/skincancer-melanoma/moreinformation/skincancerpreventionandearlydetection/index

American Cancer Society (ACS). (2011b). What are the risk factors for breast cancer? Retrieved from http://www.cancer.org/Cancer/Breast-Cancer/DetailedGuide/breast-cancer-risk-factors

American Cancer Society (ACS). (2011c). Breast cancer in men. Retrieved from http://www.cancer.org/Cancer/BreastCancer/DetailedGuide/breast-cancer-in-men-key-statistics

American Cancer Society (ACS). (2011d). Breast awareness and self-exam. Retrieved from http://www.cancer.org/Cancer/BreastCancer/MoreInformation/BreastCancerEarlyDetection/breast-cancer-early-detection-acs-recs-bse

American Cancer Society (ACS). (2011e). *Breast cancer overview*. Retrieved from http://www.cancer.org/docroot/CRI/content/CRI_2_2_1X_How_many_people_get_breast_cancer_5.asp

American Cancer Society (ACS). (2011f). What are the key statistics about ovarian cancer? Retrieved from http://www.cancer.org/Cancer/Ovarian-Cancer/DetailedGuide/ovarian-cancer-key-statistics

American College of Obstetricians and Gynecologists (ACOG). (2008). Committee opinion number 444: Alternatives to hysterectomy in the management of leiomyomas. (Reaffirmed 2012). *Obstetrics and Gynecology, 112*(2), 387–400.

American College of Obstetricians and Gynecologists (ACOG). (2010a). Committee opinion number 463: Cervical cancer in adolescents: Screening, evaluation, and management. *Obstetrics and Gynecology, 116*(1), 469–472.

American College of Obstetricians and Gynecologists (ACOG). (2010b). Committee opinion number 460: The initial reproductive health visit. *Obstetrics and Gynecology, 116*(1), 240–243.

American College of Obstetricians and Gynecologists (ACOG). (2010c). ACOG Practice Bulletin No. 114, Management of endometriosis. *Obstetrics and Gynecology, 116*(1), 223–236.

American College of Obstetricians and Gynecologists (ACOG). (2011a). Committee opinion number 483: Primary and preventive care: Periodic assessments. *Obstetrics and Gynecology, 117*(4), 1008–1015.

American College of Obstetricians and Gynecologists (ACOG). (2011b). Committee opinion number 503: Tobacco use and women's health. *Obstetrics and Gynecology, 118*(3), 746–750.

American College of Obstetricians and Gynecologists (ACOG). (2011c). Committee opinion number 502: Primary ovarian insufficiency in the adolescent. *Obstetrics and Gynecology, 118*(3), 741–745.

American College of Obstetricians and Gynecologists (ACOG). (2011d). Committee opinion number 496: At-risk drinking and alcohol dependence: Obstetric and gynecologic implications. *Obstetrics and Gynecology, 118*(2), 383–388.

American College of Obstetricians and Gynecologists (ACOG). (2011e). ACOG Practice Bulletin No. 122, Breast Cancer Screening. *Obstetrics and Gynecology, 118*(2), 372–382.

American College of Obstetricians and Gynecologists (ACOG). (2011f). Committee opinion number 482: Colonoscopy and Colorectal Cancer Screening Strategies. *Obstetrics and Gynecology, 117*(3), 766–771.

American College of Obstetricians and Gynecologists (ACOG). (2012). ACOG Practice Bulletin No. 131, Screening for cervical cancer. *Obstetrics and Gynecology, 120*(11), 1222–1238.

American Dental Association (ADA). (2013). *Fluoridation facts*. Retrieved from http://www.ada.org/4047.aspx

American Society for Colposcopy and Cervical Pathology (ASCCP). (2013). Human papillomavirus (HPV). Retrieved 10-30-13 from http://www.asccp.org/Practice-Management-3/Vulva/HPV-Infections-and-VIN

American Society on Aging. (2012). Multicultural aging. Retrieved from http://www.asaging.org/education/7

Appelbaum, H., & Nentin, F. (2010). Endometriosis in adolescents. *The Female Patient, 35*(4), 17–20.

Association of Women's Health, Obstetric and Neonatal Nurses (AWHONN). (2010a). Position Statement: Confidentiality in adolescent health care. *Journal of Obstetric, Gynecologic & Neonatal Nursing, 39*(1), 127–128.

Association of Women's Health, Obstetric and Neonatal Nurses (AWHONN). (2010b). Position Statement: HPV vaccination for the prevention of cervical cancer. *Journal of Obstetric, Gynecologic & Neonatal Nursing, 39*(1), 81–82.

Association of Women's Health, Obstetric and Neonatal Nurses (AWHONN). (2010c). Position Statement: Smoking and women's health. *Journal of Obstetric, Gynecologic & Neonatal Nursing, 39*(5), 427–429.

Association of Women's Health, Obstetric and Neonatal Nurses (AWHONN). (2010d). Position Statement: Breast cancer screening. *Journal of Obstetric, Gynecologic & Neonatal Nursing, 39*(10), 424–426.

Benzie, F., Hekman, K., Cameron, L., Wade, D., Miller, C., Smolinske, S., & Warrick, B. (2011). Emergency department visits after use of a drug sold as "bath salts"—Michigan, November 13, 2010–March 31, 2011. *Morbidity and Mortality Weekly Report (MMWR), 60*(5), 624–627.

Bonnel, W. (2011). Screening for functional deficits in older adults. *The Clinical Advisor, 14*(9), 55–60.

Braverman, P. K., & Breech, L. (2010). Gynecologic examination for adolescents in the pediatric office setting. *Pediatrics, 126*(3), 583–590. doi:10.1542/peds.2010-1564.

Burkman, R. T. (2010). New screening recommendations: Benefits and harms are in the eye of the beholder. *The Female Patient, 35*(3), 12–13.

Carr, M., & Kaplan, C. (2010). Midlife women with anorexia nervosa: A review of the literature. *The American Journal for Nurse Practitioners, 14*(6), 8–14.

Carter, J. S., & Downs, L. S. (2011). Cervical cancer tests and treatment. *The Female Patient, 361*), 34–38.

Center for the Study and Prevention of Violence (2010). *CSPV fact sheet: Ethnicity, race, class and adolescent violence*. Retrieved from http://www.colorado.edu/cspv/

Centers for Disease Control and Prevention (CDC). (2011). *HPV vaccine—questions & answers*. Retrieved from http://www.cdc.gov/vaccines/vpd-vac/hpv/vac-faqs.htm

Centers for Disease Control and Prevention (CDC). (2013a). Sudden unexpected infant death (SUID) and sudden infant death syndrome (SIDS). Retrieved from http://www.cdc.gov/sids/

Centers for Disease Control and Prevention (CDC). (2013b). Child passenger safety: Fact sheet. Retrieved from http://www.cdc.gov/motorvehiclesafety/child_passenger_safety/cps-factsheet.html

Centers for Disease Control and Prevention (CDC). (2013c). About school violence. Retrieved from http://www.cdc.gov/violenceprevention/youthviolence/schoolviolence/

Centers for Disease Control and Prevention (CDC). (2013d). Youth violence: National statistics. Retrieved from http://www.cdc.gov/violenceprevention/youthviolence/stats_at_a_glance/hr_trends_race.html

Centers for Disease Control and Prevention (CDC). (2013e). Youth physical activity guidelines toolkit. Retrieved from http://www.cdc.gov/healthyyouth/physicalactivity/guidelines.htm

Centers for Disease Control and Prevention (CDC). (2013f). Recommended immunization schedules for persons aged 0–18 years—United States, 2013. *Morbidity and Mortality Weekly Report, 62*(01), 2–8.

Centers for Disease Control and Prevention (CDC). (2013g). Recommended immunization schedule for adults aged 19 years and older, United States, 2013. *Morbidity and Mortality Weekly Report, 62*(01), 9–19.

Centers for Disease Control and Prevention (CDC). (2014). Use of 13-valent pneumococcal conjugate vaccine and 23-valent pneumococcal polysaccharide vaccine among adults aged ≥ 65 years: Recommendations of the Advisory Committee on Immunization Practices (ACIP). *Morbidity and Mortality Weekly Report, 63*(37), 822-825.

Chase, C., Wells, J., & Eley, S. (2011). Caffeine and breast pain: Revisiting the connection. *Nursing for Women's Health, 15*(4), 287–294.

Chesnut, C. H. (1989). Is osteoporosis a pediatric disease? Peak bone mass attainment in the adolescent female. *Public Health Reports, 104*(Suppl), 50–54.

Emeis, C. L. (2011). Current resources for evidence-based practice May/June, 2011. *Journal of Obstetric, Gynecologic & Neonatal Nursing, 40*(3), 329–334.

Erikson, E. H. (1959). *Identity and the life cycle*. New York, NY: International Universities Press.

Fantasia, H. C., & Fontenot, H. B. (2011). The sexual safety of adolescents. *Journal of Obstetric, Gynecologic & Neonatal Nursing, 40*(2), 217–224.

Fantasia, H. C., Fontenot, H. B., Harris, A. L., Hurd, L., & Chui, E. (2011). Ambiguity in defining adolescent sexual activity. *The Journal for Nurse Practitioners, 7*(6), 486–492.

Fong, T. G., Jones, R. N., Rudolph, J. L., Yang, F. M., Tommet, D., Habtemariam, D., . . . Inouye, S. K. (2011). Development and validation of a brief cognitive assessment tool: The sweet 16. *Archives of Internal Medicine, 171*(5), 432–437. doi:10.1001/archinternmed.2010.423

Fontenot, H. B., & Fantasia, H. C. (2011). Issues and influences on sexual violence within the adolescent population. *Journal of Obstetric, Gynecologic & Neonatal Nursing, 40*(2), 215–216.

Frey, M. K., & Gupta, D. (2011). Evaluation of women with atypical glandular cells on cervical cytology. *The Female Patient, 36*(9), 23–29.

Gies, C. E. (2011). Have we come a long way, baby? *Nursing for Women's Health, 15*(5), 413–417.

Gilliam, M. L. (2010). Cochrane update: Exercise for dysmenorrhea. *Obstetrics & Gynecology, 116*(1), 186–187.

Griffin, J. L., & Pearlman, M. D. (2010). Breast cancer screening in women at average risk and high risk. *Obstetrics & Gynecology, 116*(6), 1410–1421.

Hanson, M. J. (2010). Health behavior in adolescent women reporting and not reporting intimate partner violence. *Journal of Obstetric, Gynecologic & Neonatal Nursing, 39*(3), 263–275.

Harris, A. L. (2011). Media and technology in adolescent sexual education and safety. *Journal of Obstetric, Gynecologic & Neonatal Nursing, 40*(2), 235–242.

Hill, D. A., & Lamvu, G. (2012). Effect of lubricating gel on patient comfort during vaginal speculum examination. *Obstetrics & Gynecology, 119*(2), 227–231.

Hoffman, R. L. (2010). What lies behind the vitamin D revolution? *The Clinical Advisor, 13*(3), 31–37.

Holloway, B. W., & Moredich, C. (2011). *OB/GYN Peds Notes: Nurse's clinical pocket guide.* Philadelphia, PA: F.A. Davis.

Institute for Clinical Systems Improvement (ICSI). (2013, September). *Preventive services for adults (Guideline).* Retrieved from https://www.icsi.org/_asset/gtjr9h/

Insurance Institute for Highway Safety (IIHS). (2013). *Fatality facts: Teenagers.* Retrieved from http://www.iihs.org/iihs/topics/t/teenagers/topicoverview

Jordan, J. T., & Harrison, B. E. (2013). Bath salts ingestion: Diagnosis and treatment of substance-induced disorders. *The Journal for Nurse Practitioners, 9*(7), 402–410.

Kang, J. A., Gottlieb, A. S., Raker, C. A., Aneja, S. S., & Boardman, L. A. (2010). Interpersonal violence screening for ambulatory gynecology patients. *Obstetrics & Gynecology, 115*(6), 1159–1166.

Kanny, D., Liu, Y., & Brewer, R. D. (2011). Binge drinking—United States, 2009. Centers for Disease Control and Prevention (CDC). *MMWR Surveillance Summary 2011, 60*(Suppl), 101–104.

Kentley, D. (2011). Early-stage breast cancer treatment. *Clinical Advisor, 14*(4), 80–88.

Krowchuk, D. P. (2010). Adolescence: A metamorphosis. *North Carolina Medical Journal, 71*(4), 355–357.

Michigan Quality Improvement Consortium. (2011a, April). *Adult preventive services (ages 18–49).* Southfield, MI: Author.

Michigan Quality Improvement Consortium. (2011b, April). *Adult preventive services (ages 50–65+).* Southfield, MI: Author.

Mosher, C. E., & Danoff-Burg, S. (2010). Addiction to indoor tanning. *Archives of Dermatology, 146*(4), 412–417.

Murdoff, L. (2011). Insulin omission for weight loss: The dangers of diabulimia. *Advance for NPs & PAs, 2*(5), 35–38.

Naimi, T. S., Nelson, D. E., & Brewer, R. D. (2010). The intensity of binge alcohol consumption among U.S. adults. *American Journal of Preventive Medicine, 38*(9), 201–207.

National Alliance on Mental Illness. (2013). *Anorexia nervosa.* Retrieved from http://www.nami.org/Template.cfm?Section=By_Illness&template=/ContentManagement/ContentDisplay.cfm&ContentID=7409

National Cancer Institute (2012). *Testicular Cancer (PDQ®): Screening.* Retrieved from http://www.cancer.gov/cancertopics/pdq/screening/testicular/HealthProfessional

National Comprehensive Cancer Network. (2011). NCCN Clinical Practice Guidelines in Oncology/TM: Breast cancer. Fort Washington, PA: Author.

National Institutes of Health (NIH). (2011). Mental status testing. Retrieved from http://www.nlm.nih.gov/medlineplus/ency/article/003326.htm

National Institute of Mental Health (NIMH). (2010). NIH Publication No. 06-4594. Suicide in the U.S.: Statistics and prevention. Retrieved from http://www.nimh.nih.gov/health/publications/suicide-in-the-us-statistics-and-prevention/index.shtml

Nelson, L. M. (2010). The menstrual cycle in adolescents: A vital sign of bone health. *Contemporary OB-GYN, 55*(3), 32–37.

Office of Dietary Supplements. (2011). Dietary Supplement Fact Sheet: Vitamin D. National Institutes of Health. Retrieved from http://ods.od.nih.gov/factsheets/vitamind

Ogden, C. L., Carroll, M. D., Curtin, L. R., Lamb, M. M., & Flegal, K. M. (2010). Prevalence of high body mass index in US children and adolescents, 2007–2008. *Journal of the American Medical Association, 303*(3), 252–249.

Pearlman, M. D., & Griffin, J. L. (2010). Benign breast disease. *Obstetrics & Gynecology, 116*(3), 747–758.

Polfuss, M. L., Liebhart, J., & Greenley, R. N. (2011). Relationship between overweight/obesity and risk-taking behaviors in adolescents. *The American Journal for Nurse Practitioners, 15*(1/2), 10–24.

Polotsky, A. J. (2010). Amenorrhea caused by extremes of body mass: Pathophysiology and sequelae. *Contemporary OB/GYN, 55*(8), 18–23.

Raines, K. (2010). Diagnosing premenstrual syndrome. *The Journal for Nurse Practitioners, 6*(3), 224–226.

Ross, E. A., Watson, M., & Goldberger, B. (2011). "Bath salts" intoxication. *New England Journal of Medicine, 365*(10), 967–968.

Ruhl, C. (2011). Roadmapping health for the woman at 30. *Nursing for Women's Health, 15*(3), 235–238.

Rutecki, G. W. (2010). Think before you ink: Tattoos and the risk of hepatitis C. *Consultant, 50*(10), 449–450.

Rutecki, G. W. (2011). "Bath salts" are not for bathing anymore. *Consultant, 15*(11), 834.

Shifren, J. L., & Schiff, I. (2010). Role of hormone therapy in the management of menopause. *Obstetrics & Gynecology, 115*(4), 839–854.

Shropshire, A. M., & Thornton, K. (2011). Prevention measures for adolescent suicide: An evidence-based review. *The American Journal for Nurse Practitioners, 15*(5/6), 30–36.

Skin Cancer Foundation. (2011). Black history month reminder: Skin cancer affects everyone. Retrieved from http://www.skincancer.org/news/holidays-and-seasons/black-history-month-reminder

Speroff, L., & Fritz, M. (2010). *Clinical gynecologic endocrinology and infertility* (8th ed.). Philadelphia, PA: Lippincott Williams & Wilkins.

Stern, L. (2010). Navigating the evidence about cancer screening. *The Clinical Advisor, 13*(5), 20–34.

Substance Abuse and Mental Health Services Administration. (2012). Results from the 2011 National Survey on Drug Use and Health: Summary of national findings. Retrieved from http://www.samhsa.gov/data/nsduh/2k11results/nsduhresults2011.pdf

Sulak, P. J. (2011). Critique your caloric consumption. *The Female Patient, 36*(12), 14–19.

Sutherland, M. A. (2011). Implications for violence in adolescent dating experiences. *Journal of Obstetric, Gynecologic & Neonatal Nursing, 40*(2), 225–234.

The Nemours Foundation. (2012). *How to perform a testicular self-examination.* Retrieved from http://www.kidshealth.org/teen/sexual_health/guys/tse.html

The Nemours Foundation. (2013). *Teenshealth: Female athlete triad.* Retrieved from http://kidshealth.org/teen/food_fitness/sports/triad.html

The North American Menopause Society (NAMS). (2010a). Estrogen and progestogen use in post menopausal women: 2010 position statement of The North American Menopause Society. *Menopause: The Journal of the North American Menopause Society, 17*(2), 242–255.

The North American Menopause Society (NAMS). (2010b). *Management of osteoporosis in postmenopausal women: 2010 position statement.* Retrieved from http://www.menopause.org/docs/default-document-library/psosteo10.pdf?sfvrsn=2

The North American Menopause Society (NAMS). (2011). *Menopause practice: A clinician's guide* (4th ed.). Cleveland, OH: Author.

The Women's Health Initiative Steering Committee. (2004). Effects of conjugated equine estrogen in postmenopausal women with hysterectomy. *Journal of the American Medical Association, 291*(14), 1701–1712.

U.S. Department of Agriculture (USDA), Food and Nutrition Service. (2011). *MyPlate for kids.* Washington, DC: U.S. Government Printing Office.

U.S. Department of Health and Human Services (USDHHS). (2011). *Healthy People 2020.* Retrieved from http://www.healthypeople.gov/2020/topicsobjectives2020/default.aspx

U.S. Department of Health and Human Services (USDHHS), Office on Women's Health. (2010, August). *Breastfeeding.* Retrieved from http://www.womenshealth.gov/breastfeeding

U.S. Food and Drug Administration (FDA). (2014). *FDA approves Gardasil 9 for prevention of certain cancers caused by five additional types of HPV.* Retrieved from http://www.fda.gov/NewsEvents/Newsroom/PressAnnouncements/ucm426485.htm

U.S. Preventive Services Task Force (USPSTF). (2011a). *The guide to clinical preventive services 2011: Recommendations of the U.S. Preventive Services Task Force.* AHRQ Publication No. 10-50145, September 2010, Rockville MD. Available at http://www.ahrq.gov

U.S. Preventive Services Task Force (USPSTF). (2011b). Screening for osteoporosis: U.S. Preventive Services Task Force Recommendation Statement. *Annals of Internal Medicine, 35*(1). 466–467/

U.S. Preventive Services Task Force (USPSTF). (2012). Clinical Guideline: Screening for cervical cancer: The U.S. Preventive Services Task Force Recommendation Statement. *Annals of Internal Medicine* E-424 published ahead of print March 14, 2012.

Varghese, P., & Gray, B. P. (2011). Suicide assessment of adolescents in the primary care setting. *The Journal for Nurse Practitioners, 7*(3), 186–192.

Venes, D. (2013). *Taber's cyclopedic medical dictionary* (22nd ed.). Philadelphia, PA: F.A. Davis.

Veterans Health Administration, Department of Defense. (2011). *VHA/DoD clinical practice guideline for the management of dyslipidemia in primary care*. Washington, DC: Author.

Vulval Pain Society. (2012). *How to do vulval self-examination*. Retrieved from http://vulvalpainsociety.org/index.php?page=self-examination

Williams, D. R. (2012). Obesity in children and adolescents: Identifying eating disorders. *Consultant, 52*(2), 155–159.

Williams, E. C., Daley, A. M., & Iennaco, J. D. (2010). Assessing non-suicidal self-injurious behaviors in adolescents. *The American Journal for Nurse Practitioners, 14*(5), 18–26.

Wilton, J. M. (2011). Denosumab: New horizons in the treatment of osteoporosis. *Nursing for Women's Health, 15*.

Woo, P., & McEneaney, M. J. (2010). New strategies to treat primary dysmenorrhea. *The Clinical Advisor, 12*(11), 43–49.

Writing Group for the Women's Health Initiative Investigators (2002). Risks and benefits of estrogen plus progestin in health postmenopausal women: Principal results from the Women's Health Initiative randomized controlled trial. *JAMA, 288*(3), 321–333.

Ziegler, C. A. (2011). Self-expression through body art. *Advance for NPs & PAs, 2*(8), 43–45.

Zoller, S. (2011). Take cover: Shielding patients from skin cancer. *Advance for NPs & PAs, 2*(6), 28–31.

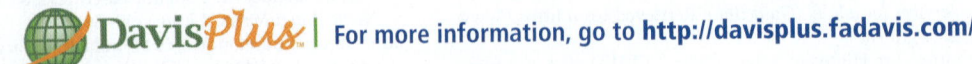

CONCEPT MAP

Caring for Women, Families, and Children Across the Life Span

Health Promotion — Disease Prevention

Infant/Child Health
Nutrition:
- Feeding: bottle vs. breast
- Solid food introduction based on developmental stage
- For greater than 3 yrs: use MyPlate for kids

Dental:
- Daily dental care

Sleep/Rest:
- Nighttime rest and naps based on developmental level

Safety:
- Home safety for injury prevention
- Control environment: crib, car, toys
- Risk-taking behavior: testing limits; sexual exploration

Activity:
- Progress through 5 types of developmental play
- Specific toys/games introduced to meet developmental goals

Immunizations:
- CDC recommendations

Sexuality:
- Child perception based on developmental level

Adolescent Health
Nutrition:
- To facilitate optimal growth/development
- Risk factors for obesity: psychological/societal/medical
- Risk for eating disorders: anorexia/bulimia

Dental:
- Checkup and cleaning twice yearly

Sleep/Rest:
- May need to decrease extracurricular activities

Safety:
- Accidents/injuries; MVA, homicides, suicides
- Risk-taking behaviors; developing own identity
- Injuries: MV, bikes, firearms, water
- Substance abuse: ETOH, drugs
- Violence/abuse
- Tattooing and piercing
- Reproductive health

Health Promotion:
- Skin cancer prevention
- Begin osteoporosis prevention
- Gynecological exams: introduction to reproductive health care
- HPV vaccination
- Manage menstrual disorders: dysmenorrhea; PMS

Family Teaching Guidelines:
- Performing vulvar self-exam
- Performing TSE

What To Say:
- Speak with respect when discussing weight issues with adolescent

Cultural Diversity:
- Influences
- Adolescent violence
- Breast cancer incidence in men and women
- Infant feeding practices
- ETOH use, disease and binge drinking
- Skin cancer risk

Young Adult Health
Safety:
- Substance use: ETOH, illicit drugs
- Safe sex

Health Promotion:
- Positive lifestyle choices
- Prevent UTIs
- Stress management
- Testicular cancer screening
- HPV Vaccination

Gynecological Disorders:
- Endometriosis
- Cervical and breast cancer
- Urinary tract infections

Nutrition:
- Promote health/prevent chronic disease

Middle Adult Health
Health Promotion:
- Screenings: BSE; mammogram; clinical breast exam; colorectal cancer screening; cholesterol/lipid screening
- Lifestyle choices: ETOH, weight, smoking

Issues with Menopause:
- Climacteric; peri-/postmenopause
  - cessation of ovulation/menstruation
  - distressing symptoms
- HT decisions

Gynecological Disorders:
- Lelomyomas
- Ovarian cysts/ovarian cancer
- Breast cancer

Older Adult Health
Health Promotion:
- Sexual functioning; physical/psychological changes affect intimacy
- Still at risk for STI/HIV
- Exercise: balance, flexibility, endurance
- Cognitive functioning: stress management/coping strategies; manage physical illnesses; attend to nutrition
- Functional ability: assess ADLs, disease impact, quality of life
- Immunizations: influenza, pneumococcal
- Climacteric; peri-/postmenopause
- Prostate cancer screening
- Osteoporosis prevention/screening and treatment

Gynecological Disorders:
- Pelvic floor dysfunction; cystocele, rectocele, enterocele, urinary stress incontinence
- Endometrial cancer

Mental/Emotional Health:
- Personality changes
- Change in ability to perform ADLs
- Requires collaborative treatment
- Death and dying issues
- Decrease in social connectedness

Nursing Insight:
- Bethesha classification system
- Diabulimia → weight loss in Type 1 DM
- Nurses can help women view menopause as a mid-life celebration

Complementary Care:
- Can use herbs for anxiety and depression: watch for S.E.
- Herbs/supplements used for menopause symptoms

Legal Alert:
- Provide accurate info on menopausal hormone therapies

Optimizing Outcomes:
- Breast self-awareness strategies to detect cancer early
- Adequate vitamin D
- Reduce sun and tanning exposure

Collaboration in Caring:
- Approach to senior care in community should be culturally sensitive

Now Can You:
- Discuss infant/child nutrition and safety issues
- List developmentally appropriate play for children
- Provide safety education for adolescents
- Discuss pelvic exam process and strategies for enhancing breast health

Across Care Settings:
- Many community resources available to keep seniors active
- Nursing → encourage, give info

one
two
three
four
five
six
seven

The Process
of Human
Reproduction

Reproductive Anatomy and Physiology

Since you are like no other being ever created since the beginning of time, you are incomparable.

—Brenda Ueland

LEARNING TARGETS *At the completion of this chapter, the student will be able to:*

- Describe gender differentiation and differences in male and female embryos including timing of anatomical sexual differences.
- Identify anatomy and explain physiological functions of the female and male reproductive systems.
- Analyze the actions and interactions of hormones from the hypothalamus, pituitary, gonads, and other hormones that affect the reproductive system.
- Describe the process of sexual maturation.
- Discuss various physiological events that accompany the menstrual cycle.
- Develop an understanding of physiological changes that occur during the menopause years.

PICO(T) Questions

The intent of evidence-based practice (EBP) is to provide nursing care that integrates the best available evidence. An initial step in EBP is to write a PICO(T) question that effectively guides the research. A PICO(T) question is an acronym that stands for population (P), intervention or issue (I), comparison of interest (C), outcome (O), and timeframe (T). Depending on the question, all or some of the question components are used in the research process. Use these PICO(T) questions to spark your thinking as you read the chapter.

1. Do (P) women with (I) early onset of menarche have an (O) earlier onset of menopause than (C) women with average age onset of menarche?

2. Do (P) postmenopausal women (I) who are treated with estrogen-only hormone therapy and receive individual education about risks of breast cancer (O) stay on the treatment for a shorter length of time (C) than those who do not receive education?

 Evidence-Based Practice

Chang, Y., Hayter, M., & Wu, S. (2009). A systematic review and meta-ethnography of the qualitative literature: Experiences of the menarche. *Journal of Clinical Nursing 19*, 447–460.

The purpose of this study was to perform a systematic review and complete a meta-ethnographical examination of the literature exploring women's reported experience with menarche. The researchers proposed to extract and synthesize key themes and concepts identified in previous qualitative studies to better organize the existing body of knowledge related to the menarche experience. The researchers posit that as a significant life event, menarche impacts a woman physically, socially, and emotionally. It is important for health-care providers to appreciate and understand the multiple domains that encompass the menarche to promote healthy adolescent development. Previous research has indicated that, as a marker of physical and sexual maturity, the

(continued)

Evidence-Based Practice (continued)

menarche can be an anxiety-producing period of difficult transition for young women, and for some, the menarcheal experience is a sociocultural event that involves secrecy, menstrual rules, and perceived regulations.

The study was designed as a systematic review and meta-ethnography. Meta-ethnography is a method used to synthesize qualitative research findings. Concepts, metaphors, and themes are extracted from existing studies and subjected to additional interpretive analysis to generate a second order of concepts. This type of analysis allows the researcher to synthesize and understand the findings of two or more qualitative studies with similar research questions or topics. A total of 14 studies met the inclusion criteria. Nine electronic databases were searched to identify qualitative studies of women's experiences with menarche. Only English language reports were considered. The original search produced 2,377 titles from which 14 were ultimately determined to meet full inclusion criteria. Two reviewers independently reviewed the articles for inclusion. Articles included consisted of sample sizes that ranged from nine to 155 participants, and the majority used convenience samples. Concepts explored in the studies included the following: the meaning of menarche, the menarche experience, women's relationships during menarche, and the menarche experience of girls whose mother was not present. For data collection, the studies used a combination of focus groups, written narratives, and face-to-face interviews. Five common themes were identified: "preparation," "significant others' response to menarche," "physical experience of menarche," "psychological experience of menarche," and "sociocultural perspective of menarche."

The investigators found that the majority of studies supported the notion that most girls do not have appropriate menstrual preparation, and this factor was associated with personal physical and emotional stress during the first menstruation. Girls reported to be better prepared were able to acknowledge and accept the physical changes that accompanied the menarche. Analysis of the studies also indicated that the primary source of preparation and information about menarche came from the girls' mothers and schoolteachers, although mothers were more likely to incorporate their own previously experienced understanding of the impact of culture and social norms versus the general facts and practical knowledge shared by schoolteachers. Data from previous studies also showed a correlation between positive experiences among females with a positive self-awareness and positive attitudes toward self-health. Interestingly, the studies underscored the importance of fathers, male classmates, and personal sociocultural background on the menarche experiences of young women. The authors concluded from the meta-ethnographic review that overall, young women do not receive appropriate menstrual preparation and highlighted the importance of expanded family support during the menarcheal experience.

1. How is this information useful to clinical nursing practice?

2. Based on these findings, what are implications for further research?

See Suggested Responses for Evidence-Based Practice on DavisPlus.

Introduction

This chapter provides an overview of the anatomy and physiology of the male and female reproductive systems. Growth and development over the life span are explored with a primary focus on females and special issues related to male development. The menstrual cycle and events that occur in the absence of fertilization as well as those that take place soon after conception are explored. A discussion of key hormones that impact the menstrual cycle enhances understanding of the symphony of cyclic events during the reproductive years.

Sexual Differentiation in the Embryo

In humans, the course of gender maturation is quite lengthy, extending from embryonic development to full maturation in later adolescence. Although the gender of an individual is determined at the moment of conception, it takes about 8 weeks of development before the reproductive system becomes differentiated as male or female. Before 8 weeks' gestation, the embryo displays no distinguishing sexual characteristics. At 5 weeks after conception, the first reproductive tissue arises from the **mesoderm**, the embryo's middle layer. The first structure formed is a **gonad** (sex gland), which is composed of an internal portion called a medulla

and an external portion known as the cortex. During the next few weeks, the gonad undergoes various developmental changes. Primitive reproductive ducts form during this undifferentiated period and include a pair of mesonephric ducts and a pair of paramesonephric ducts. The mesonephric ducts are dominant in males, and the paramesonephric ducts are dominant in females (Blackburn, 2012). Depending on the gender of the embryo, one ductal pair becomes dominant in genital development while the other genital pair regresses. Differing male/female developmental changes in the embryonic mesonephric/paramesonephric duct structure are the first gender changes that occur.

Male Gender

In a male embryo, the cortex of the gonad regresses, and the medulla develops into a testis at around the 7th to 8th week of gestation. The mesonephric ducts evolve into the efferent ductule, vas deferens, epididymis, seminal vesicle, and ejaculatory duct. Collectively, these structures become the male genital tract. This process is stimulated by the production of testosterone in the testes. The testes also secrete Müllerian regression factor, which suppresses the paramesonephric ducts. The testes do not produce **spermatozoa** (sperm) until puberty. Beginning in the

12th developmental week, androgens begin to stimulate the growth of the external genitalia (Blackburn, 2012).

Female Gender

In a female embryo, the medulla of the first primitive gonad regresses, while the cortex develops into an ovary at approximately 10 weeks. During fetal life, underdeveloped egg cells, **oogonia,** develop to become **oocytes** (primitive eggs). At the time of birth, there are 2 to 4 million oocytes present in the ovary. The process of oocyte development that results in maturation of human ova is called **oogenesis.** External female genitalia develop in the absence of androgens. At approximately 12 weeks, the clitoris is formed, and the labia majora and minora develop from the surrounding connective tissue. By 16 weeks, the paramesonephric ducts have evolved into the fallopian tubes, uterus, and vagina.

Female Reproductive System

EXTERNAL STRUCTURES (PUDENDUM MULIEBRE)

The external genital structures include the mons pubis, labia majora, labia minora, clitoris, vestibule of the vagina, urethral (urinary) meatus, Skene's glands, Bartholin's glands, vaginal introitus (opening), hymen, and the perineum (Fig. 5-1).

The **vulva** (pudendum femininum) is the portion of the female external genitalia that lies posterior to the mons pubis. It consists of the labia majora, labia minora, clitoris, vestibule of the vagina, vaginal opening, and Bartholin's glands (Venes, 2013).

Mons Pubis

The mons pubis, or mons veneris, is a layer of subcutaneous tissue anterior to the genitalia in front of the symphysis pubis. It is located in the lowest portion of the abdomen and typically is covered with pubic hair that grows in a transverse pattern. The texture and amount of pubic hair vary ethnically. In Asian women, the hair is fine and sparse. In women of African descent, the hair is thick and curly. The mons pubis is essentially a fatty pad that cushions and protects the pelvic bones, especially during intercourse.

Labia

The **labia majora** are the two folds of tissue that lie lateral to the genitalia and serve to protect the delicate tissues between them. The external labia are covered with pubic hair, while the medial surfaces, which are moist and pink, are without pubic hair. During pregnancy, the labia majora are highly vascular as a result of hormonal influences. The labia majora share an extensive lymphatic network with other vulvar structures, leading to an enhanced capacity to spread diseases such as malignant carcinomas. The labia majora become less prominent after each pregnancy.

The **labia minora** are two folds of tissue that lie within the labia majora and converge near the anus to form the **fourchette** (a tense fold of mucous membrane at the posterior opening of the vagina). Similar to but smaller than the labia majora, these structures are moist and absent of hair follicles and resemble mucous membrane. The labia minora contain a number of sebaceous glands that provide lubrication and protective bacteriocidal secretions. During puberty the labia minora enlarge. After menopause they become smaller because of declining hormonal levels. The mons, labia majora, and labia minora all function to protect the clitoris and vestibule.

Clitoris

The clitoris is located at the upper junction of the labia minora. The **prepuce,** or clitoral hood, is a small fold of skin that partially covers the glans (head) of the clitoris. Composed of erectile tissue, the clitoris is primarily the organ of sexual pleasure and orgasm in women. The clitoris contains a rich blood and nerve supply and is extremely sensitive. Sensory receptors located in the clitoris send information to the sexual response area in the brain. This message prompts the clitoris to secrete a cheese-like fatty substance with a distinctive odor called **smegma.** It is believed that smegma is a pheromone (chemical signal sent between individuals). Anatomically, the clitoral shape is similar to that of the urinary meatus, and the structural similarity of the two organs sometimes results in misguided and painful catheterization attempts.

Vestibule

The vestibule is essentially an oval-shaped space enclosed by the labia minora. It contains openings to the urethra and vagina, the Skene's glands, and the Bartholin's glands. This area of a woman's anatomy is extremely sensitive to chemical irritants. Nurses should be prepared to educate women about the potential discomforts associated with the use of dyes and perfumes found in soaps, detergents, and feminine hygiene products and encourage their discontinuation if symptoms develop.

Urethral (Urinary) Meatus

The urethral or urinary **meatus** (opening) is located in the midline of the vestibule, approximately 0.4 to 1 inch (1 to 2.5 cm) below the clitoris. The small opening is often shaped like an inverted "V." The vaginal orifice, or introitus, lies in the lower portion of the vestibule posterior to

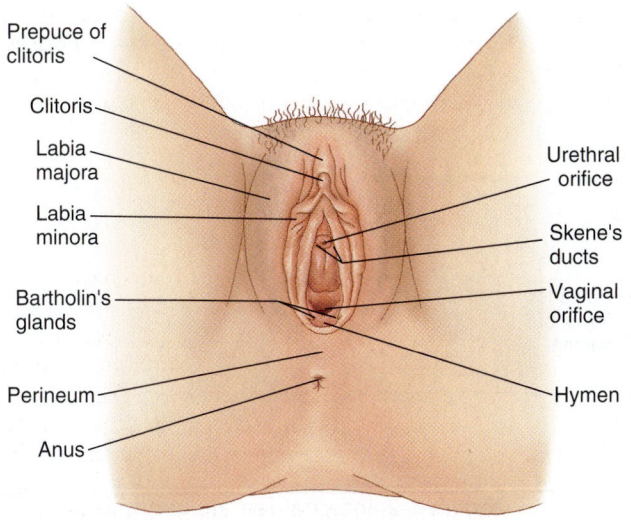

Figure 5-1 Female external genitalia.

Prepuce of clitoris

Clitoris

Labia majora

Labia minora

Bartholin's glands

Perineum

Anus

Urethral orifice

Skene's ducts

Vaginal orifice

Hymen

the urethral meatus. It is essentially a boundary between the internal and external genitals. The **hymen,** a connective tissue membrane, encircles the vaginal introitus.

Skene's Glands and Bartholin's Glands

The Skene's glands (paraurethral glands), located on each side of the urethra, produce mucus that helps to lubricate the vagina. The Skene's glands are not readily visible. To facilitate examination, the margins of the urethra are drawn apart and the mucous membrane gently everted to reveal the small glandular opening on each side of the floor of the urethra (Venes, 2013).

The Bartholin's glands, also known as the greater vestibular or vulvovaginal glands, are located deep within the posterior portion of the vestibule near the posterior vaginal introitus. These glands secrete a clear mucus that moistens and lubricates the vagina during sexual arousal.

Hymen

Surrounding the opening of the vagina is a small portion of tissue called the hymen. The hymen typically forms a border around the entrance of the vagina in premenstrual girls. Hymenal tissue does not completely cover or occlude the vagina. Ultimately the hymen becomes widened, sometimes by tearing, which may be accompanied by bleeding. Widening of the hymen may also occur following a vulvar injury, tampon insertion, or at the time of the first sexual intercourse. It is a societal myth that the hymen must be intact for a female to be considered a virgin.

Perineum

The perineum, an anatomical landmark, is the skin-covered region between the vagina and the anus. The perineal body consists of fibromuscular tissue located between the lower part of the vagina and the anus. During the labor process, as the fetus descends through the vagina, the perineum stretches and becomes very thin, sometimes tearing as the baby is born. An **episiotomy** (incision made to enlarge the perineal opening to allow delivery of a fetus) may be performed to widen the external passage (see Chapter 12 for further discussion).

 Now Can You—Discuss aspects of development of the reproductive system and identify components of the female reproductive tract?

1. Identify the developmental week when differentiation of the embryo's reproductive system occurs?
2. Name three structures that arise from the mesonephric ducts?
3. Describe the anatomical locations and functions of the labia, Skene's glands, and Bartholin's glands?

INTERNAL STRUCTURES

The internal female reproductive structures consist of the ovaries, fallopian tubes (oviducts, or uterine tubes), uterus, adjacent structures **(adnexa),** and vagina (Figs. 5-2 and 5-3). The ureters, bladder, and urethra are structures of the internal urinary system.

Ovaries

The ovaries are sometimes referred to as the essential female organ because they produce **ova** (female gametes or eggs) that are required for reproduction. They are a pair of oval structures, each measuring approximately 1.5 inches (4 cm) long, located on each side of the uterus below and behind the fallopian tubes. The ovarian ligament extends from the medial side of each ovary to the uterine wall; the broad ligament is a fold of the peritoneum that provides a covering for the ovaries. These two ligaments help to keep the ovaries in place.

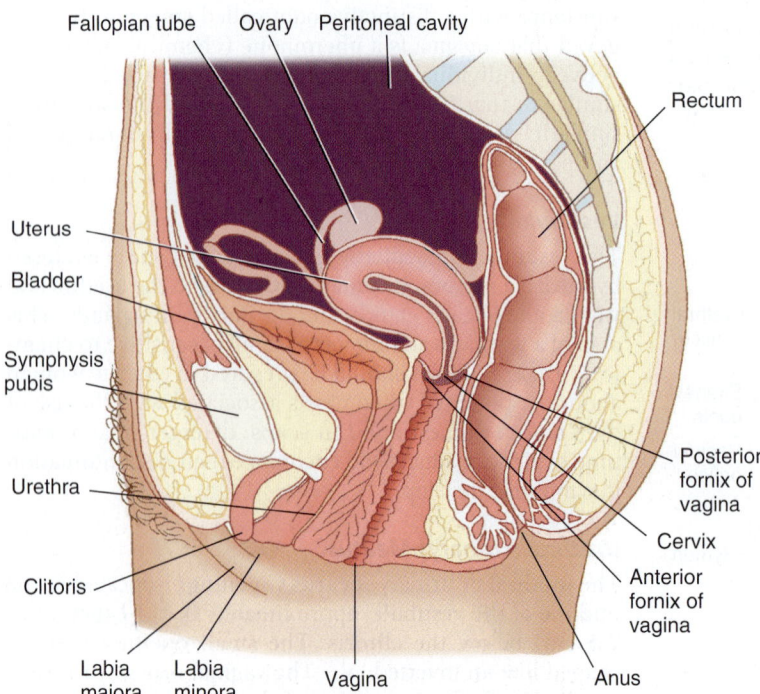

Figure 5-2 Internal female genitalia and cross section of the rectum.

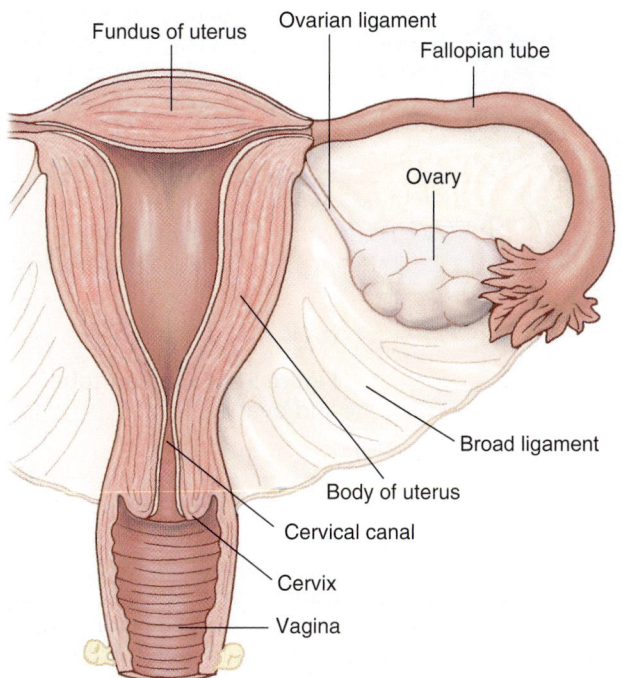

Figure 5-3 Internal structures of the adnexa.

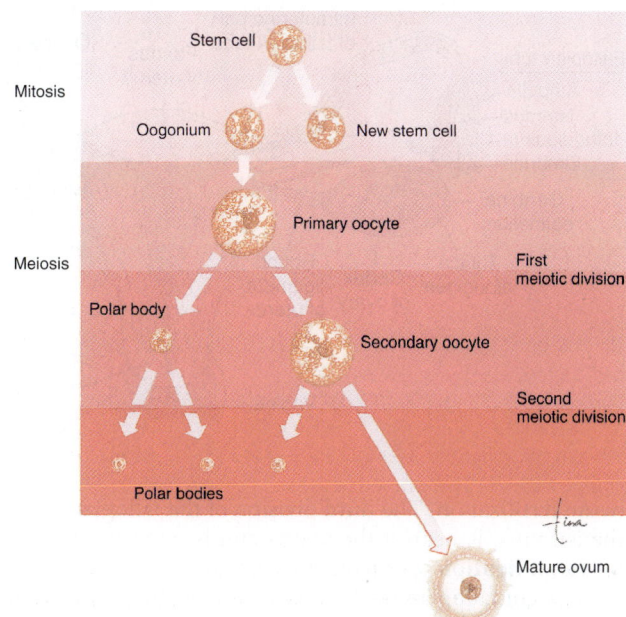

Figure 5-4 Oogenesis is the processes of mitosis and meiosis. For each primary oocyte that undergoes meiosis, only one functional ovum is formed.

The ovaries are responsible for the production of ova and the secretion of female sex hormones. Both of these functions become activated at the time of puberty. **Oogenesis** (the process of meiosis for egg cell formation) results in the formation of mature eggs within the ovary. Oogenesis is a process that occurs at regular (usually monthly) intervals. The ovaries also secrete the female sex hormones estrogen and progesterone. This important endocrine function helps to regulate the menstrual cycle.

A & P review **Oogenesis**

Oogenesis begins in the ovaries and is regulated by follicle-stimulating hormone (FSH), which initiates the growth of ovarian follicles. Each follicle contains an **oogonium**, or egg-generating cell (Fig. 5-4). FSH also stimulates the follicle cells to secrete estrogen, which promotes maturation of the ovum. For each primary oocyte that undergoes the process of meiosis, only one functional egg cell is produced. The remaining three cells, termed polar bodies, have no function and deteriorate. A mature ovarian follicle, also called a **graafian follicle**, contains the secondary oocyte, and if the egg is fertilized, the second meiotic division occurs and the ovum nucleus becomes the female pronucleus.

Microscopically, the ovarian surface is termed the germinal epithelium. Each ovary has hundreds of thousands of follicles that contain immature female sex cells. All of the follicles in a woman's ovaries develop in utero and are present at birth. During a postpubertal woman's monthly menstrual cycle, one follicle develops and releases a mature ovum. (Please refer to the menstrual cycle discussion later in this chapter for additional information.) Throughout a woman's reproductive years, only 300 to 400 follicles develop into mature ova and are released for potential fertilization by a sperm.

The ovaries are supported in their position in the pelvis by three important ligaments: the mesovarium, the ovarian ligament, and the infundibular pelvic ligament or suspensory ligament. The ovarian ligament positions the fimbriae (fingerlike projections) of the fallopian tube in contact with the lower pole of the ovary to enhance "pickup" of the ovum following ovulation. ◆

Fallopian Tubes

The (two) fallopian tubes are also called the **uterine tubes** or **oviducts.** Measuring approximately 4 inches (10 cm) in length, the lateral end of each fallopian tube encloses an ovary; the medial end opens into the uterus. Anatomically, the fallopian tubes are composed of four layers. Beginning with the external layer and progressing inward to the internal layer, these include the peritoneal (serous), which is covered by the peritoneum; the subserous (adventitial); the muscular; and the mucous layers. The blood and nerve supplies are housed in the subserous layer. The muscular layer has an inner circular and an outer longitudinal layer of smooth muscle. It provides peristalsis that assists in transporting the ovum toward the uterus for potential implantation. The mucosal layer contains **cilia** (hairlike projections) that also assist in directing the ovum toward the uterus (Venes, 2013).

The fallopian tubes are attached at the upper outer angles of the uterus and then extend upward and outward (Fig. 5-5). The diameter of each tube is approximately 6 mm. Anatomically, the tubes consist of three divisions: infundibulum, ampulla, and isthmus. The infundibulum is the funnel-shaped portion located at the distal end of the fallopian tube. The ovum enters the fallopian tube through a small opening (ostium) located at the bottom of the infundibulum. Several fingerlike processes (fimbriae) surround each ostium and extend toward the ovary. The longest fimbria, the fimbria ovarica, is attached to the ovary. The ampulla, which is the second division of the fallopian tube, is two-thirds the length of the tube and is most often the site of

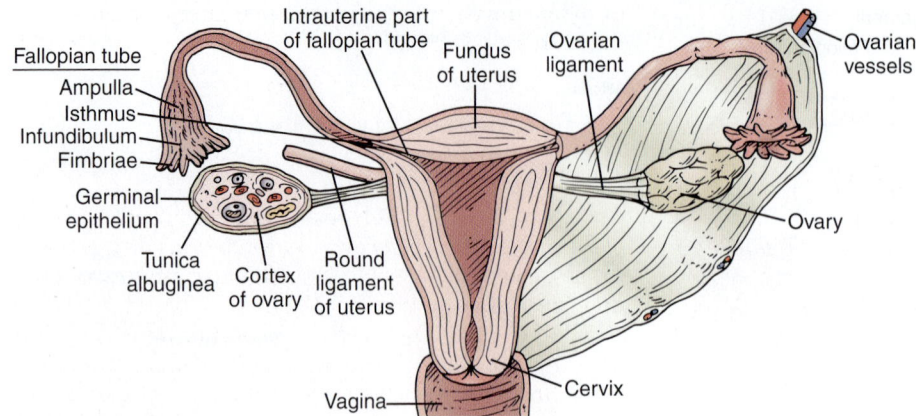

Figure 5-5 Fallopian tube and ovary.

ovum fertilization. The third division of the fallopian tube, the isthmus, is nearest the uterus and is typically the site for **tubal ligation** (permanent sterilization).

A patent fallopian tube is able to convey the ovum from the ovary to the uterus and the spermatozoa from the uterus toward the ovary. Fertilization usually occurs in the outer one-third of the fallopian tube, which provides a safe, nourishing environment for the ovum and sperm. If fertilization occurs, the fertilized ovum (termed a **zygote** until the first cell division) is slowly and gently swept into the uterus by fallopian peristalsis and cilia movement, where implantation takes place. If fertilization does not occur, the ovum dies within 24 to 48 hours and disintegrates, either in the tube or in the uterus.

Internally, each tube connects laterally with its corresponding ovary and medially with the uterus. Thus, there is a continuous route that passes from the vagina into the uterus and then on out to the tubes and ovaries. If the vagina is infected by a pathogen, the potential exists for retrograde transmission to the ovaries. Although most vaginal infections can be readily treated and cured, residual scarring from the inflammatory process can cause tubal narrowing leading to an increased risk for tubal pregnancies or infertility resulting from blockage.

Uterus

The uterus, centrally located in the pelvic cavity between the bladder (anteriorly) and rectum (posteriorly), is approximately 3 inches long by 2 inches wide (7.5 cm × 5 cm). It is a pear-shaped organ with the narrower end positioned closest to the vagina (Fig. 5-6). The uterine

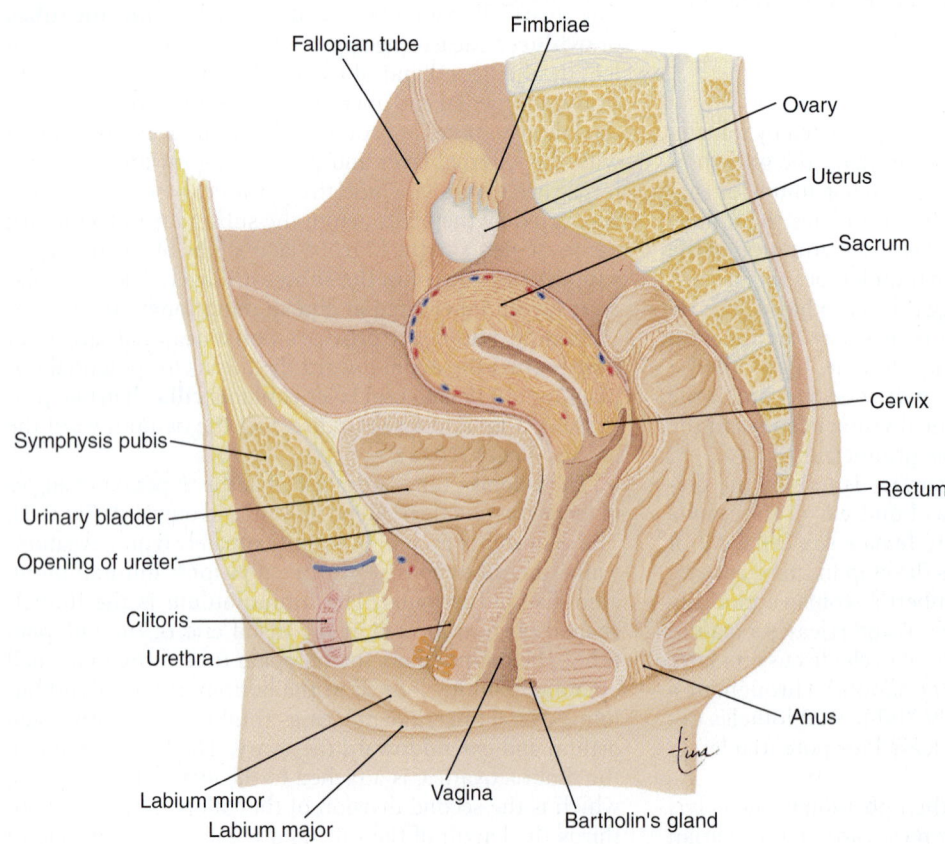

Figure 5-6 Uterus and surrounding structures of the female genitourinary system shown in a midsagittal section through the pelvic cavity.

interior is hollow and forms a path from the vagina to the fallopian tubes. Because the uterine walls are very thick and collapsed on each other, the interior cavity is, in actuality, a "potential space."

Two major functions of the uterus are to permit sperm to ascend toward the fallopian tubes and to provide a nourishing environment for the zygote until placental function begins. In addition, it provides a safe environment that protects and nurtures the growing embryo/fetus until the pregnancy has been completed. In the absence of conception, the uterus sheds the outermost layers of the inside of the endometrium (menstruation) to prepare for another menstrual cycle by regeneration of the endometrium.

The arteries of the uterus are the uterine, from the hypogastric arteries, and the ovarian, from the abdominal aorta. This rich blood supply helps to ensure ample oxygenation and nutrition to facilitate the growing uterus and fetus during pregnancy. The uterine veins drain into the internal iliac veins. The vasculature of the uterus is twisted and tortuous and as the **gravid** (pregnant) uterus expands, these vessels straighten out, allowing a continued rich blood supply throughout pregnancy.

The uterus receives its nerve supply via the afferent (sensory) and efferent (motor) autonomic nervous systems. These two systems are important in regulating both vasoconstriction and muscle contractions. The uterus also has an innate intrinsic motility as well. Thus, a patient with a spinal cord injury above level T6 may still have adequate uterine contractions to deliver a fetus vaginally.

Uterine pain nerve fibers reach the spinal cord at levels T11 and T12. Because of this location and the presence of other pain receptors there, pain from the ovaries, ureters, and uterus may all be similar and may be reported by a woman who identifies pain in the flank, inguinal, or vulvar areas. Several sensory nerve fibers that contribute to **dysmenorrhea** (painful menstruation) are housed in the uterosacral ligaments.

Uterine Anatomy

The uterus is divided into three sections: the corpus, the isthmus, and the cervix.

CORPUS. The corpus of the uterus is the upper two-thirds of the uterine body and contains the cornua portion, where the fallopian tubes enter, and the fundus or uppermost section superior to the cornua (Fig. 5-7).

The layers of the corpus of the uterus include the perimetrium, the myometrium, and the endometrium. The perimetrium is the outer, incomplete layer of the parietal peritoneum (the serous membrane that lines the abdominal wall). The **myometrium,** or middle layer, is composed of layers of smooth muscle that extend in three directions—longitudinal, transverse, and oblique—and are continuous with the supportive ligaments of the uterus (Fig. 5-8). The tridirectional formation of the muscular layers is important in facilitating effective uterine contractions during labor and birth. The endometrium is the third and innermost uterine layer. It is composed of three layers, and of these, two are shed with each menses.

ISTHMUS. The isthmus is a slight constriction on the surface of the uterus midway between the uterine body (the corpus, or upper two-thirds), and the **cervix,** or "neck." During pregnancy, the isthmus becomes incorporated into the lower uterine segment and acts as a passive or noncontractile part of the uterus during the labor process. The isthmus is the site for the uterine incision when a low-transverse cesarean section is performed.

CERVIX. The cervix is the lower, narrow end of the uterus. It is similar to a neck or tube and extends from the inside

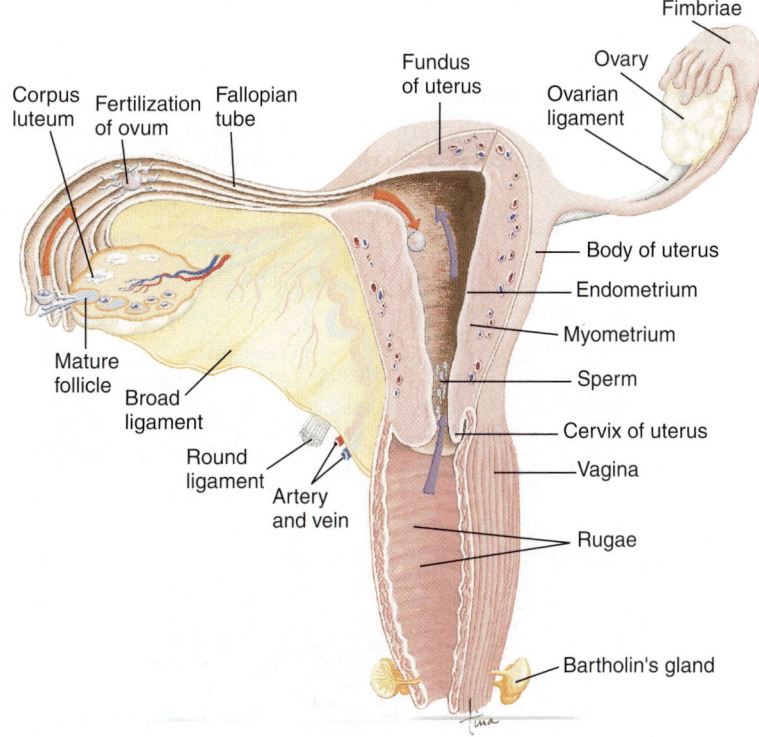

Figure 5-7 Female reproductive system shown in anterior view. The left ovary has been sectioned to show the developing follicles. The left fallopian tube has been sectioned to show fertilization. The uterus and vagina have been sectioned to show internal structures. Arrows indicate the movement of the ovum toward the uterus and the movement of sperm from the vagina toward the fallopian tube.

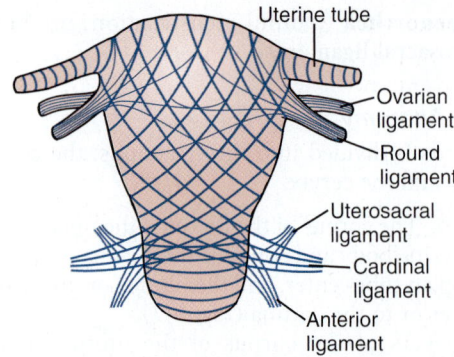

Figure 5-8 Arrangement of the directions of the smooth muscles of the myometrium. The uterine muscle fibers are continuous with the supportive ligaments of the uterus.

of the uterus, opening into the vagina. The cervix secretes mucus, which serves several functions: (1) lubricates the vaginal canal, (2) forms a barrier to sperm penetration into the uterus during nonfertile periods, (3) provides an easy-flowing pathway to facilitate sperm passage into the uterus during fertile periods, (4) provides an alkaline environment to facilitate the viability of sperm that have been deposited in the acidic vagina, (5) forms a solid plug called an **operculum** to protect a pregnancy from outside pathogens, and (6) functions as a bacteriostatic agent. The composition of cervical mucus changes during the menstrual cycle, and these changes are important in the fertility assessment.

The vaginal portion of the cervix is composed of squamous (epithelial) cells. This portion of the cervix is fleshy pink in color. The canal portion of the cervix that leads into the uterine epithelium is composed of columnar cells. This tissue is bright red in color. The juncture of these two cell types is called the **squamocolumnar junction.** After puberty, this junction is active with cellular growth activity and cell turnover, and it is the site where dysplasia (abnormal tissue development) may occur.

Uterine Support Structures

Uterine position in the body varies with age, pregnancy, and distention of related pelvic viscera. Typically, the uterus lies over the urinary bladder. The cervix points down and backward and enters the apex (the pointed extremity portion) of the vagina at a right angle. Several ligaments hold the uterus in place, but also allow for some movement.

The uterus is supported in the pelvis by several ligaments and muscles. These include the broad, round, cardinal, pubocervical, and uterosacral ligaments and the pelvic muscles (Fig. 5-9). The broad and round ligaments support the upper portion of the uterus, while the cardinal, pubocervical, and uterosacral ligaments provide support for the middle portion. The lower portion of the uterus is supported by the muscles of the pelvic floor.

The broad ligaments are supportive stretches of peritoneum that extend from the lateral pelvic sidewalls to the uterus. Within these structures are the fallopian tubes, arteries and veins, ligaments, ureters, and other tissues.

The round ligaments expand both in diameter and in length during pregnancy, and this normal physiological change may be associated with maternal discomfort termed "round ligament pain." As the uterus expands, the round ligaments become stretched tight, and sudden movements such as position changes, coughing, or stretching may result in sharp pains that can be quite concerning until the woman understands the physiology for the discomfort. The round ligaments also play an important role during labor by pulling the uterus forward and downward, thereby holding it steady to facilitate the movement of the fetal presenting part toward the cervix. The cardinal ligaments prevent uterine prolapse and are the major support structures for the uterus and cervix.

Vagina

The vagina is a tubular organ approximately 4 inches (10 cm) in length that internally extends between the uterus and perineal opening. It is located between the rectum, urethra, and bladder. The collapsible vagina is composed of smooth muscle lined with mucous membrane arranged in **rugae** (small ridges), which allow distention during childbirth. The vagina has five functions: (1) to provide lubrication to facilitate intercourse, (2) to stimulate the penis during intercourse, (3) to act as a receptacle for semen, (4) to transport tissue and blood during

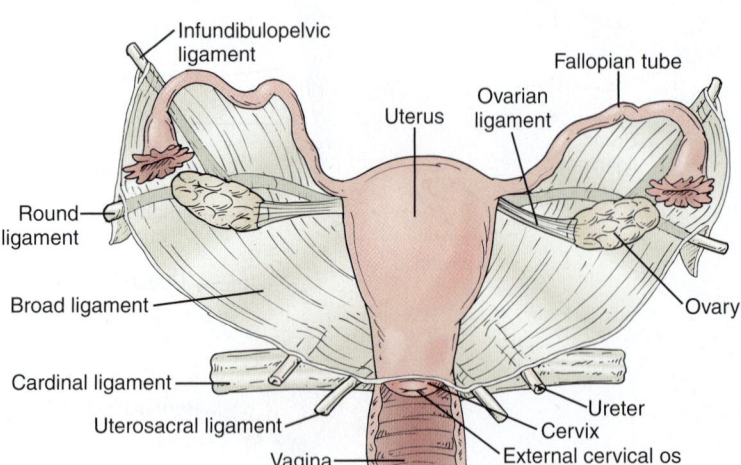

Figure 5-9 Uterine ligaments.

menses to the outside, and (5) to function as the lower portion of the birth canal during childbirth.

The apex of the vagina, also termed the vaginal vault or fornix, is the upper, recessed area around the cervix. Following intercourse, sperm pool in the fornix, where they have close contact with the cervix and its alkaline pH. The vaginal pH is typically acidic (4.5 to 5.5) during the reproductive years. The acid environment, though harmful to sperm, helps to protect the genital tract from pathogens.

Now Can You—Discuss various aspects of the female reproductive system?

1. Identify the location of the perineum and describe its importance during childbirth?
2. Describe three functions of the uterus?
3. Name the five functions of the cervix?

PELVIC ANATOMY

Bony Pelvis

The pelvis forms a bony ring that transmits body weight to the lower extremities. In women, the bony pelvis is structured to adapt to the demands of childbearing. The pelvis functions to support and protect the pelvic contents and to form a relatively fixed axis for the birth passage (Cunningham, Leveno, Bloom, Spong, Dashe, Hoffman, Casey, & Sheffield, 2014).

The bony pelvis is composed of four bones: the sacrum, the coccyx, and two innominate (hip) bones. The bilateral innominate bones are formed by the fusion of the ilium, ischium, and pubis bones (Fig. 5-10).

Pelvic Floor

The bony pelvis contains a pelvic floor of soft tissues that provides support and stability for surrounding structures. Most of the perineal support comes from the pelvic diaphragm (musculofascial layer forming the lower boundary of the abdominopelvic cavity) and the urogenital diaphragm (musculofascial sheath lying between the ischiopubic rami surrounding the female vagina). The pelvic diaphragm includes fascia and the levator ani and coccygeus muscles (Cunningham et al., 2014).

Above the pelvic diaphragm lies the pelvic cavity; below and behind is the perineum. The urogenital diaphragm includes fascia, deep transverse perineal muscles, and the urethral constrictor (Cunningham et al., 2014). The muscles of the pelvic floor include the levator ani (consists of the iliococcygeal, pubococcygeal [pubovaginal], and puborectal muscles) and the coccygeus. These structures create a "sling" that provides support for internal pelvic structures and the pelvic floor. The ischiocavernosus muscle extends from the clitoris to the ischial tuberosities on each side of the lower bony pelvis. Two transverse perineal muscles extend from fibrous tissue of the perineum to the ischial tuberosities to stabilize the perineum (Fig. 5-11).

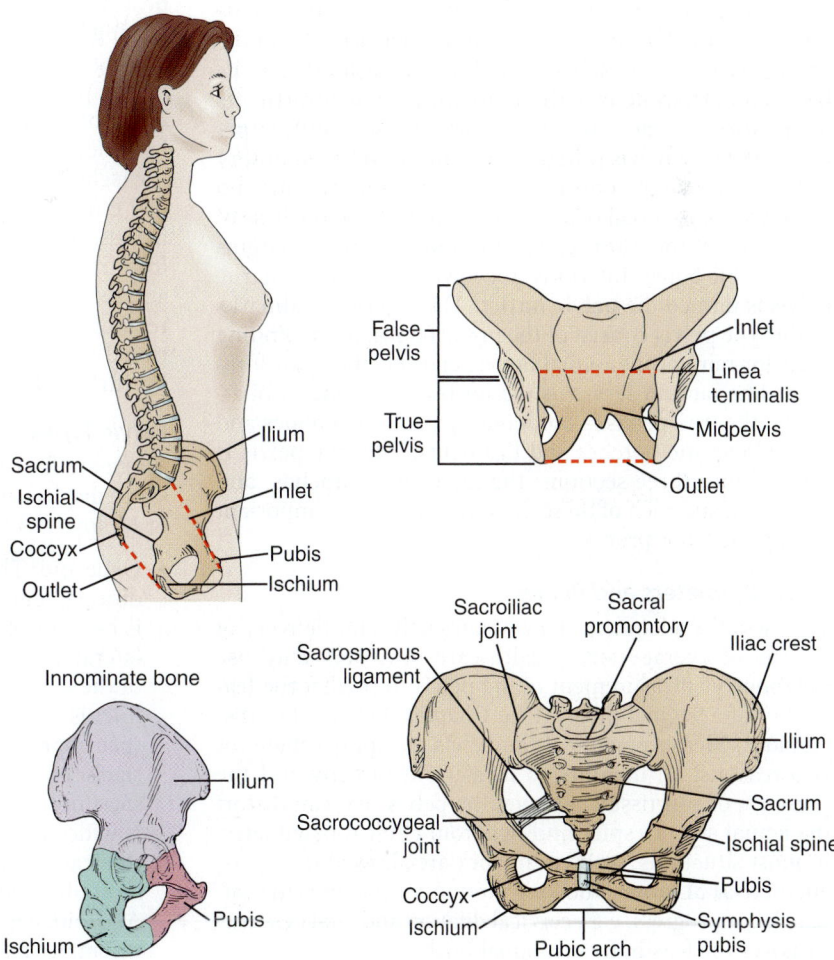

Figure 5-10 Female bony pelvis.

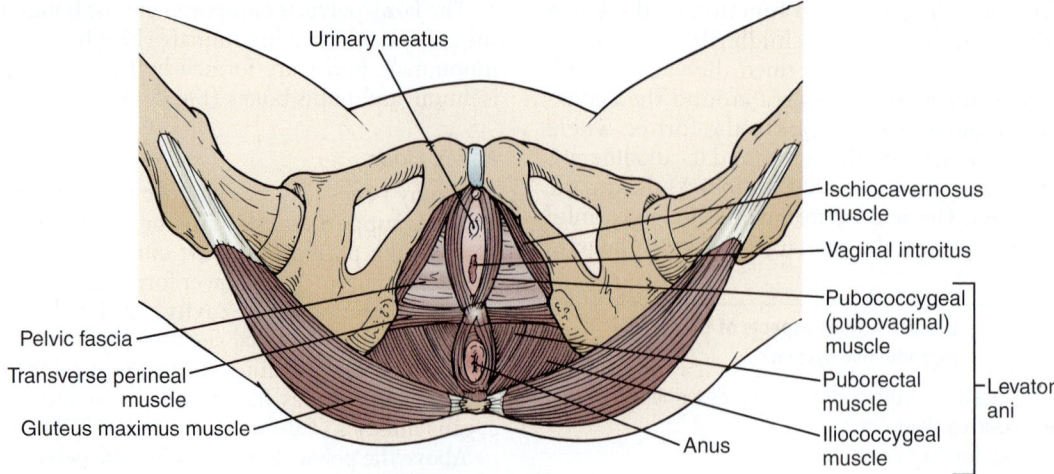

Urinary meatus

Ischiocavernosus muscle

Vaginal introitus

Pubococcygeal (pubovaginal) muscle

Puborectal muscle

Iliococcygeal muscle

Levator ani

Pelvic fascia

Transverse perineal muscle

Gluteus maximus muscle

Anus

Figure 5-11 The muscles of the female pelvic floor.

True/False Pelves

The pelvis consists of two sections known as the "false pelvis" and the "true pelvis." These sections are divided by the **linea terminalis,** or pelvic brim. The false pelvis is superior to the linea terminalis. Its anterior boundary is the abdominal wall, its posterior boundary is the lumbar vertebrae, and the lateral boundary is the iliac fossa. The false pelvis helps to support the gravid uterus and direct the fetal presenting part down toward the true pelvis.

The true pelvis, located below the linea terminalis, is important for childbearing. Its size and structure direct the fetus downward for delivery, and its dimensions must be large enough to deliver the fetus for a vaginal birth. Its boundaries are partly bony and partly ligamentous. Superiorly, the true pelvis is bounded by the sacral promontory (anterior projecting portion of the base of the sacrum) and the sacral alae (broad bilateral projections from the base of the sacrum), the linea terminalis, and the upper margins of the pubic bones. Inferiorly, the lowest portion of the true pelvis is termed the **pelvic outlet.** The anterior landmarks of the true pelvis consist of the pubic bones, the ascending superior rami of the ischial bones, and the obturator foramen. The sacrum serves as the posterior landmark. Bilaterally, the true pelvis is bordered by the ischial bones and the sacrosciatic notches and ligaments. The true pelvis is divided into three sections: the inlet, the midpelvis, and the outlet, and each of these three components is important during the labor process.

Pelvic Diameters and Planes

To assess the adequacy of a woman's pelvis for delivery of a fetus of average size, health-care providers may use **pelvimetry** (measurement of the pelvis to predict the feasibility of a vaginal birth). (See Chapter 9 for further discussion.) Measurements of the pelvis are approximate for two reasons: an inability to measure it directly and the presence of soft tissue covering the pelvis that can distort the actual size. Despite findings from clinical pelvimetry, in most situations, women in labor are allowed to experience a **trial of labor** (allowing uterine contractions to evaluate labor progress, e.g., cervical dilation and fetal descent) to assess the feasibility of vaginal birth.

Three portions of the true pelvis are measured during pelvimetry: the pelvic inlet, the midpelvis, and the pelvic outlet. The narrowest portion of the pelvic inlet is the line between the sacral promontory and the inner pelvic arch including the symphysis pubis. It is termed the **obstetrical conjugate** and should measure at least 4.5 inches (11.5 cm). Once the fetus passes this landmark, the presenting part is "engaged" in the pelvis. The midpelvis, which constitutes the area between the ischial spines, is the narrowest lateral portion of the female pelvis. This measurement needs to be at least 4.7 inches (12 cm) to allow for a vaginal birth. During labor, the ischial spines serve as a landmark for assessing the level of the fetal presenting part into the pelvis. At the pelvic outlet, two measurements are assessed: the angle of the ascending rami (pubic arch), which should be at least 90 to 100 degrees, and the distance between the ischial tuberosities, which should be at least 3.9 inches (10 cm). These are the minimal measurements deemed necessary to allow the fetus to descend through the pelvis for birth. During pregnancy the joints of the pelvis soften and become more mobile from the effects of the hormone relaxin. This important physiological change creates additional space to accommodate childbirth (see Chapter 12 for further discussion).

Pelvic Types

There are four basic bony pelvic types that have a distinct shape that has important implications for childbirth (Caldwell & Moloy, 1933) (Fig. 5-12):

- Gynecoid: The gynecoid pelvic type is the typical, traditional female pelvis (present in 50% of women) that is best suited for childbirth. The anterior/posterior and lateral measurements in the inlet, midpelvis, and outlet of the true pelvis are largest in the gynecoid pelvis. The inlet is round to oval-shaped laterally, a characteristic that improves its adequacy for childbirth. In addition, the ischial spines are less prominent; the shortened sacrum has a deep, wide curve; and the subpubic arch is wide and round. All of these characteristics enhance the feasibility for a vaginal birth. The other pelvic structures can pose problems for vaginal birth.

- Android: The android pelvis (found in 23% of women) resembles a typical male pelvis. The inlet is triangular

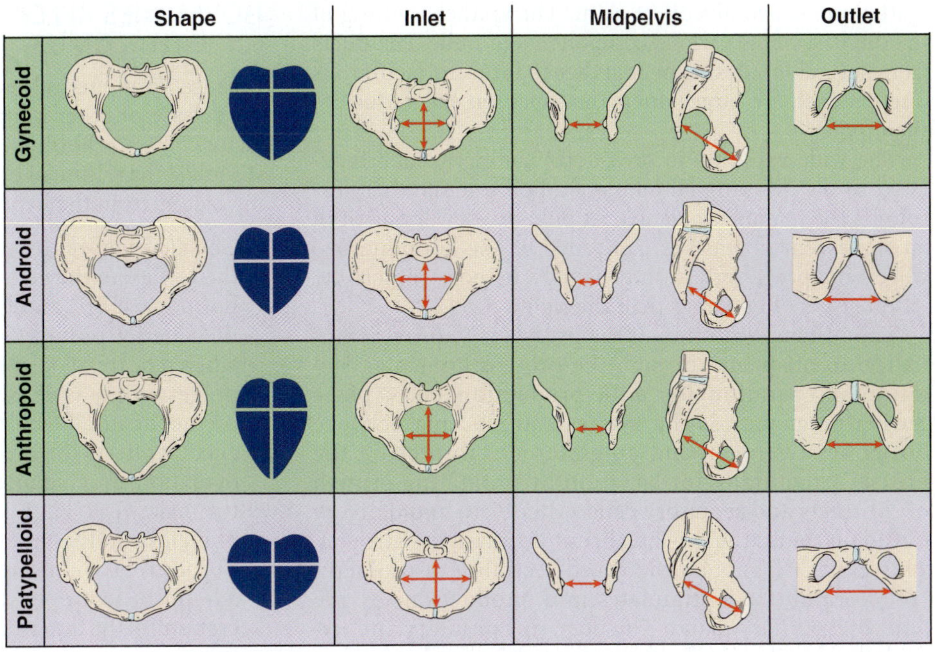

	Shape		Inlet	Midpelvis		Outlet
Gynecoid						
Android						
Anthropoid						
Platypelloid						

Figure 5-12 Comparison of the four Caldwell–Moloy pelvic types. The average woman has a gynecoid pelvis; others may have a variation or a mixture of types. Few women have pure android, anthropoid, or platypelloid types.

or heart-shaped and laterally narrow. The subpubic arch is narrow; there are more bony prominences, including the ischial spines, which are also prominent and narrow. These characteristics can cause difficulty during fetal descent.

- Anthropoid: The anthropoid pelvis (occurs in 24% of women) resembles the pelvis of the anthropoid ape. Similar to the gynecoid pelvis, the anthropoid pelvis is oval-shaped at the inlet but in the anterior–posterior, rather than lateral, plane. The subpubic arch may be slightly narrowed. Fetal descent through an anthropoid pelvis is more likely to be in a posterior (facing the woman's front) rather than anterior (facing the woman's back) presentation (see Chapter 12 for further discussion).
- Platypelloid: The platypelloid pelvis (found in 3% of women) is broad and flat and bears no resemblance to a lower mammal form. The pelvic inlet is wide laterally with a flattened anterior–posterior plane, and the sacrum and ischial spines are prominent. The subpubic arch is generally wide. Fetal descent through a platypelloid pelvis is usually in a transverse presentation and will not allow for a vaginal birth (see Chapter 12 for further discussion).

Now Can You—Discuss aspects of the female bony pelvis?

1. Differentiate between the true and false pelves?
2. Name the three components of the true pelvis that are measured during pelvimetry?
3. Identify characteristics of the gynecoid pelvis and explain why this type is best suited for vaginal birth?

Ureters, Bladder, and Urethra

The ureters, bladder, and urethra and its external opening or meatus are part of the urinary system and are not reproductive organs. The urethra is a mucous membrane–lined tube that passes from the bladder to outside the body to allow micturition. Its position is posterior to the symphysis pubis and anterior to the vagina. The urethra is approximately 1.2 inches (3 cm) in length.

Breasts

The female breasts or mammary glands are considered to be accessory organs of the reproductive system (Fig. 5-13). The two breasts lie over the pectoral and anterior serratus muscles. Breast tissue consists primarily of glandular, fibrous, and adipose tissue suspended within the conical-shaped breasts by Cooper's ligaments that extend from the deep fascia.

The glandular tissue contains 15 to 24 lobes that are separated by fibrous and adipose tissue. Each lobe contains several lobules composed of numerous alveoli clustered around tiny ducts that are layered with secretory cuboidal

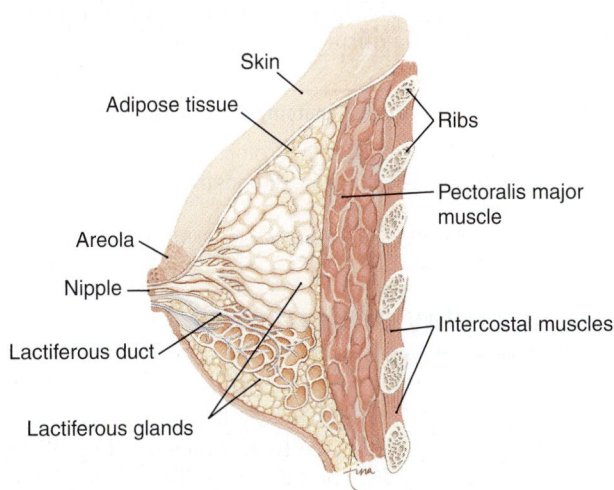

Figure 5-13 Mammary gland shown in a midsagittal section.

epithelium called alveoli or acini. The epithelial lining of the ducts secretes various components of milk. The ducts from several lobules come together to form the lactiferous ducts, which are larger ducts that open on the surface of the nipple.

The wide variation in breast size among women is related to the differing amounts of adipose tissue that surrounds the mammary glands. At puberty, development of an adolescent's breasts is controlled by the hormones estrogen and progesterone. Interestingly, in most women, the left breast is often larger than the right.

The primary function of the breasts is to provide nutrition to offspring through the process known as lactation. Preparation for milk production takes place during pregnancy as the ovaries and placenta produce hormones (estrogen and progesterone) to prepare the breasts structurally for lactation by promoting growth of the ducts and secretory cells. After birth and delivery of the placenta, there is an abrupt decrease in estrogen. This event triggers an increased secretion of prolactin (the hormone that stimulates milk production) by the anterior pituitary gland. The posterior pituitary and hypothalamus play a role in the production and secretion of oxytocin, a hormone that causes release of milk from the alveoli.

PARTS OF THE BREAST

Nipples

Centrally located on the breast, the nipples contain several pores that secrete colostrum (breast fluid that precedes breast milk) and breast milk during lactation. The nipples consist primarily of erectile tissue to assist with infant latch-on during suckling (see Chapter 15 for further discussion).

Areola

The areola is a more deeply pigmented area that surrounds the nipple. Its diameter ranges from 1 to 3.9 inches (2.5 to 10 cm).

Montgomery Tubercles

The Montgomery tubercles are papillae located on the surface of the nipple and the areola. The Montgomery tubercles secrete a fatty substance that lubricates and protects the nipple and areola during breastfeeding.

Now Can You—Discuss anatomy of the female breast?

1. Name three types of tissue that compose the breast?
2. Identify the pituitary hormone responsible for initiation of lactation?
3. Explain the function of the Montgomery tubercles?

The Interplay of Hormones and Reproduction

Knowledge of the functions of key hormones associated with reproduction is essential to an understanding of the female menstrual cycle. The following discussion centers on hormones that play a major role in the process of human reproduction.

HORMONES RELEASED BY THE HYPOTHALAMUS

Because hormones released by the hypothalamus stimulate the release of other hormones, they are termed "releasing factors." Factor hormones act on the anterior pituitary and stimulate the release of hormones from the pituitary. Releasing factors from the hypothalamus include the following:

- *Gonadotropin-releasing hormone* (GnRH): Stimulates the release of the gonadotropins follicle-stimulating hormone (FSH) and luteinizing hormone (LH) from the anterior pituitary. These hormones are released when a decrease in ovarian hormones (estrogen and progesterone) is detected by the hypothalamus. In the premenopausal female, GnRH exerts an ovarian influence: It affects the cyclic process of follicular growth, ovulation, and maintenance of the corpus luteum. In the male, GnRH affects **spermatogenesis**, the process of meiosis in the testes to produce sperm cells.
- *Corticotropin-releasing hormone* (CRH): Regulates adrenocorticotropic-stimulating hormone (ACTH) secretion by the anterior pituitary to activate the sympathetic nervous system. CRH is also released by the pregnant woman and her embryo soon after implantation. CRH appears to provide a protective action by minimizing a maternal immunological rejection that could result in a miscarriage. Other effects of CRH relate to the woman's response to stress.
- *Growth hormone-releasing hormone* (GH-RH): Stimulates the production and release of growth hormone (GH) by the anterior pituitary.
- *Growth hormone-inhibiting hormone* (GH-IH), also known as somatostatin: Inhibits the release of GH.
- *Thyrotropin-releasing hormone* (TRH): Regulates thyroid hormones (T_3 and T_4) by stimulating the anterior pituitary to release thyroid-stimulating hormone (TSH). TRH also stimulates the release of prolactin.
- *Prolactin-inhibiting factor* (PIF), also known as prolactostatin: Inhibits the synthesis and release of prolactin by the pituitary gland. Dopamine, another hormone released by the hypothalamus, also inhibits prolactin.

HORMONES RELEASED BY THE PITUITARY GLAND

The anterior pituitary produces the following hormones:

- *Thyroid-stimulating hormone* (TSH), also known as thyrotropin: Regulates the endocrine function of the thyroid gland.
- *Adrenocorticotropic hormone* (ACTH), also known as corticotropin: Controls the development and functioning of the adrenal cortex, including its secretion of glucocorticoids and androgens (Venes, 2013).
- *Prolactin* (PRL): Stimulates the maturation of the mammary glands during pregnancy; initiates milk production and provides some inhibition to the stimulation of FSH and LH.
- *Growth hormone* (GH), also known as somatotropin: Stimulates growth and cell reproduction (e.g., height growth during childhood) in humans. Growth hormone is also responsible for increased muscle mass, calcium retention and bone mineralization, the growth of various organ systems, protein synthesis, stimulation

of the immune system, reduced uptake of glucose in the liver, and the promotion of lipolysis.

- **Gonadotropins** (gonad-stimulating hormones): FSH and LH stimulate and inhibit the ovaries. These two hormones help to regulate the menstrual cycle by producing a positive and negative feedback of estrogen and progesterone by the ovaries. The feedback systems stimulate the hypothalamic secretion of releasing hormones that act on the anterior pituitary gland.

The posterior pituitary releases oxytocin. Oxytocin stimulates uterine contractions and the release of milk from milk ducts in the breasts during lactation. A synthetic form of oxytocin can be administered during labor to enhance uterine contractions and after birth to promote expulsion of the placenta and minimize uterine bleeding.

Collectively, the pituitary hormones are essential in the regulation of gonadal, thyroid, and adrenal function; lactation; body growth; and somatic development.

> **A & P review** **Hormonally Mediated Events and the Menstrual Cycle**

The menstrual cycle is hormonally mediated through events that take place in the hypothalamus, anterior pituitary gland, and the ovaries. The hypothalamus stimulates the anterior pituitary gland to produce gonadotropin. FSH, one of these hormones, stimulates the growth and development of the graafian follicle, which secretes estrogen. Estrogen stimulates proliferation of the endometrial lining of the uterus. After ovulation, the anterior pituitary gland secretes LH, which stimulates development of the corpus luteum. Progesterone secreted by the corpus luteum prompts further development of the lining of the uterus in preparation for the fertilized ovum. When pregnancy does not occur, the corpus luteum degenerates, and the levels of estrogen and progesterone decline. The decreased levels of estrogen and progesterone cause the uterus to shed its lining during menstruation. The decrease in estrogen and progesterone triggers a positive feedback to the hypothalamus, which stimulates the anterior pituitary gland to secrete FSH once again. A schema depicting the hormonal feedback mechanisms that regulate the menstrual cycle is presented in Figure 5-14. The interrelationships between the levels of hormone secretion, development of ovarian follicles, and changes in the uterine endometrium are presented in Figure 5-15. ◆

HORMONES RELEASED BY THE GONADS

The gonadal hormones are estrogen, progesterone, and testosterone. Estrogen and progesterone are primarily female hormones; testosterone is primarily a male hormone. These hormones are produced chiefly by the gonads (ovaries and testes) and have important influences on sexual characteristics and the menstrual cycle. Fluctuating levels of estrogen and progesterone stimulate or suppress the hypothalamus or pituitary gland to release or cease releasing their hormones in a complex orchestration of events that regulate the menstrual cycle.

Estrogen

Estrogen, the primary female sex hormone, is present in high levels in women of childbearing age and is also present in much smaller levels in men. In females, estrogen is responsible

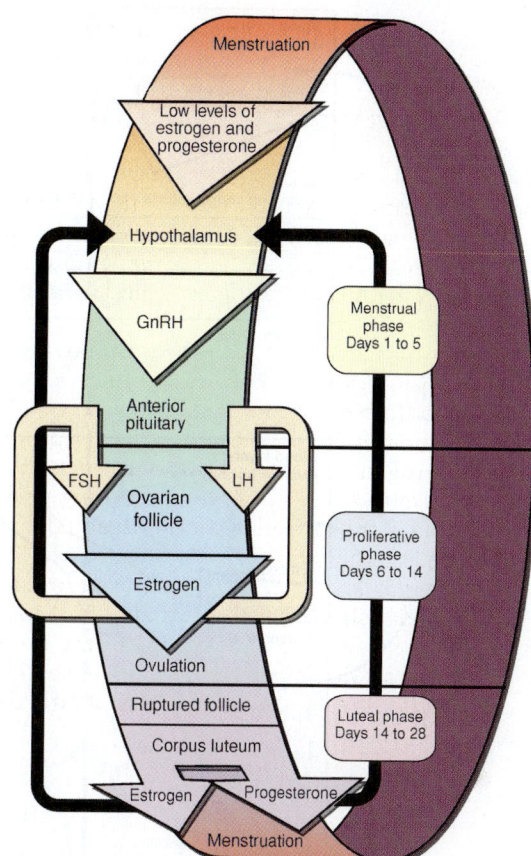

Figure 5-14 Hormonal feedback mechanisms that regulate the female menstrual cycle.

for development of the secondary sex characteristics (e.g., breast development, widening of the hips, and deposition of fat in the buttocks and mons pubis). It also helps to regulate the menstrual cycle by stimulating proliferation of the endometrial lining in preparation for a pregnancy.

Progesterone

Progesterone also plays a role in regulation of the menstrual cycle. It decreases uterine motility and contractility (caused by estrogen) and prepares the uterus for implantation after fertilization. During pregnancy, progesterone readies the breasts for lactation.

Testosterone

Testosterone, the primary male hormone, is produced by the testes (in men) and the ovaries (in women). Testosterone is responsible for the development of the male genital tract and the secondary sex characteristics (body hair distribution, growth and strength of the long bones, increase in muscle mass, and deepening of the voice through enlargement of the vocal cords). In both genders, testosterone enhances the libido, increases energy, boosts immune function, and helps protect against osteoporosis.

HUMAN CHORIONIC GONADOTROPIN, PROSTAGLANDINS, AND RELAXIN

Human chorionic gonadotropin (hCG) is an important hormone during early pregnancy. It is produced by the **trophoblast** (outermost layer of the developing blastocyst)

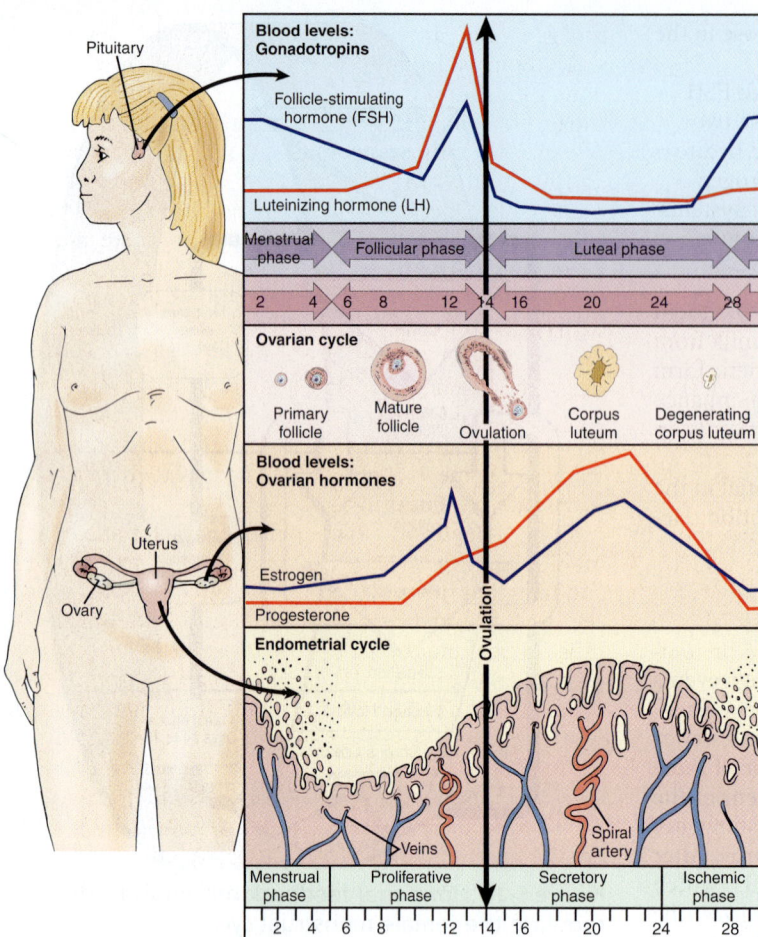

Figure 5-15 The female reproductive cycle. Levels of the hormones secreted from the anterior pituitary are shown relative to one another and throughout the cycle. Changes in the ovarian follicle are depicted. The relative thickness of the endometrium is also shown.

and maintains the ovarian **corpus luteum** (remainder of ovarian follicle after ovulation) by keeping levels of progesterone and estrogen elevated until the placenta has sufficiently developed to assume that function. Human chorionic gonadotropin may also play a role in limiting the maternal immune response to the pregnancy. Serum or urine hCG levels are measured to diagnose pregnancy.

Prostaglandins are unsaturated, oxygenated fatty acids classified as hormones. Prostaglandins are found in many body tissues, occurring in high concentrations in the female reproductive tract. Prostaglandins modulate hormonal activity and have an effect on ovulation, fertility, and cervical mucus viscosity. Premenstrually, the release of prostaglandins in the uterus causes vasoconstriction and muscle contractions that lead to the tissue ischemia and pain associated with **dysmenorrhea** (painful menses). During pregnancy, prostaglandins are believed to help maintain a reduced placental vascular resistance and most likely are involved in the biochemical process that initiates labor.

Relaxin is a hormone primarily produced by the corpus luteum during pregnancy, although the uterine decidua and the placenta are also believed to produce small amounts. Relaxin may be detected in maternal serum by the time of the first missed menstrual period. Although its role in pregnancy is not fully understood, relaxin aids in the softening and lengthening of the uterine cervix and works on the myometrial smooth muscle to promote uterine relaxation.

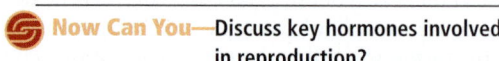 **Now Can You**—Discuss key hormones involved in reproduction?

1. Name two gonadotropins and describe their functions?
2. Explain the primary action of human chorionic gonadotropin (hCG)?
3. Identify one action of prostaglandins during pregnancy?

Sexual Maturation

PUBERTY

Puberty is the biological time frame between childhood and adulthood characterized by physical body changes that lead to sexual maturity. During this period, adolescents experience a growth spurt, develop secondary sexual characteristics, and achieve reproductive maturity. The timing of puberty onset and its progress are variable between individuals and are influenced primarily by genetics. However, other factors such as geographical location, exposure to light, nutritional status, and general health all influence the timing of puberty. It is known that the initiation of puberty is triggered by events that lead to the production of gonadotropin-releasing hormone (GnRH) in the hypothalamus. GnRH stimulates the manufacture of follicle-stimulating hormone (FSH) and luteinizing hormone (LH) in the anterior pituitary. The increasing levels of

FSH and LH initiate a gonadal response, and this response varies between males and females.

In females, sexual maturation begins with **thelarche,** the appearance of breast buds. Thelarche, which occurs at approximately 9 to 11 years, is the first signal that ovarian function has begun. It is followed by the growth of pubic hair. During thelarche, the "growth spurt," or period of peak height velocity, occurs. **Menarche,** the first menstrual period, begins approximately 1 year after the peak height velocity. It usually occurs between the ages of 9 and 15 years; the average age is 12.4 years (Chumlea et al., 2003).

Major hormonal events surrounding menarche involve the secretion of FSH from the pituitary gland. FSH stimulates the ovaries to begin follicular maturation and to produce estrogen. After maturation of an ovum, LH stimulates release of the ovum from the ovary (**ovulation**). Left behind is the **corpus luteum** ("yellow body" that remains in the ovary following ovulation), a structure that produces progesterone.

In males, LH stimulates the Leydig cells in the testicles to mature the testes and begin testosterone production. FSH and LH stimulate sperm production. Increasing levels of estrogen, progesterone, testosterone, and other circulating androgens stimulate the hypothalamus to continue to release GnRH, which perpetuates the cycle. As puberty progresses, the gonads become increasingly sensitive to hormone stimulation and begin to function. Testosterone secretion causes testicular enlargement, which is the first sign of pubertal changes in males.

Development of the secondary sexual characteristics begins around age 11 to 13, and puberty is completed when a young person reaches sexual maturity at approximately 18 to 20 years of age. The time frame from the first stages of puberty to full sexual maturation ranges from 1.5 to 9 years. In females, puberty is generally initiated about 2 years earlier in the life span than in males. Throughout the process of puberty, both genders experience a myriad of physical, psychological, and emotional changes. Alterations in body image and social interactions typically accompany these changes.

FEMALE SECONDARY SEXUAL CHARACTERISTICS

At birth, oocytes are present in the ovary as primary follicles in a state of suspended meiosis. With the onset of puberty, hormonal stimulation prompts the ovaries to secrete small amounts of estrogen. As the process of puberty progresses, estrogen levels rise, and menarche occurs. However, estrogen levels at this time are usually insufficient to stimulate ovulation, and the menstrual periods are generally unpredictable and irregular. As the gonadotropin cycles continue, the ovaries mature from sustained hormonal stimulation and eventually become capable of follicular maturation with increasing numbers of cycles. Over time, regular cyclic ovulation is established, and each menstrual period becomes increasingly more predictable. Once a female reaches a weight of 105 pounds (47.8 kg) and 16% to 23.5% body fat, there is a high correlation with menarche (Garibaldi, 2011).

In addition to the cyclic hormonal changes associated with ovulation, sexual physical changes (secondary sexual characteristics) also occur during puberty. Hormones of the hypothalamic–pituitary–ovarian axis trigger most of the changes that take place in the young woman's body during this time. (Please see the menstrual cycle discussion.) Examples of some of the pubertal changes that occur in the female are presented in Table 5-1.

Other female secondary sexual characteristic changes include growth and development of the vagina, uterus, and fallopian tubes, darkening and growth of the skin on the areola, and external genitals and widening of the hips. Appearance of the secondary sexual characteristics precedes menarche. Estrogen is primarily responsible for changes in the breasts, although progesterone, thyroxine, cortisol, insulin, and prolactin also affect glandular development. Guidelines of secondary sexual characteristic development, termed "Tanner stages" measure the predictable stages of pubertal body changes in both genders (Tanner, 1962). A sexual maturity rating concerning development of pubic hair in the female is presented in Figure 5-16.

🌀 **Now Can You**—Discuss concepts related to puberty?

1. Trace the hormonal events associated with the onset of puberty in females?
2. Explain why the first few menstrual periods are often irregular?
3. Identify six female secondary sex characteristics that precede menarche?

The Menstrual Cycle and Reproduction

Menstruation is the periodic discharge of bloody fluid from the vagina that women experience during reproductive years. Menstrual flow begins at puberty and continues for approximately three to four decades. The **menstrual cycle**

Table 5-1 Female Body Changes Associated With Puberty

Type of Body Change	Body Change	Definition	Average Age Initiated	Average Age Completed
Growth spurt	Adolescent growth spurt	Height increase 2.4–4.3 inches (6–11 cm) in 1 year	10	11.8
Secondary	Thelarche	Breast budding	9.8	14.6
	Adrenarche	↑ Adrenal androgen secretion → axillary and pubic hair	10.5	
Primary	Menarche	First menstrual period	12.8	

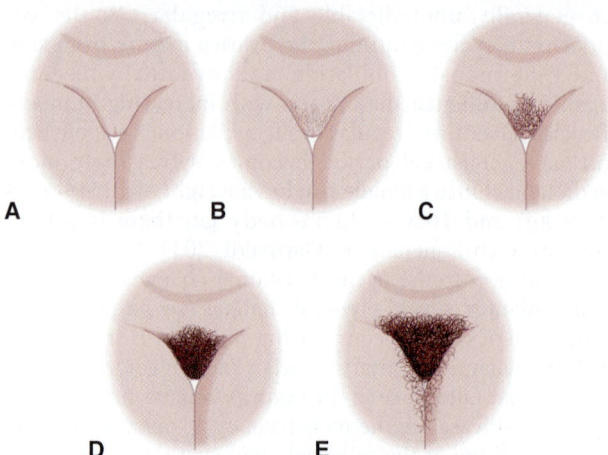

Figure 5-16 Maturation states in females. *A*, Preadolescent. No pubic hair, just fine body hair similar to hair on abdomen. *B*, Sparse growth of long, downy hair, straight or slightly curled mainly along labia. *C*, Darker, coarser, curlier hair that spreads over pubic symphysis. *D*, Hair is coarse and curly and covers more area. *E*, Adult. Hair may spread over medial surfaces of thighs but not over abdomen.

refers to the changes that occur in the uterus, cervix, and vagina associated with menstruation and during the interval between each menstruation, termed the "intermenstrual period." The average time for a menstrual cycle is 28 to 32 days, although there is considerable variation among women and monthly cycles. Factors such as stress, nutritional status, excessive exercise, fatigue, and illness can alter an individual's cycle intervals and length.

Menstruation and ovulation, key elements in the reproductive cycle, are controlled by positive and negative feedback systems associated with hormones released by the hypothalamus, pituitary, and ovaries. In synchrony, the hormones coordinate the complex biochemical events that result in the monthly menstrual cycle. Regulation of the menstrual cycle involves an overlapping of the uterine (endometrial), hypothalamic-pituitary, and ovarian cycles (see Figs. 5-14 and 5-15).

UTERINE (ENDOMETRIAL) CYCLE

The uterine, or endometrial, cycle has four phases: menstrual, proliferative, secretory, and ischemic.

Menstrual Phase

The menstrual phase is the time of vaginal bleeding (approximately days 1 to 6). The onset of menses signals the beginning of the follicular phase of the ovarian cycle. Menstruation is triggered by declining levels of estrogen and progesterone produced by the corpus luteum. The decrease in hormones results in poor endometrial support and constriction of the endometrial blood vessels. These changes lead to a decreased supply of oxygen and nutrients to the endometrium. Disintegration and sloughing of the endometrial tissue occurs. During menstruation, constriction of the endometrial blood vessels limits the likelihood of hemorrhage.

Prostaglandins also play a role in menstruation. The uterus releases prostaglandins that cause contractions of the smooth muscle and decrease the risk of hemorrhage. Prostaglandin-induced uterine contractions often produce dysmenorrhea (painful menstruation) in the days surrounding the onset of menstrual flow. Other systemic effects of prostaglandins include headache and nausea. Over-the-counter medications that inhibit prostaglandin synthesis such as nonsteroidal anti-inflammatory agents can be used to control the discomfort associated with dysmenorrhea and premenstrual syndrome.

Menstrual fluid is composed of endometrial tissue, blood, cervical and vaginal secretions, bacteria, mucus, leukocytes, prostaglandins, and other debris. The color of menstrual fluid is dark red but variable throughout the days of menses. The amount of discharge is typically 30 to 40 mL, and the duration of bleeding is 4 to 6 days ± 2 days.

Proliferative Phase

The proliferative phase is the end of menses through ovulation (approximately days 7 to 14). At the beginning of the proliferative phase, the endometrial lining is 1 to 2 mm thick. Circulating estrogen levels are low. Gradually increasing levels of estrogen, enlarging endometrial glands, and the growth of uterine smooth muscle characterize the proliferative phase. Endometrial receptor sites for progesterone are developed during this time. Systemic effects of the increasing amounts of estrogen include an increased secretion of thyroxine-binding globulin (TBG) by the liver, an increase in the breast mammary duct cells, thickening of the vaginal mucosa, and changes in cervical mucus (i.e., increased amount and elasticity) to facilitate sperm penetration at midcycle.

Secretory Phase

The secretory phase is the time of ovulation to the period just prior to menses (approximately days 15 to 26). This phase of the endometrial cycle is characterized by changes induced by increasing amounts of progesterone. Progesterone functions to create a highly vascular secretory endometrium that is suitable for implantation of a fertilized ovum. Glycogen-producing glands secrete endometrial fluid in preparation for a fertilized ovum. At this time, endometrial growth ceases, and the numbers of estrogen and progesterone receptors decrease. Other progesterone effects during the secretory phase include increased glandular growth of the breasts, thinning of the vaginal mucosa, and increased thickness and stickiness of the cervical mucus.

Ischemic Phase

The ischemic phase is from the end of the secretory phase to the onset of menstruation (approximately days 27 to 28). During the ischemic phase, estrogen and progesterone levels are low, and the uterine spiral arteries constrict. The endometrium becomes pale in color as a result of a limited blood supply, and the blood vessels ultimately rupture. Rupture of the endometrial blood vessels leads to the onset of menses (this event marks day 1 of the next cycle) and initiation of the menstrual phase of the cycle.

HYPOTHALAMIC–PITUITARY–OVARIAN CYCLE

The menstrual cycle is controlled by complex interactions between hormones secreted by the hypothalamus, anterior pituitary, and ovaries (see Fig. 5-14). Hormones from the hypothalamic–pituitary–gonadal (ovarian) axis interact with one another and influence the secretion of hormones from other sites. The hypothalamus and anterior pituitary communicate through the hypophyseal portal system (a system of venous capillary blood vessels that supplies blood and endocrine communication between the hypothalamus and pituitary). The major interacting hormones include GnRH (hypothalamus), LH, and FSH (pituitary), and estrogen and progesterone (ovaries).

Hypothalamic-Pituitary Component

The pituitary receives gonadotropin-releasing hormone (GnRH) input from the hypothalamus. GnRH stimulates the secretion of follicle-stimulating hormone (FSH) and luteinizing hormone (LH). FSH prompts the ovaries to secrete estrogen and progesterone, and these hormones inhibit the continued secretion of hypothalamic GnRH. FSH also induces the proliferation of ovarian granulosa cells. LH stimulates the growth of the ovarian follicles and prompts ovulation and luteinization (formation of the corpus luteum) of the dominant follicle. The corpus luteum produces high levels of progesterone along with small amounts of estrogen.

Ovarian Component

The ovarian portion of the hypothalamic–pituitary–ovarian axis occurs in two phases: the follicular phase and the luteal phase. The phases are distinguished by events in the ovarian cycle, especially those related to ovulation.

FOLLICULAR PHASE. Day 1 of the menstrual cycle begins with the onset of bleeding (menstruation). This event marks the beginning of the follicular phase, which lasts about 14 days but can vary from 7 to 22 days. This variance often accounts for the irregularity in menstrual cycles in some women (Cunningham et al., 2014). The follicular phase is characterized by dominance in estrogen, FSH, and LH. (Please refer to the earlier discussion concerning the role of estrogen and the endometrial cycle.)

FSH stimulates the ovary to prepare a mature ovum for release at ovulation. LH stimulates the theca cells of the ovary to produce androgens which convert to estrogen in the granulosa cells of the ovary. Immediately before ovulation, the hypothalamus secretes GnRH. This action prompts the anterior pituitary to release LH and FSH. The surge of LH stimulates the release of the ovum, and ovulation generally occurs within 10 to 16 hours after the LH surge.

Ovulation signifies the end of the follicular phase of the ovarian follicular cycle. The ovum is capable of fertilization by a sperm cell for approximately 12 to 24 hours after ovulation. The follicle that contained the mature ovum remains in the ovary and becomes the corpus luteum, a structure that plays a major role during the second half, or luteal phase, of the ovarian cycle.

LUTEAL PHASE. The luteal phase of the ovarian cycle begins at ovulation and ends with the onset of menses. When pregnancy is not achieved following ovulation, the corpus luteum dominates over the second half of the menstrual cycle. In the absence of fertilization, the life span of the corpus luteum is 14 days. Thus, the luteal phase of the uterine cycle is predictable in length and lasts for 14 days. The corpus luteum secretes estrogen and progesterone, producing a negative feedback that signals the anterior pituitary gland to decrease production of FSH and LH. As the end of the luteal phase nears (approximately 8 to 10 days), low levels of FSH and LH cause regression of the corpus luteum. Degeneration of the corpus luteum is associated with declining levels of estrogen and progesterone. The resultant low progesterone levels stimulate the hypothalamus to secrete GnRH, while the decreased levels of estrogen and progesterone trigger endometrial sloughing. The corpus albicans ("white body") forms from the remnants of the corpus luteum and eventually disappears.

BODY CHANGES RELATED TO THE MENSTRUAL CYCLE AND OVULATION

Before ovulation, several events occur to indicate that the woman's body is preparing for fertilization of the released ovum. Increased estrogen secretion by the ovaries produces changes in the cervical mucus that assist the sperm in successfully locating the ovum. There is a dramatic increase in the amount and quality of the cervical mucus. It becomes watery and clear, creating a pathway for sperm to readily swim through the cervix. The elasticity (**spinnbarkeit**) of the cervical mucus increases, and the woman can assess this change by stretching the mucus between her fingers (Fig. 5-17). Another method of assessment involves stretching the cervical mucus between two glass slides. At the time of ovulation, the cervical mucus can be stretched to 8 to 10 cm or longer. If the mucus is thin, watery, and stretchable, the woman is ready to conceive.

There is also an increase in the **ferning** capacity (crystallization) of the cervical mucus (Fig. 5-18). Ferning, an indirect indicator of estrogen production, results from a decrease in the levels of salt and water that interact with glycoproteins in the mucus during midcycle. The clinician assesses for the presence of ferning by placing a sample of cervical mucus on a glass slide, allowing it to air dry and examining it under a microscope for a fernlike pattern.

Physiological changes also accompany ovulation. The basal body temperature (BBT) increases 0.3°C to 0.6°C approximately 24 to 48 hours after ovulation, and some women experience mittelschmerz (abdominal pain that occurs at the time of ovulation, typically described as a cramping sensation) and midcycle spotting. It is still possible to become pregnant at this point in the menstrual cycle, even when spotting is present.

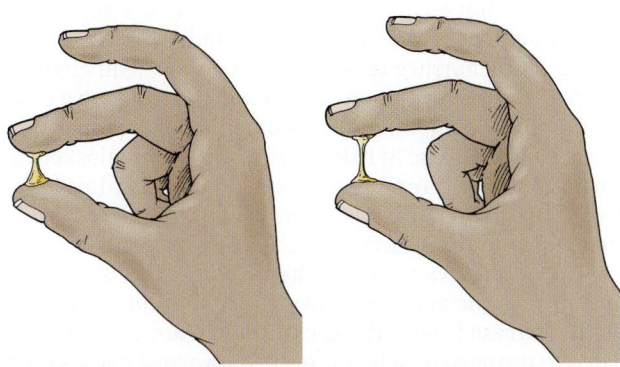

Figure 5-17 Spinnbarkeit (elasticity).

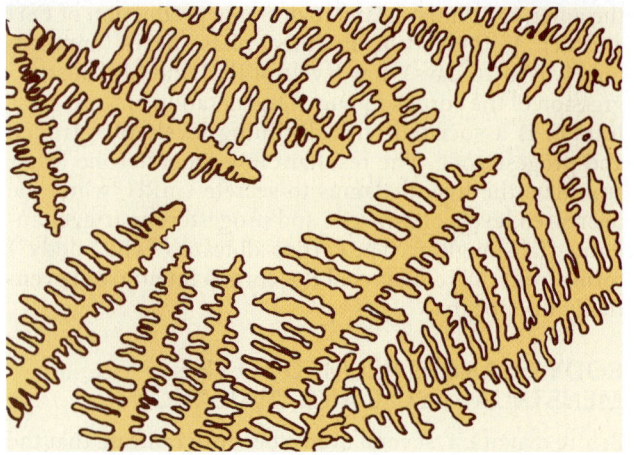

Figure 5-18 A fernlike pattern of cervical mucus occurs with high estrogen levels.

NATURAL CESSATION OF MENSES

Climacteric Phase

The **climacteric** is a phase characterized by the decline in ovarian function and the associated loss of estrogen and progesterone production.

Perimenopausal Phase

Perimenopause, the time preceding menopause, is the period associated with declining fertility for two reasons: The number of ovarian follicles responsive to gonadotropins is decreased, and the responsive follicles do not develop as quickly as before. Because of these normal changes, many cycles during perimenopause are **anovulatory** (no ova are released from the ovary). Anovulatory menstrual cycles are irregular and often variable in the amount of blood flow. Fewer functioning follicles are associated with lower estradiol (estrogen, E_2) levels. Decreased circulating estrogen levels prompt the anterior pituitary to secrete FSH. Elevated serum FSH levels combined with low estradiol levels are usually indicative of perimenopause/menopause (Fritz & Speroff, 2010).

The peri-/postmenopausal period is characterized by greatly decreased amounts of endogenous estrogen. During this time, estrone (E_1), created from the peripheral conversion of androstenedione, becomes the predominant form of estrogen. A number of physical changes may accompany the estrogen depletion. These include vasomotor instability (hot flashes and night sweats), atrophy of the urogenital sites (vaginal dryness and urinary disturbances), amenorrhea (cessation of menses), skin changes (hyper/hypopigmentation, decreased sweat and sebaceous gland activity, thinning of the epidermal and dermal skin layers, and decrease in hair distribution), musculoskeletal changes (bone thinning and osteoporosis), and psychological changes (anxiety, depression, irritability, libido changes, and insomnia).

The hot flashes associated with perimenopause usually occur at night and result from vasodilation associated with decreased estrogen levels. Vaginal atrophy, also related to estrogen deficiency, results in vaginal dryness and increased sensitivity and pain, particularly during sexual intercourse. Atrophy of the urinary tissues may cause urinary incontinence. Alterations in mood, such as depression, mood swings, and tiredness also result from decreased estrogen levels.

A number of long-term effects occur with the diminishing hormone levels during menopause. Decreased estrogen, associated with lower levels of high-density lipids and elevated levels of low-density lipids, increases the risk for cardiovascular disease. As estrogen diminishes, there is a loss in skeletal bone mass, which results in more brittle bones and leads to the development of osteoporosis and a loss of spinal flexibility.

Menopause

Menopause simply refers to the last menstrual period.

Postmenopausal Phase

Postmenopause, the time after menopause, is characterized by estrogen production solely by the adrenal glands. Although controversial, menopausal hormone therapy (HT), prescribed on a highly individual basis, may be prescribed for a short duration of time to minimize moderate to severe vasomotor symptoms (e.g., hot flashes and night sweats) and improve quality of life. HT can be provided as estrogen only or as estrogen and progestin. Estrogen-only HT reduces the symptoms of menopause. However, to reduce the risk of endometrial cancer, the continuous administration of estrogen with no progesterone to facilitate shedding of the endometrial lining should be used only after hysterectomy. Estrogen-progestin therapy increases the risk of venous thromboembolism (VTE), especially in women with a history of VTE or factor V Leiden (a hypercoagulability disorder), and breast cancer (when taken longer than 3 to 5 years) (The North American Menopause Society [NAMS], 2010).

Various nonhormonal medications have been prescribed for the relief of severe vasomotor symptoms. Antidepressant agents known as selective serotonin reuptake inhibitors (SSRIs), including fluoxetine (Prozac), paroxetine (Paxil), citalopram (Celexa), escitalopram (Lexapro), and sertraline (Zoloft), and serotonin/norepinephrine reuptake inhibitors (SNRIs), including venlafaxine (Effexor), and desvenlafaxine (Pristiq), may reduce hot flashes (Barbieri, 2013; NAMS, 2010; Pinkerton, Constantine, Hwang, & Cheng, 2013). In some women, clonidine (Catapres), an antihypertensive medication, and gabapentin (Neurontin), an anticonvulsant, have been useful in controlling hot flashes. Transdermal clonidine therapy is preferred over oral clonidine; gabapentin frequently causes nausea and other gastrointestinal side effects (Barbieri, 2013; Nelson, 2011).

Now Can You—Discuss characteristics of the uterine cycle?

1. Outline the four phases of the uterine cycle and describe the major physiological events that occur during each phase?
2. Trace the hormonal interplays that characterize the hypothalamic–pituitary–ovarian cycle?
3. Describe four physiological changes that occur in the female body around the time of ovulation?
4. Discuss the hormonal events that accompany perimenopause?

Male Reproductive System

EXTERNAL STRUCTURES

The external structures consist of the perineum, penis, and scrotum (Fig. 5-19).

Perineum

The male perineum is a roughly diamond-shaped area that extends from the symphysis pubis anteriorly to the coccyx posteriorly and laterally to the ischial tuberosity.

Penis

The penis is composed of three cylindrical masses of erectile tissue that surround the urethra. The function of the penis is to contain the urethra and serve as the terminal duct for the urinary and reproductive tracts by excreting urine and semen. During sexual arousal, the penis becomes erect to allow penetration for sexual intercourse.

The glans penis is the tip of the penis. It contains many nerve endings and is very sensitive and important in sexual arousal. The urethra is approximately 8 inches (20 cm) long and serves as a passageway for both urine and ejaculated semen. It extends from the urinary bladder to the urethral meatus at the tip of the penis. **Circumcision** is a surgical procedure in which the prepuce (epithelial layer covering the penis; foreskin) is separated from the glans penis and excised. (See Chapter 18 for further discussion.)

Scrotum

The scrotum is a two-compartment pouch covered by skin. It is suspended from the perineum and contains two testes, the epididymis, and the lower portion of the spermatic cord. The scrotum functions to enclose and protect the two testes. A large component of the protection occurs through temperature regulation of the testes (maintained at about 5°F below core body temperature), which is accomplished by the dartos and cremaster scrotal muscles. These muscles control elevation of the scrotal sac to help maintain the testes in a controlled temperature environment. When exposed to cold, the scrotal muscles contract, causing the testes to be elevated closer to the body to preserve warmth.

INTERNAL STRUCTURES

The internal male reproductive structures include the testes, epididymides, ducts (vas deferens and ejaculatory duct), urethra, spermatic cords, and accessory glands (seminal vesicles, prostate, bulbourethral glands, and urethral glands) (Fig. 5-20).

Testicles/Testes

The male testes are considered "essential organs" because they manufacture sperm, which are necessary for reproduction. The two testicles are composed of several lobules, seminiferous tubules, and interstitial cells separated by septa. They are encased in the tunica albuginea capsule. The seminiferous tubules open into a plexus (rete testis) drained by efferent ductules located on the top of the testicle that enters the head of the epididymis. The seminiferous tubules contain spermatogonia, or sperm-generating cells, that divide first by the process of mitosis to produce primary spermatocytes (Figs. 5-20 and 5-21).

One testicle is housed in each compartment of the scrotum. The function of the testicle is twofold and includes

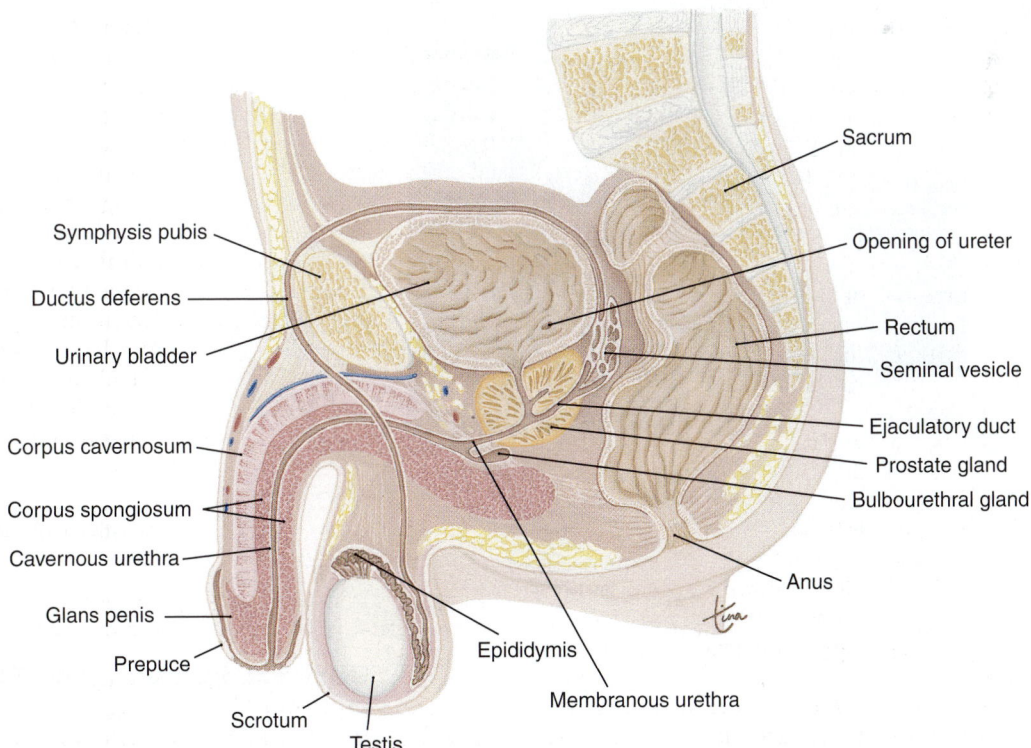

Figure 5-19 The male reproductive system shown in a midsagittal section through the pelvic cavity.

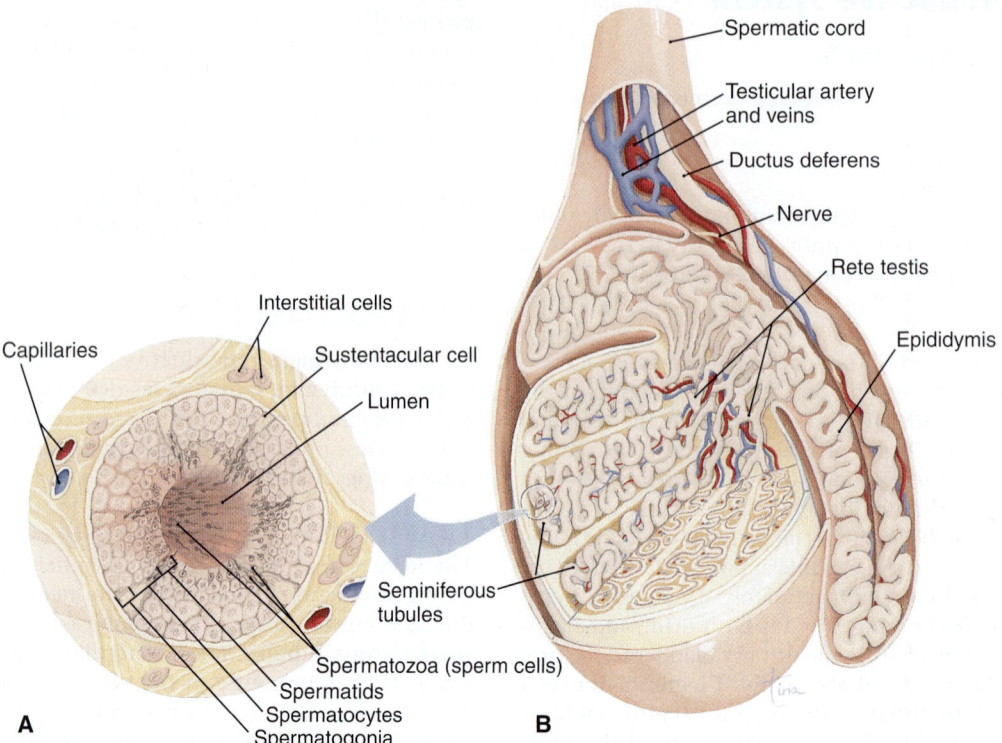

Figure 5-20 *A,* Cross section through a seminiferous tubule showing development of sperm. *B,* Midsagittal section of portion of a testis; the epididymis is on the posterior side of the testis.

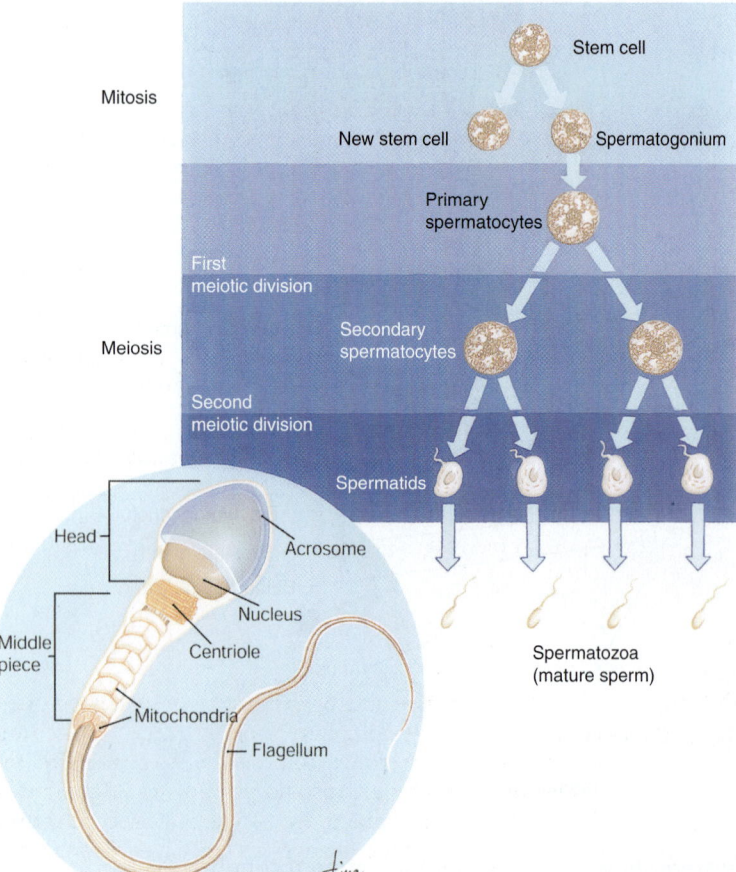

Figure 5-21 Spermatogenesis. The processes of mitosis and meiosis are shown. For each primary spermatocyte that undergoes meiosis, four functional sperm cells are formed. The structure of a mature sperm cell is also shown.

spermatogenesis and the production and secretion of the male hormone testosterone by the interstitial cells of Leydig.

A & P review **Spermatogenesis**

Spermatogenesis, the formation of mature sperm within the seminiferous tubules, is a process that occurs in the following four stages (see Figs. 5-20 and 5-21).

1. Spermatogonia, the primary germinal epithelial cells, grow and develop into primary spermatocytes. Spermatogonia and primary spermatocytes both contain 46 chromosomes; these consist of 44 autosomes and the two sex chromosomes, X and Y.
2. The primary spermatocytes divide to form secondary spermatocytes. In this stage no new chromosomes are formed; instead, the pairs only divide. Each secondary spermatocyte contains half the number of autosomes—22. One secondary spermatocyte contains an X chromosome, and the other contains a Y chromosome.
3. Each secondary spermatocyte then undergoes another division to form spermatids.
4. In the final stage, the spermatids undergo a series of structural changes that transform them into mature spermatozoa (sperm), each containing a head, neck, body, and tail. The head houses the nucleus; the tail contains a large amount of adenosine triphosphate (ATP), which provides energy for sperm motility (Dillon, 2007). ◆

Epididymis

There are two epididymides, which are tightly coiled tubes positioned on the top of each testis. The epididymides store maturing sperm cells and convey sperm to the vas deferens. They also secrete seminal fluid and serve as the site where sperm become motile.

Ducts

There are two vasa deferentia (sing. vas deferens), or ductus deferens, and two ejaculatory ducts. The vasa deferentia are two tubes that extend beyond the epididymis through the inguinal canal into the abdomen and over and behind the bladder. They serve as an excretory duct for seminal fluid. The vasa deferentia also connect the epididymis with the ejaculatory duct. The two ejaculatory ducts serve as the connection between the vasa deferentia and the seminal vesicle ducts. The ejaculatory ducts pass through the prostate gland and terminate in the urethra.

Urethra

The urethra is a mucus membrane–lined tube that passes from the bladder to the exterior of the body. It joins with the two ejaculatory ducts in the prostate gland. Its length is approximately 8 inches (20 cm). In males, the urethra functions in both the urinary and reproductive systems.

Spermatic Cords

The two spermatic cords are fibrous cylinders located in the inguinal canals. They enclose the seminal ducts, blood and lymphatic vessels, and nerves.

Accessory Glands

The accessory glands include the seminal vesicles, the prostate, the bulbourethral glands, and the urethral (Littre's) glands.

The two seminal vesicles are pouches located on the posterior surface of the bladder. They secrete the viscous nutrient-rich component of seminal fluid. This fluid, which accounts for 60% of semen volume, contains alkaline prostaglandin to help neutralize semen pH.

The prostate, located inferiorly to the bladder, is a donut-shaped structure that encircles the urethra. It secretes a thin, milky, alkaline fluid that is rich in zinc, citric acid, acid phosphatase, and calcium. Prostatic fluid helps protect sperm from the acidic environments of the vagina and male urethra and accounts for 30% of the semen volume.

Each of the two bulbourethral glands is a small pea-shaped organ that contains a 1-inch (2.5-cm) long duct leading into the urethra. These glands are located below the prostate gland, and they function to secrete fluid to lubricate the end of the penis. This fluid makes up 5% of the semen volume.

The urethral, or Littre's, glands are multiple glands located along the urethra, especially in the penile section. They secrete mucus that is incorporated into the semen.

CHARACTERISTICS OF SEMEN AND SPERM

Seminal fluid consists of secretions from the testes, the epididymides, the seminal vesicles, the prostate, the bulbourethral glands, and the urethral glands. Seminal fluid is secreted during ejaculation and is slightly alkaline with a pH of about 7.5. The typical amount present in one ejaculate is 2 to 5 mL. There are approximately 120 million sperm cells in each milliliter of ejaculate and, typically, around 40% of the sperm are motile. There are also about 5 million white blood cells in each milliliter of semen along with secretions from the testes, epididymides, seminal vesicles, prostate, and bulbourethral glands. The following pathway traces the events from the formation of sperm to the ejaculation of semen:

1. The testes produce sperm that are transported to the epididymis.
2. Sperm and seminal fluid move to the vas deferens.
3. From there the seminal fluid moves to the ejaculatory duct before exiting the body through the urethra.

Sperm are capable of surviving in optimal favorable alkaline conditions for up to 72 hours post-ejaculation in a woman's body. The average length of time for sperm to travel from the cervix to the fallopian tubes is approximately 5 minutes under favorable conditions.

MALE HORMONAL INFLUENCES

Testosterone

The testes produce androgens, the male sex hormones. Testosterone is the dominant male hormone. At the time of puberty, testosterone stimulates enlargement of the testes and accessory organs and prompts development of the secondary sex characteristics. The male secondary sex characteristics include changes in body hair (coarse hair on face, chest, and pubic area and sometimes decreased hair on the head), a deepening of the voice, thickened skin, increased upper body musculature and narrow waist, and a thickening and strengthening of bone (Shier, Butler, & Lewis, 2011). Testosterone also prompts a linear growth spurt.

FERTILITY

Male fertility is related to overall sperm number, size, shape, and motility. Decreased fertility is associated with insufficient sperm counts affected by active contact sports; smoking; and tight, constrictive clothing. Decreased fertility is also associated with an autoimmune disorder that results in the manufacture of antibodies to one's own sperm. The presence of varicose veins on the scrotum (varicocele) can cause testicular warming and adversely affect the life span of the sperm. Decreased sperm motility or "slow swimming" caused by ineffective flagella also affects male fertility.

AGE-RELATED DEVELOPMENT OF THE MALE REPRODUCTIVE SYSTEM

Similar to embryological development in the female, the male genital organs develop in the abdomen of the fetus but are immature. The testes develop near the kidneys and descend into the scrotum through the inguinal canal after 35 weeks' gestation. Scrotal examination is an important component of the male neonate's physical assessment to ensure that the testes have descended and do not remain in the inguinal canal. **Cryptorchidism** is the condition in which the testes fail to descend; sterility results unless the testes are surgically placed in the scrotum (Scanlon & Sanders, 2010) (see Chapter 18 for further discussion). It is important to locate both testes in a newborn because testicular failure to descend may indicate gonadal malgenesis, which can lead to testicular cancer and fertility issues in young adulthood.

The reproductive functions of the testes begin at the time of puberty. Once critical hormone levels have been reached, the final stages of reproductive system development take place. A gradual decline in hormone production normally occurs during late adulthood. Although the hormonal decline may be associated with a decrease in sexual desire and fertility, most men maintain the ability to reproduce into old age.

 Now Can You—Discuss aspects of the male reproductive system?

1. Identify the three external structures of the male reproductive system and describe one function for two of them?
2. Discuss the functions of the testicles, epididymis, vas deferens, and prostate gland?
3. Trace the pathway from sperm production to semen ejaculation?
4. Name five male secondary sex characteristics that result from the influence of testosterone?

Summary Points

◆ Gender is determined at the moment of conception. Identifiable sexual characteristics are apparent in the embryo at 8 weeks of gestation.

◆ Gender maturation is a lengthy process that begins during embryonic development and reaches full maturity during late adolescence.

◆ External structures of the female reproductive system include the mons pubis, labia, clitoris, vestibule, urethral meatus, Skene's and Bartholin's glands, vaginal introitus, hymen, and perineum.

◆ Internal structures of the female reproductive system include the ovaries, fallopian tubes, uterus, and vagina.

◆ The female bony pelvis supports and protects the contents of the pelvis and provides a fixed axis for the process of childbirth.

◆ The breasts or mammary glands are considered to be accessory organs of the female reproductive system.

◆ Hormones secreted by the pituitary gland are essential in the regulation of gonadal, thyroid, and adrenal function; lactation; body growth; and somatic development.

◆ Menstruation and ovulation are controlled by a complex interplay of positive and negative feedback systems associated with hormones released by the hypothalamus, pituitary, and ovaries.

◆ The male reproductive system consists of the testes, where spermatogonia and male sex hormones are formed; a series of continuous ducts that allow spermatozoa to be transported outside the body; accessory glands that produce secretions to foster sperm nutrition, survival, and transport; and the penis, which functions as the reproductive organ of intercourse.

◆ Testosterone, the dominant male hormone, is responsible for the development of secondary sex characteristics in the male.

Review Questions

Multiple Choice

1. The perinatal nurse explains to a new nurse that a female fetus has a developed ovary by
A. 8 weeks.
B. 10 weeks.
C. 12 weeks.
D. 16 weeks.

2. A perinatal nurse is conducting prenatal classes. This nurse explains that an incision for cesarean birth is normally made in which uterine segment?
A. Isthmus
B. Cervix
C. Apex
D. Corpus

3. The perinatal nurse explains to an adolescent that ova are produced and estrogen is secreted at which phase of life?
A. Puberty
B. Birth
C. The climacteric
D. Pregnancy

4. Which part of a woman's anatomy is used as the assessment landmark for the fetal presenting part?
   A. Ischial spines
   B. Sacral promontory
   C. Sacral alae
   D. True pelvis

5. A nurse is conducting prenatal classes. The nurse explains the incision made to enlarge the perineal opening for a vaginal birth. What is this incision called?
   A. Colposcopy
   B. Episiotomy
   C. Ligation
   D. Septal myotomy

6. Which hormone is responsible for regulating oogenesis?
   A. Estrogen
   B. Follicle-stimulating hormone (FSH)
   C. Gonadotropin-releasing hormone (GnRH)
   D. Progesterone

7. A pregnant woman has been advised that she has a platypelloid pelvis type. What action by the perinatal nurse is best?
   A. Advise the woman that she may need a cesarean delivery.
   B. Educate the woman that a posterior fetal presentation is possible.
   C. Instruct the woman on specific back strengthening exercises.
   D. Reassure the woman that a trial of labor will still be allowed.

8. A pediatric nurse has assessed a 13-year-old girl and notices that she is in thelarche. What situation does this term refer to?
   A. The appearance of breast buds
   B. The appearance of secondary sex characteristics
   C. The first menstrual period
   D. The growth of pubic hair

9. An adolescent in the pediatric clinic states that her vaginal secretions sometimes seem more thin, watery, and stretchable than usual. What response from the nurse is best?
   A. Advise the patient that this is related to her periods.
   B. Educate the patient that she is fertile when this occurs.
   C. Instruct the patient to douche after her periods.
   D. Screen the patient for sexually transmitted infections.

10. A perimenopausal woman complains to the nurse about the new onset of urinary stress incontinence. Which statement by the nurse is best?
   A. "A little incontinence is normal at your age."
   B. "Clonidine (Catapres) is a new treatment for this."
   C. "This is probably related to decreased estrogen."
   D. "We need to start you on estrogen therapy."

See Answers to End of Chapter Review Questions on DavisPlus.

REFERENCES

Barbieri, R. L. (2013). When estrogen isn't an option, here is how I treat menopausal symptoms. *OBG Management, 25*(6), 9–10.

Blackburn, S. T. (2012). *Maternal, fetal, and neonatal physiology: A clinical perspective* (4th ed.). St. Louis, MO: W.B. Saunders.

Caldwell, W., & Moloy, H. (1933). Anatomical variations in the female pelvis and their effect in labor with a suggested classification. *American Journal of Obstetrics and Gynecology, 26*, 479–505.

Chumlea, W. C., Schubert, C. M., Roche, A. F., Kulin, H. E., Lee, P. A., Himes, J. H., & Sun, S. S. (2003). Age at menarche and racial comparisons in U.S. girls. *Pediatrics, 11*(1), 110–113.

Cunningham, F., Leveno, K., Bloom, S., Spong, C., Dashe, J., Hoffman, B., Casey, B., & Sheffield, J. (2014). *Williams Obstetrics* (24th ed.). New York, NY: McGraw-Hill.

Dillon, P. M. (2007). *Nursing health assessment: A critical thinking, case studies approach* (2nd ed.). Philadelphia, PA: F.A. Davis.

Fritz, M. A., & Speroff, L. (2010). *Clinical gynecologic, endocrinology and infertility* (8th ed.). Baltimore, MD: Lippincott Williams & Wilkins.

Garibaldi, L. (2011). Physiology of puberty. In Kliegman, R. M., Stanton, B., St. Geme, J., Schor, N., & Behrman, R. E. (Eds.). *Nelson textbook of pediatrics* (19th ed., p. 2308). Philadelphia, PA: W.B. Saunders.

Nelson, A. L. (2011). Perimenopause, menopause, and postmenopause: Health promotion strategies. In Hatcher, R. A., Trussell, J., Nelson, A. L, Cates, W., Kowal, D., & Policar, M. S., *Contraceptive technology* (20th revised ed., pp. 737–777). Decatur, GA: Bridging the Gap Communications.

Pinkerton, J.V., Constantine, G., Hwang, E., & Cheng, J.R. (2013). Desvenlafaxine compared with placebo for treatment of menopausal vasomotor symptoms: A 12-week, multicenter, parallel-group, randomized, double-blind, placebo-controlled efficacy trial. *Menopause, 20*(1), 28–37.

Scanlon, V. C., & Sanders, T. (2010). *Essentials of anatomy and physiology* (6th ed.). Philadelphia, PA: F.A. Davis.

Shier, D., Butler, J., & Lewis, R. (2011). *Hole's essentials of human anatomy and physiology* (11th ed.). New York, NY: McGraw-Hill.

Tanner, J. M. (1962). *Growth at adolescence* (2nd ed.). Oxford: Blackwell Scientific.

The North American Menopause Society (NAMS). (2010). *Estrogen and progestogen use in postmenopausal women. 2010 position statement of The North American Menopause Society, 17*(2), 242–255.

Venes, D. (2013). *Taber's cyclopedic medical dictionary* (22nd ed.). Philadelphia, PA: F.A. Davis.

DavisPlus | For more information, go to http://davisplus.fadavis.com/

CONCEPT MAP

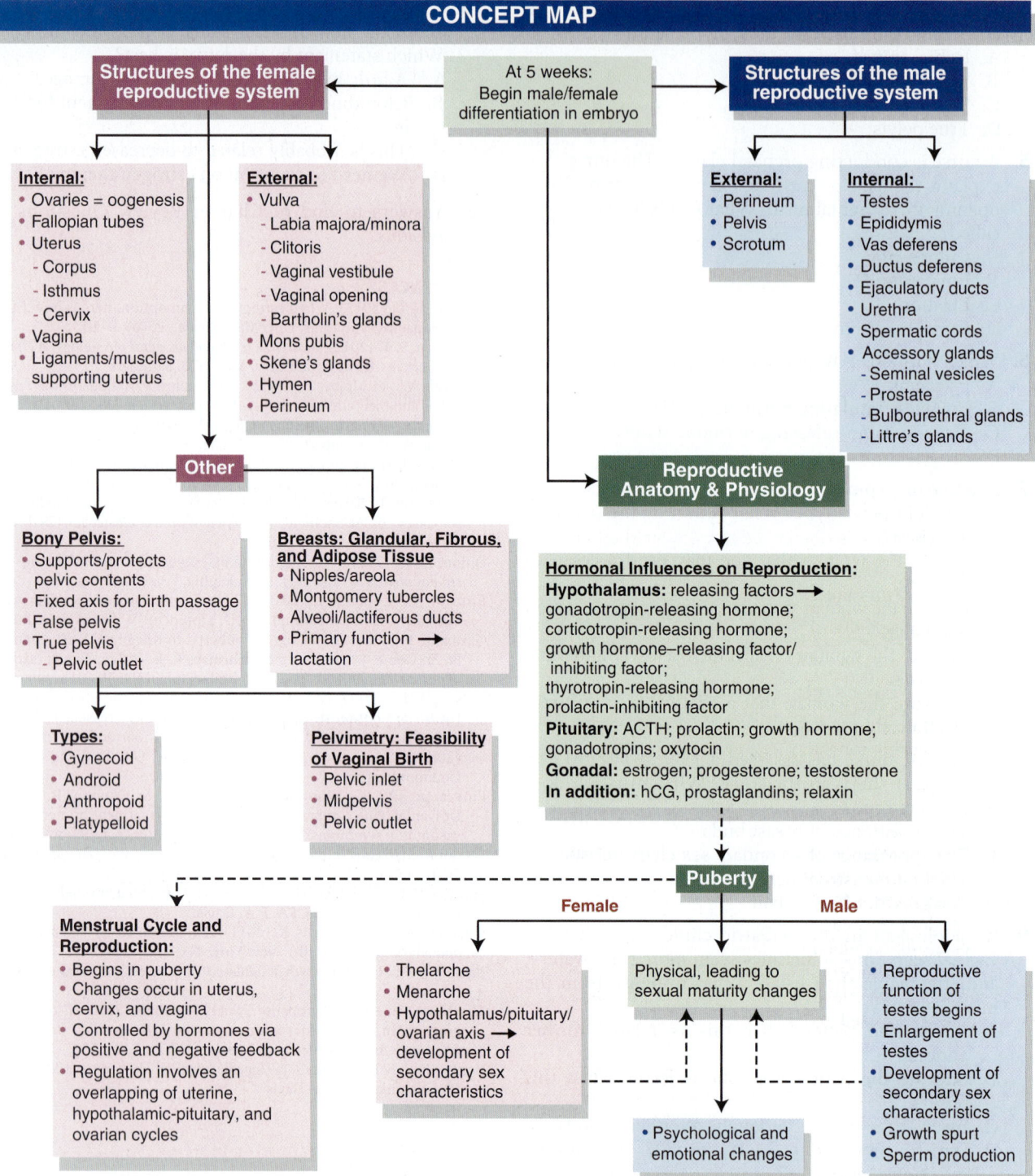

Structures of the female reproductive system

At 5 weeks: Begin male/female differentiation in embryo

Structures of the male reproductive system

Internal:
- Ovaries = oogenesis
- Fallopian tubes
- Uterus
  - Corpus
  - Isthmus
  - Cervix
- Vagina
- Ligaments/muscles supporting uterus

External:
- Vulva
  - Labia majora/minora
  - Clitoris
  - Vaginal vestibule
  - Vaginal opening
  - Bartholin's glands
- Mons pubis
- Skene's glands
- Hymen
- Perineum

External:
- Perineum
- Pelvis
- Scrotum

Internal:
- Testes
- Epididymis
- Vas deferens
- Ductus deferens
- Ejaculatory ducts
- Urethra
- Spermatic cords
- Accessory glands
  - Seminal vesicles
  - Prostate
  - Bulbourethral glands
  - Littre's glands

Other

Reproductive Anatomy & Physiology

Bony Pelvis:
- Supports/protects pelvic contents
- Fixed axis for birth passage
- False pelvis
- True pelvis
  - Pelvic outlet

Breasts: Glandular, Fibrous, and Adipose Tissue
- Nipples/areola
- Montgomery tubercles
- Alveoli/lactiferous ducts
- Primary function → lactation

Hormonal Influences on Reproduction:
Hypothalamus: releasing factors → gonadotropin-releasing hormone; corticotropin-releasing hormone; growth hormone–releasing factor/ inhibiting factor; thyrotropin-releasing hormone; prolactin-inhibiting factor
Pituitary: ACTH; prolactin; growth hormone; gonadotropins; oxytocin
Gonadal: estrogen; progesterone; testosterone
In addition: hCG, prostaglandins; relaxin

Types:
- Gynecoid
- Android
- Anthropoid
- Platypelloid

Pelvimetry: Feasibility of Vaginal Birth
- Pelvic inlet
- Midpelvis
- Pelvic outlet

Puberty

Female   Male

Menstrual Cycle and Reproduction:
- Begins in puberty
- Changes occur in uterus, cervix, and vagina
- Controlled by hormones via positive and negative feedback
- Regulation involves an overlapping of uterine, hypothalamic-pituitary, and ovarian cycles

- Thelarche
- Menarche
- Hypothalamus/pituitary/ ovarian axis → development of secondary sex characteristics

Physical, leading to sexual maturity changes

- Reproductive function of testes begins
- Enlargement of testes
- Development of secondary sex characteristics
- Growth spurt
- Sperm production

- Psychological and emotional changes

Now Can You:
?
- Discuss various aspects of the female and male reproductive systems
- Identify aspects of the bony pelvis and female breast
- Discuss key hormones involved in reproduction
- Discuss concepts related to puberty

Human Sexuality and Fertility

 Cherish your human connections: Your relationships with friends and family.

—Barbara Bush

LEARNING TARGETS *At the completion of this chapter, the student will be able to:*

◆ Discuss the nurse's role in providing sexual and reproductive health care.

◆ Identify advantages and disadvantages of barrier and hormonal contraceptive methods, intrauterine devices, and permanent sterilization.

◆ Teach patients how to use various methods of contraception.

◆ Assess a patient for short-term complications after an induced abortion.

◆ Analyze the nurse's role in infertility care.

◆ Differentiate among the various assisted reproductive technologies and identify potential alternatives to childbearing for the infertile couple.

PICO(T) Questions

The intent of evidence-based practice (EBP) is to provide nursing care that integrates the best available evidence. An initial step in EBP is to write a PICO(T) question that effectively guides the research. A PICO(T) question is an acronym that stands for population (P), intervention or issue (I), comparison of interest (C), outcome (O), and timeframe (T). Depending on the question, all or some of the question components are used in the research process. Use these

PICO(T) questions to spark your thinking as you read the chapter.

1. What (O) factors do (P) women say (I) are most important (C) when choosing a method of contraception?

2. Do (P) couples (I) who receive individual counseling as part of infertility treatments (O) stay married (or with their significant other) longer on average (C) than those whose treatment does not include counseling?

 Evidence-Based Practice

Polis, C. B., & Zabin, L. S. (2012). Missed conceptions or misconceptions: Perceived infertility among unmarried young adults in the United States. *Perspectives on Sexual & Reproductive Health, 44*(1), 30–38.

The purpose of this study was to examine perceived infertility beliefs among young adults and the potential for nonuse of contraceptives based on those beliefs. According to the researchers, approximately 50% of unintended pregnancies occur in couples who are not using contraceptives. One reason cited for nonuse of contraception is a perception that the individual is infertile regardless of medical facts. According to a national survey of reported contraceptive nonuse, 49% of women aged 15 to 24 years

experienced unintended pregnancies because they did not believe that they could become pregnant.

Participants for this study included 1,699 unmarried men and women aged 18 to 29 years of age. Participants were contacted by phone from information obtained through "The Fog Zone Data Set," a 2009 survey commissioned by the National Campaign to Prevent Teen Unplanned Pregnancy and carried out by the Guttmacher Institute. The three methods used to contact participants included

(continued)

random digit-dial sampling of landline telephones, targeted sampling of listed telephone numbers with a high probability of having an eligible respondent, and a random sampling of cell phone numbers.

Self-reported sample demographics were as follows: 60% white, 15% black, 17% Hispanic, and 7% "other." Nearly 90% were born in the United States, and 85% spoke English as their primary language. Fifty-four percent reported some college education, 44% were employed, 26% were attending school, 18% were both working and attending school, 36% were living with parents, 16% were living with a partner, 28% were living with someone else, and 19% were living alone.

The study used a descriptive analysis. Participants were provided with the following statement, "Some people are unable to become pregnant, even if they want to. How likely do you think it is that you are infertile or will have difficulty getting (a woman) pregnant when you want to?" Reponses ranged from "not at all likely," "slightly likely," and "quite likely," to "extremely likely." The researchers further grouped the last two responses ("quite likely" or "extremely likely") into one category that was labeled as those who believed they were "very likely" of being infertile. Nearly 80% of the participants had received sex education, although only 34% were aware that a woman's chance of becoming pregnant was higher at certain times during the menstrual cycle.

Twenty-five percent of the respondents reported the first heterosexual intercourse occurred at age 18 or older, and 16% of the women and 13% of the men had never experienced heterosexual vaginal intercourse. Over one-half (62%) indicated that they had friends who had experienced unplanned pregnancies.

In response to a question regarding whether they would seek medical care for sexual reasons, 84% of the women and 39% of the men responded in the affirmative. Twenty-nine percent of the women and 13% of the men reported having children, while 6% of women and 7% of men had been involved in a pregnancy but did not have children.

Nineteen percent of the women and 13% of the men reported that they believed they were very likely infertile. Of the women who expressed this belief, 41% indicated that this was based on an understanding of a physician's statement, although 20% reported never having visited a doctor regarding sexual health concerns. Other reasons cited for perceived infertility included not getting pregnant after having sexual relationships and not using contraceptives (37%), having an infertile relative (18%), and no specific reason (33%). Males who had a perception that they were infertile reported that they were more likely to have sex without using a contraceptive.

The researchers concluded that a significant number of young adults perceive that they are infertile, and this belief increases the likelihood of unintended pregnancies. They supported the notion that counseling and sex education are key strategies to increase contraceptive use and enhance understanding of the likelihood of personal infertility.

1. How is this information useful to clinical nursing practice?

2. Based on these findings, what are implications for further research?

See Suggested Responses for Evidence-Based Practice on Davis*Plus*.

Introduction

"Women's health care" is a broad term that encompasses the provision of holistic care to women within the context of their day-to-day lives. This approach to health recognizes that a woman's physical, mental, and spiritual states are interdependent, and all affect the present level of wellness. In any therapeutic setting, eliciting the woman's view of her situation and assessing her needs, values, beliefs, and supports constitute essential components in formulating an appropriate plan of care.

Nurses have an opportunity to work with women in a variety of settings. Teaching about health promotion can take place at community centers, schools, clinics, private offices, and senior centers. The majority of women's health care is delivered outside the acute care setting. Approaching women's health from a community-based perspective enables nurses to recognize each person's autonomy and provide holistic care that is sensitive to physical, emotional, sociocultural, and situational needs.

Sexuality is a multidimensional concept that encompasses one's sexual nature, activity, and interest. Influenced by ethical, spiritual, cultural, and moral factors, sexuality constitutes an important component of women's health. A

central role for nurses involves helping women to understand their sexual health and assisting them with reproductive life planning. This chapter explores the nurse's roles in various aspects of reproductive health care and concludes with a brief overview of some of the legal and ethical issues that surround methods of assisted reproductive technology.

Sexuality and Reproductive Health Care

Sexuality and its reproductive implications are woven into the fabric of human behavior. Because it is such an emotion-laden aspect of life, people have many concerns, problems, and questions about sex roles, behaviors, inhibitions, education, morality, and related components such as contraception. The reproductive implications of sexual behavior must also be considered. Some people desire pregnancy; others wish to avoid it. Health concerns are yet another issue that must be addressed. The rising incidence of sexually transmitted infections, especially HIV/AIDS and herpes virus, has prompted many individuals to modify their sexual practices. Women often ask questions and voice concerns about these issues to the nurse in the ambulatory care setting. Hence, the nurse may need to assume the role of educator, counselor, or care provider when dealing with sexual and reproductive health matters.

It is essential that nurses who practice in reproductive care settings develop an awareness and understanding of personal feelings, values, and attitudes about sexuality. These insights allow the nurse to provide sensitive, individualized care to women who have their own set of values and beliefs. Nurses must have current, evidence-based information about anatomy and physiology and about topics related to sexuality and reproductive health. Nurses must also be sensitive to the relationship dynamics they may observe when women arrive for care accompanied by their partners.

 Nursing Insight—*AWHONN advocates informed reproductive health-care decision making*

The Association of Women's Health, Obstetric and Neonatal Nurses (AWHONN) supports and promotes a woman's right to accurate and complete information and access to reproductive care services and opposes legislation and policies that may limit a health-care provider's ability to counsel patients as to their full range of treatment options and provide referrals (AWHONN, 2009a).

EXPLORING DIMENSIONS OF SEXUALITY

Sexual Orientations

Even though it constitutes an integral and normal dimension of every human being, sexuality evokes controversy when it involves alternative sexual orientation or sexual expression at either end of the age spectrum. **Heterosexual** sexual orientation is the sexual attraction to or sexual activity with a person of the opposite sex or gender. Heterosexuality is often considered the norm in America, and any other form of sexual expression is viewed as being outside the realm of "normal."

Homosexuality is the sexual attraction to or sexual activity of a person with another individual belonging to the same sex or gender. The term "gay" is often used for homosexual males; "lesbian" is used for females. An estimated 2% to 10% of women in the United States presently identify themselves as lesbian or bisexual (American College of Obstetricians and Gynecologists [ACOG], 2011a; 2012a). Although a genetic factor has been linked with male homosexuality, no such etiology has been identified for lesbians (Ridley, 2013). Thus, the origin of this sexual orientation in women remains basically unknown.

Masters and Johnson (1966) refuted the idea that homosexuality is a mental health disorder. Yet lesbians and bisexuals (individuals who are sexually active with others of both sexes) are more likely to report that they experience poor physical and mental health (Delk & Wiczyk, 2010). Although the exact etiology of diminished health status among this population is not clear, one factor may relate to homosexual/bisexual women's hesitancy in seeking health care. The mental and physical discomforts associated with seeking medical attention may translate into a failure to obtain timely professional help for health concerns or illnesses. Some lesbians may be reluctant to disclose their sexual orientation to their health-care provider because of fears related to hostility, inadequate health care, or breach of confidentiality. Also, in many health-care settings, patient heterosexuality is assumed, and interview questions are structured toward a heterosexual orientation.

Lesbians who decide to bear children often must undergo a number of medical procedures to conceive. In general, lesbian women who choose to have children are firmly committed to their decision, for they must work harder at achieving conception than other women. Significant health issues also exist for this population. Lesbians are more at risk than heterosexual women for breast cancer because of their lower rates of breastfeeding. Hormones released during pregnancy and breastfeeding may help protect women against breast, endometrial, and ovarian cancers. Also, lesbians and bisexual women are less likely than other women to have routine mammography and clinical breast exams. This may be related to a lack of health insurance, a fear of discrimination, or a history of negative experiences with health-care professionals. Women who have sex with women are also at risk for sexually transmitted infections (STIs) (including HIV) and cervical cancer. For reasons unknown, bacterial vaginosis (BV) is more common in lesbian and bisexual women than in other women. Other common STIs that can be passed between women include Chlamydia, genital herpes, human papillomavirus (HPV), and trichomoniasis (Office on Women's Health, U.S. Department of Health and Human Services 2012). However, woman-to-woman transmission of sexually transmitted infections is much lower than in heterosexual relationships. Because not all gynecological cancers are related to sexual activity, lesbian women who have never had children may be at an increased risk for endometrial and ovarian cancer. However, their risk for other cancers (e.g., lung and colon) and heart disease is not different from that of heterosexual women. It is essential that health-care providers give correct advice and conduct appropriate cancer and other disease screening for these women. The nurse should develop an approach that does not assume that all patients are heterosexual (ACOG, 2012a, 2013a; Delk & Wiczyk, 2010; Hrivnak, 2013; Office on Women's Health, U.S. Department of Health and Human Services, 2012). As is true with any group, homosexual women deserve to have their health-care concerns addressed by compassionate, nonjudgmental health-care providers who are knowledgeable about the health-care needs of women with alternative sexual preferences.

THE HUMAN SEXUAL RESPONSE

In the 1960s, the research work of Masters and Johnson (1966) helped to define sexuality as a natural component of a healthy human personality. Before that time, human sexuality was often viewed as a negative or nonexistent, sometimes shameful, aspect that needed to be shrouded in secrecy. The work of the two sexuality researchers gave new insights into the physical components of human pleasure during sexual response and orgasm.

Masters and Johnson described four human sexual response phases: excitement, plateau, orgasmic, and resolution. The *excitement phase* is characterized by physiological responses to internal and/or external cues. Women experience vaginal lubrication, breast and pelvic engorgement, and increased heart rate, respiratory rate, and blood pressure.

Clitoral and labial tissues become swollen, the nipples become erect, and the vagina becomes distended and elongated. Men experience penile engorgement with an increase in circumference and length (erection) along with scrotal thickening and elevation.

During the *plateau phase*, women experience the most heightened sense of sexual tension. The labia become more congested, the vagina becomes more fully expanded, and the uterus rises out of the pelvis in preparation for intercourse. Most women also experience sexual flushing, tachycardia, and hyperventilation. In men, the testicles enlarge and become elevated and the coronal circumference of the penis increases. Both genders experience a generalized muscular tension.

The *orgasmic phase* is characterized by an intense desire for sexual release caused by congestion of the blood vessels. Tachycardia, blood pressure, and hyperventilation are intensified. These sensations build until orgasm is reached. Muscular contractions occur in the man's accessory reproductive organs (vas deferens, seminal vesicles, and ejaculatory duct). There is a relaxation of the bladder sphincter muscles along with contractions of the urethra and perirectal muscles followed by ejaculation as orgasm occurs.

An overall release of muscular tension takes place during the *resolution phase*. Both genders experience a feeling of warmth and relaxation, and women may experience a brief refractory period or "rest time" before they are interested in sexual intercourse again. Women are capable of experiencing multiple orgasms.

Masters and Johnson were instrumental in opening the topic of human sexual response for discussion and study in the United States. The media often send the message that sexuality involves only a physical expression such as the act of sexual intercourse. In actuality, human sexuality is a multidimensional phenomenon that touches and permeates many aspects of human behavior.

A Nursing Framework for Promoting Women's Sexual and Reproductive Health

Nurses who work with women in reproductive care settings must understand what is meant by healthy sexual function before they can begin to recognize and understand how a behavior becomes dysfunctional. A newer vision of sexuality in women (Basson, 2002; Burrows & Resnick-Anderson, 2011) takes into account relationships for women by including emotional intimacy, sexual stimuli, and relationship satisfaction as a model of sexual response. Thus, women's sexual response is far more complex and complicated than the achievement of an orgasm with intercourse. Sexuality for women encompasses much more than the physical dimension of the sex act.

Sexual dysfunction for women is defined as any sexual situation that causes personal distress for the woman herself. If the woman is comfortable with a situation, there is no dysfunction. If she is distressed by any physical, emotional, or relationship aspect of her sexuality, she may be experiencing a dysfunction (Kellogg-Spadt, 2010). Dysfunction can be manifested in the form of pain, arousal disorder, orgasmic disorder, or desire disorder (American Psychiatric Association [APA], 2013).

Nursing Insight—*Toward a universal view of sexual health*

Several years ago, the World Health Organization and the World Association for Sexology convened a panel of experts to address the state of sexual health globally. The experts posited that "sexual health is a state of physical, emotional, mental, and social well-being, in relation to sexuality; it is not merely the absence of disease, dysfunction, or infirmity. Sexual health requires a positive and respectful approach to sexuality and sexual relationships, as well as the possibility of having pleasurable and safe sexual experiences, free of coercion, discrimination, and violence. For sexual health to be attained and maintained, the sexual rights of all persons must be respected, protected, and fulfilled" (World Health Organization, 2006).

ASSESSMENT

Assessment of sexuality and quality of life represents an essential component of holistic care. A first step in the sexual and reproductive health assessment involves the establishment of a trusting relationship in which the patient feels safe asking questions and sharing concerns. Discussion of sexual issues can be embarrassing for women. Nurses need to be aware of their own sexual biases and beliefs and educate themselves about the many aspects of sexuality. When assessing women for sexual concerns, it is important not to make assumptions about partner preferences or sexual activity. Misguided assumptions can bring an abrupt ending to any therapeutic communications. For example, speaking with a woman about contraceptive choices may halt further dialogue with the patient who is lesbian and has sexual concerns unrelated to a heterosexual relationship (Davis & Willoughby, 2010; Kellogg-Spadt, 2011).

Optimizing Outcomes—**A tool to help identify female hypoactive sexual desire disorder**

Generalized acquired hypoactive sexual desire disorder (HSDD) is the most common form of female sexual dysfunction (FSD). The Decreased Sexual Desire Screener (DSDS) is a sensitive, easy-to-use 5-question diagnostic tool developed to enable health-care providers who are not experts in the field of FSD to diagnose the condition with high accuracy in pre-, peri-, and postmenopausal women in only a few minutes. The use of screening tools such as the DSDS enables nurses and other members of the health-care team to quickly identify patients who may benefit from further evaluation and treatment (Clayton, Goldfischer, Goldstein, DeRogatis, Nappi, Lewis-D'Agostino, et al., 2013).

When working with very young patients, the nurse must avoid communicating personal views that adolescent sexual behavior is wrong or shameful. Regardless of involvement in sexual activity, teenagers need a reliable source of education and information. They must first feel accepted before they can ask questions and share concerns about sexuality and sexual behavior.

Optimizing Outcomes—Providing reproductive care for women with disabilities

Professionals who care for women with long-term disabilities may make the mistake of overlooking their patients' sexual identity and reproductive care needs. Longstanding societal myths regarding sexuality and disability traditionally viewed disabled women to be "different," asexual, and unable to be mothers. These myths held that those who were single were celibate and those who were intimately involved should be grateful for their sexual relationships. Nurses must reject these myths and seek to understand the impact of the disability on their patient's sexuality. Holistic reproductive care centers on validating the disabled person's sexual identity, which begins with initiating discussion of the woman's sexual function and safer sex practices (Basson, 1998).

Assessing women for current or past problems that may interfere with or contraindicate pregnancy or the use of certain types of **contraception** (products that prevent pregnancy) is an important nursing role in reproductive health care. For example, women with chronic health problems such as diabetes, stroke, multiple sclerosis, cancer, or pain may be taking medications that are contraindicated with certain contraceptives or are associated with fetal anomalies (Table 6-1). Individualized counseling, guidance, and reliable information help empower them to make informed, realistic choices about reproductive planning. Other chronic conditions, including endometriosis and polycystic ovarian disease, may interfere with fertility and create a sense of powerlessness in those who desire pregnancy. Nurses are in a unique position to listen generously to these women, make appropriate referrals, and assist them in resolving their grief and feelings of loss (ACOG, 2011b; Davis & Willoughby, 2010).

Table 6-1 Drugs That Adversely Affect the Female Reproductive System

Drug Class	Drug	Possible Adverse Reactions
Androgens	Danazol	Vaginitis, with itching, dryness, burning, or bleeding; amenorrhea
	Fluoxymesterone, methyltestosterone, testosterone	Amenorrhea and other menstrual irregularities; virilization, including clitoral enlargement
Antidepressants	Tricyclic antidepressants	Changed libido, menstrual irregularity
	Selective serotonin reuptake inhibitors	Decreased libido, anorgasmia
Antihypertensives	Clonidine, reserpine	Decreased libido
	Methyldopa	Decreased libido, amenorrhea
Antipsychotics	Chlorpromazine, perphenazine, prochlorperazine, thioridazine, trifluoperazine, haloperidol	Inhibition of ovulation (chlorpromazine only), menstrual irregularities, amenorrhea, change in libido
Beta blockers	Atenolol, labetalol hydrochloride, nadolol, propranolol hydrochloride, metoprolol	Decreased libido
Cardiac glycosides	Digoxin	Changes in cellular layer of vaginal walls in postmenopausal women
Corticosteroids	Dexamethasone, hydrocortisone, prednisone	Amenorrhea and menstrual irregularities
Cytotoxics	Busulfan	Amenorrhea with menopausal symptoms in premenopausal women, ovarian suppression, ovarian fibrosis and atrophy
	Chlorambucil	Amenorrhea
	Cyclophosphamide	Gonadal suppression (possibly irreversible), amenorrhea, ovarian fibrosis
	Methotrexate	Menstrual dysfunction, infertility
	Tamoxifen	Vaginal discharge or bleeding, menstrual irregularities, pruritus vulvae (intense itching of the female external genitalia)
	Thiotepa	Amenorrhea
Estrogens	Conjugated estrogens, esterified estrogens, estradiol, estrone, ethinyl estradiol	Altered menstrual flow, dysmenorrhea, amenorrhea, cervical erosion or abnormal secretions, enlargement of uterine fibromas, vaginal candidiasis
	Dienestrol	Vaginal discharge, uterine bleeding with excessive use
Progestins	Medroxyprogesterone acetate, norethindrone, norgestrel, progesterone	Breakthrough bleeding, dysmenorrhea, amenorrhea, cervical erosion, and abnormal secretions
Thyroid hormones	Levothyroxine sodium, thyroid USP, and others	Menstrual irregularities with excessive doses
Miscellaneous	Lithium carbonate	Decreased libido
	L-tryptophan	Decreased libido
	Spironolactone	Menstrual irregularities, amenorrhea, possible polycystic ovarian syndrome

Source: Dillon, P. M. (2007). *Nursing health assessment. Clinical pocket guide* (pp. 234–235). Philadelphia, PA: F.A. Davis. Reprinted with permission.

Women also need to be counseled about the ideal age for childbearing and the implications of delaying pregnancy too long. Those who have not conceived by the mid- to late 30s may remain childless and burdened with guilt. Outside pressures exerted by cultural influences and family expectations often compound the feelings of remorse. Providing all women with current, factual information about the natural aging process and its influence on fertility empowers women of all ages to make informed decisions that best suit their needs.

Obtaining the Sexual History

The sexual history elicits information concerning prior treatment for sexually transmitted infections (STIs), pain with intercourse **(dyspareunia),** postcoital spotting or bleeding, and frequency of intercourse. Women who have intercourse more frequently and on a regular basis are more likely to become pregnant. The probability for pregnancy with each unprotected intercourse is about 15% to 20% (Trussell & Guthrie, 2011). An important component of holistic reproductive care centers on helping women to understand their body's natural functioning in relation to the menstrual cycle, so that they can problem solve about the timing of intercourse to achieve pregnancy, if desired.

The nurse also inquires about the number of past sexual partners. This information is useful in developing an estimate of the patient's risk for STIs and guides the nurse in providing appropriate education about safe sex practices. It is estimated that 4 out of 10 Americans between 18 and 59 years of age have had five or more partners (National Health Statistics Reports, 2011). Because the risk of contracting a sexually transmitted infection increases with each sexual partner, this information is very important for women whose reproductive life plan includes future pregnancy. Sexual health promotion includes providing correct information about the implications of multiple sexual partners; this information empowers women to make knowledgeable, informed choices. Depending on the situation and purpose of the visit, other appropriate components of the patient assessment may include a physical examination and diagnostic testing (Higgins & Davis, 2011).

 Now Can You—Discuss the nurse's role in reproductive health care?

1. Explain why nurses who work in a reproductive health-care setting must be comfortable with their own sexuality?
2. Develop six questions that will assist with taking a patient's sexual history?
3. Analyze the nurse's role in the reproductive health assessment?

NURSING DIAGNOSES FOR PATIENTS SEEKING CONTRACEPTIVE CARE

Depending on the purpose of the visit and analysis of the assessment findings, a number of nursing diagnoses may be appropriate. For women seeking contraception, diagnoses may include decisional conflict regarding choice of birth control because of a health concern, contraceptive alternatives, or the partner's willingness to agree on the contraceptive method. Other possible nursing diagnoses are listed in Box 6-1.

 legal alert—Be knowledgeable of laws regarding reproductive health care for minors

Nurses who provide counseling or referrals to minors must be knowledgeable of the legal rights and restrictions in place in their practice state. State and federal laws may limit a minor's ability to access reproductive health services independent of her parents or guardian. In addition, not all states allow minors to consent to contraceptive services and prenatal care; consent by a minor to place a child for adoption or obtain abortion services also varies by state. The Guttmacher Institute Web site (www.guttmacher.org) serves as an excellent resource for state-by-state consent laws related to minors (Guttmacher Institute, 2012; Simmonds & Likis, 2011).

Where Research and Practice Meet:
Contraceptive Care for Women With Cognitive Disabilities

For years, community contraception services have assisted individuals with learning disabilities and other vulnerable adults. However, many women with learning disabilities feel that they do not have an opportunity to make their own decisions (e.g., initiating, continuing, and discontinuing a contraceptive method) regarding family planning (Rowlands, 2011).

In 2012, United Kingdom researchers Earle, Tilley, and Walmsley conducted a qualitative study of the families of women with learning disabilities and staff who work with them to examine influences on personal choice of contraception. Their findings revealed that women with learning disabilities who use contraceptives often don't get the final say over the type of contraception they use, and furthermore, are often not sexually active. Formal assessments for mental capacity had been performed for only 32% of the women taking contraceptives, 62% had been involved in contraceptive discussions, and a mere 38% had made the final decision about contraceptive type. The contraceptive implant was the most common form of contraception used, followed by the combined contraceptive pill. Interestingly, only 28% of the women were sexually active. Based on their findings, the researchers suggest that future investigation explore how practices such as prescribing contraception for a "just in case" scenario or to control menstruation are negotiated between individuals, their guardians, family members, advocates, and professionals (Earle, Tilley, & Walmsley, 2012; Tilley, Earle, Walmsley, & Atkinson, 2012).

Box 6-1 Possible Nursing Diagnoses for Reproductive Care

Ineffective Sexuality patterns related to fear of pregnancy

Knowledge Deficit related to new use of the contraceptive method of choice

Effective Therapeutic Management related to birth control method of choice

Risk for Spiritual Distress related to discrepancy between religious or cultural beliefs and choice of contraception

Risk for Infection related to use of contraceptive method or unprotected sexual intercourse

Broken skin or mucous membrane after surgery or intrauterine device (IUD) insertion

Fear related to contraceptive method side effects

Source: Bulechek, Butcher, Dochterman, & Wagner (2013); Johnson, Moorhead, Bulechek, Butcher, Maas, & Swanson (2012); Moorhead, Johnson, Maas, & Swanson (2013).

PLANNING AND IMPLEMENTATION OF CARE

Regardless of the patient's age and contraceptive method selected, the nurse must first seek the woman's confirmation that she truly wants contraception. Birth control is always an individual choice. Feelings of helplessness and manipulation may result when the woman believes that someone else has decided what is "best" for her or coerces her into contraceptive use.

One of the primary goals during the contraceptive care visit is to determine and provide the contraceptive method of "best fit" for the woman or couple. Obtaining the medical, social, and cultural history helps to safeguard the patient's health and guide discussion of the contraceptive choices available to her. Patients often come for care with a specific birth control method in mind. However, it is essential that the nurse explore the woman's knowledge and understanding of contraceptive choices, her motivations for using a method, and her level of commitment to use the method consistently. On occasion, the desired contraceptive method is contraindicated or associated with side effects that outweigh the personal benefits. Open, honest discussion where appropriate information can be provided in a nonthreatening environment empowers the patient to make an informed choice of a birth control method that is best suited to her lifestyle (Fig. 6-1).

 Across Care Settings: **Enhancing contraceptive decision making**

The choice of a contraceptive method usually rests with the individual, although certain types of birth control may not be the best fit for special populations. Methods that require planning ahead, visiting a restroom for insertion, or are considered "messy" may not be the best choice for adolescents. Combination hormonal methods may be contraindicated in women with a history of breast cancer or diabetes, and these patients need assistance in finding another method that safely suits their lifestyle and health needs. An essential nursing role centers on obtaining a comprehensive history and educating patients about options, special considerations, and side effects. Often the nurse enlists the assistance of other health professionals such as health educators, social workers, translators, and home health workers in teaching about contraception and in managing appropriate follow-up care.

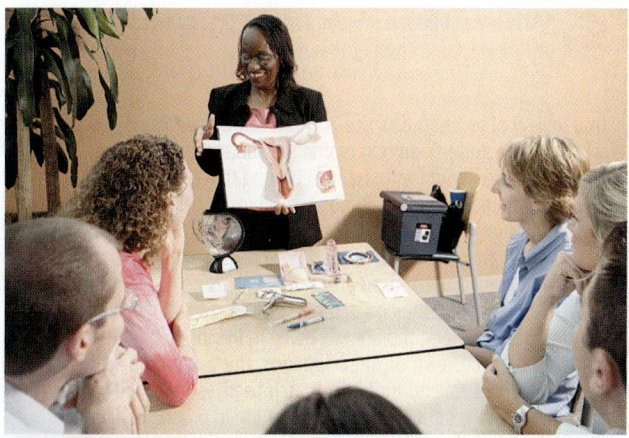

Figure 6-1 Teaching about contraception is an essential component of reproductive health care.

EVALUATION

When the purpose of the reproductive health visit is obtaining contraception, an immediate evaluation may take place at the conclusion of the patient encounter. This evaluation centers on mutually agreed on outcomes that reflect the patient's understanding of, and comfort level with, the chosen method. Examples of possible outcomes are listed below.

The patient:

- Voices understanding about the selected contraceptive method.
- Voices an understanding of all information necessary to provide informed consent.
- Voices a comfort level with use of the contraceptive method selected.

Intermediate and long-term evaluation of outcomes is especially important in the area of contraceptive care because patients who discontinue use of a birth control method are at risk for pregnancy. Primary prevention of unintended pregnancy includes an evaluation of a patient's satisfaction with her chosen contraceptive method (Taylor & James, 2011). Ideally, patients should be reassessed within a few months after initiating a new method. At this time, appropriate outcomes may include the following.

The patient:

- Has used the contraceptive method correctly and consistently.
- Has experienced no adverse side effects from use of the contraceptive method.
- Voices continued satisfaction with the selected contraceptive method.
- Consistently uses the contraceptive method without pregnancy for the following year.

 Optimizing Outcomes—**Using evidence-based guidelines to provide contraceptive care to all women, regardless of health status**

The use of evidence-based medical eligibility guidelines to prescribe contraceptive methods is pivotal in ensuring safe access to and quality of family planning services for all women. In 2010, the Centers for Disease Control and Prevention (CDC) released the first U.S. version of the World Health Organization's advisory on Medical Eligibility Criteria (MEC) for various contraceptive methods. Four numeric categories describe the acceptability of prescribing a contraceptive method in relationship to specific medical conditions (CDC, 2010, 2011a; WHO, 2010):

- Category 1—A condition for which there is no restriction for use of a given contraceptive method.
- Category 2—A condition for which the advantages of using a given method generally outweigh the theoretical or proven risks.
- Category 3—A condition for which the theoretical or proven risks of using a given contraceptive method usually outweigh the advantages.
- Category 4—A condition that represents an unacceptable health risk for use of a given contraceptive method.

In 2013, the CDC released the *U.S. Selected Practice Recommendations for Contraceptive Use,* 2013 (U.S. SPR), a companion document that offers guidance on how to use various contraceptive methods most effectively. Like the U.S. MEC[MR1], the U.S. SPR was adopted from global guidance published by the World Health Organization. Simply stated, the U.S. MEC summarizes the "who" and the U.S. SPR focuses on the "how" (ACOG, 2013b; U.S. Selected Practice Recommendations for Contraceptive Use, 2013).

Following the guidelines helps to ensure that women are not exposed to inappropriate risks, nor are they denied access to methods that are medically appropriate for them (Curtis & Peterson, 2011; Edmunds, 2011; Lockwood & Hillard, 2010).

Toward Achieving the National Goals for Reproductive Life Planning

The *Healthy People 2020* national initiative includes a number of goals that directly address reproductive health (Box 6-2). Individuals and couples who seek assistance with this aspect of their lives may need counseling about fertility and methods of contraception. Seeking guidance and making decisions about contraception are prompted by a number of influences but generally center on a desire to take control over one's reproductive life.

Nurses can be instrumental in helping the nation to achieve the objectives by assisting women who want to practice safe sex and providing effective contraception when they do not desire to become pregnant. Women of all ages are capable of responsible sexual behavior when given enough education, motivation, and opportunity. One of the challenges for nurses in the community concerns poor women who are unable to afford contraception as well as those with fertility problems who cannot afford special treatments to achieve pregnancy. Nurses must advocate for all women to ensure that reproductive care is available to all persons, regardless of socioeconomic status.

Box 6-2 *Healthy People 2020* **National Goals Related to Reproductive Life Planning**

Several of the National Health Goals are related to reproductive life planning. These include the following:

- Reduce the proportion of women experiencing pregnancy despite use of a reversible contraceptive method from a baseline of 12.4% to a target of 9.9%.
- Increase the proportion of pregnancies that are intended from a baseline of 51% to a target of 56%.
- Decrease the proportion of pregnancies conceived within 18 months of a previous birth from a baseline of 35.3% to a target of 31.7%.
- Increase the proportion of females or their partners at risk of unintended pregnancy who used contraception at most recent sexual intercourse from a baseline of 83% to a target of 91.3%.
- Increase the proportion of publicly funded family planning clinics that offer the full-range of FDA-approved methods of contraception, including emergency contraception onsite.
- Increase the proportion of sexually active males aged 15 to 44 years who received reproductive health services from a baseline of 14.9%–16.4%.

Source: U.S. Department of Health and Human Services (DHHS). (2012). *Healthy People 2020 Family Planning Objectives.* Washington, DC: DHHS.

Although the rate of unintended pregnancies in the United States has declined, the rate of unintentional pregnancy remains highest among young, less educated women with low income (Dehlendorf, Bryant, Huddleston, Jacoby, & Fujimoto, 2010). These individuals, who may be less likely to afford birth control or reach a health-care clinic, must be a major focus for education and support from nurses in the community. All women deserve holistic health care along with culturally, educationally, and developmentally appropriate information to empower them to make realistic decisions about reproductive life planning.

 Optimizing Outcomes—**Supporting legislation to mandate insurance coverage for contraception**

The Association of Women's Health, Obstetric and Neonatal Nurses (AWHONN) believes that a woman has the right to choose a particular contraceptive method based on whether it is the most appropriate one for her, not whether the method is covered by her insurance plan. Hence, AWHONN supports legislation and policies that mandate insurance coverage for the range of U.S. Food and Drug Administration-approved contraceptive drugs and devices, along with related services (AWHONN, 2009b).

Providing Contraceptive Care: Methods of Contraception

NATURAL FAMILY PLANNING AND FERTILITY AWARENESS

- *Natural Family Planning* (NFP) is a contraceptive method that involves identifying the fertile time period and avoiding intercourse during that time every cycle. It is the only method of contraception acceptable to the Roman Catholic Church.
- *Fertility Awareness-Based* methods (FAMs) identify the fertile time during the cycle and use abstinence or other contraceptive methods during the fertile periods. These methods require motivation and

---

 Where Research and Practice Meet: **Factors Associated With Unprotected Sex Among Women**

In a review of recent (i.e., since 2005) research on factors associated with unprotected sex among women in the United States, nurse researchers Paterno and Jordan (2012) found that unprotected sex has been associated with a multitude of variables including the following: increasing age, being married, establishment of trust, recent experience of intimate partner violence, contraceptive side effects, infrequent sexual intercourse, decreased arousal and pleasure caused by contraceptive use, lack of insurance, negative attitude to contraceptives, birth control sabotage, lack of planning, being in the moment, and sex with a main partner. Based on their findings, the authors identified the need for nurses to lead further research to investigate the impact of cultural factors, relationship factors, attitude to pregnancy and motherhood, and reproductive coercion on prevention of pregnancy and sexually transmitted infections.

considerable counseling to be used effectively. They may interfere with sexual spontaneity and require several months of symptom/cycle charting before they may be used effectively.

Effectiveness

The effectiveness in preventing pregnancy depends on the exact method used, but it is generally around 75% effective.

 Optimizing Outcomes—**When teaching about NFP and FAMs of contraception**

The patient and her partner need to be fully committed to use these methods successfully. There are several variations: (1) the calendar, or rhythm, method in which the fertile days are calculated; (2) the standard days method in which color-coded strung beads are used to track infertile days; (3) the cervical mucus method (also called the "ovulation detection method" or the "Billings Ovulation Method") in which the changes in cervical mucus are used to track fertile periods; (4) the basal body temperature (BBT) method in which body temperature changes are used to detect the fertile period (Fig. 6-2; Box 6-3); and (5) the symptothermal method that combines the BBT and cervical mucus methods and involves recording various symptoms such as changes in cervical mucus, mittelschmerz (abdominal pain at midcycle), abdominal bloating, and the BBT to recognize signs of ovulation (Jennings & Burke, 2011). The woman needs to realize that stress or illness can affect her cycle and cause a variation in the fertile days. These methods are not best suited for adolescents or couples who would be devastated by an unplanned pregnancy. Because the "natural" methods identify fertile periods, couples who are attempting to conceive may also wish to use them.

Ovulation predictor kits detect the surge in luteinizing hormone (LH) that occurs 24 to 36 hours before ovulation. The kits vary in price and procedure but most are similar to home pregnancy tests and are performed on the woman's urine. Intercourse can then be timed to avoid or achieve pregnancy.

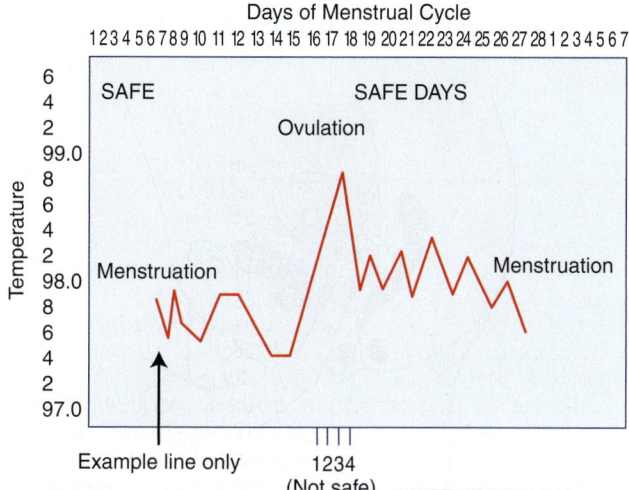

Figure 6-2 A basal body temperature chart.

Box 6-3 Basal Body Temperature as an Indicator of Ovulation

During the preovulatory phase, the basal temperature is usually below 98°F (36.7°C). As ovulation approaches, estrogen production increases. At its peak, estrogen may cause a slight drop, then a rise, in the basal temperature. Before ovulation, a surge in luteinizing hormone (LH) stimulates the production of progesterone. The LH surge causes a 0.5°F–1°F (0.3°C–0.6°C) rise in the basal temperature. These changes in the basal temperature create the biphasic pattern consistent with ovulation. Progesterone, a thermogenic, or heat-producing hormone, maintains the temperature increase during the second half of the menstrual cycle. Although the temperature elevation does not predict the exact day of ovulation, it does provide evidence of ovulation about 1 day after it has occurred. Release of the ovum probably occurs 24–36 hours before the first temperature elevation.

 Where Research and Practice Meet: **Internet-Based NFP Education Program**

In an effort to provide accurate, easily accessible natural family planning (NFP) information, a group of nurse NFP teachers developed a Web-based natural family planning (NFP) education and service program designed to help couples to either avoid or achieve pregnancy. Women who registered on the Web site were able to access an online electronic charting system, discussion forums, and have consultation from nurse NFP teachers, an obstetrician gynecologist with expertise in the use of NFP, and a bioethicist. Offered in both the English and Spanish languages, the online NFP system also notified users of possible health problems (e.g., unusual bleeding, infertility, and pregnancy) based on submitted information. The Web-based charting system recorded the results of either an electronic hormonal fertility monitor or self-observed cervical–vaginal mucus or both, and indicated the fertile phase in each user's cycle. After a 6-month pilot study to assess the program's efficacy and acceptability, the researchers concluded that the program was effective and efficient and provided an alternative method for teaching about the use of NFP methods. The researchers suggested that other women's health issues such as menstrual cycle questions could also be effectively addressed through the Internet and Web-based forums (Fehring, Schneider, & Raviele, 2011).

COITUS INTERRUPTUS

Coitus interruptus or the "withdrawal method" involves the man withdrawing his penis from the vagina before ejaculation. However, ejaculation may occur before withdrawal is complete and spermatozoa may be present in the pre-ejaculation fluid. Men with unpredictable or premature ejaculation have difficulty using this method successfully. Coitus interruptus does not eliminate the risk of sexually transmitted infections (Kowal, 2011).

Effectiveness

The typical effectiveness rate for this method is about 71%.

LACTATIONAL AMENORRHEA METHOD (LAM) (BREASTFEEDING)

Breastfeeding can be a temporary form of contraception, although it is used more effectively in underdeveloped countries where mothers breastfeed their infants exclusively. Some lactating mothers may ovulate but not menstruate. It is difficult to determine when fertility is restored.

This method works best when the mother exclusively breastfeeds, has had no menstrual period since giving birth, and whose infant is younger than 6 months of age.

Effectiveness

When the above conditions are met, the effectiveness rate for this method is about 98% (Kennedy & Trussell, 2011).

 Optimizing Outcomes—**When teaching patients about the lactational amenorrhea method**

It is important to teach women who wish to use the LAM that another method of contraception *must* be used in any of the following situations: (Kennedy & Trussell, 2011)

- Menstruation resumes
- The frequency or duration of breastfeeding is reduced
- Bottle feeding or regular food supplements are introduced
- The baby reaches 6 months of age

ABSTINENCE

Abstinence is the only contraceptive method with a 100% effectiveness rate. If a couple chooses to be **abstinent** (refrain from vaginal intercourse), intimacy and sexuality may be expressed in many other ways. Abstinence requires commitment and self-control, but success with this method can lead to increased self-esteem and enhanced communication about emotions and feelings. Abstinence can help adolescents learn negotiation skills (Santelli, Kowal, & Wheeler, 2011).

BARRIER METHODS

Barrier methods are relatively inexpensive, and some types can be used more than once. Although less effective than certain other forms of contraception, barrier methods have gained in popularity as a protective measure against the spread of sexually transmitted infections (STIs). If the woman is under 30 years of age, uses alcohol or recreational drugs, or has intercourse three or more times weekly, barrier methods are usually not as effective because of a decreased likelihood to use them consistently (Cates & Harwood, 2011).

Many women dislike barrier methods because they must be inserted or applied before intercourse. Most require a water-based lubricant, and these should never be used with an oil-based lubricant (e.g., baby oil, petroleum jelly, and vegetable oil) or vaginal yeast cream because these products cause latex deterioration. Barrier methods have few side effects, although latex allergy may lead to life-threatening anaphylaxis. There is evidence that consistent use of latex condoms reduces the rate of HIV transmission, and both condoms and diaphragms can reduce the risk of cervical STIs. Each of the barrier methods must be applied or inserted with clean hands. The key to success with these contraceptives is consistent use with every act of intercourse, and the nurse must ensure that women know how to use their barrier method correctly and that they are satisfied with their choice. Nurses should also inform patients about emergency (postcoital) contraception (EC), offer to provide it to them in advance of need, and ensure that they know how to obtain EC and also how to use it (Cates & Harwood, 2011).

 Nursing Insight—*Conditions that may make contraceptive barrier methods inadvisable*

When counseling patients about vaginal barrier contraceptives and spermicides, it is important to know about certain conditions that may make the use of one or more of them inadvisable. These conditions include (Cates & Harwood, 2011):

- Allergy to spermicide, rubber, latex, polyurethane, or ingredients in the spermicidal base
- Vaginal anatomy abnormalities (interfere with device fit, placement or retention)
- Inability to correctly insert the device
- History of toxic shock syndrome (female condom and spermicides other than the contraceptive sponge okay)
- Repeated urinary tract infections (female condom okay)
- Full-term delivery within the past 6 weeks, recent spontaneous or induced abortion, or vaginal bleeding, from any cause, including menstrual flow (for cervical cap and contraceptive sponge)

Source: Cates & Harwood (2011).

Diaphragm

The **diaphragm** is a latex or silicone dome-shaped barrier device with a spring rim that resembles half a tennis ball. It is filled with spermicide and inserted up into the vagina to cover the cervix. Diaphragms are available in several sizes and styles; the styles differ in the inner construction of the circular rim. Presently, the diaphragm must be fitted by a trained health-care professional. However, new products for over-the-counter availability are currently being tested (Cates & Harwood, 2011).

Use of the diaphragm requires some planning ahead, so this method may not be the best choice for adolescents. The diaphragm is inserted by the woman using her fingers or an inserter up to 6 hours before intercourse, and it must be filled with a spermicide applied inside and along the rim before insertion (Fig. 6-3). The diaphragm must remain in place for at least 6 hours after intercourse. If intercourse occurs again before 6 hours have elapsed, the diaphragm should be left undisturbed and another applicator-full of spermicide should be inserted into the vagina. The diaphragm should remain in place for 6 hours after the last act of intercourse. To ensure continued protection, the diaphragm should be replaced every 2 years, and it may need to be refitted after weight loss

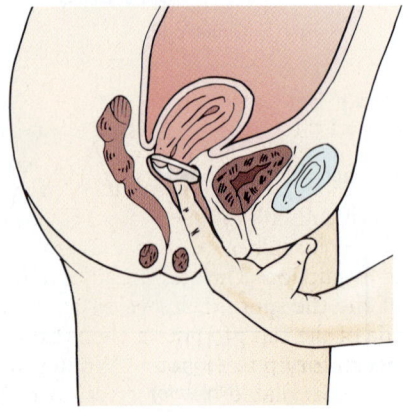

Figure 6-3 Diaphragm insertion.

or weight gain, term birth, or second trimester abortion (Hatcher, Trussell, Nelson, Cates, Stewart, & Kowal, 2011).

SIDE EFFECTS. Other than occasional allergic reactions to the diaphragm (silicone diaphragms are expected to reduce allergic adverse events experienced with latex) or spermicide, there are no side effects from a well-fitted device. There is an increased risk of urinary tract infections (UTIs) because of pressure of the diaphragm against the urethra, which may interfere with complete emptying of the bladder. Thus, women with a history of frequent UTIs should avoid this method. The diaphragm should not be used during menses, and it should not be worn for longer than 24 hours because of the risk of **toxic shock syndrome** (TSS), a rare, sometimes fatal disease caused by toxins produced by certain strains of the bacterium *Staphylococcus aureus*. Women with pelvic relaxation syndrome or a large cystocele are not suitable candidates for the diaphragm.

EFFECTIVENESS. The effectiveness in preventing pregnancy for typical use is around 84%. For this reason, the diaphragm may not be the best choice for a woman who would consider pregnancy a disaster in her life or for a woman who feels uncomfortable touching her genital area.

🅢 **Optimizing Outcomes**—When teaching patients about use of the diaphragm

The diaphragm must be in the correct position for it to be comfortable and work effectively as a contraceptive. The patient should practice insertion and removal of the diaphragm before leaving the clinic and be instructed to return with it in place for a recheck of proper fit 1 week later. Before each use, the diaphragm is carefully inspected for tears, holes, or damage. After removal, the device is cleaned with mild (nondeodorant, non-perfumed) soap and water, dried thoroughly, and stored in its case in a cool place. Talcum powder should never be used on the device or in the case, and oil-based vaginal medications or lubricants, which have a deleterious effect on the integrity of latex, should never be used with latex diaphragms (Cates & Harwood, 2011).

🅢 **legal alert**—Always inquire about latex allergy

Before dispensing latex diaphragms or latex male condoms, ask all patients about a personal or partner history of allergy to latex. Use of latex contraceptive devices is contraindicated in patients with latex sensitivity.

Cervical Cap

The **cervical cap** is a thimble-shaped silicone device that fits firmly around the base of the cervix close to the junction of the cervix and vaginal fornices (Fig. 6-4). The device has a pliable rim and is available in three sizes. It is somewhat more difficult to use than the diaphragm because it must be placed exactly over the cervix where it is held in place by suction. The seal provides a physical barrier to sperm and the spermicide placed on the inside and on the outside of the cap provides a chemical barrier. The cap may be worn for up to 48 hours. Women who choose the cervical cap, available by prescription only, should practice insertion and removal after the fitting and return

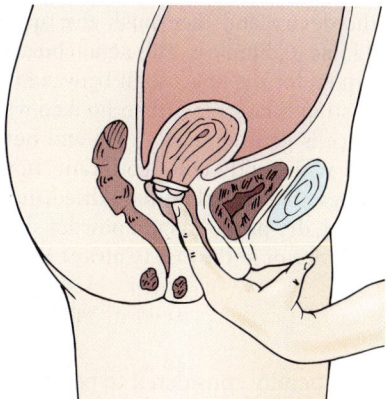

Figure 6-4 Cervical cap insertion.

in 1 week with the cap inserted to check for proper placement (Cates & Harwood, 2011).

✳ *Nursing Insight*—*When counseling patients about the cervical cap*

Certain women are not suitable candidates for the cervical cap. Patients who have a history of toxic shock syndrome, pelvic inflammatory disease (PID), cervicitis, papillomavirus infection, a previous abnormal Pap test or cervical cancer, and undiagnosed vaginal bleeding should choose another contraceptive method. Also, women who have an abnormally short or long cervix may not be able to use a cervical cap satisfactorily.

SIDE EFFECTS. There is evidence that the cervical cap can cause cervical irritation and erosion, and it is not recommended for women who are at high risk for HIV. Because the cervical cap is associated with a high failure rate, women who choose this method should receive information about emergency contraception methods.

EFFECTIVENESS. With typical use, the FemCap cervical cap failure rate ranges from 20% to 40% (after childbirth) so it may not be the best choice for the woman who would consider a pregnancy to be a disaster in her life. It is not as effective for contraception in women who have had a pregnancy. Because proper use of the cervical cap requires planning ahead and strong motivation, it may not be the best contraceptive method for adolescents.

🅢 **Optimizing Outcomes**—When teaching patients about use of the cervical cap

Before insertion, approximately one-third of the cap is filled with spermicide; a small amount of spermicide is also applied to the outside of the cap. Taking care not to spill the inner spermicide, the woman inserts the cap into the vagina and places it directly over the cervix. The woman is taught to use her finger to trace around the rim of the cap to make certain the entire cervix is covered. The cervical cap can be inserted up to 6 hours before intercourse and should remain in place for 6 hours after the last intercourse. No additional spermicide is necessary with repeated intercourse. The cap should never remain in place longer than 48 hours and it should never be used during menses or when a vaginal infection is present. To remove the cap, the woman is taught to rotate the device and then push the tip of her finger against the dome to dimple it. This action breaks the suction and allows room for the finger to fit between the dome and the removal strap. The strap is then hooked with the finger and the device is gently pulled down and out. The cap is then washed with mild (non-deodorant, non-perfumed) soap and water. The cap should be dried thoroughly and stored in a cool, dry place. Talcum powder should never be used on the device or in the case (Cates & Harwood, 2011).

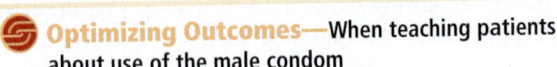

Condoms

Condoms are generally considered to be a male contraceptive device although the female condom (vaginal sheath) is also available. Male condoms may be made of latex rubber, polyurethane, or natural membranes. Latex male condoms are widely recognized for their role in preventing HIV infection and STIs. Natural skin condoms do not offer protection against HIV and STIs because they contain small pores that may permit the passage of viruses including HIV, hepatitis B, and herpes simplex. Although previous recommendations included combining condom use with the spermicide nonoxynol-9 (N-9), this practice is no longer advised, because of a higher cost, shorter shelf life, and lack of additive benefit (as compared with other lubricated condoms). Also, frequent use of condoms coated with N-9 may cause genital lesions and increase the transmission of STIs including HIV (Warner & Steiner, 2011). Condoms are nonreusable and act as a mechanical barrier between the female and male genitalia.

MALE CONDOMS. Male condoms are one of the oldest known methods of contraception. When used correctly, male condoms are placed over the erect penis before any genital, oral, or anal contact. Condoms are inexpensive, require no prescription, and are available in a variety of sizes, shapes, and colors. To prevent pregnancy and the spread of STIs, they must be used correctly at every act of intercourse.

Side Effects. Condoms may cause an anaphylactic reaction in patients who are allergic to latex. Individuals with latex allergies must choose condoms made of other materials.

Effectiveness. With typical use, male condoms are about 85% effective in preventing pregnancy.

Optimizing Outcomes—When teaching patients about use of the male condom

It is important to choose and use the correct size of condom. The condom is rolled onto the erect penis and should fit snugly. The reservoir tip should be left unobstructed or extra space at the end (of a condom with no reservoir tip) should be provided for collection of the semen. Care must be taken not to tear the condom or spill its contents during removal. When possible, patients should practice placing a condom on a penile model to enhance understanding of the proper technique. Immediately after intercourse, the man should hold the condom at the base of the penis and withdraw the penis while still erect, then check the condom for the presence of tears after removal. Expiration dates should be checked often and out-of-date condoms discarded. Condoms should always be stored in a cool, dry place and latex condoms only used with water-based lubricants (Warner & Steiner, 2011).

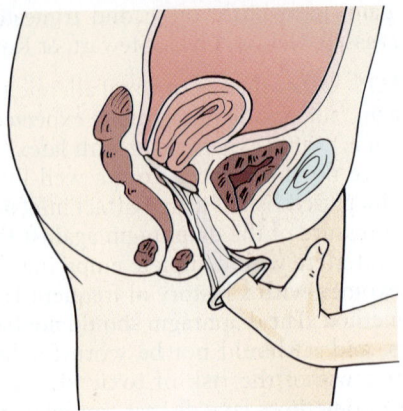

Figure 6-5 Insertion of a female condom.

FEMALE CONDOMS. Made of polyurethane in a "one size fits all," the female condom or vaginal sheath (Fig. 6-5) is less widely used than the male condom. The female condom resembles a sheath with a ring on each end: The closed end is inserted into the vagina and anchored around the cervix; the open end is placed at the vaginal introitus. The device is coated with a silicone-based lubricant, and additional (spermicide-free) lubricant for the outside is provided with the condom. Although no prescription is needed, female condoms are often difficult to find, and they are more expensive than male condoms. Because they contain no latex, female condoms are safe for use in individuals with latex allergies.

Side Effects. Common side effects associated with the female condom include allergic reactions and irritation.

Effectiveness. When used correctly and consistently, female condoms are about 79% to 95% effective in preventing pregnancy.

Optimizing Outcomes—When teaching patients about use of the female condom

Female condoms cannot be used at the same time as male condoms. The man must carefully direct his penis into the condom to keep from inserting it between the condom and the vaginal wall. The female condom can be used during oral sex. Some individuals complain that female condoms generate "noise" during intercourse, but lubricant seems to help alleviate this problem. Because it is a polyurethane-based device, the single-use female condom does not deteriorate with exposure to oil-based products; the product expiration date is 5 years from the date of manufacture (Cates & Harwood, 2011).

Spermicides

Spermicides are available in the form of gels, creams, foams, films, and suppositories. Readily available over the counter without the need for a prescription, all are inserted into the vagina or used with diaphragms or cervical caps. Spermicides act as chemical barriers that cause death of the spermatozoa before they can enter the cervix. Although spermicides can be messy, the lubrication afforded by the spermicide-based methods may improve sexual satisfaction for both partners.

Women who are at risk for HIV should not use spermicides as their only method of birth control (Hatcher et al., 2011). Because spermicidal suppositories and films require 10 to 15 minutes to become effective, women who feel they cannot comply with this time constraint may wish to use a spermicidal foam, cream, or gel instead. Because of the low effectiveness rates associated with spermicides, the woman who believes that pregnancy would be personally disastrous may wish to choose another contraceptive method.

SIDE EFFECTS. Spermicides should not be used in women with acute cervicitis because of the potential for further cervical irritation. Rarely, topical irritation may develop from contact with spermicides. When this occurs, the product should be discontinued and another contraceptive method selected.

EFFECTIVENESS. The typical use effectiveness of spermicides in preventing pregnancy is 71%.

Optimizing Outcomes—When teaching patients about the use of spermicides

The woman should wash her hands before inserting any spermicide. Spermicides are most effective when used with a diaphragm or cervical cap. Most contraceptive films and suppositories require a period of 15 minutes to elapse after insertion to become effective, and they should be inserted no longer than 1 hour before intercourse. The spermicide should be inserted deep into the vagina so that it makes contact with the cervix. Although douching is never recommended, it should be avoided for 6 hours after intercourse to avoid washing the spermicide away (Cates & Harwood, 2011). Douching in and of itself is not a reliable form of birth control.

Contraceptive Sponge

The contraceptive sponge is a single-use vaginal spermicide. Soft, round, and disposable, the polyurethane device has a concave dimple on one side that is designed to fit over the cervix; the other side contains a woven polyester loop to facilitate removal. The sponge is permeated with the spermicide nonoxynol-9.

SIDE EFFECTS. The contraceptive sponge is contraindicated in women who are allergic to the spermicide nonoxynol-9. The sponge should not be left in place for more than 30 hours (which includes the 6-hour waiting period after the last act of intercourse) because of the risk of toxic shock syndrome. It should not be used during menstruation or immediately after abortion or childbirth or if a woman has a history of toxic shock syndrome.

EFFECTIVENESS. The typical use effectiveness of the contraceptive sponge in preventing pregnancy is 84% to 87%.

Optimizing Outcomes—When teaching patients about use of the contraceptive sponge

The patient should wash her hands before inserting the sponge. The sponge is moistened thoroughly with tap water and inserted deep into the vagina prior to intercourse. It provides up to 24 hours of protection for repeated sexual intercourse. The sponge must remain in the vagina for at least 6 hours after the last act of intercourse before it is removed and discarded. The contraceptive sponge offers no protection against STIs or HIV (Warner & Steiner, 2011).

legal alert—Teach about toxic shock syndrome

Women who use the diaphragm, cervical cap, or contraceptive sponge should be aware of the possible association between these devices and toxic shock syndrome (TSS). Common signs of TSS include fever of sudden onset greater than 101.1°F (38.4°C), rash, and hypotension with a systolic blood pressure less than 90 mm Hg.

"What to say"—When talking with teens about sex, STIs, and contraception

Reproductive health-care nurses working with teens are perfectly positioned to provide counseling and factual, evidence-based information about sex, sexually transmitted infections, and methods of contraception. In any setting, it is important to allow the teen to ask questions in an atmosphere that fosters safety and comfort. To facilitate and focus the discussion, the nurse may wish to ask questions such as:

"Are you sexually active with girls, boys, or both?"

"Do you engage in vaginal, oral, or anal sex?"

"Are you using a contraceptive method?"

"What questions related to sex can I help you answer?"

When counseling about contraceptive methods, offering visual models along with written information is essential. Any time a contraceptive has been prescribed to a young patient, it is important to schedule a return visit in a few months to assess method compatibility and to provide additional counseling and support (Sullivan, 2010).

HORMONAL METHODS

Hormonal contraceptive methods include oral medications, the transdermal patch, the vaginal ring, long-acting injectables, the subdermal implant, and the progestin-releasing intrauterine device. Estrogen and progestins decrease the pituitary's release of follicle-stimulating hormone (FSH) and LH to prevent ovulation. Progestins also thicken cervical mucus to prevent sperm penetration.

Oral Contraceptives

This method, known as "the pill," or oral contraceptive pill (OCP), has been available for more than 40 years. Throughout that time, the dose of estrogen has significantly decreased and newer generation progestins have become safer with fewer side effects. It was once recommended that patients occasionally "take a break" from the pill because of the high hormonal dosages they contained. With today's formulations, however, patients can continue to take oral contraceptives into the perimenopausal years. Oral contraceptives are the most extensively studied medications in history (Hatcher et al., 2011).

Hormonal contraceptives contain a synthetic estrogen in the form of ethinyl estradiol, mestranol, or estradiol valerate; ethinyl estradiol is the most common estrogen used. Estrogens work by preventing the release of FSH from the anterior pituitary. When FSH levels are kept low, the ovarian follicle is unable to form, and ovulation is prevented (Nelson & Cwiak, 2011; Wilton, 2011).

Progestins provide effective contraception when used alone or in combination with estrogen. When combined with an estrogen, progestins inhibit the LH surge, which is required for ovulation. When used alone, progestins are believed to inhibit ovulation inconsistently. Progestin-only contraceptives are thought to function primarily by creating a thickened cervical mucus (which produces a hostile environment for sperm penetration) and by causing endometrial atrophy. These alterations inhibit egg implantation and decrease the penetration of sperm and ovum transport.

 Nursing Insight—*Progestin drospirenone and venous thromboembolism*

In 2012, the U.S. Food and Drug Administration (FDA) completed its review of earlier studies regarding the potential increased risk of blood clots in women who use oral contraceptives (OC) containing the progestin drospirenone. Based on this review, the FDA concluded that drospirenone-containing oral contraceptives might be associated with a higher risk for blood clots than other progestin-containing oral contraceptive pills. Presently, the FDA recommends that women talk with their health-care professional about their personal risk for blood clots before deciding which birth control method to use, and advises that health-care professionals consider the risks and benefits of drospirenone-containing OCs and a woman's risk for developing a clot before prescribing these drugs. Information about the studies has been added to the labels of all drospirenone-containing oral contraceptive pills (FDA, 2012).

In the United States, oral contraceptives are available in monophasic, biphasic, triphasic, and 4-phasic preparations. Monophasic formulas provide fixed doses of estrogen and progestin throughout a 21-day cycle. Biphasic preparations provide a constant amount of estrogen throughout the cycle, but there is an increased amount of progestin during the last 11 days. Triphasic formulas, designed to more closely mimic a natural cycle, provide varied levels of estrogen and progestin throughout the cycle. Triphasic preparations reduce the incidence of breakthrough bleeding (bleeding that occurs outside menstruation) in many women. The 4-phasic OCP, available in the United States since 2010, offers four progestin/estrogen dosing combinations during each 28-day cycle and is the first contraceptive to contain the "bioidentical" synthetic estrogen estradiol valerate (rather than ethinyl estradiol) (Nelson, 2010a).

Women who wish to use oral contraceptives should have their baseline blood pressure taken and recorded. Depending on the patient's history or symptoms, a breast and pelvic examination may be indicated; neither is needed before initiating OCPs in an asymptomatic woman. A Pap test is not needed prior to starting OCPs. STI testing, if indicated (based on symptoms, age, or institutional policy), may be serum or urine-based. No other screening tests are routinely needed unless the woman's history or blood pressure dictates a need for further assessment (Nelson & Cwiak, 2011). Most health-care providers schedule women for a return visit approximately 3 months after initiating the medication to confirm patient acceptance and correct use of the method and to detect any complications.

 Optimizing Outcomes—**Counseling about medications that decrease the effectiveness of oral contraceptives**

It is essential for the nurse to take a thorough history on any patient who wishes to use oral contraceptives for birth control. Certain medications such as rifampin (Rifadin, Rimactane), isoniazid, barbiturates, and griseofulvin (Fulvicin-U/F, Gris-PEG, Grifulvin V) can decrease the effectiveness of oral contraceptives, and higher doses of estrogen must be used. Vomiting and diarrhea affect the absorption of oral contraceptives, thus patients who experience these symptoms should use a backup method such as condoms. Recent research indicates that antibiotics do not affect the effectiveness of oral contraceptives (Nelson & Cwiak, 2011). Interactions with certain drugs such as acetaminophen, anticoagulants, and some anticonvulsants (e.g., phenytoin sodium, carbamazepine, primidone, and topiramate), may reduce efficacy of the OCP.

Many non-contraceptive benefits are associated with OCPs (Box 6-4). Healthy, non-obese perimenopausal women who do not smoke, who maintain a normal blood pressure, and who have a normal well-woman annual exam can safely use oral contraceptives. Oral contraceptives can moderate the irregular bleeding that often occurs during the perimenopausal period and provide contraception as well. When used on an extended cycle basis, hot flashes and vaginal dryness may also be alleviated (Nelson & Cwiak, 2011). The onset of menopause in women who use hormonal contraception may be difficult to detect.

CONTRAINDICATIONS. There are several absolute and relative contraindications to the use of combined oral contraceptive pills, and the nurse must be fully aware of them. Most contraindications to OCPs are related to the estrogen component. Relative contraindications include hypertension, migraine

---

Box 6-4 Noncontraceptive Benefits of Oral Contraceptive Pills

Oral contraceptive pills are associated with a decreased incidence of:
- Fibrocystic breast changes
- Iron-deficiency anemia, caused by a reduced amount of menstrual flow
- Colorectal, endometrial, and ovarian cancer and the formation of ovarian cysts
- Mittelschmerz and dysmenorrhea, because of the lack of ovulation
- Premenstrual dysphoric syndrome, as a result of increased progesterone levels
- Acute pelvic inflammatory disease (PID) and scarring of the fallopian tubes
- Ectopic pregnancy
- Endometriosis
- Uterine fibroids
- Osteopenia and osteoporosis

Critical Nursing Action Recognizing Contraindications to Oral Contraceptive Use

When counseling patients about oral contraceptive pills, the nurse must be aware of the following *absolute* contraindications to use:

- Cigarette smoking (at least 15 cigarettes/day) and age greater than 35 years
- Uncontrolled hypertension
- Undiagnosed abnormal vaginal bleeding
- Diabetes of more than 20 years' duration or with vascular complications
- History of pulmonary embolism or deep venous thrombosis or congestive heart failure
- Cerebrovascular disease or coronary artery disease
- Severe migraine headaches
- Estrogen-dependent neoplasia
- Known or suspected breast cancer
- Active liver disease
- Known or suspected pregnancy
- History of complications from organ transplants or presently preparing for transplant surgery
- Kidney or adrenal gland insufficiency/liver disease (drospirenone [fourth generation progestin] use only)

headaches, epilepsy, obstructive jaundice in pregnancy, gallbladder disease, surgery with prolonged immobilization, and sickle cell disease (Nelson & Cwiak, 2011; Spencer, McNamara, & Bonnema, 2011).

SIDE EFFECTS. A number of unpleasant and often troublesome side effects may accompany OCP use, especially during the first 3 months after initiation of the method. Nurses should teach patients that they might experience scanty periods, bleeding between periods (breakthrough bleeding), nausea, breast tenderness, headaches, and cyclic weight gain from fluid retention. If patients understand that these side effects may occur, they are more likely to seek health-care provider advice before arbitrarily discontinuing use of the OCP. The symptoms often subside after a few months of use, or they may be diminished with a change in routine or in the brand of contraceptive.

EFFECTIVENESS. The typical user effectiveness of combined oral contraceptives is 95% (Nelson & Cwiak, 2011).

Optimizing Outcomes—When teaching patients about use of oral contraceptive pills

The woman should identify a convenient and obvious place to keep her pills so that she will remember to take one every day. Ovulation suppressants work only when they are taken consistently and conscientiously. Several different protocols (e.g., "quick start," "first day start," and "Sunday start") are available for the initiation of OCPs. If a patient begins menstruating more than 5 days before the OCPs are started, a backup method of contraception should be used for the first 7 days. OCPs should be taken at approximately the same time each day. Many OCP formulations are available. Many are taken daily for 21 days; withdrawal bleeding usually occurs within 1 to 4 days after the last pill is taken. Some OCP packages contain seven inert or iron pills during the fourth week so that the woman never stops taking a pill. Other OCPs contain folate to reduce the risk of neural tube defects

in a pregnancy conceived while taking the product or shortly after discontinuing the product. Extended cycle oral contraceptives are also available. The extended cycle OCPs offer users the convenience of only four planned menses, each lasting about 2 to 3 days, per year. In addition to the nurse's verbal instructions, it is imperative that all women receive written information to take home with them and are encouraged to call if they have questions or experience any problems. Oral contraceptive pills offer no protection against STIs or HIV.

A major emphasis in patient teaching concerns warning signs that must be immediately reported to the health-care provider. The acronym "ACHES" can prompt the health-care provider and patient to remember the warning signs. "ACHES" uses the first letter of each sign of cardiovascular, liver, gallbladder, or thromboembolic complications that are side effects of estrogen use and can be life-threatening. If patients experience any of these signs, they must stop taking the pill and promptly contact the health-care provider. In addition to the "ACHES" signs, patients who become severely depressed or jaundiced or who develop a breast lump should notify their health-care provider.

legal alert—Teach the patient taking oral contraceptives to report ACHES

Abdominal pain (problem with liver or gallbladder)
Chest pain or shortness of breath (blood clot in lungs or heart)
Headaches: Sudden or persistent (hypertension or cardiovascular accident)
Eye problems (hypertension or vascular accident)
Severe leg pain (thromboembolism)

Nursing Insight—*OCP use in adolescents*

Teenage girls may benefit from taking OCPs to treat primary dysmenorrhea, anovulatory cycling, or acne. Because OCPs do not disrupt the orderly maturation of the hypothalamic–pituitary–ovarian axis, the adolescent's physical development will not be affected. Furthermore, the estrogen in the low-dose OCPs will not stunt the young girl's growth in height by prematurely closing the epiphyseal plates. Although adolescent girls who use OCPs do not accumulate increases in bone mineral density as rapidly as nonusers, bone changes are rapidly reversed after OCP cessation (Nelson & Cwiak, 2011; Perriera & Greenfield, 2011).

Low-Dose Progestin-Only Contraceptive Pills

Low-dose progestin-only contraceptive pills are often referred to as the "minipill" because they contain no estrogen. Although ovulation may occur, the progestins cause thickening of the cervical mucus and endometrial atrophy and reduce the activity of the cilia in the fallopian tubes. These changes inhibit implantation and decrease the penetration of sperm and ovum transport. The minipill is used primarily by women who have a contraindication to the estrogen component of the combination OCP. It must be taken continuously at the same time every day, and there are no days off between pill packs. A backup contraceptive method (or abstinence) should be used for the first 2 days after starting progestin-only contraceptive pills. The minipill may be used during breastfeeding (after the first 6 weeks postpartum) because it does not interfere with milk production. Certain drugs (e.g., rifampicin, certain anticonvulsants, some antiretroviral drugs, and Saint John's wort) may interact with progestin-only OCPs; women taking these medications should be advised to use a backup contraceptive method while taking them (Raymond, 2011a).

SIDE EFFECTS. Irregular menses frequently occur with the progestin-only pills. Also, this type of oral contraceptive may be associated with an increased number of persistent ovarian follicles.

CONTRAINDICATIONS. Women with current deep venous thrombosis or pulmonary embolus, systemic lupus erythematosus, severe cirrhosis or liver tumors, breast cancer (current or past), or a history of bariatric surgery (malabsorptive procedures) should not take the progestin-only oral contraceptive pills (Raymond, 2011a).

EFFECTIVENESS. The progestin-only contraceptive pills are 92% effective in preventing pregnancy; women should be advised to get a pregnancy test if they ever suspect they may be pregnant (Raymond, 2011a).

 Global Health Case Study Young Mexican Woman Who Believes She Is Infertile

Juanita, a 16-year-old Mexican adolescent, arrives at the family planning clinic with her 17-year-old girlfriend who has brought her in for a "checkup." During the health history, she tells the nurse that she believes she cannot have children. She confides that she has been having occasional unprotected sex with different boyfriends for the past year and has never gotten pregnant. But she believes she should use "something," just in case.

critical thinking questions

1. What are the major teaching needs for Juanita?

2. The nurse determines that this will be Juanita's first gynecological examination. What are some teaching needs and strategies?

3. In addition to specific instruction about the prescribed oral contraceptive, what other information should be emphasized?

♦ See Suggested Answers to Global Health Case Studies on Davis*Plus*.

 Where Research and Practice Meet: Text Messages and OCP Continuation

To determine if daily educational text messages had an effect on continuation of OCPs over a 6-month period, Castano and colleagues (2012) compared a group of OCP users who received routine care with a group of OCP users who received routine care plus daily educational text messages that incorporated 6 domains of OCP knowledge (i.e., risks, benefits, side effects, use, effectiveness, and mechanisms of action). The intervention was successful in increasing OCP continuation at 6 months, and continuation was enhanced most while the intervention was ongoing. Nurses who provide contraceptive counseling may wish to consider incorporating educational text messaging for OCP users as a strategy for improving patient acceptance and compliance (Castano, Bynum, Andres, Lara, & Westhoff, 2012).

Transdermal Contraceptive Patch

The transdermal contraceptive patch is applied to the abdomen, buttock, upper outer arm, or upper torso once weekly for 3 weeks, followed by one patch-free week. It should not be placed on the breasts. During the patch-free week, withdrawal bleeding occurs. The patch delivers low levels of estrogen and a progestin (norelgestromin) that are readily absorbed into the skin on a daily basis. The contraceptive patch costs slightly more than combined oral contraceptive pills.

SIDE EFFECTS. The side effects, contraindications, and warning signs for the patch are the same as for the oral contraceptive pills. However, the patch exposes patients to higher steady-state concentrations and lower peak concentrations of ethinyl estradiol (the estrogen component). There is a potential for increased adverse events in women using the patch (Nanda, 2011).

EFFECTIVENESS. The patch is about 95% effective in preventing pregnancy. Because of concerns that excessive adipose tissue may be associated with inconsistent levels of hormonal absorption, it is not recommended for women who weigh more than 198 pounds. In general, patient compliance is enhanced because of the once-weekly administration (Nanda, 2011).

 Optimizing Outcomes—When teaching patients about use of the transdermal contraceptive patch

The patch can cause skin irritation, particularly if it is placed on damp skin or in the same location every time. Thus, rotating the application site is recommended. Hypopigmentation at the site of the patch placement has been reported. Some women have complained that the patch adhesive catches fibers from their clothing; placing the patch on the buttock under the underpants may be desirable. Bathing and swimming should not interfere with the patch. If the patch becomes detached for more than 24 hours, a new one should be applied and another form of contraception used for the following 7 days. The transdermal contraceptive patch offers no protection against STIs or HIV (Nanda, 2011).

Vaginal Contraceptive Ring

The vaginal contraceptive ring contains estrogen and etonogestrel, a progestin. It is a soft, flexible ring that is inserted deep into the vagina by the fifth day of the menstrual cycle, and left in place for 3 weeks. It is removed during the fourth week to allow withdrawal bleeding, and a new ring is inserted at approximately the same time of day that the old ring was removed.

SIDE EFFECTS AND CONTRAINDICATIONS. The side effects, contraindications, and warning signs for the contraceptive ring are the same as for the oral contraceptive pills. The vaginal contraceptive ring is associated with increased vaginal discharge or wetness (not infection) when compared with other forms of hormonal contraception. Women who have significant pelvic relaxation, vaginal stenosis or obstruction, or who are uncomfortable touching their genitalia may not be suitable candidates for the vaginal contraceptive ring (Nanda, 2011).

EFFECTIVENESS. The ring slowly releases estrogen and progestin. Its effectiveness in preventing pregnancy is about 96% (Nanda, 2011).

> ### Optimizing Outcomes—When teaching patients about use of the vaginal contraceptive ring
>
> Patients are taught the following steps for insertion: wash and dry the hands; remove the ring from the foil pouch; assume a position of comfort; and squeeze the rim of the ring and place the leading edge into the vagina, sliding it into place until it is comfortable. The exact position of the ring is not critical for its function. Leave the ring in place for 3 weeks; then remove it for 7 days. To remove the ring, hook the index finger under the forward rim and pull it out. If possible, allow the patient to insert the ring in the examining room. The contraceptive ring should not be removed before, during, or after intercourse. The patient should not douche. The ring may be used concurrently with tampons. If the contraceptive ring comes out of the vagina for a time period of less than 3 hours, it should be rinsed with lukewarm water and reinserted. If the contraceptive ring is out of the vagina for over 3 hours, the ring may be rinsed and reinserted but a backup contraceptive method should be used for 7 days. Before discarding a used contraceptive ring, the patient should take care to protect the environment by placing the used ring in its original foil pouch or in a closed plastic bag. It should never be flushed down the toilet. Unopened vaginal rings must be protected from sunlight and high temperatures. The vaginal contraceptive ring offers no protection against STIs or HIV (Lindahl, 2011; Nanda, 2011).

Emergency Postcoital Contraception

Emergency contraception (EC) is available to women whose birth control methods fail or who have been the victims of sexual assault. Two forms of emergency postcoital contraception are available: hormonal methods, which include estrogen and progestin, progestin-only, and antiprogestin emergency contraceptive pills; and the insertion of a copper-releasing intrauterine device (IUD). Emergency contraception is available by prescription or office visit. The one-pill formulation of the EC Plan B One-Step is now available on drugstore shelves (i.e., without a prescription) to anyone, regardless of age or gender. Plan B is also available from generic manufacturers over-the-counter for women age 17 and older (Fine, 2011).

HORMONAL METHOD. Often referred-to as "the morning after pill," or the "emergency contraceptive pill" (ECP), there are three types of ECPs available in the United States: combined ECPs that contain both estrogen and progestin (two doses are taken 12 hours apart); one-dose progestin-only ECPs (i.e., Plan B One-Step [one tablet] and the generic formulation Next Choice [two tablets]), which contain levonorgestrel; and a one-dose ECP that contains an antiprogestin (ulipristal acetate [Ella]). Progestin-only ECPs have largely replaced the combined ECPs because they are more effective and are associated with fewer side effects. ECPs may be initiated immediately after unprotected intercourse or up to 120 hours after unprotected intercourse. Side effects (e.g., bleeding, nausea and vomiting, abdominal pain, breast tenderness, headache, dizziness, and fatigue) may occur but generally resolve within 24 hours. Although

certain ordinary OCPs can be taken for emergency contraception, the dose varies with the brand and may require taking a large number of tablets. Calculation of ECP effectiveness involves many assumptions (e.g., accurate estimates of timing of intercourse and cycle day) that are difficult to validate. Depending on the EC medication used, the efficacy in reducing pregnancy ranges from 52% to close to 100%. The antiprogestin ulipristal acetate, administered in a single 30 mg dose, is the most effective ECP option, with reported estimates of effectiveness ranging from 62% to 85%. It may be taken up to 5 days after unprotected intercourse (ACOG, 2010; Trussell & Raymond, 2012; Trussell & Schwarz, 2011).

IUD METHOD. The copper-releasing IUD can be inserted up to 5 days after unprotected intercourse to prevent pregnancy. If emergency IUD insertion is planned but cannot be carried out immediately, the patient should begin ECP treatment. The IUD is then inserted the day ECP treatment is initiated or the day after ECP treatment is completed or within 7 days of beginning the next menstrual period. If intrauterine contraception is initiated immediately after ECP use, the patient should abstain from intercourse or use a backup contraceptive method for the first 7 days. Because of the product's cost and the need for insertion by a trained professional, the IUD is used less frequently than the ECPs. The IUD is not recommended for women who have been raped or are at risk for STIs and pelvic infections (ACOG, 2010; Trussell & Raymond, 2012). IUDs are discussed in greater detail later in this chapter.

SIDE EFFECTS. Fewer side effects are associated with oral emergency contraceptive pills than with continuous oral contraceptives. The side effects for the IUD are the same whether it is being used as an emergency contraception method or as a long-term contraceptive. (See later discussion in this chapter.)

EFFECTIVENESS. Emergency insertion of a copper IUD is more effective than use of ECPs, reducing the risk of pregnancy following unprotected intercourse by more than 99% (Trussell & Raymond, 2012).

> ### Optimizing Outcomes—When teaching patients about postcoital emergency contraception
>
> Emergency contraception is sometimes confused with the medication abortion procedure. The high hormone levels in the oral contraceptive pills prevent or delay ovulation, thicken cervical mucus, alter sperm transport to prevent fertilization, and interfere with normal endometrial development. Emergency contraceptive pills may at times inhibit implantation of a fertilized egg in the endometrium. However, women should be informed that the best available evidence is that the ability of levonorgestrel and ulipristal acetate ECPs to prevent pregnancy can be fully accounted for by mechanisms that do not involve interference with post-fertilization events. Hence, ECPs do not cause abortion or harm an established pregnancy. Because ECPs can delay ovulation, women should be advised to abstain from intercourse or use a backup method of contraception for the remainder of their menstrual cycle (Trussell & Raymond, 2012; Trussell & Schwarz, 2011; WHO, 2012).
>
> Women should also be reminded that ECPs will not protect them from more than one episode of unprotected

intercourse. Patients who wish to begin OCPs as their contraceptive method may initiate a new pill pack the day after ECP treatment is completed and should abstain from intercourse or use a backup method for the first 7 days. If the patient initiates a non-OCP hormonal contraceptive method (e.g., implant, injectable, vaginal contraceptive ring, or transdermal patch) immediately after ECP treatment, she should use a backup method (e.g., condoms) for the remainder of her cycle and have a pregnancy test 3 weeks later to rule out pregnancy that may have resulted from ECP failure (Trussell & Raymond, 2012; Trussell & Schwarz, 2011; WHO, 2012).

The IUD is suitable for women who wish to have the benefit of long-term contraception. Insertion of the IUD within 5 days after intercourse causes an alteration in the endometrium to prevent implantation. With either EC method, patients should take a pregnancy test and/or contact their health-care providers if no period occurs within 3 weeks (Trussell & Schwarz, 2011). Emergency contraception offers no protection against STIs or HIV.

It is important that nurses who provide reproductive health care ensure that women and adolescents receive comprehensive contraceptive education, including information on the use, indications, side effects, and ways to obtain emergency contraceptives. Nurses can promote heightened public awareness of and access to emergency contraceptives and advocate for their availability in local health clinics and hospital emergency departments. Because of the rising rates of maternal morbidity and mortality in the United States, it is incumbent on nurses to use all possible opportunities to counsel women about strategies for planning and spacing pregnancies appropriately and to facilitate their access to emergency contraception (AWHONN, 2012; Ruhl, 2012).

Injectable Hormonal Contraceptive Methods

DEPO-PROVERA (DMPA-IM), DEPO-SUBQ PROVERA 104 (DEPOT MEDROXYPROGESTERONE). Depo-Provera (medroxyprogesterone acetate) is a progestin-only long-term contraceptive. Its effects last about 3 months, and it is injected either intramuscularly (150 mg) or subcutaneously (104 mg). The first injection should be given within the first 5 to 7 days of menstruation to ensure the patient is not pregnant. Medroxyprogesterone 150 mg is injected deeply into the deltoid or gluteus maximus muscle and functions by suppressing ovulation and altering the cervical environment. The administration site should not be massaged after injection because this action may reduce the effectiveness of DMPA (Bartz & Goldberg, 2011).

Depo-SubQ Provera 104 was the first subcutaneous hormonal contraceptive product available. It is administered into the anterior thigh or the abdomen and functions by preventing ovulation and producing thinning of the endometrium. This formulation has equivalent efficacy as the conventional intramuscular injection form, with 30% lower progestin dose because of a slower and more sustained absorption. In addition, for many, the injection is less painful than IM administration. On average, ovulation is restored within 10 months after discontinuation of the medication (both dosages) (Frederick, Voedisch, & Blumenthal, 2010).

Side Effects. Irregular bleeding is the most common side effect of Depo-Provera. Most women who use this method experience spotting during the first few months, usually until the second injection. Amenorrhea often occurs after about 6 months of use. Other side effects include weight gain, depression, headache, and breast tenderness. Although severe allergic reactions occur rarely, some clinics ask patients to remain nearby for 20 minutes after an injection. Depo-Provera may produce temporary and usually reversible decreased bone mineral density (Bartz & Goldberg, 2011; Letishock, Pariseau, Rooholamini, & Ammerman, 2011).

Effectiveness. The typical effectiveness for Depo-Provera appears to be greater than 99% (Bartz & Goldberg, 2011).

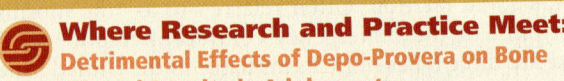

Optimizing Outcomes—When teaching patients about injectable hormonal contraception

Women who desire pregnancy within the next year may wish to choose another contraceptive method that is more easily reversible. Depo-Provera usually causes very light menstrual periods or amenorrhea, along with improvement in menstrual symptoms (e.g., ovulation pain, dysmenorrhea, and breast tenderness). However, Depo-Provera may be associated with weight gain and a temporary reduction in bone mineral density. Patients who use DMPA should include adequate vitamin D and calcium in their diet (1,200 mg/day) and perform daily weight-bearing exercise to enhance bone density maintenance and to offset weight gain. Clinic visits must be scheduled every 3 months for the contraceptive injection. Providing a reminder card that includes the date of the next injection is helpful, and some women set their PDA calendars or cell phones to alarm on the date. Because DMPA is injected, it cannot be reversed or stopped abruptly. Women who wish to hide their use of contraception from a partner or others may find this method to be particularly appealing. Because it contains no estrogen, DMPA can be safely given to breastfeeding mothers (initiated after the mature milk has come in—usually 7 days postpartum) and to women with known risk factors for venous thromboembolism, coronary artery disease, congestive heart failure, or cerebrovascular disease. DMPA has been used effectively to decrease the bleeding associated with uterine fibroid tumors, and it is associated with a reduced risk of endometrial cancer, pelvic infection, and ectopic pregnancy. Injectable hormonal contraception offers no protection against STIs or HIV (ACOG, 2006; Bartz & Goldberg, 2011).

Where Research and Practice Meet: Detrimental Effects of Depo-Provera on Bone Mineral Density in Adolescents

Findings from a 2005 prospective cohort trial established that adolescents are at increased risk for detrimental effects of Depo-Provera on bone mineral density (BMD). Study participants included 14- to 18-year-old women, in whom bone density is expected to increase as a result of continued bone growth and development. Those who used Depo-Provera experienced significant losses in bone mineral density at both the hip and spine in comparison with participants not using Depo-Provera, whose bone mineral density increased. After discontinuation of Depo-Provera, BMD significantly improved (Scholes et al., 2005). Subsequent research has revealed that the majority of BMD loss occurs in the first year of DMPA use, and near complete recovery of BMD is seen after DMPA discontinuation (Harel, Johnson, Gold, &

Cromer et al., 2010; Meier, Brauchli, Jick, Kraenzlin, & Meier, 2010; Williams, 2012). Recommendations from professional organizations including the American College of Obstetricians and Gynecologists (ACOG), the Society for Adolescent Medicine (SAM), and the World Health Organization (WHO) state that for the majority of adolescents, the benefits of DMPA use outweigh the potential risks (Bartz & Goldberg, 2011). During contraceptive counseling, nurses must empower young patients with information about decreased bone mineral density and Depo-Provera and assist them in making appropriate contraceptive choices.

SUBDERMAL HORMONAL IMPLANT NEXPLANON. Nexplanon, a second generation of Implanon, is a subdermal contraceptive that is effective for 3 years. The single-rod implant, which is inserted on the inner side of the woman's upper arm, contains etonogestrel (ENG), a progestin. Nexplanon functions to prevent pregnancy by suppressing ovulation, altering the endometrial structure, and creating a thickened cervical mucus that hinders sperm penetration. Etonogestrel is metabolized by the liver. Certain antiepileptic agents, certain antiretroviral agents and rifampicin may interfere with absorption and contraceptive effectiveness. Nexplanon contains barium to allow for localization on x-ray or CT scan. The implant may be inserted at any time during the menstrual cycle as long as pregnancy has been reasonably excluded; after childbirth, the insertion of the implant is safe at any time in non-breastfeeding women (ACOG, 2011b; Bonnema, McNamara, & Spencer, 2011; Raymond, 2011b).

Side Effects. Bleeding irregularities frequently occur during the first several months after insertion; amenorrhea becomes more common with increasing duration of use. Other reported adverse symptoms include breast pain, emotional lability, weight gain, headache, nausea, abdominal pain, loss of libido, and vaginal dryness (Raymond, 2011b).

Effectiveness. Effectiveness rates approach 100%.

⑤ Optimizing Outcomes—**When teaching patients about the contraceptive implant**

The Nexplanon contraceptive is appropriate for women who desire long-term reversible contraception and who have no objections to the insertion/removal procedures or to palpating the implant when it is in place. It must be removed and replaced by a specially trained health-care professional every 3 years if continued contraception is desired. After removal, ovulation occurs within 3 to 6 weeks. The contraceptive implant offers no protection against STIs or HIV.

Intrauterine Devices

The IUD is a small plastic device that is inserted into the uterus and left in place for an extended period of time, providing continuous contraception. The exact mechanism of action is not fully understood, although it is believed that the IUD causes a sterile inflammatory response that results in a spermicidal intrauterine environment. Few sperm are able to reach the fallopian tubes, and if fertilization does occur, the intrauterine environment is unfavorable for implantation (Dean & Schwarz, 2011; Margolis, 2010).

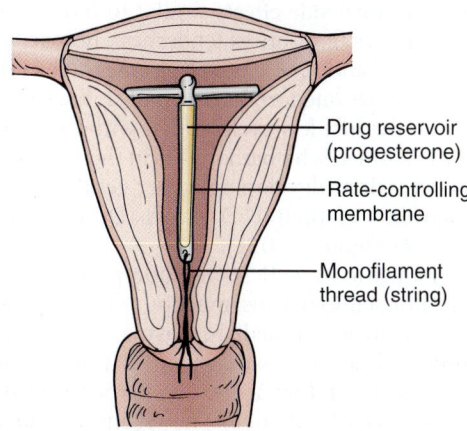

Figure 6-6 Intrauterine device (IUD) properly positioned in the uterus.

Three types of IUDs are currently available in the United States: two levonorgestrel (LNg) intrauterine systems (LNg-IUS) (Mirena; Skyla, recently approved by the FDA), which release a progestin; and the Copper T 380A (TCu380A) (ParaGard) (Fig. 6-6).

The LNg-IUS slowly releases a small amount of levonorgestrel, a progestin, into the endometrial cavity on a constant basis. Mirena must be replaced every 5 years; Skyla must be replaced every 3 years. The Copper T 380A has fine copper wire wrapped around it, and this device may remain in place for 10 years. All three types of IUDs are shaped like the letter "T." They are inserted in a collapsed position and then expand into shape in the uterus once the inserter is withdrawn. The IUD is contained wholly within the uterus and the attached plastic threads, or "tail," (which facilitates removal by the health-care practitioner), extends through the cervix and into the vagina. All types of IUDs are non-latex devices impregnated with barium sulfate for radiopacity. Mirena and ParaGard may be inserted at any time during the menstrual cycle as long as pregnancy may be reasonably excluded; they may also be inserted immediately after childbirth or first trimester abortion. Skyla should be inserted during the first 7 days of the menstrual cycle or immediately after a first trimester abortion; postpartum insertion should be postponed for a minimum of 6 weeks (ACOG, 2011c; Dean & Schwarz, 2011). Once in place, the IUD has several advantages over other methods of contraception. There is no continued expense, no daily attention is required, and the device does not interfere with sexual enjoyment. IUDs decrease the incidence of endometrial cancer and ectopic pregnancy. In addition, the Copper T 380A may be used for emergency—and then long-term—contraception, and the LNg IUS reduces dysmenorrhea and menstrual blood loss from a variety of causes (e.g., leiomyomas and adenomyosis). The IUD is appropriate for women who are at risk for developing complications related to OCPs or who desire to avoid the systemic effects of hormonal preparations. When pregnancy is desired, the IUD is removed by the health-care practitioner (Dean & Schwarz, 2011; Leslie, Thiel, & Yang, 2012; Nelson, 2010b).

Side Effects. Irregular bleeding and/or spotting may occur for about 3 months following IUD insertion (both types). Also, during the first few months, the LNg IUS (Mirena and Skyla) may be associated with lower abdominal pain, back pain, and hormonal side effects similar to those caused by oral contraceptives (e.g., breast tenderness, headache, mood changes, nausea, and acne), as well as amenorrhea after the first year of use. Dysmenorrhea and longer, heavier periods may occur in the first few cycles of use with the TCu-380A (ParaGard). Women who harbor STIs in their cervices have an increased risk of developing upper genital tract infections, regardless of their IUD status (Dean & Schwarz, 2011; Espey & Ogburn, 2011).

Contraindications to IUDs include pregnancy, active pelvic infection, endometritis, mucopurulent cervicitis, and pelvic tuberculosis. Immediate postpartum insertion is contraindicated among women in whom peripartum chorioamnionitis, endometritis, or puerperal sepsis is diagnosed. The IUD should not be newly inserted in women with cervical or endometrial cancer, and insertion may be difficult in women with severe uterine distortion from anatomical abnormalities (e.g., cervical stenosis, bicornuate uterus, and leiomyomas [fibroids] that distort the uterine cavity). It should not be used in women with gestational trophoblastic neoplasia with persistently elevated hCG levels (see Chapter 10), and the TCu380A should not be used in women with Wilson's disease, a copper allergy, or a current history of dysmenorrhea or menorrhagia. Women with current breast cancer should not use the LNg IUS (ACOG, 2011c; Bonnema, et al., 2011; Dean & Schwarz, 2011; Vickery & Madden, 2011).

Effectiveness. Both types of IUDs (i.e., LNg IUS and TCu-380A) have an effectiveness rate of 98% to 99.9% (Dean & Schwarz, 2011).

Optimizing Outcomes—**When teaching patients about the IUD**

The IUD should be considered a long-term form of contraception—it is relatively expensive if used for only a short period of time. Sharp cramping may occur at the time of insertion. If analgesia is needed, products that contain naproxen or ibuprofen work best. Although rare, perforation of the uterus can occur at the time of IUD placement. Minimal spotting may occur for a day or two after insertion, and this is normal. Patients must refrain from placing anything in the vagina for the first 24 hours after insertion (Dean & Schwarz, 2011).

Women who use the IUD may experience irregular bleeding, **menorrhagia** (heavy menstrual flow), or dysmenorrhea (painful menstruation) for several months following insertion. The progestin-releasing IUD can decrease menstrual bleeding and dysmenorrhea; the copper-bearing IUD can increase menstrual flow and cramping. Women who become pregnant using the IUD are more likely to have an ectopic pregnancy or spontaneous abortion. All IUD patients must understand warning signs ("PAINS") that may indicate infection or ectopic pregnancy (Dean & Schwarz, 2011).

Occasionally, the IUD may be expelled. The symptoms of IUD expulsion include unusual vaginal discharge, cramping, spotting, and dyspareunia. However, some IUD expulsions are asymptomatic. A vaginal "string check" should be performed each month to ensure that the IUD remains in place. If the strings are not felt or if they seem to be longer or shorter than they were previously, the woman should return to her health-care provider for evaluation. If pregnancy occurs with the IUD in place, the device is usually removed

vaginally to decrease the possibility of infection or spontaneous abortion. The IUD offers no protection against STIs or HIV (Dean & Schwarz, 2011).

Critical Nursing Action   Teach "PAINS" Warning Signs to IUD Users

Period late (pregnancy)
Abdominal pain, pain with intercourse (infection)
Infection exposure or vaginal discharge
Not feeling well, fever, or chills (infection)
Strings missing, shorter, or longer (IUD expelled)

Optimizing Outcomes—**With the IUD as a contraceptive choice**

Appropriate candidates for intrauterine contraception include nulliparas, adolescents; women with previous ectopic pregnancies, lactating women (the TCu-380A IUD may be placed immediately after delivery of the placenta; placement of either LNg IUD should be delayed until 6 to 8 weeks postpartum), women testing positive for HIV, and women immediately post first trimester abortion. The IUD may be inserted at any time during the menstrual cycle. Before insertion, patients should have a negative pregnancy test, treatment for dysplasia if present, an evaluation for abnormal uterine bleeding if present, cervical cultures to rule out STIs, and a consent form that has been signed (ACOG, 2009c, 2012b; Dean & Schwarz, 2011; Forcier & Harel, 2011; Tyler, Whiteman, Zapata, Curtis, Hillis, & Marchbanks, 2012; World Health Organization, 2010).

STERILIZATION

Sterilization should be considered a permanent and irreversible form of birth control. Although both the male and female procedures are theoretically reversible, the permanency of the method should be emphasized. An essential nursing role centers on counseling to empower the couple to make an informed decision. The nurse must also ensure that informed consent documentation has been obtained and is attached to the patient's chart.

Female Sterilization

Bilateral tubal ligation (BTL) or "tying the tubes" causes interruption in the patency of the fallopian tubes. This permanent birth control method is most easily performed during cesarean birth or in the first 48 hours following a vaginal birth because at this time the uterine fundus is located near the umbilicus and the fallopian tubes are immediately below the abdominal wall. At other times, the procedure is performed in an outpatient surgery clinic, usually under general anesthesia.

Tubal ligation may be accomplished in various ways. In the postpartum period, a minilaparotomy incision is made near the umbilicus—or just above the symphysis pubis at other times. The fallopian tubes are brought through the incision and a small segment is removed (partial salpingectomy). The remaining ends are cauterized or tied or both.

Another method of tubal ligation is accomplished with a laparoscope. The surgeon locates the fallopian tubes and obstructs them with clips or rings or destroys a portion of them with electrocoagulation (Fig. 6-7).

Two nonincisional methods of transcervical sterilization, termed "hysteroscopic tubal occlusion," are also available. These hysteroscopy-guided procedures are performed in the physician's office or as an outpatient procedure with a local anesthetic to the cervix. One method (Adiana) begins with the delivery of radiofrequency energy to produce controlled thermal damage to the lining of the fallopian tube, followed by the insertion of micro-implants into each proximal tubal ostium; the other method (Essure) involves the placement of micro-inserts into the proximal ostium of each fallopian tube (Fig. 6-8). During the following months,

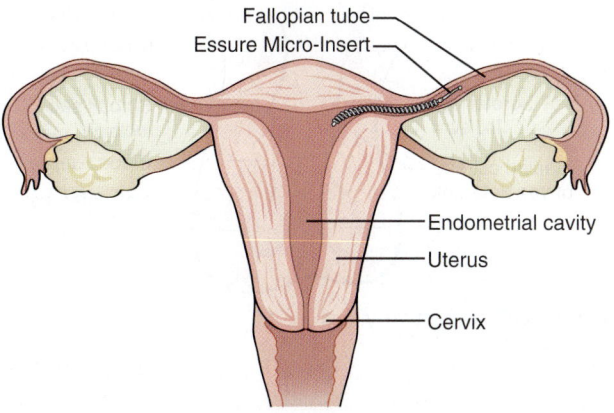

Figure 6-8 Essure Micro-Insert.

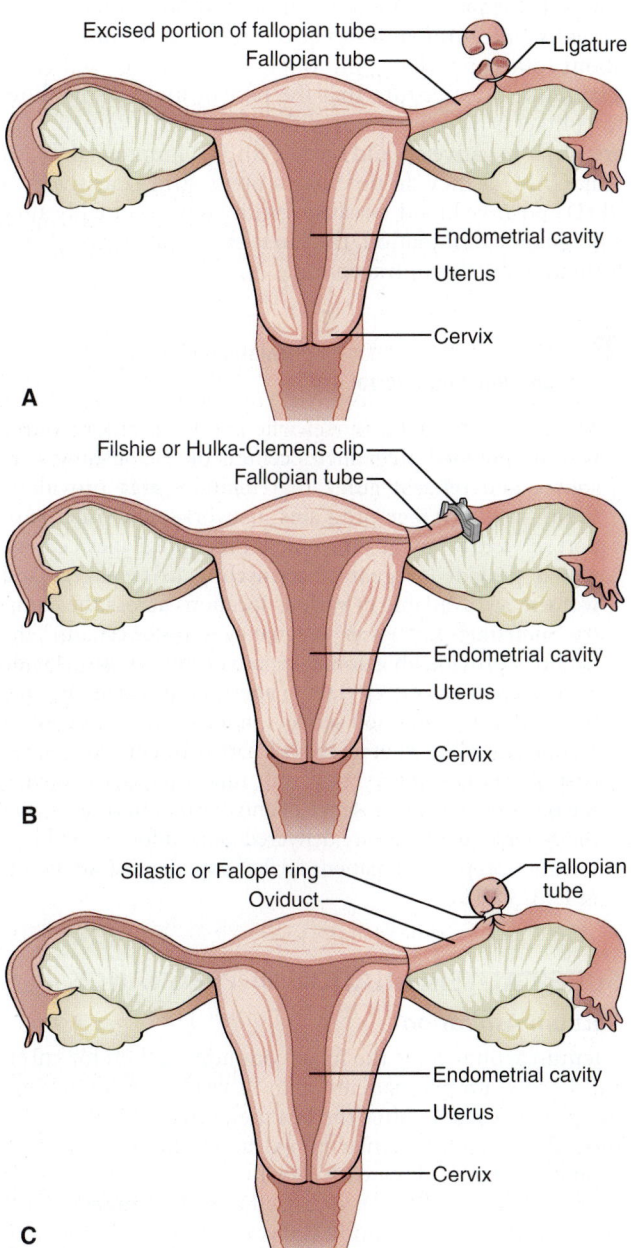

Figure 6-7 Types of tubal sterilization. *A,* Partial salpingectomy. *B,* Filshie or Hulka-Clemens Clip. *C,* Silastic or Falope ring.

scar tissue grows into the inserts, causing tubal blockage. A **hysterosalpingogram** (dye test to evaluate tubal patency) is performed at 3 months (after either method) to ensure that both tubes have been blocked. Patients are instructed to use an alternate form of contraception until bilateral tubal blockage has been confirmed (Holloway & Moredich, 2011; Roncari & Hou, 2011; Schnare & Garcia, 2010; Sufrin & Korn, 2009).

SIDE EFFECTS. As with any surgery, complications include infection, hemorrhage and blood vessel injury, damage to adjacent organs, and complications from anesthesia (Roncari & Hou, 2011).

EFFECTIVENESS. The effectiveness depends on the type of procedure used and ranges from 96.3% with the clip procedure to better than 99% with the postpartum procedure (Roncari & Hou, 2011).

🛑 legal alert—Sterilization policy and legal issues

When counseling patients about sterilization procedures, the nurse must be knowledgeable about the particular legal requirements of the practice state. Strict adherence to informed choice and consent procedures is mandatory. Partner or spousal consent in the United States is not legally required. Patients using federal or state funds for sterilization must be 21 or older and mentally competent, and they must wait 30 days after signing the consent before receiving a sterilization procedure (Roncari & Hou, 2011).

Male Sterilization

Vasectomy is a surgical procedure performed under local anesthesia that involves a small incision or puncture in the scrotum. The vas deferens is ligated, chemically occluded, cauterized, clipped, or cut to interrupt the passage of sperm into the seminal fluid (Fig. 6-9). Following vasectomy, the semen no longer contains sperm. Sexual function is unaffected. Vasectomy should be considered a permanent method of contraception.

SIDE EFFECTS. Complications following vasectomy include infection, hematoma, and excessive pain and swelling.

EFFECTIVENESS. Vasectomy is greater than 99% effective in preventing pregnancy.

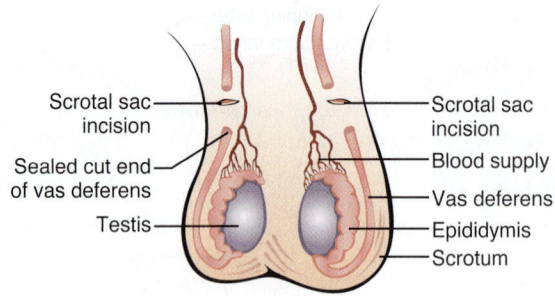

Figure 6-9 Vasectomy.

 Optimizing Outcomes—**When teaching patients about permanent sterilization**

There is a high rate of ectopic pregnancies in tubal ligation procedures that fail. Tubal sterilization has been found to decrease the risk of ovarian and endometrial cancer. Menstruation and menopause are unaffected. Patients who have nickel hypersensitivity should not use the Essure Micro-Insert. After vasectomy, the man should rest, apply ice to the scrotum, and wear snug underwear for scrotal support. Intercourse should be avoided for 2 to 3 days. Complete sterilization has not occurred until all sperm have left the system. This process may take several weeks. The man will need to submit semen specimens for analysis until two specimens show no sperm present. Permanent sterilization methods offer no protection against STIs or HIV (Al-Safi, Shavell, Katz, & Berman, 2011; Roncari & Hou, 2011).

Now Can You—**Teach about contraception?**

1. Explain what is meant by "natural family planning"?
2. Compare and contrast barrier and hormonal methods of contraception?
3. Identify five danger signs associated with OCPs and intrauterine devices?

Clinical Termination of Pregnancy

A clinical termination of pregnancy, or abortion, is a procedure performed to deliberately end a pregnancy before the fetus reaches a viable age. The legal definition of viability (usually 20 to 24 weeks) varies from state to state. Abortion has been legal in the United States since the 1973 Supreme Court decision in *Roe v. Wade.*

An abortion performed at the patient's request is termed an **elective abortion**; when performed for reasons of maternal or fetal health or disease, the term **therapeutic abortion** applies. Abortions performed during the first trimester are technically easier and safer than abortions performed during the second trimester. Methods for performing early elective abortion include vacuum aspiration and medical methods. Second-trimester abortion is associated with increased complications and costs and involves cervical dilation and removal of the fetus and placenta.

NURSING CARE RELATED TO ELECTIVE PREGNANCY TERMINATION

Holistic nursing care for women who are considering abortion includes guidance for pregnancy testing, ultrasonography to accurately determine the weeks of gestation, and individualized counseling about the available options. Any woman who is unsure of her decision deserves emotional support and time to allow her to make the choice that she feels is the appropriate one for her. The decision for nearly every woman is difficult and complicated. Once a decision has been made for an abortion, a medical history and physical examination with appropriate screening tests (e.g., complete blood count [CBC], blood typing and Rh, gonococcal smear, serological test for syphilis (STS), urinalysis, and Pap test) are obtained. Informed consent documents are signed and placed on the patient's chart. The nurse counsels the patient about potential complications such as excessive bleeding and infection, reinforces information about follow-up visits, and offers strategies for self-care. The nurse must ensure that the patient understands how to contact a health-care provider if needed. Women who are Rh$_o$D-negative should receive Rh$_o$(D) immune globulin (RhoGAM) if they do not have a preexisting sensitivity to Rh(D)-positive blood. Because fertility returns quickly after a pregnancy termination, the nurse should also provide information about contraception.

 Optimizing Outcomes—**Unintended pregnancy counseling and referral**

An important role for nurses who provide care for women with unintended pregnancies centers on establishing a resource and referral guide that includes area providers, health-care coverage programs, networks, and other support services for pregnant women. Crisis pregnancy centers, which provide pregnancy counseling to teenagers and women, are available in various locations across the country. Sometimes known as "pregnancy resource centers," the facilities provide abortion alternatives but do not provide abortion services or referrals to abortion providers. For patients who seek abortion services, nurses can provide information regarding what methods a particular clinic offers, the cost of services, the average wait time, languages spoken, the potential for the presence of antiabortion protesters, and the general quality of care delivered. Such information helps to better prepare the patient for her experience (Simmonds & Likis, 2011).

SURGICAL TERMINATION OF PREGNANCY

Vacuum Aspiration

Vacuum aspiration is the most common method for surgical abortion for pregnancies up to 12 weeks' gestation. Very early (5 to 7 weeks after the last menstrual period [LMP]) procedures, called menstrual extraction and endometrial aspiration, can be done with a small flexible plastic cannula with no cervical dilation or anesthesia. **Laminaria,** dried seaweed that swells as it absorbs moisture and mechanically dilates the cervix, may be inserted 4 to 24 hours before the pregnancy termination. Upon removal, the cervix has usually dilated two to three times its original diameter and further instrumental dilation is unnecessary.

Abortions performed between 8 and 12 weeks' gestation require mechanical cervical dilation after injection of a local anesthetic. A plastic cannula is then inserted into the uterine cavity. The contents are aspirated with negative pressure and the uterine cavity is often scraped with a curet to ensure that the uterus is empty. Patients may experience cramping for 20 to 30 minutes following the procedure. Complications include uterine perforation, cervical lacerations, hemorrhage, infection, and adverse reactions to the anesthetic agent.

Abortion during the second trimester involves cervical dilation with removal of the fetus and placenta. This procedure is termed "dilation and evacuation" (D & E). Similar to vacuum curettage, greater cervical dilation and use of a larger cannula are required because of the increased volume in the products of conception. Prior to the procedure, laminaria and/or misoprostol (a prostaglandin E1 analogue) is used to soften and dilate the cervix. D & E may be associated with long-term adverse effects from cervical trauma (ACOG, 2013c; Gilliam, 2010; Paul & Stein, 2011).

Nursing care during surgical abortion includes continued patient assessment and emotional support. The woman should be informed about what to expect: abdominal cramping and sounds emitted by the suction device. After the procedure, the patient rests in a recovery area for 1 to 3 hours to ensure that no excessive cramping or bleeding occurs. The aspirated uterine contents are inspected to ascertain that all fetal parts and adequate placental tissue have been aspirated.

Although checkup visits are usually scheduled between 2 weeks and 6 weeks postabortion, serum levels of human chorionic gonadotropin (hCG) may remain elevated even if the abortion successfully ended the pregnancy. Women whose hCG levels are still present in the urine (at the follow-up appointment) should be encouraged to return for urine hCG levels every 2 weeks until the test is negative. Persistently elevated hCG levels are associated with a delay in the return of menses.

clinical alert

Signs of short-term complications after clinical termination of pregnancy

- Fever of 40°C (104°F)
- Abdominal pain or tenderness in the abdomen
- Prolonged or heavy bleeding or passing large clots
- Foul smelling vaginal discharge
- No menstrual period within 6 weeks

Source: Paul & Stein (2011).

MEDICATION (MEDICAL) TERMINATION OF PREGNANCY

"Medication (or medical) abortion" is an alternative for the surgical form of abortion, and for some women this method is more "natural" and more closely resembles a miscarriage. A medication abortion can be performed during the first 7 to 9 weeks of pregnancy, depending on the regimen used. The woman who considers medication abortion should be carefully educated about what to expect. Specific medications are used to induce uterine contractions to end the

pregnancy. These include mifepristone (Mifeprex, originally called RU-486), an abortifacient; and methotrexate (amethopterin, Folex, Rheumatrex, Trexall), an antimetabolite used to treat certain types of cancer. (According to ACOG [2014], methotrexate is now rarely used in the United States for medication abortion because of the greater availability and efficacy of mifepristone regimens.) Both medications may be followed by the administration of misoprostol (Cytotec), a prostaglandin analogue that promotes expulsion of the pregnancy. Misoprostol, which in some situations is used alone or in combination with letrozole (a selective aromatase inhibitor used to treat estrogen-dependent breast cancer), is commonly associated with nausea, vomiting, diarrhea, and cramping (ACOG, 2013c; Gilliam, 2011; Lee, Ng, Yeung, & Ho, 2011; Paul & Stein, 2011).

Uterine cramping and bleeding begins several days after medication administration, and most patients experience a period of painless heavy bleeding along with the expulsion of tissue (the products of conception). This experience may trigger strong emotions. The nurse should advise the patient that she would most likely benefit from the presence of a caring, trusted close friend or relative who can help her through the experience and lend emotional and physical support. Follow-up visits usually include ultrasonography (to confirm that the uterus is empty) and assessment of hCG levels. In some situations, the return office visit may be replaced by telephone follow-up combined with a sensitive urine pregnancy test at home 30 days after mifepristone is given (Perriera, Reeves, Chen, Hohmann, Hayes, & Creinin, 2010). A surgical abortion procedure may be necessary if medication attempts are unsuccessful.

 Across Care Settings: **Medication abortion provided through telemedicine**

Telemedicine, the delivery of health-care services at a distance using information and communication technology, has been used to provide early access to medication abortion. In a study conducted by Grossman and colleagues (2011), women who were eligible to participate included those who were pregnant at 63 days of gestation or less, had no contraindications to medication abortion, were at least 18 years of age, and desired this pregnancy termination method. Clinical information was obtained, and ultrasonography was performed at the first clinic visit. Patients who wished to receive services through telemedicine then had a discussion with a physician (who had reviewed the medical information) using video teleconference equipment linked through a dedicated data connection. If the patient was eligible for medication abortion, the physician entered a password into her computer that remotely unlocked a drawer in front of the patient containing mifepristone and misoprostol tablets. The physician observed the patient swallow the mifepristone and gave her final instructions through the video teleconference. A follow-up visit was scheduled within 2 weeks after receiving mifepristone. At that time, pelvic ultrasonography was performed to confirm completion of the abortion. Women who chose this model of abortion service reported high levels of satisfaction, and there was no significant difference in the prevalence of adverse events among telemedicine patients compared with face-to-face patients (Grossman, Grindlay, Buchacker, Lane, & Blanchard, 2011).

Medication termination of pregnancy is probably not the ideal choice for adolescents, and for this reason, some clinics offer this method of abortion only to women 18 years of age or older. Interestingly, this method has been proven useful in evacuating pregnancies that occur in the fallopian tubes. Medication termination of a tubal pregnancy has enabled many women to avoid surgery and preserve the fallopian tubes for future pregnancy conceptions.

Medication termination during the second trimester most often includes an administration of prostaglandins via vaginal suppository, gel, or by intrauterine injection. Repeated doses are often needed, and side effects including headache, nausea, vomiting, dizziness, diarrhea, cramping, fever, and chills usually occur. Rarely used methods include the intrauterine instillation of hypertonic solutions such as saline or urea and uterotonic agents (e.g., misoprostol and dinoprostone).

COMPLICATIONS

Legal abortion is actually safer than pregnancy, especially when performed early in pregnancy. All patients should be told to expect cramping and some bleeding after an abortion. Some of the rare complications associated with abortion include infection; uterine atony; incomplete abortion (i.e., retained products of conception), hemorrhage; cervical, uterine, or abdominal organ trauma; embolism; **Asherman syndrome** (condition characterized by the presence of endometrial adhesions or scar tissue); and postabortal syndrome (occurs after first-trimester vacuum aspiration abortion procedures, manifested by severe abdominal cramping and pain from intrauterine blood clots). Patients should be cautioned to call the office should any signs of short-term complications (e.g., excessive bleeding, pain, and fever) occur. Most complications develop within the first few days after the abortion. In most clinical settings, patients are asked to return in 2 weeks for a follow-up examination (ACOG, 2013c; Paul & Stein, 2011).

The Nurse's Role in Infertility Care

THE INITIAL ASSESSMENT

Fertility requires that the sperm and the ovum can meet; that the sperm is viable, normal, and able to penetrate a viable, normal egg; and that the lining of the uterus can support the implanted embryo. **Sterility** is the term applied when there is an absolute factor that prevents reproduction. **Infertility** is diagnosed if a woman age 34 or younger has not conceived within 12 months (for women 35 and older, within 6 months) of actively attempting pregnancy. At present, 10% to 15% of heterosexual couples in the United States are infertile. Approximately 33% of cases of infertility can be attributed to female problems, 33% can be attributed to male causes, and the remaining cases of infertility are attributable to a combination of male and female factors or are undeterminable (CDC, 2013a). Delays in childbearing and increased consumer awareness of reproductive technology have prompted more heterosexual couples, single women, and same-sex couples to seek fertility assistance than ever before. The nurse's role in infertility care begins with education and counseling during the initial assessment.

 Nursing Insight—*Toward meeting the* Healthy People 2020 *national goals*

The *Healthy People 2020* goal that directly addresses infertility states, "Reduce the proportion of women aged 18 to 44 years who have impaired fecundity (i.e., a physical barrier preventing pregnancy or carrying a pregnancy to term) from a baseline of 12% to a target of 10.8%" (U.S. Department of Health and Human Services [DHHS], 2012). To help achieve this goal, nurses must be proactive in health promotion strategies for all childbearing-aged individuals. Empowering young adults with knowledge about nutrition, exercise, stress reduction, and safe sex practices helps them to make lifestyle choices that foster optimal health and preservation of fertility.

Before extensive testing for infertility, it is important to establish that the timing of intercourse and length of coital exposure are adequate. The nurse assesses the couple's understanding about the most fertile times to have intercourse during the menstrual cycle. Teaching about the signs and timing of ovulation, the most effective times for intercourse (every 48 hours around ovulation), and positions to enhance sperm retention is an important nursing intervention during the initial evaluation.

 Cultural Diversity: Obtaining a Sexual History for Infertility Care

Culturally influenced practices and taboos may create feelings of discomfort for couples when asked specific details of their intimate lives during the infertility care interview. Nurses must be sensitive to these issues and aware of cultural variations. For example, Orthodox Jewish law forbids a couple from engaging in sexual intercourse for 7 days after the menstrual period. This tenet can create an infertility problem if ovulation occurs during the early days after menstruation.

Providing an overview of what to expect during the initial and subsequent visits empowers the couple to make an informed decision about their level of commitment to the evaluation and possible treatment and affords them some sense of control over their situation. The nurse explains what is involved in the basic infertility work-up in a sensitive, unhurried manner that conveys caring and promotes a trusting, therapeutic relationship. Depending on findings from the history and physical examination, the evaluation will most likely include an assessment of ovarian function, cervical mucus (amount and receptivity to sperm), sperm adequacy, tubal patency, and the general condition of the pelvic organs.

Instructions about recording the basal body temperature are usually provided at the initial visit. An in-depth interview, preferably with both partners, may reveal medical problems (e.g., chronic illness), lifestyle patterns (e.g., tobacco use, substance abuse, and sexual orientation), or other factors such as advanced age that can adversely affect fertility. The physical examination includes evaluation of the pelvis (bimanual and rectovaginal assessment), assessment of the body mass index (BMI) and laboratory testing (Trolice, 2011).

LATER METHODS OF ASSESSMENT

A thyroid function test, glucose tolerance test, serum prolactin levels, and specific hormonal assays (e.g., estradiol, luteinizing hormone [LH], progesterone, dehydroepiandrosterone [DHEA], androstenedione, testosterone, 17 alpha-hydroxy progesterone [17-OHP]) may also be ordered along with transvaginal 3-D ultrasound and color flow Doppler to visualize the pelvic structures (and later used for follicular monitoring of women undergoing ovulation induction). Other diagnostic tests may include an endometrial biopsy to assess the endometrial response to progesterone, a hysterosalpingography (transcervical instillation of a radiopaque dye to provide visualization of the interior dimensions of the uterine cavity and fallopian tubes), and a laparoscopy to allow direct visualization of the internal pelvic structures. Selected methods of fertility evaluation in the female along with nursing implications are presented in Table 6-2.

Evaluation of the man begins with a semen analysis to assess the quality and quantity of sperm. The nurse explains the purpose of the test and advises the man to collect the semen specimen by masturbation following a 2- to 3-day abstinence. He is instructed to note the time the specimen was obtained. This information allows the laboratory to evaluate liquefaction of the semen. The specimen should be transported near the body (to preserve warmth) and should arrive at the laboratory within 1 hour after collection. Additional testing may include serum samples for evaluation of endocrine function (testosterone, estradiol, LH, and follicle-stimulating hormone [FSH]), ultrasonography, testicular biopsy, and sperm penetration assay. Referral to a urologist may be indicated. A postcoital test (PCT) may be ordered to assess the cervical mucus, sperm, and degree of sperm penetration through the cervical mucus. The test is performed on a sample of cervical mucus obtained several hours after intercourse.

Table 6-2 Common Diagnostic Methods Used in the Evaluation of Female Infertility	
Type/Name of Test	**Role of the Nurse**
PREDICTION OF OVULATION	
To identify the LH surge – precedes ovulation by 24–36 hours. Also identifies the absence of ovulation. Tests include basal body temperature (BBT), commercial ovulation predictor kits, and assessment of cervical mucus.	Teach the couple how the information helps to determine timing of intercourse to coincide with ovulation. Instruct the woman about recording the BBT and assessing cervical mucus; reinforce directions for using commercial ovulation predictor kits.
POSTCOITAL TEST (PCT); HUHNER TEST	
Assessment of the quality and quantity of cervical mucus and sperm function at the time of ovulation.	Instruct the patient to arrange to come in 6–12 hours after intercourse for evaluation of the cervical mucus.
ULTRASOUND EXAMINATION	
To evaluate structure of the pelvic organs; identify maturing ovarian follicles and the timing of ovulation.	Reassure the patient that sonography uses sound waves, not radiation, to evaluate the pelvic structures. The examination may be conducted transabdominally or transvaginally, and specific instructions are given, depending on method.
HYSTEROSALPINGOGRAM	
(See Diagnostic Tools)	
TESTS OF ENDOCRINE FUNCTION	
To evaluate the hypothalamus, pituitary gland, and ovaries. Various assays determine levels of FSH, LH, estrogen, and progesterone. Depending on the history and physical findings, additional testing may be indicated.	Inform the patient that testing is performed on serum samples, and timing is an important consideration in interpretation of the results. Explain that FSH and LH stimulate ovulation, and estrogen and progesterone make the endometrium receptive for implantation of the fertilized ovum.
ENDOMETRIAL BIOPSY	
Involves the removal of a sample of the endometrium with a small pipette attached to suction. Provides information about the effects of progesterone (produced by the corpus luteum after ovulation) on the endometrium.	Teach the patient about the purpose and appropriate timing of the test: It should be performed not earlier than 10–12 days after ovulation (2–3 days before menstruation is expected). Cramping, pelvic discomfort, and vaginal spotting may occur; a mild analgesic (e.g., ibuprofen) may be used to alleviate the discomfort.
HYSTEROSCOPY AND LAPAROSCOPY	
Procedures that involve the use of an endoscope to examine the interior of the uterus and the pelvic organs under general anesthesia. Hysteroscopy may be performed without general anesthesia in the office. Abnormalities such as polyps, myomata (fibroid tumors), and endometrial adhesions are identified.	Explain the purpose of the test and other procedures that may be done at the same time. When general anesthesia is to be used, the patient should take nothing by mouth for several hours before the planned procedure. Advise her that because carbon dioxide gas will be instilled in the abdomen to enhance organ visibility, she may experience postoperative cramping and referred shoulder pain, which can be relieved with a mild analgesic.

Labs: Basic Infertility Evaluation and Workup

Woman:	Man:
CBC	Semen analysis: sperm count should be:
Urinalysis	Volume of 2–6 mL of semen
Pap test and wet mount	
Serology	>20 million sperm per 1 mL of semen
Luteinizing-hormone-surge ovulation predictor kit	>50% forward-moving sperm
	>30% normal sperm
FSH cycle day 3 if >35 years old	
Rh factor, blood grouping	<1 million WBCs per mL of semen
Hysterosalpingogram (to reveal uterine or tubal obstruction or abnormalities)	

Diagnostic Tools Hysterosalpingography (HSG)

During hysterosalpingography, radiopaque dye is injected through the cervix. The dye enters the uterus and fallopian tubes, and through x-ray examination, any abnormalities in the uterine structure or tubal patency can be identified.

- It is performed during the follicular phase of the menstrual cycle to avoid interrupting an early pregnancy. It may exert a therapeutic effect as well: Instillation of the water-based dye may flush out debris or adhesions in the uterine cavity.
- Moderate to severe cramping and shoulder pain "referred" from the subdiaphragmatic collection of gas may occur. All patients should be warned about the possibility of pain during the test.
- The patient should be given a nonsteroidal anti-inflammatory drug (NSAID) (e.g., ibuprofen) 30 minutes to 1 hour before the procedure.
- Recurrence of pelvic inflammatory disease may result from the test; prophylactic antibiotics are recommended to prevent infection.
- The patient is instructed to report severe cramping, bleeding, fever, or malodorous discharge that develops within a week following the procedure, although spotting and slight cramping for a few days may occur. She should be advised to take an NSAID after the procedure for these symptoms.

Treatment Options for Infertility

MEDICATIONS

Depending on the cause of infertility, a number of pharmacological methods are used to induce ovulation, supplement the woman's levels of follicle-stimulating hormone (FSH) and luteinizing hormone (LH), prepare the uterine endometrium for implantation, and support the pregnancy following conception and implantation (Table 6-3).

Table 6-3 Selected Medications Used in the Treatment of Infertility

Medication	Actions	Nursing Considerations and Side Effects
Clomiphene citrate (Clomid, Serophene)	Antiestrogen that binds with estrogen receptors to trigger FSH and LH release.	Contraindicated with hepatic impairment. Patients may experience ovarian enlargement, vasomotor flushes, abdominal distention, nausea and vomiting, breast tenderness, blurred vision, headache, pelvic pain, or abnormal uterine bleeding. May cause multiple ovulation.
Bromocriptine mesylate (Parlodel)	Reduces elevated prolactin secretion by the anterior pituitary, which improves gonadotropin-releasing hormone secretion and normalizes follicle-stimulating hormone and luteinizing hormone release. Ovulation is restored, and increased progesterone by the corpus luteum supports early pregnancy.	Patients may experience nausea and vomiting, headache, dizziness, orthostatic hypotension, blurred vision, diarrhea, metallic taste, dry mouth, urticaria, and rash.
GnRH analogs (agonists): goserelin acetate (Zoladex), leuprolide acetate (Lupron), nafarelin acetate (Synarel)	Stimulates release of pituitary FSH and LH in patients with deficient hypothalamic GnRH secretion. FSH and LH stimulate ovulation (female) and testosterone and spermatogenesis (male).	Advise patients of potential side effects: headache, depression, nasal irritation (Synarel), vaginal dryness, breast swelling and tenderness, hot flashes, vaginal spotting, decreased libido, and impotence.
GnRH antagonists: cetrorelix acetate (Cetrotide), ganirelix acetate (Antagon), abarelix (Plenaxis), histrelin acetate (Supprelin)	Reduces extent of endometriosis; used with medications that stimulate ovulation by suppressing LH and FSH.	Patients are closely monitored for ovarian hyperstimulation syndrome, a rare, adverse effect of ART (symptoms include nausea and vomiting, headache, weight gain, ascites with or without pain, pleural effusion, and ruptured ovarian cysts).
Gonadotropins	Hormones used for ovulation induction. Include FSH, LH, human menopausal gonadotropin (Pergonal), (Repronex), (Humegon), human FSH (Metrodin, Fertinex, Bravelle, recombinant FSH (Gonal F, Follistim), and human chorionic gonadotropin [hCG] (Profasi, APL, Pregnyl, Novarel, Ovidrel). Ovulation usually occurs within 18 hours. Also stimulates production of progesterone by the corpus luteum.	When used with menotropins, risk for ovarian hyperstimulation and arterial thromboembolism; other side effects include headache, irritability, restlessness, and depression.
Progesterone (IM, intravaginal)	Provides luteal phase support—prepares the endometrial lining to promote implantation of the embryo.	Common side effects include nausea, weight gain, and fluid retention.

Induction of Ovulation

Medications are commonly used to stimulate follicle development in women who are anovulatory or who ovulate infrequently. Clomiphene citrate (Clomid, Serophene) is frequently prescribed. It is an antiestrogenic agent that binds to hypothalamic estrogen receptors to trigger the release of FSH and LH. Patients who will be undergoing assisted reproductive techniques including in vitro fertilization, gamete intrafallopian transfer, and tubal embryo transfer may also receive agents to induce superovulation, or the release of several ova. After adequate follicular stimulation, human chorionic gonadotropin (hCG) is administered to prompt ovulation.

Induction of ovulation increases the risk of multiple births because many ova may be released and fertilized. Depending on the medications used, daily ultrasound examinations and serum estrogen levels may be obtained to monitor ovarian response. **Ovarian hyperstimulation** is a serious complication that may result from ovulation induction. It is characterized by marked ovarian enlargement, ascites with or without pain, and pleural effusion. When detected, hCG is not given, and ovulation will not occur. The patient undergoes a "rest" period and postponement of the infertility treatment until the following cycle. Careful monitoring and medication titration are usually successful in preventing this complication as well as high-order (triplets or more) multifetal pregnancy. Throughout therapy, which often requires repeated office visits and testing, nursing interventions center on continued education and patient support. Emotional instability, anxiety, and depression are common reactions to the dramatic hormonal alterations and need for frequent surveillance.

SURGICAL OPTIONS

Surgical interventions using endoscopic techniques may be useful in correcting obstructions. Laparoscopic ablation (destruction) of endometrial implants may help patients with endometriosis achieve pregnancy, especially during the first few months immediately following the procedure. Newer laser surgical techniques are minimally invasive and useful in reducing adhesions that have resulted from infection, prior surgical procedures, and endometriosis. Microsurgical techniques may be successful in correcting obstructions in the fallopian tubes or in the male tubal structures. Transcervical tuboplasty (surgery for correction of fallopian tube abnormalities) is a minimally invasive technique that involves insertion of a catheter through the cervix into the uterus and the fallopian tube. A balloon is inflated to clear any blockage.

THERAPEUTIC INSEMINATION

Therapeutic insemination (previously termed "artificial insemination") involves the placement of semen at the cervical os or directly in the uterus (intrauterine insemination [IUI]) by mechanical means. Partner sperm (termed "therapeutic husband insemination" [THI]) or donor sperm (termed "therapeutic donor insemination" [TDI]) is used. Clomiphene citrate and ultrasound monitoring for follicle development are frequently used to ensure timing of the insemination with ovulation. Fertilization most often occurs in the fallopian tube. The technique involves the insertion of a small catheter into the vagina and through the cervix to facilitate the deposition of sperm directly into the uterus. Because seminal fluid is rich in prostaglandins, IUI prevents the nausea, cramping, abdominal pain, and diarrhea that can result from the absorption of prostaglandins by the cervical lining.

Before the IUI, the sperm are "washed": They are removed from the seminal fluid and placed in a special solution that enhances motility and improves the chances for fertilization. An added advantage of washing sperm concerns sperm antibodies. After infection or surgery, a woman's immune system may produce antibodies that cause sperm clumping and adversely affect motility and ovum penetration. Sperm washing may correct the clumping, increase sperm motility, and improve the likelihood of fertilization.

ASSISTED REPRODUCTIVE TECHNOLOGIES

Assisted reproductive technologies (ART) are procedures intended to achieve pregnancy by placing ova and sperm together to promote fertilization. ART includes gamete intrafallopian transfer (GIFT), zygote intrafallopian transfer (ZIFT), frozen embryo transfer (FET), and in vitro fertilization-embryo transfer (IVF-ET). Presently, approximately 99% of ART cycles performed are IVF-ET. Although ART methods are more common today than in the past, they are very expensive, and are often unavailable to women of lower socioeconomic status (CDC, 2013b; Society for Assisted Reproductive Technology [SART], 2012).

Gamete Intrafallopian Transfer

Gamete intrafallopian transfer (GIFT) is a technique that involves laparoscopy and ovulation induction. The patient must have at least one patent fallopian tube. Three to five oocytes are harvested from the ovary and immediately placed into a catheter along with washed, motile donor or partner sperm. The sperm and oocytes are injected into the fimbriated ends of the fallopian tube(s) through a laparoscope. Fertilization takes place in the fallopian tube, and the fertilized egg (zygote) then travels via the tube to the uterus for implantation. Because fertilization does not occur outside the woman's body, the GIFT procedure may be more acceptable to adherents of certain religious groups (e.g., Roman Catholic Church) than other procedures (e.g., ZIFT).

Zygote Intrafallopian Transfer

Zygote intrafallopian transfer (ZIFT) is a procedure that evolved from the GIFT procedure. Following ovulation induction, retrieved oocytes are fertilized outside the woman's body, and the subsequent zygotes are placed in the distal fallopian tube(s).

Tubal Embryo Transfer

Tubal embryo transfer (TET) involves placement at the embryo stage. The patient must have at least one patent fallopian tube. Exogenous progesterone is used to enhance endometrial preparation.

In Vitro Fertilization

In vitro fertilization (IVF) involves retrieval of the oocytes from the ovaries, usually via an intra-abdominal approach or a transvaginal approach under ultrasound guidance. The oocytes are then combined with partner or donor sperm in the laboratory. After fertilization, the normally developing embryos are placed in the uterus (Fig. 6-10). Success with

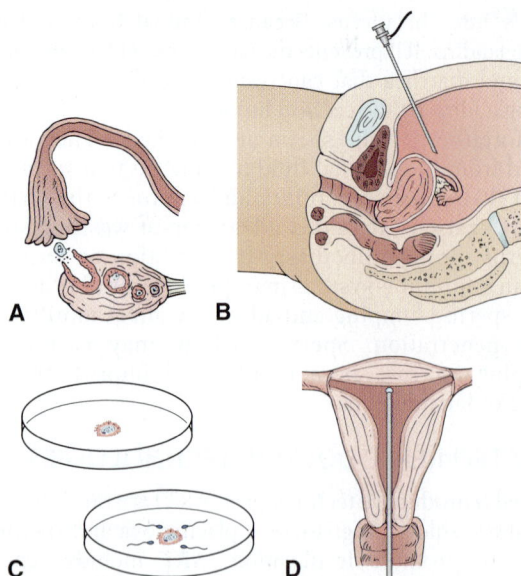

Figure 6-10 The process of in vitro fertilization. *A*, Ovulation. *B*, Intra-abdominal retrieval of the ova. *C*, Ova fertilization and growth in culture medium. *D*, Fertilized ova is placed in the uterus.

IVF is dependent on many factors, such as the woman's age and the indication for the procedure. On average, women who undergo three IVF cycles have a good chance of achieving pregnancy.

 Nursing Insight—*ART, multifetal gestation, and associated risks*

While treatment of infertility has permitted millions of couples to have their own children, of all babies born following in vitro fertilization, more than half are part of a multiple pregnancy. It is estimated that approximately 65% of twins born in the United States emanate from infertility treatments. The risks (e.g., fetal anomalies, preterm birth, death, and maternal complications) in multiple pregnancies are disproportionately larger than in singleton pregnancies (CDC, 2013b; Evans, 2010). In-depth and ongoing counseling for couples considering ART constitutes an essential component of care.

Cryopreservation

Cryopreservation, or freezing, is used in some instances to store sperm or ovarian tissue for future use or to freeze excess embryos that have resulted from an in vitro fertilization procedure. If no pregnancy results, the frozen embryos can be processed and replaced in the uterus. This option allows the couple to attempt another pregnancy without the need for ovarian stimulation and egg retrieval.

An initial fee is charged for the freezing process; additional fees are incurred for the continued preservation of the frozen reproductive tissues. One of the ethical and sociocultural issues involved with cryopreservation arises when excess embryos are no longer needed or desired by the woman or couple. In most situations, the embryos are destroyed, although a social debate presently concerns an alternate use of the embryos for research.

 Nursing Insight—*Oocyte cryopreservation*

Oocyte cryopreservation is a technique that allows women to save harvested eggs for fertilization and implantation at a future date. Cryopreservation enables excess oocytes generated during assisted reproduction to be stored, avoiding the associated ethical, moral, and religious dilemmas. Examples of situations in which oocyte cryopreservation may be used include fertility-impairing conditions (e.g., cancer treatment), premature ovarian failure (e.g., fragile X syndrome), and lack of availability of sperm at the time of oocyte harvesting (Setti & Patrizio, 2012).

Micromanipulation

Micromanipulation is a process that involves the use of micromanipulators—fine, specialized instruments—to handle individual sperm and ova. Intracytoplasmic sperm injection (ICSI) allows a sperm cell to be directly injected into an ovum. Assisted embryo hatching is used as an IVF adjunct for women in whom the normal "hatching process" is impeded because of a thickening of the zona pellucida. A small opening created in the zona pellucida facilitates the hatching process by allowing the embryo to escape from the zona pellucida to interact with the endometrium for implantation.

Preimplantation genetic diagnosis (PGD) refers to procedures performed on embryos prior to implantation. Considered an adjunct to ART, couples at risk for having a detectable single gene or chromosomal anomaly (e.g., cystic fibrosis, beta-thalassemia, or reciprocal translocation) may choose to undergo this procedure. A single cell is obtained from a six- to eight-cell embryo by a process termed "blastomere biopsy." (In some PGD centers, the biopsy is performed at the blastocyst stage—5 to 6 days after fertilization—and 2 to 9 cells are removed for analysis.) The genetic content of the cell is examined via fluorescent in situ hybridization (FISH) or polymerase chain reaction (PCR). Because results of genetic testing on the preimplantation embryos are generally available in 4 to 24 hours, unaffected embryos may still be transferred during the required biological window of time without the need for cryopreservation. An emerging application for PGD is to prevent genetic conditions (e.g., Huntington's disease and early-onset Alzheimer's disease) that manifest in adulthood (Hershberger, Schoenfeld, & Tur-Kaspa, 2011; SART, 2012).

ART and Legal Considerations

Before any ART procedure, patients must be given current, factual information about the advantages and limitations of techniques that involve the use of donor sperm or eggs for the purpose of conception. Informed consent must be obtained and documented in the patient record. Assisted reproductive technology is expensive (approximately $12,000.00 to $25,000.00 per cycle) and available only in specialized centers. Some insurance plans require women to undergo several rounds of IUI before they will pay for IVF; others do not cover IVF at all (Lee, 2011). Unfortunately, there is never a guarantee of a viable pregnancy that will result in a healthy child. Nursing responsibilities include ensuring that patients and their partners have ample opportunity to ask questions, thoughtfully explore available options, and freely express concerns. They must be able to verbalize an understanding of the chosen procedure(s), including the risks and potential complications. Ongoing support includes education, counseling, and strategies for continued follow-up.

When donor ova or sperm are to be used, patients and their partners require additional information. They need to be reassured that all gamete donors have undergone psychological and physical examinations and screening for medical and genetic disease. Clinical findings from potential donors are made available to the woman or couple to allow them to make an informed decision. The donor's and the recipient's confidentiality are closely guarded, and in most instances, their identities are not revealed without their specific permission.

Infertility, ART, and Potential Effects on the Couple's Relationship

Infertility produces a great amount of emotional stress for most couples. Societal and cultural influences may intensify the feelings of disappointment and failure. It is not unusual for the woman and her partner to experience a sense of loss: loss of perceived good health, loss of self-esteem, loss of a "normal" relationship with the spouse, loss of security and self-confidence, and loss of the potential child. Affected persons often move at their own individual pace through the stages of grieving identified by Kübler-Ross: denial, anger, bargaining, depression, and acceptance. Frequently, there are natural and individual differences in the nature, intensity, and timing of the feelings and perceptions that each partner experiences (Chachamovich, Chachamovich, Ezer, Fleck, Knauth, & Passos (2010).

For heterosexual couples, intercourse can transition from a shared loving, intimate moment into a clinical, goal-oriented procedure. Unfortunately, some relationships do not survive the stress of infertility. Even under the best of circumstances, infertile couples are subjected to a loss of privacy and often a lack of spontaneity. During treatment for infertility, menstrual periods become a regular and repeated reminder of failure. Patients are asked to share with others their most personal and emotionally laden information concerning sexual preferences and sexual practices. It is imperative that the nurse and other members of the health-care team maintain confidentiality and privacy for these patients as much as possible. The nurse's caring demeanor and expressions of genuine concern are essential qualities when dealing with the sensitive and emotional circumstances that surround infertility testing and treatment. Depending on the patient's unique situation, a number of nursing diagnoses may be appropriate (Box 6-5).

LIFESTYLE CHOICES AND INFERTILITY

Regular physical activity, adequate rest, stress reduction, and balanced nutrition are essential strategies for health promotion and are especially important during the infertility work-up and treatment. Many seek holistic and complementary alternatives to enhance therapeutic regimens or promote a sense of personal control and well-being. Yoga is an example of a lifestyle choice that combines meditation, spirituality, exercise, and relaxation to promote balance and harmony. In addition, a number of herbal alternatives to fertility medications are available, and this information may be shared with infertile couples.

Box 6-5 Potential Nursing Diagnoses for the Patient Experiencing Infertility

- Risk for ineffective coping related to infertility
- Risk for posttrauma response related to infertility
- Risk for spiritual distress related to infertility
- Risk for situational low self-esteem related to infertility

---

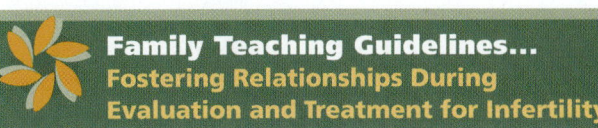

Family Teaching Guidelines...
Fostering Relationships During Evaluation and Treatment for Infertility

Couples should be encouraged to spend quality time with one another and enjoy sexual intimacy outside of the "fertile times." Professional counseling may be appropriate if one member of a couple becomes depressed or obsessed with conceiving while the other remains less involved. The nurse may suggest involvement with infertility community support groups and contact with RESOLVE, a national education/support organization that is readily available at http://www.resolve.org/.

 Complementary Care: *Herbal Supplements and Infertility*

Vitex-agnus-castus, also called Vitex, Chaste tree, Chasteberry, Abraham's Balm, or Monk's Pepper, is believed to promote ovulation; false unicorn root powder has been used to enhance fertility and prevent miscarriage. However, little research has been conducted to confirm the safety or effectiveness of these herbs, and patients should be warned about the lack of scientific data about herbal preparations. Certain herbs, including blue or black cohosh, goldenseal, poke root, pennyroyal, and aloe can be detrimental to a pregnancy and should be avoided by couples who are attempting to conceive (see Table 6-4).

ADDITIONAL OPTIONS FOR THE INFERTILE COUPLE

For patients for whom assisted reproductive technologies are unsuccessful or undesirable, surrogacy, use of a gestational carrier, or adoption may be the best option. Traditional surrogacy is an agreement by a woman to donate her egg, along with sperm of the intended father, or possible sperm donation, often accomplished through artificial insemination. The woman is considered the biological, genetic, and gestational mother, and she carries the pregnancy until delivery when she relinquishes all parental rights of the child to the intended parents. Gestational surrogates are women who undergo in vitro fertilization to carry a fetus that has no biological or genetic link to them. At birth, all parental rights are relinquished to the intended parents. The use of surrogacy is limited because of concerns about establishing legal parentage for the intended parents (Armour, 2012; Mahalingaiah & Ginsburg, 2010). A gestational carrier

Table 6-4 Herbs to Avoid When Attempting to Conceive	
Category	**Herb**
Anthraquinone Laxatives	Aloe
	Buckthorn
	Cascara sagrada
	Docks
	Meadow saffron
	Senna
Uterine Stimulants	American mandrake
	Black cohosh
	Blue cohosh
	Bloodroot
	Calamus
	Cayenne
	Fennel
	Feverfew
	Flax seed
	Goldenseal
	Lady's mantle
	Licorice
	Make fern
	Sage
	Tansy
	Thuja
	Thyme
	Wild cherry
	Wormwood
	Mayapple
	Mistletoe
	Passion flower
	Pennyroyal
	Periwinkle
	Poke root
	Rhubarb
Alkaloids/Bitter Principles	Barberry
	Bloodroot
	Celandine
	Cinchona
	Ephedra
	Goldenseal

Source: Adapted from Herbal remedies in pregnancy. *Babycenter.* Retrieved from http://www.babycentre.co.uk/a536346/herbal-remedies-in-pregnancy

contracts to carry a pregnancy that is not genetically her own offspring. Adoption may be considered after repeated attempts for pregnancy. Today, there are fewer infants and children available for adoption. Consequently, the adoptive process is often prolonged and difficult unless the couple considers a foreign-born or physically or cognitively challenged child.

Surrogacy and the use of gestational carriers involve legal as well as ethical considerations. Financial resources, personal values, and religious beliefs are all factors that may prohibit these options from being viable alternatives to a traditional pregnancy. Individuals and couples who consider these options should be advised to see an attorney to ensure that their rights, the surrogate's/carrier's rights, and the rights of the child are protected. This very important visit for legal counsel may avoid later heartbreak and legal entanglements for the patient and her family. If the surrogate/carrier changes her mind or the parents change

their minds, safeguards must be in place for all parties, including the child.

Remaining childless is another option for fertile and infertile couples. Many advantages, such as opportunity for career fulfillment, travel, and continued education make a child-free lifestyle the right choice for many couples. When working with couples who are exploring these alternative options, the nurse's role centers on education, advocacy, and empowerment. Using a framework that encompasses the cultural, spiritual, and environmental domains, the nurse provides information and guidance to community and national resources to assist the couple in dealing with these important issues.

Now Can You—Provide sensitive, appropriate care for the infertile couple?

1. Discuss emotions and stressors frequently experienced during infertility treatment?
2. Analyze the nurse's role in infertility care?
3. Create a teaching plan that describes the various reproductive technologies available?

Summary Points

- Sexuality is a multidimensional concept that is influenced by ethical, spiritual, cultural, and moral factors.

- A variety of contraceptives are available; contraceptive care should empower the patient to choose the method best suited for her.

- Tubal ligation and vasectomy are permanent sterilization procedures that have become increasingly popular.

- Infertility is the inability to conceive and carry a child when the couple wishes to do so.

- Abortion performed during the first trimester is safer than abortion performed during the second trimester.

- Reproductive alternatives include IVF, GIFT, ZIFT, oocyte/embryo donation, TDI, surrogate motherhood, and adoption.

Review Questions

Multiple Choice

1. According to Masters and Johnson's work on human sexual response phases, in which phase does a woman experience the highest sense of sexual tension?
   A. Excitement phase
   B. Plateau phase
   C. Orgasmic phase
   D. Resolution phase

2. A family planning nurse is working with an 18-year-old female who has been treated for gonorrhea in the past. In addition, the patient has a previous sexual partner who has tested positive for HIV. Which contraceptive method would probably work best for this patient?
   A. Spermicide
   B. Cervical cap
   C. Latex male condom
   D. Progestin-only pill

3. A clinic nurse schedules a patient for her initial dose of Depo-Provera (medroxyprogesterone) within
A. 24 hours of menstruation.
B. 48 hours of menstruation.
C. 3 to 4 days of menstruation.
D. 5 to 7 days of menstruation.

4. A clinic nurse is working with a woman who has been diagnosed with "sexual dysfunction." What does this nurse understand as the best explanation of this diagnosis?
A. A broad range of problems with sexual and reproductive function
B. Any sexual situation that causes personal distress for the woman
C. Psychological barriers that prevent expression of sexuality
D. Specific medical conditions that interfere with the enjoyment of sex

5. A woman has the diagnosis of "dyspareunia" on her chart. What does the nurse understand this term to mean?
A. Infrequent menstrual periods
B. Heavy menstrual bleeding
C. Lack of orgasmic ability
D. Pain with intercourse

6. A patient and her partner are in the clinic to learn about contraception options. They are especially interested in Natural Family Planning. Which of the following would be the most important for the nurse to assess?
A. Ability to use the technology
B. Commitment to the method
C. Literacy and comprehension levels
D. Regularity of the woman's cycles

7. A woman is asking the family health nurse if she needs to use contraception while she is breastfeeding. Which response by the nurse is best?
A. "It can be very effective for a short time while you are exclusively nursing."
B. "Once your baby is 1 year old, you will need to use contraception."
C. "Yes, you should use contraception; breastfeeding does not prevent pregnancy."
D. "You can rely on breastfeeding to prevent pregnancy after your period returns."

8. A young woman is being educated on the risks related to her contraceptive sponge. What symptom should the nurse advise the patient to report immediately?
A. Excessive vaginal bleeding
B. Headache and stiff neck
C. Muscle pain and weakness
D. Sudden onset of fever over 101.1°F (38.4°C)

9. A nurse is discussing contraceptive methods with a new patient. The patient is most interested in birth control pills. Which factor in her health history would be an absolute contraindication for using this method?
A. Epilepsy/Seizure disorder
B. Moderate hypertension
C. Occasional migraine headaches
D. Previous pulmonary embolism

10. A woman is being treated for infertility. The physician has prescribed a medication to stimulate follicle development. Which medication should the nurse begin teaching the patient about?
A. Clomiphene citrate (Clomid)
B. Luteinizing hormone (LH)
C. Mifepristone (Mifeprex)
D. Misoprostol (Cytotec)

See Answers to End of Chapter Review Questions on DavisPlus.

REFERENCES
Al-Safi, Z., Shavell, V. I., Katz, L. E., & Berman, J. M. (2011). Nickel hypersensitivity associated with an intratubal microinsert system. Obstetrics & Gynecology, 117(2), 461–462.
American College of Obstetricians and Gynecologists (ACOG). (2006). (Reaffirmed 2011). Practice Bulletin No.73: Use of hormonal contraception in women with coexisting medical conditions. Obstetrics & Gynecology, 107(6), 1453–1472.
American College of Obstetricians and Gynecologists (ACOG). (2009c). (Reaffirmed 2011). Committee Opinion No. 450: Increasing use of contraceptive implants and intrauterine devices to reduce unintended pregnancy. Obstetrics & Gynecology, 114(6), 1434–1438.
American College of Obstetricians and Gynecologists (ACOG). (2010). Practice Bulletin No. 112: Emergency contraception. Obstetrics & Gynecology, 115(9), 1100–1109.
American College of Obstetricians and Gynecologists (ACOG). (2011a). Primary care of lesbian and bisexual women in obstetric and gynecologic practice. In Special Issues in Women's Health, pp. 61–73. Washington, DC: Author.
American College of Obstetricians and Gynecologists (ACOG). (2011b). Practice Bulletin No. 119: Female sexual dysfunction. Obstetrics & Gynecology, 117(4), 996–1007.
American College of Obstetricians and Gynecologists (ACOG). (2011c). Practice Bulletin No. 121: Long-acting reversible contraception: Implants and intrauterine devices. Obstetrics & Gynecology, 118(1), 184–196.
American College of Obstetricians and Gynecologists (ACOG). (2012a). Committee Opinion No. 525: Health care for lesbians and bisexual women. Obstetrics & Gynecology, 119(5), 1077–1080.
American College of Obstetricians and Gynecologists (ACOG). (2012b). Committee Opinion No. 539: Adolescents and long-acting reversible contraception: Implants and intrauterine devices. Obstetrics & Gynecology, 120(4), 983–988.
American College of Obstetricians and Gynecologists (ACOG). (2013a). Committee Opinion No. 574: Marriage equality for same-sex couples. Obstetrics & Gynecology, 122(9), 729–732.
American College of Obstetricians and Gynecologists (ACOG). (2013b). Understanding and using the U.S. Selected Practice Recommendations for Contraceptive Use, 2013. Obstetrics & Gynecology, 122(5), 1132–1133.
American College of Obstetricians and Gynecologists (ACOG). (2013c). Second-trimester abortion. Practice Bulletin No. 135. Obstetrics & Gynecology, 121(6), 1394–1406.
American College of Obstetricians and Gynecologists. (ACOG). (2014). Medical management of first-trimester abortion. Practice Bulletin No. 143. Obstetrics & Gynecology, 123(3), 676–692.
American Psychiatric Association (APA). (2013). DSM-5: Diagnostic and statistical manual of mental disorders (5th ed.). Washington, DC: American Psychiatric Publishing.
Armour, K. L. (2012). An overview of surrogacy around the world. Nursing for Women's Health, 16(3), 231–236. doi:10.1111/j.1751-486X.2012.01734.x
Association of Women's Health, Obstetric and Neonatal Nurses. (AWHONN). (2009a). Position Statement: Health Care Decision Making for Reproductive Care. Journal of Obstetric, Gynecologic and Neonatal Nursing, 38(6), 523. doi:10.1111/j.1552-6909.2009.01078.x
Association of Women's Health, Obstetric and Neonatal Nurses. (AWHONN). (2009b). Position Statement: Insurance Coverage for Contraceptives. Journal of Obstetric, Gynecologic and Neonatal Nursing, 38(6), 743–744. doi:10.1111/j.1552-6909.2009.01079.x
Association of Women's Health, Obstetric and Neonatal Nurses. (AWHONN). (2012). Position Statement: Emergency Contraception. Journal of Obstetric, Gynecologic and Neonatal Nursing, 41(6), 711–713. doi:10.1111/j.1552-6909.2012.01407.x

Bartz, D., & Goldberg, A. B. (2011). Injectable contraceptives. In Hatcher, R. A., Trussell, J., Nelson, A. L, Cates, W., Kowal, D., & Policar, M. S. *Contraceptive technology* (20th revised ed., pp. 209–236). Decatur, GA: Bridging the Gap Communications.

Basson, R. (1998). Sexual health of women with disabilities. *Canadian Medical Journal Association, 159*(4), 359–362.

Basson, R. (2002). A model of women's sexual arousal. *Journal of Sex and Marital Therapy, 28*(1), 1–10.

Bonnema, R., McNamara, M. C., & Spencer, A. L. (2011). Guide to contraceptive counseling for women with medical comorbidities, Part 2: Progestin-only options. *The Female Patient, 36*(11), 23–29.

Bulechek, G. M., Butcher, H. K., Dochterman, J. M., & Wagner, C. (2013). *Nursing interventions classification (NIC)* (6th ed.). St. Louis, MO: Elsevier Mosby.

Burrows, L. J., & Resnick-Anderson, K. (2011). Female orgasmic disorder. *The Female Patient, 36*(6), 18–21.

Castano, P. M., Bynum, J. Y., Andres, R., Lara, M., & Westhoff, C. (2012). Effect of daily text messages on oral contraceptive continuation. *Obstetrics & Gynecology, 119*(1), 14–20.

Cates, W., & Harwood, B. (2011). Vaginal barriers and spermicides. In Hatcher, R. A., Trussell, J., Nelson, A. L, Cates, W., Kowal, D., & Policar, M. S. *Contraceptive technology* (20th revised ed., pp. 391–408). Decatur, GA: Bridging the Gap Communications.

Centers for Disease Control and Prevention. (2010). U.S. Medical Eligibility Criteria for Contraceptive Use, 2010. *MMWR, 59*(No. RR-4), 1–85.

Centers for Disease Control and Prevention. (2011a). Update to CDC's U.S. Medical Eligibility Criteria for Contraceptive Use, 2010: Revised recommendations for the use of contraceptive methods during the postpartum period. *MMWR, 60*(26), 878–883.

Centers for Disease Control and Prevention. (2013a). Infertility. Retrieved from http://www.cdc.gov/reproductivehealth/Infertility/

Centers for Disease Control and Prevention. (2013b). Assisted Reproductive Technology (ART). Retrieved from http://www.cdc.gov/art/

Chachamovich, J. R., Chachamovich, E., Ezer, H., Fleck, M. P., Knauth, D. R., & Passos, E. P. (2010). Agreement on perceptions of quality of life in couples dealing with infertility. *Journal of Obstetric, Gynecologic and Neonatal Nursing, 39*(5), 557–565.

Clayton, A. H., Goldfischer, E., Goldstein, I., DeRogatis, L., Nappi, R., Lewis-D'Agostino, D. J., . . . Pyke, R. (2013). Validity of the Decreased Sexual Desire Screener for diagnosing hypoactive sexual desire disorder. *Journal of Sex and Marital Therapy, 39*(2), 132–143. doi:1080/0092623X.2011.606496

Curtis, K. M., & Peterson, H. B. (2011). U.S. Medical Eligibility Criteria. In Hatcher, R. A., Trussell, J., Nelson, A. L, Cates, W., Kowal, D., & Policar, M. S. *Contraceptive technology* (20th revised ed., pp. 75–100). Decatur, GA: Bridging the Gap Communications.

Davis, S. C., & Willoughby, D. (2010). Practitioner willingness to discuss sexuality with chronic disease sufferers. *Women's Health Care: A Practical Journal for Nurse Practitioners, 9*(9), 11–20.

Dean, G., & Schwarz, E. B. (2011). Intrauterine contraceptives (IUCs). In Hatcher, R. A., Trussell, J., Nelson, A. L, Cates, W., Kowal, D., & Policar, M. S. *Contraceptive technology* (20th revised ed., pp. 147–192). Decatur, GA: Bridging the Gap Communications.

Dehlendorf, C., Bryant, A. S., Huddleston, H. G., Jacoby, V. L., & Fujimoto, V. Y. (2010). Health disparities: Definitions and measurements. *American Journal of Obstetrics and Gynecology, 202*(3), 212–213.

Delk, C., & Wiczyk, H. (2010). Approach to health care for lesbian and bisexual women. *The Female Patient, 35*(1), 26–29.

Dillon, P. M. (2007). *Nursing health assessment. Clinical pocket guide.* Philadelphia, PA: F.A. Davis.

Earle, S., Tilley, L., & Walmsley, J. (2012). Who makes crucial decisions on reproduction and contraception? *Learning Disability Practice, 15*(8), 34–35.

Edmunds, M. (2011). Contraceptive management for women with medical conditions. *The Journal for Nurse Practitioners, 7*(1), 71–72.

Espey, E., & Ogburn, T. (2011). Long-acting reversible contraceptives. *Obstetrics & Gynecology, 117*(3), 705–719.

Evans, M. I. (2010). The truth about multiples. *The Female Patient, 36*(3), 35–37.

Fehring, R. J., Schneider, M., & Raviele, K. (2011). Pilot evaluation of an Internet-based natural family planning education and service program. *Journal of Obstetric, Gynecologic & Neonatal Nursing, 40*(3), 281–291.

Fine, P. M. (2011). A new option in emergency contraception. *The Female Patient, 36*(2), 41–44.

Forcier, M., & Harel, Z. (2011). Adolescents and the IUD: An underutilized contraception for a high-risk population. *The Female Patient, 36*(6), 22–25.

Frederick, C. E., Voedisch, A. J., & Blumenthal, P. D. (2010). Hormonal contraception: New approaches for selected patients. *The Female Patient, 35*(8), 30–35.

Gilliam, M. L. (2010). Cervical preparation for first trimester surgical abortion. *Obstetrics & Gynecology, 115*(5), 1075–1076.

Gilliam, M. L. (2011). Medical methods for mid-trimester termination of pregnancy. *Obstetrics & Gynecology, 117*(5), 1223–1224.

Grossman, D., Grindlay, K., Buchacker, T., Lane, K., & Blanchard, K. (2011). Effectiveness and acceptability of medical abortion provided through telemedicine. *Obstetrics & Gynecology, 118*(2), 296–303.

Guttmacher Institute. (2012). An overview of minors' consent law. Retrieved from http://www.guttmacher.org/statecenter/spibs/spib OMCL.pdf

Harel, Z., Johnson, C. C., Gold, M. A., Cromer, B., Peterson, E., Burkman, R., . . . Bachrach, L. K. (2010). Recovery of bone mineral density in adolescents following the use of depot medroxyprogesterone acetate contraceptive injections. *Contraception, 81*(4), 281–291.

Hatcher, R. A., Trussell, J., Nelson, A., Cates, W., Stewart, F. H., & Kowal, D. (2011). *Contraceptive technology* (20th Revised ed.). Decatur, GA: Bridging the Gap Communications.

Herbal remedies in pregnancy. *Babycenter.* Retrieved from http://www.babycentre.co.uk/a536346/herbal-remedies-in-pregnancy

Herschberger, P. E., Schoenfeld, C., & Tur-Kaspa, I. (2011). Unraveling preimplantation genetic diagnosis for high-risk couples. *Nursing for Women's Health, 15*(1), 38–45.

Higgins, J. A., & Davis, A. R. (2011). Sexuality and contraception. In Hatcher, R. A., Trussell, J., Nelson, A. L, Cates, W., Kowal, D., & Policar, M. S. *Contraceptive technology* (20th revised ed., pp. 1–28). Decatur, GA: Bridging the Gap Communications.

Holloway, B., & Moredich, C. (2011). *OB/GYN Peds Notes.* Philadelphia: F.A. Davis.

Hrivnak, J. (2013). Health issues in lesbian patients. *Advance for NPs & PAs, 4*(10), 17–20.

Jennings, V. H., & Burke, A. E. (2011). Fertility awareness-based methods. In Hatcher, R. A., Trussell, J., Nelson, A. L, Cates, W., Kowal, D., & Policar, M. S. *Contraceptive technology* (20th revised ed., pp. 417–434). Decatur, GA: Bridging the Gap Communications.

Johnson, M., Moorhead, S., Bulechek, G., Butcher, H., Maas, M., & Swanson, E. (2012). *NIC and NOC linkages to NANDA-L and clinical conditions* (3rd ed.). St. Louis, MO: Elsevier Mosby.

Kellogg-Spadt, S. (2010). What's so distressing about female sexual dysfunction? *Women's Health Care: A Practical Journal for Nurse Practitioners, 9*(9), 40–41.

Kellogg-Spadt, S. (2011). Vaginal lubrication: Setting realistic expectations. *Women's Health Care: A Practical Journal for Nurse Practitioners, 10*(5), 17–18.

Kennedy, K. I., & Trussell, J. (2011). Postpartum contraception and lactation. In Hatcher, R. A., Trussell, J., Nelson, A. L, Cates, W., Kowal, D., & Policar, M. S. *Contraceptive technology* (20th revised ed., pp. 483–512). Decatur, GA: Bridging the Gap Communications.

Kowal, D. (2011). Coitus interruptus (Withdrawal). In Hatcher, R. A., Trussell, J., Nelson, A. L, Cates, W., Kowal, D., & Policar, M. S. *Contraceptive technology* (20th revised ed., pp. 409–416). Decatur, GA: Bridging the Gap Communications.

Lee, K. C. (2011). Fertility treatments and the cost of a healthy baby. *Nursing for Women's Health, 15*(1), 15–18.

Lee, V. C., Ng, E. H., Yeung, W. S., & Ho, P. C. (2011). Misoprostol with or without letrozole pretreatment for termination of pregnancy. *Obstetrics & Gynecology, 117*(2), 317–323.

Leslie, K. K., Thiel, K. W., & Yang, S. (2012). Endometrial cancer: Potential treatment and prevention with progestin-containing intrauterine devices. *Obstetrics & Gynecology, 119*(2), 419–420.

Letishock, L., Pariseau, C., Rooholamini, S., & Ammerman, S. (2011). Anaphylaxis from depot medroxyprogesterone acetate in an adolescent girl. *Obstetrics & Gynecology, 118*(2), 443–445.

Lindahl, S. H. (2011). Contraception update. *Advance for NPs & PAs, 2*(1), 31–34.

Lockwood, C. J., & Hillard, P. J. A. (2010). Use of CDC medical eligibility criteria provides evidence on contraceptive method risks and benefits. *Contemporary OB/GYN, 55*(7), 7–10.

Mahalingaiah, S., & Ginsburg, E. (2010). Trends in assisted reproductive technology. *The Female Patient, 35*(11), 18–24.

Margolis, M. B. (2010). The myths and facts of intrauterine contraception bleeding profiles. *The Female Patient, Suppl 35*(9), 1–10.

Masters, W., & Johnson, V. E. (1966). *Human sexual response.* Boston: Little Brown.

Meier, C., Brauchli, Y. B., Jick, S. S., Kraenzlin, M. E., & Meier, C. R. (2010). Use of depot medroxyprogesterone acetate and fracture risk. *Journal of Clinical Endocrinology & Metabolism, 95*(11), 4909–4916.

Moorehead, S., Johnson, M., Maas, M., & Swanson, E. (2013). *Nursing outcomes classification (NOC)* (5th ed.). St. Louis, MO: C.V. Mosby.

Nanda, K. (2011). Contraceptive patch and vaginal contraceptive ring. In Hatcher, R. A., Trussell, J., Nelson, A. L., Cates, W., Kowal, D., & Policar, M. S. *Contraceptive technology* (20th revised ed., pp. 343–370). Decatur, GA: Bridging the Gap Communications.

National Health Statistics Reports. (2011). Sexual Behavior, sexual attraction, and sexual identity in the United States: Data from the 2006–2008 National Survey of Family Growth. Retrieved from http://www.cdc.gov/nchs/data/nhsr/nhsr036.pdf

Nelson, A. L. (2010a). A new OC with a new estrogen, a new progestin, and a new indication. *The Female Patient, 35*(1), 36–38.

Nelson, A. L. (2010b). LNG-IUS: First-line therapy for idiopathic heavy menstrual bleeding. *The Female Patient, 35*(11), 39–43.

Nelson, A. L., & Cwiak, C. (2011). Combined oral contraceptives (COCs). In Hatcher, R. A., Trussell, J., Nelson, A. L, Cates, W., Kowal, D., & Policar, M. S. *Contraceptive technology* (20th revised ed., pp. 249–342). Decatur, GA: Bridging the Gap Communications.

Office on Women's Health, U.S. Department of Health and Human Services. (2012). *Lesbian and bisexual health fact sheet.* Retrieved from http://www.womenshealth.gov/publications/our-publications/fact-sheet/lesbian-bisexual-health.html

Paterno, M. T., & Jordan, E. T. (2012). A review of factors associated with unprotected sex among adult women in the United States. *Journal of Obstetric, Gynecologic & Neonatal Nursing, 41*(2), 258–274. doi:10.1111/j.1552-6909.2011.01334.x

Paul, M., & Stein, T. (2011). Abortion. In Hatcher, R. A., Trussell, J., Nelson, A. L, Cates, W., Kowal, D., & Policar, M. S. *Contraceptive technology* (20th revised ed., pp. 637-666). Decatur, GA: Bridging the Gap Communications.

Perriera, L. K., & Greenfield, M. (2011). OC therapy in teens. *Contemporary OB/GYN, 56*(5), 40–47.

Perriera, L. K., Reeves, M. F., Chen, B. A., Hohmann, H. L., Hayes, J., & Creinin, M. D. (2010). Feasibility of telephone follow-up after medical abortion. *Contraception, 81*(7), 143–149.

Raymond, E. G. (2011a). Progestin-only pills. In Hatcher, R. A., Trussell, J., Nelson, A. L, Cates, W., Kowal, D., & Policar, M. S. *Contraceptive technology* (20th revised ed., pp. 237–248). Decatur, GA: Bridging the Gap Communications.

Raymond, E. G. (2011b). Contraceptive implants. In Hatcher, R. A., Trussell, J., Nelson, A. L, Cates, W., Kowal, D., & Policar, M. S. *Contraceptive technology* (20th revised ed., pp. 145-156). Decatur, GA: Bridging the Gap Communications.

Ridley, M. (2013). *Genome: The autobiography of a species in 23 chapters.* New York: Harper Perennial.

Roncari, D., & Hou, M. Y. (2011). Female and male sterilization. In Hatcher, R. A., Trussell, J., Nelson, A. L, Cates, W., Kowal, D., & Policar, M. S. *Contraceptive technology* (20th revised ed., pp. 435–482). Decatur, GA: Bridging the Gap Communications.

Rowlands, S. (2011). Learning disability and contraceptive decision-making. *Journal of Family Planning and Reproductive Health Care, 37*(3), 173–178.

Ruhl, C. (2012). Contraception is health promotion. *Nursing for Women's Health, 16*(1), 73–77. doi:10.1111/j.1751-486X.2012.01703.x

Santelli, J., Kowal, D., & Wheeler, E. (2011). Abstinence, noncoital sex, and nonsense: What every clinician needs to know. In Hatcher, R. A., Trussell, J., Nelson, A. L, Cates, W., Kowal, D., & Policar, M. S. *Contraceptive technology* (20th revised ed., pp. 101–112). Decatur, GA: Bridging the Gap Communications.

Schnare, S. M., & Garcia, A. (2010). Essure: A nonsurgical option for female sterilization. *The American Journal for Nurse Practitioners, 14*(2), 9–17.

Scholes, D., LaCroix, A. Z., Ichikawa, L. E., et al. (2005). Change in bone mineral density among adolescent women using and discontinuing depot medroxyprogesterone acetate contraception. *Archives of Pediatric Adolescent Medicine, 159*(2), 139–144.

Setti, P. E. L., & Patrizio, P. (2012). Oocyte cryopreservation: Recent progress, future expectations. *Contemporary OB/GYN, 57*(5), 52–58.

Simmonds, K., & Likis, F. E. (2011). Caring for women with unintended pregnancies. *Journal of Obstetric, Gynecologic & Neonatal Nursing, 40*(6), 794–807.

Society for Assisted Reproductive Technology. (2012). Assisted reproductive technology. Retrieved from http://www.sart.org/detail.aspx?id=1908

Spencer, A. L., McNamara, M. C., & Bonnema, R. (2011). Guide to contraceptive counseling for women with medical comorbidities, Part 1: Combined progestin + estrogen options. *The Female Patient, 36*(10), 22–28.

Sufrin, C. B., & Korn, A. (2009). Tubal sterilization: A closer look at risk of pregnancy. *Contemporary OB/GYN, 54*(5), 50–55.

Sullivan, L. (2010). Teen contraception: Darned if you do and darned if you don't. *The Journal for Nurse Practitioners, 6*(4), 274–278.

Taylor, D., & James, E. A. (2011). An evidence-based guideline for unintended pregnancy prevention. *Journal of Obstetric, Gynecologic & Neonatal Nursing, 40*(6), 782–793.

Tilley, E., Earle, S., Walmsley, J., & Atkinson, D. (2012). The silence is roaring: Sterilization, reproductive rights and women with intellectual disabilities. *Disability and Society, 27*(3), 413–426.

Trolice, M. P. (2011). Evaluating an infertile patient: An evidence-based review. *The Female Patient, 36*(1), 25–30.

Trussell, J., & Guthrie, K. A. (2011). Choosing a contraceptive: Efficacy, safety, and personal considerations. In Hatcher, R. A., Trussell, J., Nelson, A. L, Cates, W., Kowal, D., & Policar, M. S. *Contraceptive technology* (20th revised ed., pp. 45–74). Decatur, GA: Bridging the Gap Communications.

Trussell, J., & Raymond, E. G. (2012). Emergency contraception: A last chance to prevent unintended pregnancy. Retrieved from http://ec.princeton.edu/questions/ec-review.pdf

Trussell, J., & Schwarz, E. B. (2011). Emergency contraception. In Hatcher, R. A., Trussell, J., Nelson, A. L, Cates, W., Kowal, D., & Policar, M. S. *Contraceptive technology* (20th revised ed., pp. 113–146). Decatur, GA: Bridging the Gap Communications.

Tyler, C. P., Whiteman, M. K., Zapata, L. B., Curtis, K. M., Hillis, S. D., & Marchbanks, P. A. (2012). Health care provider attitudes and practices related to intrauterine devices for nulliparous women. *Obstetrics & Gynecology, 119*(4), 762–771. doi:10.1097/AOG.0b013e31824aca.39

U.S. Department of Health and Human Services (DHHS). (2012). *Healthy People 2020 Family Planning Objectives.* Retrieved from http://www.healthypeople.gov/2020/topicsobjectives2020/objectiveslist.aspx?topicId=13

U.S. Food and Drug Administration. (2012). FDA Drug Safety Communication: Updated information about the risk of blood clots in women taking birth control pills containing drospirenone. Retrieved from http://www.fda.gov/Drugs/DrugSafety/ucm299305.htm

U.S. Selected Practice Recommendations for Contraceptive Use, 2013: Adapted from the World Health Organization selected practice recommendations for contraceptive use, 2nd edition. (2013). *Morbidity and Mortality Weekly Report, 62*(RR05), 1–46.

Vickery, Z., & Madden, T. (2011). Difficult intrauterine contraception insertion in a nulligravid patient. *Obstetrics & Gynecology, 117*(2), 391–395.

Warner, L., & Steiner, M. J. (2011). Male condoms. In Hatcher, R. A., Trussell, J., Nelson, A. L, Cates, W., Kowal, D., & Policar, M. S. *Contraceptive technology* (20th revised ed., pp. 371–390). Decatur, GA: Bridging the Gap Communications.

Williams, R. L. (2012). Long-acting reversible contraceptives for adolescents. *The Female Patient, 37*(2), 21–26.

Wilton, J. M. (2011). Oral contraception: New options. *Nursing for Women's Health, 15*(5), 431–434.

World Health Organization. (2006). *Defining sexual health: Report of a technical consultation on sexual health, 28–31 January 2002.* Geneva, Switzerland: WHO.

World Health Organization. (2010). *Medical eligibility criteria for contraceptive use* (4th ed.). Geneva, Switzerland: World Health Organization.

World Health Organization. (2012). *Emergency contraception.* (Fact sheet). Retrieved from http://www.who.int/mediacentre/factsheets/fs244/en

CONCEPT MAP

Human Sexuality and Fertility

Sexual Response:
Phases:
- Excitement
- Plateau
- Orgasmic
- Resolution

Sexual Dysfunction:
Sexual stimulation that produces personal distress:
- Pain
- Arousal disorder
- Orgasmic disorder
- Desire disorder

Sexual Orientation:
- Heterosexual
- Homosexual
  - Gay, lesbian

Nursing Assessment: Part of Holistic Care
- Establish trusting relationship
- Be aware of own biases
- Don't make assumptions about sexual partners/activity
- Avoid judgment ➞ shame
- Elicit sexual history
  - Practices
  - Partners
  - STIs

Nursing Insight:
- Certain conditions make contraceptive barrier methods inadvisable
- AWHONN supports right to accurate/complete info and access to reproductive care
- Not every woman is a candidate for cervical cap
- Be proactive with health promotion strategies
- OCP may benefit teens with dysmenorrhea, anovulatory cycling or acne

Healthy People 2020: Reproductive Life Planning
- Decrease unwanted pregnancies
- Improve contraception access/use
- Reduce proportion of women 18-44 with impaired fecundity

Across Care Settings:
- Fit birth control method to the needs of special populations
- Medication abortion can be provided through telemedicine

Infertility

Nursing Role: Infertility Care
- Assess: timing of intercourse and length of coital exposure; knowledge of fertile periods
- Assess for influencing factors: acute/chronic disease; lifestyle patterns; STIs; age
- Teach: signs of ovulation, positioning; recording basal temp
- Later assessment methods:
  - Labs: thyroid, glucose prolactin/specific hormonal assays
  - Endometrial biopsy
  - Hysterosalpingography
  - Laparoscopy
  - Semen analysis
  - Postcoital test

Managing Infertility

Fertility Treatments:
Inducing ovulation:
- Medications
- Surgery
- Therapeutic insemination
- ARTs:
  - GIFT
  - ZIFT
  - TET
  - In vitro fertilization
- Embryo cryopreservation
- Micromanipulation

- Surrogacy
- Adoption
- Childless

Preventing Conception

Methods:
- NFP: Natural family planning
- Fertility awareness base
  - Coitus interruptus
  - Breastfeeding (L.A.M.)
  - Abstinence
- Barriers
  - Diaphragm, cervical cap, male and female condoms, sponge, spermaticides
- Hormones
  - OCP, patch, vaginal ring, emergency contraceptives; subdermal implant; injected: DMPA - IM
- IUD
- Sterilization (male and female)

Clinical Termination of Pregnancy

Elective and Therapeutic Methods:
- Surgical: D&E, vacuum aspiration
- Medical:
  - Mifepristone
  - Methotrexate

Nursing:
- Emotional support
- Labs; history; exam; determine gestation
- Assess for postprocedure complications
- Teach:
  - Birth control plan
  - Importance of follow-up visits

Nursing: Assess Pt's
- Knowledge of method
- Comfort level
- Correct/consistent use of contraceptive
- Satisfaction with chosen method

Optimizing Outcomes:
- Accurate and thorough teaching about all contraceptive methods
- Specific teaching:
  - Drug/drug interactions with OCP
  - Permanent sterilization
- Support laws to mandate insurance coverage for contraception
- DSDS tool to identify H.S.D.D.
- Resource/referral guide for women with unwanted pregnancy
- Follow CDC evidence-based guidelines to prescribe contraceptives

Clinical Alert:
- Signs of short-term complications post-abortion

Complementary Care:
- Use caution when trying herbs for infertility

Critical Nursing Actions:
- Teach absolute contraindications for OCP
- Teach "PAINS" to IUD users

Where Research and Practice Meet:
- Internet-based NFP education program effective
- Depo-Provera can decrease bone density in adolescents
- Educational text messaging increases OCP compliance

Legal Alert:
- Always ask about latex allergies with condom and diaphragm use
- Teach about toxic shock syndrome
- Teach "ACHES" for OCP users
- Laws R/T reproductive health care for minors
- Legal requirements for sterilization

Now Can You:

- Develop questions that will assist with taking a sexual history
- Analyze the role of the nurse in dealing with patients seeking a contraceptive method
- Discuss the nurse's overall role in reproductive health
- Provide teaching for patients regarding various reproductive technologies

Conception and Development of the Embryo and Fetus

 You are a child of the universe no less than the trees and the stars; you have a right to be here.
And whether or not it is clear to you, no doubt the universe is unfolding as it should.
—From the poem "Desiderata"

LEARNING TARGETS *At the completion of this chapter, the student will be able to:*

◆ Explain the basic concepts of inheritance.

◆ Outline the process of fertilization, implantation, and placental development.

◆ Discuss the structure and function of the placenta and umbilical cord.

◆ Trace a drop of blood through the fetal circulatory system.

◆ Identify the time intervals and major events of the pre-embryonic, embryonic, and fetal stages of development.

◆ Discuss threats to embryo/fetal well-being and development and explain the nurse's role in minimizing threats to the developing fetus.

PICO(T) Questions

The intent of evidence-based practice (EBP) is to provide nursing care that integrates the best available evidence. An initial step in EBP is to write a PICO(T) question that effectively guides the research. A PICO(T) question is an acronym that stands for population (P), intervention or issue (I), comparison of interest (C), outcome (O), and timeframe (T). Depending on the question, all or some of the question components are used in the research process. Use these PICO(T) questions to spark your thinking as you read the chapter.

1. What are (O) the best strategies for (I) managing moderate to severe pain (P) in pregnant women while minimizing the risk to the fetus?

2. Does (I) preconception education related to teratogens and fetal health lead to (O) a lower incidence of structural or developmental anomalies (P) in newborns when provided to both men and women (C) as compared with women only?

Evidence-Based Practice

Forand, S. P., Lewis-Michl, E. L., & Gomez, M. I. (2012). Adverse birth outcomes and maternal exposure to trichloroethylene and tetrachloroethylene through soil vapor intrusion in New York State. *Environmental Health Perspectives, 120*(4), 616–621.

The purpose of this study was to investigate the prevalence of adverse outcomes among mothers exposed to trichloroethylene (TCE) and tetrachloroethylene [or perchloroethylene (PCE)] through indoor air contamination via soil vapor intrusion. Groundwater, soil, and soil gas in Endicott, New York, have been contaminated by spills of volatile organic compounds (VOCs). Previous studies have demonstrated the relationship between exposure to VOCs in drinking water and increases in adverse birth outcomes among exposed women. Cardiac defects, oral clefts, neural tube defects, and choanal atresia have all been found in infants born to women living in this area. Previous studies have associated those defects with TCE- and PCE-contaminated drinking water.

Few studies, however, have evaluated the association between contaminants and low birth weight (LBW), preterm birth, and fetal growth restriction among this population. The total exposure area included 3,002 individuals: 2,378 in the TCE area and 624 in the PCE area. Of this group, 686 were reproductive-aged females. The comparative population of New York State (excluding New York City) was 10,968,179, of which 2,297,231 were reproductive-aged women. Eighty-nine percent of the population in the contaminant exposure area were identified as Caucasian, 5% as African American, 4% as "other," 2% as multiracial, and 2% as Hispanic. Twenty-four percent of the population was described as persons living below the poverty level.

Regression analyses were used to compare birth outcomes among residents of the exposed community with those of the general New York State population. Data were obtained from existing birth certificate and birth defect registry records. All live births in the Endicott study area were included in the study population. All births for the rest of New York State excluding New York City were used for the comparison population. A record review conducted for the years 1978 to 2002 included singleton births with evidence of LBW, preterm births, and fetal growth restriction outcomes. Birth defects for all births between 1983 and 2000 were also studied because these dates most closely matched the years of exposure in which outcome data were available. Preterm and birth weight outcomes were defined as follows:

- Low birth weight (LBW) = less than 2,500 g
- Very low birth weight (VLBW) = less than 1,500 g
- Preterm birth = less than 37 weeks gestation
- Very preterm birth = less than 32 weeks of gestation

Growth restriction outcomes were defined as follows:

- Term LBW (greater than 37 weeks gestation and birth weight less than 2,500 g)
- Small for gestational age (SGA) (birth weight below the 10th percentile)

Birth records were excluded if there was any missing data, which was provided by the New York State Department of Health Congenital Malformations Registry (CMR). Specific defects were identified by using ICD-9 codes and included cardiac defects, orofacial clefts, and choanal atresia. Environmental exposure assessment was determined by sampling the indoor air of 25% of the structures in the area that were potentially affected by VOCs and/or the maternal residence at the time of birth. Each mother's age, race, education, number of previous live births, prenatal care history (number of visits and when started) and infant's gender were analyzed as covariates. Subanalysis of LBW and fetal growth restriction was also conducted in relation to maternal smoking history, which was rated as: nonsmoker, less than 0.5 pack/day, 0.5 to 1 pack/day, or greater than 1 pack/day.

Analysis of data revealed that maternal residence in the TCE area was associated with LBW (n=76), term LBW (n=117), and SGA (n=37), although this finding was not supported among those residing in the PCE exposure area. Shortened gestation was not associated with TCE exposure. Infant cardiac defects were elevated in both the PCE and TCE areas, although this finding was statistically significant only in the TCE exposure area. Sixty-one children born in the exposure areas during the designated time frame were diagnosed with at least one reportable birth defect, and this was most often a cardiac defect. There were no reported cases of orofacial clefts, neural tube defects, or choanal atresias. The investigators also noted that 39% of mothers in the study area, as compared with 14% statewide, reported smoking during pregnancy. Smoking was found to be significantly associated with LBW, SGA, and term LBW. The association was noted to increase in proportion to the number of cigarettes smoked. Several of the outcomes (i.e., LBW, term LBW, and SGA) were associated with lower socioeconomic status (SES). Maternal education was included in an attempt to control for SES differences. There was an inverse association between all birth outcomes and the mother's educational level. Incorporating race in the analysis was not found to be significantly significant.

The researchers concluded that the study added to the body of evidence linking TCE and PCE to adverse birth outcomes. Increased numbers of VLBW, term LBW, and SGA were found to occur among infants born to mothers who lived in the TCE exposure area but not in the PCE exposure area. There was also an increase in infant cardiac defects, especially conotruncal defects (malformations of the outflow tract) in both the TCE and PCE exposure areas.

1. How is this information useful to clinical nursing practice?

2. Based on these findings, what are implications for further research?

See Suggested Responses for Evidence-Based Practice on Davis*Plus*.

Introduction

The beginnings of human life occur when a female gamete (ovum) unites with a male gamete (spermatozoon). The birth of a newborn signals the completion of a successful process that begins with conception (the union of a single egg and sperm) and continues throughout a remarkable period of fetal growth and development. During this time, many complex events take place. Fertilization of an ovum by a sperm creates a zygote, which must successfully implant into the hormonally prepared uterus for continued survival. The placenta plays an essential role in the ongoing transfer of oxygen and nutrients to the developing embryo and fetus. The umbilical cord that connects the developing fetus to the placenta is another key structure that facilitates the transfer of maternal oxygen and nutrients and the removal of fetal waste products. The fetal circulatory system follows a unique pathway that allows the delivery of oxygen-rich blood from the placenta to all major organ systems while bypassing the lungs. The membranes and amniotic fluid are other important elements that are essential for successful fetal growth and development. During the gestational period, drugs, infections, and environmental hazards can have a negative impact on the developing embryo and fetus. This chapter examines the key events that take place during conception and fetal development. Threats to the embryo/fetus, influences of heredity and genetics, and the basics of multifetal pregnancy are also explored.

Basic Concepts of Inheritance

THE HUMAN GENOME PROJECT

The Human Genome Project began in 1990 with an overarching goal to identify the exact **DNA** (deoxyribonucleic acid) sequences and **genes** (segments of DNA that contain information needed to make protein) that occur in humans. The information obtained from the Human Genome Project has enabled scientists to read the complete genetic blueprint of a human being. It is anticipated that the project findings will lead to new methods of diagnosing, treating, and perhaps even preventing a host of diverse human diseases and disorders. Additional information about the Human Genome Project can be found at http://www.genome.gov/10001772 and in Chapter 2.

 Nursing Insight—*Genetics, genomics, and contemporary nursing practice*

Genetics is the study of single genes and their effects. Genomics is the study of the functions and interactions of all genes in the **genome** (a complete copy of the genetic material in an organism) (National Human Genome Research Institute, 2011). The shift from genetics to genomics may be viewed as a continuum that ranges from the concept of disease in genetics to the concept of genetic information in genomics (Khoury, Bedrosian, Gwinn, Higgins, Ioannidis, & Little, 2010). Present-day advances in genetic and genomic information has exerted an increasing influence on health-care decisions and nursing

practice. To address current health-care needs, professional nursing organizations including the Oncology Nursing Society and the International Society of Nurses in Genetics have developed position statements related to the use of genetic information and nursing practice for nurse generalists, advanced practice nurses, and those with specialty training in genetics (Loud, 2010).

CHROMOSOMES, DNA, AND GENES

Before our present understanding of DNA, scientists noticed that traits were passed down from preceding generations. In the 19th century, Gregor Mendel proposed that the "strength" of some characteristics explains the variations in patterns of inheritance. Later in the 19th century, scientists identified **chromosomes** (threadlike packages of genes and other DNA) in the nucleus of the cell and found that one-half of each pair was derived from the maternal **gamete** (mature germ cell) and one-half from the paternal gamete. A number of influences help to determine who we are. These include heredity, the process of cellular division, and environmental factors.

The fundamental unit of heredity in humans is a linear sequence of working subunits of DNA called genes. DNA carries the instructions that allow cells to make proteins and transmit hereditary information from one cell to another. Most genes are located on chromosomes found in the nucleus of cells. Genes occupy a specific location along each chromosome, known as a locus. Genes come in pairs, with one copy inherited from each parent. Many genes come in a number of variant forms, known as alleles. Different alleles produce different characteristics such as hair color or blood type. One form of the allele (the dominant one) may be more greatly expressed than another form (the recessive one).

All normal somatic (body) cells contain 46 chromosomes that are arranged as 23 pairs of **homologous** or matched chromosomes. One chromosome of each pair is inherited from each parent. Twenty-two of the pairs are **autosomes** (nonsex chromosomes that are common to both males and females), and there is one pair of the sex chromosomes that determines gender (Fig. 7-1). The autosomes are involved in the transmission of all genetic traits and conditions other than those associated with the sex-linked chromosomes. The large **X chromosome** is the female chromosome; the small male chromosome is the **Y chromosome.** The presence of a Y chromosome causes the embryo to develop as a male; in the absence of a Y chromosome, the embryo develops as a female. Thus, a normal female has a 46 XX chromosome constitution; a normal male has a 46 XY chromosome constitution. The two distinct sex chromosomes carry the genes that transmit sex-linked traits and conditions. Because the chromosomes are paired, there are two copies of each gene. If the gene pairs are identical, they are **homozygous;** if they are different, they are **heterozygous.** In the heterozygous state, if one allele is expressed over the other, this allele is considered dominant. Recessive traits can be expressed when the allele responsible for the trait is found on both chromosomes.

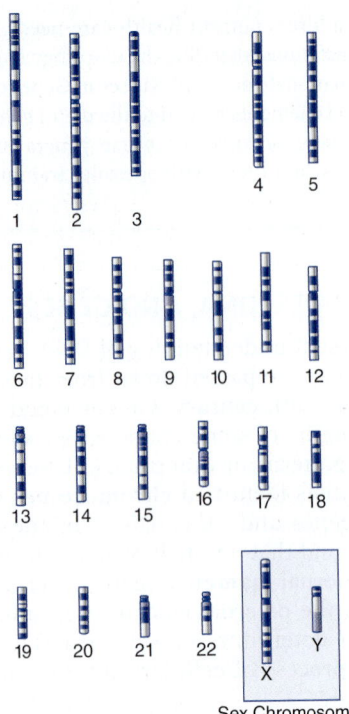

Figure 7-1 The sex chromosomes. (Courtesy of National Human Genome Research Institute.)

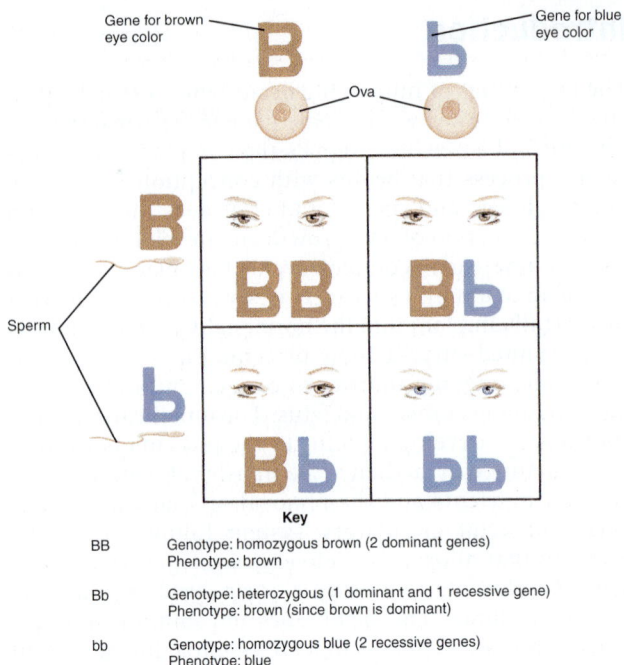

BB	Genotype: homozygous brown (2 dominant genes) Phenotype: brown
Bb	Genotype: heterozygous (1 dominant and 1 recessive gene) Phenotype: brown (since brown is dominant)
bb	Genotype: homozygous blue (2 recessive genes) Phenotype: blue

Figure 7-2 Use of a Punnett square to demonstrate inheritance of eye color.

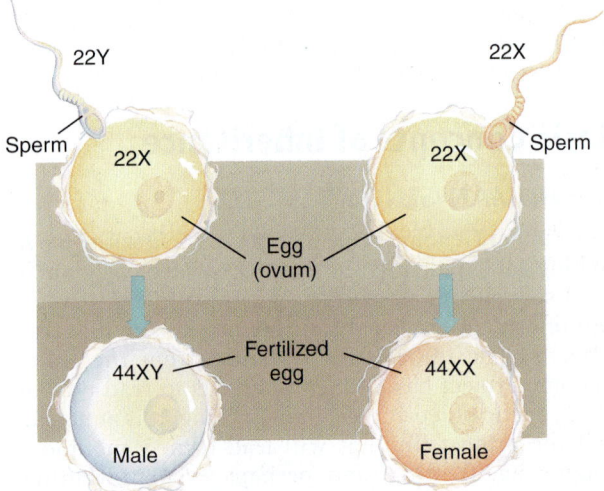

Figure 7-3 Inheritance of gender.

Nursing Insight—*Differentiating genotype from phenotype*

Although "**genotype**" refers to the genetic makeup of an individual when referring to a specific gene pair, it is sometimes used to refer to an individual's entire genetic makeup or all of the genes that a person can pass on to future generations. An individual's **genome** is the complete set of genes present (about 21,000). The term "**phenotype**" refers to the *observable* expression of a person's genotype: physical features, a biochemical or molecular trait, or a psychological trait. A trait or disorder is *dominant* if it is phenotypically apparent when only one copy of an allele associated with the trait is present. It is *recessive* if it is phenotypically apparent only when two copies of the alleles associated with the trait are present. Consider, for example, the inheritance of eye color. Although eye color is determined by many pairs of genes, with many possible phenotypes, one pair is considered the principal pair, with brown eyes dominant over blue eyes. A Punnett square (diagram drawn to determine the possible combinations of alleles in the offspring of a particular set of parents) may be used to illustrate inheritance of eye color (Fig. 7-2). Both parents are heterozygous for eye color; their genotype consists of a gene for brown eyes and a gene for blue eyes, but their phenotype is brown eyes (Scanlon & Sanders, 2011).

The sex of the embryo is determined at fertilization and is dependent on the sperm (X or Y) that fertilizes the ovum (Fig. 7-3). The union of these highly specialized cells marks the beginning of the development of each unique human being. Clinical practice is based on a calculation of pregnancy weeks, beginning with the first day of the last normal menstrual period (LNMP). However, fertilization usually occurs approximately 2 weeks after the beginning of the woman's LNMP. **Gestation** is defined as the length of time from conception to birth. The gestational period in humans ranges from 259 to 287 days. In this chapter, the weeks of gestation are calculated from the time of fertilization.

Nursing Insight—*Understanding abnormalities in sex chromosomes*

Turner syndrome, the most common sex chromosome deviation in females, is characterized by a chromosomal constitution of 45X: all or part of one X chromosome is missing (**monosomy X**). Affected females usually exhibit juvenile external genitalia, undeveloped ovaries, short stature, and webbing of the neck. When present, involvement of the cardiovascular system (e.g., bicuspid aortic valve and coarctation of the aorta) poses the most serious risk to patients (Cohen & Lynch, 2011). Intelligence may be impaired. In males, *Klinefelter's syndrome*, or trisomy XXY, is the most common sex chromosome deviation. The presence of the extra X chromosome results in poorly developed male secondary sexual characteristics, small testes, and infertility. Intelligence may be impaired as well.

Inheritance of Disease

Heritable characteristics describe those that can be passed on to offspring. The manner in which genetic material is transmitted to the next generation is dependent on the number of genes involved in the expression of the trait. A number of phenotypic characteristics can result when two or more genes on different chromosomes act together (known as multifactorial inheritance). A trait or disorder may also be controlled by a single gene (referred to as unifactorial inheritance). A family pedigree, or map of family relationships, is useful for assessing the incidence of inherited disorders.

MULTIFACTORIAL INHERITANCE

The majority of congenital malformations result from multifactorial inheritance, a combination of genetic and environmental factors. Examples include malformations such as cleft lip, cleft palate, neural tube defects, pyloric stenosis, and congenital heart disease that may range from mild to severe, depending on the number of genes for the particular defect and the amount of the environmental influence.

UNIFACTORIAL INHERITANCE

Unifactorial Mendelian or single-gene inheritance describes a pattern of inheritance that results when a specific trait or disorder is controlled by a single gene. There are many more single-gene disorders than chromosomal abnormalities. Patterns of inheritance for single-gene disorders include autosomal dominant, autosomal recessive, and X-linked dominant and recessive modes of inheritance.

Autosomal Dominant Inheritance

Autosomal dominant inheritance disorders are caused by a single altered gene along one of the autosomes. In most situations, the affected individual comes from a family of multiple

generations that have the disorder. The variant allele may also arise from a **mutation** (a spontaneous, permanent change in the normal gene structure). In this situation, the disorder occurs for the first time in the family. An affected parent who is heterozygous for the trait (i.e., has a corresponding healthy recessive gene for the trait) has a 50% chance of passing the variant allele to each offspring. Examples of autosomal dominant disorders include neurofibromatosis (a progressive disorder of the nervous system that causes the formation of nerve tumors throughout the body), Marfan's syndrome (a connective tissue disorder in which the child is taller and thinner than normal and has associated heart defects), Factor V Leiden mutation (a disorder that significantly increases the individual's risk for deep venous thrombosis and pulmonary emboli) (American College of Obstetricians and Gynecologists [ACOG], 2011a), achondroplasia (dwarfism), Huntington's disease (a progressive disease of the central nervous system characterized by involuntary writhing, ballistic or dance-like movements), and facioscapulohumeral muscular dystrophy (a form of osteogenesis imperfecta, a disorder in which the bones are extremely brittle). A typical pedigree of a family with neurofibromatosis, a dominantly inherited autosomal disorder, is shown in Figure 7-4. Several human genetic diseases, with their patterns of inheritance, are briefly described in Table 7-1.

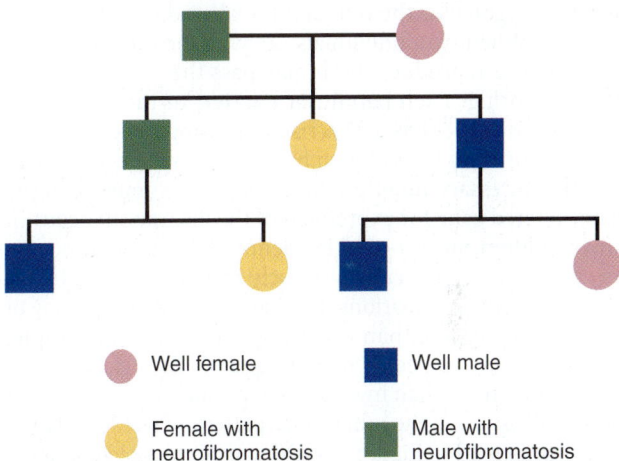

Well female Well male

Female with neurofibromatosis Male with neurofibromatosis

Figure 7-4 Family pedigree for neurofibromatosis, an autosomal dominant disorder.

Table 7-1	Human Genetic Diseases
Disease (Pattern of Inheritance)	**Description**
Sickle cell anemia (R)	The most common genetic disease among people of African ancestry. Sickle cell hemoglobin forms rigid crystals that distort and disrupt red blood cells; oxygen-carrying capacity of the blood is diminished.
Canavan disease (R)	Degenerative brain disorder that primarily affects children of eastern and central European Jewish (Ashkenazi) descent. Characterized by developmental delay, hypotonia, large head, seizures, blindness, and gastrointestinal reflux; most affected children die within the first several years of life.
Cystic fibrosis (R)	The most common genetic disease among people of European ancestry. Production of thick mucus clogs the bronchial tree and pancreatic ducts. Most severe effects are chronic respiratory infections and pulmonary failure.
Familial dysautonomia (Riley-Day syndrome (R)	Neurological disorder seen almost exclusively in individuals of eastern and central European Jewish (Ashkenazi) descent. Characterized by abnormal suck and feeding difficulties, episodic vomiting, abnormal sweating, pain and temperature sensitivity, labile blood pressure levels, absent tearing, and scoliosis.

(continued)

Table 7-1 Human Genetic Diseases (continued)	
Disease (Pattern of Inheritance)	Description
Tay-Sachs disease (R)	The most common genetic disease among people of Jewish ancestry. Degeneration of neurons and the nervous system results in death usually by the age of 4 years.
Phenylketonuria (R)	Lack of an enzyme to metabolize the amino acid phenylalanine leads to severe mental and physical retardation. These effects may be prevented by the use of a diet (beginning at birth) that limits phenylalanine.
Huntington's disease (D)	Uncontrollable muscle contractions begin between the ages of 30 and 50 years, followed by loss of memory and personality. There is no treatment that can delay mental deterioration.
Hemophilia (X-linked)	Lack of coagulation factor VIII impairs chemical clotting; may be controlled with coagulation factor VIII from donated blood.
Duchenne's muscular dystrophy (X-linked)	Replacement of muscle by adipose or scar tissue, with progressive loss of muscle function; often fatal before age 20 years because of involvement of cardiac muscle.

R = recessive; D = dominant.
Sources: ACOG, 2009; Scanlon, V. C., and Sanders, T. (2011). *Essentials of anatomy and physiology* (6th ed., p. 520). Philadelphia, PA: F.A. Davis.

Autosomal Recessive Inheritance

Autosomal recessive inheritance disorders are expressed in an individual when both members of an autosomal gene pair are altered. Although each parent carries the recessive altered gene, neither is affected by the disorder because each is heterozygous for the trait and the altered gene is not expressed. When two individuals carrying the same recessive altered gene reproduce, both may pass the altered gene to their offspring. Each parent, or **carrier,** of the autosomal recessive disorder has a 25% risk of passing the disorder to each offspring, who will then have no normal gene to carry out the necessary function. Because parents must pass the same altered gene for expression of the disorder to occur in their children, an increased incidence of the disorder occurs in consanguineous matings (closely related parents). In addition, specific populations may have a greater frequency of recessive disorders than other populations. For example, sickle cell anemia occurs more frequently in African American populations than in Caucasian populations. A Punnett square illustrating the inheritance pattern of sickle cell anemia is presented in Figure 7-5. Other examples of autosomal recessive inheritance disorders include galactosemia, phenylketonuria (PKU), maple syrup urine disease, Tay-Sachs disease, and cystic fibrosis (CF).

X-Linked Dominant Inheritance

X-linked dominant inheritance disorders are the result of an alteration in a gene located along an X chromosome (Fig. 7-6). Because females have two X chromosomes, these disorders occur twice as frequently in females as in males. When the gene is dominant, it need be present on only one of the X chromosomes for symptoms of the disorder to be expressed. X-linked dominant disorders are passed from an affected male to all of his daughters because the daughters receive the father's altered X chromosome. Conversely, none of the sons are affected because they receive only the father's Y chromosome.

A female with an X-linked dominant disorder has a 50% chance of passing the altered genes to her offspring. Each child of a female with the X-linked dominant disorder has a 1 in 2 chance of expressing the disorder. Examples of X-linked dominant disorders include hypophosphatemia

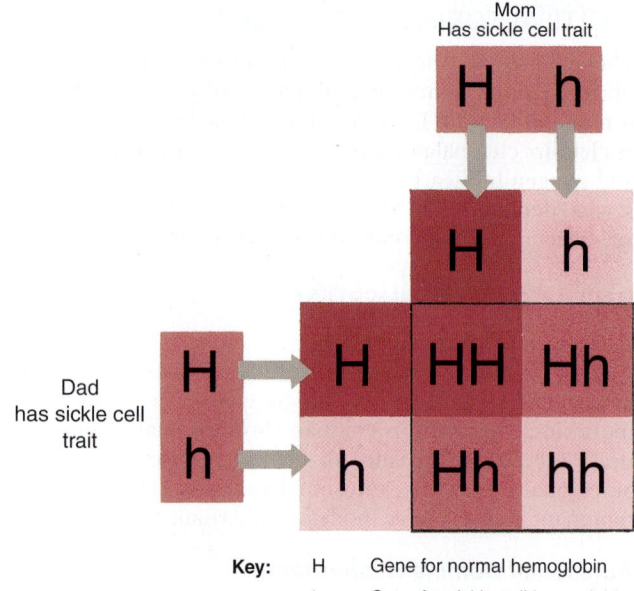

Key: H Gene for normal hemoglobin
h Gene for sickle cell hemoglobin

Figure 7-5 Inheritance of sickle cell anemia, an autosomal recessive disorder.

(vitamin D–resistant rickets) and cervico-oculo-acoustic syndrome.

X-Linked Recessive Inheritance

X-linked recessive inheritance disorders are more common than X-linked dominant disorders and occur more frequently in males. This occurs because males have a single X chromosome, and the single X chromosome carries the altered gene. Thus, when the male receives a "single dose" of the altered gene, the disorder is expressed. For the disorder to be expressed in the female, the altered gene must be present on both X chromosomes.

A female who is a carrier of a gene that causes an X-linked recessive disorder has a 50% risk of passing the abnormal gene to her male offspring. Each son has a 1 in 2 chance of expressing the disorder. The female carrier also has a 50% chance of passing the altered gene to her female offspring,

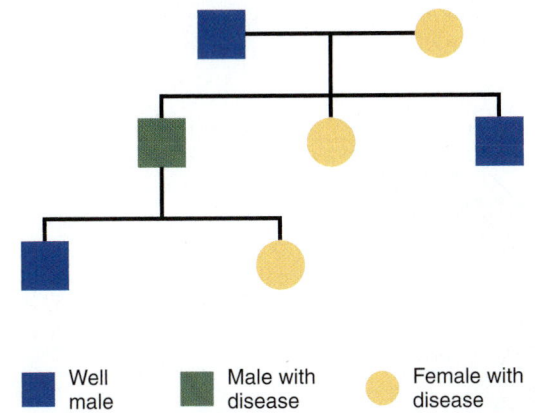

| Well male | Male with disease | Female with disease |

Figure 7-6 Family pedigree for X-linked dominant inheritance.

who will have a 1 in 2 chance of becoming carriers of the altered gene. A son who is affected by an X-linked disorder has a 100% chance of passing the variant X to his daughters because the affected father has only one X to pass on. Fathers cannot transmit the altered gene to their male offspring because they transmit the Y instead of the X chromosome to their sons. The Punnet square in Figure 7-7 illustrates the inheritance pattern for red-green color blindness, an X-linked recessive inheritance disorder. Other X-linked recessive inheritance disorders include hemophilia A, Duchenne's (pseudohypertrophic) muscular dystrophy, and Christmas disease, a blood-factor deficiency (Scanlon & Sanders, 2011).

Now Can You—Discuss aspects of patterns of inheritance?

1. Differentiate between unifactorial and multifactorial patterns of inheritance?
2. Compare and contrast autosomal dominant, autosomal recessive, and X-linked inheritance disorders?
3. Construct a Punnett square to illustrate inheritance patterns for a dominant trait?

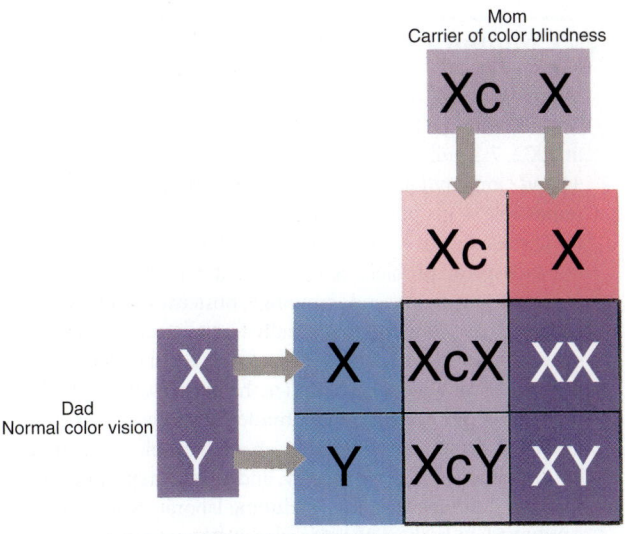

Key:
XX	X chromosome with gene for normal color vision
Y	Y chromosome (has no gene for color vision)
Xc	X chromosome with gene for red-green color blindness

Figure 7-7 Inheritance of red-green color blindness.

Cellular Division

Human cells can be categorized into either gametes (sperm and egg cells) or somatic cells (any body cell that contains 46 chromosomes in its nucleus). Gametes are haploid cells. They have only one member of each chromosome pair and contain 23 chromosomes. Somatic cells are diploid, which means that they contain chromosome pairs (a total of 46 chromosomes). One member of each pair comes from the mother, and one member comes from the father. Cells reproduce through either meiosis or mitosis. **Meiosis** is a process of cell division that leads to the development of sperm and ova, each containing half the number (haploid) of chromosomes as normal cells. **Mitosis** is the process of the formation of two identical cells that are exactly the same as the original cell and have the normal (diploid) amount of chromosomes.

Meiosis occurs during gametogenesis, the process in which germ cells, or gametes, are produced. During cell division, the genetic complement of the cells is reduced by one-half. During meiosis, a sex cell containing 46 chromosomes (the diploid number of chromosomes) divides into two, and then four cells, each containing 23 chromosomes (a haploid number of chromosomes). The resulting "daughter cells" are exactly alike, but they are all different from the original cell. The process of meiosis includes two completely different cell divisions. During the first cell division, the chromosomes replicate each of the 46 chromosomes (diploid number of chromosomes). The chromosomes then become closely intertwined and the sharing of genetic material occurs. New combinations are produced, and this process accounts for the variations of traits in individuals. Next, the chromosomes separate and the cell divides and forms two daughter cells, each containing 23 double-structured chromosomes (the same amount of DNA as a normal somatic cell).

In the second division, each chromosome divides, and each half (or chromatid) moves to opposite sides of the cell. The cells divide and form four cells containing 23 single chromosomes each, a haploid number of chromosomes, or half the number of chromosomes present in the somatic cell. Gametes must contain the haploid number of chromosomes. When the female and male gametes unite to form a fertilized ovum (zygote), the normal (diploid) number of 46 chromosomes is reestablished. The entire process results in the creation of four haploid gamete cells from one diploid sex cell.

Mitosis is the phase in the cell cycle that permits duplication of two genetically identical daughter cells, each containing the diploid number of chromosomes. The process of mitosis allows each daughter cell to inherit the exact human genome.

The Process of Fertilization

Fertilization is a complex series of events. Transportation of gametes must occur to allow the oocyte and the sperm to meet. Most often, this meeting takes place in the ampulla of the uterine (fallopian) tube (Fig. 7-8).

After completion of the first meiotic division, the secondary oocyte is expelled from the ovary during ovulation. The oocyte then makes its way to the infundibulum

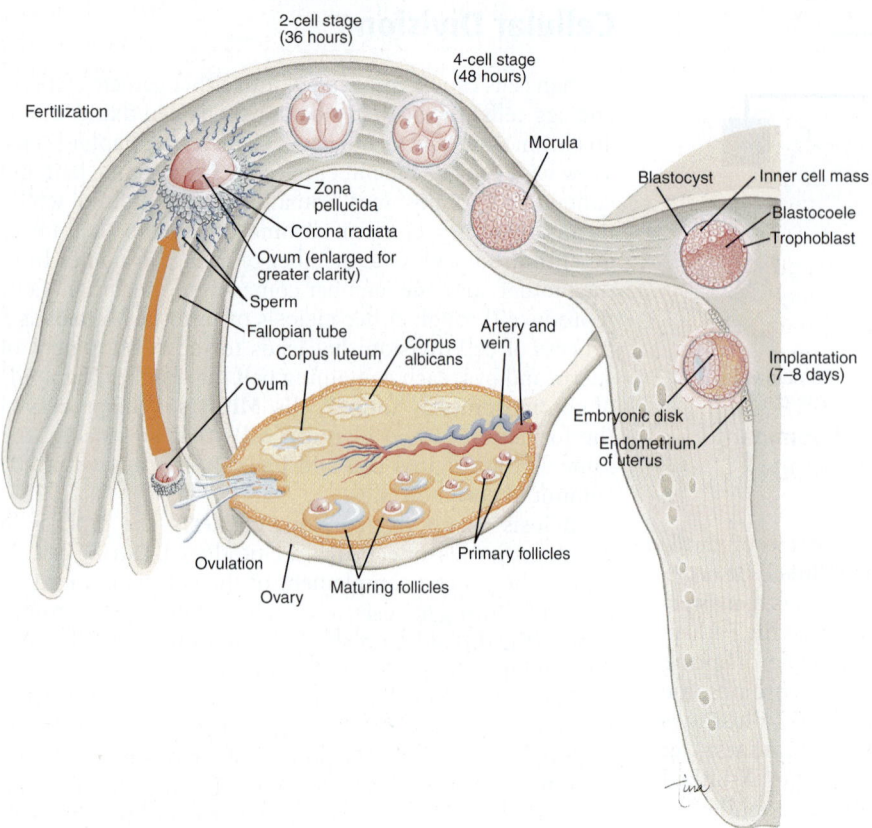

2-cell stage
(36 hours)

4-cell stage
(48 hours)

Morula

Fertilization

Zona
pellucida

Corona radiata

Ovum (enlarged for
greater clarity)

Sperm

Fallopian tube

Corpus luteum   Corpus
albicans

Ovum

Ovulation

Ovary   Maturing follicles

Primary follicles

Artery and
vein

Blastocyst   Inner cell mass

Blastocoele

Trophoblast

Implantation
(7–8 days)

Embryonic disk

Endometrium
of uterus

Figure 7-8 Ovulation, fertilization, and early embryonic development.

(funnel-shaped passage) at the end of the fallopian tube and passes into the ampulla of the tube. At the time of ejaculation, about 200 to 600 million sperm are deposited around the external cervical os and in the fornix of the vagina. During ovulation, the amount of cervical mucus increases, and it becomes less viscous and more favorable for sperm penetration. Propelled by the flagellar movement of their tails, sperm travel into the uterus and upward through the fallopian tubes. Muscular contractions of the tubal walls, believed to be enhanced by prostaglandins in the semen, facilitate the sperm movement. The fallopian tubes are lined with **cilia,** hairlike projections from the epithelial cells that serve a dual action: movement of the ovum toward the uterus and movement of the sperm from the uterus toward the ovary. Of the 200 to 600 million sperm deposited, approximately 200 actually reach the fertilization site.

Sperm must undergo a process called capacitation, whereby a glycoprotein coat and seminal proteins are removed from the surface of the sperm's acrosome (the caplike structure surrounding the head of the sperm). The sperm become more active during this process of capacitation, which takes about 7 hours and usually occurs in the fallopian tube but may begin in the uterus. An acrosomal reaction occurs when the capacitated sperm comes into contact with the zona pellucida surrounding the secondary oocyte. During the acrosomal reaction, enzymes from the sperm's head are released. This helps to create a pathway through the zona pellucida, allowing the sperm to reach the egg and fertilization to occur.

Once a sperm penetrates through the zona pellucida, a reaction takes place to prevent fertilization by other

sperm. The oocyte then undergoes its second meiotic division and forms a mature oocyte and secondary polar body. The nucleus of the mature oocyte becomes the female pronucleus. The sperm loses its tail within the cytoplasm of the oocyte and then enlarges to become the male pronucleus. Fusion of pronuclei of both the oocyte and sperm create a single zygote containing the diploid number of chromosomes. The zygote is genetically unique in that it contains half of its chromosomes from the mother and half from the father.

✳ Collaboration in Caring—*Impaired fecundity*

According to the National Center for Health Statistics (NCHS), in 2002, 7.3 million women between the ages of 15 and 44 had "impaired fecundity," meaning it was difficult or impossible to get pregnant or carry a fetus to term (Centers for Disease Control and Prevention [CDC], 2010a). Infertility is a widespread problem, and treatment may include referrals to internal medicine, endocrinology, obstetrics, urology, and psychiatry. Infertility is usually first identified by the gynecologist/obstetrician. A referral to internal medicine may be recommended to optimize the health status of both partners. A reproductive endocrinologist specializes in infertility. Treatments offered by an endocrinologist include fertility drugs, infertility surgery, and assisted reproductive therapy. Routine screening (including laboratory tests) is conducted on both partners to identify the possible cause of infertility. Abnormalities identified in the male partner may involve the care of the urologist.

The Process of Implantation and Placental Development

After conception, the fertilized ovum, or zygote, remains in the ampulla for 24 hours and then, propelled by ciliary action, travels toward the uterus. During this time, cleavage (mitotic cell division of the zygote) occurs. By 3 to 4 days after fertilization, there are approximately 16 cells. The zygote is now called a **morula** and enters the uterus. Once the morula enters the uterus, fluid passes through the zona pellucida into the intercellular spaces of the inner cell mass and forms a large fluid-filled cavity. The morula is now called a **blastocyst** and contains an inner mass of cells called the embryoblast. The embryo develops from the embryoblast and contains an outer cell layer called the trophoblast. The chorion and placenta develop from the trophoblast.

 Nursing Insight—*Understanding the origin of embryonic stem cells*

The cells of the inner cell mass are termed embryonic stem cells. In these cells, all of the DNA has the potential to develop into any of the 200 kinds of human cells that will be present at birth. As the cells continue to divide and increase in number, some DNA will be "switched off" in each cell, the genes will become inactive, and the possibilities for specialization of each cell will decrease (Scanlon & Sanders, 2011).

The uterus secretes a mixture of lipids, mucopolysaccharides, and glycogen that nourishes the blastocyst. The zona pellucida degenerates approximately 5 to 6 days after fertilization. This process allows the blastocyst to adhere to the endometrial surface of the uterus (usually in the upper posterior portion) to obtain nutrients. Implantation begins as the trophoblast cells invade the endometrium. By the 10th day after fertilization, **nidation** (implantation of the fertilized ovum into the endometrium) has occurred, and the blastocyst is buried beneath the endometrial surface.

The placenta develops from the trophoblast cells at the site of implantation. This important organ is essential for the transfer of nutrients and oxygen to the fetus and the removal of waste products from the fetus, and any alteration in its function can adversely affect growth and development. As the trophoblast cells invade the endometrium, spaces termed lacunae develop. The lacunae fill with fluid from ruptured maternal capillaries and endometrial glands. This fluid nourishes the embryoblast by the process of diffusion. The lacunae later become the intervillous spaces of the placenta. At about the same time, the trophoblast cells form primary **chorionic villi,** small nonvascular processes that absorb nutritive materials for growth. Blood vessels begin to develop in the chorionic villi around the third week, and a primitive fetoplacental circulation is established.

The trophoblast cells continue to invade the endometrium until 25 to 35 days after fertilization, when they reach the maternal spiral arterioles. Spurts of maternal blood form hollows around the villi, creating **intervillous spaces** containing reservoirs of blood that supply the developing embryo and fetus with oxygen and nutrients. The placenta has become well established by 8 to 10 weeks after conception. By 4 months, the placenta has reached maximal thickness although circumferential growth progresses as the fetus continues to grow. The placenta is responsible for providing oxygenation, nutrition, waste elimination, and hormones necessary to maintain the pregnancy (Fig. 7-9).

The placenta is a metabolic organ with its own substrate needs. Metabolic activities of the placenta include glycolysis, gluconeogenesis, glycogenesis, oxidation, protein synthesis, amino acid interconversion, triglyceride

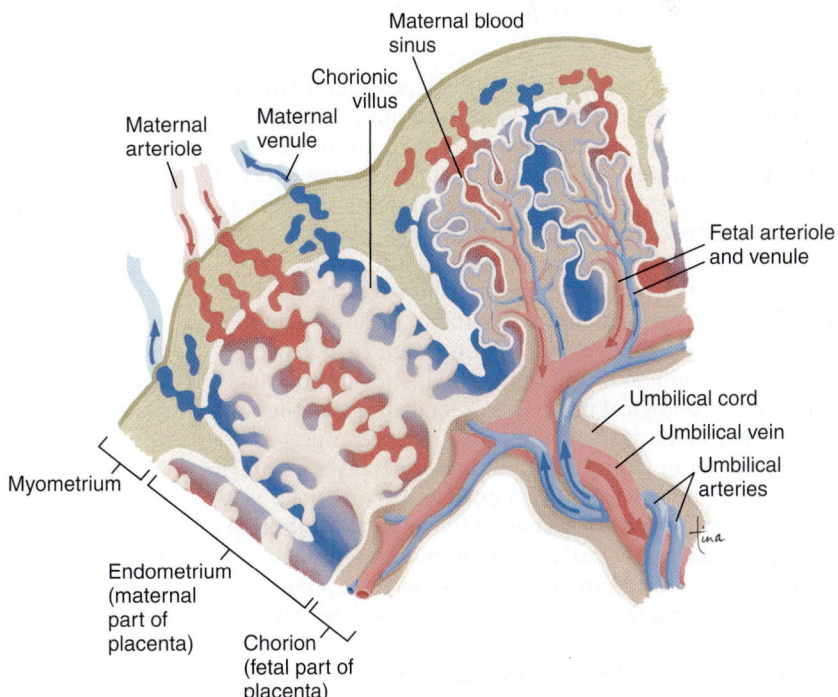

Figure 7-9 Placenta and umbilical cord.

synthesis, and lengthening or shortening of fatty acid chains. The placenta uptakes glucose, synthesizes estrogens and progesterone from cholesterol, and uses fatty acids for oxidation and membrane formation. Placental transport of gases, nutrients, wastes, and other substances occurs in a bidirectional movement from maternal to fetal circulation and from fetal to maternal circulation. Transport across the placenta increases with gestation because of the decreased distance between the fetal and maternal blood, increased blood flow, and increased needs of the developing fetus.

There are several mechanisms by which substances are transported across the placenta. These include simple (passive) diffusion, facilitated diffusion, active diffusion, pinocytosis and endocytosis, bulk flow, accidental capillary breaks, and independent movement. Pinocytosis is the process by which cells absorb or ingest nutrients and fluid; endocytosis is a method of ingestion of a foreign substance by a cell wall (Venes, 2013).

- **Simple diffusion:** Substances transported via this mechanism include water, electrolytes, oxygen, carbon dioxide, urea, simple amines, fatty acids, steroids, fat-soluble vitamins, narcotics, antibiotics, barbiturates, and anesthetics.
- **Facilitated diffusion:** Substances transported are glucose and oxygen.
- **Active transport:** Substances transported via this mechanism include amino acids, water-soluble vitamins, calcium, iron, and iodine.
- **Pinocytosis and endocytosis:** Globulins, phospholipids, lipoproteins, antibodies, and viruses use these mechanisms of transport.
- **Bulk flow and solvent drag:** Water and electrolytes use these mechanisms of transport.
- **Accidental capillary breaks:** Facilitate the transport of intact blood cells.
- **Independent movement:** Maternal leukocytes and microorganisms such as *Treponema pallidum* use this mechanism of transport.

Placental endocrine activity plays a crucial role in maintaining the pregnancy. The four main hormones produced by the placenta are human chorionic gonadotropin (hCG), human placental lactogen (hPL), progesterone, and estrogens. hCG maintains the corpus luteum (a structure that secretes progesterone) during early pregnancy until the placenta has sufficiently developed to produce adequate amounts of progesterone. hPL regulates glucose availability for the fetus and promotes fetal growth by altering maternal protein, carbohydrate, and fat metabolism. Progesterone helps to suppress maternal immunological responses to fetal antigens, thereby preventing maternal rejection of the fetus. Progesterone has a number of additional functions: decreases myometrial activity and irritability, constricts myometrial vessels, decreases maternal sensitivity to carbon dioxide, inhibits prolactin secretion, relaxes smooth muscle in the gastrointestinal and urinary systems, increases basal body temperature, and increases maternal sodium and chloride secretion.

Estrogen production increases significantly during pregnancy. This essential hormone enhances myometrial activity, promotes myometrial vasodilation, increases maternal respiratory center sensitivity to carbon dioxide, softens fibers in the cervical collagen tissue, increases the pituitary secretion of prolactin, increases serum binding proteins and fibrinogen, decreases plasma proteins, and increases sensitivity of the uterus to progesterone in late pregnancy.

The placenta also plays an important role in protecting the fetus from pathogens and in preventing maternal rejection of the pregnancy. Although many bacteria are too large to pass through the placenta, most viruses and some bacteria are able to cross the placenta. Maternal antibodies (e.g., all subclasses of IgG) transit the placenta primarily by pinocytosis; others cross by the process of diffusion. Although the fetus has a unique genetic makeup that is different from the mother's, maternal rejection of the fetus usually does not occur. The exact reason for this phenomenon is not known.

Development of the Embryo and Fetus

THE YOLK SAC

Early in the pregnancy, the embryo is a flattened disk that is situated between the **amnion** (thick membrane that forms the amniotic sac that surrounds the embryo and fetus) and the yolk sac. The yolk sac is a structure that develops in the embryo's inner cell mass around day 8 or 9 after conception. It is essential for the transfer of nutrients to the embryo during the second and third weeks of gestation when development of the uteroplacental circulation is under way. **Hematopoiesis** (formation and development of red blood cells) occurs in the wall of the yolk sac beginning in the third week. This function gradually declines after the eighth gestational week when the fetal liver begins to take over this process. As the pregnancy progresses, the yolk sac atrophies and is incorporated into the umbilical cord. Key events that take place during early development of the embryo are shown in Figure 7-10.

ORIGIN AND FUNCTION OF THE UMBILICAL CORD

During the time of placental development, the umbilical cord is also being formed. The body stalk connects the embryo to the yolk sac that contains blood vessels connecting to the chorionic villi. The vessels contract to form two arteries and one vein as the body stalk elongates and develops into the umbilical cord. Maternal blood flows through the uterine arteries and into the intervillous spaces of the placenta. The blood returns through the uterine veins and into the maternal circulation. Fetal blood flows through the umbilical arteries and into the villous capillaries of the placenta. The blood returns through the umbilical vein and into the fetal circulation. **Wharton's jelly** is a specialized connective tissue that surrounds the two arteries and one vein in the umbilical cord. This tissue, in addition to the high volume and pressure in the blood vessels, is important because it helps to protect the umbilical cord from compression. Most umbilical cords have a central insertion site into the placenta and at term are approximately 21 inches (55 cm) long with a diameter that ranges from 0.38 to 0.77 inch (1 to 2 cm).

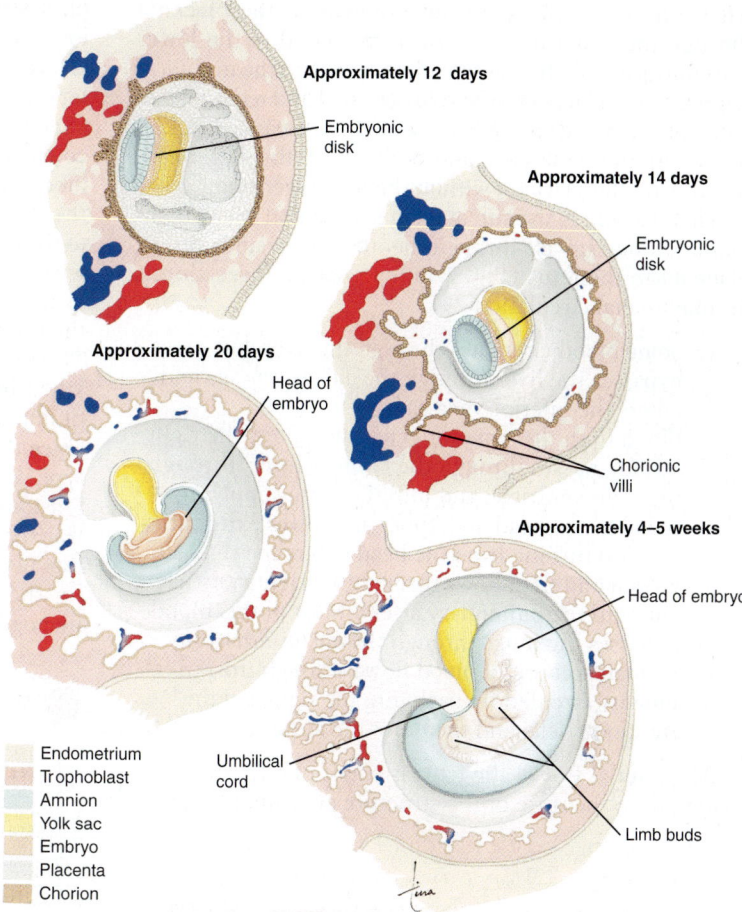

Figure 7-10 Key events during early development of the embryo.

 Now Can You—Discuss characteristics of growth in the embryo/fetus?

1. Identify where the developing embryo obtains nutrients prior to development of the feto–maternal circulatory placental unit?
2. Describe seven mechanisms used for the transport of nutrients across the placenta?
3. Discuss how human placental lactogen (hPL) promotes fetal growth?

THE FETAL CIRCULATORY SYSTEM

The embryo receives nutrition from maternal blood by diffusion through the extraembryonic coelom (fluid-filled cavity surrounding the amnion and yolk sac) and the yolk sac by the end of the second week. Blood vessels begin to develop in the yolk sac during the beginning of the third week, and embryonic blood vessels begin to develop about 2 days later. A primordial heart tube joins with blood vessels in the embryo, connecting the body stalk, chorion, and yolk sac to form a primitive cardiovascular system. The heart begins to beat, and blood begins to circulate by the end of the third week.

During the third week, capillaries develop in the chorionic villi and become connected to the embryonic heart through vessels in the chorion and the connecting stalk. By the end of the third week, embryonic blood begins to flow through capillaries in the chorionic villi. Oxygen and nutrients from maternal blood diffuse through the walls in the villi and enter the embryo's blood. Carbon dioxide and waste products diffuse from blood in the embryo's capillaries through the wall of the chorionic villi and into the maternal blood. The umbilical cord is formed from the connecting stalk during the fourth week.

Blood travels through the fetus in a unique way. The umbilical cord contains three vessels: two arteries and one vein. Blood flows through the vein from the placenta to the fetus. A small amount of blood flows through the liver and then empties into the inferior vena cava. Most of the blood bypasses the liver and then enters the inferior vena cava by way of the **ductus venosus,** a vascular channel that connects the umbilical vein to the inferior vena cava. The blood then empties into the right atrium, passes through the **foramen ovale** (an opening in the septum between the right and left atria) into the left atrium, then moves into the left ventricle and on into the aorta. From the aorta, blood travels to the head, upper extremities, and lower extremities. Blood returning from the head enters the superior vena cava, then the right atrium and the right ventricle before entering the pulmonary artery. Most of the blood that enters the pulmonary artery bypasses the lungs and enters the aorta through the **ductus arteriosus,** a vascular channel between the pulmonary artery and descending aorta. The remaining blood flows to the pulmonary circulation to support lung development. The blood then returns through the pulmonary vein to the left atrium, the left ventricle, to the aorta, and returns to the placenta through the two arteries. Most of the blood in the lower extremities enters the internal iliac artery and the umbilical arteries to the placenta to be reoxygenated and recirculated. Some of the blood in the lower extremities passes back to the ascending vena cava and is mixed with oxygenated blood from the placenta without being oxygenated.

The placenta is the site of oxygenation and waste elimination. Blood travels through the umbilical vein from the placenta to the fetus (Fig. 7-11). There are three shunts unique to fetal circulation:

1. Some blood circulates through the liver, but most bypasses the liver through the *ductus venosus* and enters the inferior vena cava.
2. Blood from the superior vena cava enters the right atrium, passes through the *foramen ovale*, through the right ventricle, and into the aorta supplying blood to the head and upper and lower extremities.
3. Blood returning from the head enters the right atrium and then flows through the right ventricle and into the pulmonary artery. Most of this blood bypasses the lungs through the *ductus arteriosus*. A small amount of blood flows through the pulmonary circulation, back into the right atrium, right ventricle, and then into the aorta.

The arterial P_{O_2} of the fetus is about one-fourth of the maternal P_{O_2} because of the structure and function of the placenta (i.e., oxygenation of fetal blood takes place at a low P_{O_2}) and because arterial blood in the fetal circulation is formed by the mixing of maternal oxygenated blood with fetal deoxygenated blood. Fetal hemoglobin has a lower oxygen content than that of the adult. The highest oxygen concentration (P_{O_2} = 30 to 35 mm Hg) is found in the blood returning from the placenta via the umbilical vein; the lowest oxygen concentration occurs in blood shunted to the placenta where reoxygenation takes place. The blood with the highest oxygen content is delivered to the fetal heart, head, neck, and upper limbs, while the blood with the lowest oxygen content is shunted toward the placenta. The low P_{O_2} level is important in maintaining fetal circulation because it keeps the ductus arteriosus open and the pulmonary vascular bed constricted. Fetal hemoglobin enables the fetus to adapt to the lowered P_{O_2}. This unique type of hemoglobin has a high affinity for oxygen at low tensions, which improves saturation and facilitates oxygen transport to the fetal tissues. The increased perfusion rate (as compared with the adult) also helps to compensate for the lower oxygen saturations and increased oxygen–hemoglobin affinity.

 Now Can You—**Discuss unique aspects of the fetal circulatory system?**

1. Name the three shunts found in the fetal circulatory system?
2. Identify where the highest and lowest fetal oxygen concentrations are found?
3. Explain how fetal hemoglobin is unique?

FETAL MEMBRANES AND AMNIOTIC FLUID

The embryonic membranes (chorion and amnion) are early protective structures that begin to form at the time of implantation. The thick **chorion,** or outer membrane, forms first. It develops from the trophoblast and encloses the amnion, embryo, and yolk sac. The chorion contains finger-like projections (chorionic villi) that may be used for genetic testing (chorionic villus sampling) during the first trimester. The villi beneath the embryo grow and branch out into depressions in the wall of the uterus, and from this structure, the fetal portion of the placenta is formed.

The amnion arises from the ectoderm during early embryonic development. This membrane is a thin, protective structure that contains the amniotic fluid. The amniotic cavity, or space between the amnion and the embryo, houses the embryo and yolk sac, except in the area where the developing embryo attaches to the trophoblast via the umbilical cord. With embryonic growth, the amnion expands and comes into contact with the chorion. The two fetal membranes are slightly adherent and form the amniotic fluid-filled sac (the **amniotic sac**), also called the bag of waters. The fetal membranes provide a barrier of protection from ascending infection.

Amniotic fluid is vital for fetal growth and development. It cushions the fetus and protects against mechanical injury, helps the fetus to maintain a normal body temperature, allows for symmetrical fetal growth, prevents adherence of the amnion to the fetus, and aids in fetal musculoskeletal development by providing freedom of movement. It is essential for normal fetal lung development. The amniotic fluid volume is dynamic, constantly

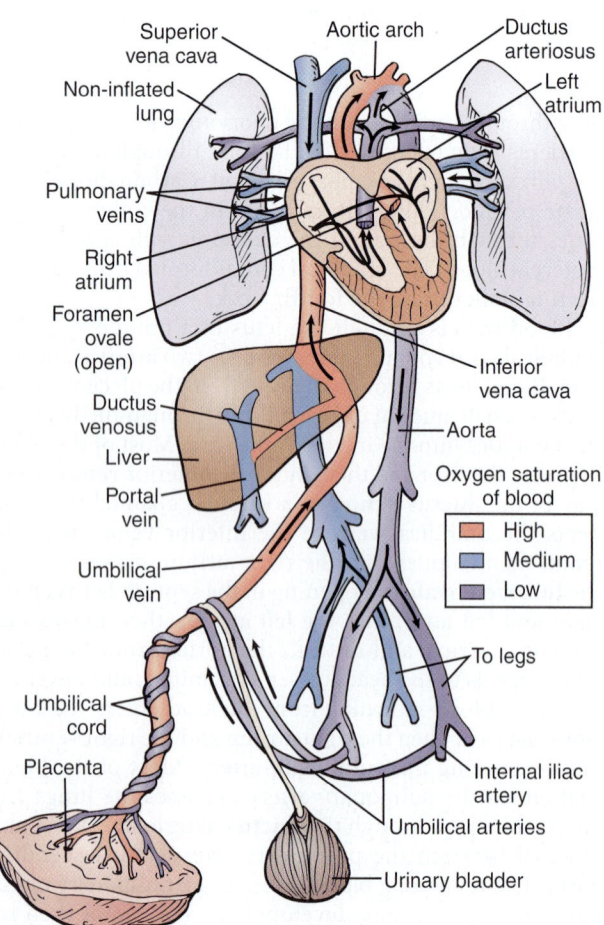

Figure 7-11 Fetal circulation.

changing as the fluid moves back and forth across the placental membrane.

Amniotic fluid first appears at about 3 weeks. Approximately 30 mL of amniotic fluid are present at 10 weeks' gestation, and this amount increases to approximately 800 mL at 24 weeks' gestation. After that time, the total fluid volume remains fairly stable until it begins to decrease slightly as the pregnancy reaches term. At term, amniotic fluid volume is estimated at 700 to 800 mL (Moore, 2010).

During late gestation, fetal urine and fetal lung secretions are the primary contributors to the total amniotic fluid volume. Fetal swallowing and absorption through the placenta are the primary pathways for amniotic fluid clearance. The fetus swallows approximately 600 mL every 4 hours, and up to 400 mL of amniotic fluid flows from the fetal lungs every 24 hours. Amniotic fluid is slightly alkaline and contains antibacterial and other protective substances similar to those found in maternal breast milk (e.g., transferrin, beta-lysin, peroxidase, fatty acids, immunoglobulins [IgG and IgA], and lysozyme). It also contains albumin, uric acid, creatinine, lecithin, sphingomyelin, bilirubin, vernix, leukocytes, epithelial cells, and **lanugo** (fine, downy hair).

 Now Can You—Discuss aspects of the amniotic sac and amniotic fluid?

1. Identify the origins of the embryonic membranes?
2. Name five functions of the amniotic fluid?
3. Discuss where amniotic fluid originates?

Human Growth and Development

Major organs are formed (organogenesis) during the first 8 weeks after fertilization. During this time, the developing organism is called an **embryo.** By the end of 8 weeks, the embryo has sufficiently developed to be called a **fetus.** Human development proceeds in a cephalocaudal pattern of maturation: motor development, control, and coordination progress from the head to the feet.

The loss of a fetus before 20 to 22 weeks' gestation (less than 500 grams) is referred to as an abortion because the fetus is considered too immature to survive the **extrauterine** (outside the uterus) environment. A fetus born before the completion of 37 weeks is considered to be preterm or premature.

PRE-EMBRYONIC PERIOD

The pre-embryonic period refers to the first 2 weeks of human development after conception. Rapid cellular multiplication, cell differentiation, and establishment of the embryonic membranes and primary germ layers occur during this time. Development takes place in a pattern that is cephalocaudal, proximal to distal, and general to specific.

EMBRYONIC PERIOD

Critical development that occurs during the embryonic period involves cleavage of the zygote, blastogenesis (early development characterized by cleavage and formation of three germ layers that later develop into tissues and organs), and

the early development of the nervous system, cardiovascular system, and all major internal and external structures. The pre-embryonic period refers to the first 2 weeks beginning at fertilization, which for most is approximately 2 weeks after the last normal menstrual period. The embryonic period is the time period beginning with the third week after fertilization and continuing until the end of the eighth week. This period is known as the organogenetic period that denotes the formation and differentiation of organs and organ systems.

Week 1

Fertilization usually occurs in the outer third portion of the uterine tube. The zygote then travels toward the uterus, while undergoing cleavage (series of mitotic cell division) and forming blastomeres (cells formed from the first mitotic division). Approximately 3 days after fertilization, a morula (a ball of 12 or more blastomeres) enters the uterus. A cavity forms within the morula, creating a blastocyst that consists of a trophoblast that encloses both the embryoblast (gives rise to the embryo and some extraembryonic tissues) and the blastocystic cavity (fluid-filled space). The trophoblast begins to invade the uterus, and the blastocyst is superficially implanted by the end of the first week.

Week 2

The trophoblast undergoes rapid proliferation and differentiation as the blastocyst continues the process of uterine implantation. The yolk sac develops, the amniotic cavity appears, and the embryoblast differentiates into the bilaminar embryonic disk. Implantation of the blastocyst is completed by the end of the second week.

Week 3

The third week is characterized by the appearance of a primitive streak (proliferation and migration of cells to the central posterior region of the embryonic disk), the development of the notochord (cellular rod along the dorsal surface that will later be surrounded by vertebrae), and differentiation of the three germ layers: embryonic **ectoderm** (outer layer, gives rise to skin, teeth, and glands of the mouth and nervous system), **endoderm** (inner layer, gives rise to epithelium of the respiratory, digestive, and genitourinary tracts), and **mesoderm** (lies between the ectoderm and endoderm; gives rise to the connective tissue) (Table 7-2).

A & P review **Formation of the Primary Germ Layers**

Implantation of the blastocyst occurs at approximately 7 to 8 days after conception. At this time, the cells of the embryonic disk are separated from the amnion by a fluid-filled space. The syncytiotrophoblast continues to erode the endometrium, and implantation is completed by the ninth day. The extraembryonic mesoderm forms a discrete layer beneath the cytotrophoblast. By the 16th day, all three germ layers are present, along with a yolk sac and the allantois, which is an outpouching of the yolk sac that forms the structural basis of the body stalk, or umbilical cord. The chorion arises from the cytotrophoblast and associated mesoderm and contains many fingerlike projections (chorionic villi) on its surface (see Figs. 7-8 and 7-10). ◆

Table 7-2 Derivatives of the Three Germ Layers

Ectoderm	Mesoderm	Endoderm
Epidermis, epithelium of mouth, oral glands, teeth, and organs of special sense	Smooth muscle coats, connective tissues, and vessels associated with tissues and organs	Epithelium of the pharynx, thyroid, thymus, parathyroid, respiratory passages, gastrointestinal tract, liver, and pancreas
Central nervous system	Blood	
Peripheral nervous system	Bone marrow	
Hypophysis	Muscular tissues	
Adrenal medulla	Skeletal tissues	
	Adrenal cortex	

Week 4

At the beginning of the fourth week, the flat trilaminar embryonic disk folds into a C-shaped, cylindrical embryo. Development continues as the three germ layers differentiate into various organs and tissues. By 28 postovulatory days, four limb buds and a closed otic vesicle (later develops into labyrinth of inner ear) are present (Fig. 7-12).

During the third and fourth weeks, development of the nervous system is well under way. A thickened portion of the ectoderm develops into the neural plate. The top portion will differentiate into the **neural tube,** which forms the central nervous system (brain and spinal cord) and the neural crest, which will develop into the peripheral nervous system. Later, the eye and inner ear develop as projections of the original neural tube. During the early period of development, the embryo's nervous system is particularly vulnerable to environmental insults.

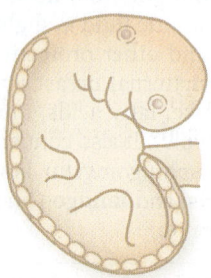

Figure 7-12 Embryo at 4 weeks' gestation (28 postovulatory days). All four limb buds are present. (Smith, B. R. [2013]. The multidimensional human embryo, Carnegie Stages. Retrieved from http://embryo.soad.umich.edu/carnStages/carnStages.html)

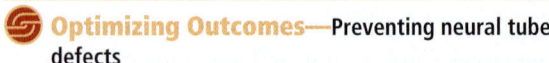

Optimizing Outcomes—**Preventing neural tube defects**

Defective closure of the neural tube during the fourth week of development results in a condition known as a **neural tube defect** (NTD). This is a malformation that involves defects in the skull and spinal column and is primarily caused by failure of the neural tube to close. Tissues overlying the spinal cord including the meninges, vertebral arches, muscles, and skin may be affected as well. Neural tube defects include rachischisis (spina bifida), myelocele, myelomeningocele, and meningocele. Immediate surgical repair is often necessary after birth, although in some situations, myelomeningocele may be repaired in utero (Adzick, Thom, Spong, Brock, Burrows, Johnson, et al., 2011). NTDs are the second most frequent structural fetal malformation and occur in 1 to 2 per 1,000 live births. Folic acid supplementation has been found to decrease the incidence of NTDs (Seibert, 2010). Currently, the United States Public Health Service recommends that all women of childbearing age who are capable of becoming pregnant consume 0.4 to 0.8 milligrams of folic acid daily to reduce the incidence of neural tube defects.

Week 8

By the end of the eighth week, there is a clear distinction between the upper and lower limbs; the external genitals are well developed, although not always well enough to distinguish the gender; and the embryo has a human appearance

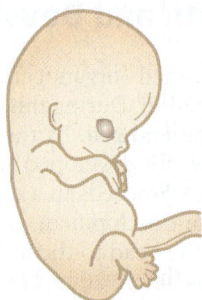

Figure 7-13 The embryo at 8 weeks (56 to 57 postovulatory days) has a human appearance. (Smith, B. R. [2013]. The multidimensional human embryo, Carnegie Stages. Retrieved from http://embryo.soad.umich.edu/carnStages/carnStages.html)

(Fig. 7-13). The main organ systems have also begun to develop by the end of 8 weeks. Except for the cardiovascular system, however, there is minimal function of most of the organ systems.

 Nursing Insight—*Ethical issues regarding embryonic stem cell research*

Embryonic stem cells are pluripotent (able to form different kinds of cells) cells found in embryonic tissue. They are derived from the inner cell mass of the blastocyst. In specialized tissue cultures, stem cells can be made to differentiate into all derivatives of the three primary germ layers (i.e., ectoderm, endoderm, and mesoderm). The specific cell types may potentially be used to treat problems such as blindness, Parkinson's and Alzheimer's diseases, traumatic spinal cord injury, and diabetes. Under specific conditions, embryonic stem cells are capable of propagating themselves indefinitely. Human embryonic stem cells may also be used as models for various human genetic disorders, such as fragile-X syndrome and cystic fibrosis. Isolating the inner cell mass, however, results in destruction of the fertilized human embryo, which raises a number of ethical issues. Central to the controversy is the ethical debate that primarily concerns the creation, treatment, and destruction of human embryos. Presently, some stem cell researchers are investigating techniques of isolating stem cells that are as potent as embryonic stem cells but do not require a human embryo. Others are using artificial viruses to reprogram human skin cells to function in a similar fashion to embryonic stem cells (National Institutes of Health, 2012).

 Now Can You—Discuss the pre-embryonic and embryonic periods of development?

1. Define the pre-embryonic period and identify the pattern of human development that occurs?
2. Identify what time frame is encompassed in the embryonic period?
3. Describe the major developmental events that have occurred by the end of the eighth week?

THE FETAL PERIOD

The beginning of the ninth week marks the beginning of the fetal period when the embryo has now developed into a recognizable human being. The fetal period is characterized by rapid body growth and differentiation of tissues, organs, and systems. The rate of head growth during this period of time slows down as compared with the rate of body growth. During the last 12 weeks of pregnancy, there is a substantial increase in fetal size: The weight triples and the body length doubles.

Weeks 9 to 12

The fetal head is half the length of the crown–rump length at the beginning of the ninth week. The face is recognizably human at 10 weeks. Body growth increases, and as a result, the crown–rump length more than doubles by the twelfth week. Head growth does not keep pace with body growth and slows considerably by the 12th week but remains proportionately large as compared with the rest of the body. Ossification centers appear in the skeleton. The intestines leave the umbilical cord and enter the abdomen. The external genitalia differentiate and are distinguishable by week 12. At 9 weeks, the liver serves as the major site for red blood cell production (erythropoiesis). However, by 12 weeks, the spleen begins to take over this process. Urine production commences between 9 and 12 weeks.

Weeks 13 to 16

There is very rapid growth during this period. Although coordinated movements of the limbs occur by the 14th week, they are too small to be felt by the mother. Ossification of the skeleton takes place, and the bones become clearly visible on ultrasound examination. The external genitalia are recognizable by 12 to 14 weeks, the ovaries are differentiated, and the primordial (primitive) ovarian follicles are present by 16 weeks.

Weeks 17 to 20

Growth continues but slows during this period. Maternal awareness of fetal movements (**quickening**) is frequently reported during this time. The skin is now covered with a thick, cheese-like material called **vernix caseosa** that protects the fetal skin from exposure to the amniotic fluid. By 20 weeks, hair appears on the eyebrows and head. Fine downy hair (**lanugo**) is usually present by 20 weeks and covers all parts of the body except the palms, soles, or areas where other types of hair are usually found. Subcutaneous deposits of **brown fat,** used by the newborn for heat production, help to make the skin less transparent in appearance. The fetal uterus is formed at 18 weeks in females, and in males, the testes have begun to descend but are still located in the abdominal wall. By 20 weeks, the fetus weighs about 300 grams and is approximately 7.3 inches (19 cm) long.

Weeks 21 to 25

The fetus gains much weight during this time. The skin appears pink or red because blood is now visible in the capillaries. Rapid eye movements begin at 21 weeks. By 24 weeks, the fetus has fingernails, and the lungs have begun to secrete **surfactant,** a substance that decreases surface tension in the alveoli and is necessary for survival following birth.

Weeks 26 to 29

A fetus may survive if born during this time because the lungs can breathe air, and the central nervous system can regulate body temperature and direct rhythmic breathing. The eyelids are open, the toenails are evident, and subcutaneous fat is present under the skin. Erythropoiesis occurs in the spleen but ends at 28 weeks when the bone marrow takes over that function.

Weeks 30 to 34

At 30 weeks, the pupillary light reflex is present.

Weeks 35 to 40

At 35 weeks, the fetus has a strong hand grasp reflex and orientation to light. At 38 to 40 weeks, the average fetus weighs 3,000 to 3,800 grams and is 17.3 to 19.2 inches (45 to 50 cm) long (Table 7-3).

 Across Care Setting: **Empowering through education**

The nurse who works in any perinatal setting can help to promote self-care and empowerment by increasing the pregnant woman's understanding of the prenatal journey and by encouraging her active involvement in safeguarding her pregnancy. Providing information regarding normal fetal growth and development is an important component of the early and ongoing bonding process for many women. Displaying fetal growth charts in visible areas and discussing developmental landmarks throughout gestation facilitate discussion and enhance understanding for the patient and her family. Other professional resources including the nutritionist, social worker, and home health worker can be instrumental in helping to ensure healthy fetal growth and development.

Table 7-3 Embryonic and Fetal Growth and Development

Weeks	Weight	Length (Crown to Rump)	Characteristics
2 weeks	?	2 mm	Blastocyst implanted in uterus.
4 weeks	0.4 g	4 mm	Embryo is curved, tail prominent. Upper limb buds and otic pits present. Heart prominence evident.
8 weeks	2 g	3 cm	Head rounded with human characteristics. Unable to determine sex. Intestines still present in umbilical cord. Ovaries and testes distinguishable.
12 weeks	19 g	8 cm	Resembles human being, with disproportionately large head. Eyes fused. Skin pink and delicate. Upper limbs almost reached final length. Intestines in the stomach. Sex distinguishable externally.
16 weeks	100 g	13.5 cm	Scalp hair appears. External ears present. Lower limbs well developed. Arm to leg ratio proportionate. Fetus active.
20 weeks	300 g	18.5 cm	Head and body hair (lanugo) present. Vernix covers skin. Quickening felt by the woman.
24 weeks	600 g	23 cm	Skin reddish and wrinkled. Some subcutaneous fat present. Some respiratory-like movements. Fingernails present. Lean body.
28 weeks	1,100 g	27 cm	Eyes open with eyelashes present. Much hair present. Skin slightly wrinkled, more fat now present.
32 weeks	1,800 g	31 cm	Skin is smooth. Increase in weight gain more than length. Toenails present. Testes descending.
36 weeks	2,200 g	34 cm	Skin pale, body plump. Body lanugo almost gone. Able to flex arm and form grasp. Umbilicus in center of body. Testes in inguinal canal, scrotum small with few rugae. Some sole creases present.
40 weeks	3200+ g	40 cm	Skin smooth and pink. Lanugo on upper back and shoulders. Ear lobes formed and firm. Chest prominent and breasts often protrude slightly. Testes with well defined rugae. Labia majora well developed. Creases cover soles of feet.

 Nursing Insight—*Birth at less than 39 weeks of gestation*

It is important to understand fetal growth and development so that the nurse can anticipate specific types of problems that may occur when infants are born prematurely. An infant born at 28 weeks will have significantly different needs from an infant born at 39⁰/⁷ weeks of gestation.

 Now Can You—**Discuss major events of the fetal period?**

1. Identify the developmental week when the fetal face becomes human in appearance?
2. Name the cheese-like substance that covers and protects the skin?
3. List three developmental events that occur from 26 to 29 weeks?

Factors That May Adversely Affect Embryonic and Fetal Development

Damage to the developing embryo/fetus may result from genetic factors or from maternal exposure to various environmental hazards. In most circumstances, the uterus provides a safe and peaceful environment for the developing embryo and fetus. However, teratogens (drugs, radiation, and infectious agents that can cause developmental or structural abnormalities in an embryo) and a variety of internal and external developmental events may cause structural and functional defects.

CHROMOSOMES AND TERATOGENS

Genetic defects and congenital anomalies usually result from genetic factors, environmental hazards (e.g., drugs and viruses), or a combination of both (multifactorial inheritance). However, the exact cause of anomalies is unknown in approximately 50% to 60% of cases. Congenital anomalies may occur singularly or in combination with other defects (multiple anomalies), and they may be of little or of great clinical significance. Single, minor anomalies occur in approximately 14% of newborns. The greater the number of anomalies present, the greater the risk of a major anomaly. Statistically, 90% of infants with three or more minor anomalies will also have one or more major anomaly. Major developmental defects are more common in early embryos that are usually spontaneously aborted. It has been estimated that approximately one-third of all birth defects are caused by genetic factors.

Before fertilization, damage may have already occurred to the chromosomes of one or both parents, or they may carry defective genes inherited from their own parents. Alterations in the development of sperm or an ovum may also cause alterations in the development of the embryo. Teratogens or environmental factors may adversely affect the process of implantation and result in loss of the zygote. Teratogens may have specific effects associated with congenital anomalies (e.g., alcohol: fetal alcohol syndrome; rubella: cataracts; and tetracycline: stained teeth), or they may produce dysmorphic (damage to the structure and form) features. The extent of the teratogenic effect depends on the developmental timing, duration, and dosage of exposure and the maternal genetic susceptibility. Greater exposure during early gestation is associated with more severe effects.

Teratogen Exposure During Organogenesis

The period of organogenesis lasts from approximately the second until the eighth week of gestation, during which time the embryo undergoes rapid growth and differentiation. During organogenesis, the embryo is extremely vulnerable to teratogens such as medications, alcohol, tobacco, caffeine, illegal drugs, radiation, heavy metals, and maternal (TORCH) infections. Structural defects are most likely to occur during this period because exposure to teratogens either before or during a critical period of development of an organ can cause a malformation.

After 11 weeks, the fetus becomes more resistant to damage from teratogens because the organ systems have been established. However, organ function can still be adversely affected. Insults that occur later in fetal life or during early infancy may cause mental and developmental disabilities, blindness, hearing loss, deafness, stillbirth, or malignancy.

The most critical time for brain development is between 3 and 16 weeks of gestation. However, the brain continues to differentiate and grow rapidly until at least the first 2 years of life. Diet and nutrition are important during this time because amino acids, glucose, and fatty acids are considered to be the primary dietary factors in brain growth.

Medications and Other Substances

It is estimated that approximately 82% of women between the ages of 18 and 44 regularly use at least one medication (prescription or over-the-counter) or vitamins, minerals, herbal supplements, topical medications, or eye drops. Forty-eight percent take a prescription medication, and the most commonly used types of drugs include analgesics, antidepressants, and cholesterol-lowering medications (National Center for Health Statistics, 2010). Many women unintentionally take medications during early pregnancy when they do not yet know they are pregnant, and approximately 59% of pregnant women receive a prescription for a medication other than a vitamin or mineral supplement. To identify drugs that are unsafe for maternal ingestion because of their teratogenic potential, the U.S. Food and Drug Administration (FDA) has established five categories of safety (Table 7-4).

A small number of medications and other substances are known or are strongly suspected to be human teratogens. These include fat-soluble vitamins, alcohol, tobacco, caffeine, cocaine, opiates, anticonvulsants (e.g., valproic acid and divalproex sodium), warfarin (Coumadin), cardiovascular agents (e.g., Lipitor, Mevacor, and Pravachol), retinoids (e.g., Soriatane, Tegison, Accutane, and Avage), certain hormones (e.g., Android, Androlone-D, and Pitressin), antineoplastic agents (e.g., Targretin, Casodex, and Emcyt), certain anti-infective agents (e.g., Penetrex, Novo quinine, and Virazole), thalidomide, and methyl mercury.

Optimizing Outcomes—Educating patients about methyl mercury risks

Methyl mercury is a known neurotoxin that is especially harmful to the fetus, infant, and child. Human exposure to mercury primarily occurs through the consumption of fish (e.g., swordfish, shark, king mackerel, orange roughy, ahi tuna, and tilefish) contaminated through atmospheric mercury releases. Exposure to low doses of methyl mercury in fetuses, infants, and children is associated with developmental delays, learning disabilities, and possibly behavioral problems. Nurses who work with women of childbearing age are perfectly positioned to educate them about the risks and benefits of fish consumption and assist them with finding alternative sources of omega-3 fatty acids essential for cardiac health and fetal/infant/child brain development (ACOG, 2013; Kuntz, Ricco, Hill, & Anderko, 2010).

Table 7-4 FDA Pregnancy Categories

Category	Interpretation
A	Adequate and well-controlled studies in pregnant women have not shown an increased risk of fetal abnormalities to the fetus in any trimester of pregnancy.
B	Animal reproduction studies have revealed no evidence of harm to the fetus; however, there are no adequate and well-controlled studies in pregnant women. OR Animal reproduction studies have shown an adverse effect, but adequate and well-controlled studies in pregnant women have failed to demonstrate a risk to the fetus in any trimester.
C	Animal reproduction studies have shown an adverse effect and there are no adequate and well-controlled studies in pregnant women. OR No animal reproduction studies have been conducted and there are no adequate and well-controlled studies in pregnant women.
D	Adequate and well-controlled or observational studies in pregnant women have demonstrated a risk to the fetus. However, the benefits of therapy may outweigh the potential risk. For example, the drug may be acceptable if needed in a life-threatening situation or serious disease for which safer drugs cannot be used or are ineffective.
X	Adequate and well-controlled or observational studies in animals or pregnant women have demonstrated positive evidence of fetal abnormalities or risks. The risk of the use of the drug in pregnant women clearly outweighs any possible benefit. The use of the product is contraindicated in women who are or may become pregnant.

FAT-SOLUBLE VITAMINS. Both high and low doses of vitamin A (Retinol) can cause fetal malformations that include anomalies of the central nervous system, microtia (deformity of the outer ear), and clefts (a fissure or elongated opening that originates in the embryo, such as a branchial or facial cleft). Vitamin D deficiency may cause poor fetal growth, neonatal hypocalcemia, rickets, and poor tooth enamel. High doses of vitamin E (α-tocopherol) may increase the risk for bleeding problems, but neither deficiency nor excess has been associated with maternal or fetal complications during pregnancy (Chalupka & Chalupka, 2010).

ALCOHOL. Ethyl alcohol is one of the most potent teratogens known. The Surgeon General's advisory on alcohol use (2005) found that, in 2003, approximately 10% of pregnant women reported drinking, and of those, 4% reported having engaged in binge drinking (CDC, 2010b).

A safe threshold level for the use of alcohol during pregnancy has never been established. Current data suggest that children of mothers who chronically ingested large amounts of alcohol or who engaged in binge drinking (five or more drinks on one occasion) during pregnancy are at greatest risk for permanent damage. (See Chapter 10 for further discussion.)

TOBACCO. Approximately 25% of women smoke while pregnant. Cigarette smoking during pregnancy is associated with an overall reduction in fetal growth, cleft lip/palate anomalies, impaired infant neurobehavior, and decreased babbling in infants (Hackshaw, Rodeck, & Boniface, 2011; Zhu & Finnell, 2010). Nicotine causes vasoconstriction of the uterine blood vessels, resulting in a decreased blood flow and supply of nutrients and oxygen to the fetus. Cigarette smoking doubles the risk of low birth weight and increases the likelihood of giving birth to a small for gestational age (SGA) infant (March of Dimes, 2011). Cessation of smoking during pregnancy is beneficial to the developing fetus, and infants born to women who stop smoking during the first trimester have birth weights similar to those of infants born to nonsmoking women (Association of Women's Health, Obstetric & Neonatal Nursing [AWHONN], 2010). (See Chapter 10 for further discussion.)

CAFFEINE. Caffeine, present in many beverages (e.g., sodas, coffee, tea, and hot cocoa) and other substances including chocolate, cold remedies, energy drinks, and analgesics, is the most popular drug in the United States. Caffeine stimulates central nervous system and cardiac function and produces vasoconstriction and mild diuresis. The half-life of caffeine is tripled during pregnancy. Although caffeine readily crosses the placenta and stimulates the fetus, it is not known to be a teratogen. However, high caffeine consumption (more than two 6-ounce cups of coffee or more than 200 mg of caffeine per day) during pregnancy may increase the risk of miscarriage (ACOG, 2010; March of Dimes, 2013). (See Chapter 10 for further discussion.)

COCAINE AND CRACK. Cocaine and crack (a form of free-base cocaine that can be smoked) use during pregnancy causes vasoconstriction of the uterine vessels and adversely affects blood flow to the fetus. Cocaine use in pregnancy is associated with spontaneous abortion, abruptio placentae, stillbirth, intrauterine growth restriction (IUGR), fetal distress, meconium staining, and preterm birth. Problems manifested in children born to women who use cocaine during pregnancy include altered neurological and behavior patterns, neonatal strokes and seizures, and congenital malformations (e.g., genitourinary anomalies, limb reduction deformities, intestinal atresia, and heart defects) (Bhuvaneswar, Chang, Epstein, & Stern, 2008; Malek, 2012). (See Chapters 9 and 10 for further discussion.)

OPIATES. Morphine, heroin, and methadone are opiates sometimes used by pregnant women. Maternal effects from these substances include spontaneous abortion, premature rupture of the membranes, preterm labor, an increased incidence of sexually transmitted infections, hepatitis, an increased potential for HIV exposure, and malnutrition. Methadone is a habit-forming synthetic analgesic drug with a potency equal to that of morphine but with a weaker narcotic action. It is frequently given to pregnant women who enter drug addiction programs. Fetal death, intrauterine growth restriction, perinatal asphyxia, prematurity, intellectual impairment, and neonatal infection are associated with maternal opiate use. Neonatal withdrawal (abstinence) syndrome, characterized by hyperirritability, gastrointestinal dysfunction, respiratory distress, and autonomic disturbances, has been reported in 50% to 80% of infants born to opiate-dependent mothers (Bhuvaneswar et al., 2008). (See Chapters 9, 11, and 19 for further discussion.)

SEDATIVES. Barbiturates and tranquilizers produce maternal lethargy, drowsiness, and CNS depression. In the neonate, these substances are associated with withdrawal syndrome, seizures, and delayed lung maturity.

AMPHETAMINES. Amphetamines are also known as "speed," "crystal," and "ice"; use of these substances during pregnancy is associated with maternal malnutrition, tachycardia, and withdrawal symptoms that include lethargy and depression. The fetus is at an increased risk for intrauterine growth restriction, prematurity, cardiac anomalies, cleft palate, and placental abruption. Following birth, affected neonates may exhibit hypoglycemia, sweating, poor visual tracking, lethargy, and difficulty feeding. (See Chapters 9 and 11 for further discussion.)

MARIJUANA. Δ-9-Tetrahydrocannabinol (THC), the active component in marijuana, passes through the placenta and may remain in the fetus for up to 30 days. The carbon monoxide levels produced with marijuana smoking are five times higher than amounts produced with cigarette smoking. Marijuana may cause intrauterine growth restriction, and research has indicated that maternal use of marijuana during pregnancy has adverse effects on neonatal neurobehavior (e.g., hyperirritability, tremors, and photosensitivity) and can affect cognitive and language development in infants up to 48 months of age. In addition, maternal marijuana use is often combined with other drugs such as cocaine and alcohol. Repeated marijuana use during pregnancy may be associated with maternal anemia and low weight gain and may increase the risk of preterm birth (Organization of Teratology Information Specialists [OTIS], 2011). (See Chapters 9 and 10 for further discussion.)

RADIATION. High levels of radiation during pregnancy may cause damage to chromosomes and embryonic cells. Radiation can adversely affect fetal physical growth and cause intellectual and developmental disabilities. Unborn babies are particularly at risk to damage from radiation exposure during the first trimester. Consequences of radiation exposure during this time include stunted growth, deformities, abnormal brain function, or cancer that may develop sometime later in life (CDC, 2011a).

LEAD. In the United States, the most common source of exposure to lead occurs from lead-based paint in older homes, lead-contaminated house dust, and soil and vinyl products. Lead passes through the placenta and has been found to be associated with spontaneous abortion, fetal anomalies, and preterm birth. The nervous system is the most sensitive target of lead exposure. Fetuses and young children are especially vulnerable to the neurological effects of lead because their brains and nervous systems are still developing and the blood–brain barrier is incomplete. Fetal anomalies associated with lead exposure include hemangiomas, lymphangiomas, hydrocele, minor skin abnormalities (e.g., skin tags and papillae), and undescended testes (CDC, 2010c; Chalupka & Chalupka, 2010).

 Optimizing Outcomes—Educating childbearing families about environmental risks

Many environmental exposures may pose significant health risks to childbearing women and their families. Some have described our present-day environment as a "toxic soup" of chemicals and hazards that exist in the air we breathe, the water we drink, and the food we eat. Synthetic chemicals found in many commonly used personal care products such as moisturizers, lotions, and nail, hair, and facial treatments may provide another potential source of exposure. Nurses must play an active role in helping to prevent long-term disease and illness in childbearing families through an informed approach to nursing practice that effectively communicates risks and offers realistic strategies to help diminish those risks (Anderko, 2010; Russ, 2009).

PESTICIDES. Pesticides, chemicals formulated to kill or repel a pest or halt a pest, are commonly found in food, water, air, soil, and at home, school, and in the workplace. Exposure to pesticides may occur via inhalation, ingestion, and dermal or ocular contact. Maternal/fetal/infant transfer may occur via amniotic fluid, transplacental transport, or during lactation. Fetal exposure to environmental contaminants after the period of cellular differentiation or during times of increased cellular proliferation can result in structural or functional defects, altered growth, and death. These particular times of increased sensitivity to environmental contaminants are referred to as "critical windows of susceptibility" (ACOG, 2013; Gilden, Huffling, & Sattler, 2010; Woodruff, Carlson, Schwartz, & Giudice, 2008). Prenatal exposure to pesticides has been linked to a number of conditions including social behavioral problems (Ribas-Fito, Cardo, Sala, Eulalia de Muga, Mazon, Verdu, et al., 2003), neurodevelopmental delays (Eskenazi, Marks, Bradman, Harley, Barr, Johnson, et al., 2007), impaired gross and fine motor skills (Guillette, Meza, Aquilar, Soto, & Garcia, 1998), otitis media, respiratory distress, asthma (Weselak, Arbuckle, Wigle, & Krewski, 2007), and acute lymphocytic leukemia, Wilms' tumor, and brain cancer (Daniels, Olshan, & Savitz, 1997; Zahm & Ward, 1998).

"What to say"—*Inquiring about substance use during the prenatal interview*

Because of the teratogenic effects of drugs and other substances on the developing embryo/fetus, prenatal screening for maternal drug use is an important component of the prenatal interview. The nurse should ask questions regarding maternal drug use in a nonjudgmental manner that conveys caring and concern. Questions should be specific and begin with inquiries that concern innocuous drug use and then progress to the most harmful substances. Examples of questions to ask include the following:

Do you drink any caffeinated beverages? How many in a day?

Do you smoke cigarettes? How many in a day?

Do you drink alcohol? What kind, and how much in a day?

Do you use substances such as marijuana, cocaine, crack, or heroin? Which ones, and how often?

Are you currently, or have you ever been, enrolled in a substance abuse program?

 Now Can You—Discuss substances that may adversely affect embryo/fetal growth and development?

1. Explain why the embryo is particularly vulnerable to teratogens during organogenesis?
2. Name two vitamins that are associated with fetal malformations?
3. List one fetal effect associated with maternal use of each of the following: tobacco, cocaine, heroin, and marijuana?

TORCH INFECTIONS

TORCH infections are a group of agents that can infect the fetus or newborn. These include **T**oxoplasmosis, "**O**ther" transplacental infections, **R**ubella virus, **C**ytomegalovirus, and the **H**erpes simplex virus. The fetal risks associated with the various TORCH infections are listed in Box 7-1; additional

Where Research and Practice Meet: Chemicals Harbored in Pregnant Women

Researchers from the University of California at San Francisco discovered that the bodies of almost all U.S. pregnant women carry multiple chemicals, including some that have been banned since the 1970s and others that exist in common products such as nonstick cookware, processed foods, and personal care products. Analyzing data for 163 chemicals, Woodruff, Zota, and Schwartz (2011) detected polychlorinated biphenyls, organochlorine pesticides, perfluorinated compounds, phenols, polybrominated diphenyl ethers, phthalates, polycyclic aromatic hydrocarbons, and perchlorate in 99% to 100% of pregnant women. To promote optimal health for childbearing women and their families, it is incumbent on nurses to heighten public awareness about the hazards of everyday chemical exposure and to actively advocate for proactive government policies to reduce people's exposure to potentially harmful chemicals.

Box 7-1 TORCH Infections

TORCH infections can cause serious harm to the embryo/fetus, especially during the first 12 weeks when developmental anomalies may occur.

TOXOPLASMOSIS
Associated with consumption of infested undercooked meat and poor hand washing after handling cat litter. Fetal infection occurs if the mother acquires toxoplasmosis after conception and passes it to the fetus via the placenta. Most infants are asymptomatic at birth but develop symptoms later.

Maternal Effects
Flu-like symptoms in the acute phase.

Fetal/Neonatal Effects
Miscarriage likely in early pregnancy. In neonates, CNS lesions can result in hydrocephaly, microcephaly, chronic retinitis, and seizures. Retinochoroiditis may appear in adolescence or adulthood.

"OTHER" INFECTIONS
Includes varicella-zoster virus, HIV, hepatitis B virus, human parvovirus B19, and syphilis.

- Varicella-zoster virus: transmitted via respiratory secretions; maternal effects include flu-like illness, lymphadenopathy, diffuse vesicular rash with crust formation. Fetal/neonatal effects include congenital varicella syndrome associated with skin lesions, ocular defects, limb abnormalities, and CNS abnormalities.
- HIV: transmitted transplacentally, intrapartally, and postpartally; maternal effects include postpartum endometritis, fever, malaise, anorexia, weight loss, opportunistic infections, and generalized lymphadenopathy. Fetal/neonatal effects include preterm birth, IUGR, perinatal mortality, and opportunistic infections.
- Hepatitis B virus: transmitted transplacentally, intrapartally; maternal effects include fever, malaise, nausea, abdominal discomfort, may be associated with liver failure. Fetal/neonatal effects include intrauterine death, preterm birth, and chronic hepatitis infection.
- Human parvovirus B19: transmitted via respiratory droplets; maternal effects include headache, mild fever, malaise, myalgia, joint pain, and red, pruritic rash on the cheeks. Fetal/neonatal effects include anemia, nonimmune hydrops, congenital anomalies, and death.
- Syphilis: transmitted transplacentally; maternal effects include primary (chancre), secondary (fever, malaise, and red, macular rash on palms or soles of feet), and lymphadenopathy. Fetal/neonatal effects include stillbirth, IUGR, prematurity, hydrops, and bone lesions.

RUBELLA (GERMAN MEASLES)
Spread by respiratory droplets; also transplacentally.

Maternal Effects
Fever, rash, and mild lymphedema.

Fetal/Neonatal Effects
Miscarriage, IUGR, cataracts, congenital anomalies, hepatosplenomegaly, hyperbilirubinemia, intellectual and developmental disabilities, and death. Other symptoms may develop later. Infants born with congenital rubella are contagious and should be isolated. Patients are instructed not to become pregnant for 1 month after receiving the immunization; a signed consent form must be obtained before administration of the vaccine.

CYTOMEGALOVIRUS (CMV)
Respiratory droplets, semen, cervical and vaginal secretions, breast milk, placental tissue, urine, feces, and banked blood (nearly 50% of adults in United States have antibodies for this virus).

Maternal Effects
Asymptomatic illness, cervical discharge, and mononucleosis-like syndrome.

Fetal/Neonatal Effects
Fetal death or severe generalized disease with hemolytic anemia and jaundice, hydrocephaly or microcephaly, pneumonitis, hepatosplenomegaly, intellectual and developmental disabilities, cerebral palsy, and deafness. The organs/tissues affected most often are blood, brain, and liver.

HERPES SIMPLEX VIRUS (HSV)
HSV II is sexually transmitted, infant usually infected during exposure to lesion in birth canal, most at risk during a primary infection in the mother (50% neonatal mortality).

Maternal Effects
Blisters, rash, fever, malaise, nausea, and headache.

Fetal/Neonatal Effects
Miscarriage, preterm birth, stillbirth, transplacental infection is rare but can cause skin lesions, IUGR, intellectual and developmental disabilities, microcephaly, seizures, and coma.

See Table 11-3 for additional information on TORCH infections.

---

information is listed in Table 11-3. (See Chapters 4, 9, and 11 for further discussion about TORCH infections.)

Toxoplasmosis

Toxoplasma gondii, a single-celled parasite, is responsible for toxoplasmosis. This parasite is found throughout the world, and although more than 60 million people in the United States may be infected, most are unaware of the disease (CDC, 2012). The majority of individuals who become infected with toxoplasmosis are asymptomatic, although when present, symptoms are described as "flu-like" and include glandular pain and enlargement (lymphadenopathy) and myalgia. Severe infection may cause damage to the brain, eyes, or organs. Toxoplasmosis is usually acquired by eating raw or poorly cooked meat contaminated with *T gondii*. This disease may also be acquired through close contact with feces from an infected animal (usually a cat) or from contact with soil that has been contaminated with *T gondii*.

Once maternal infection occurs, the *T gondii* organism crosses the placental membrane and infects the fetus, causing damage to the eyes and brain. If the infection is acquired early in gestation, there is an increased risk of fetal death. To minimize the risk of infection, pregnant women should avoid raw or poorly cooked meats and contact with animals that may be infected with the toxoplasmosis parasite.

Other Transplacental Infections

Contemporary revisions identify the "other" transplacental infections recognized as teratogens to include varicella-zoster virus (chickenpox), HIV, hepatitis B virus (HBV), human parvovirus B19, and syphilis. The varicella-zoster virus (VZV), a member of the herpes family, causes chickenpox and shingles. Infection with VZV during the first 4 months of pregnancy is associated with a number of congenital anomalies including muscle atrophy, limb hypoplasia (underdevelopment), damage to the eyes and brain, and intellectual and developmental disabilities. No proven teratogenic risks have been associated with varicella infection that occurs after 20 weeks' gestation (Moore, Persaud, & Torchia, 2011) although approximately 25% of infants born to mothers who become infected with VZV in the last 3 weeks of pregnancy will develop clinical varicella (Gershon, 2010). (See Chapter 11.)

HIV may be transplacentally transmitted to the fetus in utero. Infection may also occur intrapartally (during labor and birth) from exposure to maternal blood and body fluids and postpartally (after birth), through breast milk. Without medical intervention, the risk of perinatal transmission of HIV is approximately 25%; with appropriate treatment, the rate of perinatal transmission can be reduced to 2% (Department of Health and Human Services [DHHS], 2011). (See Chapter 11 for further discussion.)

Hepatitis B virus infection during pregnancy is associated with an increased risk for stillbirth and preterm birth. Infants may be infected transplacentally, serum to serum, or following exposure to contaminated maternal blood, urine, feces, genital secretions, or saliva. Infection occurs most commonly during birth or in the first few days of life, and the rate of transmission is highest when the mother has contracted the virus immediately before birth. Infected infants may become chronic carriers at risk for significant liver disease.

Human parvovirus B19, also known as "fifth disease," may cause miscarriage or the development of nonimmune hydrops (fetal hemolytic disorder) and intrauterine growth restriction. Transmission occurs transplacentally, and the virus may be isolated from amniotic fluid, fetal blood, and fetal tissue.

Treponema pallidum, the microorganism that causes syphilis, readily crosses the placenta. Serious fetal infection and congenital anomalies are almost always associated with primary maternal infections that occur during pregnancy. However, *T pallidum* can be destroyed with adequate treatment that will prevent placental transmission and fetal infection. Secondary infections acquired before pregnancy rarely result in fetal disease and anomalies. Left untreated, only 20% of pregnant women with primary syphilis infections will give birth to a normal term infant. Neonatal manifestations of congenital syphilis infection include prematurity, skin rash, snuffles, hydrops fetalis, failure to thrive, hepatosplenomegaly, lymphadenopathy, and bone lesions (osteochondritis, osteomyelitis, and periostitis). Late-onset manifestations of congenital syphilis infection include keratitis (inflammation of the cornea), deafness, and bowing of the shins (CDC, 2011b).

Rubella

The virus that causes rubella (also known as German measles) can cause damage to the developing embryo/fetus. The earlier in the pregnancy that the disease is contracted, the greater the risk to the developing embryo. If the pregnant woman experiences a primary rubella infection during the first trimester, there is a 20% risk that the fetus will also become infected. When maternal rubella infection occurs during the first 4 to 5 weeks after fertilization, the majority of infants will demonstrate congenital anomalies. If rubella is contracted during the second and third trimesters, the risk of congenital anomalies is decreased to 10%, but intellectual and developmental disabilities and hearing loss may result from infection that occurs late in the gestation. Birth defects associated with congenital rubella syndrome include hearing loss, eye defects causing vision loss or blindness, heart defects, and intellectual and developmental disabilities.

Cytomegalovirus (CMV)

Approximately 50% to 80% of adults have antibodies to the cytomegalovirus (CMV) (Anderson & Gonik, 2010). CMV produces no signs or symptoms of infection in the majority of affected individuals. However, CMV can cause disease in unborn babies or in persons with weakened immune systems. The cytomegalovirus is a member of the herpesvirus family and is the most common viral infection in the fetus.

Spontaneous abortion (miscarriage) may result from maternal CMV infection during the first trimester. Infection that occurs later in the pregnancy may result in fetal intrauterine growth restriction, microphthalmia, chorioretinitis, blindness, microcephaly, cerebral calcification, intellectual and developmental disabilities, deafness, cerebral palsy, and hepatosplenomegaly. In the neonate, asymptomatic CMV infections are often associated with audiological, neurological, and neurobehavioral disturbances.

Herpes Simplex Virus (HSV)

Spontaneous abortion is increased threefold if maternal infection from herpes simplex virus occurs in early pregnancy. Infection after the 20th gestational week is associated with an increased rate of prematurity. The transmission of the herpes virus occurs at the time of delivery during passage through the birth canal but may also occur transplacentally via ascending infection before labor or rupture of the membranes. Congenital anomalies associated with the herpes simplex virus include extensive dermatological scarring or bullae, microencephaly, hydranencephaly, encephalitis, microphthalmia, chorioretinitis, and hepatosplenomegaly (Schleiss & Patterson, 2011). (See Chapter 19 for further discussion.)

 Now Can You—Discuss TORCH infections?

1. Identify the components of the acronym "TORCH"?
2. Describe a teaching need for pregnant women who have indoor cats?
3. Explain why pregnant women should avoid individuals infected with chickenpox and rubella?

The Nurse's Role in Prenatal Evaluation

The clinical gestational period is divided into three trimesters that each last for 3 months. By the end of the first trimester, all major organs are developed. During the second trimester, the fetus continues to grow in size, and most fetal anomalies can be detected using high-resolution real-time ultrasound. By the beginning of the third trimester the fetus has a chance for survival, and most survive if born at or after 35 weeks' gestation.

At the initial prenatal visit, the nurse performs an assessment that includes careful consideration of cultural, emotional, physical, and physiological factors that may signal a need for genetics counseling and comprehensive fetal evaluation.

 Optimizing Outcomes—Expanding nursing roles in genetics health care

Roles for maternity, women's health, and pediatrics nurses in genetics health care have expanded significantly over the past few years as genetics education and counseling has become standard of care. Today, nurses may provide pre-conception counseling for women at risk for the transmission of a genetic disorder, prenatal care for women with genetically linked psychiatric disorders or other conditions (e.g., congenital heart disease) that require specialized care, or infant screening. Nurses may also be involved in caring for families who have children with genetic conditions or those who have lost a fetus or child affected by a genetic condition (Adamson, 2010; Hershberger & Pierce, 2010; Hershberger, Schoenfeld, & Tur-Kaspa, 2011). In 2005, nursing leaders developed the document *Essentials of Genetic and Genomic Nursing: Competencies, Curricula Guidelines, and Outcome Indicators*. This publication, updated in 2008, presents minimal genetic and genomic competencies with outcome indicators for all nurses, and may be accessed at http://www.genome.gov/Pages/Careers/HealthProfessionalEducation/geneticscompetency.pdf

Prenatal care involves ongoing medical and psychosocial support. (See Chapter 9 for further discussion.) Common prenatal screening includes blood testing and ultrasound examination. Depending on maternal and familial risk factors, advanced screening tests may be indicated. Amniocentesis, chorionic villus sampling, and percutaneous umbilical blood sampling (PUBS) are examples of specialized prenatal diagnostic methods. (See Chapters 9 and 11 for further discussion.)

 Nursing Insight—*Specific methods for gene identification and testing*

Gene identification and testing involves the analysis of human DNA, RNA (ribonucleic acid), chromosomes, or certain proteins to identify abnormalities related to an inherited condition. Through direct or molecular testing, the DNA and RNA that make up a single gene are directly examined; with linkage analysis, markers that are co-inherited with a specific gene that causes a genetic condition are analyzed; through biochemical testing, scientists examine the protein products of genes; and with cytogenetic testing, individual chromosomes are examined. Commercially available genetic tests can be accessed online at GeneTests, http://www.genetests.org./

Genetic counseling should be offered to couples with a personal or family history of a heritable genetic disorder. The nurse must be aware of, and be able to provide, education regarding the potential for an increased risk for various diseases found among certain racial and ethnic populations

(Table 7-5). Testing for many common genetic diseases is now available. For diseases in which the responsible gene has not been identified, the risk can sometimes be estimated by comparing fetal DNA with that of affected and non-affected family members.

 Cultural Diversity: Maintaining and Communicating a Caring and Accepting Attitude

It is important for the nurse to be knowledgeable of various cultural practices and beliefs that may impact on the development of the fetus. Culture and experience influence every aspect of individuals' lives and how they care for themselves and their families. For example, women from some ethnic groups choose to visit health healers and lay midwives throughout pregnancy.

The nurse should maintain an unbiased and accepting attitude when working with patients from populations with varying beliefs and practices. Awareness and understanding of personal practices and beliefs constitute the first step toward ensuring an unbiased disposition when providing patient care. Recognizing that cultural values and experiences shape an individual's likelihood to continue or discontinue familial beliefs and practices helps the nurse to develop a more accepting attitude and deliver appropriate care in a culturally sensitive manner.

Heredity and Genetics

According to the CDC, the leading cause of infant death in the United States in 2007 was related to problems associated with congenital malformations, deformations, and chromosomal abnormalities. These conditions accounted for 20% of all infant deaths (CDC, 2011c). Birth defects, or **congenital anomalies,** are structural abnormalities present at birth. Congenital anomalies may result from four different pathological processes: malformation, disruption, deformation, and dysplasia. **Malformation** is the alteration in embryonic development caused by genetic transmission, chromosomal anomalies, environmental factors, and multifactorial/unknown causes. This defect results from an intrinsic abnormal development that is present from the beginning of development, such as one that arises from a chromosomal abnormality. A disruption is caused by an external force that alters previously normal tissue and interferes with normal development. Maternal exposure to

Table 7-5 Racial and Ethnic Groups With Increased Risk for Diseases Caused by Recessive Genes	
Racial/Ethnic Group	**Disease**
African, Mediterranean, Caribbean, Latin American, or Middle Eastern descent	Hemoglobin gene mutations are more common in persons from these areas. African Americans have an increased incidence of sickle cell anemia. Southeast Asians have a greater likelihood of carrying hemoglobin E, an abnormal hemoglobin.
Mediterranean or Asian origin	These individuals have a higher risk of the hereditary anemia thalassemia.
Jewish ancestry	Individuals with Jewish ancestry have an increased risk for diseases associated with inborn errors of metabolism caused by different enzyme deficiencies (e.g., Tay-Sachs, Canavan, and Gaucher's).
Caucasian or northern European descent	The most common disorder found among this population is cystic fibrosis.

teratogens, such as drugs, viruses, or environmental hazards, may also cause a disruption. Disruptions are not inherited although an individual may be predisposed to the development of a disruption. **Deformations** are physical alterations in form, shape, or position that are caused by extrinsic mechanical factors (e.g., clubfoot that results from intrauterine fetal restraint or fetal compression defects that result from decreased amniotic fluid [**oligohydramnios**]). **Dysplasia** (an abnormal development of tissue) is caused by an abnormal organization of cells that results in abnormal tissue formation. (See Chapter 11 for further discussion.)

Damage that may alter embryological development can occur to the chromosomes of one or both parents prior to conception. During the pre-embryonic period (up to 14 days after conception), while the zygote is protected by the zona pellucida, exposure to teratogens most likely causes either no harmful effects or produces severe damage that results in loss of the pregnancy.

❝What to say❞—*Prenatal identification of a fetal anomaly*

Prenatal testing may identify a fetus with a congenital anomaly. When this occurs, families are generally faced with a flood of emotions and difficult decisions. The nurse plays an important role in providing support and education regarding options available to these couples. A nonjudgmental and caring attitude is vital at this difficult and vulnerable time.

Therapeutic communication is enhanced when the nurse uses statements such as:

"It is normal to have fear, grief, or even be angry."

"It is normal to have concerns about your ability to have a normal baby."

"I am here to answer your questions and listen to your concerns. If I do not know the answers I will either find and share them or arrange for a colleague to meet with you."

The nurse should avoid using statements such as:

"You can always have other children."

"I know how you feel."

"At least you do not know the baby yet."

⑤ Optimizing Outcomes—Including the father of the baby

Health-care providers frequently focus primarily on the pregnant woman. It is important that nurses remember to include fathers and care for the couple when providing patient education and support.

Maternal Age and Chromosomes

Advanced maternal age (age 35 and above at the time of birth) is associated with an increased risk of chromosomal abnormalities (1% risk beginning at age 35 and increasing each year, up to an 8% risk at age 46), with trisomy 21 (**Down syndrome**) accounting for half of these. The risk

of giving birth to a child with Down syndrome increases with age: The incidence is approximately 1 in 1,350 for a 25-year old woman; 1 in 350 for a 35-year-old woman; and 1 in 40 for a 44-year-old woman. However, children with Down syndrome may be born to mothers of any age: Approximately 80% of children with Down syndrome are born to mothers younger than 35 years (National Down Syndrome Society, 2012).

A **trisomy** occurs when there are three particular chromosomes instead of the normal number of two. Figure 7-14 illustrates the extra chromosome that occurs with Down syndrome. The three most common trisomies found in live newborns are trisomy 18 (Edwards syndrome), trisomy 21 (Down syndrome), and trisomy 13 (Patau syndrome).

Trisomy 13 and trisomy 18 are rare; each occurs only about once in every 5,000 live births. Trisomy 21 is the most common trisomy and occurs in approximately every 650 live births (Scanlon & Sanders, 2011). The prognosis for both trisomy 13 and 18 is very poor; approximately 70% of infants with these chromosomal disorders die within the first 3 months of life from complications associated with respiratory and cardiac abnormalities. Neonatal effects from these three most common trisomies include central nervous system abnormalities, intellectual and developmental disabilities, and hypotonia at birth. Although children with Down syndrome are intellectually challenged, there is a wide range of mental ability among this group.

Deletion and translocation describe other chromosomal abnormalities. Women younger than 35 years of age who have previously given birth to a child with a chromosomal abnormality have a 1% increased risk of having another affected child. A **deletion** is a loss of a portion of DNA from a chromosome (Fig. 7-15). This alteration can be caused by an unknown event, mutation, or exposure to radiation, or it may occur during cell division. When a gene necessary for cell function is absent, disease may result. A **translocation** occurs when all or a segment of one chromosome breaks off and attaches to the same or to a different chromosome (Fig. 7-16). Parents who have a chromosomal translocation or who have had

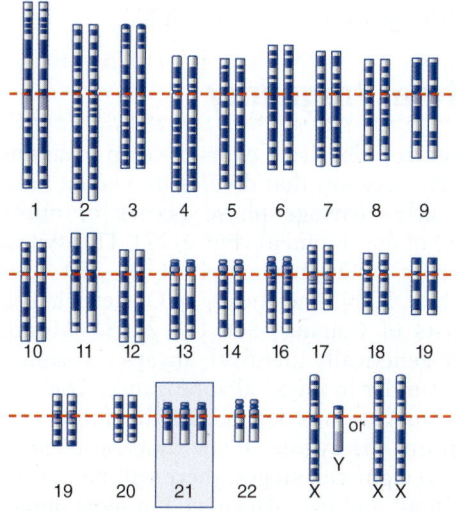

Figure 7-14 Trisomy 21. (Courtesy of National Human Genome Research Institute.)

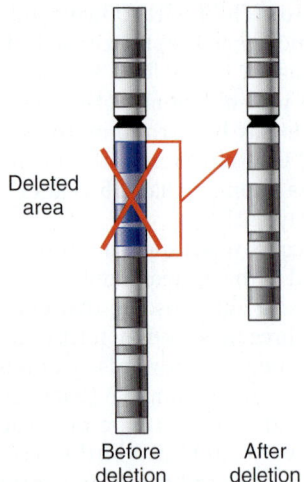

Figure 7-15 Deletion. (Courtesy of National Human Genome Research Institute.)

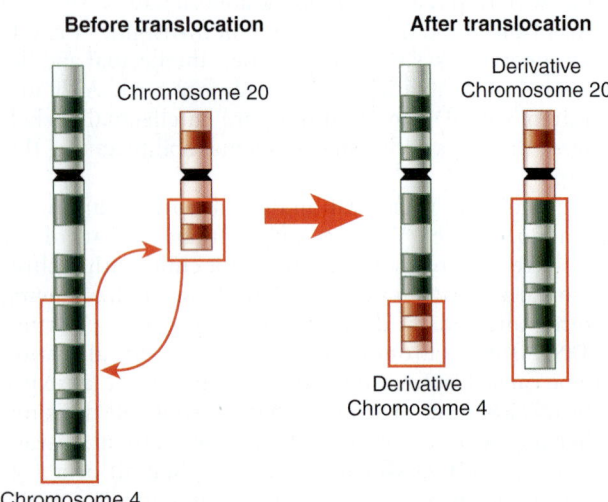

Figure 7-16 Translocation. (Courtesy of National Human Genome Research Institute.)

a child with structural malformations are at increased risk for having another affected child.

Multifetal Pregnancy

Monozygotic (identical) twins develop from one fertilized oocyte (zygote) that divides into equal halves during an early cleavage phase (series of mitotic cell divisions) of development (Fig. 7-17). This type of twinning occurs in approximately 1 of 250 live births (Benirschke, 2009; The Society of Obstetricians and Gynecologists of Canada [SOGC], 2013). Monozygotic twins are genetically identical, always the same gender, and very similar in physical appearance. The number of amnions and chorions depends on the timing of division (cleavage) of the zygote. If the division occurs during the two- to eight-cell stages, there will be two amnions, two chorions, and two placentas. For most monozygotic twins, the division occurs at the end of the first week after fertilization and results from the division of the

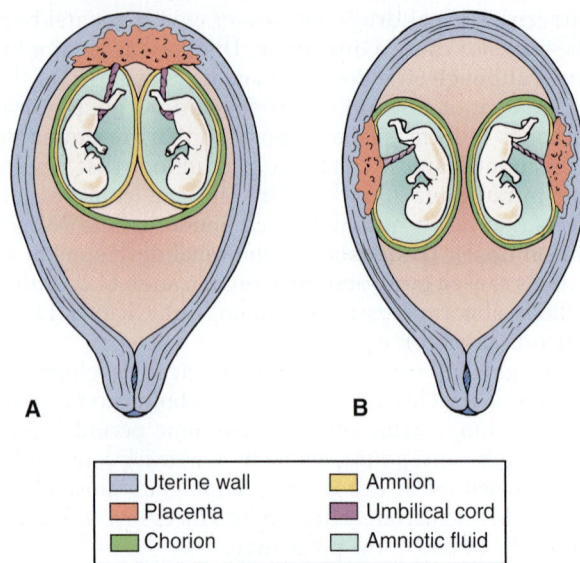

Uterine wall	Amnion
Placenta	Umbilical cord
Chorion	Amniotic fluid

Figure 7-17 Multiple gestations. *A,* Monozygotic twins with one placenta, one chorion, and two amnions. *B,* Dizygotic twins with two placentas, two chorions, and two amnions.

singular embryoblast into two embryoblasts. When the division occurs during this time, each fetus has its own amnion but resides within a single chorion and receives oxygen and nutrients from the same placenta. Depending on the timing of cleavage, the following multifetal combinations occur:

- Division that occurs during the first 72 hours after fertilization: two embryos, two amnions, and two chorions develop with two distinct placentas, or a single fused placenta.
- Division that occurs between the fourth and eighth day: two embryos, each in a separate amnion sac covered by a single chorion.
- Division that occurs approximately 8 days after fertilization after the chorion and amnion have differentiated: two embryos in a common amniotic sac.
- Division that occurs after the embryonic disk has formed: Cleavage is incomplete and conjoined twins result.

Conjoined twins occur when the embryonic disk does not divide completely or when adjacent embryonic disks fuse. Conjoined twinning occurs in approximately 1 in 50,000 to 100,000 births. Twins may be connected to one another by the skin only or by cutaneous and other tissues. In many cases, surgical separation is possible, but depending on the anatomical region of attachment and the sharing of vital organs, surgery may not be feasible.

Dizygotic (fraternal) twins develop from two zygotes and may be the same or different genders. Dizygotic twins are no more genetically similar than other siblings born to the same parents. There are separate amnions and chorions, although the chorions and placentas may be fused. The incidence of dizygotic twinning is approximately 1 in 500 Asians, 1 in 125 Caucasians, and as high as 1 in 20 in some African populations. Triplets may result from the division of a single zygote into three zygotes (one original fertilized egg), from the division of one zygote (identical twins are formed) plus another zygote (a total of two original fertilized eggs), or from three different zygotes (a total of three original fertilized eggs).

 Now Can You—Discuss maternal age-related chromosomal problems and the origins of twinning?

1. Differentiate among the terms "malformation," "disruption," "deformation," and "dysplasia"?
2. Define "trisomy" and identify two of the most common trisomies?
3. Explain how twinning occurs?

The Nurse's Role in Minimizing Threats to the Developing Embryo and Fetus

Nurses provide holistic care to the family unit. The nurse must assess for environmental and lifestyle risks that may harm the fetus or mother. According to the American College of Obstetricians and Gynecologists (2011b), all women should have a family history evaluation as a screening tool for inherited risk, and this information should be reviewed and updated on a regular basis. Ongoing evaluations should include assessment of the patient's knowledge, lifestyle patterns, environmental conditions, and physical and psychosocial well-being. Reduction of maternal–fetal risks and helping to ensure the birth of a healthy newborn to a healthy mother remains the essential goal throughout pregnancy.

 Cultural Diversity: Cystic Fibrosis Screening for All Women

Cystic fibrosis (CF), the most common life-threatening autosomal recessive condition in the non-Hispanic white population, is a progressive, multisystem disease associated with a median survival of approximately 37 years. The goal of CF carrier screening is to identify couples at risk of having a child with classic CF (i.e., significant pulmonary disease and pancreatic insufficiency). Screening is most efficacious in the non-Hispanic white and Ashkenazi Jewish populations. However, because of the fact that it is becoming increasingly difficult to assign a single ethnicity to affected individuals, the American College of Obstetricians and Gynecologists advocates that CF carrier screening be offered to all patients (ACOG, 2011c).

Ideally, counseling about strategies to promote optimal maternal and fetal health should begin before pregnancy occurs. Preconception counseling allows for the early identification of maternal risk factors and often provides an opportunity for intervention before pregnancy.

 Optimizing Outcomes—Preconception carrier screening for genetic diseases

Carrier screening for specific genetic conditions is frequently determined by an individual's ancestry. Certain autosomal recessive disease conditions are more prevalent in persons of Eastern European Jewish (Ashkenazi) descent. The American College of Gynecologists and Obstetricians Committee on Genetics recommends that routine carrier

screening for Tay-Sachs disease, Canavan disease, cystic fibrosis, and familial dysautonomia should be offered to Ashkenazi Jewish individuals before conception or during early pregnancy to allow the couple an opportunity to consider prenatal diagnostic testing options (ACOG, 2009).

Poor maternal health and illness can have a number of adverse effects on the developing fetus. In years past, women with chronic illnesses such as diabetes and hypertension were unable to conceive or were advised not to become pregnant. The advent of insulin and antihypertensive medications has allowed these women to not only contemplate pregnancy but to successfully carry a pregnancy to maturity with healthy outcomes for both the mother and her baby.

 Nursing Insight—*Karyotyping as a component of preconception counseling*

Karyotyping of the parents as well as their child with a genetic disorder may be appropriate during the preconception period. A **karyotype** is a photomicrograph of the chromosomes of a single cell; the chromosomes are then arranged in numerical order (Venes, 2013) (Fig. 7-18). Cells, obtained from a sample of peripheral venous blood or a scraping of the buccal membrane tissue, are stained and photographed following a period of growth in the laboratory. *Fluorescence in situ hybridization* (FISH) is a rapid technique that allows for immediate karyotyping without a period of cell growth.

Through preventive strategies, preconception counseling can significantly decrease the incidence of birth defects and problems associated with preterm birth along with other disorders linked to maternal illness and nutritional deficiencies. Counseling should include discussion

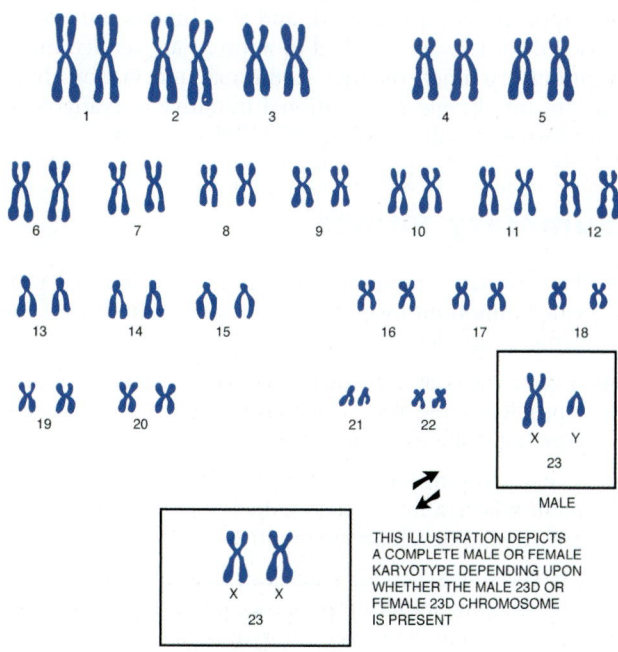

Figure 7-18 Karyotype of human chromosomes of male and female.

of possible fetal risks from exposure to teratogens. Factors that could potentially harm the developing fetus are identified, and the woman is advised of her risks. When possible, strategies to reduce or prevent risk to the fetus are discussed with the woman and her family. If exposure has occurred, every effort should be made to identify the timing of the contact and the amount of exposure. This information is essential because the calculation of risk varies according to the particular teratogen and the timing and dose of the exposure. (See Chapter 10 for further discussion.)

Optimizing Outcomes—Formulating nursing diagnoses for women and couples seeking genetic screening and assessment

Nursing diagnoses that may be applicable for genetic screening and assessment include:

- Health-seeking behaviors related to potential for genetic transmission of disease
- Deficient knowledge related to inheritance pattern of the family's inherited disorder
- Fear related to outcome of genetic screening tests
- Decisional conflict related to testing for an untreatable genetic disorder

After the infant's birth, diseases that may increase the risk for infection and cause liver damage, intellectual and developmental disabilities, or death can often be identified through newborn screening tests. Newborn screening, which was initiated in the 1960s, was the first population-based screening program to test for genetic conditions. Through screening, diagnosis and treatment for many diseases and disorders can take place before permanent damage occurs. One of the *Healthy People 2020* goals is to ensure that all newborns are screened at birth as mandated by their state-sponsored screening programs, that follow-up diagnostic testing for positive findings is performed in the appropriate time period, and that infants with diagnosed disorders are enrolled in appropriate service interventions in a timely manner. Additional information about the *Healthy People 2020* national initiative is available at http://www.healthypeople.gov/2020/default.aspx.

Summary Points

- The Human Genome Project that ended in 2003 provided important insights into our understanding of the genetic complexity of humans.

- A genotype is an individual's gene composition; a phenotype refers to the observable expression of a person's genotype; a genome is a complete copy of the genes present.

- The developing embryo/fetus lives in a unique environment where all essential elements needed for normal growth and development are provided.

- The gestational period, which lasts an average of 40 weeks from the time of fertilization, occurs in three stages: the pre-embryonic stage, the embryonic stage, and the fetal stage.

- During the embryonic stage the heart begins to beat and the body's circulation is established.

- Structural refinement and perfection of function of all systems occur during the fetal stage.

- Teratogens, substances that cause harm to the developing fetus, may be in the form of chemicals, viruses, environmental agents, physical factors, and drugs.

- By educating pregnant women about fetal developmental events and avoidance of potential hazards, nurses can help to ensure a healthy outcome for the mother and her infant.

Review Questions

Multiple Choice

1. The nurse working in reproductive health care is aware that which of the following was a goal of the Human Genome Project?
A. Identify exact human DNA sequences and genes
B. Identify human DNA and RNA sequences
C. Measure exact human DNA sequences for chromosomal diseases
D. Measure exact human DNA sequence maps for disease prevention

2. A nurse is teaching a prenatal class on fetal growth and development. In which gestational week does the nurse inform the parents that the heart begins to beat?
A. Second
B. Third
C. Fourth
D. Sixth

3. The perinatal nurse is providing information on fetal growth and development. The nurse explains that fetal urine production begins at
A. 6 to 8 weeks.
B. 9 to 12 weeks.
C. 12 to 16 weeks.
D. 15 to 18 weeks.

4. A nurse is providing preconception counseling. The nurse explains that the fetus is most vulnerable to the effects of teratogens during which time period?
A. 5 to 10 weeks
B. 2 to 8 weeks
C. 4 to 12 weeks
D. 6 to 15 weeks

5. The nurse is conducting a prenatal visit with a newly expectant mother. The woman wants to know why the nurse is concerned about her drinking habits. Which is the best response by the nurse?
A. "Alcohol has one of the strongest effects on fetal development we know of."
B. "Asking about drug and alcohol use is a normal part of a history."
C. "High amounts of drinking can lead to bleeding problems in the fetus."
D. "Women who are pregnant should limit alcohol to 2 drinks a day."

6. A woman who smokes has just learned she is 10 weeks pregnant. She does not believe that quitting will help her fetus now because she has already exposed it to the smoking. Which response by the nurse is best?
   A. "Stop now and your baby's birth weight will probably be near normal."
   B. "The effects of the carbon dioxide have already done some harm."
   C. "Tobacco exposure is worse for the fetus in the third trimester."
   D. "You are right; quitting now does not really offer any benefits."

7. A newborn nursery nurse notes that a neonate has hyperirritability and some difficulty breathing. Which response by the nurse is most appropriate?
   A. Ask the mother about opioid use during pregnancy.
   B. Inform the mother not to drink caffeinated beverages.
   C. Teach the mother infant relaxation techniques.
   D. Tell the physician about suspected maternal crack use.

8. A nurse is conducting a history on a new obstetric patient. The mother works in an animal shelter. Which instruction by the nurse is most appropriate?
   A. Avoid contact with birds and reptiles.
   B. Be sure you have a tetanus booster.
   C. Get *cytomegalovirus* antibodies drawn.
   D. Have someone else clean litter boxes.

9. A nurse is teaching a prenatal class about placental development and functions. Which information about the placenta is best?
   A. Cushions the fetus and protects it against mechanical injury
   B. Is the site of hematopoiesis during the first two gestational weeks
   C. Produces Wharton's jelly that surrounds the umbilical blood vessels
   D. Provides oxygenation, nutrition, hormones, and waste removal

10. A faculty member is teaching a nursing class about fetal circulation. The faculty member explains that most blood bypasses the liver and enters the inferior vena cava through the
   A. ductus arteriosus.
   B. ductus venosus.
   C. foramen ovale.
   D. pulmonary artery.

See Answers to End of Chapter Review Questions on Davis*Plus*.

REFERENCES

Adamson, G. D. (2010). Ethical considerations in genetic diagnosis and screening of embryos. *Sexuality, Reproduction, and Menopause, 8*(1), 21–25.

Adzick, N. S., Thom, E. A., Spong, C. Y., Brock, J. W., Burrows, P. K., Johnson, M. P., . . . Farmer, D. L. (2011). A randomized trial of prenatal versus postnatal repair of myelomeningocele. *New England Journal of Medicine, 364*(3), 993–1004. doi:10.1056/NEJMoa1014379

American College of Obstetricians and Gynecologists (ACOG). (2009). Committee Opinion Number 442. Preconception and prenatal carrier screening for genetic diseases in individuals of Eastern European Jewish descent. *Obstetrics & Gynecology, 114*(4), 950–952.

American College of Obstetricians and Gynecologists (ACOG). (2010). Committee Opinion Number 462. Moderate caffeine consumption during pregnancy. (Reaffirmed 2013). *Obstetrics & Gynecology, 116*(8), 467–468.

American College of Obstetricians and Gynecologists (ACOG). (2011a). Practice Bulletin Number 124. Inherited thrombophilias in pregnancy. *Obstetrics & Gynecology, 118*(3), 730–740.

American College of Obstetricians and Gynecologists (ACOG). (2011b). Committee Opinion Number 478. Family history as a risk assessment tool. *Obstetrics & Gynecology, 117*(3), 747–750.

American College of Obstetricians and Gynecologists (ACOG). (2011c). Committee Opinion Number 486. Update on carrier screening for cystic fibrosis. *Obstetrics & Gynecology, 117*(4), 1028–1031.

American College of Obstetricians and Gynecologists (ACOG). (2013). Committee Opinion Number 575. Exposure to toxic environmental agents. *Obstetrics & Gynecology, 122*(4), 931–934.

Anderko, L. (2010). Environmental health for childbearing women and their families. *Journal of Obstetric, Gynecologic and Neonatal Nursing, 39*(1), 82–83.

Anderson, B. L., & Gonik, B. (2010). Perinatal infections. In R. Martin, A. Fanaroff, & M. Walsh (Eds.). *Fanaroff & Martin's neonatal-perinatal medicine: Diseases of the fetus and infant* (9th ed., pp. 399–422). Philadelphia, PA: C.V. Mosby.

Association of Women's Health, Obstetric & Neonatal Nursing (AWHONN). (2010). Position Statement. Smoking and women's health. *Journal of Obstetric, Gynecologic and Neonatal Nursing, 39*(5), 427–429. doi:10.1111/j.1552-6909.2010.01178.x

Benirschke, K. (2009). Multiple gestation. The biology of twinning. In R. Creasy, R. Resnik, J. Iams, C. Lockwood, & T. Moore (Eds.), *Maternal-fetal medicine: Principles and practice* (6th ed.). Philadelphia, PA: Saunders Elsevier.

Bhuvaneswar, C. G., Chang, G., Epstein, L. A., & Stern, T. A. (2008). Cocaine and opioid use during pregnancy: Prevalence and management. *Primary Care Companion to the Journal of Clinical Psychiatry, 10*(1), 59–65.

Centers for Disease Control and Prevention (CDC). (2010a). Infertility. Retrieved from http://www.cdc.gov/nchs/fastats/infertility.htm

Centers for Disease Control and Prevention (CDC). (2010b). Alcohol use in pregnancy. Retrieved from http://www.cdc.gov/ncbddd/fasd/alcohol-use.html

Centers for Disease Control and Prevention (CDC). (2010c). Guidelines for the identification and management of lead exposure in pregnant and lactating women. Retrieved from http://www.cdc.gov/nceh/lead/publications/leadandpregnancy2010.pdf

Centers for Disease Control and Prevention (CDC), Emergency Preparedness & Response. (2011a). *Radiation and pregnancy: A fact sheet for the public.* Retrieved from http://www.bt.cdc.gov/radiation/prenatal.asp

Centers for Disease Control and Prevention (CDC). (2011b). *Sexually transmitted diseases treatment guidelines, 2010.* Retrieved from http://www.cdc.gov/std/treatment/2010/genital-ulcers.htm#syphilis

Centers for Disease Control and Prevention (CDC). National Vital Statistics Reports (2011c), Vol. 59(6). *Infant mortality statistics from the 2007 period linked birth/infant death data set.* Retrieved from http://www.cdc.gov/nchs/data/nvsr/nvsr59/nvsr59_06.pdf

Centers for Disease Control and Prevention (CDC). (2012). *Parasites–Toxoplasmosis (Toxoplasma infection).* Retrieved from http://www.cdc.gov/parasites/toxoplasmosis/

Chalupka, S., & Chalupka, A. N. (2010). The impact of environmental and occupational exposures on reproductive health. *Journal of Obstetric, Gynecologic and Neonatal Nursing, 39*(1), 84–100.

Cohen, A., & Lynch, K. A. (2011). Turner syndrome: An update for the obstetrician-gynecologist. *The Female Patient, 36*(12), 36–41.

Daniels, J. L., Olshan, A. F., & Savitz, D. A. (1997). Pesticides and childhood cancers. *Environmental Health Perspectives, 105*(10), 1068–1077.

Department of Health and Human Services (DHHS). (2011). Recommendations for use of antiretroviral drugs in pregnant HIV-1-infected women for maternal health and interventions to reduce perinatal HIV transmission in the United States. Retrieved from http://aidsinfo.nih.gov/guidelines/html/3/perinatal-guidelines/0/

Eskenazi, B., Marks, A., Bradman, A., Harley, K., Barr, D. B., Johnson, C., . . . Jewell, N. P. (2007). Organophosphate pesticide exposure and neurodevelopment in young Mexican-American children. *Environmental Health Perspectives, 115*(5), 792–798.

Gershon, A. (2010). Chickenpox, measles and mumps. In J. Remington, J. Klein, C. Wilson, & V. Nizet (Eds.), *Infectious diseases of the fetus and newborn infant* (7th ed., pp. 661–705). Philadelphia, PA: W.B. Saunders.

Gilden, R. C., Huffling, K., & Sattler, B. (2010). Pesticides and health risks. *Journal of Obstetric, Gynecologic & Neonatal Nursing, 39*(1), 103–110.

Guillette, E. A., Meza, M. M., Aquilar, M. G., Soto, A. D., & Garcia, I. E. (1998). An anthropological approach to the evaluation of preschool children exposed to pesticides in Mexico. *Environmental Health Perspectives, 106*(6), 347–353.

Hackshaw, A., Rodeck, C., & Boniface. S. (2011). Maternal smoking in pregnancy and birth defects: A systematic review based on 173,687 malformed cases and 11.7 million controls. *Human Reproduction Update, 18*(7), 1–7. doi:10.1093/humupd/dmr022

Hershberger, P. E., & Pierce, P. F. (2010). Conceptualizing couples' decision making in PGD: Emerging cognitive, emotional, and moral dimensions. *Patient Education and Counseling, 81*(1), 53–62. doi:10.1016/j.pec.2009.11.017

Hershberger, P. E., Schoenfeld, C., & Tur-Kaspa, I. (2011). Unraveling preimplantation genetic diagnosis for high-risk couples. *Nursing for Women's Health, 15*(1), 38–45.

Khoury, M. J., Bedrosian, S. R., Gwinn, M., Higgins, J. P. T., Ioannidis, J. P. A., & Little, J. (2010). *Human genome epidemiology: Building the evidence for using genetic information to improve health and prevent disease.* (2nd ed.). New York, NY: Oxford University Press.

Kuntz, S. W., Ricco, J. A., Hill, W. G., & Anderko, L. (2010). Communicating methylmercury risks and fish consumption benefits to vulnerable childbearing populations. *Journal of Obstetric, Gynecologic & Neonatal Nursing, 39*(1), 118–126. doi:10.1111/j.1552-6909.2009.01094.x

Loud, J. T. (2010). Direct-to-consumer genetic and genomic testing: Preparing nurse practitioners for genomic healthcare. *The Journal for Nurse Practitioners, 6*(8), 585–596.

Malek, A. (2012). Effects of prenatal cocaine exposure on human pregnancy and postpartum. *Pharmaceutia Analytica Acta, 3*(9), 191–199. doi:10.4172/2153-2435.1000191

March of Dimes. (2011). Smoking during pregnancy. Retrieved from http://www.marchofdimes.com/pregnancy/alcohol_smoking.html

March of Dimes. (2013). Eating and nutrition. Retrieved from http://www.marchofdimes.com/pregnancy/caffeine-in-pregnancy.aspx

Moore, K. L., Persaud, T. V. N., & Torchia, M. G. (2011). *The developing human: Clinically oriented embryology* (9th ed.). Philadelphia, PA: Saunders.

Moore, T. R. (2010). Amniotic fluid dynamics reflect fetal and maternal health and disease. *Obstetrics & Gynecology, 116*(3), 759–765.

National Center for Health Statistics (NCHS). (2010). NCHS Data Brief No. 42. Prescription Drug Use Continues to Increase: U.S. Prescription Drug Data for 2007–2008. Retrieved from http://www.cdc.gov/nchs/data/databriefs/db42.pdf

National Down Syndrome Society. (2012). Down Syndrome: Myths and truths. Retrieved from http://www.ndss.org/Down-Syndrome/Myths-Truths/

National Human Genome Research Institute. (2011). Genetic disorders, genomics, and health care. Retrieved from http://www.genome.gov/27527652

National Institutes of Health (NIH). (2012). Stem Cell Information. Retrieved from http://stemcells.nih.gov/info/basics/basics3.asp

Organization of Teratology Information Specialists (OTIS). (2011). Marijuana and pregnancy. Retrieved from www.otispregnancy.org/marijuana-r108119

Ribas-Fito, N., Cardo, E., Sala, M., Eulalia de Muga, M., Mazon, C., Verdu, A., . . . Sunyer, J. (2003). Breastfeeding, exposure to organochlorine compounds and neurodevelopment in infants. *Pediatrics, 111*(5, Pt 1), e580–e585.

Russ, K. (2009). Health effects of personal care products. *Nursing for Women's Health, 13*(5), 393–401.

Scanlon, V. C., & Sanders, T. (2011). *Essentials of anatomy and physiology* (6th ed.). Philadelphia, PA: F.A. Davis.

Schleiss, M. R., & Patterson, J. C. (2011). Viral infections of the fetus and newborn and human immunodeficiency virus infection during pregnancy. In C. A. Gleason & S. Devaskar (Eds.), *Avery's diseases of the newborn* (9th ed., pp. 468–512). Philadelphia, PA: Saunders.

Seibert, D. C. (2010). Genetics and disease prevention: Complementary or contradictory? *The Journal for Nurse Practitioners, 6*(7), 507–512.

Smith, B. R. (2013). The multidimensional human embryo, Carnegie Stages. Retrieved from http://embryo.soad.umich.edu/carnStages/carnStages.html

The Society of Obstetricians and Gynaecologists of Canada. (SOGC). (2013). Multiple birth. Retrieved from http://sogc.org/publications/multiple-birth/

Venes, D. (Ed.). (2013). *Taber's cyclopedic medical dictionary* (22nd ed.). Philadelphia, PA: F.A. Davis.

Weselak, M., Arbuckle, T. E., Wigle, D. T., & Krewski, D. (2007). In utero pesticide exposure and childhood morbidity. *Environmental Research, 103*(1), 79–86.

Woodruff, T., Carlson, A., Schwartz, J., & Giudice, L. (2008). Proceedings of the summit on environmental challenges to reproductive health and fertility: Executive summary. *Fertility and Sterility, 89*(Suppl. 1), e1–e20.

Woodruff, T. J., Zota, A. R., & Schwartz, J. M. (2011). Environmental chemicals in pregnant women in the United States: NHANES 2003-2004. *Environmental Health Perspectives, 119*(6), 878–885. doi:10.1289/ehp.1002727

Zahm, S. H., & Ward, M. H. (1998). Pesticides and childhood cancer. *Environmental Health Perspectives, 106*(Suppl. 3), 893–908.

Zhu, H., & Finnell, R. H. (2010). Update on gene-environment interactions and birth defects. *The Female Patient, 35*(4), 27–30.

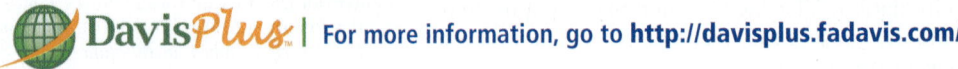

DavisPlus | For more information, go to **http://davisplus.fadavis.com/**

CONCEPT MAP

Conception and Development of the Embryo/Fetus

Factors Affecting Fetal/Embryonic Development:
- Damage to parental chromosomes
  - Advanced maternal age
  - Inheriting defective genes
- Teratogens used during organogenesis
  - Alcohol, nicotine
  - Caffeine
  - Medications/herbal supplements
  - Environmental pollutants
    - Radiation
    - Lead
    - Pesticides
  - "Street drugs"→ cocaine/crack, marijuana, opiates
- Infections
  - TORCH: toxoplasmosis, "other" infections, rubella, CMV, HSV

Potential for Inheriting a Disorder:
- Multifactorial
  - Cleft lip, cleft palate, neural tube defects, pyloric stenosis, and congenital heart disease
- Unifactorial
  - Autosomal dominant
  - Autosomal recessive
  - X-linked dominant
  - X-linked recessive

Fertilization:
- Meeting of oocyte and sperm in ampulla of fallopian tube
  - →Capacitation
  - →Acrosome reaction
  - →Zona pellucida penetration
- Zygote formation
- Potential for multifetal pregnancy

Conception

Pre-embryonic Period:
- First 2 weeks after conception
- Rapid cellular multiplication

Development:
- Cephalocaudal
- Proximal to distal
- General to specific

Implantation:
- Morula enters uterus→ blastocyst
  - Embryoblast = embryo
  - Trophoblast = placenta
- Nidation
- Formation of:
  - Chorionic villi; intervillous spaces
  - Embryonic membranes: amnion; chorion
  - Amniotic fluid

Embryonic Period:
- 3rd week after conception → end of 8th week
  - Blastogenesis
  - Development of neuro/CV systems
  - All major internal/ external structures

Nurse's Role: Minimizing Threats
- Preconception counseling
- Assessment → environmental risks, patient's knowledge, physical/psychosocial well-being
- Newborn screening→disease, genetic conditions

Cultural Diversity:
- Caring/acceptance results from knowledge about cultural practices/beliefs
- ACOG recommends CF screening offered to all pregnant women

Placental Development:
- Oxygenation
- Nutrition
- Waste elimination
- Hormone production

The Fetal Period: 9th to 40th Week
- 9–16 weeks: recognizable face; increasing body growth; ossification centers appear; distinguishable external genitalia; bones visible on ultrasound
- 17–20 weeks: quickening; vernix caseosa present; lanugo; SQ brown fat; formation of uterus/testes
- 21–25 weeks: weight gain; blood visible in capillaries; rapid eye movement; surfactant secreted
- 26–29 weeks: eyelids open; CNS regulates temp/directs breathing; may survive if born
- 30–40 weeks: pupillary light reflex; hand grasp reflex; oriented to light

Nursing Insight:
- Stage of development guides care/needs in premature infants
- Debate/ethics of using embryonic stem cells for research

Umbilical Cord Formation:
- Elongation of body stalk
- Development of 2 arteries; 1 vein from yolk sac vessels
- Wharton's jelly

Optimizing Outcomes:
- Educate re: environmental risks to childbearing women
- Use of folic acid to prevent neural tube defects
- Include father in education and support

Development of Fetal Circulation:
- Embryonic vessels → after 3rd week
- Beating heart and circulation end of 3rd week
- O_2 and nutrients from maternal blood

Unique features
- Bypasses liver and enters via ductus venosus
- Flows from right atrium to left atrium via foramen ovale
- Bypasses lungs entering aorta via ductus arteriosus

Leading Causes of Infant Death:
- Congenital anomalies: Malformation; disruption deformation; dysplasia
- Chromosomal abnormalities
  - Trisomy 13; 18

What to Say:
- Nonjudgmental and caring approach when congenital anomalies are identified
- Inquire re: substance use during prenatal interview

Across Care Settings:
- Any prenatal care setting; Education/active involvement → increases understanding and self-care

Now Can You:
- Discuss the characteristics of embryonic/fetal growth
- Identify the unique aspects of fetal circulation
- Identify the pattern of human development by periods
- Discuss substances that may adversely affect development

one
two
three
four
five
six
seven

The Prenatal Journey

Physiological and Psychosocial Changes During Pregnancy

Whether your pregnancy was meticulously planned, medically coaxed, or happened by surprise, one thing is certain—your life will never be the same.

—Catherine Jones

LEARNING TARGETS *At the completion of this chapter, the student will be able to:*

◆ Describe the physiological changes that occur during pregnancy and their etiologies.

◆ Identify nursing measures to relieve the discomforts caused by the physiological changes.

◆ Describe the psychosocial changes that occur during pregnancy and the factors that influence these changes.

◆ Identify nursing interventions to help families adapt to the psychosocial changes.

PICO(T) Questions

The intent of evidence-based practice (EBP) is to provide nursing care that integrates the best available evidence. An initial step in EBP is to write a PICO(T) question that effectively guides the research. A PICO(T) question is an acronym that stands for population (P), intervention or issue (I), comparison of interest (C), outcome (O), and timeframe (T). Depending on the question, all or some of the question components are used in the research process. Use these

PICO(T) questions to spark your thinking as you read the chapter.

1. Are (P) women's reported (I) levels of physical discomfort with pregnancy (O) changed by whether the pregnancy was planned (C) or unplanned?

2. Is there a (O) change (I) in the level or rate of acceptance of pregnancy by (P) men who are first time fathers (C) compared with men who have previously had children?

 Evidence-Based Practice

Tanninen, H., Haggman-Laitila, A., & Pietila, A. (2009). Resource-enhancing psychosocial support in family situations: Needs and benefits from family members' own perspectives. *Journal of Advanced Nursing, 65*(10), 2150–2160.

The purpose of this study was to examine a resource-enhancing family nursing intervention used to identify and meet mothers', fathers', and children's psychosocial support needs. The researchers contend that the need for psychosocial support is increasing. Previous studies demonstrate a need to identify preventive and early psychosocial services that provide attention to family needs. Specifically, services are needed to provide attention to family situations and family centeredness and to enable family empowerment. The literature also contends that regardless of the development of supplementary services, families often believe that they are alone in their problems. Recent studies have demonstrated a shift in clinical nursing practice from a

defect-based to resource-enhanced perspective, which is supported by the authors of this research.

In this study, the McGill Model of Nursing served as the theoretical basis for the nursing intervention, which used strategies such as helping the families identify internal (e.g., family members) and external resources, developing additional resources, and providing feedback. Families were also assisted in mobilizing, using, and regulating the input of external resources. Resource-enhancing discussion took place during all family meetings. The family nurse also used video guidance, creation of a family tree, network collaboration with close relatives and authorities, observations, and parent-child group activities.

(continued)

Evidence-Based Practice (continued)

Participants included 75 family members from 30 different families with young children. The families included 30 children, 26 mothers, and 19 fathers. All families had either an expectant mother or at least one child under the age of 6. The average age of the mothers was 31.4 years (range 17 to 46), the average age of the fathers was 34.6 years (range 18 to 54), and the average age of the children was 4.1 (range 0 to 9 years). On average, the families consisted of 2.5 children, with a range of 1 to 5 children per family. Participants were referred to the family-centered nursing services by public health nurses, social workers, day-care centers, psychologists, and other families. All were clients of a family nurse who was educated as a family therapist and experienced in public health.

The purpose of the family-centered nursing services was to provide psychosocial support beyond that provided in a child health clinic setting, and this provided the definition for the early psychosocial support implemented in the study. Data, collected before and after the intervention, were obtained via the "Family Situation Barometer" (FSB), a 40-item Likert scale questionnaire. In the final analysis, the responses were combined into the following two categories indicative of the amount of support needed: 1—no need of support, and 2—need of support.

Descriptive statistics and nonparametric Wilcoxon tests were used to analyze the results. The needs of the families determined the frequency of the meeting with the family nurse and ranged from 3 to 58 times. The meetings generally took place in the families' homes (81% of the time) or in other social or health-related facilities (19%). The average number of meetings was 21 per family, and the families remained in the nurse–family relationship from 2.5 to 19 months (mean of 7.5 months).

Findings for each group were as follows:

Mothers

According to results from the pre-intervention questionnaire, 65% of the mothers indicated a need for mental health support to assist in coping with daily living and in reducing the use of intoxicants. Fifty-four percent of the mothers responded that support was needed for physical health, and 58% indicated a need for support with their emotional life. Specific kinds of support requested included self-esteem building and in expressing emotions. The mothers also requested guidance and support for parenting and child care (51%) as well with supporting social relationships (58%). Post-intervention needs for support requests were as follows: support for physical health 38%, mental health 29%, desire for support in social relationships 27%, parenting and child care support 26%, and in finding outside interests 27%. The overall decrease in needs for support was found to be statistically significant for parenting and child care, mental health, emotional life, social relations, physical health, and outside interests.

Fathers

Findings from the pre-intervention questionnaire indicated that 68% of fathers expressed the need for support for mental health and in reducing the use of intoxicants, 50% for emotional life, 42% for dealing with employment situations, 37% for supporting physical health, 28% for parenting and child care needs, 26% for social relationships, and 26% for outside interests. Post-intervention results indicated that 37% of the fathers still needed support for emotional life and 34% continued to need mental health support. The decrease in need for support was statistically significant for parenting and child care, mental health, social relations, and employment needs.

Children

Pre-intervention needs for children included mental health support (87%), behavioral support (60%), sleep-related support (57%), eating issues–related support (30%), physical health support (30%), day care support (27%), and school attendance (27%). Post-intervention results were as follows: 43% continued to need additional support for issues related to behavior and mental health, 30% continued to need support for eating and sleep-related issues, and 27% continued to need support for developmental issues. The researchers found that the decrease in needed support was highly significant for social relationships, mental health, issues related to school attendance, day care, sleep, behavior, and physical health.

Families

Overall pre-intervention support needs for families included the following: 72% requested strengthening parental relationships, 51% requested support in managing daily affairs, 42% requested a need for support in parenting and child care, 33% needed support for family social relationships, 32% needed support for housing issues, and 32% needed support for financial situations. Post-intervention results indicated the following: most parents did not request any additional support with two exceptions: forty-five percent requested support for managing daily affairs, and 41% needed support for financial situations. The overall decrease in support was statistically significant for parents' relationships, parenting and child care, social relations, and family housing situations.

Based on the study findings, the researchers concluded that participant need for psychosocial support was reduced or eliminated entirely during the family nursing intervention. Parental mental health, marital relationships, and emotional lives were improved. In addition, it was noted that social support networks increased as did the participants' employment situations. The mental health and sleep-related issues initially noted in the children also demonstrated positive changes. The researchers concluded that the resource-enhancing family nursing intervention was beneficial to the health and well-being of the families.

1. How is this information useful to clinical nursing practice?

2. Based on these findings, what are implications for further research?

See Suggested Responses for Evidence-Based Practice on *DavisPlus*.

Introduction

From the time just before conception, and then for the following 10 lunar months, a woman's body undergoes many complex alterations that prepare her to nurture a new life. The physical, psychological, and emotional changes that accompany pregnancy are all focused on the growth, development, and future envelopment of the baby into a new family. The beginning of a new life is a time of awe and amazement shaped by a myriad of events that bring about unique changes for the woman and her family.

This chapter explores the physiological and psychosocial changes that occur during pregnancy and their effects on the woman, the fetus, and her family.

Physiological Preparation for Pregnancy

HORMONAL INFLUENCES

Many hormones are responsible for the changes that take place during and beyond pregnancy. Each serves a specific function in the nurturing process for the embryo, fetus, and neonate. The pituitary gland secretes hormones that influence ovarian follicular development, prompt ovulation, and stimulate the uterine lining to prepare for pregnancy and maintain it until the placenta becomes fully functional. Other pituitary hormones alter metabolism, stimulate lactation, produce pigmentation changes in the skin, stimulate uterine muscle contractions, prompt milk ejection from the breasts, allow for vasoconstriction to maintain blood pressure, and regulate water balance.

After conception, ovulation ceases. The corpus luteum produces progesterone and, to a lesser degree, estrogen. Progesterone is the hormone primarily responsible for maintaining the pregnancy. Once implantation occurs, the trophoblast secretes human chorionic gonadotrophin (hCG) to prompt the corpus luteum to continue progesterone production until this function is taken over by the placenta. The ovarian hormones work in synchrony to maintain the endometrium, provide nutrition for the developing morula and blastocyst, aid in implantation, decrease the contractility of the uterus to prevent spontaneous abortion, initiate development of the ductal system in the breasts, and prompt remodeling of maternal joint collagen.

The placenta provides hormones essential to the survival of the pregnancy and fetus. Placental hormones do the following:

- Prevent the normal involution of the ovarian corpus luteum
- Stimulate production of testosterone in the male fetus
- Protect the pregnancy from the maternal immune response
- Ensure that added glucose, protein, and minerals are available for the fetus
- Prompt proliferation of the uterus and breast glandular tissue
- Promote relaxation of the woman's smooth muscle
- Create a loosening of the pelvis and other major joints

Each of these hormones plays a vital role in the maintenance of the pregnancy, and all body systems are affected by the profound changes that prepare the woman to nurture the growing fetus and neonate.

The Major Pregnancy Hormones and Their Effects on the Reproductive System

Estrogen and progesterone are the major hormones produced by the placenta during pregnancy. The effect of estrogen is one of "growth"; the effect of progesterone is one of "maintenance."

Estrogen prompts hyperplasia and hypertrophy (growth of cells in number and size) during pregnancy. Because of the effects of estrogen, breast tissue enlarges and becomes functional and the uterus expands, a process that allows for stretching of the muscles to accommodate the growing fetus. Estrogen also enhances uterine contractility to prepare the muscles for labor.

Progesterone enables the pregnancy to thrive by its relaxation effect on the smooth muscle. Progesterone causes vasodilation and an increased blood flow to all body tissues, it slows the gastrointestinal tract to ensure absorption of essential nutrients for fetal development, and it relaxes the uterine muscle to prevent the onset of labor until term. Progesterone has been called the "pro-pregnancy hormone" (Fig. 8-1). ◆

REPRODUCTIVE SYSTEM

The reproductive system undergoes the greatest changes in size and function, and every organ within this system is affected by or focused on the needs of the growing fetus.

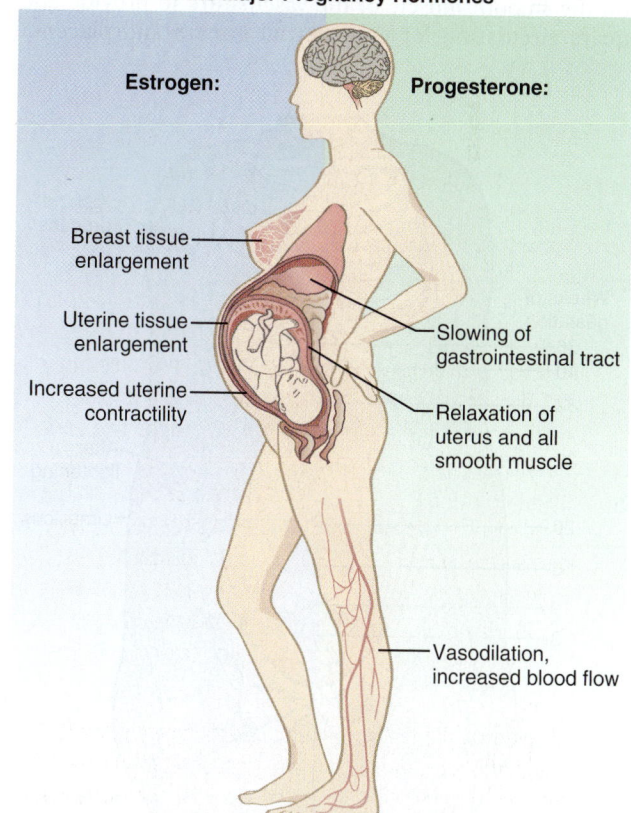

Reproductive System Effects of the Major Pregnancy Hormones

Estrogen:
- Breast tissue enlargement
- Uterine tissue enlargement
- Increased uterine contractility

Progesterone:
- Slowing of gastrointestinal tract
- Relaxation of uterus and all smooth muscle
- Vasodilation, increased blood flow

Figure 8-1 Reproductive system effects of the major pregnancy hormones.

Uterus

The uterus provides a home for the growing fetus for its 10-lunar-month stay in the woman. Its pattern of growth is very predictable for the first 20 weeks of the pregnancy. Depending on fetal size, uterine growth over the next 20 weeks varies. The shape of the uterus changes dramatically. Very early in pregnancy, the uterus is shaped like a "lightbulb" or inverted pear. By the end of the first trimester, the uterus has developed into a soft, enlarged globular structure that has risen out of the pelvis and into the abdominal cavity (Fig. 8-2). Under the influence of estrogen and progesterone, the myometrial cells and muscle fibers undergo hyperplasia and hypertrophy, processes that allow the uterus to enlarge and stretch as the fetus grows. By term, the uterine wall thins to 0.6 inch (1.5 cm) or less, and its weight will have increased from 1.8 oz to 2.2 lb (70 g to 1,100 g).

Estrogen causes the uterine muscles to contract. Braxton-Hicks contractions are irregular and painless and may begin as early as the 16th week of gestation. As the pregnancy advances and the fetal size increases, the contractions become increasingly more frequent and intense and are easily felt by the woman. Until late in the second trimester, the contractions serve to prepare the uterine muscles for the synchronized activity necessary for effective labor. As long as the contractions are irregular in frequency and last for less than 60 seconds, the patient may be reassured of their normalcy. However, if a pattern of contraction regularity is noted or if the contractions are associated with bleeding, nausea, vomiting, or intense pain, the patient should be instructed to promptly report to her health-care provider for evaluation.

Blood flow is increased from the effects of progesterone on the smooth muscle of the vasculature to provide adequate circulation for endometrial growth and placental function. The enhanced uterine circulation is important for ensuring adequate fetal nutrition and the removal of waste products.

After implantation, the endometrium lining the uterus is termed the **decidua.** The decidua consists of three layers:

> **Decidua vera** is the external layer, and it has no contact with the fetus.
> **Decidua basalis** is the uterine lining beneath the site of implantation.
> **Decidua capsularis** is the endometrial tissue that covers the embryo (Fig. 8-3).

Cervix

One of the earliest signs of pregnancy is the discoloration, or bluish purple hue, that appears on the cervix, vagina, and vulva. This color change is known as **Chadwick's sign** (Fig. 8-4). High levels of circulating estrogen cause stimulation of the cervical glandular tissue, which increases in cell number and becomes hyperactive. Increased blood flow and engorgement produces the bluish discoloration.

Stimulation from the hormones estrogen and progesterone produces cervical softening **(Goodell's sign)**. This physiological change is related to several events, including a decrease in the collagen fibers of the connective tissue,

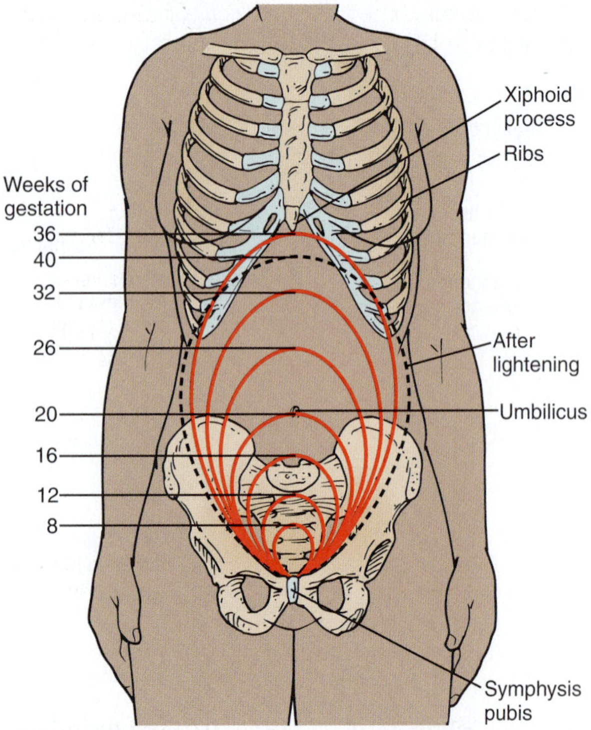

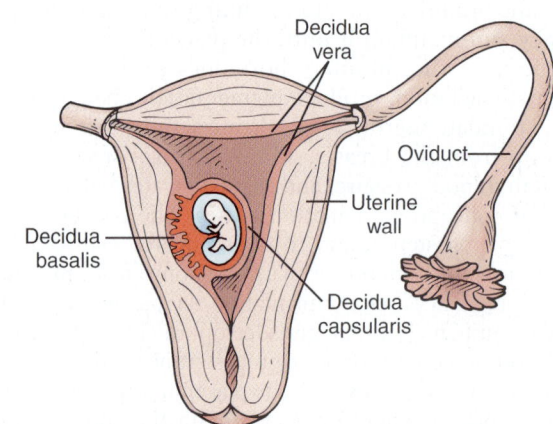

Figure 8-3 The layers of the decidua.

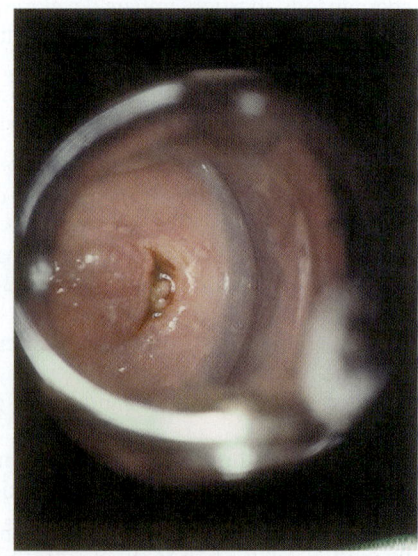

Figure 8-4 Chadwick's sign.

Figure 8-2 Pattern of uterine growth during pregnancy.

increased vascularity and edema, and slight tissue hypertrophy and hyperplasia. Before pregnancy, the cervix is firm and its texture resembles that of the tip of the nose. After conception, the cervix softens and its texture begins to resemble that of an ear lobe.

Estrogen and progesterone cause a proliferation of the mucus-producing cervical glands. Early in pregnancy, the endocervical tissue begins to take on a honeycomb appearance. Cervical mucus fills the endocervical canal and forms a mucus plug (**operculum**), which helps to keep harmful agents out of the uterus. **Leukorrhea,** an increased whitish vaginal discharge, results from hyperplasia of the vaginal mucosa and increased mucus production from the endocervical glands. The discharge is often profuse and may be worrisome. As the due date approaches, cervical effacement and dilation cause a breakdown of the mucus plug, resulting in an increased vaginal discharge. The nurse should reassure the patient about the normalcy of leukorrhea during pregnancy and instruct her to call her health-care provider if the discharge appears thicker; becomes bloody or yellowish/green; is accompanied by a foul odor; or if it causes itching, irritation, or pain in the vulvar or vaginal area.

Vagina and Vulva

Changes that occur in the vagina and vulva are similar to those that take place in the cervix. An increased blood flow (hyperemia) produces a bluish-purple hue (Chadwick's sign). Thickening of the vaginal mucosa develops, and the rugae (vaginal folds) become more prominent. The rugae deepen from hyperplasia and hypertrophy of the epithelial and elastic tissues, and this change allows for adequate stretching of the vaginal vault during childbirth. As the pregnancy progresses, the area becomes edematous from poor venous return caused by the weight of the gravid uterus. For some women, the increased pelvic congestion can lead to a heightened sexual interest and increased orgasmic experience. Leukorrhea results from increased cervical mucus along with elevated glycogen levels in the vaginal cells, which produces rapid sloughing of tissue. The increased glycogen levels also create a vaginal environment more susceptible to the growth of *Candida albicans*. Thus, during pregnancy the woman is more susceptible to the development of monilial vaginitis (yeast infections). The pH of the vaginal fluids becomes more acidic and decreases from 6.0 to 3.5. This change results from the action of *Lactobacillus acidophilus* on the increased glycogen levels in the vaginal epithelium (Cunningham, Leveno, Bloom, Spong, Dashe, & Hoffman et al., 2014). The increased acidity helps to control the growth of most pathogens in the vaginal canal.

The nurse should discuss the importance of vulvar hygiene with the patient. Gentle external cleansing with plain soap and water is adequate. Douching, or internal cleansing of the vagina, should be avoided because this practice can alter the vaginal pH and allow pathogens to grow as well as disrupt the cervical mucus plug.

Ovaries

After ovulation, the pituitary hormone luteinizing hormone (LH) stimulates the corpus luteum (functional cyst that remains on the ovary) to produce progesterone for 6 to 7 weeks. Once the placenta is developed and functional, it begins to take over the task of progesterone production. At that time, the corpus luteum ceases to function and is gradually absorbed by the ovary. The corpus luteal cyst enlarges while functioning and may reach the size of a golf ball before it begins to recede. In some cases the cyst may rupture, causing the woman some pelvic discomfort associated with bleeding into the pelvic cavity. The pain should dissipate as the cyst and blood are absorbed. If the pain is persistent or if vaginal bleeding occurs, the nurse should advise the woman to seek medical care. Ovulation ceases during pregnancy because of the high circulating levels of estrogen and progesterone, which inhibit the pituitary release of follicle-stimulating hormone (FSH) and LH.

Breasts

Estrogen and progesterone produce a number of changes in the mammary glands. Breast enlargement, fullness, tingling, and increased sensitivity occur during the early weeks of gestation. The superficial veins become more prominent from the vascular relaxation effects of progesterone. Often the venous congestion is more noticeable in primigravidas. Melanotropin, a hormone secreted by the pituitary gland, causes the nipples to become tender and more pronounced with darkening of the areola. The **Montgomery tubercles** (sebaceous glands) on and around the areola enlarge and provide lubrication for the nipple tissue. **Striae gravidarum** (stretch marks) may develop as the breast tissue stretches (Fig. 8-5).

During the second trimester, pre-colostrum, a clear thin fluid, is found in the acini cells, the smallest parts of the milk glands. Pre-colostrum becomes **colostrum,** a creamy whitish-yellow liquid that may leak from the nipples as early as the 16th week of gestation. This pre-milk substance contains antibodies, essential proteins, and fat to nourish the baby and prepare his intestines for digestion and elimination. Colostrum is converted to mature milk during the first few days after birth.

During prenatal care, the nurse should discuss the need for changes in bra size, options for infant feeding, and if

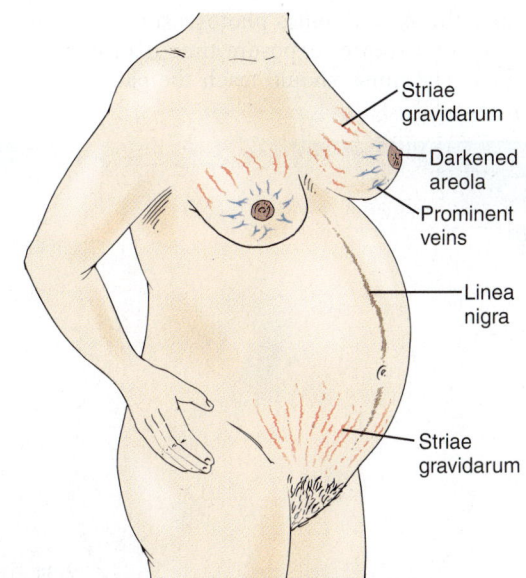

Figure 8-5 Integumentary system changes include darkening of the areolae and appearance of the linea nigra and striae gravidarum.

the patient wishes to breastfeed, strategies to help her prepare for successful breastfeeding. The process of lactation should be reviewed, and the woman should be given a list of lactation support resources. Soft cotton liners can be used to pad the bra if leaking of the nipples is troublesome.

 Now Can You—Describe major changes that occur in the reproductive system during pregnancy?

1. Identify four physiological changes that occur in the uterus and possible symptoms that may accompany these changes?
2. Explain the hormonal basis for changes in the vagina and vulva and identify patient teaching needs concerning the changes?
3. Describe three breast changes and identify the hormones responsible for the changes?

INTEGUMENTARY SYSTEM

Estrogen, progesterone, and alpha-melanocyte-stimulating hormones cause many changes in the appearance, structure, and function of the integumentary system. Though seldom serious, the outward changes in appearance may negatively affect the woman's self-concept and body image.

The skin undergoes a number of pigmentation changes related to the influence of estrogen. Moles (nevi), freckles, and recent scars may darken or appear to multiply in number. The nipples, areolae, axillae, vulvar area, and perineum also darken in color.

The linea alba, a light line that extends from the umbilicus to the mons pubis (and sometimes upward to the xiphoid process), darkens, becoming the **linea nigra** (Fig. 8-6). The linea is more noticeable in the woman with a naturally darker complexion. Melasma gravidarum, also known as **chloasma,** forms the "mask of pregnancy" (Fig. 8-7). This dark, blotchy brownish pigmentation change occurs around the hairline, brow, nose, and cheeks and often gives the appearance of "raccoon eyes." The heightened pigmentation fades after pregnancy but can recur after exposure to the sun. During pregnancy the skin becomes photosensitive, and sunburn may occur in a shorter exposure time than usual for the individual. The nurse should teach the patient about the

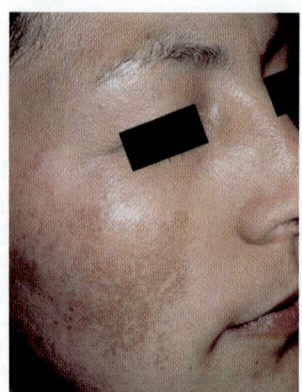

Figure 8-7 Chloasma.

importance of regular sunscreen use and decreased sun exposure time.

Alterations in hair as well as nail growth and texture may occur. The nails may become stronger and grow faster. The number of hair follicles in the dormant phase may decrease, and this change stimulates new hair growth. Once the infant is born, this process is reversed, and there is an increase in hair shedding for approximately 1 to 4 months. Although this change may be disconcerting, the nurse can reassure the patient that virtually all hair will be replaced within 6 to 12 months (Cunningham et al., 2014). During pregnancy, hair may react differently to dyes and chemicals.

Increased adrenal steroid levels cause the connective tissue to lose strength and become more fragile. This change can cause striae gravidarum, or "stretch marks," on the breasts, buttocks, thighs, and abdomen (Fig. 8-8). Striae appear as reddish, wavy, depressed streaks that will fade to a silvery white color after birth, but they do not usually disappear completely.

Increased levels of estrogen during pregnancy may cause **angiomas** and **palmar erythema.** Angiomas, also called "vascular spiders," are tiny, bluish, end-arterioles that occur on the neck, thorax, face, and arms. They may appear as star-shaped or branched structures that are slightly raised and do not blanch with pressure. More common in Caucasian women, angiomas appear most often during the

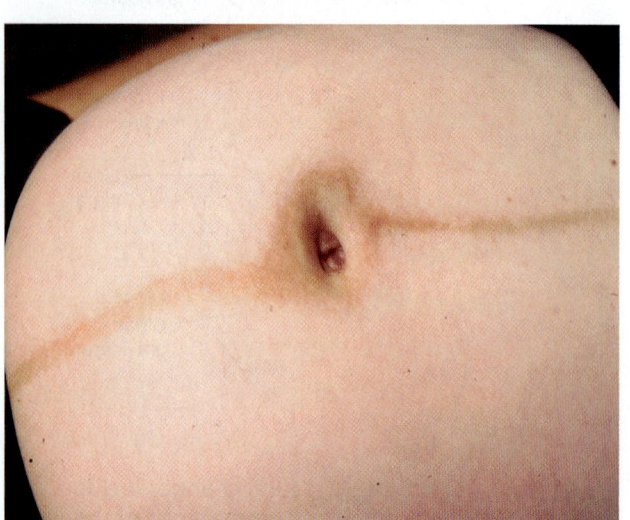

Figure 8-6 Pregnant abdomen with linea nigra.

 Where Research and Practice Meet:
Presence of Striae Gravidarum and Prediction of Perineal Trauma During Childbirth

The presence of striae gravidarum (SG), a common skin change during pregnancy, may be an indicator of poor skin elasticity. Investigating the hypothesis that women with more stretch marks would be more likely to experience perineal tissue tears (than women without SG) during vaginal childbirth, Halperin and colleagues (2010) used a previously developed numerical scoring system to determine an SG score for 385 antepartal women. The women were then examined for perineal tissue trauma 1 to 2 days after childbirth. Findings revealed that striae scores could be used as a predictor for perineal trauma during childbirth. The investigators recommended that striae scoring become a routine component of the obstetric assessment and suggested that further research be conducted to explore strategies such as perineal massage to reduce the incidence of perineal trauma in women with high antepartal SG scores.

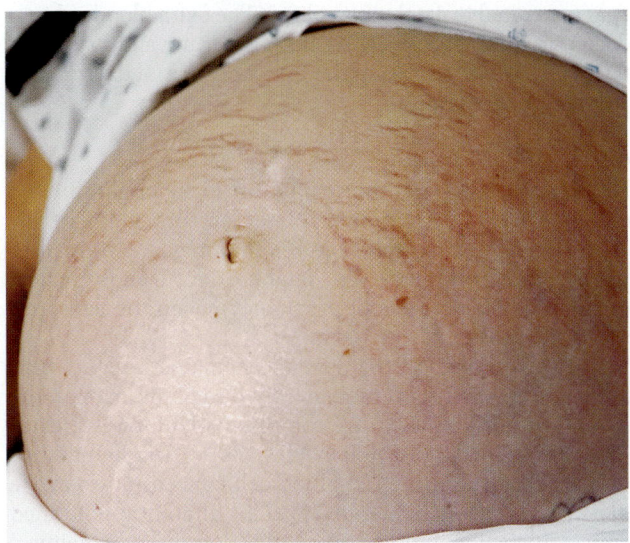

Figure 8-8 Pregnant abdomen with striae gravidarum.

second to fifth month of pregnancy and usually disappear after birth. Palmar erythema is a condition characterized by color changes over the palmar surfaces of the hands (Fig. 8-9). Approximately 60% of Caucasian women and 35% of African American women experience palmar erythema during pregnancy, which presents as a diffuse, reddish-pink mottling of the palms. Increased blood flow, along with high levels of circulating hormones, can produce other skin changes such as inflammatory pruritus and acne vulgaris, a condition seen predominately in the first trimester. Hyperactivity of the sweat and sebaceous glands may cause some women to experience excessive perspiration, night sweats, and skin changes that can range from extreme dryness to extreme oiliness.

The nurse should offer reassurance and provide anticipatory guidance as these changes occur. Recommendations to the patient include daily bathing, the liberal use of lotions or oils for dry skin, the regular use of deodorant, and limited sun exposure with the diligent use of sunscreen.

NEUROLOGICAL SYSTEM

The central nervous system appears to be affected by the hormonal changes of pregnancy, although the specific alterations other than those involving the hypothalamic–pituitary axis are less well known. Many women complain of a decreased attention span, poor concentration, and memory lapses during and shortly after pregnancy. Cunningham and colleagues (2014) identified a pregnancy

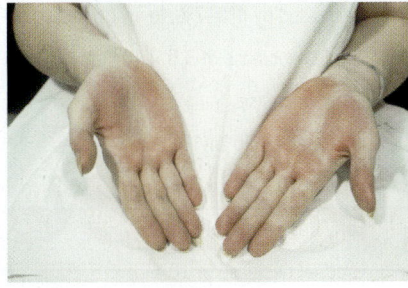

Figure 8-9 Palmar erythema.

sleep pattern phenomenon characterized by reduced sleep efficiency, fewer hours of night sleep, frequent awakenings, and difficulty going to sleep. Nurses can advise patients that afternoon napping may help alleviate the fatigue associated with the sleep alterations. Providing anticipatory guidance related to expected alterations is key in facilitating the woman's acceptance of these changes.

Edema from vascular permeability can lead to a collection of fluid in the wrist that puts pressure on the median nerve lying beneath the carpal ligament. This alteration leads to **carpal tunnel syndrome,** a condition that usually develops during the third trimester. It is manifested by pain and paresthesia (a burning, tingling, or numb sensation) in the hand that radiates to the elbow. The pain occurs in one (usually the dominant) or both hands and is intensified with attempts to grasp objects. Elevation of the hands at night may help to reduce the edema. Occasionally, a woman may need to wear a "cock-up splint" to prevent the wrist from flexing, an action that puts additional pressure on the median nerve. Carpal tunnel syndrome usually subsides after the pregnancy (and the accompanying edema) has ended although some women may require surgical treatment if symptoms persist.

Syncope (a transient loss of consciousness and postural tone with spontaneous recovery) during pregnancy is frequently attributed to orthostatic hypotension and/or inferior vena cava compression by the gravid uterus (Cunningham et al., 2014). It may also occur as increased intra-abdominal pressure from the growing uterus places pressure on the vagus nerve. Coughing, straining during bowel movements, and upward pressure from the growing fetus can trigger a vasovagal response that produces faintness or loss of consciousness. Light-headedness, sweating, nausea, yawning, and feelings of warmth are warning signs that often precede syncope. Educating the patient about signs and symptoms often helps to alleviate the fears that frequently accompany the fainting episodes. If light-headedness or other warning signs are experienced, the woman is instructed to immediately assume a sitting or lying position. A left side-lying position is preferred to avoid compression of the vena cava (which can lead to supine hypotension) from the gravid uterus.

 Now Can You—Discuss changes in the integumentary and neurological systems?

1. Identify four changes that occur in the integumentary system and discuss patient teaching needs for these changes?
2. Define carpal tunnel syndrome and identify two interventions to help alleviate the associated symptoms?
3. Discuss the physiological origins of syncope during pregnancy and patient education concerning syncope?

CARDIOVASCULAR SYSTEM

Heart

As growth of the fetus exerts pressure on the diaphragm, the maternal heart is pushed upward and laterally to the left (Fig. 8-10). Cardiac hypertrophy results from the increased blood volume and cardiac output. Exaggerated first and third heart sounds and systolic murmurs are common findings during pregnancy. The murmurs are usually asymptomatic and require no treatment. If symptomatic, the

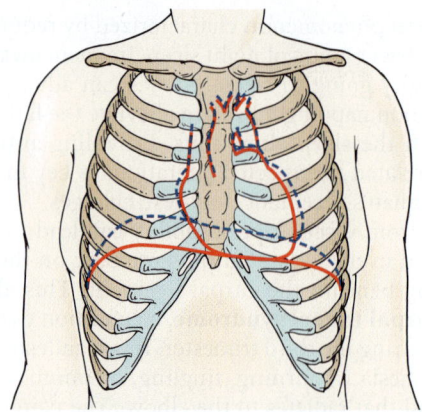

Figure 8-10 Growth of the uterus displaces the maternal heart upward and laterally to the left.

woman may experience palpitations, chest pain, shortness of breath, or a decreased tolerance to activity. The nurse should advise the patient that if these symptoms occur, she should see her health-care provider immediately for evaluation. Systolic murmurs usually resolve within the first 2 weeks postpartum after the plasma volume levels return to normal. They may recur in subsequent pregnancies.

Blood Volume

An increase in maternal blood volume begins during the first trimester and peaks at term. The increase approaches 40% to 50% and is due primarily to an increase in plasma and erythrocyte volume. Additional erythrocytes, needed because of the extra oxygen requirements of the maternal and placental tissue, ensure an adequate supply of oxygen to the fetus. The elevation in erythrocyte volume remains constant during pregnancy.

Most of the increased blood flow is directed to the uterus, and of this amount, 80% is channeled to the placenta. Blood flow to the maternal kidneys is increased by 30% to 50%, and this alteration enhances the excretion of maternal and fetal wastes. Dilation of the capillaries and increased blood flow to the skin assist the woman in eliminating the extra heat generated by fetal metabolism. The extra blood volume decreases during the first 2 weeks postpartum and a substantial amount of fluid loss in the first 3 postpartal days occurs through maternal diuresis.

Iron

Iron is necessary for the formation of hemoglobin, the oxygen-carrying component of the erythrocyte. The increased need for oxygen requires the pregnant woman to increase her iron intake. The fetal need for iron is greatest during the last 4 weeks of pregnancy, when the fetal iron stores are amassed.

During pregnancy, the woman's hematocrit values may appear low because of the increase in total plasma volume (on average, 50%). Because the plasma volume is greater than the increase in erythrocytes (30%), the hematocrit (a measurement of the red blood cell concentration in the plasma) decreases by about 7%. This alteration is termed "physiological anemia of pregnancy" or "pseudoanemia." The hemodilution effect is most apparent at 32 to 34 weeks. The mean acceptable hemoglobin level in pregnancy is 11 to 12 g/dL of blood. Some women experience symptoms of fatigue related to this phenomenon, although altered sleep patterns may also contribute to the fatigue. The nurse should teach the patient to hydrate adequately by drinking 6 to 8 glasses of water each day and also to ensure that her diet is high in protein and iron. Although gastrointestinal absorption of iron is enhanced during pregnancy, most women must add supplemental iron to meet the needs of the expanded erythrocytes and those of the growing fetus.

Leukocytes, Proteins, Platelets, Immunoglobulins

The number of leukocytes also increases, and the average white blood cell count ranges from 5,000 to 15,000/mm³. During labor and postpartum, these levels may climb as high as 25,000/mm³. Although the exact reason for this increase is unclear, it is known that leukocyte counts normally increase in response to stress and vigorous exercise (Cunningham et al., 2014). Normal laboratory values during pregnancy are presented in Table 8-1.

Table 8-1 Common Laboratory Values in Pregnancy

Laboratory Values	Usual Normal Female Value	Normal Value in Pregnancy
SERUM VALUES		
Hemoglobin	11.7–15.5 g/dL (mean Hgb is 0.5–1.0 g lower in African Americans, Mexican and Asian Americans have a higher hemoglobin and hematocrit than Caucasians)	Decreased by 1.5–2 g/dL Lowest point occurs at 30–34 weeks
Hematocrit	38%–44%	Decreased by 4%–7%, lowest point at 30–34 weeks
Leukocytes	$4.5–11.0 \times 10^3$/mm³	Gradual increase of 3.5×10^3/mm³
Platelets	$150–400 \times 10^3$/mm³	Slight decrease
Amylase	30–110 U/L	Increased by 50%–100%
CHEMISTRIES		
Albumin	3.4–4.8 g/dL	Early decrease by 1 g/dL
Calcium (total)	8.2–10.2 mg/dL	Gradual decrease of 10%

Table 8-1 Common Laboratory Values in Pregnancy (continued)

Laboratory Values	Usual Normal Female Value	Normal Value in Pregnancy
Chloride	97–107 mEq/L	No significant change
Creatinine	0.5–1.1 mg/dL	Early decrease by 0.3 mg/dL
Fibrinogen	200–400 mg/dL	Progressive increase of 1–2 g/L
Glucose (fasting)	65–99 mg/dL	Gradual decrease of 10%
Potassium	3.5–5.0 mEq/L	Gradual decrease of 0.2–0.3 mEq/L
Protein (total)	6.0–8.0 g/dL	Early decrease of 1 g/dL, then stable
Sodium	135–145 mEq/L	Early decrease of 2–4 mEq/L, then stable
Urea nitrogen	8–20 mg/dL	Decrease in first trimester by 50%
Uric acid	2.3–6.6 mg/dL	First trimester decrease of 33%, rise at term
URINE CHEMISTRIES		
Creatinine	11–20 mg/kg per 24 hr	No significant change
Protein	10–140 mg per 24 hr	Up by 250–300 mg/day by the 20th week
Creatinine clearance	75–115 mL/min/1.73 m2	Increased by 40%–50% by the 16th week
SERUM HORMONES		
Cortisol	8–21 g/dL	Increased by 20 g/dL
Prolactin	3.3–26.7 ng/mL	Gradual increase, 5.3–215.3 ng/mL, peaks at term
Thyroxine (T_4) total	5.5–11.0 mcg/dL	5.5–16.0 mcg/dL
Triiodothyronine (T_3) total	70–204 ng/dL	Early sustained increase of up to 50%
		116–247 ng/dL (last 4 months of gestation)

Sources: Adapted from Chapman, L., & Durham, R. (2013). *Maternal-Newborn nursing: The critical components of nursing care.* (2nd ed.). Philadelphia, PA: F.A. Davis; Van Leeuwen, A. M., Poelhuis-Leth, D., & Bladh, M. L. (2011). *Davis's comprehensive handbook of laboratory and diagnostic tests with nursing implications* (4th ed.). Philadelphia, PA: F.A. Davis.

Plasma proteins also increase, although because of the hemodilution effect during pregnancy, there is a decrease in protein concentrations, especially in the level of albumins. Decreased plasma albumin leads to a drop in osmotic pressure, which causes body fluids to move into the second space. This change produces edema.

Although the platelet cell count does not change significantly, fibrinogen volume has been shown to increase by as much as 50%. This alteration leads to an increase in the sedimentation rate. Blood factors VII, VIII, IX, and X are also increased, and this change causes hypercoagulability. The hypercoagulable state, coupled with venous stasis (poor blood return from the lower extremities), places the pregnant woman at an increased risk for venous thrombosis, embolism, and when complications are present, disseminated intravascular coagulation (DIC). (See Chapter 11 for further discussion.)

The production of maternal immunoglobulins (IgA, IgG, IgM, IgD, and IgE) is unchanged in pregnancy. Immunoglobulins protect the body from a variety of bacterial, viral, and parasitic infections. Three major types of immunoglobulins (IgG, IgA, and IgM) are primarily involved in immunity. Circulating levels of maternal IgG are decreased during pregnancy because of transfer across the placenta. As the only immunoglobulin transported across the placenta, IgG is active against bacterial toxins (Beckmann, Herbert, Laube, Ling, & Smith, 2013). Although transport of IgG begins around the 16th week of gestation, the fetus does not acquire a significant amount of IgG until the last 4 weeks of pregnancy. At birth, the neonate's primary immunoglobulins (IgG) have been acquired from the mother via a process termed "passive acquired immunity" (Cunningham et al., 2014). Because of its large molecular size, IgM is unable to cross the placenta. IgA, IgD, and IgE also remain in the maternal circulation. IgA, which is believed to provide protection to various secreting surfaces such as those in the respiratory tract, gastrointestinal tract, and eyes, is passed to the neonate in breast milk (Williams & Hopper, 2011). Immunoglobulins and their major actions are summarized in Table 8-2.

During pregnancy, resistance to infection is decreased as a result of depressed leukocyte function. Because of this normal physiological alteration, maternal autoimmune diseases such as lupus erythematosus may improve during pregnancy. (See Chapter 11 for further discussion.) Because of the increased susceptibility to infection, patients should be instructed to avoid crowds and individuals with active infections. Frequent, consistent hand washing and good respiratory hygiene should also be stressed.

Table 8-2 Immunoglobulins and Their Major Actions	
IgG_(75% of Total Immunoglobulin)	Appears in serum and tissues (interstitial fluid). Assumes major role in blood-borne and tissue infections. Activates the complement system. Enhances phagocytosis. Crosses the placenta.
IgA_(15% of Total Immunoglobulin)	Appears in body fluids (blood, saliva, tears, **breast milk,** and pulmonary, gastrointestinal, prostatic, and vaginal secretions). Protects against respiratory, gastrointestinal, and genitourinary infections. Prevents absorption of antigens from food. Is transferred to the neonate via breast milk.
IgM_(10% of Total Immunoglobulin)	Appears mostly in intravascular serum. Appears as the first immunoglobulin produced in response to bacterial and viral infections. Activates the complement system. No placental transfer during pregnancy.
IgD_(0.2% of Total Immunoglobulin)	Appears in small amounts in serum. Possibly influences B-lymphocyte differentiation, but its role is unclear.
IgE_(0.004% of Total Immunoglobulin)	Appears in serum. Involved in allergic and some hypersensitivity reactions. Combats parasitic infections.

Sources: Adapted from Smeltzer, S. C., Bare, B. G., Hinkle, J. L., & Cheever, K. H. (2012). *Brunner & Suddarth's textbook of medical-surgical nursing.* (12th ed.). Philadelphia, PA: Lippincott Williams & Wilkins; Van Leeuwen, A., Poelhuis-Leth, D., & Bladh, M. (2011). *Davis's comprehensive handbook of laboratory & diagnostic tests with nursing implications* (4th ed.). Philadelphia, PA: F.A. Davis.

Cardiac Output

Cardiac output increases and peaks around the 20th to 24th week of gestation at about 30% to 50% above pre-pregnancy levels. It remains increased for the duration of the pregnancy. With the increased vascular volume and cardiac output, vasodilation (related to progesterone-induced relaxation of the vascular smooth muscle) reduces blood pressure in the mid trimester. The woman's pulse rate frequently increases up to 10 to 15 beats per minute to facilitate effective circulation of the increased blood volume.

During the first trimester, blood pressure normally remains the same as pre-pregnancy levels but then gradually decreases up to around 20 weeks of gestation. After 20 weeks, the vascular volume expands and the blood pressure increases to reach pre-pregnancy levels by term. Because of the relaxed vascular resistance and stasis of blood in the lower extremities, there is an increased risk of varicose veins and hemorrhoids. The nurse should instruct the woman to elevate her lower extremities by lying on her left side with the feet higher than her heart for 15 to 20 minutes daily to improve venous return from the lower extremities. Daily walks enhance circulation and also improve intestinal peristalsis, important in facilitating regular bowel function. Patients should be advised to drink at least 8 to 10 glasses of water each day and include adequate roughage in their diet. These strategies help prevent constipation and straining with bowel movements, both of which increase the likelihood of hemorrhoids.

Supine Hypotension Syndrome

The pregnant woman may experience **supine hypotension syndrome,** or **vena caval syndrome** (faintness related to bradycardia) if she lies on her back. The pressure from the enlarged uterus exerted on the vena cava decreases the amount of venous return from the lower extremities and causes a marked decrease in blood pressure, with accompanying dizziness, diaphoresis, and pallor (Fig. 8-11). Placing the woman on her left side can relieve the symptoms. Orthostatic hypotension is another condition that occurs frequently during pregnancy and results from stagnation of blood in the lower extremities. If the woman stands for too long or arises too quickly, gravity causes the blood to flow to the lower extremities, decreasing blood flow to the brain. **Mean arterial pressure** (MAP) indicates the average

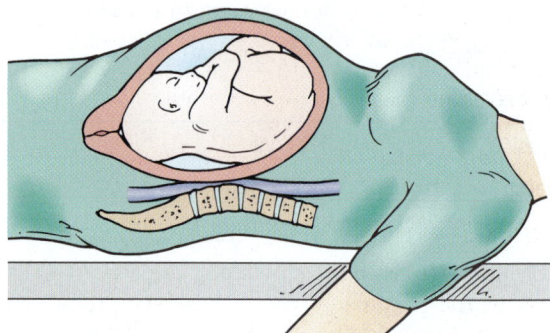

Figure 8-11 Supine hypotension, or vena caval syndrome, may occur if the pregnant woman lies on her back.

driving force for the movement of blood in the arterial system throughout the cardiac cycle (Oakes, 2010). The MAP is the same in all parts of the cardiovascular system when the patient is supine except during pregnancy, when the gravid uterus places pressure on the vena cava and produces an alteration in the blood pressure. The change in the MAP leads to decreased blood flow throughout the body, particularly in the heart, brain, and uterus.

All of the changes in the circulatory system return to normal by the second to third week postpartum as the woman's body returns to a nonpregnant state. Reassurance can be given to the patient, and she should be encouraged to arise slowly from a lying or sitting position. While standing, she should keep her feet moving to encourage adequate venous return from the lower extremities and avoid lying flat on her back.

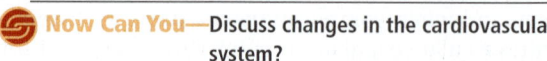

Now Can You—Discuss changes in the cardiovascular system?

1. Describe two changes in the heart and the physiological basis for these changes?
2. Discuss why there is a need for an increase in erythrocytes during pregnancy?
3. Explain what is meant by "passive acquired immunity"?
4. Differentiate between supine hypotension syndrome and orthostatic hypotension?

RESPIRATORY SYSTEM

During pregnancy, a number of changes occur to meet the woman's increased oxygen requirements. The tidal volume (amount of air breathed in each minute) increases 30% to 40%. This change is related to the elevated levels of estrogen and progesterone. Estrogen prompts hypertrophy and hyperplasia of the lung tissue. Progesterone decreases airway resistance by causing relaxation of the smooth muscle of the bronchi, bronchioles, and alveoli. These alterations produce an increase in oxygen consumption by approximately 15% to 20%, along with an increase in vital capacity (the maximum amount of air that can be moved in and out of the lungs with forced respiration).

The enlarging uterus creates an upward pressure that elevates the diaphragm and increases the subcostal angle. The chest circumference may increase by as much as 2.4 inches (6 cm). Although the "up and down" capacity of diaphragmatic movement is reduced (because of increasing pressure from the growing fetus), lateral movement of the chest and intercostal muscles accommodate for this loss of movement and keep pulmonary functions stable. Many women verbalize an increased awareness of the need to breathe and may perceive this sensation as dyspnea (difficulty breathing). The nurse should offer reassurance and educate the woman about normal alterations and symptoms. Under normal circumstances, resting with the head elevated while taking slow, deep breaths causes an improvement in the symptoms. However, certain lung diseases including asthma and emphysema may be aggravated by the normal physiological changes as the oxygen demands of the pregnancy increase. If symptoms persist or worsen, the woman should contact her health-care provider.

Eyes, Ears, Nose, and Throat

EYES. Blurred vision, the most common visual complaint in pregnant women, is caused by corneal thickening associated with fluid retention and decreased intraocular pressure. These changes begin during the first trimester, persist throughout pregnancy, and regress by 6 to 8 weeks postpartum. As part of anticipatory guidance, the nurse teaches that because the changes are only temporary, a corrective lens prescription should not be changed until the pregnancy has been completed.

EARS. No changes have been noted in auditory function during pregnancy.

NOSE. An increase in mucus production results from the combined effects of progesterone (increased blood flow to the mucus membranes of the sinus and nasal passages) and estrogen (hypertrophy and hyperplasia of the mucosa). Nasal stuffiness and congestion (rhinitis of pregnancy) are common complaints. The nurse should educate the patient about these normal changes and offer reassurance. Increasing the oral fluid intake helps to keep the mucus thin and easier to mobilize.

Edema (an effect of estrogen) of the nasal mucosa, along with vascular congestion (an effect of progesterone), may cause epistaxis (nosebleeds). The woman should be advised to use caution when blowing her nose and to avoid probing the nasal cavities with a cotton swab. The use of nasal sprays designed to relieve congestion should be avoided because of their rebound effect that causes the congestion to worsen.

Normal saline nasal sprays may be used sparingly to moisten the nasal passages.

THROAT. Hyperemia (congestion) occurs from increased blood flow and relaxation of smooth muscle. Swallowing may be difficult if food is not chewed well.

GASTROINTESTINAL SYSTEM

The gastrointestinal system is probably the source of most of the woman's discomforts during pregnancy. Nausea and vomiting during the first trimester most likely are related to rising levels of hCG and altered carbohydrate metabolism. Changes in taste and smell, because of alterations in the oral and nasal mucosa, can further aggravate the gastrointestinal discomfort. A nonspecific **gingivitis** (inflammation of the gums) occurs frequently because of the increased blood supply to the gums, along with estrogen-related tissue hypertrophy and edema. Although the gums may bleed from routine oral hygiene, the nurse should stress the importance of regular dental maintenance and its effect on good maternal nutrition.

On occasion, red, raised nodules **(epulis gravidarum)** appear at the gum line (Fig. 8-12). These growths bleed easily and usually regress within 2 months after childbirth (Beckmann et al., 2013). If associated with excessive bleeding, local excision may be necessary. **Ptyalism,** excessive saliva production often with a bitter taste, may occur and can be unpleasant or embarrassing. Its cause is uncertain, although stimulation of the salivary glands from eating starch or decreased unconscious swallowing when nauseated may be contributing factors (Cunningham et al., 2014). Limited relief can be obtained with the use of chewing gum and lozenges. Patients can also be advised to eat small, frequent meals and avoid starchy foods such as potatoes, bread, and pasta.

The effect of progesterone on smooth muscle causes relaxation of the esophagus. The movement of food is slowed and the gastroesophageal, or cardiac, sphincter (circular muscle located at the top of the stomach) weakens. This alteration prevents efficient closure when the stomach is emptying and allows the reflux of stomach contents into the esophagus, producing heartburn, or **pyrosis.** Pyrosis results from irritation to the esophageal lining by gastric secretions and acids. Eating small meals, avoiding lying down after meals for at least 1 hour, and limited use of antacids can alleviate some of these symptoms.

Nausea and vomiting of pregnancy, or "morning sickness," occurs because of high levels of hCG and relaxation of the stomach, esophagus, and gastroesophageal sphincters. Food remains in the stomach longer for enhanced digestion and moves more slowly through the small intestine to allow for complete absorption of nutrients. Because the

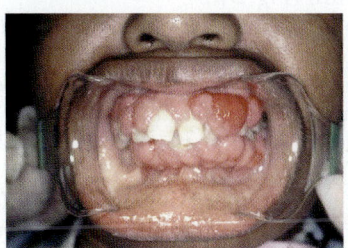

Figure 8-12 Gingival hypertrophy; epulis.

large intestine is also sluggish from the effects of progesterone on the smooth muscle, more water is reabsorbed from the bowel, and bloating and constipation can occur. Straining at defecation may cause or exacerbate hemorrhoids (vein varicosities in the lower rectum and anus).

Patients should be encouraged to drink at least 8 to 10 glasses of water each day, add fiber to their diets to produce bulk, and exercise to encourage peristalsis. They should be taught to avoid straining with bowel movements. Warm sitz baths may be helpful for hemorrhoid discomfort. (See Chapter 15 for further discussion.)

The liver, which breaks down maternal toxins, must deal with fetal waste products and toxins as well. The additional workload can lead to altered liver function tests, especially if accompanied by hepatic vessel vasoconstriction associated with preeclampsia. (See Chapter 11 for further discussion.)

The gallbladder, or storehouse for bile, is also composed of smooth muscle and becomes more relaxed, resulting in inefficient emptying. This alteration can lead to stasis of the bile (cholestasia) or inflammation and infection (cholecystitis). In addition, the progesterone-induced prolonged emptying time, combined with elevated blood cholesterol levels, may predispose the woman to gallstone formation (cholelithiasis). Pain in the epigastric region after ingestion of a high-fat meal is the major symptom of these conditions. The pain is self-limiting and usually resolves within 2 hours. Cholelithiasis occurs more often in obese individuals with fair skin and in women older than 40 years of age.

Liver functions are only slightly altered during pregnancy. Stasis of bile in the liver (intrahepatic cholestasis) occasionally occurs late in pregnancy and can cause severe itching (**pruritus gravidarum**). This condition disappears soon after birth. Patients should be advised that avoiding high-fat meals can reduce the presence or frequency of these symptoms.

URINARY SYSTEM

Pregnancy leads to changes in the structure and function of the urinary system. These changes facilitate normal waste elimination for the woman and the increasing waste products of her fetus. During the first trimester, the bladder, a pelvic organ, is compressed by the weight of the growing uterus. The added pressure, along with progesterone-induced relaxation of the urethra and sphincter musculature, leads to urinary urgency, frequency, and nocturia. In the second trimester, when the uterus becomes an abdominal organ, bladder pressure is largely relieved, along with most of the frequency and urgency. By the third trimester, the fetal presenting part descends into the pelvis. At this time, increased pressure is again exerted on the bladder, and symptoms of frequency, urgency, and nocturia return (Fig. 8-13).

Ascension of bacteria into the bladder can cause asymptomatic bacteriuria (ASB) or urinary tract infections (UTIs). These infections occur more frequently in pregnancy because of relaxation of the smooth muscle of the bladder and urinary sphincter, changes that allow bacterial ascent into the bladder.

The ureters, composed of smooth muscle, are also affected by progesterone. Elongation and dilation, especially of the right ureter, occurs. Peristalsis that normally facilitates

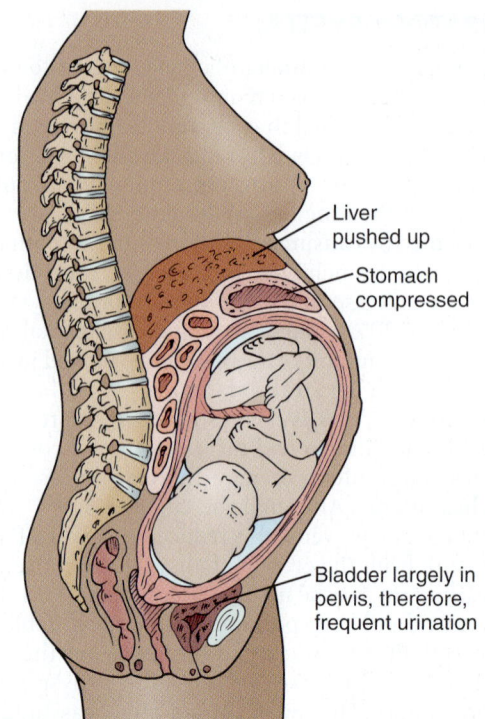

Liver pushed up

Stomach compressed

Bladder largely in pelvis, therefore, frequent urination

Figure 8-13 Compression of the bladder results from the growing uterus.

the movement of urine from the kidneys to the bladder is reduced. This change, coupled with pressure on the ureters from the enlarging uterus, causes an obstruction of urine flow. The stagnant urine becomes an excellent medium for the growth of microorganisms. Patients should be encouraged to drink at least 8 to 10 glasses of water each day and empty their bladders at least every 2 to 3 hours and immediately after intercourse. These measures help to prevent stasis of urine and the bacterial contamination that leads to infection.

The glomerular filtration rate (GFR) and renal plasma flow are increased because of hormonal changes, blood volume increases, the woman's posture, physical activity level, and nutritional intake. During the second trimester, the GFR increases up to 50% in most women. This alteration prompts an increase in renal tubular reabsorption. During pregnancy, there is a greatly increased load of glucose presented to the renal tubules. As a result, glucose excretion increases in virtually all pregnant women (Beckmann et al., 2013). Although it may be a normal finding, glucosuria should always be investigated to rule out gestational diabetes because the quantitative urine glucose does not accurately reflect blood glucose levels. (See Chapter 11 for further discussion.)

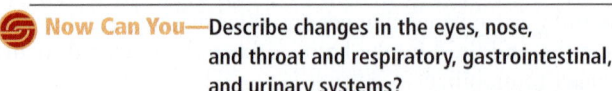 **Now Can You**—Describe changes in the eyes, nose, and throat and respiratory, gastrointestinal, and urinary systems?

1. Describe one alteration that occurs in each of the following: eyes, nose, throat and suggest interventions for relief from the accompanying symptoms?

2. Identify changes during pregnancy that compensate for the reduced diaphragmatic movement that results from the enlarging uterus?

3. Differentiate among epulis gravidarum, ptyalism, and pyrosis and delineate patient teaching needs concerning these symptoms?
4. Explain the physiological basis for glucosuria during pregnancy?

ENDOCRINE SYSTEM

Thyroid Gland

The thyroid gland changes in size and activity during pregnancy. On palpation, the increase in size is appreciated. Enlargement is caused by increased circulation from the progesterone-induced effects on the vessel walls and by estrogen-induced hyperplasia of the glandular tissue. In early pregnancy, elevated levels of thyroxine-binding globulins cause an increase in the total thyroxine (T_4) and total 3,5,3-triiodothyronine (T_3) (Beckmann et al., 2013). The active hormones free T_4 and free T_3 remain unchanged from normal nonpregnant levels. Levels of total T_4 continue to be elevated until several weeks postpartum. Increased T_4-binding capacity is noted by an increase in the serum protein-bound iodine (PBI). These changes in thyroid regulation cause a progressive increase in the basal metabolic rate (BMR) of up to 25% by term. The BMR is the amount of oxygen consumed by the body over a unit of time (mL/min). Maternal effects of the increase in BMR include heat intolerance and an elevation in pulse rate and cardiac output. Within a few weeks following birth, thyroid function returns to normal levels (Beckmann et al., 2013).

Parathyroid Glands

The parathyroid glands, which regulate calcium and phosphate metabolism, increase in size from estrogen-induced hyperplasia and hypertrophy. Maternal concentrations of parathyroid hormone increase as the fetus requires more calcium for skeletal growth during the second and third trimesters. Calcium intake is extremely important for the pregnant woman, whose daily intake should be at least 1,200 to 1,500 mg.

Pituitary Gland and Placenta

The anterior lobe of the pituitary gland, stimulated by the hypothalamus, increases in size and in weight. Pregnancy is possible because of the actions of FSH (stimulates growth of the graafian follicle) and LH, which prompts final maturation of the ovarian follicles and release of the mature ovum. If conception occurs, elevated levels of estrogen and progesterone (produced by the corpus luteum until about 14 weeks of gestation, when the placenta takes over this function) suppress production of FSH and LH. During pregnancy, ovarian follicle maturation may continue, but ovulation does not occur.

Prolactin, also produced by the anterior pituitary gland, is responsible for initial lactation. Although this hormone increases 10-fold during pregnancy, the elevated levels of estrogen and progesterone inhibit lactation by interfering with prolactin-binding to the breast tissue. Prolactin may also play a role in fluid and electrolyte shifts across the fetal membranes (Beckmann et al., 2013).

Oxytocin and vasopressin are produced in the posterior lobe of the pituitary. Oxytocin primarily causes uterine contractions, but high levels of progesterone prevent contractions until close to term. Oxytocin also stimulates milk ejection from the breasts, or the **"let down" reflex.** Vasopressin causes vasoconstriction. Vasoconstriction leads to an increase in maternal blood pressure and exerts an antidiuretic effect that promotes maternal fluid retention to maintain circulating blood volume. The increased blood volume that occurs during pregnancy, along with changes in plasma osmolarity (the fluid-pulling capacity of the plasma to retain fluids) controls the release of vasopressin.

Maternal metabolism is altered to support the pregnancy by thyrotropin and adrenotropin. These hormones, produced by the anterior pituitary gland, exert their effects on the thyroid and adrenal glands. Thyrotropin causes an increased basal metabolism, and adrenotropin alters adrenal gland function to increase fluid retention by the kidneys.

Human placental lactogen (hPL), also known as human chorionic somatomammotropin (hCS), is produced by the placental syncytiotrophoblasts. It is an insulin antagonist and acts as a fetal growth hormone. Human placental lactogen increases the number of circulating fatty acids to meet maternal metabolic needs and decreases maternal glucose utilization, which increases glucose availability to the fetus (Beckmann et al., 2013).

Adrenal Glands

The adrenal glands, located above the kidneys, change little during pregnancy. The adrenal cortex produces cortisol, a hormone that allows the body to respond to stressors. Cortisol is increased during pregnancy because of decreased renal secretion (an alteration prompted by high estrogen levels). Cortisol regulates protein and carbohydrate metabolism and is believed to promote fetal lung maturation and stimulate labor at term. Following birth, it may take up to 6 weeks for maternal cortisol levels to return to normal.

By the second trimester, the adrenal cortex secretes increased levels of aldosterone, a mineral corticoid that causes the renal reabsorption of sodium. This physiological alteration promotes the reclaiming of water and helps to enhance circulatory volume. The increase in aldosterone may be a protective response to the increased renal and excretory gland sodium excretion that occurs as a result of the effects of progesterone.

Pancreas

The pancreas secretes insulin produced by the beta cells of the islets of Langerhans. Pregnancy prompts an increase in the number and size of the beta cells. These changes are responsible for the alterations that occur in carbohydrate metabolism during pregnancy.

Prostaglandins

Prostaglandins are lipid substances found in high concentrations in the female reproductive tract and in the uterine decidua during pregnancy. Their exact function in pregnancy is unknown although they may maintain a reduced placental vascular resistance. A decrease in prostaglandin levels may contribute to hypertension and preeclampsia. At term, an increased release of prostaglandins from the cervix as it softens and dilates may contribute to the onset of labor.

MUSCULOSKELETAL SYSTEM

As the pregnancy progresses, the abdominal wall weakens, and the rectus abdominis muscles separate (**diastasis recti**) to accommodate the growing uterus. As the weight

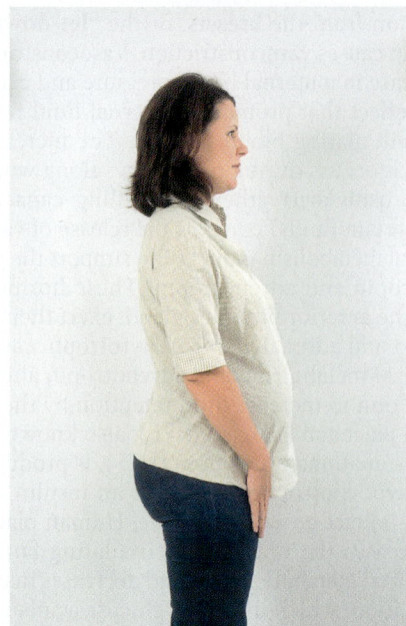

Figure 8-14 Lumbar lordosis.

of the uterus shifts upward and outward, a lumbar lordosis (anterior convexity of the lumbar spine) develops (Fig. 8-14). This alteration compensates for the changing center of gravity and allows centering to remain over the woman's legs. Low back pain usually accompanies this physiological change. Separation of the rectus abdominis muscles along with an increase in intra-abdominal pressure from the growing uterus may exacerbate an abdominal wall hernia.

Relaxin, a hormone produced by the placenta, along with the action of progesterone, causes a relative laxity of the ligaments. The pubis symphysis separates at approximately 28 to 30 weeks gestation. These changes, coupled with the change in the maternal center of gravity, result in an unsteady gait and a greater tendency toward falls. The patient's gait takes on the appearance of a "pregnancy waddle" as the bones of the pelvis shift and move. The woman should be encouraged to maintain good posture and keep the abdominal muscles toned through exercise. Sitting in a firm chair and the use of a small pillow or blanket rolled and placed in the lumbar region (lumbar roll) for support can help decrease lower back pain.

Pregnant women frequently complain of sharp pain in the lower abdominal quadrants or in the groin area. Most often, the pain is related to stretching and hypertrophy of the round ligaments that support the uterus (round ligament pain). Because of dextrorotation of the gravid uterus as it rises out of the pelvis, the right maternal side is most commonly affected. Once a serious medical condition (e.g., appendicitis) has been ruled out, the nurse should offer reassurance and instruct the patient to sit in a chair or rest on her left side. The application of heat may also be helpful. A brief review of the anatomical changes that occur during pregnancy may alleviate the patient's fear of appendicitis. Because the appendix is pushed up and posterior by the gravid uterus, the typical location of pain (McBurney's point) is not a reliable indicator for a ruptured appendix during pregnancy. The pain should gradually subside, but if it persists or is accompanied by fever, a change in bowel

habits, or decreased fetal movement, the patient should promptly contact her medical provider.

Mobilization of calcium stores occurs to provide for the fetal calcium needs necessary for skeletal grown. The total maternal serum calcium decreases, but the ionized calcium level remains unchanged from the prepregnant state. The increase in circulating maternal parathyroid hormone stimulates an increased absorption of calcium from the intestines and decreases the renal loss of calcium to maintain adequate calcium levels.

Calcitonin, a hormone important in the metabolism of calcium and phosphorus, suppresses bone resorption by inhibiting the activity of osteoclasts. Osteoclasts are a cell type that "digests" bone matrix, causing a release of calcium and phosphorus into the blood. Calcitonin is produced primarily in the thyroid gland, but it is also synthesized in a many other tissues, including the lungs and intestinal tract. The activity of calcitonin, coupled with adequate nutrition, protects the maternal skeleton from a loss of bone density despite an increase in the turnover of bone mass. Calcium intake is of major importance during pregnancy, and women should be encouraged to increase their dietary calcium through the consumption of dairy products, calcium-fortified orange juice, and dark green leafy vegetables.

Calcium supplementation may be advised for patients who are vegetarian or lactose intolerant. Pregnant women often complain of cramping in the lower extremities and calves, especially at night. The cramps, sometimes called "charley-horses," can be extremely painful and are caused by poor circulation to the extremities. They have also been associated with imbalances in calcium and phosphorus. Increasing or decreasing calcium intake may be helpful. For immediate relief of the cramping, the woman should be instructed to stand and lean forward to stretch the calf muscle or have someone gently push her toes back toward her shin and hold this position for several seconds. Daily walks can also help because ambulation improves circulation to the muscles.

NURSING ASSESSMENT OF PHYSIOLOGICAL CHANGES AND PRENATAL HEALTH EDUCATION

Nursing assessment must begin with a comprehensive history and examination at the first prenatal visit. The history should include information about the current pregnancy; the obstetric and gynecological history; a cultural assessment; and a medical, nutritional, social, and family (including the father's) medical history. A complete review of all of the physical systems should be conducted followed by a physical examination that includes appropriate nutritional assessments and diagnostic procedures. This information is essential to the formulation of appropriate nursing diagnoses (Box 8-1). Ongoing health education should focus on the current trimester and its physical changes. A trimester-by-trimester approach to teaching needs is presented in Table 8-3.

 Now Can You—Discuss major changes in the endocrine and musculoskeletal systems during pregnancy?

1. Describe maternal symptoms associated with an increased basal metabolic rate (BMR)?

2. Identify where cortisol is produced and name two important actions of this hormone?

3. Discuss two physiological alterations that produce the "pregnancy waddle" and suggest two strategies for the relief of back pain?

4. Explain why adequate calcium intake is essential during pregnancy?

Psychosocial Adaptations During Pregnancy

For many women, pregnancy is a time of turmoil that affects the ability to deal with stress and cope with the changes that will take place over many months. These

Table 8-3 Health Education Topics Related to the Physiological Adaptations to Pregnancy

Topics to Include	First Trimester	Second Trimester	Third Trimester
Physiological Changes of Pregnancy and Related Discomforts	Pain and tingling in breasts Nausea and vomiting (morning sickness) Urinary frequency Fatigue Mood swings	Enlargement of the abdomen Skin pigmentation Striae gravidarum Vascular spiders Constipation Heartburn or gastric reflux Leg cramps Groin pain from round ligament stretching Leukorrhea	Dyspnea Leg and feet cramps Constipation Indigestion, heartburn, gastric reflux Pedal edema Fatigue Vaginal discharge Urinary frequency Braxton-Hicks contractions versus true labor
Danger Signs to Report to Health-Care Provider	Vaginal bleeding Abdominal cramping or pain Severe or prolonged vomiting	Vaginal bleeding Burning or painful urination Fever, increased pulse rate Decreased or absent fetal movements Unrelenting nausea and vomiting Abdominal pain or cramping Swelling of face or fingers, headaches, visual disturbances, or epigastric pain	Visual disturbances Headache Hand and facial edema Fever Vaginal bleeding Abdominal pain; uterine contractions Premature rupture of the membranes Decreased or absent fetal movement
General Health Teaching	Schedule of return visits for routine prenatal care General hygiene Comfort measures Anticipatory guidance Sexual activity and restrictions Physical activities, exercise, and rest Nutritional guidance Avoidance of alcohol, fetal alcohol effects Effects of smoking, and smoking cessation strategies if indicated	Reinforcement and reiteration of previous teaching Comfort measures Anticipatory guidance Choices of prenatal education classes Signs and symptoms of preterm labor	Signs and symptoms of labor/preterm labor When to call the health-care provider, when to go to the birthing center or hospital Comfort measures Anticipatory guidance Reinforcement and reiteration of previous teaching Encouragement to attend a labor and birth class

Source: Adapted from Mattson, S., & Smith, J. E. (2010). *Core curriculum for maternal-newborn nursing* (4th ed.). St. Louis, MO: W.B. Saunders.

changes affect not only the woman but her partner and other family members as well. Pregnancy and childbearing constitute major developmental phases, and these events are often accompanied by ambivalence and conflicting emotions. The nurse must have a basic understanding of how the woman's progression through the developmental phases and the accompanying emotions affect her and her family's acceptance of the pregnancy and the unknown child. Nursing care for the woman and her family through each pregnancy milestone should be tailored with respect to personal and family values, cultural customs, and spiritual beliefs and health maintenance behaviors. Topics for health education related to the psychosocial adaptations to pregnancy are presented in Table 8-4.

DEVELOPMENTAL AND FAMILY CHANGES

According to Duvall's and Miller's (1984) stages of family development, the expectant family sets about the task of preparing for its new role as child care providers. The home must be reorganized to accommodate the infant, family member duties and responsibilities must often be realigned, and patterns of money management need to be altered. The couples' sexual relationship must adapt to the physical and emotional changes that accompany pregnancy. Family relationships with relatives are often reoriented as the couple gradually moves away from the former role of "child" and instead seek recognition as parents. Friendships and relationships with work associates also must adapt to the couple's changing lifestyle.

For both the expectant woman and her partner, emotional responses are often unpredictable and labile and require patience, understanding, and good communication. The couple needs to expand their knowledge about pregnancy, birth, and parenting to enhance their understanding of these life-altering events. Additional information also helps to empower them to better prepare for the major changes that will soon take place in their lives. With each subsequent pregnancy, the couple must adjust to the transitions in their relationship with one another and with each child. Each birth brings a new member who must be introduced and incorporated into the existing family structure. Sibling rivalry, or competitiveness among the children, is common and can often be diminished by parental actions that actively involve each child with the pregnancy and anticipated birth.

MATERNAL TASKS AND ROLE TRANSITION

Rubin (1975) described specific tasks that a woman must accomplish to integrate the maternal role into her personality. The "tasks of pregnancy" generally occur concurrently during the pregnancy and help the woman develop her self-concept as a mother. To be successful in accomplishing these tasks, the pregnant woman must incorporate the pregnancy into her total identity. That is, she must "accept the reality of the pregnancy" and integrate it into her self-concept, "accept the child," "reorder" her relationships, learn to "give of herself for the child," and "seek safe passage through the pregnancy, labor and birth" (Mattson & Smith, 2010). A summary of the maternal tasks of pregnancy is presented in Table 8-5.

Acceptance of the Pregnancy

The mother-to-be needs to accept the pregnancy and incorporate it into her own reality and self-concept. This process is known as "binding in." During the first trimester, the woman's focus centers on her physical discomforts (e.g., fatigue and nausea) and needs rather than on the developing child. By the second trimester, she feels

Table 8-4 Health Education Topics Related to the Psychosocial Adaptations to Pregnancy			
Topics to Include	**First Trimester**	**Second Trimester**	**Third Trimester**
Developmental Tasks of Pregnancy	Mother: Acceptance of pregnancy into her self-system	Mother: Binding-in to the pregnancy, ensuring safe passage, and differentiating the fetus from herself	Mother: Separating herself from the pregnancy and the fetus, trying various caregiving strategies
	Father: Announcement and realization of the pregnancy	Father: Anticipation of adapting to the role of fatherhood	Father: Role adaptation, preparation for labor and birth
	Couple: Realignment of relationships and roles	Couple: Realignment of roles and division of tasks	Couple: Preparation of the nursery
Psychosocial Changes During Pregnancy	Ambivalence about pregnancy	Active dream and fantasy life	Dislikes being pregnant but loves the child
	Introversion	Concerns with body image	Anxious about childbirth, but sees labor and birth as deliverance
	Passivity and difficulty with decision making	Nesting behaviors	The couple experiments with various mothering or fathering roles
	Sexual and emotional changes	Sexual behavior adjustment	Woman is introspective
	Changing self-image	Expanding to a variety of methods of expressing affection and intimacy	
	Ethical dilemmas of prenatal testing		

Source: Adapted from Mattson, S., & Smith, J. E. (2010). *Core curriculum for maternal-newborn nursing* (4th ed.). St. Louis, MO: W.B. Saunders.

Table 8-5	Maternal Tasks of Pregnancy
General Principles	Pregnancy progressively becomes part of the woman's total identity. She feels unique because she can't share her sensory experience with others. Her focus turns inward, and she is overly sensitive. She seeks the company of other women and pregnant women. Giving of self is an essential component of motherhood. She needs to feel loved and valued, and she needs to have the child accepted by her partner. Throughout pregnancy, the partner's major role is to nurture and respond to the pregnant woman's feelings of vulnerability. Absence of a female support system during pregnancy is a singular index of a high-risk pregnancy.
Acceptance of Pregnancy; Self in Maternal Role; "Binding-in"	First trimester: She accepts the idea of pregnancy but not the child. She is uncertain and ambivalent, and her primary focus is on herself, not the fetus. Although she may begin to "bind in" to the idea that she is pregnant, the baby is not yet real to her. Second trimester: With sensation of fetal movement, or "quickening," she becomes aware of the child as a separate entity. She is filled with wonder and perhaps concern over the changes taking place in her body. The fetus becomes her major focus. She experiences feelings of love and attachment and enjoys fantasizing about her new role. Third trimester: She wants the child and is tired of being pregnant. She has increasing feelings of vulnerability and often becomes more dependent on her partner during the last weeks of pregnancy.
Acceptance of the Infant by Others	First trimester: Acceptance of the pregnancy by herself and others. Securing acceptance is a process that continues throughout pregnancy. Second trimester: The family needs to relate to the fetus as a member. Acceptance from her mother is very important; many expectant women experience an increased closeness with their mothers during pregnancy. A mother's reaction to her daughter's pregnancy signifies her acceptance of the grandchild and of her daughter. Third trimester: The critical issue is the unconditional acceptance of the child; conditional acceptance may imply rejection by the mother or family members.

Reordering of Relationships, Giving of Self	First trimester: Examines what needs to be given up to assume a new role.
	  Trade-offs for having the infant.
	  May grieve the loss of a carefree life.
	Second trimester: Identifies with the child, learns how to delay her own desires.
	Third trimester: Has decreased confidence in her ability to become a good mother to her child.

Ensuring Safe Passage Throughout Pregnancy, Labor, and Birth	First trimester: Focuses on herself, not on her fetus. Second trimester: Begins to conceptualize the fetus as a separate being; develops an increasing sense of the value of her infant. Third trimester: Has concern for herself and her infant as a unit, shares a symbiotic relationship. At the seventh month, she is in a state of high vulnerability. At the end of this trimester, begins to view labor and birth as an "end point." Participating in positive self-care activities (e.g., nutrition, exercise, stress reduction, and childbirth preparation) help to accomplish this task.

Source: Adapted from Mattson, S., & Smith, J. E. (2010). *Core curriculum for maternal-newborn nursing* (4th ed.). St. Louis, MO: W.B. Saunders.

fetal movement (quickening), has most likely seen the baby on ultrasound and heard his heartbeat, and begins to conceptualize the child as an individual within her. During the third trimester, as the due date approaches, the mother-to-be wants the child and just as strongly wants the pregnancy to be over. At this point, she is tired and needs a considerable amount of emotional and physical support from her family and friends.

Acceptance of the Child

Acceptance of the child is critical to a successful adjustment to the pregnancy. Acceptance must come from the expectant woman as well as from others. During early pregnancy, announcements are made to one another and to family and friends. A positive response from those closest to the pregnant woman helps to foster her

acceptance of the child. There is a great value attached to this unborn child, and she wants and needs others in the family to accept the child as well. In the second trimester, the immediate family needs to exhibit behaviors consistent with relating to the child as a sibling, a son, or a daughter. In the third trimester, the woman must develop an unconditional acceptance of the child, or she and others may reject him for not meeting their expectations.

Reordering Relationships

To facilitate the necessary family transition, the pregnant woman must reorder her relationships to allow for the child to fit into the existing family structure and learn to give of herself to the unknown child. At this time, she becomes reflective and examines what things in her life may need to be given up or changed for the infant. If this is her first child, she may grieve the loss of her carefree life. As the pregnancy progresses, the woman begins to identify with the child and makes plans for their life together after the birth. During the last few weeks of the pregnancy, the woman must work through doubts of her ability to be a good mother. At this time, positive support from family and friends is essential in boosting her confidence and in assisting her in overcoming these feelings of self-doubt.

Seeking Safe Passage Through Pregnancy, Labor, and Birth

Seeking safe passage through the pregnancy, labor, and birth are maternal tasks that receive the most attention during the pregnancy. In the first trimester, the woman focuses on her own discomforts and places her needs before those of the fetus. Symptoms of fatigue, nausea, and breast tenderness can be overwhelming during this often difficult time. In the second and third trimesters, the woman develops an increasing sense of the value of her infant. She comes to conceptualize her fetus as a separate being (fetal distinction), and she accepts her changing body image. She becomes extremely vulnerable during her seventh month and increasingly worried about the impending labor and birth. As the due date approaches, the woman's fears about labor may diminish as she begins to view childbirth as an "end point." Participation in childbirth preparation classes can greatly assist the woman and her family in dealing with the anxiety and fears that often surround labor and birth.

Other developmental tasks take place during the passage of pregnancy as well. The woman needs to validate the pregnancy, and initial feelings of uncertainty or ambivalence are normal. When caring for expectant women, the nurse should never assume that the pregnancy was planned or wanted. Instead, the nurse should facilitate discussion of uncertainties or concerns with the patient and her family to facilitate acceptance of the pregnancy. Many women fantasize and dream about their pregnancy and how it will change their lives. The woman must incorporate the fetus into her body image, a process termed "fetal embodiment." Accomplishing this task allows her to accept the changes in her body size and shape as the pregnancy progresses. The significant other plays an important role as the woman becomes increasingly dependent on that individual for helping to meet her daily needs.

As the pregnancy advances, the woman begins to conceptualize the fetus as a separate individual. She comes to view her changing body as a "vessel of new life" and often feels closer to her own mother at this time. This deeper relationship with her mother begins as one of dependency and progresses to one in which she identifies with her mother as a peer. If her mother is not available, she may reach out to another valued maternal figure for identification and support. As she reaches the end of the third trimester, the woman begins to give up her symbiotic relationship with the fetus. She harbors feelings of anxiety about the childbirth process and begins to gather supplies and prepare for the baby's entry into the home. This process is termed "nesting." At this point in pregnancy, the woman is often impatient with the awkwardness related to her increasing size and has a strong desire to see the pregnancy end so that she can begin her next phase as a mother.

 Nursing Insight—*Building on Rubin's maternal tasks of pregnancy*

Later work by nursing researchers Ramona Mercer (1995) and Regina Lederman (1996) has greatly added to our understanding of maternal role attainment. For example, the woman's relationship with her own mother is a significant factor in the adaptation to pregnancy and motherhood. Of importance in the relationship is the mother's availability (past and present), her reactions to her daughter's pregnancy, respect for her daughter's autonomy, and the willingness to reminisce about her own childbirth and childrearing experiences (Fig. 8-15). Acceptance of the pregnancy focuses on the woman's adaptive responses to the myriad changes that occur related to normal pregnancy growth and development. The woman's partner's support during pregnancy greatly enhances her feelings of well-being and is positively associated with the initiation of early and ongoing prenatal care. Preparation for labor and birth takes place through participation in formal classes, actively fantasizing, and dreaming about labor and birth. Two factors, including loss of control over the body and loss of control over emotions, contribute to the prenatal fear of loss of control in labor (Lederman, 1996; Lederman & Weis, 2010; Mercer, 1995, 2004).

 Now Can You—Discuss the "tasks of pregnancy"?

1. Describe why it is important for the pregnant woman to successfully accomplish the tasks of pregnancy?
2. Discuss the value of ongoing family support throughout pregnancy in fostering acceptance of the child?
3. Identify what is meant by "seeking safe passage"?
4. Explain why pregnant women often feel closer to their own mothers as the pregnancy progresses?

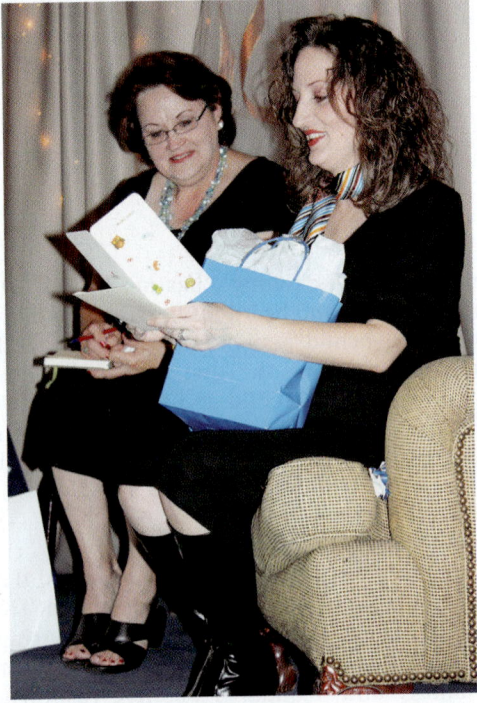

Figure 8-15 Pregnant woman and her mother enjoying a baby shower.

Developmental Tasks and the Pregnant Adolescent

For the pregnant adolescent, ongoing age-related developmental tasks can create conflict when coupled with the developmental tasks of pregnancy. Tasks associated with adolescence focus on growth and maturity. They include developing a personal value system, choosing a vocation or career, developing personal body image and sexuality, achieving a stable identity, and attaining independence from parents. Conflicts may arise when these tasks are overshadowed by the developmental tasks of pregnancy. While seeking safe passage, the adolescent may not seek prenatal care unless pressured by authority figures or peers to do so. By nature, adolescents are not future oriented. Hence, the pregnant adolescent may not be able to readily accept the reality of the unborn child. Because the adolescent's sense of identity is still incomplete, bodily changes often feel awkward. Because the family may not react positively to the pregnancy, acceptance of the pregnancy by self and others may be hindered. Many times, the adolescent's parents come to assume the role of parent. Although this may be helpful at times, this situation limits the young mother's involvement with the newborn and her ability to fully give of herself.

PATERNAL ADAPTATION TO PREGNANCY

Pregnancy is psychologically stressful for men. Expectant fathers often experience a variety of reactions to the pregnancy. Some enjoy the role of nurturer and marvel in the changes that occur in the woman. Others feel alienated and begin to stray from the relationship. Many men view pregnancy as positive proof of their masculinity and take steps to assume a dominant or more supportive role in the relationship. Others find no meaning or personal value in the pregnancy and consequently fail to develop any sense of responsibility toward the mother or the child. There are several styles of paternal involvement during pregnancy, including "observer," where the father is passive and detached; "expressive," where the expectant father attempts to experience the pregnancy as much as possible, and "instrumental," where the father is the caretaker (Callister, Matsumura, & Vehvilainnen-Julkunen, 2003; Hanson, Hunter, Bormann, & Sobo, 2009).

Couvade, in the traditional sense, is the observance of certain rituals and taboos by the male to signify his transition to fatherhood. This action affirms the man's psychosocial and biophysical relationship to his partner and the child. In recent times, couvade has come to describe the unintentional development of pregnancy-related symptoms such as weight gain, nausea, back pain, difficulty sleeping, and depression by the pregnant woman's partner. Research has shown that approximately 1 in every 10 new or prospective fathers suffers from depression, which correlates positively with its maternal counterpart (Paulson & Bazemore, 2010). Men who experience the couvade syndrome often assume a more involved paternal role during the childbearing year.

The father of the baby also experiences specific tasks of pregnancy that correspond with the trimesters. During the first trimester, the father is in an "announcement phase." Similar to the woman's experience, the father may be ambivalent at this time. He must first accept the pregnancy as "real" to begin to incorporate the future child into his life and assume the expectant father role. In the second trimester, or "moratorium phase," the man's "binding in" usually takes longer to achieve than the woman's, and this is related to his "remoteness" to the fetus. At this time, involvement in prenatal visits, listening to the baby's heartbeat, and visualization of the fetus during ultrasound can make the fetus seem more real to the father. He begins to accept the woman's changing body and the reality of the fetus as a child when he can feel fetal movement.

Optimizing Outcomes—Promoting prenatal paternal attachment

The nurse can be instrumental in promoting early paternal attachment. Encouraging the father to actively "engage" with the fetus through reflective journaling is one way to enhance prenatal bonding. One father later shared his recorded insights:

My earliest memories with Trina started the day she was born. No, they started before that. They started in the womb. I would come home and I would say, "Hello," and she would flick and flitter in the womb. She would start kicking. If I put my hand on my wife's tummy when she was carrying Trina, she would move over to where my hand was. If I put it on the other side, she would move to that side. I used to sing to her. It's always been that way and has just continued pretty much that way. I remember one night laying with my head on my wife's stomach and singing a lullaby or something, I can't remember exactly which song. She was very active but she settled down, and then I put my hand on her stomach and she moved my hand.

Source: Excerpt from Callister, L. C., Matsumura, G., & Vehvilainnen-Julkunen, K. (2003). He's having a baby. The paternal childbirth experience. *Marriage & Families.* Retrieved from http://marriageandfamilies.byu.edu/issues/2003/January/baby.aspx

The couple's sexual relationship often changes as some men deal with fears of harming the fetus. The expectant father may also feel a rivalry with a male health-care provider. Involvement of the father during examinations and tests with thorough explanations of the need for them can minimize the father's feelings of being left out. His partner's intense introspective nature may be confusing at times, and he may feel pushed away. The man also fantasizes about being a father, although his fantasies are often centered on an older child rather than on an infant.

In the third trimester, the expectant father enters a "focusing phase." During this time he negotiates what his role in labor and birth will be; prepares for the reality of parenthood; alters his self-concept to reflect that of a more mature, or fatherly figure; becomes involved in setting up the nursery; and copes with his fears of the mutilation or death of his partner or child during birth. Fears and concerns are often lessened somewhat by participation in prenatal and parenting classes. The nurse should be aware of cues (e.g., lack of participation in prenatal care or behaviors that signal lack of interest in the woman, the fetus, or the pregnancy) that may indicate paternal detachment from the mother and the pregnancy. Referral for counseling, childbirth preparation classes, or other community resources may be appropriate. Pastoral care or local fathering support groups, if available, may also assist the father with his need for involvement. Problems such as a troubled relationship with his own father, a dysfunctional couple relationship, and sociocultural factors may be barriers that prevent the man from assuming a paternal role (Callister et al., 2003; Hanson et al., 2009). Not uncommonly, the behavior associated with a "deadbeat dad" stems from feelings of being pushed away or left out by the expectant woman and her other support systems.

ADAPTATION OF SIBLINGS AND GRANDPARENTS

The psychosocial reactions of other family members to the pregnancy and childbirth must also be explored because these individuals often have a significant influence on the woman's passage through the developmental tasks of pregnancy. The reactions of siblings correlate closely to their age and level of involvement with the pregnancy. Children may express excitement, anticipation, anger, or despair. The toddler, characteristically involved in his own little world, may initially exhibit a reaction of indifference. However, the parents must be advised about the strong likelihood of a regression in age-appropriate behavior. For example, the child may want to nurse, drink from a bottle, or wear a diaper like the baby. The school-age child usually appears more interested but grasping the full reality of a baby in the family may not be realistic because the process of concrete thinking is not fully developed until around age 10. Engaging the child in family discussions about the anticipated birth, encouraging the child to feel fetal movements, and listening to the fetal heartbeat, sharing age-appropriate educational materials, and allowing him to attend sibling preparation classes are strategies that may help the child to feel that he is sharing in the pregnancy experience (Fig. 8-16).

When a child reaches early adolescence, changing sexuality associated with this developmental phase may create a barrier between him and his mother. This sort of barrier makes it difficult for the adolescent to view his parent as a pregnant woman and may give rise to feelings of resentment toward the new child about to join the family. Parents need to be aware of ways to cope with potential negative behaviors and recognize that adolescents often appear to have knowledge and understanding about pregnancy and birth but their information may be incorrect and incomplete. The nurse can suggest that the child attend prenatal visits to listen to the baby's heartbeat, and if possible, view the fetus during ultrasound examinations. Parents should be assisted in developing other strategies to include the adolescent in the changes that are taking place during pregnancy and that will occur following the birth. Older children may benefit from attending prenatal classes or touring the birthing facility.

Grandparents are very often excited and eagerly await the birth of a grandchild, although this is not always the case. The grandparents' age at the time of the birth can exert a positive or a negative effect on their reactions. For example, if they will become first-time grandparents during their 30s or 40s, they may be ambivalent or feel they are not yet ready to assume the grandparent role. Conversely, those who are already grandparents may be excited with the prospect of another grandchild. Other factors (e.g., if the pregnancy was unplanned or if the mother is very young or unwed) may prompt feelings of anger and disappointment. Along with the woman's partner, the grandparents usually harbor concerns about the health and well-being of the expectant woman and her fetus. They also may be unsure about the extent to which they should become involved in the childrearing process.

MATERNAL ADAPTATION DURING ABSENCE OF A SIGNIFICANT OTHER

If the woman has no involved significant other, she will need the presence of a strong support person to help her adapt to the pregnancy and the demands of parenting. The future she has planned for the child, such as the decision to place the child for adoption, can heavily influence her psychological needs. During prenatal visits, the nurse should ensure that the woman is given the opportunity to discuss her future plans for the child. After assessing the woman's needs, the nurse can make referrals to appropriate community resources that may include prenatal classes, psychological counseling, pastoral care, or social services.

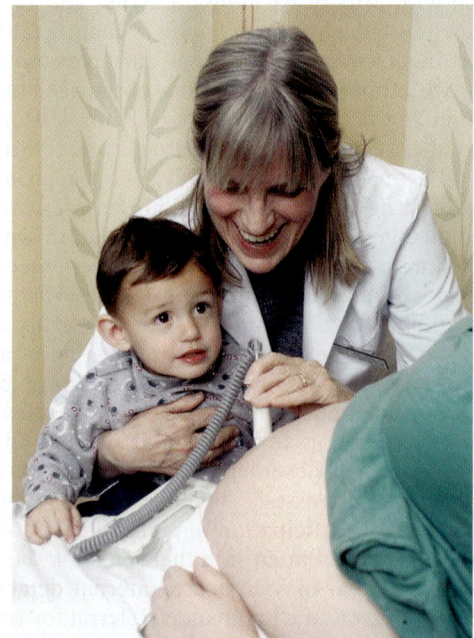

Figure 8-16 A nurse midwife listening to fetal heart tones with a pregnant mother and her child.

 Now Can You—Discuss pregnancy-related role transitions for the adolescent, father, siblings, and grandparents?

1. Describe why the adolescent may have difficulty achieving the developmental tasks of pregnancy?
2. Explain what is meant by the couvade syndrome?
3. Discuss the "focusing phase" that occurs during the third trimester and identify two behaviors that may indicate a lack of paternal attachment?
4. Contrast behaviors of toddlers, school-age, and adolescent children in response to the pregnancy?
5. Identify two factors that may influence the grandparents' ability to make role transitions in response to the pregnancy?

CULTURAL INFLUENCES AND PSYCHOSOCIAL ADAPTATIONS

Universally, some type of ritual or ceremony is attached to important life events. In pregnancy and childbirth, this ritual may involve special care of the mother and baby, events planned to welcome the new member of the family, or rigid requirements that must be met by the family and health-care providers. There are a multitude of cultural messages that may influence the woman's adaptation to pregnancy, birth, and the newborn. The nurse should explore these cultural influences with the patient and her family. By acknowledging and documenting specific beliefs and needs, the nurse can help guide the woman and her family through the prenatal and intrapartal care system more effectively. Through open discussion, erroneous or conflicting beliefs can be addressed, and a plan can be developed to ensure a satisfactory, positive experience for the childbearing year.

HAZARDS OF HIGH-TECH MANAGEMENT ON MATERNAL ADAPTATION

The technology-focused society of today can lead to an increase in the level of anxiety and number of stressors experienced by the pregnant woman and her family. Moral and ethical dilemmas may arise from positive diagnostic tests. The pregnant woman's emotional and interpersonal needs may be overlooked by those caring for her as added importance is placed on the technology that surrounds the care. Full enjoyment of the pregnancy may not be possible, as the woman instead comes to focus on each test and its results. In this situation, the pregnancy becomes a "tentative pregnancy." A conflict of interest develops between the technology and the woman's trust of her own instincts and inner feelings. These conflicts can further undermine the woman's self-confidence. Collectively, these stressors interfere with the woman's ability to move through the tasks of maternal role development and delay her preparation for parenting.

SOCIETAL AND CULTURAL INFLUENCES ON FAMILY ADAPTATION

Cultural influences often affect how pregnancy is viewed and accepted by the woman and her family. Many cultures, such as the tribal Native Americans and most Latinos, consider pregnancy to be a normal and expected life event, not a state of illness. Some African nations impose rigid taboos concerning what a woman can eat, drink, wear, and do during her pregnancy. In some Middle Eastern cultures, pregnancy is viewed as "woman's work," and the father's involvement is minimal. In Korean and other southeastern Asian cultures, a harmonious balance such as yin/yang (masculine/feminine) or hot/cold must be closely observed. In the equilibrium model of health, achievement of balance allows for the normal growth of the baby and ensures the mother's recovery from the pregnancy. Some cultures place emphasis on certain behaviors designed to protect the pregnancy, such as avoidance of particular foods and harmful substances. Immigrants to America become acculturated to Western society. In so doing, they may give up their own health-protective beliefs and behaviors and instead turn to the use of alcohol, drugs, and tobacco or consume fast foods rather than a balanced diet. The nurse's role is to assess each patient's beliefs and develop a plan of care that is individualized and incorporates the woman's customs while providing comprehensive and safe care.

 Cultural Diversity: Myths, Taboos, and "Old Wives' Tales"

In all cultures and subcultures there are myths, tales, and taboos associated with pregnancy. These have developed to explain the changes that occur during pregnancy or to link a cause to negative pregnancy outcomes. One myth concerns heartburn: If heartburn is experienced during pregnancy, the baby will be born with lots of hair. Another involves using the shape and height of the woman's belly or shape and fullness of her face as indicators to determine the baby's sex.

The Chinese and Malays believe that certain "cooling" foods—cucumber, cabbage, bananas, pineapples—and iced drinks, like coconut water and tea—are taboo during pregnancy because they contribute to poor blood circulation. For the Chinese, other taboo foods are those considered to be "acidic," such as pineapple, mango, lime, sour orange, tapai (fermented tapioca rice), and concentrated coconut milk. These foods are believed to possibly induce bleeding or miscarriage.

Many "old wives' tales" surround pregnancy. One suggests that raising the hands up over the head can cause the baby to become entangled in its cord. Another warns the pregnant woman not to take baths because germs may enter the vagina and pass to the baby. Another encourages abundant water intake so that the baby won't get dirty.

Source: Adapted from Weiss, R. E. (2012). Old Wives Tales & Pregnancy Myths. Retrieved from http://pregnancy.about.com/cs/myths/a/aa042299.htm

FACTORS THAT INTERFERE WITH PSYCHOSOCIAL ADAPTATIONS DURING PREGNANCY

Grief and loss during the perinatal period can be triggered by spontaneous abortion; elective termination; plans to relinquish the child for adoption or surrogacy; and loss of the perfect child through prematurity, illness, deformity, or less preferred gender. Parental reactions can produce a separation from the infant and delay attachment, prompt feelings of personal inadequacy concerning the inability to produce a healthy infant, and alter healthy methods of relating to the infant.

The importance of prenatal education, labor and birth preparation, and parenting classes cannot be stressed enough by the nurse. Many women bypass the courses offered by their health-care providers or hospitals in lieu of watching birth stories on television. These programs are a good adjunct but must be placed into context by information obtained at the prenatal visits and during attendance at prenatal and childbirth education classes taught by nurses and certified personnel.

NURSING ASSESSMENT OF PSYCHOSOCIAL CHANGES AND PRENATAL HEALTH EDUCATION

Nursing assessment of the psychosocial changes that occur during pregnancy must include a thorough history including the family background, past obstetric events, and the status of the current pregnancy. Each prenatal visit provides an opportunity to ask the patient about her pregnancy experience since the last visit, address current concerns, and offer anticipatory guidance of what to expect from the present visit to the next appointment. Based on this information, the nurse formulates appropriate nursing diagnoses related to the maternal psychosocial adaptation to pregnancy (Box 8-2). Health education should be focused according to the current trimester and evaluated by the patient's or couple's ability to verbalize the content presented, their efforts to seek assistance and support with psychological concerns, and indicators of satisfactory coping with the psychological transitions that are occurring. Suggested topics for health teaching during each trimester are presented in Table 8-4. Pregnancy represents a time of great physical and emotional change. The woman and her family require ongoing support and education to ensure that they safely and successfully move through the stages of pregnancy and in the end are prepared to welcome the new baby into their lives.

 Now Can You—Discuss the effects of high technology and other influences on psychosocial adaptation during pregnancy?

1. Explain how "high-tech" management can interfere with accomplishing the tasks associated with maternal role development?
2. Provide three examples of societal/cultural traditions that influence development of the maternal role?
3. Describe how assessment and education empower the pregnant woman and her family to successfully deal with the psychosocial changes that take place?

> **Box 8-2** Nursing Diagnoses Related to Psychosocial Adaptations to Pregnancy
>
> - Risk for Disturbed Body Image related to anatomical and physiological changes of pregnancy
> - Ineffective Role Performance related to taking on new roles; changes in roles
> - Risk for Situational Low Self-esteem related to pregnancy complications, changes in body image, roles
> - Ineffective Sexuality Patterns related to changes in libido during pregnancy
> - Interrupted Family Processes related to developmental stressors of pregnancy or loss
> - Anxiety related to fear of the unknown
> - Readiness for Enhanced Family Coping related to opportunity for growth/mastery
> - Risk for Impaired Parenting related to lack of knowledge, skills, support
> - Health-seeking behaviors: developmental tasks needed to prepare for parenthood
> - Dysfunctional grieving related to stillbirth, ill or preterm newborn, loss of the ideal of the perfect child, loss of pregnancy, or loss of desired labor or birth
>
> *Source:* Adapted from Mattson, S., & Smith, J. E. (2010). *Core curriculum for maternal-newborn nursing.* St. Louis, MO: W.B. Saunders.

Summary Points

- Estrogen and progesterone are the major hormones produced by the placenta during pregnancy. Estrogen's effect is one of "growth"; progesterone's effect is one of "maintenance."

- The reproductive system undergoes the greatest changes in size and function, and every organ within this system is affected by or focused on the needs of the growing fetus.

- Every system in the body experiences dramatic changes in structure and function as a result of the hormonal changes of pregnancy.

- Pregnancy is a time of turmoil in the woman's life that affects her ability to deal with stress and cope with the changes that will occur over many months. These changes affect not only the woman but also her partner and the other family members as well.

- Ethnocultural, familial, and spiritual beliefs exert a powerful influence on the woman's and her family's progress through the pregnancy and can enhance or interfere with routine prenatal care.

- The nurse's responsibility in prenatal care is to ensure that the patient and her family understand the physiological and psychosocial changes that occur because of pregnancy and equip them with strategies to cope with these changes.

Review Questions

Multiple Choice

1. The perinatal nurse knows that which of the following hormones is most responsible for maintaining pregnancy?
A. Estrogen
B. Progesterone
C. Relaxin
D. Human chorionic gonadotropin

2. A woman who is 28 weeks pregnant calls the clinic to complain of painless, irregular contractions. The clinic nurse informs her that this is related to circulating levels of which hormone?
A. Estrogen
B. Progesterone
C. Relaxin
D. Prostaglandin

3. A new patient is having a speculum exam, and the nurse notes the cervix has a bluish-purple discoloration. Which of the following does the nurse chart about this finding?
A. Goodell's sign
B. Chadwick's sign
C. Striae gravidarum
D. Linea nigra

4. During a prenatal class, the nurse explains that one of the baby's protections during pregnancy is the cervical mucus. The nurse teaches the class members that the medical term for this is
A. Linea nigra
B. Rugae
C. Striae gravidarum
D. Operculum

5. A woman who is 22 weeks pregnant calls the clinic to report painless irregular contractions. Which action by the nurse is best?
   A. Asks the woman how many pregnancies she has lost
   B. Informs the woman she needs to go to the hospital
   C. Teaches the woman that this is a normal occurrence
   D. Tells the woman to come to the clinic today

6. A pregnant woman complains of leukorrhea at her clinic visit. Which action by the nurse is best?
   A. Inform her she should abstain from sex during this time.
   B. Instruct her to buy and use perineal pads or incontinence pads.
   C. Instruct her to douche twice a week with a vinegar solution.
   D. Teach her to cleanse her vulvar area gently with soap and water.

7. A woman who is entering her third trimester complains of tingling and numb sensations that radiate up to the elbow in her dominant hand. Which action by the nurse is best?
   A. Advise her to elevate her hands at night.
   B. Have her buy a cock-up splint from the pharmacy.
   C. Instruct her on over-the-counter analgesics.
   D. Order a wrist x-ray to assess for trauma.

8. A woman in her third trimester is complaining of constipation. Which instruction by the nurse is best?
   A. "Because of the fetal location, this is difficult to treat."
   B. "Drink 8 glasses of water and increase your fiber daily."
   C. "Use little Fleets enemas when you are constipated."
   D. "You can use over-the-counter laxatives occasionally."

9. A woman complains that she feels dizzy and sweaty when she has been lying down for a few minutes. Which action by the nurse is best?
   A. Advise her to come in to the clinic today.
   B. Facilitate getting an order for an EKG.
   C. Instruct her to lie on her left side.
   D. Teach her to rest sitting in a recliner.

10. A nurse notes that a pregnant woman's chart states that she is having trouble binding in. Which action by the nurse is best?
   A. Ask the mother about preparation for the newborn at home.
   B. Demonstrate proper abdominal binding to prevent stretch marks.
   C. Discuss transition through the couvade with the woman and her partner.
   D. Talk to the mother about how she conceptualizes the child.

See Answers to End of Chapter Review Questions on *DavisPlus.*

REFERENCES

Beckmann, C. R. B., Herbert, W. N. P., Laube, D. W. Ling, F. W., & Smith, R. P. (2013). *Obstetrics and gynecology* (7th ed.). Philadelphia, PA: Lippincott Williams & Wilkins.

Callister, L. C., Matsumura, G., & Vehvilainnen-Julkunen, K. (2003). He's having a baby. The paternal childbirth experience. *Marriage & Families.* Retrieved from http://marriageandfamilies.byu.edu/issues/2003/January/baby.aspx

Chapman, L., & Durham, R. (2013). *Maternal-Newborn nursing: The critical components of nursing care* (2nd ed.). Philadelphia, PA: F.A. Davis.

Cunningham, F. G., Leveno, K. J., Bloom, S. L., Spong, C., Dashe, J., Hoffman, B., Casey, B., & Sheffield, J. (2014). Maternal physiology. In: *Williams obstetrics* (24th ed, pp. 107–135). New York, NY: McGraw-Hill Professional.

Duvall, E. M., & Miller, B. C. (1984). *Marriage and family development* (6th ed.). Philadelphia, PA: HarperCollins College Division.

Halperin, O., Raz, I., Ben-Gal, L., Or-Chen, K., & Granot, M. (2010). Prediction of perineal trauma during childbirth by assessment of striae gravidarum score. *Journal of Obstetric, Gynecologic & Neonatal Nursing, 39*(3), 292–297. doi:10.1111/j.1552-6909.2010.01137.x

Hanson, S., Hunter, L. P., Bormann, J. R., & Sobo, E. J. (2009). Paternal fears of childbirth: A literature review. *Journal of Perinatal Education, 18*(4), 12–20. doi:10.1624/105812409X474672

Lederman, R. (1996). *Psychosocial adaptation in pregnancy* (2nd ed.). New York, NY: Springer.

Lederman, R., & Weis, K. (2010). *Psychosocial adaptation to pregnancy: Seven dimensions of maternal role development* (3rd ed.). New York, NY: Springer.

Mattson, S., & Smith, J. E. (2010). *Core curriculum for maternal-newborn nursing* (4th ed.). St. Louis, MO: W.B. Saunders.

Mercer, R. (1995). *Becoming a mother.* New York, NY: Springer.

Mercer, R. (2004). Becoming a mother versus maternal role attainment. *Journal of Nursing Scholarship, 36*(3), 226–233.

Oakes, D. F. (2010). *Oakes' hemodynamic monitoring: A bedside reference manual* (5th ed.). (2010). Orono, ME: Health Educator Publications.

Paulson, J. F., & Bazemore, S. D. (2010). Prenatal and postpartum depression in fathers and its association with maternal depression. *Journal of the American Medical Association, 303*(19), 1961–1969.

Rubin, R. (1975). Maternal tasks in pregnancy. *MCN: The American Journal of Maternal-Child Nursing. 4*(3), 143–153.

Smeltzer, S. C., Bare, B. G., Hinkle, J. L., & Cheever, K. H. (2012). *Brunner & Suddarth's textbook of medical-surgical nursing.* (12th ed.). Philadelphia, PA: Lippincott Williams & Wilkins.

Van Leeuwen, A. M., Poelhuis-Leth, D., & Bladh, M. L. (2011). *Davis's comprehensive handbook of laboratory and diagnostic tests with nursing implications* (4th ed.). Philadelphia, PA: F.A. Davis.

Weiss, R. E. (2012). Old Wives Tales & Pregnancy Myths. Retrieved from http://pregnancy.about.com/cs/myths/a/aa042299.htm

Williams, L. S., & Hopper, P. D. (2011). *Understanding medical-surgical nursing* (4th ed.). Philadelphia, PA: F.A. Davis.

CONCEPT MAP

Reproductive System

Uterus/Cervix:
- Change in size/shape
  - Enlarges and stretches
- Braxton Hicks contractions
- Chadwick's sign
- Formation of operculum
- Leukorrhea
- Goodell's sign

Vagina:
- Chadwick's sign
- Change in pH

Ovaries:
- Initial progesterone from corpus luteum
- Cessation of ovulation

Breasts:
- Enlarge; increased sensitivity
- Areola darkens; presence of pre-colostrum
- Tender/pronounced nipples
- Striae

Endocrine:
- Increased BMR
- Pituitary → FSH and LH make pregnancy possible; suppressed after conception
- Lactation → oxytocin, prolactin
- Oxytocin—"let-down" reflex
- Increased PTH concentration
- hPL → acts as fetal growth hormone

Neurological:
- Decreased attention, concentration, memory
- Carpal tunnel syndrome
- Syncope
- Altered sleep pattern

Integumentary:
- Change in pigmentation
  - Linea nigra
  - Chloasma
- Hyperactive sweat and sebaceous glands
- Striae gravidarum
- Angiomas; palmar erythema
- New hair growth
- Stronger nails

Respiratory:
- Increase in tidal volume; tidal capacity
- Change in diaphragmatic excursion
- Hypertrophy and hyperplasia of lung tissue

Gastrointestinal:
- 1st trimester nausea/vomiting
- Epulis gravidarum and ptyalism
- +/– glucosuria: (abnormal finding)
- Heartburn
- Hemorrhoids
- Predisposition to cholelithiasis

Cardiovascular:
- Increased maternal blood volume/cardiac output; pseudoanemia
- Increased numbers of leukocytes; depressed function
- Dilutional hypoalbumin-emia
- Increased supine hypotension syndrome/orthostatic hypotension
- Increased need for iron
- Increased risk for varicose veins

Musculoskeletal:
- Separation of rectus abdominis
- Lumbar lordosis
  - Lower back pain
- Potential changes in serum calcium levels
- Separation of pubis symphysis

Urinary:
- Frequency, urgency, nocturia
- Increased risk for UTI
- Glucosuria

Hormonal Influences:
Major: Estrogen and Progesterone

Many Mediated By

Physiological Changes

Physiological and Psychosocial Changes During Pregnancy

Psychosocial Changes

Factors Affecting Adaptation:
- Absence of significant others
- Pregnancy in adolescence
- Cultural and societal influences
- High-tech management
- Psychosocial reactions of other family members
  - Siblings
  - Grandparents

Family Adaptations:
- Reorganization of the home; realignment of duties
- Change in money management
- Interfamily role change: child to parent
- Incorporation of each new child into existing family structure

Maternal Adaptations:
- Incorporation of pregnancy into self-concept: binding in
- Unconditional acceptance of child by 3rd trimester
- Reorder relationships → accommodate child into family structure
- Learn to give of self
- Nesting
- Seek safe passage through pregnancy, labor, and birth
- Work through post-birth doubts

Paternal Adaptations:
- Varying degrees of reaction and involvement
  - Observer; expressive; instrumental
- Corresponding tasks: by trimesters
  - Announcement phase: acceptance
  - Moratorium phase: "binding in"
  - Focusing phase: increased involvement; role clarification
- Couvade syndrome

Factors That Interfere With Adaptation:
- Termination of pregnancy
  - Spontaneous abortion/elective termination
- Plan to relinquish child
- Loss of the "perfect" child
- Parental reactions to grief and loss

Optimizing Outcomes:
- Promote early paternal attachment through reflective journaling

? Now Can You:
- Identify the major physiological and psychosocial changes that occur during pregnancy

Cultural Diversity:
- Many cultural myths/tales exist that explain changes and negative outcomes that occur during pregnancy

The Prenatal Assessment

We are weaving the future on the loom of today.

—Grace Dawson

LEARNING TARGETS *At the completion of this chapter, the student will be able to:*

◆ Outline a schedule for and describe the benefits of prenatal care.

◆ Summarize the components of the first and subsequent prenatal visits in relation to history taking, physical assessment, and ongoing risk assessment.

◆ Discuss how nurses can empower women to become shared decision makers and active participants in planning their prenatal care.

◆ Recognize lifestyle choices that may be detrimental to maternal and fetal well-being.

◆ Differentiate presumptive, probable, and positive signs of pregnancy.

◆ Discuss aspects of prenatal care for the adolescent and for women over age 35.

PICO(T) Questions

The intent of evidence-based practice (EBP) is to provide nursing care that integrates the best available evidence. An initial step in EBP is to write a PICO(T) question that effectively guides the research. A PICO(T) question is an acronym that stands for population (P), intervention or issue (I), comparison of interest (C), outcome (O), and timeframe (T). Depending on the question, all or some of the question components are used in the research process. Use these

PICO(T) questions to spark your thinking as you read the chapter.

1. What (O) reasons do (P) pregnant women give for choosing a certified nurse midwife as (C) compared with an obstetrician as (I) their care provider?

2. Do (P) womens' (I) beliefs about the necessity or value of comprehensive prenatal care (O) change based on (C) how many pregnancies they have experienced?

 Evidence-Based Practice

Ickovics, J. R., Reed, E., Margriples, U., Westdahl, C., Rising, S. S., & Kershaw, T. S. (2011). Effects of group prenatal care on psychosocial risk in pregnancy: Results from a randomized controlled trial. *Psychology and Health, 26*(2), 235–250.

The purpose of this study was to determine if a group prenatal care intervention, as compared with standard individual prenatal care, improves psychosocial outcomes. The researchers proposed that the implementation of an innovative group prenatal care model termed "*Centering Pregnancy Plus* (CP+)" would reduce negative birth outcomes, decrease sexual risk, and improve maternal psychosocial outcomes (e.g., increased self-esteem and social support and decreased stress, social conflict, and depression). It was also hypothesized that the CP+ intervention would have a greater effect

on women at high risk for adverse outcomes (e.g., younger age, African Americans, and persons reporting high levels of stress). Previous studies have found that patients who receive care using the CP+ model experienced reduced rates of pregnancy-related risks, preterm birth, rapid repeat pregnancy, and unprotected sex occasions, increased breastfeeding and condom use, and reported increased satisfaction with their prenatal care.

The framework for CP+ bundling of psychosocial health promotion within existing services has been shown to increase

(continued)

Evidence-Based Practice (continued)

accessibility and effectiveness of the intervention programs. CP+ bundling further provides a set number of regular prenatal visits, allowing for multiple interventions and opportunities to target multiple behaviors in a cost effective, sustainable manner. Target behaviors may include health promotion (e.g., nutrition, safe sex, and breastfeeding) as well as risk reduction (e.g., a decrease in depression and STD risk).

This study employed a randomized controlled trial and included 1,047 pregnant women ages 14 to 25 years of age. Participants were selected from two university affiliated public hospital prenatal clinics located in two different states. Recruitment criteria for participation included the following: English or Spanish speaking, less than 24 weeks gestation, age less than or equal to 25 years, and no evidence of medical problems that would require individual high-risk care. Maternal baseline interviews were conducted at an average of 18 gestational weeks.

Eighty percent of the participants identified themselves as African American, 13% as Latina, 6% as White, and 1% described themselves as "mixed ethnicity." The average age was 20.4 years, approximately one-half (49%) was between 14 and 19 years of age, and 51% were between 20 and 25 years of age. The participants were randomly assigned to one of three groups: standard individual care (IC), *Centering Pregnancy*—group prenatal care (CP), or *Centering Pregnancy Plus*—integrated group prenatal care intervention (CP+). Participants were randomly assigned based on an allocation goal of 40% to the IC group and 30% each to the CP and CP+ groups.

A trained prenatal care provider (certified nurse midwife or obstetrician) provided the CP+ interventions, which included the physical assessment(s), education/skills building, and support. A structured curriculum consisted of 10 sessions lasting 120 minutes each. Participants engaged in self-care activities, (i.e., weight and blood pressure assessment) and participated in discussion groups to address issues related to prenatal care, birth preparation, postpartum care, HIV prevention, and mental health or psychosocial functioning. The groups consisted of 8 to 12 women. Skill building and goal setting were important parts of the group activities. The prenatal care model used with the CP group was identical to that used with the CP+ group with one exception: the extent to which HIV prevention, assertiveness and negotiation skills were covered (i.e., these components were increased with the CP+ group). Participants assigned to the IC group met on the same prenatal care schedule and received the same number of visits as did the CP and CP+ groups. However, the IC group received "traditional"

individual prenatal care, and patient contact time for these visits averaged 10 to 15 minutes.

Structured interviews were conducted upon entry into the study using Audio-CASI, a touch screen–based, audio, computer-assisted, self-interviewing system. The literature supports and has validated the use of this type of interviewing modality to improve the quality of survey data from questionnaires and overcome respondents' limited literacy and incentives to misstate the answers to questions that may be regarded as sensitive. Follow-up interviews were conducted using the same method and occurred during the third trimester and at 6 and 12 months postpartum. The following measurement tools were also included: The Perceived Stress Scale (PSS) (assesses the degree to which participants perceive situations to be unpredictable and uncontrollable); a 10-item, self-reported, self-esteem tool; a 7-item social support subscale of the Social Relationship Scale (assesses perceived availability of support systems); a 7-item social conflict subscale of the Social Relationship Scale (assesses the perceived degree of social conflict in the person's everyday life); and a 15-item self-report scale that focused on affective components of the depressed mood and included feelings of failure, guilt, and hopelessness (assesses for current depressive symptoms). Demographics were also collected and included questions regarding both health-promoting and health-damaging behaviors.

Data analysis revealed that there were no significant differences in psychosocial function among the three groups. However, women in the top third of those who reported psychological stress at the study entry point indicated they had received a benefit from integrated group care (CP+). Those assigned to the CP+ group reported an increase in self-esteem and a decrease in stress and social conflict during the third trimester of pregnancy and a decrease in depression at the 1-year postpartum point, as compared with those in the IC group. The results showed no significant differences in intervention effectiveness when controlled for age and ethnicity. The researchers concluded that the CP+ bundled interventions have the potential to improve psychosocial outcomes when implemented with vulnerable and underserved pregnant women.

1. How is this information useful to clinical nursing practice?

2. Based on these findings, what are implications for further research?

See Suggested Responses for Evidence-Based Practice on Davis*Plus*.

Introduction

The objective of this chapter is to enhance understanding of the complexities and challenges involved in providing individualized, competent prenatal nursing care. The information presented serves as a knowledge base and introduction to clinical skills while promoting critical thinking and empathetic understanding. Framed in the nursing role,

various components of the prenatal assessment throughout pregnancy are explored.

Each prenatal visit offers an opportunity for the nurse to provide a comforting, supportive environment for the expectant woman and her family members. During these visits, educational needs can be identified and addressed, concerns can be discussed, reassurance can be provided, and problems or potential problems can be discovered.

Promoting maternal physical, psychological, and spiritual health and facilitating maternal empowerment are key to promoting and enhancing fetal well-being and a positive pregnancy outcome.

A Time of Wonder and Growth . . . and Ambivalence

For most women, pregnancy is a special time of wonder and personal growth. However, when faced with a positive pregnancy test result, many women experience ambivalence or begin to question their desire to be pregnant. This reaction is a normal response that occurs irrespective of how determined and committed the couple is to the goal of beginning or expanding a family. Part of the ambivalence relates to the sudden realization that life as it has been known is going to change dramatically and this change will be a lifelong endeavor. The woman especially can anticipate role changes in relation to her career and relationships and a need to prepare for the role of being a mother to an infant who will be dependent on her for survival. Recognizing ambivalence and its normalcy in relation to pregnancy during the first trimester and providing support and reassurance are essential in helping the woman positively embrace and celebrate her journey into motherhood.

Concerns Over Self-Preservation

Pregnancy also raises issues of maternal self-preservation. Despite tremendous improvements in perinatal care, women still die in childbirth, and it is not unrealistic for a woman to fear for her own safety. The World Health Report "Make Every Woman and Every Child Count" (World Health Organization [WHO], 2005) focuses on making pregnancy safer and asserts that reaching this goal centers on providing excellent antenatal care and constructing societies that support pregnant women. Antenatal care must be consistently accessible and responsive while incorporating patient-centered interventions, thereby removing barriers that prevent access to care. Perhaps one of the most significant roles that nurses can play in helping to achieve this important goal lies in promoting optimal prenatal care for all women (International Association for Impact Assessment, 2012).

Women who receive prenatal care experience a five-fold decrease in pregnancy-related maternal deaths and have better pregnancy outcomes than those who do not receive prenatal care. Prenatal care should offer the patient evidence-based medical and nursing care together with an educational program specifically designed to meet that patient's needs. This approach to care enables informed and shared decision making (Kirkham, Harris, & Grzybowski, 2005).

Health care should begin during the preconception period and continue throughout the pregnancy and puerperium. Firmly grounded in an understanding of the physical, emotional, and psychological changes characteristic of the childbearing period, prenatal care should be focused on the early identification of deviations from the normal. Ideally, screening procedures are conducted where warranted, health maintenance and promotion are emphasized, and psychological

support to facilitate optimal maternal and fetal outcomes is provided in a culturally sensitive setting. An integral aspect of all prenatal nursing care involves actively listening to the woman, providing individualized education, and respecting her choices. The woman has the right to expect continuity of care, clear explanations, consistent information, and the opportunity to discuss any aspect of her care at any time (Haire, 2000) (Fig. 9-1). A number of nursing diagnoses are applicable during the prenatal period. These are often related to maternal health-seeking behaviors (i.e., "health-seeking behaviors related to guidelines for activity and nutrition during pregnancy") and family support and coping (Box 9-1).

 Nursing Insight—Goals that guide nursing care of the prenatal patient

When providing care for the prenatal patient, essential nursing goals are:
- To recognize deviations from normal
- To provide individualized, evidence-based care

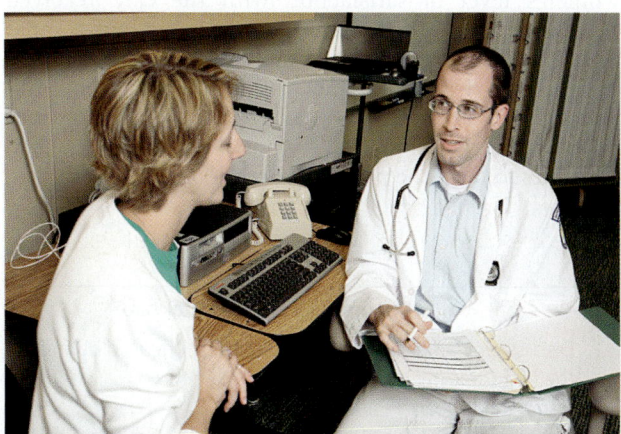

Figure 9-1 Actively listening to the patient and providing individualized education is an essential component of prenatal care.

Box 9-1 Possible Nursing Diagnoses for the Prenatal Patient

- Knowledge Deficit related to normal physiological changes of pregnancy
- Altered Nutrition Risk: less than body requirement
- Risk for Fatigue
- Risk for Disturbance in Body Image
- Risk for Altered Role Performance
- Altered sexual patterns
- Family coping
- Change in comfort level related to advancing pregnancy
- Change in sleep patterns
- Altered urinary elimination due to enlarging uterus or engagement of fetal part
- Anxiety
- Adolescent
- Family processes, altered

Source: Adapted from Doenges, Geissler-Murr & Moorhouse (2010).

- To provide culturally appropriate prenatal education designed to meet the patient's learning style and needs
- To empower women to become actively involved in their pregnancy by being informed recipients and shared decision makers

Prenatal care usually begins in the first trimester of pregnancy, when the patient is seen every 4 weeks until she reaches 28 to 32 weeks' gestation. At that time, the appointments are changed to visits every 2 weeks and then occur weekly from 36 weeks of gestation until birth. Although this schedule has to some extent become the "standard of care," it has not been possible to substantiate the necessity for such frequent visits. Interestingly, the number of total prenatal visits varies tremendously from as few as 3 to 4 visits for low-risk women in some European countries to 14 or more visits for women with uncomplicated pregnancies in the United States (Partridge & Holman, 2005).

A recent meta-analysis revealed that a reduction in the total number of prenatal visits did not negatively affect maternal or infant outcomes but did negatively affect the women's level of satisfaction with the care received (Drowswell et al., 2011). Based on these findings, a more patient-centered approach to care for low-risk women may entail fewer visits with a medical provider and more frequent visits with a nursing team who can provide continuity of care, psychological support, and individualized strategies to meet the patient's educational needs (Collins, 2012).

 Now Can You—Discuss aspects of prenatal care?

1. Discuss why ambivalence is frequently experienced during the first trimester?
2. Name three goals of prenatal care?
3. Describe the common prenatal visit schedule for a low-risk pregnancy?

Navigating the Health-Care System

A woman's initial contact with the health-care system may occur when she first seeks prenatal care. Attempts to navigate the system while becoming familiar with health insurance or Medicaid coverage can result in an overwhelming, frightening experience. Many women have no financial resources for maternity care or for health care of any kind. Despite recent changes in legislation, more than 49 million Americans remain without any source of health-care insurance at last count in 2010 (U.S. Census Bureau, 2011). For uninsured women, pregnancy can create a major financial stress because health care for a single pregnancy may well exceed $20,000, depending on the type of birth and the development of complications.

CAREing for the Patient

Throughout the childbearing experience, the nurse's primary role is to "CARE" for the patient. The "CARE" principle centers on communicating, advocating, respecting

and enabling/empowering the individual (Box 9-2). Some patients find both the health-care system and the health-care staff to be intimidating and nonreceptive when they attempt to voice concerns, doubts, or desires. There is a lack of effective communication between the patient and the nurse. When this occurs, many women adopt what is perceived as the "typical patient role"—one in which the patient simply does as requested without question. Unfortunately, nurses sometimes have a tendency to facilitate and reinforce this behavior.

The nurse's role encompasses that of being an advocate for the patient. An advocate verbalizes the patient's wishes if the patient is unable to do so herself and ensures that the patient's questions are answered in an understandable and comprehensive way. It is also the advocate's responsibility to help the patient to become an informed recipient of care. Respecting the patient involves valuing her as an individual, listening attentively, and addressing all of her concerns.

 Optimizing Outcomes—**Being an advocate for the patient**

The nurse is the ideal person to be an advocate for the pregnant patient. An advocate is a person who supports and represents the rights and interests of another individual to ensure the individual's full legal rights and access to services.

The nurse has the knowledge base to educate the patient and inform her of safe options or alternatives to meet her particular needs. The nurse also has the skills to communicate effectively with the patient, her family members, and her care provider. Thus, the nurse facilitates shared decision making and helps to promote patient satisfaction with the health-care services received.

An informed recipient of care is an individual who has been made aware of available health-care options and the possible consequences or outcomes of the choices made.

Box 9-2 CARE Principles

Communication
  The exchange of information between individuals, for example, by means of speaking, writing, or using a common system of signs or behavior
  A spoken or written message
  The communicating of information
  A sense of mutual understanding and sympathy

Advocate
  One who argues for a cause; a supporter or defender
  One who pleads in another's behalf; an intercessor: Advocates for abused children and spouses

Respect
  To feel or show admiration and deference toward somebody or something
  To pay due attention to and refrain from violating something
  To show consideration or thoughtfulness in relation to somebody or something

Enable
  To provide somebody with the resources, authority, or opportunity to do something
  To make something possible or feasible

Source: National Patient Advocate Foundation (2010).

Thus, the informed pregnant woman is able to discuss the advantages and disadvantages of various screening tools, diagnostic tests, and treatment options, and she is empowered to make an informed choice that is right for her and her family. For the nurse, an important aspect of the advocate role involves remaining nonjudgmental and able to listen and respond accurately and objectively.

As health-care professionals, nurses need to empower women by caring, actively listening, and recognizing their inner wisdom, strength, and abilities. In so doing, nurses gain insights to help them meet their patient's needs in relation to education; health promotion; and physical, psychological, emotional, and spiritual support. The pregnant woman has a journey ahead of her that should lead to greater self-understanding, enhanced feelings of self-worth, and the knowledge that she has the internal power to succeed.

Diminishing Stress and Improving Pregnancy Outcomes

Pregnancy is a developmental crisis that necessitates role adaptation and a restructuring of the tasks involved in daily living. It is a life-changing event that requires adjustments to the many physical and emotional changes that will take place. By nature, change is associated with stress. Eustress is defined as a normal, healthy level of stress. Most individuals are equipped with the resources needed to readily deal with eustress. However, when perceived stress exceeds the individual's resources, strategies, and abilities to effectively deal with it, the person moves into a state of distress.

Nursing Insight—*Diminishing maternal stress*

Women release oxytocin as a response to stress and when they engage in "tend and befriend" activities with friends. Oxytocin appears to buffer the stress response and produces a calming effect. This physiological response to engagement in friendship behaviors helps women to dissipate stress (Cardoso, Ellenbogen, Serravalle, & Linnen, 2013; Saphire-Bernstein, Way, Kim, Sherman, & Taylor, 2011). From a nursing perspective, there are a number of ways in which this information can be used. One strategy is to incorporate continuity of care, so that as the patient sees the same nursing staff throughout pregnancy, a professional relationship develops. This bond helps the patient to develop a sense of being cared for, appreciated, and known as an individual by her care providers. Ultimately, this simple action can help to reduce maternal stress.

Maternal stress during pregnancy can be associated with difficulty accessing care. Transportation problems, appointment schedules that conflict with work commitments, and personal or family member illness may prevent the woman from keeping her prenatal appointments. Communication difficulties, perceptions of staff disinterest, and a lack of understanding about the importance of frequent prenatal visits are all potential sources of stress that may diminish the patient's ability to comply with the plan of care. By using an individualized approach with a focus on communication, personalized care, and education, nurses may help to reduce the patient's stress and increase her adherence to the care plan.

Pregnancy is a time of entering the unknown. The pregnant woman faces unpredictability and quite possibly the loss of control. Because the course of the pregnancy may differ from the anticipated experience, women need to be able to adapt to unexpected situations and meet unforeseen challenges as the pregnancy advances. The new stressors associated with pregnancy can become a deterrent to seeking or continuing prenatal care. Therefore, nurses must be cognizant of the fact that women, irrespective of culture, may face different stressors and often require a variety of resources and interventions to help them deal effectively with stress and improve their utilization of prenatal care.

Racial disparities exist in the provision and use of prenatal care. The effects of these discrepancies on pregnancy outcomes have been recognized for more than 90 years. One of the goals of the *Healthy People 2020* national initiative is to address these racial disparities and to increase the uptake of prenatal care in the first trimester of pregnancy for all women to 78% (a 10% increase from the previous baseline of 71%). By using the "CARE" principles, the nurse can provide individualized support to all patients irrespective of race or culture.

As an advocate, nurses can provide information about stress management for their patients. Social support is an important and positive factor in the reduction of stress (Fig. 9-2). If the pregnant woman has a good social support system, she is much more likely to have a venue to discuss issues of concern and gain morale support. It is important to note that a support system may be lacking for women who are trying to conceal a pregnancy or for women who are trying to keep the news of their pregnancy from relatives or friends until results from genetic tests are known. These individuals may need additional support from their nurses and other health-care providers as they are placed in a powerless situation while awaiting results and face a pregnancy that may be in jeopardy.

Where Research and Practice Meet:
Text Messaging to Promote Prenatal Care for At-Risk Patients

Pelletier and colleagues (2012) conducted a small-scale pilot study to determine the usefulness of text messaging as a tool to improve at-risk patient participation in their prenatal care. A group of 25 young (average age 22 years) at-risk pregnant patients in the first or second trimester were enrolled to receive text messages throughout pregnancy. The frequency of messages was limited to no more than three per week, and messages were personalized to each patient based on date of enrollment, language preference (English or Spanish), and last menstrual period. Message content was related to fetal development and childbirth preparation and encouraged newborn and postpartum care. At the conclusion of the study, all participants indicated that they had read most or all of the messages, 84% said the program helped them learn to take care of themselves and their baby, and 100% stated that they would recommend the program to other pregnant patients. Study findings underscore the value of text messaging to provide low-cost, multilingual communication that is easily delivered between visits. Nurses in various maternity settings may wish to implement a similar program using this modality to expand care provider reach and enhance at-risk patient engagement in their prenatal care.

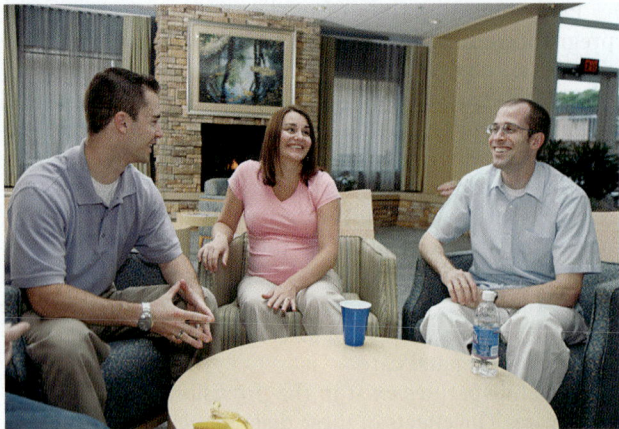

Figure 9-2 Social support helps to reduce maternal stress.

Choosing a Pregnancy Care Provider

One of the first maternal tasks of pregnancy as described by Rubin (1984) is "Ensuring safe passage." This stage encompasses the active lifestyle choices that the woman makes and the behaviors that she adopts to promote her own and her fetus's well-being. One of the early decisions the patient (and partner) makes concerns choosing a care provider. It is recommended that every patient arrange an appointment with a chosen care provider (obstetrician, family practice physician, or certified nurse midwife) to discuss the management of pregnancy and childbirth as early as possible within the first trimester. The woman may seek childbearing care from an obstetrician, a family practice physician, or a certified nurse midwife (CNM) who is educated in the disciplines of nursing and midwifery and is certified by the American College of Nurse-Midwives (Box 9-3).

Approximately 90% of pregnant women choose an obstetrician as the primary care provider. Others use a CNM who can provide a more personalized, less routine approach to a normal, uncomplicated pregnancy and birth.

Healthy women who choose a CNM are as likely as those who choose an obstetrician to have an excellent outcome, and they may also experience fewer medical interventions and a lower rate of cesarean births (Shaw-Battista, Fineberg, Boehler, Skubic, Woolley, & Tilton, 2011). Women who have complications related to the pregnancy or who are in a high-risk category should plan to meet with a perinatologist, an obstetrician with experience in managing high-risk pregnancies. The perinatologist works closely with the woman's obstetrician to determine the best plan for managing the pregnancy, labor, and birth.

A woman's journey through the pregnancy experience can have long-term effects on her self-perception and self-concept. Thus, it is especially important that the patient choose a care provider with whom she can openly relate and who shares the same philosophical views on the management of pregnancy. Continuity of prenatal care has been shown to be associated with increased maternal satisfaction and a need for fewer interventions during labor. The importance of developing a positive relationship with one's care provider and receiving personal, individualized care throughout the pregnancy is medically and psychologically advantageous (Hodnett, 2004, 2008; Hodnett, Gates, Hofmeyr, Sakala, & Weston, 2012).

During the initial interview with a care provider, it is helpful for the woman to discuss the provider's work schedule and how births that take place when the provider is not on call are managed. This is also an ideal time for the care provider to introduce the pregnant woman's Bill of Rights and to discuss the responsibilities the woman has to facilitate optimum health for herself and for her fetus (Appendix 9-1 in the Electronic Study Guide). Many pregnant women are not fully aware of their right of informed consent or of the obstetrician's legal obligation to obtain their patient's informed consent prior to treatment. The American College of Obstetricians and Gynecologists (ACOG) first publicly acknowledged the physician's legal obligation to obtain the pregnant patient's informed consent in its 1974 publication "Standards for Obstetric-Gynecological Services." The informed consent process is important in safeguarding the patient's autonomy (Box 9-4).

American patients are becoming increasingly aware that well-intentioned health professionals do not always have scientific data to support common American obstetric practices and that many of these practices are carried out primarily because they are part of medical and hospital

---

Box 9-3 Definition of Midwifery and Scope of Practice of Certified Nurse-Midwives and Certified Midwives

Midwifery as practiced by certified nurse-midwives (CNMs) and certified midwives (CMs) encompasses a full range of health-care services for women from adolescence beyond menopause. These services include the independent provision of primary care, gynecological and family planning services, preconception care, care during pregnancy, childbirth and the postpartum period, care of the normal newborn during the first 28 days of life, and treatment of male partners for sexually transmitted infections. Midwives provide initial and ongoing comprehensive assessment, diagnosis, and treatment. They conduct physical examinations; prescribe medications including controlled substances and contraceptive methods; admit, manage, and discharge patients; order and interpret laboratory and diagnostic tests, and order the use of medical devices. Midwifery care also includes health promotion, disease prevention, and individualized wellness education and counseling. These services are provided in partnership with women and families in diverse settings such as ambulatory care clinics, private offices, community and public health systems, homes, hospitals, and birth centers.

Source: American College of Nurse-Midwives (2012).

Box 9-4 Informed Consent and Communication

Informed consent is the willing and uncoerced acceptance of a medical intervention by a patient following the clinician's full disclosure of information that includes the nature of the intervention, the risks and benefits of the intervention, and the risks and benefits of any alternatives. The patient also has the right to informed refusal, that is, the right to refuse recommended medical treatment. Open, ongoing communication about relevant information empowers the patient to exercise personal choice and is central to the patient-clinician relationship.

Source: American College of Obstetricians and Gynecologists (ACOG). (2009). Informed consent. Committee Opinion No. 439. (Reaffirmed 2012). *Obstetrics & Gynecology 114*(5), 401–408.

tradition. More than 20 years ago, the distinguished obstetrician Dr. Roberto Caldeyro-Barcia articulated clearly his concerns with the medical management of low-risk pregnancy and delivery:

In the last 40 years, many artificial practices have been introduced that have changed childbirth from a physiological event to a very complicated medical procedure in which all kinds of drugs are used and procedures carried out, sometimes unnecessarily, and many of them potentially damaging for the baby and even for the mother (Haire, 2000).

A growing body of research makes it alarmingly clear that every aspect of traditional American hospital care during labor and birth must now be questioned as to its possible effect on the future well-being of both the obstetric patient and her unborn child. Care needs to be individualized to meet each patient's particular needs, and procedures performed only when the advantage to the patient outweighs any possible disadvantage.

The provision of prenatal care offers the nurse a unique opportunity to make a difference not only in the patient's life but also in the lives of her family. To truly take advantage of this opportunity, the nurse needs an expansive array of tools including the ability to communicate effectively with patients irrespective of cultural background, educational level, health-care beliefs, or age to understand family and group dynamics; and to accept diversity without prejudice or bias. Family care during the prenatal period centers on education and health promotion.

A number of issues affect a woman's willingness to use health-care services. These include personal beliefs about pregnancy, cultural expectations, previous relationships with health-care providers, and perceived benefits of prenatal care, together with the more practical issues of access to care, medical insurance, and/or financial support. By using therapeutic communication, the nurse can gain insights into the patient's belief system and manage care appropriately. Maintaining a nonjudgmental attitude is essential, for example, if the woman is a late recipient of prenatal care. Creating an atmosphere in which the patient feels accepted and valued for seeking care is a therapeutic, positive approach and one that will hopefully foster patient adherence.

Through discussion, the nurse can gain an understanding of the availability and acceptability of traditional health-care services and whether they meet the patient's individual health-care needs. Each culture embraces different customs and health practices that need to be respected, and wherever possible, accommodated. These requirements may relate to the gender of the health-care provider, the patient's clothing requirements, diet, and/or food preparation. The prenatal interview provides an opportunity to develop a positive relationship with the patient and emphasize the benefits of prenatal care for her and her unborn child.

In both the local and national arenas, nurses can empower women and their families by advocating for prenatal care that is readily available and affordable for all, especially for low-income and vulnerable populations. The "health-care safety net" is one mechanism for providing health services for the needy. Despite the availability of these types of programs, there are still women who receive inadequate or no prenatal care.

 ### *Across Care Settings:* The health-care safety net

The health-care safety net consists of a wide variety of providers who deliver care to low-income and other vulnerable populations, including the uninsured and those covered by Medicaid. Many of these providers have either a legal mandate or an explicit policy to provide services regardless of a patient's ability to pay.

Major safety net providers include public hospitals and community health centers as well as teaching and community hospitals, private physicians, and others who deliver a substantial amount of care to the targeted populations. Safety nets, which function in both metropolitan and rural settings, are locally organized and managed, serve unique local needs, and are specifically attuned to the needs of the populations they serve. Despite the recent passage of health-care legislation, it is estimated that close to 20 million people will likely remain uninsured and reliant on safety net care (Robert Wood Johnson Foundation, 2010).

 Now Can You—Discuss health promotion strategies for pregnancy?

1. Identify and describe each component of the "CARE" principle?
2. Discuss how stress adversely affects pregnancy and identify nursing interventions to help decrease patient stress?
3. Describe four important elements of a teaching plan for family health promotion during pregnancy?

The First Prenatal Visit

THE COMPREHENSIVE HEALTH HISTORY

Before initiating the interview, it is helpful for the nurse to review the paperwork to become familiar with the information to be gathered and to ensure an understanding of the relevance and appropriateness of the questions to be asked. The initial interview time with the patient should be used to build a positive, nonthreatening relationship and to gain her confidence. Strategies that are useful include active listening, validating responses when needed, maintaining eye-to-eye contact, and the use of humor as appropriate to relax the patient. Honesty is essential for effective communication. When uncertain of the answer to a question, the nurse should make a note to find the answer and report back to the patient at the end of the interview.

 Optimizing Outcomes—Employing caring communication skills to enhance the interview

The qualities of "comfort," "acceptance," "responsiveness," and "empathy" are essential components of caring communication skills. Comfort and acceptance refer to one's ability to deal with difficult topics without displaying uneasiness and accepting attitudes the patient brings to the interview without showing annoyance or intolerance. Responsiveness and empathy refer to the quality of reacting to indirect messages expressed by the patient (ACOG, 2011a). Empathetic listening helps the nurse to truly understand what the patient is actually saying. Using these skills helps to provide insights, enhances the nurse's understanding of the patient's point of view, and facilitates effective communication (Bartol, 2011).

The first prenatal visit is an extremely important one that should take place as early in pregnancy as possible. Therapeutic communication skills are of paramount importance when obtaining the prenatal history. The information requested can often be of a very personal nature, and it may be difficult for patients to disclose certain aspects of their past histories. Therefore, care must be taken to manage the environment to promote privacy and provide the patient with psychological and physical comfort.

It is important to avoid medical or technical jargon that may interfere with the patient's understanding, may intimidate her, or cause her to feel embarrassed because of a lack of comprehension. Questions should be phrased in a way to encourage the patient to discuss and share information rather than asking closed-ended questions that require only a "yes" or "no" response. The value the patient places on the care she receives and her interactions with personnel will determine whether she returns for subsequent prenatal care. Therefore, the prenatal team's objective is to provide a user-friendly service that is efficient, effective, caring, and patient centered. One major goal for this first visit is to explain the purpose of prenatal care and to establish specific goals. Care goals are determined through shared decision making with the patient and focus on promoting maternal and fetal health through assessment, education, screening, diagnosis, and treatment.

Family Teaching Guidelines...
"DEEPER CARE" for Promoting Family Health During Pregnancy

D	DIET	This is an ideal time to review the family diet and the way that foods are prepared. Encourage consumption of whole grains; dark green, yellow, and orange vegetables; dry beans and peas; a variety of fresh or dried/canned fruit; increased low-fat and fat-free foods; milk and calcium-rich foods; poultry; low-fat meats; fish that are lowest in mercury (whitefish, haddock, pollock, sole, and trout); nuts; and seeds.
E	EXERCISE	Aerobic exercise maintains physical fitness and promotes self-esteem and body image. It is a family activity that benefits all family members.
E	EDUCATION	Many childbirth education options are available to meet the needs of women and their families.
P	PLAY	Play is essential to health, happiness, and creativity. Fun family (couple) activities refresh, promote optimism, and provide an opportunity to "recharge and reconnect."
E	EXPECTATIONS	Pregnancy is a time of great expectations. Families need to know what changes are likely to occur and to be able to recognize normal from abnormal so they can recognize when to seek medical assistance.
R	RELAXATION	Relaxation benefits all family members by boosting immunity, lowering blood pressure, reducing stress, and increasing energy levels. Activities may include meditation, yoga, and visualization/positive thinking.
C	COMMUNICATION	Effective communication is essential to promote family cohesiveness. Communication includes both verbal and nonverbal language such as body posture, gestures, facial expressions, and tone of voice. Within the family, communication needs to be open and truthful and received in a nonjudgmental and accepting manner, ultimately affirming and supporting one another.
A	ATTITUDE	Positive thinking is under each individual's control but can be modeled. A positive attitude to life is associated with released stress, improved coping abilities, improved immunity, and a greater sense of well-being.
R	RESPECT	Healthy relationships require mutual respect, honesty, and trust. Compromise, negotiation, and shared responsibility are intrinsic to a positive relationship, as is equal distribution of power and control.
E	EMERGENCIES	Family members need to know the following danger signs of pregnancy and how to seek medical help:

- Reduction in fetal movements
- Signs of preterm labor such as low, dull backache, pelvic pressure feelings, uterine contractions, or menstrual cramps
- Vaginal fluid loss or vaginal bleeding
- Maternal fever over 100.5°F (38.1°C)
- Persistent headache associated with blurred vision or flashing lights in front of the eyes
- Continuous vomiting with weight loss, dehydration, weakness, dizziness, or fainting
- Couple has an "inner feeling that something is just not right." It is always better to confirm normality rather than deal with an avoidable emergency.

Biographical Data

Collection of the patient's biographical data, medical history, psychosocial history, and a medical examination are essential components of the first visit. To facilitate the collection of data, a number of prenatal forms such as the Prenatal Plus Program—Initial Assessment Form are available. This is a particularly in-depth and user-friendly tool produced by the Colorado Department of Public Health and Environment. This risk assessment form allows for the collection of information relating to the patient's pregnancy history, medical history, nutritional and exercise patterns, financial income, vocational and educational goals, living arrangements, psychosocial history (includes depression and past suicidal tendencies), and lifestyle choices. It also provides an opportunity for the patient to request educational information on a variety of topics.

Completing the prenatal history form with the patient enables the nurse to provide personalized education that focuses on risk factors pertinent to that individual. For example, it may be appropriate to discuss the maternal and fetal effects of environmental substances to which the woman is exposed at home and in the workplace. Common offenders include exposure to cigarette smoke (either directly or passively), alcohol consumption, recreational drugs, poor or inadequate diet, pollutants, viruses, and occupational hazards. It is estimated that approximately 10% of fetal malformations are related to exposure to environmental hazards (Silbergeld & Patrick, 2005).

The history should also include information concerning complementary and alternative therapies. An increasing number of individuals routinely use herbal or homeopathic remedies. Some of these substances, such as red raspberry tea, are safe and may be beneficial; others such as blue cohosh may be harmful if taken during pregnancy. Thus, it is essential to explore all nonprescription medications and supplements used.

 ### Complementary Care: *Red Raspberry and Blue Cohosh*

For centuries, the leaves of the red raspberry plant (*Rubus idaeus*) have been used as a medicinal herb for menstrual problems, pregnancy, childbirth, and breastfeeding. Safe to use during pregnancy, raspberry leaf is believed to aid fertility, ease the symptoms of morning sickness, and assist with the birth of

 Where Research and Practice Meet:
Alcohol Consumption During Pregnancy

Cheng and colleagues (2011) examined data collected from a random sample of 12,611 mothers over a 7-year period to determine the prevalence of prenatal alcohol consumption and the extent of provider screening and discussion about alcohol use during pregnancy. The researchers found that 1 out of 5 pregnant women did not get screened for alcohol consumption, and 1 out of 3 did not receive information about the effects of alcohol on the pregnancy. Interestingly, the lack of provider screening and counseling occurred most often among women who had the highest prevalence of self-reported alcohol consumption during pregnancy. Findings from this study underscore the importance of initial and ongoing prenatal screening for alcohol consumption and education regarding the harmful effects of alcohol use during pregnancy (Cheng, Kettinger, Uduhiri, & Hurt, 2011).

the baby and the placenta (Kennedy, Lupattelli, Koren, & Nordeng, 2013; Morris, 2013).

Blue cohosh (*Caulophyllum thalictroides*) belongs to the Barberry family. It also has a long history of use as a medicinal herb. It was known as "papoose root" and used by the American Indians to induce labor or abortion. Blue cohosh should be avoided during pregnancy—it has been linked with cardiovascular emergencies in the woman and anoxia in the fetus (Dugoua, 2010).

The biographical information usually includes contact information for the patient such as address, phone number(s), occupation and educational level, marital/relationship status, insurance data, and contact person information. Some forms also contain a section for recording special requests such as spiritual or cultural considerations. To ensure currency, it is important to reconfirm contact information at least every 2 months throughout the pregnancy. Maintaining a reliable and timely means for contacting the patient (e.g., to discuss screening or test results) is essential.

 Optimizing Outcomes—Caring for the woman who is a Jehovah's Witness

The Jehovah's Witnesses are a branch of Christianity whose adherents are opposed to blood transfusion. Identifying a patient as a Jehovah's Witness is an essential key step in her prenatal care. Ideally, at the first prenatal visit or soon afterward, discussion should center on blood products that are acceptable to the patient and what alternatives are available. At this time, an information package that contains a refusal of blood transfusion, health-care proxy, and a plan of care should be provided to allow the woman an opportunity to thoughtfully consider her options and discuss the information with her family. At the following return visit, the signed paperwork should be given to the patient and kept on file in the office and hospital and made accessible to all staff members at any time. The plan of care should include a complete checklist of products and alternatives (e.g., blood, fresh frozen plasma, cryoprecipitate, albumin) that she is willing to accept or decline (Mirza & Gyamfi, 2010).

The woman's age and date of birth allow for easy recognition of potential risk factors (e.g., maternal age is one of the most commonly used indicators for initiating genetic testing). Teenage girls, who fall at the opposite end of the age spectrum, often need additional support and education throughout the prenatal period.

Social History

Together with the biographical details, additional information is obtained relating to the patient's educational level and occupation. These data help to establish the patient's socioeconomic group and may provide some indication of family income, standard of housing, and nutrition. Information regarding the patient's marital status is also obtained.

 ### Nursing Insight—*Homelessness and prenatal care*

Homelessness presents a significant barrier to receiving prenatal care. Homeless women may have fears related to acceptance, judgment, costs, and the philosophies and/or expectations of health-care providers (ACOG, 2013a; Bloom, Bednarzyk, Devitt, Renaulty, Teaman, & Van Loock, 2004; Zlotnick & Zerger, 2009). Nurses, especially those working in the community, need to advocate for homeless women and their children and explore avenues for bringing prenatal and child care in a non-threatening environment to those in need.

History of Intimate Partner Violence

Intimate partner violence (IPV), formerly known as domestic violence, is the most common form of violence experienced by women worldwide. In the United States, approximately one 1 of every 4 women has been a victim of severe physical violence by an intimate partner (Centers for Disease Control and Prevention [CDC], 2011a). During pregnancy, the reported incidence of physical abuse ranges from 4% to 30% (CDC, 2013a), and up to 45% of victims of intimate partner abuse before pregnancy continue to be abused during the pregnancy (Ludermir, Lewis, Valongueiro, Barreto de Araujo, & Araya, 2010; McFarlane, Campbell, Sharps, & Watson, 2002).

Shockingly, IPV may occur for the first time during pregnancy, or the nurse may identify evidence during the physical examination that is suspicious of ongoing physical abuse. It is estimated that every day at least three women in the United States die as a result of intimate partner violence. **Femicide,** the death of a woman resulting from an act of violence against that woman, is a surprisingly common cause of death among pregnant women in the United States (Bureau of Justice Statistics, 2012).

 Nursing Insight—*Long-term consequences associated with female sexual assault*

A number of long-term health effects, such as increased patient-reported symptoms, diminished levels of functional capacity, and diminished overall quality of life, have been associated with female sexual assault. Frequently, victims are reluctant to divulge a history of childhood or adult sexual abuse but are more likely to report various emotional difficulties such as depression, anxiety, anger, and gynecological problems such as chronic pelvic pain, dysmenorrhea, and sexual dysfunction than those without a history of sexual assault (ACOG, 2011b, 2011c).

IPV is a difficult subject to discuss, and the nurse may fear insulting or psychologically hurting the patient more. A nonthreatening approach is to ask patients directly whether they feel safe going home and whether they have been hurt physically, emotionally, or sexually by a past or present partner. If the partner has accompanied the woman to the prenatal visit, these questions are postponed until the nurse is alone with the patient, for obvious reasons.

An alternative method is to use a standardized form that has valid and reliable questions concerning IPV. The form could be incorporated into the intake assessment data obtained from all patients. Women who have been sexually abused as children are at greater risk of IPV in adult relationships. Sequelae of abuse include depression, anxiety, substance abuse, and posttraumatic stress disorder. As a women's advocate, nurses have a duty to be observant, to

actively listen, and to use communication skills to gain clarification and understanding. The Centers for Disease Control and Prevention (CDC) have adopted the acronym "RADAR," a term originally developed by the Massachusetts Medical Society (Alpert, Freud, Park, Patel, & Sovak, 1992) to guide nurses as they interview patients about relationship violence:

- Routinely screen every patient
- Ask directly, kindly, and in a nonjudgmental manner
- Document your findings
- Assess the patient's safety
- Review options and provide referrals

 Nursing Insight—*Screening for intimate partner violence*

Intimate partner violence during pregnancy is more common than preeclampsia or gestational diabetes. Each year, approximately 324,000 pregnant women are abused by their intimate partner, and that number increases by a factor of 2 to 4 if the pregnancy was unplanned (CDC, 2011a; Gazmararian et al., 2000). Intimate partner violence can occur for a first time during pregnancy. Screening should be available to all pregnant women irrespective of social class or educational background.

Nurses need to promote screening for intimate partner violence so that it becomes a routine part of prenatal care. Universal screening for psychosocial factors, including partner abuse, as recommended by the ACOG (2006) has been shown to be associated with improved pregnancy outcomes. Coker and colleagues (2012) found that prenatal patients who received psychosocial screening had fewer maternal complications and were less likely to give birth to low birth weight or preterm infants.

Women may use a number of defenses to emotionally deal with abuse. One method may involve the use of recreational drugs. Irrespective of a history of intimate partner abuse, it is estimated that approximately 3% of pregnant women use

 Where Research and Practice Meet:
The SATELLITE Sexual Violence Assessment and Care Guide for Perinatal Patients

Sexual violence (SV) includes childhood sexual abuse and adult sexual assault. Noting the myriad of poor pregnancy outcomes (e.g., third trimester bleeding, preeclampsia, and preterm birth) related to SV and barriers to screening (e.g., the health-care provider's lack of comfort with or knowledge about how to screen and intervene and the patient's reluctance to disclose information), Ross and colleagues (2009) developed a tool specifically designed to overcome the barriers. The "SATELLITE Sexual Violence Assessment and Care Guide for Patients in the Perinatal Period" leads health-care practitioners through the process of setting the context for SV screening and providing the screening. The tool also offers interventions (including specific questions to ask and specific statements to make) after a positive screen finding and when providing care for an SV survivor. The use of this guide in the clinical setting enables nurses to increase their feelings of comfort and confidence as they assess and care for SV survivors during the perinatal period (Ross, Roller, Rusk, Martsolf, & Draucker, 2009).

nonprescription drugs such as cocaine, amphetamines, heroin, marijuana, or ecstasy (March of Dimes, 2011). Illegal or recreational drug use can have a number of detrimental effects (e.g., spontaneous abortion, low birth weight, placental abruption, and preterm labor) on maternal and fetal health during pregnancy. Selected recreational drugs and their effects on the pregnancy and the infant are presented in Table 9-1.

The nurse's role is to promote a healthy lifestyle for both the woman and her developing fetus. Recreational drug use puts both patients at increased risk, not only from the direct effects of the drugs, but also from the behaviors needed to procure and maintain the supply of drugs. Women using drugs are more likely to have poor nutritional status, and

they are more prone to infection because of a lack of skin integrity and increased exposure to infective agents such as those responsible for sexually transmitted infections. Sex may be used as a bargaining tool or as a means of income to support a drug habit.

Developing a therapeutic nonjudgmental relationship with a drug-addicted woman is essential to provide education, support, and guidance. The majority of expectant women wish to do the best they can for their babies, so pregnancy is an ideal time to direct the woman to drug counseling, support groups, and medical care with the goal of reducing and eventually stopping the habit. For a woman to be successful in overcoming drug addiction, she must be internally motivated. The course to success with

Table 9-1 Effects of Recreational Drug Use in Pregnancy

Name	Street Name	Route	Effect	Pregnancy	Newborn
Methamphetamines	Meth Crank	Smoked Snorted	Stimulant	Spontaneous abortion	Withdrawal Tremors
Dextroamphetamine	Speed Ice	Swallowed Injected Inhaled		Prematurity Breastfeeding not recommended	Poor muscle tone ↑SIDS
Cocaine	Coke	Inhaled	Stimulant	Spontaneous abortion	Birth defects—abnormalities of brain, skull, face, eyes, heart, limbs, intestines, genitals, and urinary tract
		Smoked		Placental abruption Preterm birth Breastfeeding not recommended	Neonatal withdrawal Visual disturbances Delay in cognitive and/or learning ability
Ecstasy	E, Adam, Roll, Bean, X, XTC, Clarity, Essence, Stacy, Lover's Speed, Eve	Pill form usually swallowed	Stimulant	Spontaneous abortion	Congenital abnormalities—cleft palate
(MDMA—compound may contain amphetamines and hallucinogens)		Crushed and Snorted	Mood enhancer	Placental abruption Preterm birth	Low birth weight
		Injected per rectum (known as "shafting") Smoked			Rats exposed to ecstasy showed memory and learning deficiencies
Marijuana Cannabis	Pot Weed Grass Mary Jane	Ingested Smoked Snorted Injected	Stimulant Psychedelic Depressant	Intrauterine growth restriction Low maternal weight gain, anemia	Adverse effects on neonatal neurobehavior (e.g., hyperirritability, tremors, photosensitivity) May cause decrease in verbal ability and memory, plus lower impulse control
Heroin	Boy, brown, china white, dragon, gear, H, horse, junk, skag, smack	Swallowed	Sedative	Spontaneous abortion Intrauterine growth restriction Preterm labor/birth Stillbirth	Neonatal withdrawal syndrome

Sources: March of Dimes (2011); Organization of Teratology Information Specialists (OTIS) (2011).

this problem is not an easy one, and the nurse can be instrumental in helping her to achieve this goal.

Psychological Assessment

Pregnancy is a time of change, and usually change of any nature is linked with additional stress. How an individual deals with stress depends on learned behaviors, coping mechanisms, and support systems. Pregnancy is a major life change or developmental phase for all women. Each woman's approach to her pregnancy encompasses cultural values and family traditions and beliefs. One's status in relation to marriage or partnership, financial security, career, or educational achievements is influential in shaping the overall childbearing experience. Past obstetric experiences including pregnancy outcomes, interactions with care providers, and level of physical health during and after pregnancy are instrumental in forming the woman's attitude toward this pregnancy. The loss of a previous pregnancy may adversely affect a woman's ability to bond with her present pregnancy. Understandably, she may be reluctant to invest in a pregnancy that she fears may not come to fruition. In other situations, acceptance of pregnancy may be delayed if it was unplanned or unwanted. Ambivalence is a normal initial reaction to pregnancy that usually diminishes as the woman accomplishes the developmental tasks of pregnancy.

Although the developmental tasks of pregnancy may be reviewed in a systematic way, it is important to remember that each woman is an individual who harbors a host of unique medical and psychological factors. For example, a woman with a history of a previous eating disorder may experience difficulty maintaining a healthy diet and achieving appropriate weight gain during pregnancy. Another woman may have struggled with anxiety and depression, alcohol or drug use, or issues related to domestic violence prior to pregnancy. These are all factors that can have a significant impact on the prenatal course. Many tools such as "The Edinburgh Postnatal Depression Scale" are available to guide the nurse in conducting the prenatal and postpartal psychological assessment. (See Chapter 16 for further discussion.)

THE OBSTETRIC HISTORY

Previous Pregnancies

One of the first steps in the prenatal interview process is to obtain an accurate and detailed obstetric history that provides the interviewer with essential information so that questions can be formulated and asked in a manner that respects and acknowledges the patient's past experiences with pregnancy. The history should cover the current pregnancy and all previous pregnancies and their outcomes because complications experienced in a prior pregnancy often reoccur in subsequent pregnancies.

A history of preterm labor and delivery, defined as a birth that occurs before the 37th completed week of pregnancy, provides one example of the importance of the obstetric history in identifying potential problems during the current pregnancy. Preterm labor is the leading cause of perinatal mortality and morbidity in the United States, where the incidence is 11%, although this figure is much lower (5%) in some European countries including France and Finland. Once a woman has experienced a preterm birth, her risk of preterm labor in subsequent pregnancies is increased

by 20% to 40%. Although the etiology for this condition remains largely unknown, there are a number of predisposing factors. Education, resources, and early interventions are important strategies because earlier diagnosis means earlier treatment and better outcomes. (See Chapter 11 for further discussion.)

A previous history of preeclampsia increases the woman's likelihood of a recurrence during subsequent pregnancies. (See Chapter 11 for further discussion.) Interestingly, if a woman did not experience preeclampsia with previous pregnancies but has a new partner for her current pregnancy, her risk of developing preeclampsia is similar to that of a woman who is pregnant for a first time. Although preeclampsia is a systemic disorder that occurs only during pregnancy, it is generally recognized via two classic symptoms: elevated blood pressure and proteinuria. The complication of preeclampsia places both the patient and her fetus at additional risk both during pregnancy and in the postpartum period.

A history of pregnancy-related diabetes or gestational diabetes mellitus (GDM) (carbohydrate intolerance that occurs during pregnancy) is also significant. GDM is estimated to affect up to 7% of pregnancies, and approximately one-half of women who have had a previous pregnancy affected by GDM will develop this condition again in a subsequent pregnancy (ACOG, 2011d). Because GDM is associated with a number of fetal and maternal complications, early screening is essential. (See Chapter 11 for further discussion.)

Patients who indicate a pattern of repeated spontaneous miscarriages most likely would benefit from genetic counseling, preferably during the preconception period. A family pedigree is often useful in determining the need for further screening and specific testing. Prenatal genetic screening questionnaires have been developed to guide counseling and intervention approaches. The Human Genome Project, completed in April 2003, provided information useful in facilitating the early diagnosis of genetic disorders and the timely initiation of medical care. For example, in April 2003, the gene for Hutchinson-Gilford Progeria Syndrome (HGPS) was identified. This finding prompted the development of a genetic test for the early diagnosis of the syndrome. In 2012, researchers identified several genes that are linked to serous endometrial cancer, one of the most lethal forms of uterine cancer. Three specific genes found in the study are frequently altered in the rare disease, suggesting that the genes prompt the development of tumors (National Human Genome Research Institute, 2013). Because of the rapid advances in the field of genetics, nurses must have a working knowledge of genetics terminology and recent findings so that they can initiate referrals when appropriate. The "Core Competencies in Genetics Essential for All Health Care Professionals" is a useful document with which all perinatal nurses should be familiar (Appendix 9-2 in the Electronic Study Guide).

🌼 **Nursing Insight**—*Preconception genetics counseling*

Birth defects affect about 1 in every 33 babies born in the United States each year. They are the leading cause of infant deaths and account for more than 20% of all infant deaths.

Although it is never possible to guarantee a family a "perfect" baby, nurses can help recognize patients who may benefit from preconception or prenatal counseling and genetic testing. Keeping abreast of advances in prenatal genetic diagnosis or knowing where to seek pertinent information is a valuable asset in providing patient-centered care (CDC, 2013b).

The loss of a previous pregnancy or the death of an infant brings a staggering cascade of emotions to a subsequent pregnancy. Fear of another fetal loss or infant death undoubtedly increases the couple's anxiety and stress. Although no couple is ever guaranteed a baby that is 100% perfect, the couple who has dealt with the death of a child or loss of a pregnancy faces the prospect of awaiting prenatal diagnostic test results with increased trepidation. Support and continuity of care are essential along with providing advice and listening to the woman's (couple's) concerns. As is true with any pregnant patient, emphasis on healthy lifestyles is of paramount importance. If the previous loss was a result of sudden infant death syndrome (SIDS), the nurse should provide the patient with information about strategies to reduce the incidence of SIDS, such as breastfeeding if at all possible, avoiding cigarette smoke, and positioning the baby on the back to sleep. Support groups may also help couples facing a new pregnancy after the loss of a previous one. (See Chapter 14 for further discussion.)

During the initial prenatal visit, it is especially important to educate the woman about the developing embryo/fetus during the first few weeks of pregnancy. This is a time when the woman needs to be particularly conscious of potential teratogens. A teratogen is a substance that adversely affects fetal development. The vulnerability of the developing embryo/fetus during the early weeks of gestation underscores the importance of a healthy body and a healthy lifestyle.

 Now Can You—**Discuss various components of the prenatal assessment?**

1. Describe biographical information to be elicited from the prenatal patient?
2. Explain how to ask the patient about intimate partner violence?
3. Discuss why the psychological assessment is an important component of the prenatal assessment?
4. Explain the importance of past pregnancies in the obstetric history?

CURRENT PREGNANCY

When obtaining the medical history, the nurse should begin with the events of the current pregnancy. For the woman, the current pregnancy is the issue of most importance to her at this time and what has brought her to the office for prenatal care. Information is gathered to assist with confirmation of the pregnancy and to determine the estimated date of birth. It is usually possible to determine from the patient's responses whether this was a planned or unexpected pregnancy. "Unexpected" does not necessarily mean "unwanted." Instead, this term refers to the fact that the pregnancy occurred when the couple was not actively trying to conceive. Often, pregnancy comes as a complete surprise when the menstrual period is missed or other signs of pregnancy appear. The diagnosis of pregnancy is based on the patient's reported symptoms and the presence of objective signs elicited by the health-care provider. The signs and symptoms are traditionally divided into three classifications: presumptive (experienced by the patient), probable (observed by the examiner), and positive (attributable only to the presence of the fetus).

Presumptive Signs of Pregnancy

The subjective signs of pregnancy are the symptoms that the patient experiences and reports. Because these symptoms may be caused by other conditions, they are the least indicative of pregnancy. In combination with other pregnancy symptoms, the following presumptive signs may serve as diagnostic clues:

- **Amenorrhea** (the absence of menses) is one of the earliest symptoms and is especially significant in a woman whose menstrual cycle is ordinarily regular. Amenorrhea may also be caused by chronic illness; infection; or endocrine, metabolic, or psychological factors.
- Nausea and vomiting ("morning sickness") may actually occur at any time, and women who experience this symptom tend to have a decreased incidence of spontaneous abortion and perinatal mortality. Nausea and vomiting may also be caused by infection or gastrointestinal or emotional disorders.
- Frequent urination (urinary frequency) is caused by pressure exerted on the bladder by the enlarging uterus. Urinary frequency may also be caused by infection, cystocele, pelvic tumors, or urethral diverticula.
- Breast tenderness results from hormonal changes during pregnancy. This symptom may also be associated with premenstrual syndrome, mastitis, and **pseudocyesis** (false pregnancy).
- Perception of fetal movement (quickening) occurs during the second trimester. The sensation of fetal movement may also result from flatus, peristalsis, and abdominal muscle contractions.
- Skin changes include stretch marks (striae gravidarum) and increased pigmentation. These changes may also result from weight gain and oral contraceptive pills.
- Fatigue may also be associated with illness, stress, or lifestyle changes.

Probable Signs of Pregnancy

The probable signs of pregnancy are objective indicators that are observed by the examiner. These signs result from physical changes in the reproductive system. However, because they may be caused by other conditions, a positive diagnosis of pregnancy cannot be based on these findings alone.

- Abdominal enlargement may also be caused by uterine or abdominal tumors.
- **Piskacek's sign** (uterine asymmetry with a soft prominence on the implantation side) may also be associated with uterine tumors.
- **Hegar's sign** (softening of the lower uterine segment) may also be caused by pelvic congestion.
- **Goodell's sign** (softening of the tip of the cervix) may also be caused by infection, hormonal imbalance, or pelvic congestion.

- **Chadwick's sign** (violet-bluish color of the vaginal mucosa and cervix) may also be caused by pelvic congestion, infection, or a hormonal imbalance.
- **Braxton Hicks contractions** (intermittent uterine contractions) may also be associated with uterine leiomyomas (fibroids) or other tumors.
- Positive pregnancy test may occur from certain medications, premature menopause, choriocarcinoma (malignant tumors that produce human chorionic gonadotropin), or the presence of blood in the urine.
- **Ballottement** (passive movement of the unengaged fetus) may be because of uterine tumors or cervical polyps instead of the presence of a fetus.

Positive Signs of Pregnancy

The positive indicators of pregnancy are attributable only to the presence of a fetus:

- Fetal heartbeat
- Visualization of the fetus
- Fetal movements palpated by the examiner

Establishing the Estimated Date of Birth

The antenatal period begins with the first day of the last normal menstrual period and ends when labor begins. This time frame is approximately 280 days in length or 40 weeks or 10 lunar months or 9 calendar months. Pregnancy is divided into three trimesters. Each trimester is approximately 14 weeks or 3 months in duration. Historically, the period from 3 weeks before until 2 weeks after the estimated date of birth was considered "term." However, neonatal outcomes (especially respiratory morbidity) vary depending on the timing of birth within the 5-week gestational age range. To address the lack of uniformity in defining "term," a workgroup of professionals convened in late 2012 to refine the definition of term pregnancy. The Defining "Term" Pregnancy Workgroup recommended that the label "term" be replaced with adoption of the following terminology:

- Early term—births between 37 weeks 0 days and 38 weeks 6 days
- Full term—births between 39 weeks 0 days and 40 weeks 6 days
- Late term—births between 41 weeks 0 days and 41 weeks 6 days
- Postterm—births 42 weeks 0 days or after

The ACOG and the Society for Maternal-Fetal Medicine endorse and encourage the uniform use of the work group's recommended new gestational age designations (ACOG, 2013b; Lowe, 2013; Spong, 2013).

The estimated date of birth (EDB) or the **estimated date of delivery** (EDD) (formerly termed the "estimated date of confinement," or EDC) is based on the date of the last normal menstrual period (LMP) with the assumption that the woman has a 28-day cycle. An important aspect of history taking involves collecting data that help to confirm the accuracy of the duration of the pregnancy. First, the date and a description of the last normal menstrual period are obtained to help determine if the LMP was a "normal" period rather than bleeding associated with implantation. The nurse should ask the patient if her last period was normal for her in relation to the

amount and duration of blood loss. The length of the menstrual cycle and its predictability are also important factors. The EDB may be calculated using **Naegele's rule.** To use Naegele's rule, add 7 days, then subtract 3 months from the date of the patient's LMP and add a year where necessary (Box 9-5). Because Naegele's rule is based on a 28-day menstrual cycle, menstrual cycle irregularity and variations in cycle length most likely invalidate the use of Naegele's rule as the sole method for estimating gestational age. A gestation wheel is a useful tool for readily determining the gestational age during pregnancy (Fig. 9-3).

Box 9-5 Naegele's Rule

Naegele's rule is used to calculate the Expected Date of Birth (EDB)—Expected Date of Delivery (EDD)

This calculation is based on the first day of the woman's last normal period.

7 days are added to the LMP, 3 months subtracted, and where necessary a year added.

For example, if the woman's LMP was June 8, 2014

Add 7 days = June 15, 2014

Subtract 3 months = March 15, 2014

Add a year = March 15, 2015; EDB = March 15, 2015

(An alternative way is to add 7 days and then add 9 months + year where needed.)

Remember to ask the woman about her last menstrual period (LMP). Did her period start on the expected date?

Was blood loss normal (the same as her usual menstrual blood loss)? Was her period different in any way?

What form of contraception had she been using and when was this method discontinued?

(Hormonal contraception may delay the return to a normal ovulation pattern.)

These questions will help you to determine an accurate date for the woman's last normal menstrual period.

Remember: Some women experience bleeding at the time of implantation, which normally occurs 7–9 days after fertilization. Care needs to be taken not to mistakenly use the date of implantation bleeding as the LMP.

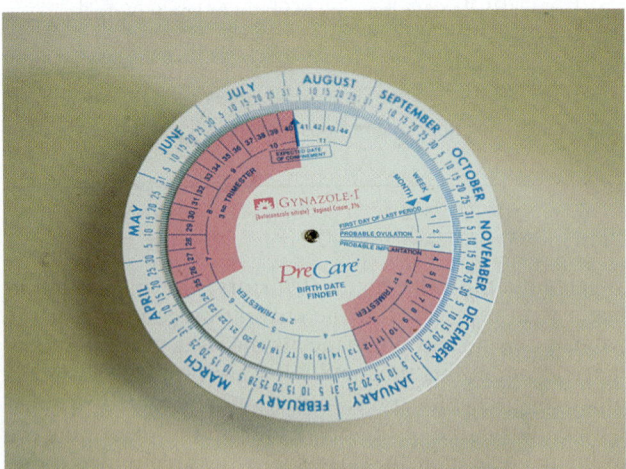

Figure 9-3 A gestation wheel is a handy tool for determining the gestational age. The arrow labeled "first day of LMP" is placed on the date of the LMP. The date at the arrow labeled "expected delivery date" is then noted.

Now Can You—Correctly calculate the EDB?

Calculate the estimated date of birth using Naegele's rule?

Lynne is a 28-year-old woman who comes to the clinic with a history of amenorrhea and a positive home pregnancy test.

Her last menstrual period began on August 26, 2014. She bled for the usual amount of time and reports that the amount of blood loss was normal. Assuming that Lynne had a 28-day cycle, use Naegele's rule to calculate her estimated date of birth.

Important to remember: The month of August has 31 days.

August 26 + 7 days = September 2
(September) ninth month – 3 = sixth month (June)
EDD/EDC/EDB = June 2

Correct calculation of the EDB is dependent on a reliable date of the LMP. Hormonal birth control methods such as combined oral contraceptive pills (OCP) and long-lasting progesterone injections can cause continued suppression of ovulation. Therefore, a discrepancy may exist between when the woman thought she ovulated and conceived and when these events actually occurred. Thus, the LMP may not be an accurate tool for estimating the due date.

Occasionally, pregnancy occurs in women who are taking oral contraceptives, usually as the result of a "pill failure" from forgotten pills or because of poor absorption that may result from various causes such as vomiting, diarrhea, or antibiotic use. Thus, contraceptive pill use may have unwittingly been continued during the early weeks of gestation. The nurse can assure the patient that prenatal hormone exposure associated with normal contraceptive use has not been shown to have any detrimental effects on the developing fetus (Nelson & Cwiak, 2011).

The Pregnancy Classification System

Another important task associated with the initial prenatal interview is to determine the patient's gravidity and parity. **Gravid** is the state of being pregnant; a **gravida** is a pregnant woman. **Gravidity** relates to the number of times that a woman has been pregnant, irrespective of the outcome. The term **nulligravida** is used to describe a woman who has never experienced a pregnancy. A **primigravida** is a woman pregnant for the first time, and a **secundigravida** is a woman pregnant for a second time. Although officially correct, this term is seldom used and instead the term multigravida is used in its place. A **multigravida** describes a woman who is pregnant for the third time (or more times). **Parity** refers to the number of pregnancies carried to a point of viability (generally accepted as 24 weeks of gestation), regardless of the outcome. For example, "para 1" indicates that one pregnancy reached the age of viability. A para 2 means that two pregnancies reached the age of viability. It is important to note that the term parity (or "para") denotes the number of pregnancies, not the number of fetuses/babies, and does not reflect whether the fetuses/babies were born alive or stillborn. Some facilities use a digital system (i.e., GTPAL) for recording the number of pregnancies and their outcomes.

G   Gravida
T   Number of **T**erm pregnancies
P   Number of **P**reterm deliveries

A   Number of **A**bortions, both spontaneous and induced
L   Number of **L**iving children

Pregnancy Testing

A detectable level of human chorionic gonadotropin (hCG) must be present in the urine or blood for a pregnancy test to be positive. hCG is produced by the syncytiotrophoblastic cells found in the outer layer of the trophoblast and secreted into the maternal plasma and then excreted in the urine. hCG levels peak between days 60 and 70 of pregnancy and then gradually decrease over approximately the next 40 days to reach a plateau that is maintained throughout the pregnancy. hCG can be detected in maternal blood as early as 1 day after implantation and in urine around day 26. The hCG molecule contains both an alpha subunit and a beta subunit. Because of the large number of commercial pregnancy tests available, women should be advised to use a home pregnancy test that is specific for the beta subunit of hCG because this marker prevents cross reactions with other hormones. The alpha subunit is very similar in molecular structure to luteinizing hormone (LH). Women with high LH levels (e.g., those experiencing perimenopause) who use a pregnancy test designed to detect the complete hCG molecule risk obtaining a false-positive result. If the over-the-counter pregnancy test used relies on urinary hCG, the patient should be advised to follow the manufacturer's recommendations carefully to avoid an unreliable result. If a home pregnancy test is negative and the signs and symptoms of pregnancy persist, the test should be repeated in a week or the woman should see her health-care provider.

A "chemical pregnancy" is a term used to describe a situation that occurs when a home pregnancy test has confirmed the presence of hCG, but a late and often heavy menstrual period follows. In these instances, conception probably occurred but for some reason the pregnancy was unable to continue and develop into a viable embryo. The frequency of this occurrence is difficult to estimate accurately, but it is thought to affect approximately 30% to 50% of all pregnancies. Before the development of sophisticated methods for detecting an early pregnancy, most of these early and unfruitful fertilizations would have gone undiagnosed.

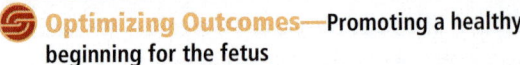 **Optimizing Outcomes**—Promoting a healthy beginning for the fetus

The first few weeks of gestation are of paramount importance to the developing fetus. During this time, the fetus is most susceptible to teratogenic substances such as alcohol, drugs, and environmental toxins. If a woman suspects that she may be pregnant despite a negative home pregnancy test, the nurse should advise her to avoid substances that could be potentially harmful to the developing fetus.

The diagnosis of a multiple gestation places the pregnancy into a "high risk" classification. An early diagnosis of a multiple gestation allows for the development of a care plan that includes more frequent visits for maternal–fetal surveillance. As with any pregnancy, early and ongoing prenatal care offers an opportunity for the timely recognition of complications (more often associated with multiple gestations) and the initiation of interventions to maintain the pregnancy as long as possible. The woman expecting a multiple birth also needs additional psychological support, practical advice, and education. She may experience more intense discomforts of pregnancy and need to deal with upsetting and extreme body changes. In addition, she also faces the financial challenges associated with a potentially complicated pregnancy, possible preterm birth, and the economic burden of providing for multiple newborns.

 Now Can You—Discuss essential aspects of the current pregnancy?

1. Differentiate among the "presumptive," "probable," and "positive" signs of pregnancy?
2. Explain how to calculate the estimated date of birth using Naegele's rule?
3. Describe the GTPAL pregnancy classification system?
4. Explain what women should be taught about home pregnancy testing?

THE MEDICAL HISTORY

To provide the patient with appropriate care to meet medical needs during pregnancy, it is essential that a detailed medical history be obtained. This information gives insights into the patient's past and present health status and use of preventative services. The nurse should obtain contact information for the primary care provider to facilitate continuity of care. Lack of a family physician may be related to financial difficulties, lack of medical insurance, or cultural/value differences. The nurse can explore these issues through sensitive and respectful questioning, and when appropriate, refer the patient and her family to local agencies that provide services such as the WIC (Women, Infants, and Children) program for nutritional support (Box 9-6).

Some European countries offer "shared" care for low-risk patients to serve as a link between the patient's primary care provider and her obstetrician. The pregnant woman visits her family physician for the majority of her prenatal care but also sees an obstetrician for two to three visits. If any complications arise, the patient is transferred for the remainder of the pregnancy to the care of the obstetrician. Because any complications that occur during pregnancy are associated

---

Box 9-6 WIC at a Glance

The WIC target population includes those who are low-income and nutritionally at risk:

- Pregnant women, and up to 6 weeks postpartum or after pregnancy ends
- Breastfeeding women (up to infant's first birthday)
- Non-breastfeeding postpartum women (up to 6 months after the birth of an infant or after pregnancy ends)
- Infants (up to first birthday). WIC serves 53% of all infants born in the United States
- Children up to their fifth birthday

BENEFITS

- Supplemental nutritious foods
- Nutrition education and counseling at WIC clinics
- Screening and referrals to other health, welfare, and social services

Source: U.S. Department of Agriculture, Food & Nutrition Service. (2013). Retrieved from http://www.fns.usda.gov/wic/about-wic-wic-glance

---

with maternal and family stress, referral to a "known" obstetrician hopefully helps to diminish some of the anxiety.

Dental Health

Together with the overall evaluation of medical well-being, it is essential to explore dental health. The initial interview is an ideal time to provide education about the benefits of preventative dental care and to dispel common myths such as "for every pregnancy, a tooth is lost." It has been well established that the hormones of pregnancy predispose women to increased plaque and the development of gingivitis, or gum inflammation (American Academy of Periodontology, 2011).

There is a link between periodontal disease in pregnancy, gingivitis, and preterm labor. It is believed that oral bacteria and their products travel via the bloodstream to the placental membranes, where an inflammatory response occurs. The inflammation may trigger the onset of preterm labor. Oral caries may also pose a greater threat during pregnancy. This is especially true during early pregnancy, when vomiting from "morning sickness" causes the mouth to harbor an acid environment that favors cariogenic activity. Other investigators suggest that women's dental health practices suffer after pregnancy because of a lack of time and result in an increase in dental caries. To promote dental health among pregnant women, some European countries such as England offer free dental care during pregnancy and for the first year following childbirth. Part of the nurse's role during the prenatal period is to promote dental hygiene to reduce the incidence of periodontal disease such as gingivitis (which is reversible). Pregnant women need to receive regular dental examinations and appropriate treatment as determined by their dental practitioner (American Academy of Periodontology, 2011; ACOG, 2013c; American Dental Association, 2011).

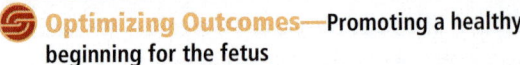 **Optimizing Outcomes**—Promoting dental health during pregnancy

- Encourage regular dental examinations.
- Promote twice daily brushing and flossing.
- Recommend the use of a fluoride toothpaste.

- Encourage a healthy diet.
- Encourage chewing gum containing xylitol after meals.

Eye Health

An ophthalmic evaluation is also recommended early in pregnancy, most often during the first trimester or at any time visual changes occur. This is especially important for women with medical conditions such as essential hypertension, Graves' disease, or diabetes mellitus and for women who wear contact lenses. During pregnancy, a number of normal physiological ophthalmic changes occur, including decreased intraocular pressure, corneal thickening, and corneal sensitivity and increased curvature of the cornea. These changes usually resolve spontaneously during the postpartum period. Medical conditions peculiar to pregnancy such as pregnancy-induced hypertension, eclampsia, and gestational diabetes can also have detrimental effects on eye health and vision (Somani, 2011).

Immunizations

Another essential component of the medical history concerns patient immunizations. Influenza causes between 3,300 and 49,000 deaths in this country each year (CDC, 2010a). Pregnant women who contract influenza have an increased risk of both needing medical care and requiring hospitalization. Vaccination against influenza is considered safe throughout pregnancy, and according to the ACOG, "preventing influenza during pregnancy is an essential element of prenatal care, and the most effective strategy for preventing influenza is annual immunization" (ACOG, 2010a, p. 1006).

Where Research and Practice Meet:
Eye Examinations During Pregnancy

During an eye examination, it is a relatively common practice to dilate the pupils to facilitate ocular assessment. Although occasional use of parasympatholytics (e.g., atropine) and sympathomimetics (e.g., epinephrine) is thought to be safe, repeated use is contraindicated because of possible teratogenic effects. Mydriatics (medications that dilate the pupils) are also contraindicated for breastfeeding mothers because they have a hypertensive and anticholinergic effect on the infant (Somani, 2011). This information is important to nurses who counsel prenatal and postpartal patients. All prenatal and breastfeeding patients should be advised that certain components of the eye examination may carry risks during pregnancy, and they should make certain their eye care professional is aware that they are pregnant (or breastfeeding).

Where Research and Practice Meet:
Electronic Record Best-Practice Alert and
Influenza Vaccination in Pregnant Women

Klatt and Hopp (2012) collaborated to estimate the effect of a best-practice alert, or reminder within the electronic medical record system, to assess the rate of vaccination of pregnant women against influenza. An electronic reminder was embedded within the electronic prenatal record to alert the health-care provider during each prenatal visit if the medical record did not contain documentation of an influenza vaccination for the current influenza season. The alert could be satisfied by ordering the vaccine, documenting that a vaccine had been given elsewhere, or by selecting "declined" and providing a reason. Once satisfied, the alert no longer appeared at subsequent visits. The researchers compared influenza vaccination rates 1 year after activation of the best practice alert (61%) with the previous year vaccination rate (42%) and found a significant improvement. Based on their findings, the investigators suggested that all users of electronic medical records consider adding a best-practice alert to the records of their pregnant patients to improve the rates of offering influenza vaccination, and because of the CDC vaccination guidelines, they also recommended that the best-practice alert could be extended to other settings and include individuals older than 6 months who do not have specific contraindications to the vaccine.

Nurses and their patients also need to be aware that some infections contracted during pregnancy can be detrimental to the developing fetus. Rubella (German measles) is one of the most commonly recognized viral infections known to cause congenital problems. If a woman contracts rubella during the first 12 weeks of pregnancy, the fetus has a 90% chance of being adversely affected. Maternal exposure to rubella later in pregnancy is associated with a decreased fetal risk. If the pregnancy is between 12 and 16 weeks when rubella infection occurs, the fetal risk decreases to 20%. Typical symptoms of congenital rubella syndrome include intrauterine growth restriction, cardiac defects, sensorineural defects, cataracts, and microcephaly (World Health Organization, 2011). It is estimated that nearly 7 million childbearing-aged women in the United States are currently susceptible to the rubella virus. A maternity patient who is not immune to rubella should be offered the rubella immunization after childbirth, ideally before hospital discharge. If possible, she should be tested greater than or equal to 3 months later to ensure immunity. After the immunization, she needs to be advised against becoming pregnant for at least 4 weeks (CDC, 2012a).

Other viruses known to cause complications during pregnancy include varicella (chickenpox) and rubeola (red measles). Information regarding the latest recommendations for immunizations can be found by visiting the Web site for the CDC: http://www.cdc.gov/vaccines/pubs/preg-guide.htm#tdap or the American Academy of Pediatrics: http://www2.aap.org/immunizationhttp://www2.aap.org/immunization/. (See Chapter 11 for further discussion.)

 Optimizing Outcomes—Maternal immunization to prevent neonatal pertussis

Pertussis, or "whooping cough," is an extremely contagious bacterial infection caused by the gram-negative coccobacillis *Bordetella pertussis*, which causes disease through the elaboration of toxins that damage respiratory epithelium. Transmitted by respiratory droplets, pertussis carries significant morbidity and mortality in newborns and young children: ninety-one percent of pertussis-associated deaths occur in children younger than 6 months of age. According to the CDC (2012a), a tetanus and diphtheria booster vaccination is indicated during pregnancy for a woman who has never received the vaccine for tetanus, diphtheria, and pertussis (Tdap) or if 10 years have elapsed since immunization.

Tdap should be administered during the third or late second trimester (after 20 weeks' gestation) of pregnancy (CDC, 2012a; Stiller, 2011).

HEPATITIS B INFECTION. The rate of new hepatitis B infections has declined by approximately 82% since 1991, when a national strategy to eliminate hepatitis B was implemented in the U.S. However, it is estimated that from 800,000 to 1.4 million Americans are chronically infected (CDC, 2012b, 2014). During the prenatal period, it is important to screen for hepatitis B because a positive diagnosis will influence both the maternal and newborn medical management. When an acute infection occurs during pregnancy, the rate of vertical transmission from mother to fetus ranges from approximately 10% in the first trimester to 80% to 90% in the third trimester (ACOG, 2007a).

Optimizing Outcomes—With universal screening for hepatitis B during pregnancy

Although the CDC and ACOG recommend universal screening of pregnant women for the marker of active hepatitis B (i.e., hepatitis B surface antigen [HbsAg]), it is important for nurses to be aware of the groups defined by CDC as being at higher risk for hepatitis B. Women should be asked about potential risk factors (e.g., persons with conditions that require immunosuppressive or immune-modifying therapy, blood or tissue donors, hemodialysis patients, and HIV-positive persons), and those at higher risk for acquiring the hepatitis B virus (HBV) should also be tested for the antibody to hepatitis B surface antigen (anti-HBs). Persons who are negative for both markers and who are at risk for infection should be vaccinated. CDC recommendations endorse vaccination during pregnancy of women who are at high risk of contracting hepatitis B (Apuzzio et al., 2012a, 2012b).

From a nursing perspective, the patient will need support and education relating to both the present and long-term implications (Box 9-7). Clinical management focuses on the potential effects of hepatitis B on the pregnancy and the long-term maternal risks, including chronic liver disease. Women with chronic hepatitis B infection may develop cirrhosis or hepatocellular carcinoma, usually after menopause, and require lifetime follow-up to treat detectable complications and determine if antiviral therapy is appropriate. It is strongly recommended that household members and intimate partners of a positive hepatitis B carrier undergo screening, and depending on the results, receive the vaccination (Appuzzio et al., 2012b; Chao, Cheung, Yang, So, & Chang, 2012; Rustgi, Carriero, Bachtold, & Zeldin, 2010).

Other populations at risk for hepatitis B infection include individuals from India, Africa, Asia, and the Pacific Isles. Because of needle sharing and a potentially high number of sexual partners (as payment for drugs), intravenous drug users are also at an increased risk for hepatitis B. Most adults in the United States contract hepatitis B through sexual contact, and it is estimated that about 25% of individuals who are sexually active with a hepatitis B infected individual will seroconvert (CDC, 2012b). **Seroconversion** is the process whereby an individual develops antibodies

---

Box 9-7 Educational Strategies for Patients Who Are Hepatitis Carriers

The nurse teaches prenatal patients who are hepatitis carriers to:

- Avoid drugs that are hepatotoxic such as acetaminophen (Tylenol).
- Avoid alcohol.
- If possible, choose noninvasive prenatal diagnosis techniques, such as ultrasound and AFP screening rather than invasive procedures such as chorionic villus sampling (CVS) and amniocentesis. However, the risk of transmission of HBV associated with amniocentesis is low.
- Make certain that the pediatrician is aware of the maternal hepatitis B status.
- Practice "daily living" precautions to prevent transmission to household members. Strategies include covering cuts or skin lesions and not sharing toothbrushes or razors.

Patients are also advised that:

- The neonate will need to receive hepatitis B immune globulin (HBIG) at birth. This action will provide antibodies to the hepatitis B virus and afford some initial protection to the newborn. The intramuscular injection must be administered within 12 hours of birth. The hepatitis B vaccine (Recombivax HB, Engerix-B), which induces protective antihepatitis B antibodies, may be administered at the same time as HBIG but at a different site. The hepatitis B vaccine is given again at 1, 2, and 12 months of age.
- In HAV-infected women, breastfeeding is permissible with appropriate hygienic precautions. Breastfeeding is not contraindicated in women chronically infected with HBV if the infant receives HBIG passive prophylaxis and vaccine active prophylaxis. Breastfeeding has not been associated with an increased risk of neonatal HCV infection.
- The method of birth does not appear to influence the incidence of mother-to-child transmission.

Sources: ACOG, 2007a; CDC, 2012b; Rustgi, Carriero, Bachtold, & Zeldin, 2010.

---

in response to an infection and subsequently tests positive when screened because of the presence of the antibodies.

Women who are considered to be at risk for hepatitis B also need to be screened for hepatitis C (HCV). The main route of transmission for this infection (previously known as "non-A, non-B hepatitis") is through intravenous drug use. Approximately 4 million Americans have HCV, which is now listed by the Institute of Medicine as an emerging infectious disease. Up to 80% of patients with acute HCV are asymptomatic, with seroconversion occurring in approximately 8 to 9 weeks. Preterm labor is the main pregnancy risk associated with HCV. However, there is a low (4% to 8%) risk of transmission to the neonate. If the mother is coinfected with HIV, the transmission rate to the newborn increases to around 13%. It is recommended that all infants born to mothers with HCV undergo testing at 12 to 18 months of age (CDC, 2010b; Hepatitis Foundation International, 2010).

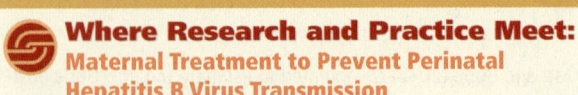

Where Research and Practice Meet:
Maternal Treatment to Prevent Perinatal Hepatitis B Virus Transmission

Perinatal transmission of hepatitis B is an important cause of chronic hepatitis B, and over 90% of perinatally infected children become chronic carriers. Although active-passive immunoprophylaxis for newborns of women positive for hepatitis B surface antigen is nearly 95%

effective in preventing perinatal transmission, women with high levels of viral replication remain at elevated risk—despite neonatal prophylaxis, perinatal transmission rates range from 13% to 62.5% (Xiao, Li, Chen, Zhu, & Miao, 2007). Unal and colleagues (2011) conducted a study to investigate the cost-effectiveness of maternal lamivudine (a medication used for the treatment of chronic hepatitis B) or hepatitis B immune globulin (HBIG) administered in the third trimester to prevent perinatal hepatitis B transmission as compared with no maternal treatment. The investigators concluded that adoption of maternal third-trimester treatment with either medication in women with high hepatitis B viral loads (e.g., 10^6 copies/mL) would be a cost-effective, cost-saving measure. Based on their findings, the researchers recommend screening all women positive for hepatitis B surface antigen at 24 to 28 weeks of gestation and initiating prophylaxis with either lamivudine or HBIG if the viral load is high.

Other Preexisting Medical Conditions

Preexisting maternal medical conditions such as diabetes, epilepsy, and phenylketonuria need to be managed appropriately to limit the risk of adverse fetal effects. For example, prenatal exposure to hydantoin (phenytoin) [Dilantin, Phenytex] has been associated with cleft lip and palate because of its folic acid antagonistic properties (Hernandez-Diaz et al., 2012). Preconception care is important. The earlier that appropriate management/treatment is implemented, the better the pregnancy outcome.

Environmental Hazards

The developing fetus is at risk from maternal exposure to a variety of environmental toxins such as pesticides and other industrial compounds (e.g., polychlorinated biphenyl [PCB], a substance widely used as a coolant and lubricant in transformers, capacitors, and other electrical equipment) that can accumulate in maternal adipose tissue and possibly be transmitted to the infant via breast milk. Although PCB manufacture was halted in this country in 1977, they remain a persistent organic pollutant that threatens our environment. The main routes of exposure today occur through dietary sources such as fish, meat, and dairy products (ACOG, 2013d; Chalupka & Chalupka, 2010).

❝What to say❞—Asking the prenatal patient about the potential for pesticide exposure

Because of the widespread use of pesticides, it is essential for nurses to assess every prenatal patient for the potential for pesticide exposures. Environmental exposure questions should be included in the comprehensive patient health history. To elicit the information, the nurse may wish to ask questions such as the following (Gilden, Huffling, & Sattler, 2010):

"Do you use pesticides in your home, lawn, or workplace?"

"Do you use pesticides on your pets?" (e.g., flea collars, dips, and once-a-month products)

"If you do use pesticides, what do you use?"; "Where and how often do you use them?"

Air pollution is one of the most common concerns for maternal and newborn health. Concentrations of air pollutants are approximately three to five times less outdoors than indoors, where the majority (up to 90%) of time is spent. Adverse birth outcomes including congenital anomalies, intrauterine growth restriction, and preterm birth have been linked to in utero exposure to various air pollutants (ACOG, 2013c; Bobak, 2000; Chalupka & Chalupka, 2010; Liu, Krewski, Shi, Chen, & Burnett, 2003; Maisonet, Bush, Correa, & Jaakkola, 2001; Pedersen, et al., 2013).

 Optimizing Outcomes—**Using an environmental and occupational health history profile**

The Environmental and Occupational Health History Profile is an easy-to-use, comprehensive tool designed to elicit specific information about potentially harmful exposures in the patient's home, community, and workplace. Composed of three broad categories ("Present Work," "Potential Workplace Exposures," and "Environmental History"), the questionnaire lists over 60 possible environmental and occupational exposures toxins that may cause harm to a developing embryo/fetus. As the nurse completes the tool in the preconceptional or antepartal setting, each affirmative response warrants additional, detailed information to quantify exposure to determine the route of exposure (inhalation, dermal, or ingestion), timing (relation of exposure to critical time windows), and duration and frequency of exposure (Chalupka & Chalupka, 2010).

Nurses can help to improve the fetal environment by educating women about the dangers of direct and passive smoking during pregnancy. The Association of Women's Health, Obstetric and Neonatal Nurses (AWHONN) supports aggressive antismoking policy initiatives, such as insurance coverage for smoking cessation products and programs. AWHONN also supports initiatives that restrict the sale of tobacco products to minors and opposes the targeted marketing of tobacco products to young persons (AWHONN, 2010). Smoking cessation programs designed for pregnant women are readily available through the CDC, the ACOG, and other professional organizations. Effects of tobacco use during pregnancy are well documented and predispose to premature rupture of the membranes, preterm labor, placental abruption, placenta previa, and infants who are small for gestational age (SGA). The detrimental effects on the fetus/neonate continue well into childhood and are associated with problems such as upper respiratory infections, childhood asthma, and wheezing (ACOG, 2010b). Because chemicals, heavy metals, and other environmental hazards that pose a threat to the embryo/fetus may be present in the home, community, or workplace, this information should be elicited and recorded in the prenatal assessment. (See Chapters 7 and 10 for further discussion.)

Where Research and Practice Meet: Secondhand Smoke Exposure During Pregnancy

Ashford and colleagues (2010) conducted a study of 210 mother-baby couplets within 48 hours of birth to examine the relationship between prenatal secondhand smoke (SHS) exposure, preterm birth, and immediate neonatal outcomes. Active maternal smoking status was confirmed by analysis of urine cotinine, a nicotine metabolite; SHS exposure was assessed via maternal hair nicotine levels. The investigators found that smoking status (i.e., nonsmoking, passive smoking, and active smoking) strongly correlated with low, medium, and high hair nicotine levels. Women exposed to prenatal SHS were at greater risk for preterm birth than nonexposed women, and infants of passive smoking mothers were at increased risk for respiratory distress syndrome and admission to a neonatal intensive care unit when compared with infants of smoking mothers. Passive smokers and/or women with hair nicotine levels greater than 0.35 ng/mL were more likely to give birth earlier (1 week), give birth to infants weighing less (a decrease of 200 to 300 g), and deliver shorter infants (a decrease of 1.1 to 1.7 cm). Based on their findings, the researchers recommended that nurses routinely inquire about SHS exposure at a patient's first prenatal appointment, provide education regarding the adverse maternal and infant health effects of SHS exposure, and encourage avoidance of SHS during and after pregnancy (Ashford, Hahn, Hall, Rayens, Noland, & Ferguson, 2010).

 Now Can You—Discuss how the prenatal patient's medical history guides care?

1. Explain why dental and eye care are important during pregnancy?
2. Identify three viruses known to adversely affect the developing fetus?
3. Name four essential guidelines that should be included in a teaching plan for pregnant women who test positive for hepatitis B?

THE GYNECOLOGICAL HISTORY

The nurse needs to obtain a concise gynecological (GYN) history primarily to determine if any event in the patient's past places the current pregnancy at risk or warrants further investigation. Women ages 35 and older and foreign-born women should be questioned about in utero exposure to **diethylstilbestrol** (DES). Diethylstilbestrol is a nonsteroidal, synthetic estrogen that is several times more potent than natural estrogens.

In the United States, diethylstilbestrol was widely prescribed during the late 1930s until the early 1970s as a preventative treatment to reduce the likelihood of spontaneous abortion (miscarriage) or preterm delivery (Smith, 1948). It is estimated that between 1 and 2 million pregnant women received this oral medication. Exposure to DES during intrauterine development produces both structural and functional gynecological abnormalities that are associated with numerous problems including infertility, increased incidence of ectopic pregnancies, preterm labor and birth, and vaginal adenocarcinoma. Male offspring may be at an increased risk of testicular and prostate cancer. Second-generational effects of in utero DES exposure include an increased incidence of ovarian cancer (granddaughters) and hypospadias (grandsons) (Cunningham, Leveno, Bloom, Spong, & Dashe, 2014; Gilden, Huffling, & Sattler, 2010; Smith, 1948).

Screening and Diagnostic Tests During Pregnancy

Before prenatal testing it is essential to determine the gestational age accurately because a number of screening and diagnostic tests have different ranges of normality based on

the maturity of the pregnancy. Before a patient is asked to consent to any investigation, she should be counseled about the purpose of the test, its reliability, and the implications of a negative or positive result. The nurse also needs to explain the difference between a screening test and a diagnostic test.

 Nursing Insight—*Educating patients about screening and diagnostic tests*

To facilitate patient understanding of care options, nurses should explain the differences between screening and diagnostic tests.

A screening test:
- Identifies patients at increased risk for developing a disorder or disease
- Identifies patients who need diagnostic testing

A diagnostic test:
- Confirms the presence of a disorder or disease

At the first prenatal visit, venous blood samples are taken so that abnormal findings can be identified and promptly treated. Blood is drawn for a number of tests: the patient's blood group and rhesus (Rh) factor; antibody screen (Kell, Duffy, rubella, varicella, toxoplasmosis, and anti-Rh), and RPR/VDRL (rapid plasma reagent/Venereal Disease Research Laboratory) screen for syphilis. If the woman has not received the hepatitis B vaccine, she is tested for hepatitis B surface antigen (HbsAG) and hepatitis B surface antibody (HbsAB). A complete blood count (CBC) with hemoglobin, hematocrit, and differential cell count is obtained and assessed using laboratory values established for pregnancy. Testing for antibody to HIV is recommended for all pregnant women (ACOG, 2011f; CDC, 2011d), and a sickle cell screen is recommended for women of African, Asian, or Middle Eastern descent. In the United States, sickle cell anemia is one of the most common genetic blood disorders and occurs most often in African American populations (CDC, 2011b). (See Chapter 11 for further discussion.) During this visit, a Tine or purified protein derivative (PPD) tuberculin test may also be administered to assess for exposure to tuberculosis.

SEXUALLY TRANSMITTED INFECTIONS

Based on the patient's risk factors, screening for sexually transmitted diseases/infections (STDs/STIs) may need to be repeated during the pregnancy. The presence of an STI can predispose to a number of adverse pregnancy outcomes including ectopic pregnancy, spontaneous abortion, preterm labor, and increased neonatal morbidity. Taking a sexual history is an important component of the prenatal nursing assessment. Self-awareness and the use of effective communication techniques foster open, honest discussion of sensitive issues in a nonthreatening environment (Box 9-8).

The sexual history should include signs or symptoms (e.g., vaginal/rectal discharge, dyspareunia, ulcers, rashes, or anogenital itching) that may be indicative of infection. Information concerning recent sexual partners is also important so that when indicated, prior contacts can be notified and offered treatment. High-risk behaviors such as intravenous drug use, acquisition of tattoos, exposure to blood or blood products, or sex with an individual from a

---

Box 9-8   Tips for Taking a Sexual History

SELF-AWARENESS

Know your own comfort level and your ease at discussing sexual issues with patients.

Acknowledge areas of discomfort.

EFFECTIVE COMMUNICATION

If you are embarrassed, this will be apparent through body language, eye-to-eye contact, tone of voice, and type of questioning chosen (e.g., closed-ended questions as opposed to exploratory questions).

Use terminology: words and terms that the patient understands.

Environment: ensure privacy and confidentiality.

Never make assumptions or be judgmental in your response or attitude.

Source: Higgins, J. A., & Davis, A. R. (2011). Sexuality and contraception. In Hatcher, R. A., Trussell, J., Nelson, A. L., Cates, W., Kowal, D., & Policar, M. S., ... *Contraceptive technology* (20th revised ed., pp. 1–28). Decatur, GA: Bridging the Gap Communications.

Where Research and Practice Meet:
Linking Maternal Bacterial Vaginosis and Vitamin D Deficiency

Bacterial vaginosis (BV) is a leading cause of vaginal infections among childbearing age women. It is a condition characterized by the loss of normal vaginal flora, especially beneficial lactobacilli, which are replaced by numerous anaerobic bacteria. Symptoms, when present, include white or gray malodorous vaginal discharge and dysuria (CDC, 2010c).

Vitamin D is important in maintaining serum calcium and phosphate concentrations for normal bone development, modulating cell growth and neuromuscular and immune function, and in reducing inflammation (Office of Dietary Supplements, 2011). Maternal vitamin D deficiency, more common in certain individuals (e.g., those with darker skin, those who cover their skin with clothing because of religious or cultural beliefs, and those who live in the northern hemisphere and receive limited sunlight exposure), can result in the limited transmission of vitamin D stores to the fetus. Neonatal and infant vitamin D deficiency may result in impaired growth and bone ossification, abnormal enamel formation, and changes in calcium formation (Harris, 2011). Two recent studies explored the possibility of a relationship between vitamin D deficiency and BV in pregnancy.

Bodnar, Krohn, and Simhan (2009) examined the prevalence of BV and vitamin D status in a group of pregnant women in their first trimester. They found that when compared with women with normal vaginal flora, the women with BV had lower concentrations of vitamin D. In the second study, Hensel, Randis, Gelber, and Ratner (2011) conducted a secondary analysis of previously collected data to assess whether BV risk factors (e.g., ethnic background, educational level, time of sexual debut, and number of lifetime sexual partners) differed among pregnant and nonpregnant women, focusing on vitamin D deficiency across subgroups. Findings revealed that certain factors (e.g., African American or Mexican American, smoking, douching, and early sexual debut) were significantly associated with BV, and vitamin D deficiency was associated with BV among the pregnant women but not among nonpregnant women.

In both studies, minority women, especially African American women, were significantly more likely to have BV and to be deficient in vitamin D. These findings suggest that being diagnosed with BV may increase the likelihood that the individual may also be deficient in vitamin D. Because both BV and vitamin D deficiency can have negative consequences for the health of mothers and babies, additional research is needed to explore the impact of BV and vitamin D deficiency in later pregnancy, the effectiveness of treatment for vitamin D deficiency and reduction of BV prevalence, and the mechanisms of action of vitamin D on vaginal flora (Aghajafari, Nagulesapillai, Ronksley, Tough, O'Beirne, & Rabi, 2013; Harris, 2011).

---

high-risk category (e.g., a sex industry worker) should also be noted.

Human Immunodeficiency Virus

Infection with HIV leads to a progressive disease that results in AIDS. (See Chapter 11 for further discussion.) Perinatal transmission may occur transplacentally, at birth from exposure to maternal blood and vaginal secretions, and via breast milk. The incidence of perinatal transmission (HIV-positive mother to her fetus) ranges from 25% to 35%. Maternal treatment with zidovudine (AZT, Retrovir) reduces the risk of perinatal transmission and the risk of infant death. Elective cesarean birth has been shown to significantly reduce the risk of transmission from the mother to the infant (AIDSinfo, 2011).

In 2011, the AWHONN and the ACOG reaffirmed a recommendation that all pregnant women be tested for HIV as part of the routine battery of prenatal tests, although patients may choose to opt out of this testing. Screening for HIV is done via an enzyme-linked immunosorbent assay (ELISA) on a blood sample. If the result from this test is positive, the finding is confirmed via a Western blot test. Repeat testing in the third trimester or rapid HIV testing should be used in labor for women with undocumented HIV status following opt-out screening. If a rapid HIV test result in labor is positive, immediate initiation of antiretroviral prophylaxis should be initiated without waiting for the results of the confirmatory test (ACOG, 2011f; AWHONN, 2011).

Nurses need to be patient advocates and ensure that patients receive individualized and informed care. One aspect of the nurse's role in this situation is to make certain that each patient receives nonjudgmental, comprehensive pre- and post-counseling in relation to HIV testing. Clearly, it is medically advantageous for the pregnant patient to be diagnosed and treated (for HIV) during pregnancy to promote maternal well-being and to reduce the incidence of perinatal HIV transmission (AWHONN, 2011; Bradley-Springer, 2010).

Syphilis

A syphilis infection during pregnancy can cause significant damage to the fetus after the 16th to 18th week of intrauterine life, when the cytotrophoblastic layer of the placental villi has atrophied and is no longer protective. Caused by the spirochete *Treponema pallidum*, syphilis is readily treated with penicillin or erythromycin. If the condition is treated before the 18th week, the fetus is rarely affected. Left untreated, transplacental transmission to the fetus is likely to occur (congenital syphilis) and may result in deafness, cognitive difficulties, osteochondritis, or fetal death.

Chlamydia Trachomatis, Neisseria Gonorrhoeae

Other routine screening tests including chlamydia and gonorrhea are obtained during the pelvic examination. Secretions from the cervix, vagina, and anus may be used to obtain samples for culture media. *Chlamydia trachomatis* is a bacterial infection that is prevalent in sexually active populations, especially those in the under-25 age group. Most patients with this infection are asymptomatic and consequently do not seek treatment. Complications of chlamydial infections include salpingitis, pelvic inflammatory disease, infertility, ectopic pregnancy, premature rupture of the membranes, and preterm birth. Transmission to the neonate may occur during birth and results in ophthalmia neonatorum and chlamydial neonatal pneumonia. During pregnancy, chlamydia is treated with oral anti-infectives or penicillin-based agents. (See Chapter 11 for further discussion.) It is recommended that pregnant women be retested 3 weeks after treatment, although the validity of this practice has not yet been established (CDC, 2010b).

Gonorrhea is caused by the gram-negative intracellular diplococcal bacteria *Neisseria gonorrhoeae*. It is readily treated with antibiotics. When left untreated, ascending maternal infection may occur after rupture of the membranes. Transmission to the fetus can occur during vaginal delivery and may result in disseminated infection and ophthalmia neonatorum. (See Chapter 11 for further discussion.) Concomitant treatment for gonorrhea and *Chlamydia* is recommended because coinfection is common (CDC, 2010b).

Herpes Simplex Virus

Herpes simplex virus type 1 (HSV-1), transmitted nonsexually, is most commonly associated with fever blisters. Herpes simplex virus type 2 (HSV-2) is usually transmitted sexually and is associated with genital lesions, although depending on sexual practices, both types are not exclusively associated with the respective sites. HSV-2 occurs more frequently in women (20.9%) than in men (11.5%), which most likely results from the greater likelihood of male-to-female transmission. Although HSV infection is not a reportable disease, it is estimated that 1 in 6 Americans between the ages of 14 and 49 are infected with herpes simplex virus type 2 (CDC, 2012c).

The initial HSV genital infection generally produces flu-like symptoms including malaise, muscle aches, and headache accompanied by dysuria and the appearance of multiple painful blister-like lesions. The symptoms may persist for several weeks. A prodromal period characterized by marked skin sensitivity and nerve pain in the affected area may precede the outbreak of lesions.

HSV-2 infection during pregnancy can have adverse effects on both the mother and her fetus. Primary infection during the first trimester is associated with congenital infection and an increased risk of pregnancy loss. In the neonate, HSV infection is associated with a 60% mortality rate, and of those who survive, approximately 50% suffer serious neurological damage. There is no cure for genital herpes. Care management centers on providing symptomatic relief. Although several antiviral agents are available, the safety of these medications during pregnancy and lactation has not been firmly established (Barclay, 2010; CDC, 2010b). (See Chapters 4, 11, and 19 for further discussion.)

CERVICAL CANCER

Cervical screening is usually a component of the first prenatal examination. Screening and treatment of cervical dysplasia (cancerous cellular changes) significantly reduce the chances that carcinoma will develop. This fact lends credence to the recommendation that screening via Papanicolaou testing be performed on all young adults, beginning at age 21. Furthermore, 50% of all women diagnosed with cervical cancer are diagnosed during the ages of young adulthood. (See Chapter 4 for further discussion.)

The Prenatal Physical Examination

PREPARING THE PATIENT

The patient should be given adequate private time to prepare for the examination and encouraged to void if needed (a urine specimen may also need to be collected). Before conducting the physical examination, it is essential to properly prepare the environment. The room should be warm, with a cover for the patient and a gown for her to wear. Ensure privacy for the patient, such as a "Do not disturb—exam in progress" sign affixed to the closed door.

Before the examination begins, the patient should receive an explanation of what the examination will involve and what she is expected to do. Obtain her consent to be examined. During a physical examination, the patient is usually scantily clothed and must remain on her back in a vulnerable position for the majority of the time. Gaining permission from the patient before proceeding gives her control, as she "allows" the examiner to continue. This action is especially important for women with a history of abuse, particularly sexual abuse. Actively engaging the patient through dialogue during the examination process provides an excellent opportunity for teaching. Also, ongoing interaction while describing the findings and their relevance empowers the patient and dispels the oft-experienced feeling that something is being "done" to her. Before beginning the physical examination, the nurse should have collected all of the equipment that may be needed, along with any teaching literature that the patient should receive. It does not inspire confidence or relieve the patient's anxiety if the nurse is constantly leaving the room to retrieve forgotten items.

---

⑤ Optimizing Outcomes—Demonstrating professionalism during the physical examination

To convey respect and minimize the transmission of infection, the nurse should:

- Ensure that the fingernails are short and all jewelry items that may cause skin trauma have been removed.
- Wash hands thoroughly in the patient's presence. This simple act demonstrates respect and an understanding of and appreciation for the risk of cross-infection.
- Develop the habit of always washing the hands when entering and leaving a patient's room.

The physical examination should proceed in the same order each time (preferably head to toe) to reduce the likelihood of unintentionally omitting any component. The examination should be organized in a manner that reduces the movements the patient must make. Also, it is less threatening to the patient when less invasive procedures are performed first. Throughout the examination, it is essential for the nurse to use good communication skills and to advocate for and treat the patient with respect. These actions empower patients to participate actively in all healthcare decisions. The time before, during, and after the examination provides the nurse with an excellent opportunity to develop a good rapport while enhancing the patient's comfort level. Proper management of the clinical environment plays an important role in facilitating the patient's feelings of safety, privacy, and security.

PERFORMING THE GENERAL ASSESSMENT

The general assessment begins by simply observing the woman. Information that can be obtained includes her overall health/nutritional status; posture; ease of movement and gait; appearance (includes clothing and cleanliness); affect and speech pattern; eye contact; and general orientation to place, person, and time. As the pregnancy advances, changes in maternal gait become apparent because of increasing lordosis (curvature of the spine) in response to the increasing weight and size of the gravid uterus that changes the woman's center of gravity.

The nurse then obtains anthropometric measurements. When obtaining the weight, it is valuable to ask the patient what her normal prepregnant weight was and to document this information (Fig. 9-4). The prepregnant weight gives an indication of how the patient is adapting to pregnancy. A dramatic, unintended weight loss can be indicative of severe nausea and vomiting (hyperemesis gravidarum). The height and weight are also recorded and used to calculate the patient's body mass index (BMI) and to determine nutritional needs. The BMI can be used to calculate whether the maternal weight is appropriate for height. (See BMI discussion in Chapter 10.) Women who are underweight before pregnancy and have a low weight gain during the pregnancy are at a greater risk for preterm labor.

Obtaining Information and Promoting Good Nutrition

An important nursing goal is to promote appropriate weight gain during pregnancy through healthy nutrition. It may be helpful to use a 24-hour diet recall form to help provide pertinent information about the patient's nutritional intake and food preparation/cooking preferences. On average, during the second and third trimesters a woman's caloric need increases by 300 per day. A well-balanced diet that contains the necessary vitamins and nutrients is essential. It is important to educate women

that prenatal vitamins are an option to ensure that their daily needs are being met, but mega-doses of vitamins can be harmful. A woman's need for folic acid doubles during pregnancy, and ideally supplementation with 400 mcg (0.4 mg) per day should be initiated prior to conception and continued at least through the first 3 months of pregnancy, to help reduce the incidence of open neural tube defects (NTDs) (CDC, 2012d). (See Chapters 7 and 10 for further discussion.)

In the mid-1970s, nutritionist Agnes Higgins developed "The Higgins Method of Nutritional Rehabilitation During Pregnancy." This program focused on the individual woman's nutritional needs based on age, prepregnant weight, activity level, pregnancy weight gain, and risk factors. The Higgins Method, still relevant today, is grounded in the philosophy that each woman has specific dietary needs, and by meeting those needs, one can promote optimal growth and development of the fetus (Higgins, 1976). (See Chapter 10 for further information about dietary needs in pregnancy.)

 Optimizing Outcomes—**Vitamin C and premature rupture of the membranes**

Low levels of vitamin C may predispose women to premature rupture of membranes. As the cellular availability of vitamin C decreases, the rate of degradation of cervical collagen increases (Casanueva et al., 2005; Osaikhuwuomwan, 2010). With decreased collagen, the cervix ripens more easily, prompting effacement and dilation. Researchers Hauth and colleagues (2010), however, were unable to demonstrate a reduction in preterm births (with or without premature rupture of membranes) following maternal supplementation with vitamins C and E beginning at 9 to 16 weeks of gestation in nulliparous women at low risk.

Recording Vital Signs

The vital signs are taken and documented. Blood pressure is a particularly important measurement and should be recorded under standardized conditions (making note of the arm used and the patient's position) and with the appropriate-size blood pressure cuff. Because the initial prenatal visit may be the patient's first adult interaction with a health-care professional, physiological indicators of anxiety (e.g., tachycardia and elevated blood pressure) may be present. In these situations, the nurse should record the first set of vital signs and then repeat the recordings later when the patient has had time to become familiar with her surroundings and is more relaxed.

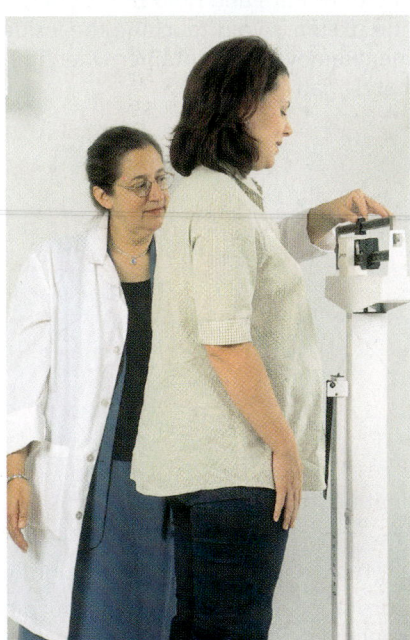

Figure 9-4 The weight is recorded and tracked throughout the pregnancy.

Cultural Diversity: Hypertension and Pregnancy

Nurses should be aware that hypertension is more prevalent in African American and Mexican American cultures, probably because of hereditary factors (Carson, Howard, Burke, Shea, Levitan, & Muntner, 2011). It is the most common medical condition affecting pregnancy and may worsen as the pregnancy progresses.

Obtaining the Urine Specimen

Before the physical examination, the nurse should ensure that the patient has had an opportunity to void, and if needed, a midstream urine sample is obtained (Procedure 9-1). A clean sample of urine should be cultured for asymptomatic bacteriuria during this first prenatal visit. As the name suggests, this type of urinary tract infection (UTI) does not cause symptoms but is present in more than 10% of pregnant women. Left untreated, a UTI may lead to a number of complications including preterm labor and pyelonephritis (Collins, 2013).

PERFORMING THE GENERAL PHYSICAL EXAMINATION

The general physical examination is then conducted with sensitivity to lifestyle choices, behaviors, and cultural beliefs. Together with physical data, the nurse should also gather information relating to the patient's usual state of health, her use of health promotion and maintenance strategies, and details of any present concerns or symptoms. The physical examination is a basic review of systems that includes ears, nose, mouth, and throat; cardio-respiratory;

 Procedure 9-1 Obtaining a Midstream Urine Sample

Purpose

To assist the woman in providing a suitable urine specimen for laboratory testing.

Preparation

1. Complete the information requested on the container label. Include the patient's full name and the date and time of collection of the specimen. If a requisition is needed, note the date and time on the requisition.

2. Explain the procedure to the woman to ensure she understands why a urine sample is requested, the purpose of any tests to be performed, and directions on how to obtain a midstream urine sample.

Equipment

- Approved empty sterile container for collection
- Towelette for cleaning in between the labia
- Tissue

Steps

Instruct the patient to do the following:

1. Wash and dry your hands thoroughly or use an alcohol-based hand-rub

   RATIONALE: *To reduce the risk of specimen contamination. Alcohol-based hand-rubs are fast acting, reduce the number of microorganisms on the skin, and may cause less skin irritation or dryness.*

2. Remove the container cap and set it on a clean, even surface with the inner surface pointing up. Do not touch the inner surface of the lid or the container.

   RATIONALE: *To reduce the risk of specimen contamination.*

3. Sit on the toilet seat and separate the labia (vaginal lips) using your nondominant hand. Clean the urogenital area from front to back with the towelette provided. Wipe for only one stroke and then discard the towelette.

   RATIONALE: *To reduce the risk of specimen contamination and to reduce the number of microorganisms on the skin. Cleansing from front to back prevents bringing rectal contamination forward.*

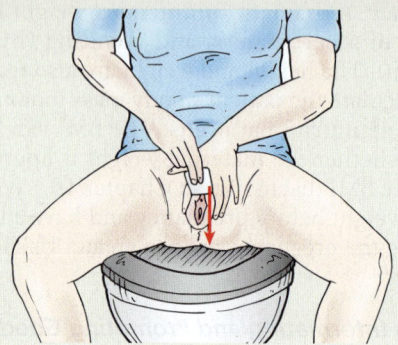

Patient cleansing labia.

4. Holding the labia apart, begin to pass urine. Allow the beginning urine to go directly into the toilet.

   RATIONALE: *The initial stream of urine washes urethral microorganisms and other debris away from the urethral meatus. The midstream collection ensures that a sterile specimen is obtained.*

5. Continue to urinate and hold the container under the urine stream. Avoid touching the inside of the container. Remove the container when it is approximately half full.

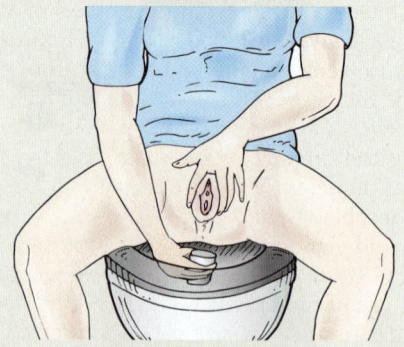

Patient urinating into specimen cup.

6. Carefully replace the cap and secure tightly.

   RATIONALE: *Placing the cap on the container prevents inadvertent spilling and possible contamination of the urine specimen.*

Procedure 9-1 Obtaining a Midstream Urine Sample (continued)

7. Wash your hands again after the specimen collection.

Clinical Alert Pregnant women are at an increased risk for developing urinary tract infections, especially if they are diabetic or have gestational diabetes. Urinary tract infections may also predispose to the onset of preterm labor.

Teach Patient

Teach the patient to recognize common signs of a urinary tract infection:

Dysuria—pain (burning sensation) on urination
Urinary frequency associated with small amounts of urine
Hematuria—blood or red blood cells in the urine

What If?

The woman is unable to obtain a urine specimen?

If the patient has no beverage with her, offer her a caffeine-free beverage (e.g., bottled water). Ask her to drink the beverage in its entirety and then remain nearby until she is able to obtain a urine specimen. Remind her that because she will be asked to supply a urine specimen at each prenatal visit, she may wish to bring a beverage with her in the future.

Documentation

1/10/13 1100 Patient educated re midstream urine collection. Patient verbalized understanding. Sample obtained, labeled with name, date, time, and type of specimen. Sent to lab at 1120 per Dr. Garner's order.
—M. D'Arcy-Evans, RN, CNM

---

musculoskeletal; and neurological function with an in-depth evaluation of the maternal physical adaptation to the pregnancy.

 Now Can You—Discuss aspects of the initial prenatal health assessment?

1. Identify five screening tests routinely performed on the patient's serum during the initial prenatal examination?
2. Briefly discuss why screening for HIV and *Chlamydia trachomatis* is recommended during pregnancy?
3. Identify four major components of the prenatal physical assessment?

THE FOCUSED OBSTETRIC EXAMINATION

Head, Neck, and Lungs

With the patient in a sitting position, the physical examination proceeds in a head to toe fashion beginning with a general evaluation of the skin and hair. Many women notice that their hair is healthier and more luxurious during pregnancy. Hair loss, common during the postpartum period, can be indicative of a vitamin or mineral deficiency. Increased levels of estrogen are responsible for a number of objective and subjective changes such as hypertrophy of the gingival tissue, nasal stuffiness, and an increased tendency for nosebleeds.

The thyroid gland is palpated while the patient remains in a sitting position. Enlargement is common during pregnancy because of increased vascularity and hyperplasia of the glandular tissue. The size and position of the thyroid are documented along with the presence of nodules or swelling. Anterior and posterior lung sounds are auscultated, and the cardiac rhythm and rate are evaluated for adventitious sounds. During pregnancy, approximately 90% of women exhibit systolic heart murmurs because of an increase in blood volume. The systolic murmur may be clearer when the woman holds her breath. Heart sounds should be evaluated with the woman in both a sitting and

lying position. Beginning late in the second trimester, the gravid uterus causes an upward and lateral displacement of the heart and the point of maximal impulse. Also, as pregnancy advances, the patient's breathing becomes thoracic in nature (rather than abdominal) because of the enlarged uterus.

The Skin

Assessment of the skin may reveal pregnancy-associated changes such as chloasma (the mask of pregnancy) and hyperpigmentation of the areolae, vulva, abdomen, and linea (linea nigra). The skin is evaluated for color consistent with the woman's ethnic background and for the presence of lesions or indicators of drug abuse (e.g., skin scratches, bruising or track marks, nasal discharge or irritated mucosa, and constricted or dilated pupils).

The Breasts

The patient is assisted to a recumbent position for the breast examination. Depending on the gestational age, it may be advisable to place a wedge under one of her hips to prevent compression of the vena cava from the gravid uterus (supine hypotension syndrome). Inspection of the breasts usually reveals pregnancy-related changes including nodularity, striae, and enlargement and hyperpigmentation of the nipples and Montgomery tubercles. Areas of indentation or skin puckering are not normal findings. Colostrum, a precursor to breast milk, may be expressed from the nipples as early as the first trimester of pregnancy. The lymph nodes should not be palpable.

 Collaboration in Caring—*Promoting breast comfort during pregnancy*

As a component of health teaching during pregnancy, the nurse should encourage patients to wear a firm, supporting bra. Some women may need a professional fitting by a brassiere specialist to find a style that promotes both comfort and support. As the breasts increase in weight, bras with wider straps may be more comfortable. Some women choose to wear a "sleeping" bra during the night for added comfort.

The Abdomen

The obstetric abdominal examination focuses on recognizing signs and changes associated with pregnancy. It is not intended to replace a comprehensive abdominal examination. The patient should be appropriately draped to maintain her privacy, comfort, and body temperature. The abdominal shape is assessed and inspected for the presence of scars (previous surgery should be documented), linea nigra, striae gravidarum, or signs of injury (e.g., bruising). As the pregnancy advances, visual inspection of the abdominal shape may reveal the fetal position, especially if transverse. Also, it may be possible to observe and palpate fetal movements. Patients generally become aware of fetal movements around the 16th to 20th week of pregnancy. A primigravida is usually able to identify fetal movements around 18 to 20 weeks; a multigravida may notice fetal movements as early as 16 weeks. This difference in awareness of fetal activity is most likely because of past experience in recognizing the movements along with a decrease in maternal abdominal muscle tone.

Uterine Size and Fetal Position

Abdominal palpation is used to evaluate the uterine size, to determine fetal position, and later in pregnancy, to determine whether the presenting part has engaged in the maternal pelvis. (See Chapter 12 for further discussion.) **Fundal height** is an indication of uterine size; periodic measurements of the fundal height should correlate strongly with fetal growth (Fig. 9-5). The relationship of the fundus (top part) of the uterus to specific maternal abdominal landmarks is used throughout pregnancy as a gauge to assess fetal growth. The fundal height measurement correlates to the weeks of gestation from approximately 22 to 34 weeks of gestation (Table 9-2). At 12 weeks of gestation, the fundus should be at the level of the symphysis pubis; at 20 weeks, the fundus should be at the umbilicus. The fundal height can be measured by using a tape measure or finger-breadths in combination with known maternal landmarks. For example, two finger-breadths above the umbilicus would be equivalent to approximately 24 weeks of gestation. Although convenient, using finger-breadths as a measuring tool is subject to variations in finger size among different examiners. This method of fundal height measurement is appropriate only if the same examiner consistently assesses uterine size.

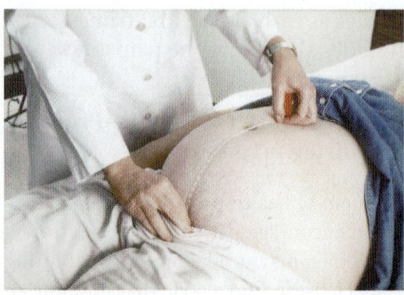

Figure 9-5 Obtaining the fundal height measurement.

Table 9-2	Approximate Fundal Height in Relation to Weeks of Pregnancy	
Weeks of Gestation	**Approximate Expected Fundal Height**
12	Level of the symphysis pubis
16	Halfway between the symphysis pubis and the umbilicus
20	1–2 finger-breadths below the umbilicus
24	1–2 finger-breadths above the umbilicus
28–30	One-third of the way between the umbilicus and the xiphoid processs
32	Two-thirds of the way between the umbilicus and the xiphoid processs
36	At the xiphoid process
38	1–2 finger-breadths below the xiphoid process
40	3–4 finger-breadths below the xiphoid process

Most often, the fundal height is measured with a tape measure. This method is usually initiated at around 22 weeks of gestation. The end of the measuring tape with the zero mark is held on the superior border of the symphysis pubis. Using the abdominal midline as guide, the tape is stretched over the contour of the abdomen to the top of the fundus (McDonald's method; see Fig. 9-5). The measurement (in centimeters) is recorded and equals the weeks of gestation. For example, at 28 weeks of gestation, the fundal height should be approximately 11 inches (28 cm; Fig. 9-6).

LEOPOLD MANEUVERS. The next step in abdominal palpation involves the use of **Leopold maneuvers**, a four-part clinical assessment method of observation and palpation to determine the lie, presentation, and position of the fetus. Steps for performing Leopold maneuvers are presented in Procedure 9-2.

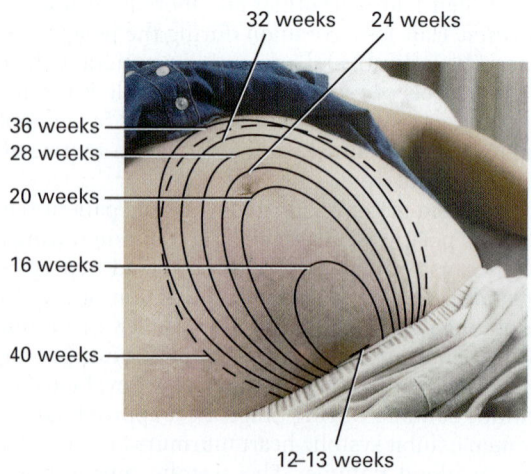

Figure 9-6 Fundal measurement should approximately equal the number of weeks of gestation.

Procedure 9-2 Performing Leopold Maneuvers

Purpose

To determine the lie, presentation, and position of the fetus and to aid in locating fetal heart sounds.

Equipment

- Gloves

Steps

Prepare the Patient:

1. Wash and dry hands and explain the procedure and purpose of the examination to the patient, noting what she will experience and what the results will indicate.

    RATIONALE: *Hand washing helps to prevent the spread of microorganisms. Explanations help to decrease anxiety and promote patient understanding and cooperation.*

2. Ask the patient to empty her bladder.

    RATIONALE: *An empty bladder facilitates the examination (e.g., the fetal contour will not be obscured by distension of the maternal bladder) and enhances patient comfort.*

3. Assess for latex allergies.

    RATIONALE: *To prevent injury from latex exposure; if the patient has a latex allergy, use non-latex gloves.*

4. Don gloves, as indicated.

    RATIONALE: *When indicated, to avoid contact with the patient's body secretions.*

5. Assist the patient to assume a supine position with the knees slightly flexed. Place a pillow under her head and a small rolled towel under one hip.

    RATIONALE: *To enhance patient comfort, to relax the abdominal muscles, and to prevent supine hypotension syndrome.*

6. Stand beside the patient, facing her head, and observe her abdomen for the longest fetal diameter and the presence of fetal movement.

    RATIONALE: *The longest fetal diameter, or axis, is the length of the fetus. The relationship of the long axis of the woman to the long axis of the fetus is known as the lie. The location of fetal movement most likely reflects the position of the fetal feet.*

7. Perform the first maneuver (fundal grip) to determine which fetal body part (head or breech [buttocks]) occupies the uterine fundus.

    Using the palmar surfaces of the hands, gently palpate the fundal region of the uterus. The breech feels soft, broad, and poorly defined. Unlike the head, the breech moves with the trunk. The head feels hard, firm, and round and moves independently of the trunk.

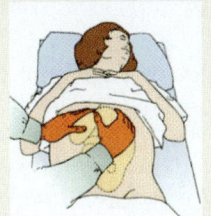

First maneuver.

8. Perform the second maneuver (umbilical grip) to determine the location of the fetal back.

    Using the palmar surface of the hands, palpate the sides of the uterus. Hold the left hand steady on one side of the uterus while using the right hand to palpate the opposite side of the uterus to determine which side the fetal back is on and which side the fetal small parts (i.e., arms and legs) are on. Repeat the palpation holding the right hand steady while palpating the opposite side of the uterus with the left hand. The fetal back feels like a firm, continuous, smooth, convex structure. The fetal arms and legs feel nodular, and may move during the palpation.

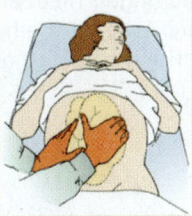

Second maneuver.

9. Perform the third maneuver ("Pawlick's grip") to confirm the presentation noted in the first maneuver and to determine if the presenting part is engaged. Engagement has occurred when the largest diameter of the presenting part reaches or passes through the maternal pelvic inlet.

    With the right hand, gently grasp the lower portion of the maternal abdomen just above the symphysis pubis between the thumb and index finger and attempt to press the thumb and finger together. If the presenting part moves upward so that the examiner's fingers can be pressed together, the presenting part is not engaged (i.e., it is not firmly settled into the maternal pelvis). If the presenting part is fixed, engagement has occurred. With the first pregnancy, engagement occurs around 37 weeks gestation; with subsequent pregnancies, engagement may not occur until labor has begun. If the presenting part is firm, it is the head; if it is soft, it is the breech.

(continued)

Procedure 9-2 Performing Leopold Maneuvers (continued)

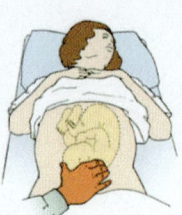

Third maneuver.

10. Perform the fourth maneuver (pelvic or inguinal grip) to determine the fetal attitude (relationship of the fetal parts to one another) and degree of fetal extension into the maternal pelvis.

Clinical Alert Omit the fourth maneuver if the fetus is in a breech presentation; this maneuver is performed only to determine if the fetal head is flexed.

Turn to face the patient's feet. Using both hands, outline the fetal head with the palmar surface of the fingertips pointed toward the pelvic inlet to determine whether the head is flexed (vertex) or extended (face). Gently slide the hands downward on each side of the uterus. On one side, the fingers easily slide to the upper edge of the maternal symphysis pubis. On the other side, the fingers meet an obstruction (i.e., the cephalic prominence). If the head is flexed, the cephalic prominence is palpated on the opposite side

Fourth maneuver.

from the fetal back. If the head is extended, the cephalic prominence is palpated on the same side as the fetal back.

11. Assist the patient to a sitting position and wash and dry hands.

12. Document the findings on the patient's medical record.

13. Inform the patient of the findings.

What If?

What if after performing Leopold maneuvers, you are still unable to determine the lie, presentation, and position of the fetus?

First, ask the patient to place her hand in the general area where she most often feels the baby's kicks. This information may guide you to the location of the fetal legs and feet. Repeat the Leopold maneuvers. If you are still unable to elicit the desired information, ask a colleague to assist you with performing the procedure.

Documentation
2-28-14 1400 Leopold maneuvers performed: fetus vertex, LOA, floating. Procedure tolerated well by patient.
S. Hisley, RN

Note: Be sure to follow your clinical practice facility's protocol for documentation.

Fetal Heart Auscultation

The information obtained during fetal palpation includes fetal presentation, lie, position, and engagement status (Table 9-3). (See Chapter 12 for further discussion.) Determining the fetal presentation facilitates fetal heart auscultation. The fetal heart rate (FHR) is heard most clearly directly over the fetal upper back (the maternal right or left lower abdominal quadrants) in a vertex presentation. The intensity of the fetal heart tones (FHT) varies according to the fetal position (Fig. 9-7). With a breech presentation, the fetal heart tones may be best heard in the patient's right or left upper abdominal quadrants. If fetal heart tones are auscultated most clearly in that location, the patient's care provider should be advised because further assessment may be indicated to confirm the fetal presentation. This is especially important when the patient is in labor. However, before approximately 32 weeks of pregnancy, it is not uncommon for the fetus to be in a breech presentation.

In most instances, by 36 to 37 weeks of gestation, the majority of fetuses will have spontaneously converted to a vertex (head down) presentation.

The normal heart rate for a fetus is approximately 110 to 160 beats per minute (bpm). If a slower heart rate is detected, the maternal pulse should first be evaluated to determine if the two heart rates are synchronous. If they are synchronous, the maternal pulse has inadvertently been auscultated through the abdomen and an attempt should be made to locate the fetal pulse. If the two pulses differ, the nurse should position the patient on her left side and seek assistance. Oxygen may be administered by mask and the patient should be instructed to take slow deep breaths. The nurse should continue to monitor the FHR and provide explanations and reassurance to the patient.

The fetal heart can be auscultated using a number of different devices. The least intrusive method involves the use

Table 9-3	**Defining Terms in Relation to Maternal Abdominal Palpations**
Lie of the Fetus	Where is the fetal spine in relation to the maternal spine? The maternal spine is always longitudinal. If the fetal spine is parallel to the maternal spine, the fetus is in a "longitudinal lie."
	If the fetal spine lies horizontally across the maternal spine, the fetus is in a "transverse lie."
	If the fetal spine lies obliquely across the maternal spine, the fetus is in an "oblique lie."
	"Lie" describes the relationship of the fetus to the long axis of the mother. Normal lie is longitudinal (the fetal long axis, or spine, is in line with the maternal long axis).
Presentation	Refers to the fetal part that would be delivered first in a vaginal birth.
	Normally, the fetal head is the part of the fetus that is presenting.
Position	The head is the most common presentation.
	When the fetus is in a well-flexed position (the fetal knees and chin against its body), the occiput area is determined to be the presenting part because this is the lowest part of the fetal head.
	To determine position, it is necessary to assess where the fetal occiput is, in relation to the maternal pelvis.
	If the fetal occiput faces toward the front near the symphysis pubis, the fetus is in an anterior position. If the occiput is on the maternal right side, the fetus is in a right occipitoanterior position (ROA). If on the maternal left side, the fetus is in a left occipitoanterior position (LOA).
	If the fetal occiput is toward the side of the maternal pelvis, the fetus is in a lateral (or transverse) position. If the occiput is on the maternal right, the fetus is in a right occipitolateral position (ROL). If on the maternal left, it is a left occipitolateral (LOL) position.
	If the fetal occiput is toward the maternal spine, the fetus is in a posterior position. If the occiput is on the maternal right, the fetus is in a right occipitoposterior position (ROP). If on the maternal left, it is a left occipitoposterior (LOP) position.
Engagement	When palpating the presenting part, is it moveable?
	If the presenting part is fixed (i.e., you are unable to move it) when palpating the maternal abdomen, the presenting part is said to be engaged.

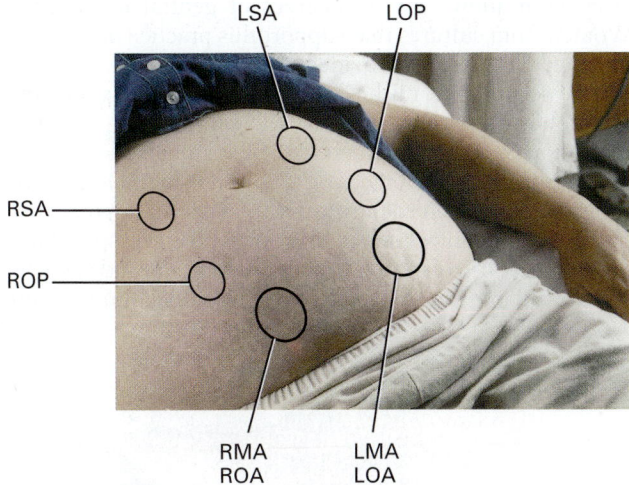

Figure 9-7 Fetal heart tone intensity varies according to the fetal position. RSA = right sacrum anterior; LSA = left sacrum anterior; ROP = right occipitoposterior; LOP = left occipitoposterior; RMA = right mentum anterior; LMA = left mentum anterior; ROA = right occipitoanterior; LOA = left occipitoanterior.

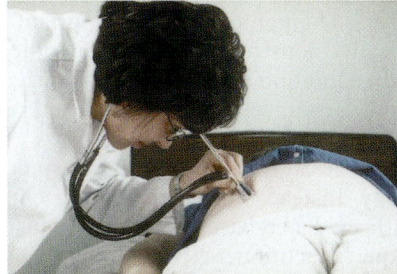

Figure 9-8 Auscultating the fetal heart tones with a fetoscope.

of a Pinard stethoscope or a fetoscope (Fig. 9-8). Both of these devices are used without any additional equipment. However, they do require the examiner's ability to be able to palpate the woman's abdomen accurately to determine the fetal position and locate the fetal shoulder to ascertain the correct location for placement of the stethoscope. This method of fetal heart auscultation is ideal if the patient has expressed a desire to avoid an ultrasound (Doppler) stethoscope. Following the invention of the Doppler ultrasound stethoscope, use of the fetoscope and Pinard stethoscopes in clinical practice has decreased. The Doppler ultrasound

stethoscope is a handheld device that uses ultrasound to locate fetal heart sounds (Fig. 9-9). Use of the Doppler stethoscope to auscultate fetal heart tones is simple and requires no special skills because placement of the instrument in the general vicinity of the fetal heart will most likely produce audible heart tones. Although this approach may provide an easy, quick assessment, the nurse who uses this method may not be performing a detailed patient examination and may miss vital information. With the Doppler stethoscope, FHT may be auscultated by 10 to 12 weeks or by 17 to 19 weeks with the fetal stethoscope.

Some sophisticated Doppler models provide a printout similar to those of the more conventional FHR monitors. Beginning in the later weeks of the second trimester, standard electronic fetal monitors may be used to record the FHR in conjunction with uterine activity. Electronic fetal monitoring during the prenatal period is generally limited to pregnancies designated as being high risk because of maternal or fetal factors. In these situations, a **nonstress test** (NST) may be ordered to provide an evaluation of the FHR in response to fetal movement and/or uterine activity. A reactive test (the desirable result), is one in which the heart

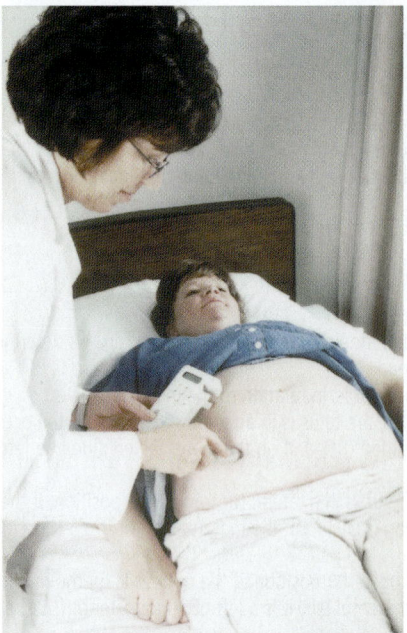

Figure 9-9 Auscultating the fetal heart tones with a Doppler ultrasound stethoscope.

rate accelerates by at least 15 beats per minute for at least 15 seconds, with at least three "acceleration episodes" in a 20-minute period of monitoring. It is important to remember that a reactive nonstress test is only an indicator of the fetus's present condition rather than a test that can be used to predict future fetal well-being. (See Chapter 11 for further discussion.)

Nurses must be cautious not to place too much reliance on technology. Instead, nurses should use clinical skills coupled with evidence-based theory to transition from novice to expert practitioner. To attain this level of expertise, it is essential to maintain hands-on patient care. Experienced clinical nurses attain a sixth sense, or "specialty intuition," that enables them to quickly recognize deviations from normal and provide expert care in a timely manner. With regard to electronic fetal monitoring and other high-tech modalities, the nurse must be careful not to rely on imperfect tools and instead use sound clinical judgment and decision making.

 Now Can You—Discuss various methods of clinical fetal assessment?

1. Describe how to perform a fundal height measurement?
2. Identify how to perform each component of Leopold maneuvers and explain what the findings indicate?
3. Compare and contrast the technique of fetal heart auscultation using a fetoscope and a Doppler ultrasound stethoscope?

The Vagina and Pelvis

A vaginal examination is usually performed at the initial prenatal visit following assessment of the maternal abdomen. Most women find this part of the examination to be intrusive and may fear being exposed, hurt, or embarrassed. An essential component of the nurse's role is to explain to the patient what to expect and to help her to

verbalize any fears. The patient's permission to conduct a vaginal assessment must always be obtained before proceeding. Demonstrating awareness of the patient's feelings can be conveyed by simple strategies: remaining gentle and respectful, showing equipment that will be used with a demonstration of how it works, and ensuring privacy with appropriate drapes. Eye-to-eye contact maintains a connection between the nurse and the patient and allows the nurse to be aware of nonverbal communication. Some women feel less anxious if they are actively involved in the examination. For example, if desired, a mirror can be placed so that the patient can view her cervix or be shown changes such as Chadwick's sign.

There are essentially four components to the examination, which begins with an assessment of the external genitalia (Fig. 9-10). Information can be obtained regarding secondary sexual characteristics by observing the pattern of hair growth. This is also an ideal time to check for the presence of **pediculosis,** or pubic lice. Signs of vaginal infection may be indicated by redness, edema, or an offensive vaginal discharge. The presence of lesions, condylomata (human papillomavirus), vesicles (herpes), ulceration (syphilitic chancre), or inflammation need to recognized and investigated. Bruising or tenderness may be present as a result of trauma or abuse. Observation of the perineal body may show evidence of a previous episiotomy or perineal tear. Women who have been subjected to female circumcision show varying degrees of genital mutilation. Women from cultures that support this practice may prefer to have a female care provider.

The second part of the examination includes visual inspection of the vaginal mucosa and cervix along with the collection of specimens such as the Papanicolaou test (Pap test), cultures for gonorrhea or *Chlamydia,* and if indicated, wet smear slides to determine the cause of vaginal discharge. The examiner selects an appropriate-size speculum. Specula may be constructed of metal or plastic and are generally available in two types: the Graves' speculum, useful

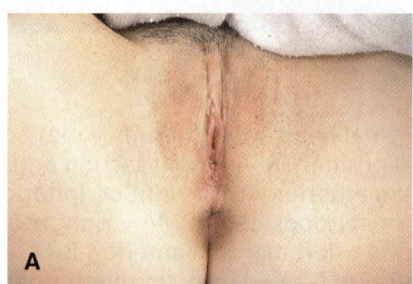

A

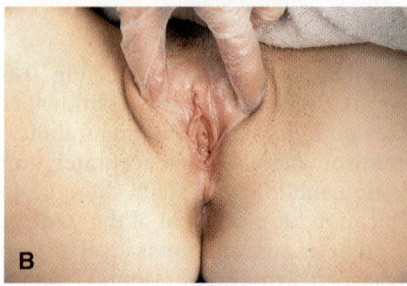

B

Figure 9-10 *A,* The vaginal examination begins with a visual inspection of the external genitalia. *B,* The fingers are used to separate the labia minora.

for examining multiparous women; and the more narrow, flat Pedersen speculum, commonly used for children, women who have never been sexually active, nulliparous women, and some postmenopausal women. The speculum is inserted into the vagina at an oblique angle, then rotated to a horizontal angle and gently advanced downward against the posterior vaginal wall. Once in position, the speculum blades are opened to allow visualization of the cervix (Fig. 9-11).

The cervix and vaginal mucosa are inspected for color and for the presence of inflammation, lesions, ulcerations, or erosion. The cervix is usually about 1 inch (2.5 cm) in length and the external cervical os is round in women who have never given birth (nulliparous) and appears "slit-shaped" in the multigravida (Fig. 9-12).

The remaining part of the assessment includes clinical pelvimetry and the bimanual examination. Bimanual examination is an evaluation of uterine shape, position, and size (Fig. 9-13). The uterus is normally anteverted (tipped forward). As it enlarges during pregnancy, the uterus becomes more midline and globular in shape. The size of the pregnant uterus should be equal to the estimated weeks of gestation. If the uterus is larger than anticipated, this finding may be associated with a number of factors including miscalculation of the date of conception, multiple pregnancy, hydatidiform mole, uterine fibroid tumors, or later in pregnancy, a condition known as **hydramnios** (an increase in the volume of amniotic fluid). A uterus smaller than expected may indicate miscalculation of dates or a missed abortion. (See Chapter 11 for further discussion.) The manual examination provides an ideal time to evaluate vaginal and perineal muscle tone and to determine the presence of a cystocele (bladder prolapse), urethrocele (urethral prolapse), or rectocele (rectal prolapse). Women should be reminded to practice Kegel exercises to help maintain perineal muscle tone.

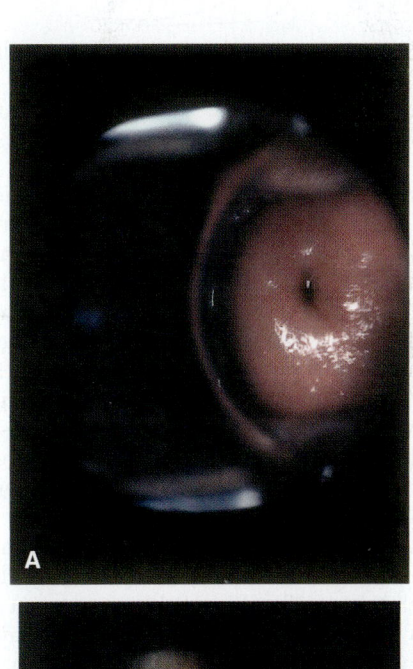

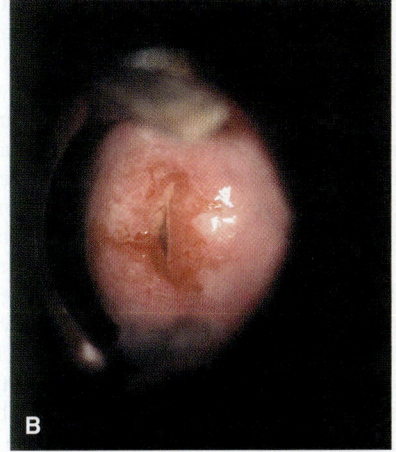

Figure 9-11 *A,* Inserting the speculum. *B,* Opening the speculum. *C,* Proper position of speculum in the vagina. *D,* View through the speculum.

Figure 9-12 *A,* Circular cervical opening: nulliparous. *B,* Slit-shaped cervical opening: multiparous.

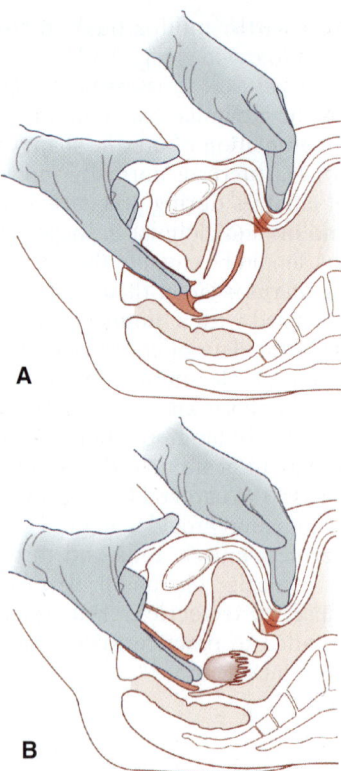

Figure 9-13 *A,* Palpating the uterus. *B,* Palpating the ovaries.

The rectovaginal examination is performed after completion of the bimanual examination. The examiner removes his or her hand from the vagina and dons a clean pair of gloves. A water-based lubricant is applied to the fingertips of the dominant hand. The index finger is reinserted into the vagina; the middle finger is inserted into the rectum. The rectal finger is advanced forward as the abdomen is depressed with the nondominant hand. Palpation of the tissue between the examining fingers allows for assessment of the strength and irregularity of the posterior vaginal wall. The fingers are withdrawn and any stool present on the glove may be tested for occult blood.

The final component of the physical examination involves the clinical evaluation of the pelvis, also known as clinical pelvimetry. The goal of this assessment is to recognize any abnormality in shape or size that may be associated with a difficult or traumatic vaginal birth. The four basic pelvic types include the gynecoid, found in more than 40% of women, the android (male), the anthropoid (most common in non-Caucasian races), and the platypelloid, which is the most rare type and is found in fewer than 3% of women. The internal pelvic measurements provide the diameters of the inlet and outlet through which the fetus must pass during birth. The measurements most commonly made include the diagonal conjugate, the true conjugate (conjugate vera), and the ischial tuberosity diameter. Clinical pelvimetry is performed by the physician, nurse midwife, or advanced practice nurse; it is generally not repeated in women who have previously given birth to an infant weighing 7 lb or more (3.18 kg) unless there is a history of pelvic trauma in the intervening period between pregnancies.

The **diagonal** conjugate is the distance between the anterior surface of the sacral prominence and the anterior surface of the inferior margin of the symphysis pubis. This measurement, performed with the patient in a lithotomy position, indicates the anteroposterior diameter of the pelvic inlet—the most narrow diameter and the one most likely to create a problem with misfit of the fetal head. If the diagonal conjugate is greater than 12.5 cm, the pelvic inlet is considered to be adequate for childbirth (Fig. 9-14).

The **true conjugate** (conjugate vera) is the measurement between the anterior surface of the sacral prominence and the posterior surface of the inferior margin of the symphysis pubis. This measurement is estimated from the dimension made of the diagonal conjugate. It cannot be measured directly. The true conjugate is the actual diameter of the pelvic inlet through which the fetal head will pass. On average, the diameter of the true conjugate ranges from 4.1 to 4.3 inches (10.5 to 11 cm).

The **ischial tuberosity** diameter (also known as the intertuberous or bi-ischial diameter) is a measurement of the distance between the ischial tuberosities (e.g., the transverse diameter of the outlet). Often assessed with a pelvimeter (a special device for measuring the pelvis), the

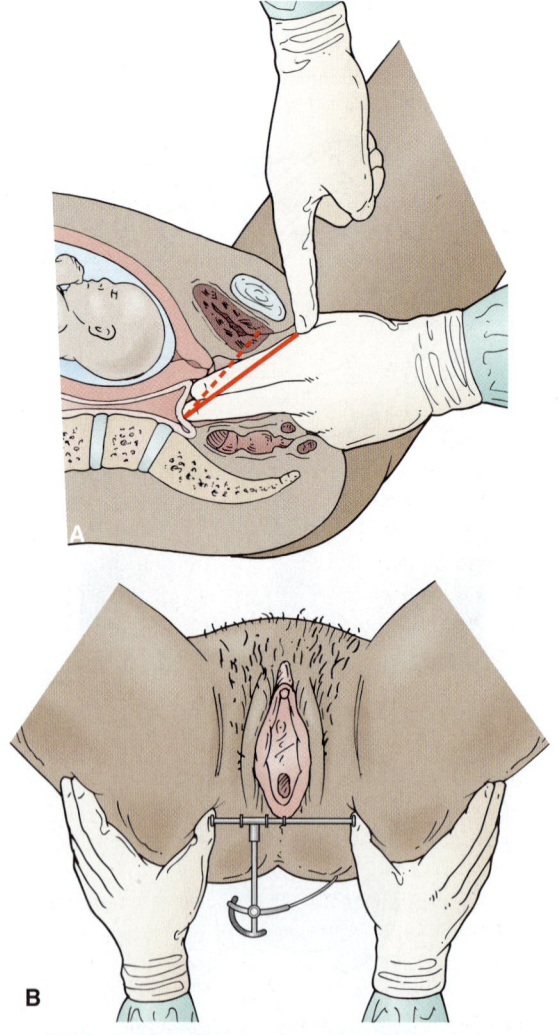

Figure 9-14 *A,* The diagonal conjugate and the true conjugate (conjugate vera). *B,* Use of a pelvimeter to measure the ischial tuberosity diameter.

diameter can also be measured with a ruler or with the examiner's clenched fist or hand span (the exact measurements of the fist and hand must be known). A diameter of 11 cm is considered adequate for passage of the widest diameter of the fetal head through the pelvic outlet. Using palpation, the examiner assesses the coccyx for mobility. A mobile nonprominent coccyx allows for some flexibility of the pelvic outlet during birth.

Subsequent Prenatal Examinations

The plan of care for the first prenatal visit should be amended to meet each individual woman's needs, based on medical, social, cultural, and individual factors. Subsequent prenatal visits are usually not as in-depth but should be designed to recognize any deviations from normal so that appropriate investigations can be ordered and care managed accordingly. Normally, patients are seen at a frequency of every 4 weeks until 28 to 32 weeks of pregnancy, then every 2 weeks until 36 weeks, and then weekly until childbirth. At each visit, standard of care includes an evaluation of the maternal weight gain, blood pressure, urine (for glucose and protein), uterine growth, fetal heart tones, fetal movements, and presentation (Box 9-9). The patient is also assessed for the presence of edema. Each prenatal appointment provides an ideal opportunity for education related to the patient's particular stage of pregnancy and what to expect before the next visit. A review of the warning signs of pregnancy is also essential, and the nurse should confirm that the woman is able to verbalize when and how to seek professional assistance.

Evaluation of fetal well-being includes documentation of the patient's perception of fetal movements. Depending

---

Box 9-9 **Essential Components of Subsequent Prenatal Visits**

REVIEW THE WOMAN'S OVERALL HEALTH STATUS
- Signs/symptoms of pregnancy
- Discomforts of pregnancy
- Changes in medications/over-the-counter/herbal/homeopathic
- Psychological assessment (emotional or psychological distress) including factors such as affect, sleep patterns, and diet

MATERNAL WELL-BEING
- Record vital signs.
  - Ensure blood pressure is recorded using an appropriately sized cuff and under the same conditions each visit (e.g., maternal position).
- Record maternal weight.
  - Weight gain is usually 1 pound per week during the second and third trimesters.
    - Excessive weight gain may be indicative of fluid retention and requires investigation.
    - Weight loss may be because of maternal disease or inadequate dietary intake: nursing assessment needed.
- Evaluate for edema: dependent edema especially in hot weather and at the end of the day is a normal finding.
- Where indicated, assess reflexes and check for clonus.
  - Any signs of preterm labor such as uterine contractions or backache.
  - Ensure patient knows indicators of preterm labor and knows how to seek medical advice.
- Assess for any signs of domestic/intimate partner abuse.

EVALUATE FETAL WELL-BEING
Listen to fetal heart tones, usually can be heard from approximately 12–14 weeks' gestation with a Doppler stethoscope: normal rate is 110–160 bpm.
- Discuss pattern and frequency of fetal movements.
  - Encourage patient to monitor and record fetal movements daily.
  - Educate patient on the importance of fetal movements as an indicator of general fetal well-being.
  - Ensure the patient knows to immediately report a decrease in fetal movements.
- Evaluate uterine growth.
  - Measure fundal height.
  - Document findings and evaluate pattern of growth.
    - Weeks of gestation are equivalent to measurement in centimeters: McDonald Method (measure from the top of the symphysis pubis to fundus, from approximately 24–34 weeks' gestation)—for example, at 30 weeks' gestation the fundal height should be 11.8 inches (30 cm).
  - Measurement less than expected could indicate intrauterine growth restriction, oligohydramnios, or incorrect dates.
  - Measurement greater than expected could indicate multiple pregnancy, macrosomic infant, hydramnios, or incorrect dates.

PATIENT TEACHING
- Provide education related to stage of pregnancy (e.g., what physical changes to expect or danger signs that need to be reported, such as vaginal bleeding or fluid loss, abdominal pain, or visual disturbances).
- Encourage attendance in prenatal education classes.
- Encourage tour of facility where patient intends to give birth.
- Later in pregnancy, focus of education needs to include preparation for care of the newborn (e.g., car seats, male circumcision, and immunizations) so that parents can make informed decisions.

Screening and laboratory testing may include:

Ultrasound	Some health-care providers offer routine ultrasound examinations in the first trimester of pregnancy to confirm dates and ensure single pregnancy; may be repeated later in pregnancy.
Prenatal screening	May be performed first trimester and/or second trimester. (See Table 9-5.)
Screening for gestational diabetes	Offered around 24–28 weeks' gestation. Patient drinks solution containing 50 g of glucose and then has blood drawn 1 hour later—results should be below 140 mg/dL.
Rh screening	Rh(D)-negative woman: Check for Rh antibodies and if negative, 300 mcg of $Rh_o(D)$ immune globulin (RhoGAM) is prescribed at 28–32 weeks' gestation.
Hemoglobin/ hematocrit	Usually repeated mid-pregnancy and then as indicated.
Group B *Streptococcus* screening	Normally offered at 37 weeks' gestation to determine whether antibiotic coverage is needed during labor.

Confirm the patient's contact information (address and telephone numbers) and ensure she has a scheduled return appointment. Always provide time for the patient to ask questions and confirm her understanding and that she has no other concerns that need to be addressed.

on the circumstances, fetal evaluation may also include electronic heart rate monitoring, ultrasonography to monitor growth patterns, and/or placental aging and a biophysical profile. In addition, the patient may be offered various screening tests during pregnancy to detect fetal genetic or structural abnormalities. (See Chapters 10 and 11 for further discussion.)

 Now Can You—Discuss the vaginal examination, clinical pelvimetry, and assessments routinely made during each prenatal visit?

1. Compare and contrast the purpose of the vaginal speculum examination and the bimanual examination?
2. Explain the purpose of clinical pelvimetry and identify three measurements that are commonly included in this assessment?
3. Name seven maternal–fetal assessments routinely performed during each prenatal visit?

Assessing Special Populations

THE ADOLESCENT

Sexual Behavior and Pregnancy

Teenage pregnancy is not a new phenomenon. The transitional period of adolescence, which spans the years from 10 to 19 (World Health Organization, 2013), marks the biological and psychological passage from childhood into adulthood. Pregnancy during adolescence has far-reaching implications for society as well as for the young woman and her family.

In the American culture, the expectation is that women marry, ideally after having completed an acceptable level of education, before the couple plans the birth of their first child. Teenage pregnancy meets none of these expectations and as such is not condoned by American society in general. Despite this stigma, adolescent pregnancies continue to occur, are often fathered by teenage males, or in some cases, by men significantly older.

Not all teen pregnancies are accidents. For some adolescents, pregnancy provides a means of escape from an unpleasant situation, a method for achieving a goal, or someone to love. Relationships with the unequal power dynamics often present between an older male and a teenage female can predispose to coercion in sexual activity. Pregnancy may also result from sexual assault, incest, and dating violence that involves sexual intercourse.

Problems that develop in the wake of teen pregnancy are not limited to the duration of the pregnancy. Instead, they appear to be much longer lasting. For example, although many teenagers who become pregnant manage to complete high school, only a small percentage continue their education to earn a college degree. Without advanced education, their earning capacity and career opportunities are somewhat limited, and this factor may become a lifelong limitation.

In addition to the many developmental, social, educational, and lifelong consequences for both the young mother and her child, the teenage patient is also at additional risk for a host of obstetric complications including anemia, preeclampsia, and preterm birth. Preterm birth and low-birth-weight infants are major causes of neonatal morbidity and mortality. Survival of a compromised infant may necessitate a lifetime of care and considerable economic resources.

 Nursing Insight—*Health issues and disparities associated with teen pregnancy*

Teen pregnancies are associated with a multitude of far-reaching issues that affect the young mothers, their infants, and society at large. For example, teen mothers are at a higher risk for sexually transmitted illnesses, and during pregnancy they experience an increased risk for hypertensive problems. Infants born to teen mothers are at a greater risk for health problems such as prematurity and/or low birth weight; these conditions place the infant at an increased risk for death, respiratory distress syndrome, intraventricular bleeding, and vision and intestinal problems. The societal impact of teen pregnancy is significant as well: Approximately 50% of teen mothers begin receiving welfare within 5 years of the birth of their first child, and approximately 25% of teen mothers will give birth to a second child within 24 months, further decreasing their ability to complete school and qualify for a well-paying job (The National Campaign to Prevent Teen and Unplanned Pregnancy, 2012).

The rate of adolescent pregnancy in the United States is almost double that of other developed countries. Clearly, teen pregnancy is a complex, multifaceted issue that must be addressed at the local, state, and national levels. One goal of the *Healthy People 2020* national health initiative directly addresses the number of pregnancies that occur in the adolescent population. It calls for a reduction in pregnancy rates among adolescent females to no more than 36.2/1,000 adolescents from a baseline of 40.2/1,000.

The Nurse's Role

Nurses can help the nation to achieve this goal by heightening public awareness of the complex personal and societal repercussions of adolescent pregnancy. Nurses can also empower women and their families with factual information and strategies to reduce unwanted pregnancies among this young population. In the community setting, nurses can advocate for responsible sexual behavior by providing educational programs for youth in schools, churches, clubs, and after-school activities. In the clinical setting, nurses can listen to, counsel, and educate young patients to help prepare them for responsible sexual decision making. Nurses can also empower mothers and fathers of young adults with methods for facilitating open, honest family discussions about sexuality and sexual behavior.

 Where Research and Practice Meet: **Nurturing Resilience in Teens at Risk for Repeat Unplanned Pregnancy**

As teens struggle with the developmental tasks of role identity, many forces affect how they respond to life stressors such as unplanned pregnancy. Because they are often the first health-care providers to interact with pregnant teens, nurses are perfectly positioned to play a pivotal role in the prevention and control of teen pregnancies.

Resilience appears to be an important factor in coping with crisis situations. The Resilience-Recoil-Rebound Theory of Teen Pregnancy Prevention (RRRTTPP), proposed by nurse researchers Porter and Holness (2011), provides a creative approach to heighten understanding of the phenomenon of repeat teen pregnancy and offers strategies for nurturing resilience in at-risk teens. For example, nurses may implement teen pregnancy prevention/intervention programs that focus on resilience-building areas such as relationships, acceptance, confidence, goals, and encouragement (Porter & Holness, 2011).

Strategies that use a holistic family approach such as promoting open communication between parents/guardians and teenagers, together with teaching self-respect, setting boundaries, and providing appropriate supervision, are essential components of any successful approach to reduce teenage pregnancy (Table 9-4).

Some groups advocate mandatory sex education for all adolescents; others support programs that only teach sexual abstinence. There is little scientific evidence to determine which approach is most effective. Because individuals' responses and actions are shaped by personality, cultural norms, and observed social patterns and behaviors, any one doctrine is rarely applicable to every group.

❝What to say❞—*Dialoging with teens about sex*

When talking with teens about sex, it is important to use language with which they can relate. For example, the nurse may say:

"You would not give your $100 mobile phone to just anyone, so do not give your body to just anyone" (Harris, 2005, p. 15).

Impact on Society

APPROACHES TO ADDRESSING THE PROBLEM OF ADOLESCENT PREGNANCY. Over the years, a variety of local and national efforts have attempted to dissuade adolescents from engaging in early sexual activity. Strategies have ranged from public awareness campaigns to public chastisement, conviction as a sex offender, and institutionalization for unacceptable moral behavior. The various approaches have met with some success, but usually on a short-term basis.

Table 9-4 A Holistic Family Approach to Preventing Teenage Pregnancies

Parental Influences	Strategies
• Parents have the strongest influence on teenage behavior.	• Promote open communication. • Foster safe and nonjudgmental environment to facilitate discussion of issues relating to vaginal and oral sex, relationships, self-esteem, self-worth, and how to say "no" to unwanted sexual contact.
• Parents/adults need to model behaviors that are respectful, honest, nonaggressive, and healthy.	• Ways to interact and communicate are learned through observation. Observing a relationship between adults in which each is given equal power and respect can help to initiate a sense of self-worth irrespective of gender.
• Promoting family values, caring behaviors, and closeness.	• Shared family activities, eating meals together, taking time to be with one another to enjoy a shared interest.
• Build a trusting, loving relationship.	• Take time to know teenagers' friends and their families. • Become involved and provide adequate supervision of activities. • Promote group activities rather than early dating.
• Providing accurate information to include both abstinence and contraception.	• Parents may need help to increase their own comfort level and knowledge before being able to confidently help their child. • Need to develop active listening skills and ensure it is a two-way conversation, not a mini lecture. • Dispel myths. • Do not promote double standards. Teenage sex is not to be encouraged irrespective of gender. Make expectations clearly known. • Use situations as they arise. For example, watching television together may provide an opportunity to discuss some relationship or sexual issue based on a program being viewed.
• Understanding developmental stages related to teenagers, such as egocentric thinking and their sense of invincibility.	• Use scenarios within the family setting to demonstrate formal reasoning—the ability to recognize alternatives and the consequences of their choices, both short and long term. • Help the adolescent to see the "whole" picture and not just focus on their immediate needs (egocentric thinking). • Teenagers are generally unable to recognize and appreciate behavioral risk; they are more likely to ignore or fail to understand the logical laws of probability. "It won't happen to me" is the opinion much more likely to be believed.
• Future plans.	• Discuss plans for the future—set goals. • Let it be known that education is essential to a bright future.

Source: The National Campaign to Prevent Teen and Unplanned Pregnancy (2012). Parent power: What parents need to know and do to help prevent teen pregnancy.

Current discussions center on the issue of whether providing sex education to children promotes early sexual activity. Rosengard and colleagues (2005) reported that although a majority of sexually active teenage boys did not intend to cause a pregnancy, they acknowledged that it was a possibility. Providing teenagers with sex education is an approach that endeavors to take the "secrecy" out of sex and instead provide basic, accurate information. It is believed that this strategy will empower adolescents with the knowledge needed to make informed decisions, or in the least, with the confidence necessary to seek guidance. When teenagers perceive sex to be a taboo subject, they are left to rely on friends, acquaintances, or peers who may not have a sound knowledge base to share. This paradigm supports the argument that knowledge reduces the need for experimentation and discovery. Experimentation without facts can lead to accidental pregnancy and sexually transmitted infections.

Teaching sexual abstinence before marriage can be effective in some cultures or populations, especially if the approach focuses on both genders. Discrepancy may exist between what is acceptable behavior or action for a teenage female and a teenage male. Interpretation of the phrase "sexual abstinence" may vary from no sexual contact of any description to simply maintaining virginity. For over two decades, the U.S. Congress has provided financial support to states that provided abstinence-only education, irrespective of the lack of substantive data demonstrating the effectiveness of this approach.

Along with a tendency to behave impulsively, adolescents lack the ability to make informed, complex decisions or to accurately compare alternatives. Neurobiological factors may be responsible for this deficit. The brain's prefrontal cortex is responsible for all "executive functions." Maturity of this area is not fully attained until an individual has reached age 20 or older. Nurses need to incorporate this information into the design of health education classes that will enable teenagers to understand better the process of making an informed decision. Ensuring that the adolescent has a realistic perception of related risks and the potential short-term and long-term outcomes is an essential component of any educational effort.

Cultural Influences on Adolescent Pregnancy

Adolescent pregnancy exists within every culture although the prevalence varies and it is not always viewed negatively. Within the sub-Saharan African region, girls often as young as 12 or 14 years of age are still sold to prospective husbands in exchange for a negotiated amount of money or in exchange for animals. In this culture, arranging a good marriage for a young teenage girl can often be a solution to family poverty.

In the United States, African American and Hispanic adolescents represent the groups most likely to engage in early sexual activity, and not surprisingly, these groups have the highest rates of teenage pregnancy, although the discrepancy among different cultures is decreasing (Box 9-10). In 2008, the teen pregnancy rate was 117 per 1,000 African American teen girls. **Pregnancy rate** is defined as the total number of pregnancies, including those that end in spontaneous abortion, elective abortion, or birth.

> **Box 9-10** Sexual Activity and Pregnancy Rates Among African American Teenagers in the United States
>
> - Have the highest pregnancy rate when compared with all major racial and ethnic groups
> - Before the age of 20, approximately 50% will have experienced at least one pregnancy
> - Have more sexual partners and are more sexually experienced
> - As a group, African American teens demonstrated one of the highest reductions (48%) in teen pregnancy during the period between 1990 and 2008. The overall teen pregnancy rate during this time fell by 42%.
> - In 2009, 97% of African American teen girls between the ages of 15 and 19 who gave birth were unmarried (The National Campaign to Prevent Teen and Unplanned Pregnancy, 2012).

 ### Cultural Diversity: Pregnancy Rates Among African American Adolescents

During the period of time from 1990 to 2008, the overall pregnancy rate in American teenagers declined 42%, and among African American teen girls, the pregnancy rate decreased 48%, from 224 to 117 pregnancies per 1,000 girls. Despite the decrease in pregnancy and birth rates among African American teen girls, the rates for this population remain higher than rates for teens overall. The pregnancy rate among African American teen girls is slightly higher than the rate among Latina teens (117 compared with 107) and is nearly three times higher than the rate for non-Hispanic teen girls (Kost & Henshaw, 2012).

During 2008, there were approximately 236,220 pregnancies in girls 15 to 17 years of age and approximately 496,780 pregnancies in girls age 18 to 19. The teen pregnancy rate among Hispanic and African American teen girls age 15 to 19 was more than two and a half times higher than the teen pregnancy rate among non-Hispanic white teen girls age 15 to 19 (The National Campaign to Prevent Teen and Unplanned Pregnancy, 2012).

Along with cultural influences, many other factors, such as education, spiritual beliefs and group support, family structure, and income also impact the occurrence of adolescent pregnancy. As educational level increases, the age at which first intercourse occurs also increases while the risk of pregnancy decreases. Teenagers from middle-class, two-parent families are more likely to delay their first sexual experience. This tendency is also documented among adolescents who report an affiliation with a church, synagogue, or other religious institution. These individuals benefit from the group support associated with their church-related activities.

Several years ago, two national organizations, The National Campaign to Prevent Teen and Unplanned Pregnancy and the National Coalition of Pastors' Spouses, produced a document intended to heighten public awareness of the issues concerning pregnancy among African American teenagers. The collaborative effort underscored the value of family and the faith community on adolescent sexual behavior. The premise of the report holds that a teenager's religious and moral beliefs, personal experiences, and perception of family love and commitment are strongly reflected in sexual behaviors.

Identifying Adolescents at Greatest Risk for Unwanted Pregnancy

Adolescents who lack the support, security, and love of a family home are more likely to engage in high-risk behaviors including sex at an early age, multiple sexual partners, failure to use contraception, and unplanned pregnancy. Incarcerated juveniles constitute the most vulnerable group, especially when placed in an environment away from family support. These teenagers often have histories of physical neglect as well as severe physical, emotional, and sexual abuse. This group is more likely to experiment with high-risk behaviors, such as tobacco and substance abuse, gang involvement, and violence. They may be more susceptible to peer pressure and are more likely to succumb to negative behaviors in an attempt to gain acceptance or peer status. Consequently, many begin sexual experimentation at a very early age and predictably experience unwanted teenage pregnancy (Vorvick & Storck, 2011).

 Across Care Settings: Reaching across the worldwide Web to encourage smoking cessation in adolescents

Nearly 20 percent of teens currently smoke, and most will continue to smoke into adulthood unless efforts are made to help them kick the habit. Many teens want to to to quit, but are unlikely to use evidence-based support resources to support their tobacco cessation attempts. To assist them in their efforts, the National Cancer Institute, part of the National Institutes of Health (NIH), has developed SmokefreeTXT, a free text message cessation service that provides 24/7 encouragement, advice, and tips geared specifically for teens who are trying to quit. Teens can sign up online at teen.smokefree.gov or text QUIT to iQUIT (47848). The Smokefree Teen initiative, which sponsors SmokefreeTXT, also offers several social media pages to connect teens with cessation tools. QuitSTART is a free smartphone application that provides an interactive quit guide for teens that delivers smoking cessation and mood management tips, tracks cravings, and monitors quit attempts. Teens who have quit smoking will continue to receive texts for up to six weeks, which is a critical time for continued cessation support (NIH, 2011).

The Impact of Pregnancy on Meeting the Developmental Tasks of Adolescence

A pregnant teenager is required to be able to make informed decisions regarding continuing the pregnancy, and if the pregnancy comes to fruition, future plans for the child. This action hinges on the premise that the adolescent has the necessary skills to appreciate the implications of these decisions as well as the potential lifelong consequences associated with these decisions. Kaiser and Hays (2004) assert that pregnant adolescents face a dual task: meeting the developmental tasks of being a teenager, coupled with the developmental tasks associated with adapting to become a mother.

 Nursing Insight—*Pregnancy and the developmental tasks of adolescence*

According to Erikson (1963), there are four developmental tasks of adolescence:
• To establish a sense of self-worth and a value system
• To establish lasting relationships
• To emancipate from parents
• To choose a vocation

Pregnancy during adolescence creates an especially vulnerable situation because the developmental tasks of pregnancy are superimposed on those of adolescence.

For a teenager to successfully adapt and fulfill the role of being a mother, she must achieve four major developmental tasks:

• Gain acceptance of pregnancy: This involves disclosing the presence of the pregnancy to her family, the father of the child, and her friends; facing family reactions; and hopefully gaining support.
• Set goals: Make realistic and attainable plans for the future. These goals will be different from her original ones and will focus on her role as a mother of a dependent child.
• View self as mother: This task addresses self-image and redefining self as a woman with a child rather than as a teenager with the freedom to explore being an adolescent and the opportunity to mature gradually.
• Grow up: Being a competent mother demands maturity with the ability to place someone else's needs before one's own. Developmentally, teenagers are typically at an egocentric stage of development. Being a mother is demanding and requires the sacrifice of being a carefree teenager (Kaiser & Hayes, 2004).

Delayed Entry Into Care

Denial, a common reaction to an unplanned and unwanted pregnancy, is often the reason why adolescents do not seek early prenatal care. In some situations, even close family members do not suspect or recognize the signs of advancing pregnancy. Unfortunately, denial and postponement of care may place the teenager and her fetus at a greater risk for medical problems. Complications such as iron-deficiency anemia, preterm labor, and preeclampsia may progress without detection and treatment. Without ongoing emotional support and education throughout pregnancy, the teenager enters labor psychologically unprepared and lacking a knowledge base to understand the natural events that surround birth. (See Chapter 11 for further discussion.)

Dulit (2000) describes three clinical types of adolescent pregnancy denial. During the first of these clinical types, the teenager realizes that pregnancy is a possibility but continues to hope that it will not come to fruition, and if it does, that it will disappear on its own accord. As the pregnancy advances, the adolescent recognizes the need to acknowledge the pregnancy and will usually seek assistance. The second type of denial is a continuation of the first except that the teenager actively conceals the pregnancy and deliberately uses whatever skills necessary to intentionally deceive and hide the changes taking place in her body. The third type is considered true denial. In this situation, the teenager is absolutely unaware of any of the physical or psychological signs or symptoms of pregnancy and experiences an unconscious denial of impending motherhood. In this situation, the onset of labor is truly an unexpected event. A teenager who experiences this type of clinical denial is displaying psychopathology coupled with a significant ego pathology. The trauma of the birth may be sufficient to trigger a psychotic episode.

Infants born to this group of teenagers are at highest risk for being victims of neonaticide because the mother fails to develop any form of attachment. Neonaticide is defined as the killing of a baby within the first 24 hours of birth. Active neonaticide is a deliberate action that occurs when the infant's death is the intended outcome of an act of violence. Passive (negligent) neonaticide results from an inability to provide the means for infant survival, for example, by maintaining an open airway, keeping the baby warm, or providing nutrition. Unfortunately, the victims are often the infants found abandoned in dumpsters or in public restrooms.

⑤ legal alert—Advocate for newborns at risk

Nurses must actively advocate for newborns at risk. One way is by becoming knowledgeable about their practice state's Safe Haven laws and programs. This information may be accessed at: http://www.adopting.org/adoptions/legalized-abandonment-state-safe-haven-laws-and-programs.html

Nursing Care of the Pregnant Adolescent

For a teenager, pregnancy presents a number of issues: deciding whether to continue with the pregnancy, securing a means for gaining access to prenatal care, planning for infant/child care in a secure home environment, and arranging for economic resources to meet the needs of a dependent new family member. Social isolation may leave the expectant teen without peer support. When this occurs, the physical, emotional, and psychological transitions associated with pregnancy are more difficult for the teenager to accomplish successfully. Because the risk of pregnancy complications (e.g., iron-deficiency anemia, preeclampsia, intrauterine growth restriction, and cephalopelvic disproportion) is increased among this group, early and ongoing prenatal care is essential. A nursing approach that is designed to meet the special needs of the adolescent patient promotes adherence and an optimal pregnancy outcome.

ASSESSMENT. Assessment of the pregnant adolescent is similar to that of older women. The initial visit includes a personal health history and family history to determine whether medical problems such as diabetes or infectious diseases may threaten maternal or fetal health. Throughout the course of pregnancy, the young patient needs to be closely monitored for iron-deficiency anemia, sexually transmitted infections, and preeclampsia. She should also be assessed for high-risk behaviors such as tobacco, alcohol, and drug use and screened for sexual abuse. Therapeutic communication with the adolescent is enhanced when the interview is conducted in a warm, conversational style that conveys caring and acceptance.

It is important to assess the young patient's knowledge and level of understanding concerning personal care during pregnancy and care of the infant following birth. An educational plan individualized to meet the adolescent's specific needs can be developed during the initial visit and refined and altered as needed throughout the pregnancy. An approach that values the patient's support persons while recognizing the need to foster her personal sense of independence is essential. A plan of care that combines the collaborative efforts of various professionals including the physician, nurse, health educator, nutritionist, school counselor, and social worker is important in optimizing the outcomes for the young patient and her fetus. Reinforcing information, allowing ample time to discuss concerns, emphasizing the need to keep return appointments, and confirming that the patient can verbalize when and how to seek help are essential components of each visit.

⑤ legal alert—Allow the pregnant adolescent to make health-care decisions

Sometimes it is difficult for parents to allow an adolescent daughter to make health-care decisions concerning her pregnancy. By law, a pregnant adolescent is an emancipated minor (a person capable of making health-care decisions), so she may sign for her own care.

Framing the physical examination in a friendly, learning context helps to diminish the young patient's anxiety and fear and reinforces the information provided at each visit. Use of the Doppler stethoscope allows the patient to hear the fetal heart tones. This action reinforces the presence of the fetus and helps the teenager to acknowledge the reality of her pregnancy. Emphasizing the progression in the fundal height measurement at each visit confirms that her fetus is growing and reinforces that she is successfully nourishing her developing child.

DIAGNOSIS AND PLANNING. Because of unawareness or denial of the pregnancy, adolescents often do not enter the prenatal care system until the second or third trimester. They may be frightened, confused, and unsure where to go for care. They are usually unaware of maternal needs, such as nutritional requirements, during pregnancy. Prenatal care is often received sporadically in the adolescent population.

⑤ Optimizing Outcomes—Formulating a nursing diagnosis for the pregnant adolescent patient

Because of a lack of information about pregnancy, "Risk for Ineffective Health Maintenance related to lack of knowledge of measures to promote health during pregnancy and family stress" is an appropriate nursing diagnosis for most pregnant adolescent patients.

Expected outcomes are based on the situation. For example, the patient will keep scheduled prenatal appointments; follow recommended strategies for health promotion; and attend childbirth and child care classes; and the family will voice emotions and concerns and provide consistent support throughout the childbearing experience.

INTERVENTIONS: STRATEGIES TO PROMOTE A HEALTHY PREGNANCY. Nursing interventions are structured to address the patient's identified needs. For example, the young patient may have difficulty accessing care because of her school schedule or transportation difficulties. The nurse helps to locate a prenatal clinic that schedules appointments in the late afternoon or evening, and when needed, works with community resources to arrange for transportation to the clinic. Many facilities offer "teen clinics" that are geared to meet the special needs of young pregnant women. Some of these provide after-school transportation to the clinic, serve nutritious snacks, encourage patient participation in certain aspects of care (e.g., checking the urine with a dipstick and recording the weight), and provide education in small peer-oriented group settings that use repetition and reinforcement of information.

In 2010, the American College of Nurse Midwives published a position statement on maternity care that advocated the implementation of group prenatal care to improve health outcomes for childbearing women and their infants. The group care model has been well supported by evidence-based research that shows improved outcomes in preterm birth, low birth weight, racial equality within the health-care system, and breastfeeding rates. Increased patient and provider satisfaction and stable costs with no increase in antenatal or childbirth care are other positive outcomes associated with the prenatal group care model (Ickovics, et al., 2007; Rotundo, 2012). In 2012, the Centers for Medicare & Medicaid Services announced *Strong Start*, a new national campaign aimed at reducing preterm birth and offering more than $40 million in grant funding to test alternative models of prenatal care, such as group prenatal care and maternity care homes (Centers for Medicare & Medicaid Services, 2012).

Optimizing Outcomes—With a CenteringPregnancy program

CenteringPregnancy is a group prenatal care program originally developed to improve pregnancy outcomes in the adolescent population. Comprehensive prenatal care is provided by a physician, certified nurse midwife, or nurse practitioner and includes risk assessment, education, and support offered in a group-focused environment. The CenteringPregnancy model incorporates a holistic approach that encourages patient involvement and empowerment in self-care activities such as blood pressure and weight checks. In CenteringPregnancy, 8 to 10 women with similar gestational ages begin their group care after their initial obstetric exam (usually around 12 to 16 weeks). Conducted in a circle, a facilitative leadership style is used to guide group discussions and provide education guided by a curriculum developed by the Centering Healthcare Institute. Women in the group are encouraged to share concerns and develop supportive relationships with one another throughout the 10 sessions (Klima, 2009; Lathrop, 2013; Moeller, Vezeau, & Carr, 2007; Rotundo, 2012). CenteringPregnancy has been shown to be beneficial in helping pregnant women in the military population cope with separation from spouses, children, and extended families because of deployment (Foster, Alviar, Neumeier, & Wootten, 2012). Additional information about CenteringPregnancy may be found at: https://www.centeringhealthcare.org/pages/centering-model/pregnancy-overview.php

Referrals to other community resources such as WIC and home health nursing may be appropriate throughout pregnancy and during the puerperium.

Nursing Insight—Adolescents and pregnancy outcomes with multiple gestations

Adolescents are at an increased risk for poor birth outcomes, particularly when multifetal pregnancies are involved. Adverse outcomes include low birth weight and very low birth weight, preterm and very preterm births, small-for-gestational-age infants, and fetal and neonatal death (Shumpert, Salihu, & Kirby, 2004).

PROMOTING OPTIMAL NOURISHMENT FOR THE PATIENT AND HER FETUS. Pregnancy during adolescence is associated with a higher risk for maternal and fetal complications. Adolescents who are still growing and those who have recently experienced menarche are at greatest risk for pregnancy complications. Growing adolescents continue to add fat to their own bodies during the third trimester, and as a result, tend to have smaller infants.

Pregnant adolescents need more calcium, magnesium, and phosphorus to help meet their own growth needs. Teens often skip meals and have a tendency to choose convenience or "fast foods" that are high in calories, fat, and sodium and low in vitamins, minerals, and fiber. Educating the young maternity patient about the importance of nutrition during pregnancy, seeking her input in making simple dietary changes, and offering nutritious snacks during prenatal visits are examples of nursing interventions that have been successful in many settings.

The Adolescent Expectant Father

Although most partners of adolescent mothers are within 2 to 3 years of their age, approximately 7% are 6 or more years older. Many become "absent" parents who rarely see or assume any responsibility in child care. The majority of adolescent fathers admit that they are not ready for fatherhood. Confusion, depression, and guilt may predominate as the young expectant father struggles with the conflicting tasks of adolescence and impending fatherhood.

The adolescent father may accompany the young woman to the clinic for pregnancy confirmation or for prenatal care. Some attend childbirth preparation classes and participate in the childbirth experience; others shy away and avoid contact with the young expectant girl. Often, support during the pregnancy and in the early months after birth diminishes as other interests and responsibilities become more important. However, nurses must guard against stereotyping young expectant fathers as being irresponsible and disinterested; many genuinely care and wish to be involved. When desired by the pregnant adolescent, the father's participation should be encouraged. It is a source of additional support for the young patient and allows the father an opportunity to work toward defining his role as a parent. Unfortunately, a large number of teenage expectant fathers come from low socioeconomic backgrounds and lack the resources, education, and job skills needed to be able to support their children (Dallas, 2009; Fletcher & Wolfe, 2011).

legal alert—Recognize the adolescent father's lack of legal rights

If the adolescent father is not married to the pregnant teenager, he has no legal rights to participate in her decision making concerning the pregnancy, elective abortion, or plans for adoption.

Evaluation

Evaluation of the interventions is reflective of the expected outcomes. For example, did the patient keep her scheduled prenatal clinic appointments? Did she adhere to suggested health-promoting strategies? Did she attend the childbirth/child classes? Did her family remain supportive throughout the pregnancy?

 Now Can You—Discuss various aspects of adolescent pregnancy?

1. Explain how pregnancy affects the developmental tasks of adolescence?
2. Develop a plan of care that is appropriate for a pregnant adolescent?
3. Identify strategies for involving the adolescent father in the pregnancy?

THE PREGNANT WOMAN OLDER THAN AGE 35

Maternal age is an important factor in the management of pregnancy. Today, more and more first pregnancies are occurring in women over the age of 35, who are no longer referred to as the "elderly primigravida." As maternal age increases, there is a greater likelihood of preexisting medical conditions such as diabetes and hypertension, which may be associated with maternal morbidity and poor fetal outcomes. Benign uterine leiomyomas (fibroid tumors) occur with greater frequency in women over age 35 and may interfere with cervical dilation during labor and cause postpartum hemorrhage. Other obstetric complications including vaginal bleeding, preeclampsia, multiple gestation, gestational diabetes, preterm labor, dysfunctional labor, and cesarean birth are also increased in older primigravidas. The fetus is at greater risk for low birth weight, macrosomia, chromosomal abnormalities, and congenital malformations.

However, the risks are considerably reduced when the patient's preconception and prenatal care is managed by a team of nurses, medical specialists, perinatologists (obstetricians with a specialty in high-risk obstetrics), nutritionists, and other health professionals. Optimal maternal–fetal outcomes result from early and ongoing care along with healthy lifestyle factors that are appropriate for women of any age: being physically, psychologically, and emotionally well; remaining physically active; having an ability to access and use health-care services; having received an adequate education; and belonging to a socioeconomic advantaged section of society.

Preconception and prenatal care for women in the over-35 age group is focused on recognizing chronic medical conditions (e.g., hypertension and diabetes) and identifying detrimental lifestyle habits such as alcohol, drug, and tobacco use. As is true with any population of women, a healthy lifestyle is an important first step toward achieving a good perinatal outcome. It is essential to listen actively to patients and their partners so that their concerns can be addressed, and where appropriate, referrals can be made for counseling and screening or prenatal diagnostic procedures. Early prenatal care affords the opportunity for timely prenatal testing. Unfortunately, the older woman may mistake a scanty or missed period for signs of early menopause rather than pregnancy. When this occurs, entry for prenatal care is often delayed.

 Optimizing Outcomes—Early prenatal care facilitates prenatal diagnosis for the expectant couple older than age 35

After age 35, there is an increased risk of conceiving a child with Down syndrome. Genetic testing is routinely offered to older expectant couples to permit the early diagnosis of chromosomal abnormalities.

Reactions to pregnancy in women 35 and older range from shock and disbelief to elation and joy. Many have reached the point in their lives where they have financial resources and economic stability, established careers, and the security of a stable interpersonal relationship. For women whose long-awaited pregnancy comes after months or years of attempts to conceive, pregnancy is a positive, exhilarating experience. Other women react with feelings of denial, uncertainty, and worry about how the pregnancy will affect their lives.

Nurses must be sensitive to each woman's situation and needs. Despite an abundance of other resources, peer support may be lacking. Often, the majority of the woman's contemporaries will have completed their childbearing many years earlier and are now the parents of almost-grown children. Effective nursing interventions include providing information and referral for genetics counseling and specialized diagnostic testing; structuring prenatal education to meet the unique needs of the older woman and her partner; and offering assistance in locating support groups, exercise, and childbirth preparation classes oriented toward the older woman. A timetable for screening for chromosomal abnormalities including those associated with advanced maternal age (e.g., trisomy 21) is presented in Table 9-5. Genetic abnormalities are also increased when the father is older than 40 years.

The physical examination should be conducted with a special focus on the identification of breast abnormalities and circulatory problems. After a careful breast examination, the patient should be encouraged to continue with monthly breast self-examination because the incidence of breast cancer is increased in the older woman. Particular attention should be paid to inspection of the lower extremities because varicosities are also more common in older women. During the first trimester, the nurse should carefully assess for the presence of fetal heart sounds because the incidence of hydatidiform mole is increased in women over age 40. (See Chapter 11 for further discussion.)

Screening for Fetal Chromosomal Abnormalities

The American College of Obstetricians and Gynecologists (ACOG) recommends that all pregnant women be offered a screening test for Down syndrome (ACOG, 2007b). The incidence of having a child affected by Down syndrome (trisomy 21) increases dramatically with maternal age

Table 9-5 Timetable for Prenatal Diagnosis

Test	Significance
First trimester combined screen: Nuchal translucency (NT) testing + pregnancy-associated plasma protein-A (PAPP-A) + free beta-human chorionic gonadotropin (free β-hCG)	NT: Fetal ultrasound examination performed between 11 and 14 weeks of pregnancy. Increased NT (>3 mm), elevated maternal serum free β-hCG and reduced PAPP-A suggest aneuploidy (e.g., trisomy 13 [Patau syndrome], trisomy 18 [Edwards' syndrome], and trisomy 21 [Down syndrome] and Turner's syndrome [gonadal dysgenesis]). When these findings are present, offer genetic counseling, and chorionic villus sampling, or amniocentesis. When combined screening results are all negative, offer second trimester maternal serum alpha-fetoprotein testing to screen for neural tube defects.
Second trimester: Maternal serum α-fetoprotein (MSAFP) screening	May be performed between 14th and 22nd weeks of pregnancy but most accurate during the 16th to 18th weeks. Higher than normal levels may be indicative of an open neural tube defect but may also result from incorrect dates, multiple gestation, or fetal demise. Lower than normal levels may indicate that the woman is at risk for trisomy 18 or trisomy 21.
Triple screen: maternal serum alpha-fetoprotein (MSAFP) + unconjugated estriol (uE3) + free beta-human chorionic gonadotropin (free β-hCG) Quadruple screen: Triple screen biochemical markers plus measurement of inhibin A	Lower than normal levels of unconjugated estriol and higher than normal levels of free β-hCG and inhibin-A (included in the quadruple screen) may indicate that a woman is at risk for trisomy 18 or trisomy 21.

(Table 9-6). Although a variety of screening and diagnostic tests are available to detect a fetus with Down syndrome, it is essential that before implementing any of these, the patient and her significant other or family support person are provided with appropriate information concerning the tests. This information is valuable in helping them to understand the reliability of the screening or diagnostic test and the implications of the results. The early diagnosis of an affected pregnancy gives the patient and her family the opportunity to determine whether termination of pregnancy is an option for her. Alternatively, early discovery of a fetal problem provides time for the parents to become informed and make preparations for rearing a child with Down syndrome. If the patient chooses an elective termination of pregnancy, the earlier the gestation, the lower the maternal morbidity associated with the procedure.

Throughout the screening and diagnosis process, the patient deserves an unbiased counselor who can provide continuity of care and up-to-date, accurate, and in-depth information. The counselor also needs to be able to facilitate open discussion whereby the patient can voice concerns related to issues such as spiritual beliefs; financial constraints; family dynamics; emotional feelings; and cultural, philosophical, and ethical values. Whatever decision the patient makes regarding the pregnancy, she needs a sound support system that will help her and her family deal with the issues that arise during pregnancy and provide the appropriate aftercare.

Screening for fetal chromosome anomalies including trisomies 13 (Patau syndrome), 18 (Edwards' syndrome), and 21 (Down syndrome) and Turner's syndrome may be initiated in the first or second trimester of pregnancy. Nuchal translucency screening, also known as nuchal testing (NT), or the nuchal fold test, is performed between 11 and 14 weeks of gestation. NT is an ultrasound-directed measurement of the translucent (clear) area directly beneath the skin on the back of the fetal neck. Fetuses with certain genetic disorders frequently have an excess accumulation of fluid at the base of the neck (an area known as the nuchal fold), and this alteration can be seen at the end of the first trimester. Findings from the nuchal translucency screening test are combined with the gestational age and the maternal age; a measurement greater than 3 mm indicates an increased risk for trisomies 13, 18, and 21. Fetuses that have a nuchal translucency measurement above the 99th percentile are also at risk for congenital heart disease and should undergo echocardiography to determine if a cardiac anomaly is present (Clur et al., 2008; Pereira, Ganapathy, Syngelaki, Maiz, & Nicolaides, 2011).

Table 9-6 Risk of Trisomy 21 (Down Syndrome) Related to Maternal Age

Maternal Age at Term	Risk of Trisomy 21 (Down Syndrome)
20	1:1,667
25	1:1,250
30	1:952
35	1:385
40	1:106
42	1:64
44	1:38
46	1:23
48	1:14
49	1:11

Sources: Egan (2004); Hook, Cross, & Schreinemachers (1983); Newberger (2001).

Nursing Insight—*Nuchal translucency testing*

The nuchal translucency screening test is a noninvasive ultrasound examination performed early in pregnancy to determine if a fetus is at risk for chromosomal disorders. The test accurately detects 70% to 80% of fetuses with Down syndrome. First trimester *combined screening*, more accurate than nuchal translucency screening alone, provides additional data obtained from maternal serum testing.

The first trimester screen combines ultrasound assessment of the thickness of the fetal nuchal fold with maternal serum testing for two biochemical "markers": Pregnancy Associated Plasma Protein-A (PAPP-A) and free β-human chorionic gonadotropin (free β-hCG). Findings suggestive of fetal aneuploidy (having less or more than the usual diploid number of chromosomes, e.g., trisomy 13, trisomy 18, and Turner's syndrome) are associated with a decreased PAPP-A (approximately one-half of the normal level), an elevated level of free β-hCG, (approximately twice the normal level), and an increased thickness of the nuchal fold. Women with these findings should be offered genetic counseling and chorionic villus sampling or second trimester amniocentesis. If the test findings are all negative, no further testing is indicated, and during the second trimester, the woman is offered a test for maternal serum alpha-fetoprotein to detect the risk of neural tube defects (ACOG, 2007b).

In the second trimester, between weeks 15 and 20, maternal serum screening can include either a "triple screen" test or a "quadruple screen" test. The triple screen test measures for three biochemical markers: α-fetoprotein (AFP), unconjugated estriol (uE3), and free beta-human chorionic gonadotropin (free β-hCG); the quadruple screen test also measures inhibin A (inhibin). Inhibin is a hormone produced by the ovarian granulosa cells that suppresses the release of follicle-stimulating hormone (FSH). It is classified into subtypes inhibin-A and inhibin-B. Levels of inhibin-A are elevated in the presence of Down syndrome (McCormick, 2011).

A diagnostic test such as an amniocentesis is usually offered if the calculated risk for Down syndrome is 1 in 150 or greater. If an open neural tube defect is suspected based on an elevated (2.5 times higher than the average for the number of gestational weeks) AFP, a diagnostic ultrasound examination can be obtained. All patients who have experienced prior pregnancies associated with fetal chromosomal abnormalities should be offered diagnostic testing such as chorionic villus sampling or amniocentesis. The risks of chorionic villus sampling are only slightly higher than those of an amniocentesis (National Institutes of Health [NIH], 2012). (See Chapter 11 for further discussion.)

Where Research and Practice Meet:
A Variety of Cultural, Medical, and Lifestyle Factors May Affect Prenatal Screening Tests

Prenatal screening test results are affected by a number of factors:

- AFP levels tend to be about 20% higher and free ß-hCG levels about 10% higher in Afro-Caribbean women than in Caucasian women.

- Free ß-hCG levels tend to be about 10% higher and uE3 (estriol) levels about 10% lower in women who have become pregnant as a result of in vitro fertilization (IVF), as compared with non-IVF pregnancies.
- Free ß-hCG levels tend to be about 20% lower and inhibin levels are about 60% higher in women who smoke, as compared with women who do not smoke.
- Second-trimester serum marker levels are increased in twin pregnancies.
- Women with insulin-dependent diabetes mellitus usually have lower levels of AFP (decreased by 18%), inhibin (decreased by 12%), and uE3 (decreased by 6%) than women without insulin-dependent diabetes.
- Vaginal bleeding that occurs immediately before a second trimester blood sample is obtained can affect the screening result because bleeding may increase the maternal serum AFP level. When bleeding has occurred, it may be advisable to delay the screening test until a week after the bleeding has stopped.
- If an amniocentesis has been attempted in the pregnancy before obtaining a second-trimester blood sample, the result cannot be correctly interpreted because of the possibility of a feto–maternal transfusion, which can increase the maternal serum AFP level.
- Nurses should use this information to appropriately counsel patients who will be undergoing prenatal screening tests.

Sources: ACOG (2007b); McCormick (2011); MOD (2013); Pereira et al. (2011).

 Now Can You—**Discuss aspects of care for the pregnant woman older than age 35?**

1. Explain why women older than age 35 may experience more pregnancy complications than younger women?
2. Identify two components of the physical examination that merit special attention?
3. Identify three tests that are useful in the prenatal diagnosis of Down syndrome?

Summary Points

◆ Education and involvement in prenatal care empowers patients and their families to make informed decisions.

◆ The first prenatal visit includes a health history, physical examination, and laboratory testing. Establishing good rapport through effective communication is essential in creating an environment to which the patient is more likely to return.

◆ Prenatal follow-up visits are shorter than the initial assessment, but they are important in monitoring maternal–fetal health and in providing anticipatory guidance for the patient and her family.

◆ Early and ongoing prenatal care is key to an optimal maternal–fetal outcome. Families should be involved in activities for health promotion and educated about strategies for self-care during the childbearing year.

◆ The diagnosis of pregnancy is based on three types of signs: presumptive, probable, and positive. Presumptive and probable signs may be caused by conditions other than pregnancy; positive signs can have no other cause.

- The teenage pregnant patient is at risk for a number of obstetric complications including anemia, preeclampsia, and preterm birth.

- Factors including education, culture, spiritual beliefs, and family support and income impact the occurrence of adolescent pregnancy.

- Preconception and prenatal care for the woman over 35 focuses on the recognition and management of chronic medical problems and strategies to promote a healthy lifestyle.

Review Questions

Multiple Choice

1. The clinic nurse is counseling a low-risk pregnant woman who is at 20 weeks' gestation. The nurse advises the woman to schedule her next routine prenatal appointment for
A. 1 week.
B. 2 weeks.
C. 3 weeks.
D. 4 weeks.

2. A woman calls the clinic to ask about taking a home pregnancy test because she has missed her last period by 2 weeks. The nurse advises her to use a home pregnancy test
A. that is specific to the beta subunit of hCG.
B. that is specific to the alpha subunit of hCG.
C. in 1 week.
D. in 2 weeks.

3. The clinic nurse knows that a probable sign of pregnancy is
A. Piskacek's sign.
B. nausea and vomiting.
C. hearing a fetal heartbeat.
D. urinary frequency.

4. A nurse is interviewing a 22-year-old primigravida. The patient's last menstrual period was December 25 and lasted 3 days (normal for her). The calculated estimated date of birth would be
A. October 1.
B. September 1.
C. October 2.
D. September 2.

5. A woman in the clinic reveals that she is experiencing high levels of stress related to her pregnancy. What action by the nurse is best?
A. Advise the woman to get plenty of sleep.
B. Encourage the woman to spend time with friends.
C. Explain why anxiolytics are not used in pregnancy.
D. Set up an exercise regimen with the woman.

6. A nurse is interviewing a woman who is in her second trimester. The woman asks the nurse if blue cohosh (*Caulophyllum thalictroides*) is safe and useful to take during pregnancy. Which response by the nurse is best?
A. Blue cohosh is safe and useful to treat morning sickness.
B. Blue cohosh used during the third trimester eases labor.
C. Blue cohosh causes fetal anoxia and should not be used.
D. Blue cohosh has not been thoroughly studied in pregnant women.

7. A nurse is reviewing a patient's chart and finds the following documentation: A 28-year-old woman complains of nausea and vomiting, breast tenderness, and frequent urination. A physical exam reveals a positive Hegar's and Chadwick's signs. The nurse interprets these findings as
A. all positive signs of pregnancy.
B. all presumptive signs of pregnancy.
C. all probable signs of pregnancy.
D. presumptive and probable signs of pregnancy.

8. A woman who is 22 weeks pregnant calls the clinic worried that her last hCG test had a lower level than the results from her initial prenatal visit. Which response by the nurse is best?
A. Ask if the woman has felt quickening.
B. Have the woman come in for an ultrasound.
C. Schedule a repeat hCG test in 1 week.
D. Reassure the woman that this is a normal finding.

9. A nurse is teaching a prenatal class. What information about cigarette exposure should the nurse provide the women?
A. Secondhand smoke is not as dangerous for the fetus.
B. Smoke exposure only affects the fetus and newborn.
C. The effects of secondhand smoke are not well documented.
D. Tobacco use can cause preterm labor and placental abruption.

10. A nurse is assessing fetal heart tones and gets a reading of 82 beats/minute. Which action by the nurse is best?
A. Take the woman's pulse for comparison.
B. Attach electronic fetal monitoring equipment.
C. Position the woman on her left side.
D. Administer oxygen to the pregnant woman.

See Answers to End of Chapter Review Questions on Davis*Plus*.

REFERENCES

Aghajafari, F., Nagulesapillai, T., Ronksley, P., Tough, S., O'Beirne, M., & Rabi, D. (2013). Association between maternal serum 25-hydroxyvitamin D level and pregnancy and neonatal outcomes: Systematic review and meta-analysis of observational studies. *British Medical Journal, 346*(3), 1169–1174. doi:http://dx.doi.org/10.1136/bmj.f1169

AIDSinfo. (2011). Recommendations for use of antiretroviral drugs in pregnant HIV-1-infected women for maternal health and interventions to reduce perinatal HIV transmission in the United States. Retrieved from http://www.aidsinfo.nih.gov/guidelines/html/3/perinatal-guidelines/150/perinatal-transmission-of-hiv-and-maternal-hiv-rna-copy-number

Alpert, E. J., Freud, K. M., Park, C. C., Patel, J. C., & Sovak, M. A. (1992). Partner violence: How to recognize and treat victims of abuse. Massachusetts Medical Society, Waltham, MA.

American Academy of Periodontology. (2011). Baby steps to healthy pregnancy and on-time delivery. Retrieved from http://www.perio.org/consumer/pregnancy.htm

American College of Nurse-Midwives (ACNM). (2010). Models of group prenatal care. Position statement. Retrieved from http://midwife.org/ACNM/files/ACNMLibraryData/UPLOADFILENAME/000000000230/Group_Prenatal_Care_12_2010.pdf

American College of Nurse-Midwives. (2012). Definition of midwifery and scope of practice of certified nurse-midwives and certified midwives. Retrieved from http://www.midwife.org/ACNM/files/ACNMLibraryData/UPLOADFILENAME/000000000266/Definition%20of%20Midwifery%20and%20Scope%20of%20Practice%20of%20CNMs%20and%20CMs%20Feb%202012.pdf

American College of Obstetricians and Gynecologists (ACOG). (2006). Psychosocial risk factors: Perinatal screening and intervention. Committee Opinion No. 343. *Obstetrics & Gynecology, 108*(4), 469–477.

American College of Obstetricians and Gynecologists (ACOG). (2007a). Viral hepatitis in pregnancy. Practice bulletin No. 86. (Reaffirmed 2012). *Obstetrics & Gynecology, 110*(4), 941–955.

American College of Obstetricians and Gynecologists (ACOG). (2007b). Screening for fetal chromosomal abnormalities. Practice Bulletin No. 77. (Reaffirmed 2013). *Obstetrics & Gynecology, 109*(3), 217–227.

American College of Obstetricians and Gynecologists (ACOG). (2009). Informed consent. Committee Opinion No. 439. (Reaffirmed 2012). *Obstetrics & Gynecology, 114*(8), 401–408.

American College of Obstetricians and Gynecologists (ACOG). (2010a). Influenza vaccination during pregnancy. Committee Opinion No. 468. *Obstetrics & Gynecology, 116*(9), 1006–1007.

American College of Obstetricians and Gynecologists (ACOG). (2010b). Smoking cessation during pregnancy. Committee Opinion No. 471. *Obstetrics & Gynecology 116*(2), 1241–1244.

American College of Obstetricians and Gynecologists (ACOG). (2011a). Effective patient-physician communication. Committee Opinion No. 492. *Obstetrics & Gynecology, 117*(5), 1254–1257.

American College of Obstetricians and Gynecologists (ACOG). (2011b). Adult manifestations of childhood sexual abuse. Committee Opinion No. 498. *Obstetrics & Gynecology, 118*(2), 392–395.

American College of Obstetricians and Gynecologists (ACOG). (2011c). Sexual assault. Committee Opinion No. 499. *Obstetrics & Gynecology, 118*(2), 396–399.

American College of Obstetricians and Gynecologists (ACOG). (2011d). Screening and diagnosis of gestational diabetes mellitus. Committee Opinion No. 504. *Obstetrics & Gynecology, 118*(9), 751–753.

American College of Obstetricians and Gynecologists (ACOG). (2011e). Vitamin D: Screening and supplementation during pregnancy. Committee Opinion No. 495. *Obstetrics & Gynecology, 118*(1), 197–198.

American College of Obstetricians and Gynecologists (ACOG). (2011f). Prenatal and perinatal human immunodeficiency virus testing: Expanded recommendations. Committee Opinion No. 418. (Reaffirmed 2011). *Obstetrics & Gynecology, 112*(6), 739–742.

American College of Obstetricians and Gyncologists (ACOG). (2013a). Health care for homeless women. Committee Opinion No. 576. *Obstetrics & Gynecology, 122*(10), 936–940.

American College of Obstetricians and Gynecologists (ACOG). (2013b). Definition of term pregnancy. Committee Opinion No. 579. *Obstetrics & Gynecology, 122*(5), 1139–1140.

American College of Obstetricians and Gynecologists (ACOG). (2013c). Oral health care during pregnancy and through the lifespan. Committee Opinion No. 569. *Obstetrics & Gynecology, 122*(2), 417–422.

American College of Obstetricians and Gynecologists (ACOG). (2013d). Exposure to toxic environmental agents. Committee Opinion No. 575. *Obstetrics & Gynecology, 122*(4), 931–934.

American Dental Association. (2011). Oral health during pregnancy. Retrieved from http://www.ada.org/~/media/ADA/Publications/Files/for_the_dental_patient_may_2011.ashx

Apuzzio, J., Block, J., Cullison, S., Cohen, C., Leong, S., London, W., . . . McMahon, B. (2012a). Chronic hepatitis B in pregnancy: A workshop consensus statement on screening, evaluation, and management, Part 1. *The Female Patient, 37*(4), 22–27.

Apuzzio, J., Block, J., Cullison, S., Cohen, C., Leong, S., London, W., . . . McMahon, B. (2012b). Chronic hepatitis B in pregnancy: A workshop consensus statement on screening, evaluation, and management, Part 2. *The Female Patient, 37*(5), 30–34.

Ashford, K. B., Hahn, E., Hall, L., Rayens, M. K., Noland, M., & Ferguson, J. E. (2010). The effects of prenatal secondhand smoke exposure on preterm birth and neonatal outcomes. *Journal of Obstetric, Gynecologic & Neonatal Nursing, 39*(5), 525–535. doi: 10.1111/j.1552-6909.2010.01169.x

Association of Women's Health, Obstetric and Neonatal Nurses (AWHONN). (2010). Smoking and women's health. Position Statement. *Journal of Obstetric, Gynecologic & Neonatal Nursing, 39*(5), 611–613. doi:10.1111/j.1552-6909.2010.01178.x

Association of Women's Health, Obstetric and Neonatal Nurses (AWHONN). (2011). HIV screening for pregnant women and infants. Position Statement. *Journal of Obstetric, Gynecologic & Neonatal Nurses, 41*(8), 154–155. doi:10.1111/j.1552-6909.2011.01325.x

Barclay, L. (2010). Acyclovir, Valacyclovir in first trimester not linked to major birth defects. *Journal of the American Medical Association, 304*(6), 905–906.

Bartol, T. (2011). Motivating patients to behavior change: Tools and techniques for patients with diabetes. *The American Journal for Nurse Practitioners, 15*(5/6), 14–24.

Bartz, D., & Goldberg, A. B. (2011). Injectable contraceptives. In Hatcher, R. A., Trussell, J., Nelson, A. L, Cates, W., Kowal, D., & Policar, M. S., . . . *Contraceptive technology* (20th revised ed.). Decatur, GA: Bridging the Gap Communications.

Bloom, K. C., Bednarzyk, M. S., Devitt, D. L., Renaulty, R. A., Teaman, V., & Van Loock, D. M. (2004). Barriers to prenatal care for homeless pregnant women. *Journal of Obstetric, Gynecologic, and Neonatal Nursing, 33*(4), 428–435.

Bobak, M. (2000). Outdoor air pollution, low birth weight, and prematurity. *Environmental Health Perspectives 108*, 173–176.

Bodnar, L., Krohn, M., & Simhan, H. (2009). Maternal vitamin D deficiency is associated with bacterial vaginosis in the first trimester of pregnancy. *Journal of Nutrition, 139*(6), 1157–1161. doi:10,3945/jn .108.103168

Bradley-Springer, L. (2010). Every nurse is an HIV nurse. *American Journal of Nursing, 110*(3), 32–39. doi:1097/01.NAJ.0000368950.95881.b1

Bureau of Justice Statistics. (2012). Homicide trends in the U.S.: *Intimate homicide.* Retrieved from http://bjs.ojp.usdoj.gov/content/intimate/ipv.cfm

Cardoso, C., Ellenbogen, M., Serravalle, L., & Linnen, A. (2013). Stress-induced negative mood moderates the relation between oxytocin administration and trust: Evidence for the tend-and-befriend response to stress? *Psychoneuroendocrinology, 38*(11), 2800–2804. doi:10.1016/j.psyneuen.2013.05.006

Carson, A. P., Howard, G., Burke, G. L., Shea, S., Levitan, E. B., & Muntner, P. (2011). Ethnic differences in hypertension incidence among middle-aged and older adults. *Hypertension, 57*(8), 1101–1107. doi:10.1161/HypertensionAHA.110.168005

Casanueva, E., Ripoll, C., Tolentino, M., Morales, R. M., Pfeffer, F., Vilchis, P., & Vadillo-Ortega, F. (2005). Vitamin C supplementation to prevent premature rupture of the chorioamniotic membranes: A randomized trial. *American Journal of Clinical Nutrition, 81*(4), 859–863.

Centers for Disease Control and Prevention (CDC). (2010a). Estimates of deaths associated with seasonal influenza- United States, 1976–2007. *Morbidity and Mortality Weekly Report, 59*(33), 1057–1062.

Centers for Disease Control and Prevention (CDC). (2010b). 2010 STD treatment guidelines. Retrieved from http://www.cdc.gov/std/treatment/2010/

Centers for Disease Control and Prevention (CDC). (2010c). Bacterial vaginosis—CDC fact sheet. Retrieved from http://www.cdc.gov/std/bv/stdfact-bacterial-vaginosis.htm

Centers for Disease Control and Prevention (CDC) Injury Center. (2011a). The national intimate partner and sexual violence survey. Retrieved from http://www.cdc.gov/ViolencePrevention/NISVS/index.html

Centers for Disease Control and Prevention (CDC). (2011b). Stay healthy with Sickle Cell Disease. Retrieved from http://www.cdc.gov/Features/SickleCell/

Centers for Disease Control and Prevention (CDC). (2011d). One test. Two lives. HIV screening for prenatal care. Retrieved from http://www.cdc.gov/Features/1Test2Lives/

Centers for Disease Control and Prevention (CDC). (2012a). Guidelines for vaccinating pregnant women. Retrieved from http://www.cdc.gov/vaccines/pubs/preg-guide.htm#tdap

Centers for Disease Control and Prevention (CDC). (2012b). Hepatitis B information for health professionals. Retrieved from http://www.cdc.gov/hepatitis/HBV/HBVfaq.htm#overview

Centers for Disease Control and Prevention (CDC). (2012c). Genital herpes – CDC Fact Sheet. Retrieved from http://www.cdc.gov/std/Herpes/STDFact-Herpes.htm

Centers for Disease Control and Prevention (CDC). (2012d). Folic Acid Recommendations. Retrieved from http://www.cdc.gov/ncbddd/folicacid/recommendations.html

Centers for Disease Control and Prevention (CDC). (2013a). Facts about intimate partner violence. Retrieved from http://www.cdc.gov/reproductivehealth/violence/intimatepartnerviolence/sld001.htm

Centers for Disease Control and Prevention (CDC). (2013b). Birth defects. Retrieved from http://www.cdc.gov/ncbddd/birthdefects/index.html

Centers for Disease Control and Prevention (CDC). (2014). Hepatitis B FAQS for health professionals. Retrieved from http://www.cdc.gov/hepatitis/HBV/HBVfaq.htm#overview

Centers for Medicare & Medicaid Services. (2012). Strong start for mother and newborns. Retrieved from http://innovations.cms.gov/initiatives/strong-start/

Chao, S., Cheung, C., Yang, E., So, S., & Chang, E. (2012). Low levels of knowledge and preventive practices regarding vertical hepatitis B transmission among perinatal nurses. *Journal of Obstetric, Gynecologic & Neonatal Nursing, 41*(4), 494–505. doi:10.1111/j.1552-6909.2012.01379.x

Chalupka, S., & Chalupka, A. N. (2010). The impact of environmental and occupational exposures on reproductive health. *Journal of Obstetric, Gynecologic & Neonatal Nursing, 39*(1), 84–102. doi:10.1111/j.1552-6909.2009.0109.x

Cheng, D., Kettinger, L., Uduhiri, K., & Hurt, L. (2011). Alcohol consumption during pregnancy. *Obstetrics & Gynecology, 117*(2), 212–217. doi:10.10097/AOG.0b013e3182078569

Clur, S. A., Mathijssen, I. B., Pajkrt, E., Cook, A., Laurini, R. N., Ottenkamp, J., & Bilardo, C. M. (2008). Structural heart defects associated with an increased nuchal translucency: 9 years experience in a referral centre. *Prenatal Diagnosis, 28*(4), 347–354.

Coker, A. L., Garcia, L. S., Williams, C. M., Crawford, T. N., Clear, E. R., McFarlane, J., & Ferguson II, J. E. (2012). Universal psychosocial screening and adverse pregnancy outcomes in an academic obstetric clinic. *Obstetrics & Gynecology, 119*(6), 1180–1189. doi:10.1097AOG.0b013e318253d76c

Collins, M. (2012). Extended interval schedule for prenatal visits. *The Journal for Nurse Practitioners, 8*(6), 488–489. doi:org/10.1016/j.nurpra.2012.04.004

Collins, M. (2013). To dip or not? That is the question. *The Journal for Nurse Practitioners, 9*(8), 544–545. doi:org/10.1016/j.nurpra.2013.06.001

Cunningham, F. G., Leveno, K. J., Bloom, S. L., Spong, C. & Dashe, J. (2014). Maternal physiology. In *Williams Obstetrics* (24th ed, pp. 141–168). New York, NY: McGraw-Hill Professional.

Dallas, C. M. (2009). Interactions between adolescent fathers and health care professionals during pregnancy, labor, and early postpartum. *Journal of Obstetric, Gynecologic & Neonatal Nursing, 38*(3), 290–299. doi:10.1111/j.1552-6909.2009.01022.x

Doenges, M. E., Geissler-Murr, A., & Moorhouse, M. F. (2010). *Nurse's pocket guide: Diagnoses, prioritized interventions and rationales* (12th ed.). Philadelphia, PA: F.A. Davis.

Drowswell, T., Carroli, G., Duley, L., Gates, S., Gulmezoglu, A. M., Khan-Neelofur, D., & Piaggio, G. G. P. (2011). Alternative versus standard packages of antenatal care for low-risk pregnancy. *Cochrane Database of Systematic Reviews, 10*(CD000934. doi:10.1002/14651858.CD000934.pub2

Duguoa, J. J. (2010). Herbal medicines and pregnancy. *Journal of Population Therapeutics and Clinical Pharmacology, 17*(3), e370–e378.

Dulit, E. (2000). Girls who deny a pregnancy. Girls who kill the neonate. *Adolescent Psychiatry, 25*(4), 219–235.

Egan, J. F. (2004). Down syndrome births in the United States from 1989 to 2001. *American Journal of Obstetrics and Gynecology, 191*(3), 104–108.

Erikson, E. H. (1963). *Childhood and society*. New York, NY: W.W. Norton.

Fletcher, J. M., & Wolfe, B. L. (2011). The effects of teenage fatherhood on young adult outcomes. *Economic Inquiry, 50*(1), 182–201. doi:10.1111/j.1465-7295.2011.00372.x

Foster, G. A., Alviar, A., Neumeier, R., & Wootten, A. (2012). A tri-service perspective on the implementation of a CenteringPregnancy model in the military. *Journal of Obstetric, Gynecologic & Neonatal Nursing, 41*(2), 315–321.

Gazmararian, J.A., Lazorick, S., Spitz, A., Ballard, T.J., Saltzman, L.E., & Marks, J.S. (2000). Violence and reproductive health: Current knowledge and future research directives. *Maternal and Child Health Journal, 4*(2), 79–84.

Gilden, R. C., Huffling, K., & Sattler, B. (2010). Pesticides and health risks. *Journal of Obstetric, Gynecologic & Neonatal Nursing, 39*(1), 103–110. doi:1111/j.1552-6909.2009.01092.x

Haire, D. (2000). Prepared for: American Foundation for Maternal and Child Health by Doris Haire. Alliance for the Improvement of Maternity Services (AIMS). The Pregnant Patient's Bill of Rights. Retrieved from http://www.aimsusa.org/ppbr.htm

Harris, A. L. (2011). Vitamin D deficiency and bacterial vaginosis in pregnancy. *Nursing for Women's Health, 15*(5), 423–430. doi:10.1111/j.1751-486X.2011.01667.x

Harris, S. (2005). Under-12s have sex one night and play with Barbie dolls the next. *Nursing Standard, 19*(39), 14–16.

Hauth, J. C., Cliffon, R. G., Roberts, J. M., Spong, C. Y., Myatt, L., Leveno, K. J., et al. (2010). Vitamin C and E supplementation to prevent spontaneous preterm birth: A randomized controlled trial. *Obstetrics & Gynecology, 116*(3), 653–658.

Hensel, K., Randis, T., Gelber, S., & Ratner, A. (2011). Pregnancy-specific association of vitamin D deficiency and bacterial vaginosis. *American Journal of Obstetrics & Gynecology, 204*(1), e1–e9. doi:10.1016/j.ajog.2010.08.013

Hepatitis Foundation International. (2010). The ABC's of hepatitis. Retrieved from https://ethnomed.org/patient-education/hepatitis/GRID_ABC.pdf

Hernandez-Diaz, S., Smith, C. R., Shen, A., Mittendorf, R., Hauser, W., Yerby, M., . . . North American AED Pregnancy Registry. (2012). Comparative safety of antiepileptic drugs during pregnancy. *Neurology, 78*(21), 1692–1699. doi:10.1212/WNL.0b013e3182574f39

Higgins, A. C. (1976). Nutritional status and the outcome of pregnancy. *Journal of the Canadian Diet Association, 37*, 17.

Higgins, J. A., & Davis, A. R. (2011). Sexuality and contraception. In Hatcher, R. A., Trussell,J., Nelson, A. L, Cates, W., Kowal, D., & Policar, M. S., . . . *Contraceptive technology* (20th revised ed., pp. 1–28). Decatur, GA: Bridging the Gap Communications.

Hodnett, E. D. (2004). Continuity of caregivers for care during pregnancy and childbirth. *Cochrane Database of Systematic Reviews* (Issue 2), CD000062

Hodnett, E. D. (2008). Withdrawn: Continuity of caregivers for care during pregnancy and childbirth. *Cochrane Database of Systematic Reviews* (Issue 4), CD000062.

Hodnett, E. D., Gates, S., Hofmeyr, G. J., Sakala, C., & Weston, J. (2012). Continuous support for women during childbirth. *Cochrane Database of Systematic Reviews* (Issue 10), CD003766. doi:10.1002/14651858.CD003766.pub4

Hook, E. B., Cross, P. K., Schreinemachers, D. M. (1983). Chromosomal abnormality rates at amniocentesis and in live-born infants. *Journal of the American Medical Association, 249*(15), 2034-2038.

Ickovics, J. R, Kershaw, T. S, Westdahl, C., Magriples, U., Massey, Z., Reynolds, H., & Rising, S. S. (2007). Group prenatal care and perinatal outcomes: a randomized controlled trial. *Obstetrics & Gynecology, 110*(4), 330–339.

International Association for Impact Assessment. (2012). Eliminating health inequities: Every woman and every child counts. Retrieved from http://healthimpactassessment.blogspot.com/2012/01/eliminating-health-inequities-every.html

Kaiser, M. M., & Hays, B. J. (2004). The adolescent prenatal questionnaire: Assessing psychosocial factors that influence transition to motherhood. *Health Care for Women International, 25*, 5–19.

Kennedy, D., Lupattelli, A., Koren, G., & Nordeng, H. (2013). Herbal medicine use in pregnancy: results of a multinational study. *BMC Complementary and Alternative Medicine, 13*(3), 355–365. doi: 10.1186/1472-6882-13-355

Kirkham, C., Harris, S., & Grzybowski, S. (2005). Evidence-based prenatal care: Part I. General prenatal care and counseling issues. *American Family Physician, 71*(7), 32–41.

Klatt, T. E., & Hopp, E. (2012). Effect of a best-practice alert on the rate of influenza vaccination of pregnant women. *Obstetrics & Gynecology, 119*(2), 301–305.

Klima, C. (2009). CenteringPregnancy: The benefits of a group prenatal care. *Contemporary OB/GYN, 54*(5), 40–49.

Kost, K., & Henshaw, S. (2012). U.S. Teenage pregnancies, births and abortions, 2008: National trends by age, race, and ethnicity. Retrieved from http://www.guttmacher.org/pubs/USTPtrends08.pdf

Lathrop, B. (2013). A systematic review comparing group prenatal care to traditional prenatal care. *Nursing for Women's Health, 17*(2), 118–130. doi:10.1111/1751-486X.12020

Liu, S., Krewski, D., Shi, Y., Chen, Y., & Burnett, R. T. (2003). Association between gaseous ambient air pollutants and adverse pregnancy outcomes in Vancouver, Canada. *Environmental Health Perspectives, 111*, 1773–1778.

Lowe, N. K. (2013). A new take on term pregnancy. *Journal of Obstetric, Gynecologic & Neonatal Nursing, 42*(6), 617. doi:10.1111/1552-6909.12257

Ludermir, A. B., Lewis, G., Valongueiro, S. A., Barreto de Araujo, T. V., & Araya, R. (2010). Violence against women by their intimate partner during pregnancy and postnatal depression: A prospective cohort study. *The Lancet, 376*(9744), 903–910. doi:10.1016/S0140-6736(10)60887-2

Maisonet, M., Bush, T. J., Correa, A., & Jaakkola, J. J. (2001). Relation between ambient air pollution and low birth weight in the northeastern United States. *Environmental Health Perspectives 109*(Suppl 3), 351–358.

March of Dimes. (2011). Illicit drug use during pregnancy. Retrieved from http://www.marchofdimes.com/pregnancy/alcohol_illicitdrug.html

March of Dimes. (2013). Down syndrome. Retrieved from http://www.marchofdimes.com/baby/down-syndrome.aspx#

McCormick, M. J. (2011). Ethical concerns about genetic screening: The Down's dilemma. *The Journal for Nurse Practitioners, 7*(4), 316–320.

McFarlane, J., Campbell, J., Sharps, P., & Watson, K. (2002). Abuse during pregnancy and femicide: Urgent implications for women's health. *Obstetrics and Gynecology, 100*(1), 27–36.

Mirza, F. G., & Gyamfi, C. (2010). Management of pregnancy in the Jehovah's Witness. *Contemporary OB/GYN, 55*(12), 41–48.

Moeller, A. H., Vezeau, T. M., & Carr, K. C. (2007). CenteringPregnancy: A new program for adolescent prenatal care. *The American Journal for Nurse Practitioners, 11*(6), 48–58.

Morris, T. (2013). Red raspberry tea and fertility. Retrieved from http://www.livestrong.com/article/381672-red-raspberry-tea-fertility/

National Human Genome Research Institute. (2013). News release archive. Retrieved from http://www.genome.gov/27552138

National Institutes of Health (NIH). (2011). Smokefree teen. Retrieved from http://teen.smokefree.gov/

National Institutes of Health (NIH). (2012). Chorionic villus sampling. Retrieved from http://www.nlm.nih.gov/medlineplus/ency/article/003406.htm

National Patient Advocate Foundation. (2010). CARE Principles. Retrieved from http://www.npaf.org

Nelson, A. L., & Cwiak, C. (2011). Combined oral contraceptives (COCs). In Hatcher, R. A., Trussell, J., Nelson, A. L, Cates, W., Kowal, D., & Policar, M. S., . . . *Contraceptive technology* (20th revised ed.). Decatur, GA: Bridging the Gap Communications.

Newberger, D. (2001). Down Syndrome: prenatal risk assessment and diagnosis. *American Family Physician, 62*(4), 825-832.

Office of Dietary Supplements. (2011). Dietary supplement fact sheet: Vitamin D. Retrieved from http://ods.od.nih.gov/factsheets/VitaminD-HealthProfessional/

Organization of Teratology Information Specialists (OTIS). (2011). Marijuana and pregnancy. Retrieved from www.otispregnancy.org/marijuana-r108119

Osaikhuwuomwan, J. A. (2010). Preterm rupture of membranes: The vitamin C factor. *African Journals Online, 12*(1), 60–68.

Partridge, C. A., & Holman, J. R. (2005). Effects of a reduced-visit prenatal care clinical practice guideline. *The Journal of the American Board of Family Practice, 18*, 555–560. doi:10.3122/jabfm.18.6.555

Pedersen, M., Giorgis-Allemand, L., Bernard, C., Aguilera, I., Andersen, M., Ballester, F., . . . et al. (2013). Ambient air pollution and low birthweight: A European cohort study (ESCAPE). *The Lancet Respiratory Medicine, 1*(9), 695–704. doi:10.1016/S2213-2600(13)70192-9

Pelletier, A., McDermott, L., Myint-U, & Kvedar, J. C. (2012). *The Female Patient, 37*(1), 36–38.

Pereira, S., Ganapathy, R., Syngelaki, A., Maiz, N., & Nicolaides, K. H. (2011). Contribution of fetal tricuspid regurgitation in first-trimester screening for major cardiac defects. *Obstetrics & Gynecology, 117*(6), 1384–1391.

Porter, L. S., & Holness, N. A. (2011). Breaking the repeat teen pregnancy cycle: How nurses can nurture resilience in at-risk teens. *Nursing for Women's Health, 15*(5), 369–381.

Robert Wood Johnson Foundation. (2010). Health care safety nets. Retrieved from http://www.rwjf.org/coverage/product.jsp?id=49869

Rosengard, C., Phipps, M. G., Adler, N. E., & Ellen, J. M. (2005). Psychosocial correlates of adolescent males' pregnancy intention. *Pediatrics, 116*(3), e114–e119.

Ross, R., Roller, C., Rusk, T., Martsolf, D., & Draucker, C. (2009). The SATELLITE Sexual Violence Assessment and Care Guide for Perinatal Patients. *Women's Health Care: A Practical Journal for Nurse Practitioners, 8*(11), 25–31.

Rotundo, G. (2012). CenteringPregnancy: The benefits of group prenatal care. *Nursing for Women's Health, 15*(6), 510–517. doi:10.1111/j.1751-486X.2011.01678.x

Rubin, R. (1984). *Maternal Identity and maternal experience.* New York, NY: Springer.

Rustgi, V., Carriero, D., Bachtold, M., & Zeldin, G. (2010). Update on chronic hepatitis B. *The Journal for Nurse Practitioners, 6*(8), 631–639.

Saphire-Bernstein, S., Way, B. M., Kim, H. S., Sherman, D. K., & Taylor, S. E. (2011). Oxytocin receptor gene (OXTR) is related to psychological resources. *Proceedings of the National Academy of Sciences of the United States of America, 108*(37), 15118–15122. doi:10.1073/pnas.1113137108

Shaw-Battista, J., Fineberg, A., Boehler, B., Skubic, B., Woolley, D., & Tilton, Z. (2011). Obstetrician and nurse-midwife collaboration. *Obstetrics & Gynecology, 118*(3), 663–670.

Shumpert, M. N., Salihu, H. M., & Kirby, R. S. (2004). Impact of maternal anemia on birth outcomes of teen twin pregnancies: A comparative analysis with mature young mothers. *Journal of Obstetrics and Gynecology, 24*, 16–21.

Silbergeld, E., & Patrick, T. (2005). Environmental exposures, toxicologic mechanisms, and adverse pregnancy outcomes. *American Journal of Obstetrics and Gynecology, 192*(5), S11–S21.

Smith, O. W. (1948). Diethylstilbestrol in the prevention and treatment of complications of pregnancy. *American Journal of Obstetrics and Gynecology, 56*, 821–834.

Somani, S. (2011). Pregnancy: Special considerations. Retrieved from http://emedicine.medscape.com/article/1229740-overview

Spong, C. Y. (2013). Defining "term pregnancy: Recommendations from the Defining "Term" pregnancy workgroup. *Journal of the American Medical Association, 309*(23), 2445–2446. doi:10.1001/jama.2013.6235

Stiller, R. J. (2011). Preventing neonatal pertussis through maternal immunization. *Contemporary OB/GYN, 56*(3), 38–42.

The National Campaign to Prevent Teen and Unplanned Pregnancy. (2012). Teen pregnancy, birth, and sexual activity data. Retrieved from http://www.thenationalcampaign.org/national-data/teen-pregnancy-birth-rates.aspx

Unal, E. R., Lazenby, G. B., Lintzenich, A. E., Simpson, K. N., Newman, R., & Goetzl, L. (2011). Cost-effectiveness of maternal treatment to prevent perinatal hepatitis B virus transmission. *Obstetrics & Gynecology, 118*(3), 655–662. doi:10.1097/AOG.0b013e31822ad2c2

U.S. Census Bureau. (2011). Income, poverty and health insurance coverage in the United States: 2010. Retrieved from http://www.census.gov/newsroom/releases/archives/income_wealth/cb11-157.html

U.S. Department of Agriculture, Food & Nutrition Service. (2013). Retrieved from http://www.fns.usda.gov/wic/about-wic-wic-glance

Vorvick, L. J., & Storck, S. (2011). Adolescent pregnancy. Retrieved from http://www.nlm.nih.gov/medlineplus/ency/article/001516.htm

World Health Organization (WHO). (2005). Report: *Make every woman and every child count.* Retrieved from http://www.who.int/whr/2005/whr2005_en.pdf

World Health Organization (WHO). (2011). Rubella and congenital rubella syndrome. Retrieved from http://www.who.int/immunization_monitoring/diseases/rubella/en/index.html

World Health Organization (WHO). (2013). *Adolescent development*. Retrieved fromhttp://www.who.int/maternal_child_adolescent/topics/adolescence/dev/en/

Xiao, X. M., Li, A. Z., Chen, X., Zhu, Y. K., & Miao, J. (2007). Prevention of vertical hepatitis B transmisson by hepatitis B immunoglobulin in the third trimester of pregnancy. *International Journal of Gynaecology & Obstetrics, 96*(3), 167–170.

Zlotnick, C., & Zerger, S. (2009). Survey findings on characteristics and health status of clients treated by the federally funded (US) Health Care for the Homeless Programs. *Health & Social Care in the Community, 17*(1), 18–26.

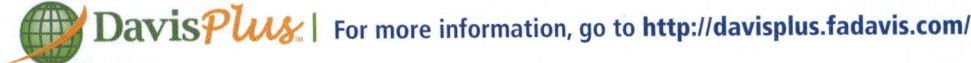

DavisPlus | For more information, go to **http://davisplus.fadavis.com/**

CONCEPT MAP

The Prenatal Assessment

Pregnancy:
- Wonder/growth
- Ambivalence
- Self-preservation concerns

For Best Outcomes

Prenatal Care:
- Begins in first trimester
- Visits: once every 4 wks for 28–32 wks → q2wks
- Focus: early identification of deviations from the norm
- Facilitate health promotion/ health maintenance via screenings
- Psychosocial support
- Culturally appropriate education

First Visit

Comprehensive Health History:
- Biographical data/social history
- History of intimate partner violence
- Psychological assessment
- OB history/previous pregnancy
- Gynecological history

Current Pregnancy:
- Presumptive, probable and positive symptoms
- Establish estimated date of birth
- Determine gravidity and parity
- Complete pregnancy testing
- Identify multiple gestation

Medical History:
- Identifies past and present health status
- Dental and eye health
- Status of maternal immunizations
- Educate re: environmental hazards
- Manage maternal preexisting conditions

Cultural Diversity:
- HTN more prevalent in African American and Hispanic women
- Teen pregnancy/birth rates increased in African American teens

What To Say:
- Use language a teen can relate to during discussions about sex
- Ask re: pesticide exposure

Across Care Settings:
- Health-care safety net of providers for vulnerable populations
- Use teen.smokefree.gov website

Family Teaching Guidelines:
- DEEPERCARE acronym to promote family health

Nursing Insight:
- Continuity of care decreases maternal stress
- Homelessness is a barrier to prenatal care
- Intimate partner violence is more common than preeclampsia or gestational diabetes during pregnancy
- Identify couples who would benefit from genetic testing
- Educate re: difference between screening and diagnostic testing
- Adolescents have greater health risks with multiple gestation
- Developmental tasks of pregnancy superimposed on those of adolescence

Complementary Care:
- Avoid use of blue cohosh during pregnancy

Assist Patient With

Nursing Role: CARE ing
- **C**ommunicating
- **A**dvocating
- **R**especting
- **E**nabling/empowering

- Choosing a care provider
  - Management of pregnancy/childbirth
  - Individualized care

Eustress:
- Role adaptation
- Restructuring of tasks

Distress:
- Accessing care
- Unknown/loss of control
- Lack of social support

- Navigating the health-care system
- Coping with financial concerns

Prenatal Physical Exam:
- Explain; obtain consent
- Ensure privacy
- Actively engage patient
- Same order each visit

Includes:
- General assessment → i.e., observation, weight, VS, urine
- Focused OB exam → skin; breasts, abdomen, uterine size, fetal position, fetal heart auscultation, vagina, pelvis, fundal height

Pregnant Adolescents:
- Long-term social and developmental consequences R/T pregnancy

Nursing:
- Heighten public awareness; ID those teens at greatest risk
- Advocate for responsible sexual behavior
- Empower families with information: provide age-appropriate health education classes
- Be aware of denial of pregnancy → neonaticide
- Assess in a caring/accepting manner; frame exam in a learning context
- Assist with access to prenatal care
- Promote optimal nutrition

Screening and Diagnostic Tests:
- Blood tests: blood type, Rh, antibody screens, RPR, VDRL, hepatitis, CBC, HIV, sickle cell anemia, PPD
- STI screening: HSV, syphilis, chlamydia, gonorrhea
- Cervical cancer

Woman Older Than 35 Yrs:
- Increased risk of preexisting medical conditions/obstetric complications

Nursing:
- Be aware of varying responses to pregnancy
- Structure prenatal education to meet unique needs
- Special assessment for breast/circulatory abnormalities
- Education re: screening tests for chromosomal abnormalities

Where Research and Practice Meet:
- Increase Ca+/weight-bearing exercise when Depo-Provera used pre-pregnancy
- Screen for alcohol consumption during pregnancy
- Assess for SV using SATELLITE Care Guide
- Should screen for Hep B and begin prophylactic tx for high viral load
- EMR best practice alerts increase flu vaccine rates
- Women exposed to SHS have increased risk of preterm birth
- Use resilience-recoil-rebound theory to nurture resilience in pregnant teens

Optimizing Outcomes:
- Be an advocate for pregnant patient's rights/access
- Use CenteringPregnancy Model to enhance patient outcomes
- Demonstrate professionalism during physical exams
- Follow CDC immunization guidelines for maternal pertussis
- Use caring communication skills to enhance patient interview
- Identify Jehovah Witness patient and develop plan for OB care/delivery
- Offer routine testing for Down syndrome for those older than 35 yrs

Legal Alert:
- Advocate for newborns at risk
- Allow adolescents to make health-care decisions
- Recognize rights of adolescent fathers

Now Can You:
- Discuss goals of prenatal care
- Discuss health-promotion strategies for pregnancy
- Discuss components of prenatal assessment and various methods of clinical fetal assessment
- Discuss aspects of care for pregnant adolescents and women older than 35 yrs

Promoting a Healthy Pregnancy

 Little Seth, Precious One

What a miracle to be
A new life formed
Created from our deep love
And blessed by everyone above.
Our love combined as one
Creating a miracle of joy
Filling our hearts completely
Producing a baby boy.
Even though we have never seen your face
Or even heard your first cry
A special bond has been formed
Well deep from inside.
A bond that will never be broken
For as long as life shall be
Love will last forever
Far beyond than anyone can see.

As each day passes on
Your beginning edging nearer
We shield you from harm and
Pray for your well being
Until we may protect you in our arms.
You are our miracle soon to behold
For life is a beauty sometimes unseen
Ten tiny fingers, ten tiny toes
Perfection only to be seen.
You are so tiny, so small
So fragile, so sweet
A life not yet known
And yet loved so complete.
With all our love,
Mommy and Daddy
—Tamera and Daniel Ayriss

LEARNING TARGETS *At the completion of this chapter, the student will be able to:*

♦ Discuss holistic approaches for empowering women in planning for a healthy pregnancy.

♦ Describe factors that must be integrated to achieve optimal nutrition and weight gain during pregnancy.

♦ Develop an exercise plan for women in the first, second, and third trimesters of pregnancy.

♦ Identify the signs of pregnancy and methods to manage the common associated discomforts.

♦ Recognize signs of impending complications of pregnancy and discuss interventions to decrease morbidity and mortality.

♦ Discuss the various methods of childbirth education and assist a pregnant patient in developing a birth plan.

PICO(T) Questions

The intent of evidence-based practice (EBP) is to provide nursing care that integrates the best available evidence. An initial step in EBP is to write a PICO(T) question that effectively guides the research. A PICO(T) question is an acronym that stands for population (P), intervention or issue (I), comparison of interest (C), outcome (O), and timeframe (T). Depending on the question, all or some of the question components are used in the research process. Use these

PICO(T) questions to spark your thinking as you read the chapter.

1. Does (I) changing pregnant women's diets to avoid peanut consumption, (O) decrease the incidence of peanut allergies (P) in infants?

2. Do (P) women whose pregnancy was not planned have (O) a higher incidence of (I) clinical depression (C) than women who were actively trying to conceive?

Evidence-Based Practice

O'Connor, P. J., Poudevigne, M. S., Cress, M. E., Motl, R. W., & Clapp, J. F. (2011). Safety and efficacy of supervised strength training adopted in pregnancy. *Journal of Physical Activity and Health 8*, 309–320.

Previous studies have found that physical inactivity predisposes to reduced fitness and increased fetal and maternal risks during pregnancy. Maternal fitness and several aspects of fetal and maternal health have previously been found to improve through the use of low- to moderate-intensity exercise during pregnancy. The purpose of this study was to describe the progression of supervised, low- to moderate-intensity strength training program implemented among a sample of pregnant women. A further purpose was to explore the incidence of associated musculoskeletal injuries, lumbar endurance, blood pressure changes, and the occurrence of problematic symptoms (e.g., swelling in hands or feet; headache or visual disturbance; chest, pelvic, or abdominal pain; irregular heartbeats or dizziness; and unexpected vaginal bleeding or leaking).

The sample was composed of 32 healthy pregnant women who were primarily recruited through midwives and obstetricians. The participants were between 21 and 25 weeks of gestation and their ages ranged from 18 to 38 years of age. They were at low risk for any pregnancy-related complications and free from back pain or a history of back pain. Women who reported use of regular strength training and those who reported uncontrolled psychiatric conditions and orthopedic or cardiovascular limitations were excluded.

Prior to initiating the exercise program, experienced trainers taught and supervised participants on the use of strength training and specific types of exercises. The participants were then expected to implement strength training twice a week for a 12-week period. Data recorded included blood pressure, extension endurance exercise test, and report of symptoms or musculoskeletal injuries. Participants were instructed to complete a warm-up that included 5 minutes of walking on a treadmill. Following the warm-up, participants performed six resistance exercises: dual leg extension, dual leg press, dual arm lat pull, dual leg curl, lumbar extensions, and a transverse abdominis muscle (abdominal) exercise. Using the Universal Gym and Cybex Eagle for the first five exercises, the number of sets and repetitions were constant throughout the

training at a low to moderate velocity with scheduled rest periods between exercises. Participants were instructed to rate exercise intensity using a rated perceived exertion (RPE) scale. A rating of 13 represented moderate intensity, 11 represented fairly light, and ratings of 10 or less represented low intensity. External load was progressively increased based on RPE responses to each exercise. Participants usually performed the abdominal exercise from a standing position and were asked to draw in their abdominal muscles as if trying to reach the spine. Repetitions were held at 8 throughout the training. Five minutes after completing the training, the blood pressures were measured, and participants were asked about potential problematic symptoms and back pain.

The researchers stated that no musculoskeletal injuries were reported for women at risk for low back pain. No chest palpitations or chest pains were reported. Symptoms were reported 13 times and included dizziness (8/13) and abdominal/pelvic pain (4/13). One person reported a headache. Most symptoms were reported within the first 3 weeks of the study. The percentage of increase in the external load across the 12 weeks was found to be statistically significant and reported as follows: leg presses (36%), leg curl (39%), lat pull down (39%), lumbar extension (41%), and leg extensions (56%). The researchers reported that exercises were performed at a low to moderate perceived intensity with a mean RPE of 10.5 to 12.9, which did not change significantly throughout the 12-week period. A 14% increase in lumbar endurance was reported. No significant changes in blood pressure were reported during and at the conclusion of the 12-week training. The researchers concluded that use of supervised, low- to moderate-intensity strength training during pregnancy is safe and efficacious.

1. How is this information useful to clinical nursing practice?

2. Based on these findings, what are implications for further research?

See Suggested Responses for Evidence-Based Practice on Davis*Plus*.

Introduction

This chapter focuses on health promotion of childbearing women during preconception and throughout pregnancy. Counseling is an essential component of preconception care and provides information and education to women and families, which enables them to plan for their pregnancy and to develop a healthy body and a healthy mind surrounding the pregnancy.

Another important facet of health promotion during pregnancy concerns adequate nutrition and weight gain. Women need to have an understanding of essential elements required for a healthy pregnancy and of how to incorporate them into their daily diets. Along with diet and nutrition, exercise, work, and rest must be balanced to

achieve an optimal pregnancy outcome. Health-care providers must provide guidelines for safe and beneficial exercise, which include teaching pregnant women about the effects of exercise and work.

This chapter also discusses the effects of medications during pregnancy and provides information concerning safe versus unsafe medications. Included in this section is information about over-the-counter medications, herbal therapies, and prescription medications. Certain medications are considered to be safe for use during pregnancy, and these are incorporated into the discussion about the common discomforts of pregnancy.

Nurses and other health-care providers can teach patients about common pregnancy discomforts to help alleviate anxiety and fear. Prenatal education also promotes empowerment that encourages women to manage pregnancy in a healthy manner. Pregnant women must also be knowledgeable about signs and symptoms of danger, including interventions that can be incorporated at home along with an understanding of when to seek professional care.

The course of a normal pregnancy, along with information concerning prenatal visits, is discussed in this chapter. Included in this section is a schedule for prenatal visits, information to be covered by the nurse at each visit, and laboratory tests that are completed with each visit. The nursing diagnosis: *"health seeking behaviors related to interest in maintaining optimal health during pregnancy"* is usually appropriate for women who regularly engage in prenatal care. Examples of other nursing diagnoses that address health promotion of the pregnant woman and her fetus are presented in Box 10-1.

Lastly, this chapter presents information about childbirth education, including a comparison of methods and strategies for finding information about various prenatal and childbirth education classes. As an integral part of promoting a healthy pregnancy and incorporating a holistic approach to care, women should be encouraged to develop a birth plan, which includes their preferences for care during the labor and birth of their child.

Planning for Pregnancy

Healthy People 2020 targets women of childbearing age with the goal of improving the health and well-being of women, infants, children, and families (U.S. Department of Health and Human Services [USDHHS], 2012). To meet this goal, specific objectives are identified, focusing on the number of women receiving preconception and prenatal care, attendance at prepared childbirth education classes, delivery of low-birth-weight and very-low-birth-weight infants, preterm delivery, and maternal weight gain. One of the most important ways to facilitate meeting these objectives is for nurses and health-care providers to promote healthy pregnancies in women through preconception counseling, individualized prenatal care, and identification and treatment of medical concerns and problems throughout the pregnancy.

Pregnancy care is a continuum that begins in adolescence. Once a female reaches menarche and is capable of reproduction, she should be cognizant of the fact that she could become pregnant and strive to achieve the best level of health that is possible. This time frame, which represents the earliest stage of the pregnancy continuum, is called **preconception**. The pregnancy continuum spans across the childbearing years and encompasses the prenatal period, birth, postpartum, and parenthood. **Periconception** is a term that generally refers to the time immediately before conception through the period of organogenesis, while **interconception** is the time period between the end of one pregnancy and the beginning of the next pregnancy. It is considered to be an optimal time to address problems that occurred with the previous pregnancy to minimize the likelihood of a repeated poor pregnancy outcome (ACOG, 2005).

PRECONCEPTION COUNSELING: A TOOL TO HELP PROMOTE A POSITIVE PREGNANCY OUTCOME

It is during preconception that a woman builds the foundation for a healthy pregnancy long before she may ever even think of becoming pregnant. When a woman accesses her care provider during this time, it is known as preconception care. Ideally, health promotion for the pregnant woman should begin during the preconception period. Working with her health-care provider during this time provides opportunities for empowering the woman for planning and carrying out a healthy pregnancy and birth.

The purpose of preconception care is to identify conditions, whether physical, psychological, environmental, or social, that could adversely affect a future pregnancy. By identifying these conditions early, interventions can be initiated to reduce or prevent potential complications that may be associated with them. Although certain conditions cannot be ameliorated, it may be possible to manage or treat them so that they have the smallest impact possible on future pregnancies.

 Nursing Insight—Identifying potential environmental threats during preconception

Preconception care provides an ideal opportunity for the nurse to explore environmental threats that may potentially cause harm to an embryo/fetus. Parental exposure to various environmental contaminants (e.g., metals, solvents, petrochemicals, and pesticides) may be associated with a plethora of adverse reproductive effects (e.g., infertility and spontaneous abortion) and genetic damage in the fetus. Oogonia (primordial germ cells that differentiate into oocytes) develop completely during fetal life, and oocytes undergo their first meiotic division in utero and remain dormant until puberty. Environmental insults to fetal oocytes may result in impaired fertility. Similarly, environmental injury to stem-cell spermatogonia may result in infertility (Chalupka & Chalupka, 2010; Gilden, Huffling, & Sattler, 2010).

Each time a woman of childbearing age presents to her care provider for an annual gynecological exam, preconception counseling should be included, regardless of whether or not the woman is planning a pregnancy now or

---

Box 10-1 Possible Nursing Diagnoses Related to Health Promotion of the Pregnant Woman and Her Fetus

- Anxiety related to minor symptoms of pregnancy
- Disturbed Body Image related to change of appearance with pregnancy
- Fatigue related to metabolic changes of pregnancy
- Risk for Deficient Fluid Volume related to nausea and vomiting of pregnancy
- Constipation related to reduced peristalsis during pregnancy
- Deficient Knowledge related to inadequate information regarding nutritional needs during pregnancy
- Health-seeking Behaviors related to a lack of information about childbirth and newborn care
- Ineffective Coping related to lack of support people
- Risk for Fetal Injury related to maternal substance abuse

at any time in the foreseeable future. Use of a tool such as a reproductive life plan (RLP) is beneficial for women, men, and couples. The RLP is a reflection of a person's intentions about the number and timing of pregnancies in the context of their personal values and life goals, and it may serve as the starting point of focused, personalized counseling to directly address the individual's plan. Especially useful in populations at risk for adverse outcomes, the RLP serves as a comprehensive strategy that can be incorporated into nursing practice at all levels to improve birth outcomes (Barry, 2011; Malnory & Johnson, 2010).

 Optimizing Outcomes—Endorsing preconception care

The past decade has shown a growing trend among clinicians in women's health to expand the definition of prenatal care to include preconception counseling. National organizations such as the American College of Obstetricians and Gynecologists (ACOG), the March of Dimes, and the Centers for Disease Control and Prevention (CDC) endorse preconception counseling as an important component of care for women contemplating pregnancy or at risk of unintended pregnancy (ACOG, 2005). Nurses play a major role in endorsing preconception care for all women of childbearing age, and as part of preconception care, nurses should encourage patients to recognize their pregnancies early. Educational strategies (e.g., one-to-one or group teaching, brochures, and videos) about signs and symptoms of pregnancy should take place in all health-care settings in which women of childbearing age are likely to receive care (Ayoola, Nettleman, & Strommel, 2010).

THE HEALTHY BODY

Preparing for pregnancy before becoming pregnant is the ideal because it empowers women to become educated about the workings of their bodies and the benefits gained from pregnancy planning. During the preconception visit, the provider reinforces the importance of early and ongoing prenatal care and counsels the woman about establishing realistic expectations for pregnancy and its outcomes (ACOG, 2005) (Fig. 10-1).

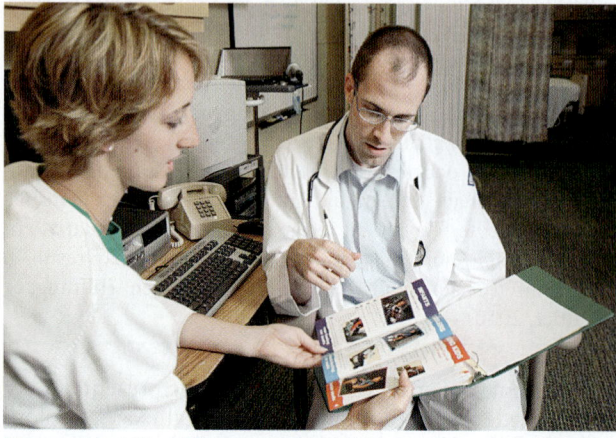

Figure 10-1 Health promotion for pregnancy begins during the preconception visit.

 Collaboration in Caring—*Preconception dental care*

According to the American Academy of Periodontology (2011) and the American Dental Association (2011), women who are considering pregnancy should be counseled to undergo a dental examination during the preconception period. This health promoting strategy offers the opportunity for the identification and subsequent treatment of dental conditions that may be associated with adverse pregnancy outcomes related to periodontal disease (ACOG, 2013c).

Menstrual and Medical History

When pregnancy is desired, the nurse can be instrumental in empowering the woman to take charge of her conception care by embracing a healthy lifestyle to ensure the best possible outcome. During the preconception visit, a review of the menstrual history guides the nurse in identifying specific needs so that an individualized conception plan can be developed. Determining the frequency and length of menstrual periods is essential information for teaching about the fertile period and how to enhance the likelihood of conception. The patient should be educated about the value of keeping an accurate menstrual calendar. She can be instructed to mark the first and every successive day of her menstrual periods on the calendar (Fig. 10-2). This information will help her to determine the length of each cycle and when to time sexual intercourse in succeeding months to increase the likelihood of conception. When pregnancy does occur, one of the first questions she will be asked is, "What was the first day of your last normal menstrual period (LNMP)?" If she has recorded this information, she can easily refer to her calendar for the accurate date.

There are times when charting a menstrual calendar also provides clues to menstrual and, perhaps, fertility problems. Some women have irregular cycles that are too close together or too far apart. This information, documented in a calendar, may signal the need for referral to a reproductive specialist.

A review of the family history is another important component of the preconception visit. Through the information gained, the woman's and her partner's extended families can be assessed for potential illnesses or diseases that tend to run in families. For this reason, it is desirable for the patient's partner to be present at the preconception visit so that he can accurately provide information about his family.

Complementary Care: *Ayurveda to Enhance the Preconception Period*

Ayurveda is a term derived from the words *ayur*, or life, and *veda*, or science. Developed hundreds of years ago in ancient India, Ayurveda is a system of natural and medical healing that includes diet, herbs, massage, exercise, music therapy, meditation, yoga, and aromatherapy. Practitioners of this modality believe that Ayurveda is beneficial during the preconception period in promoting optimal maternal and fetal health. According to Ayurveda, a healthy lifestyle is achieved by maintaining a mutually satisfying, harmonious emotional relationship while avoiding stress, tobacco, alcohol, and drugs and consuming a vegetarian diet that includes alternate sources of protein and calcium.

INSTRUCTIONS: Shade in the appropriate box for every date of menstrual bleeding																														
January	1	2	3	4	5	6	7	8	9	10	11	12	13	14	15	16	17	18	19	20	21	22	23	24	25	26	27	28	29	30	31
February	1	2	3	4	5	6	7	8	9	10	11	12	13	14	15	16	17	18	19	20	21	22	23	24	25	26	27	28	{29}		
March	1	2	3	4	5	6	7	8	9	10	11	12	13	14	15	16	17	18	19	20	21	22	23	24	25	26	27	28	29	30	31
April	1	2	3	4	5	6	7	8	9	10	11	12	13	14	15	16	17	18	19	20	21	22	23	24	25	26	27	28	29	30	
May	1	2	3	4	5	6	7	8	9	10	11	12	13	14	15	16	17	18	19	20	21	22	23	24	25	26	27	28	29	30	31
June	1	2	3	4	5	6	7	8	9	10	11	12	13	14	15	16	17	18	19	20	21	22	23	24	25	26	27	28	29	30	
July	1	2	3	4	5	6	7	8	9	10	11	12	13	14	15	16	17	18	19	20	21	22	23	24	25	26	27	28	29	30	31
August	1	2	3	4	5	6	7	8	9	10	11	12	13	14	15	16	17	18	19	20	21	22	23	24	25	26	27	28	29	30	31
September	1	2	3	4	5	6	7	8	9	10	11	12	13	14	15	16	17	18	19	20	21	22	23	24	25	26	27	28	29	30	
October	1	2	3	4	5	6	7	8	9	10	11	12	13	14	15	16	17	18	19	20	21	22	23	24	25	26	27	28	29	30	31
November	1	2	3	4	5	6	7	8	9	10	11	12	13	14	15	16	17	18	19	20	21	22	23	24	25	26	27	28	29	30	
December	1	2	3	4	5	6	7	8	9	10	11	12	13	14	15	16	17	18	19	20	21	22	23	24	25	26	27	28	29	30	31

Figure 10-2 The menstrual calendar provides an accurate record for recording menstrual periods.

 Now Can You—Discuss preconception care?

1. Differentiate among preconception, periconception, and interconception?
2. Identify the purpose of preconception care?
3. Describe how to create a menstrual calendar?

The Physical Examination

Using the patient history as a guide to help identify problems or special needs, the health-care provider performs a complete physical examination. Along with the general physical assessment, a complete pelvic examination is also performed to evaluate the organs and bony structures of the pelvis. Abnormalities in this region can be crucial during pregnancy and childbirth. A Papanicolaou test (Pap test), cultures for sexually transmitted infections (STIs), and cultures for other infections are often obtained during this exam as well. (See Chapter 9 for further discussion.)

Laboratory Evaluation

Every pregnant woman who presents for prenatal care is tested for various potential problems during the first visit and periodically throughout the antepartal period. The complete blood count (CBC) serves as the primary test for anemia via analysis of the hemoglobin and hematocrit. If the woman is anemic, the indices can aid in identifying the type of anemia (e.g., iron-deficiency, etc.). The patient can also be screened for infection by the white blood cell (WBC) count. If the WBCs are elevated, more information can be ascertained via the differential analysis. Platelets, essential components of the clotting mechanism, are also evaluated in a CBC.

Blood is also drawn for the identification of the woman's blood type, Rh status, and the presence of irregular antibodies. The blood type and Rh status are important in determining if the woman is at risk for developing isoimmunization during her pregnancy. This problem can occur if the woman's blood is Rh(D)-negative and the fetus she is carrying is Rh(D)-positive. Screening identifies the presence of antibodies that have been produced in response to exposure to fetal blood or other irregular antibodies that could potentially cause problems. (See Chapter 11 for further discussion.)

Exposure to Childhood Illnesses

Some of the routine maternal laboratory tests screen for childhood diseases that are known to cause congenital anomalies or other pregnancy complications if contracted during early pregnancy. Rubella, or German measles, was once a common childhood disease. Today, most women of childbearing age received rubella immunization during childhood. When contracted during the first trimester, rubella causes a number of fetal deformities. Therefore, all pregnant women are screened for rubella. A positive rubella screening test is indicative of immunity, and the woman cannot contract the disease. If the screening test is negative, the patient is advised to stay away from children who could possibly have the disease, and she is immunized for rubella after the infant is born.

Varicella (chickenpox) is another common childhood disease that may cause problems in the developing embryo and fetus. At present, an immunization for chickenpox is available and given to most children. If a woman presents for a preconception visit and her history reveals no prior chickenpox infection, she should be immunized before attempting pregnancy. Pregnant women should be questioned about childhood chickenpox, and a varicella titer may be obtained to confirm immunity. If nonimmune, the patient should be advised to avoid children who could potentially expose her to the chickenpox virus.

Finally, all adults should receive a tetanus booster immunization at least every 10 years. A booster can be given to the woman during the preconception period if she has not been immunized within the previous 10 years.

Exposure to Sexually Transmitted Infections

Sexually transmitted infections (STIs) may cause maternal and fetal complications during pregnancy. Routine screening for STIs aids in early detection and treatment. The Venereal Disease Research Laboratory (VDRL) test is a screening titer for syphilis that measures antibodies produced in mid-disease but can produce a false positive result in women who are pregnant or who have rheumatoid arthritis or systemic lupus erythematosus. For these patients, a rapid plasma reagin (RPR) screening test may be used to confirm the presence of antibodies. In the event of a positive result, further testing is needed to confirm the findings and to determine whether the infection is in an active or latent phase.

In addition to screening for syphilis, all women should be screened for HIV as early as possible during each pregnancy (ACOG, 2008a). If positive, therapy can be initiated to decrease the likelihood of transplacental viral transmission to the fetus. An important nursing role includes educating all women about HIV and the methods for decreasing the risk of infection.

Gonorrhea and chlamydia are cervical infections that can ascend through the cervix and increase the risk of premature rupture of the membranes and preterm labor. A cervical sample obtained during a speculum examination can be tested to determine if either of the pathogens is present. If no speculum examination is performed, chlamydia testing may be conducted via vaginal swab or urine specimen (Tao, Hoover, & Kent, 2010).

Hepatitis B virus (HBV) is a bloodborne infection that is acquired primarily by sexual contact or through exposure to infected blood. The hepatitis B surface antigen (HBsAg) is used to screen for this infection. If the screening test is positive, further testing is indicated. (See Chapter 9 for further discussion.)

 Now Can You—Identify essential laboratory tests during preconception planning?

1. Discuss components of the CBC?
2. Explain the importance of identifying the woman's blood type and Rh status?
3. Identify routine screening tests performed for childhood diseases?
4. Describe the processes for sexually transmitted infection screening?

Genetic Testing

During the patient's first interview and visit, the nurse should ask questions that relate to the patient's and family's genetic history. Depending on the information gained, further blood work and testing may be indicated. For example, a positive family history of sickle cell disease or trait should be followed up with a maternal hemoglobin electrophoresis. If the patient tests positive, her partner should also be tested.

All women should be offered screening with ultrasonography and maternal serum markers. Several different tests are available, such as Pregnancy Associated Plasma Protein-A (PAPP-A) and free β-human chorionic gonadotropin (free β-hCG) during the first trimester, and the Triple Screen and the Quadruple Screen during the second trimester. Depending on the specific test, biochemical markers (e.g., maternal serum alpha-fetoprotein [MSAFP], unconjugated estradiol [uE3], and free β-human chorionic gonadotropin [β-hCG]) are measured to screen for potential neural tube defects, trisomy 13, trisomy 18, and trisomy 21. If the screen is positive, the woman should be referred to a genetics specialist for counseling, and further testing, such as chorionic villus sampling (CVS) or amniocentesis, should be performed (ACOG, 2007). (See Chapter 9.)

While it is not possible to inquire about every inheritable disease or disorder, those most frequently encountered are addressed in Table 10-1.

 Optimizing Outcomes—Prenatal genetic testing

Prenatal nursing care is enhanced with the implementation of interventions for early diagnosis and treatment for the prevention of complications related to birth defects. It is essential that nurses provide prenatal interventions, including folic acid supplementation for all women of reproductive age, conduct rubella screening and immunization, teach women to avoid alcohol consumption during preconception and pregnancy, offer screening and detection of prenatal genetic disorders and early treatment of disorders when possible, and offer termination of pregnancy for severe defects.

Exposures Related to Lifestyle Choices

Several factors related to lifestyle choices can have detrimental effects on the developing fetus, including use of tobacco, alcohol, caffeine, artificial sweeteners, marijuana, and cocaine.

TOBACCO. Smoking during pregnancy causes a plethora of problems for the woman and the developing fetus. Carbon monoxide in the cigarette smoke binds more readily than oxygen to hemoglobin, thereby decreasing the oxygen-carrying capacity of the red blood cells. This alteration decreases the amount of oxygen traveling to the placenta, thereby decreasing the amount of oxygen available to the fetus for growth and development of tissues and organs.

The nicotine in the cigarette smoke also poses a significant risk to the developing fetus. Depending on the amount and the frequency of smoking, nicotine can act as either a stimulant or a relaxant. Nicotine causes the release of epinephrine, stimulating the "fight or flight" response that results in tachycardia, hypertension, and tachypnea. This response occurs in both the woman and her fetus. The stimulation of the sympathetic nervous system also prompts the release of cortisol from the adrenal glands, increasing blood glucose levels and altering the body's immune response. Vasoconstriction results from stimulation of the sympathetic nervous system, causing decreased blood flow through the arteries and decreased oxygen transport to the placenta and the developing fetus.

Smoking is associated with spontaneous abortion, low birth weight, intrauterine growth restriction, preterm labor and birth, placenta previa, placental abruption, and premature rupture of the membranes. Infants born to mothers who smoke are more likely to be small for gestational age (SGA). Each of these complications predisposes the fetus to complications related to growth and physical and cognitive development. In fact, babies born to mothers who smoked during pregnancy are 1.4 to 3.0 times more likely to die from sudden infant death

Table 10-1 Genetics Screening During Pregnancy

Disorder	Population Affected	Pathology	Pregnancy and Newborn Complications
Sickle cell disease	African Americans Persons of Mediterranean descent	• Autosomal recessive hemolytic disease • Involves an abnormal substitution of an amino acid in the structure of hemoglobin • Red blood cells assume abnormal, sickle shape in response to triggers, including hypoxia, infection, dehydration • Results in inability to oxygenate tissues • Leads to occlusion and rupture of blood vessels	• Spontaneous abortion • Preterm labor • Intrauterine growth restriction • Stillbirth
Tay-Sachs disease	Ashkenazi Jews Jewish people from eastern or central Europe French Canadians Cajuns	• Lipid storage disorder that results from a deficiency in the enzyme *beta-hexosaminidase A* (necessary for the biodegradation of acidic fatty materials known as "gangliosides"). • Both parents must carry and pass on the trait to the child	• Infants appear normal at birth, until about 3–6 months of age • Nerve cells become distended with fatty material; muscles atrophy; neurological system deteriorates • Death usually occurs between the ages of 2 and 4 years
Thalassemia	Greeks Italians Southeast Asians Filipinos	• Disorder of hemoglobin synthesis • Thalassemia minor: person is heterozygous for the trait; experiences fewer symptoms • Thalassemia major: person is homozygous for the trait; experiences more severe symptoms	• Children appear normal at birth • During first 2 years, become pale, lethargic, and develop jaundice • Results in enlarged liver, spleen, and heart • Death results from heart failure and infection
Hemophilia	Males affected Females are carriers	• Mutation in the gene for coagulation factor VIII • Causes a defect in blood clotting • Leads to frequent bleeding episodes and hemorrhage	• Males can have excessive bleeding when circumcised • Increased incidence of intracranial hemorrhage • Easy bruising and bleeding with injuries
Glucose-6-phosphate dehydrogenase (G6PD) deficiency	African Americans Seen mostly in males	• Causes drug-induced destruction of red blood cells when taking certain medications (e.g., sulfonamides)	• Increased incidence of pathological jaundice or hyperbilirubinemia caused by destruction of red blood cells
Cystic fibrosis	Caucasians	• Autosomal recessive genetic disorder • Causes exocrine gland dysfunction	• Results in chronic obstructive lung disease from thick mucous secretions in the lungs • Frequent lung infections occur • Causes a deficiency in pancreatic enzymes that prevents normal digestion

Sources: Data from: Cunningham, Leveno, Bloom, Spong, & Dashe (2014); National Institutes of Health (NIH) (2011d); U.S. National Library of Medicine (2012).

syndrome (SIDS) than babies born to women who do not smoke (Centers for Disease Control and Prevention [CDC], 2012a).

Pregnancy is an ideal time to offer smoking cessation interventions because during the prenatal period women generally have an increased concern for their fetus as well as for themselves. Smoking cessation programs are 50% to 70% effective in assisting and empowering women who smoke to be successful in quitting (Albrecht, 2010; March of Dimes Birth Defects Foundation, 2010). Smoking cessation during pregnancy reduces perinatal complications, even if the woman does not quit until the second or third trimester. (See Chapter 7 for further discussion.)

 Optimizing Outcomes—**The SUCCESS program for smoking cessation during pregnancy**

The Association of Women's Health, Obstetric and Neonatal Nurses (AWHONN) developed an evidence-based practice program, "Setting Universal Cessation Counseling Education and Screening Standards" (SUCCESS) to educate nurses and other health-care professionals about smoking cessation interventions, to increase the number of health professionals who provide smoking cessation interventions, and to implement the program to childbearing women who smoke. Outcomes of the program revealed that health-care practitioners represented an ideal group to provide smoking cessation interventions. The SUCCESS program was shown to be valuable in educating nurses and other health-care providers about smoking and smoking cessation, in reducing the number of women who smoke during pregnancy, and in improving birth outcomes (Albrecht, Kelly-Thomas, Osborne, & Ogbagaber, 2011).

ALCOHOL. Alcohol consumption during pregnancy can cause physical and mental abnormalities in the developing fetus. Each year, more than 40,000 babies are born with complications resulting from alcohol use during pregnancy (March of Dimes Birth Defects Foundation, 2008). The current recommendation is that no alcohol consumption during pregnancy is safe because no safe level has been determined.

Alcohol passes quickly through the placenta and reaches the fetal bloodstream much more rapidly than it does in adults. Fetal body system functions are immature and unable to metabolize alcohol, resulting in elevated alcohol levels and damage to developing organs and tissues. The resulting problems are manifested in the facial features associated with fetal alcohol syndrome (FAS): a low nasal bridge, short nose, flat midface, and short palpebral fissures. FAS is one of the most common causes of intellectual disability. Body organs affected include the heart and the brain. Children born with lesser damage are diagnosed with fetal alcohol effects (FAEs), fetal alcohol spectrum disorder (FASD), or alcohol-related birth defects (ARBDs). (See Chapter 19 for further discussion.)

Heavy maternal drinking can result in spontaneous abortion or a low-birth-weight infant. In fact, heavy drinkers are 2 to 4 times more likely to have a spontaneous abortion than are nondrinkers (CDC, 2012b). While drinking alcohol should be discouraged for the duration of the pregnancy, many women do not know they are pregnant during the first few weeks. During this time, occasional alcohol consumption is not believed to harm the fetus. (See Chapter 7 for further discussion.)

 Optimizing Outcomes—**The Screening, Brief Intervention, and Referral to Treatment Tool**

Developed by the Emergency Nurses Association (ENA), the Screening Brief Intervention and Referral to Treatment (SBIRT) program may be useful in treating patients who have alcohol use disorders during pregnancy. Readily available from the ENA Web site (http://www.ena.org), the SBIRT toolkit assists nurses with strategies to conduct patient-centered motivational interviewing designed to make patients aware of their alcohol problems and to help them get started on a regimen of responsible behavior (Keough & Jennrich, 2009).

 Now Can You—**Discuss complications related to alcohol consumption during pregnancy?**

1. Identify facial anomalies associated with FAS?
2. Identify fetal body organs affected by alcohol exposure?
3. Describe pregnancy complications related to alcohol consumption?

CAFFEINE. Caffeine acts as a central nervous system (CNS) stimulant, causing tachycardia and hypertension. Because caffeine readily passes through the placenta to the fetus, the effects of caffeine affect fetal heart rate and movement. It has been thought that high caffeine intake during pregnancy increases the rate of miscarriage and is harmful to the fetus because it stresses the fetus's immature metabolic system and decreases blood flow to the placenta (ACOG, 2010; Guilbeau, 2012; Sengpiel et al., 2013).

The primary sources of caffeine for most pregnant women include coffee, tea, and sodas. Energy drinks, the latest fad in the caffeine market, are loaded with caffeine and sugar and infused with herbal additives. Ingredients added to energy drinks may include ginseng, guarana, bitter orange, and taurine. Other lesser known sources include chocolate, over-the-counter medications that contain caffeine as an ingredient, and dietary supplements. Women should be counseled that coffee and tea labeled "caffeine-free" still contain small amounts of caffeine (Guilbeau, 2012; Pohler, 2010).

 Where Research and Practice Meet: **Posttraumatic Stress, Coping, and Tobacco Use in Pregnancy**

Lopez and colleagues (2011) investigated the relationship between trauma history, posttraumatic stress disorder (PTSD), coping, and smoking in 1,547 pregnant women who were classified as nonsmokers, quitters (those who stopped smoking during pregnancy), and active smokers. They found that smokers differed from nonsmokers on all demographic risk factors (e.g., being African American, being pregnant as a teen, having lower income and less education, and living in high-crime areas), had higher rates of current and lifetime PTSD, and were more likely to report abuse as their worst trauma. Participants who continued to actively smoke during pregnancy had lower levels of education, were more likely to classify their worst trauma as "extremely troubling," and were more likely to exhibit PTSD hyperarousal symptoms (e.g., irritability, difficulty sleeping, and difficulty concentrating). Data analysis revealed that for these women, smoking to help cope with problems and emotions doubled the odds of continuing to smoke while pregnant. The researchers concluded that smoking behavior in pregnancy (e.g., a form of self-medicating) may be influenced by the need to cope with abuse-related PTSD symptoms. Nurses can use this information to guide the use of trauma-informed interventions (as defined by the Substance Abuse and Mental Health Services Administration) that consider tobacco use as a form of self-medication for posttraumatic stress when caring for tobacco-using patients (Lopez, Konrath, & Seng, 2011).

Nurses should assess all patients for their daily intake of caffeine during preconception and early pregnancy visits and can advise them that based on research findings by Savitz and colleagues (2008), small amounts (less than 2 cups) of caffeine daily do not increase the odds of miscarriage. Data from an investigation by Sengpiel et al. (2013) revealed that caffeine intake is associated with decreased birth weight and an increased risk for an SGA infant. Hence, women should be counseled to limit caffeine to 2 cups a day or less or change to decaffeinated sources. (See Chapter 7 for further discussion.)

ARTIFICIAL SWEETENERS. Aspartame (Nutrasweet, Equal), acesulfame potassium (Sunett), and sucralose (Splenda) have not been shown to have any negative effects associated with the developing fetus. However, because aspartame consists of two naturally occurring amino acids, women who have phenylketonuria (PKU) should not use this product. Saccharin, another artificial sweetener, is considered to be unsafe for use during pregnancy and should be avoided altogether.

 ### Nursing Insight—*Maternal phenylketonuria*

Phenylketonuria (PKU) is an autosomal recessive disorder of phenylalanine (Phe) metabolism characterized by a deficiency of phenylalanine, a hepatic enzyme responsible for the conversion of phenylalanine to tyrosine, and elevated levels of Phe and Phe metabolite. Nurses should ensure that all women with PKU or hyperphenylalaninemia are strongly encouraged to receive family planning and preconception counseling. Women with either of these conditions should begin appropriate, medically directed dietary phenylalanine restriction before attempting to conceive. Left untreated, PKU can result in fetal growth failure, microcephaly, seizures, and intellectual disability (ACOG, 2009a).

MARIJUANA. Marijuana may be associated with adverse effects on neonatal neurobehavior, producing symptoms such as hyperirritability, tremors, and photosensitivity. Also, women who use marijuana may engage in other high-risk behaviors (e.g., alcohol and tobacco use) and the combination of effects may be associated with poor fetal outcomes. (See Chapters 7 and 9 for further discussion.)

COCAINE. It is difficult to determine the effects of cocaine use in pregnancy because of the high potential that the woman may be using other drugs and engaging in additional high-risk behaviors. Fetal exposure to cocaine is associated with an increased risk for congenital anomalies that involve the brain, skull, face, eyes, heart, limbs, intestines, genitals, and urinary tract. The pregnant woman who uses cocaine is at risk for pregnancy complications that include stillbirth, abruptio placentae, preterm labor, preterm birth, and giving birth to an infant who is SGA (National Institute on Drug Abuse, 2012). (See Chapters 7, 9, and 11 for further discussion.)

 Now Can You—Discuss substances to be avoided during pregnancy?

1. Name one harmful effect of caffeine during pregnancy?
2. Identify women who should be counseled to avoid the artificial sweetener aspartame?
3. Name three maternal–fetal complications that can result from cocaine use during pregnancy?

THE HEALTHY MIND

Maternal attachment to the fetus is an important area to assess and can be useful in identifying families at risk for maladaptive behaviors (Youngkin, Davis, Schadewald, & Juve, 2012). The nurse should assess for indicators such as unintended pregnancy, intimate partner violence, difficulties in the partner relationship, sexually transmitted infections, limited financial resources, substance use, adolescence, poor social support systems, low educational level, and the presence of mental conditions that might interfere with the patient's ability to bond with and care for the infant. It is important to remember that, depending on what is going on in her life at the time of the pregnancy, any woman has the potential for maladaptive behaviors.

Readiness for Motherhood

Motherhood is not necessarily instinctive for the pregnant woman. Each woman must work through the "process" of becoming a mother. Much of the woman's reservoir of beliefs about motherhood relate back to how she was parented as a child (Attrill, 2002). The pregnant woman must be able to see herself as a mother. To do so, she relies on her life experiences of how she was nurtured as a child and the types of relationships that she has developed over the years with other women (Lederman & Weis, 2010). The relationship with her own mother plays a significant role in how she views motherhood. If the woman's mother is available, accepting the pregnancy and respect for her daughter's autonomy play an integral role in assisting the woman to become a successful mother. Absence of some of these components may impede the pregnant woman's ability to develop into the motherhood role.

One way that a pregnant woman can demonstrate a positive attitude toward her pregnancy is by educating herself

---

 ### Where Research and Practice Meet:
Sociodemographic Factors, Coping Styles, and Spirituality in Pregnancy

Borcherding (2009) used two coping tools to examine the influence of sociodemographic factors on various coping styles used by healthy primigravidae pregnant women. Prayer (i.e., praying for an uncomplicated birth and a healthy baby) and task coping (a problem-focused strategy) were the most frequently used coping styles, while avoidance and emotion coping (using emotions as a response to stressful situations) were used least frequently. Non-white race was associated with frequent use of prayer, task, and distraction coping (e.g., sleeping and watching TV). An important role for nurses who care for antepartal women centers on assessment of personal coping styles and the development of educational and community-based programs that promote healthy coping.

Other investigators have examined the domain of spirituality in childbearing women. Callister and Khalaf (2010) conducted a secondary analysis of two decades of cross-cultural studies to explore the meaning of birth to diverse childbearing women. Data analysis revealed the following themes: childbirth as a time to grow closer to God, the use of religious beliefs and rituals as powerful coping mechanisms, childbirth as a time to make religiosity more meaningful, the significance of a Higher Power in influencing birth outcomes, and childbirth as a spiritually transforming experience. Because an understanding of the spiritual dimensions of childbirth is an essential component of holistic care, the investigators suggest that nurses should routinely inquire about spiritual beliefs that may better guide care.

about maternal changes during pregnancy, fetal growth and development, and motherhood (Fig. 10-3). Many helpful books, brochures, online resources, and community programs on pregnancy and parenting are available for mothers-to-be.

Psychological Changes During Pregnancy

Hormone levels during pregnancy often play havoc with the pregnant woman's psyche. Progesterone exerts a depressant effect. Physical changes, changes in body image and fears related to becoming a mother, the impending labor and birth, and the increased responsibilities that accompany pregnancy and parenthood often produce anxiety or heighten depression during pregnancy (Younkin et al., 2012). Providers must be aware of this potential and remain cognizant for signs and symptoms of mental illness in the pregnant woman. Referral to a mental health professional may be necessary.

The Healthy Relationship

The incidence of intimate partner violence (IPV) during pregnancy is high, and statistically, as many as 20% of pregnant

Where Research and Practice Meet:
Qi Exercise to Enhance Maternal–Fetal Interaction and Maternal Well-Being

Rooted in yoga, Qi exercise is an intervention based on mind and body interconnectedness that incorporates gentle stretching, relaxed controlled breathing, and meditation to lead to preparation of physical strength-flexibility-energy, a state of body-mind relaxation and development of self-awareness. Nurse researchers Ji and Han (2010) implemented a 90-minute Qi exercise program (twice a week for 12 weeks) with 70 pregnant women in Korea to promote maternal–fetal interaction and maternal psychological and physical well-being. Based on study findings, the investigators concluded that Qi exercise has positive effects on maternal–fetal interaction, maternal depressive symptoms, and physical discomfort among healthy pregnant women in Korea and recommend that Qi exercise is beneficial as a prenatal nursing intervention to improve the quality of maternal and child health care. Nurses who work with prenatal patients may wish to suggest Qi exercise as a holistic, beneficial strategy for improving maternal–fetal interaction and maternal well-being during pregnancy.

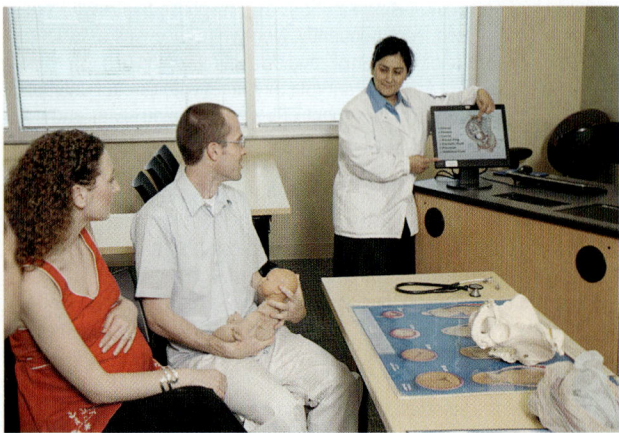

Figure 10-3 Learning about maternal changes, fetal growth and development, and motherhood fosters a positive attitude toward the pregnancy.

Where Research and Practice Meet:
Recognizing Factors Associated With Childbirth Fear

Hall and colleagues (2009) designed a descriptive survey to explore women's levels of childbirth fear, sleep deprivation, anxiety, and fatigue and their relationships during the third trimester of pregnancy. Based on their findings, the nurse researchers concluded that women who have high childbirth fear were likely to have significantly less help available, more daily stressors, and more anxiety and fatigue than those with moderate or low childbirth fear. The investigators propose that health-care providers could improve their caring and support of women during pregnancy by attending equally to their psychological, emotional, and physiological states.

women experience violence in the home (ACOG, 2012a). Every woman should be screened for IPV during the initial visit and then as necessary (e.g., if bruises or other injuries are present) throughout the pregnancy. (See Chapter 9 for further discussion.)

Maternal stress also has a negative effect on the developing fetus. Women who are anxious or stressed during their pregnancy are more likely to deliver preterm or to give birth to smaller babies. The nurse should assess all pregnant women for stressors and coping skills during pregnancy. (See Chapter 9 for further discussion.)

 Complementary Care: *Promoting Stress Management during Pregnancy*

There are several complementary therapies that can safely be used during pregnancy, often recommended by nurse midwives and obstetricians:

- Massage therapy: Increases blood flow to maternal and fetal tissues; increases relaxation
- Chiropractic care: Treats lower back pain and headaches related to increased hormone levels
- Acupuncture and acupressure: Treat many physical ailments during pregnancy without the introduction of medications
- Relaxation exercises, meditation, and breathing techniques: Increase blood flow to maternal and fetal tissues; increase relaxation
- Light therapy: Enhances mood and treats depression
- Reflexology: Stimulates nerve pathways to increase blood flow and energy flow to corresponding areas of the body
- Aromatherapy: Increases relaxation
- Mindfulness-based yoga: Enhances physical well-being and diminishes psychological stress (Beddoe, Yang, Kennedy, Weiss, & Lee, 2009)

Readiness for Fatherhood

In preparation for parenthood, the male partner moves through a series of developmental tasks. During the first trimester, the father begins to deal with the reality of the pregnancy. At this time, he may worry about financial strain and his ability to be a good father. Feelings of confusion and guilt often surface with the recognition that he is not as excited about the pregnancy as is his partner. Couvade syndrome, the experience of maternal signs and symptoms, may develop. (See Chapter 8 for further discussion.)

In the second trimester, the pregnancy becomes more real for the father. The pregnancy begins to "show," and he is able to identify fetal movement through the maternal abdomen. Because there is an increased paternal willingness to learn about fetal growth and development during this time, the second trimester is the best time to provide prenatal education for the expectant couple.

During the third trimester, both parents are preparing for their new roles. Many of the father's early concerns regarding financial demands, personal parenting skills, and partner safety during birth return during this time. Conflicting feelings may emerge between excitement over the prospect of a new baby and the major lifestyle changes that will accompany the presence of a new family member. Most couples attend prenatal classes in preparation for the birth experience during the third trimester. The father may fear for the safety of his partner. How well the couple progresses through the developmental tasks of pregnancy has a major influence on their level of adaptation once the baby is born.

 Now Can You—Discuss common paternal reactions and educational needs during pregnancy?

1. Name two overriding concerns sometimes harbored by fathers during the first trimester?
2. Explain why pregnancy becomes more "real" for fathers during the second trimester?
3. Identify the trimester when education is likely to be most beneficial for the expectant couple?

Nutrition and Weight Gain

Nutrition and weight management play an essential role in the development of a healthy pregnancy. Not only does the patient need to have an understanding of the essential nutritional elements, but she must also be able to assess and modify her diet for the developing fetus and her own nutritional maintenance. To facilitate this process, it is the nurse's responsibility to provide education and counseling concerning dietary intake, weight management, and potentially harmful nutritional practices (Fig. 10-4).

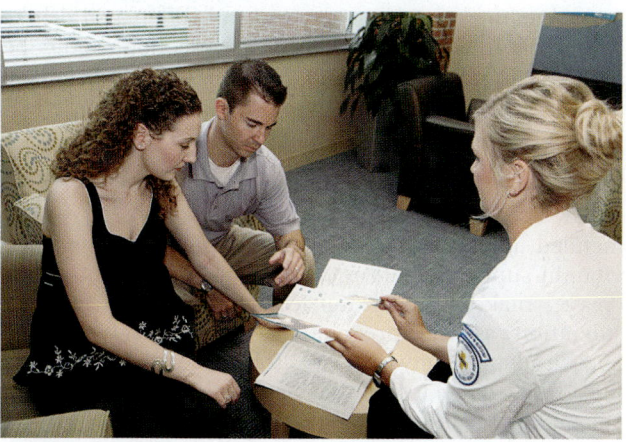

Figure 10-4 Nutritional counseling is an important component of prenatal care.

 Optimizing Outcomes—Resources for optimal nutritional counseling

The document *Dietary Guidelines for Americans 2010* is an evidence-based resource guide for professionals and consumers that offers strategies for promoting health and reducing the risk for chronic diseases through diet and physical activity. Dietary guidelines, food composition, the food guide pyramid, dietary supplements, and resource lists are included in the guide (U.S. Department of Health & Human Services [USDHHS], 2011).

The nurse should obtain a nutritional history on all pregnant patients and patients of childbearing age. Information that is gained in a general nutritional assessment includes questions regarding eating patterns; changes in appetite, chewing, swallowing, and taste; presence of vomiting, diarrhea, or constipation; food allergies and intolerances; and self-care behaviors. In addition to these questions, the nurse needs to gain specific information related to the pregnancy, including:

- Foods that are preferred during pregnancy, which may provide information about cultural and environmental dietary factors
- Special diets, which will assist the nurse in planning for education or interventions for risk factors associated with dietary practices
- Cravings or aversions to specific foods

 Cultural Diversity: Orthodox Jewish Patients and Dietary Laws

To provide culturally appropriate care, nurses should be familiar with and inquire about religious and cultural rituals such as adherence to dietary laws. For example, Orthodox Jewish women adhere to a strict kosher diet, and all food must be prepared with cookware, utensils, and in ovens that have never been used with non-kosher food. Only certain categories of animals, fish, and fowl may be consumed, and dietary law requires that they be slaughtered and prepared in a specific way. Meat and dairy may not be prepared or eaten together, and there is a 3- to 6-hour waiting period after the consumption of meat or fowl before dairy may be eaten again. (Zauderer, 2009).

IMPORTANT NUTRITIONAL ELEMENTS

Many elements combine to facilitate a healthy pregnancy. Often pregnant women are told to eat as much as they want because "they are eating for two." However, this is not necessarily accurate advice. Practitioners must evaluate the amount as well as the nutritional value of the food consumed. Calories are an important consideration when planning the patient's daily food intake. Other essential nutritional elements are protein, water, iron, folic acid, and calcium. Maternal dietary practices that may exert a negative influence on the pregnancy must also be addressed.

Calories

A calorie, or unit of heat, signifies the energy expenditure of food. A kilocalorie (kcal) is equivalent to 1,000 calories. It is the basic unit of measurement that more accurately defines the amount of energy needed to metabolize food and provide an energy source from this food (Venes, 2013). The body's energy needs are met by carbohydrate, fat, and protein in the diet.

The Recommended Daily Allowance (RDA) for caloric intake for nonpregnant women ranges from 1,200 to 2,400 kcal/day, depending on activity level. Women who are sedentary and who exercise less than 30 minutes per day should have a daily intake of 1,200 kcal/day. Women who exercise vigorously for at least 30 minutes per day, 5 to 7 days per week, and engage in cardiovascular and strength training activities should consume 2,000 to 2,400 kcal/day.

During pregnancy, the RDA for caloric intake increases only slightly and requires only a 300 kcal/day increase from prepregnant needs. Growth during the first and second trimesters occurs primarily in the maternal tissues; during the third trimester, growth occurs mostly in the fetal tissues. An increase in maternal caloric intake is most important during the second and third trimesters. In the first trimester, the average maternal weight gain is 1 to 2.5 kg, and thereafter the recommended weight gain for a woman of normal weight is approximately 0.4 kg per week. For overweight women, the recommended weekly weight gain during the second and third trimesters is 0.3 kg; for underweight women, it is 0.5 kg.

Pregnant women should be counseled about healthy ways to incorporate the additional 300 kcal needed in their daily diets. For example, adding an additional serving from each of the major food groups (skim milk, yogurt or cheese; fruits; vegetables; and bread, cereal, rice, or pasta) meets this need. It is essential for health-care providers to stress to patients that the additional kilocalories should not be met through an increased intake of "empty calories" such as soda, candy, or simple carbohydrates.

Protein

Protein is necessary for tissue growth and repair. For pregnant women, protein is important for growth of maternal tissues, including the uterus and the breasts, and for development of fetal tissues and organs. Only a modest increase in protein is required; increasing intake of milk and dairy products by one or two servings per day meets the daily requirement for protein.

Protein is typically found in animal sources, specifically in meat, poultry, and fish. However, other protein sources are also available. Dairy products are a great source of protein and include eggs, milk, cheese, and yogurt. For women who do not prefer dairy sources of protein, or who may be lactose intolerant, soy milk and soy cheese are available as protein-rich substitutes. In addition, beans and legumes provide a rich source of protein and fiber to the diet and can be substituted for protein servings in many meals. Peanut butter is another source rich in protein, but potentially high in fat. Beans and legumes are combined protein sources that provide carbohydrates with protein to supply the essential amino acids that may be missing when insufficient protein from animal sources is consumed.

Optimizing Outcomes—Prevention of foodborne illness

It is important for nurses to educate pregnant women about strategies to prevent foodborne illness, which occurs as a result of the consumption of microorganisms (bacteria,

parasites, and viruses) or chemical contaminants found in some foods and drinking water. Raw, or unpasteurized, milk, as well as partially cooked eggs and foods containing raw or partially cooked eggs should be avoided altogether. Meat, poultry, fish, and eggs should be thoroughly cooked and temperature-checked with a food thermometer. Deli meats, luncheon meats, and frankfurters should be heated before consumption. Foods must be stored properly at 40°F or below, and prepared foods should be eaten within 4 days. In addition, raw shellfish and fish high in mercury, including shark, swordfish, tilefish, and king mackerel should be avoided. Fresh or frozen (non-albacore) tuna, red snapper, and orange roughy contain moderate amounts of mercury and women who are pregnant or planning to become pregnant should limit their intake of these products to 12 ounces per week. Remind patients that consistent, thorough hand washing is paramount to the prevention of foodborne infection (USDHHS, 2011; U.S. Department of Veterans Affairs, 2013).

Water

Water is necessary for all body tissues and all body system functions. It is essential for the maintenance of life and must be consumed in sufficient quantity to sustain homeostasis. All persons should consume six to eight (8-oz) glasses of fluid daily; however, pregnant women should have an intake of eight to ten (8-oz) glasses of fluid per day. The increased amount needed during pregnancy is necessary to meet the changing physiology of the maternal cardiovascular system and to maintain adequate blood flow to the fetus.

During pregnancy, blood volume increases about 1,500 mL, which represents a 40% to 50% increase from the prepregnancy blood volume. The increase in maternal blood volume occurs for three primary reasons: to meet the needs of the hypertrophied vascular system of the enlarged uterus, to adequately hydrate maternal and fetal tissues, and to provide a fluid reserve for blood loss during childbirth. In addition, adequate blood flow to the fetus is necessary for oxygenation of body tissues and maintenance of a normal acid-base balance.

Water intake can be in the form of many different types of fluids, including fruit juice and vegetable juice. However, at least four to six glasses of the fluid consumed each day should be water. Patients should be cautioned to consume certain beverages, such as diet sodas (high in sodium and contain artificial sweeteners) and caffeinated drinks (promote diuresis) in moderation. Alcohol should be avoided entirely throughout the pregnancy because no safe amount has been determined.

Minerals and Vitamins

Women who eat a balanced diet that includes recommended servings and serving sizes may meet the recommended nutritional needs during pregnancy without vitamin supplementation. However, the need for an increased intake of specific nutrients must be taken into consideration as the pregnant woman plans her diet. Specifically, the daily intake of calcium, iron, and folic acid must be adequate to meet the maternal–fetal needs for adequate growth and development.

CALCIUM AND VITAMIN D. The RDA for calcium is 1,000 mg/day in pregnant and prepregnant women.

Calcium requirements are increased in pregnant adolescents (ages 13 to 18), who need an intake of 1,300 mg/day. Without supplementation, most women fail to consume adequate amounts of dietary calcium. Calcium is essential for maintaining bone and tooth mineralization and calcification. During pregnancy, calcium must be available to the fetus for the growth and development of the skeleton and teeth.

Dairy products, especially milk and milk products, constitute the best nutritional sources of calcium. Three daily servings of dairy products are recommended for women; one to two additional daily servings of milk are recommended during pregnancy (National Institutes of Health [NIH], 2011a). Other rich sources of calcium include legumes, dark green leafy vegetables, dried fruits, and nuts.

Optimizing Outcomes—Teaching patients to avoid bone meal supplements

Bone meal, sometimes used as a calcium source, should be avoided during pregnancy. This supplement is frequently contaminated with lead, a toxin that readily crosses the placenta and can result in high levels in the fetus.

Vitamin D, a fat-soluble vitamin obtained largely from consuming fortified milk or juice, fish oils, and dietary supplements, is important in the absorption and metabolism of calcium. During pregnancy and lactation, the RDA for vitamin D is 600 IU (15 mcg)/day. Severe maternal vitamin D deficiency has been associated with biochemical evidence of disordered skeletal homeostasis, congenital rickets, and fractures in the neonate. While there is insufficient evidence for the recommendation for screening all pregnant women for vitamin D deficiency, it is important to educate women about the need for vitamin D–fortified foods or supplements (ACOG, 2011a; Harris, 2011). Fortified milk and ready-to-eat cereals constitute the major food sources of vitamin D, which is also produced in the skin by the action of sunlight. Women who do not include milk in their diets should be taught about other vitamin D sources such as cereals, egg yolks, liver, and fatty fish such as salmon, sardines, and trout. Sunscreens with a recommended SPF rating of 8 appear to block vitamin D–producing UV rays. In practice, however, most people do not apply adequate amounts, cover all sun-exposed skin, or reapply sunscreen regularly. Most likely, the skin synthesizes some vitamin D even when it is protected by sunscreen as typically applied (NIH, 2011b).

Cultural Diversity: Maternal Vitamin D Deficiency

African Americans and other women with naturally dark skin whose melanin affects UV penetration are at the greatest risk for vitamin D deficiency. Women who habitually cover most of their skin with clothing for religious or cultural purposes, vegetarians, and those who live in northern latitudes with limited exposure to sunlight are also more likely to be deficient in vitamin D. Because newborn vitamin D levels are largely dependent on maternal vitamin D status, infants of mothers with or at high risk of vitamin D deficiency are also at risk for vitamin D deficiency (ACOG, 2011a).

IRON AND VITAMIN C. As blood volume increases during pregnancy, the number of circulating red blood cells also increases. Maternal iron intake must be increased to maintain the oxygen-carrying capacity of the blood and to provide an adequate number of red blood cells. Fetal iron needs are increased during the last trimester. At this time, iron is stored in the immature liver for use during the first 4 months of life while the liver matures and liver enzymes are being produced. The newborn uses the stored iron to compensate for insufficient amounts of iron in the breast milk and in non-iron-fortified infant formula.

The iron RDA for prepregnant women ages 14 to 18 is 15 mg/day, for women age 19 and older, 18 mg/day, and for pregnant women, this amount increases to 27 mg/day, starting by 12 weeks of gestation (Institute of Medicine, 2001). Iron can be found in a variety of food sources. Many individuals may not be aware that adequate amounts of iron are found in fortified ready-to-eat cereals, white beans, lentils, spinach, kidney beans, lima beans, soybeans, shrimp, and prune juice. Red meats, including beef, duck, and lamb, contain moderate amounts of iron as well. Some of the best food sources for iron include oysters, organ meats (e.g., liver and giblets), and fortified instant cooked cereals. Interestingly, canned, drained clams provide the highest amount of iron per serving, with 23.8 mg of iron in each 3-ounce serving (NIH, 2012).

While most other necessary nutrients can be met through a balanced diet, it is almost impossible to meet the maternal daily requirements for iron without a dietary supplement. Consideration must be given, however, to the gastrointestinal side effects of supplemental iron, which include constipation, black tarry stools, nausea, and abdominal cramping. These side effects may exacerbate other pregnancy-related gastrointestinal discomforts. Daily iron supplementation is often initiated at around 12 weeks of gestation to avoid compounding the nausea commonly prevalent during the first trimester. Adequate water intake helps to decrease constipation, and patients may take the iron at bedtime if abdominal discomfort is experienced when taking iron between meals. A systematic review published by the Cochrane Collaboration (Pena-Rosas, De-Regil, Dowswell, & Viteri, 2012) shows that taking iron supplements one to three times per week is just as effective at preventing anemia as taking them every day, and the intermittent dosing schedule is associated with fewer side effects.

Nursing Insight—When teaching about iron supplements

Nurses can teach patients about substances known to decrease the absorption of iron. Women should be taught to avoid consuming bran, tea, coffee, milk, oxylates (found in Swiss chard and spinach), and egg yolk at the same time as they take the iron supplement. Also, iron is best absorbed when taken between meals with a beverage other than tea, coffee, or milk.

Vitamin C (ascorbic acid), important in tissue formation, also enhances the absorption of iron. Women who take iron supplements should consume foods or beverages that contain vitamin C. Food sources rich in vitamin C include red and green sweet peppers, oranges, kiwi fruit,

Medication: Ferrous Sulfate

(**fer**-us **sul**-fate)

Pregnancy Category: B

Indications: Prevention/treatment of iron-deficiency anemia

Actions: An essential mineral found in hemoglobin, myoglobin, and many enzymes. Prevents iron deficiency.

Therapeutic Effects: Prevents/treats iron deficiency

Pharmacokinetics:
ABSORPTION: Therapeutically administered PO iron may be 60% absorbed; absorption is an active and passive transport process.

Contraindications and Precautions:
Use cautiously in peptic ulcer, ulcerative colitis; indiscriminate chronic use may lead to iron overload.

Adverse Reactions and Side Effects: Constipation, dark stools, diarrhea, epigastric pain, gastrointestinal bleeding

Route and Dosage:
(for vitamin/mineral supplementation during pregnancy/lactation): 325 mg orally once a day.

Nursing Implications:
1. Assess nutritional status and dietary history to determine possible cause of anemia and need for patient teaching.
2. Assess bowel function for constipation or diarrhea; notify care provider and use appropriate nursing measures if these symptoms occur.

Source: Data from Vallerand, A. H., & Sanoski, C. A. (2014). *Davis's drug guide for nurses* (14th ed.). Philadelphia, PA. F.A. Davis.

grapefruit, strawberries, Brussels sprouts, cantaloupe, broccoli, sweet potatoes, tomato juice, cauliflower, pineapple, and kale. Most pregnant women are able to meet the recommended daily allowance (80 to 85 mg) by including at least one daily serving of citrus fruit or juice or vitamin C-rich food source, although women who smoke need more (NIH, 2011c).

Optimizing Outcomes—Counseling pregnant patients to avoid pomegranates

Although rich in vitamin C, magnesium, potassium, and folate, the pomegranate fruit is a potent stimulant of uterine contractions and is unsafe for use during pregnancy (Sego, 2010).

Inadequate iron intake can lead to anemia, a decrease in the oxygen-carrying capacity of the blood. Physiological anemia, common during pregnancy, occurs when the plasma volume increases more than the red blood cell mass, producing a modest decrease in the hemoglobin concentration and hematocrit. True anemia, or iron-deficiency anemia, occurs when the hemoglobin level drops below 10 g/dL. The blood's decreased oxygen-carrying capacity causes a reduction in oxygen transport to the developing fetus. Decreased fetal oxygen transport has been associated with intrauterine growth restriction (IUGR) and preterm birth.

Cultural Diversity: Anemia During Pregnancy

In the United States, maternal anemia occurs most commonly among adolescents, African American women, and women of lower socioeconomic status (ACOG, 2008b).

In recent years, there has been some controversy surrounding the value of iron supplementation during pregnancy. According to ACOG (2008b), there is good and consistent scientific evidence that iron supplementation decreases the prevalence of maternal anemia at the time of childbirth. However, limited scientific data exist to indicate that iron deficiency anemia during pregnancy is associated with an increased risk of low birth weight, preterm delivery, and perinatal mortality. Based on consensus and expert opinion, ACOG recommends that all pregnant women should be screened for anemia, and those with iron deficiency anemia be treated with supplemental iron, in addition to prenatal vitamins (ACOG, 2008b).

FOLIC ACID. Vitamin B_9, or folic acid (folate), is a water-soluble vitamin that is closely related to iron. Working with vitamin B_{12}, folic acid helps to regulate red blood cell development and facilitates the oxygen-carrying capacity of the blood. Folic acid is essential in the production of DNA and RNA and helps to maintain normal brain function and to stabilize mental and emotional health. Folic acid also works with vitamins B_6 and B_{12} to control blood levels of homocysteine, an amino acid that, in elevated amounts, has been linked to heart disease, depression, and Alzheimer's disease.

Increased estrogen production during pregnancy alters the absorption and metabolism of folic acid, producing an increased maternal susceptibility for folic acid deficiency. Folic acid deficiency is primarily responsible for the development of neural tube defects (NTDs), including spina bifida, cleft lip and palate, and anencephaly. The neural tube, an embryonic structure that develops during the first 4 weeks after conception, divides during embryo-fetal development to form the CNS, including the spinal cord and the brain. (See Chapter 7 for further discussion.)

During the early developmental weeks of pregnancy, the majority of women do not yet know that they have conceived. Because of the strong connection between folic acid deficiency and the subsequent development of neural tube defects, folic acid supplementation is important, even in women who are not actively attempting to conceive. The U.S. Public Health Service (USPHS) and the CDC recommend that all women of childbearing age consume 0.4 mg (400 mcg) of synthetic folic acid daily, from supplements and/or fortified foods, to reduce NTD risk. During pregnancy, a minimum of 800 mcg/day of folic acid is recommended, and this amount is usually provided through supplementation. Childbearing-aged women who have previously given birth to an infant with a neural tube defect should consume 0.4 mg of folic acid daily when not planning to become pregnant. When these women do plan to become pregnant, they should be advised to consult with their health-care provider about the desirability of following the 1991 USPHS guideline that called for the consumption of 4 milligrams (4,000 mcg) of folic acid daily beginning 1 month before attempting conception and continuing through the first 3 months of pregnancy (ACOG, 2003; CDC, 2012c).

Optimizing Outcomes—Educating childbearing-age women about folic acid supplementation

Nurses who work with childbearing-age women in a variety of settings have the responsibility to educate them about the benefits of folic acid consumption. Wellness and contraceptive care visits, for example, provide the perfect opportunity to remind patients about the protective effects of a folate-rich diet combined with synthetic folic acid, provide information about how this can be achieved, and teach them that up to 70% of NTDs can be prevented by consuming 400 mcg of folic acid every day from good sources including a daily multivitamin supplement (AWHONN, 1999).

Foods that are rich in folic acid include dark leafy greens, asparagus, broccoli, citrus fruits, beans, peas and lentils, avocado, okra, Brussels sprouts, seeds and nuts, fortified breakfast cereals, and calf liver. In 1998, the Food and Drug Administration (FDA) mandated the addition of 140 mcg of folic acid to every 100 grams of certain grain products, such as flour, breakfast cereals, and pasta. Current recommendations include consuming folic acid with vitamin C to enhance the absorption of iron and folic acid.

 Now Can You—Discuss aspects of good nutrition during pregnancy?

1. Identify two protein sources for women who wish to avoid dairy products?
2. Identify three calcium sources for women who wish to avoid dairy products?
3. Explain why adequate intake of vitamin C and folic acid are important during pregnancy?

WEIGHT GAIN DURING PREGNANCY

Weight gain is expected during pregnancy and results from a combination of maternal physiological changes and fetal growth. During early pregnancy, maternal weight gain is related to an increased blood volume, necessary to supply the enlarging uterus and support fetal growth and development. Dilation of the renal pelvis and ureters from increased blood flow adds volume to the bladder and results in an increased production of urine. Essential nutrients provided through the maternal blood supply enable fetal growth and development. As the pregnancy progresses, enlargement of the placenta and fetal body add to the woman's increase in weight. By term, maternal extracellular fluid, blood, uterine tissue, and breast tissue account for 35% of the gestational weight gain; the maternal reserves account for 27%; fetal tissue accounts for 27%; and placental fluid accounts for 11% of the total maternal weight gain (Cunningham, Leveno, Bloom, Spong, & Dashe, 2014).

Factors Affecting Weight Gain

In addition to maternal–fetal physiological factors, social influences are also important predictors of gestational weight gain. Social factors related to an insufficient maternal weight gain may include an inability to purchase food, inadequate dairy intake, unplanned pregnancy, intimate partner violence, anorexia nervosa, shortened time period between pregnancies, and lack of prenatal care. Factors that may influence an excessive maternal weight gain during pregnancy include inadequate or inconsistent physical activity, a high carbohydrate or fat intake, excessive consumption of sweets, and lack of prenatal care.

An adverse outcome may result when the woman gains too much or too little weight during her pregnancy. Healthcare providers need to assess the patient's weight during the first prenatal visit and monitor the weight gain closely throughout the pregnancy. The amount of weight that is gained during the gestational period results from a combination of influences, including biological and social factors. Biological factors include genetic alleles that affect phenotypes responsible for regulating energy and fat metabolism. These, in turn, affect maternal weight and fat gain during pregnancy. High levels of insulin and leptin (a protein hormone that regulates energy metabolism and appetite) during the first trimester are also associated with higher maternal weight and fat gain during pregnancy (Institute of Medicine, 2009).

Women who gain too much weight during pregnancy are at an increased risk for gestational diabetes. This complication places the infant at risk for macrosomia (large body size), congenital anomalies, birth trauma, perinatal asphyxia, respiratory distress syndrome, hypoglycemia, hypocalcemia, cardiomyopathy, hyperbilirubinemia, and polycythemia. Gestational diabetes also increases the risk for cesarean birth and maternal **preeclampsia**. Preeclampsia is a condition associated with a decreased blood supply to the maternal organs and to the developing fetus and may result in preterm birth, premature rupture of membranes, maternal organ damage, thrombocytopenia, IUGR, and an altered acid-base balance in the fetus (ACOG, 2013a, 2013b). (See Chapter 11 for further discussion.)

Management of Weight During Pregnancy

Classification of weight is often based on **body mass index** (**BMI**), which is a method of evaluating the appropriateness of weight for height. The BMI is calculated using the formula:

$$BMI = \frac{Weight}{Height^2}$$

where the weight is recorded in kilograms and the height is in meters. For example, the calculated BMI for a woman who weighed 52 kg before pregnancy and is 1.58 m tall is:

$$BMI = \frac{52}{1.58^2} = 20.8$$

Persons with a BMI less than 18.5 are underweight, those with a BMI between 18.5 and 24.9 are of normal weight, and those with a BMI between 25.0 and 29.9 are overweight. Persons with a BMI between 30 and 34.9 are classified at Level 1 obesity; those with a BMI between 35 and 39.9 are classified at Level 2 obesity. Extreme obesity, or Level 3 obesity, includes persons with a BMI of 40 or above. Given the increase in obesity in the United States, one of the *Healthy People 2020* goals (USDHHS, 2012) is to increase the number of women who attain a recommended weight gain (Institute of Medicine, 2009) during their pregnancies, in consultation with their health-care provider (Table 10-2).

 Nursing Insight—*Perinatal risks associated with obesity*

Obesity is a risk factor for a number of pregnancy complications such as gestational diabetes mellitus, hypertension, congenital anomalies, fetal macrosomia, adverse birth outcomes, and low Apgar scores. As the BMI increases, the risk for cesarean delivery increases and is almost 3 times higher for women with Level 2 obesity as compared with women with a normal BMI. Higher BMI is associated with an increased risk for wound infection and breakdown (Bennett & McDonald-Mosley, 2011; Ovesen, Rasmussen, & Kesmodel, 2011; Walters & Smith-Taylor, 2010).

Optimizing Outcomes—The "5-A's" model to assist weight reduction prior to conception

Women who are overweight and obese are at risk for developing numerous complications (e.g., spontaneous abortion, stillbirth, thromboembolism, sleep apnea, asthma exacerbations, abnormal labor, and uterine rupture) during pregnancy. During preconception counseling, the evidence-based "5-A's" model may be useful in helping patients to achieve weight reduction. Nurses can:

- *Ask* the patient about her current diet/exercise habits, and self-perception of her present weight as compared with her ideal weight
- *Advise* the patient of the health issues associated with obesity and emphasize the value of weight reduction as a strategy to reduce the risks
- *Assess* the patient's willingness to take action
- *Assist* the patient with her weight loss efforts (e.g., identify support systems)
- *Arrange* follow-up through regular counseling appointments and weight checks

(Gebhardt & Truehart, 2012)

Nurses should be aware that following bariatric surgery for weight loss, pregnant patients might experience perinatal complications associated with decreased nutrition intake. Patients who have undergone a gastric banding procedure should be closely monitored by their bariatric surgeon throughout pregnancy to assess for the need to adjust the gastric band so that the woman can eat enough to foster fetal growth. The Roux-en-Y gastric bypass (RYGB) procedure involves sectioning off a small area of the stomach and reconnecting it to the jejunum, where the absorption of important nutrients (i.e., iron, calcium, vitamin A, vitamin B_{12}, vitamin K, and folate) occurs. In rare situations, the increased intra-abdominal pressure that occurs

during pregnancy may be associated with obstruction after intestinal modifications related to RYGB. Women are also at risk for intestinal herniations, which are more likely to occur during the intra- and postpartal periods. During preconception and prenatal counseling, patients who have had (or are considering) bariatric surgery should be educated about the changes in nutrient absorption and the potential impact on a fetus. Referral to a registered dietitian who can offer specific advice about supplementation is beneficial, and an important nursing role centers on determining the patient's level of compliance with the nutritional plan (Conrad, Russell, & Keister, 2011; Kominiarek, 2013).

The recommended weight gain ranges for short women and for racial or ethnic groups are the same as those for the whole population. Pregnant adolescents should use the adult BMI categories to determine their weight gain range until further research is conducted to determine whether special categories are indicated for them. Women pregnant with twins should be given provisional guidelines. Those in the normal BMI category should aim to gain 37 to 54 pounds, overweight women 31 to 50 pounds, and obese women, 25 to 42 pounds (Institute of Medicine, 2009).

Ideally, weight management begins before the pregnancy. At the preconception visit, women should be screened for height and weight, with the BMI calculated as a beginning point for determining an appropriate weight gain during pregnancy (Institute for Clinical Systems Improvement [ICSI], 2011). The BMI and weight are then monitored at each prenatal visit. Throughout the pregnancy, counseling, educational interventions, and prophylaxis are provided (Table 10-3). Because excess weight gain during early pregnancy is associated with an increased incidence of gestational diabetes, current recommendations indicate that complications can be decreased if screening for gestational diabetes in women at high risk takes place during the first trimester (National Diabetes Information Clearinghouse, 2011). Gestational weight gain recommendations should be individualized, especially for obese women, who should be encouraged to participate in healthy lifestyle modifications (e.g., exercise, modified diets, and limited weight gain) during pregnancy (Artal, Lockwood, & Brown, 2010; Flick & Artal, 2013). It is important for health-care providers to be proactive throughout the course of pregnancy to help the woman maintain a sense of self-efficacy and control (Walters & Smith-Taylor, 2010). During the postpartal period, obese women should be encouraged to lose weight to prevent the successive weight gain that is common with each pregnancy (Chescheir, 2011).

Table 10-2 Recommended Total Weight Gain During Pregnancy for a Single Birth	
Prepregnancy BMI	**Recommended Total Weight Gain**
Underweight (<18.5)	28–40 lb
Normal weight (18.5–24.9)	25–35 lb
Overweight (25.0–29.9)	15–25 lb
Obese (> 30.0)	11–20 lb

Source: From the Institute of Medicine (2009). *Weight gain during pregnancy: Reexamining the guidelines.* Available at http://www.iom.edu/~/media/Files/Report%20Files/2009/Weight-Gain-During-Pregnancy-Reexamining-the-Guidelines/Report%20Brief%20-%20Weight%20Gain%20During%20Pregnancy.pdf

Where Research and Practice Meet: Gestational Weight Gain Restriction in Obese Women

Numerous studies (Dodd, Grivell, Crowther, & Robinson, 2010; Guelinckx, Devlieger, Mullie, & Vansant, 2010; Quinlivan, Lam, & Fisher, 2011; Streuling, Beyerlein, Rosenfeld, Hofmann, Schulz, & Kries, 2011; Thornton, Smarkola, Kopacz, & Ishoof, 2009; Wolff, Legarth, Vangsaard, Toubro, & Astrup, 2008) have suggested that at the time of presentation for prenatal care, 30% to 40% of pregnant women have a BMI higher than 25. Quinlivan, Julania, and Lam (2011) conducted a meta-analysis to determine if antenatal dietary interventions to restrict maternal weight gain in obese pregnant women had an adverse effect on

Table 10-3 Recommendations for Weight Management During Pregnancy			
Time Frame	**Screening**	**Education**	**Prophylaxis**
Preconception Visit	Height Weight BMI calculation	Nutrition and weight	Folic acid supplementation
Initial Prenatal Visit: First Trimester	Height Weight BMI calculation	Lifestyle education on nutrition	Nutritional supplements
Subsequent Visits Up to 22 weeks	Weight	Follow-up on risk factors	Nutrition evaluation
Visit at Approximately 22 weeks	Weight	Gestational diabetes	Nutrition evaluation
Visits from 28 to 36 weeks	Weight	Follow-up on risk factors	Nutrition evaluation
Visits from 38 to 41 weeks	Weight	Follow-up on risk factors	Discussion of postpartum nutrition

Source: Adapted from Institute for Clinical Systems Improvement (ICSI). (2011). Prenatal care, Routine. Available at http://www.icsi.org/guidelines_and_more/gl_os_prot/womens_health/prenatal_care_4/prenatal_care_routine_3.html

newborn birth weight. The results suggested that antenatal dietary intervention programs (e.g., individual counseling sessions, food diary, and educational brochures) were effective in reducing the total maternal gestational weight gain but did not alter newborn birth weight. The investigators noted that the time of pregnancy represents an ideal time for a weight intervention in women who are overweight or obese and suggest that it may be effective for these women to gain less weight than that advised in the 2009 Institute of Medicine recommendations. Results from Bloomberg's (2011) analysis of over 45,000 obese pregnant women suggested that obese women (classes II and III) who lose weight during pregnancy seem to have a decreased or unaffected risk for cesarean delivery, large for gestational age, preeclampsia, excessive postpartum bleeding, instrumental delivery, low Apgar score, and fetal distress. Nurses who work with overweight and obese pregnant patients may wish to offer various antenatal dietary interventions to achieve maternal gestational weight restriction and reduce the potential for numerous maternal–fetal complications associated with excessive weight gain in pregnancy.

PLANNING DAILY FOOD INTAKE

While planning daily food intake is based on individual preferences, consideration must be given to ensure that adequate nutrients are provided without an excessive increase in caloric intake. New guidelines indicate strategies for daily food consumption (USDHHS, 2011). The primary recommendations include the following:

- Including a variety of nutrient-dense foods and fluids while limiting saturated and trans fats, cholesterol, excessive sugar, salt, and alcohol
- Developing a balanced daily eating pattern, using the USDA Food Guide or the DASH Eating Plan (see Table 10-4).

Specific recommendations for women who are capable of becoming pregnant incorporate the following strategies:

- Eating foods that supply heme iron and iron-fortified foods
- Including vitamin C–rich foods to enhance the absorption of iron
- Consuming 400 mcg per day of synthetic folic acid through consumption of fortified foods and/or

supplements in addition to food forms of folate from a varied diet
- Consuming 8 to 12 ounces of seafood per week (women who are pregnant or breastfeeding), while limiting white (albacore) tuna to 6 ounces per week and avoiding tilefish, shark, swordfish, and king mackerel (because of their methyl mercury content)

The *USDA Food Guide* visualized by the new ChooseMyPlate, which replaces the Food Pyramid, is based on individual factors, including age, gender, and activity level. The Daily Food Plan for Moms is based on the guiding principles of overall health, up-to-date research, total diet, usefulness, realism, flexibility, practicality, and evolution. This easy-to-use tool shows the foods and amounts that are recommended for each stage of pregnancy and during the breastfeeding period. An added feature is the SuperTracker's MyPlan, which focuses the patient on developing an individual approach to daily dietary planning. A Web site (http://www.choosemyplate.gov/supertracker-tools/supertracker.html) is available for more information on how to develop a personalized nutrition and physical activity plan.

The DASH (Dietary Approaches to Stop Hypertension) Eating Plan resulted from a study designed to investigate whether the typical American diet affected blood pressure (USDHHS, 2006). The diet plan includes the daily consumption of whole grain products, fish, poultry, and nuts. There is also a focus on reducing lean red meat, sweets, and added sugar found in foods and beverages. The DASH Eating Plan encourages an increased intake of potassium, magnesium, calcium, protein, and fiber. Table 10-4 compares the daily servings and serving sizes between the USDA Food Pattern and the DASH Eating Plan.

Now Can You—**Plan a daily menu for a woman who is pregnant?**

1. Identify proteins that meet pregnancy needs?
2. Suggest foods to increase daily intake of potassium, magnesium, calcium, protein, and fiber?
3. Describe foods that should be avoided by women who are pregnant?

Table 10-4 USDA Food Pattern and the DASH Eating Plan

Food Groups	USDA Food Pattern Amount	DASH Eating Plan Amount
Fruits	2 cups (4 servings)	2–2.5 cups (4–5 servings)
Vegetables	2.5 cups (5 servings)	2–2.5 cups (4–5 servings)
Dark Green Vegetables	1.5 cups/week	
Red and Orange Vegetables	5.5 cups/week 1.5 cups/week	
Beans and Peas	5 cups/week	
Starchy Vegetables	4 cups/week	
Other Vegetables		
Grains	6 ounce-equivalents	6–8 ounce-equivalents (6–8 servings)
Whole Grains	3 ounce-equivalents	
Enriched Grains	3 ounce-equivalents	
Protein Foods Seafood Meat, Poultry, Eggs Nuts, Seeds, Soy Products	5.5 ounce-equivalents 8 ounces/week 26 ounces/week 4 ounces/week	6 ounces or less of meat, poultry, and fish 4-5 servings per week of nuts, seeds, beans, or lentils
Dairy	3 cups	2–3 cups
Oils	27 grams (6 tsp)	8–12 grams (2–3 tsp)
Maximum "Empty" Calories from Solid Fats and Added Sugars	258 calories (13%)	2 tsp (5 tbsp or less per week)
Maximum Sodium Limit		2300 mg/day

Source: Department of Health and Human Services/U.S. Department of Agriculture. Dietary Guidelines for Americans (2010). Available at https://www.nhlbi.nih.gov/health/educational/wecan/downloads/intake.pdf

FACTORS AFFECTING NUTRITION DURING PREGNANCY

Several additional factors affect nutrition during pregnancy and may lead to potentially adverse effects. These factors include eating disorders and certain cultural variations.

Eating Disorders

PICA. **Pica,** the consumption of nonnutritive substances or food, is a common eating disorder that can affect pregnancy. Substances that are most often ingested include clay, dirt, cornstarch, and ice (Fig. 10-5). Some individuals engage in poly-pica, the practice of consuming more than one of the nonnutritive substances. Pica occurs with greater frequency in developmentally disabled persons. There is also a cultural link that is considered nonpathological and is seen more commonly in African Americans and persons of Middle-Eastern lineage (Young, 2012).

Causes of pica are believed to include nutritional deficiencies, cultural and familial factors, stress, low socioeconomic status, and biochemical disorders. Specific nutritional deficiencies associated with pica include deficiencies in iron, calcium, zinc, thiamine, niacin, vitamin C, and vitamin D. The consumption of clay and starch is most commonly seen in southern, rural, African American communities, and it is believed that this practice, especially the practice of eating

Global Health Case Study   Excessive Weight Gain During Pregnancy

Eliana, a 24-year-old Hispanic primigravida at 26 weeks gestation, has presented for a routine second-trimester prenatal visit. During the interview with the nurse, Eliana voices no complaints. Her vital signs and laboratory data are assessed and all are within normal limits. However, her weight today is 155 pounds, which represents a 30-pound weight gain from her prepregnancy weight. Eliana has no preexisting health conditions. She is married and lives in a mobile home. She works part time at a local fast food restaurant and readily admits that she enjoys eating the food served in her restaurant.

critical thinking questions

1. What are the major health concerns regarding Eliana at this time?

2. What patient education should the nurse provide for Eliana?

3. What additional care should be provided for Eliana?

◆ See Suggested Answers to Global Health Case Studies on Davis*Plus.*

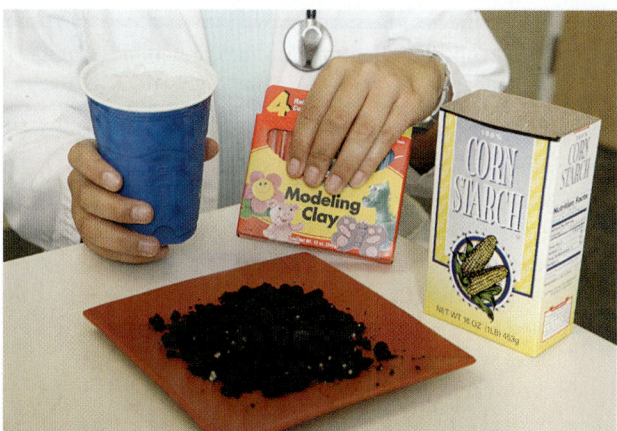

Figure 10-5 Common sources of pica.

starch, was first initiated to alleviate the discomfort of nausea in early pregnancy.

Treatment of pica focuses on the diagnosis and treatment of underlying nutritional deficiencies. The practice usually subsides after the birth of the baby.

 ### *Cultural Diversity: Consuming Nonnutritive Substances*

Health-care providers need to have an understanding of the cultural and religious factors associated with pica. In some cultures, nonnutritive food substances are thought to bring health or have positive spiritual effects for those who consume them. Some cultures believe that the consumption of specific nonnutritive substances plays a role in enhancing fertility or promoting luck within the family. The health-care provider's knowledge and understanding about pica can provide opportunities for assessing complications in patients, providing education to reduce the behavior when harmful, or discussing alternatives for meeting the patient's needs.

ANOREXIA NERVOSA AND BULIMIA NERVOSA. Anorexia nervosa and bulimia nervosa are conditions characterized by a distorted body image. Both involve an intense fear of becoming obese and can have a major impact on the person's physical and psychological well-being. Patients with **anorexia nervosa** lose weight either by excessive dieting or by purging themselves of calories they have ingested. Patients with **bulimia nervosa** engage in recurrent episodes of binge eating, self-induced vomiting and diarrhea, excessive exercise, strict dieting, or fasting and display an exaggerated concern about body shape and weight (Venes, 2013).

Both of these eating disorders pose potentially harmful effects on the woman and the developing fetus because nutrients are either not consumed or are quickly eliminated from the body. The health-care practitioner needs to address the nutritional history of patients with these disorders and work closely with them and other appropriate resources to achieve a healthy pregnancy. Prenatal care should center on a team approach that includes nutritional counseling, psychological counseling, stress management, and active participation in support groups for individuals with eating disorders.

 ### *Nursing Insight—Pregnancy and anorexia nervosa*

Because of advances in reproductive health care, women with anorexia nervosa may achieve pregnancy with induced ovulation through hormonal therapy. It is essential that they be closely monitored throughout the childbearing year because the emotional and physical demands of pregnancy may further compromise their already delicate physical state. Although pregnancy typically intensifies anorexic symptoms, the patient's concern for the health of her fetus may prevent her from engaging in eating-disordered behaviors (Carr & Kaplan, 2010).

Cultural Factors

Health-care providers need to identify and address special cultural considerations in pregnant women from various ethnic backgrounds. The practitioner must possess an understanding of different dietary habits and knowledge of preparation and cooking methods and the basic ingredients commonly used in cooking.

For many cultures and religions, food items have a symbolic or special meaning, especially during pregnancy. Persons from different backgrounds need to be encouraged to continue their practices as long as there is adequate nutrition for the patient and her fetus. Food cravings during pregnancy are considered normal by most cultures although the specific foods craved are culturally influenced. In most cultures, women crave nutritionally acceptable foods. As the woman and her family become more integrated into the dominant culture, cultural influences on food usually lessen.

 ### *Cultural Diversity: Mexican Women and Food Fearfulness*

Pregnant Mexican women may harbor fears that personal or fetal harm may result from eating pork when taking medications such as prenatal vitamins. These women may also have been warned that lemons and limes thin the blood and that the consumption of chili causes "chincual" (red spots on a newborn's face or bottom) or colic. Nurses who care for these patients should be aware of culturally influenced beliefs about diet and nutrition and take time to openly explore these misconceptions about food safety and cultural dietary taboos (Cox & Phelan, 2009).

Vegetarian Diets

Most vegetarian diets include vegetables, fruits, legumes, nuts, seeds, and grains. However, there are many variations. For example, semivegetarian diets include fish, poultry, eggs, and dairy products but no beef or pork, and ovolactovegetarians consume plant and dairy products. Pregnant women who adhere to these diets may consume inadequate amounts of iron and zinc. Because strict vegetarians (vegans) consume only plant products, their diets are deficient in vitamin B_{12}, found only in foods of animal origin. Pregnant women who are strict vegetarians should be counseled to regularly consume vitamin B_{12}-fortified foods such as soy milk or to take a vitamin B_{12} supplement.

Other essential elements that may be deficient in women on this diet include iron, calcium, zinc, vitamin B$_6$, calories, and protein. Nutritional counseling, along with ongoing assessment of maternal weight gain and laboratory testing for evidence of anemia, are important strategies in ensuring optimal maternal–fetal well-being.

 Nursing Insight—*Teaching about vitamin B$_{12}$ deficiency*

When counseling patients who are vegetarians, nurses should educate them about vitamin B$_{12}$ deficiency. Vitamin B$_{12}$ deficiency is associated with maternal problems that include megaloblastic anemia, glossitis, and neurological deficits. Infants born to mothers with vitamin B$_{12}$ deficiency are also more likely to have megaloblastic anemia and to exhibit neurodevelopmental delays.

 Now Can You—**Discuss various factors that may affect nutrition during pregnancy?**

1. Define pica and provide two examples of pica?
2. Describe a team approach to prenatal care for women with anorexia nervosa or bulimia?
3. Develop a teaching plan for prenatal patients who are vegetarians?

Exercise, Work, and Rest During Pregnancy

The demands of daily life can create significant stressors during pregnancy as well as opportunities for incorporating facets of health promotion into a woman's life. Balancing these demands requires an understanding of the physical and emotional changes that occur during pregnancy and developing strategies to relieve the stress that may result from these changes. Activity and exercise benefit both the mother and her fetus, but consideration must be given to the current level of activity and precautions that are required as a result of the pregnancy. Work demands often create additional stress during a woman's pregnancy, requiring decisions of employment versus unemployment and maternity leave. For women not employed outside the home, responsibilities of caring for the home and family must also be balanced. Rest becomes an important component of managing a healthy pregnancy, and patients need to understand how fatigue will impact their daily life and how to manage this fatigue throughout the pregnancy.

EXERCISE AND TRAVEL

Exercise can provide women who are pregnant with many benefits, whether they are just beginning to exercise to facilitate a healthy pregnancy or whether they are already active in an exercise program. Unless there are absolute contraindications to aerobic exercise (Box 10-2), pregnant women should be encouraged to engage in regular, moderate-intensity physical activity for 30 minutes or more each day. The exercises practiced during pregnancy should focus on strengthening muscles without rigorous

---

> **Box 10-2** **Absolute Contraindications to Aerobic Exercise During Pregnancy**
>
> - Hemodynamically significant heart disease
> - Restrictive lung disease
> - Cervical insufficiency/incompetence
> - Multiple gestation at risk for premature labor
> - Persistent second- or third-trimester bleeding
> - Placenta previa after 26 weeks of gestation
> - Premature labor during the current pregnancy
> - Ruptured membranes
> - Preeclampsia/pregnancy-induced hypertension
>
> *Source:* ACOG (2002).

> **Box 10-3** **Safety Guidelines for Muscle Strengthening Exercise During Pregnancy**
>
> Healthy pregnant women aged 18 to 45 years of age may perform 8 to 10 muscular strength exercises for one to two sessions per week on nonconsecutive days, using the following safety guidelines:
>
> - Use lighter weights and more repetitions (heavy weights may overload the "loosened" joints)
> - Avoid walking lunges (lunges may injure connective tissue in the pelvic area)
> - Use caution with free weights, to avoid hitting the abdomen (use resistance bands instead)
> - Avoid lifting from a supine position (to prevent vena caval syndrome and decreased placental perfusion—tilt the bench to an incline)
> - Avoid the Valsalva maneuver (may decrease placental perfusion)
> - Avoid heavy weightlifting and reduce the frequency of workouts if fatigue or muscle strain develop
>
> *Source:* Zavorsky & Longo (2011).

---

aerobic activity that may cause complications. As long as basic safety guidelines are followed, muscle strengthening will benefit the woman as she copes with the physical changes of pregnancy, including weight gain and postural changes, and will decrease the chances of ligament and joint injury (Box 10-3). Pregnant women gain many additional benefits from exercise such as an increased energy level, improved posture, relief from back pain, enhanced circulation, increased endurance, decreased muscle tension, increased feelings of well-being, and strengthened muscles to prepare for labor and birth (Loprinzi, Fitzgerald, & Cardinal, 2012) (Fig. 10-6). Also, physical activity before and during pregnancy may help to decrease mood disorders during the puerperium (Demissie, Siega-Riz, Evenson, Herring, Dole, & Gaynes, 2011).

When traveling for long distances, the pregnant woman should plan periods of activity combined with rest. While sitting, the woman can engage in slow, deep breathing, make circling motions with her feet and practice alternately contracting and relaxing different muscle groups. Automobile restraints that consist of a combination lap belt and shoulder harness should always be used. The shoulder harness is placed above the gravid uterus and below the woman's neck to avoid irritation. The woman should

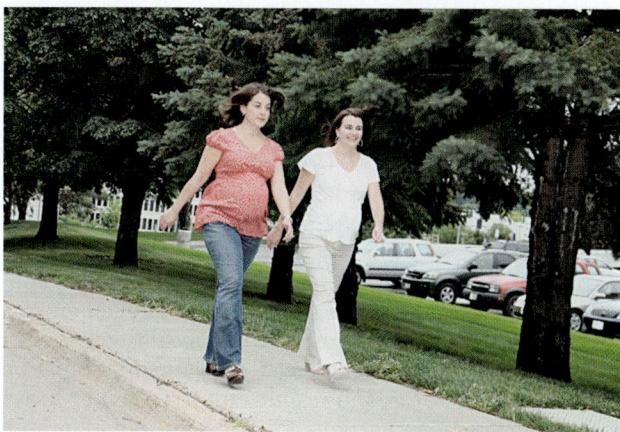

Figure 10-6 Exercise during pregnancy has many benefits and enhances the woman's sense of well-being.

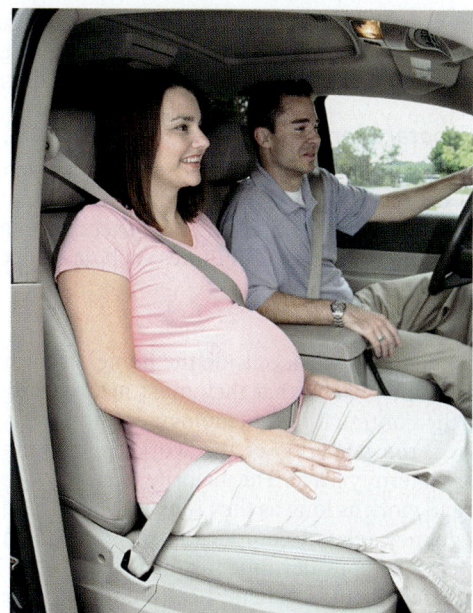

Figure 10-7 Proper use of the seat belt and headrest during pregnancy.

Where Research and Practice Meet:
Exercise During Pregnancy

According to the *Physical Activity Guidelines for Americans* (USDHHS, 2008), pregnant women who are not already highly active should get at least 150 minutes of moderate-intensity aerobic activity per week during pregnancy. Participation in vigorous-intensity exercise is not recommended for previously inactive women or women who engage in only moderate-intensity exercise. Women who are currently vigorously active may continue this level of activity during pregnancy according to the guidelines. Szymanski and Satin (2012) studied 45 healthy pregnant women between 28 and 33 weeks of gestation to evaluate acute fetal responses to individually prescribed exercise (e.g., progressive treadmill) according to USDHHS guidelines for active and inactive pregnant women. The findings revealed that exercise according to the current USDHHS guidelines was well tolerated by the mothers and their fetuses. The investigators suggest that health-care providers should feel reassured in recommending that pregnant women can exercise during pregnancy when following existing exercise recommendations.

assume an upright position and ensure the headrest is properly aligned to avoid a whiplash injury (Fig. 10-7).

Occasional air travel is generally safe but is not recommended at any time during pregnancy for women who have medical or obstetric conditions that may be exacerbated by flight or that could require emergency care. Most commercial airlines allow pregnant women to fly up to 36 weeks of gestation. The metal detectors used at security checkpoints are not harmful to the fetus. Because the airline cabin humidity is typically maintained at a low level, the nurse should advise the pregnant woman to drink plenty of water to remain hydrated throughout the flight. Also, the use of support stockings, periodic movement of the lower extremities, avoidance of restrictive clothing, and occasional ambulation are important strategies to minimize the risk of superficial and deep vein thrombophlebitis. Seat belts should be worn continuously while seated (ACOG, 2009b).

Now Can You—Discuss guidelines for exercise during pregnancy?

1. Name five absolute contraindications to aerobic exercise during pregnancy?

2. Describe two ways that muscle-strengthening exercises are beneficial during pregnancy?

3. Identify four benefits that may result from any form of physical exercise during pregnancy?

General Safety Guidelines for Exercise

Although exercise provides significant benefits during pregnancy, women should adhere to some basic safety guidelines when formulating their exercise program. The most important consideration involves monitoring the breathing rate and ensuring that the ability to walk and talk comfortably is maintained during physical activity. Exercise must be stopped when the woman becomes tired, and she must be taught to never exercise to the point of exhaustion. Exercises that can cause any degree of trauma to the abdomen or those that include rigorous bouncing, arching of the back, or bending beyond a 45-degree angle should be avoided. Adequate fluid intake must be maintained before, during, and after exercise to prevent dehydration. Activities that require balance and coordination should also be avoided, especially during later pregnancy when the center of gravity shifts and the joints and ligaments soften and relax (ACOG, 2002).

Limiting strenuous aerobic exercise and engaging in low-impact aerobics, swimming, and cycling are strategies to ensure protection against increased metabolism and overheating. Increased maternal body temperature can cause reduced oxygen saturation and is associated with the development of fetal neural tube defects during early pregnancy. Decreased oxygen saturation in the maternal circulation directly affects fetal blood flow and oxygenation and can result in delayed or improper growth and development. Also, as the pregnant woman's body temperature increases, the fetal body temperature increases as well. The fetus is unable to reduce body temperature through perspiration or other means and instead must rely on the mother's body for temperature regulation. Other adverse effects that may result from maternal overheating during exercise include spontaneous abortion, preterm labor, and fetal distress.

Basic Prenatal Exercises

Women who are pregnant can safely engage in several basic prenatal exercises designed to generate energy, improve balance, and increase flexibility. These exercises can be accomplished in as little as 10 minutes each day (Box 10-4).

WORK

Many women who work outside the home discover rather early in the pregnancy that they must make decisions regarding the continuation of employment, the safety of the workplace, the demands of the work environment, and plans for maternity leave. The majority of employed women continue to work as long as they remain healthy and free of any pregnancy-related complications. Some factors that women need to consider, in consultation with the health-care provider, include general health and well-being, the overall progression of the pregnancy, present age, prior pregnancy complications, the type of work performed, the number of hours worked, and the environmental and safety risk factors associated with the work.

Evaluation of Work and Its Impact on the Pregnancy

The pregnant woman may be advised to reduce the number of hours worked if the job requires heavy lifting, prolonged standing, extensive walking, or physical exertion. When the nature of the work is physically demanding, safety concerns may require that she stop working altogether. The potential for maternal exposure to toxic substances such as chemotherapeutic agents, lead, and ionizing radiation (found in laboratories and health-care facilities) or heavy machinery and other hazardous equipment should prompt reassignment to a different work area. If reassignment is not possible, the woman may need to stop working until the pregnancy has been completed. Women who are currently experiencing pregnancy complications and those who have a history of pregnancy complications or other preexisting health disorders may be required to reduce their hours or stop working as well. Examples of problems and pregnancy complications that may necessitate a change in work hours include diabetes, kidney disease, heart disease, back problems, hypertension, and a history of spontaneous abortion or preterm labor.

Planning for Maternity Leave

Maternity leave provides the woman with time off from work during the pregnancy and after the birth of the child. While some companies may allow up to 6 weeks of paid time off, other companies may require that their pregnant employees use a combination of short-term disability, vacation time, sick time, and unpaid leave time. Health-care providers can help women plan how much time they may need or wish to be away from work and can provide them with options that may be available to them. All women who are employed outside the home should be encouraged to meet with their employers to discuss the options that are provided by the workplace and to determine a satisfactory plan for their leave.

The Family and Medical Leave Act of 1993 (U.S. Department of Labor, 1995) guarantees most women, as well as men, 12 weeks of unpaid family leave following the birth or adoption of a child. By law, the employer is required to allow the family member to return to his or her job or a similar job with the same salary and benefits, without a reduction in seniority. Family members qualify for this benefit if they work for the federal, state, or local government or if the company has 50 or more employees working within 75 miles of the workplace. In addition, the family member must have worked for the employer at least 12 months or for at least 1,250 hours in the previous year.

REST

Fatigue and tiredness are common symptoms associated with pregnancy. As the pregnancy progresses from one trimester to the next, the woman's level of fatigue changes along with the need for rest. An understanding of the expected alterations in maternal anatomy and physiology empowers the woman to anticipate and make changes in her daily routine to accommodate the necessary rest. Nurses should provide education about the

---

Box 10-4 **Basic Prenatal Exercises**

Basic prenatal exercises to help generate energy, diminish discomfort, and improve balance and stamina:

- **Arm and upper back stretch:** Raise your arms above your head, keeping the elbows straight, palms facing one another and hold for 20 seconds. Lower your arms to your sides. Bring the backs of your hands together behind your back and stretch.
- **Pelvic tilt:** Lie on your back with your knees slightly bent. Inhale through your nose while tightening your stomach muscles and buttocks. Flatten your back against the floor and tilt your pelvis slightly upward. Slowly exhale through your mouth while counting to 5. Relax.
- **Sit-ups:** Lie on your back with your knees slightly bent. Inhale through your nose. While breathing out slowly through pursed lips, raise your head with your hands placed behind your head. Tuck your chin toward your chest and slightly lift your shoulders off the floor.
- **Kegels:** Before beginning this exercise for the first time, isolate the pubococcygeal (PC) muscle, which is the muscle used to start and stop the flow of urine. Practice stopping the flow of urine a few times; do not continue to do this as this may lead to a urinary tract infection. If you have difficulty isolating the muscle in this fashion, insert a clean finger into the vaginal opening and squeeze. This is the muscle that will tighten as the exercise is done properly. Kegel exercises will help to support the growing baby by strengthening the pelvic floor, assist during the birth process, decrease urinary problems during postpartum, and help to prevent hemorrhoids.
  - Squeeze the PC muscle for 5 seconds, then relax for 5 seconds. Repeat for a total of 10 repetitions each day.
  - Squeeze and release the PC muscle as rapidly as possible for a total of 10 times.
  - Increase this exercise up to 100 repetitions each day.
- **Squatting:** Move to a squatting position, with the knees located directly over the toes. Keeping your heels flat on the floor, stretch the back of the thighs. Hold for 20 to 30 seconds. Increase time to 60 to 90 seconds. Remember to keep your head and arms relaxed during this exercise.
- **Calf stretch:** Lean against a wall or flat surface with your hands against the surface. Move one leg behind you, keeping your heel flat on the floor. Lean into the wall to stretch the calf muscles. Hold for 20 to 30 seconds. Repeat with the other leg. This exercise will help to reduce leg cramps experienced during pregnancy.

anticipated need for additional rest and suggest strategies for managing fatigue and for promoting rest and relaxation.

Contributors to Fatigue During the First Trimester

During the first trimester, the woman's body begins to undergo changes that will support the developing fetus. One of the major changes is an increase in the production of progesterone, a hormone that causes increased fatigue and feelings of tiredness, especially during the day. The maternal blood volume also begins to increase and frequently results in physiological anemia. Women with decreased iron stores may develop "true" (iron-deficiency) anemia. As the fetus grows, oxygen requirements increase and cause an increased workload on the woman's body systems. These changes, along with the emotional stress often associated with adjustment to the news of the pregnancy, combine to produce fatigue. Strategies for coping with pregnancy-related fatigue should routinely be discussed with patients early in the pregnancy.

Contributors to Fatigue During the Second Trimester

During the second trimester the rapid physiological changes that occurred in the first trimester come into balance with the body's workload demands. Pregnant women experience increased energy and endurance during this time and are able to focus more on planning for the upcoming birth. Some women, however, may continue to experience fatigue that persists into the second trimester. Potential causes of the fatigue include depression, external stressors, and anemia. Other underlying medical causes may also be a factor and should be investigated by the woman's health-care provider.

Contributors to Fatigue During the Third Trimester

The pregnant woman's level of fatigue increases as the fetus continues to grow and develop. The maternal weight-bearing load associated with the fetus is compounded by a corresponding increase in extracellular fluid and blood volume, maternal reserves, placental mass, and amniotic fluid. The enlarging fetus causes the maternal diaphragm to be upwardly displaced, decreasing lung expansion. Increased bladder pressure from the gravid uterus causes increased voiding, especially at night, when the woman is trying to sleep. Each of these factors plays a role in the overwhelming fatigue common during the third trimester.

Through education, the health-care provider can empower the expectant mother throughout the pregnancy to better manage her rest demands and cope with fatigue. Planning and making healthy choices concerning rest enables the woman to feel more relaxed and energetic and better able to cope with and manage this common discomfort of pregnancy.

Now Can You—Discuss work and fatigue during pregnancy?

1. Identify three situations in which women may need to stop working during pregnancy?
2. Name two reasons why fatigue is especially pronounced during the first and third trimesters?
3. Identify three strategies to help women cope with fatigue during pregnancy?

Medications

Medication use during pregnancy must be handled very carefully, and the needs of the patient and her fetus should always be considered on an individual basis. Nurses need to be aware that their patients may be taking over-the-counter (OTC) medications and herbal preparations and often do not readily report this information during the prenatal interview. Thus, the nurse should ask specific questions regarding prescription and OTC medications and the use of any herbal therapies.

SAFE VERSUS TERATOGENIC MEDICATIONS

A **teratogen** is anything that adversely affects the normal cellular development in the embryo or fetus (Venes, 2013). Although some medications are safe, others are known teratogens or the safety of their use during pregnancy has not been demonstrated. The fetus is most vulnerable to the effects of teratogens from the third week of gestation through the third month. However, the risk for fetal developmental anomalies continues to exist throughout the pregnancy. The third trimester is the most vulnerable time for cognitive impairment from a teratogenic insult.

Over-the-Counter Medications

Nonprescription medications such as acetaminophen (Tylenol) and guaifenesin (Robitussin) are often taken for minor problems such as headaches, coughs, and colds. It is commonly assumed that a medication that requires no prescription must be safe to take. However, all medications, whether available by prescription or over the counter, have side effects, and many have adverse effects. The nurse needs to counsel women who are planning to become pregnant and those who are already pregnant not to

Where Research and Practice Meet:
Medication Use During Pregnancy

Working from data on medication use during pregnancy of more than 30,000 women, Mitchell and colleagues (2011) reported a widespread and growing use of medications among pregnant women and also found that medication use varied by socioeconomic status, maternal age, race/ethnicity, and state of residence. The findings included information on both prescription and OTC medications. During the first trimester of pregnancy, 70% to 80% of women reported taking at least one medication, and by 2008, approximately 50% of women reported taking at least one prescription medication. Over the past 30 years, first trimester use of prescription medications increased by more than 60%, the use of four or more medications during the first trimester tripled, and antidepressant use during the first trimester increased significantly. The researchers also found that medication use increased with a woman's age and education level, use was higher among non-Hispanic white women compared with women of other races or ethnicities that were studied, and use during pregnancy varied by state of residence (Mitchell, Gilboa, Werler, Kelley, Louik, & Hernandez-Diaz, 2011). The findings underscore the importance of the nurse's role in providing preconception and prenatal counseling about the potential hazards associated with any medication use during pregnancy.

take any medications (prescription or nonprescription) without first consulting with the primary health-care provider. The provider will make a determination regarding the safety and necessity of the medication. Additional information (including a physical assessment) may need to be obtained, and an alternate medication or therapy may be advised. When possible, all nonprescription drugs should be avoided during preconception and throughout pregnancy.

Herbal and Homeopathic Preparations

One of the most important facts about herbal and homeopathic preparations is that the U.S. Food and Drug Administration (FDA) has not approved these drugs and does not regulate or control them. Further, there are major drawbacks to the use of these substances. There is no regulation that controls product development, the dosages are not consistent between brands, and additives used in their composition may differ in type and amount. Also, because herbal and homeopathic products have not been subjected to rigorous research to determine their efficacy, effectiveness, side effects, therapeutic dosages, and adverse effects, there is no guarantee that the claims made about them are true. Although herbal and homeopathic treatments are considered to be "natural" because they have been developed from plants and other natural sources, many of these products are dangerous and toxic and may cause effects that have not yet been discovered (Shane-McWhorter & Martinez, 2011).

Several herbal products are recognized to be dangerous; others are known to have specific teratogenic effects. These substances need to be completely avoided during the periods of preconception and pregnancy. Nurses should warn patients about the use of these products, provide written information that can be taken home, and reinforce the teaching at each visit.

Prescription Medications

Certain prescription medications may be necessary during preconception and pregnancy. Women who suffer from life-threatening illnesses, such as seizure disorders, heart disease, respiratory disorders, or infections need to continue or initiate treatment to maintain their own health and safety. The health-care practitioner must be aware of all prescription medications currently being taken to evaluate the safety of their continued use. In some instances, dosages can be adjusted or the medications can be replaced with safer medications.

Prenatal vitamins are usually given during preconception or at the beginning of a pregnancy. Prenatal vitamins provide the RDA for most vitamins and minerals as well as the additional calcium, iron, and folic acid needed during pregnancy.

Certain prescription medications must be avoided completely. Isotretinoin (Accutane), prescribed primarily for the treatment of acne, is associated with spontaneous abortions and congenital anomalies when taken early in pregnancy. Some antimicrobials cause altered fetal growth and development and should be avoided during the later months of gestation. Sulfonamides, for example, are associated with delayed fetal skeletal development while prenatal exposure to tetracycline causes staining of the child's teeth.

Family Teaching Guidelines...
Common Herbs to Avoid During Preconception and Pregnancy

During preconception counseling and pregnancy, nurses should educate couples to avoid the following common herbs:

- Uterine stimulants that may cause preterm labor
  - Barberry
  - Black cohosh
  - Feverfew
  - Goldenseal
  - Mugwort
  - Pennyroyal leaf
  - Yarrow root
- Blood thinners and anticoagulants that may cause miscarriage
  - Dong quai
- Laxatives that may overstimulate digestion and metabolism and cause fluid and electrolyte imbalance
  - Blessed thistle
  - Cascara sagrada
  - Drug aloe
  - Senna
- Cardiovascular stimulants that may elevate blood pressure or cause abnormal heart rhythms
  - Ephedra
  - Licorice root
- Others that may damage the fetus during development
  - Gotu kola
  - Juniper berries

Nursing Insight—*Teaching childbearing-aged women about isotretinoin*

Isotretinoin (Accutane, Amnesteem, Claravis, Sotret) is an extremely successful medication in the treatment of acne, and research demonstrates a successful remission (of acne) after only one treatment. However, there are significant adverse and teratogenic effects associated with the use of this medication. Isotretinoin is labeled as a pregnancy category X medication. Use of isotretinoin or other high-dose vitamin A medications such as etretinate (Tegison) and acitretin (Soriatane) during pregnancy may result in spontaneous abortion or stillbirth, and over 35% of exposed infants are affected by a pattern of birth defects that include physical deformities of the face, ears, heart, and brain; abnormal formation of internal organs; and moderate to severe intellectual and developmental disabilities. Isotretinoin is approved for marketing only under a special restricted distribution program called iPLEDGE that is approved by the FDA. Isotretinoin users MUST adhere to all requirements of the iPLEDGE program. Requirements of iPLEDGE include signing an informed consent statement, completing two negative pregnancy tests prior to beginning the medication, having a pregnancy test every month during treatment, and a negative test a month after treatment, and using 2 different forms of birth control at all times (Organization of Teratology Information Specialists [OTIS], 2010). Additional information about the iPLEDGE program is available at https://www.ipledgeprogram.com.

FDA CLASSIFICATION SYSTEM FOR MEDICATIONS USED DURING PREGNANCY

To determine the safety of medication use during pregnancy, the FDA devised a classification system according to known fetal risk, based on research findings. The following list summarizes the categories and associated fetal risk (see Chapter 7):

- Category A: Controlled studies in pregnant women have demonstrated no associated fetal risk
- Category B: No associated fetal risk in animals, but no controlled studies in pregnant women; or animal studies indicate a risk, but controlled human studies fail to demonstrate a risk
- Category C: Evidence of adverse effects in animal fetuses, but no controlled studies in pregnant women; or no adequate animal or human reproduction studies are available
- Category D: Evidence of adverse effects and fetal risk in humans; benefits and risks must be considered before prescribing
- Category X: Evidence of fetal risk and congenital anomalies in humans; risks outweigh the benefits; not prescribed during pregnancy

There are no absolutes when using any prescription or nonprescription drug during pregnancy. Each situation is different and requires individualized decision making that must be a mutual endeavor between the patient and her care provider. Cultural considerations, benefits, risks, and goals of all therapies must be assessed before any decisions are reached. Nurses play an essential role in gathering information for assessment and evaluation and in providing patient education and counseling.

⊘ Now Can You—Discuss the use of herbal preparations and prescription medications in pregnancy?

1. Identify two major concerns related to the use of herbal and homeopathic preparations?
2. Name four herbs that should be avoided during pregnancy?
3. Identify two types of prescription medications that should not be used during pregnancy?
4. Discuss what is meant by a Category B medication?

Common Discomforts During Pregnancy

Common discomforts experienced during pregnancy are caused by the major hormonal and anatomical changes that take place in the woman's body. (See Chapters 8 and 9 for further discussion.) As the pregnancy progresses, most patients report at least some of the common discomforts, which are presented in Table 10-5. Anticipatory guidance includes educating women about the normal physiological changes that occur during pregnancy, symptoms that frequently accompany the changes, and strategies for dealing with the discomfort (Fig. 10-8).

NAUSEA

Nausea is often one of the first symptoms of pregnancy experienced. Although commonly known as "morning

Table 10-5	Common Discomforts During Each Trimester of Pregnancy
Trimester	**Common Discomforts**
First	Nausea
	Vomiting
	Fatigue
	Urinary frequency
	Nocturia
Second	Dyspepsia
	Gum hyperplasia and bleeding
	Dependent edema
	Leg varicosities
	Hyperventilation and shortness of breath
	Numbness and tingling of fingers
	Supine hypotensive syndrome
Third	Fatigue
	Urinary frequency
	Dyspepsia
	Flatulence
	Gum hyperplasia and bleeding
	Leg cramps
	Dependent edema
	Leg varicosities
	Dyspareunia
	Nocturia
	Round ligament pain
	Supine hypotensive syndrome
All Trimesters	Ptyalism
	Nasal congestion
	Back pain
	Leukorrhea
	Constipation
	Insomnia

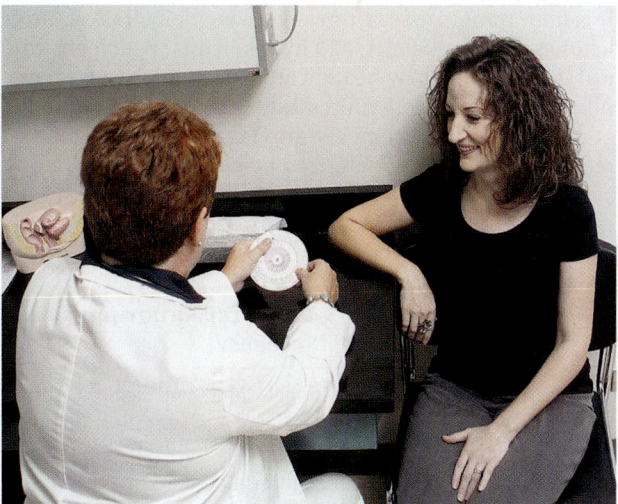

Figure 10-8 Nurse counseling pregnant woman.

sickness," nausea can occur at any time of the day or night. While the exact cause of nausea is unknown, it most probably is related to the increased levels of the pregnancy hormones. Nausea is primarily noted during the first trimester of the pregnancy and usually resolves by 13 to 14 weeks, although it may persist throughout the pregnancy. Nausea during the early weeks of pregnancy is believed to be a reassuring indicator of embryo/fetal development with adequate hormonal support. Complaints of nausea should never be dismissed without further assessment to rule out pregnancy-related complications such as hyperemesis gravidarum, multiple gestation, gestational trophoblastic disease, or maternal gastrointestinal or eating disorders. (See Chapter 11 for further discussion.)

Nurses can suggest strategies to help offset the nausea, such as the avoidance of "trigger foods" (foods that cause nausea from sight or smell) and tight clothing that constricts the abdomen. The use of relaxation techniques (e.g., slow, deep breathing and mental imagery) can also help to decrease nausea. Other techniques that are often helpful include consuming plain, dry crackers or sucking on peppermint candy before arising; adhering to small, frequent meals; consuming liquids and solids separately, avoiding cold, acidic, or sweet beverages, and remaining in an upright position after eating. Women should also be advised to decrease daily activities and get plenty of rest.

Medication is usually not necessary for the nausea of early pregnancy, although some women have found that taking vitamin B_6 or ginger tablets helps to lessen nausea. These oral supplements can be purchased over the counter and should be taken with meals. Acupressure bracelets, often used for the prevention of motion sickness, can also be purchased without a prescription and may be beneficial in reducing nausea during early pregnancy (King, Brucker, Kriebs, & Fahey, 2013).

VOMITING

Vomiting in early pregnancy often accompanies the nausea, although it is important to ascertain that the amount vomited is not excessive. During the assessment, nurses should question patients about vomiting frequency and amount and their ability to consume and retain foods and liquids. It is important to assess for weight loss, dehydration, urine ketones, blood alkalosis, and hypokalemia, which are clinical findings that may be indicative of a more serious complication known as hyperemesis gravidarum (Youngkin et al., 2012). **Hyperemesis gravidarum** is a pregnancy-related condition characterized by persistent, continuous, severe nausea and vomiting, often accompanied by dry retching. (See Chapter 11 for further discussion.)

 Complementary Care: *Acupuncture for Nausea and Back Pain during Pregnancy*

A treatment modality of traditional Chinese medicine, acupuncture involves stimulation of specific points by the manual insertion and manipulation of fine needles into the skin. During pregnancy, acupuncture stimulation at the PC6 point (*Neiguan*) located 3 finger-width breadths above the wrist crease may be effective in relieving symptoms of nausea and vomiting. Acupuncture may also be beneficial in relieving pregnancy-related pelvic girdle pain and lower back pain (Malshe & Wiczyk, 2011).

PTYALISM

Ptyalism, or excessive salivation, can be quite distressing for the pregnant woman, who must frequently wipe her mouth or spit into a cup. Although the cause of ptyalism is unknown, it is most likely related to increased hormone levels. Ptyalism can also be a symptom of hyperemesis gravidarum, and when extreme, may be associated with maternal dehydration. While little can be done to reduce the amount of saliva, it is important to rule out dental abnormalities, upper gastrointestinal problems, and pica. Nurses can counsel patients to consume small, frequent meals; avoid starchy foods; drink plenty of water in small sips; suck on hard candies; and brush their teeth frequently (Youngkin et al., 2012).

FATIGUE

Fatigue occurs primarily during the first and third trimesters of pregnancy. In the first trimester, the fatigue is most likely related to physiological and hormonal changes. Psychological concerns may also lead to insomnia. During the third trimester, fatigue is usually related to physical discomforts and an increasing inability to sleep. Nurses can counsel patients to take naps during the day when possible, establish a bedtime "ritual" that includes going to bed at approximately the same time each night, increase daytime exercise, and practice relaxation techniques. If these strategies are not effective or the patient exhibits signs of psychosocial stress or depression, she should be referred for additional evaluation (Youngkin et al., 2012).

NASAL CONGESTION

Nasal congestion, a common maternal complaint, is known as rhinitis of pregnancy. Increased levels of estrogen and progesterone cause swelling of the nasal mucus membranes and produce symptoms of excess mucus and congestion. It is important to rule out colds and allergies. The nurse can suggest relief measures such as increasing fluids; taking a hot, steamy shower; using a vaporizer or humidifier; and the occasional administration of nasal saline drops. Decongestants should be avoided during the first trimester.

UPPER AND LOWER BACKACHE

Back pain during pregnancy results from the change in the center of gravity as the uterus enlarges. It is also related to high levels of progesterone, which cause a relaxation and softening of the connecting cartilage and joints. Low backache can be exacerbated by activities that require prolonged standing, walking, bending, or lifting. It is important to rule out other causes of backache, such as kidney stones, pyelonephritis, pancreatitis, ulcers, muscle sprain or strain, and preterm labor. For some women, a referral for physical therapy may be indicated (King et al., 2013).

 Optimizing Outcomes—Relief of backache during pregnancy

Nurses should educate all patients about strategies that may prevent or relieve backache. Women can be taught to wear supportive, low-heeled shoes; use proper body mechanics; perform back strengthening and pelvic rock exercises; take frequent rest periods; sleep on a firm, supportive mattress; and wear a well-fitting, supportive bra. Body massage and warm tub baths may also be helpful.

LEUKORRHEA

High levels of estrogen stimulate vascularity and hypertrophy of the cervical glands, causing an increase in vaginal discharge. The discharge is usually yellow to white in color, thin, and more acidic than normal. It is important to rule out vaginal and sexually transmitted infections and rupture of membranes. The nurse can counsel the patient to wear cotton underwear, avoid tight-fitting clothing, and follow strict hygiene to prevent infection. If a panty liner or sanitary pad is worn to absorb moisture, it should be changed frequently to prevent dampness and odor.

URINARY FREQUENCY

In early pregnancy, urinary frequency is caused by pressure exerted by the enlarging uterus on the bladder. During the second trimester, bladder pressure lessens once the uterus becomes an abdominal organ. In the third trimester, a number of physiological events cause urinary frequency. The fetal presenting part once again exerts pressure on the bladder. Progesterone relaxes the muscles of the urethra and may lead to incontinence, while an increase in the glomerular filtration rate causes increased urine production. It is important to rule out urinary tract infection, rupture of the membranes, kidney stones, gestational diabetes, and stress urinary incontinence. The nurse can suggest relief measures, including intake of adequate hydration, Kegel exercises, use of panty liners, frequent voiding, and decreasing fluid intake 2 to 3 hours before bedtime.

DYSPEPSIA

Dyspepsia, or heartburn, results from reflux of acidic gastric contents into the lower esophagus. Dyspepsia is caused by the progesterone-induced relaxation of the cardiac sphincter and delayed gastric emptying. Because of these changes, stomach contents remain in the stomach for a longer period of time and can reflux into the esophagus. As the pregnancy advances, the enlarging uterus pushes up on the stomach and compresses it, causing a reduced capacity. Making changes in the diet and eating patterns may be helpful in reducing heartburn although it is unlikely to disappear until after the baby is born.

 Nursing Insight—*Relief measures for dyspepsia*

Nurses can suggest a number of relief measures for dyspepsia, a common complaint during pregnancy. Patients can be taught to consume small, frequent meals to avoid overloading the stomach, maintain good posture, remain upright after meals, and avoid greasy and fatty foods and very cold foods and consuming beverages with meals. Drinking cultured or sweet milk and using over-the-counter antacids may also be helpful (King et al., 2013).

FLATULENCE

Flatulence (excessive gas in the stomach and intestines) is caused by decreased gastric motility that results from elevated levels of progesterone during pregnancy. Pressure of the enlarging uterus on the abdominal contents also contributes to the formation of gas. When excessive or particularly disturbing, other causes, such as irritable bowel syndrome or lactose intolerance should be ruled out. Patients can be counseled to avoid gas-forming foods, constipation, gum chewing, consuming large meals, and swallowing air.

CONSTIPATION

Elevated levels of progesterone relax the smooth muscles, causing decreased contractility of the lower gastrointestinal tract and slowed movement of the stool. As the uterus enlarges, the large intestines become compressed, further slowing movement of stool through the intestines. Supplemental iron may also be a contributor to the development of constipation. All patients should be taught about the importance of regular physical exercise and bowel habits, consuming a high-fiber diet with increased liquids, and to avoid straining at defecation and the use of mineral oil and bulk-forming laxatives.

DENTAL PROBLEMS

Elevations in pregnancy hormones cause the gums to become edematous and friable, which can lead to bleeding during brushing. Open lesions and other dental problems, such as caries, can open a direct pathway for pathogens to enter the bloodstream. Meticulous dental care during pregnancy is important to prevent infections and other dental complications. The dentist should be informed of the pregnancy so that an abdominal shield can be used if x-ray films are needed. If treatment is indicated, most local anesthetics can be used safely during pregnancy (ACOG, 2013c).

LEG CRAMPS

The actual cause of leg cramps is unknown, although decreased levels of calcium and phosphorus have been implicated. As the uterus enlarges, pressure is exerted on the major blood vessels, causing impaired circulation to the lower extremities. It is important to rule out thrombosed blood vessels, muscular strain, and other injuries to the lower extremities. The patient should be advised to engage in regular exercise and maintain good body mechanics; elevate the legs above the heart several times throughout the day; dorsiflex the foot; and consume a diet that includes adequate amounts of calcium and phosphorus (King et al., 2013; Youngkin et al., 2012).

DEPENDENT EDEMA

Edema in the lower extremities is caused by relaxation of the blood vessels (an effect of increased progesterone) and the increased pressure placed on the pelvic veins by the enlarging uterus. Tight, restrictive clothing that inhibits venous return from the lower extremities increases the edema. Once pathological conditions such as gestational hypertension, renal disease, liver disease, cardiac disease, vascular disorders, trauma, and infection have been ruled out, the nurse can suggest relief measures. These include avoiding constrictive clothing, elevating the legs periodically throughout the day, and assuming a side-lying position when resting.

VARICOSITIES

A positive family history, coupled with the normal physiological changes of pregnancy, predisposes the patient to the development of varicose veins. Physiological changes of pregnancy include vascular relaxation from the effects of progesterone and impaired venous circulation from pressure exerted by the enlarged uterus. Constrictive clothing also increases the risk for varicose veins. Nursing care for patients with varicosities includes regular assessment of lower extremity peripheral pulses and education. Patients should be taught to avoid crossing their legs and the use of constrictive clothing such as knee-high stockings. They should also be encouraged to elevate their legs above the level of the heart at least twice a day. For some women, a maternity girdle may provide relief (King et al., 2013; Youngkin et al., 2012).

DYSPAREUNIA

Dyspareunia, or painful intercourse, may result from pelvic congestion and impaired circulation caused by the enlarging uterus. Also, as the pregnancy advances, finding a position of comfort for intercourse may become increasingly difficult because of the enlarging abdomen. Concerns that intercourse will harm the fetus may also interfere with sexual enjoyment and increase the likelihood of dyspareunia. Unless a medical condition contraindicates intercourse, the patient and her partner should be reassured that intercourse is safe during pregnancy. Education about sexual intimacy should include suggestions for comfortable positions for intercourse and alternative methods for mutual sexual satisfaction (King et al., 2013; McDaniel, 2010).

"What to say"—*When asked about sexual activity during pregnancy*

Couples have many questions regarding sexual activity during pregnancy. These questions relate to the safety of sexual intercourse, potential complications, when to stop having intercourse, and sexual positions that facilitate comfort. It is important for the health-care provider to address sexual activity early in the pregnancy in an honest, open manner and to encourage the couple to communicate with each other. The nurse can address the couple's concerns with the following statements:

"It is perfectly safe to continue sexual activity throughout your pregnancy unless your doctor or nurse midwife identifies risk factors that may preclude your activity (e.g., a risk for preterm labor). With no risk factors, sexual activity is safe for you and your baby as long as you continue to practice safe sex behaviors as you would if you were not pregnant. As you gain pregnancy weight, some sexual positions may be less comfortable; for comfort, you can try woman on top and side-lying positions. A sexual activity to avoid during pregnancy includes oral sex during which water or air is placed in the vagina."

NOCTURIA

Nocturia, or excessive nighttime urination, is more common during the first and third trimesters. When the woman assumes a recumbent position, the gravid uterus no longer compresses the pelvic vessels, and blood flow to the kidneys is enhanced. This factor, combined with an increased glomerular filtration rate, increases the need to urinate. Although there is no remedy for nocturia, the nurse can teach the patient about the cause of nocturia and advise her that limiting fluids in the few hours before bedtime may be helpful.

INSOMNIA

Insomnia may have a variety of causes, including physical discomfort, nocturia, caffeine, or stress. The nurse can suggest strategies to enhance relaxation and comfort before bedtime. For example, the woman may incorporate sleep-inducing nighttime rituals such as taking a warm bath, enjoying a warm drink such as milk, engaging in a restful activity like reading, practicing meditation and other forms of relaxation, and arranging the bed covers and pillows in an inviting way that promotes rest.

ROUND LIGAMENT PAIN

The round ligaments support the uterus as it enlarges during pregnancy. These structures attach to the fundus on each side, pass through the inguinal canal, and insert into the upper portion of the labia majora. As the uterus enlarges, the round ligaments stretch and produce a painful sensation in the lower quadrants. Once pathological conditions such as preterm labor, rupture of an ovarian cyst, ectopic pregnancy, appendicitis, gallbladder disease, and peptic ulcer disease have been ruled out, the nurse can educate the patient about the cause of the pain and make suggestions for relief measures. Taking a warm bath, applying heat, supporting the uterus with a pillow when resting, and using a pregnancy girdle may help to diminish the discomfort (King et al., 2013; Youngkin et al., 2012).

HYPERVENTILATION AND SHORTNESS OF BREATH

Increased metabolic activity during pregnancy increases the amount of carbon dioxide in the maternal respiratory system. Hyperventilation decreases the amount of carbon dioxide and may trigger a feeling of "air hunger." Patients may also experience shortness of breath related to uterine enlargement and the upward pressure exerted on the diaphragm. Once pathological conditions such as upper respiratory infection, asthma, cardiac problems, and anemia have been ruled out, the nurse should explain the cause of hyperventilation to the patient and suggest that she consciously attempt to regulate her breathing. Other measures that may be helpful include breathing into a paper bag to decrease the symptoms of hyperventilation, maintaining good posture, and stretching the arms above the head (King et al., 2013; Youngkin et al., 2012).

NUMBNESS AND TINGLING IN THE FINGERS

Numbness and tingling in the fingers may be associated with hyperventilation or from nerve compression in the median and ulnar nerves in the arm. Pregnancy is one of the most frequent physiological conditions associated with carpal tunnel syndrome (compression of the median nerve, where it travels down to the transverse carpal ligament). Maintaining good posture, elevating the hands on a pillow while sleeping, or wearing a wrist brace when sleeping may provide symptomatic relief. A thermoskin carpal tunnel glove with heat therapy and support to help relieve pain and inflammation and prevent wrist movements is also available (O'Donnell, Elio, & Day, 2010).

SUPINE HYPOTENSIVE SYNDROME

Supine hypotension is caused by pressure of the enlarging uterus on the inferior vena cava while the woman is in a supine position. Vena caval compression impedes venous blood flow, reduces the amount of blood in the heart, and decreases cardiac output, causing dizziness and syncope. Pathological causes of supine hypotension include cardiac or respiratory disorders, anemia, hypoglycemia, dehydration, anxiety, and stress. Once these conditions have been ruled out, the nurse should educate the patient about the causes of supine hypotension and advise the woman to rest on her side and slowly move from a lying to a sitting to a standing position to minimize changes in blood pressure.

 Now Can You—Discuss common discomforts of pregnancy?

1. Name four strategies to alleviate nausea during early pregnancy?
2. Identify four pathological causes of backache during pregnancy?
3. Explain how you would counsel couples regarding sexual intercourse during pregnancy?

Recognizing Signs and Symptoms of Danger

Complications can occur at any time during the pregnancy. Nurses need to educate the pregnant woman and her family about danger signs and symptoms, teach them about interventions that can be initiated at home, and provide specific instructions about when to notify the health-care provider.

FIRST TRIMESTER

Nausea and Vomiting

During the first trimester, nausea and vomiting are common discomforts. However, when vomiting becomes severe, weight loss and dehydration can occur and place both the woman and her fetus at risk. Severe, persistent vomiting is indicative of hyperemesis gravidarum. Causes of hyperemesis gravidarum include multiple gestation; thyroid disorder; and **hydatidiform mole**, which is the growth of abnormal tissue that results from conception but does not give rise to a viable fetus. Nausea and vomiting are managed with oral fluids; small, frequent meals; and emotional support. Dehydration may require intravenous fluids and hospitalization. (See Chapter 11 for further discussion.)

Abdominal Pain and Vaginal Bleeding

Abdominal cramping and vaginal spotting or bleeding may indicate spontaneous abortion, or miscarriage. **Spontaneous abortion** is the termination of pregnancy by natural causes before 20 weeks' gestation. The majority of spontaneous abortions are related to chromosomal defects. Approximately 15% to 20% of clinically recognized pregnancies end in spontaneous abortion. A woman may assume she is having a heavy period when she is actually experiencing a miscarriage. (See Chapter 11 for further discussion.) Treatment includes bedrest and emotional support. If bleeding and/or pain are excessive, the patient should contact her primary health-care provider or report to the emergency department.

Infection

Generalized symptoms of infection include chills, fever, malaise, and anorexia. Burning on urination may indicate a urinary tract infection, which is treated with antibiotics. Patient education to prevent a urinary tract infection includes advising the woman to use white, unscented toilet paper; to avoid bubble baths or the addition of "additives" in the bath; to wear underwear with cotton crotches; to drink at least 8 to 12 glasses of liquid each day; and to urinate before going to bed and before and after sexual intercourse. Diarrhea may indicate a gastrointestinal infection, which may be treated with antibiotics if bacterial in origin.

SECOND TRIMESTER

Maternal Complications

Preeclampsia is one of the most common pregnancy complications during the second trimester. It is a pregnancy-specific systemic syndrome that is clinically defined as an increase in blood pressure (greater than or equal to 140 mm Hg systolic or greater than or equal to 90 mm Hg diastolic on 2 occasions at least 4 hours apart) after 20 weeks' gestation accompanied by proteinuria (National High Blood Pressure Education Program Working Group, 2000). Early signs and symptoms of preeclampsia include headache, vision changes, elevated blood pressure, and edema. Patients who experience any of these symptoms should promptly notify their health-care provider. Bedrest is the first intervention implemented in an effort to reduce blood pressure and alleviate the myriad of other problems that can be associated with this disorder. (See Chapter 11 for further discussion.)

Premature rupture of the membranes, which is rupture of the membranes before the onset of labor, can also occur during the second trimester. Patients are taught to promptly seek advice from their health-care provider if vaginal discharge is present. Although increased vaginal discharge is normal during pregnancy, the provider will determine if the vaginal discharge is normal, is associated with a vaginal infection, or results from the leakage of amniotic fluid. Women who have experienced premature rupture of membranes must be closely monitored for signs of infection. (See Chapter 11 for further discussion.)

The presence of uterine contractions during the second trimester may indicate preterm labor (PTL). **Preterm labor** is defined as regular uterine contractions and cervical dilation before the end of the 36th week of gestation (ACOG, 2012b). All pregnant women are taught the signs and symptoms of preterm labor and instructed to contact their health-care provider if the symptoms appear. True labor must be differentiated from Braxton Hicks contractions (disorganized tightenings of the uterine muscles as they stretch to prepare for labor) so that appropriate interventions may be initiated. (See Chapters 11 and 12 for further discussion.)

Fetal Complications

During the second trimester the fetus is assessed for well-being. The fundal height measurement should correlate to the weeks of gestation from approximately 22 to 34 weeks of gestation. A decreased fundal height may indicate intrauterine growth restriction, while increased fundal height is suggestive of multiple gestation, fetal macrosomia, or hydramnios. The gestational age is also determined from a variety of sources that include the patient's menstrual history, contraceptive history, pregnancy test results, first documentation of fetal heart sounds, and ultrasonography. (See Chapters 9 and 11 for further discussion.)

A number of potential fetal problems may occur during the second trimester. These include hypoxia from maternal hypertension, irregular or absent heart rate, preterm birth, infection from premature rupture of membranes, and absence of fetal movements after quickening. If the woman experiences an absence of fetal movements, she is instructed to drink 2 full glasses of water, rest on her left side for 2 hours, and assess for fetal movements once again. If fewer than 10 fetal movements are noted after the liquid intake, the patient must be evaluated by her health-care provider. (See Chapter 11 for further discussion.)

THIRD TRIMESTER

Maternal Complications

During the third trimester, the patient may develop the same problems that can occur during the second trimester, such as preeclampsia, premature rupture of the membranes, and preterm labor. Also, gestational diabetes may develop during this time. A Glucose Challenge Test (Glucola screening) is performed between 24 and 28 weeks of gestation, and a positive test warrants further screening with a 3-hour oral glucose tolerance test (OGTT). A positive OGTT indicates the presence of gestational diabetes, and patient care involves education and a team approach that usually includes the obstetrician, internist, endocrinologist, diabetes educator, neonatologist, dietitian, and nurse. (See Chapter 11 for further discussion.)

Hemorrhagic disorders may also develop during the third trimester. **Placenta previa** is an implantation of the placenta in the lower uterine segment, near or over the internal cervical os. The abnormal location of the placenta can cause painless, bright red vaginal bleeding as the lower uterine segment stretches and thins during the third trimester. Depending on the placental location, the patient may need to adhere to strict bedrest, and a cesarean birth may be necessary. **Abruptio placentae,** or placental abruption, is the premature separation of a normally implanted placenta from the uterine wall. An abruption results in hemorrhage between the uterine wall and the placenta, causing abdominal pain and vaginal bleeding. Interventions may include hospitalization, bedrest, Trendelenburg position, intravenous fluids, and delivery. (See Chapter 11 for further discussion.)

Fetal Complications

Leopold maneuvers are used to determine the lie, presentation, and position of the fetus. (See Chapter 9 for further discussion.) To monitor fetal growth, the fundal height is measured and compared with the estimated date of delivery at each prenatal visit during the second and third trimesters. During the third trimester, nonstress tests may be performed to evaluate fetal well-being. (See Chapter 11 for further discussion.) Fetal complications during the third trimester are the same as for the second trimester although hypoxia related to poor placental perfusion may become more of a threat during this time.

 Optimizing Outcomes—Fetal activity and well-being

Maternal involvement in activities to monitor fetal well-being is an important component of prenatal care. Beginning in the second trimester, the patient should consistently assess fetal movements. Reassuring findings include a count of at least four movements within 1 hour, during rest after meals.

Best outcome: Fetal well-being is maintained during the third trimester, labor, and birth. The neonate is full term and appropriate for gestational age. Normal physiological transitions in the neonate occur without difficulty.

 Now Can You—Identify danger signs during pregnancy?

1. Discuss the significance of abdominal cramping and vaginal bleeding during the first trimester?
2. Identify two actions the pregnant woman should take if she experiences an absence of fetal movements?
3. Name two placental problems that can cause hemorrhage, especially during the third trimester?

Using a Pregnancy Map to Guide Prenatal Visits

A prenatal care map that includes a timetable for prenatal visits helps to ensure consistency of care, especially when many health-care professionals are involved in the woman's care. The care map can be placed in the patient's chart during the initial visit, and an abbreviated version that outlines the schedule for prenatal care visits may be given to the patient. Some facilities add a grid that provides additional space for entering scheduled appointment dates. An example of a prenatal care map is presented in Table 10-6. In other institutions, the care map consists of a comprehensive guide with check boxes and identifies counseling and education needs throughout pregnancy and during the postpartum period (Fig. 10-9).

 Across Care Settings: **Prenatal care coordination to enhance healthy birth outcomes**

Prenatal Care Coordination (PNCC), a benefit of the federal Medicaid program, targets women perceived to be at highest risk for poor birth outcomes by assisting women with accessing prenatal care and obtaining health information to improve their pregnancy outcomes. PNCC services are delivered based on a mutually created care plan and may include various interventions such as strategies to diminish barriers associated with prenatal care attendance, support for continued education or job training, strategies to reduce the use of tobacco or other substances, and referral to other community resources (e.g., the Special Supplemental Nutrition Program for Women, Infants, and Children (WIC). A recent (2010) study conducted by Van Dijk and colleagues (2011) found PNCC to be an effective strategy in reducing the incidence of adverse birth outcomes for at-risk women who received the service.

Table 10-6 Example of a Prenatal Care Map

Trimester	Schedule for Return Visits	Components of the Nursing Interview	Lab Tests to Be Obtained
First	Every 4 weeks	• Reason for seeking care • Presumptive signs • Review of systems • Medical history • Family history • Gynecological and obstetric history • Nutritional history • Social history • Drug use • Assessment of abuse risk • Birth plan	• CBC with differential • Blood type and Rh • Rubella titer • VDRL or RPR • HbsAG and HbsAB if indicated • HIV • Hemoglobin electrophoresis (sickle cell, thalassemia) • Urinalysis • Pap test if indicated • Vaginal smear • Nuchal translucency test or combined screening
Second	Every 4 weeks	• Summary of relative events since last visit • General emotional state • Complaints/problems/questions • Vital signs • Weight • Presence of edema	• Hematocrit • Urinalysis • Urine culture • Triple screen or quadruple screen
Third	Every 4 weeks through weeks 28–32 Every 2 weeks through week 36 Every week thereafter	• Primary concerns • Attendance at childbirth education classes • Physical assessment • Psychosocial responses • Vital signs • Weight • Presence of edema • Confirmation of gestational age	• Hematocrit • Urinalysis • Urine culture • Glucose tolerance test • Repeat, if needed: VDRL or RPR, HIV, CBC, sickle cell prep, vaginal smears

Childbirth Education to Promote a Positive Childbearing Experience

Childbirth education provides a wealth of information to parents who are having a baby for the first time as well as to parents who have already experienced childbirth. The difficulty often lies in finding the right class to meet the specific needs of the expectant parents. Traditionally, childbirth education focused on managing labor and birth. Contemporary classes focus on a wide variety of topics, with the primary goal centered on facilitating a positive childbearing experience, including pregnancy, childbirth, postpartum care, and newborn care. Topics typically discussed in childbirth classes include anatomy and physiology related to pregnancy; comfort measures during each trimester of pregnancy; the labor and birth process; relaxation and pain management, including pharmacological and nonpharmacological measures; complications related to pregnancy, labor, and birth; vaginal and cesarean births; postpartum care; newborn care; and newborn feeding, including bottle feeding and breastfeeding (Fig. 10-10).

Optimizing Outcomes—Breast care during pregnancy

The preconceptional and antepartal periods present nurses with an ideal opportunity to educate patients about the health benefits of breastfeeding for the woman and her infant. Nursing care should be focused on the history (e.g., maternal surgery or injury, infertility, and previous problems with breastfeeding), assessment (e.g., identify changes and assess for nipple tattoos or piercings), and referrals (e.g., International Board Certified Lactation Consultant) (Johnson & Strube, 2011).

METHODS OF CHILDBIRTH PREPARATION

Expectant parents can choose from a variety of available childbirth education classes. Ideally, they will select one that is in harmony with their beliefs and values about the childbearing experience and be able to engage in the educational process without reservation and with complete commitment. While different, all childbirth preparation classes incorporate a holistic approach to childbearing, which encompasses the biological, psychological, and social factors related to the experience. For many expectant parents, the experience of childbearing is more than just a physical and biological one; the experience can have emotional, mental, and spiritual meaning. This holistic approach to having a child allows the parents to assimilate all aspects of the experience to be prepared physically and mentally for becoming a parent.

Many childbirth education programs in the community combine aspects from the traditional stand-alone methods of childbirth preparation. Combining philosophies and activities into the classes allows the couple to identify more strongly with features that fit their individual and collective needs. The most common childbirth methods include the Lamaze and the Bradley methods of natural childbirth.

INDIANA PERINATAL NETWORK
Lead/Convene/Collaborate
FOR MOTHERS & BABIES

INDIANA PRENATAL CARE GUIDE
Screening, Education & Counseling
2008

This Guide is intended as a resource for clinicians involved in the design and implementation of prenatal care services. This information should not be interpreted as excluding other acceptable course of care based upon medical judgement and patient preferences. The Guide reflects the current opinion of IPN for a standard approach to prenatal care. The use of pre-printed standardized antenatal record is recommended to reduce errors of omission.

Note: It is strongly recommended that prenatal care begin in the first trimester.

INITIAL VISIT	EACH VISIT	8-18 WEEKS	24-28 WEEKS	35-37 WEEKS	POSTPARTUM
HISTORY & PHYSICAL					
☐ Assess for intent of pregnancy: "How are you/your partner feeling about being pregnant?" ☐ Medical and reproductive history ☐ Current pregnancy history ☐ Family history (including genetic history) ☐ Sexual History/practices ☐ Counsel and provide HIV information (required by IN law) ☐ Social history (including drugs, substance use, smoking, alcohol) ☐ Work history (including occupational hazards) ☐ Physical activity ☐ Domestic violence (physical, sexual, emotional abuse) ☐ Psychosocial stressors ☐ Dietary/nutritional assessment ☐ Physical examination (including dental, height, weight) ☐ Assign pregnancy risk status ☐ Other genetic counseling if needed ☐ Transportation availability ☐ Screen for health literacy	☐ History since last visit; questions and problems ☐ Smoking status ☐ Weeks gestation ☐ Blood pressure ☐ Weight ☐ Cumulative weight gain/loss ☐ Fundal height (in cm) ☐ Fetal heart tones ☐ Edema ☐ Fetal presentation (when appropriate) ☐ Fetal movement ☐ Cervical exam (if indicated) ☐ Other physical exam as indicated Ask regarding: ☐ Uterine contractions/cramping ☐ Pain/pressure ☐ Change in vaginal discharge ☐ Vaginal bleeding ☐ Dysuria	☐ Document beginning of fetal movement ☐ Document auscultation of fetal heart tones with fetoscope	☐ Re-evaluate pregnancy risk status		☐ Physical exam ☐ Nutritional assessment ☐ Lactation assessment if appropriate ☐ Psychosocial stressors ☐ Smoking status ☐ Perinatal Mood Disorders ☐ Family planning
ROUTINE BIOCHEMICAL EVALUATION					
☐ Blood type ☐ Rh type ☐ Antibody screen ☐ CBC ☐ Rubella titre ☐ Syphilis screening (required by IN law) ☐ HbsAG* ☐ Offer/recommend HIV testing ☐ Cervical cytology ☐ Gonorrhea culture ☐ Chlamydia culture ☐ Urinalysis and culture ☐ Wet mount for bacterial vaginosis, if symptomatic or previous preterm delivery	Urine dipstick: ☐ Protein ☐ Sugar ☐ Leukocytes ☐ Nitrites ☐ Ketosis	☐ Offer Maternal Multiple Marker at 15-18 weeks (labs may vary on timing of tests) ☐ Ultrasound as indicated	☐ One hour GCT (if indicated) ☐ Hct/Hgb Syphilis screening > or = 28 weeks (as required by IN law)	☐ Group B Beta Strep Culture (unless already plan to treat due to risk factors)	☐ Cervical cytology
OTHER BIOCHEMICAL EVALUATION (when indicated)					
If indicated: ☐ Diabetes screen ☐ Hgb electrophoresis (sickle cell) ☐ Tay Sachs screen ☐ TB skin test ☐ TORCH titers ☐ Group B Beta Strep culture ☐ Toxoplasmosis titer ☐ Varicella titer ☐ Urine drug screen	*Other tests as indicated:* e.g. Antepartum Fetal Surveillance, wet prep for bacterial vaginosis, STD cultures and urine cultures as appropriate	☐ Ultrasound as indicated	*If indicated:* ☐ Antibody screen (if Rh-) ☐ RhoGAM given (28 weeks if indicated) ☐ GTT	*If indicated:* ☐ GC/Chlamydia ☐ Herpes culture (if active lesion) ☐ Hepatitis B* ☐ HIV test	*If indicated:* ☐ Rubella immunization ☐ RhoGAM ☐ Varicella vaccine ☐ dt ☐ Hgb/Hct ☐ Gtt: 2 hour post 75 grams clucola if GDM during pregnancy

© 2008 Indiana Perinatal Network   www.indianaperinatal.org

* If positive, notify OB department at delivering hospital and physician caring for infant.

See reverse ▶

INITIAL VISIT & EACH VISIT (AS NEEDED)	20-24 WEEKS	24-28 WEEKS	34-40 WEEKS	POSTPARTUM
COUNSELING & EDUCATION BY PROVIDER, PRENATAL CARE COORDINATOR OR OTHER EDUCATOR				
☐ Emotional adaptation to pregnancy ☐ Screen for perinatal mood disorders (Edinburgh Postpartum Depression Scale) ☐ Physical changes during pregnancy ☐ Fetal growth and development ☐ Available options; Preference/plans for birth ☐ Benefits of and preparation for breastfeeding ☐ Violence-free environment ☐ Prenatal diagnosis ☐ "Smoke-free" pregnancy education ☐ Effects of drugs and alcohol ☐ Teratogen exposures ☐ Nutrition/prenatal vitamins/folate/calcium/iron ☐ Safety (seat belt, smoke detector) ☐ Communicable diseases/STDs/HIV ☐ Weight gain appropriate for body mass ☐ Minor discomforts ☐ Exercise and rest ☐ When to call, numbers to call, emergency plan ☐ Danger signs ☐ Adoption information if indicated	☐ Preterm birth prevention education ————	Repeat as needed to 37 weeks ————▶ ☐ Signs and symptoms of pre-eclampsia —— Repeat as needed ——▶ Repeat as needed ————————▶ Repeat as needed ————————▶ Repeat as needed ————————▶		☐ Parenting and coping with a new baby ☐ Crying strategies ☐ Never shake a baby (Happiest Baby skills) ☐ Perinatal mood disorders (signs and symptoms) ☐ Domestic violence (physical, sexual, emotional abuse) ☐ Breastfeeding support ☐ If HIV positive, do not breastfeed ☐ Back to work/school ☐ Siblings ☐ Family planning/Tubal sterilization ☐ Safe sleep education ☐ "Smoke-free" home ☐ Car seat ☐ Safety/CPR ☐ Immunizations ☐ Feeding ☐ When to call health care provider ☐ ASK about tobacco exposure ☐ Developmental issues ☐ Child care arrangements
Referrals as indicated for: ☐ WIC ☐ Dietician/Nutritionist ☐ Medicaid/managed care ☐ Prenatal care coordination ☐ Childbirth education ☐ Smoking cessation ☐ HIV care coordination ☐ High risk management or pregnancy consultation ☐ Alcohol and drug cessation ☐ Home care ☐ Genetic counseling ☐ Food and housing assistance		☐ Fetal movement/kick counts ☐ Preparation for labor and delivery- VBAC, counseling, labor signs and symptoms, pain management for labor, begin childbirth classes, induction of labor	**Consents signed:** ☐ VBAC, C-section, tubal (at least 30 days prior to EDD if on Medicaid)	☐ Referral to early intervention as indicated
		Initiate Postpartum Education: ☐ Evaluate plans ☐ Preparation for breastfeeding/Lactation Consultant ☐ Home preparation ☐ Choosing/meeting a health care provider for baby ☐ Family planning ☐ Circumcision information	**Preparing to bring baby home:** ☐ Safe sleep education ☐ "Smokefree" home ☐ Car seat ☐ Breastfeeding/feeding ☐ Assistance after going home ☐ Safety/CPR ☐ Jandice ☐ Rashes ☐ Cord Care ☐ Circumcised/Uncircumcised Care ☐ Immunizations ☐ Crying strategies ☐ Never shake a baby ☐ Temperature taking ☐ When to call health provider ☐ Back to school/work ☐ Newborn hearing screening ☐ Newborn metabolic screening ☐ Family planning ☐ Touching/holding/cuddling	

This document reflects the consensus of the Indiana Perinatal Network (IPN) State Perinatal Advisory Board—a constituency of professional organizations (i.e. ACOG, AAP) and individuals (i.e. CNMs, MDs, consumers). It is intended to serve as recommendations—not as established standards or rigid rules. Health care providers must make the best decisions possible within the limitations of the particular situation.

© 2008 Indiana Perinatal Network   www.indianaperinatal.org

Figure 10-9 Prenatal Care Guide.

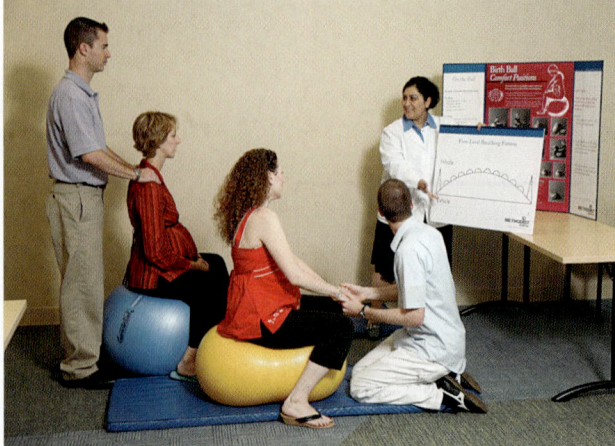

Figure 10-10 Childbirth education classes help to prepare the expectant couple for many aspects of the childbearing year.

Lamaze Method

The Lamaze childbirth experience was started in 1960 by the American Society for Psychoprophylaxis in Obstetrics (ASPO) as a way to bring families together in the labor and delivery process while focusing on the normality of birth. The concepts were founded on principles and techniques used by Dr. Fernand Lamaze, giving rise to the familiar labeling of the association as ASPO/Lamaze. It was not until the 1970s that the organization officially changed its name to Lamaze International, becoming known as such throughout the United States.

The heart of the Lamaze method is empowerment, recognizing the woman's innate ability to give birth, while finding strength and support from her family and the members of the health-care team during the labor and birth process. The Lamaze Approach to Birth (Box 10-5) identifies the core ideals of the organization and provides the template for the classes. The Lamaze Fundamentals for Parenting (Box 10-6) is another of the organization's many resources designed to help support and prepare expectant parents during the childbearing year. Historically, Lamaze has focused on breathing techniques during labor and birth. As the philosophy indicates, this method incorporates the ideology of

---

Box 10-5 Lamaze Approach to Birth

- Birth is normal, natural, and healthy.
- The experience of birth profoundly affects women and their families.
- Women's inner wisdom guides them through birth.
- Women's confidence and ability to give birth is either enhanced or diminished by the care provider and place of birth.
- Women have a right to give birth free from routine medical interventions.
- Birth can safely take place in homes, birth centers, and hospitals.
- Childbirth education empowers women to make informed choices in health care, to assume responsibility for their health, and to trust their inner wisdom.

Source: Lamaze International. (2012). *The Lamaze Approach to Birth.* Retrieved from http://www.lamaze.org/WhoWeAre/AboutLamaze/tabid/105/Default.aspx

---

Box 10-6 Lamaze Fundamentals for Parenting

- Good parenting is vital to the physical, emotional, and spiritual health of our children, ourselves, and our society.
- Parenting is joyful, important, challenging, and deeply satisfying work that is worthy of everyone's best efforts.
- Parenting begins before birth. The intimate connection between children and their parents must be respected and protected from the moment of birth throughout life.
- Mothers and fathers play unique, irreplaceable roles in their children's lives.
- Babies and children thrive in close, consistent interaction with their parents.
- Parenting is a learned art; our most important teachers are our own parents, our family, and our children.
- Good parenting requires the support of family, friends, and community.
- Knowledge and support enhance parents' confidence and ability to make informed decisions that meet the needs of their children and themselves.

Source: Lamaze International (2012). *Fundamentals for Parenting.* Retrieved from http://www.lamaze.org/ApproachToParenthood

---

empowerment into the entire experience, providing much more than just instruction on breathing.

As the Lamaze method has evolved over the years, many myths have continued to prevail regarding this method of childbirth preparation. The organization identified and addressed these myths (Lamaze International, 2012), and they include:

- *Lamaze is all about breathing*: In fact, Lamaze classes provide education on movement and position, massage, relaxation, and use of heat and cold in addition to the traditional focused-breathing techniques.
- *Lamaze promises painless childbirth*: Pain is a natural and normal part of childbirth. Instead of attempting to alleviate the pain, women are taught strategies for coping with the pain associated with labor and birth in positive ways. The strategies provide the woman with education to understand and respond to the pain signals and to facilitate the process of labor and birth.
- *Lamaze childbirth means you cannot have an epidural*: Education on epidural use is provided during Lamaze education in addition to education on natural pain relief. Lamaze educators stress that women need to make the decision that is personally best for them, with the knowledge that elimination of the pain makes it difficult to respond appropriately to contractions. In addition, after an epidural is placed, hospitals usually require that women remain in bed, have continuous fetal monitoring, and use medication to augment their contractions. The addition of these added procedures takes away from the philosophy that childbirth is a natural process.
- *Lamaze does not work*: When the woman has a complete understanding of the process of birth, the strategies for coping with the pain of the birth process, and the support of her family and members of the health-care team, she is able to experience the birth of her baby as a normal and natural experience.
- *Lamaze is not for everyone*: The strategies used by Lamaze educators stress the natural process of childbearing. The

philosophy of birth according to Lamaze International provides education and strategies for coping with labor and delivery that can be used by anyone who chooses this method.

Conscious breathing is the primary coping strategy used by proponents of the Lamaze method. Different breathing techniques and continued childbirth partner coaching facilitate each stage of labor. During the first stage of labor, breathing is used to relax the abdominal muscles and enlarge the abdominal cavity to enhance fetal descent. The woman inhales slowly, expanding her chest and abdominal cavity, and focuses on energy entering her body. As she exhales slowly, she focuses on tension leaving her body.

As the woman enters the second phase of the first stage of labor, known as transition, contractions become stronger and more frequent. Often it becomes difficult to concentrate on breathing. During this time, the woman's partner watches for signs of hyperventilation and helps her to focus on slow-paced breathing. During the second stage of labor, the active or pushing stage, the woman should be encouraged to bear down while exhaling and to take deep cleansing breaths before and after each contraction. She should be encouraged to take breaths between bearing-down efforts and avoid breath holding for more than 5 to 7 seconds at a time, as this practice decreases maternal and fetal oxygen flow. Once the fetal head crowns (distends the vulva), the partner or nurse may coach the woman to take panting breaths or to exhale slowly through pursed lips. These breathing patterns help to ensure a slow, controlled birth of the fetal head. (See Chapters 12 and 13 for further discussion.)

The Bradley Method of Natural Childbirth

While the Lamaze method uses techniques that focus the woman on recognizing the signals of labor and using controlled breathing and muscle relaxation to facilitate the birth, the Bradley method uses techniques that focus the woman on inward relaxation, by means of breathing control, abdominal breathing, and general relaxation. The partner facilitates the implementation of these techniques through coaching, giving rise to the term "husband-coached childbirth." To assist the partner in coaching the laboring woman to relax, there is an emphasis on darkness, solitude, and quiet to reduce stimulation and enhance the calm and comfort needed to conserve energy that will be required for birth and to decrease anxiety and tension in the woman. The Bradley method teaches that the woman should breathe normally throughout the labor and birth process to maintain her state of relaxation and to oxygenate the baby adequately. Medication is discouraged (Bradley, 1965).

Dr. Robert Bradley developed this method of childbirth in the 1960s after a decision that radically changed the traditional delivery room. Bradley became the first obstetrician to allow fathers into the delivery room and to seek out methods to involve them in the labor and birth of their child to provide the woman with another individual who could provide her with support. After noting the dramatic effects of having the father present during the labor and birth, educational programs were developed to teach the fathers to be labor coaches and have an active role in the experience. It is through this active participation by the fathers that the woman is able to remain relaxed, assume positions that are most comfortable, and experience the childbirth as a more natural and spiritual event.

Other Methods

While the Lamaze and Bradley methods remain the top childbirth education formats, with training to prepare educators to teach parents the strategies, other methods for childbirth exist. Prepared childbirth classes incorporate approaches from diverse methods to assist expectant couples in developing coping skills that will work best for them. Additional methods and techniques include the following:

- Dick-Read: The underlying philosophy in Dick-Read's approach to childbirth still focuses on the natural aspect of giving birth. After witnessing a birth in the 1920s, without the use of the traditional chloroform to render the laboring woman unconscious, he discovered that it was possible for women to experience pain-free birth. Through his study of physiology, he hypothesized that the pain associated with childbirth was caused by fear and tension, stimulating the sympathetic nervous system. This physiological event decreased blood flow to the uterus and created uterine muscle cell hypoxia. Through various relaxation techniques that consist of conscious and progressive relaxation of different muscle groups, the tension is reduced and blood flow to the uterus is restored. Although Dick-Read did not advocate the use of pharmacological pain management during labor and delivery, he approved of its use when the woman was unable to relax or was experiencing complications (Dick-Read, 1987).
- HypnoBirthing (Mongan Method): Classes using this method are based on Dick-Read's fear-tension-pain philosophy. Couples are taught, in four sessions, relaxation techniques to eliminate the pain associated with the fear and tension. Deep, total relaxation is key.
- LeBoyer method: Using this method, the baby is born in a dimly lit room that is conducive to relaxation and facilitates a tranquil entrance into the world. Immediately after birth, the newborn is placed in a warm water bath to enhance the transition from the intrauterine to the extrauterine environment. The infant is then moved to the mother's abdomen to initiate bonding. Through the gentle handling and the quiet, smooth transition, the newborn is able to open her eyes and breathe with minimal external stimulation.
- Odent method: This method arose from the LeBoyer method and includes moving the woman into a warm water bath for the birth. In addition to reducing labor pain, the warm water provides a comforting atmosphere to transition the newborn to extrauterine life. The underlying concept is that the infant can safely be born while submersed in water, without fear of drowning, because the fetus has lived in fluid for the duration of the pregnancy. Not all women are candidates for hydrotherapy. It is not an option for women who have rupture of the membranes or other complications that require continuous fetal monitoring.
- Birthing From Within: This method views childbirth as a rite of passage for parents and their infant. The underpinnings of this method focus on the psychological and spiritual aspects of birth, using art, writing, painting, and sculpting to encourage self-discovery. The focus is not on the birth process, but on the experience of birth.

Where Research and Practice Meet:
Benefits/Risks of Underwater Birth

Using various electronic databases, Simpson (2013) reviewed articles related to research about underwater birth published from 1966 to April 2013. Two randomized controlled trials comparing underwater birth to traditional birth served as the primary focus of the analysis. Overall results suggested minimal maternal benefit of underwater birth and no benefit for neonates. Although both studies were underpowered to adequately evaluate risk of neonatal harm, a number of cases of neonatal morbidity were identified. Neither the American College of Obstetricians and Gynecologists nor the American Academy of Pediatrics supports underwater birth outside the context of a randomized controlled trial. Based on these findings, the investigator concluded that underwater birth requires further investigation.

FINDING INFORMATION ON CHILDBIRTH EDUCATION

There are many ways that expectant mothers and their partners can locate information on childbirth education. The best strategy is to begin with the health-care provider, who can provide information about potential birth locations and childbirth education provided by the individual facilities. Internet sources can also assist couples in finding classes that are available to them locally. Expectant couples can engage in online childbirth education classes as well as home education through the purchase of comprehensive childbirth programs (Theroux, 2011).

In determining the childbirth preparation class that will meet the individual needs of the parents, the following questions should be considered:

- Who sponsors the class?
- How many classes will we be expected to attend?
- How many couples are in the class?
- Can I bring more than one support person to the class?
- What types of teaching and learning strategies are used?
- What topics are covered in the course?
- Where will the classes be held?
- Is there a cost involved?
- Is the instructor certified? If so, with what organization is the instructor affiliated?

With the abundance of childbirth methods available and the different certifications that exist for childbirth educators, it is important for expectant parents to identify the approaches and methods that best meet their needs to make the childbirth experience as meaningful as possible to them. It is helpful not only to examine the questions listed above, but also to consider what the most important factors are with regard to personal values and beliefs. Using the list below, nurses can direct parents to the appropriate education program to meet their needs. The woman should identify which four of the following factors are most important in selecting a childbirth education class:

- Familiarize me with hospital routines
- Prepare me for a natural, nonmedicated birth
- Teach me breathing patterns and distraction techniques
- Give my partner the skills necessary to be an active and informed labor coach

- Teach us as parents to be childbirth consumers and to take responsibility for our child's birth
- Follow current medical policies
- Represent the most common type of childbirth education class in our area
- Teach relaxation and natural breathing
- Stress good nutrition and exercise
- Discuss medication options without making value judgments

CREATING A BIRTH PLAN

From the moment a woman discovers that she is pregnant, she begins to consider ideas for her birth experience. Although the birth is usually not imminent, previous knowledge and experience, along with information shared by friends and family, prompt her to seek out information on options that are available and choices that she can make to prepare for the birth. While the birth plan is not a concrete document from which to outline every step of the labor and birth, it provides written information that identifies preferences for labor and birth, empowering the expectant couple with the control that is needed to reduce the anxiety associated with labor. When creating the birth plan, the couple should understand that while it reflects their desires and preferences, the plan may need to be altered during the childbirth experience to ensure safety for the mother and her fetus. Birth plans can be tailored to meet the needs of expectant couples that anticipate a hospital delivery, a birthing center delivery, a home delivery, a cesarean delivery, or a multiple delivery. Developing a birth plan in conjunction with the health-care provider ensures that the woman's individual situation is considered, especially important for high-risk pregnancies.

Nursing Insight—*Planning for umbilical cord blood banking*

Nurses must be aware of the latest information about umbilical cord blood banking to provide the latest evidence-based care to families during the childbearing year. Following childbirth, umbilical cord blood is painlessly collected and sent for processing and cryopreservation at the parents' selected private (for-profit) or public (not-for-profit) cord blood bank. Stem cells from the umbilical cord blood may be used at a later time to treat conditions such as leukemia, lymphoma, aplastic anemia, hemoglobinopathies, myelodysplasia, and metabolic storage diseases. It is important to make parents aware, however, that the chances are remote that the stem cells from their baby's banked cord blood will be used to treat that same child, or any other family member in the future (ACOG, 2008c; Brown, 2012)

Birth Plan Choices

There are many issues to consider when developing a personal birth plan. One concerns the presence of additional people in the birthing room. The woman may wish to include her partner, friends, relatives, a **doula** (a woman who is experienced in childbirth and provides physical and emotional support to the mother during the prenatal period, during labor, during birth, and during the postpartum period) or birthing coach, and children. She may desire to personalize the experience by wearing her own clothes, listening to music, and taking pictures or videotaping the birth. Fluids and food preferences can be noted, along with the woman's desire for a saline or heparin lock or an intravenous line. While most hospitals use continuous fetal monitoring, the woman can identify her wish for intermittent monitoring or no monitoring at all, unless an emergency develops. Preferences for laboring and birthing positions can also be noted. Choices regarding strategies for pharmacological and non-pharmacological pain management are identified, with the understanding that the woman has the right to change her mind and alter her plan at any time.

The woman who anticipates a vaginal birth should identify her preference regarding an episiotomy and the use of medication to augment labor contractions. The partner's desired level of involvement in the birth should also be identified. The woman can decide if she would like to hold her baby immediately after birth, and if she plans to breast-feed, whether she wishes to do so at that time (Anderson & Kilpatrick, 2012).

Women who anticipate a cesarean birth or who discover that they need a cesarean birth can usually maintain some degree of control over this procedure as well. They may be allowed to have their partner present during the surgery. The partner may be permitted to hold the newborn during the first moments of life if there are no immediate health concerns. The mother may also choose to initiate breast-feeding in the recovery room. Other preferences regarding infant feeding, rooming-in, and circumcision should be noted in the birth plan.

Choosing a Health-Care Provider

Selecting a health-care provider for the preconception, pregnancy, and birth experience is an essential first step that empowers the woman and her partner to become actively involved in care during the childbearing year. Approximately 90% of pregnant women choose an obstetrician as the primary care provider. Others use a certified nurse-midwife (CNM), who is trained in both nursing and midwifery and can provide a more personalized, less routine approach to a normal, uncomplicated pregnancy and birth. It is especially important that the patient choose a care provider with whom she can openly relate and who shares the same philosophical views on the management of pregnancy. (See Chapter 9 for further discussion.)

Choosing a Birth Location

A hospital is the most common birth location. In this setting, health-care providers and patients have access to technology and individuals trained to manage any complications that may arise. Obstetricians and CNMs attend and facilitate childbirth in the hospital setting. When choosing the facility that best meets their needs, the expectant couple should identify the type of setting provided by the hospital. For example, some institutions have separate labor, delivery, recovery, and postpartum rooms. This arrangement requires the family to be moved from one location to another during their hospital stay. The newest facility models place emphasis on family-centered care and offer large, comfortable rooms where the woman remains for the duration of the childbirth experience.

Freestanding birthing centers were first opened in 1974 to provide women with a more homelike atmosphere in which to give birth. Although these facilities are located

near the hospital in the event of an emergency, they are recommended for women with low-risk pregnancies. A major benefit of the birthing centers is that they have fewer restrictions and generally allow the parents more freedom to make personal decisions regarding labor and birth.

Home births are returning as an option for women with low-risk pregnancies and no known labor complications. The ACOG recently (2011b) released an updated statement of policy regarding home births (Box 10-7). Although obstetricians will not deliver babies at home, many CNMs are willing to do so. Many expectant couples believe that giving birth at home enriches the childbirth experience and allows them to better integrate the birth as a normal and natural event in their lives. However, the parents must be open to transfer to a hospital if complications arise.

 Now Can You—Discuss childbirth preparation, birth plans, and doulas?

1. Compare and contrast the Lamaze, Bradley, and LeBoyer methods of childbirth preparation?
2. Discuss the purpose of a birth plan?
3. Describe the role of a doula?

 Where Research and Practice Meet:
Safety of Home Births in the United States

Using 2007–2010 data from the CDC's National Center for Health Statistics on singleton term births, researchers Cheng and colleagues (2013) found that infants delivered at home were roughly 10 times more likely to be stillborn and 4 times more likely to develop neonatal seizures or other neurological dysfunction than were their hospital-born counterparts. Both home births and freestanding birth center deliveries had a significantly higher risk of a 5-minute Apgar score (a numeric expression [range 0 = worst to 10 = best] of the condition of a newborn obtained by assessment at 1 and 5 minutes of age) of 0 than hospital births attended by either a physician or a midwife. A higher risk for neonatal seizures or neurological dysfunction was also seen with home deliveries and freestanding birth center deliveries. The researchers concluded that maternity health-care providers should inform patients about these findings and use patient concerns about the hospital deliveries to make hospitals more desirable places to give birth (Cheng, Snowden, King, & Caughey, 2013; Norwitz, 2013).

Box 10-7 **ACOG Statement on Planned Home Birth**

In 2007, the American College of Obstetrics and Gynecology (ACOG) wrote: "Monitoring of both the woman and the fetus during labor and delivery in a hospital or accredited birthing center is essential because complications can arise with little or no warning" (p. 275). In 2011 ACOG revised the opinion, still noting that the Committee on Obstetrics Practice "believes that hospitals and birthing centers are the safest setting for birth" but now adding that the committee also "respects the right of a woman to make a medically informed decision about delivery" (p. 427). The committee also recommends that "women inquiring about planned home birth should be informed of its risks and benefits based on recent evidence" and should be informed that "assurance of safe and timely transport to nearby hospitals are critical to reducing perinatal mortality rates and achieving favorable home birth outcomes" (p. 427).

Sources: American College of Obstetricians and Gynecologists, 2011b; Ecker & Minkoff, 2011.

Summary Points

◆ Preconception counseling empowers families to plan for pregnancy and develop healthy bodies and minds to optimize birth outcomes.

◆ Nurses and other health-care providers must collaboratively provide families with prenatal education and incorporate interventions for a holistic approach to pregnancy.

◆ A balance of diet and nutrition, exercise, work, and rest enhances the development of a healthy pregnancy.

◆ To determine safety of use during pregnancy, all medications, including prescription, over-the-counter, and herbal preparations, must be carefully evaluated. It is essential that the nurse obtain a comprehensive medication history during each prenatal visit.

◆ Ongoing prenatal education regarding pregnancy danger signs and symptoms and appropriate home interventions is key in reducing complications.

◆ Nurses can help to empower families by providing information about childbirth education programs and other community resources.

◆ A holistic approach to a healthy pregnancy and birth includes all members of the family and the health-care team. Encouraging the family to develop a birth plan is an important step in helping to create a positive, satisfying birth experience.

Review Questions

Multiple Choice

1. The perinatal nurse knows that the most ideal time to address issues related to a poor outcome in a past pregnancy is
A. Postpartum.
B. Prenatally.
C. Preconception.
D. Interconception.

2. The prenatal nurse provides nutritional counseling during pregnancy to ensure adequate weight gain. The nurse teaches that the additional daily calories required are the equivalent of
A. 1 glass of skim milk.
B. 2 servings of yogurt.
C. 2 apples.
D. 3 ounces of cheese.

3. The perinatal nurse knows that the blood volume in pregnancy increases on average by
A. 20% to 30%.
B. 30% to 40%.
C. 40% to 50%.
D. 50% to 60%.

4. The prenatal nurse counsels a woman to stop smoking prior to conceiving. Which of the following does the nurse advise is a potential complication of smoking during pregnancy?
A. Gestational diabetes mellitus
B. Intellectual and developmental disabilities
C. Intrauterine growth restriction
D. Hyperirritability

5. A nurse is reviewing the chart of a woman being seen for a routine prenatal visit. The chart documents concerns with Couvade syndrome. The nurse understand this includes
A. The partner experiencing maternal signs and symptoms.
B. A history of prior problems with preterm labor.
C. A history of multidrug abuse in the pregnant female.
D. A history of extreme pregnancy-related nausea and vomiting.

6. An obese pregnant woman is in the clinic for nutritional counseling. What weight gain should the nurse recommend to this woman in her second and third trimesters?
A. 0.1 kg/week
B. 0.3 kg/week
C. 0.4 kg/week
D. 0.5 kg/week

7. A pregnant woman is concerned about the possibility of her baby being born with a neural tube defect (NTD). Which response by the nurse is best?
A. "I can ask the physician to order genetic screening for you if you like."
B. "Be sure to take your iron supplement each day with a glass of orange juice."
C. "You need to be sure to get at least 1,000 mg of calcium and 600 IU of vitamin D daily."
D. "About 70% of NTDs can be prevented by getting 400 mcg of folic acid each day."

8. A woman in her first trimester of pregnancy complains of nausea. Which suggestion by the nurse is best?
A. "Try eating plain, dry crackers before you get out of bed."
B. "You may be constipated; try some senna tablets."
C. "I have heard that licorice root is good for nausea."
D. "Don't worry unless you start vomiting continuously."

9. A woman in her second trimester calls the perinatal clinic and reports having two large cavities that the dentist wants to fill. Which response by the nurse is best?
A. "You should wait until your third trimester to have dental work done."
B. "It is safe to use most local anesthetics for dental work during pregnancy."
C. "You will need to wait until after you have given birth to your baby."
D. "You can have them filled, but you will have to avoid the anesthetics."

10. A pregnant woman and her partner are preparing her birth plan. It is the couple's wish that the woman give birth in warm water. The nurse recognizes this style of birthing as the
A. Lamaze method.
B. LeBoyer method.
C. Odent method.
D. Dick-Read method.

See Answers to End of Chapter Review Questions on Davis*Plus*.

REFERENCES

Albrecht, S. A. (2010). Smoking cessation in pregnancy. *Nursing for Women's Health, 14*(3), 177–179.

Albrecht, S., Kelly-Thomas, K., Osborne, J., & Ogbagaber, S. (2011). The SUCCESS program for smoking cessation for pregnant women. *Journal of Obstetric, Gynecologic and Neonatal Nursing, 40*(5), 520–531. doi:10.1111/j.1552-6909.2011.01280.x

American Academy of Periodontology. (2011). Baby steps to healthy pregnancy and on-time delivery. Retrieved from http://www.perio.org/consumer/pregnancy.htm

American College of Obstetricians and Gynecologists (ACOG). (2002). Exercise during pregnancy and the postpartum period. Committee Opinion No. 267. (Reaffirmed 2009). *Obstetrics & Gynecology, 99*(1), 171–173.

American College of Obstetricians and Gynecologists (ACOG). (2003). Neural tube defects. Practice Bulletin No. 44. (Reaffirmed 2013). *Obstetrics & Gynecology, 102*(7), 203–213.

American College of Obstetricians and Gynecologists (ACOG). (2005). The importance of preconception care in the continuum of women's health care. Committee Opinion No. 313. (Reaffirmed 2012). *Obstetrics & Gynecology, 106*(5), 665–666.

American College of Obstetricians and Gynecologists (ACOG). (2007). Screening for fetal chromosomal abnormalities. Practice Bulletin No. 77. (Reaffirmed 2013). *Obstetrics & Gynecology, 109*(3), 217–227.

American College of Obstetricians and Gynecologists (ACOG). (2008a). Prenatal and perinatal Human Immunodeficiency Virus testing: Expanded recommendations. Committee Opinion No. 418. (Reaffirmed 2011). *Obstetrics & Gynecology, 112*(9), 739–742.

American College of Obstetricians and Gynecologists (ACOG). (2008b). Anemia in pregnancy. Practice Bulletin No. 95. (Reaffirmed 2013). *Obstetrics & Gynecology, 112*(7), 201–207.

American College of Obstetricians and Gynecologists (ACOG). (2008c). Umbilical cord blood banking. Committee Opinion No. 399. (Reaffirmed 2012). *Obstetrics & Gynecology, 111*(2), 475–477.

American College of Obstetricians and Gynecologists (ACOG). (2009a). Maternal phenylketonuria. Committee Opinion No. 449. *Obstetrics & Gynecology, 114*(6), 1432–1433.

American College of Obstetricians and Gynecologists (ACOG). (2009b). Air travel during pregnancy. Committee Opinion No. 443. *Obstetrics & Gynecology, 114*(10), 954–955.

American College of Obstetricians and Gynecologists (ACOG). (2010). Moderate caffeine consumption during pregnancy. Committee Opinion No. 462. *Obstetrics & Gynecology, 116*(2), 467–468.

American College of Obstetricians and Gynecologists (ACOG). (2011a). Vitamin D: Screening and supplementation during pregnancy. Committee Opinion No. 495. *Obstetrics & Gynecology, 118*(1), 197–198.

American College of Obstetricians and Gynecologists (ACOG). (2011b). Planned home birth. Committee Opinion No. 476. (Reaffirmed 2013). *Obstetrics & Gynecology, 117*(2), 425–428.

American College of Obstetricians and Gynecologists (ACOG). (2012a). Intimate partner violence. Committee Opinion No. 518. *Obstetrics & Gynecology, 119*(2), 412–417.

American College of Obstetricians and Gynecologists (ACOG). (2012b). Management of preterm labor. Practice Bulletin No. 127. *Obstetrics & Gynecology, 119*(6), 1308–1317.

American College of Obstetricians and Gynecologists (ACOG). (2013a). Gestational diabetes mellitus. Practice Bulletin No. 504. *Obstetrics & Gynecology, 122*(8), 406–416.

American College of Obstetricians and Gynecologists (ACOG). (2013b). Weight gain during pregnancy. Committee Opinion No. 548. *Obstetrics & Gynecology, 121*(1), 210–212.

American College of Obstetricians and Gynecologists (ACOG). (2013c). Oral health care during pregnancy and through the lifespan. *Obstetrics & Gynecology, 122*(2), 417–422.

American Dental Association. (2011). Oral health during pregnancy. Retrieved from http://www.ada.org/~/media/ADA/Publications/Files/for_the_dental_patient_may_2011.ashx

Anderson, C. J., & Kilpatrick, C. (2012). Supporting patients' birth plans: Theories, strategies & implications for nurses. *Nursing for Women's Health, 16*(3), 211–218. doi:10.1111/j.1751-486X.2012.01732.x

Artal, R., Lockwood, C. J., & Brown, H. L. (2010). Weight gain recommendations in pregnancy and the obesity epidemic. *Obstetrics & Gynecology, 115*(1), 152–155.

Association of Women's Health, Obstetric and Neonatal Nurses (AWHONN). (1999). *Preconceptional Consumption of Folic Acid.* Position Statement. (Reaffirmed 2007). Retrieved from: https://www.awhonn.org/awhonn/content.do?name=07_PressRoom/7C1_FolicAcidAware.htm

Attrill, B. (2002). The assumption of the maternal role: A developmental process. *Australian Journal of Midwifery, 15*, 21–25.

Ayoola, A. B., Nettleman, M. D., & Strommel, M. (2010). Time from pregnancy recognition to prenatal care and associated newborn outcomes. *Journal of Obstetric, Gynecologic & Neonatal Nursing, 39*(5), 550–556. doi:10.1111/j.1552-6909.2010.01167.x

Barry, M. (2011). Preconception care at the edges of the reproductive life span. *Nursing for Women's Health, 15*(1), 68–74.

Beddoe, A. E., Yang, C. P., Kennedy, H. P., Weiss, S. J., & Lee, K. A. (2009). The effects of mindfulness-based yoga during pregnancy on maternal psychological and physical distress. *Journal of Obstetric, Gynecologic & Neonatal Nursing, 38*(3), 310–319. doi:10.1111/j.1552-6909.2009.01023.x

Bennett, W. L., & McDonald-Mosley, R. (2011). Management of severe obesity in pregnancy. *The Female Patient, 36*(7), 23–28.

Bloomberg, M. (2011). Maternal and neonatal outcomes among obese women with weight gain below the new Institute of Medicine recommendations. *Obstetrics & Gynecology, 117*(5), 1065–1079. doi:10.1097/AOG.0b013e318214f1d1

Borcherding, K. E. (2009). Coping in healthy primigravidae pregnant women. *Journal of Obstetric, Gynecologic & Neonatal Nursing, 38*(4), 453–462. doi:10.1111/j.1552-6909.2009.01041.x

Bradley, R. (1965). *Husband-coached childbirth.* New York, NY: Harper-Collins.

Brown, H. L. (2012). Obstetricians' role critical in increasing patients' access to cord blood. *Contemporary OB-GYN, 57*(7), 10–11.

Callister, L. C., & Khalaf, I. (2010). Spirituality in childbearing women. *Journal of Perinatal Education, 19*(2), 16–24. doi:10.1624/10581240XX495514

Carr, M., & Kaplan, C. (2010). Midlife women with anorexia nervosa: A review of the literature. *The American Journal for Nurse Practitioners, 14*(6), 8–15.

Centers for Disease Control and Prevention (CDC). (2012a). Tobacco use and pregnancy. Retrieved from http://www.cdc.gov/reproductive-health/tobaccousepregnancy/index.htm

Centers for Disease Control and Prevention (CDC). (2012b). Alcohol and public health. Retrieved from http://www.cdc.gov/alcohol/fact-sheets/womens-health.htm

Centers for Disease Control and Prevention (CDC). (2012c). Folic acid recommendations. Retrieved from http://www.cdc.gov/ncbddd/folicacid/recommendations.html

Chalupka, S., & Chalupka, A. N. (2010). The impact of environmental and occupational exposures on reproductive health. *Journal of Obstetric, Gynecologic & Neonatal Nursing, 39*(1), 84–102. doi:10.1111/j.1552-6909.2009.0109.x

Cheng, Y. W., Snowden, J. M., King, T. L., & Caughey, A. B. (2013). Selected perinatal outcomes associated with planned home births in the United States. *American Journal of Obstetrics & Gynecology, 209*(4), 325.e1–e8. doi:10.1016/j.ajog.2013.06.022

Chescheir, N. C. (2011). Global obesity and the effect on women's health. *Obstetrics & Gynecology, 117*(5), 1213–1222. doi:10.1097/AOG.0b013e3182161732

Conrad, K., Russell, A. C., & Keister, K. J. (2011). Bariatric surgery and its impact on childbearing. *Nursing for Women's Health, 15*(3), 228–234.

Cox, J. T., & Phelan, S. T. (2009). Food safety in pregnancy: Putting risks into perspective. *Contemporary OB/GYN, 54*(11), 44–54.

Cunningham, F. G., Leveno, K. J., Bloom, S. L., Spong, C., & Dashe, J. (2014). *Williams Obstetrics* (24th ed.). New York, NY: McGraw-Hill Professional.

Demissie, Z., Siega-Riz, A., Evenson, K., Herring, A., Dole, N., & Gaynes, B. (2011). Associations between physical activity and postpartum depressive symptoms. *Journal of Women's Health, 20*(7), 1025–1034. doi:10.1089/jwh.2010.2091

Dick-Read, G. (1987). *Childbirth without fear* (5th ed.). New York, NY: Harper & Collins.

Dodd, J. M., Grivell, R. M., Crowther, C. A., & Robinson, J. S. (2010). Antenatal interventions for overweight or obese pregnant women: A systematic review of randomised trials. *British Journal of Obstetrics & Gynecology, 117*(3), 1316–1326.

Ecker, J., & Minkoff, H. (2011). Home birth: What are physicians' ethical obligations when patient choices may carry increased risk? *Obstetrics & Gynecology, 117*(5), 1179–1182.

Flick, A., & Artal, R. (2013). Obesity and weight gain in pregnancy. *Contemporary OB/GYN, 58*(7), 26–28.

Gebhardt, J. G., & Truehart, A. (2012). Obesity in pregnancy: A systematic approach to decrease complications. *The Female Patient, 37*(1), 28–34.

Gilden, R. C., Huffling, K., & Sattler, B. (2010). Pesticides and health risks. *Journal of Obstetric, Gynecologic & Neonatal Nursing, 39*(1), 103–110. doi:1111/j.1552-6909.2009.01092.x

Guelinckx, I., Devlieger, R., Mullie, P., & Vansant, G. (2010). Effect of lifestyle intervention on dietary habits, physical activity, and gestational weight gain in obese pregnant women: A randomized controlled trial. *American Journal of Clinical Nutrition, 91*(3), 373–380.

Guilbeau, J. R. (2012). Health risks of energy drinks: What nurses and consumers need to know. *Nursing for Women's Health, 16*(5), 423–428. doi:10.1111/j.1751-486X.2012.01766.x

Hall, W. A., Hauck, Y. L., Carty, E. M., Hutton, E. K., Fenwick, J., & Stoll, K. (2009). Childbirth fear, anxiety, fatigue, and sleep deprivation in pregnant women. *Journal of Obstetric, Gynecologic & Neonatal Nursing, 38*(5), 567–576. doi:10.1111/j.1552-6909.2009.01054.x

Harris, A. L. (2011). Vitamin D deficiency and bacterial vaginosis in pregnancy. *Nursing for Women's Health, 15*(5), 423–430.

Institute for Clinical Systems Improvement (ICSI). (2011). Prenatal care, routine. Bloomington, MN: Author.

Institute of Medicine. (2001). Food and Nutrition Board. *Dietary Reference Intakes for Vitamin A, Vitamin K, Arsenic, Boron, Chromium, Copper, Iodine, Iron, Manganese, Molybdenum, Nickel, Silicon, Vanadium and Zinc.* Washington, DC: National Academies Press.

Institute of Medicine. (2009). *Weight gain during pregnancy: Reexamining the guidelines.* Retrieved from http://www.iom.edu/~/media/Files/Report%20Files/2009/Weight-Gain-During-Pregnancy-Reexamining-the-Guidelines/Report%20Brief%20-%20Weight%20Gain%20During%20Pregnancy.pdf

Ji, E. S., & Han, H. (2010). The effects of Qi exercise on maternal/fetal interaction and maternal well-being during pregnancy. *Journal of Obstetric, Gynecologic & Neonatal Nursing, 39*(3), 310–318. doi:10.1111/j.1552-6909.2010.01135.x

Johnson, T. S., & Strube, K. (2011). Breast care during pregnancy. *Journal of Obstetric, Gynecologic & Neonatal Nursing, 40*(2), 144–148. doi:10.1111/j.1552-6909.2011.01227.x

Keough, V. A., & Jennrich, J. A. (2009). Including a screening and brief alcohol intervention program in the care of the obstetric patient. *Journal of Obstetric, Gynecologic & Neonatal Nursing, 38*(6), 715–722. doi:10.1111/j.1552-6909.2009.01073.x

King, T. L., Brucker, M. C., Kriebs, J. M., & Fahey, J. O. (2013). *Varney's midwifery.* (5th ed.). Burlington, MA: Jones & Bartlett Learning.

Kominiarek, M. (2013). Assessing nutritional needs in pregnant patients with prior bariatric surgery. *Contemporary OB/GYN, 28*(10), 45–50.

Lamaze International. (2012). *About Lamaze.* Retrieved from http://www.lamazeinternational.org/p/cm/ld/fid=1

Lederman, R., & Weis, K. (2010). *Psychosocial adaptation in pregnancy: Seven dimensions of maternal role development* (3rd ed.). New York, NY: Springer Publishing Company.

Lopez, W. D., Konrath, S. H., & Seng, J. S. (2011). Abuse-related posttraumatic stress, coping, and tobacco use in pregnancy. *Journal of Obstetric, Gynecologic & Neonatal Nursing, 40*(4), 422–431.

Loprinzi, P. D., Fitzgerald, E. M., & Cardinal, B. J. (2012). Physical activity and depression symptoms among pregnant women from the National Health and Nutrition Examination Survey 2005-2006. *Journal of Obstetric, Gynecologic & Neonatal Nursing, 41*(2), 227–234.

Malnory, M. E., & Johnson, T. S. (2010). The reproductive life plan as a strategy to decrease poor birth outcomes. *Journal of Obstetric, Gynecologic & Neonatal Nursing, 40*(1), 109–121. doi:10.1111/j.1552-6909.2010.01203.x

Malshe, A., & Wiczyk, H. (2011). Acupuncture stimulation and obstetrics: "To stick or not to stick?—That is the question." *The Female Patient, 36*(2), 16–19.

March of Dimes Birth Defects Foundation. (2008). *Alcohol and drugs.* Retrieved from http://www.marchofdimes.com/pregnancy/alcohol_indepth.html

March of Dimes Birth Defects Foundation. (2010). *Smoking during pregnancy.* Retrieved from http://www.marchofdimes.com/pregnancy/alcohol_smoking.html

McDaniel, M. L. (2010). Counseling on sexuality in pregnancy. *The Female Patient, 35*(1), 42–44.

Mitchell, A. A., Gilboa, S. M., Werler, M. M., Kelley, K. E., Louik, C., & Hernandez-Diaz, S. (2011). Medication use during pregnancy, with particular focus on prescription drugs: 1976–2008. *American Journal of Obstetrics & Gynecology, 205*(1), 51–58.

National Diabetes Information Clearinghouse. (2011). *What I need to know about gestational diabetes.* NIH Publication No. 06-5129. Retrieved from http://diabetes.niddk.nih.gov/dm/pubs/gestational/#4

National High Blood Pressure Education Program Working Group. (2000). *Working group report on high blood pressure in pregnancy.* NHBPEP Publication No. 00-3029. Washington, DC: National Heart Lung and Blood Institute.

National Institute on Drug Abuse. (2012). Medical consequences of drug abuse. Retrieved from http://www.drugabuse.gov/publications/medical-consequences-drug-abuse/prenatal-effects

National Institutes of Health (NIH). (2011a). Dietary supplement fact sheet: Calcium. Retrieved from http://ods.od.nih.gov/factsheets/calcium-HealthProfessional/

National Institutes of Health (NIH). (2011b). Dietary supplement fact sheet: Vitamin D. Retrieved from http://ods.od.nih.gov/factsheets/vitamind-HealthProfessional/

National Institutes of Health (NIH). (2011c). Dietary supplement fact sheet: Vitamin C. Retrieved from http://ods.od.nih.gov/factsheets/vitaminc-HealthProfessional/

National Institutes of Health (NIH). (2011d). NINDS Tay-Sachs Disease information page. Retrieved from http://www.ninds.nih.gov/disorders/taysachs/taysachs.htm

National Institutes of Health (NIH). (2012). Dietary supplement fact sheet: Iron. Retrieved from http://ods.od.nih.gov/factsheets/iron-HealthProfessional/

Norwitz, E. R. (2013). What do the latest data reveal about the safety of home birth in the United States? *OBG Management, 25*(11), 24–26.

O'Donnell, M. J., Elio, R., & Day, D. (2010). Carpal tunnel syndrome: Coping during pregnancy and breastfeeding. *Nursing for Women's Health, 14*(4), 318–321.

Organization of Teratology Information Specialists (OTIS). (2010). *Isotretinoin (Accutane) and Pregnancy.* Retrieved from http://www.mothertobaby.org/files/Isotretinoin.pdf

Ovesen, P., Rasmussen, S., & Kesmodel, U. (2011). Effect of prepregnancy maternal overweight and obesity on pregnancy outcome. *Obstetrics & Gynecology, 118*(2), 305–312. doi:10.10987/AOG.0b013e3182245d49

Pena-Rosas, J., De-Regil, L. M., Dowswell, T., & Viteri, F. E. (2012). Intermittent oral iron supplementation during pregnancy. *Cochrane Database of Systematic Reviews 2012,* Issue 7. Art. No.:CD009997. doi:10.1002/14651858.CD009997

Pohler, H. (2010). Caffeine intoxication and addiction. *The Journal for Nurse Practitioners, 6*(1), 49–52.

Quinlivan, J. A., Julania, S., & Lam, L. (2011). Antenatal dietary interventions in obese pregnant women to restrict gestational weight gain to Institute of Medicine recommendations. *Obstetrics & Gynecology, 118*(6), 1395–1401.

Quinlivan, J. A., Lam, L. T., & Fisher, J. A. (2011). A randomized trial of a four-step multidisciplinary approach to the antenatal care of obese pregnant women. *Australian and New Zealand Journal of Obstetrics & Gynaecology, 51*(4), 141–146.

Savitz, D., Chan, R., Herring, A., Howards, P., & Hartmann, K. (2008). Caffeine and miscarriage risk. *Epidemiology, 19*(1), 55–62.

Sego, S. (2010). Pomegranate. *The Clinical Advisor, 13*(2), 101–105.

Sengpiel, V., Elind, E., Bacelis, J., Nilsson, S., Grove, J., Myhre, R., . . . Brantsaeter, A-L. (2013). Maternal caffeine intake during pregnancy is associated with birth weight but not with gestational length: Results from a large prospective observational cohort study. *BMC Medicine, 11*(42), 701–718. doi:10.1186/1741-7015-11-42

Shane-McWhorter, L., & Martinez, L. (2011). Dietary supplements for women. *Obstetrics & Gynecology, 117*(5), 1170–1174. doi:10.1097/AOG.0b13e3182107192

Simpson, K. R. (2013). Underwater birth. *Journal of Obstetric, Gynecologic & Neonatal Nursing, 42*(5), 588–594. doi:10.1111/1552-6909.12235

Streuling, I., Beyerlein, A., Rosenfeld, E., Hofmann, H., Schulz, T., & Kries, R. (2011). Physical activity and gestational weight gain: A meta-analysis of intervention trials. *British Journal of Obstetrics & Gynecology, 118*(9), 278–284.

Szymanski, L. M., & Satin, A. J. (2012). Exercise during pregnancy: Fetal responses to current public health guidelines. *Obstetrics & Gynecology, 119*(3), 603–610. doi:10.1097/AOG.0b13e31824760b5

Tao, G., Hoover, K. W., & Kent, C. K. (2010). 2009. Cervical cytology guidelines and Chlamydia testing among sexually active young women. *Obstetrics & Gynecology, 116*(6), 1319–1324.

Theroux, R. (2011). Media as a source of information on pregnancy and childbirth. *Nursing for Women's Health, 15*(1), 62–67.

Thornton, Y. S., Smarkola, C., Kopacz, S. M., & Ishoof, S. B. (2009). Perinatal outcomes in nutritionally monitored obese pregnant women:

A randomized clinical trial. *Journal of the National Medical Association,* *101*(2), 569–577.

U.S. Department of Health & Human Services (USDHHS). (2006). *Your guide to lowering your blood pressure with DASH* (NIH Publication No. 06-4082). Washington, DC: U.S. Government Printing Office.

U.S. Department of Health & Human Services (USDHHS). (2008). *2008 Physical Activity Guidelines for Americans.* Washington, DC: U.S. Government Printing Office.

U.S. Department of Health & Human Services (USDHHS). (2011). *U.S. Department of Agriculture Dietary Guidelines for Americans, 2010.* Washington, DC: U.S. Government Printing Office.

U.S. Department of Health & Human Services (USDHHS). (2012). *Introducing Healthy People 2020.* Retrieved from http://www.healthypeople .gov/2020/about/default.aspx

United States Department of Labor. (1995). Wage and Hour Division: *The Family and Medical Leave Act of 1993.* Retrieved from http://www .dol.gov/whd/fmla/

U.S. Department of Veterans Affairs. (2013). *Food-borne illness.* Retrieved from http://www.publichealth.va.gov/infectiondontpassiton/womens-health-guide/food-borne-illness/index.asp

United States National Library of Medicine. (2012). Genetics home reference: Heomphilia. Retrieved from http://ghr.nlm.nih.gov/condition/hemophilia

Vallerand, A. H., & Sanoski, C. A. (2014). *Davis's drug guide for nurses* (14th ed.). Philadelphia, PA: F.A. Davis.

Van Dijk, J. A., Anderko, L., & Stetzer, F. (2011). The impact of Prenatal Care Coordination on birth outcomes. *Journal of Obstetric, Gynecologic & Neonatal Nursing, 40*(1), 98–108.

Venes, D. (Ed.). (2013). *Taber's cyclopedic medical dictionary* (22nd ed.). Philadelphia, PA: F.A. Davis.

Walters, M. R., & Smith-Taylor, J. (2010). Maternal obesity: Consequences and prevention strategies. *Nursing for Women's Health, 13*(6), 488–494. doi:10.1111/j.1751-486X.2009.01483.x

Wolff, S., Legarth, J., Vangsaard, K., Toubro, S., & Astrup, A. (2008). A randomized trial of effects of dietary counseling on gestational weight gain and glucose metabolism in obese pregnant women. *International Journal of Obesity (London), 32*(1), 495–501.

Young, S. (2012). *Craving earth: Understanding pica.* New York, NY: Columbia University Press.

Youngkin, E. Q., Davis, M. S., Schadewald, D., & Juve, C. (2012). *Women's health: A primary care clinical guide* (4th ed.). Upper Saddle River, NJ: Prentice Hall.

Zauderer, C. (2009). Maternity care for Orthodox Jewish couples. *Nursing for Women's Health, 13*(2), 113–120.

Zavorsky, G. S., & Longo, L. D. (2011). Adding strength training, exercise intensity, and caloric expenditure to exercise guidelines in pregnancy. *Obstetrics & Gynecology, 117*(6), 1399–1402. doi:10.1097/AOG.0b013e31821b1f5a

DavisPlus | For more information, go to **http://davisplus.fadavis.com/**

CONCEPT MAP

Promoting a Healthy Pregnancy

Preconception Counseling

Healthy Body: assess →
- Medical/menstrual history
- Findings from physical/lab exams
- Exposure to STIs/childhood illness
- Lifestyle choices
- Patient/family genetic history

Healthy Mind: assess →
- Readiness for motherhood/fatherhood
- Healthy relationship
- Social support
- Educational level
- Mental illness

Nutrition

Factors Affecting:
- Eating disorders: pica, anorexia/bulimia
- Cultural influences/ religious beliefs
- Being vegan

Nursing:
- Obtain nutritional hx.
- Assess for nutritional elements: calories, proteins, water, minerals, vitamins, calcium, iron, vitamin C
- Assess folic acid supplement use
- Teach "daily food plan for moms"

Medications

- Encourage consultation with PCP to determine drug safety
- Know teratogens and FDA classifications for meds used during pregnancy
- Assess for use of herbal/homeopathic preparations and OTCs

Activity

Work: assess impact
- What is the nature of the work?
- Is there exposure to toxins?
- What is the number of hours?
- Are there complications with pregnancy?
- Plan for maternity leave

Exercise:
- Focus on muscle strengthening
- Maintain adequate breathing rate; fluid intake during exercise
- Limit strenuous aerobics and increased body temperature
- Avoid exhaustion

Rest: tending to fatigue caused by
- Increased progesterone production
- Physiological anemia
- Increased fetal oxygen needs
- Emotional stress
- Decreased maternal lung expansion
- Nocturia

Common Discomforts

Anticipatory guidance/care strategies for:
GI: nausea, vomiting, constipation, flatulence, dyspepsia, ptyalism
CV: dependent edema, varicosities, supine hypotensive syndrome
GU: frequency, nocturia
Pain: round ligament, paresthesias, backache, leg cramps
Other: leukorrhea, fatigue, shortness of breath, dyspareunia, dental issues, insomnia

Recognize signs of complications: Differentiate from discomforts

- Hyperemesis gravidarum
- Spontaneous abortion
- Infection
- Preeclampsia
- PROM
- Absence of fetal movement
- Placenta previa/abruptio placentae

Weight Gain

Factors Affecting:
Genetic/social hx.
Enlarging placenta
- Increased bladder volume
- Increased blood volume
- Fetal growth

Nursing:
- BMI screening
- Conscious planning of food intake: Choose MyPlate and DASH plans
- Patient education/ counseling

Childbirth Education

- Class → harmonious with beliefs/values
- Goal → facilitate positive birth experience
- Topics: A&P, comfort measures, labor and birth process, childbirth methods, relaxation/pain management, types of births, postpartum care, newborn care/feeding
- Create a birth plan

Complementary Care:
- Ayurveda beneficial during preconception period
- Stress management → massage, light and aromatherapy, reflexology, relaxation, mindfulness-based yoga
- Acupuncture for nausea and back pain

Nursing Insight:
- Some foods decrease iron absorption
- Identify potential environmental threats to embryo
- Women with PKU should receive family planning counseling
- Obesity is a risk factor for an increased number of pregnancy complications
- Isotretinoin can have significant teratogenic effects

Optimizing Outcomes:
- Use prenatal interventions to prevent birth defects
- Encourage preconception care counseling
- Use SUCCESS program to educate about smoking/smoking cessation strategies
- Use SBIRT program interventions to treat women with alcohol use disorders during pregnancy
- Teach health benefits of breastfeeding

Where Research and Practice Meet:

- Maternal smoking behavior influenced by need to cope with abuse-related PTSD symptoms
- Qi exercise beneficial prenatal nursing intervention
- Antenatal dietary intervention programs do not negatively alter newborn birth weight
- Pregnant women can exercise following existing recommendations
- Many factors influence increased medication use by pregnant women

Cultural Diversity:

- Higher maternal anemia in pregnant adolescents, African American women, and women of low-socioeconomic status
- Higher vitamin D deficiency rates in African Americans
- Pica associated with some cultural, religious beliefs
- Mexican women may have culturally influenced fears R/T diet and fetal harm

Now Can You:
- Discuss preconception care
- Identify substances to be avoided
- Discuss aspects of good nutrition
- Discuss work, fatigue, and medication use
- Identify common discomforts of pregnancy
- Identify danger signs in pregnancy

Caring for the Woman Experiencing Complications During Pregnancy

 Apprehension, uncertainty, waiting, expectation, fear of surprise, do a patient more harm than exertion.

—Florence Nightingale, 1860

LEARNING TARGETS *At the completion of this chapter, the student will be able to:*

◆ Describe the roles of the perinatologist, neonatologist, obstetric nurse, visiting nurse, diabetes educator, chaplain, nutritionist, and social worker in caring for the family experiencing complications during a pregnancy.

◆ Discuss the importance of understanding and respecting the cultural differences the nurse may encounter when caring for a diverse population experiencing a high-risk pregnancy.

◆ Plan nursing assessments and interventions for the woman experiencing complications of pregnancy.

◆ Discuss the importance of complete and accurate documentation in caring for the patient experiencing an obstetric emergency.

◆ Identify complications of pregnancy that require fetal surveillance, and describe various fetal surveillance modalities.

◆ Relate the effects of antenatal bedrest to the physical, psychological, and social adjustment of a high-risk pregnancy.

PICO(T) Questions

The intent of evidence-based practice (EBP) is to provide nursing care that integrates the best available evidence. An initial step in EBP is to write a PICO(T) question that effectively guides the research. A PICO(T) question is an acronym that stands for population (P), intervention or issue (I), comparison of interest (C), outcome (O), and timeframe (T). Depending on the question, all or some of the question components are used in the research process.

Use these PICO(T) questions to spark your thinking as you read the chapter.

1. Are (P) women with multifetal pregnancies (I) at greater risk for (O) gestational diabetes than (C) women who are pregnant with a single fetus?

2. Are (P) women who have a miscarriage with their first pregnancy (I) more likely to (O) have another miscarriage (C) than women who have a miscarriage with their second pregnancy?

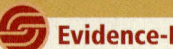

Evidence-Based Practice

Loprinzi, P. D., Fitzgerald, E. M., & Cardinal, B. J. (2012). Physical activity and depression symptoms among pregnant women from the National Health and Nutrition Examination Survey 2005–2006. *Journal of Obstetric, Gynecologic, and Neonatal Nursing, 41,* 227–235.

The purpose of this study was to examine objectively measured physical activity and the occurrence of depression symptoms in a national sample of pregnant women. According to the literature review, the rate of depression among pregnant women is approximately 20%. Most women are unlikely to be routinely screened for depression during pregnancy or receive effective treatment for the condition. Previous research has indicated that women who experience depression during pregnancy have a greater risk for postpartum depression. While antidepressant mediations can reduce the rate of depression in the general population, the safe use of antidepressants during pregnancy has generally not been well established. Hence, alternate strategies such as physical activity should be explored as a modality to complement or supplement traditional therapies for maternal depression. The American Congress of Obstetricians and Gynecologists (ACOG) recommends a pregnancy regimen of at least 30 minutes of physical activity each day on most if not all days of the week.

The study sample included 141 pregnant women selected from data obtained through the National Health and Nutrition Examination Survey (NHANES) 2005–2006. The NHANES data obtained on each participant included results from an accelerometer (a device that provides an objective measure of the frequency, intensity, and duration of physical activity); this information served to overcome the limitations of participant self-report.

Participants were asked to wear the accelerometer during a 7-day period. Daily physical activity recommendations were based on those recommended by the U.S. Department of Health and Human Services and included 150 minutes of moderate intensity activity plus 75 minutes of vigorous intensity activity, or a combination of both. To be included in the analysis, participants must have logged at least 4 days with 10 or more hours of accelerometer monitoring per day.

The participants were also asked to complete the Patient Health Questionnaire-9 (PHQ-9), which is a self-administered 9-item depression-screening module that includes a 4-point Likert-type scale. The PHQ-9 depression scale is composed of the nine criteria on which the diagnosis of *DSM-IV* depressive disorders is based. Possible responses are *not at all* (0), *several days* (1), *more than half the days* (2), and *nearly every day* (3) and when summed, a range of 0 to 27 points are possible. Severity of depression was defined as *no depression* (0–4), *mild depression* (5–9), *moderate depression* (10–14), *moderately severe depression* (15–19), and *severe depression* (20–27). None of the participants were classified as having severe depression; two were determined to have moderately severe depression, three were determined to have moderate depression, and 22 were determined to have mild depression.

Descriptive statistics were used to compare population characteristics. No significant differences were found among the demographic data of the women determined to have some depression, as compared with those having none. Demographic characteristics included height, weight, BMI, race-ethnicity, smoking status, marital status, and weeks of gestation. Women classified as not having depressive symptoms (n=114) spent more time involved in moderate-intensity and moderate to vigorous intensity physical activity than those found to have some depression (n=27). Nineteen percent of the participants were found to have some depression symptoms. The researchers reported that their findings are consistent with previously completed research and demonstrated an inverse association between physical activity and depression symptoms.

1. How is this information useful to clinical nursing practice?
2. Based on these findings, what are implications for further research?

See Suggested Responses for Evidence-Based Practice on Davis*Plus.*

Introduction

Pregnancy is a normal physiological function of all living species. People who have chosen to become parents look forward to having a healthy, happy, and bright newborn enter their lives. They anticipate the arrival of a baby whom they will be able to love and nurture over the years to grow into a happy, healthy, productive adult. However, pregnancies do not always progress smoothly, and the pregnant woman and her family or significant other may experience a complication at some point during the childbearing year. Complications that arise during this time are often challenging and demanding for the perinatal nurse. The nurse must apply skills, knowledge, and expertise combined with the nursing process to first identify the pregnant patient at risk and then formulate, implement, and evaluate an appropriate, holistic plan of care. Identification and activation of appropriate community resources are also essential components of the care plan. Throughout the entire process, the nurse must remain cognizant of the unique individuality of the patient and her family and deliver care that is respectful of their diversity and culture.

Interviewing is a skill basic to nursing. A carefully conducted interview is a tool that enables nurses to collect data, recognize signs and symptoms of emerging problems, identify risks, and formulate nursing diagnoses and counseling strategies. The signs and symptoms of the complications that may arise during pregnancy can be subtle. The nurse's need to elicit information from the patient through the interview and to process that information cannot be overemphasized. Anticipatory nursing care is invaluable in preventing a complication from becoming a major health crisis. Notifying the primary health-care provider immediately of signs or symptoms of alterations from the expected clinical progression during pregnancy can facilitate early intervention and guide an appropriate management plan.

The complications described in this chapter can be extremely serious to both the patient and her fetus and result in severe morbidity or even death. It is essential that women feel comfortable and confident with the care they receive. Maternal health care often represents the first point of contact between immigrant women and the U.S. health-care system. Because many do not speak and/or read English, the nurse must facilitate an interview in the woman's primary language. Use of the woman's native language greatly increases her level of comfort and acceptance and is paramount to establishing an accurate diagnosis and appropriate plan of care. When indicated, every effort should be made to secure a female interpreter who is not a member of the family. In most cases, children are not suitable translators, because many assessment questions involve subjects that women may not wish to discuss with their children or with men. Friends and family members who serve as interpreters are not bound by a code of conduct and may breach confidentiality, editorialize, omit information they find threatening or embarrassing, or jeopardize the woman's privacy. By providing culturally competent nursing care to childbearing families, many potential complications can be identified in a timely manner to allow for effective treatment and improved outcomes.

EARLY PREGNANCY COMPLICATIONS

Perinatal Loss

Perinatal loss can be divided into two major types: death of the fetus or newborn or birth of a less than perfect child. The perinatal period encompasses the total embryonic, fetal, and neonatal life span. Because there is a greater danger to life during this period than at any other time during the life cycle, adverse outcomes can be expected. Loss of a child,

whether it is an embryo, fetus, or neonate, can be totally devastating not only to the woman but to the entire family. Supporting the family through a perinatal loss can be very challenging to the obstetric nurse who must be in touch with personal feelings to help understand the family's response to their loss (see Chapter 14 for further discussion).

"What to say"—*Communicating with the family who has experienced a perinatal loss*

The nurse approaches the family with compassion and sincerity. Expressions of caring are conveyed in the following statements:

"I understand this is a very difficult time for you and your family, but I want you to know that I am here and willing to listen if you want to talk. You let me know if and when you are ready."

"It is normal for you to be sad, and you will probably feel like this for some time. Losing a baby, no matter how far along in your pregnancy, is very difficult. I can recommend some support groups if you think you might be interested." If the patient says she does not want the information at this time, continue with "Please do not hesitate to call us if you change your mind. We can always give you the information."

"Does your baby have a name?" The nurse would then refer to the fetus by name. Do not use the term "fetus" with the patient. To her, the deceased fetus was her baby.

ECTOPIC PREGNANCY

An ectopic pregnancy is one where the fertilized egg implants outside the uterine cavity. Implantation may occur in the fallopian tube (99%), on the ovary, on the cervix, on the outside of the fallopian tube, on the abdominal wall, or on the bowel (Fig. 11-1). Patients who present with vaginal bleeding, a missed period, or abdominal tenderness or pain should always be evaluated for an ectopic pregnancy. Pain increases after rupture of the ectopic pregnancy, and the woman may experience referred shoulder

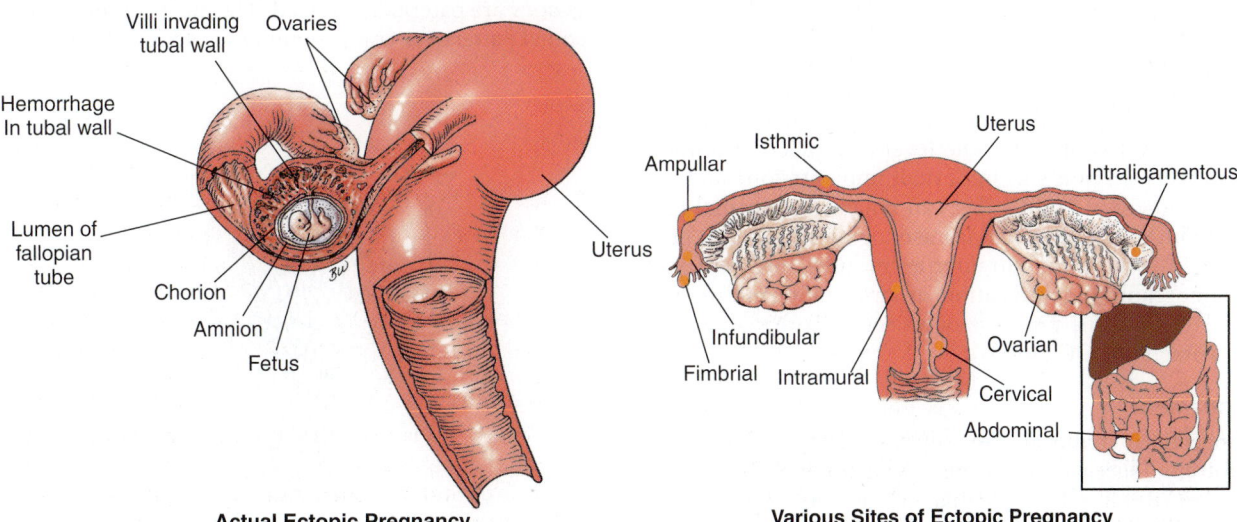

Actual Ectopic Pregnancy

Various Sites of Ectopic Pregnancy

Figure 11-1 Ectopic pregnancy.

pain from diaphragmatic irritation caused by blood in the peritoneal cavity.

A number of factors place a woman at risk for experiencing an ectopic pregnancy. These include past and current medical and gynecological problems such as:

- History of sexually transmitted infections or pelvic inflammatory disease
- Prior ectopic pregnancy
- Previous tubal, pelvic, or abdominal surgery
- Endometriosis
- Current use of exogenous hormones (e.g., estrogen and progesterone)
- Use of an intrauterine device
- In vitro fertilization or other method of assisted reproduction
- In utero diethylstilbestrol (DES) exposure with abnormalities of the reproductive organs

 Nursing Insight—*Heterotopic pregnancy*

Heterotopic pregnancy (HP) is the existence of two (or more) simultaneous pregnancies with separate implantation sites, one of which is ectopic. HP occurs in approximately 1 in 10,000 to 30,000 pregnancies, as compared with ectopic pregnancy, which occurs in about 2% of all pregnancies in the United States. The incidence of HP is higher in recipients of assisted reproductive technology, women with a history of pelvic inflammatory disease, and those who have undergone reconstructive tubal surgery. Although most cases of HP occur in the fallopian tube, other sites include the cervix and the cesarean delivery scar (Pippitt & Stoesser, 2011).

Diagnosis

To prevent major morbidity or death, an ectopic pregnancy should be diagnosed before the onset of hypotension, bleeding, pain, and overt rupture. The patient's history (e.g., unilateral, bilateral, or diffuse abdominal pain and missed period) and physical exam (a palpable mass is present on bimanual examination in approximately 50% of women) should alert the health-care professional to the possible presence of an ectopic pregnancy. Active bleeding is associated with rupture; other symptoms of this complication may include hypotension, tachycardia, vertigo, and shoulder pain. Diagnostic laboratory tests include a beta-human chorionic gonadotropin (β-hCG) that is low for gestational age (because an ectopic pregnancy has a poorly implanted placenta, the level of β-hCG does not double every 48 hours as in normal implantation) and a white blood count (WBC) that can range from normal to 15,000/mm^3. Transvaginal ultrasonography should be performed to confirm intrauterine or tubal pregnancy. Ultrasonographic identification of an intrauterine pregnancy rules out the presence of an ectopic pregnancy in most women (ACOG, 2008a).

Management

Salpingectomy (removal of the ruptured fallopian tube) by **laparotomy** (surgical procedure in which the abdomen is opened to visualize the abdominal organs) has long offered an almost 100% cure for the treatment of an ectopic pregnancy. However, current clinical emphasis is aimed not only on prevention of maternal death but also on the

prompt restoration of health through a rapid recovery with preservation of fertility. To achieve this goal, **laparoscopy** (visualization of the reproductive organs using a laparoscope inserted into the pelvic cavity through a small incision in the abdomen), **salpingostomy** (incision into the fallopian tube to remove the pregnancy), and partial salpingectomy are replacing laparotomy as the treatment mode of choice. At present, laparotomy is performed only when a laparoscopic approach is too difficult, the surgeon is not trained in operative laparoscopy, or the patient is hemodynamically unstable.

Methotrexate, a chemotherapeutic drug and folic acid inhibitor that stops cell production and destroys remaining trophoblastic tissue, is used in the management of uncomplicated, non–life-threatening ectopic pregnancies. Patients are considered to be eligible for methotrexate therapy if the ectopic mass is unruptured and measures 1.6 in. (4 cm) or less on ultrasound examination. Patients with larger ectopic masses, embryonic cardiac activity, or clinical evidence of acute intra-abdominal bleeding (acute tender abdomen, hypotension, or falling hematocrit) are not eligible for this mode of treatment (ACOG, 2008a; Skubisz & Tong, 2011).

GESTATIONAL TROPHOBLASTIC DISEASE

Gestational trophoblastic disease (GTD) is a clinical diagnosis that includes the histological diagnoses of hydatidiform mole ("molar pregnancy"), locally invasive mole, metastatic mole, and choriocarcinoma. It is a disease characterized by an abnormal placental development that results in the production of fluid-filled grapelike clusters (instead of normal placental tissue) and a vast proliferation of trophoblastic tissue (Fig. 11-2). It is associated with loss of the pregnancy and, rarely, the development of cancer. GTD occurs in 1 in 1,200 pregnancies (Cohn, Ramaswamy, & Blum, 2013).

Pathophysiology

The cause of molar pregnancy is unknown, but it is thought that complete moles result from the fertilization of an empty ovum (one whose nucleus is missing or nonfunctional) by a normal sperm. Because the ovum contains no maternal genetic material, all chromosomes in a molar pregnancy are paternally derived. The most common chromosomal pattern for complete moles is 46 XX. A complete

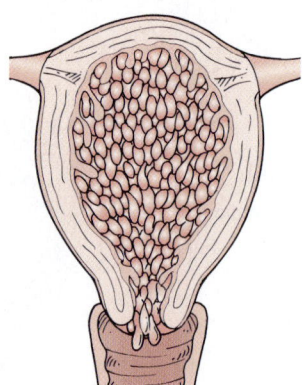

Figure 11-2 A hydatidiform mole pregnancy is one in which the chorionic villi degenerate into a mass of fluid-filled grapelike clusters.

mole is characterized by trophoblastic proliferation and the absence of fetal parts. Incomplete moles often appear with a coexistent fetus that has a triploid genotype (69 chromosomes) and multiple anomalies. Most fetuses associated with incomplete moles survive only several weeks in utero before being spontaneously aborted. Incomplete moles are almost always benign and have a much lower malignancy potential than complete moles. An invasive mole is similar to a complete mole but has invaded the myometrium layer of the uterus. Invasive moles rarely metastasize. Choriocarcinoma is an invasive, malignant trophoblastic disease that is usually metastatic and can be fatal (ACOG, 2004a; Cohn et al., 2013; Genovese, 2011; Marcus, 2011).

Risk Factors

The incidence of hydatidiform mole, whether complete or partial, increases with maternal age (especially in women 50 or older) and in those with a history of a previous molar pregnancy. The risk for a second molar pregnancy is 1% to 2%, whereas the risk for a third molar pregnancy after two previous molar pregnancies is approximately 2.5%. Higher incidences have been found in geographical areas where the maternal diet is low in beta-carotene, animal fats, and folic acid and also in women with blood type A whose partners are of blood type O. There is also a higher incidence among women who have experienced prior miscarriages and in those who have undergone ovulation stimulation with clomiphene (Clomid) (ACOG, 2004a; Genovese, 2011).

Signs and Symptoms

More than 95% of patients experience vaginal bleeding that may be scant or profuse and ranges in color from dark brown to bright red. In early pregnancy, there is often a discrepancy between uterine size and dates. Uterine enlargement results from the rapidly proliferating trophoblastic tissue and the large accumulation of clotted blood. Anemia may result from the blood loss. Also, the patient may complain of excessive nausea and vomiting (hyperemesis gravidarum) and abdominal pain caused by uterine distention. Preeclampsia may occur earlier in pregnancy, usually between 9 and 12 weeks of gestation, but any symptoms of gestational hypertension before 24 weeks of gestation may be indicative of hydatidiform mole. Clinical and laboratory findings include an absence of fetal heart sounds, a markedly elevated quantitative serum hCG (may be greater than 100,000 mIU/mL), and very low levels of maternal serum α-fetoprotein (MSAFP). Hyperthyroidism and trophoblastic pulmonary emboli are less common but serious complications of hydatidiform mole (Cunningham, Leveno, Bloom, Spong, & Dashe, 2014).

Diagnosis

The diagnosis of a molar pregnancy is made by an ultrasound examination. The placental tissue appears in a "snowstorm" pattern because of the profuse swelling of the chorionic villi. When a complete mole is present, no fetus is identified in the uterus.

Management

Clinical management involves removal of the uterine contents with meticulous follow-up that includes serial ß-hCG levels. A sensitive marker, hCG is secreted by the molar cells. The amount of this hormone measured in maternal serum is directly related to the number of viable molar cells. The hCG levels should be assessed every 1 to 2 weeks until hCG is undetectable on two consecutive determinations. Thereafter, hCG should be measured every 1 to 2 months for at least a year (ACOG, 2004a; Cunningham et al., 2014). Effective contraception is needed during this time to prevent pregnancy and the resulting confusion about the cause of changes in the hCG levels. In addition, pregnancy could mask an hCG rise associated with malignant GTD. The perinatal nurse should carefully counsel the patient about different methods of contraception and stress the importance of avoiding pregnancy for a year. During a subsequent pregnancy, first trimester sonography should be performed to confirm that the pregnancy is normal (Goldstein, Baron, & Berkowitz, 2010).

 Collaboration in Caring—*Dealing with a molar pregnancy*

With any pregnancy loss, a challenging situation exists. However, the couple experiencing a molar pregnancy not only must realize that there will be no baby, but attempts at becoming pregnant must be delayed for at least a year. There is also the fear of malignant sequelae. The perinatal nurse's role is to support the couple, educate them regarding their contraceptive options, encourage them to voice their fears and concerns, and answer their questions appropriately. Involving community resources such as social services, support groups, and spiritual advisors can be of significant benefit.

Chemotherapy is initiated immediately if the hCG titer rises or plateaus during follow-up or if **metastases** (movement of cancer cells from the original site to another site) are detected at any time. Surgery may be indicated if chemotherapy is not successful or for patients who have completed their childbearing. Radiation therapy is usually reserved for treating brain and liver metastases (Cunningham et al., 2014).

Prognosis

Invasive moles are generally not metastatic and respond well to single-agent chemotherapy. Choriocarcinoma spreads to the lungs, vagina, pelvis, brain, liver, intestines, and kidneys. Because choriocarcinoma can occur weeks to years after any type of gestation, patients usually present with signs and symptoms of active metastases. The long-term prognosis depends on the degree of metastases and the patient's response to the chemotherapy.

SPONTANEOUS ABORTION

Not all conceptions result in a live-born infant. Of all clinically recognized pregnancies, 12% to 15% are lost, and approximately 22% of pregnancies detected on the basis of hCG assays are lost before the appearance of any clinical signs or symptoms. By definition, an early pregnancy loss occurs before 12 weeks of gestation; a late pregnancy loss is one that occurs between 12 and 20 weeks of gestation.

A **spontaneous abortion** (SAB) or miscarriage is a pregnancy that ends before 20 weeks gestation. The type of SAB that occurs is defined by whether any or all products of conception (POC) have been passed and whether or not the cervix is dilated.

Terminology/classifications associated with spontaneous abortions include the following:

- **Abortus**: Fetus lost before 20 weeks of gestation, less than 17.5 oz (500 g), or less than 9.8 in. (25 cm) in size
- **Complete abortion**: Complete expulsion of all POC before 20 weeks of gestation
- **Incomplete abortion**: Partial expulsion of some but not all POC before 20 weeks of gestation
- **Inevitable abortion**: No expulsion of products, but bleeding and dilation of the cervix such that continuation of a pregnancy is unlikely
- **Threatened abortion**: Any intrauterine bleeding before 20 weeks of gestation, without dilation of the cervix or expulsion of any POC
- **Missed abortion**: Death of the embryo or fetus before 20 weeks of gestation with complete retention of the POC; these often proceed to a complete abortion within 1 to 3 weeks, but occasionally they are retained much longer.
- **Septic abortion**: POC become infected during the abortion process
- **Recurrent abortion**: Two or more successive pregnancies have ended in spontaneous abortion

Etiology

It is estimated that 60% to 80% of all SABs in the first trimester are associated with chromosomal abnormalities. Infections (e.g., bacteriuria and *C trachomatis*), maternal anatomical defects, and immunological and endocrine factors have also been identified as causes of early pregnancy loss, although many have no obvious cause. Second-trimester spontaneous abortions (12 to 20 weeks) have been linked to chronic infection, recreational drug use, maternal uterine or cervical anatomical defects, maternal systemic disease, exposure to fetotoxic agents, and trauma (Cunningham et al., 2014).

Diagnosis

A woman who is experiencing an SAB usually presents with bleeding and may also complain of cramping, abdominal pain, and decreased symptoms of pregnancy; cervical changes (dilation) may be present on vaginal examination. An ultrasound is performed for placental evaluation and to determine fetal viability. Laboratory tests include a quantitative level of ß-hCG, which should show a lower value than when associated with a viable pregnancy (Fig. 11-3); hemoglobin and hematocrit levels; blood type and Rh status determination; and indirect Coombs' screen (Cunningham et al., 2014).

Management

Incomplete, inevitable, and missed abortions are usually managed via a dilation and curettage (D and C: the cervix is dilated and a curette is inserted and used to scrape the uterine walls and remove the uterine contents). In the case of an incompetent cervix, an emergent **cerclage** (placement of ligature to close the cervix) may be performed. An unsensitized, Rh(D)-negative woman should be given Rh$_o$(D) immune globulin (RhoGAM) to prevent antibody formation. (See discussion later in this chapter.)

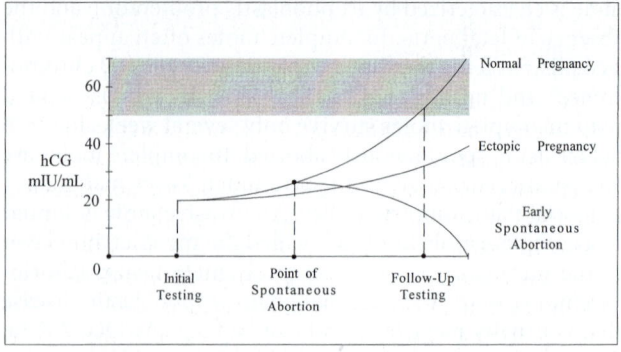

Figure 11-3 hCG levels.

Depending on the circumstances, the nurse can provide counseling or make an appropriate referral. Not all couples who suffer a pregnancy loss require formal assessment, but all couples should be offered a formal evaluation after several losses. The nurse should also allow the family to express as much grief as they are feeling at the moment and are willing to share, allow them to talk freely of what their hopes and expectations had been for this new life, and acknowledge that this is a very difficult time for them. The nurse may offer to enlist the assistance of social services, a chaplain, a rabbi, or appropriate support groups if the couple so desires.

> **⟲ Optimizing Outcomes**—Follow-up for women who experience habitual abortions
>
> Patients who experience habitual (three or more) abortions may be offered these tests:
>
> - A karyotype obtained from the POC and from both parents
> - Examination of maternal anatomy, beginning with a hysterosalpingogram; if abnormal, hysteroscopy or laparoscopy
> - Screening tests for maternal hypothyroidism, diabetes mellitus, antiphospholipid syndrome (APS; an acquired hypercoagulable state that involves venous and arteriole thrombosis) and systemic lupus erythematosus (SLE)
> - Serum progesterone level during the luteal phase of the menstrual cycle
> - Cultures of the cervix, vagina, and endometrium
> - Endometrial biopsy during the luteal phase of the menstrual cycle (Cunningham et al., 2014)

CERVICAL INSUFFICIENCY/CERVICAL INCOMPETENCE

The American College of Obstetricians and Gynecologists (ACOG) (2014) defines cervical insufficiency as "the inability of the uterine cervix to retain a pregnancy to term." Historically, cervical incompetence was defined as passive, painless cervical dilation in the second trimester of pregnancy, with no labor, bleeding, or chorioamnionitis (infection). Patients with cervical insufficiency/incompetence frequently give a history of repeated second trimester losses with no apparent etiology. Incompetent cervix is estimated to cause approximately 15% of all second trimester losses (Cunningham et al., 2014).

Nursing Insight—*Identifying clues when taking the patient history*

The importance of knowing your patient's history cannot be overemphasized. Remember to read the prenatal records and also question your patient about all previous pregnancies and their outcomes. Because we live in such a mobile society, prenatal records may not always be available. A woman who is visiting on vacation or who has recently moved into the community often has no prenatal records with her. Many communities regularly see pregnant women seeking refuge from a war-torn country who arrive at the hospital with no records or who have had no prenatal care. You may also need to work with a medical interpreter to obtain an accurate history that can provide insights into present problems.

Etiology and Diagnosis

Reduced cervical competence can be acquired (i.e., after trauma or surgery) or congenital (i.e., resulting from uterine anomalies or a history of DES exposure). The patient may provide a typical history of recurrent mid-pregnancy deliveries without presenting contractions, membrane rupture, or infection. Sometimes women experience painless cervical dilation in the first and every subsequent pregnancy; others experience a progressively earlier delivery with each pregnancy until a typical "incompetent" history occurs (Berghella, 2010a).

Because the current ACOG criteria for cervical insufficiency requires a history of multiple pregnancy losses, some experts have advocated that transvaginal ultrasound (TVU) cervical length (CL) assessment could be used to aid in the diagnosis of this condition. The presence of both criteria—one or more prior early preterm births and/or second-trimester losses along with TVU CL less than 25 mm, *or* cervical dilation (e.g., greater than or equal to 1 cm) on digital vaginal examination before 24 weeks in the current pregnancy—may arouse suspicion of cervical insufficiency. TVU is also useful in demonstrating funneling and shortening of the CL or effacement of the internal cervical os (ACOG, 2012b, 2014; Berghella, 2010; Berghella & Mackeen, 2011).

 Nursing Insight—*Appreciating the dynamic characteristics of the cervix during pregnancy*

In modern times, the pregnant cervix has come to be viewed as a dynamic organ, with incompetence occurring along a continuum as a result of multiple factors such as infection, hormonal changes, inflammation, and genetic predisposition. Transvaginal ultrasonography has become the "gold standard" for cervical evaluation. During pregnancy, the cervix follows a predictable pattern of effacement and dilation. Effacement begins at the internal cervical os and progresses in a "funneling" manner toward the external cervical os. On ultrasound examination, this process initially appears as a Y-shaped "beaking" of the cervical canal sidewalls that develops into a U-shaped space. The CL normally remains stable until the early third trimester and shortens progressively thereafter (Thompson & Keehbauch, 2009).

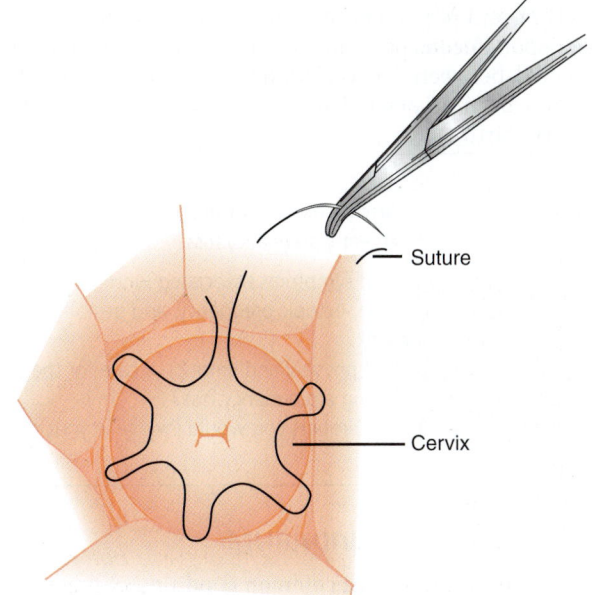

Figure 11-4 Cerclage.

Management

Management may include TVU CL screening and/or the vaginal placement of a cerclage, or pursestring suture, that is put beneath the cervical mucosa either at the cervical–vaginal junction (a McDonald cerclage) (Fig. 11-4) or at the internal cervical os (a Shirodkar cerclage). The intent of the cerclage is to close the cervix. The cerclage is usually removed in the office or clinic at 37 weeks of gestation to facilitate vaginal birth. A new cerclage will need to be placed with subsequent pregnancies. The cerclage may also be left in place, necessitating a cesarean delivery. Sometimes a cerclage is placed via an abdominal incision. It may be placed electively before pregnancy or at 12 to 14 weeks of gestation or as an emergency procedure.

Patients who have an abdominal cerclage must give birth via cesarean section. Before and after cerclage placement, prophylactic **tocolytics** (medications used in an attempt to stop labor) may be given to prevent uterine contractions. Bedrest is an important part of the expectant management, and patients may also be placed on home uterine activity monitoring, although according to ACOG (2012c), the U.S. Preventive Services Task Force (1996), and the National Institute of Child Health and Human Development (2002), portable monitors that detect uterine contractions do not appear to be useful for identifying women likely to have a preterm delivery. Depending on the gestational age and imminence of delivery, patients may receive betamethasone, a glucocorticoid shown to decrease the chance of respiratory distress syndrome in premature infants.

Based on findings from a recent (2011) meta-analysis, Berghella and Mackeen concluded that singleton gestations in women with prior preterm birth might be monitored safely with TVU CL screening. The researchers also suggested that cerclage placement be reserved for the minority of women who actually develop a short CL. According to a 2014 ACOG practice bulletin, ". . . short cervical length has been shown to be a marker of preterm birth in general rather than a specific marker of cervical insufficiency"

(p. 372), and placement of a cerclage in women without a prior spontaneous preterm birth and a CL less than 25 mm detected between 16 weeks and 24 weeks of gestation has not been associated with a significant reduction in preterm birth.

 Now Can You—Discuss the care of the patient experiencing an early pregnancy loss?

1. Name three signs and symptoms associated with spontaneous abortion, ectopic pregnancy, and gestational trophoblastic disease?
2. Describe your plan of physical and emotional care for the patient who is suffering a pregnancy loss?
3. Identify other team members you would involve in your plan of care?

HYPEREMESIS GRAVIDARUM

Nausea and vomiting is a common condition of pregnancy that affects 70% to 85% of pregnant women and usually resolves by the 16th week of gestation. **Hyperemesis gravidarum** represents the extreme end of the nausea/vomiting spectrum in terms of severity. Criteria for the diagnosis of hyperemesis gravidarum include persistent vomiting unrelated to other causes, a measure of acute starvation (usually large ketonuria), and some discrete weight loss, most often 5% of the prepregnancy weight. Hyperemesis gravidarum is the most common indication for admission to the hospital during the first part of pregnancy and is second only to preterm labor as the most common reason for hospitalization during pregnancy (ACOG, 2004b).

Etiology and Risk Factors

Although the exact etiology of nausea and vomiting of pregnancy is unknown, several theories have been proposed. Hyperemesis gravidarum may be related to the elevated levels of estrogen or hCG, or it may be associated with the transient elevation of thyroid hormone during pregnancy. Others have hypothesized a relationship between hyperemesis and the intrinsic hormones of the gastrointestinal tract (Cunningham et al., 2014). Psychological and metabolic causes have also been explored, and recent research suggests an inherited genetic component to this poorly understood condition (Zhang, Cantor, MacGibbon, Romero, Goodwin, Mullin, et al., 2011).

Risk factors include an increased placental mass associated with multiple gestation and molar pregnancy, a history of hyperemesis gravidarum in a previous pregnancy, and a history of motion sickness or migraine headaches. Daughters and sisters of women who experienced hyperemesis gravidarum and women who are pregnant with a female child are also considered to be at risk (ACOG, 2004b).

Maternal and Fetal Effects

In contrast to the early part of the 1900s, maternal mortality is rare today with very few cases reported. Serious complications of hyperemesis gravidarum for the woman and fetus arise in the group of women who cannot maintain their weight despite antiemetic therapy. In addition to increased hospital admissions, some women experience psychosocial morbidity of such significance that they feel compelled to terminate the pregnancy. Depression, **somatization** (the conversion of mental experiences into physical symptoms), and hypochondriasis can also be a problem for some women (ACOG, 2004b). The effects on the embryo and fetus depend on the severity of the condition. Significant maternal weight loss may be associated with fetal intrauterine growth restriction (IUGR).

 Nursing Insight—*Intrauterine growth restriction/fetal growth restriction*

Intrauterine growth restriction (IUGR), also known as fetal growth restriction, refers to the inability of a fetus to achieve full growth potential while in utero. A common complication of pregnancy, IUGR has been associated with a variety of adverse perinatal outcomes. Around the world, various definitions of IUGR are accepted: abdominal circumference below the 10th or 5th pecentile; weight at birth less than 2500 g; and estimated fetal weight less than 10th percentile. IUGR may be related to genetic factors (e.g., trisomy 13 and trisomy 18), congenital anomalies (e.g., 2-vessel umbilical cord), infection (e.g., cytomegalovirus, rubella, and toxoplasmosis), multiple gestation, maternal malnutrition, environmental toxins (e.g., maternal cigarette smoking and excessive alcohol ingestion), placental factors (e.g., uteroplacental insufficiency), and maternal vascular disease related to medical conditions (e.g., diabetes, chronic hypertension, and morbid obesity). A primary goal for fetal specialists who care for the growth-restricted fetus centers on ensuring fetal well-being and determining the optimal timing for delivery (ACOG, 2013a; Tate & Mari, 2013).

Management

Women with a history of nausea and vomiting in a previous pregnancy are advised to regularly take multivitamins before the next conception. Rest is encouraged. The nurse should counsel the woman to avoid foods and sensory stimuli that provoke symptoms (e.g., some women become nauseous when they smell certain foods being prepared) and also to eat small frequent meals of dry, bland foods and include high-protein snacks in their diet. Spicy foods should be avoided. Eating crackers before arising in the morning may be of benefit, and ginger capsules have been shown to be effective. If the patient requires hospitalization, IV fluids containing dextrose and vitamins are given, and the patient is placed on a nothing by mouth status and treated with antiemetics (Box 11-1). Parenteral or enteral feedings may be ordered if the patient is unable to take oral nourishment and if normal weight gain parameters for the gestation of pregnancy are not being achieved (ACOG, 2004b).

 Complementary Care: *Nausea and Vomiting of Pregnancy*

Ginger, a perennial native to many Asian countries, has been found to be effective in treating nausea and vomiting during pregnancy. The antiemetic effect of this root (taken in a dosage of 250 mg 4 times daily) is related to its ability to increase gastrointestinal motility. Ginger is available in tablet, capsule, and syrup form. Some concerns about taking ginger during pregnancy have been raised, but to date no significant side effects have been documented. For some women, behavioral therapy such as relaxation, hypnosis, and psychotherapy may be beneficial.

Elasticized wristbands (e.g., Sea-Bands®) that use a firm object to place pressure on the Neiguan point (acupressure P6 point) are a nonpharmacological, noninvasive method that may lessen the frequency and severity of nausea and vomiting during pregnancy. A similar modality, acu-stimulation, is delivered by a bracelet-type, battery-operated device that also stimulates the skin at the P6 acupressure point. Marketed as the "Reliefband," the FDA-approved device allows users to adjust the intensity of the electrical stimulation via a rotary dial on the band (Nayeri, 2012).

Hemorrhagic Disorders

Hemorrhagic disorders constitute an obstetric emergency and are a leading cause of maternal death in the United States. Third-trimester vaginal bleeding occurs in 3% to 4% of all pregnancies and may be obstetric or nonobstetric in nature (Cunningham et al., 2014). Examples of nonobstetric causes include severe cervicitis, benign and malignant neoplasms, lacerations, and varices.

 clinical alert

Early identification of maternal hemorrhage

During pregnancy, the woman's blood volume increases 50%, and in the case of multiple gestation, it increases as much as 100%. Because of this expanded blood volume, the patient may be asymptomatic and exhibit vital signs that remain within normal parameters despite a large amount of blood loss. Blood pressure is a very poor indicator of blood volume deficit. The maternal pulse (tachycardia) and/or fetal heart rate (bradycardia or tachycardia) may be the first indicators of maternal instability.

Obstetric Causes of Vaginal Bleeding

PLACENTA PREVIA

Placenta previa is an implantation of the placenta in the lower uterine segment, near or over the internal cervical os. This condition accounts for 20% of all antepartal hemorrhages. There are three recognized variations of placenta previa. With a **complete (total) placenta previa**, the placenta covers the entire cervical os. Because it is associated with the greatest amount of blood loss, a complete placenta previa presents the most serious risk. A **partial placenta previa** describes a placenta that partially occludes the cervical os. A **marginal placenta previa** is characterized by the encroachment of the placenta to the margin of the cervical os, and a low-lying placenta is one that is implanted in the lower uterine segment in close proximity to the internal cervical os (Fig. 11-5). **Placenta accreta**, **placenta percreta**, and **placenta increta** are placentas with abnormally firm attachments to the uterine wall. Unusual placental adherence may accompany a placenta previa (ACOG, 2012a).

Placenta previa may be associated with conditions that cause scarring of the uterus such as a prior cesarean birth or previous abortions with curettage. A placenta previa may also occur with a large placental mass as seen in multiple gestations, diabetes, and erythroblastosis fetalis. Other risk factors include smoking, cocaine use, a prior history of placenta previa, closely spaced pregnancies, African or Asian ethnicity, and maternal age greater than 40 years (Genovese, 2011; Hull & Resnik, 2013).

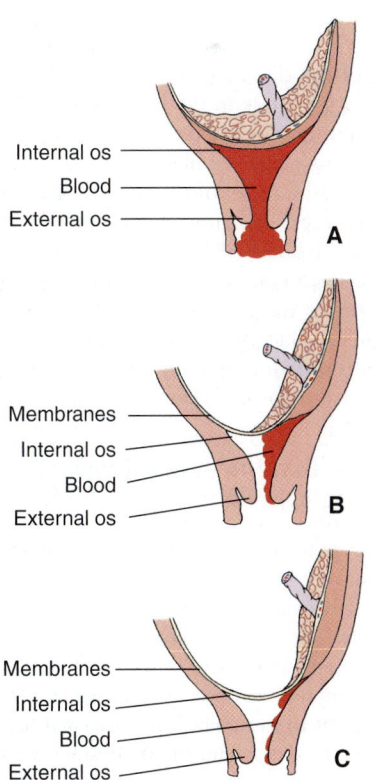

Figure 11-5 Placenta previa. *A,* Complete (Total). *B,* Partial. *C,* Marginal/Low lying.

Signs and Symptoms

The most common symptom is painless vaginal bleeding. This is believed to occur from small disruptions in the placental attachment during normal development and the subsequent stretching and thinning of the lower uterine segment during the third trimester. Initially, the bleeding is usually a small amount that stops as the uterus contracts to close the open blood vessels. However, bleeding can reoccur at any time and may be associated with profuse hemorrhage and shock that leads to significant maternal and fetal morbidity and mortality. The blood is bright red. Painful bleeding may occur if the placenta abrupts away from the uterine tissue (Cunningham et al., 2014; Genovese, 2011).

Maternal and Fetal Morbidity and Mortality

Premature delivery is responsible for 60% of perinatal deaths associated with placenta previa. Other fetal risks include preterm premature rupture of the membranes, IUGR, malpresentation, congenital anomalies, and **vasa previa.** Vasa previa is a condition in which the umbilical cord is implanted into the membranes rather than the placenta. The vessels traverse within the membranes and cross the cervical os before reaching the placenta. The umbilical blood vessels are at risk for laceration. The appearance of bright red blood at the time of rupture of the membranes should alert the nurse to the possibility of a vasa previa. Maternal risks associated with placenta previa are uterine rupture, the potential for emergency hysterectomy, postpartum hemorrhage (caused by placental implantation in the less muscular, lower uterine segment, which contracts poorly and lacerates easily during delivery and manual removal of the placenta), shock (from significant blood loss), and death (Cunningham et al., 2014; Genovese, 2011; Pacheco, Saade, Tyner, Clark, & Hankins, 2012).

Diagnosis

The timing of the diagnosis of placenta previa has undergone significant change in the last decade. Although third-trimester bleeding was often the first indicator of placenta previa, today most cases of placenta previa are detected antenatally before the onset of significant bleeding. The common practice of second-trimester abdominal ultrasound for the detection of fetal anomalies has led to this change. However, because most cases of placenta previa diagnosed in the second trimester tend to resolve as the uterus enlarges, management of placenta previa diagnosed in the second trimester differs from that for the same diagnosis made during the third trimester (Pacheco et al., 2012).

 Nursing Insight—*Second trimester ultrasonography for the diagnosis of placenta previa*

The widespread use of second trimester ultrasound for screening purposes may lead to a finding of placenta previa or low-lying placenta in otherwise asymptomatic women. Often, this finding is actually a false-positive because the maternal bladder filling used in transabdominal ultrasound may exaggerate the length of the cervix and compress the lower uterine segment. Thus, exact locations of the internal os and the lower placental edge are not accurately viewed on transabdominal sonography. The true diagnosis of placenta previa or low-lying placenta should be made by transvaginal ultrasound (TVU) on a patient whose bladder is empty. As an alternative, the TVU is delayed and the placental location is reevaluated at 28 to 32 weeks with a follow-up abdominal ultrasound. Approximately 80% of women with a placenta previa or low-lying placenta on TVU in the second trimester will no longer have the condition at term (Oyelese, 2010).

In patients diagnosed before 24 weeks' gestation, a repeat ultrasound should be scheduled between 24 and 28 weeks' gestation to confirm the diagnosis of placenta previa. However, if patients experience vaginal bleeding during this interval, they should be managed as presumed cases of placenta previa. Placenta previa should be suspected in all patients who present with bleeding after 24 completed weeks of gestation. Because of the risk of placental perforation, vaginal examinations are not performed. The nurse should advise any patient with a known or suspected placenta previa to inform medical personnel that vaginal exams are prohibited. Abdominal examination generally shows a nontender, soft uterus with normal tone. Leopold maneuvers often reveal the fetus to be in a breech or oblique position or transverse lie because of the abnormal location of the placenta.

Management of the pregnant woman who is experiencing active bleeding associated with a placenta previa requires astute assessment skills so that there is no delay in treatment. Delay can mean the difference between an optimal or poor outcome for the patient and her fetus. Stabilization involves the administration of IV fluids and a laboratory work-up that includes a complete blood count, prothrombin time, partial thromboplastin time, fibrin split products, and fibrinogen. A blood type and crossmatch should be obtained in anticipation of the need for a transfusion. A maternal **Kleihauer–Betke** blood test may be ordered to determine if there has been a transfer of fetal blood cells into the maternal circulation. If the patient is Rh negative and unsensitized, $Rh_o(D)$ immune globulin (RhoGAM) should be administered even if the blood type of the baby cannot be determined; RhoGAM will cause no harm to the woman or her fetus if the fetus is Rh(D)-negative. (See discussion later in this chapter.) The patient is placed on bedrest and the fetus is continuously assessed by electronic fetal monitoring. If time permits, betamethasone (a long-acting corticosteroid) may be administered (to the woman) to promote fetal lung maturity. Labor that cannot be halted, fetal compromise, and life-threatening maternal hemorrhage are indications for immediate delivery regardless of gestational age (Cunningham et al., 2014; Genovese, 2011; Wylie & D'Alton, 2010).

 Nursing Insight—*Recognizing maternal stress factors associated with placenta previa*

The nurse caring for women with placenta previa should recognize various manifestations of maternal stress associated with the diagnosis (e.g., anxiety, feelings of helplessness, fear of pregnancy loss, fear for self, confusion and panic, and difficulty in making decisions). Nurses can be instrumental in helping to assuage anxiety by speaking calmly to the patient and her support persons; carefully explaining her condition (using pictures, images, and other resources of the health-care team); describing planned interventions and why they are being performed; providing preparatory educational videotapes and reading materials regarding pregnancy, childbirth, infant care, and postpartum self-care; and offering reassurances and instructions for home care (when appropriate) (Genovese, 2011).

PLACENTAL ABRUPTION

Placental abruption (**abruptio placentae**) is the premature separation of a normally implanted placenta from the decidual lining of the uterus after 20 weeks' gestation. An abruption results in hemorrhage between the uterine wall and the placenta. Fifty percent of abruptions occur before labor and after the 30th week, 15% occur during labor, and 30% are identified only on inspection of the placenta after delivery (Cunningham et al., 2014).

Etiology, Risk Factors, and Classifications

At the initial point of placental separation, nonclotted blood courses from the site of injury. The enlarging collection of blood may cause further separation of the placenta. Bleeding can be either concealed (internal) or revealed (apparent). A concealed hemorrhage occurs in 20% of cases and describes an abruption in which the bleeding is confined within the uterine cavity. The most common abruption is associated with a revealed or external hemorrhage, in which the blood dissects downward toward the cervix (Fig. 11-6).

Risk factors include maternal hypertension (chronic, gestational, preeclampsia/eclampsia), cigarette smoking, multiparity, abortions (spontaneous, elective), illicit drug use (cocaine, methamphetamine), short fetal umbilical cord, maternal abdominal trauma, rupture of the membranes, and uterine leiomyoma (fibroids) located behind the placenta (Cunningham et al., 2014; Genovese, 2011). Placental abruption may be broadly classified into three grades that correlate with clinical and laboratory findings (Box 11-2).

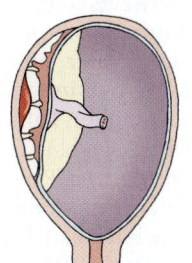 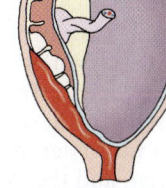 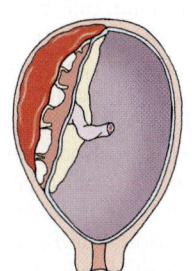

| Partial separation (concealed hemorrhage) | Partial separation (apparent hemorrhage) | Complete separation (concealed hemorrhage) |

Figure 11-6 Abruptio placentae.

Box 11-2 Classifications of Abruptio Placentae

Grade 1: Slight vaginal bleeding and some uterine irritability are usually present. Maternal blood pressure is unaffected, and the maternal fibrinogen level is normal. The fetal heart rate pattern is normal.

Grade 2: External uterine bleeding is absent to moderate. The uterus is irritable and tetanic, or very frequent contractions may be present. Maternal blood pressure is maintained, but the pulse rate may be elevated and postural blood volume deficits may be present. The fibrinogen level may be decreased. The fetal heart rate pattern often shows signs of fetal compromise.

Grade 3: Bleeding is moderate to severe but may be concealed. The uterus is tetanic and painful. Maternal hypotension is frequently present, and fetal death has occurred. Fibrinogen levels are often reduced or are less than 150 mg/dL; other coagulation abnormalities (e.g., thrombocytopenia and factor depletion) are present.

Source: Cunningham et al. (2014).

Perinatal and Maternal Morbidity and Mortality

Maternal mortality from abruptio placentae varies from 0.5% to 5%. The degree of hemorrhage that results from the torn placental vessels can vary from maternal anemia in mild cases to shock, acute renal failure, and maternal death in severe cases. Thirty-five percent of infants whose mothers require an antepartal transfusion will themselves be anemic and require a transfusion after birth. Fetal mortality occurs in about 35% of all placental abruptions and can be as high as 50% to 80% when associated with severe placental abruption. Death results from hypoxia that is related to the decreased placental surface area and maternal hemorrhage (Cunningham et al., 2014).

Signs and Symptoms

The classic presenting sign is third-trimester bleeding associated with severe abdominal pain. Other signs include uterine tenderness and abdominal or back pain, a boardlike abdomen and no vaginal bleeding, abnormal contractions and increased uterine tone, fetal compromise as evidenced by late fetal heart rate (FHR) decelerations, bradycardia and lack of variability on the electronic fetal monitor, and fetal demise.

Diagnosis

Vaginal bleeding in the third trimester of pregnancy is the hallmark of placental abruption or placenta previa and should always prompt an investigation to determine its etiology. Diagnosis is made by clinical findings and, when available, ultrasound examination. Recent advances in ultrasound imaging and interpretation have greatly improved the diagnosis rate. On ultrasound examination, more than 50% of patients with a confirmed placental abruption will demonstrate evidence of hemorrhage. However, during the acute phase of placental abruption, ultrasound findings may not be reliable, so a thorough clinical evaluation of any pregnant woman who presents with bleeding or acute abdominal pain is always indicated (Cunningham et al., 2014).

Management

The potential for rapid deterioration (hemorrhage, disseminated intravascular coagulation [DIC], fetal hypoxia) necessitates delivery in some cases of placental abruption. However, most abruptions are small and noncatastrophic, and therefore do not necessitate immediate delivery. Certain actions, including hospitalization, laboratory studies, continuous monitoring, and ongoing patient support should be initiated when placental abruption is suspected (Box 11-3).

⊛ Optimizing Outcomes—Religious beliefs and blood transfusions

Members of Jehovah's Witnesses do not receive blood products or their derivatives. When bleeding occurs during pregnancy and blood is deemed necessary to save the woman's and/or fetus' life, a very challenging situation exists. Non-blood products (e.g., crystalloids and colloids) may be given but are not always successful. Sometimes a court order is obtained so that blood can be administered to save the life of the woman and/or fetus. The delivery of a Jehovah's Witness should be planned to take place at a

Box 11-3 Care for the Patient Experiencing an Abruptio Placentae

- Hospitalization.
- IV placement with a large-bore catheter (16-gauge).
- Labwork: Includes CBC, coagulation studies (fibrinogen, PT, PTT, platelet count, and fibrin degradation products), type and screen for 4 units of blood, Kleihauer–Betke for Rh(D)-negative patients. A "clot test" may be performed: A red top tube of blood is drawn, set aside, and checked for clotting. If a clot does not form within 6 minutes or if it forms and lyses within 30 minutes, a coagulation defect is probably present and the fibrinogen level is less than 150 mg/dL.
- Betamethasone may be given to the woman to promote fetal lung maturity when delivery is not imminent.
- Rh(D)-negative patients should receive RhoGAM to prevent isoimmunization.
- Continuous evaluation of intake and output.
- Continuous electronic fetal monitoring.
- Delivery (cesarean or vaginal birth) may be initiated depending on the status of the mother and the fetus.
- Nursing care is centered on continuous maternal–fetal assessment, with ongoing information and emotional support for the patient and her family.

Source: Cunningham et al. (2014).

tertiary care center where resources are available to combat a potential massive hemorrhage. The perinatal nurse must be able to respect the family's beliefs and support them during this very difficult time when the health of both the woman and her fetus as well as their religious beliefs are being challenged (Braithwaite, Chichester, & Reid, 2011; Mirza & Gyamfi, 2010).

 Now Can You—Discuss the management of bleeding during pregnancy?

1. Describe the difference between placenta previa and abruptio placentae?
2. Name three initial steps in the management of the bleeding pregnant patient?
3. Explain why it may be difficult to identify an early maternal hemorrhage?

Preterm Labor

Preterm labor (PTL) is defined as cervical changes and regular uterine contractions occurring between 20 and 37 weeks of pregnancy. Many patients present with preterm contractions, but only those who demonstrate changes in the cervix are diagnosed with PTL (ACOG, 2012c).

INCIDENCE

Preterm birth, which is a birth that occurs between $20^{0/7}$ weeks of gestation and $36^{6/7}$ weeks of gestation, is considered the most acute problem in maternal–child health (ACOG, 2012c; American College of Obstetricians and Gynecologists [ACOG]/American Academy of Pediatrics

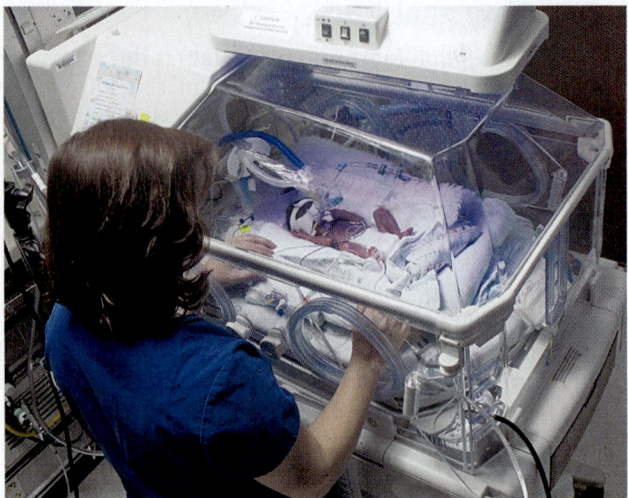

Figure 11-7 Premature infant in the neonatal intensive care unit (NICU).

[AAP], 2013) (Fig. 11-7). The sequelae of preterm birth have a profound effect on the survival and health of about one in every eight infants born in the United States each year. From 1981 to 2001, the rate of preterm births in the United States increased by 27%. In 2001, more than 476,000 infants were born at least 3 weeks before their due date (National Center for Health Statistics [NCHS], 2012).

In 2009, however, the preterm birth rate declined for the third straight year to 12.18 percent of all births. Declines were reported in both early (less than 34 weeks) and late (34 to 36 weeks) preterm births between 2008 and 2009 (Martin, Hamilton, Sutton, Ventura, Osterman, Kirmeyer, et al., 2011). Despite progress in this area, much work remains. Today, in the United States, one in eight babies is born prematurely; worldwide, 13 million babies are born too soon each year (March of Dimes, 2011). The prematurity report *Born Too Soon: The Global Action Report on Preterm Birth,* published by the March of Dimes Foundation, the Partnership for Maternal, Newborn & Child Health, Save the Children, and the World Health Organization (2012), ranks the United States 131st in the world in terms of its preterm birth rate of 12.0 per 100 live births, almost tied with Somalia, Thailand, and Turkey. Preterm birth is the leading cause of neonatal morbidity and mortality worldwide (Doyle, 2011). The U.S. government estimates that caring for premature infants costs more than $26 billion a year (CDC, 2013; Lee, 2011). According to ACOG (2011a, 2012d), there has been a shift away from prevention to the early detection of PTL to allow the administration of corticosteroids (to facilitate fetal lung maturity) and delivery at a site capable of providing the acute care needed for the neonate.

 Cultural Diversity: Ethnicity and Preterm Birth

According to the March of Dimes (2012), the rate of preterm birth is highest for African American infants (18.4%), followed by Native Americans (14.2%), Hispanics (12.2%), whites (11.6%) and Asians (10.8%).

MORBIDITY AND MORTALITY

As a result of high-tech neonatal intensive care, advanced technology, and improved medications, the morbidity of babies born after 34 to 35 weeks has decreased, and the definition of viability has changed dramatically throughout the past several decades (ACOG, 2002b). The limits of viability keep moving downward in gestation time, and this factor contributes to the increasing numbers of preterm births.

With appropriate medical care, neonatal survival dramatically improves as gestational age increases, with more than 50% of neonates surviving at 25 weeks' gestation and more than 90% at 28 to 29 weeks' gestation. Short-term neonatal morbidities associated with preterm birth are numerous and include respiratory distress syndrome, intraventricular hemorrhage, periventricular leukomalacia, necrotizing enterocolitis, bronchopulmonary dysplasia, sepsis, and patent ductus arteriosus. Long-term morbidities include cerebral palsy, intellectual and developmental disabilities, and retinopathy of prematurity. The risk of these morbidities is directly related to the infant's gestational age and birth weight (ACOG, 2002b, 2012c).

ETIOLOGY AND RISK FACTORS

The defining physiological mechanism that triggers the onset of PTL is largely unknown but may include decidual hemorrhage (abruption), mechanical factors (uterine overdistention or cervical incompetence), hormonal changes (perhaps mediated by fetal or maternal stress), and bacterial infections (ACOG, 2012c). However, a number of risk factors have been associated with PTL (Box 11-4).

 Collaboration in Caring—*Increasing public awareness of the problems of prematurity*

The Association of Women's Health, Obstetric and Neonatal Nurses (AWHONN), ACOG, and AAP have partnered with the March of Dimes in a multi-million-dollar research, education, and awareness campaign to address the problem of prematurity. Educating all women of childbearing age about preterm labor is a crucial component of prevention (March of Dimes, 2011).

RISK SCREENING FOR PRETERM BIRTH

Fetal Fibronectin Testing

Fetal fibronectin (fFN) is a glycoprotein produced by the fetal membranes. It is normally present in the cervicovaginal fluid until 16 to 20 weeks of gestation. Fetal fibronectin may be described as the "glue" that attaches the fetal membranes to the underlying uterine decidua. When uterine contractions occur, the adherence is disrupted and fFN is released. It has been suggested that fFN is a marker for the disruption of the chorioamnion and underlying decidua caused by inflammation with or without infection; a positive fFN test result between 24 and 34 weeks has been associated with subsequently diagnosed maternal and fetal infection. fFN testing is done when the membranes are not ruptured and the patient is not bleeding. The patient should not have had a pelvic exam, vaginal ultrasound, or vaginal intercourse within the 24 hours prior to collection

---

Box 11-4 Various Risk Factors Associated With Preterm Labor and Birth

- History of preterm birth, especially in the second trimester
- Preterm premature rupture of the membranes (PPROM)
- Uterine or cervical anomalies
- Multiple gestation
- Hypertensive disorders of pregnancy
- Diabetes (especially inadequately controlled)
- Low prepregnancy weight
- Clotting disorders
- Bacterial infections (e.g., mycoplasma of the genital tract, pyelonephritis, asymptomatic bacteriuria, pneumonia)
- Fetal anomalies
- Uterine overdistension (e.g., multiple gestation, hydramnios)
- Vaginal bleeding, especially in the second trimester or in more than one trimester
- Late or no prenatal care
- Alcohol or drug use
- Smoking
- Cervical injury (e.g., related to surgery or elective abortion)
- Diethylstilbestrol (DES) exposure
- Trauma including intimate partner violence
- Non-Hispanic African American race
- Maternal age extremes (i.e., less than 16 years or greater than 40 years)
- Low socioeconomic and educational status
- Stress
- Long working hours with long periods of standing
- Periodontal disease

Sources: ACOG (2012b), (2012c); Allen & Founds (2013); Gilbert (2011); Iliodromiti, Antonakopoulos, Sifakis, Tsikouras, Danillidis, Dafopoulos, et al. (2012); Lachat, Solnik, Nana, & Citron (2011).

(ACOG, 2012c, 2014). To test for the presence of fFN, a sterile cotton-tipped swab is placed in the posterior vaginal fornix or in the ectocervical region of the external cervical os for a minimum of 10 seconds. The collection swab is then removed, placed in a manufacturer-supplied medium, and sent to a laboratory that performs the test. Results are reported in 24 to 48 hours. For women whose fetal fibronectin test is negative (i.e., no fFN is detected), the likelihood of giving birth in the following week is less than 1% (Simhan, Berghella, & Iams, 2013). According to ACOG (2001), fFN testing may be useful in women with symptoms of PTL to identify those with negative values (and thus a reduced risk of preterm birth), thereby avoiding unnecessary hospitalization and medical intervention.

Assessment of Cervical Length and Funneling

A number of studies have confirmed the association of cervical shortening (less than 15 to 25 mm, depending on gestational age) with preterm birth, particularly if associated with a positive fFN test result. Cervical length (CL) measurements are performed, preferably with TVU or with the FDA-approved CervilLenz CL measuring device. The risk of preterm delivery increases as the CL in the second trimester declines. According to ACOG (2001, 2012b), CL measurement has limited clinical application and, because of the lack of proven treatments affecting outcomes, the routine use of ultrasound for CL assessment cannot be recommended. When a short CL is incidentally detected during transabdominal ultrasound scanning of the lower uterine segment, a subsequent transvaginal "confirmatory" ultrasound examination should be performed. If short CL is present, the patient's risk factors for preterm birth should be reviewed to determine appropriate clinical management (ACOG, 2012c).

Nursing Insight—Enhancing transvaginal ultrasonography for cervical length assessment

It is important to ask the patient to empty her bladder before undergoing a transvaginal ultrasound for assessment of CL. A full bladder may cause discomfort and can stretch the lower uterine segment, making the cervix appear to be longer than it actually is (B. Taylor, 2011).

In addition to CL assessment, other lower uterine segment and cervical characteristics can be assessed by mid-trimester ultrasound. One of these is the presence of cervical funnel, defined as protrusion of the amniotic membranes greater than 5 mm into the internal os. It has been demonstrated that the presence of funneling is a significant risk factor for an adverse perinatal outcome and that it is best measured as either "present" or "absent." Methods of cervical funneling assessment include observation of the shape of the funnel (U or V), percentage of funneling, and the depth and width of the funnel. In high-risk women with a prior spontaneous preterm birth and short cervix, the progression to a U-shaped funnel has been associated with an increased risk of preterm delivery (Mancuso, Szychowski, Owen, Hankins, Iams, Sheffield, et al., 2010).

Optimizing Outcomes—Interventions to possibly prevent preterm labor

Research has demonstrated that the following interventions appear to be beneficial in decreasing the risk of preterm labor: preconception control of chronic medical conditions (e.g., diabetes, seizures, asthma, and hypertension); smoking cessation; routine prenatal screening and treatment for asymptomatic bacteriuria; and the use of laminaria for women undergoing second trimester pregnancy termination via dilation and evacuation. Women at risk for preterm labor may benefit from progesterone supplementation: Micronized progesterone vaginal gel or suppositories (every night from weeks 16 to 20 through 36) may reduce preterm labor, especially in women with a history of preterm birth and a short CL verified by vaginal ultrasound (Fontenot & Fantasia, 2012; Gilbert, 2011). A landmark clinical trial conducted by the National Institute of Child Health and Human Development Maternal-Fetal Medicine Units Network demonstrated that weekly injections of 17-α-hydroxyprogesterone caproate (17P) significantly reduced the risk of preterm birth prior to 37, 35, and 32 weeks (Meis, Klebanoff, Thom, Dombrowski, Sibai, Moawad, et al., 2003). According to ACOG (2008b), progesterone supplementation for the prevention of recurrent preterm birth should be offered to all women with a singleton pregnancy and a prior spontaneous preterm birth because of spontaneous preterm labor or premature rupture of the membranes. In 2011, the FDA approved the use of progesterone supplementation (i.e., hydroxyprogesterone caproate injection [Makena]) to reduce the risk of recurrent preterm birth in women with a singleton pregnancy with a history of at least one prior spontaneous preterm birth. However, the optimal progesterone formulation, route of delivery, and dose for the prevention of preterm birth has not yet been determined (Norwitz & Caughey, 2011).

DIAGNOSIS

The diagnosis of PTL can be very challenging, because many of the symptoms are subtle and common during pregnancy. For example, women experiencing PTL may complain of backache, pelvic aching, menstrual-like cramps, increased vaginal discharge, pelvic pressure, urinary frequency, and intestinal cramping with or without diarrhea.

A diagnosis of PTL is made when the following criteria are met (ACOG/AAP, 2013):

- A gestation of 20 to 37 weeks
- Documented persistent uterine contractions (4 every 20 minutes or 8 in 1 hour)
- Documented cervical effacement of 80% or greater
- Cervical dilation of more than 0.4 in. (1 cm) or a documented change in dilation

Infection has been implicated as a contributing factor in PTL. Prostaglandin production by the amnion, chorion, and decidua is stimulated by cytokines (extracellular factors) that are released by activated macrophages. Group B streptococci, chlamydia, and gonorrhea have been associated with PTL and preterm premature rupture of the membranes (Cunningham et al., 2014). It is always prudent for the nurse to obtain a clean-catch, midstream, or catheterized urine specimen to identify and treat infection if the patient presents with signs of PTL or preterm premature rupture of the membranes.

MANAGEMENT

The two major goals in the management of PTL are to inhibit or reduce the strength and frequency of contractions, thus delaying the time of delivery, and to optimize the fetal status before preterm delivery (ACOG, 2012d; Cunningham et al., 2014). **Tocolysis** is the use of medications ("tocolytics") to inhibit uterine contractions. It is important to note that no medication has been identified to effectively stop PTL, and no one drug is approved in the United States or has been proven superior as a tocolytic agent. Medication selection is individualized based on efficacy, risks, contraindications (Box 11-5), and side effects. Because tocolytic therapy generally is effective for up to 48 hours, only women whose fetuses would benefit from a 48-hour delay in delivery should receive tocolytic therapy. In general, tocolytics are not indicated for use before neonatal viability; the upper limit for use is 34 weeks of gestation (ACOG, 2012b; Gilbert, 2011).

Optimizing Outcomes—Antenatal corticosteroids to improve neonatal outcomes

The administration of antenatal corticosteroids is the most beneficial intervention for improvement of neonatal outcomes among women who give birth preterm. A single course of corticosteroids is recommended for pregnant women between 24 and 34 weeks of gestation who are at risk

---

Box 11-5 Contraindications to the Use of Tocolytics in Preterm Labor

- Preeclampsia with severe features or eclampsia
- Maternal bleeding with hemodynamic instability
- Maternal contraindications to tocolysis (agent specific)
- Nonreassuring fetal status
- Fetal demise or lethal anomaly
- Chorioamnionitis
- Preterm premature rupture of the membranes
- In the absence of infection, tocolytics may be considered for the purposes of maternal transport, steroid administration, or both

Sources: ACOG (2012b); Cunningham et al. (2014).

Box 11-6 Nursing Care of the Patient Receiving Tocolytic Therapy

- Explore the woman's understanding of what is taking place.
- Include the woman's partner in all discussions about medications and their effects.
- Provide anticipatory guidance regarding what is likely to happen during medication administration.
- Position the woman on her side for better placental perfusion.
- Explain the side effects and contraindications of the medication(s).
- Assess blood pressure, pulse, and respirations regularly according to hospital policies (in many institutions every 15 minutes).
- Notify the health-care provider if systolic blood pressure is greater than 140 mm Hg or less than 90 mm Hg.
- Notify the health-care provider if diastolic blood pressure is greater than 90 mm Hg or less than 50 mm Hg.
- Assess for signs of pulmonary edema (chest pain and shortness of breath).
- Assess for the presence of deep tendon reflexes (DTRs).
- Monitor intake and output; avoid volume overload.
- Provide continuous external fetal monitoring for FHR pattern and frequency, duration, and approximate intensity of uterine contractions.
- Palpate the maternal abdomen to assess strength of uterine contractions.
- Provide psychosocial support and opportunities for the patient to express anxiety.
- Administer tocolytic therapy as ordered to delay delivery long enough to administer therapy: corticosteroids to accelerate fetal lung maturity; complete maternal transport to a Level III center prior to delivery; maternal antibiotic therapy to prevent neonatal Group B streptococcus (GBS) infection.

Source: Gilbert (2011).

---

of preterm delivery within 7 days. A single course of antenatal corticosteroids should also be administered to women with premature rupture of the membranes before 32 weeks of gestation. According to a Cochrane review, a single course of antenatal corticosteroids should be considered routine for all preterm deliveries. Neonates whose mothers receive antenatal corticosteroids have significantly lower severity, frequency, or both, of respiratory distress syndrome, intracranial hemorrhage, necrotizing enterocolitis, and death, compared with neonates whose mothers did not receive the medication (ACOG, 2012b; Roberts & Dalziel, 2006). According to ACOG (2011a), either of the following corticosteroid courses is appropriate: betamethasone (12 mg) IM 24 hours apart for 2 doses, or dexamethasone (6 mg) IM every 12 hours for 4 doses. Maternal risks associated with steroid administration include infection, pulmonary edema, hyperglycemia, and diabetic ketoacidosis (Myles, 2011).

According to ACOG (2012b), evidence supports the use of first-line tocolytic treatment with beta-adrenergic receptor agonists (e.g., terbutaline sulfate), nonsteroidal anti-inflammatory drugs (e.g., indomethacin), and calcium channel blockers (e.g., nifedipine) for the short-term prolongation (i.e., up to 48 hours) of pregnancy to allow an opportunity to begin the administration of antenatal corticosteroids to accelerate fetal lung maturity. Also, delaying the birth provides time for maternal transport to a facility equipped with a neonatal intensive care unit. Magnesium sulfate ($MgSO_4$), a central nervous system (CNS) depressant, has also been used to inhibit acute PTL. Magnesium sulfate has limited effect as a tocolytic agent and is associated with severe maternal risk factors including pulmonary edema and cardiovascular problems. However, $MgSO_4$ may exert a neuroprotective benefit, protecting the brain of the very preterm infant by possibly reducing the risk of cerebral palsy (ACOG, 2010a; Magee, Sawchuck, Synnes, & von Dadelszen, 2011). According to ACOG (2012b), long-term maintenance therapy with any tocolytic medication is ineffective for preventing preterm birth and improving neonatal outcomes and is not recommended for this purpose. Caring for the patient receiving tocolytic therapy requires the nurse to be cognizant of not only the safety aspects of administering the medication to the pregnant woman but also to the emotional needs of the patient as attempts to halt the PTL are being made (Box 11-6).

 clinical alert

Avoid combining nifedipine with certain other medications

Nifedipine, a calcium channel blocker used to inhibit preterm labor, works primarily by blocking the flow of calcium ions through the cell membrane (thereby decreasing the activation of smooth muscle contractile proteins). If nifedipine is given with magnesium sulfate or erythromycin, sudden cardiac arrest can occur (Gilbert, 2011; Vallerand & Sanoski, 2014).

 Now Can You—Care for the patient experiencing preterm labor?

1. Identify five symptoms of preterm labor?
2. Discuss the use of tocolytics in preterm labor?
3. Develop a teaching plan about preterm labor for pregnant women?

Premature Rupture of the Membranes

To facilitate an understanding of premature rupture of the membranes (ROM), it is helpful to first define the various terms used:

- **Premature** rupture of the membranes (PROM) is defined as rupture of the membranes before the onset of labor at any gestational age.

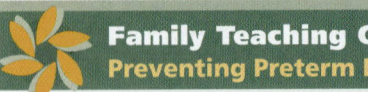

Family Teaching Guidelines...
Preventing Preterm Birth

Perinatal nurses must be proactive by educating women and their families about preterm labor, teaching them to recognize warning signs and symptoms, and actions to take if symptoms occur.

ESSENTIAL INFORMATION:

You may be experiencing preterm labor if you experience:

◆ Uterine contractions, cramping, or low-back pain
◆ A feeling of pelvic fullness, pressure, or pain
◆ A change in the amount or character of vaginal discharge
◆ Gastrointestinal symptoms: nausea, vomiting, diarrhea
◆ A general sense of discomfort or unease

To check for contractions, try these steps:

◆ Sit up from a reclining position and immediately place your hands on your abdomen—this action will often induce a uterine contraction.

◆ If you are unsure, try flexing your arm and feel the contraction of the biceps muscle to get an understanding of what a muscle contraction feels like.

If you believe you are having symptoms of preterm labor, take the following actions:

◆ Empty your bladder
◆ Lie down on your side
◆ Drink two to three glasses of a caffeine-free beverage
◆ Feel for uterine contractions
◆ Call your health-care provider or go to the hospital for further evaluation if your symptoms persist or if you experience four or more contractions in 1 hour.

Sources: Gilbert (2011); March of Dimes (2014); Nagtalon-Ramos (2011).

- **Preterm** rupture of membranes is defined as rupture of the membranes before 37 completed weeks of gestation. It complicates 8% of all pregnancies and is a common cause of PTL, preterm delivery, and chorioamnionitis (ACOG, 2013b).
- **Preterm premature** rupture of the membranes (PPROM) is defined as a combination of both terms—rupture occurs before the 37th completed week of gestation and in the absence of labor. PPROM accounts for 25% of all cases of premature rupture of the amniotic membranes and is responsible for 30% to 40% of all preterm deliveries (Cunningham et al., 2014).

PATHOPHYSIOLOGY

PROM is multifactorial. Choriodecidual infection or inflammation appears to play an important role in the etiology of PPROM, especially at early gestational ages. Other factors include decreased amniotic membrane collagen, lower socioeconomic status, cigarette smoking, sexually transmitted infections, prior preterm delivery, prior PTL during the current pregnancy, uterine distention (e.g., multiple gestation and hydramnios), cervical cerclage, amniocentesis, and vaginal bleeding in pregnancy (Gilbert, 2011). In many cases, the cause is not known.

DIAGNOSIS

Most often, the patient reports a gush or leakage of fluid from the vagina. However, any increased vaginal discharge should be evaluated. The diagnosis is based on the patient's history of leaking vaginal fluid and the finding of a pooling of fluid on sterile speculum examination. The nitrazine, AmniSure, or fern test can confirm the diagnosis of PROM. Easily performed, these tests are used to discriminate between vaginal discharge and amniotic fluid (see Procedure 12-2). Ultrasound examination of amniotic fluid volume may be useful in documenting **oligohydramnios** (decreased amniotic fluid), but is not considered diagnostic. When the clinical history or physical examination is unclear, membrane rupture can be diagnosed unequivocally with the ultrasound-guided transabdominal instillation of indigo carmine (a blue dye), followed by observation for passage of blue fluid from the vagina (ACOG, 2013b).

MANAGEMENT

The risk of perinatal complications changes dramatically according to the gestational age when rupture of the membranes occurs. Clinical practice varies, and, at present, considerable controversy exists concerning the optimal management of PPROM. However, there is general consensus in regard to the following factors:

- Gestational age should be established based on clinical history and prior ultrasound assessment when available.
- Ultrasound should be performed to assess fetal growth, position, and residual amniotic fluid.
- The woman should be assessed for evidence of advanced labor, chorioamnionitis (intrauterine infection), abruptio placentae, and fetal distress.
- Patients with advanced labor, intrauterine infection, significant vaginal bleeding, or nonreassuring fetal testing are best delivered promptly, regardless of gestational age.

There is further debate over the use of tocolytics, corticosteroids, and antibiotics in patients with PPROM. Tocolysis appears to be of little benefit in PPROM and may be harmful when chorioamnionitis is present. However, in many hospitals, tocolytic therapy is instituted for 48 hours, especially with earlier gestational ages, to administer a course of corticosteroids to enhance fetal lung maturity (Cunningham et al., 2014).

Conservative management includes inpatient observation unless the membranes reseal and the leakage of fluid stops. This approach initially consists of prolonged continuous fetal and maternal monitoring combined with modified bedrest to promote amniotic fluid reaccumulation and spontaneous membrane sealing. Delivery of the fetus should be accomplished if signs of infection are present: maternal temperature of 100.4°F (38°C) or greater, foul-smelling vaginal discharge, elevated white blood count, uterine tenderness, and maternal and/or fetal tachycardia.

Without intervention, approximately 50% of patients who have ROM will go into labor within 24 hours, and up to 75% will do so within 48 hours. These rates are inversely correlated to the gestational age at the time of rupture of the membranes. Thus, patients with ROM before 26 weeks' gestational age are more likely to gain an additional week than those greater than 30 weeks' gestation. Whereas maintaining the pregnancy to gain further fetal maturity can be beneficial, prolonged PPROM has been correlated with an increased risk of chorioamnionitis, placental abruption, and cord prolapse (Cunningham et al., 2014).

The nurse's role in caring for the patient with PPROM includes explaining to the patient that she will be on full or modified bedrest and her vital signs will be checked at least every 4 hours to detect early signs of a developing infection. If the patient does not exhibit signs of labor, intermittent fetal monitoring is appropriate. Frequent ultrasound examinations are performed to assess amniotic fluid levels. An important component of the nursing care plan centers on providing emotional support to the patient who is understandably worried about the outcome for her baby. The nurse should encourage the woman and her family members to ask questions and express fears and concerns. When the nurse does not have enough information to respond adequately, another health team member who can appropriately answer the patient's questions and address her concerns should be contacted (Moran, 2011a).

 Now Can You—Discuss the care of the patient with premature rupture of the membranes?

1. Name three factors associated with premature rupture of membranes?
2. Discuss three major complications that accompany premature rupture of membranes?
3. Describe the nitrazine, AmniSure, and fern tests?
4. Formulate a plan of care for the patient who has experienced premature rupture of the membranes?

Hypertensive Disorders of Pregnancy

Hypertensive disorders are the most common medical complication of pregnancy. The incidence of hypertensive disorders is between 5% and 10%, and this complication is the second leading cause of maternal death in the United States (embolic events are the leading cause) (Martin et al., 2011). Hypertensive disorders contribute significantly to stillbirth and neonatal morbidity and mortality (National High Blood Pressure Education Program Working Group [NHBPEP], 2000; Sibai, 2012) and can result in maternal cerebral hemorrhage, disseminated intravascular coagulation (DIC), hepatic failure, acute renal failure, pulmonary edema, adult respiratory distress syndrome, aspiration pneumonia, and abruptio placentae (ACOG, 2002a; ACOG 2012e).

CLASSIFICATIONS AND DEFINITIONS

The terminology used to describe the hypertensive disorders of pregnancy is generally associated with imprecise usage. This misuse of terminology often creates confusion for health-care professionals who care for women who experience hypertensive complications during pregnancy and childbirth (ACOG, 2013c; Sibai, 2012). Numerous attempts have been made to accurately describe pregnancy-related hypertensive disorders. The NHBPEP (2000) and the ACOG Task Force on Hypertension in Pregnancy (2013c) recommend the following classifications:

- Chronic hypertension
- Preeclampsia/eclampsia
- Preeclampsia superimposed on chronic hypertension
- Gestational hypertension
- Transient hypertension

Clinically, there are two basic types of hypertension during pregnancy. Distinction between chronic hypertension and pregnancy-induced hypertension (PIH) is based on the timing of the onset of the hypertension. However, NHBPEP (2000) advocates discarding the term pregnancy-induced hypertension because it does not differentiate between gestational hypertension, a relatively benign disorder, and the more serious condition of preeclampsia (Lockwood, 2013).

Chronic Hypertension

Chronic hypertension is defined as hypertension that is present and observable before pregnancy or hypertension that is diagnosed before the 20th week of gestation and persists beyond the 84th day postpartum. Hypertension is defined as a systolic pressure greater than or equal to 140 mm Hg and a diastolic pressure greater than or equal to 90 mm Hg (ACOG, 2013c; Lockwood, 2013; Roberts & Funai, 2013).

 Optimizing Outcomes—Accurate assessment of maternal blood pressure

Although aneroid and oscillometric devices are widely available, the mercury sphygmomanometer is still considered the "gold standard" for blood pressure measurement. It is important to use an appropriate-sized cuff (length 1.5 times the upper arm circumference or a cuff with a bladder that encircles 80% or more of the arm) to ensure accurate readings. Blood pressure should be measured only after the patient has rested (preferably 10 minutes or more) and is seated (feet flat) with the cuff positioned at the level of her heart. Automated systems for blood pressure measurement have been shown to be unreliable in severe preeclampsia and tend to under-record the true value (ACOG, 2012c; Lockwood, 2013).

Preeclampsia/Eclampsia

Preeclampsia is a pregnancy-specific systemic syndrome clinically defined as an increase in blood pressure (i.e., systolic and diastolic blood pressures greater than or equal to 140 and greater than or equal to 90 mm Hg, respectively, occurring twice, 4 hours apart) after 20 weeks' gestation accompanied by proteinuria (excretion of greater than or equal to 300 mg protein/24 hours) (ACOG, 2013c; Lockwood, 2013; NHBPEP, 2000). This increase in blood pressure represents a change from the usual blood pressure findings during pregnancy. Under normal conditions, the blood pressure increases during the first trimester, decreases in the second trimester, and then returns to nonpregnant values by the end of the third trimester.

At one time, the presence of edema was included in the definition of preeclampsia, but this criterion has been removed because edema is common during pregnancy. However, the sudden onset of severe edema always warrants close evaluation to rule out preeclampsia or other pathological processes such as renal disease. **Eclampsia** is the presence of new-onset grand mal seizures (and/or unexplained coma) in a woman with preeclampsia who has no other cause for seizure (ACOG, 2002a; Dix, 2011; Roberts & Funai, 2013).

 Nursing Insight—*Recognizing variations in the onset of eclampsia*

Approximately one-third of cases of eclampsia develop during pregnancy, one-third during labor, and one-third within 72 hours postpartum (Al Safi, Imudia, Filetti, Hobson, Bahado-Singh, & Awonuga, 2011).

Preeclampsia Superimposed on Chronic Hypertension

There is ample evidence that preeclampsia can occur in women who are already hypertensive and that the prognosis for the woman and her fetus is worse for these patients than when either condition exists alone. Distinguishing superimposed preeclampsia from worsening chronic hypertension tests the skills of the clinician and the obstetric nurse. The following criteria are necessary to establish a diagnosis of superimposed preeclampsia (NHBPEP, 2000; Roberts & Funai, 2013):

- Hypertension and *no* proteinuria prior to 20 weeks' gestation and new-onset proteinuria, (defined as the urinary excretion of 0.3 g of protein in a 24-hour specimen)

or

- Hypertension and proteinuria before 20 weeks' gestation:
  1. A sudden increase in protein—urinary excretion of 0.3 g protein or more in a 24-hour specimen, or two dipstick test results of 2+ (100 mg/dL), with the values recorded at least 4 hours apart, with no evidence of urinary tract infection
  2. A sudden increase in blood pressure after a period of good control
  3. Thrombocytopenia (platelet count lower than 100,000/mm^3)
  4. An increase in the liver enzymes alanine transaminase (ALT) or aspartate transaminase (AST) to abnormal levels

Gestational Hypertension

This is a temporary diagnosis that refers to blood pressure elevation occurring after mid-pregnancy but without proteinuria. This term is used only *during* pregnancy until a more specific diagnosis can be assigned postpartum.

Transient Hypertension

This diagnosis, used only *after* pregnancy, describes women who develop gestational hypertension but have no preeclampsia and whose blood pressure returns to normal within 12 weeks postpartum (women with gestational hypertension who remain hypertensive postpartum are diagnosed as having chronic hypertension) (NHBPEP, 2000; Roberts & Funai, 2013).

PREECLAMPSIA

Pathophysiology

The normal physiological adaptations to pregnancy are altered in the woman who develops preeclampsia. Preeclampsia is a multisystem, vasopressive disease process that targets the cardiovascular, hematological, hepatic, renal, and central nervous systems.

Preeclampsia is associated with a clinical spectrum of events that range from mild to severe with a potential endpoint of eclampsia. Patients do not suddenly "catch" severe preeclampsia or develop eclampsia but rather progress in a fairly predictable course through the clinical spectrum. In most cases, the progression is relatively slow, and the disorder may never proceed beyond a mild form. In other situations, the disease can progress more rapidly and change from a mild to a severe form in a matter of days or weeks. In the most serious cases, the progression can be rapid: Mild disease at the time of diagnosis evolves to preeclampsia with severe features or eclampsia over hours or days (ACOG, 2013c; Roberts & Funai, 2013). Hence, the nurse must alert the patient to signs and symptoms that signal a worsening condition and continuously assess the patient for any change.

Although the pathophysiology is poorly understood, it is clear that the blueprint for its development is laid down early in pregnancy. Preeclampsia is a disease of the placenta because it has been documented in pregnancies that involve trophoblastic tissue but no fetus (i.e., a molar pregnancy). In a normal pregnancy, the endovascular trophoblast cells of the placenta transform uterine spiral arteries to accommodate an increased blood flow. In the presence of preeclampsia, the arterial transformation is incomplete. Women with preeclampsia have a distinctive lesion in the placenta termed "acute atherosis" (fat accumulation in the placental arteries). Their placentas also exhibit a greater degree of infarction (necrosis related to decreased blood supply) than are found in placentas of normotensive women. These pathological changes can lead to decreased placental perfusion and placental hypoxia (Cunningham et al., 2014; NHBPEP, 2000).

Vasospasm and endothelial cell damage are the major underlying pathophysiological events in preeclampsia. Vasospasm may be associated with an elevation in arterial blood pressure and resistance to blood flow. It is unclear whether vasospasm produces damage to the vessels or if damage to the vessels produces vasospasm. Regardless, the restriction of blood flow is associated with endothelial cell damage, and this tissue insult prompts the systemic utilization of platelets and fibrinogen. The widespread vascular changes alter blood flow and result in hypoxic damage to vulnerable organs. Over time, the alterations produce widespread maternal vasospasm that results in decreased perfusion to virtually all organs, including the placenta. Associated physiological events include decreased plasma volume, activation of the coagulation cascade, and alterations in the glomerular endothelium. The increased platelet activation and markers of endothelial activation can predate clinically evident preeclampsia by weeks or even months (Cunningham et al., 2014; Sibai, 2012) (Fig. 11-8).

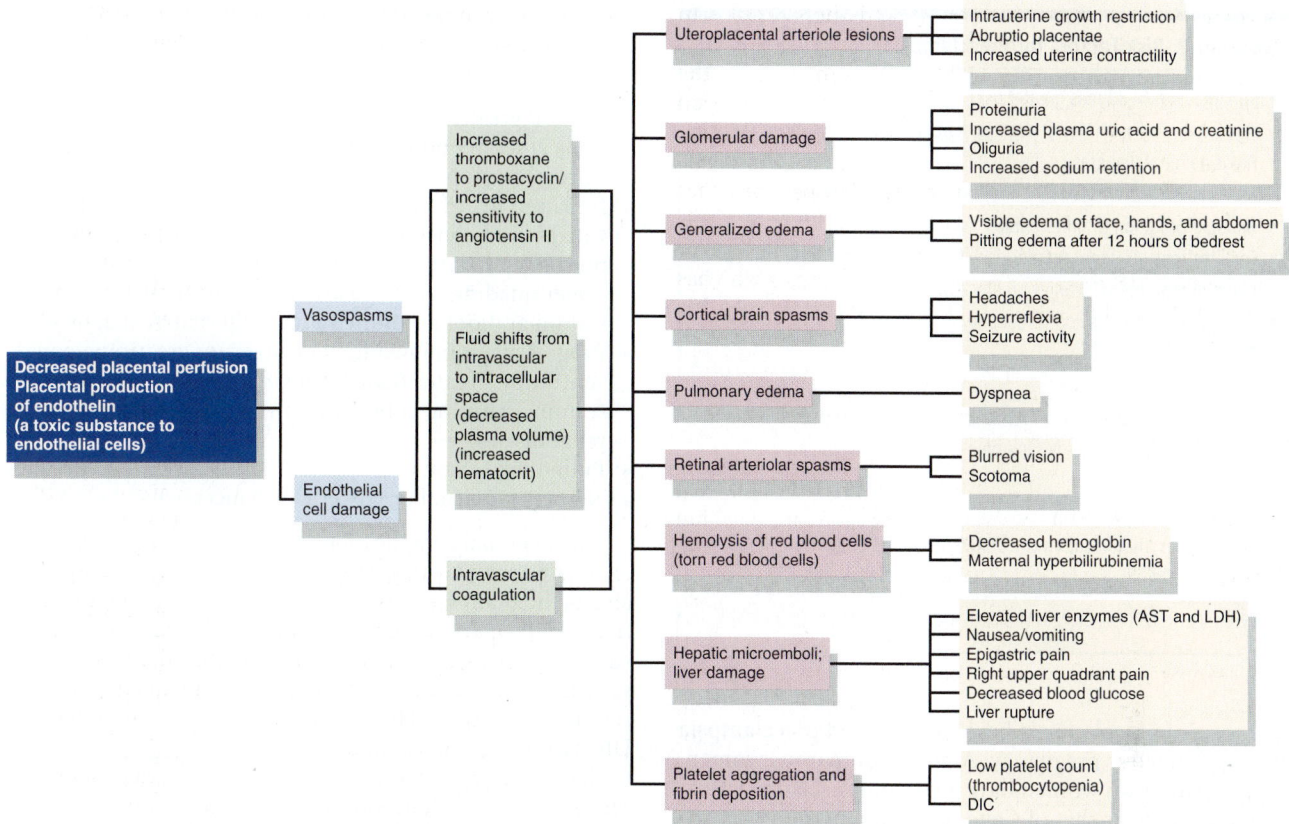

Figure 11-8 Pathophysiological changes of preeclampsia.

In addition to endothelial damage and vasospasm, women with preeclampsia show an exaggerated response to angiotensin II. Angiotensin II is produced by the renin-aldosterone pathway in the kidney when enzymes are released to convert angiotensin I to angiotensin II. Angiotensin II is a potent vasoconstrictor that can trigger arterial hypertension. During a normal pregnancy, the patient's physiological response to angiotensin II is blunted or decreased. In women with preeclampsia, the normal "blunting" does not occur (Cunningham et al., 2014; Sibai, 2012).

Pregnancy is normally associated with a low sensitivity to pressor agents, which increase blood pressure. Women with preeclampsia, however, demonstrate an exaggerated response to pressor agents. An imbalance between prostacyclin (a prostaglandin and potent vasodilator) and thromboxane (a compound synthesized in platelets from a prostaglandin) is also thought to occur. Prostacyclin exerts a direct effect on the tone of the arterial smooth muscles. It decreases blood pressure, prevents platelet aggregation (clumping), and promotes uterine blood flow. Thromboxane exerts the opposite effect. It is a potent vasoconstrictor that causes an increase in blood pressure and platelet aggregation (Cunningham et al., 2014; NHBPEP, 2000; Sibai, 2012).

 Nursing Insight—SPASMS: A memory enhancer when caring for a patient with preeclampsia

S   Significant blood pressure changes may occur without warning.
P   Proteinuria is a serious sign of renal involvement.

A   Arterioles are affected by vasospasms that result in endothelial damage and leakage of intravascular fluid into the interstitial spaces. Edema results.
S   Significant laboratory changes (most notably, liver function tests [LFTs] and the platelet count) signal worsening of the disease.
M   Multiple organ systems can be involved: cardiovascular, hematological, hepatic, renal, and central nervous system.
S   Symptoms appear after 20 weeks of gestation.

Risk Factors for Preeclampsia/Eclampsia

In the United States, the incidence of preeclampsia is rising, most likely caused by an increased prevalence of predisposing disorders such as obesity, diabetes, and chronic hypertension. Preeclampsia is a subtle and insidious disease process. Signs and symptoms become apparent relatively late in the course of the disease, usually during the third trimester of pregnancy. Preeclampsia occurs in about 5% to 8% of pregnancies, and there is no truly "typical" patient (ACOG, 2002a; Martin et al., 2011).

Risk factors associated with preeclampsia are presented in Box 11-7. Throughout the world, an estimated 50,000 women die each year from preeclampsia. Preeclampsia is more likely to develop in women whose mothers had preeclampsia than in women whose mothers did not. Nulliparity has been confirmed as a risk factor in both large-scale epidemiological studies and in detailed clinical studies. Approximately 35% of multiparous women with a

Box 11-7 Risk Factors for Preeclampsia

- Primigravida (6–8 times greater risk)
- Age extremes (less than 19 years and greater than 40 years)
- Pregestational diabetes
- Preexisting hypertension, renal disease, or collagen disease
- Multiple gestation (5 times greater risk)
- Fetal hydrops (10 times greater risk)
- Hydatidiform mole (10 times greater risk)
- Preeclampsia in a previous pregnancy
- Family history
- Obesity
- Periodontal disease
- Antiphospholipid antibody syndrome
- Rh incompatibility
- African American ethnicity
- Pregnancies that result from donor insemination, oocyte donation, embryo donation

Sources: ACOG (2002a); Dix (2011); Sibai (2012).

diagnosis of preeclampsia have experienced preeclampsia during a previous pregnancy. Among nulliparous women, African American women have a risk of preeclampsia that is twice as high as that of Caucasian women; they are also more likely to have hypertension that is independent of pregnancy. Obese women (a body mass index of 29 or greater) are three times more likely than nonobese women to develop preeclampsia (Sibai, 2012).

Immunological factors, genetic disposition, and environmental factors may also contribute to the development of preeclampsia. The high incidence of preeclampsia in many poor countries suggests that an inadequate diet may constitute a risk factor. Dietary inadequacies that have been proposed as relevant to the development of preeclampsia include deficiencies of calcium, magnesium, zinc, vitamins C and E, and n-3 essential fatty acids, although to date, large clinical trials have shown a lack of support for the role of dietary supplementation of magnesium or vitamins C and E in preventing or reducing the severity of preeclampsia (ACOG, 2002b; Dix, 2011; Sibai, 2012).

According to the ACOG Task Force on Hypertension in Pregnancy (2013c), low-dose aspirin (i.e., 60–80 mg/day, starting in the late first trimester) should be offered as primary prevention of preeclampsia to the following: women with a history of early-onset preeclampsia and delivery before 34 weeks' gestation, women with a history of preeclampsia in multiple pregnancies, and other high-risk patients (e.g., chronic hypertension and diabetes). No other treatments (e.g., vitamin C or E, salt restriction, or bedrest) are recommended for the prevention of preeclampsia, although calcium supplementation may be recommended for women with a low baseline dietary intake of calcium.

Classification of Preeclampsia and Maternal and Fetal Morbidity and Mortality

A number of maternal and fetal complications are likely to develop as the condition progresses from preeclampsia without severe features (formerly termed "mild" preeclampsia) to preeclampsia with severe features (formerly termed "severe" preeclampsia). According to ACOG (2013c), signs of severe disease include any of the following:

- Systolic BP greater than or equal to 160 mm Hg or diastolic BP greater than or equal to 110 mm Hg on 2 occasions at least 4 hours apart while the patient is on bedrest
- Thrombocytopenia (platelets less than $100 \times 10^9/L$)
- Impaired liver function, as indicated by abnormally elevated blood concentrations of liver enzymes (to twice normal concentration) and/or severe, persistent right upper quadrant or epigastric pain unresponsive to medication and not accounted for by alternative diagnoses
- Progressive renal insufficiency (serum creatinine concentration greater than 1.1 mg/dL or a doubling of the serum creatinine concentration in the absence of other renal disease
- Pulmonary edema
- New-onset visual or CNS disturbances

The maternal complications associated with preeclampsia are related to the widespread arteriolar vasoconstriction that affects the brain (seizure and stroke), kidneys (oliguria and renal failure), liver (edema and subcapsular hematoma), and small blood vessels (small ruptures within the walls of the vessels use up large amounts of platelets in an effort to correct the bleeding). This results in thrombocytopenia and DIC (Cunningham et al., 2014).

The perinatal outcome in preeclampsia is dependent on one or more of the following factors: the gestational age at the onset of the disease process, the presence of a multiple gestation, and the presence of underlying maternal hypertension or renal disease. In patients with preeclampsia without severe features at term, the perinatal mortality, incidence of fetal growth restriction, and neonatal morbidity are similar to those associated with normotensive pregnancies. In contrast, both perinatal and maternal morbidity are increased when the disease is severe, particularly when disease develops in the second trimester, and the fetus is quite immature. Maternal death and severe complication rates from preeclampsia are also lowest among women who receive regular prenatal care and are managed by experienced physicians in tertiary centers (ACOG, 2013c; Cunningham et al., 2014; Sibai, 2012).

Management of Preeclampsia/Eclampsia

Once the diagnosis of preeclampsia has been made, delivery of the fetus is the only cure. The primary considerations of therapy must always be the safety of the patient and the delivery of a live, mature newborn who will not require intensive and prolonged neonatal care. According to ACOG (2013c), preeclampsia without severe features, which presents as a maternal blood pressure of greater than or equal to 140 mm Hg systolic or greater than or equal to 90 mm Hg diastolic (on 2 occasions at least 4 hours apart after 20 weeks of gestation) and proteinuria (greater than or equal to 300 mg/24 hours *or* protein/creatinine ratio greater than or equal to 0.3 *or* dipstick reading greater than or equal to 1+), can often be managed at home after the patient has had a careful assessment of her signs and symptoms, a physical examination, laboratory tests, and evaluation of fetal well-being.

However, the NHBPEP recommends that, for patients with new-onset preeclampsia, the initial examination be performed in the hospital. Ongoing education (e.g., rationales for various tests and instructions for fetal activity monitoring) and the provision of a supportive environment are important nursing interventions at this time. If the woman's blood pressure and laboratory test results indicate that her care may be safely managed at home, the nurse must make certain that the patient fully understands the signs and symptoms associated with a worsening of the condition. The effects of illness, language, age, culture, beliefs, and support systems must be considered for each patient, and appropriate community resources should be explored (Bell, 2010; Dix, 2011) (Fig. 11-9).

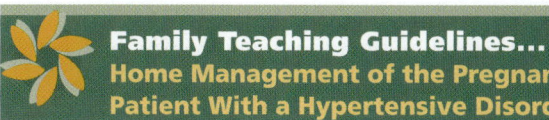

Family Teaching Guidelines...
Home Management of the Pregnant Patient With a Hypertensive Disorder

Before discharge, it is important to ascertain that the home environment is conducive to rest and the patient will be able to rest frequently throughout the day. It is essential that the patient can verbalize understanding of the importance of keeping all prenatal appointments and that she must immediately notify her physician or midwife at the first appearance of:

- Blood pressure values greater than those at the time of hospital discharge—MD or certified nurse-midwife should provide parameters
- Visual changes
- Epigastric pain
- Nausea and vomiting
- Bleeding gums
- Headaches
- Increasing edema, especially of the hands and face
- Decreasing urinary output
- Decreased fetal movement
- "Just not feeling right"

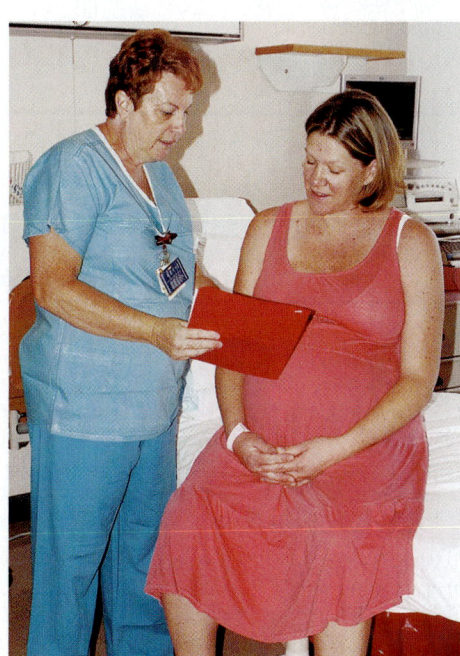

Figure 11-9 Nurse provides discharge teaching to a patient with preeclampsia.

Across Care Settings: Promoting rest at home

Obtaining an adequate amount of rest is not always easy, especially for women who have other children at home and no extended family to help. The nurse may offer suggestions for getting adequate rest, such as lying down and resting while the other children nap, bringing young children into bed and reading them a story, or asking a neighbor to watch the children. The woman's partner should also be involved in formulating a plan to help facilitate rest. Church groups may be able to help out with child care, running errands, or preparing meals for the family. When friends ask what they can do to help, suggest that the woman have a prepared "wish list" of specific actions that would make it easier for her to maintain a calm, restful home environment. The hospital's social services department should also be contacted and asked for assistance. They are a useful resource that can share information about organizations that can be called on to help.

Because lying in the lateral side position decreases pressure on the vena cava, the woman is instructed to maintain this position as much as possible. This position also increases venous return, circulatory volume, and placental and renal perfusion. Improving renal blood flow helps decrease angiotensin II levels, promotes diuresis, and lowers blood pressure. Antihypertensive medications have not been shown to improve perinatal outcomes in preeclampsia without severe features and should not be routinely prescribed (NHBPEP, 2000).

Critical Nursing Action Facilitating Effective CPR for the Pregnant Patient

Always instruct pregnant patients to never lie on their backs and explain that the weight of their baby exerts pressure on the large blood vessels and impedes blood flow back to the heart. If the pregnant patient experiences a cardiac arrest, this information is essential. Cardiopulmonary resuscitation (CPR) will not be effective if the fetus remains on the large blood vessels. One nurse must take responsibility to displace the uterus to the left while the cardiac compressions are being performed.

Where Research and Practice Meet:
Lack of Evidence for "Therapeutic" Bedrest in Pregnancy

Based on results from six Cochrane systematic reviews of bedrest in pregnancy, McCall, Grimes, and Lyerly (2013) concluded that although widely prescribed, "therapeutic" bedrest in pregnancy carries no benefits and is associated with known harms. According to the investigators' findings, evidence is insufficient to support bedrest for threatened abortion, hypertension, preeclampsia, preterm birth, multiple gestations, or impaired fetal growth. In addition to the lack of demonstrable benefit, potential harms from bedrest include venous thrombosis, bone demineralization, muscle atrophy, maternal weight loss, and maternal psychological problems such as depression, anxiety, and self-blame.

The clinical course of preeclampsia with severe features may be characterized by a progressive deterioration in both maternal and fetal conditions. Pregnancies complicated by preeclampsia with severe features have been associated with increased rates of perinatal mortality and significant risks for maternal morbidity and mortality. Because of this, there is universal agreement that delivery should be prompt if the disease develops after 34 weeks' gestation or earlier if there is evidence of maternal or fetal compromise. Management of preeclampsia with severe features includes the following clinical actions (Cunningham et al., 2014; Sibai, 2012):

1. Seizure prophylaxis with magnesium sulfate, which has been universally accepted as the drug of choice because of its CNS-depressant action.
2. Antihypertensive medications (Tables 11-1 and 11-2)
   - The use of antihypertensive agents in severe preeclampsia is generally indicated when diastolic blood pressures reach or exceed

Table 11-1 Medications Used to Treat Chronic Severe Hypertension in Pregnancy

Agent (Trade Name)	Class	Dose	Maternal Adverse Effects	Breastfeeding
alpha-methyldopa	Central alpha-adrenergic inhibitor	0.5–3.0 g PO per day in 2–3 divided doses	Sedation, elevated liver function tests, depression, dry mouth, lethargy, hemolytic anemia	Safe
labetalol (Trandate)	Alpha-/beta-adrenergic blocker	200–2,400 mg PO per day in 2–3 divided doses	Headache, dizziness, orthostatic hypotension, nausea/vomiting, sweating, bronchospasm, dyspnea, scalp tingling, tremulousness, flushing	Safe
nifedipine (Adalat, Procardia)	Calcium channel blocker	30–120 mg PO per day of aslow-release preparation	Headache, orthostatic hypotension, flushing, tachycardia	Safe
Adjunctive Agents				
hydralazine hydrochloride	Peripheral arteriolar vasodilator	50–300 mg PO per day in 2–4 divided doses	Tachycardia, dizziness, headache, palpitations. Use with methyldopa or labetalol to prevent reflex tachycardia; risk of neonatal thrombocytopenia	Safe
hydrochlorothiazide	Loop diuretic	12.5–50 mg PO per day	Dizziness, drowsiness, lethargy, weakness, hypotension, volume depletion, electrolyte disorders (e.g., hypokalemia, hypercalcemia, hypomagnesemia, hyponatremia, hypophosphatemia)	Risk is remote, but there are concerns about potential thrombocytopenia in infants.

Sources: ACOG (2011b), (2012e); Dix (2011); Vallerand & Sanoski (2014).

Table 11-2 Medications Used for Urgent Control of Severe Acute Hypertension in Pregnancy

Agent (Trade Name)	Class	Dosage	Maternal Adverse Effects
labetalol hydrochloride (Normodyne, Trandate)	Alpha-/beta-adrenergic blocker	20 mg IV, then 20–80 mg every 5–15 minutes, up to a maximum of 300 mg; or constant infusion of 1–2 mg/min	See above. Probably less risk of tachycardia and arrhythmia than with other vasodilators; increasingly preferred as first-line agent. May cause neonatal bradycardia and should be avoided in women with asthma or heart failure.
hydralazine	Peripheral/arterial vasodilator	5 mg IV or IM, then 5–10 mg every 20–40 minutes; or constant infusion of 0.5–10 mg/hr	See above. Long experience of safety and efficacy; risk of delayed maternal hypotension (systolic BP $\leq$ 90 mm Hg) and fetal bradycardia. Considered a first-line agent.

Table 11-2 Medications Used for Urgent Control of Severe Acute Hypertension in Pregnancy (continued)

Agent (Trade Name)	Class	Dosage	Maternal Adverse Effects
nifedipine (Adalat, Procardia)	Calcium channel blocker	10–30 mg PO, repeat in 45 minutes if needed	See hydralazine. Possible interference with labor; use caution if the patient is also receiving magnesium sulfate.
sodium nitroprusside (Nitropress)	Vasodilator	0.25 mcg/kg/min (increase by 0.25 mcg/kg/min every 5 minutes) to a maximum of 5 mcg/kg/min	Should be reserved for extreme emergencies and used for the shortest amount of time possible because of concerns about cyanide and thiocyanate toxicity in the mother and fetus or newborn and of cerebral edema in the mother

Sources: ACOG (2011b), (2012e); Dix (2011); Vallerand & Sanoski (2014).

110 mm Hg. The goal of therapy is to reduce the risk of cerebral vascular accident while maintaining uteroplacental perfusion. A decrease in the diastolic pressure to less than 90 mm Hg in the patient with severe hypertension will decrease placental blood flow, often with a decrease in the fetal heart rate (FHR). Management is directed at reducing the diastolic blood pressure to a value of less than 110 mm Hg but greater than 95 to 100 mm Hg.

3. Invasive hemodynamic monitoring may be required if any of the following are present:
   - Oliguria unresponsive to a fluid challenge
   - Pulmonary edema
   - Hypertensive crisis refractory to conventional therapy
   - Cerebral edema
   - Disseminated intravascular coagulation (DIC)
   - Multisystem organ failure

Nursing Assessments

Nursing care centers on extremely accurate, astute observations and assessments. An in-depth understanding of the pharmacological regimens, management plans, and potential complications associated with this disease is also essential. The clinical manifestations of preeclampsia are directly related to the presence of vascular vasospasms. Vasospasms cause endothelial injury, red blood cell destruction, platelet aggregation, increased capillary permeability, increased systemic vascular resistance, and renal and hepatic dysfunction. Hypertension and proteinuria are the most significant indicators of preeclampsia (Dix, 2011).

Identifying Hypertension

Preventing hypertension-induced problems in pregnancy requires nurses to use their assessment, advocacy, and counseling skills. Assessment begins with accurate blood pressure measurements. Checking blood pressures should never be treated as a routine, mundane task.

In the past, hypertension indicative of preeclampsia had been defined as an elevation of more than 30 mm Hg systolic or more than 15 mm Hg diastolic above the patient's

 Medication: Magnesium Sulfate

(mag-**nee**-zhum **sul**-fate)

Pregnancy Category: D

Indications: Anticonvulsant in severe preeclampsia or eclampsia

Unlabeled Use: Preterm labor
(Note: Magnesium sulfate is not FDA-approved for the treatment of preterm labor)

Actions: Plays an important role in neurotransmission and muscular excitability

Therapeutic Effects: Resolution of eclampsia

Pharmacokinetics:
ABSORPTION: IV administration results in complete bioavailability; well absorbed from IM sites
DISTRIBUTION: Widely distributed; crosses the placenta and is present in breast milk
METABOLISM AND EXCRETION: Excreted primarily by the kidneys
HALF-LIFE: Unknown

Contraindications and Precautions:
CONTRAINDICATED IN: Hypermagnesemia/hypocalcemia/anuria/heart block/active labor or within 2 hours of labor (unless used for preeclampsia or eclampsia)
USE CAUTIOUSLY IN: Any degree of renal insufficiency

Adverse Reactions and Side Effects:
Central nervous system: Drowsiness
Respiratory system: Decreased respirations
Cardiovascular system: Arrhythmias, hypotension, bradycardia
Gastrointestinal system: Diarrhea
Dermatology system: Flushing, sweating
Metabolic: hypothermia

Interactions: Potentiates neuromuscular blocking agents

Route and Dosage (Eclampsia/Preeclampsia): Piggyback a solution of 40 g of magnesium sulfate in 1,000 mL of lactated Ringer's solution—use an infusion control device (pump) at the ordered rates: loading dose, initial bolus of 4 to 6 g over 15 to 30 min; maintenance dose, 1 to 3 g/hr. IM: 4 to 5 g given in each buttock; can be repeated at 4-hour intervals; use Z-track technique. (Note: IM route rarely used because the absorption rate cannot be controlled and injections are painful and may result in tissue necrosis.)

Time/Action Profile for Anticonvulsant Effect:
IM: Onset is 60 minutes with peak unknown, and duration is 3 to 4 hours;
IV: Onset is immediate with peak unknown and duration is 30 minutes.

Nursing Implications: Remember that this is a very potent, high-alert drug!

1. Explain purpose and side effects of the medication to the patient and her companion.
2. Explain that she may feel very warm and become flushed and experience nausea and vomiting, visual blurring, and headaches.
3. Magnesium sulfate must never be abbreviated (i.e., MgSO4 is not acceptable) and requires a written order by the physician for administration.
4. Always use an infusion pump for administration and run the medication piggyback, not as the main line.
5. Monitor pulse, blood pressure, respirations, and ECG frequently throughout parenteral administration. Respirations should be at least 16/min before each dose.
6. Monitor neurological status before and throughout therapy.
7. Institute seizure precautions.
8. Keep the room quiet and darkened to decrease the likelihood of triggering seizure activity.
9. Patellar reflexes should be tested before each parenteral dose of magnesium sulfate. If absent, no additional dose should be administered until a positive response returns.
10. Monitor intake and output. Urine output should be maintained at a level of at least 100 mL/4 hr.
11. Serum magnesium levels and renal function should be monitored periodically throughout administration of parenteral magnesium sulfate (Box 11-8).
12. Have 10% calcium gluconate available should toxicity occur. Administer 10 mL IV over 1 to 3 minutes until signs and symptoms are reversed.
13. After delivery, monitor the newborn for hypotension, hyporeflexia, and respiratory depression.

Source: Data from Vallerand, A. H., & Sanoski, C. A. (2014). *Davis's drug guide for nurses* (14th ed.). Philadelphia, PA: F.A. Davis.

Box 11-8 Serum Magnesium Levels

Serum Magnesium Levels	(mEq/L)
Normal	1.5–2
Therapeutic	4–7
ECG changes	5–10
Loss of reflexes	8–12
Respiratory distress	15
Cardiac arrest	25

Sources: Dix (2011); Vallerand & Sanoski (2014).

- Implement periodic magnesium sulfate overdose drills with airway management and calcium administration with the physician and nurse team members participating together.
- Maintain the calcium antidote in the patient's room in a locked box.

---

baseline blood pressure. However, this definition has not been a good prognostic indicator of outcome. The frequently cited "30–15" rule is not part of the criteria for preeclampsia according to the National High Blood Pressure Education Program Working Group. Instead, women who demonstrate a blood pressure elevation of more than 30 mm Hg systolic or more than 15 mm Hg diastolic above the prepregnancy baseline "warrant close observation" (ACOG, 2002a; Dix, 2011).

The nurse needs to remember that blood pressure presents differently in women with preeclampsia. Preeclamptic patients often demonstrate labile (unstable) pressures and a flattening or reversal of normal circadian blood pressure rhythms, with the highest values recorded at night (Cunningham et al., 2014). Because of this variation, hospitalized patients should routinely have a nocturnal blood pressure assessment unless otherwise ordered by the physician. A daily cardiovascular assessment is also an important monitoring component for the hospitalized patient.

 clinical alert

Preventing magnesium sulfate accidents

Accidental overdose of magnesium sulfate administration can pose a significant risk to both mother and newborn.

Current recommendations to prevent magnesium sulfate accidents:

- A standardized unit protocol should be consistent and include standing orders addressing the initial bolus and maintenance dose to be administered; how the pump should be programmed; the maintenance IV solutions that will be used; and the frequency that the fetus and mother will be assessed.
- Administer IV magnesium sulfate (including the initial bolus) only through a controlled infusion device with free-flow protection.
- Use universal standardized dose prepackaged magnesium sulfate.
- Have a second nurse check the initial magnesium sulfate IV bag and pump settings (and every magnesium sulfate IV bag that is added and each subsequent rate change).
- Use a 100-mL (4 g) or 150-mL (6 g) IV piggyback for the initial bolus instead of bolusing from the main bag with a rate change on the pump.
- Use color-coded tags on the lines as they go into the pumps and into the IV ports.
- Provide 1:1 nursing care for women in labor who are receiving magnesium sulfate.
- When care is transferred to another nurse, have both nurses together at the bedside to review the pump settings for both the magnesium sulfate and mainline IV fluids and to review written physician orders for magnesium sulfate infusion orders.

legal alert—Perform a daily cardiovascular assessment on patients with preeclampsia

During the assessment, the nurse should include the following parameters:

- Auscultation of heart sounds, lungs, and breath sounds
- Presence and degree of edema
- Early signs or symptoms of pulmonary edema, such as tachycardia and tachypnea
- Daily weight taken at the same time of the day and on the same scale
- Skin color, temperature, and turgor
- Capillary refill, which may indicate decreased perfusion or vasoconstriction if greater than 3 seconds

Significance of Proteinuria

Proteinuria is defined as the excretion of 300 mg or more of protein every 24 hours. If 24-hour urine samples are not available, proteinuria is defined as a protein concentration of 300 mg/L or more (greater than or equal to 1+ on dipstick) in at least two random urine samples taken at least 4 to 6 hours apart and no more than 7 days apart. However, studies have shown that urinary dipstick determinations and random protein to creatinine ratios correlate poorly with the amount of protein found in a 24-hour sample of women with gestational hypertension. Therefore, the definitive test to diagnose proteinuria should be quantitative protein excretion over 24 hours (ACOG, 2002a; Lindheimer & Kanter, 2010).

The purpose of the renal assessment is to identify renal compromise. As a result of the vasospasm that accompanies preeclampsia, the expected increases in the glomerular filtration rate and renal blood flow may not occur, nor the expected decrease in serum creatinine, especially if the disease is severe. Preeclampsia may be associated with a profuse swelling in the kidney glomerular endothelial cell cytoplasm. This pathological change causes glomerular endotheliosis, a lesion that correlates with proteinuria (ACOG, 2002a; Lindheimer & Kanter, 2010).

As an important component of hospital care, the nurse assesses urine output every 1 to 4 hours to confirm adequate renal perfusion and oxygenation. A urine output of 25 to 30 mL/hr or 100 mL/4 hr is normal; a downward trend in output should be reported immediately. A urimeter attached to the Foley catheter tubing is useful in the accurate assessment of the hourly urine output. A 24-hour urine test for total protein may be ordered to monitor for an increase in the excretion of protein, a finding indicative of increasing kidney impairment. The nurse should be aware that if the 24-hour urine specimen (for total protein) shows the presence of protein, a dipstick is not appropriate. Once protein is evident in a 24-hour urine collection, protein will always be present when the urine is tested by the dipstick. Therefore, no new information is obtained. The 24-hour urine sample yields more accurate information because it shows whether or not the urine protein is increasing, decreasing, or remaining the same. When indicated, a high-protein diet may be needed to replace the protein excreted in the urine.

Assessing Edema

At one time, edema was an important component of the triad considered along with hypertension and proteinuria to diagnose preeclampsia. However, edema is a common finding in pregnancy. Dependent edema in the absence of hypertension or proteinuria is generally related to changes in the interstitial and intravascular hydrostatic pressures that facilitate the movement of intravascular fluid into the tissues. When preeclampsia is present, continuous capillary leakage combined with a decreased colloidal pressure can lead to pulmonary edema. In this situation, intravascular fluid leaks out through holes (caused by vasospasms) in the endothelial lining of the blood vessels. Pulmonary edema can occur very suddenly, especially if the patient receives an overload of IV fluid. Because of the potential for rapid development of this life-threatening complication, the nurse must frequently perform a careful assessment of the patient's pulmonary status and meticulously monitor the total intake and output.

Central Nervous System Alterations

Preeclampsia may quickly develop into eclampsia, the convulsive phase of preeclampsia. Before the onset of seizure activity, the patient may complain of headaches, visual disturbances, blurred vision, scotomata (specks or spots in the vision where the patient cannot see; "blind spots"), and, in rare cases, cortical blindness. These symptoms can be indicators of increased CNS irritability that precedes the onset of seizures. A retinal examination often reveals vascular constriction and narrowing of the small arteries. These changes are reflective of the widespread vasoconstriction that is occurring throughout the body. Deep tendon reflexes (DTRs) are also routinely assessed for evidence of irritability and clonus (rapidly alternating muscle contraction and relaxation), two additional signs of increased CNS irritability (Cooray, Edmonds, Tong, Samarasekera, & Whitehead, 2011) (Figs. 11-10 and 11-11).

⬤ Optimizing Outcomes—Grading reflexes and checking for clonus

During the assessment, grade maternal reflexes on a 0 to 4+ scale:

4+ Very brisk, hyperactive; often indicative of disease; often associated with clonus

3+ Brisker than average; possibly but not necessarily indicative of disease

2+ Average; normal

1+ Somewhat diminished

0   No response

If the reflexes are hyperactive, test for ankle clonus. Support the knee in a partly flexed position. With your other hand, dorsiflex and plantar flex the foot a few times while encouraging the patient to relax, and then sharply dorsiflex

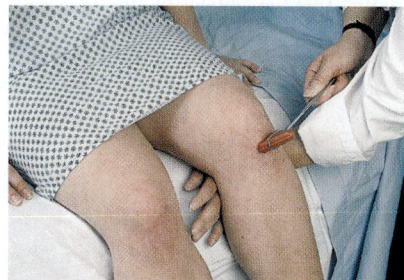

Figure 11-10 Assessing deep tendon reflexes.

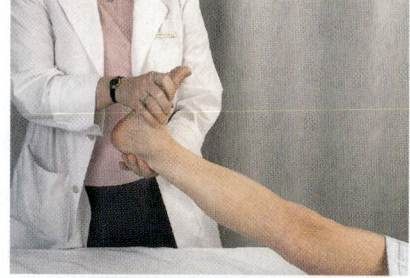

Figure 11-11 Testing for clonus.

the foot and maintain it in dorsiflexion. Look and feel for rhythmic oscillations between dorsiflexion and plantar flexion. Normal is no reaction to this stimulus. Sustained clonus indicates upper motor neuron disease. The ankle plantar flexes and dorsiflexes repetitively and rhythmically (see Fig. 11-11) (Dillon, 2007). Clonus is usually noted as "absent" or "present" but it may be rated as:

- Mild (2 movements)
- Moderate (3 to 5 movements)
- Severe (6 or more movements)

A neurological assessment of the patient with preeclampsia includes establishing her level of consciousness (LOC). Determining if the patient is alert and oriented can be accomplished by asking if she knows why she is in the hospital and if she can correctly identify the name of the hospital. It is also important for the nurse to assess for any change in the patient's behavior or personality. Preeclampsia is an insidious condition, and symptoms associated with worsening of the disease can be very subtle. Maintaining a quiet, darkened environment reduces stimuli that may trigger seizure activity. Ensure that seizure precautions (e.g., suction equipment, oxygen administration equipment, and emergency medication tray) are in place.

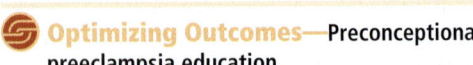

Optimizing Outcomes—Preconceptional preeclampsia education

Women who experience preeclampsia during pregnancy are at greater risk for developing cardiovascular disease, and their offspring are at increased risk for developing cardiovascular disease as an adult. It is well known that obesity constitutes a significant risk factor for many complications such as cardiovascular disease, diabetes, and preeclampsia. During preconception, nurses can provide counseling about lifestyle factors that may affect the likelihood of developing preeclampsia. Discussing the importance of maintaining or establishing healthy weight control is especially important with patients whose prepregnancy body mass index is greater than 25 (Alfonso, 2009).

ECLAMPSIA

Eclampsia is the occurrence of grand mal seizures in women who have either gestational hypertension or preeclampsia. It is the most common CNS complication of hypertension, and most maternal deaths attributable to hypertension occur in women with eclampsia. Although patients with severe preeclampsia are at the greatest risk for developing seizures, eclampsia-related seizures have been reported in women with preeclampsia without severe features. Women developing eclampsia exhibit a wide spectrum of signs and symptoms, ranging from extremely high blood pressure, 4+ proteinuria, generalized edema, and 4+ patellar reflexes to minimal blood pressure elevation, no proteinuria or edema, and normal reflexes (Sibai, 2012, 2013).

Maternal complications of eclampsia include cerebral hemorrhage, aspiration pneumonia, hypoxic encephalopathy, coma, thromboembolic events, and maternal death

(incidence 0.4% to 14%). The perinatal death rate in pregnancies complicated by eclampsia is 9% to 23%. Perinatal deaths are closely related to gestational age and most often result from premature delivery, abruptio placentae, and intrauterine asphyxia (Cunningham et al., 2014).

The exact cause of eclamptic seizures is unknown, but many etiologies, including cerebral vasospasm with local ischemia, hypertensive encephalopathy with hyperperfusion, vasogenic edema, and endothelial damage, have been proposed (Cunningham et al., 2014). Eclamptic seizures are clonic–tonic in nature and are almost always self-limiting. They seldom last longer than 3 to 4 minutes.

Critical Nursing Action Care of the Pregnant Patient Post Seizure

- Do not attempt to shorten or abolish the initial seizure. Attempts to administer anticonvulsants IV without secure venous access can lead to phlebitis and venous thrombosis.
- Prevent maternal injury. Pad the side rails.
- Maintain adequate oxygenation; administer oxygen via face mask at 10 L/min.
- Minimize the risk of aspiration. Position the patient on her side to facilitate drainage. Suction equipment should be ready and working. Insert an oral airway.
- Give adequate magnesium sulfate to control seizures. As soon as possible following the seizure, venous access should be secured with a 4- to 6-g loading bolus of magnesium sulfate given over 15 to 20 minutes. If the patient seizes following the loading dose, another 2-g bolus may be given IV over 3 to 5 minutes.
- Correct maternal acidemia. Blood gas analysis allows monitoring of oxygenation and pH status. Respiratory acidemia is possible after a seizure.
- Avoid polytherapy. Maternal respiratory depression, respiratory arrest, or cardiopulmonary arrest is more likely in women who receive polytherapy to arrest a seizure. Remember that anticonvulsants are respiratory depressants and may interact.
- *Be sure to check the fetus or fetuses* (all must be accounted for). After a seizure, there may be loss of FHR variability and bradycardia on the fetal monitoring tracing.
- Assess for ruptured membranes, contractions, cervical dilation, and signs of placental abruption.
- Prepare for delivery as indicated.
- Support the patient and her family. This is a very frightening event for them, and they will need reassurance and to be kept aware of the plan of care and the well-being of their baby (Dix, 2011; Sibai, 2013).

legal alert—Document after a patient seizure

- Time and length of seizure
- Associated symptoms
- Vital signs, including fetal heart assessment
- Presence or absence of uterine contractions
- Any untoward results such as rupture of the membranes or signs of placental abruption
- Medications that were given. Remember to have the physician write or cosign any verbal orders that were given during the emergency (Dix, 2011).

Global Health Case Study Rosa Garcia

Rosa Garcia is a 25-year-old married Mexican immigrant who is pregnant with her first child. Rosa's family practice physician has been caring for her since her first prenatal visit at 11.4 weeks' gestation. During the initial prenatal visit, the following data were obtained:

Vital signs: temperature: 98.6°F (37.0°C); pulse: 78 beats/min; respirations: 20 breaths/min; blood pressure: 110/70; weight: 146 lb (66.4 kg)

A complete physical exam was performed with normal findings, and prenatal labs including a thyroid-stimulating hormone level (TSH, because of a positive family history for hypothyroidism) were drawn. During the interview, the nurse inquired about any other family medical problems. Rosa reported that both her sister and her mother had experienced preeclampsia during pregnancy.

An ultrasound was ordered for pregnancy dating because Rosa had experienced irregular menstrual periods since discontinuing oral contraceptives.

Rosa kept her regular prenatal appointments every 4 weeks and the pregnancy progressed uneventfully until 4 months later, when she presented to the office with increased blood pressure and swollen legs. Rosa had noticed an increased swelling that extended up to the knees of both legs. She denied hand or facial swelling, headaches, visual problems, or right upper quadrant (RUQ) pain. Her sister, a chiropractor, had been checking her blood pressure and noted it to be as high as 160 to 170/100 to 110 mm Hg. At this prenatal visit, the following data were obtained:

Blood pressure: 144/96 (sitting). Repeat on left side: 140/90.
Weight: 172.5 lb (78.4 kg)
Urine dipstick reading: 1+
Physical exam: General—in no acute distress; abdomen: nontender; fundus at 28–11.8 in. (30 cm) above the symphysis pubis; FHR 150 bpm; cardiovascular: 1+ pedal edema; neurological: reflexes 3+ with no clonus.
Assessment: Preeclampsia without severe features.

The following lab tests were ordered: CBC with platelet count; liver enzyme determination (AST, ALT, LDH), alkaline phosphatase (ALP); prothrombin time (PT); a chemistry panel (electrolytes: Na^+, K^+, Cl^-, HCO_3^-, Ca^{2+}, Mg^{2+}), blood urea nitrogen (BUN), creatinine (Cr), uric acid, and a 24-hour urine collection for protein and creatinine clearance. A sonogram (ultrasound) was also ordered to monitor the status of the fetus.

Rosa was instructed to go home, rest on her left side as much as possible, and call the nurse if she experienced increased edema, headaches, visual disturbances, or RUQ pain. She was told to continue with fetal kick counts and twice daily blood pressure monitoring, record all findings and symptoms, and return to the office in 1 week.

On her next office visit 8 days later, Rosa reported that she had been adhering to frequent rest periods at home and had noticed that her leg edema was improved. She exclaimed: "I can see my ankle bones again!" Her sister had continued to monitor the blood pressure. According to the blood pressure log, Rosa's systolic blood pressure measurements had been in the 160s and the diastolic measurements were in the 80 to 90 range. Rosa denied headaches, visual disturbances, or abdominal pain and remarked that the fetus had been active. At this visit, the following data were obtained:

Blood pressure: 160/98 (sitting); 162/100 (left side); weight: 160 lb (72.7 kg); fundal height: 27 cm; FHR: 150 to 170 bpm; reflexes: 3 to 4+ with no clonus; urinary protein: 4+ (2000+ mg/dL) on dipstick
Assessment: Preeclampsia with severe features at $29^{4/7}$ weeks' gestational age

At this point, Rosa's physician consulted with a maternal fetal medicine specialist, who advised transferring Rosa to a tertiary care center 50 miles away. Rosa was promptly transferred to the tertiary care center and admitted to the obstetric service.

critical thinking questions

1. What are Rosa's risk factors for developing preeclampsia?

2. Why did the nurse ask Rosa about headaches, blurred vision, and RUQ pain?

3. What signs and symptoms prompted Rosa's physician to consult with the maternal–fetal specialist and arrange for a transfer to a tertiary care center?

◆ See Suggested Answers to Global Health Case Studies on Davis*Plus*.

HELLP SYNDROME

HELLP is an acronym for **H**emolysis and **E**levated **L**iver enzymes and **L**ow **P**latelet levels. As a result of the arteriolar vasospasms in the cardiovascular system that occur in preeclampsia, the circulating red blood cells (RBCs) are destroyed as they try to navigate through the constricted vessels (Hemolysis). Vasospasms decrease blood flow to the liver, resulting in tissue ischemia and hemorrhagic necrosis (Elevated Liver enzyme level). In response to the endothelial damage caused by the vasospasms (small openings develop in the vessels), platelets aggregate at the site and a fibrin network is set up, leading to a decrease in the circulating platelets (Low Platelet level).

HELLP syndrome is a rare (5% of women with preeclampsia), serious complication of preeclampsia that can manifest itself at any time during pregnancy and the puerperium, but like preeclampsia, it is rare before 20 weeks' gestation. However, unlike preeclampsia, HELLP syndrome occurs more often in Caucasians, multiparas, and in women older than 35 years. One-third of all cases of HELLP syndrome occur postpartum, and only 80% of these patients are diagnosed with preeclampsia before delivery (Dix, 2011; Sibai, 2012, 2013).

HELLP syndrome is actually a laboratory diagnosis for a variant of preeclampsia with severe features. The primary presentation is consistent with hepatic dysfunction evidenced by findings from the patient's liver function tests (ACOG, 2002a; Dix, 2011). Signs of HELLP syndrome usually develop in the third trimester, or within 48 hours after birth. HELLP syndrome is characterized by rapidly deteriorating liver function and thrombocytopenia. Liver capsule distention often produces epigastric pain. Though rare, liver rupture is one of the most ominous consequences of severe preeclampsia/HELLP syndrome, with a reported maternal death rate of more than 30%. The precise cause of liver rupture is unknown, but the prevailing theory postulates that the increased hepatic pressure leads to rupture. It is theorized that endothelial dysfunction with intravascular fibrin deposits and hepatic sinusoidal obstruction leads to intrahepatic vascular congestion, increased intrahepatic pressure, and distention of Glisson's capsule. This pathological process progresses to the development of a subcapsular hepatic hematoma and subsequent liver rupture. Other maternal signs and symptoms include malaise with influenza-like complaints, nausea or vomiting, headache, shoulder pain, and bruising or hematuria (ACOG, 2002a; Cunningham et al., 2014; Dix, 2011; Grand'Maison, Sauve, Weber, Dagenais, Durand, & Mahone, 2012).

Therapy for HELLP syndrome centers on improving the platelet count by transfusion of fresh-frozen plasma or platelets and delivery as soon as feasible by vaginal or cesarean birth. Intrapartum nursing care involves continuous maternal–fetal monitoring. Measurement of central venous pressure or pulmonary arterial wedge pressure (Swan–Ganz catheter) may be required to monitor fluid status accurately when pulmonary edema or acute renal failure is present (ACOG, 2002a).

 Now Can You—Discuss HELLP syndrome?

1. State what the acronym HELLP stands for?
2. Describe the basic pathology of HELLP syndrome?
3. Discuss the significance of epigastric pain in the patient with HELLP syndrome?

 Now Can You—Discuss hypertensive complications of pregnancy?

1. Differentiate among the following conditions: chronic hypertension, preeclampsia, eclampsia, chronic hypertension with superimposed preeclampsia, and gestational hypertension?
2. Describe the pathophysiology of preeclampsia?
3. Discuss the indications for use, action, dosage, and side effects of magnesium sulfate?
4. State the specific nursing actions required when caring for the patient receiving magnesium sulfate?

Disseminated Intravascular Coagulopathy

Disseminated intravascular coagulopathy (DIC) is a hematological disorder characterized by a pathological form of clotting that is diffuse and consumes large amounts of clotting factors. DIC causes widespread external or internal bleeding or both (Cunningham et al., 2014). The most common causes of DIC in pregnancy are excessive blood loss with inadequate blood component replacement, placental abruption, amniotic fluid embolism, and severe preeclampsia/HELLP syndrome. Because DIC is a consumptive coagulopathy that results in depletion of the platelets and clotting factors, early diagnosis and prompt and appropriate management are critical in reducing maternal and perinatal death and complication rates (Cunningham et al., 2014; Genovese, 2011).

NURSING CARE

Nursing care includes continued meticulous assessment for signs of bleeding (e.g., petechiae, oozing from injection sites, and hematuria). Use of an indwelling catheter for monitoring urinary output is essential because renal failure is a potential consequence of DIC. Vital signs and fetal assessments are monitored frequently, and the patient is maintained in a side-lying tilt to enhance blood flow to the uterus. Oxygen may be administered through a rebreathing mask at 8 to 10 L/min, and blood and blood products are

administered according to physician orders (Cunningham et al., 2014; Genovese, 2011). The patient and her family are emotionally supported and kept informed about the maternal–fetal status. (See Chapters 14, 16, and 33 for further discussion.)

Multiple Gestation

Multiple gestation refers to a pregnancy in which two or more fetuses are present in the uterus, and the majority of multiples are twins. Twinning occurs when ovulation produces two separate ova and each is fertilized (dizygotic, or fraternal twins), or if a single fertilized ovum (zygote) splits early in pregnancy and develops into two fetuses (monozygotic, or identical twins) (Fig. 11-12). Assisted reproductive technologies such as assisted embryo hatching and intracytoplasmic sperm injection have resulted in increased monozygotic twinning by as much as eightfold; monozygotic pregnancies account for only 30% of spontaneously conceived twins. In monozygotic twins, the timing of the twinning process determines the type of placenta and membranes that develop (Cunningham et al., 2014; Moise, Kugler, & Jones, 2012):

- *Dichorionic/diamniotic:* Two chorions (outer membrane) and two amnions (inner membrane); division of the embryo takes place during the first 3 days of development; occurs in approximately 25% to 30% of monozygotic twins.
- *Monochorionic/diamniotic:* One chorion (outer membrane) and two amnions (inner membrane) and a single, shared placenta. Division of the embryo takes place between 4 to 8 days of development; occurs in approximately 70% to 75% of monozygotic twins. Each twin has its own amnion, but the fetuses are surrounded by one chorion.
- *Monochorionic/monoamniotic:* One chorion and one amnion—the fetuses share the same living quarters.

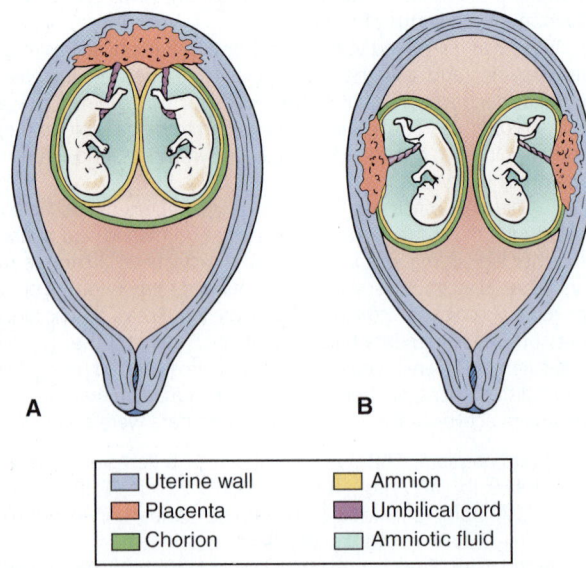

Uterine wall	Amnion
Placenta	Umbilical cord
Chorion	Amniotic fluid

Figure 11-12 Multiple gestations. *A,* Monozygotic twins with one placenta, one chorion, and two amnions. *B,* Dizygotic twins with two placentas, two chorions and two amnions.

The zygotic division occurs later than the first week of development. Associated with a very high (40% to 60%) mortality rate as a result of cord accidents from entanglement.

 Nursing Insight—*Conjoined twins*

Conjoined twins are identical twins, usually female, whose bodies are joined in utero. The twins share a common chorion, amnion, and placenta. Two theories have been proposed to explain the origin of this rare phenomenon (University of Maryland Medical Center, 2014):

- Fission—the fertilized egg splits partially
- Fusion—the fertilized egg separates completely, but stem cells find corresponding stem cells on the other twin and fuse the twins together. This theory is more generally accepted than fission.

INCIDENCE

Multiple gestation (also known as multifetal pregnancy) has increased significantly during the past 10 years and is largely a result of advanced maternal age at childbirth and the widespread availability of assisted reproductive technology. "Multiples" account for 3% of all live births in the United States. During the past decade there has been a 25% increase in the number of twin births, a 116% increase in triplets, a 149% increase in quadruplets, and a 250% increase in the number of quintuplet or higher order births (Malone & D'Alton, 2008; Martin et al., 2011). Dizygotic twins tend to run in families and are more common in people of African descent. Around the world, the rate of dizygotic twins ranges from 1 in 1,000 in Japan to 1 in 20 in several tribes in Nigeria (Cunningham et al., 2014).

ASSOCIATED COMPLICATIONS

Because multiple gestations are associated with a number of maternal and fetal complications, they are considered to be high-risk pregnancies. Complications may occur during the antepartal, intrapartal, or postpartal period. Preterm labor (PTL) often results from uterine overdistension and frequently necessitates an early operative delivery. Other complications include PTL, gestational diabetes, increased urinary tract infections, preeclampsia/eclampsia, acute fatty liver, pulmonary embolism, placenta previa, fetal intrauterine growth restriction (IUGR), abnormal presentation, and umbilical cord prolapse (ACOG, 2004c; Cunningham et al., 2014).

MATERNAL AND FETAL MORBIDITY AND MORTALITY

Maternal morbidity is higher in women with multiple gestations and seems to be related to the number of fetuses present. Twin pregnancies are associated with significantly higher risks of hypertension, placental abruption, anemia, and UTIs than singleton pregnancies (ACOG, 2004c; Malone & D'Alton, 2008). Monochorionicity, growth restriction, and prematurity pose the main risks to fetuses and neonates in a multiple gestation. The mean duration of a twin gestation is 35 weeks; for triplets and quadruplets the mean duration of gestation is 32 and 30 weeks, respectively. The mean gestational age at delivery for multiple gestations can be misleading because the classification does not reveal the true incidence of extreme prematurity, which has great clinical significance. The incidence of preterm delivery prior to 28 weeks for singletons is 0.7% in the United States. For twins, the incidence increases to 5%, and the incidence for triplet gestations is 14%. The perinatal mortality rate for twins is at least threefold higher than with singletons (Malone & D'Alton, 2008).

Perinatal morbidity is also more likely in a multiple gestation. The incidence of a severe handicap in neonatal survivors of multiple gestation is increased from 19.7 per 1,000 for singleton survivors to 34.0 and 57.5 per 1,000 twin and triplet survivors, respectively. Cerebral palsy occurs 17 times more often in triplet pregnancies and more than 4 times more often in twin pregnancies than in singleton pregnancies (ACOG, 2004c; Malone & D'Alton, 2008).

DIAGNOSIS AND DETERMINATION OF CHORIONICITY

A positive diagnosis of a multiple gestation can be confirmed by ultrasound examination. Sonography reveals multiple gestational sacs with yolk sacs by 5 weeks of gestation and multiple embryos with cardiac activity by 6 weeks of gestation (Malone & D'Alton, 2008). Rapid uterine growth, excessive maternal weight gain, or palpation of three or more fetal large parts (cranium and breech) on Leopold maneuvers are clinical findings suggestive of multiple gestation. Laboratory tests show elevated levels of human chorionic gonadotropin (hCG), human placental lactogen (hPL), and maternal serum α-fetoprotein (MSAFP) (Cunningham et al., 2014).

Ultrasound determination of chorionicity (an examination of the chorion), best performed around 10 to 13 weeks' gestation, constitutes an important component of modern management. The presence of placental tissue between the layers of the intervening twin membrane near the placenta is indicative of a dichorionic/diamniotic (DC/DA) gestation, whereas the absence of intervening placental tissue between the membranes is indicative of a single chorion (a monochorionic/diamniotic [MC/DA] twin gestation). As a group, twins contribute disproportionately to the overall perinatal morbidity/mortality rate, and MC/DA twins demonstrate higher mortality rates than DC/DA twins. Twin-to-twin transfusion syndrome, a complication of monochorionic twins, results from vascular connections or anastomoses (i.e., artery-to-vein, artery-to-artery, vein-to-vein) within the single, monochorionic placenta. In most cases, the vessels carry blood from one fetus to the other without creating an imbalance of flow. However, if an imbalance of blood flow occurs, one fetus receives a reduced blood volume (eventually leading to oligohydramnios) while the other twin receives an increased blood volume (eventually leading to polyhydramnios). Without intervention, fetal death eventually occurs in one or both fetuses. Selective IUGR and twin-reversed arterial perfusion sequence are other complications that may affect monochorionic twins; management depends on the underlying cause and the gestational age at the time of diagnosis (Moise et al., 2012; Squires, 2013).

MANAGEMENT

Because multiple gestation pregnancies are considered to be high risk, ideally an appropriately trained specialist should manage the obstetric care. Delivery should be planned to take place at a Level III facility that has trained personnel who are prepared to deal with maternal or neonatal complications. When a pregnancy is complicated by a multiple gestation, the normal maternal physiological adaptations to pregnancy are heightened. Complications that are associated with these changes help to guide the clinical management. Consideration of maternal–fetal physiological parameters along with ongoing surveillance is essential in developing an appropriate plan of care.

NURSING IMPLICATIONS

Caring for the patient with a multiple gestation pregnancy can be challenging, especially when complications arise. Hospitalization may be needed because of the increased risk of complications, and the nurse needs to remain cognizant of this. There is an increased risk of pulmonary edema caused by the expanded plasma volume and increased cardiac output. Also, nutritional requirements are increased. Maternal caloric needs are approximately 40% greater for a woman expecting twins and 80% greater for a woman pregnant with triplets or higher multiples (Gilbert, 2011). Early in the pregnancy, the patient may suffer from severe hyperemesis gravidarum as a result of higher levels of pregnancy hormones found in multiple pregnancies as compared with singleton pregnancies. This condition can lead to dehydration and poor nutrient intake and require hospitalization for rehydration. At this time, the nurse can refer the patient to a nutritionist and also review foods that might be more appealing to the patient. Providing ongoing counseling about the importance of regular prenatal care and the identification of signs and symptoms of PTL and other complications constitutes a critical nursing action throughout the pregnancy.

The nurse must also remain aware that the patients being cared for are the woman (the primary patient) as well as each individual fetus. Serial ultrasounds, nonstress tests, and biophysical profiles will be part of the ongoing assessment for fetal well-being and growth. Fetal surveillance with electronic fetal monitoring may be difficult, especially when there are more than two fetuses. Triplet monitors are available that allow for the tracing of three separate FHRs on a single channel, or two heart rate tracings and a digital readout for the third fetus. It is best to monitor all fetuses simultaneously, and the nurse should label which line corresponds to which ultrasound transducer so that it is clear which fetus is being monitored. The presenting twin is always "A," with the remaining fetuses ("B," "C," etc.) identified by relative ascending positions. Although not common, late pregnancy changes in fetal positions (e.g., male fetus B now in the position of female fetus A) should be noted in the patient record. If no recent ultrasound has been obtained, the nurse should identify each FHR by the appropriate abdominal quadrant (Gilbert, 2011).

A multifetal pregnancy can cause many concerns for the family. They often fear for the well-being of the babies, especially because PTL is a major complication with multiples. The thought of the everyday rigors of caring for several newborns at one time can constitute another major cause of stress. If there are other children in the household, the expectant couple may question how they are going to be able to give the older siblings the care and time they will also need. Family finances can be a great concern as well as the affordability of child care when it is necessary for the mother to return to work. The nurse can be supportive in encouraging families to voice their concerns and address them as appropriately as possible. Helping the family to prepare for the birth of the babies can be of great benefit. The nurse may offer suggestions that include giving the older children household chores appropriate for their age; alerting the partner's employer of a potential need to adjust the work schedule to help out at home; or finding someone to help with housekeeping, grocery shopping, laundry, cleaning, and/or child care. Other team members such as social services can also provide valuable solutions to these concerns. Referring the couple to a "multiples" support group may also be appropriate and welcomed.

 Now Can You—Discuss care of the pregnant patient with a multiple gestation?

1. Name five complications associated with a multiple gestation?
2. Describe your plan of care, taking into consideration the maternal fetal physiological parameters of the multiple gestation pregnancy?
3. Identify other team members you would include in your plan of care?

Infections

URINARY TRACT INFECTION

Urinary tract infection (UTI) is the most common bacterial infection in pregnancy. The three most common clinical syndromes associated with UTI are asymptomatic bacteriuria, acute cystitis, and acute pyelonephritis.

Pathophysiology

The physiological dilation of the urinary collecting system that occurs normally during pregnancy is associated with an increase in ascending urinary infections. Mechanical and hormonal changes may lead to hydroureter, decreased peristalsis, bladder distention, and incomplete emptying. These events can result in urine stasis or reflux in the bladder and ureters (Cunningham et al., 2014; Moran, 2011a).

The most common infecting organism is *Escherichia coli* (*E coli*), which is responsible for 75% to 90% of all bacteriuria during pregnancy. Other organisms frequently responsible for UTIs include *Klebsiella, Proteus, Pseudomonas, Chlamydia, Enterobacter,* Group B streptococcus, and coagulase-negative staphylococci (Thadhani & Maski, 2013).

Morbidity

Bacteriuria in pregnancy predisposes the patient to the development of acute pyelonephritis, a condition that poses significant risk to the woman and her fetus. Asymptomatic and untreated bacteriuria has been associated with a number of complications during pregnancy including low birth-weight, intrauterine death, preeclampsia, and maternal anemia (Thadhani & Maski, 2013).

Asymptomatic Bacteriuria

Asymptomatic bacteriuria is defined as the presence of at least 10^5 colony-forming units of bacteria per milliliter of clean, voided, midstream urine in specimens obtained on two separate occasions. As the name implies, the patient does not express any symptoms of a UTI. Asymptomatic bacteriuria occurs in 2% to 11% of pregnancies, and if left untreated, approximately 40% of those infected will develop an acute symptomatic UTI. Treatment includes anti-infectives such as ampicillin (Marcillin) for a 7- to 10-day period, although 3-day courses may be as effective. See the CDC Guidelines for Treatment (http://www.cdc.gov/std/treatment/2010/toc.htm) for current treatment regimens. Screening women for asymptomatic bacteriuria on the first prenatal visit constitutes a standard of obstetric care (Moran, 2011a; Thadhani & Maski, 2013).

Acute Cystitis

Symptomatic lower UTI occurs in 1.3% to 3.4% of pregnant women. Symptoms include urinary frequency, urgency, dysuria, and suprapubic pain. The treatment is the same as for asymptomatic bacteriuria (Thadhani & Maski, 2013).

 Nursing Insight—*Anti-infective medication use for UTI during pregnancy*

Commonly used antibiotics, including penicillins, erythromycin, and cephalosporins, are safe to use during pregnancy. The evidence regarding an association between the nitrofuran and sulfonamide classes of antibiotics and birth defects is mixed; these medications should be used during the first trimester only when no other suitable alternative antibiotics are available. During the second and third trimesters, sulfonamides and nitrofurantoins may continue to be used as first-line agents for the treatment and prevention of UTIs (ACOG, 2011c).

Acute Pyelonephritis

Pyelonephritis, an inflammation of the kidney substance and pelvis, occurs in 1% to 2% of pregnant women. This condition presents as flank tenderness on the affected side and is associated with nausea, vomiting, fever, and chills along with the symptoms of a lower UTI. Significant pyuria and bacteriuria are present. Pyelonephritis is treated aggressively with hospitalization and IV antibiotics. If left untreated or inadequately treated, septic shock, adult respiratory distress syndrome, and/or PTL may result (Cunningham et al., 2014; Thadhani & Maski, 2013).

 Optimizing Outcomes—**When caring for the patient with an UTI**

During pregnancy, a urine specimen is more likely to be contaminated by bacteria that originate in the urethra, vagina, or perineum. This occurs because of a change in pH during pregnancy: the urine becomes more alkaline as a result of the maternal excretion of bicarbonate; the vagina also becomes alkaline and the vaginal secretions have increased glycogen content, which aids bacterial growth. Before collecting a midstream specimen, the nurse should instruct the patient about the importance of proper cleansing.

A urinalysis and urine culture and sensitivity should be obtained on all patients who present with signs of preterm labor, and the nurse must remember that signs of UTI often mimic normal pregnancy complaints (i.e., urgency, frequency). It is important to remind the patient to take *all* the medication that has been prescribed, even if the symptoms subside and she feels better. A Test of Cure (repeat urine test to evaluate whether bacteria are still present) should be obtained once the treatment has been completed.

 Now Can You—**Discuss the significance of a UTI in the pregnant patient?**

1. Describe anatomical and physiological renal system changes during pregnancy that place women at risk for UTIs? Identify the most common organism responsible for a UTI?
2. Explain why pyelonephritis must be treated aggressively?
3. Discuss nursing responsibilities when obtaining a urine specimen from a pregnant patient and identify instructions that should be given to the patient who is treated for a UTI?

Group B Streptococcal Infection

Group B streptococcus (GBS) is a frequent cause of UTIs and chorioamnionitis during pregnancy and a significant cause of endometritis after pregnancy has ended. It is a major pathogen in neonatal sepsis that can result in significant neonatal morbidity and mortality. Women harbor GBS as part of the normal fecal and vaginal flora. It is estimated that 10% to 30% of women are asymptomatic carriers of the organism. However, the rates vary according to the culture technique used, the number of samples cultured, and the nature of the populations studied. When maternal GBS colonization is present, transmission to the neonate is estimated to occur in approximately 60% of cases. The incidence is approximately 1.8 per 1,000 live births (ACOG, 2011d; Cunningham et al., 2014).

The onset of neonatal infection may be early (within the first 6 days of life) or late. Infants with early-onset infection generally develop signs (i.e., respiratory distress, septic shock) during the first 12 hours of life. Exposure to the organism occurs either in utero or during labor as the fetus travels down the colonized birth canal. Risk factors for contracting the infection include prematurity, low birth weight, premature rupture of the membranes (PROM), prolonged labor, maternal chorioamnionitis, multiple gestation, and GBS bacteremia during pregnancy. The overall rate of neonatal mortality from early onset GBS has declined from 50% in 1977 to approximately 6% currently, although infants of low birth weight continue to be at a substantial risk. Late-onset GBS is community acquired (the route of transmission is less clear and can be nosocomial [acquired while in the hospital], environmental, or maternal) and presents more than a week after birth. The majority of infants with community-acquired GBS are full term, and 85% exhibit signs and symptoms of meningitis (ACOG, 2011d).

In an effort to protect infants from GBS infections, the Centers for Disease Control and Prevention (CDC) has issued guidelines (available at http://www.cdc.gov/groupbstrep/guidelines/guidelines.html) that advocate obtaining vaginal and rectal cultures from all pregnant women between 35 and 37 weeks of pregnancy. Women with positive cultures and those with unknown GBS status at the onset of labor and any of the following: delivery at less than 37 weeks of gestation; ruptured membranes greater than or equal to 18 hours; or an intrapartum temperature greater than or equal to 100.4°F (38.0°C) are treated with a penicillin-based anti-infective agent (ACOG, 2011d; Verani, McGee, & Schrag, 2010).

Cultural Diversity: Group B Streptococcal Infection in Infants

Between the years 2003 and 2006, the incidence of early-onset neonatal group B streptococcal (GBS) disease rates increased significantly among term African American infants (0.56 to 0.86/1,000) compared with the rates among Caucasian infants, which remained essentially unchanged (0.26 to 0.29/1,000). The cause of this racial disparity is largely unexplained (Lockwood, 2011).

TORCH INFECTIONS

TORCH refers to a group of maternal infectious diseases that cause harm to the embryo–fetus (see Table 11-3). The TORCH acronym stands for **T**oxoplasmosis, **R**ubella, **C**ytomegalovirus (CMV), and **H**erpes simplex virus type 2 (HSV-2). (Some sources identify the "O" as "other" infections, such as hepatitis B, syphilis, and HIV.) Maternal exposure to the TORCH infections during the first 12 weeks of gestation is associated with fetal developmental anomalies.

SEXUALLY TRANSMITTED INFECTIONS

Sexually transmitted infections (STIs) can cause serious morbidity and, in some cases, mortality in the mother, fetus, and infant. Following perinatal exposure, newborns are at risk for a number of minor and major complications that include congenital anomalies, mental impairment, and death. Women exposed to STIs are at risk for infertility, ectopic pregnancy, and pregnancy complications (Cunningham et al., 2014). See the CDC website (www.cdc.gov/std/treatment/) for the latest STI treatment guidelines.

Chlamydia Trachomatis

Chlamydia trachomatis is the most prevalent sexually transmitted infection in the United States. An estimated 3 million cases occur annually, and approximately 30% of pregnant women are infected. *C trachomatis* causes genital infections that are frequently asymptomatic and thus difficult to treat. However, infected women who do experience symptoms usually complain of vaginal discharge, dysuria, and, on occasion, abnormal vaginal bleeding. On speculum examination, the cervix exhibits a distinct mucopurulent discharge along with marked inflammation of the endocervix. Some women also experience an acute urethral syndrome manifested by dysuria, urinary frequency, and the presence of pyuria in a sterile urine specimen. Oral anti-infectives such as erythromycin or penicillin-based agents are used to treat *C trachomatis* during pregnancy (CDC, 2010c).

Neonatal infection, most commonly manifested as conjunctivitis and pneumonia, results from exposure to the pathogen during birth. Typically, conjunctivitis occurs during the first 5 to 12 days of life, whereas pneumonia does not develop until 1 to 3 months after birth. Topical antibiotic therapy, routinely administered during the immediate neonatal period, is inadequate for the treatment of a chlamydial infection. Because treatment with erythromycin is only about 80% effective, the newborn requires careful follow-up by the pediatrician (Anderson & Gonik, 2010).

Neisseria Gonorrhoeae

Neisseria gonorrhoeae (gonococci [GC], gonorrhea), a gram-negative diplococcus, is one of the oldest known sexually transmitted infections. It often coexists with chlamydia. The most common site of infection is the genitourinary tract. Infection sites unique to women include the Skene's and Bartholin's glands, endocervix, endometrium, and fallopian tubes. Symptoms of infection include vaginal discharge, dysuria, and abnormal vaginal bleeding. A speculum examination often reveals an inflamed, friable (easy to bleed) cervix. The treatment regimen may include ceftriaxone IM, or cefixime PO, or an injectible cephalosporin, plus azithromycin PO or doxycycline PO (log on to www.cdc.gov/std/gonorrhea for the most up-to-date recommendations) (CDC, 2010c). Infants born to untreated, infected mothers are at risk for disseminated infection (bacteremia) and **ophthalmia neonatorum** (an eye inflammation) that can result in permanent blindness from perforation of the globe of the eye.

The amniotic infection syndrome is an additional manifestation of gonococcal infection in pregnancy. This entity manifests as placental, fetal membrane, and umbilical cord inflammation that occurs after PROM and is associated with infected oral and gastric aspirate, leukocytosis, neonatal infection, and maternal fever. Characteristics of the syndrome include PROM, premature delivery, and a high rate of infant morbidity (Duff, 2013; Moran, 2011a).

Syphilis

Syphilis is an acute and chronic infection caused by the spirochete *Treponema pallidum*. It has a long clinical course that begins with an incubation period followed by primary, secondary, and tertiary infection. Throughout this time, there is progressive damage to the CNS, cardiovascular system, and musculoskeletal system. Syphilis is transmitted primarily through sexual contact, or fetal infection may occur transplacentally. During pregnancy, syphilis usually occurs in women who are young and unmarried and in those who receive little or no prenatal care (CDC, 2010c).

The onset of primary syphilis is usually heralded by the appearance of a chancre, a painless, round, ulcerated lesion with a raised border and indurated (hardened) base. In women, the chancre most commonly appears on the vulva, cervix, and vagina. Penicillin is the treatment of choice for all stages. If left untreated, the disease progresses, becomes chronic, and may lead to death.

Prompt maternal treatment eliminates most fetal syphilis infections, but delayed treatment or failure to obtain treatment may result in fetal effects that range from minor anomalies to preterm birth or fetal death. Damage to the fetus depends on when during gestation the infection occurred and the amount of time elapsed before treatment. Neonatal infection may be present at birth but not expressed for up to 2 years ("silent infection"). Manifestations of congenital syphilis include rhinitis (snuffles), macular rash on the palms and soles of the feet, osteochondritis (inflammation of the bony epiphysis), perichondritis (inflammation of the membrane that covers the surface of cartilage), hepatosplenomegaly, jaundice, anemia, and thrombocytopenia (Patterson & Davies, 2011).

Human Papillomavirus Infection

Human papillomavirus (HPV) is a sexually transmitted virus that causes **condylomata acuminata** (genital warts) and is the primary cause of cervical neoplasia. Approximately 70% of cervical cancers result from infection with HPV (ACOG, 2010b). Risk factors associated with HPV infection include early onset of sexual activity, multiple sex partners, cigarette smoking, and long-term use of oral contraceptives (Duff, 2013).

The prevalence of genital warts is highest among the 16- to 25-year-old age-group, which is also the age-group with the highest rate of pregnancy. The warts grow more rapidly during pregnancy and may involve the cervix, vagina, or vulva so extensively that vaginal delivery is precluded. The reason for the increase in size and number of the lesions is not known but has been postulated to be the decrease in cell-mediated immunity that occurs during pregnancy. Management of these lesions in pregnancy presents difficult problems, and treatment includes trichloroacetic acid, dichloroacetic acid, cryotherapy, and surgical excision. None of these therapies has been shown to be superior to the others. The best approach to treatment during pregnancy may be the excision of the lesions by laser, electrocautery, or cryosurgery. Care must be taken to prevent extensive scarring or sloughing of tissue (CDC, 2010c; Duff, 2013; Moran, 2011a).

The risk for transmission of the virus from maternal condylomata acuminata to the neonate has not been established. HPV is present in maternal blood and can be transmitted transplacentally to the fetus, but the incidence is very low according to reported studies (Porterfield, 2011).

✿ Nursing Insight—*Preventing HPV through vaccination*

Nurses can be instrumental in preventing infection caused by the human papillomavirus. The American Congress of Obstetricians and Gynecologists (ACOG) Committee on Adolescent Health Care and the ACOG Working Group on Immunization recommend that females 9 to 26 years of age receive vaccination against HPV. (The CDC Advisory Committee on Immunization Practices also recommends routine quadrivalent HPV vaccination for boys aged 11 or 12 years, and for others up to age 21 years who haven't already received the vaccine). Although obstetricians/gynecologists are not likely to care for many girls in this initial vaccination group, ACOG has recommended that the first adolescent reproductive health-care visit take place between 13 and 15 years of age. These visits are a strategic time to discuss HPV and the potential benefit of the HPV vaccine and to offer vaccination to those who have not already received it (ACOG, 2010b; CDC, 2011).

HIV and AIDS

HIV type 1 (HIV-1) infection, with rare exception, causes a slow but relentless destruction of the immune system that ultimately results in AIDS. HIV type 2 (HIV-2) infection has a more variable and benign course. HIV-2 has remained largely confined to West Africa, whereas HIV-1 strains are causing increasing epidemics around the world (CDC, 2012).

HIV-1 infection is an increasing problem among women of childbearing age. AIDS is the fifth leading cause of death among women 25 to 44 years of age and has become a leading cause of death for young children in many parts of the world. Without identification of HIV-infected women and the aggressive use of preventive therapy, 20% to 30% of these children will become infected with HIV (CDC, 2012; Moran, 2011a; National Institutes of Health [NIH], 2012). Ideally, HIV testing is offered preconceptionally; if not, testing should take place as early in the pregnancy as possible. Repeat testing in the third trimester, or rapid HIV testing during labor or birth as indicated (i.e., women living in areas with high HIV prevalence), or both also are recommended as additional strategies to further reduce the rate of perinatal HIV transmission (ACOG, 2008c). Screening with a rapid HIV test is recommended for women who present in labor with an unknown HIV status; if reactive, immediate antiretroviral prophylaxis should be recommended (AWHONN, 2011).

TRANSMISSION. Heterosexual unprotected sexual contact now poses the greatest risk to women. Because vaginal mucus can harbor the retrovirus, women are more likely than men to contract HIV infection through heterosexual activity. Factors that increase the risk of transmission include (Moran, 2011a):

- Unprotected sexual intercourse (no condom is used)
- Sexual contact with an uncircumcised man
- Increased number of sexual contacts
- Presence of genital sores
- Advanced disease state
- Presence of other sexually transmitted infections, especially those that cause genital ulcers (e.g., herpes, syphilis, and chancroid)

The risk of vertical transmission to the fetus or newborn is proportional to the concentration of virus in maternal plasma (viral load). Vertical transmission occurs antepartally when the virus crosses the placenta, intrapartally when it travels (via the bloodstream) from the vagina up into the uterus during labor or following rupture of the membranes, or postpartally through transfer in the breast milk (Lawrence & Lawrence, 2010). Transmission of HIV to the fetus or infant is believed to most often occur late in pregnancy or during labor and birth. Increased rates of transmission also occur with advanced maternal disease and ruptured membranes and after events during labor and delivery that increase fetal exposure to maternal blood (ACOG, 2000b). In 2000, ACOG established guidelines to prevent HIV transmission; these guidelines were updated in 2004 and reaffirmed in 2010 (Box 11-9).

⊖ Optimizing Outcomes—**Decreasing the incidence of STIs in women and children**

Nurses should be aware of the signs and symptoms of STIs so as to recognize them and appropriately counsel patients about them.

- Alert the pediatrician to the patient's positive history of an STI.
- Counsel women in a nonjudgmental and compassionate manner about safe sex habits (i.e., the use of condoms).

Table 11-3 TORCH Infections

Infection/Agent/ Transmission	Detection	Maternal Effects
Toxoplasmosis *Toxoplasma gondii* **Single-celled protozoan parasite. Transmitted transplacentally.**	Serological antibody testing IgM-specific antibody IgG seroconversion from negative to positive. Active infection indicated by a rise in IgG titer in two appropriately spaced tests. After 20 weeks of gestation, fetal blood samples can be tested for the presence of specific IgM. Ultrasonography can demonstrate severe congenital toxoplasmosis (e.g., ventriculomegaly, intracranial calcifications, microcephaly, ascites, hepatosplenomegaly, intrauterine growth restriction).	Most infections are asymptomatic but may cause fatigue, muscle pains, penumonitis, myocarditis, and lymphadenopathy.
Other Hepatitis B DNA virus Transmitted via direct contact with blood or body fluids from an infected person.	HBsAG identified 7–14 days after exposure HBsAb present with HBsAG indicates non infectious stage	Course of the disease is not altered during the pregnancy, and 30%–50% of infected women are asymptomatic. When present, symptoms include low-grade fever, nausea, anorexia, jaundice, hepatomegaly, malaise, preterm labor, and preterm birth.
Rubella (German measles) Caused by the rubella virus. Transmitted via nasopharyngeal secretions; also transplacentally	Rubella-specific IgM antibodies Rubella antibody titer of 1:8 or more indicates immune status	Erythematous maculopapular rash on face, neck, arms, and legs lasting 3 days. Also, lymph node enlargement, slight fever, malaise, headache, and arthralgia.
Cytomegalovirus (CMV) DNA virus of the herpes group. Transmitted by droplet infection and contact with infected secretions (saliva, urine, breast milk, cervical mucus, semen); also transplacentally	Serology of CMV-specific IgM antibody	Most infections are asymptomatic, but when present (15% of adults), include a mononucleosis-like syndrome (e.g., fever, pharyngitis, lymphadenopathy, polyarthritis).

Fetal/ Neonatal Effects	Management	Nursing Considerations
Severity varies with gestational age (i.e., the earlier the fetus is infected, the more severe the disease); congenital infection can result if acute toxoplasmosis occurs during pregnancy (especially likely in third trimester). Can cause spontaneous abortion, low birth weight, hepatosplenomegaly, icterus, anemia, neurological disease, and chorioretinitis	Pregnant women who acquire toxoplasmosis should be treated with spiramycin. If fetal infection is established, treatment consists of a combination of pyrimethamine, sulfadiazine, and folinic acid, alternating with spiramycin to eradicate parasites in the placenta and in the fetus.	Teach women: avoid consuming raw or poorly cooked meat, especially pork, lamb, or venison and do not touch the hands or mouth after handling undercooked meat; avoid contact with cat feces; peel or thoroughly wash fruits and vegetables. Approximately 50% of adults have an antibody to this organism. ACOG (2000a) does not recommend routine screening except for women with HIV infection.
Stillbirth Neonates may be infected following exposure to maternal blood, genital secretions at birth. 1 in 1,000–8,000 infants have a 90% chance of becoming chronically infected, HBV carrier and a 25% risk of developing significant liver disease; 95% can be prevented with prophylaxis at birth; 90%–95% of those infected are symptomatic and become chronic hepatitis B carriers	Mother: No specific treatment, but may include bedrest and a high-protein, low-fat diet Infant: HBIG HBV vaccine recommended (three doses)	Women at risk include: Pregnant women from China, Southeast Asia, Africa, Philippines, and Indonesia Eskimos Prostitutes Homosexuals IV drug users Hemophiliacs Transfusion recipients People with other sexually transmitted diseases or multiple sex partners CDC recommends universal screening of all prenatal patients. Hepatitis B vaccine can be safely given in pregnancy at 0, 1, and 6 months (standard schedule), or at 0, 1, and 4 months (accelerated schedule) (Sheffield et al., 2011). Mother to child transmission of HBV occurs in 10%–20% of women who are seropositive for HBsAG and in 90% of women who are seropositive for both HBsAG and HBcAg.
Overall risk of congenital rubella syndrome is 20% for primary maternal infection in the first trimester; 50% if maternal infection occurs during the first 4 weeks of gestation; and 25% if the infection occurs in the 2nd 4-week period after conception. Congenital spectrum anomalies include: Deafness (60%–75%) Eye defects (10%–30%) CNS anomalies (10%–25%) Cardiac malformation (10%–20%)	Women with rubella require no special therapy other than mild analgesics and rest. Infants born with congenital rubella may shed virus for many months and thus be a threat to other infants, as well as to susceptible adults.	Occurs most often in the springtime, and an estimated 6%–25% of women are susceptible. Inquire about history of exposure 3 weeks earlier. Vaccine is contraindicated during pregnancy. Patient counseling: If nonimmune (i.e., absence of rubella antibody), she should be vaccinated immediately postpartum and use contraception for a minimum of 1 month after vaccination.
Infection to fetus most likely with primary maternal infection and timing: first and second trimester exposure associated with more severe effects: low birth weight, IUGR, microcephaly CNS abnormalities, mental and motor retardation, intracranial calcifications, sensorineural deafness, blindness with chorioretinitis, intellectual and developmental disabilities, hepatosplenomegaly, jaundice	Mother: treat symptoms Infant: no satisfactory treatment is available; isolate the infant. Ganciclovir may prevent hearing loss and developmental outcomes in infants born with symptomatic congenital CMV infection with CNS involvement, but this antiviral medication has serious side effects.	Factors associated with increased risk of maternal infection include history of abnormal cervical cytology, lower socioeconomic status, birth outside North America, first pregnancy at younger than 15 years, and history of STI. Day care centers can be a common source of infection. Counsel patients at high risk (e.g., those with young children or who work with young children): carefully handle potentially infected articles (e.g., diapers), practice safe-handling techniques such as rigorous hand washing and the use of latex gloves, avoid high risk behaviors (e.g., IV drug use, sharing of needles), use condoms. Maternal immunity does not eliminate the possibility of fetal infection. Routine serological screening is not recommended by ACOG (2000a). Vaccine is available but more research is needed. Counsel patients: maintain rigorous personal hygiene throughout pregnancy.

(continued)

Table 11-3 TORCH Infections (continued)

Infection/Agent/ Transmission	Detection	Maternal Effects
Herpes simplex virus (HSV) **Double-stranded DNA virus, associated with chronic infection.** **Transmitted via viral exposure at time of birth and ascending infection, also transplacental transmission is possible if initial infection occurs during pregnancy.**	Tissue culture (swab specimen from vesicles) Immunofluorescent staining of the cell can differentiate HSV-1 from HSV-2	Painful genital vesicle lesions (may be present on the cervix, vagina, or external genitalia). The primary infection is commonly associated with fever, malaise and myalgia, numbness, tingling, burning, itching, and pain. May also have lymphadenopathy and urinary retention.

ACOG, American College of Obstetricians and Gynecologists; CDC, Centers for Disease Control and Prevention; DNA, deoxyribonucleic acid; HBV, hepatitis B virus; HIV, human immunodeficiency virus; HbsAb, surface antibody to hepatitis B; HBsAG, surface antigen to hepatitis B; HBcAg, core antigen to HBV; HBIG, hepatitis B immune globulin; IgG, immunoglobulin G; IgM, immunoglobulin M; IUGR, intrauterine growth restriction

Sources: ACOG (2000a), (2007a), (2007b), (2008c); CDC (2010a), (2010b); Moran (2011a); Sheffield, Hickman, Tang, Moss, Kourosh, Crawford, et al. (2011).

Box 11-9 **Management to Prevent Transmission of HIV Infection**

- Patients should be counseled that in the absence of antiretroviral therapy, the risk of vertical transmission is approximately 25%. With zidovudine (ZDV) therapy, the risk is reduced to 5%–8%. When care includes both ZDV therapy and scheduled cesarean delivery, the risk is approximately 2%. A risk of 2% or less is seen in those women with viral loads of less than 1,000 copies per milliliter even without delivery via cesarean section.

- Plasma viral loads should be determined at baseline and then every 3 months or following changes in therapy. The patient's most recently determined viral load should be used to direct counseling regarding the mode of delivery.

- Women infected with HIV whose viral loads are greater than 1,000 copies per milliliter should be counseled as to the benefits of a scheduled cesarean section in reducing the risk of vertical transmission to the infant.

- Patients should receive antiretroviral chemotherapy during pregnancy according to the accepted guidelines for adults. This therapy should not be interrupted around the time of cesarean delivery. For those patients receiving ZDV, adequate levels of the drug in the blood should be achieved if the infusion is begun 3 hours preoperatively.

- Best clinical estimates of gestational age should be used for planning cesarean delivery. Amniocentesis to determine fetal lung maturity should be avoided whenever possible.

- All women should be clearly informed of the risks associated with cesarean delivery, because the preoperative maternal health status affects the degree of the risk of maternal morbidity associated with cesarean delivery.

- The patient's autonomy in making the decision regarding the route of delivery must be respected. A patient's informed decision to undergo vaginal delivery must be honored, with cesarean delivery performed only for other accepted indications and with patient consent.

Source: ACOG (2008c).

Fetal/ Neonatal Effects	Management	Nursing Considerations
Transmission rate of 30%–50% among women who first acquire genital herpes near time of delivery and is less than 1% among women with recurrent genital herpes. Mortality of 50% if neonatal exposure is with active primary infection. Neurological morbidity associated with chorioretinitis, microcephaly, intellectual and developmental disabilities, seizures, and apnea.	Maternal prophylactic treatment with oral acyclovir, valacyclovir, or famciclovir may be prescribed for women with frequent recurrent infections. Women with active recurrent genital herpes should be offered suppressive viral therapy at or beyond 36 weeks of gestation. Intrapartally, avoid routine invasive monitoring (e.g., fetal scalp electrodes), which increases the risk of neonatal infection. However, may be used if indicated.	Routine antepartal genital HSV cultures in asymptomatic patients with recurrent disease are not recommended; routine HSV screening of pregnant women is not recommended. In early pregnancy, inquire about symptoms, including prodromal symptoms (e.g., vulvar pain, burning, and tingling). Teach patients: use condoms to decrease risk of exposure; avoid all genital contact when male partner has penile lesions. HSV risk factors: Female gender, history of a prior STI, early age for first sexual intercourse, unprotected sex and having an intimate partner with genital herpes, poor socioeconomic status, and a high number of sexual partners. Women with compromised immune systems are at very high risk for HSV. During pregnancy, transabdominal invasive procedures (e.g., chorionic villus sampling, amniocentesis, and percutaneous umbilical cord blood sampling) may be performed even when genital lesions are present. In patients with active HSV infection and ruptured membranes at or near term, current recommendations call for cesarean delivery. Counsel patients: if prodromal symptoms or active genital lesions are present, cesarean birth will be the recommended mode of delivery. However, cesarean delivery does not completely prevent vertical transmission to the neonate. Breastfeeding is not contraindicated, but it is essential to consistently practice rigorous hand washing. When active lesions are present, use extreme caution when handling the infant. Also, be aware that neonatal infection may be acquired from family members (other than the mother) and from sites other than the genital tract.

- Encourage women to obtain routine checkups and promptly report any signs or symptoms of an STI to their provider.
- Instruct the woman undergoing treatment that she must take all the medication prescribed and keep any follow-up appointments.
- Remind the patient that her partner must also be treated, and if he refuses, she must abstain from sex with him until he is treated.
- Remember to always use standard precautions.

TUBERCULOSIS

Tuberculosis (TB) is an infectious, communicable disease caused by the tubercle bacillus, *Mycobacterium tuberculosis*. The disease causes inflammatory infiltrations most commonly in the respiratory tract, although TB may also affect the gastrointestinal and genitourinary tracts, bones, joints, nervous system, lymph nodes, and skin. TB is the most common infectious disease in the world. Since 1992, the number of cases of TB has decreased. However, health-care professionals caring for pregnant women and newborns are challenged to remain skilled in screening, identifying, and treating TB infection because the disease remains at epidemic levels in certain areas of the country and in certain populations. Women who are homeless, infected with HIV, or IV drug users or those who have emigrated from countries with a high rate of TB (e.g., Latin America, Asia, and Africa) are at highest risk (Cunningham et al., 2014; Yancy, 2011).

Although maternal TB does not appear to cause congenital malformations, it may lead to fetal infection. TB can spread to the fetus from the maternal blood if the bacilli cross the placenta and enter the umbilical vein. Fetal blood then passes through the liver, and this organ serves as the primary focus for the disease in the fetus and newborn. If the bacilli bypass the fetal liver, the lungs may become the primary infection site. Neonates may become infected at the time of birth by aspiration of infected amniotic fluid or by aspiration of infected blood and tissue if the mother has tuberculosis endometritis. They may also become infected through the traditional airborne route if individuals in the infant's environment have pulmonary tuberculosis (Cunningham et al., 2014; Yancy, 2011).

Initial treatment of active TB in pregnancy includes isoniazid, ethambutol, and rifampin, medications that are considered to be safe during pregnancy. Therapy should be continued for 9 months. Breastfeeding is not contraindicated and can begin or can continue during anti-TB therapy, because the medications do not cross into the breast milk. However, if the infant is concurrently taking oral antituberculosis therapy, excessive drug levels may be reached in the neonate, and breastfeeding should be avoided (Cunningham et al., 2014; Yancy, 2011).

⊙ Optimizing Outcomes—Immunizations during pregnancy

The ideal time to immunize women to prevent the spread of disease to the fetus is during the preconceptional period. However, the maternal and fetal benefits of immunization during pregnancy usually outweigh the theoretical risks of adverse effects. The risk for exposure to disease and its deleterious effects on the pregnant woman and the fetus must be balanced against the efficacy of the vaccine and any beneficial effects that may result from it. The American College of Obstetricians and Gynecologists Advisory Committee on Immunization Practices guidelines recommends that health-care providers administer a dose of tetanus toxoid, reduced diphtheria toxoid, and acellular pertussis vaccine (Tdap) during each pregnancy, irrespective of the patient's prior history of receiving Tdap. To maximize the maternal antibody response and passive antibody transfer and levels in the newborn, the optimal timing for Tdap administration is between 27 weeks and 36 weeks of gestation, although Tdap may be given at any time during pregnancy (ACOG, 2013d). Nurses can educate their patients regarding the importance of immunizations, and documentation of the patient's immunization status should be a part of the permanent medical record.

Systemic Lupus Erythematosus

Systemic lupus erythematosus (SLE) is a chronic multisystem inflammatory disorder. It is characterized by an autoimmune antibody production that results in an inflammation of the connective tissue in various organs or systems in the body. The disease tends to affect young women in the second, third, and fourth decades of life but may occur in any age-group. The prevalence of SLE is approximately 1 per 1,000 in the general population, and 90% of cases occur in women during their childbearing years (Cunningham et al., 2014; Yancy, 2011).

PATHOPHYSIOLOGY

The immune system is composed of specialized cells that destroy invading organisms by phagocytosis and antibody and lymphocyte production. When a foreign organism or antigen enters the body, it is consumed by macrophages and then passed on to lymphokines, which present the

antigens to the T and B lymphocytes. The B lymphocytes are activated, resulting in the production of an increased number of circulating antibodies that target their specific antigen. The antigen–antibody complex either promotes destruction of the antigen or activates the normal inactive proteins in the complement system. With SLE, the body fails to recognize its own proteins. The clinical manifestations result from inflammation of multiple organ systems, especially the joints, skin, kidneys, nervous system, and serous membranes (Lockshin, Salmon, & Erkan, 2013).

EFFECTS DURING PREGNANCY

Adverse pregnancy outcome is more common in SLE than in any other rheumatic disease. In the pre-steroid era, it was common practice to terminate pregnancy in patients with active SLE. However, with successful treatment of active disease with corticosteroids, this practice has become less frequent. Patients are more likely to have inactive SLE at the onset of pregnancy because of earlier disease diagnosis and more effective prepregnancy therapy, as well as appropriate prepregnancy counseling (Lockshin et al., 2013). Pregnancy outcome is improved in the following circumstances: SLE has been in remission for at least 6 months; there is no active renal involvement; superimposed preeclampsia does not develop; and there is no evidence of antiphospholipid antibody activity (Cunningham et al., 2014).

The patient with SLE should be seen frequently by both an internist-rheumatologist and a perinatologist specializing in high-risk cases. Assessment of the signs and symptoms of an impending SLE flareup should be elicited on the patient's history and physical examination, and blood samples obtained for serological evaluation. A rise in the anti-dsDNA antibody titer and a decrease in complement may be predictive of an exacerbation of SLE. The onset of edema and hypertension in pregnancy in these patients is characteristic of both preeclampsia and active SLE-associated nephritis. Because the treatment of these conditions is very different, the importance of an accurate diagnosis is essential (Lockshin et al., 2013).

PERINATAL MORBIDITY AND MORTALITY

When SLE complicates the pregnancy, there is an increased risk of spontaneous abortion (SAB), PROM, PTL, preterm birth, stillbirth, and neonatal death (Lockshin et al., 2013; Yancy, 2011). Congenital heart block or congestive heart failure of the fetus or newborn is of particular concern. Maternal autoantibodies may cross the placenta and form immune complexes with fetal autoantigens, promoting fetal tissue destruction. Autoantibodies may initiate injury to fetal cardiac tissue, resulting in conduction disturbances that may be temporary or permanent (Lockshin et al., 2013).

MANAGEMENT

Management of SLE is aggressive and includes immunosuppression of lupus flare with corticosteroid therapy, nonsteroidal anti-inflammatory drugs, antimalarial agents, azathioprine, and careful fetal surveillance. If the disease flares during the pregnancy, treatment must be implemented as quickly as possible. The physician assesses the manifestations and extent of the disease exacerbation and selects the safest, most effective therapy. The patient's health must be deemed the first priority, and the treatment is planned accordingly (Lockshin et al., 2013). When caring for patients with SLE, nurses should offer support and remain alert for early indicators of SLE exacerbation and pregnancy complications. Patients and their families should be educated about the plan of care, the need for close surveillance, and the importance of effective family planning after the birth.

Hemoglobinopathies of Pregnancy

The major function of the red blood cell (RBC) is to carry hemoglobin, which transports oxygen from the lungs to the tissues. The ability of hemoglobin to bind to oxygen is determined by its structural composition. Normal hemoglobin consists of a heme molecule, which is an iron protoporphyrin, combined with two pairs of globin chains. Significant shortening of RBC survival occurs because of alterations in the structure (i.e., sickle hemoglobin) or quantity (i.e., thalassemia) of the hemoglobin chains. These alterations result from inherited disorders. In their most severe forms, these disorders are associated with hemolytic anemia and progressive multi-organ failure (Cunningham et al., 2014).

SICKLE CELL DISEASE

Sickle cell disease is the most common hemoglobinopathy in the United States. It is of recessive inheritance and occurs when the gene for the production of hemoglobin S (HbS) is inherited from both parents (homozygous). It is seen most frequently in those of African and Mediterranean descent. Sickle cell anemia (SCA) is the most prevalent and severe form of the sickle cell diseases (Yancy, 2011).

Pathophysiology

Patients with sickle cell anemia suffer from lifelong complications, in part as a result of the markedly shortened life span of their RBCs. When HbS is exposed to low oxygen tension, it precipitates into long crystals, or polymers, within the RBC. With the lowered or absent amount of oxygen, the sickle cell hemoglobin molecule becomes rigid and dehydrated and assumes an abnormal crescent (sickled) shape (Fig. 11-13). The sickled erythrocytes cannot change their shape and are unable to squeeze through the microcirculation. Obstruction results, leading to hypoxia. Progressive tissue and organ damage occur along with painful vaso-occlusive crises and an increased susceptibility to infection. The signs and symptoms, which are related to vascular occlusion, hemolysis (lysis of the RBCs), and infection, are associated with a number of laboratory and clinical findings. Hemoglobin levels usually fall within the range of 6 to 8 g/dL; there is an increase in bilirubin levels caused by hemolysis; and folate, or iron deficiency, results from bone marrow suppression. Clinical signs may include hepatomegaly, cardiomegaly, conjunctival vessel changes, systolic murmurs, and arthritis (ACOG, 2007c; Kilpatrick, 2013).

Effects During Pregnancy

Many pregnancies complicated by SCA are associated with poor perinatal outcomes. Severe anemia and frequent vaso-occlusive crises may occur during pregnancy, and these problems are associated with an increased maternal and perinatal morbidity and mortality. Although maternal mortality is rare

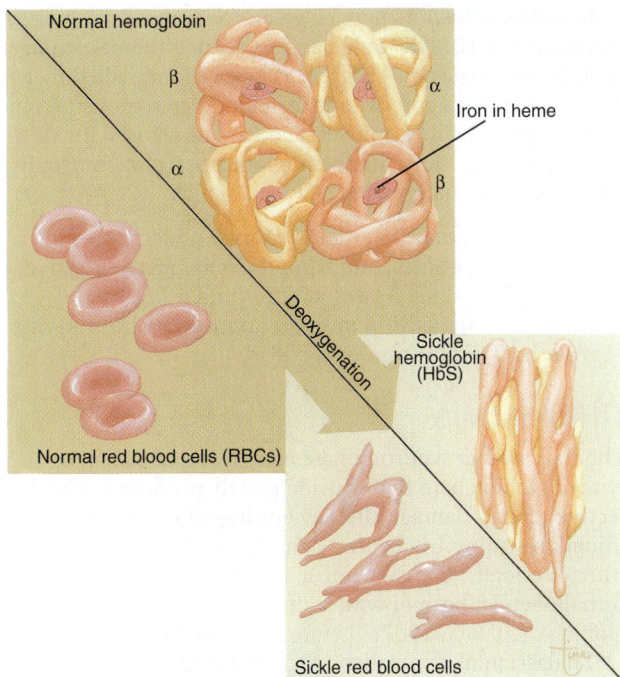

Figure 11-13 Comparison of normal hemoglobin and normal red blood cells to sickle hemoglobin (Hb S) and sickle red blood cells.

in patients with SCA, maternal morbidity is great. Infections are common and occur in 50% to 67% of affected women. The respiratory and urinary tracts are the most common sites of infection, and all infections must be promptly treated because fever, dehydration, and acidosis results in further sickling and painful crises (Cunningham et al., 2014).

The rate of SAB in pregnancies complicated by SCA may be as high as 25%, and stillbirth rates have been reported to reach 8% to 10%. Poor perinatal outcome is related to an increased frequency of PTL, PROM, preterm birth, intrauterine infection, preeclampsia, poor placental perfusion with IUGR, and maternal postpartum infection (ACOG, 2007c; Cunningham et al., 2014).

Management

The care of the maternity patient with SCA must be individualized. Ideally, care should be provided in a medical center experienced in treating the multitude of problems that can complicate these pregnancies. Management of care includes the following (ACOG, 2007c; Kilpatrick, 2013):

- Promotion of good dietary habits with a folate supplement of at least 4 mg/day. Iron supplements are not routinely given, but serum iron and ferritin levels should be checked monthly and iron supplementation initiated only when the levels are diminished. Of note, the incidence of pica appears to be significantly increased in sickle cell patients. This nonnutritional practice may compromise the iron available for hemoglobin synthesis.
- Early detection of infection and treatment. Urine cultures are performed routinely to detect asymptomatic bacteriuria.
- Prevention of dehydration; IV fluids may be indicated.
- Prompt treatment of sickle cell crisis with oxygen, fluids, and pain management; IV morphine is usually the drug of choice.

Blood transfusions may be given to increase the hemoglobin to the 10 g/dL range and to reduce the percentage of sickle hemoglobin. This goal is best accomplished by an exchange transfusion: 2 units of blood are removed from the patient and 3 to 4 units of blood are transfused in. With this maneuver, the sickle hemoglobin percentage usually falls to approximately 40%.

- Fetal surveillance: Fetal kick counts, nonstress tests, biophysical profiles, and Doppler velocimetry begin as early as 26 weeks. Assessment of fundal height and ultrasound are used to monitor appropriate intrauterine growth (Cunningham et al., 2014).

THALASSEMIA

The thalassemia syndromes are named and classified by the type of globin chain that is inadequately produced. The defective chains damage the developing RBCs by oxidative injury, resulting in chronic hemolysis and, ultimately, in iron overload. The two most common types are α- or β-thalassemia, both of which affect the synthesis of hemoglobin A (ACOG, 2007c; Leung & Lockwood, 2013).

Thalassemia, also called "Mediterranean anemia," predominately affects African Americans and individuals of Italian, Greek, Middle Eastern, Indian, Asian, and West Indies descent. However, with the increased interethnic mixing and increasing immigration patterns of today, the at-risk populations are changing (ACOG, 2007c; Kilpatrick, 2013).

β-*Thalassemia*

β-Thalassemia is the most common form of thalassemia. The homozygous state of β-thalassemia is known as "thalassemia major" or "Cooley's anemia." Patients with this disorder are transfusion dependent and have marked hepatosplenomegaly and bone changes secondary to increased hematopoiesis. Death generally is caused by infectious or cardiovascular complications before the third decade of life. Female infants who survive to puberty usually have amenorrhea and severely impaired fertility (Kilpatrick, 2013).

Heterozygous β-thalassemia minor results in various degrees of illness, depending on the rate of β-chain production. The characteristic findings of this disorder include a relatively high RBC count, moderate to marked microcytosis, and a peripheral smear that resembles iron deficiency. However, there may actually be a severe overload of iron because of the increased iron absorption that results from ineffective erythropoiesis (ACOG, 2007c; Kilpatrick, 2013).

β-THALASSEMIA AND PREGNANCY. The thalassemia syndromes constitute a group of inherited hemoglobinopathies that require close maternal and fetal surveillance during pregnancy. Ongoing consultations and appropriate treatment by maternal–fetal medicine and hematology specialists are essential throughout the pregnancy. The management is similar to care of patients with sickle cell disease. As with sickle cell disease, iron supplementation should be given only if necessary because indiscriminate use of iron can lead to hemochromatosis (ACOG, 2007c; Cunningham et al., 2014; Kilpatrick, 2013).

Rh$_o$(D) Isoimmunization

Hemolytic disease of the fetus and newborn is a condition in which the life span of the fetal or neonatal RBCs is shortened by the action of maternal antibodies against antigens present on the fetal and neonatal RBCs. Antigens provoke an immune reaction if an incompatible blood cell enters the circulation. The RBCs are agglutinated and destroyed. The two most problematic types are those of the Rh (rhesus) system and the ABO system. Maternal antibodies form in the Rh(D)-negative mother after exposure to Rh(D)-positive fetal blood. Theoretically, no mixing of fetal and maternal blood occurs during pregnancy and childbirth. In reality, however, drops of fetal blood most likely enter the maternal circulation after small placental "accidents." The development of maternal antibodies, which destroy the fetus' Rh(D)-positive blood, is termed **isoimmunization, alloimmunization,** or **sensitization.** In addition to the Rh (rhesus) system, there are more than 400 different antigens found on the surface of RBCs. The incidence of hemolytic disease in the newborn has dramatically declined with the advent of Rh$_o$(D) immune globulin (RhoGAM) in the 1960s (Moise, 2013).

PATHOPHYSIOLOGY

For Rh(D) maternal isoimmunization to occur, at least three circumstances must exist:

- The fetus must have Rh(D)-positive erythrocytes, and the mother must have Rh(D)-negative erythrocytes.
- A sufficient number of fetal erythrocytes must gain access to the maternal circulation. This amount can be as little as 0.1 mL.
- The mother must have the immunogenic capacity to produce antibodies directed against the D antigen.

Fetal RBCs gain access to the maternal circulation during pregnancy, childbirth, and in the immediate postpartum period. Clinical factors such as cesarean birth, multiple gestation, bleeding placenta previa or abruption, manual removal of the placenta, and intrauterine manipulation may increase the chance of substantial hemorrhage.

Rh$_o$(D) immune globulin (such as RhoGAM) works by coating and destroying fetal cells in the maternal circulation. Rh$_o$(D) immune globulin *must* be given within 72 hours, and its effects last for 3 months. To ensure that the correct amount of Rh$_o$(D) immune globulin (sometimes more than one 300-mcg vial is required) is given to the patient, a fetal screen or Kleihauer–Betke blood test is performed on the woman's blood after it has been determined that the baby is Rh(D) positive. This test estimates the number of fetal RBCs in the mother's circulation. In most situations, exposure of maternal blood to fetal blood occurs during the third stage of labor at the time of placental separation. The woman's first child is usually unaffected because the maternal antibodies form after the infant's birth. However, subsequent Rh(D)-positive fetuses may be affected unless the woman receives Rh$_o$(D) immune globulin to prevent antibody formation. Rh$_o$(D) immune globulin must be given after the birth of *every* Rh(D)-positive infant (Fig. 11-14). The information presented in Box 11-10 helps to simplify what can be a very confusing clinical situation.

When antibodies to the Rh factor are present in the pregnant patient's blood (i.e., the woman is sensitized), they freely cross the placenta and destroy the RBCs of the Rh(D)-positive fetus. Over time, the fetus develops an RBC deficiency, the fetal bilirubin levels rise ("icterus gravis"), and severe neurological disease ("bilirubin encephalopathy") may result. In the fetus, this pathological process triggers a rapid production of erythroblasts (immature RBCs)

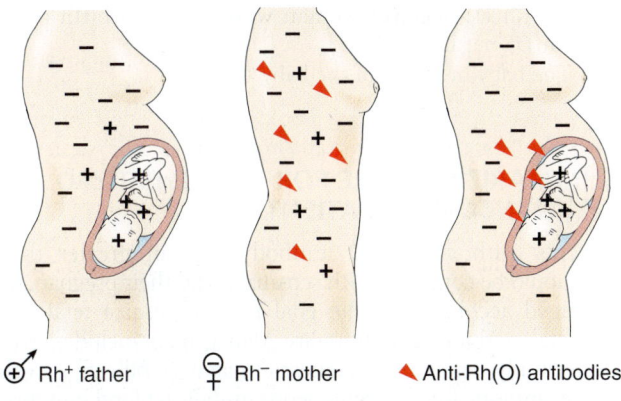

⊕♂ Rh+ father   ♀ Rh- mother   ▲ Anti-Rh(O) antibodies

Figure 11-14 The Rh isoimmunization sequence. Rh+ father and Rh- mother; Rh+ fetus. During pregnancy or childbirth, a small amount of fetal blood enters the mother's circulation. The mother's immune system produces anti-Rh_o(D) antibodies (triangles). In subsequent pregnancies with an Rh+ fetus, the antibodies cross the placenta, enter the fetal circulation, and attack the fetal red blood cells, causing hemolysis.

Box 11-10 Simplifying and Understanding the Rh Factor

RH FACTOR

Rh(D)-positive: Persons who have the D genotype: The Rh antigen is present on their erythrocytes

Rh(D)-negative: Persons who DO NOT possess the antigen on their red blood cells

Anti-Rh antibodies do not spontaneously occur and are only formed if there is sensitization by Rh(D)-positive cells entering the circulation of the Rh(D)-negative person. The Rh(D)-negative person develops antibodies against the Rh(D)-positive cells. This is why the first pregnancy is not affected, UNLESS the mother was previously sensitized during a miscarriage, amniocentesis, or antepartum hemorrhage.

EXAMPLE

Rh(D)-negative mother gives birth to an Rh(D)-positive baby and some of the baby's blood enters the mother's system at the time of delivery. (It takes only 0.1 mL.) Mother develops antibodies against any future Rh(D)-positive babies.

---

that are unable to carry oxygen. The syndrome associated with this hemolytic process is termed **erythroblastosis fetalis.** Fetal anemia and generalized edema ("hydrops fetalis") develop and lead to fetal congestive heart failure. (See Chapter 19 for further discussion.)

During the prenatal period, all Rh(D)-negative women receive an antibody titer (indirect Coombs' test) to determine whether they are sensitized from a previous exposure to Rh(D)-positive blood. If the test is negative, another antibody titer is obtained at 28 weeks of gestation to rule out sensitization that may have occurred later in the pregnancy. If the woman remains unsensitized, Rh_o(D) immune globulin is given as a preventive measure to prevent formation of active antibodies during the remainder of pregnancy. After birth, if the infant is Rh(D) positive, another dose of Rh_o(D) immune globulin is administered. If the infant is Rh(D) negative, no Rh_o(D) immune globulin is necessary.

If the prenatal patient's indirect Coombs' test is positive, sensitization has occurred and antibodies against Rh(D)-positive erythrocytes are present in the maternal circulation. In this situation, the patient's antibody titer is repeated

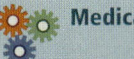 **Medication:** Rh_o(D) Immune Globulin (RhoGAM, HypRho-D, BayRho-D, Gamulin Rh, Rhophylac)

(**arr** aych oh dee im-**yoon glob**-yoo-lin)

Pregnancy Category: C

Indications: Administered to Rh(D)-negative women who have been exposed to Rh(D)-positive blood by:
Delivering an Rh(D)-positive infant
Aborting an Rh(D)-positive fetus
Having chorionic villus sampling (CVS), amniocentesis, or intra-abdominal trauma while carrying an Rh(D)-positive fetus
Accidental transfusion of Rh(D)-positive blood

Action: Prevents production of anti-Rh_o(D) antibodies in Rh(D)-negative patients who were exposed to Rh(D)-positive blood by suppressing the immune reaction of the Rh(D)-negative woman to the antigen in the Rh(D)-positive blood.

Therapeutic Effects: Prevents antibody response and subsequently prevents hemolytic disease of the newborn (erythroblastosis fetalis) in future pregnancies of women who have conceived an Rh(D)-positive fetus. Prevention of Rh_o(D) sensitization following transfusion accident.

Pharmacokinetics:
ABSORPTION: Well absorbed from IM sites.

Contraindications and Precautions:
CONTRAINDICATED IN: Rh_o(D)- or Du-positive patients; patients previously sensitized to Rh_o(D) or Du.

Adverse Reactions and Side Effects: Pain at IM site

Route and Dosage: One vial *standard* dose (300 mcg) administered IM:
- At 28 weeks of pregnancy and within 72 hours of delivery.
- Within 72 hours after the termination of a pregnancy of 13 weeks or more of gestation.
- After an accidental transfusion, dosage is calculated based on the volume of blood that was erroneously administered.

One vial *MICRhoGAM (microdose)* (50 mcg) within 72 hours after chorionic villus sampling (CVS) or the termination of a pregnancy of less than 13 weeks of gestation.

Note: (1) More than 300 mcg of RhoGAM may be indicated after a large transplacental hemorrhage or after a mismatched blood transfusion; (2) Rhophylac can be given IM or IV (prefilled syringes are available).

Nursing Implications:
1. Do not give to infant, to Rh(D)-positive individual, or to Rh(D)-negative individual previously sensitized to the Rh_o(D) antigen. Note: There is no more risk than when given to a woman who is not sensitized—if in doubt, administer Rh_o(D) immune globulin.
2. Administer into the deltoid muscle. Should be given within 3 hours but may be given up to 72 hours after delivery, miscarriage, abortion, or transfusion.
3. Explain to the patient the purpose of this medication to protect future Rh(D)-positive infants; prior to administering, obtain a signed consent form if required by the agency.
4. Special considerations may be indicated for women who are members of Jehovah's Witnesses because this medication is made from human plasma.

Source: Data from Vallerand, A. H., & Sanoski, C. A. (2014). *Davis's drug guide for nurses* (14th ed.). Philadelphia, PA: F.A. Davis.

frequently throughout pregnancy to identify a rising level. A rise in the maternal antibody titer is indicative of ongoing antibody formation and an increased likelihood of fetal erythrocyte destruction.

When sensitization has occurred, an amniocentesis may be performed periodically throughout pregnancy to assess change in the optical density (ΔOD_{450}) of amniotic fluid. The ΔOD_{450} reflects the amount of bilirubin (bile pigment that remains after RBC destruction) in the amniotic fluid. When the fluid optical density remains low, it could indicate (1) that the fetus is Rh(D) negative (and thus in no jeopardy) or (2) that the fetus is Rh(D) positive and is presently in no jeopardy. If the ΔOD_{450} is elevated, the fetus is experiencing RBC destruction and is in jeopardy.

Ultrasound evaluations may also be performed to assess for evidence of severe fetal anemia that has occurred because of hemolysis: edema, ascites, an enlarged heart, and hydramnios. An invasive procedure such as percutaneous umbilical blood sampling (discussed later in this chapter) may be performed to quantitatively determine the amount of fetal erythrocyte destruction. When necessary, an intrauterine transfusion of O-negative blood through the umbilical cord may be carried out or, as an alternative, erythrocytes may be transfused into the fetal abdominal cavity for absorption into the circulation.

 legal alert—Administer and document RhoGAM when clinically indicated

Administering and properly documenting $Rh_o(D)$ immune globulin (RhoGAM) is an important nursing action.

If the mother is Rh negative and unsensitized and the baby is Rh positive, always check to be sure the patient has received $Rh_o(D)$ immune globulin (RhoGAM) if indicated before discharge. Make certain that she has received the appropriate dose.

Patients who have miscarried also must be treated. In cases in which it is not possible to determine the fetus' or baby's blood type, $Rh_o(D)$ immune globulin (RhoGAM) is still given. Question if an order has not been written.

MANAGEMENT

Prevention of isoimmunization (a rising anti-Rh antibody titer in an Rh(D)-negative woman) is the goal throughout pregnancy. All pregnant women should be tested for ABO and $Rh_o(D)$ type along with an antibody screen during their first prenatal visit. It is essential that these determinations be made during each subsequent pregnancy, as previous maternal antibody screening is not an adequate assessment. $Rh_o(D)$ immune globulin (RhoGAM) should also be given at any time during the pregnancy when a possibility exists that a patient may be exposed to fetal blood (e.g., CVS, amniocentesis, miscarriage, vaginal bleeding, abortion, and ectopic pregnancy).

 Optimizing Outcomes—Safe administration of $Rh_o(D)$ immune globulin (RhoGAM)

In an Rh(D)-negative woman who is *non*sensitized, RhoGAM should be given:

After delivery of an Rh(D)-positive infant. In the United States, the standard dose is 300 mcg and it is given within 72 hours of delivery.

Remember to educate your patient as to the reason she is receiving RhoGAM.

Be sure to give your patient documentation that she has received RhoGAM.

Never give RhoGAM to:

- An Rh(D)-positive woman
- A sensitized Rh(D)-negative woman

- An Rh(D)-negative woman who has given birth to an Rh(D)-negative baby
- The baby or father of the baby!

SUMMARIZING CARE FOR THE SENSITIZED $RH_O(D)$-NEGATIVE PATIENT

Patients with an anti-D antibody titer of greater than 1:4 should be considered Rh sensitized and their pregnancies managed accordingly. The goal is to minimize fetal and neonatal morbidity and mortality. Management includes serial ultrasounds, serial amnioceneses to analyze bilirubin levels in the amniotic fluid, percutaneous umbilical blood sampling (PUBS) to obtain a fetal hematocrit, and intrauterine blood transfusions for a fetal hematocrit less than 30% (Moise, 2013). A delayed manifestation of Rh isoimmunization is neonatal **kernicterus**, a condition characterized by CNS damage after exposure of the infant brain to hyperbilirubinemia (see Chapter 19). The nurse's identification of infants at risk anticipates this danger after birth and allows for early intervention with phototherapy or exchange transfusion before any damage may occur (ACOG, 1999a; Cunningham et al., 2014; M. Taylor, Uhlmann, Meyer, & Mari, 2011).

ABO

In this condition the *mother is blood group O,* and the *baby is either A or B.* This form of blood incompatibility is unrelated to the Rh factor. It is important for nurses to remember that blood group O carries no antigens; group A carries A antigen, and group B carries B antigen. Because the mother already has anti-A and anti-B antibodies present during the first pregnancy, the first child may be affected. IgG antibodies (immunoglobulins that respond to a specific antigen (in this case, A or B) can cross the placenta and cause hemolysis of the fetal RBCs.

The Coombs' test is performed on the baby's cord blood obtained at the time of birth. A **direct Coombs'** test identifies the presence of maternal antibodies in the neonate's blood and hemolysis or lysis of RBCs, whereas the **indirect Coombs'** test detects antibodies against RBCs in the maternal serum. The results are reported as either positive or negative. A positive direct Coombs' test must be reported to the pediatrician.

 Now Can You—Discuss $Rh_o(D)$ and ABO isoimmunization?

1. Describe the pathophysiology of Rho(D) isoimmunization?
2. Discuss the importance of preventing maternal isoimmunization?
3. Discuss the action of RhoGAM and the nursing responsibilities required in administering this medication?
4. Explain why ABO sensitization may occur during a first pregnancy?

Respiratory Complications

Pulmonary diseases have become more prevalent in the general population and, therefore, in pregnant women. The normal physiological changes of pregnancy can cause a woman with a history of compromised respirations to develop significant problems. The outcome for a pregnant woman with respiratory complications depends on the adequacy of ventilation and oxygenation and the early detection of respiratory compromise. Hypoxia poses a major threat to the fetus (Yancy, 2011).

PNEUMONIA

Although pneumonia is a rare complication of pregnancy, it is the most common nonobstetric infection that causes maternal mortality during the peripartum period. The overall frequency of pneumonia during pregnancy ranges from approximately 1 per 400 to 1 per 1,200. The incidence may be increasing primarily as a reflection of the declining general health status of certain segments of the childbearing population (i.e., individuals with AIDS, cystic fibrosis, obesity, and those who smoke) (Cunningham et al., 2014).

Etiology

Streptococcus pneumoniae, *Mycoplasma pneumoniae*, *Chlamydia pneumoniae*, and viruses (e.g., influenza A and varicella) are the major causative agents.

Effects on Pregnancy

Pneumonia can complicate pregnancy at any time during gestation. Maternal bacteremia, empyema, a need for mechanical intervention, and death have all been reported. Pneumonia may be associated with poor fetal growth (IUGR), preterm birth, and perinatal loss (Cunningham et al., 2014).

Management

The normal physiological changes in the respiratory system that occur during pregnancy result in a loss of ventilatory reserve. These changes, coupled with pregnancy-related immunosuppression, place the woman and her fetus at an increased risk for respiratory infection. Any pregnant patient suspected of having pneumonia should be managed aggressively with appropriate laboratory testing, clinical surveillance, and medications.

 Nursing Insight—*Maternal morbidity associated with influenza during pregnancy*

Among healthy individuals, two groups are especially vulnerable to serious illness and hospitalization with influenza infection: pregnant women and their infants. Alterations in the maternal immune system, along with pregnancy-related physiological factors in the cardiovascular and respiratory systems (e.g., increased heart rate, stroke volume, and oxygen consumption, and decreased lung capacity) are believed to contribute to an increased susceptibility and severity of the illness. To prevent seasonal flu, it is recommended that pregnant women receive the inactivated vaccine. An important role for nurses centers on counseling childbearing-age patients about the importance of influenza vaccine to reduce febrile influenza-like illness in themselves and in their young infants (ACOG, 2010c).

ASTHMA

Asthma is the most common form of lung disease that affects pregnancy; from 0.5% to 8% of pregnant women have this condition. Asthma is characterized by a limitation of airflow that is generally more marked during expiration than during inspiration. The obstruction associated with asthma is a reversible process caused by airway inflammation and an increased responsiveness of the airways to a variety of stimuli (e.g., dust, pollen, grass, and cold temperature). The airway response to the stimuli involves contraction of the bronchial smooth muscle, hypersecretion of mucus, and edema of the mucosal surfaces. Collectively, these events contribute to the pathophysiological processes associated with the reversible airway obstruction characteristic of asthma (ACOG, 2008d).

Effects on Pregnancy

Asthma is associated with significant risks for both the patient and her fetus. Maternal complications reported among asthmatics include hyperemesis, vaginal bleeding, hypertensive disorders, a predisposition to infections, gestational diabetes, preterm rupture of the membranes and PTL, and delivery of a low-birth-weight infant. There is little risk to the fetus with well-controlled maternal asthma, and it is safer for pregnant asthmatics to be treated with appropriate medications than to have asthma symptoms and exacerbations. Exacerbations that cause hypoxia and decreased uterine blood flow increase the incidence of IUGR, preterm birth, and neonatal mortality (ACOG, 2008d; Yancy, 2011).

Signs and Symptoms

A number of classic symptoms are associated with an exacerbation of asthma. These include dyspnea, coughing, wheezing, voice changes, chest tightening, and the presence of scant or copious clear sputum. Lung auscultation usually reveals bilateral expiratory wheezing.

Management

Careful monitoring and appropriate adjustments in therapy may be required to maintain maternal lung function and ensure an adequate oxygen supply to the fetus. Failure to control asthma during pregnancy may result in hypoxia in both the patient and her fetus. A PO_2 of less than 60 mm Hg places the fetus in jeopardy. Guidelines for asthma management have been developed to help ensure maternal–fetal safety and well-being during pregnancy. Goals of therapy include optimal control of asthma symptoms, attainment of normal pulmonary function, prevention and reversal of asthma attacks, and prevention of maternal and fetal complications. Asthma therapy is based on a stepwise classification system designed to control symptoms, avoid acute attacks, and help patients achieve unhampered lifestyles (ACOG, 2008d; National Heart, Lung, and Blood Institute, 2007; Whitty & Dombrowski, 2013).

Medications currently used for asthma are generally well tolerated during pregnancy and appear to be safe for the fetus. Therefore, the management of asthma in the pregnant woman differs little from management in the nonpregnant patient. It is also widely accepted that the fetal risk is higher with poorly controlled maternal asthma than with medications necessary to gain optimal symptom control. Nevertheless, nurses must be aware of available data concerning the use of these drugs during pregnancy.

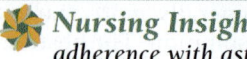

> ### Nursing Insight—*Importance of patient adherence with asthma medications*
>
> Interestingly, noncompliance with asthma medication is the primary cause of worsening asthma symptoms during pregnancy. During every patient visit, nurses should reinforce the importance of taking asthma medications as prescribed to promote maternal–fetal well-being.

CYSTIC FIBROSIS

Cystic fibrosis (CF) is a chronic, progressive, genetic multisystem disease. It affects nearly 30,000 children and young adults and occurs in approximately one out of every 3,200 Caucasian live births. One thousand new cases are diagnosed each year, usually by the age of 3; however, nearly 10% of newly diagnosed cases involve individuals age 18 or older. Because CF is a recessive disorder, a child must inherit a defective gene from each parent. Each time two CF carriers conceive, there is a 25% chance that the child will have CF, a 50% chance that the child will be a carrier, and a 25% chance the child will be a noncarrier. One in 20 Americans (more than 20 million total) is an unknowing carrier of the defective gene for CF (Cystic Fibrosis Foundation, 2012).

The last several decades have witnessed a dramatic increase in the survival of patients with CF. This trend is attributable in large part to earlier diagnosis and intervention, the introduction of pulmonary therapies such as dornase-alpha and high-dose ibuprofen, new airway clearance techniques, effective antipseudomonal antibiotics such as tobramycin for inhalation, improved nutritional management, and dietary recommendations (ACOG, 2011e). In the United States, the median survival age for persons with CF has increased to 31.1 years for men and 28.3 years for women (Cystic Fibrosis Foundation, 2012). An increasing number of women with CF are now surviving into the reproductive years and, with meticulous management of their pulmonary function, usually maintain their fertility.

Pathophysiology

The major CF gene product is the protein cystic fibrosis transmembrane regulator (CFTR). When CFTR is not produced or is altered in structure or function as a result of mutations in the CF gene, viscid secretions are produced that primarily affect the respiratory and gastrointestinal systems. An absence or abnormality of the protein results in a blocked or altered chloride channel in the epithelial cell membranes. Chloride ions are trapped within the cell and cause sodium ions and water to diffuse back into the cell, leading to dehydration of the mucus secretions.

Effects on Pregnancy

Factors that may predict a poor outcome for a pregnant woman with CF include prepregnancy evidence of poor nutritional status, significant pulmonary disease with hypoxemia, and pulmonary hypertension. The risk of maternal mortality for those with cor pulmonale and deteriorating pulmonary function in the first trimester is exceptionally high, and the couple may be advised to consider termination of the pregnancy. Risks to the fetus include preterm birth, growth restriction caused by uteroplacental insufficiency, and CF. The couple must also consider the long-term psychosocial and physical assistance needs that may ensue because of the potential for maternal physical deterioration and/or premature death (Whitty & Dombrowski, 2013).

> ### Optimizing Outcomes—Counseling women with cystic fibrosis
>
> Preconception counseling is essential for women with CF. Because of extremely thick cervical mucus, fewer than one in five women with CF are able to conceive. Women who achieve pregnancy should be advised of the risks, according to their health status. If possible, women should be 90% of their ideal body weight before conception (ACOG, 2011e).

Management

When caring for a pregnant woman with CF, it is important for the nurse to recognize that the fetus is at risk for uteroplacental insufficiency and IUGR. The maternal nutritional status and weight gain during pregnancy greatly affect fetal growth. Ongoing collaboration with the nutritionist is essential, and close attention must be paid to the patient's nutritional status because maldigestion, malabsorption, and malnutrition are all complications of CF (Whitty & Dombrowski, 2013). An early nutritional consultation should be included in the nursing care plan developed for every CF patient. Throughout pregnancy, the nurse and other members of the care team must work closely with the nutritionist to ensure that the caloric requirements are being met. This component of care is especially important when the pregnant patient with CF experiences hyperemesis gravidarum.

Early recognition and prompt treatment of pulmonary infections are also important in the management of the pregnant woman with CF. Diagnostic tests that are helpful for assessing and guiding therapy with CF patients include sputum and culture sensitivity, chest films, spirometry, pulse oximetry, and complete blood counts with a chemistry panel (Whitty & Dombrowski, 2013).

Respiratory management during the preconception and the antenatal period includes baseline pulmonary function tests such as forced vital capacity (FVC), forced expiratory volume (FEV_1), lung volumes, pulse oximetry, and arterial blood gases as indicated. Laboratory values are closely monitored during pregnancy, and any deterioration in pulmonary function is promptly addressed. Fetal growth should be monitored by fundal height measurements and serial ultrasound evaluations of fetal growth and amniotic fluid volume. Doppler flow studies are also used to assess fetal growth and development and general health status. Maternal kick counts should begin at 28 weeks and nonstress tests initiated at 32 weeks to assess fetal well-being (Whitty & Dombrowski, 2013). Management of the pregnant woman with CF requires the involvement of an entire team of professionals: the perinatologist, pulmonologist, neonatologist, nutritionist, social worker, and nurse. When difficulties arise and the family is further challenged, spiritual guidance can be of great comfort and support to the family.

Maternal and, consequently, fetal oxygenation is of paramount importance during labor and birth. Continuous monitoring of maternal oxygen saturation using pulse oximetry is used to gauge the need for and response to supplemental oxygen therapy. Respiratory depressants, anticholinergic drugs, and inhalation anesthesia should be avoided. Lumbar epidural analgesia is the preferred mode of labor pain relief. The fetal heart rate (FHR) should be continuously monitored during labor, and any signs of fetal intolerance (i.e., decelerations and/or a lack of FHR variability) must be promptly addressed (Whitty & Dombrowski, 2013). A critical intrapartal nursing issue centers on the recognition that high-risk couples may have depleted their coping skills because of perinatal complications. The nurse needs to be aware that the anxiety coupled with the stress of labor may be extremely difficult for the patient and her family. The nurse can provide assistance by encouraging the couple to express their emotional concerns, keeping them informed of changes as the labor progresses, and encouraging them to freely ask questions.

⬤ Now Can You—Discuss respiratory complications during pregnancy?

1. Describe the normal anatomical and physiological changes in the respiratory system during pregnancy and how they affect the patient with asthma and cystic fibrosis?
2. Discuss the fetal effects of maternal oxygen deprivation?
3. Formulate a plan of care for the pregnant patient with a respiratory complication?

Cardiovascular Disease

Cardiovascular disease in women affects 1% to 4% of all pregnancies and remains the primary cause of nonobstetric maternal mortality in the United States (Foley, Rokey, & Belfort 2011). Care of the patient with cardiovascular disease continues to be a great challenge to the obstetric team despite advances in surgical techniques, medications, and technology, because of three broad trends (Simpson, 2012):

- Successful treatment of congenital heart disease has created a new population of clinically complex patients who are able to reach childbearing age.
- There is an increasing trend toward pregnancies in older women who are susceptible to heart diseases acquired in adulthood.
- Immigration from underdeveloped nations has reacquainted Western medicine with a cohort of young childbearing patients who have rheumatic heart disease.

Signs and symptoms of cardiac disease can be similar to physiological changes that normally occur during pregnancy. For example, the pregnant patient may experience heart palpitations associated with the normal increase in blood volume. Women with heart disease may experience heart palpitations caused by an arrhythmia. Fatigue, a common complaint during pregnancy, may result from poor cardiac output and myocardial ischemia in patients with heart disease. The incidence of maternal and fetal morbidity and mortality associated with cardiac disease during pregnancy depends on the specific cardiac lesion, the functional abnormality produced by the lesion, and the development of pregnancy-related complications, such as infection, hemorrhage, or preeclampsia (Yancy, 2011).

Categories of cardiac disease during pregnancy include congenital cardiac disease (e.g., atrial septal defect, ventricular septal defect, pulmonic stenosis, congenital aortic stenosis, coarctation of the aorta, tetralogy of Fallot, and Eisenmenger's syndrome) and acquired cardiac disease (e.g., lesions that are rheumatic in origin and valvular lesions such as mitral and aortic stenosis). Rheumatic mitral stenosis is the most common clinically significant valvular abnormality in pregnant women and may be associated with pulmonary congestion, edema, and atrial arrhythmias during pregnancy and soon after childbirth. Ischemic cardiac disease (coronary artery disease and myocardial infarction) is rare in pregnancy.

The New York Heart Association (NYHA) classification system is often used to assess the functional ability of the pregnant cardiac patient (Criteria Committee of the NYHA, 1994). Patient cardiac function is divided into four classes:

Class I	The patient is asymptomatic and there is no limitation on physical activity.
Class II	The patient is asymptomatic at rest, symptomatic with heavy physical activity, and requires slight limitation of activity.
Class III	The patient is asymptomatic at rest, symptomatic with minimal physical activity, and physical activity is considerably limited.
Class IV	The patient may be symptomatic at rest, is symptomatic with any activity, and has severe limitations on physical activity.

Patients classified as NYHA I and II generally do well during pregnancy, but those classified as III or IV have a significantly increased risk of morbidity and mortality with pregnancy. However, it must be remembered that any patient with a cardiac history, regardless of classification, must be thoroughly assessed for any signs of decompensation at each prenatal visit.

MANAGEMENT

Management of cardiac disease in pregnancy is frequently complicated by unique social and psychological concerns. Patients with congenital heart disease may have experienced multiple hospitalizations over the years and be fearful of the medical environment. Some of them never expected to bear children. Often, women with a history of rheumatic heart disease have lived outside the traditional medical care system because of conditions of poverty and cultural differences. Not uncommonly, they are recent immigrants. When caring for any patient with special needs, it is imperative for the nurse to collaborate with other health professionals and community support systems to facilitate the patient's access to care and to ensure her comfort with the health-care environment (Easterling & Otto, 2012).

 Optimizing Outcomes—Caring for the pregnant woman with cardiac disease

Antepartally, continuity of care with a single provider, frequent prenatal visits, routine screening for bacteriuria, and prophylaxis against anemia are essential. Intrapartal care includes the induction of labor when cervical favorability is present and the avoidance of prolonged labor, second stage pushing, and maternal blood loss. Infective endocarditis prophylaxis is no longer recommended for vaginal or cesarean births in the absence of infection irrespective of the type of maternal heart disease. According to current recommendations from the American Heart Association, patients with high-risk cardiac lesions should receive intrapartum prophylaxis only when childbirth is associated with infection. Postpartal care centers on strict management of blood volume and careful but aggressive diuresis (Easterling & Otto, 2012; Simpson, 2012).

Labor, birth, and the immediate postpartum period provide a time of increased risk because of the rapid volume changes that occur. During labor and birth, epidural anesthesia may be used for most patients with cardiac disease, but care must be taken to avoid hypotension. Effective pain control is important in decreasing the cardiac workload. Positioning the patient in a lateral recumbent position and careful administration of IV fluids will help to balance the patient's blood pressure. Continuous invasive hemodynamic monitoring is beneficial in evaluating rapid changes in heart rate, cardiac output, and pulmonary capillary wedge pressure (an estimation of left atrial pressure) so that fluid, diuretic, vasodilator, or pressor therapy may be guided (Simpson, 2012; Yancy, 2011).

Medications that may be indicated for the pregnant cardiac patient include diuretics (e.g., Lasix) to prevent congestive heart failure, digitalis, nitrates (to reduce afterload, the resistance the ventricles must overcome to eject blood during systole), antiarrhythmic agents (e.g., lidocaine), beta blockers (e.g., labetalol), calcium channel blockers (e.g., nifedipine), antibiotics, and anticoagulants (heparin–warfarin [Coumadin] is contraindicated because it crosses the placenta). As with any medication being considered for the pregnant patient, a thorough investigation of side effects and potential fetal harm must be evaluated before administration.

 Nursing Insight—*Adverse effects of various cardiac medications used in pregnancy*

Cardiovascular medications commonly used during pregnancy can have adverse maternal–fetal effects. For example, diuretics may exacerbate preeclampsia by reducing uterine blood flow; vasodilators, which produce maternal hypotension, may jeopardize placental perfusion; and ACE inhibitors have been associated with fetal renal development abnormalities. Antiarrhythmic agents (e.g., quinidine) may potentially cause fetal dysrhythmias, and beta-blocking agents have been associated with IUGR and neonatal bradycardia, hypotension, hypoglycemia, and respiratory depression (Gelson, Curry, Gatzoulis, Swan, Lupton, Steer, et al., 2011; Yancy, 2011).

Vaginal birth is advisable for most patients with cardiac disease with care taken to avoid causing stress on the heart during the second stage of labor (pushing). The nurse should encourage gentle pushing to avoid erratic venous return associated with the Valsalva maneuver. Elective low or outlet forceps may be used to shorten this stage. Cesarean section may limit the stress of vaginal birth in patients with cardiac disease, but this method involves major surgery, blood loss, and the possibility of maternal

stress from intubation. Cesarean birth is reserved for situations such as fetal compromise and failure of labor progression (Yancy, 2011).

NURSING IMPLICATIONS FOR THE PREGNANT CARDIAC PATIENT

Because of the intense cardiovascular demands of pregnancy, care of the pregnant cardiac patient presents one of the greatest challenges to the obstetric nurse. Nursing care should focus on assessment, early detection of problems, and treatment and prevention of complications to both mother and baby. Ideally, these women are cared for in a tertiary care center, but when this is not possible, there should be collaboration between critical care nurses and obstetric nurses. Nursing interventions include:

- Antenatal assessment of weight gain to ensure proper fetal growth while avoiding excessive weight gain, which causes increased cardiac workload
- Nutritional counseling (a diet high in iron to prevent anemia and low in sodium to prevent fluid retention)
- Education to avoid/reduce stress and anxiety
- Encouragement of adequate nighttime sleep and frequent daytime rest periods
- Explanation of fetal surveillance testing
- Stressing the importance of taking medications and keeping prenatal appointments
- Education regarding the signs and symptoms of complications; when to call the provider

 Nursing Insight—*Understanding hemodynamic changes in pregnancy*

A patient with a cardiac disorder is at greatest risk when hemodynamic changes reach their maximum, between the 28th and 32nd weeks of gestation. The nurse must have knowledge of the disease process and be able to assess the hemodynamic changes that occur during pregnancy.

Intrapartal interventions focus on assessing the patient and fetus for decreased cardiac output and oxygenation and intervening as needed.

 Critical Nursing Action Assessing the Cardiac Patient During Labor and Birth

The nurse needs to assess the patient for signs and symptoms of decreased cardiac output:

- Decreased and/or irregular pulse
- Increased respiratory rate
- Dyspnea
- Chest pain
- Abnormal breath sounds: crackles at the base of the lungs
- Decreased blood pressure
- Decreased urinary output (less than 30 mL/hr)
- Edema of the hands, face, and feet
- Abnormal heart sounds: diastolic murmur at the heart's apex
- Signs of air hunger: anxiety
- Decreased oxygen saturation: less than 95%
- Cool, clammy, cyanotic skin
- Increased capillary refill time: greater than 3 seconds
- EKG changes
- Mental changes: disorientation; fatigue; syncope

Oxygen, if required, should be supplied via a rebreather mask at 10 L per minute, IV fluids are administered via a pump, and intake and output are meticulously monitored throughout labor. Antibiotic prophylaxis may be indicated for selected patients with cardiac disease because of their increased risk for developing endocarditis as a result of invasive procedures (e.g., invasive hemodynamic monitoring, intrauterine pressure catheter, and fetal scalp electrode). Continuous fetal monitoring during labor is also a nursing responsibility. With decreased maternal cardiac output, the fetus will show signs of poor placental perfusion, as evidenced by late heart rate decelerations and/or the loss of baseline variability (see Chapter 12 for further discussion). Should these indicators develop, improved oxygenation must be delivered to the fetus by giving oxygen to the woman, who should be maintained in a lateral position. IV fluids should be increased with caution to avoid maternal fluid overload.

After delivery of the baby and placenta, large quantities of fluid are rapidly mobilized. The patient with cardiac disease must be continually assessed for decompensation (inability of the heart to maintain a sufficient cardiac output) during the puerperium. Ambulation should be encouraged, as ordered, as soon as possible after birth to prevent deep vein thrombosis. If the mother who is receiving cardiovascular medications chooses to breastfeed, careful clinical observation of the newborn is warranted. Digoxin and beta-adrenergic blockers are generally regarded to be safe during lactation (Simpson, 2012).

MITRAL VALVE PROLAPSE

Mitral valve prolapse (MVP) is a common condition that affects 2% to 3% of reproductive-aged women; however, it generally does not affect pregnancy (Cunningham et al., 2014). The hemodynamic changes associated with pregnancy may alleviate the murmur of MVP and its symptoms. In rare cases, patients experience chest discomfort or rhythm disturbances and should be managed with reassurance. Therapy with beta-adrenergic blockers may be initiated in highly symptomatic patients. If a murmur is audible, antibiotic prophylaxis should be administered at the time of childbirth (Cunningham et al., 2014; Simpson, 2012).

PERIPARTUM CARDIOMYOPATHY

Peripartum cardiomyopathy is a rare syndrome of heart failure that occurs in late pregnancy or within the first 5 months postpartum. The patient typically has no history of cardiac disease and presents with dyspnea, fatigue, and peripheral or pulmonary edema. Radiological findings are consistent with cardiomegaly. Acute treatment is directed at improving cardiac function. Treatment includes diuretics to decrease preload and relieve pulmonary congestion, digoxin to improve contractility and facilitate rate control when atrial fibrillation is present, beta-adrenergic blockers, anticoagulation with heparin if the woman is antepartum and Coumadin if postpartum, and fluid and sodium restriction (Easterling & Otto, 2012; Simpson, 2012).

The mortality rate associated with peripartum cardiomyopathy is reported to be 25% to 50%. Within 6 months after childbirth, half the patients will demonstrate resolution of left ventricular dilation. Of those who do not, 8.5% will die within 4 to 5 years. Death is usually a result of progressive heart failure, arrhythmia, or thromboembolism (Simpson, 2012).

 Now Can You—Discuss cardiac complications during pregnancy?

1. Describe the normal anatomical and physiological changes that occur in the cardiovascular system during pregnancy and their impact on the pregnant woman with a cardiac disease?
2. State three important factors in the management of cardiac disease in pregnancy?
3. Identify team members you would include in your plan of care?

Diabetes in Pregnancy

Diabetes during pregnancy encompasses a range of disease entities that include gestational diabetes mellitus (GDM) and overt diabetes mellitus. Diabetes complicates approximately 7% of all pregnancies each year in the United States (ACOG, 2013e; Van Otterloo, 2011a). Diabetes is a complex health-care problem that requires a comprehensive, multidisciplinary approach to ensure a healthy outcome for both the patient and her infant. When working with this population, perinatal nurses are challenged to provide care and education that incorporates diabetes management principles into obstetric care during all phases of childbearing, from preconception through the postpartum period.

DEFINITION AND CLASSIFICATION OF DIABETES MELLITUS

Pregestational Diabetes Mellitus

Pregestational diabetes mellitus is a chronic metabolic disease characterized by hyperglycemia that results from limited or absent insulin production, deficient insulin action, or a combination of the two (Expert Committee on the Diagnosis and Classification of Diabetes Mellitus [ECDCDM], 2007). Diabetes is divided into two broad categories—type 1 and type 2—that are differentiated according to the primary underlying etiology. Type 1 diabetes (formerly termed "insulin-dependent diabetes mellitus") is characterized by an autoimmunity directed at the pancreatic beta cells. With Type 1 diabetes, there is an absolute insulin deficiency, and the following characteristics are typically present (ECDCDM, 2007):

- It is usually diagnosed in those younger than 30 years of age.
- Acute symptoms precede the diagnosis and include polyuria, polydipsia, and significant weight loss.
- It has an abrupt onset that requires emergency medical attention.
- It accounts for approximately 5% to 10% of those diagnosed with diabetes.

Type 2 diabetes, the most prevalent form of the disease, is characterized by a combination of insulin resistance and inadequate insulin production (ECDCDM, 2007). Characteristics of type 2 diabetes include:

- It is diagnosed primarily in adults older than age 30, but with the current obesity epidemic, it is now seen in children.
- The disease is typically symptom free for many years, with a slow onset and a gradual progression of symptoms.

- Individuals with type 2 are not ketosis prone.
- It does not always require insulin and can often be treated with diet, exercise, and/or oral hypoglycemic agents.

 Optimizing Outcomes—Preconception care for pregestational diabetes mellitus

Nurses who care for childbearing-age women with diabetes mellitus are perfectly positioned to offer preconceptional counseling during every patient contact. Women should be taught about the adverse obstetric and maternal outcomes that may result from poorly controlled diabetes and the importance of euglycemic control before pregnancy. Depending on the situation, testing to assess for vascular changes may include a retinal examination, 24-hour urine collection for protein excretion and creatinine clearance, and electrocardiography. Thyroid function studies may also be indicated, and all women who contemplate pregnancy should receive a multivitamin containing at least 400 mcg of folic acid, especially important in women with diabetes, who have an increased risk for offspring with neural tube defects (ACOG, 2011f).

Gestational Diabetes Mellitus

GDM is an impairment in carbohydrate metabolism that first manifests during pregnancy. This category may include a small number of previously undiagnosed type 1 and type 2 diabetic women. The following characteristics apply (ACOG, 2013e; ECDCDM, 2007; Gabbe, Landon, Warren-Boulton, & Fradkin, 2012a; Landon & Gabbe, 2011; Van Otterloo, 2011a; Yehuda, Nagtalon-Ramos, & Trout, 2011):

- Estimated to occur in approximately 4% to 7% of pregnancies; however, the prevalence may range from 1% to 14%, depending on the population studied and the diagnostic test used. Accounts for 90% of diabetic pregnancies; incidence has been increasing in the United States along with the obesity epidemic.
- Develops in the latter half of pregnancy as a result of the altered hormonal milieu.
- Symptoms are usually mild and not life threatening.
- May be treated by diet and exercise (classified as A1), or requires the addition of oral medications and/or insulin (classified as A2), depending on the blood glucose levels.
- Women diagnosed with GDM are at an increased risk for developing diabetes later in life; ACOG and the American Diabetes Association recommend testing women with a history of GDM at 6 to 12 weeks postpartum.

 Nursing Insight—*Preconception bariatric surgery and gestational diabetes*

Preconception bariatric surgery is associated with a reduction in gestational diabetes in subsequent pregnancies. However, because of the potential for maternal malnutrition or intestinal malabsorption, bariatric surgery may be associated with adverse neonatal outcomes, including small for gestational age (SGA) neonates, preterm delivery, and perinatal mortality (ACOG, 2009a; Lesko & Peaceman, 2012).

RISK FACTORS FOR GESTATIONAL DIABETES

- Women older than age 25 years
- Obesity
- Insulin resistance
- Polycystic ovary syndrome
- History of pregnancy-related diabetes mellitus
- History of a large for gestational age infant, hydramnios
- Stillbirth, miscarriage, or an infant with congenital anomalies during a previous pregnancy
- Family history of type 2 diabetes (first-degree relative)
- Ethnicity

 Cultural Diversity: Gestational Diabetes

An increased incidence of gestational diabetes occurs in Native Americans, African Americans, Hispanic Americans, Asian Americans, and Pacific Islanders (ECDCDM, 2007).

PATHOPHYSIOLOGY

The body requires a constant source of energy, provided mainly by glucose. Once glucose enters a cell, it may undergo oxidative (glycolysis) or nonoxidative (glycogen synthesis) metabolism. In response to glucose ingestion, the pancreatic beta cells of the islets of Langerhans secrete insulin, a hormone that promotes the uptake of glucose into the cells. The regulation of plasma glucose levels and the entry of glucose into the cells are of critical importance.

Changes in carbohydrate, protein, and fat metabolism in normal pregnancy are profound, mediated in part by the developing fetus and the production of placental hormones. The first half of pregnancy is considered an "anabolic phase." It is associated with an increased storage of fat and protein, along with an increase in the secretion of estrogen and progesterone. These physiological events lead to maternal hyperplasia and hyperinsulinemia. The increased insulin production prompts an increased tissue response to insulin and the increased uptake and storage of glycogen and fat in the liver and tissues.

The second half of pregnancy is characterized by a "catabolic phase" associated with the breakdown of protein and

 Where Research and Practice Meet:
Maternal Vitamin D Status and Gestational Diabetes

Evidence suggests that vitamin D exerts an effect on pancreatic beta cells, modulating insulin secretion (Alfonso, Liao, Busta, & Poretsky, 2009; Lapillonne, 2010). Nurse researchers Senti, Thiele, and Anderson (2012) reviewed six studies that examined maternal vitamin D during pregnancy, GDM, glucose tolerance, and insulin resistance and concluded that maternal vitamin D deficiency and insufficiency is prevalent among pregnant women and is associated with markers of altered glucose homeostasis. While there is a need for further research, nurses can use this information to encourage pregnant women to follow current guidelines for vitamin D intake of at least the minimum daily requirement 600 IU/day during pregnancy (Heaney & Holick, 2011), although evidence suggests there is a need for additional supplementation to reduce the risk for GDM.

fat. During this time there is also an increased insulin resistance caused by the heightened production of placental hormones (insulinase and human placental lactogen), cortisol, and growth hormones. These hormones are diabetogenic and act as insulin antagonists. In women who cannot meet the increasing needs for insulin production, this change leads to an altered carbohydrate metabolism and progressive hyperglycemia.

During this time, the developing fetus continuously removes glucose and amino acids, substances that can easily cross the placenta, from the maternal circulation. Because insulin does not cross the placenta, the fetus must increase its own insulin production. Fetal hyperinsulinemia develops and acts as a growth hormone that contributes to an increase in fetal size (macrosomia), and a decrease in pulmonary surfactant production. Macrosomia occurs in 20% to 25% of diabetic pregnancies. When the pregnant woman's blood glucose levels remain abnormally elevated, there is a constant transport of maternal glucose across the placenta. This "glucose load" prompts the fetus to produce insulin at a greater rate to use the glucose.

 Nursing Insight—*Anticipating changes in insulin needs during pregnancy*

During the first trimester, maternal blood glucose levels are normally reduced and the insulin response to glucose is enhanced. The woman with well-controlled pregestational diabetes may need a decrease in her insulin dosage to avoid hypoglycemia. During the second and third trimesters, as the insulin requirements steadily increase, the insulin dosage must be adjusted to prevent hyperglycemia. Maternal insulin resistance begins around 14 weeks of gestation and continues to increase until it stabilizes during the final weeks of pregnancy.

MATERNAL AND PERINATAL MORBIDITY AND MORTALITY

The changes in the maternal milieu that characterize the diabetic state can have profound effects on the growth and development of the fetus, increase the risk of perinatal morbidity and mortality, and exert adverse effects throughout life. The physiological adaptations induced by pregnancy can unmask latent maternal diabetes or result in transient worsening of preexisting vascular compromise. Diabetic women are four times more likely to develop preeclampsia or eclampsia than are nondiabetic women and twice as likely to experience a spontaneous abortion. The rates of infection, hydramnios, postpartum hemorrhage, and cesarean birth are increased. In the long term, GDM is also associated with impaired insulin tolerance and the manifestation of diabetes in later life (ACOG, 2013e; Cunningham et al., 2014; Van Otterloo, 2011a).

Major fetal effects associated with diabetes include a fivefold increase in perinatal death and a two- to threefold increase in the rate of congenital malformations. Early in pregnancy, the fetus is at risk for congenital malformations and poor fetal growth. The risk of major congenital defects is 4% to 8% greater with type 1 or 2 diabetes. Congenital defects result from the teratogenic effects of hyperglycemia during the time of organogenesis during the early gestational weeks. Late in pregnancy, the fetus is at risk for growth

abnormalities and sudden intrauterine death (ACOG, 2013e; Cunningham et al., 2014; Fleming & Corbett, 2010).

Control of maternal glucose levels is an important factor in determining fetal outcome. The **glycosylated hemoglobin A_{1c}** (HbA_{1c}) level is commonly assessed to guide adjustments in the treatment plan throughout pregnancy. Because the maternal serum HbA_{1c} reflects the degree of glycemic control during the preceding 5 to 6 weeks, the test is repeated every trimester. Good diabetic control is reflected by an HbA_{1c} value of 2.5% to 5.9%; an HbA_{1c} value greater than 8% is indicative of poor diabetic control. In the absence of prepregnancy and prenatal care, the rate of perinatal mortality for the diabetic patient and her fetus may be as high as 40%. However, with close, meticulous care, the perinatal mortality rate can be reduced to 3% to 5% (ACOG, 2005; Cunningham et al., 2014).

Ketoacidosis

Diabetic ketoacidosis (DKA) is an accumulation of ketones in the blood that results from hyperglycemia. DKA can lead to metabolic acidosis; however, this has become a less common occurrence because of the implementation of meticulous antenatal care and protocols that stress the strict metabolic control of maternal blood glucose levels. Early recognition of the signs and symptoms of DKA helps to improve both maternal and fetal outcome. As occurs in the nonpregnant state, clinical signs of volume depletion follow the symptoms of hyperglycemia, which include polydipsia and polyuria. Malaise, headache, nausea, and vomiting are common patient complaints. A distinctive feature of DKA during pregnancy is that it can occur with remarkably low blood glucose levels (barely exceeding 200 mg/dL, compared with 300 to 350 mg/dL in the nonpregnant state) and requires emergency management (i.e., aggressive hydration and IV insulin) to prevent maternal coma or death. Ketoacidosis that occurs at any time during pregnancy may result in fetal death, and it is a common cause of preterm labor (PTL) (ACOG, 2013e; Cunningham et al., 2014; Hood, 2012; Sibai & Viteri, 2014).

"What to say"—*Teaching patients about hypoglycemia*

Hypoglycemia occurs more frequently in pregnancy than at other times, especially in patients with type 1 pregestational diabetes mellitus. When teaching about hypoglycemia, the nurse should include the following information (ACOG, 2013e):

- Hypoglycemia is a condition that occurs when your blood sugar levels decrease to less than 60 mg/dL.

- It is more common during pregnancy.

- Symptoms include light-headedness, shaking, headache, sweating, confusion, hot flashes, nervous and anxiety attacks, intense hunger, sudden irritability, and changes in vision.

- It is important that you and your family are able to immediately recognize and respond to hypoglycemia.

- Drinking a glass of milk is better than a glass of juice that contains high levels of glucose.

- Always keep glucagon on hand for severe hypoglycemia or loss of consciousness.

clinical alert

Maternal diabetes and preterm labor

Magnesium sulfate is the drug of choice for diabetic women who experience preterm labor. The use of antenatal corticosteroids to accelerate fetal lung maturation can cause significant maternal hyperglycemia and precipitate DKA. Patients must be closely followed in an acute care setting for at least 48 to 72 hours after corticosteroids have been given. An IV insulin infusion will usually be required and is adjusted on the basis of frequent capillary glucose measurements (Landon, Catalano, & Gabbe, 2012).

SCREENING AND DIAGNOSIS

Since 1970, much has been learned about the important relationship between maternal glycemic control before and during pregnancy and its effects on fetal outcomes. The perinatal mortality rate has simultaneously improved as an intensive approach to the diabetic pregnancy has become standard. In 2014, the U.S. Preventive Services Task Force (USPSTF) released a recommendation statement advising that all women be screened for gestational diabetes after 24 weeks of pregnancy. According to ACOG (2013e), all pregnant women should be screened for GDM, whether by patient history, clinical risk factors, or a 50-g, 1-hour loading test to determine blood glucose levels at 24 to 28 weeks of gestation. Women with high risk factors (previous medical history of GDM, known impaired glucose metabolism, obesity [body mass index greater than or equal to 30]) should be screened earlier in pregnancy; if diabetes mellitus is not diagnosed, blood glucose testing should be repeated at 24 to 28 weeks of gestation.

In the United States, most centers use the following diagnostic recommendations and criteria established by the National Diabetes Data Group:

- The Glucose Challenge Test (Glucola screening): A 50-g oral glucose solution is administered to the woman and a blood sample is taken 1 hour after it is consumed. Patients with a 1-hour plasma glucose value that exceeds 130 to 140 mg/dL (depending on the lab used) should be further evaluated with the formal 3-hour oral glucose tolerance test (OGTT).
- The 3-hour OGTT requires the fasting patient to ingest 100 g of glucose with blood drawn at 1-hour intervals. Before the test, the woman should avoid caffeine (it may increase glucose levels) and refrain from smoking at least 12 hours before and during the test. The diagnosis of GDM is made when two values or more of the threshold are above the norm. According to the American Diabetes Association (ADA) (2010), the normal plasma values are:

Fasting blood sugar	<95 mg/dL
1 hour	<180 mg/dL
2 hour	<155 mg/dL
3 hour	<140 mg/dL

In early 2011, the International Association of Diabetes in Pregnancy Study Group (IADPSG) published recommendations for the diagnosis and classification of hyperglycemia during pregnancy. IADPSG recommended a simplified "one-step" approach to the screening and diagnosis of GDM with a 75-g, 2-hour glucose tolerance test

(Metzger, Gabbe, Persson, Buchanan, Catalano, Damm, et al., 2010). According to ACOG (2013e), adoption of the guidelines would result in GDM being diagnosed in approximately 18% of all pregnant women. Because there is no evidence that diagnosis using the IADPSG guidelines criteria leads to clinically significant improvements in maternal or newborn outcomes and would lead to a significant increase in health-care costs, ACOG does not recommend adoption of the guidelines at this time. The updated (2013e) ACOG practice bulletin on gestational diabetes recommends the two-step approach to testing: the 1-hour test with either 135 or 140 mg/dL acceptable as a cutoff, and the 3-hour test using the National Diabetes Data Group criteria: 105, 190, 165, and 145 mg/dL.

MANAGEMENT

The goal of modern glycemic management during the diabetic pregnancy is to maintain blood glucose levels as close to normal (euglycemia) as possible. Euglycemia is a normal blood glucose level in the range of 65 to 105 mg/dL preprandially. Two-hour postprandial blood glucose levels should be less than 120 mg/dL (ADA, 2013). Metabolic monitoring during pregnancy is directed at detecting hyperglycemia and making all necessary pharmacological, dietary, or activity adjustments to minimize any adverse effects to the fetus. Home blood glucose monitoring with a glucose reflectance meter or biosensor monitor is a widely accepted method for monitoring blood glucose levels and an essential tool for helping the woman to assess her degree of blood glucose control (Fig. 11-15). Patients monitor their blood glucose levels daily, record the findings, and bring their blood glucose logs with them to each prenatal appointment.

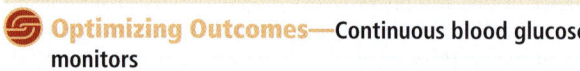

Optimizing Outcomes—Continuous blood glucose monitors

Self-monitoring of blood glucose (SMBG) via the intermittent monitoring of capillary blood has brought significant improvements to the care of patients with diabetes. Recently, continuous glucose monitoring (CGM) has become available. This modality, which provides real-time glucose data, offers patients and providers a tool to use along with

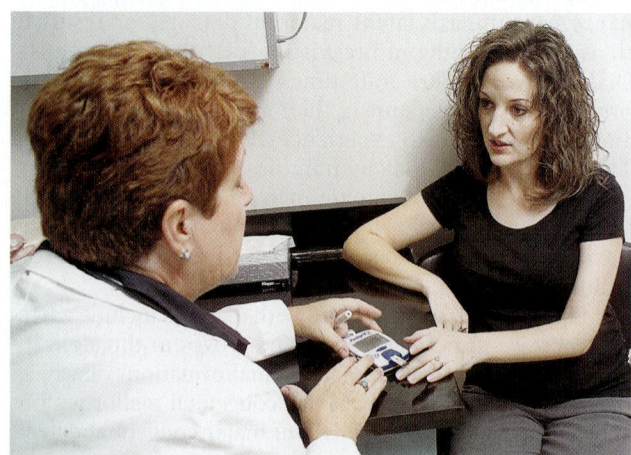

Figure 11-15 Blood glucose monitoring is an essential component of care for the pregnant patient with diabetes.

SBGM to achieve a more complete picture of 24-hour blood glucose patterns. CGM can identify sudden blood glucose drops, hyperglycemia and postprandial changes in glucose levels that cannot be identified with intermittent glucose monitoring. Pregnant women may especially benefit from this added information because glycemic goals during pregnancy are more stringent (Pereira & Nicollerat, 2011).

Ongoing fetal surveillance is of utmost importance. Maternal care requires the cooperative efforts of a clinical team that includes the obstetrician, internist, endocrinologist, diabetes educator, neonatologist, dietitian, and nurse. Ultrasound examinations throughout the pregnancy are useful in determining viability and accurately establishing the gestational age early in pregnancy, diagnosing fetal cardiac and central nervous system (CNS) malformations, monitoring fetal growth and obtaining amniotic fluid volume measurements, predicting maternal and fetal complications, and assisting with timing and mode of delivery (Yehuda et al., 2011). Patient education is essential to ensure that the woman understands her diabetic state and the need to adhere to treatment so that an optimal outcome is achieved. Social services, home nursing visitation, and spiritual support are often involved as well.

 Optimizing Outcomes—Diet and exercise for the patient with GDM

It has been demonstrated that women who develop GDM have higher gestational weight gain, especially in early pregnancy. Gestational weight gain is a significant risk factor for GDM in the overweight or obese patient but not in patients who were underweight or had a normal BMI before pregnancy (Gibson, Waters, & Catalano, 2012; Hedderson, Gunderson, & Ferrara, 2010). Diet and exercise are important components of care for the woman with GDM. Typically, the patient is placed on a standard diabetic diet that is calculated to include 30 kcal/kg per day, based on a normal preconceptional weight. For the obese woman, the diet may be calculated to include up to 25 kcal/kg per day. Approximately 40% to 50% of calories should come from complex, high-fiber carbohydrates, 20% should come from protein, and 30% to 40% should come from primarily unsaturated fats. Bedtime snacks are recommended to help reduce nocturnal hypoglycemia (ACOG, 2013e; ADA, 2009, 2010). Ongoing nutritional counseling is essential, and patients should be encouraged to maintain a food intake log several days each week to help guide management. Physical activity such as walking, cycling on stationary bikes, and swimming is also important for the woman with GDM. Exercise helps to lower blood glucose levels and may decrease the need for insulin (Elkins & Taylor, 2013; Landon et al., 2012).

Nursing Insight—*Planning care for the woman with GDM*

Optimal glycemic goals for GDM include a fasting venous plasma glucose concentration less than or equal to 95 mg/dL and a one-hour postprandial plasma glucose of less than or equal to 140 mg/dL. Blood glucose self-monitoring is recommended. Although diet and exercise are the mainstays of care for the woman

with GDM, up to 20% will require insulin during pregnancy to maintain euglycemia. If fasting blood glucose levels exceed 105 mg/dL, insulin therapy is initiated (ADA, 2009).

INSULIN AND ORAL HYPOGLYCEMIC THERAPY

Most insulin used to treat pregestational diabetes mellitus is biosynthetic human insulin such as lispro or aspart, which are short- or rapid-acting insulin analogs that mimic physiological insulin action. The analogs can be given closer to a meal (i.e., 5–10 minutes vs. 30–45 minutes) than regular insulin, but patients must be warned that significant hypoglycemia can occur if they do not eat promptly after administering the medication. Often, a four-dose regimen that combines a short-acting (preprandial) with a long-acting (bedtime dosing) insulin is used. Patients who are highly motivated and compliant may wish to use an insulin pump, which delivers a continuous subcutaneous infusion of a rapid-acting insulin such as lispro, which has been shown to be more effective in maintaining desired glucose levels and in reducing the risk of fetal macrosomia (ACOG, 2013e; Hurst, 2011).

Oral hypoglycemic agents, which cross the placenta and have not been well studied in pregnancy, are generally not used. However, glyburide (Glynase, Micronase), a second-generation oral sulfonylurea, does not cross the placenta and has been used to treat GDM. Glyburide has been found to be comparable to insulin in improving glucose control without evidence of adverse maternal and neonatal complications. According to ACOG (2013e), the use of oral agents for the control of type 2 diabetes mellitus during pregnancy should be limited and individualized until the safety and efficacy of these medications have been confirmed.

 Now Can You—Discuss diabetes management during pregnancy?

1. State three risk factors for gestational diabetes?
2. Discuss the effects of maternal diabetes on fetal growth and development?
3. Describe how you would educate the pregnant patient about the importance of diabetes screening?

The Thyroid Gland and Pregnancy

Thyroid disorders are relatively common among pregnant women. The hormonal changes and increasing metabolic demands of pregnancy bring about complex compensatory alterations in maternal thyroid function. Human chorionic gonadotropin (hCG), which is at its highest levels in early pregnancy, possesses intrinsic, weak thyroid-stimulating activity. Thyroid-stimulating hormone (TSH) levels fall during the first trimester, and this decrease parallels the rise in the production of hCG.

HYPERTHYROIDISM

Signs and Symptoms

The signs and symptoms of mild to moderate hyperthyroidism are common during pregnancy (heat intolerance, diaphoresis, fatigue, anxiety, emotional lability, tachycardia,

Nursing Care Plan Gestational Diabetes Mellitus

Nursing Diagnosis: Nutrition, Imbalanced: Less than Body Requirements related to impaired carbohydrate metabolism during pregnancy

Measurable Short-Term Goal: The patient will plan a balanced diet and exercise program to follow during pregnancy.

Measurable Long-Term Goal: The patient will obtain and metabolize sufficient nutrients for maternal and fetal needs and to maintain appropriate blood glucose levels during pregnancy.

NOC Outcomes:

Diabetes Self-Management (1619) Personal actions to manage diabetes mellitus and prevent disease progression.

Nutritional Status: Nutrient Intake (1009) Adequacy of usual pattern of nutrient intake

NIC Interventions:

Nutrition Therapy (1120)
Nutrition Counseling (5246)

Nursing Interventions:

1. Assess the patient's understanding of gestational diabetes and provide additional information as needed about changes in carbohydrate metabolism during pregnancy and how these may affect the patient and her fetus.

   RATIONALE: Teaching is based on the patient's need for information to help promote active participation in self-care.

2. Refer patient to a registered dietitian and reinforce the recommended diet parameters with patient at each visit: An additional 300 calories per day are needed in the second and third trimesters; 40% to 50% from complex carbohydrates, 10% to 20% from protein, and 30% from fats; avoid concentrated sweets; nutrients should be divided each day between three meals and three snacks.

   RATIONALE: The diet is planned to maintain a normoglycemic state during pregnancy based on the patient's lifestyle and individual food preferences.

3. Encourage the patient to engage in 30 minutes of daily exercise appropriate for her pregnancy such as walking or swimming.

   RATIONALE: Regular exercise helps maintain lower blood glucose levels.

4. Ask patient to keep a daily log of her diet and exercise. Review at each prenatal visit and offer support and encouragement to continue regimen.

   RATIONALE: A written log allows the patient to monitor her own progress and provides a record of interventions to compare with blood glucose levels.

5. Inform patient that she will need to have her blood glucose checked weekly in the office, and if it is still high after about 2 weeks of diet and exercise, she may need to begin insulin therapy.

   RATIONALE: Dietary changes and exercise may not be enough to maintain carbohydrate balance. Anticipatory guidance helps motivate the patient and prepare her for possible change.

6. Monitor fetal growth and well-being. Instruct patient in a method for fetal kick counts beginning at 28 weeks and prepare her for weekly nonstress tests from 34 weeks until birth.

   RATIONALE: Maternal hyperglycemia may result in fetal macrosomia. The fetus of a diabetic mother is at higher risk for complications.

and a wide pulse pressure). However, weight loss, tachycardia greater than 100 beats per minute, and diffuse goiter (enlargement of the thyroid gland) are clinical features suggestive of hyperthyroidism. Because of an increased risk for malignancy during pregnancy, it is essential to investigate all thyroid nodules. Gastrointestinal symptoms (i.e., severe nausea, excessive vomiting, and diarrhea), cardiomyopathy, lymphadenopathy, and congestive heart failure can also accompany thyrotoxicosis (excessive thyroid activity) in pregnancy (Cunningham et al., 2014; Nader, 2013). Establishing a diagnosis of maternal hyperthyroidism can be challenging because of the myriad of metabolic and hormonal changes that normally take place during pregnancy. However, a depressed maternal serum TSH concentration and an elevated free thyroxine (T_4) level are useful in confirming the diagnosis. Although difficult, prompt diagnosis of hyperthyroidism is imperative because of the potential for serious maternal and fetal complications. Research suggests that uncontrolled hyperthyroidism during pregnancy may be associated with congestive heart failure, increased preeclampsia, PTL, postpartum hemorrhage, low birth weight, and neonatal mortality (Abel, 2011a; Cunningham et al., 2014; Nader, 2013; Van Otterloo, 2011a).

Treatment

Treatment for hyperthyroidism includes the use of antithyroid medications such as the thioamides, propylthiouracil (PTU—the drug of choice), or methimazole (Tapazole). Symptomatic improvement usually occurs within 2 weeks after the initiation of therapy, although the medication does not become fully effective for 6 to 8 weeks. During treatment, the patient's free T_4 levels are obtained on a monthly basis, and the findings are used to taper the dosage to achieve the smallest effective level to prevent unnecessary fetal hypothyroidism. When unresponsive to drug therapy, surgery (subtotal thyroidectomy) may be necessary. Because the surgery is associated with an increased risk of pregnancy loss and PTL, it is performed only for cases of severe hyperthyroidism. The use of radioactive iodine for diagnosis or treatment of hyperthyroidism is contraindicated during pregnancy because it may adversely affect the fetal thyroid (Abel, 2011a). When caring for patients with hyperthyroidism, it is important that the nursing assessment include the maternal pulse rate (less than 100 bpm), reflexes (2+ to 3+), weight gain, and fetal growth. Patient education should focus on complications of antithyroid therapy (i.e., purpuric skin rash, pruritus, fever, and nausea) and dietary needs (i.e., increased calories and protein) (Van Otterloo, 2011a).

HYPOTHYROIDISM

Symptoms

Caused by an inadequate production of thyroid hormone, the symptoms of hypothyroidism are insidious and can be masked by the hypermetabolic state associated with pregnancy. Maternal symptoms can include modest weight gain, a decrease in exercise capacity, lethargy, cold intolerance, constipation, hoarseness, hair loss, brittle nails, and dry skin. Laboratory confirmation is made from an elevated TSH level and low to normal T_3 and T_4 values. Patients with hypothyroidism have an increased likelihood of having another autoimmune disease (Abel, 2011b; Cunningham et al., 2014; Nader, 2013; Sullivan, 2011; Van Otterloo, 2011a).

Treatment

During early gestation, thyroid hormones cross the placenta in small amounts. The fetus is dependent on the hormones until fetal production begins at 12 weeks. Maternal hypothyroidism must be treated promptly, because there is an increased risk for preeclampsia, placental abruption, preterm birth, low birth weight, and stillbirth. Fetal neurological development can be severely affected by decreased levels of thyroid hormone. Treatment involves the use of a thyroid hormone supplement (e.g., levothyroxine [Synthroid]) with the dose adjusted every 4 weeks until the TSH level reaches the lower end of the normal range for pregnancy. Radioactive iodine (^{131}I) is contraindicated in pregnancy (Abel, 2011b; Nader, 2013; Van Otterloo, 2011a).

Venous Thrombosis and Pulmonary Embolism

Venous thromboembolic diseases, which complicate approximately 1 in 1,600 births, include superficial and deep vein thrombophlebitis (DVT), pulmonary embolus (PE), septic pelvic thrombophlebitis, and thrombosis. These conditions account for one-half of all obstetric morbidity. Pulmonary embolism, the leading cause of maternal mortality, accounts for 9% of all maternal deaths in the United States (ACOG, 2011f, 2013d). Pregnant and postpartum women are about 4 to 5 times more likely to develop venous thromboembolism than nonpregnant, age-matched women. The most common form of thrombosis that occurs during pregnancy involves veins of the calf, thigh, and pelvis. The most important aspect of lower extremity and pelvic venous thrombosis is that it can lead to pulmonary embolism, which poses a major threat to the pregnant woman (Bowman & Branch, 2012; Cunningham et al., 2014).

PATHOPHYSIOLOGY

Thrombosis is thought to be the consequence of alterations in the vessel wall, slowing of blood flow (or stasis), and changes in blood components. Pregnancy presents the ideal state in which all three of these components may exist. Trauma to the vessel wall may occur during childbirth with alterations in the clot-inhibiting endothelial surface. Blood flow from the legs and pelvic veins are slowed during pregnancy because of pressure exerted on the iliac veins by the gravid uterus and by the relaxation of the smooth muscles in response to increased progesterone.

Finally, changes in blood components occur during pregnancy whereby some clotting factors are increased while other anticoagulant and fibrinolytic system factors are decreased.

INCIDENCE AND RISK FACTORS

When compared with nonpregnant women of similar age, the likelihood of venous thromboembolism during normal pregnancy and the puerperium is increased by a factor of five. Venous thromboembolism (VTE) occurs in 0.5 to 2.0 per 1,000 pregnancies. An untreated DVT is associated with a 15% to 25% incidence of pulmonary embolus, which is associated with a 12% to 15% maternal mortality rate. The most important individual risk factor for venous thromboembolism in pregnancy is a personal history of thrombosis. Medical factors (e.g., hemoglobinopathies, obesity, hypertension, smoking, advanced age, and increased parity) and pregnancy complications (e.g., preeclampsia, multiple gestation, and dehydration) place women at high risk for thromboembolic disease during pregnancy (ACOG, 2011g, 2013f). When assessing the pregnant patient, the nurse must be aware of the characteristic signs and symptoms associated with thromboembolic disease.

The diagnosis can be very challenging, because some of the signs and symptoms are normal during pregnancy (e.g., lower extremity edema). Doppler ultrasound technique has become the diagnostic study of choice in cases of proximal vein occlusion. When results are negative and iliac vein thrombosis is suspected, confirmatory imaging with magnetic resonance imaging (MRI) is recommended. If there is a suspicion of PE, ventilation–perfusion scanning or computed tomographic (CT) angiography results in minimal radiation exposure to the fetus. Management involves a combination of strategies including medications (i.e., anticoagulant therapy with heparin), bedrest with elevation of the involved extremity, and the application of warm, moist heat. (ACOG, 2011g).

Critical Nursing Action Recognizing Thromboembolism

During the examination, the nurse assesses for the presence of the following signs and symptoms that may be indicative of thromboembolism (Cunningham et al., 2014):

- Pain, tenderness, warmth.
- Swelling of the lower extremity, which is asymmetric with a difference of greater than 0.8 in. (2 cm) between the normal and affected leg. Swelling of the thigh is especially relevant because the risk of pulmonary embolism is associated with femoral or iliac phlebitis.
- Color change, especially in the left leg.
- A palpable cord underlying the region of pain and tenderness.

Symptoms of a pulmonary embolism:

- Tachypnea
- Dyspnea
- Pleuritic chest pain
- Atelectatic rales
- Cough
- Fever
- Diaphoresis
- Tachycardia
- Hemoptysis
- Cyanosis
- Heart gallop or murmur
- Anxiety
- Apprehension

Now Can You—Discuss thromboembolism during pregnancy?

1. Describe why pregnancy is an ideal state for the development of thromboembolism?
2. Name five signs and symptoms to consider when assessing your pregnant patient for thromboembolism?
3. Formulate a plan of care for the patient with a diagnosis of thromboembolism?

Psychiatric Complications During Pregnancy

The recognition and management of depression and psychoses during pregnancy and the puerperium are of critical importance. Particularly in the United States, these disorders often are underrecognized and undertreated, and this factor potentially contributes to the likelihood of devastating effects on the child, the mother, the family, and society.

CONSULTING WITH THE PREGNANT PSYCHIATRIC PATIENT

Psychiatric complications during pregnancy can represent an exacerbation of an ongoing psychiatric disorder, a resurgence of previously remitted symptoms, or the onset of a new illness. Millions of women suffer from mental illness during their childbearing years, and more than 50% of pregnancies are unplanned in this population. These facts highlight the importance of prenatal counseling with regard to the natural history of various psychiatric disorders during pregnancy and the potential associated with fetal exposure to psychotropic agents and/or maternal mental illness.

Consultations with pregnant women who suffer from a psychiatric disorder, regardless of the diagnosis, should include discussion of the following facts (ACOG, 2007d, 2009b):

- Psychoactive medications readily cross the placenta.
- There are potential risks associated with untreated maternal psychiatric illness as well as exposure to psychotropic medications. (Risks may include poor attention to prenatal care, substance abuse, and deliberate self-harm).
- Many women experience relapse or worsening of symptoms if pharmacological treatment is not continued or instituted when necessary. (Maternal anxiety and stress have been shown to have adverse effects on pregnancy outcome, infant/child neurodevelopment, and maternal postnatal mental health.)
- Use of a single medication at a higher dose is preferable to the use of multiple medications for the treatment of psychiatric illness during pregnancy. (Changing medication increases the exposure to the fetus.)
- Patient care is optimized when provided by a multidisciplinary team composed of the obstetrician, mental health clinician, primary health-care provider, and pediatrician.

Depression

The incidence of depression during pregnancy is estimated to be 10% to 13%. Women at risk for antepartum and/or postpartum depression are those with a personal or family history of affective disorders (unipolar and bipolar), young age, few social supports, high psychosocial stress, intimate partner violence, marital conflict, or significant life events. Antenatal depression may increase the risk of preterm birth, low birth weight and abnormal stress responses in offspring (ACOG, 2009b; Melville, Gavin, Guo, Fan, & Katon, 2010; Shade, Miller, Borst, English, Valliere, Downs, et al., 2011). Psychotherapeutic counseling is beneficial for mild to moderately ill women with unipolar major depressive disorder, but medication is frequently required for women with severe major depressive disorder or bipolar disorder (Yonkers, Vigod, & Ross, 2011). Also, electroconvulsive therapy is an effective treatment for major depression and is safe to use during pregnancy (ACOG, 2009b).

Medications prescribed for depression include selective serotonin reuptake inhibitors (SSRIs), such as fluvoxamine, sertraline, citalopram, and fluoxetine, and tricyclic antidepressants (TCAs) including amitriptyline, clomipramine, doxepin, and protriptyline. Presently, there are conflicting data regarding first trimester SSRI exposure and the risk for fetal malformations; late pregnancy exposure has been associated with neonatal abstinence syndrome, persistent pulmonary hypertension, cardiac dysrhythmias, and transient neonatal complications (e.g., jitteriness, weak cry, poor tone, and mild respiratory distress). Breastfeeding is generally considered safe for women using SSRIs. Effects associated with TCA exposure include transient withdrawal symptoms, hypertonia, irritability, tachypnea, and tachycardia (Abel, 2013; ACOG, 2007d).

Across Care Settings: Community strategies to address perinatal depression

In 2006, the U.S. Department of Health and Human Services, Health Resources and Services Administration's Maternal and Child Health Bureau granted funding to six states for 2-year projects to develop, launch, and evaluate new strategies to improve awareness, detection, and treatment of perinatal depression and anxiety disorders. The projects, implemented in rural, urban, and disaster-impacted areas, successfully engaged large numbers of diverse women's health-care providers in training related to perinatal depression and anxiety disorders. Innovative strategies, which included screening programs and public awareness campaigns, and addressing barriers to perinatal mental health screening and treatment are expected to positively impact the health of women and their families in the targeted states (Shade, Miller, Borst, English, Valliere, Downs, et al., 2011).

Bipolar Disorder

Bipolar disorder is commonly characterized by distinct periods of abnormally and persistently elevated, expansive, or irritable mood and separate distinct periods of depressed mood or anhedonia (inability to gain pleasure from normally pleasurable experiences). Women are more likely than men to experience depressive episodes of bipolar disorder, rapid cycling, and mixed episodes. Early prenatal exposure to lithium, the mainstay of treatment, may be associated with congenital cardiac malformations; later exposure has been associated with fetal and neonatal cardiac arrhythmias, hypoglycemia, polyhydramnios, and preterm birth. Fetal assessment with fetal echocardiography is appropriate when exposure occurs during the first trimester (ACOG, 2007d).

The course of bipolar disorder is particularly unpredictable during pregnancy. Maternal physiological alterations affect the absorption, distribution, metabolism, and elimination of lithium, and current recommendations call for frequent monitoring of serum lithium levels throughout the perinatal period. The decision to discontinue lithium therapy during pregnancy because of the concern for fetal risk must be balanced against the maternal risks of exacerbation of illness. There have been reports of heightened risk of depressive or manic relapse in women who rapidly discontinued lithium treatment, in comparison with those who underwent a slow, controlled tapering off over 4 weeks. Regardless of how rapidly lithium doses are tapered, the risk of relapse illness during pregnancy and the puerperium is significantly high. Anticonvulsants including valproate, carbamazepine, and lamotrigine are also used in the treatment of bipolar disorder. Valproate and carbamazepine are associated with adverse effects when used during pregnancy and should be avoided, especially during the first trimester (ACOG, 2007d; Pigarelli, Kraus, & Potter, 2011).

Schizophrenia

Schizophrenia is defined as a psychotic disorder that lasts for at least 6 months and includes a 1-month duration of two or more of the following symptoms: delusions, hallucinations, disorganized speech, grossly disorganized or bizarre behavior, and symptoms involving loss of behaviors such as avolition (lack of motivation), affective blunting (reduced emotional expression) or alogia (empty verbal response) (American Psychiatric Association, 2013). During pregnancy, women often experience worsening of their symptoms, and, because of the potential teratogenic effects on the fetus, the prescribed psychotropic medication may need to be discontinued or changed (Tormoehlen &

Lessick, 2011). No significant teratogenic or toxic effects have been documented with typical antipsychotic drugs including haloperidol, perphenazine, and chlorpromazine. However, reproductive safety data on the commonly used atypical antipsychotics (e.g., risperidone, clozapine, and aripiprazole) are extremely limited, and the routine use of the atypical antipsychotics during pregnancy and lactation is not recommended (ACOG, 2007d).

Maternal high-risk symptoms of schizophrenia include psychotic denial of pregnancy (the woman denies she is pregnant despite clear evidence that she is), self-mutilation, fetal abuse, and neonaticide. Nurses caring for pregnant women with schizophrenia should assess for delusions and coexisting health problems such as depression, eating disorders, sexually transmitted infections, alcohol or drug abuse, and chronic conditions including diabetes mellitus and hypertension. An important nursing role centers on prenatal patient education and on ensuring that community support services and referrals to community agencies are in place for the patient and her family members during the antepartal period (Tormoehlen & Lessick, 2011).

Anxiety Disorders

Anxiety disorders including panic disorder, generalized anxiety disorder, obsessive–compulsive disorder (OCD), and posttraumatic stress disorder (PTSD) are common during the childbearing years. Childbearing has been associated with the onset or worsening of panic disorder or OCD, and women are at greatest risk for exacerbation of both disorders during the postpartum period. Benzodiazepines (alprazolam, diazepam, and clorazepate), anxiolytic medications often used in the treatment of anxiety disorders, may be associated with a small risk of fetal oral cleft, and the long-term impact of prenatal benzodiazepine exposure is unclear. If discontinuation of benzodiazepine therapy during pregnancy is considered, the medication should not be abruptly withdrawn. Infants exposed to maternal benzodiazepine use shortly before birth require close monitoring for "floppy infant syndrome," characterized by hypothermia, lethargy, poor respiratory effort, and feeding difficulties (ACOG, 2007d; Avni-Barron & Wiegartz, 2011).

Eating Disorders

Eating disorders in pregnant women have both physiological and psychological effects on the outcome of the pregnancy and on subsequent infant development. Anorexia nervosa has been associated with higher rates of perinatal mortality, obstetric complications, and congenital anomalies. Bulimia nervosa has been associated with extreme maternal weight gain, preeclampsia, and eclampsia.

MANAGEMENT

The importance of the detection of psychiatric problems in the pregnant population cannot be overemphasized. The health and welfare of not only the mother is at stake but also that of the entire family. Nurses are often the first care providers to recognize indicators of psychiatric difficulties in their patients. Strategies to help identify mental health problems during pregnancy may include (Townsend, 2011; Yonkers, 2013):

- Placing psychoeducational materials throughout all patient areas

- Routinely inquiring about the patient's and her family's psychiatric history during the initial interview
- Administering the Edinburgh Postnatal Depression Scale, the Beck Depression Inventory, the Postpartum Depression Screening Scale, or a similar tool
- Assessing the woman's access to social and family supports
- Referring the woman to community resources such as home health visitation and the local mental health agency

"What to say"—*When screening for depression during pregnancy*

The U.S. and Canadian Task Forces on Preventive Health Care recommend using the following two "probe questions" to screen women for depression during pregnancy:

- "Over the past 2 weeks have you felt down, depressed, or helpless?"
- "Over the past 2 weeks have you felt little interest or pleasure in doing things?" (Stewart, 2011).

Substance Abuse in Pregnancy

Alcohol and drug use during pregnancy is a common phenomenon and a significant public health issue. Studies of substance abuse during pregnancy have documented a high incidence of adverse and, sometimes, catastrophic perinatal outcomes associated with intrauterine drug and alcohol exposure. Risk factors for maternal alcohol use in pregnancy include poverty, homelessness, substance abuse by one's partner, and preconception substance use (Velasquez, Ingersoll, Sobell, Floyd, Sobell, & von Sternberg, 2010). Nurses are responsible for having up-to-date knowledge of the effects of alcohol, tobacco, and other drugs in pregnancy and for performing skilled and compassionate assessments of pregnant and postpartum women without criticizing their behavior or alienating them from their sources of health care.

Because of increased public education and awareness or the decrease in self-reporting (related to accompanying social stigma), rates of alcohol use in pregnancy have decreased over the past decade. In multiple surveys prior to 2001, 20% of all women reported consuming some alcohol during pregnancy. Combined 2011 to 2012 data from the National Survey on Drug Use and Health revealed that 8.5% of pregnant women aged 15 to 44 drank alcohol in the past month and 2.7% binge drank. Most alcohol use by pregnant women occurred during the first trimester, and alcohol use was lower during the second and third trimesters (Substance Abuse and Mental Health Services Administration, Office of Applied Studies [SAMHSA], 2013).

SUBSTANCE ADDICTION

Pregnancy does not occur in a vacuum but rather it is an event that is superimposed on the context and circumstances of women's lives. Substance-abusing women have a high incidence of social (intimate partner violence and risk-taking sexual behaviors) and psychological (low self-esteem) conditions that affect their health status, their ability to engage in prenatal care, and their ability

to succeed in drug abuse treatment. These social and psychological conditions become more important considerations when the biological and psychological stresses of pregnancy are added to an already fragile system (ACOG, 2012f).

Opioid Abuse

Opioid abuse in pregnancy includes the use of heroin and the misuse of prescription opioid analgesic medications such as codeine, fentanyl, methadone, oxycodone, merperidine, and hydrocodone. Maternal chronic untreated heroin use is associated with an increased risk of fetal growth restriction, abruptio placentae, fetal death, PTL, and the intrauterine passage of meconium. Neonatal abstinence syndrome, characterized by CNS hyperirritability, gastrointestinal dysfunction, respiratory distress, and various autonomic symptoms (e.g., yawning, sneezing, and fever), follows prenatal exposure to opioids (ACOG, 2012f; Moran, 2011b; Pritham, Paul, & Hayes, 2012).

To lessen health risks, pregnant women who are opioid dependent have been treated with methadone maintenance therapy (MMT). Dispensed by a registered substance abuse treatment program, MMT is part of a comprehensive inpatient package of prenatal care, chemical dependency counseling, family therapy, nutritional education, and other medical and psychosocial services. In 2002, the U.S. Food and Drug Administration (FDA) approved buprenorphine hydrochloride for treatment of opioid-dependent patients but not for pregnant patients. Buprenorphine acts on the same receptors as heroin and morphine. Although clinicians are reluctant to prescribe buprenorphine for pregnant women, emerging evidence supports the use of buprenorphine for opioid-assisted treatment during pregnancy. When compared with MMT, buprenorphine is associated with a lower risk of overdose, fewer drug interactions, the ability to be treated on an outpatient basis without the need for daily visits to a licensed treatment program, and evidence of less severe neonatal abstinence syndrome (ACOG, 2012f; Pritham, Paul, & Hayes, 2012).

Methamphetamine Abuse

Methamphetamine is a powerful stimulant that can be smoked, snorted, injected, or ingested orally or anally. It is the only illegal drug that can be easily made from legally obtained ingredients found in over-the-counter cold medications or decongestants. Use during pregnancy is associated with adverse neonatal outcomes including small for gestational age, low birth weight, and neonatal and childhood neurodevelopmental abnormalities (ACOG, 2011g; Good, Solt, Acuna, Rotmensch, & Kim, 2010).

Pregnant women who use methamphetamines should be encouraged to immediately seek care at a residential treatment center. Comprehensive prenatal care, including nutritional assessment and social support services is essential, along with STD/HIV testing. Fetal monitoring for growth restriction involves baseline ultrasonography with follow-up ultrasound examinations for growth determination in the third trimester. Use of amphetamines inhibits prolactin release and can reduce breast milk supply. The concentration of amphetamines found in breast milk is higher than that found in maternal plasma, and infants who ingest the breast milk of women using amphetamines exhibit increased irritability, agitation, and crying. Hence, women who are actively using amphetamines should not breastfeed (ACOG, 2011g).

Nurses face difficult ethical dilemmas when caring for pregnant and parenting women who use harmful substances. The conflict may be viewed as one that exists between the women's right to autonomy over her body and behavior and the nurse's obligation to prevent harm to the fetus or child (Kearney, 2008). Nurses in prenatal care and acute care settings are responsible for thoroughly assessing psychosocial risks and conducting mutual goal setting with pregnant patients to minimize the harm associated with these risks. Support and respect should be offered regardless of the woman's decisions about her health care or self-care. A nonjudgmental, concerned, and empathetic environment should be provided so that the patient feels encouraged to express her feelings and concerns about herself, her drug use, and her unborn child (Kearney, 2008; Moran, 2011b).

 Now Can You—Discuss issues associated with substance abuse during pregnancy?

1. Name five behaviors that may signal a substance abuse problem?
2. Discuss how substance abuse can affect the course and outcome of pregnancy?
3. Discuss the ethical dilemmas faced by the perinatal nurse who is caring for the pregnant woman with a substance abuse problem?

Antepartum Fetal Assessment

Fetal assessment is an integral component of prenatal care. Careful assessment of fetal well-being enhances perinatal outcome through early identification and intervention for fetal compromise. The goals of antepartum fetal surveillance are to prevent permanent fetal injury or death, to help ensure the best possible fetal outcome, and to identify fetuses that are "healthy" (thus preventing unnecessary intervention). A number of tests can be performed during pregnancy to monitor fetal growth, development, and well-being. Antenatal assessment during the first and second trimester is directed primarily at the diagnosis of fetal congenital anomalies, whereas the goal of third trimester assessment is to determine the quality of the intrauterine environment for the maturing fetus (ACOG, 1999b, Torgersen, 2011).

CHORIONIC VILLUS SAMPLING

Chorionic villus sampling (CVS) is an invasive procedure that can be used to obtain a fetal karyotype. Because the villi arise from trophoblast cells, their chromosome structure is identical to that of the fetus. CVS is performed between 10 and 12 weeks' gestation and results are available quickly because of the rapid proliferation of the chorionic villi cells. Using ultrasound guidance to locate the chorion cells, a thin catheter is inserted vaginally into the intrauterine cavity (Fig. 11-16). An alternative technique involves the abdominal or intravaginal insertion of a biopsy needle. A small quantity of chorionic villi is then aspirated from the placenta. The risk of complications associated with CVS is 1 in 200. Risks

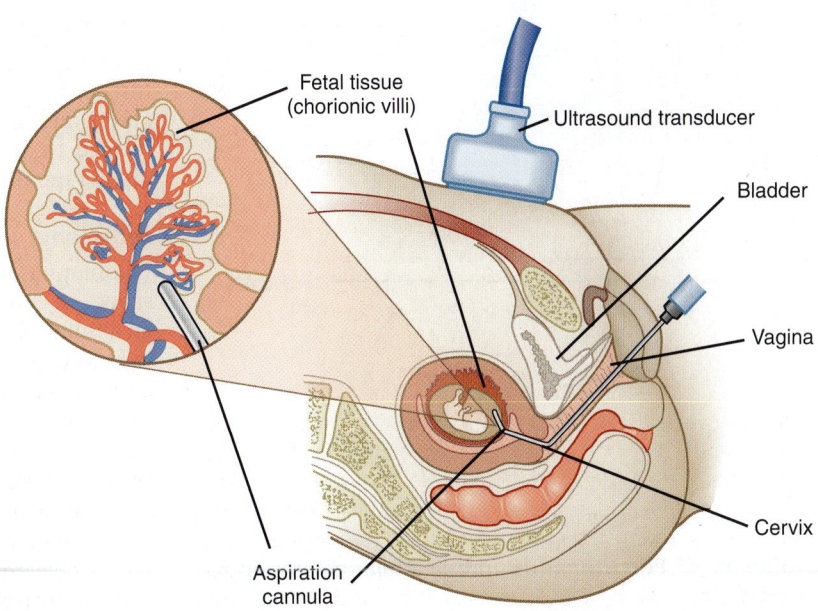

Figure 11-16 Chorionic villus sampling procedure.

include infection (in 0.5% of cases), fetal loss (in 0.3% of cases), rupture of membranes (in 0.1% of cases), Rh isoimmunization, and possible fetal limb reduction (Gilbert, 2010).

PERCUTANEOUS UMBILICAL BLOOD SAMPLING

Percutaneous umbilical blood sampling (PUBS) is an invasive procedure that is performed to obtain a sample of fetal blood for karyotyping and to test for anemia, isoimmunization, metabolic disorders, and infection. Under ultrasound guidance, a needle is inserted through the maternal abdomen and into the fetal umbilical cord (Fig. 11-17). Use of a fetal blood sample for karyotyping allows for more rapid test results than when fetal skin cells are used, as with amniocentesis. Complications include cord laceration, thromboembolism, PTL, PROM, and infection (Wapner, 2013).

AMNIOCENTESIS

Amniocentesis is an invasive procedure that involves the removal of amniotic fluid. Under ultrasound guidance, a needle is inserted through the maternal abdomen and into the amniotic sac (Fig. 11-18). Amniocentesis may be performed beginning at 12 weeks' gestation. Components of the amniotic fluid, including fetal cells, may be analyzed for chromosomal abnormalities, fetal lung maturity, infection, and the presence of bilirubin in Rh-sensitized pregnancies. Later in the pregnancy, amniotic fluid reduction (via amniocentesis) may be performed for temporary alleviation of maternal symptoms associated with hydramnios (excessive amniotic fluid). Complications associated with amniocentesis include rupture of the membranes, PTL, infection, fetal injury, and fetal death. If the woman has Rh(D)-negative blood, $Rh_o(D)$ immune globulin should be administered following the amniocentesis to prevent isoimmunization.

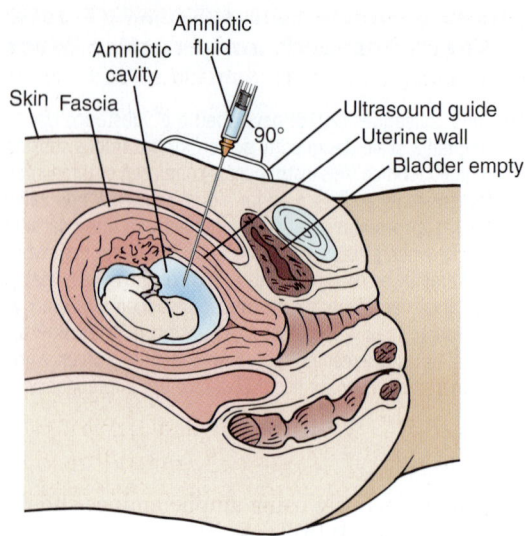

Figure 11-18 Amniocentesis.

Amniocentesis is frequently performed late in pregnancy to provide information concerning fetal lung maturity. **Lecithin** and **sphingomyelin** are the protein components of surfactant, the lung enzyme that is formed by the alveoli beginning around the 22nd week of gestation. After amniocentesis, the **lecithin/sphingomyelin ratio** (L/S ratio) may be quickly determined by a "shake test" or sent to the laboratory for a quantified analysis. An L/S ratio of 2:1, which typically occurs by 35 weeks' gestation, is traditionally accepted as lung maturity (a ratio of 3:1 in the infant of a diabetic mother).

Phosphatidylglycerol and **desaturated phosphatidylcholine** are two other compounds that are found in surfactant after approximately 35 to 36 weeks of gestation. Because these two substances are present only with lung maturity, their presence in the amniotic fluid sample is another indicator that respiratory distress syndrome will not occur in the neonate.

ADDITIONAL INVASIVE PROCEDURES

Amnioscopy

Amnioscopy involves the use of an amnioscope (a small fetoscope) to visually inspect the amniotic fluid through the cervix and membranes. Most often this procedure is performed to detect meconium staining. It carries a risk of membrane rupture.

Fetoscopy

Fetoscopy is a method of visualizing the fetus with a fetoscope, an extremely narrow, hollow tube inserted through an amniocentesis technique. It is sometimes used to assess fetal well-being, obtain fetal tissue and blood samples, and perform fetal surgery, but not before 17 weeks of gestation. The procedure carries a risk of PTL and infection.

Fetal Surgery

Intrauterine fetal surgery is performed to correct anatomical lesions such as myelomeningocele that, if left untreated, are associated with significant morbidity/mortality. Performed during the second trimester before viability, open

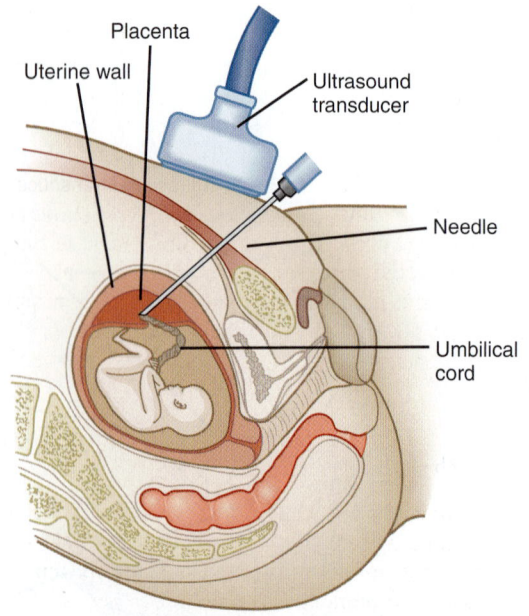

Figure 11-17 Percutaneous umbilical blood sampling procedure.

fetal surgery involves uterine hysterotomy (opening the uterus), surgical repair, and fetal replacement back into the uterus. Intrauterine surgery is associated with significant maternal and fetal risks, and because the upper, active segment of the uterus is entered, the mother is committed to a cesarean birth for this and all future pregnancies. It is essential that the woman and her family be extensively educated about the surgical procedure, the accompanying maternal/fetal risks (e.g., PROM and PTL and birth), the commitment to cesarean birth, and alternatives to the treatment. To safeguard the interests of both the pregnant woman and the fetus, ACOG and the American Academy of Pediatrics (AAP) (2011) published recommendations regarding informed consent, the multidisciplinary nature of fetal intervention teams, the oversight of fetal care centers, and the need to accumulate maternal and fetal outcome data (Farrell & Howell, 2012; Spinner, Miesnik, Koh, & Howell, 2012).

 Nursing Insight—The fetal surgical patient

The past two decades have brought significant advances in imaging modalities such as fetal echocardiography, Doppler assessment, ultrafast MRI, and computed tomography, which are used to diagnose fetal anomalies. Techniques for open fetal surgery and devices for fetal surgical intervention have been developed as well. Today, certain fetal interventions (e.g., ultrasound-guided fetoamniotic shunt placement) have become standard of care, and the number of physicians and hospitals performing these procedures is increasing (Gregory, Wright, Schwarz, & Rakowski, 2012; Miesnik, 2012).

Ultrasonography

Ultrasonography is the use of high-frequency (greater than 20,000 Hz) sound waves to detect differences in tissue density and visualize outlines of structures in the body. Widely used in modern obstetrics, ultrasonography is an important component of antepartum fetal assessment and surveillance. The examination can be done abdominally (after application of a transmission gel, a transducer is moved over the skin) or transvaginally (a lubricated transducer probe is placed in the vagina) during pregnancy. The abdominal technique is more useful after the first trimester when the gravid uterus becomes an abdominal organ (Fig. 11-19). The sound frequencies that bounce back from the uterus are displayed on an oscilloscope screen as a three-dimensional visual image. During the painless examination, the patient should be positioned so that she (and her support person, if present) can observe the images, if they wish to do so.

 Nursing Insight—Levels of ultrasonography

There are three levels of ultrasonography examinations: standard, limited, and specialized.

Ultrasonographers or other health-care professionals who have received special training may perform the *standard* examination, which is used to detect fetal viability, assess the gestational age, determine the presentation of the fetus, locate the

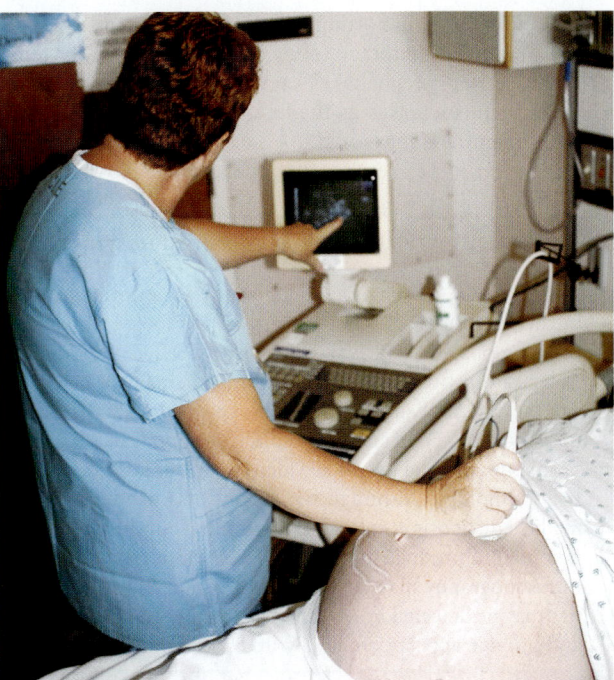

Figure 11-19 An abdominal ultrasound is more useful after the first trimester when the gravid uterus becomes an abdominal organ.

placenta, assess amniotic fluid volume (AFV), and examine the fetus for certain anatomical abnormalities. The *limited* examination is performed for a specific indication, such as determining the fetal presentation during labor or evaluating fetal heart activity when it cannot be detected by other methods. The *specialized* examination is performed to evaluate a fetus suspected to have an anatomical or physiological abnormality. This level of examination is generally performed by specialists in high-risk perinatal centers (ACOG, 2009c; AWHONN, 2010).

During the first trimester, ultrasound may be used to confirm the viability and age of the pregnancy, determine the number, size, and location of the gestational sacs, identify uterine abnormalities (and rule out an ectopic pregnancy), and locate the presence of an intrauterine contraceptive device. Fetal heart rate (FHR) activity can be observed as early as 6 to 7 weeks via real-time echo sonography. In the second and third trimesters, ultrasound is frequently used to confirm fetal viability and gestational age, monitor fetal growth, AFV, placental location and maturity, and assess uterine fibroid tumors and CL. Serial measurements are useful in providing an accurate determination of fetal age. Ultrasound is an essential component of the biophysical profile and fetal Doppler studies (discussed later).

 Optimizing Outcomes—Accurately determining fetal age with ultrasonography

Ultrasonography examinations provide an accurate estimate of fetal age during the first 20 weeks of gestation because most normal fetuses grow at approximately the same rate. Throughout the gestational period, fetal age determination may be made by the following sonographic measurements: (1) gestational sac dimensions (around

8 weeks); (2) crown–rump length (around 7 to 12 weeks); (3) biparietal diameter (after 12 weeks); and (4) femur length (after 12 weeks). The accuracy of gestational age assessment increases as the fetus ages because more than one structure is measured.

Nursing Insight—*Keepsake fetal imaging*

"Keepsake" fetal imaging (sonography) is performed in non-medical settings (e.g., shopping malls) to provide women with photographs and videos of the fetus. ACOG (2004d) and the American Institute of Ultrasound in Medicine (2012) discourage the use of obstetric ultrasonography for nonmedical purposes, and the Food and Drug Administration (2008) views the production of fetal keepsake videos as an "unapproved use" of the technology. Although the general use of ultrasound for medical diagnosis is considered safe, ultrasound energy has the potential to produce biological effects. Moreover, nonmedical ultrasonography may falsely reassure women, and abnormalities may be detected in settings that are not prepared to discuss and provide appropriate follow-up (Lockwood, 2010).

KICK COUNTS

Counting fetal movements, or "kick counts," has been proposed as a primary method of fetal surveillance for all pregnancies (Fig. 11-20). This method of fetal assessment has many benefits. It is easy to perform, readily available to the woman, and has no associated costs. The patient is instructed to lie on her side and count the number of times that she feels the fetus move. Many variations have been developed, but there are two major methods for performing kick counts:

- The first method is done while the woman lies on her side. She counts and records 10 distinct movements in

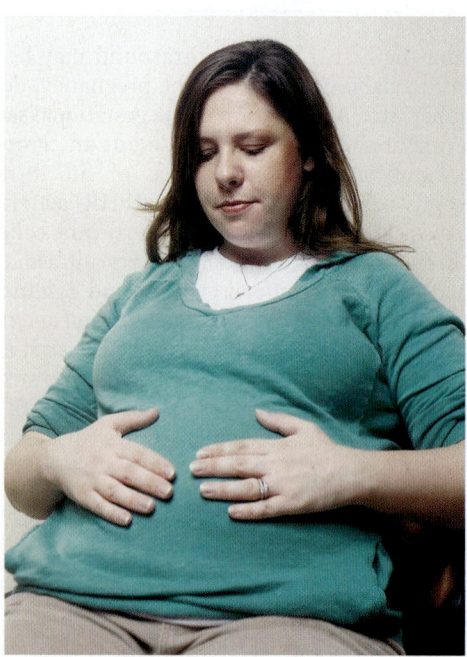

Figure 11-20 Counting fetal movements is easy to perform and constitutes an important method of fetal surveillance.

a period of up to 2 hours. Once 10 movements have been perceived, the count may be discontinued.
- With the second method, the patient counts and records fetal movements for 1 hour three times per week. The count is to be considered reassuring if it equals or exceeds the woman's previously established baseline.

DOPPLER ULTRASOUND BLOOD FLOW STUDIES (VELOCIMETRY)

Doppler ultrasound is used to study blood flow in the umbilical vessels of the fetus, placental circulation, fetal cardiac motion, and maternal uterine circulation. This technology is useful in managing pregnancies at risk because of hypertension, diabetes mellitus, intrauterine growth restriction (IUGR), multiple fetuses, or PTL. A noninvasive Doppler wave measures the velocity of red blood cell movement through the uterine and fetal vessels. Assessment of the blood flow through the uterine vessels is useful in determining vascular resistance in women at risk for developing placental insufficiency. Decreased velocity is associated with poor neonatal outcome (Torgersen, 2011).

FETAL BIOPHYSICAL PROFILE

The fetal **biophysical profile** (BPP) is a noninvasive "fetal physical examination" that is more accurate in predicting fetal well-being than any single assessment. It combines electronic FHR monitoring with ultrasonography to evaluate fetal well-being. The fetus responds to central hypoxia by alterations in movement, muscle tone, breathing, and heart rate patterns. A finding of normal fetal biophysical parameters indicates that the CNS is functional and therefore the fetus is not hypoxemic. The BPP comprises the following five components and is based on a 30-minute time period (Kaimal, 2013):

- Nonstress test (NST)
- Fetal breathing movements (one or more episodes of rhythmic fetal breathing movements for 30 seconds)
- Fetal movement (three or more discrete body or limb movements)
- Fetal tone (one or more episodes of extension of a fetal extremity with return to flexion, or opening or closing of a hand)
- Determination of the amniotic fluid volume

Sonographic methods for determining amniotic fluid volume include subjective assessment, three-dimensional techniques with ultrasonography or MRI, and measurement of amniotic fluid pockets (amniotic fluid index [AFI] and maximal vertical pocket). The widely used AFI is calculated by summing the deepest vertical amniotic fluid pockets in each of four quadrants of the uterus. At term, an AFI less than 5 cm has been used as a common cutoff value to define oligohydramnios; to reduce measurement error, current recommendations call for AFI measurements performed in triplicate and averaged. Hydramnios, which arises from overproduction or under-removal of amniotic fluid, is described sonographically as an AFI of greater than 24 cm or maximal vertical pocket greater than 8 cm (ACOG, 1999b; Moore, 2010).

Each of the five BPP components is assigned a score of 2 (normal or present) or 0 (abnormal). A score of 8 to 10 is reassuring whereas a score of 6 is considered "equivocal," and the test should be repeated within 24 hours in the case of a preterm infant; the term infant should be promptly delivered. When the score is 0 to 4/10, especially in the fetus with IUGR that has reduced amniotic fluid and in whom serial observations have previously been normal, delivery should commence without any delay (ACOG, 1999b; Kaimal, 2013).

⊘ Optimizing Outcomes—The modified fetal biophysical profile

During the late second and throughout the third trimester, amniotic fluid volume is indicative of fetal urine production. Placental dysfunction may result in decreased fetal renal perfusion, leading to oligohydramnios. Hence, amniotic fluid volume assessment can be used to evaluate long-term uteroplacental function. Because of this observation, the "modified biophysical profile" has come to be used as a primary mode of antepartum fetal surveillance. The modified BPP combines the NST as a short-term indicator of fetal acid-base status, with the amniotic fluid index (AFI) as an indicator of long-term placental function. An AFI greater than 5 cm generally is considered to be representative of an adequate volume of amniotic fluid. Thus, the modified BPP is considered normal if the NST is reactive and the AFI is more than 5 and abnormal if either the NST is nonreactive or the AFI is 5 or less (ACOG, 1999b).

NONSTRESS TEST

The nonstress test (NST) is one of the most common methods of antenatal screening. It involves the use of electronic fetal monitoring (EFM) for approximately 20 minutes. The NST is based on the premise that a normal fetus moves at various intervals and that the CNS and myocardium responds to movement. The response is demonstrated by an acceleration of the FHR (the FHR "reacts"). Loss of heart rate reactivity is associated most commonly with a fetal sleep cycle but may result from any cause of CNS depression, including fetal hypoxia, acidosis, and some congenital anomalies (ACOG, 1999b; Kaimal, 2013; Miller, Miller, & Tucker, 2012).

Reactivity is also based on gestational age; 32 to 34 weeks is considered to be the appropriate age for reactivity to occur. Before this gestational age, a very large percentage of fetuses will not meet the acceptable criteria: a FHR acceleration of 15 beats per minute (bpm) that lasts for 15 seconds (ACOG, 1999b). Fetuses less than 32 weeks are more likely not to meet the criteria for a reactive NST. When the preterm fetus is monitored, consideration should be given to the effect of the gestational age on the size of the accelerations: A FHR acceleration of 10 bpm that lasts for 10 seconds is acceptable at 32 weeks. Once a fetus has a reactive tracing, however, it should remain reactive. Nonstress testing is performed once or twice weekly for women with certain risk factors (Box 11-11) (ACOG, 1999b; Cunningham et al., 2014).

To prepare the patient for an NST, the nurse explains the procedure and asks her to void. The patient is then assisted into a semi-Fowler's or lateral tilt position, and the nurse performs Leopold maneuvers to determine fetal position and to guide proper placement of the external fetal heart ultrasound transducer (U/S) and tocodynamometer (toco),

Box 11-11 Selected Indications for Nonstress Testing/Biophysical Profile	
Maternal	**Pregnancy-related**
Hyperthyroidism (poorly controlled)	Intrauterine growth restriction
Trauma/bleeding	Polyhydramnios
Diabetes mellitus (type 1 or type 2)	Oligohydramnios
Chronic renal disease	Multiple gestation
Prior stillbirth or intrauterine fetal demise (IUFD)	Isoimmunization
Hemoglobinopathies (Hgb SS, SC, S-thalassemia) Cyanotic heart disease	Postterm gestation (greater than 42 weeks)
Systemic lupus erythematosus	Decreased fetal movement
Hypertensive disorders	Hypertensive disorders

Sources: ACOG (1999b); Torgersen (2011).

a pressure-sensitive device. Next, the nurse applies the external U/S and toco on the maternal abdomen (Fig. 11-21) and obtains baseline maternal vital signs. The tracing is then observed for evidence of FHR accelerations of at least 15 bpm above the baseline heart rate. During this time, the patient may or may not be aware of fetal movement (ACOG, 1999b; Miller et al., 2012; Torgersen, 2011).

In a term fetus, at least two FHR accelerations sustained for at least 15 seconds (from beginning to end of the acceleration) should occur over a 20-minute time period. If these criteria are met, the test is considered normal or reassuring and is termed a "reactive test." The test may be extended for another 40 minutes if needed. For a preterm fetus, a reactive test is one in which two or more FHR accelerations of at least 10 bpm above the baseline occur; the accelerations must last for more than 10 seconds (from beginning

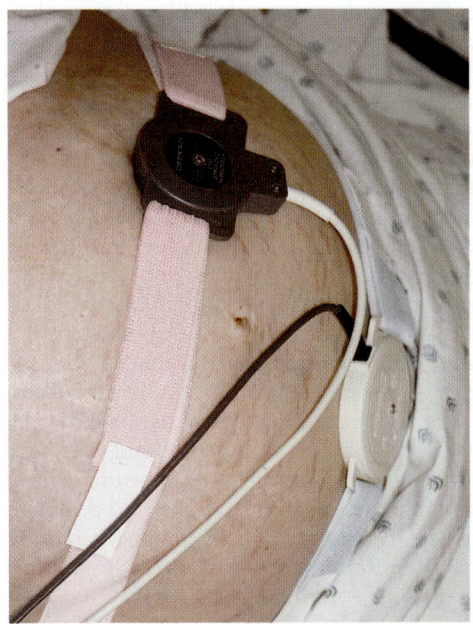

Figure 11-21 Placement of the fetal heart ultrasound transducer and tocodynamometer for a nonstress test.

to end of acceleration) within a 20-minute period. Testing time may be increased to 60 to 90 minutes. For fetuses over 30 weeks of gestation, an FHR greater than 160 bpm is considered tachycardia. FHR accelerations that occur as a result of acoustic stimulation (see discussion below) are considered reassuring (ACOG, 1999b; Miller et al., 2012; Torgersen, 2011).

If the reactive criteria are not met (i.e., no FHR accelerations or the accelerations do not reach 15 bpm or do not last for 15 seconds) over a 40-minute period in a term fetus or over a 90-minute period in a preterm fetus (no FHR accelerations or the accelerations do not reach 10 bpm or do not last for 10 seconds), the test is considered to be "nonreactive." Depending on the fetal age, a nonreactive NST result should be followed by a contraction stress test or a BPP. An "unsatisfactory" NST result occurs if there is inadequate fetal activity or if the data cannot be interpreted (ACOG, 1999b; Miller et al., 2012; Torgersen, 2011).

ACOUSTIC STIMULATION/VIBROACOUSTIC STIMULATION

Acoustic (sound) **stimulation** and **vibroacoustic** (vibration and sound) **stimulation** may be used as an adjunct to the NST to elicit an acceleration of the FHR. A handheld instrument such as an artificial larynx (especially designed for this purpose) is positioned on the maternal abdomen near the fetal head (Leopold maneuvers are performed to determine location), and a low-frequency vibration and a buzzing sound are emitted. The stimulus is applied for 1 to 2 seconds in an attempt to awaken the fetus and may be repeated up to three times with a 1-minute rest period between attempts. Once a fetal response (i.e., FHR accelerations) is achieved, additional stimuli are not required. A fetus that shows no response to the applied stimulus may be neurologically compromised or acidotic and requires further evaluation (ACOG, 1999b; Torgersen, 2011).

CONTRACTION STRESS TEST

The **contraction stress test (CST)** evaluates the FHR response to uterine contractions. The CST is based on the premise that fetal oxygenation that is only marginally adequate with the uterus at rest is transiently worsened by uterine contractions. The nurse uses the electronic fetal monitor to obtain a baseline FHR tracing for 20 minutes. If spontaneous uterine contractions do not occur during this time, uterine stimulation is produced through IV oxytocin infusion (beginning with 0.5 milliunits/min and increasing the dose by 0.5 milliunits/min at 15- to 30-minute intervals) or patient nipple self-stimulation until three contractions of at least 40 seconds' duration occur within a 10-minute time frame. CSTs are evaluated according to the presence or absence of late FHR decelerations. A late deceleration, associated with fetal hypoxia, is one that begins at the peak of the contraction and persists after the conclusion of the contraction. Episodic patterns (i.e., accelerations, variable decelerations, and prolonged decelerations) are FHR patterns that do not have a direct relation to uterine contractions (ACOG, 1999b; Kaimal, 2013; Torgersen, 2011) (see Chapter 12).

The test is considered negative (normal) if there is no evidence of late or significant variable decelerations. A positive CST (abnormal) is one in which there are late decelerations

with 50% of contractions, even if the frequency is less than three in 10 minutes. An equivocal/suspicious result indicates the presence of either intermittent late decelerations or significant (severe) variable decelerations. An equivocal/hyperstimulatory result indicates the presence of one of the following: late decelerations occurring with uterine contractions that are more frequent than 5 contractions in 10 minutes, late decelerations occurring with uterine contractions that are more frequent than every 2 minutes, or late decelerations occurring with uterine contractions lasting longer than 90 seconds. An unsatisfactory or equivocal/unsatisfactory result occurs when there are fewer than 3 uterine contractions within a 10-minute period or when a poor quality FHR data tracing occurs that is perceived as uninterpretable or indeterminate (ACOG, 1999b; Kaimal, 2013; Torgersen, 2011).

Because the CST is based on the presence of uterine contractions, there are several contraindications to the test. Patients who have experienced third trimester bleeding from placenta previa or marginal abruptio placentae, women who have had extensive uterine surgery (including classical cesarean section), those at high risk for PTL, and those with PROM are not candidates for a CST (ACOG, 1999b; Torgersen, 2011).

> **"What to say"**—*Patient teaching to facilitate nipple stimulation*
>
> Nipple stimulation is often successful in inducing an adequate contraction pattern for the CST, and allows completion of the testing in a faster, noninvasive manner than when oxytocin is given. Nipple stimulation occurs in four cycles of 2 minutes on and 2 to 5 minutes off. To facilitate nipple stimulation, the nurse first applies warm packs to the breasts for approximately 10 minutes to enhance comfort and circulation and then provides the following instructions (Torgersen, 2011):
>
> - You may perform nipple stimulation through your clothing or skin-to-skin (if skin to skin, provide a drape and apply mineral oil to the patient's fingers to facilitate the stimulation).
> - Brush your palm across one nipple or roll the nipple using the palmar surface of your index finger and your thumb.
> - Stimulate the nipple until contractions begin or 2 minutes have passed.
> - If a uterine contraction occurs during the stimulation, stop the stimulation; you will restart the stimulation after the contraction ends.
> - If no contractions have occurred after 4 cycles, you will rest for 5 to 10 minutes and then begin bilateral (or alternating nipples) continuous stimulation for 5 to 10 minutes. Stop when a contraction begins; restart the stimulation when the contraction ends.

ELECTRONIC FETAL HEART RATE MONITORING

Electronic fetal heart rate monitoring (EFM) uses electronic techniques to give an ongoing assessment of fetal well-being. EFM provides information related to the response of the fetal heart rate in the presence or absence of uterine contractions. Electronic monitoring of the fetal heart rate can be accomplished by either external or internal means. EFM is discussed in greater detail in Chapter 12.

 Now Can You—Discuss methods of antepartum fetal surveillance?

1. Differentiate among chorionic villus sampling, percutaneous umbilical sampling, and amniocentesis?
2. Identify two methods for conducting kick counts?
3. List the fetal parameters assessed in a BPP?
4. Discuss how the NST is performed and describe what is meant by a "reactive" and a "nonreactive" test result?

Special Conditions and Circumstances That May Complicate Pregnancy

THE PREGNANT WOMAN WHO REQUIRES BEDREST

The patient whose antenatal course is compromised by medical or obstetric complications that require bedrest faces even more challenges. Maloni (2002, 2010) has written extensively about the deleterious effects of bedrest on body systems and addresses problems such as muscle wasting, bone loss, failure to gain weight, and cardiovascular and psychological difficulties. Lack of weight bearing and inactivity make muscles weak. Dizziness, difficulty regulating blood pressure, and fainting are common symptoms in the patient confined to bedrest.

 Optimizing Outcomes—Identifying emotional needs in the pregnant patient on bedrest

Nurses have a professional responsibility to assess the mental well-being of their patients. This is especially important with the hospitalized pregnant woman who is confined to bedrest, because her emotional health will have a profound effect on the pregnancy and family dynamics throughout the childbearing year. To facilitate the emotional assessment, a tool such as the Abbreviated Scale for the Assessment of Psychosocial Status in Pregnancy can be used upon admission; rescreening (and appropriate interventions) can occur as needed (Doyle, 2011).

In most situations, regular home visitation by a community health nurse is an important component of care (Fig. 11-22). The nurse caring for the patient with a high-risk pregnancy needs to remain cognizant of the fact that, depending on the circumstances, the woman's libido is often unaffected and she and her partner will need guidance regarding "safe" practices that promote intimacy without threatening the pregnancy. Also, as the pregnancy progresses, the woman on bedrest is presented with the same maternal tasks (Rubin, 1976) as any other woman who is approaching motherhood. The woman's physical condition may cause difficulty in mastering the tasks. For example, Rubin observed that a pregnant woman is drawn to the company of other pregnant women, not only for acceptance

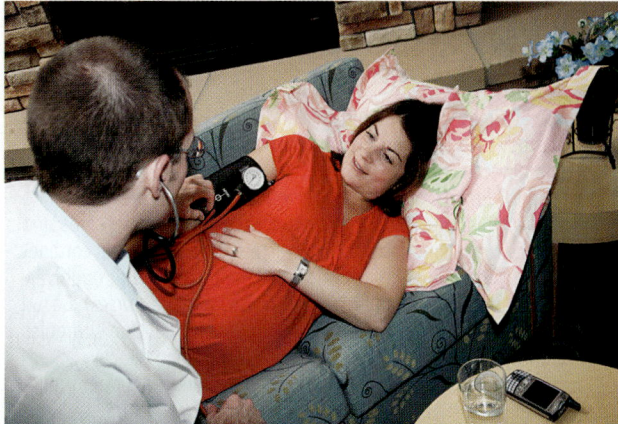

Figure 11-22 Visiting patients confined to bedrest at home is an important nursing intervention.

but also to promote a greater understanding of interpersonal behavior during this special stage of her life. These normal feelings and activities can be jeopardized by hospitalization and the woman's subsequent removal from the comforting patterns and rhythm of day-to-day life. Hospitalization, especially when prolonged, can create many additional problems, because hospitalized patients often suffer from loneliness, boredom, powerlessness, anxiety, anger, and depression (Bauer, Victorson, Rosenbloom, Barocas, & Silver, 2010).

Maloni, Brezinski-Tomasi, and Johnson (2001) reported that women confined to bedrest felt like prisoners and often experienced guilt over the extra responsibilities foisted on their partners. In addition, child care, with the necessary involvement of multiple providers and the disruption of usual routines, was viewed as a major concern. Financial strain and its impact on family well-being was also an issue. Referral to social services and other community resources may be helpful in assisting the couple with financial matters and other aspects of home care.

Nursing interventions that can be instituted to help the family adjust to the stress of a complicated pregnancy include the involvement of high-risk pregnancy or other specialty support groups, professional counseling when appropriate, and religious support when desired. The educational needs of the pregnant woman who is experiencing a high-risk pregnancy are essentially the same as those of any childbearing woman. Whenever possible, nurses should encourage their patients to participate in prenatal classes, seek lactation counseling, learn about infant care, and attend self-care classes. The nurse may arrange for the couple to attend childbirth education classes in either a group or private setting. For most, participating in a group promotes a feeling of normalcy. Family members, particularly the woman's partner, should be included, because they can share infant care responsibilities and provide emotional support.

"Sidelines," a national support group, provides resources such as a helpful bedside checklist that describes a variety of activities for women confined to bedrest. This organization may be contacted at www.sidelines.org.

The recognition that high-risk couples may have depleted their coping skills as a result of perinatal complications

Where Research and Practice Meet:
Enhancing the Experience of Antepartum Bedrest

Nurse researcher Rubarth and colleagues (2012) conducted a qualitative study to explore the lived experience of 11 high-risk hospitalized pregnant women on bedrest. Three major themes were identified: "the war within" (internal conflicts and emotions faced each day), "fighting each battle" (struggles such as endurance of the physical signs and symptoms of the pregnancy, activity restriction, and hospital confinement), and "bringing in reinforcements" (help provided through various supports, such as family, friends, physicians, and nurses). Based on their findings, the authors suggest that nurses develop strategies (e.g., allowing the patient to make choices concerning the daily schedule, providing liberal and open visiting hours, and celebrating milestones and the passage of time) to help empower women whose situations often offer little control.

Box 11-12 **Examples of Nursing Diagnoses for Selected Complications of Pregnancy**

- Risk for injury, maternal or fetal related to inadequate prenatal care and screening
- Fear related to uncertain outcome of the pregnancy
- Risk for deficient fluid volume related to bleeding during pregnancy
- Risk for infection related to preterm rupture of the membranes
- Risk for injury to fetus related to uteroplacental insufficiency
- Ineffective tissue perfusion related to hypertension
- Risk for injury to self and fetus related to chronic substance abuse
- Interrupted family processes related to adolescent pregnancy
- Deficient diversional activity related to imposed bedrest

---

constitutes an important nursing issue, especially during the intrapartal period. The nurse needs to be aware that the anxiety and stress of labor may be extremely difficult for the couple. The nurse can assist and empower the patient and her partner by encouraging them to express their emotional concerns, keeping them informed of changes in the woman's condition, and encouraging them to ask questions.

Depending on the circumstances, the postpartum period may be very difficult as well because of physical and emotional exhaustion, especially if antenatal hospitalization was required. Adverse symptoms associated with weeks of bedrest are often not resolved by 6 weeks postpartum (Maloni & Park, 2005). The woman may not be able to care for her infant as she would like, and this situation can quickly lead to feelings of helplessness, frustration, and disappointment. The nurse needs to remain supportive, conduct an ongoing assessment of the family's coping skills, monitor the extent of maternal–infant attachment, and engage the appropriate hospital and community resources.

Now Can You—Discuss care for the patient on antenatal bedrest?

1. State six complications of antenatal bedrest?
2. Formulate a plan of care to meet the physiological, psychological, and social needs of the pregnant patient on bedrest?
3. Identify team members to be included in your plan of care when caring for the pregnant patient on bedrest?
4. Describe how antenatal bedrest can affect the patient after childbirth (postpartum)?

THE ADOLESCENT PREGNANT PATIENT

Although teen pregnancies have been decreasing steadily during the past decade, the United States still has the highest teen pregnancy rate among all developed countries (CDC, 2014). With early and thorough prenatal care, adolescents older than age 15 years experience no greater risks than those of the general pregnant population. Although the incidence of certain complications may be higher because of age extremes, the nursing diagnoses, interventions, and evaluations remain relatively unchanged from those for the general pregnant population with the same complications (Von Kohler, 2011).

Examples of nursing diagnoses for several complications of pregnancy are presented in Box 11-12.

Prenatal medical and behavioral risk factors can severely complicate adolescent pregnancy and result in poor birth outcomes, particularly when late or inadequate prenatal care occurs. Prenatal medical and behavioral risks for the adolescent population include (Barry, 2011; Porter & Holness, 2011):

- PTL and birth—especially when combined with low socioeconomic status, single parent, smoker, illicit drug use, prepregnant weight less than 100 lb (45.5 kg), poor weight gain during pregnancy, and inadequate prenatal care
- Anemia
- Preeclampsia/eclampsia
- Repeated exposure to sexually transmitted infections
- Chronic or asymptomatic urinary tract infections
- Acute pyelonephritis
- IUGR/low birth weight infants (less than 2,500 g)
- Social issues: poverty, unmarried status, low educational levels, smoking, and drug use

The nurse's need for good communication skills when working with adolescents cannot be overstated, because these young women often lack trust in medical personnel and fear that their behaviors might be judged. Without good communication, the nurse is unable to make an accurate assessment of the adolescent's knowledge about the importance of quality, consistent prenatal care. Without good communication, the professional nurse–patient relationship is neither established nor developed, and the prenatal plan of care is jeopardized (Broussard & Broussard, 2010; Katz, 2011).

THE ADVANCED AGE PREGNANT PATIENT

Many women are now choosing to delay childbirth until later years. The implementation of infertility technology has broadened the boundaries of the reproductive age. Both socioeconomic circumstances and the nature of the older mother have changed with time. The older maternity patient today is at significantly lower risk than her contemporary of two decades ago, who tended to be the mother of many children, having commenced childbearing many years earlier. However, the nurse must be aware of special considerations such as an increased likelihood of chronic diseases (e.g., diabetes and hypertension) when planning care for the woman who has become pregnant after the age of 35 years (see Chapter 9 for further discussion).

 Nursing Insight—*Recognizing potential problems associated with mature mothers*

Pregnant women older than age 35 are more likely to experience obstetric complications such as placenta previa, abruptio placentae, prolonged labor, cesarean birth, and mortality. The fetus is at a greater risk for low birth weight, macrosomia, chromosomal abnormalities, congenital malformations, and neonatal mortality.

THE PREGNANT PATIENT WHO HAS SUFFERED TRAUMA

Trauma is the fourth leading cause of death worldwide and the leading nonobstetric cause of maternal death during pregnancy. Motor vehicle accidents account for more than one-half of maternal trauma incidents. About 50% of fetal deaths result from maternal trauma, and most of these result from motor vehicle accidents (Poole & Thompson, 2013; Robbins, Martin, & Wilson, 2013). Blunt trauma is caused by the following conditions (Van Otterloo, 2011b):

- Motor vehicle collisions in which force is applied to the abdomen from direct impact or as a result of secondary injury from abdominal organs. Abruption of the placenta and/or PTL may result from the trauma.
- Accidental falls are usually more common in the third trimester as the woman's center of gravity becomes increasingly displaced.
- Assaults involving intimate partner violence (the incidence increases during pregnancy) and gunshot and stabbing wounds.

 Optimizing Outcomes—**Considerations when caring for the obstetric trauma patient**

Maternal stabilization is the initial goal in resuscitation. Resuscitation during pregnancy proceeds as with any other trauma. Trauma in pregnancy involves at least two patients (more in the case of multiple gestation). Minor injuries in the woman may cause significant or fatal injury to the fetus. Maternal outcome in trauma corresponds to the injury; fetal outcome depends on the injury and the maternal physiological response. The fetal heart rate is often the first vital sign to change. All pregnant trauma patients need continuous fetal monitoring. Risk factors predictive of fetal death include ejection during an automobile crash (preventable with proper seat belt use), motorcycle and pedestrian collisions, abnormal heart fetal heart rate patterns, maternal tachycardia, and maternal death (Robbins et al., 2013; Van Otterloo, 2011b).

 legal alert—**Take care with documentation**

Document your nursing care by writing accurate and factual notes. Make certain you have described your assessment, plan of care, interventions, and evaluation for your plan of care. Frequently, trauma cases involve litigation. Well-documented records protect both the patient and the health-care system.

SURGERY DURING PREGNANCY

Surgery for nonobstetric reasons occurs in about 1% to 2% of pregnant women. This figure is most likely an underestimated number, because many women may not know that they are pregnant at the time of surgery (Callahan, 2011).

Maternal and Fetal Risks During Surgery

Anesthetic considerations are of prime importance when surgery becomes necessary during pregnancy. General anesthesia is a more complex issue during pregnancy because of the increase in maternal blood volume and cardiac output. Surgery risks are related to the possibility of increased maternal morbidity associated with pregnancy-induced changes in the cardiovascular, respiratory, hematological, and gastrointestinal systems. Normal physiological changes that occur during pregnancy can adversely affect the use of anesthesia and the safety of the surgical procedure. Surgery carries a possibility of increased fetal risks because of an intraoperative decrease in uteroplacental blood flow (leading to fetal hypoxia), along with possible teratogenic effects from the anesthetic agents. The risk of spontaneous abortion (SAB) associated with maternal surgery is approximately 8% during the first trimester and 6.9% in the second trimester. Extra-abdominal surgery is less likely to be complicated by SAB (Callahan, 2011).

CANCER DURING PREGNANCY

The incidence of cancer is low during the childbearing years. During pregnancy, the incidence of cancer is similar to that of nonpregnant women of childbearing age. Cancer complicates 1 out of 1,000 pregnancies and accounts for 5% of deaths that occur during pregnancy. Because more women today choose to delay childbearing, the co-occurrence of pregnancy and cancer may increase. The prognosis best correlates with the anatomical extent of the disease at the time of diagnosis. Cancer in the pregnant woman does not appear to metastasize to the fetus because of the placenta's effectiveness as a barrier against spread and also because the fetus may be capable of resisting the invasion of malignant cells (Cunningham et al., 2014).

During pregnancy the diagnosis of cancer can be difficult for the following reasons: Many of the presenting symptoms of cancer are often attributed to the pregnancy; many of the physiological and anatomical alterations of pregnancy can compromise the physical examination; many serum tumor markers (e.g., β-hCG, *a*-fetoprotein, and CA 125) are normally increased during pregnancy; and the ability to perform either imaging studies or invasive diagnostic procedures is often altered (Gabbe, Niebyl, Galan, Jauniaux, Landon, Simpson, et al., 2012b).

Care of the pregnant patient with cancer is related to a number of factors:

- Gestational age of the pregnancy
- Stage of the cancer and the associated prognosis
- Potential for the cancer treatment to have adverse effects on the fetus, including the potential for long-term occult problems

- Risk to the patient of delaying therapy to permit fetal viability
- Risk to the fetus of early delivery to allow more timely cancer therapy, and the possible need to terminate an early pregnancy to allow an optimal opportunity to treat the patient and cure the malignancy

It is important to recognize that women who receive a diagnosis of cancer during pregnancy are extremely vulnerable. Nurses who care for them should encourage an open dialogue that provides current, evidence-based information, offers support, and encourages expression of concerns and feelings. Other aspects of holistic care include identifying positive social support systems, making referrals when appropriate, and carefully monitoring for indicators of depression throughout the childbearing year (Harrison, 2013).

OBESITY

Obesity has reached epidemic proportions in the United States, and nearly two-thirds of reproductive-aged women are currently overweight or obese (Flegal, Carroll, Ogden, & Curtin, 2010). In pregnancy, obesity is associated with a higher incidence of antepartum complications, such as diabetes and hypertension, and with peripartum complications, including fetal macrosomia, very low birthweight, prolonged labor, shoulder dystocia, higher cesarean birth rates, and increased postpartum infection. Cesarean delivery is often complicated by excessive operative blood loss (greater than 1,000 mL), difficult anesthesia intubations, and operative times greater than 2 hours duration. Postoperative wound complications, including infection, delayed healing, operative injury, the need for blood transfusions, thromboembolism, and hysterectomy are also increased in obese women, resulting in prolonged hospitalization and increased costs (ACOG, 2013g).

 Nursing Insight—*Differentiating between "overweight" and "obese"*

A pregnant woman is considered *overweight* if she is 20% above ideal weight or has a BMI of 25 to 29.9; she is considered *obese* if her weight exceeds 200 lb (91 kg), if she is 50% over ideal body weight for height, or if her BMI is above 30.

Dieting for weight loss during pregnancy is not recommended because if carbohydrates are restricted too much, the body will burn fat and protein for energy. This can result in inadequate protein available for the fetus and lead to ketoacidosis. Dietary counseling should focus on reduced carbohydrates (daily caloric intake should not go below 1,500 to 1,800 calories per day), education to recognize nutritious food choices, and the value of daily exercise. During the postpartum period, the woman should receive continued nutritional counseling and support with realistic goals for weight loss.

 legal alert—**Voice concerns about difficulties with FHR monitoring**

As a nurse using electronic fetal monitoring, you must be able to obtain an FHR strip that can be interpreted. Monitoring the obese patient can be very challenging. If you are having difficulty monitoring the fetal heart rate and/or uterine contractions, bring your concerns to the physician or midwife. In the event of a malpractice claim, the fetal monitoring strips can be used as evidence as to whether the standard of care was met.

Obese patients often suffer from low self-esteem and are embarrassed by their size. Health-care providers must always strive to preserve the patient's dignity and treat her with respect. Remarks should never be made as to the need for a bigger bed or blood pressure cuff. Requesting that extra personnel be available in the labor room to aid with a fetal shoulder dystocia or to help the patient to get out of bed postpartum should be made discreetly.

THE PATIENT WITH A DISABILITY

The pregnant woman with a disability often faces two major concerns: her ability to maintain her own health and her fetus' health throughout pregnancy, childbirth, and during the postpartum period. In addition, she may fear being unable to physically care for her baby. The first concern, universally shared by all mothers, has added significance for the woman with a disability because of the possible interactions between the pregnancy and her disability. The disabled woman's experience of pregnancy, birth, and postpartum is shaped by what she brings to this period of transition and her prior experiences with the health-care system. The woman's specific disability, her resources, and her unique approach to pregnancy and birth are all factors that help shape her overall childbearing experience (Signore, Spong, Krotoski, Shinowara, & Blackwell, 2011).

While pregnancy and childbirth can be very challenging for the woman with a disability, it provides the nurse with a wonderful opportunity to help make this event a special, memorable time in her life. Care must be well planned and individualized because many women with disabilities face unpredictability in their symptoms and in their day-to-day abilities. The nurse can develop a well-organized plan of care by ensuring that there is documentation of the patient's specific needs, concerns, and desires for her labor and birth and that this information is readily available to all appropriate personnel.

Early in the pregnancy, a referral to the clinical nurse specialist or nurse manager on the birth unit allows the care plan and specific needs to be noted and prepared. Special equipment (e.g., mattress and commode) may need to be ordered, and if there are mobility issues, a notation made that this patient will need assignment to a handicap accessible room. Staff nurses may also need to be educated about how to appropriately care for the patient. Advance notice may facilitate development of a nursing schedule that allows the same team to provide continuity of care throughout the woman's hospital stay. Other members of the health team (e.g., physical therapist, occupational therapist, lactation consultant, and visiting nurse) should also be involved in the plan of care and kept aware of the patient's needs. If the patient has a service dog, all staff should be aware that it is permissible for the dog to be in the hospital. Furthermore, the staff should understand that the dog provides an important service for the patient and is "working" and should not be played with. While the woman and her dog are in the hospital, a family member should assume responsibility for the dog's needs. Many special devices are available to assist new mothers who have hearing or mobility impairments, and adaptive equipment for infant care helps to facilitate independent parenting by women with disabilities.

INTIMATE PARTNER VIOLENCE DURING PREGNANCY

Intimate partner violence (IPV), family violence, battering, and spousal abuse are all terms used to describe a pattern of assaultive and coercive behaviors. The true incidence of IPV perpetuated against women in the United States is unknown because much of it remains undetected and unreported. However, it is estimated that battered women account for up to 35% of all women seeking care in an emergency room. Pregnancy is often the trigger for the beginning or escalation of violence in a relationship, and many chronically abused women report an increase in violence directed at them during pregnancy. There are many theories to account for this behavior. For example, the stress of pregnancy may strain a troubled relationship beyond normal coping abilities. The abuser may harbor jealousy against the fetus. Physical violence may be an attempt to end the pregnancy, and frequently, the battered pregnant woman is unlikely to have a strong social support network on which she can rely (Fontenot & Fantasia, 2011; Records, 2011). Studies within the past two decades have shown that maternal homicide is a leading cause of pregnancy-associated death (i.e., a death from any cause occurring during pregnancy or within 1 year of pregnancy delivery or pregnancy termination) (Cheng & Horon, 2010).

Characteristically, the abuser targets different maternal body parts during pregnancy. Pregnant women are likely to have more multiple injury sites than nonpregnant women, and the abuse is often directed to the breasts, genitalia, and abdomen. The risk of injury to the fetus is very high because of the chance of placental injury that can result in an abruption.

Pregnant teenagers are particularly vulnerable because of their need to rely on others for the basics of life. Often those whom they rely on are their abusers. Incest, rape, child abuse, gang (group) fighting, stalking, and IPV from both male and female partners have been described. Nurses can help teenagers with violence only if they know that the teenagers are experiencing it. Thus, nurses need to be able to gain their young patients' trust and confidence so that they feel comfortable sharing their problems. Assessment, safety planning, documentation, and follow-up are all essential components of providing care for women who are experiencing violence, no matter what their age. The medical record is often the source of information that can raise suspicions of abuse, and a number of assessment forms specifically designed to elicit information regarding patterns of abuse have been developed (see Chapter 9 for further discussion).

Now Can You—Discuss abuse during pregnancy?

1. Explain why pregnancy is often the trigger for the beginning or escalation of intimate partner violence?

2. Describe the body areas that are usually targeted during pregnancy?

3. Discuss your nursing plan of care when you suspect that your patient has been abused?

Summary Points

◆ Complications that arise during pregnancy are often challenging and demand the perinatal nurse's skills, knowledge, and expertise, combined with the nursing process, to first identify the pregnant patient at risk and then formulate, implement, and evaluate an appropriate, holistic plan of care.

◆ Anticipatory nursing care is invaluable in preventing a complication from becoming a major health crisis.

◆ Alterations of signs and symptoms from the expected clinical progression during pregnancy must be immediately conveyed to the primary health-care provider so that an appropriate management plan may be activated.

◆ The nurse must always remain cognizant of the important role the patient's family, culture, language, and religious beliefs play in her adjustment to motherhood and overall well-being.

◆ By providing culturally competent care to childbearing families, many potential complications can be identified in a timely manner to allow for effective treatment and improved outcomes.

◆ Meticulous documentation of the patient's plan of care and response to the plan of care cannot be overemphasized.

Review Questions

Multiple Choice

1. A woman and her partner have experienced a miscarriage at 11 weeks' gestation. They desire information about miscarriages. The nurse explains that the most common cause of miscarriage is
   A. nausea and vomiting in early pregnancy.
   B. prenatal stress.
   C. chromosomal abnormalities.
   D. umbilical cord accidents.

2. The perinatal nurse uses the acronym "SPASMS" to teach a new nurse about preeclampsia. What does the "P" refer to?
   A. Pregnancy
   B. Proteinuria
   C. Pelvic circulation
   D. Pressure

3. A woman is making an appointment in the perinatal clinic after suffering a spontaneous abortion. The nurse schedules extra time for this patient because it is critical to provide what nursing action at this time?
   A. Time to listen to her grief
   B. Information about risk factors
   C. A referral to a high-risk obstetrician
   D. Appropriate contraceptive information

4. A nurse is reviewing a patient's chart and notes that she has a history of "TORCH infection—T." What infection has this woman had?

A. Toxoplasmosis

B. Trigeminal neuralgia

C. Tricuspid insufficiency secondary to rheumatic fever

D. Tetanus

5. A nurse is teaching a woman who is considering pregnancy in the near future. The woman lives with her husband who smokes; she drinks 2 glasses of wine a day and has both cats and dogs in the house. What action should the nurse suggest to prevent acquiring a TORCH infection?

A. Ask the husband to smoke only outside.

B. Stop drinking and avoid secondhand smoke.

C. Avoid changing the kitty litter.

D. Avoid blood and body fluids of other people.

6. A woman is discussing becoming pregnant at the age of 42. What important information should the nurse provide to this woman?

A. Women older than 35 are more likely to experience obstetric complications.

B. Women older than 40 have SABs at four times the normal rate.

C. Women do not have more pregnancy-related problems until they reach their 50s.

D. Women older than 40 should not consider having a vaginal birth.

7. A patient is scheduled to have a salpingostomy to treat an ectopic pregnancy. What information should the nurse teach this patient?

A. The operation will prevent any further ectopic pregnancies.

B. It is an incision into the fallopian tube to remove the pregnancy.

C. You will have your entire fallopian tube removed in this procedure.

D. This operation has a high risk of causing infertility.

8. A nurse notes that a pregnant patient has 3+ reflexes noted on her chart. How would the nurse describe this finding to a nursing student?

A. Average or normal

B. Presence of clonus

C. Brisker than average

D. No response

9. A woman presents to the OB unit in active labor. She has had no prenatal care and tells the nurse that the baby's father has gonorrhea. She has not been treated. For what complication is the newborn at most risk?

A. Pneumonia

B. Skin lesions

C. Blindness

D. Intellectual disability

10. A woman with systemic lupus erythematosus (SLE) is being seen for her first prenatal visit. What information about SLE should the nurse provide to this patient?

A. Cardiac problems in the newborn present the biggest concern.

B. Labor and delivery will most likely exacerbate your disease.

C. If the disease flares during pregnancy, elective abortion is needed.

D. Medications for SLE are all contraindicated in pregnancy.

See Answers to End of Chapter Review Questions on Davis*Plus*.

REFERENCES

Abel, D. E. (2011a). Thyroid disease during pregnancy. Part 2: Hyperthyroidism. *The Female Patient, 36*(2), 23–28.

Abel, D. E. (2011b). Thyroid disease during pregnancy. Part 1: Thyroid function testing and hypothyroidism. *The Female Patient, 36*(1), 16–22.

Abel, D. E. (2013). SSRIs in pregnancy: Weighing benefits and risks. *Contemporary OB/GYN, 58*(8), 46–54.

Alfonso, H. (2009). Preventing preeclampsia: The evidence of nutrients. *Nursing for Women's Health, 13*(5), 419–421.

Alfonso, B., Liao, E., Busta, A., & Poretsky, L. (2009). Vitamin D in diabetes mellitus – a new field of knowledge poised for Development. *Diabetes/Metabolism Research Review, 25*, 417–419. doi:10.1002/dmrr.927

Allen, C. M., & Founds, S. A. (2013). Genetics and preterm birth. *Journal of Obstetric, Gynecologic & Neonatal Nursing, 42*(6), 730–736. doi:10.1111/1552-6909.12246

Al Safi, Z., Imudia, A., Filetti, L., Hobson, D., Bahado-Singh, R., & Awonuga, A. (2011). Delayed postpartum preeclampsia and eclampsia: Demographics, clinical course, and complications. *Obstetrics & Gynecology, 118*(5), 1102–1107. doi:10.1097/AOG.0b013e318231934c

American College of Obstetricians and Gynecologists (ACOG). (1999a). *Prevention of Rh D Alloimmunization*. Practice Bulletin No. 4. (Reaffirmed 2010). Washington, DC: Author.

American College of Obstetricians and Gynecologists (ACOG). (1999b). *Antepartum fetal surveillance*. Practice Bulletin No. 9. (Reaffirmed 2012). Washington, DC: Author.

American College of Obstetricians and Gynecologists (ACOG). (2000a). *Perinatal viral and parasitic infections*. Practice Bulletin No. 20. (Reaffirmed 2011). Washington DC: Author.

American College of Obstetricians and Gynecologists (ACOG). (2000b). Scheduled cesarean delivery and the prevention of vertical transmission of HIV infection. Committee Opinion No. 234. (Reaffirmed 2010). Washington, DC: Author.

American College of Obstetricians and Gynecologists (ACOG). (2001). Assessment of risk factors for preterm birth. Practice Bulletin No. 31. (Reaffirmed 2010). *Obstetrics & Gynecology, 98*(10), 709-716.

American College of Obstetricians and Gynecologists (ACOG). (2002a). Diagnosis and management of preeclampsia and eclampsia. Practice Bulletin No. 33. (Reaffirmed 2010). *Obstetrics & Gynecology, 99*(1), 159–167.

American College of Obstetricians and Gynecologists (ACOG). (2002b). Prenatal care at the threshold of viability. Practice Bulletin No. 38. (Reaffirmed 2010). *Obstetrics & Gynecology, 100*(9), 617–624.

American College of Obstetricians and Gynecologists (ACOG). (2004a). Diagnosis and treatment of gestational trophoblastic disease. Practice Bulletin No. 53. (Reaffirmed 2012). *Obstetrics & Gynecology, 103*(6), 1365–1377.

American College of Obstetricians and Gynecologists (ACOG). (2004b). Nausea and vomiting of pregnancy. Practice Bulletin No. 58. (Reaffirmed 2013). *Obstetrics & Gynecology, 103*(4), 803–815.

American College of Obstetricians and Gynecologists (ACOG). (2004c). Multiple gestation: complicated twin, triplet, and high-order multifetal pregnancy. Practice Bulletin No. 56. (Reaffirmed 2010). *Obstetrics & Gynecology, 104*(10), 869–883.

American College of Obstetricians and Gynecologists (ACOG). (2004d). Nonmedical use of ultrasonography. Committee Opinion No. 297. (Reaffirmed 2012). *Obstetrics & Gynecology, 104*(2), 423–424.

American College of Obstetricians and Gynecologists (ACOG). (2005). Pregestational diabetes mellitus. Practice Bulletin No. 60 (Reaffirmed 2010). *Obstetrics & Gynecology, 105*(3), 675–685.

American College of Obstetricians and Gynecologists (ACOG). (2007a). Viral hepatitis in pregnancy. Practice Bulletin No. 86. (Reaffirmed 2012). *Obstetrics & Gynecology, 110*(10), 941–955.

American College of Obstetricians and Gynecologists (ACOG). (2007b). Management of herpes in pregnancy. Practice Bulletin No. 82. (Reaffirmed 2012). *Obstetrics & Gynecology, 109*(6), 1233–1248.

American College of Obstetricians and Gynecologists (ACOG). (2007c). Hemoglobinopathies in pregnancy. Practice Bulletin No. 78. (Reaffirmed 2013) *Obstetrics & Gynecology, 109*(1), 229–237.

American College of Obstetricians and Gynecologists (ACOG). (2007d). Use of psychiatric medications during pregnancy and lactation. Practice Bulletin No. 92. (Reaffirmed 2012). *Obstetrics & Gynecology, 111*(4), 1001–1020.

American College of Obstetricians and Gynecologists (ACOG). (2008a). Medical management of ectopic pregnancy. Practice Bulletin No. 84. (Reaffirmed 2010). *Obstetrics & Gynecology, 111*(6), 1479–1485.

American College of Obstetricians and Gynecologists (ACOG). (2008b). Use of progesterone to prevent preterm birth. Committee Opinion No. 419. (Reaffirmed 2011). *Obstetrics & Gynecology, 112*(10), 963–965.

American College of Obstetricians and Gynecologists (ACOG). (2008c). Prenatal and perinatal human immunodeficiency virus testing: Expanded recommendations. Committee Opinion No. 418. (Reaffirmed 2011). *Obstetrics & Gynecology, 112*(9), 739–742.

American College of Obstetricians and Gynecologists (ACOG). (2008d). Asthma in pregnancy. Practice Bulletin No. 90. (Reaffirmed 2012). *Obstetrics & Gynecology, 111*(2), 457–464.

American College of Obstetricians and Gynecologists (ACOG). (2009a). Bariatric surgery and pregnancy. Practice Bulletin No. 105. (Reaffirmed 2013). *Obstetrics & Gynecology, 113*(6), 1405–1413.

American College of Obstetricians and Gynecologists (ACOG). (2009b). Screening for depression during and after pregnancy. Committee Opinion No. 453. (Reaffirmed 2012). *Obstetrics & Gynecology, 115*(4), 394–395.

American College of Obstetricians and Gynecologists (ACOG). (2009c). Ultrasonography in pregnancy. Practice Bulletin No. 101. (Reaffirmed 2011). *Obstetrics and Gynecology, 113*(2), 451–461.

American College of Obstetricians and Gynecologists (ACOG). (2010a). Magnesium sulfate before anticipated preterm birth for neuroprotection. Committee Opinion No. 455. *Obstetrics & Gynecology, 115*(3), 669–671.

American College of Obstetricians and Gynecologists (ACOG). (2010b). Human papillomavirus vaccination. Committee Opinion Number 344. *Obstetrics & Gynecology, 116*(9), 800–803.

American College of Obstetricians and Gynecologists (ACOG). (2010c). Influenza vaccination during pregnancy. Committee Opinion No. 468. *Obstetrics & Gynecology, 116*(10), 1006–1007.

American College of Obstetricians and Gynecologists (ACOG). (2011a). Antenatal corticosteroid therapy for fetal maturation. Committee Opinion No. 475. *Obstetrics & Gynecology, 117*(2), 422–424.

American College of Obstetricians and Gynecologists (ACOG). (2011b). Emergent therapy for acute-onset, severe hypertension with preeclampsia or eclampsia. Committee Opinion No. 514. *Obsteetrics & Gynecology, 118*(6), 1465–1468.

American College of Obstetricians and Gynecologists (ACOG). (2011c). Sulfonamides, nitrofurantoin, and risk of birth defects. Committee Opinion No. 494. *Obstetrics & Gynecology, 117*(6), 1484–1485.

American College of Obstetricians and Gynecologists (ACOG). (2011d). Prevention of early-onset Group B Streptococcal Disease in newborns. Committee Opinion No. 485. *Obstetrics & Gynecology, 117*(4), 1019–1027.

American College of Obstetricians and Gynecologists (ACOG). (2011e). Update on carrier screening for cystic fibrosis. Committee Opinion No. 486. *Obstetrics & Gynecology, 117*(4), 1028–1031.

American College of Obstetricians and Gynecologists (ACOG). (2011f). Thromboembolism in pregnancy. Practice Bulletin No. 123. *Obstetrics & Gynecology, 118*(8), 718–729.

American College of Obstetricians and Gynecologists (ACOG). (2011g). Methamphetamine abuse in women of reproductive age. Committee Opinion No. 479. *Obstetrics & Gynecology, 117*(3), 751–755.

American College of Obstetricians and Gynecologists (ACOG). (2012a). Placenta accreta. Committee Opinion No. 529. *Obstetrics & Gynecology, 120*(7), 207–211.

American College of Obstetricians and Gynecologists (ACOG). (2012b). Incidentally detected short cervical length. Committee Opinion No. 522. *Obstetrics & Gynecology, 119*(4), 879–882.

American College of Obstetricians and Gynecologists (ACOG). (2012c). Prediction and prevention of preterm birth. Practice Bulletin No. 130. *Obstetrics & Gynecology, 120*(10), 964–973.

American College of Obstetricians and Gynecologists (ACOG). (2012d). Management of Preterm Labor. Practice Bulletin No. 127. *Obstetrics & Gynecology, 119*(6), 1308–1317.

American College of Obstetricians and Gynecologists (ACOG). (2012e). Chronic hypertension in pregnancy. Practice Bulletin No. 125. *Obstetrics & Gynecology, 119*(2), 396–408.

American College of Obstetricians and Gynecologists (ACOG). (2012f). Opioid abuse, dependence, and addiction in pregnancy. Committee Opinion No. 524. *Obstetrics & Gynecology, 119*(5), 1070–1076.

American College of Obstetricians and Gynecologists (ACOG). (2013a). Fetal growth restriction. Practice Bulletin No. 134. *Obstetrics & Gynecology, 121*(5), 1122–1133.

American College of Obstetricians and Gynecologists (ACOG). (2013b). Premature rupture of membranes. Practice Bulletin No. 139. *Obstetrics & Gynecology, 12210*), 918–930.

American College of Obstetricians and Gynecologists (ACOG). (2013c). Hypertension in pregnancy: Report of the American College of Obstetricians and Gynecologists' Task Force on Hypertension in Pregnancy. *Obstetrics & Gynecology, 122*(5), 1122–1133.

American College of Obstetricians and Gynecologists (ACOG). (2013d). Update on immunization and pregnancy: Tetanus, diphtheria, and pertussis vaccination. *Obstetrics & Gynecology, 121*(6), 1411–1414.

American College of Obstetricians and Gynecologists. (ACOG). (2013e). Gestational diabetes mellitus. Practice Bulletin No. 137. *Obstetrics & Gynecology, 122*(2), 406–416.

American College of Obstetricians and Gynecologists (ACOG). (2013f). Inherited thrombophilias in pregnancy. Practice Bulletin No. 138. *Obstetrics & Gynecology, 122*(3), 706–717.

American College of Obstetricians and Gynecologists (ACOG). (2013g). Obesity in pregnancy. Committee Opinion No. 549. *Obstetrics & Gynecology, 121*(1), 213–217.

American College of Obstetricians and Gynecologists (ACOG). (2014). Cerclage for the management of cervical insufficiency. Practice Bulletin No. 142. *Obstetrics & Gynecology, 123*(2), 372–379.

American College of Obstetricians and Gynecologists & American Academy of Pediatrics (ACOG/AAP). (2011). Maternal-fetal intervention and fetal care centers. Committee Opinion No. 501. *Obstetrics & Gynecology, 118*(2), 405–410.

American College of Obstetricians and Gynecologists & American Academy of Pediatrics (ACOG/AAP). (2013). *Guidelines for perinatal care* (6th ed.). Washington, DC: Author.

American Diabetes Association. (2009). Prepregnancy counseling and management of women with preexisting diabetes or previous gestational diabetes. In *Medical management of pregnancy complicated by diabetes*. (4th ed., pp. 4–27). Alexandria, VA: ADA.

American Diabetes Association. (2010). Diagnosis and classification of diabetes mellitus. *Diabetes Care, 33*(1), S62–S69. doi:10.2337/dc10-S062

American Diabetes Association. (2013). Standards of medical care in diabetes–2013. *Diabetes Care, 36*(Suppl1):S11–S66. doi:10.2337/dc13-S011

American Institute of Ultrasound in Medicine (AIUM). (2012). Keepsake fetal imaging. Retrieved from http://www.aium.org/officialStatements/31

American Psychiatric Association, (2013). *Diagnostic and statistical manual of mental disorders*. (5th ed.). Arlington, VA: American Psychiatric Publishing.

Anderson, B., & Gonik, B. (2010). Perinatal infections. In R. Martin, A. Fanaroff, & M. Walsh (Eds.). *Fanaroff & Martin's neonatal-perinatal medicine: Diseases of the fetus and infant* (9th ed., pp. 399–422). Philadelphia, PA: C.V. Mosby.

Association of Women's Health, Obstetric and Neonatal Nurses. (2010). *Ultrasound examinations performed by nurses in obstetric, gynecologic, and reproductive medicine settings: Clinical competencies and education guide* (3rd ed.). Washington, DC: Author.

Association of Women's Health, Obstetric and Neonatal Nurses (2011). HIV screening for pregnant women and infants. *Journal of Obstetric, Gynecologic & Neonatal Nursing 41*(6), 88–89. doi:10.1111/j.1552-6909.2011.01325.x

Avni-Barron, O., & Wiegartz, P. S. (2011). Issues in treating anxiety disorders in pregnancy. *Psychiatric Times, 28*(9), 47–51.

Barry, M. (2011). Preconception care at the edges of the reproductive lifespan. *Nursing for Women's Health, 15*(1), 68–74.

Bauer, C. L., Victorson, D., Rosenbloom, S., Barocas, J., & Silver, R. K. (2010). Alleviating distress during antepartum hospitalization: A randomized controlled trial of music and recreation therapy. *Journal of Women's Health, 19*(3), 523–531. doi:10.1089/jwh.2008.1344

Bell, M. J. (2010). A historical overview of preeclampsia-eclampsia. *Journal of Obstetric, Gynecologic & Neonatal Nursing, 39*(5), 510–518. doi:10.1111/j.1552-6909.2010.01172.x

Berghella, V. (2010). Cervical cerclage for the woman with prior adverse pregnancy outcome. *Contemporary OB/GYN, 55*(6), 18–20.

Berghella, V., & Mackeen, A. D. (2011). Cervical length screening with ultrasound-indicated cerclage compared with history-indicated cerclage for prevention of preterm birth: A meta-analysis. *Obstetrics & Gynecology, 118*(1), 148–155. doi:10.1097/AOG.0b013e31821fd5b0

Bowman, Z., & Branch, D. W. (2012). Thromboprophylaxis in pregnancy. *Contemporary OB/GYN, 57*(6), 46–58.

Braithwaite, P., Chichester, M., & Reid, A. (2011). When the pregnant Jehovah's Witness patient refuses blood: Implications for nurses. *Nursing for Women's Health, 4*(6), 464–470. doi:10.1111/j.1751-486X.2010.01593.x

Broussard, A. B., & Broussard, B. S. (2010). Pregnant teens: Lessons learned. *Nursing for Women's Health, 14*(2), 105–111. doi:10.1111/j.1751-486X.2010.01523.x

Callahan, L. (2011). Surgery in pregnancy. In S. Mattson & J. Smith (Eds.), *Core curriculum for maternal-newborn nursing* (4th ed., pp. 556–572). Philadelphia, PA: W.B. Saunders.

Centers for Disease Control and Prevention (CDC). (2010a). Toxoplasmosis (Toxoplasma infection). Retrieved from http://www.cdc.gov/parasites/toxoplasmosis/health_professionals/index.html

Centers for Disease Control and Prevention (CDC). (2010b). Cytomegalovirus (CMV) and congenital CMV infection. Retrieved from http://www.cdc.gov/cmv/congenital-infection.html

Centers for Disease Control and Prevention (CDC). (2010c). Sexually transmitted diseases treatment guidelines 2010. *MMWR Morbidity and Mortality Weekly Report, 59*(RR12), 1–110.

Centers for Disease Control and Prevention (CDC). (2011). *HPV vaccine—questions & answers.* Retrieved from http://www.cdc.gov/vaccines/vpd-vac/hpv/vac-faqs.htm

Centers for Disease Control and Prevention (CDC). (2012). HIV/AIDS Update: A glance at the epidemic. Retrieved from http://www.cdc.gov/hiv/

Centers for Disease Control and Prevention (CDC). (2013). Preterm birth. Retrieved from http://www.cdc.gov/reproductivehealth/maternalinfanthealth/pretermbirth.htm

Centers for Disease Control and Prevention (CDC). (2014). *Teen pregnancy.* Retrieved from http://www.cdc.gov/teenpregnancy/

Cheng, D., & Horon, I. L. (2010). Intimate-partner homicide among pregnant and postpartum women. *Obstetrics & Gynecology, 115*(6), 1181–1186.

Cohn, D., Ramaswamy, B., & Blum, K. (2013). Malignancy and pregnancy. In R. Creasy, R. Resnik, J. Iams, C. Lockwood, T. Moore, & M. Greene, *Creasy & Resnik's maternal-fetal medicine: Principles and practice* (7th ed., pp. 932–948). Philadelphia, PA: W.B. Saunders.

Cooray, S. D., Edmonds, S. M., Tong, S., Samarasekera, S. P., & Whitehead, C. L. (2011). Characterization of symptoms immediately preceding eclampsia. *Obstetrics & Gynecology, 118*(5), 995–999. doi:10.1097/AOG.0b013e3182324570

Criteria Committee of the New York Heart Association. (1994). Nomenclature and criteria for diagnosis of diseases of the heart and great vessels (9th ed.). New York, NY: Little, Brown & Company.

Cunningham, F., Leveno, K., Bloom, S., Spong, C., & Dashe, J. (2014). *Williams obstetrics* (24th ed.). New York, NY: McGraw-Hill Professional.

Cystic Fibrosis Foundation. (2012). What is CF? Retrieved from http://www.cff.org:80/AboutCF/

Dillon, P. M. (2007). *Nursing health assessment* (2nd ed.). Philadelphia, PA: F.A. Davis.

Dix, D. (2011). Hypertensive disorders in pregnancy. In S. Mattson & J. Smith (Eds.), *Core curriculum for maternal-newborn nursing* (4th ed., pp. 432–448). St. Louis, MO: W.B. Saunders.

Doyle, C. S. (2011). When delivery expectations change. *Nursing for Women's Health, 15*(6), 465–469.

Duff, P. (2013). Maternal and fetal infections. In R. Creasy, R. Resnik, J. Iams, C. Lockwood, T. Moore, & M. Greene, *Creasy & Resnik's maternal-fetal medicine: Principles and practice* (7th ed., pp. 802–851). Philadelphia, PA: W.B. Saunders.

Easterling, T., & Otto, C. (2012). Heart disease. In S. Gabbe, J. Niebyl, H. Galan, E. Jauniaux, M. Landon, J. Simpson, & D. Driscoll (Eds.), *Obstetrics: Normal and problem pregnancies* (6th ed., pp. 1081–1116). Philadelphia, PA: W.B. Saunders.

Elkins, D., & Taylor, J. S. (2013). Evidence-based strategies for managing gestational diabetes in women with obesity. *Nursing for Women's Health, 17*(5), 421–430. doi:10.1111/1751-486X.12065

Expert Committee on the Diagnosis and Classification of Diabetes Mellitus. (2007). Report of the expert committee on the diagnosis and classification of diabetes mellitus. *Diabetes Care, 27*(Supplement 5), S5–S20. doi:10.2337/diacare.27.2007.S5

Farrell, J., & Howell, L. J. (2012). An overview of surgical techniques, research trials, and future directions of fetal therapy. *Journal of Obstetric, Gynecologic & Neonatal Nursing, 41*(3), 419–425. doi:10.1111/j.1552-6909.2012.01356.x

Flegal, K. M., Carroll, M. D., Ogden, C. L., & Curtin, L. R. (2010). Prevalence and trends in obesity among U.S. adults, 1999–2008. *Journal of the American Medical Association, 303*(3), 235–241.

Fleming, S. E., & Corbett, C. (2010). Promoting stringent glycemic control before and during pregnancy. *Nursing for Women's Health, 14*(4), 281–288. doi:10.1111/j.1751-486X.2010.01558.x

Foley, M., Rokey, R., & Belfort, M. (2011). Cardiac disease. In G. M. Belfort, G. Saade, M. Foley, J. Phelan, & G. Dildy III (Eds.), *Critical care obstetrics* (5th ed., pp. 256–282). Hoboken, NJ: Wiley-Blackwell.

Fontenot, H. B., & Fantasia, H. C. (2011). Do women in abusive relationships have contraceptive control? *Nursing for Women's Health, 15*(3), 239–243.

Fontenot, H. B., & Fantasia, H. C. (2012). Vaginal progesterone to prevent preterm birth in high-risk women. *Nursing for Women's Health, 16*(3), 237–241. doi:10.1111/j.1751-486X.2012.01735.x

Food and Drug Administration. (FDA). (2008). Avoid fetal "keepsake" images, heartbeat monitors. Retrieved from http://www.fda.gov/downloads/ForConsumers/ConsumerUpdates/ucm095602.pdf

Gabbe, S. G., Landon, M. B., Warren-Boulton, E., & Fradkin, J. (2012a). Promoting health after gestational diabetes. *Obstetrics & Gynecology, 119*(1), 171–176. doi:10.1097/AOG.0b013e3182393208

Gabbe, S. G., Niebyl, J. R., Galan, H. L., Jauniaux, E. R., Landon, M. B., Simpson, J. L., et al. (Eds.). (2012b). *Obstetrics: Normal and problem pregnancies* (6th ed.). Philadelphia, PA: W.B. Saunders.

Gelson, E., Curry, R., Gatzoulis, M., Swan, L., Lupton, M., Steer, P., et al. (2011). Effect of maternal heart disease on fetal growth. *Obstetrics & Gynecology, 117*(4), 886–891. doi:10.1097/AOG.0b013e31820cab69

Genovese, S. K. (2011). Hemorrhagic disorders. In S. Mattson & J. Smith (Eds.), *Core curriculum for maternal-child nursing* (4th ed., pp. 478–499). Philadelphia, PA: W.B. Saunders.

Gibson, K. S., Waters, T. P., & Catalano, P. M. (2012). Maternal weight gain in women who develop gestational diabetes mellitus. *Obstetrics & Gynecology, 119*(3), 560–565. doi:10.1097/AOG.0b013e31824758e0

Gilbert, E. (2010). *Manual of high risk pregnancy and delivery* (5th ed.). St. Louis, MO: C.V. Mosby.

Gilbert, E. (2011). Labor and delivery at risk. In S. Mattson & J. Smith (Eds.), *Core curriculum for maternal-child nursing* (4th ed., pp. 624–649). Philadelphia, PA: W.B. Saunders

Goldstein, D. P., Baron, E., & Berkowitz, R. S. (2010). Managing molar pregnancy. *Contemporary OB/GYN, 55*(4), 48–56.

Good, M. M., Solt, I., Acuna, J. G., Rotmensch, S., & Kim, M. J. (2010). Methamphetamine use during pregnancy. *Obstetrics & Gynecology, 116*(2), 330–334.

Grand'Maison, S., Sauve, N., Weber, F., Dagenais, M., Durand, M., & Mahone, M. (2012). Hepatic rupture in hemolysis, elevated liver enzymes, low platelets syndrome. *Obstetrics & Gynecology, 119*(3), 617–625. doi:10.1097/AOG.0b013e318245c283

Gregory, C. L., Wright, J., Schwarz, J., & Rakowski, L. (2012). A review of fetal thoracoamniotic and vesicoamniotic shunt procedures. *Journal of Obstetric, Gynecologic & Neonatal Nursing, 41*(3), 426–433. doi:10.1111/j.1552-6909.2012.01354.x

Harrison, P. (2013). Psychosocial impact of a cancer diagnosis during pregnancy. *Nursing for Women's Health, 17*(5), 437–442. doi:10.1111/1751-486X.12067

Heaney, R. P., & Holick, M. F. (2011). Why the IOM recommendations to vitamin D are deficient. *Journal of Bone and Mineral Research: The Official Journal of the American Society for Bone and Mineral Research, 26*(3), 455–457. doi:10.1002/jbmr.328.10.1002/jbmr.328

Hedderson, M. M., Gunderson, E. P., & Ferrara, A. (2010). Gestational weight gain and risk of gestational diabetes mellitus. *Obstetrics & Gynecology, 115*(3), 597–604.

Hood, D. G. (2012). Continuous subcutaneous insulin infusion for managing diabetes. *Nursing for Women's Health, 16*(4), 308–318. doi:10.1111/j.1751-486X.2012.01749.x

Hull, A. D., & Resnik, R. (2013). Placenta previa, placenta accreta, abruptio placentae, and vasa previa. In R. Creasy, R. Resnik, J. Iams, C. Lockwood, T. Moore, & M. Greene, *Creasy & Resnik's Maternal-fetal medicine: Principles and practice* (7th ed., pp. 732–742). Philadelphia, PA: W.B. Saunders.

Hurst, H. (2011). Insulin revisited: Safety in the maternity setting. *Nursing for Women's Health, 15*(3), 244–248.

Iliodromiti, Z., Antonakopoulos, N., Sifakis, S., Tsikouras, P., Danillidis, A., Dafopoulos, K., et al. (2012). Endocrine, paracrine, and autocrine placental mediators in labor. *Hormones, 11*(4), 397–409.

Kaimal, A. J. (2013). Assessment of fetal health. In R. Creasy, R. Resnik, J. Iams, C. Lockwood, T. Moore, & M. Greene, *Creasy & Resnik's maternal-fetal medicine: Principles and practice* (7th ed., pp. 473–487). Philadelphia, PA: W.B. Saunders.

Katz, A. (2011). Adolescent pregnancy: The good, the bad, and the promise. *Nursing for Women's Health, 15*(2), 149–152.

Kearney, M. (2008). *Tobacco, alcohol and drug use in childbearing families.* White Plains, NY: March of Dimes.

Kilpatrick, S. J. (2013). Anemia and pregnancy. In R. K. Creasy, R. Resnik, J. D. Iams, C. J. Lockwood, T. Moore, & M. F. Greene, *Creasy and Resnik's maternal-fetal medicine: Principles and practice* (7th ed., pp. 906–917). Philadelphia, PA: W.B. Saunders.

Lachat, M. F., Solnik, A. L., Nana, A. D., & Citron, T. L. (2011). Periodontal disease in pregnancy: Review of the evidence and prevention strategies. *Journal of Perinatal and Neonatal Nursing, 25*(4), 312–319.

Landon, M., Catalano, P., & Gabbe, S. (2012). Diabetes mellitus complicating pregnancy. In S. Gabbe, J. Niebyl, J. Simpson, M. Landon, H. Galan, E. Jauniaux, & D. Driscoll, *Obstetrics: Normal and Problem Pregnancies* (6th ed.). Philadelphia, PA: W.B. Saunders.

Landon, M. B., & Gabbe, S. G. (2011). Gestational diabetes mellitus. *Obstetrics & Gynecology, 118*(6), 1379–1391. doi:10.1097/AOG.0b013e31823974e2.

Lapillonne. A. (2010). Vitamin D deficiency during pregnancy may impair maternal and fetal outcomes. *Medical Hypotheses, 74*(1), 71–75. doi:10.1016/j.mehy.2009.07.054

Lawrence, R., & Lawrence, R. (2010). *Breastfeeding: A guide for the medical professional* (7th ed.). Philadelphia, PA: W.B. Saunders.

Lee, K. C. (2011). Fertility treatments and the cost of a healthy baby. *Nursing for Women's Health, 15*(1), 15–18. doi:10.1111/j.1751-486X.2011.01606.x

Lesko, J., & Peaceman, A. (2012). Pregnancy outcomes in women after bariatric surgery compared with obese and morbidly obese controls. *Obstetrics & Gynecology, 119*(3), 547–554. doi:10.1097/AOG.0b013e318239060e

Leung, A. N., & Lockwood, C. J. (2013). Thromboembolic disease. In R. K. Creasy, R. Resnik, J. D. Iams, C. J. Lockwood, T. Moore, & M. F. Greene, *Creasy and Resnik's maternal-fetal medicine: Principles and practice* (7th ed., pp. 906–917). Philadelphia, PA: W.B. Saunders.

Lindheimer, M. D., & Kanter, D. (2010). Interpreting abnormal proteinuria in pregnancy. *Obstetrics & Gynecology, 115*(2), 365–375.

Lockshin, M., Salmon, J., & Erkan, D. (2013). Pregnancy and the rheumatic diseases. In R. K. Creasy, R. Resnik, J. D. Iams, C. J. Lockwood, T. Moore, & M. F. Greene, *Creasy and Resnik's maternal-fetal medicine: Principles and practice* (7th ed., pp. 1092–1099). Philadelphia, PA: W.B. Saunders.

Lockwood, C. J. (2010). Keepsake fetal ultrasounds. *Contemporary OB/GYN, 55*(11), 8–12.

Lockwood, C. J. (2011). Understanding the new CDC group B streptococcal guidelines. *Contemporary OB-GYN, 56*(1), 6–8.

Lockwood, C. J. (2013). ACOG task force on hypertension in pregnancy: A step forward in management. *Contemporary OB-GYN, 58*(12), 10–13.

Magee, L., Sawchuck, D., Synnes, A., & von Dadelszen, P. (2011). SOGC clinical practice guideline. Magnesium sulphate for fetal neuroprotection. *Journal of Obstetrics & Gynaecology Canada, 33*(5), 516–529.

Malone, F., & D'Alton, M. (2013). Multiple gestation: Clinical characteristics and management. In R. K. Creasy, R. Resnik, J. D. Iams, C. J. Lockwood, T. Moore, & M. F. Greene, *Creasy and Resnik's maternal-fetal medicine: Principles and practice* (7th ed., pp. 578–598). Philadelphia, PA: W.B. Saunders.

Maloni, J. A. (2002). Astronauts & pregnancy bed rest: What NASA is teaching us about inactivity. *AWHONN Lifelines, 6*(4), [318–319], 320–323.

Maloni, J. A. (2010). Antepartum bed rest for pregnancy complications: Efficacy and safety for preventing preterm birth. *Biological Research for Nursing, 12*(2), 106–124. doi:10.1177/1099800410375978

Maloni, J. A., Brezinski-Tomasi, J. E., & Johnson, L. A. (2001). Antepartum bed rest: Effect upon the family. *JOGNN: Journal of Obstetric, Gynecologic and Neonatal Nursing, 30*(2), 165–173.

Maloni, J., & Park, S. (2005). Postpartum symptoms after antepartum bedrest. *Journal of Obstetric, Gynecologic and Neonatal Nursing, 34*(2), 163–171.

Mancuso, M., Szychowski, J., Owen, J., Hankins, G., Iams, J., Sheffield, J., et al. (2010). Cervical funneling: Effect on gestational length and ultrasound-indicated cerclage in high risk women. *American Journal of Obstetrics & Gynecology, 203*(3), 259.e1–259.e5. doi:10.1016.j.ajog.2010.07.002

March of Dimes. (2011). *March of Dimes prematurity campaign.* Retrieved from http://www.marchofdimes.com/mission/prematurity_campaign.html

March of Dimes. (2012). *Peristats: 2012 Premature birth report card.* Retrieved from http://www.marchofdimes.org/peristats/pdflib/998/us.pdf

March of Dimes. (2014). *Preterm labor.* Retrieved from http://www.marchofdimes.com/pregnancy/signs-and-symptoms-of-preterm-labor-and-what-to-do.aspx

March of Dimes Foundation, the Partnership for Maternal, Newborn & Child Health, Save the Children, & the World Health Organization. (2012). *Born Too Soon: The Global Action Report on Preterm Birth.* Retrieved from http://www.marchofdimes.com/mission/globalpreterm.html

Marcus, P. (2011). Gestational trophoblastic neoplasms: A century of progress. *The Female Patient, 36*(2), 35–38.

Martin, J., Hamilton, B., Sutton, P., Ventura, S., Osterman, J., Kirmeyer, S., et al. (2011). Births: Final data for 2009. *National Vital Statistics Report,* Vol. 60, No. 1. Hyattsville, MD: National Center for Health Statistics.

McCall, C. A., Grimes, D. A., & Lyerly, A. D. (2013). "Therapeutic" bed rest in pregnancy: Unethical and unsupported by data. *Obstetrics & Gynecology, 121*(6), 1305–1308. doi:10.1097/AOG.0b013e318293f12f

Meis, P., Klebanoff, M., Thom, E., Dombrowski, M., Sibai, B., Moawad, A., et al. (2003). Prevention of recurrent preterm delivery by 17 alpha-hydroxyprogesterone caproate. *New England Journal of Medicine, 348*(24), 2379–2385.

Melville, J. L., Gavin, A., Guo, Y., Fan, M. Y., & Katon, W. J. (2010). Depressive disorders during pregnancy. *Obstetrics & Gynecology, 116*(5), 1064–1070.

Metzger, B. E., Gabbe, S. G., Persson, B., Buchanan, T. A., Catalano, P. A., Damm, P., et al. (2010). International Association of Diabetes and Pregnancy Study Groups recommendation on the diagnosis and classification of hyperglycemia in pregnancy. International Association of Diabetes and Pregnancy Study Groups Consensus Panel. *Diabetes Care, 33*(1), 676–682.

Miesnik, S. R. (2012). The fetus as patient. *Journal of Obstetric, Gynecologic and Neonatal Nursing, 41*(3), 417–418. doi:10.1111/j.1552-6909.2012.01356.x

Miller, L. A., Miller, D., & Tucker, S. M. (2012). *Mosby's pocket guide to fetal monitoring: A multidisciplinary approach.* (7th ed.). Maryland Heights, MO: Mosby.

Mirza, F. G., & Gyamfi, C. (2010). Management of pregnancy in the Jehovah's Witness. *Contemporary OB/GYN, 55*(12), 41–48.

Moise, K. (2013). Hemolytic disease of the fetus and newborn. In R. K. Creasy, R. Resnik, J. D. Iams, C. J. Lockwood, T. Moore, & M. F. Greene, *Creasy and Resnik's maternal-fetal medicine: Principles and practice* (7th ed., pp. 578–598). Philadelphia, PA: W.B. Saunders.

Moise, K. Y., Kugler, L., & Jones, T. (2012). Contemporary management of complicated monochorionic twins. *Journal of Obstetric, Gynecologic & Neonatal Nursing, 41*(3), 434–444. doi:10.1111/j.1552-6909.2012.01355.x

Moore, T. R. (2010). Amniotic fluid dynamics reflect fetal and maternal health and disease. *Obstetrics & Gynecology, 116*(3), 759–765.

Moran, B. (2011a). Maternal infections. In S. Mattson & J. Smith (Eds.), *Core curriculum for maternal-newborn nursing* (4th ed., pp. 449–477). St. Louis, MO: W.B. Saunders.

Moran, B. (2011b). Substance abuse in pregnancy. In S. Mattson & J. Smith (Eds.), *Core curriculum for maternal-child nursing* (4th ed., pp. 573–586). Philadelphia, PA: W.B. Saunders.

Myles, T. D. (2011). Steroids-plenty of benefits, but not without risk. *Obstetrics & Gynecology, 117*(2), 429–430.

Nader, S. (2013). Thyroid disease in pregnancy. In R. K. Creasy, R. Resnik, J. D. Iams, C. J. Lockwood, T. Moore, & M. F. Greene, *Creasy and Resnik's maternal-fetal medicine: Principles and practice* (7th ed., pp. 1022–1037). Philadelphia, PA: W.B. Saunders.

Nagtalon-Ramos, J. (2011). Counseling pregnant patients at high risk for a preterm birth. *Women's Health Care: A Practical Journal for Nurse Practitioners, 10*(9), 21–27.

National Center for Health Statistics (NCHS). (2012). *Births: Final data for 2009.* Retrieved from http://www.cdc.gov/nchs/fastats/births.htm/

National Heart, Lung, and Blood Institute. (2007). *Expert Panel Report 3 (EPR-3): Guidelines for the diagnosis and management of asthma.* Retrieved from http://www.nhlbi.nih.gov/guidelines/asthma/asthgdln.htm

National High Blood Pressure Education Program Working Group (NHBPEP). (2000). Working group report on high blood pressure in pregnancy. NHBPEP Publication No. 00-3029. Washington, D.C.: National Heart Lung and Blood Institute.

National Institute of Child Health and Human Development. (2002). Home uterine monitors not useful for predicting premature delivery. Retrieved from https://www.nichd.nih.gov/news/releases/Pages/uterine.aspx

National Institutes of Health. AIDSinfo. (2012). *Recommendations for use of antiretroviral drugs in pregnant HIV-1-infected women for maternal health and interventions to reduce perinatal HIV transmission in the United States.* Retrieved from http://aidsinfo.nih.gov/guidelines/html/3/perinatal-guidelines/0/

Nayeri, U. A. (2012). Hyperemesis in pregnancy: Taking a tiered approach. *Contemporary OB-GYN, 57*(7), 22–31.

Norwitz, E. R., & Caughey, E. B. (2011). Progesterone supplementation and the prevention of preterm birth. *Reviews in Obstetrics & Gynecology, 4*(2), 60–72.

Oyelese, Y. (2010). Evaluation and management of low-lying placenta or placenta previa on second-trimester ultrasound. *Contemporary OB-GYN, 55*(12), 30–33.

Pacheco, L. D., Saade, G., Tyner, J., Clark, S. L., & Hankins, G. D. V. (2012). Obstetric hemorrhage: New insights. *Contemporary OB/GYN, 57*(6), 30–38.

Patterson, M. J., & Davies, H. D. (2011). Syphilis (*Treponema pallidum*). In R. M. Kliegman, B. M. Stanton, J. St. Geme, N. F. Schor, & R. E. Behrman, *Nelson textbook of pediatrics.* (19th ed.), pp. 1662–1685. Philadelphia, PA: W.B. Saunders.

Pereira, K., & Nicollerat, J. (2011). Continuous glucose monitors: A GPS for blood sugar control? *Advance for NPs & PAs, 2*(2), 40–48.

Pigarelli, D., Kraus, C., & Potter, B. (2011). Pregnancy and lactation: Therapeutic considerations. In J. DiPiro, R. Talbert, G. Yee, & G. Matzke (Eds.), *Pharmacotherapy: A pathophysiologic approach* (8th ed., pp 1297–1312). New York, NY: McGraw-Hill.

Pippitt, K., & Stoesser, K. (2011). Woman with heterotopic pregnancy after natural conception. *Consultant, 51*(5), 289–291.

Poole, J., & Thompson, J. (2012). Obstetric emergencies. In B. Hammond, & P. Zimmermann (Eds.), *Sheehy's manual of emergency care* (7th ed., pp. 483–496). Philadelphia, PA: Mosby.

Porter, L. S., & Holness, N. A. (2011). Breaking the repeat teen pregnancy cycle. *Nursing for Women's Health, 15*(5), 369–381. doi:10.1111/j.1751-486X.2011.01661.x

Porterfield, S. P. (2011). Vertical transmission of human papillomavirus from mother to fetus: A literature review. *JNP-The Journal for Nurse Practitioners, 7*(8), 665–670.

Pritham, U. A., Paul, J. A., & Hayes, M. J. (2012). Opioid dependency in pregnancy and length of stay for neonatal abstinence syndrome. *Journal of Obstetric, Gynecologic & Neonatal Nursing, 41*(2), 180–190. doi:10.1111/j.1552-6909.2011.01330.x

Records, K. (2011). Intimate partner violence. In S. Mattson & J. Smith (Eds.), *Core curriculum for maternal-child nursing* (4th ed., pp. 417–431). Philadelphia, PA: W.B. Saunders.

Robbins, K. S., Martin, S. R., & Wilson, W. C. (2013). Intensive care considerations for the critically ill parturient. In R. K. Creasy, R. Resnik, J. D. Iams, C. J. Lockwood, T. Moore, & M. F. Greene, *Creasy and Resnik's maternal-fetal medicine: Principles and practice* (7th ed., pp. 1182–1214). Philadelphia, PA: W.B. Saunders.

Roberts, D., & Dalziel, S. R. (2006). Antenatal corticosteroids for accelerating fetal lung maturation for women at risk of preterm birth. *Cochrane Database of Systematic Reviews 2006.* Issue 3. Art. No.: CD004454. doi:10.1002/14651858. CD004454.pub2.

Roberts, J. M., & Funai, E. F. (2013). Pregnancy-related hypertension. In R. K. Creasy, R. Resnik, J. D. Iams, C. J. Lockwood, T. Moore, & M. F. Greene, *Creasy and Resnik's maternal-fetal medicine: Principles and practice* (7th ed., pp. 756–784). Philadelphia, PA: W.B. Saunders.

Rubarth, L. B., Schoening, A. M., Cosimano, A., & Sandhurst, H. (2012). Women's experience of hospitalized bed rest during high-risk pregnancy. *Journal of Obstetric, Gynecologic & Neonatal Nursing, 41*(3), 398–407. doi:10.1111/j.1552-6909.2012.01349.x

Rubin, R. (1976). Maternal tasks of pregnancy. *Journal of Advanced Nursing, 1,* 367–376.

Senti, J., Thiele, D., & Anderson, C. (2012). Maternal vitamin D status as a critical determinant in gestational diabetes. *Journal of Obstetric, Gynecologic & Neonatal Nursing, 41*(3), 328–338. doi:10.1111/j.1552-6909.2012.01366.x

Shade, M., Miller, L., Borst, J., English, B., Valliere, J., Downs, K., et al. (2011). Statewide innovations to improve services for women with perinatal depression. *Nursing for Women's Health, 15*(2), 128–136.

Sheffield, J. S., Hickman, A., Tang, J., Moss, K., Kourosh, A., Crawford, N. M., et al. (2011). Efficacy of an accelerated hepatitis B vaccination program during pregnancy. *Obstetrics & Gynecology, 117*(5), 1130–1135. doi:10.1097/AOG.0b013e3182148efe

Sibai, B. M. (2012). Hypertension. In S. G. Gabbe, J. R. Niebyl, J. L. Simpson, M. B. Landon, H. L. Galan, E. R. Jauniaux, & D. A. Driscoll, *Obstetrics: Normal and problem pregnancies* (6th ed., pp. 631–666). Philadelphia, PA: W.B. Saunders.

Sibai, B. M. (2013). A stepwise approach to managing eclampsia and other hypertensive emergencies. *OBG Management, 25*(10), 35–48.

Sibai, B. M., & Viteri, O. A. (2014). Diabetic ketoacidosis in pregnancy. *Obstetrics & Gynecology, 123*(1), 167–177. doi:10.1097/AOG.000000000000060

Signore, C., Spong, C. Y., Krotoski, D., Shinowara, N. L., & Blackwell, S. C. (2011). Pregnancy in women with physical disabilities. *Obstetrics & Gynecology, 117*(4), 935–947. doi:10.1097/AOG.0b013e3182118d59

Simhan, H., Berghella, V., & Iams. J. (2013). Preterm labor and birth. In R. Creasy, R. Resnik, J. Iams, C. Lockwood, T. Moore, & M. Greene, *Creasy & Resnik's maternal-fetal medicine: Principles and practice* (7th ed., pp. 624–653). Philadelphia, PA: W.B. Saunders.

Simpson, L. L. (2012). Maternal cardiac disease. *Obstetrics & Gynecology, 119*(2), 345–364. doi:10.1097/AOG.0b013e318242e260

Skubisz, M. M., & Tong, S. (2011). Of leaves and butterflies: How methotrexate came to be the savior of women. *Obstetrics & Gynecology, 118*(5), 1169–1173. doi:10.1097/AOG.0b013e31822fcc0d

Spencer, R. (2003). *Conjoined twins: Developmental malformations and clinical implications.* Baltimore, MD: The Johns Hopkins University Press.

Spinner, S. S., Miesnik, S. R., Koh, J. G., & Howell, L. J. (2012). Maternal, fetal, and neonatal care in open fetal surgery for myelomeningocele. *Journal of Obstetric, Gynecologic & Neonatal Nursing, 41*(3), 447–455. doi:10.1111/j.1552-6909.2012.01357.x

Squires, L. S. (2013). A case study of recipient twin surviving complications of twin-to-twin transfusion syndrome. *Nursing for Women's Health, 17*(5), 390–398. doi:10.1111/1751-486X.12062

Stewart, D. E. (2011). Depression during pregnancy. *New England Journal of Medicine, 365*(10), 1605–1611.

Substance Abuse and Mental Health Services Administration, Office of Applied Studies. (2013). *The National Survey on Drug Use and Health Report—Data Spotlight Pregnancy and Alcohol.* Retrieved from http://www.samhsa.gov/data/spotlight/spot123-pregnancy-alcohol-2013.pdf

Sullivan, S. A. (2011). Subclinical hypothyroidism: Identification and treatment in pregnancy. *Contemporary OB/GYN, 37*(6), 46–53.

Tate, D. L., & Mari, G. (2013). Detection and surveillance of IUGR. *Contemporary OB/GYN, 28*(10), 28–38.

Taylor, B. K. (2011). Sonographic assessment of cervical length and the risk of preterm birth. *Journal of Obstetric, Gynecologic & Neonatal Nursing, 40*(5), 617–631. doi:10.1111/j.1552-6909.2011.01284.x

Taylor, M., Uhlmann, R. A., Meyer, N. L., & Mari, G. (2011). Hemolytic disease: Diagnosis, counseling, and management. *Contemporary OB/GYN, 56*(6), 34–45.

Thadhani, R. I., & Maski, M. R. (2013). Renal disorders. In R. K. Creasy, R. Resnik, J. D. Iams, C. J. Lockwood, T. Moore, & M. F. Greene, *Creasy and Resnik's maternal-fetal medicine: Principles and practice* (7th ed., pp. 949–964). Philadelphia, PA: W.B. Saunders.

Thompson, K. B., & Keehbauch, J. (2009). Cervical incompetence update. *The Female Patient, 34*(11), 14–19.

Torgersen, K. L. (2011). Antepartum fetal assessment. In S. Mattson & J. Smith (Eds.), *Core curriculum for maternal-child nursing* (4th ed., pp. 128–162). Philadelphia, PA: W.B. Saunders.

Tormoehlen, K., & Lessick, M. (2011). Schizophrenia in women: Implications for pregnancy and postpartum. *Nursing for Women's Health, 14*(6), 484–495.

Townsend, M. (2011). *Psychiatric mental health nursing: Concepts of care in evidence-based practice* (7th ed.). Philadelphia, PA: F.A. Davis.

U.S. Preventive Services Task Force. (1996). Screening for home uterine activity monitoring. Topic page. U.S. Preventive Services Task Force. Retrieved from http://www.uspreventiveservicestaskforce.org/uspstf/uspshuam.htm (Accessed 1-28-14).

U.S. Preventive Services Task Force. (2014). Screening for gestational diabetes mellitus: U.S. Preventive Services Task Force recommendation statement. *Annals of Internal Medicine,* published online 14 January 2014. doi:10.7326/M13-2905

University of Maryland Medical Center. (2014). Conjoined twins. Retrieved from http://umm.edu/programs/conjoined-twins/facts-about-the-twins

Vallerand, A. H., & Sanoski, C. A. (2014). *Davis's drug guide for nurses* (14th ed.). Philadelphia, PA: F.A. Davis.

Van Otterloo, L. R. (2011a). Endocrine and metabolic disorders. In S. Mattson & J. E. Smith (Eds.). *Core curriculum for maternal-newborn nursing* (4th ed). New York, NY: Saunders Elsevier.

Van Otterloo, L. R. (2011b). Trauma in pregnancy. In S. Mattson & J. E. Smith (Eds.). *Core curriculum for maternal-newborn nursing* (4th ed.). New York, NY: Saunders Elsevier.

Velasquez, M., Ingersoll, K., Sobell, M., Floyd, R., Sobell, L., & von Sternberg, K. (2010). A dual-focus motivational intervention to reduce the risk of alcohol-exposed pregnancy. *Cognitive and Behavioral Practice, 17*(2), 203–212.

Verani, J. R., McGee, L., & Schrag, S. J. (2010). Prevention of perinatal group B streptococcal disease-revised guidelines from CDC, 2010. Division of Bacterial Diseases, National Center for Immunization and Respiratory Diseases, Centers for Disease Control and Prevention (CDC). *MMWR Recommendations and Reports 2010, 59*(RR-10): 1–36.

Von Kohler, C. S. (2011). Age-related concerns. In S. Mattson & J. E. Smith (Eds.). *Core curriculum for maternal-child nursing* (4th ed., pp. 117–127). Philadelphia, PA: W.B. Saunders.

Wapner, R. (2013). Prenatal diagnosis of congenital disorders. In R. K. Creasy, R. Resnik, J. D. Iams, C. J. Lockwood, T. Moore, & M. F. Greene, *Creasy and Resnik's maternal-fetal medicine: Principles and practice* (7th ed., pp. 417–464). Philadelphia, PA: W.B. Saunders.

Whitty, J., & Dombrowski, M. (2013). Respiratory diseases in pregnancy. In R. K. Creasy, R. Resnik, J. D. Iams, C. J. Lockwood, T. Moore, & M. F. Greene, *Creasy and Resnik's maternal-fetal medicine: Principles and practice* (7th ed., pp. 965–987). Philadelphia, PA: W.B. Saunders.

Wylie, B. J., & D'Alton, M. E. (2010). Fetomaternal hemorrhage. *Obstetrics & Gynecology, 115*(5), 1039–1051.

Yancy, M. (2011). Other medical complications. In S. Mattson & J. Smith (Eds.), *Core curriculum for maternal-newborn nursing* (4th ed., pp. 587–623). Philadelphia, PA: W.B. Saunders.

Yehuda, I., Nagtalon-Ramos, J., & Trout, K. (2011). Fetal growth scans and amniotic fluid assessments in pregestational and gestational diabetes. *Journal of Obstetric, Gynecologic & Neonatal Nursing, 40*(5), 603–616. doi:10.1111/j.1552-6909.2011.01283.x

Yonkers, K. A. (2013). Management of depression and psychoses in pregnancy and in the puerperium. In R. K. Creasy, R. Resnik, J. D. Iams, C. J. Lockwood, T. Moore, & M. F. Greene, *Creasy and Resnik's maternal-fetal medicine: Principles and practice* (7th ed., pp. 1122–1131). Philadelphia, PA: W.B. Saunders.

Yonkers, K. A., Gotman, N., Kershaw, T., Forray, A., Howell, H., & Rounsaville, B. (2010). Screening for prenatal substance use: Development of the Substance Use Risk Profile-Pregnancy Scale. *Obstetrics & Gynecology, 116*(4), 827–833.

Yonkers, K. A., Vigod, S., & Ross, L. E. (2011). Diagnosis, pathophysiology, and management of mood disorder in pregnant and postpartum women. *Obstetrics & Gynecology, 117*(4), 961–977. doi:10.1097/AOG.0b013e31821187a7

Zhang, Y., Cantor, R. M., MacGibbon, K., Romero, R., Goodwin, T. M., Mullin, P. M., & Fejzo, M. S. (2011). Familial aggregation of hyperemesis gravidarum. *American Journal of Obstetrics & Gynecology, 204*(3), 226–236.

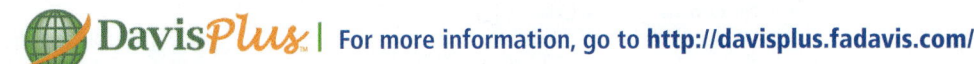

DavisPlus | For more information, go to **http://davisplus.fadavis.com/**

CONCEPT MAP

Caring for the Woman Experiencing Complications During Pregnancy

Complications of Early Pregnancy

- Hyperemesis gravidarum
- Spontaneous abortion/ miscarriage
- Gestational trophoblastic disease
- Ectopic pregnancy
- Perinatal loss
  - Fetal death
  - Less-than-perfect child

Miscellaneous Complications

- Multiple gestation
- Premature rupture of membranes
- Preterm labor
- Cervical insufficiency/ incompetence

Endocrine

- Pregestational diabetes
  - Type I & II
- Gestational
  - DKA
- Hyper/hypothyroid

Unique Conditions That Complicate Pregnancy

- Antenatal bedrest
- Adolescence/Advanced age
- Blunt abdominal trauma
- Surgery
- Cancer
- Obesity
- Physical disability
- Intimate partner violence
- Rh sensitization
- Systemic lupus

Cardiovascular/ Hematological

C/V:
- Mitral valve prolapse
- Peripartum cardiomyopathy
- Venous thromboem- bolic disease

Hematological
- Sickle cell anemia
- Thaassemia syndrome

Hypertensive disorders:
- Chronic hypertension
- Preeclampsia/eclampsia
  - Proteinuria, edema, CNS alterations, HELLP syndrome
- Preeclampsia superim- posed on chronic HTN
- Gestational hypertension
- Transient HTN

Bleeding Disorders

- Placenta previa
- Placental abruption
- DIC

Psychiatric

Exacerbation; Resurgence; New Onset
- Depression
- Anxiety
- Eating disorder
- Substance abuse or addiction
- Bipolar disease
- Schizophrenia

Infections

- UTIs acute asymptomatic
  - Bacteriuria, cystitis pyelonephritis
- Group B strep
- TORCH
- STIs
  - Chlamydia, gonorrhea, syphilis, HPV, HIV/AIDS
- TB

Respiratory

- Pneumonia
- Asthma
- Cystic fibrosis

Family Teaching Guidelines:
- Teach symptoms of preterm labor
- Preventing preterm birth
- Home care for patient with hypertensive disorder

Critical Nursing Actions:
- Maternal positioning in CPR
- Correct maternal/fetal care post maternal seizure
- Assess for decreased cardiac output during labor in maternal cardiovascular disease hx

Nursing Insight:
- Transvaginal ultrasound is gold standard to evaluate dynamic changes in the cervix
- Use pneumonic SPASMS when caring for patient with preeclampsia
- Vaccine can prevent HPV
- Be aware of CV meds that can have negative maternal/fetal effects
- Recognize signs of maternal stress in placenta previa and intervene
- Pregnant women and their infants are vulnerable to serious illness/hospitalization due to having the flu
- Preconception bariatric surgery associated with reduced gestational diabetes

Cultural Diversity:
- Beliefs related to pregnancy itself
- Preferences for provider's gender
- Culturally significant foods
- Need for interpreter
- Gestational diabetes ➞ more prevalent in certain ethnic groups

Optimizing Outcomes:
- Use research-based interventions to prevent preterm labor
- In preterm births, antenatal steroids improve neonatal outcomes
- Offer testing to women with hx of habitual spontaneous abortions
- Support religious beliefs about transfu- sions
- Use correct technique/equipment to obtain maternal BP
- Correctly administer and document when giving RhoGAM
- Decrease incidence of STIs by recogniz- ing and teaching signs/sx
- Use CGM to achieve better glycemic control during pregnancy

Clinical Alert:
- Expanded volume in pregnancy can mask sx of hemorrhage
- Serious consequences occur with overdose of magnesium sulfate
- Have calcium gluconate (antidote) at bedside
- Do not combine nefedipine with magnesium sulfate or erythromycin

Now Can You:
- Discuss the management of bleeding during pregnancy
- Identify 3 symptoms of preterm labor/PROM
- Discuss Rho(D) and ABO isoimmuni- zation
- Discuss major disease processes that affect maternal health during pregnancy
- Identify how unique conditions complicate pregnancy

Complementary Care:
- For nausea/vomiting of pregnancy ➞ use ginger, relaxation, hypnosis

Collaboration in Caring:
- Educating all women of childbearing age about preterm labor is crucial component of prevention
- Involve community resource groups for the couple having experienced a molar pregnancy

Legal Alert:
- Perform daily CV assessments on woman with preeclampsia
- Document correctly following a maternal seizure

one
two
three
four
five
six
seven

The Birth Experience

The Process of Labor and Birth

 To my labor and delivery nurse:

On February 24th you helped us welcome our darling daughter into the world. In fact you practically delivered her yourself. My labor and delivery moved along quite quickly. Through it all you somehow managed to always say and do the right thing. I have taken great pleasure in telling people what a really good labor and birth experience I had. You played a key role in that. While we know it's your job and all that, we thought you still deserved to know that your contribution to our daughter's birth was important and will always be a part of our memory. Years from now when we are telling her about her birth, your name is sure to come up. Thanks again!

—Anonymous

LEARNING TARGETS *At the completion of this chapter, the student will be able to:*

- ◆ Discuss various theories concerning the onset of labor, and describe signs and symptoms of impending labor.
- ◆ Contrast advantages and disadvantages of various childbirth settings.
- ◆ Describe the "5 Ps" and how each influences labor and birth.
- ◆ Differentiate among the four stages of labor according to the duration and work accomplished, contraction patterns, and maternal behaviors.
- ◆ Discuss methods of fetal assessment during labor.
- ◆ Identify nursing interventions for each stage of labor.

PICO(T) Questions

The intent of evidence-based practice (EBP) is to provide nursing care that integrates the best available evidence. An initial step in EBP is to write a PICO(T) question that effectively guides the research. A PICO(T) question is an acronym that stands for population (P), intervention or issue (I), comparison of interest (C), outcome (O), and timeframe (T). Depending on the question, all or some of the question components are used in the research process.

Use these PICO(T) questions to spark your thinking as you read the chapter.

1. Are (P) women over age 30 (O) at a higher risk of (I) uterine hemorrhage in the fourth stage of labor (C) than women under age 30?

2. In the absence of known risks, do more (P) women in active labor (O) prefer (I) intermittent auscultation (IA) of the fetal heart rate (C) or continuous electronic fetal monitoring (EFM)?

Evidence-Based Practice

Selby, C., Valencia, S., Garcia, L., Keep, D., Overcash, J., & Jackson, J. (2012). Activity level during a one-hour labor check evaluation: Walking versus bed rest. *The American Journal of Maternal/Child Nursing (MCN), 37*(2), 101–107.

The purpose of this study was to compare patient activity levels during a 1-hour labor check in relation to changes in cervical dilation and progression of labor. Additional purposes included determining the mother's comfort level in relation to her activity level and to determine the predictive value of a 1-hour labor check in relation to delivery within 24 hours of the initial assessment. Determination of the progress of labor was based on the policy of the institution where the study was conducted. Progression of labor is described as evidence of cervical dilation increased by greater than or equal to 1 cm at the 1-hour assessment with vaginal birth determined to be likely within the next 24 hours. Women whose 1-hour cervical dilation status remained similar to the initial evaluation with intact membranes and infrequent or irregular contractions were usually sent home with the assumption that delivery was unlikely within the next 24 hours.

The study participants included a convenience sample of 63 nulliparous full-term, low-risk women whose initial assessment was negative for active labor. Additional inclusion criteria included an ability to speak and understand the English language, gestational age from 37 to 42 weeks, single pregnancy, cephalic presentation, intact amnion, cervical dilation less than 4 cm, blood pressure less than 140/90 mm Hg and fetal heart rate tracing at a category I. Patients who were unable to walk were not included.

The study design was described as a randomized controlled trial. Patients were randomly assigned by a computer-generated system to either the bedrest or the walking group during a 1-hour labor check period. Informed consent and baseline demographic data were obtained along with a determination of the woman's comfort level as measured by a visual analog scale (VAS). The VAS measured various symptoms by instructing the patient to mark her perceived level of pain on a 100-mm vertical scale with the lowest point indicating "extremely comfortable" and the highest point indicating "extremely uncomfortable." The patients were taught how to use the scale and were given an opportunity to practice using the VAS at the beginning of the study. According to the researchers, the VAS scores have previously been determined to be a valid and reliable method of measuring various symptoms including pain.

At the time of admission, initial and 1-hour vaginal examinations were performed by the same investigator (as a means to control for measurement error). Thirty-two women were assigned to the bedrest group and instructed to remain in bed for 1 hour, with the exception of trips to the bathroom. Thirty-one women were assigned to the walking group and instructed to walk around the nursing unit as desired during the 1 hour period of time. Participants assigned to the walking group were provided with a pedometer (device that counts each step taken). At the completion of the 1-hour period, cervical dilation and patient comfort level were determined.

Descriptive statistics were used to summarize the data, and a *t*-test was performed to determine differences in cervical dilation changes and comfort levels between the two groups. Changes in cervical dilation were described as at least a 1-cm increase at the 1-hour check, which was interpreted as a high likelihood that delivery would occur within 24 hours. The average change in cervical dilation that occurred during the 1-hour check period was 0.38 cm for the bedrest group and 0.33 cm for the walking group, a finding that was not statistically significant. Eight patients in the bedrest group and seven patients in the walking group experienced a greater than or equal to 1 cm cervical dilation increase during the 1-hour time period. Fifty-seven percent (36 women) delivered within 24 hours; of these 17 women were in the bedrest group and 19 women were in the walking group. The findings were not significantly different. A cervical dilation of greater than or equal to 1 cm increase at the 1-hour assessment was found to be predictive of delivery within 24 hours 88% of the time. Comfort scores were reported as similar and small between the two groups and were not significantly different.

1. How is this information useful to clinical nursing practice?

2. Based on these findings, what are implications for further research?

See Suggested Responses for Evidence-Based Practice on Davis*Plus*.

Introduction

The journey from conception to birth is one of ongoing development and adaptation for the woman, the fetus, and the family. Physiological, psychological, and emotional changes that take place during pregnancy help to prepare the woman for labor and birth. Near the end of the pregnancy, the fetus continues to develop physiological abilities that facilitate successful adaptation for the transition from in utero life to the outside environment.

Each woman's labor and birth experience is uniquely shaped by a myriad of factors. Throughout this journey,

the actions of nurses play a vital role in supporting the patient, the fetus, and the family. This chapter presents the processes of labor and birth and the important roles of nurses during each stage.

Theories Concerning Labor Onset

For the majority of women, the onset of labor usually occurs between the 38th and 42nd weeks of pregnancy. For most of the pregnancy, the uterus stays in a relaxed state and the cervix remains closed and firm to maintain the

---

Box 12-1 Theories Regarding the Onset of Labor

MATERNAL FACTORS

- **Uterine muscle stretching**, which causes a release of prostaglandins.
- **Pressure on the cervix**, which stimulates the release of oxytocin by the maternal posterior pituitary gland.
- **Oxytocin stimulation** increases significantly during labor and works together with prostaglandins to activate uterine contractions. Endogenous oxytocin, a neuropeptide released from the posterior pituitary, is also synthesized locally by the amnion, chorion, and decidua. Shortly prior to the onset of labor, the uterus is primed with a dramatic increase in the number of oxytocin receptors, which causes it to become markedly sensitive to increases in endogenous oxytocin that normally occur during spontaneous labor.
- **Increase in the ratio of estrogen to progesterone**: As term approaches, biochemical changes cause a decreased availability of progesterone (relaxes smooth muscle) to the uterine myometrial cells. With rising estrogen levels, the uterus becomes more excitable and contractions begin.

FETAL FACTORS

- **Placental aging** and deterioration triggers the initiation of contractions.
- **Fetal cortisol concentration** increases. This results in a decrease in the production of placental progesterone and an increase in the release of prostaglandins.
- **Fetal membranes** produce prostaglandins, which aid in the stimulation of uterine contractions.

Sources: Cunningham et al. (2014); Lowe (2012); Simpson & Creehan (2013).

---

pregnancy. Toward the end of pregnancy, there is a complete reversal in which the uterus becomes more excitable, and cervical softening (ripening) occurs. The cervical changes result from the breakdown of collagen fibers, which produce a decrease in the binding capacity. This change, coupled with an increase in cervical water content, causes weakening and softening. Although many theories regarding the origin of labor have been proposed, no one theory can account for the onset of labor in all women. Instead, a combination of maternal and fetal factors most likely interacts to bring about the initiation of labor (Box 12-1).

The Process of Labor and Birth

A number of forces affect the progress of labor and help to bring about childbirth. These critical factors are often referred to as the "Ps" of labor:

- Powers (physiological forces)
- Passageway (maternal pelvis)
- Passenger (fetus and placenta)
- Passageway + Passenger and their relationship (engagement, attitude, position)
- Psychosocial influences (previous experiences, emotional status)

Position of the laboring patient is sometimes designated as a separate critical "P." In this chapter, maternal positions to facilitate labor and enhance comfort are included in the discussion under promoting comfort during labor. The coordination of the various factors that affect labor is essential for the labor and birth to progress in a successful manner.

POWERS

The powers are the physiological forces of labor and birth that include the uterine contractions and the maternal pushing efforts. The uterine muscular contractions, primarily responsible for causing cervical effacement and dilation, also move the fetus down toward the birth canal during the first stage of labor. Uterine contractions are considered the primary force of labor. Once the cervix is fully dilated, the maternal pushing efforts serve as an additional force. During the second stage of labor, use of the maternal abdominal muscles for pushing (the *secondary force* of labor) adds to the primary force to facilitate childbirth.

Characteristics of Uterine Contractions

Contractions are a rhythmic tightening of the uterus that occurs intermittently. Over time, this action shortens the individual uterine muscle fibers and aids in the process of cervical effacement and dilation, birth, and postpartal **involution** (the reduction in uterine size after birth). Each contraction consists of three distinct components: the **increment** (building of the contraction), the **acme** (peak of the contraction), and the **decrement** (decrease in the contraction).

Between contractions, the uterus normally returns to a state of complete relaxation. This rest period allows the uterine muscles to relax and provides the woman with a short recovery period that helps her to avoid exhaustion. In addition, uterine relaxation between contractions is important for fetal oxygenation because it allows for blood flow from the uterus to the placenta to be restored.

Contractions bring about changes in the uterine musculature. The upper portion of the uterus becomes thicker and more active. The lower uterine segment becomes thin-walled and passive. The boundary between the upper and lower uterine segments becomes marked by a ridge on the inner uterine surface, known as the "physiological retraction ring."

With each contraction, the uterus elongates. Elongation causes a straightening of the fetal body so that the upper body is pressed against the fundus and the lower, presenting part is pushed toward the lower uterine segment and the cervix. The pressure exerted by the fetus is called the fetal axis pressure. As the uterus elongates, the longitudinal muscle fibers are stretched upward over the presenting part. This force, along with the hydrostatic pressure of the fetal membranes, causes the cervix to dilate (open).

Assessment of Uterine Contractions

Contractions are often described in terms of their frequency, duration, and intensity. The **frequency** of a contraction is measured from the beginning of one contraction to the beginning of the next contraction. The **duration** of a contraction is measured from the start of one contraction to the end of the same contraction. The **intensity** of a contraction is most frequently measured by uterine palpation and is described in terms of mild, moderate, and strong (Fig. 12-1).

Palpation is a noninvasive procedure and requires the nurse to place the fingertips of one hand on the fundus of the uterus where most contractions can be felt. The nurse applies gentle pressure and keeps the hand in the same place (moving the hand over the uterus may stimulate additional contractions, therefore interfering with the ability to accurately assess labor progress). Gentle palpation of

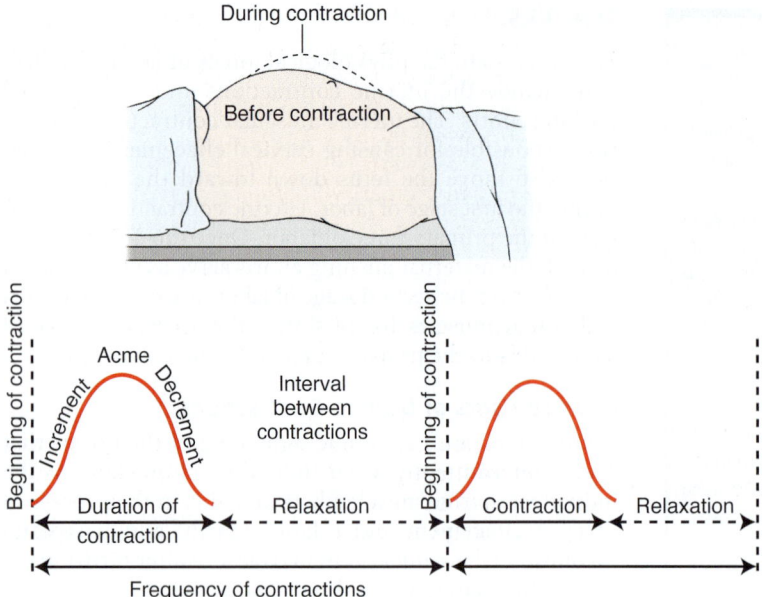

During contraction

Before contraction

Beginning of contraction

Acme

Increment   Decrement

Interval
between
contractions

Beginning of contraction

Duration of
contraction

Relaxation

Contraction

Relaxation

Frequency of contractions

Figure 12-1 Counting contractions. Contraction frequency is the time from the beginning of one contraction to the beginning of the next contraction. Contraction duration is the time from the beginning to the end of the same contraction.

the uterine fundus can determine the firmness of the uterus and whether there is an ability to indent the uterus at the acme (peak) of the contraction. Palpating the intensity of contractions is often compared with palpating one's nose (mild intensity), chin (moderate intensity), or forehead (strong intensity). When the uterine fundus remains soft at the acme of a contraction, the contraction intensity is described as "mild." Conversely, when there is an inability to indent the uterus at the acme of a contraction, the contraction intensity is described as "strong." "Moderate" contraction intensity falls somewhere in between and is characterized by a firm fundus that is difficult to indent with the fingertips. Several contractions must be evaluated to accurately determine the frequency, duration, and intensity.

Contractions may also be measured via electronic monitoring. Monitoring may be external or internal, and this modality can provide a continuous assessment of uterine activity. External contraction monitoring uses a **tocodynamometer**, which is a pressure-sensitive device that is applied against the uterine fundus. When the uterus contracts, the pressure that is exerted against the "toco" is measured and recorded on graph paper. External monitoring may be continuous or intermittent. It provides information about the frequency and duration of contractions. However, it may not give accurate data regarding the intensity of contractions because there are many variables (e.g., maternal position, obesity, and the placement of the monitor on the uterus) that can affect the tracing. Contraction intensity is best assessed with palpation.

Another method to measure the intensity of uterine contractions is an invasive procedure that involves the use of an internal monitor. If the amniotic membranes have ruptured, an internal pressure catheter is inserted through the cervix and into the uterus to measure the internal pressure generated during the contraction. Normally, the resting pressure (or resting tone) in the uterus (between contractions) is 10 to 12 mm Hg. During the acme, contraction intensity ranges from 25 to 40 mm Hg during early labor, 50 to 70 mm Hg during active labor, 70 to 90 mm Hg

during transition, and 70 to 100 mm Hg during maternal pushing in the second stage. Internal uterine pressure monitoring is most often used with high-risk pregnancies when accurate measurement of uterine activity is required. Because internal monitoring is an invasive procedure, it is associated with a slight risk of infection. (See Chapter 14 for further discussion.)

During early labor, uterine contractions are characteristically weak and irregular. They usually last for about 30 seconds and occur every 5 to 7 minutes. As the labor pattern becomes established, the uterine contractions typically become regular in frequency, longer in duration, and increased in intensity. The duration of contractions increases to about 60 seconds, and they occur every 2 to 3 minutes. The contractions are involuntary and are most efficient when there is a regular, rhythmic, coordinated labor pattern. The woman in labor is unable to control contraction frequency, duration, or intensity.

Uterine contractions also bring about changes in the pelvic floor musculature. The forces of labor cause the levator ani muscles and fascia of the pelvic floor to draw the rectum and vagina upward and forward. During descent, the fetal head exerts increasing pressure and causes thinning of the perineal body from 5 cm to less than 1 cm in thickness. Continued pressure causes the maternal anus to evert, and the interior rectal wall is exposed as the fetal head descends forward (Cunningham, Leveno, Bloom, Spong, & Dashe, 2014).

Now Can You—Evaluate uterine contractions?

1. Discuss what is meant by the "powers" of labor?
2. Describe the terms used to evaluate contractions?
3. Identify two methods used to assess the intensity of contractions?

The coordinated efforts of the contractions help to bring about effacement and dilation of the cervix. **Effacement** is the process of shortening and thinning of the cervix. As contractions occur, the cervix becomes progressively shorter until the cervical canal eventually disappears. The amount of cervical effacement is usually expressed as a percentage related to the length of the cervical canal, as compared with a noneffaced cervix. For example, if a cervix has thinned to half the normal length of a cervix, it is considered to be 50% effaced. **Dilation** is the opening and enlargement of the cervix that progressively occurs throughout the first stage of labor. Cervical dilation is expressed in centimeters, and full dilation is approximately 10 cm. With continued uterine contractions, the cervix eventually opens large enough to allow the fetal head to come through. At this point, the cervix is considered fully dilated, or completely dilated, and measures 10 cm (Fig. 12-2).

The first stage of labor, which begins with the onset of true labor, concludes when cervical effacement and dilation are complete. Effacement and dilation occur concurrently but at different rates. In a nulliparous patient, most cervical effacement is completed early during the process of cervical dilation, whereas the multiparous cervix is often patulous (distended) before effacement begins.

Effacement and dilation are evaluated by a vaginal examination performed by a qualified practitioner such as a maternity nurse who has received specialized training in this procedure (Procedure 12-1). The vaginal examination provides important information regarding the diameter of the opening of the cervix, which ranges from 1 cm (not dilated) to 10 cm (fully dilated), the status of the amniotic membranes (ruptured or intact), and the fetal presentation and the station, or the extent of the fetal descent through the maternal pelvis. Once the cervix is fully dilated and retracted up into the lower uterine segment, it can no longer be palpated.

Maternal Pushing Efforts

After the cervix has become fully dilated, the laboring woman usually experiences an involuntary "bearing down" sensation that assists with the expulsion of the fetus. At this time, the woman can use her abdominal muscles to aid in the expulsion. It is important to remember that the cervix must be fully dilated before the patient is encouraged to push. Bearing down on a partially dilated cervix can cause cervical edema and damage and adversely affect the progress of the labor. For most women, the urge to bear down generally occurs when the fetal head reaches the pelvic floor. Women who have a strong urge to push often do so more effectively than women who force themselves to push without experiencing any sensations of pressure.

PASSAGEWAY

The passageway consists of the maternal pelvis and the soft tissues. The bony pelvis through which the fetus must pass is divided into three sections: the inlet, midpelvis (pelvic cavity), and outlet. Each of these pelvic components has a unique shape and dimension through which the fetus must maneuver to be born vaginally. In human females, the four classic types of pelvis are the gynecoid, android, platypelloid, and anthropoid. (See Chapter 5 for further discussion.)

PASSENGER

The passenger comprises the fetus and the fetal membranes. In the majority (96%) of pregnancies, the fetus presents in a head-first position. The fetal skull, usually the largest body structure, is also the least flexible part of the fetus. However, because of the sutures and fontanelles, there is some flexibility in the fetal skull. These structures allow the cranial bones the capability of movement and they overlap in response to the powers of labor. The overlapping or overriding of the cranial bones is called **molding**.

A & P review   The Fetal Skull

The fetal skull, or cranium, consists of three major components: the face, the base of the skull, and the vault of the cranium (roof). The facial bones and the cranial base are fused and fixed. The cranial base is made up of two temporal bones, and each has a sphenoid and ethmoid bone.

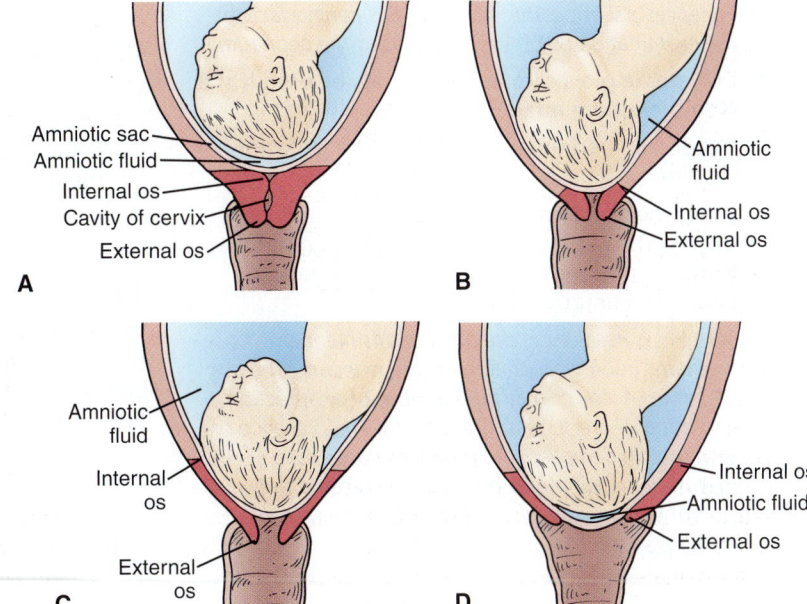

Figure 12-2 Cervical effacement and dilation. The membranes are intact. *A,* Before labor. *B,* Early effacement. *C,* Complete (100%) effacement; the fetal head is well applied to the cervix. *D,* Complete dilation (10 cm); note overlapping of the cranial bones.

Procedure 12-1 Performing the Intrapartal Vaginal Examination

Purpose

Vaginal examination may be performed during the intrapartal period for many reasons including: assessment of cervical dilation, effacement and station, fetal position and presentation, rupture of the membranes, prolapse of the umbilical cord, and to perform fetal scalp stimulation.

Equipment

- Sterile examination gloves (clean gloves may be used if the membranes are intact)
- Sterile lubricant
- Antiseptic solution and light source (if required)
- Disposable wipes

Steps

1. Wash and dry your hands. Explain the procedure and purpose of the examination to the patient.

    RATIONALE: *Hand washing helps to prevent the spread of microorganisms. Explanations help to decrease anxiety and promote patient understanding and cooperation.*

2. Assess for latex allergies.

    RATIONALE: *To prevent injury from latex exposure; if patient has a latex allergy, use nonlatex gloves.*

3. Ensure privacy.

    RATIONALE: *Privacy promotes comfort and self-esteem.*

4. Assemble necessary equipment including clean gloves (if the membranes are intact) or sterile examination gloves (if the membranes are ruptured), sterile lubricant, antiseptic solution (if required).

5. Position the patient in a supine position with a small pillow or towel under her hip to prevent supine hypotension. Instruct the patient to relax and position herself with her thighs flexed and abducted.

    RATIONALE: *Relaxation decreases muscle tension and enhances patient comfort. Proper positioning facilitates the examination by providing access to the perineum.*

6. Don sterile gloves (clean gloves may be used if the membranes are intact).

7. Inspect the perineum for any redness, irritation, or vesicles.

8. Using the nondominant hand, spread the labia majora and continue assessment of the genitalia. Note the presence of any discharge including blood or amniotic fluid.

    RATIONALE: *Positioning the hand in this manner facilitates good visualization of the perineum. The presence of lesions may be indicative of an infection and possibly preclude a vaginal birth. The presence of amniotic fluid implies that the membranes have ruptured. Bleeding may be a sign of placenta previa. Do not perform a vaginal examination if a placenta previa is suspected.*

9. Gently insert the lubricated gloved index and third fingers into the vagina in the direction of the posterior wall until they touch the cervix. The uterus may be stabilized by placing the nondominant hand on the woman's abdomen.

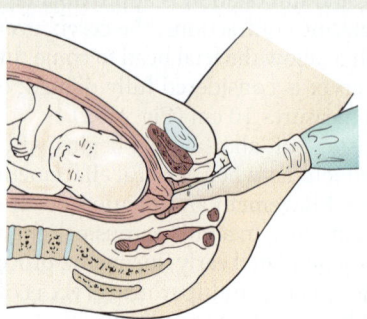

RATIONALE: *This position facilitates the examination by allowing the fingertips to point toward the umbilicus and find the cervix.*

10. Assess the cervix for effacement and the amount of dilation.

11. Assess for intact membranes; if fluid is expressed, test for amniotic fluid.

12. Palpate the presenting part.

    RATIONALE: *It is necessary to determine the presenting part to assess fetal position and evaluate fetal descent.*

13. Assess fetal descent and station by identifying the position of the posterior fontanelle.

14. Withdraw the fingers. Assist the patient in wiping her perineum from front to back to remove lubricant or secretions. Help her to resume a comfortable position.

    RATIONALE: *Wiping from front to back prevents the transfer of rectal contamination toward the vagina.*

15. Inform the patient of the findings from the examination.

16. Wash hands.

17. Document the procedure on the patient's chart and on the fetal monitor strip (if a fetal monitor is being used). Include the assessment findings and the patient's tolerance of the procedure.

    RATIONALE: *Documentation provides a record for communication and evaluation of patient care.*

What If?

What if you are performing a vaginal exam in a patient with ruptured membranes and you palpate a pulsating umbilical cord below the level of the presenting part (fetal head)?

You should take the following steps:

- Call for assistance; notify the primary care provider
- Use two fingers to exert upward pressure against the fetal head to relieve compression of the cord

Procedure 12-1 Performing the Intrapartal Vaginal Examination (continued)

- Assist the woman into an extreme Trendelenburg, modified Sims, or knee-chest position
- Administer oxygen at 10 L/min by face mask
- Increase the IV fluid rate
- Continuously monitor the FHR
- Provide information to the woman and her support person
- Prepare for immediate birth (vaginal if the cervix is fully dilated or cesarean if it is not)

Documentation

6/8/09. 1235: Vaginal examination performed for assessment of labor. Cervix 4 cm dilated, 100% effaced, station 0. No membranes felt, patient leaking clear fluid from the vagina, position OA. Procedure tolerated well by patient, fetal heart rate 152 bpm post examination.

–L. Lopez, RN

The cranial vault is composed of five bones: two frontal bones, two parietal bones, and the occipital bone. These bones, which are not fused, meet at the **sutures**. The sutures of the fetal skull are composed of strong but flexible connective tissue that fills the spaces that lie between the cranial bones.

The sagittal suture lies between the parietal bones and runs in an anteroposterior direction between the fontanelles, dividing the head into a right and a left side. The lambdoidal suture extends from the posterior fontanelle and separates the occipital bones from the parietal bones. The coronal sutures are located between the frontal and parietal bones. They extend from the anterior fontanelle laterally and separate the parietal from the frontal bones. The frontal (mitotic) suture lies between the frontal bones and extends from the anterior fontanelle to the prominence between the eyebrows.

Two membrane-filled spaces are present where the suture lines meet. These spaces are referred to as the anterior and posterior **fontanelles**. The anterior fontanelle is the larger of the two and measures approximately 0.8 × 1.2 inches (2 × 3 cm). It is diamond shaped and is positioned where the sagittal, frontal, and coronal sutures intersect. The anterior fontanelle remains open until approximately 18 months of age to allow normal brain growth to occur. The posterior fontanelle is triangular in shape and is much smaller than the anterior fontanelle. It measures approximately 0.8 inch (2 cm) at its widest point. The posterior fontanelle is positioned where the lambdoidal and sagittal sutures meet. Shaped like a small triangle, it closes at approximately 6 to 8 weeks after birth. The location of the fontanelles assists the examiner in determining the position of the fetal skull during a vaginal examination. Important landmarks of the fetal skull are presented in Figure 12-3. ◆

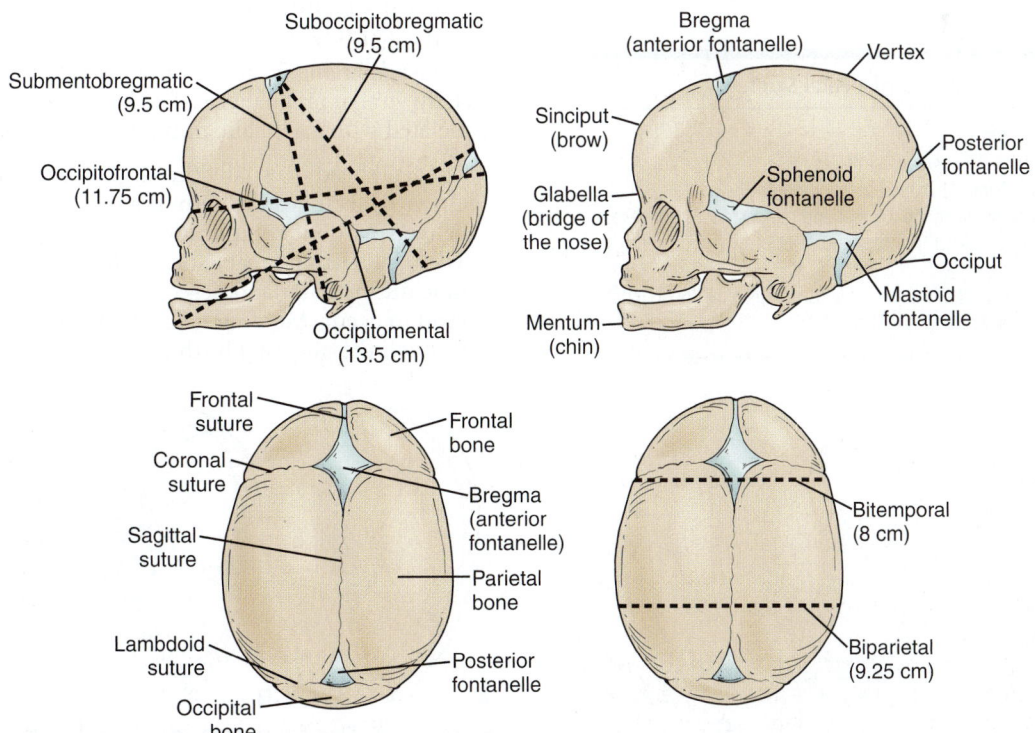

Figure 12-3 Bones, fontanelles, and sutures of the fetal head. An understanding of the placement and relationships of these structures is essential in making an accurate assessment during the labor process.

The fetal skull contains several important landmarks (Box 12-2). There is much variation among skull diameters. As molding occurs during labor, some skull diameters shorten while others lengthen. The head diameters are measured between the various skull landmarks. Most fetuses enter the maternal pelvis in the cephalic presentation, but a number of variations are possible. The biparietal diameter is the major transverse diameter of the fetal head. It is measured between the two parietal bones and averages 3.7 inches (9.5 cm) in a term fetus. The anteroposterior diameter of the fetal head varies according to the degree of flexion. During labor, the most favorable situation occurs when the head becomes fully flexed and the anteroposterior diameter is the suboccipitobregmatic, which averages 3.7 inches (9.5 cm).

 Now Can You—Discuss various factors associated with the process of labor?

1. Define effacement and dilation?
2. Explain what is meant by the "passageway"?
3. Describe anatomical landmarks of the fetal skull?

Fetal Lie

The **fetal lie** refers to the relationship of the long axis of the woman to the long axis of the fetus (Fig. 12-4). If the head to tailbone axis of the fetus is the same as the woman's, the fetus is in a **longitudinal lie**. In more than 99% of pregnancies, the lie is longitudinal. In the longitudinal lie, either the fetal head or the fetal buttocks enter the pelvis first. If the head to tailbone axis of the fetus is at a 90-degree angle to the woman, the fetus is in a **transverse** (horizontal) **lie**. A transverse lie occurs in fewer than 1% of pregnancies. An **oblique lie** is one that is at some angle between the longitudinal and the transverse lie.

Box 12-2 Landmarks of the Fetal Skull

Mentum: fetal chin
Sinciput: anterior area known as the "brow"
Bregma: large, diamond-shaped anterior fontanelle
Vertex: the area between the anterior and the posterior fontanelles
Posterior fontanelle: the intersection between the posterior cranial sutures
Occiput: the area of the fetal skull that is occupied by the occipital bone, beneath the posterior fontanelle (Fig. 12-3).

Fetal Attitude

The fetal **attitude** describes the relationship of the fetus' body parts to one another. The fetus normally assumes an attitude of flexion. In this attitude, the fetal head is flexed so that the chin touches the chest, the arms are flexed and folded across the chest, the thighs are flexed on the abdomen, and the calves are flexed against the posterior aspects of the thighs. This is commonly referred to as the "fetal position."

In moderate flexion, the fetal chin is not touching the chest but is in an alert, or "military position." This position causes the occipital frontal diameter to present to the birth canal. An attitude of moderate flexion usually does not interfere with labor because during descent and flexion the fetal head flexes fully. The fetus in partial extension presents the brow or face of the head to the birth canal.

Flexion of the fetal head (in which the chin touches the chest) is the preferred position for birth because it allows the smallest anteroposterior diameter of the fetal skull to enter into the maternal pelvis. Any other position of the fetal head (other than that of complete flexion) will present with a larger anteroposterior diameter, which can ultimately contribute to a longer, more difficult labor (Fig. 12-5).

Fetal Presentation

The fetal **presentation** refers to the fetal part that enters the pelvic inlet first and leads through the birth canal during labor. The fetal presentation may be cephalic, breech, or shoulder. The part of the fetal body first felt by the examining finger during a vaginal examination is the "**presenting part.**" The presenting part is determined by the fetal lie and attitude.

CEPHALIC PRESENTATION. A **cephalic presentation** identifies that the fetal head will be first to come into contact with the maternal cervix. Cephalic presentations constitute the most desirable position for birth and occur in approximately 95% of pregnancies. The following advantages are associated with a cephalic presentation:

- The fetal head is usually the largest part of the infant. Once the fetal head is born, the rest of the body usually delivers without complications.
- The fetal head is capable of molding. There is sufficient time during labor and descent for molding of the fetal head to occur. Molding helps the fetus to maneuver through the maternal birth passage.

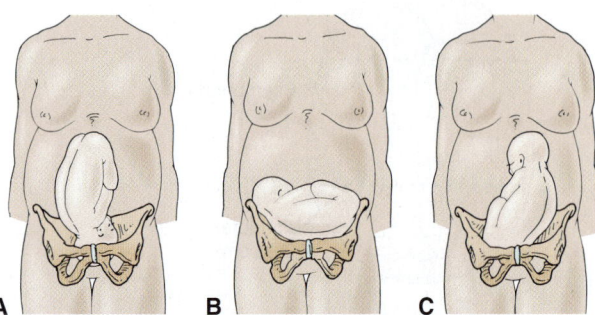

Figure 12-4 The fetal lie refers to the relationship of the long axis of the woman to the long axis of the fetus. *A,* Longitudinal lie. *B,* Transverse lie. *C,* Oblique lie.

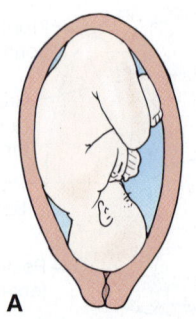 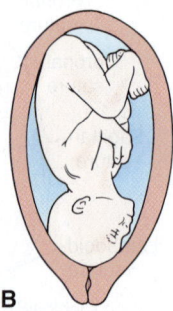 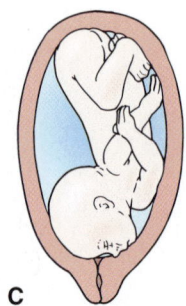

Figure 12-5 The fetal attitude describes the relationship of the fetal body parts to one another. *A,* Flexion (vertex). *B,* Moderate flexion (military). *C,* Extension.

- The fetal head is smooth and round, which is the optimal shape to apply pressure to the cervix and aid in dilation.

There are four types of cephalic presentations: vertex, military, brow, and face (Fig. 12-6):

Vertex. The fetal head presents fully flexed. This is the most frequent and optimal presentation because it allows the smallest suboccipitalbregmatic diameter to present. It is called a "vertex presentation."

Military. In the military position, the fetal head presents in a neutral position, which is neither flexed nor extended. The occipitofrontal diameter presents to the maternal pelvis and the top of the head is the presenting part.

Brow. In the brow position, the fetal head is partly extended. This is an unstable presentation that converts to a vertex if the head flexes or to a face presentation if the head extends. The occipitomental diameter (the largest anteroposterior diameter) presents to the maternal pelvis and the sinciput (fore and upper part of the cranium) is the presenting part.

Face. In the face presentation, the fetal head is fully extended and the occiput is near the fetal spine. The submentobregmatic diameter presents to the maternal pelvis, and the face is the presenting part.

Other presentations (e.g., breech and shoulder) are associated with difficult, prolonged labor and often require cesarean births. They are called malpresentations.

 Now Can You—Discuss passenger characteristics important during labor?

1. Define "fetal lie" and identify three types of fetal lie?
2. Explain what is meant by "fetal attitude"?
3. Describe three advantages associated with a cephalic presentation?

BREECH PRESENTATION. A **breech** presentation occurs when the fetal buttocks enter the maternal pelvis first. Breech presentations occur in approximately 3% of births and are classified according to the attitude of the fetal hips and knees. Breech presentations are more likely to occur in preterm births or in the presence of a fetal abnormality such as hydrocephaly (head enlargement caused by fluid) that prevents the head from entering the pelvis. They are also associated with abnormalities of the maternal uterus or pelvis. Because many factors can compromise the normal labor and birth process associated with breech presentations, delivery is usually accomplished via cesarean section. Several disadvantages are associated with a breech presentation:

- An increased risk for umbilical cord prolapse because the presenting part may not be covering the cervix (i.e., footling breech)
- The presenting part (buttocks or feet) is not as smooth and hard as the fetal head and is less effective in dilating the cervix
- Once the fetal body (abdomen) is delivered, the umbilical cord can become compressed. The fetus must then be delivered expeditiously to prevent hypoxia. Rapid delivery may be difficult because the fetal head is usually the largest body part, and in this situation, there is no time to allow for molding.

There are three types of breech presentations: frank, complete (full), and footling (Fig. 12-7):

Frank. The frank breech is the most common of all breech presentations. In the frank breech position, the fetal legs are completely extended up toward the fetal shoulders. The hips are flexed, the knees are extended, and the fetal buttocks present first in the maternal pelvis.

Complete (Full). The complete, or full, breech position is the same as the flexed position with the fetal buttocks presenting first. The legs are typically flexed. Essentially, this position is a reversal of the common cephalic presentation.

Footling. In the footling breech position, one or both of the fetal legs are extended with one foot ("single footling") or both feet ("double footling") presenting first into the maternal pelvis.

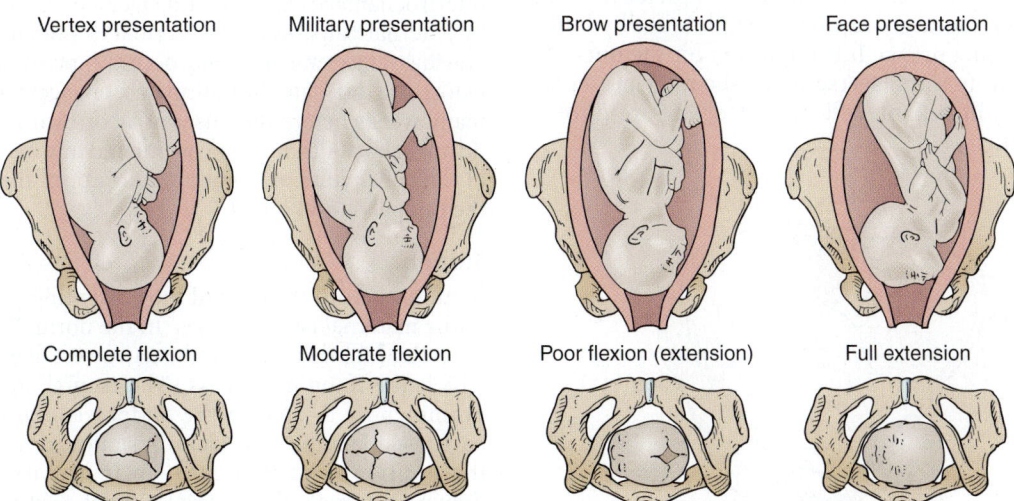

Vertex presentation   Military presentation   Brow presentation   Face presentation

Complete flexion   Moderate flexion   Poor flexion (extension)   Full extension

Figure 12-6 There are four types of cephalic presentation; the vertex presentation with complete flexion is optimal. Fetal presentation refers to the fetal body part that first enters the maternal pelvis.

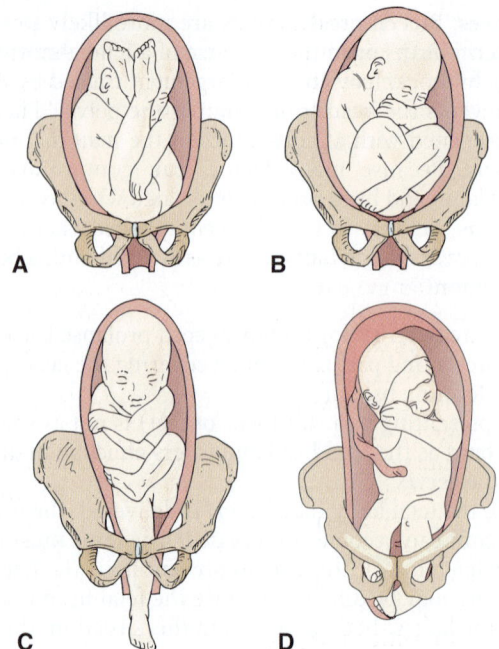

Figure 12-7 There are three types of breech presentation. *A,* Frank. *B,* Complete or full. *C,* Footling (single). *D,* Footling (double).

In response to adverse outcomes that have been associated with vaginal breech births, the American College of Obstetricians and Gynecologists (ACOG, 2006a) has published a Committee Opinion concerning planned breech deliveries.

SHOULDER PRESENTATION. The shoulder presentation is a transverse lie (Fig. 12-8). This presentation is rare and occurs in fewer than 1% of births. When a transverse lie is present, the maternal abdomen appears large from side to side, rather than up and down. In addition, the woman may demonstrate a lower than expected (for the gestational age) fundal height measurement. Although the shoulder is usually the presenting part, the fetal arm, back, abdomen, or side may present in a transverse lie. This presentation occurs most often with preterm birth, high parity, prematurely ruptured membranes, hydramnios, and placenta previa. It is important for the nurse to promptly identify a transverse lie or shoulder presentation because the infant will almost always require a cesarean birth.

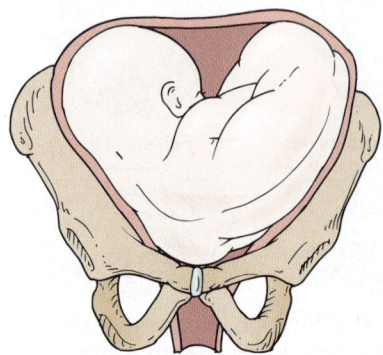

Figure 12-8 Shoulder presentation.

Where Research and Practice Meet:
Optimizing the Breech Birth

The American College of Obstetricians and Gynecologists (ACOG) published a Committee Opinion in 2006 (reaffirmed in 2012) advising that in light of published studies that further clarify the long-term risks of vaginal breech delivery, "the mode of delivery should depend on the experience of the health-care provider. . . . Cesarean delivery will be the preferred mode for most physicians because of the diminishing expertise in vaginal breech delivery" (p. 235). Several investigators (Hannah et al., 2000; Reitberg, Elferink-Stinkens, & Visser, 2005; Su, Hannah, Willan, Ross, & Hannah, 2004) have found that perinatal mortality, neonatal mortality, or serious neonatal morbidity was significantly lower for the planned cesarean section group than for the planned vaginal birth group. Currently, the standard of care in most practices is to deliver all breeches by cesarean section to avoid the potential complications of vaginal breech deliveries such as cord prolapse, head entrapment, birth asphyxia, and birth trauma.

Now Can You—Discuss the breech and shoulder presentations?

1. Identify three types of breech presentations?
2. Explain three disadvantages of a breech presentation?
3. Describe how the nurse could identify a shoulder presentation?

PASSAGEWAY + PASSENGER

The passageway and the passenger have been identified as two of the factors that affect labor. The next "P" is the relationship between the passageway (maternal pelvis) and the passenger (fetus and membranes). The nurse assesses the relationship between the two when determining the engagement, station, and fetal position.

Engagement

Engagement is said to have occurred when the widest diameter of the fetal presenting part has passed through the pelvic inlet. In a cephalic presentation, the largest diameter is the biparietal; in breech presentations, it is the intertrochanteric diameter. Engagement can be determined by external palpation or by vaginal examination. In primigravidas, engagement usually occurs approximately 2 weeks before the due date. In multiparas, engagement may occur many weeks before the onset of labor or it may take place during labor. Although engagement confirms the adequacy of the pelvic inlet, it is not an indicator of the adequacy of the midpelvis and outlet.

Station

Station refers to the level of the presenting part in relation to the maternal ischial spines. In the normal female pelvis, the ischial spines represent the narrowest diameter through which the fetus must pass. The ischial spines, blunted prominences located in the midpelvis, have been designated as a landmark to identify station zero. To visualize the location of station zero, an imaginary line may be drawn between the ischial spines. Engagement has occurred when the presenting part is at station zero. When the presenting part lies above the maternal ischial spines, it is at a minus station. Therefore, a station of minus 5

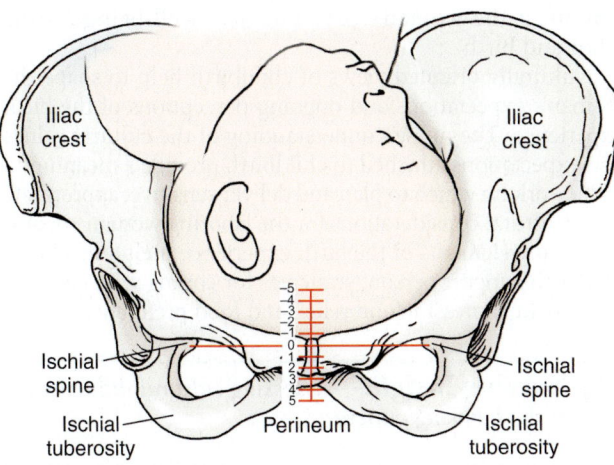

Figure 12-9 Station.

(–5) cm indicates that the presenting part is at the pelvic inlet. Positive numbers indicate that the presenting part has descended past the ischial spines. A presenting part below the level of the ischial spines is considered to be a positive station. A station of +4 cm indicates that the presenting part is at the pelvic outlet (Fig. 12-9). During labor, the presenting part should continue to descend into the pelvis, indicating labor progress. As labor advances and the

presenting part descends, the station should also progress to a numerically higher positive station. If the station does not change in the presence of strong, regular contractions, this finding may indicate a problem with the relationship between the maternal pelvis and the fetus ("cephalopelvic disproportion").

Position

Position refers to the location of a fixed reference point on the fetal presenting part in relation to a specific quadrant of the maternal pelvis (Fig. 12-10). The presenting part can be right anterior, left anterior, right posterior, and left posterior. These four quadrants designate whether the presenting part is directed toward the front, back, right, or left of the passageway.

Four landmarks of the fetus are used to describe the relationship of the presenting part to the maternal pelvis. In a vertex presentation, the occiput (O) is used. For a face presentation, the chin (M for mentum) is used. In a breech presentation, the sacrum (S) is used, and for a shoulder presentation, (A) for acromion process of the shoulder is used. Fetal position may be described as:

- Right (R) or left (L) side of the maternal pelvis
- The landmark of the presenting part: occiput (O), mentum (M), sacrum (S), or acromion process (A)
- Anterior (A), posterior (P), transverse (T): This designation depends on whether the landmark is in the front, back, or side of the maternal pelvis

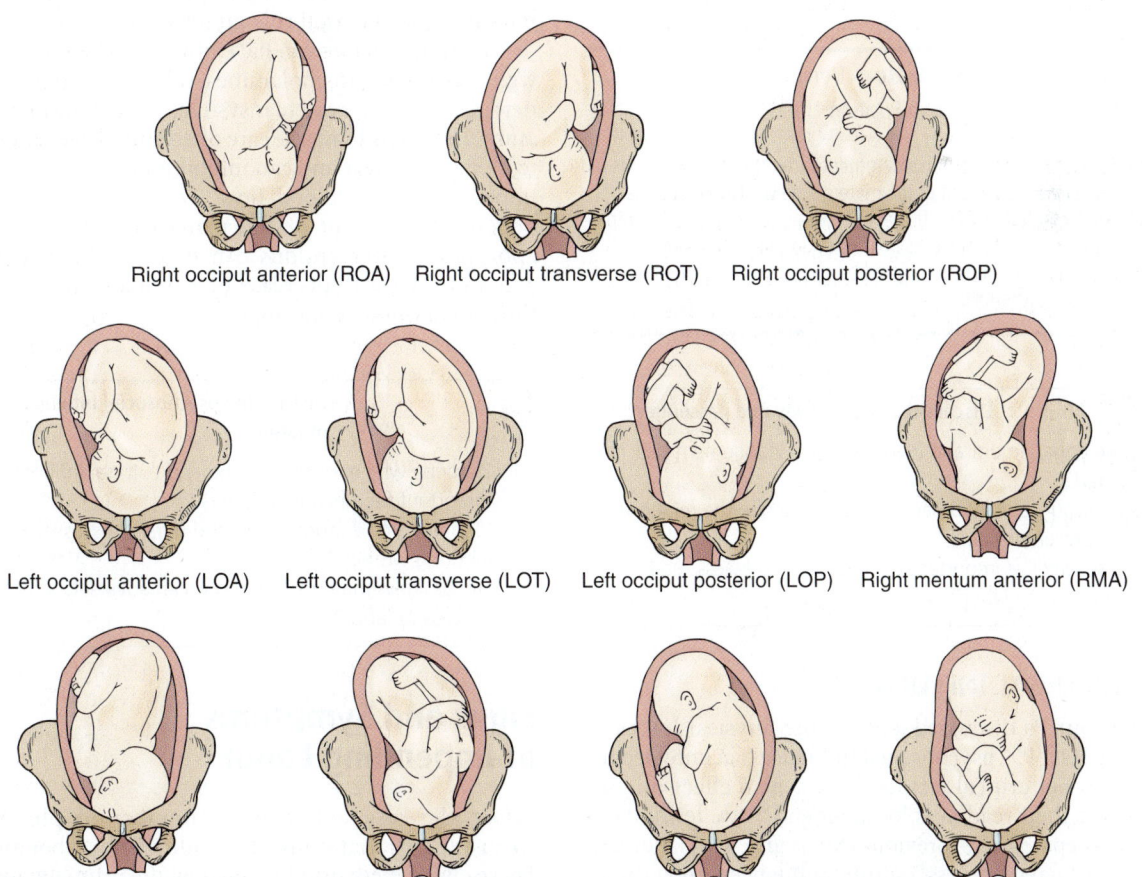

Right occiput anterior (ROA) Right occiput transverse (ROT) Right occiput posterior (ROP)

Left occiput anterior (LOA) Left occiput transverse (LOT) Left occiput posterior (LOP) Right mentum anterior (RMA)

Right mentum posterior (RMP) Left mentum anterior (LMA) Left sacrum anterior (LSA) Left sacrum posterior (LSP)

Figure 12-10 Fetal presentations and positions. The position refers to how the presenting fetal part is positioned in relation to a specific quadrant of the maternal pelvis: front, back, or side.

It is important for the nurse to assess the position of the fetus to identify whether the fetus is in an optimal position for a vaginal birth. To do so, the nurse uses inspection and palpation of the maternal abdomen and vaginal examination. Use of the abbreviated notations (listed earlier) helps to convey essential information to other members of the health-care team. For example, when the fetal occiput is directed toward the maternal back (a posterior lie) and to the right of the birth passageway, the nurse would chart "ROP," to indicate right occiput–posterior. The fetal position most common, and most favorable for birth, is the right occiput–anterior (ROA). Identification of a malpresentation such as a footling breech or transverse lie is important because the presence of a malpresentation may signal the need for a cesarean delivery. Identification of a posterior lie may identify the potential for a longer labor because the fetus may attempt to rotate to an OA position. In addition, the nurse must be aware that the fetal position will vary as the fetus changes position to move through the different diameters of the maternal pelvis.

In some situations, the physician may have the option to attempt a fetal rotation. Prenatally, an external cephalic version may be performed in an attempt to rotate an identified breech presentation. A forceps rotation from a transverse or posterior position to an anterior position may also be indicated during a prolonged second stage of labor. However, as with any procedure, these maneuvers are associated with risks and benefits that must be presented to the patient for informed consent. (See Chapter 14 for further discussion.)

Critical Nursing Action Determining and Documenting Fetal Position

During the assessment, the nurse determines that the fetal occiput is in the right anterior quadrant of the maternal pelvis. The position is correctly documented as ROA. If the fetus were presenting in the frank breech position with the buttocks positioned to the left maternal posterior quadrant, the position would be correctly documented as LSP (left sacrum posterior).

 Now Can You—Discuss the passageway and passenger?

1. Define engagement and identify when engagement has occurred?
2. List the four fetal landmarks used to describe the relationship of the presenting part?
3. Discuss why it is important for the nurse to assess fetal position during labor?

PSYCHOSOCIAL INFLUENCES

The first four Ps discussed address the physical forces of labor. The last "P" (psychosocial influences) acknowledges the many other critical factors that have an effect on parents such as their readiness for labor and birth, level of educational preparedness, previous experience with labor and birth, emotional readiness, cultural influences, and ethnicity. Transition into the maternal role, and most likely, also into the paternal role, is facilitated by a positive childbirth experience. A number of internal and external influences can affect the woman's psychological well-being during labor and birth.

Culturally oriented views of childbirth help to shape the woman's expectations and ongoing perceptions of the birth experience. The nurse's understanding of the cultural values and expectations attached to childbirth provide a meaningful framework on which to plan and deliver sensitive, appropriate care. Cultural considerations for the laboring woman encompass many elements of the birth experience including choice of a birth support person, strategies for coping with contractions, pain expression and relief, and food preferences.

 Nursing Insight—*Assessing cultural influences of the laboring patient*

To provide culturally sensitive care to the laboring patient, the nurse should consider:

- The patient's and family's level of comfort with the nurse's "language" and whether an interpreter is needed
- Who is the designated birth support person and what will be the extent of this person's role
- The patient's level of comfort with touch
- If any special rituals or practices will be used during the childbirth experience

Studies have revealed that marked anxiety, fear, and fatigue can adversely affect the woman's ability to cope with the demands of labor. A negative childbirth experience can have far-reaching implications, interfering with bonding and maternal role attainment.

Emotional factors can have physiological implications as well. Maternal catecholamines (chemicals that affect the nervous and cardiovascular systems, metabolic rate, temperature, and smooth muscle) are often stimulated as a response to anxiety and fear and can inhibit uterine contractions and impede placental blood flow. During labor, the nurse's ongoing assessment of the maternal psyche along with appropriate interventions can help facilitate therapeutic communication to decrease or eliminate anxiety and fear through discussion and support.

 Now Can You—Discuss the psychosocial influences of labor?

1. Describe why maternal psyche and cultural influences are important factors during labor?
2. Identify three culturally oriented nursing assessments for the laboring woman?
3. Discuss how maternal emotions can adversely affect the process of labor?

Signs and Symptoms of Impending Labor

Before the onset of labor, a number of physiological changes occur that signal the readiness for labor and birth. These changes are usually noted by the primigravid woman at about 38 weeks of gestation. In multigravidas, they may not take place until labor begins. It is important for nurses to empower pregnant women and their families by teaching them about the signs and symptoms of impending labor. Providing guidelines about when to contact the health-care provider or come to the birth facility helps to demystify the sometimes confusing events that surround birth and lessen the anxieties that can accompany the onset of labor.

LIGHTENING

At about 38 weeks in the primigravid pregnancy, the presenting part (usually the fetal head) settles downward into the pelvic cavity, causing the uterus to move downward as well. This process, called **lightening**, marks the beginning of engagement. As the uterus moves downward, the woman may state that her baby has "dropped." She may also report changes in the appearance of her abdomen such as a flattening of the upper area and an enhanced protrusion of the lower area. This downward settling of the uterus may decrease the upward pressure on the diaphragm and result in easier breathing. The downward settling may also lead to the following maternal symptoms:

- Leg cramps or pains
- Increased pelvic pressure
- Increased urinary frequency
- Increased venous stasis, causing edema in the lower extremities
- Increased vaginal secretions because of congestion in the vaginal mucosa

BRAXTON HICKS CONTRACTIONS

As the pregnancy approaches term, most women become more aware of irregular contractions called Braxton Hicks contractions. As the contractions increase in frequency (they may occur as often as every 10 to 20 minutes), they may be associated with increased discomfort. Braxton Hicks contractions are usually felt in the abdomen or groin region, and patients may mistake them for true labor. It is believed that these contractions contribute to the preparation of the cervix and uterus for the advent of true labor. Braxton Hicks contractions do not lead to dilation or effacement of the cervix, and thus are often termed "**false labor.**"

CERVICAL CHANGES

In the nonpregnant woman, the cervix is normally rigid. In preparation for passage of the fetus, the cervix undergoes many physiological changes. The cervix softens ("cervical ripening"), stretches, and thins and eventually is taken up into the lower segment of the uterus. This softening and thinning is called cervical effacement.

BLOODY SHOW

During pregnancy the cervix is plugged with mucus. The mucus plug acts as a protective barrier for the uterus and its contents throughout the pregnancy. As the cervix begins to soften, stretch, and thin through effacement, there may be rupture of the small cervical capillaries. The added pressure created by engagement of the presenting part may lead to the expulsion of a blood-tinged mucus plug, called **bloody show.** Its presence often indicates that labor will begin within 24 to 48 hours. Late in pregnancy, vaginal examination that involves cervical manipulation may also produce a bloody discharge that can be confused with bloody show.

RUPTURE OF THE MEMBRANES

About 12% of pregnant women experience spontaneous rupture of the amniotic sac ("ruptured membranes" or "ruptured bag of waters") prior to the onset of labor. In the majority of pregnancies, the amniotic membranes rupture once labor is well established, either spontaneously or by **amniotomy**, the artificial rupture of the membranes by the primary care provider. Rupture of the membranes is a critical event in pregnancy. Assessment by the woman if rupture occurs at home, or by the nurse if it occurs in the birthing unit, is essential. If the membranes do rupture at home, the woman should be taught to immediately contact the nurse at the provider's office or at the birthing center who will advise her to report for an examination. It is important for the woman to note the color, amount, and odor of the amniotic fluid. The fluid should be clear and odorless. Often it contains white specks (vernix caseosa) and fetal hair (lanugo). A yellow-green tinged amniotic fluid may indicate infection or fetal passage of meconium, and this finding always signals the need for further assessment and fetal heart rate monitoring. Urinary incontinence (frequently associated with urgency, coughing, and sneezing) is sometimes confused with ruptured membranes. The presence of amniotic fluid can be confirmed by a Nitrazine tape test, an AmniSure test, or by a fern test (Procedure 12-2).

ENERGY SPURT

Toward the end of the pregnancy, some women experience a sudden increase in energy coupled with a desire to complete household preparations for the new baby. Some refer to this energy spurt as "nesting." The energy spurt may be related to an increase in the hormone adrenaline, which is needed to support the woman during the work of labor. Women should be cautioned not to overexert themselves doing household chores and instead to "store up" their energy for the childbirth process.

WEIGHT LOSS

Before the onset of labor, changes in the levels of estrogen and progesterone can lead to electrolyte shifts and may result in a reduction in fluid retention. The increased fluid loss can lead to a weight loss of up to 3 pounds (0.5 to 1.5 kg).

GASTROINTESTINAL DISTURBANCES

Some women experience gastrointestinal disturbances (diarrhea, nausea, vomiting, or indigestion) as a sign of impending labor. The etiology of the gastrointestinal disturbances is generally unknown.

Distinguishing True Labor From False Labor

Recognizing the difference between true and false labor is important for the pregnant woman and her nurse (Table 12-1). True labor contractions lead to progressive dilation and effacement of the cervix. True labor contractions occur with regularity and increase in frequency, duration, and intensity. The pain of true labor usually begins in the woman's lower back region and radiates to the abdomen. The pain often intensifies with activity such as walking. In contrast, false labor contractions are irregular

Procedure 12-2 Assessing for Amniotic Fluid

Purpose

Assessing for the presence of amniotic fluid helps determine whether the membranes have ruptured. There are three tests that may be used to detect amniotic fluid: the Nitrazine tape test, the AmniSure test, and the fern test.

Equipment

- Nitrazine test tape or the AmniSure kit (contains the test strip, sterile swab, and test vial)
- Sterile gloves
- Sterile speculum
- Sterile cotton swab and glass slide
- Microscope

Steps

1. Gather the necessary supplies. Confirm the patient's identity, using at least two patient identifiers according to the institutional policy. Explain the procedure and purpose of the examination to the patient, noting what she will experience and what the results will indicate. Ensure privacy. Wash and dry hands and position the patient in a dorsal lithotomy position.

   RATIONALE: *Hand washing helps to prevent the spread of microorganisms. Explanations help to decrease anxiety and promote patient understanding and cooperation. The dorsal lithotomy position facilitates collection of a specimen that is least likely to be contaminated.*

2. Assess for latex allergies.

   RATIONALE: *To prevent injury from latex exposure; if the patient has a latex allergy, use nonlatex gloves.*

3. Ask the patient if she has noticed any leakage of fluid from her vagina.

4. Assess for the presence of amniotic fluid before other tests that require the use of lubricant (such as vaginal examination).

   RATIONALE: *Lubricant may alter the pH of amniotic fluid and contaminate the test result.*

5. Don sterile gloves. With one hand, spread the labia to expose the vaginal opening.

   For the Nitrazine tape test:

   With the other hand, place a 2-inch (5 cm) piece of Nitrazine tape against the vaginal opening, ensuring contact with enough fluid to wet the tape. Alternately, a sterile cotton-tipped applicator may be used to obtain fluid from the vagina. The applicator is then touched to the Nitrazine tape.

6. Remove the tape. Compare the color of the tape with the color guide on the Nitrazine tape container. If the tape turns blue-green, gray, or deep blue, amniotic fluid is present. If the tape remains beige, no amniotic fluid has been detected.

   RATIONALE: *Amniotic fluid is alkaline, with a pH of 6.5 to 7.5. Urine and vaginal secretions are usually acidic.*

Caution: Blood, *Trichomonas vaginalis*, and other substances may also turn the Nitrazine test strip alkaline or blue.

For the AmniSure test:

a. Hold the cap secure on the solvent vial and shake the vial to ensure that all the liquid in the vial has reached the bottom of the vial.

b. Remove the cap and place the vial upright on a flat, secure surface.

c. Carefully remove the sterile swab from the package.

d. Grasp the swab in the middle of the stick and insert the swab tip into the vagina until the fingers make contact with the patient's skin (no more than 2" to 3" [5 to 7 cm]).

e. Hold the swab in the vagina for 1 minute and then remove it.

f. Carefully place the tip of the swab in the vial and rotate it in the solvent for 1 minute to ensure that the vaginal secretions are thoroughly mixed with the solvent.

g. Remove the swab and discard it in an appropriate receptacle.

h. Open the foil packet containing the test strip.

i. Insert the white end of the test strip into the vial with the solvent, making sure the arrows are within the solvent. Hold the test strip in the solvent for no less than 5 minutes and no more than 10 minutes.

j. Remove the test strip from the vial if 2 stripes appear clearly on the strip (no earlier than 5 minutes) or after 10 minutes sharp.

k. Place the test strip on a clean, dry, flat surface to read the result.

   1. If only one line (a "control line") is visible, there is no rupture of membranes (negative result).

   2. If two lines ("control line" and "test line") are visible, rupture of membranes has occurred (positive result).

   3. If no lines are visible, the test result is invalid and may need to be repeated.

   RATIONALE: *The AmniSure test detects trace amounts of placental alpha-1-microglobulin (PAMG-1), one of the amniotic fluid proteins that appears in vaginal discharge after rupture of the membranes.*

Caution: The AmniSure test may not be accurate after digital cervical examinations (perform the test before digital examination). AmniSure test results may not be reliable for patients with placenta previa (i.e., a significant amount of blood on the swab may cause inaccurate test results; a trace amount of blood on the swab may still produce accurate results). Avoid performing the AmniSure test less than 6 hours after the use of vaginal medication.

Procedure 12-2 Assessing for Amniotic Fluid *(continued)*

For the fern test:

a. When the Nitrazine tape or AmniSure tests are unavailable or have not confirmed the presence of amniotic fluid, the nurse may insert a speculum and sterile cotton swab to collect a sample of fluid from the posterior vagina. The swab is smeared on a glass slide and allowed to dry. The glass slide is then placed on the microscope. The presence of a ferning pattern confirms the presence of amniotic fluid. The fern test is often indicated if premature rupture of the membranes (PROM) is suspected.

   RATIONALE: *Dried amniotic fluid shows a fern pattern because of its high estrogen content.*

b. Properly discard all disposable equipment in a biohazard container and perform hand hygiene.

c. Document the findings on the admission or labor record.

d. Inform the patient of the findings.

What If?

What if you have performed both a Nitrazine tape test and a fern test and have obtained the following findings:

Nitrazine test—positive

Fern test—negative

You may:

- Assess for the presence of infection—bacterial vaginosis (BV) and *Trichomonas vaginalis* thrive in an alkaline environment and the presence of these microorganisms may account for the Nitrazine tape color change.
- Inquire about recent sexual intercourse—seminal fluid is alkaline; its presence may account for the Nitrazine tape color change.
- Perform an AmniSure test—which specifically tests for an amniotic fluid protein.

> **Documentation**
>
> 8/30/09. 0430 Sterile speculum exam performed, large amount of clear, nonmalodorous fluid noted in vagina. Specimen obtained, fern test positive. Procedure tolerated well by patient, fetal heart rate 148 bpm by auscultation.
>
> —L. Lopez, R.N.

Table 12-1 Distinguishing True From False Labor	
True Labor	**False Labor**
• Contractions are at regular intervals.	• Contractions are irregular.
• Contractions increase in frequency, duration, and intensity.	• Usually there is no increase in frequency, duration, or intensity of contractions.
• Pains usually begin in lower back, radiating to the abdomen.	• Pains usually occur in the abdominal region.
• Dilation and effacement of the cervix are progressive.	• There is no change in the cervix.
• Activity such as walking usually increases labor pains.	• Walking may lessen the pain.

and usually do not change in intensity and duration. False labor does not lead to dilation and effacement of the cervix. The pain of false labor is usually felt in the abdominal region, and often stops with activities such as walking, position changes, and hot showers or other comfort measures.

Depending on the assessment findings, the nurse can help validate the next steps the woman should take. Any pregnant woman who arrives at the birth unit complaining of contractions must be carefully evaluated. After the assessment, if the maternity nurse confirms normal findings and intact membranes, the woman is sent home. For many, this can be a disappointing and frustrating experience. It is important for the nurse to provide reassurance that distinguishing true from false labor is difficult. Signs and

symptoms of true labor should be reviewed in a sensitive, supportive manner, and the patient should be instructed about when to return to the birth unit.

"What to say"—*Questions to ask the patient who calls the birth unit*

A pregnant woman calls the birth unit to determine if she should come in for an evaluation or remain at home. The nurse conducts the telephone assessment by asking the following questions:

- "What is your due date?"
- "Are your membranes ruptured?" or "Did your water break?" and "Are you having any bleeding or vaginal discharge?"
- "Describe your contractions: When did they start? How frequent? How long? How strong?"
- "Is the fetus active?"
- "What helps with the discomfort?"
- "Who is with you?"

Now Can You—Identify true labor?

1. List four signs that may signify impending labor?
2. Compare and contrast signs of true labor versus false labor? Discuss how they can be differentiated?
3. Explain when a woman experiencing contractions at term should be instructed to go to the hospital?

Childbirth Settings and Labor Support

The decision about where to give birth is influenced by several factors: geographical location, socioeconomic status, the patient's preference, and the absence or presence of pregnancy complications. The size of the community often dictates the type and number of maternity health-care facilities and the available primary care providers who may include family physicians, obstetricians, and certified nurse midwives (CNMs).

Large urban centers have hospitals with birthing units or birthing centers. Some of the units may offer labor options such as whirlpool baths. Other settings may provide a home-like environment for the expectant couple. Taking a tour of the available birth settings as part of prenatal education classes can help the pregnant woman and her partner develop an understanding of what to expect during the childbirth experience.

The woman's socioeconomic status and whether or not she has health insurance also affect the choices available for labor and birth. Some pregnant women who have no pregnancy complications may choose to have their prenatal care and birth managed by a CNM, and they may also plan for a home birth.

The patient usually determines whether or not a support person accompanies her to the birthing unit and remains throughout the labor and birth. This decision is based on personal preferences and may reflect cultural or religious practices. The woman's partner or the baby's father is the most common labor support person, although the woman's mother or friend may also serve as a support person, especially if the patient is single. The nurse can identify the patient's preference for a support person by asking a question such as, "Who is the main person whom you want to stay with you during labor?"

In some centers, women may use a **doula** as a labor support person. The doula is a woman who has received professional training and is experienced in childbirth. The doula's role is to provide continuous information and physical and emotional support to the woman and her partner before, during, and immediately after the birth. She does not function in a clinical role but instead specializes in providing comfort measures to decrease the woman's anxiety. Breathing techniques, application of hot and cold, and massage are strategies often used to enhance comfort and the progress of labor (Klaus, Kennell, & Klaus, 2012).

 Where Research and Practice Meet:
Alternative Institutional Birth Settings

In this Cochrane review of alternative institutional (home-like) versus conventional institutional settings for birth (in women who preferred and required little or no medical intervention), Hodnett and colleagues (2010) reviewed nine trials of over 10,000 women. The findings revealed a number of benefits associated with alternative institutional settings for childbirth: increased maternal satisfaction with the intrapartum care, increased initiation and continuation of breastfeeding, an increased incidence of spontaneous vaginal births, and a reduced likelihood of medical interventions including analgesia/anesthesia and episiotomies.

The doula assists the family in gathering information concerning the labor process and available options before childbirth. If a cesarean birth is required, the doula may accompany the laboring woman into the surgical suite. Doulas also provide some postpartum services. In some situations, the family hires the doula. Doulas can be paid hospital employees, or volunteer doulas may be available in certain settings. When needed, the bilingual doula can be an essential team member in helping to promote a positive childbirth experience for the woman and her family (Maher, Crawford-Carr, & Neidigh, 2013).

 Now Can You—Discuss childbirth settings and support persons?

1. Discuss various childbirth settings and factors that may influence the woman's choice?
2. Describe the role of a doula?

Routine Hospital and Birth Center Admission Procedures

In the third trimester it is important for the prenatal care nurse to explain the differences between true and false labor and to teach the patient about when to go to the birthing center. Table 12-2 summarizes the circumstances that warrant going to the birthing center. The nurse should reinforce this information during each prenatal visit.

---

 legal alert—Understand federal regulations that relate to obstetric care

The federal regulation known as *The Emergency Medical Treatment and Active Labor Act (EMTALA)* was created to ensure that all women receive emergency treatment or active labor care whenever such treatment is sought. Under the EMTALA regulation, true labor is considered to be an emergency medical condition. Thus the nurse working in a birthing unit must be familiar with the full range of responsibilities included in the EMTALA regulations: (1) provide services to pregnant women when an urgent pregnancy problem such as labor, rupture of the membranes, decreased fetal movement, or recent trauma is experienced and (2) fully document all relevant information to include assessment findings, interventions implemented, and the patient's response to the care provided. Any pregnant woman who presents to an obstetric triage is considered to be experiencing "true labor" until a qualified health-care provider determines that she is not (ACOG, 2013).

Once the woman arrives at the birthing center, the role of the nurse is twofold: to establish a positive relationship with the patient and her family and support person and to assess the status of the patient and her fetus.

ESTABLISHING A POSITIVE RELATIONSHIP

The onset of labor is a time of many emotions for the woman and her family. There can be excitement, fear, and anxiety. The role of the nurse in recognizing these emotions and creating a caring, trusting relationship is

Table 12-2 Providing Patient Guidelines for Reporting to the Birthing Center

Questions to Ask the Patient	Guidelines for Admission
Describe your contractions: frequency, duration, and intensity?	Primigravida: Contractions are regular, occur about every 5 minutes for at least 1 hour. Multipara: Contractions are regular, occur about every 10 minutes for at least 1 hour.
Have your membranes ruptured?	*Any* gush of fluid needs to be evaluated, even if there are no contractions.
Is there any vaginal bleeding?	The mucus plug or "bloody show" is usually pink or dark red. Any bright red bleeding requires immediate evaluation.
Has there been a decrease in the movement of the baby?	Any decrease in fetal movement signals the need to report to the birthing center.
Has there been any change in your health?	Any cause for worry or anxiety in the pregnant woman needs to be explored by the nurse and may lead to admission.

paramount to a positive birth experience. The nurse needs to respect individual differences in the woman's knowledge and understanding of childbirth and recognize the cultural or religious practices that may influence the experience. The nurse needs to remain nonjudgmental, particularly with patients who have not had adequate prenatal care or who have made unhealthy lifestyle choices during the pregnancy.

To foster a positive and therapeutic relationship, the nurse creates a patient-centered atmosphere that encourages questions and the sharing of information (Box 12-3). Some women have prepared written childbirth plans that describe their expectations of the experience. If the patient doesn't have a birth plan, the nurse may wish to use a template with simple questions about her particular preferences, and this information can be used to guide care. Getting to know each patient's expectations for her childbirth experience constitutes an important element in the relationship, and understanding and supporting the birth plan fosters patient autonomy and may lead to enhanced satisfaction with the childbirth experience (Anderson & Kilpatrick, 2012; Association of Women's Health, Obstetric & Neonatal Nurses [AWHONN], 2009). The nurse must also recognize when an interpreter is needed to assist in the understanding and exchange of information.

Touch is an integral aspect of the nurse–patient relationship during labor and birth. Touch can convey caring and provide comfort. The nurse continuously assesses the patient's response to touch and provides intimate care that is culturally sensitive.

COLLECTING ADMISSION DATA

The nurse uses multiple sources and data collection methods to compile a comprehensive database to plan and deliver individualized care to the woman in labor. The prenatal record provides data regarding the current pregnancy and previous pregnancies and birth outcomes for the multiparous woman. Measurements such as maternal weight gain, fundal height, blood pressure, fetal heart rate patterns; laboratory values such as blood type and Rh factor; results from diagnostic tests such as amniocentesis; non-stress tests; and ultrasound examinations provide the basis for determining intrapartal risk.

The admission interview provides the nurse with information about the woman's reason for coming to the birthing center, her understanding and expectations of the labor and birth process, her subjective experience of the labor, and psychosocial and cultural factors that can impact her birth experience. The fetal assessment, including presentation, fetal heart rate (FHR), and movement, provides essential data regarding fetal well-being. Maternal vital signs, particularly blood pressure and temperature, and the assessment of current labor status (uterine contraction patterns, cervical dilation and effacement, fetal station, and rupture of membranes) provide important baseline labor data. A systematic physical assessment provides the nurse and other care providers with overall health data, and various laboratory tests, such as hematocrit, blood glucose, and HIV status, give further direction for the individual plan of care.

Initial Admission Assessments

For women who have received prenatal care, the prenatal care record is sent to the birthing center prior to the expected due date. The information is stored and readily available when the laboring patient reports there for care. Women without a prenatal care record require a more extensive assessment upon admission to the birth setting.

THE FOCUSED ASSESSMENT

On admission to the birthing unit, the nurse initiates a focused assessment to determine the condition of the mother and fetus and the progression of the labor. The data collected answer these critical questions and help the nurse to establish priorities for care:

- Is this true labor, and if so, is birth imminent?
- Are there any factors that increase risk to the mother or fetus?

Box 12-3 Characteristics of Patient-Centered Care for Childbearing Families

In a "Call to Action" statement on quality patient care in labor and delivery, the Association of Women's Health, Obstetric and Neonatal Nurses (AWHONN) (2011a) described the nature of "patient-centered" care: Health-care providers and the system they practice within "accept that the values, culture, choices, and preferences of a woman and her family are relevant within the context of promoting optimal health outcomes" (p. 151). Treating all childbearing women with kindness, respect, dignity, and cultural sensitivity throughout the maternity care experience serve as the overarching principles of patient-centered care, which is enhanced when women are provided with supportive resources (e.g., education and skilled attendants). Patient-centered care requires a balance between "maternal-child safety and well being with the woman's needs and desires" (p. 151).

The nurse assesses the fetus' well-being by recording the fetal heart rate (FHR) and noting the FHR in response to uterine contractions. Uterine contractions are quantified as the number of contractions present in a 10-minute window, averaged over 30 minutes, and notes other factors such as duration, intensity, and relaxation time between the contractions (Macones, Hankins, Spong, Hauth, & Moore, 2008).

The nurse also assesses fetal movement. If the woman reports that her membranes have ruptured, the nurse validates the presence of amniotic fluid (see Procedure 12-2) and examines the amniotic fluid for color and odor. The nurse assesses the patient's vital signs to establish a baseline for comparison during the labor and birth. An elevation in blood pressure may be a sign of pregnancy-induced hypertension (PIH). An elevated temperature may signal infection. The nurse also assesses the progression of the labor by monitoring the pattern of uterine contractions for frequency, duration, and intensity. The nurse further assesses the labor status by evaluating cervical dilation and effacement and fetal station, presentation, and position.

A patient who states "I feel like pushing" may be indicating that the birth is imminent. Important questions to ask this patient upon admission include the following:

- What is your name? Your support person's name?
- Have you received prenatal care? Who is your care provider?
- How many pregnancies and births have you had? Were the deliveries vaginal or cesarean? Were there any difficulties with previous deliveries?
- What is your due date? When was your last normal menstrual period?
- Have your membranes ruptured? What time? Describe the fluid.
- Have you had any complications with this pregnancy?
- Do you have any allergies?
- Describe your contractions—mild, moderate, or intense. When did your contractions begin? How are you coping?
- Are you taking any medications—prescribed and/or over-the-counter? Do you use illegal/street drugs? Do you smoke? Do you drink alcoholic beverages?
- When did you last eat or drink anything and what was it?
- Have you prepared a birth plan? Do you have any cultural preferences related to your labor and birth?

If the nurse determines that the fetal or maternal assessments are not normal, or that the birth is imminent, the physician or primary care provider is notified immediately. If the assessments are normal, and birth does not appear to be imminent, the nurse can then complete a more thorough admission assessment, which would include a systematic physical assessment.

THE PSYCHOSOCIAL ASSESSMENT

An important, yet sometimes challenging part of the data collection is the psychosocial assessment. Understanding the woman's behavioral responses to the pregnancy and childbirth experience allows the nurse to support and strengthen the identified coping mechanisms. Obtaining information that addresses questions such as "What was the previous birth experience like?" "How is the patient handling the labor pain?" and "Who is providing labor support for her?" helps the nurse to better meet the patient's and her support person's needs.

The nurse completes a social assessment, collecting information about the woman's family and support systems and living conditions. Questions about family violence can be particularly difficult. If the nurse suspects partner abuse, the patient should be interviewed alone in a private place where she feels safe.

Assessing the woman's social and lifestyle habits can also be difficult. Questions about drug and alcohol use and sexually transmitted infections are often embarrassing. The nurse can facilitate the sharing of this information through the establishment of a caring and nonjudgmental relationship with the patient.

❝What to say❞—*Asking the difficult questions*

Asking closed-ended questions such as "Do you drink alcohol?" may elicit a quick "No" response. Asking more directed and open questions such as "How many drinks do you have each day?" may encourage a more detailed response. The nurse should remember that a caring and nonjudgmental attitude, in a private, nonthreatening environment, helps to foster a trusting nurse–patient relationship.

THE CULTURAL ASSESSMENT

To provide care that is culturally relevant, the nurse must assess the patient's cultural preferences, practices, and values related to labor and childbirth. Issues such as care provider gender preference, comfort level with intimate touch, and the presence or absence of a labor support person may be culturally determined. The woman's responses to the labor pain, her acceptance or rejection of labor support interventions, and her emotional responses to the newborn can be culturally based.

LABORATORY TESTS

Laboratory testing is a routine component of the admission process. Tests for blood type and Rh factor, complete blood count, hemoglobin and hematocrit, and blood glucose are generally obtained. Blood tests for syphilis, hepatitis B, and HIV are also collected. The urine specimen is tested for the presence of protein, glucose, and ketones.

Documentation of Admission

Each birth setting has documentation forms and set protocols to be completed with patient admissions (Figs. 12-11 and 12-12). Collecting a complete health and childbirth history and performing a physical examination of the patient and her fetus provide an essential foundation for the care and support to be given during labor and birth. Once the admission assessments have been completed, the nurse documents the information using the birth setting's recording procedures, notifies the patient's primary care provider of the admission status, and

Labor and Delivery Admission Record

PT. NAME: _____   AGE: _____   CARE PROVIDER: _____

ADMIT DATE/TIME: _____

EDC	LMP	Weeks of Gestation	Gravida	Para	Term	Preterm	Spontaneous Abortion	Elective Abortion	Living	Stillborn	C-Section	VBAC

T	P	R	BP	Height	Weight	Pre-Pregnant weight	Weight Gain	How Admitted		Accompanied By	

Date/Time Care Provider Notified	Date/Time Seen by Care Provider	Reason for Admission

---

Onset of Labor   **Contraction Frequency (Min)**

Dilatation (cm)   **Effacement (%)**   **Station**

Contraction Duration (Sec)   **Contraction Quality**
                   None   Mild   Moderate   Strong

Pelvic Exam By:

Pain Level Assessment: *Pain scale 0–10*

Admission Membranes: Intact   Ruptured   Bulging   Unknown

Fern: N/A   Negative   Positive   Equivocal

AROM/SROM (Date/Time):

Amniotic Fluid:

Amount: None N/A Copious Large Moderate Small Scant
Color: N/A Clear Bloody Meconium Heavy Light Particulate
Odor: None   N/A   Normal   Foul
Amniotic Fluid Comments:

Vaginal Bleeding: None   Normal   Frank bleeding

Describe Vaginal Bleeding:

Mental Status: Alert   Anxious   Confused

Feeding Preference: Breast Bottle Breast/bottle Undecided

Support Person: None   Husband   Partner   Other

Support Person(s) Name:

Anesthesia Plans: None Local Epidural Spinal General Pudendal
                   Paracervical
Anesthesia Plans Other:

Anesthesia Class: Yes   No   Yes, Previous Pregnancy

Attended Prenatal Class: Yes   No   Yes, Previous Pregnancy

Labor Teaching Initiated: Yes   No   N/A
  Fetal Well-being   Yes   No   N/A
  Labor Progress   Yes   No   N/A
  Pain Relief Measures   Yes   No   N/A
  Other

Nutritional Screen:
[ ] N/A
[ ] History of Diabetes/Gestational Diabetes
[ ] History of Eating Disorder
[ ] Multiple Pregnancy
[ ] Special Diet/Vegetarian Diet
[ ] Pt. is 18 Years Old or Younger
[ ] Failure to Gain at Least 1/2 lb. per
    Wks. of Gestation
[ ] Food Allergies
[ ] Other _____

Describe Last Solid Intake (Include Date/Time):

Describe Last Fluid Intake (Include Date/Time):

In-Pt. Dietary Referral Entered in Computer: Yes No N/A	In-Pt. Dietary Referral Entered in Computer: Yes No N/A

Medication Allergy: Yes   No
Medication Allergy Detail:

Food Allergies: Yes   No
Food Allergy detail:

Latex Allergy: Yes   No
Describe Latex Reaction:

Allergy Sticker on Chart: Yes N/A	Allergy Band on Patient: Yes N/A

Prenatal Vitamins This Pregnancy:	Anticoagulants Describe: This Pregnancy:
Yes No	Yes No

For current prescription/over the counter medications taken during pregnancy see Home Medication Order Sheet.

Prescription/over the counter medications previously taken during pregnancy:

Addressograph

Figure 12-11 Labor and delivery admission record.

(continued)

Labor and Delivery Admission Record (continued)

PT. NAME: _____

GBS Yes Results: Negative Results	**Drug Use:** Denies Yes If Yes, Describe:
Tested: No Positive Date:	**Drug Use Comments:**
Unknown	

GBS Tested: Yes No   Results: Negative Positive Unknown   Results Date: _____

Blood Type/Rh: | **Rhogam** | **This Pregnancy:** N/A Yes No No Record

Rubella: Immune Non-immune Unknown   **HBsAg:** Negative Positive Unknown   **RPR:** Nonreactive Reactive Unknown

Hemoglobin = _____ g/dl   **Initials:** _____
Reference Range: 11–14 g/dl (pregnancy)   **HIV:** Nonreactive Reactive

Heart Disease: Yes No   **Hypertension:** Yes No

MVP: Yes No   **Diabetes:** Yes No

Asthma: Yes No   **DVT:** Yes No

Blood Transfusion: Yes No
Blood Transfusion Reason/Yr: _____

Sexually Transmitted Diseases: Denies Chlamydia Syphilis Gonorrhea HIV HPV/Genital Warts Herpes Other _____

Exposure to Infectious Disease This Pregnancy: Denies Measles Mumps HIV/AIDS Chicken Pox TB Hepatitis Other _____

Cervical Procedures: Denies D & C LEEP Cervical biopsy Laser Cryo/Cautery Other _____

History of Major Illness or Surgery: _____

Patient History Detail: _____

Past Pregnancy Complications: None PIH Cystitis Pyelitis Preterm Labor Preterm Birth Anemia Rh Sensitization Positive GBS Other _____
Comments:

Complications Current Pregnancy: None PIH Cystitis Preterm Labor Anemia Rh sensitization Placental abnormalities _____ Other _____
Comments:

Fetal Assessments Done This Pregnancy: None Non-Stress Test OCT CVS BPP US Amnio

Previous Labor Durations: _____

Sibling History: _____

Family History: N/A Adopted Heart Disease HTN Diabetes Cancer Bleeding Disorder Other _____
Family History Comments:

Smoke Use/Frequency: Denies <5 per day 5–10 per day >10 per day >20 per day

Alcohol Use: Denies Occasional 3–5 Drinks/Week 6 or More Drinks/Week

Contact Lenses: Yes No Soft Lenses Hard Lenses Lenses In Lenses Out

Glasses: Yes No   **Dentures:** Yes No

Body Piercing: Yes No   **Body piercing Location/Removed:**

Support System After Birth: Family Friends Community None
If None, Social Service Referral Entered In Computer: Yes No N/A

History of Abuse: Denies Emotional Physical Sexual Other _____   If Other, Describe

Social Service Referral Entered in Computer: Yes No N/A

Special Needs: None Spiritual Cultural Emotional Other _____   Hearing/vision impaired: Yes No   If Other, Describe

Social Service Referral Entered in Computer: Yes No N/A   **Pastoral Service Referral Entered in Computer:** Yes No N/A

Interpreter needed? Yes No Primary language: _____

Psychosocial Comments:

Room Orientation: EFM Bed Phone Call Light Visitors Computer

Does the Patient Have an Advance Directive?
Yes — **If Yes, Is Copy in Chart?** Yes No — **If No Copy on Chart, Remind Pt. to Have Family Member Bring Copy AND Send Advance Directive Referral to Pastoral Services** — **Referral Entered in Computer:** Yes No
No — **If No, Does Pt. Want Additional Information or Assistance?** Yes No — **If Yes, Was Referral Sent to Pastoral Care?** Yes No — **Referral Entered in Computer:** Yes No

Disposition of Valuables: Sent Home Kept with Pt. Valuables in Security Office Pt. Encouraged to Take Valuables Home Other _____
Valuables Comments:

Pt. Wants Other Physician or Family Notified: Yes No

Other Physician/Family Notified: _____

Morse Fall Scale Score:
[ ] < 45, low fall risk; initiate appropriate interventions
[ ] > 50, high fall risk; initiate appropriate interventions
[ ] ≥ 4 medications associated with increased fall risk; high fall risk; initiate appropriate interventions

Initiate Care Plan If:
[ ] Anticipated physiological fall risk
[ ] Unanticipated physiological fall risk
[ ] Accidental fall risk

Immunization History
Vaccines:				
Influenza	Yes	No	Date	_____
Pneumonia	Yes	No	Date	_____
Tetanus	Yes	No	Date	_____
PPD	Yes	No	Date	_____

Requests cord blood banking: Y N
Cord blood banking type: [ ] NA
[ ] St. Louis Cord Blood Bank
[ ] Private cord blood bank

Nursing Assessment Summary: _____

Addressograph

Figure 12-11 (continued)

Patient Name:		Physician/CNM:			KEY
	DATE:				**Variability**
	TIME:				Ab = Absent (undetectable)
Cervix	Dilation				Min = Minimal (>0 out ≤5 bpm)
Cervix	Effacement				Mod = Moderate (6–25 bpm) Mar = Marked (>25 bpm)
Cervix	Station				**Accelerations**
Fetal Heart	Baseline Rate				+ = Present and appropriate for gestational age
Fetal Heart	Variability				Ø = Absent
Fetal Heart	Accelerations				**Decelerations** E = Early
Fetal Heart	Decelerations				L = Late V = Variable
Fetal Heart	STIM/pH				P = Prolonged **Stim/pH**
Fetal Heart	Monitor Mode				+ = Acceleration in response to stimulation
Uterine Activity	Frequency				Ø = No response to stimulation Record number for scalp pH
Uterine Activity	Duration				**Monitor mode** A = Auscultation/Palpation
Uterine Activity	Intensity				E = External u/s or toco
Uterine Activity	Resting Tone				FSE - Fetal spiral electrode IUPC = Intrauterine pressure catheter
Uterine Activity	Monitor Mode				**Frequency of uterine activity**
Uterine Activity	Oxytocin milliunits/min				Ø = None Irreg = Irregular
	Pain				**Intensity of uterine activity** M = Mild
	Coping				Mod = Moderate Str = Strong
	Maternal Position				By IUPC = mm Hg
	O2/LPM/Mask				**Resting tone** R = Relaxed
	IV				By IUCP = mm Hg
	Nurse Initials				**Coping** W = Well
Narrative notes:					S = Support provided For pain use 0–10 scale
					Maternal position A = Ambulatory
					U = Upright SF = Semi-Fowler's
					RL = Right lateral LL = Left lateral MS = Modified Sims'

Figure 12-12 Labor documentation record.

receives orders. Critical information to relay to the physician or nurse-midwife includes:

- Patient's name and age
- Gravidity and parity
- Gestational age and estimated date of delivery
- Labor status: pattern of contractions, cervical dilation and effacement, fetal presentation and station
- Status of membranes
- Fetal heart rate and response to contractions
- Patient's vital signs, especially blood pressure and temperature
- Any identified risk to maternal or fetal well-being
- Patient's coping ability in response to labor

After admission, the patient and her fetus are assessed frequently to monitor both the progression of labor and the responses of both to the labor. Throughout each stage of

labor, ongoing maternal assessments include vital signs, intake and output, pattern of contractions, cervical dilation and effacement, and response to labor. Fetal assessments, which primarily center on the response to labor, involve intermittent or continuous FHR monitoring.

First Stage of Labor

The first stage of labor is often referred to as the stage of dilation. This stage begins with the onset of regular uterine contractions and ends with complete dilation of the cervix. The onset of labor is often made retrospectively because the woman may not always recognize when true labor actually begins. The contractions often start slowly and are fairly tolerable. Over time, contractions tend to increase in frequency, duration, and intensity as the first stage of labor progresses. The first stage of labor is most often the longest stage, and its duration can vary considerably among women. The first stage of labor is divided into three distinct phases: latent, active, and transition. Multiparous women tend to progress through the childbirth process much more rapidly than do nulliparous women. Factors such as analgesia, maternal and fetal position, the woman's body size, and her level of physical fitness can also affect the length of labor.

LATENT PHASE

The **latent phase** of labor begins with the establishment of regular contractions (labor pains). Labor pains are often initially felt as sensations similar to painful menstrual cramping and are usually accompanied by low back pain. Contractions during this phase are typically about 5 minutes apart, last 30 to 45 seconds, and are considered to be mild. During this phase, the woman is usually excited about labor commencing, and she remains chatty and sociable. Often this phase of labor is completed at home. During the latent phase cervical effacement and early dilation (0 to 3 cm) occur. The latent phase of labor can last as long as 10 to 14 hours because the contractions are mild and cervical changes occur slowly.

ACTIVE PHASE

The **active phase** of labor is characterized by more active contractions. The contractions become more frequent (every 3 to 5 minutes), last longer (60 seconds), and are of a moderate to strong intensity. During the active labor phase, the woman becomes more focused on each contraction and tends to draw inward in an attempt to cope with the increasing demands of the labor. Cervical dilation during this phase advances more quickly because the contractions are often more efficient. While the length of the active phase is variable, nulliparous women generally progress at an average speed of 1 cm of dilation per hour and multiparas at 1.5 cm of cervical dilation per hour. A 2010 review of cervical dilation rates among nulliparous women revealed that, for low-risk, nulliparous women with spontaneous labor onset, cervical dilation is likely slower than 0.5 cm/hour in earlier active labor and faster in more advanced active labor (Neal, Lowe, Patrick, Cabbage, & Corwin, 2010).

TRANSITION PHASE

The **transition phase** is the most intense phase of labor. Transition is characterized by frequent, strong contractions that occur every 2 to 3 minutes and last 60 to 90 seconds on average. Fortunately, this phase often does not take long because dilation usually progresses at a pace equal to or faster than active labor (1 cm/hr for a nullipara and 1.5 cm/hr for a multipara). During the transition phase, the laboring woman may feel that she can no longer continue or she may question her ability to cope with much more. Other sensations that a woman may feel during transition include rectal pressure, an increased urge to bear down, an increase in bloody show, and spontaneous rupture of the membranes (if they have not already ruptured). Table 12-3

Table 12-3	Characteristics of the First and Second Stages of Labor	
	First Stage	**Second Stage**
Definition	Commences with the onset of regular contractions and ends with full dilation (10 cm) of the cervix.	Begins with full dilation of the cervix (10 cm) and ends with the expulsion (birth) of the fetus.
Contractions	Latent: 5–10 minutes, may be irregular in frequency, duration 30–40 seconds, mild to moderate strength. Active: Regular pattern established (2–5 minutes apart), 40–60 seconds duration and moderate to strong by palpation. Transition: 2–3 minutes apart lasting 60–90 seconds, strong by palpation.	Contractions continue at a similar rate as during the transition phase; 2–3 minutes apart lasting 60 seconds and strong by palpation.
Dilation	Latent: 0–3 cm Active: 4–7 cm Transition: 8–10 cm	Fully dilated
Physical discomforts	Latent: Contractions often begin as painful menstrual-like cramps or low backache. Active: Increasing discomfort as contractions become stronger and more regular. May have backache. Transition: Increasing discomfort because contractions are very strong with little time for relaxation in between. As the fetal head descends there may be an increase in rectal pressure and the urge to push.	May have an urge to push that increases as the fetal head descends. Many women prefer to push so that they can use the contractions and work with them. When head is crowning may feel intense pain, burning.
Maternal behaviors	Latent: Pain often well controlled; various behaviors may be present: excited, talkative, confident, anxious, withdrawn. Stage may be completed at home. Active: Needs to focus more on staying in control and managing the pain; often requires coaching at this stage; quieter and more inwardly focused. Transition: Most intense phase. Often difficult to cope; may experience various emotions: irritable, agitated, hopeless ("can't do it"); tired (sleeps between contractions).	Often during this stage many women get a "second wind" as they see that they are making progress and are embarking on a new (labor) phase. Intense concentration with pushing efforts.

presents a summary of the characteristics of the first and second stages of labor.

A labor curve assessment tool, often referred to as a "Friedman curve," is a graph used to help identify whether a patient's labor is progressing in a normal pattern (Fig. 12-13). Composite normal labor patterns are graphically presented for the multiparous and nulliparous patient. The labor curve assessment tool contains categories that include the time of day, amount of cervical dilation and effacement, and hours of labor that have elapsed. The patient's own labor progress is plotted on the graph to allow a comparison between her progress and the norm.

 Now Can You—Identify characteristics of the first and second stages of labor?

1. Define the characteristics of the first and second stages of labor including contractions, dilation, and maternal response?
2. Describe the three phases of the first stage of labor and the changes that occur during each phase?
3. Explain the value of using a labor curve assessment tool?

 Where Research and Practice Meet:
Maternal Obesity Lengthens the Labor Curve

Norman and co-investigators (2012) examined labor progression patterns in over 5,200 women with singleton term pregnancies and vertex presentation who had completed the first stage of labor. Two comparison groups were identified as defined by body mass index (BMI): less than 30 (n=2,413); or, 30 or more (n=2,791). The labor curves indicated longer duration and slower progression of the first stage of labor among women with BMIs of 30 or more for both nulliparous and multiparous women. These findings suggest that obesity should be considered in defining norms for the management of labor, and the researchers assert that the use of a single "normal" labor curve may lead to overdiagnosis of labor dystocia (difficult or abnormal labor).

NURSING CARE DURING THE FIRST STAGE OF LABOR

Cunningham and associates (2014) noted that there are two opposing priorities in the ideal management of labor:

- Birthing should be recognized as a normal physiological process and should be treated as such.
- Intrapartum complications can arise quickly and unexpectedly and therefore should be anticipated.

There are several key roles for the nurse who is providing care for the woman in labor. It is essential that the nurse continually assess the patient and her fetus to ensure a safe delivery, help to facilitate a positive birth experience, assist in the satisfactory management of pain, and advocate for the patient's needs.

It is important to remember that nursing interventions must first be safe and consistent with the current standard of care. Interventions are also tailored to meet the individual needs and preferences of the woman in labor. The patient's needs may quickly change throughout the process of labor. For example, during early labor the woman may be very independent and in little need of assistance. During active labor or transition, the needs often become very different. Research has shown that, during labor, support by nurses has a positive effect on maternal and fetal outcomes.

Labor Support

Whenever possible, continuous labor support should be given to women in labor. Providing this level of care has been associated with positive outcomes for mothers and infants, and there have been no documented harmful or adverse effects. Continuous labor support can be provided by professional nurses or by lay people. In 2011, the Association of Women's Health, Obstetric and Neonatal Nurses (AWHONN) published a position statement, *Nursing Support of Laboring Women,* that underscores the importance of continuously available labor support from a registered nurse in helping to achieve improved birth outcomes.

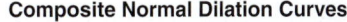
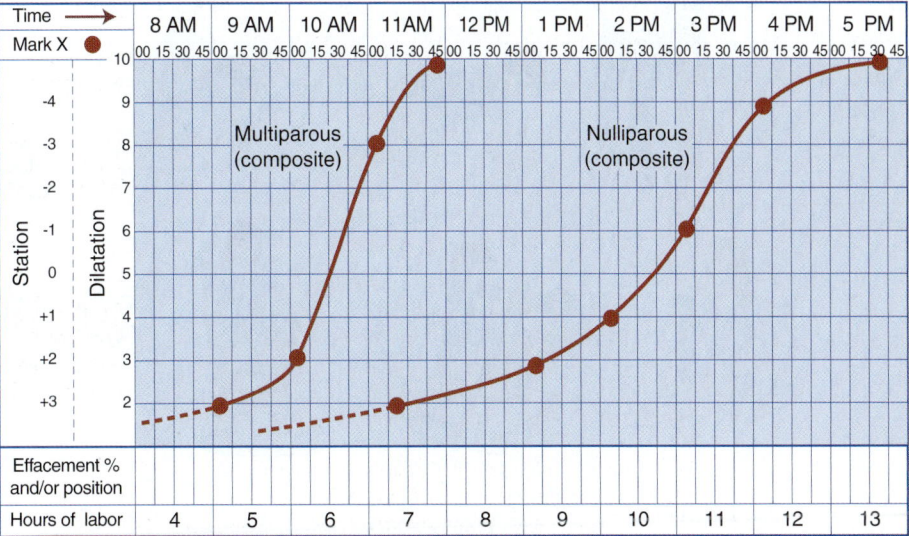

Figure 12-13 A labor curve assessment tool, often referred to as a "Friedman Curve," helps to identify whether a patient's labor is progressing in a normal pattern.

According to AWHONN, labor care and labor support are powerful nursing functions that should include assessment and management of the physiological and psychological processes of labor, facilitation of normal physiological processes, provision of physical comfort measures, emotional support, instruction, role modeling and advocacy, evaluation of fetal well-being, and direct collaboration with other members of the health-care team (AWHONN, 2011b).

PRESENCE

Presence is one method of providing continuous support. Offering one's presence in labor can be defined simply as "physically being with the woman." Women find that having a nurse present can be reassuring because they recognize that assistance is available when needed. Studies have

demonstrated that "women want the nurse to be available, to be emotionally involved, to help create a special moment, to hear and respond to their concerns, to share the responsibilities for keeping them safe, and to act as a go-between for their family and the medical institution" (MacKinnon, McIntyre, & Quance, 2005, p. 32). Unfortunately, other studies have demonstrated that nurses may not be actually providing this type of care for several different reasons such as inadequate staffing, lack of time, lack of training, hospital practices that emphasize technological care, and resistance from physicians. Nurses are especially adept in providing therapeutic labor support because their educational background emphasizes a caring, holistic approach that centers not only on knowledge of the labor process and supportive techniques but also on empowerment of the woman experiencing childbirth (Barrett & Stark, 2010; Simkin, Bolding, Keppler, Durham, & Whalley, 2010).

SPIRITUALITY

Spirituality or faith may serve as a source of inner strength and comfort for the laboring woman. The nurse can support the patient by providing spiritual care that may include prayer, meditation, chanting, reading or reciting from scriptures, and the use of rituals or sacraments. Creating a serene, respectful environment is conducive to prayer or meditation, and, depending on the woman's wishes, the nurse can offer to read scripture or prayers or seek the assistance of clergy who typically administer rituals or sacraments (Adams & Bianchi, 2008).

PROMOTION OF COMFORT

Position Changes

In labor, frequent position changes are beneficial in helping to promote the descent of the fetus. The nurse may assist the laboring woman to various positions and activities such as walking, standing, sitting, squatting, leaning over a piece of furniture, or assuming a hands and knees position (Fig. 12-14). Maternal preferences can guide the nurse in

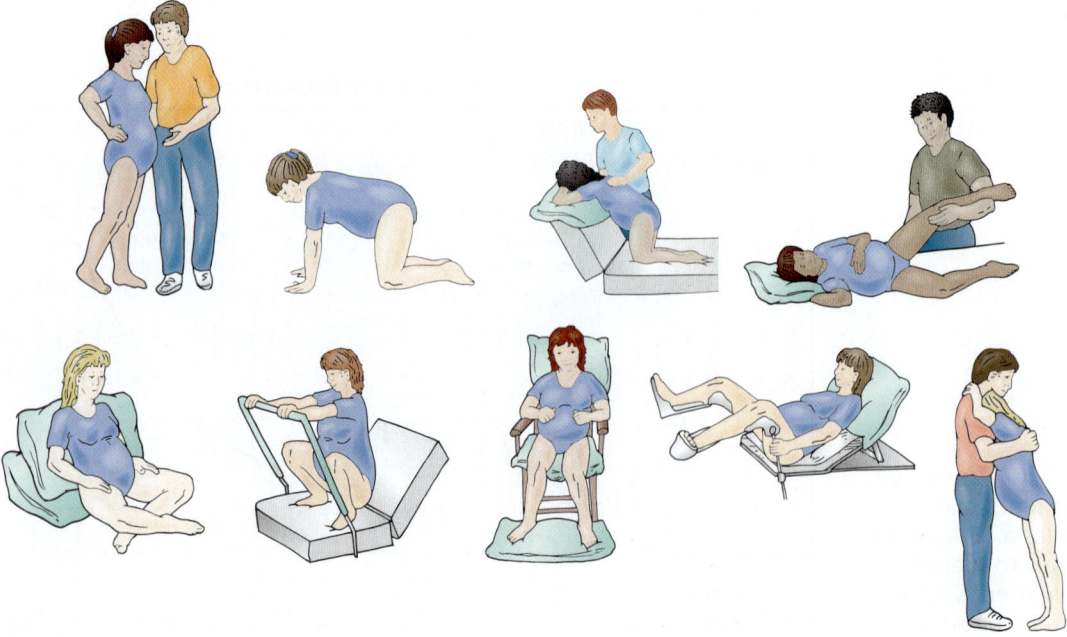

Figure 12-14 Various positions for labor and birth.

assessing which positions or activities the woman finds most comfortable. Each position is associated with advantages and disadvantages (Box 12-4). During early labor, women are often encouraged to remain ambulatory because activity has been shown to enhance the normal progression of labor (Fig. 12-15).

As labor advances, the woman may feel tired and in need of some relaxation between contractions. Sitting in a chair and reclining on the side are two positions that often bring comfort. Changes in the patient's status such as continuous fetal monitoring, premature rupture of the membranes, or epidural analgesia may necessitate a need for bedrest. In these situations, the nurse should encourage the laboring woman to rest on her left side to facilitate optimal uteroplacental blood flow. In addition, position changes should be encouraged even if the woman must remain in bed. If bedrest is necessary, the nurse may be able to assist the woman into a variety of positions in bed. Sitting, getting on hands and knees, or resting on alternate sides may be desirable, depending on the patient's condition and preferences. It is important to avoid the supine position because the pressure of the uterus on the maternal spine can cause compression of the inferior vena cava and lead to decreased blood pressure and diminished uteroplacental blood flow.

Personal Comfort Measures

Nurses can provide personal comfort measures for the laboring woman based on her preferences and needs. For example, assistance with basic hygiene, back rubs, ice chips, or application of a cold cloth may be quite comforting (Fig. 12-16). Family members and support persons should be encouraged to remain with the woman and help to meet her personal comfort needs.

ENVIRONMENT. The woman or her family may prefer to have the lights dimmed to create a relaxing atmosphere. Conversely, other women and families may prefer to have the sun streaming into the room. During active labor the woman may verbalize heat intolerance (being too hot) because of the physical work and energy expenditure required in labor. An electric fan may be beneficial in providing a cooling breeze. Nurses must remember to turn off the fan or assess the room temperature during childbirth to ensure that the infant does not get unnecessarily chilled.

PERSONAL HYGIENE. As needed, the nurse can help promote the patient's sense of cleanliness and well-being by changing pads, linens, or gown especially if the woman is

---

Box 12-4 Advantages and Disadvantages of Various Positions for Labor

WALKING/STANDING
Uses gravity, facilitates descent, places fetus in alignment with pelvis, may decrease the length of labor by enhancing the effect of contractions.
  May be tiring, requires telemetry for continuous electronic fetal monitoring, may not be possible with regional anesthesia.

SITTING
Uses gravity, increases pelvic diameter and shortens second-stage labor, avoids supine hypotension syndrome, decreases back pain, enhances communication with partner and allows for ready access to back and sacrum for massage and counterpressure.
  Labor may be slowed if not alternated with other positions, may intensify suprapubic pain and cause edema of the vulva or cervix.

HANDS AND KNEES POSITION
Stimulates rotation of fetus from a posterior to an anterior position, relieves backache and rectal pressure, facilitates pelvic rocking and pelvic mobility.
  May be tiring or embarrassing, difficult to keep external fetal monitor in place, may not be possible with regional anesthesia.

SQUATTING
Uses gravity, increases pelvic diameter, relieves backache, promotes fetal descent and rotation, facilitates second-stage pushing.
  May impede descent before engagement has occurred, may be tiring, uncomfortable, or embarrassing, may increase perineal and cervical edema.

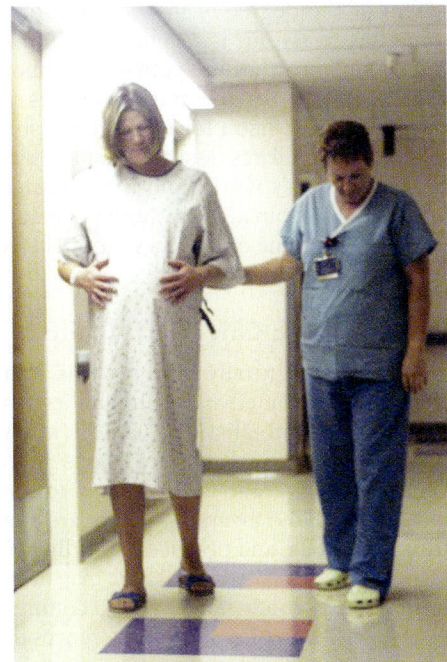

Figure 12-15 Laboring woman walking with her nurse.

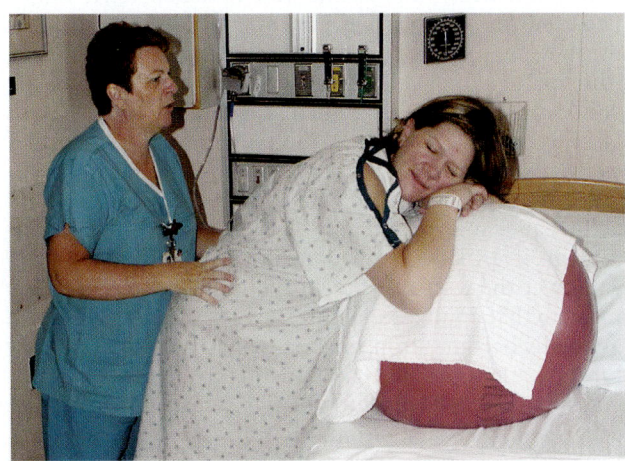

Figure 12-16 Woman receiving labor support from her nurse.

leaking amniotic fluid or bloody show. Many women who remain ambulatory are able to perform their own personal care. However, if the laboring woman is confined to bed or exhausted from the exertion of labor, full assistance should be provided.

Frequent mouth care should be encouraged because dry mouth is common during labor. Providing fluids to drink, ice chips, popsicles, or hard candy may help to alleviate the symptoms. In addition, the use of mouthwash or brushing the teeth may be especially beneficial following vomiting. Nurses should be aware that different institutional policies exist regarding oral intake in labor and remain knowledgeable of the policies and procedures that affect their practice.

ELIMINATION. A full bladder can inhibit the descent of the fetus and contribute to increased pain with contractions. Encouraging and assisting the woman to the toilet (or bedpan) to void at least every 2 hours is recommended. If the woman is unable to void and has a distended bladder, a urinary catheter may be required.

SUPPORTIVE RELAXATION TECHNIQUES. During labor, the nurse may encourage, assist, or teach the woman about different interventions to help decrease pain and relieve anxiety. Relaxation techniques may include visualization, focal points, imagery, hydrotherapy, and breathing techniques. In addition, patients may bring items from home to enhance relaxation such as music, a picture, or a stuffed animal. (See Chapter 13 for further discussion.)

Now Can You—Provide comforting nursing care during labor?

1. List four examples of nursing interventions that patients have identified as helpful in promoting comfort and relaxation?
2. Identify three beneficial positions for the laboring woman who is confined to bedrest?
3. Describe what is meant by "presence"?

ANTICIPATORY GUIDANCE

Providing anticipatory guidance for the woman and her family constitutes an essential role of the obstetric nurse. Regardless of whether they have attended prenatal classes, most women and their families have many questions. Anticipatory guidance should be provided throughout the childbirth experience. Women and families usually want to know what to expect. While the nurse cannot predict exactly what will happen, helpful information can be provided in general terms. For example, a woman in early active labor may comment: "These contractions are getting stronger. How strong will they get?" The nurse can empower the woman by identifying the progress she has made to that point. Explaining how the contractions have gradually become stronger and emphasizing how successful the patient has been in adjusting to the changes provides factual feedback and positive reinforcement of the progress made. In addition, the nurse may suggest comfort measures such as relaxing in a whirlpool bath or shower for later on when the contractions become stronger.

"What to say"—*Positive, encouraging words during labor*

During labor the patient needs encouragement with positive words regarding what she is doing well even when she may not be coping at her optimal ability. Nurses must be careful not to use language that may be discouraging for the woman such as "This is just the beginning. It is going to get much worse." Instead, nurses should offer comments such as "Try focusing on one contraction at a time" or "See if you can concentrate on relaxing more between the contractions" followed by "That is really great, keep going, excellent, now let's try that again with the next one."

Keeping the woman and her family informed about the process of labor and birth is a constant and ever-changing task. For example, during the transition phase the nurse may be teaching the woman breathing techniques to avoid pushing with a partially dilated cervix. In a matter of minutes, the patient can reach full cervical dilation. The nurse then teaches her how to push and may need to assist the woman into an effective pushing position.

CARING FOR THE BIRTH PARTNER

Obviously, most of the nurse's attention focuses on the woman in labor. Efforts also should be made to help the support person feel welcome and included whenever possible according to the woman's wishes. Awareness of the support person's emotional status and taking action to help reduce stress (e.g., offering information about labor progress and demonstrating supportive measures) is important in alleviating maternal stress. Labor support behaviors include expressions of encouragement, praise, reassurance, and nursing presence (Adams & Bianchi, 2008; Felton, 2011). Orientation to the birth unit is helpful in identifying where to locate items such as towels and washcloths, kitchen supplies (ice chips), and the restroom.

Assessment of the degree of involvement the support person would like to assume is also important. It is helpful to determine whether or not the patient and labor partner have attended childbirth preparation classes and give respect to the support person for identified wishes and or limitations. In some cultures, assistance at the birth might be considered "woman's work" and the laboring woman instead seeks support from a sister, mother, and aunt while the husband stays at home or assumes more of an observational role.

ENSURING CULTURE-CENTERED CARE

Providing care that is culturally appropriate is as important in caring for laboring women and their families as with any other patients. It is unrealistic to expect nurses to be knowledgeable about the cultural traditions and customs of all patients. However, it is important for nurses to remain open minded and aware that there are a myriad of values, attitudes, beliefs, and practices regarding childbearing that vary among cultures just as there may be wide variations within cultures. Body language and communication approaches provide examples of how differences in cultural practices can be applied when caring for a woman and her family during the childbirth experience.

Cultural Diversity: Cultural Differences in Communication

Eye contact: North American nurses have been taught that eye contact is an integral part of the communication process when communicating with patients. Some cultures do not maintain eye contact because they consider eye contact to be impolite or aggressive.

Silence: Some individuals find silence to be uncomfortable and may make efforts to communicate when there are gaps in a conversation. However, labor may be a time where it is inappropriate to be carrying on a conversation. Silence can be seen as a sign of respect for the laboring woman and the effort that she may be using to stay focused.

Touch: Often during the care of laboring women, nurses will use touch as a sign of caring and empathy. Wide variations in meaning can be attributed to touch among cultures. It is recommended to always ask the patient prior to touching her and assess her response to being touched.

Space: The concept of personal space varies among individuals and cultures. An awareness of personal space boundaries is essential; the individual patient will help the nurse to identify what she finds acceptable.

Care provider and labor support gender: Variations exist within cultures regarding norms relating to gender. Some cultures require a female care provider for the woman in labor. Other cultures require that a female labor companion accompany the woman in labor while the husband assumes a passive role.

Sick role behavior: Sick role behavior can vary among individuals and cultures. In some cultures it may be unacceptable to shout out during labor, and the woman may be very stoic even though she is in extreme pain. Other cultures consider the childbearing year to be a time that requires intense assistance. In these situations, it is appropriate for the mother or sister to come live with the family to help care for the mother and infant.

Assessment of the Fetus During Labor and Birth

Assessment of the fetus during labor and birth is a fundamental component of caring for a woman in labor. Intrapartal assessment of the fetus should be included in the maternal assessments at admission and remain ongoing throughout the intrapartal period. Fetal assessments include the identification of fetal position and presentation and the evaluation of fetal status. A healthy fetus is able to withstand the mechanical and hemodynamic changes that occur during normal labor without adverse effects. Various fetal physiological responses to labor are presented in Box 12-5.

Nurses use a variety of assessment techniques including observation, palpation, and auscultation. When assessing a woman in labor, the nurse is able to use observation and interview skills from the moment the woman comes through the door. Astute observation assists the nurse in assessing the patient's level of pain, her coping abilities, her contraction frequency, and the effectiveness of her support person. However, the nurse is unable to use direct observation skills to assess the status of the fetus. Therefore, it is critical that fetal assessment be a priority when the patient enters the intrapartal unit.

FETAL POSITION

There are four central ways to identify fetal position, and some methods are more accurate than others. The nurse may attempt to identify the fetal presentation in the following ways:

- Abdominal palpation (Leopold maneuvers)
- Location of the point of auscultation of the fetal heart rate (FHR)
- Vaginal examination
- Ultrasound

Leopold Maneuvers and Point of FHR Auscultation

Leopold maneuvers are a systematic way of palpating the maternal abdomen to assess the fetal position. In addition, through the identification of fetal position, Leopold maneuvers can also assist the nurse to identify the location in which to auscultate the fetal heart tones. Performing Leopold maneuvers is a skill that requires practice and is not always accurate in identifying fetal position. Factors such as maternal obesity, hydramnios, and multiple gestation can increase the difficulty of identifying fetal position by Leopold maneuvers. (See Chapter 9 for further discussion.)

 Critical Nursing Action Prevent Supine Hypotension

Much of the fetal assessment involves the maternal abdomen. Avoid positioning the patient flat on her back. Instead, slightly elevate the head of the bed or place a wedge under the patient's hip to prevent compression of the maternal vena cava caused by the gravid uterus.

Vaginal Examination

Another method of assessing the fetal position is by vaginal examination (see Procedure 12-1). The examiner may be able to palpate the fontanelles or cranial suture to identify that the fetus is in a cephalic presentation. The landmarks may also be used to further identify the degree of flexion and the specific presentation such as vertex. If the membranes are intact or if the cervix is minimally dilated, the examiner may not be able to identify the position of the fetus.

 Where Research and Practice Meet: **Intrapartal Cervical Examinations and Maternal Fever**

Cahill and colleagues (2012) reviewed intrapartum data from approximately 2,400 women to determine if there was an association between the number of digital cervical examinations and the risk of maternal fever (temperature greater than or equal to 38.0°C on at least one occasion during labor, delivery, or during the first 6 hours postpartum). Women were examined between one and 14 times, and those who developed a fever underwent two more digital cervical examinations on average than those who remained afebrile. Extensive data analysis revealed no significant association between the number of cervical examinations and the risk of maternal fever, even when multiple cervical examinations were performed after rupture of membranes. Based on their findings, the investigators suggested that clinicians could be reassured that increasing the number of cervical examinations in term labor does not place patients at increased risk of peripartum fever.

Nursing Care Plan   Young Primigravida in Labor

Allison is a 16-year-old gravida 1 para 0 who presents to the birth unit in early active labor accompanied by her mother. Allison appears quite fearful as she frequently asks, "what is that for?," "what are you going to do with that?," and "will it hurt?" On further questioning the nurse determines that Allison did not attend prenatal classes and has never been hospitalized.

Nursing Diagnosis: Deficient Knowledge related to hospitalization for labor and birth as manifested by frequent questions, no prenatal classes, and no previous hospitalizations.

Measurable Short-Term Goal: The patient will obtain increased knowledge about labor, birth, and hospital procedures.

Measurable Long-Term Goal: The patient will actively participate in her labor and birth.

NOC Outcome:

Knowledge: Labor and Delivery (1817) Extent of understanding conveyed about labor and vaginal delivery

NIC Interventions:

Childbirth Preparation (6760)
Teaching: Individual (5606)

Nursing Interventions:

1. Establish rapport with the patient and her significant other(s).

   RATIONALE: The support and understanding of the nurse will help decrease the patient's anxiety to facilitate learning. Including significant other(s) in teaching provides an additional source of information and comfort for the patient.

2. Describe the admission process and standard care for labor patients with rationales.

   RATIONALE: Explaining to the patient what will occur and the reasons why they are important will increase the patient's knowledge and may alleviate some of her anxiety.

3. Orient the patient to the unit/room/birthing area including how to change lighting and temperature and use of audiovisual equipment.

   RATIONALE: Orientation to the hospital environment empowers the patient to feel more comfortable with her surroundings.

4. Describe any procedures before performing them, including rationales, sensations, risks, and benefits.

   RATIONALE: This allows the patient to participate in her own care and make decisions based on knowledge.

5. Explain the nature of uterine contractions, cervical dilation, labor progress, and fetal monitoring.

   RATIONALE: This knowledge will reduce the patient's anxiety, which may also reduce perceived pain.

6. Teach the patient and significant other(s) simple breathing and relaxation techniques that may be used as labor advances.

   RATIONALE: Anticipatory guidance provides the patient with tools to use during labor.

7. Teach support person(s) measures to comfort the patient during labor (specify, e.g., back rub, cool cloth, position changes, massage, imagery, and use of birthing ball).

   RATIONALE: Providing presence conveys support and respect for the patient. Continuous support should be ongoing to prevent the patient from being left alone during labor.

8. Offer encouragement, praise, and suggestions for coping strategies as labor advances.

   RATIONALE: Empowers the patient to gain better control over her situation and helps to diminish fear and anxiety.

(Bulechek, Butcher, Dochterman, & Wagner, 2013)

Ultrasound Examination

Ultrasound may be used when the practitioner is unable to identify the position by abdominal palpation or when it is necessary to determine the fetal position with the most accuracy. If a breech presentation is suspected during labor, an ultrasound examination may be performed to confirm the fetal presentation prior to performing a cesarean section.

 Now Can You—Discuss determination of fetal position during labor?

1. Identify and describe three methods used to determine fetal position?
2. Outline the major steps involved in performing an intrapartal vaginal examination?

ASSESSMENT OF THE FETAL HEART RATE

Much debate exists regarding the optimal method for evaluating the FHR in labor with the use of continuous or intermittent electronic fetal monitoring (EFM) and intermittent auscultation (IA). IA, which promotes the "high touch, low-tech" approach to care, has been found to be as effective as the electronic method for fetal surveillance, and research evidence supports the use of IA for low-risk pregnant women. However, in practice, many low-risk women continue to be electronically monitored during labor. The use of continuous electronic fetal monitoring has been shown to increase the rate of cesarean deliveries and operative vaginal deliveries (ACOG, 2009; Feinstein, Sprague, & Trepanier,

---

Box 12-5 Various Fetal Physiological Responses to Labor

Changes in heart rate
- Decelerations may occur with increased intracranial pressure as the head presses against the maternal cervix. The early decelerations are thought to result from hypoxic depression of the central nervous system, which is under vagal control.

Changes in acid-base status
- Decreased fetal blood flow, which occurs at the peak of the contraction, leads to a slow decrease in pH.
- This process is accelerated during the second stage of labor, as a result of longer, stronger contractions and maternal pushing efforts.

Changes in hemodynamic status
- Fetal blood pressure, necessary for the adequate exchange of nutrients and gases in the fetal capillaries and intervillous spaces, protects the fetus during the anoxic periods that normally occur during uterine contractions.

Awareness of sensation
- By 37 weeks, the fetus is able to experience sensations of light, sound, and touch.
- During labor, the term fetus is aware of pressure sensations (e.g., head pressure during contractions and vaginal examination).

Sources: Blackburn (2012); Cunningham et al. (2014); Torgersen (2011).

2009; Torgersen, 2011). Over the years, various professional organizations have published and updated recommendations for fetal monitoring during labor (Table 12-4).

 Across Care Settings: **Variations in practice environments for perinatal nurses**

Because diverse policies are found in different practice environments, nurses are encouraged to seek relevant policies and procedures within their individual health-care organizations to guide their practice. It is important that the nurse practice within the standards set by the employer institution. The nurse is professionally accountable and has a legal responsibility to be knowledgeable of the current standards that affect practice. Perinatal nurses should be fully cognizant of the institutional policies concerning fetal heart surveillance during labor. Pertinent information generally includes the method of assessment, qualifications for those performing the technique, nurse to patient ratio, frequency and duration of assessment for specific stages of labor and defined risk categories, indications for specific methods, when to notify the primary care provider, and documentation (Torgersen, 2011).

Table 12-4 Professional Organizations and Fetal Monitoring Recommendations

Professional Organization	Recommendations

AWHONN (Association of Women's Health, Obstetric and Neonatal Nurses, 2008a)	Supports the assessment of the laboring woman through the use of auscultation, palpation, and/or EFM. Recognizes that the fetal auscultation and palpation of uterine activity and the judicious application of intrapartum EFM are appropriate and effective methods to assess and promote maternal–fetal well-being. Does not "support the use of EFM as a substitute for appropriate professional nursing care and support of women in labor" (p. 1); does recommend a 1:1 nurse-to-patient ratio during the second stage of labor. Recommends ongoing education in the interpretation of fetal assessment, the development of guidelines in facilities that specify modes and frequency of fetal assessment, and policies that address communication and collaboration essential to providing quality care and optimizing patient outcomes. Standards for frequency of FHR assessment Intermittent auscultation (IA) recommendations
	
	• No risk factors present
	  • Every 1 hour during the latent phase
	  • Every 5–15 minutes during the active phase
	  • Every 5–15 minutes during the second stage
	• Risk factors present
	  • Continuous EFM
	
	Note: IA can only interpret Category I and Category II FHR characteristics—all Category III patterns include assessment of FHR variability (which is not possible with IA). FHR assessment frequency increases if:
	
	• Indeterminate or abnormal FHR characteristics
	• ROM or administration of medication (before and after either event)
	
	When indeterminate or abnormal characteristics are heard, EFM of the FHR is used to:
	
	• Clarify pattern interpretation
	• Assess variability
	• Further assess fetal status
	
	When risk factors are present, continuous EFM recommended and the FHR should be evaluated:
	
	• Every 30 minutes during the latent phase
	• Every 15 minutes during the active phase
	• Every 5 minutes while pushing
	
	It is common practice for all women to at least have a baseline EFM tracing (≥ 20 minutes duration) when first evaluated in labor. Routine continuous FHR monitoring remains controversial.

(continued)

Table 12-4	Professional Organizations and Fetal Monitoring Recommendations (continued)
Professional Organization	**Recommendations**
ACOG (American College of Obstetrics and Gynecology, 2009)	States that IA may not be appropriate for all pregnancies and there are no comparative data regarding the optimal frequency for performing IA; one method is to evaluate and record the FHR at least every 15 minutes in the active phase of the first stage of labor and at least every 5 minutes in the second stage. The labor of women with high-risk conditions should be monitored with continuous FHR monitoring.
SOGC (Society of Obstetricians and Gynaecologists of Canada, 2007)	Recommends IA following an established protocol of surveillance and response as the preferred method of fetal surveillance of low-risk pregnancies; when compared with EFM, it has lower intervention rates without evidence of compromising neonatal outcome. EFM is recommended for pregnancies at risk of adverse perinatal outcome.

FHR = fetal heart rate; IA = intermittent auscultation; EFM = electronic fetal monitoring; ROM = rupture of membranes.

Auscultation of Fetal Heart Sounds

Fetal heart sounds are best heard over the fetal back when the fetus is in the flexed position because this is the part in closest contact with the uterine wall. Where to auscultate the fetal heart sounds depends on the fetal position (e.g., back to maternal left or right side and breech versus cephalic) (Fig. 12-17). Finding the best location to auscultate fetal heart sounds facilitates another method to identify or confirm fetal position. Typically, with a cephalic presentation, the fetal heart sounds are heard below the level of the maternal umbilicus. In an ROA position, the heart sounds are heard loudest in the right lower quadrant. Conversely, with a breech presentation, the fetal heart sounds are often auscultated above the level of the umbilicus. In an LSA position, the fetal heart sounds should be heard loudest in the upper left quadrant.

Regardless of the method used to assess fetal well-being in labor, nurses need to be extremely attentive to the fetal heart sounds. In addition, nurses must be knowledgeable regarding the identification of various FHR patterns and the appropriate interventions that may be required.

INTERMITTENT AUSCULTATION. Intermittent auscultation (IA) of the FHR is frequently the recommended method for evaluating fetal status in women who have been identified as low risk. The FHR can be auscultated with a fetoscope or Doppler instrument and should be assessed for the baseline FHR, regular or irregular rhythm pattern, and the presence of accelerations (discussed later). In addition, the nurse should be able to identify normal and abnormal FHR patterns and recognize the implications and interventions that may be required. Intermittent auscultation is conducted using a fetoscope or Doppler instrument (Procedure 12-3). IA does not provide a continuous printout of information on the FHR. According to AWHONN (2008a), when no risk factors are present, the suggested frequencies for FHR auscultation are within the range of every 60 minutes during the latent phase of labor and every 5 to 15 minutes during the active phase and the second stage of labor.

 legal alert—Use appropriate terminology during documentation of FHR auscultation

When documenting the findings from FHR auscultation, descriptive terms associated with EFM such as "marked variability" or "variable deceleration" should be avoided because these terms reflect visual descriptions of the patterns produced on the monitor tracing. Terms that are *numerically* defined (e.g., bradycardia and tachycardia) may be used. When auscultated, FHR must be described as a baseline number or range and as having a regular or irregular rhythm. The presence or absence of accelerations or decelerations that occur during and after contractions should be noted (AWHONN, 2000, 2009).

 Now Can You—Assess FHR by auscultation?

1. Describe situations in which intermittent auscultation of the FHR is indicated?
2. Demonstrate how to auscultate FHR during labor?

Electronic Fetal Heart Rate Monitoring

Electronic fetal monitoring (EFM) may be conducted on an intermittent or continuous basis. In a large number of American and Canadian hospitals, women are routinely monitored on admission for a short period of time to assess fetal well-being and then the monitoring is conducted periodically throughout labor. This practice is referred to

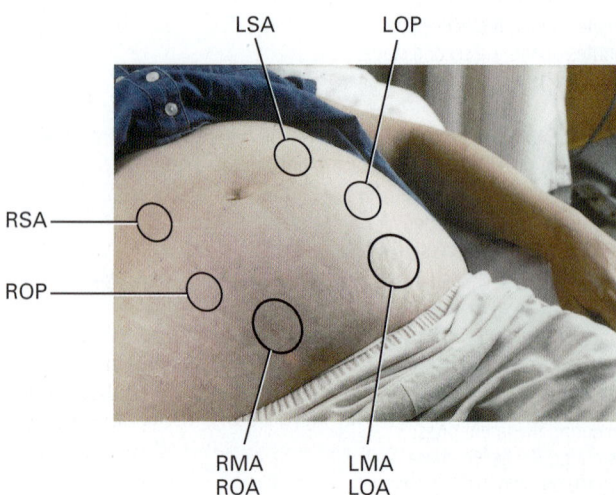

Figure 12-17 Location of fetal heart sounds on the maternal abdomen.

Procedure 12-3   Auscultating the Fetal Heart Tones During Labor

Purpose

Auscultation, an auditory method of monitoring the fetal heart tones, is performed intermittently during labor to assess the fetus. Auscultation allows the laboring woman greater freedom because she is not attached to a machine and does not have to wear belts to secure the ultrasound transducer and the toco-transducer. Intermittent auscultation does not provide a printed record of the fetal heart rate (FHR) for other members of the health-care team to review. Auscultation also does not provide an assessment of FHR variability or of other subtle changes in the FHR.

Equipment

- Fetoscope or handheld Doppler ultrasound with gel ("Doppler")
- Disposable wipes

Steps

a. Wash and dry hands and explain procedure and purpose of the examination to the patient.

   RATIONALE: *Hand washing helps to prevent the spread of microorganisms. Explanations help to decrease anxiety and promote patient understanding and cooperation.*

b. Help the patient assume a comfortable position that provides access to the abdomen.

c. Palpate the maternal abdomen using Leopold maneuvers to identify the fetal position to aid in obtaining the location of the fetal heart tones. Note that the fetal heart tones are heard most loudly over the fetal back.

d. Palpate the fundus of the uterus for the presence of uterine contractions. At the end of a uterine contraction, place the fetoscope or Doppler over the location of the fetal back. Adjust the fetoscope or Doppler if necessary to obtain a clearly audible FHR. Depending on fetal position, the fetal heart sounds may be soft and muffled or loud and clear.

e. Listen for audible fetal heart sounds. Note that two distinctly different sounds can be heard: fetal heart tones that result from blood moving through the placenta and umbilical cord (funic

souffle) and the uterine souffle, which is the same rate as the maternal pulse.

f. Palpate the maternal radial pulse to ensure that the auscultated fetal heart sounds are at a different rate than the maternal pulse.

g. Auscultate the fetal heart sounds for the rate and rhythm. The greatest accuracy for assessment of the FHR occurs when listening for 1 minute.

Note: During active labor, 30-second intervals may be more feasible.

h. Count the FHR for 30–60 seconds between contractions to determine the baseline rate.

   RATIONALE: *The baseline rate can be assessed only during the absence of uterine activity.*

i. Interpret the FHR: Is the baseline normal between 110 and 160 bpm? Is there tachycardia (baseline greater than 160 [MR7] bpm) or bradycardia (baseline less than 110/bpm)? Is the rhythm regular or irregular? Can you note the presence of accelerations or decelerations?

j. Repeat the procedure as indicated according to agency policy.

k. Inform the patient of the findings.

l. Document the FHR according to agency policy.

What If?

What if you have carefully applied the Doppler in several locations over the area of the fetal back, yet you are unable to hear any fetal heart tones?

   Immediately notify the primary care provider, who will most likely perform an ultrasound assessment.

Documentation

5/5/09 1030: FHR obtained by fetoscope at 144 bpm and regular. Acceleration of the FHR noted. Patient coping well in active labor. Contractions 3 min apart, 60-second duration with moderate intensity.

　　　　　　　　　　　　　　　　　　　-L. Lopez, RN

---

as "intermittent" fetal monitoring. However, the evidence base supporting this practice has not demonstrated improved outcomes. EFM, as compared with IA, has not been associated with a decrease in neonatal mortality or morbidity although EFM has been associated with increased rates of cesarean section, operative vaginal birth, and the use of obstetric anesthesia. Despite recommendations from professional organizations, approximately 3.4 million low-risk laboring women in the United Sates are monitored electronically for at least part of their labor. The continued use of EFM (which provides a continuous printout of information on the FHR) over intermittent

FHR auscultation is believed to be related to concerns about liability and the increased nurse-to-patient ratio required with IA (Grimes & Peipert, 2010).

The professional perinatal nursing association AWHONN issued a clinical position statement (2008a) regarding the frequency of fetal assessment with EFM. In the absence of risk factors, the FHR should be evaluated every 30 minutes during the active phase of the first stage of labor and every 15 minutes during the active pushing phase of the second stage of labor (AAP & ACOG, 2013). In Canada, the FHR is evaluated every 5 minutes in the active phase of the second stage of labor (Society of Obstetricians and Gynaecologists of Canada (SOGC) (2007). When risk factors are present, continuous EFM is recommended during the active phase of the first stage of labor, and the FHR should be determined and evaluated every 15 minutes (AAP & ACOG, 2013). During the active pushing phase of the second stage of labor, the FHR should be determined and evaluated at least every 5 minutes. A full description of the EFM tracing requires a qualitative and quantitative description of baseline FHR, variability, accelerations, decelerations, changes in FHR patterns, and uterine contractions (AWHONN, 2008a).

Situations in which EFM is recommended continuously for assessing fetal well-being include history of a stillbirth (in utero fetal death at greater than or equal to 38 weeks' gestation), the presence of a complication of pregnancy (e.g., preeclampsia-eclampsia, placenta previa, abruptio placentae, multiple gestation, and prolonged or premature rupture of the membranes), induction of labor with oxytocin, when IA identifies a need for more detailed information about the FHR, or if the institution is unable to provide IA. EFM can be performed externally or internally. The external EFM involves a process that is very similar to the nonstress test (NST) (see Chapter 11). The external monitor is composed of a Doppler ultrasound transducer and tocodynanometer that is applied to the maternal abdomen to monitor and display the FHR and contractions (Fig. 12-18). Although the use of an external transducer requires that the woman remain confined to a bed or chair, portable telemetry units allow patients to ambulate during electronic monitoring. The nurse is able to observe the FHR and uterine contraction patterns at a centrally located electronic display station. Some facilities are equipped with monitoring units that can be used when the woman is submerged in water.

The internal fetal monitor is composed of a spiral electrode (fetal spiral electrode, or FSE) that must be inserted into the fetal scalp or presenting part during a vaginal examination (Fig. 12-19). The cardiac signal is transmitted through the spiral electrode and a fetal electrocardiogram tracing is produced. Uterine activity is assessed by a solid or fluid-filled intrauterine pressure catheter (IUPC) that is introduced into the uterine cavity. The IUPC can measure contraction frequency, duration, and intensity. The internal method is a more accurate form of fetal monitoring.

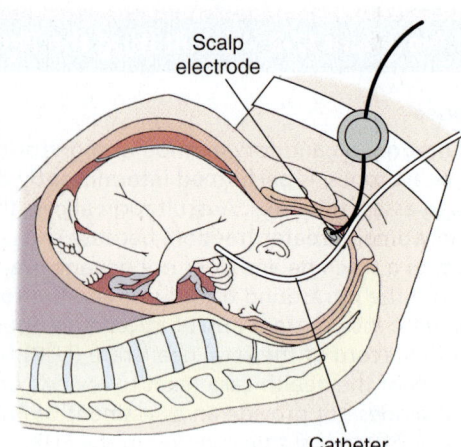

Figure 12-19 Internal fetal monitor.

However, because of the invasive nature of the procedure, internal EFM is often reserved for high-risk pregnancies (situations in which external fetal monitoring is insufficient in obtaining the FHR or in situations in which there is evidence of a non-reassuring fetal heart rate). The application of an internal electrode requires that the membranes be ruptured and that the cervix has sufficiently dilated.

The interpretation of the fetal heart rate pattern requires a holistic assessment of the maternal risk factors, uterine activity, and FHR patterns including baseline, variability and the presence of accelerations, and the identification of any decelerations. The primary objective of intrapartal FHR monitoring interpretation is to assess the adequacy of fetal oxygenation during labor. An understanding of FHR physiology and the various influences on the FHR is useful in interpreting FHR patterns (Box 12-6). Members of the obstetric team must maintain close communication and reach mutual consensus regarding interpretation of fetal heart patterns. Often, nurses who practice in labor and delivery units obtain advanced training and education regarding fetal monitoring to aid in accurate interpretation.

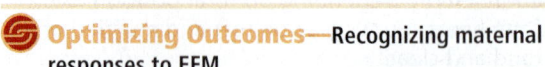

Optimizing Outcomes—Recognizing maternal responses to EFM

Unless they have experienced EFM with a previous pregnancy or learned about it in a childbirth preparation class, many women may have little knowledge and understanding about the modality. Reactions to EFM vary: some women view the intervention as a means of reassurance that the fetus is tolerating the labor well and find comfort in knowing that potential problems can be identified promptly. Others view the monitor as an unnecessary intrusion that interferes with the natural birth process and creates undue anxiety related to the wires, sounds, and position restrictions. Holistic nursing practice for the laboring woman and her birth partner centers on education and empowerment to help ensure a safe, satisfying, and positive birth experience.

Baseline Fetal Heart Rate

The **baseline fetal heart rate** (FHR) is referred to as the average fetal heart rate observed between contractions over a 10-minute period (Fig. 12-20). The recorded baseline

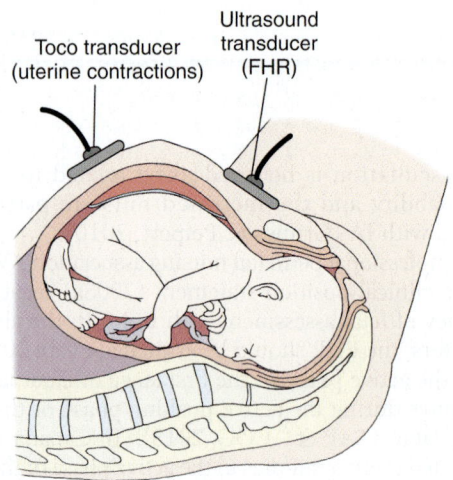

Figure 12-18 External fetal monitor.

Box 12-6 Various Influences on the Fetal Heart Rate

UTERO-PLACENTAL UNIT

- Transfer of oxygen and carbon dioxide between the maternal and fetal circulation (depends on adequate uterine blood flow, sufficient functional placental mass, and umbilical cord patency)
- Adequate fetal oxygenation (depends on adequate maternal oxygenation, placental blood flow, uteroplacental circulation, umbilical circulation, and innate ability of the fetus to initiate compensatory mechanisms to regulate the FHR)
- Other fetal environmental factors that influence oxygenation (uteroplacental function, uterine activity, umbilical cord patency, and maternal physiological functioning)
- Adequate placental reserve (reserve oxygen available to the fetus to withstand the transient changes in blood flow and oxygen during labor)
  - The placenta normally provides oxygen and nutrients over and above fetal baseline needs
  - In periods of decreased oxygen, blood flow is deferred to vital fetal organs (heart, brain, and adrenal glands) to compensate
  - If placental reserves are decreased or depleted, the fetus may not be able to adapt to or tolerate the decreased oxygen that occurs during a uterine contraction
  - The fetus adapts to the stresses of labor through homeostatic mechanisms

AUTONOMIC NERVOUS SYSTEM

Parasympathetic Nervous System

- Primarily mediated by the vagus nerve innervating the sinoatrial (SA) and atrioventricular (AV) nodes in the heart
- Parasympathetic stimulation decreases the heart rate
- Stimulation of the vagus nerve slows the FHR and helps to maintain variability (develops around 28–30 weeks of gestation)

Sympathetic Nervous System (SNS)

- SNS stimulation increases the FHR
- Stimulation of nerves (located throughout the fetal heart) produces an increase in the strength of the fetal heart contraction
- SNS is responsible for long-term baseline variability

- Action occurs through the release of norepinephrine
- SNS may be stimulated during periods of fetal hypoxemia

BARORECEPTORS

- Stretch receptors present in the aortic arch and the carotid arch; detect pressure changes
- Maintain homeostasis: regulate the heart rate by stimulating a vagal response and decreasing the FHR, fetal blood pressure, and cardiac output

CENTRAL NERVOUS SYSTEM (CNS)

- The integrative center responsible for variations in the FHR and baseline variability related to fetal activity
- Regulates and coordinates autonomic activities
- Mediates cardiac and vasomotor reflexes
- Responds to fetal movement

CHEMORECEPTORS

- Located in the aortic arch and the CNS
- Respond to changes in fetal O_2, CO_2 and pH levels: decreased O_2 and increased CO_2 cause peripheral chemoreceptors to stimulate the vagal nerve and slow the FHR; central chemoreceptors respond to an increased FHR and an increased blood pressure

HORMONAL REGULATION

- The fetus responds to a decrease in O_2 or in uteroplacental blood flow by releasing hormones that maximize blood flow to vital organs (heart, brain, and adrenal glands)
- Epinephrine, norepinephrine, catecholamines, and vasopressin prompt hemodynamic changes in response to changes in fetal oxygenation; fetal hypoxia triggers a release of epinephrine and norepinephrine that increases FHR and blood pressure
- Renin-angiotensin (secreted by the kidneys) produce vasoconstriction in response to fetal hypovolemia

Sources: Chapman & Durham (2014); Cunningham et al. (2014); Miller (2010); Torgersen (2011).

---

excludes periodic FHR changes that are evidenced by increased variability or accelerations. The normal baseline fetal heart rate at term is 110 to 160 beats per minute (bpm). There are two abnormal variations of the baseline: tachycardia (baseline above 160 bpm) and bradycardia (baseline below 110 bpm).

TACHYCARDIA. **Tachycardia** is generally defined as a sustained baseline fetal heart rate greater than 160 beats per minute for a duration of 10 minutes or longer (Fig. 12-21). A number of conditions are associated with fetal tachycardia:

- Fetal hypoxia: The fetus attempts to compensate for reduced blood flow by increasing sympathetic stimulation of the central nervous system (CNS).
- Maternal fever: An increase in maternal temperature accelerates fetal metabolism, thus increasing the FHR. This situation may be seen in a laboring woman who becomes dehydrated or has an increased temperature following prolonged exposure in a warm bath or whirlpool.
- Maternal medications: Both parasympathetic drugs (e.g., atropine and scopolamine) and beta-sympathetic drugs (tocolytic drugs used to halt contractions) can have a stimulant effect and increase the fetal heart rate.

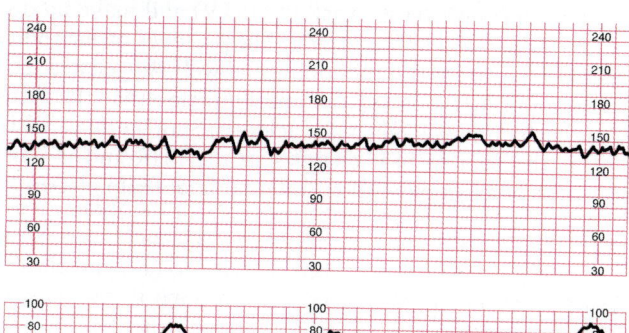

Figure 12-20 The normal baseline fetal heart rate at term is 110 to 160 bpm. (Top: fetal heart rate; Bottom: uterine contractions)

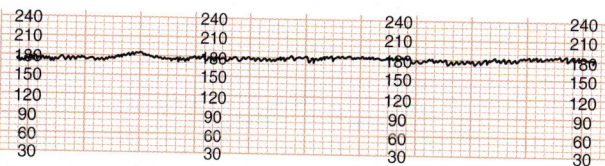

Figure 12-21 Fetal tachycardia.

- Infection: Tachycardia may be an initial sign of uterine infection (amnionitis) and may precede an increased maternal temperature by 1 to 2 hours.
- Fetal anemia: In response to a decrease in hemoglobin, the FHR increases to compensate and improve tissue metabolism.
- Maternal hyperthyroidism: Thyroid-stimulating hormone (TSH) may cross the placenta and stimulate the fetal heart rate (Cunningham et al., 2014).

BRADYCARDIA. **Bradycardia** is defined as a sustained (greater than 10 minutes) baseline FHR of less than 110 bpm (Fig. 12-22). Fetal bradycardia may be associated with the following (Cunningham et al., 2014):

- Late fetal hypoxia: Myocardial activity becomes depressed and lowers the fetal heart rate.
- Medications: Beta-adrenergic blocking drugs (e.g., propranolol [Inderal]).
- Maternal hypotension: Results in decreased blood flow to the fetus and can lower the FHR. Maternal hypotension can result from positioning (i.e., supine hypotension) and is a common side effect associated with an epidural or spinal anesthetic.
- Maternal or fetal hypothermia and dehydration
- Prolonged umbilical cord compression: Stimulates fetal baroreceptors that cause vagal stimulation and a decreased FHR.
- Fetal bradyarrhythmias: With complete heart block, the FHR baseline is often as low as 70 to 90 bpm.
- Uterine tachysystole (hyperstimulation)
- Abruptio placentae
- Uterine rupture or vasa previa
- Vagal stimulation during the second stage (fetal recovery is possible because this condition does not involve hypoxia)
- Chronic fetal head compression

When bradycardia is observed, the nurse first confirms that the EFM is monitoring the FHR, rather than the maternal heart rate, then assesses for fetal movement and the fetal response to fetal scalp stimulation (performed when the FHR is between contractions). A vaginal exam is performed to assess for umbilical cord prolapse. Assessment of maternal vital signs and hydration status with prn fluid

administration may be useful in reducing contractions and in promoting fetal oxygenation. Depending on other parameters (e.g., FHR variability), other actions that may be appropriate include changing the maternal position, discontinuing oxytocin, administering oxygen (8–10 L/min by mask), modifying the patient's pushing pattern, and notifying the primary care provider.

 Critical Nursing Action Recognizing and Responding to Uterine Tachysystole

Sometimes referred to as hyperstimulation, uterine tachysystole is a condition of excessively frequent contractions with the following characteristics: greater than 5 uterine contractions in 10 minutes (averaged over a 30-minute window) with contractions occurring within 1 minute of each other, and a uterine resting tone greater than 20 to 25 mm Hg with a peak pressure greater than 80 mm Hg (Fig. 12-23). Tachysystole may occur in spontaneous or stimulated labor and is most commonly caused by cervical ripening agents, induction, and augmentation of labor. (See Chapter 14). Medical management centers on addressing the cause of tachysystole (e.g., discontinuing oxytocin or removing cervical ripening medication). Nursing interventions center on reducing uterine activity with intrauterine resuscitative actions such as maternal position change, increasing hydration, relieving maternal anxiety and pain, and administering a tocolytic medication as ordered.

BASELINE VARIABILITY

Variability of the FHR is manifested by fluctuations in the baseline fetal heart rate observed on the fetal monitor. The pattern denotes an irregular, changing FHR rather than a straight line that indicates few changes in the rate. The variability of the FHR is a result of the interplay (a "push and pull" effect) between the fetal sympathetic nervous system, which assists to increase the heart rate and the parasympathetic nervous system, which acts to decrease the heart rate. Baseline variability, which is the fluctuations in the baseline FHR that are irregular in amplitude and frequency, is the most important predictor of adequate fetal oxygenation during labor. Reduced variability is the best single predictor for determining fetal compromise. The fluctuations are visually quantified as the amplitude of the peak and trough in bpm (Alfirevic, Decane, & Gyte, 2013; Cunningham et al., 2014).

Current guidelines from NICHD (Macones et al., 2008) describe variability as a summation of long-term variability (LTV) and short-term variability (STV) and make no distinction between LTV and STV. The presence of variability is reflective of a well-functioning and well-oxygenated fetal autonomic nervous system and confirms that the fetus is not experiencing metabolic acidosis. Short-term variability is the beat to beat changes in the FHR and is most accurately assessed with an internal fetal scalp electrode.

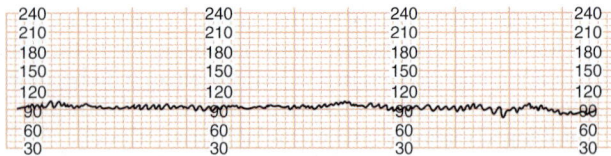

Figure 12-22 Fetal bradycardia.

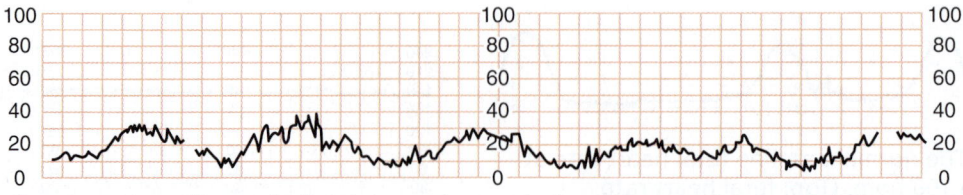

Figure 12-23 Tachysystole (inadequate interval of resting tone between UC).

Long-term variability refers to the changes in fetal heart rate over a longer period of time such as 1 minute. The absence of or undetected variability is considered a warning sign of non-reassuring fetal status. Reduced variability may be associated with fetal dysrhythmias or anomalies affecting the heart, central nervous system, or autonomic nervous system, a previous neurological insult, tachycardia, or prematurity (less than 32 weeks' gestation). If decreased variability is noted with an external modality, application of an internal fetal scalp electrode should be considered to obtain more accurate information. Variability may be described as absent, minimal, moderate, or marked (ACOG, 2010) (Table 12-5) (Figs. 12-24 to 12-27).

Table 12-5 Classifications of FHR Variability and Possible Causes

Variability	Amplitude of FHR Changes	Causes
Absent	Undetectable	May represent fetal cerebral asphyxia. Warrants immediate evaluation.
Minimal	>2–<5 beats per minute (bpm)	May be related to narcotics, tranquilizers, magnesium sulfate, barbiturates, anesthetic agents, supine hypotension, cord compression, uterine tachysystole, prematurity, or fetal sleep.
Moderate	6–25 bpm	Indicative of fetal well-being.
Marked	>25 bpm	Marked variability is believed to be a less common response to fetal hypoxia.

Source: Macones et al. (2008).

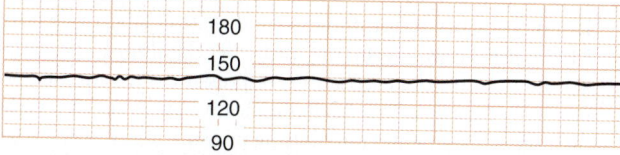

Figure 12-24 Absent variability.

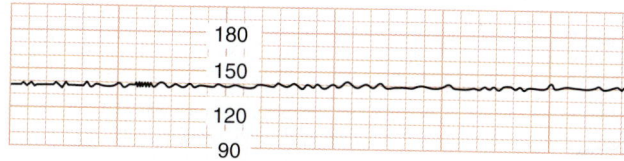

Figure 12-25 Minimal variability.

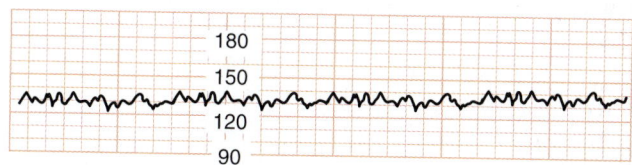

Figure 12-26 Moderate variability.

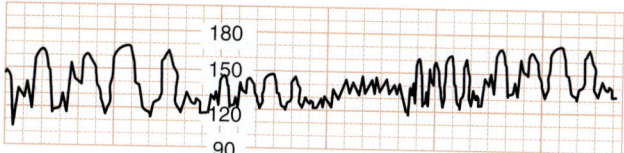

Figure 12-27 Marked variability.

 Nursing Insight—Appreciating the concepts of acidemia, acidosis, and asphyxia

Under normal circumstances, carbon dioxide (CO_2), an acidic waste product of cell metabolism during aerobic metabolism, is carried away on the hemoglobin and efficiently eliminated from the fetal circulation through the placenta. Maternal conditions such as diabetes and hypertension may impair placental circulation, resulting in a reduced oxygen supply, which is worsened with uterine contractions. When the oxygen supply is low, the cell converts to an inefficient anaerobic metabolism and produces lactic acid (rather than CO_2) as a waste product. Without oxygen, *acidemia* (increased concentration of hydrogen ions [acidity] in the fetal blood) progresses to *acidosis*, a more perverse acidity deep within the fetal tissues. *Asphyxia* (lack of O_2, excess of CO_2) follows acidosis, the fetal metabolic and adaptive processes are interrupted and fail, and without improvement in oxygenation, myocardial depression and brain ischemia result (Blackburn, 2012; Simpson & O'Brien-Abel, 2013).

The presence of adequate (moderate) variability is an important indicator of fetal well-being. FHR variability is indicative of an adequately oxygenated neurological pathway in which impulses are transmitted from the fetal brain to the cardiac conduction system. An electronic fetal monitor tracing that records the FHR as a changing, jagged line is reflective of an adequately oxygenated, responsive fetal brain and fetal heart (Freeman, Garite, Nageotte, & Miller, 2012).

Conversely, the absence of variability may indicate normal variations such as fetal sleep (the sleep state should not last longer than 30 minutes), a response to certain drugs that depress the CNS (e.g., analgesics: meperidine [Demerol]; tranquilizers: diazepam [Valium]; barbiturates: secobarbital [Seconal] and pentobarbital [Nembutal]; and ataractics: promethazine [Phenergan]) and general anesthetics or a pathological condition such as hypoxia, a CNS abnormality, or acidemia.

 Critical Nursing Action When Minimal or Absent Variability Is Detected

Minimal or absent variability that does not appear to be associated with a fetal sleep cycle or the administration of maternal medications may signal fetal hypoxia or acidosis. When detected, nurses should take the following actions (Freeman et al., 2012; Simpson & Creehan, 2013; Simpson & O'Brien-Abel, 2013):

- Assist the patient into a position that promotes enhanced fetal oxygenation
- Assess the fetal response to fetal scalp stimulation or vibroacoustic stimulation
- Assess maternal hydration: administer an IV bolus to reduce uterine activity and promote increased uterine perfusion

- Discontinue oxytocin to reduce uterine activity
- Administer oxygen (8–10 L/min by mask) to promote fetal oxygenation
- Consider more invasive monitoring (i.e., internal fetal scalp electrode)
- Offer support to the patient and her birth partner
- Notify the primary care provider

PERIODIC AND EPISODIC CHANGES

Periodic changes are accelerations and decelerations in the FHR that occur in relation to uterine contractions and persist over time. Periodic changes include FHR accelerations and four types of FHR decelerations: early, variable, late, and prolonged.

Episodic changes are FHR acceleration and deceleration patterns that are not associated with uterine contractions. FHR accelerations are the most common episodic change.

ACCELERATIONS

An **acceleration** is defined as an increase in the FHR of 15 bpm above the fetal heart baseline that lasts for at least 15 seconds to less than 2 minutes. Accelerations are visually abrupt and transient—the onset to peak is less than 30 seconds. Before 32 weeks of gestation, accelerations are defined as an acceleration greater than or equal to 10 bpm over the baseline FHR for greater than or equal to 10 seconds. A prolonged acceleration is greater than or equal to 2 minutes but less than or equal to 10 minutes. Accelerations are considered a sign of fetal well-being when they accompany fetal movement. Thus, when a fetus is active in utero, accelerations (caused by a sympathetic response to fetal movement) are normally present. Consequently, when the fetus is sleeping or not moving, limited FHR accelerations may be noted.

When contractions are present, accelerations are often noted as a response to the contraction. This type of periodic FHR acceleration with contractions is thought to be a compensatory accelerative response to a transient decrease in blood flow (e.g., umbilical vein compression) to the fetus. Accelerations may occur before, during, or after a contraction. Accelerations are often associated with a normal FHR baseline and normal variability (Fig. 12-28). The presence of FHR accelerations should be recorded in the patient's labor chart.

DECELERATIONS

Decelerations are defined as any decrease in FHR below the baseline FHR. They are classified according to their shape, timing, and duration in relation to the uterine contraction (UC). Recurrent decelerations occur with at least 50% of UCs over a 20-minute period. Intermittent decelerations occur with fewer than 50% of UCs over a 20-minute period. Decelerations are further defined according to their onset and are characterized as early, variable, late, and prolonged (Fig. 12-29). Appropriate nursing actions for variable, late, and prolonged decelerations are presented in Table 12-6.

Early Decelerations

An early deceleration is defined as a visually apparent, usually symmetrical, gradual decrease and return of the FHR associated with a uterine contraction (Macones et al., 2008). Early decelerations are characterized by a deceleration in the FHR that resembles a mirror image to the contraction. Therefore, the onset of the deceleration begins near the onset of the contraction, the lowest part of the deceleration (nadir) occurs at the peak of contraction, and the FHR returns to baseline by the end of the contraction. Early decelerations are usually repetitive and are commonly observed during active labor and descent of the fetus (Fig. 12-30).

Early decelerations are considered benign and are usually well tolerated by the fetus. They are believed to be related to transient fetal head compression and the resulting vagal stimulation that slows the FHR. When present, early decelerations usually occur during the first stage of labor. They may also occur during vaginal examinations as a result of fundal pressure and during placement of the internal mode of fetal monitoring. Early decelerations are viewed as an indicator of fetal well-being and adequate oxygen reserve and no nursing intervention is needed.

Nursing Insight—*Repetitive early decelerations may signal labor progress*

Repetitive early decelerations may signal advanced cervical dilation or the beginning of the second stage of labor. When the EFM strip shows recurring early decelerations, the nurse should inquire about sensations of pressure. Pressure that occurs only during contractions is indicative of advanced cervical dilation, while intense, unremitting pressure may signal the beginning of the second stage. A vaginal exam may be performed to confirm the cervical status.

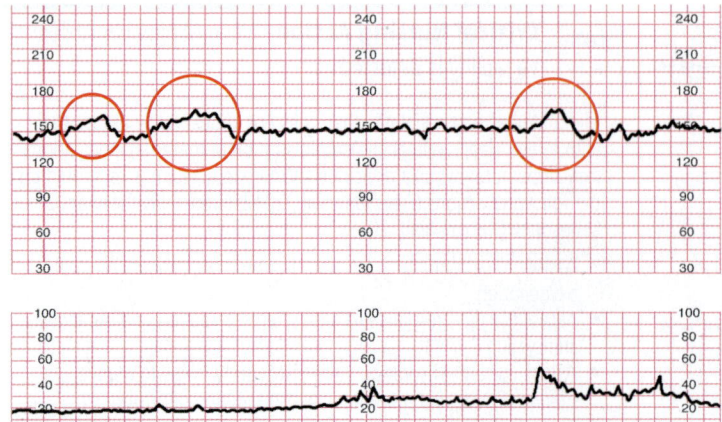

Figure 12-28 FHR accelerations.

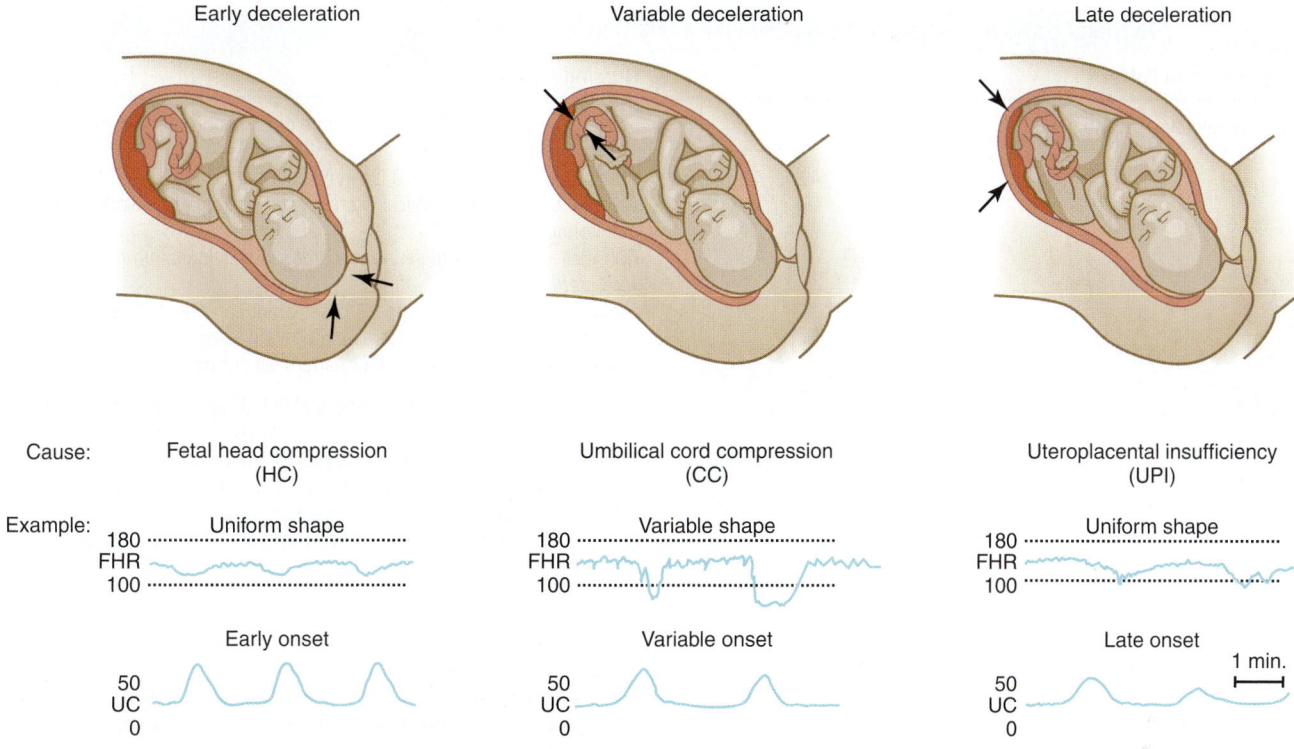

Figure 12-29 Causes and examples of periodic decelerations.

Table 12-6 Nursing Actions for Variable, Late, and Prolonged FHR Decelerations	
Deceleration Pattern	**Nursing Actions**
Variable decelerations: Normal (transient) (duration less than 60 seconds, rapid return to baseline, normal baseline and variability)	Explain finding and offer support to patient and her birth partner *to decrease anxiety or pain, and to enhance uterine blood flow and fetal oxygenation.*
Variable decelerations: Indeterminate or abnormal (prolonged return to baseline, persistence to less than 60 bpm and greater than 60 seconds, presence of overshoots tachycardia, repetitive overshoots, and absent variability)	Change the maternal position (side to side, knee chest) *to minimize or correct cord compression and promote fetal oxygenation.* Decrease or discontinue oxytocin if infusing *to decrease uterine contractions.* Note: A tocolytic (e.g., terbutaline) may be given *to promote uterine relaxation.* Administer oxygen at 8 to 10 L/min (via tight face mask) *to improve fetal oxygenation.* Assist with/perform sterile vaginal examination *to assess for umbilical cord prolapse, to assess labor progress, and to perform fetal scalp stimulation.* Assist with amnioinfusion (if ordered) *to alleviate umbilical cord compression by increasing the intrauterine fluid volume.* Alter the maternal pushing technique (open glottis, shorter duration of pushes) *to enhance uteroplacental blood flow.* Consider internal monitoring *to obtain a more accurate fetal and uterine assessment.* Explain finding and offer support to the patient and her birth partner. Prepare for birth: If FHR pattern cannot be corrected, expect cesarean or operative vaginal delivery (e.g., forceps, vacuum extraction).
Late decelerations	Position patient on her side. Assess for maternal hypotension; to correct—increase IVF rate, administer an IVF bolus (at least 500 mL Ringer's lactate), elevate maternal legs *to increase blood volume and raise the blood pressure.* Continue adequate maternal hydration (IVF—normal saline or Ringer's lactate) *to maximize maternal intravascular volume and enhance uteroplacental perfusion.* Palpate the uterus *to assess for tachysystole.*

(continued)

Table 12-6 Nursing Actions for Variable, Late, and Prolonged FHR Decelerations (continued)

Deceleration Pattern	Nursing Actions
Late decelerations (continued)	Discontinue oxytocin if infusing and late decelerations persist. Note: Terbutaline may be ordered. Administer oxygen at 8 to 10 L/min (via tight face mask). Assess labor progress (cervical dilation, fetal station); consider internal monitoring. Consider fetal scalp stimulation or vibroacoustic stimulation *to assess fetal status.* Explain finding and offer support to the patient and her birth partner. Prepare for birth – expect cesarean or operative vaginal delivery (e.g., forceps, vacuum extraction) if FHR pattern cannot be corrected.
Prolonged decelerations	Assess baseline variability preceding and following the deceleration *to observe for accompanying FHR pattern changes.* Assist patient into a position that improves FHR pattern. Discontinue oxytocin if infusing (terbutaline may be ordered). Administer oxygen at 8 to 10L/min (via tight face mask). Increase IVF rate prn; consider administering an IVF bolus (500 mL Ringer's lactate). Assist with/perform sterile vaginal examination and fetal scalp stimulation. Assist with amnioinfusion (if ordered). Consider internal monitoring. Explain finding and offer support to the patient and her birth partner. Prepare for birth – expect cesarean or operative vaginal delivery (e.g., forceps, vacuum extraction) if FHR pattern cannot be corrected.

Sources: Freeman, Garite, Nageotte, & Miller (2012); Simpson & Creehan (2013); Torgersen (2011).

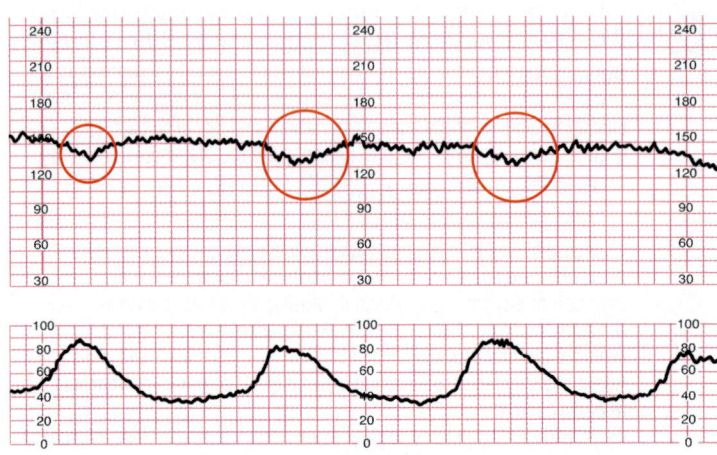

Figure 12-30 Early decelerations.

Variable Decelerations

Variable decelerations, as the name implies, are decelerations that are variable in terms of their onset, frequency, duration, and intensity. The visually abrupt decrease in FHR below the baseline is 15 bpm or more, lasts at least 15 seconds, and returns to the baseline in less than 2 minutes from the time of onset (Macones et al., 2008) (Fig. 12-31). Variable decelerations occur at any time during the uterine contracting phase and may appear in the shape of a "U," "W," or "V." Sometimes a variable deceleration is preceded and followed by brief acceleration of the FHR, known as "shouldering." A shoulder is a compensatory response to hypoxemia and is an increase in the FHR of 20 bpm for less than 20 seconds. An "overshoot" or "rebound overshoot" is a gradual smooth acceleration in FHR of 10 to 20 bpm for more than 60 to

90 seconds (Miller, Miller, & Tucker, 2012; Simpson & O'Brien-Abel, 2013).

The most common deceleration pattern seen in labor, variable decelerations, are thought to be a result of umbilical cord compression, which triggers a vagal response that slows the FHR. Umbilical vein compression is accompanied by decreased PO_2 and chemoreceptor stimulation, then compression of the more muscular umbilical arteries. Thus, the degree by which the cord is compressed (partially versus completely) can affect the severity of the deceleration. For example, a cord that is briefly compressed by the fetus may manifest as a very abrupt decrease in the FHR with a rapid return to baseline. Conversely, a cord that is tightly wrapped around the fetal neck (**nuchal cord**) progressively becomes more compressed as the fetus descends into the maternal pelvis. This situation is most

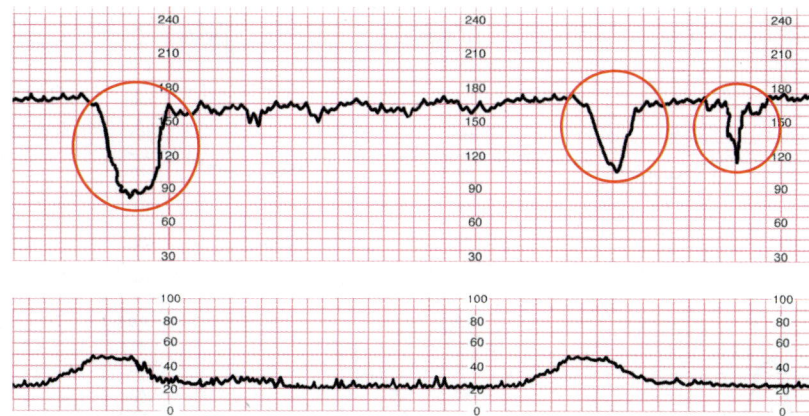

Figure 12-31 Variable decelerations.

likely to result in longer, more severe decelerations. Variable decelerations may also occur with sudden descent of the fetal head late in the active phase of labor. When related to head compression, variable decelerations are usually non-repetitive and irregular in shape (ACOG, 2010; Miller, Miller, & Tucker, 2012).

In general, brief, occasional decelerations are often considered benign, whereas repetitive, worsening variable decelerations are cause for concern and always warrant further investigation. Nursing actions center on efforts directed at intrauterine resuscitation: assessment of cervix (prolapsed cord and labor progress), uterine activity (tachysystole), maternal vital signs (fever and hypotension), interventions (position changes, IV fluids, oxygen, and medications), and maternal/birth partner support (see Table 12-6). These actions maximize intravascular volume, uterine perfusion, placental exchange, and the delivery of oxygen to the fetus (Simpson & O'Brien-Abel, 2013).

- To summarize, "normal" variable decelerations are less than 60 seconds in duration, have a rapid return to the baseline, and are accompanied by a normal baseline and variability. Characteristics of "abnormal" or "indeterminate" variable decelerations include the following: slow return to the baseline, persistence to less than 60 bpm and greater than 60 seconds, presence of overshoots, tachycardia, and repetitive overshoots and absent variability.

 Nursing Insight—*Understanding the oxygen pathway*

Both late and variable decelerations are reflective of a fetal reflex autonomic response to an interruption of oxygen transfer along the oxygen pathway. The oxygen pathway includes the maternal lungs, heart, vasculature, uterus, placenta, and umbilical cord. Miller (2012) proposes the following guide for evaluation and correction of interruptions to the oxygen pathway:

- Lungs: Assess maternal respiratory rate, airway, and breathing; give supplemental oxygen
- Heart and vasculature: Assess maternal heart rate and rhythm, blood pressure, and volume status; change maternal position, administer IV fluid bolus, correct hypotension
- Uterus and placenta: Assess uterine activity and rule out uterine rupture, check for bleeding and rule out

abruption; stop or reduce any labor-stimulating agent, consider administration of a uterine relaxant
- Umbilical cord: Perform a vaginal exam and rule out cord prolapse; consider amnioinfusion

 Optimizing Outcomes—**Amnioinfusion to relieve cord compression**

Amnioinfusion is the transcervical instillation of warmed normal saline into the uterus via sterile catheter (IUPC). The infusion of saline provides additional intraamniotic fluid to cushion the umbilical cord and help lessen cord compression. Amnioinfusion may be used in an attempt to reduce the severity of repetitive variable decelerations caused by cord compression (ACOG, 2006b). The nurse assists with the procedure by assembling the equipment; monitoring the FHR, contraction status, and maternal temperature; and verifying and documenting that the infused fluid is exiting the uterus.

Late Decelerations

A late deceleration of the FHR is a visually apparent, gradual decrease in and return to baseline FHR associated with uterine contractions. The patterns of late decelerations typically mirror the contraction, and this characteristic is similar in appearance to early decelerations. With late decelerations, the deceleration has a late onset and begins around the peak of the contraction (Fig. 12-32). This type of deceleration does not resolve until after the contraction has ended. Late decelerations indicate the presence of **uteroplacental insufficiency,** a decline in placental function. Normally, the fetus can withstand repeated contractions with sufficient oxygenation. However, in this circumstance a decrease in blood flow from the uterus to the placenta results in fetal hypoxia and late decelerations.

Late decelerations require prompt attention and reporting. The presence of persistent and repetitive late decelerations is usually indicative of fetal hypoxemia that may progress to hypoxia and metabolic acidemia. The longer the late decelerations persist, the more serious they become. Immediate attempts should be made to correct the cause of the late decelerations if possible. For example, late decelerations in the presence of an oxytocin

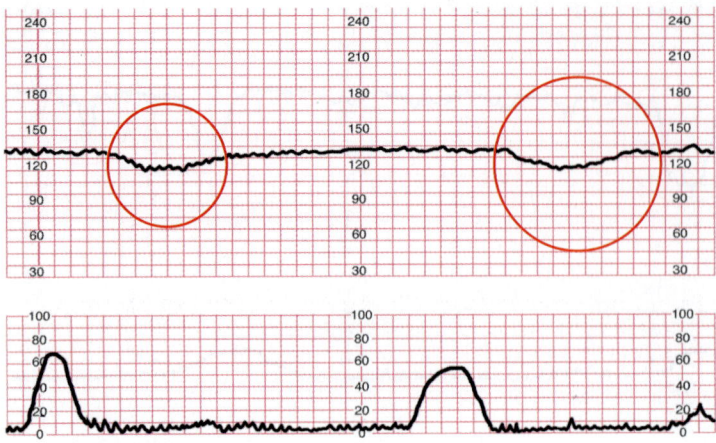

Figure 12-32 Late decelerations.

infusion may signal a need to immediately discontinue the oxytocin infusion, especially if uterine hyperstimulation is suspected. Nursing interventions that should be implemented immediately center on intrauterine resuscitation (see Table 12-6).

It is important to note that late decelerations can present very obviously or very subtly. In addition, late decelerations are often accompanied by other non-reassuring fetal heart patterns such as a loss of or decrease in variability. Decelerations may be further classified as recurrent or intermittent. Recurrent decelerations occur with greater than 50% of uterine contractions; intermittent decelerations occur with less than 50% of uterine contractions (Lyndon, O'Brien-Abel, & Simpson, 2013; Miller, 2012; Miller, Miller, & Tucker, 2012).

 ### Nursing Insight—*Potential causes of uteroplacental insufficiency*

Late decelerations that are caused by uteroplacental insufficiency may be related to uterine hyperstimulation with oxytocin, placental changes that affect gas exchange (e.g., postmaturity), preterm pregnancy, amnionitis, preeclampsia, small for gestational age (SGA) fetus, placenta previa, abruptio placentae, maternal diabetes, hypotension related to hemorrhage, conduction anesthesia, or supine positioning, maternal cardiopulmonary disease, hypertension, and severe maternal anemia.

Prolonged Decelerations

A prolonged deceleration is an abrupt decrease in the FHR below the baseline that is greater than or equal to 15 bpm and lasts greater than or equal to 2 minutes but less than 10 minutes (Fig. 12-33). Prolonged decelerations may be abrupt or gradual, and when they are non-recurrent and preceded and followed by normal baseline and moderate variability, prolonged decelerations are not associated with fetal hypoxemia. The following events can cause prolonged decelerations: any mechanism that produces a profound change in the fetal O_2, interruption of uteroplacental perfusion (e.g., tachysystole [hyperstimulation], maternal hypotension, or abruptio placentae), interruption of umbilical blood flow (e.g., cord compression or cord prolapse), or vagal stimulation (e.g., profound head compression or rapid fetal descent). If prolonged decelerations are observed, the nurse must immediately initiate appropriate interventions (see Table 12-6) and promptly notify the primary care provider.

INTERPRETATION OF FHR TRACINGS

A systematic approach to the interpretation of FHR tracings ensures that all possibilities are considered. When assessing FHR tracings, nurses should consider factors such as contraction frequency and intensity, stage of labor, and the earlier FHR pattern. Most institutions have established protocols to guide electronic fetal heart monitoring methods and to maintain consistency in the interpretation of FHR patterns.

In 1997, the National Institute of Child Health and Human Development (NICHD) published a proposed nomenclature system for EFM interpretation. Standardized definitions for FHR monitoring were presented. In 2004, the Society of Obstetricians and Gynaecologists in Canada (SOGC) adopted the NICHD nomenclature as their standard in the interpretation of FHR tracings; the American Congress of Obstetricians and Gynecologists (ACOG), the American College of Nurse-Midwives (ACNM), and the Association for Women's Health, Obstetric, and Neonatal Nurses (AWHONN) followed suit and also adopted the NICHD nomenclature (Torgersen, 2011). In 2008, a group of fetal monitoring experts convened under the auspices of

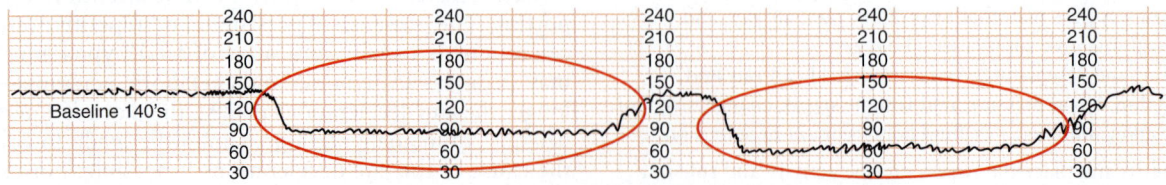

Figure 12-33 Prolonged decelerations.

the NICHD, ACOG, and the Society for Maternal-Fetal Medicine (SMFM) to expand the intrapartal fetal heart rate (FHR) monitoring guidelines to include interpretive categories (Hankins & Miller, 2011; Macones et al., 2008). None of the previously defined FHR terms were changed, but new terms for defining uterine activity were added and a categorization of FHR patterns, termed the "Three-Tier Fetal Heart Rate Interpretation System," was recommended (Box 12-7). A schema to guide decision making in FHR assessment is presented in Figure 12-34.

 Critical Nursing Action Interpreting Fetal Monitor Tracings

To aid in the interpretation of EFM tracings, the nurse should consider the following parameters:

- **Uterine activity:** What is the frequency, duration, and intensity of contractions?
- **Labor progress:** What is the stage of labor? What is the dilation, effacement, station, presentation, and position?
- **Baseline FHR:** What is the baseline FHR? Is tachycardia or bradycardia present?
- **Baseline variability:** What is the variability of the FHR (absent, minimal, moderate, marked, or other)?
- **Periodic changes in FHR:** Are there any FHR changes from the baseline? Are accelerations present? Are any decelerations present? If decelerations are present, are they early, variable, late, or prolonged?
- **Maternal history and condition:** Are there any preexisting conditions that increase risk for this pregnancy? Are there any intrapartal high-risk factors (e.g., meconium) that should be noted?

Fetal monitoring documentation, usually recorded on a standard form, should include all the critical elements including characteristics of the FHR, UC, and monitor mode (Fig. 12-35).

Box 12-7 **Fetal Heart Rate Terms and Interpretation of FHR Patterns (NICHD, 2008)**

In 2008, the National Institute of Child and Human Development (NICHD) added two new terms for defining uterine activity:

Normal: Less than or equal to 5 contractions in 10 minutes, averaged over a 30-minute window.

Tachysystole: Greater than 5 contractions in 10 minutes, averaged over a 30-minute window.

- Tachysystole should always be qualified as to the presence or absence of associated FHR decelerations.
- The term "tachysystole" applies to both spontaneous or stimulated labor. The clinical response to tachysystole may differ, depending on whether contractions are spontaneous or stimulated.
- The terms "hyperstimulation" and "hypercontractility" are not defined and should be abandoned.

The NICHD also recommended a categorization of FHR patterns, the "Three-Tier Fetal Heart Rate Interpretation System," which is based on the association between each FHR pattern and fetal acidemia:

CATEGORY 1

Category 1 fetal heart rate tracings include all of the following:

- Baseline rate: 110–160 beats per minute (bpm)
- Moderate baseline FHR variability
- Late or variable decelerations are absent
- Early decelerations may be present or absent
- Accelerations may be present or absent

Category I FHR tracings are normal and strongly predictive of normal fetal acid-base status at the time of observation. Category I FHR tracings may be followed in a routine manner and no specific action is required.

CATEGORY II

Category II FHR tracings include all FHR tracings not categorized as Category I or Category III. Category II tracings may represent an appreciable fraction of those encountered in clinical care. Examples of Category II FHR tracings include any of the following:

BASELINE RATE

- Bradycardia not accompanied by absent baseline variability
- Tachycardia

Baseline FHR Variability

- Minimal baseline variability

- Absent baseline variability not accompanied by recurrent decelerations
- Marked baseline variability

Accelerations

- Absence of induced accelerations after fetal stimulation

Periodic or Episodic Decelerations

- Recurrent variable decelerations accompanied by minimal or moderate baseline variability
- Prolonged deceleration greater than or equal to 2 minutes but less than 10 minutes
- Recurrent late decelerations with moderate baseline variability
- Variable decelerations with other characteristics, such as slow return to baseline, "overshoots," or "shoulders"

Category II FHR tracings are indeterminate. Category II FHR tracings are not predictive of abnormal fetal acid-base status; there is a lack of adequate evidence to classify these tracings as Category I or Category III. Category II FHR tracings require evaluation and continued surveillance and reevaluation, taking into account the entire associated clinical circumstances.

CATEGORY III

Category III FHR tracings include either:

- Absent baseline FHR variability and any of the following:
  - Recurrent late decelerations
  - Recurrent variable decelerations
  - Bradycardia
- Sinusoidal pattern

Category III FHR tracings are abnormal. Category III tracings are predictive of abnormal fetal acid-base status at the time of observation. Category III FHR tracings require prompt evaluation. Depending on the clinical situation, efforts to expeditiously resolve the abnormal FHR pattern may include, but are not limited to, provision of maternal oxygen, change in maternal position, discontinuation of labor stimulation, and treatment of maternal hypotension.

Sources: Macones G. A., Hankins G. D., Spong C. Y., Hauth J., & Moore T. (2008). The 2008 National Institute of Child Health and Human Development Research Workshop Report on Electronic Fetal Heart Rate Monitoring: Update on Definitions, Interpretation, and Research Guidelines. *Obstetrics & Gynecology 112*(3), 661–666, *Journal of Obstetric, Gynecologic, & Neonatal Nursing, 37*(5), 510–515.

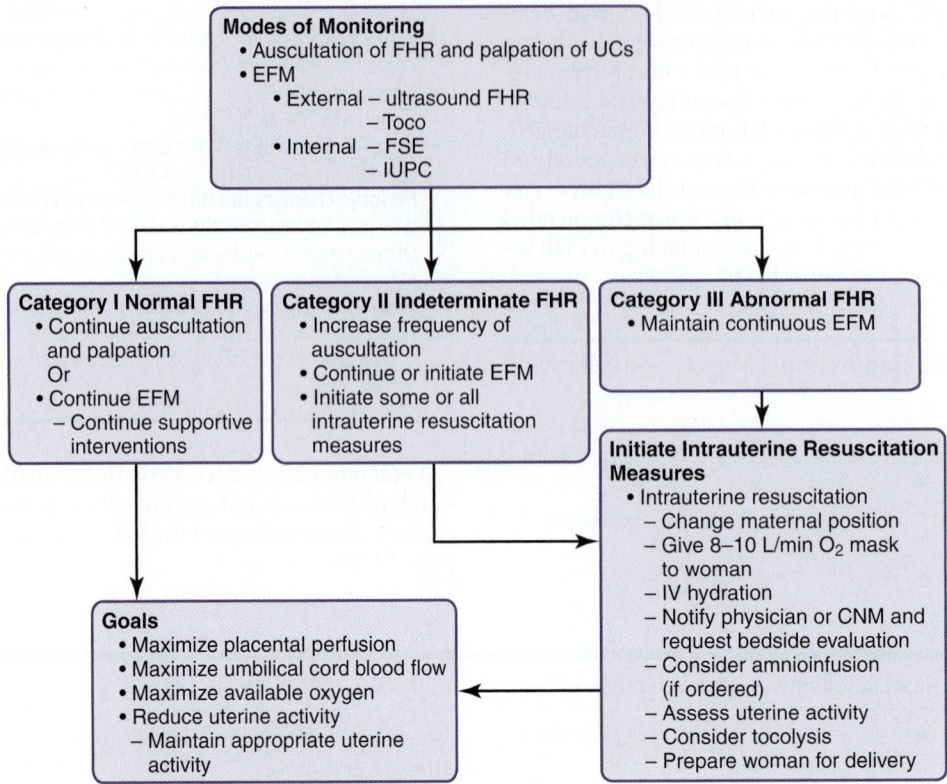

Figure 12-34 Decision making in FHR assessment.

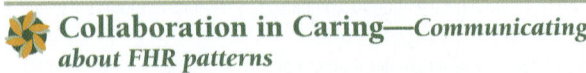

Collaboration in Caring—*Communicating about FHR patterns*

In clinical practice, various guidelines exist concerning the management of FHR tracings. Accurate, consistent, and timely communication among health-care providers is crucial in optimizing outcomes for the patient and her fetus. Burkman and Fennell (2010) suggest use of the SBAR tool to efficiently convey key information:

- Situation (what is happening with the patient now?)
- Background (what is the clinical background or context?)
- Assessment (what is the problem?)
- Recommendation (what can be done to correct it?)

ADDITIONAL METHODS OF FETAL ASSESSMENT

Other methods of fetal assessment have been developed to use in conjunction with EFM to provide additional information about the fetal status when non-reassuring FHR patterns are observed. These methods include FHR response to stimulation, fetal scalp blood sampling, and umbilical cord acid-base sampling (performed in the neonate).

Fetal Heart Rate Response to Stimulation

Fetal stimulation is performed to elicit an acceleration of the FHR of 15 bpm for at least 15 seconds and/or to improve FHR variability. Presently, two methods of fetal stimulation are in practice: scalp stimulation (the use of digital pressure during a vaginal examination) and vibroacoustic stimulation (the use of an artificial device [artificial larynx or fetal acoustic stimulation device] positioned over the fetal head for 1 to 2 seconds). Fetal stimulation procedures may be performed with or without ruptured membranes. However, they should only be performed when the FHR is at baseline, and neither stimulation method should be instituted if FHR decelerations or bradycardia is present. Acceleration of the FHR is usually indicative of fetal well-being; absence of an acceleration is usually indicative of a need to conduct further fetal evaluation.

Fetal Scalp Blood Sampling

A sample of fetal scalp blood is obtained through the dilated cervix after rupture of the membranes. Seldom used in the United States, this procedure is associated with many limiting factors: the requirement for cervical dilation and membrane rupture, the technical difficulty of the procedure, the need for repeated pH determinations, and the uncertainty surrounding the interpretation and application of results.

Umbilical Cord Acid-Base Assessment

During the immediate assessment of the newborn, a sample of cord blood is a useful adjunct to the Apgar score. Blood is withdrawn from the umbilical artery and tested for pH, PCO_2, and PO_2. Arterial values are reflective of the fetal condition; venous blood values are reflective of placental function. Umbilical cord gas measurements reflect the acid-base status of the neonate at birth; if acidemia is present, the type (respiratory, metabolic, or mixed) is determined by an analysis of the blood gas values (Miller, Miller & Tucker, 2012).

Patient Name:		Physician/CNM:			KEY
DATE:					
TIME:					**Variability** Ab = Absent (undetectable) Min = Minimal (>0 out ≤5 bpm) Mod = Moderate (6–25 bpm) Mar = Marked (>25 bpm)
Cervix	Dilation				
	Effacement				
	Station				**Accelerations** + = Present and appropriate for gestational age ∅ = Absent
Fetal Heart	Baseline Rate				
	Variability				**Decelerations** E = Early L = Late V = Variable P = Prolonged
	Accelerations				
	Decelerations				
	STIM/pH				**Stim/pH** + = Acceleration in response to stimulation ∅ = No response to stimulation Record number for scalp pH
	Monitor Mode				
Uterine Activity	Frequency				**Monitor mode** A = Auscultation/Palpation E = External u/s or toco FSE - Fetal spiral electrode IUPC = Intrauterine pressure catheter P = Palpation T = Telemetry
	Duration				
	Intensity				
	Resting Tone				
	Monitor Mode				**Frequency of uterine activity** ∅ = None Irreg = Irregular
	Oxytocin milliunits/min				**Intensity of uterine activity** M = Mild Mod = Moderate Str = Strong By IUPC = mm Hg
	Pain				
	Coping				**Resting tone** R = Relaxed By IUCP = mm Hg
	Maternal Position				**Coping** W = Well S = Support provided For pain use 0–10 scale
	O2/LPM/Mask				
	IV				**Maternal position** A = Ambulatory U = Upright SF = Semi-Fowler's RL = Right lateral LL = Left lateral MS = Modified Sims'
	Nurse Initials				
Narrative notes:					

Figure 12-35 Example of FHR documentation.

NURSING INTERVENTIONS AND DIAGNOSES

Early decelerations are considered to be benign, and no action is necessary. However, it is important to identify them so that they can be differentiated from variable or late decelerations. Depending on the cause, interventions for variable and late decelerations include lateral position changes (to displace the weight of the gravid uterus off the inferior vena cava), oxygen administration at 8 to 10 L per minute by face mask, palpation of the uterus for hyperstimulation (excessive uterine activity, also referred to as **tachysystole**), discontinuation of oxytocin if infusing, increasing the rate of the maintenance intravenous solution, and assisting with fetal oxygen saturation monitoring if ordered. Possible nursing diagnoses include impaired fetal gas exchange related to umbilical cord compression or placental insufficiency, decreased maternal cardiac output related to supine hypotension secondary to position, and anxiety related to lack of knowledge concerning fetal monitoring/fetal well-being during labor.

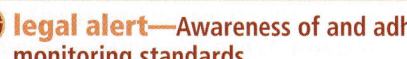 **legal alert**—Awareness of and adherence to fetal monitoring standards

Nurses who care for women during childbirth are legally responsible for the correct interpretation of FHR patterns, the timely initiation of appropriate nursing interventions based on those patterns, and full documentation of the outcomes of all interventions. In the event of non-reassuring FHR patterns that signal the need for intervention or expeditious birth, perinatal nurses are responsible for the timely notification of the primary care provider (physician or certified nurse-midwife), and they are also responsible for instituting the institutional chain of command if differences in opinion arise among care providers regarding the interpretation of the FHR pattern and appropriate interventions.

Now Can You—Assess FHR patterns detected by EFM?

1. Describe situations when electronic fetal monitoring instead of intermittent auscultation is indicated?
2. Define the following frequently used terminology: baseline fetal heart rate, variability, acceleration, and deceleration?
3. Describe the assessment of a Category II indeterminate FHR and a Category III abnormal fetal heart rate?
4. List four nursing interventions for variable and late decelerations?

Second Stage of Labor

The second stage of labor commences with full dilation of the cervix and ends with the birth of the infant. Often the woman or nurse may suspect that the woman has entered the second stage of labor because of the patient's urge to push or the presence of involuntary bearing down efforts. The contractions often remain very similar to those experienced during the transition stage. They continue to occur frequently and are very intense. The woman may exhibit varying emotions during the second stage. Some patients may get a spurt of energy or a "second wind" to help them get through the second stage. Others may be nervous or fearful of the new sensations that they are feeling. Encouragement and support from the labor nurse and support person are crucial at this stage. The woman is not to be left alone during this time, and continuous support should be provided. It is important to encourage the patient to rest between pushing to maintain her energy throughout the second stage.

PROMOTING EFFECTIVE PUSHING

Women push most effectively when they experience the urge to bear down and push. The urge to push is believed to be stimulated by the Ferguson reflex as the presenting part stretches the pelvic floor muscles. Thus, the maternal urge to push may be more related to the station of the presenting part rather than to the dilation of the cervix.

Differing practices exist regarding the promotion of pushing during the second stage. Many practitioners believe that pushing should be encouraged only when the woman has the urge to push, instead of when full cervical dilation has been reached. Some women (e.g., those with an epidural analgesia or other types of anesthesia) may have no urge to bear down. When this situation occurs, a process called "laboring down" may be used. "Laboring down" allows the woman to rest as the fetus descends. Pushing is postponed until the urge to push is experienced. Research suggests that there is a decrease in maternal fatigue and an increase in fetal oxygenation when women delay pushing until they feel the urge. It has been proposed that the decision concerning when to initiate pushing should be based on the individual maternal response rather than on standardized routine practices. Furthermore, the duration of active maternal pushing is more closely related to the neonate's condition at birth than the duration of the second stage of labor (AWHONN, 2008b; Prins, Boxem, Lucas, & Hutton, 2011; Simpson & O'Brien-Abel, 2013). In a recent (2012) systematic review of studies to date, Tuuli and colleagues found few clinical differences in outcomes with immediate compared with delayed pushing in the second stage of labor.

There are generally two methods of pushing during the second stage of labor: closed-glottis and open-glottis pushing. With closed-glottis pushing, also referred to as "directed pushing," the woman begins pushing at full cervical dilation regardless of the urge to bear down. The nurse should avoid instructing the patient to hold her breath and bear down as in a Valsalva maneuver while pushing as hard and as long as she is able throughout the contraction. This pushing method leads to a prolonged second stage of labor and adverse fetal effects such as hypoxia, acidemia, and lower neonatal Apgar scores. The poor outcomes are believed to result from prolonged maternal breath holding that ultimately affects uteroplacental blood flow (Prins et al., 2011; Simpson & Creehan, 2013; Simpson & O'Brien-Abel, 2013; Turley, 2011).

Open-glottis pushing, also referred to as "involuntary pushing," is the recommended method of pushing. With this technique, air is released during pushing so that no intrathoracic pressure builds up. The laboring woman is encouraged to hold her breath for only 5 to 6 seconds during pushing and to take several breaths between each bearing down effort. In addition, women are allowed to exhale throughout the bearing down attempts. This process facilitates maternal/fetal circulation and gradual fetal descent and is believed to be associated with fewer maternal and fetal adverse effects (Simpson & O'Brien-Abel, 2013; Turley, 2011).

Variations in pushing techniques are found in clinical practice. Regardless of the process used for second-stage pushing, laboring women require continuous support and encouragement from their health-care provider(s). It is important to calmly provide easy-to-understand, consistent information to avoid confusion. It is also important to remember that the patient and her partner can become anxious and confused if several people attempt to give directions at the same time.

ACHIEVING A POSITION OF COMFORT

During the second stage, comfort measures remain equally important, and many of the interventions and positioning identified for the first stage of labor can be implemented during the second stage as well. Many factors (e.g., the woman's personal preferences, the use of analgesia or anesthesia, the preferences of the health-care practitioner, and the imminence of birth) have an influence on the optimal maternal position during this stage. When pushing, women are encouraged whenever possible to maintain an upright or semi-upright position, such as squatting, sitting, standing, kneeling, on all fours, or sitting on the toilet.

Pushing when in an upright position allows the use of gravity to promote fetal descent and has been associated with a shortened labor. Positions such as squatting and kneeling may also help to increase the dimensions of the maternal pelvis. Assuming a hands and knees position or leaning over a table or chair helps to take pressure off the maternal spine and often reduces backache commonly associated with a fetal occipital–posterior position (see Fig. 12-14).

 Now Can You—Discuss comfort measures and pushing techniques for the second stage of labor?

1. List three comfort measures used during the first stage of labor that would also be effective during the second stage of labor?
2. Discuss how the nurse can advocate for a patient who does not have the urge to push in the second stage?
3. List two positions for pushing and provide one advantage of each?

PREPARATION FOR THE BIRTH

As the fetus descends, the woman experiences an increasing urge to bear down because of pressure of the fetal head on the sacral and obturator nerves. As the patient pushes, contraction of the abdominal muscles exerts intra-abdominal pressure. With the maternal bearing down efforts and further descent of the fetus, the nurse may notice bulging of the perineum and rectum. As the fetal head progresses downward, the perineum begins to stretch, thin out, and move anteriorly. The amount of bloody show may increase at this time, and the labia begin to part with each contraction. The fetal head, which may be observable at the vaginal introitus, often appears to recede between contractions. As the contractions and maternal pushing efforts continue, the presenting part descends farther.

Crowning, which means that birth is imminent, occurs when the fetal head is encircled by the vaginal introitus (Fig. 12-36). Some women may complain of a burning sensation as the perineum is stretched. This experience can be frightening for the woman, and it is important for the nurse to identify it as a normal sensation. The woman may also feel intense pressure in the rectum and a need to evacuate her bowels. Again, the nurse should confirm the normalcy of these sensations and continue to offer encouragement and support. If the woman does pass stool, she should be cleaned in a timely manner. Some women may feel as though they are losing control, and a variety of emotions (e.g., irritability, fear, embarrassment, and helplessness) may be displayed. These behaviors also can be frightening to the support person. The nurse needs to continue to

encourage and reinforce to the woman and her support person that these reactions are normal and that progress is being made.

LACERATIONS

Every birth is associated with damage to the soft tissues of the vagina and adjacent structures. Nulliparous women tend to experience more pronounced damage because the tissues are firmer and more resistant than those of multiparous women. Lacerations may occur in the cervix, vagina, and perineum (Fig. 12-37). Perineal lacerations, which usually occur when the fetal head is being born, are defined in terms of their depth:

- First degree—involve the perineal skin and vaginal mucous membrane
- Second degree—involve the skin, mucous membrane, and fascia of the perineal body
- Third degree—involve the skin, mucous membrane, and muscle of the perineal body and extend to the rectal sphincter
- Fourth degree—extend into the rectal mucosa and expose the lumen of the rectum

Immediately after birth, the cervix, vagina, and perineum are carefully inspected to assess for tissue damage. Rapid repair promotes healing and comfort, limits residual damage (e.g., fistulas, dyspareunia, cystocele, and rectocele), and decreases the possibility of infection.

EPISIOTOMY

Episiotomy is a surgical incision of the perineum that is performed to enlarge the vaginal orifice during the second stage of labor. The frequency of routine episiotomy has decreased over the last 20 years as the benefits of performing routine episiotomy began to be questioned. In the 1980s, the episiotomy rate was reported to be approximately 64 out of 100 births. At that time, many physicians routinely performed episiotomies based on the belief that surgical enlargement of the vaginal opening would prevent intrapartal complications such as protracted second stage

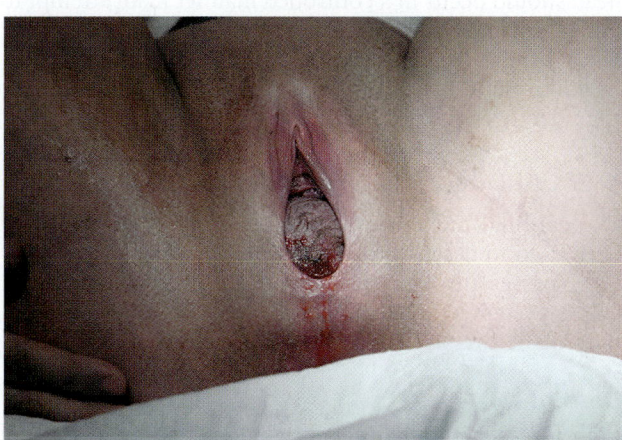
Figure 12-36 Crowning.

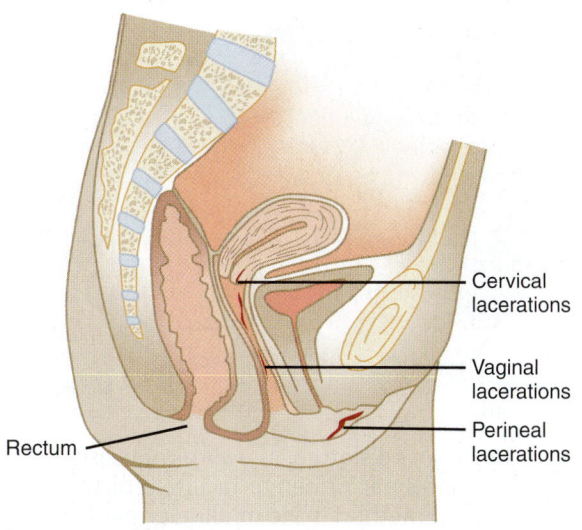
Figure 12-37 Potential locations of lacerations associated with childbirth.

Cervical lacerations

Vaginal lacerations

Perineal lacerations

Rectum

of labor, fetal trauma, and severe lacerations, and later maternal problems such as cystocele, rectocele, dyspareunia, and uterine prolapse (ACOG, 2006c).

Many women questioned the use of routine episiotomy, and current practices have changed to reflect existing evidence that routine episiotomy has not been associated with better outcomes over selective episiotomy. In studies in which episiotomy had been performed for medical indications, the results demonstrated positive benefits. When medically indicated, episiotomy was associated with decreased posterior perineal trauma and suturing and fewer complications. No differences were found in maternal pain experience or the incidence of severe vaginal or perineal trauma when routine and selective episiotomies were compared. There was an increased risk of anterior perineal trauma associated with selective episiotomy. Many practitioners currently reserve the use of episiotomy for medical indications, which include instrumentation during birth (forceps or vacuum), a need to expedite the birth (evidence of fetal compromise), or in the event of maternal exhaustion.

Two different methods are used for the episiotomy. The most common method is the midline or median episiotomy. An incision is made from the vaginal opening downward toward the rectum. A midline episiotomy is easily repaired, heals quickly, and is associated with less postoperative pain than a mediolateral episiotomy. However, the primary disadvantage of a midline episiotomy is the risk of third- and fourth-degree lacerations with extension through the rectal sphincter. The mediolateral episiotomy is less common. An incision is made from the vagina to the 5 o'clock or 7 o'clock position (the maternal left mediolateral or right mediolateral position). Compared with a midline incision, the mediolateral episiotomy is associated with a smaller risk of fourth-degree lacerations although third-degree lacerations may occur. The amount of blood loss is usually greater, the surgical repair is more difficult, and there is increased pain postpartum (Fig. 12-38).

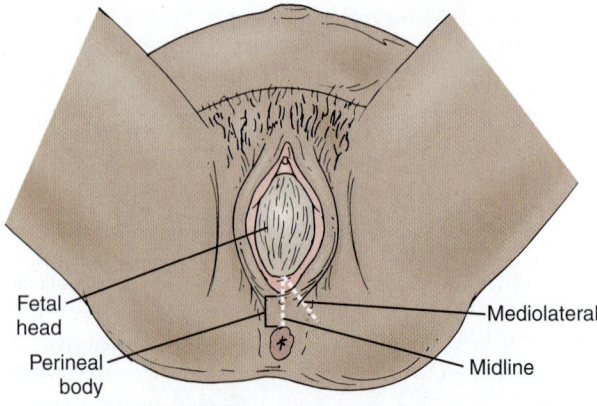

Figure 12-38 An episiotomy is a surgical incision of the perineum that is performed to facilitate birth. The most common method is the midline or median episiotomy—an incision is made from the vaginal opening downward toward the rectum.

 Complementary Care: *Methods to Decrease Perineal Trauma*

Various strategies to decrease the risk of perineal trauma during the second stage of labor have been implemented and evaluated. These include perineal massage (antenatal and intrapartal), application of warm compresses, use of lubricating oils, and manual support. However, research has demonstrated variable results, and further investigation is indicated. Maternal positioning for birth has also shown variable results regarding its effect on perineal trauma. Soong and Barnes (2005) found that women who gave birth in a semirecumbent position had an increased need for sutures for perineal lacerations than women who gave birth in an "all fours" position. In addition, women who received regional anesthesia also demonstrated an increased need for suturing than women who gave birth in a lateral position. Findings from a 2012 Cochrane review (Gupta, Hofmeyr, & Shehmar) of different positions during the second stage of labor in women without epidural anesthesia suggested various benefits (e.g., reduction in assisted births and episiotomies) for upright posture but revealed an increased risk for perineal tears with blood loss greater than 500 mL.

Nurses should be aware of the potential benefits and risks associated with various techniques intended to help minimize perineal trauma. It is important for nurses to remain open-minded, encouraging, and supportive of patients who wish to use alternate methods to help facilitate perineal stretching.

 Now Can You—Discuss factors associated with impending childbirth?

1. Explain the significance of crowning?
2. Discuss the controversies surrounding routine episiotomy?
3. Identify three strategies that may be effective in reducing perineal trauma during childbirth?

Birth

As the fetal head is crowning, the perineum is stretched very thin and the anus stretches and protrudes. With continued maternal pushing efforts, the fetal head extends under the symphysis pubis and is born. The practitioner assisting at the birth may prefer to coach the patient regarding pushing and breathing because the birth of the head should occur in a controlled manner in an attempt to limit injury to the perineum. Once the anterior shoulder reaches the pelvic outlet, it rotates to the midline and is delivered from under the pubic arch. The posterior shoulder is guided over the perineum, and the body follows.

THE CARDINAL MOVEMENTS

The **cardinal movements**, or mechanisms of labor, have been used to describe how the fetus (in a vertex presentation) passes through the birth canal and the positional changes required to facilitate birth (Fig. 12-39). The cardinal movements are presented in the order in which they occur.

Descent

Four forces facilitate **descent**, which is the progression of the fetal head into the maternal pelvis: (1) pressure of the

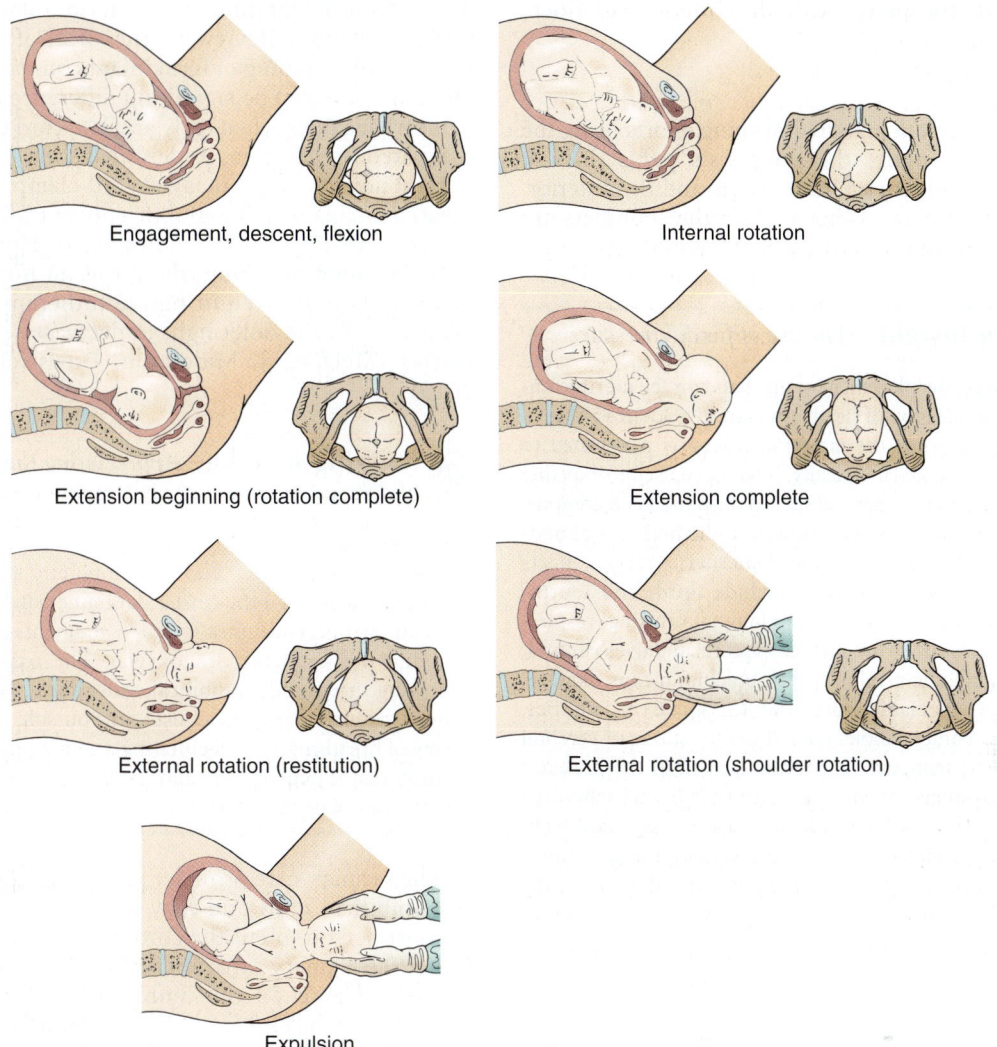

Engagement, descent, flexion

Internal rotation

Extension beginning (rotation complete)

Extension complete

External rotation (restitution)

External rotation (shoulder rotation)

Expulsion

Figure 12-39 The cardinal movements, or mechanisms of labor.

amniotic fluid, (2) direct pressure of the uterine fundus on the fetal breech, (3) contraction of the maternal abdominal muscles, and (4) extension and straightening of the fetal body. The fetal head enters the maternal inlet in the occiput transverse or the oblique position because the pelvic inlet is widest from side to side. The sagittal suture is equidistant from the maternal symphysis pubis and sacral promontory. The degree of fetal descent is measured by stations.

Flexion

Flexion occurs as the fetal head descends and comes into contact with the soft tissues of the pelvis, the muscles of the maternal pelvic floor, and the cervix. The resistance encountered with these structures causes the fetal chin to flex downward onto the chest. This position allows the smallest fetal diameters to enter the maternal pelvis.

Internal Rotation

To fit into the maternal pelvic cavity, which is widest in the anteroposterior diameter, the fetal head must rotate. As the occiput of the fetal head comes into contact with the levator ani muscles and surrounding fascia, it meets with resistance. This causes the occiput to rotate, usually from left to right, and the sagittal suture aligns with the

long axis of the maternal pelvis (the anteroposterior pelvic diameter).

Extension

As the fetal head passes under the maternal symphysis pubis, it meets with resistance from the pelvic floor. The head pivots and extends with each maternal pushing effort. The head is born in extension as the occiput slides under the symphysis and the face is directed toward the rectum. The fetal brow, nose, and chin then emerge.

Restitution

Internal rotation causes the fetal shoulders to enter the maternal pelvis in an oblique position. After the head is delivered in the extended position, it rotates briefly to the position it occupied when it was engaged in the inlet. This movement is termed restitution. The 45-degree turn of the fetal head facilitates realignment with the long axis of the body.

External Rotation

As restitution continues, the shoulders align in the antero-posterior diameter, causing the head to continue to turn farther to one side (external rotation). The fetal trunk moves through the pelvis with the anterior shoulders descending first.

Expulsion

After external rotation, maternal pushing efforts bring the anterior shoulder under the symphysis pubis. Lateral flexion of the shoulder and head occurs and the anterior, then posterior, shoulder is born. Once the shoulders are delivered, the rest of the body quickly follows.

 Nursing Insight—The use of fundal pressure

Fundal pressure, the placement of one hand on the uterine fundus with the application of steady pressure at a 30- to 45-degree angle directed toward the maternal pelvis, is performed to facilitate vaginal birth. Historically, it has been used to expedite childbirth when the woman's ability to push has been compromised by exhaustion or medication or in the presence of non-reassuring fetal heart patterns. Maternal adverse effects associated with fundal pressure include third- and fourth-degree lacerations, hypotension, abdominal bruising, respiratory distress, fractured ribs, uterine rupture, and liver rupture; fetal injuries include cerebral palsy, brachial plexus damage, humerus and clavicular fractures, thoracic spinal cord injuries, and asphyxial complications related to alterations in cerebral blood flow. The maneuver is contraindicated in the presence of shoulder dystocia, previous cesarean birth, and when the fetal station is above +2. Because of a lack of a standard technique for the maneuver, along with the lack of legal, professional, or regulatory standards in many clinical settings, the use of fundal pressure by nurses is not advised (Hoogsteder & Pijnenborg, 2010; Tongate & Gibbs, 2010).

CLAMPING THE UMBILICAL CORD

Much controversy exists concerning the issue of when and how to clamp the umbilical cord. When the newborn is held above the level of the placenta, a transfer of blood occurs from the newborn back to the placenta. Conversely, delaying the umbilical cord clamping and holding the newborn below the level of the placenta can result in a transfer of 50 to 100 mL of blood from the placenta to the newborn. The additional blood may be beneficial in reducing infant iron deficiency anemia and improved hematocrit and ferritin levels for up to 6 months. For the term infant, clamping should be delayed for at least 60 seconds, probably for 120 seconds, or until cord pulsation ceases. For the preterm infant, especially one who does not require resuscitation in the first minute, delaying cord clamping from 60 to 120 seconds is beneficial in improving circulatory and respiratory function and in reducing the need for blood transfusion and the risk for intraventricular hemorrhage. Because of concerns of neonatal hypervolemia or polycythemia or maternal postpartum hemorrhage, delayed cord clamping has not become a standard of practice. However, while there is a slight increase in the risk of polycythemia with a delay in cord clamping in the term infant, no other adverse effects have been found (Bell, 2011). According to ACOG (2012), insufficient evidence exists to support or to refute the benefits of delayed umbilical cord clamping for term infants born in settings with rich resources, while evidence does support delayed cord clamping in preterm infants. A recent (2013) Cochrane Review on the effect of timing of umbilical cord clamping of term infants on mother and baby outcomes revealed no significant difference in postpartum hemorrhage rates when early and late cord clamping were compared. In addition, it identified some potentially important advantages of delayed cord clamping such as increased neonatal hemoglobin concentrations and iron reserves up to 6 months after birth. However, in the delayed-clamping group, there was an increased risk of neonatal jaundice requiring phototherapy (therapeutic exposure to ultraviolet light to decrease serum bilirubin levels) (McDonald, Middleton, Dowswell, & Morris, 2013).

 Nursing Insight—Appreciating the benefits of delayed umbilical cord clamping

Delayed umbilical cord clamping provides more blood volume, red blood cells, and hematopoietic stem cells to the neonate than when the cord is cut immediately. Also, placental circulation continues for a few moments after birth, supplying the neonate with oxygen. The oxygen-rich blood flowing through the umbilical cord allows the neonate additional protected time to adjust to the outside world and a new way of breathing, thus facilitating a gentle physiological transition that is beneficial to all infants and especially to vulnerable ones (Coggins, 2009).

The primary care provider places two Kelly clamps on the umbilical cord and may invite the father or birth support person to cut the cord between the two clamps. Either the primary care provider or the nurse then places a plastic clamp on the umbilical cord approximately 0.5 to 1 inch (1.2 to 2.5 cm) from the newborn's abdomen, being careful to not catch the abdominal skin in the clamp. The nurse observes the cut cord for the presence of three blood vessels: two arteries and one vein. Samples of cord blood are collected for laboratory analysis. Some parents request to have their newborn's cord blood "banked" in the event that the stem cells in the cord blood may be required in the future for the treatment of a family illness. A vaginal birth sequence is presented in Figure 12-40.

 Nursing Insight—Significance of single umbilical artery

Single umbilical artery (SUA), which results from atrophy or agenesis of one of the arteries, occurs in 0.25% to 1% of all singleton pregnancies and in up to 4.6% of twin gestations. SUA may occur as an isolated event (i.e., with no other structural or chromosomal abnormalities) or with other anomalies in the renal, cardiovascular, gastrointestinal, and central nervous systems. Genetic syndromes that may feature an SUA include VATER complex (a group of congenital anomalies consisting of vertebral defects, imperforate anus, tracheoesophageal fistula, and radial and renal dysplasia), Meckel-Gruber syndrome, and Zellweger syndrome. In addition, certain teratogenic exposures (e.g., maternal hyperglycemia and phenytoin) have also been associated with SUA (Mandujano & Wilkins, 2010).

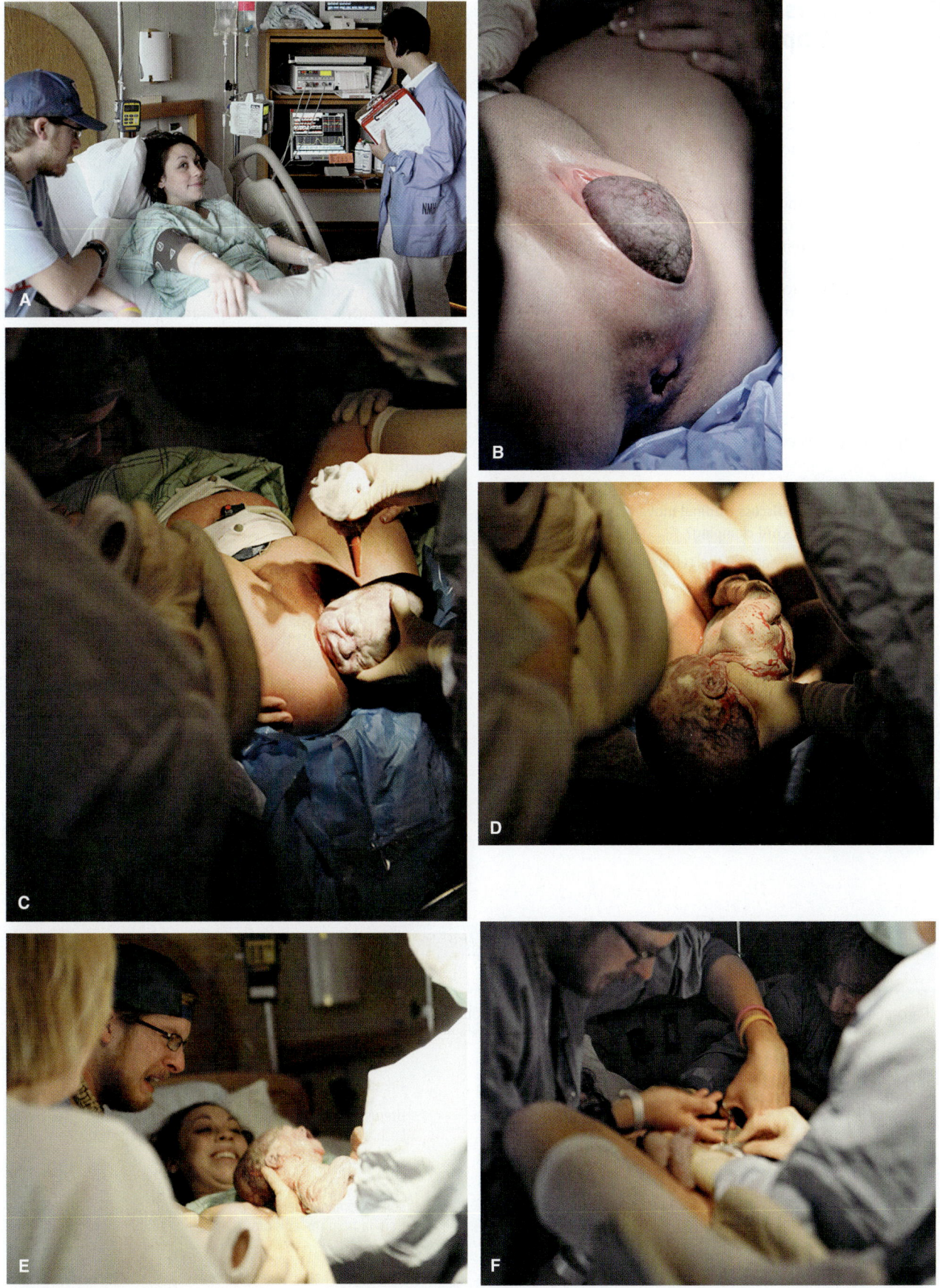

Figure 12-40 Vaginal birth sequence. *A,* Pushing in an upright position allows the use of gravity to promote fetal descent. *B,* Crowning. *C.* Birth of the head. *D,* Birth of the shoulders. *E,* The infant is shown to the new parents. *F,* The baby's father cuts the cord.

Possible Nursing Diagnoses for the Intrapartal Patient

Examples of common nursing diagnoses during labor and birth are listed below. It is important to be cognizant of individual differences among patients. While these are common nursing diagnoses, they will vary among individuals and stages of labor.

- Pain related to increasing frequency, duration, and intensity of contractions
- Knowledge deficit related to pain management techniques for active labor
- Anxiety related to the previous birth experience
- Fatigue related to a prolonged latent phase labor
- Risk for infection related to prolonged rupture of membranes
- Impaired fetal gas exchange related to umbilical cord compression
- Deceased maternal cardiac output related to supine hypotension secondary to maternal position

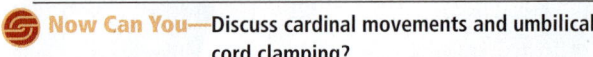

Now Can You—Discuss cardinal movements and umbilical cord clamping?

1. Describe what is meant by the cardinal movements?
2. Compare and contrast early versus late clamping of the umbilical cord?

Third and Fourth Stages of Labor

Nursing care during the third and fourth stages of labor is focused on providing immediate care for the newborn in the adjustment to extrauterine life, assisting with the delivery of the placenta, monitoring and assisting the mother with the physiological adjustments of labor and birth, and

facilitating the attachment between the mother and baby. Characteristics of the third and fourth stages of labor are presented in Table 12-7.

THIRD STAGE OF LABOR

The third stage of labor is the period of time from the birth of the baby to the complete delivery of the placenta. This stage usually lasts 5 to 10 minutes, and may last up to 30 minutes. Once the baby is born, the uterine cavity immediately becomes smaller. The change in the interior dimension of the uterus results in a reduction in the size of the placental attachment site. This event leads to the separation of the placenta from the uterus. The following clinical indicators signal that separation of the placenta from the uterus has occurred:

- The uterus becomes spherical in shape.
- The uterus rises upward in the abdomen as a result of the descent of the placenta into the vagina.
- The umbilical cord descends further through the vagina.
- A gush of blood occurs once the placenta detaches from the uterus.

The placenta is expelled in either the Schultze or Duncan manner (Fig. 12-41). The **Schultze mechanism** ("shiny Schultze") occurs when the placenta separates from the inside to the outer margins with the shiny, fetal side of the placenta presenting first. It is the most common method of placental expulsion. The **Duncan mechanism** occurs when the placenta separates from the outer margins inward, rolls up, and presents sideways. Because the placental surface is rough, the Duncan mechanism is commonly called "dirty Duncan" (Fig. 12-42).

As the placenta separates from the uterine wall, it is important that the uterus continues to contract. The contractions minimize the bleeding that results from

Table 12-7 Characteristics of the Third and Fourth Stages of Labor		
	Third Stage	**Fourth Stage**
Description	Begins with the birth of the infant and ends with the delivery of the placenta. Usually takes 5–10 minutes, and may take up to 30 minutes.	A time of physiological adaptation that begins following delivery of the placenta and lasts 1–2 hours.
Contractions	The uterus should be firmly contracted.	The uterus should be firmly contracted.
Assessment	Uterus becomes globelike. Uterus rises upward. Umbilical cord descends further. Gush of blood as placenta detaches.	Uterus remains firmly contracted. Lochia rubra, bright red blood flow with occasional small clots. Vital signs return to prelabor values.
Physical discomforts	Some discomfort or cramping as the placenta is expelled.	Some women experience perineal discomfort usually related to trauma from the episiotomy or tearing, or hemorrhoids.
Maternal behaviors	Focus on infant well-being. Crying common. Expressions of relief. Culturally influenced.	Excited, tired. Bonding and attachment with infant. Initiation of breastfeeding. Culturally influenced.

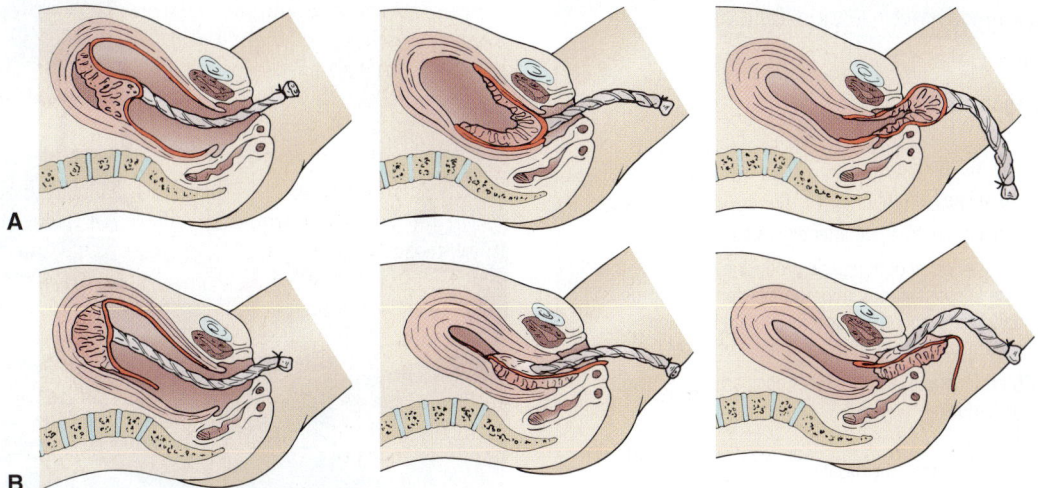

Figure 12-41 Third stage of labor: separation and expulsion of the placenta. *A,* Schultze mechanism. *B,* Duncan mechanism.

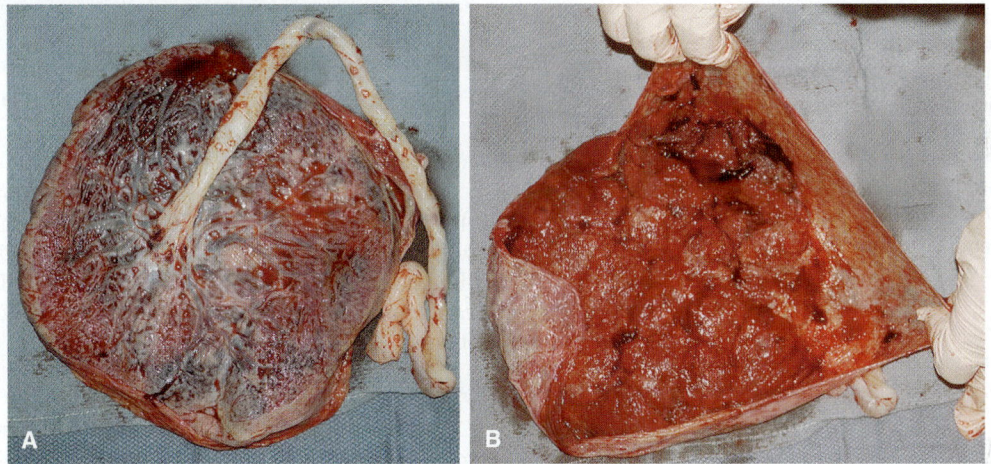

Figure 12-42 The delivered placenta. *A,* Fetal side. *B,* Maternal side.

the open blood vessels left at the placental attachment site. Failure of the uterus to contract adequately with separation of the placenta can result in excessive blood loss or hemorrhage. To enhance the uterine contractions after expulsion of the placenta, oxytocic medications are often given. Oxytocin is administered either by IV or IM.

Nursing Care of the Mother During the Third Stage of Labor

After the birth of the infant, the nurse observes for signs that the placenta has separated from the wall of the uterus. The uterus is palpated to determine the rise upward and the characteristic change in shape from one resembling a disk to that of a globe. The nurse may ask the woman to push again to facilitate in the delivery of the placenta. If 30 minutes have elapsed from completion of the second stage of labor and the placenta has not yet been expelled, it is considered to be "retained." (See Chapter 14 for further discussion.)

Oxytocic medications such as Pitocin and Syntocinon are often administered at the time of the delivery of the placenta. These drugs are used to stimulate uterine contractions, thereby minimizing the bleeding from the placental attachment site and reducing the risk of postpartum hemorrhage. The nurse administers oxytocic medications according to institutional protocol. If a peripheral intravenous infusion has been established, oxytocin 10 to 20 units may be added to the intravenous infusion. If no intravenous infusion is present, 10 units of oxytocin may be administered intramuscularly. In situations where there is excessive blood loss, the physician may order up to 40 units of oxytocin per liter of intravenous infusion fluid. Other medications such as methylergonovine maleate (Methergine) or carboprost tromethamine (Hemabate) may be given intramuscularly to control blood loss. During this time the nurse continues to assess the volume of blood loss and monitor the patient's vital signs, paying close attention to the blood pressure and heart rate.

Medication: Oxytocin (Pitocin, Syntocinon)

(ox-i-**toe**-sin)

Pregnancy Category: X

Indications:

IV: Induction of labor at term

IV: Facilitation of threatened abortion

IV, IM: Control of postpartum bleeding after expulsion of placenta

Actions: Stimulates uterine smooth muscle producing uterine contractions similar to those in spontaneous labor (administered intravenously). Stimulates mammary gland smooth muscle facilitating lactation (administered intranasally). Has vasopressor and diuretic effects.

Therapeutic Effects: Induces labor. Reduces postpartum bleeding. Induces breast milk letdown.

Pharmacokinetics:

ABSORPTION: Well-absorbed from the nasal mucosa when administered intranasally.

DISTRIBUTION: Through extracellular fluid. Small amounts reach fetal circulation.

METABOLISM: Metabolized rapidly in kidneys and liver.

EXCRETION: Small amounts excreted in urine, half-life 3 to 9 minutes.

Contraindications and Precautions:

CONTRAINDICATED IN: CPD or deliveries that require conversion (e.g., transverse lie). Use with caution in first and second stages of labor.

Adverse Reactions and Side Effects:

Maternal adverse reactions are associated with IV use only. Painful contractions and increased uterine motility most common. May contribute to maternal coma, seizures, and hypotension. May contribute to fetal asphyxia or arrhythmias.

Route and Dosage:

May be added to IV for labor induction or given IV or IM to control postpartum bleeding (do not administer IM and IV routes simultaneously). (See Chapters 14 and 16.)

Nursing Implications:

1. Fetal maturity, presentation, and maternal pelvic adequacy should be assessed before administration to induce labor.
2. Monitor contractions and resting uterine tone frequently.
3. Monitor maternal BP and pulse frequently and FHR continuously throughout administration.
4. Monitor uterus for firmness and early detection of bogginess.
5. Monitor lochia for signs of excessive bleeding.
6. Monitor patient for signs and symptoms of water intoxication (drowsiness, listlessness, confusion, headache, and anuria) and monitor electrolyte (hypochloremia and hyponatremia) status.

Source: Adapted from Vallerand, A. H., & Sanoski, C. A. (2014). *Davis's drug guide for nurses* (14th ed.). Philadelphia, PA: F.A. Davis.

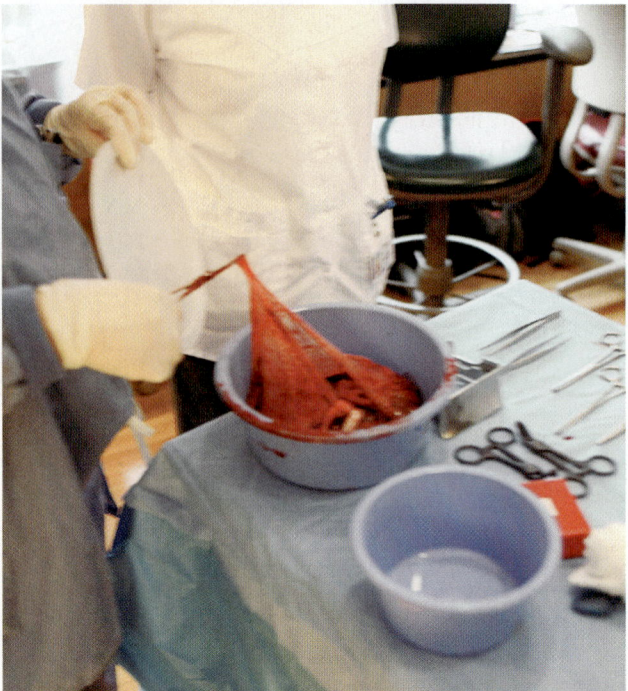

Figure 12-43 Examination of the placenta.

the mother and her birth partner by promoting contact with the infant. The stable newborn can be placed on the maternal abdomen, and as soon as possible, the nurse can help the mother into a comfortable position to hold the infant.

Initiating Infant Attachment

Once the birth has taken place, the time that immediately follows is ideal for fostering attachment between the mother, her birth partner, and the newborn. The infant is in a stage of alertness during the first hour after birth and is responsive to voice, touch, and gaze. The nurse can facilitate eye-to-eye contact between the patient and her neonate by dimming the room lights. This occasion also provides an excellent time to initiate breastfeeding if the mother wishes to do so.

 Optimizing Outcomes—Facilitating the breast crawl

The breast crawl is when a newborn, when left undisturbed and placed skin-to-skin on the mother's trunk following birth, moves toward the maternal breast for the purpose of locating and self-attaching for the first feeding (Gangal, Bhagat, Prabhu, & Nair, 2007; Klaus, 1998). With a mature and high-functioning nervous system, the healthy newborn possesses the necessary senses and motor skills, tone, and reflexes to complete the breast crawl. Nurses can help to facilitate the breast crawl by educating expectant mothers, promoting maternal/neonatal comfort and safety, ensuring privacy, delaying non-time sensitive practices, and conducting time-sensitive interventions (e.g., neonatal IM injections) while the infant is in skin-to-skin contact with the mother (Henderson, 2011).

Once the placenta has been delivered, the nurse carefully examines it to ensure that all cotyledons are intact (Fig. 12-43). If any part of the placenta is missing, the nurse immediately reports this finding to the attending physician. Because retained placental fragments can contribute to postpartum hemorrhage or infection, the physician may perform a manual exploration of the uterus to remove any remaining placental tissue.

Emotional Support

The birth of the newborn is an emotional experience for the patient and her support person. Hearing the infant's first cry can evoke tears, laughter, and feelings of relief, accomplishment, and amazement. The nurse can support

IMMEDIATE NURSING CARE OF THE NEWBORN

Once the newborn has been born, the primary care provider (physician or certified nurse midwife) places the infant on the mother's abdomen (if the infant is stable) in a modified Trendelenburg position. This immediate "birth skin-to-skin contact" between mother and newborn provides reassurance to the mother regarding the overall well-being of the baby and begins the attachment process. According to the American Academy of Pediatrics, all healthy infants should remain in skin-to-skin contact with their mothers immediately after birth until the first feeding occurs (Henderson, 2011).

 Nursing Insight—*Appreciating the advantages of maternal-infant skin-to-skin contact*

Considered a recommended best practice for healthy term newborns, skin-to-skin contact (SSC), especially during the first hour after birth, holds numerous benefits for mothers and their infants. For example, SSC at birth has been associated with decreased crying, grimacing, and heart rate surges in the neonate, enhanced mother–infant interaction, stabilization of the infant's temperature, and successful initiation of breastfeeding (Haxton, Doering, Gingras, & Kelly, 2012; Takahashi, Tamakoshi, Matsushima, & Kawabe, 2011).

Birth signals the transition from fetus to newborn. Several physiological adaptations must occur to facilitate the adjustment of the newborn to the extrauterine environment. Of primary importance is the initiation of the newborn's respirations, a process that results in the replacement of fetal lung fluid with air. In most situations, the actions of drying the newborn and performing nasopharyngeal suctioning, if needed, provide adequate stimulation to initiate the newborn's respiratory effort. While respirations are being established, the newborn's cardiovascular system is also undergoing major adaptations to allow the flow of deoxygenated blood into the lungs for gas exchange. Fetal circulation transitions to neonatal circulation after closure of the ductus arteriosus, the foramen ovale, and the ductus venosus. (See Chapter 17 for further discussion of the physiological transitions in the newborn.)

The modified Trendelenburg position facilitates the drainage of mucus from the newborn's nasopharynx and trachea. The nurse suctions the newborn's nose and mouth with a bulb syringe as needed. Preventing heat loss in the neonate constitutes an important nursing role. Before the infant is placed on the mother's abdomen, the nurse dries the infant, discards the wet linens, and applies warm blankets. Skin-to-skin contact between the mother and baby also helps to maintain the newborn's temperature.

The Apgar Scoring System

The nurse assesses this transition stage at 1 minute and again at 5 minutes after birth, using the **Apgar Scoring System** (Apgar, 1953), which provides a standardized assessment for infants. The Apgar scoring system evaluates five signs of newborn cardiopulmonary adaptation and neuromuscular function: heart rate, respiratory effort, muscle tone, reflex irritability, and color (Table 12-8).

Table 12-8 The Apgar Scoring System

Physiological Parameter	Score		
	0	1	2
Heart rate	Absent	Slow: below 100	Above 100
Respiratory effort	Absent	Slow: irregular, weak cry	Good; strong cry
Muscle tone	Flaccid	Some flexion of extremities	Well flexed
Reflex irritability	No response	Grimace	Vigorous cry
Color	Blue, pale	Pink body, blue extremities	Completely pink

Range of Apgar Score: from 0 to 10

A 5-minute Apgar score of 7 to 10 is considered normal. Scores of 4, 5, and 6 are intermediate and not markers of increased risk of neurological dysfunction because such scores may be the result of physiological immaturity, maternal medications, the presence of congenital malformations, and other factors (ACOG, 2006d).

HEART RATE. The priority assessment of the newborn is the heart rate. On auscultation or palpation, the nurse recognizes an absent heart rate or heart rate less than 100 bpm as a signal for resuscitation.

RESPIRATORY EFFORT. The newborn's vigorous cry best indicates adequate respiratory effort, the next most important assessment after birth. A weak or absent cry is a signal for intervention.

MUSCLE TONE. The nurse determines the newborn's muscle tone by assessing the response to the extension of the extremities. Good muscle tone is noted when the extremities return to a position of flexion.

REFLEX IRRITABILITY. The nurse assesses reflex irritability by observing the newborn's response to stimuli such as a gentle stroking motion along the spine or flicking the soles of the feet. When this stimulation elicits a cry, the score is 2. A grimace in response to stimulation scores 1, and no response is a score of 0.

COLOR. The nurse assesses skin color for pallor and cyanosis. Most newborns exhibit cyanosis of the extremities at the 1-minute Apgar check, and this normal finding is termed **acrocyanosis**. A score of 2 indicates that the infant's skin is completely pink. Newborns with darker pigmented skin are assessed for pallor and acrocyanosis.

 Nursing Insight—*Appreciating limitations of the Apgar score*

The Apgar score is an expression of the neonate's physiological condition, has a limited time frame, and includes subjective components. It is important to remember that certain elements of the score (i.e., tone, color, and reflex irritability) partially depend on the physiological maturity of the infant. Many factors, such as maternal medications, trauma, infection, congenital anomalies, hypovolemia, preterm birth, and hypoxia may influence an Apgar score (ACOG, 2006d).

Identification of the Newborn

Another important nursing action involves placing matching identification bands on the infant and the mother. Some hospitals also provide identification bands for the father or other designated birth support person. The infant's identification bands are placed snugly enough so that when the initial weight loss occurs, the ID band does not fall off. Agency protocols may also direct the nurse to footprint the newborn. (See Chapter 18 for further discussion.)

While the newborn rests on the mother's abdomen, the nurse performs a head-to-toe assessment to detect any abnormalities. The nurse observes the infant's overall size relative to the gestational age, noting the shape and size of the head and chest. The color of the skin, presence of vernix and lanugo, and any evidence of trauma are also noted. (See Chapter 18 for further discussion.)

 Now Can You—Discuss essential nursing actions during the third stage of labor?

1. Name three clinical indicators that signal placental separation during the third stage of labor?
2. Explain what is meant by "shiny Schultze" and "dirty Duncan"?
3. Describe essential nursing actions concerning the oxytocin infusion, placenta inspection, and immediate newborn care?

FOURTH STAGE OF LABOR

The fourth stage of labor is the period of maternal physiological adjustment that occurs from the time of delivery of the placenta through the first 1 to 2 hours after birth. Monitoring of the mother and infant takes place frequently during this time.

Nursing Care During the Fourth Stage of Labor

While the physician or certified nurse midwife examines the mother's perineum, cervix, and vagina for evidence of tears, the nurse assesses the uterus for firmness, height, and position. To perform fundal palpation, the left hand is placed directly above the symphysis pubis and gentle downward pressure is exerted. The right hand is cupped around the uterine fundus (Fig. 12-44). On palpation, the uterus is expected to feel firm and be positioned in the midline, at or just below the umbilicus. It can be described as closely approximating the size of a grapefruit. A full bladder or excessive blood in the uterus may cause it to be displaced from the midline.

A finding of a soft or "boggy" uterus on palpation may indicate that excessive blood and/or clots have pooled in the uterus. The nurse immediately begins to massage the uterus until it becomes firm. To perform uterine fundal massage correctly, the nurse uses two hands. One hand applies firm pressure to the fundus to express the blood clots; the other hand supports the lower aspect of the uterus to protect the ligaments from damage.

While monitoring the firmness and position of the uterus, the nurse also assesses the bloody vaginal discharge or **lochia**, noting the color, amount, and presence of clots. The first lochia that appears is bright red and is called **lochia rubra**. The amount of lochia is determined by examining the soaking of the perineal pads and the frequency of pad changes required. One soaked pad within the first

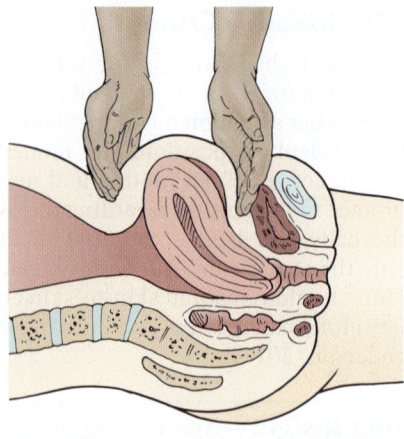

Figure 12-44 Fundal palpation during the fourth stage of labor. The left hand is placed directly above the symphysis pubis and exerts gentle downward pressure; the right hand is cupped around the uterine fundus.

postpartal hour is considered the normal maximum flow. Small blood clots are common; large clots are not normal. A steady trickle of blood or blood pooling under the mother's buttocks can be a sign of trauma to the perineum or birth canal.

The nurse also assesses the mother's vital signs frequently, generally every 5 to 15 minutes. The blood pressure should return to the prelabor level, and the pulse rate should be slower than that recorded during the labor experience. A rising pulse rate or a decreasing blood pressure is an indicator of excessive blood loss. The temperature is also assessed at the beginning of the fourth stage of labor and on transfer from the birthing room to the postpartum area. A rise in temperature and an increase in the pulse may be early indicators of postpartum infection.

The nurse monitors maternal urine output. A full, distended bladder can displace the uterus and impede its ability to contract adequately, potentially leading to hemorrhage. Trauma to the urethra or bladder during childbirth may impair the mother's perception of the urge to void. A complete documentation of the birth (labor summary, maternal-newborn delivery summary, newborn information including resuscitation, and all personnel in attendance) constitutes another important nursing action at this time (Fig. 12-45).

 Critical Nursing Action Fourth-Stage Signs of Danger

The nurse must be alert to the following risk signs that may occur during the fourth stage of labor: hypotension, tachycardia, excessive bleeding, or a boggy noncontracting uterus. These signs are associated with hemorrhage and must be reported immediately. If the uterus is boggy, the nurse must immediately initiate fundal massage and continue until the uterus becomes firm.

Comfort

It is not unusual for the mother to experience extreme shivering during the fourth stage of labor. The nurse can offer a heated blanket or warm beverage as comfort measures.

Delivery/Newborn Record

LABOR SUMMARY

Time   Date

Regular contractions began: _____ _____
Time of Oxytocin start: _____ _____
BOW ruptured: _____ _____
(best estimate) 4cm: _____ _____
10cm: _____ _____

Labor description:
- ☐ spontaneous
- ☐ augmented, oxytocin
- ☐ induced, oxytocin
- ☐ AROM for induction
- ☐ no labor

Fetal monitoring in labor:

- ☐ Cervical ripening agent _____
- ☐ **IUPC**
- ☐ **Amino infusion**

Previous C/S: ☐ No   **VBAC** ☐ No
☐ Yes   **attempted:** ☐ Yes

Fetal monitoring in labor:
- ☐ Auscultation only
- ☐ External monitor
- ☐ Internal monitor
- ☐ Both
- ☐ IFM site

Amniotic fluid rupture:
- ☐ Spontaneous
- ☐ Artificial

Color:
- ☐ Clear
- ☐ Light mec. (stain)
- ☐ Medium mec.
- ☐ Thick mec.
- ☐ Cloudy
- ☐ Bloody

Analgesics: before delivery

drug	dose	time

Labor analgesia:
- ☐ none
- ☐ narcotic
- ☐ epidural
- ☐ both
- ☐ _____ cervical dil@epid

Steroids for lung maturity: Date _____ Time _____ Date _____ Time _____
Antibiotic started: (prior to birth): ☐ <4 hrs ☐ ≥4 hrs ☐ >24 hrs
Why: ☐ GBS ⊕ Pending / Preterm   # Doses before birth _____
- ☐ Cardiac prophylaxis
- ☐ Fever / Chorioamnionitis
- ☐ Other: _____

Peak maternal temp ☐ <99.5   ☐ 99.5–101.9   ☐ ≥102

GROUP B STREP SCREEN

Universal Risk Factors
- ☐ Previous GBS infected infant
- ☐ ⊕ urine cx for GBS in current pregnancy

Culture Based
- ☐ negative
- ☐ positive
- ☐ not available

Risk Based (Intrapartum)
- ☐ No risk factors
- ☐ < 37 weeks
- ☐ ROM ≥ 18 hours
- ☐ Maternal temp ≥ 100.4

APGAR SCORE

	1 min	5 min
Heart Rate		
Respiratory Effort		
Muscle Tone		
Reflex Irritability		
Color		
TOTAL		

Cord around neck X ☐

Umbilical Vessel Number: ☐

- ☐ Voided in DR
- ☐ Stool in DR

DELIVERY–MOTHER

Method of Delivery:
- ☐ Vertex, Vaginal
- ☐ Breech, Vaginal
- ☐ Cesarean Section
- ☐ Vacuum
- ☐ Forceps

Episiotomy/Laceration:
- ☐ None
- ☐ Median
- ☐ Mediolateral
- ☐ Laceration
- ☐ Repaired

PLACENTA:
- ☐ Spontaneous
- ☐ Assist
- ☐ Manual

Abnormalities:

Medications at Delivery:

drug	dose	time
Pitocin IV IM	units	

PEDIATRICIAN:

DELIVERY SUMMARY

Baby [____] of a [____] gestation
    Birth Order   Plurality

	Time	Date
DELIVERY:	_____	_____
PLACENTA:	_____	_____
C/S start time:	_____	
Uterine incis. time:	_____	
C/S finish time:	_____	

INFANT   (circle)   Boy   Girl

Weight	_____ lb	_____ gm
Length	_____ in	_____ cm
Head circ	_____ in	_____ cm

Delivery Outcomes:
- ☐ live birth admitted for regular care
- ☐ live birth admitted to trans. nursery
- ☐ live birth admitted to NICU
- ☐ neonatal death in delivery room
- ☐ fetal death before admission
- ☐ fetal death after admission

Feeding:
- ☐ Breast
- ☐ Bottle

Gest. Age @ Delivery

I.D. BAND #: [____]
Bands Checked by:
_____ RN   _____ RN

Cord Blood to Lab: ☐ Yes   ☐ No
Cord Gases Sent: ☐ Yes   ☐ No
Specimen to Lab: ☐ Type _____
Culture to Lab: ☐ Type _____

RESUSCITATION

Check ALL that apply:
- ☐ suction
- ☐ oxygen
- ☐ mask vent
- ☐ intubation for resuscitation
- ☐ chest compression
- ☐ medications
- ☐ volume

Respirations: ☐ Spontaneous
☐ Delayed _____ min
☐ Narcan Given
Time: _____
Dose: _____
Route: _____
By whom: _____

For Meconium Babies:
- ☐ Not intubated
- ☐ Intubated – ∅ Below Cords
- ☐ Intubated – Meconium noted

Note: _____
_____
_____
_____

Newborn attended by _____ RN/MD
☐ Newborn admitted time: _____ am/pm
MR # _____   Pat # _____
Pediatrician notified of delivery: K # _____
    Name _____ MD
    Date _____ Time _____ am/pm
    Via _____ by _____

DELIVERING PHYSICIAN/CNM:	APN/NICU STAFF AT DELIVERY:	ANESTHESIOLOGIST:
ASSIST MD/CNM:	OB/RN AT DELIVERY:	RN SIGNATURE DATE/TIME:

Patient's Data/Addressograph

Figure 12-45 Documentation of the birth.

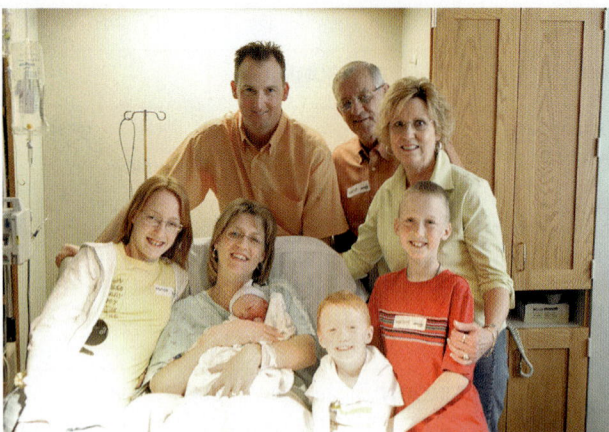

Figure 12-46 Family members share a special time with the newborn.

The work of labor has expended considerable maternal energy, and providing a light meal and fluids can help replace lost calories. The process of labor is also extremely fatiguing, and the nurse can encourage both the mother and her birth partner to rest.

Promoting Attachment and Breastfeeding

The first hour after the birth is an ideal time to promote parent–infant attachment. During this time the stable newborn is in a state of alertness and is responsive to voice and touch. The nurse can support this attachment by completing many maternal and newborn assessments while the infant is held by the parents. Providing a private, quiet environment enhances the opportunity for parent–infant eye contact. Some parents may wish to include siblings or other family members in this experience (Fig. 12-46).

The mother may wish to initiate breastfeeding at this time. The nipple stimulation associated with maternal breastfeeding is beneficial in two ways: It initiates the process of lactation and assists in the process of uterine involution by triggering the release of endogenous oxytocin. As with any interactions with childbearing families, it is important for the nurse to be aware of and respect the family's cultural practices.

Now Can You—Discuss the fourth stage of labor?

1. Explain what is meant by the fourth stage of labor?
2. Describe essential nursing assessments and appropriate interventions during the fourth stage of labor?
3. Name two nursing actions to promote infant attachment during the fourth stage of labor?

 Global Health Case Study The Birth Experience of a Multigravida

Tina Sanchez is a 26-year-old Mexican-American gravida 2 para 1 who comes to the birthing unit with her husband Jose. On arrival, Tina describes her contractions as starting approximately 2 hours earlier, regular and of moderate strength. You note that while she is walking to her room she has two contractions that are approximately 4 minutes apart and 60 seconds long. Tina is coping well with the contractions. Between contractions, she tells you that with her first baby 3 years ago she was induced and confined to bed with an electronic monitor and does not want that constraint this time if at all possible.

critical thinking questions

1. What type of information do you need to obtain from Tina and her husband?

2. What are your priority nursing assessments?

3. How would you respond to Tina's request not to be confined to bed?

   The nurse completes the assessment of Tina and the admission history between contractions. Tina has experienced a healthy pregnancy and is considered low risk. The institution policy promotes intermittent auscultation for low-risk patients in active labor. Tina's contractions are growing longer in duration and becoming stronger in intensity. Tina states: "I don't know how long I am going to be able to do this, it is getting harder."

4. What evaluation of the FHR would you make during intermittent auscultation?

5. How would you respond to Tina, considering that at this time she appears to be coping well?

6. What type of comfort measures could you suggest?

   While ambulating in the room, Tina experiences a large gush of greenish-brown fluid from her vagina.

7. What are your priority nursing assessments?

8. Are these findings normal or pathological? What further interventions are required?

   Thirty minutes later Tina is fully dilated and begins to push with each contraction. The FHR is now decreasing with each contraction and resembles the mirror image of the contraction.

9. What stage of labor has Tina now entered?

10. What is your interpretation of the FHR at this time?

11. What type of nursing interventions would you anticipate for Tina?

   Tina gives birth to a healthy baby girl 20 minutes later. The infant is suctioned well at the perineum and examined by the pediatrician because of the presence of meconium in the amniotic fluid. The infant is pink with acrocyanosis and does not demonstrate any signs of respiratory difficulties and is quickly returned to the proud parents.

12. Considering that the newborn infant has acrocyanosis, what is the highest possible Apgar score this infant could receive?

13. What are your priority nursing interventions for the newborn, Tina, and the family?

◆ See Suggested Answers to Global Health Case Studies on Davis*Plus*.

Summary Points

◆ Each patient's labor and birth experience is unique, and nurses play a vital role in facilitating a positive outcome for the patient, infant, and family.

◆ Nurses recognize that the labor and birth experience is influenced by a myriad of factors such as maternal age and well-being, social support, and cultural and religious beliefs and practices.

◆ Nurses need a strong knowledge base about the physiological processes of labor and birth to provide safe and effective care.

◆ In each of the four stages of labor, the nurse uses well-developed assessment skills to recognize the normal progression of labor, to identify potential risks to the patient and fetus, and to identify how and when to intervene and consult with other health-care providers.

◆ The overall goal of intrapartal nursing care is to promote comfort and safety of the patient, the fetus, and the newborn infant.

◆ A positive nurse–patient relationship in which the woman feels cared for and informed will empower her in coping with her labor.

◆ Nurses include the patient and her support person(s) in the planning and delivery of care.

◆ The nursing care given throughout labor and birth is an important determinant of the woman's overall perception of her childbirth experience.

Review Questions

Multiple Choice

1. When describing the "powers" of labor to a new nurse, the perinatal nurse discusses the uterine contractions and the
   A. Woman's pushing efforts.
   B. Unique musculature of the uterus.
   C. Position of the fetus.
   D. Hormonal influences regulating labor.

2. The perinatal nurse assesses a primigravida who has just arrived at the birth facility for labor assessment. The woman describes contractions that are 7 to 10 minutes apart and felt in the abdomen. She states the contractions feel better when she is walking. This is most likely
   A. True labor.
   B. Transition.
   C. Early labor.
   D. False labor.

3. The perinatal nurse describes for the student nurse the lettering used to designate fetal position. The correct use includes
   A. "P" indicating fetal pelvis location.
   B. "P" indicating posterior maternal pelvis.
   C. "M" indicating fetal mandible.
   D. "A" indicating maternal anus.

4. A nurse is told in a hand off report that a woman's cervix is not yet ripened. What does the nurse understand about this patient?
   A. She is ready to deliver.
   B. Her cervix has not yet softened.
   C. Vaginal delivery will not be possible.
   D. This change begins labor in all women.

5. The nurse explains to a laboring woman that the relaxation periods between contractions are important for which of the following reasons?
   A. Avoids uterine rupture
   B. Allows fetal oxygenation
   C. Permits fetal assessment
   D. Prevents uterine ischemia

6. Which of the following is considered the primary force of labor?
   A. Pushing by the mother
   B. Uterine contractions
   C. Contraction decrement
   D. Uterine elongation

7. A nurse assesses the intensity of a woman's contractions. At the acme of her contraction, the nurse is unable to indent the uterus. How would the nurse document this finding?
   A. Mild contraction
   B. Moderate contraction
   C. Strong contraction
   D. Intense contraction

8. A nurse assesses the level of a fetal presenting part in a laboring woman at station 0. What does this finding indicate?
   A. Engagement has occurred.
   B. The presenting part is above the maternal ischial spines.
   C. Labor is not progressing.
   D. The presenting part is at the pelvic outlet.

9. A nurse reads in a patient's chart that she has employed a doula. What does the nurse understand about this role?
   A. Provides physical and emotional support during labor
   B. Performs continuous patient assessment during labor
   C. Performs private duty nursing care during labor and birth
   D. Assists the surgeon during a cesarean delivery

10. A nurse assesses a woman in labor and finds that her contractions are occurring once every 1 to 1 and one-half minutes with a uterine resting tone greater than 30 mm Hg. How does the nurse document this finding?
    A. First stage labor, active phase
    B. First stage labor, transition
    C. Second stage labor
    D. Uterine tachysystole

See Answers to End of Chapter Review Questions on DavisPlus.

REFERENCES

Adams, E. D., & Bianchi, A. L. (2008). A practical approach to labor support. *Journal of Obstetric, Gynecologic & Neonatal Nursing, 37*(1), 106–115. doi:10.1111/J.1552 6909.2007.00213.x

Alfirevic, Z., Decane, D., & Gyte, G. (2013). Continuous cardiotocography (CTG) as a form of electronic fetal monitoring (EFM) for fetal assessment during labour. *Cochrane Database of Systematic Reviews 2013*, Issue 5. Art. No.: CD006066. doi:10.1002/14651858.CD006066.pub2

American Academy of Pediatrics and American College of Obstetricians and Gynecologists. (2013). *Guidelines for Perinatal Care,* (7th ed.). Elk Grove Village IL: Author.

American College of Obstetricians and Gynecologists (ACOG). (2006a). Mode of term singleton breech delivery. Committee Opinion No. 340. (Reaffirmed 2012). *Obstetrics & Gynecology, 108*(7), 235–237.

American College of Obstetricians and Gynecologists (ACOG). (2006b). Amnioinfusion does not prevent meconium aspiration syndrome. Committee Opinion No. 346. (Reaffirmed 2012). *Obstetrics & Gynecology, 108*(10), 1053–1055.

American College of Obstetricians and Gynecologists (ACOG). (2006c). Episiotomy. Practice Bulletin No. 71. (Reaffirmed 2013). *Obstetrics & Gynecology, 107*(4), 957–962.

American College of Obstetricians and Gynecologists (ACOG). (2006d). The Apgar Score. Committee Opinion No. 333. (Reaffirmed 2010). *Obstetrics & Gynecology, 107*(5), 1209–1212.

American College of Obstetricians and Gyneologists (ACOG). (2009). Intrapartum fetal heart rate monitoring: Nomenclature, interpretation, & general management principles. Practice Bulletin No. 106. (Reaffirmed 2013). *Obstetrics & Gynecology, 114*(7), 192–202.

American College of Obstetricians and Gynecologists (ACOG). (2010). Management of intrapartum fetal heart rate tracings. Practice Bulletin No. 116. (Reaffirmed 2013). *Obstetrics & Gynecology, 116*(11), 1232–1240.

American College of Obstetricians and Gynecologists (ACOG). (2012). Timing of umbilical cord clamping after birth. Committee Opinion No. 543. *Obstetrics & Gynecology, 120*(12), 1522–1526.

American College of Obstetricians and Gynecologists (ACOG). (2013). *Guidelines for women's health care: A resource manual* (3rd ed.). Washington, DC: Author.

Anderson, C. J., & Kilpatrick, C. (2012). Supporting patients' birth plans: Theories, strategies & implications for nurses. *Nursing for Women's Health, 16*(3), 212–218. doi:10.1111/j.1751-486X.2012.01732.x

Apgar, V. (1953). A proposal for a new method of evaluation of the newborn infant. *Current Researches in Anesthesia and Analgesia, 32,* 260–267.

Association of Women's Health, Obstetric and Neonatal Nurses (AWHONN). (2000). *Fetal Assessment (position statement).* Washington, DC: Author.

Association of Women's Health, Obstetric and Neonatal Nurses (AWHONN). (2008a). *Fetal Heart Monitoring.* Clinical Position Statement. Washington, DC: Author.

Association of Women's Health, Obstetric and Neonatal Nurses (AWHONN). (2008b). *Nursing care and management of the second stage of labor: Evidence-based clinical practice guideline* (2nd ed.). Washington, DC: Author.

Association of Women's Health, Obstetric & Neonatal Nurses (AWHONN). (2009). *Standards for professional nursing practice in the care of women and newborns* (7th ed.). Washington, DC: Author.

Association of Women's Health, Obstetric and Neonatal Nurses (AWHONN). (2011a). Call To Action: Quality patient care in labor and delivery: A call to action. *Journal of Obstetric, Gynecologic & Neonatal Nursing, 41*(6), 151–153. doi:1111/j.1552-6909.2011 .01317.x

Association of Women's Health, Obstetric and Neonatal Nurses (AWHONN). (2011b). Clinical Position Statement: Nursing support of laboring women. *Journal of Obstetric, Gynecologic & Neonatal Nursing, 40*(11), 665–666. doi:10.1111/j.1552-6909.2011.01288.x

Barrett, S. J., & Stark, M. A. (2010). Factors associated with labor support behaviors of nurses. *Journal of Perinatal Education, 19*(1), 12–18. doi:10.1624/105812410X481528

Bell, E. F. (2011). Increasing the placental transfusion for preterm infants. *Obstetrics & Gynecology, 117*(2), 203–204.

Blackburn, S. (2012). *Maternal, fetal, & neonatal physiology: A clinical perspective.* (4th ed.). Philadelphia, PA: Saunders.

Bulechek, G. M., Butcher, H. K., & Dochterman, J. M., & Wagner (2013). *Nursing interventions classification (NIC)* (6th ed.). St. Louis, MO: Elsevier Mosby.

Burkman, R. T., & Fennell, J. L. (2010). Fetal heart tracing: Why communication and documentation are essential. *The Female Patient, 135*(9), 38–40.

Cahill, A. G., Duffy, C. R., Odibo, A. O., Roehl, K. A., Zhao, Q., & Macones, G. A. (2012). Number of cervical examinations and risk of intrapartum maternal fever. *Obstetrics & Gynecology, 119*(6), 1096–1101. doi:10.1097/AOG.0b013e318256ce3f

Chapman, L., & Durham, R. (2014). *Maternal-newborn nursing: The critical components of nursing care.* (2nd ed.). Philadelphia, PA: F.A. Davis.

Coggins, M. (2009). Delayed cord clamping: Advantages for infants. *Nursing for Women's Health, 13*(2), 133–139. doi:10.1111/j.1751-486X .2009.01404.x

Cunningham, F., Leveno, K., Bloom, S., Spong, C., & Dashe, J. (2014). *Williams obstetrics* (24th ed.). New York, NY: McGraw-Hill Professional.

Feinstein, N., Sprague, A., & Trepanier, M. (2009). *Fetal heart rate auscultation.* (2nd ed.). Washington, DC: Association of Women's Health, Obstetric and Neonatal Nurses.

Felton, M. B. (2011). Normal childbirth. In S. Mattson & J. E. Smith (Eds.), *Core curriculum for maternal-newborn nursing* (4th ed., pp. 225–247). Philadelphia, PA: W.B. Saunders.

Freeman, R. K., Garite, T. J., Nageotte, M. P., & Miller, L. A. (2012). *Fetal heart rate monitoring* (4th ed.). Philadelphia, PA: Lippincott Williams & Wilkins.

Gangal, P., Bhagat, K., Prabhu, S., & Nair, R. (2007). *Breast crawl: Initiation of breastfeeding by the breast crawl.* Retrieved from http://www.breastcrawl.org/

Grimes, D. A., & Peipert, J. F. (2010). Electronic fetal monitoring as a public health screening program. *Obstetrics & Gynecology, 116*(6), 1397–1400.

Gupta, J. K., Hofmeyr, G. J., & Shehmar, M. (2012). Position in the second stage of labour for women without epidural anaesthesia. *Cochrane Database of Systematic Reviews, 2013*(5): CD002006. doi:10.1002/ 14651858.CD02006.pub3

Hankins, G. D., & Miller, D. A. (2011). A review of the 2008 NICHD Research Planning Workshop: Recommendations for fetal heart rate terminology and interpretation. *Clinical Obstetrics & Gynecology, 54*(1), 3–7. doi:10.1097/GRF.0b013e31820a015b

Hannah, M., Hannah, W., Hewson, S., Hodnett, E., Saigal, S., & Willan, A. R. (2000). Planned cesarean section vs vaginal birth for breech presentation at term: A randomized multicenter trial. *Lancet, 356,* 1375–1383.

Haxton, D., Doering, J., Gingras, L., & Kelly, L. (2012). Implementing skin-to-skin contact at birth using the Iowa Model. *Nursing for Women's Health, 16*(3), 222–230. doi:10.1111/j.1751-486X .2012.01733.x

Henderson, A. (2011). Understanding the breast crawl: Implications for nursing practice. *Nursing for Women's Health, 15*(4), 296–307. doi:10.1111/j.1751-486X.2011.01650.x

Hodnett, E. D., Downe, S., Walsh, D., & Weston, J. (2010). Alternative versus conventional institutional settings for birth. *The Cochrane Library.* Retrieved from http://summaries.cochrane.org/CD000012/ alternative-versus-conventional-institutional-settings-for-birth doi:10.1002/14651858.CD000012.pub3

Hoogsteder, P., & Pijnenborg, J. (2010). Use of uterine fundal pressure maneuver at vaginal delivery and risk of severe perineal laceration. *Archives of Gynecology and Obstetrics, 281*(3), 579–580. doi:10 .1007/s00404-009-1229-3

Klaus, M. (1998). Mother and infant: Early emotional ties. *Pediatrics, 102*(5), 1244–1246.

Klaus, M., Kennell, J., & Klaus, P. (2012). The doula book: How a trained labor companion can help you have a shorter, easier, and healthier birth. (3rd ed.). Cambridge, MA: Da Capo Lifelong Books.

Lowe, N. K. (2012). The persistent problem of postpartum hemorrhage. *Journal of Obstetric, Gynecologic & Neonatal Nursing, 41*(4), 459–460. doi:10.1111/j.1552-6909.2012.01397.x

Lyndon, A., O'Brien-Abel, N., & Simpson, K. R. (2013). Fetal assessment during labor. In K. R. Simpson, & P. Creehan (Eds.), *Perinatal nursing* (4th ed., pp. 445–492). Philadelphia, PA: Lippincott.

MacKinnon, K., McIntyre, M., & Quance, M. (2005). The meaning of the nurse's presence during childbirth. *Journal of Obstetric, Gynecologic and Neonatal Nursing, 34*(1), 28–36.

Macones G. A., Hankins G. D., Spong C. Y., Hauth J., & Moore T. (2008). The 2008 National Institute of Child Health and Human Development Research Workshop Report on Electronic Fetal Heart Rate Monitoring: Update on Definitions, Interpretation, and Research Guidelines. *Obstetrics & Gynecology 112*(3), 661–666.

Maher, S., Crawford-Carr, A., & Neidigh, K. (2013). The role of the interpreter/doula in the maternity setting. *Nursing for Women's Health, 16*(6), 472–481. doi:10.1111/j.1751-486X.2012.01775.x

Mandujano, A., & Wilkins, I. (2010). Single umbilical artery: What you need to know. *Contemporary OB/GYN, 55*(10), 26–29.

McDonald, S. J., Middleton, P., Dowswell, T., & Morris, P. S. (2013). Effect of timing of umbilical cord clamping of term infants on maternal and neonatal outcomes. *Cochrane Database of Systematic Reviews, 2013,* Issue 7. Art. No.: CD004074. doi:10.1002/14651858.CD004074 .pub3

Miller, D. A. (2010). Intrapartum fetal monitoring: Maximizing benefits and minimizing risks. *Contemporary OB-GYN, 55*(2), 26–36.

Miller, D. A. (2012). Late and variable decelerations: Ominous or benign? *Contemporary OB-GYN, 57*(7), 18–20.

Miller, L. A., Miller, D., & Tucker, S. M. (2012). *Mosby's pocket guide to fetal monitoring: A multidisciplinary approach* (7th ed.). Maryland Heights, MO: Mosby.

National Institute of Child Health and Human Development (NICHD) Research Planning Workshop. (1997). Electronic fetal heart rate monitoring: Research guidelines for interpretation. *American Journal of Obstetrics and Gynecology, 177*(6), 1385–1390.

Neal, J. L., Lowe, N. K., Patrick, T. E., Cabbage, L. A., & Corwin, E. J. (2010). What is the slowest-yet-normal cervical dilation rate among nulliparous women with spontaneous labor onset? *Journal of Obstetric, Gynecologic & Neonatal Nursing, 39*(4), 361–369. doi:10.1111/j.1552-6909.2010.01154.x

Norman, S., Tuuli, M., Odibo, A., Caughey, A., Roehl, K., & Cahill, A. (2012). The effects of obesity on the first stage of labor. *Obstetrics & Gynecology, 120*(1), 130–135. doi:10.1097/AOG.0b013e318259589c

Prins, M., Boxem, J., Lucas, C., & Hutton, E. (2011). Effect of spontaneous pushing versus Valsalva pushing in the second stage of labour on mother and fetus: A systematic review of randomised trials. *British Journal of Obstetrics & Gynecology, 118*(6), 662–670. doi:10.1111/j.1471-0528.2011.02910.x

Reitberg, C. C., Elferink-Stinkens, P. M., & Visser, G. H. (2005). The effect of the Term Breech Trial on medical intervention behaviour and neonatal outcome in The Netherlands: An analysis of 35,453 term breech infants. *British Journal of Obstetrics & Gynecology, 112*(6), 205–209.

Simkin, P., Bolding, A., Keppler, A., Durham, J., & Whalley, J. (2010). *Pregnancy, childbirth, and the newborn* (4th ed.). Minnetonka, MN: Meadowbrook Press.

Simpson, K. R., & Creehan, P. A. (2013). *AWHONN Perinatal Nursing* (4th ed.). Philadelphia, PA: Lippincott Williams & Wilkins.

Simpson, K. R., & O'Brien-Abel, N. (2013). Labor and birth. In K. R. Simpson & P. Creehan (Eds.), *Perinatal nursing* (4th ed., pp. 343–444). Philadelphia, PA: Lippincott Williams & Wilkins.

Society of Obstetricians and Gynaecologists of Canada (SOGC). (2007). Fetal health surveillance: Antepartum and intrapartum consensus guideline. *Journal of Obstetrics and Gynaecology Canada, 29*(9), Supplement 4, S1–S56.

Soong, B., & Barnes, M. (2005). Maternal position at midwife-attended birth and perineal trauma: Is there an association? *Birth, 32*(3), 164–169.

Su, M., Hannah, W. J., Willan, A., Ross, S., & Hannah, M. E. (2004). Planned cesarean section decreases the risk of adverse perinatal outcome due to both labour and delivery complications in the Term Breech Trial Collaborative Group. *British Journal of Obstetrics & Gynecology, 111*(6), 1065–1074.

Takahashi, Y., Tamakoshi, K., Matsuhima, M., & Kawabe, T. (2011). Comparison of salivary cortisol, heart rate, and oxygen saturation between early skin-to-skin contact with different initiation and duration times in healthy, full-term infants. *Early Human Development, 87*(3), 151–157. doi:10.1016/j.earlhumdev.2010.11.012

Tongate, S., & Gibbs, J. D. (2010). Nurses, physicians and disagreements about fundal pressure. *Nursing for Women's Health, 14*(2), 137–142. doi:10.1111/j.1751-486X.2010.01527.x

Torgersen, K. L. (2011). Intrapartum fetal assessment. In S. Mattson & J. E. Smith (Eds.), *Core curriculum for maternal-newborn nursing* (4th ed., pp. 248–298). Philadelphia, PA: W.B. Saunders.

Turley, G. M. (2011). Essential forces and factors in labor. In S. Mattson & J. E. Smith (Eds.), *Core curriculum for maternal-newborn nursing* (4th ed., pp. 191–224). Philadelphia, PA: W.B. Saunders.

Tuuli, M., Frey, H., Odibo, A., Macones, G., & Cahill, A. (2012). Immediate compared with delayed pushing in the second stage of labor. *Obstetrics & Gynecology, 120*(3), 660–668. doi: 10.1097/AOG.0b013e3182639fae

Vallerand, A. H., & Sanoski, C. A. (2014). *Davis's drug guide for nurses* (14th ed.). Philadelphia, PA: F.A. Davis.

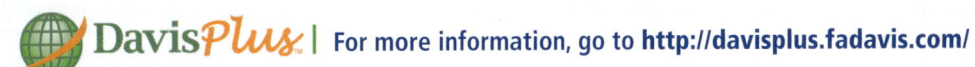

DavisPlus | For more information, go to **http://davisplus.fadavis.com/**

CONCEPT MAP

The 5 Ps of Labor

Powers
Uterine Contractions:
- Increment; acme; decrement
- Responsible for cervical:
  - Effacement
  - Dilation

Maternal Pushing:
- Facilitates expulsion of fetus

Passageway
- Maternal bony pelvis
  - Inlet
  - Midpelvis
  - Outlet
- Pelvic soft tissue

Passenger/Passageway: Relationship Between
- Determined by assessing
  - Engagement
  - Station
  - Position

Passenger: Fetus and Fetal Membranes
Fetal Considerations:
- Fetal lie
- Fetal attitude
- Fetal presentation
  - Cephalic
  - Breech
  - Shoulder

Psychosocial Influences
- Readiness for labor/birth
- Level of educational preparedness
  - Prior experience
  - Emotional readiness
  - Culture

The Process of Labor and Birth

Complementary Care:
- Perineal massage, warm compresses, lubricating oils, semi-recumbent position ➞ potentially decrease perineal trauma

Where Research And Practice Meet:
- Planned vaginal delivery of singleton term breech may no longer be appropriate
- Various labor support strategies enhance physical/emotional maternal comfort
- Alternative institutional birth settings linked to maternal benefits/satisfaction
- Maternal obesity lengthens the labor curve
- Optimize breech birth by doing cesarean section

Critical Nursing Actions:
- Determine/document fetal position
- Assess for 4th-stage signs of hemorrhage danger
- Prevent maternal supine hypotension
- Interpret fetal monitor tracings correctly
- Recognize and respond to uterine tachysystole

Fetal Assessment: Labor/Birth
- Fetal position
  - Leopold maneuvers
  - FHR and patterns
  - Vaginal exam/ultrasound
- Fetal heart rate
  - Baseline variability
  - Accelerations/decelerations
  - Interpret FHR pattern ➞ requires holistic assessment
  - Interpret FHR tracings: use protocol
- Fetal heart sounds
- Electronic fetal monitoring
- FHR response to stimuli
- Fetal scalp blood sampling
- Cord acid/base sampling

Stages of Labor:
1st Stage: regular contractions to complete cervical dilation
  - Latent phase
  - Active phase
  - Transition
2nd Stage: full dilation to birth
  - Urge to push/"bearing down"
  - Duration variable
Birth: fetal cardinal movements
  - Descent; flexion; internal rotation; extension; restitution; external rotation; expulsion
3rd Stage: birth to delivery of placenta
  - Decrease in uterine size
  - Placenta separates from uterus
4th Stage: delivery of placenta through first 4 hours post birth

Impending Labor: Signs/Symptoms
- Lightening
- Braxton-Hicks contractions
- Cervical ripening
- Bloody show/ruptured membranes
- Energy spurt
- Weight loss/GI disturbances

Nursing Considerations: Labor
- Stage 1: continual monitoring mother/fetus; facilitate positive experience; manage pain
- Stage 2: promote effective pushing; position for comfort
- Stage 3: facilitate delivery of placenta; promote infant bonding; immediate infant care; ID infant
- Apgar score
- Stage 4: promote comfort, attachment, and breastfeeding
- Establish a positive relationship

General Labor Support:
- Offering presence
- Promote comfort/position changes/relaxation
- Provide relaxed environment
- Attend to hygiene/elimination needs
- Provide anticipatory guidance
- Support birth partner

True Labor vs. False Labor: ➞ Differences In
- Regularity, intensity, duration; whether effacement/dilation occurs
- Back pain that radiates and worsens with activity vs. abdominal pain that eases with activity
- Assess for amniotic fluid

What to Say:
- Questions for telephone assessment of a laboring woman
- Use direct, open questions for difficult topics ➞ drug, alcohol use
- Use positive and encouraging statements during labor

Legal Alert:
- Understand EMTALA
- Use appropriate terms during FHR documentation and interpretation

Now Can You:
- Evaluate uterine contractions
- Identify and discuss the 5 Ps of labor
- Identify the characteristics of nursing care for each stage of labor
- Identify the critical elements of fetal assessment during and after labor

Promoting Patient Comfort During Labor and Birth

 The pains of childbirth were altogether different from the enveloping effects of other kinds of pain. These were pains one could follow with one's mind.

—Margaret Mead

LEARNING TARGETS *At the completion of this chapter, the student will be able to:*

- Describe the unique characteristics of pain associated with childbirth.
- Discuss sociocultural factors that shape the woman's pain experience during labor and childbirth.
- Identify nonpharmacological methods to promote comfort during labor and birth.
- Compare pharmacological interventions used for discomfort and pain during different stages of labor.
- Summarize the possible complications associated with regional and general anesthesia.
- Discuss the nurse's role in ensuring maternal–fetal safety while promoting comfort during labor and birth.

PICO(T) Questions

The intent of evidence-based practice (EBP) is to provide nursing care that integrates the best available evidence. An initial step in EBP is to write a PICO(T) question that effectively guides the research. A PICO(T) question is an acronym that stands for population (P), intervention or issue (I), comparison of interest (C), outcome (O), and timeframe (T). Depending on the question, all or some of the question components are used in the research process.

Use these PICO(T) questions to spark your thinking as you read the chapter.

1. Do (P) pregnant women (I) who have regional anesthesia during labor (O) report a higher satisfaction with their labor experience (C) than women who choose analgesia or nonpharmacological measures?

2. Are (P) women who had a positive first experience with the birthing process (O) less likely to try (I) a different birth plan with subsequent pregnancies?

Evidence-Based Practice

Hidaka, R., & Callister, L. C. (2012). Giving birth with epidural analgesia: The experience of first-time mothers. *The Journal of Perinatal Education, 21*(1), 24–35.

The purpose of this qualitative descriptive study was to describe and better understand the birth experiences of women who used epidural analgesia for pain control. Previous studies have identified that the anticipated pain during childbirth is a major concern of pregnant women. Researchers have also predicted that the use of epidural anesthesia has increased in the past five years. Though risks have been associated with the use of epidural anesthesia, it has been found to be an effective method of pain control during labor. Previous research has suggested that women's satisfaction with childbirth is associated with personal expectations, personal sense of control, caregiver support, quality of the relationship with the caregiver, and active involvement in decision making, and that pain relief does not necessarily relate to a positive birth experience.

Study participants included nine primiparas who were recruited from childbirth education classes and from the mother-baby unit of a hospital with an annual birth census of 800. All of the participants were Caucasian. Their ages ranged from 19 to 37 years (mean age 27.7); the majority (n=7) were married, had greater than a high school education (n=6), and were employed (n=8). All women received epidural anesthesia and experienced a vaginal birth of a full-term infant. The first and second stages of labor combined ranged from 4 to over 20 hours and the length of labor after receiving epidural anesthesia ranged from 3 to 10 hours. Nonpharmacological pain relief strategies implemented before administration of the epidural anesthesia included walking, hydrotherapy, and massage. Cervical dilation at the time of epidural administration ranged from 4 to 8 centimeters. Eight of the nine participants had singleton births, and one gave birth to twins. Four of the participants were induced with Pitocin, and three required Pitocin augmentation after receiving the epidural. Only one of the nine women had planned on having an epidural. Six of the participants stated they had no difficulty in deciding to receive the epidural although two women expressed ambivalent feelings.

The researchers believed that the qualitative descriptive design this research method used in this study provided a richer understanding of the women's perceptions of their childbirth experiences as well as their satisfaction with pain control during the birthing process. Participants were asked what the experience was like for them and how the epidural anesthesia contributed to the overall experience. Participants were interviewed in their homes 4 to 6 weeks postpartum. The interviews, which lasted from 60 to 90 minutes, were recorded and transcribed verbatim. The participants were provided with the narrative to verify accurate understanding and interpretation.

Sentences were examined and clustered and labeled based on suggested emerging themes. Themes generated from the narratives included (a) "coping with pain before opting for an epidural," (b) "finding epidural administration uneventful,"

(c) "feeling relief using an epidural," (d) "experiencing joy," and (e) "being left with unsettled feelings of ambivalence" (p. 26). Study findings related to each theme were as follows:

- *Coping with pain*: Women did not anticipate nor were they prepared for the intensity of discomfort experienced during the birthing process. Participants coped with the pain as long as possible before agreeing to the epidural anesthesia. The pain of labor left them feeling exhausted.
- *Finding epidural administration uneventful:* The participants worried about receiving the epidural and considered it an unknown experience. One participant was aware of a friend who had experienced complications related to an epidural. After receiving the epidural, all of the women indicated that the experience was positive and did not cause discomfort.
- *Feeling relief using an epidural*: The participants reported significant relief after receiving the epidural. Seven participants rated their labor pain at "zero" after receiving the epidural. Participants indicated that the epidural had a positive effect on the birth experience. The epidural provided an opportunity for women to remain in control during the birthing process.
- *Experiencing joy:* All of the participants reported feeling joy at completing the birth and seeing their child.
- *Being left with unsettled feelings:* Participants expressed ambivalence, having insufficient information, and concern over the care providers' attitudes toward them and the labor process. Three of the participants rated their satisfaction at less than 10 (10 = most satisfied). Reasons for this rating were related to how the participants were treated by the health-care providers and the fact that procedures were frequently not explained, leaving them with anxiety and fear. One participant noted that options for the birth were not discussed with her nor were her questions answered. She reported that her experience was traumatic because of the attitudes of the providers.

The researchers concluded that their findings correspond to those of previous studies that suggest that women underestimate the extent of pain related to childbirth. Women in general held unrealistic expectations and were not prepared for the intensity of the pain. Actions that may help to ensure a positive birth experience include strategies to provide the patient with a sense of connection and control and conveying a caring attitude.

1. How is this information useful to clinical nursing practice?

2. Based on these findings, what are implications for further research?

See Suggested Responses for Evidence-Based Practice on Davis*Plus*.

Introduction

When a laboring woman experiences discomfort and pain, there are many interventions that nurses can implement to help reduce anxiety and promote comfort. There is an increasingly accepted perspective that certain physiological processes are normally associated with a certain level of pain and that the pain serves a useful purpose. The pain of childbirth, for example, may serve to warn the woman to seek a safe haven and obtain help. Ideally, these actions help to ensure that the birth takes place in safe surroundings and facilitate a positive outcome, whether childbirth takes place at home, in a free-standing birth center, or at a hospital. However, this perspective should not be confused with the belief that childbirth should not be painful. To deny that discomfort or pain exists during childbirth is patently unrealistic. According to the American College of Obstetricians and Gynecologists (2006), labor causes severe pain for many women, and a woman's request is sufficient justification for pain relief. The nurse, the laboring woman, and her support person(s) all benefit from an understanding of the physiological and psychological processes that underlie the experience of pain. Becoming familiar with strategies for managing or diminishing the pain of childbirth empowers the laboring woman to make informed decisions about the various pain management measures she will use. This chapter discusses the physiology of childbirth pain, theories related to pain perception, cultural and psychological factors that affect childbirth pain, nonpharmacological and pharmacological pain management interventions, and implications for nursing care.

 Optimizing Outcomes—Helping to achieve *Healthy People 2020* national goals

Because the use of anesthesia and analgesia during childbirth can increase maternal mortality, several of the *Healthy People 2020* national goals relate to pain relief during labor. One such goal is:

- Reduce the maternal mortality rate to no more than 11.4 per 100,000 live births from a baseline of 12.7 maternal deaths in 2007 (U.S. Department of Health and Human Services, 2012).

Nurses can help the nation achieve this goal by educating women about the benefits of prepared childbirth. During labor, nurses can educate, reassure, and continuously monitor patients and assist them in the use of nonpharmacological pain relief methods to enhance comfort and reduce the total amount of analgesics needed.

The Physiology of Pain During Labor and Birth

DEFINING PAIN

Pain is a complex, multidimensional experience. According to Padfield and colleagues (2003), pain is defined as whatever the person who is experiencing it says it is. The International Association for the Study of Pain defines pain as an unpleasant sensory and emotional experience arising from actual or potential tissue damage or described in terms of such damage. Pain includes not only the perception of an uncomfortable stimulus but also the response to that perception (Venes, 2013). The expression of pain is influenced by a number of psychosocial and cultural factors. For example, in some cultures it is permissible for the woman in labor to freely verbalize her pain. In others, the laboring woman must be stoic and keep her emotions to herself.

The pain experienced during childbirth is an unpleasant sensation that is usually localized to the back and the abdomen. For most, the pain associated with childbirth intensifies an already highly emotional experience for both the laboring woman and her support person. How well the laboring woman is able to cope with her pain significantly affects the overall birth experience.

During the assessment, the nurse may identify physiological and psychological changes that are indicative of maternal pain. These include an increased pulse rate and blood pressure, changes in mood, increased anxiety and stress, marked agitation, confusion, decreased urine output, decreased intestinal motility, and guarding of the target area of discomfort. Pain affects the patient's physiological, behavioral, sensory, and cognitive responses. It is frequently intensified by fear, anxiety, and fatigue.

The experience of pain is shaped by many factors such as the patient's age, educational background, state of wellness, prior experiences, sociocultural background, degree of family and social support, and mastery of coping mechanisms. Nurses must simply accept what the patient says about her pain experience. The pain is real for each woman and occurs wherever she reports it to hurt. Despite the presence or absence of physiological indicators of pain, only the patient can validate with certainty her present level of discomfort.

 Nursing Insight—*Recognizing the unique characteristics of childbirth pain*

When caring for laboring women, nurses must recognize that unlike other sources of pain, childbirth pain:
- Is part of a normal process (not associated with illness or injury)
- Can be anticipated and thus prepared for (through childbirth education and the practice of distraction techniques and comfort measures)
- Has an end point (the baby's birth brings relief on a physical and emotional level)

PHYSICAL CAUSES OF PAIN RELATED TO LABOR AND BIRTH

Pain Neurology

The pain associated with labor and birth has both visceral and somatic origins (Lowe, 2002). Uterine contractions during the first stage of labor bring about cervical dilation and effacement. During each contraction, arteries that supply the myometrium are compressed, causing uterine ischemia (oxygen deficit that results from decreased blood flow). During the first stage of labor, pain impulses are transmitted via the T11 and T12 spinal nerve segments and accessory lower thoracic and upper lumbar sympathetic nerves. These nerves originate in the uterus.

Visceral pain describes the predominant discomfort experienced during the first stage of labor. It is related to changes in the cervix (i.e., dilation and effacement), distention of the lower uterine segment, and uterine ischemia. Visceral pain is a slow, deep, poorly localized pain that occurs over the lower abdomen. It is commonly described as a dull aching pain. Laboring women may also experience **referred pain**. Referred pain describes pain that originates in the uterus and then radiates to the abdominal wall, the lumbosacral area of the back, the iliac crests, the gluteus maximus, and down the thighs. Usually, the discomfort is felt only during contractions. A period of pain relief occurs between contractions although some women report continued unremitting pain even during the interval between contractions (Labor & Maguire, 2008; Lowe, 2002).

Somatic pain, a faster, well-localized intense, sharp, burning, prickling pain, occurs during the second stage of labor. Somatic pain is associated with stretching and distention of the perineal body to allow for birth. It is also related to distention and traction placed on the peritoneum and uterocervical supportive tissue during contractions and can result from soft tissue lacerations that frequently occur in the cervix, vagina, or perineum. Somatic pain may also occur from the maternal expulsive forces during the second, or "pushing," stage of labor or by fetal pressure on the bladder, bowel, or other pelvic structures. During the second stage of labor, pain impulses are transmitted via the pudendal nerve through S2 to S4 spinal nerve segments and the parasympathetic system (Labor & Macguire, 2008; Lowe, 2002).

During the third stage of labor, and in the early postpartum period, discomfort is associated with uterine contractions. The pain experienced during this time is similar to that associated with the first stage of labor.

PAIN PERCEPTION AND EXPRESSION

Although pain is a universal experience, how a woman reacts to and expresses pain is highly personal and subjective. One's perception of and response to pain is colored by many factors including gender, culture, ethnicity, and past experiences. Research from the disciplines of psychology, anthropology, and sociology has offered insights into the influence of one's primary social group on the meaning of pain and verbal and nonverbal expressions of pain.

Optimizing Outcomes—Recognizing cultural influences on the experience of pain

When providing care, nurses must recognize that culture strongly influences how one perceives and copes with pain. Women from certain cultures seek pain relief through prayer; others rely on herbal remedies, the application of cold or warmth, acupuncture, the "laying on of hands," and therapeutic massage. Assessment of cultural beliefs and practices, questions to identify specific needs and encouragement, and support to use safe interventions is key in providing culturally sensitive care that empowers the patient to maintain her sense of control over her labor and childbirth experience.

For example, a primigravid Haitian woman may respond to painful uterine contractions with crying, loud screams, and hysteria. Laboring Cambodian women, usually attended by a female relative rather than the male partner, tend to be quiet and sedate during labor and birth. The Mexican American woman in labor is likely to be very vocal. Family members other than the baby's father frequently assist with emotional and verbal support. In any clinical setting, it is helpful for the nurse to identify the ethnic groups most often cared for and develop an awareness of culturally specific childbirth practices and pain behaviors. However, the nurse should be cautious not to stereotype patients and must remain sensitive to individual variations in women's choices for dealing with pain during the childbirth process. Approaching each woman's response to her labor and pain with acceptance and support is key to a therapeutic nursing relationship (Purnell, 2014).

Cultural Diversity: Realities of the Cultural Model

When caring for women, nurses must be aware that a potential limitation of relying solely on a cultural perspective comes from neglecting to recognize women's individuality in how they conform to traditional values and norms. Cultural models of health care frequently stereotype women who share the same cultural heritage. In so doing, they may immobilize health providers who seek to change unfavorable health-care situations in the name of protection of the cultural heritage (Meleis, 2003).

Pain is expressed in a number of physiological and affective ways. During labor and childbirth, the sympathetic nervous system responds to pain with increased levels of catecholamines (e.g., epinephrine and norepinephrine—biologically active substances that produce a marked effect on the nervous and cardiovascular systems, metabolic rate, temperature, and smooth muscle). There is a rise in blood pressure and heart rate. Increased maternal oxygen consumption results in an altered respiratory pattern that may produce hyperventilation and respiratory alkalosis. The woman may become diaphoretic, and nausea and vomiting are common during the active phase of labor. Throughout this process, decreased placental perfusion and uterine activity can potentially prolong labor and adversely affect fetal well-being.

Visceral and somatic pain has been described as burning, prickling, stabbing, heavy, pulling, pointing, sharp, stinging, and throbbing. On an emotional, or affective, level, maternal pain during childbirth has been characterized as exhausting, nauseating, annoying, and sickening (Lowe, 2002). Outward signs of suffering tend to be universal and are exhibited in varying degrees. Patients in pain cry, scream, clench and wring their hands, moan, groan, clench their jaws, and in other ways demonstrate increasing anxiety with a reduced perceptual field.

FACTORS THAT AFFECT MATERNAL PAIN RESPONSE

Physical, physiological, and psychological influences affect the laboring woman's perception and tolerance of pain. Physical factors include labor intensity, cervical readiness, fetal position, pelvic dimensions, fatigue, and medical interventions.

Physical Factors

A brief, intense labor is often associated with a greater level of discomfort and pain because the contractions are highly efficient in accomplishing cervical changes (effacement and dilation) and fetal progress (descent). Also, a shortened labor may diminish the woman's options for pharmacological methods of pain relief. When cervical changes (softening, some dilation and effacement) have occurred before the onset of labor, the cervix opens more readily. Theoretically, fewer contractions are needed to achieve dilation and effacement.

When the fetus is in an unfavorable position, the labor is likely to be longer and associated with a greater amount of discomfort. For example, when the fetus is in an occiput posterior position, the woman experiences intense pain during contractions as the fetal occiput is pressed against the maternal sacrum. The pain associated with "back labor" persists between contractions and is unremitting until the fetus rotates to a more favorable position (e.g., occiput anterior). The size and shape of the maternal pelvis influences the progress and thus the level of discomfort and pain associated with the labor. Structural abnormalities may cause the labor to be prolonged and may contribute to fetal malpresentation.

Maternal fatigue adversely affects the ability to tolerate pain and the effective use of coping techniques and strategies to remain in control. Fatigue can hamper the woman's ability to concentrate and prevent her from using imagery, focal points, breathing techniques, and other methods of distraction. While a lack of refreshing sleep is not unusual during the last weeks of pregnancy, even a well-rested woman who experiences a prolonged labor can quickly become exhausted long before the birth takes place.

Certain care provider interventions, such as intravenous and fetal monitoring equipment, can intensify the discomfort naturally associated with labor. At times, these methods may also interfere with maternal mobility and the ability to assume a position of comfort. Labor induction and augmentation, amniotomy, and vaginal examinations may also be associated with intensifying labor discomfort.

Physiological Factors

Physiological forces influence the laboring woman's pain response. If there is a history of dysmenorrhea, increased childbirth pain may be related to higher levels of circulating prostaglandins. Laboring in an upright, instead of supine, position may help alleviate discomfort. Freedom to ambulate and assume a position of comfort during labor has been shown to be beneficial in reducing pain and muscle tension. Furthermore, the opportunity to choose positions for labor empowers the woman with a greater sense of control over her situation. In addition, the fetal size in relation to the maternal pelvic dimensions may also affect the level of pain intensity (Felton, 2011; Lowe, 2002; Simkin, Bolding, Keppler, Durham, & Whalley, 2010).

Although the physiological role is not well understood, the level of circulating endorphins is believed to have an important effect on the laboring woman's sense of well-being. **Endorphins** are endogenous opioids secreted by the pituitary gland. Endorphins act as opiates and produce analgesia by binding at opiate receptor sites involved in pain perception. In this manner, endorphins increase the threshold for pain. Beta-endorphin is the most active compound. When present in higher levels, endorphins are believed to increase the laboring woman's ability to tolerate pain; increased endorphin levels have been demonstrated with spontaneous, natural childbirth.

Psychological Factors

A number of psychological forces such as anxiety, fear, previous experiences, support systems, and childbirth preparation influence perception of and response to pain. Maternal anxiety during labor triggers the release of catecholamines, which increase the amount of pelvic pain stimuli sent to the brain, resulting in an intensified perception of pain (Lowe, 2002). As muscle tension increases, the effectiveness of the uterine contractions decreases and maternal discomfort and pain are intensified. Over time, the cycle of anxiety → tension → pain diminishes the progress of labor. At the same time, the woman's self-confidence in her ability to cope with the pain erodes, and therapeutic interventions to help reduce pain and discomfort become less effective.

The woman's previous experience with pain and childbirth also influences her pain perception and ability to cope during labor. For most young, healthy women, childbirth often represents the first exposure to prolonged, intense pain. During early labor, sensory pain tends to be more pronounced in the nulliparous patient because the reproductive tract structures are less pliant and flexible. Multiparous patients may experience greater sensory pain during the transition phase of the first stage of labor because their pliable reproductive tract structures allow for a more rapid fetal descent accompanied by a heightened intensity in pain. During the first stage of labor, affective pain is usually greater for nulliparous women but is decreased for both nulliparous and multiparous women during the second stage (Labor & Maguire, 2008; Lowe, 2002).

The patient's personal experience with a previous childbirth also influences her pain perception. A prior negative experience marked by misery and pain may produce an expectation of a repeated negative experience that is filled with fear and dread. A woman whose prior childbirth experience was satisfying is more likely to approach the present birth with a positive attitude and confidence in her ability to cope with the pain and discomfort (Nilsson, Bondas, & Lundgren, 2010).

The physical environment that envelops the birth experience should be considered as well. *Environment* encompasses those present as well as the physical space where the labor takes place. When indicated, labor support persons should be encouraged to serve as the patient's advocate in communicating desires, expectations, and concerns and in providing physical comfort measures. Women prefer to be cared for in a home-style setting by trusted, familiar caregivers (Hodnett, Gates, Hofmeyr, Sakala, & Weston, 2011).

 Nursing Insight—*Environmental strategies to enhance comfort during labor*

The labor environment should provide privacy, comfort, and a sense of security. Allowing patients to determine the amount of noise, light, and temperature in their room fosters relaxation and a sense of control over their situation. Ideally, the room has an abundance of space that freely allows for patient and staff mobility, equipment (preferably hidden from view unless needed), and comfort measures such as birth balls, reclining chairs, tubs, and showers.

Now Can You—Discuss characteristics of pain during labor and birth?

1. Identify three distinct characteristics of childbirth pain?
2. Differentiate among visceral, somatic, and referred pain and discuss when these pain types are most likely to occur during labor?
3. Discuss the physical, physiological, and psychological factors that influence the laboring woman's experience of pain?

THE EFFECTS OF PREPARED CHILDBIRTH ON PAIN PATHWAYS

Prepared childbirth provides the patient and her partner with an understanding of what to expect during childbirth and empowers them to become knowledgeable consumers of health care who can make informed choices concerning their childbearing experience. Accessible through many avenues, childbirth education is offered by most care providers and may also be obtained in written or online materials or through participation in formal childbirth education classes. In most areas, a variety of classes are available to provide general or specialized information. Prenatal classes focus on fetal growth and maternal changes and often place emphasis on health promotion through nutrition, exercise, stress reduction, and adequate rest. Other classes are intended to prepare the expectant couple for the labor process, and much time is spent exploring nonpharmacological and pharmacological measures for pain relief. These classes generally focus on educating the woman and her support person(s) about strategies such as position changes, breathing techniques, massage, and other methods to achieve relaxation and enhance comfort during labor. Classes for women with a planned cesarean birth are also available, and for those who wish to breastfeed, hospital maternity programs and local lactation support groups frequently provide focused breastfeeding classes.

To enhance understanding of how methods learned through prepared childbirth work to promote comfort during labor, it is helpful to review pain pathways and the gate control theory of pain. Pain may be viewed as a multidimensional phenomenon that encompasses the following five dimensions: affective, physiological, behavioral, sensory, and cognitive. The neural pathway for pain involves four processes: transduction, transmission, perception, and modulation. Transduction is the conversion of a mechanical, thermal, or chemical stimulus into a neuronal action potential. Transduction occurs at the nociceptors, nerves that receive and transmit painful stimuli. Stated another way, incoming noxious stimuli are converted to electrical activity at the sensory endings of the peripheral nerves. Transmission is the movement of the pain impulse from the site of transduction (e.g., uterine contractions) to the brain. Perception is the development of the sensory, subjective, and emotional experience identified by the individual as pain. Perception occurs when the patient feels the pain and responds to it, and modulation involves the activation of descending pathways that exert either inhibitory or facilitatory effects on the transmission of pain (Labor & Maguire, 2008; Lowe, 2002).

Sometimes it is possible for painful stimuli to be ignored. Groups of certain nerve cells located in the spinal cord, brainstem, and cerebral cortex have the ability to modulate, or alter, pain impulses through a blocking mechanism. According to the **gate-control theory** of pain control (Melzack & Wall, 1965), pain sensations travel along sensory nerve pathways to the brain—but only a certain number of sensations, or "messages" can pass through the nerve pathways at one time. Methods of distraction learned and practiced in prepared childbirth classes such as breathing patterns, massage, music, and the use of focal points and imagery reduce or completely block the capacity of the nerve pathways to transmit pain. It is believed that these physical and psychological distractions work by "shutting the gate" in the spinal cord so that pain signals are unable to reach the brain.

When the laboring woman is actively involved in neuromuscular and motor activity, there is an increase in spinal cord activity that further modifies the transmission of pain. For example, the cognitive effort channeled into concentration on breathing patterns, focal points, and imagery requires selective and directed cortical activity that activates and closes the gating mechanism. The gate-control theory helps to explain how methods such as hypnosis and the various pain relief techniques taught in childbirth education classes help to diminish the laboring woman's perception of pain.

BENEFITS OF COMFORT AND SUPPORT ON PAIN PERCEPTION

In the traditional medical model, pain and discomfort during labor have largely been viewed as a negative component that should be eliminated. An alternative approach views labor as a natural process that challenges women to seek activities of comfort that will allow them to transcend the pain to achieve the satisfaction and contentment of birth. Feeling safe, secure, comforted, and in control empowers the laboring woman to find strength in dealing with her discomfort and pain. Nurses can facilitate comfort by providing a caring, supportive, therapeutic presence.

Support during labor and birth has a major impact on the woman's birth experience. Support includes both non-pharmacological and pharmacological measures. The nurse's attitude, expressions of caring, and supportive actions play a significant role in the woman's perception of pain and in her overall childbearing experience. Patients who feel they have control over their situation (self-efficacy) and who are actively engaged in the decision-making process concerning interventions and pain relief measures during labor and birth report a greater sense of satisfaction with their birth experience (Hodnett, 2002). When support is perceived to be ongoing and individualized throughout labor, women require fewer pain medications and interventions and experience improved outcomes such as shorter labors, increased likelihood of breastfeeding, and increased satisfaction with the overall childbirth experience (AWHONN, 2011a; Hodnett et al., 2011; Simkin et al., 2010). Spending as much time as possible at the patient's bedside (e.g., charting in the room and assessing the woman's comfort level and satisfaction with her birth plan) is an important nursing strategy. Offering verbal support, touch, and eye contact can help keep the woman centered and in control (Anderson & Kilpatrick, 2012).

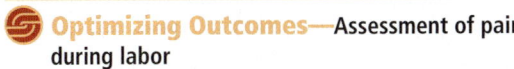 **Optimizing Outcomes**—Assessment of pain during labor

Throughout the process of labor and birth, the nurse continuously assesses the patient and addresses her needs for comfort measures. Conducting an initial and ongoing pain assessment lays the foundation for intrapartal nursing care. Once the beginning assessment has been completed, the nurse uses the information to develop an individualized plan of care that includes pain relief interventions acceptable to the patient. A number of tools have been developed to facilitate pain assessment during labor; these may be modified or adapted as needed (Fig. 13-1).

Providing Comfort and Pain Relief

Methods to provide comfort and relieve pain are of paramount importance for the childbearing couple. The woman's perception of her overall birth experience is greatly influenced by her ability to cope with pain in whatever manner is acceptable to her. Nonpharmacological pain relief measures are for the most part inexpensive, easy to use, safe, and readily available. They also allow the patient to gain an enhanced sense of control over her childbirth experience. Despite their effectiveness, however, none of the various techniques are more effective than methods of epidural analgesia. Nurses play a key role in educating women and their support persons about the various nonpharmacological and pharmacological pain relief methods available. During labor, women should be encouraged to try a variety of pain relief measures, including pharmacological methods, if needed. Factual information and ongoing support empower the patient to make informed choices and to participate fully in the decision-making process.

Another important component of childbirth preparation concerns the choice of the birth setting. Many communities offer several options for where the childbirth will take place. Often during the first prepared childbirth class, expectant couples are encouraged to explore community options for the childbirth setting that best "fits" with their desired childbirth experience.

 Across Care Settings: **Childbirth options in the local community**

Encouraging expectant couples to explore options for the childbirth setting is an important component of prenatal education. As consumers of health care, patients should seek a primary care provider and facility that will safely meet their childbirth needs. Depending on the locale, the community may have a large city hospital, a small community hospital, a birth center, or a practicing group of certified nurse midwives (CNMs) that provides care during home births. When considering a birth facility, the woman may wish to ask about the availability of hydrotherapy, birth balls, aromatherapy, and transcutaneous electrical nerve stimulation units.

 Now Can You—Discuss a pain control theory, pain perception, and considerations for the childbirth setting?

1. Discuss the basic premise of the gate control theory of pain control?
2. Explain how comfort and support during labor decrease the woman's perception of discomfort and pain?
3. Formulate four questions the expectant couple may wish to ask to help determine their choice of childbirth setting?

NONPHARMACOLOGICAL PAIN RELIEF MEASURES

Maternal Position and Movement

One way the nurse can facilitate relaxation is by helping the patient to find a position of comfort. Movement and changes in maternal position are important strategies for facilitating labor and childbirth (Evans-Lynn, 2012; Lothian & DeVries, 2010). As the patient changes positions, gravity assists the fetus's descent down the birth canal. Slow dancing during labor is an activity that the expectant couple may enjoy. Most find slow dancing to special music from their own collection to be comforting and relaxing. When the couple assumes the slow dance position, the woman can lean on her coach (this helps to support her), and they can sway and dance together through the contractions.

Laboring women may also wish to use a "squatting bar" or assume a squatting position at the edge of the bed. The squatting position helps to open the pelvic outlet, which facilitates the fetus's downward movement. Assuming a hands and knees position is comforting for women who have back labor or whose fetus is in a posterior position. The hands and knees position decreases the patient's back pressure and helps the fetus to rotate into an anterior position. Many hospital birthing suites offer wireless telemetry units that provide continuous monitoring while the patient ambulates at her leisure (Fig. 13-2).

The "birth ball" may be also used to promote comfort during labor. Essentially, the birth ball is a large, firm yet pliable physical therapy ball or gymnastic ball that provides support for the laboring woman. With assistance from the nurse, doula, or support person, the patient carefully sits on the birth ball and rhythmically rocks back and forth or moves the ball around in a circular motion. Assuming a sitting position on the birth ball facilitates a supported squatting position that opens the pelvis to allow fetal descent in preparation for birth. Warm compresses applied to the back and perineum while balancing on the ball enhance relaxation and promote comfort (Fig. 13-3). The birth ball should be large enough to allow the woman to sit comfortably on it with her knees bent at a 90-degree angle with her feet flat on the floor and approximately 2 feet apart (Perez, 2000). The woman may also place the birth ball against the wall behind the small of her back and gently lunge from side to side to open the pelvis. When needed, assuming a kneeling position while leaning forward on the birth ball may encourage the rotation of the fetus from a posterior to an anterior position. Researchers Taavoni and colleagues (2011) found that while this complementary treatment had no effect on the duration of the active phase of labor, the duration of uterine contractions, or the interval between

Pain Assessment During Labor

Patient's Name _____

Date _____ Age _____ Room_____

Diagnosis_____

Physician/Midwife _____

Gravida _____ Para _____

Location of Pain_____

Intensity of Pain (scale of 1–10) _____

Present Pain _____

The Worst the Pain Has Been _____

Quality _____

Onset and Duration _____

What Has the Patient Done at Home to Cope With the Pain?_____

_____

What Comfort Measures Would the Patient Like to Use Now? _____

_____

How Is the Pain Affecting the Patient?_____

_____

Other _____

_____

Nurse's Plan for Pain Management _____

_____

_____

Signature of Nurse Completing Form _____

Figure 13-1 Example of a tool used for the assessment of pain during labor.

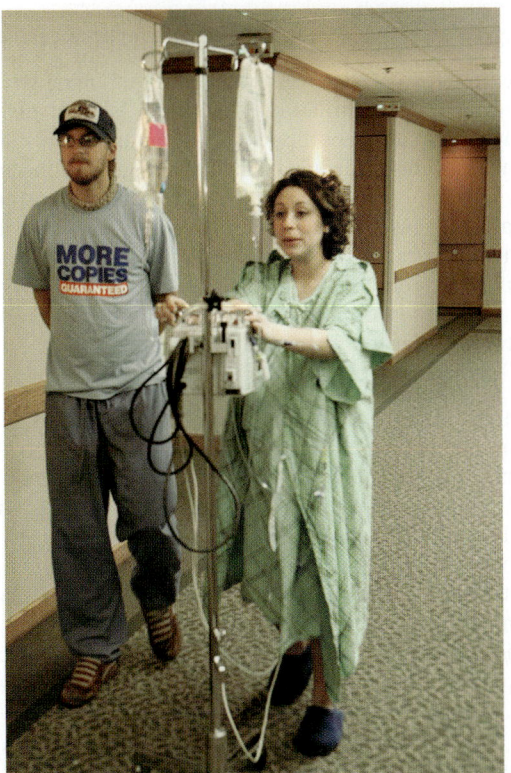

Figure 13-2 Use of a wireless telemetry unit allows the woman to ambulate during labor.

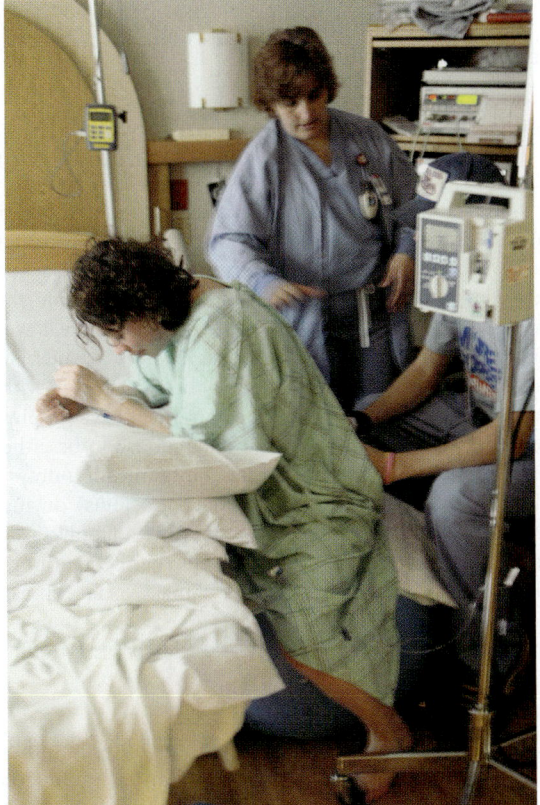

Figure 13-3 The coach applies counterpressure and warm compresses to the woman's lower back as she balances on the birth ball.

contractions, the birth ball could reduce the intensity of pain during the active phase of labor.

Breathing Techniques

During childbirth education classes, the pregnant woman and her labor coach learn about conscious breathing patterns that involve slowed respirations to enhance relaxation. Specific breathing methods are also taught as attention-focusing and distraction techniques to help relieve discomfort and pain during labor. Distraction helps to reduce the woman's perception of pain. The labor "coach," or support person, assists the woman by learning to palpate her body to identify muscle tenseness, by signaling the onset of contractions, and by monitoring her effective use of the breathing techniques. Techniques learned in class are practiced at home so that when labor begins, the couple is prepared to use relaxation and breathing patterns as a strategy to help diminish discomfort and pain (Fig. 13-4).

The woman is instructed to take a slow, deep cleansing breath in through the nose and out through the mouth at the beginning of every contraction. During early labor, when the woman is no longer able to walk or talk through contractions, she may wish to begin using *slow-paced* breathing. With this pattern, following a cleansing breath, the woman begins to slowly breathe in and out through her mouth while her coach slowly counts out loud. The breathing rate is approximately half the woman's normal breathing rate—6 to 8 breaths per minute. With this pattern, she is prompted to slowly breathe in while the coach counts "one, two, three, four," and then slowly breathe out to the same rhythm as the coach counts "one, two, three, four."

As the labor progresses and the contractions increase in frequency and intensity, the patient may need to change to a *modified-paced* breathing pattern. This breathing technique is shallower and approximately twice the woman's normal rate of breathing—32 to 40 breaths per minute. After a deep cleansing breath, the woman inhales slowly, but exhales at faster pace. For example, the coach may instruct her to take a cleansing breath, then breathe in to a count of one, two, three, four and breathe out to a count of one, two, three. All contractions should end with another deep cleansing breath. The modified-paced breathing

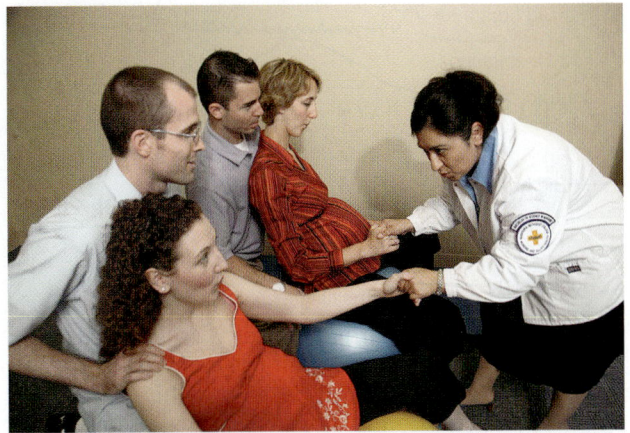

Figure 13-4 Practice of relaxation techniques and breathing exercises help to prepare the couple for labor and birth.

pattern requires more concentration and is believed to block more painful stimuli than the slow-paced breathing pattern (Perinatal Education Associates, 2012). The woman may wish to combine the slow and modified-paced breathing: use the slow-paced breathing at the beginning and end of the contractions and the modified-paced breathing during the contraction intensity. Combining the patterns helps to conserve maternal energy and lessens fatigue and the likelihood of hyperventilation (Fig. 13-5).

During the transition phase of labor, when contractions are most intense, patients usually find it difficult to concentrate on breathing techniques. At this time, the *pattern-paced* breathing technique, which requires increased concentration, is helpful. With this breathing pattern, following a cleansing breath, the woman begins with a 3:1 pattern: breathe in, breathe out; breathe in, breathe out; breathe in, then blow (as if blowing out a candle). This sequence is repeated throughout the contraction. As needed, the ratio may be increased to 4:1. As with the other breathing patterns, a cleansing breath is taken at the end of the contraction. The patient can use and modify any of the breathing techniques that work best for her at any stage of her labor.

❝What to say❞—*When the patient needs assistance refocusing during labor*

While in the transition phase of labor, the laboring patient screams out "I quit, I cannot do this anymore, I have no more energy, I can't do this." At this point, comfort measures are ineffective. Instead, the nurse can help the patient stay focused on dealing with each contraction by offering words of support and encouragement with statements such as:

"You are doing a great job!"
"You are almost there!"
"I can see your baby's head—reach down and feel it!"
"You can do it!"

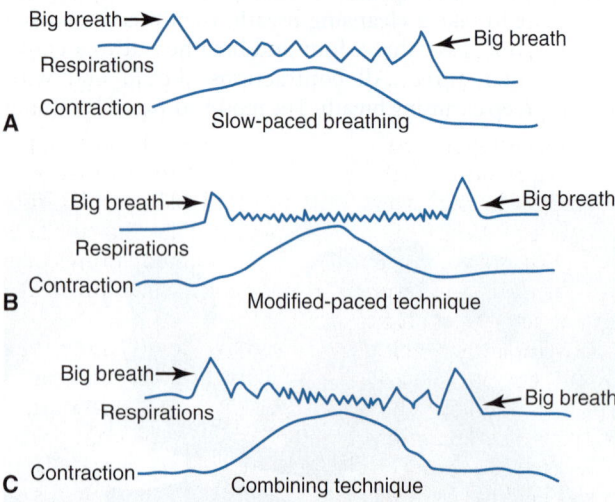

Figure 13-5 Labor breathing patterns. *A,* Slow-paced breathing is approximately half the woman's normal breathing rate. *B,* Modified-paced breathing is approximately twice the woman's normal breathing rate. *C,* Combined breathing: Slow-paced pattern at the beginning of the contraction and then the modified-paced pattern during the contraction's peak.

ⓢ Optimizing Outcomes—Recognizing hyperventilation

The pattern-paced breathing technique may result in maternal hyperventilation. The nurse should alert the patient and her support person to symptoms of respiratory alkalosis: light-headedness, dizziness, tingling of the fingers, or circumoral numbness. Strategies to eliminate respiratory alkalosis focus on replacement of the bicarbonate ion by rebreathing carbon dioxide. This can be accomplished by instructing the woman to breathe into a paper bag held tightly around the mouth and nose or, if no bag is available, instructing her to breathe into her cupped hands.

During the second-stage pushing phase of labor, patients should be encouraged to use whatever breathing pattern is comfortable and relaxing. To ensure optimal blood flow to the fetus, prolonged breath holding during pushing should be avoided. When needed, the urge to push may be controlled by a breathing pattern that consists of repeated puffing air in and out as if blowing out a candle (Perinatal Education Associates, 2012).

It is important for the pregnant woman and her coach to practice all breathing techniques before the onset of labor. The practice helps to increase their comfort level with the techniques and increases the likelihood that they will be able to use them effectively during labor. The breathing and relaxation techniques can be practiced together at home and at any time to reduce stress. When necessary, couples who are unfamiliar with breathing strategies can be taught during labor. Breathing techniques offer a form of distraction because the woman who is concentrating on slow-paced breathing cannot focus on her pain. The breathing patterns are also beneficial in increasing blood flow to the fetus.

✿ Cultural Diversity: *Caring for the Orthodox Jewish Couple in Labor*

Orthodox Jewish women are encouraged to learn breathing techniques to help them cope with the pain of labor; pain medication is allowed when absolutely necessary. Nurses who provide maternity care for the Orthodox Jewish couple should understand the laws of *niddah* (a ritual impure state; a woman is in *niddah* whenever blood is discharged from her uterus) and modesty (the woman's husband may be in the room with her only when she is properly covered and may have no physical contact with her). The husband may choose to be either an active participant (offering verbal communication only) or a religious participant (reciting a book of psalms) during the labor and birth. Nurses can offer support without physical contact with verbal communication (help with breathing and relaxation) and body language (eye contact, facial expression) (Zauderer, 2009).

Music

Music can help to create a relaxing environment and boost spirits. During labor, music provides comfort and decreases maternal anxiety by stimulating the release of endorphins. For most couples, quiet, soothing music works best. Music players are often available in hospital birthing suites and freestanding birth centers, and patients are encouraged to supply music of their choice. A headset or earphones used with the compact disc player or patient's personal iPod may be even more effective because environmental sounds are tuned out. Comforting music during labor promotes maternal relaxation, thereby increasing oxygen intake. Some women find that music enhances their ability to remain focused during contractions. Music alone may also provide pain relief during labor, although further research is needed (Smith, Levett, Collins, & Crowther, 2011). In some birth settings, patients are allowed to bring personal videos or DVDs from home to enjoy as another strategy for distraction during labor.

Relaxation

Various relaxation techniques are used to help decrease anxiety during labor. When the nurse, patient, and her labor support person(s) are successful in diminishing the patient's level of anxiety, stress and tension are also reduced. When tension is reduced, the woman breathes more deeply, resulting in improved maternal and fetal oxygenation. When the laboring woman experiences increased anxiety, stress levels and tension build and trigger a cascade of events that heighten the sensation of pain. Pain also impedes the patient's ability to relax. The nurse's ongoing assessment of maternal pain should be conducted throughout labor and birth. The use of a standardized pain assessment tool facilitates the evaluation and allows for an easy reassessment of pain following therapeutic interventions. Use of a patient self-assessment tool is preferable because it ensures that the management of pain is based on the subjective nature of the woman's pain rather than on the nurse's judgment alone.

 Nursing Insight*—Use of a visual analog scale for the assessment of pain*

A visual analog scale for pain assessment is helpful because the patient is able to indicate on a line how intense she perceives her pain to be: The choices range from "no pain" to "pain as bad as it could possibly be." Other scales that present drawings that range from happy, smiling faces to sad, crying faces are also available. The nurse should ask the woman to rate her pain on the scale before and after pain-relief measures to evaluate their effectiveness.

Other Attention-Focusing Strategies

Guided imagery is a state of intense, focused concentration that one uses to create persuasive mental images. Guided imagery distracts the laboring woman and transports her to a place that is special to her. The nurse or labor support person assists with guided imagery by asking the laboring woman to focus on a place where she likes to be. Many patients choose the beach or the mountains as their special locale. Next, the nurse or the labor support person verbalizes sights and sounds of that unique place in an attempt to relax and distract the patient. Often, the labor support person can describe the special place in a meaningful, calming way. For example, the coach may say:

> Close your eyes, get comfortable in your chair (or bed), take yourself to the beach. You are standing on the edge of the water. You hear the sounds of the waves rolling in. The water

gently laps at your feet. The waves roll in, and the waves roll out. You smell the salty air. Feel the warm sun on your face, the sun is getting warmer and warmer. The waves roll in and out, and the sun is getting warmer. Listen, the sea gulls are flying overhead, you hear them crying out, and you hear the peaceful sound of the waves rolling in and out. You glow with the warm sun on your face, and you feel the gentle breezes against your skin. The waves roll in and out.

Focal points, or visual stimuli, also distract the patient. A focal point may be a picture, photograph, stuffed animal, or piece of needlework. The laboring woman concentrates or "focuses" on the object while breathing during the contractions. Patients are encouraged to bring the object that will serve as a focal point with them to the hospital or birth center. An "internal" focal point may be a thought or visual image—the laboring woman closes her eyes and focuses on the mental image. Focal points enhance concentration and help distract from the discomfort associated with contractions (Simkin et al., 2010).

Massage and Touch

Massage and touch are techniques that have long been used to facilitate comfort and relaxation during labor. The patient's labor support person or nurse can perform simple hand massage to help decrease tension. Back massage is especially beneficial for the discomfort of back labor. Current evidence suggests that massage may be beneficial in reducing pain and improving women's emotional experience of labor; however, further study is indicated (Smith, Levett, Collins, & Jones, 2012).

Effleurage, taken from the French word *effleurer* (to touch lightly), is a gentle stroking technique performed in rhythm with contractions. The patient or her labor support person massages the abdomen using light circular motions. Effleurage is helpful in distracting the patient from her contractions. Massage of the hands, feet, and back may be effective in diminishing tension and in enhancing comfort. Throughout the labor experience, patients and their partners should be encouraged to experiment with various techniques to determine what methods work best for them.

Counterpressure is often effective in enhancing the woman's ability to cope with discomfort from internal pressure and lower back pain. This technique involves use of the labor support person's fist or heel of the hand to apply steady pressure to the sacral area. Counterpressure is especially helpful when maternal back pain results from pressure of the occiput against spinal nerves when the fetal head is in a posterior position. This technique brings pain relief as the counterpressure lifts the occiput off of the spinal nerves (Smith et al., 2012).

Therapeutic touch is based on the use of "prana," the body's energy fields. Prana is believed to be deficient in some individuals who experience pain. Specially trained persons use laying-on of hands to provide therapeutic touch to redirect the energy fields thought to be associated with the pain (Krieger, 1979). Although the benefits of therapeutic touch in enhancing relaxation and in reducing anxiety and pain have been documented, the effectiveness of this modality for pain relief during labor is not known (Smith et al., 2012).

Healing touch is also based on use of the body's energy fields. This modality employs a combination of techniques from multiple disciplines. Persons trained in healing touch are taught energetic diagnosis and treatment forms and how to document the patient's response and progress. It is believed that the various techniques align and balance the human energy field, enhancing the body's ability to heal itself. Although healing touch has been used during labor, no studies have been published to document its effectiveness (Hover-Kramer, 2011).

Hydrotherapy

Hydrotherapy (water therapy) is the use of warm water to promote comfort and relaxation. Hydrotherapy may involve showering or soaking in a regular tub or whirlpool bath. When showering is the selected method of hydrotherapy, the patient stands in a warm shower and allows the water to gently glide over her abdomen. Alternatively, she may wish to sit in a shower chair. The nurse or labor coach may use a handheld sprayer to direct a steady stream of water over the abdomen or back. Throughout this time, the support person provides reassurance and encouragement, assists with breathing techniques during contractions, and offers touch and massage. The flow of warm water enhances feelings of relaxation and helps to decrease muscle tension. Reduced discomfort and increased relaxation often empowers the woman to have more control over her labor (Cluett & Burns, 2009).

Immersion in a tub of warm water filled up to shoulder level is also beneficial in promoting comfort and relaxation. For most, the buoyancy provided by the water provides welcomed relief from labor discomfort and pain. The production of maternal catecholamines is decreased, prompting an increase in the release of oxytocin (stimulates uterine contractions) and endorphins (reduces the perception of pain). If the woman is experiencing "back labor" from a fetal occiput posterior or transverse position, she may be assisted into a side-lying or hands-and-knees position in the tub. These positions enhance comfort and help to facilitate fetal rotation into an occiput anterior position.

Whirlpool tubs ("jet hydrotherapy") are available in many birth settings, although some institutions require prior approval for use from the patient's primary care provider. The pulsating flow of warm water from the whirlpool jets is soothing and delivers continuous massage to the patient's legs, abdomen, and back. The rhythm of the water flowing in the shower or whirlpool tub provides a soothing sound that aids in relaxation.

During hydrotherapy, fetal heart rate (FHR) monitoring may be intermittent or continuous. It may be conducted via Doppler technique, fetoscope, or use of a wireless external monitor device. Internal electrode placement may not be used with whirlpool baths. In some settings, women with ruptured membranes are allowed to use jet hydrotherapy, provided that the amniotic fluid is clear.

Patients may stay in the tub as long as desired; most remain for 40 to 60 minutes. During that time, if the maternal temperature or FHR increase, if the labor slows or becomes too intense, or if the comforting effects of the water are diminished, patients may come out of the tub and return at a later time. For many, repeated immersions are more effective in relieving pain than a long, continuous exposure to the water. During tub hydrotherapy, the nurse or labor partner can offer comforting, cool washcloths for the face and fluids to promote hydration. To avoid overheating, the water temperature should be maintained at 96.8°F to 100.4°F (36°C to 38°C) (Simkin et al., 2010).

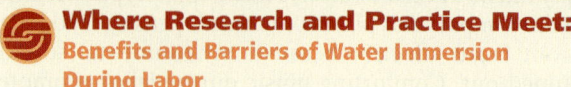

Where Research and Practice Meet:
Benefits and Barriers of Water Immersion During Labor

A Cochrane review of 12 randomized trials (3,243 women) evaluated the safety and efficacy of water immersion during labor and/or birth in women who were considered to be at low risk of complications. Water immersion during the first stage of labor significantly reduced maternal pain and the need for epidural/spinal analgesia and duration of the first stage. One trial showed that water immersion during the second stage of labor increased the women's reported satisfaction with their birth experience. There was no evidence of increased adverse effects to the fetus/neonate or woman from laboring or giving birth in water. The reviewers suggested that further research is needed to assess the effect of water on neonatal and maternal morbidity (Cluett & Burns, 2009).

Other researchers (Stark & Miller, 2009; Youness & Moustafa, 2012) explored nurses' perceived barriers to the use of hydrotherapy in labor. Stark and Miller (2009, 2010) developed, tested, and administered a 30-item survey to 401 intrapartum nurses to identify specific barriers encountered in providing the complementary therapy to laboring women. The instrument comprised four subscales, including health-care environment, knowledge and beliefs, personal concerns, and effort required for hydrotherapy. The investigators concluded that the culture of the birthing unit in which nurses provide care influences perception of barriers to the use of hydrotherapy in labor. The use of this complementary modality requires a supportive environment, adequate nursing policies and staffing, and collaborative relationships among the health-care team.

Hypnotherapy

Hypnotherapy is a structured technique that enables the patient to achieve a state of heightened awareness and focused concentration that can be used to alter the perception of pain. With this modality, emphasis is placed on promoting maternal relaxation while decreasing fear, anxiety, and the perception of pain. To accomplish this, the woman may be given direct suggestions about pain relief or indirect suggestions that she is experiencing decreased discomfort. Teaching expectant women about the method and encouraging continued practice during the prenatal period are essential strategies for the successful use of hypnotherapy during labor and birth. Hypnotherapy involves the induction of a state of great mental and physical relaxation that can be therapeutic in the management of pain control (Landolt & Milling, 2011; Tuschhoff, 2014).

Aromatherapy

Aromatherapy is the use of essential oils, derived from plants, flowers, herbs, and trees, whose aroma is thought to have a therapeutic effect in treating illnesses and promoting health and well-being. The fragrances of rose, lavender, frankincense, and bergamot oils are believed to promote comfort and relaxation and decrease pain. Patients may use the scented oils by adding a few drops to a warm tub bath, to body compresses and massage lotions, or to an aromatherapy lamp used to add fragrance to the room. Drops of lavender and other essential oils may also be massaged into the woman's temples or forehead or placed on a pillow to induce relaxation (Simkin et al., 2010). While the use of aromatherapy is associated with beneficial effects for some women, further research is needed to determine the efficacy of this complementary modality for pain management in labor (Smith, Collins, & Crowther, 2011).

Where Research and Practice Meet:
Physiological and Psychological Effects of Self-Hypnosis

Hypnosis is an innovative low-technology modality that may contribute to stress reduction and health promotion. Using a convenience sample of 30 healthy, nonpregnant women, nurse researchers VandeVusse, Hanson, Berner, and Winters (2010) conducted a quasi-experimental study designed to examine the physiological and psychological effects of hypnosis. Participants listened to a 30-minute recording of relaxing, affirming hypnotic suggestions while comfortably positioned in a recliner chair. Hypnotizability and trait anxiety were measured at baseline; tension-anxiety was measured at baseline and following the hypnotic induction. Heart rate, respiratory rate, and heart rate variability were collected before, during, and following the hypnotic experience. Data analysis revealed significantly reduced heart rates, respiratory rates, low-to-high frequency heart rate variability ratios and tension-anxiety, findings that provide support for the physiological and psychological benefits from relaxation associated with a hypnotic experience. The investigators suggest that the technique of hypnosis may be especially useful in noisy conditions such as labor and birthing units and surgical environments and encourage nurses to consider recommending hypnosis as an additional technique to help achieve relaxation and reduction of stress.

clinical alert

When using aromatherapy

Nurses must be aware that the essential oils used in aromatherapy should never be applied to the skin in a full-strength form. Instead, the oils must be diluted, usually in a vegetable oil base, before application. Patients should be cautioned that not all aromatherapy oils are safe to use during pregnancy; some oils, when inhaled, cause side effects such as nausea and headache (Weiss, 2014).

Complementary Care: *Yoga to Reduce Discomfort During Labor*

Prenatal yoga classes, which focus on breathing techniques and enhanced relaxation, are becoming increasingly popular. Physiologically, yoga increases the efficiency of the heart, slows the respiratory rate, and lowers blood pressure. For many, yoga helps decrease stress and anxiety during the prenatal period and provides coping strategies that can be used during labor. The practice of yoga during pregnancy helps women learn to decrease the urge to tighten muscles in response to pain. This response promotes the release of oxytocin to enhance the progress of labor. Poses used in prenatal yoga also facilitate the descent of the fetus and often decrease back pain. Women should always check with their primary care provider before beginning prenatal yoga. For many, attending a prenatal yoga class in the community is a healthy way to meet other women who are beginning a new chapter in their life.

Application of Heat and Cold

The application of heat and cold can promote comfort and help decrease pain during labor and birth. The two modalities may be used alternately to enhance their effects. Heat exerts a therapeutic effect by relieving muscle ischemia and increasing blood flow to the area of discomfort. Warm washcloths applied to the perineum help to relieve the discomfort associated with stretching and may also help to prevent tearing during the second stage of labor. Socks or bags that are sewn from cloth can be filled with uncooked rice and heated in a microwave oven. Once warmed, the bags radiate soothing heat that helps to diminish pain. The rice bags may be placed on the patient's neck, lower back, or wherever the discomfort is felt. When desired, lavender oil, a comforting aroma to many, may be added to the homemade rice bag before heating (March of Dimes, 2012; Simkin et al., 2010).

Cold washcloths or ice packs placed on the forehead, chest, or face may be comforting to laboring women who feel warm (Fig. 13-6). Cold packs may also be applied to areas of pain where they exert a therapeutic effect by reducing muscle temperature and relieving muscle spasms. During contractions, ice massage to the acupuncture point on the hand (Hoku point) may help reduce pain. The nurse should be aware that some patients' cultural beliefs may not permit the use of cold therapy during labor (Simkin et al., 2010).

 ## Optimizing Outcomes—When using heat and cold for pain relief during labor

Nurses should avoid the application of heat or cold over body areas that have been anesthetized because of the risk for tissue damage. Hot and cold packs should be used only after one to two layers of cloth have been placed between the pack and the patient's skin (Simkin et al., 2010).

Biofeedback

Biofeedback has been used for many years to enhance relaxation and help patients to gain control over their pain. It is based on the concept that the mind controls the body: If one can recognize physical signals, certain internal physiological events can be changed. During the prenatal period, the woman is taught body awareness, how to recognize responses to stimuli, and various relaxation techniques. She practices using strategies such as concentration, focal points, and breathing to control her response to uncomfortable stimuli. The labor partner learns to recognize cues (e.g., grimacing, tensing, frowning, moaning, and breath holding) indicative of pain and uses verbal feedback and touch to help the woman to achieve relaxation. Formal biofeedback,

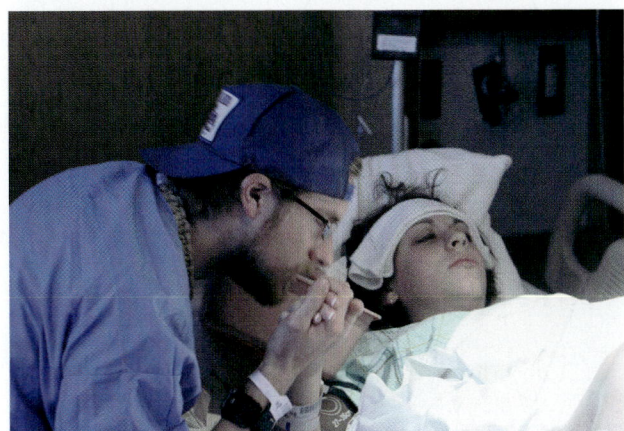

Figure 13-6 A cool washcloth placed on the forehead provides comfort during labor.

which involves the use of a recording device to measure physiological responses, requires special training by a skilled biofeedback therapist. Body signals (e.g., skin temperature, blood flow, and muscle tension) that indicate pain and stress are sent via attached electrodes back to the biofeedback unit. The unit then alerts the patient who uses various techniques to decrease the tension and discomfort.

Transcutaneous Electrical Nerve Stimulation

Transcutaneous electrical nerve stimulation (TENS) involves the delivery of an electric current through electrodes that are applied to the skin over the painful region of a peripheral nerve (Simkin et al., 2010). The TENS unit relieves pain by producing counterirritation on the nociceptors. Normally, two pairs of flat electrodes are placed on either side of the patient's thoracic and sacral spine. Continuous low-intensity electrical impulses are delivered through a battery-operated device. During a contraction, patients are instructed to turn the knobs on the unit to increase the degree of stimulation from a low intensity to a high intensity. High-intensity levels maintained for at least 1 minute facilitate the release of endorphins. Most women report a pleasant buzzing or tingling sensation that offsets the pain. The TENS unit is especially beneficial for relief of ante- and intrapartal low-back pain, and does not appear to be associated with any adverse maternal–fetal effects (Bedwell, Dowswell, Neilson, & Lavender, 2011; Keskin, Onur, Keskin, Gumus, Kafali, & Turhan, 2012). The doctor or certified nurse midwife prescribes the use of a TENS unit, which may initially be applied by a physical therapist. The nurse explains the use of the device, assists with its application, and evaluates its effectiveness.

Intradermal Water Block

Intradermal water block is a technique that involves the use of a small (e.g., 25-gauge) needle to inject small amounts (e.g., 0.05 to 0.1 mL) of sterile water into four locations (two over each posterior superior iliac spine and two 3 cm below and 1 cm medial to each of the first sites) on the patient's lower back to relieve back pain (Fig. 13-7). Preferably, two people perform the injections

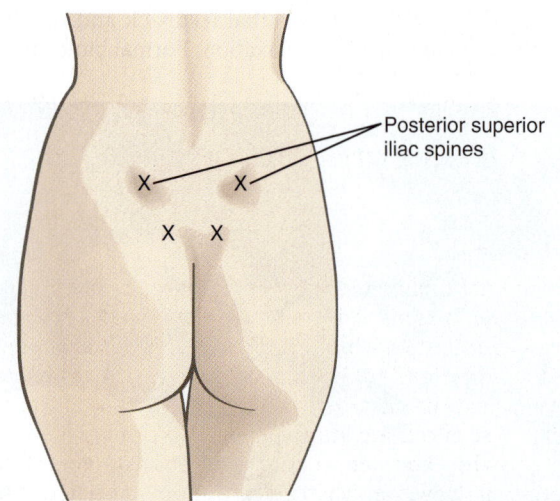

Figure 13-7 Intradermal water block involves the intracutaneous injection of sterile water into four locations on the lower back; four small blebs should be formed.

simultaneously (to decrease the pain of the injections). This method may be used during early labor to delay the initiation of pharmacological pain relief methods. Patients experience a brief, intense stinging sensation immediately after the injections, but the back pain is generally relieved for 45 minutes to 2 hours. Although the mechanism of action is not fully understood, the technique is believed to work by producing counterirritation (pain in one specific area is reduced while skin in close proximity is irritated), gate control, or by increasing circulating endorphins. Once the beneficial effects have diminished, the treatment may be repeated or another pain relief method may be instituted (Simkin et al., 2010; Wong, 2010).

 Global Health Case Study Intradermal Water Block for Labor Discomfort

Sato is a 32-year-old Asian primigravida at 41 weeks gestation who is experiencing back labor from a posterior presentation. She and her husband-coach are in the birthing suite. Sato has declined pain medication but complains of increasing back pain and states she is now having difficulty staying focused on her relaxation and breathing techniques. Sato's friend, who recently gave birth at this hospital, experienced noticeable pain relief from an intradermal water block during labor. Sato states that she and her husband would like to know more about this modality and "give it a try."

critical thinking questions

1. What patient education should the nurse provide for Sato and her husband?

2. After the intradermal water block has been administered, how can the nurse assess if this intervention has been effective?

◆ See Suggested Answers to Global Health Case Studies on Davis*Plus*.

Acupressure and Acupuncture

Acupressure, sometimes called "Chinese massage," involves the application of pressure, or heat or cold to identified acupuncture points to decrease the sensation of pain. The points contain an increased density of neuroreceptors and increased electrical conductivity. It is believed that the technique's effectiveness is related to the gate-control theory of pain and an increased release of endorphins. Pressure may be applied by the support person's hands, tennis balls, or by the application of pressure bands—cloth-covered elastic bands that contain rigid plastic inserts—to provide the pressure. During labor, pressure is applied to various acupressure points, which are located on the neck, shoulders, wrists, lower back, hips, area below the kneecaps, ankles, toenails, and soles of the feet. A commonly identified point used for women in labor is Co4 (Hoku or Hegu point), which is located between the first and second metacarpal bones on the back of the hand. Another acupressure point is located between the inner anklebone and the Achilles' tendon. Applying pressure for 1 minute on each ankle is believed to be beneficial in relieving labor pain.

Acupuncture is a therapy used in traditional Chinese medicine for healing and comfort. It is based on the theory that illness results from an imbalance of energy. This method involves the insertion of fine, sterile, stainless steel needles into specific points in the body (e.g., those associated with labor pain) to control the flow of "chi," or life energy. Activation of the insertion points is believed to trigger the release of endorphins. Acupuncture should be performed only by a trained, certified acupuncturist. Although acupuncture is considered to be safe, it is an invasive therapy that carries a risk of infection (Smith, Collins, Crowther, & Levett, 2011). A 2010 meta-analysis by Cho, Lee, and Ernst found little convincing evidence that women receiving acupuncture were more likely to experience less labor pain than those who did not receive the modality. However, acupuncture did have a transient (30 minutes, on average) effect on pain relief, and there was a reduction in maternal use of meperidine and other analgesics (Malshe & Wiczyk, 2011).

 Collaboration in Caring—*Acupressure and acupuncture as modalities for labor pain relief*

Not as widely accepted in the United States as in some countries, interest in acupressure and acupuncture as a method of inducing labor and relieving labor pain is increasing as more individuals seek holistic practices and alternative medicine. Today, there are more than 40 schools and colleges of acupuncture that offer training in the technique. While the practice of acupuncture requires a considerable amount of education and training, the certified nurse midwife may work with an acupressurist/acupuncturist to become skilled in the manual massage of acupuncture and acupressure points, as well as shiatsu (the application of pressure to acupuncture sites) and other touch therapies.

 Now Can You—Discuss nonpharmacological methods of pain relief during labor?

1. Demonstrate three breathing patterns for labor and explain when each is likely to be of most benefit?
2. Identify four signs of hyperventilation and describe nursing interventions to facilitate restoration of the patient's oxygen–carbon dioxide balance?
3. Briefly discuss the use of guided imagery, touch, hydrotherapy, application of heat and cold, and transcutaneous electrical nerve stimulation as nonpharmacological methods to reduce discomfort and pain during labor?

Pharmacological Pain Relief Measures

Pharmacological methods of pain control should be initiated before the pain intensifies to the point that catecholamines are released and labor is prolonged. A combination of nonpharmacological and pharmacological measures provides pain relief, enhances the patient's comfort and sense of control over her situation, and promotes a positive childbearing experience for the woman and her family. During early labor, nonpharmacological methods alone are often satisfactory for relaxation and pain relief. As labor progresses, contractions and discomfort intensify, often necessitating the addition of pharmacological agents for pain control. Because nonpharmacological measures promote relaxation and potentiate the effects of analgesic agents, less pharmacological intervention is usually required (Smith et al. 2012).

 legal alert—Ensure the patient is informed about available pharmacological methods of pain relief

The nursing role of patient advocate includes ensuring that the woman understands the alternative methods of pain relief that are available in the birth facility and, when indicated, by asking the primary care provider for further details or clarification. Obtaining an informed consent for interventions means that the procedure and its advantages and disadvantages are fully explained, the patient must agree with the plan of care as it is described to her, and the patient's consent must be given freely without coercion or manipulation from her health-care provider (Lowe, 2004).

SEDATIVES AND ANTIEMETICS

Sedatives are agents that relieve anxiety and induce sleep. They are primarily used during the early latent phase of labor, when the cervix is long, closed, and thick and rest has been prescribed for the patient. Sedatives may also be used to augment analgesics and reduce nausea after the administration of opioids. Sedatives induce sleep for a few hours. Once the woman awakens, either the contractions have ceased (i.e., the patient had experienced false labor) or regular, effective contractions that produce cervical change occur. Sedatives should not be used during active labor because they can cause respiratory depression in the neonate.

 legal alert—Assess and reassess during the intrapartal period

During the intrapartal period, it is important to assess the laboring patient and her fetus following each intervention to promote comfort. Specifically, nurses should:

- Assess for risk factors: bleeding, infection, ruptured membranes, fetal presentation, prolapsed cord, precipitous labor, meconium-stained amniotic fluid, postmaturity, prematurity, or fetal heart rate irregularities.
- Assess maternal vital signs per facility protocol.
- Assess the patient's anxiety level, coping mechanisms, and labor support.
- Assess the progress of labor.
- Assess the fetal heart rate, lie, and presentation.
- Assess the maternal and fetal response to each comfort measure.
- Carefully document all findings.

Barbiturates

Secobarbital sodium (Seconal) is the most commonly used barbiturate in labor. It is a fast-acting oral agent that produces mild sedation within 15 minutes after administration; its effects last for 3 to 4 hours. Undesirable effects include maternal and neonatal respiratory and vasomotor depression. These effects are intensified if a barbiturate is administered with another central nervous system (CNS) depressant. However, when given without an analgesic to a woman experiencing pain, the pain is increased. For these reasons, barbiturates are rarely used in labor (Cunningham, Leveno, Bloom, Spong, & Dashe, 2014).

Nursing Care Plan Patient Who Plans to Use Nonpharmacological Methods of Pain Relief During Labor

Ann is a 28-year-old gravida 2, para 1, who was admitted 45 minutes ago. Ann's cervix is 4 cm dilated and 100% effaced, the station is −2, and her membranes are intact. Uterine contractions occur every 3 minutes, last 45 to 50 seconds and are of moderate intensity. The fetal heart rate averages 140 to 145 beats per minute and demonstrates category 1 characteristics. Ann complains of low-back pressure and pain. She and her husband Raul have prepared a birth plan; they attended childbirth preparation classes and state they feel comfortable with using the methods learned.

Nursing Diagnosis: Coping, Readiness for Enhanced related to intention and preparation to meet the demands of childbirth

Measurable Short-Term Goal: Ann will demonstrate a relaxed facial and body posture during contractions.

Measurable Long-Term Goal: Ann will successfully use relaxation and breathing techniques learned in childbirth class throughout her labor.

NOC Outcomes:
Personal Well-Being (2002) Extent of positive perception of one's current health status
Coping (1302) Personal actions to manage stressors that tax an individual's resources

NIC Interventions:
Coping Enhancement (5230)
Support System Enhancement (5440)

Nursing Interventions:

1. Review the birth plan with Ann and Raul, answering any questions and providing additional information as needed. Inform other caregivers of the couple's plans for their labor and birth.

   RATIONALE: Appraisal of the couple's expectations allows the opportunity to provide factual information and offer support in an accepting environment.

2. Ensure a comforting environment: offer warmed blankets, an electric or handheld fan; adjust lighting and the room thermostat as needed.

   RATIONALE: A comfortable environment enhances relaxation and increases the patient's ability to focus on her coping skills.

3. Provide nonpharmacological pain relief methods as preferred by Ann; hydrotherapy; music of her choice; aromatherapy; ensure the focal point is within easy view; avoid conducting assessments and procedures during contractions; ensure that bed linens are soft, clean, and dry.

   RATIONALE: Hydrotherapy promotes relaxation and stimulates endorphin release and listening to favorite music may distract the patient from discomfort and external noises. Environmental distractions and unnecessary stimulants interfere with the successful use of learned techniques to manage labor discomfort.

4. Assist Raul in helping Ann to find a position of comfort; encourage position changes every 30 to 60 minutes, and unless contraindicated, encourage ambulation, sitting in a chair, or use of a birth ball.

   RATIONALE: Assistance empowers Raul to participate actively in the labor and birth experience. Position changes enhance maternal comfort by reducing muscle tension and facilitate fetal descent.

5. Encourage Raul to perform back rubs or provide counterpressure as learned in childbirth classes, according to Ann's desires.

   RATIONALE: Back rubs and counterpressure provide some relief from pain associated with back labor by interfering with the transmission of pain impulses to the brain.

6. Keep Ann and Raul informed of the progress of labor.

   RATIONALE: Ongoing information helps to decrease anxiety and fear, which increase the perception of pain and decrease pain tolerance; news of labor progress provides an incentive to continue with efforts to cope with labor.

Benzodiazepines

Benzodiazepines are agents primarily used to treat anxiety (e.g., diazepam [Valium] and lorazepam [Ativan]). Their mechanism of action is similar to that of barbiturates. When given with an opioid analgesic, benzodiazepines enhance pain relief and decrease nausea and vomiting, although some have an amnesic effect that may be unacceptable for women in labor (Lehne, 2012).

 clinical alert

Flumazenil to reverse the effects of benzodiazepine sedatives

Flumazenil (Romazicon) is an agent that reverses the effects of benzodiazepine sedatives. This intravenously administered medication should be readily available in any childbirth setting where benzodiazepines are used.

H₁-Receptor Antagonists

H₁-receptor antagonists are medications that block the action of histamines at the receptor sites. These medications produce sedative, anti-Parkinson, and antiemetic effects. They cause drowsiness and are often used during early labor to promote sleep and decrease anxiety. During labor, the H₁-receptor antagonists commonly used include promethazine (Phenergan), hydroxyzine (Vistaril), and diphenhydramine (Benadryl) (Gabbe, Niebyl, Galan, Jauniaux, Landon, Simpson, et al., 2012).

Promethazine (Phenergan), a phenothiazine, produces marked sedation and has strong antiemetic effects. It is frequently combined with opiates because it potentiates their effects. Phenothiazines readily cross the placenta and may produce decreased FHR beat-to-beat variability. They also bind to bilirubin binding sites in the neonate and may cause increased hyperbilirubinemia and jaundice in term infants who were exposed to the drug during the intrapartal period (Gabbe et al., 2012).

Hydroxyzine (Vistaril), a piperazine subtype, is used during early or prodromal labor to decrease nausea and anxiety. It also exerts a sedative effect. Often, women who receive this intramuscular medication awaken to increased contraction intensity that produces cervical changes (i.e., active labor).

Diphenhydramine (Benadryl) is a nonprescription medication with sedative and antiemetic properties that is given during early labor. Because the drug is readily available, nurses can advise women to use it at home although it may cause agitation in some patients. The half-life of diphenhydramine is 1 to 4 hours and its effects may last up to 8 hours.

 Nursing Insight—*Recognizing the anxiety–tissue anoxia–pain connection*

Pain can trigger the body's general stress response, called the "fight or flight" reaction. The release of epinephrine causes peripheral and uterine vasoconstriction, which results in tissue anoxia and increased pain. Decreasing the patient's anxiety through assistance with relaxation techniques or administration of antianxiety medications reduces vasoconstriction and helps to decrease pain.

 Now Can You—Discuss informed consent and the use of sedatives and antiemetics during labor?

1. State the three components of an informed consent that must be ensured before instituting pharmacological interventions for pain relief during labor?
2. Describe the indications for the use of sedatives and antiemetics during labor and identify two commonly prescribed H1-receptor antagonists?
3. Explain how diminishing maternal anxiety helps to relieve pain?

DIFFERENTIATING ANALGESIA FROM ANESTHESIA

To enhance understanding of the pharmacological methods of pain relief, it is important to distinguish between the concepts of analgesia and anesthesia. **Analgesia** is relief, to some degree, from pain. Pain may be entirely eliminated or only lessened. Analgesia may be accomplished via many methods, including medications, the application of heat or cold, massage, or electrical stimulation. **Anesthesia** is the partial or complete loss of sensation with or without the loss of consciousness. There are many types of analgesia and anesthesia and a number of methods for administering them. The analgesic or anesthetic selected is determined, to some degree, by the patient's stage of labor and by the method of birth anticipated (Boxes 13-1 and 13-2). When given too early, analgesia may prolong the labor and cause fetal depression. When administered too late, analgesia provides no benefit to the woman and may cause depression in the neonate.

The nurse's role involves continuous patient assessment to monitor the progress of labor and to identify cues that indicate that the patient would benefit from the administration of analgesic medications prescribed by the physician, certified nurse-midwife (CNM), or certified registered nurse-anesthetist (CRNA). Depending on institutional policy, the CNM or physician may evaluate the woman in

---

Box 13-1 Pharmacological Interventions for Intrapartal Pain Control According to Stage of Labor

FIRST STAGE OF LABOR
Systemic Analgesia
Opioid agonists (e.g., hydromorphone hydrochloride [Dilaudid]; meperidine hydrochloride [Demerol]; fentanyl citrate [Sublimaze]; sufentanil citrate [Sufenta])
    Opioid agonist–antagonists (e.g., butorphanol [Stadol]; nalbuphine [Nubain])

Nerve Block Analgesia
Epidural
Combined spinal–epidural

SECOND STAGE OF LABOR
Nerve Block Analgesia and Anesthesia
Local infiltration
Pudendal block
Spinal block
Epidural block
Combined spinal–epidural

Box 13-2 Pharmacological Interventions for Intrapartal Pain Control According to Birth Method

VAGINAL BIRTH
• Local infiltration anesthesia
• Pudendal block
• Epidural block analgesia/anesthesia
• Spinal block anesthesia
• Combined spinal–epidural analgesia/anesthesia

CESAREAN BIRTH
• Spinal block anesthesia
• Epidural block anesthesia
• General anesthesia

the birthing facility or rely on the nurse's assessment and instruct the nurse to administer the ordered medications. In most facilities, the CRNA monitors analgesia-related complications and conducts continuous monitoring for patients who receive epidural anesthesia. In some institutions, an anesthesiologist (physician who specializes in the administration of anesthesia) is available to provide these services.

SYSTEMIC ANALGESIA

Systemic analgesic agents provide central analgesia to the patient and fetus because they readily cross the placenta. Although this method of pain control during labor has declined, it is still used in facilities where specialists trained in administering regional analgesia (e.g., epidural analgesia) are not available. Fetal–neonatal effects include respiratory depression, decreased alertness, and delayed sucking, depending on the agent used, the dosage given, and the route and timing of administration. Intravenous administration is preferred over intramuscular injection because the onset of action is more rapid and predictable, pain relief is obtained with smaller doses of the drug, and the duration of the effect is more predictable (ACOG, 2002). The medication is administered into the intravenous tubing port nearest the patient while the IV solution is stopped.

 Optimizing Outcomes—When administering intravenous medications during labor

Intravenous analgesics are given slowly, in small doses during a contraction. When necessary, the medication may be given over a period of four to five consecutive contractions to complete the dose. Administering the medication during a contraction decreases fetal exposure to the drug because uterine blood vessels are constricted during contractions and the medication remains in the maternal vascular system for several seconds before the uterine blood vessels reopen.

In many institutions, patient-controlled analgesia (PCA) is available. The laboring woman self-administers small amounts of an opioid analgesic using a pump previously programmed for dose and frequency. As a result, a smaller amount of medication is required, and women are generally pleased with the level of pain control achieved. Analgesic agents available for the intrapartum period include opioid (narcotic) agonists and opioid (narcotic) agonist–antagonists (ACOG, 2002).

 Nursing Insight—*Differentiating between agonist agents and antagonist agents*

Analgesic medications used intrapartally include opioid agonists and opioid antagonists.

Agonist agents stimulate receptors to act. Antagonist agents block receptors or medications designed to activate receptors.

Opioid Agonist Analgesics

Opioid agonist analgesics include hydromorphone hydrochloride (Dilaudid), meperidine hydrochloride (Demerol), fentanyl citrate (Sublimaze), and sufentanil citrate (Sufenta) (Table 13-1). These agents work by stimulating the major opioid receptors mu and kappa. They promote feelings of euphoria and exert no amnesic effects. Because they delay gastric emptying time, nausea and vomiting are common side effects; bladder and bowel elimination may also be diminished. Ideally, opioid agonist analgesics should be given either less than 1 hour or greater than 4 hours before birth to minimize neonatal depression. Fentanyl citrate and sufentanil citrate require more frequent administration because of their relatively short duration of action (30 to 60 minutes, compared with 2 to 4 hours for hydromorphone hydrochloride and meperidine hydrochloride). Consequently, these agents are often administered intrathecally or epidurally, alone or in combination with a local anesthetic medication (Lehne, 2012).

Optimizing Outcomes—Safety measures for women who receive opioid analgesics

Opioid analgesics may cause bradycardia/tachycardia, hypotension, and respiratory depression and should be

Table 13-1 Opioid Agonist Analgesics		
Opioid–Agonist Analgesic	**Route and Dosage**	**Nursing Considerations**
Hydromorphone hydrochloride (Dilaudid)	IV: 1 mg q3h prn IM: 1–2 mg q3–6h prn	Monitor vital signs, FHR pattern and uterine activity prior to and during administration; observe for maternal respiratory depression; encourage voiding q2h, palpate for bladder distention; if birth occurs within 1–4 hours after administration, observe neonate for respiratory depression
Meperidine hydrochloride (Demerol)	IV: 25 mg q1–3h prn IM: 50–100 mg q1–3h prn	Common side effects include pruritus, dizziness, sedation, nausea, constipation
Fentanyl citrate (Sublimaze)	IV: 25–50 mcg IM: 50–100 mcg Epidural: 1–2 mcg with 0.125% bupivacaine at a rate of 8–10 mL/hr	Contraindications: Hypersensitivity to the drug, convulsive disorders
Sufentanil (Sufenta)	Epidural: 1 mcg with 0.125% bupivacaine at a rate of 10 mL/hr	

administered cautiously in women with respiratory or cardiovascular disorders (Lehne, 2012). Because patients may experience sedation and dizziness following administration, nurses should assist with ambulation and observe for adverse effects.

Opioid Agonist–Antagonist Analgesics

Opioid agonist–antagonist agents include butorphanol (Stadol) and nalbuphine (Nubain), which are agonists at kappa opioid receptors and either antagonists or weak agonists at mu opioid receptors. During labor, these medications provide satisfactory pain control; the incidence of respiratory depression is similar to that associated with morphine. They are also associated with less nausea and vomiting and are used more often during labor than the opioid agonist analgesics. They may be administered intravenously or intramuscularly; the parenteral route is preferred. Opioid agonist–antagonists should not be given to women with an opioid dependence because the antagonist activity may precipitate maternal/neonatal withdrawal symptoms. Symptoms of hypersensitivity, which include pruritus, urticaria, and/or burning sensation, may be treated with naloxone or diphenhydramine (Lehne, 2012; Vallerand & Sanoski, 2014).

Optimizing Outcomes—Special needs for opioid-dependent patients

During the intrapartum and postpartum periods, special considerations are needed for women who are opioid dependent to provide appropriate pain management, prevent relapse during postpartum and a risk of overdose, and ensure adequate contraception to prevent unintended pregnancy. Laboring women who are receiving opioid-assisted therapy (e.g., methadone and buprenorphine) should receive pain relief as if they were not taking opioids because the maintenance dosage does not provide adequate analgesia for labor. Epidural or spinal anesthesia should be offered as needed for pain during labor and birth. In general, patients undergoing opioid maintenance treatment will require higher doses of opioids to achieve analgesia than other patients. Narcotic agonist–antagonist drugs (e.g., butorphanol, nalbuphine, and pentazocine), which may precipitate acute withdrawal, should be avoided. Postpartal patients who are receiving opioid therapy should be closely monitored for symptoms of oversedation, and it is important to encourage them to continue in their treatment and addiction support (ACOG, 2012).

 Critical Nursing Action When Combining Butorphanol With Other CNS Depressants

Butorphanol is associated with respiratory depression in both the mother and fetus. When administering butorphanol with other CNS depressants (e.g., hypnotic agents, phenothiazines, sedatives, other tranquilizers, and general anesthetics), the nurse should closely monitor the patient's respiratory and cardiac status for signs of respiratory depression. Ongoing observation of the maternal level of consciousness, vital signs, and pulse oximetry as well as continuous electronic FHR monitoring is recommended. Naloxone (Narcan), the specific antagonist for this medication, should be readily available to reverse the drug effects if needed.

 Medication: Fentanyl (Sublimaze)

(**fen**-ta-nil)

Schedule II Pregnancy Category: C

Indications: Supplement to regional/local anesthesia; often administered epidurally or intrathecally to relieve moderate to severe labor pain and postoperative pain after cesarean birth.

Actions: Binds to opiate receptors in the CNS, alters the response to and perception of pain; produces CNS depression

Therapeutic Effects: Supplement to anesthesia; decreased pain

Contraindications and Precautions:
CONTRAINDICATED IN: Hypersensitivity; known intolerance; opioid dependency

Adverse Reactions and Side Effects: Bradycardia, hypotension, confusion, drowsiness, dizziness, rash, maternal and fetal/neonatal respiratory depression, nausea and vomiting, urinary retention

Route and Dosage: 50 to 100 mcg IM q2h; 25 to 50 mcg IV q2h; 1 to 2 mcg with 0.125% bupivacaine at a rate of 8 to 10 mL/hr epidurally

Nursing Implications: Assess for respiratory depression; naloxone should be readily available as antidote.

Source: Adapted from Vallerand, A. H., & Sanoski, C. A. (2014). *Davis's drug guide for nurses* (14th ed.). Philadelphia, PA: F.A. Davis.

 Medication: Butorphanol (Stadol)

(byoo-**tor**-fa-nole)

Schedule IV Pregnancy Category: C

Indications: Moderate to severe labor pain; postoperative pain after cesarean birth

Actions: Stimulates kappa opioid receptors and blocks or weakly stimulates mu opioid receptors; alters pain perception, produces generalized CNS depression

Therapeutic Effects: Decreased severity of pain

Contraindications and Precautions:
CONTRAINDICATED IN: Hypersensitivity; patients dependent on opioids (may precipitate withdrawal), women with chronic hypertension, preeclampsia

Adverse Reactions and Side Effects: Confusion, drowsiness, sedation, blurred vision, headache, dizziness, dysphoria, hallucinations, hypotension, hypertension, sweating, maternal palpitations/tachycardia or bradycardia, respiratory depression, transient nonpathological sinusoidal-like FHR rhythm, urinary retention and urgency

Route and Dosage: 2 mg (range 1–4 mg) IM every 3 to 4 hours as needed; 1 mg (range 0.5–2 mg) IV every 3 to 4 hours as needed

Nursing Implications: May precipitate withdrawal symptoms in woman/neonate. Protect medication from light and store at room temperature.

Source: Adapted from Vallerand, A. H., & Sanoski, C. A. (2014). *Davis's drug guide for nurses* (14th ed.). Philadelphia, PA: F.A. Davis.

Opioid Antagonists

Opioid antagonists, such as naloxone (Narcan), reverse the CNS depressant effects of opioids. Administered intravenously or intramuscularly, they are of benefit when labor progresses more rapidly than anticipated and birth is expected to occur when the opioid is at its peak effect. Placental transfer of naloxone is variable; the neonate may not require treatment with an opioid antagonist (Lehne, 2012).

Nursing Insight—*Nitrous oxide for labor analgesia*

Nitrous oxide (N_2O), a colorless, nearly odorless and tasteless gas made for inhalation, was first used in the United States for labor pain management from the 1930s until the 1970s, when regional anesthesia became a more popular analgesic modality. Today, self-administered nitrous oxide provided in a 50-50 blend of nitrous oxide and oxygen allows women to experience pain relief, decreased anxiety, and euphoria while remaining awake and alert, with complete motor and sensory function throughout its use. Maternal adverse effects include nausea and vomiting, restlessness, anxiety, and feelings of unpleasantness; in the neonate, N_2O is associated with neither central nervous system nor respiratory depression or altered Apgar scores. In 2010, the American College of Nurse-Midwives (ACNM) published a position statement on nitrous oxide that supports and encourages the promotion of additional labor and analgesic options to methods currently available. Presently, the reintroduction of nitrous oxide has been pursued in some facilities as a viable analgesic option during labor, birth, and the immediate postpartum period. However, a recent (2012) review by the Agency for Healthcare Research and Quality (AHRQ) concluded that, because of a paucity of literature on the aspects of use of nitrous oxide for labor analgesia, further research is needed (ACNM, 2010; Likis, Andrews, Collins, Lewis, Seroogy, Starr et al., 2012; Stewart & Collins, 2012).

 Now Can You—Discuss characteristics of systemic analgesia used during labor?

1. Explain how systemic analgesia should be administered during labor?
2. Identify three advantages and one major disadvantage associated with the use of opioid agonist agents during labor?
3. Explain specific precautions that should be taken when administering opioid agonist–antagonists to a woman in labor?

NERVE BLOCK ANALGESIA AND ANESTHESIA

Local anesthetics used in obstetrics may produce regional analgesia, which provides some degree of pain relief and motor block, and anesthesia, which provides complete pain relief and motor block. Regional analgesia may be obtained by the injection of a narcotic agent such as fentanyl along with a small amount of a local anesthetic agent. **Regional anesthesia,** a temporary and reversible loss of sensation, is produced by the injection of an anesthetic agent (a local anesthetic) into an area that brings the medication into direct contact with nervous tissue. Regional anesthetic agents block sodium and potassium transport in the nerve membrane, causing stabilization of the nerve(s) in a polarized resting state, which prevents the initiation and transmission of nerve impulses. Rarely, serious reactions (e.g., respiratory depression and hypotension) to local anesthesia may occur from one or more anesthetic agents. The nurse should ensure that emergency measures, including epinephrine, antihistamines, and oxygen, are readily available in all patient areas where these medications are used. When caring for patients receiving analgesia/anesthesia by catheter, nurses must be aware of institutional policy and national standards. The Association of Women's Health, Obstetric and Neonatal Nurses (AWHONN) has developed a clinical position statement (2012; available at awhonn.org) to guide safe practice.

 ### Nursing Insight—*Recognizing local anesthetic agents*

Because most local anesthetic agents are chemically related to cocaine, their names end with the suffix *-caine.* Examples of such medications include lidocaine, mepivacaine, bupivacaine, ropivacaine, and chloroprocaine.

The regional anesthetic blocks commonly used in obstetrics include epidural, spinal, or combined epidural–spinal. Epidural blocks may be administered for analgesia during labor and vaginal birth and for anesthesia during cesarean birth. Alternately, a combined epidural–spinal block may be used—the epidural provides analgesia for labor; the spinal provides anesthesia for birth or analgesia after the birth. During the first stage of labor, an epidural relieves pain by blocking the sensory nerves that supply the uterus. Pain experienced during the second stage of labor and with birth can be alleviated with epidural, combined epidural–spinal, and pudendal blocks. A summary of commonly used regional blocks is presented in Table 13-2.

Local Perineal Infiltration Anesthesia

Local perineal infiltration anesthesia is used to provide pain control when an episiotomy is to be performed or when suturing of lacerations is necessary in a patient who does not have regional anesthesia. Epinephrine, which causes vasoconstriction, may be added to the anesthetic agent to intensify the anesthesia effect and to minimize bleeding and prevent systemic absorption (Lehne, 2012).

 ### Nursing Insight—*Recognizing the value of natural pressure anesthesia*

Pressure anesthesia is the natural numbing effect caused by pressure of the fetal head against the woman's stretched perineum. For some, pressure anesthesia is adequate enough to allow an episiotomy to be performed without feeling the sensation of the actual surgical cut. Others require additional medication to help reduce the pain associated with childbirth.

Pudendal Nerve Block

A pudendal nerve block provides pain relief in the lower vagina, vulva, and perineum (Fig. 13-8). It should be administered 10 to 20 minutes before perineal anesthesia is needed and may be used late in the second stage of labor if an episiotomy is to be performed or if forceps or vacuum extraction will be used to facilitate birth. The anesthetic effect diminishes or completely removes the maternal bearing-down reflex. It may also be used during the third stage of labor for laceration repair (Cunningham et al., 2014; Hawkins & Bucklin, 2012).

Spinal Anesthesia Block

Spinal anesthesia block involves the injection of a solution containing a single local anesthetic or an anesthetic

Table 13-2 Commonly Used Regional Blocks for Labor and Birth

Type of Block; Areas Affected	When Used During Labor and Birth	Nursing Implications
Local Perineal Infiltration *Affected area:* Perineum	Immediately before birth for episiotomy; after birth for repair of lacerations.	Assess patient's knowledge and understanding; provide information as needed. Observe perineum for bruising, discoloration, hematoma, or signs of infection during the recovery period.
Pudendal Nerve Block *Affected areas:* Perineum and lower vagina	Late in the second stage for episiotomy, forceps, or vacuum extraction; during third stage for repair of episiotomy or lacerations.	Assess patient's level of knowledge and understanding; provide additional information as needed. Monitor for signs of infection, urinary retention.
Spinal Anesthesia Block *Affected areas:* Uterus, cervix, vagina, and perineum	First stage for both elective and emergent cesarean births; low spinal anesthesia block may be used for vaginal birth—not suitable for labor.	Assess patient's level of knowledge and understanding and level of pain relief; provide additional information as needed. Monitor maternal vital signs (hypotension most common complication) and FHR status. Assess for urinary retention, itching, nausea, vomiting, headache. Monitor site for leakage of spinal fluid or development of a hematoma.
Lumbar Epidural Block *Affected areas:* Uterus, cervix, vagina, and perineum	First and second stages.	Assess patient's level of knowledge and understanding and level of pain relief; provide additional information as needed. Monitor maternal blood pressure—major complication is hypotension—and FHR status. Provide ongoing support. Assess for urinary retention, itching, nausea, vomiting, headache.
Combined Spinal–Epidural *Affected areas:* Uterus, cervix, vagina, and perineum	Spinal analgesia may be administered during the latent phase for pain relief. Epidural is given when active labor begins.	Perform patient assessments as listed above for spinal and epidural anesthesia.

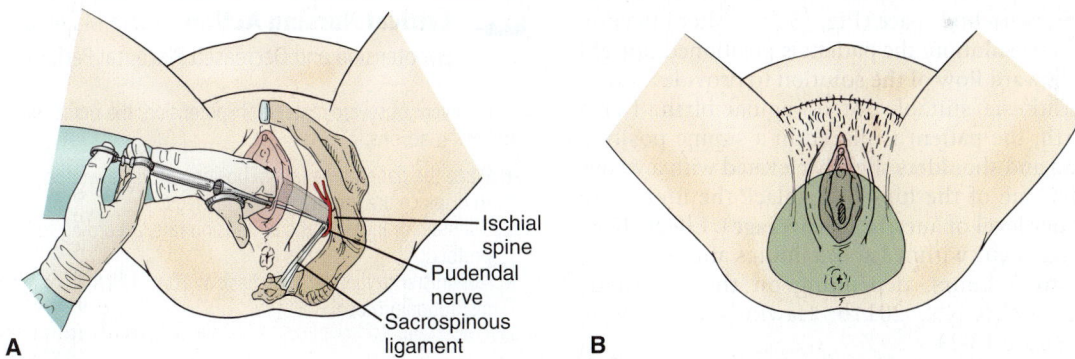

A   Ischial spine
 Pudendal nerve
 Sacrospinous ligament

B

Figure 13-8 *A,* Administration of a pudendal block. *B,* The areas of the perineum affected by a pudendal block.

combined with fentanyl through the third, fourth, or fifth lumbar interspace into the subarachnoid space, where it mixes with cerebrospinal fluid. The subarachnoid space is a fluid filled area located between the dura mater and the spinal cord. Used for elective or emergent cesarean births, the differences in the levels of spinal anesthesia for vaginal and cesarean birth are created by the dosage of the anesthetic agent administered and the position of the patient after placement of the medication in the dural sac. For vaginal birth, a low spinal anesthesia block provides anesthesia from level T10 (hips) to the feet; patients remain in a sitting position for a brief period of 1 to 2 minutes after administration to facilitate downward migration of the anesthetic solution toward the sacral area. For cesarean birth, the level of anesthesia coverage extends from the nipples (T6) to the feet; after administration of the anesthetic solution, patients are immediately assisted to a supine position with a left lateral tilt to enhance a cephalad spread of the anesthesia (and a higher level of sensory blockade). The anesthetic agent may be "weighted" with glucose to make it heavier than CSF. This prevents the medication from rising too high in the spinal canal and interfering with motor control of the uterus or with the maternal respiratory muscles (Fig. 13-9).

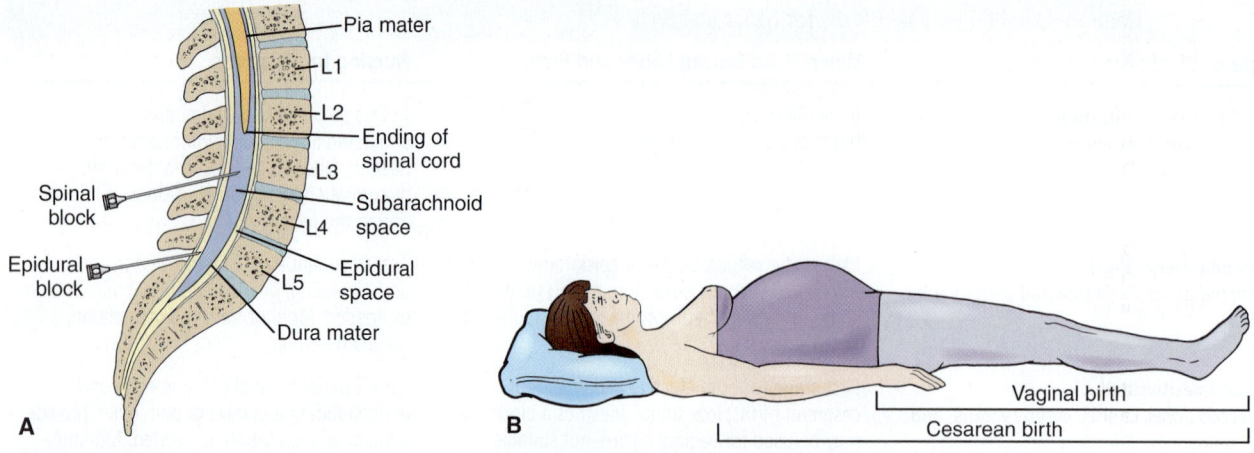

Figure 13-9 *A,* The spinal column: levels of the sacral, lumbar, and thoracic nerves. *B,* Levels of anesthesia necessary for vaginal and cesarean births.

Spinal anesthesia block has several advantages: It is easy to administer, has an immediate onset of anesthesia, requires a smaller volume of medication, produces excellent muscular relaxation, allows for maintenance of maternal consciousness, and is associated with minimal blood loss. However, because uterine contraction sensation is lost, the patient must be instructed when to bear down during a vaginal birth. Because voluntary maternal expulsive efforts are compromised, there is an increased likelihood of an operative (e.g., episiotomy, forceps-assisted, or vacuum-assisted) birth. After childbirth, there is an increased incidence of bladder and uterine atony and post–dural puncture headache.

Nursing care during administration of a spinal anesthesia block includes proper positioning of the patient in a lateral or sitting position with the back curved outward to widen the intervertebral space (Fig. 13-10). After injection of the anesthetic solution, the patient is positioned upright to allow downward flow of the solution to provide a lower level of anesthesia suitable for a vaginal birth. For a cesarean birth, the patient is placed in a supine position with the head and shoulders slightly elevated with a wedge placed under one of the hips to displace the uterus (to obtain a higher level of anesthesia coverage). Effects from the anesthesia occur within 1 to 2 minutes after injection and last 1 to 3 hours, depending on the anesthetic agent used (AWHONN, 2011b; Hawkins & Bucklin, 2012) (Procedure 13-1).

Complications that may occur with spinal anesthesia block include maternal hypotension, decreased placental perfusion, and an ineffective breathing pattern. Before administration, the patient's fluid balance is assessed, and intravenous fluids are administered to reduce the potential for sympathetic blockade (decreased cardiac output that results from vasodilation with pooling of blood in the lower extremities). After administration of the anesthetic, the patient's blood pressure, pulse, and respirations and FHR must be taken and documented every 5 to 10 minutes. If indicators of severe maternal hypotension (e.g., a drop in the baseline blood pressure of more than 20%) or fetal compromise (e.g., bradycardia, decreased variability, or late decelerations) develop, emergency measures must be instituted.

 Critical Nursing Action Severe Maternal Hypotension and Decreased Placental Perfusion

In the event of severe maternal hypotension, the nurse takes the following actions:

- Place the patient in a lateral position or use a wedge under the hip to displace the uterus; elevate the legs.
- Maintain or increase the IV infusion rate, according to institution protocol.
- Administer oxygen by face mask at 10 to 12 L/min or according to institution protocol.

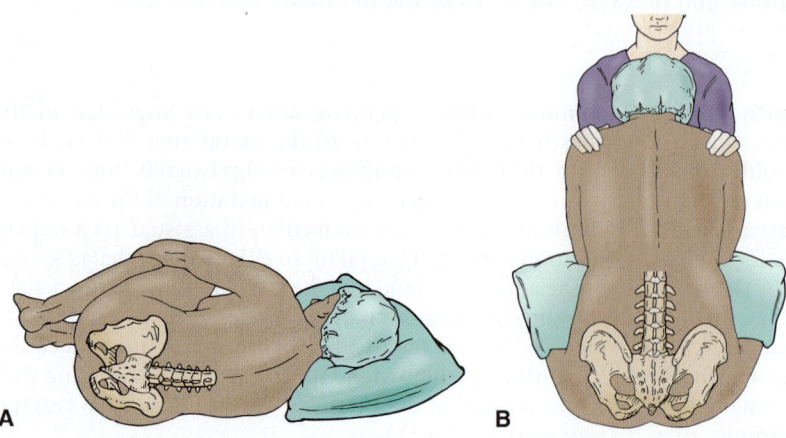

Figure 13-10 *A,* Lateral position for spinal and epidural blocks. *B,* Sitting position for spinal and epidural block.

Procedure 13-1 Assisting With the Administration of Spinal Anesthesia

Purpose

To facilitate administration of a spinal anesthesia block for the relief of pain during labor and birth.

Equipment

- Blood pressure cuff
- Stethoscope
- Fetal monitor

Steps

1. Wash and dry your hands. Explain the procedure and purpose of the examination to the patient.

   RATIONALE: *Hand washing helps to prevent the spread of microorganisms. Explanations help to decrease anxiety and promote patient's understanding and cooperation.*

2. Assist the patient to a sitting position on the edge of the bed or operating table (as directed by the nurse anesthetist or anesthesiologist).

3. Provide support, promote comfort, and limit motion during the procedure.

   RATIONALE: *Proper positioning (e.g., head bowed so that the back arches outward to widen the intervertebral space) and restricted movement are essential to successful anesthesia administration. Support prevents the patient from falling forward (she is "top heavy" from the gravid uterus).*

4. Check the intravenous infusion for patency.

   RATIONALE: *Hypotension from sympathetic blockage in the lower extremities may occur immediately after anesthesia administration. For this reason, IV fluids such as lactated Ringer's solution (500–1,000 mL) are usually given before the injection to ensure maternal hydration; confirming the patency of IV tubing ensures that the fluid is infusing well before the anesthesia is administered and facilitates the rapid infusion of fluids if needed for postadministration hypotension.*

5. Assist the patient to lie down on her back after anesthesia administration (as directed by the nurse anesthetist or anesthesiologist).

6. Place a pillow under her head and a wedge under her right hip.

   RATIONALE: *Remaining in an upright position for too long prevents the anesthetic from rising high enough up the spinal canal to achieve pain relief. Conversely, lying down too soon allows the anesthetic to rise too high in the spinal canal. Lying with a pillow under the head helps to ensure that the anesthesia will be confined to the lower spinal canal. A wedge placed under the right hip displaces the uterus and helps to prevent compression of the vena cava.*

7. Monitor the pulse, blood pressure, and respirations every 1 to 2 minutes for the first 10 minutes, then every 5 to 10 minutes. Use electronic monitoring to continuously monitor the FHR.

   RATIONALE: *Frequent assessment of maternal vital signs is essential for recognizing hypotension (from sympathetic blockage in the lower extremities) or an adverse reaction. Ongoing assessment of the fetal heart rate and pattern provides evidence of fetal well-being.*

8. Document the procedure on the patient's chart.

   RATIONALE: *Documentation provides a record for communication and evaluation of patient care.*

Nursing Consideration The nurse informs the nurse anesthetist or anesthesiologist when a contraction is beginning so that the anesthetic will not be administered during a contraction.

What If?

What if you detect a drop in the FHR while the anesthesiologist is administering the spinal anesthesia? You should take the following steps:

- Immediately alert the anesthesiologist
- Immediately alert the obstetrician or certified nurse midwife
- Assist the patient into a left side-lying position
- Administer oxygen at 10 L by face mask
- Increase the IV fluid rate
- Continuously monitor the FHR
- Provide information to the woman and her support person
- Prepare for birth

Documentation

8/30/13. 0425: Spinal anesthesia administered by J. Chen, CRNA. 1,000 mL lactated Ringer's solution infused IV prior to administration per protocol. Procedure tolerated well by patient. Vital signs: Preanesthesia administration, BP: 116/78 mm Hg, Pulse: 84 bpm, Respirations: 14 breaths/min, FHR: 146 bpm and regular; Postanesthesia administration, BP: 110/72 mm Hg, Pulse: 80 bpm, Respirations: 12 breaths/min, FHR: 148 bpm and regular.

—S. Rinaldi, RNC

- Alert the primary care provider, anesthesiologist, or nurse anesthetist.
- Administer an IV vasopressor (e.g., ephedrine 5–10 mg) according to institutional protocol, if the above measures are ineffective.
- Remain calm, offer reassurance, and continue to assess maternal blood pressure and FHR every 5 minutes until stable or per order from the primary care provider.

Post–dural puncture headache, a complication that may develop within 48 hours after the puncture, is believed to occur from leakage of cerebrospinal fluid (CSF) from the puncture site in the dura mater. Typically, the headache is intensified when the patient assumes an upright position and relieved when she assumes a supine position. Accompanying symptoms include auditory (tinnitus) and visual (blurred vision or photophobia) problems. Interventions usually center on oral analgesics, bedrest in a darkened room, caffeine, and hydration. If these measures are not effective, an autologous epidural blood patch may be administered. Approximately 10 to 20 mL of the patient's blood is slowly injected into the lumbar epidural space. A clot forms in the tear or hole in the dura mater around the spinal cord, effectively sealing the area from further CSF leakage (Fig. 13-11).

❝What to say❞—*Providing discharge instructions after autologous epidural blood patch*

Discharge planning after administration of an autologous epidural blood patch is an essential component of care. The nurse provides the following instructions:

- Maintain bedrest for 24 to 48 hours.
- Apply cold packs to the area as needed for pain relief.
- Increase oral fluids.
- Avoid the use of analgesics that affect platelet aggregation (e.g., nonsteroidal anti-inflammatory drugs) for 2 days.
- Observe for signs of infection at the site.
- Observe for signs of neurological complications (e.g., pain, numbness, tingling in the legs, and difficulty with ambulation).

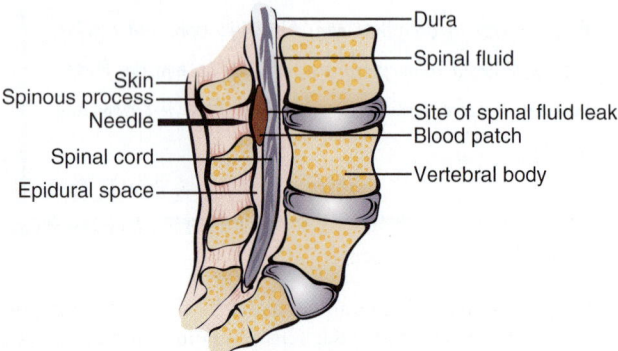

Figure 13-11 Autologous epidural blood patch.

 Now Can You—Discuss local infiltration, pudendal nerve block, and spinal block anesthesia?

1. Discuss the indications for and timing of administration for local infiltration anesthesia and a pudendal nerve block?
2. Name four advantages and two disadvantages associated with spinal block anesthesia?
3. Describe the immediate nursing actions to be taken for severe maternal hypotension with decreased placental perfusion?

Epidural Anesthesia or Analgesia Block

Injection of a local anesthetic such as bupivacaine, an opioid analgesic such as fentanyl or sufentanil, or both into the epidural space (between L4 and L5) provides pain relief from uterine contractions and vaginal or cesarean birth. The degree of analgesic or anesthetic effect obtained is related to the specific medication used. Combining an opioid with a local anesthetic agent reduces the total amount of anesthetic required and helps to preserve a greater amount of maternal motor function (Gabbe et al., 2012; Hawkins & Bucklin, 2012).

A & P review The Epidural Space

The nerves located in the spinal cord are covered and protected by several tissue layers. The pia mater is the membrane that adheres to the nerve fibers. It is surrounded by CSF. The next layer is the arachnoid membrane; the dura mater is the protective covering that lies outside this membrane. An anesthetic agent administered into the CSF in the subarachnoid space is called *spinal anesthesia*. The epidural space is a vacant space located outside the dura mater; beyond the epidural space, the ligamentum flavum, which extends from the base of the skull to the end of the sacral canal, provides another protective layer. With *epidural anesthesia*, an anesthetic agent is placed just inside the ligamentum flavum in the epidural space (Figs. 13-12 and 13-13). ◆

Nursing Insight—*Methods for administering an epidural block*

Epidural blocks, administered by a nurse anesthetist or anesthesiologist, may be given in different ways. For analgesia and anesthesia during labor, the block may be administered as a single dose with an epidural needle. It may also be administered as a single dose through an epidural catheter, with additional doses ("top-offs") given as needed, or given as a continuous epidural. Patients may be required to remain in bed; other blocks allow ambulation ("walking epidural").

LUMBAR EPIDURAL ANESTHESIA AND ANALGESIA BLOCK. The lumbar epidural anesthesia and analgesia block is the most commonly used method of pain control during labor; nearly two-thirds of women in the United States incorporate this intervention for discomfort and pain into their birth plan. Advantages of this method include maternal relaxation, enhanced comfort and pain relief, and an ability to remain alert and participate in the birth. Also, there is little blood loss, the respiratory reflexes remain intact, there is no delay

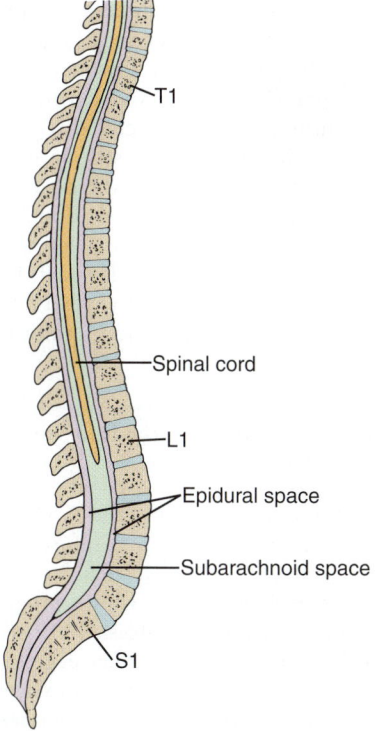

Figure 13-12 The epidural space is located between the dura mater and the ligamentum flavum.

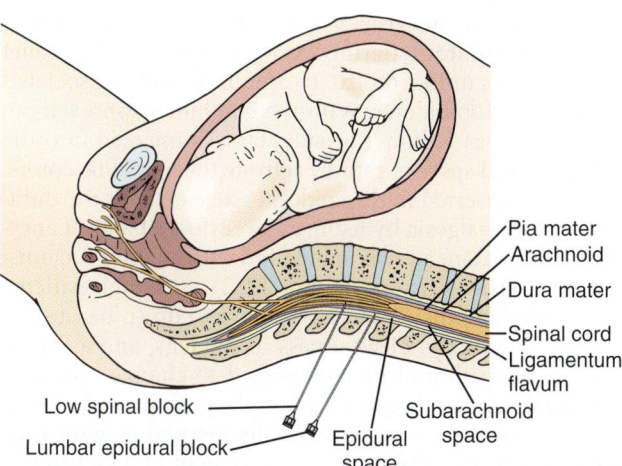

Figure 13-13 The spinal canal: injection sites for regional anesthesia.

in gastric emptying, and only a partial degree of motor paralysis occurs. Fetal complications are rare and are related to maternal hypotension or effects from the rapid absorption of the medication. Post–dural puncture headaches, caused by leakage of CSF, rarely occur because with epidural anesthesia, the CSF space is not entered (ACOG, 2002).

Optimizing Outcomes—**Emotional care for women with epidurals**

Although epidurals usually provide effective pain relief, laboring women may experience stress from other sources.

For example, during the second stage, unusual sensations such as difficulty breathing or extreme numbness may trigger acute anxiety or panic. After an epidural, the birth partner may become less attentive, and the labor nurse may offer less presence, leaving the woman with feelings of vulnerability and abandonment. Providing emotional care for all patients during labor constitutes an essential nursing action, and nurses are ideally positioned to provide it (AWHONN, 2011a, 2011b; Simkin et al., 2010).

Epidural blocks are advantageous for patients with diabetes, heart disease, pulmonary disease, and, in some cases, gestational hypertension because they essentially eliminate the pain associated with labor and thus reduce the maternal stress associated with labor discomfort. The patient's energy level is preserved because she does not feel the contractions. Epidural blocks may be used with preterm pregnancies because there is minimal effect on the fetus. A gentle, controlled birth is associated with minimal trauma to the immature fetal skull, and there are no systemic narcotic analgesics to cause depression in the premature neonate.

Maternal hypotension is the most common complication of epidural anesthesia. Preloading the patient with a rapid infusion of intravenous fluids, which increases the blood volume and cardiac output, can usually prevent this complication. Intravenous fluids are then infused continuously. Most institutions use dextrose-free solutions because dextrose can cause fetal hyperglycemia with rebound hypoglycemia during the first several hours after birth. The nurse should be in continuous attendance after administration of an epidural anesthetic. To detect hypotension, blood pressure should be continuously monitored for at least the first 20 minutes and after each new injection of the anesthetic. Blood pressure should be monitored during the entire time the anesthetic is in effect to ensure that the systolic pressure does not fall below 100 mm Hg or decrease 20 mm Hg in a hypertensive patient. A drop greater than this may be life-threatening to the fetus unless effective interventions (e.g., maternal position change or administration of antihypotensive agents) are instituted.

Other disadvantages include lengthened duration of labor and increased requirements for oxygen and oxytocin and limited mobility because of medical interventions such as the intravenous infusion and electronic monitoring equipment. Patients may experience orthostatic hypotension, dizziness, sedation, and lower extremity weakness. The accidental injection of a local anesthetic into a blood vessel can cause CNS effects including bizarre behavior, disorientation, excitation, and convulsions. Severe maternal hypotension resulting from sympathetic blockade can cause a significant decrease in uteroplacental perfusion and the delivery of oxygen to the fetus (ACOG, 2002; Anim-Somuah, Smyth, & Jones, 2011; Kukulu & Demirok, 2008).

Nursing Insight—*Shiver response after epidural block administration*

The patient may exhibit a shiver response after administration of epidural block anesthesia. This physiological reaction can result from heat loss related to increased peripheral blood flow. It may also be related to an alteration of thermal input to the

CNS when warm but not cold sensations have been suppressed. Essentially, the body believes that the temperature is lower than the true temperature and raises the "thermostat" to generate heat by shivering. The nurse should apply warm blankets for comfort and offer reassurance.

The nurse must perform frequent assessments of the maternal bladder to avoid bladder distention. Although the patient may be unable to void and require catheterization, the bedpan should always be offered initially to minimize the potential for a urinary tract infection. Nursing actions to facilitate voiding include assisting the patient to an upright position on the bedpan, raising the head of the bed to support the back, and providing privacy. Urinary retention and stress incontinence may also occur immediately postpartum. Intense pruritus is a common side effect of opioid use; this symptom is usually treated with diphenhydramine (Benadryl), 25 mg IV or 50 mg IM. A temporary elevation in temperature may occur after administration of epidural anesthesia (AWHONN, 2011b; DeSevo & Semeraro, 2010; Hawkins & Bucklin, 2012).

Optimizing Outcomes—During the second stage of labor after administration of an epidural block

The patient who has received an epidural block may require assistance with pushing because of an inability to feel the contractions or experience the urge to push. She may also need someone to hold or control her legs to push. After birth, the nurse must ensure that full sensation has returned and the patient is able to control her legs before ambulation is permitted. Depending on the agent used and the dose administered, this may take several hours.

For relief of labor pain and a vaginal birth, a block from T10 to S5 is performed, usually when the cervix has dilated to 5 to 6 cm. For a cesarean birth, a block from T8 to S1 is required. The patient is positioned on her side with her legs slightly flexed, or she is asked to sit on the edge of the bed.

 Where Research and Practice Meet:
Delaying Pushing After Epidural Administration

Previous research has suggested that nulliparous patients with epidurals, more than multiparas, are at increased risk of muscular fatigue related to increased lengths of labor and stronger pushing efforts during the second stage. Using a convenience sample of 77 nulliparous laboring women with epidural anesthesia, nurse researchers Gillesby and colleagues (2010) conducted a randomized clinical trial to determine if the use of delayed (i.e., 2 hours) pushing after the onset of the second stage of labor decreased the time of active pushing and decreased maternal fatigue. The investigators found that by delaying the onset of active pushing for 2 hours after the beginning of the second stage of labor, the time that nulliparous women with epidural anesthesia spent in active pushing was significantly decreased by 27%. Although the delayed pushing group rested for up to 2 hours, the total time in the second stage of labor averaged only 59 minutes longer than the immediate pushing group. No significant differences were found in fatigue scores between the immediate and delayed pushing groups. Based on their findings, the investigators recommended that increased emphasis be placed on the practice of delayed pushing during prenatal education.

She is instructed to drop her shoulders, round out the small of her back ("arch the back like a cat"), and put her chin into her chest. The medication is injected between contractions to minimize the risk of tachycardia that can occur if the drug is unintentionally injected directly into a vessel. The diffusion of the epidural anesthesia is dependent on the placement of the catheter tip, the dose and volume of medication used, and the patient's position (e.g., horizontal or upright). Once the epidural has been administered, a side-lying position (alternating sides each hour) is maintained to prevent compression of the vena cava. Depending on the degree of motor impairment, ambulation may be encouraged.

Nursing Insight—Methods for epidural anesthesia block

Most often, a continuous epidural anesthesia block, a method achieved by the use of a pump to infuse solution into an indwelling catheter, is used. In many areas, patients are allowed to control the dosing with a programmed pump (patient-controlled epidural analgesia [PCEA]). This method empowers the patient to achieve some degree of control over her labor comfort and has been shown to decrease the total amount of medication needed. A lock-out period after each self-administration prevents overdosage. Less commonly, an intermittent block that relies on repeated injections of anesthetic solution is performed.

COMBINED SPINAL–EPIDURAL ANALGESIA.   A combination of spinal–epidural analgesia may be used to block pain transmission without interfering with motor ability. Pain relief is immediate, unlike the 20- to 30-minute delay associated with an epidural alone. With the combined approach, an opioid such as fentanyl or sufentanil is injected into the subarachnoid space to rapidly activate the opioid receptors. A catheter inserted in the epidural space extends the duration of the analgesia by using a lower dose of a local anesthetic agent alone or in combination with an opioid agonist analgesic (Hawkins & Bucklin, 2012). Although patients may ambulate, they often choose not to do so because of fatigue, sensations of weakness in the legs, and a fear of falling. They should be encouraged to change positions frequently and assisted to an upright position to enhance bearing-down efforts. Because this method is associated with puncture of the dura and placement of a catheter in the epidural space, there is a greater risk for infection and post–dural puncture headache (ACOG, 2002; Hawkins & Bucklin, 2012). A combined spinal–epidural block may be used for both labor analgesia and for cesarean birth; the anesthetic and analgesic agents used vary according to the purpose of the procedure. Additional medication may be added to increase its effectiveness or if an instrument-assisted or cesarean birth is needed.

EPIDURAL AND INTRATHECAL OPIOIDS.   Another approach for nerve block analgesia/anesthesia involves the use of opioids alone. This method eliminates the effects of a local anesthetic. Advantages of epidural or intrathecal (injected into the subarachnoid space) opioids without local anesthetics include the following: There is no maternal hypotension or alteration in vital signs; the patient is aware of contractions but does not feel pain—thus she is able to bear down during the second stage of labor; and her motor power remains intact.

Opioids such as fentanyl, sufentanil (short-acting agents—effects last 1.5 to 4 hours) and preservative-free morphine (long-acting—effects last up to 7 hours) may be used. A drawback of this method concerns the potential need for a pudendal nerve block or local perineal infiltration anesthesia because intrathecal opioids do not provide adequate anesthesia for second-stage labor pain, episiotomy, or birth for most women (Cunningham et al., 2014). More often, epidural and intrathecal opioids are used for postoperative pain control. After cesarean birth, women are comfortable enough to freely ambulate and care for their newborns. Early ambulation is associated with enhanced bladder emptying, more rapid return of peristalsis, and a decreased risk of respiratory complications and thrombophlebitis. Side effects are more common when preservative-free morphine is used. These include nausea and vomiting, pruritus, urinary retention, and delayed respiratory depression.

 Optimizing Outcomes—**When epidural and intrathecal opioids are administered**

The nurse should monitor and record the patient's respiratory rate every hour for 24 hours (or per institutional protocol) after administration of epidural or intrathecal opioids. Naloxone (Narcan) should be administered if the maternal respiratory rate decreases to less than 10 breaths per minute or if the maternal oxygen saturation rate decreases to less than 89%. Oxygen may be administered by face mask and the anesthesiologist should be notified.

 Now Can You—**Discuss epidural and intrathecal anesthesia?**

1. Name six advantages of epidural anesthesia and identify the most common complication associated with this method?

 Where Research and Practice Meet: **A Systematic Review of Pain Management in Labor**

A recent (2012) systematic review was conducted to provide an overview of available evidence from previous reviews that address the efficacy and safety of various pharmacological and nonpharmacological methods of pain management for women during labor. Fifteen Cochrane reviews and 3 non-Cochrane reviews with a total of 310 trials were included. Effective methods of pain management in labor included epidural anesthesia, combined spinal–epidural anesthesia, and inhaled anesthesia, each of which was noted to have potential adverse effects. There was limited evidence to suggest that water immersion, relaxation, acupuncture, massage, local anesthetic nerve blocks, and non-opioid medications were beneficial in improving women's perception of labor pain, and these modalities were associated with fewer side effects. Relaxation and acupuncture were associated with fewer assisted vaginal births. There was insufficient evidence that hypnosis, biofeedback, sterile water injections, aromatherapy, transcutaneous electrical nerve stimulation, and parenteral opioids are more effective than placebo or other interventions in labor. The authors concluded that despite the limited data for efficacy, many of the nonpharmacological methods of labor pain management appear to be safe for mother and baby (Jones et al., 2012).

2. Describe the benefits of combined spinal–epidural anesthesia?
3. Identify an essential component of nursing assessment after the administration of epidural or intrathecal opioids?

GENERAL ANESTHESIA

General anesthesia (induced unconsciousness) may be used for unplanned, rapid (emergency) cesarean birth, when there are contraindications to an epidural or spinal block, or when surgical intervention is required for certain obstetric complications (Box 13-3). The major risks associated with general anesthesia administered for childbirth are increased maternal blood loss related to uterine relaxation, hypoxia, and the possible inhalation of vomitus during administration. Pregnant women are particularly prone to gastric reflux because of increased stomach pressure from the gravid uterus beneath it. In addition, the gastroesophageal valve may be displaced, allowing the upward passage of stomach contents. The aspiration of stomach contents that have an acid pH may cause chemical pneumonitis and secondary infection of the respiratory tract (Gaiser, 2012; Munnur & Suresh, 2012).

Fetal depression is directly related to the depth and duration of the anesthesia. Most general anesthetic agents reach the fetus in approximately 2 minutes. General anesthesia is not recommended when the fetus is considered to be high risk, especially in preterm birth. Measures to reduce respiratory depression in the neonate include reducing the time from induction of the anesthesia until the umbilical cord is clamped and using a minimum of sedating drugs and anesthetics until after the cord has been clamped.

To prepare the patient for general anesthesia, the nurse ensures that an IV infusion is in place, and if time permits, premedicates her with an oral antacid (e.g., sodium citrate, citric acid/sodium citrate, or effervescent aspirin/citric acid) to neutralize the acidic contents of the stomach. Some anesthesiologists order ranitidine hydrochloride (Zantac) IV or cimetidine (Tagamet) to decrease the production of stomach acid; metoclopramide (Reglan) may also be prescribed to increase gastric emptying (Gaiser, 2012; Hawkins & Bucklin, 2012). Before administration of the anesthesia, a wedge is placed under the right hip to displace the uterus (to prevent aortocaval compression and decreased placental perfusion). When possible, the patient is preoxygenated with 3 to 5 minutes of 100% oxygen.

Thiopental sodium (Pentothal), an ultra-short-acting barbiturate, is usually given. This agent causes rapid induction

---

Box 13-3 **Contraindications to Spinal/Epidural Block Anesthesia**

- Maternal refusal
- Local or systemic infection
- Coagulation disorders
- Actual or anticipated maternal hemorrhage
- Allergy to specific anesthetic agents
- Lack of trained staff available (Cunningham et al., 2014)

of anesthesia and minimal postpartal bleeding. Succinyl choline (Anectine) is a muscle relaxant used to facilitate passage of the endotracheal tube. To prevent gastric reflux and aspiration before the woman fully loses consciousness, the nurse may be asked to assist with applying cricoid pressure. This maneuver seals off the esophagus by compressing it between the cricoid cartilage and the cervical vertebrae. The cricoid ring, which is the only tracheal cartilage that forms a complete ring, is located immediately above the thyroid isthmus. The cricoid cartilage is depressed 2 to 3 cm posteriorly, and pressure is maintained until the cuffed endotracheal tube is securely in place (Fig. 13-14). While applying pressure, the nurse should use the other hand to support the patient's neck.

After intubation, a 50:50 mixture of oxygen and nitrous oxide is usually administered. Small amounts of a halogenated agent such as isoflurane or methoxyflurane may also be given to enhance pain relief and to reduce maternal awareness and recall (Hawkins & Bucklin, 2012). The halogenated agents produce rapid uterine relaxation to facilitate intrauterine manipulation and extraction. However, at high concentrations they readily cross the placenta and can produce fetal narcosis and an increased risk for postpartal maternal hemorrhage because of uterine relaxation.

Recovery room care is focused on maintenance of an open airway, continuous monitoring of cardiopulmonary function, and the prevention of postpartum hemorrhage. Postpartal care should be arranged to facilitate parent–infant bonding as soon as possible. The nurse offers emotional support, answers questions concerning the birth, provides updates regarding maternal/neonatal status, and assesses the patient's readiness to interact with her newborn.

Now Can You—Discuss implications of general anesthesia used during childbirth?

1. Identify two major risks associated with the use of general anesthesia for childbirth?
2. Demonstrate how to apply cricoid pressure and explain the importance of this intervention?
3. Describe two major nursing responsibilities for recovery room patient care following the use of general anesthesia?

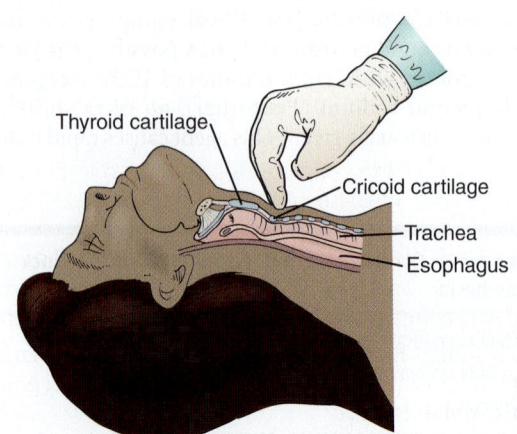

Thyroid cartilage

Cricoid cartilage

Trachea

Esophagus

Figure 13-14 Correct position for applying cricoid pressure until endotracheal tube placement has been completed.

Nursing Care for the Patient Receiving Interventions to Promote Comfort During Labor and Birth

The patient's methods of pain relief are influenced by several factors: her wishes and desires, the phase and stage of labor, the availability of the chosen modalities in the birth center, and the knowledge and expertise of the health-care team with the various pharmacological and nonpharmacological methods.

NURSING ASSESSMENT AND DIAGNOSES

Assessment during labor is an ongoing process that requires a collaborative approach from the primary care provider, the nurse, the patient, and her labor support person(s). Factors such as maternal–fetal status, the progress of labor, and the patient's level of comfort must be taken into consideration before a decision is made concerning whether nonpharmacological methods, pharmacological methods, or a combined approach will be used. The nurse never assumes that all pain experienced during labor is uterine in origin. Instead, a physical assessment that includes an evaluation of the characteristics of the patient's pain (location, intensity, quality, frequency, duration, and effectiveness of all relief measures) must be performed. The patient's prenatal record is reviewed to identify pertinent obstetric information; drug allergies; a history of tobacco, alcohol, or other substance abuse; and spinal or neurological disorders.

The patient interview focuses on information concerning the onset of labor: the most recent oral intake (time and amount), present illnesses, allergies, and events that have occurred since her last visit with her primary care provider. She is asked about attendance in childbirth education classes and preferences for intrapartum comfort measures. When available, the birth plan is reviewed and updated or modified as needed.

The physical examination includes assessment of maternal vital signs, fetal heart rate and pattern, uterine contractions, amniotic membranes and fluid, cervical effacement and dilation, and fetal descent. The nurse also evaluates the patient's hydration status and palpates for bladder distention. After the administration of pharmacological agents, the nurse provides ongoing assessment of the patient, fetus, and labor progress according to institutional policy and professional standards (Association of Women's Health, Obstetric and Neonatal Nurses [AWHONN], 2012). Maternal assessment for evidence of allergic reaction to medications includes monitoring vital signs, respiratory status, platelet, and white blood cell count and observing for integumentary changes. Laboratory data are analyzed to identify anemia, coagulopathy or bleeding disorders, or infection. Fetal status is also assessed and non-reassuring changes in heart rate or pattern are promptly reported to the patient's primary health-care provider.

A number of nursing diagnoses are relevant to anxiety, discomfort, and pain relief during labor and birth:

- Anxiety related to lack of knowledge about the labor experience
- Ineffective coping related to the combination of uterine contractions and anxiety
- Acute pain related to the processes of labor and birth

Expected outcomes of nursing interventions include:

- The patient verbalizes understanding of what is happening with her labor; she is able to identify the beginning and ending of contractions and demonstrates confidence instead of confusion with the labor process.
- The patient verbalizes confidence in her ability to participate actively in her labor experience; she demonstrates effective breathing techniques, guides her labor support person in providing effective comfort measures, readily engages in position changes and other strategies to enhance comfort and remain in control, and expresses confidence in her labor nurse and other care providers.
- The patient verbalizes that with the methods used, her pain has been relieved to a tolerable level; she is responsive to questions and suggestions and demonstrates an ability to deal with her contractions

A plan of care individualized to each patient is developed and modified as needed. A collaborative approach that includes the patient, her primary care provider, and labor support person is important in ensuring that safe, effective care is provided that promotes a positive childbirth experience for the woman and her family.

Summary Points

- Pain during labor is unique in that it is normal, can be anticipated and prepared for, and ends with a birth.
- Although a universal phenomenon, every individual perceives pain differently.
- The better prepared a woman is for childbirth, the less likely is the need for analgesia and anesthesia.
- Relaxation, massage, breathing techniques, and other nonpharmacological strategies should be encouraged in conjunction with prescribed analgesics.
- The type of analgesic or anesthetic to be used depends, in part, on the stage of labor and the method of birth.
- Sedatives are used during a prolonged early labor when there is a need to decrease anxiety or promote rest.
- Regional anesthesia can be extremely effective for pain; the nurse must ensure adequate maternal hydration and normal blood pressure before administration.
- General anesthesia is rarely used for vaginal birth because of risks for both the woman and her neonate.

Review Questions

Multiple Choice

1. In the first stage of labor, the perinatal nurse is aware that pain impulses are transmitted via which route?
   A. T11, T12 spinal nerve segments
   B. T9, T10 spinal nerve segments
   C. L4, L5 spinal nerve segments
   D. Sacral spinal nerve segments

2. The perinatal nurse is aware that a woman's history of past painful experiences with labor and birth are part of which neural pathway process for pain?
   A. Transduction
   B. Transmission

C. Perception
D. Modulation

3. A laboring woman was given promethazine (Phenergan) and meperidine hydrochloride (Demerol) for pain. The nurse is aware that during the first 24 hours of life, the newborn will have an increased risk for which of the following problems?
   A. Hyperbilirubinemia
   B. Tachypnea
   C. Irritability
   D. Tremors

4. A nurse is studying therapeutic touch and is explaining it to family and friends. What description is most accurate?
   A. It is a gentle stroking massage of the patient's abdomen.
   B. It redirects the patient's energy fields to diminish pain.
   C. It uses a focal point on which the laboring woman can concentrate.
   D. It is well documented as a tool to diminish pain during labor.

5. What information about aromatherapy for labor discomfort should the nurse provide the patient?
   A. Full strength oils on the skin are most effective.
   B. Aromatherapy does not offer any benefits.
   C. Not all aromatherapy oils are safe to use in pregnancy
   D. Oils are only placed on the pillowcase, never the skin.

6. The nurse is applying a hot pack to a laboring woman's perineum. The student nurse asks about the purpose of this intervention. What explanation by the nurse is best?
   A. Relieves muscle spasms
   B. Helps regulate temperature
   C. Prevents tissue trauma
   D. Relieves muscle ischemia

7. A nursing faculty member is explaining the women's health goals of *Healthy People 2020* to a class of nursing students. Which of the following is a goal in this document?
   A. Reduce the mortality rate to no more than 11/100,000 live births
   B. Increase the percentage of women using pharmacological pain control
   C. Decrease the numbers of community-based childbirth education classes
   D. Increase the number of women referred to a tertiary health-care center

8. A woman in labor complains of back pain and a headache. What action by the nurse is best?
   A. Call for an epidural or spinal analgesic/anesthesia
   B. Perform a complete pain assessment on the woman
   C. Document the findings and reassure the woman
   D. Ask the support person to provide massage therapy

9. A woman near term expresses fears of not being able to tolerate the pain of childbirth. What response by the nurse is best?
   A. "Remember that pain in childbirth is normal and expected."
   B. "Choose your support person carefully so he or she can really help you."

C. "Be sure to get plenty of sleep in the weeks leading up to the birth."

D. "I wouldn't worry too much; most women end up doing just fine."

10. What instruction by the nurse will help give the woman a sense of control over her childbirth experience?

A. Tour different birthing facilities

B. Only use a certified nurse midwife

C. Request an elective cesarean birth

D. Ask your friends how they handled their birth experiences

See Answers to End of Chapter Review Questions on Davis*Plus*.

REFERENCES

American College of Nurse-Midwives. (2010). Nitrous oxide for labor analgesia. *Journal of Midwifery & Women's Health, 55*(3), 292–296. doi:10.1016/j.jmwh.2010.03.003

American College of Obstetricians and Gynecologists (ACOG). (2002). Obstetric analgesia and anesthesia. Practice Bulletin No. 36. (Reaffirmed 2013). *Obstetrics & Gynecology, 100*(7), 177–191.

American College of Obstetricians and Gynecologists (ACOG). (2006). Analgesia and cesarean delivery rates. Committee Opinion No. 339. (Reaffirmed 2013). *Obstetrics & Gynecology, 107*(6), 1487–1488.

American College of Obstetricians and Gynecologists (ACOG). (2012). Opioid abuse, dependence, and addiction in pregnancy. Committee Opinion No. 524. *Obstetrics & Gynecology, 119*(5), 1070–1076.

Anderson, C. J., & Kilpatrick, C. (2012). Supporting patients' birth plans: Theories, strategies & implications for nurses. *Nursing for Women's Health, 16*(3), 212–218. doi:10.1111/j.1751-486X.2012.01732.x

Anim-Somuah, M., Smyth, R., & Jones, L. (2011). Epidural versus non-epidural or no analgesia in labor. *Cochrane Database of Systematic Reviews 2011,* Issue 12. Art. No.: CD000331. doi:10.1002/14651858 .CD000331.pub3

Association of Women's Health, Obstetric, and Neonatal Nurses (AWHONN). (2011a). Clinical Position Statement: Nursing support of laboring women. *Journal of Obstetric, Gynecologic, & Neonatal Nursing, 40*(11), 665–666. doi:10.1111/j.1552-6909.2011.01288.x

Association of Women's Health, Obstetric, and Neonatal Nurses (AWHONN). (2011b). *Nursing care of the woman receiving regional analgesia/anesthesia* (2nd ed.). Washington, DC: Author.

Association of Women's Health, Obstetric, and Neonatal Nurses (AWHONN). (2012). Clinical Position Statement: Role of the registered nurse (RN) in the care of the pregnant woman receiving analgesia and anesthesia by catheter techniques. *Journal of Obstetric, Gynecologic & Neonatal Nursing, 41*(3), 455–457. doi:10.1111/j.1552-6909 .2012.01364.x

Bedwell, C., Dowswell, T., Neilson, J. P., & Lavender, T. (2011). The use of transcutaneous electrical nerve stimulation (TENS) for pain relief in labour: A review of the evidence. *Midwifery, 27*(5), 141–148. doi:10.1016/j.midw.2009.12.004

Bulechek, G. M., Butcher, H. K., & Dochterman, J. M., & Wagner, C. (2013). *Nursing interventions classification (NIC)* (6th ed.). St. Louis, MO: Elsevier Mosby.

Cho, S. H., Lee, H., & Ernst, E. (2010). Acupuncture for pain relief in labour: A systematic review and meta-analysis. *British Journal of Obstetrics & Gynaecology, 117*(8), 907–920.

Cluett, E. R., & Burns, E. (2009). Immersion in water in labour and birth. *Cochrane Database of Systematic Reviews 2009,* Issue 2. Art. No.: CD000111. doi:10.1002/14651858.CD000111.pub3

Cunningham, F. G., Leveno, K. J., Bloom, S. L., Spong, C., & Dashe, J. (2014). *Williams Obstetrics* (24th ed.). New York, NY: McGraw-Hill Professional.

De Sevo, M. R., & Semeraro, P. (2010). Urinary catheterization during epidural anesthesia. *Nursing for Women's Health, 14*(1), 11–13. doi:10.1111/j.1751-486X.2010.01502.x

Evans-Lynn, C. J. (2012). Labor limits: Does restricting movement result in higher cesarean section rates? *Advance for NPs & PAs, 3*(10), 29–31.

Felton, M. B. (2011). Normal childbirth. In S. Mattson & J. E. Smith (Eds.), *Core curriculum for maternal-newborn nursing* (4th ed., pp. 225–247). Philadelphia, PA: W.B. Saunders.

Gabbe, S., Niebyl, J., Galan, H., Jauniaux, E., Landon, M., Simpson, J., & Driscoll, D. (2012). *Obstetrics: Normal and problem pregnancies* (6th ed.). Philadelphia, PA: W.B. Saunders.

Gaiser, R. (2012). Anesthesia for cesarean delivery. In B. A. Bucklin, D. R. Gambling, & D. Wlody (Eds.). *A practical approach to obstetric anesthesia* (pp. 185–208). Philadelphia, PA: Lippincott Williams & Wilkins.

Gillesby, E., Burns, S., Dempsey, A., Kirby, S., Mogensen, K., Naylor, K., et al. (2010). Comparison of delayed versus immediate pushing during second stage of labor for nulliparous women with epidural anesthesia. *Journal of Obstetric, Gynecologic & Neonatal Nursing, 39*(6), 635–644. doi:10.1111/j.1552-6909.2010.01195.x

Hawkins, J. L., & Bucklin, B. A. (2012). Obstetric analgesia and anesthesia. In S. G. Gabbe, J. R. Niebyl, H. L. Galan, E. R. Jauniaux, M. B. Landon, J. L. Simpson, & D. A. Driscoll, *Obstetrics: Normal and problem pregnancies* (6th ed., pp. 362–387). Philadelphia, PA: Saunders.

Hodnett, E. (2002). Pain and women's satisfaction with the experience of childbirth: A systematic review. *American Journal of Obstetrics and Gynecology, 186*(5), S160–S172.

Hodnett, E. D., Gates, S., Hofmeyr, G. J., Sakala, C., & Weston, J. (2011). Continuous support for women during childbirth. *The Cochrane Database of Systematic Reviews,* 2011 Feb 16(2): CD003766. doi:10 .1002/14651858.CD003766.pub3

Hover-Kramer, D. (2011). *Healing touch: Essential energy for yourself and others.* Louisville, CO: Sounds True, Inc.

Jones, L., Othman, M., Dowswell, T., Alfirevic, Z., Gates, S., Newburn, M., et al. (2012). Pain management for women in labour: An overview of systematic reviews. *Cochrane Database of Systematic Reviews 2012,* Issue 3. Art. No.: CD009234. doi:10.1002/14651858. CD009234.pub2

Keskin, E. A., Onur, O., Keskin, H. L., Gumus, I. L., Kafali, H., & Turhan, N. (2012). Transcutaneous electrical nerve stimulation improves low back pain during pregnancy. *Gynecologic and Obstetric Investigation, 74*(1), 76–83. doi:10.1159/000337720

Krieger, D. (1979). *The therapeutic touch.* New York, NY: Touchstone.

Kukulu, K., & Demirok, H. (2008). Effects of epidural analgesia on labor progress. *Pain Management Nursing, 9*(1), 10–16.

Labor, S., & Maguire, S. (2008). The pain of labour. *British Journal of Pain, 2*(2), 15–19. doi:10.1177/204946370800200205

Landolt, A. S., & Milling, L. S. (2011). The efficacy of hypnosis as an intervention for labor and delivery pain: A comprehensive methodological review. *Clinical Psychology Review, 31*(6), 1022–1031.

Lehne, R. (2012). *Pharmacology for nursing care* (8th ed.). Philadelphia, PA: Saunders.

Likis, F. E., Andrews, J. A., Collins, M. R., Lewis, R. M., Seroogy, J. J., Starr, S. A., et al. (2012). *Nitrous oxide for the management of labor pain. Comparative effectiveness review No. 67.* Rockville, MD: Agency for Healthcare Research and Quality.

Lothian, J., & DeVries, C. (2010). *The official Lamaze guide: Giving birth with confidence* (4th ed.). Minnetonka, MN: Meadowbrook Press.

Lowe, N. (2002). The nature of labor pain. *American Journal of Obstetrics and Gynecology, 186*(5), S16–S24.

Lowe, N. (2004). Context and process of informed consent for pharmacologic strategies in labor pain care. *Journal of Midwifery & Women's Health, 49*(3), 250–259.

Malshe, A., & Wiczyk, H. (2011). Acupuncture stimulation and obstetrics: "To stick or not to stick?—That is the question." *The Female Patient, 36*(2), 16–19.

March of Dimes. (2012). Natural relief for labor pain. Retrieved from http://www.marchofdimes.com/pregnancy/vaginalbirth_naturalrelief .html

Meleis, A. (2003). Theoretical considerations of health care for immigrant and minority women. In St. Hill, P., Lipson, J. G., & Meleis, A. I. (Eds.), *Caring for women cross-culturally* (pp. 1–10). Philadelphia, PA: F.A. Davis.

Melzack, R., & Wall, P. (1965). Pain mechanisms: A new theory. *Science, 150*(2), 971–982.

Munnur, U., & Surresh, M. S. (2012). Difficult airway management in the pregnant patient. In B. A. Bucklin, D. R. Gambling, & D. Wlody (Eds.). *A practical approach to obstetric anesthesia* (pp. 209–222). Philadelphia, PA: Lippincott Williams & Wilkins.

Nilsson, C., Bondas, T., & Lundgren, I. (2010). Previous birth experience in women with intense fear of childbirth. *Journal of Obstetric, Gynecologic & Neonatal Nursing, 39*(3), 298–309. doi:10.1111/j.1552-6909.2010.01139.x

Padfield, D., Hurwitz, B., & Pither, C. (2003). *Perceptions of pain.* Stockport, England: Dewi Lewis Publishing.

Perez, P. (2000). *Birthballs: The use of physical therapy balls in maternity care.* Johnson, VT: Cutting Edge Press.

Perinatal Education Associates. (2012). *Breathing*. Retrieved from http://www.birthsource.com/scripts/article.asp?articleid=211

Purnell, L. D. (2014). *Guide to culturally competent health care* (3rd ed.). Philadelphia, PA: F.A. Davis.

Simkin, P., Bolding, A., Keppler, A., Durham, J., & Whalley, J. (2010). *Pregnancy, childbirth, and the newborn* (4th ed.). Minnetonka, MN: Meadowbrook Press.

Smith, C., Collins, C., & Crowther, C. (2011). Aromatherapy for pain management in labour. *Cochrane Database of Systematic Reviews 2011*, Issue 7. Art. No. doi:10.1002/14651858.CD009215

Smith, C., Collins, C., Crowther, C., & Levett, K. (2011). Acupuncture or acupressure for pain management in labour. *Cochrane Database of Systematic Reviews 2011*, Issue 7. Art. No.: CD009232. doi:10.1002/14651858.CD009232

Smith, C., Levett, K., Collins, C., & Crowther, C. (2011). Relaxation techniques for pain management in labour. *Cochrane Database of Systematic Reviews 2011*, Issue 12. Art. No.: CD009514. doi:10.1002/14651858.CD009514

Smith, C., Levett, K., Collins, C., & Jones, L. (2012). Massage, reflexology and other manual methods for pain management in labor. *Cochrane Database of Systematic Reviews 2012*, Issue 2. Art. No.: CD009290. doi:10.1002/14651858.CD009290.pub2

Stark, M. A., & Miller, M. G. (2009). Barriers to the use of hydrotherapy in labor. *Journal of Obstetric, Gynecologic & Neonatal Nursing, 38*(6), 667–675. doi:10.1111/j.1552-6909.2009.01065.x

Stark, M. A., & Miller, M. G. (2010). Development and testing of nurses' perceptions of the use of hydrotherapy in labor questionnaire. *Journal of Nursing Measurement, 18*(1), 36–48.

Stewart, L. S., & Collins, M. (2012). Nitrous oxide as labor analgesia: Clinical implications for nurses. *Nursing for Women's Health, 16*(5), 400–409. doi:10.1111/j.1751-486X2012.01763.x

Taavoni, S., Abdolahian, S., Haghani, H., & Neysani, L. (2011). Effect of birth ball usage on pain in the active phase of labor: A randomized controlled trial. *Journal of Midwifery and Women's Health, 56*(2), 137–140. doi:10.1111/j.1542-2011.2010.00013.x

Tuschhoff, K. (2014). Hypnosis for childbirth: What is it and does it work? Retrieved from http://www.pregnancy.org/article/hypnosis-childbirth-what-it-and-does-it-work

U.S. Department of Health and Human Services (USDHHS). (2012). *Healthy People 2020*. Retrieved from http://www.healthypeople.gov/2020/topicsobjectives2020/default

Vallerand, A. H., & Sanoski, C. A. (2014). *Davis's drug guide for nurses* (14th ed.). Philadelphia, PA: F.A. Davis.

VandeVusse, L., Hanson, L., Berner, M., & Winters, J. (2010). Impact of self-hypnosis in women on select physiologic and psychological parameters. *Journal of Obstetric, Gynecologic & Neonatal Nursing, 39*(2), 159–168. doi:10.1111/j.1552-6909.2010.01103.x

Venes, D. (Ed.). (2013). *Taber's cyclopedic medical dictionary* (22nd ed.). Philadelphia, PA: F.A. Davis.

Weiss, R. E. (2014). Aromatherapy: Pregnancy & birth. Retrieved from http://pregnancy.about.com/cs/laborbirth/a/aa042098.htm

Wong, C. A. (2010). Advances in labor analgesia. *International Journal of Women's Health, 1*(4), 139–154.

Youness, E. M., & Moustafa, M. F. (2012). Nurses' knowledge about using hydrotherapy as a non-pharmacological pain relief method in labor and its barriers to use. *Medical Journal of Cairo University, 80*(2), 151–160.

Zauderer, C. (2009). Maternity care for Orthodox Jewish couples. *Nursing for Women's Health, 13*(2), 110–120. doi:10.1111/j.1751-486X.2009.01402.x

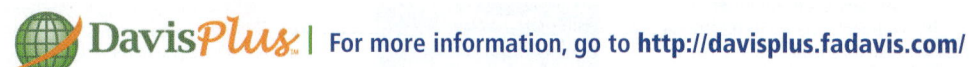

DavisPlus | For more information, go to **http://davisplus.fadavis.com/**

CONCEPT MAP

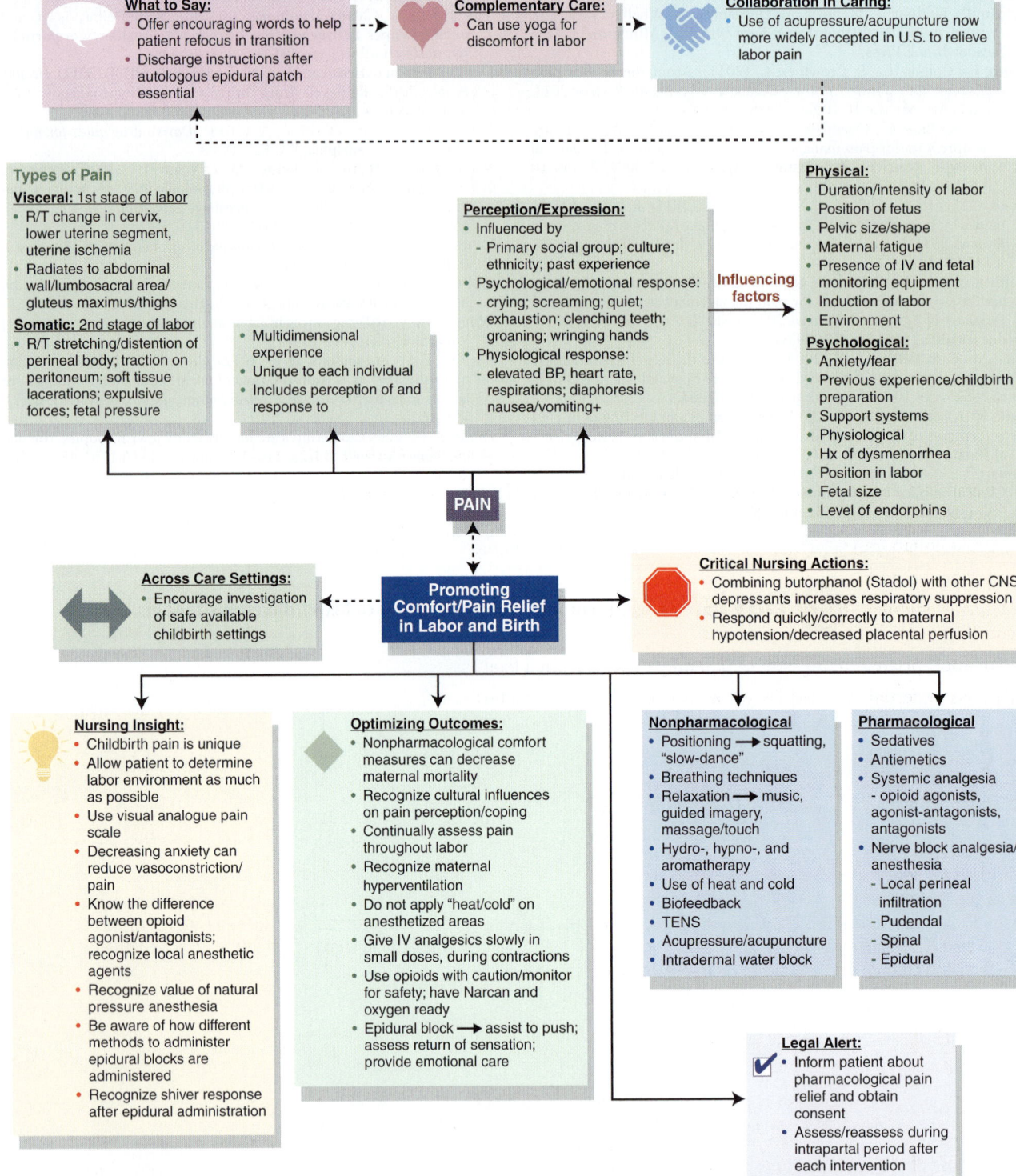

What to Say:
- Offer encouraging words to help patient refocus in transition
- Discharge instructions after autologous epidural patch essential

Complementary Care:
- Can use yoga for discomfort in labor

Collaboration in Caring:
- Use of acupressure/acupuncture now more widely accepted in U.S. to relieve labor pain

Types of Pain
Visceral: 1st stage of labor
- R/T change in cervix, lower uterine segment, uterine ischemia
- Radiates to abdominal wall/lumbosacral area/gluteus maximus/thighs

Somatic: 2nd stage of labor
- R/T stretching/distention of perineal body; traction on peritoneum; soft tissue lacerations; expulsive forces; fetal pressure

- Multidimensional experience
- Unique to each individual
- Includes perception of and response to

Perception/Expression:
- Influenced by
  - Primary social group; culture; ethnicity; past experience
- Psychological/emotional response:
  - crying; screaming; quiet; exhaustion; clenching teeth; groaning; wringing hands
- Physiological response:
  - elevated BP, heart rate, respirations; diaphoresis nausea/vomiting+

Influencing factors

Physical:
- Duration/intensity of labor
- Position of fetus
- Pelvic size/shape
- Maternal fatigue
- Presence of IV and fetal monitoring equipment
- Induction of labor
- Environment

Psychological:
- Anxiety/fear
- Previous experience/childbirth preparation
- Support systems
- Physiological
- Hx of dysmenorrhea
- Position in labor
- Fetal size
- Level of endorphins

PAIN

Across Care Settings:
- Encourage investigation of safe available childbirth settings

Promoting Comfort/Pain Relief in Labor and Birth

Critical Nursing Actions:
- Combining butorphanol (Stadol) with other CNS depressants increases respiratory suppression
- Respond quickly/correctly to maternal hypotension/decreased placental perfusion

Nursing Insight:
- Childbirth pain is unique
- Allow patient to determine labor environment as much as possible
- Use visual analogue pain scale
- Decreasing anxiety can reduce vasoconstriction/pain
- Know the difference between opioid agonist/antagonists; recognize local anesthetic agents
- Recognize value of natural pressure anesthesia
- Be aware of how different methods to administer epidural blocks are administered
- Recognize shiver response after epidural administration

Optimizing Outcomes:
- Nonpharmacological comfort measures can decrease maternal mortality
- Recognize cultural influences on pain perception/coping
- Continually assess pain throughout labor
- Recognize maternal hyperventilation
- Do not apply "heat/cold" on anesthetized areas
- Give IV analgesics slowly in small doses, during contractions
- Use opioids with caution/monitor for safety; have Narcan and oxygen ready
- Epidural block → assist to push; assess return of sensation; provide emotional care

Nonpharmacological
- Positioning → squatting, "slow-dance"
- Breathing techniques
- Relaxation → music, guided imagery, massage/touch
- Hydro-, hypno-, and aromatherapy
- Use of heat and cold
- Biofeedback
- TENS
- Acupressure/acupuncture
- Intradermal water block

Pharmacological
- Sedatives
- Antiemetics
- Systemic analgesia
  - opioid agonists, agonist-antagonists, antagonists
- Nerve block analgesia/anesthesia
  - Local perineal infiltration
  - Pudendal
  - Spinal
  - Epidural

Legal Alert:
- Inform patient about pharmacological pain relief and obtain consent
- Assess/reassess during intrapartal period after each intervention

Now Can You:
- Discuss characteristics of pain during labor/birth
- Discuss a pain control theory
- Discuss nonpharmacologic/pharmacologic pain-relief methods and all of the nursing implications
- Discuss different types of blocks/anesthetics and associated nursing considerations

Where Research and Practice Meet:
- Water immersion during labor/birth is safe and may be beneficial
- Maternal self-hypnosis is an additional technique to achieve relaxation and decrease stress
- Delaying pushing in nulliparous women after epidural administration can decrease active labor time

Caring for the Woman Experiencing Complications During Labor and Birth

And when our baby stirs and struggles to be born it compels humility, what we began is now its own.

—Anne Ridler

LEARNING TARGETS *At the completion of this chapter, the student will be able to:*

- ◆ Differentiate critical factors associated with nursing care of women experiencing dysfunctional labor patterns.
- ◆ Discuss collaborative care of the woman experiencing an induction of labor.
- ◆ Describe the management of selected maternal complications during the intrapartal period.
- ◆ Describe emergency nursing care for various uterine, placental, umbilical, and amniotic complications during labor and birth.
- ◆ Plan appropriate nursing care for a family experiencing a fetal loss.
- ◆ Discuss maternal and fetal factors associated with cesarean birth.

PICO(T) Questions

The intent of evidence-based practice (EBP) is to provide nursing care that integrates the best available evidence. An initial step in EBP is to write a PICO(T) question that effectively guides the research. A PICO(T) question is an acronym that stands for population (P), intervention or issue (I), comparison of interest (C), outcome (O), and timeframe (T). Depending on the question, all or some of the question components are used in the research process.

Use these PICO(T) questions to spark your thinking as you read the chapter.

1. Do (P) infants (I) delivered with forceps assistance (O) have a higher rate of injury at birth (C) than infants delivered with vacuum assistance?

2. What (I) nursing interventions do (P) parents who experience perinatal fetal loss say are (O) most meaningful in coping with this event?

 Evidence-Based Practice

Madan, J., Chen, M., Goodman, E., Davis, J., Allan, W., & Dammann, O. (2010). Maternal obesity, gestational hypertension, and preterm delivery. *The Journal of Maternal-Fetal and Neonatal Medicine, 23*(1), 82–88.

The purpose of this study was to explore obesity as a factor associated with preterm delivery. Recent national surveys on health and nutrition have estimated that presently, 66% of U.S. adults are overweight or obese. In the past 10 years, the percentage of adults classified as obese has increased from 23% to 32%. An increased risk of maternal antenatal, intrapartum, and postpartum complications has been identified in large population-based studies of obese women. Past research has shown an association between preeclampsia, an elevated maternal body mass index (BMI), and increased rates of medically induced preterm births. Other pregnancy complications associated with an elevated BMI include gestational diabetes, hypertension, cesarean delivery, eclampsia, and adverse fetal and neonatal outcomes. Moreover, breastfeeding is less likely to be successful in obese women.

The population for this study, which used a cohort design, included 58,112 non-Hispanic white mother-infant pairs from births

(continued)

Evidence-Based Practice (continued)

that occurred over a 10-year period. Data (excluding stillbirths, fetal demise, and neonatal deaths) from the vital statistics records of a northeastern state (comprised of 97% non-Hispanic white individuals) were studied and analyzed. Of this population, 8% (n=4,653) gave birth to preterm infants, defined as a birth occurring before 37 completed weeks of gestation. Maternal BMI was calculated during an antenatal visit that took place between 13 to 18 weeks of gestation. For study purposes, categories of BMI were defined as follows: normal weight (BMI less than 25), overweight (BMI 25 to less than 30), obese (BMI 30 to less than 40), and morbidly obese (BMI greater than or equal to 40). Other data included maternal age, education, the presence of gestational hypertension (BP greater than 140/90 mm Hg, proteinuria, and edema), diabetes (existing or gestational with glucose greater than 130 mg/dL on at least two occasions), chronic hypertension, smoking, previous small for gestational age infant (SGA), and previous preterm infant with a birth weight at less than the 10th percentile or born at less than 37 completed weeks of gestation. Additional information available included information about the labor process, the development of complications during labor and delivery, and details about the neonate.

Data were analyzed to determine the relationship between maternal BMI and the risk of preterm delivery and also the relationship between maternal obesity and the risk of prematurity. Of the total cohort population, 43% was identified as normal weight, 29% was classified as overweight, 23% were classified as obese, and 5% were classified as morbidly obese. Of the cohort that experienced preterm labor, 42% were of normal weight, 27% were overweight, 25% were obese, and 6% were morbidly obese. Thirteen percent of the cohort that experienced preterm labor had a diagnosis of gestational hypertension, 3% had chronic hypertension, 5% had gestational diabetes, 2% had pre-existing diabetes, and 5% had a history of a previous preterm or SGA birth. Twenty percent of this population was identified as smokers. It was noted that the maternal BMI increased with advancing age and parity. The incidence of pregnancy and labor and delivery complications also increased with the women designated as obese or morbidly obese. The most significant variable noted in the multivariable regression analysis was the development of gestational hypertension/preeclampsia.

The researchers reported that an association was also found between maternal obesity and preterm delivery. They concluded that as the maternal BMI increases, the risk of preterm delivery increases. Other complications such as diabetes and chronic hypertension, conditions that can be associated with obesity, also increase the risk of preterm delivery.

1. How is this information useful to clinical nursing practice?

2. Based on these findings, what are implications for further research?

See Suggested Responses for Evidence-Based Practice on Davis*Plus*.

Introduction

The nurse who cares for women and their families experiencing complications during labor and birth is responsible for creating a supportive environment that provides complex nursing care. Under normal circumstances labor and birth place stress on the family unit, and when problems are superimposed during this time frame, another layer of complexity is added. The woman often needs to respond rapidly to changing health conditions for which she might not be prepared. The nurse has to be proactive and reassuring in support of the woman and her family unit. It is critical to empower the woman and encourage her to take control as much as possible. The nurse acts as her advocate in collaborative care when the woman is unable to have her voice.

Complications arise from a variety of factors. Women experience problems with uterine dysfunction often referred to as the powers of labor. The presentation and position of the fetus is integral to a positive labor outcome. When the fetus is not in a favorable lie, the labor process may lengthen, require instrumentation assistance, or necessitate an operative birth. Multiple fetuses are more prone to these issues because of their locations within the uterus. Placenta obstruction or an inadequate bony pelvis may hinder fetal progress through the birth canal and require more extensive medical intervention. Medical emergencies and complications from maternal disease also place the patient at increased risk for a complicated and intervention-driven labor and birth.

Cesarean or operative birth is one of the outcomes associated with a complicated labor. In the United States, the cesarean birth rate has steadily increased. Controversy surrounds this statistic while at the same time more women are requesting an elective cesarean birth. The nurse working in perinatal care has to be concerned with ethical issues and be prepared to foster evidence-based research studies to examine the multiple factors involved with cesarean deliveries.

Perinatal loss necessitates a collaborative response from all professionals involved in the care of the patient. Nurses can lead others in providing support. Spiritual, emotional, psychological, and physical needs are important considerations that need to be met during this time. Although this situation cannot be normalized, the nurse can encourage the woman to hold her infant, give her a baby picture, and provide a memory book to acknowledge the existence of the child.

The nurse serves in many capacities when managing the care of patients experiencing a complicated labor and birth. Use of the nursing process combined with a strong theoretical background provides a foundation for the critical decision making that exists in the clinical unit. Nursing diagnoses specific to the woman experiencing a complication during the intrapartal period refer to specific problems and often relate to the broad concepts of fear, anxiety, coping,

---

Box 14-1 Possible Nursing Diagnoses for the Woman Experiencing Complications During Labor and Birth

- Fear related to unknown high-risk condition of labor
- Anxiety related to loss of control during labor
- Coping, Ineffective related to inadequate opportunity to prepare for high-risk labor
- Fatigue related to increased physical exertion during a long labor
- Powerlessness related to lack of control over decisions in a complicated birth
- Deficient Knowledge related to unknown high-risk condition
- Communication, Verbal Impaired related to cultural differences
- Risk for Spiritual Distress related to emotional response to high-risk labor and birth
- Risk for Ineffective Tissue Perfusion related to excessive loss of blood
- Risk for Injury related to damage of tissue during a complicated birth
- Pain, Acute related to tissue damage
- Fluid Volume, Deficit related to decreased urinary output
- Fluid Volume, Excess related to compromise of the cardiovascular system
- Risk for Trauma related to instrumentation-assisted birth
- Anticipatory Grieving related to fetal demise

---

and fatigue. Examples of possible nursing diagnoses are presented in Box 14-1. The nurse has the unique opportunity to empower the woman and assist her in taking control as much as possible in these difficult situations. Because patients are unique in their responses, it is incumbent on the nurse to be sensitive to all individuals and be culturally competent. Finally, the nurse must constantly examine practice and promote research initiatives that give evidence to optimal outcomes in complex perinatal care.

 Optimizing Outcomes—Helping to meet *Healthy People 2020* national goals

Nurses who work with birthing mothers can be instrumental in helping the nation to meet *Healthy People 2020* goals that address intrapartal complications (U.S. Department of Health and Human Services [USDHHS], 2012):

- Reduce the maternal mortality rate to no more than 11.4 per 100,000 live births from a baseline of 12.7 per 100,000.
- Reduce cesarean births among low-risk women giving birth for the first time to no more than 23.9% from a baseline of 26.5% by carefully monitoring laboring women to identify early signs of potentially life-threatening events (e.g., placental abruption and uterine rupture) and by assisting women with fetal malpresentations amenable to rotation with positional changes to help reduce the number of cesarean births.

Dystocia

Dystocia, defined as a long, difficult or abnormal labor, is a term used to identify poor labor progression. Dystocia may arise from any of the three major components of the labor process—the powers (uterine contractions), the passenger

(fetus), or the passageway (maternal pelvis). In addition, various medical interventions used during labor and birth may create problems that complicate the birth process.

Dystocia may be related to maternal positioning during labor, as well as fetal malpresentation, anomalies, macrosomia, and multiple gestation. Also, maternal psychological responses to the labor based on past experiences, cultural influences, and the woman's present level of support may play a role in the normal progress of labor.

 Nursing Insight—*Recognizing indicators of dystocia*

Nurses should suspect dystocia when there is a lack of progress in the rate of cervical dilation, fetal descent and expulsion, or an alteration in the pattern of normal uterine contractions.

DYSFUNCTIONAL LABOR PATTERNS

Dysfunctional labor patterns are deviations from the normal pattern of labor as illustrated by a labor curve (see Chapter 12). Labor alterations occur more frequently during the first stage of labor (cervical dilation and effacement) than during the second stage (maternal expulsive efforts). Nulliparous women have a higher incidence of abnormalities than do multiparous women. Dysfunctional labor is the fourth most common complication of labor and birth, and several factors may increase a woman's risk for dystocia (Box 14-2). There are two general types of labor dysfunction: hypertonic and hypotonic (Fig. 14-1). These contraction patterns are classified according to when they occur in labor and the nature of the uterine contractions.

Hypertonic Labor

Hypertonic labor contractions are strong and often painful but are ineffective in producing cervical effacement and dilation. An increase in maternal catecholamine release (e.g., epinephrine and norepinephrine) can result in poor uterine contractility (Cunningham, Leveno, Bloom, Spong, & Dashe, 2014). Uterine pacemakers (the energy source of contractions located in the uterine wall) do not initiate a good myometrial response needed for progressive cervical

---

Box 14-2 Factors Associated With an Increased Risk for Uterine Dystocia

- Uterine abnormalities, such as congenital malformations and overdistention (e.g., hydramnios and multiple gestation)
- Fetal malpresentation or malposition
- Cephalopelvic disproportion (CPD)
- Maternal body build (greater than 30 lb [13.6 kg] overweight, short stature)
- Uterine overstimulation with oxytocin
- Inappropriate timing of administration of analgesic/anesthetic agents
- Maternal fear, fatigue, dehydration, electrolyte imbalance

Sources: American College of Obstetricians and Gynecologists (ACOG) (2003a); Gilbert (2010).

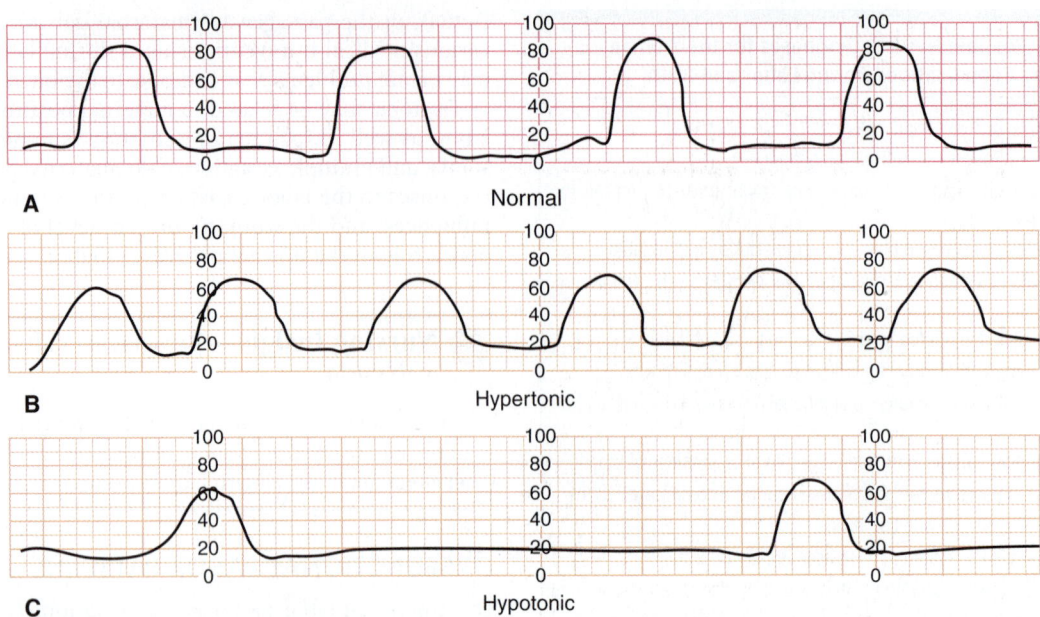

Figure 14-1 Uterine contraction patterns. *A,* Normal uterine contraction pattern. *B,* Hypertonic uterine contraction pattern. *C,* Hypotonic uterine contraction pattern.

change. Instead, irregular spasmodic episodes occur that do not result in effective contractions or assist in bringing the fetus into a more favorable downward position (Gilbert, 2010).

Maternal anxiety plays a major role in hypertonic labor. Anxiety is known to produce high levels of catecholamines. Many factors contribute to a woman's fear related to labor and birth:

- Primiparous labor
- Loss of control
- Sexual abuse
- Lack of support
- Cultural differences
- Fear of pain

An occiput–posterior malposition of the fetus, which occurs in approximately 15% of labors, also leads to hypertonic labor contractions. In approximately one-half of all cases of hypertonic labor patterns, however, there is no apparent cause (Gilbert, 2010).

Although the management of hypertonic labor contractions varies, in general, the emphasis is on establishing a more effective labor pattern. Rest, hydration, and sedation reduce the irritability of the uterus and help to diminish the ineffective contractions. Medications that may be prescribed to induce therapeutic rest include meperidine (Demerol), hydromorphone (Dilaudid), and morphine (Cunningham et al., 2014). Natural labor with effective contractions often resumes after this simple intervention. Nonpharmacological techniques to reduce anxiety such as relaxation techniques, massage, a warm shower or tub bath, and increased emotional support are also helpful for some women.

For a woman whose fetus is in an occiput–posterior position, the major goal of care is to facilitate rotation of the fetal head into a more favorable position. The nurse can encourage the laboring woman to walk and change positions frequently throughout the course of labor. The descent of

the fetus into an anterior lie creates a better environment for normal labor progression.

Nursing care begins with a thorough assessment. It is critical to identify factors that contribute to increased maternal anxiety. Careful monitoring of contractions may provide early information regarding poor labor progression and lead to timely interventions. While frequent checks for cervical dilation are not advisable, this assessment, when performed at proper intervals, provides a strong indicator of labor progression. Along with continued assessment of the contraction pattern, the nurse can use this information to validate the finding of hypertonic labor. Once any intervention has occurred, the nurse evaluates the plan of care, and depending on the results, initiates appropriate measures.

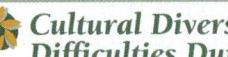 ### *Cultural Diversity: Communication Difficulties During Labor*

Nurses need to be sensitive to cultural differences among women experiencing hypertonic labor—those who are unable to speak or understand the English language may have difficulty communicating their feelings.

Hypotonic Labor

Hypotonic labor is a more common type of uterine dysfunctional pattern that contributes to poor labor progression. With hypotonic dystocia, the uterine contractions decrease in frequency and intensity. A hypotonic labor pattern usually occurs during the active phase of labor. It is defined as fewer than two to three contractions during a 10-minute period. The uterus can be easily indented, even at the peak of the contraction, and the intrauterine pressure (IUP) is insufficient for the progression of cervical effacement and dilation (Gilbert, 2010).

Hypotonic labor may be associated with a number of maternal and fetal factors that produce excessive uterine stretching and overdistention. For example, fetal macrosomia, anomalies, malpresentation, multiple gestation, and hydramnios are all risk factors for hypotonic labor. Grand multiparity may also be a contributing cause.

Fetal **macrosomia** occurs in one-fourth of all pregnancies and is the leading cause of uterine hypotonia. Macrosomia, defined as a fetus whose birth weight is above the 90th percentile on an intrauterine growth chart for that gestational age, often results from a fetal imbalance between glucose and insulin in women diagnosed with any type of diabetes. Over time, as increased amounts of glucose are absorbed from the mother, the fetus produces pancreatic insulin which results in an increase in fat deposits.

Maternal obesity unaccompanied by diabetes also contributes to a larger fetus. A pregnant woman is considered obese if her weight exceeds 200 lb (91 kg), if she is 50% over ideal body weight for height, of if her body mass index (BMI) is above 30. Direct links between maternal obesity and fetal macrosomia have been established, and other obesity-related peripartum complications include shoulder dystocia, high cesarean birth rates, and postpartum infection.

Pharmacological agents used to alleviate pain during labor may also contribute to the risk of uterine hypotonia. If a labor pattern is not well established, these medications often halt or significantly slow down the progress of labor. Various studies have produced conflicting data concerning a clear link between the use of analgesia, anesthesia, and the progress of labor. After administration of epidural anesthesia, some women may experience a longer second stage of labor. The effects of the epidural may make it difficult for the patient to identify when to push and how long to push because the contractions are not always detected. However, nulliparous women who experience long and painful labors are more likely to choose epidural anesthesia for pain relief. Often it is difficult to document which factors contribute most significantly to a protracted labor.

 Nursing Insight—*Recognizing negative maternal effects of hypotonic labor*

As an ineffective labor pattern continues, the woman is likely to become fatigued and may be at an increased risk for infection. She is also likely to experience increased anxiety and discomfort and difficulty coping with pain.

Depending on the cause, labor hypotonia is managed in different ways. Careful, ongoing assessments are key. If a diagnostic modality such as ultrasound examination has demonstrated that the woman's pelvis is adequate for vaginal birth, measures to produce effective contractions are implemented. Walking and position changes in labor assist in fetal descent through the maternal pelvis and therefore need to be encouraged. The use of relaxation techniques, massage, and water treatments can decrease the need for pharmacological agents for pain.

Augmentation of labor contractions is considered when either the natural measures are unsuccessful or when it is deemed the best approach. At certain points in the labor, an amniotomy, or artificial rupture of the membranes, may be successful in increasing uterine contractility. Other measures to enhance the progress of labor include membrane stripping, nipple stimulation, and oxytocin infusion. Maternal and fetal assessments including vital signs, contraction patterns, and cervical changes need to be documented on a regular basis.

PRECIPITOUS LABOR AND BIRTH

Contrary to both hypertonic and hypotonic labor, **precipitous labor** contractions produce very rapid, intense contractions. By definition, a precipitous labor lasts less than 3 hours from the beginning of contractions to birth. Multiparous women with little soft tissue resistance are at the greatest risk for this labor pattern. Patients often progress through the first stage of labor with little or no pain and may present to the birth setting already advanced into the second stage. In a nulliparous patient, cervical dilation that occurs faster than 5 cm per hour is defined as precipitous labor. In a multiparous woman, cervical dilation may occur as rapidly as 10 cm in 1 hour. Precipitous labor may result from hypertonic uterine contractions that are tetanic in their intensity (Cunningham et al., 2014; Wing & Farinelli, 2012) (Fig. 14-2).

Complications from a precipitous labor pattern result from trauma to maternal tissue and to the fetus because of the rapid descent. Hemorrhage may occur from uterine rupture and vaginal lacerations. Most women are ill prepared for the rapid advancement of their labor and become alarmed, highly anxious, and fearful. The fetus may suffer from hypoxia related to the decreased periods of uterine relaxation between the contractions and intracranial hemorrhage related to the rapid birth (Cunningham et al., 2014).

Nursing Considerations

Initial assessments are paramount to establishing the pattern of precipitous labor. A multiparous patient with a previous history of rapid labors needs to alert her physician or certified nurse midwife (CNM) as soon as she recognizes any signs of labor. Her prenatal record should include this information and be readily accessible to nursing personnel managing her care. In a nulliparous patient, careful examination for cervical dilation and effacement is required. Because a previous labor pattern is an unknown variable in the nulliparous patient, the nurse must be alert in recognizing signs of abnormally rapid cervical dilation (Wing & Farinelli, 2012).

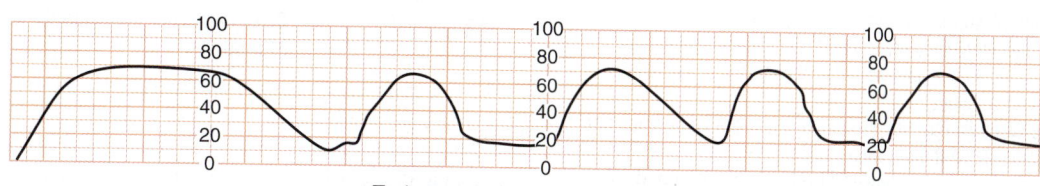

Tachysystole (tetanic contractions)

Figure 14-2 Tetanic uterine contractions.

The woman and her support person need reassurance throughout the rapidly advancing labor. Breathing and relaxation techniques are helpful tools that the nurse can use to assist the woman to cope with labor. If the patient and her family do not speak or understand the English language, it is incumbent on the nurse to request a translator. Precipitous labor is an anxiety-producing situation that can be compounded by the woman's inability to understand what is happening to her body. Although some precipitous labors occur with little or no pain, the patient is nevertheless aware of contractions that are occurring more quickly than normal. This experience can be frightening. The woman may also have concerns regarding a loss of control over her labor. Continuous surveillance, frequent updates on her status, and reassurance about her condition can help to allay the patient's anxiety. Medical management includes readiness on the part of the entire health team for the birth, particularly when the patient has a history of rapid labor. In most circumstances, a planned induction is part of the plan. Small dosages of intravenous analgesics may be used to help decrease pain.

The nurse can assist the woman in breathing through her contractions to avoid pushing and to help prevent tearing. If the nurse is alone with the patient during a precipitous delivery, the nurse follows delivery protocols when assisting in the birth of the infant. At the same time, the nurse uses the call bell to alert others for assistance. The nurse supports the perineum, assists the fetal head as it emerges, and checks for the umbilical cord as the head rotates. The newborn's nose and mouth are suctioned; the shoulders and then the rest of the newborn's body are supported during the birthing process. The nurse assesses the neonate's respiratory and cardiac rates.

After birth, whether assisted by the nurse or physician, the maternal soft tissue and placenta need to be carefully examined. The patient may require suturing of the cervix or vagina for lacerations. During the immediate postpartum period, the woman must be continuously monitored for hemorrhage. Providing ongoing information and support assists the patient and helps her support person cope with this unexpected event (Cunningham et al., 2014; Wing & Farinelli, 2012).

Critical Nursing Action Assisting With a Precipitous Birth

The nurse who assists with a precipitous birth should take the following actions:

- Request a translator to interpret for patients unable to speak or understand English.
- Assist the laboring woman to breathe through each contraction to prevent pushing.
- Provide continuous emotional support.
- Provide perineal support with warm cloths.
- Frequently monitor the maternal and fetal vital signs and immediately report any abnormal findings to the physician or certified nurse midwife.
- After birth, carefully monitor the patient for signs of hemorrhage; assess for trauma to the perineum.
- Assess the neonate for evidence of trauma and report and document all findings.

PELVIC STRUCTURE ALTERATIONS

Pelvic Dystocia

Pelvic dystocia occurs when contractures of the pelvic diameters reduce the capacity of the bony pelvis, the midpelvis, the outlet, or any combination of these planes. Contractures of the maternal pelvis may result from malnutrition, neoplasms, congenital abnormalities, traumatic spinal injury, or spinal disorders. In addition, immaturity of the pelvis may predispose some adolescent mothers to pelvic dystocia. During labor, contractures of the inlet, midplane, or outlet can cause interference in engagement and fetal descent, necessitating cesarean birth (Cunningham et al., 2014).

Soft Tissue Dystocia

Soft tissue dystocia occurs when the birth passage is obstructed by an anatomical abnormality other than that involving the bony pelvis. The obstruction, which prevents the fetus from entering the bony pelvis, may be caused by placenta previa, uterine fibroid tumors (leiomyomas), ovarian tumors, or a full bladder or rectum. **Bandl ring** is a pathological retraction ring that develops between the upper and lower uterine segments. It is associated with protracted labor, prolonged rupture of the membranes, and an increased risk of uterine rupture (Cunningham et al., 2014).

TRIAL OF LABOR

A **trial of labor** (TOL) is the surveillance of a woman and her fetus for a set amount of time (usually 4 to 6 hours) during spontaneous active labor to assess the safety of a vaginal birth. Indications for a trial of labor include situations when the maternal pelvis is of questionable size or shape, when the fetus is in an abnormal presentation, and when the woman desires to have a vaginal birth after a previous (low-segment transverse) cesarean birth. Before the TOL, an assessment of the adequacy of the maternal pelvis for vaginal birth (to rule out cephalopelvic disproportion [CPD]) is conducted with sonography or maternal pelvimetry. The cervix must be favorable (soft, dilatable), and throughout the TOL, the woman is assessed for the presence of adequate contractions, engagement and descent of the fetal presenting part, and cervical dilation and effacement.

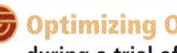

Optimizing Outcomes—Providing support during a trial of labor

Nursing responsibilities during a TOL include assessment of maternal vital signs and FHR and pattern. If complications arise, the nurse notifies the primary health-care provider, and evaluates and documents the maternal–fetal responses to the interventions. Offering support and encouragement to the woman and her labor partner and ongoing information about labor progress are essential components of care.

Now Can You—Discuss factors that impede the progress of labor?

1. Describe why maternal anxiety contributes to a lack of labor progression?
2. List three ways the nurse can reduce maternal anxiety?
3. Identify which synthesizing enzymes are significant to the lack of myometrial contractility?

Obstetric Interventions

AMNIOINFUSION

Pregnancy outcome in patients experiencing variable fetal heart rate (FHR) decelerations caused by cord compression is improved through the use of amnioinfusion, which is the instillation of normal saline or lactated Ringer's solution into the uterine cavity. Amnioinfusion is used to supplement the amniotic fluid volume in patients with oligohydramnios caused by uteroplacental insufficiency, premature rupture of the membranes, and postmaturity. Although previously advocated as a technique to reduce the incidence of neonatal meconium aspiration syndrome, evidence shows that a large proportion of women with meconium-stained amniotic fluid have infants who have taken meconium into the trachea or bronchioles before meconium passage has been detected. According to the American College of Obstetricians and Gynecologists (2006), prophylactic amnioinfusion for meconium-stained amniotic fluid is not recommended. Risks of the procedure include infection, overdistention of the uterus, and increased uterine tone.

In most circumstances, the fluid is instilled through an intrauterine pressure catheter (IUPC); the amniotic membranes must be ruptured for catheter placement. The fluid may be warmed with a blood warmer before administration and the infusion may be given by bolus or continuous flow. When possible, a double-lumen IUPC is used because the intrauterine pressure can be monitored without stopping the amnioinfusion.

Nursing considerations include careful monitoring of the infusion, the intensity and frequency of uterine contractions, and the maternal vital signs. In some institutions, patients are required to sign an informed consent prior to the intervention. It is important for the nurse to educate the woman and her support person regarding the need for the infusion and its purpose. Nurses must document the amount of the solution infused and the presence of any vaginal discharge (Gilbert, 2010).

 Critical Nursing Action When Caring for a Patient Undergoing Amnioinfusion

When caring for a patient undergoing amnioinfusion, the nurse must:

1. Assess the patient's response to the fluid infusion.
2. Continually monitor the frequency and intensity of uterine contractions.
3. Stop the infusion if the following signs and symptoms are noted: maternal shortness of breath, an overdistended uterus, hypotension, or tachycardia.

AMNIOTOMY

Amniotomy, or the artificial rupture of membranes (AROM), is a nonpharmacological intervention that may be done to augment or induce labor or to facilitate the placement of internal monitors during labor. According to the Association of Women's Health, Obstetric and Neonatal Nurses (AWHONN) (2009), because of the risk of complications that may necessitate emergency medical intervention, perinatal nurses should not routinely, independently perform amniotomy. However, registered nurses who have received specialized education, training, and competence validation may apply a fetal spiral electrode through intact membranes for the purpose of obtaining additional assessment data and continuing treatment under certain circumstances.

AROM is a procedure that involves the insertion of an Amnihook or other sharp instrument into the lower segment of the fetal membranes; following rupture, the fluid is allowed to drain slowly (Fig. 14-3). The rupture of the membranes causes a release of arachidonic acid, which converts to prostaglandins, known inducers of labor through the stimulation of oxytocin in the uterus (Gilbert, 2010). Labor usually commences within 12 hours after artificial rupture. However, if labor does not ensue, there is an increased risk of infection; other risks include fetal injury and umbilical cord prolapse. Because of the risk for infection, amniotomy is frequently used in combination with oxytocin induction to facilitate delivery.

The nurse carefully monitors the patient who will undergo an amniotomy. Vital signs, cervical effacement and dilation, station of the presenting part, FHR, and contractions are documented. The presenting part must be engaged and well applied to the cervix to prevent **umbilical cord prolapse** (protrusion of the umbilical cord in advance of the presenting part). There should be no evidence of active infection of the genital tract (e.g., herpes) or HIV infection (Kilpatrick & Garrison, 2012).

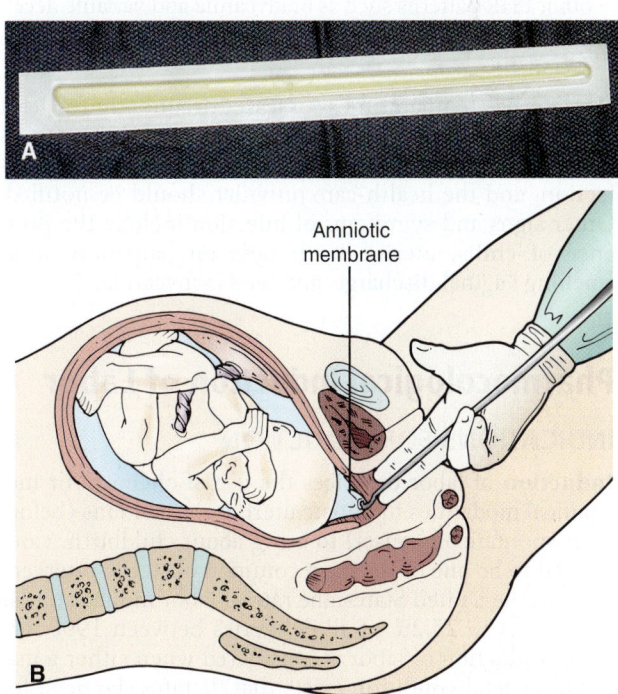

Figure 14-3 *A,* An Amnihook. *B,* An Amnihook is used to rupture the membranes.

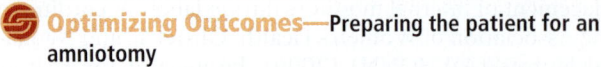

Optimizing Outcomes—Preparing the patient for an amniotomy

The nurse provides information, assesses the woman's understanding of the procedure, and assures her that the membrane rupture will be painless to her and her fetus although she may experience some discomfort when the instrument is inserted through the vagina and cervix. The nurse ensures that the necessary equipment has been assembled: sterile gloves, lubricant, and the Amnihook or Allis clamp. After placing hip pads under the buttocks to absorb the fluid, the nurse positions the woman on a padded bedpan or with rolled up linens to elevate the hips. The nurse assists the health-care provider performing the procedure by unwrapping and passing the equipment.

Immediately after the artificial rupture, the nurse notes and records the FHR and pattern. The color, odor, consistency, and clarity (and amount, if unusual) of the amniotic fluid are also documented, along with the time of rupture and the indication for the amniotomy. The patient may request analgesia or epidural anesthesia before the procedure. If she has not requested any medication, the nurse assists her with relaxation and breathing techniques during the contractions following the amniotomy because they are likely to be stronger.

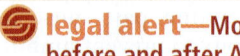

legal alert—Monitor and document FHR before and after AROM

Immediately before AROM, the nurse should assess the FHR and characteristics, perform a vaginal examination to palpate for umbilical cord, and determine fetal station and presentation. The FHR should also be assessed immediately after AROM (AWHONN, 2009). Changes such as transient fetal tachycardia may occur and are common. However, other FHR patterns such as bradycardia and variable decelerations may be indicative of cord compression or prolapse.

Maternal temperature is assessed frequently (at least every 2 hours) after amniotomy to rule out infection. A temperature of 100.4°F (38°C) may be indicative of an infection, and the health-care provider should be notified. Other signs and symptoms of infection include the presence of chills, uterine tenderness on palpation, foul-smelling vaginal discharge, and fetal tachycardia.

Pharmacological Induction of Labor

INDICATIONS FOR INDUCTION

Induction of labor describes the use of chemical or mechanical modalities to initiate uterine contractions (before their spontaneous onset) to bring about childbirth. Considered to be one of the most common obstetric interventions in the United States, the rate of labor induction rose from 9.5% to 23.2% of all deliveries between 1990 and 2010. Induction of labor is considered when either a maternal or fetal condition exists that dictates the need for medical intervention in the labor process. Labor induction often leads to an increase in interventionist care including

the use of intravenous therapy, amniotomy, internal monitoring, epidural anesthesia, and a longer stay in the labor unit. Interestingly, non-Hispanic Caucasian women experience the highest rate of inductions, as compared with Hispanic women, who experience the lowest induction rates (U.S. Census Bureau, 2012; Zhang & Kramer, 2012).

According to the American College of Obstetricians and Gynecologists (ACOG) (2009), the following maternal–fetal conditions serve as some of the indications for induction:

- Postterm pregnancy
- Maternal medical conditions (e.g., diabetes mellitus, renal disease, chronic pulmonary disease, chronic hypertension, or antiphospholipid syndrome)
- Gestational hypertension
- Fetal demise
- Chorioamnionitis
- Premature rupture of membranes
- Fetal compromise (e.g., severe fetal growth restriction, isoimmunization, or oligohydramnios)
- Preeclampsia, eclampsia

Because induction carries certain risks, it is not performed without careful consideration and evaluation of the maternal–fetal status. However, because of the rise in the U.S. cesarean rate over the last two decades, medical management of labor is commonly practiced in many hospitals to prevent the need for surgical delivery. This practice often involves admission of the patient with complete cervical effacement, rupture of the membranes, or expulsion of the mucus plug who is begun on a series of protocols that frequently include amniotomy combined with oxytocin infusion.

Induction of labor is more successful when the cervix is "favorable," or inducible. The **Bishop score** is a rating system that may be used to determine the level of cervical inducibility. A series of points is awarded to cervical dilation, effacement, station, consistency, and position (Table 14-1). In general, labor induction is more likely to be successful with a higher score (9 or more for nulliparous women; 5 or more for multiparous women) (Bishop, 1964; Cunningham et al., 2014). A recently developed simplified Bishop score composed of three components (cervical dilation, station, effacement) has been shown to attain a similarly high predictive ability of successful induction as the original score (Laughon, Zhang, Troendle, Sun, & Reddy, 2011).

Cervical Ripening Agents

If it is determined that the cervix is not favorable for oxytocin induction, a chemical cervical ripening agent using prostaglandin E_1 (PGE_1) (Misoprostol) or prostaglandin E_2 (PGE_2) (Dinoprostone) may be prescribed (Table 14-2). These agents are most beneficial when the patient's Bishop score is greater than 6, although they are commonly used when the Bishop score is 4 or less. Before administration, informed consent may be required, according to agency protocol.

Misoprostol (Cytotec), an analogue of PGE_1, can be administered intravaginally, orally, or sublingually and is used for both cervical ripening and induction of labor. In 2002, the U.S. Food and Drug Administration (FDA) approved a new label on the use of misoprostol during pregnancy for cervical ripening (effacement and dilation) and for the induction of labor. The labeling does not contain

Table 14-1 The Bishop Score

Component	Score			
	0	1	2	3
Dilation	0	1–2 cm	3–4 cm	>5cm
Effacement	0%–30%	40%–50%	60%–70%	>80%
Station	−3	−2	−1 to 0	+1, +2
Cervical consistency	Firm	Medium	Soft	
Cervical position	Posterior	Midposition	Anterior	

Each component is given a score of 0–2 or 0–3; the highest possible score is 13.

Table 14-2 Cervical Ripening Agents

Medication	Action	Adverse Effects	Dosage
prostaglandin E_1 misoprostol (Cytotec)	Ripens the cervix (causes softening and initiates dilation and effacement). Stimulates uterine contractions	Diarrhea, nausea and vomiting, headaches, fever, tachysystole (>5 uterine contractions in 10 minutes averaged over a 30-minute window without alteration of FHR or pattern), uterine hyperstimulation (tachysystole with non-reassuring FHR or patterns), fetal passage of meconium.	Intravaginally: 25 to 50 mcg—repeat every 3 to 6 hours (maximum of 300 to 400 mcg in a 24-hour period) until Bishop score equals 8 or greater. The tablet is placed into the posterior fornix using the tips of the index and middle fingers; no lubricant is used. Note: Misoprostol is available as a 100-mcg tablet. One-quarter of an unscored 100-mcg tablet is considered as the initial dose for cervical ripening and labor induction. The tablet must be cut in the pharmacy to ensure dosing accuracy.
prostaglandin E_2 dinoprostone gel (Prepidil Gel; Prostin E_2) dinoprostone vaginal insert (Cervidil)	Ripens the cervix (causes softening and initiates dilation and effacement). Stimulates uterine contractions	Diarrhea, nausea and vomiting, headache, back pain, fever, hypotension, tachysystole (>5 uterine contractions in 10 minutes averaged over a 30-minute window without alteration of FHR or pattern), uterine hyperstimulation (tachysystole with non-reassuring fetal heart rate or patterns), fetal passage of meconium. *Adverse effects are more common with intracervical administration.*	Prepidil Gel: (2.5-mL syringe containing 0.5 mg of dinoprostone). Repeat gel insertion in 6 hours as needed (maximum = 1.5 mg or 3 doses/24 hr). Allow gel to reach room temperature before administration; do not heat. Continue administration until maximum dose is reached, or uterine contractions are established (3/10 min) or Bishop score equals 8 or greater or adverse reactions occur. Cervidil Insert: (10 mg dinoprostone gradually released over 12 hours). Remove after 12 hours or at labor onset. Keep insert frozen until ready to use.

Teaching: Patient Education

- Assess knowledge of the medication.
- Explain purpose of medication and side effects.
- Discuss comfort options to offset side effects.
- Instruct the patient to void before insertion.
- Instruct the patient to maintain a supine position with a lateral tilt or side-lying position for 30 minutes to 2 hours (depending on medication used) after insertion.

Sources: Simpson (2009); Simpson & Creehan (2013); Simpson & O'Brien-Abel (2013); Vallerand & Sanoski (2014).

claims regarding the efficacy or safety of the medication. At least 4 hours after the last dose, oxytocin may be initiated for the induction of labor if cervical ripening has occurred and labor has not begun.

Two FDA-approved PGE_2 preparations are commercially available for cervical ripening in women at or near term: dinoprostone vaginal gel (Prepidil and Prostin E_2), available in a 2.5 mL syringe containing 0.5 mg, 10 mg, and 20 mg of dinoprostone; and dinoprostone vaginal insert (Cervidil), which contains 10 mg of dinoprostone. The vaginal insert releases prostaglandins at a slower rate than the gel. Cervical ripening agents make the cervix softer, causing it to begin to dilate and efface and stimulate uterine contractions. PGE_2 is used for preinduction cervical ripening when the Bishop score is 4 or less. The dinoprostone vaginal insert is applied into the posterior vaginal fornix; the dinoprostone gel is inserted through a syringe into the cervical canal just below the internal cervical os or into the posterior fornix. Uterine contractions usually begin in 5 to 7 hours after administration. When necessary, induction with oxytocin can be initiated 30 to 60 minutes after removal of the dinoprostone insert. When using Prepidil gel, oxytocin induction must be delayed until 6 to 12 hours after the last instillation of the medication. Cervidil has an added advantage—the insert can be removed if uterine tachysystole occurs.

Contraindications to the PGE_1 and PGE_2 cervical ripening agents include the presence of a non-reassuring fetal heart rate (FHR) or pattern, maternal fever, infection, vaginal bleeding, hypersensitivity, regular, progressive uterine contractions, and a history of cesarean birth or uterine scar. The medications should be cautiously used in women with a history of asthma, glaucoma, or renal, hepatic, or cardiovascular disorders. After insertion, the nurse should clearly document all assessment findings and administration procedures.

 Optimizing Outcomes—When cervical ripening agents are administered

Prior to administration of a prostaglandin cervical ripening agent, the nurse explains the procedure to the woman and her support person, ensures that informed consent has been obtained per institutional policy, and asks her to void. Maternal vital signs and FHR and pattern are assessed before each medication insertion and periodically throughout treatment, according to agency protocol. After placement of the medication, the nurse assists the woman to maintain a supine position with lateral tilt or a side-lying position (30 to 40 minutes after misoprostol; 30 to 60 minutes after dinoprostone gel; 2 hours after placement of dinoprostone insert). In the event of adverse reactions, the nurse uses saline-soaked gauze wrapped around the fingers to swab the vagina (or grasps the pull string attached to the insert) to remove remaining medication and prepares to administer terbutaline, 0.25 mg subcutaneously or intravenously.

Mechanical Methods

Mechanical methods provide another approach to cervical ripening. Dilators placed in the cervix cause cervical ripening by stimulating the release of endogenous prostaglandins. A balloon catheter (e.g., Foley) placed into the intracervical canal causes cervical ripening by increasing pressure exerted on the lower uterine segment. Compared with prostaglandins, a transcervical catheter decreases the risk of uterine tachysystole and offers the advantage of lower cost, reversibility, and stability at room temperature (Esakoff & Kilpatrick, 2013; Salin, Zafran, Nachum, Garmi, Kraiem, & Shalev, 2011). Hydroscopic dilators (those that enlarge as they absorb moisture from

the surrounding tissue) such as laminaria tents (made from desiccated seaweed) and synthetic dilators containing magnesium sulfate (Lamicel) may be inserted into the endocervix without rupturing the membranes. The dilators remain in place for 6 to 12 hours before removal for assessment of cervical dilation. Fresh dilators may then be inserted if necessary. Nursing care includes careful documentation of the number of dilators inserted (and later removed) and assessment for urinary retention, rupture of membranes, uterine tenderness and contractions, vaginal bleeding, and fetal distress (Gilbert, 2010; Simpson, 2009; Simpson & O'Brien-Abel, 2013). Amniotomy and membrane stripping or "sweeping" (the physician or midwife inserts a gloved finger into the internal cervical os and rotates it 360 degrees to gently "strip" or separate the amniotic membranes in the lower uterine segment) can also be used to ripen the cervix.

Oxytocin

Oxytocin, a hormone produced by the pituitary gland, stimulates uterine contractions (see Chapter 12). It can be used to induce labor or augment a labor that is progressing slowly because of ineffective uterine contractions. Administration of the medication (via electronic infusion device) is closely monitored according to institutional protocols; use of a checklist-driven protocol for the monitoring of oxytocin infusion improves patient safety. Some institutions have established low- and high-dose regimens for oxytocin infusion:

- Low-dose oxytocin regimen:
  - Begin at 2 milliunits per minute
  - Increase by 2 milliunits per minute every 30 minutes until less than or equal to 5 contractions lasting 45 to 90 seconds in 10 minutes averaged over 30 minutes
  - Maximum dose is 20 milliunits per minute
- High-dose oxytocin regimen:
  - Begin at 4 milliunits per minute
  - Increase by 4 milliunits per minute every 30 minutes until less than or equal to 5 contractions lasting 45 to 90 seconds in 10 minutes averaged over 30 minutes
  - Maximum dose is 20 milliunits per minute

The patient should be reevaluated if the dose reaches 20 milliunits per minute; oxytocin may exceed 20 milliunits per minute with provider discretion and documentation of rationale for exceeding the protocol (ACOG, 2009; Mandel, Pirko, Grant, Kauffman, Williams, & Schneider, 2009; Vallerand & Sanoski, 2014; Wing & Farinelli, 2012). According to findings from a recent meta-analysis (Zhang, Branch, Ramirez, Laughon, Reddy, Hoffman et al., 2011), a high-dose oxytocin regimen is associated with a shorter duration of first-stage labor for all parities without increasing the cesarean delivery rate or adversely affecting perinatal outcomes.

 Optimizing Outcomes—Through the safe administration of oxytocin

First, the patient's primary health-care provider writes an order for oxytocin for labor induction or augmentation. After an explanation and assessment of the patient's level of understanding, the nurse assists the woman to a side-lying or upright position. Assessment of the patient and fetus is conducted and documented. The solution is prepared and administered with a pump delivery system according to the prescribed orders. The piggyback solution is flagged with a medication label and connected to the intravenous infusion at the port nearest the point of venous insertion (Fig. 14-4). The medication is administered as ordered; ongoing assessments are conducted according to institutional protocol. The nurse documents the medication (kind, amount, time of beginning infusion, increasing the dose, maintaining the dose, and discontinuing the infusion), maternal–fetal reactions (FHR and pattern, maternal vital signs, pattern and progress of labor, nursing interventions, and maternal response) and when notification of the primary health-care provider takes place (Simpson & Creehan, 2013; Simpson & O'Brien-Abel, 2013).

Oxytocin acts on receptors in the myometrium to create an increase in the strength, duration, and frequency of the contractions. These same receptors are susceptible to uterine tachysystole (sometimes referred to as hyperstimulation), which constitutes a major risk associated with the medication. Signs of uterine hyperstimulation include the following:

- Uterine contractions that last greater than 90 seconds and occur more frequently than every 2 minutes
- Uterine resting tone greater than 20 to 25 mm Hg with a peak pressure greater than 80 mm Hg
- Non-reassuring FHR and pattern (baseline less than 100 or greater than 160 beats per minute; absent variability; repeated late decelerations or prolonged decelerations)

Higher doses are associated with an increased incidence of uterine tachysystole; however, low dosages result in an increased rate of cesarean births because of failure of labor progression. Uterine tachysystole causes reduced blood flow through the placenta and results in FHR decelerations, fetal asphyxia, and neonatal hypoxia. Because of the potential for

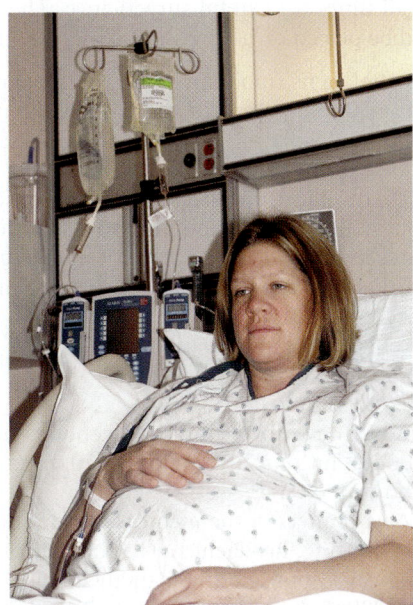

Figure 14-4 Administration of intravenous oxytocin.

life-threatening adverse complications associated with the use of oxytocin during the intrapartal period, the FDA has issued a number of restrictions to its use (ACOG, 2009; Simpson, 2009; Simpson & O'Brien-Abel, 2013; Wing & Farinelli, 2012).

 clinical alert

Contraindications to the use of oxytocin to stimulate labor

Nurses should be aware of contraindications to labor induction, which include, but are not limited to, the following (ACOG, 2009):

- Vasa previa or complete placenta previa
- Transverse fetal lie
- Umbilical cord prolapse
- Previous classical cesarean delivery
- Active genital herpes infection
- Previous myomectomy (surgical excision of a fibroid) entering the endometrial cavity

Conditions that necessitate special precaution during oxytocin administration include:

- Breech presentation
- Multifetal pregnancy
- Presenting part above the pelvic inlet
- Severe hypertension
- Maternal heart disease
- Polyhydramnios
- One or more previous low-transverse cesarean deliveries
- Abnormal FHR patterns not necessitating emergent delivery

 legal alert—Ensuring patient safety and risk management in the perinatal setting

Nurses in perinatal care settings must be well educated about the interpretation of FHR tracings and the risks associated with oxytocin; they must also be mindful of practice areas commonly identified in malpractice claims as contributors to adverse birth outcomes. These include inaccurate interpretation of FHR tracings and lack of timely, appropriate responses to non-reassuring FHR tracings, failure to reduce administration rates/discontinue oxytocin or other induction agents in the presence of non-reassuring FHR tracings, and incomplete/inaccurate documentation. In the courtroom, multimillion dollar malpractice lawsuit payouts related to adverse perinatal outcomes are commonly associated with evidence of permanent brain damage and the estimated costs of providing lifelong medical care for the damaged child, as well as compensation for the parents' emotional suffering related to lost dreams and the "loss" of their perfect child (Doyle, Kenny, Burkett, & von Gruenigen, 2011; Miller, Miller, & Tucker, 2012; Simpson, 2009; Pearson, 2011).

Augmentation of labor is used to stimulate uterine contractions after labor has begun spontaneously but is not progressing satisfactorily. It is most commonly indicated for the management of hypotonic uterine dysfunction. Labor augmentation may be accomplished with amniotomy, oxytocin infusion, and nipple stimulation. Noninvasive approaches include ambulation, hydration, relaxation, and hydrotherapy, and these methods should be attempted before the initiation of invasive measures.

Nipple stimulation has been used for labor augmentation and induction. The action of nipple rolling produces an increase in the release of oxytocin from the anterior pituitary gland. The nurse instructs the woman to roll her nipple through her clothing for 10 minutes on one side and then proceed to the other side, resting during a contraction. A breast pump may also be used. Nipple stimulation rarely causes uterine tachysystole. However, the results of nipple stimulation are less predictable than the administration of specified dosages of oxytocin. Sexual intercourse has also been helpful as a method of induction because semen contains prostaglandins (Gilbert, 2010). Both of these methods require additional evidence-based research before their endorsement as viable alternatives for labor induction.

 Complementary Care: *Alternative Methods for Induction of Labor*

Several nonpharmacological methods or alternative methods have been used to induce labor. Herbal remedies such as black haw, primrose oil, black and blue cohosh, chamomile, and red raspberry leaves are prescribed as labor inducers in some cultures. Technically these substances are medicinal agents with some properties similar to those of oxytocin. Use of these agents creates problems because of the lack of scientific research and validation of their effectiveness. Much of the information about how they work is anecdotal, which also makes it difficult to evaluate the risks and the benefits, critical information for patients and their health-care providers. Nonherbal methods include acupuncture, the ingestion of a laxative (e.g., castor oil), a soapsuds enema, and the stripping of membranes (Agency for Healthcare Research and Quality [AHRQ], 2013).

ELECTIVE INDUCTION AND EARLY TERM BIRTH

Defined as a birth that occurs at 37 to 38 weeks of gestation, early term birth is frequently elective and accompanied by a host of health risks (e.g., need for specialized neonatal care, respiratory complications, feeding and learning difficulties, and death) to infants who are born 1 to 3 weeks short of term. Many early term births occur because of preventable elective induction, despite the recommendation from the American College of Obstetricians and Gynecologists (ACOG) (2009) that no elective delivery occur prior to 39 weeks of gestation. In a 2014 AWHONN position statement, AWHONN advocated for the implementation of policies that limit non-medically indicated induction and augmentation of labor, that support spontaneous labor when the mother and fetus are healthy, and that increase funding for research and education related to spontaneous and induced labor.

In many settings, however, it is common practice for providers to offer elective induction to pregnant women who have reached term gestation. For some, early term delivery is viewed as a convenience of modern life, and women who eagerly accept it may be unaware of the potential short- and long-term risks to their infants. Women may also be confused about what constitutes "full term." In one study (Goldenberg,

McClure, Bhattacharya, Groat, & Stahl, 2009), slightly more than half of the participants believed that full term was 37 to 38 weeks, and only one-fourth considered 39 to 40 weeks' gestation as full term. It is incumbent on nurses who work with childbearing-age women to educate them about fetal development, the risks of early term birth, and the prevention of non–medically indicated delivery before 39 weeks (AWHONN, 2014; Craighead, 2012; Simpson, 2010; Simpson, Kortz, & Knox, 2009; Simpson, Newman, & Chirino, 2010). Development and implementation of an institutional induction scheduling procedure and consent form has been shown to be an important strategy for eliminating elective induction of labor at less than 39 weeks of gestation (Doyle, Kenny, von Gruenigen, Butz, & Burkett, 2012).

 Across Care Settings: **AWHONN's GoTheFull40 campaign to promote full-term births**

In 2012, the Association of Obstetric, Gynecologic and Neonatal Nurses (AWHONN) launched an educational campaign (www.GoTheFull40.com) to help women understand why it is important to carry their babies to term. The "40 Reasons to Go the Full 40" are divided into three different categories: "Finish healthy and well"; "Manage your risks"; and "Enjoy this time"—with important related tips in each category. AWHONN encourages nurses and other health-care providers and mother/baby advocates to share the campaign with women.

NURSING CONSIDERATIONS

The nurse's responsibilities during labor induction or augmentation begins with obtaining informed consent for the procedure after physician explanation. Patient education regarding the procedure and its consequences is critical. Monitoring of the labor is essential because uterine tachysystole may lead to uterine rupture. Oxytocin protocols in many institutions require that the nurse remain at the patient's bedside at all times for careful surveillance. The following data should be placed on a flow sheet in the patient record:

- Patient's vital signs (blood pressure, pulse, and respirations every 30 to 60 minutes and with every increment in medication dose)
- FHR (via electronic monitoring)
- Frequency, duration, and strength of contractions (note contraction pattern and uterine resting tone every 15 minutes and with every increment in medication dose during first stage; then monitor every 5 minutes during second stage)
- Cervical effacement and dilation
- Fetal station and lie
- Rate of oxytocin infusion
- Intake and urine output (limit intravenous fluid intake to 1,000 mL/8 hr; output should be 120 mL or more every 4 hours)
- Any untoward effect of the medication administration (nausea, vomiting, headache, or hypotension)
- Psychological response of the patient (ACOG, 2009; Felton, 2011; Gilbert, 2010; Simpson & Creehan, 2013).

Critical Nursing Action Recognizing and Responding to Problems During Labor Induction With Oxytocin

According to the AWHONN (2010a), patients receiving the high-alert medication oxytocin should have a 1:1 nurse-to-patient ratio. During induction of labor with oxytocin, the nurse remains critically alert to signs indicative of complications such as uterine tachysystole, especially when coupled with a non-reassuring FHR pattern, and suspected uterine rupture. Management of tachysystole generally involves efforts to reduce uterine activity to minimize the risk of evolving fetal hypoxemia or acidemia. Immediate emergency measures include discontinuing the oxytocin per institutional protocol, positioning the patient on her side, IV fluid bolus and/or increasing the primary IV rate up to 200 mL/hr (unless there is evidence of water intoxication—in this situation, the rate is decreased to one that keeps the vein open), administering oxygen by face mask at 8 to 10 L/min or per physician order or institutional protocol, and preparing to administer tocolytic medications (e.g., terbutaline) per physician order or institutional protocol (ACOG, 2010; Doyle et al., 2011).

The nurse needs to discuss pain relief options with the patient before oxytocin administration. The information presented should include prescribed medications as well as natural options. If the woman declines pharmacological analgesia or anesthesia, the nurse must work closely with her and her support person in the effective use of relaxation and breathing techniques. The woman placed on bedrest as a result of the induction needs frequent position changes. Massage may enhance her comfort during the procedure. The nurse should keep the patient and her support person informed of her progress because this information reassures the patient and gives her confidence.

 Now Can You—Discuss labor induction?

1. Identify eight indicators for labor induction?
2. Explain the relationship between the Bishop score and induction of labor?
3. Identify and discuss the implications of pertinent data recorded on the maternal flow sheet during labor induction with oxytocin?

Where Research and Practice Meet:
Normal Progress of Induced and Augmented Labor

Harper and colleagues (2012) conducted a retrospective cohort study of over 5,000 women who experienced spontaneous (n=2,000), augmented (n=1,700), or induced labor (n=1,650) at term to compare the progress of labor for each group. Their findings revealed that nulliparous and multiparous women who undergo induction of labor and reach complete cervical dilation are in labor for a longer period of time than women in spontaneous labor, as a result of a slower rate of cervical dilation between 4 and 6 cm. Interestingly, after 6 cm, women have similar rates of cervical dilation. The labor progress for women who are augmented with oxytocin closely resembles the induction of labor group before 6 cm, and these women also progress more slowly through labor as compared with the spontaneous labor group. Nurses can use this information to guide patient care and education for women undergoing labor induction and augmentation.

ASSISTED/OPERATIVE VAGINAL DELIVERY

Forceps and vacuum extraction are used to decrease the length of the second stage of labor when indicated because of maternal exhaustion or epidural anesthesia, suspected fetal distress, and the need to rotate the fetal head. In the United States, there has been a decrease in the overall use of instrumentation as a birth assist while there has been an increase in operative deliveries. Speculation as to the reason for this trend has been attributed to a fear of malpractice related to complications associated with the methods as well as a lack of physicians' training in the use of delivery instrumentation (Nielson & Galan, 2012).

According to the ACOG (2000, reaffirmed 2012), the following indications for operative vaginal delivery apply when the fetal head is engaged and the cervix is fully dilated.

- Prolonged second stage:
  - Nulliparous women: lack of continuing progress for 3 hours with regional anesthesia or 2 hours without regional anesthesia
  - Multiparous women: lack of continuing progress for 2 hours with regional anesthesia or 1 hour without regional anesthesia
- Suspicion of immediate or potential fetal compromise
- Shortening of the second stage for maternal benefit

Forceps-Assisted Birth

A forceps-assisted birth is one in which a steel instrument with two curved blades is used to facilitate the birth of the infant's head. **Forceps** is an instrument consisting of cephalic-curved blades similar to the shape of the fetal head (Fig. 14-5). The two blades slide together at the shaft to form a handle. The first blade is inserted into the maternal vagina next to the fetal head. The second blade is then inserted and applied to the opposite side of the fetal head. The shafts of the forceps are brought together in the midline and secured to form a handle. Forceps prevent pressure from being exerted on the fetal head and facilitate birth.

Maternal indications for a forceps-assisted birth include a need to shorten the second stage of labor for the following reasons: dystocia, an inability to push with contractions (e.g., because of exhaustion, spinal or epidural anesthesia, or spinal cord injury), and to prevent worsening of serious medical complications such as cardiac compensation. Fetal indications include an abnormal presentation, arrest of rotation, immaturity, and distress from a complication such as prolapsed cord.

There are various applications and several different types of forceps for forceps-assisted birth. Outlet forceps are used when the fetal scalp is visible on the maternal perineum without manual separation of the labia. Low forceps are used when the fetal head is at a +2 station or more. Midforceps are used when the fetal head is engaged but at less than a +2 station. Because birth trauma has been associated with the use of midforceps, this procedure has been largely replaced by cesarean birth, which poses less risk to the fetus. Forceps are never applied to an unengaged presenting part. Piper forceps are used to facilitate delivery of the head in a breech birth. Some form of anesthesia is administered before forceps application to achieve pelvic relaxation and decrease pain. An episiotomy is usually performed

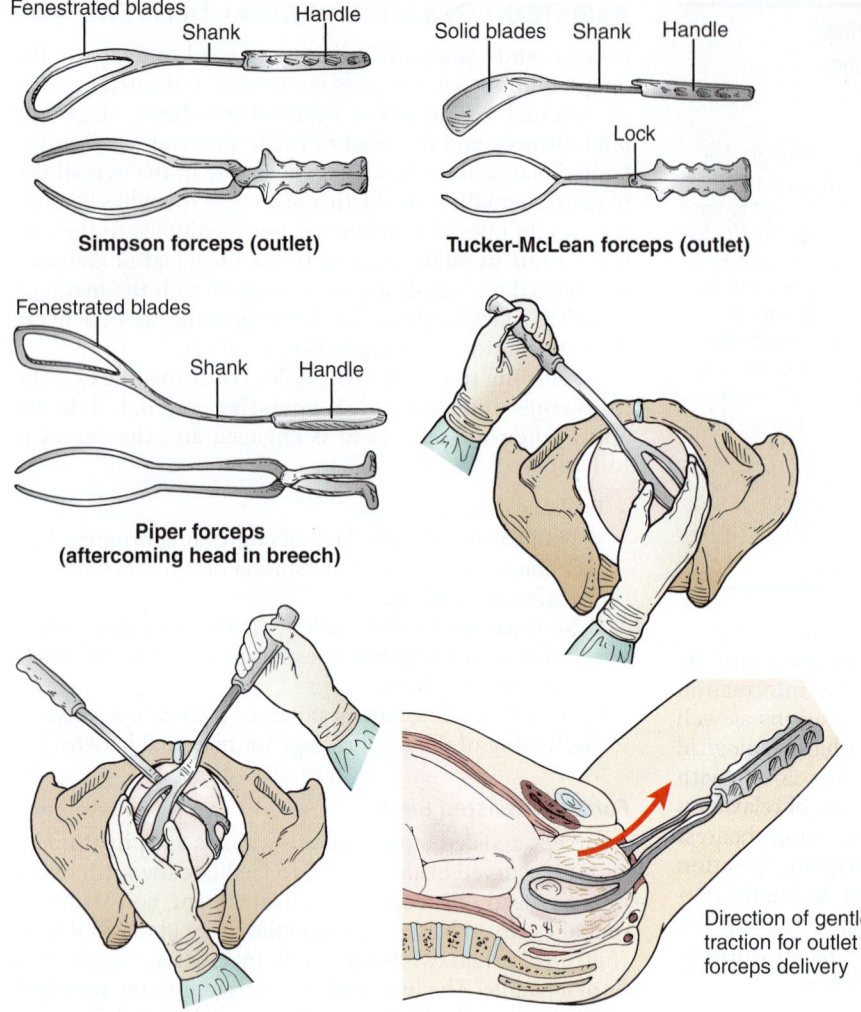

Simpson forceps (outlet)

Tucker-McLean forceps (outlet)

Piper forceps
(aftercoming head in breech)

Direction of gentle traction for outlet forceps delivery

Figure 14-5 Forceps are instruments with curved blades that are used to facilitate the birth of the fetal head.

to prevent perineal tearing. Before forceps application, the following criteria must be met:

- The cervix must be fully dilated; bladder empty; presenting part engaged
- The membranes must be ruptured
- Cephalopelvic disproportion (CPD) must not be present
- Informed consent must be obtained

 Critical Nursing Action When Attending a Forceps-Assisted Birth

The FHR and pattern is assessed and recorded before the forceps application. When the forceps are applied, there is a danger of compression of the cord between the fetal head and the forceps blade. Cord compression causes a decrease in FHR. Therefore, assess and record the FHR and pattern again *immediately* after the forceps application.

Perineal trauma is one of the major complications associated with the use of forceps. Because hemorrhage may result from cervical lacerations and vaginal tearing, the woman requires close observation during the postpartum period. To rule out maternal bladder injury, the nurse documents the time and amount of the first postbirth voiding. Some women have reported fecal incontinence following forceps injury. Women who experience forceps-related problems may suffer

fear and anxiety regarding the birth experience in subsequent pregnancies (Nielson & Galan, 2012).

Fetal morbidity occurs in direct response to occipital trauma. Superficial scalp and facial markings are the most common complications and are rarely significant. However, it is important for the nurse to clearly discuss this possibility with the family. Once the parents understand that the trauma marks gradually disappear, they are usually more accepting of the baby's (usually) superficial injuries. Other forceps-related complications that rarely occur include facial nerve injury, cephalhematoma (or cephalohematoma), retinal hemorrhage, and ocular trauma. Neonatal intracranial bleeding is a major concern, but it is often difficult to ascertain whether the hemorrhage resulted from the forceps or was related to the difficult birth (ACOG, 2000; Nielson & Galan, 2012).

Now Can You—Discuss issues surrounding the use of forceps?

1. Identify three maternal indications and three fetal indications for a forceps-assisted birth?
2. Describe maternal–fetal complications associated with the use of forceps instrumentation?
3. Discuss key information the nurse provides the parents regarding a forceps-assisted birth?

Vacuum-Assisted Birth

Vacuum-assisted birth, also termed vacuum extraction, is an alternative method used in an assisted vaginal delivery. The vacuum extractor consists of a soft plastic cup that is attached to the fetal head over the posterior fontanelle and a suction apparatus that uses negative pressure to facilitate the birth of the head (Fig. 14-6). This modality is used for a patient who is unable to voluntarily push during the second stage of labor (most often because of exhaustion or pharmacological agents), fetal distress, or failure to progress. The same conditions apply to the use of the vacuum as for forceps: vertex presentation, ruptured membranes, and absence of CPD. Vacuum-assisted birth has certain advantages over forceps-assisted birth: little anesthesia is required (the fetus is less depressed at birth), and it is associated with fewer lacerations of the maternal birth canal. Vacuum extraction should not be used following fetal scalp blood sampling. The suction pressure can cause excessive bleeding at the sampling site. It is also not recommended for preterm fetuses whose skulls are extremely soft (ACOG, 2000).

To prepare the patient for a vacuum-assisted birth, the nurse provides education and support and encourages the woman's continued participation in childbirth by pushing during contractions. The FHR and pattern are assessed before and throughout the procedure. The nurse assists the woman to a lithotomy position to allow sufficient traction. The primary care provider applies the cup to the fetal head, and a caput (swelling of the soft tissue) develops inside the cup as the pressure is initiated (Fig. 14-7). Gentle traction is applied to facilitate descent of the fetal head. An episiotomy may be performed as the head crowns.

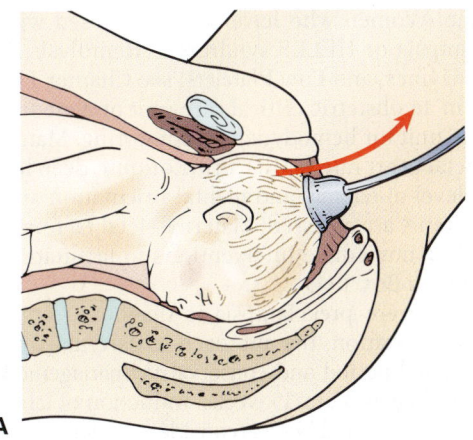

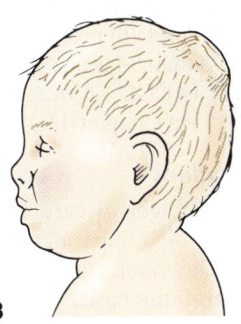

Figure 14-7 *A,* Vacuum extractor is applied with a downward and outward traction. *B,* A caput succedaneum, or chignon, is formed from the suction cup.

> 🅢 **legal alert—Assume nursing responsibilities associated with a vacuum-assisted birth**
>
> The nurse is responsible for patient education and support during a vacuum-assisted procedure. The perinatal team must communicate frequently during the procedure as they each assess progress or the lack of progress. The nurse, following protocols, can advocate for cesarean birth if maternal exhaustion and/or failure of descent indicates that the vacuum assistance is not effective. If the nurse fails to communicate concerns and there is an untoward event, the nurse can be held liable. Liability is also incurred if the nurse fails to document a detailed sequence of events (e.g., number of applications, number of pulls, occurrence of *pop-offs*, and maximum amount of suction applied) during the vacuum assistance along with the maternal–fetal response. After an assisted birth, the nurse who assesses the neonate is also liable with regard to the documentation of vital signs and the neonatal assessment.

The caput that has formed on the neonate's scalp begins to disappear in several hours but may persist for up to 7 days after birth. Appropriate education of the parents before the vacuum application helps them to understand that the caput swelling is not harmful to the infant and the markings will decrease rapidly. Potential neonatal complications include cephalhematoma (or cephalohematoma), subgaleal hematoma, subdural hematoma, intracranial hemorrhage, scalp lacerations, and retinal hemorrhage. The infant should be carefully observed for signs of trauma and infection at the application site, and jaundice may develop as tissue damage resolves (ACOG, 2000).

Maternal Conditions That Complicate Childbirth

HYPERTENSIVE DISORDERS

Management of hypertensive disorders during parturition is based on two goals: preventing further deterioration of affected organs and fostering a positive maternal–infant

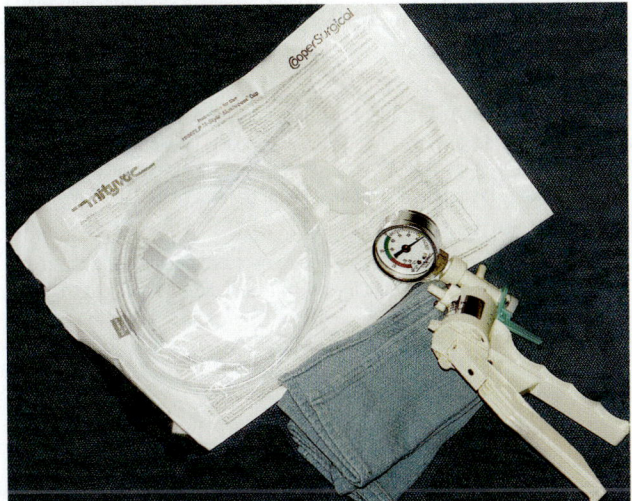

Figure 14-6 Vacuum device.

outcome. Women who have been diagnosed with severe preeclampsia or HELLP syndrome (**H**emolysis, **E**levated **L**iver enzymes, and **L**ow **P**latelets; see Chapter 11) may be placed in an obstetric critical care unit or a medical intensive care unit for hemodynamic monitoring. Maternal vital signs, fetal heart rate (FHR), urine output, deep tendon reflexes, level of edema, and mental orientation and neurological status are assessed. Maternal–fetal factors that may necessitate immediate interventions to facilitate birth are presented in Box 14-3.

When severe preeclampsia is diagnosed at less than 34 weeks' gestation, the approach to care may include an observational period and conservative management. If the gestational age is 32 to 35 weeks, induction of labor is usually initiated. Vaginal birth is considered safer than cesarean birth and is attempted if cervical favorability is present. Antenatal glucocorticoids such as betamethasone may be given (12 mg IM 24 hours apart) to promote lung maturity if the gestational age is less than 34 weeks and delivery can be delayed for 48 hours (ACOG, 2002a; Cunningham et al., 2014; Sibai, 2012). (See Chapter 11.)

Nursing Considerations

The nurse is the manager of care for the woman with preeclampsia during the intrapartal period. Careful assessments are critical. The nurse plans and evaluates all interventions on a continuous basis. The patient with severe preeclampsia is in an extremely fragile condition. Because any change in condition may require an emergency intervention, the nurse must be prepared to provide the necessary care immediately. The nurse is responsible for the continuous monitoring of several key parameters (Box 14-4). Laboratory tests include a complete blood count (CBC) with platelets, coagulation profile to assess for disseminated intravascular coagulation (DIC), metabolic studies for determination of liver enzymes (aspartate aminotransferase [AST], alanine aminotransferase [ALT], and lactate dehydrogenase [LDH]) and electrolyte studies to establish renal functioning (ACOG, 2002a). (See Chapter 11 for further discussion.)

Box 14-3 **Factors That May Necessitate Immediate Intervention to Facilitate Birth in Patients With Hypertensive Disorders**

- Uncontrolled severe hypertension
- Eclampsia
- Persistent oliguria (greater than 500 mL/24 hr)
- Abruptio placentae
- Platelet count less than 100,000/mm³
- Elevated liver enzyme levels with epigastric pain or right upper quadrant tenderness
- Pulmonary edema
- Persistent severe headache or visual changes
- Spontaneous labor
- Fetal death
- Rupture of the membranes
- Gestational age less than 34 weeks (an observational period may be initially attempted as a conservative management approach)
- Evidence of fetal compromise

Box 14-4 Intrapartal Nursing Care for Patients With Preeclampsia

BLOOD PRESSURE

The blood pressure is taken every 4 hours or more frequently according to physician orders or institutional protocol. Blood pressure should be taken in the same arm at each assessment. Encourage the patient to assume a side-lying position to enhance uterine perfusion. Record the data. Notify the physician of an increase in blood pressure.

MEDICATION ADMINISTRATION

Administer medication as ordered and evaluate its effect. Adhere to hospital protocol for magnesium sulfate infusion. Monitor maternal vital signs, FHR & pattern, urine output, deep tendon reflexes (DTRs), IV flow rate, and serum magnesium levels to assess for magnesium sulfate toxicity (e.g., depressed respirations, hyporeflexia, sudden onset of hypotension, oliguria, and indicators of fetal compromise). Administer calcium gluconate (the antidote for magnesium sulfate toxicity) for respirations below 12 breaths/min and discontinue the magnesium sulfate infusion.

RENAL BALANCE

Edema is rated on a scale of 1 to 4. A score of 4 is generalized massive edema that includes the face, abdomen, and sacrum. Assess and record urinary output. An indwelling urinary catheter may be inserted to more accurately measure urinary output. A urine output less than 30 mL/hr is indicative of oliguria, and the physician must be notified. A dipstick measurement is performed every 4 hours or more frequently to assess urinary protein on a scale of 1–4. A dipstick reading over 2+ is indicative of a worsening condition.

NEUROLOGICAL STATUS

DTRs are assessed every 4 hours (or more frequently) and rated on a scale of 1 to 4. Reflexes greater than 2+ signify worsening status. If dorsiflexion of the foot produces clonus (convulsive spasm), this finding provides an additional indication of a deteriorating maternal condition.

PULMONARY STATUS

Auscultation of the lungs is performed every 4 hours (or more frequently) to assess for dyspnea, crackles, and diminished breath sounds, which may be indicative of pulmonary edema. The respiratory rate is assessed every 4 hours (or more frequently, according to institutional protocol). Patients who are receiving magnesium sulfate require more frequent respiratory assessments because a respiratory rate below 12 is an indicator of magnesium toxicity. Hemoglobin oxygen saturation can be assessed with a pulse oximeter.

PSYCHOLOGICAL STATUS

Assess the woman for indicators of anxiety and fear. Provide information to the patient and family about the treatment protocols and status of the maternal condition. Assess their level of understanding and provide updates when indicated.

ADVANCING SYMPTOMS

Headaches, blurred vision, severe right upper quadrant epigastric pain, and restlessness are all indicators of impending eclampsia. Prepare for immediate delivery.

SEIZURES

Protect the patient. Keep the airway patent: turn head to one side and place a pillow or folded linen under one shoulder or back. Call for assistance. Ensure that the side rails have been raised. Observe and document all seizure activity. Notify the physician and prepare for delivery. Administer oxygen.

FETAL STATUS

Monitor the FHR and pattern every 4 hours or more frequently as indicated. Assess fetal movements. Notify the physician if indicators of fetal compromise are noted.

The nurse must also monitor the laboratory values for impending HELLP syndrome during labor. The nurse follows the plan of care for the patient with severe preeclampsia.

Where Research and Practice Meet:
Magnesium Sulfate and Fetal Heart Rate
Patterns

Duffy and colleagues (2012) conducted a 4-year retrospective cohort study of over 5,300 consecutive term deliveries to examine the effect of maternal exposure to magnesium sulfate on FHR characteristics during active labor. FHR tracings of women exposed to magnesium for severe preeclampsia (n=248) were compared with FHR tracings of women not exposed to magnesium (n=5,139). Data analysis revealed that maternal exposure to magnesium is associated with a lower fetal heart rate baseline within the accepted normal range (110–160 beats per minute [bpm]), decreased variability, and fewer prolonged decelerations without evidence of adverse effect on neonatal outcome. Based on their findings, the investigators suggested that magnesium, a CNS depressant, blunts the fetal response toward tachycardia, marked variability, and prolonged decelerations and may mask signs of fetal distress.

Special precautions need to be considered to prevent adverse outcomes in a patient with the HELLP syndrome who requires a cesarean birth. The nurse is responsible for administering 5 to 10 units of platelets on the physician's order before the birth to prevent thrombocytopenia. Providing ongoing information to the patient and her family is an essential nursing intervention to help decrease anxiety and fear (Sibai, 2012).

CARDIAC DISEASE

Recent years have shown a decline in the traditional causes of maternal death: hemorrhage, hypertension, and pulmonary embolism but an ominous increase in cardiac-related deaths. Heart disease now complicates more than 1% of pregnancies and is the leading cause of indirect maternal deaths. This trend is most likely related to several factors: the dramatic improvement in survival of young girls who received surgical correction for congenital heart disease and are now of reproductive age; delayed childbearing, which has produced increased numbers of mothers over the age of 40 years; and the rising epidemic of obesity among children and adults (Lockwood, 2011; Simpson, 2012).

The physiological demands that accompany normal intrapartum events make this an especially critical time for patients with cardiac disease. During labor, pain and anxiety combined with uterine contractions result in further increases in maternal heart rate, stroke volume, cardiac output, and blood pressure. Because of the risk of vena cava compression and decreased venous return from the weight of the gravid uterus, nurses should avoid placing the patient in a supine position for procedures such as cervical examinations or bladder catheterization. Increased hemodynamic and oxidative cardiac stress occur during the second stage of labor, and the 500 mL maternal autotransfusion that occurs after delivery of the placenta may not be tolerated. As a result, the patient's fluid balance must be closely monitored during the immediate postpartum period, which frequently is a time of acute decompensation (Harris, 2011; Simpson, 2012)

DIABETES MELLITUS

Women with the metabolic disorder of diabetes mellitus that is under control may safely give birth spontaneously at term provided there are no indications of severe cephalopelvic

disproportion (CPD). When a possibility of CPD exists, the diabetic woman may be given a trial of labor. If successful, a cesarean birth, which always presents a higher risk than a vaginal birth for the fetus, has been avoided.

Nursing Insight—*Recognizing medical indications for elective preterm birth in women with diabetes mellitus*

As long as she remains in good metabolic control and all parameters of fetal surveillance are within normal limits, the woman whose pregnancy is complicated by diabetes may safely carry the pregnancy to 38.5 to 40 weeks of gestation. However, the presence of poor metabolic control, a worsening hypertensive disorder, fetal macrosomia (often defined as weight greater than 4,000 g), or fetal growth restriction are all indications for elective preterm birth (ACOG, 2013a; Cunningham et al., 2014).

The physician may plan an elective induction of labor between 38 and 40 weeks of gestation. An amniocentesis performed between 37 and 38.5 weeks of gestation is performed to confirm fetal lung maturity. In the pregnancy complicated by diabetes mellitus, an amniotic fluid phosphatidyl glycerol level greater than 3% is a better predictor of fetal lung maturation than an amniotic fluid lecithin/sphingomyelin ratio (3:1). If the fetal lungs are immature, birth may be delayed as long as all parameters of the maternal and fetal assessment remain reassuring (Moore, Hauguel deMouzon, & Catalano, 2013). (See Chapter 11.)

Intrapartum management for the woman with pregestational diabetes centers on the close surveillance of maternal hydration and blood glucose levels to prevent complications associated with dehydration, hypoglycemia, and hyperglycemia. An intravenous infusion of a maintenance fluid such as lactated Ringer's solution or 5% dextrose in lactated Ringer's solution may be ordered. Insulin is usually administered by continuous infusion; only regular insulin may be administered intravenously. In some situations, patients who use continuous subcutaneous insulin infusion (insulin pump) are closely monitored and allowed to continue the therapy throughout labor and birth. Blood glucose levels are assessed every hour and fluid/insulin adjustments are made as needed to maintain maternal blood glucose levels between 80 and 120 mg/dL. It is essential that maternal hyperglycemia during the intrapartal period be avoided to prevent neonatal metabolic problems such as hypoglycemia (deValk & Visser, 2011; Hood, 2012).

The laboring patient is maintained in an upright or side-lying position with continuous FHR monitoring. Nursing care involves close surveillance for indicators of normal labor progression along with a stable maternal–fetal unit. Failure to progress may be related to fetal macrosomia or CPD and necessitate a cesarean birth. Diabetes-related complications such as hyperglycemia, ketosis, and ketoacidosis may develop and must be promptly managed. Shoulder dystocia associated with fetal macrosomia may complicate the second stage of labor. A team that consists of the obstetrician and neonatologist, pediatrician, or neonatal nurse practitioner should attend the birth to provide immediate neonatal assessment and care.

When a cesarean birth has been planned, the surgery is scheduled for the early morning to achieve optimal glycemic control. Depending on physician orders, the nurse may be instructed to withhold the morning insulin. Other protocols allow administration of an intermediate-acting insulin in the morning and every 8 hours until surgery. The patient is allowed nothing by mouth. Epidural anesthesia is preferred because hypoglycemia can be detected earlier if the woman remains awake. After the surgery, maternal blood glucose levels are assessed at least every 2 hours; target plasma levels are between 80 and 160 mg/dL (deValk & Visser, 2011; Hood, 2012).

The first 24 hours postpartum are remarkable for the dramatic decrease in insulin requirements that occurs after removal of the placenta. Depending on the amount of food consumed, women with type I diabetes may require only one-fourth to one-third of the prenatal insulin dose. Some women may not require insulin for 24 to 72 hours postpartum. Throughout the postpartal period, blood glucose levels continue to be monitored, and insulin dosage adjustments are made as needed, often using a sliding scale (deValk & Visser, 2011).

 Nursing Insight—*Increased risk of postpartal complications in diabetic women*

Women whose pregnancies have been complicated by diabetes have an increased risk for complications such as preeclampsia/eclampsia, hemorrhage, and infection (e.g., endometritis) during the postpartal period. Hemorrhage is more likely if the uterus was overdistended because of fetal macrosomia or hydramnios (see Chapter 16).

The nurse should encourage mothers with pregestational and gestational diabetes to breastfeed. However, because glucose levels are lower, especially during early postpartum, breastfeeding women are at an increased risk for hypoglycemia. Also, the mother with poor metabolic control may have a delay in lactogenesis that results in decreased milk production.

Discharge planning for women with diabetes should include discussion about contraceptive information as appropriate. Because women with gestational diabetes are at increased risk for developing diabetes later in life, the nurse should counsel them about the importance of maintaining a healthy weight and undergoing glucose testing during routine health maintenance visits.

PRETERM LABOR AND BIRTH

Preterm labor that is not arrested leads to preterm birth. In the United States, preterm birth has increased over the last decade despite the use of preventive pharmacological therapies. Approximately 12% of all live births occur before term, and preterm labor precedes over half of them. Preterm births account for around 70% of neonatal deaths, 36% of infant deaths, and up to 50% of cases of long-term neurological impairment in children (ACOG, 2012a).

 Cultural Diversity: Preterm Labor and Birth

Race and ethnicity cannot be disregarded in any discussion of preterm labor. African American women are at a higher risk for preterm birth than are Caucasian women. When preterm birth rates of married, educated African American women are compared with those of matched Caucasian women, a disparity continues to be noted in the African American women. The increase in cases of preterm labor results in a greater percentage of infant mortality in the African American population (Simhan, Iams, & Romero, 2012).

The causes for preterm birth are often a series of overlapping conditions such as premature rupture of membranes combined with cervical insufficiency. Premature rupture of the membranes accounts for approximately 3% of all preterm births. In many cases, patients experience "silent" (asymptomatic) uterine contractions throughout pregnancy that contribute to progressive cervical effacement and dilation (see Chapter 11).

Although interventions including bedrest, hydration, and tocolytic therapy (for up to 48 hours to allow for administration of antenatal steroids) are used to inhibit contractions, in many situations the labor cannot be halted. If the woman's membranes have ruptured or if the cervix is greater than 50% effaced and 3 to 4 cm dilated, it is unlikely that the labor can be stopped. If the fetus is very immature and birth is deemed to be inevitable, a cesarean birth may be planned to reduce pressure on the fetal head and decrease the possibility of a subdural or intraventricular hemorrhage.

Nursing Considerations

In addition to careful maternal monitoring, FHR monitoring is one of the most important nursing responsibilities when caring for a patient in preterm labor. A number of perinatal complications such as preeclampsia, intra-amniotic infection, oligohydramnios, umbilical cord compression, placental abruption, intrauterine growth restriction, uteroplacental insufficiency, and multiple gestation occur more often with preterm labor. This combination of complications may result in FHR patterns that differ from the norm. Because of the increased incidence of neurological deficits in premature infants, it is essential that the nurse be able to identify and report data suggestive of hypoxia as early as possible (Simpson & O'Brien-Abel, 2013).

Best clinical practice for fetal monitoring begins with correct application of the tocodynamometer and the fetal heart monitor. Leopold maneuvers are used to identify the fetal back and presenting part. Because multiple gestations are often associated with preterm labor, it is important to identify and monitor each fetus. The tocodynamometer needs to be placed at the height of fundus to ensure the best interpretation of the labor contractions (Simpson & O'Brien-Abel, 2013).

 Optimizing Outcomes—**Providing pain relief during preterm labor and birth**

The length of the first stage of labor for a woman who is preterm is essentially the same as for a woman with a full-term gestation although the second stage may be shorter—the smaller fetal size can be pushed through the dilated cervix more easily. Maternal analgesia is used cautiously because of the immaturity of the fetus, who may have considerable difficulty breathing without the additional burden of sedative effects from maternal analgesic agents. If the patient desires analgesia, the nurse can explain why epidural pain relief is most likely preferable. An episiotomy is often performed at the time of birth to lessen trauma on the fragile fetal head; forceps may also be used.

Because of the patient's medical complications and related fetal issues, she and her support person often experience increased anxiety and fear during the labor and birth. The nurse is there to offer clinical expertise; provide a calming presence; and inform, support, and assist the patient and her partner throughout the birth experience. A careful assessment of the patient's psychological status can help direct the care. Expressions of caring coupled with dialog that includes specific questions help to identify the patient's main concerns.

 Optimizing Outcomes—**Exploring concerns of the woman experiencing preterm labor**

The nurse should use active listening and remain nearby. The patient should be encouraged to participate in decision making as much as possible throughout the labor process. Women who have anticipated an uncomplicated labor and birth experience often feel out of control when events occur that differ from their expectations. The nurse can play a vital role in keeping the patient informed and helping her to remain an active participant throughout the birth process. One approach involves teaching the patient and her partner what to expect during each phase and how they can help one another throughout the process. If the patient so wishes, the nurse involves the support person in the care as much as possible.

 Cultural Diversity: Minority Women and Level of Care Received

The Agency for Healthcare Research and Quality (2010) reported that minorities do not receive the same level of quality care as do Caucasian Americans. A nurse working in the birth unit needs to be attentive to this problem. It is incumbent on all nurses to advocate for patients any time there appears to be an ethnic bias in treatment. The nurse also must be aware of any personal prejudices that could affect care. In institutions that serve minority populations, it is essential that all hospital staff members undergo frequent in-service educational offerings that focus on heightening cultural sensitivity.

 Now Can You—**Discuss aspects of various maternal conditions that complicate childbirth?**

1. Discuss critical aspects of intrapartal care for the woman with diabetes mellitus?
2. Describe one critical nursing responsibility in the patient experiencing a non-arrested preterm labor?
3. Identify three teaching needs for the patient experiencing preterm labor and birth?

Complications of Labor and Birth Associated With the Fetus

FETAL MALPRESENTATION

Malpresentations are all presentations of the fetus other than vertex. Fetal malpresentation is the second most commonly reported complication of labor and birth. The fetal occiput is the most favorable presenting part for a vaginal birth, and in most situations, the fetal head engages in the occipito-anterior position. Face, brow, shoulder, compound, and breech constitute malpresentations. A breech presentation in which the buttocks or legs present first occurs in approximately 3% of all births and is considered the most common malpresentation (see Chapter 12). It is important that these conditions be identified during the antepartum period because a malpresentation may place the woman and fetus at risk for complications during labor and birth. Diagnosis is made by abdominal palpation (i.e., Leopold maneuvers) and vaginal examination and is usually confirmed by ultrasonography.

During labor, descent of the fetus in a breech presentation may be slow (Fig. 14-8). This is because the breech is not as effective as a dilating wedge as the fetal head. There is an increased risk of prolapsed cord if the membranes rupture during early labor.

 Nursing Insight—*Breech presentation and meconium in the amniotic fluid*

When the fetus is in a breech presentation, the presence of meconium in the amniotic fluid may not be indicative of fetal distress. Pressure exerted on the fetal abdomen during the birth process may cause the passage of meconium. It is important to assess the fetal heart rate (FHR) and pattern to ensure there are changes indicative of fetal hypoxia. When the fetus is in a breech position, the FHR is best auscultated at or above the maternal umbilicus.

During the vaginal birth of a fetus in a breech presentation, the physician uses labor mechanisms that manipulate the buttocks and lower extremities. Piper forceps are sometimes applied to facilitate delivery of the head. Before the birth, the physician may attempt an external cephalic version to rotate the fetus to a vertex presentation (see later discussion). Cesarean birth is commonly performed when the following circumstances exist: The fetus is estimated to be larger than 3,800 g or smaller than 1,500 g, the labor is ineffective, this is the woman's first pregnancy, or there are additional maternal–fetal complications.

Face and brow presentations are examples of **asynclitism** (the fetal head is presenting at a different angle than expected). Face and brow presentations hyperextend the neck and increase the overall circumference of the presenting part. These presentations are uncommon and are usually associated with fetal anomalies (e.g., anencephaly), macrosomia, cephalopelvic disproportion (CPD), and contractures of the maternal pelvis. Vaginal birth may be accomplished if the fetus flexes to a vertex presentation. Forceps are often used. Cesarean birth is indicated if the presentation persists, if there is evidence of fetal compromise, or if there is an arrest in the progression of labor. Shoulder and compound presentations (e.g., a hand combined with the head) contribute to fetal and vaginal trauma and usually require cesarean birth (Cunningham et al., 2014).

Version

Version (turning of a fetus from one presentation to another) may be done either externally or internally by the physician.

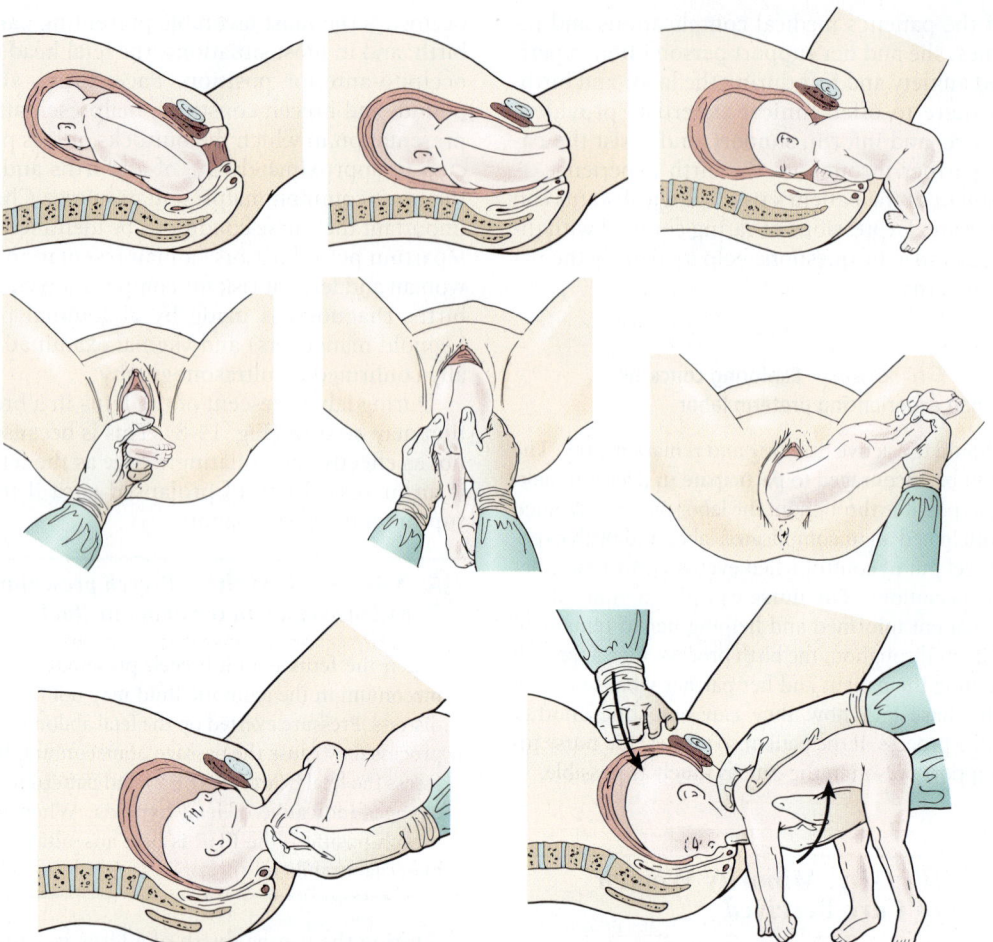

Figure 14-8 The mechanisms of labor in a breech presentation—the aftercoming fetal head delivers last.

EXTERNAL CEPHALIC VERSION. An external cephalic version (ECV) is used as an attempt to turn the fetus from a breech presentation to a vertex presentation to allow a vaginal birth (Fig. 14-9). Because cesarean birth is a major surgical procedure associated with numerous maternal and fetal risks, ECV may offer an alternative to surgery. The procedure, performed in a birth unit, may be attempted after 37 weeks of gestation. Contraindications to ECV include previous cesarean birth, uterine anomalies, CPD, placenta previa, multifetal gestation, and oligohydramnios (Cunningham et al., 2014).

Before the version, ultrasonography is obtained to confirm the fetal position; locate the umbilical cord; rule out placenta previa; and assess the maternal pelvic dimensions and the amniotic fluid volume, fetal size and gestational age, and the presence of anomalies. Before the version, a nonstress test (NST) is performed to confirm fetal well-being, or the FHR and pattern may be electronically monitored for a brief period (e.g., 10–20 minutes). Some experts have proposed the use of regional anesthesia, which relaxes the maternal abdominal wall and improves maternal tolerance of the procedure, to enhance the success of ECV. Ultrasound guidance is used as the physician slowly applies gentle, steady pressure over the fetal head and buttocks to rotate the position. Complications associated with version include umbilical cord compression, placental abruption, maternal

hemorrhage, and fetal bradycardia (Goetzinger, Harper, Tuuli, Macones, & Colditz, 2011; Vadhera & Locksmith, 2011).

The procedure of rotating the fetus (version) requires uterine relaxation. Tocolytic agents such as magnesium sulfate or terbutaline are used to facilitate this process. Acoustic stimulation of the fetus has also resulted in successful versions (Vadhera & Locksmith, 2011).

Optimizing Outcomes—Assisting with ECV

The nurse is responsible for obtaining written informed consent from the patient after physician explanation, providing teaching regarding the procedure, administering medications as ordered, and conducting constant surveillance of the maternal–infant dyad. The patient needs to know not only that the version attempt might not be successful; she must also be aware of the associated complications that may occur such as rupture of the membranes, fetal bradycardia, and discomfort. During the version, if there is any indication of significant fetal or maternal compromise, the nurse prepares the woman for a cesarean birth. Women who are Rh(D)-negative are given $Rh_o(D)$ immune globulin because the manipulation may cause feto-maternal bleeding (Vadhera & Locksmith, 2011).

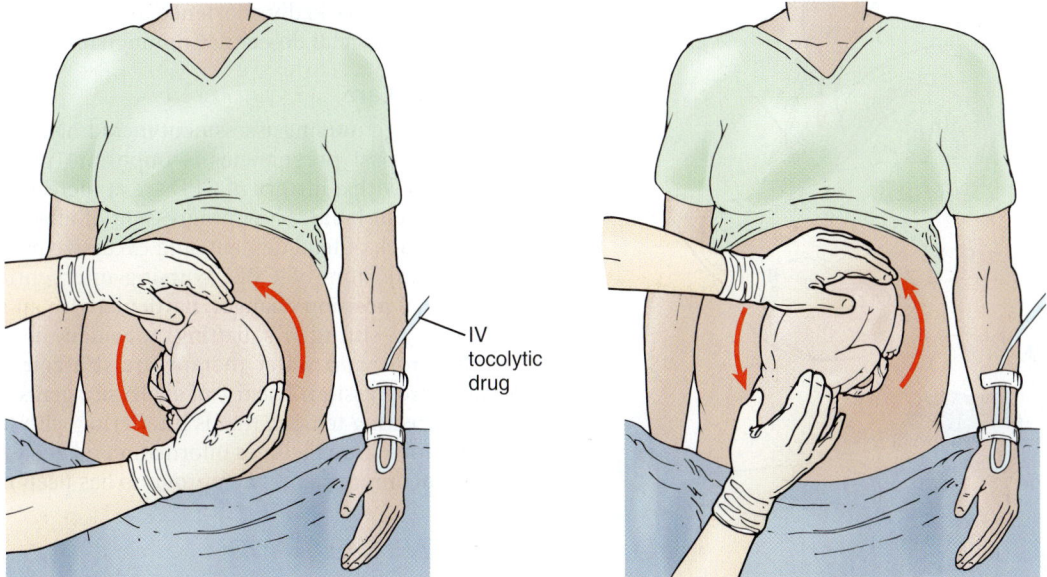

IV tocolytic drug

Figure 14-9 External cephalic version is a maneuver performed through the maternal abdominal wall in an attempt to change the fetal position from a breech to a cephalic presentation.

INTERNAL VERSION. With internal version, the physician rotates the fetus by inserting a hand into the uterus and changes the fetal presentation to cephalic (head) or podalic (foot). Internal version is used with multifetal gestations to deliver the second fetus. However, the safety of this procedure has not been documented. Cesarean birth is usually performed for malpresentation in multiple gestations. Nursing responsibilities center on maternal–fetal monitoring and providing support to the woman.

SHOULDER DYSTOCIA

Shoulder dystocia is an uncommon obstetric emergency that occurs in 0.2% to 3.0% of all births. In this type of dystocia, the head is born, but the anterior shoulder cannot pass under the maternal pubic arch. The problem is often not identified until the head is born. Risk factors for shoulder dystocia include maternal pelvic abnormalities, a history of shoulder dystocia in a previous pregnancy, obesity, diabetes, short stature, prolonged labor, postdate pregnancy, and fetal macrosomia (greater than 4,000 g) (Antoniewicz & Hollier, 2011; Ashmead, 2012; Paris, Greenberg, Ecker, & McElrath, 2011).

Although there are no methods to predict or prevent shoulder dystocia, the nurse should be alert to clinical indicators: slowed labor progression and formation of a caput succedaneum that increases in size. When the fetal head emerges on the perineum (crowning), it retracts instead of protruding with subsequent contractions (termed the *turtle sign*), and external rotation does not occur (ACOG, 2002b; Ashmead, 2012). Fetal/neonatal injuries are related to birth asphyxia, damage to the brachial plexus (e.g., Duchenne-Erb paralysis or Klumpke's paralysis), and fractures, usually of the humerus or clavicle. Maternal injury is most commonly associated with excessive blood loss that results from uterine atony or rupture; other risks include lacerations, extension of the episiotomy, rectovaginal fistula, symphyseal separation, and postpartum endometritis (Leung, Stuart, Suen, Sahota, Lau, & Lao, 2011).

A number of maneuvers have been attempted to free up the anterior shoulder and facilitate delivery. The McRoberts maneuver is one approach. The woman is placed in a dorsal lithotomy position, and her thighs are sharply flexed on her abdomen. This position increases the angle between the symphysis pubis and the sacral promontory, allowing for greater room in fetal descent. Suprapubic pressure applied immediately above the symphysis pubis may be needed along with the McRoberts maneuver to loosen the trapped shoulders (Ansell Irving, McAra-Couper, & Smythe, 2012; Ashmead, 2012; Leung et al., 2011) (Fig. 14-10).

Other methods of delivery assistance for shoulder dystocia center on maternal positional changes: a hands-and-knees position, a squatting position, or a lateral recumbent position. The use of fundal pressure is contraindicated in shoulder dystocia (Simpson & Creehan, 2013).

> **Optimizing Outcomes**—**When birth is complicated by shoulder dystocia**
>
> When childbirth is complicated by shoulder dystocia, the nurse's role is to assist the woman in assuming the positions, assist the physician with the maneuvers, and to document all procedures. The nurse also provides careful instruction to the patient to facilitate cooperation and understanding. After birth, the woman is closely observed for signs of hemorrhage and soft tissue trauma of the birth canal; the neonate is assessed for fracture of the clavicle or humerus, brachial plexus injuries, and asphyxia.

CEPHALOPELVIC DISPROPORTION

Although there are true problems that create issues between the head of the fetus and the pelvis of the mother, in the United States, **cephalopelvic disproportion** (CPD) (sometimes termed fetopelvic disproportion) is often used to describe unsuccessful attempts at vaginal birth. When CPD is present, the fetus cannot fit through the maternal

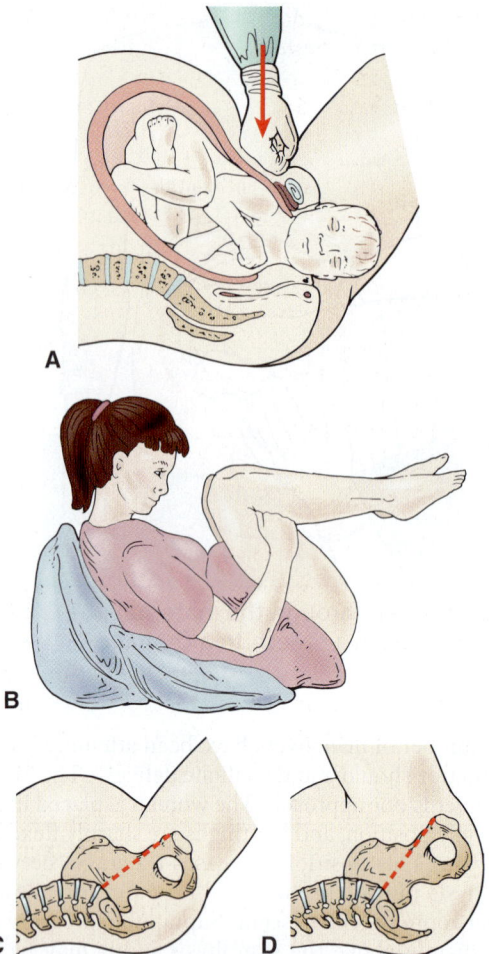

Figure 14-10 Methods to relieve shoulder dystocia. *A,* Pressure is applied immediately above the maternal symphysis pubis to push the fetal anterior shoulder downward. *B,* McRoberts maneuver: The woman's thighs are sharply flexed on her abdomen to straighten the pelvic curve. *C,* Angle of pelvis before maneuver. *D,* Angle of pelvis after maneuver.

pelvis to allow a vaginal birth. CPD is often related to excessive fetal size (macrosomia), a condition that may be associated with maternal diabetes mellitus, obesity, and multiparity. A macrosomic infant (birth weight greater than 4,000 g) is likely to have a large head that can prevent descent into the mother's pelvis.

Despite ultrasound evaluation, it is difficult to predict the safest mode of birth for the macrosomic infant. A trial of labor is suggested if the woman is nulliparous. Women with a previous history of cesarean birth for CPD may also be offered a trial of labor although a prompt cesarean birth is recommended at the earliest sign of maternal or fetal compromise.

The maternal pelvis is assessed before the onset of labor to determine type and size. A gynecoid pelvis is considered to be the most common female pelvic type and most amenable to vaginal birth although markedly small dimensions may preclude a vaginal birth. Other pelvic types are the android, anthropoid, and platypelloid (see Chapter 5 for further discussion). Although the other types of pelvises may not contraindicate a trial of labor, vaginal birth may not be possible for the woman with a platypelloid pelvis

because its markedly shortened anterior–posterior diameter prevents fetal descent (Cunningham et al., 2014).

Nursing Care

A thorough nursing assessment including a review of present and past pregnancies is important in guiding care. Women with a history of CPD are at increased risk during the present labor. Slow progression of effacement and dilation, lack of fetal descent, and excessive pain are all possible indicators of CPD. Nursing interventions such as maternal position changes, particularly to an upright posture (e.g., sitting or squatting) to widen the pelvic girdle, relaxation, and water therapy are strategies to facilitate labor progression. The use of analgesic agents may alleviate pain-creating tension that is interfering with fetal descent. Supportive care includes information related to labor status and encouragement when progress has been made.

MULTIPLE GESTATION

Managing the births of more than one fetus is complex and requires the expert collaboration of medical and nursing personnel. The gestational age, number, health, and presentation of the fetuses determine the mode of birth, whether vaginal or cesarean.

 Nursing Insight—*Fetal presentations with multiple gestations*

Both fetuses present in the vertex position (most favorable for vaginal birth) in only one-half of all twin pregnancies. In one-third of multifetal pregnancies, one twin may present in the vertex position and one in the breech position (Cunningham et al., 2014).

Multiple births are associated with more complications than singleton births. The woman's health status may be compromised by problems such as gestational hypertension, pregnancy, anemia, or gestational diabetes. She is also at increased risk for hemorrhage related to atony from uterine overdistention, abruptio placentae, and multiple or adherent placentas. Because of the multiple fetuses, abnormal fetal presentation may occur. Increased fetal/newborn complications are related primarily to problems associated with low-birth-weight infants because of preterm birth and intrauterine growth restriction. Intrapartal fetal distress may result from cord prolapse and the onset of placental separation after the birth of the first fetus. Because of these problems, the risk for long-term disabilities such as cerebral palsy is greater among multiple births (Malone & D'Alton, 2013).

Women who present at 38 weeks with a twin pregnancy are less likely than women with higher-order multiples to experience fetal morbidity and mortality and may be appropriate candidates for a vaginal birth. It is recommended, although it is not always possible, that women with a multiple gestation, particularly triplets or higher-order multiples, deliver at a tertiary care center where facilities are available in the event of an emergency. Birthing centers must have transport ready for infant transfer to neonatal intensive care units. Patients who will undergo labor or a trial of labor require careful monitoring. Ultrasound is used to determine position and presentation of the fetal parts. Electronic fetal monitoring (EFM) is applied. It is important to identify each of the individual FHRs, and the use of a separate monitor for each fetus is preferable. Interventions, such as analgesia, anesthesia, and intravenous infusions are determined on a case-by-case basis. The stimulation of labor with oxytocin, and epidural anesthesia, forceps, vacuum assistance, and fetal version may all be used to facilitate the vaginal birth of twins. Women in good health and with no evidence of fetal distress should be given the opportunity to participate in medical decision management.

When the woman is fully dilated and ready to push, she is moved to the birthing suite, where personnel, equipment, and supplies are readily available in the event there is a need for a cesarean birth. The woman may safely give birth in a labor, delivery, recovery, postpartum (LDRP) suite provided there is quick access to the surgical area. The nurse prepares the woman and her support for the possibility that she may experience both a vaginal and a cesarean birth depending on the fetal presentation. The nurse also explains the external version procedure in case this intervention is necessary. Patient education is carried out in a timely manner when the patient is capable of participation.

The majority (approximately 80%) of vertex twins are delivered with success vaginally. The first infant born is identified as "A" and neonatal care is initiated. In some settings, each infant has its own team of neonatal care providers present at the birth. In the vertex breech presentation, an external version of the second twin is attempted provided that the conditions are favorable. If the second fetus is a footling breech, has a hyperextended head, or exhibits signs of compromise, a cesarean birth is considered the better option. The birth of the second twin normally occurs within 15 minutes of the birth of the first twin. Although there has been concern over complications associated with a longer time period between births, studies have shown that with proper fetal monitoring and maternal surveillance, a safe vaginal birth can take place in an indefinite amount of time (Cunningham et al., 2014; Vadhera & Locksmith, 2011). The nurse documents the time of birth for the first infant and all subsequent infants who are born.

✿ *Across Care Settings:* Planning the multifetal birth

Together, the obstetrician, anesthesiologist, and patient discuss the anesthetic options available for childbirth. This collaborative meeting is best done in an office visit before the onset of labor. Epidural anesthesia is considered a safe method for providing relief of pain, and it allows prompt intervention in case the second twin requires an external version or a cesarean birth (Vadhera & Locksmith, 2011). The woman may experience an unmedicated birth provided she understands that if it is necessary to proceed to a cesarean birth, she will receive a general anesthetic to facilitate uterine relaxation.

Triplets and higher-order multiples generally require a cesarean birth. This mode of birth decreases the risk that the second fetus will experience anoxia as well as other complications such as cord entanglement and premature placental separation. While there are reports of triplet vaginal births, these successes are tempered with the strong possibility that both the second and third neonates may be in breech presentations and require operative

interventions. If it is deemed possible for the woman to give birth to triplets vaginally, the medical team must be on ready standby for an immediate cesarean surgery (Cunningham et al., 2014).

 Now Can You—Discuss birth options for a woman with a multifetal pregnancy?

1. Identify the factors that determine whether a woman with multiple gestation may be allowed to attempt a vaginal birth?
2. Describe the primary recommendations concerning the childbirth options available for a woman with a multifetal pregnancy?
3. Discuss controversies that surround the medical management of twin births?

NON-REASSURING FHR PATTERNS

Fetal heart monitoring is one type of assessment that provides the nurse, the patient, and her support(s) feedback concerning the well-being of the fetus. Families often request to increase the volume of the fetal monitor so that they hear the reassurance of a strong heartbeat. It is essential that the nurse understand actions that should be taken when decelerations or other ominous FHR patterns are detected (see Chapter 12).

Depending on the situation, watchful waiting with continuous monitoring conducted by the nurse may provide the best option for assessment of fetal well-being. Because non-reassuring FHR patterns constitute a risk indicator for cesarean birth, the nurse and all members of the healthcare team must be ready for this outcome at all times. It is important to provide ongoing support for the laboring woman and keep her informed of her labor progress and fetal status.

❝What to say❞—*When a non-reassuring FHR pattern is detected via electronic monitoring*

When electronic monitoring reveals a non-reassuring FHR pattern, the nurse needs to maintain a calming presence and offer factual, simple explanations for all actions. For example, the nurse may say:

"We are concerned about your baby's heart rate pattern."

"I am going to change your position to your side to increase oxygen flow to your baby."

"I am also going to place this oxygen mask on your face to increase the oxygen flow to you and to your baby, and increase your IV rate."

"Do you have any questions?"

"I am here to help in any way, and I will stay here with you. Please let me know what concerns you have."

⟳ **Optimizing Outcomes**—The STAN (ST-interval ANalysis) S31 fetal heart monitor

Developed as an adjunct to standard FHR monitoring, STAN S31 technology permits visualization of changes in fetal electrocardiographic (ECG) waveforms (obtained via a fetal scalp electrode) indicating that a fetus is experiencing oxygen deficiency. The STAN S31 fetal heart monitor is indicated for use in patients who are greater than 36 weeks' gestation with a singleton fetus in a vertex presentation, planned vaginal delivery in the first stage of labor, and ruptured membranes. Combining the visual assessment of FHR patterns with STAN S31 is intended to improve identification of cases in which acute intervention would be necessary for suspected metabolic acidosis. Changes in the ST interval on the fetal ECG are indicators of the fetal response to the stress of labor, and combining the STAN S31 with EFM provides additional information about the fetus and has been shown to improve maternal–fetal outcomes (Huerta-Bogdan, 2011; Neoventa, 2012).

NUCHAL CORD

Nuchal cord (a cord that is wrapped around the infant's neck) and cords with true knots are observed in approximately 1% of all births. Nuchal cord, which rarely causes hypoxia, occurs most often in fetuses with long umbilical cords. When a tight knot is present in the cord, variable heart rate decelerations associated with fetal asphyxia may be noted on EFM. Nursing interventions follow protocols used for other abnormal variations of the fetal heart tracing.

Once the head is born, gentle palpation is used to feel for the cord. If the cord is present, it is loosened and carefully slipped over the head. If it is too tightly coiled to allow this intervention, the cord is clamped twice, cut between the clamps, and unwound from around the neck before the shoulders are delivered. Otherwise, the cord could tear and interfere with the fetal oxygen supply.

Amniotic Fluid Complications

Oligohydramnios (less than 300 mL of amniotic fluid), **hydramnios** (polyhydramnios) (greater than 2 L of amniotic fluid), and the presence of **meconium** (the first stools of the infant) in the amniotic fluid complicate labor and birth.

OLIGOHYDRAMNIOS

Oligohydramnios may result from fetal renal abnormalities, poor placental perfusion, or premature rupture of the membranes. During labor, the absence of the amniotic fluid buffer may lead to cord compression during contractions and decreased fetal blood flow as evidenced by variable heart rate decelerations. Women with pregnancies complicated by oligohydramnios require careful nursing and medical surveillance; amnioinfusion may be indicated to replace the cushion of fluid for the cord and relieve the frequency and intensity of variable decelerations (see Chapter 12).

HYDRAMNIOS

Hydramnios occurs in multiple gestations, fetal anomalies, and as a complication of maternal disease such as diabetes. During labor, the nurse needs to be aware that the excessive volume of fluid may obscure the fetal heart tracings. Hydramnios can cause fetal malpresentation because of the extra uterine space that it provides for the fetus to turn. The mother is also at risk for prolapse of the umbilical cord

because the increased amount of fluid pushes the fetus high into the uterine cavity. Preterm rupture of the membranes, another complication associated with hydramnios, increases the risks of both infection and prolapsed cord.

MECONIUM

Meconium-stained amniotic fluid during the intrapartal period is an indication for careful fetal surveillance by electronic fetal monitoring and possibly fetal scalp blood sampling. Although not always a sign of fetal distress, its presence, which occurs during fetal loss of sphincter control, is highly correlated with its occurrence. Reasons for the passage of meconium during labor include:

- Hypoxia-related peristalsis and sphincter relaxation
- Breech presentation or normal physiological function that occurs with fetal maturity
- Following umbilical cord compression-induced vagal stimulation in the mature fetus

Meconium staining, which occurs in approximately 20% of births, is observed more frequently in prolonged pregnancies. A decrease in amniotic fluid (oligohydramnios) increases the viscosity of the meconium and the risk of neonatal aspiration during delivery. The nurse must carefully document the presence of meconium stained fluid at the time of rupture of the membranes. In addition, the nurse should note the occurrence of variable decelerations and immediately notify the physician or certified nurse midwife regardless of whether meconium is present. Amnioinfusion has been shown to be effective in decreasing the fetal mortality associated with variable fetal heart rate (FHR) decelerations.

 Optimizing Outcomes—Intrapartal neonatal suctioning and meconium-stained amniotic fluid

The nasopharynx and oropharynx of the neonate born in the presence of meconium-stained amniotic fluid are often suctioned before the first breath (after the head is born but before the shoulders are born) to reduce the incidence and severity of meconium aspiration syndrome (MAS). However, because research does not support the efficacy of routine intrapartum suctioning to prevent MAS, this practice is no longer recommended (Vain, Szyld, Prudent, Wiswell, Aguilar, & Vivas, 2004). According to the International Liaison Committee on Resuscitation (2006), tracheal suctioning for meconium-stained depressed neonates should be performed immediately after birth; this intervention is not recommended for non-depressed meconium-stained full-term neonates.

Complications Associated With the Placenta

Critical nursing actions are required when the woman's intrapartum course is complicated by bleeding related to placenta previa (a low implantation of the placenta) or abruptio placentae (a premature separation of the placenta). (See Chapter 11.) Either condition places the woman at risk for hemorrhage and shock. A deteriorating physiological status of the mother impacts the fetus and often results in hypoxia. The nurse faces the challenge of helping to manage this intrapartal emergency. Guidelines for nursing care of the patient experiencing an intrapartal hemorrhage are presented in Table 14-3.

PLACENTA PREVIA

With placenta previa, bleeding occurs when the lower uterine segment begins to differentiate from the upper segment late in pregnancy and the cervix begins to dilate. If the bleeding has stopped, the maternal vital signs are stable, the fetal heart sounds are of good quality, and the fetus has not yet reached 36 weeks, the woman is usually managed by expectant watching. If the woman is near term (greater than 37 weeks of gestation) and in labor or bleeding persistently, immediate birth by cesarean is almost always indicated. Women diagnosed with partial or marginal placenta previa who have no bleeding or minimal bleeding may be allowed to attempt a vaginal birth.

 Collaboration in Caring—*Prenatal planning for patients likely to hemorrhage*

Advanced planning and interdisciplinary collaboration are essential for the management of patients who are at risk for intrapartal hemorrhage. Women with placenta previa, placenta accreta, or significant leiomyomas (fibroids) should be started on prenatal iron and folic acid as needed to maintain normal hemoglobin values, and, ideally, referred to a tertiary care center with capacities (e.g., maternal–fetal medicine, general surgery, urology, vascular surgery, and neonatology) to care for them. According to the Society for Maternal-Fetal Medicine, patients with placenta previa, previous myomectomies, and previous classic cesarean surgery should be delivered at 36 to 37 weeks, and those with suspected placenta accreta should be delivered at 34 to 35 weeks (Clark & Hankins, 2012; Eller, Bennett, Sharshiner, Masheter, Soisson, Dodson, et al., 2011; Pacheco, Saade, Tyner, Clark, & Hankins, 2012; Spong, Mercer, D'Alton, Kilpatrick, Blackwell, & Saade, 2011).

Table 14-3 Care of the Patient Experiencing an Intrapartal Hemorrhage

Assessment	Plan	Intervention	Evaluation
Vital signs	Establish maternal stability.	Take every 5 minutes if unstable, or every 15 minutes if stable. Use pulse oximetry. Auscultate respirations.	Vital signs are within normal range. Pulse is between 60 and 120 beats/min. Respirations are between 14 and 26 breaths/min. Temperature is less than 100.4°F (38.0°C). Blood pressure is greater than 90/60 mm Hg.
Bleeding	Resolve hemorrhage. Prevent shock.	Start two large-bore IV sites. Infuse normal saline and lactated Ringer's solution. Estimate blood loss (1 g = 1 mL) for replacement. Infuse blood products as necessary. Monitor circulatory volume using CVP/Swan-Ganz catheter as needed for extreme bleeding. Send blood sample to lab for analysis of gases. Document blood loss.	Bleeding is minimized. Homeostasis is established.
Intake/Output	Prevent volume depletion.	Insert indwelling urinary catheter. Measure and record output every hour. Measure and record input every hour.	Urine output will be greater than 30 mL/hr.
Fetal status	Prevent fetal injury.	Continuous electronic fetal monitoring.	FHR tracings remain between 120 and 160 beats/min. No evidence of abnormal FHR tracings.
Emotional response	Assist patient to cope with condition.	Educate the patient regarding all procedures. Inform the patient of her status throughout the bleeding crisis. Provide relaxation and breathing techniques. Provide spiritual support as necessary.	Patient verbalizes an understanding of her condition. Face displays no grimace. Muscles remain relaxed.
Pain	Reduce pain.	Provide relaxation and breathing techniques. Use guided imagery. Offer massage. Monitor contractions. Offer limited pain medication as ordered.	Patient reports pain on a scale of 1–10 as between 3 and 5.

Sources: Adapted from Francois & Foley (2012); Harvey & Dildy (2012); MacMullen, Dulski, & Meagher (2005).

When cesarean birth is planned, nursing responsibilities include continuous maternal–fetal assessment while preparing the woman for surgery. Maternal vital signs are assessed for indicators of hemorrhage (decreasing blood pressure, tachycardia, changes in the level of consciousness (LOC), and oliguria). Continuous electronic fetal monitoring (EFM) is used to assess the fetus for signs of hypoxia.

There is an increased risk for postpartal hemorrhage because the placental site is in the lower uterine segment, which does not contract as efficiently as the upper segment. Also, because the uterine blood supply is less in the lower uterine segment, the placenta tends to grow larger than when implanted in the upper segment. Thus, a larger denuded surface area is exposed after removal of the placenta. Nursing care throughout the intrapartal course centers on providing emotional support for the woman and her family and collaborating with and supporting medical management.

PLACENTAL ABRUPTION

Placental abruption (abruptio placentae), which tends to occur in late pregnancy, may occur as late as the first or second stage of labor. Although the primary cause of premature placental separation is unknown, predisposing factors include maternal hypertension, cocaine use (associated with vasoconstriction), direct trauma, and a history or previous placental abruption.

Treatment for abruptio placentae depends on the severity of maternal blood loss and the fetal maturity and status. If the abruption is mild and the fetus is less than 36 weeks and not in distress, expectant management may be implemented (see Chapter 11). When the fetus is at term gestation or if the bleeding is moderate to severe and the woman or fetus is in jeopardy, delivery is facilitated. Nursing care includes continuous maternal–fetal monitoring and emotional support. The patient is maintained in a lateral position to prevent pressure on the vena cava and to facilitate placental blood flow. To avoid further damage to the injured placenta, no vaginal or pelvic examinations are performed and no enemas are administered.

Blood and fluid volume replacement are implemented to maintain the urine output (assessed by indwelling Foley catheter) at 30 mL/hr or more and the hematocrit at 30% or more. Hemodynamic monitoring may be necessary. If the premature placental separation occurs during active labor, the physician may elect to rupture the membranes or augment the labor with intravenous oxytocin to hasten birth. Rupturing the membranes prevents large amounts of blood from collecting in the myometrium, which can interfere with uterine contractions. Artificial rupture of the membranes allows a slow, steady escape of amniotic fluid, preventing a sudden change in intrauterine pressure that may encourage further placental separation. Vaginal birth is desirable, especially in cases of fetal death. If birth does not appear to be imminent, a cesarean birth is the delivery method of choice. However, cesarean birth should be reserved for cases of fetal distress or other obstetric indications and should not be attempted if the woman has severe and uncorrected coagulopathy (e.g., disseminated intravascular coagulation [DIC]).

The patient with unresolved bleeding from a placental abruption is most vulnerable to severe complications. Maternal problems resulting from abruptio placentae include a **Couvelaire** uterus (the accumulation of blood between the separated placenta and the uterine wall) and DIC. Although a Couvelaire uterus is rare, its implications are severe. The uterus takes on a bluish tinge as blood extravasates from the clot into the myometrium. Contractility is lost. The condition is so severe that a hysterectomy may be necessary to control the bleeding (Cunningham et al., 2014).

If DIC has developed, surgery poses a major maternal risk because of the possibility of hemorrhage during surgery and later from the incisional site. The administration of intravenous fibrinogen or cryoprecipitate (which contains fibrinogen) may be given to increase the maternal fibrinogen level.

The maternal prognosis depends on how quickly interventions are initiated and how effective they are in halting the hemorrhage. Death can occur from massive hemorrhage that leads to shock or renal failure from circulatory collapse. The fetal prognosis depends on the extent of the abruption and the severity of the accompanying hypoxia.

 Optimizing Outcomes—**After the onset of hemorrhage**

Intraoperative cell salvage may be used for obstetric hemorrhage. With this technique, blood is salvaged from the surgical wound and filtered into a collecting reservoir. Filters in the device remove certain molecules (e.g., tissue factor, alpha-fetoprotein, platelets, and circulating procoagulants). After filtration, packed red blood cells with a hematocrit of 55% to 80% will be obtained and can be administered to the patient (Pacheco et al., 2012). Another intervention involves the use of recombinant activated factor VII (rFVIIa), a synthetic product that is not derived from blood (and is acceptable to many Jehovah's Witnesses). rFVIIa is increasingly being used for off-label indications including obstetric hemorrhage. However, the product has been associated with an increased incidence of thromboembolic complications, and the optimal dose is unknown (Braithwaite, Chichester, & Reid, 2011; Mirza & Gyamfi, 2010; Pacheco et al., 2012).

 Global Health Case Study A Pregnant Adolescent in the Emergency Department

Maria Selles is a 14-year-old Latina who arrives in the emergency department (ED) complaining of severe abdominal pain. She is pale and diaphoretic. A small amount of bright red blood is slowly trickling from her vagina. On assessment, her blood pressure is 120/70; pulse, 100; respirations 22 breaths/minute; temperature 99°F (37.2°C). Her physical examination reveals an enlarged abdomen, which is rigid and boardlike with extreme tenderness. Maria is known to the ED because of a history of repeated drug abuse including cocaine. She has been living on the street since she was kicked out of her house several months ago.

critical thinking questions

1. Based on this initial information, what is the nurse's assessment of the possible problem?

2. Because Maria is in such extreme distress, the nurse is aware of a need to limit the number of questions asked. What critical questions should be asked at this point?

3. What laboratory tests would be important to check?

The nurse's further assessment reveals dark red vaginal bleeding and clinical signs consistent with pregnancy (the presence of abdominal enlargement, deeply pigmented areolae, linea nigra, and striae gravidarum). The young patient has said very little in response to the questions, but Maria does admit to sexual intercourse and no recent menstrual periods.

Given this information, the nurse formulates the care priorities for Maria. Although her physical condition and that of the fetus warrant immediate priority, the nurse needs to support this young girl psychologically to proceed with any plan. Any support people who have come with her to the ED should be identified. If there is no one with her, the nurse explains the plan of care and describes what she should expect. The nurse places Maria on the electronic fetal monitor and immediately notifies the physician of her condition. Because cocaine is associated with placental abruption, the nurse must identify any recent drug use. The care plan should be developmentally oriented. The nurse implements strategies to keep Maria warm, provides emotional support and a calming presence, and continues to monitor her vital signs and her vaginal flow until the physician arrives.

◆ See Suggested Answers to Global Health Case Studies on DavisPlus.

DISSEMINATED INTRAVASCULAR COAGULATION

Disseminated intravascular coagulation (DIC) is an acquired disorder of blood clotting. Affected individuals can experience widespread internal and external bleeding and clotting. Clinical symptoms may include easy bruising, the appearance of multiple petechiae, and bleeding from intravenous sites. DIC is most often triggered by the release of large amounts of tissue thromboplastin, which occurs in abruptio placentae and in retained dead fetus (the fetus has died and is retained in the uterus for 6 or more weeks) and amniotic fluid syndromes (Cunningham et al., 2014).

 Optimizing Outcomes—Prompt identification of clinical signs that may indicate DIC

When conducting a physical assessment of the pregnant woman at risk for DIC, the nurse must be alert to the following clinical signs:

* Bleeding from multiple sites (e.g., intravenous access site, venipuncture site, and site of urinary catheter insertion)
* Spontaneous bleeding from the gums and nose
* Widespread petechiae and bruising
* Gastrointestinal bleeding
* Tachycardia
* Diaphoresis

With DIC, the anticoagulation and procoagulation factors are activated simultaneously. Thromboplastin (a clotting factor) is released into the maternal circulation as a result of placental bleeding and the consequent clot formation. Circulating levels of thromboplastin activate widespread clotting throughout the microcirculation. This process consumes, or *uses up*, other clotting factors such as fibrinogen and platelets. The condition is complicated further by the activation of the fibrinolytic system to lyse (destroy) the clots. As a result, there is a simultaneous decrease in clotting factors and an increase in circulating

anticoagulants, leaving the circulating blood unable to clot. Laboratory results reveal low hemoglobin, hematocrit, platelets, and fibrinogen and elevated fibrin split/degradation products.

The priority in treatment of DIC is to correct the underlying cause and replace fluids and essential clotting factors. When premature placental separation has triggered the coagulopathy, delivery of the fetus and placenta must be accomplished so that the production of thromboplastin, which is driving the process, is halted. This is accomplished with intravenous administration of heparin to stop the clotting cascade. Heparin is cautiously given close to the time of birth to decrease the likelihood of postpartum hemorrhage after the delivery of the placenta. The administration of blood and platelets is usually delayed until after completion of the heparin therapy so that the newly infused blood factors are not consumed by the widespread coagulation process. Depending on the clinical setting, antithrombin III factor, fibrinogen, or cryoprecipitate may also be used to restore blood clotting (Francois & Foley, 2012; Gilbert, 2011).

Nursing care includes continuous maternal–fetal assessment; administering the prescribed fluids, blood, and blood products; and assessing for signs of complications from the replacement products. The woman is positioned in a side-lying tilt to maximize placental perfusion, and oxygen may be administered via rebreathing mask at 8 to 10 L/min or according to physician or institutional protocol. Because renal failure may result from DIC, urinary output is closely monitored; it should be maintained at more than 30 mL/hr. The patient and her family should be provided with ongoing information and emotional support (Francois & Foley, 2012; Genovese, 2011). (See Chapters 11, 16, and 33 for further discussion on DIC.)

RUPTURE OF THE UTERUS

Rupture of the uterus during labor is a rare but life-threatening obstetric complication that occurs in 1 in 1,500 to 2,000 births (Fig. 14-11). It is most often associated with the tearing of a uterine scar (usually from a previous classic

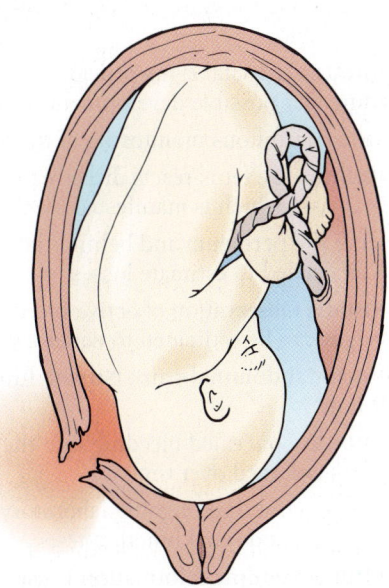

Figure 14-11 Rupture of the uterus in the lower uterine segment.

cesarean birth), uterine trauma (e.g., accidents or surgery), and a congenital uterine anomaly. Rupture of the uterus occurs more often in multigravidas than in primigravidas. Intrapartal uterine rupture may result from overdistention (e.g., multiple gestation), tachysystole (e.g., oxytocin and prostaglandin), external or internal version, malpresentation, or a difficult forceps-assisted birth (Mirza, Devine, & Gaddipati, 2010).

 Nursing Insight—Understanding types of uterine rupture

Uterine rupture may be classified as complete or incomplete (also known as uterine scar dehiscence; occurs when a previous scar begins to separate). A complete rupture extends through the endometrium, myometrium, and peritoneum. When this occurs, uterine contractions stop. The woman complains of sudden, severe abdominal pain during a strong contraction followed by cessation of the pain. There is bleeding into the abdominal cavity and possibly into the vagina and protrusion of fetal parts and/or placenta into the abdominal cavity. An incomplete rupture (scar dehiscence) extends into the peritoneum but not into the peritoneal cavity or broad ligament. Bleeding is usually internal, and the woman may be asymptomatic (a "silent" rupture) or complain of localized tenderness and aching pain over the lower uterine segment.

Changes in fetal heart tracings such as sudden bradycardia or prolonged late or variable decelerations are the most common signs and symptoms and frequently precede the onset of abdominal pain or bleeding. Maternal signs and symptoms may include faintness, vomiting, abdominal tenderness, hypotonic uterine contractions, and lack of labor progress. As blood loss continues, the woman may exhibit signs of hypovolemic shock (hypotension; tachypnea; pallor; and cool, clammy skin). Fetal parts may be readily palpable through the abdomen (Gilbert, 2011).

Rupture of the uterus constitutes an obstetric emergency; the type of medical management depends on the severity. A small rupture may be safely managed with a laparotomy and birth of the infant, repair of the tear, and volume replacement with fluids and blood transfusions if needed. A complete uterine rupture requires hysterectomy and blood replacement.

 Nursing Care Plan The Patient With Abruptio Placentae

Nursing Diagnosis: Deficient Fluid Volume related to active losses from premature separation of the placenta.

Measurable Short-Term Goal: The patient and her fetus will maintain fluid balance during the intrapartal period.

Measurable Long-Term Goal: The patient and newborn will demonstrate homeostasis prior to discharge.

NOC Outcomes:
Fluid Balance (0601) Water balance in the intracellular and extracellular compartments of the body
Blood Loss Severity (0413) Severity of signs and symptoms of internal or external bleeding
Fetal Status Intrapartum (0112) Extent to which fetal signs are within normal limits from onset of labor to delivery

NIC Interventions:
Fluid Management (4120)
Bleeding Reduction: Antepartum Uterus (4021)
Electronic Fetal Monitoring: Intrapartum (6772)

Nursing Interventions:

1. Monitor blood pressure, pulse, and respirations every 5 to 15 minutes with active bleeding or if the vital signs are not stable.

   RATIONALE: The vital signs provide important information about the response of the cardiac system to active bleeding and possible development of shock.

2. Provide continuous monitoring of the fetal heart rate and pattern.

   RATIONALE: The fetus reacts directly to an assault on the mother's system. Bleeding from the placenta places the fetus at risk, which is manifested by changes in the fetal heart rate pattern.

3. Observe the perineum and behind the patient's back at least every hour for signs of active bleeding. Weigh pads as needed to estimate losses.

   RATIONALE: Observation of active bleeding may indicate the need for an emergency cesarean delivery. One gram of weight can be estimated to equal 1 mL of blood lost.

4. Assess for abdominal pain, palpate fundal tone, and measure abdominal girth at the umbilicus at least each hour.

   RATIONALE: Concealed bleeding into the myometrium may result in a painful, rigid, boardlike uterus that becomes enlarged over time.

5. Review baseline and ongoing laboratory data including complete blood count (CBC), clotting studies, serum electrolytes, and renal function tests.

   RATIONALE: Baseline information is used to alert the care providers to changes in the patient's condition as additional lab tests are obtained.

Nursing Care Plan The Patient With Abruptio Placentae (continued)

6. Maintain intravenous access with a large-bore catheter and administer isotonic intravenous fluids as directed.

   RATIONALE: Intravenous access is required to maintain and replace fluid volume. Large catheters facilitate the infusion of large volumes of fluid quickly.

7. Administer blood replacement products in a timely manner as directed.

   RATIONALE: The hematocrit level should be 30% or greater to prevent severe shock.

8. Assess hourly intake and output with an indwelling urinary catheter.

   RATIONALE: A decrease in urine output below 30 mL/hr indicates poor organ perfusion and that the patient may be developing shock.

9. Monitor for development of abnormal clotting studies, bleeding from gums, oozing from injection sites, bruising, or petechiae and notify caregiver.

   RATIONALE: The patient is at risk for developing DIC because of excessive bleeding.

10. Facilitate delivery as necessary to prevent maternal–fetal injury.

    RATIONALE: If the patient is actively bleeding, or there is any indication that she has concealed bleeding, she must be delivered to prevent hemorrhage, shock, and death.

Nursing responsibilities include administering intravenous fluids, blood products, and oxygen and helping to prepare the woman for immediate surgery. Because the patient is anxious and fearful, it is important for the nurse to attempt to provide emotional support for the woman and her support person throughout the process. The nurse must maintain a calm demeanor while organizing critical care for the patient. As much as possible, the patient and her support person should be involved in decision making and informed of all procedures. Depending on the circumstances, it may be appropriate to provide information about chaplain support services. The associated fetal mortality rate ranges from 50% to 75%, and the maternal mortality rate may be high if treatment is not initiated immediately (Cunningham et al., 2014).

UTERINE INVERSION

Uterine inversion (uterus is turned inside out) is a rare but potentially life-threatening complication that most often results from excessive pulling on the umbilical cord in an attempt to hasten the third stage of delivery. Other contributing factors include fundal implantation of the placenta, vigorous fundal pressure, uterine atony, macrosomic infants, magnesium sulfate, precipitous labor, congenital uterine malformations, and abnormally adherent placental tissue (Mirza, Devine, & Gaddipati, 2010). When complete inversion occurs, a large, red, globular mass (that may contain the still-attached placenta) protrudes 20 to 30 cm outside the vaginal introitus. A partial or incomplete inversion is not visible; instead, a smooth mass is palpated through the dilated cervix. Maternal symptoms include pain, hemorrhage, and shock. Management involves manual replacement of the fundus (under general anesthesia) by the physician, followed by oxytocin to facilitate uterine contractions and antibiotic therapy to prevent infection. Prevention (by not pulling strongly on the cord until the placenta has fully separated) is the safest and most effective therapy (Cunningham et al., 2014).

UMBILICAL CORD PROLAPSE

Umbilical cord prolapse occurs when a loop of the umbilical cord slips down below the presenting part of the fetus (Fig. 14-12). Prolapse of the umbilical cord may be *occult* (hidden; not visible) at any time during labor whether or not the membranes have ruptured—the cord lies beside the presenting part in the pelvic inlet. With a *complete* cord prolapse, the cord descends into the vagina, where it is felt as a pulsating mass on vaginal

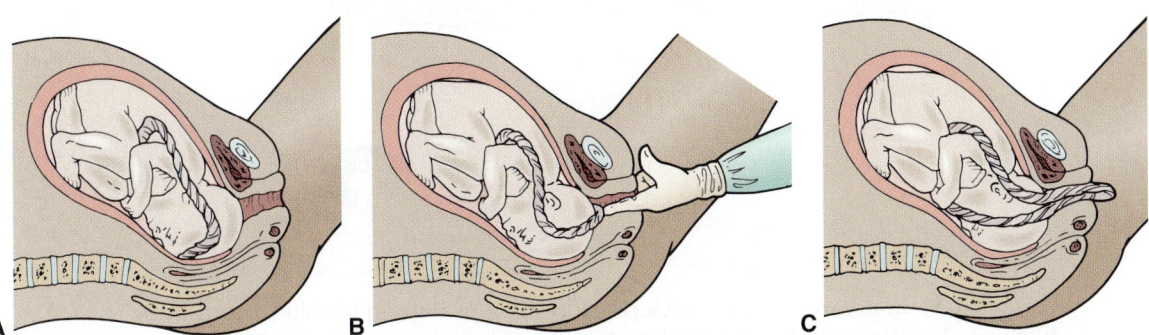

A   B   C

Figure 14-12 Umbilical cord prolapse. *A,* Occult—the cord cannot be seen or felt during a vaginal examination. *B,* Complete—during a vaginal examination, the cord is felt as a pulsating mass. *C,* Frank—the cord precedes the fetal head or feet and can be seen protruding from the vagina.

examination. It may or may not be seen. Frank (visible) prolapse most commonly occurs immediately after rupture of membranes as gravity washes the cord in front of the presenting part. Risk factors associated with cord prolapse include a long (greater than 100 cm) cord, malpresentation (e.g., breech), transverse lie, hydramnios, preterm or low-birth-weight infant, multiple gestation, and an unengaged presenting part (Cunningham et al., 2014). If the presenting part does not fit snugly into the lower uterine segment, the sudden gush of amniotic fluid that accompanies rupture of the membranes may cause the cord to be displaced downward.

Optimizing Outcomes—Actions to reduce the risk of umbilical cord prolapse

If spontaneous rupture of the membranes (SROM) has occurred, the woman should be kept on bedrest until the fetal presenting part is engaged. Artificial rupture of the membranes (AROM) should not be attempted until engagement has occurred. To rule out umbilical cord prolapse, the nurse should assess the fetal heart sounds immediately after spontaneous or artificial rupture of the membranes.

It is imperative that the nurse recognizes indicators of umbilical cord prolapse: fetal bradycardia with variable decelerations during contractions, observing or palpating the cord in the vagina, and the woman's statement that she "feels the cord" after membrane rupture. Prolonged cord compression causes fetal hypoxia; occlusion of blood flow to and from the fetus for greater than 5 minutes is likely to result in central nervous system damage or fetal death.

To relieve pressure on the cord, the examiner places a sterile gloved hand into the vagina and manually lifts the presenting part off the umbilical cord. The patient is assisted into a position such as a modified Sims, extreme Trendelenburg, or knee–chest position, which uses gravity to cause the presenting part to fall back from the cord (Fig. 14-13). The nurse administers oxygen at 10 L/min by face mask to improve oxygenation to the fetus; the physician may order administration of a tocolytic agent to reduce uterine activity and relieve pressure on the fetus. If the cord is protruding from the vagina, the exposure to room air will cause drying, which leads to atrophy of the umbilical vessels. No attempts should be made to place the cord back into the vagina. Instead, the nurse should cover the exposed segment of umbilical cord with warm, sterile saline compresses to prevent drying. Prompt delivery, often with forceps assistance, is facilitated if the cervix is fully dilated. Otherwise, the nurse or other care provider continues to manually maintain upward pressure on the presenting part (using a hand in the vagina) until a cesarean birth can be accomplished.

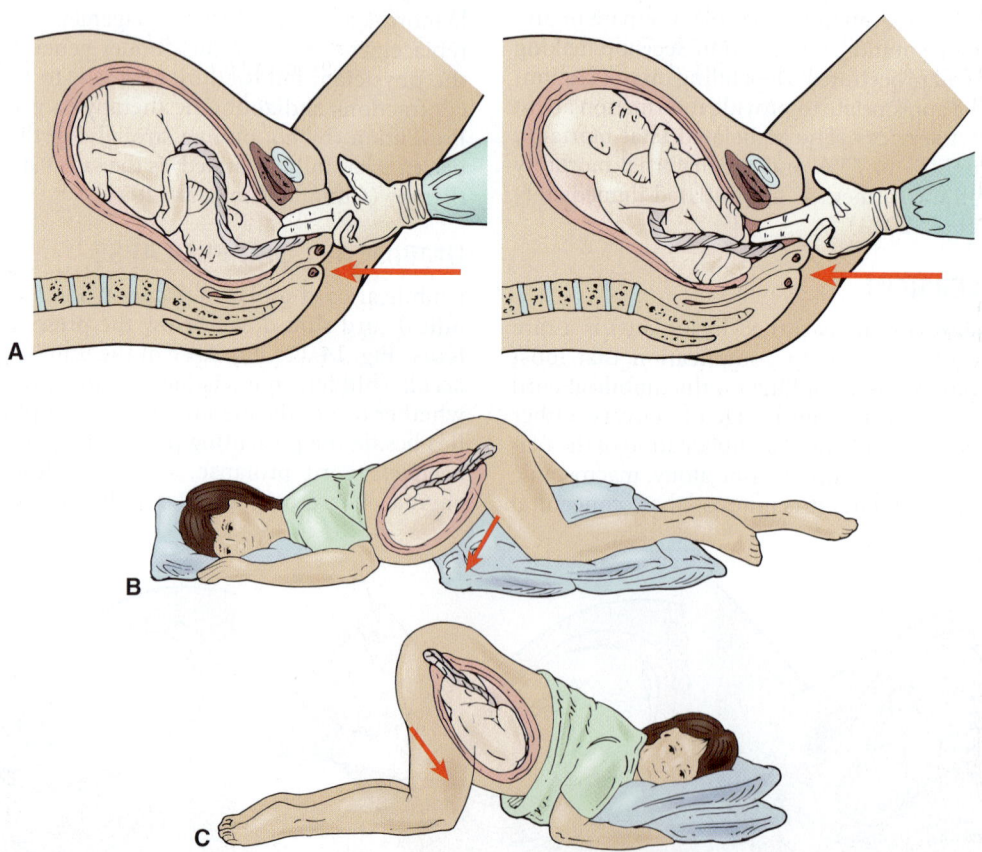

Figure 14-13 Interventions to relieve pressure on a prolapsed umbilical cord until birth can be effected. *A,* A gloved hand is placed in the vagina to lift the presenting part off the cord. *B,* The maternal hips are elevated with two pillows; this intervention is often combined with a Trendelenburg position. *C,* The knee–chest position uses gravity to shift the fetus out of the maternal pelvis.

Critical Nursing Action After Prolapse of the Umbilical Cord

After prolapse of the umbilical cord, immediate nursing interventions are essential:

- Call for assistance; notify the primary health-care provider.
- Using the gloved examining hand, insert two fingers into the vagina to the cervix. Place one finger on either side of the cord or both fingers to one side and quickly exert upward pressure against the presenting part to relieve compression of the cord.
- Assist the woman into an extreme Trendelenburg, modified Sims, or knee–chest position.
- If the cord is protruding from the vagina, wrap it loosely in a sterile towel saturated with a warmed, sterile normal saline solution.
- Administer oxygen at 10 L/min by face mask.
- Increase the IV fluid rate; administer a tocolytic agent as ordered.
- Continuously monitor the fetal heart rate (FHR) by internal fetal scalp electrode if possible.
- Provide information and support to the woman and her birth partner.
- Prepare for an immediate vaginal birth if the cervix is fully dilated or for cesarean birth if it is not.

VARIATIONS RELATED TO UMBILICAL CORD INSERTION AND THE PLACENTA

Velamentous Cord Insertion/Vasa Previa

A *velamentous* insertion of the umbilical cord occurs when the fetal vessels separate at the distal end of the cord and insert into the placenta at a distance away from the margin (Fig. 14-14). The vessels are not protected by Wharton's jelly and are subject to compression, rupture, and thrombosis, major complications that may lead to severe fetal distress and death. This form of cord insertion most frequently occurs with placenta previa and multiple pregnancies; it may also be associated with fetal anomalies. Rupture of the membranes or traction on the umbilical cord may tear the fetal vessels. This event produces rapid, usually fatal, fetal hemorrhage. **Vasa previa** occurs when the unprotected fetal vessels cover the cervical os and precede the fetus. It is usually seen with a velamentous insertion of the umbilical

cord. Because the vessels are not covered with Wharton's jelly, the examiner may be able to feel pulsations of the umbilical cord. Lacerations of the vessels, which can occur at any time, cause sudden fetal blood loss. The onset of sudden, painless bleeding at the beginning of cervical dilation or during rupture of membranes (ROM) may signal the presence of vasa previa; diagnosis may be confirmed by sonogram (Cunningham et al., 2014; Hull & Resnik, 2013).

Without ultrasound assessment, velamentous cord insertion is not easily detectable. The nurse may note a drop in FHR during a vaginal exam. A ready FHR return to the baseline after the exam may be indicative of a velamentous cord insertion. With any episode of vaginal bleeding, the alum-precipitated toxoid (APT) test may be used to determine the presence of fetal blood cells. After the rupture of blood vessels, fetal blood leaks into the vagina and can be readily sampled for examination. Despite the rarity of this condition, velamentous cord insertion should always be suspected and ruled out via a careful vaginal exam with cervical palpation for detection of exposed vessels. Immediate action by the medical team, prompted by the nurse's critical assessments, can result in an emergency cesarean birth; best outcomes occur with early prenatal diagnosis and cesarean birth at 35 weeks or earlier (Genovese, 2011).

Circumvallate, Succenturiate, and Battledore Placenta

Other placental variations and problems related to the umbilical cord insertion site include **circumvallate** placenta (placenta circumvallata), **succenturiate** placenta (placenta succenturiata), and **battledore** placenta. These conditions are associated with variations that occurred during placentation (formation and attachment of the placenta). The circumvallate placenta is one in which a ring composed of a double fold of amnion and chorion has formed near the fetal surface. This placental aberration has been reported to be associated with antepartum hemorrhage, preterm delivery, and fetal malformations. The succenturiate placenta contains one or two separate lobes, each with its own circulation. After childbirth, one of the separate lobes may be retained in the uterus and impede contractions, resulting in severe maternal hemorrhage. The remaining lobes must be manually removed from the uterus to prevent hemorrhage.

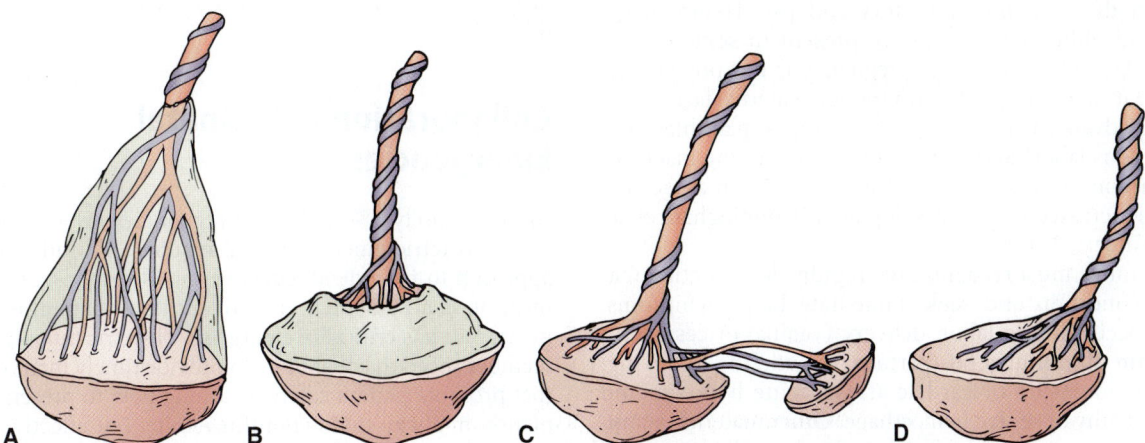

Figure 14-14 Variations related to umbilical cord insertion on the placenta. *A,* Velamentous insertion of the umbilical cord. *B,* Circumvallate placenta. *C,* Succenturiate placenta. *D,* Battledore placenta.

Battledore insertion of the cord describes a condition in which the umbilical cord is implanted near the margin of the placenta. Battledore placenta may be associated with fetal hemorrhage, especially after marginal separation of the placenta (Cunningham et al., 2014).

Placenta Accreta, Placenta Increta, Placenta Percreta

Abnormal adherence of the placenta is rare, and its causes are unknown. After birth, the usual maneuvers to remove the placenta are unsuccessful, and laceration or perforation of the uterine wall may result. When this occurs, the woman is at high risk for hemorrhage and infection. The placental adherence may be partial or complete. **Placenta accreta** describes a slight penetration of the myometrium by the trophoblast. **Placenta increta** describes a deep placental penetration of the myometrium, and **placenta percreta** describes placental perforation of the uterus. Depending on the degree of placental adherence (and the severity of the hemorrhage), the patient will require blood replacement, and a vaginal hysterectomy may be indicated (Cunningham et al., 2014; Hull & Resnik, 2008).

ANAPHYLACTOID SYNDROME OF PREGNANCY

Anaphylactoid syndrome of pregnancy (formerly known as amniotic fluid embolism; obstruction of a blood vessel by amniotic fluid) is a rare complication of the intra- and postpartum periods that is associated with a high incidence of maternal and fetal death. For mothers, the mortality rate is as high as 80%, and most survivors have neurological deficits; approximately 50% of neonates who survive this event have neurological impairment. The origins of the problem are not clear, but it is hypothesized that amniotic fluid containing particles of fetal debris (meconium, hair, vernix, or skin cells) escapes into the maternal circulation, and in certain patients, triggers an anaphylactic reaction and the release of endogenous mediators such as histamine, prostaglandins, and thromboxane. However, it should be noted that fetal material is not always found in the maternal circulation in patients with anaphylactoid syndrome of pregnancy, and material of fetal origin is often found in women who do not develop the condition. When the complication does occur, obstruction of the pulmonary vessels leads to respiratory distress and circulatory collapse. Hemorrhage, DIC, and pulmonary edema are present to some extent. Anaphylactoid syndrome of pregnancy is not preventable because it cannot be predicted although maternal factors (including advanced age, multiparity, abruptio placentae, and tumultuous labor) and fetal problems (including macrosomia, meconium passage, and death) have been associated with an increased risk for development (Cunningham et al., 2014; Gilbert, 2011).

The nurse must recognize the rapidly deteriorating maternal condition and seek immediate help. Symptoms, which occur during labor, delivery (vaginal or cesarean), or within 30 minutes postpartum, include the following: acute hypotension or cardiac arrest, acute hypoxia, and coagulopathy or severe hemorrhage. Other maternal symptoms include restlessness, facial erythema, cough, cyanosis, chest pain, uterine atony, seizures, pulmonary edema, tachycardia, respiratory arrest, shock, and cardiac arrest (Gilbert, 2011).

 Critical Nursing Action When Anaphylactoid Syndrome of Pregnancy Develops

The immediate management includes the administration of oxygen by face mask or cannula at a rate of 8 to 10 L/min or resuscitation bag to deliver 100% oxygen. Nursing interventions center on support of resuscitation efforts:

- Prepare for intubation and mechanical ventilation.
- Initiate or assist with cardiopulmonary resuscitation (CPR). Position the pregnant woman in a 30-degree lateral tilt to displace the uterus.
- Administer intravenous fluids and blood (e.g., packed cells or fresh frozen plasma); because circulatory collapse is a possibility, consider having two IV lines in place. Caution: Do not overload with fluids because of the threat of pulmonary edema resulting from developing adult respiratory distress syndrome (ARDS).
- Have emergency medications to assist in patient stabilization (e.g., dopamine, digoxin, hydrocortisone, and uterotonics).
- Prepare for and assist with placement of a central line.
- Insert indwelling urinary catheter; measure hourly urine output.
- Continuously monitor maternal–fetal status.
- Prepare for emergency birth once the woman is stable.
- Provide ongoing information and emotional support to the woman and her family.

The maternal prognosis depends on the size of the embolism and speed and skill of the responding perinatal team. If the woman survives, she will most likely be transferred to a critical care unit for hemodynamic monitoring, blood replacement, and coagulopathy treatment. Although rapid delivery is paramount to save the fetus, a delay in delivery usually occurs to stabilize the mother. In the event of maternal cardiopulmonary arrest, for optimal fetal survival, a perimortem cesarean delivery should occur within 5 minutes (Cunningham et al., 2014).

This type of a situation is very difficult for all health professionals involved in the care of the patient. An ethical conflict may arise when the health of the mother is given consideration over the fetus. While there are no easy answers to these dilemmas, the nurse can serve as a leader by organizing regular meetings during which issues of this nature can be discussed in a calm, open manner. The nurse is in a key position to help create an environment where health professionals can resolve or work through difficult dilemmas.

Collaboration in Perinatal Emergencies

Approximately 1% to 2% of pregnancies are complicated by an obstetric emergency and require a multidisciplinary approach to provide an effective, rapid response. Communication is an essential component in all patient environments, but it is critical in emergency obstetric nursing. Team members need to collaborate to provide timely interventions that promote patient safety. Learning how to present information in a way that is nonthreatening but effective is key to promoting positive communication patterns (ACOG, 2011, 2012b; Pettker & Funai, 2011).

Miller (2005) identifies the hierarchical communication that often exists between physicians and nurses as detrimental to good perinatal outcomes. The need to employ healthy communication patterns to effect safe and healthy outcomes for the patient is tantamount. Effective communication does not mean that there are no followers of orders or directives. Instead, it is important for both the leaders and the followers to employ critical thinking skills. Use of the word "we" promotes collaboration and underscores the nurse's role as a patient advocate in this effective communication style (Burkman & Fennell, 2010).

"What to say"—*Communicating concerns with members of the health-care team*

Simpson (2005) emphasizes the critical need for effective communication among the health-care team. Problems in care are encountered when people fail to collaborate or communicate. Teamwork is enhanced when everyone knows the expectations of their role in the obstetric emergency (Box 14-5). Standardization of protocols allows everyone to function more effectively and prevent poor outcomes.

 ### Collaboration in Caring—*Family-witnessed resuscitation*

In recent times, there has been a growing trend toward allowing family members to be present during resuscitation, including resuscitation of the neonate. Family-witnessed resuscitation (FWR), or family presence during resuscitation (FPDR), is becoming increasingly more common, and evidence suggests that there are benefits for family members, who treasure the opportunity to be with their child during their final precious moments (Scheans, 2009). The American College of Critical Care Medicine includes neonatal intensive care in its recommendations, and this document extrapolates to newborns at any birthing center (Davidson, Powers, Hedayat, Tieszen, Kon, Shepard et al., 2007). The development and implementation of a policy to achieve FWR requires the collaboration of a multidisciplinary team that endorses a family-centered holistic model of care. As traditional patient advocates, nurses are well situated to foster this caring approach to resuscitation (Scheans, 2009).

Box 14-5 **Collaborative Care Principles in Perinatal Nursing**

To facilitate the team process when providing care in emergency situations, the perinatal nurse should:

- Employ effective communication techniques.
- Advocate for the patient through assertive statements.
- Conduct interdisciplinary reviews of all cases to identify risks.
- Promote team collaboration by rotating leadership roles in the case reviews.
- Assist in the evaluation process of all emergency cases.
- Use outcome measurements to evaluate safe and effective care.

COLLABORATION IN EMERGENCY PREPAREDNESS

In 2012, The Association of Women's Health, Obstetric and Neonatal Nurses (AWHONN) published a position statement regarding the nurse's role in emergency preparedness for natural, accidental, or deliberate emergencies and disasters. In this document, AWHONN acknowledged that institutional hazard plans do not always address the special needs of pregnant and postpartum women and their infants and recognized the importance of women's health and neonatal nurses in responding to these needs. Critical considerations for pregnant and postpartum women and officials at all stages of disaster planning and response are included, along with guidelines for nursing education about emergency preparedness information.

Perinatal Loss

Perinatal loss is the death of a fetus or infant from the time of conception through the end of the newborn period 28 days after birth. A perinatal loss can occur during the antepartal, intrapartal, or postpartal periods. A variety of causes may lead to the death of the fetus or the newborn, and these are often related to obstetric complications such as placental abruption or neonatal prematurity related to genetic disorders or congenital malformations. Many believe perinatal death to be a rare phenomenon because the majority of the childbearing population consists of young healthy women who expect to give birth to healthy babies. This prevailing expectation among the general population is a major reason why it is so difficult for all involved when a perinatal death occurs.

Nursing practice has changed over the years in regard to caring for families who are dealing with a perinatal loss. From the 1960s through the 1980s, women who experienced a perinatal loss were often placed on a medical–surgical unit to prevent them from hearing the sounds of infants crying. One problem with this approach lies in the fact that the most experienced professionals in perinatal nursing are not located in the medical–surgical areas. The patient who has suffered a loss still requires all assessments and interventions involved in normal postpartum care. A nurse in the perinatal practice area can better focus on therapeutic interventions to assist the woman and her family in the grieving process.

The nurse organizes and coordinates a team approach to bereavement. Different members may participate, but there should be key individuals such as spiritual or religious representatives, social workers, and physicians, in addition to the nurse. It is important to identify which hospital routines associated with perinatal death might interfere with allowing the family to have options concerning decisions made regarding their infant. As an example, in some cases, the infant's body might be moved to the funeral home before the family has had the opportunity to hold him or her. Many parents wish to hold their child prior to an autopsy, and they should be encouraged to do so. Before presenting the parents with their infant, the nurse should make certain the infant has been cleaned and is wrapped in a soft blanket. Some institutions use a commercially developed presentation/handling system that includes a basket for infant presentation and a carrier component designed to discreetly transport the infant to the morgue.

Depending on the cause of death, it may also be prudent to give the parents an idea of their infant's appearance. Usually, parents' preconceived perception of how their infant will look is much worse than the reality. Individuals from the hospital morgue or a funeral home who are involved with regular bereavement team meetings can be instrumental in developing a perinatal bereavement plan that is grounded in compassion and sensitivity.

When healthy infants are discharged, it is common practice to take their picture. Photographs should also be taken when an infant has died. Parents should always be encouraged to view, touch, and hold the deceased infant. However, if they do not wish to see the infant while in the hospital, the picture provides a way for them to see their infant at a future time when they are ready. Photographs can be stored with the patient's medical record and given to the parents upon their request. Use of an experienced photographer is preferred, because the infant may not always be in the most favorable condition. The maternity unit should always have a supply of clothing and new blankets available for these infants.

Where Research and Practice Meet:
Providing Perinatal Palliative Care

Based on their literature search, Kauffman, Hauck, and Mandel (2010) developed a perinatal palliative care team (PPCT) in their institution to provide support for pregnant women and their families who were facing a lethal prenatal diagnosis. The goal of the program is to educate and empower the patient and her family to make decisions concerning fetal/neonatal care and their delivery/birth experience. Women are referred to the Perinatal Palliative Care Program by perinatologists, obstetricians, family doctors, staff nurses, chaplains, and family members. All members of the PPCT (neonatologist, chaplain, labor and delivery nurse, neonatal intensive care nurse, and social worker) received training through the Resolve Through Sharing Bereavement Program and are equipped with communication skills that foster helpful conversations with the woman and her family to help them formulate a birth plan that addresses expectations during pregnancy, delivery, and the time following birth. At least one team member is available for the woman and her family upon admission and remains present during the delivery. The PPCT works with the bereavement team to provide bereavement care (e.g., photographs, footprints, and memory boxes) after the neonate's death and attends the funeral or memorial service if desired by the family. A member of the PPCT contacts patients following discharge to assess postpartum needs and grief response. The PPCT addresses the emotional needs of staff after each case, provides an opportunity for debriefing about the experience, and offers family feedback about their experience. Community resources for families receiving perinatal palliative care provide additional support such as professional photography services and handcrafted infant clothing and blankets.

Various other researchers have also contributed to our understanding of the state of the science on perinatal palliative care. English and Hessler (2013) discussed the value of an Advance Care Birth Plan as a framework in assisting families facing a serious fetal diagnosis; Vesely and Beach (2013) described a model for providing an alternate site of care, known as an inpatient pediatric palliative care center. Based on her findings regarding palliative care for parents who choose to continue pregnancies with life-limiting fetal diagnoses, Wood (2013) suggested that additional nursing research be undertaken to determine factors that will benefit parents in need of perinatal palliative care programs and also to identify the needs, perceptions, and willingness of the professionals who will provide this care.

To provide the family as much privacy as possible from hospital workers who might not know that the family has experienced a loss, it is best to have some sort of indicator outside the room. One hospital unit places a single red rose across the door. Another places a special "remembrance card" outside the doorframe. Both provide an immediate identification to any hospital worker entering the room that the patient and her family have experienced a loss.

All of these practices stem from the development of hospital protocols regarding bereavement. The team develops a list of critical actions and specific plans to respond to each point. There is flexibility to allow the parents to be active participants in the decision making, but it is also organized so that as nursing and hospital personnel change, there is consistency in the approach.

Communication is another critical factor in providing care for the family who has experienced a fetal or neonatal loss. Parents report that comforting words, touch, and directed speech are helpful to them. Nurses need to avoid using phrases such as:

- "It's God's will."
- "You can always have another."
- "There was a problem with this baby."
- "There's always next time."

Parents respond better to acknowledgment of the infant's death than to avoidance. It is essential that nursing interventions focus on healing communication. A simple "I'm sorry" and a touch of the hand can convey the nurse's care and concern when the right words are hard to find. It is also important for the nurse to sit and listen and offer presence rather than avoidance. Parents often have multiple feelings, which they need to share. The nurse, as the objective individual, can help interpret feelings and recommend resources to assist the family as they deal with their grief. It is essential that the perinatal care team remain sensitive to the cultural and spiritual beliefs and practices of the bereaved parents and families (Phillips & Bulmer, 2013). (See Chapter 11 for further discussion.)

❝What to say❞—*To the mother whose newborn has died*

When caring for the mother whose infant has died, the nurse conveys compassion by simply being available. Often, the mother finds comfort in talking about the birth experience, her infant, and how she will cope with her loss. The nurse can gain insights into the mother's support systems by asking the following questions:

"What are you most worried or fearful about?"

"How supportive is the baby's father and your family or friends?"

"What coping techniques have been helpful for you in the past?"

(Gilbert, 2010)

A perinatal loss might be the first experience a family has with death. It is a confusing, anxiety-provoking time that often creates a fear that it will happen again. Death of a child of any age is also viewed as unnatural. Parents expect their children to die after them—not before them. Dreams and expectations for the lost child will now never be realized. A resource guide given to the family on discharge is an important tool to help them cope with their loss. Because much of the grieving work is done after the hospitalization, family members need to know where to call for help.

A support group that includes someone from the bereavement team can offer the parents a connection to the hospital. Some parents find this helpful in acknowledging the existence of their child while others feel more comfortable with the support of a close family network. The key is that the family is supported through their loss and is able to move through the grief process toward resolution. It is important to understand that many families will never totally come to terms with the untimely death of a child, regardless of the age of the infant or fetus.

Optimizing Outcomes—Holistic care for families experiencing perinatal loss

Families with young children who experience perinatal loss face unique challenges. Research indicates that young children need parents who are emotionally available to help them sort through their feelings and come to an understanding of the baby's death. Nurses can provide guidance to help parents anticipate questions that their child may ask and practice the words they will use to tell the child about the baby's death. Holistic care that is based on a family-centered model allows children to participate in seeing and holding a sibling who has died and in taking part in various family rituals such as a blessing or baptism (Limbo & Kobler, 2009).

CULTURAL ASPECTS OF LOSS

In a cultural context, death has many views. There are different ways of grieving. Tears and emotional outbursts are common to some cultures while others are quiet and introspective. The nurse needs to have an awareness and understanding of how different cultural groups interpret the

meaning of death and the factors that govern their response to death. The Hispanic culture that includes Mexicans, Puerto Ricans, and Cubans views children as their future. The loss of a child denies that future. They welcome touch from others and expect health-care professionals to respect their need for extended family during this time frame. All cultures should be treated with sensitivity, respect, and caring (Gilbert, 2010).

Cultural Diversity: Disparities in Risk of Stillbirth

In the United States, the chance that a pregnancy will end in a stillbirth is about 1 in 200 for Caucasian women and 1 in 87 for African American women. Interestingly, stillbirth is 10 times more common than sudden infant death syndrome and is more common than infant deaths related to congenital anomalies. It has been estimated that 40% of all stillbirths are significantly growth restricted, and preterm stillbirths (especially from 20 to 24 weeks of gestation) are more likely to be growth restricted and occur in black women (Fretts, 2010; Hogue & Silver, 2011).

Now Can You—Discuss issues concerning perinatal loss?

1. Identify significant members of the bereavement team?
2. Discuss interventions for families experiencing a perinatal loss?
3. Voice some comments that would be helpful for a grieving family?

Cesarean Birth

DEFINITION AND INCIDENCE

Cesarean birth is the birth of a fetus through an abdominal incision into the uterus; it is performed to preserve the life of the mother and her fetus. Today, cesarean delivery is the most common operation in the United States, and nearly one-third of all births occur in this manner (Blanchette, 2011). In 1965, the rate of cesarean births in the United States was less than 5%. The cesarean section rate in 2010 was 32.8%, slightly down from 32.9% in 2009. This figure, which has held steady in 2012, represented the first decline in cesarean births since 1996. Overall, since 1996, the number of cesarean births has increased by 46%, driven by both an increase in the percentage of all women having a first cesarean and a decline in the percentage of women who gave birth vaginally after a previous cesarean birth (Hamilton, Martin, Ventura, & Division of Vital Statistics, 2011; U.S. National Center for Health Statistics, 2013). Modern surgical advances and the use of antibiotics have resulted in a decrease in maternal and fetal morbidity and mortality. However, despite these advances, cesarean birth is a major surgical procedure that poses threats to the health of the mother and her infant.

INDICATIONS

Cesarean birth is performed when the health of the mother or her fetus is jeopardized. Maternal medical risk factors most closely associated with cesarean birth include hypertensive disorders, active genital herpes, positive HIV status, and diabetes. Fetal complications most closely associated with cesarean birth include cephalopelvic disproportion, malpresentations (i.e., breech or shoulder), placental abnormalities (e.g., abruptio previa), dysfunctional labor patterns, fetal distress, multiple gestation, and umbilical cord prolapse. In actuality, few absolute indications exist for cesarean birth, and most are primarily performed for the benefit of the fetus (Hamilton et al., 2011).

Elective cesarean births have been on the rise since 1985. In contemporary society, women are requesting cesarean births for reasons other than medical, obstetric, or fetal complications. One reason is related to a fear of vaginal birth, or tocophobia. Others are concerned about labor pain, fetal death or injury, and the potential for future problems with pelvic support or sexual dysfunction related to perineal or rectal injury. Some women view cesarean birth to be an empowering experience and wish to choose the birth method and date rather than have it selected for them. At issue is the question of whether an elective cesarean birth is more beneficial or harmful to a woman and her baby than a vaginal birth. The Association of Women's Health, Obstetric and Neonatal Nurses (AWHONN) supports the need to learn more about the nature of elective cesarean birth. AWHONN calls for continued research into strategies to decrease traumas associated with vaginal birth and subsequently decrease the need for elective cesarean birth because of maternal fear. Both the American College of Nurse-Midwives (ACNM) and the International Federation of Gynecology and Obstetrics (FIGO) have published statements stating that the practice of elective cesarean birth for nonmedical reasons is not ethically justified (ACNM, 2010; Campbell, 2011; FIGO, 2009).

Cultural Diversity: Cesarean Birth Rates Among Ethnic Groups and Predictors of Increased Cesarean Birth Rates

Among the five largest ethnic groups, cesarean birth rates are as follows: African Americans: 34%, Caucasians: 32%, Asians/Pacific Islanders: 31%, Hispanics: 30%, and Native Americans: 28%. Among all women, four medical risk factors increase the likelihood of cesarean birth: pregnancy weight gain greater than 40 pounds, diabetes, pregnancy-associated hypertension, and chronic hypertension (Centers for Disease Control and Prevention [CDC], 2012; Menacker & Hamilton, 2010). For both nulliparous and multiparous women, the main predictors of medically indicated and elective cesarean birth (including elective repeat cesarean delivery) include the following: labor induced before 39 weeks, maternal age over 35 years, use of assisted reproductive technology, and multiple gestation pregnancies (Campbell, 2011).

Cesarean birth is a major surgical procedure that carries risks and complications. It is associated with a host of potential postoperative problems such as hemorrhage, thromboembolism, and infection during the postpartum period. The surgery can result in chronic pain from scar tissue, urinary tract injury, adhesions, dehiscence of the wound, and problems with the placenta in subsequent pregnancies (Cunningham et al., 2014). Women face a higher incidence of death during a surgical procedure with

the use of general anesthesia and are at greater risk for intraoperative surgical complications such as lacerations of the uterus and bladder. In addition, there is a greater likelihood for hysterectomy associated with cesarean birth than with vaginal birth. The risk associated with previous cesarean delivery increases as the number of previous cesarean deliveries rises. Knight and colleagues (2008) found women undergoing hysterectomy at delivery were 18 times more likely to have had 2 or more previous cesarean births (Matthews & Rebarber, 2010). Furthermore, neonates born by cesarean section are at increased risk for respiratory problems, which can lead to asthma in childhood and adulthood (Azad, Konya, Maughan, Guttman, Field, Chari, et al., 2013; Collard, Diallo, Habinsky, Hentschell, & Vezeau, 2009).

Nursing Insight—*Impact of surgical adhesions on subsequent cesarean birth*

Tissue adhesions, band-like structures that form as a result of a defect in the healing process, can lead to significant morbidity, chronic pelvic pain, and complications of future surgery such as cesarean delivery. Adhesion interference originating from a primary cesarean birth prolongs repeat cesarean surgery, and the operative time (required for tissue dissection) is extended with each subsequent birth. Delayed delivery may negatively impact neonates (especially when urgent delivery is required) and mothers, whose anesthesia time is also prolonged (Burke, 2012; Greenberg, Daniels, Blumenfeld, Caughey, & Lyell, 2011).

ETHICAL CONSIDERATIONS OF ELECTIVE CESAREAN BIRTH

If it is more dangerous to have an elective cesarean birth than a vaginal birth, is it ethical to allow the woman to select this as her birth method of choice? One must consider the ethical principles of beneficence (the principle of doing good), non-maleficence (the physician's responsibility to do no harm), and the patient's right to autonomy (the capacity for self-determination). Autonomy requires the physician to assist the woman in integrating her own priorities, values, and fears while taking care not to impose personal beliefs into the decision-making process. The American College of Obstetricians and Gynecologists (ACOG) Committee on Ethics maintains that if a patient requests a cesarean birth, and the physician believes that the overall health of the mother and fetus will benefit, then the elective cesarean delivery has merit. If the physician does not think a cesarean method of birth is in the best interest of the patient (i.e., in the absence of maternal or fetal indications for cesarean delivery), the patient should be informed and given the right to select another physician (ACOG, 2003b, 2013b, 2013c). However, the issue is far more complex than this simple example.

Williams and Shah (2003) plead for a return to common sense. Birth is a normal and natural event. These authors raise the following questions: "Have we become a nation so obsessed with expediency and control that we are willing to relinquish our humanity to technology? Are we truly willing to sacrifice our health and future childbearing for the lure of 'birth by appointment'? Are our demands for perfection or compensation unnecessary interventions (p. 284)?" All women are entitled to unbiased information and a safe, supportive environment. Continued studies that examine the myriad issues concerning aspects of benefit versus harm including the economic ramifications of elective cesarean birth are in order, and nurses are perfectly positioned to contribute to this ongoing research and discussion (Campbell, 2011).

Optimizing Outcomes—Empowering women with elective cesarean birth education

In the advocate role, nurses should encourage women to enter into lengthy dialogs with their physicians about elective cesarean birth, exploring fully the advantages, disadvantages, misperceptions, and complications of their birth options. Long-term consequences should be discussed, and the woman should be informed that elective cesarean birth brings no significant benefit to pelvic or sexual health but does increase the likelihood of another cesarean birth with subsequent pregnancies. In the teacher role, nurses should assess the woman's understanding of different modes of birth and provide evidence-based information and resources (e.g., brochures and decision aids) so that women feel informed and prepared to enter into a dialog about birth choice. Ongoing exploration of feelings and education about expectations are essential elements of holistic care (Collard et al., 2009; Eden, Denman, Emeis, McDonagh, Fu, Janik, et al., 2012).

SURGICAL PROCEDURES

There are two main types of cesarean operations: the classic (vertical) incision and the lower-segment transverse (LST) incision (Fig. 14-15). The surgeon chooses the incision type based on the patient's condition and the fetal status. Rarely used today, the classic cesarean incision is reserved for some cases of shoulder presentation, placenta previa, and when birth must take place immediately. Because this type of uterine

incision is associated with complications including considerable blood loss, infection, and uterine rupture with subsequent pregnancies, women who undergo classic cesarean births may not attempt future vaginal births.

The lower segment cesarean (preferred by women for cosmetic reasons) may involve either a vertical or a transverse uterine incision. The transverse incision, more commonly performed, is associated with less blood loss, fewer postoperative infections, and a decreased likelihood of uterine rupture during subsequent pregnancies (Cunningham et al., 2014). The skin incision made into the abdomen is either transverse (sometimes called a "Pfannenstiel" or "bikini" incision) or vertical (sometimes called a "midline" incision). The skin incision may or may not be the same type of incision that is made into the abdomen. After the skin incision, the surgeon carefully moves through the tissue layers to the uterus. An incision is made into the uterus and the fetal head is gently elevated through the opening. A patent airway is established and the rest of the fetus is delivered. The cord is clamped and the newborn is placed, depending on the circumstances, either in the arms of the parent or in the neonatal warmer. After removal of the placenta, the incision is sutured at each layer, and a sterile bandage is placed over it (Cunningham et al., 2014).

The nurse documents all components of patient care including the time of birth and offers ongoing encouragement and support to the mother. Once the birth has taken place, the nurse facilitates attachment with the new family. Keeping mothers and their newborns together after cesarean birth promotes family-centered care and is associated with increased satisfaction among patients, nurses, and physicians (Elliott-Carter & Harper, 2012). When complications are present, the nurse provides information including a description of the newborn to the family. If the newborn requires resuscitation or a transfer to the neonatal intensive care unit, the family is allowed to view the neonate in the isolette before transport. When the newborn's condition is satisfactory, the newborn is presented to the parent or support person to hold. Although the mother is restrained by surgical equipment, the parent or support person can hold the baby close to the mother's face so that she can see her child (Fig. 14-16). This initial bonding experience can usually take place while the surgeon completes the suturing process. The family is then moved to the recovery room for postsurgical care.

NURSING CARE

In most instances, the patient scheduled for a planned cesarean birth is admitted on the day of surgery (Fig. 14-17). When the need for an emergency or unplanned cesarean arises, the patient undergoes the same procedures but in a more timely manner. Blood work, including type and cross match and a complete blood count, is obtained before admission, and the results are entered in the chart. The woman has been instructed to remain NPO since midnight before admission. The nurse orients the patient to the unit, reviews the prenatal history, and responds to any questions or concerns. An informed consent is signed. A fetal monitor is placed on the patient's abdomen for a 20- to 30-minute baseline assessment. Vital signs are taken and charted. In preparation for the surgery, the abdomen is cleaned and shaved, an intravenous line is placed, and an

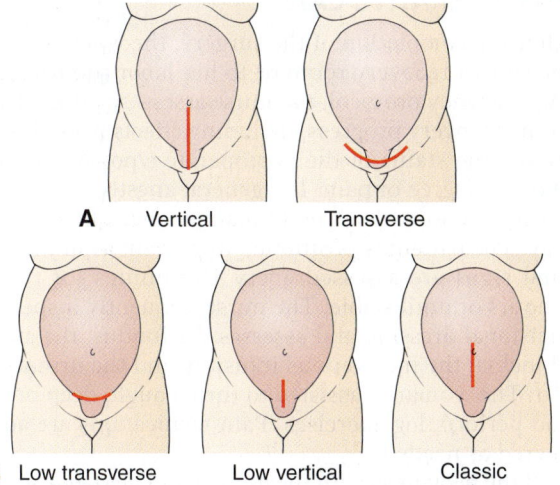

A Vertical   Transverse

B Low transverse   Low vertical   Classic

Figure 14-15 Abdominal wall and uterine incisions for cesarean births. *A,* Skin (abdominal wall) incisions. 1. Vertical, 2. Transverse (Pfannenstiel). *B,* Uterine wall incisions. 1. Low transverse, 2. Low vertical, 3. Classic.

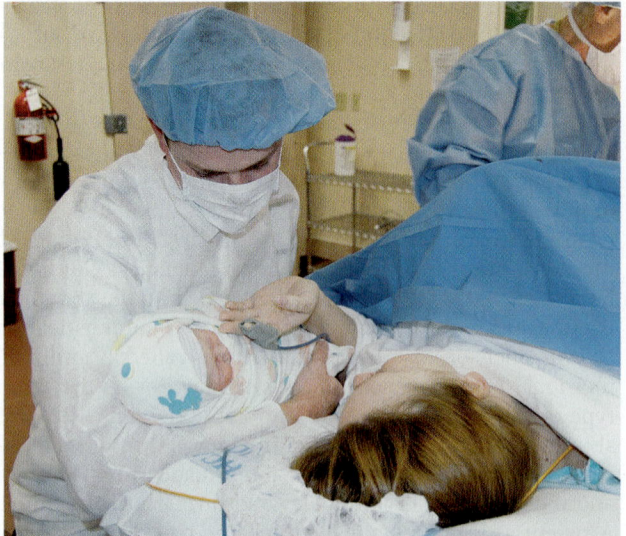

Figure 14-16 Family in cesarean birth.

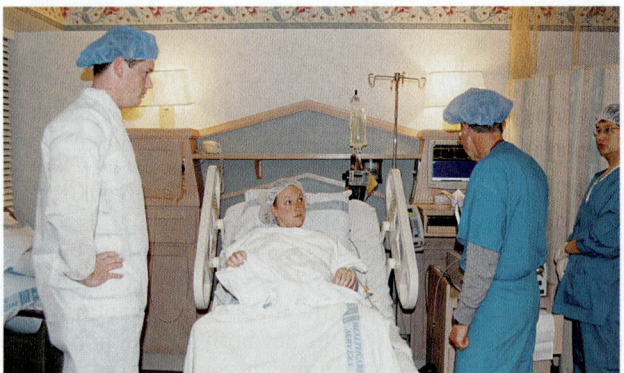

Figure 14-17 Couple awaiting scheduled cesarean section.

indwelling urinary catheter is inserted to keep the bladder empty during the operation. Medications are administered according to the physician's orders. If an epidural anesthetic is to be used, the nurse properly positions the patient and supports her during its administration. If a general anesthetic is to be used, an oral antacid may be prescribed to neutralize gastric secretions in the event of aspiration. The woman is then transported to the operative suite (Simpson & Creehan, 2013).

> **Optimizing Outcomes**—Enhancing maternal anesthesia knowledge and choice
>
> Spinal, epidural, and general anesthesia are used for cesarean births. Although epidural anesthesia is a popular choice because the woman may remain awake during the birth experience, the type of anesthesia used depends on factors such as the maternal medical history and current status and how quickly the birth needs to take place. In addition, the woman is a factor—she may harbor fears about having an anesthetic injected into her back. Patients should be given information including the risks and benefits associated with the different types of anesthesia to empower them to make an informed decision whenever there is a choice.

SURGICAL CARE

The nurse's role varies during the surgical procedure. Depending on the hospital setting and protocols, one nurse assists the physician during the procedure while another nurse circulates. A team consisting of a neonatal nurse and a neonatologist or nurse skilled in neonatal resuscitation is in attendance to provide care for the infant. The patient is placed on the surgical table with a hip wedge to slightly elevate the hips. The fetal heart rate (FHR) is continuously monitored until the patient's abdomen is ready for surgical preparation according to hospital protocol. The support person, dressed in appropriate surgical attire, may be present at any point in the process but is usually asked to wait until the surgical drapes are in place before being seated by the patient's head. The anesthesiologist monitors the maternal vital signs and the intravenous solutions.

When the woman remains awake during the procedure, the nurse and other members of the care team provide information about the events taking place and sensations that the woman may be experiencing. Continued support and explanations help to decrease anxiety, enhance feelings of comfort, and help the woman to maintain a sense of control in the unfamiliar and perhaps frightening, environment. A cesarean birth sequence is presented in Figure 14-18.

> **Optimizing Outcomes**—Maintaining competence in basic life support
>
> The AWHONN (2010b) supports the Joint Commission recommendation that all nurses achieve and maintain competence in basic life support. Because perinatal complications (e.g., medical, surgical, obstetric, and anesthetic) may develop, the AWHONN maintains that competence in assessment skills specific to these areas are important for nurses who provide care to women during the obstetric postanalgesia and postanesthesia periods.

POSTOPERATIVE CARE

After the completion of the surgery, the woman is transferred to a recovery room or to her labor room. According to agency protocol, the nurse assesses various aspects of the recovery progress, including effects from the anesthesia, the status of the postoperative/postbirth uterus, and the degree of pain. If a general anesthetic was used, special attention is given to maintenance of a patent airway. The patient is positioned to prevent aspiration, and vital signs are assessed every 15 minutes for the first 2 hours or until stable. The nurse frequently inspects the incisional dressing and assesses the fundus, the amount of lochia, the intravenous infusion, and the urinary output. The woman is assisted to turn, cough, deep breathe, and perform leg exercises. Pain medications are administered as needed.

If the neonate is with the mother and her labor support, time is provided to facilitate family bonding and attachment. If the woman wishes to breastfeed, she is encouraged to do so. Patients generally remain in the recovery area for 1 to 2 hours before transfer to the postpartum unit for continued care (see Chapter 15).

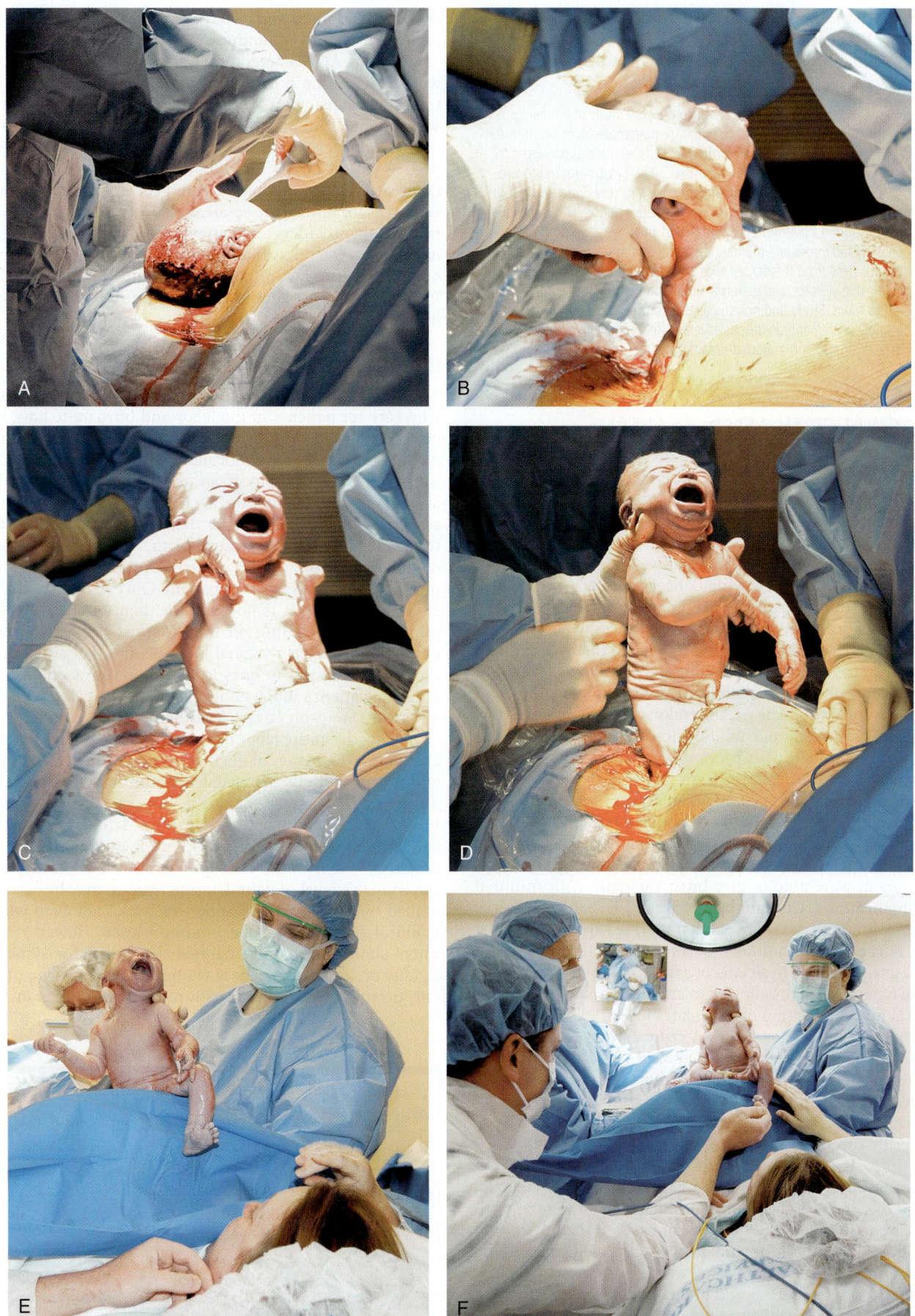

Figure 14-18 Cesarean birth. *A,* Delivery of the head. The nose and mouth are suctioned. *B,* Delivery of the shoulders. *C, D,* Delivery of the body. *E, F,* The newborn is presented to her parents.

Where Research and Practice Meet:
Minimizing Maternal–Infant Separation After Cesarean Birth

Noland and Lawrence (2009) conducted a pilot study of a nursing intervention protocol designed to minimize maternal–infant separation after elective, repeat cesarean birth. The "Nursing Intervention Protocol to Minimize Maternal-Infant Separation" (NIMS) was created to promote sustained, close maternal–infant proximity and direct contact in the intraoperative and immediate postoperative period. NIMS components included environmental intra- and postoperative preparation, unobstructed maternal–infant visualization and maintenance of spatial distance (less than 8 feet), *en face* presentation, cheek-to-cheek and skin-to-skin contact, and maternal–infant mutual transfer from the operating room. Study findings suggested that the NIMS protocol could be safely implemented without adverse effects and shows promise for positively improving maternal–infant outcomes after cesarean birth.

VAGINAL BIRTH AFTER CESAREAN

There is an old adage, "once a cesarean, always a cesarean." During the 1970s and 1980s, women challenged this rule and fought for the opportunity to attempt a **vaginal birth after a cesarean birth** (VBAC). Research conducted during that time provided evidence that a VBAC was safe and a more cost-effective birth alternative. This movement also coincided with the growing concern in the United States over the dramatic increase in cesarean birth rates, especially among women requiring a repeat cesarean birth.

In 1988, the ACOG, having concluded that women with a low transverse incision could safely be allowed a trial of labor and possible vaginal birth, released a statement in support of VBAC. The ACOG endorsed the practice of oxytocin administration, epidural anesthesia, and early ambulation for women with previous cesarean births who met certain criteria. A standby team prepared to perform a cesarean birth in the event of an emergency was to be available at all times. Numerous studies supported the success of VBAC. During the 1990s, approximately 60% to 80% of women who underwent a trial of labor following a previous cesarean were able to give birth vaginally with minimal complications (Cunningham et al., 2014). Safety concerns arose although data showed that uterine rupture, the most serious of complications, was a rare event. In response to these concerns, physicians began to more closely restrict the types of patients allowed to attempt a trial of labor. Criteria for the selection of candidates for a trial of labor have been developed (Box 14-6). A critical point confirmed by the studies was that VBACs needed to be performed in large hospitals or tertiary level centers because these institutions offer continued 24-hour anesthesia coverage necessary to prevent perinatal mortality and morbidity if uterine rupture occurs (Cunningham et al., 2014).

In 2010, both a National Institutes of Health (NIH) Consensus Development Panel on vaginal birth after cesarean and the ACOG issued updated statements on vaginal birth after cesarean delivery. Placing emphasis on shared decision making among informed patients and providers, the NIH Consensus Development Panel wrote: "information, including risk assessment, should be shared with the woman at a level and pace that she can understand. When both trial of labor and elective repeat cesarean delivery are medically equivalent options, a shared decision-making process

should be adopted and, whenever possible, the woman's preference should be honored" (NIH, 2010, p. 33).

Current ACOG recommendations state that most women with one previous cesarean delivery with a low transverse incision are candidates for and should be counseled about VBAC and offered a trial of labor after previous cesarean delivery (TOLAC), that epidural analgesia may be used as part of TOLAC, and that TOLAC should be undertaken at facilities capable of emergency deliveries. When resources for immediate cesarean delivery are not available, health-care providers and patients should discuss the facility's resources and availability of staff (e.g., obstetric, pediatric, anesthetic, and operating room), and once fully informed, patients should be allowed to accept increased levels of risk (ACOG, 2010).

NURSING IMPLICATIONS

To provide safe, effective care, it is essential that nurses who care for patients in the labor and birth suite have received extensive training in fetal monitoring interpretation. At the first sign of any abnormality in the FHR tracing, the nurse must alert the physician or certified nurse midwife. Meticulous documentation is critical because it provides essential information to other members of the health-care team. For the elective cesarean birth, informed consent is obtained in the physician's office before admission, and the nurse confirms this with the patient. Once patients actually experience labor, it is possible for them to change their minds, and depending on the circumstances, they may choose not to have a vaginal birth. As in other situations, the nurse responds to questions and concerns and ascertains the patient's understanding of the associated benefits and risks (Simpson & O'Brien-Abel, 2013).

During the entire labor process the nurse is alert for any changes in the maternal–fetal condition. The FHR pattern and uterine activity are usually monitored electronically during the active phase of labor. Non-reassuring FHR patterns such as prolonged decelerations, late decelerations, and variable decelerations may precede uterine rupture or herald its occurrence. The nurse continuously evaluates the woman's level of pain. Uterine rupture may be accompanied by abdominal, shoulder, or back pain even when epidural anesthesia has been administered. However, the nurse should frequently palpate the uterus for signs of rigidity because the patient may report no pain. When present, uterine or abdominal pain most often occurs in the

Box 14-6 Selection Criteria for Vaginal Birth After Cesarean Birth (VBAC)

- One previous low-transverse cesarean birth (if two prior cesarean births, only those who have also had a vaginal birth as well should be considered candidates for a spontaneous labor)
- Clinically adequate pelvis in relation to fetal size
- No other uterine scars, anomalies, or previous rupture
- Physician immediately available throughout active labor capable of monitoring labor and performing an emergency cesarean birth
- Availability of anesthesia and personnel for emergency cesarean birth

Source: American College of Obstetricians and Gynecologists (ACOG) (2010).

area of the previous incision and can range from mild to a "tearing" sensation. Uterine contractions may diminish in intensity and frequency, accompanied by loss of station of the presenting part. Vaginal or intra-abdominal bleeding may be accompanied by symptoms of anxiety, restlessness, weakness, dizziness, and gross hematuria. Because there is always the possibility of an emergency at any time, the nurse must be prepared to react in a calm manner. As the labor progresses, the patient and her support(s) should receive reassurance and information regarding any change in the plan of care (Scott, 2011).

⊖ **Now Can You**—Discuss VBAC?

1. Name five criteria for a patient to be allowed to attempt a vaginal birth after a previous cesarean birth?
2. Discuss possible patient concerns regarding VBAC and how the nurse should appropriately respond to them?
3. List three specific nursing implications associated with the care of the woman who is experiencing a VBAC?

CESAREAN BIRTH: AREAS FOR CONTINUED RESEARCH

The rising rate of cesarean births and the decrease in the number of vaginal births after cesarean births (VBAC) are related. The higher the number of first-time mothers who experience a cesarean delivery, the higher the number of women who may not have a choice for a vaginal delivery the next time if their physician is reluctant to attempt a VBAC. Medical studies currently question the rising cesarean birth rate. The adverse consequences of higher cesarean birth rates contribute to an increase in maternal morbidity and mortality. In addition, there are significant economic costs related to the prolonged hospital stays and the increased need for expensive surgery-related technologies. Although the greatest concern centers on the health and safety of the mother and her fetus, burgeoning health-care costs cannot be discounted as a problem.

Nurse researchers should continue to examine evidence to provide a better understanding of the factors that impact the cesarean birth rate. A few of the modifiable variables include maternal obesity, fear of labor and delivery, physiological pushing techniques, fear of injury, and convenience in planning a birth. Nurses need to engage in clinical research designed to offer evidence identifying the myriad of factors that contribute to the rise in cesarean births. The results of such studies may lead to a decrease in the overall cesarean birth rate, which has risen steadily throughout the last decade. Nurse educators in the community can provide supportive interventions for all of these issues. Counseling during the prenatal period to allay anxieties and fears is critical. Families also need realistic plans for the childbirth along with thorough explanations of procedures and what they should expect (Collard et al., 2009).

Prepared childbirth classes have increased in numbers and variety in the United States. Although many health educators serve an important role, the nurse with a clinical practice in obstetrics and women's health is in an ideal position to offer constructive guidance to families. Families need to learn to advocate for themselves through increased knowledge and understanding of the issues surrounding operative deliveries. If women's fears concerning childbirth are lessened, they become more open to teaching and can begin to function as collaborators in their own care. For example, perinatal education and selective tension-reducing labor techniques may reduce the woman's fear of labor and birth. Perhaps women who are able to overcome their fear of labor will choose to attempt vaginal birth instead of an elective cesarean birth. Nurses who serve as childbirth educators have a unique opportunity to empower women and their families through education, and this new knowledge and self-confidence may translate into a reduction in the rate of cesarean births.

Postterm Pregnancy/Prolonged Pregnancy

A **postterm pregnancy** is defined as one that extends beyond 294 days or 42 weeks past the first day of the last normal menstrual period. According to the American College of Obstetricians and Gynecologists (2013d), a postterm pregnancy is one at $42^{0/7}$ weeks and beyond. A similar term, **postdate,** identifies a pregnancy that has gone past the estimated date of birth. It is estimated that postterm pregnancies occur in approximately 3% to 12% of all pregnancies.

Prolonged pregnancies are at risk for a number of problems including fetal macrosomia associated with shoulder dystocia and fetal injury, oligohydramnios, meconium aspiration, intrapartum fetal distress, and stillbirth. Neonatal problems may include asphyxia, meconium aspiration syndrome, hypoglycemia, polycythemia, respiratory distress, and dysmaturity syndrome (Gilbert, 2010, 2011).

Maternal risks such as trauma, hemorrhage, infection, and labor abnormalities are also associated with postterm pregnancy. Labor interventions including induction with prostaglandins or oxytocin, forceps- or vacuum-assisted birth, and cesarean birth are more likely to be needed. In addition, the woman may experience fatigue and psychological responses such as depression, frustration, loss of control, and feelings of inadequacy as the pregnancy extends beyond the estimated date of birth (ACOG, 2013d; Simhan et al., 2012).

The exact cause of postterm pregnancy is unknown. However, a possible cause may be related to a deficiency of placental estrogen and the continued secretion of progesterone. Low levels of estrogen may result in a decrease in prostaglandin precursors and the reduced formation of myometrial oxytocin receptors (Gilbert, 2010). A woman with a history of one postterm pregnancy is more likely to experience another with subsequent pregnancies (Rampersad & Macones, 2012).

Because the placenta ages rapidly past the 40th week of gestation, it becomes inefficient and cannot adequately support the fetus. Areas of infarction coupled with calcium and fibrin deposits result in reduced placental reserves (Fig. 14-19). The decrease in oxygen and nutrients results in fetal hypoxic episodes. Hypoxic events that occur on a regular basis stress the fetus. When labor commences, the postterm compromised fetus is at a greater risk for severe distress than the nonstressed term infant (Gilbert, 2010).

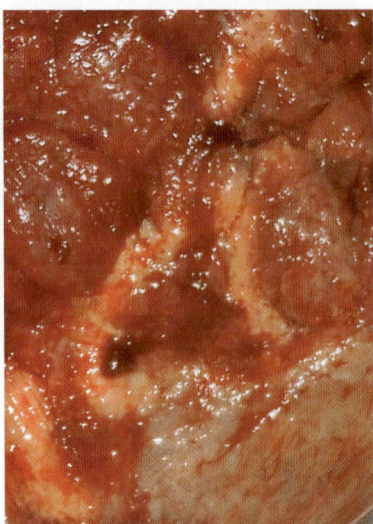

Figure 14-19 Calcifications appear as white areas in the placenta.

Antenatal testing combined with careful expectant management is used to monitor fetal status beyond the 40th week of gestation. Antenatal testing is not viewed as a predictor of an untoward event but as a way to identify the fetus that demonstrates signs of compromise. The antenatal assessments most often obtained include nonstress tests, biophysical profiles, amniotic fluid volume measurements, and maternal daily fetal movement counts. Other tests include the contraction stress test, which relies on oxytocin-stimulated contractions to identify fetal heart rate (FHR) decelerations associated with fetal hypoxia, and Doppler flow measurements. The tests are usually performed on a weekly or twice-weekly basis (Cunningham et al., 2014; Rampersad & Macones, 2012). (See Chapter 11 for further discussion.)

MEDICAL MANAGEMENT

If a woman does not experience spontaneous labor by the 42nd week (sometimes earlier), induction is considered the primary medical management choice. Expectant management, including daily kick counts, weekly monitoring of the amniotic fluid index, and nonstress testing, provide information regarding fetal well-being but are not always conclusive. If the gestational age is documented by ultrasound to be beyond 42 weeks and the cervix is favorable, most physicians proceed with labor induction. A cervix that is favorable (i.e., one that has begun to efface and dilate) is more conducive to the induction. If the cervix is not favorable, a cervical ripening agent (e.g., prostaglandin insert or gel) may be administered, followed by oxytocin induction (ACOG, 2009; Cunningham et al., 2014). Some women with an unfavorable cervix may choose to continue with careful daily monitoring instead of the induction. As long as the physician considers the surveillance to be a safe option, the patient may be allowed to continue with the process of expectant management. However, if spontaneous labor does not begin by the 42nd or 43rd week, most physicians proceed with induction (Beckman, Herbert, Laube, Ling, & Smith, 2013).

NURSING IMPLICATIONS

The nurse conducts the nonstress and nipple stimulation contraction stress tests in the antepartum clinical setting, interprets information for the patient, and provides reassurance. The nurse must be cautious in providing only the factual information. Because there is a possibility of false readings, the nurse must avoid offering unfound reassurances and immediately notify the physician if test results are not normal. Understandably, patients often experience increased anxiety when their due date has passed and they are still pregnant. The nurse is in a position to provide a consistent presence and respond to any questions or concerns. If induction is decided as the treatment option, the nurse explains the procedure to the patient and again responds to questions and concerns.

Intrapartal nursing care centers on close maternal–fetal surveillance and continued emotional support. During labor, the fetus should be monitored electronically to obtain an accurate assessment of the FHR and pattern. Umbilical cord compression, which is more likely to occur in the presence of decreased amniotic fluid, results in fetal hypoxia. Variable or prolonged deceleration patterns and the passage of meconium are reflective of fetal hypoxia. If oligohydramnios is present, amnioinfusion may be performed to restore the amniotic fluid volume to provide a fluid cushion for the umbilical cord (Cunningham et al., 2014).

Summary Points

- The nurse serves in many capacities when managing the care of women experiencing a complicated labor and birth; a strong theoretical background provides a foundation for the necessary critical decision making.

- Dystocia—a long, difficult, or abnormal labor—may arise from any of the three major components of the labor process: the powers, passenger, or passageway.

- During a trial of labor, nursing responsibilities center on assessment of maternal vital signs and FHR and pattern.

- Oxytocin used during labor induction and augmentation should always be administered as a *piggyback* solution, and a uterine and FHR monitor should be used continuously during the infusion.

- Forceps and vacuum extraction are methods to assist birth; the mother and the infant require special observation during and after these procedures.

- The management of hypertensive disorders during intrapartum is focused on preventing further deterioration of affected organs and fostering a positive maternal–fetal outcome.

- Cesarean birth, which may be a scheduled or emergency procedure, is associated with increased risk for the mother and her infant and should be undertaken only when medically necessary.

- Perinatal loss necessitates a collaborative response from all professionals involved in the care of the patient.

Review Questions

Multiple Choice

1. A nurse is reviewing hypotonic labor with a student nurse. The nurse explains to the student that which of the following is the most common cause of this dysfunctional labor pattern?
A. Fetal macrosomia
B. Maternal android pelvis
C. Inadequate uterine pacemakers
D. Fetal occiput–posterior position

2. The perinatal nurse is aware that complications arising from amnioinfusion include which of the following?
A. Infection
B. Halt in labor
C. Neonatal hydrocephalus
D. Fluid overload

3. The perinatal nurse understands that one of the risks of oxytocin infusion includes FHR changes related to which of the following?
A. Decreased placental perfusion
B. Oligohydramnios
C. Maternal hypotonic contractions
D. Maternal hypotension

4. A nurse reads in a woman's chart that she has a history of dystocia. Based on this information, the nurse assesses the woman for what condition?
A. Fetal abnormalities
B. Long, difficult labor
C. Prior fetal demise
D. Bleeding abnormalities

5. A patient has an order for a prostaglandin E_2 preparation. What does the nurse understand about this medication?
A. Only used when delivery is imminent
B. Cervical ripening agent
C. Has a high rate of adverse reactions
D. Is only given subcutaneously

6. The perinatal nurse is aware that recommendations for elective deliveries specify induction no earlier than what gestational age?
A. 30 weeks
B. 35 weeks
C. 37 weeks
D. 39 weeks

7. The perinatal nurse knows that which of the following conditions must be met before assisting at a forceps delivery?
A. Presenting part must be engaged
B. Membranes must still be intact
C. Patient's bladder should be full
D. Cervix at least 50% dilated

8. A nurse hears a health-care provider describe a pregnant woman as having tocophobia. What does the nurse understand this to mean?
A. Allergy to tocolytics
B. Fear of childbirth
C. Fear of pain
D. Atonic uterus

9. A woman has a history of placenta increta. What does the nurse understand about this condition?
A. Slight penetration of the myometrium by the trophoblast
B. Placental perforation of the uterus
C. Deep placental penetration of the myometrium
D. Abnormal implantation of the placenta

10. A woman has a history of a bilobed placenta, each with its own circulation. What condition does this describe?
A. Battledore placenta
B. Circumvallate placenta
C. Succenturiate placenta
D. Placenta percreta

See Answers to End of Chapter Review Questions on Davis*Plus*.

REFERENCES

Agency for Healthcare Research and Quality (AHRQ). (2010). *Health care for minority women: Recent findings*. Program Brief. AHRQ Pub. No. 11-P005. Rockville, MD: Author.

Agency for Healthcare Research and Quality (AHRQ). (2013). Induction of labour. Retrieved from http://www.guideline.gov/content.aspx?id=14308

American College of Nurse-Midwives. (2010). *ACNM responds to ACOG 2010 VBAC recommendations*. Retrieved from http://midwife.org/acnm/files/ccLibraryFiles/Filename/000000000075/ACNMResponse-toVBACBulletin_082610FINAL.pdf

American College of Obstetricians and Gynecologists (ACOG). (2000). Operative vaginal delivery. Practice Bulletin No. 17. (Reaffirmed 2012). Washington, DC: Author.

American College of Obstetricians and Gynecologists (ACOG). (2002a). Diagnosis and management of preeclampsia and eclampsia. Practice Bulletin No. 33. (Reaffirmed 2010). *Obstetrics & Gynecology, 99*(1), 159–167.

American College of Obstetricians and Gynecologists (ACOG). (2002b). Shoulder dystocia. Practice Bulletin No. 40. (Reaffirmed 2013). *Obstetrics & Gynecology, 100*(11), 1045–1050.

American College of Obstetricians and Gynecologists (ACOG). (2003a). Dystocia and augmentation of labor. Practice Bulletin No. 49. (Reaffirmed 2013). *Obstetrics & Gynecology, 102*(12), 1445–1454.

American College of Obstetricians and Gynecologists (ACOG). (2003b). *New ACOG opinion addresses elective cesarean controversy*, ACOG news release, October 31, 2003. Washington, DC: Author.

American College of Obstetricians and Gynecologists (ACOG). (2006). Amnioinfusion does not prevent meconium aspiration syndrome. Committee Opinion No. 346. (Reaffirmed 2012). *Obstetrics & Gynecology, 108*(10), 1053–1055.

American College of Obstetricians and Gynecologists (ACOG). (2009). Induction of labor. Practice Bulletin No. 107. (Reaffirmed 2013). *Obstetrics & Gynecology, 114*(8), 387–397.

American College of Obstetricians and Gynecologists (ACOG). (2010). Vaginal birth after previous cesarean delivery. Practice Bulletin No. 115. (Reaffirmed 2013). *Obstetrics & Gynecology, 116*(8), 450–463.

American College of Obstetricians and Gynecologists (ACOG). (2011). Preparing for clinical emergencies in obstetrics and gynecology. Committee Opinion No. 487. *Obstetrics & Gynecology, 117*(4), 1032–1034.

American College of Obstetricians and Gynecologists (ACOG). (2012a). Management of preterm labor. Practice Bulletin No. 127. *Obstetrics & Gynecology, 119*(6), 1308–1317.

American College of Obstetricians and Gynecologists (ACOG). (2012b). Disclosure and discussion of adverse events. Committee Opinion No. 520. (Reaffirmed 2013). *Obstetrics & Gynecology, 119*(3), 686–688.

American College of Obstetricians and Gynecologists (ACOG). (2013a). Gestational diabetes mellitus. Practice Bulletin No. 137. *Obstetrics & Gynecology, 122*(8), 406–416.

American College of Obstetricians and Gynecologists (ACOG). (2013b). Cesarean delivery on maternal request. Committee Opinion No. 559. *Obstetrics & Gynecology, 121*(4), 904–907.

American College of Obstetricians and Gynecologists (ACOG). (2013c). Elective surgery and patient choice. Committee Opinion No. 578. *Obstetrics & Gynecology, 122*(11), 1134–1138.

American College of Obstetricians and Gynecologists (ACOG). (2013d). Definition of term pregnancy. Committee Opinion No. 579. *Obstetrics & Gynecology, 122*(11), 1139–1140.

Ansell Irving, L., McAra-Couper, J., & Smythe, E. (2012). Shoulder dystocia: A qualitative exploration of what works. *Midwifery, 28*(4), 64–69. doi:10.1016/j.midw.2011.05.007

Antoniewicz, L., & Hollier, L. (2011). Strategies for reducing adverse patient outcomes in obstetrics. *The Female Patient, 36*(5), 39–47.

Ashmead, G. G. (2012). Shoulder dystocia. *The Female Patient, 37*(2), 32–40.

Association of Women's Health, Obstetric and Neonatal Nurses (AWHONN). (2009). Amniotomy and placement of internal fetal spiral electrode through intact membranes. AWHONN Position Statement. *Journal of Obstetric, Gynecologic & Neonatal Nursing, 13*(6), 521. doi:10.1111/j.1552-6909.2009.01076.x

Association of Women's Health, Obstetric and Neonatal Nurses (AWHONN). (2010a). *Guidelines for professional registered nurse staffing for perinatal units.* Washington, DC: Author.

Association of Women's Health, Obstetric and Neonatal Nurses (AWHONN). (2010b). Advanced cardiac life support in obstetric settings. AWHONN Position Statement. *Journal of Obstetric, Gynecologic & Neonatal Nursing, 39*(5), 422–423. doi:10.1111/j.1552-6909.2010.01176.x

Association of Women's Health, Obstetric and Neonatal Nurses (AWHONN). (2012). The role of the nurse in emergency preparedness. AWHONN Position Statement. *Journal of Obstetric, Gynecologic & Neonatal Nursing, 41*(5), 170–172. doi:10.1111/j.1552-6909.2011.01338.x

Association of Women's Health, Obstetric and Neonatal Nurses (AWHONN). (2014). Non-medically indicated induction and augmentation of labor. AWHONN Position Statement. *Journal of Obstetric, Gynecologic & Neonatal Nursing, 43*(5), 678-681. doi:10.1111/1552-6909.12499

Azad, M., Konya, T., Maughan, H., Guttman, D., Field, C., Chari, R., et al. (2013). Gut microbiota of healthy Canadian infants: Profiles by mode of delivery and infant diet at 4 months. *Canadian Medical Association Journal, 185*(5), 373–375. doi:10.1503/cmaj.130147

Beckman, C., Herbert, W., Laube, D., Ling, F., & Smith, R. (2013). *Obstetrics and Gynecology* (7th ed.). Philadelphia, PA: Lippincott Williams & Wilkins.

Bishop, E. H. (1964). Pelvic scoring for elective induction. *Obstetrics & Gynecology, 24*(9), 266–268.

Blanchette, H. (2011). The rising cesarean delivery rate in America: What are the consequences? *Obstetrics & Gynecology, 118*(3), 687–690. doi:10.1097/AOG.0b013e318227b8d9

Braithwaite, P., Chichester, M., & Reid, A. (2010). When the pregnant Jehovah's Witness patient refuses blood: Implications for nurses. *Nursing for Women's Health, 14*(6), 464–470.

Bulechek, G. M., Butcher, H. K., Dochterman, J. M., & Wagner, C. (2013). *Nursing interventions classification (NIC)* (6th ed.). St. Louis, MO: Elsevier Mosby.

Burke, C. (2012). Surgical adhesions: Implications for women's health. *Nursing for Women's Health,* Suppl., February-March, S4–S22.

Burkman, R. T., & Fennell, J. L. (2010). Fetal heart tracing: Why communication and documentation are essential. *The Female Patient, 35*(9), 38–40.

Campbell, C. (2011). Elective cesarean delivery: Trends, evidence and implications for women, newborns and nurses. *Nursing for Women's Health, 15*(4), 310–319. doi:10.1111/j.1751-486X.2011.01651.x

Centers for Disease Control and Prevention (CDC). (2012). *Assisted reproductive technology (ART).* Retrieved from http://www.cdc.gov/art/

Clark, S. L., & Hankins, G. D. (2012). Preventing maternal death: 10 clinical diamonds. *Obstetrics & Gynecology, 117*(2 Pt 1), 360–364.

Collard, T. D., Diallo, H., Habinsky, A., Hentschell, C., & Vezeau, T. M. (2009). Elective cesarean section: Why women choose it and what nurses need to know. *Nursing for Women's Health, 12*(6), 481–488. doi:10.1111/j.1751-486X.2008.00382.x

Craighead, D. V. (2012). Early term birth: Understanding the health risks to infants. *Nursing for Women's Health, 16*(2), 138–144. doi:10.1111/j.1751-486Z.2012.01719.x

Cunningham, F. G., Leveno, K. J., Bloom, S. L., Spong, C., & Dashe, J. (2014). *Williams Obstetrics* (24th ed.). New York, NY: McGraw-Hill Professional.

Davidson, J., Powers, K., Hedayat, K., Tiedszen, M., Kon, A., Shepard, E., et al. (2007). Clinical practice guidelines for the support of the family in the patient-centered intensive care unit: American College of Critical Care Medicine Task Force 2004–2005. *Critical Care Medicine, 35*(2), 605–622.

deValk, H. W., & Visser, G. H. A. (2011). Insulin during pregnancy, labour, and delivery. *Best Practice & Research Clinical Obstetrics and Gynaecology, 25,* 65–76.

Doyle, J., Kenny, T., Burkett, A., & von Gruenigen, V. (2011). A performance improvement process to tackle tachysystole. *Journal of Obstetric, Gynecologic & Neonatal Nursing, 40*(5), 512–519. doi:10.1111/j.1552-6909.2011.012875.x

Doyle, J. L., Kenny, T. H., von Gruenigen, V. E., Butz, A. M., & Burkett, A. M. (2012). Implementing an induction scheduling procedure and consent form to improve quality of care. *Journal of Obstetric, Gynecologic & Neonatal Nursing, 41*(4), 462–473. doi:10.1111/j.1552-6909.2012.01380.x

Duffy, C. R., Odibo, A. O., Roehl, K. A., Macones, G. A., & Cahill, A. G. (2012). Effect of magnesium sulfate on fetal heart rate patterns in the second stage of labor. *Obstetrics & Gynecology, 119*(6), 1129–1136. doi:10.1097/AOG.0b013e318257181e

Eden, K. B., Denman, M. A., Emeis, C. L., McDonagh, M. S., Fu, R., Janik, R. K., et al. (2012). Trial of labor and vaginal delivery rates in women with a prior cesarean. *Journal of Obstetric, Gynecologic & Neonatal Nursing, 41*(5), 583–598. doi:10.1111/j.1552-6909.2012.01388.x

Eller, A. G., Bennett, M. A., Sharshiner, M., Masheter, C., Soisson, A. P., Dodson, M., & Silver, R. M. (2011). Maternal morbidity in cases of placenta accreta managed by a multidisciplinary team compared with standard obstetric care. *Obstetrics & Gynecology, 117*(2 Pt 1), 331–337.

Elliott-Carter, N., & Harper, J. (2012). Keeping mothers and newborns together after cesarean. *Nursing for Women's Health, 16*(4), 291–295. doi:10.1111/j.1751-486X.2012.01747.x

English, N. K., & Hessler, K. L. (2013). Prenatal birth planning for families of the imperiled newborn. *Journal of Obstetric, Gynecologic & Neonatal Nursing, 42*(3), 390–399. doi:10.1111/1552-6909.12031

Esakoff, T. F., & Kilpatrick, S. J. (2013). The transcervical Foley balloon. *Contemporary OB/GYN, 58*(11), 34–41.

Felton, M. B. (2011). Normal childbirth. In S. Mattson & J. E. Smith (Eds.), *Core curriculum for maternal-newborn nursing* (4th ed., pp. 225–247). Philadelphia, PA: W.B. Saunders.

Francois, K. E., & Foley, M. R. (2012). Antepartum and postpartum hemorrhage. In S. G. Gabbe, J. R. Niebyl, J. L. Simpson, M. B. Landon, H. L. Galan, E. R. Jauniaux, & D. A. Driscoll, *Obstetrics: Normal and problem pregnancies* (6th ed., pp. 415–444). Philadelphia, PA: W.B. Saunders.

Fretts, R. C. (2010). The study of stillbirth and the "12 steps" toward prevention. *The Female Patient, 35*(3), 38–41.

Genovese, S. K. (2011). Hemorrhagic disorders. In S. Mattson, & J. Smith (Eds.), *Core curriculum for maternal-child nursing* (4th ed., pp. 478–499). Philadelphia, PA: W.B. Saunders.

Gilbert, E. S. (2010). *Manual of high risk pregnancy and delivery* (5th ed.). St. Louis, MO: C.V. Mosby.

Gilbert, E. S. (2011). Labor and delivery at risk. In S. Mattson, & J. Smith (Eds.), *Core curriculum for maternal-child nursing* (4th ed., pp. 624–649). Philadelphia, PA: W.B. Saunders.

Goetzinger, K. R., Harper, L. M., Tuuli, M., Macones, G. A., & Colditz, G. A. (2011). Effect of regional anesthesia on the success rate of external cephalic version. *Obstetrics & Gynecology, 118*(5), 1137–1144. doi:10.1097/AOG.0b013e3182324583

Goldenberg, R. L., McClure, E. M., Bhattacharya, A., Groat, T. D., & Stahl, P. J. (2009). Women's perceptions regarding the safety of births at various gestational ages. *Obstetrics & Gynecology 114*(6), 1254–1258.

Greenberg, M. B., Daniels, K., Blumenfeld, Y. J., Caughey, A. B., & Lyell, D. J. (2011). Do adhesions at repeat cesarean delay delivery of the newborn? *American Journal of Obstetrics and Gynecology, 205,* 380.e1–380.e5.

Hamilton, B., Martin, J., Ventura, M., & Division of Vital Statistics. (2011). Births: Preliminary data from 2010. *National Vital Statistics Reports, 60*(2). Hyattsville, MD: National Center for Health Statistics.

Harper, L. M., Caughey, A. B., Odibo, A. O., Roehl, K. A., Zhao, Q., & Cahill, A. G. (2012). Normal progress of induced labor. *Obstetrics & Gynecology, 119*(6), 1113–1118. doi:10.1097/AOG.0b013e318253d7aa

Harris, I. S. (2011). Management of pregnancy in patients with congenital heart disease. *Progress in Cardiovascular Diseases, 53*(4), 305–311. doi:10.3410/f.9378962.10007061

Harvey, C., & Dildy, G. A. (2012). In N. Troiano, C. Harvey, & B. Chez. *AWHONN High-risk & critical care obstetrics* (3rd ed, pp. 246–273). Philadelphia, PA: Lippincott Williams & Wilkins.

Hogue, C., & Silver, R. (2011). Racial and ethnic disparities in the United States: Stillbirth rates: Trends, risk factors, and research needs. *Seminars in Perinatology, 35*(4), 221–233. doi:10.1053/j.semperi.2011.02.019

Hood, D. G. (2012). Continuous subcutaneous insulin infusion for managing diabetes. *Nursing for Women's Health, 16*(4), 310–318. doi:10.1111/j.1751-486X.2012.01749.x

Huerta-Bogdan, B. I. (2011). Improving interpretation of electronic fetal heart monitoring. *Women's Health Care: A Practical Journal for Nurse Practitioners, 10*(9), 52–56.

Hull, A. D., & Resnik, R. (2013). Placenta previa, placenta accreta, abruptio placentae, and vasa previa. In R. Creasy, R. Resnick, J. Iams, C. Lockwood, T. Moore, & M. Greene, *Creasy & Resnik's Maternal-fetal medicine: Principles and practice* (7th ed., pp. 732–742). Philadelphia, PA: W.B. Saunders.

International Federation of Gynecology and Obstetrics (FIGO). (2009). *Recommendations on ethical issues in obstetrics and gynecology.* Retrieved from http://www.figo.org/about/guidelines

International Liaison Committee on Resuscitation (ILCOR). (2006). The International Liaison Committee on Resuscitation (ILCOR) consensus on science with treatment recommendations for pediatric and neonatal patients: Neonatal resuscitation. *Pediatrics, 117*(5), e978–e988.

Kauffman, S. G., Hauck, C. B., & Mandel, D. A. (2010). Perinatal palliative care: The nursing perspective. *Nursing for Women's Health, 14*(3), 189–197. doi:10.1111/j.1751-486X.2010.01540.x

Kilpatrick, S., & Garrison, E. (2012). Normal labor and delivery. In S. G. Gabbe, J. R. Niebyl, J. L. Simpson, M. B. Landon, H. L. Galan, E. R. Jauniaux, & D. A. Driscoll, *Obstetrics: Normal and problem pregnancies* (6th ed., pp. 267–286). Philadelphia, PA: W.B. Saunders.

Knight, M., Kurinczuk, J., Spark, P., & Brocklehurst, P. (2008). Cesarean delivery and peripartum hysterectomy. *Obstetrics & Gynecology, 111*(1), 97–105. doi:10.1097/01.AOG.0000296658.83240.6d

Laughon, S. K., Zhang, J., Troendle, J., Sun, L., & Reddy, U. M. (2011). Using a simplified Bishop score to predict vaginal delivery. *Obstetrics & Gynecology, 117*(4), 805–811. doi:10.1097/AOG.0b013e3182114ad2

Leung, T. Y., Stuart, O., Suen, S. S., Sahota, D. S., Lau, T. K., & Lao, T. T. (2011). Comparison of perinatal outcomes of shoulder dystocia alleviated by different type and sequence of manoeuvres: A retrospective review. *British Journal of Obstetrics & Gynaecology, 118*(8), 985–990.

Limbo, R., & Kobler, K. (2009). Will our baby be alive again? Supporting parents of young children when a baby dies. *Nursing for Women's Health, 13*(4), 303–311. doi:10.1111/j.1751-486X.2009.01440.x

Lockwood, C. J. (2011). The changing face of maternal mortality. *Contemporary OB/GYN, 56*(3), 8–11.

MacMullen, N., Dulski, L., & Meagher, B. (2005). RED ALERT: Perinatal hemorrhage. *The American Journal of Maternal Child Health, 30*(1), 46–51.

Malone, F. D., & D'Alton, M. E. (2013). Multiple gestation. Clinical characteristics and management. In R. Creasy, R. Resnick, J. Iams, C. Lockwood, T. Moore, & M. Greene, *Creasy & Resnik's Maternal-fetal medicine: Principles and practice* (7th ed., pp. 578–598). Philadelphia, PA: W.B. Saunders.

Mandel, D., Pirko, C., Grant, K., Kauffman, T., Williams, L., & Schneider, J. (2009). A collaborative protocol on oxytocin administration. *Nursing for Women's Health, 13*(6), 480–485. doi:10.1111/j.1751-486X .1009.01482.x

Matthews, G., & Rebarber, A. (2010). Postpartum uterine wound dehiscence leading to secondary postpartum hemorrhage. *Contemporary OB/GYN, 55*(5), 30–36.

Menacker, F., & Hamilton, B. E. (2010). *Recent trends in cesarean delivery in the United States, NCHS data brief no. 35* (DHHS Publication No., PHS 2010-1209). Washington, DC: U.S. Government Printing Office.

Miller, L. (2005). Patient safety and teamwork in perinatal care: Resources for clinicians. *The Journal of Perinatal & Neonatal Nursing, 19*(1), 46–51.

Miller, L. A., Miller, D., & Tucker, S. M. (2012). *Mosby's pocket guide to fetal monitoring: A multidisciplinary approach* (7th ed.). Philadelphia, PA: Mosby.

Mirza, F. G., Devine, P. C., & Gaddipati, S. (2010). Update on obstetric emergencies. *The Female Patient, 35*(2), 31–33.

Mirza, F. G., & Gyamfi, C. (2010). Management of pregnancy in the Jehovah's Witness. *Contemporary OB/Gyn, 55*(12), 41–48.

Moore, T., Hauguel deMouzon , S., & Catalano, P. (2013). Diabetes in pregnancy. In R. Creasy, R. Resnick, J. Iams, C. Lockwood, T. Moore, & M. Greene, *Creasy & Resnik's Maternal-fetal medicine: Principles and practice* (7th ed., pp. 988–1021). Philadelphia, PA: W.B. Saunders.

National Institutes of Health. (2010). National Institutes of Health Consensus Development Conference Statement: Vaginal birth after cesarean: New insights March 8–10, 2010. *Obstetrics & Gynecology, 115*(6), 1279–1295. doi:10.1097/AOG.0b013e3181e459e5

Neoventa. (2012). ST analysis: The STAN method. Retrieved from http://www.neoventa.com/US/

Nielson, P. E., & Galan, H. L. (2012). Operative vaginal delivery. In S. G. Gabbe, J. R. Niebyl, J. L. Simpson, M. B. Landon, H. L. Galan, E. R.

Jauniaux, & D. A. Driscoll (Eds.), *Obstetrics: Normal and problem pregnancies* (6th ed., pp. 311–329). Philadelphia, PA: W.B. Saunders.

Noland, A., & Lawrence, C. (2009). A pilot study of a nursing intervention protocol to minimize maternal-infant separation after cesarean birth. *Journal of Obstetric, Gynecologic & Neonatal Nursing, 38*(4), 430–442. doi:10.1111/j.1552-6909.2009.01039.x

Nowak, E. W., & Stevens, P. E. (2010). Vigilance in parents' experiences of fetal and infant loss. *Journal of Obstetric, Gynecologic & Neonatal Nursing, 40*(1), 122–130. doi:10.1111/j.1552-6909.2010.01207.x

Pacheco, L. D., Saade, G., Tyner, J., Clark, S. L., & Hankins, G. D. (2012). Obstetric hemorrhage: New insights. *Contemporary Ob-Gyn, 57*(6), 30–38.

Paris, A. E., Greenberg, J. A., Ecker, J. L., & McElrath, T. F. (2011). Is an episiotomy necessary with a shoulder dystocia? *American Journal of Obstetrics & Gynecology, 205*(3), e1–e3.

Pearson, N. (2011). Oxytocin safety: Legal implications for perinatal nurses. *Nursing for Women's Health, 15*(2), 111–117.

Pettker, C. M., & Funai, E. F. (2011). Managing obstetric risk: Is your L & D ready? *Contemporary OB/GYN, 35*(2), 40–45.

Phillips, C., & Bulmer, J. (2013). Splenic artery aneurysm rupture during pregnancy. *Nursing for Women's Health, 17*(6), 509–518. doi:10.1111/1751-486X.12079

Rampersad, R., & Macones, G. A. (2012). Prolonged and postterm pregnancy. In S. G. Gabbe, J. R. Niebyl, J. L. Simpson, M. B. Landon, H. L. Galan, E. R. Jauniaux, & D. A. Driscoll (Eds.), *Obstetrics: Normal and problem pregnancies* (6th ed., pp. 769–776). Philadelphia, PA: W.B. Saunders.

Salin, R., Zafran, N., Nachum, Z., Garmi, G., Kraiem, N., & Shalev, E. (2011). Single-balloon compared with double-balloon catheter for induction of labor. *Obstetrics & Gynecology, 118*(1), 79–86. doi:10.1097/ AOG.0b013e318220e4b7

Scheans, P. (2009). Family-witnessed resuscitation in the perinatal arena. *Nursing for Women's Health, 13*(3), 209–214. doi:10.1111/j .1751-486Z.2009.01421.x

Scott, J. R. (2011). Vaginal birth after cesarean delivery: A common-sense approach. *Obstetrics & Gynecology, 118*(2), 342–350. doi:10 .1097/AOG.0b013e3182245b39

Sibai, B. M. (2012). Hypertension. In S. G. Gabbe, J. R. Niebyl, J. L. Simpson, M. B. Landon, H. L. Galan, E. R. Jauniaux, & D. A. Driscoll (Eds.), *Obstetrics: Normal and problem pregnancies* (6th ed., pp. 631–666). Philadelphia, PA: W.B. Saunders.

Simhan, H. N., Iams, J. D., & Romero, R. (2012). Preterm birth. In S. G. Gabbe, J. R. Niebyl, J. L. Simpson, M. B. Landon, H. L. Galan, E. R. Jauniaux, & D. A. Driscoll (Eds.), *Obstetrics: Normal and problem pregnancies* (6th ed., pp. 627–658). Philadelphia, PA: W.B. Saunders.

Simpson, K. (2005). Failure to rescue: Implications for evaluating quality of care during labor and birth. *Journal of Perinatology & Neonatal Nursing, 19*(1), 24–36.

Simpson, K. (2009). *Cervical ripening and induction and augmentation of labor* (3rd ed.). [Monograph]. Washington, DC: Association of Women's Health, Obstetric and Neonatal Nurses.

Simpson, K. (2010). Reconsideration of the cost of convenience: Quality, operational, and fiscal strategies to minimize elective induction. *Journal of Perinatal and Neonatal Nursing, 24*(1), 43–52.

Simpson, K., & Creehan, P. A. (2013). (Eds.) *AWHONN Perinatal Nursing* (4th ed.). Philadelphia, PA: Lippincott Williams & Wilkins.

Simpson, K., Kortz, C., & Knox, G. (2009). A comprehensive perinatal patient safety program to reduce preventable adverse outcomes and costs of liability claims. *The Joint Commission Journal on Quality and Patient Safety, 35*, 565–574.

Simpson, K., Newman, G., & Chirino, O. (2010). Patient education to reduce elective inductions. *Maternal Child Nursing, 35*(4), 188–194.

Simpson, K., & O'Brien-Abel, N. (2013). Labor and birth. In K. R. Simpson, & P. Creehan (Eds.), *Perinatal nursing* (4th ed., pp. 343–444). Philadelphia, PA: Lippincott Williams & Wilkins.

Simpson, L. L. (2012). Maternal cardiac disease. *Obstetrics & Gynecology, 119*(2), 345–364. doi:10.1097/AOG.0b013e318242e260

Spong, C. Y., Mercer, B. M., D'Alton, M., Kilpatrick, S., Blackwell, S., & Saade, G. (2011). Timing of indicated late-preterm and early-term birth. *Obstetrics & Gynecology, 118*(2), 322–323.

U.S. Census Bureau. (2012). *Statistical abstract of the United States: 2012.* Retrieved from http://www.census.gov/compendia/statab/2012/ tables/12s0088.pdf

U.S. Department of Health & Human Services (USDHHS). (2012). *Introducing Healthy People 2020.* Retrieved from http://www.healthypeople .gov/2020/about/default.aspx

U.S. National Center for Health Statistics. (2013). *Births – method of delivery.* Retrieved from http://www.cdc.gov/nchs/fastats/delivery.htm

Vadhera, R., & Locksmith, G. (2011). Breech presentation, malpresentation, and multiple gestation. In S. Datta (Ed.), *Anesthetic and obstetrics management of high-risk pregnancy* (3rd ed., pp. 67–86). Boston, MA: Springer.

Vain, N., Szyld, E., Prudent, L., Wiswell, T., Aguilar, A., & Vivas, N. (2004). Oropharyngeal and nasopharyngeal suctioning of meconium-stained neonates before delivery of their shoulders: Multicentre, randomized, controlled trial. *Lancet, 364*(9434), 597–602.

Vallerand, A. H., & Sanoski, C. (2014). *Davis's drug guide for nurses* (14th ed.). Philadelphia, PA: F.A. Davis.

Vesely, C., & Beach, B. (2013). One facility's experience in reframing non-feeding into a comprehensive palliative care model. *Journal of Obstetric, Gynecologic & Neonatal Nursing, 42*(3), 383–388. doi:10.1111/1552-6909.12027

Williams, D., & Shah, M. (2003). Soaring cesarean section rates: A cause for alarm. *Journal of Obstetric, Gynecologic and Neonatal Nursing, 32,* 283–284.

Wing, D. A., & Farinelli, C. K. (2012). Abnormal labor and induction of labor. In S. G. Gabbe, J. R. Niebyl, J. L. Simpson, M. B. Landon, H. L. Galan, E. R. Jauniaux, & D. A. Driscoll, *Obstetrics: Normal and problem pregnancies* (6th ed., pp. 287–310). Philadelphia, PA: W.B. Saunders.

Wood, C. (2013). State of the science on perinatal palliative care. *Journal of Obstetric, Gynecologic & Neonatal Nursing, 42*(3), 372–382. doi:10.1111/1552-6909.12034

Zhang, J., Branch, D., Ramirez, M., Laughon, S., Reddy, U., Hoffman, M., et al. (2011). Oxytocin regimen for labor augmentation, labor progression, and perinatal outcomes. *Obstetrics & Gynecology, 118*(2), 249–256. doi:10.1097/AOG.0b013e3182220192

Zhang, X., & Kramer, M. S. (2012). The rise in singleton preterm births in the USA: The impact of labour induction. *British Journal of Obstetrics & Gynecology, 119*(11), 1309–1315. doi:10.1111/j.1471-0528.2012.03453.x

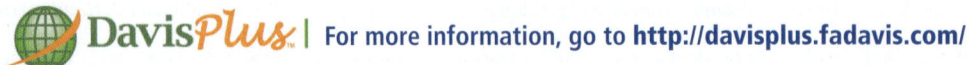

DavisPlus | For more information, go to http://davisplus.fadavis.com/

CONCEPT MAP

Caring for the Woman Experiencing Complications During Labor and Birth

Complications of Labor

Dysfunctional Labor Patterns:
- Hypertonic labor
- Hypotonic labor
- Precipitous labor

Pelvic Structure Alerations:
- Pelvic dystocia
- Soft tissue dystocia

Nursing Interventions
Hypertonic Labor:
- Establish effective labor pattern; rest; hydration; sedation; medication; facilitate fetal rotation

Hypotonic Labor:
- Careful, ongoing assessment; maternal walking/position changes; document contraction pattern/cervical changes

Precipitous Labor:
- Recognize sx of rapid cervical dilation; manage anxiety/fear/pain; post delivery assess/monitor → maternal soft tissue for hemorrhage

Placental Complications

Placenta Previa:
- Collaborate with medical treatment plan

Placental Abruption:
- Continuous fetal monitor
- Frequent vital signs
- Assess perineum, urine output, labs

May necessitate

Obstetric Interventions:
- Amnioinfusion
- Amniotomy
- Complementary measures
- Assisted/operative vaginal delivery

Pharmacological Induction of Labor:
- Cervical ripening agents; mechanical methods; oxytocin

Nursing Interventions:
- Tailored to the intervention
- Obtain consent
- Monitor vs, fetal heart tones, contractions, cervical changes, fetal station/lie
- Monitor rate of oxytocin, side effects, urine output
- Pain management
- Maternal positioning

Maternal Conditions Complicating Childbirth

Preeclampsia:
- Manage HTN
- Fetal monitoring
- Vitals/neurological
- Urine output/edema
- Watch labs for HELLP
- MgSO₄ monitoring

Cardiac Disease:
- Acute monitoring of fluid status

Diabetes Mellitus:
- FSBG q 2 hours
- Possible insulin drip
- Prepare for C-birth

Preterm Labor and Birth:
- Maternal and fetal monitoring
- Correct application of monitoring equipment and interpretation of tracings

Perinatal Loss:
- Often due to obstetric complications
- Team approach to bereavement: organized, culturally sensitive, flexible plan
- Allow parental decisions
- Communication
- Support groups

Fetal Complications

Fetal Malpresentation:
- Consent for version
- Prep for C-birth

Cephalopelvic Disproportion:
- Position changes
- Relaxation, water therapy
- Pain management

Multiple Gestation:
- Careful monitoring
- Assess individual fetal heart rates

Fetal Compromise:
- Immediate MD notification
- Assess acid/base
- Position change

Amniotic Fluid Complications:
- Oligohydramnios, hydramnios, presence of meconium

Cesarean Birth:
- When health of mother/fetus in jeopardy
- Major surgical procedure
- Involves care of the postoperative patient
- Ethical concerns re: nonmedical reason
- VBAC → use NIHR and ACOG recommendations

Other Complications
- Uterine rupture
- Uterine inversion
- Prolapse of the umbilical cord
- Vasa previa/velamentous insertion
- Anaphylactoid syndrome of pregnancy

Legal Alert:
- Monitor/document FHR before/after AROM
- Accurately interpret FHR tracings during oxytocin administration
- Communication/documentation critical in vacuum-assisted birth

Critical Nursing Actions:
- Assisting with precipitous birth
- Caring for the patient undergoing amnioinfusion
- Responding to umbilical cord prolapse immediately
- Assess/record FHR in forceps delivery

Cultural Diversity:
- Level of quality of care differs between Caucasian and non-Caucasian populations
- African American → higher risk of preterm and stillbirths

Across Care Settings:
- Collaborative care for multifetal birth
- AWHONN → Go-Full-40 campaign

What to Say:
- For preterm labor: active listening, explore concerns
- Calm, factual explanation during fetal distress
- Effective team communication during obstetric emergencies
- Conveying compassion in fetal loss

Now Can You:
- Identify factors that impede labor progression
- Explain the difference between labor induction and augmentation
- Explain correct procedure for application of the fetal monitor
- Discuss care and medical management of twin births
- Discuss issues and appropriate communication concerning perinatal death

Care of the
New Family

Caring for the Postpartal Woman and Her Family

Within a period of one day, most of what has been carefully accumulated over nine months is eliminated as no longer necessary by the body.

—Rubin, 1984, p. 753

LEARNING TARGETS *At the completion of this chapter, the student will be able to:*

- ◆ Assess the physiological and psychosocial status of the postpartal woman.
- ◆ Plan holistic nursing care for the postpartal woman and her family that includes strategies for home follow-up.
- ◆ Implement nursing interventions to promote positive breast and formula feeding outcomes for the mother and her infant.
- ◆ Discuss methods for assessing and treating pain in the postpartal period.
- ◆ Conduct appropriate nursing assessments and plan interventions for the patient who has experienced a cesarean birth.
- ◆ Plan holistic postpartal nursing care with interventions to assess and foster maternal/infant/family bonding.

PICO(T) Questions

The intent of evidence-based practice (EBP) is to provide nursing care that integrates the best available evidence. An initial step in EBP is to write a PICO(T) question that effectively guides the research. A PICO(T) question is an acronym that stands for population (P), intervention or issue (I), comparison of interest (C), outcome (O), and timeframe (T). Depending on the question, all or some of the question components are

used in the research process. Use these PICO(T) questions to spark your thinking as you read the chapter.

1. Do (I) breastfeeding benefits (P) for babies (O) change after the first 12 months of age?

2. What (I) nursing strategies are (O) most effective to assist (P) fathers in bonding with their newborn child?

 Evidence-Based Practice

Kuo, S., Yang, Y., Kuo, P., Tseng, C., & Tzeng, Y. (2012). Trajectories of depressive symptoms and fatigue among postpartum women. *Journal of Obstetric, Gynecologic, and Neonatal Nursing, 41*(2), 216–225.

The purpose of this study was to identify and describe patterns of depression and fatigue symptoms in postpartum women, and determine the relationship between the patterns and predictors of the symptoms. Previous research has indicated that the prevalence of depressive symptoms occurring at 1 week postpartum ranges from 24.7% to 29.5%; the prevalence of fatigue is 79.8%. Both conditions are considered common in postpartum women and may impact the woman's transition to motherhood. Earlier studies have identified a relationship between fatigue and depression and supported a need to screen for fatigue and depressive symptoms before hospital discharge. Certain risk factors (e.g., unemployment, low education, lack of exercise, and type of birth) have been shown to be associated with symptoms of depression and fatigue.

(continued)

This prospective longitudinal study utilized a convenience sample of 121 low-risk childbearing women. All participants received prenatal care in one prenatal clinic, and inclusion criteria included the following: married, singleton pregnancy, no perinatal complications, and no history of a chronic medical condition. The women provided baseline information during the third trimester and completed follow-up questionnaires on the first and third postpartum days. A phone interview was conducted on the seventh postpartum day.

Instruments used included the Edinburgh Postnatal Depression Scale (EPDS), the Fatigue Continuum Form (FCF), and the Pittsburgh Sleep Quality Index (PSQI); the investigators also collected demographic data and information concerning health status. The EPDS consists of 10 items related to depressive symptoms; it uses a 4-point scale that ranges from 0 (no symptoms) to 3 (most of the time). For the purpose of analysis, the depressive symptoms were grouped and based on the total score for all 10 items: low level (0–9), high level (10–30).

The FCF is a 30-item questionnaire designed to assess for fatigue symptoms; it uses a 4-point scale that ranges from 1 (not at all) to 4 (very much so). For the purpose of analysis, the responses were grouped and based on the total score for all 30 items: low (30–38.5), moderate (38.6–64.4), and high (64.5–120).

The PSQI is a 19-item questionnaire designed to assess for sleep quality, duration, habits, disturbances, use of medication and daytime dysfunction related to fatigue. The results are based on a cumulative score using a rating that ranges from 0 (good sleep) to 21 (very poor sleep). For the purpose of analysis, cumulative scores greater than 5 were indicative of sleep difficulty.

The mean age of the participants was 31.2 years (range 19 to 40 years), and 48% were primiparas. Fifty-five percent experienced a spontaneous vaginal birth. Sixty-seven percent reported sleep disturbances prior to labor, and 33% reported participation in prenatal exercises. The overall depressive symptoms score was 10.1 (high level category) in the third trimester assessment; this score decreased between the first and third postpartum days, and then rose to 8.9 (low level category) on the seventh postpartum day.

The fatigue scores rose from the third trimester through the first postpartum day and then decreased between the third and seventh postpartum days. The researchers concluded that women in the high-risk depressive symptoms group were most likely to fall into the high-risk fatigue group.

Based on their scores, the majority of participants were identified as being at low risk for both depression and fatigue. Approximately 33% of women reported depressive symptoms, and 54% reported fatigue symptoms, a finding comparable to previous studies. Participants with high and persistent depressive symptoms were more likely to follow high fatigue patterns, and the researchers were able to differentiate between the participants with depressive-related postpartum fatigue and those with non-depressive-related fatigue. The participants in the non-depressive group reported less depression once their fatigue had been relieved. No statistically significant differences were associated with the variables related to participation in prenatal exercise, mode of birth, parity, or prenatal employment.

1. How is this information useful to clinical nursing practice?

2. Based on these findings, what are implications for further research?

See Suggested Responses for Evidence-Based Practice on Davis*Plus*.

Introduction

Postpartum care begins immediately after childbirth. During this time, the nurse assists the new mother in learning how to care for herself and her baby. This 6-week period of time, also known as the **puerperium**, is filled with a myriad of changes that require careful nursing assessments for the mother, the newborn, and the family. The nurse's knowledge and care provided during this "**fourth trimester**" of pregnancy can have a lifelong impact in shaping the future plans and choices for the new family.

The *Healthy People 2020* national initiative includes several goals that encompass the time period of the early puerperium:

- Reduce the maternal mortality rate to no more than 11.4/100,000 live births from a baseline of 12.7/100,000.
- Reduce the proportion of births conceived within 18 months of a previous birth to 31.7% from a baseline of 35.3%.
- Increase to 46.2% the proportion of infants who are breastfed exclusively through 3 months of life from a baseline of 33.6% (U.S. Department of Health & Human Services [USDHHS], 2012).

Nursing actions to help the nation achieve these goals center on close observation to identify hemorrhage and related complications during the critical first hour after childbirth and ongoing education and support for women and families. Teaching about normal physiological changes during the puerperium, signs of danger, contraceptive methods, and benefits of breastfeeding empowers them to make informed decisions and choices.

Current trends reflect a shortened hospital stay for the new mother and her infant. However, there are several drawbacks to this approach. A longer (greater than 24 hours) hospital stay provides more rest and recuperation time for the mother; a greater opportunity for postpartal education about self and infant care; and time for infant observation and assessment for anomalies, defects, or other problems and improved maternal outcomes. Early hospital discharge has advantages as well. These include a decreased risk of nosocomial infections for the mother and infant, reduced medical expenses, and an opportunity for enhanced infant–family bonding.

Providing care during this period requires knowledge of the physiological and psychosocial aspects of the puerperium. The transitions that occur as the changes of pregnancy are reversed are considered to be a normal, but distinct, process. Protecting this process requires the nurse who cares for the postpartum patient to be equipped with special knowledge and skills. This chapter will discuss the physiological and psychosocial adaptations that occur during the postpartum period and the nursing assessments and interventions required to promote positive, healthy outcomes.

Ensuring Safety for the Mother and Infant

Early newborn discharge began as a consumer-initiated movement and as an alternative to home births in the 1980s. In the 1990s, third-party payers began to refuse reimbursement for hospital stays that extended beyond 24 hours, particularly after an uncomplicated vaginal birth. Congress responded to the growing concern over the safety of this practice by signing into law the Newborns' and Mothers' Health Protection Act of 1996. This legislation prohibits third-party payers from restricting benefits for hospital stays of less than 48 hours after a vaginal birth or less than 96 hours after a cesarean birth. Forty-eight hours is an incredibly short amount of time to assess, assist, and educate new mothers about matters concerning personal, newborn, and family health. Information provided by the postpartum nurse can protect the newborn and his family from unnecessary morbidity and mortality.

Fears surrounding infant abductions have long been a common concern among hospital staff and families. These concerns have created the need for the electronic tracking of infants. The growing need for fail-proof mechanisms to ensure infant safety has prompted the development of a variety of systems designed to foil infant abduction attempts. In response to increased litigation and pressure from The Joint Commission, it has become mandatory for hospitals to offer state-of-the-art security protection for their patients, mother/baby units, and visitors.

To meet The Joint Commission mandatory infant safety requirements, hospitals have instituted policies and procedures that nurses and mothers must follow to ensure their newborn's safety. Infant security experts agree that an informed mother is the baby's first line of defense while in the hospital as well as after returning home. It is essential that nurses educate new mothers about measures designed to protect their newborns from potential abductors.

legal alert—Check identification bracelets

The safety and security of the infant must be maintained at all times during hospitalization. This process involves the placement of identification bands on both the mother and infant shortly after birth. On bringing the infant to the mother, it is essential for the nurse to verify that the bracelets match. At discharge, it may be necessary for the nurse to retain both the infant's and parent's identification bracelets as part of the permanent record. This safety measure serves a twofold purpose: to prevent the unauthorized removal of the infant from the hospital unit and to prevent the inadvertent mix-up or switching of newborns.

legal alert—Protect the infant from abduction

Protecting the infant from abduction is an extremely important consideration during hospitalization. Personnel, parents, and significant others must be educated regarding the various measures implemented to protect the safety of the infant. Any time the infant is transported from the nursery to the mother's room, it is essential for staff to follow the hospital's protocol. In most facilities, infants may be transported only in a bassinet and parents are prohibited from carrying the infant in the halls. When identification bracelets are used, they are matched before giving the infant to the mother. Mothers should be instructed to release the infant only to properly identified hospital personnel. After birth, admission photographs and footprints are most likely taken and affixed to the permanent record. Some facilities use an umbilical cord clamp equipped with an embedded infant security alarm (Fig. 15-1). The clamp, which remains in place until discharge, activates an alarm if the infant is removed from the hospital unit or if the clamp is cut or disengaged. Another system involves use of an infant electronic radio transmitter tag; a matching maternal tag is also available to ensure that the mother is correctly matched with her infant. When two or more infants have a similar or same last name, it is common practice for the infants' cribs and charts to indicate the mother's first name and bear a label that designates a "NAME ALERT." When there are multiple births, the infants' cribs may be

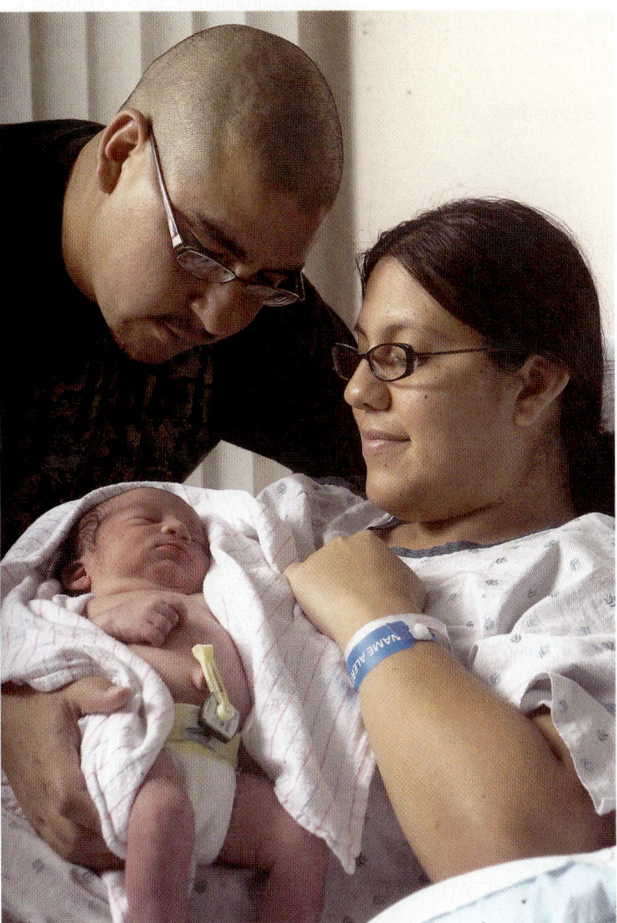

Figure 15-1 Umbilical cord clamp equipped with an infant security alarm.

labeled with the infant's name followed by a letter of the alphabet (e.g., A, B, C, or D). Some facilities use a color-coding system for infants of multiple births; colored bands are placed on each infant's ankle, and the patient labels and charts are also color-coded to additionally assist in identification (Salera-Vieira & Tanner, 2009).

Hospital personnel are typically required to wear visible photo identification when working in the maternal child unit. All employee photo badges should be similar in appearance to facilitate the ready identification of individuals posing as hospital employees. Visitors may be required to wear identification badges while on the unit. Hospital staff should be empowered to question any suspicious activity or individuals who are present on the maternal child unit.

> ⟳ **Now Can You—Discuss strategies to ensure maternal–infant safety?**
>
> 1. Identify three measures the hospital nurse can implement to ensure the safety of both the infant and the mother?
> 2. Suggest a strategy to decrease the potential for confusing infants whose last names are similar or identical?
> 3. Describe two actions that hospital personnel can take to help prevent infant abduction?

Early Maternal Assessment

VITAL SIGNS

During the postpartum period, vital signs are a reflection of the body's attempts to return to a prepregnant state. Vital signs can alert the nurse to the presence of hemorrhage or infection and should be monitored according to hospital policy. After a vaginal birth, vital signs are typically monitored every 15 minutes during the first hour after childbirth, then every 30 minutes during the second hour, once during the third hour, and then every 8 hours until discharge or until they are stable. A different protocol is followed for vital sign assessment after a cesarean birth (e.g., every 30 min × 4 hours; then every hour × 3; then every 4 to 8 hours). The nurse may wish to use a postpartum guide such as the rapid assessment tool presented in Table 15-1 to record and store critical information during the early postpartal period.

Table 15-1 Postpartum Rapid Assessment Tool: First 24 Hours After Birth

Critical Indicators	Normal Findings	Alterations/Possible Causes
Temperature (Oral)	Within normal range: 98.6°F–100.4°F (37°C–38°C)	>101.0°F (38.3°C) (Infection)
Pulse	Within normal range: 50–90 beats/min; bradycardia (50–70 beats/min) may be present	Tachycardia (Difficult labor/birth; hemorrhage)
Respirations	Within normal range: (12–20 respirations/min)	Marked tachypnea (Pulmonary disease) Note: Decreased respiratory rate may occur after an extremely high spinal block or epidural narcotic after a cesarean birth
Blood pressure (BP)	Consistent with baseline BP during the first trimester	Elevated (Anxiety, preeclampsia, essential hypertension, renal disease) Low (Hemorrhage) Note: This is a late sign; assess for increased pulse rate; cool, clammy skin
Fundus	Immediately after birth: midline, firmly contracted and palpable through the abdominal wall midway between the umbilicus and the symphysis pubis. One hour after birth: approximately at the level of the umbilicus × 24 hours	Boggy (Full bladder, uterine bleeding)
Lochia	Normal progression: lochia rubra (1- to 2-inch stain on pad, may contain small clots), consistent with a heavy menstrual period for the first 2 hours, then should steadily decrease, fleshy odor	Large amounts, clots (Hemorrhage) Foul-smelling (Infection)
Episiotomy or incision	No redness, edema, ecchymosis, or discharge; edges well approximated	Redness, edema, ecchymosis, discharge, non-approximated edges (Infection)
Hemorrhoids	None, or if present, small	Tender, enlarged and tense (Inflamed hemorrhoids)
Bladder	Able to spontaneously empty bladder within 6 to 8 hours, urine output at least 150 mL/hour; bladder not palpable after voiding	Unable to empty bladder (Urinary retention) Presence of urgency, frequency, dysuria (Urinary tract infection)
Costovertebral angle tenderness (CVAT)	None	Present (Kidney infection)
Lower extremities Homans' sign	No pain with palpation; no warmth, tenderness; negative Homans' sign	Positive findings (Thrombophlebitis)

Table 15-1 Postpartum Rapid Assessment Tool: First 24 Hours After Birth (continued)		
Critical Indicators	**Normal Findings**	**Alterations/Possible Causes**
Mood	Range of emotions; passive or talkative; may need to converse about her birth experience	Extremely quiet and passive (Fatigue, disappointment about her birth experience)
Bonding/Attachment	Taking-in; maternal–infant en face position, cuddles infant	Apprehensive; refuses to care for infant, no demonstration of bonding behaviors (Attachment difficulty)

Temperature

During the first 24 hours postpartum, some women experience an increase in body temperature up to 100.4°F (38°C). The exertion and dehydration that accompany labor are the primary causes for the temperature elevation, and increased fluids usually return the temperature to a normal range. Increased breast vascularity may also cause a transient increase in temperature. After the first 24 postpartal hours have passed, however, the patient should be afebrile. A temperature above 100.4°F (38°C) at this time may be indicative of infection. (See Chapter 16 for further discussion.)

Pulse

Heart rates of 50 to 70 beats per minute (bradycardia) commonly occur during the first 6 to 10 days of the postpartum period. During pregnancy, the weight of the gravid uterus causes a decreased flow of venous blood to the heart. After childbirth, there is an increase in intravascular volume. The elevated stroke volume leads to a decreased heart rate. Postpartal tachycardia may result from a complication, prolonged labor, blood loss, temperature elevation, or infection.

Blood Pressure

Postpartal blood pressure values should be compared with blood pressure values obtained during the first trimester. Decreased blood pressure may result from the physiological changes associated with the decrease in intrapelvic pressure, or it may be indicative of uterine hemorrhage. An increase in the systolic blood pressure of 30 mm Hg or 15 mm Hg in the diastolic blood pressure, especially when associated with headaches or visual changes, may be a sign of gestational hypertension. Further assessment is indicated.

In the puerperium, plasma renin and angiotensin II levels return to normal, nonpregnant levels. These physiological changes produce a decrease in vascular resistance. Orthostatic hypotension may occur when the patient moves from a supine to a sitting position. Otherwise, maternal blood pressure should remain stable (Cunningham, Leveno, Bloom, Spong, & Dashe, 2014).

Respirations

The respiratory rate should remain within the normal range of 12 to 20 respirations per minute. However, slightly elevated respirations may occur because of pain, fear, excitement, exertion, or excessive blood loss. Careful nursing assessment for causes of an elevated respiratory rate is indicated, along with appropriate interventions. Tachypnea, abnormal lung sounds, shortness of breath, chest pain, anxiety, or restlessness are abnormal findings that must be reported immediately. These signs and symptoms may be indicative of pulmonary edema or emboli. (See Chapter 16 for further discussion.)

Pain

Pain, sometimes considered the fifth "vital sign," must be recognized as an important assessment focus immediately and throughout the postpartum period. Nurses play an important role in assessing, planning, and implementing interventions to manage maternal pain effectively. Pain should be recognized and treated in a timely manner. The failure to manage pain effectively has been associated with numerous complications, including prolonged recovery, increased length of hospital stay, depression, anxiety, poor coping, and altered sleep patterns.

 Nursing Insight—*Promoting comfort during the immediate postpartum period*

It is not unusual for women to experience shaking chills during the time immediately after childbirth. This physiological response results from: (1) pressure changes in the abdomen after the reduction in the bulk of the uterus and (2) temperature readjustments after the diaphoresis of labor. Feelings of excitement and exhaustion may also play a role. Nurses should reassure patients of the normalcy of this temporary reaction and offer warm blankets and beverages as comfort measures.

FUNDUS, LOCHIA, PERINEUM

Within a few minutes after birth, the firmly contracted uterine fundus should be palpable through the abdominal wall halfway between the umbilicus and the symphysis pubis. Approximately 1 hour later, the fundus should have risen to the level of the umbilicus, where it remains for the following 24 hours.

 Optimizing Outcomes—**Uterine assessment crucial during the first hour postpartum**

Because the first postpartal hour represents the most dangerous time for the patient, it is essential that the nurse conduct frequent uterine assessments during this time. Relaxation of the uterus (atony) results in rapid, life-threatening blood loss because no permanent thrombi have yet formed at the placental site.

The fundus then descends 1 fingerbreadth (1 cm) per day in size. The fundus, **lochia** (puerperal discharge of blood, mucus, and tissue), and perineum need to be assessed every 15 minutes during the immediate postpartum period. To facilitate the perineal assessment, the nurse assists the patient into a Sims' (side-lying) position with her back facing the nurse.

Nursing Insight—*Perineal assessment*

Protecting the patient's privacy and ensuring adequate lighting are essential components of the perineal assessment. Although some edema of the vulva and perineum is a common finding during the first few postpartum days, excessive swelling, discoloration, incisional separation, or discharge other than lochia should be reported, along with the patient's complaints of pain or discomfort.

With adequate lighting in place, the nurse gently lifts the buttock cheeks to visualize the perineum. Use of the acronym REEDA guides the nurse to assess for *R*edness, *E*dema, *E*cchymosis, *D*rainage or discharge, and *A*pproximation of the episiotomy if present (Table 15-2). The episiotomy and/or laceration repairs should appear intact with the tissue edges closely approximated. Hemorrhoids may also be present. The nurse should note and document the number, appearance, and size (in centimeters) of the hemorrhoids.

HEMORRHOIDS

Hemorrhoids that may be present before pregnancy or develop during pregnancy can become enlarged because of pressure on the lower bowel during the second stage of labor. The application of ice packs and/or pharmaceutical preparations such as topical anesthetic ointments or witch hazel pads helps to relieve discomfort. Frozen tea peripads may also be used as a comfort measure for hemorrhoids and labial swelling. The tannic acid decreases edema and is soothing. Other actions to minimize hemorrhoidal discomfort include assisting the patient to a side-lying position in bed and teaching her to sit on flat, hard surfaces and to tighten her buttocks before sitting. Soft surfaces and pillows such as donut rings should be avoided because they separate the buttocks and decrease venous flow, intensifying the pain. If the hemorrhoids are severe, the patient can be taught how to manually reposition the hemorrhoids back into the rectum. Hemorrhoids that developed during pregnancy generally disappear within a few weeks after childbirth.

Now Can You—Discuss postpartum vital signs and perineal assessment?

1. Describe the expected vital sign findings during the postpartum period?

2. Identify potential causes for increased blood pressure, pulse, and respirations during the postpartum period?

3. Explain what is meant by the REEDA acronym to facilitate the perineal assessment?

A Concise Postpartum Assessment Guide to Facilitate Nursing Care

THE BUBBLE-HE MNEMONIC

Use of a systematic assessment process helps the nurse ensure that the special needs of postpartum patients are met. As with all nursing care, a complete head-to-toe assessment must be completed for the postpartum patient who has unique needs not found in any other nursing environment. To assist with the postpartum assessment, the mnemonic BUBBLE-HE is commonly used to guide nursing practice. BUBBLE-HE reminds the nurse to assess the breasts, uterus, bladder, bowel, lochia, and episiotomy. Assessment of maternal pain, lower extremities, the patient's emotional status and initiation of infant bonding are other important components to be included in the postpartum evaluation (Table 15-3). Medications commonly prescribed during the puerperium are presented in Table 15-4.

Breasts

A number of physiological changes occur during pregnancy to prepare the breasts for the process of lactation. The mammary glands, or milk-producing system, are unlike any other organ system. Throughout the woman's growth and development, no other human organ undergoes the dramatic changes in size, shape, and function that take place in the breasts (Riordan & Wambach, 2009). Essentially, the breasts serve no function other than to nourish the child. Breast size has no bearing on the woman's ability or capacity to nourish her infant. Instead, the infant's appetite and frequent emptying of the breasts dictate the quantity of milk produced.

A & P review　Hormonal Changes to Prepare the Breasts for Lactation

Up until the onset of puberty, the breasts are much the same in males and females and their internal structure is similar: They consist of a collection of ducts that empty into the nipple. In the female, breast tissue responds to the release of

Table 15-2　The REEDA Acronym to Guide the Perineal Assessment

Points	Redness	Edema	Ecchymosis	Discharge	Approximation
0	None	None	None	None	Closed
1	Within 0.25 cm of incision bilaterally	Less than 1 cm from incision	1–2 cm from incision	Serum	Skin separation 3 mm or less
2	Within 0.5 cm of incision bilaterally	1–2 cm from incision	0.25–1 cm bilaterally or 0.5–2 cm unilaterally	Serosanguineous	Skin and subcutaneous fat separated
3	Beyond 0.5 cm of incision bilaterally	Greater than 2 cm from incision	Greater that 1 cm bilaterally or 2 cm unilaterally	Bloody, purulent	Skin, subcutaneous fat and fascial separation

Table 15-3 BUBBLE-HE(B): Components of a Postpartum Assessment

Letter	Assess	Assessment Includes
B	Breasts	Inspection of nipples: everted, flat, inverted? Breast tissue: soft, filling, firm? Temperature and color: warm, pink, cool, red streaked?
U	Uterus	Location (midline or deviated to right or left side) and tone (firm, firm with massage, boggy)
B	Bladder	Last time the patient emptied her bladder (spontaneously or via catheter)? Palpable or nonpalpable? Color, odor, and amount of urine?
B	Bowels	Date/time of last BM; presence of flatus and hunger (unless the colon was manipulated, do not need to auscultate for bowel sounds)
L	Lochia	Color, amount, presence of clots, any free flow?
(I) E	(Incision) Episiotomy	Type as well as other tissue trauma (lacerations, etc.); assess using REEDA
L/H	Legs (Homans' sign)	Pain, varicosities, warmth or discoloration in calves; presence of pedal pulses; sensation and movement (after cesarean birth)
E	Emotions	Affect, patient-family interaction, effects of exhaustion
(B)	Bonding	Interaction with infant—"taking in" phase—presence of finger tipping, gazing, enfolding, calling infant by name, identifying unique characteristics

Table 15-4 Commonly Used Medications in the Postpartum Period

Classification	Medication	Dose Safety of Use in Breastfeeding	Indication for Use in Postpartum Period
Stool softener	docusate sodium (Colace)	50 mg to 500 mg by mouth daily until bowel movements are normal. Not contraindicated in breastfeeding mother.	Used in the treatment of constipation
Stimulant laxative	bisacodyl (Dulcolax)	10 mg to 30 mg by mouth until bowel movements are normal. Not contraindicated in breastfeeding mother.	Used in the treatment of constipation
Topical anesthetic	lidocaine spray	Spray to perineal area after sitz bath or perineum care. Not contraindicated in breastfeeding mother.	Used on the skin to relieve pain and itching
Hemorrhoid care	witch hazel (Tucks)	Apply to perineal area after sitz bath or perineum care. Not contraindicated in breastfeeding mother.	Used on the skin to relieve the itching, burning, and irritation associated with hemorrhoids
Nonsteroidal anti-inflammatory drugs	ibuprofen (Motrin)	400 mg by mouth every 4–6 hours as needed for pain. Not contraindicated in breastfeeding mother.	Used for the treatment of mild to moderate pain
Opioid analgesics	Percocet (oxycodone and acetaminophen)	Take one to two tablets every 4–6 hours as needed for pain. Not contraindicated in breastfeeding mother.	Used for the treatment of moderate to severe pain

Source: Vallerand & Sanoski (2014).

the female sex hormones estrogen and progesterone during puberty. Estrogen stimulates the formation of additional ducts, the elongation of existing ducts, and the formation of a system of milk-secreting glands. These changes are associated with an increase in volume and elasticity of connective tissue, deposition of adipose tissue, and increased vascularity. Progesterone stimulates the formation of lobules, the glands in the breast that produce milk (Fig. 15-2).

By the time the breasts are fully formed, typically by the age of 15, breast tissue extends medially from the second or third rib to the sixth or seventh rib, and laterally from the breastbone to the edge of the axillae. Although genetic factors, body size, and ethnicity account for some variations, on average, the breasts weigh approximately 200 grams. During pregnancy, each breast increases in size and weight to reach approximately

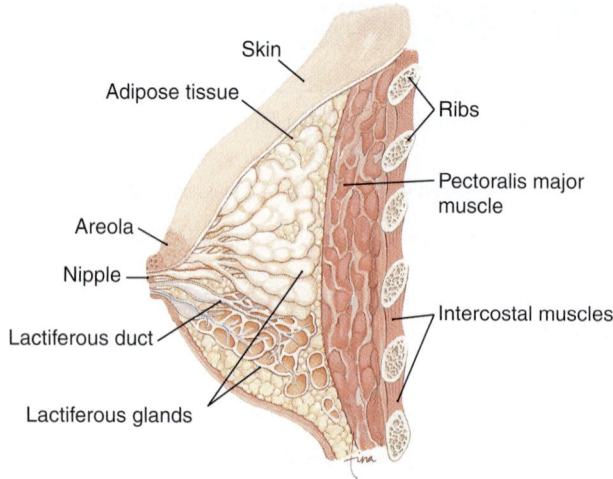

Skin

Adipose tissue

Ribs

Pectoralis major muscle

Areola

Nipple

Intercostal muscles

Lactiferous duct

Lactiferous glands

Figure 15-2 Mammary gland shown in a midsagittal section.

600 grams and 600 to 800 grams during lactation (Lawrence & Lawrence, 2010).

Until menopause, when menstrual periods cease, the woman's breast tissue continues to respond to the changing hormonal environment that accompanies each menstrual cycle. Throughout the majority of the woman's life, the breasts remain in a resting state except for the time during pregnancy and lactation. ◆

Regardless of whether the woman plans to breast- or bottle-feed, the breasts require careful assessment. After ensuring privacy, the nurse asks the patient to remove her bra. The chest area is covered with a sheet or towel, and the woman is instructed to raise her arms and rest her hands on her head. The nurse inspects and palpates each breast for size, shape, tenderness, and color. During the first 2 postpartal days, the breast tissue should feel soft to the touch. By the third day, the breasts should begin to feel firm and warm. This change is described as "filling." On the fourth and fifth days postpartum, breastfeeding mothers' breasts should feel firm before infant feeding, then become soft once the baby is satiated. The noticeable changes in breast firmness are indicative of milk transfer.

The process of lactation is established in all postpartum women, regardless of their intention to breast or formula feed. Tense, painful breasts in a breastfeeding mother are indicative of poor transfer of milk to the infant. This finding should prompt a breastfeeding assessment, and when appropriate, referral to an international board-certified lactation consultant (see discussion later in this chapter).

Occasionally, small, firm nodules can be palpated in the filling breasts. The nodules result from incomplete emptying of the breasts during the previous feeding. Usually, a nodule arises from a blocked milk duct or from milk contained in a gland that is not flowing forward to the nipple. Although the nodules typically disappear after a satisfactory feeding, their location should be noted and monitored. Persistence of any breast mass may be indicative of fibrocystic disease or malignant growths unrelated to the pregnancy. The nurse also documents the appearance of the nipples, noting the presence of fissures, cracks, blood, or dried milk and whether they are erect or inverted.

Uterus

Involution is a term that describes the process whereby the uterus returns to the nonpregnant state. The uterus undergoes a dramatic reduction in size although it will remain slightly larger than its size before the first pregnancy. Immediately after expulsion of the placenta, the uterus rapidly contracts to prevent hemorrhage. The uterus weighs approximately 1,000 g in the immediate postpartal period, and by the end of the first week, its weight has diminished to 500 g. Uterine size and weight continue to decrease, and on average, the uterus weighs 300 g by the end of the second week. Thereafter, the weight decreases to 100 g or less (Cunningham et al., 2014).

After the birth of the infant, placental expulsion spontaneously occurs within 15 minutes in approximately 90% of women. To prevent hemorrhage, rapid uterine contractions seal off the placental site, effectively pinching off the massive network of maternal blood vessels that were attached to the placenta (Cunningham et al., 2014).

The original site of placental implantation covers a surface area that is approximately 8 to 10 cm in size. By the end of the second postpartal week, the site has shrunk to about 3 to 4 cm; complete healing takes approximately 6 to 7 weeks. The uterus is predominantly composed of a muscle layer, the myometrium. The myometrium is covered by serosa and lined by the decidua basalis. The process of uterine involution results from a decrease in the *size* of the myometrial cells rather than from a decrease in the *number* of myometrial cells. The decrease in cell size results in myometrial thickening and ischemia from reduced blood flow to the contracted uterus.

Phagocytosis (the engulfment and destruction of cells) contributes to the process of uterine involution by removing elastic and fibrous tissue from the uterus. The process is further hastened by autolysis (self-digestion) that results from migration of macrophages to the uterus.

Subinvolution is the failure of the uterus to return to the nonpregnant state. Uterine involution may be inhibited by multiple births, hydramnios, prolonged labor or difficult birth, infection, grand multiparity, or excessive maternal analgesia. In addition, a full bladder or retained placental tissue may prevent the uterus from sustaining the contractions needed to prevent hemorrhage or to facilitate involution. (See Chapter 16 for further discussion.)

The placental site heals by a process called exfoliation. Exfoliation is the scaling off of dead tissue. New endometrial tissue is generated at the site from the glands and tissue that remain in the lower layer of the decidua after separation of the placenta. This physiological process results in a uterine lining that contains no scar tissue, which could impede implantation in future pregnancies. Regeneration of the endometrium is complete by the 16th postpartum day, except at the placental site, where regeneration is usually not complete until approximately 6 weeks after childbirth.

To perform the uterine assessment, the nurse assists the patient to a supine position so that the height of the uterus is not influenced by an elevated position. The patient's abdomen is observed for contour to detect distention and the presence of striae or a diastasis (separation), which appears as a slightly indented groove in the midline. When present, the width and length of a diastasis are recorded in fingerbreadths. The uterine fundus is palpated by placing one

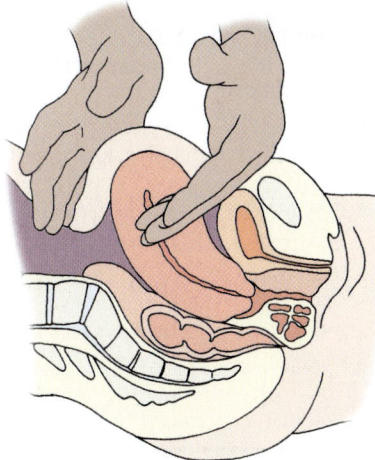

Figure 15-3 To palpate the uterus, the upper hand is cupped over the fundus; the lower hand stabilizes the uterus at the symphysis pubis.

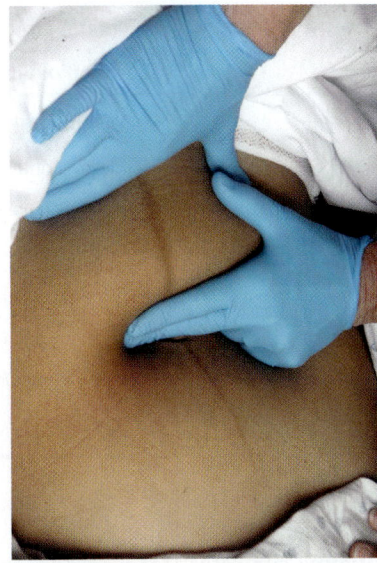

Figure 15-4 The fundus is palpated in the midline, at the level of the umbilicus.

hand immediately above the symphysis pubis to stabilize the uterus and the other hand at the level of the umbilicus (Fig. 15-3). The nurse presses inward and downward with the hand positioned on the umbilicus until the fundus is located. It should feel like a firm, globular mass located at or slightly above the umbilicus during the first hour after birth.

clinical alert

Proper technique for uterine palpation

The uterus should never be palpated without supporting the lower uterine segment. Failure to do so may result in uterine inversion and hemorrhage.

FUNDUS. Immediately after childbirth, the uterus rapidly contracts to facilitate compression of the intramyometrial blood vessels. The uterine fundus can be palpated midline, midway between the umbilicus and symphysis pubis. Within an hour, the uterus settles in the midline at the level of the umbilicus (Fig. 15-4). Over the course of days, the uterus descends into the pelvis at a rate of about 1 cm/day (1 fingerbreadth) (Fig. 15-5). After 10 days, the uterus has descended into the pelvis and is no longer palpable.

The fundus is assessed for consistency (firm, soft, or boggy), location (should be midline), and height (measured in fingerbreadths). During the fundal assessment, the nurse notes whether it is located midline or deviated to one side. On occasion, the fundus can be palpated slightly to the right because of displacement from the sigmoid colon during pregnancy. Assessment of the fundus should be made shortly after the patient has emptied her bladder. A full bladder prevents the uterus from contracting and instead pushes the uterus upward and may deviate it from the midline because of laxness of the uterine ligaments. A flabby, noncontracted, boggy uterus is associated with increased bleeding. A well-contracted fundus is firm, round, and midline. The nurse documents the location of the fundus according to fingerbreadths above or below the umbilicus (Table 15-5).

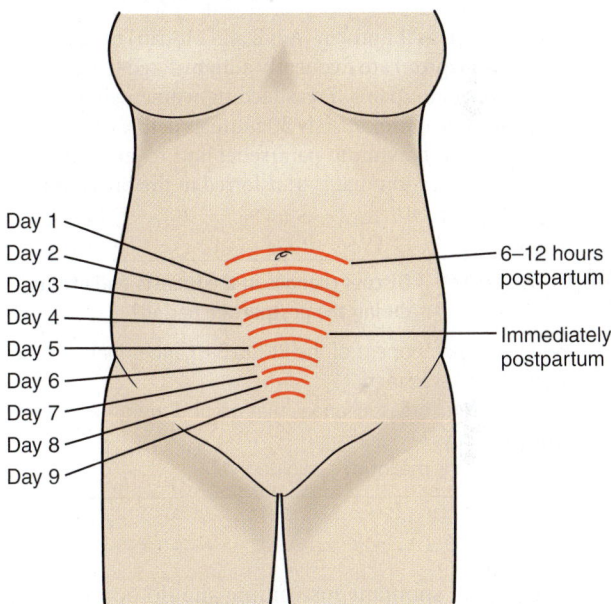

Figure 15-5 Fundal heights postpartum.

Afterpains (afterbirth pains) are intermittent uterine contractions that occur during the process of involution. Patients often describe the sensation as a discomfort similar to menstrual cramps. The primiparous woman typically has mild afterpains, if she notices them at all, because her uterus is able to maintain a contracted state. Multiparas and patients with uterine overdistention (e.g., large baby, multifetal gestation, or hydramnios) are more likely to experience afterpains because of the continuous pattern of uterine relaxation and vigorous contractions. When the uterus maintains a constant contraction, the afterpains cease. Breastfeeding and the administration of exogenous oxytocin usually produce pronounced afterpains because both cause powerful uterine contractions. Afterbirth pain is often severe for 2 to 3 days after childbirth. Nursing interventions for discomfort include assisting the patient into

Table 15-5 Assessment and Documentation of Uterine Involution		
Time	**Location of Fundus**	**Documentation**
Immediately after birth	Midline, midway between umbilicus and symphysis pubis	
1–2 hours	At the level of the umbilicus	at U (umbilicus)
12 hours	1 cm above umbilicus (1 fingerbreadth)	U + 1
24 hours	1 cm below umbilicus	U − 1
2 days	2 cm below umbilicus (2 fingerbreadths)	U − 2
3 days	3 cm below umbilicus (3 fingerbreadths)	U − 3
7 days	Palpable at the symphysis pubis	
10 days	Not palpable	

a prone position with a small pillow placed under her abdomen, initiating sitz baths (for warmth), encouraging ambulation, and administrating mild analgesics.

 Optimizing Outcomes—Breastfeeding and afterpains

Analgesics such as ibuprofen (Advil and Motrin) or naproxen (Aleve and Anaprox) are frequently administered to lessen the discomforts of afterpains. Breastfeeding women should take pain medication approximately 30 minutes before nursing the baby to achieve maximum pain relief and to minimize the amount of medication that is transferred in the breast milk.

 Now Can You—Discuss changes in the breasts and uterus during the postpartum period?

1. Name each component of the BUBBLE-HE mnemonic for the postpartum assessment?
2. Explain normal breast changes that occur during the first few postpartal days?
3. Explain what is meant by "involution"?

Bladder

After childbirth, spontaneous voiding should occur within 6 to 8 hours, and the first few voiding amounts should be monitored. Urinary output of at least 150 mL/hr is necessary to avoid urinary retention, or stasis. Generalized edema is often present in the early puerperium. It is related to the fluid accumulation that normally occurs during pregnancy combined with intravenous fluids frequently administered

during labor and birth. Maternal diuresis occurs almost immediately after birth and urinary output reaches up to 3,000 mL each day by the second to fifth postpartum days.

Decreased bladder tone is normal during pregnancy, and results from the effects of progesterone on the smooth muscle, edema from pressure of the presenting part, and mucosal hyperemia from the increase in blood vessel size. Prolonged labor, the use of forceps, analgesia, and anesthesia may intensify the changes in the immediate postpartum period. Pressure caused by the fetal head pressing on the bladder during labor can result in trauma and a transient loss of bladder sensation during the first few postpartal days or weeks. These changes can result in incomplete bladder emptying and overdistention.

Bladder and urethral trauma is not uncommon during the intrapartal period and may be associated with a decreased flow of urine immediately after a vaginal birth. An increase in the voided volume, the total flow time (how long it takes to empty the bladder), and the time to peak urine flow (the maximum urinary flow rate) begins to occur during the first postpartum day. Urine volume and flow time should return to prepregnant levels by 2 to 3 days after childbirth. Epidural anesthesia, catheterization before birth, and an instrument-facilitated birth are associated with an increased risk of postpartum urinary retention. Urethral and bladder trauma and lacerations may accompany vaginal or cesarean birth.

Urinary retention can also result from bladder hypotonia after childbirth because the weight of the gravid uterus no longer limits bladder capacity. Assessment of the maternal bladder is an extremely important component of the nursing evaluation (Table 15-6). An overdistended bladder, which

Table 15-6 Nursing Assessment and Interventions for the Urinary System	
Patient's Signs and Symptoms	**Nursing Interventions**
• Location of fundus above baseline level • Fundus displaced from midline • Excessive lochia • Bladder discomfort • Bulge of bladder above symphysis pubis • Frequent voiding of less than 150 mL of urine; urinary output disproportionate to fluid intake	• Promote hydration • Promote ambulation • Administer an analgesic before voiding, as prescribed • Place ice on perineum to reduce swelling and pain • Encourage the use of a sitz bath • Provide privacy • Turn on the bathroom faucet

displaces the uterus above and to the right of the umbilicus, can cause uterine atony and lead to hemorrhage. Other assessment findings may include presence of the bladder palpated as a hard or firm area just above the symphysis pubis and a urinary output that is disproportionate to the fluid intake. Bladder percussion enhances the assessment. To percuss the bladder, the nurse places one finger flat on the patient's abdomen over the bladder and taps it with the finger of the other hand. A full bladder produces a resonant sound. An empty bladder has a dull, thudding sound. Patients may express an urge to void but be unable to void. Fortunately, spontaneous voiding typically returns within 6 to 8 hours after childbirth. Until this time, the nurse should support and enhance the woman's attempts to void. Nursing interventions may include assisting the patient to the toilet, providing privacy and an unhurried environment, turning on the lavatory faucet, and assisting the patient into a sitz bath.

Bowel

The gastrointestinal system becomes more active soon after childbirth. The patient often feels hungry and thirsty after the food and fluid restrictions that usually accompany the intrapartal experience. The peptide hormone relaxin, which reaches high circulating levels during pregnancy, depresses bowel motility (Cunningham et al., 2014). The relaxed condition of the intestinal and abdominal muscles, combined with the continued effects of progesterone on the smooth muscles, diminishes bowel motility. These factors commonly result in constipation during the early puerperium. After childbirth, bowel movements are typically delayed until the second or third puerperal day and hemorrhoids (distended rectal veins), perineal trauma, and the presence of an episiotomy may be associated with painful defecation. Early ambulation, abundant fluids, and a high-fiber diet are a few strategies to help prevent constipation (Box 15-1).

Lochia

Separation of the placenta and membranes occurs in the spongy or outer layer of the decidua basalis. The uterine decidua basalis reorganizes into the basal and superficial layers. The inner basal layer becomes the foundation from which new layers of endometrium will form. The superficial layer becomes necrotic and sloughs off in the uterine discharge, called lochia. Lochia is composed of erythrocytes; epithelial cells; blood; and fragments of decidua, mucus, and bacteria (Cunningham et al., 2014). The characteristics of the lochia are indicative of the woman's status in the process of involution.

During the first few days postpartum, the lochia consists mostly of blood, which gives it a characteristic red color known as **lochia rubra.** Lochia rubra also contains elements of amnion, chorion, decidua, vernix, lanugo, and meconium if the fetus had passed any stool in utero. These components cause the fleshy odor associated with lochia rubra.

After 3 to 4 days, the lochia becomes the pinkish-brownish **lochia serosa.** Lochia serosa contains blood, wound exudates, erythrocytes, leukocytes, and cervical mucosa. After approximately 10 to 14 days, the uterine discharge has a reduced fluid content and is largely composed of leukocytes. This combination produces a white or yellow-white thick discharge known as **lochia alba.** Lochia alba also contains decidual cells, mucus, bacteria, and epithelial cells. It is present until about the third week after childbirth but may persist for 6 weeks.

The pattern of lochia flow, from lochia rubra to serosa to alba, should not reverse. A return of lochia rubra after it has turned pink or white may indicate retained placental fragments or decreased uterine contractions and new bleeding. Lochia should contain no large clots, which may indicate the presence of retained placental fragments that are preventing closure of maternal uterine blood sinuses. The odor of lochia is similar to that of menstrual blood. An offensive odor is indicative of infection.

After assessment of the lochia, the nurse may find it difficult to document the findings correctly. Lochia is typically documented in amounts described as *scant, small, moderate,* or *heavy.* The amount of vaginal discharge is not a true indicator of the lochia flow unless the time factor is also considered. For example, a perineal pad (peripad) that accumulates less than 1 cm of lochia in 1 hour is associated with scant flow (Fig. 15-6). Nurses must also be certain to take into account the specific type of peripad used because some are more absorbent than others. At times, visually assessing the amount of lochia flow can be difficult and inaccurate.

Box 15-1 Nursing Interventions to Facilitate Normal Bowel Function During the Puerperium

To facilitate the return of normal bowel function in the puerperium, the nurse should:

- Encourage the patient to drink at least six to eight 8-oz glasses of water every day to help keep the stool soft.
- Encourage the patient to eat a high-fiber diet that includes an abundance of fruits and vegetables, oat and bran cereal, whole-grain bread, and brown rice.
- Encourage the patient to avoid ignoring the urge to defecate.
- Encourage the patient to avoid straining to have a bowel movement.
- Encourage the patient to initiate early ambulation.
- Administer stool softeners and/or laxatives as ordered.
- Explain that after hospital discharge, over-the-counter medications may be helpful for hemorrhoidal symptoms of pain, itching, or swelling but encourage the patient to consult with her caregiver before using such medications.

Optimizing Outcomes—**Abnormal findings in a postpartal patient**

During a routine postpartal assessment conducted 2 hours after childbirth, the nurse records the following vital signs: pulse = 102 beats/minute; blood pressure = 130/86 mm Hg; respirations = 21 breaths/minute; temperature = 98.9°F (37.1°C). The nurse's first action is to assess the fundus. With the cupped palm placed directly over the uterine fundus, the nurse uses palpation to assess for the state of contraction (e.g., soft, boggy, or firmly contracted), along with the location and height of the fundus. If soft, the fundus is massaged in a circular motion with the cupped palm until the uterus is well contracted. The nurse inspects the peripad for the lochia amount and color and the presence of odor. The physician or nurse midwife is notified of the findings. If excessive blood loss has occurred or if the uterus is not well contracted, the nurse administers appropriate as needed (prn) medication(s) as ordered.

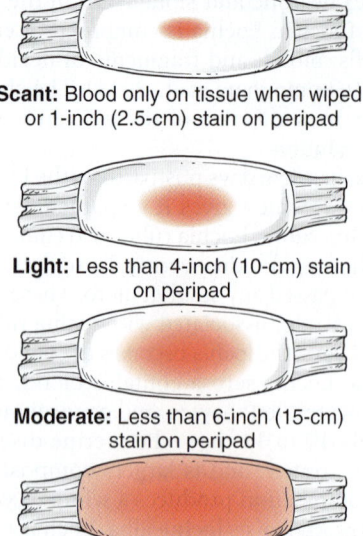

Scant: Blood only on tissue when wiped or 1-inch (2.5-cm) stain on peripad

Light: Less than 4-inch (10-cm) stain on peripad

Moderate: Less than 6-inch (15-cm) stain on peripad

Heavy: Peripad saturated within 1 hour

Figure 15-6 Assessment of lochia flow in 1 hour.

Episiotomy

An episiotomy is a 1- to 2-inch surgical incision made in the muscular area between the vagina and the anus (the perineum) to enlarge the vaginal opening before birth. The midline episiotomy is a straight incision extending toward the anus. A mediolateral episiotomy extends downward and to the side. (See Chapter 12.) Typically, the episiotomy edges have become fused (the edges have sealed) by the first 24 hours after birth. Although the patient's perineal folds may interfere with full visualization of a midline episiotomy, it is important for the nurse to carefully assess the episiotomy for redness, edema, ecchymosis, discharge, and approximation (REEDA) and then document all findings.

 clinical alert

Hematoma after an episiotomy

Severe hemorrhage after an episiotomy is possible. Maternal complaints of excessive perineal pain should alert the nurse to the possibility of a perineal, vulvar, vaginal, or ischiorectal **hematoma** (a blood-filled swelling that occurs from damage to a blood vessel).

To assess for perineal hematoma, the nurse should:

1. Look for discoloration of the perineum.
2. Listen for the patient's complaints or expression of severe perineal pain.
3. Observe for edema of the area.
4. Listen for the patient's expression of a need to defecate (the hematoma may cause rectal pressure).
5. Don sterile gloves, gently palpate the area, and observe for the patient's degree of sensitivity to the area by touch.
6. Call the physician or nurse-midwife to report the findings immediately. The bleeding that has produced the hematoma must be promptly identified and halted.

 Optimizing Outcomes—Early episiotomy care

The nurse should apply an ice bag or commercial cold pack to the perineum during the first 24 hours after childbirth. The ice bag should be wrapped in a towel or disposable paper cover to prevent a thermal injury. Application of cold provides local anesthesia and promotes vasoconstriction while reducing edema and the incidence of peripheral bleeding. Later (after 24 hours), the nurse encourages the use of moist heat (sitz bath) between 100°F and 105°F (37.8°C–40.5°C) for 20 minutes three to four times per day. The sitz bath increases circulation to the perineum, enhances blood flow to the tissues, reduces edema, and promotes healing. Dry heat, in the form of a commercial perineal "hot pack," may also be used. The packs are "cracked" to generate heat. Women should be cautioned to apply a washcloth or gauze square between the hot pack and their skin to prevent a potential burn.

CONTINUED ASSESSMENT OF PAIN. Discomfort and pain may occur from several sources. Afterpains, which most commonly occur in the multiparous patient, can be quite intense, especially after breastfeeding. Analgesics such as acetaminophen (e.g., Tylenol) or nonsteroidal anti-inflammatory agents (NSAIDs) such as ibuprofen (e.g., Motrin and Advil) are effective and safe for use. Heat is not applied to the abdomen because of the potential for uterine relaxation and bleeding.

Muscular aches and cramps related to the physical exertion expended during labor and birth may be relieved with back rubs and massage. When necessary, acetaminophen (e.g., Tylenol) may be used to alleviate the discomfort. Pain occurring in the calf of the leg must be carefully evaluated for thromboembolic disease. Episiotomy pain and discomfort may be associated with sitting, walking, bending, urinating, and defecating. It may interfere with the woman's ability to comfortably hold and feed her infant. Interventions to decrease discomfort from the episiotomy include the application of cold (first 24 hours) and heat, and the use of topical anesthetic creams, sprays, and sitz baths. The **sitz bath** is a portable unit with a reservoir that fits on the toilet. When filled with warm water, the swirling action of the fluid soothes the tissue, reduces inflammation by promoting vasodilation to the area, and provides comfort and healing. The nurse prepares and assists the patient to the sitz bath, which should be used for 20 minutes three to four times a day (Procedure 15-1).

 Optimizing Outcomes—Enhancing comfort and healing with a sitz bath

A sitz bath is a warm-water bath taken in the sitting position that covers only the perineum and buttocks. It can be placed in the toilet, with the seat raised. Other mechanisms for taking a sitz bath include sitting in a tub filled with 4 to 6 inches of warm water or the use of a nonportable sitz bath unit (similar to a toilet that fills up with warm water). A sitz bath may be used for either healing or hygiene purposes. The water may contain medication. Sitz baths are used to relieve pain, itching, or muscle spasms.

Procedure 15-1 Preparing a Sitz Bath

Purpose
To facilitate healing through the application of moist heat.

Equipment
- Sitz bath tub/toilet insert with water receptacle
- Medications to be added to water or saline, as ordered
- Towels for drying the perineal area after the treatment
- Clean perineal pad to be applied after the treatment

Steps
1. Wash your hands, identify the patient, and explain the procedure.

   RATIONALE: *Hand washing helps to prevent infection. Patient identification ensures that the procedure is performed on the correct patient. Providing an explanation educates the patient and helps to alleviate anxiety.*

2. Assess the patient to confirm that she is able to ambulate to the bathroom.

   RATIONALE: *A sitz bath can cause dizziness and increase the potential for injury. It is important to ascertain that the patient can safely ambulate to the bathroom before initiating the procedure.*

3. Assemble equipment and ensure that all equipment is clean.

   RATIONALE: *Gathering all equipment before the procedure enhances efficiency.*

4. Raise the toilet seat in the patient's bathroom.

5. Insert the sitz bath apparatus into the toilet. The overflow opening should be directed toward the back of the toilet.

6. Fill the collecting bag with water or saline, as directed, at the appropriate temperature (105°F [41°C]).

7. Test the water temperature. It should feel comfortably warm on the wrist.

   RATIONALE: *Ensuring a correct water temperature reduces the chance of thermal injury. The flow of warm water to the perineum promotes healing by increasing circulation and reducing inflammation.*

8. If prescribed, add medications to the solution.

9. Hang the bag overhead to allow a steady stream of water to flow from the bag, through the tubing, and into the reservoir.

10. Assist the ambulating patient to the bathroom. Help with removal of the perineal pad from front to back. Assist the patient to sit in the basin.

    RATIONALE: *Assistance with ambulation reduces the chance for patient injury. Removal of the pad from front to back decreases the risk for infection transmission. Proper placement on the seat ensures comfort and effectiveness of the treatment.*

11. Instruct the patient to use the tubing clamp to regulate the flow of water. Ensure that the patient is adequately covered with a robe or blankets to prevent chilling.

    RATIONALE: *The swirling warm water helps to reduce edema and promote comfort. Clothing and extra blankets for warmth prevent chilling and enhance patient comfort.*

12. Verify that the call bell is within reach and provide for privacy.

    RATIONALE: *Easy access to the call bell reassures the patient that prompt assistance is readily available when needed.*

13. Encourage the patient to remain in the sitz bath for approximately 20 minutes.

    RATIONALE: *After 20 minutes, vasoconstriction occurs and heat is no longer therapeutic.*

14. Provide assistance with drying the perineal area and applying a clean perineal pad by grasping the pad by the ends or bottom side.

    RATIONALE: *Holding the pad correctly decreases the risk for contamination and subsequent infection.*

15. Assist the patient back to the room.

    RATIONALE: *After the procedure, the patient may be fatigued or light-headed from the warm water; assistance minimizes the risk of injury.*

16. Assess the patient's response to the procedure. Reinforce teaching about continued perineal care at home.

    RATIONALE: *Assessment helps to determine the effectiveness of the procedure; teaching enhances understanding and promotes continuity of care after discharge.*

17. Record completion of the procedure, the condition of the perineum, and the patient's tolerance.

    RATIONALE: *Documentation provides evidence of the intervention and an additional opportunity for evaluation of care and the patient's tolerance of the procedure.*

Clinical Alert The warm environment associated with a sitz bath may cause the patient to feel light-headed or dizzy. It is important to monitor the patient frequently throughout the intervention to ensure safety and tolerance.

Teach the Patient
1. The benefits of using the sitz bath, which include enhanced hygiene, comfort, and improved circulation

2. To use the sitz bath as often as recommended—usually three to four times per day or as needed for discomfort

3. To contact the nursing staff immediately if she becomes light-headed or dizzy

(continued)

Procedure 15-1 Preparing a Sitz Bath (continued)

4. To check the temperature of the solution before use; applying water or solution that is too warm may result in local trauma or burns to the area

Note

A specific sitz bath device is more effective for local treatment than a regular bathtub because the application of heat to the extremities causes vasodilation and draws blood away from the perineal area. However, if the patient prefers to prepare a sitz bath in the bathtub at home, she should be instructed not to use the same water for bathing. Instead, fresh water should be drawn for washing to diminish the potential for infection.

Caution: The nurse must check the temperature of the water before administration of the sitz bath to ensure that it is not too warm.

What If?

What if you are assisting a patient back to bed after a sitz bath, and she suddenly complains of dizziness? You should take action to maintain safety and prevent falling: provide physical support, offer reassurance, and assist her to the bed (or chair if more convenient). Once she is in bed, raise the guardrails and check her vital signs. Place the call bell within easy reach. Offer an explanation of why the dizziness occurred (hypotension) and reinforce the need to ask for assistance before attempting to ambulate. Before leaving the room, ensure that the dizziness

has subsided, and continue to check on her frequently for the next 2 hours.

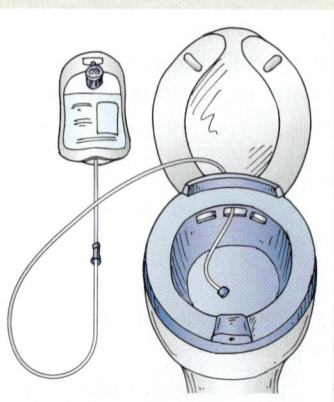

Documentation

6/29/13 1500 Patient reported perineal discomfort. Mild perineal edema noted. Patient assisted into bathroom for sitz bath. Tolerated sitz bath with warm water for 20 minutes. She denied any discomfort or syncope throughout treatment. Perineal care was provided and a new peri-pad was applied. The patient was assisted back into bed. She denies perineal pain at present.

–Olga Sanchez, RN

The patient likely has expectations regarding pain management during the postpartum phase. She should be encouraged to express her requests or concerns regarding pain control. Education regarding the available modalities is essential and will likely enhance the patient's perception of control, as well as her level of satisfaction with the nursing care received. The nurse should regularly assess for pain and medication side effects and actively involve the patient in her pain management regimen. Use of a standardized pain rating scale enhances the assessment by allowing the patient to select the pain intensity level being experienced.

The nurse assesses and documents the patient's pain behavior regarding the:

- Location of the pain
- Type of pain: stabbing, burning, throbbing, or aching
- Duration of pain: intermittent or continuous

Nursing interventions include the administration of analgesics and patient education about other measures to promote comfort.

- Suggest nonpharmacological methods for pain relief such as imagery, therapeutic touch, relaxation, distraction, and interaction with the infant.
- Provide pain relief by administering prescribed agents such as ibuprofen, propoxyphene napsylate/

acetaminophen (Darvocet-N), or oxycodone/acetaminophen (Percocet).

- Suggest over-the-counter medications and alternative therapies such as tea tree oil for self-care after hospital discharge. Teach the patient that medications such as acetaminophen or ibuprofen may be equally as effective as narcotic analgesics.
- Reassure the patient that the pain and discomfort should not persist beyond 5 to 7 days and that because the episiotomy sutures are made of an absorbable material, they will not need to be removed.

 Complementary Care: *Tea Tree Oil to Facilitate Episiotomy Healing*

Tea tree (*Melaleuca alternifolia*) oil applied to the perineum is believed to be beneficial in facilitating healing of the episiotomy site. *Melaleuca alternifolia* oil has been in use as a botanical medicine in various forms for centuries. For hundreds of years, the Australian aboriginal people have used tea tree oil as an antiseptic, antimicrobial, and anti-inflammatory agent. The anti-inflammatory properties are believed to be particularly helpful in promoting incisional healing although allergic contact dermatitis may occasionally occur (Stonehouse & Studdiford, 2011).

Postpartum women with episiotomies may be taught to fill an applicator with tea tree oil and then apply the oil directly to the wound. A few drops of the oil provide cooling to the wound, relieve pain, enhance comfort, and promote healing. Some individuals may experience an allergic reaction or sensitivity to *M alternifolia*. If redness, increased swelling, burning, or other signs of allergic reaction occur, application of tea tree oil should be discontinued immediately.

Homans' Sign

Homans' sign is used as a screening tool in the assessment for deep venous thrombosis (DVT) in the leg. To assess for Homans' sign, the patient's legs should be extended and relaxed with the knees flexed. The examiner grasps the foot and sharply dorsiflexes it. A positive sign is present when there is resistance or discomfort in the calf or popliteal region. The other leg is assessed in the same manner. If resistance or discomfort in the calf is elicited, a positive Homans' sign is present. The pain occurs from inflammation of the blood vessel and may be associated with the presence of a thrombosis. However, there are other causes of calf pain upon dorsiflexion such as strained muscles and contusions, and a positive Homans' sign is indicative of DVT in approximately 50% of patients. Thus, a negative Homans' sign does not rule out DVT. A diagnosis based solely on the evaluation of clinical signs that include pain in the calf, erythema, warmth greater in one calf than the other, and unequal calf circumference has proven to be unreliable. Instead, specific diagnostic procedures (e.g., venography and real-time and color Doppler ultrasound) should be performed when DVT is suspected (American College of Obstetricians and Gynecologists [ACOG], 2011). (See Chapter 16 for further discussion.) In some facilities, Homans' sign is no longer a component of the nursing assessment because of its limited diagnostic reliability and fear that performance of the maneuver could lead to emboli if the clot is dislodged during the assessment. However, there are no published reports of emboli resulting from performance of a Homans' sign.

❝What to say❞—*Suggestions to help prevent postpartum thrombophlebitis*

During postpartum care, the nurse can offer the following strategies to improve peripheral circulation and decrease the risk for thrombophlebitis (Rhode, 2011):

- Early ambulation is important—but ask for assistance the first few times you walk.
- If ambulation is not possible, perform active and passive leg exercises and do not place pillows under your knees (sharp flexion at the knees and pressure on the popliteal space cause pooling of blood in the lower extremities).
- Avoid sitting in one position or standing for a prolonged period of time.
- When you sit, elevate your legs and do not cross them.
- Drink plenty of fluids (10–12 8-ounce glasses) to prevent dehydration.

Emotional Status

The birth of a child is associated with a range of emotional experiences in the new mother. During the early puerperium, it is not unusual for patients to have periods of happiness that are intermingled with sadness, insecurity, and depression. Continued assessment of the woman's emotional status is an important nursing action that begins immediately after childbirth and continues throughout the hospital stay. The nurse should offer support to the new mother, which may include listening to her share her labor experience or reassuring her about her ability to effectively care for the newborn. The nurse should also provide information regarding the "baby blues," and emphasize that these feelings are common and temporary.

 Now Can You—**Discuss essential components of postpartum nursing care?**

1. Identify three types of lochia and explain the characteristics and duration of each?
2. Describe nursing interventions to promote healing, enhance comfort, and prevent infection in the patient with an episiotomy?
3. Discuss the nurse's role in pain assessment of the postpartal patient?

Maternal Physiological Adaptations and Continued Assessment of the Patient

HEMATOLOGICAL AND METABOLIC SYSTEMS

During the immediate postpartum period, a decrease in blood volume correlates with the blood loss experienced during delivery. During the next few days after childbirth, the maternal plasma volume decreases even further as a result of diuresis. The 500-mL blood loss that typically accompanies a vaginal birth (1,000 mL for a cesarean birth) usually results in a 1 gram (2 grams for a cesarean birth) drop in hemoglobin. It is important for the nurse to remember that as the body's excess fluid is excreted, the hematocrit may rise because of hemoconcentration. However, the hematocrit should have returned to prepregnancy levels by 4 to 6 weeks postpartum.

The white blood cell (WBC) count, which increases during labor and in the immediate postpartum period, returns to normal values within 6 days. Levels of plasma fibrinogen tend to remain elevated during the first few postpartal weeks. Although this alteration exerts a protective effect against hemorrhage, it increases the patient's risk of thrombus formation. Overall, the hematological system has usually returned to a nonpregnant status by the third to fourth postpartal week.

Circulating levels of estrogen and progesterone decrease dramatically after delivery of the placenta. The decline in these two hormones signals the anterior pituitary gland to produce prolactin in readiness for lactation. In nonlactating (formula feeding) women, prolactin levels return to normal by the third to fourth postpartal week.

After childbirth and expulsion of the placenta, circulating levels of other hormones, including human placental lactogen, cortisol, growth hormone, and insulinase, also fall. During the early postpartum period, the decline in the serum levels of these substances reduces the anti-insulin effects that occur during pregnancy. Hence, insulin requirements

Nursing Care Plan Acute Pain/Discomfort in the Postpartal Patient

Nursing Diagnosis: Acute Pain related to tissue damage secondary to childbirth

Measurable Short-Term Goal: The patient will report decreased pain to a level that is acceptable to her.

Measurable Long-Term Goal: The patient will report minimal or no pain upon discharge from the hospital.

NOC Outcomes:
Pain Level (2102) Severity of observed or reported pain
Pain Control (1605) Personal actions to control pain

NIC Interventions:
Pain Management (1400)
Analgesic Administration (2210)
Heat/Cold Application (1380)

Nursing Interventions:

1. Perform routine, comprehensive pain assessments (specify frequency) to include onset, location, intensity, quality, characteristics, and aggravating and alleviating factors of the discomfort. Note verbal and nonverbal indications of discomfort.

   RATIONALE: Assessments enable the nurse to provide interventions in a timely manner to enhance effectiveness of medications and ensure early identification of complications resulting in painful stimuli.

2. Assess for complications that may be causing additional pain such as hematomas, wound dehiscence, or beginning infection.

   RATIONALE: Complications may manifest with unusual pain and should be ruled out before treating pain.

3. Identify cultural or personal beliefs about the experience of pain and the use of pain interventions, including prescribed medications.

   RATIONALE: Expression of pain and use of pain relief interventions may vary according to culture and personal beliefs. Patients may prefer a stoic response to pain or fear becoming addicted to narcotics.

4. Provide factual, nonjudgmental information regarding pain interventions that are available to the patient. Encourage use of culturally based comfort measures when appropriate.

   RATIONALE: Accurate information and respect for the individual's experience and preferences empowers the patient and reduces psychic discomfort.

5. Offer an ice pack to the perineum if the patient experienced perineal trauma or episiotomy. Apply for 20 minutes followed by removal for 10 minutes.

   RATIONALE: Cold therapy causes vasoconstriction and reduces edema resulting in decreased pain. Periodic removal avoids thermal injury.

6. Assist the patient with a cool or warm sitz bath as ordered if the patient experiences perineal discomfort.

   RATIONALE: Cool water in the sitz bath decreases pain associated with edema while warm water promotes vasodilation and increased circulation to promote healing and provide comfort.

7. Teach the patient to apply topical medications for perineal or hemorrhoid pain as ordered.

   RATIONALE: Topical anesthetics, such as Dermoplast spray, produce localized pain relief by inhibiting conduction of sensory nerve impulses. Tucks pads contain witch hazel, which has astringent properties to shrink hemorrhoids and reduce perineal edema.

8. Teach the patient about the sources of pain and the effects of prescribed medications and interventions. Encourage her participation in developing a pain management plan.

   RATIONALE: Information and involvement increases the patient's perception of control and increases her personal satisfaction with postpartum pain management.

---

are reduced for insulin dependent women during this time, sometimes termed a "honeymoon phase." For many insulin-dependent diabetics, glucose levels remain in a normal range (without intervention) during the first few days after childbirth (Chan, 2011).

NEUROLOGICAL SYSTEM

Fatigue and discomfort are common complaints after childbirth. The demands of the newborn frequently create altered sleep patterns that contribute to increased maternal fatigue. Anesthesia and analgesia received during labor and birth may cause transient maternal neurological changes such as numbness in the legs or dizziness. When these changes are present, the nursing priority is to safeguard the patient and her infant and prevent injury from falls.

Complaints of headaches require further nursing assessment. Patients who received epidural or spinal anesthesia may experience headaches, especially when they assume an upright position. After spinal or epidural anesthesia, headaches may result from the leakage of cerebrospinal fluid into the extradural space. Labor-induced stress or gestational hypertension may also cause headaches. It is essential that the nurse assess the quality and location of the headache and carefully monitor maternal vital signs. Headaches that are accompanied by double or blurred vision, photophobia, epigastric or abdominal pain, and proteinuria may be signs of a developing or worsening preeclampsia. Report these findings immediately to the primary health-care provider. Implement environmental interventions such as reducing the room lighting and noise levels and limiting visitors. The physiological edema of pregnancy is dramatically reversed during postpartum diuresis. Patients who experienced medial nerve compression and carpal tunnel syndrome during pregnancy often obtain relief of symptoms.

RENAL SYSTEM, FLUID, AND ELECTROLYTES

The renal plasma flow, glomerular filtration rate, plasma creatinine, and blood urea nitrogen return to prepregnant levels by the second to third month after childbirth. Urinary glucose excretion increases in pregnancy by 100-fold over nonpregnant values. These values return to nonpregnant levels after the first postpartal week. Pregnancy-associated proteinuria (up to 1– on a urine dipstick or less than 300 mg in 24 hours) is common during pregnancy and generally returns to prepregnancy values by 6 weeks postpartum (Cunningham et al., 2014).

During the postpartum period, there is a rapid, sustained natriuresis (excessively large amount of sodium in the urine) and diuresis as the sodium and water retention of pregnancy is reversed. The physiological reversal is particularly pronounced during the second to fifth puerperal days. In most women, the body's fluid and electrolyte balance has been restored to a nonpregnant homeostatic state by the third postpartal week.

After childbirth, a decrease in levels of oxytocin and estrogen naturally occurs and contributes to diuresis. As the serum levels decline, the diuresis becomes more pronounced. Nurses often note a maternal urinary output that reaches 3,000 mL excreted in a 24-hour period. For the postpartum patient, a single voiding may contain 500 to 1,000 mL of urine.

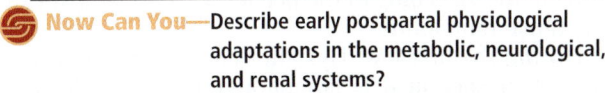 **Now Can You**—Describe early postpartal physiological adaptations in the metabolic, neurological, and renal systems?

1. Explain what is meant by the "honeymoon phase" and why this may occur?
2. Identify possible causes and describe appropriate nursing assessments for patients who complain of headache?
3. Discuss physiological adaptations in the renal system and identify one patient teaching need related to these adaptations?

RESPIRATORY SYSTEM

Respiratory alkalosis and compensated metabolic acidosis occur during labor and may persist into the postpartum period. In most situations, however, after delivery of the placenta and the decline in levels of progesterone, the respiratory system quickly returns to a prepregnant state. In addition, the immediate decrease in intra-abdominal pressure associated with the birth of the baby allows for increased expansion of the diaphragm and relief from the dyspnea usually associated with pregnancy. By the third postpartal week, the respiratory system has returned to a prepregnant state.

INTEGUMENTARY SYSTEM

Changes in the skin during pregnancy and in the postpartum period are related to the major alterations in hormones. Women may experience alterations in pigmentation, connective and cutaneous tissue, hair, nails, secretory glands, and pruritus. Most pregnancy-related skin changes disappear completely during the postpartum period although some, such as striae gravidarum (stretch marks) fade but may remain permanently.

 ### Cultural Diversity: Pregnancy-Related Skin Changes in the Puerperium

Although abdominal stretch marks (striae gravidarum) appear more pronounced immediately after childbirth, they tend to fade over the following 6 months. In light-skinned women, striae generally appear pinkish; in dark-skinned women, they appear lighter than the surrounding skin.

CARDIOVASCULAR SYSTEM

During pregnancy, the heart is displaced slightly upward and to the left. As involution of the uterus occurs, the heart returns to its normal position. Dramatic changes in the maternal hemodynamic system result from birth of the baby, expulsion of the placenta, and loss of the amniotic fluid. These abrupt alterations can create cardiovascular instability during the immediate postpartum period. Despite the usual blood loss (500 mL with a vaginal birth; 1,000 mL with a cesarean birth), the maternal cardiac output is significantly elevated above prelabor levels for 1 to 2 hours postpartum and remains high for 48 hours postpartum. The cardiac output returns to prepregnant levels within 2 to 4 weeks after childbirth.

On average, a 3-kg weight loss occurs during the first postpartal week. Diuresis takes place between the second and fifth day. A major fluid shift involves the movement of extracellular fluid back into the venous system for excretion through urine and perspiration. If the physiological diuresis does not occur, there is an increased risk of pulmonary edema. The cardiac output and stroke volume remain elevated for at least 48 hours after childbirth. Within 2 weeks, the cardiac output has decreased by 30% and then reaches prepregnant values by 6 to 12 weeks postpartum in most women (Cunningham et al., 2014).

IMMUNE SYSTEM

The WBC count is increased during labor and birth and remains elevated during the early postpartum period, gradually returning to normal values within 4 to 7 days after childbirth. Depending on the patient's blood type and immune status, administration of RhoGAM (see next page) may be indicated. Women who are rubella susceptible during pregnancy should receive the MMR (measles–mumps–rubella) vaccine at the time of hospital discharge; varicella vaccine should also be encouraged (American College of Obstetricians and Gynecologists [ACOG], 2013a), along with the tetanus/diphtheria/acellular pertussis (Tdap) vaccine, now available for use in adults as an important disease-prevention measure for adults who have close contact with infants (Tracey, 2012).

$Rh_o(D)$ Immune Globulin

Nonsensitized women who are Rh(D)-negative and have given birth to an Rh(D)-positive infant should receive 300 mcg of $Rh_o(D)$ immune globulin (RhoGAM) within 72 hours after giving birth. RhoGAM should be given whether or not the mother received RhoGAM during the antepartum period. In some situations, depending on the extent of hemorrhage and exchange of maternal–fetal blood, a larger dose of RhoGAM may be indicated. (See Chapter 11 for further discussion.)

Rubella Vaccine

Before discharge, the patient needs to be assessed for rubella immunity. If nonimmune (rubella titer less than 1:8, or antibody negative on the enzyme-linked immunosorbent assay [ELISA]), the MMR vaccine should be administered. The nurse should counsel the patient about the need to avoid pregnancy for 1 month after receiving the vaccine (because of the teratogenic effects associated with congenital rubella syndrome) and advise her that she may briefly experience rubella-type symptoms such as lymphadenopathy, arthralgia, and a low-grade fever. The vaccine may be safely given to breastfeeding mothers. A signed consent form must be obtained before administration of the vaccine (Centers for Disease Control and Prevention [CDC], 2012a).

REPRODUCTIVE SYSTEM

The uterus undergoes a rapid reduction in size (involution) and returns to its prepregnant state in about 3 weeks. The former site of the placenta heals by the process of exfoliation, which ensures that the placental site heals without leaving a fibrous scar. Formation of scar tissue would limit areas for future implantation and adversely affect the potential for future pregnancies. After a vaginal birth, the vagina often appears edematous or bruised, and superficial lacerations may be present. Although swelling is resolved during the healing process, the vagina does not return to its nulliparous size, and the labia majora and labia minora remain more flaccid in the multiparous woman (Cunningham et al., 2014).

During the postpartum phase, the return of ovulation and menstruation varies according to the individual. Menstruation usually resumes within 6 to 8 weeks after childbirth in women who are not breastfeeding. Seventy-five percent menstruate by the 12th postpartal week. The first cycle is often anovulatory. The return of ovulation and menstruation is typically prolonged in lactating women. Those who exclusively breastfeed may not ovulate or menstruate for 3 or more months. It is important to educate patients that because ovulation can precede menstruation, breastfeeding is not a reliable method of contraception.

GASTROINTESTINAL SYSTEM

Because of hormonal effects, gastric motility is decreased during pregnancy. It is further decreased during labor and in the first few postpartal days because of decreased abdominal wall

---

> **Box 15-2** Common Nursing Diagnoses During the Puerperium
>
> - Breastfeeding, ineffective/effective
> - Risk for constipation
> - Sleep-pattern disturbed
> - Fatigue
> - Pain, acute
> - Activity intolerance
> - Skin integrity, risk for impaired
> - Knowledge, deficient regarding self-care or care of infant
> - Risk for infection
> - Family processes parenting impaired
> - Risk for situational low self-esteem related to body image changes
> - Risk for urinary retention

---

tone. Abdominal discomfort results from gaseous distention related to decreased motility and abdominal muscle relaxation. Constipation, a common nursing diagnosis for the postpartal patient, is associated with abdominal discomfort and decreased hunger. Straining to pass hard stool can cause hemorrhoids and tear episiotomy sutures. Although spontaneous bowel movements usually resume by the second or third day after childbirth, it is important to educate the patient about strategies to prevent constipation. Stool softeners may be necessary. Additional nursing diagnoses for the postpartal patient focus on a variety of other problems such as pain, fatigue, and sleep disturbances, infant feeding difficulties, and knowledge deficit (Box 15-2).

MUSCULOSKELETAL SYSTEM

During pregnancy, the pelvic joints and ligaments have increased laxity. The hormones relaxin and progesterone are believed to contribute to the relaxation of the soft tissues (muscles, ligaments, and connective tissue) in the maternal pelvis to create room for the birthing process. In some women, the loosening of the pelvic joints causes pain and functional limitations.

During the first few days after childbirth, the woman may experience muscle fatigue and general body aches from the exertion of labor and delivery of the baby. Muscle fatigue can be exacerbated by the extended lack of nutrition and fluids throughout the course of labor. The maternal expenditure of glucose during **parturition** (the act of giving birth) can also add to muscle fatigue and may interfere with the patient's ability to ambulate and initiate postpartum exercises. The nurse needs to assure the patient that the muscular discomforts are temporary and not indicative of a serious medical problem.

During pregnancy, the abdominal walls are stretched to accommodate the growing fetus. The progressive stretching causes a decrease in the muscle tone of the rectus muscles of the abdomen and results in the soft, flabby, and weak muscles experienced after birth. Diastasis recti abdominis (abdominal separation) is a conventional term used to define the separation between the two rectus abdominis muscles that can occur from pregnancy (Fig. 15-7). Women should be aware that during the early postpartal period, the abdominal wall may not be sufficiently protected to

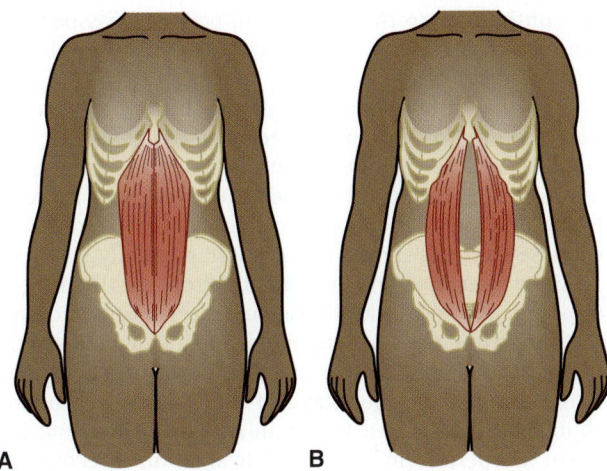

A   **B**

Figure 15-7 Diastasis recti abdominis *A,* Normal location of the rectus muscles of the abdomen. *B,* Diastasis recti—there is separation of the rectus muscles.

withstand additional stress from increased activities. Nurses should teach them to maintain correct posture when performing activities such as lifting, carrying, and bathing the baby for at least 12 weeks after birth. Performing modified sit-ups during this time is beneficial in helping to strengthen the abdominal muscles.

 Now Can You—Describe postpartal physiological adaptations in the respiratory, cardiovascular, and reproductive systems?

1. Explain why pregnancy-related dyspnea is relieved in the early postpartal period?
2. Describe three intra-postpartal events that cause dramatic changes in the maternal hemodynamic system?
3. Identify when ovulation and menstruation usually occur in the postpartal woman and explain specific information that should be given to lactating mothers?

Care for the Multicultural Family

ENHANCING CULTURAL SENSITIVITY

According to the United States Census Bureau (2010), ethnic and racial diversity in the U.S. population has reached new levels. At present, the population includes 72.4% Caucasians, 12.6% African Americans, 16.3% Hispanics, 4.8% Asians, 1.7% Native Americans/Alaska Natives, 0.4% Native Hawaiian/other Pacific Islanders, and 2.9% as persons who describe themselves as members of other races. Diversity in the population reaches into the health-care sector and has prompted emphasis on cultural awareness in nursing education curricula and mandatory in-service offerings for hospital staff.

Culturally competent care involves knowledge of the various dimensions of care, including moving beyond the biomedical needs of the patient. Rather, a holistic approach is one that expands knowledge, changes attitudes, and enhances clinical skills. To provide optimal care in a variety of clinical settings, it is important for health-care professionals

to conduct cultural assessments and expand their knowledge and understanding of culturally influenced beliefs, common health-care practices, customs, and rituals (Mattson, 2011). In preparation for the cultural assessment, health-care providers should:

- Assess their own cultural beliefs, identifying personal biases, stereotypes, and prejudices.
- Make a conscious commitment to respect and value the beliefs of others.
- Learn the customs and rituals of the common cultural groups within the community.
- Seek input from patients regarding health-related traditions and practices.
- Evaluate if what is about to be taught is really better than what the patient is already doing for herself.
- Adapt care to meet the special needs of the patient and her family, as long as standards of health and safety are not compromised.
- Include cultural assessment as a routine part of perinatal health care.

CULTURAL INFLUENCES ON THE PUERPERIUM

In certain multicultural populations such as India, Thailand, and China, the woman's postpartum confinement lasts for 40 days. During this time, prolonged rest with restricted activity is believed to be essential. The postpartum period is an important time for ensuring future good health; thus great emphasis is placed on allowing the mother's body to regain balance after the birth of a child.

During the 40-day confinement, support for the mother is provided by the female family members, usually the woman's mother, sister(s), and mother-in law, who perform household chores such as cooking and caring for the siblings and new baby. The woman's mother or older female relative often prescribes cultural remedies to aid in recovery and promote good health in the future. The female family members also provide the new mother with information on caring for herself and activities to avoid. Lack of adequate rest and poor diet are believed to result in poor eyesight, varicose veins, digestive disorders, headache, and backache (Giger, 2012).

Certain beliefs regarding hot and cold exist among several multicultural groups. Blood is considered "hot," and because the postpartum woman loses blood, she is considered to be in a "cold" state. To avoid illness, the mother must restore her health status by moving from a cold to hot state. The mother accomplishes this by:

- Adopting a diet that includes drinking/eating hot foods (foods such as black pepper, ginger, and garlic are believed to improve blood circulation). Sour foods such as lemons, grapefruits, and oranges are discouraged because they are thought to cause urinary incontinence later in life if eaten too early during the puerperium.
- Avoiding the consumption of ice water or cold water. These cold beverages are believed to cause weakness and delay healing.
- Avoiding cold temperatures, which are thought to be detrimental to the mother's recovery. To maintain warmth, the mother dresses warmly and stays in bed for several days. Bathing, showering, and washing the hair is delayed for 40 days because water cools the body.

• Avoiding drafts by keeping doors and windows closed and avoiding fans and air-conditioning.

 Cultural Diversity: Postpartum Practice of La Cuarentena

Waugh (2011) conducted a qualitative study to examine underlying beliefs that motivate the observed behaviors of *la cuarentena*, which refers to the 40 days of postpartum recovery observed by Mexican immigrant women in the United States. Data were collected from 40 Spanish-speaking individuals from 19 different Mexican immigrant families that were observed and interviewed in their homes during pregnancy and the puerperium. Families described perceptions of the body as "open" and vulnerable to drafts or *aire*. The women reported that the cultural traditions of *la cuarentena* served to "close" the body, and this was viewed as the central purpose of postpartum recovery. Because a lack of awareness of *la cuarentena* among health-care providers represents a barrier for many women seeking professional care, nurses and clinicians should seek to increase their understanding of the underlying fears associated with *la cuarentena* so that they can better support immigrant families during their postpartum recovery.

CLINICAL IMPLICATIONS OF CULTURALLY APPROPRIATE CARE

To provide sensitive, appropriate care, nurses need to adopt a flexible approach when caring for women who embrace non-Western health beliefs and practices. Inquiring about cultural beliefs, and, when possible, incorporating the beliefs into the plan of care are important strategies to help achieve this goal. For example, to demonstrate sensitivity to beliefs regarding hot and cold, the nurse may offer a warm sponge bath instead of a shower, adjust the thermostat in the room and provide extra blankets for warmth, offer warm drinks instead of cold beverages, and allow female family members as much access to the mother as possible (Mattson, 2011).

 Now Can You—Provide culturally sensitive postpartal care?

1. Identify at least five ways that health-care providers can enhance cultural sensitivity before conducting a cultural assessment?
2. Describe several cultural beliefs concerning "hot" and "cold" and identify specific nursing interventions that allow women to adhere to these beliefs?

Promoting Recovery and Self-Care in the Puerperium

ACTIVITY AND REST

In the postpartum period, it is important for the new mother to begin ambulating as soon as her condition permits. Despite recent advances in diagnosis and treatment, deep vein thrombosis after birth continues to be a leading cause of maternal morbidity and mortality. Venous stasis and hypercoagulation, conditions that exist in pregnancy,

are continued into the postpartum period. Early postpartum ambulation is key in preventing maternal thromboembolic events.

The type of birth and overall health status determine how soon the patient is allowed to resume exercise. The woman should be taught to begin with mild exercises, such as Kegel exercises, to strengthen the pelvic floor muscles. Nonambulating patients may begin with leg exercises. All exercise methods should be increased gradually.

Many women enter labor fatigued from the discomforts of pregnancy and lack of satisfying sleep associated with the third trimester. The length of labor and demands of the new mothering role further increase the feelings of exhaustion. During the hospital stay and later at home, all patients should be encouraged to obtain adequate sleep and frequent rest periods to help facilitate an optimal recovery.

NOURISHMENT

A weight loss of approximately 10 to 12 lb (4.5 to 5.5 kg) occurs immediately after childbirth, and this amount is directly related to the collective weights of the baby, placenta, and amniotic fluid. An additional 5 lb (2.3 kg) is lost over the following week as a result of puerperal diuresis and uterine involution. How quickly the woman returns to her prepregnancy weight depends on her physical activity level, eating habits, and lifestyle. In general, women whose weight increase is within the recommended limit of 25 to 30 lb (11.4 to 13.6 kg) during pregnancy can anticipate a return to the prepregnancy weight by 6 to 8 weeks postpartum. Factors associated with weight changes during the postpartum period include gestational weight gain, frequency of exercise, dietary intake, and breastfeeding for longer than 1 year.

Because of the restriction of food during labor, most patients demonstrate a hearty appetite after childbirth. All parturient women should be encouraged to eat a balanced, nutritious diet with multivitamin supplements. Iron is recommended only if the patient's hemoglobin is low.

ELIMINATION

Voiding should occur within 4 hours of childbirth. Patients should be encouraged to empty the bladder every 4 to 6 hours and to expect to excrete large volumes of urine. In addition to the extra- to intravascular fluid shift that follows childbirth, there is a decrease in the production of the adrenal hormone aldosterone. Declining levels of aldosterone are associated with a decrease in sodium retention and an increase in urinary output.

An intake and output record should be maintained to monitor the volume of urine passed during the first 24 hours. The woman who has recently given birth is prone to urinary stasis and retention. Incomplete bladder emptying or urinary retention may result from trauma to urethral tissue sustained during the "pushing phase" of a vaginal birth. Also, patients who were catheterized or who received regional anesthesia during childbirth sometimes experience an absence of the sensation to void. Bladder hypotonia during labor may also lead to postpartal urinary retention or stasis, factors that increase the risk of infection.

Incomplete emptying of the bladder is suspected when the patient experiences urinary frequency and passes 100 to 150 mL of urine with each voiding. The nurse's assessment includes careful palpation of the lower abdomen to identify a distended or displaced uterus. The uterine fundus is felt above the symphysis pubis with a lateral displacement of the uterus. The nurse also notes an increase in the amount of lochia because the uterus is unable to contract effectively. The bladder is displaced, bulges above the symphysis pubis, and feels "boggy" on palpation. Patients experiencing urinary retention because of absence of the urge to void can be helped by assisted early ambulation to the toilet and other measures such as running the water from the lavatory faucet. If ambulation is not possible, the nurse can pour warm water over the vulva and perineal area to help relax the urethral sphincter. Because of the risk of urinary infection associated with urinary stasis, catheterization may be necessary if the patient is unable to void.

Constipation commonly occurs because of slowed peristalsis associated with pregnancy hormones and childbirth anesthesia. In addition, perineal discomfort, fear of suture separation at the episiotomy site, and incisional pain (after a cesarean birth) may contribute to decreased frequency in bowel movements. To prevent constipation, nurses should encourage patients to consume foods high in fiber and roughage. Adequate fluid intake that includes drinking at least six to eight glasses of water or juice daily is another important strategy to prevent constipation. Early ambulation is also encouraged to improve peristalsis and relieve abdominal gas pain. If these measures are not effective, the primary care provider may prescribe a stool softener, suppository, or enema to alleviate the symptoms.

 Nursing Insight—*Postpartum care after bariatric surgery*

Nurses must be particularly alert to the possibility of complications in women who have undergone bariatric surgery. Patel, Patel, Thomas, Nelms, and Colella (2008) noted that maternal intestinal herniations and obstructions, post-bariatric surgery complications are more likely to develop with the increased pressure that occurs during childbirth. Left undiagnosed and untreated, these acute intestinal complications can lead to bowel dissection and potentially maternal death (Conrad, Russell, & Keister, 2011).

PERINEAL CARE

The perineum is susceptible to infection because of impaired tissue integrity resulting from bruising, laceration, or an episiotomy. The proximity of the perineum to the anus increases the risk of the incision becoming contaminated with fecal material; continuous drainage of blood creates a favorable medium for the proliferation of bacteria. To minimize infection, patients should be taught about perineal hygiene. A teaching approach that incorporates a return demonstration, encouragement, and positive reinforcement is most likely to be successful. Instructions should be given about properly cleansing the perineal area and the value of sitz baths, which not only cleanse but also provide relief from discomfort during the first 24 to 48 hours postpartum.

Patients should be educated about the importance of cleansing the perineum after each voiding and bowel movement. Hand washing before and after perineal care ("pericare") is essential for the prevention of infection. The nurse instructs the patient to gently rinse her perineum with fresh warm water after use of the toilet and before a new perineal pad is applied. The patient is taught to fill the peri-bottle (handheld squirt bottle) with warm tap water and gently squirt the water toward the front of the perineum and allow the water to flow from front to back. Consistent use of the peri-bottle is soothing, cleansing, and helps to relieve discomfort. Peri-pads should be changed often and secured in the underwear to allow for free drainage of the lochia. Tampons are contraindicated because of the risk of infection.

The nurse provides pericare for patients recovering from cesarean births until they are ambulatory and able to perform personal self-care. To provide pericare for the bed-bound patient, a plastic-covered pad is placed under the patient's buttocks to protect the bed during the procedure. With the woman in a supine position, the nurse carefully removes the perineal pad in a front-to-back direction. This prevents the portion of the pad that touched the rectal area from sliding forward and contaminating the vagina. Next, a bedpan is positioned under the buttocks. The movement associated with lifting the buttocks helps to expel clots and/or pooled blood in the vaginal canal. This also serves as a good time to assess the fundus for tone. Uterine palpation may be beneficial in helping the patient expel additional blood or clots. The nurse uses a peri-bottle filled with warm water (or other solution used according to hospital policy) and gently squirts the perineum from front to back while allowing the water to collect in the bedpan. The labia are not separated because they prevent the solution from entering the vagina. The perineal area is then gently dried and a clean peri-pad is applied from front to back (Whitmer, 2011).

"What to say"—*Teaching about perineal care*

To enhance the patient's understanding about proper perineal care, the nurse provides the following instructions:

1. Fill the squeeze/peri-bottle with tap water. The water should feel comfortably warm on your wrist.

2. Sit on the toilet with the bottle positioned between your legs so that water can be squirted directly on the perineum. Aim the bottle opening at your perineum and spray so that the water moves from front to back. Do not separate the labia and do not spray the water into your vagina. Empty the entire bottle over the perineum—this should take approximately 2 minutes.

3. Gently pat the area dry with toilet paper or cotton wipes. Move from front to back, use each wipe once, then drop it in the toilet.

4. Grasping the bottom side or ends of a clean perineal pad, apply it from front to back.

5. Stand before flushing the toilet to prevent the water from the toilet from spraying onto your perineum.

Ice Packs

To reduce perineal swelling and pain that result from bruising, ice packs may be applied every 2 to 4 hours. Application of cold is beneficial because of its vasoconstriction and numbing effects. The ice pack should always be covered and applied from front to back. It should be left in place for no longer than 20 minutes to minimize the complications associated with prolonged vasoconstriction. Patients obtain the most relief when ice packs are applied within the first 24 hours after childbirth.

SPECIAL CONSIDERATIONS FOR WOMEN WITH HIV/AIDS

Women who have HIV or AIDS require special precautionary care during the puerperium. All personnel who come in close contact with the patient should wear latex gloves (unless the patient has a latex allergy). In that situation, nonlatex gloves are used, as well as safety glasses to prevent the transmission of blood and body fluids. Patients need to be taught to avoid contact of personal body fluids with the infant's mucous membranes and open skin lesions. Breastfeeding is not advised because of the risk of transmission of HIV to the infant. (See Chapter 11 for further information.)

 Now Can You—Promote recovery and self-care in the puerperium?

1. Identify factors that determine how quickly patients should return to the prepregnant weight?
2. Describe the essential components of patient teaching about perineal care?
3. Describe special precautions that should be taken for postpartal HIV-positive women?

Care of the Postpartal Surgical Patient

PERMANENT STERILIZATION (TUBAL LIGATION)

A postpartum tubal ligation is a procedure that blocks the fallopian tubes to prevent the woman from becoming pregnant. When requested, the procedure, called a minilaparotomy, is performed after childbirth while the mother is still hospitalized. The size and position of the uterus during the early puerperium facilitates the surgical procedure. When a cesarean birth has been performed, the tubal ligation may be done at the same time. Patients need to be informed that while it is typically considered to be a permanent form of fertility control, there is a small chance that a future pregnancy may occur. (See Chapter 6 for further discussion.)

Patients scheduled for a tubal ligation receive nothing by mouth (NPO) before the surgical procedure. If epidural anesthesia was used for childbirth, the catheter is often left in place so that the patient can be re-anesthetized easily. When no epidural was previously placed, general anesthesia will most likely be used during surgery.

 Collaboration in Caring—*Removing barriers to access postpartum sterilization*

According to the American College of Obstetricians and Gynecologists (ACOG) (2012), postpartum tubal sterilization is one of the safest and most effective methods of contraception. However, not all women who desire postpartum sterilization actually undergo the procedure, and women with unfulfilled requests for postpartum sterilization have a high rate (approaching 50%) of repeat pregnancy within the following year. Potentially correctable barriers to obtaining the surgical procedure include patient and health-care provider factors, along with hospital and health-care system issues. Differences in requirements surrounding consent for sterilization procedures are based on the woman's particular type of insurance; those with government insurance face additional barriers to sterilization procedures based on cumbersome consent requirements. Nurses and other health-care professionals must advocate for policies and procedures to remove barriers and increase efficiency in accomplishing desired postpartum sterilization.

CARE OF THE PATIENT AFTER A CESAREAN BIRTH

Nursing care of the postoperative postpartum patient is similar to the care provided to all postoperative patients. The nurse must complete the breasts, uterus, bladder, bowel, lochia, and episiotomy (BUBBLE-HE) assessment previously discussed. Because the woman is confined to bed until full sensation has returned to the lower extremities, interventions for the prevention of deep vein thrombosis (DVT) must be implemented. Preventive strategies include leg exercises (flexion and extension of the knee) and the application of graduated compression stockings or use of an intermittent pneumatic compression device as ordered by the physician.

How the patient reacts to her surgery is often tied to the circumstances surrounding the birth—that is, whether the cesarean section ("c-section") was a planned procedure or an emergency event. Women who experience an emergency or unplanned cesarean birth may suffer from extreme disappointment, feelings of inadequacy, guilt, and personal failure. They may also harbor hostilities directed toward the medical and nursing staff. (See Chapter 16 for further discussion.)

After a cesarean birth, especially when unplanned, nurses must be aware of the myriad of potential psychological issues that may arise. Research suggests that women may perceive unplanned cesarean birth to be a less positive experience than a vaginal birth. Historically, vaginal birth has been shown to be associated with enhanced maternal satisfaction and perceptions of greater personal control over the birth. Women who experience vaginal birth describe feelings of empowerment, elation, and achievement. However, recent findings by Blomquist, Quiroz, MacMillan, Maccullough, and Handa (2011) revealed that women experiencing planned cesarean birth had higher birth satisfaction scores than women who planned a vaginal birth. For women with unplanned or emergent cesarean deliveries, the experience of cesarean birth may be associated with more negative perceptions of the birthing experience. However, research regarding the psychological outcomes associated with cesarean birth remains mixed.

The benefits of maternal–child interaction during the early postpartal hours are well documented. The first few hours after childbirth are a critical time for the initiation of a healthy maternal–infant interaction. For most mothers, a successful vaginal birth is psychologically better tolerated and avoids the need for additional recovery time that is necessary after a cesarean birth. In addition, early breast-feeding (for those who wish to breastfeed) is more easily implemented after a vaginal birth.

Additional challenges faced by patients during recovery from a cesarean birth include recovery from the anesthesia, a need to cope with incisional and gas pain, and slow ambulation. Mother–infant bonding may be delayed, and patients are at an increased risk for hemorrhage, surgical wound infection, urinary tract infections, and DVT. (See Chapter 16 for additional information.)

CARE OF THE INCISIONAL WOUND

The surgical incision requires ongoing nursing assessment after a cesarean birth. The nurse should assess for approximation of the wound edges, and make note of any redness, discoloration, warmth, edema, unusual tenderness, or drainage. If a dry sterile dressing has been applied, the surrounding tissue should be carefully evaluated for evidence of a reaction to the tape used to secure the dressing. Assessing for and effectively treating incisional pain is also of paramount importance.

RECOVERY FROM ANESTHESIA

Ambulation is encouraged as soon as the patient's vital signs are stable. If a spinal or epidural anesthesia was used, ambulation is delayed until full sensation has returned to the lower extremities. Common side effects of anesthesia include paresthesias (sensation of pins and needles in the legs) and headache. Assistance is required when the patient gets out of bed for the first time. Nurses should administer pain medication 30 minutes before the patient attempts ambulation. To minimize dizziness from orthostatic hypotension, the nurse should instruct the patient to sit on the side of her bed for several minutes before moving into a standing position.

Respiratory Care

Incisional pain and abdominal distension often cause patients to adopt shallow breathing patterns that can lead to decreased gas exchange and a reduced tidal volume. To facilitate adequate lung functions, patients should be taught how to perform pulmonary exercises. After being placed in a high Fowler's position, the patient is shown how to use a pillow to support her incision and instructed to take a deep breath and cough. Respiratory therapists are often included in the team approach to care for postoperative patients. Expectoration of secretions and deep breathing help prevent common complications including atelectasis and pneumonia. The nurse should administer pain medication 15 to 30 minutes before the patient begins her respiratory exercises.

Abdominal distension and gas pains are common after abdominal surgery and result from delayed peristalsis. Breakdown of digested food in the colon produces a buildup of gas that results in distension and discomfort. Anesthesia also causes a delay in the return of peristalsis, and it usually takes several days for the intestinal function to return.

Until bowel sounds are present, the nurse should offer the patient ice chips and small sips of water only. The diet is slowly advanced as tolerated. To minimize gas pains and stimulate the return of peristalsis, frequent ambulation is encouraged.

An indwelling Foley catheter connected to a closed drainage system remains in place for approximately 24 hours after a cesarean birth. While the catheter is in place, the nurse must assess for urine output of at least 150 mL/hr and maintain appropriate perineal care to reduce the risk of urinary tract infection. Once the catheter has been removed, the patient is at risk for urinary retention, and her output must be closely monitored. The nurse can help facilitate the return of normal voiding patterns by encouraging early ambulation to the toilet, ensuring privacy, allowing water to run in the lavatory, and pouring warm water on the perineum. If the patient is unable to void within 6 hours, a diagnosis of urinary retention should be considered and catheterization may be necessary.

 Now Can You—Provide nursing care for the surgical postpartal patient?

1. Identify nursing assessments appropriate for the postoperative postpartal patient?
2. Describe maternal psychological issues that may accompany a cesarean birth?
3. Discuss nursing interventions to facilitate ambulation and lung expansion?

Facilitating Infant Nourishment: Educating Parents to Make Informed Choices

Holistic care during the puerperium includes educating women and their partners about infant nutrition and providing support to facilitate success with the feeding method chosen. By the time they enter the postpartum phase of childbearing, most women have already made a decision about infant feeding. Providing current, evidence-based information, offering clinical guidance, and identifying appropriate resources when needed empowers patients to achieve success in nourishing and nurturing their newborn.

 Where Research and Practice Meet:
Analgesia, Post-Cesarean Pain, and Breastfeeding

Woods, Crist, Kowalewski, Carroll, Warren, and Robertson (2012) conducted a review of medical records of over 600 women with cesarean births to assess patient-controlled epidural analgesia (PCEA) versus patient controlled analgesia (PCA) for post-cesarean analgesia and to determine the impact of analgesic modality on breastfeeding in the first 24 hours postpartum. Study findings revealed that, consistent with the literature, PCEA provided greater pain control post-cesarean birth than PCA. Also, women with greater pain were less likely to breastfeed six or more times within the first 24 hours, a factor that could potentially affect duration of breastfeeding. The investigators suggest that the collaborative approach of an intraprofessional team consisting of perinatal administrators, nurses, lactation consultants, obstetricians, nurse anesthetists, and anesthesiologists, especially during the first 12 hours post-cesarean birth, may improve initial pain management postoperatively and subsequently facilitate early initiation of breastfeeding, decrease or eliminate supplemental feedings, and increase the frequency of breastfeeding.

Optimizing Outcomes—Encouraging breastfeeding in women with diabetes mellitus

During the intrapartal and postpartal periods, insulin requirements decrease rapidly, and experts recommend that the maternal insulin dose be decreased to 25% to 40% of the predelivery dose to avoid hypoglycemia in women who give birth both vaginally and via cesarean section. Nurses should encourage breastfeeding and be aware that insulin requirements decrease with lactation. Mother–baby nurses should be alert to the signs and symptoms of hypoglycemia; a maternal snack before breastfeeding may help prevent it (de Valk & Visser, 2011; Hood, 2012).

Breastfeeding, a vital preventive health practice, has long been established as the optimal method of infant feeding, and current trends are reflective of the public's awareness of its value. In 2008, the U.S. Preventive Services Task Force (USPSTF) released recommendations for primary care interventions during pregnancy and after childbirth (e.g., breastfeeding education and support for mothers and staff training) to encourage and support breastfeeding. Today, more women in the United States are breastfeeding their babies than at any time in modern history. While the rate of breastfeeding has increased in all demographic groups, certain populations of women are less likely to breastfeed. These include women younger than 25 years of age; those with a lower income; primiparas; African Americans; those who participate in the special Supplemental Nutrition Program for Women, Infants, and Children (WIC); those with a high school education or less; and those who are employed full time outside the home (Labbok, Taylor, & Parry, 2013; National Initiative for Children's Healthcare Quality, 2013; Office of the Surgeon General, 2011; USPSTF, 2008).

In 2011, Surgeon General Regina Benjamin issued a "Call to Action" to support breastfeeding. According to Dr. Benjamin, actions to help increase the number of children who are breastfed in this country include increased community- and hospital-based educational programs, encouragement and support from family members, and commitment from employers to provide time and space for breastfeeding mothers to nurse or pump (U.S. Department of Health and Human Services, 2011). The *Healthy People 2020* objectives will continue to track national breastfeeding rates, but new objectives will also address recognized barriers to breastfeeding success. According to the Centers for Disease Control and Prevention (2012b), 75% of new mothers initiate breastfeeding, but only 13% of breastfed infants are breastfed exclusively for 6 months and 22% continue some breastfeeding to 1 year. The *Healthy People 2020* initiative aims to increase these rates to 81.9% initiating breastfeeding, 23.7% breastfeeding exclusively through 6 months, and 31.4% continuing at 1 year. To help facilitate this goal, the American College of Obstetricians and Gynecologists (2013b) calls for a multidisciplinary approach that involves community, family, patients, and the health-care team.

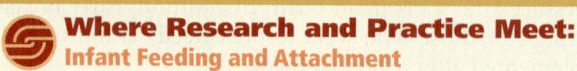 **Where Research and Practice Meet:**
Infant Feeding and Attachment

Recent nursing research has addressed various dimensions of infant feeding and attachment. The work of Reyna and Pickler (2009) focused on synchrony, described as an interactive pattern of behavior where the responses of one guide the responses of the other. Examination of synchrony during feedings of high-risk infants provides one way to assess the development of attachment at a very early stage. Brown, Thoyre, Pridham, and Schubert (2009) described the Mother-Infant Feeding Tool, an observational system that enables description of the process involved in mother–infant feeding interactions and permits description of the sequence of mother and infant feeding interactive behaviors in relation to each other. Pate (2009), who conducted a review of breastfeeding intervention delivery methods, found that breastfeeding promotion programs delivered via the Internet might be an appealing alternative to time-consuming and expensive provider-based breastfeeding education and support. McQueen, Dennis, Stremler, and Norman (2011) pilot tested an intervention (three individualized one-on-one nurse-patient sessions) designed to increase primiparous mothers' breastfeeding self-efficacy and concluded that such an intervention was feasible and acceptable. Tenfelde, Finnegan, and Hill (2011) examined predictors of breastfeeding exclusivity in low-income women who received the services of the Special Supplemental Nutrition Program for Women, Infants and Children Program (WIC). Findings revealed that women who received first-trimester prenatal care were more likely to exclusively breastfeed than women who entered prenatal care in later trimesters; women who declared intentions prenatally to exclusively breastfeed were more likely to exclusively breastfeed than women who did not intend to breastfeed; and overweight/obese women were less likely to exclusively breastfeed than normal/underweight women. Albert and Heinrichs-Breen (2011), who implemented use of a breastfeeding privacy sign in a hospital maternity unit, found that use of the sign significantly decreased the number of interruptions during breastfeeding sessions and was associated with the mothers' agreement that their breastfeeding sessions had been successful. The work of Lewallen and Street (2010), who used focus groups to explore issues related to initiating and sustaining breastfeeding in African American women, revealed that women need to be taught early in their pregnancies about the benefits of breastfeeding and offered ongoing support once breastfeeding is established. Based on their findings, the investigators encouraged the establishment of peer support groups for breastfeeding African American women. Thulier and Mercer (2009) conducted a review of data to identify the variables associated with breastfeeding duration. Their findings revealed that the following demographic factors influence breastfeeding duration: race, marital status, education, socioeconomics, and WIC. Biological variables included insufficient milk supply, infant health problems, maternal obesity and the physical challenges of breastfeeding, maternal smoking, parity, and method of delivery. Social factors included paid work, family support, and professional support, and psychological variables consisted of maternal intention, interest, and confidence in breastfeeding. Grassley and Sauls (2011) developed and evaluated the effect of an intrapartum nursing intervention (Supportive Needs of Adolescents during Childbirth [SNAC]) on adolescents' childbirth satisfaction and breastfeeding rates. The intervention included four maternity care practices: age-specific professional labor support, age-specific intrapartum breastfeeding support, help with initiating breastfeeding in the first hour after birth, and immediate skin-to-skin contact between mother and infant. Their findings suggest that learning the SNAC intervention may help nurses positively influence adolescents' childbirth experience and timing of breastfeeding initiation.

Cultural Diversity: Breastfeeding Practices in Orthodox Jewish Women

Viewed as the ultimate source of nourishment for the infant and the ultimate maternal–infant bonding experience, breastfeeding is the infant feeding method chosen by most Orthodox Jewish women. Breastfeeding is also encouraged for maternal benefits such as the enhancement of uterine involution. Maintaining modesty is an important consideration, and Orthodox Jewish women generally choose not to breastfeed in public. When necessary, however, the woman uses a blanket or towel to cover herself completely. Contraception is usually not permitted in the Orthodox Jewish religion although breastfeeding may be used as a method of delaying ovulation. It is important for the nurse to educate the woman that breastfeeding does not constitute a reliable method of contraception, and pregnancy may occur during lactation (Zauderer, 2009).

Human breast milk is the ideal infant food choice. It is bacteriologically safe, fresh, readily available, and balanced to meet the infant's needs. According to the American Academy of Pediatrics (2012), "breastfeeding and the use of human milk confer unique nutritional and nonnutritional benefits to the mother and, in turn, optimize infant, child, and adult health as well as child growth and development" (p. 837). When discussing infant feeding options with parents, nurses can share factual information about the physiological and psychological benefits of breastfeeding (Davis, Stichler, & Poeltler, 2013; Kim & Froh, 2012) (Box 15-3). There are economic benefits as well: Breastfeeding reduces the cost of feeding and preparation time. Providing such information may reinforce the mother's decision to breastfeed or help women and their partners in the decision-making process. The partner's level of support with the infant feeding method is an important factor in the woman's decision and success. There are only a few situations in which breastfeeding is contraindicated:

- Infants with galactosemia (because of an inability to digest the lactose in the milk)
- Mothers with active tuberculosis or HIV infection
- Mothers with active herpes lesions on the nipples
- Mothers who are receiving certain medications, such as lithium or methotrexate
- Mothers who are exposed to radioactive isotopes (e.g., during diagnostic testing)

Despite knowledge of the benefits of breastfeeding, some women choose to formula feed. Concerns about convenience, opportunity to involve the father in the baby's care, and modesty and embarrassment may be factors that influence the mother's decision. An unsuccessful breastfeeding experience during a previous pregnancy may also play a role. Some women anticipate that breastfeeding will interfere with plans to return to work. Whatever the reasons, the nurse must provide information and support in a caring, nonjudgmental manner. Postpartal women who planned to bottle-feed may still benefit from education about the benefits of breast milk over formula. The nurse's offer of breastfeeding support and assistance may encourage some women to change their chosen feeding method. The importance of the nurse's role in the promotion of breastfeeding has been underscored in an Association of Women's Health, Obstetric and Neonatal Nurses (AWHONN) (1999) clinical position statement.

 Optimizing Outcomes—Supporting women in their infant feeding choice

Although breast milk provides the best nutrition choice for infants, the decision to breastfeed is always one that must be made by the woman. She should make the choice based on what pleases her and makes her feel most comfortable. If the woman is pleased and comfortable with her choice, the infant will also be pleased and comfortable and both will benefit from the experience.

ENHANCING UNDERSTANDING OF THE PROCESS OF LACTATION

Normal Structure of the Breast

The breast is composed of glandular, connective, and fatty tissue. The lactating breast contains lobes that house the milk production cells called alveoli (singular: alveolus), fatty tissue, and a series of small and main ducts. The ducts converge into 9 to 10 duct openings in the nipple (Fig. 15-8). According to most published literature, each breast contains 15 to 20 lobes although ultrasound studies have demonstrated variations that range from 4 to 18 lobes per breast. Each lobe has a small duct that unites with others to form a main duct. The lobes are connected by areolar tissue and blood vessels. The ducts function to collect milk from the alveolus and transport it toward the nipple. The Cooper's ligaments, along with the fatty adipose tissue, give shape to the breasts and provide support to the ductal system (Fig. 15-9).

Box 15-3 Selected Breastfeeding Benefits

FOR MOTHERS
- Decreased risk of breast, ovarian, and uterine cancer
- Decreased risk of type 2 diabetes mellitus
- Lactational amenorrhea (LAM) (although breastfeeding is not considered an effective form of contraception)
- Enhanced involution (caused by uterine contractions triggered by the release of oxytocin) and decreased risk of postpartum hemorrhage
- Enhanced postpartum weight loss
- Increased bone density
- Enhanced bonding with infant

FOR INFANTS
- Enhanced immunity through the transfer of maternal antibodies; decreased incidence of infections including otitis media, pneumonia, urinary tract infections, bacteremia, and bacterial meningitis
- Enhanced maturation of the gastrointestinal tract
- Decreased risk of sudden infant death syndrome (SIDS)
- Decreased likelihood of developing insulin-dependent (type 1) diabetes
- Decreased risk of childhood obesity
- Enhanced jaw development
- Protective effects against certain childhood cancers

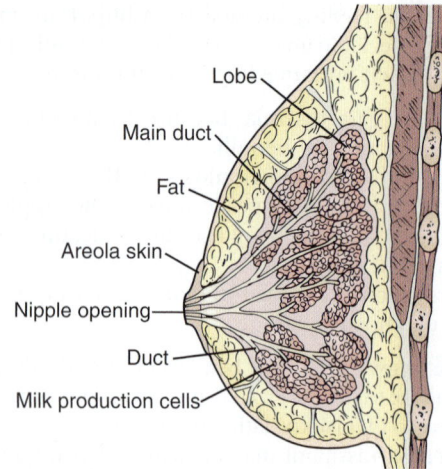

Figure 15-8 Cross section of a lactating breast.

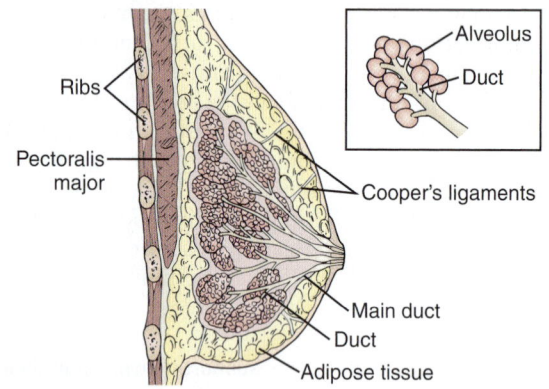

Figure 15-9 The ductal system of the breast.

The areola, a 15- to 16-mm circular pigmented structure, darkens and enlarges with pregnancy. The Montgomery tubercles are small sebaceous glands in the areola that enlarge during pregnancy. They secrete a waxy substance that acts as a lubricant and contains anti-infective properties that protect the nipples. The nipple, a mass of conical erectile tissue, is located in the center of the areola and projects a few millimeters from the center of the breast. Circular smooth muscles surround the areola and cause the nipple to become erect with stimulation. The main ducts converge and open into the nipple (Riordan & Wambach, 2009).

Blood and Nerve Supply and Lymphatic Drainage

There is an abundant vascular supply to the breasts. Approximately 60% of the blood supply to the breasts comes from the internal mammary artery. The remainder is supplied by branches of the intercostal, subclavian, and axillary arteries (Lawrence & Lawrence, 2010). Branches from the mammary arteries anastomose around the nipples and areolae and provide blood to those structures.

The fourth, fifth, and sixth intercostal nerves provide innervation to the breasts. The fourth nerve enters into the posterior aspect of the breast (anatomically, in the position of 4 o'clock on the left breast; 8 o'clock on the right breast) and provides maximum sensation to the nipple and the areola. The areola is the most sensitive area of the breast; the nipple itself is the least sensitive area. Damage to the intercostal nerves can result in some loss of sensation to the

breast (Riordan & Wambach, 2009). Loss of sensation may prevent the nipple from protruding and becoming erect in preparation for a baby's latching-on to breastfeed.

The breasts contain an extensive lymphatic network. The skin covering the breasts houses superficial lymph channels that serve the chest wall and are continuous with the superficial lymphatics of the neck and abdomen. A rich network of lymphatics is also present deep in the breasts. The primary deep lymphatics drain laterally toward the axillae.

The Physiology of Lactation

MILK PRODUCTION AND LET-DOWN. Lactogenesis, the process by which the breasts secrete milk, is dependent on the release of the hormones prolactin and oxytocin. The process of milk synthesis begins after the delivery of the placenta. This event results in a dramatic decrease in plasma progesterone and estrogen and an increase in the secretion of prolactin from the anterior lobe of the pituitary gland. Prolactin stimulates the alveoli, or milk-producing cells, to secrete milk. Stimulation from infant suckling or pumping the breasts triggers the release of oxytocin from the posterior lobe of the pituitary gland. Oxytocin prompts contraction of the smooth muscle myoepithelial cells surrounding the alveoli to eject milk from the alveoli into the lactiferous (main) ducts (Fig. 15-10). Movement of milk into the large lactiferous ducts for removal is called the "**milk ejection reflex**" or the "**let-down**" reflex. Lactating mothers describe "let-down" as a tingling or pins and needles sensation that occurs immediately before or during breastfeeding. Frequent stimulation and release of milk from the breasts are necessary for the continued release of prolactin (Kent, Prime, & Garbin, 2012).

The initiation of milk production is divided into three stages. Stage 1 occurs in late pregnancy and is characterized by the maturation of the alveoli, the proliferation of the secretory alveoli ductal system, and the increase in size and weight of the breast. Stage 2 begins during the postpartum period. The transition from colostrum (a sticky white-yellow

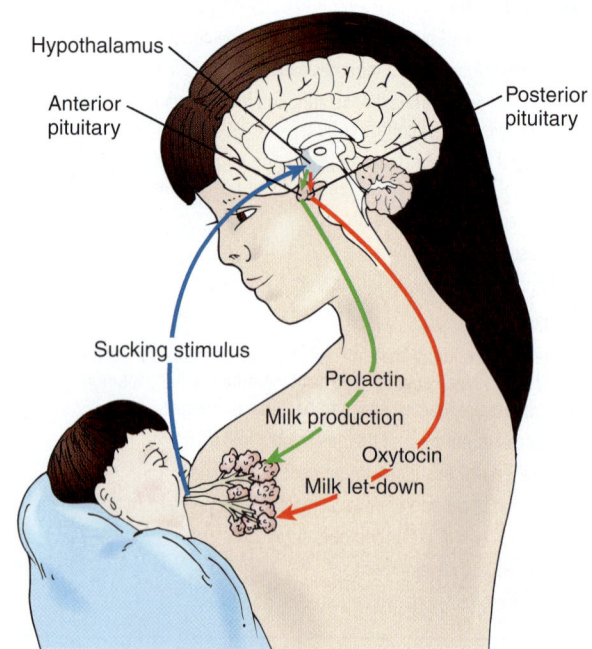

Figure 15-10 Mechanism for milk production.

fluid secreted by the breasts before the breast milk comes in) to mature milk occurs approximately 30 to 40 hours after birth, which allows time for secretory immunoglobulin (IgA) and other protective proteins present in the colostrum to coat the neonate's gastrointestinal and respiratory tracts. Reduced plasma progesterone levels lead to an increase in prolactin levels that cause a copious milk production by the fourth to fifth postpartal day. Stage 3, the establishment and maintenance of the milk supply, is governed by a principle of "supply and demand" and continues until breastfeeding ceases. The "weaning" stage, sometimes referred to as "Stage 4," begins when breast stimulation ceases. This stage is characterized by a significant reduction in milk volume (Stuebe, 2014).

A lack of breastfeeding (in breastfeeding or non-breastfeeding mothers), or a failure to empty the breasts by pumping, results in an accumulation of inhibiting peptides, or hormones released from the hypothalamus. Inhibiting peptides act on the breast secretory cells, causing a gradual decrease in milk volume and the eventual death of the epithelial cells.

ASSISTING THE MOTHER WHO CHOOSES TO BREASTFEED: STRATEGIES FOR BREASTFEEDING SUCCESS

The most important information that the nurse can give to a mother is that breastfeeding should not be painful. When the baby is feeding at the breast, the woman should experience a strong tugging sensation and occasional mild discomfort. However, pain associated with breastfeeding is not a normal finding. The nurse should refer women who experience breastfeeding pain or other difficulties to a board-certified lactation consultant (IBCLC) for help and assistance. Although the pediatrician is responsible for the health care of the infant, the IBCLC is a lactation expert who offers the most current, up-to-date, accurate information on breastfeeding using a "hands-on" approach. Mothers should be encouraged to consult with an IBCLC when they have any questions, are having difficulty with the latch-on process, or express concerns about their milk production. Ideally, all breastfeeding mothers should be discharged with an appointment to an IBCLC.

 Collaboration in Caring—*Partnering with an IBCLC and other community resources*

An IBCLC is a health-care professional who specializes in the clinical management of breastfeeding. IBCLCs are certified by the International Board of Lactation Consultant Examiners Inc. under the direction of the U.S. National Commission for Certifying Agencies. IBCLCs work in a variety of health-care settings including hospitals, pediatric offices, public health clinics, and private practice. The IBCLC credential is primarily an add-on qualification that brings together health professionals from different disciplines who share a common knowledge base in human lactation. Among those who become IBCLCs are midwives, nurses, family practitioners, pediatricians, obstetricians, educators, dietitians, and occupational, speech, and physical therapists. Most of these health-care professionals have spent at least 4 years acquiring the experience and education required for certification.

Costs for services provided by IBCLCs depend on the environments in which they work. Charges for inpatients are typically incorporated into the hospital stay. Follow-up visits in a hospital-based lactation department may or may not be included as a benefit for giving birth at that facility. Other consultations are fee-for-service. Most insurance companies do not pay for lactation services unless the service is provided within a physician's office under the supervision of the physician. Under these circumstances, the office visit charges may apply.

Many government-sponsored health programs such as WIC provide breastfeeding support services that are staffed by breastfeeding peer counselors. A mother who indicates that she is breastfeeding and is part of the WIC program will be provided with a special food package for herself and for her newborn. The La Leche League, an international support organization for breastfeeding mothers, is another resource that may be available in the community.

 Optimizing Outcomes—**Care of the breasts during lactation**

The nurse should teach breastfeeding mothers to wash the nipples with warm water. Soap, which can have a drying effect and cause cracked nipples, should be avoided. Breast creams are also to be avoided. They may block the natural oil secreted by the Montgomery tubercles on the areolae; others contain alcohol, a drying agent. Creams or oils that contain vitamin E should also be avoided because the infant may absorb toxic amounts of the fat-soluble vitamin.

Initiating the Feeding

The optimal time to breastfeed is when the baby is in a quiet alert state. Crying is usually a late sign of hunger and achieving satisfactory latch-on at this time is difficult. **Latch-on** is proper attachment of the infant to the breast for feeding. The neonate is most alert during the first 1 to 2 hours after an unmedicated birth, and this is the ideal time to put the infant to the breast. Bathing the neonate before the first breastfeeding should be avoided. The smell of the amniotic fluid on the infant matches the smells of the mother and serves as a "homing device" for the baby. Evidence shows that newborns engaged in skin-to-skin contact have improved suckling reflexes, breastfeed more easily immediately after birth, and have more stable temperatures than those swaddled in blankets, possibly because of extra tactile, odor, and thermal cues provided by proximity to the mother's breast (American Academy of Pediatrics, 2013; Anderson, Moore, Hepworth, & Bergman, 2003; Bramson, Lee, Moore, Montgomery, Neish, Bahjri, et al. 2010; Bystrova, Ivanova, Edhborg, Matthiesen, Ransjo-Arvidson, Mukhamedrakhimov, et al., 2009; Haxton, Doering, Gingras, & Kelly, 2012; Moore, Anderson, & Bergman, 2007; Mori, Khanna, Pledge, & Nakayama, 2010). Flacking, Ewald, and Wallin (2011) demonstrated the empowering effects of Kangaroo Mother Care (continuous and intermittent skin-to-skin contact in a Kangaroo position) on the process of breastfeeding in very preterm infants. Cesarean deliveries and medicated births, including those with epidural anesthesia, may require more mother–infant skin-to-skin contact before a successful latch-on occurs.

Optimizing Outcomes—Benefits of the breast crawl

The primary benefit of the breast crawl (TBC) (when placed skin-to-skin on the mother's trunk, the newborn's movement toward the maternal breast) is the initiation and establishment of effective breastfeeding. When the newborn is allowed to breastfeed right after birth, feeding is more effective than if TBC is interrupted before the first feeding takes place. When facilitated immediately after delivery, TBC promotes the physical stabilization (i.e., temperature regulation, heart and respiratory rates, and blood glucose) of the healthy newborn (Henderson, 2011).

To assist the breastfeeding mother, the nurse must understand that a baby latched-on to the breast is not necessarily transferring milk. A baby that breastfeeds effectively cues (shows readiness) for feedings, is in a good feeding position, latches-on (attaches) deeply at the breast, and moves milk forward from the breast and into the mouth. When the infant is properly latched-on to the breast, the tip of his nose, cheeks and chin should all be touching the breast (Fig. 15-11).

To feed effectively, the infant must awaken and let his mother know that he wants to eat. When possible, mother–baby rooming-in creates an optimal situation for breastfeeding. When the infant is in the mother's room at all times, she is able to observe "feeding-readiness cues" that signal the infant's readiness to feed (Box 15-4).

"What to say"—To assist the mother whose infant will not awaken to breastfeed

During hospitalization, nurses provide much information and coaching regarding breastfeeding. One new mother

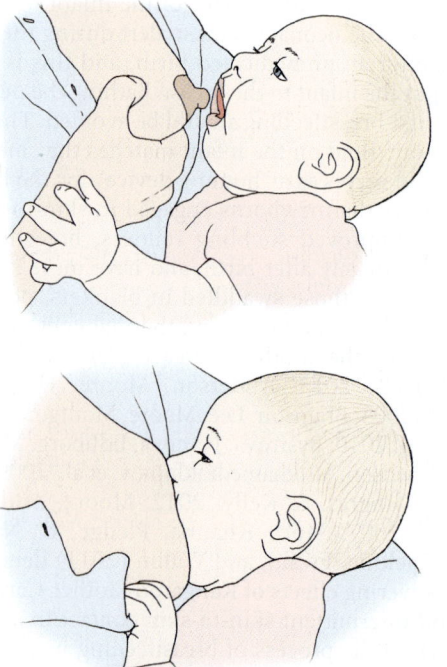

Figure 15-11 When properly latched-on, the tip of the infant's nose, cheeks, and chin should all be touching the breast.

Box 15-4 Infant Feeding-Readiness Cues

The infant demonstrates readiness for feeding when she:
- Begins to stir.
- Bobs the head against the mattress or mother's neck/shoulder.
- Makes hand-to-mouth or hand-to-hand movements.
- Exhibits sucking or licking.
- Exhibits rooting.
- Demonstrates increased activity; arms and legs flexed; hands in a fist.

expresses her concern that her infant is too sleepy to breastfeed.

The nurse may ask:

- Have you tried to unwrap the baby's swaddling? Doing this will increase skin-to-skin contact and help to awaken the infant and promote feeding.

- Have you tried to rest with the baby by your breast? Doing this may allow the infant to feel and/or smell the breast, which may promote feeding.

- Are you familiar with feeding cues? Watching for feeding cues may help you to recognize when your baby is ready to breastfeed. Examples of infant feeding cues are vocalizations, movements of the mouth, and moving the hand toward the mouth. Hunger-related crying is a late sign of hunger and should not be used as the cue for feeding.

An optimal breastfeeding experience begins with the mother's prompt response to her infant's feeding readiness cues. The mother should hold the baby so that his nose is aligned with the nipple and watch for an open mouth gape. At the height of the gape, when the mouth is open widest, the mother should aim the bottom lip as far away as possible from the base of the nipple. With this action, the infant's chin and the lower jaw meet the breast first and the nipple is pointed to the roof of the mouth. To facilitate a proper latch-on, it is desirable that the nipple be aligned with the baby's nose. This position allows the baby to tilt his head upward slightly so that the chin and lower jaw drops, creating the wide open gape desired. Next, the infant's mouth should be placed 1 to 2 inches beyond the base of the nipple. Depending on the areola size, most of the areola should be visible from the infant's top lip but not from the bottom lip. The top and bottom lips should be flanged outward. When properly positioned, there should be no slurping or clicking sounds or dimpling of the cheeks. Also, the mother should report a tugging sensation but no pain or pinching. If any of these are present, the infant should be removed from the breast by instructing the mother to insert her finger into the corner of the baby's mouth to break the seal. As an alternative, the mother can gently lift up and push back on the baby's upper lip (Fig. 15-12).

Optimizing Outcomes—Assessing for milk let-down

The nurse assesses for cues that indicate that the milk let-down reflex has occurred:

- The mother reports a tingling sensation in the nipples (not always present).

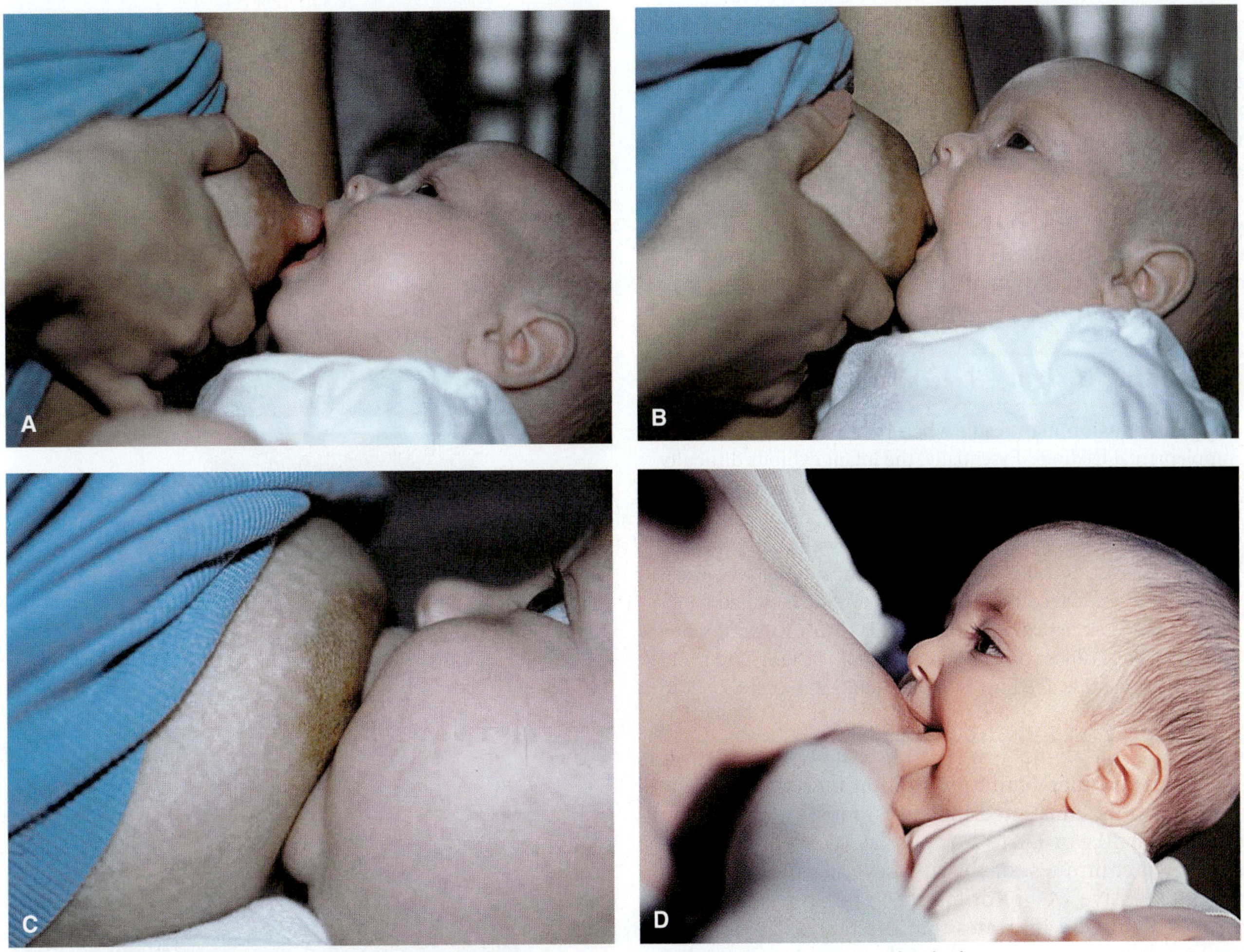

Figure 15-12 Infant latch-on. *A.* Nipple is aligned with the baby's nose. *B, C.* As the baby latches-on to the nipple, the baby's mouth is placed 1 to 2 inches beyond the base of the nipple. *D.* To remove the baby from the breast, the mother inserts her finger into the corner of the baby's mouth to break the seal.

- The infant's quick, shallow sucking pattern transitions to a slower, more drawing pattern.
- The infant exhibits audible swallowing.
- The mother reports uterine cramping; increased lochia may be present.
- The mother states she feels extremely relaxed during the feeding.
- The opposite breast may leak milk.

Once the baby is latched-on correctly, he must suckle and transfer milk. There should be a 2:1 or 1:1 suck/swallow ratio with audible swallowing to indicate that milk transfer is occurring. A 5:1 or higher suck/swallow ratio is indicative of non-nutritive suckling. Non-nutritive suckling can result in poor milk supply and lead to poor infant weight gain. Feedings that last less than 10 minutes or continue for longer than 40 minutes are not satisfactory and require consultation and assessment by a lactation consultant.

Optimal feeding results in the infant coming off the breast without assistance. Once the feeding has ended, the infant should be in a relaxed state with hands open; he may or may not be asleep. After a successful breastfeeding experience, mothers often describe their baby as having a "drunken stupor" look. The nipple should be everted and round, never flat or pinched on any side. The mother should report no pain, and the infant should appear satiated.

Collaboration in Caring—*Facilitating breastfeeding in the mother with a physical disability*

Mothers with physical disabilities, especially those that affect the upper extremities, may need special assistance and strategies for infant care and breastfeeding. Interventions to facilitate breastfeeding include the following: early contact with skilled lactation and occupational therapy consultants with relevant experience, adaptive equipment such as the use of a wheelchair lap tray for positioning the infant near the breast, networking with breastfeeding role models, and consultation and training in the hospital and at home (Phillips & Bulmer, 2012; Signore, Spong, Krotoski, Shinowara, & Blackwell, 2011).

EVALUATION OF NOURISHMENT: INFANT WEIGHT GAIN

All newborns are expected to lose weight during the early days of life. A newborn who is feeding frequently and effectively, in general, may lose an average of 5% of his birth weight (American Academy of Pediatrics [AAP] Committee on Fetus and Newborn, 2010). Any infant who loses more than 7% of his birth weight should be carefully evaluated to make sure that he is being fed frequently enough and that the feeding technique is effective in transferring milk from the mother's breast.

An infant weight loss of greater than 7% is not an "automatic" reason to supplement breastfeedings with formula. The administration of formula may interfere with the baby's interest in feeding at the breast and his ability to learn appropriate breastfeeding techniques.

 Nursing Insight—*Preventing nipple confusion*

Nipple confusion may result when breastfed infants receive supplemental feedings. Essentially, the infant exhibits difficulty in knowing how to latch-on to the breast. Nipple confusion occurs because breastfeeding and bottle feeding require different skills. Sucking and swallowing patterns as well as the way the tongue, cheeks, and lips are used vary considerably between breast- and bottle feeding. The infant's tongue is pulled backward when sucking from the breast; it is thrust forward when sucking from a rubber nipple. Parents should be taught to avoid bottles until breastfeeding is well established (usually 3 to 4 weeks).

Once the mother's milk production increases and the volume of milk consumed increases, most infants begin to gain 15 to 30 g or 1/2 to 1 oz per day (AAP, 2010). This rate of gain continues for the first several months of life. Loss of excessive weight or failure to begin a steady pattern of weight gain indicates that the mother is not producing adequate milk or the infant is not ingesting adequate milk, or, much less commonly, the infant has other organic problems. In most instances, correcting latch-on difficulties and proper positioning improves milk transfer from the breast to the baby. As long as the baby continues to feed well and is gaining weight, the mother can be reassured not to worry.

POSITIONS FOR BREASTFEEDING

Common positions for nursing a baby include cradle hold, cross-cradle hold, football, and side-lying (Fig. 15-13). In the cradle hold position, the infant is cradled in the arm, close to the maternal breast. The infant's abdomen is placed against the mother's abdomen with the mother's other hand supporting the breast. The cross-cradle hold is similar to the cradle hold, although in this hold, the infant is laying in the opposite direction. In the football hold, the infant's back and shoulders are held in the palm of the mother's hand. The infant is tucked up under the mother's arm, keeping the infant's hip, shoulder, and ear in alignment. The mother supports the breast to touch the infant's lips. Once the infant's mouth is open, the mother pulls the infant toward the breast. In the side-lying position, both the mother and the infant lay on their sides. Facing one another, the mother should place a pillow behind the infant's back for support. The nipple should be placed within easy reach for the infant with the mother guiding the nipple into the infant's mouth (Lawrence & Lawrence, 2010). Because of reports of apparent accidental infant suffocation during side-lying

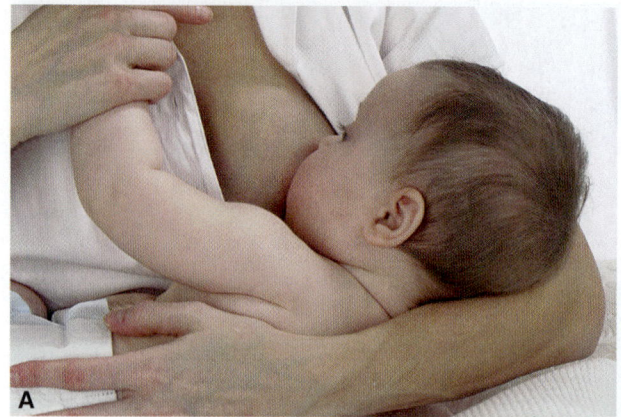

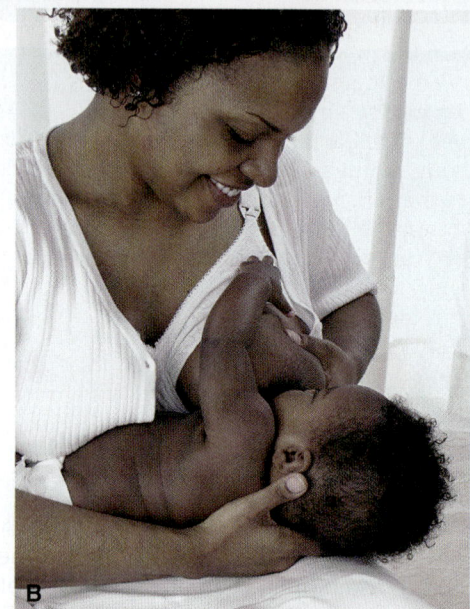

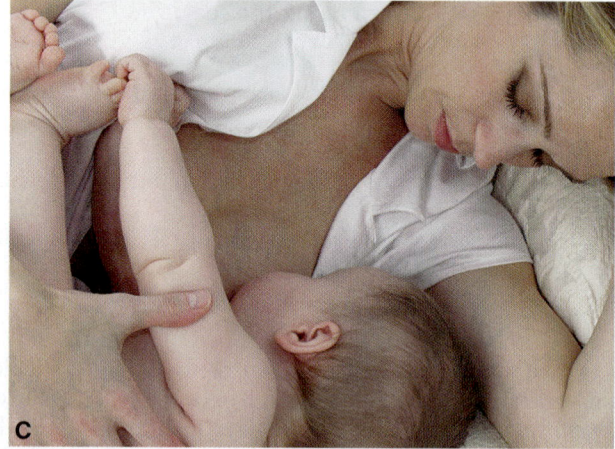

Figure 15-13 Common positions for breastfeeding. *A*, Cradle hold position. *B*, Football hold position. *C*, Side-lying position.

breastfeeding, frequent mother–baby checks during breastfeeding and skin-to-skin interventions constitute important nursing actions. Also, nurses should ensure that newborns not be left with their fatigued mother in a side-lying position for prolonged periods of time (Feldman & Whyte, 2013).

Now Can You—Discuss the physiology of lactation and assist the breastfeeding mother?

1. Describe the four stages involved in the process of lactation?
2. Discuss techniques the breastfeeding mother can use to promote proper "latch-on"?
3. Explain what the mother should be taught regarding the infant's weight?
4. Demonstrate four common breastfeeding positions?

PROBLEMS THAT RESULT IN INEFFECTIVE BREASTFEEDING

Sore nipples are related to an incorrect latch-on and positioning of the infant at the breast. If a mother complains of pain when the infant is nursing, it is important to observe the baby for correct latch-on during feeding. The nurse can assess for proper latching-on by making the following observations when the infant is at the breast: Maternal–infant positioning is optimal for feeding; the infant exhibits a flanged lower lip, a good seal between the mouth and nipple, and an audible swallow. Successful latch-on is essential to prevent trauma to the nipple. The shape of the nipple at the conclusion of the feeding also provides a good indicator for correct latching-on. If the nipple shape has changed at the end of the feeding, the nurse should troubleshoot for specific problems and teach the mother about correct latch-on and positioning techniques.

 Optimizing Outcomes—Breast shells for flat, inverted, or sore nipples

Breast shells, which are plastic "nipple cups," or inserts that fit into the bra, are sometimes recommended for women with flat or inverted nipples because they may help the nipples to become more protuberant. They may also be used to prevent sore nipples from making contact with the woman's clothing or bra.

Breast **engorgement** is described as excessive swelling and overfilling of the breast and areola and is a physiological response to an increase in blood flow and an increase in milk production. Engorgement, which may occur from infrequent feeding or ineffective emptying of the breasts, results in congestion and overdistention of the collecting ductal system and obstruction of lymphatic drainage. It typically lasts about 24 hours. Symptoms of engorgement usually occur between the third and fifth day after childbirth (when the milk "comes in") and vary from minimally engorged (patients complain of breast fullness and discomfort) to severe engorgement, characterized by symptoms of pain, tenderness, hardness, and warmth to the touch. With severe engorgement, swelling of the breasts is profuse and extends from the clavicle to the tail of Spence (an extension of the tissue of the breast that extends into the axilla) and the lower rib cage. The breasts may have a shiny, taut appearance. The areolae become very firm, and the nipples may flatten, making it difficult for the infant to latch-on. Back pressure exerted on full milk glands inhibits milk production. Thus, if milk is not removed from the breasts, the milk supply may decrease. Treatment involves relieving the patient's discomfort by removal of the milk (via breastfeeding

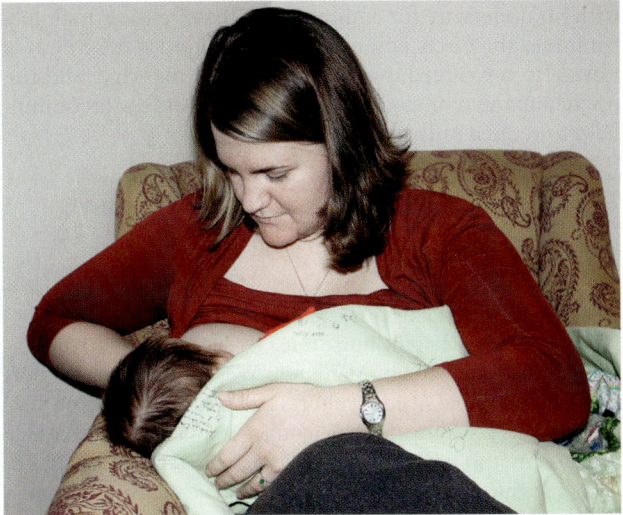

Figure 15-14 The infant should feed at each breast for at least 15 to 20 minutes.

or pumping) to decrease stasis, which reduces the swelling and discomfort.

Because the infant is very efficient in the removal of milk, frequent feeding (at least every 2 to 3 hours) is advised to minimize the stasis of milk. The infant should feed at each breast at least 15 to 20 minutes until at least one breast softens after the feeding (Fig. 15-14). To help reduce the swelling and enhance milk flow, the nurse should instruct the mother to use warm compresses and perform hand expression before nursing. This action softens the areola, initiates the let-down reflex, and allows the infant to more easily grasp the areola. Massaging the breasts during feedings is also beneficial. Other methods to enhance milk flow and help facilitate infant latch-on include taking a warm shower or leaning over a bowl of warm water and hand-expressing some milk before nursing. Because breast swelling is related to increased blood flow, cold ice packs may be used after breastfeeding or pumping to constrict blood flow and reduce the edema (Orr, 2011).

 Complementary Care: *Cabbage Leaves to Diminish Breast Swelling*

Patients can be taught to place raw cabbage leaves over their breasts between feedings to help reduce swelling. First, several large cabbage leaves are washed, then stored in the refrigerator until they become cool. The leaves are then crushed and placed directly on the breasts for 20 to 30 minutes. This process may be repeated three to four times only; frequent application of the cabbage leaves may decrease the milk supply. Women who are allergic to cabbage, sulfa drugs, or who develop a skin rash should not use cabbage leaves (Davis, 2010).

A nonprescription anti-inflammatory medication such as ibuprofen (e.g., Motrin or Advil) may be taken for the pain and swelling related to engorgement. It may be particularly helpful for the mother to take the medication before breastfeeding in anticipation of postfeeding discomfort. Because of the significant increase in breast size during lactation, patients should be advised to wear well-fitting supportive bras with no underwire for comfort. Bras that are too small may compress the ducts and obstruct milk flow. If the infant is unable to breastfeed, warm soaks, breast massage, and the use of a manual or electric pump for the expression of milk help to reduce milk stasis and swelling.

Cultural Diversity: Cultural Influences and Interventions for Breastfeeding Discomfort

When educating mothers regarding management of breastfeeding-related discomfort, the nurse must consider the cultural background of the patient. Many non-Western cultures such as Asian, Latin, and African cultures embrace a hot and cold "humoral theory." Breastfeeding mothers from these cultures may choose not to use a cold modality for the relief of breast engorgement or discomfort. Although the nurse may explain the clinical rationale for applying ice packs to the breasts, the patient is culturally bound to adhere to her beliefs. Nurses must remain sensitive to culturally influenced customs and allow patients to use relief measures that do not conflict with their personal beliefs.

COLLECTING AND STORING BREAST MILK

Collecting and storing breast milk is a necessity for mothers who are separated from their infants because of problems such as prematurity or illness. In other situations, women may elect to return to school or work and wish to have breast milk available for feeding by another individual. Freshly pumped breast milk can be safely stored at room temperature for 4 hours or refrigerated at 34°F (1.11°C) to 39°F (3.89°C) for 5 to 7 days after collection. Milk kept in a deep freezer at 0°F (−19°C) can be stored for 6 to 12 months (Lawrence & Lawrence, 2010).

The oldest milk should be used first, unless the pediatrician recommends the use of recently expressed milk. Women should be taught to thaw breast milk by placing the collection container in the refrigerator. The thawing process may be accelerated by holding the collection container under warm running water or by placing it in a cup, pot, bowl, or basin of warm water. Breast milk should not be allowed to thaw at room temperature, in very hot water, or in the microwave oven. Microwaving the breast milk container can create "hot spots" and use of the microwave oven or heating the container in very hot water may decrease the milk's anti-infective properties. Breast milk separates during storage. The cream rises to the top because breast milk is not homogenized. To mix the milk after storage, the collection container should be gently swirled, or rotated; vigorous shaking should be avoided. After the feeding, any milk that remains in the feeding container should be discarded and not saved for a later feeding. Thawed milk should never be refrozen (Murray, 2013).

Optimizing Outcomes—With manual (hand) and electric expression of breast milk

Performing manual or electric expression of breast milk is sometimes necessary because of medical complications or for occupational reasons. During the early postpartum period, the woman should be encouraged to frequently express her breast milk. This action helps to establish and increase the milk supply for later breastfeeding needs. Recent research suggests that hand expression is more effective than pump suction in early milk removal—this may be related to colostrum viscosity (Flaherman, Gay, Scott, Avins, Lee, & Newman, 2012; Morton, Hall, & Pessl, 2014; Ohyama Watabe, & Hayasaka, 2010). Once lactation has been established, the mother should be encouraged to express milk, either manually or with an electric breast pump, whichever method is most convenient or effective for her (Lawrence & Lawrence, 2010).

Electric Expression of Breast Milk

Women should be encouraged to avoid pumping the breasts until the infant is breastfeeding comfortably. Although the mother can help her baby learn to take a bottle once breastfeeding has been well established, it is best to wait for 3 to 4 weeks before introducing bottle feeding. The American Academy of Pediatrics (2012) recommends exclusive breastfeeding, with no supplements, for the first 6 months of life.

The nurse teaches the woman to use hot, soapy water to wash her hands, all components of the breast pump that will touch her breasts, and all collecting bottles before proceeding. Most equipment may also be safely cleaned in an automatic dishwasher. If soap and water are not available, many "quick clean" products may be safely used instead. Collecting bottles should be allowed to air dry on a clean towel.

The woman is encouraged to carefully read the instruction manual and practice pumping when she is rested, relaxed, and when her breasts feel full. The nurse can teach employed mothers to begin to pump and store breast milk 2 to 3 weeks before returning to work. The breasts should be pumped once a day, every day, 7 days a week. The first morning pumping usually produces the largest quantity of milk. If possible, the woman should nurse the baby on one breast while pumping the other breast. The breast milk may be stored in the refrigerator or freezer. The 7-day-a-week pumping schedule should continue even after the woman has returned to work (Lawrence & Lawrence, 2010).

Many employed mothers use the fresh breast milk they pump while at work for infant feedings the following day. For example, the breast milk pumped at work on Monday should be refrigerated and used on Tuesday. Mothers should be counseled to breastfeed the infant before leaving for work and then adhere to a set schedule of pumping and feeding each day. Breast milk collected (by pumping) on Friday and Saturday can be frozen for future use. Ideally, mothers should pump the breasts for each missed feeding, but two pumpings per work day during an 8-hour work shift is realistic for most women. The breasts should be pumped for 15 to 20 minutes or until the milk flow stops. Breastfeeding should be resumed during the evening and throughout weekends (Lawrence & Lawrence, 2010).

Types of Breast Pumps

A variety of manual and electric breast pumps are available, and, for most women, the choice is made according to needs, preferences, and financial resources. Hospital-grade electric breast pumps are designed for complete mother–baby separation. In these situations, the infant will not be able to breastfeed for an indeterminate period of time because of problems such as prematurity, surgery, or illness. Hospital-grade electric pumps are typically considered to be multiple-user

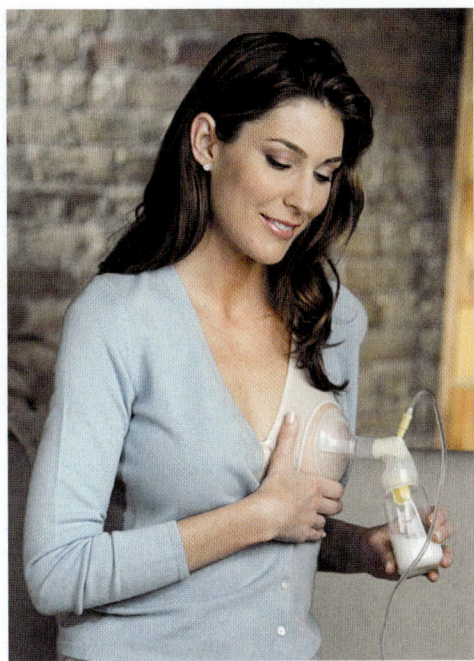

Figure 15-15 Personal use electric breast pump.

rental equipment. Retail or "personal use" electric breast pumps are excellent alternatives to the rented hospital-grade pump (Fig. 15-15). These single-user electric breast pumps usually work well for the working mother or in situations in which consistent pumping is needed. Occasional-use, battery-powered or manual breast pumps are designed for the mother who needs to have extra milk only once in a while.

Optimizing Outcomes—Donor breast milk

When a mother is unable to provide breast milk or does not have a sufficient supply, pasteurized donor milk is an important option. Processed through a Human Milk Banking Association of North America, donor breast milk maintains many of the benefits of breastfeeding and is safer than formula for preterm and low-birth-weight infants. Before donation, potential donors undergo serological screening (e.g., HIV, Hepatitis B and C, syphilis, and human T-cell lymphotropic virus) and complete an interview and lifestyle questionnaire to evaluate their suitability. Mothers and infants must receive care provider confirmation that there are no contraindications to breast milk donation. Donors are not reimbursed for their milk, which is shipped frozen to a donor milk bank where it is thawed, pooled with other breast milk, pasteurized, and refrozen for shipment (Arslanoglu, Corpeleijn, Moro, Braegger, Campoy, Colomb, et al., 2013; Rosenbaum, 2012).

INFANT WEANING

When a mother decides to wean the baby from the breast, it is recommended that she begin by eliminating one feeding at a time. Usually the least favorite nursing time is the first one that is discontinued (Cadwell, Turner-Maffei, O'Conner, Cadwell-Blair, Arnold, & Blair, 2006). After waiting for a few days, an alternate feeding time (not the one immediately before or after the one already discontinued) may be eliminated. Mothers should be advised to carefully observe the baby for signs of emotional or physical reactions (e.g., cow's milk allergy if formula is introduced). Babies sometimes choose to stop nursing although this does not usually occur with infants younger than 1 year of age. The American Academy of Pediatrics (2012) currently recommends breastfeeding for the first 12 months of life.

"What to say"—*Caffeine, alcohol, and breastfeeding*

When asked about caffeine, alcohol, and breastfeeding, the nurse can offer the following information (American Academy of Pediatrics, Meek, & Yu, 2011; Bowen & Tumback, 2011; Guilbeau, 2012):

- Breast milk usually contains less than 1% of the caffeine that you ingest. It is best to drink no more than 3 cups of a caffeinated beverage spread throughout the day. If your baby becomes fussy or restless, consider decreasing your caffeine intake.
- Alcohol does pass through you to your breast milk.
- Alcohol does not improve the quality or the quantity of your breast milk.
- Neither you nor your baby receives any sleep benefits when you drink alcohol.
- Drinking alcohol during breastfeeding may have long-term negative effects on your child.
- The amount of alcohol you drink may be more than you realize because there are many variations in the alcohol content of drinks.
- If you wish to go out and drink alcohol, you may pump and store your breast milk beforehand so that it will be available when you return home. Then, pump again after at least 2 hours have passed since drinking alcohol and discard that milk.

ASSISTING THE MOTHER WHO CHOOSES TO FORMULA-FEED HER INFANT

Information regarding formula choices should be offered to mothers who choose not to breastfeed. Formula preparations come in ready-to-feed cans that can be poured directly into a bottle, liquid concentrates that require dilution before feeding, and powder formulas that are mixed with water. When counseling parents about formula preparation, it is essential to stress that all water used must come from a safe and tested source. Water obtained from rural wells may be contaminated with nitrates (from fertilizer) or bacteria that can cause significant infant morbidity. Also, boiling well water does not ensure its safety; boiling causes the nitrates (if present) to become more concentrated (Murray, 2013).

Optimizing Outcomes—Reducing the likelihood of formula-related fluorosis

Community water fluoridation is widely used to prevent and control tooth decay. According to the CDC (2013), fluoride intake from water and other fluoridated substances (e.g., toothpaste and mouth rinses) during tooth development (from birth through age 8) can result in changes in the appearance of the tooth's surface, a condition known as "dental fluorosis." In the United States, most dental fluorosis is mild and appears as faint white lines or spots on the permanent teeth. Recent evidence suggests that regularly mixing powdered or liquid infant formula concentrate with fluoridated water may increase the chance of mild enamel fluorosis. To reduce the likelihood of dental fluorosis, nurses can teach parents to use low-fluoride bottled water (labeled as "de-ionized," "purified," "demineralized," or "distilled") some of the time to mix the infant formula.

A variety of bottles and nipples are also available, and selection is usually based on the parent's preference. For example, the mother may choose from glass bottles or plastic bottles with angled or straight nipples or convenience bottles with disposable liners. Nurses can assist parents in making informed decisions about a bottle/nipple system by suggesting that they gather enough information to consider the evidence critically and realize that no one product is best (Dowling & Tycon, 2010). The nurse should remind the parents to periodically check the nipple integrity to ensure that the formula flows freely one drop at a time. If the formula flows too quickly, the nipple should be discarded because it poses a risk for infant choking and aspiration.

Parents should also be advised to read and follow the manufacturer's instructions explicitly when preparing the formula. For example, no water should be added to the ready-to-feed preparations, and care should be taken to correctly dilute the concentrate and powder preparations. Poorly prepared formula that is too concentrated (from adding an incorrect amount of water) may result in infant hypernatremia and dehydration. Formula that is too dilute may cause the infant to demonstrate symptoms of undernourishment and water intoxication.

Bottles and nipples must be thoroughly washed in hot soapy water with dishwashing detergent and then rinsed in hot clean water. They may also be cleaned in an automatic dishwasher. Some parents prefer to sterilize their equipment, and a variety of commercial sterilizers that can be placed in a microwave oven are available for purchase at most baby stores. If boiling is the preferred cleaning method, parents should be instructed to wash the bottles, nipples, rings, discs, and all other equipment used to prepare the formula in hot soapy water. The items are then well rinsed in hot, clean water, placed in a pot filled with enough water to cover the equipment, and boiled for 5 to 10 minutes.

Although formula can be fed to the baby at room temperature, if warmed formula is preferred, the parents are instructed to place the prepared bottle of formula in a bowl of hot (not boiling) water for a few minutes. Alternatively, the prepared bottle of formula can be warmed in an electric bottle warmer available at most baby stores. It is important to emphasize to parents the need for testing the temperature of warmed formula before feeding. Parents are instructed to shake a few drops of formula on the inside of the wrist. The liquid should feel warm but not hot.

When feeding the baby, parents should choose a comfortable chair and hold the baby in their arms close to them with the baby's head higher than the rest of the body to prevent aspiration and minimize ear infection (Fig. 15-16). Holding the baby skin-to-skin and maintaining full eye

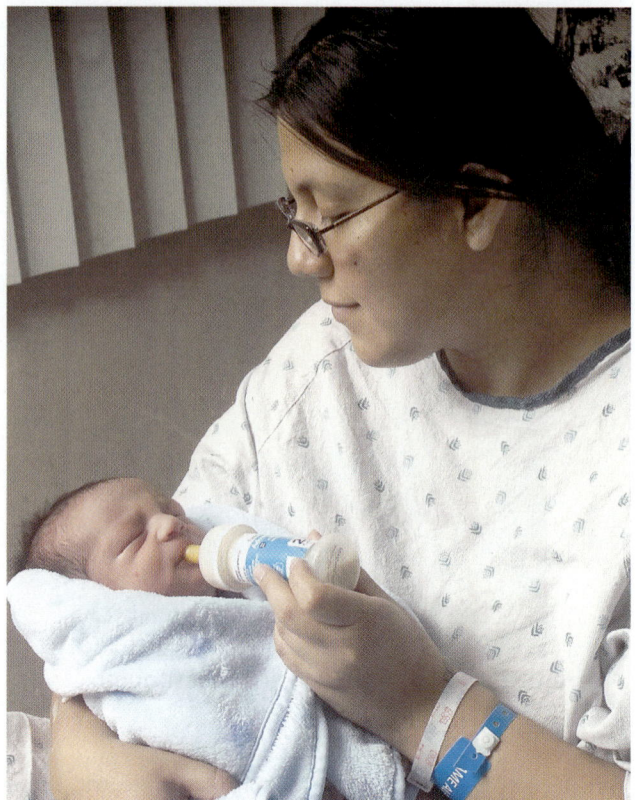

Figure 15-16 When formula feeding, parents should choose a comfortable chair and hold the baby close with the head higher than the rest of the body to prevent aspiration.

contact throughout the feeding helps to facilitate the bonding process. To prevent the baby from swallowing too much air, the bottle should be kept in an angled position with the nipple continuously filled with formula. Burping is usually performed midway and at the end of the feeding to remove excess air from the infant's stomach. To burp the baby properly, parents are taught to either hold the baby over their shoulder or on their lap with the baby's head supported. The baby's back is gently rubbed until air is expelled (Fig. 15-17).

Parents should be advised that babies usually spit up during burping and that this is normal, regardless of whether the infant is breastfed or bottle-fed. However, the pediatrician must be consulted if the baby vomits a large amount of formula with burping or after feeding. Because babies eat more efficiently and take in the desired amount of formula when they are hungry, a "baby-driven" demand feeding schedule rather than a regimented feeding schedule is desirable. The pediatrician can provide guidelines regarding the volume of formula the baby needs.

Safe Practices for Bottle Feeding

When informing parents about the safety of formula, it is important for health-care professionals to be aware that liquid formulas have been subjected to high temperatures to make the product sterile. Powdered formulas are not sterile because high temperatures destroy vital nutrients. The microorganism *Enterobacter sakazakii*, known to cause meningitis, has been identified in powdered formula. To minimize

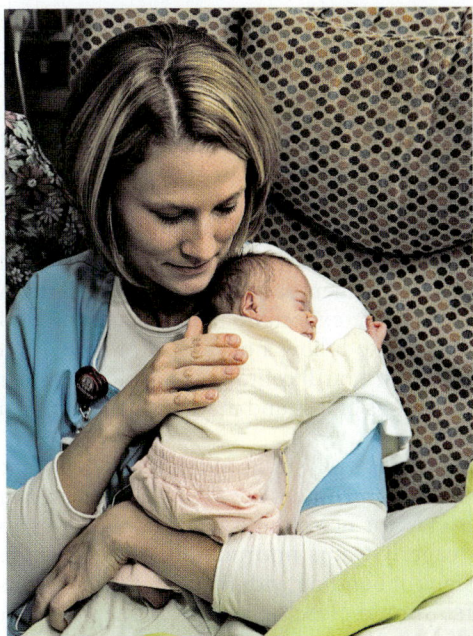

Figure 15-17 One infant burping technique.

the risk of infection, health-care professionals must provide accurate instructions to parents regarding the correct procedure for formula preparation, storage, and reconstitution. Instructions given should emphasize the importance of good hand washing techniques before handling the equipment that is to be used to reconstitute the powder. The formula should never be mixed in a blender or stored in large amounts for longer than 24 hours. Cold water should be used to mix the powder, only the amount to be used for each feeding should be prepared, and any unused formula should be discarded. Parents should be cautioned not to use a microwave oven to prepare or warm the formula because of the potential for "hot spots" that can burn the infant's mouth. They should also be taught to never prop the bottle to allow the infant to feed alone or put the infant to bed with a bottle. These practices may result in choking, ear infections, and tooth decay (Hancock & Brown, 2010).

 Optimizing Outcomes—Safely preparing infant formula

Nurses can provide the following safety instructions to parents who plan to formula feed their infant:
- Wash hands before beginning to prepare formula and after any interruptions.
- Always shake and wash tops of liquid formula cans before opening.
- Reconstitute the formula according to the manufacturer's recommendations.
- Store the ready-to-feed formula according to the manufacturer's recommendations.
- Shake the bottle well before feeding.
- Discard any formula that the infant does not drink.
- Wash thoroughly/sterilize all equipment used to prepare the infant formula and use a bottle and nipple brush to remove milk residue.
- Replace the nipples regularly.

 Now Can You—Discuss breast milk storage and assist the mother who is bottle feeding her infant?

1. Explain what the breastfeeding mother should be taught about pumping and storing breast milk?
2. Discuss appropriate cleaning techniques for bottles and nipples?
3. Describe special precautions to be used with powdered formulas?

Promoting Family and Infant Bonding

FACILITATING THE TRANSITION TO PARENTHOOD

The transition to parenthood can be an especially difficult and challenging time for primiparous mothers with limited experience in infant care and for new parents who are experiencing social isolation from family or friends. Feelings of anxiety and inadequacy regarding parenting skills, lack of knowledge and confidence about providing baby care, emotional concerns, depression, and detachment toward the infant are all symptoms not infrequently expressed by first-time mothers. This information underscores the importance patients place on nurses and other health-care professionals to provide emotional support and accurate information about self-care and baby care.

An essential goal of nursing care at this time is to create a supportive teaching environment that increases the parents' knowledge and confidence in caring for themselves and their infants. Using the principles of Family-Centered Care as a guideline, nurses can help parents cope with the emotional and physical changes that accompany the childbearing year. To create a supportive teaching environment, the nurse can:

- Perform a needs assessment to identify the parents' knowledge/skill deficits.
- Use good communication and listening skills to provide support.
- Empower the parents by assisting them in recognizing their own strengths.
- Facilitate parents' actions to participate in the decision-making process.
- Provide learning opportunities that move the parents from dependence to independence and self-reliance.

Nursing Insight—*Parent–infant bonding behaviors*

"En face" (face-to-face) is a position in which the mother's face and the infant's face are aproximately 8 inches apart and on the same plane. Research shows that mothers seek eye-to-eye contact and that they instinctively move the baby to an en face position (Fig. 15-18). New fathers exhibit signs of intense interest and absorption in their newborn. These behaviors have been identified as "engrossment." Engrossment has been defined as an absorption, preoccupation, and interest in the newborn, and new fathers can be observed gazing at their infants for prolonged periods of time, as if they are in a hypnotic trance (Greenberg & Morris, 1974) (Fig. 15-19).

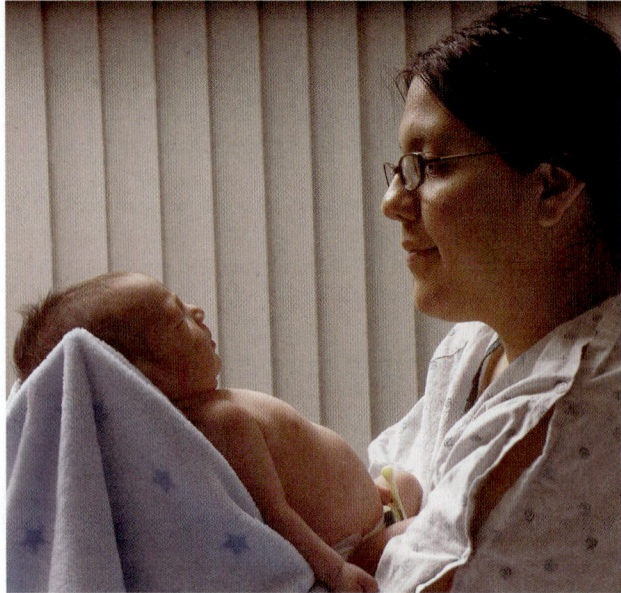

Figure 15-18 Mother and son engaged in en face position.

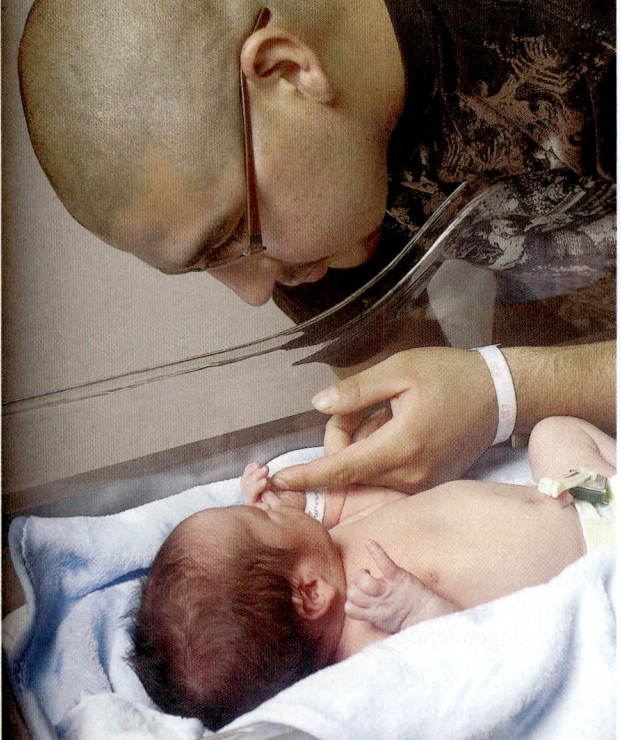

Figure 15-19 By gazing intently at his new son, a father exhibits a sign of engrossment.

ASSUMING THE MOTHERING ROLE

Rubin (1975) described three distinct phases that are associated with the woman's assuming the mothering role. She labeled these phases "Taking-in," "Taking-hold," and "Letting-go" (Table 15-7). At the time of Rubin's work, women were traditionally hospitalized for 5 to 7 days after childbirth, and nurses could readily observe their patients' transitions through each phase. Today, however, with shortened hospital stays, women seem to move through the transitions much more rapidly, and often there is overlapping of the phases.

In the first day or two after birth, the mother is exhausted and should be encouraged to rest. During this time she is reflecting and clarifying, or "*taking-in*" her birth experience. Many mothers want to talk about their labor, discuss with family members the detailed events of the labor, seek clarification if unexpected events occurred, and share joys or disappointments associated with the birth. Mothers who hold specific expectations for their birth experience and are unable to follow a birth plan or who are required to transfer from a birth center to a hospital setting may experience feelings of loss and mourn for the hoped for birth experience.

As the mother's physical condition improves, she begins to take charge and enters the *taking-hold* phase where she assumes care for herself and her infant. At this time, the mother eagerly wants information about infant care and shows signs of bonding with her infant. During this phase, the nurse should closely observe mother–infant interactions for signs of poor bonding, and if present, implement actions to facilitate attachment.

 Critical Nursing Action Assessing for Maternal–Infant Attachment

When observing the mother with her newborn, the nurse should look for clues that indicate successful bonding. The nurse should assess for the following indicators:

Does the mother show eagerness to care for her infant?

What is her response when the baby cries?

Does she make eye contact when holding and feeding her baby?

In the *letting-go phase*, seen later in the mother's recovery, the woman begins to see the infant as an individual separate from herself. At this point, she can leave the baby with a sitter, set aside more time for herself, become more involved with her partner, and begin adapting to the realities of parenthood. Maladjustment during this phase may occur with an overprotective mother who has difficulty accepting help with infant care from others and who excludes the partner from her affections.

 Across Care Settings: Successful maternal transition into the letting-go phase

During the letting-go phase, the mother may have difficulty with the tasks associated with viewing the infant as a separate individual. This phase occurs after the mother has been discharged from the hospital or birthing center. Postpartum and community health nurses who suspect that patients may have difficulty making a successful transition into this phase must communicate their concerns with the infant's pediatric care team so that appropriate assessments and interventions can be carried out.

Mercer (2004) proposed replacing the term "maternal role attainment" (the process by which a woman learns mothering behaviors and becomes comfortable with her identity

Table 15-7 Phases Associated With the Mothering Role		
Phase 1: Taking-In	**Phase 2: Taking-Hold**	**Phase 3: Letting-Go**
FIRST 1–2 DAYS	SECOND AND/OR THIRD DAY	FIRST 2–6 WEEKS POSTPARTUM
The mother is recovering from the immediate exhaustion of labor. She is relatively dependent on others to meet her physical needs. Characteristics of her behavior include: 1. Physical exhaustion 2. Elation, excitement, and/or anxiety and confusion 3. Reliving, verbally and mentally, the events of her labor and birth	The mother starts to initiate action and to begin some of the tasks of motherhood. She may: 1. Ask for help with self-care 2. Begin caring for the baby 3. Be anxious about her mothering abilities	This is the time during which the mother redefines her new role. She: 1. Moves beyond the mother–infant symbiosis of pregnancy and early postpartum and begins to see her infant as an emerging individual 2. Starts to focus on issues larger than those associated directly with herself and her newborn (She begins to focus on her partner, other children, and family issues.)

Source: Adapted from Rubin R. (1975). Maternal tasks in pregnancy. *MCN: The American Journal of Maternal-Child Nursing, 4*(3), 143–153.

as a mother) with the term "becoming a mother," which is reflective of the dynamic transformation and evolution of a woman's persona. Nurses can help facilitate the transition process of becoming a mother and assist the childbearing family in adjusting to their new and changing roles with strategies such as education about infant care, activities to foster maternal–infant attachment and interaction, and interactive maternal/social role preparation (Mercer & Walker, 2006).

Bonding and Attachment

Bonding is described by Klaus (1982) as the promotion of a unique and powerful relationship between the parent and the infant. **Attachment** refers to the tie that exists between the parent and infant and is recognized as a feeling that binds one person to another.

MATERNAL

Bonding begins at the moment the pregnancy is confirmed and continues through the birth experience, during the postpartal period, and throughout the early years of the child's life. Bonding is critical for the infant's survival and development. Providing parents with a model of caring during labor, birth, and in the early postpartum period enhances the bonding process and helps to lay the foundation for the nurturing care that the child will later receive.

Touch is recognized as an important communication tool between humans. Touch is an essential element in the creation of a loving relationship and lasting attachment between the parents and their child. Nurses can be instrumental in enhancing the bonding process by minimizing the time that the infant is separated from the mother. Fostering a positive mother–child relationship begins in the delivery/birthing room when the infant is placed directly on the mother's chest and is held skin-to-skin. The nurse should encourage the mother to initiate early eye contact during the first 30 minutes after childbirth when both the mother and her baby are alert (Fig.15-20). This special quiet time provides an opportunity for connecting and communicating with one another. Early initiation of breastfeeding for mothers who wish to breastfeed and utilizing a

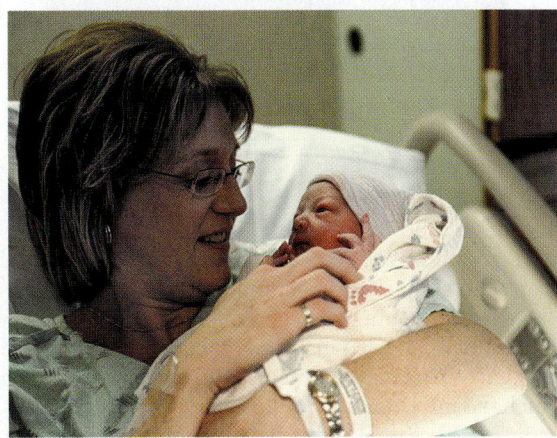

Figure 15-20 Bonding is enhanced with mother–infant eye-to-eye contact.

rooming-in protocol are important nursing interventions that contribute to a positive maternal–child relationship (Dabrowski, 2007).

Optimizing Outcomes—Mother–baby care

Mother–baby care is defined as care of the postpartum mother and her newborn by the same nurse. This model of care centers on treatment of the mother and baby as an inseparable unit; mother and baby should remain unseparated except in extreme circumstances. The mother–baby model promotes continuity of care, enhances patient education, enriches communication and teamwork, and improves nursing competency and patient and nurse satisfaction. In the AWHONN's *Guidelines for Professional Registered Nurse Staffing for Perinatal Units* (2010), it was reported that the majority of perinatal units practice within a mother–baby model of care (Waller-Wise, 2012).

PATERNAL

Historically, mothers have been considered to be the major nurturer of children. By tradition, the mother took care of the child's needs while the father, in the "breadwinner"

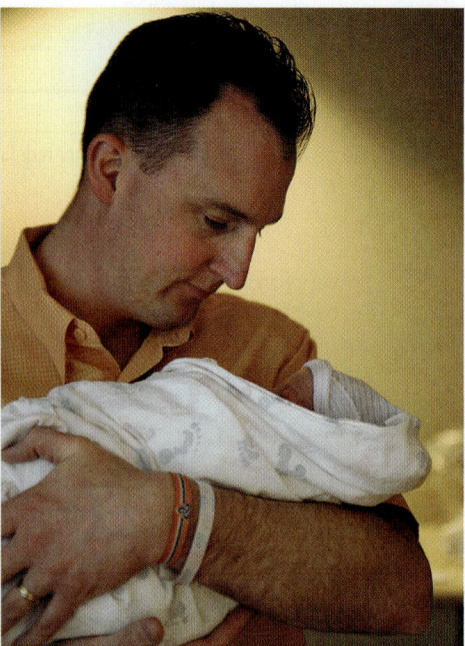

Figure 15-21 The father gets acquainted with his newborn.

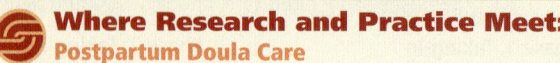

Where Research and Practice Meet:
Postpartum Doula Care

Recent research has explored various domains of doula care during the postpartum period. A doula is a lay birth attendant who provides non-medical support to women and their partners. During the puerperium, doulas facilitate the transition to parenthood by providing evidence-based education (e.g., infant feeding and soothing, recovery from childbirth, and coping skills) and emotional support for the new family (Doula Organization of North America, 2014). McComish and Visger (2009) conducted a qualitative study of 13 women and their infants who received postpartum doula care from 4 postpartum doulas to describe the domains of postpartum doula care and gain insights into how doulas facilitate development of maternal responsiveness and competence. The following 11 domains were identified: emotional support, physical comfort, self-care, infant care, information, advocacy, referral, partner/father support, support mother/father with infant, support mother/father with sibling care, and household organization. Activities in all of the domains were used to facilitate the development of maternal responsiveness and maternal competence with resolution of infant feeding, integration of the infant into the family, and support of developmental care and attachment. Based on their findings, the investigators suggest that by using the 11 domains of care, postpartum doulas facilitate maternal responsiveness and competence.

Nommsen-Rivers, Mastergeorge, Hansen, Cullum, & Dewey (2009) examined the associations between doula care, early breastfeeding outcomes, and breastfeeding duration. Study participants, low-income full gestation primiparae receiving doula care (n=44) or standard care (n=97), were interviewed at 3 days after birth (to record the timing of onset of lactogenesis and breastfeeding behavior) and at 6 weeks (to obtain current breastfeeding status). Study findings revealed that doula care was associated with improved childbirth outcomes (i.e., shorter labor analgesia exposure, shorter stage 2 labor, and unassisted vaginal delivery) and timely onset of lactogenesis, a factor that significantly increased the odds of breastfeeding at 6 weeks postpartum.

role, worked and formed little attachment during the infant's early years. Changes in women's roles, couples' participation in childbirth preparation classes, allowing fathers in the delivery room, and encouraging early contact with the infant have all been instrumental in promoting and fostering early paternal–infant bonding. Other researchers (Ramchandani, Domoney, Sethna, Psychogiou, Vlachos, & Murray, 2013; Yu, Hung, Chan, Yeh, & Lai, 2012) have documented the benefits of early and ongoing contact between fathers and infants (Fig. 15-21). When the primary caregiver is able to touch, hold, and attach with the newborn infant, this special interaction helps to build the foundation for a nurturing and protective relationship. Fathers should be encouraged to assume an active role in infant bonding by participating in the caregiving activities. For example, fathers can change diapers, engage in skin-to-skin holding and infant massage, and feed the bottle-fed infant.

FACTORS THAT MAY INTERRUPT THE BONDING PROCESS

Stress associated with insufficient finances to purchase infant supplies, a chaotic home life, concerns about child care if the mother must return to work, lack of family support, and substance abuse may negatively interfere with the bonding process. An essential nursing role involves identifying obstacles to optimal bonding and coordinating with appropriate community resources such as social services to explore the mother's eligibility for Medicaid, the Women's Infants and Children's (WIC) program, and Healthy Start. Other resources may include counseling and support services, financial aid, and pastoral care (Herrman, 2010).

Adolescent mothers may not demonstrate attachment behaviors because they have unrealistic expectations of the infant's level of functioning and may not be aware of the infant's vulnerability. It is important for nurses to create a supportive environment that allows the young mother close and frequent interaction with her infant. The nurse must also provide anticipatory guidance and education about infant care that includes how to recognize and respond appropriately to infant cues. With today's shortened hospital stays, it becomes imperative that appropriate home follow-up and social work referrals are established before discharge for this vulnerable population.

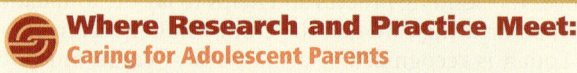

Where Research and Practice Meet:
Caring for Adolescent Parents

Because teen mothers tend to have less healthy relationships with their infants than adult mothers, it is essential that nurses plan interventions that encourage mother–infant synchrony, infant attachment, and maternal sensitivity (Grassley, 2010a). Recent nursing research has explored the special needs of adolescent parents. Dallas (2009) conducted home interviews of 25 sets of adolescent parents, grandmothers (n=50), and grandfathers (n=11) to examine interactions between adolescent fathers and health-care professionals from the perspectives of the families of the adolescent fathers during pregnancy and early postpartum. Supportive (information, emotional, and material support), distancing (denigration of the adolescent father), and neutralizing (failure to recognize the adolescent father in his father role) interactions between health-care professionals and adolescent fathers were identified. While most interactions were perceived as supportive, distancing and neutralizing interactions could potentially have long-term adverse effects for these vulnerable families and contribute to health-care disparities. In an effort to identify and describe the labor support needs of adolescents that promote a positive childbirth experience, Sauls (2010) administered the Bryanton Adaptation of the Nursing Support in Labor Questionnaire-Adolescents to 185 adolescents in the immediate postpartum period. Interestingly, the most helpful supportive behavior was to provide pain medication. Early adolescents (ages 12–14) perceived the nurse's praise to be most helpful; middle (ages 15–16) and late (ages 17–19) adolescents perceived the provision of pain medication the most helpful. Identification and implementation of adolescents' desired supportive behavior in labor might guide nurses in improving the overall childbirth experience for adolescent patients. Grassley (2010b), who examined aspects of social support that adolescents need when initiating breast-feeding in the early postpartal period, concluded that through their support (informational, instrumental, emotional, esteem, and network), nurses could promote the long-term health of adolescents and their children. Stiles (2010) conducted a case study to examine the efficacy of a teen parenting home intervention on maternal sensitivity in a teen mother–infant dyad by exploring the changes from pre- to postintervention in parenting stress, depression, and social support, all of which influence maternal sensitivity. At the conclusion of the intervention, which included nine 1-hour bi-weekly sessions, the adolescent mother's levels of maternal sensitivity and self-concept had improved, and her overall stress score on the parenting domain had decreased. Based on study findings, the investigator suggested that assessment and intervention related to maternal sensitivity should be incorporated into the care of adolescent mothers in all settings.

Global Health Case Study Adolescent Primipara With a Possible Bonding Difficulty

Shenice is a 16-year-old African American primipara who lives at home with her mother and 4 siblings. She gave birth to a healthy 7 lb, 8 oz (3.4 kg) baby boy yesterday. Although Shenice has been pleasant during her hospitalization, she has expressed little interest in her infant. When the nurses offer to bring the infant to the room, Shenice typically asks them to keep the infant in the nursery so that she can "relax and sleep." She plans to bottle-feed her son but has repeatedly found excuses not to feed the baby. The nursery personnel have been feeding the infant instead. The nurses are becoming very concerned because Shenice is to be discharged home with the infant tomorrow.

critical thinking questions

1. How would you initially respond to the situation? Based on your understanding of the developmental tasks of adolescence, how will you initiate dialog with Shenice?

2. How can the nurse help Shenice begin to feel comfortable holding her baby and also promote maternal–infant bonding?

3. What other nursing actions are indicated?

◆ See Suggested Answers to Global Health Case Studies on DavisPlus.

Women from diverse cultural groups who reside in extended families may be comfortable enlisting the help of their mother, mother-in-law, or a female relative in caring for the infant while they recuperate from childbirth. It is important for the nurse to explore the mother's cultural values and mores before reporting a lack of bonding and attachment between the mother and her infant.

An interruption in the bonding process may occur when infants must be separated from their parents for medical or surgical interventions. To promote optimal bonding in these special circumstances, it is important to allow the parents early and frequent access to the infant. The staff in the neonatal intensive care unit can enhance parental attachment and bonding by encouraging the parents to touch, speak to, and hold their neonate skin-to-skin as soon as is medically safe. If the mother is unable to visit, photographs of the infant should be sent to her as soon as possible and frequent telephone calls made to keep her advised of the infant's status. The mother must be reassured that the bonding process is ongoing and that lack of early contact will not interfere with the development of a positive relationship with her infant.

ADJUSTMENT OF SIBLINGS TO THE NEWBORN

The arrival of a new baby into the family results in many emotional changes for the siblings. Feelings of hurt and jealousy, sibling rivalry, and behavioral regression are all common among younger siblings. For example, a toilet-trained toddler may once again require diapers or a 2-year-old who has been weaned may now wish to breastfeed.

Parents should be prepared for these common emotional upheavals and formulate strategies that will help the sibling(s) adjust and accept the baby. Many hospitals offer sibling classes for young (ages 2 to 8) children that introduce the concept of having a new addition to the family and provide parents with specific information about how to make the transition easier (Fig. 15-22).

ADJUSTMENT OF GRANDPARENTS TO THE NEWBORN

Grandparents can provide much support to the new family, and the degree of their involvement is often linked to cultural expectations. Many cultures (e.g., Hispanics, Asians, and Caribbeans) strongly value the extended family. In these settings, the grandparents are intimately involved in the fabric of family dynamics and frequently exert a strong influence on child-rearing practices. Grandparents' classes, offered by most hospitals and family centers, usually focus

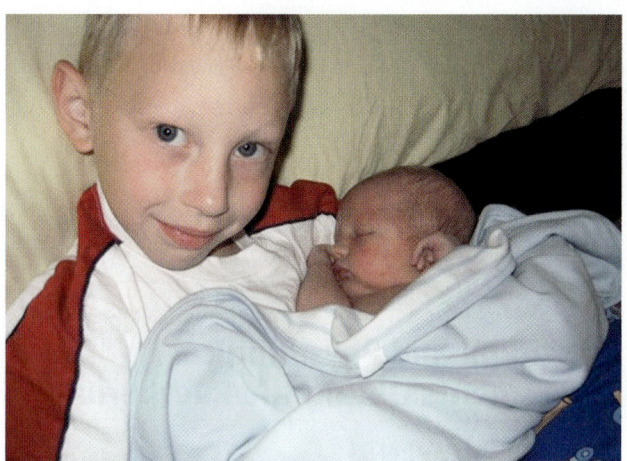

Figure 15-22 Providing an opportunity for the sibling to spend time with the newest family member facilitates sibling adjustment.

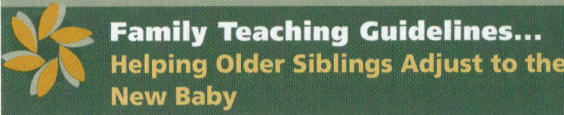

Family Teaching Guidelines...
Helping Older Siblings Adjust to the New Baby

Nurses can be instrumental in arming parents with strategies to help their children accept and adjust to a new infant. The following tips may be useful:

- Talk with the child(ren) about their feelings regarding the new baby. Listen and validate their feelings.
- Teach the older sibling how to play with the new baby; encourage gentleness.
- Help develop the child's self-esteem by giving him or her special jobs, for example, bringing the diaper when you are changing the baby. Praise each contribution.
- Praise age-appropriate behaviors and do not criticize regressive behaviors.
- Set aside a special time each day for you to be alone with the older child; remind the child that he or she is loved very much.

TOPIC: Warning Signs Indicative of Poor Sibling Adjustment

Professional help may be needed when the child:
- Continually avoids or ignores the baby
- Shows the baby no affection
- Is consistently angry, taunting, or demonstrating aggressive behavior toward the baby or other family members
- Experiences nightmares and sleeping difficulties

Source: Adapted from International Childbirth Education Association (2012).

on defining grandparenting roles such as helping with sibling care during the mother's hospitalization and providing assistance with household activities and cooking and shopping during the first few postpartal weeks. Other class themes include current recommendations concerning infant positioning, feeding and clothing, responding to behavior cues, and positive strategies for assuming a supportive, rather than a parenting role.

 Now Can You—Facilitate family bonding with the newborn?

1. Identify and describe Rubin's three phases associated with assuming the mothering role?
2. Describe strategies to facilitate maternal and paternal bonding?
3. Discuss five specific activities that parents can use to help older siblings adjust to the newborn?

Emotional and Physiological Adjustments During the Puerperium

EMOTIONAL EVENTS

Many mothers experience a roller coaster of emotions after childbirth. These feelings stem from a number of influences and are often linked to perceptions concerning the fulfillment of expectations surrounding the childbirth experience. A complicated birth, a premature birth or a sick infant, and the woman's parity, age, marital status, and stability of family finances are some of the many factors known to shape emotions experienced during the postpartum period.

The first 3 months after birth are recognized as the most vulnerable emotional period for mothers. Insecurity about infant care, the constant demands associated with caring for the baby, sleep deprivation, and minimal social support create the potential for frequent and dramatic mood changes. Rapid hormonal changes during the first few postpartal days and weeks may give rise to mood disorders. The most common of these is often termed "the blues." Other less common puerperal mood disorders include postpartum depression and postpartum psychosis. (See Chapter 16 for further discussion.)

Maternity Blues/Baby Blues/Postpartum Blues

The "maternity blues" are considered to be a normal reaction to the dramatic changes that occur after childbirth including abrupt withdrawal of the hormones estrogen, progesterone, and cortisol. Women experience a range of symptoms that include tearfulness, mood swings, insomnia, fatigue, anxiety, difficulty concentrating, irritability, and poor appetite. The symptoms usually begin during the first few postpartal days, peak on the fifth day, and then subside over the next several days. Blues do not affect the woman's ability to care for herself or her newborn and family.

The "blues" are treated with support and reassurance (Beck, 2006, 2008; Beck, Records, & Rice, 2006). Proactive education to prepare the woman and her family for the possibility of postpartum blues is important. The nurse needs to explore what resources the new mother will have available when she goes home. The discussion should focus on whether the patient has adequate food, clothing, shelter, and transportation and whether there are relational concerns that need to be addressed before discharge. Incorporating community resources such as the woman's church, a Mother's Day Out group, a hobby club, or La Leche League can help the new mother realize she is not alone in the experience of nurturing a newborn, while also caring for herself and her family. Referral to a health-care provider is appropriate for women whose symptoms persist for more than 10 days because this pattern is suggestive of postpartum depression.

Postpartum Depression

Postpartum depression, which affects 10% to 13% of women, usually appears around 2 weeks after childbirth. The symptoms associated with this condition are often insidious and include sleep disturbances, guilt, fatigue, and feelings of hopelessness and worthlessness. In severe instances, suicidal ideation may occur. Patients who demonstrate symptoms of postpartum depression must be promptly referred for evaluation and intervention. (See Chapter 16 for further discussion.)

Postpartum Psychosis

Postpartum psychosis develops in approximately one or two women for every 1,000 births and is unlikely to manifest itself during the early postpartum period. Symptoms include delusions; hallucinations; agitation; inability to sleep; and bizarre, irrational behavior. Before hospital discharge, patients with a history of mood disorders or depression

Where Research and Practice Meet:
Maternal–Infant Skin-to-Skin Contact and Depression

Bigelow, Power, MacLellan-Peters, Alex, & McDonald (2012) collected longitudinal data on 90 mothers to investigate the effect of mother–infant skin-to-skin contact (SSC) on mothers' postpartum depressive symptoms during the first 3 postpartum months and their physiological stress during the first postpartum month. Mothers in the SSC group (n=30) provided approximately 5 hours per day of SSC with their infants in the newborn's first week and then more than 2 hours per day until the infants reached 1 month of age. Mothers in the control group (n=90) provided little or no SSC. All infants were full term. Data were collected during home visits via self-reported depression scales collected when the infants were 1 week, 1 month, 2 months, and 3 months of age. Study findings revealed that compared with mothers in the control group, mothers in the SSC group had lower scores on the depression scales when the infants were 1 week; marginally lower scores when the infants were 1 month, and when the infants reached ages 2 and 3 months, there were no differences between groups in the mothers' depression scores. Over their infants' first month, mothers in the SSC group had a greater reduction in their salivary cortisol (a marker of physiological stress). The investigators suggest that mother–infant SSC be promoted as an easy to use, cost-free, readily available and effective intervention strategy to lessen depressive symptoms and anxiety, improve maternal mood, and enhance the psychophysiological connection between mothers and infants.

should be referred to appropriate resources for community support and follow-up. (See Chapter 16 for further discussion.)

PHYSIOLOGICAL RESPONSES TO EMOTIONAL EVENTS

Tiredness and Fatigue

Postpartum tiredness and fatigue have long been considered a natural physiological and psychological response to the stresses of labor and childbirth coupled with the additional responsibilities of motherhood. Although new mothers are often confident that tiredness will improve upon returning home, this phenomenon is not supported by the nursing literature. Rather, the multiplicity of demands associated with motherhood augments the experience of physical and mental exhaustion. While changes in societal trends in the care of children suggest that fathers are taking a more active role, mothers continue to hold the main responsibility for care. Thus, it is essential for the nurse to encourage new mothers to enlist the support and assistance of family and friends in an effort to promote time for rest and recovery (Hunter, Rychnovsky, & Yount, 2009; Whitmer, 2011).

Nursing Insight—*Persistent fatigue during the puerperium*

Feelings of fatigue that extend beyond the 6-week postpartal period may be indicative of a more serious condition. Persistent, pervasive fatigue may be indicative of postpartum depression. The woman and her family should be provided with guidelines about normal feelings and reactions during the puerperium and encouraged to report excessive tiredness or fatigue to the health-care provider.

Contributors to fatigue and tiredness in the postpartum period include physical, psychological, and situational variables. Physical contributors include the length of labor, maternal hormone shifts, maternal anemia, episiotomy or surgical incision healing, breastfeeding, and pain. Psychological contributors include difficulty sleeping, depression, and a non-supportive partner. The challenge of managing multiple roles, cultural influences and expectations, a lack of assistance with housework or child care, having more than one child under the age of 5 in the home, and returning to outside employment are situational variables that can readily lead to fatigue. Insights into the multiple contexts that shape the patient's environment allow nurses to provide anticipatory guidance regarding fatigue and its relationship with diminished quality of life in the postpartum period (Hunter et al., 2009).

Postpartal Discharge Planning and Teaching

PROMOTING MATERNAL SELF-CARE

Because of early postnatal discharge, all postpartal women must be taught strategies for self-care. A self-assessment sheet completed before discharge helps to identify areas of deficits. When possible, parents are encouraged to attend a discharge teaching class. Topics reviewed usually include infant feeding and bathing, breastfeeding, perineal hygiene, physical activity, rest, and expected emotional changes. This information is useful because it empowers the family to identify normal events and to promptly recognize complications that should be reported to the health-care provider. Many institutions also distribute home care booklets that provide written information about maternal and newborn care and available community resources. Often, home visitation by a community health nurse is arranged before the patient's discharge. The community health nurse visit typically includes an examination of the mother and infant, an opportunity for discussion about problems or concerns, and breastfeeding or formula feeding support. Additional areas of focus during the postpartal visit include education regarding basic maternal and infant care, plans for follow-up visits, and contraception counseling (Smith & Waller-Wise, 2011) (Fig. 15-23).

 Optimizing Outcomes—**When early postpartum discharge is planned**

Women and their families may have the option of early discharge with postpartum home care. Maternal criteria for early discharge includes an uncomplicated perinatal course, no evidence of premature rupture of membranes, no difficulties with voiding or ambulation, normal vital signs, hemoglobin greater than 10 g, and no significant vaginal bleeding. The infant must also meet certain criteria (e.g., full term, normal vital signs and physical examination, feeding, urinating, stooling, and laboratory/screening tests completed). Early follow-up visits are an essential component of safe care for mothers and their infants (AAP Committee on Fetus and Newborn, 2010).

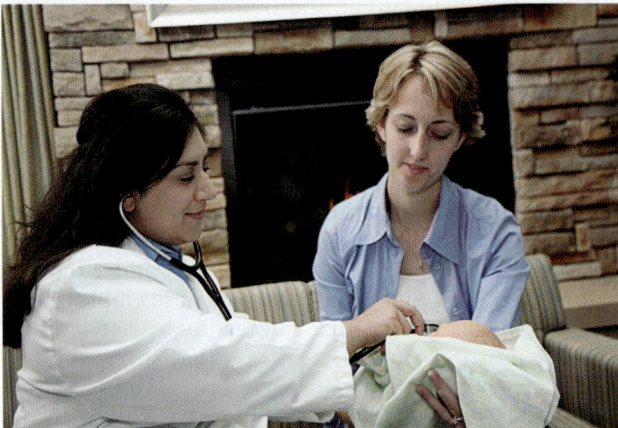

Figure 15-23 The postpartum home visit usually involves an examination of the mother and baby. It provides an opportunity for teaching and promotes continuity of care.

COMPONENTS OF MATERNAL SELF-ASSESSMENT

Fundus

The woman is taught how to locate and palpate the fundus and how to determine the progression of the fundal height as it involutes into the pelvis. After months of abdominal enlargement, many women are delighted to be able to rest in a prone position. Nurses can explain that lying on the abdomen is beneficial because this position supports the abdominal muscles and aids involution because the uterus is tipped into its natural forward position.

 clinical alert

Avoiding the knee–chest position

The nurse teaches the patient to avoid a knee–chest position until at least the third postpartal week. This position causes the vagina to open. Because the cervical os is still open to some extent, there is a danger that air can enter the vagina, pass into the cervix, and enter the open blood sinuses inside the uterus. Entry of air into the circulatory system can cause an air embolus.

Lochia

The nurse reinforces to the patient that the lochia (vaginal discharge) may continue for 3 to 6 weeks after birth. During this time, it is important for her to examine the peri-pads for color, amount, and odor each time she visits the toilet. The woman should be provided with guidelines concerning the anticipated color and amount of the lochia and reminded to promptly report abnormal findings such as heavy bleeding, the passing of large clots, and foul smelling odor.

Hygiene

The patient is advised to continue to use her perineal squeeze bottle until the bleeding stops and to use the pre-scribed medications and/or sitz bath for episiotomy discomfort. She is reminded to carefully wipe from front to back after each visit to the toilet and thoroughly wash her hands before and after changing the peri-pads.

Abdominal Incision

Nurses should instruct the postoperative patient to shower as normal and to carefully pat the incision dry. If staples were applied at the incision site, the obstetrician will inform her when to come into the office for removal. Steri-strips used for incision closure should remain undisturbed until they eventually fall off. The woman is advised to avoid the application of cream or powder to the incision site and to notify her obstetrician if she experiences fever or develops signs of incisional infection such as redness, offensive odor, or discharge.

Body Temperature

Some women experience a transient increase in body temperature along with breast heaviness on the third to fourth postpartum day when the milk supply is established. They should be reminded that temperatures above 100.4°F (38.0°C) and flu-like symptoms (e.g., chills, body aches, or severe pain) may indicate infection and should be promptly reported to the health-care provider.

Urination

Before discharge, all patients should be able to pass urine without difficulty. Women should be taught the signs and symptoms of a urinary tract infection (UTI). Specifically, burning on urination (dysuria), frequent voiding with only a small amount of urine passed, the presence of a "fishy" odor to the urine and lower abdominal or flank pain are symptoms that must be reported to the health-care provider. To reduce the likelihood of a UTI, patients are advised to drink at least eight 8-oz glasses of water each day, avoid delays in emptying the bladder, wipe the perineum from front-to-back after each use of the toilet, change peri-pads after toileting, and to wash their hands frequently.

Bowel Function

The nurse teaches about the importance of maintaining good hydration and consuming a healthy diet abundant in fiber and roughage. An exploration of the woman's dietary preferences facilitates discussion about specific types of foods (e.g., fruits, vegetables, and whole-grain cereals) that promote bowel regularity. The patient should consult with her obstetrician or certified nurse-midwife if laxatives or other medications become necessary. Stool softeners are usually prescribed for women with third- or fourth-degree episiotomies or vaginal lacerations.

Nutrition

Most women are concerned about weight increase during the pregnancy and how quickly they can expect to return to their prepregnancy weight. A well-balanced diet that includes high-energy foods is essential to recovery in the puerperium. Patients should be counseled about the need for adequate protein to promote tissue repair and healing and encouraged to select a healthy, low-fat diet that contains protein along with carbohydrates, fruits, and vegetables.

Fatigue

Patients should be reminded that because the first six postpartal weeks are devoted to infant care and recovery from childbirth, energy depletion, usually manifested as extreme tiredness and fatigue, often occurs. They should be encouraged to limit visitors and whenever possible to rest when the baby sleeps. Patients may wish to cook easily prepared meals in advance and freeze foods for later use. When possible, the new mother should solicit help from her partner, family members, and friends to assist with the household chores, shopping, and child care.

Weight Loss

Weight loss at the time of childbirth is precipitous. Within minutes after birth, the parturient woman loses half of the weight gained during the previous 9 months. On average, the weight loss amounts to 10 to 12 lb (4.5 to 5.5 kg). This loss comes from the infant, the placenta, amniotic fluid, and blood. Rapid diuresis and diaphoresis occur during the second to fifth postpartum days and result in an additional weight loss of about 5 lb (2.3 kg). By the sixth to eighth postpartal week, many women will have returned to their prepregnant weight. The amount of weight lost during the puerperium is primarily related to the amount of weight gained during pregnancy and the woman's level of physical activity.

Exercise

The patient is advised to resume activities gradually, beginning with Kegel exercises to strengthen the pelvic-floor muscles. After a vaginal birth, patients may begin modified sit-ups to strengthen the abdominal muscles and perform knee and leg roll exercises to firm the waist. Modified sit-ups are especially beneficial for women with diastasis recti.

 Optimizing Outcomes—Postnatal exercises to promote physical fitness

Teaching patients about exercises to help return the body to its prepregnant state is an important component of postpartal care. Exercises to strengthen the back, abdominal muscles, thighs, and shoulders are particularly beneficial at this time.

Supple Spine
Begin on all fours. Inhale. Lift your head, keeping your back straight or arching slightly (avoid strain). Then exhale, round your back, tighten abdominals, tuck in tail and head. Repeat the sequence eight times. This exercise strengthens the back and abdominals.

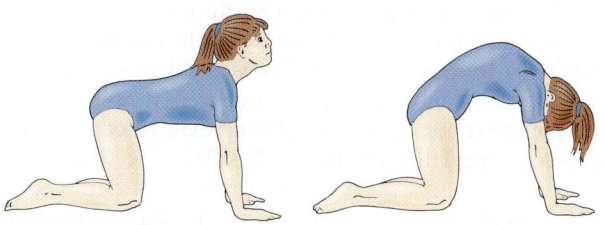

Tighter Abdominals
Lie on your back in a straight line. Then exhale, lowering the back, vertebra by vertebra. Repeat sequence five

times. This exercise helps develop a strong back and abdominals.

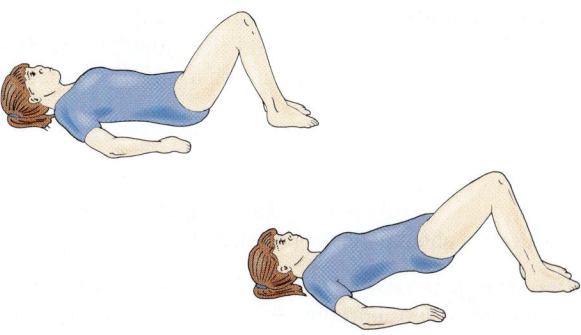

Stronger Back
Sit upright, knees bent, feet flat on the floor, back straight, arms forward at shoulder level. Inhale, then exhale and lean back halfway. Inhale again and sit up slowly. Repeat five times. This exercise strengthens the back and abdominals.

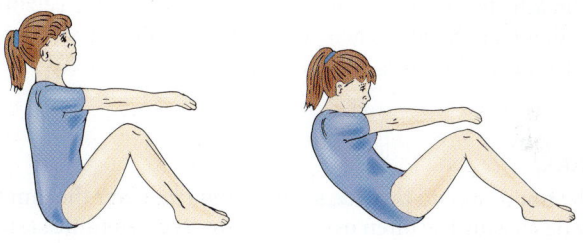

Flexible Body
Stand upright with arms raised, elbows slightly relaxed. Inhale, then exhale and bend forward, keeping back straight and swinging arms down and back. Then relax your head and stretch your arms up behind you. Inhale as you swing arms and body up again, returning to your original position. Repeat eight times. Go carefully and do not strain. This exercise is good for thighs, hips, back, arms, shoulders, and neck.

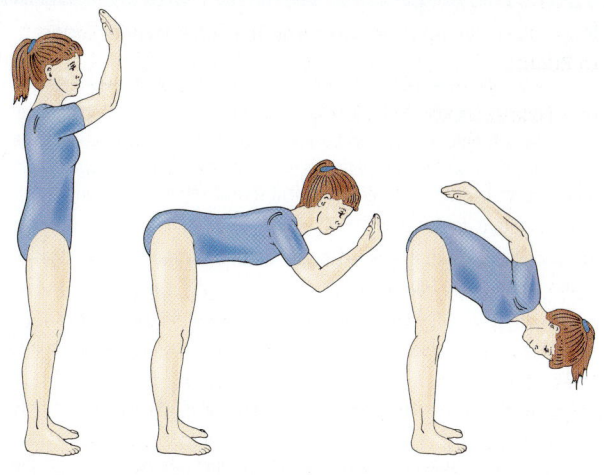

Pain Management

Medications for pain relief (nonsteroidal anti-inflammatory medications or analgesics) may be prescribed, especially for postoperative patients. The nurse should ensure that medications prescribed for breastfeeding patients are not contraindicated. Information regarding therapeutic modalities such as ice packs, sitz baths, or topical anesthetics may be helpful for the relief of perineal discomfort from hemorrhoids or the episiotomy incision. Patients are instructed to notify their health-care provider if pain persists or increases in intensity, and the nurse also reviews other danger signs and symptoms that must be promptly reported (Box 15-5).

 Optimizing Outcomes—Providing postpartum education about perinatal preeclampsia

Preeclampsia is associated with major maternal and perinatal morbidity and mortality. Because the condition abates following delivery of the placenta, most obstetric units tend to discontinue seizure prophylaxis within 48 hours postpartum. However, up to 26% of eclamptic seizures occur beyond 48 hours and as late as 6 weeks after childbirth. Prior to discharge, an important nursing intervention centers on teaching patients about prodromal symptoms that may herald preeclampsia-eclampsia: headache, shortness of breath, blurry vision, nausea, vomiting, edema, seizure, other neurological deficit, and epigastric pain (Al-Safi, Imudia, Filetti, Hobson, Bahado-Singh, & Awonuga, 2011).

Mood

The nurse should provide support and empower the family by discussing the often overwhelming responsibilities associated with newborn care. Information shared with the mother and her partner includes the emotional changes such as feelings of sadness and weepiness that often appear on the second or third postpartal day. Patients can be assured that "mood swings" and periods of unexpected crying, moodiness, or anxiety are common and occur in 70% to 80% of women. If the following symptoms persist for more than 2 weeks after childbirth, the woman, her partner, a family member, or a support person should contact the health-care provider for assistance:

- Crying excessively
- Significant changes in appetite
- Feeling helpless
- Experiencing extreme worry, concern
- Unable to sleep/wanting to sleep all the time
- Unable to care for herself or the baby
- Panic attack
- Fear of harming self or the baby

Sexual Activity and Contraception

To maximize healing and prevent infection, patients are discouraged from resuming sexual activity until after the 6-week postpartum checkup with the obstetrician or midwife. It is important for the nurse to inform the woman and her partner that because ovulation may resume as early as 2 weeks after childbirth, pregnancy can occur if no contraceptive is used.

Although advised to abstain from sexual intercourse until the postpartum examination, many couples wish to resume intimate relations before this time. Coitus is safe once the woman's lochia has transitioned to alba and the episiotomy (if present) has healed. This usually occurs after the first week after childbirth. The patient should be warned that she may experience vaginal discomfort because the cells lining the vagina may not be as thick as before because of a hormone imbalance. Breastfeeding may alter sexual function as a result of vaginal dryness produced by the high levels of prolactin and lowered estrogen levels. A contraceptive foam or lubricating jelly may be used to enhance comfort (Leeman & Rogers, 2012).

Exploring previously used methods of contraception may be helpful in identifying a starting place for the discussion. The couple's religion and cultural background often dictates their contraceptive choice. Discussing contraception options with the patient and her partner (if present) before discharge allows the couple time to make informed decisions before resuming sexual intercourse. The breastfeeding mother should be warned that she can become pregnant during lactation and that breastfeeding is not a substitute for birth control. If the breastfeeding patient wishes to use an oral contraceptive, the nurse must inform the health-care provider so that a progesterone-only pill can be prescribed. (See Chapter 6 for further information.) According to the Centers for Disease Control and Prevention (2011), postpartum women should not use combined hormonal oral contraceptives during the first 21 days after childbirth because of a high risk for venous thromboembolism. Progestin-only and nonhormonal contraceptive methods can be safely initiated by both breastfeeding and non-breastfeeding women before 21 days postpartum. Women who are breastfeeding and who have no risk factors for venous thromboembolism may use COC after the first postpartum month, when hypercoagulability is decreased and milk flow is established. The World Health Organization (2010) discourages progesterone-only contraception before 6 weeks and COC before 6 months (Stuebe, 2014; Tilley & Mishell, 2013).

PLANNING FOR THE FOLLOW-UP EXAMINATION

Most health-care providers schedule a 6-week follow-up appointment ("postpartal check"). Women who have had cesarean births are often scheduled for a return visit to the

---

Box 15-5 Postpartum Discharge Teaching: Danger Signs to Report

An important component of discharge teaching focuses on alerting patients to signs and symptoms that must be reported to the health-care provider. The nurse should ensure that the patient is given written information and knows how to reach her care provider. The patient should immediately report:

- Temperature greater than 100.4°F (38.0°C), chills, or flu-like symptoms.
- Abdominal incision that is red, tender to touch, or painful or if edges of the incision have separated.
- Difficulty initiating urination, urinary frequency, or painful urination.
- Increased vaginal bleeding with or without clots, or foul-smelling vaginal discharge.
- Persistent pain or marked swelling at the site of a perineal laceration or episiotomy.
- Swelling or masses in the breasts, red streaks, shooting pain in the breasts, or cracked, bleeding nipples.
- Swelling, warmth, tenderness, or painful areas in the legs.
- Blurred vision or persistent headache that is not relieved by pain medication.
- Overwhelming feelings of sadness or an inability to care for self or the baby.

physician's office 2 weeks after hospital discharge. It is helpful to indicate the date and time of the return appointment in the patient's discharge instructions.

The nurse can explain that during the 6-week follow-up visit, fundal palpation and a vaginal examination will be performed to evaluate the size of the uterus. The episiotomy or abdominal incision site will be evaluated for healing, and a breast examination will be performed. If desired, a contraceptive method or prescription will also be given. The nurse should encourage the patient to discuss any concerns during this visit. According to recommendations published by the National Diabetes Education Program and the American College of Obstetricians and Gynecologists, the postpartum visit should also include testing for glucose intolerance in women whose pregnancies were complicated by gestational diabetes mellitus (Gabbe, Landon, Warren-Boulton, & Fradkin, 2012). A fasting plasma glucose or a 75-g oral glucose tolerance test can be used for screening (ACOG, 2013c). The parents should also schedule a newborn follow-up appointment before hospital discharge. Most physicians and clinics wish to see the infant within the first week or by age 2 weeks.

 Now Can You—Promote self-care for the puerperium?

1. Outline postpartal teaching guidelines that include information about self-assessment of the fundus, lochia, hygiene, incisional site, body temperature, and elimination?

2. Demonstrate appropriate exercises for the postpartal patient?

3. Identify at least six symptoms indicative of poor emotional adjustment that, if present for more than 2 weeks, should be reported to the health-care provider?

Patients with Special Needs During the Puerperium

CARE OF THE ADOLESCENT

The period of adolescence is a time to form important relationships with peers; these close connections help to facilitate self-growth and development. Adolescents who are thrust into an untimely motherhood role must also deal with their own personal and social development. Adjusting to pregnancy and impending motherhood can be emotionally and physically challenging for a mature woman; the adolescent requires special assistance from the nurse.

Many adolescents enter motherhood with unrealistic expectations. They lack mothering and child care skills. Fatigue and sleep deprivation, common in all new mothers, coupled with the responsibility of caring for an infant who requires constant attention, often result in limited time for social activities and subsequent social isolation from their peers.

Nurses who care for the adolescent mother must be cognizant of personal prejudices or feelings of disapproval and avoid expressing negative feelings toward the teen mother. It is important for the nurse to provide emotional support for the postpartum adolescent that will help her adjust to role changes, foster feelings of positive self-esteem, and assist her in developing a new identity and sense of self. The nurse must create a supportive environment by recognizing the adolescent as the infant's primary caregiver, irrespective of her age. The nurse models and facilitates infant caring behaviors that will promote bonding and teaches about infant care and child safety. Before discharge, arrangements should be made for a community health nurse follow-up visit within a week (Grassley, 2010a; Sauls, 2010; Stiles, 2010).

❝What to say❞—*When planning the adolescent mother's hospital discharge*

The adolescent mother has unique needs for discharge planning. The nurse can best explore the young patient's immediate plans for herself and the baby by initiating dialog in a supportive, nonthreatening environment. Examples of appropriate questions that the nurse may ask include the following:

"Do you have someone available to offer you help and/or support?"

"Do you feel a sense of closeness or attachment to your baby?"

"After you leave the hospital, will anyone be helping you to care for your baby?"

"Will anyone be taking care of the baby so that you can go back to school?"

"Where will you take the baby for follow-up care?"

To facilitate a supportive home and family environment, the community health nurse will conduct a social support assessment to identify the significant family member or other person who will be assisting with parenting responsibilities and financial support. If the adolescent's mother is identified as the primary support person, the nurse explores the mother's and grandmother's expectations in caring for the newborn to provide anticipatory guidance regarding each person's new role before discharge.

A supportive family environment is the single most important element in facilitating the adolescent mother's successful transition to motherhood. When appropriate, referrals should be made for social services and other community resources such as home health nursing care, pastoral care, teen parent support groups, and economic assistance. Guidance and support provided by these professionals help to reinforce infant care skills and identify additional resources to enable the young mother to complete her education. Professional and family support has proven to be effective in helping adolescents delay a subsequent pregnancy, stay enrolled in school, find work, and complete the developmental tasks of adolescence (Sauls, 2010; Yozwiak, 2010).

THE WOMAN WHO IS PLACING HER INFANT FOR ADOPTION

The relinquishment of an infant triggers a host of emotions for the woman and her family. Nurses must be sensitive to the myriad of psychological stressors and social stigmas associated with placing a child for adoption. Depending on hospital policy, the patient may be admitted to the postpartum unit where she can be attended to by nurses who are experienced in perinatal care. The nurse should offer support, a "listening ear," and a compassionate environment where the patient feels safe in expressing her feelings. The woman will likely experience a range of emotions such as grief, loneliness, and guilt. After birth, the patient should have access to her newborn if she so desires. The opportunity to see, hold, and feed the infant may help her to accept the reality that she has given birth to a healthy child. This affirmation may foster feelings of self-esteem and provide a foundation for emotional healing. Postpartum care may continue well beyond hospital discharge for women who choose to give up the infant. Referrals to various community resources may be appropriate (Cunningham et al., 2014). In some cases, the adoptive couple may come into the hospital to meet the new infant. The new parents will need the same instruction in infant care and safety as the biological parents.

THE OLDER WOMAN

Today, it is not uncommon for women over age 35 to experience their first pregnancy, and when pregnancy occurs among this population, it is deemed "advanced maternal age."

The older patient may have preexisting medical conditions (e.g., hypertension or diabetes) and experience greater health risks and pregnancy complications such as gestational diabetes and preeclampsia. In these situations, pregnancy and puerperal care involve a collaborative approach that includes a physician with special training in high-risk obstetrics (perinatologist) and medical specialists (e.g., endocrinologist, rheumatologist, and cardiologist).

Women experience pregnancy after the age of 35 for a number of reasons. Some postpone pregnancy to make advancements in careers; others have struggled with infertility and become pregnant following advanced reproductive techniques while others report contraceptive failure. There is a wide range of attitudes and emotions that accompany parenthood during midlife. Some women believe that delaying motherhood enhances the adaptation to the parental role. They cite qualities such as maturity, patience and understanding, and greater life experiences as positive influences for assuming the parental role. For others, parenthood at an older age can be disruptive to intimate relationships, interfere with career goals, and create a perception of loss of control. Reassurance, support, and referral, when appropriate, help to facilitate transitions during the puerperium for the older couple.

Community Resources for the New Family

SUPPORT GROUPS

The birth of a newborn is a major life transition. For the new parent, attending a support group can provide a venue for sharing experiences and challenges with other new parents. Information about "essential" parenting topics, such as infant feeding and nutrition, behavior, sleeping patterns, and strategies for fostering family relationships, is readily available during the meetings. Specific support groups may also be available for unique populations, such as single parents, working mothers, and parents of infants with special needs. Parents who participated in childbirth education classes together often reunite to form a support group after childbirth.

HOME VISITS

Some facilities routinely schedule home visits for maternal and baby assessment. This visit provides the nurse with an opportunity to assess bonding, conduct patient teaching, answer questions, correct learning deficits, reinforce hospital discharge instructions, and make appropriate community referrals.

 Across Care Settings: CenteringParenting group health-care visits

CenteringParenting is an innovative model of centering health care in which 5 to 6 mother–infant dyads continue group care throughout the baby's first year of life. The model incorporates 10 postpartum and well-baby examinations and provides an avenue of continued support for the woman's transition to motherhood. In keeping with the centering model of care, mothers are actively engaged with tasks such as weighing the baby, plotting the baby's growth on an appropriate chart, and assisting with developmental screens. Educational themes focus on health, safety, growth and development, and mother–baby attachment (Morse, 2009).

TELEPHONE FOLLOW-UP

Facilities that offer home follow-up services usually call parents approximately 2 to 3 days after discharge. Making personal contact with the family provides early support and reassurance and allows for questions to be answered and discharge instructions to be reviewed and clarified.

OUTPATIENT CLINICS

Outpatient clinics provide another option for facilities that do not offer home visitation. The clinics are often nurse-managed and allow the mother and her baby to receive further information about maternal–infant care. The patient's additional questions or concerns can also be dealt with at this time.

 Where Research and Practice Meet: **Use of Communication Technologies to Provide Postpartum Information**

Walker, Im, and Vaughn (2012) described findings from a health survey completed by 145 White (n=67), African American (n=37), and Hispanic (n=41) women of higher and lower incomes who had given birth approximately 5 to 10 months earlier. The investigators wished to determine the women's access, perceived skill, confidence, and use of Internet and mobile technologies, their views about receiving health information about postpartum weight and parenting, and whether those factors varied by race/ethnicity or income level. Study results revealed that women with a lower income were more likely to express high interest in receiving health information related to parenting by mail than those of higher incomes, and women of higher incomes were more likely to express high interest in receiving weight loss and parenting information through the Internet. The researchers concluded that their findings underscore the importance of considering the characteristics of the population being served when designing health communications and resources.

A list of community resources and phone numbers is often provided to the couple before discharge. These services may include professional lactation services, nursing mother's support groups, "Mommy and Me" classes, postnatal exercise classes, parenting education and support groups, medical care, crisis lines/counseling, emergency and financial assistance, and bereavement support.

Cultural Diversity: Family and Community Care for the Orthodox Jewish Mother

The provision of care and support to a new mother is an important cultural expectation in the Orthodox Jewish community. A mother receives special treatment after childbirth, and for the first 7 days, she is considered to be "dangerously ill" and is cared for by family members. From the eighth day to the 30th day, she is considered to be non-seriously ill and is observing a period of convalescence. Most new mothers rely on family or the community for help; others may be sent to a friend, relative, or in-law. A number of convalescent homes have been established throughout Israel and the United States, specifically meant for Orthodox Jewish women to recuperate after childbirth (Zauderer, 2009).

 Now Can You—Care for postpartal patients with special needs and identify community resources for the postpartal family?

1. Identify nursing interventions that foster the postpartal adolescent's self-esteem and empower her to bond with and care for her infant?
2. Describe nursing interventions to provide appropriate emotional support for the woman who chooses to place her infant for adoption?
3. Identify at least three sources of community support for the postpartal family and discuss the benefits of each?

Summary Points

◆ During the postpartum period, the nurse assumes the responsibility of facilitating the integration of the newborn into the family unit.

◆ The postpartum patient has unique assessment needs that include physical and psychosocial considerations.

◆ The new mother should be given the opportunity to discuss her birth experience.

◆ The postpartum woman who has experienced a cesarean birth is also considered to be a surgical patient who has special needs for additional nursing care.

◆ Effective pain management should be an integral component of the postpartal nursing assessment.

◆ The breastfeeding mother should be provided with sufficient support to facilitate success.

◆ The nurse should provide anticipatory guidance that includes family members whenever possible.

Review Questions

Multiple Choice

1. In the preadmission clinic, the perinatal nurse describes the advantages to a short hospital stay as including which of the following?
   A. Decreased risk of nosocomial infection
   B. Increased rest and recuperation
   C. Increased opportunity to initiate successful breastfeeding
   D. Increased teaching about infant care

2. In the immediate postpartum period, the perinatal nurse knows that the postpartum woman most often has
   A. Bradycardia.
   B. Tachycardia.
   C. A pulse within the normal adult range.
   D. Tachycardia with a return of normal pulse within 4 hours.

3. The postpartum nurse expects a postpartum woman's bladder function to return to normal within what length of time?
   A. 2 to 4 hours
   B. 4 to 6 hours
   C. 6 to 8 hours
   D. 8 to 12 hours

4. A student nurse in the perinatal clinic sees a notation on the chart of a patient describing her as being in the "puerperium." What explanation does the registered nurse provide the student?
   A. Time period when breastfeeding inhibits ovulation
   B. Time period when the infant loses weight after birth
   C. Time period from childbirth through 6 weeks postpartum
   D. Time period when risk of the "baby blues" is highest

5. A nurse performing a perineal assessment on a postpartum woman assists her into which position?
   A. Sim's
   B. Prone
   C. Supine
   D. Knee–chest

6. The perinatal nurse understands the term "subinvolution" to mean which of the following?
   A. Inverted uterus
   B. Abnormally small uterus
   C. Uterus not returned to prepregnant state
   D. Uterus with retained placental tissue

7. A nurse notes a postpartum woman's vaginal drainage as red fluid with a fleshy odor. How should the nurse document this finding?
   A. Lochia maxima
   B. Lochia alba
   C. Lochia serosa
   D. Lochia rubra

8. The nurse knows that during what time frame is a woman most likely to experience heart failure?
   A. First trimester
   B. Second trimester
   C. Third trimester
   D. Postpartum

9. The perinatal nurse understands the concept of attachment as which of the following?
- A. Promotion of a unique and powerful relationship between parent and baby
- B. The tie that exists between parent and baby; recognized as a feeling that binds
- C. Learning to care for the infant and knowing him or her well enough to anticipate needs
- D. An urge to protect the infant against the world, which may lead to overprotectiveness

10. During which time frame is the new mother most vulnerable to emotional difficulties?
- A. First 10 days postpartum
- B. First 3 months postpartum
- C. First 6 months postpartum
- D. First year postpartum

See Answers to End of Chapter Review Questions on Davis*Plus.*

REFERENCES

Albert, J., & Heinrichs-Breen, J. (2011). An evaluation of a breastfeeding privacy sign to prevent interruptions and promote successful breastfeeding. *Journal of Obstetric, Gynecologic & Neonatal Nursing, 40*(3), 274–280. doi:10.1111/j.1552-6909.2011.01233.x

Al-Safi, Z., Imudia, A. N., Filetti, L. C., Hobson, D. T., Bahado-Singh, R. O., & Awonuga, A. O. (2011). Delayed postpartum preeclampsia and eclampsia. *Obstetrics & Gynecology, 118*(5), 1102–1107. doi:10.1097/AOG.0b013e318231934c

American Academy of Pediatrics (AAP). (2012). Policy Statement: Breastfeeding and the use of human milk. *Pediatrics, 129,* e827–e841.

American Academy of Pediatrics (AAP). (2013). Early skin contact linked to higher breastfeeding rates. *ScienceDaily, 28*(2), 2–4.

American Academy of Pediatrics (AAP) Committee on Fetus and Newborn. (2010). Hospital stay for healthy term newborns. *Pediatrics, 125*(2), 405–409. doi:10.1542/peds.2009-3119

American Academy of Pediatrics (AAP), Meek, J. Y., & Yu, W. (2011). *The American Academy of Pediatrics new mother's guide to breastfeeding,* (2nd ed.). New York, NY: Bantam.

American College of Obstetricians and Gynecologists (ACOG). (2011). Practice Bulletin No. 123. Thromboembolism in pregnancy. *Obstetrics & Gynecology, 118*(3), 718–729.

American College of Obstetricians and Gynecologists (ACOG). (2012). Committee Opinion No. 530. Access to postpartum sterilization. *Obstetrics and Gynecology, 120*(1), 212–215.

American College of Obstetricians and Gynecologists (ACOG). (2013a). Update on immunization and pregnancy tetanus diphtheria and pertussis vaccination. Committee Opinion No. 566. *Obstetrics and Gynecology, 121*(6), 1411–1414.

American College of Obstetricians and Gynecologists (ACOG). (2013b). Breastfeeding in underserved women: Increasing initiation and continuation of breastfeeding. Committee Opinion No. 570. *Obstetrics and Gynecology, 122*(2), 423–428.

American College of Obstetricians and Gynecologists (ACOG). (2013c). Gestational diabetes mellitus. Committee Opinion No. 137. *Obstetrics and Gynecology, 122*(2), 406–416.

Anderson, G. C., Moore, E., Hepworth, J., & Bergman, N. (2003). Early skin-to-skin contact for mothers and their healthy newborn infants. *Birth, 30*(3), 206–207.

Arslanoglu, S., Corpeleijn, W., Moro, G., Braegger, C., Campoy, C., Colomb, V., et al. (2013). Donor human milk for preterm infants: Current evidence and research directions. *Journal of Pediatric Gastroenterology and Nutrition, 57*(4), 535–542. doi:10.1097/MPG.0b013e3182a3af0a

Association of Women's Health, Obstetric and Neonatal Nurses (AWHONN). (1999). Clinical position statement. *Breastfeeding.* (Reaffirmed 2007). Washington, DC: Author.

Association of Women's Health, Obstetric and Neonatal Nurses (AWHONN). (2010). *Guidelines for professional registered nurse staffing for perinatal units.* Washington, DC: Author.

Beck, C. T. (2006). Postpartum depression: It isn't just the blues. *American Journal of Nursing, 106*(5), 40–50.

Beck, C. T. (2008). *Postpartum mood and anxiety disorders: Case studies, research, and nursing care.* (2nd ed.). Washington, DC: Association of Women's Health, Obstetric and Neonatal Nurses.

Beck, C., Records, K., & Rice, M. (2006). Further development of the postpartum depression predictors inventory-revised. *Journal of Obstetric, Gynecologic & Neonatal Nursing, 35*(6), 735–745.

Bigelow, A., Power, M., MacLellan-Peters, J., Alex, M., & McDonald, C. (2012). Effect of mother/infant skin-to-skin contact on postpartum depressive symptoms and maternal physiological stress. *Journal of Obstetric, Gynecologic & Neonatal Nursing, 41*(3), 369–382. doi:10.1111/j.1552-6909.2012.01350.x

Blomquist, J. L., Quiroz, L. H., MacMillan, D., Maccullough, A., & Handa, V. L. (2011). Mothers' satisfaction with planned vaginal and planned cesarean birth. *American Journal of Perinatology, 28*(5), 383–388. doi:10.1055/s-0031-1274508

Bowen, A., & Tumback, L. (2011). Alcohol and breastfeeding: Dispelling the myths and promoting the evidence. *Nursing for Women's Health, 14*(6), 455–461. doi:10.1111/j.1751-486X.2010.01592.x

Bramson, L., Lee, J. W., Moore, E., Montgomery, S., Neish, C., Bahjri, K., & Melcher, C. L. (2010). Effect of early skin-to-skin mother-infant contact during the first 3 hours following birth on exclusive breastfeeding during the maternity hospital stay. *Journal of Human Lactation, 26*(2), 130–137. doi:10.1177/0890334409355779

Brown, L. F., Thoyre, S., Pridham, K., & Schubert, C. (2009). The Mother-Infant Feeding Tool. *Journal of Obstetric, Gynecologic & Neonatal Nursing, 38*(4), 491–503. doi:10.1111/j.155206909.2009.01047.x

Bulechek, G. M., Butcher, H. K., & Dochterman, J. M., & Wagner, C. (2013). *Nursing interventions classification (NIC)* (6th ed.). St. Louis, MO: Elsevier Mosby.

Bystrova, K., Ivanova, V., Edhborg, M., Matthiesen, A.S., Ransjo-Arvidson, A.B., Mukhamedrakhimov, R., et al. (2009). Early contact versus separation: Effects on mother-infant interaction one year later. *Birth, 36*(2), 97–109. doi:10.1111/j.1523-536X.2009.00307.x

Cadwell, K., Turner-Maffei, C., O'Conner, V., Cadwell-Blair, A., Arnold, L., & Blair, E. (2006). *Maternal and infant assessment for breastfeeding and human lactation: A guide for the practitioner* (2nd ed.). Sudbury, MA: Jones and Bartlett.

Centers for Disease Control and Prevention (CDC). (2011). U.S. medical eligibility criteria for contraceptive use, 2011. *Morbidity and Mortality Weekly Report, 60,* 878–883.

Centers for Disease Control and Prevention (CDC). (2012a). *Immunization schedules.* Retrieved from http://www.cdc.gov/vaccines/schedules/index.html

Centers for Disease Control and Prevention (CDC). (2012b). *Breastfeeding report card – United States, 2012.* Retrieved from http://www.cdc.gov/breastfeeding/data/reportcard.htm

Centers for Disease Control and Prevention (CDC). (2013). *Infant formula and fluorosis.* Retrieved from http://www.cdc.gov/fluoridation/safety/infant_formula.htm

Chan, P. (2011). *Gynecology and obstetrics: Current clinical strategies, 2011 Edition.* Laguna Hills, CA: CCS Publishing.

Conrad, K., Russell, A. C., & Keister, K. J. (2011). Bariatric surgery and its impact on childbearing. *Nursing for Women's Health, 15*(3), 228–234. doi:10.1111/j.1751-486X.2011.01637.x

Cunningham, F. G., Leveno, K. J., Bloom, S. L., Spong, C., & Dashe, J. (2014). *Williams Obstetrics* (24th ed.). New York, NY: McGraw-Hill Professional.

Dabrowski, G. A. (2007). Skin to skin contact: Giving birth back to mothers and babies. *Nursing for Women's Health, 11*(1), 64–71.

Dallas, C. M. (2009). Interactions between adolescent fathers and health care professionals during pregnancy, labor, and early postpartum. *Journal of Obstetric, Gynecologic & Neonatal Nursing, 38*(3), 290–299. doi:10.1111/j.1552-6909.2009.01022.x

Davis, M. (2010). Engorgement: The cabbage cure. Retrieved from http://www.lactationconsultant.info/cabbagecure.html

Davis, S. K., Stichler, J. F., & Poeltler, D. M. (2013). Increasing exclusive breastfeeding rates in the well-baby population. *Nursing for Women's Health, 16*(6), 461–470. doi:10.1111/j.1751-486X.2012.01774.x

deValk, H. W., & Visser, G. H. A. (2011). Insulin during pregnancy, labour, and delivery. *Best Practice & Research Clinical Obstetrics and Gynaecology, 25,* 65–76.

Doula Organization of North America (DONA). (2014). *The postpartum doula's role in maternity care.* Position paper. Retrieved from http://www.dona.org/PDF/positionpaper_PPdoula_083011.pdf

Dowling, D. A., & Tycon, L. (2010). Bottle/nipple systems: Helping parents make informed choices. *Nursing for Women's Health, 14*(1), 61–66. doi:10.1111/j.1751-486X.2010.01508.x

Feldman, K., & Whyte, R. K. (2013). Two cases of apparent suffocation of newborns during side-lying breastfeeding. *Nursing for Women's Health, 17*(4), 337–341. doi:10.1111/1751-486X.12053

Flacking, R., Ewald, U., & Wallin, L. (2011). Positive effect of Kangaroo Mother Care on long-term breastfeeding in very preterm infants. *Journal of Obstetric, Gynecologic & Neonatal Nursing, 40*(2), 1990–1997. doi:10.1111/j.1552-6909.2011.01226.x

Flaherman, V., Gay, B., Scott, C., Avins, A., Lee, K., & Newman, T. (2012). Randomised trial comparing hand expression with breast pumping for mothers of term newborns feeding poorly. *Archives of Diseases of Children: Fetal and Neonatal Edition, 97*(1), F18–F23. doi:10.1136/adc.2010.209213

Gabbe, S. G., Landon, M. B., Warren-Boulton, E., & Fradkin, J. (2012). Promoting health after gestational diabetes: A National Diabetes Education Program call to action. *Obstetrics & Gynecology, 119*(1), 171–176. doi:10.1097/AOG.0b013e3182393208

Giger, J. N. (2012). *Transcultural nursing: Assessment and intervention* (6th ed.). St. Lous, MO: C.V. Mosby.

Grassley, J. S. (2010a). Promoting health among childbearing adolescents and their infants. *Journal of Obstetric, Gynecologic & Neonatal Nursing, 39*(6), 694–695. doi:10.1111/j.1552-6909.2010.01183.x

Grassley, J. S. (2010b). Adolescent mothers' breastfeeding social support needs. *Journal of Obstetric, Gynecologic & Neonatal Nursing, 39*(6), 713–722. doi:10.1111/j.1552-6909.2010.01181.x

Grassley, J. S., & Sauls, D. J. (2011). Evaluation of the Supportive Needs of Adolescents during Childbirth intrapartum nursing intervention on adolescents' childbirth satisfaction and breastfeeding rates. *Journal of Obstetric, Gynecologic & Neonatal Nursing, 41*(1), 33–44. doi:10.1111/j.1552-6909.2011.01310.x

Greenberg, M., & Morris, N. (1974). Engrossment: The newborn's impact upon the father. *American Journal of Orthopsychiatry, 44*, 520–531.

Guilbeau, J. R. (2012). Health risks of energy drinks. *Nursing for Women's Health, 16*(5), 423–428. doi:10.1111/j.1751-486X.2012.01766.x

Hancock, M. E., & Brown, J. (2010). Formula-feeding safety. *Nursing for Women's Health, 14*(4), 304–309. doi:10.1111/j.1751-486X.2010.01560.x

Haxton, D., Doering, J., Gingras, L., & Kelly, L. (2012). Implementing skin-to-skin contact at birth using the Iowa Model. *Nursing for Women's Health, 16*(3), 221–230. doi:10.1111/j.1751-486X.2012.01733.x

Henderson, A. (2011). Understanding the breast crawl: Implications for nursing practice. *Nursing for Women's Health, 15*(4), 296–307. doi:10.1111/j.1751-486X.2011.01650.x

Herrman, J. W. (2010). Assessing the teen parent family. The role for nurses. *Nursing for Women's Health, 14*(3), 214–221. doi:10.1111/j.1751-486X.2010.01542.x

Hood, D. G. (2012). Continuous subcutaneous insulin infusion for managing diabetes. *Nursing for Women's Health, 16*(4), 310–318. doi:10.1111/j.1751-486X.2012.01749.x

Hunter, L., Rychnovsky, J., & Yount, S. (2009). A selective review of maternal sleep characteristics in the postpartum period. *Journal of Obstetric, Gynecologic & Neonatal Nursing, 38*(1), 60–68.

International Childbirth Education Association (ICEA). (2012). *Siblings and the new baby.* (Brochure). Minneapolis, MN: Author.

Johnson, M., Moorhead, S., Bulechek, G., Butcher, H., Maas, M., & Swanson, E. (2012). *NOC and NIC Linkages to NANDA-I and clinical conditions: Supporting critical reasoning and quality care* (3rd ed.). St. Maryland Heights, MO: Elsevier Mosby.

Kent, J. C., Prime, D. K., & Garbin, C. P. (2012). Principles for maintaining or increasing breast milk production. *Journal of Obstetric, Gynecologic & Neonatal Nursing, 41*(1), 114–121. doi:10.1111/j.1552-6909.2011.01313.x

Kim, J. H., & Froh, E. B. (2012). What nurses need to know regarding nutritional and immunobiological properties of human milk. *Journal of Obstetric, Gynecologic & Neonatal Nursing, 41*(1), 122–137. doi:10.1111/j.1552-6909.2011.01314.x

Klaus, M. (1982). *Parent-infant bonding* (2nd ed.). St. Louis, MO: C.V. Mosby.

Labbok, M., Taylor, E., & Parry, K. (2013). *Clinics in human lactation: Achieving exclusive breastfeeding.* Amarillo, TX: Hale Publishing.

Lawrence, R., & Lawrence, R. (2010). *Breastfeeding: A guide for the medical profession* (7th ed.). Philadelphia, PA: Saunders.

Leeman, L. M., & Rogers, R. G. (2012). Sex after childbirth. *Obstetrics & Gynecology, 119*(3), 647–655. doi:10.1097/AOG.0b013e3182479611

Lewallen, L. P., & Street, D. J. (2010). Initiating and sustaining breastfeeding in African American women. *Journal of Obstetric, Gynecologic & Neonatal Nursing, 39*(6), 667–674. doi:10.1111/j.1552-6909.2010.01196.x

Mattson, S. (2011). Ethnocultural considerations in the childbearing period. In S. Mattson & J. Smith (Eds.), *Core curriculum for maternal-newborn nursing* (4th ed., pp. 61–79). Philadelphia, PA: W.B. Saunders.

McComish, J. F., & Visger, J. M. (2009). Domains of postpartum doula care and maternal responsiveness and competence. *Journal of Obstetric, Gynecologic & Neonatal Nursing, 38*(2),148–156. doi:10.1111/j.1552-6909.2009.01002.x

McQueen, K. A., Dennis, C., Stremler, R., & Norman, C. D. (2011). A pilot randomized controlled trial of a breastfeeding self-efficacy intervention with primiparous mothers. *Journal of Obstetric, Gynecologic & Neonatal Nursing, 40*(1), 35–46. doi:10.1111/j.1552-6909.2010.01210.x

Mercer, R. T. (2004). Becoming a mother versus maternal role attainment. *Journal of Nursing Scholarship, 36*(3), 226–232.

Mercer, R. T., & Walker, L. O. (2006). A review of nursing interventions to foster becoming a mother. *Journal of Obstetric, Gynecologic & Neonatal Nursing, 35*(5), 568–582.

Moore, E. R., Anderson, G. C., & Bergman, N. (2007). Early skin-to-skin contact for mothers and their healthy newborn infants. *Cochrane Database of Systematic Reviews (Online),* (3), CD003519. doi:10.1002/14651858.CD003519.pub2

Moorhead, S., Johnson, M., Maas, M. L., & Swanson, E. (2013). *Nursing outcomes classification (NOC)* (5th ed.). St. Louis, MO: Elsevier Mosby.

Mori, R., Khanna, R., Pledge, D., & Nakayama, T. (2010). Meta-analysis of physiological effects of skin-to-skin contact for newborns and mothers. *Pediatrics International, 52*(2), 161–170. doi:10.1111/j.1442-200X.2009.02909.x

Morse, S. L. (2009). Group healthcare visits: Current models of care. *The American Journal for Nurse Practitioners, 13*(10), 52–58.

Morton, J., Hall, J., & Pessl, M. (2014). Five steps to improve bedside feeding care. *Nursing for Women's Health, 17*(6), 479–488. doi:10.1111/1751-486X.12076

Murray, N. (2013). Counseling parents on the avoidance of feeding-associated infections. *The Clinical Advisor, 16*(9), 45–52.

National Initiative for Children's Healthcare Quality (NICHQ). (2013). *Confronting cultural barriers to breastfeeding.* Retrieved from http://breastfeeding.nichq.org/stories/cultural%20barriers%20to%20breastfeeding

Nommsen-Rivers, L. A., Mastergeorge, A. M., Hansen, R. L., Cullum, A. S., & Dewey, K. G. (2009). Doula care, early breastfeeding outcomes, and breastfeeding status at 6 weeks postpartum among low-income primiparae. *Journal of Obstetric, Gynecologic & Neonatal Nursing, 38*(2), 157–173. doi:10.1111/j.1552-6909.2009.01005.x

Office of the Surgeon General. (2011). *Barriers to breastfeeding in the United States.* Retrieved from http://www.ncbi.nlm.nih.gov/books/NBK52688/

Ohyama, M., Watabe, H., & Hayasaka, Y. (2010). Manual expression and electric breast pumping in the first 48 h after delivery. *Pediatrics International, 52*(1), 39–43.

Orr, S. S. (2011). Breastfeeding. In S. Mattson & J. Smith (Eds.), *Core curriculum for maternal-newborn nursing* (4th ed., pp. 315–334). Philadelphia, PA: W.B. Saunders.

Pate, B. (2009). A systematic review of the effectiveness of breastfeeding intervention delivery methods. *Journal of Obstetric, Gynecologic & Neonatal Nursing, 38*(6), 642–653. doi:10.1111/j.1552-6909.2009.01068.x

Patel, J., Patel, N., Thomas, R., Nelms, J., & Colella, J. (2008). Pregnancy outcomes after laparoscopic Roux-en-Y gastric bypass. *Surgery for Obesity and Related Diseases, 4*(1), 39–45.

Phillips, C., & Bulmer, J. (2012). Postpartum care of a woman with cerebral palsy and deep vein thrombosis. *Nursing for Women's Health, 16*(1), 38–44.

Ramchandani, P., Domoney, J., Sethna, V., Psychogiou, L., Vlachos, H., & Murray, L. (2013). Do early father-infant interactions predict the onset of externalising behaviours in young children? Findings from a longitudinal cohort study. *The Journal of Child Psychology and Psychiatry, 54*(1), 54–64. doi:10.1111/j.1469-7610.2012.02583.x

Reyna, B. A., & Pickler, R. H. (2009). Mother-infant synchrony. *Journal of Obstetric, Gynecologic & Neonatal Nursing, 38*(4), 470–477. doi:10.1111/j.1552-6909.2009.01044.x

Rhode, M. A. (2011). Postpartum complications. In S. Mattson & J. Smith (Eds.), *Core curriculum for maternal-newborn nursing* (4th ed., pp. 650–665). Philadelphia: W.B. Saunders.

Riordan, J., & Wambach, K. (2009). *Breastfeeding and human lactation* (4th ed.). Sudbury, MA: Jones and Bartlett Publishers.

Rosenbaum, K. (2012). Implementing the use of donor milk in the hospital setting: Implications for nurses. *Nursing for Women's Health, 16*(3), 200–208. doi:10.1111/j.1751-486X.2012.01731.x

Rubin, R. (1975). Maternal tasks in pregnancy. *MCN: The American Journal of Maternal-Child Nursing, 4*(3), 143–153.

Rubin, R. (1984). *Maternal identity and the maternal experience.* New York: Springer.

Salera-Vieira, J., & Tanner, J. (2009). Color coding for multiples. *Nursing for Women's Health, 13*(1), 83–84. doi:10.1111/j.1751-486X.2009.01385.x

Sauls, D. J. (2010). Promoting a positive childbirth experience for adolescents. *Journal of Obstetric, Gynecologic & Neonatal Nursing, 39*(6), 703–712. doi:10.1111/j.1552-6909.2010.01182.x

Signore, C., Spong, C. Y., Krotoski, D., Shinowara, N. L., & Blackwell, S. C. (2011). Pregnancy in women with physical disabilities. *Obstetrics & Gynecology, 117*(4), 935–947. doi:10.1097/AOG.0b013w3182118d59

Smith, T., & Waller-Wise, R. (2011). Creating an obstetric preadmission and discharge clinic. *Nursing for Women's Health, 15*(2), 115–125. doi:10.1111'j.1751-486X.2011.01620.x

Stiles, A. S. (2010). Case study of an intervention to enhance maternal sensitivity in adolescent mothers. *Journal of Obstetric, Gynecologic & Neonatal Nursing, 39*(6), 723–732. doi:10.1111/j.1552-6909.2010.01183.x

Stonehouse, A., & Studdiford, J. (2011). Allergic contact dermatitis from tea tree oil. *Consultant, 51*(12), 914.

Stuebe, A. M. (2014). Enabling women to achieve their breastfeeding goals. *Obstetrics & Gynecology, 123*(3), 643–652. doi:10.1097/AOG.0000000000000142

Tenfelde, S., Finnegan, L., & Hill, P. D. (2011). Predictors of breastfeeding exclusivity in a WIC sample. *Journal of Obstetric, Gynecologic & Neonatal Nursing, 40*(2), 179–189. doi:10.1111/j.1552-6909.2011.01224.x

Thulier, D., & Mercer, J. (2009). Variables associated with breastfeeding duration. *Journal of Obstetric, Gynecologic & Neonatal Nursing, 38*(3), 259–268. doi:10.1111/j.1552-6909.2009.01021.x

Tilley, I., & Mishell, Jr., D. (2013). How to choose a contraceptive for your postpartum patient. *Clinician Reviews, 23*(8), 32–36.

Tracey, P. M. (2012). Tdap vaccination for postpartum women. *The American Journal for Nurse Practitioners, 16*(11/12), 28–33.

U.S. Census Bureau. (2010). 2010 Census Brief. Retrieved from http://www.census.gov/

U.S. Department of Health & Human Services (USDHHS). (2011). *The Surgeon General's Call to Action to Support Breastfeeding.* Washington, DC: U.S. Department of Health and Human Services, Office of the Surgeon General.

U.S. Department of Health & Human Services (USDHHS). (2012). *Introducing Healthy People 2020.* Retrieved from http://www.healthypeople.gov/2020/about/default.aspx

U.S. Preventive Services Task Force (USPSTF). (2008). Primary care interventions to promote breastfeeding: U.S. Preventive Services Task Force Recommendation Statement. *Annals of Internal Medicine, 149*(3), 560–564.

Vallerand, A. H., & Sanoski, C. (2014). *Davis's drug guide for nurses* (14th ed.). Philadelphia, PA: F.A. Davis.

Walker, L. O., Im, E., & Vaughan, M. W. (2012). Communication technologies and maternal interest in health-promotion information about postpartum weight and parenting practices. *Journal of Obstetric, Gynecologic & Neonatal Nursing, 41*(2), 201–214. doi:10.1111/j.1552-6909.2011.01333.x

Waller-Wise, R. (2012). Mother-baby care: The best for patients, nurses and hospitals. *Nursing for Women's Health, 16*(4), 273–278. doi:10.1111/j.1751-486X.2012.01744.x

Waugh, L. J. (2011). Beliefs associated with Mexican immigrant families' practice of *La Cuarentena* during postpartum recovery. *Journal of Obstetric, Gynecologic & Neonatal Nursing, 40*(6), 732–741. doi:10.1111/j.1552-6909.2011.01298.x

Whitmer, T. (2011). Physical and psychologic changes. In S. Mattson & J. Smith (Eds.), *Core curriculum for maternal-newborn nursing* (4th ed., pp. 301–314). Philadelphia, PA: W.B. Saunders.

Woods, A. B., Crist, B., Kowalewski, S., Carroll, J., Warren, J., & Robertson, J. (2012). A cross-sectional analysis of the effect of patient-controlled epidural analgesia versus patient controlled analgesia on postcesarean pain and breastfeeding. *Journal of Obstetric, Gynecologic & Neonatal Nursing, 41*(3), 339–346. doi:10.1111/j.1552-6909.2012.01370.x

World Health Organization (WHO). (2010). *Medical eligibility criteria for contraceptive use: A WHO family planning cornerstone.* (4th ed.). Geneva, Switzerland: WHO.

Yozwiak, J. A. (2010). Postpartum depression and adolescent mothers: A review of assessment and treatment approaches. *Journal of Pediatric & Adolescent Gynecology, 23*(3), 172–178.

Yu, C.-Y., Hung, C.-H., Chan, T.-F., Yeh, C.-H., & Lai, C.-Y. (2012). Prenatal predictors for father-infant attachment after childbirth. *Journal of Clinical Nursing, 21*(3), 1577–1583. doi:10.1111/j.1365-2702.2011.04003.x

Zauderer, C. (2009). Maternity care for Orthodox Jewish couples. *Nursing for Women's Health, 13*(2), 110–120. doi:10.1111/j.1751-486X.2009.01402.x

DavisPlus | For more information, go to **http://davisplus.fadavis.com/**

CONCEPT MAP

Physiological Adaptations/Con't Assessments:
- Decreased blood volume/elevated cardiac output; CV instability; physiologic diuresis
- WBC: increased with labor, decreased after 6 days
- Estrogen/progesterone decrease; prolactin released
- Fatigue/discomfort: further assess headaches
- GFR/creatinine/BUN decreased by 2–3 months
- Decreased urine protein and glucose
- Natriuresis/diuresis/possible urinary retention
- Involution/uterine contractions; in 6–8 wks resumption of menstruation and ovulation
- Muscle/body aches; rectus abdominus diastasis
- GI-prevent constipation
- RhoGam or rubella vaccine may be indicated

Promoting Maternal Recovery/Self-Care:
- Early ambulation; adequate sleep/frequent rest; balanced and nutritious diet
- Promote bowel and bladder function: monitor for urinary retention, possible catheterization prn, stool softeners/enemas prn
- Peri-care: ice packs, sitz bath
- Analgesics for afterpains
- Routine post-op care for patient having sterilization/cesarean birth: wound care, anesthesia recovery, pain control, Foley catheter; psychological issues with cesarean

Discharge: Planning/Teaching
- Maternal self-care
- Infant bathing, breastfeeding, activity/rest, perineal hygiene, emotional changes
- Teach physical self-assessment
- Teach: nutrition, weight loss, exercise, pain management, sexual activity, emotional changes, follow-up exams
- Identify community resources

Postpartal Maternal Assessments:
- Vital signs
- Fundus; lochia; perineum: REEDA acronym
- Hemorrhoids
- BUBBLE-HE: breasts, uterus, bladder, bowel, lochia, episiotomy, lower extremities, emotions
- Pain assessment

Nursing Insight:
- Engrossment = positive bonding behavior
- Perineal assessment: lighting/privacy
- Prevent nipple confusion
- Persistent fatigue may indicate depression
- Possible postpartum complications in women after bariatric surgery

Clinical Alert:
- Proper uterine palpation technique
- Avoid knee–chest position until 3rd postpartal week
- Identify post-episiotomy hematoma

Emotional Adjustments:
- Linked to childbirth preconceptions, parity, age, maturity, finances, complications
- Insecurity
- Potential mood changes
- Postpartum blues
- Refer for indicators of postpartum depression or psychosis

Maternal Care

Complementary Care:
- Tea tree oil for episiotomy healing
- Cabbage leaves to decrease breast swelling

Caring for the Postpartal Woman and Her Family

Infant

Family–Infant Bonding:
- Create positive environment
- Provide emotional support/accurate information
- Maternal: taking in/taking hold/letting go; promote bonding/attachment
- Paternal: encourage participation
- Siblings: formulate strategies to increase acceptance
- Grandparents: involvement linked to culture

Multicultural Family Care:
- Holistic and flexible approach
- Know and understand rites/customs/beliefs
- Cultural assessment
- Affects: longevity of confinement/activity during/degree of family involvement
- Hot/cold beliefs: affect diet and environmental temperature

Nutrition

Legal Alert:
- Check ID bands: mother and infant
- Prevent abduction

Critical Nursing Action:
- Assessing for maternal–infant attachment

Promoting Breastfeeding:
- Teach: lactation/lactogenesis
- Success strategies: IBCLC
- ID feeding readiness cues
- Facilitate latching-on/suckling
- Proper positioning
- Care: sore nipples/breast engorgement
- Teach about collection/storage of breast milk and weaning

Formula Feeding:
- Correct, safe preparation
- Cleaning bottles/nipples
- No microwaving or propping
- Skin-to-skin/full eye contact
- Watch for large emesis of formula

Optimizing Outcomes:
- Uterine assessment critical in 1st hr
- Deal quickly with abnormal postpartum findings
- Early episiotomy care: ice pack
- Teaching peri-care
- Support feeding choice
- Breast care during lactation
- Preparing formula safely
- Couplet care
- Provide breastfeeding mother private room and a snack
- Facilitate TBC immediately after birth
- Mother—baby care

Cultural Diversity:
- Striae color varies among races
- Use culturally appropriate methods for breastfeeding discomfort

Collaboration in Caring:
- IBCLCs/LaLeche League
- WIC program
- Remove barriers postpartum sterilization

Across Care Settings:
- Community health nurse should refer patient if "letting go" becomes an issue

Now Can You:
- Discuss important physiological changes in the postpartum period and essential components of postpartum nursing care
- Discuss physiological adaptations during the postpartum period
- Provide care to the surgical postpartal patient
- Promote recovery and self-care
- Support and care for the breastfeeding mother
- Care for postpartal mothers with special needs

16

Caring for the Woman Experiencing Complications During the Postpartal Period

Hope is the thing with feathers that perches in the soul—and sings the tunes without the words—and never stops at all.

—Emily Dickinson

LEARNING TARGETS *At the completion of this chapter, the student will be able to:*

- Describe the causes and collaborative management of postpartum hemorrhage.
- Discuss the signs and symptoms of postpartum hematoma; describe nursing care for a patient experiencing a postpartum hematoma.
- Discuss the collaborative management of venous thromboembolic conditions in postpartum women.
- Describe the collaborative management for infections during the puerperium.
- Summarize important interventions in meeting psychosocial needs of postpartum women and their families.
- Describe current community and governmental services that are available to vulnerable postpartum women and their families.

PICO(T) Questions

The intent of evidence-based practice (EBP) is to provide nursing care that integrates the best available evidence. An initial step in EBP is to write a PICO(T) question that effectively guides the research. A PICO(T) question is an acronym that stands for population (P), intervention or issue (I), comparison of interest (C), outcome (O), and timeframe (T). Depending on the question, all or some of the question components are used in the research process.

Use these PICO(T) questions to spark your thinking as you read the chapter.

1. Is late (I) postpartum hemorrhage (O) more prevalent in (P) Caucasian women (C) than in African American women?

2. What (I) strategies best assist (P) family members to (O) help and support women with postpartum depression?

 Evidence-Based Practice

Oswalt, K. L., & Biasini, F. J. (2012). Characteristics of HIV-infected mothers associated with increased risk of poor mother–infant interactions and infant outcomes. *Journal of Pediatric Health Care, 26*(2), 83–91.

The purpose of this study was to explore the relationship between individual and familial characteristics of HIV-infected mothers and their psychological health as it relates to parenting and their parenting beliefs and abilities. Literature supports the concern that depressed mothers have poorer infant interaction than do non-depressed mothers. There is an increased risk for depression in HIV-infected mothers who also have a greater need for interventions to strengthen the mother–child relationship. Previous research has suggested that, compared with non-HIV-infected mothers, HIV-infected mothers have higher levels of poverty, experience poorer mental health, report increased stress, demonstrate difficulty performing parenting tasks, and engage in risky behaviors such as drug use. In addition, children of HIV-infected parents tend to exhibit behavior problems (e.g., inferior

Evidence-Based Practice (continued)

development and externalizing behaviors) and demonstrate significantly lower gains in weight and height than their peers. Previous studies have found that the majority of HIV-infected mothers serve as their child's primary caretaker.

Participants included 17 HIV-infected mothers and their infants; mothers identified as drug abusers and those with premature infants were excluded. The mothers' ages ranged from 17 to 35 years of age; the infants' ages ranged from 5 to 10 weeks of age and their weights ranged from 2.38 to 3.4 kg (5.24–7.48 lb). Eighty-eight percent of the mothers were African American. Significant symptoms of depression (as reflected by scores on the Beck Depression Inventory-II [BDI-II]) were found in 35% of the participants. Forty-three percent of the women were at or below the federal poverty level; 22.6% were uninsured; and 39.9% were enrolled in the Medicaid health program.

The study utilized a descriptive correlation design. Demographic information was obtained, and maternal screening questionnaires were administered during the infant's 6-week clinic appointment. The questionnaires included the BDI-II, the Maternal Confidence Questionnaire (MCQ), the Parental Stress Index-Short Form (PSI-SF), and the Questionnaire About Physical Contact. Predictive Analytics Software was used to explore the relationship between demographics and data from the various maternal questionnaires.

A significant positive correlation was found between infant weight and maternal confidence—as maternal confidence increased, infant weight also increased. Maternal depression and parental distress were increased when there were more children in the family. Maternal stress was higher where there were increased levels of parental distress, dysfunctional parent–child relationships, and the presence of children considered to have a difficult temperament. A negative correlation was found between comfort level with the importance of physical contact and difficult child temperament—as difficult child temperament increased, the mother's level of comfort with physical contact decreased. These findings were consistent with previous research demonstrating that HIV-infected mothers exhibit high levels of stress and an increased risk for depression, both of which can negatively impact parenting and child development.

1. How is this information useful to clinical nursing practice?

2. Based on these findings, what are implications for further research?

See Suggested Responses for Evidence-Based Practice on *DavisPlus*.

Introduction

Most childbearing women have healthy babies and recover from the physiological and psychological adaptations to pregnancy without difficulty. Physiological complications and psychosocial complications are rare, especially in industrialized nations such as the United States, Japan, Australia, and in European countries. Because perinatal care focuses on wellness, health promotion-maintenance, and education for healthy women in multiple settings across the childbearing cycle, the danger of minimizing or misinterpreting pathological signs and symptoms is ever present. A lack of attention to signs of danger, combined with poor provider communication can lead to suboptimal outcomes for women and their families.

When prenatal care begins, whether in a private practice or clinic setting, nurses can serve as liaisons between patients, families, care providers, and community agencies. In this role, the nurse is often the first health-care provider to identify physiological signs and symptoms or recognize psychosocial concerns that need to be addressed by the health-care team. Synthesizing knowledge with clinical data and thinking critically about the meaning of these data are vitally important.

This chapter describes postpartum physiological and psychosocial complications and concerns from a nursing process perspective. The nurse's role in the collaborative treatment of patients and their families who experience these complications is multifaceted and cannot be overly emphasized. More than any other health-care team member, the nurse uses vigilance to apply nursing knowledge and implement informed nursing actions. Vigilance involves combining careful observation, knowledge, and expectations with cues from the patient and her family (Meyer & Lavin, 2005) and is a critical component of nursing care, particularly in the perinatal area where patients are assumed to be healthy. Whether functioning as an independent practitioner or as a member of the health-care team, the nurse's judgments and actions affect both present and future generations for years to come.

Postpartum Hemorrhage

INCIDENCE AND DEFINITION

Postpartum hemorrhage (PPH) is a leading cause of maternal morbidity and mortality in the United States and around the world. Approximately 5% of all women who give birth vaginally experience a postpartum hemorrhage. Internationally, postpartum hemorrhage accounts for one of the three major causes of maternal mortality. According to The World Health Organization, 25% of all pregnancy-related deaths result from postpartum hemorrhage, and more than 50% of the hemorrhage-related deaths have been shown to be preventable (Berg, Callaghan, Syverson, & Henderson, 2010; Cunningham, Leveno, Bloom, Spong, & Dashe, 2014; Della Torre et al., 2011). Historically, practitioners have defined postpartum hemorrhage as a blood loss greater than 500 mL after a vaginal birth and 1,000 mL or more after a cesarean birth (American College of Obstetricians and Gynecologists [ACOG], 2006). Hematocrit levels that decrease 10% from pre- to postbirth measurements are also included in the definition (Cunningham et al., 2014), along with a need for a red blood cell transfusion because of anemia or hemodynamic instability. Cunningham and colleagues (2014) emphasize that postpartum hemorrhage is a description "of an event, not a diagnosis" (p. 772).

Critical Nursing Action Recognizing Additional Indicators of Hemorrhage

To recognize obstetric hemorrhage in a timely manner, nurses should begin to quantify blood loss immediately after birth and remain alert to indicators that may point to ongoing obstetric hemorrhage: maternal heart rate greater than 110 beats per minute, 15% drop in blood pressure, or oxygen saturation less than 95% (Lyndon, Lagrew, Shields, Melsop, Bingham, & Main, 2010).

As is often the case with other clinical events, most definitions of postpartum hemorrhage contain a subjective component. Caregivers rarely measure actual blood loss after childbirth. Instead, the physician, nurse-midwife, or nurse attendant estimates the amount of blood soaked on the bedding and pads or collected in the placenta basin and suction canister. This nonscientific method is frequently inaccurate and may lead to an underestimation of actual blood loss by as much as 40% to 50% (Cunningham et al., 2014). Accuracy in determining true blood loss is possible if a member of the health-care team carefully weighs the placenta basin and all bloody items such as pads, linens, and clothing with a gram scale (1 mL = 1 gram in fluid volume) (Al Kadri, Anazi, & Tamim, 2011). The use of graduated drapes and volume measuring containers are more accurate at quantifying blood loss than unmarked drapes. Calibrated drapes manufactured specifically for the obstetric setting are readily available. If in doubt, the nurse should err on the side of safety until objective data can be obtained and confirmed (Gabel & Weeber, 2012).

Critical Nursing Action Accurately Determining Blood Loss

After childbirth, the nurse carefully weighs all pads, linens, clothing, and clots in the placenta basin on a gram scale to accurately determine the patient's blood loss. A worksheet can be used to facilitate the process of tracking cumulative blood loss (Gabel & Weeber, 2012).

EARLY VERSUS LATE POSTPARTAL HEMORRHAGE

Although the criteria for a diagnosis of postpartum hemorrhage may vary from practitioner to practitioner, the definition of an early and a late postpartum hemorrhage is straightforward. An early (primary) postpartal hemorrhage occurs within the first 24 hours after childbirth. A late (secondary) postpartal hemorrhage occurs from 24 hours to 12 weeks after childbirth. The greatest likelihood for occurrence of an early hemorrhage is within the first 4 postpartum hours. During this time, the blood flow to the uterus is between 500 and 800 mL/minute, and the placental site contains multiple exposed venous areas and

low resistance. In clinical practice, the 4 "Ts" serve as a reminder of factors associated with PPH: tone, trauma, tissue, and thrombin. A lack of uterine tone (**atony**) and genital tract trauma are the most common conditions that cause postpartum hemorrhage (ACOG, 2006; Cunningham et al., 2014; Francois & Foley, 2012).

Cultural Diversity: Maternal Mortality From Obstetric Hemorrhage

Government researchers Tucker, Berg, Callaghan, and Hsia (2007) examined black-white disparity in prevalence and maternal mortality from five specific pregnancy complications including postpartum hemorrhage. They found that although black women did not have significantly higher prevalence rates of obstetric hemorrhage than white women, they were 2 to 3 times more likely to die from the complication. According to Bingham and Jones (2012), "women who die from obstetric hemorrhage must be honored by ensuring that their deaths will be counted and reviewed accurately and that lessons learned will prevent injury and the possibility of other deaths" (p. 537). Nurses can be instrumental in the development and implementation of quality improvement initiatives to ensure that all women have equal access to effective treatments.

UTERINE ATONY

Uterine atony, the leading cause of early PPH, is a failure of the uterine myometrium to contract and retract following birth. Normally, the uterine muscle fibers contract firmly around the blood vessels during placental separation. A lack of contraction and retraction results in noncompression of the uterine arteries and veins at the placental implantation site, thereby preventing hemostasis. The hallmark of uterine atony is a soft uterus filled with clots and blood (Brown & Smrtka, 2011). Multiple factors place the childbearing woman at risk for hemorrhage from uterine atony. An understanding of the factors that increase the risk of uterine atony allows the nurse to anticipate hemorrhage and intervene to prevent excessive blood loss (Box 16-1).

Box 16-1 Risk Factors for Uterine Atony

- Uterine overdistention (associated with multifetal gestation, hydramnios, and macrosomia)
- Dysfunctional or prolonged labor (indicator that the uterus is not contracting normally)
- Previous history of uterine atony/PPH
- Trauma during birth (e.g., forceps-assisted birth, vacuum-assisted birth, and cesarean birth)
- Labor induction/augmentation with oxytocin
- Chorioamnionitis
- High parity (stretched uterine musculature has decreased contractility)
- Retained placental fragments
- Use of anesthesia/analgesia, especially halogenated anesthetic agents or other drugs (e.g., magnesium sulfate and nifedipine) that promote uterine relaxation
- Prolonged/mismanaged third stage of labor

TRAUMA

During the second stage of labor, soft tissue trauma from a number of causes (e.g., rapid labor, operative delivery, and episiotomy) can result in genital tract lacerations (Box 16-2). While PPH from uterine atony is evident from a soft, blood-filled uterus, if the source of hemorrhage is genital tract lacerations, the uterus remains firm and midline. Because one large or several small lacerations can adversely affect hemodynamic stability, it is essential to frequently monitor vital signs. Perineal inspection may reveal either a steady stream or a small trickle of bright red blood.

clinical alert

Postpartal blood loss

The nurse and other practitioners must remember that in the presence of a firm uterus, continual vaginal bleeding in a slow but steady trickle, with or without clots, can result in significant blood loss, and most maternal deaths from postpartal hemorrhage result from ineffective management of slow, steady blood loss.

Lacerations are usually internal and are not visible when the nurse examines the perineum. Identifying either a vaginal wall or cervical laceration usually requires that the physician or midwife examine the patient while she is in the lithotomy position. Not infrequently, the physician locates and repairs a laceration before the patient's transfer to the postpartum unit.

TISSUE

Careful examination of the placenta after delivery is a component of standard care. Hence, retained placental tissue is an uncommon cause of early PPH. If the pregnancy included problems with placental implantation (e.g., placenta previa or placenta accreta), the primary care provider is aware of these risks before the birth takes place. Should the practitioner note that lobes of the placenta are missing during the placental examination, the physician or certified nurse-midwife explores the patient's uterus to remove them. More often, a soft uterus with bright red bleeding

later in the postpartum course identifies the source of a late postpartum hemorrhage (Cunningham et al., 2014).

Optimizing Outcomes—Recognizing causes of retained placenta

Retained placenta, which occurs as a complication of childbirth in approximately 3% of vaginal deliveries, can result in fatal hemorrhage and is the second leading cause of postpartum hemorrhage (after uterine atony). Bedside transabdominal ultrasound may be used to locate the retained products, and manual removal under anesthesia is usually required, increasing the patient's risk for postpartum endometritis and blood loss. Nurses should be alert to the following factors that are associated with retained placenta: previous retained placenta, preterm birth, grand multiparity, previous dilation and curettage, small placental weight, previous cesarean delivery, previous abortions, induced labor, older maternal age, preeclampsia, and oxytocin use (Endler, Grunewald, & Saltvedt, 2012). With retained placenta, the risk for uterine inversion (the descent of the uterine corpus through the uterine cervix) is also increased. This complication, which can be associated with major hemorrhage, requires immediate recognition and replacement of the uterus to the normal position (Brown & Smrtka, 2011).

THROMBIN

Thrombin refers to problems with maternal coagulation. Disorders of the coagulation system and platelets do not usually result in excessive bleeding during the immediate postpartum period. Preexistent maternal factors such as low fibrinogen levels and idiopathic thrombocytopenia (ITP) and acquired pathology such as HELLP syndrome (condition characterized by **H**emolysis, **E**levated **L**iver enzymes, and **L**ow **P**latelet count), disseminated intravascular coagulation (DIC), sepsis, and abruptio placentae require vigilant care and anticipation of possible hemorrhage after birth.

LATE (SECONDARY) POSTPARTUM HEMORRHAGE

Late postpartum hemorrhage occurs in only 1% to 2% of all childbearing women, usually within the first 2 weeks after birth. Retained placental fragments are the most common cause of late PPH. Other causes include subinvolution (failure of the uterus to return to its prepregnant size), uterine infection, and less commonly, inherited coagulation defects such as von Willebrand (vW) disease.

Nursing Insight—Congenital clotting defects and women: von Willebrand disease

von Willebrand disease is caused by a deficiency of von Willebrand factor, a protein required for platelet adhesion. Although vW disease is rare, it is the most common of all hereditary bleeding disorders. vW disease results from a factor VIII deficiency and is transmitted as an incomplete autosomal dominant trait to both sexes. Symptoms include a familial bleeding tendency, reports of previous bleeding episodes, prolonged bleeding time, factor VIII deficiency, and bleeding from

---

Box 16-2 Risk Factors for Postpartum Hemorrhage From Tissue Trauma

- Rapid second stage labor
- Rapid/precipitous labor (less than 3 hours from onset to delivery)
- Operative vaginal deliveries (forceps- or vacuum-assisted)
- Fetal manipulation (extrauterine or intrauterine version, corkscrew maneuver for shoulder dystocia [corkscrew maneuver: a progressive 180-degree manual rotation of the baby's posterior shoulder to release the impacted anterior shoulder])
- Large episiotomies, including extensions
- Fetal macrosomia
- Cesarean birth
- Uterine rupture (increased incidence with previous uterine surgery, tetanic contractions, labor stimulation, versions, and placental attachment abnormalities—placenta accreta, placenta increta, and placenta percreta)

the mucous membranes. Although pregnancy is associated with an increase in factor VIII, the patient with vW disease remains at risk for PPH as the levels of vW factor begin to decrease; the risk for bleeding may persist for up to 4 weeks postpartum. Treatment usually involves the administration (orally, nasally, or IV) of desmopressin, which promotes the release of vW factor and factor VIII; other treatment modalities include the transfusion of plasma products treated for viruses that contain factor VIII and vW factor and the IV administration of antihemophiliac factor-vW factor complex (Humate-P and Alphanate) (Rooger & Silver, 2013).

Regardless of the cause, treatment usually includes ergonovine medication (Ergotrate or Methergine 0.2 mg orally every 4 hours for 48 hours), antibiotics, and, if necessary, dilation and curettage to remove placental fragments. After birth and before discharge, the nurse is responsible for educating the patient and her family about the signs and symptoms of subinvolution. Signs and symptoms of subinvolution include lower abdominal (uterine) tenderness with or without fever, continuation of red vaginal drainage beyond 1 week, and foul-smelling vaginal drainage, regardless of color.

 Nursing Insight—Recognizing characteristics that point to the source of postpartal bleeding

The color and character of the blood and the consistency of the uterus can often identify the source of postpartal bleeding. When bleeding is associated with uterine atony or retained placental fragments, the blood is dark red with clots and the uterus is soft and boggy. When bleeding is associated with lacerations from the perineum, cervix, or vagina, the blood is bright red, often without clots, and the uterus remains firmly contracted.

HYPOVOLEMIC SHOCK

Hypovolemic (hemorrhagic) shock can result if PPH is not managed aggressively. Most women can tolerate a 1,000 mL blood loss because they are healthy, have a 35% to 45% increase in the plasma and red blood cell (RBC) volume (2 pints of blood), and give birth in positions that "pool blood" in the pelvis (Cunningham et al., 2014).

 clinical alert

Blood loss and vital signs

Normal physiological adaptations in pregnancy mean that a large loss of blood can occur before changes in vital signs (decreased blood pressure and increased pulse) are evident. The lack of objective signs and symptoms may lead to a delay in treatment.

The nurse, physician, or midwife may not see the usual signs of shock—restlessness; anxiety; pallor; cool, clammy skin; increased pulse; tachypnea; shaking; and decreased blood pressure—until 30% to 40% of the patient's total circulating blood volume has been lost.

COLLABORATIVE MANAGEMENT OF PPH

After birth, standard care requires frequent measurement of vital signs and fundal massage to check the location and condition of the uterine fundus. Most hospitals and birthing centers require that the registered nurse perform these checks at least every 15 minutes for the first postpartal hour. Thereafter, the frequency of assessment varies from one institution to another. As the primary caregiver and the one completing these assessments, the registered nurse may be the first person to identify excessive blood loss. When identified, immediate actions are necessary. While another member of the team calls the physician or nurse-midwife, the nurse can obtain some important assessment data. The nurse must be cognizant of risk factors in the patient's history. After locating the uterine fundus and initiating fundal massage, the nurse can also begin frequent vital sign measurements with an automatic device. The nurse should also palpate the bladder for distention. The length of time it takes for blood loss to saturate a perineal pad is an important parameter to record, as is a measurement of total intake and output up to that point. Keeping in mind that the pulse and blood pressure may remain unchanged until a large volume of blood has been lost, the nurse must pay particular attention to the mean arterial pressure (MAP). A decrease in this measurement may be the first indicator of hypovolemia (Cunningham et al., 2014). Of importance, also, is to note the patient's behavior, in particular her level of consciousness, the presence of restlessness, vague complaints, and her pain level. Possible nursing diagnoses and goals for postpartum hemorrhage are listed in Boxes 16-3 and 16-4.

 Optimizing Outcomes—**Using time intervals and weight to improve accuracy of the estimate of perineal pad saturation**

It is difficult to estimate the amount of blood required to saturate a perineal pad. When fully saturated, a perineal

---

Box 16-3 Possible Nursing Diagnoses for Postpartum Hemorrhage

Fluid volume deficit related to decreased circulating blood volume secondary to uterine atony (genital tract trauma, uterine rupture, retained placental fragments, and inversion of the uterus)

- Altered tissue perfusion related to hypovolemia
- Fear related to threat to health and powerlessness
- Pain related to uterine massage and invasive procedures
- Risk for infection related to invasive procedures

Box 16-4 Possible Goals for the Patient Experiencing a Postpartum Hemorrhage

- The patient's circulating blood volume will be maintained and/or the blood volume will be restored to a physiologically adequate level.
- Peripheral pulses and oxygenation will be maintained.
- The patient/family will express their fears.
- The patient's pain will be managed at a level acceptable to her.
- The patient will maintain normal vital signs and laboratory values.

Source: Adapted from Ackley & Ladwig (2013).

pad can hold between 50 and 80 mL. The nurse can use distinct time intervals for measurement, such as every 15 or 30 minutes, to increase the accuracy of the estimated blood loss. For example, six pads saturated in 30 minutes is much more alarming than six pads saturated in 6 hours. It is also essential to differentiate between the terms "saturated" and "used" when performing a pad count. An accurate way to measure vaginal blood loss is to weigh the perineal pad before and after use and subtract the difference. One gram (1 g) in weight equals 1 milliliter (1 mL) in volume of blood because grams and milliliters are comparable measures. The woman should be positioned on her side when observing for blood loss. Otherwise, large amounts of pooled blood under her buttocks may go undetected.

Once the physician or nurse identifies a postpartum hemorrhage, interventions quickly follow. If the cause of the hemorrhage is uterine atony, continual fundal massage *with lower uterine segment support* is mandatory (Procedure 16-1). While one member of the team massages the fundus, another nurse establishes IV access with a large-bore needle (usually an 18-gauge or larger) and administers oxytocic drugs.

 ### Procedure 16-1 Performing Fundal Massage

Purpose

Fundal massage is used as an emergency measure to contract the uterus that is soft and boggy because of atony. It is performed to promote uterine tone and consistency and minimize the risk of hemorrhage. Uterine atony may result from prolonged labor, rapid or precipitous labor and birth, high parity, medications during labor (e.g., oxytocin, magnesium sulfate, or inhalation anesthesia), intra-amniotic infection, operative delivery and uterine overdistention from multiple gestation, hydramnios, or macrosomia.

Equipment

- Clean examination gloves
- Disposable cleansing wipes
- Two clean peri-pads

Preexamination Preparation

1. Wash and dry hands, explain the procedure and its purpose to the patient; ensure privacy.

   RATIONALE: *Hand washing helps to prevent the spread of microorganisms. Explanations help to decrease anxiety; providing privacy helps to promote the patient's comfort and self-esteem.*

2. Assemble necessary equipment, including clean examination gloves, disposable cleansing wipes, and clean peri-pads.

3. Ask the patient to void, unless fundal massage must be performed immediately because of excessive bleeding.

   RATIONALE: *An empty bladder prevents uterine displacement and facilitates an accurate assessment of uterine tone.*

4. Assist the woman to a supine position with the knees flexed and the feet placed together.

   RATIONALE: *Proper positioning facilitates easy visualization and enhances the effectiveness of the procedure.*

Steps

1. Don gloves, remove the peri-pad, and inspect the perineum. Observe the character and amount of drainage on the pad and the presence of clots. Apply a clean peri-pad.

RATIONALE: *Gloves serve as a barrier against possible infection from the vaginal drainage. Obtaining a baseline assessment provides information for future assessments; it also provides a means for evaluating the effectiveness of the procedure.*

2. Place one hand on the abdomen, just above the symphysis pubis.

   RATIONALE: *This location provides support for the lower uterine segment.*

3. Place the other hand around the top of the fundus.

   RATIONALE: *This location helps to locate and assess the fundus and the fundal height.*

4. With the lower hand maintained in a stable position, rotate the upper hand and massage the uterus until it is firm. Avoid overmassaging the uterus.

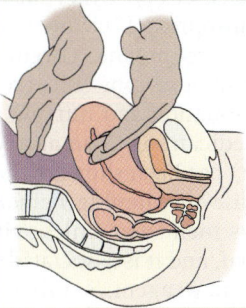

RATIONALE: *The uterus should be massaged only when it is not firm. Massaging a firm uterus may result in muscle fatigue and uterine relaxation. Overly aggressive fundal massage may result in uterine prolapse.*

5. Once the uterus has become firm, *gently* press the fundus between the hands. Apply a slight downward pressure against the lower hand.

   RATIONALE: *Gentle squeezing with downward pressure assists in the expulsion of blood or clots that have collected in the uterine cavity.*

6. Observe the perineum for the passage of clots and the amount of bleeding.

   RATIONALE: *This action helps to assess the presence of clots and the degree of bleeding.*

(continued)

Procedure 16-1 Performing Fundal Massage (continued)

7. Once the uterus remains firm, cleanse the perineum and apply a clean peri-pad. Dispose of the soiled gloves and pads according to institutional policy.

RATIONALE: *This action promotes maternal comfort and hygiene and reduces the risk for infection.*

8. Document the findings. Continue to assess the fundus and vaginal drainage according to institutional protocol.

RATIONALE: *Documentation serves as a means for evaluation. Continued assessment allows for the early identification of problems and facilitates timely intervention with additional measures such as medications (e.g., oxytocin) to prevent hemorrhage.*

What If?

What if the fundus does not remain contracted or heavy bleeding persists despite a contracted uterus?

After ensuring that the bladder is empty (ask the patient to void; palpate for bladder fullness), alert the physician or nurse-midwife, ensure IV access, continue to provide ongoing maternal surveillance, and prepare for an intervention (e.g., examination, medication, or bimanual compression).

Documentation

7/27/10 0550: Fundal massage performed with a moderate amount of bright red lochia and small clots expressed. Uterus remained firm and contracted below the umbilicus. Procedure tolerated well by the patient.

—Sejal Patel, RNC

Medical management of PPH begins with administration of uterotonics starting with oxytocin (Pitocin). International guidelines recommend 10 units of oxytocin IM or IV as one acceptable uterotonic for active management of the third stage of labor (Begley, Gyte, Devane, McGuire, & Weeks, 2011). Other medications that may be used include misoprostol (Cytotec), methylergonovine (Methergine) or ergonovine (Ergotrate), carboprost (Hemabate), and dinoprostone (Prostin E₂). See Table 16-1 for further information and nursing implications concerning these medications. Human recombinant factor VIIa (NovoSeven) has been shown to be effective in controlling severe, life-threatening hemorrhage. However, this medication is ineffective unless vital clotted factors have been replaced, and it is associated with thromboembolism. Another new agent, synthetic fibrinogen (RiaSTAP), has been approved for congenital fibrinogen deficiency. Extremely expensive and associated with maternal morbidities, further investigation is needed to establish the role of these two medications in the treatment of PPH (ACOG, 2006; Brown & Smrtka, 2011; Pacheco, Saade, Tyner, Clark, & Hankins, 2012).

Medication: Methylergonovine (Methergine)

(meth-ill-er-goe-**noe**-veen)

Pregnancy Category: C

Indications: Prevention and treatment of postpartum and postabortion hemorrhage caused by uterine atony or subinvolution

Actions: Directly stimulates uterine and vascular smooth muscle

Therapeutic Effects: Uterine contraction

Pharmacokinetics:
ABSORPTION: Well absorbed after oral or IM administration

ONSET OF ACTION: Oral: 5 to 10 minutes; IM: 2 to 5 minutes; IV: Immediately
DISTRIBUTION: Oral: 3 hours; IM: 3 hours; IV: 45 minutes. Enters breast milk in small quantities.
METABOLISM AND EXCRETION: Probably metabolized by the liver
HALF-LIFE: 30 to 120 minutes

Contraindications and Precautions:

CONTRAINDICATED IN: Hypersensitivity. Should not be used to induce labor.
USE CAUTIOUSLY IN: Hypertensive or eclamptic patients (more susceptible to hypertensive and arrhythmogenic side effects); severe hepatic or renal disease; sepsis
EXERCISE EXTREME CAUTION IN: Third stage of labor

Adverse Reactions and Side Effects:
Central nervous system: Dizziness, headache
Eyes, ears, nose, throat: Tinnitus
Respiratory: Dyspnea
Cardiovascular: Hypotension, arrhythmias, chest pain, hypertension, palpitations
Gastrointestinal: Nausea, vomiting
Genitourinary: Cramps
Dermatological: Diaphoresis

Route and Dosage:
PO: 200 to 400 mcg (0.4–0.6 mg) q6 to 12h for 2 to 7 days
IM, IV: 200 mcg (0.2 mg) after delivery of fetal anterior shoulder, after delivery of the placenta, or during the puerperium; may be repeated as required at intervals of 2 to 4 hours up to five doses.

Nursing Implications:
1. Physical assessment: Monitor blood pressure, heart rate, and uterine response frequently during medication administration. Notify the primary health-care provider if uterine relaxation becomes prolonged or if character of vaginal bleeding changes.
2. Assess for signs of ergotism (cold, numb fingers and toes; chest pain; nausea; vomiting; headache; muscle pain; and weakness)

Source: Data from Vallerand, A. H., & Sanoski, C. (2014). *Davis's drug guide for nurses* (14th ed.). Philadelphia, PA: F.A. Davis.

Table 16-1 Medications and Nursing Considerations for Postpartum Hemorrhage

Name	Classification/Action	Dosage/Route	Contraindications	Nursing Considerations
oxytocin (Pitocin)	Oxytocic Stimulates uterine smooth muscle and produces contractions similar to those that occur during spontaneous labor	10 units IM if no IV access; 10–40 units in 1,000 cc crystalloid IV fluid (lactated Ringer's solution or normal saline)	Hypersensitivity	Monitor uterine response. DO NOT administer a bolus of undiluted oxytocin, because it can cause hypotension and cardiac arrhythmias. Consider administration of pain medication for uterine cramping.
methylergonovine maleate (Methergine)	Ergot alkaloid Causes uterine contractions by stimulating uterine and vascular smooth muscles	0.1–0.2 mg IM q2–4h; followed by 0.2 mg PO q4–6h × 24 hours (for 6 doses)	Hypersensitivity History of, or current elevation of blood pressure	Keep refrigerated. DO NOT add it to IV solutions or mix in a syringe with other medications. Take precautions to prevent inadvertent administration to the newborn.
carboprost tromethamine (Hemabate)	Prostaglandin analogue Stimulates contractions of the myometrium	0.25 mg (250 mcg) IM or directly into the uterus (by MD or CNM) q 15–90 min; 8 doses maximum	Asthma, hepatic, renal, and cardiac disease	Do not administer if patient demonstrates shock because it will not be well absorbed. Keep refrigerated. This medication is VERY expensive.
misoprostol (Cytotec)	Prostaglandin analogue; stimulates powerful contractions of the myometrium	800–1000 mcg rectally (single dose)	Hypersensitivity to prostaglandins	Stable at room temperature. Rectal absorption is likely slower than IV medication.
dinoprostone (Prostin E₂)	Prostaglandin analogue; stimulates powerful contractions of the myometrium	20 mg suppository vaginally or rectally q2h	Hypersensitivity to prostaglandins Avoid in severe hypotension	Monitor uterine response. If vaginal bleeding is brisk, the use of vaginal suppositories is not likely to be effective. Fever is common. Stored frozen, it must be thawed to room temperature.

Sources: Data from ACOG (2006); Adams et al. (2013); Brown & Smrtka (2011); Cunningham et al. (2014); Vallerand & Sanoski (2014).

 Nursing Insight—*Maternal morbidity associated with severe PPH survival*

Women who survive severe PPH are likely to experience significant morbidity, including exposure to blood products, intensive care admission, additional surgeries, infection, and prolonged hospitalization, which may lead to thromboembolism (Zelop, 2011).

 Critical Nursing Action   Immediate Intervention for Uterine Atony

As soon as excessive blood loss is noted, the nurse's most important intervention is to begin fundal massage. Support the lower uterine segment by placing a hand in a slight "C" position just above the symphysis pubis. *Do not* express clots if the uterus does not become firm with massage. The clots may protect the patient from an even greater blood loss.

 Collaboration in Caring—*In situ drill programs to enhance emergency response*

In situ drills (simulation that occurs in the patient care area) involving the multidisciplinary health-care team serve as a key adjunct to evidence-based protocols and established educational programs. Held every few months, the drills are instrumental in reinforcing important educational concepts concerning high-risk events such as maternal hemorrhage, allow the team to develop skills to improve performance, and identify areas that warrant further work and collaboration. Videotaping the simulation enhances the participant debriefing process and allows for an accurate review of factors that increased and reduced efficiency in the emergency situation (ACOG, 2014; Hansen & Arafeh, 2012), and use of a project-designed checklist with a trained debriefing facilitator accelerates the overall improvement process for the team (Corbett, Hurko, & Vallee, 2012).

If the patient has a distended bladder, an indwelling urinary catheter needs to be inserted and all intake and output carefully recorded. The nurse also needs to weigh pads, linens, and other bloody items on a gram scale to obtain an accurate picture of blood loss. It may be necessary to administer oxygen at 10 to 12 L/min to treat compromised tissue perfusion. Additional baseline information that should be obtained includes a complete blood count (CBC) and coagulation studies (PT [prothrombin time] partial thromboplastin time [PTT], fibrinogen, and fibrin degradation products). The physician or nurse-midwife orders the blood tests, along with a type and cross match for replacement blood as an anticipatory measure in the event a transfusion is necessary. The patient is carefully assessed for indicators of DIC.

DIC is a diffuse clotting pathology that involves the consumption of large amounts of clotting factors including platelets, fibrinogen, prothrombin, and factors V and VII. The pathological process may cause both internal and external bleeding. Vascular occlusion of small vessels occurs as small clots form in the microcirculation. Although DIC may occur during the postpartum period, it is most likely to be associated with abruptio placentae, severe preeclampsia, amniotic fluid embolism, septicemia, cardiopulmonary arrest, hemorrhage, and dead fetus syndrome (a complication that may occur when the fetus has died and is retained in the uterus for 6 or more weeks). Diagnosis is made according to clinical findings and laboratory results. (See Chapters 11, 14, and 33 for further discussion.)

The physician or midwife may also perform bimanual compression in an effort to empty the uterus of clots and restore its tone. To perform this procedure, the physician inserts one hand in the vagina while pushing against the fundus through the abdominal wall with the other hand (Fig. 16-1). If these conservative measures fail to stabilize the patient by restoring tone to the uterus and decreasing the blood loss, surgical intervention is indicated. Invasive procedures include the placement of uterine packing (used less often today because of concerns of concealed hemorrhage), uterine balloon tamponade, ligation of the uterine arteries, which provide approximately 90% of the uterine blood flow, hypogastric artery ligation (rarely used in contemporary practice), uterine suture techniques, radiographic-guided pelvic arterial embolization, and hysterectomy, a last resort to life-threatening hemorrhage (ACOG, 2006; Brown & Smrtka, 2011).

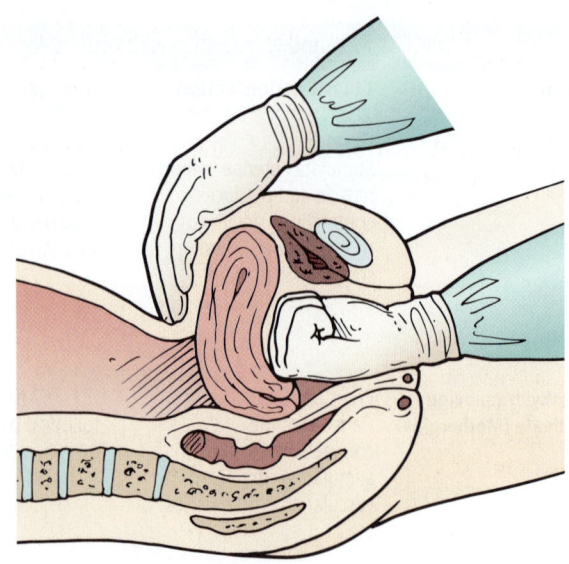

Figure 16-1 Bimanual compression.

Collaborative interventions for hemorrhage from genital tract lacerations are essentially the same. Patients who are experiencing hemorrhage from genital tract lacerations need a large-bore IV site, frequent recording of vital signs, accurate measurements of intake and output from all sources (including blood), lab work, an indwelling urinary catheter, oxygen, and pain medication. In addition, the physician or nurse-midwife examines the perineum, vagina, and cervix in an attempt to locate the source of bleeding. The postpartum nurse needs to help the patient assume a lithotomy position, obtain bright lighting and examination instruments, and prepare suction equipment. The nurse continually provides support and reassurance to the patient and her family. Most physicians or midwives choose to repair lacerations in the operating room with an anesthesiologist present and the patient anesthetized.

Once the crisis has passed and immediate interventions have been completed, a debriefing of the health-care team's response to the situation can be helpful as a learning opportunity. The patient's outcomes will be evident as she recovers from the postpartum hemorrhage event. Of significance is to note the family's response to the unforeseen events and include them, as appropriate, in the discussion. Because most families expect childbirth to be uneventful, a postpartum hemorrhage can provoke widely differing emotional responses. The prudent and compassionate clinician takes the time to let both the patient and the family express their feelings and affirm their concerns. The nurse must be sure to include care of and bonding with the newborn in the recovery process (Foreman, 2014).

Optimizing Outcomes—Holistic care during management of a PPH

Best outcome: The nurse provides physiological care in a timely manner and also serves as an advocate for the patient's pain control and reassures the patient and her family by explaining interventions as they occur. These actions help control not only the blood loss but also the patient's pain and the patient's and family's anxiety.

Collaboration in Caring—*AWHONN's Postpartum Hemorrhage Project*

In late 2013, the Association of Women's Health, Obstetric and Neonatal Nurses (AWHONN) launched the Postpartum Hemorrhage (PPH) Project designed to achieve the following goals: increase clinician recognition of women at greatest risk of obstetric hemorrhage, increase early recognition of which women are bleeding too much, increase the readiness of clinical team preparedness to

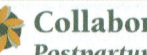

Labs: Findings With DIC

Low hemoglobin	Low fibrinogen
Low hematocrit	Elevated fibrin split/degradation products
Low platelets	

successfully respond to obstetric hemorrhage, and track clinician response to obstetric hemorrhage for improving future performance. Additional practice improvements include the identification of barriers to treating obstetric hemorrhage and methods for effectively implementing similar improvements in all hospitals in the United States.

 Now Can You—Discuss postpartum hemorrhage?

1. State the four "Ts" that lead to postpartum hemorrhage?
2. Describe five standard nursing interventions for managing postpartum hemorrhage?
3. Discuss holistic care in the management of a woman/family experiencing a postpartum hemorrhage?

Hematomas

DEFINITION, INCIDENCE, AND RISK FACTORS

A **hematoma** is a localized collection of blood in connective or soft tissue under the skin that follows injury of or laceration to a blood vessel without injury to the overlying tissue. At the time of injury, pressure necrosis and inadequate hemostasis occurs. This complication can result in a large amount of blood loss and patient discomfort if not recognized rapidly. Risk factors for hematoma formation include genital tract lacerations, episiotomies, operative vaginal deliveries, a difficult or prolonged second stage of labor, and nulliparity. Hematomas occur most frequently in the vulva, but they can also occur in the vagina and in the retroperitoneal area (Figs. 16-2 and 16-3).

SIGNS AND SYMPTOMS

The most common sign or symptom of a hematoma is unremitting pain and pressure. The pain and pressure worsen if active bleeding continues; the uterus remains firm. When located in the vaginal area, the patient often complains

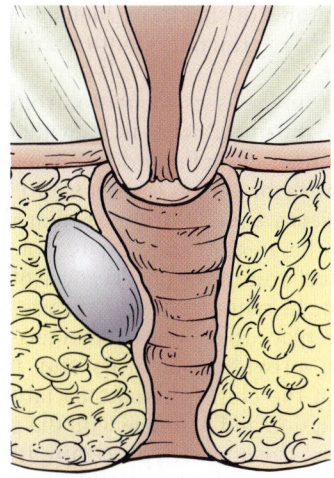

Figure 16-3 Vaginal wall hematoma.

of a sensation of "heaviness" in the vagina and/or rectal pressure. On examination of the perineal or vulvar areas, the nurse may notice a bluish discoloration and bulging of the tissue at the hematoma site. If touched, the patient complains of severe tenderness, and the clinician generally describes the tissue as "full." If the hematoma is large, signs of shock (e.g., tachycardia and hypotension) may be evident, and the patient may exhibit an absence of lochia and an inability to void. Possible nursing diagnoses and goals for a patient experiencing a hematoma are presented in Box 16-5.

COLLABORATIVE MANAGEMENT

Assessment for the presence of a hematoma involves listening to the patient's subjective complaints, measuring vital signs, and examining the perineal and vulvar areas to identify a bulging mass. To examine the perineal and vulvar areas, the nurse assists the patient to a side-lying position, gently lifts the upper buttock, and asks her to bear down. The nurse also needs to watch for behavioral

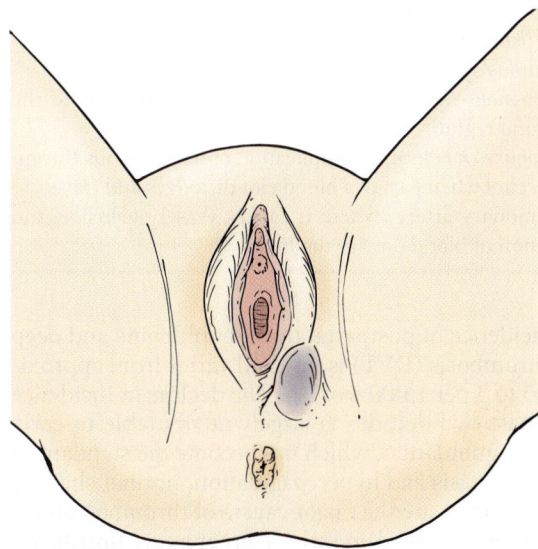

Figure 16-2 Vulvar hematoma.

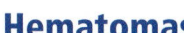

Box 16-5 Possible Nursing Diagnoses and Goals for Patients With a Postpartum Hematoma

Pain related to tissue trauma and pressure.

Patient's pain will be managed to an acceptable level.

Anxiety and/or fear related to knowledge deficit of procedures and plan of care.

Patient will express her fears.

Altered family processes related to physiological crisis.

Patient and her family will support one another verbally and behaviorally.

Powerlessness related to loss of control of physiological functions.

Patient will make choices over which she has control.

At risk for infection related to invasive procedures.

Patient will remain afebrile and her WBC will be within normal limits.

Patient's perineum will heal without evidence of drainage or separation.

At risk for fluid volume deficit.

Patient's blood loss will be minimized.

At risk for altered attachment related to separation from infant.

Patient will demonstrate concern for and care of infant before discharge.

signs and symptoms of shock (previously described) and assess the patient's and family's understanding of what is occurring.

If findings from the assessment are strongly suggestive of a hematoma, the nurse needs to immediately notify the physician or nurse-midwife and implement pain relief measures. If the hematoma is less than 3 to 5 cm in diameter, the physician usually orders palliative treatments such as ice to the area for the first 12 hours along with pain medication and close observation of the area for extension of the hematoma. After 12 hours, sitz baths are prescribed to replace the application of ice. Sitz baths are therapeutic in providing comfort and in facilitating reabsorption of the clot. A hematoma larger than 5 cm may require incision and drainage with the possible placement of a drain. This invasive procedure is performed in the operating room while the patient is sedated with an anesthetic.

The health-care team must be particularly sensitive to the fact that large hematomas can lead to shock. In this case, the physician orders aggressive treatment that includes IV fluids, oxygen, frequent measurement of vital signs, urinary catheter placement, and strict intake and output measurements to stabilize the patient before taking her to the operating room.

In the midst of the important interventions implemented to deal with the hematoma, the nurse needs to remember that the family is watching and responding to events as they unfold. Neither the patient nor the family may understand what they are seeing or experiencing. As the various treatments and medications are administered, the nurse should explain each action, along with the rationale for it. If the patient and her family can be involved, it is important to allow them to make choices, so that they do not feel as powerless. The nurse can assist the family by encouraging them to care for and bond with the infant as much as possible.

? **Global Health Case Study** Patient Experiencing a Vulvar Hematoma

Francisca is a 20-year-old Mexican American gravida 1, para 1 who gave birth to a term, healthy baby boy, weighing 9 lb 1 oz (4.1 kg) at 23:32 hours. She received an epidural for labor pain control, pushed for 3 hours, and required a vacuum-assisted delivery. Her perineum required repair of a third-degree laceration. After birth, the nurse discontinued the continuous epidural pump, placed ice on the perineum, completed the required 15-minute checks (× 5), helped Francisca breastfeed, and assisted Francisca's boyfriend in holding the baby and taking pictures. On arrival to the mother–baby unit, Francisca requests pain medication and states that the ice is helping some but that she wants to "stay on top of it." She rates the pain as a 5 on a 10-point scale. The admission vital signs and fundal location are within normal limits. An examination of Francisca's perineum reveals mild swelling and a normal amount of vaginal bleeding. Francisca is tired and asks that she be allowed to sleep. Her boyfriend goes home to sleep, and the baby is taken to the nursery.

Two hours later, Francisca calls for her nurse and complains of intense burning, pain, and pressure "where I had my stitches." You examine her perineum and note an 8-cm bulging mass on her left vulva. When you touch it with a gloved hand, Francisca says, "Oh, that is so tender! That hurts!"

---

critical thinking questions

1. What factors during birth placed Francisca at risk for development of a hematoma?
2. Name two appropriate nursing diagnoses for Francisca.
3. What are the expected outcomes for Francisca?
4. List four nursing interventions along with rationales.

◆ See Suggested Answers to Global Health Case Studies on *DavisPlus*.

 Now Can You—Discuss implications of a postpartum hematoma?

1. Describe the classic signs and symptoms of a puerperal hematoma?
2. Identify the most common anatomical locations for a postpartum hematoma?
3. Differentiate between the collaborative management for a small and a large hematoma?

Thrombophlebitis and Thrombosis

DEFINITION, INCIDENCE, AND RISK FACTORS

Thrombophlebitis and **thrombosis** are terms that describe an inflammation of the venous circulation and blood clot formation that typically occur in the lower extremities. The depth of the inflammation and the location of the involved veins determine the severity of this complication. Veins located above the fascia, such as the saphenous vein system, are superficial, and distend easily, while veins below the fascia, such as the popliteal system, are deep and less elastic.

 Nursing Insight—*Differentiating among three thromboembolic conditions*

During pregnancy and the puerperium, three thromboembolic conditions are of concern:

Superficial venous thrombosis involves the superficial saphenous venous system.

Deep venous thrombosis may extend from the foot to the ileofemoral region.

Pulmonary embolism, a complication of deep venous thrombosis, occurs when part of a blood clot dislodges and travels to the pulmonary artery, where it causes vessel occlusion and obstruction of blood flow to the lungs.

The incidence of postpartal thrombophlebitis and deep venous thrombosis (DVT) is low and varies from approximately 0.5 to 3 per 1,000 women. The decline in incidence over the past two decades is largely attributable to early postpartum ambulation, which has become the standard of care. Venous stasis and hypercoagulation, normal changes during pregnancy, are the major causes of thromboembolic disease. After the third month of pregnancy, fibrinogen levels increase, and in the second half of pregnancy, clotting factors VII, VIII, IX, and X increase in preparation for minimizing normal blood loss during birth. A decreased breakdown of fibrin, which forms the protein mesh of a clot, also occurs (Cunningham et al., 2014).

Lower extremity venous stasis results from the weight of the gravid uterus on the maternal inferior vena cava and pelvic veins. If the woman smokes, is obese, older (greater than 35 years), immobile, or a grand multigravida, the risk of DVT also increases. Chronic health problems such as inflammatory bowel disease, lupus erythematosus, antiphospholipid syndrome, varicose veins, and pregnancy-related conditions such as preeclampsia, an operative vaginal delivery, cesarean birth, hemorrhage, and sepsis are all possible precursors to the development of DVT. A woman with a positive history of DVT is also at greater risk than one with no DVT history, and the risk of venous thromboembolism is higher during the puerperium than it is during pregnancy, especially during the first week postpartum (ACOG, 2011a; Cunningham et al., 2014; Rhode, 2011).

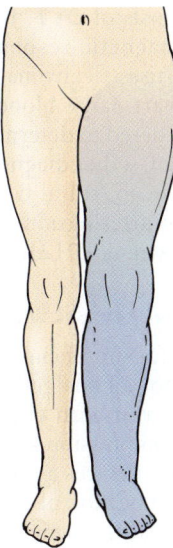

Figure 16-4 Deep venous thrombophlebitis.

 Cultural Diversity: Ethnicity and Factor V Leiden Mutation

Ethnicity influences coagulation patterns. Approximately 5% to 7% of North American Caucasians, 2% of Hispanics, and 1% of African Americans have a deficiency of coagulation inhibitors, termed the factor V Leiden mutation. Individuals need factor V to convert prothrombin to thrombin. Protein C inhibits the conversion of prothrombin to thrombin. Normally, protein C levels remain constant during pregnancy. When a factor V Leiden mutation occurs, protein C is lower than normal, and the body converts prothrombin to thrombin more readily. Women with factor V Leiden mutation have an increased risk for the development of a DVT during the puerperium (ACOG, 2011b; Cunningham et al., 2014).

PATHOPHYSIOLOGY

DVT develops from several key factors: a hypercoagulable state, venous stasis, and vein injury (Virchow's triad). A hypercoagulable state and venous stasis routinely exist in a normal pregnancy. Vessel injury can occur from trauma to an extremity, from birth events such as operative vaginal deliveries or cesarean births, and from simple invasive procedures such as an IV catheter insertion or venous blood sampling. Once vessel injury occurs, platelets begin to clump, then stick to one another. Thrombus formation follows.

SIGNS AND SYMPTOMS

Superficial venous thrombosis involves the superficial saphenous venous system. The most common form of postpartum thrombophlebitis, superficial venous thrombosis is characterized by pain and tenderness in the lower extremity. Deep venous thrombosis is more common during pregnancy and may extend from the foot to the iliofemoral region. It is associated with unilateral leg pain, calf tenderness, and swelling. However, up to 50% of all individuals with a DVT are asymptomatic. Signs and symptoms depend on the size, location, degree of vessel occlusion, and development of collateral circulation around the clot. The classic presentation of DVT involves pain, tenderness,

edema, redness, and localized heat. The presence of a palpable cord, changes in skin color ("milk" or "blue leg"), a decreased peripheral pulse, and a circumference that is 2 cm larger (or more) in the affected extremity assists in the DVT diagnosis (Fig. 16-4). Dorsiflexing the woman's foot while her knee is extended may elicit a positive Homans' sign (resistance or discomfort in the calf or popliteal region) in the presence of thrombophlebitis and thrombosis. However, there are other causes of calf pain upon dorsiflexion such as strained muscles and contusions, and a positive Homans' sign is indicative of DVT in only around 50% of patients. Thus, a negative Homans' sign does not rule out DVT (Cunningham et al., 2014).

 Nursing Insight—Recognizing signs and symptoms indicative of DVT

Additional signs and symptoms that may be associated with DVT include elevated temperature, cough, tachycardia, hemoptysis, pleuritic chest pain, and increasing apprehension. The presence of dyspnea and tachypnea may signal pulmonary embolism. Pulmonary embolism is a complication of DVT that occurs when part of a blood clot breaks away and travels to the pulmonary artery, where it occludes the vessel and obstructs blood flow to the lungs. Iliofemoral venous thrombosis is manifested by coolness of the entire extremity, associated with edema and pain.

DIAGNOSTIC TESTS

Because pregnancy and the early postpartum period are frequently accompanied by various aches and lower extremity edema, the clinical presentation of thrombophlebitis and DVT may be difficult to identify. The venogram, an invasive test used to confirm deep vein thrombosis, is contraindicated in pregnancy. D-dimer (a product of the degradation of fibrin by the circulating enzyme plasmin) assays may be ordered, along with non-invasive diagnostic methods such as venous duplex ultrasonography (real-time imaging and Doppler flow studies) to establish the diagnosis of DVT. If the results of these tests are equivocal, **magnetic resonance imaging** (MRI) (a diagnostic test that uses electromagnetic energy to provide images of the heart, large blood vessels, brain, and soft tissues) may be ordered to determine the extent of any pelvic vein involvement. Other diagnostic tests include the ventilation-perfusion scan, spiral computed tomography scan, and pulmonary arteriogram (Cunningham et al., 2014, Pettker & Lockwood, 2012).

COLLABORATIVE MANAGEMENT

Routine interventions for superficial venous thrombosis include the administration of analgesics (nonsteroidal anti-inflammatory agents); rest with elevation of the affected extremity; graduated compression stockings or intermittent pneumatic compression devices along with increased fluid intake; and the local application of moist, warm packs. The nurse should ensure that the weight of the warmed pack does not rest on the leg, causing obstruction of blood flow.

clinical alert

Avoiding extremity massage when DVT is suspected

If DVT is present or suspected, it is essential to refrain from massaging the affected area. This action could loosen the clot and result in a pulmonary or cerebral embolism.

Possible nursing diagnoses and goals for the patient with DVT are presented in Box 16-6. The patient usually is given bathroom privileges for elimination needs. If the thrombosis is located in a deep vein, hospitalization for either IV or subcutaneous heparin therapy is generally required. The patient is usually placed on complete bedrest until the anticoagulation therapy is effective. IV heparin therapy is administered via infusion pump. Currently, the Activated Partial Thromboplastin Time (aPTT) is the laboratory test most commonly used to monitor unfractionated heparin therapy. The pregnant patient has a greater plasma volume and an increased renal clearance (because of increased blood flow to the kidneys). The combination of normally occurring heparin-binding proteins along with the breakdown of heparin often results in the need for higher doses of heparin during pregnancy. The primary purpose of heparin therapy is to prevent extension of the current clot and to prevent new clot formation (Meguid, 2011).

During hospitalization, the nurse needs to monitor the patient for any signs of unusual bleeding and make certain

that the antidote for heparin (protamine sulfate) is readily available. Vital signs should be measured at least every 4 to 6 hours, analgesics administered as needed, and circulation to the affected extremity checked during every nursing shift. The circumference of the affected extremity should be measured and recorded daily. As the therapy continues, the nurse should assist the patient in increasing her level of activity and in assuming self-care activities. Equally as important, the nurse must assess the patient and her family for signs and symptoms of depression, anger, or decreased attachment to the newborn. Many insurance companies require that the infant be discharged, even if her mother needs to stay in the hospital. Some families may choose to care for the infant at home during the first few postpartum days while the mother is acutely ill. This decision may negatively impact the new mother's ability to feed, care for, and bond with her infant and may also create family conflicts that require the assistance of a spiritual advisor, financial counselor, social worker, home health nurse, lactation consultant, or family therapist. All members of the health-care team need to encourage family involvement in the patient's care. If a family member can bring the infant to the hospital daily, the patient can be assisted in holding and caring for her infant, and maternal attachment can be promoted.

Warfarin sodium (Coumadin), an oral anticoagulant, is introduced before the patient's discharge, and during this time, the heparin therapy is tapered. The oral anticoagulant therapy (warfarin sodium) is continued for a minimum of 3 months after birth and is safe for lactating mothers. Use of this long-term therapy regimen mandates specific patient–family education and support from a variety of health-care providers. An important component of the discharge teaching conducted by the nurse, dietitian, or pharmacist includes a discussion about all medications, side effects, and potential interactions.

Optimizing Outcomes—Teaching patients about aspirin and anticoagulants

During discharge teaching, the nurse cautions the patient on anticoagulant therapy to avoid medications that contain aspirin (acetylsalicylic acid) and nonsteroidal agents such as naproxen and ibuprofen. Aspirin, which acts as an antiplatelet agent and prevents blood clotting, can lead to a prolonged clotting time and an increased risk of bleeding.

Collaboration in Caring—*Education about food–drug interactions*

The nurse, pharmacist, or dietitian can initiate patient and family education about food and drug interactions. Nurses do not always feel comfortable providing education on dietary topics, and the dietitian has the knowledge to discuss this information with the patient and her family. Likewise, the pharmacist has greater knowledge than the nurse about drug effects and side effects. A team approach works well with topics such as this one. Be sure to obtain an interpreter if needed and have written information available that the patient and her family can take home.

Box 16-6 **Possible Nursing Diagnoses for Thrombophlebitis and Thrombosis**

- Pain
- At risk for injury
- Altered peripheral tissue perfusion
- Altered family processes
- Self-care deficit
- Fear
- Altered individual/family coping

The nurse should emphasize the importance of follow-up care for laboratory tests and medication dosage adjustments. Avoiding trauma that may result in extensive bruising, using safe care practices to avoid bleeding, and instructing the patient and her family to be alert for signs that indicate the anticoagulation therapy is excessive are also important topics for instruction. Short-term referral to a home health nurse should be considered; the hospital nurse may need to mention the need for this referral to the physician.

Medication: Warfarin sodium (Coumadin)

(**war**-fa-rin)

Pregnancy Category: X

Indications: Prophylaxis and treatment of: venous thrombosis, pulmonary embolism, atrial fibrillation with embolization

Action: Interferes with hepatic synthesis of vitamin K-dependent clotting factors (II, VII, IX, and X)

Therapeutic Effects: Prevention of thromboembolic events

Pharmacokinetics: Well absorbed from the GI tract after oral administration. Crosses the placenta but does not enter breast milk. Protein binding: 99% binds to plasma proteins, thereby delaying the effects of warfarin.

Route and Dosage: Orally; dosage adjusted on the basis of international normalized ratio (INR) results (range is 2.5 to 10 mg daily)

Contraindications and Precautions: Drug–drug interactions occur with NSAIDs, diuretics, antidepressants, steroids, some antibiotics and antifungals, vaccines, vitamin K, and aspirin, which may increase the response to warfarin and increase the risk of bleeding. Chronic alcohol ingestion may decrease the action of warfarin; acute alcohol ingestion may increase the action of warfarin.

Cranberry products and herbal supplements such as anise, arnica, chamomile, clove, dong quai, fenugreek, feverfew, garlic, ginger, ginkgo, Panax ginseng, and licorice may increase the risk of bleeding; Saint John's wort decreases the effect of the medication. Ingestion of large quantities of foods high in vitamin K (e.g., green leafy vegetables, liver, and green tea) may antagonize the anticoagulant effect of warfarin.

Even after the drug is discontinued, its effects may continue for up to 10 days. Warfarin dosage must be individualized on the basis of prothrombin time results. The INR is now used for dosage adjustments. A normal INR is 2.0 to 3.5.

Adverse Reactions and Effects: Overdosage leads to excessive blood loss that may appear via gastrointestinal bleeding, bleeding from the gums, nosebleeds, petechiae, excessive bruising, excessive menstrual flow, hematuria, etc. The patient begins with heparin therapy for anticoagulation and transitions to warfarin. Because normal clotting factors circulate in the patient's bloodstream routinely, several days of both heparin and warfarin therapy may be required for the anticoagulant effect

Nursing Implications:
1. This drug is dangerous. The patient and family must receive detailed information regarding follow-up care and drug–drug, drug–herb, and food–drug interactions.
2. Instruct the patient to notify the doctor of excessive bruising, take warfarin at the same time each day, and to avoid activities that could result in a bleeding injury.
3. Be sure the patient receives instructions on foods to minimize or avoid. (Involve the dietitian.)
4. Instruct the patient to carry identification describing medication regimen at all times and to inform all health-care personnel caring for the patient before lab tests, treatment, or surgery.
5. Emphasize the importance of frequent lab tests to monitor coagulation factors.

Source: Data from Vallerand, A. H., & Sanoski, C. (2014). *Davis's drug guide for nurses* (14th ed.). Philadelphia, PA: F.A. Davis.

---

legal alert—Document family education

The importance of clear, concise, complete chronological documentation of all patient and family education cannot be overly emphasized. The current litigious society in the United States lends itself to lawsuits against all health-care providers. The nurse has primary responsibility for both routine/standard patient and family education as well as specialized education. If another health-care provider, such as a dietitian, social worker, or pharmacist, is involved in any aspect of patient and family education, the nurse should note this collaboration in the medical record as soon as possible.

PULMONARY EMBOLUS

The abrupt onset of chest pain, dyspnea, shock, diaphoresis, syncope, and anxiety in a patient with DVT signals a major complication, pulmonary embolus (PE). PE is a life-threatening emergency that results from the breakup of the clot with migration of pieces through the heart to the lungs. Emergency treatment for this potentially fatal complication involves the "ABC" response used for any cardiorespiratory event. The nurse should immediately call for assistance, administer oxygen, obtain the crash cart, and begin cardiopulmonary resuscitation if necessary. Both the physician and respiratory therapist are important responders. Assuming that chest compressions are not needed, the nurse should elevate the head of the bed and apply an automatic blood pressure machine, cardiorespiratory monitor, and pulse oximeter. If not already in place, a large-bore IV line must be started immediately, so that fluids, heparin, and pain medication (usually morphine) can be readily administered. Once stabilized, patients with a PE are routinely transferred to a critical care unit for further care.

If the PE occurs while the patient is still recovering from childbirth, ensuring care for the newborn and support for the patient's family are paramount. Until the patient's condition improves, limitations are placed on visitors. This arrangement usually means that the family can remain with the infant. In this situation, the postpartum nurse can debrief and provide explanations to the family about events and possible future care requirements. If the patient survives, both she and her family will need detailed instructions concerning the prevention of thrombus reoccurrence. They also need to understand that the patient is at a much greater risk for the subsequent development of a DVT, even in the absence of another pregnancy.

Now Can You—Discuss deep venous thrombosis?

1. Describe why the postpartum patient is at risk for development of deep venous thrombosis?
2. Discuss routine nursing care for the postpartum patient hospitalized with deep venous thrombosis? (Remember to include the baby and family in this answer.)
3. Develop a teaching plan for the postpartum patient who is discharged on warfarin?

Puerperal (Postpartum) Infections

DEFINITION AND INCIDENCE

Puerperal infection refers to a bacterial infection, usually of the endometrium (**endometritis/metritis**), that occurs within 28 days after miscarriage, induced abortion, or childbirth. The presence of fever often indicates puerperal infection. According to the U.S. Joint Commission on Maternal Welfare, postpartum febrile morbidity is defined as an oral temperature of greater than or equal to 100.4°F (38°C) on any two of the first 10 days postpartum or 101.6°F (38.7°C) or higher during the first 24 hours, taken by a standard technique at least four times a day. A fever of 102.2°F (39°C) or greater within the first 24 hours is often associated with severe pelvic sepsis, usually resulting from Group A or B *Streptococcus* (Cunningham et al., 2014) (Table 16-2).

Throughout the world, puerperal infection probably constitutes the major cause of maternal morbidity and mortality; in the United States, the postpartum infection rate is 1% to 8%, with a mortality of 4% to 8% from complications. Cesarean birth mothers have a greater incidence (5% to 15%) of postpartum infection than do mothers who give birth vaginally (1% to 3% incidence). If a cesarean birth mother experiences a prolonged labor prior to delivery, the incidence of postpartum infection increases to 30% to 35% (Duff, 2013).

 Optimizing Outcomes—**Educating patients about risk factors for puerperal infection**

The prevailing practice of shorter hospital stays after birth makes the nurse's role in educating the new mother and her family about signs and symptoms of postpartum infection vitally important. The nurse should alert the patient about antepartum or intrapartum events that are risk factors for the development of a postpartum infection and make certain the family understands the importance of promptly notifying their care provider if any symptoms occur.

TYPES OF PUERPERAL INFECTIONS

Infections during the puerperium most commonly involve the endometrium (endometritis), operative wound (cesarean incision; episiotomy), urinary tract, and breasts (**mastitis**). Septic pelvic thrombophlebitis may also occur.

Endometritis (Metritis)

During the immediate postpartum period, the most common site of infection is the uterine endometrium (Fig. 16-5). This infection usually starts at the placental site and spreads to encompass the entire endometrium (Duff, 2012). It presents with a temperature elevation over 101°F (38.4°C), often within the first 24 to 48 hours after childbirth, followed by tachycardia, uterine tenderness, subinvolution, and malaise. Heavy, foul-smelling lochia (a later sign that occurs when the entire endometrium is involved) is noted when anaerobic organisms are present; scant, odorless lochia is noted when beta-hemolytic *Streptococcus* is present. Because urinary tract infections can occur during any part of the pregnancy and puerperium, differentiating the various signs and symptoms is important. As noted in Tables 16-2 through 16-6, other infections are more likely to occur following discharge from the hospital. Therefore,

Table 16-2 Postpartum Infection: Endometritis			
Type of Infection	**Risk Factors**	**Onset**	**Signs and Symptoms**
Endometritis (inflammation and infection of the inner lining of the uterus) Incidence: vaginal birth 1%–3% and cesarean birth 10%–20%	Cesarean birth, prolonged labor, prolonged rupture of the membranes, PPH, multiple vaginal examinations, internal electronic FHR monitoring, low socioeconomic status, poor nutrition, young age, diabetes, prior genital infection, lapse in aseptic technique, anemia, smoking, nulliparity, operative vaginal delivery, poor postpartum perineal care	2–4 days following childbirth	Prolonged fever >100.4°F (38°C), heavy, foul-smelling lochia (later sign; signals anaerobic organisms) or scant, odorless lochia (signals beta-hemolytic *Streptococcus*), uterine or abdominal tenderness, chills, poor appetite, malaise, increased pulse rate, cramping pain, increased white blood cell count (WBC) (above 20,000–30,000 mm^3)

Sources: American Academy of Pediatrics & American College of Obstetricians and Gynecologists (2013); Cunningham et al. (2014); Duff (2013); Giraldo-Isaza, Jaspan, & Cohen (2011).

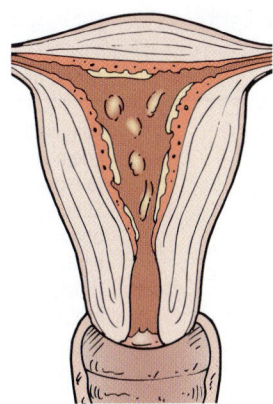

Figure 16-5 Postpartum endometritis.

follow-up in the home or clinic by a nurse or primary care provider may offer the first opportunity to identify infectious processes.

Mastitis

Mastitis is usually unilateral and develops after the flow of milk has been established. The most common causative organism is the hemolytic *Staphylococcus aureus*, introduced from the infant's mouth through a fissure in the nipple. Other, less common causes include *Haemophilus parainfluenzae*, *Haemophilus influenzae*, *Escherichia coli*, and *Streptococcus*. The infection involves the ductal system, causing inflammatory edema, enlarged axillary lymph nodes, and breast engorgement with obstruction of milk flow (see Fig. 16-6). Without treatment, mastitis may progress to a breast abscess. Symptoms include fever, malaise, and localized breast tenderness. Management centers on antibiotic therapy (e.g., cephalosporins and vancomycin), application of heat or cold to the breasts, hydration, and analgesics. To maintain lactation, the woman may empty the breasts every 2 to 4 hours by breastfeeding, manual expression, or breast pump. Because mastitis usually occurs after hospital discharge, an important component of nursing care includes teaching the breastfeeding mother about signs of mastitis and strategies to prevent cracked nipples.

 ### Nursing Insight—*Mastitis and methicillin-resistant Staphylococcus aureus (MRSA)*

Community-associated methicillin-resistant *Staphylococcus aureus* (CA-MRSA) infections have become increasingly more common in the United States. MRSA colonization is a frequent finding with pregnant women and is associated with cesarean and episiotomy incision infections and mastitis. Postpartum mastitis associated with MRSA is more likely to produce abscess and require longer recovery times, possibly because of the virulence of MRSA. Women who do not respond to first-line antibiotic therapy (e.g., trimethoprim-sulfamethoxazole, clindamycin, and rifampin) may require incision and drainage of the breast abscess, along with breast milk culture. Breastfeeding should continue on the affected breast although MRSA transmission via breast milk has been documented in term and preterm infants. Antibiotic treatment should be initiated in infants who test positive for MRSA (Guilbeau & Broussard, 2010; Harris & Fantasia, 2010; Rubolino-Gallego, 2010; Stuebe, 2014).

Causative Organisms	Diagnosis Based On	Collaborative Treatment	Prognosis and Complications
Normal vaginal flora, enteric bacteria, Herpes simplex virus, cytomegalovirus (in immunocompromised women), *Aerobes*: Group A, B, D streptococcus; enterococcus, *Staphylococcus* species, *Escherichia coli*; *Klebsiella pneumoniae*; *Proteus mirabilis* Anaerobes: *Chlamydia trachomatis*; *Peptostreptococcus;* Genital *mycoplasma; Clostridium* species; *Bacteroides* species	Clinical signs and symptoms Vaginal and bimanual examination Laboratory test results: culture of lochia; leukocytosis (white blood cell [WBC] count >20,000/mm³) (Must also rule out urinary tract infection)	1. MD/CNM: order antibiotics: a. broad-spectrum cephalosporin or penicillin is frequently used in mild to moderate cases; administered by IV route and changed to PO route 24 hours after there has been no temperature elevation. 2. Treat symptoms: a. Rest b. Antipyretics c. Increase fluid intake d. Encourage high protein, high vitamin C foods e. Promote uterine drainage via ambulation and Fowler's position f. Instruct in perineal care g. Surgical intervention (extreme cases) 3. Explain treatments to patient/family. 4. Home antibiotic therapy may need to be arranged with follow-up by a home care nurse. 5. Promote infant attachment	90%–95% improvement within 48–72 hours after treatment. May be discharged on oral antibiotics. *Complications:* Extension of infections via lymphatic system to connective tissues (pelvic infection) Dehiscence of cesarean section incision or episiotomy Peritonitis

Table 16-3 Postpartum Infection: Wound Infections

Type of Infection	Risk Factors	Onset	Signs and Symptoms for ALL
Wound infections Perineal Incidence: 0.35%–10% Cesarean incision Incidence: 3%–5%	Endometritis (infected lochia), poor hygiene, fecal contamination, hematoma ALL wound infections: obesity, diabetes, hypertension, immunosuppression, malnutrition, anemia, hemorrhage, prolonged labor, chorioamnionitis, prolonged rupture of the membranes, hematoma	Early: 48 hours Late: 6–8 days	Pain, foul-smelling discharge, edema, low-grade fever Sudden chills, high fever, abdominal tenderness, erythema, edema, warmth of incision, drainage from the incision

*Secondary intention: healing from the inside of the wound out to the skin.
Sources: Cunningham et al. (2014); Duff (2013); Harris & Fantasia (2010); Rhode (2011).

Table 16-4 Postpartum Infection: Urinary Tract Infections (UTI)

Type of Infection	Risk Factors	Onset	Signs and Symptoms
Urinary tract infections Incidence: 2%–4%	Catheterization, multiple vaginal exams, poor postpartum hygiene, genital tract trauma, epidural anesthesia, cesarean birth, premature rupture of the membranes, poor nutritional status, history of UTIs during pregnancy, diabetes, decreased bladder sensation following birth	Any time during pregnancy or after childbirth	May have none Dysuria (painful urination), frequency, burning on urination, difficulty voiding and/or urinary retention, costovertebral angle tenderness (CVAT), back or suprapubic pain, hematuria (blood in the urine); fever, fatigue, nausea, vomiting

Sources: Cunningham et al. (2014); Duff (2013).

Causative Organisms	Diagnosis Based On	Collaborative Treatment	Prognosis and Complications
Polymicrobial, normal vaginal flora *Staphylococcus aureus,* MRSA, aerobic streptococci, aerobic and anaerobic bacilli	Clinical signs and symptoms, subjective complaints. Clinical signs and symptoms, along with a poor response to antibiotics given for endometritis. Laboratory test results: leukocytosis	1. Antibiotics per order. 2. May require incision and drainage with placement of drain to facilitate healing by secondary intention.* If packing has been placed in the wound to keep it open and maintain drainage, alert the patient to exercise caution when changing her perineal pads to avoid dislodging the packing. 3. Perineal: sitz baths; instruct in perineal care. 4. Cesarean: wet to dry dressing changes 3+ times/day. 5. Pain medication per order (usually nonsteroidal anti-inflammatory drugs [NSAIDs]). 6. Instructions to patient and family about wound care. 7. Possible referral for home health or community health nurse visits.	Improvement usually within 24–48 hours; may require long-term antibiotic therapy. Complication: necrotizing fasciitis, abscess, wound dehiscence

Causative Organisms	Diagnosis Based On	Collaborative Treatment	Prognosis and Complications

Most common: *Escherichia coli* (60%–90% of all UTIs); *Proteus mirabilis, Klebsiella pneumoniae,* Group B hemolytic streptococcus, *Staphylococcus saprophyticus*	Clinical signs and symptoms. Laboratory test results: urine C&S, presence of leukocytes and blood on urine dipstick	1. Antibiotics per order (usually sulfonamides, aminopenicillins, anti-infectives, nitrofurantoin, or cephalosporins × 3–10 days depending on symptoms). Teach importance of taking all medication.
		2. Measure voidings for the first 24 hours, assessing for complete emptying of the bladder (each voiding should be ≥150 mL)
		3. Change peri-pads every 3 to 4 hours
		4. Encourage voiding every 3 to 4 hours; increased fluid intake (3,000 mL/day); and consumption of foods that increase acidity in the urine (e.g., cranberry juice, apricots, and plums).
		5. Encourage rest.
		6. Instruct in perineal care.
		7. Instruct in monitoring temperature, bladder function, normal appearance of urine.
		8. Instruct in/administer antipyretics, antispasmodics, analgesics, and antiemetics.
		9. Educate patient to avoid recurrence:
		  a. When intercourse resumes, void following.
		  b. Clean from front to back.
			Improvement within 48–72 hours following initiation of antibiotic therapy. Can reoccur with bacteremia and scarring of the kidney followed by hypertension and kidney damage

Table 16-5 Postpartum Infection: Mastitis

Type of Infection	Risk Factors	Onset	Signs and Symptoms
Mastitis	Milk stasis, plugged milk duct, infrequent breastfeeding, fatigue, nipple trauma, primiparity	2 to 4 weeks postpartum	Warm, tender, hardened area on breast (usually only one), a triangular flush underneath the affected breast is an early sign, enlarged axillary lymph nodes, fever (up to 102°F [38.9°C]), chills, generalized aching, headache, malaise

Source: Lawrence & Lawrence (2010).

Table 16-6 Postpartum Infection: Septic Pelvic Thrombophlebitis

Type of Infection	Risk Factors	Onset	Signs and Symptoms
Septic pelvic thrombophlebitis	Cesarean birth, prolonged labor with potential pelvic vein endothelial damage, lower extremity trauma, genital tract lacerations, history of varicosities, immobility, operative vaginal delivery, obesity, multiple vaginal exams, advanced age, infection/septicemia, inherited or acquired hypercoagulation condition	48 hours to 4–6 weeks postpartum; ovarian vein thrombophlebitis onset usually within 1 week	Fever >102.2°F (39°C) with spikes after initiation of antibiotic therapy, abdominal and/or back pain, chills, increased pulse (resting tachycardia), few or absent bowel sounds

Sources: Cunningham et al. (2014); Duff (2012).

Causative Organisms	Diagnosis Based On	Collaborative Treatment	Prognosis and Complications
Most common: *Staphylococcus aureus*; also: *Haemophilus parainfluenzae* (from infant's mouth and nose), *Candida albicans*, *Streptococcus viridans*	Clinical signs and symptoms Laboratory test results: culture of breast milk	1. Notify MD/CNM. 2. Initiate 10-day course of antibiotics 3. Continue breastfeeding (offer affected breast first) or manual/electrical expression of milk to maintain lactation, promote complete emptying, and prevent clogged ducts. May be instructed to discard the milk. 4. Promote rest. 5. Increase fluid intake. 6. Pump breast after infant feeding to ensure breast is empty. 7. Warm compress or ice to breast for comfort. 8. Antipyretics. 9. Instruct in high-protein, high-vitamin C diet. 10. Educate regarding hygiene and prevention of future recurrence. 11. Assess the infant's mouth for signs of thrush (oral *Candida*), an overgrowth of fungal organisms related to the mother's antibiotic therapy. 12. Isolate patient and infant from other nursing mothers and infants to prevent spread of infection.	Improvement within 24–48 hours following initiation of antibiotics Complication: breast abscess If breast abscess occurs: must discontinue breastfeeding on the affected side—may lead to decreased maternal–infant attachment, low self-esteem, and feelings of disappointment and guilt Frank abscesses require incision and drainage.

Causative Organisms	Diagnosis Based On	Collaborative Treatment	Prognosis and Complications
Normal vaginal flora and enteric bacteria—is usually an extension of endometritis	Clinical signs and symptoms Pelvic CT, MRI to confirm the clinical presentation Laboratory test results: CBC; coagulation profile; D-dimer assays; blood chemistries	1. MD/CNM: prescribe antibiotics. 2. Add heparin therapy to increase APTT (activated partial thrombo-plastin time) to 1.5–2 times the normal value. 3. Rest in Fowler's position 4. High-protein, high-vitamin C diet. 5. Increased fluids. 6. Comfort measures: pain medications, antipyretics. 7. Complementary therapies: heat, cold, relaxation, music, touch, etc. 8. Explain treatments. 9. Promote infant attachment.	Improvement usually within 48–72 hours of heparin initiation; may need to continue anticoagulant therapy for 6 months (7–10 days of heparin followed by warfarin [Coumadin]) Complication: Pulmonary embolism Possible decreased infant attachment; prolonged hospitalization

NURSING ASSESSMENT

Assessment is central to the delivery of safe, effective postpartal nursing care. Ongoing, careful attention must be paid to the patient's mental status and to her vital signs, breasts, fundus, lochia, incisions, and urinary status. Temperature elevation may be the first indication of an infection. If an elevated temperature is combined with any of the following signs and symptoms, the nurse must notify the primary care provider immediately: tachycardia, uterine or fundal tenderness or pain, foul-smelling lochia, an absence or decrease in lochia, chills, decreased appetite, malaise, elevated white blood cell count (WBC), back pain (costovertebral angle tenderness [CVAT]), generalized aching, headache, dysuria, urinary frequency or retention, wound drainage, erythema, and edema. Early, ongoing collaborative treatment can then be initiated.

 Optimizing Outcomes—Laboratory analysis to help identify a postpartum infection

To detect sources of puerperal infection, the nurse can anticipate that the following samples are likely to be obtained:

- Complete blood count (CBC) with differential
- Blood cultures if sepsis is suspected
- Urinalysis with culture and sensitivity
- Cervical, uterine, or wound culture as needed

COLLABORATIVE MANAGEMENT

All bacterial puerperal infections require treatment with antibiotics. The nurse can encourage rest and increased fluid intake and instruct the patient about the importance of increasing protein and vitamin C in her diet. In many hospitals, a nurse can refer a patient to a dietitian for instruction without a physician's order.

Comfort measures are as important in facilitating the patient's full recovery as the administration of antibiotics. Cool showers, sitz baths, warm compresses applied to the breasts, therapeutic touch and massage, soothing music, relaxation techniques, pain medications, and antipyretics are all strategies to promote patient well-being. Because of their anti-inflammatory effect, many physicians order a nonsteroidal anti-inflammatory medication to serve as an antipyretic and analgesic. Throughout the course of treatment, health-care team members also need to provide education to the patient and her family regarding her diagnosis and prognosis, treatment plan, measures to promote good hygiene, and follow-up care.

Although the infection may be easily treated and short lived, any postpartum complication can psychosocially affect a patient and her family. Prolonged treatment or hospitalization may create financial hardships, negatively impact family relationships and attachment with the infant, or result in psycho-emotional or spiritual crises. Referrals to the social worker, hospital chaplain or pastor, financial counselor, lactation consultant, community health nurse, or counselor need to be considered as an essential component of holistic care. As the health-care team member who is most consistently present, the nurse has a responsibility to help the patient and her family

Family Teaching Guidelines...
Prevention of Infection

- Wash your hands before and after going to the bathroom, when changing pads, changing the baby's diaper, etc. Hand washing with friction removes infection-causing microorganisms.
- Use a squeeze bottle with warm water to cleanse the perineum, pat the perineum dry, and remove and replace peri-pads from front to back. Front to back patting and peri-pad removal/application prevents bringing rectal organisms forward to the perineum and vagina.
- Change your peri-pad at least every 3 to 4 hours. A soiled peri-pad can encourage the growth of bacteria that can enter the urethra or vagina.
- Drink extra fluids (eight 8-ounce glasses of water) to increase urine production. The increased blood flow and urine production will decrease the stagnation of microorganisms in the urinary tract.
- Wash incisions with soap and water. Be sure to dry the incision completely. If necessary, use a hair dryer set on low heat to be sure the incision is dry. A dry incision is less likely than a wet one to promote bacterial growth.
- If breastfeeding, feed the infant every 2 to 3 hours and alternate feeding positions. Be sure the baby gets as much of the nipple and areola in his mouth as possible. These actions reduce the likelihood of injury to the nipple.
- For a breast infection to occur, a cracked or blistered nipple is necessary. To prevent this complication, wash the nipples with warm water and avoid soap, which can have a drying effect. Also avoid breast creams, which may block the natural oil secreted by the Montgomery tubercles on the areolae (the darkened area around the nipple). After breastfeeding the infant, allow your nipples to air dry and leave some breast milk behind on the nipples—the milk contains natural skin softeners.

ESSENTIAL INFORMATION:

- Notify your health-care provider if you develop pain, redness, or swelling at the site of any incision.
- Notify your health-care provider if you develop a fever of 100.4°F (38°C). (If you are breastfeeding, a temperature elevation to 100.4°F [38°C] may occur when your milk production begins).

identify when such referrals would be beneficial and to serve as an advocate to ensure that the patient receives these services.

 Across Care Settings: Care collaboration to prevent postpartum infection after discharge

If the postpartum patient is at risk for the development of a postpartum infection, the nurse needs to communicate this information to health-care providers and family members who may be involved in helping her after she goes home. Some hospitals routinely follow new mothers into the home

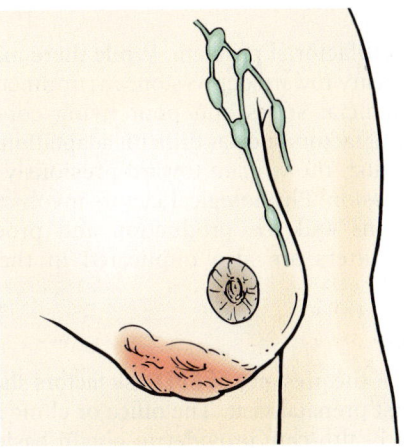

Figure 16-6 Mastitis usually occurs several weeks after childbirth. The axillary lymph nodes are enlarged, and there is a warm, tender, hardened area on the affected breast.

with a postpartum and newborn visit by a registered nurse. The lactation consultant or breastfeeding support group, newborn's physician, or public health nurse should also be notified of events during labor, birth, or postpartum that they should address the first time they see the new mother following discharge.

 Now Can You—Discuss infections that may occur during the puerperium?

1. List six risk factors for the development of a postpartum infection?
2. Describe nursing assessment findings that should be reported to the physician or nurse-midwife that indicate the patient has an infection?
3. Discuss ways the nurse can promote healthy family dynamics for the woman hospitalized with a postpartum infection?

Postpartum Psychosocial Complications

The focus on physiological recovery and health in the childbearing woman and her infant can easily result in an inaccurate assumption that all is well with the new family. Beyond the physical needs of the new mother lies a gamut of emotional, spiritual, relational, and socioeconomic concerns to which the nurse must be sensitive. Because most people consider childbearing a joyful time in life, the new mother who experiences negative emotions or who cannot cope with new demands on her time, energy, or priorities may struggle to recognize her need for help. Moreover, even if she recognizes her limitations and knows she needs help, the new mother may be reluctant to ask for help. Whether working in the hospital, in home care, in a clinic, or in a physician's office, the nurse can be a lifeline for the woman who experiences postpartum psychosocial complications. These complications include postpartum blues, depression, psychosis, panic disorder, and the long-term

sequelae from abusive relationships, homelessness, and access to care.

POSTPARTUM BLUES

Postpartum blues are common. Fifty to eighty percent of all postpartum women experience some degree of postpartum blues within the first 2 weeks after childbirth. Blues are usually self-limiting, last several days, and often peak by the end of the first week. Signs and symptoms include tearfulness, mood swings, anxiety, fatigue, sadness, insomnia, forgetfulness, and confusion (American Academy of Pediatrics [AAP] & American College of Obstetricians and Gynecologists [ACOG], 2013; Beck, 2008). Often, extra rest, reassurance, and therapeutic listening help to alleviate many of these issues. (See Chapter 15 for further discussion.)

POSTPARTUM DEPRESSION

Incidence, Definition, and Risk Factors

Fortunately, most postpartum women recover from the blues and are able to enjoy their newborns and families. However, 9% to 15% of postpartal women progress to postpartum depression (PPD). According to the American Psychiatric Association (2014), a diagnosis of depression requires that one of two symptoms exist most or all of the day: a depressed mood or decreased interest/pleasure in previously enjoyable activities. Recognized risk factors for PPD include an undesired/unplanned pregnancy, a history of depression, recent major life changes such as the death of a family member or moving to a new community, lack of family or social support, financial stress, marital discord, adolescent age, low self-esteem, and homelessness (Beck, 2001; Doucet, Dennis, Letourneau, & Blackmore, 2009).

 Collaboration in Caring—*Resources for the postpartal patient*

A woman who presents to the hospital with no prenatal care, gives birth, and prepares to go home should be closely screened for and warned about PPD. Often these women do not have the financial resources for perinatal care. They could also be homeless or lack social support. The nurse should ensure that the social worker is involved in the screening process. To facilitate ongoing care and follow-up for the new mother and her infant, appropriate community resources should be contacted and arrangements made before discharge.

Signs and Symptoms and Diagnosis

According to the American Psychological Association (2014), postpartum depression is a form of major depressive disorder that develops within 4 weeks postpartum, and the diagnostic criteria are otherwise identical to those applied to major depression. However, most experts now consider PPD to be any major depressive disorder occurring within the first 2 to 6 months postpartum, and some authorities extend this to 1 year postpartum. Symptoms of PPD resemble those of other depressions (Box 16-7). The difference between PPD and other types is that the depression affects not only the woman and her adult family

Box 16-7 Signs and Symptoms of Postpartum Depression	
Anorexia or weight loss	Excessive fears about the infant's health/safety
Insomnia/fragmented sleep	Feelings of worthlessness or excessive guilt
Fatigue or loss of energy	Negativity, irritability
Inability to concentrate	Complaints about "loss of self" and a "sense of loneliness" (Clemmens et al., 2004)
Anhedonia	
Withdrawal	Psychomotor retardation/agitation
Decreased self-esteem	Decreased interest and functioning in both self and infant care
Suicidal thoughts	Depressed mood almost every day for at least 2 weeks
Infant neglect or abuse	Recurrent thoughts of death

members, but also her newborn. The woman may have a decreased interest in the baby or may be overly concerned that "something bad" is going to happen to the baby. These fears may be expressed in a panic attack with hyperactivity and an inability to make decisions or prioritize. Male partners of women suffering from PPD report feelings of being anxious, depressed, overwhelmed, inadequate, fearful, isolated, stigmatized, and extremely frustrated. The combined negative effects of maternal and paternal depression on infant development place the child at risk (Beck, Records, & Rice, 2006; Paulson & Bazemore, 2010; Yawn, 2010a).

Children of depressed mothers have a greater likelihood of delayed psychological and cognitive development, and are at higher risk of avoidance and distressed behavior. Infants of depressed mothers who exhibit withdrawn, unresponsive, or negative behavior are more likely to be fussier, vocalize less, and make fewer positive facial expressions than infants of mothers who are not depressed. Because of the limited stimuli provided by the depressed mother and the restricted responses allowed to the infant, abnormal maternal–infant interactions can slow neurological growth and motor development. Children younger than 1 year whose mothers have experienced untreated PPD display cognitive and behavioral problems such as regressive and neurotic behaviors and insecure maternal attachment, and these difficulties continue through ages 4 to 8 years (Beck, Records, & Rice, 2006; Morgan, 2012; Yates, 2014; Yawn, 2010a).

The greatest barrier in diagnosing PPD lies in differentiating it from other types of major depression. Because the presenting symptoms are similar to those of other types of depression, and the onset of the symptoms varies within the first year after childbirth, PPD is often underdiagnosed. The reasons for this are varied. Many women believe that labile feelings are a normal part of adjusting to parenthood. They fear the stigma associated with a diagnosis of depression, as well as the possible negative consequences, such as the involvement of local Child Protective Services. In addition, the emphasis on physiological recovery frequently results in an unwillingness on the part of health-care providers and the woman's support systems to explore psychosocial concerns (Clemmens, Driscoll, & Beck, 2004; Doucet, et al., 2009; Weinberg, 2013; Yawn, 2010a).

Etiology

PPD is a multifactorial problem. While there may be a genetic propensity toward depression, environmental factors such as financial stress and poor living conditions or psychological factors such as difficult adaptation to parenthood may push the woman toward previously unexperienced depression. Physiological factors involving changes in endorphins and the production and processing of neurotransmitters are also implicated in the onset of depression.

Assessment

Screening for the presence of PPD risk factors should begin with the first prenatal visit. The office or clinic nurse may be the first health-care provider to obtain basic information, such as educational level, living conditions, financial stressors, whether the pregnancy was planned or unplanned, support systems available for the pregnant woman, and family involvement and attitudes of its members toward the pregnancy. If the nurse, physician, social worker, or other health-care team member identifies risk factors, these should be noted in detail on the prenatal record. If prenatal support groups are available, the woman should be referred to one of them in an attempt to minimize the risk for PPD.

The postpartum nurse needs to be aware of previously identified risk factors. A personal history of a mood disorder or a family history of a mood disorder, mood or anxiety symptoms during the prenatal period, and postpartum blues are factors that increase the risk for PPD. Moreover, as the nurse carefully assesses the new mother and her interaction with the baby, other risk factors may be noted. Some of these may include unmet pregnancy or labor and birth expectations resulting in feelings of failure, a delay in a prolonged sleep and rest period, and a demanding newborn without the presence of family members to help. A new mother's continued dependency on caregivers despite adequate sleep and apparent control of postpartum discomforts may constitute another signal that requires close observation. If the new mother does not respond to her infant's needs or demonstrate bonding or attachment behaviors, these actions require follow-up. The hospital nurse's primary responsibility is to detect comments or behaviors that need to be referred to the social worker, home health nurse, physician, chaplain, lactation consultant, and community agencies. It is important to recognize that, because of concerns that her lack of interest in her baby, sadness, and inability to cope may suggest that she is not a "good mother," the patient may be reluctant to discuss her symptoms (Yawn, 2010a).

If a home health nurse does not visit the newborn and mother within the first week, the well-baby checkup that follows 1 to 2 weeks after the hospital discharge may offer the first opportunity to assess the mother–baby dyad. In this setting, the nurse needs to be alert for subtle cues from the new mother, such as making negative comments about the baby or herself, ignoring the baby's or other children's needs, and the mother's physical appearance. Does she look unkempt or exhausted? Is the baby clean and dry? Does the new mother say something about needing more help at home? Did she come to the office or clinic with the baby (and other children) or by herself?

"What to say"—*Exploring the new mother's feelings*

In a private area, the nurse should take time to explore the new mother's feelings. A non-threatening way to open the dialogue might be to say: "Tell me how the first few days at home have gone." This statement provides the new mother with an opportunity to share both positive and negative impressions. Do not "fill the silence" if the new mother does not respond immediately. She may need to process her thoughts before speaking. Be aware, too, of nonverbal cues and body language, such as affect, eye contact, and open or closed posture.

If the nurse believes that the new mother is demonstrating signs and symptoms of PPD, several depression screening tools are available. These include the Edinburgh Postnatal Depression Scale, the Postpartum Depression Screening Scale, the Patient Health Questionnaire, and Beck Depression Inventory II. Because they are highly predictive, these scales are valuable tools that can be combined with the informal interview during a routine postbirth checkup (Beck et al., 2006; Schaar, 2011; Yates, 2014; Yawn, 2010b). Nursing diagnoses for PPD may incorporate psychological, circumstantial, and physiological factors (Box 16-8).

Collaborative Management

An important first step in the collaborative management of PPD involves ruling out a physical cause such as hypothyroidism. Once a physical cause has been eliminated, both traditional and complementary therapies can begin. Cognitive behavioral therapy (CBT) and interpersonal psychotherapy (IPT) have been shown to be beneficial in treating perinatal depression. CBT is an action-oriented approach that treats maladaptive thinking as the cause of pathological behavior and "negative" emotions. IPT is a treatment in which the woman is educated about depression and its symptoms and her relation to the environment, especially social functioning. Unlike some forms of psychotherapy, IPT does not focus on underlying personality structures (Yates, 2014). If the depressive symptoms are moderate to severe and do not respond to nonpharmacological treatment, the physician often prescribes a selective serotonin reuptake inhibitor (SSRI) or serotonin-norepinephrine reuptake inhibitor (SNRI) antidepressant. If the woman is experiencing sleep disturbances, tricyclic antidepressants may be useful (Cunningham et al., 2014; Weinberg, 2013; Yonkers, Vigod, & Ross, 2011) (Box 16-9).

Box 16-9 Medications Used to Treat Postpartum Depression

SSRIs	SNRIs	TRICYCLICs
fluoxetine (Prozac)	venlafaxine (Effexor)	nortriptyline (Pamelor)
paroxetine (Paxil)	duloxetine (Cymbalta)	imipramine (Tofranil)
sertraline (Zoloft)	doxepin (Sinequan)	

 Where Research and Practice Meet:
Mood Disorders During the Puerperium

Recent research has focused on various aspects of postpartum mood disorders. Horowitz and colleagues (2010, 2013) conducted a community-based, postpartum depression (PPD) screening initiative and nursing intervention (Communicating And Relating Effectively [CARE]) that included over 5,000 postpartum women. The Edinburgh Postnatal Depression Scale was used to screen the women at 4 to 6 weeks postpartum; those whose scores indicated risk for PPD and/or self-harm were referred for mental health referral and safety evaluation. The mothers were receptive to PPD screening (conducted by telephone and by mail), and the investigators suggested that their screening approach might be adapted to other methods such as an online implementation. Baisch, Carey, Conway, and Mounts (2010) discussed the benefits of a health marketing campaign targeted toward the general public and health professionals to improve screening for perinatal depression. Throughout their state, routine assessment of maternal mental health status was integrated into pediatric visits, an interdisciplinary collaboration was established between primary care providers, and a pathway for recommended screening, treatment, and support services for women experiencing prenatal and postpartum depression was developed and successfully implemented. Kuo, Yang, Kuo, Tseng, and Tzeng (2012), who investigated the trajectories of depressive and fatigue symptoms, found that mothers in the high-risk depressive symptoms group (determined by scores on the Edinburgh Postnatal Depression Scale) were most likely to fall into the high-risk group for fatigue (determined by scores on the Fatigue Continuum Form). Their findings supported the concept that depressive symptoms and fatigue are related, but distinct symptoms. Kurth et al. (2010) found that maternal health (physical complications) and mood problems (psychological decompensation and depression) in the immediate postpartum period were significantly associated with midwife-reported infant crying problems. The investigators recommended the development and implementation of clinical- and policy-level strategies to reduce maternal stress after birth, especially for first-time mothers. Foulkes (2011) conducted a qualitative study to explore the barriers and enablers identified by women (n=10) experiencing a postpartum mood disorder (PPMD) that preclude and facilitate their help-seeking behaviors. The women identified four main stressors that contributed to their development of a PPMD, two barrier categories, and an enabler category that influenced their help-seeking behaviors. The investigator concluded that pregnancy, birth, and becoming a mother represent a critical period of physical and emotional upheaval in a woman's life, and a holistic care approach that supports the emotional and physical health of the maternal–infant dyad is essential. Watkins, Meltzer-Brody, Zolnoun, and Stuebe (2011) found a significant relationship between negative early breastfeeding experiences and depressive symptoms at 2 months postpartum. Shade et al. (2011) summarized various statewide innovations to improve services for women with perinatal depression, McQueen, Montgomery, Lappan-Gracon, Evans, and Hunter (2008) in Canada described the development process of an evidence-based practice guideline for postpartum depression, and Schaar and Hall (2013) conducted a nurse-led initiative to improve obstetricians' screening for postpartum depression.

Box 16-8 Possible Nursing Diagnoses for Postpartum Depression

Ineffective coping	Situational low self-esteem
Compromised family coping	Compromised family coping
Anxiety	Injury to the newborn
Impaired parent/infant attachment	
Impaired parenting	
Hopelessness	
Impaired sleep pattern	

Each of the medication groups is associated with side effects, and all antidepressants pass into the breast milk. If the woman is breastfeeding, the physician and nurse must monitor both the desired effects on the mother and any possible undesired effects on the baby. Medication dosage adjustments may be necessary, and the pharmacological treatment needs to continue for at least 6 months, even if rapid improvement occurs. If the woman does not respond to medications or psychotherapy, electroconvulsive therapy (ECT) may be used for the most severe cases of PPD (Cunningham et al., 2014; Yonkers et al., 2011).

Complementary therapies for PPD are not to be discounted. These therapies enhance the effects of traditional treatments, but Snyder and Lindquist (2001) assert that "merely adding additional therapies to a system of care without implementing a holistic, caring approach to the care of patients will do little to improve health" (p. 1). Because many complementary therapies can be used without a physician's prescription, they can also empower the woman and her family in self-care and help them to feel that they are actively involved in the treatment plan.

Complementary Care: *Therapies for Postpartum Depression*

The nurse may be asked about various complementary therapies that may help new mothers and their families deal with PPD. Hypnosis enhances relaxation and an ability to focus on daily tasks. Exercise has been shown to increase levels of neurotransmitters that communicate with brain cells to increase feelings of euphoria. Saint John's wort (*Hypericum perforatum*) is an herb that has been approved in Germany for the treatment of anxiety and depression, skin inflammation, blunt injuries, wounds, and burns. It is believed to bind with neuroreceptors in the brain to prevent a response to the "depression" neurotransmitters. *Saint John's wort cannot be used in combination with SSRI antidepressants.* Biofeedback promotes relaxation and decreases anxiety; meditation helps the woman to focus on "being rather than doing," thereby relieving stress and tension; and humor has been shown to decrease anxiety, fear, tension, anger, and frustration and stimulate the immune system. Acupuncture, aromatherapy, bright light therapy, massage, and dietary calcium are other complementary therapies that may be beneficial for women with mild depressive illness (National Center for Complementary and Alternative Medicine, 2013; Yonkers et al., 2011).

Prognosis

The earlier that PPD is recognized and treatment begun, the better the prognosis for a full recovery. However, the woman must be prepared for a relapse should she choose to have another baby. A previous history of any type of depression places a woman at a 25% risk of PPD; those who experienced PPD with a previous birth have a 50% to 90% recurrence rate. Preconception counseling with a physician, nurse, social worker, or spiritual advisor and the initiation of antidepressants early in the pregnancy (after the first trimester) are preventative strategies (Yawn, 2010b).

POSTPARTUM PSYCHOSIS

Definition, Incidence, and Onset

Postpartum psychosis is a rare but severe form of mental illness that seriously affects not only the new mother but also the entire family. The incidence is low, occurring in 1 to 2 women per 1,000 births worldwide. Though rare, postpartum women have a 10 to 15 times greater risk of psychosis than they do at any other time in their lives. Its onset may be dramatic, often occurring within the first 24 to 48 hours following birth, but it always appears within the first 8 postpartum weeks. Women with preexisting psychosis, especially bipolar disorder, are at the greatest risk for postpartum psychosis, and there is increasing evidence to support the role of genetics in this mood disorder. First-time mothers, especially those who are older (ages 40–44) appear to be at increased risk of experiencing postpartum psychosis (Doucet et al., 2009; Monzon, Lanza di Scalea, & Pearlstein, 2014; Weinberg, 2013).

Postpartum psychosis may present with symptoms of PPD. However, the distinguishing signs of psychosis are hallucinations, delusions, agitation, confusion, disorientation, sleep disturbances, suicidal and homicidal thoughts, and a loss of touch with reality. This condition may also resemble a sudden manic attack. Mothers who are in a manic state require constant supervision when caring for their infant; they are frequently too preoccupied to tend to their infant's needs (Doucet, Letourneau, & Blackmore, 2012; Tormoehlen & Lessick, 2011).

Across Care Settings: Recognizing behavioral cues that signal postpartum psychosis

When providing hospital and community care for postpartum women, the nurse and other health-care professionals should be alert to behavioral cues that may signal psychosis:

- Demonstrates hyperactivity, agitation, confusion, or suspiciousness
- Reports auditory hallucinations to inflict harm to the infant
- Voices delusions that the infant is dead or defective or the birth did not occur
- Voices excessive complaints
- Exhibits obsessive concerns about the baby's health and welfare

Collaborative Management

Infanticide (the killing of an infant) is as high as 4% in women with postpartum psychosis. Because of this danger and the loss of touch with reality, postpartum psychosis is a true emergency. The woman must be hospitalized, and mental health experts must become involved in her care as quickly as possible. Immediate treatment usually includes a mood stabilizer (e.g., lithium and valproic acid), antipsychotic medications (e.g., chlorpromazine, thioridazine, and trifluroperazine), and anti-anxiety medications (benzodiazepines—alprazolam, chlordiazepoxide, diazepam). If required, ECT often leads to rapid improvement. Long-term psychotherapy and pharmacological treatment follows the immediate care (Adams, Holland, & Urban, 2013; American College of Obstetricians & Gynecologists [ACOG], 2007; Doucet et al., 2009; Rhode, 2011).

Women who are taking mood stabilizers need extensive counseling about the side effects associated with these medications. Patients on lithium must have serum lithium

Nursing Care Plan The Woman Experiencing Postpartum Depression

Nursing Diagnosis: Ineffective Coping related to multiple factors, including hormonal changes, addition of a newborn to the family, and time management constraints

Measurable Short-Term Goal: The patient will acknowledge that she is depressed and agree to participate in individual and family therapy.

Measurable Long-Term Goal: The patient will participate in activities she previously enjoyed and her affect will demonstrate positive feelings.

NOC Outcomes:
Depression Level (1208) Severity of melancholic mood and loss of interest in life events.
Depression Self-Control (1409). Personal actions to minimize melancholy and maintain interest in life events.

NIC Interventions:
Coping Enhancement (5230)
Counseling (5240)
Medication Management (2380)

Nursing Interventions:

1. Approach the patient in a calm, nonthreatening, and concerned manner.

   RATIONALE: This approach may encourage the patient to be open about her thoughts and feelings.

2. Ask open-ended questions and wait for a response.

   RATIONALE: Open-ended questions require more than a one-word answer, which may encourage verbalization. Waiting for an answer indicates that what she says is worth the silence.

3. Affirm the woman's feelings and allow her to cry should she desire.

   RATIONALE: These responses demonstrate genuine concern.

4. Notify the patient's primary caregiver about the patient's depressed affect.

   RATIONALE: Postpartum depression may require medication or therapy.

5. Provide information about postpartum depression and gently correct any misinformation or misconceptions the patient has about depression.

   RATIONALE: Correct information may instill hope and encourage the woman to continue therapy.

6. Provide instructions about medications (antidepressants) that may be ordered including effects on breastfeeding.

   RATIONALE: The patient needs to know the effects and side effects of medications so that she can report unusual symptoms and make an informed decision about breastfeeding.

7. Ask the patient what activities she no longer enjoys that were previously enjoyable.

   RATIONALE: This baseline information allows the nurse and the patient to establish some goals for therapy.

8. Involve the family in helping the patient cope with her feelings and assisting with infant care.

   RATIONALE: Involvement of the patient's support system helps the patient to know that she is not alone in her struggle with depression.

9. Help the patient/family establish an activity goal that she can achieve within the next week.

   RATIONALE: This intervention involves the patient in her care, allows her some control, and encourages her to focus on a positive action/behavior.

---

levels drawn every 6 months. Most antipsychotic medications can cause orthostatic hypotension and sedation, side effects that pose a major risk for mothers providing child care. Because the woman's thought processes may be altered, the nurse should share specific information about medication side effects with a close family member. If the mother wishes to breastfeed, some sources recommend that no pharmacological agents be prescribed, while others advise caution when prescribing some medications. Current recommendations are that although most medications pass into breast milk, there are very few instances in which breastfeeding must be discontinued (Pigarelli, Kraus, & Potter, 2011). The infant's daily dose of medications is less than the maternal daily dose. With lithium, however, serum concentrations in the infant may reach 50% of maternal levels. Thus, breastfeeding is usually discouraged in mothers who are taking lithium; the American Psychiatric Association considers lithium incompatible with breastfeeding (Fankhauser & Freeman, 2011). Long-term neurobehavioral effects on the infant related to exposure to psychotropic medications in breast milk are unknown.

Prognosis

Women with postpartum psychosis have a 15% to 50% chance of reoccurrence in future pregnancies (Monzon et al., 2014). These women are also at greater risk for a future psychotic event unrelated to pregnancy. Counseling and educational roles of the health-care team for these patients and their families are paramount to health promotion and maintenance.

 Nursing Insight—Posttraumatic stress disorder during the puerperium

Posttraumatic stress disorder (PTSD) is a psychological reaction occurring after experiencing a highly stressful event (e.g., wartime combat, physical violence, or natural disaster) that may be characterized by depression, anxiety, flashbacks, recurrent nightmares, and avoidance of reminders of the event. According to Beck (2004), childbirth can qualify as a stressful, traumatic event; recent studies (Ayers, Harris, Sawyer, Parfitt, & Ford, 2009; Lev-Wiesel, Chen, Daphna-Tekoah & Hod, 2009; Polachek, Harari, Baum, & Strous, 2012) suggest that a prior history of life trauma can have an adverse effect on women's health and their childbearing experiences. Routinely screening all childbearing women for a past history of trauma can aid in the early identification of those who may be at increased risk of PTSD after childbirth and facilitate the initiation of early treatment.

 Now Can You—Discuss postpartum blues, depression, and psychosis?

1. State the difference between postpartum blues and postpartum depression?
2. Discuss what you would tell a woman with a history of postpartum depression about future pregnancies and the probable plan of care?
3. Describe the signs and symptoms of postpartum psychosis?

SUMMARIZING POSTPARTUM PSYCHOSOCIAL NURSING CARE

Perinatal nursing offers an opportunity to develop a therapeutic relationship with a woman and her family during one of the most vulnerable times in their lives. Most pregnancies are both planned and desired, but physiological and psychosocial adaptations to the pregnancy, birth, and expanded family present challenges that require maturity and flexibility. The nurse can become involved with the childbearing family during the first prenatal visit. As the pregnancy progresses, the nurse becomes increasingly familiar with the woman and her family's lifestyle, stressors, successes, disappointments, and challenges. The postpartum nurse is at a distinct disadvantage because of the limited time a woman remains hospitalized after birth. However, any nurse, regardless of care setting or time constraints, can develop an attentive ear and sensitivity. By doing so, the nurse is then able to promote health and well-being for the new mother, her newborn, and the family.

During the postpartum period, the nurse can provide information that stresses the importance of asking for help if the patient feels overwhelmed. Promoting care and activities that allow the new mother and her family to attach to the infant is vitally important. Examples of bonding-oriented nursing care include rooming-in, decreasing sensory stimuli so that the family can focus on one another, and limiting visitors (if the patient desires). The postpartum nurse should note negative comments the patient makes about herself, her family, or the newborn and encourage the patient to talk about her expectations for both herself and the family. If the pregnancy and birth were difficult, the patient may be disappointed in herself and "blame" the baby for the difficulties.

Moreover, if the patient is exhausted and requires extra rest, the nurse can help her inform her friends and family about this need. The nurse should give the patient permission to send her newborn to the nursery without feeling guilty, so that when she awakens, she can enjoy the newborn rather than becoming frustrated by his demands. It is paramount for the nurse to remain sensitive to patients who are not coping well in the hospital, and advocate for follow-up by a home health nurse or social worker.

After discharge, the nurse in the office or clinic can use waiting time for conversation and make note of any physical characteristics that may indicate the need for some respite time from the demands and responsibilities of parenthood. The nurse should become familiar with available community support services such as a Mother's Day Out to which the mother can be referred. It is also important to involve the collaborative team—the physician, lactation consultant, social worker, and spiritual advisor—in the patient's care.

Postpartum Nursing for Vulnerable Populations

While caring for women and their families after birth, the postpartum nurse may be informed about or discover that special needs exist. If the woman received prenatal care, the prenatal history and physical examination may contain information that indicates the patient is in an abusive relationship, is living in a homeless shelter, has no transportation, is a migrant worker, or did not initiate care until the second or third trimester. These social risk factors are of concern and always require follow-up. In addition, a woman who gives birth with no prenatal care requires support from health-care professionals to ensure that both she and her newborn will have their basic needs of food,

 Where Research and Practice Meet:
Supporting Mothers Who Experience Puerperal Psychosis

Doucet, Letourneau, and Blackmore (2012) conducted a qualitative study to explore the perceived support needs and preferences of women (n=9) with postpartum psychosis and their partners (n=8). Participant interviews revealed that couples that experienced postpartum psychosis looked to health professionals to provide reassurance and information on the illness, its management, and prognosis. The quality of support and interactions with staff varied, and the couples reported difficulty identifying and obtaining professional support upon discharge. All participants believed that support groups for postpartum illnesses would be beneficial in normalizing their experiences and in dissipating their feelings of isolation. Fathers were reluctant to identify personal support needs and had difficulty in asking for help from professionals and their own support network. The investigators suggested that clinical interventions are needed to address the support needs and aid in the recovery of families affected by puerperal psychosis.

clothing, and shelter met. Though many in the world view the United States as an international social welfare agency and wish to live here, some American citizens, visitors, and undocumented immigrants live in fear, poverty, poor health, or oppression. The nurse caring for childbearing women and their families has a mandate to address these needs whether these patients are in a hospital, clinic, or private physician's office.

VICTIMS OF ABUSE

Abuse can take several forms: physical, emotional, verbal, or sexual. Unfortunately, most often someone the woman loves is the perpetrator, and the abuse may take more than one form. Physical violence during pregnancy has far-reaching effects for the infant as well as the mother. Battery during pregnancy is associated with a greater incidence of low-birth-weight neonates, preterm birth, and neonatal death (ACOG, 2012). (See Chapters 9 and 11 for further discussion.) No stereotypes exist for women who are abused because the problem crosses all socioeconomic, ethnocultural, and educational lines. The National Network to End Domestic Violence and other researchers list multiple factors that place an individual at risk for committing intimate partner abuse and for being a victim of intimate partner abuse (Tables 16-7 and 16-8).

❝What to say❞—*Inquiring about intimate partner violence during pregnancy*

Physicians routinely screen pregnant women for gestational diabetes and pregnancy-induced hypertension. However, more pregnant women are battered by their intimate partners than the combined total of pregnant women who develop these physiological complications (National Network to End Domestic Violence, 2012). Regardless of the setting, the nurse caring for perinatal patients at any time before or after birth can initiate a conversation about intimate partner violence. Many victims want to tell someone about the

violence they are experiencing, but they must be asked directly. After establishing privacy, the nurse should be direct and say, "In this office, a part of our routine care is to ask about domestic violence. Do you currently feel safe with your partner? Have you been kicked, hit, slapped, or otherwise physically hurt within the last year? Do you have concerns about how your partner treats you emotionally or treats you sexually?" *Be sure to wait for the answer to each question. Do not rush the answers.*

Cultural Diversity: Women of Color and Intimate Partner Violence

For women of color, many factors such as high rates of poverty, poor education, limited job resources, language barriers, and fear of deportation heighten their difficulty in finding help and support services. Underreporting of intimate partner violence and a failure to seek assistance may be related to various commonalities among women of color, such as the following (Women of Color Network, 2006):

- A strong personal identification based on familial structure or hierarchy, patriarchal elements, and cultural identity
- Religious beliefs that reinforce the woman's victimization and legitimize her abuser's behavior
- A fear of isolation and alienation
- A strong loyalty to the immediate and extended family; loyalty to race and culture
- A guarded trust and prevailing reluctance to discuss personal, private matters
- A fear of rejection from family, friends, the congregation and the community at large
- A mindset that personal needs should defer to family unity and strength
- An overall distrust of law enforcement

Table 16-8 Risk Factors for Being a Victim of Intimate Partner Abuse

Individual Factors	Relationship Factors
History of child abuse	Marital conflict
History of physical abuse	Marital instability
History of sexual abuse	Male dominance in the family
Prior injury from the same partner	Poor family functioning
Having a verbally abusive partner	Partner history of alcohol or drug abuse
Economic stress, low income	
Tobacco, alcohol, and illicit drug use	
Depression or suicide attempts	
History of sexually transmitted infections	
Young age (less than 24 years, especially adolescents)	
Lack of high school diploma	
Unplanned pregnancies (often as a result of birth control sabotage)	

Table 16-7 Risk Factors for Committing Intimate Partner Violence

Individual Factors	Relationship Factors
Young age	Marital conflict
Low self-esteem	Marital instability
Low income	Male dominance in the family
Low academic achievement	Poor family functioning
Aggressive or delinquent behavior as a child	Emotional dependence and insecurity
Alcohol or drug use	Belief in strict gender roles
Witnessing or experiencing childhood violence	Desire for power and control in relationships
Social isolation	Angry or hostile behavior toward a partner
Unemployment	

- A prevailing skepticism and distrust that shelter and intervention services are not culturally or linguistically competent
- A fear of the threat of deportation or separation from children

When a postpartum nurse determines that a postpartum patient and her infant are possibly returning to an abusive environment, several interventions can occur. The nurse must first confirm the suspicions by asking direct questions. If the patient confirms that she is a victim of intimate partner violence (regardless of the form), the nurse needs to immediately enlist the help of a social worker and a chaplain. These professionals are more knowledgeable about community resources such as safe houses, churches, and child protective services to which the patient can be referred. The health-care team can help empower the patient to have an action plan to escape the abuse at a later time, should she choose to delay this decision.

It is important to remember that if the patient chooses to return to the abusive environment, the nurse's role does not end. Follow-up after discharge may include a home visit or a well-baby checkup, during which time further interventions can occur. When a patient has only herself to think about, she may be less likely to take protective action. However, maternal instincts may empower the woman to protect her baby and other children from abuse or violence. Even if the nurse is only able to be a therapeutic listener, this role may allow the patient to rehearse her action plan, ask questions, share information, and affirm her decisions regarding the future.

Lack of personal contact does not mean that interventions cannot occur. McFarland et al. (2004) used telephone interviews to conduct a longitudinal study on abused women. After an initial personal contact with abused women to ask about inclusion in the study and to obtain informed consent, researchers contacted the women with either six intervention and four follow-up calls (experimental group) or four follow-up calls only (control group). During the phone calls, the interviewers asked women in the experimental group to answer yes or no to a series of safety-promoting behaviors. These behaviors included such actions as hiding money, hiding house and car keys, removing weapons from the house, asking neighbors to call police if violence begins, establishing a code with family and friends, and obtaining items such as birth certificates, important phone numbers, identification cards, and rent and utility receipts. The research findings indicated that women in the intervention group (those who received six additional phone calls) practiced more safety-promoting behaviors than did those in the control group and that the required nursing time was minimal. Such research findings are significant in supporting the important role that nurses and other members of the health-care team can have in helping victims of intimate partner violence take control of their environments and practice positive behaviors that can break the cycle of abuse.

UNDOCUMENTED IMMIGRANTS AND MINORITY HEALTH CARE

As a nurse provides care for postpartum women and their families, ethical and legal concerns inevitably arise. One of these issues often concerns undocumented immigrants and minority health. The United States continues to attract a cosmopolitan population and to be viewed as a haven for those in search of a better life. Not all who come to the United States seek American citizenship or a legal visa for employment purposes. In particular, citizens in states that border Mexico (i.e., Texas, New Mexico, Arizona, and California) routinely fund and provide care for undocumented immigrants. Wrongly, many Americans believe that the primary reason Latinos come to the United States is to receive free medical care, which can include delivering a baby in this country to have a United States citizen in the family. Findings from a Latino Decisions study of 400 undocumented Latinos (Latino Decisions/NALEO Educational Fund, 2013) revealed that more than 75% of undocumented Latinos identify one of two primary reasons for immigrating to the United States: economic opportunity or to build a better life for their families. Approximately 52% of Latinas said they migrated to the United States either to build a better life for their families or to reunite with loved ones.

Signed into law in 2010, the Patient Protection and Affordable Care Act calls for nearly universal health coverage for Americans but fails to extend such coverage to undocumented immigrants. The new legislation prohibits undocumented immigrants from purchasing private health insurance in newly formed state exchanges at full costs and receiving premium tax credits or cost-sharing reductions to help purchase insurance. Undocumented immigrants may still receive emergency care under the Emergency Medical Treatment and Active Labor Act (EMTALA) and Emergency Medicaid, but neither program provides adequate care. Beyond screening and stabilizing patients, EMTALA imposes no additional obligations on health-care facilities to provide care. Emergency Medicaid is only available to individuals who are so acutely ill that failure to receive medical attention would place their health in serious jeopardy. Both of these programs focus on providing care only when individuals are at their sickest and when the cost of treatment is at its highest (Elrington, 2010).

In response to passage of the health-care reform legislation, the American Nurses Association (ANA) leadership (2010) reaffirmed its position that all individuals living in the United States, including documented and undocumented immigrants, have access to health care and resolved that the ANA will educate nurses regarding the wideranging social, economic, and political ramifications of undocumented immigrants' lack of access to health-care services. The ANA continues to advocate that health reform be expanded so that all immigrants will have access to affordable care. Statistically, immigrant and minority women continue to have higher rates of disability and mortality, and their overall health status is lower than that of Caucasian women (Agency for Healthcare Research and Quality, 2010).

The nurse needs to provide unbiased, excellent care to all patients, regardless of immigration or minority status. A new mother and her family's immigration status or nationality does not change her needs or her family's need for compassionate, holistic, and quality care. If the patient has received minimal or no prenatal care, physical and psychosocial needs may be greater and may result in complications that require greater skill on the part of every involved individual. Direct care nurses are not primarily policy experts, nor do many desire this role. A vital factor in being able to provide ongoing perinatal care is to assure women and their families that they can trust those with whom they share information and concerns. While the United States and individual state politicians debate the financial implications and resources required to provide health care for those in this country who need it, the mandate for nurses is that they be one of the most valuable resources available to meet the needs of all new mothers and families for whom they care. Nursing is as much a "calling" as it is a profession.

 Now Can You—Discuss issues related to the care of minority and undocumented immigrant women?

1. State the most common reason undocumented immigrants come into the United States?
2. Describe a major nursing role when caring for immigrant and minority women?
3. State some potential outcomes for women and their babies who obtain minimal or no prenatal care?

HOMELESSNESS AND LIMITED ACCESS TO CARE

Women and newborns who are homeless and without an established health-care provider for follow-up constitute a particularly vulnerable population after childbirth. Better health-care outcomes are positively correlated with having a usual or principal source of care. African American and Hispanic American women are much less likely than others to have a primary source of care, and this population is also more likely to be uninsured (Partnership for the Homeless, 2012).

Often these same women are those who are homeless. Whether migrant workers who follow the crops they help to harvest or individuals with socioeconomic and interpersonal challenges, homeless women and their children represent a population that requires sensitive, skilled discussions, so that they can receive appropriate follow-up care. The fact that the pregnancy rate among homeless women is almost twice that of the general population (National Network for Youth, 2012) is a statistic that requires action. The *Healthy People 2020* (2012) indicators include access to prenatal care for all women as a major initiative.

Studies designed to address barriers to perinatal care have noted similar findings. The research of both Mikhail (1999) and Bloom, Bednarzyk, Devitt, Renault, Teaman, and Van Loock (2004) examined barriers among homeless, pregnant women (in California and Florida, respectively). There are several barriers pregnant, homeless women face when considering whether to begin or continue prenatal care (e.g., waiting time to see a practitioner, especially when compared with the time the practitioner actually spends with the patient; lack of transportation, care for older children, or encouragement to get prenatal care from family members; concern about having their children removed from their care; and finances). Women who give birth with late or no prenatal care are more likely to be teen-aged, multiparous, living with at least one child, less educated, uninsured, and

tobacco or recreational drug users. Most pregnant, homeless women surveyed did not intend to become pregnant. Ethnically, more American Indian, Alaska Native, African American, and Hispanic women are likely to bypass prenatal care than are their Caucasian counterparts (ACOG, 2013; Child Trends Data Bank, 2012).

If a woman presents to a hospital in labor and has not received prenatal care, EMTALA requires that a physician and hospital staff members deliver her baby and provide her and her newborn with care until they can be safely discharged. If it is determined that the mother is homeless, once again the nurse must solicit the help of the interdisciplinary team, including the social worker and chaplain. The physician caring for the mother and baby needs to satisfy legal requirements before discharging the patient and newborn. Often, the nurse needs to collect newborn urine and/or meconium samples for drug screening. If the hospital or birthing center employs a nurse who conducts a follow-up visit to check on the new mother and baby and immediate housing is available, the physician may elect to discharge them with an early visit arranged.

If the woman has absolutely nowhere to go after discharge, the nurse and others have an ethical and legal responsibility to ensure that the newborn is adequately fed and clothed. Child Protective Services, the United Way Agency, or church-affiliated social programs may be sources of help for this family. Immediate solutions are required. Longer-term arrangements will take additional resources and time. Ultimately, because the newborn is completely dependent on others for his needs to be met, the best situation for the baby often drives the final decisions.

POSTPARTUM CARE OF VULNERABLE POPULATIONS

Most commonly, postpartum nurses care for women and families who are functional and healthy (physically, psychosocially, and spiritually). If the nurse knows a couple or family who is unable to have children and who is exploring the option of adoption, handling dilemmas such as abuse or homelessness may be especially difficult. When a childbearing woman faces difficult challenges and requires additional support, her only source of this support may be the health-care community. Regardless of personal impressions, the nurse needs to be receptive to lessons that can be learned from this patient's situation. Most new mothers want the best life possible for their newborns. Armed with this fact, nurses can grow in their ability to understand and respond with sensitivity to all families for whom they care.

 Now Can You—Discuss strategies in caring for vulnerable populations?

1. List important members of the health-care team to involve in the continuum of care for vulnerable pregnant women or new mothers and their babies?
2. State a *Healthy People 2020* goal for pregnant women?
3. List characteristics of pregnant women who are most unlikely to get prenatal care?

Summary Points

◆ Postpartum hemorrhage may occur early (within the first 24 hours after birth) or late (after the first 24 hours but within 12 weeks after childbirth).

◆ Thrombophlebitis is an inflammation of the venous circulation and blood clot formation that typically occurs in the lower extremities. Treatment involves analgesia, bedrest with elevation of the affected extremity, compression stockings or devices, application of moist heat, and anticoagulant therapy. If thromboembolic disease is suspected, the affected area should never be massaged because this action may cause dislodgement of the clot and the potential for a pulmonary embolism.

◆ Puerperal infections may involve the uterus, urinary system, incisions, and breasts. Each type of infection has common and unique risk factors, onset, signs and symptoms, causative organisms, and complications.

◆ Postpartum "blues" are common and usually self-limiting. Postpartum depression is a multifactorial problem that requires prompt assessment and intervention.

◆ Vulnerable populations include homeless, minority, and undocumented immigrant women, as well as those who are victims of abuse. Providing holistic, quality postpartal nursing care for vulnerable populations requires self-examination, sensitivity, and compassion.

Review Questions

Multiple Choice

1. As part of a postpartum woman's assessment, the perinatal nurse observes for signs and symptoms of hematoma formation. Which of the following is the most common anatomical site for a hematoma to form?
   A. Rectum
   B. Vulva
   C. Cervix
   D. Episiotomy site

2. The perinatal nurse promotes postpartum health and prevents infection with the inclusion of information about which concept?
   A. Good hand washing
   B. Early ambulation
   C. Minimal fluid intake
   D. Restricted protein intake

3. The perinatal nurse is providing information to a postpartum woman being discharged from the hospital on warfarin (Coumadin) therapy. Which drug would the nurse instruct the patient to restrict?
   A. Acetaminophen (Tylenol)
   B. Ibuprofen (Motrin)
   C. Prenatal vitamins
   D. Docusate sodium (Colace)

4. The perinatal nurse understands that a puerperal infection occurs within how many days after giving birth?
   A. 10 to 14
   B. 15 to 30
   C. Within 28 days
   D. Within 6 months

5. A nurse reads on a patient's chart that she has a clot in her superficial saphenous venous system. What condition should the nurse be prepared to treat?
   A. Pulmonary embolism
   B. Superficial venous thrombosis
   C. Deep venous thrombosis
   D. Uterine thrombophlebitis

6. A nurse is caring for a patient on IV heparin for a deep vein thrombosis. Which lab value should the nurse monitor as the priority?
   A. Hemoglobin
   B. INR
   C. PTT
   D. Platelet count

7. The nurse caring for postpartum patients understands that which of the following is the most common type of psychosocial disturbance seen in this population?
   A. Postpartum blues
   B. Postpartum depression
   C. Postpartum psychosis
   D. Postpartum mania

8. What teaching is important for the woman being treated with lithium for postpartum psychosis?
   A. Dental visits every 4 months
   B. Lithium levels drawn every 6 months
   C. Do not drink any citrus juices
   D. Use two types of birth control

9. The perinatal nurse is aware of the physical effects that maternal battering can have on a newborn. Which of the following is inconsistent with this knowledge?
   A. Low-birth-weight infant
   B. Preterm birth
   C. Neonatal death
   D. Prolonged labor

10. A perinatal nurse screens all patients for intimate partner violence. What technique is best when performing this screening?
    A. Asking direct questions about abuse
    B. Having the woman fill out a survey
    C. Scheduling a social worker to visit all new patients
    D. Distributing flyers that encourage reporting abuse

See Answers to End of Chapter Review Questions on DavisPlus.

REFERENCES

Ackley, B. J., & Ladwig, G. B. (2013). *Nursing diagnosis handbook: An evidence-based guide to planning care* (10th ed.). St. Louis, MO: Mosby.

Adams, M., Holland, L., & Urban, C. (2013). *Pharmacology for nurses: A pathophysiologic approach* (4th ed.). Upper Saddle River, NJ: Prentice Hall.

Agency for Healthcare Research and Quality (AHRQ). (December, 2010). *Health care for minority women: Recent findings.* Program Brief (AHRQ Publication No. 11-P005). Rockville, MD.

Al Kadri, H., Anazi, B., & Tamim, H. (2011). Visual estimation versus gravimetric measurement of postpartum blood loss: A prospective cohort study. *Archives of Gynecology and Obstetrics, 283,* 1207–1213.

American Academy of Pediatrics (AAP) & American College of Obstetricians and Gynecologists (ACOG). (2013). *Guidelines for perinatal care.* (7th ed.) Washington, DC: Author.

American College of Obstetricians and Gynecologists (ACOG). (2006). Postpartum hemorrhage. Practice Bulletin No. 76. (Reaffirmed 2013). *Obstetrics & Gynecology, 108*(4), 1039–1047.

American College of Obstetricians and Gynecologists (ACOG). (2007). Use of psychiatric medications during pregnancy and lactation. Practice Bulletin No. 92. (Reaffirmed 2012). *Obstetrics & Gynecology, 111*(4), 1001–1020.

American College of Obstetricians and Gynecologists (ACOG). (2011a). Thromboembolism in pregnancy. Practice Bulletin No. 123. *Obstetrics & Gynecology, 118*(3), 718–729.

American College of Obstetricians and Gynecologists (ACOG). (2011b). Inherited thrombophilias in pregnancy. Practice Bulletin No. 124. *Obstetrics & Gynecology, 118*(3), 730–740.

American College of Obstetricians and Gynecologists (ACOG). (2012). Intimate partner violence. Committee Opinion No. 518. *Obstetrics & Gynecology, 119*(2), 412–417.

American College of Obstetricians and Gynecologists (ACOG). (2013). Health care for homeless women. Committee Opinion No. 576. *Obstetrics & Gynecology, 122*(4), 936–940.

American College of Obstetricians and Gynecologists (ACOG). (2014). Preparing for clinical emergencies in obstetrics and gynecology. Committee Opinion No. 590. *Obstetrics & Gynecology, 123*(3), 722–725.

American Nurses Association. (2010). Nursing beyond borders: Access to health care for documented and undocumented immigrants living in the U.S. Retrieved from http://nursingworld.org/MainMenu Categories/Policy-Advocacy/Positions-and-Resolutions/Issue-Briefs/Access-to-care-for-immigrants.pdf

American Psychiatric Association. (2014). Depression. Retrieved from http://www.psychiatry.org/depression

American Psychological Association. (2014). *Postpartum depression.* Retrieved from http://www.apa.org/pi/women/programs/depression/postpartum.aspx#

Ayers, S., Harris, R., Sawyer, A., Parfitt, Y., & Ford, E. (2009). Posttraumatic stress disorder after childbirth: Analysis of symptom presentation and sampling. *Journal of Affective Disorders, 119*(3), 200–204.

Baisch, M .J., Carey, L. K., Conway, A. E., & Mounts, K. O. (2010). Perinatal depression: A health marketing campaign to improve screening. *Nursing for Women's Health, 14*(1), 21–33. doi:10.1111/j.1751-486X.2010.01504.x

Beck, C. T. (2001). Predictors of postpartum depression: An update. *Nursing Research, 50,* 275–285.

Beck, C. T. (2004). Birth trauma: In the eye of the beholder. *Nursing Research, 53,* 28–35.

Beck, C. T. (2008). *Postpartum mood and anxiety disorders: Case studies, research, and nursing care.* (2nd ed.). Washington, DC: Association of Women's Health, Obstetric and Neonatal Nurses.

Beck, C. T., Records, K., & Rice, M. (2006). Further development of the Postpartum Depression Predictors Inventory-Revised. *Journal of Obstetric, Gynecologic & Neonatal Nursing, 35*(6), 735–745.

Begley, C. M., Gyte, G. M. L., Devane, D., McGuire, W., & Weeks, A. (2011). Active versus expectant management for women in the third stage of labour. *Cochrane Database of Systematic Reviews,* 11. Art. No: CD007412. doi:1002/14651858. CD007412.pub3

Berg, C. J., Callaghan, W. M., Syverson, C., & Henderson, Z. (2010). Pregnancy-related mortality in the United States, 1998 to 2005. *Obstetrics & Gynecology, 106*(6), 1302–1309.

Bingham, D., & Jones, R. (2012). Maternal death from obstetric hemorrhage. *Journal of Obstetric, Gynecologic & Neonatal Nursing, 41*(4), 531–539. doi:10.1111/j.1552-6909.2012.01372.x

Bloom, K. C., Bednarzyk, M. S., Devitt, D. L., Renault, R. A., Teaman, V., & Van Loock, D. M. (2004). Barriers to prenatal care for homeless pregnant women. *Journal of Obstetric, Gynecologic and Neonatal Nursing, 33*(4), 428–435.

Brown, H. L., & Smrtka, M. (2011). Postpartum hemorrhage: Emergency management and treatment. *The Female Patient, 36*(9), 16–22.

Bulechek, G. M., Butcher, H. K., & Dochterman, J. M., & Wagner, C. (2013). *Nursing interventions classification (NIC)* (6th ed.). St. Louis, MO: Elsevier Mosby.

Child Trends Data Bank. (2012). Late or no prenatal care. Retrieved from http://www.childtrendsdatabank.org/?q=node/214

Clemmens, D., Driscoll, J. W., & Beck, C. T. (2004). Postpartum depression as profiled through the postpartum depression screening scale. *The American Journal of Maternal/Child Nursing, 29*(3), 180–185.

Corbett, N., Hurko, P., & Vallee, J. T. (2012). Debriefing as a strategic tool for performance improvement. *Journal of Obstetric, Gynecologic and Neonatal Nursing, 42*(4), 572–579. doi:10.1111/j.1552-6909.2012.01374.x

Cunningham, F. G., Leveno, K. J., Bloom, S. L., Spong, C., & Dashe, J. (2014). *Williams obstetrics* (24th ed.). New York, NY: McGraw-Hill Professional.

Della Torre, M., Kilpatrick, S. J., Hibbard, J. U., Simonson, L, Scot, S., Koch, A., et al. (2011). Assessing preventability for obstetric hemorrhage. *American Journal of Perinatology, 28*(10), 753–760. doi:10.1055/s .0031.1280856

Doucet, S., Dennis, C., Letourneau, N., & Blackmore, E. (2009). Differentiation and clinical implications of postpartum depression and postpartum psychosis. *Journal of Obstetric, Gynecologic & Neonatal Nursing, 38*(3), 269–279. doi:10.1111/j.1552-6909.2009.01019.x

Doucet, S., Letourneau, N., & Blackmore, E. (2012). Support needs of mothers who experience postpartum psychosis and their partners. *Journal of Obstetric, Gynecologic & Neonatal Nursing, 41*(2), 236–245. doi:10.1111/j.1552-6909.2011.01329.x

Duff, P. (2012). Maternal and perinatal infection–bacterial. In S. G. Gabbe, J. R. Niebyl, H. L. Galan, E. R. Jauniaux, M. B. Landon, J. L. Simpson, & D. A. Driscoll (Eds.), *Obstetrics: Normal and problem pregnancies* (6th ed., pp. 1140–1155). Philadelphia, PA: W.B. Saunders.

Duff, P. (2013). Maternal and fetal infections. In R. Creasy, R. Resnik, J. Iams, C. Lockwood, T. Moore, & M. Greene (Eds.), *Creasy & Resnik's Maternal-fetal medicine: Principles and practice* (7th ed., pp. 802–851). Philadelphia, PA: W.B. Saunders.

Elrington, S. (2010). Health Justice NYC: Leaving undocumented immigrants behind. Retrieved from http://healthjustice.wordpress.com/2010/07/27/leaving-undocumented-immigrants-behind/

Endler, M., Grunewald, C., & Saltvedt, S. (2012). Epidemiology of retained placenta. *Obstetrics & Gynecology, 119*(4), 801–809. doi: 10.1097/AOG.0b013e31824acb3b

Fankhauser, M., & Freeman, M. (2011). Bipolar disorder. In J. DiPiro, R. Talbert, G. Yee, G. Matzke, B. Wells, & M. Posey (Eds.), *Pharmacotherapy: A pathophysiologic approach* (8th ed., pp. 216–233). New York, NY: McGraw-Hill.

Foreman, S. (2014). Developing a process to support perinatal nurses after a critical event. *Nursing for Women's Health, 18*(1), 61–65. doi:10 .1111/1751-486X.12094

Foulkes, M. (2011). Enablers and barriers to seeking help for a postpartum mood disorder. *Journal of Obstetric, Gynecologic & Neonatal Nursing, 40*(4), 450–457. doi:10.1111/j.1552-6909.2011.01264.x

Francois, K. E., & Foley, M. R. (2012). Antepartum and postpartum hemorrhage. In S. Gabbe, J. Niebyl, H. Galan, E. Jauniaux, M. Landon, J. Simpson, & D. Driscoll (Eds.), *Obstetrics: Normal and problem pregnancies* (6th ed., pp. 415–478). Philadelphia, PA: W.B. Saunders.

Gabel, K. T., & Weeber, T. A. (2012). Measuring and communicating blood loss during obstetric hemorrhage. *Journal of Obstetric, Gynecologic & Neonatal Nursing, 41*(4), 551–558. doi:10.1111/j.1552-6909 .2012.01375.x

Giraldo-Isaza, M. A., Jaspan, D., & Cohen, A. W. (2011). Postpartum endometritis caused by herpes and cytomegaloviruses. *Obstetrics & Gynecology, 117*(2), 466–467. doi:10.1097/AOG.0b013e3181f73805

Guilbeau, J. R., & Broussard, L. P. (2010). Community-associated methicillin-resistant *Staphylococcus aureus* (MRSA): An overview for nurses. *Nursing for Women's Health, 14*(4), 311–316. doi:10.1111/j.1751-486X .2010.01561.x

Hansen, S. S., & Arafeh, J. (2012). Implementing and sustaining in situ drills to improve multidisciplinary health care training. Debriefing as a strategic tool for performance improvement. *Journal of Obstetric, Gynecologic and Neonatal Nursing, 41*(4), 559–570. doi:10.1111/j .1552-6909.2012.01376.x

Harris, A. L., & Fantasia, H. C. (2010). Community-associated MRSA infections in women. *The Journal for Nurse Practitioners, 6*(6), 435–441.

Horowitz, J. A., Murphy, C. A., Gregory, K. E., & Wojcik, J. (2010). A community-based screening initiative to identify mothers at risk for postpartum depression. *Journal of Obstetric, Gynecologic & Neonatal Nursing, 40*(1), 52–61. doi:10.1111/j.1552-6909.2010.01199.x

Horowitz, J. A., Murphy, C. A., Gregory, K. E., Wojcik, J., Pulcini, J., & Solon, L. (2013). Nurse home visits improve maternal/infant interaction and decrease severity of postpartum depression. *Journal of Obstetric, Gynecologic & Neonatal Nursing, 42*(3), 287–300. doi:10 .1111/1552-6909.12038

Johnson, M., Moorhead, S., Bulechek, G., Butcher, H., Maas, M., & Swanson, E. (2012). *NOC and NIC Linkages to NANDA-I and clinical conditions: Supporting critical reasoning and quality care* (3rd ed.). St. Maryland Heights, MO: Elsevier Mosby.

Kuo, S., Yang, Y., Kuo, P, Tseng, C., & Tzeng, Y. (2012). Trajectories of depressive symptoms and fatigue among postpartum women. *Journal* of Obstetric, Gynecologic & Neonatal Nursing, 41(2), 216–226. doi:10.1111/j.1552-6909.2011.01331.x

Kurth, E., Spichiger, E., Cignacco, E., Kennedy, H., Glanzmann, R., Schmid, M., et al. (2010). Predictors of crying problems in the early postpartum period. Journal of Obstetric, Gynecologic & Neonatal Nursing, 39(3), 250–262. doi:10.1111/j.1552-6909.2010.01141.x

Latino Decisions/National Association of Latino Elected and Appointed Officials (NALEO) Educational Fund. (2013). America's Voice Education Fund Undocumented immigrant survey, March, 2013. Retrieved from http://www.latinodecisions.com/blog/2013/05/10/gender-and-undocumented-immigrant-experiences/

Lawrence, R., & Lawrence, R. (2010). Breastfeeding: A guide for the medical profession (7th ed.). Philadelphia, PA: Saunders.

Lev-Wiesel, R., Chen, R., Daphna-Tekoah, S., & Hod, M. (2009). Past traumatic events: Are they a risk factor for high-risk pregnancy, delivery complications, and postpartum posttraumatic symptoms? Journal of Women's Health, 18, 119–125.

Lyndon, A., Lagrew, D., Shields, L., Melsop, K., Bingham, D., & Main, E. (2010). A California toolkit to transform maternity care: Improving health care response to obstetric hemorrhage. Sacramento, CA: California Department of Public Health.

McFarland, J., Malecha, A., Gist, J., Watson, K., Batten, E., Hall, I., & Smith, S. (2004). Original research: Increasing the safety promoting behaviors of abused women. American Journal of Nursing, 104(3), 40–51.

McQueen, K., Montgomery, P., Lappan-Gracon, S., Evans, M., & Hunter, J. (2008). Evidence-based recommendations for depressive symptoms in postpartum women. Journal of Obstetric, Gynecologic & Neonatal Nursing, 37(2), 127–136. doi:10.1111/j.1552-6909.2008.00215.x

Meguid, C. (2011). Best practice for deep vein thrombosis prophylaxis. The Journal for Nurse Practitioners – JNP, 7(7), 582–587. doi:10.1016/j.nurpra.2011.04.002

Meyer, G., & Lavin, M. A. (2005). Vigilance: The essence of nursing. The Online Journal of Issues in Nursing, 10(1). doi:10.3912/OJIN.Vol10No03PPT01

Mikhail, B. I. (1999). Perceived impediments to prenatal care among low-income women. Western Journal of Nursing Research, 21(3), 335–348.

Monzon, C., Lanza di Scalea, T., & Pearlstein, T. (2014). Postpartum psychosis: Updates and clinical issues. Retrieved from http://www.psychiatrictimes.com/special-reports/postpartum-psychosis-updates-and-clinical-issues

Moorhead, S., Johnson, M., Maas, M. L., & Swanson, E. (2013). Nursing outcomes classification (NOC) (5th ed.). St. Louis, MO: Elsevier Mosby.

Morgan, J. P. (2012). Postpartum depression in a primary-care setting. Clinical Advisor, 15(12), 28–40.

National Center for Complementary and Alternative Medicine (NCCAM). (2013). St. John's Wort and depression. Retrieved from http://nccam.nih.gov/health/stjohnswort/sjw-and-depression.htm

National Network for Youth. (2012). Pregnant and parenting unaccompanied youth. Retrieved from http://www.nn4youth.org/system/files/IssueBrief_Pregnancy_and_parenting.pdf

National Network to End Domestic Violence. (2012). About domestic violence. Retrieved from http://www.nnedv.org/resources/stats.html

Pacheco, L. D., Saade, G., Tyner, J., Clark, S. L., & Hankins, G. D. (2012). Obstetric hemorrhage: New insights. Contemporary Ob-Gyn, 57(6), 30–38.

Partnership for the Homeless. (2012). The Partnership's programs work to break the cycle of homelessness. Retrieved from http://www.partnershipforthehomeless.org/

Paulson, J. F., & Bazemore, S. D. (2010). Prenatal and postpartum depression in fathers and its association with maternal depression: A meta-analysis. Journal of the American Medical Association, 303(19), 1961–1969.

Pettker, C. T., & Lockwood, C. J. (2012). Thromboembolic disorders. In S. Gabbe, J. Niebyl, H. Galan, E., Jauniaux, M. Landon, J. Simpson, & D. Driscoll (Eds.), Obstetrics: Normal and problem pregnancies (6th ed., pp. 980–993). Philadelphia, PA: W.B. Saunders.

Pigarelli, D., Kraus, C., & Potter, B. (2011). Pregnancy and lactation: Therapeutic considerations. In J. DiPiro, R. Talbert, G. Yee, G. Matzke, B. Wells, & M. Posey (Eds.), Pharmacotherapy: A pathophysiologic approach (8th ed., pp. 1297–1312). New York, NY: McGraw-Hill.

Polachek, I. S., Harari, L. H., Baum, M., & Strous, R. D. (2012). Postpartum Post-Traumatic Stress Disorder symptoms: The uninvited birth companion. Israel Medical Association Journal, 14(6), 46–55.

Rhode, M. A. (2011). Postpartum complications. In S. Mattson & J. Smith (Eds.), Core curriculum for maternal-newborn nursing (4th ed., pp. 650–665). Philadelphia, PA: W.B. Saunders.

Rooger, M. A., & Silver, R. M. (2013). Coagulation disorders in pregnancy. In R. Creasy, R. Resnik, J. Iams, C. Lockwood, T. Moore, & M. Greene (Eds.), Creasy & Resnik's Maternal-fetal medicine: Principles and practice (7th ed., pp. 878–905). Philadelphia, PA: W.B. Saunders.

Rubolino-Gallego, M. L. (2010). Mastitis and MRSA. Advance for Nurse Practitioners, 18(3), 31–36.

Schaar, G. L. (2011). Is your new mom depressed (did you ask)? The Journal for Nurse Practitioners, 7(10), 879–880. doi:10.1016/j.nurpra.2011.08.001

Schaar, G. L., & Hall, M. (2013). A nurse-led initiative to improve obstetricians' screening for postpartum depression. Nursing for Women's Health, 17(4), 307–316. doi:10.1111/1751-486X.12049

Shade, M., Miller, L., Borst, J., English, B., Valliere, J., Downs, K., et al. (2011). Statewide innovations to improve services for women with perinatal depression. Nursing for Women's Health, 15(2), 127–136. doi:10.1111/j.1751-486X.2011.01621.x

Snyder, M., & Lindquist, R. (2001). Issues in complementary therapies: How we got to where we are. Online Journal of Issues in Nursing, 6(2), 1–7.

Stuebe, A. M. (2014). Enabling women to achieve their breastfeeding goals. Obstetrics & Gynecology, 123(3), 643–652. doi:10.1097/AOG.0000000000000142

Tormoehlen, K., & Lessick, M. (2011). Schizophrenia in women: Implications for pregnancy and postpartum. Nursing for Women's Health, 14(6), 484–495. doi:10.1111/j.1751-486X.2010.01595.x

Tucker, M. J., Berg, C. J., Callaghan, W. M., & Hsia, J. (2007). The Black-White disparity in pregnancy-related mortality from 5 conditions: Differences in prevalence and case-fatality rates. American Journal of Public Health, 97(2), 247–251. doi:10.2105/AJPH.2005.072975

U.S. Department of Health & Human Services (USDHHS). (2012). Introducing Healthy People 2020. Retrieved from http://www.healthypeople.gov/2020/about/default.aspx

Vallerand, A. H., & Sanoski, C. (2014). Davis's drug guide for nurses (14th ed.). Philadelphia, PA: F.A. Davis.

Watkins, S., Meltzer-Brody, S., Zolnoun, D., & Stuebe, A. (2011). Early breastfeeding experiences and postpartum depression. Obstetrics & Gynecology, 118(2), 214–221. doi:10.1097/AOG.0b013e3182260a2d

Weinberg, K. (2013). Postpartum depression. Advance for NPs & PAs, 4(10), 25–27.

Women of Color Network. (2006). Facts & Stats: Domestic violence in communities of color. Retrieved from http://womenofcolornetwork.org/docs/factsheets/fs_domestic-violence.pdf

Yates, J. (2014). Perinatal depression: What you can do to reduce its long-term effects. OBG Management, 26(2), 48-58.

Yawn, B. P. (2010a). Postpartum depression: Prevalence and considerations in screening. The Female Patient, 35(2), 41–45.

Yawn, B. P. (2010b). Postpartum depression: Office interventions. The Female Patient, 35(10), 48–54.

Yonkers, K. A., Vigod, S., & Ross, L. E. (2011). Diagnosis, pathophysiology, and management of mood disorders in pregnant and postpartum women. Obstetrics & Gynecology, 117(4), 961–977. doi:10.1097/AOG.0b013e3182118a7

Zelop, C. M. (2011). Postpartum hemorrhage: Becoming more evidence-based. Obstetrics & Gynecology, 117(1), 3–5. doi:10.1097/AOG.0b013e31820209bb

CONCEPT MAP

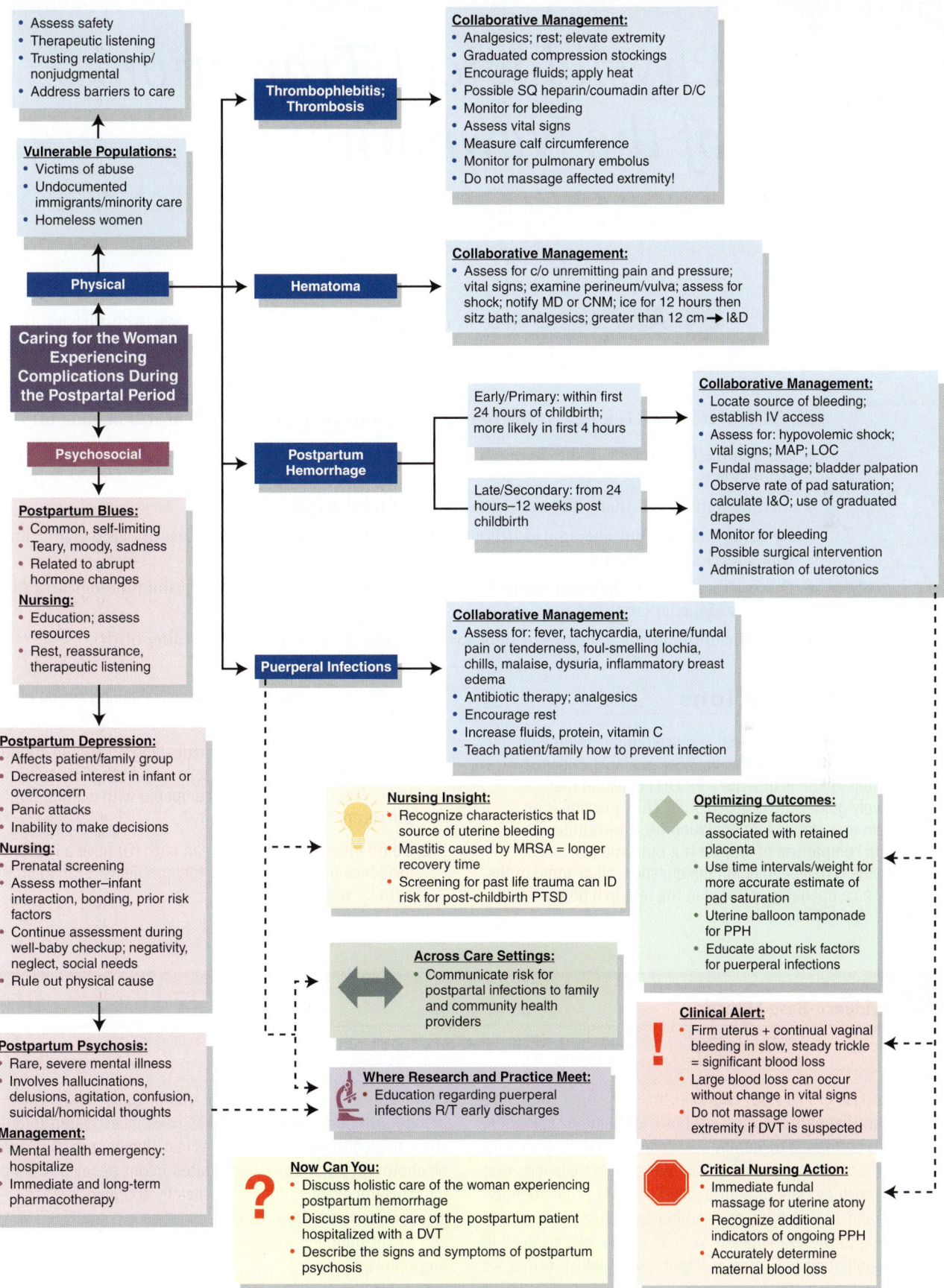

- Assess safety
- Therapeutic listening
- Trusting relationship/nonjudgmental
- Address barriers to care

Vulnerable Populations:
- Victims of abuse
- Undocumented immigrants/minority care
- Homeless women

Physical

Caring for the Woman Experiencing Complications During the Postpartal Period

Psychosocial

Postpartum Blues:
- Common, self-limiting
- Teary, moody, sadness
- Related to abrupt hormone changes

Nursing:
- Education; assess resources
- Rest, reassurance, therapeutic listening

Postpartum Depression:
- Affects patient/family group
- Decreased interest in infant or overconcern
- Panic attacks
- Inability to make decisions

Nursing:
- Prenatal screening
- Assess mother–infant interaction, bonding, prior risk factors
- Continue assessment during well-baby checkup; negativity, neglect, social needs
- Rule out physical cause

Postpartum Psychosis:
- Rare, severe mental illness
- Involves hallucinations, delusions, agitation, confusion, suicidal/homicidal thoughts

Management:
- Mental health emergency: hospitalize
- Immediate and long-term pharmacotherapy

Thrombophlebitis; Thrombosis

Collaborative Management:
- Analgesics; rest; elevate extremity
- Graduated compression stockings
- Encourage fluids; apply heat
- Possible SQ heparin/coumadin after D/C
- Monitor for bleeding
- Assess vital signs
- Measure calf circumference
- Monitor for pulmonary embolus
- Do not massage affected extremity!

Hematoma

Collaborative Management:
- Assess for c/o unremitting pain and pressure; vital signs; examine perineum/vulva; assess for shock; notify MD or CNM; ice for 12 hours then sitz bath; analgesics; greater than 12 cm → I&D

Postpartum Hemorrhage

Early/Primary: within first 24 hours of childbirth; more likely in first 4 hours

Late/Secondary: from 24 hours–12 weeks post childbirth

Collaborative Management:
- Locate source of bleeding; establish IV access
- Assess for: hypovolemic shock; vital signs; MAP; LOC
- Fundal massage; bladder palpation
- Observe rate of pad saturation; calculate I&O; use of graduated drapes
- Monitor for bleeding
- Possible surgical intervention
- Administration of uterotonics

Puerperal Infections

Collaborative Management:
- Assess for: fever, tachycardia, uterine/fundal pain or tenderness, foul-smelling lochia, chills, malaise, dysuria, inflammatory breast edema
- Antibiotic therapy; analgesics
- Encourage rest
- Increase fluids, protein, vitamin C
- Teach patient/family how to prevent infection

Nursing Insight:
- Recognize characteristics that ID source of uterine bleeding
- Mastitis caused by MRSA = longer recovery time
- Screening for past life trauma can ID risk for post-childbirth PTSD

Across Care Settings:
- Communicate risk for postpartal infections to family and community health providers

Where Research and Practice Meet:
- Education regarding puerperal infections R/T early discharges

Now Can You:
- Discuss holistic care of the woman experiencing postpartum hemorrhage
- Discuss routine care of the postpartum patient hospitalized with a DVT
- Describe the signs and symptoms of postpartum psychosis

Optimizing Outcomes:
- Recognize factors associated with retained placenta
- Use time intervals/weight for more accurate estimate of pad saturation
- Uterine balloon tamponade for PPH
- Educate about risk factors for puerperal infections

Clinical Alert:
- Firm uterus + continual vaginal bleeding in slow, steady trickle = significant blood loss
- Large blood loss can occur without change in vital signs
- Do not massage lower extremity if DVT is suspected

Critical Nursing Action:
- Immediate fundal massage for uterine atony
- Recognize additional indicators of ongoing PPH
- Accurately determine maternal blood loss

Physiological Transition of the Newborn

 A new baby is like the beginning of all things—wonder, hope, a dream of possibilities.

—Edna J. LeShan

LEARNING TARGETS *At the completion of this chapter, the student will be able to:*

- Explain the importance of the development of surfactant and its role in the successful transition of the neonate.

- Identify four factors that influence the initiation of respirations.

- Describe how the four anatomical structures that enable in utero survival must undergo significant transition following birth.

- Discuss thermogenic, hematopoietic, hepatic, gastrointestinal, genitourinary, immunological, and psychosocial adaptations in the neonate.

- Describe normal neonatal patterns of behavior during the first several hours after birth.

PICO(T) Questions

The intent of evidence-based practice (EBP) is to provide nursing care that integrates the best available evidence. An initial step in EBP is to write a PICO(T) question that effectively guides the research. A PICO(T) question is an acronym that stands for population (P), intervention or issue (I), comparison of interest (C), outcome (O), and timeframe (T). Depending on the question, all or some of the question components are used in the research process. Use these PICO(T) questions to spark your thinking as you read the chapter.

1. Do (I) initial attempts at breastfeeding (P) infants during the first period of reactivity following birth (O) result in fewer feeding issues (C) as compared with waiting until the second period of reactivity?

2. Do (P) infants born by cesarean birth (O) have a higher incidence of (I) initial respiratory problems (C) than infants born by vaginal birth?

 Evidence-Based Practice

Ganda, A. J., Ibrahim, L. F., Natchimutu, K., & Ryan, A. A. (2011). No more tears? Maternal involvement during the newborn screening examination. *Clinical Pediatrics, 50*(8), 753–756.

The purpose of this study was to examine the effect of maternal participation during the newborn screening examination, which is performed to identify abnormalities requiring medical intervention prior to discharge. Current evidence supports that factors such as state of arousal, feeding status, room temperature, and the amount of handling influence a newborn's response to the examination. Various procedures involved in the examination may prompt infant crying, which can upset the parents and interfere with the overall quality of the examination. Although previous studies have investigated infant stress related to painful procedures (e.g., lumbar puncture and phlebotomy), none have investigated infant behavior during the newborn examination. It is generally accepted that strategies such as nonnutritive sucking, speaking in a soothing voice, and infant bundling provide comfort to the newborn during procedures.

Evidence-Based Practice (continued)

Participants in this study included 34 full-term newborn infants whose births were uncomplicated. The pre-intervention group (n=20) was observed while receiving a traditional newborn examination; the post-intervention group (n=14) was observed after implementation of a pediatric residents' training session on the use of comforting techniques and maternal involvement. Specifically, the residents were taught about the use of comforting techniques to support the infant during the examination and instructed how to involve the infants' mothers throughout the examination. The mothers were shown how to provide support for the infant's head and encourage nonnutritive sucking, and instructed to speak in a soothing voice.

All of the 34 newborn examinations were video recorded by one independent observer. Two observers then examined the video recordings while using a modified Neonatal Behavioral Assessment Scale. The evaluations were completed independently and then compared for discrepancies in scoring; afterwards, average scores were determined. The length and duration of newborn crying during the examinations were recorded. The mothers of the infants in both groups also completed a 13-item questionnaire designed to evaluate their satisfaction with the performance of the newborn examination. Specific items included the appropriateness and length of the exam, the doctors' responses toward the mother (i.e., caring, respectful, and courteous), the mothers' feelings of calm and security during the examination, and the mothers' level of involvement in the exam and perceived ability to comfort the infant during the examination.

Data analysis revealed the following findings:

- The pre-intervention group was composed of 10 male and 10 female infants with a mean birth weight of 3,492 grams (7 lb 11 oz); the post-intervention group was composed of 5 male and 9 female infants with a mean birth weight of 3,660 grams (8 lb 1 oz).
- The average age of each group at the time of the examination was 15.8 hours (pre-intervention group) and 30.1 hours (post-intervention group).
- The mean duration of the examination was 10 minutes for the pre-intervention group; 9 minutes for the post-intervention group.

- On average, pre-intervention group infants cried for 82 + 56 seconds; post-intervention group infants cried for 18 + 34 seconds.
- The number and percentage of infants crying during specific portions of the exam were as follows: red reflex examination—5 infants (25%) (pre-intervention group); no infants (0%) (post-intervention group); auscultation of the heart—5 infants (25%) (pre-intervention group); 1 infant (7%) (post-intervention group); palpation of femoral pulses—8 infants (40%) (pre-intervention group); 4 infants (29%) (post-intervention group), Barlow-Ortolani hip test—8 infants (40%) (pre-intervention group); 4 infants (29%) (post-intervention group).
- Results of overall maternal satisfaction with the physicians' performance were equal in both groups: The physicians were perceived as friendly, courteous, and caring.
- Fifty-five percent of the pre-intervention group described their infants as "calm" during the examination; 86% of the post-intervention group described their infants as "calm" during the examination.
- Fewer than 45% of the mothers in the pre-intervention group agreed that they felt involved in the newborn examination, as compared with 100% in the post-intervention group, who stated that they felt involved in their infant's examination.
- Twenty percent of the mothers in the pre-intervention group reported that they felt that they had learned how to comfort their infant during the examination, as compared with 80% of mothers in the post-intervention group who believed that they had learned how to provide infant comfort during the examination.

The researchers concluded that when mothers are provided guidance on infant comforting techniques and the opportunity to actively support their infant during the newborn examination, maternal satisfaction is enhanced, and their infants cry less during the examination.

1. How is this information useful to clinical nursing practice?
2. Based on these findings, what are implications for further research?

See Suggested Responses for Evidence-Based Practice on Davis*Plus*.

Introduction

Once the umbilical cord is clamped and the infant takes the first breath, the transition from intrauterine to extrauterine life begins. Transition is one of the most intense and dynamic periods in the human life cycle. The transition from total dependence on another for every life-sustaining need from oxygenation and nutrition to total independence requires dramatic changes. For the neonate, the transitional phase may take minutes, hours, or days.

This chapter explores the physiological changes that take place in the newborn during the process of transition. Alterations that occur in each major body system are discussed, with emphasis on nursing assessment and interventions to facilitate a normal transition.

A & P review Normal Respiratory Function

The primary function of the respiratory system is twofold: the exchange of oxygen and carbon dioxide through respiration and maintenance of the acid-base balance.

The mechanical process of respiration is accomplished via the exchange of air between the lungs and the atmosphere (pulmonary ventilation). The two phases of pulmonary ventilation are inspiration and exhalation.

The physiological processes involved in pulmonary ventilation take place on three levels: external, internal, and cellular. External respiration is the exchange of gases (oxygen and carbon dioxide) between the alveoli and the blood through the alveolar–capillary membrane. Internal respiration is the exchange of gases between the systemic capillaries and the tissue at the cellular level. The cellular physiological process is the exchange of gases within the cell (Dillon, 2007). ◆

Adaptations of the Respiratory System

INTRAPULMONARY FLUID, FETAL BREATHING MOVEMENTS, AND SURFACTANT

After birth, the initiation of respirations is the first important step in neonatal transition. Many forces that occur during pregnancy and childbirth facilitate this essential process. The amniotic fluid plays an important role in fetal lung development. Inhalation of the amniotic fluid into the lungs helps to promote growth and differentiation of the lung tissue. Normal pulmonary functioning is dependent on two factors: the alternating in and out fetal breathing movements and the formation of intrapulmonary fluid.

 Nursing Insight—*Fetal breathing movements*

Breathing efforts are first initiated in utero as the fetus spends months practicing coordinated inhalation and exhalation movements. Fetal breathing movements can be observed by ultrasonography as early as 11 weeks of gestation. The breathing movements serve as an important mechanism that helps to develop the muscles of the chest wall and the diaphragm.

As the fetus approaches term, there is a decrease in the secretion of intrapulmonary fluid. The absorption of fetal lung fluid is accelerated during labor and delivery and for up to a few hours after birth. This fluid shift is an important physiological event: It assists in reducing the pulmonary resistance to blood flow (necessary while in utero) and facilitates the initiation of air breathing (Rozance & Rosenberg, 2012). During a vaginal birth, approximately one-third of the fetal lung fluid is expelled as a result of the "thoracic squeeze" that occurs during passage through the birth canal. Infants of cesarean births are at a higher risk for pulmonary transitional difficulties because they do not receive the lung compression benefits associated with a vaginal birth.

Lung expansion after birth stimulates the release of **surfactant**, a slippery, detergent-like lipoprotein. Surfactant causes a decreased surface tension within the alveoli, which allows for alveolar re-expansion after each exhalation. Under normal circumstances, by the 34th to 36th weeks of gestation, surfactant is produced in sufficient amounts to maintain alveolar stability (Goldsmith, 2010).

Many factors such as acidemia, hypoxia, shock, mechanical ventilation, and hypercapnia (an increased level of serum carbon dioxide) may interfere with surfactant metabolism. Surfactant production is decreased in infants of diabetic mothers (White's classification A, B, and C), infants with hemolytic disorders (e.g., erythroblastosis fetalis), and in multiple gestations. Conversely, surfactant production may be accelerated in other infants such as those of mothers with White's classification D, F, and R diabetes, hypertension, and heroin addiction. Fetal exposure to maternal infections and placental insufficiency may also accelerate the production of surfactant.

THE FIRST BREATH

Four factors influence the initiation of the newborn's first breath. These include internal stimuli: the chemical changes; and external stimuli: the sensory, thermal, and mechanical changes (Fig. 17-1). Each factor stimulates the respiratory center located within the medulla of the brain.

Chemical Factors

Chemical factors that initiate respirations are hypercarbia, acidosis, and hypoxia. These conditions, brought about by the stress of labor and birth, stimulate the respiratory center in the brain to initiate breathing. Hypoxia causes blood oxygen levels (P_{O_2}) and pH to drop. Subsequently, blood

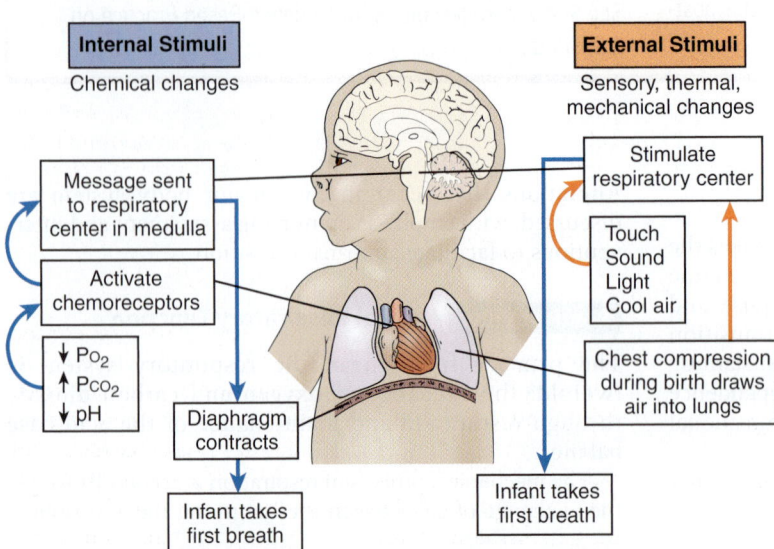

Figure 17-1 Chemical, sensory, thermal, and mechanical factors involved in the initiation of respirations.

carbon dioxide levels (P_{CO_2}) begin to rise and prompt the respiratory center within the medulla to initiate breathing. This brief period of asphyxia occurs in all newborns during the birth process. However, prolonged asphyxia that accompanies a traumatic birth is abnormal and may cause a central nervous system–mediated respiratory depression.

Sensory Factors

The newborn experiences a vast amount of stimuli when leaving a familiar, comfortable, warm environment to enter into an extremely sensory-overloaded one—filled with a multitude of tactile, visual, and auditory stimuli. These sensory experiences aid in the initiation of respirations.

Thermal Factors

After months of development in a warm (98.6°F [37°C]) fluid-filled environment, the newborn abruptly enters into a thermal environment that ranges from 70°F to 75°F (21°C–23.9°C). The drastic change in temperature helps to stimulate the initiation of respirations. Sensors in the skin respond to the temperature changes and send signals to the respiratory system in the brain. Physiological changes in the neonate's temperature may occur, and as long as the temperature remains within the normal range of 97.7°F to 98.6°F (36.5°C–37.0°C), no problems related to the thermal environment should develop. However, to prevent cold stress and respiratory depression, it is imperative for the nurse to immediately dry and either place the infant (skin-to-skin) with the mother or in a radiant warmer.

Mechanical Factors

Removal of fluid from the lungs with the subsequent replacement of air constitutes the primary mechanical factors involved in the initiation of respirations. The fetal chest compression that occurs during a vaginal birth increases the intrathoracic pressure and helps to push fluid out of the lungs. Recoil of the chest wall after delivery of the neonate's trunk creates a negative intrathoracic pressure. This facilitates a small, passive inspiration of air, which replaces the fluid that has been squeezed out.

 Nursing Insight—*Recognizing normal neonatal lung sounds during early auscultation*

Continuation of respirations occurs when the pressure within the neonate's lungs increases and pushes the remaining fetal lung fluid into the lymphatic and circulatory systems. Most of the fluid is reabsorbed within the first few hours, but in some infants this process may take up to 24 hours (Fig. 17-2). The neonate's lung sounds may sound moist during early auscultation but should become clear as the fluid is absorbed.

 Now Can You—**Discuss elements of pulmonary function in the neonate?**

1. Discuss why intrapulmonary fluid and fetal breathing movements are important for normal pulmonary functioning?

2. Explain why surfactant is important for respirations and identify two prenatal conditions that may be associated with a decrease in surfactant production?

3. Describe the four factors that are essential for the initiation of respirations?

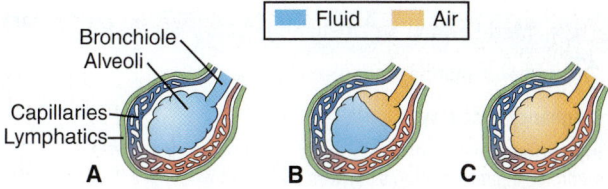

Figure 17-2 The process of absorption of fetal lung fluid once breathing has been initiated after birth. *A,* Before labor, alveolar fluid fills the lungs and circulates with amniotic fluid. During labor, air sacs and airways remain filled with fluid. *B,* During vaginal birth, the fetal thorax is compressed (thoracic squeeze) and approximately one third of the lung fluid is expelled. *C,* After vaginal birth, the neonate's first breath expands the lungs and fluid is displaced. Spontaneous respirations happen over the next 24 hours. Air displaces the remaining fluid, which is removed by the capillaries and lymphatics.

FACTORS THAT MAY INTERFERE WITH INITIATION AND MAINTENANCE OF RESPIRATIONS

A number of factors may interfere with the neonate's ability to initiate respirations. Conditions such as prematurity or birth asphyxia can adversely affect lung compliance (elasticity) and surfactant production. Childbirth events including trauma, maternal medications, and the mode of delivery can interfere with normal pulmonary transition.

Because of the low levels of surfactant normally present in infants less than 36 weeks' gestation, preterm infants are more likely to develop **respiratory distress syndrome** (RDS). RDS is a developmental disorder of the respiratory system that begins at birth or very soon afterward. It occurs most frequently in infants born with immature lungs. Lack of adequate surfactant leads to the sequelae associated with RDS: progressive atelectasis, loss of functional residual capacity, alterations in the ventilation perfusion ratio, and poor lung compliance (Cheffer & Rannalli, 2011; Thilo & Rosenberg, 2012). (See Chapters 18 and 19 for further discussion.)

When there is a strong likelihood that a preterm delivery will occur, the pregnant patient may receive tocolytic medications (inhibit uterine contractions) to postpone birth. The delay allows for the administration of glucocorticoids (e.g., betamethasone) to boost fetal lung maturation in an effort to improve the neonate's outcome. Betamethasone is given to the woman at least 24 hours before birth, if possible, to prompt the production of fetal surfactant and hopefully improve respiratory functioning in the neonate.

CARDIOPULMONARY TRANSITIONS

Cardiopulmonary adaptations must also occur during the transition from fetal to neonatal pulmonary functioning. As air enters the lungs, the P_{O_2} rises in the alveoli. This normal physiological response causes pulmonary artery relaxation and results in a decrease in pulmonary vascular resistance. As the pulmonary vascular resistance decreases, pulmonary blood flow increases, reaching 100% by the first 24 hours of life. The increased pulmonary blood volume contributes to the conversion from fetal to newborn

Medication: Betamethasone, Dexamethasone

(bay-ta-**meth**-a-sone), (dex-a-**meth**-a-sone)

Pregnancy Category: C

Indications: To prevent or reduce the severity of respiratory distress syndrome in preterm infants between 24 and 34 weeks of gestation (unlabeled use).

Action: Stimulates fetal lung maturation by promoting the release of enzymes that induce the production or release of lung surfactant.

Classification(s):
Therapeutic: Stimulates fetal lung maturation
Pharmacological: Glucocorticoids (corticosteroids)

Pharmacokinetics:
ABSORPTION: Preferred method of absorption is via injection.
DISTRIBUTION: Crosses the placenta; enters the breast milk.
METABOLISM AND EXCRETION: Metabolized in the liver and excreted by the kidneys
HALF-LIFE: 6.5 hours

Contraindications and Precautions: Contraindicated in women in whom there is a medical indication for delivery (e.g., severe preeclampsia/eclampsia, cord prolapse, chorioamnionitis, and abruptio placentae) and in women with systemic fungal infection.

Adverse Reactions and Side Effects: Seizures, headache, vertigo, hypertension, increased perspiration, petechiae, ecchymoses, facial erythema, maternal infection, pulmonary edema (if administered with beta-adrenergic medications). May worsen certain maternal conditions such as diabetes and hypertension.

Route and Dosage: Betamethasone 12 mg IM q24h × 2 doses
Dexamethasone 6 mg IM q12h × 4 doses

Nursing Implications:
1. Inform the woman of the benefit of medication and the need to administer to prevent RDS in her preterm infant.
2. Teach the woman the signs and symptoms of pulmonary edema; assess lung sounds.
3. Shake the suspension well; prolonged exposure to heat and light must be avoided.
4. Administer the medication into a large muscle; avoid the deltoid to prevent local atrophy.
5. Vital signs must be monitored frequently, and fetal monitoring should be performed according to institution policy.
6. Accurate intake and output must be monitored and recorded.
7. Monitor blood sugars if the woman is diabetic or at risk for diabetes.
8. Do not administer if the woman has an infection.
   NOTE: The FDA has not approved the medication for this use.

Source: Data from Vallerand, A. H., & Sanoski, C. A. (2014). *Davis's drug guide for nurses* (14th ed.). Philadelphia, PA: F.A. Davis.

provides one of the most important indicators of how well the neonate is making the transition to extrauterine life. Caucasian infants typically exhibit a central pink hue with **acrocyanosis**, a bluish coloration of the hands and feet that may persist for up to 24 hours until peripheral circulation improves. In dark-skinned infants, the mucus membranes provide a better indication of cyanosis than skin color.

The normal respiratory rate for a healthy term newborn is 30 to 60 breaths per minute. The breathing pattern is often shallow, diaphragmatic, and irregular. Abdominal movements should be synchronous with the chest movements. The breathing pattern may include brief pauses that last 5 to 15 seconds. Termed **periodic breathing**, this pattern is usually not associated with any change in skin color or heart rate, and it has no prognostic significance. **Apnea** is cessation of breathing that lasts more than 20 seconds. It is abnormal in the term neonate and may or may not be accompanied by changes in skin color or a decrease in the heart rate less than 100 beats per minute. Apnea should be reported immediately. Other indicators of respiratory difficulties include expiratory grunting and retractions when the neonate is at rest or a breathing rate that is outside the normal range.

Global Health Case Study Baby Girl Asta

Baby girl Asta is a 2-hour-old infant born at 40 weeks' gestation via a normal spontaneous vaginal birth. Her mother is a 20-year-old Scandinavian primipara who experienced an uneventful pregnancy and has a strong support system, which includes her 25-year-old Scandinavian husband. Baby Asta has remained with her parents in the birthing suite since her birth. Her mother expresses concern about Asta's hands and feet and asks the nurse why they are "bluish" in appearance, when the rest of Asta's body is nice and pink. She also states that, at times, Asta seems to "stop breathing."

critical thinking questions

1. What would you tell Asta's parents about the bluish appearance of Asta's hands and feet?

2. What would you tell the parents about Asta's breathing pattern?

♦ See Suggested Answers to Global Health Case Studies on Davis*Plus*.

Cardiovascular Adaptation

CHANGES AFTER PLACENTAL EXPULSION

Expulsion of the placenta following childbirth triggers important physiological events in the transition process. In utero, the placenta serves as the exchange organ for oxygen and nutrients and for the excretion of fetal waste products such as carbon dioxide. Maternal oxygenated blood enters the fetal circulation via the umbilical vein. Approximately 40% to 60% of the blood perfuses the fetal liver while the remaining volume of blood passes through the ductus venosus and enters the right atrium via the inferior vena cava.

During gestation, the placenta is the organ primarily responsible for gas exchange in the fetus although there is a small amount of blood flow to the lungs. As a "low resistance circuit," the placenta receives approximately 50% of the fetal circulation (Rozance & Rosenberg, 2012).

circulation (Fig. 17-3). Once the pulmonary circulation has been functionally established, blood is distributed throughout the lungs.

Although a variety of hemoglobins are present in the fetus and newborn, the most significant types are fetal hemoglobin (HbF) and adult hemoglobin (HbA). Because HbF has a greater affinity for oxygen than does HbA, the newborn's blood oxygen saturation is greater than that found in adults. However, there is less oxygen available to the tissues. Before birth, this situation is beneficial—the fetus must maintain an adequate oxygen uptake despite low oxygen tension levels because the umbilical venous Po_2 cannot exceed the uterine venous Po_2.

Assessment of the neonate's cardiopulmonary system must occur immediately after birth. Overall skin color

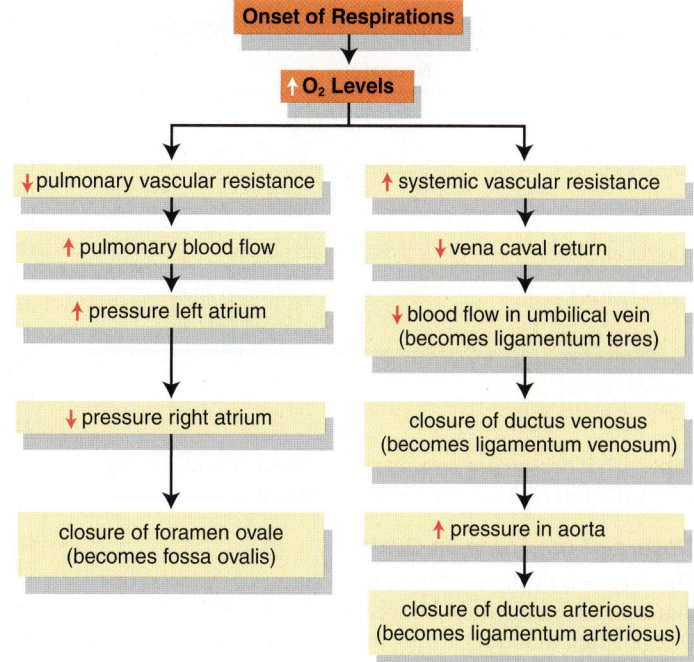

Figure 17-3 Major events that occur during the transition from fetal to neonatal circulation include closure of the foramen ovale, the ductus arteriosus, and the ductus venosus.

The fetal pulmonary circulation is a low flow, "high pulmonary resistance circuit" that receives only approximately 10% of the ventricular output (Thilo & Rosenberg, 2012). (See Chapter 7 for further discussion.)

After placental separation at birth, the umbilical arteries and vein constrict as the fetal circulatory system is interrupted. Successful cardiopulmonary adaptation in the neonate involves five major changes: an increased aortic pressure and decreased venous pressure; an increased systemic pressure and decreased pulmonary pressure; and closure of the foramen ovale, the ductus arteriosus, and the ductus venosus (Rozance & Rosenberg, 2012) (Fig. 17-4).

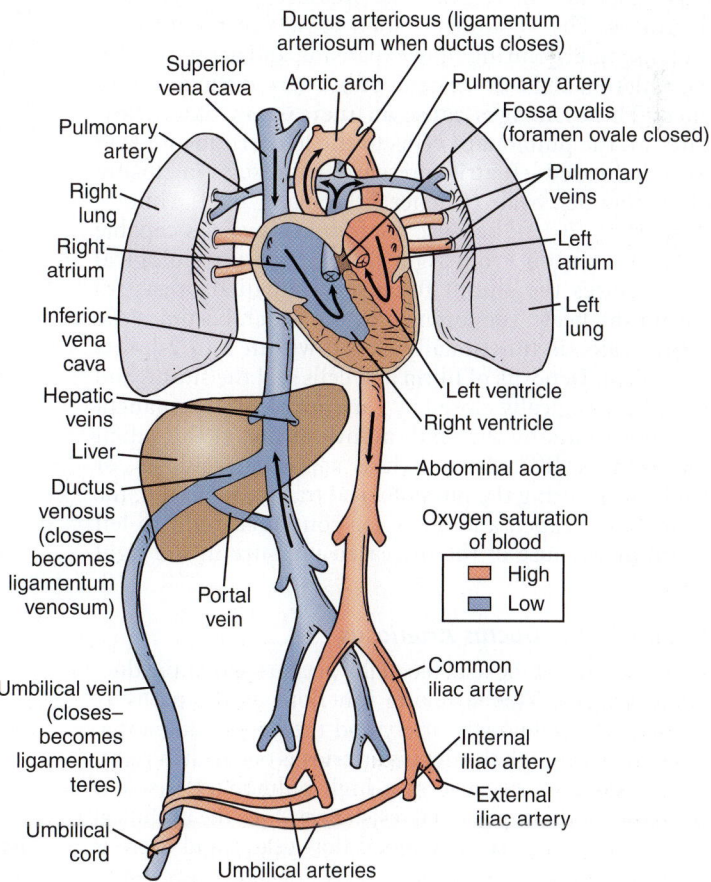

Figure 17-4 Neonatal circulation.

Table 17-1 Structural Changes in Circulation After Birth	
Fetus	**Neonate**
Umbilical vein	Ligamentum teres
Ductus venosus	Ligamentum venosum
Foramen ovale	Closed atrial septum
Ductus arteriosus	Ligamentum arteriosum
Umbilical artery	Superior vesical (bladder) artery Lateral vesicoumbilical ligaments

Table 17-1 presents a summary of the structural changes in circulation that take place in the neonate.

Closure of the Foramen Ovale

The foramen ovale is a flap in the septum of the fetal heart that allows blood flow between the left and right atria. Oxygen-rich blood returning to the heart from the inferior vena cava crosses from the right atria to the left atria across the foramen ovale. This pathway allows most of the oxygenated blood to bypass the nonfunctioning lungs and supply the aorta and vessels of the heart and head with oxygen. Blood flowing through the foramen ovale accounts for approximately one-third of the fetal cardiac output; less than 10% is used for lung perfusion (Beckmann, Herbert, Laube, Ling, & Smith, 2013).

The right-to-left shunting ceases once the umbilical cord has been clamped. The ventricular and aortic pressures in the left side of the heart rise. The systemic vascular resistance increases while pressure in the right side decreases. The pulmonary blood vessels respond to the increase in Po_2 during lung expansion and aeration with vasodilation and a decrease in pulmonary vascular resistance. These changes cause an increase in blood flow through the pulmonary veins to the left atrium and lead to an increased left atrial pressure that results in closure of the foramen ovale (Cheffer & Rannalli, 2011; Thilo & Rosenberg, 2012). Because the foramen ovale is capable only of shunting from right to left, this physiological event closes the shunt. Because of unequal pressures within the heart, the foramen ovale, which becomes the fossa ovalis, is functionally closed within 1 to 2 hours after birth. Deposits of fibrin and cells seal the shunt, and it is physiologically closed by 1 month of age. Permanent closure occurs by the sixth month of life. If the infant experiences difficulties such as asphyxia, acidosis, or cold stress during the physiological transition period, the shunt may reopen and allow for continued right to left shunting because of the increased pressure in the right atria.

Closure of the Ductus Arteriosus

In utero, most of the fetal blood flow occurs across the ductus arteriosus. This structure functions as the pathway between the pulmonary artery and the descending aorta. Blood flow through the ductus arteriosus occurs in a right-to-left direction because of a high pulmonary vascular resistance and low placental resistance. Once the umbilical cord is clamped, placental blood flow ceases and there is an increase in the systemic blood pressure and vascular resistance. At this point, the lungs oxygenate the blood and the increased PaO_2 stimulates the closure of the ductus arteriosus.

During pregnancy, the placenta produces prostaglandin E_2 (PGE_2), a hormone-like substance that causes vasodilation of the ductus arteriosus. After birth, declining PGE_2 levels contribute to the closure of the ductus arteriosus. In the neonate, a small amount of blood flowing through the ductus arteriosus may produce a soft murmur. When present, it can be auscultated at the left sternal border in the area of the second intercostal space. Considered innocent, the functional murmur occurs in the absence of any cardiac anomalies and is generally asymptomatic (Taylor, Wright, & Woodrum, 2011).

Functional closure of the ductus arteriosus in a term infant typically occurs within the first 72 hours of life. Once permanent closure occurs at 3 to 4 weeks, the structure is termed the **ligamentum arteriosum**. Permanent closure results from endothelial destruction, connective tissue formation, and subintimal proliferation (Thilo & Rosenberg, 2012).

The infant whose birth transition has been complicated by factors such as asphyxia or prematurity has an increased risk of a return to fetal circulation. This event results from continued blood flow through the partially opened ductus arteriosus (Fig. 17-5). Low levels of oxygenated blood flowing through the shunt cause it to dilate, creating a serious transitional complication (Thilo & Rosenberg, 2012).

Closure of the Ductus Venosus

The ductus venosus links the inferior vena cava with the umbilical vein. The umbilical vein delivers approximately 50% of the placental blood flow through the ductus venosus into the inferior vena cava and then mixes with the systemic venous drainage from the lower body. Blood flow through the left hepatic vein mixes with blood in the inferior vena cava and flows toward the foramen ovale. Oxygenated blood traveling through the umbilical vein enters the left ventricle and

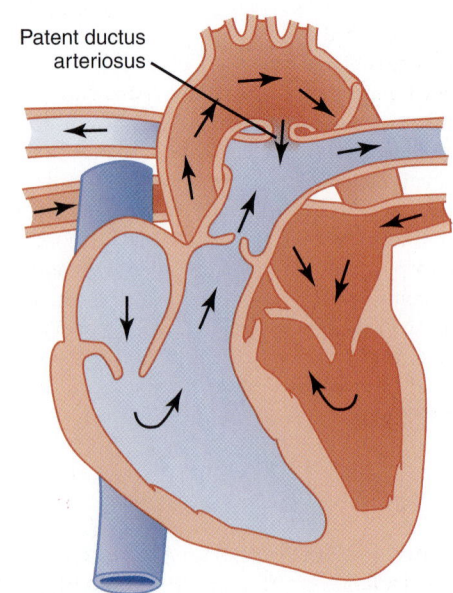

Figure 17-5 Patent ductus arteriosus.

supplies the carotid arteries with oxygen (Beckmann et al., 2013). Once the umbilical cord is clamped, cessation of umbilical venous blood return, along with mechanical pressure changes, leads to closure of the ductus venosus. Closure of the bypass route forces enhanced blood flow to the liver. Fibrosis occurs in the nonfunctional ductus venosus, and the structure, which is termed the **ligamentum venosum**, usually closes by the end of the first week.

 Now Can You—Discuss cardiopulmonary transitions in the neonate?

1. Explain characteristics of periodic breathing in the neonate?
2. Identify when the ductus venosus functionally closes?
3. Describe the physiological event that causes closure of the foramen ovale?

ASSESSING THE CARDIOVASCULAR TRANSITION

It is important to continually monitor the newborn's cardiovascular status during transition. Immediately after birth, the newborn's pulse rate may reach 160 to 180 beats per minute but during the first 30 minutes of life, the rate should decline to 120 to 160 beats per minute. This normal fluctuation occurs in response to the cardiovascular transition and the newborn's behavioral states.

On assessment, the systemic circulation is deemed adequate if the newborn exhibits a brisk capillary refill and stable blood pressure. Capillary refill in less than 3 seconds is considered adequate. A refill time greater than 4 seconds may be indicative of an underlying condition such as sepsis, hypoxia, or cardiovascular or central nervous system compromise.

 Across Care Settings: **Facilitating newborn transition in a birth center**

It is essential that the nurse who assists with an unexpected birth in a nonhospital setting such as a minor care clinic or physician office be able to recognize behaviors associated with normal and abnormal physiological transition in the newborn. Because resources outside the hospital are usually limited, the nurse must be alert to signs of transitional difficulties. As much as is possible, the environment should be manipulated to provide immediate care for the newborn during transition from the intra- to the extrauterine environment. After ensuring effective respirations, facilitating a neutral thermal environment is an essential nursing action. Ideally, a supply of warm, dry linens should be available to prevent neonatal cold stress. In the optimal situation, the nurse has time to evaluate the mother prior to delivery and can be alert to any potential maternal complications during childbirth. A reliable mechanism for the safe transport of the mother and her newborn to the hospital should be established as soon as possible. The nurse must manage care of the neonate and the mother until the transport team arrives.

Thermogenic Adaptation

Neonatal thermoregulation is essential for life-sustaining physiological adaptation. The newborn's ability to maintain a normal body temperature after birth is dependent on factors in the external environment as well as internal physiological processes. Newborns are characteristically **homeothermic**—that is, they attempt to regulate and maintain their internal core temperature regardless of varying external environmental temperatures.

THE NEUTRAL THERMAL ENVIRONMENT

Thermogenic adaptation is closely related to the infant's rate of oxygen consumption and metabolism. The **neutral thermal environment** (NTE) is the range of temperature in which the newborn's body temperature can be maintained with minimal metabolic demands and oxygen consumption. To maintain an NTE, the neonate may need to make certain vasomotor adjustments, such as vasoconstriction to conserve heat or vasodilation to release heat.

Factors such as the infant's body size and gestational age can affect the ability to maintain an NTE. Although the term newborn's protective subcutaneous fat helps to maintain a barrier for prevention of heat loss, neonates have less than half of the amount of subcutaneous fat normally present in adults. Preterm infants are born with very little adipose tissue and lack the muscle development needed to maintain a flexed position for heat conservation. Although full-term newborns have a large body area in relation to the total body mass, their normal position of flexion facilitates maintenance of body heat.

As the newborn transitions to extrauterine life, the core body temperature decreases in response to the environmental temperature. A term infant's core temperature can fall by approximately 0.5°F (0.3°C) per minute up to a total of 5.4°F (3°C) before ever leaving the birthing area. However, most term newborns are able to restore the initial decline in body temperature and stabilize at a normal (axillary) temperature of 97.7°F (36.5°C) to 98.6°F (37°C) within 2 to 3 hours after birth (Cheffer & Rannalli, 2011; Rozance & Rosenberg, 2012).

FACTORS RELATED TO COLD STRESS

Exposure to low environmental temperatures, especially for a prolonged period of time, causes an increase in oxygen consumption and an increased rate of metabolism. These metabolic events lead to cold stress. All newborns are at high risk for cold stress and ineffective thermal regulation because of the following factors:

- Large body area in relation to body mass
- Limited subcutaneous fat
- Limited ability to shiver
- Their skin is thin and their blood vessels are close to body surface

PHYSIOLOGICAL ADAPTATIONS FOR HEAT PRODUCTION

When the infant is exposed to a cold environment, several physiological adaptations help him to increase heat production. These include increasing the basal metabolic rate and muscle activity to generate heat, peripheral vasoconstriction to conserve heat, and **nonshivering** (or chemical) **thermogenesis** (NST) (heat production). Unlike children and adults, newborns are unable to shiver to generate heat. Instead, they must produce heat via NST, and this process becomes the key mechanism for maintaining a neutral thermal environment.

The sympathetic nervous system responds to skin receptors programmed to recognize a drop in the environmental temperature. Once low temperatures are detected, the receptors alert the sympathetic nervous system. Nonshivering thermogenesis uses the newborn's stores of **brown adipose tissue** (BAT) to provide heat in the cold-stressed newborn. Formation of BAT in the fetus begins at around 26 to 30 weeks of gestation. The deposits of BAT steadily increase until 2 to 5 weeks after birth unless they have been depleted by cold stress. Stores of brown adipose tissue are located in the midscapular area, around the neck, and in the axillae. Deeper deposits are found around the trachea, esophagus, abdominal aorta, kidneys, and adrenal glands (Fig. 17-6).

BAT, also known as "brown fat," is a unique highly vascular fat found only in newborns. BAT derives its name from the rich abundance of blood vessels, cells, and nerve endings that cause it to appear dark in color. The masses of brown fat cells accelerate triglyceride metabolism, triggering a process that produces heat. Rapid metabolism, along with the generation of heat, quickly sends heat to the peripheral circulation. However, fatty acids are released from metabolized BAT and can cause a life-threatening metabolic acidosis. When the elevated fatty acids are released into the bloodstream, the infant is at risk for jaundice caused by interference with the transport of bilirubin to the liver (Sedin, 2010).

⊖ **Optimizing Outcomes**—**Preventing cold stress in the newborn**

An important factor in neonatal resuscitation is the prevention of cold stress. Several body systems are affected when the infant has difficulty maintaining a normal temperature and becomes hypothermic. During nonshivering thermogenesis, the newborn metabolizes brown fat, a process that increases the metabolic rate and oxygen consumption. Over time, the newborn uses all available glucose and glycogen stores while attempting to maintain a neutral thermal environment. Utilization of the brown fat stores places the infant at risk for metabolic acidosis. Decreased oxygen causes peripheral vasoconstriction and increases the likelihood of respiratory distress. Peripheral vasoconstriction can lead to

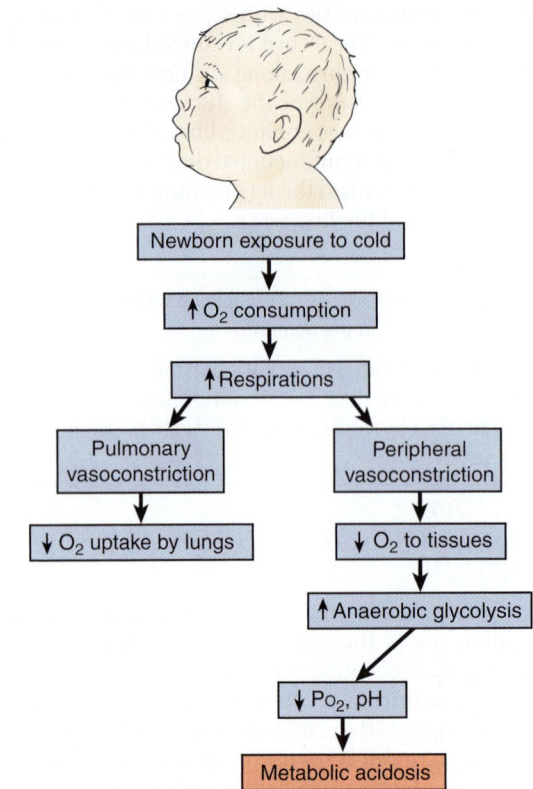

Figure 17-7 Metabolic events associated with cold stress in the neonate.

increased pulmonary vascular resistance and a return to fetal circulation as a compensatory mechanism. Elevated fatty acids can interfere with the transport of bilirubin to the liver and increase the risk of jaundice (Sedin, 2010) (Fig. 17-7).

MECHANISMS FOR NEONATAL HEAT LOSS

The nurse's role in preventing neonatal cold stress is critical. Supporting thermoregulation after birth allows the newborn to have a successful transition from intrauterine to extrauterine life. Thorough assessments of all of the newborn's systems should be aimed at maintaining a neutral thermal environment. The newborn has four mechanisms by which heat is lost after birth: evaporation, conduction, convection, and radiation (Fig. 17-8).

Evaporation

Evaporation is the loss of heat that occurs when water is converted into a vapor. If not adequately dried after birth, the neonate loses heat through the evaporation of amniotic fluid on the skin. This invisible process is termed **insensible water loss** (IWL). Nursing interventions geared toward preventing evaporative heat loss include thoroughly drying the neonate after birth, promptly removing wet linens, and immediately placing a hat on the head to prevent evaporation through the scalp.

Conduction

Conduction is the loss of heat to a cooler surface via direct skin contact. Conductive heat loss occurs when the infant

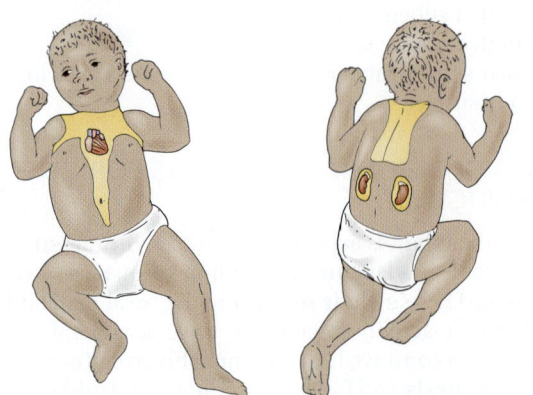

Figure 17-6 Sites of brown adipose tissue stores in the newborn.

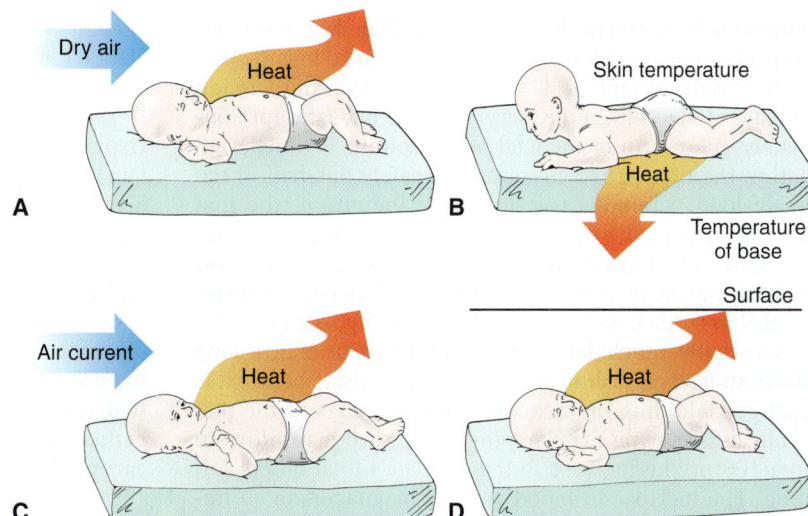

Figure 17-8 The four mechanisms of heat loss in the newborn. *A,* Evaporation. *B,* Conduction. *C,* Convection. *D,* Radiation.

is placed on a cold surface, such as a cold scale, mattress, or examining table. Nursing interventions to minimize conductive heat loss include placing the infant on a pre-warmed radiant warmer, using warmed blankets, covering scales with blankets prior to weighing, and avoiding the use of cold instruments (e.g., stethoscope). The newborn can also be placed skin-to-skin with the mother to facilitate body warming and bonding.

Convection

Convection is the loss of heat from the warm body surface to the cooler air currents. Convective heat loss occurs when the neonate is exposed to drafts and cool circulating air. The nurse can help minimize neonatal heat loss through convection by preventing drafts in the birth area (e.g., no ceiling fans) and by placing the newborn away from doors or windows. Also, depending on the environment, the neonate should be warmly clothed and possibly swaddled to prevent cooling from air currents.

Radiation

Radiation heat loss occurs when there is a transfer of heat between objects that are not in direct contact with each other. The walls of the nursery or the incubator may serve as potential sources of heat loss through radiation. Nursing interventions to prevent heat loss through radiation include having a prewarmed radiant warmer present at the birth, avoiding placement of the crib or incubator by a cold window, and keeping cold objects well away from the neonate.

PREVENTING HYPERTHERMIA

It is also important to prevent neonatal **hyperthermia** (elevated core body temperature). Although sweating is the full-term infant's initial response to elevated body temperature, the sweat glands are not fully functional until after the first month of life. Before that time, the body loses heat through peripheral vasodilation and the evaporation of IWL. An increase in oxygen consumption and the metabolic rate are associated with hyperthermia, and when severe, brain damage or death may result.

During the first few minutes of life, neonatal hyperthermia is most often associated with maternal fever. An elevated core body temperature can also result from an ambient environment that is too hot for the newborn to successfully maintain a neutral temperature. Other causes of hyperthermia include infection, central nervous system impairment, dehydration, and medications (Thilo & Rosenberg, 2012).

Radiant warmers, essential equipment in the birth area, must be monitored closely to ensure they are in proper working order with reliable heating mechanisms. Caution must be exercised with the use of servo-controlled radiant warmers because they may cause an undesirable elevation in the neonate's temperature if not monitored correctly. In addition, if programmed to maintain a set temperature, these units may mask the signs and symptoms of an infection if the neonate is not appropriately assessed. On discharge, the nurse needs to teach parents to closely monitor body temperature when placing the newborn in a sunny location to decrease elevated bilirubin levels. (See Chapters 18 and 19 for further discussion.)

Now Can You—Discuss thermoregulation in the newborn?

1. Define nonshivering thermogenesis and discuss its effect on thermoregulation in the newborn?
2. Identify three nursing interventions to prevent heat loss by evaporation and convection after birth?
3. Explain how depletion of the brown adipose tissue stores places the term newborn at risk for respiratory distress?

Hematopoietic Adaptation

As with most of the neonate's other body systems, the hematopoietic system is not fully mature at birth. Instead, in the days following birth, the neonate's hematopoietic system transitions from an in utero oxygenation pathway to an extrauterine perfusion pathway.

BLOOD VOLUME

The full-term infant's average blood volume ranges from 80 to 90 mL/kg of body weight as compared with a blood volume of 90 to 105 mL/kg of body weight in the preterm infant. The neonate's blood volume is determined in large part by the timing of umbilical cord clamping. At birth there is a transfer of blood from the placenta to the neonate: approximately one-fourth of the fetal blood volume is transferred within the first 15 seconds; approximately one-half of the fetal blood volume is transferred by the end of the first minute of life. The umbilical vessels carry approximately 75 to 125 mL of blood at birth, and the neonate's total blood volume may be increased by as much as 61%, depending on a delay in cord clamping (Thilo & Rosenberg, 2012).

Currently, much debate surrounds the issue of how long the umbilical cord should be allowed to pulsate before it is clamped. Holding the neonate below the level of the placenta and delaying the clamping of the cord may allow up to a 100 mL/kg increase in the neonate's total blood volume. The increase in blood volume may facilitate an improved transition because of enhanced pulmonary perfusion and the gain of additional iron stores. A disadvantage of this practice concerns the increased risk of jaundice caused by the higher volume of erythrocytes and possible resultant polycythemia.

Blood volume in the newborn varies according to gestational age, a factor that determines the amount of circulating volume, and the occurrence of prenatal or postnatal hemorrhage. Maternal prenatal or perinatal hemorrhage can have a dramatic impact on the infant's hematopoietic system; following a significant hemorrhage the infant may exhibit decreased hemoglobin and hematocrit levels along with a risk of hypovolemia (Cunningham, Leveno, Bloom, Spong, & Dashe, 2014).

BLOOD COMPONENTS

Erythrocytes and Hemoglobin

At birth, the neonate has a greater number of erythrocytes and higher hemoglobin and hematocrit levels than those found in an adult. During early fetal development, erythropoiesis (formation of red blood cells) occurs primarily in the liver. At approximately 6 months of gestation, the bone marrow becomes the site for hematopoiesis (formation of blood cells). During the later stages of fetal development, fetal hemoglobin (HbF) is slowly replaced by adult hemoglobin (HbA). Fetal hemoglobin carries 20% to 50% more oxygen than adult hemoglobin (Thilo & Rosenberg, 2012).

The process of erythropoiesis is stimulated by the renal hormone erythropoietin. Red blood cell (RBC) production increases in response to a rise in erythropoietin after low fetal oxygen saturation. This physiological event facilitates adequate tissue perfusion and oxygenation. After the initiation of normal respirations at birth, the neonate's oxygen saturation rises, causing an inhibition in the secretion of erythropoietin. This event inhibits the production of RBCs. The neonate's erythrocytes (fetal RBCs) have a shorter life span (90 days) than do adult RBCs (120 days). As the neonate's RBC count decreases from deterioration of the fetal RBCs, physiological anemia of infancy may develop and persist for 2 to 3 months. The life span of RBCs in the full-term neonate is 60 to 70 days; for the preterm neonate, the RBC life span is only 35 to 50 days. In the event of hemolysis, the hemoglobin is broken down, and bilirubin is released into the systemic circulation. If large numbers of RBCs are involved, blood levels of bilirubin rise and the newborn becomes jaundiced (Van Leeuwen, Poelhuis-Leth, & Bladh, 2011). (See Chapter 19 for further discussion.)

Hematocrit

Hematocrit is defined as a percentage of RBCs within a certain unit volume of blood. Normal neonatal blood values vary according to gestational age and the volume of placental blood that was transfused at the time of birth (i.e., delayed cord clamping) (Table 17-2). Hematocrit levels are generally higher in peripheral blood samples because of peripheral vasoconstriction and the stasis of blood cells. A peripherally drawn hematocrit for a normal infant ranges from 46% to 68%. If the hematocrit drawn from a central site is greater than 65%, the infant is considered to be polycythemic. **Polycythemia**, an abnormally high RBC count, is a condition that can place the infant at high risk for jaundice and organ

Table 17-2 Laboratory Values for the Normal Term Neonate: Blood	
Blood Component	**Normal Range**
Albumin	2.8–5.4 g/dL
Bilirubin, total	
Newborn	≤3.0 mg/dL (peripheral blood)
1–2 days	3.4–11.5 mg/dL (peripheral blood)
3–5 days	1.5–12.0 mg/dL (peripheral blood)
Bleeding time	2 minutes
Arterial blood gases Birth, cord, full term	
pH	7.35–7.45
P_{CO_2}	32–66 mm Hg
P_{O_2}	8–24 mm Hg
Venous blood gases Birth, cord, full term	
pH	7.35–7.45
P_{CO_2}	27–49 mm Hg
P_{O_2}	17–41 mm Hg
Calcium, ionized	4.20–5.84 mg/dL
Glucose (birth)	30–60 mg/dL
Hematocrit	42%–62% (cord blood)
	46%–68% (0–1 week)
Hemoglobin	13.5–20.7 g/dL (cord blood)
	15.2–23.6 g/dL (0–1 week)
Platelets	150,000–350,000/mm³
Immunoglobulins, total	660–1,439 mg/dL
Iron	100–250 mcg/dL
Erythrocytes	4,800,000–7,100,000/mm³
Leukocytes	9,000–30,000/mm³

Source: Adapted from Van Leeuwen, Poelhuis-Leth, & Bladh (2011).

damage caused by increased viscosity of the blood cells. Polycythemic infants are also at an increased risk for hypoglycemia and respiratory distress. Under routine circumstances, unless the infant exhibits signs and symptoms associated with transitional difficulties, hematocrit and hemoglobin levels are not routinely assessed (Van Leeuwen et al., 2011).

Leukocytes

Leukocytes (white blood cells [WBCs]) serve as the major defense against infection in the neonate. The WBCs are classified into five categories: neutrophils, eosinophils, basophils, lymphocytes, and monocytes. Neutrophils act as phagocytes that ingest and destroy small particles of bacteria and cellular debris. Eosinophils perform similar duties but are less effective. However, eosinophils survive for longer periods of time and are important mediators in allergic and anaphylactic responses. Basophils play an important role as responders to allergic and inflammatory reactions. Lymphocytes respond to graft versus host allergic diseases and allergic reactions. Monocytes clean up old blood cells and cellular debris and remove activated clotting factors from the circulation.

An elevated leukocyte count in a normal newborn does not always indicate infection. During the first 12 hours after birth, the leukocyte count typically remains elevated before it begins to decline. The average white blood cell count in the term newborn is 18,000/mm³, but ranges from 9,000 to 30,000/mm³ are considered to be within normal limits. Infection is usually associated with a decrease in the leukocyte count. Neonatal sepsis is accompanied by an increased number of immature leukocytes along with a decrease in the total platelet count (Roberts & Murray, 2012). (See Chapter 19 for further discussion.)

Platelets

Because of the absence of vitamin K at birth, the neonate is at risk for developing a blood-clotting deficiency during the first few days of life. To facilitate clotting, the following blood factors must be present: factor II (prothrombin) and factors VII, IX, and X. Vitamin K, synthesized in the infant's intestinal tract, is not produced in the intestines until food and normal intestinal flora are present.

The infant is given an IM injection of vitamin K_1 phytonadione (AquaMEPHYTON) during the initial care and assessment to prevent hemorrhagic disease of the newborn. (See Chapter 19 for further discussion.) The normal newborn's platelet (thrombocyte) levels range from 150,000 to 350,000/mm³ and are essentially the same as in adults. Small for gestational age (SGA) infants may have platelet counts up to 25% lower than those found in appropriate for gestational age neonates. Circulating platelets are hypoactive during the first few days of life. Although this physiological phenomenon prevents the newborn from developing thrombosis, there may be an increased risk for bleeding and coagulopathy (Van Leeuwen et al., 2011).

Hepatic Adaptation

The newborn's liver is a large organ that accounts for about 40% of the total abdominal area. It is palpable approximately 2 to 3 cm below the right costal region. An essential organ, the liver is responsible for the regulation of blood glucose, iron storage, bilirubin conjugation, and coagulation of the blood.

GLYCOGEN AND BLOOD GLUCOSE MAINTENANCE

Throughout pregnancy, the fetus receives glucose by way of the placenta. During the last 4 to 8 weeks of gestation, the glucose is stored as glycogen in the fetal liver and skeletal system for use after birth. Glucose is used more rapidly in the newborn than in the fetus because of the metabolic events that occur during the normal transitional phase. The newborn requires added energy to accomplish several essential tasks to offset the stress of birth, to initiate breathing, to activate muscular activity, and to produce heat.

The stressful events associated with the birth process prompt the conversion of fats and glycogen to glucose. After delivery, an increase in circulating catecholamines triggers the release of glycogen from the neonate's liver. Glycogen provides a ready source of glucose to the brain and other vital organs. During the first 3 hours of life, a healthy term newborn may use up to 90% of his liver's glycogen stores (Rozance & Rosenberg, 2012). Although the brain's primary source of fuel is glucose, it can also use ketones, lactic acids, fatty acids, and glycerol if necessary to maintain an adequate supply of energy. The liver's ability to adequately convert glycogen to glucose for fuel is essential for a successful physiological transition.

The blood glucose of a term infant should be 70% to 80% of the maternal blood glucose level. The maternal glucose level is influenced by a number of factors including the timing and contents of the last meal consumed, the duration and mode of delivery, and the components of any intravenous fluids or medications administered during labor and birth.

During the first 4 to 6 hours of life, the newborn's main source of energy is glucose. The serum blood glucose level drops during the first 3 hours of life and then gradually rises over the next 3 to 4 hours to reach a steady state of 40 to 60 mg/dL. **Glycogenolysis**, the breakdown of glycogen into the more usable glucose within the body tissues, can occur if the newborn does not receive any exogenous glucose before the initial hepatic and skeletal glycogen stores have been depleted. This process prompts the release of glucose into the bloodstream as needed to maintain normal blood levels.

Hypoglycemia

Hypoglycemia can occur after any stressful events (e.g., hypothermia or hypoxia) that increase metabolic demands. Nurses must be aware of risk factors associated with neonatal hypoglycemia (Box 17-1). For example, preterm and SGA infants may not have accumulated the glycogen stores necessary to maintain serum glucose levels required for energy needs. Large for gestational age (LGA) infants and infants of diabetic mothers (IDM) may produce too much insulin postnatally and rapidly metabolize their glucose stores (Fig. 17-9) (Kalhan & Devaskar, 2010). Postterm or intrauterine growth restricted (IUGR) fetuses can develop hypoglycemia related to poor intrauterine nourishment from a deteriorating placenta. Consequently, they have depleted glucose stores before birth. Neonates exposed to postbirth stressors such as asphyxia, infection, or cold stress rapidly use their glucose stores to assist with the transition process (Thilo & Rosenberg, 2012). (See Chapter 19 for further discussion.)

Box 17-1 **Risk Factors for Hypoglycemia in the Neonate**

- Prematurity
- Postmaturity
- Intrauterine growth restriction (IUGR)
- Large or small for gestational age (LGA or SGA)
- Asphyxia
- Difficult transition at birth
- Cold stress
- Maternal diabetes mellitus or preeclampsia-eclampsia
- Maternal intake of terbutaline (Brethine)
- Infection
- Congenital malformations

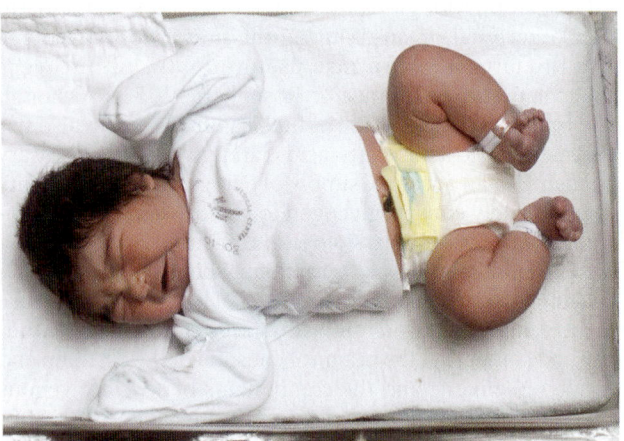

Figure 17-9 The large for gestational age neonate is at risk for postnatal hypoglycemia.

Critical Nursing Action Recognizing Hypoglycemia in the Neonate

When assessing the neonate during the transitional period, the nurse should be alert to signs and symptoms of hypoglycemia. These include jitteriness, diaphoresis, poor muscle tone, poor sucking reflex, temperature instability (low temperature), respiratory distress, tachycardia, dyspnea, apnea, high-pitched cry, irritability, lethargy, seizures, or coma. However, the infant may be asymptomatic. Therefore, awareness of prenatal and perinatal risk factors that may predispose to postnatal hypoglycemia is essential.

Labs: Neonatal Blood Glucose Assessment

Capillary blood obtained from the neonate's heel is commonly used to assess blood glucose. When available, a heel warmer is used to increase blood flow to the sample site. The area is cleansed with a sterile alcohol pad, and the heel is gently punctured, taking care to avoid the middle area where there is a risk for nerve damage or puncture of the plantar artery. A large drop of blood is placed on the test strip, and a sterile bandage is used to apply pressure on the sample site.

IRON STORAGE

During the last few weeks of pregnancy, iron is stored in the fetal liver, and at birth, the neonate's iron store is proportional to the total body hemoglobin and length of gestation. As red blood cells (RBCs) are destroyed after birth, the neonatal liver stores additional iron until needed for the production of new RBCs. At term, the newborn has approximately 270 mg of iron, and of this amount, 140 to 170 mg of iron is contained in the hemoglobin. Adequate maternal iron intake during pregnancy ensures that a sufficient amount of iron is available in the infant to last up to 6 months of age. Term infants who are exclusively breastfed do not need additional iron until at least 6 months of age. However, formula-fed infants should be given an iron-fortified formula, and beginning at 6 months, all infants should receive iron supplements or iron-rich foods to prevent anemia (Blackburn, 2012; Luchtman-Jones & Wilson, 2010).

CONJUGATION OF BILIRUBIN

Conjugation of bilirubin is a major function of the newborn's liver. Conjugation is a process that converts the yellow lipid-soluble (nonexcretable) bilirubin pigment (present in bile) into a water-soluble (excretable) pigment. **Jaundice** is a condition characterized by a yellow (icteric) coloration of the skin, sclera, and oral mucous membranes. First noticed in the head, jaundice gradually progresses to the thorax, abdomen, and extremities. However, it is important to recognize that visual assessment does not provide an accurate assessment of the serum bilirubin level. Jaundice results from the accumulation of bile pigments associated with an excessive amount of bilirubin in the blood **(hyperbilirubinemia).** This condition occurs in approximately 60% of full-term infants and in up to 80% of preterm infants. The presence of jaundice is directly related to the liver's maturity and its ability to conjugate bilirubin (Thilo & Rosenberg, 2012).

Bilirubin is produced from the hemolysis (breakdown) of RBCs. Removal of bilirubin begins in the reticuloendothelial system, where mononuclear phagocytes remove aging RBCs from the circulation. Heme, the oxygen-carrying component of hemoglobin, is broken down into three elements: iron, carbon monoxide, and biliverdin. Iron, stored in the hemoglobin, is used for a number of essential bodily functions. Carbon monoxide is exhaled through the lungs as a waste product, and biliverdin is further broken down into lipid-soluble bilirubin.

During the process of normal conjugation, bilirubin attaches to the blood albumin and is transported to the liver. In the liver, the unbound bilirubin detaches from the albumin and is conjugated with glucuronide in the presence of the enzyme glucuronyl transferase. This process produces water-soluble **direct bilirubin**, which is excreted into the common duct and duodenum. Normal intestinal flora reduce the direct bilirubin into urobilinogen and stercobilinogen. This product is then excreted as a yellow-brown pigment in the stools, and a small amount is excreted through the kidneys. The physiological pathway for the excretion of bilirubin is presented in Figure 17-10.

The breakdown of 1 gram of hemoglobin yields approximately 34 mg of bilirubin. The normal term newborn produces 6 to 10 mg of bilirubin per kilogram per day.

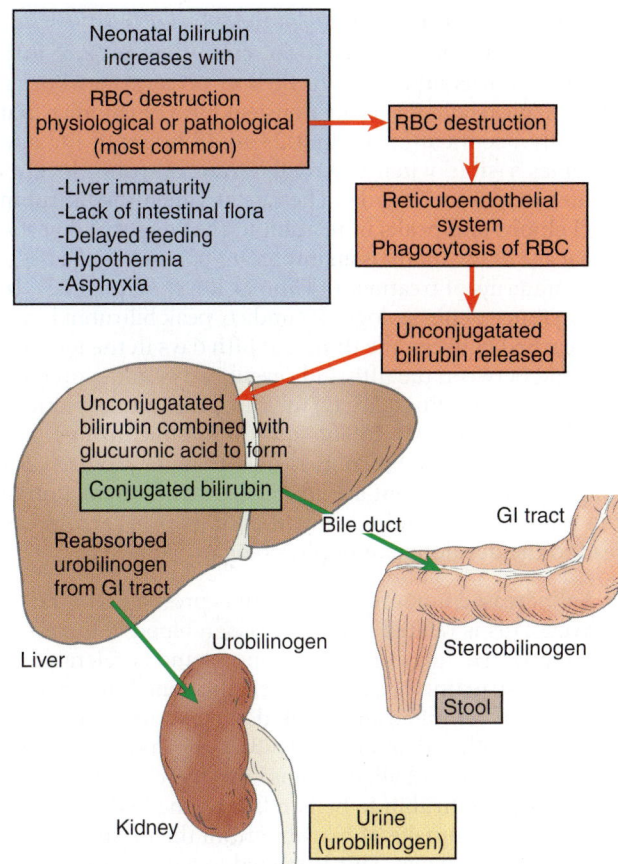

Neonatal bilirubin increases with

RBC destruction physiological or pathological (most common)

-Liver immaturity
-Lack of intestinal flora
-Delayed feeding
-Hypothermia
-Asphyxia

RBC destruction

Reticuloendothelial system Phagocytosis of RBC

Unconjugatated bilirubin released

Unconjugatated bilirubin combined with glucuronic acid to form

Conjugated bilirubin

Reabsorbed urobilinogen from GI tract

Bile duct

GI tract

Liver

Urobilinogen

Stercobilinogen

Stool

Kidney

Urine (urobilinogen)

Figure 17-10 Physiological pathway for the excretion of bilirubin.

In comparison, adults produce 3 to 4 mg of bilirubin per kilogram per day. The increased bilirubin production in the newborn is related to the high concentration of RBCs at birth and the shortened life span of fetal RBCs (Rozance & Rosenberg, 2012).

Conjugated or "direct" bilirubin has been converted from a lipid-soluble, nonexcretable pigment into a water-soluble, excretable pigment. Unconjugated, or "indirect," bilirubin is fat-soluble and nonexcretable. The newborn's liver must be able to convert the fat-soluble (nonexcretable) bilirubin into a water-soluble (excretable) form by way of conjugation. Bilirubin is a highly neurotoxic substance. Elevated blood levels of unconjugated bilirubin can result in **kernicterus** ("yellow nucleus"), which refers to the deposition of unconjugated bilirubin in the basal ganglia of the brain and to the permanent neurological sequelae of untreated hyperbilirubinemia (elevated bilirubin level). (See Chapter 19 for further discussion.)

 Nursing Insight—Kernicterus and acute bilirubin encephalopathy

According to the American Academy of Pediatrics (AAP), Subcommittee on Hyperbilirubinemia (2004), the term "acute bilirubin encephalopathy" should be used to describe the acute manifestations of bilirubin toxicity (e.g., lethargy, hypotonia, and poor suck) seen in the first weeks after birth. The term "kernicterus" should be reserved for the chronic and permanent clinical sequelae of bilirubin toxicity (e.g., cerebral palsy, auditory dysfunction, paralysis of upward gaze, coma, and death).

The total serum bilirubin level (TSB) is a measurement of both the conjugated and unconjugated bilirubin. At birth, the normal TSB is 3 mg/dL or less. Before birth, the fetus does not need to conjugate bilirubin; instead, unconjugated bilirubin is transferred across the placenta for maternal excretion. After birth, the neonate's liver must be able to satisfactorily conjugate bilirubin (Thilo & Rosenberg, 2012).

Nursing Insight—Maternal medications may decrease neonatal albumin-binding sites

Maternal ingestion of medications such as aspirin and sulfa drugs may reduce the number of albumin-binding sites in the infant and result in neonatal hyperbilirubinemia.

Risk Factors for Hyperbilirubinemia

Neonatal jaundice that occurs during the first week of life most often results from excessive levels of unconjugated bilirubin. Unlike pathological jaundice (present at birth or occurring during the first 24 hours), the signs of physiological jaundice do not occur until *after* the first 24 hours of life. Jaundice is usually first noted on the face and sclera when the serum bilirubin levels reach approximately 4 to 6 mg/dL. The yellow coloration then progresses caudally as the TSB rises to 6 to 7 mg/dL (Ives, 2012). Many maternal and neonatal factors such as ethnicity, diabetes, prematurity, and delay in feeding place the infant at risk for hyperbilirubinemia (Box 17-2). Charts (nomograms) are available that graphically display the rise and fall of bilirubin and the degree of risk for various levels of TSB according to the age of the infant in hours. (See Chapter 19 for further discussion.)

> **Box 17-2 Factors That May Influence Bilirubin Levels in the Neonate**
>
> - Cultural background: Chinese, Japanese, Korean, Alaska Native, and Native American neonates exhibit higher bilirubin levels than do European and American Caucasian neonates. The elevated levels of bilirubin persist for a longer period of time and cause no apparent adverse effects.
> - Perinatal events (e.g., delayed cord cutting, breech presentation, the use of Pitocin)
> - Prematurity
> - Maternal diabetes
> - Excess bilirubin production (e.g., hemolytic diseases such as Rh(D) isoimmunization and ABO incompatibility; sepsis; metabolic disorders)
> - Delayed feedings
> - Liver immaturity (e.g., prematurity or glucose-6-phosphate dehydrogenase deficiency)
> - Birth trauma
> - Family history of jaundice or previous child with jaundice
> - Neonatal complications (e.g., asphyxia neonatorum, cold stress, and hypoglycemia)

Optimizing Outcomes—Use of a postnatal bilirubin nomogram

The American Academy of Pediatrics (AAP), Subcommittee on Hyperbilirubinemia (2004) recommends use of hour-specific serum bilirubin levels to predict term newborns at risk for rapidly rising levels. Healthy neonates at 35 weeks of gestation or greater should be monitored before discharge from the hospital. The nomogram displays three levels (high, intermediate, or low risk) of rising total serum bilirubin values to assist in the determination of which newborns may need further evaluation before hospital discharge. The AAP recommends that healthy infants (35 weeks or greater) receive follow-up care and assessment of bilirubin within 3 days of discharge, if discharged at less than 24 hours, and a risk assessment with tools such as the hour-specific nomogram. Infants discharged at 24 to 47.9 hours should receive follow-up evaluation within 4 days; infants discharged between 48 and 72 hours should receive follow-up within 5 days.

Cultural Diversity: Neonatal Jaundice and RBC Enzyme Defects

Jaundice occurs with greater frequency in infants of Chinese, Japanese, Korean, Alaska Native, Native American, and Greek descent. In these populations, there is an increased incidence of RBC enzyme defects, including glucose-6-phosphate dehydrogenase (G6PD) deficiency and pyruvate kinase deficiency. G6PD deficiency, an X-linked recessive disorder, represents one of the most common autosomal recessive traits. It occurs most frequently in Mediterranean, Middle-Eastern, Southeast Asian, and African infants. An estimated 11% to 13% of African American infants who are born in the United States are affected as well (Rozance & Rosenberg, 2012). Pyruvate kinase deficiency, also an autosomal recessive trait, is the next most common enzyme deficiency. Affected infants typically display symptoms of jaundice, anemia, and reticulocytosis (Thilo & Rosenberg, 2012).

Perinatal events, such as delayed clamping of the umbilical cord, increase the volume of circulating RBCs and predispose the neonate to an increased breakdown of RBCs and the subsequent development of jaundice. Traumatic births that involve the use of forceps or vacuum extraction, and fetal presentations that increase the likelihood of bruising, all lead to RBC destruction. Although the mechanism is unclear, there is evidence to suggest that the use of oxytocin and epidural medications may lead to hemolysis of RBCs and serve as an increased source of jaundice (Verklan & Walden, 2014).

Infants who begin feeding early and are feeding well soon establish normal intestinal flora and the regular passage of meconium, which contains large amounts of bilirubin. Infants with delayed or poor feedings have a prolonged exposure to the enzyme beta-glucuronidase, which converts conjugated bilirubin back into deconjugated bilirubin, which is then reabsorbed into the blood. Premature infants, whose livers and blood–brain barriers are immature, do not yet produce the enzymes necessary for bilirubin conjugation and thus are at an increased risk for jaundice (Thilo & Rosenberg, 2012).

Development of Physiological (Neonatal) Jaundice

Physiological jaundice occurs in more than 60% of full-term newborns and in up to 80% of preterm newborns. Physiological jaundice is the transient form of jaundice that typically occurs after the first 24 to 48 hours of life and becomes visible when the total serum bilirubin level is greater than 5 to 7 mg/dL. The rate at which the bilirubin level climbs and peaks in relation to the weight and gestational age of the infant is an important parameter of assessment in terms of treatment (Thilo & Rosenberg, 2012). In the presence of physiological jaundice, peak bilirubin levels are reached between the third and fifth days in the term infant and between the fifth and seventh days in the preterm infant. These values apply to European and American Caucasian newborns; infants of other ethnic groups normally have higher bilirubin levels that may persist for longer periods without adverse effects. The interaction of the following physiological and pathological factors can lead to the development of physiological jaundice:

- An increased amount of bilirubin is presented to the liver. This is related to an increase in blood volume (following a delay in cord clamping) and accelerated RBC destruction because of their shortened life span. Newborns produce and break down two to three times more bilirubin than do adults. Bruising and other birth trauma (e.g., cephalhematoma) can increase the amount of bilirubin to be handled by the liver.
- The hepatic uptake of bilirubin from the plasma is impaired in neonates. This is related to a deficiency of ligandin, the primary bilirubin-binding protein in hepatocytes.
- The hepatic circulation is inadequate. This condition, which may result from neonatal hypoxia or congenital heart disease, is associated with decreased liver oxygenation and increased bilirubin levels.
- Increased amounts of unconjugated bilirubin are reabsorbed from the intestines. This is related to the lack of intestinal bacteria, decreased gastrointestinal motility, and increased beta-glucuronidase (a deconjugating enzyme).
- Defective bilirubin conjugation related to a decrease in glucuronyl transferase activity (as occurs in hypothyroidism, for example), coupled with inadequate caloric intake may cause saturation of the intracellular binding proteins and result in increased blood levels of unconjugated bilirubin. Also, fatty acids present in breast milk are believed to compete with bilirubin for albumin binding sites and interfere with bilirubin metabolism.
- A defect in bilirubin excretion may result from a congenital infection. A delay in the introduction of normal bacterial flora coupled with decreased intestinal motility may cause delayed excretion and increase the bilirubin deconjugation process via the enterohepatic circulation (Blackburn, 2012; McGrath & Hardy, 2011; Thilo & Rosenberg, 2012).

Several nursing interventions can help to decrease the probability of elevated bilirubin levels in the neonate. For example, the nurse should ensure that the infant's skin temperature is maintained at 97.8°F (36.5°C) or greater because cold stress causes acidosis. Acidosis decreases the available serum albumin-binding sites, diminishes

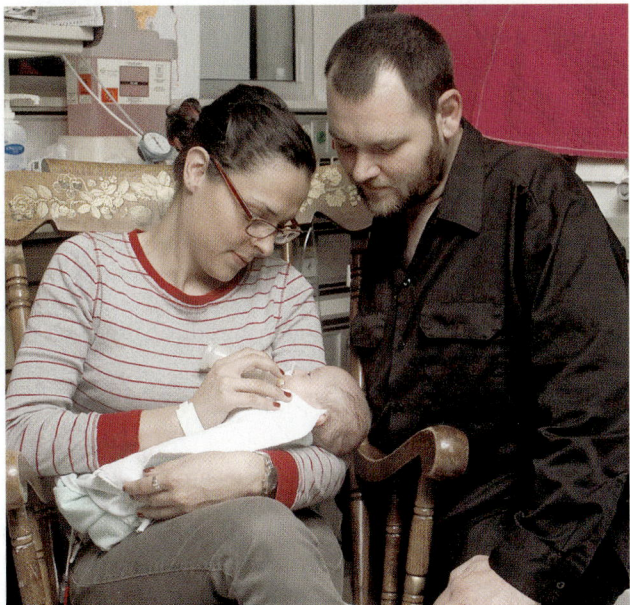

Figure 17-11 Early feedings help to decrease the probability of elevated bilirubin levels in the neonate.

albumin-binding powers, and causes elevated unconjugated bilirubin levels. Because bilirubin is eliminated in the feces, it is important to monitor the infant's stool for amount and characteristics. Inadequate stooling can prompt the recycling and reabsorption of bilirubin. Mothers should be encouraged to initiate early breastfeeding because colostrum exerts a laxative effect that increases meconium excretion. For all healthy infants, early feedings promote intestinal elimination and bacterial colonization and provide calories essential for the formation of hepatic binding proteins (Fig. 17-11).

🌸 Nursing Insight—*Potential benefits of physiological jaundice*

When associated with physiological jaundice, neonatal hyperbilirubinemia may actually confer certain biological benefits at the molecular level. For example, neonates have deficient levels of most antioxidants; bilirubin exerts a potent antioxidant effect (McGrath & Hardy, 2011).

Development of Nonphysiological or Pathological Jaundice

Pathological jaundice occurs within the first 24 hours of life. The infant may exhibit a TSB that increases by 0.5 mg/dL per hour or 5 mg/dL per day. The diagnosis is usually made when TSB concentrations climb greater than 12.9 mg/dL in a term infant and greater than 15 mg/dL in a preterm infant. Pathological jaundice results from disorders that cause excessive hemolysis of RBCs, leading to an increased production of bilirubin. Excessive blood cell breakdown may result from polycythemia or increased bruising after a traumatic delivery. Infections, metabolic disorders, and incompatibilities between the mother's and newborn's blood (Rh incompatibility) may also cause pathological jaundice (McGrath & Hardy, 2011). (See Chapter 19 for further discussion on pathological jaundice.)

Breastfeeding-Associated Jaundice (Early-Onset Jaundice)

Breastfeeding-associated jaundice is a condition that occurs when there is a decreased intake of breast milk and a decreased passage of meconium. Breastfed infants tend to have higher bilirubin levels than bottle-fed infants. Breastfeeding jaundice generally occurs between the second and fourth days of life. The total serum bilirubin levels peak at 15 to 19 mg/dL by 72 hours of life. Breastfeeding jaundice is believed to be associated with poor feeding practices and is not related to the composition of the breast milk. Early and frequent feedings (10–12 times per day) with avoidance of formula and glucose supplementation constitutes the primary therapy for breastfeeding jaundice (Blackburn, 2012; McGrath & Hardy, 2011; Thilo & Rosenberg, 2012).

Breast Milk Jaundice (Late-Onset Jaundice)

Breast milk jaundice typically occurs in the full-term infant, with an incidence of approximately 2% to 4%. This condition has a later onset than breastfeeding jaundice and usually appears after the first week of life and peaks around day 10. Unlike physiological jaundice, a condition characterized by declining bilirubin levels within the first week, bilirubin levels associated with breast milk jaundice continue to rise and peak at 2 to 3 weeks of life. Meanwhile, infants typically are thriving, stooling appropriately, and gaining weight without any evidence of hemolysis (Thilo & Rosenberg, 2012).

At one time, it was thought that breast milk jaundice was related to an enzyme in the breast milk that inhibited the action of glucuronyl transferase. Today, the appearance of breast milk jaundice is believed to be related to factors in human milk that inhibit the conjugation or decrease the excretion of bilirubin. In most circumstances, no intervention is necessary. If the infant continues to breastfeed, the TSB gradually declines over the course of a few weeks. Some experts recommend temporarily halting breastfeeding for 48 hours to allow the serum bilirubin levels to decline. It is important to carefully monitor infants and provide phototherapy or supplemental nutrition when needed (Fig. 17-12) (Blackburn, 2012; McGrath & Hardy, 2011; Verklan & Walden, 2014). (See Chapter 19 for further discussion.)

In 2010, the Association of Women's Health, Obstetric and Neonatal Nurses (AWHONN) published a position paper in support for universal screening for hyperbilirubinemia. Emphasizing the importance of screening as a key intervention in the prevention of acute bilirubin encephalopathy and kernicterus, the perinatal organization encourages facilities to aggressively develop mechanisms to educate all clinical staff that visual infant inspection should not be the sole means of determining elevated bilirubin levels. Instead, best practice should include documentation through the use of an hour-specific bilirubin nomogram prior to infant discharge to assess risk of severe hyperbilirubinemia. AWHONN advocates for nursing authority to independently order total serum bilirubin levels or perform transcutaneous bilirubin assessments based on identified risk factors for jaundice and emphasizes the importance of the nursing role in providing parental education about newborn jaundice (AWHONN, 2010).

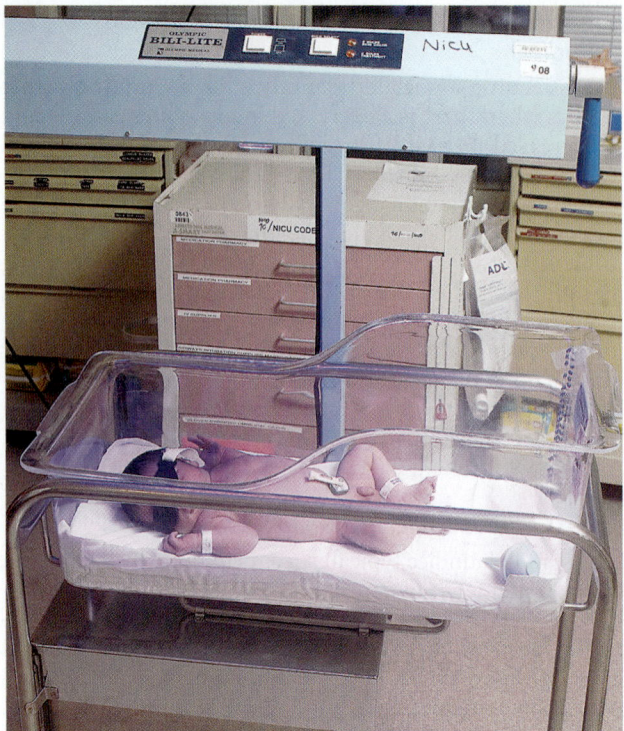

Figure 17-12 Infant receiving phototherapy via fluorescent "bili lights."

COAGULATION OF BLOOD

Another important function of the liver involves the production of coagulation factors to enable the newborn to effectively clot blood after birth. The coagulation factors are activated by vitamin K (AquaMEPHYTON), given to the newborn within 1 hour following birth. An IM injection of vitamin K (AquaMEPHYTON) given prophylactically within this first hour of life prevents hemorrhagic diseases of the newborn. Coagulation factors synthesized in the liver include prothrombin and factors II, VII, IX, and X. Circulating levels of the coagulation factors vary according to the gestational age of the infant (Thilo & Rosenberg, 2012).

 Now Can You—Discuss neonatal jaundice?

1. Identify two factors that may place an infant at risk for physiological jaundice?
2. Explain why infants of Mediterranean descent are at a higher risk for jaundice?
3. Discuss why delayed cord clamping at birth can affect the development of jaundice?

Gastrointestinal Adaptation

STOMACH AND DIGESTIVE ENZYMES

The neonate's stomach capacity is approximately 6 mL/kg at birth, and by the end of the first week of life, the capacity has increased to hold approximately 90 mL. In utero, the fetal gastrointestinal system reaches maturity around 36 to 38 weeks of gestation when there is sufficient enzymatic

activity for digestion and the transport of nutrients throughout the body. To nutritionally thrive, newborns must be able to digest essential carbohydrate disaccharides that include lactose, maltose, and sucrose. Lactose, the primary carbohydrate in breast milk, is easily digested and readily absorbed (Thilo & Rosenberg, 2012). A deficiency of pancreatic amylase, the only enzyme lacking at birth and during the first few months of life, makes it difficult for infants to digest fats efficiently. Newborns also have a decreased production of pancreatic lipase and bile acids, which further limits their ability to absorb fats. Production of pancreatic lipase gradually increases during the first few weeks of life.

INTESTINAL PERISTALSIS

Fetal peristalsis can be influenced by anoxia, which triggers the expulsion of meconium into the amniotic fluid. Immediately after birth, air enters the stomach and reaches the small intestine within 2 to 12 hours. Bowel sounds are present within the first 15 to 30 minutes of life because of the air that has entered the stomach and small intestines. The gastrocolic reflex is stimulated when the stomach fills, and this process helps to enhance intestinal peristalsis. The stomach empties intermittently, usually at the beginning of a feeding and up until 2 to 4 hours after a feeding. The salivary glands are immature at birth; little saliva is produced for the first 3 months of life. The cardiac sphincter (located between the esophagus and the stomach) is immature, and it is not unusual for newborns to regurgitate small amounts following feedings (Thilo & Rosenberg, 2012).

Compared with the overall body size, the newborn's intestines are long, a feature that provides an increased surface area for the absorption of nutrients. However, if diarrhea occurs, the additional surface area places the infant at an increased risk for dehydration and water loss. Infants born at term generally pass their first meconium stool within 8 to 24 hours of life. An important nursing function includes documentation of the first meconium stool. Absence of passage of a bowel movement by 72 hours of age may be indicative of an obstructive bowel problem (Taylor, Wright, & Woodrum, 2011).

Meconium consists of particles found in the amniotic fluid such as vernix, skin cells, hair, and cells that have been shed by the intestinal tract. Meconium stools, which are characteristically greenish-black and viscous, gradually change to transitional stools that are thinner and greenish-brown to yellowish-brown. The newborn may pass stools from one to ten times a day over a 24-hour period. Following the transitional stools, stool appearance and frequency varies, depending on whether the infant is breast- or bottle-fed.

 Now Can You—Discuss gastrointestinal functioning in the newborn?

1. Describe the fetal to newborn transition process that takes place in the gastrointestinal tract?
2. Identify the enzymes that aid in digestion and those that are deficient at birth?
3. Identify when bowel sounds become present in the newborn?

Genitourinary Adaptation

KIDNEY FUNCTION

In the term newborn, the following three major physiological factors enable the kidneys to manage bodily fluids and excrete urine:

- The nephrons are fully functional by 34 to 36 weeks of gestation.
- The glomerular filtration rate is lower than that of the adult.
- There is a limited capacity for the reabsorption of HCO_3^- and H^+.

Although the fetal kidneys contain working nephrons by 34 to 36 weeks of gestation, the kidneys are not mature and fully functional until after birth when the newborn becomes responsible for the elimination of waste products. The neonate's elevated hematocrit (related to the high concentration of red blood cells) and low blood pressure may lead to a decreased glomerular filtration rate (GFR) (the volume of glomerular filtrate that is formed over a specific period of time). With a low GFR, the newborn's kidneys are unable to dispose of fluid rapidly and tend to reabsorb excess sodium. As the kidneys mature and enlarge, the GFR rapidly increases during the first 4 months of life. Adult GFR values are reached at around 2 years of age (Rozance & Rosenberg, 2012).

In the neonate, urine specific gravity normally ranges from 1.002 to 1.010. Term newborns are unable to adequately concentrate urine (reabsorb water back into the blood) because the kidney tubules are short and narrow. This alteration may lead to an inappropriate loss of substances such as amino acids and glucose. By 3 months of age, infants are able to fully concentrate their urine (Modi, 2012). Table 17-3 presents normal laboratory values for components in the neonate's urine.

Along with the lungs and circulatory system, the kidneys perform an important function in helping the body maintain a normal acid-base balance. Several factors can interfere with the newborn's ability to maintain homeostasis in this system. The limited capacity for tubular reabsorption of HCO_3^- and H^+ can lead to a loss of essential substances (e.g., amino acids, bicarbonate, glucose, and sodium) in the filtrate. Because of immaturity of the newborn's kidneys, there is a greater capacity for glomerular filtration than for tubular reabsorption and secretion (Cloherty, Eichenwald, Hansen, & Stark, 2011).

It is important for the nurse to carefully monitor the newborn's intake and output to prevent overhydration and/or dehydration. Most newborns void immediately after birth or within the first few hours, although some may not void for up to 24 hours. On average, approximately 68% of normal newborns void within the first 12 hours, 93% by 24 hours, and 100% will have voided by 48 hours. Recording the neonate's first voiding is an important nursing action. If voiding has not occurred by 24 hours of life, the nurse must alert the pediatrician or neonatal nurse practitioner. The infant may be experiencing hypovolemia related to an insufficient fluid intake. Failure to void during the first 24 hours of life may also indicate the presence of an obstruction in the urinary outflow system, and the infant should be carefully assessed for bladder distention, restlessness, and symptoms of pain (Rozance & Rosenberg, 2012).

Initially, the newborn's bladder capacity ranges from 6 to 44 mL of urine. During the first 2 days of life, infants normally void two to six times in a 24-hour period, with a total output of 15 to 60 mL of urine per kilogram per day. Urine output is significantly higher in infants with edema. By the fourth day, the frequency of voiding should have increased to more than six voids in a 24-hour period. Because the kidneys have difficulty concentrating urine and removing waste products from the blood immediately after birth, small amounts of protein and glucose are frequently present in the urine. Urate crystals, which are pink-red in color, are excreted in the urine and can be mistaken for blood. The crystals (sometimes referred to as "brick dust spots") disappear after the first few days of life as kidney function matures.

During the first 24 to 48 hours, full-term newborns require 60 to 80 mL/kg of fluids to maintain an adequate fluid balance. This requirement increases to 100 to 150 mL/kg per day after the first few days, and a urine output of 1 to 3 mL/kg per hour is indicative of adequate fluid maintenance (Thilo & Rosenberg, 2012). Because the neonate's kidneys are unable to tolerate large changes in volume, careful monitoring of fluid balance is essential. Large changes in fluid balance can create a problem if the infant becomes ill and needs to receive IV fluids during that time. Nursing diagnoses for the neonate experiencing difficulty during the transitional period may be related to the specific organ system(s) involved, environmental factors, or medical interventions (Box 17-3).

Assessing the appearance of the newborn's urine is important when evaluating genitourinary system function. When necessary, the nurse may need to apply a urine collection bag to obtain a urine sample from the infant. After the first voiding, the urine may be cloudy (from mucus) and contain (innocuous) urate crystals. The urine should be odorless and straw colored to clear in appearance as the newborn's fluid intake increases.

Table 17-3	Laboratory Values for Urine in the Normal Term Neonate
Urine Component	**Normal Range**
Osmolality (maximum concentration ability)	75–300 mOsm/kg
pH	4.5–8.0
Phenylketonuria	No color changes
Specific gravity	1.001–1.010
Protein	May be present during the first 2–4 days
Glucose	Negative
Blood	Negative
Leukocytes	Negative

Source: Adapted from Van Leeuwen, Poelhuis-Leth, & Bladh (2011).

> **Box 17-3** Possible Nursing Diagnoses Related to Newborn Physiological Transitions
>
> - Altered Health Maintenance related to separation from the maternal support system.
> - Risk for Infection related to the newborn's immature immunological system.
> - Risk for Ineffective Airway Clearance related to excessive fluid present in lungs during neonatal transition.
> - Risk for Pain related to increased environmental stimuli.
> - Risk for Ineffective Thermoregulation related to the newborn's immature temperature regulation systems.
> - Altered Nutrition: Less than Body Requirements related to limited nutritional and fluid intake and increased caloric expenditure.

Immunological Adaptation

The newborn's immunological system remains immature after birth and may not adequately react to an infectious process. Signs of infection in the newborn can be very subtle and often are not as obvious as they would be in an older child. The newborn receives immunity through two types of methods: active acquired immunity and passive acquired immunity. The pregnant woman's exposure to illness and immunizations prompts the development of antibodies in a process termed **active acquired immunity**. The infant receives **passive acquired immunity** through antibodies that have been passed through the placenta by way of the IgG immunoglobulins.

There are three primary immunoglobulins: IgG, IgA, and IgM. These immunoglobulins, also referred to as humoral antibodies, are proteins that are synthesized in response to a specific antigen. Humoral immunity is important in protecting the newborn against bacterial and viral infections. Low levels of immunoglobulins and immature leukocyte function in destroying pathogens render the newborn especially vulnerable to infections.

IgG is the only immunoglobulin able to pass through the placenta before birth. Placental transfer of this immunoglobulin occurs primarily during the third trimester. At birth, full-term infants have already acquired immunity to tetanus, diphtheria, smallpox, measles, mumps, poliomyelitis, and a host of other bacterial and viral diseases. Preterm infants born before 34 weeks of gestation are at a greater risk for infection. Passive acquired immunity typically disappears by 6 months of age. The infant continues to develop antibodies by active acquired immunity either by direct exposure to an infection with the subsequent development of antibodies or through the immunization schedule recommended by the American Academy of Pediatrics (AAP) and the Centers for Disease Control and Prevention (CDC) (Bedford & Isaacs, 2012; Kapur, Yoder, & Poplin, 2010).

IgA is important in protecting the infant against gastrointestinal and respiratory infections. Colostrum and breast milk are important sources of IgA, and this factor is yet another benefit of breastfeeding. IgA is not detectable in the newborn's system until at least 2 to 3 weeks of life, unless elevated levels are present from a viral infection (Bedford & Isaacs, 2012).

IgM immunoglobulins are produced in response to blood group antigens, gram-negative enteric pathogens, and certain maternal viruses. This immunoglobulin is synthesized early in utero, beginning at approximately 10 to 15 weeks of gestation. Detectable levels are reached by 30 weeks of gestation, and IgM serum concentrations increase rapidly after birth. Elevated levels at birth may result from placental leaks or, more likely, from antigenic stimulation that occurred in utero. Thus, an increased IgM titer is suggestive of exposure to an intrauterine infection such as syphilis or one of the TORCH infections (toxoplasmosis, rubella, cytomegalovirus, and herpes virus) (Kapur et al., 2010). (See Chapter 11 for further discussion.)

 Nursing Insight—*Preventing newborn infections*

Newborns are especially susceptible to infections because of their immature immune system and their poor ability to fight infections. During the birth process, the neonate is exposed to a vast number of potential infectious agents, such as *Staphylococcus* and group B *Streptococcus*. Newborns do not exhibit signs and symptoms of infection in the same manner as do older infants and children. Instead, they may demonstrate subtle behavior changes and poor feeding patterns, develop respiratory distress, or become hypothermic. Maintenance of skin integrity is crucial, especially in the preterm infant, because the skin is thin and fragile. The nurse's awareness of potential risk factors (e.g., maternal group B *Streptococcus* exposure) and thorough assessment skills are essential in the prevention and early detection of newborn infections. Circumcision sites, healing heel sticks, and umbilical stumps are all potential areas for infection that can challenge the newborn's immature immune system. Providing parents with thorough discharge instructions regarding infant hygiene, proper skin care, and awareness of signs and symptoms of infection is an important component of the nursing care plan.

 Now Can You—Discuss aspects of the genitourinary and immunological systems?

1. Identify three physiological factors that enable the newborn's kidneys to produce and excrete urine?
2. Explain the origin and significance of "brick dust spots" in the neonate's urine?
3. Describe what is meant by "humoral immunity"?

Psychosocial Adaptation

EARLY STAGES OF ACTIVITY

Full-term infants experience several "activity" stages during the early hours after birth. It is important to educate parents about normal neonatal behavior during this period and encourage them to enjoy this opportunity to become acquainted with their newest family member. An understanding of normal neonatal activities during the first hours of life provides reassurance and empowers parents to promptly recognize and seek assistance for any signs of difficulty. The infant's psychosocial adaptation begins with two stages of activity followed by a period of sleep.

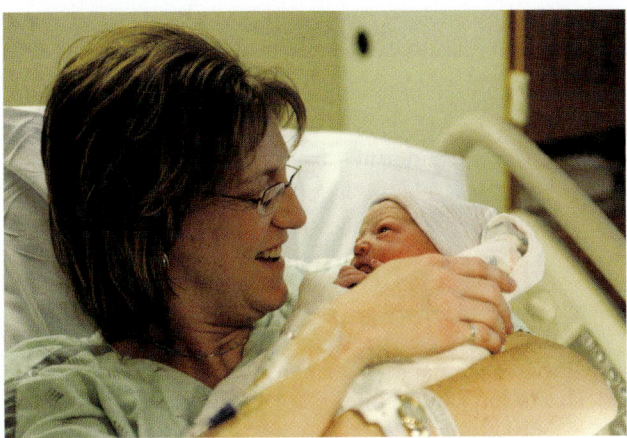

Figure 17-13 The mother and her newborn become acquainted during the first period of reactivity.

The First Period of Reactivity

This stage is the first period of active, alert wakefulness that the infant displays immediately after birth (Fig. 17-13). It lasts approximately 30 minutes and is a wonderful time for parents to get to know their baby. The newborn is very alert during this stage and moves around energetically while taking in the new surroundings. The heart rate and respirations are rapid, and the infant may exhibit occasional nasal flaring and grunting that can last for up to 15 minutes. Muscle tone and motor activity are increased. Body temperature is decreased. Bowel sounds tend to be absent during this period, and there is minimal saliva production (Rozance & Rosenberg, 2012). This first period of reactivity is an opportune time for the mother to initiate breastfeeding if she wishes to do so.

 Optimizing Outcomes—Promoting initial bonding in the breastfeeding mother

Best outcome: The nurse places the infant on the mother's chest for skin-to-skin contact and eye-to-eye contact for early bonding. The infant nuzzles the mother's breast, smells colostrum, and attempts to latch-on to the breast during the first period of reactivity.

The Period of Inactivity and Sleep

After the first period of reactivity, the neonate settles into the sleep phase. At this time, the infant displays decreased muscle activity and is difficult to awaken, instead resting quietly and recovering from the stress of birth. The heart rate and respirations return to a normal range. Central perfusion and general coloring should be excellent at this time, although acrocyanosis is not unusual (Rozance & Rosenberg, 2012). The sleep period may last from a few minutes to 2 to 4 hours.

The Second Period of Reactivity

At this time, the newborn awakens and becomes alert once again. Most infants show signs for feeding readiness (e.g., sucking and rooting) and are eager to begin feeding if not previously fed. During the second period of reactivity, the newborn becomes increasingly more responsive to exogenous and endogenous stimulation, which can cause the heart rate to become labile. The infant may exhibit brief periods of tachycardia, tachypnea, and rapid changes in color and muscle tone. The nurse needs to be aware of normal newborn behaviors during this period that may last for minutes up to several hours. Careful and ongoing assessment allows for differentiation between normal reactions and symptoms that signal difficulty with transition (Rozance & Rosenberg, 2012).

Bowel sounds are usually present, and the infant may have increased oral mucus, causing transient episodes of gagging and vomiting. The nurse should monitor the infant closely, assess for a clear airway, and have suctioning equipment readily available. Parents should be taught how to use a bulb syringe correctly in the event of gagging or vomiting episodes (Thilo & Rosenberg, 2012). (See Chapter 18 for further discussion.) The gastrointestinal system becomes more active during the second period of reactivity, and it is not unusual for newborns to pass their first meconium stool or void if they have not already done so.

Newborn Behavioral States

SLEEP STATES

According to Brazelton (2005), newborn behavior can be divided into the sleep state and the alert state. Two sleep states are exhibited: the deep or quiet sleep and the period of active rapid eye movement (REM). The length of time spent in each sleep cycle is dependent on the newborn's age. At term, REM active and quiet sleep occurs in intervals of approximately 50 minutes. Approximately one-half of the infant's total sleep is "active" sleep. Forty-five percent is "quiet" sleep, and 10% is transitional sleep occurring between the two periods. It has been suggested that REM sleep is instrumental in promoting growth of the neural system. As the infant matures, the sleep-wake cycle adjusts to a diurnal pattern of sleeping during the night and remaining awake during the day.

 Nursing Insight—*Recognizing sleep states in the neonate*

Nurses who care for newborns should be aware of behaviors typically exhibited during deep, quiet sleep and active REM sleep. During deep sleep, the infant's eyes are closed, no eye movements occur, and breathing is regular and even. Jerky motions are common although behavioral responses to external stimuli are delayed. The heart rate ranges from 100 to 120 beats per minute.

During REM sleep, the infant's respirations are irregular, the eyes are closed with REMs visible through the lids, and irregular sucking motions are common. There is minimal activity. Environmental and internal stimuli may prompt a startle reaction and a change of state.

ALERT STATES

The quiet alert state, which generally occurs during the first 30 minutes after birth, characterizes the first period of reactivity and is an excellent time for parents to enjoy bonding with their infant. The periods of alertness are fairly brief

Nursing Care Plan Normal Newborn Transition

Nursing Diagnosis: Readiness for Enhanced Organized Infant Behavior related to effective modulation of the physiological and behavioral systems of functioning

Measurable Short-Term Goal: The newborn will transition to necessary extrauterine cardiorespiratory, feeding, and elimination functions without complications.

Measurable Long-Term Goal: The newborn and mother (family) will experience successful interactions and psychosocial adaptation to each other.

NOC Outcomes:
Newborn Adaptation (0118): Adaptive response to the extrauterine environment by a physiologically mature newborn during the first 28 days.
Parent–Infant Attachment (1500): Parent and infant behaviors that demonstrate an enduring affectionate bond.

NIC Interventions:
Infant Care: Newborn (6824)
Environmental Management (6480)
Lactation Counseling (5244) or Bottle Feeding (1052)
Attachment Promotion (6710)

Nursing Interventions:

1. Before birth, review maternal record for antenatal or intrapartal complications, events, or medications that may affect the neonate. Prepare room and equipment for the birth.

   RATIONALE: Review allows anticipation and preparation for complications that may occur at birth.

2. Dry newborn quickly with pre-warmed blankets while on mother's abdomen. Assess respiratory effort, clear airway and stimulate as needed. Discard wet blankets, cover mother and infant with a warm, dry blanket, and place a cap on the infant's head.

   RATIONALE: Prevents heat loss by evaporation and convection and helps open the airway and initiate respirations.

3. Assess newborn's heart rate and color. Complete Apgar scoring at 1 and 5 minutes of age. If the score is 7 or greater, continue to monitor infant in mother's arms.

   RATIONALE: Heart rate and color provide information about cardiovascular transition to extrauterine function. Infants with Apgar scores of 7 or higher are considered stable.

4. Once the umbilical cord has been cut, assess the number of cord vessels and encourage mother to place the baby in kangaroo care (skin-to-skin) at the breast.

   RATIONALE: It is easiest to note the cord vessels in a freshly cut cord. Kangaroo care helps the newborn maintain temperature and facilitates breastfeeding.

5. Offer instruction about breastfeeding if needed and give praise and encouragement. Provide time and space for first feeding.

   RATIONALE: During the first period of reactivity, the unmedicated infant is alert and ready to breastfeed. The mother should not be overwhelmed with teaching and nursing activity but encouraged to get to know her baby.

6. Continue to monitor infant's vital signs per protocol. Encourage stable infant to remain with mother in kangaroo care for first period of reactivity.

   RATIONALE: The stable infant benefits most from maternal contact. Vital signs can be monitored in the mother's arms.

7. At a convenient time during the first 2 hours, place the infant under a radiant warmer with a servo-controlled skin probe in place. Perform a brief physical exam and administer vitamin K and eye prophylaxis as ordered. Place identification bands on the infant and mother.

   RATIONALE: The radiant warmer and probe provide a safe source for external heat as the infant is examined. Vitamin K prevents neonatal hemorrhage and eye prophylaxis is required to prevent eye infection. Two forms of identification applied before separation help ensure that the right mother and infant are together.

8. Monitor for passage of urine and first meconium and document. Teach parents about elimination and diapering as needed.

   RATIONALE: The passage of urine and meconium provides information about the normal newborn's anatomy and physiology. Every opportunity for teaching should be appreciated during the short hospital stay.

9. Observe the parents' interactions with the newborn: eye contact, stroking, and talking to baby. Point out attractive features and infant's responses to parents. Offer encouragement to fathers to touch and hold their newborn.

   RATIONALE: Observation helps the nurse identify appropriate behaviors related to attachment and bonding with the newborn. Encouragement provides the novice father with "permission" to parent.

during the first 2 days of life as the infant recovers from the events associated with birth. After that time, the infant's alert states result from choice or necessity. Stimuli that may prompt wakefulness include hunger, cold, and heat. Once the triggering stimuli are removed, the infant tends to fall back asleep. The alert state has been subcategorized into four distinct phases: drowsy or semidozing, quiet alert or wide-awake, active alert, and crying (Brazelton, 2005).

Drowsy or Semidozing State

Physical manifestations include open or closed eyes; fluttering eyelids; semidozing appearance; and slow, regular movement of the extremities. There is a delayed response to external stimuli.

Quiet Alert or Wide-Awake State

The infant is alert and follows and fixates on attractive objects, faces, or auditory stimuli. There is minimal motor activity and a delayed response to external stimuli.

Active Alert State

The eyes are open, motor activity is intense, and the infant displays thrusting movements of the extremities. Environmental stimuli increase the motor activity.

Crying State

Jerky movements accompany intense crying. Crying often serves as a distraction from unpleasant stimuli such as hunger and pain. It allows the infant to discharge energy and elicits a helpful response from the parents.

Now Can You—Discuss psychosocial adaptation in the newborn?

1. Compare and contrast the first period of reactivity and the period of inactivity/sleep?
2. Identify two behavioral characteristics associated with deep, quiet sleep and REM sleep?
3. Name four subcategories of the alert state and identify two behavioral characteristics of each phase?

Summary Points

◆ Surfactant, a lipoprotein that reduces surface tension, is essential in keeping the lungs expanded during expiration.

◆ Initiation of the neonate's first breath is influenced by chemical, sensory, thermal, and mechanical factors.

◆ Successful cardiopulmonary adaptation in the neonate is dependent on five major changes related to aortic, venous, and pulmonary pressures and closure of the foramen ovale, ductus arteriosus, and ductus venosus.

◆ A number of factors, including body size and gestational age, affect the neonate's ability to maintain a neutral thermal environment.

◆ Heat loss may occur through the processes of evaporation, conduction, convection, and radiation.

◆ The neonate's liver has essential roles in iron storage, carbohydrate metabolism, bilirubin conjugation, and blood coagulation.

◆ The neonate receives immunity through active acquired immunity and passive acquired immunity.

◆ The newborn exhibits two periods of reactivity and two behavioral states that may be divided into sleep states and alert states.

Review Questions

Multiple Choice

1. The labor and delivery nurse knows that the newborn transition can take how long?
   A. Minutes to hours
   B. Minutes to days
   C. Several hours
   D. Several weeks

2. The labor and delivery nurse notes the term "acrocyanosis" on a newly born infant's chart. What action should the nurse take?
   A. Stimulate the infant
   B. Apply oxygen to the infant
   C. Continue to monitor
   D. Warm the baby more

3. The pediatric nurse knows that the foramen ovale is permanently closed in infants by what time frame?
   A. 24 hours
   B. 7 days
   C. 4 weeks
   D. 6 months

4. A new mother asks why her neonate prefers a flexed position. What information does the nurse provide?
   A. It is the baby's habit to get in that position.
   B. It helps to conserve heat.
   C. It is easy on the joints.
   D. It helps muscle development.

5. A nurse assesses a polycythemic infant for complications related to this condition. What finding would be inconsistent with neonatal polycythemia?
   A. Jaundice
   B. Hypoglycemia
   C. Respiratory distress
   D. Infection

6. What term does the nurse use to describe an infant who has chronic neurological problems associated with poorly treated infant jaundice?
   A. Kernicterus
   B. Cerebral palsy
   C. Minimal brain damage
   D. Acute bilirubin encephalopathy

7. A student nurse in the mother–baby unit is concerned because a neonate has passed a blackish-green, thick, sticky stool. What action by the registered nurse is best?
   A. Ask the student to document the stool.
   B. Perform a thorough gastrointestinal assessment.
   C. Notify the health-care provider.
   D. Ask if the mother is breast- or bottle-feeding.

8. The perinatal nurse explains to a student that an infant receives passive acquired immunity in which of the following ways?
   A. Immunizations and antibiotics
   B. Antibodies passing through the placenta
   C. Mother's exposure to illness
   D. Infusion of gamma-globulins

9. What purpose does REM sleep serve in the neonate?
   A. Allows for complete rest
   B. Promotes neural development
   C. Facilitates digestion
   D. Improves immunity

10. The perinatal nurse knows that the fetal ductus arteriosus closes and becomes what structure?
   A. Ligamentum teres
   B. Superior vesical artery
   C. Closed atrial septum
   D. Ligamentum arteriosum

See Answers to End of Chapter Review Questions on DavisPlus.

REFERENCES

American Academy of Pediatrics (AAP), Subcommittee on Hyperbilirubinemia. (2004). Clinical Practice Guideline: Management of hyperbilirubinemia in the newborn infant 35 or more weeks of gestation. *Pediatrics, 114*(1), 297–316. doi:10.1542/p3ew.114.1.297

Association of Women's Health, Obstetric and Neonatal Nurses (AWHONN). (2010). Universal screening for hyperbilirubinemia. *Journal of Obstetric, Gynecologic & Neonatal Nursing, 39*(1), 83–84. doi:10.1111/j.1552-6909.2009.01098.x

Beckmann, C., Herbert, W., Laube, D., Ling, F., & Smith, R. (2013). *Obstetrics and gynecology* (7th ed.). Philadelphia, PA: Lippincott Williams & Wilkins.

Bedford. A., & Isaacs, D. (2012). Infection in the newborn. In J. Rennie (Ed.), *Rennie & Roberton's textbook of neonatology* (5th ed., pp. 1013–1064). Philadelphia, PA: Churchill Livingstone.

Blackburn, S. T. (2012). *Maternal, fetal, & neonatal physiology: A clinical perspective* (4th ed.). St. Louis, MO: Saunders.

Brazelton, T. B. (2005). Behavioral competence. In M. G. MacDonald, M. D. Mullett, & M. K. Seshia (Eds.), *Avery's neonatology: Pathophysiology and management of the newborn* (6th ed., pp. 321–332). Philadelphia, PA: Lippincott Williams & Wilkins.

Bulechek, G. M., Butcher, H. K., & Dochterman, J. M., & Wagner, C. (2013). *Nursing interventions classification (NIC)* (6th ed.). St. Louis, MO: Elsevier Mosby.

Cheffer, N. D., & Rannalli, D. A. (2011). Transitional care of the newborn. In S. Mattson & J. Smith (Eds.), *Core curriculum for maternal-newborn nursing* (4th ed., pp. 346–361). Philadelphia, PA: W.B. Saunders.

Cloherty, J., Eichenwald, E., Hansen, A., & Stark, A. (2011). *Manual of neonatal care* (7th ed.). Philadelphia, PA: Lippincott Williams & Wilkins.

Cunningham, F. G., Leveno, K. J., Bloom, S. L., Spong, C., & Dashe, J. (2014). *Williams obstetrics* (24th ed.). New York, NY: McGraw-Hill Professional.

Dillon, P. M. (2007). *Nursing health assessment: A critical thinking, case studies approach* (2nd ed.). Philadelphia, PA: F.A. Davis.

Goldsmith, J. P. (2010). Delivery room resuscitation of the newborn: Part 1: Overview and initial management. In R. Martin, A. Fanaroff, & M. Walsh (Eds.), *Fanaroff and Martin's neonatal-perinatal medicine: Diseases of the fetus and infant* (9th ed., pp. 449–457). Philadelphia, PA: C.V. Mosby.

Ives, N. K. (2012). Neonatal jaundice. In J. Rennie (Ed.), *Rennie & Roberton's textbook of neonatology* (5th ed., pp. 672–692). Philadelphia, PA: Churchill Livingstone.

Johnson, M., Moorhead, S., Bulechek, G., Butcher, H., Maas, M., & Swanson, E. (2012). *NOC and NIC Linkages to NANDA-I and clinical conditions: Supporting critical reasoning and quality care* (3rd ed.). St. Maryland Heights, MO: Elsevier Mosby.

Kalhan, S., & Devaskar, S. (2010). Metabolic and endocrine disorders. In R. Martin, A. Fanaroff, & M. Walsh (Eds.), *Fanaroff and Martin's neonatal-perinatal medicine: Diseases of the fetus and infant* (9th ed., pp. 1497–1522). Philadelphia, PA: C.V. Mosby.

Kapur, R., Yoder, M., & Poplin, R. (2010). Developmental immunology. In R. Martin, A. Fanaroff, & M. Walsh (Eds.), *Fanaroff and Martin's neonatal-perinatal medicine: Diseases of the fetus and infant* (9th ed., pp. 761–792). Philadelphia, PA: C.V. Mosby.

Luchtman-Jones, L., & Wilson, D. (2010). Hematologic problems in the fetus and neonate. In R. Martin, A. Fanaroff, & M. Walsh (Eds.), *Fanaroff and Martin's neonatal-perinatal medicine: Diseases of the fetus and infant* (9th ed., pp. 1303–1359). Philadelphia, PA: C.V. Mosby.

McGrath, J. M., & Hardy, W. (2011). The infant at risk. In S. Mattson & J. Smith (Eds.), *Core curriculum for maternal-newborn nursing* (4th ed., pp. 362–414). Philadelphia, PA: W.B. Saunders.

Modi, N. (2012). Fluid and electrolyte balance. In J. Rennie (Ed.), *Rennie & Roberton's textbook of neonatology* (5th ed., pp. 331–344). Philadelphia, PA: Churchill Livingstone.

Moorhead, S., Johnson, M., Maas, M. L., & Swanson, E. (2013). *Nursing outcomes classification (NOC)* (5th ed.). St. Louis, MO: Elsevier Mosby.

Roberts, I., & Murray, N. (2012). Haematology. In J. Rennie (Ed.), *Rennie & Roberton's textbook of neonatology* (5th ed., pp. 755–790). Philadelphia, PA: Churchill Livingstone.

Rozance, P. J., & Rosenberg, A. A. (2012). The neonate. In S. G. Gabbe, J. R. Niebyl, H. L. Galan, E. R. Jauniaux, M. B. Landon, J. L. Simpson, & D. A. Driscoll (Eds.), *Obstetrics: Normal and problem pregnancies* (6th ed.), pp 481–516). Philadelphia, PA: W.B. Saunders.

Sedin, G. (2010). Physical environment: Part 1. The thermal environment. In R. Martin, A. Fanaroff, & M. Walsh (Eds.), *Fanaroff and Martin's neonatal-perinatal medicine: Diseases of the fetus and infant* (9th ed., pp. 555–569). Philadelphia, PA: C.V. Mosby.

Taylor, J. A., Wright, J. A., & Woodrum, D. (2011). Routine newborn care. In C. Gleason & S. Devaskar, *Avery's diseases of the newborn* (9th ed., pp. 300–315). Philadelphia, PA: W.B. Saunders.

Thilo, E. H., & Rosenberg, A. A. (2012). The newborn infant. In W. Hay, M. Levin, R. Deterding, & M. Abzug, *Current pediatric diagnosis & treatment* (21st ed., pp. 9–72). New York, NY: McGraw-Hill Professional.

Vallerand, A. H., & Sanoski, C. A. (2014). *Davis's drug guide for nurses* (14th ed.). Philadelphia, PA: F.A. Davis.

Van Leeuwen, A., Poelhuis-Leth, D., & Bladh, M. (2011). *Davis's comprehensive handbook of laboratory & diagnostic tests with nursing implications* (4th ed.). Philadelphia, PA: F.A. Davis.

Verklan, M., & Walden, M. (2014). *Core curriculum for neonatal intensive care nursing* (5th ed.). St Louis, MO: Saunders.

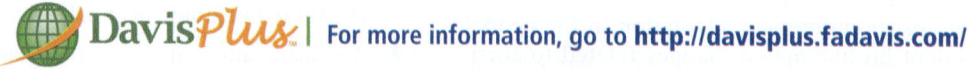

CONCEPT MAP

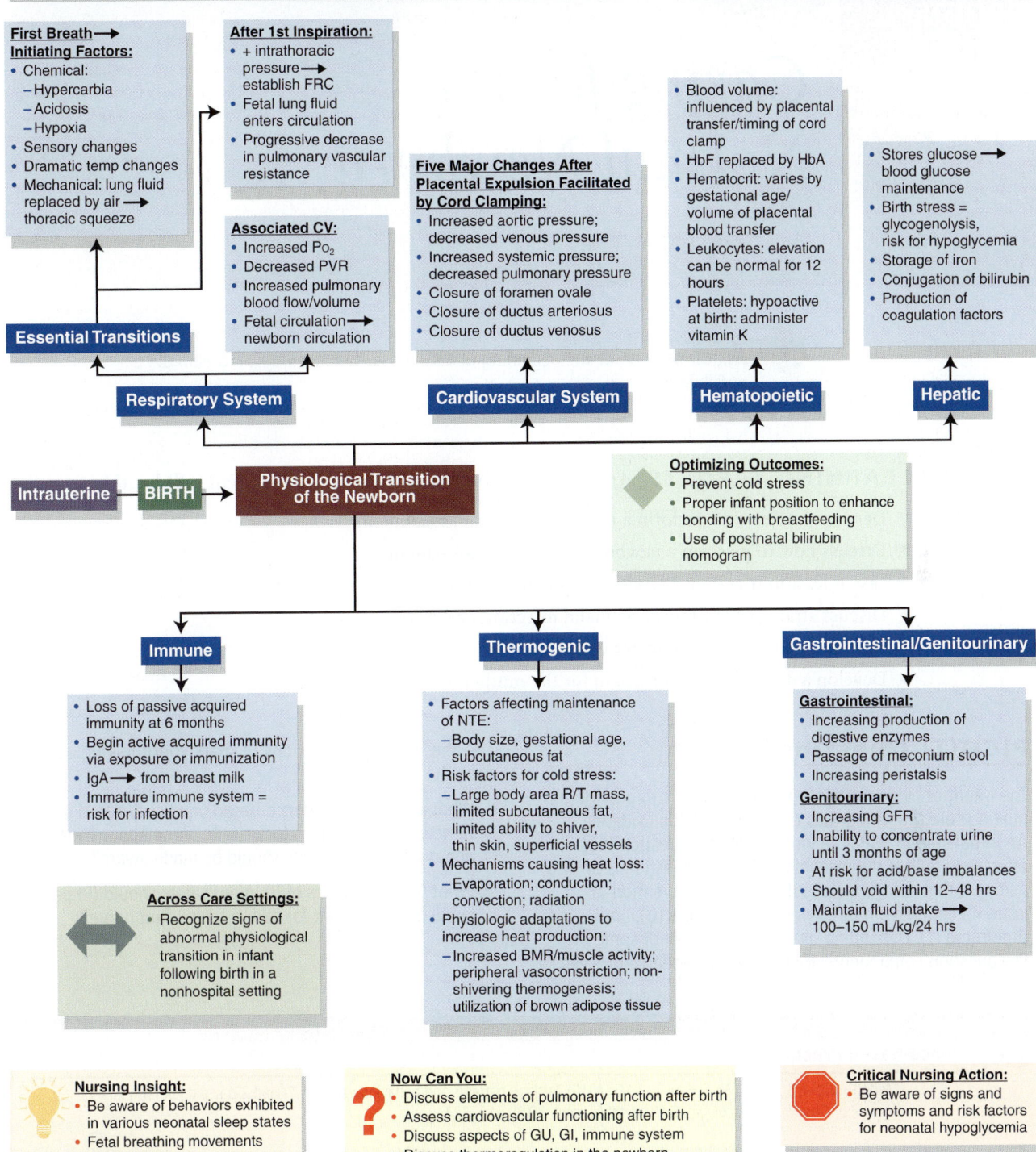

First Breath ➝
Initiating Factors:
• Chemical:
  – Hypercarbia
  – Acidosis
  – Hypoxia
• Sensory changes
• Dramatic temp changes
• Mechanical: lung fluid replaced by air ➝ thoracic squeeze

After 1st Inspiration:
• + intrathoracic pressure ➝ establish FRC
• Fetal lung fluid enters circulation
• Progressive decrease in pulmonary vascular resistance

Associated CV:
• Increased Po₂
• Decreased PVR
• Increased pulmonary blood flow/volume
• Fetal circulation ➝ newborn circulation

Five Major Changes After Placental Expulsion Facilitated by Cord Clamping:
• Increased aortic pressure; decreased venous pressure
• Increased systemic pressure; decreased pulmonary pressure
• Closure of foramen ovale
• Closure of ductus arteriosus
• Closure of ductus venosus

• Blood volume: influenced by placental transfer/timing of cord clamp
• HbF replaced by HbA
• Hematocrit: varies by gestational age/ volume of placental blood transfer
• Leukocytes: elevation can be normal for 12 hours
• Platelets: hypoactive at birth: administer vitamin K

• Stores glucose ➝ blood glucose maintenance
• Birth stress = glycogenolysis, risk for hypoglycemia
• Storage of iron
• Conjugation of bilirubin
• Production of coagulation factors

Essential Transitions

Respiratory System   **Cardiovascular System**   **Hematopoietic**   **Hepatic**

Intrauterine — **BIRTH** ➝ **Physiological Transition of the Newborn**

Optimizing Outcomes:
• Prevent cold stress
• Proper infant position to enhance bonding with breastfeeding
• Use of postnatal bilirubin nomogram

Immune

• Loss of passive acquired immunity at 6 months
• Begin active acquired immunity via exposure or immunization
• IgA ➝ from breast milk
• Immature immune system = risk for infection

Across Care Settings:
• Recognize signs of abnormal physiological transition in infant following birth in a nonhospital setting

Thermogenic

• Factors affecting maintenance of NTE:
  – Body size, gestational age, subcutaneous fat
• Risk factors for cold stress:
  – Large body area R/T mass, limited subcutaneous fat, limited ability to shiver, thin skin, superficial vessels
• Mechanisms causing heat loss:
  – Evaporation; conduction; convection; radiation
• Physiologic adaptations to increase heat production:
  – Increased BMR/muscle activity; peripheral vasoconstriction; non-shivering thermogenesis; utilization of brown adipose tissue

Gastrointestinal/Genitourinary

Gastrointestinal:
• Increasing production of digestive enzymes
• Passage of meconium stool
• Increasing peristalsis

Genitourinary:
• Increasing GFR
• Inability to concentrate urine until 3 months of age
• At risk for acid/base imbalances
• Should void within 12–48 hrs
• Maintain fluid intake ➝ 100–150 mL/kg/24 hrs

Nursing Insight:
• Be aware of behaviors exhibited in various neonatal sleep states
• Fetal breathing movements begin in utero
• Differentiate kernicterus from acute bilirubin encephalopathy
• Be aware of risk factors for infection in the newborn

Now Can You:
• Discuss elements of pulmonary function after birth
• Assess cardiovascular functioning after birth
• Discuss aspects of GU, GI, immune system
• Discuss thermoregulation in the newborn

Critical Nursing Action:
• Be aware of signs and symptoms and risk factors for neonatal hypoglycemia

Caring for the Normal Newborn

 A new baby is like the beginning of all things—wonder, hope, a dream of possibilities.

—Eda J. Le Shan

LEARNING TARGETS *At the completion of this chapter, the student will be able to:*

◆ Demonstrate how to perform a newborn physical assessment.

◆ Discuss how to perform a newborn behavioral assessment.

◆ List at least four actions to assess the neonate's transition to extrauterine life.

◆ Discuss strategies to prevent neonatal infection and injury.

◆ Describe four activities to foster early infant attachment.

◆ Develop a discharge teaching plan for the mother and her newborn infant.

PICO(T) Questions

The intent of evidence-based practice (EBP) is to provide nursing care that integrates the best available evidence. An initial step in EBP is to write a PICO(T) question that effectively guides the research. A PICO(T) question is an acronym that stands for population (P), intervention or issue (I), comparison of interest (C), outcome (O), and timeframe (T). Depending on the question, all or some of the question components are used in the research process.

Use these PICO(T) questions to spark your thinking as you read the chapter.

1. What are (O) the evidence-based practices related to (I) newborn screenings for genetic or metabolic conditions about which (P) parents should be made aware?

2. What (O) key aspects of (I) infant safety should (P) parents know in preparation for taking their infant home?

 Evidence-Based Practice

Medoff-Cooper, B., Bilker, W., & Kaplan, J. M. (2010). Sucking patterns and behavioral state in 1- and 2-day-old full-term infants. *Journal of Obstetric, Gynecologic, & Neonatal Nursing, 39*(5), 519–524.

The purpose of this study was to analyze the temporal structure of sucking in full-term infants during the first 48 hours of life and to determine whether changes in sucking patterns during this period are related to changes in infant behavioral states. It is well known that infants suck less on the first day of life than they do on the second day. This behavior is most often associated with the infant's state of alertness; it does not always take into consideration maturation and experience. Previous studies have documented the effects of factors including degree of arousal, birth weight, gestational age, maternal sedation, length of labor, Apgar

score on sucking and feeding over various time frames (e.g., the second to third days of life and the first four days of life), and changes in sucking, breathing, and swallowing during the first 6 months of life. However, none of the research describes transition of the sucking patterns during the first 2 days of feeding.

The participants consisted of a cohort of healthy infants (n=56) who were part of a larger sample of infants (n=315) in a research project at a large university. All infants were full term and appropriate for gestational age, they were between 10 hours of age (first day of 5-minute sucking assessment) and 48 hours of age (second day of 5-minute sucking assessment), and none were subjected to an invasive procedure before being fed. During labor, 58% (n=33) of the mothers had received epidural or pudendal anesthesia, 27% (n=15) had received no anesthesia, 0.05% (n=3) had received local anesthesia, and 0.08% (n=5) had received general anesthesia. The mothers' average age was 24 years. The average gestational age of the infants was 39 weeks with a range of 37 to 42 weeks. The average birth weight was 3,128 grams (6 lb 14 oz). African American descent was represented by 98% of the infants, and there were an equal number of males and females. All of the mothers indicated that they planned to bottle-feed their infants.

To ensure consistency in data collection, all infants were given their morning feeding by the mother or a nurse at 6:00 a.m. on the day of testing. Measurement of sucking efforts was performed 30 minutes before the second morning feeding. To prepare for the test, the infants were lightly wrapped in a blanket. The researcher held the infant for the duration of the testing period, which involved a 5-minute sucking test. The sucking test was preceded and followed by a 5-minute rest period. A 12-item behavioral scale was used to assess the infants' behavioral states, which were assessed at the first and fifth minutes of both the preceding and following 5-minute periods. The scale ranged from 1 (regular quiet sleep) to 12 (hard crying). For the purpose of data analysis, the 12 scales were collapsed into three groups: sleeping, awake, and crying. A sucking apparatus measured the negative pressure generated by sucking; the pressure signal was then entered into a computer software program that displayed the pattern of sucks.

This generated a "range of session summary parameters including number of sucks, number of bursts, sucks per burst, interburst intervals (time between bursts), suck width (length of time for an individual suck), mean maximum sucking pressure, and intersuck interval" (p. 520).

Regression analysis revealed that the number of sucks, intersuck width, and interburst width were significantly different between the first and second days of life. Significantly more sucks were generated on the second day of life, with a decrease in interburst and intersuck width. These changes were determined to be independent of the number of hours that had elapsed after birth and the infant's amount of feeding experience. Also, there was a significant difference in infant sucking patterns between the first and second days of life and an increase in the presence of an alert behavioral state from the first to second sucking assessment.

The researchers concluded that their findings show that sucking analysis is sensitive to infant status and suggest that the development of sucking methodology can be considered as a useful clinical tool to assess the normal developmental course of sucking patterns.

1. How is this information useful to clinical nursing practice?

2. Based on these findings, what are implications for further research?

See Suggested Responses for Evidence-Based Practice on Davis*Plus*.

Introduction

Most nurses who care for newborns and their families view their specialty to be the most exhilarating and rewarding of any area in nursing. Childbirth marks the beginning of profound changes in the lives of the mother, her infant, and the family. From the moment of the parents' first interaction with their newborn, a journey of growth and exploration begins for each of them. After ensuring that the neonate is physiologically stable, the infant's nurse plays a pivotal role in preserving and protecting this most special time by not intruding or allowing any interruptions as the new family becomes acquainted.

During the transitional period after birth, nursing care focuses primarily on two goals: to safeguard and support the neonate's physical well-being and to promote the establishment of a healthy family unit. The first goal is met by close observation coupled with skilled assessment throughout the time the infant remains in the health-care facility. The nurse meets the second goal by educating the family about care of their newborn. Ongoing interaction with the parents provides insights concerning the family's ethnic influences and cultural values, and this information helps to direct and guide the teaching plan. By providing culturally appropriate education along with

expressions of support of parenting efforts, the nurse empowers the parents with information and knowledge about their infant's needs. Furthermore, the nurse's teaching efforts can be instrumental in heightening parents' awareness of family adjustments that may need to occur during this time of family transition and role changes. This chapter focuses on the healthy neonate. A system-by-system guide to physical assessment of the infant is provided along with a discussion of nursing measures intended to meet the newborn's needs. Methods to determine the neonate's gestational age are presented. The chapter concludes with infant discharge planning; Box 18-1 presents a list of possible nursing diagnoses for the healthy neonate.

The Immediate Neonatal Assessment

The newborn infant's physical condition is assessed immediately at the time of birth. If necessary, suctioning of the oral, pharyngeal, or endotracheal area is conducted according to the health facility's policy, procedure, and protocol (Fig. 18-1) (Procedure 18-1). The infant is carefully handed to the nurse, who receives the neonate into a sterile baby blanket and, in the ideal situation, places him on the

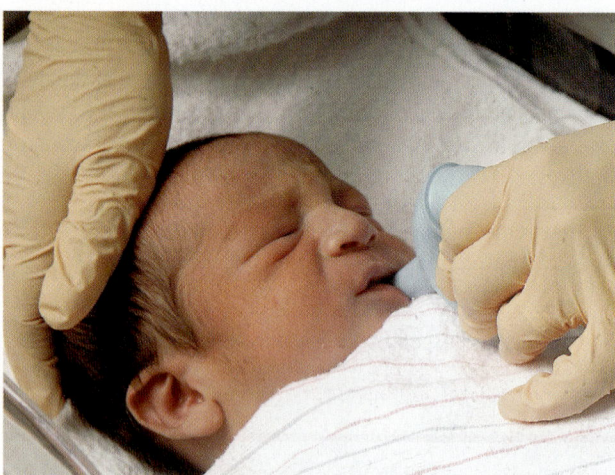

Figure 18-1 A bulb syringe is used to remove mucus.

mother's abdomen. For most, this simple action is a deeply satisfying source of comfort for the mother and her infant, and the warmth of the mother's body helps to maintain the neonate's body temperature. In addition, heated blankets placed over the neonate minimize heat loss by evaporation. In other situations, the nurse places the infant in an incubator or directly beneath a radiant heater unit to prevent evaporative heat loss. After being carefully dried off, a cap is placed on the head for extra warmth.

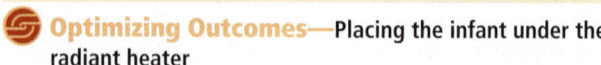 **Optimizing Outcomes—Placing the infant under the radiant heater**

Best outcome: The nurse dries the infant before placing him unclothed on a clean, dry blanket under the radiant-heater unit. Because the generated heat from the unit warms only the outer surface of objects, it is counterproductive to cover or clothe the infant because he will get no benefit from the radiant heat.

While performing these actions, the nurse observes the infant's respiratory effort, color, and muscle tone and makes sure that the activities under way are stimulating the neonate to breathe deeply and cry. If needed, lightly flicking the infant's soles prompts a crying response.

 Nursing Insight—*Observing standard precautions when handling the neonate*

Because there is a possibility of transmission of viruses such as hepatitis B (HBV) and HIV from maternal blood and blood-stained amniotic fluid, the neonate is considered a potential contamination source. Nurses must observe standard precautions by wearing gloves when handling the neonate until blood and amniotic fluid are removed by bathing.

Procedure 18-1 Suctioning the Infant's Oral and Nasal Passages

Purpose
To clear secretions from oral and nasal passages

Equipment
- One bulb syringe
- Tissue

Steps for Oral Suctioning

1. Assess the infant for oral secretions.
2. Position the infant's head to the side or downward if he is vomiting or gagging.
3. Compress the bulb syringe.

   RATIONALE: *Removing the air prevents forcing secretions deeper into the respiratory tract.*

4. Insert the bulb syringe approximately 1 inch into one side of the infant's cheek. Avoid contact with the roof of the mouth and the back of the throat.

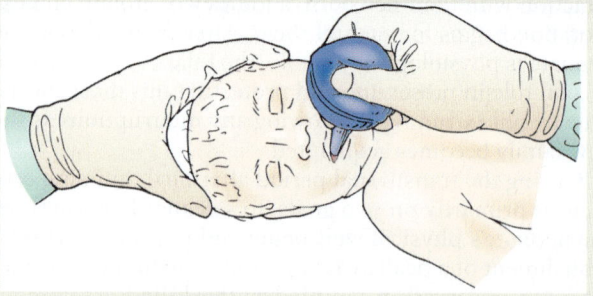

RATIONALE: *To prevent stimulation of the gag reflex.*

5. Gently release compression of the bulb syringe and allow it to fill with oral secretions.
6. Gently remove the bulb syringe; expel drainage into a tissue.

Procedure 18-1 Suctioning the Infant's Oral and Nasal Passages (continued)

7. Repeat the process on the other side of the infant's cheek.

8. Repeat as needed.

Clinical Alert Always suction the mouth before suctioning the nares because fluids and secretions that could obstruct the respiratory tract may be present in the mouth or the nares or both. Placing the syringe in the nares first may trigger an inspiratory gasp, causing the infant to pull mucus further into the respiratory tract.

Steps for Nasal Suctioning

1. Assess the infant for nasal congestion.

2. Position the infant's head to the side or downward if he is vomiting or gagging.

3. Compress the bulb syringe.

   RATIONALE: *Removing the air prevents forcing secretions deeper into the respiratory tract.*

4. Insert the bulb syringe into the tip of the infant's nostril. Avoid obstructing the nasal passageway.

   RATIONALE: *To prevent respiratory distress.*

5. Gently release the compression of the bulb syringe to allow it to fill with mucus or nasal drainage.

6. Gently remove the bulb syringe; expel drainage into a tissue.

7. Repeat as needed.

Clinical Alert An increasing respiratory rate is often the first sign of respiratory compromise or obstruction. If this occurs, measures must be initiated to maintain effective ventilation.

Teach Parents

- Proper technique for use of the bulb syringe; ask for return demonstration.
- Proper care of the bulb syringe: wash in warm, soapy water each day and after each use.
- Store the bulb syringe at the infant's bedside.

Note

Instruct the parents to position the infant's head to the side or downward if he is vomiting or gagging.

Caution: The nurse must emphasize to the parents that the bulb syringe must be compressed first and then inserted into the infant's nostril or mouth. If they insert the bulb syringe and then compress the bulb syringe, they may actually force secretions further back into the nose or throat and possibly cause an obstruction.

What If?

What if the infant gags as you attempt to perform oral suctioning with a bulb syringe?

You should remove the bulb syringe and position the infant's head to the side or downward. Once the gagging has ceased, perform oral suctioning with the bulb syringe, taking care to avoid any contact with the roof of the mouth or the back of the throat.

Documentation

6/29/10 0300 Baby boy Smith had a small amount of clear thick mucus draining from both nares, respirations 40 per minute, breathing without difficulty, and no retractions noted. Both nares suctioned with bulb syringe with a return of a small amount of clear thick mucus, procedure tolerated without difficulty.

—S. Chang, RN

During the initial assessment, the nurse remains alert for any signs of respiratory difficulty, such as rib or sternal retractions, "grunting" sounds, or nasal flaring. To check the heart rate, the nurse places the thumb and two fingers at the base of the umbilical cord and counts the pulsations. The infant's body temperature may be assessed by recording the axillary temperature or by attaching a thermoprobe and recording monitor to the skin. At this time, the infant is usually crying and turning pink, although the hands and feet remain slightly blue because of acrocyanosis, a condition related to vasomotor insufficiency and poor peripheral perfusion. If necessary, respiratory support is initiated according to hospital protocol. Oxygen may be administered via bag or mask. Obvious abnormalities are noted, and the nurse also checks and records the number of vessels in the umbilical cord, which should have two arteries and one vein. If the cord contains only two vessels (one artery and one vein), the physician should be notified immediately because this finding may be associated with renal and cardiac anomalies. Further testing is indicated. A two-vessel cord may be indicative of renal agenesis, a condition in which one kidney fails to develop normally during the gestational

period. The infant's weight and length are determined and recorded. Table 18-1 presents normal newborn parameters.

A numerical expression of the neonate's well-being, the Apgar score, is assigned at 1 and 5 minutes after birth. This score provides an objective means for assessing the neonate's immediate adaptation to extrauterine life. Five categories, including respiratory effort, heart rate, muscle tone, reflex irritability, and skin color are assessed, and each component is given a score ranging from 0 to 2. If neonatal resuscitation is required, it should be initiated before the 1-minute Apgar score (American College of Obstetricians and Gynecologists & American Academy of Pediatrics [ACOG/AAP], 2013; ACOG, 2006). (See Chapter 12 for further discussion.)

Various newborn laboratory tests may be routinely ordered according to hospital protocol. One test may be a sample of the cord blood if the mother is Rh(D)-negative or has type O blood group. The cord blood for the infant's blood type and Rh factor is obtained by the birth attendant while awaiting placental separation. If the infant's Apgar score is low, cord blood gas analysis may be ordered as well.

When the Apgar score is less than 9 at 5 minutes of life, it is important to stabilize the infant rather than allowing him

Table 18-1 Normal Neonatal Parameters at Birth	
Parameter	**Normal Finding**
Respirations	Rate 30–60 breaths per minute, irregular No retractions or grunting
Apical pulse	Rate 120–160 beats per minute
Temperature	97.7°F–99.3°F (36.5°C–37.4°C)
Skin color	Pink body, blue extremities
Umbilical cord	Contains two arteries and one vein
Gestational age	Full term: >37 completed weeks (should be 38–42 weeks to remain with parents for an extended time period)
Weight	2,500–4,300 grams
Length	45–54 cm

to remain with his mother in the birthing unit. Other conditions that would necessitate immediate infant stabilization include observations of nasal flaring, grunting respirations, rib retractions, heart rate less than 120 beats per minute or greater than 160 beats per minute, pallor, serious congenital anomalies (such as a neural tube defect), preterm infant (less than 38 weeks' gestational age), infant of a diabetic mother, or an infant who appears to be small for gestational age.

 Critical Nursing Action Recognizing Immediate Neonatal Respiratory Distress

During the neonatal assessment, the nurse is alert to the following signs and symptoms that are indicative of respiratory distress. If any of these symptoms are present, the nurse must immediately notify the physician:

- Generalized cyanosis
- Tachycardia (heart rate greater than 160 beats per minute)
- Tachypnea (respiratory rate greater than 70 breaths per minute)
- Rib retractions
- Expiratory grunting
- Flaring nostrils

IDENTIFICATION

After the Apgar evaluation, the nurse completes the mother–infant identification process according to hospital policy. This procedure usually includes obtaining infant footprints and a fingerprint and thumbprint of the mother along with appropriate labeling. Most institutions employ a system of waterproof matching identification bracelets that show the mother's name, the baby's gender, the name of the physician or nurse-midwife of record, and the date and time of birth. Two bracelets are worn by the neonate while the mother and her partner wear the others. Careful and continuous monitoring

 Nursing Care Plan Maintaining Newborn Thermoregulation

Nursing Diagnosis: Ineffective Thermoregulation related to immature regulatory systems

Measurable Short-Term Goal: The newborn will maintain a body temperature between 97.7°F and 99.3°F (36.5°C–37.4°C) in the first 24 hours post-birth.

Measurable Long-Term Goal: The newborn will maintain a body temperature between 97.7°F and 99.3°F (36.5°C–37.4°C) (wrapped in blankets in an open crib) after the first 24 hours post-birth.

NOC Outcome:
Thermoregulation: Newborn (0801) Balance among heat production, heat gain, and heat loss during the first 28 days of life

NIC Interventions:
Infant Care: Newborn (6824)
Temperature Regulation (3900)

Nursing Interventions:

1. Place newborn skin-to-skin with mother or under pre-warmed radiant warmer after birth. Dry well, discarding wet linens.

   RATIONALE: The maternal skin or radiant warmer provides a heat-gaining environment. Drying the infant reduces heat loss from evaporation.

2. Monitor newborn's axillary temperature per protocol (specify frequency) until stabilized.

   RATIONALE: Monitoring the temperature will assess the effectiveness of the therapy.

3. Apply stockinet cap and instruct parents to keep infant's head covered.

   RATIONALE: A cap helps prevent heat loss by convection from the large surface area of the head to the cooler room air.

4. Place the newborn under the radiant warmer with temperature probe attached and alarms turned on as needed to maintain temperature between 97.7°F and 99.3°F (36.5°C–37.4°C).

   RATIONALE: The radiant warmer provides a heat-gaining environment and prevents heat loss from contact with a cool surface (conduction). Active alarms and use of the temperature probe ensure the infant will not be under- or overheated.

5. When the temperature stabilizes, wrap the infant in two blankets and place him in an open crib. Instruct the parents to keep the crib away from windows and drafts.

   RATIONALE: Keeping the crib away from windows and drafts helps to prevent heat loss by radiation and convection.

of infants is essential to prevent misidentification, baby switching, or abduction. Alerting staff about mothers who share identical last names helps to decrease the likelihood of mistakes, and special security measures such as sensing devices, video cameras, and door alarms on all mother–baby units helps allay parents' concerns about their infants' safety. (See Chapter 15 for further discussion.)

INFECTION AND INJURY PREVENTION

The prevention of infection and injury constitute important aspects of newborn care. Hand washing is essential in preventing cross-contamination by all individuals caring for the newborn. In many facilities, nursery personnel are required to wear scrub clothes, remove nail polish, and keep fingernails trimmed. Other measures to prevent infection include infant bathing, umbilical cord care, care of the circumcision, and eye care. Soon after birth, the newborn receives a prophylactic ophthalmic agent to prevent ophthalmia neonatorum, eye inflammation from gonorrheal or chlamydial infection contracted during passage through the mother's birth canal. Medications most often used are erythromycin, tetracycline, or silver nitrate.

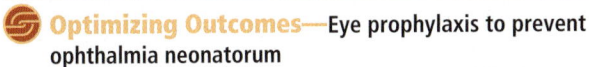

Optimizing Outcomes—**Eye prophylaxis to prevent ophthalmia neonatorum**

In some birth facilities, neonatal eye prophylaxis is delayed up to an hour to allow eye contact to facilitate parent–infant bonding. However, the Centers for Disease Control and Prevention (CDC) recommends that the medication be administered as soon as possible after birth. If instillation is delayed, the facility should have a monitoring system in place to ensure that all infants receive the prophylaxis (CDC, 2010).

During the first few days of life, the newborn has low levels of vitamin K because of sterile intestinal contents. Vitamin K acts as a catalyst to synthesize prothrombin, needed for blood clotting, in the liver. To prevent neonatal injury caused by hemorrhage, a single dose (0.5–1.0 mg) of vitamin K_1 phytonadione (AquaMEPHYTON) is administered via an IM injection in the vastus lateralis (preferred) or the ventrogluteal muscle (American Academy of Pediatrics, 2006) (Fig. 18-2).

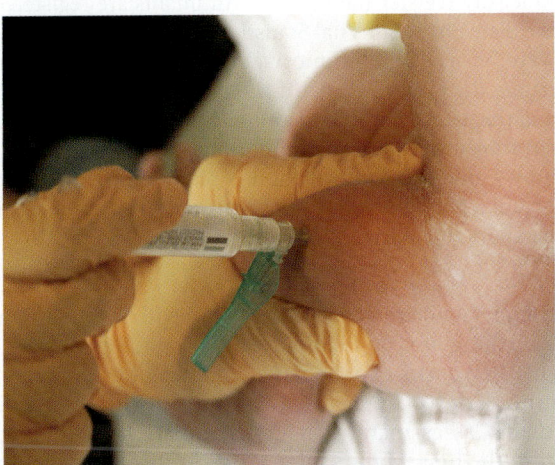

Figure 18-2 Newborn IM injection.

 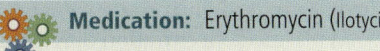 **Medication:** Erythromycin (Ilotycin)

(eh-**rith**-roe-**mye**-sin)

Pregnancy Category: B

Indications:

Infants: Prophylaxis of ophthalmia neonatorum

Actions: Suppresses protein synthesis at the level of the 50S ribosome

Therapeutic Effects: Bacteriostatic action against susceptible bacteria spectrum: Streptococci, staphylococci, gram-positive bacilli

Pharmacokinetics:

ABSORPTION: Minimal absorption may follow topical or ophthalmic use.

Contraindications and Precautions:

CONTRAINDICATED IN: Hypersensitivity

Adverse Reactions and Side Effects: Irritation

Route and Dosage: Apply a thin strip to each eye as a single dose.

Nursing Implications:

1. Inform parents of medication administration.
2. Prepare to administer the eye ointment to the infant 1 hour after birth.
3. Apply a thin strip to each eye as a single dose.
4. Start at the inner canthus and move to the outer canthus.
5. Dab excess medication off gently; do not wash away the medicine.

Source: Adapted from Vallerand, A. H., & Sanoski, C. A. (2014). *Davis's drug guide for nurses* (14th ed.). Philadelphia, PA: F.A. Davis.

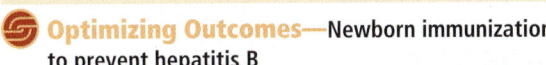

Optimizing Outcomes—**Newborn immunization to prevent hepatitis B**

Vaccination for hepatitis B, given in a series of three doses beginning at birth, is recommended for all infants. The vaccine must be given within 12 hours of birth. Before administration, the nurse obtains written parental consent. According to the American Council on Immunization Practices, aspiration for blood return with IM injections is unnecessary because there are no large blood vessels located within the recommended vaccination sites (Kroger, Sumaya, Pickering, & Atkinson, 2011). After injection of hepatitis B vaccine (Recombivax HB or Enerix-B) into the vastus lateralis muscle, the nurse massages the site with a gauze square to decrease pain sensation and to enhance absorption. Additional doses are administered at 1 and 6 months of age (Hensel & Springmyer, 2011).

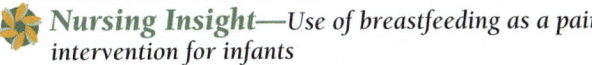

Nursing Insight—*Use of breastfeeding as a pain intervention for infants*

Evidence has shown that infants perceive and remember painful procedures such as immunizations, venipunctures, and heel sticks. Breastfeeding, an act that encompasses taste, suckling, and skin-to-skin contact, may be used as a natural, safe, and cost-effective intervention to help decrease the infant's perception of pain. Nurses can educate mothers about the beneficial use of breastfeeding to decrease painful stimuli (Tansky & Lindberg, 2010).

Assessment of blood glucose helps to prevent newborn injury related to hypoglycemia. In healthy term infants after an uneventful pregnancy and delivery, blood glucose monitoring often takes place within the first hour after birth. During the early newborn period of a term infant, hypoglycemia is defined as a blood glucose concentration of less than 35 mg/dL or a plasma concentration of less than 40 mg/dL. Infants with a low blood glucose level or those who exhibit signs and symptoms of hypoglycemia (jitteriness, apnea, seizures, or lethargy) require immediate attention to prevent brain cell damage. Hypoglycemia is usually resolved with feeding. If the newborn continues to display signs and symptoms of hypoglycemia along with low blood glucose laboratory results, transfer to the neonatal intensive care unit for IV administration of glucose may be necessary.

A heel stick blood sample for hematocrit and hemoglobin may be performed to detect anemia or polycythemia (an excess number of red blood cells). Anemia can result from hypovolemia associated with complications such as placenta previa, abruptio placentae, or cesarean birth. Polycythemia may be related to excessive blood flow from the umbilical cord into the infant at birth. A normal hematocrit at 1 hour of life is 46% to 55%. A normal hemoglobin is 15.2 to 22.5 g/dL. Early detection of abnormal laboratory results can ensure immediate treatment.

 Medication: AquaMEPHYTON (Phytonadione, Mephyton, vitamin K)

(fye-**toe**-na-dye-one)

Classification(s):
THERAPEUTIC: Antidotes, vitamins
PHARMACOLOGICAL: Fat-soluble vitamins

Pregnancy Category: UK

Indications: Prevention and treatment of hypoprothrombinemia, which may be associated with excessive doses of oral anticoagulants, salicylates, certain anti-infective agents, nutritional deficiencies, and prolonged total parenteral nutrition. Prevention of hemorrhagic disease of the newborn.

Action: Required for hepatic synthesis of blood coagulation factors II (prothrombin), VII, IX, and X.

Therapeutic Effects: Prevention of bleeding because of hypoprothrombinemia

Pharmacokinetics:
ABSORPTION: Well absorbed after oral or subcutaneous administration
DISTRIBUTION: Crosses the placenta; does not enter breast milk.
METABOLISM AND EXCRETION: Rapidity metabolized in the liver
HALF-LIFE: Unknown

Contraindications and Precautions:
CONTRAINDICATED IN: Hypersensitivity, hypersensitivity or intolerance to benzyl alcohol (injection only)
USE CAUTIOUSLY IN: Impaired liver function
EXERCISE EXTREME CAUTION IN: Severe life-threatening reactions have occurred after IV administration; use other routes unless IV is justified.

Adverse Reactions and Side Effects:
GASTROINTESTINAL: Gastric upset, unusual taste
DERMATOLOGICAL: Flushing, rash, urticaria
HEMATOLOGICAL: Hemolytic anemia
LOCAL: Erythema, pain at injection site, swelling
MISCELLANEOUS: Allergic reactions, hyperbilirubinemia (large doses in very premature infants), kernicterus

Route and Dosage: IV use of phytonadione should be reserved for emergencies.

Prevention of Hemorrhagic Disease of the Newborn:
IM (NEONATES): 0.5 to 1 mg, given within 1 to 2 hours after birth; may repeat in 6 to 8 hours if needed. May be repeated in 2 to 3 weeks if the mother received previous anticonvulsant/anticoagulant/anti-infective/antitubercular therapy. 1 to 5 mg may be given IM to the mother 12 to 24 hours before delivery.

Nursing Implications:
1. Inform parents of medication administration; invite them to offer comfort to their infant.
2. Prepare to administer the injection to the infant within 2 hours after birth: follow the six rights (i.e., the right patient, the right medication, the right dose, the right route, the right time, and the right documentation) of medication administration.
3. Draw up the medication in a 1-mL syringe.
4. Don gloves; unfasten the diaper to allow full visualization of the leg; identify and cleanse the injection site with an alcohol (or other skin antiseptic) swab.
5. Stabilize the knee with the heel of the hand and grasp the muscle between the thumb and forefinger.
6. Using a 25-gauge, 5/8-inch to 7/8-inch needle inserted at a 90-degree angle, slowly administer the medication into the middle third of the vastus lateralis muscle.
7. After removing the needle, use a dry gauze square to gently rub the injection site to promote absorption and decrease discomfort. Place a small dressing over the site and document date, time, and location of the injection.
8. Report any symptoms of unusual bleeding or bruising (bleeding gums; nosebleed; black, tarry stools; hematuria; or bleeding from the base of the umbilical cord or other open wounds).
9. A decrease in hemoglobin and hematocrit levels or any bleeding may indicate that the effects of the medicine have not been achieved and that more vitamin K may be necessary. Call the physician for further instruction.

Source: Adapted from Vallerand, A. H., & Sanoski, C. A. (2014). *Davis's drug guide for nurses* (14th ed.). Philadelphia, PA: F.A. Davis.

 legal alert—Document appropriate birth information

After the baby's birth, many pieces of important information are collected during the nursery admission process. The nurse records the actual time of birth, the status of infant's respirations—whether spontaneous or assisted, the 1- and 5-minute Apgar scores, the birth weight in pounds and kilograms, the axillary temperature, and the number of vessels in the umbilical cord. Also documented is the type and amount of medication instilled for eye prophylaxis, the injection sites for vitamin K and hepatitis B vaccine administration, the findings from the general physical assessment, observations of voiding or stooling, and all laboratory testing obtained, such as blood glucose or cultures. It is the responsibility of the physician, midwife, or the birth facility to legally register the neonate. All infants are registered at the State Bureau of Vital Statistics in the state in which they were born. Essential information including the mother's name; the father's name (if the mother gives permission); and the date, time, and place of birth is required. Birth registration information is important, because as the child grows older, this information is required to enter school, obtain a Social Security card, register to vote, and obtain a passport and a driver's license.

Infants who are stable may remain with their parents in the birthing area to facilitate family bonding and attachment. Newborns experiencing complications are taken to the nursery for further evaluation. After the immediate neonatal assessment, a later examination is conducted within the first 4 hours after birth. At this time, the nurse performs a brief physical assessment to estimate the infant's gestational age and evaluate the neonate's transition to extrauterine life (AAP & ACOG, 2012). Problems that place the neonate at risk are identified and evaluated. At some point before the infant's discharge, a complete physical examination and behavioral assessment are conducted to detect any emerging or potential problems. Depending on birthing facility protocol, this evaluation may be performed by the nurse, with certain components completed by a physician, certified nurse-midwife, or nurse practitioner.

 Now Can You—Discuss components of the neonate's initial adaptation?

1. Recognize what constitutes normal vital signs in the infant?
2. Use the following information to calculate Baby O'Leary's Apgar score. At 1 minute of life, Baby O'Leary is crying quietly in a radiant warmer. Her hands and feet are blue, and her extremities are floppy. Her heart rate is 122 beats per minute, and her respiratory rate is 28 breaths per minute and irregular. The Apgar score at 1 minute is _____?
3. Identify six indicators of neonatal respiratory distress?

The Later Neonatal Assessment

The neonate is usually greeted with a whirlwind of activities immediately after birth. However, many other activities and assessments will take place later in the newborn nursery. In the initial setting, the nurse conducts a brief physical assessment, carefully making note of body position, skin color, overall body size and symmetry, and level of interaction with the environment.

BODY POSITIONING

Not surprisingly, many infants seek comfort and security by resuming their dominant in utero position following birth. The normal newborn baby assumes a position of flexion of the upper and lower extremities. Flexed arms enable infants to use their hands to touch their faces, suck their fingers, and explore their world (Fig. 18-3).

The legs may be extended, arranged in the position assumed at the time of birth, or flexed. Most often, the infants' body positioning is symmetrical. Nurses should recognize that asymmetrical positioning at the time of the assessment might indicate injury from birth trauma. An infant's failure

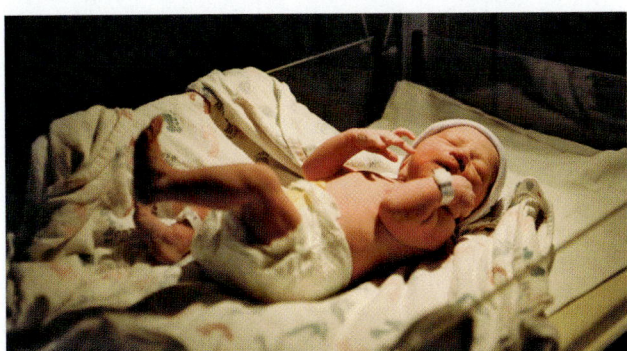

Figure 18-3 The full-term infant assumes a flexed position.

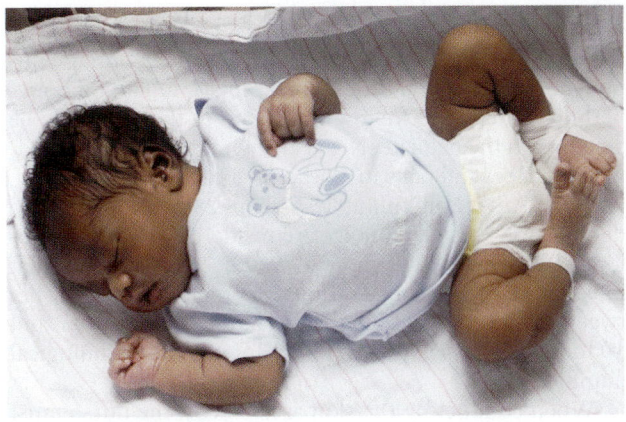

Figure 18-4 The infant is placed on his back to sleep.

to move one or more extremities also signals that further investigation is warranted. When positioning the infant, nurses must be sure to follow the guidelines established by the American Academy of Pediatrics (2011a) to prevent sudden infant death syndrome (SIDS) (Fig. 18-4). (See Chapter 19.)

 Critical Nursing Action Safe Positions to Prevent SIDS

- All infants should be placed for sleep in a supine position (wholly on the back) for every sleep by every caregiver until 1 year of life.
- Side sleeping is not safe and is not advised.

 Nursing Insight—Helping to meet the Healthy People 2020 national goals

One national goal directly addresses the reduction in SIDS-related infant deaths: "reduce the rate of infant deaths from sudden infant death syndrome" with a target of 0.50 infant deaths per 1,000 live births" (a 10% improvement) (U.S. Department of Health and Human Services [USDHHS], 2011). Nurses can help to meet this goal by teaching parents and all infant care providers the advantages of placing the newborn on the back to sleep. Teaching about infant safe sleep practices should extend beyond the hospital to include postnatal clinics, child care centers, churches, and community centers (Hoogsteen, 2010; Shaefer, Herman, Frank, Adkins, & Terhaar, 2010). According to the American Academy of Pediatrics Task Force on Sudden Infant Death Syndrome (2011a), other actions to help reduce SIDS-related infant deaths include use of a firm sleep surface (i.e., a firm mattress covered by a fitted sheet), room-sharing without bed-sharing, removal of soft objects and loose bedding from the crib, breastfeeding, offering a pacifier at nap time and bed time, avoidance of overheating exposure to tobacco smoke, use of commercial devices marketed to reduce the risk of SIDS, and compliance with recommended immunization schedules. In late 2012, the National Institutes of Health (NIH) expanded and renamed the original "Back to Sleep" campaign as the "Safe to Sleep" campaign, which now encompasses all sleep-related sudden unexpected infant deaths and includes those from SIDS as well as those from other causes such as accidental suffocation and entrapment (Hellwig, 2013; Hitchcock, 2012; NIH, 2012).

SKIN COLOR

Assessment of the infant's skin color is an essential component of the general physical examination. Jaundice (hyperbilirubinemia), a yellow coloration of the skin, may be apparent in the neonate. Normally, jaundice develops gradually over several days in a head-to-toe, or cephalocaudal, pattern. Any term infant less than 24 hours old who demonstrates visual jaundice is considered to have "pathological jaundice" or "hemolytic jaundice," a condition that most often results from a serious blood incompatibility between the mother and her newborn. (See Chapters 17 and 19 for further discussion of physiological and pathological jaundice.)

When conducting the skin assessment, the nurse must remember that certain characteristics of the nursery or mother's postpartum room can affect the accuracy of the exam. For example, pink walls and artificial lighting may mask the early detection of jaundice and interfere with an accurate assessment of the degree of severity of the condition. It is best to examine the neonate's skin in natural daylight, if possible. When jaundice is suspected, the nurse can readily assess the skin coloring by pressing on the infant's forehead or nose with a finger. When blanching occurs, the nurse can observe for the yellow coloration associated with jaundice.

"Physiological jaundice" or "nonhemolytic" jaundice describes the more commonly occurring yellowing of the skin in neonates that becomes apparent after the first 24 hours of life and usually peaks by the third to fifth day. Physiological jaundice often has a nonhemolytic cause and frequently results from a failure to adequately process bilirubin because of inadequate intake or elimination, birth trauma, or minor blood incompatibilities.

Breastfed infants may develop early-onset or "breastfeeding-associated jaundice," which is associated with insufficient feeding and infrequent stooling. Because colostrum has a natural laxative effect that stimulates the passage of meconium, frequent breastfeeding during the early days of life is beneficial in reducing the neonate's serum bilirubin levels. Late-onset or "breast milk jaundice" sometimes affects breastfed infants during the second week of life. This type of jaundice usually develops around the fourth day when the mother's mature breast milk comes in and peaks around day 10. Breast milk jaundice is thought to be related to factors in human milk that inhibit the conjugation or decrease the excretion of bilirubin. Although usually no treatment is necessary, some physicians advise mothers to discontinue breastfeeding for 12 to 24 hours to allow the infant's bilirubin levels to decrease (Verklan & Walden, 2014).

Nurses can implement several actions to decrease the likelihood of high bilirubin levels in the neonate. Maintaining the infant's skin temperature at or greater than 97.7°F (36.5°C) is beneficial because cold stress can cause acidosis, a condition linked with an elevated serum bilirubin. Also, careful monitoring of the infant's intake and output, with special attention to stool characteristics and frequency is important. Because bilirubin is excreted in the feces, inadequate elimination can result in the reabsorption and recycling of bilirubin. Finally, the nurse should encourage early (within the first hour of life) feedings when possible to promote rapid and continuous intestinal evacuation and provide the calories necessary for the production of hepatic binding proteins.

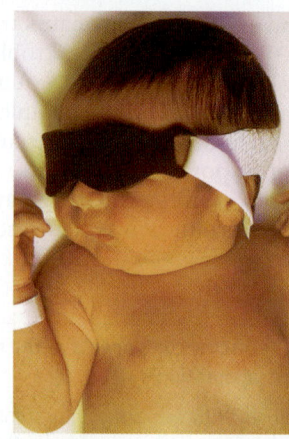

Figure 18-5 The jaundiced infant undergoing phototherapy. The eyes are covered to prevent retinal damage.

Understandably, the presence of physiological jaundice in the infant can be distressing for parents. Nurses can address these concerns by providing ongoing emotional support and accurate explanations of the condition. Parents should be taught about the importance of adequate hydration and how to assess the infant for signs of jaundice. If the baby undergoes phototherapy (exposure to high-intensity lights) for treatment, additional days of hospitalization may be required, and the mother may have to leave the birth center without her baby (Fig. 18-5). Parents should be encouraged to help meet their infant's emotional needs by holding, feeding, touching, and interacting with the baby. When the mother must leave the hospital without her infant, the nurse can support the bonding process by providing the nursery telephone number and name(s) of the baby's primary caregiver(s). Mothers should also be encouraged to call for updates and return for feedings as often as possible. Breastfeeding mothers may wish to remain in the hospital until the infant is released. In other situations, initiation of home phototherapy for the jaundiced infant may be an option. When the infant is treated in the home, nurses monitor the phototherapy regimen and obtain serum bilirubin levels as dictated by hospital or agency policy (Seagraves, Brulte, McNeely, & Pritham, 2013). (See Chapter 19.)

Infants with congenital heart defects often exhibit skin pallor that does not improve with time. All infants should exhibit pink skin, which is an important indicator of satisfactory perfusion to the extremities. Acrocyanosis, a common finding, is confined to the hands and feet (Fig. 18-6). Neonates with central cyanosis may demonstrate a blue tint

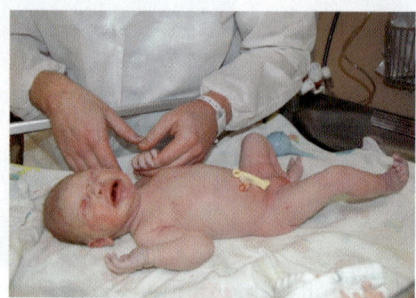

Figure 18-6 Acrocyanosis.

to the lips, gums, tongue, fingertips, and toes, as well as pallor under the eyes and on the cheeks. These findings are indicative of a circulatory problem and warrant immediate investigation into the suspected cause of the cyanosis. The diagnostic work-up for infants with central cyanosis may include echocardiography and cardiac catheterization. Depending on the findings, treatment may involve medical or surgical intervention. (See Chapters 19 and 26.)

When stimulated by physical contact, infants should demonstrate a rapid pinking of the skin that progresses to a red color. These changes are reflective of an increased respiratory and heart rate. Observing how long it takes for the infant to return to the previous skin color after stimulation is an important component of the nurse's visual assessment of the neonate's cardiovascular system. Making an accurate assessment of the infant's "true" skin color is of paramount importance when observing for color changes related to pathological conditions. For the nurse to accurately assess the color of the neonate's skin, it is necessary to know the "normal" skin color for that individual. It is important to remember that skin color is influenced by ethnicity. For example, the natural skin colors of African American and Hispanic infants may be infused with yellow tones that make it difficult for the nurse to determine normal skin color.

 Optimizing Outcomes—**Obtaining an accurate assessment of the infant's true skin color**

- Use a variety of light sources (helps to ascertain the "true" color).
- Examine the infant's entire skin surface.
- Carefully inspect the palms, soles of the feet, lips, and areas behind the ears.
- Gently palpate bony prominences (nose, sternum, sacrum, wrists, and ankles).
- Apply slight pressure for 1 second ("blanching").
- Observe for true skin color, reflective of the infant's ethnic heritage.
- Record true skin color; yellow is indicative of jaundice; white is indicative of pallor.

BODY SIZE

At the time of birth, the neonate's weight and length are measured and recorded. The nurse also visually inspects the infant for symmetry of head-to-toe length along with abdominal girth. Later, the neonate's actual body measurements are correlated with a development graph to ascertain appropriateness of the physical size. As a component of the visual inspection, the nurse confirms that the infant's head appears to be the largest body part.

 Now Can You—**Discuss essential nursing actions associated with newborn safety and skin color assessment?**

1. Describe and demonstrate how the infant should be positioned to prevent SIDS?
2. Name three nursing actions that can help minimize physiological jaundice?
3. Discuss four techniques that should be used to assess the infant's true skin color?

LEVEL OF REACTIVITY

The infant's reaction to the environment is an important indicator of the level of neuromuscular development. The nurse routinely assesses the infant's state of responsiveness and reactivity. During the exam, it is helpful to consider these questions, designed to ensure a thorough assessment:

"Is the neonate awake and quiet, or restless and crying?"
"Does the infant respond by looking and moving all extremities?"
"Is the infant's sleep pattern best characterized by quiet slumber or agitated restlessness?"

According to Brazelton (1973), neonates exhibit several discrete behavioral levels or "states" of awareness and normally progress or regress smoothly from one to the other. The sleep states include deep sleep and rapid eye movement sleep; the alert states include drowsy, quiet alert, active alert, and crying. The neonatal behavioral assessment is an important component of the overall evaluation because it validates a mature neurological–organizational system that allows the term infant to readily transition from one behavioral state to another. Certain conditions such as in utero exposure to cocaine disrupt this normal development; affected neonates exhibit erratic, disorganized behavior, an excessive response to stimuli, and lengthy or absent transition periods between behaviors. (See Chapter 19 for further discussion.)

The nurse may assess the infant's response to voices and physical presence to confirm the level of responsiveness and behavioral organization. An infant who displays irritability and an overreaction to voices, touch, or movement needs to be comforted, and special care must be taken to provide calming measures such as swaddling the neonate in blankets, cuddling, rocking, and gentle holding. It is best to postpone the physical examination because the manipulation and handling will most likely cause further disruption and behavioral disorganization.

 Optimizing Outcomes—**The Behavioral Observation of the Newborn Education Trainer**

Nurses play an important role in teaching parents about their newborns and facilitating emotional bonds between parents and infants. The Behavioral Observation of the Newborn Educational Trainer (BONET) is a learning aid designed to educate clinicians about newborn behavioral organization, self-regulation skills, and interactive capabilities. The BONET, which contains 19 behavioral items and 8 newborn reflexes, was largely adapted from the Neonatal Behavioral Assessment Scale originally developed by Brazelton and Nugent (1995). By showing newborn behavior as a series of increasingly mature systems that the newborn must master, the BONET guides understanding of this behavior and enables the nurse to help parents understand the systematic, purposeful, and seldom random pattern of their newborn's behavior and how to appropriately respond to various newborn cues (Karl & Keefer, 2011).

OBTAINING MEASUREMENTS AND DETERMINING THE GESTATIONAL AGE

Routine assessment of the neonate's vital signs is important before the physical examination and throughout the infant's hospital stay. It is essential that the nurse recognize the normal parameters for temperature, pulse, respirations, and blood pressure so that any change in the neonate's status can be readily identified.

Critical Nursing Action Recognizing Normal Newborn Vital Signs

When assessing newborn vital signs, the nurse must be aware of the following normal parameters:

Temperature:
Rectal: 98.6°F to 100.0°F (37.0°C–37.8°C)
Axillary: 97.7°F to 99.3°F (36.5°C–37.4°C)

Heart rate:
120 to 160 beats per minute (count heart rate for 1 full minute)
During sleep, the heart rate can be as low as 80 beats per minute.
During crying the heart rate can be as high as 180 beats per minute.

Respirations:
30 to 60 respirations per minute (count respiratory rate for 1 full minute)
Abdominal breathing is normal. Periodic breathing is considered normal and classified as short pauses in the breathing of the newborn that last only approximately 3 seconds. Apneic episodes are significant if they last more than 15 to 20 seconds; they may be accompanied by abrupt pallor, hypotonia, cyanosis, and bradycardia. Apnea must be differentiated from periodic breathing, which is normal in the newborn.
Caution: Withhold oral feeding if the respiratory rate is greater than 60 respirations per minute.

Blood pressure:
Systolic: 60 to 80 mm Hg; diastolic: 40 to 50 mm Hg at birth
Systolic: 95 to 100 mm Hg; diastolic: slight increase at 10 days of age

The neonate's weight, recorded in grams, and the length, recorded in centimeters, are measured in the birthing room and again during the transitional period (Figs. 18-7 and 18-8). On average, a term newborn infant weighs 3,400 grams, with a normal range of 2,500 to 4,300 grams. Recumbent length is a crown-to-heel measurement taken with the infant in a supine position (Procedure 18-2). The recumbent length is recorded on a regular basis until the infant reaches 24 months of age. Normal length parameters for newborns are approximately 18 to 22 inches (45–55 cm).

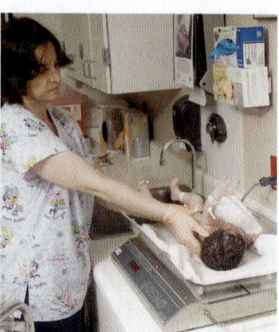

Figure 18-7 Weighing the infant.

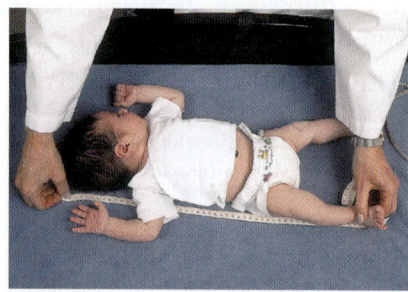

Figure 18-8 Measuring the infant's body length.

Procedure 18-2 Measuring the Newborn's Body Length

Purpose
To establish and document the newborn's body length

Equipment
- Standard paper tape measure

Steps
1. Place the infant on a paper-covered flat surface.
2. Fully extend the infant's body by holding the head midline.

   RATIONALE: *The newborn normally assumes a flexed position and must be fully extended to obtain an accurate measurement.*

3. Gently grasp the knees and place them together.
4. Push down gently on the knees until they are fully extended and flat against the table surface.
5. Measure the crown-to-heel recumbent length by placing the paper tape measure beside the infant with the 0 end of the tape at the top of the head.

Keep the infant's body in alignment and carefully extend one leg. Ensure that the tape measure remains straight. Note the length and record it in the infant's chart. As an alternate measurement method, make a slash mark with a pen at the end points by the top of the infant's head and the heels of the foot. While providing continuous support, gently roll the infant to the side and measure between the two points with a paper tape measure that has increments designated in tenths.

RATIONALE: *Careful body positioning and use of a tape measure gradated in tenths ensures an accurate measurement. Measurements are taken and recorded to note abnormalities and to provide a baseline value.*

Documentation

3/4/10 0800 – Infant length: 50 cm.

—J. Yamoto, RN

The nurse also obtains and records the frontal–occipital circumference (FOC), or head measurement (Fig. 18-9). A paper tape measure with increments marked in tenths of a centimeter is used to ensure an accurate measurement. To obtain the head circumference, the tape measure is placed on the area immediately above the eyebrows and pinna of the ears and then wrapped around to the occipital prominence at the back of the head. This location represents the area of the greatest head circumference. After obtaining the head measurement three times, the nurse records the largest finding. The normal head circumference for a full-term neonate ranges from 13 to 15 inches (33–38 cm). Measurement of the head circumference is repeated at subsequent physical exams until the infant reaches 36 months of age.

To obtain the chest measurement, the paper tape measure is placed on the nipple line and then wrapped around the entire thoracic area (Fig. 18-10). The head and chest measurement may be equal during the first few days of life. A normal chest measurement is 12 to 13 inches (30.5–33 cm). The abdominal circumference may be obtained by encircling the infant's body with the paper tape measure placed directly above the umbilicus (Fig. 18-11). The abdomen should be approximately the same size as the chest (Dillon, 2007). Once all measurements have been obtained, the nurse plots the weight, length, and head circumference against the infant's gestational age to determine the appropriate size category (Fig. 18-12). Size categories are small for gestational age (SGA), appropriate for gestational age (AGA), and large for gestational age (LGA). If at any time the physical measurements fall outside the normal growth parameters, the physician should be notified. Information concerning normal growth parameters for infants, children, and adults is available at the CDC National Center for Health Statistics Web site: http://www.cdc.gov/growthcharts/

 Nursing Insight—*Understanding classifications for newborn weight*

Large for gestational age (LGA): Weight is above the 90th percentile at any week.

Appropriate for gestational age (AGA): Weight falls between the 10th and 90th percentiles for the infant's age.

Small for gestational age: (SGA): Weight falls below the 10th percentile for the infant's age.

In 1967, the American Academy of Pediatrics recommended that all newborns be classified by birth weight and gestational age. Since that time, a scoring system developed by Ballard and colleagues (1991), which represents a modification of the Dubowitz system, has been the most commonly used method for determining the neonate's gestational age. With this assessment system, the infant examination yields a score of neuromuscular and physical maturity that can be extrapolated onto a corresponding age scale to reveal the infant's gestational age in weeks. Additional methods used to determine gestational age are fundal height measurement before delivery, ultrasonography, and eye lens vascularity. A rough approximation of the gestational age at birth can be calculated according to the date of the mother's last normal menstrual period. Because these other sources of age determination are not as accurate as the neonatal physical examination, gestational age assessments are frequently performed by the nurse and recorded on the infant's chart.

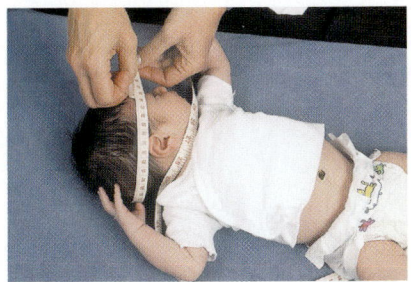

Figure 18-9 Measuring the head circumference.

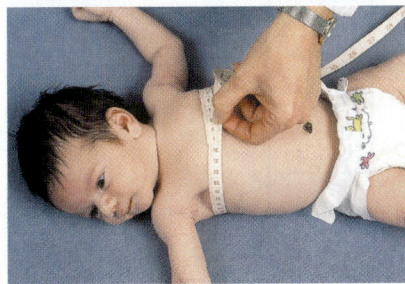

Figure 18-10 Measuring the chest circumference.

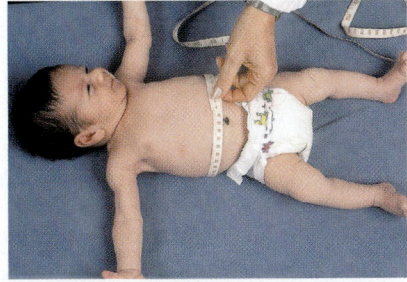

Figure 18-11 Measuring the abdominal circumference.

Optimizing Outcomes—Use of the Ballard Gestational Age by Maturity Rating tool

The Ballard Gestational Age by Maturity Rating tool includes a neuromuscular maturity and a physical maturity component (Fig. 18-13) that contains six characteristics to be assessed. At the conclusion of the examination, the scores from each component are added together, then mathematically extrapolated onto the maturity rating scale to determine the infant's gestational age by examination. The scoring system is designed to identify the decreased levels of muscle and joint flexibility characteristic of the premature infant, as well as the mature term infant's ability to return to the original position after movement. The nurse usually performs this assessment within the first 12 hours of the infant's life. The Ballard scoring system is more accurate when conducted on term infants who are between 10 and 36 hours of life. The order in which the assessment is conducted is unimportant.

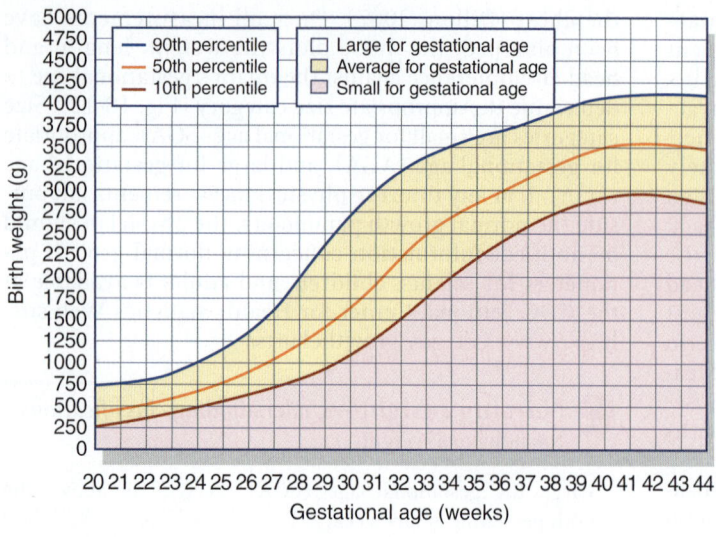

Figure 18-12 Gestational age assessment.

Neuromuscular Maturity

	-1	0	1	2	3	4	5
Posture							
Square Window (Wrist)	-90°	90°	60°	45°	30°	0°	
Arm Recoil		180°	140°-180°	110°-140°	90°-110°	<90°	
Popliteal Angle	180°	160°	140°	120°	100°	90°	<90°
Scarf Sign							
Heel to Ear							

Physical Maturity

Skin	Sticky Friable Transparent	Gelantinous Red Translucent	Smooth pink Visible veins	Superficial Peeling or rash, few veins	Cracking Pale areas Rare veins	Parchment Deep cracking No vessels	Leathery Cracked Wrinkled
Lanugo	None	Sparse	Abundant	Thinning	Bald areas	Mostly bald	
Plantar Surface	Heel-toe 40–50 mm:-1 <40 mm:-2	>50 mm No crease	Faint red marks	Anterior transverse crease only	Creases ant. 2/3	Creases over entire sole	
Breast	Imperceptible	Barely perceptible	Flat areola No bud	Stippled areola 1–2 mm bud	Raised areola 3–4 mm bud	Full areola 5–10 mm bud	
Eye/ear	Lids fused loosely:-1 tightly:-2	Lids open Pinna flat Stays folded	Sl. Curved pinna; soft; slow recoil	Well-curved pinna; soft but ready recoil	Formed and firm Instant recoil	Thick cartilage Ear stiff	
Genitals (Male)	Scrotum flat, smooth	Scrotum empty Faint rugae	Testes in upper canal Rare rugae	Testes descending Few rugae	Testes down Good rugae	Testes pendulous Deep rugae	
Genitals (Female)	Clitoris prominent Labia flat	Prominent clitoris Small labia minora	Prominent clitoris Enlarging minora	Majora and minora equally prominent	Majora large Minora small	Majora cover clitoris and minora	

Maturity Rating

Score	Weeks
-10	20
-5	22
0	24
5	26
10	28
15	30
20	32
25	34
30	36
35	38
40	40
45	42
50	44

Figure 18-13 Ballard Gestational Age Assessment Tool.

Interestingly, gestational age maturity may occur at different rates among the various categories. For example, a score of 4 (full maturity) in one category does not indicate that all subsequent categories must also reflect a score of 4. "Half-scores" are often recorded if the examiner believes that the infant exhibits a characteristic that falls between two scoring options during the assessment. It is important to remember that the infant's maturity scoring does not directly translate to the gestational age in weeks.

Now Can You—Obtain neonatal measurements
and determine gestational age?

1. Describe and demonstrate how to obtain neonatal body measurements?
2. Identify two maturity components that are assessed in the Ballard tool? Describe when and why the Ballard assessment should be performed?
3. Discuss whether or not the Ballard maturity score should be identical to the gestational age of the neonate?

Conducting and Documenting the Neonatal Physical Assessment

The nurse conducts the neonatal physical examination with the review of systems following the general nursing assessment of the newborn. This examination should not be initiated if the infant is crying or appears to be upset. Instead, it is best to postpone the assessment until the infant is calm. Infant registration and documentation of findings from the physical examination, along with other pertinent information (e.g., site and dosage of the vitamin K and hepatitis B vaccine injections and instillation of medication for eye prophylaxis) must be completed for each infant before hospital discharge.

> *Nursing Insight—Differentiating between the terms "major" and "minor" congenital anomaly*
>
> The majority of congenital anomalies occur during early embryogenesis. A *major* congenital anomaly is a structural defect, present at birth, that has a significant effect on function or social acceptability. A *minor* congenital anomaly occurs in less than 4% of the normal population and has minimal effect on function but may have cosmetic or social significance (Askin, 2009).

ASSESSMENT OF THE NEONATE: A SYSTEMS APPROACH

Once the assessment of the infant's general physical growth parameters and gestational age has been completed, the nurse systematically examines each body system, beginning with the skin and proceeding in a head-to-toe direction. This assessment may take place in the nursery with the infant resting comfortably in a crib, under a radiant warmer (to maintain temperature stability), or if stable, in the mother's room. Carrying out the assessment by the mother's bedside has several advantages. For most, the bedside is a nonthreatening environment where the mother and the nurse can "explore" the baby's special and unique characteristics. Also, conducting the evaluation in this relaxed setting gives the nurse an opportunity to observe the mother's ease in interacting with and touching and holding her infant. Appropriate positive reinforcement by the nurse affirms and validates the mother's actions, enhances her sense of maternal worthiness, and strengthens the bonding relationship. For the infant, the evolving sense of trust and perception of a secure environment are two essential developmental milestones first established during these early

contacts with caregivers. These experiences lay the foundation for the child's lifelong development of self-esteem and self-love. A spiritual health promotion strategy for the family with a newborn centers on encouraging the parents and caregivers to shower their infants and toddlers with love and comfort (Bowden, 2012).

With the infant in a supine position, the nurse follows the steps of inspection, light palpation, deep palpation, and auscultation to facilitate the examination. When assessing the abdomen, the proper sequence is inspection, auscultation, and light palpation followed by deep palpation.

Assessment of the Integumentary System

Wearing gloves, the nurse examines the neonate's skin, scalp and body hair, and nails for color, texture, distribution, disruptions, eruptions, and birthmarks. It is important that the assessment take place in a well-lit room, and additional light sources may be needed to confirm accuracy of findings. The infant's skin should be pink, a finding that indicates adequate peripheral cardiac perfusion. Blanching the skin over bony prominences should yield a pink-white color before returning to natural pigmentation.

As previously described, acrocyanosis, a bluish coloration to the hands and feet, is a normal condition related to vasomotor instability and poor peripheral circulation. To differentiate between acrocyanosis and true cyanosis, the nurse can vigorously rub the sole of the neonate's foot. If the sole turns pink, the diagnosis is acrocyanosis. If the sole remains blue, it is true cyanosis. Also, acrocyanosis disappears when the infant cries. Visual inspection of the infant's mouth, tongue, and gums confirms the skin color assessment because these areas should be pink-red in color and darken to bright red with crying. True cyanosis produces a bluish coloration and pallor (paleness) of the lips and on the area around the mouth.

Careful, daily assessment of the newborn's skin is an important nursing action that may lead to early detection of potential problems. If pallor, **plethora** (a deep purplish color related to an increased number of circulating red blood cells), **petechiae** (pinpoint hemorrhagic areas), central cyanosis, or jaundice is detected, further evaluation is warranted. The nurse describes and records in the infant's medical chart the location of any birth injuries such as forceps marks or fetal monitoring lesions. Infants born with a nuchal cord (umbilical cord around the neck) or those who assumed a face presentation commonly exhibit bruises or petechiae on the head, neck, and face. If extensive bruising is present, the infant's bilirubin level may be elevated. Although focal petechiae may be related to injury from increased pressure, the presence of petechiae scattered throughout the infant's body can be indicative of an underlying problem such as a low platelet count or infection. Periauricular papillomas, or skin tags, are a benign common finding that often run in families and usually are insignificant and require no intervention.

The term infant's skin should feel smooth and soft. Lanugo (fine, downy hair) may be noted on the neonate's back, shoulders, and head, and vernix caseosa may be present in the axillary and genital areas (Figs. 18-14 and 18-15). In the postterm infant, the skin is often tough and leathery, with cracking and peeling. Disruptions or breaks in the skin may be related to electrode marks or lacerations. Infants delivered by forceps or vacuum extraction may have skin disruptions or bruising on the scalp and face. Often,

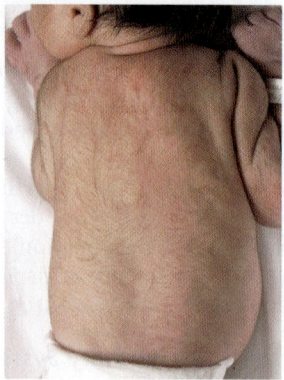

Figure 18-14 Lanugo.

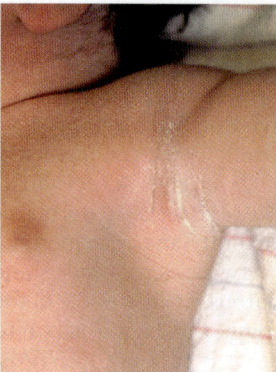

Figure 18-15 Vernix caseosa.

infants are born with pustular melanosis, a condition in which small pustules are formed prior to delivery. As the pustule disintegrates, a small residue or "scale" in the shape of the pustule is formed. This lesion later develops into a small (1- to 2-mm) macule, or flat spot. Macules, which are brown in color, appear similar to freckles and are frequently located on the chest and extremities. Pustular melanosis occurs more commonly on African American infants than on Caucasian infants (Association of Women's Health, Obstetric and Neonatal Nurses [AWHONN], 2013; Taylor, Wright, & Woodrum, 2011).

Another common skin condition is **milia**, small white papules or sebaceous cysts on the infant's face that resemble pimples (Fig. 18-16). Inclusion cysts may be seen singularly or in pairs on the penis or scrotum of male infants or on the areola of female infants. Acne, a skin condition common in adolescents, may also be present in newborns and is related to excessive amounts of maternal hormones. Over time, neonatal acne disappears spontaneously from the infant's cheeks and chest. **Erythema toxicum**, a transient rash that covers the face and chest with spread to the entire body, is the most common normal skin eruption in term neonates. It is also called "erythema neonatorum," "newborn rash," or "flea bite" dermatitis. Typically, the rash consists of small, irregular, flat red patches on the cheeks that develop into singular, small yellow pimples appearing on the chest, abdomen, and extremities. The cause of this skin condition is unknown, and it may persist for up to 1 month of life. There is no treatment available to hasten the resolution of the rash, which, because of its frequently unsightly appearance, can be quite disturbing to parents.

Blisters related to repetitive sucking may form on the fingers, wrists, and upper lips of infants who often perpetuate a habit begun in utero. Although these lesions may appear to be serious, parents can be assured that they will resolve over time without intervention.

Many neonatal skin variations are characterized by color changes that are different from normal pigmentation. For example, **Mongolian spots** are areas that appear gray, dark blue, or purple and are most commonly located on the back and buttocks, although they may also be found on the shoulders, wrists, forearms, and ankles (Fig. 18-17). Mongolian spots are seen most often in infants whose ethnic backgrounds include the Mediterranean area, Latin America, Asia, or Africa. Parents can be assured that these skin changes will fade and disappear as the infant grows older. Because they may be mistaken for bruises, it is important that the nurse document Mongolian spots on the infant's chart. Another condition, "cutis marmorata," or mottling, is common in neonates and is most often caused by the infant's vasomotor response to the lower environmental temperature outside the uterus. Mottling may also be related to prolonged apnea. Usually, the mottling disappears once the newborn adjusts to the extrauterine environment. A deepened coloration of the genital skin in males and females may occur because of the influence of maternal hormones. This color change also diminishes over time.

Birthmarks are distinct areas of color that may be tan, brown, white, or red. Their appearance varies but generally these lesions are small and flat. It is important to distinguish birthmarks from skin lesions that result from birth trauma. The nurse documents the location, size, and color of the birthmark, and if the lesion contains hair or is located along

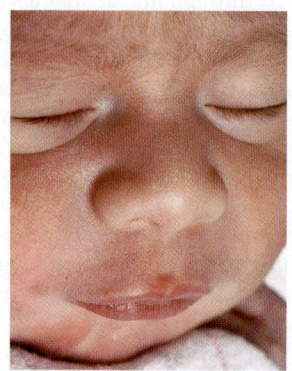

Figure 18-16 Milia.

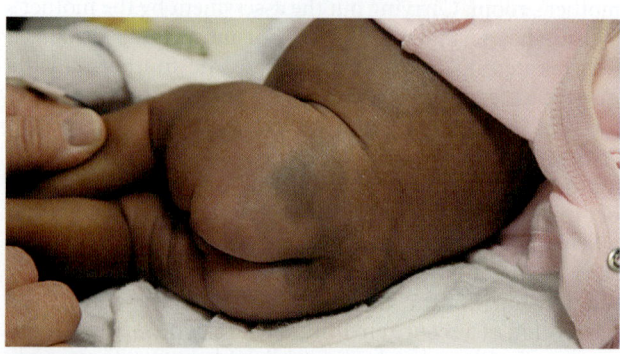

Figure 18-17 Mongolian spots.

the anterior or posterior midline, further investigation is warranted to rule out underlying tissue involvement.

Café-au-lait birthmarks are flat, tan spots that are quite common and insignificant unless the infant exhibits six or more marks that are greater than 1 cm in diameter. In this circumstance, the neonate should be carefully evaluated during infancy for tumors that develop beneath the skin because he may be at risk for developing type 1 neurofibromatosis. The nurse should be aware that because café-au-lait spots and other skin pigment variations can be very difficult to identify in African American infants, extra care must be taken when performing the integumentary system assessment (Taylor et al., 2011).

Brown **nevi** (from Latin naevi, for "birthmark") are brown skin marks whose color can vary from brown to deep black. Because a nevus may represent a very early form of a precancerous lesion, the nurse should teach parents to routinely check the lesion for changes in color, shape, size, or elevation from the skin surface. The careful observation of this skin lesion should be ongoing and continuous throughout the child's lifetime.

A **nevus flammeus**, a birthmark often referred to as a "port wine stain," is a capillary angioma located directly below the epidermis. Usually apparent at birth, the nevus flammeus is a non-elevated, red to purple network of dense capillaries that varies in size, shape, and location, although it commonly appears on the face. It does not blanch on pressure, disappear, or grow in size. Sturge-Weber syndrome, a clinical condition involving the fifth cranial nerve, may be present when a nevus flammeus is accompanied by convulsions or other indicators of neurological problems (Taylor et al., 2011).

A **telangiectatic nevus** is a red birthmark often seen at the nape of the neck and commonly referred to as a "stork bite" or "angel kiss" (Fig. 18-18). This lesion may also occur on the face between the eyebrows or on the eyelids, nose, or upper lip. It is usually irregular in shape and pale red, often turning bright red when the infant cries. The telangiectatic nevus tends to fade as the infant grows older and usually disappears by the second birthday. A **nevus vasculosus**, or "strawberry mark," is a red, raised capillary

hemangioma that can occur anywhere on the neonate's body. This birthmark usually has sharp borders and a rough surface that resembles a strawberry. Although often alarming because of its appearance, the nurse can reassure parents that over time this lesion will eventually undergo a process of involution and disappear during the first year of life. Unless they interfere with a vital organ system or are located on the face, surgical removal of capillary hemangiomas is not recommended. The blue nevus appears as a distinct blue or blue-black birthmark often found on the buttocks, hands, and feet. Although sometimes mistaken for a Mongolian spot when it appears on the buttocks, nurses can differentiate the blue nevus by noting its distinct borders and brighter color, as compared with the Mongolian spot, which covers a larger area. The blue nevus is usually 1 cm or less in size.

Hypopigmentation refers to a white or pale area of skin. When it occurs as a single lesion, hypopigmentation is not a cause for worry. However, if multiple hypopigmented areas, including lesions in a leaf pattern, are present, the infant should be referred for further evaluation. These lesions, which sometimes appear on the chest, back, extremities, and axillae, may be associated with tuberous sclerosis, a neurological condition.

CONDITIONS THAT MAY WARRANT FURTHER ASSESSMENT. Blemishes and other marks on an infant's skin that are related to birth trauma most often mirror the traumatizing instrument such as forceps or scalp electrodes. Characteristically, the color of these lesions progresses through the various skin color changes commonly associated with bruising. When assessing for birth injuries, the nurse pays close attention to the scalp, face, shoulders, arms, legs, and feet. Large infants frequently exhibit marks from trauma sustained during a difficult vaginal birth. Infants born with a nuchal cord (umbilical cord around the neck) may demonstrate considerable bruising of the neck and face. Also, neonates whose presenting part was the legs, feet, or buttocks may have extensive edema or bruising of the lower extremities. Sometimes the full extent of tissue damage cannot be appreciated by routine inspection and palpation. Instead, the nurse may note that the infant responds to positional changes and other gentle manual manipulation with excessive crying or irritability. In these circumstances, further assessment should be conducted with the infant placed in the supine and prone positions. Because excessive bruising may be associated with elevated bilirubin levels, the infant should be closely observed for signs of jaundice. Widespread petechiae or petechiae unrelated to birth trauma should be reported to the pediatrician because these findings may be associated with infection, low platelets, or congenital problems such as rubella.

Abnormally pigmented skin lesions and variations in hair patterns are other findings that may signal underlying problems. Infants who exhibit hairy pigmented skin lesions containing two distinct areas of color should be evaluated by a dermatologist. Because these findings may be related to an underlying structural defect, diagnostic ultrasound is often performed to evaluate the tissue beneath the skin surface. Hairy nevi describe skin nevi that contain individual hairs or a full tuft of hair. The presence of hairy nevi located in the posterior midline area near the spinal column may indicate a vertebral defect. When present, ultrasound

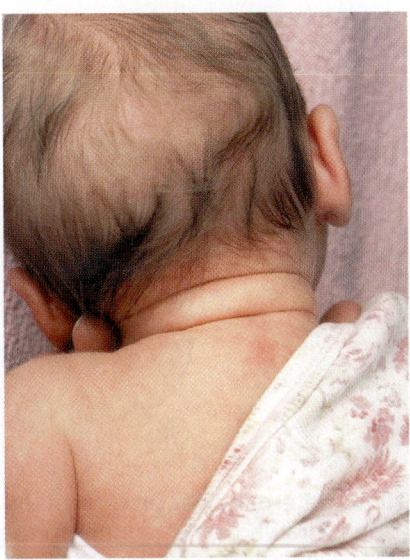

Figure 18-18 Stork bite.

examination of the spinal column is necessary to confirm any defects related to spina bifida or spina bifida occulta.

The nurse may identify an infant whose skin color remains deep pink or red during quiet rest or sleep. This finding may indicate plethora, a condition most often caused by polycythemia vera or hyperthermia. Polycythemia vera, a condition characterized by an excessive number of red blood cells, occurs from the transfer of maternal blood into the neonate's circulation during the time when the umbilical cord was cut. Polycythemia vera can be confirmed by a capillary hematocrit value of 65 or greater or a venous hematocrit of 60 or more. Treatment for this condition usually involves a partial exchange transfusion. (See Chapter 19 for further discussion of neonatal exchange transfusions.) Hyperthermia can be detected by checking the infant's body temperature.

Careful examination of the infant's hair pattern is another essential component of the nursing assessment. Special attention should be paid to the hair texture, color, and distribution, noting any disruptions to the hair distribution or areas of asymmetry on the scalp. Hair that covers the forehead and creates a shortened distance between the hairline and the eyebrows may be indicative of a congenital syndrome. The nurse notes any variations such as hair that is lighter in color than the surrounding hair or hair that appears to grow in a circular pattern or whorl. Sections of white hair embedded in darker scalp hair may indicate an underlying structural defect or the presence of a congenital syndrome.

Ongoing observation and assessment of the neonate's skin allows the nurse an opportunity to confirm normalcy, identify potential problems, and prepare for possible interventions. It also provides an opportunity to educate and reassure parents about normal neonatal skin characteristics and findings that might indicate problems. Parents are often fearful about "body marks," and the nurse can allay anxieties and stress the importance of conducting routine skin observations throughout childhood.

Now Can You—Discuss neonatal skin conditions?

1. Explain what parents should be taught about treatment for their infant's erythema toxicum?
2. Identify when the presence of café-au-lait spots in the neonate warrants further investigation?
3. Discuss the significance of hairy, pigmented skin lesions in the newborn?
4. Describe why the nurse should carefully assess the neonate's hair pattern?

Assessment of the Infant's Head

Following the skin assessment, the infant's head, eyes, ears, nose, and throat are evaluated next. The nurse methodically assesses the face for symmetry, noting the placement of the eyes, nose, lips, mouth, and ears (Fig. 18-19). Eye shape and size are noted along with assessment for coordinated movement of the lids. Eye color and placement on the forehead are recorded. The lips are also assessed for movement. Birth-related damage to the seventh cranial (facial) nerve can result in a number of findings such as unilateral drooping of the tongue or mouth, unequal movement of the cheek muscles, or inappropriate eyelid movement.

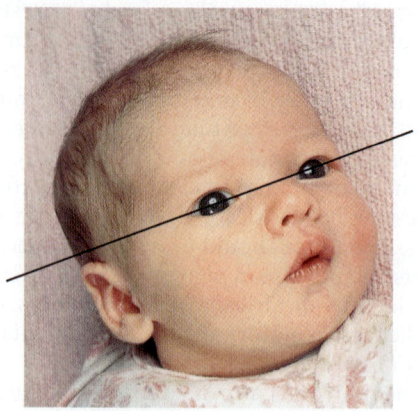

Figure 18-19 The face is examined for symmetry, noting placement of the eyes, nose, lips, mouth, and ears.

Special attention is paid to the shape, size, and placement of the ears. Low-set ears may signal the need for further assessment and evaluation for chromosomal abnormalities (Fig. 18-20). Placement of one ear slightly lower than the other is a common finding that generally has no clinical significance. Nostrils should be open bilaterally, and the nasal bridge should be centered with no lateral deviations. Lip color should be consistent with the tongue and buccal mucosa of the mouth. The upper and lower lips should be approximately uniform in size. The infant's chin should be readily apparent when viewed in a profile position. Micrognathia, or small jaw, may interfere with tooth development, sucking, swallowing, and tongue movement inside the mouth during speech (Dillon, 2007).

The nurse carefully palpates the infant's head to assess the fontanelles, the cranial suture lines, and the presence of any birth-related edema. The anterior fontanelle is readily

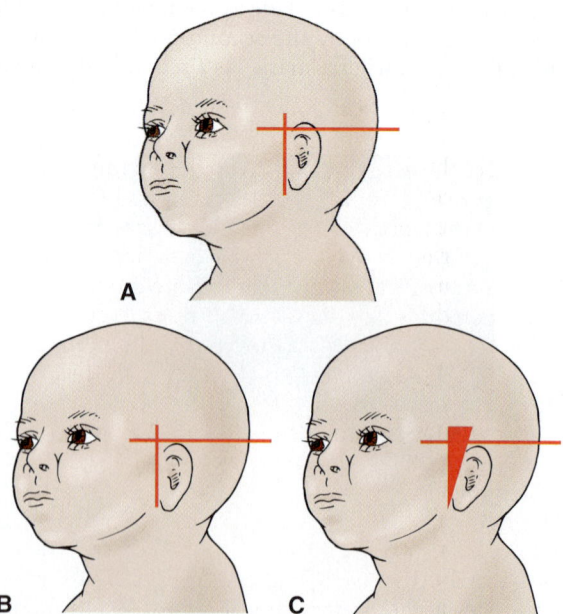

Figure 18-20 To determine ear placement, an imaginary line is drawn from the inner to the outer canthus of the eye and then to the ear. *A,* Normal ear position. *B,* Low-set ear. *C,* Slanted low-set ear.

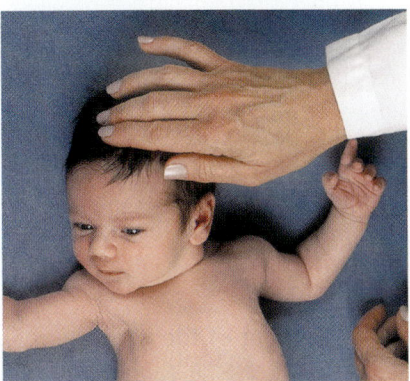

Figure 18-21 Palpating the fontanelle borders.

identifiable as a diamond-shaped open space formed by the anterior–posterior sagittal and frontal sutures and the lateral coronal suture (Fig. 18-21). Assessment of the fontanelle includes an estimation of the overall fontanelle size. The nurse can readily determine this dimension by palpation of the fontanelle borders with use of the finger for measurements (the distance from the tip of the finger to the first finger joint is roughly 1 in., or 2.5 cm). Variations in anterior fontanelle size are common and range from 0.4 to 2.8 inches (1–7 cm). The posterior fontanelle, located toward the back of the cranium, is a small, triangular-shaped space formed by the sagittal suture and the posterior lateral suture. At its widest point, the posterior fontanelle is usually only 0.4 inch (1 cm) and may be closed at initial examination. The anterior fontanelle must remain open during the first year of life to accommodate skull bone expansion that accompanies normal brain growth. Open spaces between the suture lines result from cranial molding during the birth process. Assessment of the fontanelles for intracranial pressure is an important component of the examination. Normal intracranial pressure is characterized by a finding of fontanelle fullness without bulging, either on visual inspection or palpation. Bulging, tense fontanelles in an infant with a large head circumference are indicative of increased intracranial pressure, often associated with hydrocephalus.

The nurse may note the presence of swelling or soft tissue edema of the head that has resulted from trauma during the birth process. **Caput succedaneum** is diffuse edema that crosses the cranial suture lines and disappears without treatment during the first few days of life. **Cephalhematoma**, a more serious condition, results from a subperiosteal hemorrhage that does not cross the suture lines (Fig. 18-22). It appears as a localized swelling on one side of the infant's head and persists for weeks while the tissue fluid is slowly broken down and absorbed. During this time, the infant may exhibit signs of jaundice related to the metabolism of damaged red blood cells from the subperiosteal hemorrhage.

The nurse next palpates the neonate's eyes, ears, and nose to confirm shape and size. The eyelids are manually opened and the iris, sclera, and conjunctiva are examined. It is not unusual to detect tiny pinpoint scleral hemorrhages (related to birth trauma) in the outer canthus of the eyes. Swollen eyelids and a yellow discharge that adheres to the eyelashes may provide evidence of eye prophylaxis medication. The nurse uses an ophthalmoscope to check

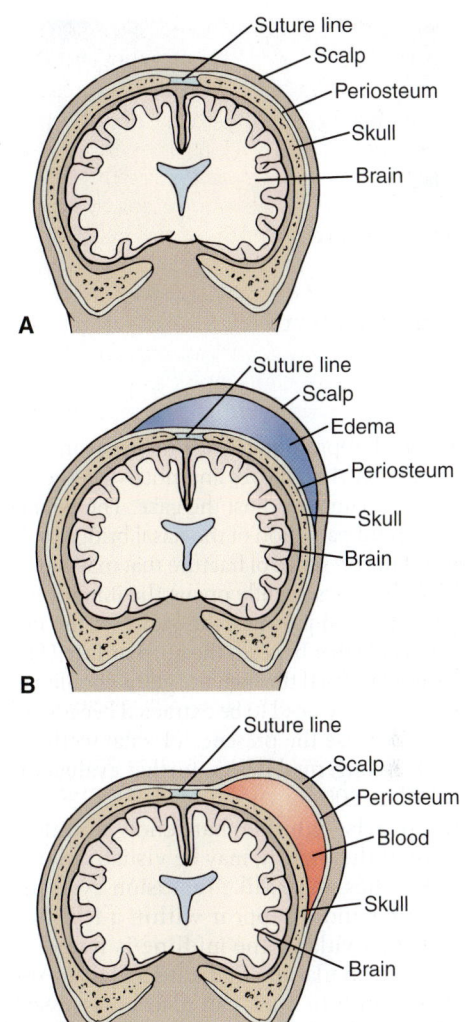

Figure 18-22 A, Normal head. B, Caput succedaneum—localized soft tissue edema present at birth; does not increase in size; swelling crosses the suture lines. C, Cephalhematoma—collection of blood from a subperiosteal hemorrhage, appears after birth; increases in size; swelling does not cross the suture lines.

for bilateral red reflexes and records the findings on the infant's chart. Absence of bilateral red reflexes is a medical emergency; this finding warrants immediate attention.

The nurse may assess the infant's gross vision by determining the infant's ability to direct his or her gaze at the examiner

 Critical Nursing Action Recognizing an Ophthalmic Emergency in the Infant

When using an ophthalmoscope to examine an infant's eyes, the nurse notes the following finding: Right eye: red reflex present. Left eye: red reflex absent.

What is the significance of these findings? What action should the nurse take next?

Absence of the red reflex indicates an interference with the transmission of light to the retina. This finding is an ophthalmic emergency that requires immediate medical attention because optic nerve suppression from obstructed light pathways may result in permanent blindness. The nurse must immediately notify the physician.

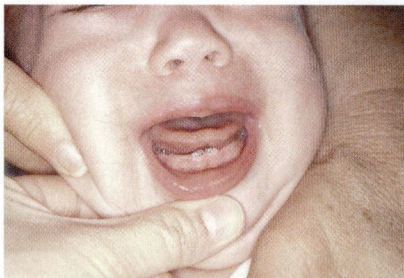

Figure 18-23 Natal teeth.

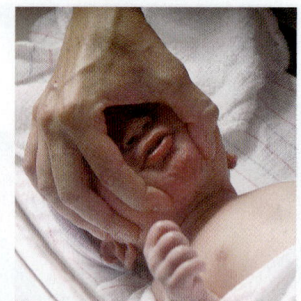

Figure 18-25 Assessment of the neck.

when positioned approximately 10 inches from the infant's face. The examiner then moves and notes whether the infant is able to appropriately readjust the gaze. The infant's nose is assessed by careful palpation of the nasal bridge to determine symmetry and the presence of fracture that may have occurred during birth. The nurse gently opens the infant's mouth and visually inspects, then palpates, the gums for the presence of neonatal teeth above or beneath the gum surface (Fig. 18-23). Teeth that have emerged through the gums should be checked for looseness and may need to be extracted because of the risk of aspiration. Because the presence of natal teeth may be associated with a congenital defect, further evaluation may be indicated (Dillon, 2007).

Epstein pearls, whitish hardened nodules on the gums or roof of the mouth, may be visualized or palpated (Fig. 18-24). These pearl-like inclusion cysts are not an unusual finding and disappear within a few weeks. The presence of the uvula in the midline is noted; a bivalve or double lobed uvula may indicate a cleft in the palate. The infant's ability to suck can also be assessed during the oral examination. The nurse inserts a gloved finger into the infant's mouth and notes and records the strength of the sucking motion. Also, at this time the hard and soft palates can be examined for size, shape, and cleft formations. When present, a cleft defect is felt as an open space or as a notched ridge. A high, arched palate may be associated with difficulty swallowing or with later speech development. Next, the gag reflex is elicited, and the back of the throat, tongue, and uvula are visualized. The infant's throat is also externally palpated to check for enlargement of the thyroid gland and to ensure that the trachea is located in the midline. The chin is lifted to assess the neck area; the neck is short with skin folds (Fig. 18-25). The nurse checks for neck rotation

by observing the infant's head movement and by gently turning the head from side to side. Torticollis is a deviation of the neck to one side caused by a spasmodic contraction of neck muscles. In the neonate, a torticollis is apparent when the head is positioned on one side while the chin points to the opposite side. Torticollis or the presence of a congenital cervical spine defect are two serious conditions that may produce limitations in neck movement and should be reported immediately.

The nurse palpates and inspects the neonate's ears to determine the thickness of the ear lobe and pinna. Ear pits and ear tags are common preauricular ear malformations. Ear pits, tiny pinholes found near the upper curved border of the pinna, arise from the imperfect fusion of the tubercles of the first and second brachial arches during early fetal development. Because they may signal a small sinus tract between the skin and underlying structures, they should be carefully evaluated to determine whether a layer of skin covers the opening or if the pit is open at the bottom. When signs of infection (e.g., redness, edema, or draining fluid) are present, the ear pits should be surgically repaired. Ear tags, fleshy bulb-shaped growths that project from the surface of the skin, should be removed for cosmetic purposes by a plastic surgeon because they frequently contain microcapillaries that bleed when cut. The ear canals are assessed for patency, and gross hearing may be evaluated by softly ringing a bell near each ear.

Most states in the United States require routine hearing screening before a newborn's discharge from the hospital. The goal of newborn screening is to identify congenital hearing loss and to refer those affected for early intervention. Most universal hearing-screening programs use the otoacoustic emissions (OAEs) test and/or the automated auditory brainstem response (AABR) test (National Institute on Deafness and Other Communication Disorders, 2011).

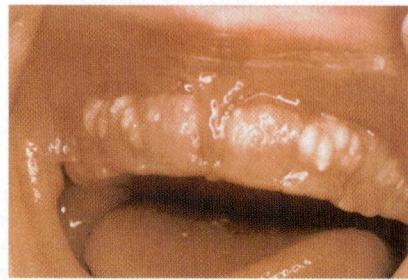

Figure 18-24 Epstein pearls usually disappear within a few weeks.

 Diagnostic Tool Newborn Hearing Screening

Otoacoustic emissions (OAEs): Painless test performed when the neonate is sleeping. Assesses cochlear function for the 500 to 6,000 Hz frequency range. A tiny, flexible earplug that contains a microphone is inserted into the infant's ear and records responses of the outer hair cells of the cochlea to clicking sounds coming from the microphone. Testing effectiveness is reduced by ambient noise in the nursery, vernix, blood, and amniotic fluid in the ear canal or any middle ear pathology.

Automated auditory brainstem response (AABR): Painless test performed when the neonate is sleeping. Assesses auditory function from the eighth

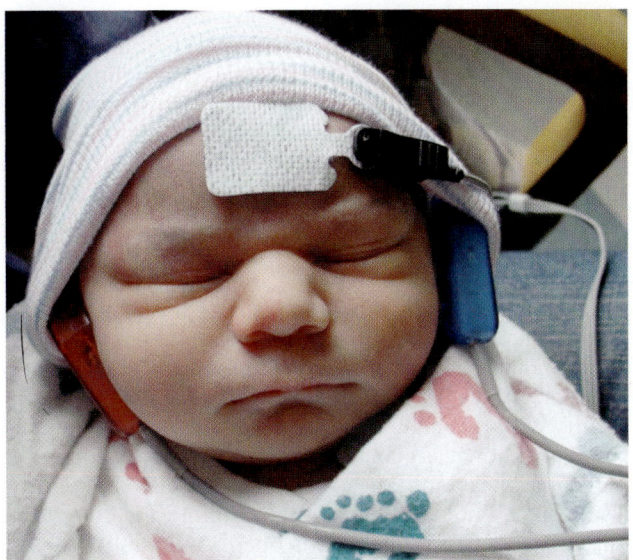

Figure 18-26 Neonatal hearing screening.

nerve through the auditory brainstem. Disposable surface electrodes are placed high on the forehead, on the mastoid, and on the nape of the neck (Fig. 18-26). The click stimulus is delivered to the neonate's ear via small disposable earphones; the test assesses electrical activity of the cochlea, auditory nerve, and brainstem in response to the sound stimuli and can be conducted in the presence of background noise.

Infants who do not pass an initial hearing screening at birth should return for follow-up testing within 1 month.

Optimizing Outcomes—The *Healthy People 2020* hearing screening national objective

The *Healthy People 2020* national objective related to newborn hearing screening states: "Increase the proportion of newborns who are screened for hearing loss by no later than age 1 month, have audiological evaluation by age 3 months, and are enrolled in appropriate intervention services no later than age 6 months." Nurses can help the nation achieve this goal by educating parents about the importance of newborn hearing screening; ensuring that newborn hearing screening is completed prior to hospital discharge, if possible, and that appropriate referral is made, if indicated; and by advocating for universal newborn hearing screening.

Assessment of the nose begins with an observation of the placement of the nose, normally located in the middle of the face. The nurse can draw an imaginary line from the center of the bridge of the nose downward to the notch of the upper lip. The nose should lie exactly vertical to this line. Each side of the nose should be symmetrical. It is important to note any deviation to one side, as well as asymmetry in relation to the size and dimensions of the nostrils. Remember that the bridge of the nose in African American or Asian children is normally flat.

CONDITIONS THAT MAY WARRANT FURTHER ASSESSMENT. When conducting an assessment of the head, ears, eyes, nose, and throat, the nurse is alert to findings of asymmetry, unusual shape or evidence of defects in underlying structures, or congenital syndromes. Generally, findings that are immediately apparent to the nurse examiner pose the greatest problems for the neonate. For example, Down syndrome is frequently identified during the assessment of the head when the nurse notes a flattened (instead of round) occiput, a broad nasal bridge, upward slanted eyes with epicanthal folds, low-set ears, an enlarged tongue, high arched palate, and a small chin. Open separations of the lip, mouth, nose, and hard or soft palate are indicative of cleft lip or cleft palate. Because facial disfigurement accompanies these defects, nurses should be extremely sensitive to the feelings of parents and other family members who interact with the infant.

The eye examination may provide an early indicator of several conditions that can affect the infant's well-being. For example, sclera, normally white, may appear to be blue or yellow in color. Bluish colored sclera may signal a congenital condition known as osteogenesis imperfecta, which is characterized by a loss of bone structure and integrity. Infants with this condition must be handled with extreme gentleness and may have already suffered fractures during the birth process. Yellowing of the sclera, related to elevated bilirubin levels, is a late manifestation of jaundice in the neonate. The nurse should seek immediate medical assistance for the infant and plan for rapid intervention such as IV fluids and phototherapy. A disruption in the iris, called a coloboma, appears as a keyhole in the circle of the iris and pupil and will affect vision in that eye. Congenital cataracts are noted when white or pale yellow tissue covers the pupil and iris and occludes the red reflex. This finding warrants prompt referral. Occasionally, the red reflex (normally red or reddish orange in color) appears to be white, a finding that requires immediate attention because it may signal the presence of a neuroblastoma. Congenital glaucoma is an ophthalmic emergency that requires the timely instillation of eye drops to prevent blindness caused by increased intraocular pressure. This condition is characterized by protuberant eyes that appear to extend beyond the orbits and feel firm on gentle palpation.

Careful examination of the infant's facial features may provide evidence of birth defects associated with maternal alcohol use. Characteristic findings include short palpebral fissures; a flattened nasal bridge with a small, upturned nose; and a flat midface, thin upper lip, and smooth philtrum. Alcohol-related birth defects (ARBD) also include poor growth, intellectual disabilities (often associated with **microcephaly**, or small head), and small chin (micrognathia). This condition, also called fetal alcohol syndrome (FAS) or fetal alcohol effects (FAE), describes the range of physical and mental effects that are related to the mother's alcohol use during fetal growth and development. After birth, affected infants are often jittery, irritable, and poor feeders. Nursing interventions focus on providing a calming, quiet, nurturing environment with minimal stimulation. (See Chapter 19 for further discussion.)

The nurse's careful assessment of the infant's head, face, eyes, ears, nose, and throat constitutes an essential component of the neonatal physical examination. Because infants are frequently bundled in blankets when presented to parents and loved ones, initial impressions are often formed based on the appearance of the neonate's face and head. Because many congenital malformations affect these body parts, the nurse must be sensitive to parents' feelings and approach the initial "viewing" prepared to provide immediate emotional support and subsequent referral to appropriate resources as indicated. It is important to remember that a wide range of normal variations (e.g., birthmarks; hair patterns; and large eyes, nose, or ears) commonly occurs and results from familial characteristics and inheritance patterns rather than from congenital syndromes.

 Now Can You—Describe the assessment related to the infant's head?

1. Describe the location of the fontanelles? Explain why it is important to assess them?
2. Differentiate between caput succedaneum and cephalhematoma and discuss how each is treated?
3. Describe how to conduct an assessment of the neonate's mouth and explain why this assessment is important?
4. Identify neonatal features that are characteristic of Down syndrome and maternal alcohol use?

 Global Health Case Study Baby Boy Goldman

Baby Boy Goldman was born via a normal spontaneous vaginal birth 4 hours ago. His parents are of eastern Mediterranean descent. His mother's prenatal care was initiated during the third month of gestation, and the pregnancy was uncomplicated. He is awake and resting quietly in the nursery bassinet. During a review of the infant's medical record, the nurse notes the following information, recorded approximately 1 hour earlier: axillary temperature: 98.0°F (36.7°C); heart rate: 136 beats per minute; respirations: 40 breaths per minute; weight: 8 lb 2 oz (17.7 kg); and length: 20.5 inches (8.1 cm). At birth, Baby Goldman's heart rate was 92 beats per minute, and he was crying and moving all extremities. The nurse now observes that the infant's hands and feet are bluish in color, and his face contains several white "bumps" that are scattered over his nose and forehead. Dark gray areas are seen on his lower back and buttocks. On palpation of Baby Goldman's head, the nurse notes a small degree of swelling that is symmetrical and crosses the suture lines.

critical thinking questions

1. Are these findings normal or pathological?

2. What actions should the nurse take?

◆ See Suggested Answers to Global Health Case Studies on Davis*Plus*.

Assessment of the Respiratory System

When assessing the neonate's respiratory efforts, the nurse first observes for symmetry in chest movement and at the same time notes the placement and size of breast tissue. Enlargement of the breasts in male infants is common and only a temporary condition because it is related to maternal hormones. The breast tissue and nipples should be located in the midclavicular line. This anatomical landmark is actually an imaginary line that is one-half of the distance from the midline (the lower border of the sternum) to the lateral border of the chest wall formed by the rib cage. If the breast

tissue is located between the midclavicular line and the lateral chest wall, the nurse documents this finding as "wide-spaced nipples." The presence of wide-spaced nipples may signal a congenital syndrome, such as Down syndrome. Extra or "accessory" nipples may be located above or below the primary nipples. This finding is not associated with a congenital syndrome, and parents can be assured that the accessory nipples will not enlarge during puberty, and if desired, may be safely removed at a later date (Dillon, 2007).

To assess for nasal patency, the nurse carefully occludes one naris while the infant's mouth is closed. A rise in the infant's chest confirms that the nasal passageway is open and air has been inhaled. The assessment may be repeated with the other naris. If the infant demonstrates difficulty with this maneuver, he may have a developmental anomaly known as **choanal atresia** (a malformation of the bucconasal membrane). When present bilaterally, cyanosis is noted when the infant's mouth is closed but disappears when the mouth is open. An inability to pass a small catheter into the nares confirms the diagnosis. Because choanal atresia may be associated with other developmental anomalies, a positive finding should be reported immediately.

With the infant in a supine position, the nurse can readily assess his ease with overall breathing efforts. Respirations are counted, and the pattern and any use of accessory muscles are noted. Slight sternal retractions may occur; this is a normal finding. Prominence of the xiphoid process is not unusual, and with normal growth and development, the prominence will diminish. The lungs are auscultated anteriorly and posteriorly (Fig. 18-27). Infants may exhibit irregular breathing patterns accompanied by periods of

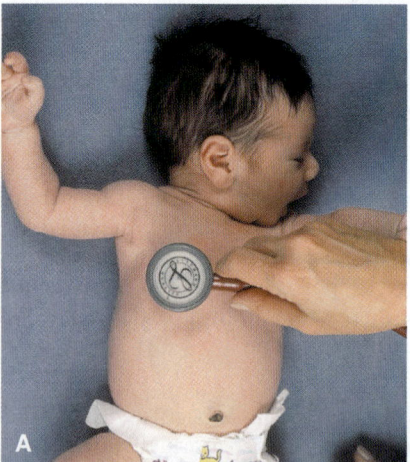
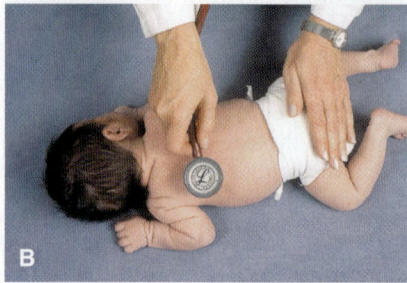

Figure 18-27 *A,* The lungs are auscultated anteriorly. *B,* The lungs are auscultated posteriorly.

apnea that can persist for up to 15 to 20 seconds. While not worrisome, it is important to alert parents that a brief cessation in respirations is common in neonates. The nurse also teaches the infant's caregivers how to recognize signs of respiratory distress: flaring of the nares, **retractions** (indrawing of tissues between the ribs, below the rib cage, or above the sternum and clavicles), or grunting with expirations. For healthy full-term neonates, a respiratory rate less than 60 breaths per minute is considered normal. To obtain an accurate respiratory rate, it may be necessary to count the infant's respirations at several different times during the physical assessment. If the respiratory rate remains greater than 60 to 70 breaths per minute during rest, further evaluation is warranted.

CONDITIONS THAT MAY WARRANT FURTHER ASSESSMENT. If the infant appears to be expending considerable energy to breathe or shows other signs of breathing difficulty, prompt evaluation of the respiratory status must be immediately sought. Signs of respiratory distress may be manifested by marked sternal or intercostal retractions. During the assessment, the nurse should gently palpate the anterior lung field to identify birth injuries, such as fractures of the clavicle or ribs. These injuries can cause an increased respiratory rate as a result of pain. Asymmetry of the chest wall during respirations may also signal the presence of a rib fracture. The nurse next inspects the chest wall to confirm symmetry and shape. Anatomical deformities such as pectus carinatum (pigeon chest) and pectus excavatum (funnel chest) arise from abnormal development of the ribs and sternum and may interfere with normal lung expansion. All lung fields should be auscultated anteriorly and posteriorly, and the respiratory rate is counted from the auscultation, rather than from observation of abdominal movements (Dillon, 2007). Auscultation of the infant's nose can help differentiate upper airway congestion (from mucus or amniotic fluid) from lower airway congestion. When the nasal passages, throat, or upper bronchus is congested, noisy breath sounds are often detected. Using a bulb syringe, the nurse gently removes fluid and mucus from the infant's nasal and throat passages to facilitate easy respirations. After this intervention, any retractions should disappear.

If the infant continues to exhibit retractions and other signs of breathing difficulty, prompt investigation is warranted because this finding may constitute a life-threatening event. Respiratory distress is associated with a number of conditions that may be related to the lungs or heart. Narrowing of the airways is associated with many congenital respiratory conditions while congenital heart defects often interfere with the lungs' capacity to oxygenate the blood. Congenital or acquired infection in the neonate may also cause respiratory distress. If the infant's respiratory rate remains elevated (60–70 breaths per minute) during periods of rest, the nurse must provide continuous observation. While the increased respiratory rate may represent a transitional period of adjustment to extrauterine life, the development of other symptoms such as nasal flaring, grunting, or intercostal retractions is indicative of respiratory distress. (See Chapter 19 for further discussion.) To complete the assessment, the nurse should also note the infant's skin color and assess the capillary refill of his extremities, actions that provide additional information concerning the status of respiratory system functioning.

Now Can You—Discuss components of the neonatal respiratory system assessment?

1. Discuss what parents should be told about breast enlargement in their male infant?
2. Describe the significance of wide-spaced or accessory nipples in a neonate?
3. Discuss why palpation is an important component of the neonatal respiratory assessment?
4. Identify the indicators of neonatal respiratory distress?

Assessment of the Cardiovascular System

The nurse assesses the neonate's circulatory system by visual inspection and auscultation. Careful inspection of the skin, lips, gums, and buccal mucosa provides reliable evidence of cardiac perfusion. At rest, the infant's skin should be pink in color and progress to red during crying or physical activity. The nurse palpates the chest to detect any thrills or heaves and the point of maximum impulse, which is auscultated at the apex of the heart near the third or fourth left intercostal space (Dillon, 2007) (Fig. 18-28). For infants, the normal heart rate should be between 120 and 160 beats per minute. A heart rate greater than 160 beats per minute is termed tachycardia.

To assess capillary refill in the extremities, the nurse gently pinches the end of the infant's finger or toe and then counts the number of seconds required for the skin to return to its normal color. The average refill time is 3 seconds. If more than 3 seconds lapse, there may be shunting of blood from the periphery toward the infant's trunk.

Family Teaching Guidelines...
How to Recognize Breathing Difficulties

As a component of newborn care, the nurse provides the following information to parents:

Your baby may be experiencing breathing difficulty if she:
- Has above normal respirations.
- Has prolonged (greater than 15 seconds) periods of breath holding.
- Shows sucking-in and seesaw movements around her rib cage.
- Flares her nostrils.
- Makes grunting sounds.

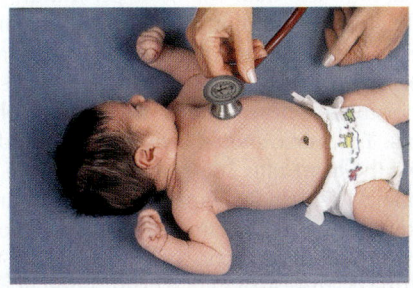

Figure 18-28 Auscultating the heart.

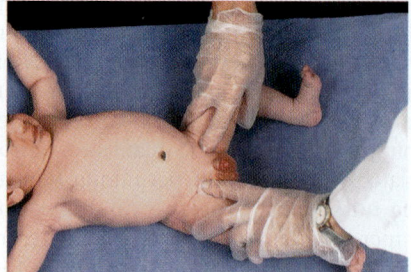

Figure 18-29 Palpating the femoral pulse.

The nurse palpates all peripheral pulses for bilateral symmetry, strength, and rate. The femoral pulses on each side are carefully checked and compared with the brachial pulses (Fig. 18-29). If a decrease in the strength of the pulse between the brachial pulses and femoral pulses is noted, this finding may be indicative of coarctation of the aorta, a cardiac condition associated with a narrowing of the aortic arch. Because the aorta is the main vessel for transporting oxygenated blood to the upper and lower body, a narrowing of the aortic arch produces a compromise in blood flow and should be suspected when decreased femoral pulses are detected. (See Chapter 19 for further discussion of coarctation of the aorta.)

Optimizing Outcomes—**Critical congenital heart disease screening in the newborn**

Critical congenital heart disease (CCHD) is a heterogenous group of disorders affecting 1.2 infants per 1,000 live births in the United States in which surgical or catheter-based therapy within the first year of life is mandatory for survival. CCHD screening in the first 24 to 48 hours of life with the use of pulse oximetry (the device is applied to the right hand and either foot to obtain oxygen saturation readings) is a safe, simple, noninvasive strategy for improving the early identification of newborns with CCHD. Supported by the American Academy of Pediatrics, the American Heart Association, the American College of Cardiology Foundation, and other advocacy organizations, evidence-based guidelines are available to guide clinicians in the use of universal screening for CCHD (Martin, Kemper, & Bradshaw, 2012).

COMMON FINDINGS. The nurse carefully auscultates all areas of the heart, including the aortic, pulmonic, tricuspid, and mitral valves, along with the base and apex. Because the normal infant heart rate is between 110 and 160 beats per minute, rates greater than 160 beats per minute are consistent with tachycardia; rates less than 100 beats per minute are termed bradycardia. Either condition, if persistent, warrants further investigation. Heart rate auscultation in the neonate is often difficult because of the thinness of the chest wall combined with the noisiness of heart sounds that are often obscured by respirations. The nurse should listen carefully and take time in counting the heart rate. It is not uncommon to hear murmurs in infants less than 24 hours old. The murmurs are characterized by a sound (best heard near the sternal border at the second or third intercostal space on the left side) that grows louder during systole. Although a heart sound arising from a patent ductus arteriosus may be heard initially, the sound

disappears within 2 to 3 days when the ductus closes. If a murmur remains audible after the second day of life and intensifies to a "whoosh" sound, further investigation is warranted because this finding is not characteristic of a patent ductus and may indicate the presence of another type of heart lesion.

CONDITIONS THAT MAY WARRANT FURTHER ASSESSMENT. Ventricular septal defect (VSD), a condition in which a small hole exists in the ventricle wall between the right and left chambers of the heart, is the most common heart murmur in infants. The VSD produces a sound created by the leaking of blood through the small defect. Interestingly, smaller defects are associated with louder murmurs because of the buildup of pressure in the heart chambers as the blood leaks through with each contraction. Large defects are associated with softer murmurs because the ease with which blood flows through the opening produces little pressure buildup. Most ventral septal defects close with normal cardiac growth during the first year of life and require no surgical intervention. (See Chapter 19 for further discussion.)

Cardiac insufficiency describes a condition that occurs when an infant cannot adequately oxygenate and circulate blood. This condition is characterized by pallor, rapid breathing, and cyanosis around the lips. Pulse oximetry readings should be obtained immediately. Readings of less than 94% oxygen saturation are of major concern, and if an infant's oxygen saturation drops below 90%, rapid transfer to an intensive care unit for continuous respiratory and cardiac monitoring should be accomplished. Cardiac evaluation is carried out, and depending on the findings, treatment may be medical, surgical, or both.

Infants who demonstrate cardiac instability within the first 2 days of life are usually those with a genetic karyotype of trisomy 13, 18, or 21 or **tetralogy of Fallot.** Tetralogy of Fallot is a congenital heart defect that involves four distinct cardiac anomalies: transposition of the aorta and pulmonary artery, right ventricular hypertrophy, pulmonary stenosis, and ventricular septal defect. Infants born with tetralogy of Fallot demonstrate no difficulties until the ductus begins to close after the first 24 hours of life. At that point, the infant experiences severe cardiac instability and develops central cyanosis. Transfer to an intensive care unit allows for IV fluids, medications, and continuous cardiac monitoring to be carried out until surgical and medical evaluation can take place. (See Chapter 19 for further discussion.) When any infant is diagnosed with a cardiac problem, the nurse should be sensitive to the parents' frequently overwhelming feelings of fear and inadequacy and be prepared to offer reassurance, support, and accurate information.

Now Can You—**Identify cardiac problems in the neonate?**

1. Demonstrate how to assess capillary refill and discuss why this assessment is important?
2. Identify when auscultation of a heart murmur in a neonate is considered to be a normal finding?
3. Describe a ventricular septal defect and discuss the treatment for this condition?

Assessment of the Gastrointestinal System

The nurse begins the assessment by placing the infant in a supine position to facilitate the abdominal inspection. The abdomen should be round and bilaterally symmetrical. The

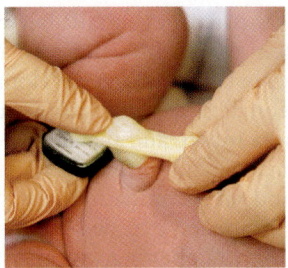

Figure 18-30 Assessing the umbilical cord.

clamped umbilical cord should show no evidence of active bleeding or oozing (Fig. 18-30). It is inspected to confirm the presence of three vessels: two arteries and one vein. If fewer than three vessels are seen, the nurse documents the findings and notifies the physician because this finding may be associated with congenital anomalies. Wharton's jelly, the gelatinous substance that prevents compression of the blood vessels, may appear as areas of varying amounts of thickness. The abdomen may appear distended because of stool that has not yet been emptied from the bowel. The nurse carefully auscultates all four quadrants of the abdomen for bowel sounds (Fig. 18-31). To facilitate thorough auscultation, each quadrant is divided into small sections to lessen the likelihood that any one area is overlooked. Bowel obstruction in the neonate is often first identified by an absence of bowel sounds in a small, distinct section of the intestines. The nurse completes the assessment with auscultation of the upper abdomen for the gastric bubble and the heart sounds of the abdominal aorta.

COMMON FINDINGS. The nurse uses light, then deep, palpation of the abdomen to assess the structure and contents of the abdomen. Light palpation is initiated at the lower sternal border and proceeds along the midline down to the umbilicus. Diastasis rectus, a thinning of the abdominal wall, may be detected. Diastasis rectus can also be identified by the presence of a long, raised "lump" along the midline that becomes prominent when the infant is crying. The nurse assesses the area surrounding the umbilicus for the

presence of an umbilical hernia. Using the fingertips to determine the hernia size, the nurse notes whether it appears to be large or small and documents this information in the medical record. Small umbilical hernias are common in newborns and often close without surgical intervention as the infant grows. The nurse continues palpation along the midline toward the symphysis pubis to detect any inferior extension of the hernia. Light palpation from the midline is then extended laterally toward the rib cage to assess for masses or enlarged organs.

Deep palpation facilitates examination of the organs. The border of the liver should be smooth and firm and located just below the right costal margin. The spleen, which lies beneath the left costal margin, should be palpable only at the tip. If a larger segment of spleen is palpated, this finding is reason for concern because it is indicative of organ enlargement. Because of their small size, the kidneys may be difficult to detect. They are located approximately 1 to 2 cm above the umbilicus and are at a right angle to the umbilicus at the midline. The bladder should be present as a smooth organ in the midline below the umbilicus.

CONDITIONS THAT MAY WARRANT FURTHER ASSESSMENT. Findings indicative of a serious abdominal problem in the neonate include the following: abdominal distention, absence of bowel sounds, discharge from the umbilical cord or cord site, and palpation of an abdominal mass. Abdominal distention may involve the entire abdomen, or it may be confined to small areas. Abdominal blood vessels may be readily visible in the distended abdomen. The presence of stool in the intestines is frequently detected, and this finding is not a cause for concern. Abdominal bulging that shifts when the infant's position is changed may be indicative of fluid in the abdomen. Absence of bowel sounds indicates an area of bowel that is not functioning; this finding must be immediately reported.

Necrotizing enterocolitis is a life-threatening condition that occurs when a lack of blood flow to the bowel results in destruction of the intestinal mucosa. Loss of bowel function results and toxins are released from the damaged, necrotic tissue. Immediate surgical intervention is required. (See Chapter 19 for further discussion.)

Discharge from the umbilical cord or cord site indicates the presence of infection. Unless a bacteriostatic dye has been used to paint the area, the cord should be pale yellow in appearance. An extra clamp may be applied if blood is actively leaking from the umbilical cord. If meconium was passed in utero, the cord may be stained a gray-green color. The area around the base of the cord should be kept clean and dry. During diapering, care must be taken not to allow stool or urine to come in contact with the cord or the cord base. If this occurs, the nurse should carefully clean and dry the site. The tissue surrounding the base of the cord should be inspected for redness, a finding that may indicate **omphalitis** (an infection that is readily treated with antibiotics).

Palpation to detect an abdominal mass or enlarged organ is usually facilitated by the infant's small abdominal girth. Positive findings require immediate referral for evaluation. Often, an ultrasound examination is conducted to determine the source of the clinical findings and to guide the management. In infancy, abdominal masses are frequently a form of neuroblastoma, a type of tumor that is confirmed by biopsy. The kidneys, liver, and spleen are the

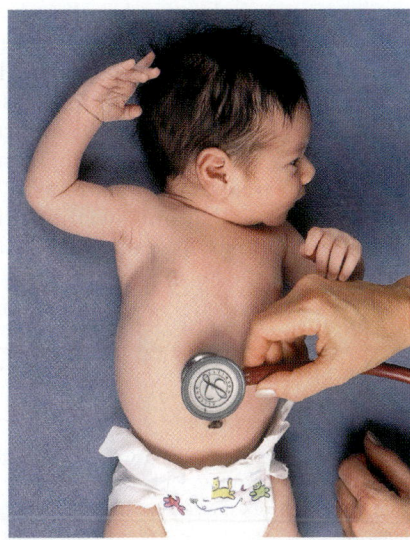

Figure 18-31 Auscultating bowel sounds.

organs most commonly enlarged, and these findings can be confirmed with ultrasound. Enlargement may result from obstruction, or it may be associated with a congenital malformation.

Critical Nursing Action Recognizing Acute Abdomen in the Neonate

During the neonatal assessment, the nurse is alert to the following symptoms that may indicate acute abdomen:

• Rigid, boardlike abdomen
• Inability to palpate abdominal organs
• Indicators of pain (continuous crying, facial changes, or gross motor movements)

 Now Can You—**Identify gastrointestinal problems in the neonate?**

1. Demonstrate how to perform the abdominal assessment on the neonate?
2. Identify findings that are associated with serious abdominal problems?
3. Describe two nursing interventions to minimize the risk of infection at the umbilical cord site?

Assessment of the Genitourinary System

The nurse begins the assessment by placing the infant in a supine position with the hips abducted. With the male neonate, the scrotum is examined to confirm that both testicles have descended. If flat or depressed areas are identified, this finding may indicate that a testis has not descended. Palpation of the scrotum is accomplished by placement of the examiner's second finger at the posterior scrotal midline with the thumb on the anterior midline (Fig. 18-32). Using the index finger and the thumb, the nurse palpates the left side of the scrotum for the presence of a testis and then uses the third finger and thumb to palpate for a testis on the right side of the scrotum. Proceeding in this pattern helps to ensure that one testis is not mistakenly being "counted" twice. If a testis is not detected, the nurse can softly stroke the inguinal canal in an attempt to locate an undescended testis. Warm soapy water applied to the inguinal area may enhance testicular prominence and help it to be more easily identified. Any infant older than 35 weeks' gestation who has undescended testicles should be referred for a urological consultation (Dillon, 2007).

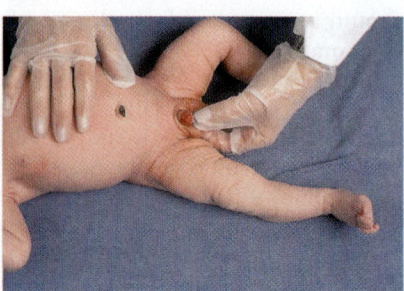

Figure 18-32 Palpating the scrotum.

Inspection of the female genitalia begins with the labia majora. The extent to which the labia cover the surrounding tissues corresponds with the developmental maturity of the female neonate. For most term infants, the borders of the labia majora touch, and the clitoris is covered completely. Occasionally, a full-term infant has delayed genital development, and on examination, the nurse can easily view the labia minora and exposed clitoris.

The anus and anal opening are also assessed at this time. While stooling confirms anal patency, it is beneficial to actually witness the passage of meconium because it provides an opportunity for the nurse to confirm that the stool passes through only one opening. Stool in the vagina indicates the presence of a rectovaginal fistula, an opening between the rectum and vagina. To palpate the anus, the nurse gently touches the tissue around the anal opening and assesses the musculature surrounding the opening. Tiny rectal tears from the passage of stool in the anal ring are noted, and the anal wink reflex is assessed. The infant is placed in a prone position and, using the index finger, the nurse gently strokes the buttocks from side to side. In response, the buttocks draw together and "wink" at the point of the anal opening. This response validates the correct anatomical position of the anal opening. In females, the anal wink reflex is useful in assessing anal openings that are positioned less than 1 cm from the vaginal opening. When the anal opening is located too close to the vaginal opening, proper muscle strength needed to evacuate the rectum as the child grows older does not develop. The wink reflex is also useful in facilitating proper placement of the anal opening during future surgical correction (Dillon, 2007).

COMMON FINDINGS. Careful assessment of genitalia is essential in both males and females. First, the nurse visually inspects, then palpates, the male genitalia. Infants of various ethnic backgrounds, especially those of African American heritage, have dark-colored scrotal skin. Scrotal swelling may interfere with an accurate palpation. If swelling is present, it is important to auscultate the scrotum to ensure that it does not hold entrapped bowel.

If no bowel sounds are heard, transillumination can be used to verify the presence of fluid in the scrotal sac. The nurse secures a penlight or ophthalmoscope, which will be used as a light source; darkens the room; and gently presses the light source against the scrotum. Fluid appears as a reddish yellow reflection. Masses do not transilluminate, and if detected, must be reported immediately. Scrotal fluid is slowly reabsorbed during the first weeks of life, and no treatment is necessary. The nurse can reassure the parents that any swelling will resolve over time and the scrotum will gradually take on a more normal appearance.

clinical alert

Bowel sounds in the scrotum

To confirm that no bowel is entrapped in the scrotum, the nurse carefully auscultates the scrotum for bowel sounds. If bowel sounds are present, immediate assistance must be obtained. This is a medical emergency.

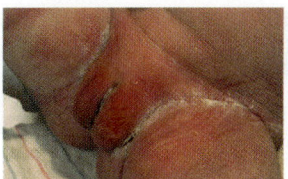

Figure 18-33 Assessing the female genitalia.

The penis is palpated to estimate the approximate length. Penile length in the full-term newborn male is approximately 2 cm. The nurse gently retracts the prepuce, or foreskin, to inspect the urethral opening and to determine the location of the opening on the glans. Smegma, a waxy substance, may be present on the glans beneath the foreskin. Instead of the normal round urethral opening, or meatus, a vertical opening may be seen. When present on the ventral (instead of central) surface, this finding is indicative of **hypospadias.** Hypospadias requires surgical repair by a physician. Because excess foreskin is used to create a properly positioned meatus, males with suspected hypospadias should not be circumcised. **Epispadias** is a similar condition. When present, the vertical urinary opening is located on the dorsal surface of the penis instead of on the glans. Epispadias is also repaired surgically with the use of excess foreskin.

During the inspection of the female genitalia, the nurse may identify vernix caseosa, a whitish, cheesy substance, covering the tissue between the labia (Fig. 18-33). This is a normal finding. The hymenal tag, a small piece of triangle-shaped tissue, may also be present between the labia. The nurse gently palpates the labia majora and labia minora, an action that facilitates examination of the hymenal area. Small amounts of blood and whitish mucoid discharge ("pseudomenstruation"), related to the maternal hormones, may be noted in the vaginal area. Parents can be assured that this discharge is normal and will disappear in about a week. Smegma may also be present between the labia.

CONDITIONS THAT MAY WARRANT FURTHER ASSESSMENT. When examining the male genitalia, the nurse may note the presence of bruising or swelling, especially if the infant was delivered in a breech presentation. Careful palpation facilitates the scrotal assessment, conducted to confirm that both testes have descended. Inspection and palpation of the penis includes assessment of the penile length. Micropenis, a penis that is less than 2 cm in length, may be associated with a pituitary tumor. Ambiguous genitalia describes a condition in which the male has genital structures that mimic labia or the female has a structure similar to a penis. If the definite genitalia cannot be determined, the infant is referred for genetic studies and evaluated for adrenal gland insufficiency. In situations of ambiguous genitalia, the nurse must be careful not to prematurely label an infant as a "boy" or "girl" to avoid compounding the parents' confusion. It is important that the nurse approach the parents with sensitivity and compassion.

❝**What to say**❞—*Infant with ambiguous genitalia*

Despite the initial birthing room determination of the neonate's gender, careful later examination of the genitalia may prompt concerns regarding the true sex assignment. It is important to promptly alert parents of the need for further testing for gender determination. The nurse can address the parents' concerns with reassuring statements such as:

"Because there is some question regarding your baby's sex organs, the doctor has asked a specialist to examine your baby. Additional testing may be indicated. You may want to wait to name your baby until we know for sure. For now, it is important to spend as much time as possible with the baby as you get to know one another."

In the assessment of the female genitalia, most concerns center around the presence of an enlarged clitoral hood and the finding of an imperforate hymen. Although maternal hormones may produce slight clitoral enlargement, a hood-shaped, grossly enlarged clitoris may be related to excessive androgen production. Because this condition may signal congenital adrenal hyperplasia, further evaluation and testing should be performed. The infant's genitalia may also be edematous from birth trauma, making the examination difficult. The nurse should gently separate the labia and inspect the area for the location of the urethral and vaginal openings. Imperforate hymen is present when tissue obstructs the vaginal opening, necessitating later surgical correction to allow for the discharge of menstrual blood.

Male and female infants may have anal ring skin tags or an anal ring that has no opening. The skin tags are hemorrhoid-like tissues that can cause discomfort or bleeding when the infant stools. The absence of an opening in the anal ring is a condition known as **imperforate anus.**

The finding of imperforate anus is a medical emergency because the infant is unable to pass stool through the anus. In approximately half of the infants with this condition, the imperforate anus occurs as an isolated event unrelated to any congenital syndrome. In the other half of occurrences, the imperforate anus is a part of a congenital syndrome associated with anal malformations, called the VATER association. At least three of the major abnormalities must be present for diagnosis. The overall prognosis is improved following the surgical correction of each anomaly. Characteristics of VATER association in the newborn include:

V = vertebral abnormalities
A = anal abnormalities (imperforate anus)
T = tracheal abnormalities
E = esophageal abnormalities (tracheoesophageal fistulas)
R = renal and radial abnormalities

 Critical Nursing Action Recognizing the Infant With Imperforate Anus

The nurse observes that Infant Gracie has not passed a meconium stool since her birth 26 hours ago. Infant Gracie has been breastfed several times, and her mother reports that her baby is a "ready feeder" who is "always hungry." The mother states that she has not changed her baby's diaper. The infant's abdomen appears distended and feels firm on palpation. The nurse recognizes that these clinical findings may be indicative of imperforate anus and immediately notifies the physician.

The nurse's careful assessment of the neonate's genitalia has far-reaching implications. The findings from this examination form the foundation for future parental interaction with their newborn. While gender determination is briefly addressed at the time of birth, the nurse who later conducts the thorough assessment is responsible for identifying any problems and seeking appropriate consultation. The nurse must remain sensitive to the parents' concerns and be ready to correct any misinformation that might affect the parents' ability to relate to their infant in a positive manner.

 Now Can You—Identify genitourinary conditions in the neonate?

1. Describe how to assess for undescended testes in the male infant and discuss the significance of this finding?
2. Describe the procedure for performing a transillumination of the scrotum and identify when this examination is used?
3. Name the two most common problems that affect the female genitalia?
4. Discuss how the infant is assessed for imperforate anus and describe the treatment for this condition?

Assessment of the Musculoskeletal System

The nurse can readily assess the functioning of the musculoskeletal system by observing the newborn in the crib where the infant has the freedom to continue and expand movements first initiated in utero. By flexing and extending the arms and legs, sucking on the fingers, and moving the head from side to side, the neonate provides a visual display of his musculoskeletal status. Any compromise in movement alerts the nurse to the location of possible birth trauma or other injury. Inspection of the extremities for differences in length or size is an important component of the assessment. Positive findings may be indicative of achondroplasia, a congenital condition characterized by a small thoracic area, an inability to extend the elbows, and a marked shortening of the femurs and humerus. Often referred to as "dwarfs" or "little persons," individuals with achondroplasia frequently have neurological and respiratory problems in addition to their skeletal deformities.

To assess muscle tone and strength, the nurse first places the infant in a supine position and then in a prone position. If the infant is unable to move the lower extremities, damage to the spinal cord is suspected. Asymmetry in movement suggests nerve damage or fracture related to birth trauma. If the infant does not move or appears floppy when repositioned, the nurse suspects hypotonia, or diminished muscle tone. Hypotonia may be related to an episode of anoxia, either during birth or while in utero. Increased muscle tone, or hypertonia, is characterized by muscle tremors, twitches, or jerkiness, and this finding is often associated with neonatal abstinence syndrome. Symptoms of drug withdrawal are manifest through the increased muscular movements.

COMMON FINDINGS. After the visual inspection, the nurse begins palpation of the musculoskeletal system. Starting with the shoulders, the examination progresses downward toward the lower extremities. The muscles and joints are assessed for symmetry, and gentle passive range of motion is used to evaluate joint rotation. Rotation of the neck is

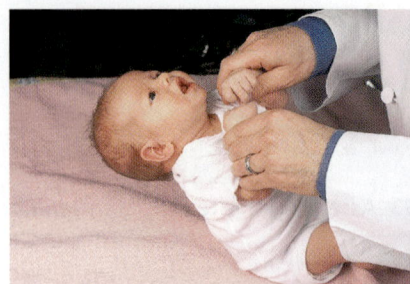

Figure 18-34 To assess head lag, the infant is gently pulled up as the nurse observes his head fall back.

the first and most important rotation assessed. Passive range of motion should confirm the infant's ability to accomplish full rotation of the neck. Failure to achieve full rotation may be related to torticollis or to the congenital absence of portions of the cervical vertebrae. Normal growth and development in infants is enhanced by their ability to turn the head toward the location of sound and then follow the auditory cue with their eyes. Thus, normal neck rotation plays an important role in the refinement of hearing and in the development of sight. To assess head lag, the nurse carefully pulls the infant up while watching the head gently fall back (Fig. 18-34). This maneuver also provides an opportunity to inspect the neck for bulging of the thyroid gland and for assessing the muscle tone of the upper body along with shoulder and arm strength.

The nurse's attention is next directed toward assessment of the hip joint, the second most important joint evaluation in the neonate. **Developmental dysplasia of the hip** (DDH) is a congenital condition that, if left untreated, can affect the infant's future ability to walk and maintain balance. It occurs when the acetabulum is flat, rather than round and cuplike in shape. DDH most often results when the developing fetus assumed a dominant breech position with upwardly extended legs during the period of bone growth. The assessment begins with inspection of the skin folds on the infant's thighs in both the prone and supine positions (Fig. 18-35).

Asymmetry of the skin folds may signal the presence of hip dysplasia. The nurse also assesses the leg length and knee height for unevenness. Next, the nurse slowly moves the infant's lower extremities in a kicking motion while observing for signs of pain or distress. The nurse's hands are placed on the infant's thigh with the fingertips around the femur head while the thumb and index finger stabilize the knee joint. While maintaining this position, the nurse performs the Barlow test by exerting a downward pressure on the head of the femur in an attempt to dislodge the femur head from the acetabulum (Procedure 18-3). The Ortolani

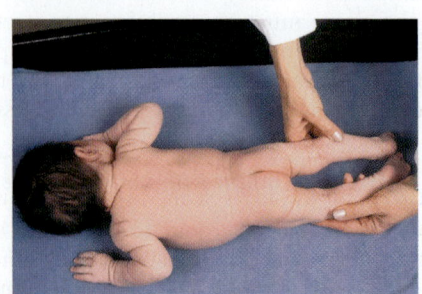

Figure 18-35 Inspecting gluteal skin folds.

Procedure 18-3 Performing the Barlow Test (Steps 2 and 3) and the Ortolani Maneuver (Step 4)

Purpose

To assess for developmental dysplasia of the hips

Equipment

None

Steps

1. Place the infant supine on a flat surface.
2. Place your thumbs on the infant's inner thighs and your fingers on the outside of the greater trochanters of the hips.

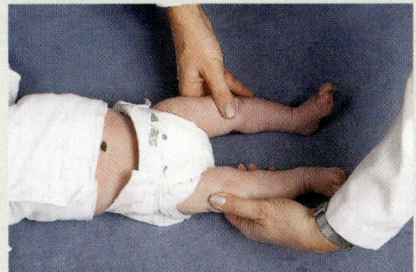

3. Flex the infant's knees and move the legs inward until your fingers touch.

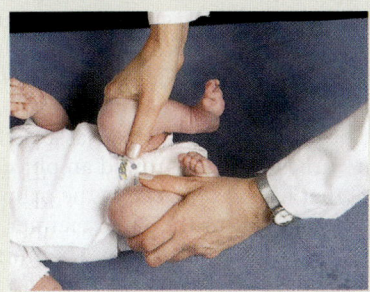

4. Using gentle but firm pressure, rotate the hips outward so that the knees touch the flat surface. No clicking or crepitus should be detected.

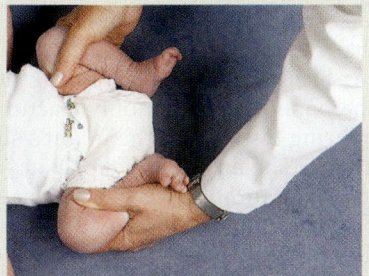

RATIONALE: *The presence of clicking or crepitus indicates joint instability.*

Documentation

3/4/10 1500 – Barlow Test and Ortolani maneuver negative

–J. Yamoto, RN

---

maneuver involves a circular rotation of the femoral head or an inward–outward action that attempts to reposition the femur head that was displaced by the Barlow test. In the normal neonate, the hip joints move easily, and it is not uncommon to detect crepitus, or a slight grinding (known as a "hip click") when the femur head is manipulated in the socket (Dillon, 2007).

It is not unusual to detect hip dysplasia in infants who maintained a breech position in utero or who were delivered vaginally in a breech position. Hip dysplasia can be confirmed by a noticeable difficulty when moving the leg in the hip joint and also by feeling the head of the femur pop out of the hip socket, sometimes referred to as a "hip clunk." Often, infants who were in a breech position in utero have hyperextended knee joints that can give the appearance of hip dysplasia. However, subsequent examination confirms that the head of the femur remains firmly secured in the acetabulum. Parents can be assured that over time, the infant's legs will return to the normal flexed position. The nurse may also detect a "looseness" in the infant's hip joint despite a normal evaluation that shows no evidence of hip dysplasia. This finding is related to the maternal hormones that create a joint flexibility not only in mothers but in their infants as well.

Developmental dysplasia of the hip, once confirmed by ultrasound or computed tomography, is managed by the placement of a special splint to keep the infant's legs in a position of abduction. The Pavlik harness, the most widely used device, does not rigidly immobilize the hip but acts to prevent hip extension or abduction. The harness is worn continuously for approximately 3 to 6 months, until new bone growth has formed around the head of the femur and a normal cup-shaped hip joint has been created.

To assess the remaining joints, the nurse performs passive range of motion and also continues to observe the infant's spontaneous movements in his crib. It is not uncommon to identify unusual positions of the foot, and these findings are most often related to the infant's position in utero. Pronation, or inward turning, of both feet is common, and the nurse can demonstrate to the parents how gentle stroking of the infant's insoles prompts a ready return to a normal position. When the foot is severely pronated, spontaneous normal alignment may be unattainable. In this instance, an evaluation of the posterior alignment of the infant's heel and knee is conducted. Club foot, suspected when there is a medial displacement of the heel from the posterior knee alignment, can be confirmed by x-ray exam. Soon after a diagnosis of clubfoot, a cast is placed on the affected extremity to restore proper alignment. The nurse should demonstrate how to safely stabilize the cast when holding the infant and teach the parents how to care for the cast.

CONDITIONS THAT MAY WARRANT FURTHER ASSESSMENT. Before performing the musculoskeletal assessment, the nurse first must determine that there are no broken bones. It is important that the infant not be moved or repositioned until this has been accomplished. In the neonate, the clavicle is the bone most commonly fractured. The injury occurs during birth when the infant's shoulders do not readily rotate. The nurse should palpate the clavicles to check for a separation between the bone ends or for the presence of crepitus. Signs and symptoms of fractures include swelling at the fracture site, bruising, or discoloration of the affected area and the infant's expression of discomfort when moved. Other common sites for neonatal fractures are the ribs, humerus, and skull. An x-ray exam is used to confirm the diagnosis. Clavicular fractures heal over time without intervention, and the nurse can teach the parents to position the infant on the side opposite the injury and how to hold and support the infant's head and shoulders until healing is complete. Casts are usually applied to humeral fractures, while rib fractures are generally wrapped. Infants with skull fractures are most often cared for in the intensive care unit where they can be continuously monitored.

Sometimes, infants are born with extra digits (fingers) and toes (**polydactyly**) or with what appears to be webbing of the skin between the digits and toes (**syndactyly**). On the hand, the extra digits often are located below the fourth finger and are attached to the palm by a thin line of skin. They may resemble the fourth finger and may even contain a fingernail. The nurse should palpate all extra digits for the presence of bone, which must be surgically removed. If no bone is present, the digit may be tied off with suture silk to occlude the capillary to cause necrosis and loss of the digit. Polydactyly is often a family characteristic, and parents may recall other family members who were born with extra digits or toes. Webbing of the toes does not interfere with balance or walking, and parents may not wish to have their infant's toes surgically released from one another. Webbing of the fingers is often surgically corrected to facilitate dexterity and for cosmetic reasons.

The nurse inspects the palms of the hands for the presence of palmar creases. The hands of a normal neonate usually contain three or four curved palmar creases. A **simian crease** is a single, straight crease that appears in the middle of the palm on one or both hands (Fig. 18-36). When unaccompanied by other findings, the simian crease is insignificant. However, when detected along with other symptoms, a simian crease may be associated with other syndromes, such as Down syndrome.

Now Can You—Complete a neonatal musculoskeletal assessment?

1. Identify the most important joints to assess in the neonate and describe how the assessments are performed?
2. Discuss the management options for an infant with developmental dysplasia of the hip?

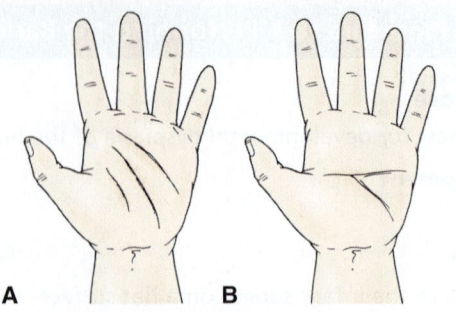

Figure 18-36 *A*, Normal palmar crease. *B*, Simian crease.

3. Describe the significance of polydactyly and syndactyly?
4. Recognize why the discovery of a simian crease prompts further investigation?

Assessment of the Neurological System

The physical assessment of the neonate concludes with the nervous system and reflexes. During this assessment, the nurse focuses on the reflexes and other movements that provide an indication of the infant's level of neurological function. It is helpful to divide the reflexes into two broad categories: major reflexes (reflective of normal neurological function) and minor reflexes (finger grasp, toe grasp, rooting, sucking, head righting, stepping, and tonic neck). The major reflexes include the gag, Babinski, Moro, and Galant reflexes. Table 18-2 displays methods for assessing the various reflexes.

The finger or palmar grasp reflex is assessed by observing the infant curl the fingers around an object (often the nurse's finger) that has been placed in the palm. The toe or plantar grasp is assessed in the same manner, by placing an object across the sole of the foot. The nurse observes the rooting and sucking reflexes by stroking the infant's cheek and watching him turn toward the finger, open the mouth, and suck on an object placed in the mouth. The head righting reflex is elicited by lifting the neonate in the prone position and then gently stroking the back in the midline, along the spinal cord. With this action, the normal infant attempts to raise the head and arch the back at the same time. To assess the stepping reflex, the nurse holds the infant in an upright position with the legs flexed. The soles of the feet are lightly brushed against a flat surface. In response to the stimulation, the infant lifts his feet and then places them back down in a stepwise pattern that imitates walking. The tonic neck or "fencing" reflex is observed with the infant in a supine position. The nurse observes the infant extend the arm and leg on the side to which the head and jaw are turned while flexing the arm and leg on the opposite side.

To assess the major reflexes, the nurse progresses methodically, taking care to document and record each finding. For the infant to successfully eat and move fluid away from the back of the throat without choking, the gag reflex must be intact. The Babinski reflex is demonstrated by lightly stroking the plantar surface of the foot from the heel toward the toes. The infant responds to this stimulation by first incurving the toes, then uncurling and stretching them out. The nurse can assess the **Moro reflex** at the same time as the head righting reflex is elicited. As the infant's head is lifted, the nurse mimics a release and watches for extension

Table 18-2 Newborn Reflexes

Palmar Grasp

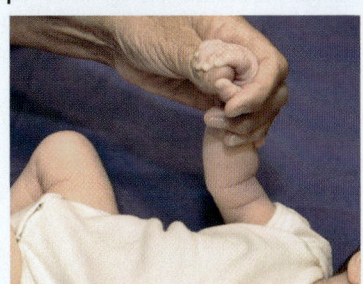

The infant curls his fingers around an object.

Toe or Plantar Grasp

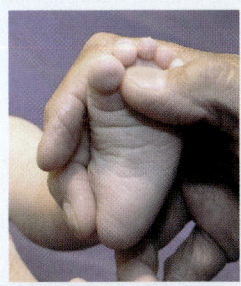

The infant curls his toes around an object that has been placed at the sole of the foot.

Rooting and Sucking Reflexes

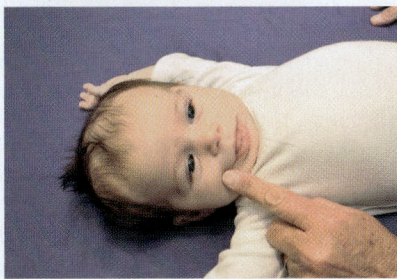

Stroke the infant's cheek and watch him turn toward the finger, open his mouth, and suck on an object placed in his mouth.

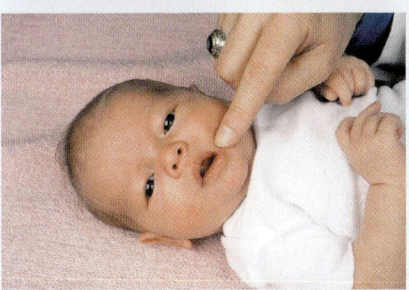

Extrusion Reflex

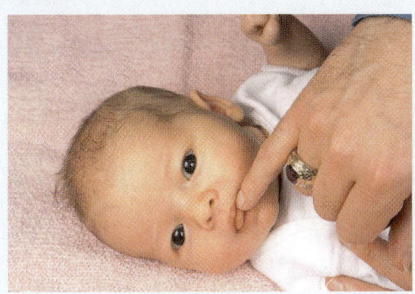

Touch the tip of the infant's tongue and the tongue will protrude outward.

(continued)

Table 18-2 Newborn Reflexes (continued)

Stepping Reflex

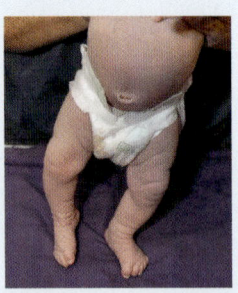

Hold the infant in an upright position with the legs flexed. The soles of the feet are lightly brushed against a flat surface. In response to the stimulation, the infant lifts his feet and then places them back down in a stepwise pattern that imitates walking.

Tonic Neck or Fencing Reflex

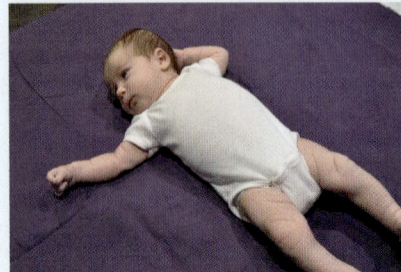

Observe the infant, in a supine position, extend his arm and leg on the side to which his head and jaw is turned while flexing his arm and leg on the opposite side.

Glabellar Reflex

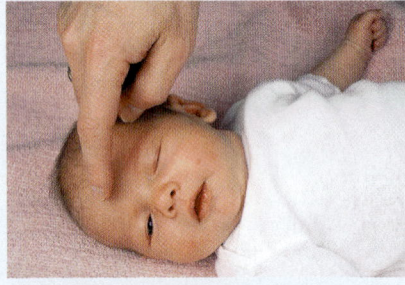

Tap on infant's forehead and observe him blink for the first few taps.

Babinski Reflex

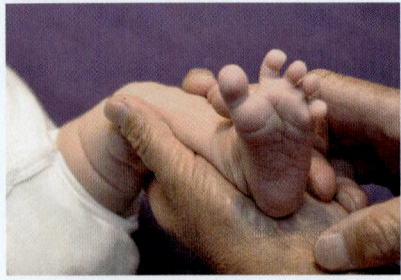

Lightly stroke the plantar surface of the foot from the heel toward the toes. The infant responds to this stimulation by first incurving the toes, then uncurling and stretching them out.

Moro Reflex

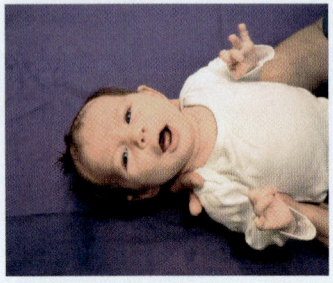

Observe the infant's head as it is lifted while the nurse mimics a release and watches for extension of both arms along with flexion of the legs.

Table 18-2 Newborn Reflexes (continued)

Magnet Reflex

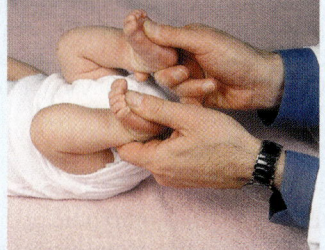
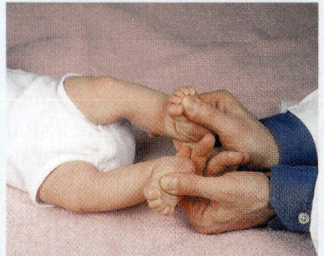

With the infant in a supine position, flex the leg and apply pressure to the soles of the feet. Observe the infant extend his legs against the pressure.

Galant Reflex or Trunk Incurvation Reflex

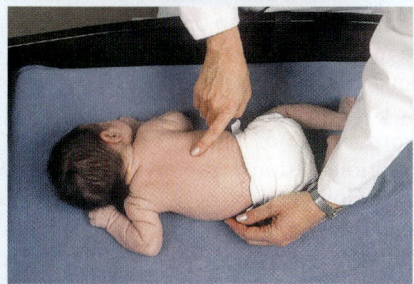

Observe the infant while supported in a prone position. Stroke one side of the vertebral column. The infant responds to this stimulus by moving his buttocks in a curving motion toward the side that is being stroked.

Crawling Reflex

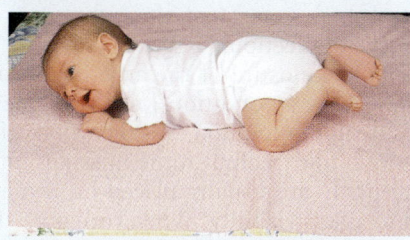

Place infant on his abdomen; observe him attempt to crawl.

Crossed Extension

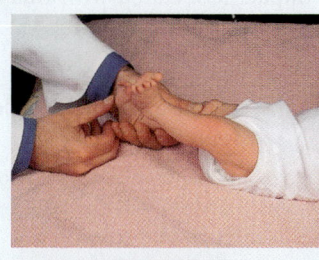
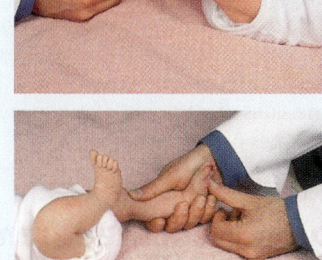

With the infant in a supine position, stimulate one foot; observe flexion, adduction, and then extension of the opposite leg.

of both arms along with flexion of the legs, movements that confirm the Moro reflex. In the past, the examiner often assessed the Moro reflex by creating a loud clapping sound near the infant in an attempt to startle him. This method of assessment is not reliable. The infant's response to the clapping stimulus may not be consistent with the Moro movements because the infant could be reacting to the movement of air across his body as the examiner makes the clapping sound, or to the sound of the clap itself. The Galant reflex, also called the trunk incurvation reflex, is elicited as the infant is held or supported in a prone position. One side of the vertebral column is then stroked. The infant responds to this stimulus by moving the buttocks in a curving motion toward the side that is being stroked.

CONDITIONS THAT MAY WARRANT FURTHER ASSESSMENT. The most frequently seen neurological injuries in the neonate involve the brachial plexus and are related to difficulties with shoulder rotation and delivery at the time of birth. The nurse must differentiate these injuries from shoulder dystocia, which is identified by a temporary decrease in the movement and muscle tone of a shoulder and upper arm. Injury related to shoulder dystocia rapidly improves after delivery.

Erb's palsy is one form of brachial plexus injury that is readily identified from the positioning of the infant's arm while in the supine position. When Erb's palsy is present, one or both arms and hands are extended and do not move into a flexed position. On palpation, the nurse notes a decrease in muscle tone, a decreased grasp reflex, and an absence of arm recoil on the affected side. Sometimes called the "waiter's position," the position is reminiscent of a waiter who keeps one arm by the side while the other is held out for a tip.

Most injuries involving the brachial plexus resolve in approximately 2 weeks without treatment. The infant should be positioned with the arm in a gently flexed position and when held, care should be taken to support the arm on the affected side. The nurse should teach parents how to use gentle exercise to facilitate the healing process. Simple arm strengthening exercises that passively flex and extend the infant's arm can be practiced during each parent–infant interaction.

Infants with major neurological problems that have occurred during embryonic or fetal development or result from events during the birthing process are assessed in the neonatal intensive care unit. Severe damage that affects the brain or muscle movement may be associated with periods of anoxia (lack of oxygen) that occurred during fetal growth or during the birth process. Cerebral palsy is one condition that results from oxygen deprivation. Infants with cerebral palsy often demonstrate a number of motor difficulties, such as difficulty swallowing, breathing, or moving. The length of the anoxic period corresponds with the severity of brain damage. When caring for infants with cerebral palsy, the nurse may deal with a spectrum of difficulties that ranges from minimal limitation to a total loss of reflexes and controlled body movements.

 Optimizing Outcomes—The neurobehavioral assessment of the high-risk neonate

In the neonate, "neurobehavior" refers to the concept that physiological and behavioral systems dynamically influence each other, and their quality is dependent on neural feedback (Lester & Tronick, 2004). Nurses who care for high-risk full-term and preterm infants can use a comprehensive assessment tool such as the NICU Network Neurobehavioral Scale to provide an assessment of neurological integrity and the behavioral function of infants at risk. Such advanced assessment specifically identifies the nature of infant instability and helps to ensure timely intervention (Sullivan, Miller, Fontaine, & Lester, 2012).

In utero development of the brain and spinal cord is a process initiated during the embryonic period. During the first 30 days of gestation, the primitive neural tube closes. A failure of the tube to close at the posterior end results in an open area that may be filled with fluid or with a section of the spinal cord. This condition, called spina bifida, is usually detected during routine maternal–fetal antenatal testing. When the infant is born, the lesion of spina bifida resembles a skin-covered sac (termed a **meningocele**—it may contain the dura mater and spinal fluid) located between the fifth lumbar and first sacral vertebrae. This condition usually does not cause any loss of motor function, or paralysis, below the waist. Treatment of spina bifida is related to the location and extent of the lesion. Most often, the sac is surgically closed to prevent infection. Spina bifida occulta is a mild variation of spina bifida. In this condition, there is a small defect in the spinal vertebrae. However, because there is no protrusion of the dura mater, spinal fluid, or spinal cord, all motor activity remains intact.

A more serious lesion is the **myelomeningocele.** When present, a myelomeningocele is a sac that contains dura mater, spinal fluid, and a portion of the spinal cord. Individuals with a myelomeningocele have no bladder or bowel control, and there is a loss of motor function below the waist. Treatment of spina bifida is related to the location and extent of the lesion. Most often, the sac is surgically closed to prevent infection.

An incomplete closure of the anterior portion of the neural tube causes a condition known as **anencephaly.** Lack of closure in this location causes portions of the brain, forehead, skull, and occiput to be missing. Infants born with anencephaly are usually placed on respirators and monitored to assess viability. When caring for the mother and her family, the nurse must be extremely sensitive to the emotional impact associated with this condition and offer the parents privacy and support.

 Now Can You—Complete a neonatal neurological assessment?

1. Identify the major and minor reflexes in a neonate?
2. Demonstrate how the Moro reflex is elicited and describe why this assessment is performed?
3. Recognize the signs of a brachial plexus injury?
4. Describe two types of neural tube defects?

Enhancing the Neonate's Transition to Extrauterine Life

The newborn's adaptation to extrauterine life is an amazing and complex process. In the early days of adjustment as well as through infancy, newborns need significant

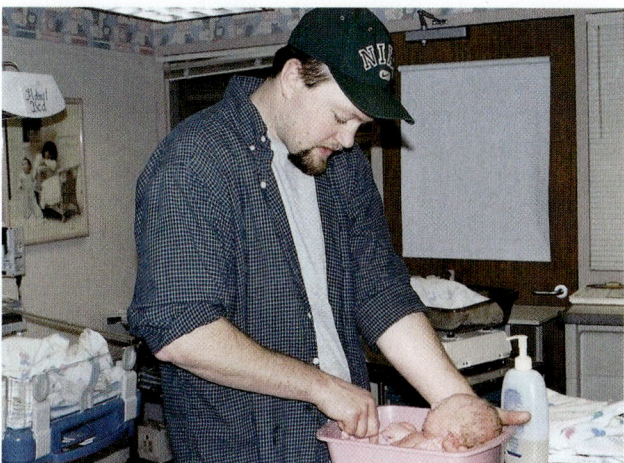

Figure 18-37 A new father bathes his infant.

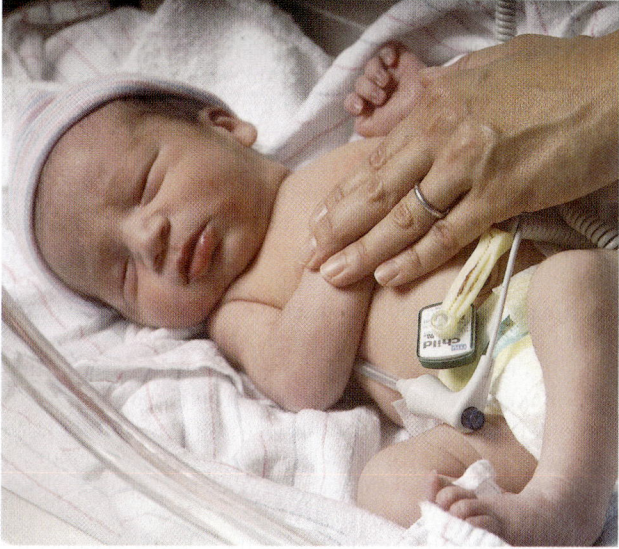

Figure 18-38 Proper technique for taking the axillary temperature.

physical, emotional, and spiritual care. Mothers and other caregivers must learn the essential aspects of newborn care to promote optimal infant growth and development. Critical aspects of physical care include feeding, clothing, diapering, and bathing the infant (Fig. 18-37). It is also important that parents' discharge instructions provide easy to understand information about the proper care of the infant's nails, umbilical cord, and, when appropriate, the circumcision. Bonding with the newborn is essential for emotional care, and the beginnings for spiritual development are established by building trust through relationships with the primary caregiver. Parents must be educated about the importance of timely metabolic screening for the newborn because many life-threatening problems can be detected early enough for effective intervention.

TEMPERATURE ASSESSMENT

To prevent dangerous heat loss in the infant, nurses, mothers, and other caregivers need to understand how to protect the infant from extreme temperature fluctuations during bath time. In the hospital before the bath is given, it is important to take the newborn's temperature to ensure stability.

Temperature may be assessed by several methods. The axillary skin method, which is reflective of the infant's core temperature and the body's compensatory response to the environment, is the preferred noninvasive method that provides a close estimation of the rectal temperature (Fig. 18-38). Although rectal temperature represents the closest approximation of core temperature, this route is not recommended because of the possibility of transmission of stool-borne pathogens and irritation and perforation of the rectal mucosa. The infant's temperature may also be assessed with a continuous skin probe (especially useful with small newborns or infants placed in incubators or under radiant warmers) or via tympanic thermometer, a portable sensor probe that is placed in the ear canal. This method employs infrared technology to measure the temperature of the internal carotid artery blood flow. As long as the body temperature is maintained between 97.7°F and 99.3°F (36.5°C–37.4°C), the bath can be given. At home, it is not necessary to take the temperature before bath time.

 Where Research and Practice Meet:
Comparison of Temporal Artery and Axillary Temperatures in Healthy Newborns

Haddad and colleagues (2012) conducted a descriptive study to compare temperature readings of axillary and temporal artery thermometers in 125 healthy late preterm and term infants. Axillary temperature measurement, a noninvasive method, is time consuming (taking from 15 seconds to 3 minutes) and may be associated with infant heat loss and disruption. Also, axillary temperatures might be the least accurate of any noninvasive techniques, and the findings consistently vary from core pulmonary artery temperatures (Lee, Flannery-Bergey, Randall-Rollins, Curry, Rowe, Teague, et al., 2011). Temporal artery thermometry is another noninvasive method that takes about 6 seconds and involves placing a device on the neonate's forehead and sweeping it laterally to the temporal hairline area. An infrared scanner collects multiple temperature measurements and calculates the core temperature based on the readings, providing an accurate temperature with minimal disruption to the infant. Study findings revealed that the temporal temperatures were consistently significantly higher than the axillary temperatures although the findings did not result in the infants being treated differently clinically. Citing the importance of accuracy in temperature readings, the investigators concluded that clinicians can feel confident in using temporal artery thermometry as a noninvasive method of temperature measurement (Haddad, Smith, Phillips, & Heidel, 2012).

BATHING THE NEWBORN

When bathing the newborn, the bath should take place in a warm area free from drafts. The newborn can be given a sponge bath using only warm water for the first few days of life. After the cord stump has dried completely and fallen off in approximately 2 weeks, the infant can be immersed in a small tub filled with about 4 to 5 inches of water.

 Nursing Insight—The NIH Human Microbiome Project and Maternal-Child Nursing

The Human Microbiome Project (HMP) is a United States National Institutes of Health initiative designed to identify and characterize the microorganisms that are found in association with healthy and diseased humans (the Human microbiome). Launched in 2008, the five-year project focuses on the microbiology of five body sites (oral, skin, vaginal, gut, nasal/lung) and includes deep sequencing of bacterial 16S rRNA. The HMP has been described as an extension of the Human Genome Project.

Information stemming from the HMP initiative has fostered a deeper understanding of the importance of the physiological role of human microbiota (formerly called gut flora) in the maturation of the immune system and in the developmental regulation of intestinal physiology. Infants first come into contact with microbes provided by the maternal microbiota. Certain factors (e.g., mode of birth, type of infant feeding) can influence the establishment of the infant microbiota. Hence, exposure to adequate microbes during gestation and the early neonatal period may play an important role in health (Collado, Cernada, Bauerl, Vento, & Perez-Martinez, 2012).

While research is essential before the following practices may be considered evidence-based, information emerging from the HMP initiative may have important implications for maternal-child health. For example, mothers should achieve and maintain a healthy biodome, both pre- and post-natally (e.g., consume a healthy diet, minimize stress, avoid pharmaceutical drugs and tobacco). Suggestions for promoting a healthy infant biodome include placing the naked neonate on the maternal chest immediately after birth and during the first few days, avoiding bathing for at least 24 hours after birth, minimizing skin-to-skin contact by non-family members during the first few weeks of life and exclusive breastfeeding (Reed & Johnson-Cash, 2014).

⑤ Optimizing Outcomes—Ensuring safety for the newborn

It is paramount to remember that wet newborns are slippery! The nurse and parents must keep a firm hold on the baby, and continuously support the head up out of the water. When instructing new parents about the bath, it is important that they understand that it is never acceptable to leave any child unattended near water, even a small amount of water. Submersion injury is the second leading cause of accidental death in children.

Newborns do not require a daily bath; bathing them three times a week is adequate. However, the face and hands can be wiped off daily. The infant's bottom and genital area should be cleansed several times during the day. Because the newborn's skin may be sensitive, a mild, unscented soap is recommended for the bath. The initial bath after birth takes place after temperature stabilization. The procedure for the bath after birth and at home is fairly simple. The bath should proceed from head to toe. Parents must understand that good hygiene, including clean clothes, hair, nails, and teeth is important in promoting proper growth and development for their infant. At home, newborns can be placed in 4 to 5 inches of water in a small nonskid surface infant bathtub. Infants who are immersed in water for bathing have a tendency to be calmer and quieter and experience less heat loss than infants who are sponge bathed. Immersing

the infant's body with water facilitates thorough distribution of the water to ensure even temperature and decreased evaporative heat loss. Benefits of immersion include a soothing feeling, hydration to the skin, and tactile stimulation.

If dry skin is a problem, baths may be given less frequently, and a moisturizing lotion can be applied after the infant is dried. Because the newborn's skin can be sensitive to scented lotion, it is best to use an unscented product. Bath time is an ideal time for the nurse to assess the newborn's physical condition, muscular activity, behavior, and state of arousal and alertness, and the act of showing parents how to properly bathe their infant provides a perfect opportunity to observe and encourage maternal and family bonding.

NAIL CARE AND UMBILICAL CORD CARE

Newborn nails are rarely trimmed in the hospital or birthing center in the initial days of life because of the increased potential for injury to surrounding tissue that may result in infection. After about a week, the nails more readily separate from the skin and often break off naturally. In the early days, to prevent the infant's nails from scratching the face, filing the nails with a fine emery-textured board or covering the infant's hands with a cuffed T-shirt or mittens are safer options. However, covering the hands should be avoided if possible because this action prevents the infant from sucking on the fingers for self-consolation. In the home, parents may continue to file their newborn's nails, or they may be taught how to carefully trim them, often while the infant sleeps.

The umbilical cord appears as a gelatinous white stump with two arteries and one vein. Immediately after birth, the cord is cut with a sterile scissors and clamped. Goals of cord care center on the prevention and early detection of hemorrhage or infection. Because it provides an excellent medium for bacterial growth, the cord stump is a potential source of infection (Taylor et al., 2011). The Association of Women's Health, Obstetric and Neonatal Nurses (AWHONN) recommends that the cord initially be cleaned with sterile water or a neutral pH cleanser and thereafter with water (AWHONN, 2013). The cord begins to dry out in approximately 1 to 2 hours. The cord clamp must remain in place for 24 hours when it can be removed with a special cord clamp remover. By the third day, the cord appears to be discolored and shrunken. By 10 to 14 days, the cord has usually detached completely, and parents often find the remnants in the infant's diaper or on the bedding.

⑤ Optimizing Outcomes—Teaching parents about umbilical cord care

Information regarding umbilical cord care should be included as a component of discharge teaching. Parents are taught about the cord's normal appearance and shown how to fold and position the diaper below the cord stump (Fig. 18-39). Remind parents to keep the area free from urine and wetness during bathing and when to expect complete cord detachment. It is also helpful to alert them to potential danger signs such as bleeding or a foul odor.

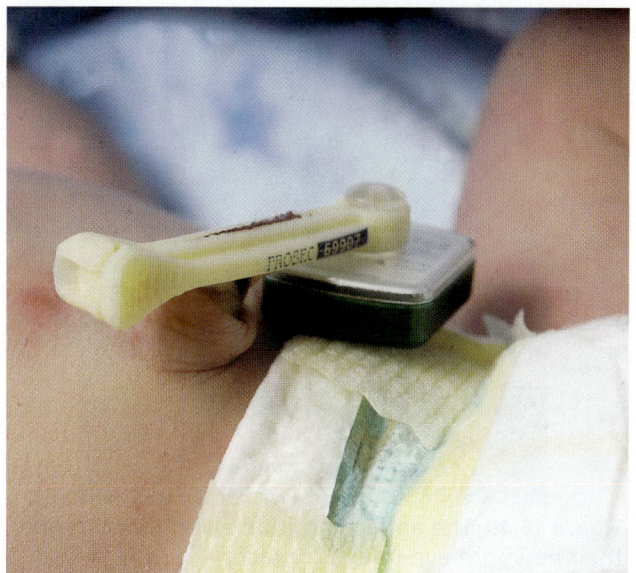

Figure 18-39 The diaper is positioned below the cord stump.

CLOTHING

Understanding the concepts of thermoregulation is also important when clothing the newborn. In the hospital or birthing center, the infant often wears a T-shirt, diaper, and booties. Frequently, two or three blankets and a hat are required to help the newborn maintain body temperature within a normal range.

 Nursing Insight—*Importance of temperature assessment*

If the newborn's body temperature drops below normal parameters (97.7°F–99.3°F [36.5°C–37.4°C]), it is essential that the nurse immediately initiate temperature stabilization measures such as skin-to-skin contact by placing the infant directly on the mother's unclothed arms, chest, or abdomen or move him to a radiant warmer. When the newborn's body temperature reaches a normal level, he can safely be dressed in a T-shirt and hat and covered with two or three blankets.

At home, the type and amount of clothing for the newborn is dependent on the local climate and temperature. The infant can be dressed like other family members are dressed; that is, appropriate for the temperature and season. Special attention should be given when the newborn is outdoors. A cap or bonnet decreases body heat loss and protects the newborn from dangerous sun rays and wind drafts to the ears. During warm weather, babies should be covered in lightweight clothing and placed in shady spots when outdoors.

 clinical alert

Protecting the infant from the sun
While specially formulated sunscreens especially made for infants are available, it is important to advise parents to check with their health-care provider about use of these products. Many health-care providers do not recommend use of sunscreens until the infant is at least 6 months of age.

DIAPERING

Many families prefer the convenience of disposal diapers, which vary in style, size, functionality, and cost. It is important to remember that the infant's sensitive skin may react adversely to the perfume in the diaper. If diaper rash or dermatitis occurs, parents can be advised to try another brand of diaper but should contact their health-care professional if the problem persists. Other parents prefer cloth diapers, which may be provided by a commercial diapering service or personally purchased and laundered. Parents need to be taught that cloth diapers must be laundered separately from other clothing articles, using 1/4 cup of detergent. Presoaking is often necessary to remove stains. When teaching parents about the advantages of breastfeeding, remember to include information that a breastfed baby's stools do not have an odor or cause diaper stains.

 Cultural Diversity: Diapering Practices

While diapering practices vary widely according to personal preference, custom, or culture, the nurse can teach the caregiver from any culture how to prevent diaper rash:
- Keep the baby's diaper area clean and dry.
- Change the baby's diaper often.
- Carefully clean the baby's bottom between diaper changes, using a mild soap and plain warm water.
- During a wet or soiled diaper change, allow the baby's skin to dry completely before putting on another diaper.
- Allow the baby to go without a diaper whenever possible to let the air dry the skin.
- If diaper rash persists, contact the health-care provider.

FOSTERING ATTACHMENT

Attachment describes a mutually reciprocal relationship that takes place between the parents and their infant during the moments after birth. Attachment is critical to the child's ongoing optimal growth and development. One of the nurse's most important roles is observing for healthy attachment behaviors and helping the family to establish a good relationship with their infant. By observing parental behaviors and engaging in meaningful dialogue with the mother and father, the nurse may uncover important cues that could have an impact on the infant's growth and development. Remember that after 9 months of pregnancy and perhaps a difficult labor and birth, parents often feel tired and overwhelmed with the realization that their newborn is totally dependent on them. They may be too embarrassed to ask questions or clarify information previously given to them. The nurse must create a nonthreatening and nonjudgmental environment in which parents can openly express ideas and ask questions. An important concept for the nurse, mother, and other caregivers to understand is that healthy bonding is essential for adequate physical, emotional, and spiritual growth. Early infancy is an ideal time to establish a trusting relationship between the newborn and the primary caregiver.

"What to say"—*Questions the nurse can ask the mother to assess attachment*

On the first day after giving birth, a mother states that she doesn't want to hold her baby. The nurse responds by asking:

- Can you tell me more? Are you in pain? Are you feeling sleepy? Are you afraid?
- Does your baby have a name yet?
- Do you have any concerns about basic care for your baby such as holding, feeding, diapering, or bathing?
- How will you respond when your baby fusses or cries?

Minutes after the infant's birth, most parents are given an opportunity to spend quality bonding time with their newborn. To accurately assess this first expression of parent–infant attachment, it is important for the nurse to watch for and understand the behaviors commonly observed. Mothers and fathers usually begin with an exploration of their infant's physical characteristics. Often, they begin by examining each tiny fingertip. Next, they carefully explore their baby's extremities. Finally, they view and softly stroke the full length of the infant's trunk. During this entire process, the parents assume the **en face** position where they establish and maintain direct visual contact with their infant (Fig. 18-40). This initial exploration of gentle touch, coupled with reciprocal eye contact, helps to lay the foundation for a loving bond between the parents and their infant.

Nurses can be instrumental in facilitating a healthy parent–infant attachment. Taking time to teach, providing assistance when needed, and listening to concerns help encourage and foster healthy parenting skills and enhance the newborn's potential for optimal growth and development.

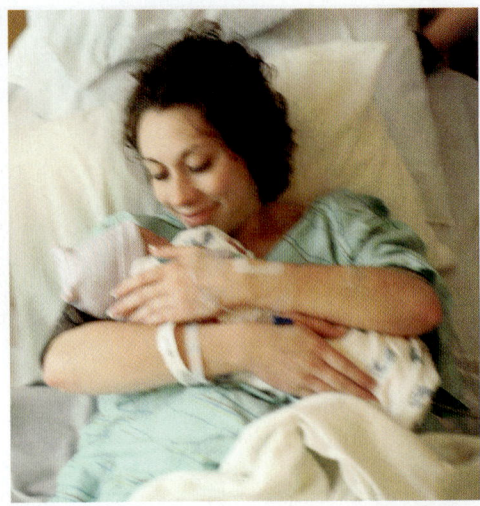

Figure 18-40 The en face position allows parents and their newborn eye-to-eye contact.

Cultural Diversity: Accepting Customs and Traditions

It is important for nurses who work with childbearing families from various ethnic backgrounds to be aware of differences in cultural beliefs and practices related to pregnancy and newborn care. While many facets of the Western lifestyle may be readily adopted, families from other countries often wish to preserve certain customs and traditions brought from their native countries. Not surprisingly, valued health beliefs frequently extend to the area of infant care. For example, persons of the Latin American or Filipino cultures may apply an abdominal binder or protective "belly band" to the infant's umbilical stump to protect against dirt, injury, or hernia. Cradle boards may be used by Native American mothers, notably the Navajos, to carry the infant and maintain close contact. Persons of Iranian heritage may breastfeed female infants longer than male infants. Some Asians, Hispanics, Eastern Europeans, and Native Americans delay the initiation of breastfeeding because of the belief that colostrum is "bad" (Andrews, 2011; D'Avanzo, 2007).

Family Teaching Guidelines...
Promoting Family Attachment

Nurses can promote family attachment in many ways:

- Provide time in the first few hours after birth for privacy and time for the new family to get to know one another.
- Delay any unnecessary procedures immediately after birth, such as measurements and other admission procedures. Instead, allow the family adequate time alone after birth to spend time getting to know one another.
- Encourage early breastfeeding by providing proper education and support.
- Teach parents about infant behavioral cues for feeding (rooting, sucking on fingers or fist, increasing motor activity, or crying) and how to respond to their infant.
- Help parents understand that crying is the infant's way of communicating, and all newborns have distinguishable cries for hunger, pain, tiredness, fussiness, or getting attention.

- Teach parents that newborns have a built-in capacity to console themselves and do so by sucking, motion, and distraction.
- Help parents to recognize the joys and frustrations that go along with ongoing parenting. Assure them it takes time to feel comfortable in meeting their newborn's unique needs.
- Introduce the concept of anticipatory guidance to help prepare parents for important developmental milestones that will occur.
- Encourage the parents to invite siblings and other family members to visit for short periods of time to share the joy and to provide support.
- Provide consistent nurses during the hospital or birthing center stay.

CIRCUMCISION

Circumcision is a surgical procedure that involves removal of the foreskin on the glans penis. Although commonly done to promote hygiene and easier cleaning, circumcision may primarily be requested because of family tradition or social and cultural factors. Historically based on a religious rite of passage from the Jewish and Muslim traditions, circumcision has gained widespread acceptance in the United States.

According to the American Academy of Pediatrics (AAP) Circumcision Policy Statement (2012), "evaluation of current evidence indicates that the health benefits of newborn male circumcision outweigh the risks and that the procedure's benefits justify access to this procedure for families who chose it" (p. 585). Benefits of circumcision include prevention of urinary tract infections, penile cancer, and transmission of some sexually transmitted infections, including HIV. The American College of Obstetricians and Gynecologists (ACOG) (2001) has endorsed this statement.

While the health benefits are not great enough to recommend routine circumcision for all male newborns, the AAP maintains that the benefits of circumcision are sufficient to justify access to the procedure for families who choose it and to warrant third-party payment for male newborn circumcision. It is important that parents be knowledgeable about this surgical procedure. The AAP policy advises that physicians give parents correct and impartial information about the benefits and risks of male newborn circumcision in an unbiased and accurate manner. Parents need to have the opportunity to examine all of the facts surrounding circumcision, ask questions, and weigh medical information in the context of their own religious, ethical, and cultural beliefs and practices. The AAP further recommends that if parents choose to circumcise their infant, appropriate analgesia be provided. Bleeding, infection, dehiscence (separation of the approximated edges of skin), and trauma are complications that can be associated with the procedure.

 Nursing Insight—Factors that may influence the parental decision for infant circumcision

The American Academy of Pediatrics Task Force on Circumcision (2012) concludes that although there are associated risks (i.e., hemorrhage, infection, and penile injury), circumcision provides health benefits that outweigh the risks. For parents, additional reasons for choosing infant circumcision may include a desire to ensure that their son's body likeness is consistent with that of peers from the same area, region, or country and to avoid complications that are associated with circumcision performed on a child who is older than 1 month of age.

While the surgical removal of the foreskin is a fairly simple procedure that can take place in either the hospital or community setting, it must be performed using sterile technique. The infant is restrained on a board or chair and warmed blankets may be placed on the upper body to enhance comfort and prevent heat loss. Hospitalization is necessary if the infant is older than 1 month. The newborn must be stable and a physical examination by a physician or other health-care provider, along with a signed permit, should have been completed before the circumcision. The procedure involves removing the prepuce, which is the epithelial layer of skin on the penis. This small piece of skin is separated and removed from the glans penis. Newborn circumcision is frequently performed with the use of a surgical device such as the Gomco (Yellen) clamp or a Mogen clamp. Once the procedure is completed, a petrolatum gauze dressing or a generous amount of petrolatum is applied to the penis for 1 to 2 days to prevent the diaper from adhering to the surgical site. Another method involves use of the PlastiBell device, which is fitted over the glans. A suture is tied around the bell's rim, the excess prepuce is cut away and the plastic rim remains in place until it falls off in approximately 5 to 7 days (Fig. 18-41). No petrolatum gauze dressing is used after circumcision with a PlastiBell device (Zderic & Lambert, 2011).

Nursing care for the circumcised newborn focuses on alleviation of pain and the prevention of infection. The circumcision should be assessed every 30 minutes for at least 2 hours following the procedure, and it is important to observe for the first voiding after a circumcision to evaluate for urinary obstruction related to penile injury or edema. Parent/caregiver education is also an important component of care. Parents should be taught to continue to apply

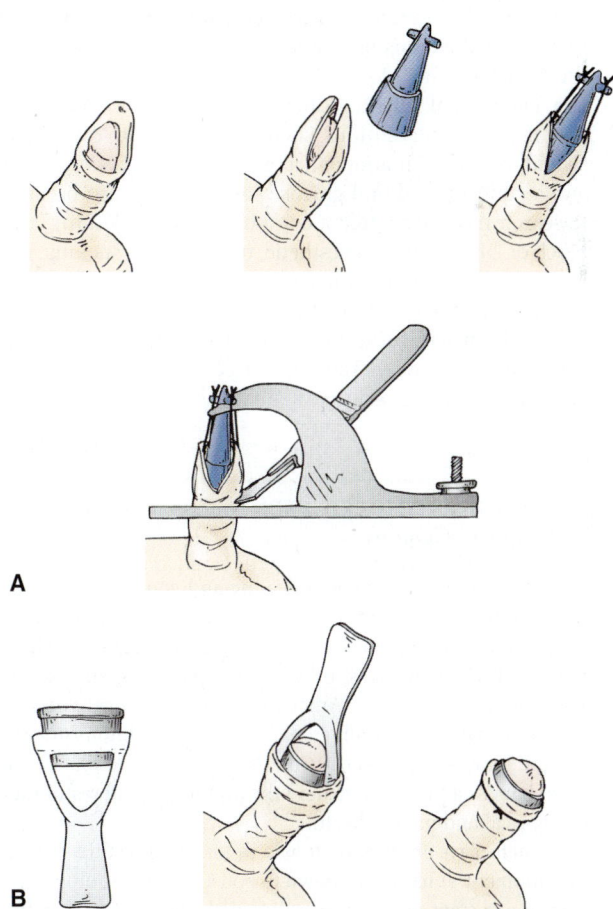

Figure 18-41 Removal of the prepuce during a circumcision. *A,* Yellen clamp procedure. *B,* PlastiBell procedure.

a petroleum ointment as directed by the physician, report bleeding or signs and symptoms of infection (e.g., increased swelling, pus, or cessation of urination), and to take care during diapering to ensure that the diaper is neither too loose (causes rubbing with movement) nor too tight (causes pain). Therapeutic touch is a beneficial comfort measure for all infants and is especially useful following painful procedures.

Optimizing Outcomes—Providing pain management during circumcision

The American Society for Pain Management Nursing (2011) holds the position that nurses and other health-care professionals must provide optimal pain management throughout the circumcision process and parents must be prepared for the procedure and educated about infant pain assessment and pharmacological and integrative pain management therapies. Three types of pain management can be used for circumcision. A subcutaneous penile ring block is considered the most effective method (buffered lidocaine is subcutaneously injected on each side of the penile shaft). Alternatively, a dorsal penile nerve block (DPNB) (buffered lidocaine is subcutaneously injected at the 2 o'clock and 10 o'clock positions at the base of the penis) may be administered, or the DPNB and the ring block may be used together. In other settings, a topical anesthetic such as prilocaine-lidocaine cream (i.e., eutectic mixture of local anesthetic [EMLA]) is applied to the base of the penis 1 hour before the procedure. Although all three techniques reduce surgical pain, the subcutaneous anesthetics are more effective than the EMLA cream (Morris, Wodak, Mindel, Schrieber, Duggan, Dilley, et al., 2012; Ridings & Amaya, 2007). Nonpharmacological interventions such as non-nutritive sucking, swaddling, and containment, along with oral acetaminophen and a concentrated oral glucose solution may also be used. Research has shown that a combination of swaddling, ring block or DPNB, topical anesthetic, non-nutritive sucking, oral acetaminophen, and a concentrated solution of oral sucrose given during the procedure by syringe or applied to a pacifier or nipple provides the most effective pain relief (Anand, Johnston, Oberlander, Taddio, Lehr, & Walco, 2005; Morris et al., 2012; Ridings & Amaya, 2007).

Complementary Care: *Therapeutic Touch Enhances Comfort*

The use of touch to promote healing and comfort dates back to more than 5,000 years ago, when Asian therapists used a variety of touching methods as an important strategy in the healing ritual. Over the ages, other ancient cultures, such as the East Indians and Native Americans, also found value in the power of "hands on" healing. Many spiritual traditions, including the Judeo–Christian doctrine, view healing by the "laying on of hands" as a key element in the promotion and restoration of physical and mental health.

Touch plays an important role in fostering healthy human development. It has been shown to boost the functioning of the immune system and enhance overall feelings of well-being. Touch is a basic human expression that conveys caring and nurturing. The mother intuitively places a comforting hand to her child's feverish head, pinched finger, or scraped knee.

Friends instinctively reach out to touch one another in an expression of caring and compassion. Nurses have long recognized and embraced the value of touch as an important therapeutic tool useful with patients of all ages.

For the neonate, life's initial impressions, wrapped in a halo of warmth, love, and pleasure, are all conveyed through touch. The infant's growing knowledge and awareness of those around him are directly shaped by the way in which he is handled. His sense of comfort, security, and well-being are powerfully influenced by the nature of his mother's or caregiver's touch. Touch experiences occurring during the hours and days after birth, and the infant's feelings that are shaped by these experiences, serve to set the foundation for feelings about people throughout life. Premature and sick infants in the intensive care unit can also benefit from a light, calming touch that promotes a sense of security and warmth.

Reasons for not circumcising a newborn may be related to the surgical risks and/or pain associated with the procedure. If the parents choose not to have their son circumcised, they need to receive information about how to keep their son's penis clean.

"What to say"—*Teaching parents who choose not to have their son circumcised*

When parents who have decided against infant circumcision inquire about personal hygiene for their son, the nurse may offer the following information:

"The foreskin and glans of the penis are actually two similar layers of cells that separate from each other. The separation process begins before the baby is born and is normally completed between ages 3 and 5. During the separation process, sterile sloughed cells build up between the layers; this is harmless."

"Clean your son's penis with water each time you change his diaper and at bath time. Take care not to force the foreskin back over the penis; over time (it may take 3 to 5 years), the foreskin will retract normally."

"Around the age of 4 to 5 years, when the foreskin fully retracts, boys should be taught how to wash underneath the foreskin every day. Teach your son to clean his foreskin by gently pulling it back away from the head of the penis and then rinsing the head of the penis and inside fold of the foreskin with soap and warm water. After washing, the foreskin should be pulled back over the head of the penis."

Now Can You—Discuss aspects of circumcision?

1. Discuss the benefits and risks of circumcision?
2. Explain how to promote parents' increased knowledge and understanding about circumcision?

ENSURING OPTIMAL NUTRITION

Most parents begin to consider feeding options for their baby during the prenatal period. How to feed a newborn after birth is an important decision with implications for the entire family. Two feeding choices are available for newborns: breastfeeding with the mother's natural milk or bottle-feeding with a commercially prepared cow's milk formula. It is paramount that the infant's diet be sufficient to optimally meet his rapidly changing physical and psychosocial needs and adhere to the current recommended dietary allowances. The diet must include essential nutrients such as protein to support rapid cellular growth; carbohydrates to provide energy; and fat to supply the needed calories, regulate fluid and electrolyte balance, and sustain development of the brain and neurological system. Water intake, essential for tissue hydration, should amount to 140 to 160 mL/kg per day. Because the bioavailability of iron in breast milk is much greater than in formula preparations, full-term infants who are breastfed do not need supplemental iron until they reach 6 months of age. At that time, breastfed babies require iron-fortified formula in combination with the breast milk. Infants who are bottle-fed should be given a commercial formula fortified with iron from the beginning. Adequate calories are also necessary, and daily requirements of 105 to 108 kcal/kg per day have been established. (See Chapter 15 for further discussion about infant feeding.)

Discharge Planning for the Infant and Family

The new family is discharged from the hospital or birthing center as early as 24 hours after birth, so early initiation of the discharge planning process is crucial. If this is the couple's first child, discharge planning becomes even more important. The nurse must use every opportunity, beginning during the prenatal period, to teach the family about newborn care. The astute nurse gathers cues about family adaptation to the new baby by observing how the members interact with one another and their level of comfort when holding, feeding, diapering, and dressing the newborn. Questions such as "Tell me how you will care for your new baby?" or "Who is available to help you care for your new baby?" may give the nurse insight as to the type of information the family may need.

 Across Care Settings: **Providing parenting information**

Offering essential information in any setting through individual instruction, educational videos, or parenting classes about such topics as health promotion, growth and development, handling, nasal and oral suctioning, hygiene, diapering, dressing, comforting, nutrition and elimination, rest and sleep, safety, and anticipatory guidance may help the mother and family gain confidence about caring for their baby. It is also helpful to educate parents about routine laboratory screening tests that may be performed in the hospital, home, doctor's office, or community clinic (Cheffer & Rannalli, 2011).

Discharge from the hospital or birthing center is an ideal time to discuss and implement car seat safety measures because automobile accidents are a safety concern for new parents. In moving vehicles, infants and older children must always be transported in a safe seating device. According to the American Academy of Pediatrics (2011b), all infants and toddlers should ride in a rear-facing car safety seat (CSS) until they are 2 years of age or until they reach the highest weight or height allowed by the manufacturer of their CSS. Infants must not be placed in the front seat because inflating front seat air bags may cause suffocation. Information about specific child passenger safety laws for each state has been published by the Governors Highway Safety Association and is available at http://www.ghsa.org/html/stateinfo/laws/childsafety_laws.html.

 Across Care Settings: **Car seat safety**

The nurse can assist the new family by providing information and guidance to resources on car seat safety:

- When purchasing a car seat, parents need to be aware that the seat must meet certain federal guidelines. A label on the seat tag or packaging box states whether the product has met these guidelines. The AAP Web site (www.AAP.org) also lists the guidelines. Another resource,"2011 Car Safety Seats: A Guide for Families" includes data on products, prices, and height/weight limits (www.healthychildren.org/carseatlist). It is important to emphasize that the car seat instructions must be followed when installing the car seat.
- Several community resources are available to the family that will rent or loan a car seat for the infant's discharge home. The hospital or birthing center may have a car seat program. Other resources include the American Red Cross, the Local Health and Safety Council, and the State Department of Health.
- The infant must be dressed so that the clothing facilitates ease of positioning and strap placement. To ensure correct fit, the infant can wear a single layer of clothing, preferably pants, so that the strap can fit between the legs. Sack sleepers are not recommended, and bundling is discouraged because the strap may not fit snugly. Head support is recommended. Parents can use a commercially made product or place a rolled-up receiving blanket around the head and neck area. To protect the infant from burns and overheating in warm weather, parents should check the temperature of the car seat by touching the surface.
- Trained professionals may be available to perform safety checks to help parents with proper car seat installation and use. The National Child Passenger Safety Certification program offers a searchable link to local technicians and inspection sites (http://cert.safekids.org/).
- New cars are required to be equipped with tethers and lower anchors to ensure child safety. Technicians trained to fit safety seats for children with special health-care needs can be found at the Riley Hospital for Children Automotive Safety Program Web site: www.preventinjury.org/specNeeds.asp.

CHILD CARE

When the new family arrives home, they have many decisions to make about the new baby. One important decision is who will care for the child when the parent(s) return to work.

Over the past 35 years, caring for children has shifted from home care to care away from the home. It is essential that the child care facility offer an environment of trust along with safe and competent care. In addition, the child care provider must offer ways to stimulate growth and development as well as meet the physical and psychosocial needs of the developing child. The nurse's responsibility is to help guide the family when choosing a child care facility. There are several options available for families today. In-home care refers to a child care provider such as a nanny, babysitter, family member, or friend who comes into the family home. Work-based group care occurs when the child is placed in a facility that is directly associated with the parent(s)' employment. Another child care option involves placement of the child in another family's home. This type of care can be licensed or unlicensed and may be considered more informal. Established business day care centers offer more formal licensed care settings that comply with set standards and follow state regulations. These day care centers have specific policies that include minimum child to worker ratios. Sick-child care may also be available to the family in times of illness. These care facilities are often offered in community or hospital settings.

Collaboration in Caring—*Child care for new families*

The nurse can encourage the family to:

- Communicate their needs and express their concerns about child care.
- Interview the facility director along with other individuals who may be involved in the child's care.
- Evaluate the educational programs related to qualification of teachers and structure of the learning environment (structured or unstructured).
- Investigate the provision of meals, nutrition, and related sanitation.
- Visit the child care facility on a few occasions, announced and unannounced.
- Identify practical aspects of child care such as location, hours of operation, fee requirements and payment schedule, child to worker ratio, environmental safety, indoor and outdoor space, sick day policies, and availability of care during a holiday or inclement weather.
- Evaluate the infection control and injury prevention measures.
- Gain broader information about the facility related to breast feeding, discipline, nurturing, diapering/toileting, stimulating growth and development, play, nap/rest time, and field trips.
- Discover state regulations and read the care facility's policies and related public records.
- Become familiar with early childhood programs that offer voluntary accreditation such as the National Academy of Early Childhood Program.

Newborn Metabolic Screening Tests

Newborn screening, designed to identify newborns with genetic, metabolic, and/or infectious conditions, is an essential part of preventative care. Approximately four million newborns are screened in the United States each year (Rose &

Dolan, 2012). Through screening, many life-threatening problems can be detected early enough for effective intervention. Conditions commonly discovered through early screening include biotinidase deficiency, hemoglobinopathies, medium-chain acyl Co-A dehydrogenase deficiency, galactosemia, cystic fibrosis, congenital adrenal hyperplasia, congenital hypothyroidism, sickle cell anemia, and phenylketonuria (PKU). PKU, which occurs in approximately 1 in 10,000 to 25,000 births, is a genetic metabolic disorder. It is characterized by a deficiency of the enzyme phenylalanine hydroxylase, which the body needs to convert phenylalanine to tyrosine. A lack of proper conversion results in a buildup of toxic blood levels of phenylalanine, a condition that causes central nervous system damage (AAP, Committee on Genetics, 2008; ACOG, 2009, 2011; AWHONN, 2011; Sparks, 2013). (See Chapter 19 for further discussion.)

Under state law requirements, screening of neonates has been routinely performed in the United States since the 1960s. However, no universal screening policy has been in place to ensure uniformity. Instead, policies concerning routine neonatal screening vary from state to state and are frequently based on local demographics, cost, reimbursement, politics, and ready availability of resources. To address the lack of uniformity in screening practices, the American Academy of Pediatrics (AAP) convened a national Task Force on Newborn Screening in 2000. An important outcome of this work was the directive that each newborn have a medical home. A medical home means that every newborn should receive the benefit of a pediatrician or other primary care health professional who works in partnership with the newborn's family to ensure that appropriate screening is completed, test results are reported, and appropriate follow-up is conducted (AAP, 2000; AAP, Newborn Screening Authoring Committee, 2008).

Nursing Insight—*The National Center for Medical Home Implementation*

The National Center for Medical Home Implementation is a cooperative agreement between the Maternal and Child Health Bureau and the AAP with a mission to ensure that every child and youth has access to a medical home. Developed by the AAP, the medical home model was created to deliver primary care that is accessible, continuous, comprehensive, family-centered, coordinated, compassionate, and culturally effective to all children and youth.

Across Care Settings: Web site enhances exchange of newborn screening data

The National Library of Medicine developed the Newborn Screening Coding and Terminology Guide (http://newbornscreeningcodes.nlm.nih.gov/) to enhance efficient electronic exchange of standard newborn screening data. The goal of the Guide is to provide a standard framework for reporting the results of newborn screening tests whose contents can be accurately interpreted by recipient electronic systems for use in care, follow-up, and analysis; the standard framework also enables the use and comparison of data from different laboratories.

It is essential that nurses recognize that early detection of various disorders allows for timely intervention that can prevent or minimize complications. Before mothers and their infants are discharged from the hospital or birthing center, the nurse should educate the family about the importance of newborn screening. Emphasis should be placed on the long-term benefits of neonatal screening because early detection can allow for the initiation of timely treatment and the development of a plan for ongoing follow-up care. From a community perspective, universal screening and timely intervention can lead to a national reduction in infant disabilities, morbidity, and mortality.

While a positive screening test may indeed indicate that the newborn has a disorder, a diagnosis is generally not made from a single laboratory result. Instead, subsequent testing is conducted because "false positives" (a positive finding although the infant does not have the disorder) can occur. A false-negative result can occur if the specimen was collected at too young of an age or if the quality of the specimen was in some way jeopardized.

 Optimizing Outcomes—**Newborn metabolic screening**

The American College of Obstetricians and Gynecologists, the U.S. Human Resources and Service Administration, the American College of Medical Genetics, and the American Academy of Pediatrics all stress the importance of communication about newborn screening at some point during the prenatal period. An important nursing role centers on understanding the effects of various disorders detected by metabolic screening and advocating for the universal routine screening of all newborns. At present, all states presently screen for at least 26 conditions, and some states screen for 50 or more diseases (Rose & Dolan, 2012). A current list of conditions screened for in each state is maintained online by the National Newborn Screening and Genetic Resource Center, available at http://genes-r-us.uthscsa.edu/resources/consumer/statemap.htm In Canada, newborn screening testing varies by province (Canadian Agency for Drugs and Technologies in Health, 2012), and expanded screening programs are becoming more likely (Etchegary, Dicks, Hodgkinson, Pullman, Green, & Parfey, 2012).

Diagnostic Tools Newborn Metabolic Screening

Approximately 24 hours following birth, a small sample of blood is taken from the infant's heel and placed on special filter paper. The specimen should be obtained as close to the time of the infant's hospital discharge as possible and not later than 7 days. A blood sample taken before 24 hours of age may be unreliable in detecting several conditions. However, if the newborn is discharged from the hospital or birthing center before completing the first 24 hours of life, a sample must be obtained, and the infant's parents must be instructed to contact the physician within 2 weeks to arrange to have another specimen drawn (Drake & Gibson, 2010; Tluczek & DeLuca, 2013).

Neonates born at home must also be screened for disease. The parents or the person registering the birth must make the proper arrangements with a doctor or health-care provider to have the tests completed prior to completion of the first week of life. If the 1-week time period is missed, the infant should be tested anyway because he may still benefit from early intervention for certain disorders.

Now Can You—**Discharge the new family?**

1. Identify cues that may indicate how the family is adapting to the newborn?
2. Develop a discharge teaching plan for the family of a normal neonate?
3. Counsel parents about metabolic screening for their new baby?

Summary Points

◆ Key components of the immediate nursing assessment of the neonate center on ensuring adequate respiratory function and the prevention of heat loss.

◆ The later assessment of the newborn is conducted in a systematic manner that includes careful evaluation of each body system.

◆ Important aspects of newborn care focus on the prevention of infection and injury.

◆ The nurse provides newborn care in an environment that is safe and protective, enhances the transition to extrauterine life, and fosters parent–infant bonding.

◆ Parents must be given correct and impartial information that includes the risks and benefits of circumcision, an elective surgical procedure.

◆ Neonatal pain must be readily identified, assessed, and appropriately managed.

◆ An essential role for nurses involves teaching and discharge planning for the new family.

Review Questions

Multiple Choice

1. The nurse uses pre-warmed blankets to wrap the newborn at birth to prevent heat loss by which mechanism?
A. Evaporation
B. Convection
C. Conduction
D. Radiation

2. During the reflex assessment, the nurse places the infant in the prone position and strokes one side of the vertebral column. The nurse is assessing which reflex?
A. Moro
B. Galant
C. Babinski
D. Stepping

3. The perinatal nurse notes diffuse, soft tissue edema of an infant's head. How will the nurse chart this finding?
A. Caput succedaneum
B. Cephalhematoma
C. Subperiosteal hemorrhage
D. Periorbital edema

4. A newborn has the differential diagnosis of polycythemia after a heel stick was obtained at 1 hour of life. What result would the nurse correlate with this condition?
   A. Hemoglobin: 15.5 g/dL
   B. Hemoglobin: 23 g/dL
   C. Hematocrit: 54%
   D. Hematocrit: 68%

5. The perinatal nurse is caring for an infant with a minor congenital anomaly. What does the nurse understand about this type of defect?
   A. Affects one or more minor body systems only
   B. Structural defect impacting only social acceptability
   C. Defect that only has cosmetic or social significance
   D. Anomaly that can be corrected with minor surgery

6. A nurse reads the diagnosis "plethora" on an infant's chart. What assessment finding correlates with this condition?
   A. Pinpoint hemorrhagic areas on the skin
   B. Tough, leathery, cracked and peeling skin
   C. Deep purple color caused by too many red blood cells
   D. Blue discoloration of the soles and palms

7. A nurse sees that an infant's chart has a notation concerning Epstein pearls. What assessment technique does the nurse use to assess for this finding?
   A. Gently palpates the anterior and posterior fontanelles
   B. Shines a penlight into the infant's open mouth
   C. Palpates the skin for evidence of small nodules
   D. Inspects the skin for tiny, white, raised lesions

8. During hand-off report, the off-going nurse reports that a newborn is tachycardic. What heart rate does the nurse expect to find on assessment?
   A. 80 to 100 beats/minute
   B. 100 to 120 beats/minute
   C. Greater than 140 beats/minute
   D. Greater than 160 beats/minute

9. A nurse notes that a male infant's urinary meatus is located on the ventral surface of the penis. Which action by the nurse is best?
   A. Inform the parents that the planned circumcision cannot proceed.
   B. Have the urologist explain the modifications to the circumcision that are needed.
   C. Have the parents sign a consent form for an emergency surgical repair.
   D. Place an indwelling urinary catheter to facilitate bladder emptying.

10. A nurse assessing a newborn for birth injuries knows that the bone most often fractured during delivery is which of the following?
    A. Clavicle
    B. Femur
    C. Wrist
    D. Ankle

See Answers to End of Chapter Review Questions on *DavisPlus.*

REFERENCES

American Academy of Pediatrics (AAP). (2000). Serving the family from birth to the medical home: Newborn screening: A blueprint for the future: Executive summary: newborn screening task force report. *Pediatrics, 106*(2) (Supplement), 389–427.

American Academy of Pediatrics (AAP). (2006). Controversies concerning vitamin K and the newborn: Committee on fetus and newborn: Policy statement. (Reaffirmed 2009). *Pediatrics 118*(3), 1266. doi:10 .1542/peds.2006-1697

American Academy of Pediatrics (AAP). (2011a). Policy Statement: SIDS and other sleep-related infant deaths: Expansion of recommendations for a safe infant sleeping environment. *Pediatrics, 128*(11), 1030–1039. doi:10.1542/peds.2011-2284

American Academy of Pediatrics (AAP). (2011b). Committee on injury, violence, and poison prevention. Policy Statement: Child passenger safety. *Pediatrics, 127*(4), 788–793. doi:10.1542/peds.2011-0213

American Academy of Pediatrics (AAP) Committee on Genetics. (2008). Policy Statement: Maternal phenylketonuria. (Reaffirmed 2013). *Pediatrics, 122*(2), 445–449. doi:10.1542/peds.2008-1485

American Academy of Pediatrics (AAP) Newborn Screening Authoring Committee. (2008). Newborn screening expands: Recommendations for pediatricians and medical homes—implications for the system. *Pediatrics, 121*, 192–217.

American Academy of Pediatrics (AAP) Task Force on Circumcision. (2012). Circumcision policy statement. *Pediatrics, 130*(3), 585–586. doi:10.1542/peds.2012-1989

American College of Obstetricians and Gynecologists (ACOG). (2001). Circumcision. Committee Opinion No. 260. (Reaffirmed 2011). *Obstetrics & Gynecology, 98*(10), 707–708.

American College of Obstetricians and Gynecologists (ACOG). (2006). The Apgar Score. Committee Opinion No. 333. (Reaffirmed 2010). *Obstetrics & Gynecology, 107*(5), 1209–1212.

American College of Obstetricians and Gynecologists (ACOG). (2009). Maternal phenylketonuria. Committee Opinion No. 449. *Obstetrics & Gynecology, 114*(6), 1432–1433.

American College of Obstetricians and Gynecologists (ACOG). (2011). Newborn screening. Committee Opinion No. 481. *Obstetrics & Gynecology, 117*(3), 762–765.

American College of Obstetricians and Gynecologists & American Academy of Pediatrics (ACOG/AAP). (2012). *Guidelines for perinatal care* (7th ed.). Washington, DC: Author.

American Society for Pain Management Nursing. (2011). Position Statement. *Male infant circumcision pain management.* Retrieved from http://www.aspmn.org/documents/Circumcision.pdf

Anand, K., Johnston, C., Oberlander, R., Taddio, A., Lehr, V., & Walco, G. (2005). Prevention and management of pain and stress in the neonate. *Pediatrics, 27*(6), 844–876.

Andrews, M. M. (2011). Transcultural perspectives in the nursing care of children. In M. M. Andrews & J. S. Boyle, *Transcultural concepts in nursing care* (6th ed., pp. 116–145). Philadelphia, PA: Lippincott Williams & Wilkins.

Askin, D. F. (2009). Physical assessment of the newborn. *Nursing for Women's Health, 13*(2), 141–149. doi:10.1111/j.1751-486X.2009 .01405.x

Association of Women's Health, Obstetric and Neonatal Nurses (AWHONN). (2011). Position Statement: Newborn screening. *Journal of Obstetric, Gynecologic & Neonatal Nursing, 40*(1), 86–87. doi:10.1111/j.1552-6909.2010.01213.x

Association of Women's Health, Obstetric and Neonatal Nurses (AWHONN). (2013). *Neonatal skin care* (3rd ed.). Washington, DC: Author.

Ballard, J. L., Khoury, J. C., Wedig, K., Wang, L., Eilers-Waisman, B. L., & Lipp, R. (1991). New Ballard score, expanded to include extremely premature infants. *Journal of Pediatrics, 119*, 417–423.

Bowden, P. (2012). Promoting mother, infant and toddler health. In J. A. Maville, & C. G. Huerta (Eds.), *Health promotion in nursing* (3rd ed., pp. 162–195). Albany, NY: Delmar Cengage Learning.

Brazelton, T. B. (1973). *Neonatal behavioral assessment scale.* Philadelphia, PA: Lippincott.

Brazelton, T. B., & Nugent, J. K. (1995). *Neonatal behavioral assessment scale* (3rd ed.). London, UK: MacKeith Press.

Bulechek, G. M., Butcher, H. K., & Dochterman, J. M., & Wagner, C. (2013). *Nursing interventions classification (NIC)* (6th ed.). St. Louis, MO: Elsevier Mosby.

Canadian Agency for Drugs and Technologies in Health. (2012). Newborn screening for disorders and abnormalities in Canada. Retrieved from http://www.cadth.ca/products/environmental-scanning/environmental-scans/newborn-screening

Centers for Disease Control and Prevention (CDC). (2010). Sexually transmitted disease treatment guidelines, 2010. *MMWR Morbidity and Mortality Weekly Report, 59*(No. RR-12), 1–94.

Cheffer, N. D., & Rannalli, D. A. (2011). Transitional care of the newborn. In S. Mattson & J. Smith (Eds.), *Core curriculum for maternal-newborn nursing* (4th ed., pp. 346–361). Philadelphia, PA: W.B. Saunders.

Collado, M. C., Cernada, M., Bauerl, C., Vento, M., & Perez-Martinez, G. (2012).Microbial ecology and host-microbiota interactions during early life stages. *Gut Microbes, 3*(4), 352-365. doi:10.4161/gmic.21215

D'Avanzo, C. (2007). *Pocket guide to cultural health assessment* (4th ed.). St. Louis, MO: C.V. Mosby.

Dillon, P. M. (2007). *Nursing Health Assessment: A critical thinking, case studies approach* (2nd ed.). Philadelphia, PA: F.A. Davis.

Drake, E., & Gibson, M. E. (2010). Update on expanded newborn screening. *Nursing for Women's Health, 14*(3), 199–211. doi:10.1111/j.1751-486X.2010.01541.x

Etchegary, H., Dicks, E., Hodgkinson, K., Pullman, D., Green, J., & Parfey, P. (2012). Public attitudes about genetic testing in the newborn period. *Journal of Obstetric, Gynecologic & Neonatal Nursing, 41*(92), 191–200. doi:10.1111/j.1552-6909.2012.01341.x

Haddad, L., Smith, S., Phillips, K., & Heidel, R. (2012). Comparison of temporal artery and axillary temperatures in healthy newborns. *Journal of Obstetric, Gynecologic & Neonatal Nursing, 41*(3), 383–388. doi:10.1111/j.1552-6909.2012.01367.x

Hellwig, J. P. (2013). "Safe to Sleep Campaign": Preventing sudden unexpected infant death. *Nursing for Women's Health, 16*(6), 505. doi:10.1111/j.1751-486X.2012.01799.x

Hensel, D., & Springmyer, J. (2011). Do perinatal nurses still check for blood return when administering the Hepatitis B vaccine? *Journal of Obstetric, Gynecologic & Neonatal Nursing, 40*(5), 589–594. doi:10.1111/j.1552-6909.2011.01277.x

Hitchcock, S. (2012). Endorsing safe infant sleep: A call to action. *Nursing for Women's Health, 16*(5), 387–395. doi:10.1111/j.1751-486X.2012.01762.x

Hoogsteen, L. (2010). Safe infant sleeping: What is the ideal sleeping environment? *Nursing for Women's Health, 14*(2), 121–129. doi:10.1111/j.1751-486X.2010.01525.x

Johnson, M., Moorhead, S., Bulechek, G., Butcher, H., Maas, M., Moorhead, S., & Swanson, E. (2011). *NOC and NIC Linkages to NANDA-I and clinical conditions: Supporting critical reasoning and quality care* (3rd ed.). St. Louis, MO: Mosby Elsevier.

Karl, D. J., & Keefer, C. H. (2011). Use of the behavioral observation of the newborn educational trainer for teaching newborn behavior. *Journal of Obstetric, Gynecologic & Neonatal Nursing, 40*(1), 75–83. doi:10.1111/j.1552-6909.2010.01202.x

Kroger, A. T., Sumaya, C. V., Pickering, L. K., & Atkinson, W. L. (2011). General recommendations on immunization practices: Recommendations of the Advisory Committee on Immunization Practices (ACIP). *Morbidity and Mortality Weekly Report, 60*(RR02), 1–60.

Lee, G., Flannery-Bergey, D., Randall-Rollins, K., Curry, D., Rowe, S., Teague, M., et al. (2011). Accuracy of temporal artery thermometry in neonatal intensive care infants. *Advances in Neonatal Care, 11*(1), 62–70. doi:10.1097/ANC.0b013e3182087d2b

Lester, B. M., & Tronick, E. Z. (2004). NICU Network Neurobehavioral Scale (NNNS). *Pediatrics (Supplement), 113,* 631–669.

Martin, G. R., Kemper, A. R., & Bradshaw, E. A. (2012). CCHD screening guidelines: Implementation of standardized protocols. *The Clinical Advisor, 15*(10), 29–36.

Moorhead, S., Johnson, M., Maas, M. L., & Swanson, E. (2013). *Nursing outcomes classification (NOC)* (5th ed.). St. Louis, MO: Elsevier Mosby.

Morris, B., Wodak, A., Mindel, A., Schrieber, L., Duggan, K., Dilley, A., et al. (2012). Infant male circumcision: An evidence-based policy statement. *Open Journal of Preventive Medicine, 2*(3), 79–92. doi:10.4236/ojpm.2012.21012

National Institute on Deafness and Other Communication Disorders. (2011). *It's important to have your baby's hearing screened.* NIH Publication No. 11-4968. Bethesda, MD: Author.

National Institutes of Health. Child Health & Human Development. (2012). *Safe to Sleep public education campaign.* Retrieved from http://nichd.nih.gov/sids/Pages/sids.aspx

Reed, R., & Johnson-Cash, J. (2014). The human microbiome: Considerations for pregnancy, birth and early mothering. Retrieved from http://midwifethinking.com/2014/01/15/the-human-microbiome-considerations-for-pregnancy-birth-and-early-mothering/

Ridings, H., & Amaya, M. (2007). Male neonatal circumcision: An evidence-based review. *Journal of the American Academy of Physician Assistants, 20*(2), 32–34.

Rose, N. C., & Dolan, S. M. (2012). Newborn screening and the obstetrician. *Obstetrics & Gynecology, 120*(4), 908–916. doi:http://10.1097/AOG.0b013e31826b2f03

Seagraves, K., Brulte, A., McNeely, K., & Pritham, U. (2013). Supporting breastfeeding to reduce newborn readmissions for hyperbilirubinemia. *Nursing for Women's Health, 17*(6), 498–507. doi:10.1111/.1751-486X.12078

Shaefer, S., Herman, S., Frank, S., Adkins, M., & Terhaar, M. (2010). Translating infant safe sleep evidence into nursing practice. *Journal of Obstetric, Gynecologic & Neonatal Nursing, 41*(1), 17–23. doi:10.1111/j.1552-6909.2011.01322.x

Sparks, S. E. (2013). Update on newborn screening. *North Carolina Medical Journal, 74*(6), 514–521.

Sullivan, M. C., Miller, R. J., Fontaine, L. A., & Lester, B. (2012). Refining neurobehavioral assessment of the high-risk infant using the NICU Network Neurobehavioral Scale. *Journal of Obstetric, Gynecologic & Neonatal Nursing, 39*(6), 618–626. doi:10.1111/j.1552-6909.2010.01194.x

Tansky, C., & Lindberg, C. E. (2010). Breasfeeding as a pain intervention when immunizing infants. *JNP: The Journal for Nurse Practitioners, 6*(4), 287–295.

Taylor, J. A., Wright, J. A., & Woodrum, D. (2011). Routine newborn care. In C. Gleason & S. Devaskar (Eds.), *Avery's diseases of the newborn* (9th ed., pp. 300–315). St Louis, MO: W.B. Saunders.

Tluczek, A., & DeLuca, J. M. (2013). Newborn screening policy and practice issues for nurses. *Journal of Obstetric, Gynecologic & Neonatal Nursing, 42*(6), 718–728. doi:10.1111/1552-6909.12252

U.S. Department of Health and Human Services (USDHHS). (2011). *Healthy People 2020.* Retrieved from http://www.healthypeople.gov/2020/topicsobjectives2020/default.aspx

Vallerand, A. H., & Sanoski, C. A. (2014). *Davis's drug guide for nurses* (14th ed.). Philadelphia, PA: F.A. Davis.

Verklan, M., & Walden, M. (2014). *Core curriculum for neonatal intensive nursing* (5th ed.). St. Louis, MO: Saunders.

Zderic, S. A., & Lambert, S. M. (2011). Developmental abnormalities of the genitourinary system. In C. Gleason & S. Devaskar (Eds.), *Avery's diseases of the newborn* (9th ed., pp. 1191–1205). St Louis, MO: W.B. Saunders.

CONCEPT MAP

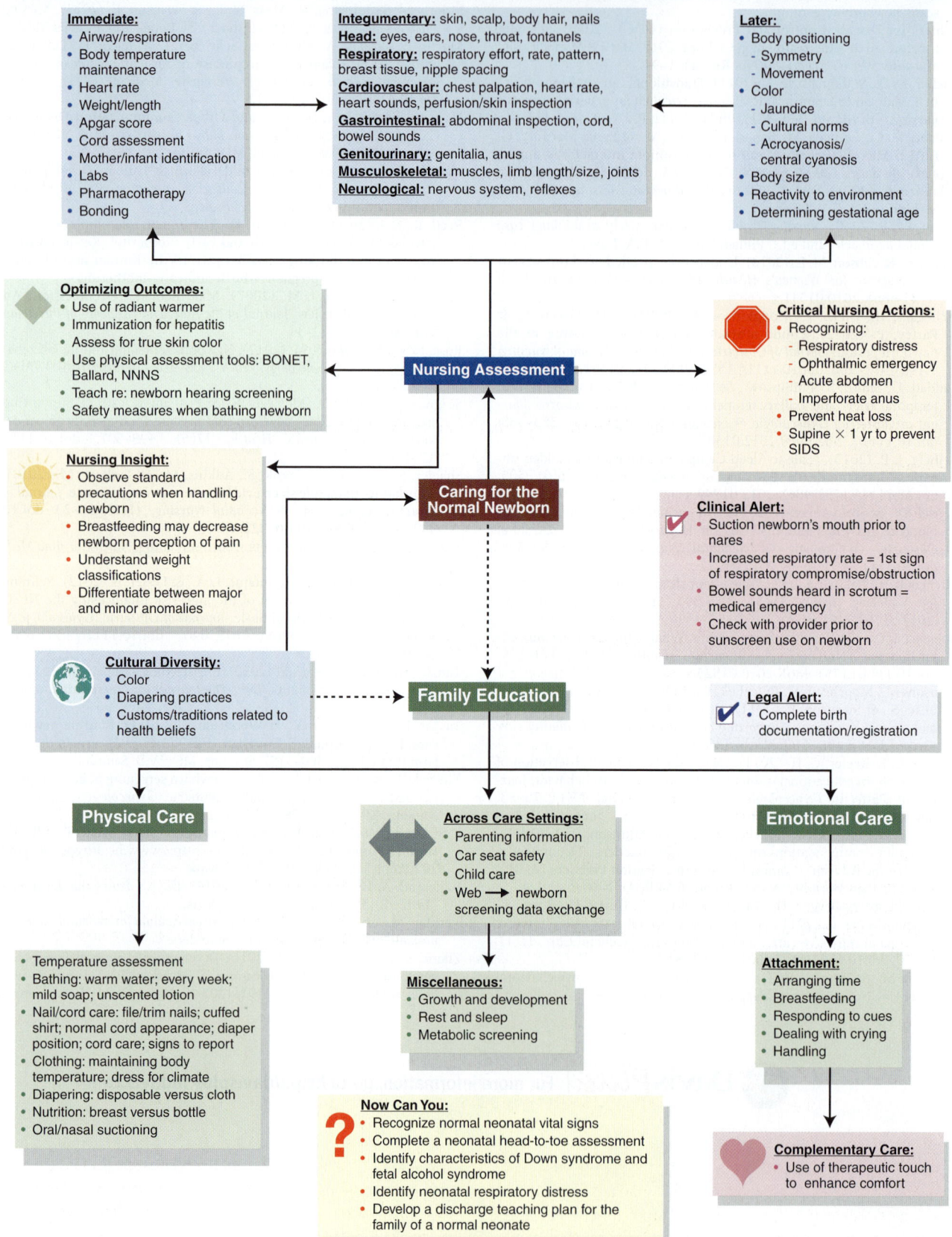

Immediate:
- Airway/respirations
- Body temperature maintenance
- Heart rate
- Weight/length
- Apgar score
- Cord assessment
- Mother/infant identification
- Labs
- Pharmacotherapy
- Bonding

Integumentary: skin, scalp, body hair, nails
Head: eyes, ears, nose, throat, fontanels
Respiratory: respiratory effort, rate, pattern, breast tissue, nipple spacing
Cardiovascular: chest palpation, heart rate, heart sounds, perfusion/skin inspection
Gastrointestinal: abdominal inspection, cord, bowel sounds
Genitourinary: genitalia, anus
Musculoskeletal: muscles, limb length/size, joints
Neurological: nervous system, reflexes

Later:
- Body positioning
  - Symmetry
  - Movement
- Color
  - Jaundice
  - Cultural norms
  - Acrocyanosis/ central cyanosis
- Body size
- Reactivity to environment
- Determining gestational age

Optimizing Outcomes:
- Use of radiant warmer
- Immunization for hepatitis
- Assess for true skin color
- Use physical assessment tools: BONET, Ballard, NNNS
- Teach re: newborn hearing screening
- Safety measures when bathing newborn

Nursing Assessment

Critical Nursing Actions:
- Recognizing:
  - Respiratory distress
  - Ophthalmic emergency
  - Acute abdomen
  - Imperforate anus
- Prevent heat loss
- Supine × 1 yr to prevent SIDS

Nursing Insight:
- Observe standard precautions when handling newborn
- Breastfeeding may decrease newborn perception of pain
- Understand weight classifications
- Differentiate between major and minor anomalies

Caring for the Normal Newborn

Clinical Alert:
- Suction newborn's mouth prior to nares
- Increased respiratory rate = 1st sign of respiratory compromise/obstruction
- Bowel sounds heard in scrotum = medical emergency
- Check with provider prior to sunscreen use on newborn

Cultural Diversity:
- Color
- Diapering practices
- Customs/traditions related to health beliefs

Family Education

Legal Alert:
- Complete birth documentation/registration

Physical Care

Across Care Settings:
- Parenting information
- Car seat safety
- Child care
- Web → newborn screening data exchange

Emotional Care

- Temperature assessment
- Bathing: warm water; every week; mild soap; unscented lotion
- Nail/cord care: file/trim nails; cuffed shirt; normal cord appearance; diaper position; cord care; signs to report
- Clothing: maintaining body temperature; dress for climate
- Diapering: disposable versus cloth
- Nutrition: breast versus bottle
- Oral/nasal suctioning

Miscellaneous:
- Growth and development
- Rest and sleep
- Metabolic screening

Attachment:
- Arranging time
- Breastfeeding
- Responding to cues
- Dealing with crying
- Handling

Now Can You:
- Recognize normal neonatal vital signs
- Complete a neonatal head-to-toe assessment
- Identify characteristics of Down syndrome and fetal alcohol syndrome
- Identify neonatal respiratory distress
- Develop a discharge teaching plan for the family of a normal neonate

Complementary Care:
- Use of therapeutic touch to enhance comfort

Caring for the Newborn at Risk

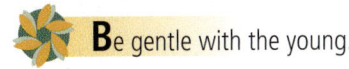

Be gentle with the young.

—Juvenal, *Roman poet and satirist (55 A.D.–127 A.D.)*

LEARNING TARGETS *At the completion of this chapter, the student will be able to:*

- Describe the anatomy and physiology of the high-risk infant.
- Identify the criteria for classification of high-risk newborns using gestational age and birth weight.
- Examine conditions related to the small-for-gestational-age and large for gestational-age infants.
- Prioritize developmentally appropriate and holistic nursing care for the high-risk newborn.
- Explain common complications affecting the premature and postterm newborn.
- Discuss the high-risk newborn physical assessment.
- Describe additional conditions that place all newborns at high risk.
- Develop teaching plans and discharge criteria for parents whose children have various high-risk conditions.

PICO(T) Questions

The intent of evidence-based practice (EBP) is to provide nursing care that integrates the best available evidence. An initial step in EBP is to write a PICO(T) question that effectively guides the research. A PICO(T) question is an acronym that stands for population (P), intervention or issue (I), comparison of interest (C), outcome (O), and timeframe (T). Depending on the question, all or some of the question components are used in the research process. Use these PICO(T) questions to spark your thinking as you read the chapter.

1. What role might (O) nurses' play related to (I) ethical decision-making for (P) newborns with uncertain viability?

2. What are the best (I) evidence-based practices for (O) early identification of sepsis in (P) neonates?

3. What are the benefits (O) of olfactory stimulation (I) during gavage feedings for (P) premature neonates?

 Evidence-Based Practice

Yidiz, A., Arikan, D., Gözüm, S., Taştekin, A., & Budancamanak, I. (2011). The effect of the odor of breast milk on the time needed for transition from gavage to total oral feeding in preterm infants. *Journal of Nursing Scholarship, 43*(3), 265–273.

The purpose of this study was to investigate the effect of olfactory stimulation with breast milk in gavage-fed preterm infants. Prematurity is defined as infants born at or before the 37th week of gestation. Feeding methods for premature infants are often determined by gestational age, birth weight, sucking ability, muscle tone, vital signs, and gastrointestinal development.

Feeding the premature infant is often difficult requiring the use of enteral or parenteral feeding. To tolerate oral feedings there needs to be coordination among sucking, swallowing, and respiration. Infants born at or before the 34th week often have poor coordination between sucking and swallowing leading to a potential for aspiration. Feeding the infant by gavage limits the

(continued)

Evidence-Based Practice (continued)

infant's opportunity to develop self-feeding sucking behaviors. Premature infants have fully developed olfactory capacity; hence, maternal odors stimulate breastfeeding behaviors (e.g., sucking movements).

A total of 80 preterm infants were included in this study with 40 in the control group and 40 in the experimental group. All infants were patients in the same university hospital neonatal intensive care or premature units. Criteria for inclusion included born between 28 and 34 weeks of gestation, medically stable in the first 24 hours, having no congenital malformations that could affect breathing, and tolerating gavage feedings with breast milk. Additional criteria included birth weight of 1,000 g, Apgar scores with a mean of greater than 6, neonatologist designation of being without sucking reflex when born, and no evidence of cranial bleeding or hyperbilirubinemia.

A prospective experimental study design was used. Written parent consent was obtained and demographic data collected by semi-structured questionnaire. No one but the researchers knew which group the infants were assigned to. Data were collected by the researchers at three feeding time intervals daily (i.e., 9:00 a.m.,

noon, and 3:00 p.m). Infants were weighed daily before the 9:00 a.m. feeding. All infants received a gavage feeding of breast milk from their own mother's milk using gravity flow through a suspended feeding device and without applying pressure. The control group received no interventions. The study group was stimulated during gavage feeding by the placement of a sterile pad soaked in breast milk approximately 2 cm from the infant's nose. This procedure was repeated with each of the three feedings daily until the infants were placed on oral feedings.

Results of the study indicated that preterm infants who received olfactory stimulation with breast milk during gavage feeding transitioned to oral feedings 3 days sooner than that of the control group and were discharged from the hospital 4 days sooner than the control group.

1. How is this information useful to clinical nursing practice?
2. Based on these findings, what are implications for further research?

See Suggested Responses for Evidence-Based Practice on Davis*Plus*.

Introduction

This chapter provides essential information about newborns at risk. The anatomy and physiology of the respiratory, circulatory, and neurological systems of the fetus and newborn are reviewed. These three systems present the greatest challenges when a newborn is born preterm or postterm. The anatomy and physiology review is followed by a discussion of how newborns at risk are classified according to weight and gestational age.

An examination of newborn conditions that are common for newborns at different weights and gestational ages is presented. Many of the conditions are commonly seen in different populations of newborns. Teaching plans and discharge criteria for parents whose children have various gastrointestinal conditions are included.

Congenital (conditions present at birth) health-care conditions are also presented in this chapter. Information about the condition is broken down into signs and symptoms, diagnostic tests, medications prescribed, appropriate nursing interventions, and information regarding family education. High-risk newborns are a vulnerable population, and the nursing care provided to these special patients makes all the difference in their initial health-care outcomes and subsequent life, including any long-term developmental disabilities.

A & P review **The Newborn at Risk**

High-risk newborns can have conditions that affect any body system, but the three systems that are commonly affected because of maturational interruption or insult are the respiratory, circulatory, and neurological systems.

Respiratory system: Fetal lung maturity develops in utero progressively until term. Fetal lung maturity is

Growth and Development

The high-risk newborn is extremely vulnerable because of intrauterine or extrauterine factors and immaturity. The high-risk newborn requires tedious nursing care to promote lung, circulatory, and neurological maturity. Developmental care should focus on promoting healthy growth and development while minimizing debilitating consequences of immaturity. Developmental delays are common in the high-risk newborn. Frequent assessment of growth and developmental milestones is important. The nurse must provide an optimal healing environment with special attention to noise, light, and infant handling and positioning.

Many successful strategies have been identified that consider the physical, psychological, and emotional vulnerabilities of the infant (Coughlin, Gibbins, & Hoath, 2009). Protected sleep is vital for the high-risk newborn. Often the immature newborn is not prepared to live outside the womb. Adequate sleep is necessary for recovery and growth. The environment should be one of healing. A dark and quiet environment is best to promote sleep and rest. Pain and stress management is essential for high-risk newborns because they are unable to handle high amounts of stress. Pain management and stress-reducing interventions promote comfort. The nurse should frequently assess the infant for pain and stress, and the nurse understands that minimal handling of the high-risk infant is necessary to reduce stressful events experienced by the infant. The high-risk newborn may have difficulties regulating temperature and blood sugar. The nurse should ensure that temperature and blood sugar are frequently measured and within normal ranges to decrease stress experienced by the infant. Developmental activities of daily living for the high-risk newborn include positioning, feeding, and skin care (Coughlin, Gibbins, & Hoath, 2009). The nurse should place the infant in a position that promotes comfort. The high-risk newborn should be repositioned to reduce the risk of skin breakdown. Gel pads may be appropriate to relieve pressure on the infant's head. The high-risk newborn has increased metabolic needs. These increased needs must be met through a variety of nursing interventions including enteral and parenteral feedings when appropriate. The nurse should monitor the weight of the infant daily to ensure adequate weight gain.

Source: Coughlin, M., Gibbins, S., & Hoath, S. (2009). Core measures for developmentally supportive care in neonatal intensive care units: theory, precedence and practice. *Journal of Advanced Nursing, 65*(10), 2239–2248. Blackwell Publishing Ltd.

determined by the **L/S ratio** (lecithin to sphingomyelin) and **PG** (phosphatidylglycerol) values, which are essential **phospholipids** in promoting oxygenation of the lung alveoli. They act on the pulmonary surface to decrease surface tension and are needed to keep the alveoli open when the newborn exhales. L/S ratio and PG values are often mature at 35 to 36 weeks' gestation; before this time newborns are at risk for **respiratory distress syndrome (RDS)**. Between 24 and 40 weeks' gestation, the lungs continue to develop additional alveolar ducts and alveoli, as well as further develop the pulmonary vasculature. These physiological changes continue past term with alveoli continuing to increase in number, size, and shape.

Circulatory system: Fetal circulation functions in utero to oxygenate the organs needed for intrauterine growth. Fetal blood is shunted away from the lungs and liver because the placenta performs the functions of those organs. Increased blood is circulated to the brain and heart to accommodate rapid growth. The circulatory system of the fetus also develops strength and resiliency with increasing gestational age. At birth, the three fetal shunts (ductus arteriosus, foramen ovale, and ductus venosus) close, and circulation converts to adult circulation to accommodate oxygen intake by the lungs and filtering of blood by the liver. If the shunts fail to respond to extrauterine oxygen and pressure levels, there is a structural deformity in the circulatory system, and the newborn is at risk. The preterm newborn is at increased risk because of a fragile circulatory system that is overexerted by the stress of the extrauterine environmental pressures that can easily damage the fragile blood vessels.

 Nursing Insight—Increasing oxygen to organs

What if a newborn needed to increase oxygen to the organs? The newborn's ability to alter cardiac output is limited. The myocardium of newborns is not as adaptable as the adult myocardium, and they cannot increase stroke volume. The physiological mechanism used to increase circulation of oxygen to the organs is an increase in the infant's heart rate (Watson, 2012).

Neurological system: The neurological system, including the central and peripheral nervous systems and the parasympathetic and sympathetic nervous systems, are underdeveloped at birth. Neurologically, newborns are immature because of limited synaptic and dendritic interconnections in the brain and immature myelination of the nerve cells. The preterm newborn has an increased risk for neurological immaturity resulting in the inability to cope with the extrauterine stimuli at birth. Neurological deficits are experienced both short and long term in newborns at risk as a result of interrupted neuronal development (Martin, Fanaroff, & Walsh, 2011) (Fig. 19-1). ◆

The Neonatal Intensive Care Unit

The **neonatal intensive care unit** (NICU) is a frightening place for parents. The first visit to the NICU is extremely difficult, and the parents must be prepared for what they are about to experience. The rules of the unit must be outlined and the expectations gently discussed. The newborns

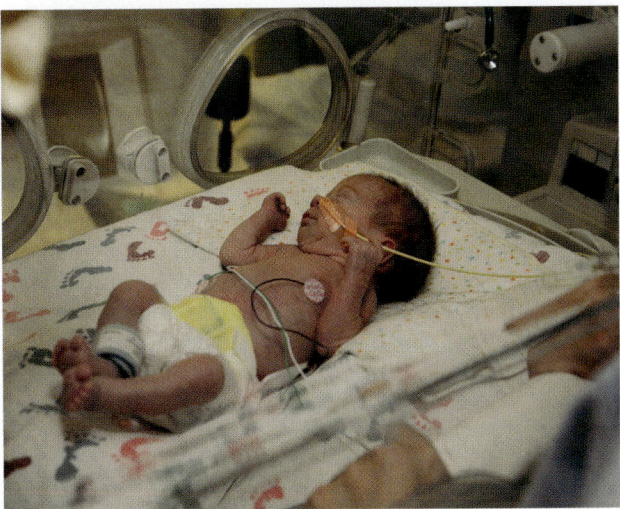

Figure 19-1 A high-risk newborn in the neonatal intensive care unit.

are extremely small and fragile, and there are several pieces of highly technical equipment, all with alarms. The nurse can explain that the NICU keeps the lighting dimmed and voices low to increase rest for the newborn to promote developmental care. Care is done in clusters, and the nurse tries to schedule all the procedures needed on the newborn during the assessment period, which is usually every 1 to 3 hours depending on the acuity of care for the threatened newborn. The nurse can also explain that NICU tries to simulate an intrauterine environment as much as possible. This means decreasing the stimulus to the newborn as much as possible to allow normal growth and development.

Some of the NICU care concepts create a difficult adjustment for parents. Most parents are back to work long before their newborn is discharged. Many parents have an overwhelming desire to interact with their newborn but are not available during the care times. Creating partnership in care between the NICU staff and family benefits the newborn and every effort needs to be made to communicate and collaborate with parents. The family of the NICU newborn is encouraged to bond with their newborn just as if it was in the newborn nursery. NICU nurses encourage them to visit and assist with care whenever possible.

Parents of NICU newborns actually go through some developmental phases until they can become partners with the staff in their newborn's care. First, the environment of the NICU is overwhelming, but most parents are able, after a short time, to focus on the baby and keep the environmental distractions in the background. Second, the parents begin to develop a relationship with the newborn and take ownership of their newborn. This is less difficult today with the current philosophy of family-centered care. Parents are partners in the care of their newborns and become the voice of the newborn. This stage lends itself to parents as partners in providing the best individual developmental care for the newborn (Reis, Rempel, Scott, Brady-Fryer, & Van Aerde, 2010).

Most NICUs practice primary care nursing so the parents can have a consistent contact person to ask questions and to call when they are home. Some NICU staffs make routine phone calls to the family to give updates.

From the very first visit onward, the parents are encouraged to touch the newborn. Touch is a very important act for bonding with the newborn. Kangaroo Care (see Family Teaching Guidelines—Kangaroo Care) is also encouraged as soon as the newborn is stable enough to be taken out of the incubator. Many parents have the need to stay at the bedside for extended periods of time. The NICU nurse must assist the parents in finding a realistic routine that enhances the newborn's health-care needs. Fathers are included in the educational and care process of the newborn. Discharge planning includes education about developmental care and continuity of care that includes home care that is most important to the high-risk newborn.

Collaboration in Caring—*Parents and the NICU*

Nurses and parents work collaboratively in caring for the newborn.

- Orient the parents to the NICU environment, policies, and procedures and the Health Insurance Portability and Accountability Act regulations.
- Assign one primary care nurse as the main contact for the parents.
- Explain the rationale for policies and procedures.
- Listen to the parents' expectations of their role in the NICU.
- Explain the integration of caretaking roles between parents and nurse.
- Use a whiteboard at the newborn's bed to relay messages back and forth.
- Encourage parents to call the NICU and inquire about their newborn 24/7.
- Encourage parents to bring in the newborn's personal clothing for use when allowed.
- Encourage parents to verbalize dissatisfaction with newborn's care.
- Incorporate parent's suggestions and wishes in the care routine.

legal alert—Health Insurance Portability and Accountability Act (HIPAA)

Explain to parents that HIPAA (Health Insurance Portability and Accountability Act of 1996 from the U.S. Department of Health and Human Services [HHS]) is taken seriously within the NICU unit and is addressed during parent orientation to the unit including:

- Parents may be asked to step out of the unit during medical rounds, nursing report times, and possibly in emergencies to protect the privacy of all newborns.
- Phone inquiries can only be done by the parents after they identify themselves by the newborn's medical record or bracelet number and they have signed a consent permitting nursing and medical personnel to discuss information on the phone with them.
- Nurses and physicians will not answer questions regarding the condition of other newborns in the unit.
- Pictures of their own newborn are allowed, but they cannot photograph other newborns in the unit.

CLASSIFICATION OF THE NEONATAL INTENSIVE CARE UNIT

NICUs are classified according to level of care. Regionalization is a concept in care that arose in the 1980s to conserve health-care dollars, consolidate services, and improve outcomes. Today, hospitals often compete within the same geographic area to have the largest and most recognized services in specialty care areas. Level I nursery care is for well newborns and can stabilize high-risk newborns for transport. Level II nurseries can provide the same care as Level I nurseries plus provide premature care, give oxygen by hood, and start IV therapy. Level III NICUs are the most sophisticated of the nurseries because they ventilate newborns (Martin et al., 2011).

The High-Risk Newborn

Nursing care of the high-risk newborn has become an extremely technologically enhanced specialty over the past 50 years and has rapidly evolved into a dynamic field of nursing care. Advances in NICUs are steadily increasing the survival rate of newborns at risk, but this population still has a significantly higher mortality and morbidity rate when compared with uncomplicated, full-term newborns.

Newborns can be put at risk any time during their intrauterine (in utero), intrapartum (from the beginning of the first stage of labor to the end of the third stage of labor), or **extrauterine** development (once the newborn is born). They can be placed at risk in their prenatal or intrauterine environment by **genetic disorders** (associated with inheritance), congenital anomalies, or maternal factors such as disease states, trauma, and drug use. Newborns are at risk based on a stressful intrapartum environment resulting in conditions of **asphyxia** (lack of oxygen) and **birth injuries** (trauma associated with delivery), or they can be placed at risk in the immediate neonatal or extrauterine environment as a result of conditions such as **hypothermia** (low body temperature), poor oxygenation, or prematurity. Review Table 19-1 for conditions that place a newborn at risk.

The majority of newborns who are cared for in NICUs are preterm newborns (newborns born at 37 weeks of gestation or earlier). In the United States, 1 in 8 deliveries will be preterm (CDC, 2011a). This is a rate of 11.99%, which is a decline from previous decades (March of Dimes, 2011). The primary risk factor for preterm birth is having a previous preterm birth. Other risk factors are presented in Box 19-1.

TRANSPORTING THE HIGH-RISK NEWBORN

Newborn transport is done if more technologically advanced care is needed than can be safely provided at the institution (Fig. 19-2). Most Level III NICUs have a specially trained transport team who go to the referring institution, stabilize the newborn, and bring the high-risk newborn back to the regional Level III center by ambulance or helicopter. The terrain, location, and weather of each referring NICU determine the safest transport mode. Transport of newborns is traumatic for the newborn and family and is avoided when at all possible (Thear & Wittmann-Price, 2008).

Table 19-1 Risk Factors That Compromise the Newborn

Intrauterine	Intrapartum	Extrauterine
Genetic disorders such as trisomy 13, 18, and 21	Asphyxia	Hypothermia
Congenital anomalies	Birth injuries	Poor oxygenation
Maternal disease such as diabetes, thyroid disease, renal disease, epilepsy, and systemic lupus erythematosus	Complications of labor	Prematurity
Trauma	Multiple gestation	Congenital anomalies
Drugs such as phenytoin (Dilantin) or illicit drugs such as alcohol, cocaine, or nicotine	Poor presentation	Metabolic disorders
	Maternal infection such as group B streptococcal or rubella	

Box 19-1 Risk Factors for Preterm Birth

Maternal smoking

Maternal age: older than 35 years at delivery and younger than 20 years

Maternal drug abuse

Female partner abuse

Multiple gestations

Maternal uterine abnormalities

Fetal anomalies

Maternal infection (especially chlamydia, gonorrhea, and bacterial vaginosis)

Maternal cervical anomalies

History of previous preterm birth (carries twice the risk)

African American descent

Genetic susceptibility

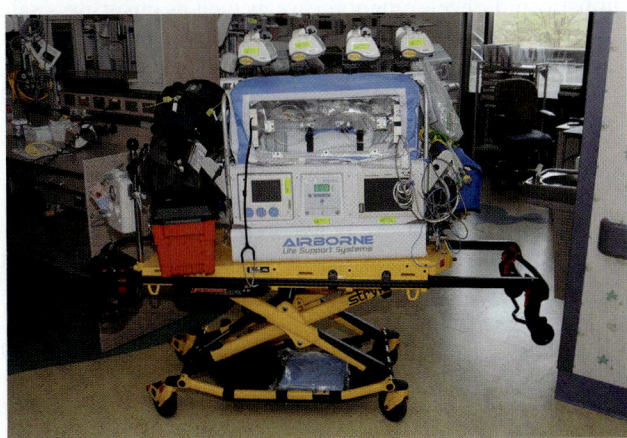

Figure 19-2 Neonatal transporter.

Box 19-2 Steps Emphasized in the S.T.A.B.L.E. Program

S Sugar

T Temperature

A Airway

B Blood pressure

L Lab work

E Emotional support

Source: STABLE Program. (2012). http://www.stableprogram.org/

The Transport Team

Neonatal transport teams are composed of a physician or nurse practitioner from the Level III nursery along with nursing and respiratory staff who are educated in stabilizing the newborn. Specific protocols are followed, and the team contacts the referring neonatologist during transport for any updates and further information.

The **S.T.A.B.L.E. Program** is a program designed to assist health-care professionals in the postresuscitation/pretransport phase of neonatal care. It is an acronym for aspects critical to stabilization of the high-risk newborn (Box 19-2). It is a program promoted by the March of Dimes and American Academy of Pediatrics as an adjunct to neonatal resuscitation to improve neonatal outcomes (STABLE program, 2012).

"What to say"—*Parents ask if it is necessary to transport the newborn*

Parents often ask if it is necessary for the newborn to be transported. The nurse can explain the advantages of treatment offered at the referring hospital and make sure the parents have a direct number to the unit and the name and number of the admitting neonatologist and nurse.

CLASSIFICATION OF HIGH-RISK NEWBORNS

High-risk newborns are classified according to two main criteria: **gestational age** (GA; length of time in utero) and **birth weight** (recorded in grams in the NICU).

Gestational Age (GA)

Term newborns are neonates delivered any time from 38 to 41 completed weeks of gestation. This GA produces optimal fetal developmental time for adjustment to the extrauterine environment. A neonate born at or before the completion of 37 weeks of gestation is considered **preterm** and behaves differently and has different nursing care needs than a full-term newborn. A newborn delivered on or after 42 weeks of gestation is **postterm** and also has different nursing care needs than a full-term newborn. Review Table 19-2 for other terms used to describe gestational age.

Birth Weight

Previously, newborns were classified as high-risk solely on the basis of birth weight. Now birth weight is considered along with GA for a more accurate assessment of risk factors and growth patterns. Newborns with a weight between

Table 19-2	Definitions of Newborn Age
Gestational age or formerly referred to as menstrual age	Counted from the first day of the woman's last period to the day of birth of the newborn
Chronological age (formerly referred to as postnatal age)	Time after birth (e.g., days, weeks, months, or years)
Postmenstrual age	Time from the first day of the woman's last menstrual period plus the time the newborn has been alive after birth
Corrected age (formerly referred to as adjusted age)	The corrected age is calculated by subtracting the number of weeks born before 40 weeks' gestation from the chronological age
Conceptual age or postconceptual age	Time from conception to birth (this is inaccurate and not often used)

Source: Adapted from American Academy of Pediatrics (AAP). (2004, 2009). Reaffirmation of Policy statement: *Age Terminology During the Perinatal Period. Pediatrics, 123*(1), 188.

the 10th and 90th percentile on the developmental growth chart for their GA have less mortality and morbidity than those above the 90th percentile or below the 10th percentile. Table 19-3 shows newborn classification by birth weight compared with GA.

There are other classification systems that use newborn weight as a criterion for classifying premature newborns but do not consider the gestational age in relation to weight. This clinical terminology uses **low birth weight (LBW)**, **very low birth weight (VLBW)**, or **extremely low birth weight (ELBW)**. Low birth weight refers to a newborn weighing less than 2,500 grams (7.8% of all births), and very low birth weight refers to a newborn weighing less than 1,500 grams (1.46% of all births). Extremely low birth weight refers to newborns who weigh less than 1,000 grams (Watson, 2012).

 Nursing Insight—*Understanding newborn classification*

Gestational age is many times written in weeks with days indicated by a fraction. If a newborn is 34 weeks and 4 days of gestation, how would this gestational age be documented? It would be documented as $34^{4/7}$.

Table 19-3	Newborn Classification by Birth Weight and Gestational Age
SGA: Small for Gestational Age	Weight below the 10th percentile for gestational age
AGA: Appropriate for Gestational Age	Weight between the 10th and 90th percentiles for gestational age
LGA: Large for Gestational Age	Weight above the 90th percentile for gestational age

 focus on safety

Recording newborn weight in kilograms

Safety standards demand that newborn weight is recorded in kilograms to decrease potential medication errors when needing to determine medication dosage based on standard mg/kg formulations.

"What to say"—*Intrauterine growth restriction*

If a health-care professional uses the term "intrauterine growth retardation," you can remind them that the correct term is intrauterine growth restriction and denotes a lack of intrauterine fetal growth that usually results in a small-for-gestational-age newborn. The older term previously used in clinical practice, "intrauterine growth retardation," is no longer used because the lay person may equate the word "retardation" with cognitive (intellectual) development, whereas in fact it was a reference to somatic (body) development of the newborn.

Mortality rates for preterm newborns have also been decreasing with the use and invention of technological advances. The more premature the newborn, the higher the mortality rate will be.

Very preterm newborns present moral dilemmas regarding resuscitation. **Resuscitation** of very-low-birth-weight newborns is an emotional and difficult topic for both health-care providers and families. One recent recommendation concerning newborns from $22^{0/7}$ weeks to $23^{6/7}$ weeks is selective resuscitation, which considers the parental decision (Nuffield Council on Bioethics, 2013). The International Liaison Committee on Resuscitation considers newborns less than 23 weeks' gestation or less than 400 grams not candidates for resuscitation and additionally that parental decisions be supported in cases where there is substantial concern regarding prognosis and survival (Batton, 2009).

Care of the High-Risk Newborn

Providing nursing care for the high-risk newborn is multifaceted and complex. The nurse provides general care measures, interventions tailored to specific conditions, and holistic and developmental care as well as ensuring a safe nurturing environment. A thorough physical assessment is completed, and vital signs are monitored frequently. Vital signs include temperature, pulse, respiration, blood pressure, pulse oximetry reading, and pain assessment.

BLOOD PRESSURE

Blood pressure measurements are an indicator of cardiovascular function. Systolic, diastolic, and **mean arterial pressure (MAP)** are assessed on the high-risk newborn. MAP is the average pressure during the entire cardiac cycle, and it is reported on cardiac monitors and differs by birth weight. MAP can also be calculated by internal blood pressure monitoring done through an umbilical vessel. **Pulse pressure** is the difference between the systolic and diastolic pressures and is another cardiac indicator. A wide pulse pressure is sometimes indicative of a patent ductus arteriosus (the average values are 25 to 30 mm Hg in term newborns and 15 to 25 mm Hg in preterm newborns).

Most NICUs use oscillometry methods to take noninvasive blood pressure readings in the newborn. Studies have shown that noninvasive blood pressure readings by oscillation are consistent with invasive blood pressure readings.

To take a blood pressure reading accurately on a newborn, several things need to be considered. The equipment needs to be reliable and calibrated correctly for newborns. The appropriate cuff size needs to be chosen. The correct size is 40% to 50% of the circumference of the extremity (Watson, 2012). Blood pressures can be greatly affected by the newborn's temperature, activity, or posture (newborns who are awake and sucking average 10 to 20 mm Hg higher). Single- and four-extremity blood pressures can be done (Table 19-4).

Low-birth-weight newborns are prone to hypotension (16% to 52%), which jeopardizes organ blood perfusion. Hypotension is usually treated with fluid boluses to boost

Table 19-4	Normal Blood Pressures by Newborn Weight
<2,000 g	50/35 mm Hg
2,000–3,000 g	60/35 mm Hg
>3,000 g	51/40 mm Hg

blood volume (Raju, Stevenson, Higgins, & Stark, 2009). Single blood pressure reading is done for all high-risk newborns on a regular basis. In the NICU, blood pressures are recorded on the C-R monitor along with the other vital signs of the infant (Fig. 19-3). Four-extremity blood pressures are done if a cardiac murmur is heard to determine if the MAP of the upper and lower extremities are similar. Blood pressure is normally slightly greater in the lower extremities. A difference (15 mm Hg or higher) in the upper extremities may indicate aortic coarctation (Watson, 2012). Procedure 19-1 illustrates the method for taking a newborn's blood pressure.

Procedure 19-1 Taking a Newborn's Blood Pressure

Purpose

Taking the blood pressure is an indicator of a newborn's state of health. It measures the amount of pressure needed to force the blood as it is forced through the arteries during a cardiac contraction.

Equipment

- Appropriate-size cuff
- Blood pressure (B/P) machine
- Method to record results

Steps

1. Choose the appropriate-size cuff by measuring the midpoint of the limb.

   RATIONALE: *Cuffs that are either too narrow or too small affect the accuracy of the blood pressure measurement. Choose a cuff that has a width that is approximately 40% of the arm's circumference. A properly fitting cuff will cover about two-thirds or entire upper arm (or other extremity). The blood pressure machine is calibrated frequently (Keijzer-Veen, Dülger, Dekker, Nauta, & van der Heijden, 2010).*

2. Do not use an extremity that has an IV.

   RATIONALE: *This prevents trauma or damage to the IV site.*

3. Do not apply to broken skin areas.

   RATIONALE: *This prevents further damage to the skin.*

4. Do not extend cuff over a joint.

   RATIONALE: *This prevents an inaccurate measurement.*

5. Inspect the cuff for intactness and decompress it to ensure it is not leaking.

   RATIONALE: *Properly functioning equipment is essential for accurate blood pressure measurement.*

6. If the cuff has an arterial mark, palpate the artery and line up the mark.

7. Wrap cuff snugly.

   RATIONALE: *A properly fitting cuff is essential for accurate blood pressure measurement.*

8. Connect the cuff to the air hose.

9. Start the blood pressure device.

10. Remove the cuff and inspect the skin.

 focus on safety

Attempt to take blood pressure while the newborn is sleeping or use a pacifier to quiet the newborn for the procedure.

Note

The B/P is usually slightly higher in the legs.

Caution: A wide pulse pressure may indicate atrioventricular malformation, truncus arteriosus, or patent ductus arteriosus. A narrowed pulse pressure may indicate peripheral vasoconstriction and cardiac failure. A systolic pressure in the arms that is 20 mm Hg or higher may indicate aortic coarctation.

Teach Parents

The nurse can teach the parents that the blood pressure is an indicator of a newborn's state of health.

Documentation
2/17/10 1300 Murmur auscultated, HR 160 BPM, pulse O₂ = 97%, 4 extremity B/Ps done. R. Wittmann-Price, RN

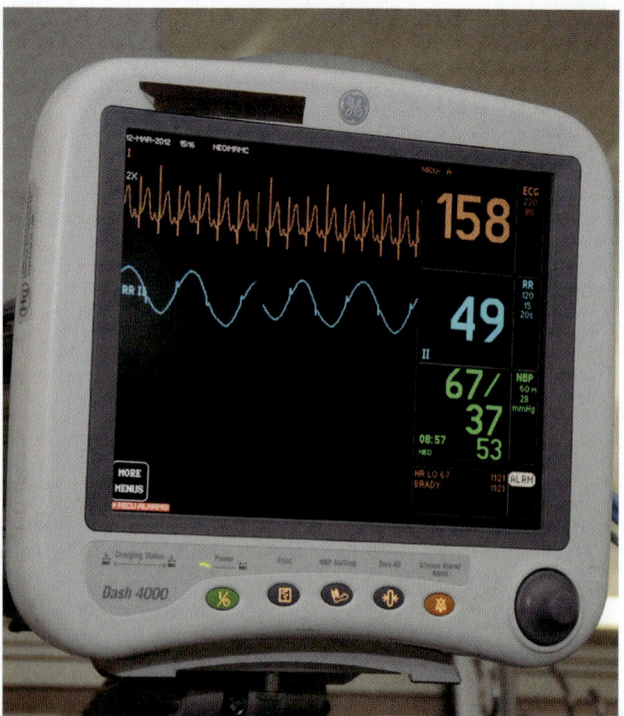

Figure 19-3 Blood pressure of 67/37 with an MAP.

NUTRITIONAL CARE OF THE HIGH-RISK NEWBORN

Intravenous Feedings

Initially, parenteral fluids are provided to the high risk newborn. Peripheral lines are used for shorter periods of time, and most preterm newborns are placed on parenteral fluids for the first few days of life. The goal for the newborn in the first few days of life is to provide sufficient fluid to result in a urine output of 1 to 3 mL/kg per hour and a urine specific gravity of no greater than 1.012.

A central line placed in the umbilical artery or vein is used for longer periods of time and provides the high-risk newborn with fluids, nutrients, blood components, and medications. Another type of line called a **peripherally inserted central catheter** line is also used for long-term parenteral therapy.

Total Parenteral Nutrition (TPN)

TPN is the initial essential nutritional support for high-risk newborns and is used to establish positive nitrogen and energy balance to promote growth. TPN also increases protein synthesis and reversal of any negative nitrogen effects that may take place in the first days of life.

The TPN solution is a calculated combination of glucose, amino acids, and electrolytes. TPN is usually started by the third or fourth day. After the first days of TPN, IV lipid emulsions are added to the parenteral therapy as a piggy-backed, or secondary, solution in concentrations of 10% to 20% over a slow continuous infusion. This is done to reverse fatty acid deficiency and provide energy for tissue healing and growth. TPN, although needed to keep high-risk newborns in positive nitrogen balance, is associated with complications. Long-term TPN is associated with liver dysfunction and catheter infections (Izquierdo-García,

Fernández-Ferreiro, Gomis-Muñoz, Herreros de Tejada, & Moreno-Villares, 2011).

Enteral Feedings

Enteral feedings of prescribed formula or breast milk given through either a nasogastric or orogastric tube are started as soon as the preterm newborn is stable to prevent gastrointestinal damage. Enteral feeding is provided by continuous infusion pump method or bolus delivery. As the newborn grows and becomes more stable, bolus feedings every 3 hours are eventually started because the newborn can now tolerate this kind of feeding. As the feedings are increasingly tolerated by the preterm newborn, the parenteral therapy can be decreased (Amendolia, 2011).

Bottle and Breastfeeding

Once the newborn reaches 32 weeks of gestational age and is stable, bottle and/or breastfeeding is attempted, usually once a day and increased as tolerated. The feedings start slowly and advance over several days. Breast milk is the "gold standard" (Amendolia, 2011, p. 88) because it decreases the incidence of necrotizing enterocolitis and increases the preterm newborn's immunological function.

 focus on safety

Aspiration

Newborns with greater than 60 respirations/minute must *never* be fed orally because they have an increased risk of aspiration pneumonia.

There are many different types of formulas used for newborns. Each type of formula has a different nutritional goal. Preterm newborn formula has increased protein, calcium, phosphorus, and medium-chain triglycerides than full-term newborn formula. When preparing a formula feeding for high-risk newborns, the procedure is done on a clean surface with only one formula preparation being done at a time with proper labeling.

Breastfeeding is encouraged for families who choose this method of feeding as soon as the newborn is able to spend limited amounts of time out of the incubator and is more than 32 to 34 weeks postconceptual age. Preterm newborns can be successfully taught to breastfeed if there is a planned approach that supports the family's decision (Yildiz, Arikan, Gözüm, Taştekın, & Budancamanak, 2011). Before the newborn can successfully breastfeed, mothers should be taught to pump their milk at regular intervals to maintain breast milk supply. Pumped breast milk can be given via a bottle.

Nonnutritive Sucking (NNS)

Nonnutritive sucking (NNS) is promoted for the preterm and high-risk newborn for physiological and psychological reasons. Using a pacifier promotes comfort, and NNS may promote breastfeeding in the high-risk newborn. Pacifiers are made in different sizes to accommodate the size of the newborn.

Intake and Output

High-risk newborns are maintained on strict intake and output (I&O) until they are growing adequately. Adequate

Where Research and Practice Meet:
Music

Music therapy has been shown to increase NNS when a lullaby was used to stimulate the newborns (Standley, Cassidy, Grant, Cevasco, Szuch, Nguyen, et al., 2010).

Where Research and Practice Meet:
Other Nutrients Needed for High-Risk Newborn Growth

Calcium phosphate and magnesium are needed to prevent undermineralization of bones, fractures, and rickets. Calcium is given at 185 to 200 mg/kg per day, phosphorus at 100 to 113 mg/kg per day, and magnesium 5.3 to 6.1 mg/kg per day as the recommended doses and is usually started after the first day or so of TPN. Vitamin D is also required for metabolism of calcium, phosphate, and magnesium for the preterm newborn. Trace elements of copper, zinc, selenium, manganese, and chromium are also added to TPN to prevent deficiencies.

Vitamin intake for the preterm newborn is calculated on weight and can be delivered in the TPN or lipid solution. Vitamin A is also placed in the TPN. Protein intake is approximately 3 to 4 g/kg/day (Watson, 2012).

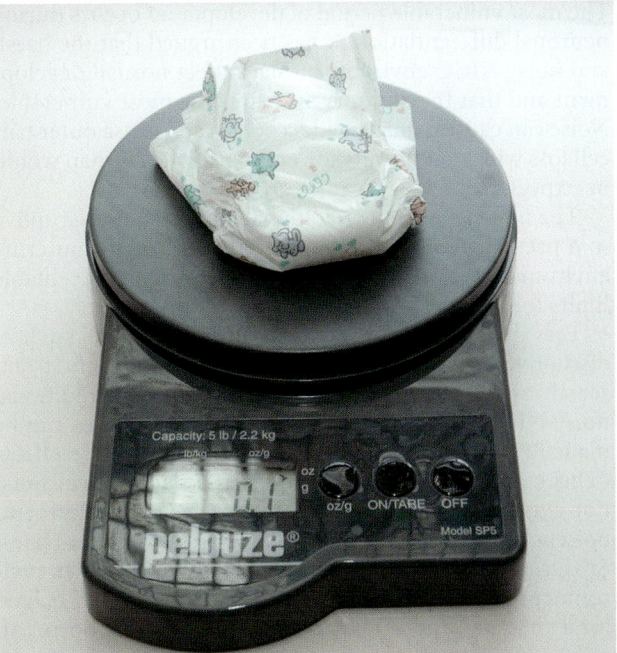

Figure 19-4 Newborn output is calculated by weighing the diaper on a gram scale.

growth means a sustained pattern of weight gain, approximately 20 to 30 grams per day (Martin et al., 2011). The actual intake of a newborn is calculated on total daily amount of calories (kcal/kg per day) and fluid requirements (mL/kg per day). To maintain adequate growth, preterm newborns need a caloric intake of 105 to 120 kcal/kg per day and a fluid intake of 120 to 180 mL/kg per day (Watson, 2012).

focus on safety

Calculating standard newborn formulas

$$\text{kcal/kg/day} = \frac{\text{kcal/mL} \times \text{Total mL of formula}}{\text{Weight}}$$

The normal output for a preterm newborn is 1 to 3 mL/kg per hour with a specific gravity of approximately 1.08 to 1.012. Oliguria is defined as less than 0.5 to 1 mL/kg per hour (Fig. 19-4).

SKIN CARE

The care of a preterm newborns skin is extremely important. Skin breakdown will increase the risk of nosocomial infection. Routine bathing of high-risk newborns is not done every day; it is usually done every third day to avoid drying out the skin. Plain water is used rather than soap for very preterm newborns. Tape and adhesive are removed carefully with warm water, and solvents are not used (Watson, 2012). The Braden Q skin risk assessment tool is found at http://www.marthaaqcurley.com/braden-q.html.

DEVELOPMENTAL CARE

Although more preterm newborns are surviving, many still have negative consequences, including developmental disabilities and delays, as well as vision and hearing deficits (Watson, 2012). Appropriate developmental care in the neonatal intensive care unit (NICU) is key to decreasing long-term developmental disabilities for the preterm newborn. There is increasing evidence in the literature that environmental issues, such as excessive noise and uncontrolled lighting, are detrimental to the developing preterm newborn (Thear & Wittmann-Price, 2006). The NICU environment must be a smooth transition from the intrauterine environment and limit excessive stimuli to ensure maximum developmental growth. NICU environments are beginning to change and try to replicate a natural milieu for the newborn, which includes parents and decreasing stress and pain (Als & McAnulty, 2011).

Preterm newborns do not have the neurological and social development needed to deal with the sudden stimuli of extrauterine life. Cortical organization in the preterm newborn is immature, and preterm newborns are poorly equipped to self-modulate their behavior. Overstimulation from environmental factors can have long-term detrimental developmental effects.

Providing an environment for optimal growth is the primary philosophy of developmental care. Developmental care assists to modulate the preterm newborn's behavioral states. Some of the environmental issues that can be controlled by the nurse to promote developmental growth include noise, lighting, handling, and positioning.

Noise

Sensory systems of the fetus develop in sequences. The sensory modalities develop in the third trimester. Premature birth exposes the newborn to excessive stimuli before this sensory sequencing is established. The preterm newborn is suddenly in an unnatural environment that demands use of the different systems out of sequence and ultimately becomes a source for developmental problems.

The most vulnerable period of development occurs during neuronal differentiation. It has been argued that the harsh and noisy NICU environment may affect normal development and that the auditory system is the most vulnerable. Noise can cause damage to the cochlea and cause outer hair cell loss with significantly lower intensity levels than would be expected.

The noise level in the traditional NICU can be disruptive to a premature newborn compared with the intrauterine environment. Noise in NICUs can easily exceed acceptable limits for optimal growth and development.

Prevalent neurological and behavioral deficits such as disruptive sleep, poor motor function, attention deficit, and sensorineural hearing loss could result from the traditional noisy NICU environment. Environmental changes can be made to decrease the noise level and offset adverse effects (Thear & Wittmann-Price, 2006). The noise level must not exceed 45 decibels, and the greatest contributor to noise is the human voice (Gardner, Carter, Enzman-Hines, & Hernandez, 2011). The nurse can provide a quiet environment to prevent hearing loss, neurological and behavioral deficits, and stress in the high-risk newborn. All newborns must be screened for hearing loss. Preterm newborns have a secondary follow-up screening.

Sleep

Preterm newborns sleep the majority of the day and preventing interruption of sleep cycles in very important for neurodevelopment. If at all possible, newborns should not be woken up; care is done when they are naturally awake (Watson, 2012).

Lighting

Most NICUs use ambient lighting. Studies are now showing that newborns with light-dark cycles imposed in the external environment have better weight gain and better sleep patterns then those newborns cared for in continuous light or dark. The nurse can provide an environment that promotes a natural sleep-wake cycle for the newborn to help regulate the newborn's circadian rhythm. Much more research is needed about proper lighting in the NICU and the light's effect on the development of retinopathy of prematurity (Antonucci, Porcella, & Fanos, 2009).

Handling

Overstimulation of high-risk newborns can be detrimental to the newborn's development. This has prompted most NICUs to organize nursing care into "cluster care." Cluster care is a concept in which all the nursing care for a high-risk newborn is done at one time, usually at 3-hour intervals. With cluster care there are several hours of undisturbed time in between vital signs, feedings, and treatments. Although overstimulation can be detrimental, gentle newborn touch can be therapeutic and soothing and can actually decrease oxygen consumption, so a balance between overstimulation and therapeutic stimulation calls for nursing judgment in a family-centered care environment (Watson, 2012). Organization and collaboration of multidisciplinary care to enhance minimal disturbance of the high-risk newborn is a goal in NICU.

Current philosophy, such as the information being taught by the Newborn Individualized Developmental Care and Assessment Program (NIDCAP), views the newborn as an active participant in care. Care is regulated not by task and time but by the behavioral assessment of the newborn. Care is based on parents as partners and Kangaroo Care (see Family Teaching Guidelines Box—Kangaroo Care) included in the NIDCAP program (Als & McAnulty, 2011).

Positioning

Positioning is done with the goal of providing comfort and modulation. Premature newborns have normally extended extremities compared with flexed full-term newborns. "Nesting" is a concept in which the linen is used to safely contain the newborn in a flexed position. Specially made bean bag rolls and "frogs" are used to provide security to body parts and keep them in position. Proper positioning not only provides comfort to the newborn but affects ventilation, neuroevolutive development, and prevention of **occipital plagiocephaly** (flattening of the occiput) (Giometti, Baroni, Artese, & Davidson, 2009).

Small-for-Gestational-Age (SGA) Newborns

SGA newborns are those born at any gestational age (GA) who have a birth weight that falls below the 10th percentile on the

---

Family Teaching Guidelines...
Kangaroo Care

TOPIC: The nurse will teach parents about the importance and technique of Kangaroo Care

ESSENTIAL INFORMATION:

- The nurse communicates to parent that **Kangaroo Care** is skin-to-skin holding of the baby who is dressed only in a diaper.
- The newborn is held next to the mother's or father's chest, preferably with an ear over the parent's heart to allow the baby to hear the familiar heartbeat.

- KC is an effective way of maintaining newborn temperature and is recommended for a growing newborn who is stable and can tolerate periods of time out of the incubator.
- KC has been found to produce benefits for both the mother or father and the baby by enhancing mother or father baby interaction and promoting bonding and newborn growth and development.

Source: Ludington-Hoe (2011).

Box 19-3 Conditions That Can Produce SGA Newborns

Genetic factors	Maternal diabetes
Chromosomal factors	Maternal systemic lupus erythematosus
Maternal fibroids	Intrauterine factors
Maternal asthma	Twin to twin transfusion
Maternal hypertension	Abnormal uterine anatomy
Drug use	TORCH infections
Maternal congenital heart disease	

Box 19-4 Symmetrical and Asymmetrical SGA Newborns

SGA newborns are small because they have suffered a nutritional or oxygenation deficit in utero as a result of maternal causes, fetal causes, or a placental or cord malfunction. If the fetus experienced the deficit in the first trimester, the newborn is usually symmetrically SGA, but if the deficit started after the 20th week of gestation, the result is more likely to be asymmetrically SGA. Interestingly, in developed countries, such as the United States, one of the most common factors related to intrauterine fetal growth restriction is maternal smoking. In developing countries, the leading causes are maternal nutritional deficits and infections such as malaria.

---

growth charts. Box 19-3 lists some conditions that can produce an intrauterine environment leading to an SGA newborn.

The SGA condition is a result of intrauterine growth restriction (IUGR) and can be classified into two categories: **asymmetrical** and **symmetrical**. Asymmetrically small newborns have an appropriate-size head circumference that measures between the 10th and 90th percentile for their GA when plotted on the head circumference chart but their weight falls below the 10th percentile. Asymmetrical SGA is sometimes called "brain sparing" SGA. Symmetrically small newborns are not only below the 10th percentile for weight but also have a small head circumference that measures below the 10th percentile for their GA. Symmetrical SGA is sometimes called "nonbrain-sparing." To further understand the difference between symmetrical and asymmetrical newborns, review Box 19-4.

 Collaboration in Caring—*Neighborhood deprivation*

Another influence on SGA births is neighborhood deprivation. Recent studies reveal that mothers who live in high-risk neighborhoods are more likely to have SGA newborns because of their economic status. These mothers are less likely to receive adequate prenatal care. Neighborhood deprivation can include a multitude of negative influences such as abandoned housing, graffiti, empty lots, and poor school systems (Sundquist, Sundquist, Johansson, Li, & Winkleby, 2011). Nurses must collaborate with other health-care professionals and community leaders to provide a wide variety of services to these underserved neighborhoods to decrease the percentage of SGA newborns born.

CHARACTERISTICS OF AN SGA NEWBORN

SGA newborns are smaller and often have a characteristic appearance. In asymmetrical SGA newborns, the head appears large in relation to the body. The characteristics of both types (symmetrical and asymmetrical) of SGA newborns may include:

- Wasted muscle tissue
- Lack of brown fat
- Abdomen is often *scaphoid (sunken in)*
- Eyes appear large with a "wise old man" look
- Fingernails are often long
- Meconium-stained thin cord is often present (Martin et al., 2011)

CONDITIONS AFFECTING THE SGA NEWBORN

Morbidity and mortality are significantly higher for SGA newborns. Delivery problems include asphyxia and low **Apgar scores** (Chapter 18). The following discussion highlights common conditions found in SGA newborns who are nursing concerns. These conditions may also be found in other high-risk infants, and they include:

- Cold stress (a consequence of prolonged hypothermia)
- Pain
- Hypoglycemia
- Polycythemia (Martin et al., 2011)

Cold Stress

Cold stress is more likely in SGA and preterm newborns because these infants have less brown fat, are less flexed, and have thinner skin. In very-low-birth-weight (VLBW) newborns, water loss can be 8 to 10 times greater than in an adult and heat loss 5 to 6 times greater. Cold stress increases metabolic needs and places the newborn at further risk for respiratory distress and metabolic acidosis. Keeping SGA and preterm newborns warm and reducing evaporative heat loss is a nursing priority (Lyon & Freer, 2011).

Signs and Symptoms

Cold stress occurs when the baby becomes cold and loses heat at a faster rate than the body can create heat, and it is reflected in the following signs and symptoms:

- Hypothermia or a body temperature less than 96.6°F (35.8°C)
- Cold, pale, or bluish skin
- Poor feeding
- Lethargy
- Respiratory distress
- Bradycardia

Diagnosis

Diagnosis is based on nursing assessment of the newborn's temperature and other clinical manifestations. Although normally a newborn's temperature is taken with an axillary thermometer to reduce the risk of vagal stimulation and rectal perforation, when the newborn is hypothermic, a rectal temperature is needed for accuracy.

Prevention

Provide a **neutral thermal environment** (NTE), an environment that provides for minimal heat loss or expenditure, at all times. Hypothermia is assessed in at-risk newborns and is continuously monitored while using

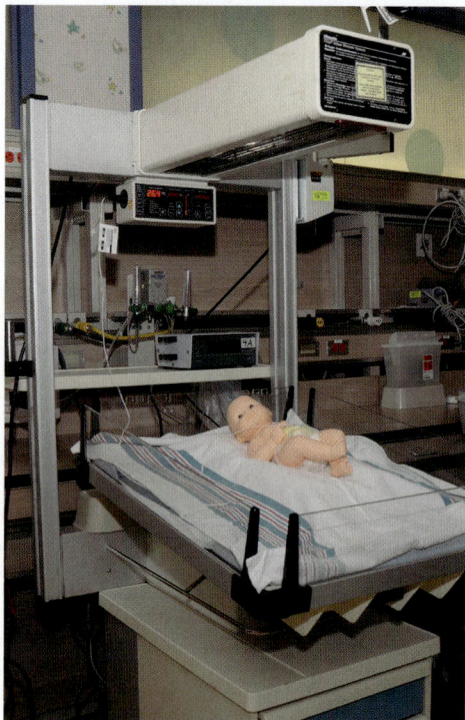

Figure 19-5 Radiant warmer.

radiant warmers for extremely-low-birth-weight babies in incubators (Fig. 19-5).

 focus on safety

Chemical warming packs

Chemical warming packs are sometimes used in the delivery room to warm an SGA or preterm newborn (Pinheiro, Boynton, Furdon, Dugan, & Reu-Donlon, 2011). These warming packs should not be placed directly on the newborn's skin but between the skin and a blanket to prevent burning the skin. Only products specifically made for this purpose are used to guard against burns from products not designed for newborn temperature maintenance.

Collaborative Care

Nursing Care.

- Use an artificial heat source (radiant warmers and incubators).
- A radiant warmer that is used in the normal newborn nursery is an overhead heater that accommodates an open crib underneath. The nurse can assess and bathe a normal newborn under the warmer and then remove the crib from the warmer once the newborn's body temperature is stable. The radiant warmers used primarily in the NICU have a flat table-like mattress with low sides that can be taken down for easy accessibility to the newborn. During warming, the newborn's temperature is monitored continuously with a skin probe. Review Box 19-5 for normal temperature readings.

 Box 19-5 Normal Temperature Readings in Children

Normal skin temperature: 97°F–98°F (36.2°C–36.8°C)
Normal axillary temperature: 97.7°F–99.5°F (36.5°C–37.5°C)
Normal rectal temperature: 97.9°F–100.4°F (36.6°C–38°C)

Critical Nursing Action Skin Probes

- The skin probe is attached to the newborn with a reflective insulated adhesive to help the heat source record the temperature of the skin. The probe is positioned on the newborn's body so the adhesive piece is exposed to the heat source above. Skin probes are placed on the abdomen avoiding bone and the liver border for an accurate reading.
- Incubators are used to provide longer periods of artificial heat. They are double-walled containers with portholes that are covered in plastic to allow caregiver access. They can also be set on two different modes: skin (servo) or air (ambient). The skin mode works via the same mechanism as the radiant warmer servo mode. The servo mode uses a skin probe on the newborn. The air mode maintains a set temperature within the incubator, and the newborn regulates her body temperature in the warmer environment. The newest models of incubators open from the top, thereby maintaining some of the heat, as does a radiant warmer. Incubators are often covered with a baby blanket or coverlet to protect the newborn from excessive light (Fig. 19-6). At times a plastic covering is placed over an open warmer (Watson, 2012).

 Optimizing Outcomes—**Weaning the newborn from the incubator**

When the newborn is being "weaned" from the servo (skin) mode of the incubator, the temperature is decreased gradually every few hours while the infant's body temperature is checked. Once the newborn can maintain his temperature above 96.6°F (35.8°C) axillary, the newborn is switched to air mode and dressed. The newborn's temperature, weight gain, and behavioral status are observed closely during and after the weaning process.

If the newborn is in an open crib and develops a temperature below 97.7°F (36.5°C) axillary, re-warm the infant then double wrap her and keep her head covered with a stockinette cap. Another way to provide a temporary heat source is to wrap the newborn in blankets that were warmed in a blanket warmer. This is a temporary method because the blankets cool fairly rapidly.

Medical Care. The primary care provider will prescribe the type of environment the newborn is to be in such as an incubator or open crib.

 focus on safety

Artificial heat source

Any use of an artificial heat source needs frequent nursing monitoring to prevent overheating or infant burns.

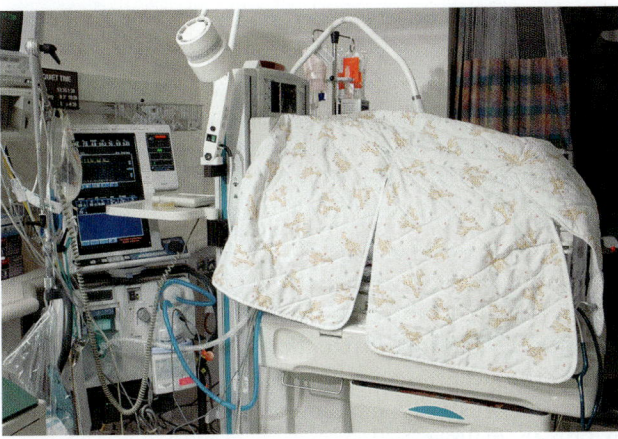

Figure 19-6 Incubator used in the NICU.

Education/Discharge Instructions

Parents are taught that by the time their newborn is discharged, they will be able to regulate her temperature. Overdressing is not necessary, and hyperthermia can be detrimental because it increases metabolism and increases the need for oxygen.

Pain

High-risk newborns undergo life-saving interventions, many of which can produce pain. Pain is assessed during both procedural and routine care. An appropriate assessment tool is used to assess newborn pain. Because newborns cannot verbalize their pain, the assessment tool will measure physiological symptoms such as heart rate, respirations, movement, and facial expression. Pain has detrimental physiological short- and long-term effects on the newborn's cardiovascular, respiratory, endocrine, metabolic, immunological, and coagulation systems.

Signs and Symptoms

- Increased heart rate
- Increased blood pressure
- Increased respiratory rate
- Shallow respirations
- Pallor
- Flushing
- Diaphoresis
- Palmar sweating
- Decreased oxygen saturation
- Change in facial expressions:
  - Lowering the brows and drawing them together

- Crunching the forehead and revealing vertical furrows between the brows
  - Closing the eyes tightly
  - Squaring off the mouth while holding the lips tight
- High-pitched cry with long pauses in breathing before it eventually becomes a rhythmic rising and falling pattern of crying
- Body movements include:
  - Limb withdrawal from touch
  - Rigidity or flaccidity
  - Clenched fists
- Altered sleep-wake cycles

Diagnosis

A pain diagnosis is based on nursing assessment using a neonatal pain scale. There are many different pain scales available for assessing newborn pain. Most pain scales assess four parameters: facial expression, cry, state of arousal, and body activity (Liu, Lin, Chou, & Lee, 2010). Some pain assessment scales are for the term newborn while others are specific to the preterm newborn. A commonly used pain assessment in the NICU is the Premature Infant Pain Profile (Stevens, Johnston, Taddio, Gibbins, & Yamada, 2010) (Fig. 19-7). The Neonatal Pain, Agitation, and Sedation Scale is also a valid tool used to assess acute and chronic pain in neonates and can be found online at http://www.anestesiarianimazione.com/2004/06c.asp (Hummel, Lawlor-Klean, & Weiss, 2010; Hummel, Puchalski, Creech, & Weiss, 2008).

Prevention

Pain prevention is an important nursing consideration in the NICU. Pain is considered the fifth vital sign and is assessed per protocol or with nursing care. Pain can be accurately assessed using a verified pain scale. The important pain prevention nursing care is to consistently use a pain scale to detect increases in the neonatal pain level so the pain can be treated before it becomes intense.

Collaborative Care

Nursing Care. Many NICUs have protocols to treat a newborn once the pain assessment scale reaches a specific score on the scale (Fig. 19-8). Nursing care to decrease pain includes maintaining a neutral thermal environment (NTE), swaddling the newborn, decreasing environmental stimuli, and providing non-nutritive sucking (NNS) (Liu et al., 2010).

Premature Infant Pain Profile (PIPP)

	0	1	2	3
GA	>/= 36 wks	32–36 6/7 wks	28–31 6/7 wks	</= 28 wks
Behavioral state	Active/awake	Quiet/awake	Active/sleep	Quiet/sleep
HR	0–4 beats/ minute Inc	5–14 beats/ minute Inc	15–24 beats/ minute Inc	25 beats or > Inc
O₂% sats	0%–2.4% decrease	2.5%–4.9% decrease	5%–7.4% decrease	7.5% or decrease
Brow bulge	None	Minimum	Moderate	Maximum
Eye squeeze	None	Minimum	Moderate	Maximum
Nasolabial furrow	None	Minimum	Moderate	Maximum

Figure 19-7 A commonly used pain assessment in the NICU is the Premature Newborn Pain Profile (PIPP).

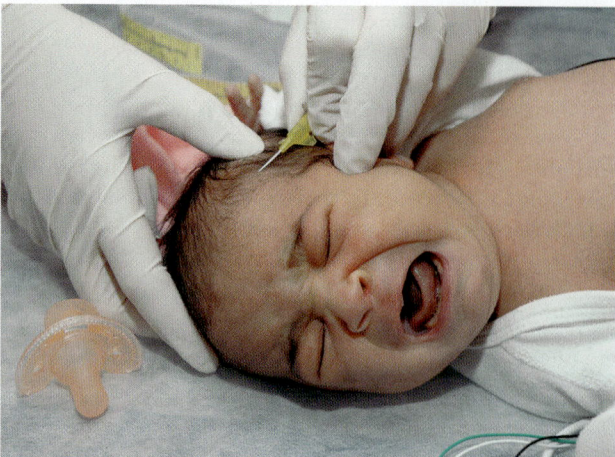

Figure 19-8 Many NICUs have protocols that treat a newborn for a PIPP score higher than 6 or 7. A score of 12 indicates severe pain and needs immediate attention.

Medical Care. Medical care of pain includes treating the newborns with analgesia using oral sucrose solutions. "Sucrose/glucose administration is the installation of 0.05 to 0.5 mL of 24% solution of sucrose/glucose into a neonate's mouth followed by immediately inserting a pacifier 2 minutes prior to, during, and sometimes 1 to 2 minutes after a minor procedure such as heel stick, venipuncture, and subcutaneous injection for the purpose of preventing pain" (Matteucci, Grose, & Pravikoff, 2011, p. 1).

Other categories of medications used for neonatal pain include nonsteroidal antiinflammatory drugs, opiates, sedatives, and local anesthetics. Appropriate pain medication is determined by the level of pain experienced. Postsurgical pain will commonly be treated with opiates. Common opiates include:

- Fentanyl (Sublimaze), which has a peak effect in 3 to 4 minutes
- Morphine (Astramorph), which has a peak effect in 45 minutes (Watson, 2012)

All opiates depress respiration so care is taken to closely monitor the medication level and the newborn's response (Crescencio, Zanelato, & Leventhal, 2009). For pain that is less severe, acetaminophen (children's Tylenol) or ibuprofen (children's Advil) can be safely administered.

 Complementary Care: *Mechanical Vibration During Painful Procedures*

Another method of pain relief being studied with good results is mechanical vibration used during minor painful procedures, such as a heel stick. The device is placed on the heel for 7 seconds prior to the procedure (Baba, McGrath, & Liu, 2010).

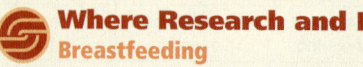 **Where Research and Practice Meet:**
Breastfeeding

Breastfeeding during minor painful procedures such as immunization or blood draws, has been shown to decrease the painful stimuli effect (Razek & El-Dien, 2009). Some parents may be uncomfortable with this intervention; it is essential to educate parents on the benefits of this practice to allow them to make an educated choice.

 focus on safety

Unrelieved pain

Newborns experiencing unrelieved pain have increased body activity that puts them at risk for injury. Increased vigilance in securing incubator portholes, radiant warmer sides, and maintaining open cribs in the flat position is important. Skin breakdown caused by rubbing and shearing is also a common occurrence with unrelieved pain and warrants frequent assessment.

Education/Discharge Instructions

Parents of newborns who experience pain are taught to recognize the signs and symptoms of pain so they can respond in a timely manner.

Hypoglycemia (Low Blood Glucose)

Hypoglycemia occurs rapidly in newborns. SGA newborns have higher glucose needs than term newborns. Approximately 15% of SGA newborns are hypoglycemic (Watson, 2012). In utero, glucose is provided by continuous placental transfer from maternal circulation. In utero fetal glucose levels are maintained at 60% to 70% of the maternal level. After the umbilical cord is cut and the glucose supply is halted, the newborn has to use liver glycogen and adipose tissue stores to supply glucose. Gluconeogenesis and ketogenesis are underdeveloped, and glucose levels can fall rapidly after birth. Glucose is the main source of energy for the newborn's brain, and levels lower than 30 mg/dL result in shunting of increased blood volumes to the brain to compensate. Besides SGA newborns, other at-risk newborns for hypoglycemia include:

- Preterm newborns
- LGA newborns
- Stressed newborns:
  - Newborns with a diabetic mother, sometimes referred to as an infant of a diabetic mother or an infant of an insulin-dependent diabetic mother
- Newborns who are poor feeders

Signs and Symptoms

Hypoglycemic symptoms in the newborn may be asymptomatic or manifest by the following:

- Lethargy
- Jitteriness
- Poor feeding
- Cyanosis
- Apneic episodes
- Tachypnea
- High-pitched or weak cry
- Eye rolling
- Seizures
- Prolonged hypoglycemia can produce neurological damage
  (American Academy of Pediatrics [AAP], 2011a; Jain, Agarwal, Sankar, Deorari, & Paul, 2010)

Diagnosis

Blood glucose levels are obtained by heel sticks. Each nursery has its own policy on what value constitutes hypoglycemia. Often there are different values for preterm and term newborns because preterm newborns cannot tolerate glucose levels as low as term newborns because of their lack of fat stores.

It is not abnormal for healthy newborn glucose to be as low as 30 mg/dL within 1 to 2 hours after birth but then stabilize above 40 to 60 mg/dL within 12 hours after birth (Van Leeuwen, Poelhuis-Leth, & Bladh, 2011). Many nurseries consider a value of 40 mg/dL as the cut-off point for low-risk newborns (Jain et al., 2010). Often, preterm newborns or high-risk newborns are considered hypoglycemic when blood glucose levels fall below 50 to 60 mg/dL.

Prevention

The most effective way to assist a newborn to maintain **nor-moglycemic** blood values is maternal regulation of glucose levels in utero. A high maternal glucose level while the fetus is in utero stimulates the fetal pancreas to produce insulin. After birth, the maternal glucose is no longer available to the newborn yet the pancreas is still secreting insulin to produce a **hyperinsulinemia** and hypoglycemic state in the newborn. Recognizing newborns who are at risk for hypoglycemia and feeding the newborn as soon as possible after delivery will assist them to maintain normal glucose blood levels.

Collaborative Care

Nursing Care. Glucose levels are monitored carefully in all high-risk newborns. Glucose testing is done by heel stick (capillary blood sampling). A heel stick is done by pricking the heel and scooping the dripping blood into the appropriate neonatal laboratory tubes that require approximately 1 mL of blood for testing (Fig. 19-9).

Follow the established nursery protocol, which requires blood glucose levels at specific intervals for high- and low-risk newborns. Many nurseries have protocols that continue to check newborn glucose levels at birth and 1, 2, 4, and 8 hours of age. Some NICUs even repeat glucose levels at 12 and 24 hours of age to ensure that glucose levels are being maintained.

For newborns on IV therapy, because a basic component of the parenteral fluid is glucose, nurseries maintain routine blood glucose checks. IV therapy to treat hypoglycemia consists of providing glucose at a prescribed rate according to the health-care provider.

If a stable newborn is found to be hypoglycemic on routine blood glucose check, enteral feedings are started immediately. After the feeding, the glucose level is rechecked at 30 minutes.

Medical Care. Medical care of a newborn whose blood glucose level is not responding to oral feedings will be started on IV glucose concentrate. The glucose level and IV will be carefully monitored to maintain the newborn's glucose within normal limits. Once the newborn is beginning to regulate blood glucose, the IV glucose solution will be weaned until the newborn is normoglycemic without the parenteral therapy.

focus on safety

Hypoglycemia of the newborn

Hypoglycemia of the newborn is a common condition and can be asymptomatic; therefore, nursing care must include accurate documentation of a newborn's I&O. A deficit in a newborn's intake may indicate a risk for hypoglycemia and the need for a more focused assessment.

Education/Discharge Instructions

Parents are taught the signs and symptoms of hypoglycemia and to provide frequent feedings based on the cues of the newborn. Frequent feedings are done to prevent any future occurrences of hypoglycemia.

Polycythemia

Polycythemia is a condition consisting of too many circulating red blood cells (RBCs) in the newborn and can have several causes. Newborns who experience oxygen deprivation in utero produce additional RBCs to increase the circulation of oxygen. Polycythemia greatly increases the viscosity of the circulating volume of blood, which can produce multiple organ damage. Complications of polycythemia are:

- Necrotizing enterocolitis (NEC)
- Pulmonary hypertension
- Thrombocytopenia
- Jaundice
- Neurological sequelae including central nervous system irritability, seizures, and cerebral infarction (Morag, Strauss, Lubin, Schushan-Eisen, Kenet, & Kuint, 2011)

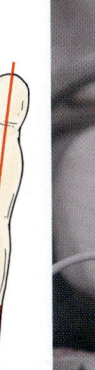

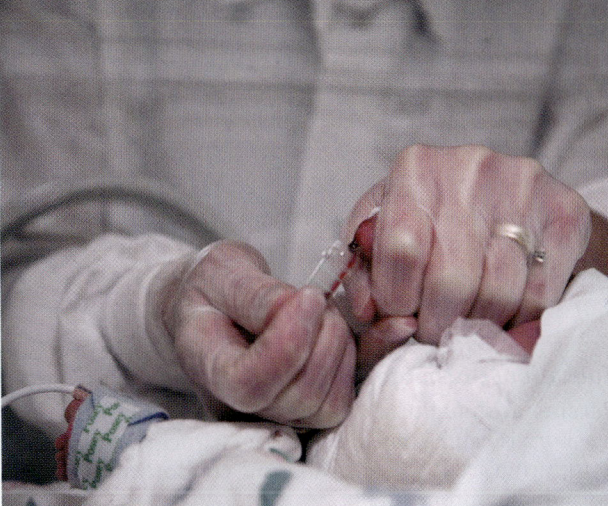

Figure 19-9 A heel stick is done by pricking the heel and scooping the dripping heel blood into the appropriate neonatal laboratory tubes that require approximately 1 mL of blood for testing.

In addition to SGA, other common conditions in utero that produce polycythemia in the newborn are:

- Multiples
- Newborns with a diabetic mother (Sankar, Agarwal, Deorari, & Paul, 2010)

Polycythemia may also occur when a newborn is exposed to an intrapartum environment that allows the blood in the cord and placenta to enter his circulation by gravity or "milking the cord" at delivery.

Signs and Symptoms

Polycythemia may be asymptomatic (Sankar et al., 2010), but clinical signs can include:

- (Ruddy) **plethoric** skin
- Delayed capillary refilling
- Hematuria
- Proteinuria

Diagnosis

Diagnosis of polycythemia is made by obtaining a complete blood count, which reveals a venous hematocrit of 65% or greater (Sankar et al., 2010).

Prevention

Polycythemia is prevented by good prenatal care of mothers to decrease intrauterine stressors for the fetus because this has been linked to the development of polycythemia. This condition can also be prevented by maintaining the newborn parallel to the maternal perineum until the umbilical cord is clamped so the blood flow through the cord is similar to that in utero.

Collaborative Care

Nursing Care. Hematocrit levels peak at 2 hours of age; therefore, high-risk newborns are screened at 2, 12, and 24 hours of age (Sankar et al., 2010). Hemoglobin, hematocrit, and bilirubin levels can be assessed by peripheral blood drawing or heel stick. Initiating oral feedings or parenteral therapy may decrease the blood viscosity (Morag et al., 2011).

Medical Care. Severe polycythemia (hematocrit greater than 70%) is usually treated with a **partial exchange transfusion** (PET). PET refers to manually phlebotomizing a percentage of the patient's whole blood prior to or concomitantly with a packed red blood cell transfusion (Morag et al., 2011).

 focus on safety

Monitoring bilirubin levels
Close monitoring of bilirubin levels is needed because of the anticipated breakdown of the excessive red blood cells, which will overload the newborn's system with heme, the precursor of bilirubin.

Education/ Discharge Instructions

Parents are taught about the condition for which the newborn is being treated so they can participate in the care by offering frequent feedings and comforting the newborn during procedures.

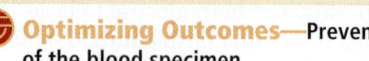 **Optimizing Outcomes**—Preventing hemolysis of the blood specimen

To prevent hemolysis of the blood specimen, avoiding excessive squeezing with capillary heel sticks and transporting the blood specimen to the lab as soon as possible promote the best outcome. Hemolysis has been known to falsely decrease the bilirubin levels.

 Nursing Diagnoses The SGA Newborn

- Nutritional imbalance related to hypoglycemia
- Caregiver role strain related to increased care needs
- Risk for activity intolerance related to increased metabolic needs
- Risk for ineffective feeding pattern related to increased metabolic needs
- Risk for impaired parenting related to increased care needs
- Risk for growth and developmental delays related to intrauterine nutritional and oxygenation status
- Risk for imbalanced body temperature related to decreased subcutaneous tissue and brown fat

Source: Doenges, Moorhouse, & Murr (2010).

 Now Can You— Discuss the SGA newborn?

1. Identify SGA newborns by assessing clinical characteristics?
2. Describe the probable reasons for the newborn being SGA?
3. Discuss the complications that are common to the SGA newborn?

Large-for-Gestational-Age (LGA) Newborns

Newborns who are large for gestational age (LGA) are over the 90th percentile on the growth chart (e.g., a newborn who weighs approximately 3,750 grams [8 lb 4 oz] at 40 weeks' gestational age [GA]). A macrosomic newborn who weighs more than 4,050 grams (8 lb 14.85 oz) is always LGA. LGA newborns have a higher morbidity rate than appropriate-for-gestational-age (AGA) newborns.

There are two reasons why newborns may grow to a larger than average size in utero. They can be genetically large or, more commonly, they are exposed to an imbalance of nutrients in utero. The most common energy and growth source in utero is glucose. It is easily transported by diffusion across the placental barrier. If the maternal circulation contains excessive glucose levels, the fetus's circulation will have a higher than normal glucose level also. Box 19-6 lists the intrauterine conditions that place a newborn at risk for LGA. Box 19-7 lists delivery complications of an LGA newborn.

Newborns with a diabetic mother are often LGA and are at risk after delivery for:

- Transient tachypnea because of delayed lung development
- Hypoglycemia because of insulin overproduction
- Hypocalcemia from decreased parathyroid production
- Hypomagnesemia because of metabolic abnormalities

Conditions common to LGA conditions can also occur in other high-risk newborns (Larkin, Speer, & Simhan, 2011).

Box 19-6 Maternal Risk Factors Contributing to LGA Newborns

- Increased parity
- Increased maternal age
- Increased maternal height
- History of other LGA newborns
- Prolonged pregnancy
- Maternal obesity
- Maternal glucose intolerance
- Large pregnancy weight gain

Box 19-7 Complications Associated With LGA or Macrosomic Newborns

- Shoulder dystocia at delivery
- Brachial nerve plexus injury
- Asphyxia
- Hyperinsulinemia and hypoglycemia
- Hypocalcemia

CONDITIONS AFFECTING THE LGA NEWBORN

Newborns With a Diabetic Mother

Newborns with a diabetic mother may experience a chronic hyperglycemic state in utero because of elevated maternal glucose levels. The effects of the maternal glucose levels on the newborn depend on several factors such as the maternal glucose control, the onset of the diabetic state, and the length of gestation. Glucose readily passes through the placenta but insulin, because of its molecular size, does not. Therefore, the fetus produces larger than normal amounts of insulin (**hyperinsulinemia**) to keep up with the extra glucose. This makes the glucose accessible to the cells, producing a large newborn. When the cord is cut at delivery, the glucose supply is abruptly stopped but the newborn's pancreas is still hyperstimulated and producing insulin. This results in a severe hypoglycemic state (review the previous section on hypoglycemia). Hypoglycemia can occur rapidly in newborns with a diabetic mother, often within 15 to 20 minutes; therefore, early frequent glucose monitoring is necessary.

 Nursing Insight—*Hyperglycemia*

Hyperglycemia is rarer than hypoglycemia but is still significant. Hyperglycemia often occurs when glucose is administered parenterally because enteral feedings are delayed. A blood glucose level above 150 mg/dL is considered hyperglycemia and can cause dehydration and weight loss. Severe hyperglycemia may also cause cerebral hemorrhage and be a factor in accelerating retinopathy of prematurity (Kaempf, Kaempf, Wu, Stawarz, Niemeyer, & Grunkemeier, 2011).

 Nursing Diagnoses The Newborn With a Diabetic Mother

- Pain related to possible birth injuries
- Impaired gas exchange related to transient tachypnea of the newborn
- Infection, at-risk or related to increased hospital procedures

- Impaired physical mobility related to possible fractures
- Nutrition: Imbalanced, less than body requirements related to somatic size and glucose needs
- Parenting: Impaired related to newborn with special needs

Source: Doenges et al. (2010).

Transient Tachypnea of the Newborn

Respiratory distress syndrome type II, or **transient tachypnea of the newborn (TTN)**, is common in newborns with a diabetic mother. TTN is a delayed clearance of fetal lung fluid (which differs from amniotic fluid). There is fetal lung fluid in the alveoli, and air is trapped in the alveoli resulting in hypoxia because of poor lung ventilation. The onset of labor appears to be the mechanism by which the lungs reabsorb fluid, which puts newborns who have not experienced labor (cesarean births) at even greater risk for TTN. Newborns at risk for TTN are:

- LGA newborns
- Newborns with a diabetic mother who are delivered by cesarean birth or a precipitous delivery
- Late preterm infants—between 34 and 36 completed gestational weeks

Signs and Symptoms

Clinical signs and symptoms of TTN include:

- A high respiratory rate of 60 to 120 breaths/minute
- Grunting
- Retractions
- Cyanosis may be present
- Nasal flaring
  (Ma, Huang, Lou, Lv, Su, Tan, et al., 2009) (Fig. 19-10)

 Assessment Tool Retractions

Retractions in newborn are a result of increased chest compliance and respiratory pressure. Also, the chest muscles of the newborn are immature, so increasing retraction depth means that the respiratory disease is worsening (Watson, 2012).

Diagnosis

Blood gases usually show respiratory acidosis (Table 19-5).

 Diagnostic Tools Acid-Base Calculators

Acid-base calculators can be found online and are another assessment tool that nurses can use to support a plan of care (http://www.medcalc.com/acidbase.html).
    X-rays of the chest show bilateral streakiness caused by the interstitial and alveolar fluid (Watson, 2012).

 Nursing Insight—*Metabolic acidosis*

Metabolic acidosis increases pulmonary resistance. Bicarbonate therapy as a treatment is now used less often because oxygenation treatments of newborns have improved. Bicarbonate is given IV push 1 to 2 mEq/kg in a maximum concentration of 0.5 mL. If the newborn weighs 1,000 g, administer 1 to 2 mEq bicarbonate.

Prevention

Prevention of TTN may be accomplished by maintaining maternal glucose levels within normal limits and only performing elective cesarean births after 39 weeks' gestation.

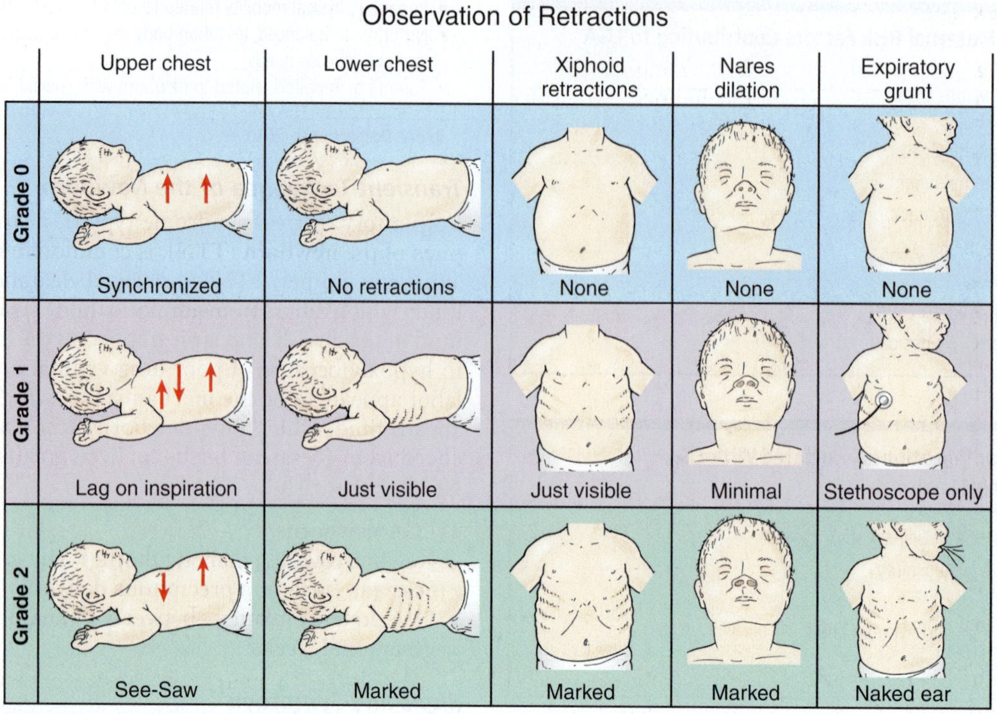

Observation of Retractions

	Upper chest	Lower chest	Xiphoid retractions	Nares dilation	Expiratory grunt
Grade 0	Synchronized	No retractions	None	None	None
Grade 1	Lag on inspiration	Just visible	Just visible	Minimal	Stethoscope only
Grade 2	See-Saw	Marked	Marked	Marked	Naked ear

Figure 19-10 The Silverman and Andersen Index Evaluation of Respiratory Status.

Table 19-5 The Relationship Between pH and Concentration of Arterial Blood Gases

	pH	Pco$_2$	Pao$_2$	P$_{HCO_3^-}$
	Measures blood acidity.	Partial pressure of carbon dioxide in blood	Partial pressure of oxygen in blood	Partial pressure of bicarbonate (alkaline or base) in blood
Normal Neonatal Values	pH = 7.25–7.45	Pco$_2$ = 35–40 mm Hg	Pao$_2$ = 50–80 mm Hg	P$_{HCO_3^-}$ = 20–22 mEq/L
Respiratory Acidosis (caused by poor ventilation)	↓ pH	↑ Pco$_2$	WNL	WNL
Metabolic Acidosis (anaerobic metabolism from hypoxia, diarrhea, or kidney disease)	↓ pH	WNL	WNL	↓ P$_{HCO_3^-}$
Respiratory Alkalosis (hyperventilation)	↑ pH	↓ Pco$_2$	↑ Pao$_2$	WNL
Metabolic Alkalosis (vomiting, diarrhea, or hypocalcemia)	↑ pH	WNL	WNL	↑P$_{HCO_3^-}$

WNL = within normal limits.

Source: Adapted from Noerr, B. (2000). Neonatal respiratory disease and management strategies, May 18. A continuing education service of Penn State's College of Medicine at the Milton S. Hershey Medical Center. Hershey, PA.

Cesarean births before 39 weeks' gestation increase the risk for TTN. Vaginal delivery allows for extra fluid to be squeezed from the infant's lungs, therefore decreasing the risk of TTN (Tutdibi, Gries, Bücheler, Misselwitz, Schlosser, & Gortner, 2010).

Collaborative Care

Nursing Care. Perform accurate assessment of the respiratory system immediately after birth and during the transitional period (within 1–2 hours). The newborn's respiratory rate should be below 60 with *no* retractions, nasal flaring, or grunting and a peripheral oximeter reading of greater than 92%. If any of these clinical signs appear immediately after birth or persist into the transitional period, immediate attention and supplemental oxygen are warranted.

Nursing care of a newborn with TTN also includes holding oral feeding for respirations over 60 to decrease the risk of aspiration. Maintain a neutral thermal environment to decrease the expenditure of energy and maintain peripheral oxygen levels within normal limits.

Medical Care. The treatment is often continuous positive airway pressure at 40% oxygen for 24 to 48 hours. Complete resolution of TTN takes 2 to 3 days. TTN is self-limiting with no reported long-term complications (Martin et al., 2011).

focus on safety

Continuous positive airway pressure

Continuous positive airway pressure (CPAP) is oxygen most often delivered through nasal prongs to avoid intubation with an endotracheal tube. CPAP maintains the patency of the upper airway and is usually set at pressures of 2 to 6 cm H_2O. The nasal prongs fit snugly into the newborn's nose and are usually held in place by pinning the tubing to a stockinette cap. If the prongs are not placed correctly or too much pressure is applied, nasal septal damage and necrosis can occur (Helou, Birenbaum, Blue, Pane, & Marinkovich, 2011).

Hypocalcemia

Calcium levels should be greater than 7.5 mg/dL in preterm newborns and 8 mg/dL in term newborns. Low calcium level can produce seizures in the newborn and may be present along with **hypoglycemia**. Reasons for hypocalcemia in the newborn are trauma, hemolytic disease, asphyxia, and maternal hypocalcemia. Lack of oxygen stimulates calcitonin release, which inhibits calcium release from the bone. Newborns at risk for hypocalcemia are:

- Newborns with a diabetic mother
- Preterm newborns
- Newborns with perinatal asphyxia (Jain et al., 2010)

Signs and Symptoms

Signs and symptoms of hypocalcemia can range from asymptomatic to manifestations that include:

- Jitteriness
- Hyperalertness
- Increased tone
- Poor feeding
- High-pitched cry
- Seizures

Diagnosis

The diagnosis of hypocalcemia is made by laboratory study, wherein the calcium level is below 7.5 mg/dL in preterm newborns and 8 mg/dL in term newborns. Calcium levels are the lowest at 24 to 48 hours after birth; if levels remain low at 72 hours, the newborn requires treatment (Jain et al., 2010).

Prevention

Decreasing intrauterine and intrapartum stress to the fetus and newborn, maintaining normal maternal glucose and calcium levels, and decreasing birth trauma are the preventative measures.

Collaborative Care

Nursing Care. Feeding the newborn soon after birth can facilitate normal calcium levels.

Medical Care. Medical care includes physiological correction of maternal hypoparathyroidism, administration of calcium supplements, and in severe cases, the administration of 10% calcium gluconate.

Hypomagnesemia

Magnesium is necessary for proper parathyroid function. **Hypomagnesemia** frequently coexists with hypocalcemia.

Signs and Symptoms

The decreased magnesium in the blood is usually accompanied by:

- Increased neuromuscular irritability or hypotonia
- Poor feeding
- Respiratory distress

Diagnosis

Hypomagnesemia is present when the magnesium levels are below 1.5 mg/dL (normal newborn range is 1.5–2.8 mg/dL). It can be caused by low maternal magnesium levels, SGA or LGA growth patterns, and hypoparathyroidism.

Prevention

Maternal levels of calcium and magnesium should be maintained during pregnancy.

Collaborative Care

Nursing Care. Nursing care consists of neuromuscular assessment (active and passive muscle tone), maintaining normoglycemic blood levels, and when indicated, monitoring calcium and magnesium levels every 24 hours until stable.

Medical Care. Replacement magnesium in the form of magnesium sulfate is administered orally in the form of citrate, gluconate, and chloride (Martin et al., 2011).

Education/Discharge Instructions

Hypomagnesemia and its treatment are explained to the parents so they can participate in the care of the newborn.

BIRTH INJURIES

A thorough physical assessment is warranted for the LGA newborn to assess for birth injuries related to difficult deliveries. Birth injuries or traumas are usually one of two types: neurological injuries (e.g., brachial plexus injury) or bone fractures (e.g., clavicle fracture).

Diagnosis

Diagnosis of birth injuries is made by a thorough nursing assessment, x-ray exam, or appropriate laboratory studies.

Brachial Plexus Injuries (BPI)

The brachial plexus is a complex nerve supply that is responsible for the movement of the shoulders, chest, and arms. The nerve innovation starts at C5 to T1 nerve roots, and BPI or palsy occurs when these nerves are stretched and leave the arm without function. Nerve injury to C5 to C7 results in **Duchenne-Erb's paralysis** while injury to C8 to T1 results in **Klumpke's paralysis**. BPI affects 2 in every 1,000 newborns in the United States each year (Box 19-8).

Risk factors for BPI include:

- LGA or macrosomic newborns
- Newborns with a diabetic mother
- Instrument delivery
- Prolonged labor
- Shoulder dystocia
- Multiparity

Signs and Symptoms

The manifestations of brachial plexus injuries include:

- Lack of movement of an arm, elbow, wrist, or hand
- Lack of Moro reflex on affected side

Diagnosis

Diagnosis of BPI is made through a complete neurological assessment to determine the exact damage including the type and degree as well as the extent of nerve impairment. Diagnostic tests such as myelography, computed tomography myelography, and magnetic resonance imaging are used to confirm the diagnosis (Abzug & Kozin, 2010).

Prevention

Prevention is dependent on good prenatal care. LGA newborns are often the result of uncontrolled gestational diabetes. Adequate prenatal care would allow for earlier diagnosis of gestational diabetes, which may allow for better control of maternal blood sugar and, ultimately, a newborn who does not experience sequelae. Because BPI is often the result of birth trauma, decreasing intrapartum trauma is essential.

Collaborative Care

Nursing Care. Nursing of BPI care focuses on assessment, resolution of the trauma, and preventing further joint damage. The nurse can assess the Moro, biceps, and radial reflexes. Initially the arm is rested to allow swelling to decrease. Then, after 5 to 10 days, passive **range-of-motion (ROM)** exercises are done multiple times a day with consultation of a physical therapist. Tactile stimulation is provided for the limb to identify feeling (Abzug & Kozin, 2010).

Surgical Care. Microsurgery is done if nerve repair is indicated. Types of surgery used are direct nerve repair, neurolysis, nerve grafting, and nerve transfer (Abzug & Kozin, 2010).

 focus on safety

Nerve damage

Nerve damage limits the newborn's ability to move an extremity away from danger.

Education/Discharge Instructions

Parents are taught to do passive ROM multiple times a day to keep the joints of the affected extremity from developing contractures.

Fractures

Fractures are also common birth injuries and usually involve the clavicle. Other fractures may occur in the long bones of the humerus or femur, but these are much less common.

CLAVICLES. Broken clavicles are the most common birth fractures (0.4%–10% of all vaginal births) (Mavrogenis, Mitsiokapa, Kanellopoulos, Ruggieri, & Papagelopoulos, 2011). Fractured clavicles can occur alone, with brachial plexus injury, or with a fractured humerus. Risk factors for a broken clavicle include:

- LGA newborns
- Instrument delivery
- Shoulder dystocia

Signs and Symptoms

Symptoms of a broken clavicle include:

- Asymmetrical arm movement
- Asymmetrical Moro reflex
- Swelling
- Pain
- **Crepitus** detected on palpation of the bone if the bone is displaced. Crepitus describes the assessment of bone rubbing against bone, which can be felt and sometimes even heard on examination. This is often described as having "rice crispies" under the skin.

Diagnosis

An x-ray exam will confirm the diagnosis.

Prevention

To prevent clavicle fractures, intrapartum (birth trauma) and postpartum (falls or abuse) trauma must be avoided.

Collaborative Care

Nursing Care. The newborn's T-shirt is sometimes pinned to produce a loose splint so that the affected arm is immobilized (National Institutes of Health [NIH], 2011). Pain management is needed if the newborn appears uncomfortable. Keep the newborn off the injured side to decrease pain and promote alignment.

Medical Care. Most clavicle fractures heal spontaneously without medical intervention (Shannon, Hart, & Grottkau, 2011). Pain management must be addressed to decrease the pain the newborn experiences, especially with handling.

Surgical Care. Surgical treatment with open reduction and internal fixation is done only in severe cases that threaten the newborn's full ROM of the affected extremity (Shannon et al., 2011).

 focus on safety

Gentle handling of newborns

Gentle handling of newborns with fractures is necessary to maintain alignment of the bones. Avoid picking up the newborn under the arms because this increases the pain the newborn feels.

Education/Discharge Teaching

Parental teaching includes proper handling of the newborn, assessing the newborn for pain, and administering pharmacological and nonpharmacological pain interventions.

Long Bone Fractures

The incidence of a fractured humerus is significantly less than that of clavicle fractures. When long bone fractures occur, they are often treated with soft splinting to immobilize the arm for approximately 2 weeks. Healing is rapid and complete in most cases. Radial fractures are the second most frequent fractures, and femoral fractures are the third. Risk factors for long bone fractures are:

- Breech presentation
- Multiples
- Prematurity
- Osteoporosis

Signs and Symptoms

Some of the symptoms to observe for any birth fractures include:

- Crepitus on palpation
- Pain on palpation
- Asymmetrical movement or Moro reflexes
- Swelling and discoloration
- Malalignment of the extremity

Diagnosis

All long bones are examined by inspection and palpation. Definitive diagnosis is made by x-ray exam (Martin et al., 2011).

Prevention

To prevent long bone fractures, intrapartum and postpartum trauma (birth-related injuries, falls, or abuse) must be avoided.

Collaborative Care

Nursing Care. The nurse understands a fractured humerus must be immobilized immediately. Neurovascular checks are completed frequently, and the extremity is elevated above the level of the heart to facilitate return circulation. Initial cold therapy for 30 minutes can help reduce swelling, and pain assessment and appropriate interventions, such as medication administration, are essential. The nurse must remember to communicate the newborn's condition to parents and what care measures will be implemented.

Medical Care. Medical care of fractures includes immobilization done by an orthopedic specialist. Femoral fractures can be treated with a Pavlik harness, which immobilizes the hip and leg and allows the femur to heal.

Surgical Care. Surgical repair of the fracture is done if function of the extremity is in jeopardy.

focus on safety

Circulation

Circulation to the injured extremity is assessed frequently. The injury may obstruct and decrease the ability of blood to circulate below the level of the injury.

Education/Discharge Instructions

Parental teaching includes proper handling of the newborn (not picking up under the affected arm) and assessing and treating the newborn for pain.

focus on Safety

Newborn falls

Close physical contact between mother and newborn is important in the postpartum period. The challenge is to support these important interactions in the hospital while ensuring the safety of the newborn. Newborn falls, or drops, occurring in the hospital is a topic that is now coming to the forefront of the literature. It is estimated that 600 to 1,600 newborns experience a fall in a U.S. hospital each year (Helsey, McDonald, & Stewart, 2010).

Now Can You—Discuss SGA and LGA?

1. Describe the physiology of glucose utilization in LGA newborns?
2. Discuss conditions affecting LGA newborns?
3. Identify important nursing assessments for the LGA newborn?

The Premature Newborn

Premature delivery at or before 37 weeks of gestation is still a major health problem in the United States because each year 11.99% of newborns are premature (March of Dimes, 2011). Prematurity is classified by the weeks of gestation. Severe prematurity is classified as birth at 23 to 26 weeks. Moderate prematurity is classified as birth at 26 to 34 weeks, and late pretermaturity is classified as 34 to 37 weeks' gestation. The risk factors increase as the size and gestational age of the newborn decrease. A newborn can have size variation as well as being preterm; for example, a preterm newborn who is 32 weeks' gestation but above 90% on the growth chart is a large-for-gestational-age (LGA) preterm newborn. Premature newborns are at risk for any number of short-term and long-term complications; the most common conditions are discussed in the following sections.

PHYSICAL ASSESSMENT OF THE PREMATURE NEWBORN

The preterm newborn is not only smaller than a term newborn but also has specific characteristics because of the abbreviated development in utero (Table 19-6).

Global Health Case Study The Premature Newborn

Ms. Jones, an 18-year-old G-1, comes into the labor and delivery suite at 6 cm cervical dilation. She is 33 weeks' gestation by last menstrual period. Baby girl Jones is delivered within the hour and weighs 2,000 grams. She breathes spontaneously, and her heart rate is 166 beats per minute. She is thoroughly dried, suctioned with a small-size bulb syringe for excessive nasal pharyngeal fluid, placed under the radiant warmer, and an initial assessment is done. Her rectal temperature is 98.2°F (36.8°C). Her Premature Infant Pain Profile score is 2 (1 for gestational age and 1 for increased heart rate). The skin assessment reveals no skin lesions, birthmarks, or reddened areas. Respirations are 70 breaths per minute with slight nasal flaring, intercostal retractions, and an expiratory grunt. Her extremities have full range of motion but poor flexion and reduced tone **(hypotonic)**.

critical thinking questions

1. What classification by gestational age is baby girl Jones?

2. What condition is associated with her respiratory assessment?

3. What are the priority nursing interventions for baby girl Jones?

4. What task would be safe to delegate to the unlicensed assistive personnel in the delivery room?

- See Suggested Answers to Global Health Case Studies on Davis*Plus*.

Table 19-6 Assessment of the Preterm Newborn

Skin	Head	Chest	Cardiac
Skin tags	Irregular-shaped head, molding after delivery, caput succedaneum, cephalhematoma	Funnel or pigeon chest	Apical heart rate is assessed for a full minute and is in the fourth intercostal space slightly left of the mid-clavicular line.
Translucent	Large anterior and posterior fontanelles present Fused sutures Bulging or depressed fontanelles	Supernumerary nipples or nipples are flat on the chest wall	The heart rate may normally be above 160 bpm but not above 180 bpm
Lanugo covering the shoulders, back, thighs, forehead, and ears	Ear pinnae are flat and readily fold on themselves	Ribs are visible	Heart auscultation is done in the second and fourth right and left intercostal spaces as well as the apex and axillae area
Little subcutaneous fat	Eyes are fused before 24 weeks' gestation	Grunting, nasal flaring, or retractions (subcostal, sternal, or suprasternal) are signs of respiratory distress	Auscultation of heart sounds are done routinely to detect murmurs, which may or may not be innocent
Fragile and easily injured	Nose flattened or bruised Nasal patency Low placement of ears	Auscultate anterior, posterior, and at the sides of the chest	Blood pressures on all four extremities are done to determine any wide variations that are indicative of a ductal defect
Mottled related to poor peripheral perfusion	Facial anomalies	Auscultate respiratory rate for a full minute	Persistent central cyanosis
Prominent veins		Respiratory rate is between 60 and 80 respirations per minute	Displacement of apex
Covered in vernix		Respiratory rate above 80 respirations per minute are not within normal limits	Cardiomegaly
Pale (pallor) related to anemia from blood loss		Asymmetrical chest movement may suggest respiratory conditions such as pneumothorax or diaphragmatic hernia	
Congenital strawberry hemangiomas		Excessive secretions will affect the oxygen intake	
Diaper rash is common related to the increase in irritation of the stool when the newborn is on antibiotics and because of the fragility of the skin			
Soles of the feet are smooth			

CONDITIONS AFFECTING THE PREMATURE NEWBORN

Premature newborns are at risk for cold stress and hypoglycemia as is the small-for-gestational-age (SGA) newborn. Other conditions common to preterm newborns that will be discussed in order of priority are:

- Respiratory distress syndrome (RDS)
- Apnea of prematurity
- Bronchopulmonary dysplasia (BPD)
- Jaundice
- Anemia of prematurity
- Necrotizing enterocolitis (NEC)

- Gastroesophageal reflux disease (GERD)
- Retinopathy of prematurity (ROP)
- Intraventricular/periventricular hemorrhage (IVH/PVH)

Respiratory Distress Syndrome (RDS)

RDS is a developmental respiratory disorder affecting preterm newborns because of lack of lung surfactant and underdeveloped alveolar saccules. In RDS there is diffuse **atelectasis** (parts of the lung are not expanded), with congestion and edema in the lung spaces. Lecithin-sphingomyelin (L/S) ratio and phosphatidylglycerol (PG) levels are low and inadequate to keep the immature alveoli

Abdomen	Musculoskeletal	Genitalia	Neurological/Sensory
Cord does not have two arteries and one vein	No flexion of extremities, resulting in increased susceptibility to heat loss and skin breakdown	Male scrotum has no rugae and the testes are often undescended	Marked head lag in all positions
Palpate for masses	Assess for fractures or developmental hip dysplasia or fractured clavicle	Female clitoris is often prominent and not covered by the labia minora; the labia majora are also small	Consistent caregivers read the cues and notice subtle changes
Auscultate bowel sounds		Inguinal hernias are common	Sucking and gagging reflexes are often absent until 32 to 34 weeks' gestation
Abdominal circumference is done to assess for distention that may indicate necrotizing enterocolitis (NEC)		Female absence of vaginal opening or male urethral opening covered by prepuce	Moro reflex may be absent to weak
		Meconium found in the vaginal opening	Any signs or symptoms of increased intracranial pressure is related to cerebral insults
Enlarged liver or spleen		Ambiguous genitalia	Hypotonia or hypertonia
		Bladder exstrophy	Twitches or jittery, myclonic jerks
			Eyelids edematous, drainage present, minimal reactivity to light, congenital cataracts, absence of red reflex, inability to follow object or bright light
			Eyes have nystagmus, strabismus, or ruptured capillaries

of the lungs open. Lung compliance is diminished and significantly adds to the infant's work of breathing.

 Nursing Insight—*Respiratory distress syndrome*

Respiratory distress syndrome (RDS) affects 50% of premature newborns between the weights of 501 grams and 1,500 grams. The smaller and more preterm the newborn is, the higher the risk for RDS (Oretti, Marino, Mosca, Colnaghi, De Iudicibus, Drigo, et al., 2009). Respiratory distress syndrome was formerly referred to as hyaline membrane disease, surfactant deficiency, or idiopathic respiratory distress. When the nurse is

called to a delivery for a premature newborn, ensure there is proper ventilation and oxygenation equipment, an infant warmer, the "crash cart" and adequate transport to the neonatal intensive care unit (NICU).

Signs and Symptoms

The clinical signs and symptoms of RDS begin shortly after birth and include:

- Expiratory grunting
- Nasal flaring
- Cyanosis in room air
- Rapid breathing (tachypnea)

- Labored breathing with retractions
- Decreased breath sounds, often with rales

Diagnosis

If untreated, the arterial blood gas values show oxygenation deficits with hypercarbia and metabolic acidosis. A pulse oximetry can assist with diagnosis to determine hypoxia.

 Collaboration in Caring—*Radiology*

The x-ray findings of RDS reveal a reticulogranular pattern that looks like "ground glass"; possible atelectasis, which looks like "whiteout"; and obscure heart borders (Martin et al., 2011).

Prevention

Preventative nursing care includes proactive health-care teaching to prevent preterm birth. If preterm birth is inevitable, the mother is given betamethasone (Celestone or Soluspan) in an attempt to increase surfactant production.

Collaborative Care

Nursing Care. Airway maintenance and oxygenation are the priority interventions for the newborn with RDS. There are many types of oxygen therapy, and they include:

- Humidified oxygen
- Continuous positive airway pressure
- Conventional mechanical ventilation
- Bilevel ventilators
- High-frequency oscillating ventilation
- High-frequency jet ventilation
- Nitric oxide (for patients with subsequent persistent pulmonary hypertension)
- Extracorporeal membrane oxygenation (in the worst cases) (Valenza, 2009)

Medical Care. The first action to promote the neonate's stability has historically been to promote oxygenation with mechanical ventilation via endotracheal intubation. More health-care providers are using **continuous positive airway pressure** (CPAP) *initially* because it is less damaging to lung tissue. If CPAP is not adequate enough to oxygenate the newborn, then mechanical ventilation with positive end-expiratory pressure is needed.

To mechanically ventilate a newborn, an endotracheal tube is placed by a clinician certified in intubations and neonatal resuscitation. Endotracheal intubation is done by inserting an endotracheal tube orally to create an open secure airway to which the ventilator can be attached.

Newborns are generally "weaned" from mechanical ventilation or CPAP as soon as possible to avoid complications of oxygen such as bronchopulmonary dysplasia (BPD) and retinopathy of prematurity (ROP).

An oxygen hood is often used to keep a baby in an oxygen-rich environment for a short period of time. Oxygen hoods are easy to use and provide easy access to the newborn for procedures and assessment (Fig. 19-11). The newborn with RDS requires blood gas monitoring to determine whether adequate oxygenation is occurring as well as blood analysis for electrolytes, calcium, and glucose levels. Newborns who are working harder to oxygenate often have issues maintaining appropriate electrolyte, calcium, and glucose levels.

Another mode of delivering oxygen is via nasal cannula, which is continuous flow of low-level oxygen (1–2 L/min)

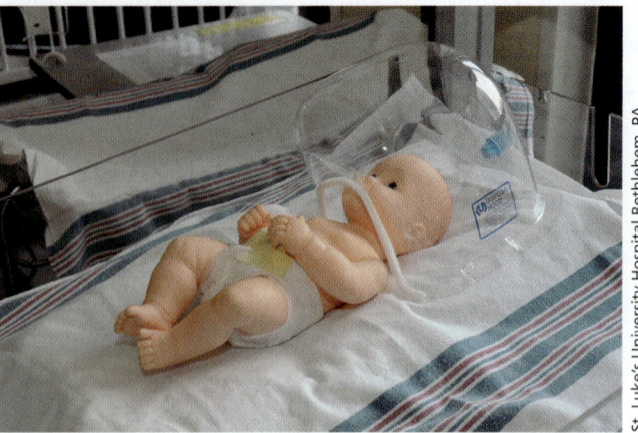

St. Luke's University Hospital Bethlehem, PA

Figure 19-11 Oxygen hood.

to supplement the newborn's own intake. Oxygen by mask is an unreliable method for a newborn.

Medications. After an airway has been established, the administration of synthetic surfactant within 15 to 30 minutes of birth is required. The synthetic surfactant is administered through a catheter in the endotracheal tube. For newborns less than 1,000 g, it is given to coat the alveoli to keep them open so that they can perfuse with oxygen. Newborns greater than 1,000 g benefit from surfactant therapy at any time during the first 2 to 6 hours of life. Continued mechanical ventilation after administration helps the medication to be spread throughout the lung tissue.

 Optimizing Outcomes—Pulse oximeter

The best outcome to ensure adequate oxygenation (above 92%) is to keep the newborn on a pulse oximeter whenever oxygen is being used.

 Medication: Beractant (Survanta)

(be-**rak**-tant)

Classification(s): Sterile nonpyrogenic pulmonary surfactant.

Indications: Lowers minimum surface tension and increases pulmonary compliance and oxygenation in preterm newborns. Prevents and treats RDS in newborns (Valenza, 2009).
Action: Lowers surface tension at alveoli level.
Storage: Refrigerate and protect from light.

Pharmacokinetics:
ABSORPTION: Absorbed only in lungs.
DISTRIBUTION: Does not get absorbed systemically.

Contraindications and Precautions: Monitor heart rate and respiration.

Adverse Reactions and Side Effects: Transient bradycardia, hypotension, oxygen desaturation, endotracheal tube blockage, pulmonary hemorrhage, and possible increased nosocomial infections.

Route and Dosage: Intratracheal 4 mL/kg q6h × 4 (maximum of four doses in first 48 hours)

Nursing Implications:
1. Give within 15 minutes of birth to premature newborns.
2. Naso-oral suction before administration.
3. Warm vial 20 minutes to room temperature.
4. Do not suction for 1 hour after administration.
5. Discard vial after use—do not re-refrigerate once it is warmed.

Source: Vallerand & Sanoski (2014).

Apnea of Prematurity (AOP)

Apnea, a spontaneous pause in breathing, is a common occurrence in preterm newborns. The inspiratory center in the medulla oblongata of the brainstem, the central and peripheral chemoreceptors, and the neuroregulators are immature and do not provide the normal negative feedback loop to **hypoxia** and **hypercapnia**. Prolonged apnea leads to hypoxemia and bradycardia, which may not respond to tactile stimulation and may require positive pressure ventilation (PPV; bag and mask) (Henderson-Smart & De Paoli, 2010).

 Nursing Insight—Apnea versus periodic breathing

Apnea of prematurity must be differentiated from periodic breathing, which is normal in the newborn. Periodic breathing is classified as short pauses in the breathing of the newborn that only last approximately 3 seconds. The incidence of apnea increases as the gestational age of the newborn decreases. Many times, the apneic spells are accompanied by a **bradycardic** episode, which has led to the clinical term "A&B spell."

Signs and Symptoms

Apneic spells or episodes are significant if they last more than 20 seconds and many times are accompanied by:

- Abrupt pallor
- Hypotonia
- Cyanosis
- Bradycardia
- Oxygen desaturation

Diagnosis

Apnea is diagnosed if there is absence of respiration that lasts more than 20 seconds.

Prevention

To prevent apneic spells, nurses must assist the preterm newborn to conserve energy by keeping the newborn neutral thermal and reducing environmental stress.

Collaborative Care

Nursing Care. Most preterm newborns are on a **cardiorespiratory (C-R) monitor** (Fig. 19-12). The C-R monitor is attached to the newborn by three electrodes. Two electrodes are placed on either side of the chest and the third on the abdomen. The electrodes are changed often based on NICU protocol. Every time the electrodes are changed, they are applied to a new area of skin to prevent breakdown from the adhesive. The C-R monitor is set to alarm if the newborn fails to breathe spontaneously for 20 seconds, the respiratory rate falls below a certain rate (usually 20 respirations/min) or the heart rate drops below a certain rate (usually 80 to 100 beats per minute). An alarm notifies the nurse of an impending apnea or bradycardic spell or combined A&B episode.

 Diagnostic Tools Pulse Oximeter

The pulse oximeter used in conjunction with the C-R monitor is a small plastic light-emitting probe that is noninvasive and can be secured to the newborn's extremity. The newborn is maintained on continuous pulse oximetry to guard against desaturation episodes. Oxygen saturation is calculated from the

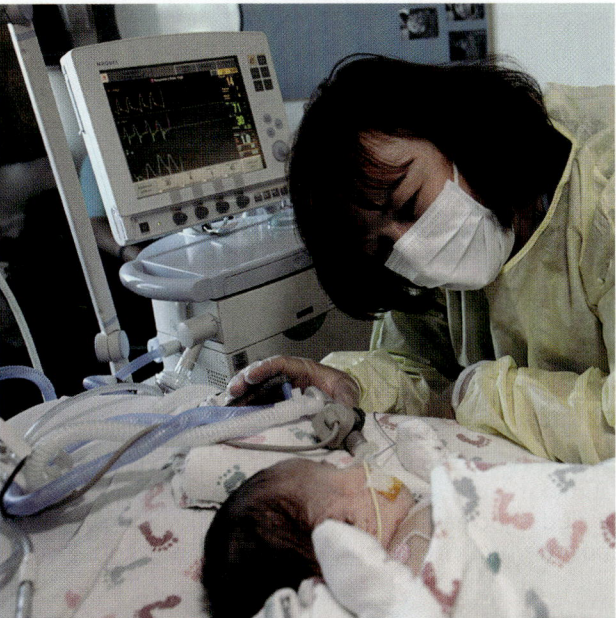

Figure 19-12 Most preterm newborns are on a cardiorespiratory monitor.

hemoglobin flowing under the light, and then the percentage is displayed on the monitor. It is easy to use, and the saturation measurements are fairly reliable when compared with arterial samples of blood. The oxygen saturation is maintained above 92% (Mathew, 2011).

The pulse oximeter is also set to alarm during a low peripheral O_2 saturation (usually below 88%). If the newborn desaturates without a corresponding A&B spell, it is called a desaturation episode.

 focus on safety

Apneic, bradycardic, or desaturation episode

An apneic, bradycardic, or desaturation episode requires immediate attention. There are different severities of A&B spells. Some newborns take a deep breath and regulate themselves back into a normal cardiorespiratory pattern without intervention, which is often called a self-limiting episode. Some newborns continue the apnea, bradycardia, and/or desaturation spell and need mild stimulation to induce them to take a deep breath and regain a normal cardiorespiratory pattern. Stimulation is done by rubbing their backs or flicking their feet. Periodically, newborns need aggressive stimulation to regain cardiorespiratory control, which includes increasing existing oxygen flow or using positive pressure through bag and mask ventilation (Fig. 19-13).

Medical Care. Initially theophylline (Aerolate) or aminophylline (Phyllocontin) is used to stimulate respirations, but caffeine (Cafcit) is the most widely used medication for long-term treatment.

Medication: Caffeine Citrate (Cafcit)

Caffeine citrate (Cafcit) loading dose is 20 mg/kg IV or orally, and the maintenance dose is 5 mg/kg/day. The therapeutic caffeine level, which is drawn approximately once a week, is in the range of 5 to 20 mcg/mL (Martin et al., 2011).

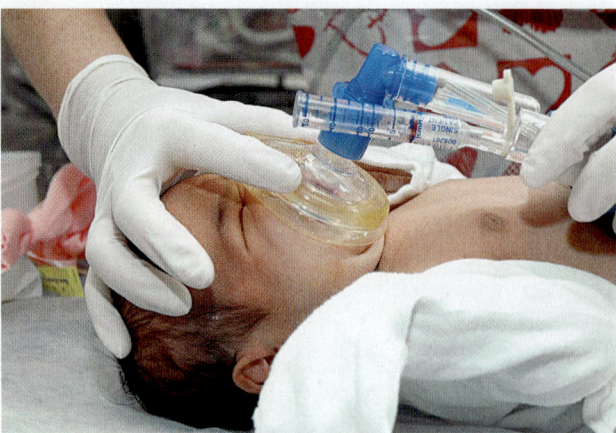

Figure 19-13 Some newborns need aggressive stimulation to regain cardiorespiratory control that includes increasing existing oxygen flow or using positive pressure through bag and mask ventilation.

focus on safety

Caffeine citrate (Cafcit)

Caffeine is never withdrawn abruptly from the newborn. Once the newborn does not require therapeutic levels to control AOP, the newborn is allowed to grow out of the dosage and withdrawal takes place slowly.

Education/Discharge Instructions

Parents are taught to give caffeine citrate (Cafcit) to their newborn if it is going to be maintained after discharge. AOP usually resolves at 37 to 38 weeks postconceptual age but may last longer. Many preterm newborns are sent home on home C-R monitoring systems that alarm if respirations stop longer than 20 seconds or the heart rate drops below the set parameters. If newborns are discharged without monitors, they usually need to be A&B spell free in the hospital for at least 5 to 7 days prior to discharge.

Bronchopulmonary Dysplasia (BPD)

Bronchopulmonary dysplasia (BPD), or chronic lung disease, is a condition in which the newborn becomes oxygen dependent past 36 weeks' gestation. BPD is a complication produced by long-term oxygen use, especially with mechanical ventilation therapy. Although oxygen is needed by the preterm infant to maintain proper tissue perfusion until the maturing lungs can resume that function, supplemental oxygen can also damage lung tissue by suppressing compliance. Because oxygen is administered, the lungs fail to develop the normal compliance needed to force adequate levels of air in and out. Sometimes the preterm newborn ends up with noncompliant lungs with fibrosis that need oxygen via cannula for an extended period of time, sometimes up to a few years, to properly oxygenate their growing bodies. Newborns with BPD are often sent home on O_2 after the parents have been educated in oxygen administration. The amounts of oxygen needed through the cannula vary with the severity of the BPD, but often it is a small flow at anywhere from 1/4 to 1 liter flow rate with anywhere from 21% to 30% of oxygen (Deakins, 2009).

Signs and Symptoms
• Inability to wean off oxygen completely

Diagnosis
Chest x-ray in BPD can show changes consistent with cyst formation, increased density, and progressive hyperinflation.

Prevention
When treating preterm newborns with oxygen, use the lowest amount possible to maintain acceptable oxygen saturations levels. High levels of oxygen and long-term ventilation have both been linked with the development of BPD.

Collaborative Care
Nursing Care. Wean newborns from oxygen as soon as possible. Prevent erratic oxygen levels during delivery, maintaining at a constant level of oxygen delivery.
Medical Care. Management often includes medications to treat the symptoms of BPD. Bronchodilators, such as beta-2-agonists, anti-cholinergics, and theophyllines and inhaled and systemic steroids, to decrease inflammation, have been used to try to increase lung compliance. Other medical management includes the use of oxygen therapy, diuretics, and nutritional therapy.

focus on safety

Newborns discharged on oxygen therapy

Newborns discharged on oxygen therapy need a home care nurse to evaluate the home for oxygen safety and teach parents how to care for the child receiving oxygen therapy. The parents and other primary caregivers will also need training on the use of a pulse oximeter and CPR training prior to discharge.

Education/Discharge Instructions

Parents are taught to care for the oxygen-dependent newborn and how to secure an oxygen supply for the home. Parents are taught newborn positioning and care of the oxygen prongs and equipment and receive C-R monitor training.

Critical Nursing Action Infant Car Seat Challenge

Newborns who are born at or before 37 weeks' GA need an Infant Car Seat Challenge (ICSC). The test is done by placing the newborn in the car seat that will be used to transport him home for 80 to 120 minutes (or longer if the distance to their home will take more than 120 minutes).
The test is failed if there is apnea longer than 20 seconds, bradycardia less than 80 beats per minute, or desaturation recorded on the pulse oximeter of less than 93% (Bass, 2010). Newborns who fail the ICSC on multiple occasions may require a car bed rather than a car seat for transportation.

Jaundice

Newborn physiological jaundice (**hyperbilirubinemia**) is common and occurs because of the newborn's immature liver (especially the preterm newborn). The liver cannot conjugate the bilirubin as quickly as needed. The excess bilirubin in the circulatory system moves into the skin, sclerae, nails, body fluids, and other body tissues, resulting in jaundice. Jaundice that appears on the second or third day of life usually peaks on day 4 and then declines on day 5.

Nursing Insight—*Jaundice in breastfeeding newborns*

Early jaundice in breastfed newborns begins at 2 to 4 days and most likely results from decreased fluid intake and caloric intake. After the milk supply is well established, this type of jaundice resolves.

Late jaundice in breastfed newborns begins at 4 to 7 days and can peak during the second week of life. Factors in the breast milk are thought to inhibit the conjugation or decrease the excretion of excess bilirubin. This type of jaundice usually resolves on its own.

What if parents told the nurse 2 days after delivery that they were going to discontinue breastfeeding because their baby was jaundiced and a friend told them it was from the breast milk? The nurse instructs parents about the different types of jaundice and encourages the mother to continue to breastfeed.

Signs and Symptoms

The signs and symptoms of jaundice include:

- Visible jaundice (a yellowish discoloration) is seen at a level of 5 mg/dL within the first 24 hours of birth.

Diagnosis

Hyperbilirubinemia is diagnosed if the serum bilirubin level is rising faster than 5 mg/dL in 24 hours; or the direct bilirubin is greater than 2 mg/dL; or in a healthy neonate the serum bilirubin concentration is greater than 15 mg/dL and that for preterm infants, "sick" infants, or those with hemolytic disease, the serum bilirubin level for hyperbilirubinemia would be lower than that of the full-term neonate. The level of concern varies with gestational age and postnatal age in hours (Fig. 19-14).

Without appropriate screening and treatment of hyperbilirubinemia in the newborn, complications can occur. Bilirubin encephalopathy describes the clinical findings when the serum bilirubin level is so elevated that the central nervous system is affected. The newborn becomes lethargic, hypotonic, and has feeding difficulty. This is a severe hyperbilirubinemic condition that warrants exchange transfusions to prevent a condition called **kernicterus** (AAP, 2004). Refer to Box 19-9 for further explanation.

Box 19-9 Kernicterus

A newborn with untreated jaundice is at risk for kernicterus. If bilirubin crosses the blood–brain barrier, it can permanently damage a newborn's brain. Not all newborns with bilirubin encephalopathy progress to kernicterus, and the exact level of serum bilirubin required to cause damage is not yet known. The damage caused by kernicterus can be cerebral palsy, auditory dysfunction, dental-enamel dysplasia, and upward gaze as well as intellectual and other disabilities.

Prevention

The best method to prevent physiological jaundice is frequent and early feedings to stimulate the release of meconium stool by which the bilirubin is excreted.

Collaborative Care

Nursing Care. Treatment of jaundice in the newborn is based on the underlying cause. Newborns who are plotted on the graph in the high-risk zone on the bilirubin risk chart undergo phototherapy (bilirubin lights). Phototherapy uses daylight, cool white, blue, or "special blue" fluorescent light tubes. Fluorescent lights are the most effective form of phototherapy and are placed around and above the newborn. The level of bilirubin in the blood determines if the newborn is placed under single, double, or triple phototherapy. Fiber-optic systems (Biliblanket) can also deliver phototherapy in a blanket form placed under or around the newborn.

Critical Nursing Action Care of the Jaundiced Newborn

The nurse must remember that when a newborn is under phototherapy, the eyes must be shielded by an opaque mask. The nurse assesses the newborn's eyes often to assess for discharge or corneal irritation. It is important to remove the mask during feedings so the newborn can receive visual stimulation. The newborn's genital area must also be covered (Fig. 19-15).

During phototherapy or use of the biliblanket, the newborn is kept warm. The newborn is susceptible to hypothermia because of skin exposure, and the temperature needs to be monitored closely. In addition, it is important that the newborn receive proper nutrition to ensure the clearance of the bilirubin. The breast- or formula-feeding mother can be encouraged to feed the child as often as every 2 hours.

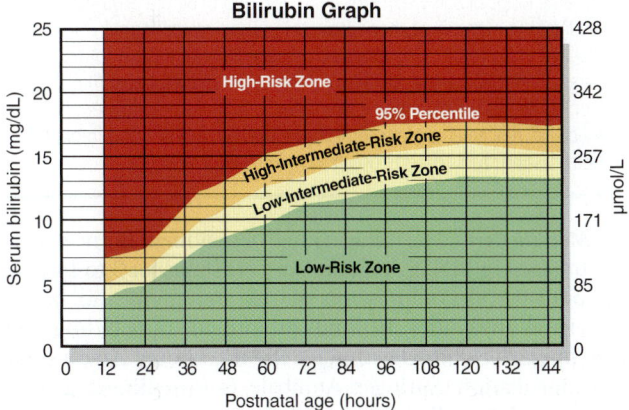

Figure 19-14 Laboratory evaluation of the jaundiced newborn of 35 or more weeks' gestation.

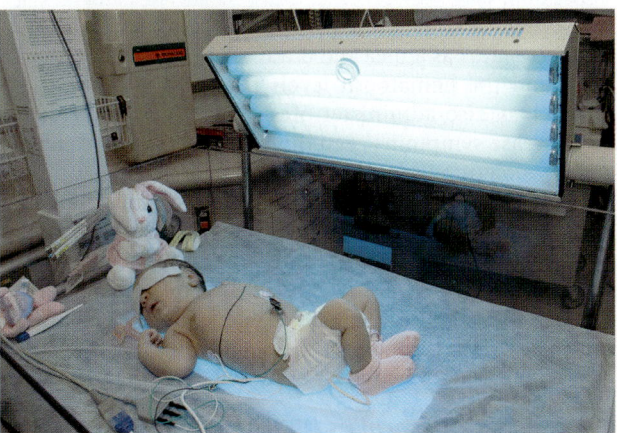

Figure 19-15 The eyes and genitalia of the newborn are always covered to prevent tissue and retinal damage.

Medical Care. Other treatments for hyperbilirubinemia may include hydration with an electrolyte solution if the newborn shows signs of dehydration such as dry skin and mucus membranes, poor intake, concentrated urine, or limited urine output and irritability (AAP, 2004).

❝What to say❞—*Hyperbilirubinemia*

Treatment measures must be explained to parents to help decrease their anxiety. Parents need to report any changes in the newborn's condition such as an increase in jaundice, poor feeding, lethargy, or vomiting.

Anemia of Prematurity (AOP)

Newborn red blood cells (RBCs) have a life span of only 60 to 70 days compared with 100 to 120 days for adult RBCs. Premature newborns are often anemic for several compounding reasons. One reason is that the newborn undergoes many blood serum evaluations. Even though small amounts of blood are taken for each study, multiple studies are done and it reduces circulatory volume. A second reason for anemia is the rapid growth a preterm newborn undergoes in a short period of time. A third reason has to do with erythropoietin release. Erythropoietin is not released until 34 to 36 weeks of gestation and then responds when hematocrit levels are low. There is an approximate 1-week delay between erythropoietin release and the production of reticulocytes (Bishara & Ohis, 2009).

Signs and Symptoms

Typical signs and symptoms of anemia of prematurity include:

- Fatigue
- Respiratory distress
- Pale skin

Diagnosis

A drop in hemoglobin below the average hematocrit value (between 35% and 45%) is the definitive sign of anemia.

Prevention

Laboratory tests are limited as much as possible, and the least amount of blood is drawn for the blood analysis. Frequent blood draws have been associated with anemia of prematurity.

Collaborative Care

Nursing Care. The nurse assesses skin color, cardiopulmonary status as apnea and bradycardia increase with anemia, and the hematocrit levels per hospital policy. The nurse may also administer prescribed blood transfusions to decrease symptoms even though they actually delay the erythropoietin mechanisms.

Medical Care. Management includes treating the symptoms of anemia of prematurity. Often this will require prescribing blood transfusions and appropriate medications.

Medications. Anemia of prematurity is treated with recombinant human erythropoietin subcutaneous to stimulate erythropoiesis. Erythropoietin or epoetin (Epogen or EPO) is given until 34 to 35 weeks of gestation (Martin et al., 2011).

Necrotizing Enterocolitis (NEC)

NEC is another complication that affects mostly preterm newborns. It is caused by an ischemic episode of the bowel. When a lack of oxygen occurs in any human, blood is shunted from the nonessential organs (e.g., bowel) to the essential organs: lungs and brain. If the ischemic attack is severe, it can decrease the circulation to the bowel to the point of **ischemia**. The extent that any portion of the bowel is affected depends on the severity of the ischemic attack. Once the bowel is necrotic or the tissue dies from lack of O_2, there is no peristalsis to move food or gas and it builds up in that section of the bowel. NEC is dangerous because it can easily produce septicemia in the preterm newborn (full-term newborns who experience a severe asphyxia can also experience NEC).

Signs and Symptoms

Necrotizing enterocolitis is suspected if there is:

- Lack of bowel movements
- Emesis
- Prefeeding aspirates
- Abdominal distention
- Increase of 1 to 2 cm in abdominal circumference from the last feed
- Irritability
- Lethargy
- Observable loops of bowel (late symptom)

Diagnosis

Necrotizing enterocolitis is diagnosed via x-ray exam when a sausage-shaped dilation of the intestine is present. A dangerous sign is free air in the abdomen that may indicate perforation of the bowel. Laboratory findings show leukopenia, metabolic acidosis, anemia, electrolyte imbalance, and leukocytosis.

Prevention

The nurse keeps oxygen saturation levels at acceptable values and decreases excessive environmental stress. Hypoxemia and environmental stress cause blood to be shunted away from the bowel and to the heart and brain.

Nursing Care. When providing care to a newborn suspected with NEC, enteral feedings are stopped immediately and the physician or neonatal nurse practitioner is notified.

 Critical Nursing Action Necrotizing Enterocolitis (NEC)

When caring for a child recovering from necrotizing enterocolitis, the nurse must measure and record abdominal circumferences, auscultate bowel sounds before every feeding, and observe for abdominal distention (observable loops or shiny skin indicating distention). Before any gastric tube feeding, the nurse must check aspirates for undigested formula or breast milk. If excessive (20%) undigested breast milk or formula is found, the nurse must follow the hospital's protocol, which may suggest that the next feeding be held and the physician or neonatal nurse practitioner notified. All bowel movements are recorded: amount, consistency, and frequency. Hematesting stools detects occult (non-visible) fecal blood.

Medical Care. The initial course of treatment for newborns with stage I or II NEC includes an NPO status for 3 to 14 days, nasograstric decompression of the abdomen, and broad-spectrum antibiotics. IV fluids are provided, including TPN and lipids. Newborns with stage III NEC should have a surgical consultation (Springer, Annibale, & Rosenkranz, 2012).

Surgical Care. If only a small portion of the bowel is affected, a rest period may reinstate enough circulation for future functioning. If a large section of the bowel is affected, a surgical bowel resection is warranted, and sometimes it can lead to an ostomy (or ostomies) that may or may not be permanent.

Education/Discharge Instructions

Parents are taught about the condition and all the interventions being completed to avoid complications (e.g., gavage feedings and special formulas such as Pregestimil) and promote long-term health for the infant. Specifically, parents must be taught about caring for the ostomy.

Gastroesophageal Reflux Disease (GERD)

GERD is a frequent and sometimes normal occurrence in high-risk newborns. It is treated as a disease when excessive amounts of formula or breast milk are being regurgitated or it causes complications such as failure to gain weight (Martin et al., 2011). Residual formula from prior feedings is common in preterm newborns because of their small stomach capacity and immature gastrointestinal mobility (Watson, 2012).

Signs and Symptoms

- Frequent spitting up or vomiting
- Irritability when feeding
- Refusing to eat
- Only eating small amounts
- Arching the back while feeding
- Regurgitation
- Frequent hiccups or cough
- Frequent waking during sleep
- Respiratory problems

Diagnosis

It is a more serious form of gastroesophageal reflux in which the lower esophageal sphincter does not close properly or spontaneously opens, which results in retrograde flow of gastric contents into the esophagus.

Prevention

While GERD cannot be prevented, there are interventions that can be implemented to decrease episodes of reflux from occurring. These include holding the newborn in an upright position when bottle feeding and for 30 minutes after feeding to decrease reflux; placing the infant at a 30-degree angle while sleeping; smaller, more frequent feedings; adding rice cereal to formula or pumped breast milk; diet modifications for mothers who breastfeed; and frequent burping to minimize gastric pressure (Gillson, 2008).

Collaborative Care

Nursing Care. The nurse assesses aspirates from nasogastric or orogastric tubes for the amount and color prior to each feeding. Use thickened formula or breast milk as prescribed. Place the newborn with the head of the bed at a 30-degree angle for sleeping. Observe the infant often for signs of aspiration (e.g., respiratory changes, leakage of food or saliva from mouth or tracheostomy, excess secretions, shortness of breath, or choking).

Medical Care. A proton-pump inhibitor (PPI) is used to neutralize stomach acidity, or prokinetic agents are used to increase gastric emptying (Watson, 2012). PPIs include omeprazole (Prilosec), lansoprazole (Prevacid), pantoprazole (Protonix), or rabeprazole (Aciphex). Prokinetic agents include metoclopramide (Reglan) and cisapride (Propulsid).

Education/Discharge Instructions

During the newborn's hospital stay, the family-centered care includes teaching parents about upright feedings and

focus on safety

Preventing aspiration

Slow feedings and upright positioning of the newborn is necessary to prevent aspiration of gastric contents that can occur with emesis.

sleeping where the infant is placed on his back and the head of the bed is elevated at a 30-degree angle for sleeping. Education should be tailored to meet the specific needs of the newborn and may include information on prescribed medications and special formulas.

Retinopathy of Prematurity (ROP)

The retinal vessels of the preterm newborn are frail and immature. **Retinopathy of prematurity (ROP)** is a result of immature retinal vasculature followed by hypoxia. The concentration and duration of supplemental oxygen are thought to play a role in the development of ROP. Retinopathy of prematurity is inversely related to gestational age. Therefore, the earlier the gestational age, the greater the likelihood of developing this condition. Risk factors for ROP include:

- Gestational age of less than 32 weeks
- Birth weight of less than 1,500 g
- Respiratory distress syndrome
- Patent ductus arteriosus that needs surgery
- Hypothermia
- Sepsis and meningitis
- High-intensity lighting

The extent of retinal damage in the preterm newborn is dependent on three criteria: (1) the gestational age of the newborn, (2) the length of exposure to oxygen, and (3) arterial pressure. Damage is classified according to stages (Box 19-10).

Signs and Symptoms

Signs and symptoms of ROP are limited to those that can be assessed by expert exam of the retina by ophthalmological procedures. During the neonatal period, a newborn who has visual impairment might not react to a human face.

Diagnosis

Retinopathy of prematurity is diagnosed by examination of the retina by an ophthalmologist based on five stages, ranging from mild to severe.

Prevention

Preventing retinopathy of prematurity can be accomplished by preventing premature birth. Preventing other complications of prematurity (such as neonatal RDS) may also help prevent ROP. The more premature a newborn is, the more

---

Box 19-10 Stages of Retinopathy of Prematurity (ROP)

Stage I—abnormal blood vessel growth is mild

Stage II—abnormal blood vessel growth is moderate

Stage III—abnormal blood vessel growth is severe

Stage IV—the retina is partially detached

Stage V—completely detached retina. This is the end stage of the disease

likely the development of ROP. If premature birth cannot be avoided, monitoring the amount of oxygen the premature infant is exposed to decreases the risk of developing ROP (NIH, 2013).

Collaborative Care

Nursing Care. During oxygen administration, fluctuations in arterial concentrations of oxygen must be prevented. The Pao_2 is not set greater than 80 mm Hg, and the preterm newborn is weaned off oxygen as soon as possible. In addition, the nurse can decrease the constant bright lights in the newborn's environment. A blanket, to provide shading, can be placed over the incubator during the day. Nap time can be designated in the NICU during which the lights are lowered and other environmental stimuli are decreased. Treatment and follow-up care is imperative to the newborn's maintenance of sight, and the nurse is the coordinator of care (Scott, Wittmann-Price, & Thear, 2008).

Medical Care. The preterm newborn is checked routinely for signs of ROP by an ophthalmologist. Examinations are started at 4 to 6 weeks of age and continue until vascularization of the retina is complete to reduce the risk of visual impairment (usually myopia) and blindness. Most babies who develop retinopathy of prematurity have stages I or II. If ROP is left untreated, it will destroy the newborn's vision.

Surgical Care. Cryotherapy is used to treat ROP (Kumar, Sankar, Deorari, Azad, Chandra, Agarwal, et al., 2011). Additional surgical options include laser surgery, and for detached or partially detached retinas, scleral buckling surgery and/or vitrectomy is performed.

 Complementary Care: *Sucrose Use for Eye Examinations*

Newborns in the NICU receive routine eye examinations that are uncomfortable. The use of sucrose has been shown to decrease desaturation and bradycardic episodes if used before the procedure to decrease pain (O'Sullivan, O'Connor, Brosnahan, McCreery, & Dempsey, 2010).

 Critical Nursing Action Retinopathy of Prematurity

Because retinopathy of prematurity (ROP) may be a complication of oxygen therapy, the nurse must maintain the lowest level of oxygen as possible to maintain the pulse oximeter reading above 92%.

Acute Intracranial Hemorrhage (ICH)

Classifications of Intraventricular Hemorrhage (IVH) and Periventricular Leukomalacia (PVL) are hemorrhages, which are bleeding into the epidural, subdural, or subarachnoid areas of the brain. Most bleeds occur within the first 72 hours of life. One cause of IVH is attributed to rapid volume expansion in preterm newborns. An ICH can be minimal or extensive and present clinically from asymptomatic to seizure activity, depending on the stage of involvement (Box 19-11). Neurological sequelae related to IVH and PVL are associated with the severity of the bleed. Severe bleeds can lead to seizures, mental deficiencies, and cerebral palsy. Head ultrasounds are done routinely in the

---

> **Box 19-11** Classifications of Intraventricular Hemorrhage (IVH) and Periventricular Leukomalacia (PVL)
>
> - Grade I hemorrhages bleed into the subependyma only.
> - Grade II hemorrhages bleed into the subependyma, and the ventricles but do not produce distention of the ventricles.
> - Grade III hemorrhages bleed into the ventricles and produce dilation of the ventricles that can lead to hydrocephalus.
> - Grade IV hemorrhages produce the same bleeding as in grade III, but the bleeding extends to the parenchyma.

NICU, usually every week to evaluate the presence of IVH and PVL in the preterm population. If the bleed causes obstruction of cerebrospinal fluid, a shunt is needed to prevent **hydrocephalus.**

Signs and Symptoms

Symptoms of intracranial hemorrhages can be asymptomatic to profound neurological impairment:

- Decreased tone or change in activity level
- Seizures
- Sudden drop in hematocrit
- Full anterior fontanelle

Diagnosis

Intracranial hemorrhages are diagnosed by cerebral ultrasound and followed up with magnetic imaging or computed tomography scan. Diagnosis can also be made by observing behavioral changes and altered states of consciousness in the preterm newborn. In addition, an enlarging head circumference needs immediate attention and is indicative of a worsening IVH or PVL.

Prevention

Treatment of RDS and resuscitation by a neonatal team proficient in caring for low-birth-weight newborns decreases the incidence of intracranial hemorrhages. Also, gentle nursing care of the low-birth-weight newborn and providing a neutral thermal environment may decrease the risk of low-birth-weight newborns developing ICH (Martin, 2011).

Collaborative Care

Nursing Care. The nurse monitors the newborn's behavior and assesses head circumference and fontanelles. Decrease intracranial pressure by placing the newborn in a supine position at a 30-degree angle. Priority nursing care centers on recognition of newborn seizures so treatment can begin immediately.

 Critical Nursing Action Intraventricular (IVH) and Periventricular Leukomalacia (PVL)

When caring for a newborn with either intraventricular or periventricular hemorrhage, the nurse must observe for neurological symptoms, including poor oxygenation readings on pulse oximeter, poor feeding (if the newborn is being fed), and lethargic behavior. Increased apnea, bradycardic spells, and seizures may also occur. Critical nursing actions include keeping accurate and frequent measurements of head circumference in centimeters, reporting any sudden increase in head circumference, and monitoring fontanelles to ensure they are soft, flat, and open on palpation.

Medications. Medications are given to prevent and treat seizure activity that accompanies IVH. Phenobarbital (Luminal Sodium is the drug of choice) and phenytoin (Dilantin) are prescribed to prevent seizure activity and are considered maintenance medications. Lorazepam (Ativan) and diazepam (Valium) are often given to stop seizure activity and are considered emergency medications.

Education/ Discharge Instructions

Parents need ongoing information about their newborn's status and subsequent care. Education should be provided on how to keep the newborn safe during seizure activity and proper medication administration.

NUTRITIONAL CARE OF THE PRETERM NEWBORN

Preterm newborn nutrition is also a challenge because they are born without the full development of the gastrointestinal enzymes needed for digestion. The goal of preterm nutrition is to simulate a growth pattern in the NICU similar to what would have been if the newborn was still in utero. Feeding readiness in preterm newborns is determined by each individual newborn's behavioral states. Alert states around feeding time are assessed to determine newborn feeding readiness. Preterm newborns spend less time in wake states than full-term newborns.

The nutritional needs of the preterm newborn are complicated for several reasons:

1. They have not had the time in utero to build up nutritional stores.
2. They have lost 10% of their body weight after birth.
3. They have extrauterine complications such as RDS which increases their metabolic expenditure.
4. They need to be gaining weight daily at rates double those of a full-term newborn. In addition, the preterm newborn may not be able to feed because of regurgitating the feeding, losing weight, or cold stress. If a newborn is not ready to feed by mouth, the nurse uses alternative ways to ensure proper nutrition such as IV or enteral feeding. Nutritional therapy for preterm infants has lifelong effects on their physical and neurological development (Wiedmeier, Joss-Moore, Lane, & Neu, 2011).

 Now Can You—Discuss preterm newborns?

1. Describe different conditions that affect preterm newborns?
2. Discuss nursing interventions to minimize effects of conditions specific to the preterm newborn?
3. Evaluate lab values for conditions that affect the preterm newborn?

The Postterm Newborn

Postterm newborns, delivered on or after 42 weeks of gestation, are also considered high-risk. Although fewer pregnancies are carried to postterm today because of elective inductions, there are still incidences where a newborn is born after 42 weeks of gestation. Postterm newborns may or may not be large for gestational age (LGA). The newborn may have actually lost weight in utero because of declining placental ability to transport nutrients and oxygen. Postterm newborns are at risk for passing meconium stool in utero, which increases their chances of **meconium aspiration syndrome (MAS)** and persistent pulmonary hypertension (PPHN).

Signs and Symptoms

Clinical signs displayed by many postterm newborns include:

- Meconium-stained cord
- **Desquamation** or peeling of the skin
- Parchment-like skin that is often cracked on the abdomen and extremities
- Fingers appear long and are often peeling
- General muscle wasting may be evident

CONDITIONS AFFECTING THE POSTTERM NEWBORN

Meconium Aspiration Syndrome (MAS)

MAS occurs when a newborn is delivered through meconium stained amniotic fluid (MSAF). Approximately 10% to 12% of all newborns are delivered through MSAF, and 3% to 10% develop MAS (Wiswell, 2011). The passage of meconium in utero is believed to be either a response to intrauterine hypoxia or a maturational occurrence for the newborn. Meconium can be aspirated at birth if it is not removed from the trachea at delivery. Meconium in the lungs causes obstruction in the small airways and hyperinflation with areas of atelectasis (collapse of a portion or the entire lung because of blockage of air passage) leading to hypoxia. Some newborns with meconium aspiration pneumonia have elevated pulmonary arterial pressures and develop **persistent pulmonary hypertension (PPHN)** (Wiswell, 2011).

Signs and Symptoms

Signs and symptoms of MAS include:

- Meconium-stained skin, nails, and umbilical cord
- Initial respiratory distress
- Barrel-shaped chest from overinflated lungs
- Rales and rhonchi are heard on auscultation

The respiratory symptoms get progressively worse over the first 12 to 24 hours (Watson, 2012). MAS is often complicated by **pneumothorax** (collection of gas in the space surrounding the lungs) and **pneumomediastinum** (condition in which air is present in the space in the chest between the two lungs). Pneumothorax is an emergency situation and requires chest tubes. Chest tubes require frequent monitoring to ensure tube patency and prevent air leaks.

Diagnosis

Diagnosis is confirmed through a chest x-ray exam which shows bilateral diffuse opacities with areas of atelectasis and hyperinflation from trapped air (Whitfield, Charsha, & Chiruvolu, 2009).

Prevention

In the past, every newborn who was being delivered through MSAF had nasopharynx suctioning before the delivery of their shoulders and were then intubated and suctioned before being stimulated to breathe. Intubation is now only done if the newborn demonstrates signs of respiratory distress (Whitfield et al., 2009). Delivering an infant prior to 42 weeks' gestation is also a preventive measure because increased gestational age is associated with MAS. Continuous fetal monitoring for intrapartum fetal stress would indicate if the fetus is experiencing stress, which is associated with passing meconium in utero and MAS.

Collaborative Care

Nursing Care. Nursing care of newborns with MAS consists of chest physiotherapy (PT) and oxygen administration. Chest PT can be done by percussion with a small cup, base of a feeding nipple, or specifically made neonatal chest PT device or by vibration by a battery-operated vibrator. Chest PT is done every 3 to 4 hours to help maintain a clear airway. Postural drainage with percussion or vibration is followed by suctioning the nasopharynx.

Medical Care. Continuous positive airway pressure is frequently used to provide oxygen. Oxygen by noninvasive means such as hood or cannula is often not sufficient. Oxygen hoods require a flow meter and blender to deliver the amount of oxygen concentration prescribed. If the newborn cannot maintain a PaO_2 of 50 mm Hg or higher in 100% oxygen, then mechanical ventilation is used.

Medications. Because many newborns with MAS are postterm and neurologically more mature than ventilated preterm newborn, neuromuscular medications such as pancuronium (Pavulon) or vecuronium (Norcuron) are used to increase the effectiveness of ventilation efforts. Analgesic and sedative medications are also used (e.g., fentanyl [Sublimaze] or lorazepam [Ativan]). Morphine sulfate (Astramorph) is used to prevent the newborn from "fighting" the ventilator (Martin et al., 2011).

Persistent Pulmonary Hypertension of the Newborn (PPHN)

PPHN was once termed persistent fetal circulation because there is right-to-left shunting of blood across the foramen ovale and through the ductus arteriosus. PPHN is vascular resistance in the pulmonary system that can be caused by sepsis or pneumonia, but the most common cause of newborn PPHN is meconium aspiration pneumonia. This occurs when pulmonary vascular resistance does not decrease after birth so the transition to normal adult-type circulation to the pulmonary system is resisted, forcing fetal circulation to persist. PPHN produces a right ventricular overload and poor left ventricular filling. PPHN occurs in approximately 2 per 1,000 newborns (Oishi, Sanjeev, & Fineman, 2011). Other causes of PPHN can be because of abnormalities in the newborn's pulmonary circulation, surfactant deficiency, or abnormal lung development such as the case in diaphragmatic hernias. (Oishi et al., 2011). Figure 19-16 shows the critical cycle of PPHN.

Signs and Symptoms

PPHN usually affects term or postterm newborns because they frequently are born through meconium-stained amniotic fluid. The newborn usually demonstrates brief respiratory distress at birth and then responds normally. By 12 hours after birth, the signs and symptoms of PPHN are displayed and include:

- Central cyanosis and tachypnea
- Grunting and retractions
- Possible audible murmur because of tricuspid insufficiency
- Blood pressure usually remains normal

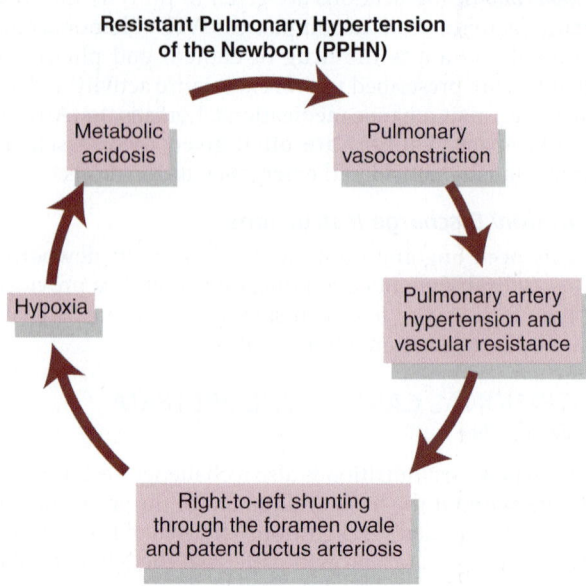

Figure 19-16 Persistent pulmonary hypertension of the newborn.

Diagnosis

Diagnosis of PPHN is confirmed from the clinical signs and symptoms and chest x-ray exam. Serum blood tests show hypoglycemia and hypocalcemia. Arterial blood gases show oxygen desaturation. Ultrasonography of the heart is done to rule out cardiac anomalies and to visualize any right-to-left shunting (Martin et al., 2011).

Prevention

Newborns who are delivered through MSAF and show signs of respiratory distress in the delivery room are intubated and suctioned. All newborns who deliver through MSAF need frequent assessment of respiratory status.

Collaborative Care

Nursing Care. See Nursing Care Plan: Persistent Pulmonary Hypertension (PPHN) of the High-Risk Newborn.

Medical Care. Newborns with PPHN are oxygenated with nitric oxide because it dilates the pulmonary vessels (Valenza, 2009). If inhaled nitric oxide (iNO) treatment (which is a potent vasodilator) is not successful (30% of newborns with PPHN), then extracorporeal membrane oxygenation (ECMO) is used (Shah & Ohlsson, 2011).

ECMO has only an 80% success rate, and it is used as a last resort for respiratory support. Delivering ECMO is a complicated procedure and is a heart and lung bypass procedure used mainly for newborns with meconium aspiration pneumonia, neonatal pneumonia, and congenital diaphragmatic hernias. The use of ECMO is expanding, and it is being considered for other pediatric conditions (Hornik, Hartman, Markert, Lodge, Cheifetz, & Turner, 2011). Newborns less than 34 weeks' gestation or 2,000 g are usually not candidates because of the need for heparinization of the blood, which can cause a cerebral hemorrhage in small or preterm newborns. ECMO is accomplished by inserting a catheter into the right internal jugular vein that extends into the right atrium and another catheter inserted into the right carotid artery into

Nursing Care Plan Persistent Pulmonary Hypertension (PPHN) of the High-Risk Newborn

Nursing Diagnosis: Ineffective Tissue Perfusion: Cardiopulmonary related to pulmonary hypertension and right-to-left shunting

Measurable Short-Term Goal: The newborn will maintain peripheral oxygen saturation levels of 92% to 95%.

Measurable Long-Term Goal: The newborn will maintain adequate tissue perfusion on room air.

NOC Outcomes:

Tissue perfusion: Pulmonary (0408): Adequacy of blood flow through pulmonary vasculature to perfuse alveoli/capillary unit

Respiratory status: Gas Exchange (0402): Alveolar exchange of carbon dioxide and oxygen to maintain arterial blood gas concentrations

NIC Interventions:

Respiratory Monitoring (3350)
Oxygen Therapy (3320)

Nursing Interventions:

1. Monitor respiratory rate, rhythm, breath sounds, effort of respirations, color, and oxygen saturation frequently (specify how often) for 24 to 48 hours after delivery.

   RATIONALE: PPHN sometimes develops after the first 12 to 24 hours of life.

2. Notify the caregiver of signs of respiratory distress: tachypnea, grunting, nasal flaring, retracting, cyanosis, or decreased oxygen saturation.

   RATIONALE: Respiratory distress related to PPHN can occur rapidly.

3. Record a preductal (right radial) pulse oximeter reading and postductal (left radial or either foot) pulse oximeter reading simultaneously.

   RATIONALE: A difference of 5% may indicate a right-to-left shunt produced by PPHN.

4. Take four extremity blood pressures.

   RATIONALE: A difference of greater than 10 to 15 mm Hg preductal and postductal may suggest a right-to-left shunt.

5. Provide and monitor warm, humidified oxygen and respiratory support as prescribed by the health-care provider (specify) to maintain a pulse oximetry reading of greater than 92%.

   RATIONALE: Oxygen therapy is needed to maintain adequate saturation levels.

6. Maintain newborn in a neutral thermal environment (NTE) without excessive noise or stimulation. Cluster care.

   RATIONALE: An NTE decreases metabolic needs, and decreased environmental stimuli may avoid excess neurological stimulation.

7. Administer sedation as prescribed by the health-care provider (specify drug, dose, route, and time).

   RATIONALE: (Specify action of the drug.) Sedation may reduce metabolic needs.

8. Closely monitor intake and output. Restrict fluids as prescribed by the health-care provider (specify).

   RATIONALE: Excessive fluids can increase pulmonary workload and increase respiratory distress.

9. Provide information and support to the family.

   RATIONALE: These newborns can become critically ill and are often transferred out to the most technologically advanced Level III NICU for extracorporeal membrane oxygenation (ECMO) support.

---

the aortic arch. The system drains venous blood and replaces arterial blood with oxygenated packed red blood cells, platelets, and fresh frozen plasma. The procedure is expensive, work intensive, and carries a multitude of complications including infection. It is available only at select Level III neonatal centers (Agar & Berkowitz, 2011) (Fig. 19-17).

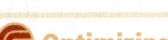 **Optimizing Outcomes**—**The newborn with PPHN**

Nursing care of the newborn with PPHN is critical with the best outcome of good oxygen saturation as well as overall stabilization.

 Now Can You—**Discuss the postterm newborn?**

1. Describe the risk factors for postterm newborns?
2. Discuss the importance of airway clearance if meconium is present at birth?
3. Implement nursing care to postterm newborns who are compromised because of MAS?

Additional Conditions Affecting the High-Risk Newborn

Many conditions of the high-risk newborn are now diagnosed prenatally with an ultrasound. High-risk newborns

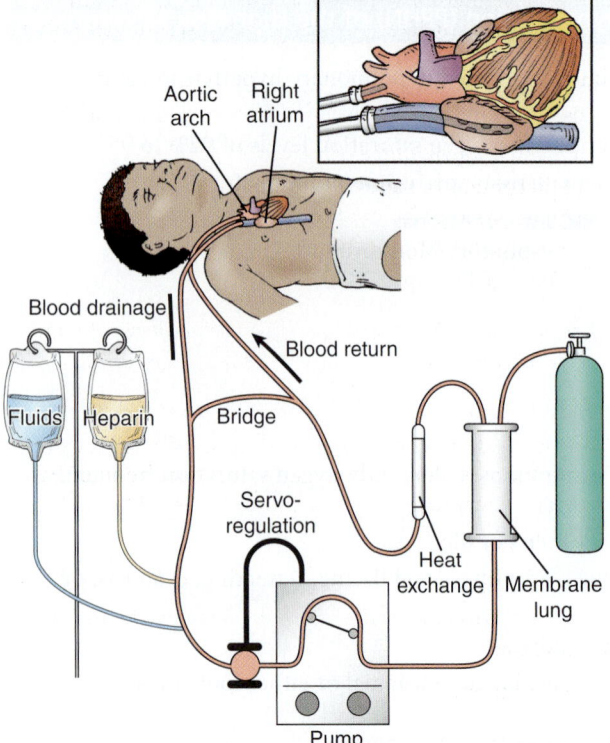

Aortic arch

Right atrium

Blood drainage

Blood return

Fluids

Heparin

Bridge

Servo-regulation

Heat exchange

Membrane lung

Pump

Figure 19-17 Extracorporeal membrane oxygenation (ECMO) is used for newborns who are not responding to conventional or high-frequency ventilation.

> **Box 19-12** Newborn Screening
>
> All 50 states (and Puerto Rico) screen for phenylketonuria (PKU) and hypothyroidism; 46 states screen for galactosemia and 45 for hemoglobinopathy. Maple syrup urine disease is included in the screening for 25 states. Other disorders are screened for in various states such as homocystinuria, biotinidase deficiency, congenital adrenal hyperplasia, cystic fibrosis, and toxoplasmosis. Screening for these conditions can promote early intervention, thereby decreasing devastating complications. States vary greatly among the different screening tests, and new tests that can be included in regular screening are being discovered on a regular basis. Nurses working with newborns need to know the tests that are done within her or his state of employment. This information can be located on the CDC Web site (2011b) at http://genes-r-us.uthscsa.edu/nbsdisorders.htm . The AAP has the following fact sheets that are easily accessible on the Web (www.pediatrics.org/cgi/content/full/118/3/e934) (AAP, 2011) for the following inborn disorders:
>
> - Biotinidase deficiency
> - Congenital adrenal hyperplasia
> - Congenital hearing loss
> - Congenital hypothyroidism
> - Cystic fibrosis
> - Galactosemia
> - Homocystinuria
> - Maple syrup urine disease (branched-chain ketoaciduria)
> - MCAD deficiency
> - PKU
> - Sickle cell disease and other hemoglobinopathies
> - Tyrosinemia

may have several conditions that impact their health. Any compromising condition can be devastating for the family and may require prompt treatment after birth. Some significant conditions include metabolic, neurological, and gastrointestinal anomalies; infections; and conditions that cause developmental delays. Examples of common conditions in the aforementioned systems are discussed in the next section. These conditions can be present at any gestational age and are not dependent on newborn weight classifications.

NEWBORN SCREENING

Every year, 4 million babies are screened for inborn disorders that can lead to permanent disability or death if left untreated. Four thousand identified newborns are then diagnosed with metabolic disorders and another 1,000 go undetected (AAP, 2011). Screening is used for three groups of disorders, and they include metabolic disorders (such as **phenylketonuria [PKU]**), hematological disorders (such as sickle cell disease), and **endocrinopathies** (such as hypothyroidism).

There are over 30 disorders that can be screened with the dried-blood patch method using **tandem mass spectrometry**, which can fragment blood elements checking for any number of deficiencies. All newborn screening tests as well as any supplemental tests for that particular state are done from this one dried blood spot test (CDC, 2001).

A heel stick blood testing method must be done after the newborn is 24 hours old for enough formula or breast milk intake to have occurred. If the infant was on nothing by mouth status for any reason, the test may need to be redone at a later date. Blood is collected by heel stick and is

soaked into a special absorbent paper that is left to dry and then mailed to a state-approved laboratory. In the future, newborn screening may be done by DNA sampling. Further information about newborn screening can be found in Box 19-12.

Prevention

Nursing care for prevention and education of various inborn conditions is discussed below. Genetic counseling for parents with a known inborn disorder is imperative.

Education/Discharge Instructions

Parents can find information about these inborn conditions and associated diets at the Centers for Disease Control and Prevention Web site (http://www.cdc.gov/ncbddd/pediatric-genetics/newborn_screening.html). Additionally, parents can be referred to specialists for genetic testing and nutritional counseling.

METABOLIC DISORDERS

Phenylketonuria (PKU)

PKU disorder is the inability to convert an essential amniom acid, phenylalanine, to tyrosine because of the lack of an enzyme. It was the first metabolic disease that prompted universal screening for metabolic diseases, and it is currently screened for in all U.S. states and territories. It is a disease transmitted by an autosomal recessive gene. The incidence varies greatly by race from 1:6,000 in Caucasians to 1:60,000 in newborns of Japanese descent (Kids Health, 2012).

Signs and Symptoms

There are no signs or symptoms of PKU at birth. Untreated PKU produces an accumulation of phenylalanine that may eventually cause:

- Developmental delays
- Intellectual disabilities (ID)
- Seizures

Collaborative Care

Nursing Care. PKU is controlled by a phenylalanine-free diet with the elimination of proteins (including breast milk and formula). The diet is continued for the child's entire life.

Galactosemia

Galactosemia is screened in 46 U.S. states and territories. The incidence is 1:60,000 to 1:80,000. It is an inherited metabolic deficiency. Children with galactosemia cannot metabolize galactose.

Signs and Symptoms

The signs and symptoms of galactosemia are caused by the inability to use galactose to produce energy and are usually noted in the first few weeks of life. They include:

- Failure to thrive
- Vomiting
- Liver disease (hepatomegaly)
- Cataracts
- Intellectual disabilities (ID)
- Death

Nursing Care. Children diagnosed with galactosemia are placed on a galactose-free diet that needs to be maintained for life (AAP, 2011).

Maple Syrup Urine Disease (Branched-Chain Ketoaciduria)

Maple syrup urine disease is screened for in 25 U.S. states and territories. It is an autosomal recessive disorder that results in high body fluid levels of ketoacids and can lead to lethargy, irritability, and then progress to coma and death. This specific metabolic deficiency has a high incidence in the Mennonite population (1 in 760) and is considered for any newborn with severe acidosis in the first 10 days of life.

Signs and Symptoms

There are no signs or symptoms of maple syrup urine disease at birth. However, they usually are noted in the first few weeks of life. They include:

- Urine has a characteristic odor (sweet smelling like brown sugar or maple syrup)
- Poor feeding
- Vomiting
- Increased reflexes
- Seizures

Collaborative Care

Nursing Care. A low-protein diet is initiated, and thiamine supplements are given. The dietary treatment must begin as soon as possible and continued throughout life (AAP, 2011).

Homocystinuria

Homocystinuria is screened for in 22 U.S. states and territories. The incidence is 1:50,000. It is an autosomal recessive genetic transmission. There is a deficiency in cystathionine beta-synthase which causes high levels of serum methionine.

Signs and Symptoms

Signs and symptoms of homocystinuria can include:

- Skeletal abnormalities
- Displacement of the eye lens
- Increase risk for blood clots
- Learning and developmental delays

Collaborative Care

Nursing Care. Diet therapy includes high doses of vitamin B_6 and methionine and cystine restriction (AAP, 2011).

Biotinidase Deficiency

Biotinidase deficiency is screened for in 21 U.S. states and territories. It is an autosomal recessive metabolic disorder that leads to carboxylase deficiency because of faulty biotin recycling.

Signs and Symptoms

Without treatment, symptoms show at 7 weeks to 3 years and include:

- Developmental delay
- Hypotonia
- Uncoordinated movement
- Alopecia
- Rash
- Hearing loss
- Optic nerve atrophy
- Seizures
- Intellectual disabilities (ID)
- Metabolic acidosis can lead to death

Nursing Care. The nurse communicates to the family that the newborn must receive pantothenic acid or biotin (types of B vitamins). These vitamins must be replaced every day because they are essential to growth and help the body break down and use food. Pantothenic acid and biotin are also found in foods such as eggs, fish, milk and milk products, whole grain cereals, lean beef, legumes, and broccoli (AAP, 2011).

Nutrition. Many newborns with metabolic or structural disorders need special diets lifelong. For example, a high-risk infant diagnosed with PKU needs a phenylalanine-free diet for life.

ENDOCRINE CONDITIONS

Congenital Hypothyroidism (CH)

CH is an endocrine disorder that produces a lack of thyroid hormone and if left untreated can cause ID. It affects 1 in 3,000 to 4,000 newborns and is screened for in most states.

Signs and Symptoms

Clinical signs and symptoms of CH include:

- Lethargy
- Poor feeding
- Constipation
- Prolonged jaundice
- Hoarse cry
- Hypotonia
- Slow reflexes
- Delayed linear growth and neurodevelopment

Diagnosis

Lab values reveal low thyroxine (T_4) and triiodiothyronine (T_3) levels (Watson, 2012). The thyroid hormone levels must remain in a determined range (Boxes 19-13 and 19-14) to promote normal brain development and growth of the child. Thyroid-stimulating hormone assists in the diagnosis of congenital hypothyroidism (Box 19-15) (Van Leeuwen et al., 2011).

Collaborative Care

Nursing Care. A thorough newborn assessment may alert health-care providers to subtle signs, but the manifestations increase as the child grows.

Medical Care. Medical management includes lifelong thyroid hormone replacement therapy.

Medications. Levothyroxine (Synthroid) tablets starting at a dose of 10 to 15 mcg/kg/day is the treatment of choice.

Education/Discharge Instructions

Parents are taught to administer the medication and instructed about the importance of lifelong therapy (Sahai & Marsden, 2009).

NEUROLOGICAL CONDITIONS

Several neurological conditions can affect newborns of any gestational age and weight classification. These defects are multifaceted and prevention may not be possible, but mothers can follow guidelines for thorough preconceptual and prenatal care and have adequate folic acid intake. Education and discharge instructions will depend on the prognosis, but families need follow-up by a nurse liaison and referrals to the appropriate support groups.

Spina bifida is the overriding term for common neural tube defects. These defects include anencephaly, encephalocele, microcephaly, and holoprosencephaly (Sandler, 2010). Anencephaly is not compatible with life while encephalocele has a high mortality rate, depending on the severity.

Anencephaly

Anencephaly is a condition in which the skull and cerebrum is malformed but the anterior lobe of the pituitary is intact. These newborns can be born alive, but the condition is lethal so they die in a short period of time. Anencephaly has a higher incidence in girls than boys. The defect is visually disturbing because most of the skull is not present (Wiggs, 2011).

Signs and Symptoms

The overt sign and symptom of anencephaly is the malformed cerebrum or absence of the skull and brain. Other signs include:

- Facial feature abnormalities
- Heart defects

Diagnosis

Diagnosis of anencephaly is made by visualization and assessment of the defect. Other tests that may be helpful in the diagnosis include:

- Amniocentesis (assessing for increased levels of alpha-fetoprotein because increased levels suggest a neural tube defect)
- Urine estriol level

Prevention

Prevention of this condition includes adequate amount of prepregnancy serum folic acid levels. Folic acid supplements (400 mcg/day) are recommended for all women of childbearing age.

Collaborative Care

Nursing Care. Nurses provide palliative and spiritual care with no effort at resuscitation. The ethical consideration for these newborns is to Allow a Natural Death (AND) (Wittmann-Price & Celia, 2010). The family requires emotional support to cope with the newborn's devastating condition (Wiggs, 2011). For more information on perinatal loss, see Chapter 11.

Encephalocele

Encephalocele is a neural tube defect that is noticeable at birth because there is protrusion of the brain through the skull. It occurs in the occipital area 60% to 80% of the time, but it can also occur in the parietal, frontal, or nasal regions. The mortality rate is higher than 30%, and many of the survivors have neurological deficits. Encephalocele requires care that is directed at the defect, including the neurological and developmental effects (Sandler, 2010).

Signs and Symptoms

Signs and symptoms of encephalocele are noted when the infant's brain comes through an opening in the skull. Sometimes, part of the membrane that covers the brain and

---

Box 19-13	Thyroxine, Total (T_4)
AGE IN DAYS, WEEKS, MONTHS, AND YEARS	**THYROXINE, TOTAL (T_4)**
1–3 days	11.8–22.6 mcg/dL
1–2 weeks	9.8–16.6 mcg/dL
1–4 months	7.2–14.4 mcg/dL

Source: Van Leeuwen, A. M., Poelhuis-Leth, D. J., & Bladh, M. L. (2011). *Davis's comprehensive handbook of laboratory and diagnostic tests with nursing implications* (4th ed., p. 1101). Philadelphia, PA: F.A. Davis.

Box 19-14	Triiodothyronine, Free (T_3)
AGE	**TRIIODOTHYRONINE, FREE (T_3)**
Children and adults	260–480 pg/dL

Source: Van Leeuwen, A. M., Poelhuis-Leth, D. J., & Bladh, M. L. (2011). *Davis's comprehensive handbook of laboratory and diagnostic tests with nursing implications* (4th ed., p. 1112). Philadelphia, PA: F.A. Davis.

Box 19-15	Thyroid-Stimulating Hormone
Age in months and years	Thyroid-stimulating hormone (TSH)
Neonates to 3 days	Less than 20 microinternational units/mL

Source: Van Leeuwen, A. M., Poelhuis-Leth, D. J., & Bladh, M. L. (2011). *Davis's comprehensive handbook of laboratory and diagnostic tests with nursing implications* (4th ed., p. 1093). Philadelphia, PA: F.A. Davis.

spinal cord also come through an opening in the skull. Other areas where the brain can protrude include:

- From the top of the skull around to the back of the skull
- The base of the skull
- In the area around the nose, sinuses, and forehead

Diagnosis

Diagnosis of encephalocele is made by visualization and assessment of the defect.

Collaborative Care

Nursing Care. Nursing care will depend on the extent of the defect and the prognosis.

The immediate nursing care is to cover the defect with warm sterile gauze to decrease the chance of infection.

Medical Care. This defect often accompanies other congenital anomalies, and surgical repair is attempted to close the defect and prevent infection.

Microcephaly

Microcephaly may be caused by an autosomal recessive disorder, toxic stimulus during prenatal development, or a chromosomal abnormality. Microcephaly means the newborn has a smaller than normal head circumference. Microcephalic newborns may have other congenital malformations but in many cases do not show a recognizable syndrome (Szabo, Pap, Kobar, Svekus, Turi, & Sztriha, 2009). There is no treatment for microcephaly.

Signs and Symptoms

Microcephaly is defined as head circumference 2 standard deviations below the mean for gestational age and is identified by progressive head circumference measurements.

Diagnosis

Microcephaly is diagnosed at birth or during routine well-baby examinations when the infant's height, weight, and head circumference are measured.

Nursing Care. Nursing care for microcephaly is supportive and ongoing.

focus on safety

Microcephaly

It is critical to maintain accurate and consistent head circumference measurements by plotting on the growth chart and monitoring the newborn for neurological symptoms.

 Nursing Insight—*Holoprosencephaly*

Holoprosencephaly is a condition in which the cerebral matter fails to form as two distinct hemispheres. There is no fissure between the brain's hemispheres, and often the ventricular system of the brain is malformed. These newborns often have facial deformities from the midline. These defects can be as severe as having one eye or nostril. These newborns are often stillborn or die shortly after birth. Nursing care includes the perinatal bereavement nurse who is sensitive to the grieving needs of the family.

GASTROINTESTINAL CONDITIONS

Cleft Lip and Cleft Palate

Cleft lip (CL), cleft palate (CP), or both is a multifactorial congenital defect that has genetic and environmental predispositions. It is the fourth most common congenital birth defect that occurs in 1:500 to 1:10,000 births. During intrauterine fetal life the primary palate does not fully fuse, and any one of several variations of clefts can occur depending on the timing of the insult. CL is sometimes detected prenatally on ultrasound (Gabrielli, Piva, Perolo, DeSantis, Bevini, Bonasoni, et al., 2009).

Signs and Symptoms

- Unilaterally or bilaterally cleft lip
- Can occur with or without a cleft of the hard and/or soft palate
- Both or either of the palates can have a cleft without the lip
- Uvula can also contain a cleft

Diagnosis

CL is obvious, but CPs call for a thorough examination of the newborn's mouth with a good light source.

Nursing Care. The focus of nursing care for CL or CP (or both) is on maintaining adequate nutrition. The nurse understands that newborns with CL and CP can be successfully breastfed. Breastfeeding may be interrupted for a period of time based on the need for surgical repair. Bottle feeding is initiated with a special nipple that is longer than a regular nipple to help prevent aspiration. Another type of nipple is the **Haberman feeder** (Fig. 19-18), which is longer and has a reservoir to regulate the flow of formula. Newborns with clefts are fed in an upright position to decrease the incidence of regurgitation and aspiration.

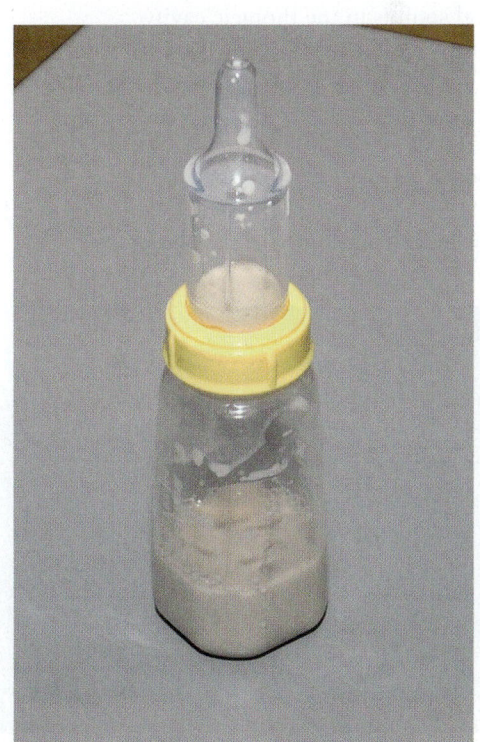

Figure 19-18 Haberman feeder.

Surgical Care. Surgical repair of CL is typically done at 3 months of age, and CPs are usually repaired before 18 months. Some clefts require more than one surgical procedure to reconstruct.

Education/ Discharge Instructions

Parents must be supported by having all the treatments, feeding methods, and care measures explained. Emotional support is needed to assist in the grieving process of dealing with the reality of the "non-perfect" child with possible ongoing surgical needs and feeding problems. Later in life the infant may experience psychosocial problems because of facial deformity.

 Across Care Settings: **The child with cleft lip or cleft palate**

The nurse provides parents with emotional support related to their newborn's cleft lip and palate repair. The nurse can also refer parents to reputable Web sites that contain valuable information. Some Web sites provide the parents with suggestions on wording for the birth announcement so that family and friends are informed about this issue prior to seeing the baby.

RESPIRATORY CONDITIONS

Congenital Diaphragmatic Hernia (CDH)

CDH is a condition in which the diaphragm is not developmentally complete, and abdominal organs displace into the thoracic cavity taking up the room needed for proper lung development. It occurs in approximately 1 in 2,200 newborns. Survival rate is 50% (Watson, 2012).

Signs and Symptoms

Signs and symptoms of CDH include respiratory distress at birth with diminished breath sounds and difficulty in ventilating the newborn. Additional signs and symptoms include:

- Bowel sounds in the thoracic cavity
- Cyanosis
- Bradycardia
- Barrel chest
- Scaphoid abdomen

Diagnosis

In CDH a chest x-ray shows bowel loops in the thoracic cavity and displaced heart (Fig. 19-19).

Prevention

There is no prevention for CDH. Early detection of CDH in utero can assist the family to deliver at a Level III neonatal intensive care unit (NICU) center that is capable of extracorporeal membrane oxygenation (ECMO) and other emergency care measures needed for the infant's survival.

Collaborative Care

Nursing Care. The priority nursing intervention is to maintain the newborn's airway and oxygenation. It is also important to ensure a nasogastric tube is in place to decrease bowel distention (Watson, 2012).

Medical Care. Respiratory support and possibly ECMO is needed to stabilize the newborn for impending surgery.

Surgical Care. The newborn's diaphragm is surgically closed once the bowel is returned to the abdomen (Martin et al., 2011).

ABDOMINAL WALL DEFECTS

Gastroschisis and Omphalocele

Gastroschisis is a congenital anomaly that is usually diagnosed during a prenatal ultrasound. In gastroschisis, the stomach and intestine herniate through the abdominal wall (Fig. 19-20).

Omphalocele (exomphalos) is a congenital condition in which the intestines protrude into the umbilical cord region of the abdominal wall. It is often associated with trisomy 13 and 18 and urinary tract anomalies.

Signs and Symptoms

Signs and symptoms in gastroschisis include:

- The abdominal wall fails to close, usually on the right side of the umbilicus, and the intestines are exposed (Kemp, 2011).

Signs and symptoms in omphalocele include:

- The intestines are covered only by a thin layer of tissue and can be easily seen (the abdominal wall defect is greater than 4 cm). Note: if the defect is less than 4 cm it is usually considered an umbilical hernia and does not usually require repair.

Diagnosis

Diagnosis of either defect is made by visualization and assessment of the defect.

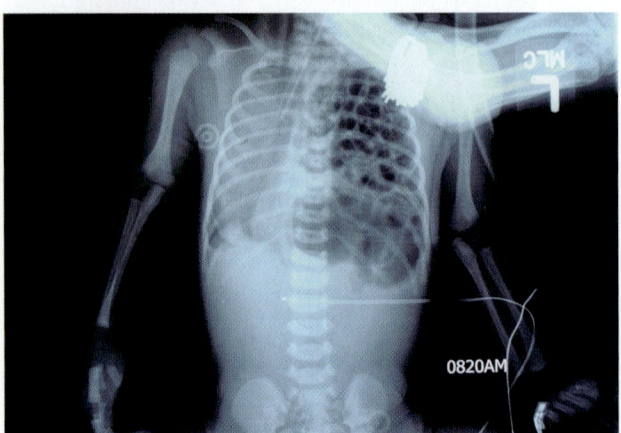

Figure 19-19 X-ray of infant with congenital diaphragmatic hernia (CDH), note bowel loops in the left side of the chest and the displaced heart.

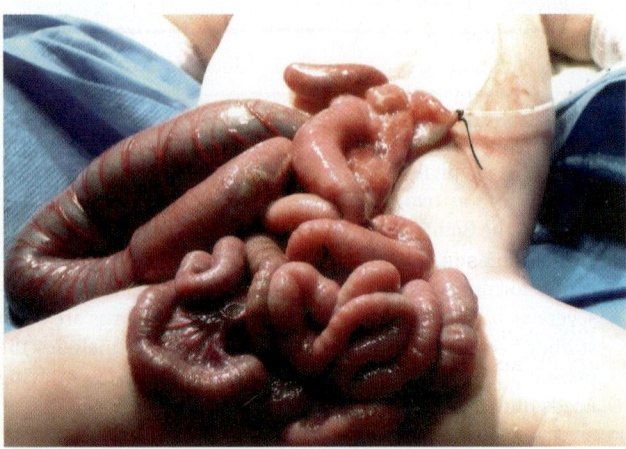

Figure 19-20 The newborn with gastroschisis.

Prevention

Although gastroschisis and omphalocele cannot be prevented, early detection in utero can occur with good prenatal care. Good prenatal nutrition has been linked with better outcomes for newborns who experience these conditions.

Collaborative Care

Nursing Care. For a newborn with gastroschisis, the nurse keeps the abdominal contents sterile by covering them with moist gauze and wrapped in plastic. The intestines are positioned above the level of the defect to maintain a sterile environment. Often the bowel is placed in a silo and reduced back into the abdomen over a few days. Extreme care is taken to position the newborn supine and prevent the mesenteric vessels from kinking so adequate blood supply continues to flow to the bowel. Both conditions (gastroschisis and omphalocele) may require either a nasogastric or orogastric tube placement to eliminate air in the bowel.

Medical Care. Fluids are replaced IV at 1.5 times the normal maintenance volume because of insensible water loss from the exposed bowel in gastroschisis. Antibiotics are started preoperatively to prevent against infection. For larger bowel exposure, a silo device is used to cover the abdominal contents, and they are pushed back into the abdominal cavity gradually over 7 to 10 days. Then repair is accomplished.

Surgical Care. Surgery is performed as soon as possible to prevent intestinal atresia, which could result in obstruction. Many times, surgical repair is done within 2 to 4 hours of birth if the repair can be accomplished in one stage. The amount of displaced intestines determines the course of treatment of an omphalocele. Postoperative care for either condition focuses on fluid and electrolyte balance, nutritional support with **total parental nutrition (TPN)** through a central line, infection protection, and pain management.

Education/Discharge Instructions

Parents must be kept informed about the newborn's condition and treatment regimens while the newborn is hospitalized and then taught how to care for the infant at home.

INFECTIONS IN THE NEWBORN

Herpes Simplex

Genital herpes simplex virus (HSV-2) is one of the fastest growing sexually transmitted infections in the United States. Mothers who contract a primary infection in the third trimester are more likely to transmit the infection to the newborn than those who had primary cases preconceptually. Most infections are transferred during vaginal delivery. A small percentage of newborns can acquire an HSV-2 infection transplacentally in utero or through reoccurring genital infections. Newborns can acquire HSV type 1 infections from people in the environment with herpes lesions of the mouth. Disseminated infections (involving multiple organs) carry a high mortality rate and chance for neurological sequelae. HSV-2 can be disseminated or localized involving brain, skin, eyes, or mouth.

Signs and Symptoms

Genital herpes simplex virus has signs and symptoms that include:

- Vesicular rash over the infant's presenting part at delivery (Watson, 2012)

Diagnosis

HSV-2 can be cultured from the stool, urine, cerebrospinal fluid, conjunctivae, nasopharynx, and skin.

Prevention

Mothers with active genital herpes have a cesarean birth to decrease the likelihood the newborn will come in contact with a genital lesion. There is no guarantee that newborns born by cesarean birth will not develop herpes virus.

Collaborative Care

Nursing Care. Nursing care for the newborn involves the administration of acyclovir (Avirax) for a minimum of 14 days after birth (Martin et al., 2011). For newborns who develop lesions, it is important to keep them clean and dry to prevent a secondary bacterial infection. Pain management for newborns who develop lesions is also essential.

Education/Discharge Instructions

The emphasis of teaching is to decrease the newborn's contact with any active herpes lesions. Parents should be taught to avoid newborn contact with individuals with active lesions on the face or lips.

Neonatal Sepsis

The incidence of neonatal sepsis is 1:1,000 to 10:1,000 for newborns but is increased in the high-risk newborn population to 13:1,000 to 27:1,000. Mortality rates can be anywhere from 13% to 50%. Newborn sepsis is a systemic infection and can be a result of any number of causes. The most common causes include preterm delivery, prolonged labor, rupture of membranes greater than 18 hours, maternal fever, amnionitis, or maternal group B streptococcal infection. Sepsis is classified according to the time of onset. Early onset occurs within the first 5 to 7 days of life and can progress rapidly. Late-onset sepsis is most common after a week of life, and it often results in meningitis. **Nosocomial sepsis** occurs in high-risk newborns who have extended periods of stay in the NICU. Table 19-7 lists the most common causes of neonatal sepsis according to onset of symptoms.

Signs and Symptoms

Sepsis in the newborn may be asymptomatic, so risk factors and maternal history need to be evaluated carefully. When symptoms do appear, the first indications of sepsis may include:

- Behavioral changes, which is a good reason to have consistent nursing care in the nursery and NICU because a nurse who "knows the newborn" may pick up subtle changes earlier than someone who has not previously cared for the newborn
- Hypothermia
- Lethargy
- Hypoglycemia

Table 19-7 Most Common Causes of Neonatal Sepsis Broken Down Into Onset of Symptoms	
Early Onset and Late Onset	**Nosocomial Onset**
Group B streptococci (GBS)	*Staphylococci epidermidis*
Listeria monocytogenes	*Pseudomonas*
Staphylococcus	*Klebsiella*
Streptococci	Serratia
Haemophilus influenzae	Proteus

- Poor feeding
- Apnea
- Bradycardia

Diagnosis

The diagnostic work-up includes a complete blood count with differential, C-reactive protein level, platelet count, and blood culture. Some "septic work-ups" may also include a spinal tap and urinalysis. No one test is sensitive, so an evaluation of all the data is important. Neutropenia (low neutrophils in the blood) is a significant sign because neutrophils battle bacterial infections and are depleted if the newborn has an infection. Many nurseries use a formula that analyzes the ratio of immature to total neutrophils (I/T ratio) in the white blood cell count. Most neutrophils should be segmented (SEGS) or mature cells. When 20% to 25% of the neutrophils are immature or there are bands (sometimes called juveniles or stabs) or unsegmented neutrophils, it is suspicious of an infection. If a shift of 0.3 or greater is detected, the newborn is treated for sepsis.

Prevention

Good hand washing and minimization of invasive procedures when possible is effective in preventing neonatal sepsis.

Collaborative Care

Nursing Care. Nursing care measures include:

- Maintaining accurate intake and output
- Administering antibiotics on time
- Monitoring cardiorespiratory status
- Minimizing the newborn's energy expenditure

Medical Care. Antibiotic treatment is started for a minimum of 48 hours at which time the reports on the cultured specimens are known. A broad-spectrum antibiotic or a combination of antibiotics is started as soon as possible.

Medications. The usual antibiotics of choice are ampicillin (Marcillin) and gentamicin (Garamycin) (Martin et al., 2011).

 Nursing Insight—*Group B streptococcus (GBS) infection in the newborn*

Group B streptococcus (GBS) is the leading cause of neonatal sepsis in the United States. One in three women has colonized GBS in the vagina, and it can be spread to the newborn during the labor process, which is called vertical transmission. Before the recognition of GBS as a cause of newborn sepsis in the 1970s, the mortality rate was 55%. Today, mortality rate is less than 5% of those newborns contracting GBS because of protocols in place to treat women in labor or to treat the newborn if the woman was not adequately treated in labor. All women should be screened for GBS at 35 to 37 weeks of gestation.

 Labs: Differential White Blood Cell Count

The formula for an I/T ratio is bands divided by segs + bands or

$$\frac{bands}{segs + bands}$$

$$\frac{7\ bands}{54 + 7} = 0.11\ shift$$

Example:
This is less than 0.3 shift and is not indicative of an infection.

Table 19-8	Drugs That Can Cause Withdrawal Symptoms	
Opiates	**Barbiturates**	**Others**
Codeine	Butalbital	Alcohol
Heroin	Phenobarbital	Amphetamine
Meperidine	Secobarbital	Chlordiazepoxide
Methadone		Clomipramine
Morphine		Cocaine
Pentazocine		Desmethylimipramine
Propoxyphene		Diazepam
		Diphenhydramine
		Ethchlorvynol
		Fluphenazine
		Glutethimide
		Hydroxyzine
		Imipramine
		Meprobamate
		Phencyclidine

What if the newborn is born prematurely and a GBS culture on the mother was never done? For newborns delivered in which the maternal GBS status is unknown because of premature delivery or inadequate prenatal care, the newborns are carefully observed for signs of sepsis including poor feeding, inability to maintain body temperature, inability to maintain blood glucose level over 60 mg/dL, lethargy, and seizure activity (Edmond & Zaidi, 2010).

DEVELOPMENTAL DELAYS

Neonatal Abstinence Syndrome (NAS)

There are 250,000 to 300,000 female IV drug abusers in the United States. More than 50% of them are in the childbearing age group. An infant of a drug-abusing mother (IDAM) is a newborn who has been exposed to drugs in the intrauterine environment, which can cause withdrawal symptoms in the extrauterine environment (Table 19-8). Drugs that are abused have low molecular weight and transfer easily across the placenta. These drugs have a long half-life in the fetus and bind to central nervous system receptors, causing fetal cell damage. Some drugs such as cocaine are vasoconstrictors and affect blood flow to the fetus. Newborns exposed to heroin usually display symptoms about 48 hours after delivery, and newborns exposed to alcohol begin symptoms 12 hours after delivery (Watson, 2012). Newborns who require sedation and long-term narcotic pain management may also experience NAS once the narcotics are withdrawn from care.

Signs and Symptoms

Box 19-16 lists the signs and symptoms of withdrawal or neonatal abstinence syndrome (NAS) to determine if a newborn is an IDAM.

Box 19-16 Signs of Neonatal Abstinence Syndrome

Irritability	Hypertonia
Tremors	Seizures
Wakefulness	Exaggerated rooting reflex
Uncoordinated feeding pattern	Regurgitation and vomiting
Loose stools	Tachypnea or apnea
Yawning or hiccups	Sneezing and stuffy nose
Poor weight gain	Lacrimation and profuse sweating

---

 focus on safety

Neonatal abstinence syndrome (NAS)

Intrauterine stress (hypoxia) accelerates lung maturity (Watson, 2012). Respiratory distress syndrome is a condition not to be expected in a heroin-addicted newborn.

Diagnosis

Laboratory tests are often done to reveal if the drugs are in the newborn's system. Urine tests are most frequently done but reflect only the last few days of intrauterine environmental exposure. The newborn's meconium stool and hair specimens are being used more and more to test for drugs in the newborn's system. These specimens can be obtained up to 3 days and reflect a longer period of time of intrauterine exposure than urine testing.

Prevention

To prevent NAS, good prenatal care is needed with referral to substance abuse treatment center.

Collaborative Care

Nursing Care. Newborns with NAS are a nursing challenge because they sleep very little and are very irritable. Providing a quiet and dark environment helps the infant sleep. Gently rock and hold the infant to provide comfort and security. Some infants prefer not to be held. Newborns who have tested positive for drugs or display signs and symptoms of NAS are assessed using a neonatal abstinence scoring tool approximately every 3 hours.

Newborns with neonatal abstinence scores greater than 7 for three consecutive scorings are uncomfortable and need to be treated with medication to decrease the severity of the withdrawal effects. Mothers addicted to methadone are sometimes encouraged to breastfeed to offset withdrawal symptoms in the newborns (McQueen, Murphy-Oikonen, Gerlach, & Montelpare, 2011).

 Nursing Insight—Using naloxone (Narcan) in a newborn with neonatal abstinence syndrome

Naloxone (Narcan) use may increase the severity of drug withdrawal in an infant of a drug-abusing mother. If the mother is a suspected drug abuser, it should not be used. If an infant of a drug-abusing mother is in respiratory distress at the time of delivery, use positive pressure oxygen to resuscitate the newborn.

Medications. Box 19-17 lists the medications used to treat an infant of a drug-abusing mother.

Box 19-17 Medications Used to Treat an Infant of a Drug-Abusing Mother

paregoric (Camphorated Tincture of Opium)	chlorpromazine (Thorazine)
phenobarbital (Luminal)	diazepam (Valium)
clonidine (Catapres)	methadone (Dolophine)

Sudden Infant Death Syndrome

"Back to Sleep" is the American Academy of Pediatrics' (AAP, 2011b) campaign to educate parents and families who are involved in newborn care to prevent sudden newborn death syndrome (SIDS) by positioning all newborns supine to sleep. Since U.S. public education started in the early 1990s, there has been a 50% reduction rate in SIDS deaths, but the decrease has leveled off and a new campaign has been initiated that includes educating the public on safe sleep environments that can reduce the risk of not only SIDS but also suffocation, asphyxia, and entrapment. Sudden unexpected newborn death is the term used for the death of a newborn that can not be explained nor the cause can be determined and unexplained such as SIDS. Premature newborns are at an increased risk for SIDS (AAP, 2011b).

Prevention

The recommendations from the AAP (2011b) for a safe sleep environment include:

- "Back to Sleep" for every sleep
- Firm mattress
- Keep the newborn in parent's room, NOT in the parent's bed
- Remove all soft objects and loose bedding from the crib
- No smoking during pregnancy or in the house of a newborn
- Offer a pacifier at nap time and bedtime
- Do not let the newborn get overheated (AAP, 2011b)

Education/Discharge Instructions

Priority nursing care includes education about sudden newborn death. The following recommendations are

---

 Global Health Case Study Underdeveloped Country

The nurse is working on a mission to an underdeveloped country. Many of the families at the set-up clinic have multiple children, many of whom are under the age of 1. As the missionary nurse, you are educating parents to safely sleep newborns. Most of the families do not own a crib. Many families use family beds. Two families have told you that they have cribs that are family heirlooms that were passed down from their grandparents. Another family tells you they "papoose" their babies so they sleep better.

critical thinking questions

1. What is the priority educational piece to enforce while teaching?

2. How would you approach the subject of the family bed?

3. How would you teach families about using old cribs?

4. Would you discuss with families the culture of using a blanket to tightly wrap their newborns at night?

◆ See Suggested Answers to Global Health Case Studies on DavisPlus.

incorporated into the care of the preterm newborn in the NICU. Newborns who have been in the NICU and are preparing for discharge in the near future must be taught to sleep on their backs even though the prone position may have been used as a care intervention to increase gastric motility. Home monitors are not recommended for SIDS prevention although preterm newborns may be sent home on monitoring for other reasons. Most preterm newborns are well acquainted with a pacifier long before their discharge date to assist with their sucking and swallowing coordination, so this practice is continued.

 Now Can You—Discuss conditions that affect the newborn?

1. Describe different congenital conditions that may affect the newborn?
2. Plan nursing care for newborns with specific congenital conditions?
3. Educate parents on high-risk newborn care?

Discharge Planning

Discharge planning must be started as soon as the newborn is admitted to the neonatal intensive care unit (NICU). Most NICUs use standards for discharge such as respiratory stability, consistent weight gain, and successful oral feedings as discharge criteria. Nursing follow-up and phone calls decrease parental anxiety and increase follow-up (Nehra, Pici, Visintainer, & Kase, 2009). Parents have to assimilate large amounts of information including selecting a pediatrician and preparing the home for the infant. Not all parents report feeling ready and having confidence in their child's health and maturity and their readiness for their newborn's needs (Smith, Young, Pursley, McCormick, & Zupancic, 2009). Discharge instructions for NICU newborns are extensive and include parental education on:

- Cardiopulmonry resuscitation
- Environmental and sleep safety
- Car seat training
- Monitor training
- Recognition of danger signs and illness
- Medication administration
- Oxygen therapy
- Skin care
- Formula preparation or breastfeeding instructions
- Vitamin administration

The newborn at risk may have immediate and long-term disabilities. Newborns are extremely resilient, but the lack of neurological development associated with interrupted intrauterine growth affects them not only physically but socially and developmentally. NICU "graduates" often need intensive follow-up care. They are sometimes referred to specialists for sight and hearing follow-up (Wittmann-Price & Pope, 2002). Other follow-up appointments may include:

- Ophthalmologist
- Physical therapy
- Occupational therapy
- Developmental specialist
- Neurologist
- Registered Dietitian
- Speech Pathologist

 legal alert—Ophthalmologist appointments

Be sure that ophthalmologist appointments are made before the family is discharged because retinopathy of prematurity is a time-sensitive condition, and poor scheduling has resulted in newborn blindness (Scott et al., Wittmann-Price, & Thear, 2008).

 Collaboration in Caring—*Nurse case managers*

Nurse case managers are an invaluable resource in the NICU when coordinating follow-up efforts with families and issues regarding insurance reimbursement plans.

 Complementary Care: *Social Events*

Many NICU units host social events that increase parent-to-parent support after discharge.

Summary Points

- Newborns can be put at risk any time during their intrauterine or extrauterine development, by genetic disorders, congenital anomalies, maternal factors, asphyxia, or birth injuries resulting from conditions such as hypothermia, poor oxygenation, prematurity, or congenital anomalies.

- Small-for-gestational-age (SGA) newborns can be born at any gestational age and have a birth weight that falls below the 10th percentile on the growth chart and have suffered a nutritional or oxygenation deficit in utero because of maternal causes, fetal causes, or a placenta or cord malfunction.

- Newborns who are large for gestational age (LGA) are over the 90th percentile on the growth chart because of genetics or, more commonly, have been exposed to an imbalance of nutrients in utero.

- Newborns with a diabetic mother are often LGA. LGA newborns are also at risk for transient tachypnea, hypoglycemia, hypocalcemia, hypomagnesemia, birth injuries, brachial plexus injuries, and fractures.

- Postterm newborns are at high risk for complications such as meconium aspiration pneumonia and persistent pulmonary hypertension.

- Premature newborns are at risk for respiratory distress syndrome, apnea of prematurity, jaundice, retinopathy of prematurity, anemia of prematurity, and sudden infant death syndrome.

- Appropriate developmental care in the NICU is key to decreasing long-term developmental disabilities for the preterm newborn.

- Discharge planning includes respiratory stability, consistent weight gain, and successful oral feedings.

Discharge planning must be started as soon as the newborn is admitted to the NICU.

◆ Newborns with metabolic disorders are screened after they are 24 hours old and if diagnosed are placed on therapeutic diets for life.

◆ Surgical emergencies occur in the newborn, and when organs are outside the body, nursing priority is to cover them with warm, sterile, wet dressings.

Review Questions

Multiple Choice

1. Immediate conditions that pose nursing concerns for the small-for-gestational-age (SGA) newborn include which of the following?
   A. Long-term chronic or end-of-life care
   B. Bronchopulmonary dysplasia and ischemia
   C. Muscle contractures and hyperthermia
   D. Hypothermia and pain management

2. Upon assessing the newborn, the nurse notes shallow rapid respirations, palmar sweating, decreased oxygen saturation, and a high-pitched cry. These clinical assessments are indicative of which of the following?
   A. A neurological problem
   B. Hypoglycemia
   C. Pain
   D. Transient tachypnea of the newborn (TTN)

3. A 24-hour-old newborn is being treated for hyper-bilirubinemia with phototherapy bilirubin lights. The patient is in an incubator fully undressed. Which of the following nursing actions are inconsistent with best practice for this type of infant?
   A. Apply eye patches and a covering over the genital area
   B. Administer proper nutrition to ensure the clearance of bilirubin
   C. Apply a head covering (stockinet hat) to prevent heat loss
   D. Maintain adequate hydration to promote excretion of bilirubin

4. A 42-week gestational-aged newborn is assessed 20 hours after delivery by the nurse. On assessment, the nurse auscultates rales and rhonchi and notes the newborn is tachypneic and has meconium-stained nails. The nurse suspects that the newborn has
   A. sepsis.
   B. meconium aspiration pneumonia.
   C. transient tachypnea of the newborn (TTN).
   D. respiratory distress syndrome (RDS).

5. A 30-week gestational-aged neonate has anemia of prematurity. The neonatologist has ordered recombinant human erythropoietin 250 units/kg subcutaneous 3 times a week. Which intervention does the nurse implement related to this medication?
   A. Administering the medication prior to feedings
   B. Applying pressure to the injection site for 5 min
   C. Assessing hematocrit levels as per hospital policy
   D. Assessing electrolyte levels weekly

6. A nurse is caring for a premature infant in the neonatal intensive care unit (NICU). When does the nurse begin discharge planning?
   A. On the baby's admission to the NICU
   B. 1 week prior to planned discharge
   C. When parents are able to learn about care
   D. When the baby is medically stable

7. A premature infant has frequent apnea episodes, and the physician orders mild stimulation when these occur. To perform this intervention correctly, what does the nurse do?
   A. Flick the heels of the infant's feet
   B. Increase the oxygen flow rate
   C. Shake the baby by the shoulders
   D. Speak loudly to the infant

8. A premature infant born at 35 weeks' gestational age is being discharged pending the results of an Infant Care Seat Challenge. During the testing, the infant has three episodes of apnea lasting longer than 20 seconds. Which action by the nurse is best?
   A. Arrange for the parents to get an apnea-bradycardia monitor for the trip
   B. Have the parents bring a different car seat to try with the infant
   C. Instruct the parents to use supplemental oxygen on the trip home
   D. Support the parents as they cope with the delay in the baby's discharge

9. A nurse assessing an infant notes the baby has been constipated, is lethargic, and is hypotonic. Which laboratory tests does the nurse anticipate being ordered?
   A. Complete blood count
   B. Direct bilirubin
   C. Hemoglobin and hematocrit
   D. Thyroxine and triiodothyronine

10. The charge nurse in the neonatal intensive care unit wants to create an atmosphere that is more conducive to developmental growth of their premature infants. Which nursing care action by the staff would best accomplish that goal?
    A. Instruct the nurses to use quiet gentle voices
    B. Maintain low, soothing lighting at all times
    C. Position infants with limbs in an extended position
    D. Wake the babies up every hour to stimulate them

See Answers to End of Chapter Review Questions on Davis*Plus*.

REFERENCES

Abzug, J. M., & Kozin, S. H. (2010). Current concepts: Neonatal brachial plexus palsy. *Orthopedics, 33*(6), 430–437. doi:10.3928/01477447-20100429-25

Agar, N. J. M., & Berkowitz, R. G. (2011). Airway complications of pédiatrie extracorporeal membrane oxygénation. *Annals of Otology. Rhinology & Laryngology l20*(6), 353–357.

Als, H., & McAnulty, G. B. (2011). The Newborn Individualized Developmental Care and Assessment Program (NIDCAP) with Kangaroo Care: Comprehensive care for preterm infants. *Current Women's Health Reviews, 7*(3), 288–301.

Amendolia, B. (2011). An integrative review of feeding intolerance in preterm infants: State of the science. *Clinical Scholars Review, 4*(2), 82–90.

American Academy of Pediatrics (AAP). (2004). Clinical Practice Guidelines. Management of Hyperbilirubinemia in the Newborn 35 or More Weeks of Gestation, Subcommittee on Hyperbilirubinemia. *Pediatrics, 114*(1), 297–316.

American Academy of Pediatrics (AAP). (2011a). Committee on Fetus and Newborn: Clinical Report: Postnatal Glucose Homeostasis in Late-Preterm and Term Newborns. *Pediatrics, 127*(3) 575–579. doi:10.1542/peds.2010-3851

American Academy of Pediatrics (AAP). (2011b). SIDS and other sleep-related newborn deaths: Expansion of recommendations for a safe newborn sleeping environment. *Pediatrics, 128*(5), e1341–e1367. doi:10.1542/peds.2011-2284

American Academy of Pediatrics (AAP). (2004, 2009). Reaffirmation of Policy statement: *Age Terminology During the Perinatal Period. Pediatrics, 123*(1), 188.

Antonucci, R., Porcella, A., & Fanos, V. (2009). The infant incubator in the neonatal intensive care unit: Unresolved issues and future developments. *Journal of Perinatal Medicine, 37*(6), 587–598. doi:10.1515/JPM.2009.109

Baba, L. R., McGrath, J. M., & Liu, J. (2010). The efficacy of mechanical vibration analgesia for relief of heel stick pain in neonates: A novel approach. Journal of Perinatal & *Neonatal Nursing, 24*(3), 274–283. doi:10.1097/JPN.0b013e3181ea7350

Bass, J. L. (2010). The Infant Car Seat Challenge: Determining and managing an "abnormal." *Pediatrics, 125*(3), 597–598. doi:10.1542/peds.2009-3344

Batton, D. (2009). Clinical Report—Antenatal counseling regarding resuscitation at an extremely low gestational age, AAP. *Pediatrics, 124*(1), 422–427. doi:10.1542/peds.2009-1060

Bishara, N., & Ohis, R. K. (2009). Current controversies in the treatment of anemia of prematurity. *Seminars in Perinatology, 33*(1), 29–34. doi:10.1053/j.semperi.200810.006

Bulechek, G. M., Butcher, H. K., Dochterman, J. M., & Wagner, C. (2013). *Nursing interventions classification (NIC)* (6th ed.). St. Louis, MO: Elsevier Mosby.

Centers for Disease Control and Prevention (CDC). (2001). Using Tandem Mass Spectrometry for Metabolic Disease Screening Among Newborns. Retrieved from http://www.cdc.gov/mmwr/preview/mmwrhtml/rr5003a1.htm

Centers for Disease Control and Prevention (CDC). (2011a). *Premature Birth*. Retrieved from http://www.cdc.gov/Features/PrematureBirth/

Centers for Disease Control and Prevention (CDC). (2011b). National Newborn Screening Status Report. Retrieved from http://genes-r-us.uthscsa.edu/nbsdisorders.htm .

Crescencio, E. P., Zanelato, S. & Leventhal, L. C. (2009). Assessment and pain relief in newborns. *Revista Eletrônica de Enfermagem, 11*(1), 64–69.

Deakins, K. M. (2009). Bronchopulmonary dysplasia. *Respiratory Care, 54*(9), 1252–1262.

Doenges, M., Moorhouse, M., & Murr, A. (2010). *Nursing diagnosis manual: Planning, individualizing, and documenting client care*. Philadelphia, PA: F.A. Davis.

Edmond, K., & Zaidi, A. (2010). New approaches to preventing, diagnosing and treating newborn sepsis. *PLOS Medical, 7*(3), 2–8.

Gabrielli, S., Piva, M., Perolo, T., DeSantis, A., Bevini, M., Bonasoni, P., et al. (2009). Bilateral cleft lip and palate maxillary protrusion is associated with lethal aneuploides. *Ultrasound in Obstetrics and Gynecology, 34*(4), 416–418. doi:10.1002/uog.6451

Gardner, S. L., Carter, B. S., Enzman-Hines, M., & Hernandez, J. A. (2011). *Merenstein & Gardner's Handbook of neonatal intensive care* (7th ed.). St. Louis, MO: Mosby.

Gillson, S. (2008). *Preventing infant reflux*. Retrieved from http://heartburn.about.com/od/infantschildrenandreflux/a/infantreflux.htm

Giometti, E., Baroni, L., Artese, C., & Davidson, A. (2009). Postural care of newborns in the NICU: A study on nurses' education needs. *Children's Nurses: Italian Journal of Pedia tric Nursing Science, 1*(3), 95–100.

Helou, R., Birenbaum, H. J., Blue, D., Pane, M. A., & Marinkovich, G. A. (2011). The velcro mustache: A potential barrier to effective bag-and-mask ventilation in neonates on nasal CPAP: Two case reports. *Respiratory Care, 56*(7), 1040–1042.

Helsey, L., McDonald, J. V., & Stewart, V. T. (2010). Addressing in-hospital "falls" of new borns. *Joint Commission Journal on Quality & Patient Safety, 36*(7), 327–333.

Henderson-Smart, D. J. & De Paoli, A. G. (2010). Prophylactic methylxanthine for prevention of apnoea in preterm newborns. *Cochrane Database of Systematic Reviews, 12.*

Hornik, C. P., Hartman, M. E., Markert, M. L., Lodge, A. J., Cheifetz, I. M., & Turner, D. A. (2011). Successful extracorporeal membrane oxygenation for respiratory failure in a newborn with DiGeorge anomaly, following thymus transplantation. *Respiratory Care, 56*(6), 866–870. doi:10.4187/respcare.01051

Hummel, P., Lawlor-Klean, P., & Weiss, M. G. (2010). Validity and reliability of the N-PASS assessment tool with acute pain. *Journal of Perinatology, 30*(7), 474–478. doi:10.1038/jp.2009.185

Hummel, P., Puchalski, M., Creech, S. D., & Weiss. M. G. (2008). Clinical reliability and validity of the N-PASS: Neonatal Pain, Agitation and Sedation Scale with prolonged pain. *Journal of Perinatology, 28*(1), 55–60.

Izquierdo-García, E., Fernández-Ferreiro, A., Gomis-Muñoz, P., Herreros de Tejada, A., & Moreno-Villares, J. M. (2011). Liver disease associated with short-term total parenteral nutrition in a pediatric hospital through the course of the year 2008. Nutritional *Therapy & Metabolism, 29*(3), 134–138.

Jain, A., Agarwal, R., Sankar, M. J., Deorari, A., & Paul, V. K. (2010). Hypocalcemia in the newborn. *Indian Journal of Pediatrics, 77*(10), 1123–1128. doi:10.1007/s12098-010-0176-0

Kaempf, J. W., Kaempf, A. J., Wu, Y. Stawarz, M., Niemeyer, J., & Grunkemeier, G. (2011). Hyperglycemia, insulin and slower growth velocity may increase the risk of retinopathy of prematurity. *Journal of Perinatology, 31*(4), 251–257. doi:10.1038/jp.2010.152

Keijzer-Veen, M. G., Dülger, A., Dekker, F. W., Nauta, J., & van der Heijden, B. J. (2010). Very preterm birth is a risk factor for increased systolic blood pressure at a young adult age. *Pediatric Nephrology, 25*, 509–516. doi:10.1007/s00467-009-1373-9

Kemp, J. E. (2011). SASPEN case study. *South African Journal of Clinical Nutrition, 24*(1), 47–48.

Kids Health. (2012). Newborn Screening Tests. Retrieved from http://kidshealth.org/parent/system/medical/newborn_screening_tests.html#

Kumar, P., Sankar, M. J., Deorari, A., Azad, R., Chandra, P., Agarwal, R., & Paul, V. (2011). Risk factors for severe retinopathy of prematurity in preterm low birth weight neonates. *Indian Journal of Pediatrics, 78*(7), 812–816.

Larkin, J. C., Speer, P. D., & Simhan, H. N. (2011). A customized standard of large size for gestational age to predict intrapartum morbidity. *American Journal of Obstetrics & Gynecology, 204*(6), 499.e1–499.e10.

Liu, M., Lin, K., Chou, Y., & Lee, T. (2010). Using non-nutritive sucking and oral glucose solution with neonates to relieve pain: A randomized controlled trial. *Journal of Clinical Nursing, 19*(11–12), 1604–1611. doi:10.1111/j.1365-2702.2009.03014.x

Ludington-Hoe, S. M. (2011). Thirty years of kangaroo care science and practice. *Neonatal Network. 30*(5), 357–362.

Lyon, A. J., & Freer, Y. (2011). Goals and options in keeping preterm babies warm. *Archives of Disease in Childhood—Fetal & Neonatal Edition, 96*(1), F71–F74. doi:10.1136/adc.2009.161158

Ma, X., Huang, C., Lou, S., Lv, Q., Su, W., Tan, J., et al. (2009). The clinical outcomes of late preterm infants: A multi-center survey of Zhejiang, China. *Journal of Perinatal Medicine, 37*(6), 695–699. doi:10.1515/JPM.2009.130

March of Dimes (2011). US Preterm Birth Rate Under 12 Percent, the Lowest Level in Nearly a Decade. Retrieved from: http://www.marchofdimes.com/news/10289.html

Martin, J. B. (2011). Prevention of intraventricular hemorrhages and periventricular leukomalacia in the extremely low birth weight infant. *Newborn and Infant Nursing Review, 11*(3), 141–152. doi:10.1053/j.nainr.2011.07.006

Martin, R. J., Fanaroff, A. A., & Walsh, M. C. (2011). *Fanaroff and Martin's neonatal-perinatal medicine: Diseases of the fetus and newborn* (9th ed.). Philadelphia, PA: Mosby.

Mathew, O. P. (2011). Apnea of prematurity: Pathogenesis and management strategies. *Journal of Perinatology, 31*(5), 302–310. doi:10.1038/jp.2010.126

Matteucci, R., Grose, S., & Pravikoff, D. (2011). Sucrose/glucose administration in newborns with pain. *Cinahl Information Systems, evidence-based care sheet*, 1–2.

Mavrogenis, A. F., Mitsiokapa, E. A., Kanellopoulos, A. D., Ruggieri, P., & Papagelopoulos, P. J. (2011). Birth fracture of the clavicle. *Advances in Neonatal Care, 11*(5): 328–331.

McQueen, J. A., Murphy-Oikonen, K., Gerlach, A. & Montelpare, W. (2011). The impact of infant feeding method on neonatal abstinence scores of methadone exposed infants. *Advances in Neonatal Care, 11*(4), 282–290. doi:10.1097/ANC.0b013e318225a30c

Moorhead, S., Johnson, M., Maas, M. L., & Swanson, E. (2013). *Nursing outcomes classification (NOC)* (5th ed.). St. Louis, MO: Elsevier Mosby.

Morag, I., Strauss, T., Lubin, D., Schushan-Eisen, I., Kenet, G., & Kuint, J. (2011). Restrictive management of neonatal polycythemia. *American Journal of Perinatology, 28*(9), 677–682.

National Institutes of Health (NIH). (2011). *Fractured clavicle in the newborn.* Retrieved from http://www.nlm.nih.gov/medlineplus/ency/article/001588.htm

National Institutes of Health (NIH). (2013). *Retinopathy of prematurity.* Retrieved from http://www.nlm.nih.gov/medlineplus/ency/article/001618.htm

Nehra, V., Pici, M., Visintainer, P., & Kase, J. S. (2009). Indicators of compliance for developmental follow-up of infants discharged from a regional NICU. *Journal of Perinatal Medicine, 37*(6), 677–681. doi:10.1515/JPM.2009.135

Noerr, B. (2000). Neonatal respiratory disease and management strategies, May 18. A continuing education service of Penn State's College of Medicine at the Milton S. Hershey Medical Center. Hershey, PA.

Nuffield Council on Bioethics. (2013). Critical care and decisions in fetal and neonatal medicine: Ethical issues. London, England. Retrieved from www.nuffieldbioethics.org/go/ourwork/neonatal/introduction

Oishi, P., Sanjeev, A. D., & Fineman, J. R. (2011). Advances in the management of pediatric pulmonary hypertension. *Respiratory Care, 56*(9), 1314–1340. doi:10.4187/respcare.01297

Oretti, C., Marino, S., Mosca, F., Colnaghi, M. R., De Iudicibus, D., Drigo, I., et al. (2009). Glutathione-S-transferase-P1I105V polymorphism and response to antenatal betamethasone in the prevention of respiratory distress syndrome. *European Journal of Clinical Pharmacology, 65,* 483–491. doi:10.1007/s00228-009-0617-8

O'Sullivan, A., O'Connor., M, Brosnahan, D., McCreery, K. & Dempsey, E. M. (2010). Sweeten, soothe and swaddle for retinopathy of prematurity screening: A randomised placebo controlled trial. *Archives of Disease in Childhood — Fetal & Neonatal Edition, 95*(6): F419–F422. doi:10.1136/adc.2009.180943

Pinheiro, J., Boynton, S., Furdon, S. A., Dugan, R., & Reu-Donlon, C. (2011). Use of chemical warming packs during delivery room resuscitation is associated with decreased rates of hypothermia in very low-birth-weight neonates. *Advances in Neonatal Care, 11*(5), 357–362.

Raju, T. N. K., Stevenson, D. K., Higgins, R. D. & Stark, A. R. (2009). Safe and effective devices and instruments for use in the neonatal intensive care units. *Biomedical Instrumentation & Technology, 43*(5), 408–418. doi:10.2345/0899-8205-43.5.408

Razek, A. A., & El-Dien, A. Z. (2009). Effect of breast-feeding on pain relief during newborn immunication injections. *International Journal of Nursing Practice, 15*(2), 99–104. doi:10.1111/j.1440-172X.2009.01728.x

Reis, M. D., Rempel, G. R., Scott, S. D., Brady-Fryer, B. A., & Van Aerde, J. (2010). Developing nurse/parent relationship in the NICU through negotiated partnership. *JOGNN, 39,* 675–683. doi:10.1111/j.1552-6909.2010.01189.x

Sahai, I., & Marsden, D. (2009). Newborn screening. *Critical Reviews in Clinical Laboratory Science, 46*(2), 55–82. doi:10.1080/10408360802485305

Sandler, A. D. (2010). Children with spina bifida: Key clinical issues. *Pediatric Clinics of North America, 57*(4), 879–892. doi:10.1016/j.pcl.2010.07.009

Sankar. M. J., Agarwal, R., Deorari, A., & Paul, V. K. (2010). Management of polycythemia in neonates. *Indian Journal of Pediatrics, 77*(10), 1117–1121. doi:10.1007/s12098-010-0177-z

Scott, C., Wittmann-Price, R. A., & Thear, G. (2008). Keeping a watchful eye on retinopathy of prematurity. *Neonatal Network, 27*(5) 355–357.

Shah, P. S., & Ohlsson, A. (2011). Sildenafil for pulmonary hypertension in neonates. *Cochrane Database of Systematic Reviews, 2011*(8).

Shannon, E. G., Hart, E. S., & Grottkau, B. E. (2011). Clavicle fractures in children: The essentials. *Orthopaedic Nursing, 28*(5): 210–216. doi:10.1097/NOR.0b013e3181b57a27

Smith, V. C., Young, S., Pursley, D. M., McCormick, M. C., & Zupancic, J. A. F. (2009). Are families prepared for discharge from the NICU? *Journal of Perinatology, 29*(9), 623–629. doi:10.1038/jp.2009.58

Springer, S. C., Annibale, D. J., & Rosenkranz, T. (2012). *Necrotizing entercolitis.* Retrieved from http://emedicine.medscape.com/article/977956-overview

STABLE Program. (2012). Retrieved from http://www.stableprogram.org/

Standley, J. M., Cassidy, J., Grant, R., Cevasco, A., Szuch, C., Nguyen, J., et al. (2010). The effect of music reinforcement for non-nutritive sucking on nipple feeding of premature infants. *Pediatric Nursing, 36*(3), 138–146.

Stevens, B., Johnston, C., Taddio, A., Gibbins, S., & Yamada, J. (2010). The premature infant pain profile: Evaluation 13 years after development. *Clinical Journal of Pain, 26*(9), 813–830. doi:10.1097/AJP.0b013e3181ed1070

Sundquist, J., Sundquist, K., Johansson, S. E., Li, X., & Winkleby, M. (2011). Mothers, places and small for gestational age births: A cohort study. Archives of Disease in *Childhood, 96*(4), 380–385.

Szabo, N., Pap, C., Kobar, J., Svekus, A., Turi, S., & Sztriha, L. (2009). Primary microcephaly in Hungary: Epidemiology and clinical features. *Acta Peadiatrica, 99,* 690–693. doi:10.1111/j.651-2227.2009.01666x

Thear, G., & Wittmann-Price, R. A. (2006). Project Noise Buster in the NICU. *AJN, 106*(5), 64AA-64EE.

Thear, G., & Wittmann-Price, R. A. (2008). And two become one: Unit integration. *Nursing Management, 39*(1), 20–23.

Tutdibi, E., Gries, K., Bücheler, M., Misselwitz, B., Schlosser, R. L., & Gortner, L. (2010). Impact of labor on outcomes in transient tachypnea of the newborn: Population-based study. *Pediatrics, 125*(3), e577–e583. doi:10.1542/peds.2009-0314

Valenza, T. (2009). Alls quiet in the NICU: Newborn RDS. *The Journal for Respiratory Care Practitioners (RT), 22*(1), 26–29.

Vallerand, A. H., & Sanoski, C. A. (2014). *Davis's drug guide for nurses* (14th ed.). Philadelphia, PA: F.A. Davis.

Van Leeuwen, A. M., Poelhuis-Leth, D. J., & Bladh, M. L. (2011). *Davis's comprehensive handbook of laboratory and diagnostic tests with nursing implications* (4th ed.). Philadelphia, PA: F.A. Davis.

Watson, R. L. (Ed.). (2012). *Certification and core review for neonatal intensive care nursing* (4th ed.). Philadelphia, PA: Elsevier.

Whitfield, J. M., Charsha, D. S., & Chiruvolu, A. (2009). Prevention of meconium aspiration syndrome: An update and the Baylor experience. *Baylor University Medical Center Proceedings, 22*(2), 128–131.

Wiedmeier, J. E., Joss-Moore, L. A. Lane, R. H., & Neu, J. (2011). Early postnatal nutrition and programming of the preterm neonate. *Nutritional Reviews, 69*(2), 76–82. doi:10.1111/j.1753 4887.2010.00370.x

Wiggs, C. M. (2011). Baby John – Nursing reflections on moral agent. *Nursing Ethics, 18*(4), 606–612. doi:10.117/09973301140407

Wiswell, T. E. (2011). Resuscitation in the delivery room: Lung protection from the first breath. *Respiratory Care, 56*(9), 1360–1368.

Wittmann-Price, R. A., & Celia, L. M. (November, 2010). Exploring perceptions of "Do not resuscitate" and " Allowing natural death" among physicians and nurses. *Holistic Nursing Practice, 24*(6), 333–337.

Wittmann-Price, R. A., & Pope, K. A. (2002). Universal newborn hearing screening. *AJN, 102*(11), 71–77.

Yildiz, A., Arikan, D., Gözüm, S., Taştekın, A. & Budancamanak, İ. (2011). The effect of the odor of breast milk on the time needed for transition from gavage to total oral feeding in preterm infants. *Journal of Nursing Scholarship, 43*(3), 265–273. doi:10.1111/j.1547-5069.2011.01410.x

CONCEPT MAP

Nursing Considerations:
- Neutral thermal environment/artificial heat source
- Use pain management protocols
- IV or enteral therapy
- Swaddling/decrease stimuli
- Heel stick blood glucose monitoring
- Correct process for incubator weaning
- Accurate physical assessment
- Monitor lab results

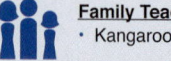
Family Teaching Guidelines:
- Kangaroo care

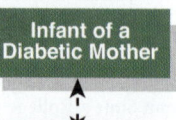
Collaboration in Caring:
- Providing services in high-risk neighborhoods decreases % of SGA infants

Nursing Considerations:
- Monitor blood glucose, serum calcium, magnesium
- Accurate respiratory assessment
- Use of CPAP for TTN
- Positioning for fractures; pinned T-shirt to splint
- Neurovascular checks; assess reflexes and behavior

Infant of a Diabetic Mother

- Cold stress
- Pain
- Hypoglycemia
- Polycythemia

SGA: Small for Gestational Age

LGA: Large for Gestational Age

- Hypoglycemia
- Hypocalcemia
- Hypomagnesemia
- Transient tachypnea
- Birth injuries
  - Brachial plexus
  - Fractures

Preterm Infant

Caring for the Newborn at Risk

Postterm Infant

- Respiratory distress syndrome
- Apnea/anemia of prematurity
- Bronchopulmonary dysplasia
- Jaundice
- Necrotizing enterocolitis
- GERD
- Intracranial hemorrhage
  - Intraventricular
  - Periventricular leukomalacia
- Retinopathy of prematurity

Other Conditions → High-Risk Newborn:
- Metabolic: e.g., PKU, galactosemia
- Endocrine: C.H.
- Neurological: e.g., anencephaly; microcephaly
- GI: cleft lip/palate
- Infections/neonatal sepsis
- SIDS
- Developmental delays

- Meconium aspiration pneumonia
  - Pneumothorax
  - Pneumonmediastinum
- Persistent pulmonary hypertension

Nursing Considerations:
- Chest physiotherapy
- O_2 administration/CPAP/mechanical ventilation
- Inhaled nitric oxide (iNO)
- Last resort: ECMO

Nursing Considerations:
- Thorough ongoing assessment
- Airway maintenance/oxygenation → cannula, CPAP, mechanical ventilation, ECMO
- C-R monitor; BP; pulse ox: prevent O_2 fluctuation
- Phototherapy per bilirubin level
- Nutritional support
- Monitory hydration status; I&O
- Ophthalmologist consult ROP

Critical Nursing Action:
- Proper placement of skin probes
- Infant car seat challenge for < 37 wks gestational age
- NEC: abdominal circumference, bowel sounds, residual check, record stools
- ROP prevention: lowest O_2 level for sat of 92%
- Assess head circumference/fontanel: report sudden changes; neuro assessment IVH + PVL
- Phototherapy: cover eyes/genitalia; monitor temp, bilirubin; adequate hydration/nutrition

Where Research and Practice Meet:
- Breastfeeding decreases effect of painful stimuli during painful procedures
- Lullaby music therapy increases NNS

Nursing Insight:
- The smaller, more preterm → high RDS risk
- Metabolic acidosis increases pulmonary resistance
- Differentiate between apnea and periodic breathing
- Group B-strep is leading cause of neonatal sepsis
- Naloxone may increase severity of withdrawal in infants of drug-abusing mother
- Jaundice in breastfeeding infants often resolves on its own

Focus on Safety:
- Use warming packs specifically for SGA
- Hypoglycemia: may be asymptomatic → accurate I&O
- Place CPAP nasal prongs properly
- Handle newborn with fractures gently
- Increasing concerns with newborn falls
- Immediate attention needed for apneic/bradycardic/desaturation episodes
- Slow feeding in upright position to prevent aspiration in GERD

Now Can You:
- Identify SGA, LGA, pre- and postterm infants by clinical characteristics
- Safely care for the high-risk newborn using evidence-based practices

one
two
three
four
five
six
seven

Caring for the Child and Family

Caring for the Developing Child

chapter

20

> "It is when we include caring and love in our science, we discover our caring-healing professions and disciplines are much more than a detached scientific endeavor, but a life-giving and life-receiving endeavor for humanity."
>
> —Watson, 2005 p. 3

LEARNING TARGETS *At the completion of this chapter, the student will be able to:*

- ◆ Describe the principles inherent in the developmental process.
- ◆ Identify and explain the theories of growth and development.
- ◆ Discuss the components for each developmental stage.
- ◆ Address anticipatory guidance for each developmental stage.
- ◆ Develop a developmental care plan for the child and family.

PICO(T) Questions

The intent of evidence-based practice (EBP) is to provide nursing care that integrates the best available evidence. An initial step in EBP is to write a PICO(T) question that effectively guides the research. A PICO(T) question is an acronym that stands for population (P), intervention or issue (I), comparison of interest (C), outcome (O), and timeframe (T). Depending on the question, all or some of the question components are used in the research process. Use these

PICO(T) questions to spark your thinking as you read the chapter.

1. Does (I) being raised in a single-parent household (O) impact behavioral development (P) in toddlers?

2. Do (P) preschool-age children without siblings who attend group day care (I) develop physical skills (O) at the same rate on average as (C) preschool children with siblings who do not attend group day care?

Evidence-Based Practice

Bigbee, J. L., Musil, C., & Kenski, D. (2011). The health of caregiving grandmothers: A rural-urban comparison. *The Journal of Rural Health 27*, 289–296.

The purpose of this study was to compare the characteristics of rural and urban caregiving grandmothers to include physical and mental health. The study compares demographic data and differences in physical and mental health between these populations. According to national statistics, the past two decades have seen an increase in the number of grandparents raising or providing care for their grandchildren. It is estimated that over 2.4 million grandparents are responsible for grandchildren in their homes.

Factors impacting these numbers include incarcerated parents, mental illness, substance abuse, death, and child abuse or neglect. Statistics indicate the following:

- One in ten grandparents provide child care for at least 6 months or more.
- Two-thirds of grandparents providing care are under the age of 60.

(continued)

Evidence-Based Practice (continued)

- Over half of the grandparents providing care are non-Hispanic white.
- Two-thirds of the grandparents providing care are female.
- 70% of the grandparents providing care are employed.
- 30% of the grandparents providing care are disabled.

Previous research has examined the health of grandparents in the parenting role with mixed findings though some have implied that grandparents experience higher rates of depression, anxiety, diabetes, hypertension, insomnia, and limitations to activity. Those studies have speculated that these findings may be related to the physical demands, financial stress, social isolation, cramped housing, and time needed for child care. Other studies have disputed these findings and noted that, though some grandparents indicate an initial decline in their health, this disappears over time. Inconsistent results have been found in studies comparing self-assessed physical health and incidence of anxiety and depression when comparing the caregiving grandparent or custodial grandparents with non-caregiving grandparents as well as inconsistent findings among grandparents of various ethnicities. The authors cite a recently completed small pilot study of 11 caregiver grandparents from one rural, northwestern state and found health problems to include diabetes (36%), hypertension (36%), hyperlipidemia (18%), and fibromyalgia (18%). The authors further state that little research has been done comparing caregiving grandparents living in rural and urban settings.

Participants in this study included 485 caregiving grandmothers from one northeastern state. All of the grandmothers were part of a larger longitudinal study. The participants in the study had at least one grandchild younger than 16 years of age. Participants were assigned to one of three groups: primary, multigenerational, or traditional. Primary caregivers refers to grandmothers raising grandchildren without the parents living in the residence. The multigenerational arrangement includes the grandmother, one or more grandchildren, and the parent(s) of the grandchild or grandchildren. The traditional arrangement refers to families in which the grandmother lives within an hour's drive, retains close contact with the family, and provides less than 20 hours of care to the grandchildren per week. Participants were recruited through a random digit dialing system. Participants were placed into either rural or urban groups based on their zip codes. Based on this classification, there were 388 (80%) participants in the urban group and 97 (20%) of the participants in the rural group, which the researchers indicated was a fair representation of the state's population.

This study was a comparative retrospective study and included a secondary analysis of data reported from an earlier large longitudinal study. Participants were mailed a consent form and the SF-36 survey along with a stamped return envelope. Those who returned the survey received a $15.00 incentive when the survey was returned. The SF-36 survey contained 36 items, which measured physical and mental health status as self-reported. The SF-36 survey had previously been used in more than 200 studies and found to be reliable and valid. Items were rated using an 8-point scale. An additional 20-item CES-D (Center for Epidemiological Studies Depression Scale) depressive symptoms survey was also included. This survey used a four-point scale with responses ranging from 0 to 4 (0, 1, 2, 3, 4). Total scores of 16 or higher on this scale indicated an increased risk for clinical depression. Demographic variables including race, marital status, age, and work status were also compared.

The mean age for the grandmothers in the rural setting was 56.6 years and in the urban setting 57.1 years. Significant differences were noted in the demographics between the urban and rural participants. The urban participant population was 59.6% white and 36.6% African American versus 89.7% white and 4.1% African American in the rural setting. Other racial groups represented very small percentages. Sixty-seven percent of the rural grandmothers were married compared with 52.1% of the urban grandmothers. Grandmothers in both settings had similar levels of employment (51.1% in the rural setting and 46.1% in the urban setting). Approximately half of the participants in both groups had completed post-high school study.

No significant differences were found between the two groups in relation to physical health as noted on the SF-36 survey. Composite physical health scores from the SF-36 were below adult norms for both groups with means of 43.5 for rural and 42.9 for urban. Composite mental health scores from the SF-36 survey were also not significantly different with a mean of 47.9 for both groups. There were also no significant differences between the two groups in relation to specific health conditions. The most common conditions reported by both groups included arthritis, diabetes, poor circulation, hypertension, and chronic lung disease. Similar numbers in both groups reported no known conditions (14.1% rural and 15.7% urban). The mean scores from the CES-D depression index also did not vary significantly and were reported as 12.9 for the rural group and 13.5 for the urban group. Significant differences were found between the two groups in the caregiver category and are as follows: traditional caregiver 48.3% rural and 34.9% urban, multigenerational 16.1% rural and 32.8% urban, and primary caregiver 35.6% rural and 32.3% urban.

The researchers concluded that there was no significant difference between rural and urban grandmother caregivers in relation to physical and mental health.

1. How is this information useful to clinical nursing practice?

2. Based on these findings, what are implications for further research?

See Suggested Responses for Evidence-Based Practice on Davis*Plus*.

Introduction

This chapter presents the major theories and important milestones of childhood growth and development. It is important for the pediatric nurse to have a thorough understanding of growth and development to tailor care to the specific needs of the child and help the family understand normal limits. While it is impossible to divide the stages of development into discrete age groups, the following groupings are acceptable standards. *Newborn* refers to the stage immediately after birth until 1 month. *Infancy* is the period from 1 to 12 months of age. The *toddler* stage is from 12 months until approximately 3 years. The next developmental stage, ages 3 to 6 years, is interchangeably referred to as *early childhood or preschool-age*. *School-age* children are 6 to 12 years old. *Adolescence* is the period of time between 12 and 18 years of age.

Influences on Growth and Development

The debate over nature versus nurture is longstanding. Which is the more powerful influence in the formation of a person's essence? Nature describes the traits inherent in the infant at birth: biologically imposed idiosyncratic factors that create what and how each person "is." Nurture, on the other hand, refers to the influence of external events such as parenting received, culture, or the "times" in which a child lives. It appears that both are intrinsically influential. "Generally speaking, genes are responsible for the basic wiring plan—for forming all of the cells (neurons) and general connections between different brain regions—while experience is responsible for fine-tuning those connections, helping each child adapt to the particular environment (geographical, cultural, family, school, peer-group) to which he belongs. Genetic potential is necessary, but DNA alone cannot teach a child to talk" (Zero to Three Brainwonders, n.d.).

Principles of Childhood Growth and Development

It is inherently pleasurable to watch a baby grow and develop. Each child grows and develops at his or her own pace. One child may move quickly through physical tasks, only to be slower with words. Another child may be emotionally tuned into the needs of others while peers are still very self-focused. Despite these differences, development occurs in an orderly sequence, and each child should progress through the predictable stages within a certain time frame. Growth refers to the continuous adjustment in the size of the child, internally and externally. Development refers to the ongoing process of adapting throughout the life span. Growth and development is a continuous process from conception to death. For the child, growth "spurts" tend to be followed by periods of relative "rest" because it takes plenty of energy to continue the growth process. The periods of rest allow the child to incorporate the new growth or the newly developed skill into his or her personal repertoire more completely before attempting the next level.

There are three primary considerations related to growth and development. First, development proceeds in a cephalocaudal direction. **Cephalocaudal** is a progression from head to toe—top to bottom. For example, the baby's brain develops quickly; therefore, the head grows first in comparison to the rest of the body. The child gains head and neck control before learning to grasp or sit up. Second, development proceeds **proximodistally**. This means children develop from near to far and midline to periphery. For example, the torso develops before the arms and legs, and development proceeds to the hands and feet and then to the fingers and toes. The third consideration is that development proceeds from gross motor skills to fine motor skills. Gross motor skills such as running, jumping or riding a bike provide the foundation for fine motor developments such as eating, coloring, or buttoning a shirt.

T. Barry Brazelton, a renowned pediatrician, developed the Touchpoints model of child development. Brazelton described **Touchpoints** as "periods during the first 3 years of life during which childrens' spurts in development result in pronounced disruption in the family system" (Brazelton, 2006, p. xvii). An early Touchpoint is noted in the 4-month-old infant who becomes increasingly aware of surroundings. This interest in the environment will disrupt meals as the infant searches out the sounds that are heard. Sleep may also be disrupted because of this new awareness, and the infant may awaken at night. Brazelton mapped the psychological development of children, focusing on the periods of regression that occur just prior to periods of growth; "the cost of each new achievement can temporarily disrupt the child's and even the whole family's progress"

Growth and Development

Child development has been described through various theories, stages, principles, and models. Regardless of theory or model, child development is typically an organized sequence of advancing milestones including posture, dexterity, and locomotion from birth to adolescence (Vereijken, 2010). Nursing care promoting normal growth and development must be individualized to each child and incorporated into the nursing plan of care. The nurse must assess the developmental age and stage of the child to anticipate normal growth and development expectations. This should include measurement of height, weight, head circumference, and body mass index. By plotting measurements on a standardized growth chart, the nurse can track and identify alterations in normal growth and development. The nurse should assess for achieved developmental milestones and identify specific needs of each child based on his or her stage of development. The nurse can assist the family to understand developmental needs of the child and provide direction in ways to promote healthy growth and development (Ward & Hisley, 2009).

The nurse must understand that growth and development is an individualized and unique process for each child and that variability in ages of achievement of milestones may exist from child to child. Children can skip stages of development and master more advanced milestones before less advanced milestones or can skip back and forth between milestones (Vereijken, 2010). The nurse should provide appropriate education including anticipatory guidance to the parents about the normal trajectory of growth and development emphasizing the uniqueness of each child. Once the nurse and family members have identified developmental goals for the child, age appropriate toys, stimulation, play, nutrition, and sleep should be provided to facilitate normal growth and development.

Source: Vereijken, B. (2010). The complexity of childhood development: Variability in perspective. *Physical Therapy, 90*(12), 1850–1859.

Box 20-1 Touchpoint Examples: Birth to Three Years

PREGNANCY TO 7 MONTHS
Parents are concerned with who the child will be. Choice time to develop a rapport with the parents before the child is born.

NEWBORN
Soon after birth the newborn is assessed for his ability to habituate, or remain calm in a chaotic environment.

3 WEEKS
Infant starts to learn to self-calm. Parents debate use of pacifier versus thumb.

6 TO 8 WEEKS
Infant reacts differently to each parent through facial expression and physical movements.

4 MONTHS
Infant cycles through light and deep sleep several times a night as he learns to sleep through the night. This is important to avoid sleep problems.

7 MONTHS
Naps and bedtime are interrupted by the constant practice of new physical skills, such as sitting and crawling.

9 MONTHS
Increasing independence (e.g., crawling and cruising) makes the infant more dependent as separation anxiety takes hold.

12 MONTHS
All foods become finger foods. Parents must often give up on the idea of a "rounded diet" because the child now controls what is eaten and when.

15 MONTHS
The word "no" becomes prevalent. Toddlers demonstrate frustration at not being able to talk.

18 MONTHS
The child tests the limits of parents and caregivers and learns appropriate behavior through consistent limit-setting and consequences.

2 YEARS
The child has now developed gender identity and behaves accordingly.

3 YEARS
Learning to handle anger and aggression is paramount. Children may regress and exhibit temper tantrums as they process these emotions.

Source: Brazelton, T. B. (2006). *Touchpoints: Birth to three: Your child's emotional and behavioral development.* Cambridge, MA: Perseus.

Box 20-2 A Paradigm Shift

FROM	TO
• Deficit model	• Positive model
• Linear development	• Multidimensional development
• Prescriptive	• Collaborative
• Objective involvement	• Empathic involvement
• Strict discipline boundaries	• Flexible discipline boundaries

Source: Reprinted with permission from Brazelton, T. B. (2002). *Touchpoints: Birth to three: Your child's emotional and behavioral development.* Cambridge, MA: Perseus.

 Optimizing Outcomes—Understanding growth and development

To achieve the best outcome, the nurse can use the multidimensional developmental framework of Drs. Brazelton and Sparrow (2002) to anticipate developmental transition points to help both families and caregivers deal with the difficulties that may arise during these times.

Growth and Development Theories

Growth and development can be discussed in terms of theoretical approaches or developmental domains. A theoretical approach explains, describes, and predicts the various aspects of growth and development. A developmental domain refers to a way of understanding the total child in relation to the mind, body, and spirit. Understanding both the theoretical and developmental aspects is important because each contributes to a broader understanding about the child. A variety of theories are discussed as well as the following developmental domains: physical, psychosocial (emotional, psychological, and social), cognitive (including language and intelligence), moral/spiritual, and family development. Some of the theories are stage related, meaning that the theorist identified specific stages and ages through which a child progresses.

Each child develops at an individualized pace, and the stages are not rigid. It is also important to note that there is developmental variability within each child. For example, a child may be ahead or behind physically and within normal cognitive and emotional limits, or any combination of these patterns. Growth and development takes energy. How each child expends that energy is a result of individual, family, and social variables. In contrast to the stage theories that are described, the non-stage theories are less concerned with specific ages or time frames but are focused on the process or trajectory of developing maturity.

PSYCHOSOCIAL DEVELOPMENT THEORIES

The psychosocial domain refers to the psychological and emotional progression of the child and the relationships with others who are involved in the child's life. Although there are many psychosocial theorists, this chapter describes the well-known theories of Sigmund Freud and Erik Erikson.

(Brazelton, 2006, p. xvii) (Box 20-1). Brazelton also tracked the variations in these Touchpoints and offered anticipatory guidance for parents and professionals who are moving with the child through the stages of development.

Brazelton and Sparrow (2002) went on to develop specific aspects about the Touchpoints that related to temperament, learning, moral development, relationships, independence, and separation issues for each of the years from ages 3 to 6. Responding to these Touchpoints gives parents the tools to help the child develop in a healthy manner.

It is important to know that Touchpoints represents a positive and well-integrated way of conceptualizing developmental progress. Its perspective assumes, among other things, that parents know their child better than anyone else (Brazelton & Sparrow, 2002). With that in mind, the nurse works with the family at the various Touchpoints to help them anticipate and move through the periods of disequilibrium (Box 20-2).

ORAL STAGE (BIRTH–1 YEAR)

The infant is fixated on oral curiosity (whatever he can put in the mouth). The infant derives pleasure from, and relieves anxiety through, oral sensations (e.g., the infant sucks on his mother's breast or bottle and is fed and pleasured). The infant puts his fist in his mouth or uses a teething ring. Children at this stage often use pacifiers or thumbs to decrease anxiety and increase comfort.

ANAL STAGE (1–3 YEARS)

By the time the child reaches this stage, the child is ready to control elimination. Some children readily use the "big kid" potty; others resist. This is a time of increasing control in other areas of the child's life. The child recognizes that this newfound control can run a collision course with the world, and hence the term "the terrible twos." For example, the child explores, asserts, and learns boundaries about where to play safely. The child may struggle against these boundaries by escaping the backyard and running down the street.

PHALLIC STAGE (3–6 YEARS)

By early childhood, sexual difference is discovered. The child begins to compare both the male and female bodies simply out of curiosity. For example, the child notices that girls are physically different from boys. During this time, a girl child wants to push mommy aside and marry daddy, or vice versa.

LATENCY STAGE (6–12 YEARS)

Freud believed that the child "takes a break" psychosexually during this period of development. This allows the child to focus more intently on other aspects of growth and learning. For example, the child spends time with his or her same-gender friends, excelling in sports or video games. At this age, the child presumably has little interest in issues of sexuality.

GENITAL STAGE (12–18 YEARS)

By the time the child reaches puberty, sexuality and relationships are the focus. For example, this is a time for exploring relationships and developing a sense of romanticism.

Sigmund Freud, Psychosexual

Sigmund Freud (1856–1939) believed that development was most influenced by biological instincts. Freud observed that these instincts were psychosexual in nature, meaning that a child progresses through developmental stages based on resolution of conflicts surrounding urges and rules (Box 20-3). Through observation, Freud developed a framework that is widely known today and that set the stage for modern psychoanalysis.

Freud also described the development of three essential aspects of the human personality: the id, the ego, and the superego. The initial aspect, the id, is the emotional part of the personality. The id is present at birth and is predominantly unregulated. For instance, the infant responds to all stimuli emotionally. The infant cries, laughs, or coos automatically and without thought. The id is the part of the personality that relies solely on instinct.

During the baby's first year, the ego begins to develop to provide balance between the competing id and reality. The ego provides a sense of identity separate from others and promotes the ability of the child to function individually. During infancy, the ego helps the baby begin to learn that the mother is not simply an extension of his body.

Between the ages of 3 and 6, a superego, which serves to help regulate behavior, is developed. In this stage, the child develops cognitively and learns about rules and the needs of others. The superego functions as not only a center for conscience, but as a sense of what and how the child

perceives self. An example of the superego is the young child obeying the parents' rules by picking up toys even though the child would rather continue playing. The child is learning that there is a difference between right and wrong and that the child is not the "center of the universe" as previously believed. The child knows that a "good" boy or girl obeys his or her parents.

During adolescence, the ego again provides a balance, this time between the id and the superego. When the adolescent refuses to drink alcohol with friends because it is against the child's conscience and the law, it shows that the ego has prevailed.

Erik Erikson

Erik Erikson (1902–1994) was a contemporary of Freud's. Unlike Freud, who attributed personality formation only to the interplay within a person's family of origin, Erikson focused on the influence of social interaction. Erikson identified seven stages of development. Mastery of each stage requires that the individual achieve a balance between two tasks (conflicting variables). Each stage represents a crisis that must be resolved to move on to the next stage in a healthy manner. Erikson's stages (listed and explained in the following sections) are well known and are used often in tracking the development of children.

TRUST VERSUS MISTRUST. Trust versus mistrust occurs between birth and 1 year. The task of this stage is for the infant to recognize that there are people, generally parents, who can be trusted to take care of basic needs. The infant's struggle becomes evidenced in the recognition that not everyone or every situation is "safe." Through trust, the infant learns to have confidence in personal worth and well-being along with connectedness to others. Failure to master this stage leaves a sense of hopelessness and disconnectedness. Examples of this disconnect can be seen in infants with failure to thrive or with attachment disorders. Difficulty in trusting can be seen even in adults who have problems maintaining significant relationships.

AUTONOMY VERSUS SHAME AND DOUBT. Autonomy versus shame and doubt occurs between 1 and 3 years of age. The task of this stage is for the child to balance independence and self-sufficiency against the predictable sense of uncertainty and misgiving when placed in life's situations. It is the time for the child to establish willpower, determination, and a can-do attitude about self. An example of this stage happens when the toddler wants to choose clothing and dress independently. The struggle happens when the parents allow the child to make personal choices yet expect the choices to be socially acceptable. At this age, the child is able to do many new things and wants to explore everything. This newfound independence is accompanied by new rules that may cause internal conflict. The child must develop personal abilities while struggling with both fears and wishes. The child has self-doubt later in life if this stage is not successfully met.

INITIATIVE VERSUS GUILT. Initiative versus guilt occurs between 3 and 6 years of age. The child's task during this stage is to develop the resourcefulness to achieve and learn new things without receiving self-reproach. It is difficult for a young child to resolve the conflict between wanting to be independent and needing to stay attached to parents. The child's learning of new songs, games, or jokes are good examples of initiative. The child feels confident to try new ideas. It is important that parents and teachers encourage this initiative to help the child develop a sense of purpose. If initiative is discouraged or ignored, the child may feel guilt and lack of resourcefulness.

INDUSTRY VERSUS INFERIORITY. Industry versus inferiority occurs between the ages of 6 and 12. In this stage, the child develops a sense of confidence through mastery of tasks. This sense of accomplishment can be counterbalanced by a sense of inadequacy or inferiority that comes from not succeeding. The realization that the child is competent is one of the important building blocks in the development of self-esteem. Industry is evident when the child is able to do homework independently and regulate social behavior. Performing the prescribed tasks at school or home also shows industry. If the child cannot accomplish realistic expected tasks, the feeling of inferiority may result.

IDENTITY VERSUS ROLE CONFUSION. Identity versus role confusion occurs between the ages of 12 and 18. This is a time of forging ahead and acquiring a clear sense of self as an individual in the face of new and at times conflicting demands or desires. During this stage, the adolescent wants to define "what to be when I grow up." The adolescent concentrates on goals and life plans separate from those of peers and family. At this point, the adolescent child has the ability to think about self as well as others and proceeds accordingly. An adolescent who is unable to make decisions about possible career choices, a personal belief and value system, and sexual orientation, for example, may develop a weak sense of self and be incapable of committing to an identity. This indecision leads to role confusion.

> **"What to say"**—*When a parent inquires about the development of her child*
>
> When parents ask the nurse about a delay in their child's development, the nurse can respond by saying "It is important to note that your child may not have reached the 'appropriate' developmental stage based on chronological age alone. There may be events or variables that delay your child's attempts to move forward, such as an illness."

ATTACHMENT THEORIES

Attachment refers to the bond or emotional and physical connection that develops between an infant and caregiver that tends to endure (Ainsworth, 1978). Early theorists associated attachment with the mother who met the infant's innate drive to be fed and nurtured. Other examples of attachment behaviors are dressing, bathing, diapering, cuddling, loving, playing, and comforting.

John Bowlby and Mary Ainsworth

In 1978, psychologists John Bowlby (1907–1990) and Mary Ainsworth (1913–1999) wanted to expand on early attachment theories by focusing on the attainment of and subsequent quality of the bonding relationship between the infant and caregiver. Both the infant and the caregiver rely on the quality of the interaction between them. In other words, a healthy mother–infant relationship is contingent on the characteristic value of the communication between them. Most researchers generally concentrated on the birth

mother as the primary attachment figure in the infant's world, but Bowlby (1978) also referred to attachment with a "mother-substitute" (p. xxvii).

Bowlby viewed attachment as a biological and evolutionary adaptation. The infant develops an attachment to the mother or mother-substitute as a means of surviving the vulnerability of infancy, rather than as a simple response to having biological needs met. As the infant begins to explore the world and the other people in it, the mother or mother-substitute is perceived as "home base." When the infant becomes frightened or threatened, home base is found. If the infant feels secure in the knowledge that the home base is reliable, the infant can move on to develop additional relationships and attachments.

Separation

Bowlby was not only fascinated with the attachment of mother and child, but also with the influence that separation had on their ability to bond with their caregivers. Bowlby became particularly interested in the impact of separation of young children from their mothers, and he identified three phases of response to that separation: *protest* (in response to the anxiety produced by separation), *despair* (related to the grief and mourning caused by prolonged separation), and *detachment* (a defense against the feelings associated with despair).

Types of Attachment

Ainsworth added to Bowlby's work with studies about infants in unfamiliar situations. Through the use of the "strange situation" room, the researcher introduced infants and toddlers, ages 10 to 24 months old, to a series of situations that tested the strength of their attachment to their mothers. The situations demonstrated three patterns:

- *Secure attachment*: Baby cries when the mother leaves and is happy when the mother returns.
- *Avoidant attachment*: Baby rarely cries when the mother leaves and avoids the mother upon return.
- *Ambivalent attachment*: Baby becomes anxious prior to the mother leaving, is very upset when the mother leaves, and seeks contact with her while pushing her away on return.

Ainsworth's research in Uganda, and later in Baltimore, was important because it was the first truly empirical research related to Bowlby's original attachment theory (see Table 20-1).

 Cultural Diversity: Attachment

> Infants from various cultures bond with parents and caregivers in the manner appropriate to each culture. Some cultures are more comfortable with physical touch and others with verbal exchange. Infants respond based on the cultural norms.

LEARNING THEORIES

Beginning with Ivan Pavlov's work in 1890 about "classical conditioning," learning theorists began to understand development as a cognitive or learning process. There were two main types of learning theorists: behavioral and social learning scientists. Behavioral scientists saw the learner as passive, while social learning scientists

Nursing Care Plan Delayed Growth and Development

Nursing Diagnosis: Delayed growth and development, related to chronic illness

Measurable Short-Term Outcome: Child will maintain current weight and participate in age-appropriate activities, as possible.

Measurable Long-Term Outcome: Child will reach age-appropriate growth and developmental milestones.

NOC Outcomes:

Growth (0110) Normal increase in bone size and body weight during growth years

Child Development: Middle Childhood (0108) Milestones of physical, cognitive, and psychosocial progression from 6 through 11 years of age (specify other age groups as appropriate)

Play Participation (0116) Use of activities by a child from 1 year through 11 years of age to promote enjoyment, entertainment, and development

NIC Interventions:

Nutrition Management (1100)
Developmental Enhancement: Child (8274)
Normalization Promotion (7200)
Activity Therapy (4310)

Nursing Interventions:

1. Build a trusting, supportive relationship with child and caregivers by taking time, actively listening to concerns, and offering information and encouragement.

   RATIONALE: A trusting relationship facilitates implementation of developmental interventions.

2. Monitor child's height and weight (specify frequency) and record on a continuous flow sheet.

   RATIONALE: A flow sheet provides a continuous record of the child's growth over time.

3. Monitor attainment of age-appropriate developmental milestones.

   RATIONALE: Provides information about the child's developmental needs.

4. Collaborate with child, caregivers, and dietitian as needed to provide healthy high-calorie and high-protein meals, snacks, and drinks that the child enjoys.

   RATIONALE: Collaboration ensures that the diet will be appealing to the child and provide the necessary nutrients for growth and development.

5. Encourage caregivers to view the child as "a child with an illness" rather than "an ill child."

   RATIONALE: Encouraging normalcy within the bounds of what is physically possible assists the child to reach maximal growth and development.

6. Assist caregivers to identify the child's special needs and make environmental adaptations to promote normalcy. Refer to community resources as needed (specify).

   RATIONALE: A supportive, adaptive environment may downplay the child's disabilities and enhance normal development.

7. Refer caregivers to appropriate support groups (specify).

   RATIONALE: The support of other families and children may provide additional information and ideas to foster growth and development.

8. Encourage caregivers to hold the same expectations and use the same parenting techniques for the child as they would for other children in the family, as appropriate.

   RATIONALE: Consistent caregiver expectations and parenting techniques help the child view himself or herself as a normal child.

9. Provide anticipatory guidance to caregivers about age-appropriate developmental tasks and milestones for the child.

   RATIONALE: This provides information for goal-setting in development enhancement.

10. Encourage caregivers to provide age-appropriate activities and normal childhood experiences for the child whenever possible (e.g., school, scouting, and camp).

    RATIONALE: Participation in usual activities and experiences for age facilitates the child's physical, emotional, and social development.

11. Assist the caregivers to provide for and encourage the child's interaction with other children.

    RATIONALE: Interaction with peers promotes the child's social development.

12. Collaborate with care provider to enlist the assistance of a Child Development Specialist when the child is hospitalized.

    RATIONALE: This provides professional developmental support specifically for the hospitalized child.

(continued)

Nursing Care Plan Delayed Growth and Development (continued)

13. Provide age-appropriate explanations to the child about the illness, treatments, and procedures.

    RATIONALE: It provides information at a developmentally appropriate level.

14. Encourage and facilitate the child's participation in activities of daily living and self-care during hospitalization.

    RATIONALE: Participation enhances motor development and self-esteem.

15. Provide age-appropriate materials and play activities for the hospitalized child (specify).

    RATIONALE: Play enhances motor and psychological development.

16. Assist the caregivers to arrange for the child's continuation of schoolwork during hospitalization, as appropriate.

    RATIONALE: This prevents the child from falling behind in school during illness.

17. Assist the child and caregivers to set a preferred daily schedule for activities while hospitalized.

    RATIONALE: A regular schedule promotes normalcy, and participation enhances the child's self-esteem.

18. Provide developmentally appropriate incentives and rewards for the child's accomplishments (specify for child).

    RATIONALE: Incentives and rewards bolster the child's self-esteem and encourage further development.

19. Encourage caregivers to obtain needed rest and respite from child care. Make referrals as needed.

    RATIONALE: Fatigue and stress during chronic illness may interfere with optimum caregiving for the child.

emphasized the interplay of the individual within the specific environment.

J. B. Watson, a behavioral scientist, sought to understand observable behavior. B. F. Skinner, also a behavioral scientist, described growth and development is a process of responding to stimuli within the environment (positive and negative reinforcement) that created new learning along with adaptive behaviors. Although both types of scientific investigation are important, this chapter discusses the theories of the social learning theorists, Albert Bandura, Lev Vygotsky, and Urie Bronfenbrenner.

Social Learning Theories

ALBERT BANDURA. Albert Bandura's (1925–present) theory of development does not rely on predetermined stages.

Bandura proposed that learning occurs within a social context through observation and modeling. The child pays attention to a new concept or task, retains that image, and then reproduces the action physically. Each successful approximation (reproduction) of the action increases the child's perception of personal effectiveness, which then contributes to the development of new social skills. For example, a newborn has no sense of self as separate from others. As the infant develops new skills, inadvertently at first, the infant becomes motivated to continue learning. Bandura also describes **self-efficacy** (sense of self) and refers to several foundations for developing self-efficacy. They are mastery (being successful), modeling by others (imitation), "social persuasion" (pairing situations in which success is likely to occur after positive feedback),

Table 20-1 Phases of Attachment

Phase	Bowlby (1978)	Ainsworth (1978)	Manifestation
Phase I (birth–2 months)	Orientation and signals without discrimination of figure	The initial pre-attachment phase	The infant responds to everyone in his or her environment without discrimination.
Phase II (8–12 weeks)	Orientation and signals directed toward one or more discriminated figures	Attachment-in-the-making phase	The infant responds most to those significant caretakers in his or her life.
Phase III (6–7 months)	Maintenance of proximity to a discriminated figure by locomotion and signals	Clear-cut attachment	The baby attaches to his or her caretaker by crawling toward the caregiver, reaching for or cooing at the caregiver.
Phase IV (around age 3)	Implications of the partnership for the organization of attachment behavior during the preschool years	Goal-corrected partnership	The preschool child begins to develop an understanding of the caregiver's goals. The child knows that a tantrum might get the mother to fulfill demands.

Source: Ainsworth, M. (1978). *Patterns of attachment: A psychological study of the strange situation.* Hillsdale, NJ: Lawrence Erlbaum Associates.

and being able to decrease the perception of stress and threat (a conscious willingness to continue using the senses for learning rather than simply for surviving).

As the infant acquires this sense of self and begins to differentiate self from others, the infant develops new skills, and, hopefully, resilience in the face of life's difficulties, along with adaptations to surviving developmental transitions. Conversely, children who have not had adequate positive modeling, or who have not had access to success-inducing experiences, may suffer negative consequences and lack good self-efficacy.

LEV VYGOTSKY. Vygotsky (1896–1934) was a Russian psychologist who studied the influence of culture on development. Vygotsky was a contemporary of Albert Bandura. He emphasized that culture and certain factors within the child's environment have a dramatic impact on language development. He believed that development occurs on two levels: personal (intrapsychological) and social (interpsychological). Vygotsky coined the term "zone of proximal development," which means that one learns much more successfully when assisted by another person. In other words, a child left alone to her own devices would accomplish fewer developmental tasks and not nearly to the degree that would be achieved if the child had received the assistance of another person.

URIE BRONFENBRENNER. Urie Bronfenbrenner (1917–2005) studied the effects that social environment has on a child's development (1979). Within this ecological approach, Bronfenbrenner defined three systems in each child's life. The *microsystem* refers to the systems in which the child is actively involved. Typically, in a child's life, the microsystem would be family, school, and peer group. *Mesosystem* refers to the interaction between two microsystems, such as the interplay between a child's home and school. The *exosystem* refers to those systems that may have an impact on the child, but with which the child is not intimately involved—for instance, the parent's work. The parent's work affects the child's life, yet the child is not directly involved in it.

COGNITIVE THEORIES

Cognitive theory focuses on how an individual thinks and how thinking influences worldview. The capacity to think develops over time and with experience. Jean Piaget discussed cognition (thought) and how it influences development.

JEAN PIAGET. Jean Piaget (1896–1980), a Swiss psychologist, studied the development of cognition in children. In Piaget and Inhelder's book, *The Psychology of the Child* (1969), information was presented about how children think and learn. Thinking and learning for children take place through four distinct stages. The initial period, the *sensorimotor stage*, takes place from birth to age 2. During this time, the primary means of cognition is through the senses. The child takes in and processes information strictly on a physiological or emotional level.

At the age of 2, the child begins to use cognitive processes to respond to the world physically. The *preoperational stage* (ages 2–7 years) takes into account the development of motor skills and is divided into two substages: *preconceptual* and *intuitive*. The child is still not capable of logical thinking, but because of an increased ability to use words and actions together, the child is increasingly able to connect cognitively with the world.

The third stage is the *concrete operational stage*. At this stage, the 7- to 11-year-old child is able to organize thoughts in a logical order. The child is able to categorize and label objects. It is also possible at this stage for the child to solve concrete problems.

Piaget's final stage of cognitive development is the *formal operational stage* during which the 11- to 15-year-old child uses abstract reasoning to handle difficult concepts and can analyze both sides of an issue.

INTELLIGENCE THEORIES

Intelligence is the capacity for learning, abstract thought, problem solving, and self awareness. It is measured by objective criteria such as tests (Venes, 2013). Intelligence has been studied primarily in terms of how it is measured. As in all other developmental dimensions, intelligence does not exist in a vacuum. The ability to bring in and retain new information and skills relies on the interconnectedness of cognitive, emotional, and environmental factors. Traditional standardized measures of intelligence have relied on assessing cognitive abilities, most specifically math and verbal. Many of these measures are criticized for not taking into account varying cultural and socioeconomic factors. In other words, a child may test as less intelligent than the norm when, in fact, his test responses are based on his cultural experience. Standardized IQ tests have also been criticized for not measuring varying learning styles and experiences.

In the early 1980s, psychologist Howard Gardner argued that intelligence cannot be measured by a single number from an IQ test. In his book, *Frames of Mind* (2011), he describes eight forms of intelligence: bodily-kinesthetic, interpersonal, intrapersonal, linguistic, logical-mathematical, musical, naturalistic, and spatial. Every child possesses the ability to use all eight of these intelligences. However, over time, children develop one or more to a greater degree than the others. While the particular form of intelligence possessed by a child may vary, Gardner believes that the multiple intelligences are all equally important. Thomas Armstrong (2009) applied Gardner's work to the classroom to describe how a child learns depending on the form(s) of intelligence for which the child demonstrates a tendency (Table 20-2).

Nurses are responsible for teaching children, and their families, as part of the implementation phase of the nursing process. The nurse uses information from learning and intelligence theories to assess a child's ability to learn. Assessment includes questioning the child's hobbies and interests, which provides the nurse information about how the child learns.

The nurse then uses this information to plan appropriate teaching interventions and to assist the family in understanding how the child learns best. The nurse advises the family about opportunities that will stimulate learning at home. Empowering the family with information about the child's favored methods of learning also allows the parents to advocate for the child within the school system.

Table 20-2	Eight Ways of Learning		
Children Who Are Highly . . .	**Think . . .**	**Love . . .**	**Need . . .**
Linguistic	in words	reading, writing, telling stories, playing word games	books, tapes, writing tools, paper, diaries, dialogue, discussion, debate, stories
Logical-Mathematical	by reasoning	experimenting, questioning, figuring out logical puzzles, calculating	materials to experiment with, science materials, manipulatives, trips to planetariums and science museums
Spatial	in images and pictures	designing, drawing, visualizing, doodling	art, Legos™, videos, movies, slides, imagination games, mazes, puzzles, illustrated books, trips to art museums
Bodily-kinesthetic	through somatic sensations	dancing, running, jumping, building, touching, gesturing	role-play, drama, movement, building things, sports and physical games, tactile experiences, hands-on learning
Musical	via rhythms and melodies	singing, whistling, humming, tapping feet and hands, listening	sing-along time, trips to concerts, playing music at home and school, musical instruments
Interpersonal	by bouncing ideas off other people	leading, organizing, relating, manipulating, mediating, partying	group activities, social events, sports
Intrapersonal	in relation to their needs, feelings, and goals	setting goals, meditating, dreaming, planning, reflecting	secret places, time alone, self-paced projects, choices
Naturalist	through nature and natural forms	playing with pets, gardening, investigating nature, raising animals, caring for planet Earth	access to nature, opportunities for interacting with animals, tools for investigating nature (e.g., magnifying glasses, binoculars)

Source: Reprinted with permission from the Association of Supervision and Curriculum Development.

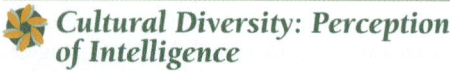

Cultural Diversity: Perception of Intelligence

When providing nursing care, it is important to understand that culture or ethnicity can influence perception of intelligence. For example, a Hispanic immigrant child in grade school may not understand his food choices in the school cafeteria based on his cultural knowledge about food. The child may be misinterpreted as unintelligent rather than recognizing that he has grown up with different food choices than his peers.

MORAL DEVELOPMENT THEORIES

Study of moral development deals with a child's perception about right and wrong. Jean Piaget, Lawrence Kohlberg, and Carol Gilligan are three of the most well-known theorists in this area. Of these, Kohlberg is the writer most often cited for his understanding of moral development in children.

Piaget studied the progression of moral thinking in children based on the ability to reason and understand the environment. Piaget identified two stages of moral judgment. The first stage describes the way in which children younger than 11 years old experience right and wrong as concrete, black-and-white concepts. Simply put, the child understands that an act is good or bad, right or wrong. The second stage coincides with Piaget's Formal Operational Stage of cognitive development during which the child is better

able to think abstractly. Rules are important but are not always absolute or "carved in stone."

LAWRENCE KOHLBERG. Lawrence Kohlberg (1927–1987) based the theory of moral development (1984) on the thinking processes involved when making moral decisions. Kohlberg identified three levels of moral development: preconventional, conventional, and postconventional. Each level of moral development represents a major modification in the child's thinking and is further separated into stages (Table 20-3).

Within Level I, the *Preconventional Level*, the child's thinking is concrete and egocentric. Obedience and punishment are unquestioned and understood as either good or bad. The child's behavior is based on which actions are rewarded or punished. Individualism and exchange occur when the child begins to define right and wrong and develops an individual sense of fairness and personal justification. As the child matures and is confronted with opposing views, he begins to recognize that not everything is black and white. The child's sense of morality is still concrete, but the child begins to take into account personal reasoning. If the child can justify an action, then, in his mind, it is acceptable to bend or break rules.

Transition to Level II, the *Conventional Level* for the child, is marked by the child's incorporation of social and interpersonal relationships. The interpersonal and relationships stage is where the child's actions are justified by personal motivation to "do good" for family members or other

Table 20-3 Lawrence Kohlberg's States of Moral Development

Level I. Preconventional Morality Morality is determined by external sources—rules, laws, possibility of punishment.	Stage 1: Obedience and Punishment—The child will obey to avoid being punished. Stage 2: Individualism and Exchange—The child thinks that it may be okay to do something wrong if good comes from it (in other words, the end justifies the means).
Level II. Conventional Morality Morality is determined by being a "good person." The intent is to please others and to do the "right thing."	Stage 3: Good interpersonal relationships—The child's moral decisions are based on the "goodness" of motivation and on what others expect. Stage 4: Maintaining the social order—The child's good moral decisions are those that preserve the needs of society.
Level III. Postconventional Morality	Stage 5: Social contract and individual rights—The individual's thinking is characterized by a deeper questioning of social order versus an individual's personal rights. A person in this stage works tirelessly to change unjust laws. Stage 6: Universal principles—An individual incorporates a deep awareness of justice. An example would be breaking an unjust law to save the lives of innocent people.

individuals. The child understands that maintaining the social order means that society as a whole may benefit by his actions.

Level III, *Postconventional Morality*, is divided into social contract and individual rights and universal principles, both of which require significant degrees of personal deliberation and maturity. These stages are sequential and require a level of cognitive development; they are not necessarily age related. In fact, because progression through the levels is influenced by a variety of factors, such as experience, health, socioeconomic status, family structure, and culture, an adult may have reached only the preconventional level of moral development and not the postconventional level of moral development.

CAROL GILLIGAN. Carol Gilligan (1936–present) initially worked with Kohlberg as a research assistant. Gilligan became concerned that Kohlberg's studies of moral development were based only on norms for males. When girls were compared with boys using Kohlberg's framework, girls appeared morally weaker or slower to develop than their male counterparts. In Gilligan's book, *In a Different Voice* (1982), previously held beliefs about female moral development were questioned by interviewing both women and men about their life experiences. Gilligan identified two tracts of moral development. One was based on autonomy and justice, as seen in Kohlberg's interviews with men. The other was based on caring and relationship, which Gilligan attributed to women. Gilligan's work helped to define moral development for women in a different way than men. Even though Gilligan later withdrew the charge of gender bias, Gilligan continued to champion the study of female moral development (Box 20-4).

SPIRITUAL DEVELOPMENT THEORIES

James Fowler (1981–present) identified seven stages related to faith and spiritual development. Fowler defined faith outside the usual "religious" definition. Fowler believed that faith is commonly experienced and that it is the individual's striving for something "more than the self." The development of faith depends on a certain level of cognitive achievement. Deepening levels of belief rely on the ability to think abstractly. Understanding Fowler's stages

Box 20-4 Gilligan's Three Levels of Moral Development

Level 1: *Orientation of individual survival.* As the girl *transitions* through this level, she moves from *selfishness to responsibility,* where she considers other people.

Level 2: *Goodness as self-sacrifice.* This level involves looking at the world through the needs of others. The girl sacrifices her own needs and considers herself responsible for others.

Level 3: *The transition level.* This level requires movement from goodness to truth. In other words, the woman recognizes that choice is important when doing for herself or others rather than focusing on being good for the sake of being good.

is important in providing complementary care to children and their families (see Complementary Care: Understanding spirituality).

 Complementary Care: *Understanding Spirituality*

Stage 0: Undifferentiated (infancy): Prestage during which the infant is learning "fundamentals of basic trust and the relational experience of mutuality with the one(s) providing primary love and care" (Fowler, 1981, p. 121). This foundation of trust sets the stage for developing a spiritual faith.

Stage 1: Intuitive-projective (ages 2 to 6 or 7): Corresponds with the child's imaginative period in which beliefs and faith are unquestioning. It is a time of fantasy and magical thinking.

Stage 2: Mythical-literal (ages 6–12): The child retells the spiritual stories and takes them literally and concretely.

Stage 3: Synthetic-convention (typically begins around 12 or 13 years): The young person begins to personalize beliefs. The youth looks beyond her family to include values encountered in relationships, in school, and in society in general. Sometimes adults remain in this stage.

Stage 4: Individuating–reflexive (may begin in late adolescence or early adulthood or not at all): The individual takes responsibility for personal beliefs and commitments. The individual invests personal energy in what spiritually makes sense, regardless of what others believe.

Fowler goes on to describe two additional stages of faith that may occur in adulthood, *Conjunctive Faith* and *Universalizing Faith.*

FAMILY DEVELOPMENT THEORIES

There are many theories describing family interaction. Duvall's (1977) 8-stage theory is based on Erikson's individual stages of psychosocial development and is the most well known. This theory is based on the oldest child as the marker for transition into the next stage. The family development stages are:

- *Marriage.* The task of couples in this stage is to establish themselves as a pair and to prepare for parenting. This is also a time for realigning with both families of origin from the position of a new family.
- *Family With Infants.* During this stage, a child is born and the family adjusts to its new structure while the couple begins to adjust to their new role as parents. Grandparents and others in the child's life adjust to their new role, too.
- *Family With Preschool Children.* As the oldest child enters the stage of early childhood, the family functions to socialize the children, helping them to cope with separation involved in starting school.
- *Family With School Children.* As the children develop friendships and launch socially outside the family, the system must adjust.
- *Family With Adolescent.* The oldest child turns toward launching and independence. At this point, the parents begin to refocus on their marriage.
- *Family Launching Young Adult.* This stage begins when the oldest child leaves home. If there are other children, it ends when the youngest leaves home. Family tasks during this stage center on the development of individual and independent identities of both the children and the parents. The marriage continues to be a major area of energy.
- *Middle-Age Family.* The family continues to focus on reinvesting in the couple's relationship. Relationships with extended family are realigned.
- *Aging Family.* During this stage, the family copes with the process of, and losses involved in, retirement and aging.

 Nursing Insight—*Applying Duvall's theory*

Duvall's theory provides a framework for observing the development of families. It is important to understand that this framework applies to specific family types and styles such as those families with children who remain married and whose children leave home in the appointed time frame. Remember, when caring for children from other family types, the nurse must consider family makeups such as divorced families, single-parent families, child-free families, families with same-sex parents, children who return home after launching, and culturally diverse families. The nurse needs to consider a multitude of factors, approach families using a nonjudgmental demeanor, and help the family understand and explore solutions based on the unique aspects of their family.

 Collaboration in Caring—*The health-care team*

Various members of the health-care team oversee growth and development across care settings, throughout the life of a child. Nurses and physicians assess a newborn while in the hospital, and a lactation consultant may be involved if the newborn is breastfed. Well-child visits to the primary health-care provider at regular intervals help track a child's growth and development and intervene if problems arise. Public health nurses may also assess the child, particularly at times of immunizations. Complementary and alternative health-care providers such as chiropractors, massage therapists, and naturopaths may also play a role in caring for a child.

When providing nursing care to a child and her family, the nurse must be cognizant that none of these theories stand alone but are interconnected. It is essential that the nurse and all health-care providers base their care on the knowledge of growth and development based on the theories presented thus far (Table 20-4).

Temperament

Children come in all shapes and sizes and represent all temperamental profiles and personality styles. Children are not simply "miniature adults." They require professional assessment and attention across care settings based on their level of development.

Temperament refers to those characteristics present at birth that govern the way in which an infant responds to his surroundings. There is a strong biological and environmental basis for temperament. Likewise, the baby's temperament generally has a profound influence on her interactions with caretakers and the environment.

Thomas and Chess (1977) studied temperament and identified nine temperamental traits present at birth that persist throughout life (see Across Care Settings: Child temperament). These traits exist on a continuum depending on the infant's reaction to the environment. To help ensure effective parenting, the nurse can teach parents about their infant's temperament traits.

 Across Care Settings: **Child temperament**

During a normal daily routine, the child may be exposed to a variety of settings and exposed to several people: a day care center, visiting extended family, the physician's office, or in public places in the community. Understanding an infant's temperament is essential in the care of the child to help both the parent and child adapt to these experiences. Based on the work by Thomas, Chess, and Birch (1968), the following descriptors are used to help recognize the infant's unique personality.

- *Regularity:* The child needs regularity in sleeping, eating, and bowel habits. A child who is "easy" is one who can adapt to relatively flexible schedules. A child who is "difficult" has difficulty when the schedule has been disrupted.
- *Reaction to new people and situations:* The "easy" child responds easily to new people in their environment. Another child may stand back or withdraw when something or someone new is present.
- *Adaptability to change:* This trait refers to a child's willingness to change routine. An "easy" child makes transitions with little or no discomfort. A slow-to-adapt child will become distressed with even the smallest changes, for instance, taking a different route home from school.
- *Sensory sensitivity:* An "easy" child with lower sensitivity will appear much less meticulous or disturbed by her

Table 20-4 Summary of Theorists

Theorist(s)	Key Points
PYSCHOSOCIAL DOMAIN	
Sigmund Freud	Psychosexual stages • Oral (birth–1 year) • Anal (1–3 years) • Phallic (3–6 years) • Latency (6–12 years) • Genital (12–18 years)
Erik Erikson	Psychosocial stages • Trust Versus Mistrust (birth–1 year) • Autonomy Versus Shame and Doubt (1–3 years) • Initiative Versus Guilt (3–6 years) • Industry Versus Inferiority (6–12 years) • Identity Versus Role Confusion (12–18 years)
John Bowlby	Three phases of responses to separation • Protest • Despair • Detachment
Mary Ainsworth	Patterns of attachment • Secure attachment • Avoidant attachment • Ambivalent attachment
LEARNING DOMAIN	
Ivan Pavlov (mentioned)	Classical conditioning
J. B. Watson (mentioned)	Observable behavior
B. F. Skinner (mentioned)	Stimulus-response
Albert Bandura	Social context of learning • Approximation • Self-efficacy • Mastery • Modeling • Social persuasion • Decreased perception of stress and threat
Lev Vygotsky	Levels of development • Personal (intrapsychological) • Social (interpsychological) • Zone of proximal development
Urie Bronfenbrenner	Ecological definition of development • Microsystem • Mesosystem • Exosystem
COGNITIVE DOMAIN	
Jean Piaget	Stages of cognitive development • Sensorimotor (birth–2 years) • Use of reflexes • Primary circular reactions • Secondary circular reactions • Coordination of secondary schemes • Tertiary circular reactions • Mental combinations • Preoperational (2–7 years) • Preconceptual (2–4 years) • Intuitive (4–7 years) • Concrete Operational (7–11 years) • Formal Operational (11–15 years)

(continued)

Table 20-4 Summary of Theorists (continued)

Theorist(s)	Key Points
INTELLIGENCE DOMAIN	
Howard Gardner	Multiple intelligences • Bodily–kinesthetic • Interpersonal • Intrapersonal • Linguistic • Logical–mathematical • Musical • Naturalistic • Spatial
MORAL DOMAIN	

Lawrence Kohlberg	Moral development
	 • Preconventional Morality
	    • Obedience and punishment
	    • Individualism and exchange
	 • Conventional Morality
	    • Good interpersonal relationships
	    • Maintaining the social order
	 • Postconventional morality
	    • Social contract and individual rights
	    • Universal principles

Carol Gilligan	Moral development • Orientation of individual survival • Goodness as self-sacrifice Shift from goodness to truth
SPIRITUAL DOMAIN	
James Fowler	Spirituality stages • Undifferentiated (infancy) • Intuitive–projective (2–6 or 7 years) • Mythical–literal (6–12 years) • Symbolic–convention (12 years) • Individuation–reflexive (late adolescence through adulthood)
FAMILY DOMAIN	
E. R. Duvall	Family development • Marriage • Family with infants • Family with preschool children • Family with school-age children • Family with adolescent • Family launching young adult • Middle-age family • Aging family

senses. A "difficult" child with high sensitivity may react strongly when exposed to sensory stimuli. The child may become irritated with certain textures, tastes, smells, or sounds.

- *Emotional intensity:* An "easy" child shows little or no response to a situation. An intense child reacts dramatically and profoundly, whether that reaction is loud or withdrawn.
- *Level of persistence:* This trait refers to the child's willingness to stay engaged regardless of setbacks. A persistent child has difficulty giving up until the goal is reached. A less persistent child is more flexible and may give up more easily.

- *Activity level:* An "easy" child will generally be less frenetic with activity. A "difficult" child has difficulty with inactivity, preferring to always be on the move.
- *Distractibility:* The distractible child has difficulty concentrating on tasks in which they are not immersed—this is not the same as the entity known as attention deficit disorder (ADD). A less distractible child stays with a task longer.
- *Mood:* An "easy" child tends to see the world in a more positive way. A "difficult" child tends to react in a more negative manner.

The ability to recognize these traits is helpful for determining the strength of the fit between the caregiver, family members, and the child, along with helping families strategize to improve the fit. This way of understanding the child takes into account that each person in the child's life also has a unique temperamental style, which complements, becomes enmeshed with, or antagonizes that of the child.

 Now Can You—Apply theories to nursing practice?

1. Describe the importance of using theory-based knowledge in the care of children and families?

2. Discuss the different types of theories used in the care of children and families?

3. Describe the importance of understanding a child's temperament and his interaction with his surroundings and caregivers?

Growth and Development Milestones

An understanding of normal growth and development assists the nurse to assess that the child is meeting expected milestones for each stage of development. Early detection of alterations in growth and development is important in the life of the child and family. The following is a discussion of the predictable growth and development at each of the accepted age divisions.

NEWBORN AND INFANT

The entire infant period of development encompasses the time between birth and 12 months of life. During this time there is rapid change in all aspects of development. It is important for the nurse to remember that while each infant moves at his own pace through the developmental stages, these stages occur in a somewhat sequential fashion that can be anticipated (Table 20-5).

Reflexes and Neurological Development

Primitive reflexes are those adaptive and innate mechanisms that protect the developing infant while the brain is maturing. The reflexes are controlled by the lower brain centers. There are several reflexes present at birth or shortly after and help determine normal or altered neurological development. The reflexes present at birth naturally disappear by 9 months (see Focus on Safety, next page).

Table 20-5 Developmental Milestones of the Infant (0–12 Months)

Physical Growth	Gross Motor Skills	Fine Motor Skills	Cognitive, Sensory, and Language	Psychosocial and Play
		NEWBORN: BIRTH–1 MONTH		
Height: 19–21 inches Weight: 7.5 pounds Head circumference: 13–14 inches Chest circumference: 12–13 inches	Reflexes present Absence of head control, but can momentarily hold the head in midline Head lag when the newborn is pulled from a lying to a sitting position Assumes flexed position When supine assumes tonic neck flex position Kicks legs and waves arms Rounded back when sitting Rolls over accidentally	Hands predominately closed Strong palmar and plantar grasp reflexes	Uses all five senses to explore the world; Touch: First sense to develop Smell: Recognizes mother and has a taste preference for sweets Hearing well developed: Becomes quiet when hears a familiar voice Limited visual acuity 20/100, fascinated with faces, follows moving objects, contrasting colors (black and white) Language: Cries to express unmet needs Smiles during sleep	Psychosocial: Learns to relieve anxiety through oral sensations (breastfeeding, sucking on fist); begins to learn to trust caregivers Play: Interaction with parents and caregivers; mobiles
		INFANT: 1–2 MONTHS		
Weight: Increases 1.5 pounds per month Height: Increases 1 inch per month Head circumference: Increases 0.5 inches per month	Less head lag when pulled to sitting position When prone can slightly lift head off floor Improved head control, turns and lifts head from side to side when prone, some head control when upright	Holds hands open Grasp reflex absent Can pull at clothes and blanket, bats at object	When supine follows dangling toys Visually searches for sounds When crying, can be consoled easily by being held or spoken to Turns head to sound Language: Coos, has social smile	Psychosocial: Same as above; learns to calm self Play: Solitary play stimulates sensorimotor development with simple imitative games Interaction with parents and caregivers through games such as: • Patty-cake • Peek-a-boo

(continued)

Table 20-5 Developmental Milestones of the Infant (0–12 Months) (continued)

Physical Growth	Gross Motor Skills	Fine Motor Skills	Cognitive, Sensory, and Language	Psychosocial and Play
		INFANT: 3–6 MONTHS		
Weight: Double the birth weight by 6 months Height: Increases by 1 inch per month	Can hold head more erect when sitting, still some bobbing, by 6 months sturdy head control Only slight head lag, by 6 months no head lag Raises head to 45°–90° off floor In sitting position (tripod) back is straight and balances head well, sits alone by 8 months When held in a standing position can bear some weight, by 8 months readily bears weight Rolls from back to side and then abdomen to back When supine puts feet to mouth Begins to creep on hands and knees	Plays with toes Clutches own hands, inspects and plays with hands Pulls blanket over face Rakes objects Grasps objects with both hands (palmar grasp) Shakes rattle and holds bottle Eventually able to put objects in container and bang them together Carries objects to mouth Transfers objects from hand to hand Reaches and bangs toys on table Likes mirror images	Follows object 180° Develops binocular vision Locates sound by turning head Beginning eye–hand coordination Pursues dropped object visually Sees small objects Responds to name Recognizes parent's voice and touch; by 6 months differentiates between parents Language: Coos, babbles, laughs By 6 months may say "dada" and "baba" Begins to distinguish emotion based on tone of voice	Psychosocial: Same as above Play: Solitary play stimulates sensorimotor development with simple imitative games Interaction with parents and caregivers through games such as: • Patty-cake • Peek-a-boo • Songs
		INFANT: 9–12 MONTHS		
Weight: Triple the birth weight Height: Increases 1 inch per month Head and chest circumference are the same at 1 year of age	Creeps on hands and knees Pulls self to standing position Stands while holding onto furniture and begins to cruise Stands alone Changes from prone to sitting position Can reach backwards while sitting Can sit down from standing position alone Begins to walk holding hand and then independently, takes first step	Uses pincer grasp Hand dominance now evident Releases and rescues an object When sitting, purposely reaches around back to retrieve object Can randomly turn pages in a book Can make a simple mark on paper Waves bye-bye and plays patty-cake Begins to feed self finger foods	Increasing depth perception Moves toward sound Thoroughly explores and experiences objects Points to simple objects Language: Says "mama," "dada," and "uh-oh" Understands a few words Responds to own name Exhibits stranger anxiety Begins to distinguish colors Increasing ability to see things in the distance	Psychosocial: Completes Erikson's stage of trust versus mistrust; able to calm self Play: Solitary play stimulates sensorimotor development with simple imitative games; interaction with parents and caregivers through games such as: • Patty-cake • Peek-a-boo • Songs • Finger painting • Ball rolling • High chair fishing

 focus on safety

Reflexes

As the nurse performs an assessment, it is imperative to note important infant reflexes:

• Rooting: Infant's head turns and he begins to suck when his cheek or lower lip is stroked.

• Sucking: Sucking motion of lips, mouth, and tongue allows the infant to take in sustenance.

• Moro: Startle response with sudden jarring causes extension of the head. The arms abduct and move upward. The hands form a "C."

• Grasping: This is noted when the palms of the hands or soles of the feet are stroked causing fingers or toes to curl inward.

• Babinski: This is the turning in of the foot and fanning out of the toes when the sole of the foot is stroked.

At birth, the lower portions of the nervous system, the spinal cord and the brainstem, are already developed. These structures are necessary for the infant to sustain basic body functions and primitive reflexes. As the infant matures, the higher sections of the nervous system become more developed. For instance, the limbic system and the cerebral cortex are responsible for ongoing learning that occurs during the life span.

Sensory Development

Touch is an extremely important sense and is the first sense to develop. The ability to feel objects, textures, and other people opens up the newborn's world of learning. It is important for the infant to experience soft, comforting textures. The ability to experience pain is also an extremely important element, particularly as a protective device. If the infant has a pain experience, he reacts to pain with the whole body by quickly extending and then retracting the extremities. Along with this reaction, the infant cries.

Smell and taste begin developing in utero and are intrinsically connected. Infants respond to smells within the first few days and have an innate preference for sweet tastes. The nurse is aware that infants can recognize their mother's smell long before they achieve visual recognition.

Hearing is well developed at birth. A newborn can immediately recognize the difference between male and female voices and will generally turn toward the female voice. By the second week, the newborn can recognize the sound of the mother's voice. A newborn's ability to discriminate sounds develops quickly, contributing to language development. By the time the infant is 3 months old, the infant jabbers and begins to imitate sounds. During the next few months, the infant becomes more adept at responding to and imitating familiar sounds by smiling and cooing.

Vision is the least developed of the senses at birth. Newborns are fascinated with faces and with designs or objects that resemble faces. A newborn is able to remember an object but only in the exact form originally seen (e.g., if the child sees his sister in pigtails, the child does not recognize the sister with her hair down). Infants are most attracted to bright colors and to black and white because of the limited nature of their vision. The newborn generally has poor peripheral vision until 10 weeks of age. Within the first 3 months, the infant will watch faces intently, follow moving objects, and recognize familiar objects and people at a distance. There will also be the beginnings of eye–hand coordination. Binocular vision (ability to use both eyes to see) develops at about 4 or 5 months of age. The capacity to distinguish colors and to see things in the distance develops throughout the first 7 to 12 months.

Physical Development

Growth is rapid. Infants gain 1.5 pounds (680 g)/month, double their weight by 6 months, and triple it by 1 year. Height increases by 1 inch (2.5 cm)/month for the first 6 months and slows during the second 6 months. A newborn's head is proportionally larger than the rest of the body, which is in keeping with the cephalocaudal course of development. The newborn's head grows rapidly during the first month as the brain grows. By the time the infant reaches 1 year of age, the head and chest circumferences are about the same.

For the infant to move or to perform actions (motor skills), the infant must have adequate muscle development. At birth, the newborn's movement is involuntary. It takes the infant time to mature physically to be able to demonstrate motor skills. Gross motor skills (the ability to use large muscles for movement) are the first to develop in the newborn and infant. Generally, by the end of the first 3 months of life, the infant can raise his head and chest while lying on his belly and stretch the legs out and kick from a prone position, and roll from side to side (Fig. 20-1). The infant can turn over completely at about 6 or 7 months of age. By 8 to 9 months of age, the infant begins to crawl and then, by using high objects, the infant can begin pulling up. Once the infant has mastered an upright position, he may begin to cruise (walking

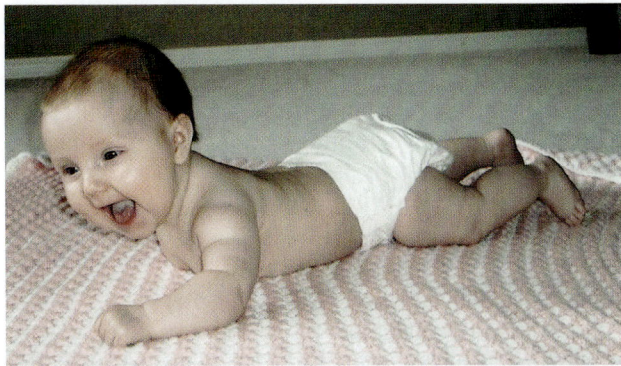
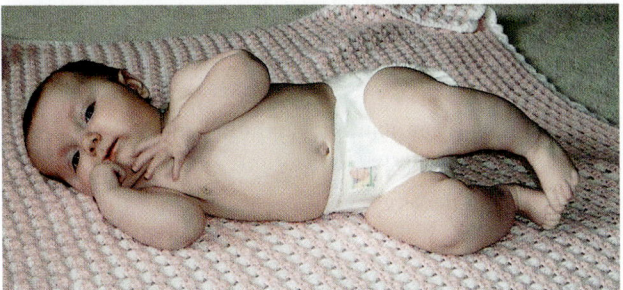

Figure 20-1 At 3 months of age, an infant can lift his or her head and chest while on his or her belly (top) and roll on his or her side (bottom).

while holding on to furniture) or even attempt to walk unaided. It is important to remember that every child develops at his own pace. One child may be walking before his first birthday, while another does not walk until months later.

Fine motor skills (the use of muscles to accomplish minute tasks like pinching or picking up food) build on the gross motor skills (Fig. 20-2). Those fine motor skills that develop between 6 and 12 months include the ability to stack large objects, scribble, bang on pots and pans, and transfer objects from one hand to another and back again.

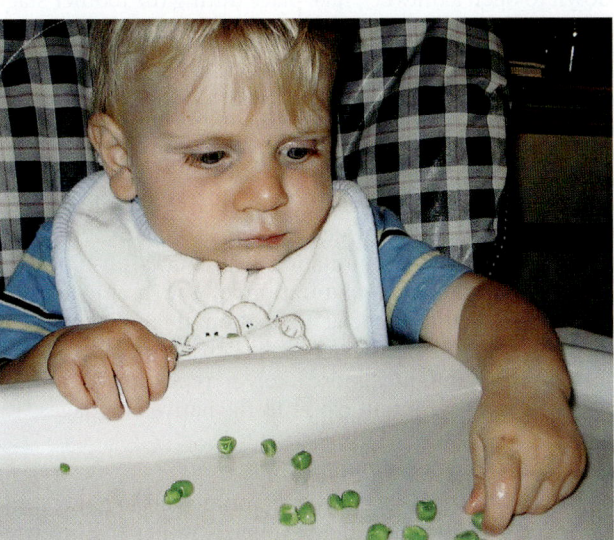

Figure 20-2 One of the first fine motor skills to develop is the ability to pinch to pick up small objects like food.

Cognitive Development

Infancy corresponds to Piaget's sensorimotor stage of development. The infant uses the five senses to explore and to learn about the world. For instance, the infant learns that lip smacking when hungry leads to a full stomach. When the infant's belly is full, physical needs are met, and the infant can then begin to explore the environment. Ultimately, the infant learns that he can have an impact within that environment. The infant must achieve three major tasks during this phase of development:

- *Separation.* The infant recognizes that there is no merging with or attachment to familiar people (family members).
- *Object Permanence.* The infant knows that an object or person still exists even if covered up or removed from sight; this is why infants respond so strongly to peek-a-boo.
- *Mental Representation.* The infant has the ability to use symbols to communicate.

Piaget also identified six substages within the sensorimotor stage that describe mental representation. It is important to note that four of these substages occur during the first year of life. The first substage, *use of reflexes,* is present at birth. The majority of the reflexes are necessary for survival and disappear during the first 9 months. The second substage, *primary circular reactions* (1–4 months), takes place when the infant responds to things that give pleasure. The infant's response encourages caregivers to continue providing pleasurable experiences. The third substage, *secondary circular reactions,* begins when the infant recognizes cause and effect. For example, the actions that the infant can perform independently begin to capture his attention (e.g., shaking a rattle). The fourth substage begins around 8 to 12 months when the infant becomes deliberate with his actions. During substage 4, *coordination of secondary schemes,* the infant intentionally seeks out objects. The infant now knows that pushing a button starts the music on a toy. During this substage, the infant also develops object permanence. The remaining substages, *tertiary circular reactions* (making interesting things last such as hitting a drum with a stick and making the rat-a-tat-tat sound) and *mental combinations* (problem solving such as putting a toy down to open a drawer), take place during the toddler stage of development.

Language Development

Infants initially communicate through the universal language of crying to indicate physical discomfort or loneliness. As a mother or father responds to the cries, the infant learns to communicate more deliberately. The nurse must recognize that an infant's early speech is characterized by crying, babbling, and imitation. Influences on language development include maturation of the brain and the degree and quality of social interaction. If families respond favorably to the infant's sounds, like "ba" for bottle or "da" for daddy, the infant is more likely to repeat these sounds, thus bringing the infant closer to the native language.

Psychosocial Development

In infants, the first displays of emotions, crying and smiling, are related to physiological needs rather than to psychological stimuli. For example, the newborn wails loudly when physically uncomfortable and smiles involuntarily during sleep. However, by the time the baby is 2 weeks of age, the smiles begin to signify contentment and elicit a positive family response. The infant's smile then becomes social, and interaction with the environment occurs.

Corresponding with Erikson's psychosocial stage of trust versus mistrust, the nurse recognizes that this is a critical time for the newborn to absorb the whole environment along with its related experiences. The caretaker's task is to respond to the infant in such ways as to engender a sense of security and well-being. Essentially, the infant's mission is to develop a sense that his caretakers are reliable and present.

Ainsworth described four stages of attachment. During the first stage (birth to 2 months), the newborn and infant randomly respond to anyone. By the second stage (8–12 weeks), the infant begins to respond more to the mother than to anyone else, but the infant continues to respond indiscriminately to others. It is not until the third stage (6 or 7 months) that the infant demonstrates a strong connection to the mother and possibly develops a fear of strangers. Not all infants develop stranger anxiety. Throughout the first year, the infant develops attachments to all of the important people in the family. Achieving the necessary milestones is essential for the infant to move on to the next stage of psychosocial development. An example of psychosocial development is the infant becoming more aware of others and responding to people or animals that are physically on the same eye-level (Fig. 20-3).

Discipline

Discipline plays an important role in the psychosocial development of the infant because it helps correct misbehavior and molds moral character. Infants learn about safe boundaries and trusting relationships through effective discipline. The nurse helps parents determine how they plan to discipline their child now and later on as the child grows and develops. The American Academy of Pediatrics (2011) indicates that early forms of discipline take place when the caregiver molds and structures the infant's daily routines and responds to the infant's needs. Limit-setting functions to acclimate the infant to the world and to keep the infant

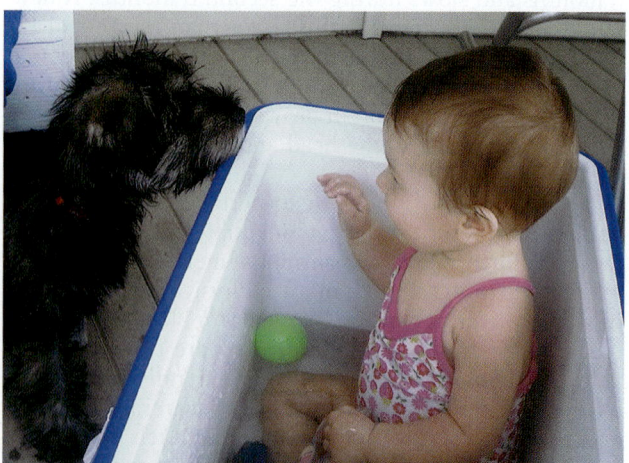

Figure 20-3 An example of psychosocial development is when an infant becomes more aware of others by responding to people or animals that are physically on the same eye-level.

out of harm's way. It is important to note that parents often learn how to discipline from their own experiences as children. It is essential that parents be taught what to expect at each of the developmental stages and how to recognize appropriate strategies for teaching and limit setting.

Anticipatory Guidance

Infancy is a period of tremendous growth and development. As infants acquire new skills at a rapid rate, parents are in need of information to know what to expect at each stage. In the first year, infants see a health-care provider at regular intervals for physical assessment and immunizations. Nurses are in a unique position to provide anticipatory guidance during each of these visits. It is important to provide teaching regarding nutrition, health promotion, safety, sleep-wake patterns, growth and development, and discipline (Box 20-5). Health promotion and safety are priority topics to approach with parents. They need to know the signs and symptoms of illness, when to call the health-care provider, and emergency procedures. Infants require a safe environment—from cribs and car seats to a child-proofed home. Nurses must also promote the idea that parents need to take care of themselves. Parents are often so busy learning how to be parents that they do not recognize that they need time to be a couple.

Critical Nursing Action Anticipatory Guidance

Anticipatory guidance is a way of providing caregivers with information and examples about what to expect in the future regarding their child's next developmental phase (e.g., discipline, nutrition, safety, schooling, elimination, immunizations, or play). It is important that the nurse teach parents that infants do not misbehave on purpose. Exploration and crying are normal behaviors for infants. The purpose of discipline at this age is to keep the child safe. Parents can use a firm tone of voice or facial expression while telling the child "no" or "stop" as she reaches for the stove; this helps the infant know that there are limits to her actions. The infant can then be redirected to a similar experience, such as reaching instead for a toy off a countertop.

TODDLER (1–3 YEARS)

Physical Development

By the time the infant reaches 1 year of age, physical growth has slowed. For each year between the ages of 1 and 3, the typical toddler gains 3 to 5 pounds (1.3–2.6 kg) and grows 3 inches (7.6 cm) taller. Most of the toddler's energy during this period is directed to other realms of development. As the physical growth rate slows, the toddler develops physical, cognitive, and emotional skills that help her to become more independent. As the toddler develops mobility, she explores how things work and her senses become more refined. The toddler uses newly acquired gross motor skills to run, jump, and move up and down stairs with increasing ease. Around age 3, the toddler may learn to ride a tricycle or slide down the slide in the park without help. This newfound freedom and movement create many opportunities for danger as the toddler moves quickly from one new experience to another.

Fine motor skills continue to develop rapidly in this age group. The toddler can hold a spoon or a large crayon appropriately and continues to make artwork that is more

Box 20-5 Anticipatory Guidance for Infants

Nutrition: Review breast- and bottle feeding guidelines; introduction of solid foods (4–6 months); encourage self-feeding when appropriate; finger foods; weaning to cup (9–12 months); family meal time; change to whole milk at 12 months

Health Promotion: Signs and symptoms of illness: vomiting, diarrhea, fever, dehydration, and jaundice; immunizations (see immunization schedules at http://www.cdc.gov/vaccines/schedules/); recommend CPR training; review emergency procedures; oral health—brushing with non-fluoride toothpaste after eruption of first tooth, schedule first dentist appointment

Focus on Safety: Safety guidelines for crib; place car seat in back of car in a rear-facing position; position on back for sleeping to decrease risk of sudden infant death syndrome, do not leave infant unattended, install smoke detectors; lower crib mattress and childproof environment as child becomes more mobile; close supervision; discourage use of baby walkers

Sleep-Wake Patterns: Expected patterns at each month of age; expectations for sleeping through the night, naps; establishment of nighttime rituals (see *Family Teaching Guidelines: Sleep/Rest*)

Cognitive and Emotional Development: Age-appropriate toys and interactive games; talk and sing to infant; read stories; respond to infant cries; face to face time

Motor Development: Support head and neck; supervised "tummy time" to increase neck, arm, and torso strength; provide safe space for child to move about; provide opportunities for sitting, crawling, and walking

Discipline: Discuss discipline versus punishment; limit-setting; apply rules consistently

representative of the object she is trying to depict. The toddler is increasingly able to manipulate smaller toys (Table 20-6).

Cognitive Development

Early toddlerhood corresponds with Piaget's fifth substage of cognitive development, *tertiary circular reactions*, during which time the toddler experiments and learns new behaviors. The toddler then transitions into Piaget's sixth substage, *mental combinations*, when she begins to understand cause and effect and is able to imitate others and problem solve.

The toddler loves to imitate the people around her. Much of the toddler's behavior is replication of what she sees and hears. The toddler also learns through repetition. This is why a toddler may want the same book to be read over and over, staying engrossed in the story every time.

A toddler also likes order and often responds with difficulty to any disruption in routine. The level of response is related to the temperament of the child. Some toddlers may revolt with temper tantrums, and others will calmly transition into an experience. Regardless of temperament, most children at this stage respond favorably to predictable routines.

Language Development

With increasing cognitive development, toddlers are able to listen to and understand short explanations. This is a time when the child develops a more understandable language system. Language is about fulfilling needs: "I do" or "want drink." The toddler moves from using single words to short phrases. Some parents worry when their child does not fall exactly within what are considered normal language parameters. The nurse can reassure parents that it is important to assess what the child understands and what the child is able to communicate, with or without words, rather than exact correctness in pronunciation.

Table 20-6 Developmental Milestones of the Toddler (1–3 years)

Physical Growth	Gross Motor Skills	Fine Motor Skills	Cognitive, Sensory, and Language	Psychosocial and Play
Weight: 3–5 pounds per year Height: 3 inches per year	Stands without support Walks independently Walks backwards Creeps up stairs Pulls toys while walking Runs with wide stance Jumps in place with both feet Climbs Throws a ball; eventually kicks the ball Rides a tricycle by 3 years of age Begins to stand on one foot momentarily; may be able to hop on one foot Can walk up and down stairs with alternate feet Blows kisses	Holds a pencil or a large crayon Makes artwork that is more representative of the object Copies a circle and cross by age 3 years Knows colors Feeds self with a spoon and drinks from a cup Constantly throws objects on floor Builds tower of 3 to 4 cubes, eventually building tower of 7 to 8 cubes Screws/unscrews Turns pages in a book one page at a time Turns knobs Removes shoes and socks, learns to undress self Begins toilet training around 3 years of age	Experiments and learns new behaviors Begins to learn cause and effect Imitates behaviors of parents and caretakers Well-developed vision Can identify geometric objects Intense interest in picture books and listens to stories Distinguishes food preferences based on senses Language: Single words and simple phrases, " I do" or "Want drink"; by 15 months knows 15 words; 20 words by 2 years Follows simple instructions	Psychosocial: Increases control of self and environment; explores; learns about safety and boundaries, but may test those boundaries; shows affection Play: Parallel play (play alongside another child) helps children make the transition from solitary play to associative play by stimulating sensorimotor and psychosocial development; activities include: • Matching games • Simple puzzles • Blowing bubbles • Bean bag toss • Catching fireflies • Ring around the rosy • London Bridge • Duck-duck-goose • Hide and seek • Coloring • Drawing

Psychosocial Development

Toddlers typically exemplify characteristics of Freud's *anal stage*. The child begins to develop a sense of self as separate from her mother. The toddler's task is to move away from the primary caregiver while in some way maintaining enough connection to feel secure. This process, called rapprochement, is healthy and expected.

Toddlerhood also corresponds with Erikson's stage of autonomy versus shame and doubt. It is a time when the child makes every effort to "do it myself." Mastery is an extremely important task of this stage of development. Because the toddler's abilities begin to surpass cognitive judgment, it is also a time of potential hazard for the developing child. Caregivers must walk the fine line between allowing exploratory independence and "mastery" on one hand and vigilance on the other. It is often a time of bumps and "booboos."

Often dubbed as the "terrible twos," this entire stage can be a tumultuous time for both caregivers and toddlers. The child must begin to internalize behavioral standards at a time when establishing independence is important. The nurse can help parents understand that the toddler does not set out to make life miserable. The toddler simply has few internal mechanisms in place to accomplish what needs to be done safely. It is frustrating to the toddler when confronted with blocks to budding mastery. The word "no" begins to signify the toddler's simple response to frustrated emotions encountered.

Moral Development

Cognitively, the toddler is still a very concrete thinker and knows that something is "good" or "bad" but does not know why. At this stage, the toddler identifies good and bad and right and wrong by virtue of whether or not it is rewarded or punished. This corresponds to Kohlberg's preconventional level of moral development.

Discipline

The purpose of discipline is to teach the child socialization and safety. It is the responsibility of the parent to provide a firm structure so the toddler can explore the world while offering safe limits (Box 20-6). Many children repeatedly test rules, while also unconsciously learning to rely on the security those limits provide. Having a structured environment for the child does not necessarily mean rigid or inflexible. Parents must learn to structure the toddler's surroundings to allow enough flexibility to test limits.

A child at this stage needs guidance to determine how to act appropriately. The toddler thinks concretely and must

---

Box 20-6 Discipline Strategies

Distraction: Provide a toy to divert the child's attention.
Time-Out: Move the child to a "cooling-off" place where the child can calm down.
Removal of Privileges: Withhold a favorite toy until the child's behavior is appropriate.
Verbal Reprimands: Give spoken warnings or disapprovals without berating the child or judging the child as "bad."
Corporal Punishment (e.g., spanking, swatting, and grabbing): Not recommended.

rely on others to help give realistic parameters. Some parameters may create a great deal of conflict when what the toddler is allowed to do does not match what the toddler wants to do, which may result in a temper tantrum. Praise becomes an excellent component of discipline because most children want to please the parent.

Temper Tantrums

Because this is a time of intense exploration and discovery and a time when the toddler is establishing a sense of herself as a competent doer, there will be "bumps in the road" (Fig. 20-4). A tantrum is a normal way of working things out internally for the toddler. Parents and caregivers need to know that tantrums are normal for the toddler. It may be possible for parents to anticipate when tantrums are most apt to occur (e.g., when the toddler is tired, hungry, or overwhelmed by new situations, reserves are low, and therefore, the toddler may be more likely to explode or "melt down").

Tantrums may be avoided or minimized if anticipated. Get a tired child to rest or feed a hungry child to decrease her frustration level. If a tantrum does develop, there are coping strategies that a nurse can teach a parent. When the child is wailing and thrashing, but not doing any harm, ignore her. Often this is not possible, and it may be necessary for the parent to intervene quickly and decisively to remove the child to a quieter or safer place. Touching and distractions may help soothe a tantrum for one child. Another child may need to continue the tantrum under the watchful eye of the parent. The latter requires that the parent be present but not engaged in direct communication with the child. The goal is for the child to feel (and be) safe without being negatively or positively reinforced for having a tantrum.

When faced with the sometimes daunting task of caring for a "willful" toddler (one who is regularly asserting her power), parents are often confused. It is indeed difficult to know how and when to avoid the power struggles inherent in a clash of wills. It is essential to be able to create boundaries that limit the toddler's scope of power. Inevitably, there are times when the toddler must be disciplined, so seeking help from a professional child counselor is essential.

❝What to say❞—*Tips for effective discipline*

During effective discipline, allow for negotiation and flexibility, which can help build the child's social skills. Also, allow the child to experience the consequences of behavior.

- Speak to the child as you would want to be spoken to if someone were reprimanding you.
- Never resort to name-calling, yelling, or disrespect.
- Be clear about what you mean.
- Be firm and specific.

Whenever possible, the consequences must be delivered immediately, relate to the rule broken, be short enough in duration, and emphasize the positives. In addition, the consequences must be fair and appropriate to the situation and the child's age.

Anticipatory Guidance

The increasingly mobile toddler presents challenges to parents and caregivers to keep the child safe at all times. Constant supervision is required. As the toddler actively explores his environment, he does so with little understanding of the consequences of his actions. Cabinet doors need to have child-safe locks, mini-blind cords must be secured above the reach of the toddler to prevent asphyxiation, and windows and doors must be locked. As the older toddler learns to ride a tricycle, teach the importance of wearing a helmet. The toddler is beginning to learn about rules and consequences. Consistency in how those rules and consequences are applied is very important. Discipline must be appropriate to the rule broken. Providing a toddler with a brief time-out is a very effective disciplinary tool. It is important to choose a safe place for the time-out, such as a chair in a visible area of a room. A general rule of thumb for time-outs with toddlers is 1 minute per year of age. Box 20-7 discusses additional anticipatory guidance guidelines for the toddler.

EARLY CHILDHOOD (PRESCHOOLER) (3–6 YEARS)

Physical Development

Children at this age come in various sizes, shapes, and body types. As a rule, the preschooler begins to grow taller and thinner. Her abdomen will flatten as she grows. The abdominal muscles strengthen, and the pelvis straightens. The physical growth rate for this stage of development is slow but steady. The average weight gain of the preschooler is about 5 pounds (2 kg), and growth is 2.5 to 3 inches (6.3–7.6 cm) per year. By age 4, the child's posture straightens and the child is able to move around in a more balanced fashion. As muscles become more developed, the preschooler becomes stronger. Her face narrows, the nose enlarges, and the skin becomes more adult-like.

The preschooler is much more agile. At age 4, the preschooler can ride her tricycle and climb up and down the

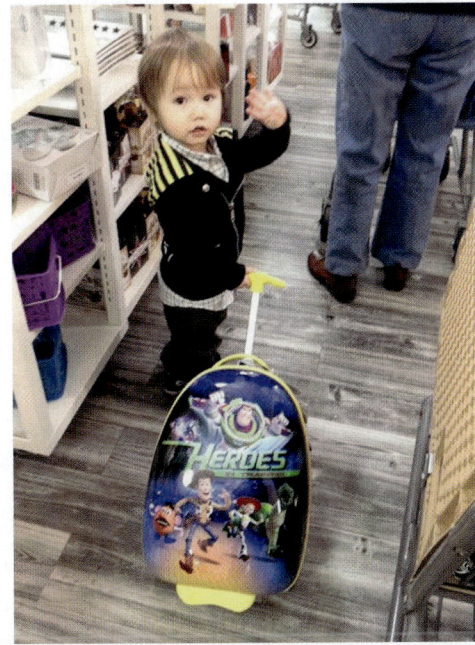

Figure 20-4 Toddlers enjoy doing for themselves.

stairs comfortably using alternating feet. The preschooler can also skip and hop and is much more coordinated on the balance beam.

Fine motor skills rely on the use of the forefinger and the thumb. As the brain becomes more developed, she is better able to pick things up with the fingers. Hand dominance begins to develop around the age of 3 when the preschooler may show a preference in using one hand over the other. By the age of 4, that preference is established (Table 20-7).

Cognitive Development

This period of development corresponds with Piaget's pre-operational stage (2–4 years). During this time, the preschooler increases the ability to verbalize. The preschooler can symbolically use language to represent concepts that need to be conveyed. The young child is still egocentric (focused only on her own sense of things) and therefore is limited socially. This is in large part because of concrete thinking processes and the inability to abstractly shift focus from self to others. The preschooler is also not able to transfer attention from one aspect of an object to another (e.g., a child at this stage can identify a dog's collar but is not able to describe its texture) (Fig. 20-5).

Language Development

The preschooler has increased ability to verbalize; vocabulary increases from 1,500 to 2,000 words between the ages 3 and 5. The preschooler uses sentences and is much more able to convey an intended message. When the young child is able to use words, tantrums generally begin to subside. The preschooler loves silly words and rhymes and asks many questions, generally those that begin with "why?" To meet the needs of the preschooler, keep answers simple and avoid giving too much information. Bombarding the preschooler with overwhelming answers can be quite disconcerting for the child. The nurse can tell the parent that a preschooler may stutter as he or she tries to get out all of the words faster than she is able to speak them. Stuttering generally resolves quickly.

Table 20-7 Developmental Milestones of Early Childhood (Preschooler) (3–6 years)

Physical Growth	Gross Motor Skills	Fine Motor Skills	Cognitive, Sensory, and Language	Psychosocial and Play
Weight: Increases 5 pounds per year Height: Increases 2.5–3 inches per year	Dresses self Throws and catches ball Pedals tricycle Kicks ball forward Stands on one foot for 5 to 10 seconds Skips and hops on one foot Walks down steps with alternate feet Jumps from bottom step Balances on alternate feet with eyes closed	Moves around in a more balanced fashion Builds tower of 9 to 10 cubes Draws stick figure with 6 parts Uses scissors to cut outline of picture Copies and traces geometric patterns Ties shoelaces Uses fork, spoon, and knife with supervision Colors, prints letters Mostly independent toileting and dressing	Focus is on self Uses language to convey concepts Concrete thinking Well-developed senses Preferences based on the use of senses Learns address and phone number Language: Recognizes most letters; vocabulary has increased from 1,500 to 2,000 words, eventually speaks in complete sentences with increasing fluency Sings songs Enjoys silly words and rhymes Asks many "Why" questions	Psychosocial: Begins to regulate own behavior; learns about rules; increases confidence to try new things; recognizes differences between boys and girls Play: Associative play helps children learn how to share, play in small groups, and learn simple games with rules, concepts of language, and social rules; activities include: • Memory • Chutes and Ladders • Candyland • Hokey Pokey • Hot Letters • Alphabet games • Color games • Checkers • Make believe play

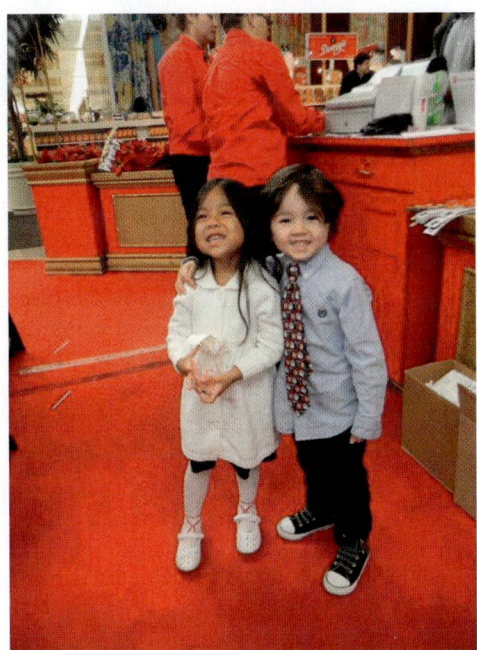

Figure 20-5 Preschoolers discover what it means to be kind.

Case Study   Early Childhood Development

Mrs. James brings Steven, her 3-year-old son, into the clinic for a well-child visit. She states she is concerned because Steven does not talk as well as his peers. She describes how, at play group, the other 3-year-olds talk more than Steven, and she states that Steven barely says a word. When asked how Steven communicates what he wants, Mrs. James states that he points to things and sometimes says single words such as "more" or "juice." Mrs. James added that Steven often gets frustrated when his parents do not understand what he wants. A review of his medical history reveals that Steven was born at 39 weeks, weighed 8 lb 1 oz (3.7 kg), and had an unremarkable birth. He has had no difficulties with feeding or sleep. He began babbling at 6 months but did not speak his first word until 14 months. By 19 months he could say "mama," "dada," and "juice." Presently, Mrs. James states he uses approximately 10 words but does not combine them.

critical thinking questions

1. What further assessments would you complete for Steven?

2. What would you say to Mrs. James about Steven?

3. What nursing interventions would be appropriate at this time?

◆ See Suggested Answers to Case Studies on Davis*Plus*.

Psychosocial Development

Early childhood is a wonderful time marked by the exploration of new skills and the ability to finally be able to figure out how to get and do things for oneself. As the preschooler develops, she is presented with many situations where she can truly excel. The preschooler has learned many new skills and is becoming a "big kid." The preschooler enjoys positive feedback for accomplishments. The fact that the preschooler is able to do many new things creates a dilemma, and the preschooler must decide which

things are most important. Parents may not approve of the decisions made by the preschooler, and she may become conflicted when limits are set. Often the preschooler ponders about doing "the right thing" or doing "the wrong thing" and risking the parent's dismay. Conscience develops and begins to guide the child through the maze of "wants" versus "cans."

The preschool child has a good deal of magical thinking. In a preschooler's desire to do what she wants to do, she may angrily wish something bad would happen to another person, often a parent. If something bad actually does happen, the preschooler will believe that her thinking caused the outcome.

Freud described this period as the phallic or oedipal period. The child is becoming more aware of gender differences. The preschooler may want to marry dad or the boy in preschool, rather than relate to her best female friend.

Family is very important to the preschooler. However, the preschooler is now discovering the joys of friendships. The young child looks to her peers for new ideas and information and begins to develop an understanding of what it means to be kind. The preschooler is more social and is often more willing to share toys with others than when she was a toddler.

Moral Development

Early childhood typically corresponds with Kohlberg's preconventional morality stage when the major impetus for moral judgment is to avoid punishment. It is common for the child in this age group to tell lies to avoid consequences. A child at this age may judge an action to be wrong only if caught. The young child is only guilty if the parent has seen the actions.

Discipline

Because the preschooler is beginning to understand that actions have consequences, caregivers can take advantage of this understanding. The preschooler is able to understand that there are rules and that not obeying those rules leads to consequences. It is best if rules are explained before infractions occur. At the very least, they are addressed before disciplining the child. This helps the preschool child learn more clearly how to behave. Consequences can, as much as possible, follow naturally and fit the behavior being punished (e.g., having the child clean up her own mess or miss a favorite television show if she dawdles).

As with toddlers, a typical discipline strategy instituted with preschoolers is providing the child with a time-out. A rule of thumb is a minute time-out per year of age. Whether that time-out is in a specified chair or section of the room, it is important to help the child know that the purpose of the time-out is to calm herself and to shift gears and act appropriately.

Many parents begin using behavioral charts at this age to praise positive behavior and to help the preschooler understand what is expected and to be rewarded when "good" behavior is shown. For many preschoolers, simply getting a star or sticker on the chart is reward enough to encourage good behavior. For others, a more sophisticated measure of rewards is needed, such as allowing additional television time or a favorite activity. The goal of discipline and limit-setting at this stage of development is to begin teaching the preschooler to regulate her own behavior.

Anticipatory Guidance

The preschooler has much to learn in these years. Parents can assist in language development and comprehension by reading and singing to the preschooler each day. It is important to praise the child's accomplishments to build confidence and a sense of achievement. Parents can expect the preschooler to test limits. It becomes increasingly important for parents to set and maintain consistent limits on behavior and provide appropriate discipline (Box 20-8).

Many parents ask how they will know that their preschooler is ready to begin kindergarten. Mastery of skills previous to, and including, the preschool years assists the child in becoming ready to start school. Preschools and child care programs provide opportunities for the preschooler to interact with other children, learn cooperative play, and enhance cognitive, language, social, and physical skills. Working closely with the teachers in these early childhood programs provides parents with the information they need to assess when their child is ready to begin school.

SCHOOL-AGE CHILD (6–12 YEARS)

Physical Development

Early in this stage (ages 6–9), boys and girls follow similar growth trajectories. Both begin to grow taller, reducing their "baby fat" even more. Children at this age gain about 4 to 6 pounds (1.8–2.7 kg) and grow 2 inches (5 cm) per year. As their abdominal muscles strengthen, their posture straightens. Facial features become more refined. Still, there are many variations in size and shape of children in this period. These variations are influenced not only by familial and cultural genetics, but also by environmental factors (e.g., diet and exercise).

Box 20-8 Anticipatory Guidance for Early Childhood (Preschooler)

Nutrition: Family meal times should be pleasant; provide 3 meals and 2 nutritious snacks per day; allow child to make nutritious choices

Health Promotion: Signs and symptoms of illness: vomiting, diarrhea, fever, dehydration; immunizations (see immunization schedules at http://www.cdc.gov/vaccines/schedules/); recommend CPR training; oral health: brushing, routine cleanings

Focus on Safety: Car seat (see guidelines at safercar.gov: http://www.safercar.gov/parents/CarSeats.htm); update home childproofing (secure matches, guns, outlets, medications, poisons); sunscreen; bike helmet; water and playground safety; teach about stranger safety; continue close supervision

Sleep-Wake Patterns: Dreams and nightmares are evident now; develop strategies to handle them; naps start to disappear; maintain consistent bedtime routine (see *Family Teaching Guidelines: Sleep/Rest*)

Cognitive and Emotional Development: Offer praise; show affection; expect fantasy play as child tries new roles; address fears as they occur; read, sing, and talk to child to develop language skills; creative toys; expose child to various places within the community; encourage assertiveness, not aggression; teach how to solve conflicts; encourage self-expression; expect sexual exploration and answer questions; assign simple chores; encourage self-care: toileting, dressing

Motor Development: Encourage peer play and physical activities; may want to join an organized sport; bike safety; water safety

Discipline: Continue with consistent rules; teach right from wrong; teach respect for authority; continue with time-outs

---

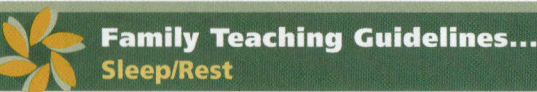

Family Teaching Guidelines...
Sleep/Rest

TOPIC:

Sleep and rest are the body's way of providing renewed energy and a feeling of well-being. It provides not only physical renewal but also mental renewal. It is also a time for essential brain development in young children, facilitating growth, healing, and learning. If a person is deprived of sleep, problems can occur with concentration and emotional functioning. Sleep and rest impact many body cycles such as temperature regulation and heart, lung, kidney, and digestive functions. The sleep-awake cycle of persons varies with age.

HOW TO: Promote Age-Appropriate Sleep

- Establish a household schedule that provides for the appropriate amount of sleep for the child.
- Determine signs of sleepiness or fatigue, such as yawning, increased activity, temper tantrums, rubbing eyes, fussiness, and/or crying.
- Decide on a bedtime agreed on by both parents.
- Establish a pre-night or nap-time ritual, such as bathing, bottle- or breastfeeding, toileting, and/or story time.
- Encourage quiet play activities prior to bedtime.
- Avoid excess stimuli, such as action and/or frightening television programs.
- Consider quieting behaviors, such as rocking, walking, and/or use of a pacifier/feeding.
- Provide a consistent nighttime room environment appropriate for the child's age, which may include the child's own bed/crib, quiet environment, comfortable room temperature, use of a night-light, and/or restful music.
- Avoid exposing children to environmental smoke and avoid overheating of infants.
- Ensure that the mattress used in a crib is firm and that there is no soft or loose bedding or toys in the crib.

ESSENTIAL INFORMATION:

Because children use a lot of energy growing and learning, it is important that they receive adequate rest. Newborns sleep an average of 17 to 20 hours in a 24-hour period. A 6- month-old child needs approximately 12 to 16 hours of sleep in a 24-hour period. The average 2- year-old needs approximately 12 to 14 hours of sleep in a 24-hour period, and the average preschool-aged child needs about 10 to 12 hours of sleep in a 24-hour period. Sleep problems are not unusual during the preschool years. Children of this age (3–6 years old) may have nightmares and trouble falling asleep because of their imaginations and immaturity. Because of the immaturity and imagination, children of this age frequently have a difficult time distinguishing between fantasy and reality and believe that monsters and creatures lurk in their rooms after the lights are turned out. A familiar environment, comfort with a hug, and verbal reassurance are provided and repeated to reassure the child.

Most school-age children begin to develop axillary sweating. In girls, hips begin to broaden and the pelvis widens in preparation for childbearing. Breasts begin to enlarge and become tender. The vaginal pH changes from alkaline to acidic, and the vagina develops a thick mucoid lining. Pubic hair begins to develop between the ages of 8 and 14. While menarche can begin as early as 8 to 10 years of age, the average age in the United States is 12 years of age.

Boys also begin sexual development at these ages. Their bodies become more muscular. Between 10 to 12 years of age, the testes become more sensitive to pressure, the skin of the scrotum darkens, and pubic hair begins to develop. Boys often experience gynecomastia, a temporary enlargement of breasts as a result of hormonal shifts. This can be embarrassing, and the child and family need reassurance of its transient nature.

Both males and females are assessed at well-child visits using the Tanner staging of development of secondary sex characteristics (see Chapter 21 for more information). Tanner staging is done to document evidence of normal pubertal development for the age of the child, and it is an important assessment to detect signs of sexual abuse and precocious puberty (Table 20-8).

focus on safety

Privacy

At this age, it is important to guard the child's privacy. As a nurse, be aware of self-conscious behavior related to physical changes occurring in the body. Along with privacy, the nurse must be aware of other issues affecting the child and family related to menstruation, secondary sexual characteristics, hormone imbalances, mood swings, and social needs, as well as other specific areas identified by the child and family.

Cognitive Development

The school-age child is better able than the younger child to use logical thinking. This logic in thinking corresponds with Piaget's Concrete Operations stage of cognitive development. While the child's thinking is still quite concrete, he can begin to solve problems. During this childhood stage, he begins to replace the ever-present "why?" question with "how?" Mastery is focused on figuring out how things work. The school-age child builds on experience and begins to recognize consequences of actions. In school, he works on tasks requiring awareness of space (where things are in relation to other things), causality (logical consequences), categories (how things fit together), conservation (physical quantity can remain constant even when state is altered), and numbers. He is also capable of metacognition, the ability to think about thinking. At this age, the child is aware of his own thinking and is able to assess how he came to conclusions, a process that eventually leads to critical thinking.

Memory deepens as the child grows. He becomes more adept at processing and working through information. Memory improves because the brain retains more information. A child in this age group is also better able to determine what is important to remember and what is not. This helps him filter out irrelevant data, leaving memory space available.

Language Development

Language improves considerably. The child uses words more accurately, particularly verbs, metaphors, and similes. The child is able to elaborate on concepts that he wants to get across.

Table 20-8	Developmental Milestones of the School-Age Child (6–12 years)				

Physical Growth	Gross Motor Skills	Fine Motor Skills	Cognitive, Sensory, and Language	Psychosocial and Play
Weight: Increases 4–6 pounds per year Height: Increases 2 inches per year	Gradual increase in dexterity and becomes limber Improves coordination, strength, balance, and rhythm Climbs, bikes, skips, jumps rope, and swings Learns to swim, dance, do somersaults, and skate	Good eye–hand coordination Balance improves Can sew, draw, make arts and crafts, build models, play video games Handwriting improves Prints and writes Likes activities that promote dexterity such as playing a musical instrument and building models	Increased logical thinking leads child to be able to solve problems Wants to know "how" things work Understands that actions have consequences Aware of own thinking and how conclusions were reached 20/20 Visual acuity Color discrimination fully developed Mature sense of smell Hearing deficits may be discovered as language develops Language: Accelerated, vocabulary expands to 8,000 to 15,000 words; as comprehension expands children engage in long conversations on a variety of topics; enjoy jokes; may experiment with profanity	Psychosocial: Increases peer group involvement as peers influence values and beliefs; same-sex friends; masters skills; increases confidence and self esteem Play: Cooperative play teaches children how to bargain, cooperate, and compromise to develop logical reasoning, which increases social skills; activities include: • Baseball • Soccer • Gymnastics • Swimming • Dodge ball • Board games • Simple card games • Computer games • Video games • Puzzles • Crosswords • Word search puzzles

Psychosocial Development

There is vast emotional growth during the middle child years. Erikson described this stage as one of industry versus inferiority. Unlike the younger child who believes he can do almost anything, the 6- to 10-year-old child begins to assess what he can and cannot accomplish. School-age children need and seek praise. They have a more definite sense of self-esteem or competence based on the ability or lack of ability to perform.

Early in the middle childhood period (ages 6–9), the child is still self-focused. The school-age child continues to exhibit magical thinking, in that he still may feel responsible for bad things that happen. Later in this stage (ages 9–12); the child is increasingly independent, although he wants approval and validation. Throughout this stage, sorting, collecting, and board games are common activities. Competing and winning become important in the growing sense of self-competence. Friendships are exceptionally important at this stage. The school-age child looks more to friends than family, but family is still important. Best friends tend to be of the same gender, although mixed gender groups of school-age children become common as they reach the preteen and early teen years (Fig. 20-6).

Moral Development

For the first several years, the school-age child is still operating within preconventional morality. The younger child sees things as black and white and as self-referenced, rather than connected with more generalized rules and concepts. By the age of 10, the child enters Kohlberg's conventional morality stage. During this time, the child has internalized rules and is intently gaining approval. The older child operates within a morality of cooperation that implies recognition of the interaction between the self and a "bigger" worldview. Most children at this age are motivated to adhere to laws as a way to keep order.

Discipline

Because the child in this stage of development is beginning to internalize rules, it is important to allow the child more independence and thus more awareness of the natural consequences of behavior. An effective parental technique is to refrain from "rescuing" the child from the consequences of his behavior (e.g., rushing home to retrieve a forgotten piece of homework whenever the child calls rather than allowing him to learn a valuable lesson).

While many school-age children respond appropriately to natural consequences, some do not yet understand responsibility. In fact, most children opt at some time to ignore the natural consequences. Parents may need to impose the previously discussed time-out strategy (e.g., grounded for a period of time or privileges restricted).

Anticipatory Guidance

The school-aged child experiences many physical changes that can be confusing and frightening. Many parents are uncomfortable discussing, or unsure how to discuss, pubertal changes and need information to help them explain these changes to their child. Educating the parents and child about these changes before they occur is important. Many elementary and middle schools invite parents to view the materials taught in health classes regarding puberty and physical changes. Nurses can encourage parents to review those materials and give permission for their child to receive that information in class and then reinforce it at home (Box 20-9).

ADOLESCENCE (12–19 YEARS)

Physical Development

Adolescence technically begins with the onset of puberty when the pituitary gland relays messages to sex glands to

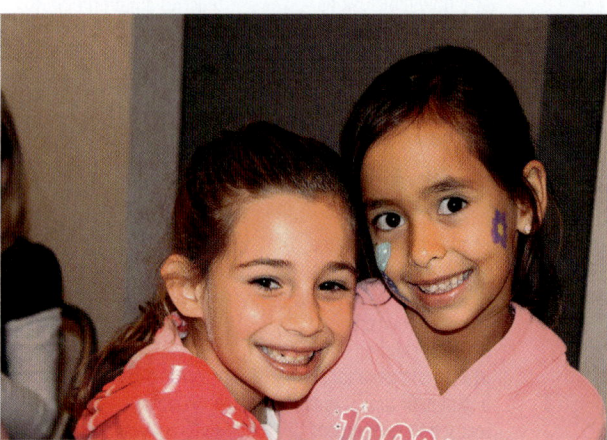

Figure 20-6 Establishing strong friendships is very important to school-age children.

Box 20-9 Anticipatory Guidance for School-Age Children

Nutrition: Family meals; provide 3 healthy meals and two to three nutritious snacks per day; teach child how to make nutritious choices; avoid high-fat, processed, and "fast" foods; manage weight through exercise and healthy nutrition

Health Promotion: Immunizations (see immunization schedules at http://www.cdc.gov/vaccines/schedules/); recommend CPR and Heimlich maneuver training (see Chapter 23); oral health: brushing, routine cleanings; be alert to mood changes, stress; discuss smoking and substance abuse avoidance; discuss sexual feelings and how to say "no" to sex

Focus on Safety: Seat belt and car safety (use seat belt safety information based on the state of residence; see general guidelines at safercar.gov: http://www.safercar.gov/parents/index.htm); sunscreen; safe home environment: secure matches, guns; bike helmet; water, sports, and playground safety; check smoke detectors; protective equipment for sports; review rules for being home alone

Sleep-Wake Patterns: Require 8 to 12 hours of sleep a night; night terrors may occur

Physical Development: Discuss physical changes related to secondary sex characteristics in later childhood; body odor; some girls may start menstruation in late childhood

Cognitive and Emotional Development: Stimulate thinking; praise academic achievement; provide regular time and space for homework; teach organizational skills; teach and encourage problem-solving skills; implement goal-setting through calendars or charts; assign regular chores; provide for family-centered activities and trips; assist child to recognize and handle new emotions; teach social skills; demonstrate acceptance, love, concern for the child; support participation in hobbies, clubs, and extracurricular activities; discuss ways to handle peer pressure; encourage taking on new responsibilities: volunteering in the community

Motor Development: Daily regular exercise; support participation in organized sports

Discipline: Clearly defined limits; restriction of privileges

Where Research and Practice Meet:
Prevention of Unintentional Injuries

Many studies have been done to examine the reasons that more than 3 million children between the ages of 1 and 7 years are seen annually in emergency rooms and clinics for unintentional injuries (UI). Many legislative and educational initiatives have attempted to improve the number of UI with varying degrees of success.

In an integrative literature review of unintentional early childhood injuries, Rosales and Allen (2012) noted that injuries occur frequently because of parental optimism bias. Simply stated, optimism bias is the feeling that unintentional injuries "won't happen to my child," and it is this bias that leads to poor implementation of safety measures by caregivers, such as installing car seats. The authors concluded that the most effective way to address UI with families lies with the primary health-care providers and nurses. Strategies identified to improve child safety and address optimism bias are:

- Provide age-appropriate anticipatory guidance on child safety and unintentional injuries.
- Discuss with parents or caregivers optimism bias and the common belief that bad things will not happen to their child. Use of fear information may be beneficial.
- Ask parents or caregivers about unintentional injuries to other children in their families to personalize the potential for injury.
- Identify dangerous behaviors exhibited by the child in the examination room that could result in injury. Apply to home setting (Rosales and Allen, 2012, p. 78).

manufacture hormones necessary for reproduction. It is a period of great growth, second only to infancy. While the growth rate is not as dramatic as that of the earlier stage, it is still significant. It is not unusual for girls to gain 15 to 55 pounds (6.8–25 kg) and grow 2 to 8 inches (5–20 cm) and boys to gain 15 to 66 pounds (6.8–30 kg) and grow 4 to 12 inches (10–30 cm) before they reach maturity. Girls develop earlier than boys and tend to have a smaller overall physical structure. Both boys and girls develop primary and secondary sex characteristics at this stage. The timing of development is variable (Table 20-9).

Cognitive Development

Adolescence corresponds with Piaget's Formal Operational stage. The adolescent is able to think abstractly and uses logic to solve problems and to test out hypotheses. In addition, she uses deductive reasoning and can think about thinking. She begins to be concerned with such things as philosophy, morality, and social issues. The adolescent is able to project her thoughts over the long term, thus making plans and setting life goals. She often compares her beliefs with those of her peers.

Language Development

By adolescence, the child has highly developed and sophisticated language skills. She has the ability to speak and write correctly. The adolescent is also able to communicate and debate alternative points of view.

Psychosocial Development

According to Erikson, the adolescent crisis is concerned with identity versus role confusion. The adolescent must begin to identify who she is and who she will be in life. One of the major sources of influence over an adolescent is the peer group (Fig. 20-7). Members of the peer group offer differing viewpoints, allow for the establishment of strong relationships, and provide the opportunity for the adolescent to practice adult behaviors by becoming active within a social group and increasingly self-sufficient.

Table 20-9	Developmental Milestones of the Adolescent (12–18 years)			
Physical Growth	**Gross Motor Skills**	**Fine Motor Skills**	**Cognitive, Sensory, and Language**	**Psychosocial and Play**
Variable Girls: Weight: Increases 15–55 pounds Height: Increases 2–8 inches Boys: Weight: Increases 15–66 pounds Height: Increases 4–12 inches Both genders develop secondary sex characteristics	Begins to develop endurance Increases speed, accuracy, and coordination Develops the necessary skills for an identified interest (sports, hobbies)	Manipulates complicated objects High skill level playing video games and using computer Good finger dexterity for writing and other intricate tasks Precise eye–hand coordination	Abstract thought well developed Uses logic to solve problems Projects thoughts over long term to develop future plans Increased concentration so can follow complicated instructions Senses tied into body image Develops adult preferences based on senses Language: Continues to develop and refine with increased vocabulary up to 50,000 words Improved communication skills; converses with increasing abstract thought and analysis	Psychosocial: Peer group primary social environment; desires parent involvement yet pushes parent away at same time; begins to explore romantic relationships; concentrates on goals and life plans Play: Cooperative play continues within peer group, team sports, school or community activities, and dating; enjoys solitary time

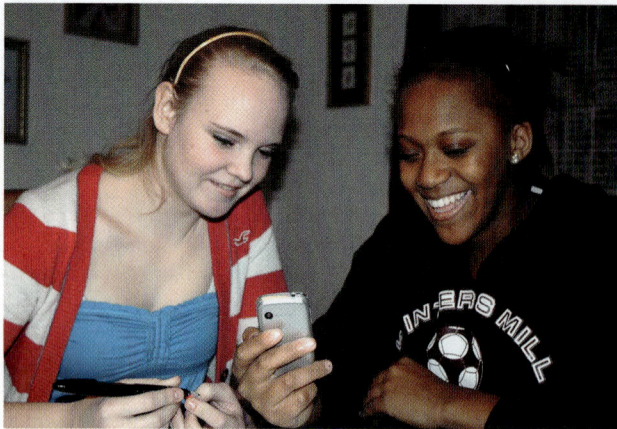

Figure 20-7 Development of strong peer relationships provides adolescents the opportunity to practice adult behaviors.

There are three major issues that must be confronted by the adolescent: selecting an occupation, establishing and subscribing to a set of values, and developing a satisfactory sexual identity. As the adolescent makes these important decisions, she becomes more confident in her abilities and gradually develops a sense of who she is becoming.

 legal alert—Include the adolescent in the informed consent process

An **informed consent** is a way to elicit permission that is given freely that protects a person's right to autonomy and self-determination. Informed consent is given when the person understands the usual procedures, their rationales, and associated risks. A parent or legal guardian customarily gives informed consent on behalf of the child. As children gain critical thinking skills, they can become more active in the consent process. Depending on state law, children under the age of 18 can give legal informed consent under these circumstances: when they are minor parents of the child patient; when they are seeking birth control, counseling, or help for substance abuse; or when they are self-supporting (emancipated). In many states, a pregnant teen is considered emancipated and can provide informed consent. The physician is ultimately responsible for explaining the procedure and related risks, and the nurse's role is to serve as a witness to the signature of a parent for the minor child or an emancipated adolescent. The nurse is responsible for notifying the physician if the parent (or legal guardian) does not understand the procedure or related risks.

Moral Development

At this stage, conflicts emerge between what the adolescent has believed to be right or wrong and what others may believe. This is a time of great questioning and consternation as the adolescent learns that it is possible for several views of morality to exist. Kohlberg defined this stage as postconventional morality.

"What to say"—*Helping the adolescent make good decisions*

The nurse can be influential in helping the adolescent make healthy decisions. This can be accomplished by employing these techniques:

- Listen: Pay close attention not only to what the adolescent is saying, but also to her nonverbal cues. Try to understand her view of the world and stay open minded.
- Discuss without judging: The nurse can share a personal understanding of the issues and various perspectives while respecting those of the adolescent.
- Encourage critical thought: Allow the adolescent to explore and further develop her options.

Discipline

The adolescent is at the stage where she begins to internalize responsibility for behavior. She still needs parental input and guidance in terms of rules (e.g., curfew, homework, chores, etc.) and possible consequences for infractions, but she is much more able than in any previous stage to monitor and regulate her own actions based on her own critical thinking. It is important in this stage, as in all others, that the parent focus on the positives of the adolescent's behavior. Natural consequences are powerful motivators, but by this time, the adolescent may have learned that she can avoid consequences by being crafty. Removing privileges may be an effective consequence for the adolescent's poor decision making.

Anticipatory Guidance

The adolescent is deeply influenced by the peer group. She spends a great deal of time with her peers, often foregoing family activities in favor of time with friends. Depending on the peer group, there may be peer pressure to drink alcohol, smoke, experiment with illicit drugs, or engage in sexual activity. Parents must keep the lines of communication with their adolescent open and teach her how to resist peer pressure. It is important for the adolescent to identify a trusted adult with whom she can talk about sensitive issues and from whom to get advice (Box 20-10).

 Global Health Case Study　Senglui Nguyen

Senglui Nguyen is a 14-year-old Korean American girl born to parents who emigrated from South Korea. Mrs. Nguyen brings her daughter to the Asian Health Clinic for an annual exam. In keeping with clinic practice with adolescents, the nurse asks, and receives, permission from Mrs. Nguyen to speak to Senglui alone for a few minutes before the mother joins her daughter in the exam room. In private, Senglui shares that she has been feeling sad and alone and is tearful much of the time but cannot explain why. Senglui is involved in her high school's volleyball and softball teams but has been skipping practices. She is doing "okay" academically. She shares that she is normally a straight A student but is struggling to maintain a B average this semester. She is part of a multicultural peer group but has not been spending much time with her friends lately, not even her best friend. When asked how things are at home, Senglui states that her parents are "constantly criticizing" her and putting a lot of pressure on her about her grades. They are considering making her give up school sports.

critical thinking questions

1. Based on what Senglui has said, what are you most concerned about?

2. What additional questions would you ask Senglui?

3. What nursing interventions are appropriate at this time?

◆ See Suggested Answers to Global Health Case Studies on Davis*Plus*.

 Nursing Diagnoses The Developing Child

1. Growth and Development, altered related to inadequate caretaking, environmental or stimulation deficiencies.
2. Injury, high risk for related to lack of awareness of environmental hazards.
3. Self-esteem, chronic low related to ineffective relationship with parents or peers.

 Now Can You—Describe normal growth and development?

1. Educate families about what to expect during growth and development at each developmental stage?
2. Educate families regarding anticipatory guidance at each developmental stage?
3. Describe effective discipline for each age group?

Box 20-10 Anticipatory Guidance for Adolescents

Nutrition: Provide 3 healthy meals and two to three healthy snacks per day; avoid high-fat, processed, and "fast" foods; manage weight through exercise and healthy nutrition
Health Promotion: Immunizations (see immunization schedules at http://www.cdc.gov/vaccines/schedules/); oral health; discuss sex, sexual feelings, protection against sexually transmitted infections; abstinence as the best way to prevent pregnancy and sexually transmitted infections; if having sex, discuss birth control and safe sex practices; discuss smoking and substance abuse avoidance; symptoms of stress and how to deal with it
Focus on Safety: Seat belts; driving safety; sports and water safety; sunscreen; avoid tanning salons
Sleep-Wake Patterns: Require 8 to 10 hours of sleep per night
Physical Development: Explain development of secondary sex characteristics; females: explain menstruation and masturbation; males: explain masturbation and nocturnal emissions
Cognitive and Emotional Development: Praise academic success; monitor for academic struggles; encourage new challenges; model respect for differing opinions and needs of others; model conflict resolution strategies; expect increasing independence from family; peer groups and activities with peers are increasingly important; provide for some privacy at home; development of intimate relationships; teach to balance school, work, and peer group participation; begin planning for the future
Motor Development: Daily regular exercise; support participation in organized sports
Discipline: Increase levels of responsibility at home to foster movement to adulthood; restriction of privileges

Summary Points

◆ Prominent theories of development allow the nurse and family to have a deeper understanding of the "why'" behind developmental tasks and stages.

◆ Each child possesses his own way of learning about the world around him.

◆ Information about growth and development, newborn through adolescence, is important for the nurse and family.

◆ Principles of growth and development can assist the nurse when teaching the family about their child.

◆ It is important for the nurse to recognize cultural influences on growth and development.

◆ Even though all children grow and develop in their own manner, each child typically follows a designated pattern or trajectory.

◆ Identifying the specific characteristics that define the temperament of a child can help the nurse and family understand the uniqueness of the child.

◆ Families must adjust to new skills and tasks at each stage of development.

◆ Understanding growth and development provides the nurse with tools to develop a plan of care for the family across care settings.

◆ Anticipatory guidance is an important aspect of the teaching provided to parents by nurses.

Review Questions

Multiple Choice

1. The pediatric nurse assesses the toddler's fine motor skills by observing which task?
  A. Buttoning a shirt
  B. Writing with a pencil
  C. Holding a spoon to eat
  D. Using the pincer grasp

2. According to Piaget, an infant uses his or her senses to learn and explore the environment. Which action is the most appropriate for the nurse to implement to determine object permanence?
  A. Playing the game of peek-a-boo
  B. Encouraging the infant to shake a rattle
  C. Pushing a button on an overhead mobile
  D. Placing the child in a stroller and going for a walk

3. The pediatric nurse is promoting anticipatory guidance about safety to the mother of a 10-month-old infant. Which statement is not appropriate for the nurse to include in the teaching session?
  A. "Do not leave small objects on the floor because your baby will be crawling soon."
  B. "Keep the side rails up to prevent your baby from falling out of the crib."
  C. "Put safety locks on all cabinets to prevent accidents."
  D. "Allow your baby to stay alone for short periods of time to promote independence."

4. The mother of a 26-month-old toddler tells the pediatric nurse that she is having trouble disciplining her daughter. The mother states, "She really knows how to push me to my limit. I don't know what to do with her!" Which response by the nurse is the most therapeutic?
   A. "The terrible twos are a difficult time. You have to show her that you are the boss!"
   B. "When she does something wrong, tell her she is a bad girl and has to be punished for her actions."
   C. "A 2-minute time-out combined with praise for good behavior is very effective for this age group."
   D. "Take away her favorite doll and tell her that she cannot have it back until she changes her behavior."

5. The parents of a toddler ask the nurse how to best prepare the toddler for a planned medical procedure. What should the nurse recognize when answering the toddler's parents?
   A. The toddler is too young to understand what will happen and does not need an explanation.
   B. The use of short explanations can best help the toddler understand the planned procedure.
   C. Allowing the toddler to explore the procedure room may be helpful.
   D. It is beneficial for the nurse to demonstrate the upcoming procedure to the toddler.

6. The father of a 4-year-old is concerned about his son's reaction to an injury of his friend. He told the nurse that the child stayed in his room over the weekend and cried himself to sleep. When the pediatric nurse questioned the child, he described an argument that he and his friend had about a week prior to his friend's injury. Based on the assessment, what is this preschool child exhibiting?
   A. Magical thinking
   B. Inferiority
   C. Guilt complex
   D. A morality issue

7. What is not a key aspect in a teen's environment that helps when making good decisions?
   A. Ability to think abstractly
   B. Ability to use deductive reasoning
   C. Ability to make long-term plans
   D. Ability to use logical thinking

8. A nurse is planning an educational class for new families based on Duvall's family development theory. Based on the theory, how are family stages determined?
   A. Number of children in the family
   B. The oldest child in the family
   C. The youngest child in the family
   D. Years the couple has been married

9. A mother is complaining to the nurse that her 3-year-old child often has difficulty falling and staying asleep. The following day, the child is cranky and uncooperative. Which action by the nurse is the most appropriate?
   A. Assess the child's usual nighttime routine.
   B. Assure mom that sleep and behavior are not related.
   C. Encourage active play before bedtime.
   D. Have mom put the child to bed only when sleepy.

10. A nurse is providing anticipatory guidance to the parents of a preschool-aged child regarding discipline. Which information is most beneficial?
    A. Children at this age lie frequently and without reason.
    B. Consequences should be natural and fit the behavior.
    C. Explaining the rules is not as important as discipline.
    D. Taking away privileges is a powerful tool for this age group.

See Answers to End of Chapter Review Questions on Davis*Plus.*

REFERENCES

Ainsworth, M. (1978). *Patterns of attachment: A psychological study of the strange situation.* Hillsdale, NJ: Lawrence Erlbaum Associates.

American Academy of Pediatrics (AAP) Policy Statement. (2011). Guidance for effective discipline. *Pediatrics, 101*(4), 723–728. Retrieved from http://www.aap.org

Armstrong, Thomas. (2009). *Multiple intelligences in the classroom* (3rd ed.) Alexandria, VA: Association for Supervision & Curriculum Development.

Bowlby, J. (1978). *Attachment and loss.* Harmondsworth, UK: Penguin Education.

Brazelton, T. B. (2006). *Touchpoints: Birth to Three: Your child's emotional and behavioral development.* Cambridge, MA: Perseus.

Brazelton, T. B., & Sparrow, J. (2002). *Touchpoints: Three to Six: Your child's emotional and behavioral development.* Cambridge, MA: Perseus.

Bronfenbrenner, U. (1979). *The ecology of human development.* Cambridge, MA: Harvard University Press.

Bulechek, G., Butcher, H. M., & Dochterman, J. (2013). *Nursing interventions classification (NIC)* (6th ed.). St. Louis, MO: C.V. Mosby.

Duvall, E. R. (1977). *Marriage and family development.* Philadelphia, PA: Lippincott.

Fowler, J. W. (1981). *Stages of faith: The psychology of human development and the quest for meaning.* San Francisco, CA: Harper & Row.

Gardner, H. (2011). *Frames of mind: The theory of multiple intelligences.* New York, NY: Basic Books.

Gilligan, C. (1982). *In a different voice: Psychological theory and women's development.* Cambridge, MA: Harvard University Press.

Kohlberg, L. (1984). *Essays on moral development.* San Francisco, CA: Harper & Row.

Moorehead, S., Johnson, M., Maas, M., & Swanson, E. (2013). *Nursing outcomes classification (NOC)* (4th ed.). St. Louis, MO: C.V. Mosby.

Piaget, J., & Inhelder, B. (1969). *The psychology of the child.* New York, NY: Basic Books.

Rosales, P. R., & Allen, P. L. J. (2012). Optimism bias and parental views on unintentional injuries and safety: Improving anticipatory guidance in early childhood. *Pediatric Nursing, 38*(2), 73–79.

Thomas, A., & Chess, S. (1977). *Temperament and development.* New York, NY: Brunner/Mazel.

Thomas, A., Chess, S., & Birch, H. G. (1968). *Temperament and behavior disorders in children.* New York, NY: New York University Press.

Venes, D. (2013). *Taber's cyclopedic medical dictionary* (22nd ed.). Philadelphia, PA: F.A. Davis Company.

Ward, S., & Hisley, S. (2009). *Maternal-child nursing care. Optimizing outcomes for mothers, children & families.* Philadelphia, PA: F.A. Davis Company.

Watson, J. (2005). *Caring Science as Sacred Science.* Philadelphia, PA: F.A. Davis.

Zero To Three Brainwonders. (n.d.). *Brain development: Frequently asked questions.* Retrieved from http://www.zerotothree.org/brainwonders/FAQ–body.html.

CONCEPT MAP

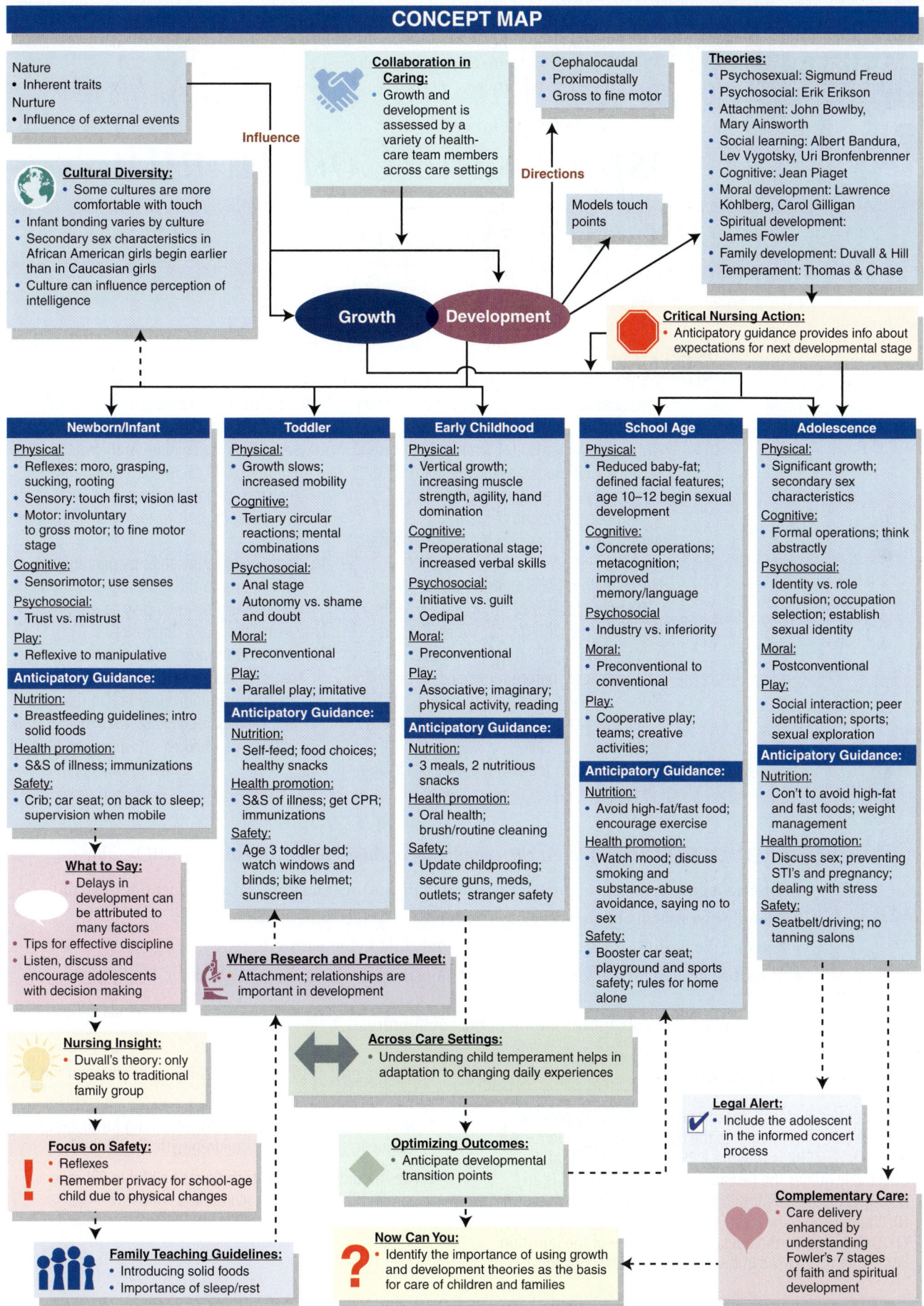

Nature
• Inherent traits
Nurture
• Influence of external events

Influence

Cultural Diversity:
• Some cultures are more comfortable with touch
• Infant bonding varies by culture
• Secondary sex characteristics in African American girls begin earlier than in Caucasian girls
• Culture can influence perception of intelligence

Collaboration in Caring:
• Growth and development is assessed by a variety of health-care team members across care settings

• Cephalocaudal
• Proximodistally
• Gross to fine motor

Directions

Models touch points

Theories:
• Psychosexual: Sigmund Freud
• Psychosocial: Erik Erikson
• Attachment: John Bowlby, Mary Ainsworth
• Social learning: Albert Bandura, Lev Vygotsky, Uri Bronfenbrenner
• Cognitive: Jean Piaget
• Moral development: Lawrence Kohlberg, Carol Gilligan
• Spiritual development: James Fowler
• Family development: Duvall & Hill
• Temperament: Thomas & Chase

Growth **Development**

Critical Nursing Action:
• Anticipatory guidance provides info about expectations for next developmental stage

Newborn/Infant
Physical:
• Reflexes: moro, grasping, sucking, rooting
• Sensory: touch first; vision last
• Motor: involuntary to gross motor; to fine motor stage
Cognitive:
• Sensorimotor; use senses
Psychosocial:
• Trust vs. mistrust
Play:
• Reflexive to manipulative
Anticipatory Guidance:
Nutrition:
• Breastfeeding guidelines; intro solid foods
Health promotion:
• S&S of illness; immunizations
Safety:
• Crib; car seat; on back to sleep; supervision when mobile

Toddler
Physical:
• Growth slows; increased mobility
Cognitive:
• Tertiary circular reactions; mental combinations
Psychosocial:
• Anal stage
• Autonomy vs. shame and doubt
Moral:
• Preconventional
Play:
• Parallel play; imitative
Anticipatory Guidance:
Nutrition:
• Self-feed; food choices; healthy snacks
Health promotion:
• S&S of illness; get CPR; immunizations
Safety:
• Age 3 toddler bed; watch windows and blinds; bike helmet; sunscreen

Early Childhood
Physical:
• Vertical growth; increasing muscle strength, agility, hand domination
Cognitive:
• Preoperational stage; increased verbal skills
Psychosocial:
• Initiative vs. guilt
• Oedipal
Moral:
• Preconventional
Play:
• Associative; imaginary; physical activity, reading
Anticipatory Guidance:
Nutrition:
• 3 meals, 2 nutritious snacks
Health promotion:
• Oral health; brush/routine cleaning
Safety:
• Update childproofing; secure guns, meds, outlets; stranger safety

School Age
Physical:
• Reduced baby-fat; defined facial features; age 10–12 begin sexual development
Cognitive:
• Concrete operations; metacognition; improved memory/language
Psychosocial
• Industry vs. inferiority
Moral:
• Preconventional to conventional
Play:
• Cooperative play; teams; creative activities;
Anticipatory Guidance:
Nutrition:
• Avoid high-fat/fast food; encourage exercise
Health promotion:
• Watch mood; discuss smoking and substance-abuse avoidance, saying no to sex
Safety:
• Booster car seat; playground and sports safety; rules for home alone

Adolescence
Physical:
• Significant growth; secondary sex characteristics
Cognitive:
• Formal operations; think abstractly
Psychosocial:
• Identity vs. role confusion; occupation selection; establish sexual identity
Moral:
• Postconventional
Play:
• Social interaction; peer identification; sports; sexual exploration
Anticipatory Guidance:
Nutrition:
• Con't to avoid high-fat and fast foods; weight management
Health promotion:
• Discuss sex; preventing STI's and pregnancy; dealing with stress
Safety:
• Seatbelt/driving; no tanning salons

What to Say:
• Delays in development can be attributed to many factors
• Tips for effective discipline
• Listen, discuss and encourage adolescents with decision making

Where Research and Practice Meet:
• Attachment; relationships are important in development

Nursing Insight:
• Duvall's theory: only speaks to traditional family group

Across Care Settings:
• Understanding child temperament helps in adaptation to changing daily experiences

Legal Alert:
• Include the adolescent in the informed concert process

Focus on Safety:
• Reflexes
• Remember privacy for school-age child due to physical changes

Optimizing Outcomes:
• Anticipate developmental transition points

Complementary Care:
• Care delivery enhanced by understanding Fowler's 7 stages of faith and spiritual development

Family Teaching Guidelines:
• Introducing solid foods
• Importance of sleep/rest

Now Can You:
• Identify the importance of using growth and development theories as the basis for care of children and families

Caring for the Child in the Hospital, the Community, and Across Care Settings

 A Link in the Chain

Nurses assist in making the lives of children better.

Nurses work in hospitals, in intensive care units with alarms everywhere, in clinics with toys all around, in community settings, or behind desks in offices.

Nurses assist in making the lives of children better.

Nurses help repair children's bodies when they are broken or not made just right.

Nurses help children smile when they are receiving medication that might make them sicker before they become better.

Nurses deliver treatments to open up their airways, change dressings, and deliver IV fluids.

Nurses assist in making the lives of children better.

Nurses must be creative and make medical situations fun rather than frightening.

Nurses cradle the children in their hearts and hands to help them feel secure and safe in a strange environment.

Nurses assist in making the lives of children better.

Nurses give of themselves by opening up their hearts to the families—letting them know that they genuinely care.

Nurses truly make a difference.

Nurses together are a long and strong chain that embraces many children.

Each nurse is an individual link in that chain.

—Megan Connelly, MSN, APRN, CCRN, CPNP-AC, Children's Hospital and Medical Center in Omaha, Nebraska

LEARNING TARGETS *At the completion of this chapter, the student will be able to:*

- Discuss a developmental approach to gathering the history and physical assessment of the child.
- Identify assessment and management issues related to the child in pain.
- Explore the health-care needs of the family and child living with a disability.
- Prioritize developmentally appropriate and holistic nursing care for the child and family across care settings.
- Examine ways to care for the family in the community.

PICO(T) Questions

The intent of evidence-based practice (EBP) is to provide nursing care that integrates the best available evidence. An initial step in EBP is to write a PICO(T) question that effectively guides the research. A PICO(T) question is an acronym that stands for population (P), intervention or issue (I), comparison of interest (C), outcome (O), and timeframe (T). Depending on the question, all or some of the question components are used in the research process. Use these

PICO(T) questions to spark your thinking as you read the chapter.

1. What is the (O) best method for screening for (I) caregiver fatigue in (P) parents of children with disabilities?

2. Are (I) guided imagery techniques helpful in (O) reducing pain in (P) hospitalized school-age children?

Evidence-Based Practice

Murphy, K. L., Kobayashi, D., Golden, S. L., & Nageswaran, S. (2012). Rural and nonrural differences in providing care for children with complex chronic conditions. *Clinical Pediatrics, 51*(5), 498–503.

The purpose of this study was to better understand the challenges of providing care for children with complex chronic conditions (CCC) as faced by primary care providers. National statistics indicate that close to 14% of children in the United States have special health-care needs. Households with at least one special needs child include more than one-fifth of the homes in the United States of which children with CCC are considered a subgroup. Murphy, Kobayashi, Golden, and Nageswaran (2012) describe this subgroup as including "children who are medically fragile, technology dependent, or medically complex" (p. 498). Children in this category are living longer and account for a large portion of hospitalizations, hospital days, and hospital charges than they did 10 years ago. Previous studies have noted access to care in rural settings is more difficult to obtain because of a lack of providers and other resources as well as transportation issues. Providing family-centered, comprehensive, and coordinated care for this population is also encompassed by the *Healthy People 2020* Objective 31. The medical home model, which was developed by the American Academy of Pediatrics, addresses the care of special needs children living in rural areas although it is currently not available to all children with CCC. Murphy, Kobayashi, Golden, and Nageswaran (2012) contend that understanding the challenges faced in providing care to CCC children better equips the medical community in meeting those needs.

Of the initial 316 surveys that were sent to primary care providers, 132 responded (42%) and agreed to participate. This included a total of 132 physicians, nurse practitioners, and physician assistants in pediatric and family practice settings located in six counties of one southeastern state, which was further divided into cohorts of 94 physicians and 37 midlevel providers. Five of the six counties in the study were classified as rural. The participants were placed in either rural or non-rural cohorts, which were broken into physician and midlevel provider groups and are as follows: rural physicians n=31 (67%) and midlevel providers n=15 (33%); non-rural physicians n=63 (74%) and midlevel providers n=22 (26%). The practice settings were as follows: a total of 58 (47%) pediatric practices of which 13 (29%) were in rural settings and 45 (57%) were in non-rural settings; family practice or other groups a total of 66 (53%) of which 31 (71%) were in rural settings and 34 (43%) were in non-rural settings.

Data were gathered using a cross-sectional survey of primary care providers, which included physicians, nurse practitioners, and physician assistants. The survey was composed of 41 questions. The content of the survey was further divided into questions related to communication between hospital-based and primary care providers and care provided for children with CCC. Demographic questions included location, number, and nature (i.e., physician, NP, or PA) of the providers in the office, number of office staff, and portion of children with CCC needs. Providers were also asked about the perceived level of difficulty in caring for children with CCC as well as barriers to providing care and availability of a care coordinator. Level of difficulty in providing the care had four options to select from (i.e., very difficult, somewhat difficult, not difficult, and does not apply). For

the purpose of analysis, the responses were collapsed into two categories (i.e., very/somewhat difficult and not difficult/does not apply). Providers were also asked to respond by yes or no to the question regarding perceptions about whether a care coordinator would improve the ease of caring for the children with CCC.

Data were examined using univariate and bivariate analysis. The open-ended responses were reviewed and organized into themes by two independent investigators. Analysis of data concluded that pediatric practices were more likely to be found in non-rural areas (57%) than in rural areas (29%). Rural practices were more likely to have a smaller number of staff and providers than non-rural practices. The researchers further stated that rural practices were three times more likely to have a smaller portion of children with CCC than non-rural practices (52% vs. 26%, respectively). Seventy-seven percent (n=97) of the total participants in the study reported that providing care for children with CCC was very/somewhat difficult. This was further divided into rural and non-rural participants with responses as follows: n=32 (70%) versus n=65 (81%), respectively. A total of 97 (81%) participants responded that a care coordinator would improve the ease of providing care. This was further expanded into rural and non-rural responses as follows: n=35 (78%) versus n=62 (83%), respectively. The researchers extrapolated five main themes from participant responses to the question regarding difficulties faced in providing care for children with CCC: "(1) poor communication between providers (specialists and other agencies), (2) delay or difficulty in obtaining referrals to specialists, (3) difficulty coordinating care with multiple providers, (4) lack of services or resources in the community for CCC, and (5) lack of knowledge about issues related to CCC and resources in the community for children with CCC" (p. 500). Themes that emerged describing how a care coordinator would help included "(1) helping coordinate care between multiple specialists and agencies, (2) making access to specialists easier, (3) helping families with logistics (e.g., making appointments, transportation, etc.), and (4) improving communication between multiple specialists" (p. 501).

The researchers concluded that providers in rural practices were less equipped to provide care for children with CCC. Primary care providers in both rural and non-rural settings experienced difficulties in caring for children with CCC. Location, smaller numbers of staff and providers, and availability of community resources contribute to the difficulty in providing care to this population in rural settings. Lack of care coordination was found to be a constant theme throughout the study. The researchers also concluded that the addition of a care coordinator could increase the efficiency, reduce the barriers, and decrease the costs of providing care to children with CCC.

1. How is this information useful to clinical nursing practice?

2. Based on these findings, what are implications for further research?

See Suggested Responses for Evidence-Based Practice on Davis*Plus*.

Introduction

The standards of nursing practice describe a competent level of care for the nursing profession (American Nurses Association [ANA], 2010). Several themes that are fundamental to many of the standards include providing age-appropriate and culturally sensitive care, maintaining a safe environment, educating patients about healthy practices, and ensuring continuity of care (ANA, 2010). For a pediatric nurse, these themes are fundamental to a holistic and caring practice (Fig. 21-1).

Registered nurses are held accountable for thinking critically through conclusions derived in the course of their practice. The judgments made and actions taken are based on a core body of knowledge. This chapter provides the basis of that core in several areas.

First, the chapter presents a complete assessment of the child and family. Age-appropriate and culturally sensitive topics are interspersed throughout the chapter in relation to history-taking and the physical assessment of the child.

How children perceive and respond to pain depends on many factors. The nurse must take into account the child's developmental level, type and severity of pain, and psychological considerations. Pain assessment tools and common pain management strategies are described.

The child with a disability presents additional challenges for the pediatric nurse. The child living with a disabling condition often requires the involvement of several medical specialties. The pediatric nurse is in a unique position to assist the family in learning about complex medical issues and providing support when needed.

Medical care and, therefore, nursing care is accessed in a variety of settings. Pediatric nurses in all settings must have a sound understanding of normal growth and development to be better able to assess when there are disturbances in progress, including regression because of hospitalization or loss of previously attained milestones. The nurse becomes acquainted with the norms of pediatric nursing practice in the context of caring for the child across care settings and understands that the nurse's practice must be individualized for the unique needs of the child. Because each child has a personal story to share, nurses are in a privileged position to guide and educate the child and the family.

Finally, the chapter presents the fundamentals of general care measures the nurse provides in the hospital, clinic, and community settings. Maintaining a safe environment is an essential component for some general care practices, such as the use of restraints and infection control measures. Explaining procedures gives nurses the opportunity to educate the patient about healthy practices, to relieve anxiety, and to promote well-being.

Gathering the Child's Health History

ESTABLISHING A RELATIONSHIP WITH THE PATIENT AND THE FAMILY

Assessing a child's health history can be a daunting task. Children vary in language skills, clarity of speech, cognitive abilities, and social skills. Some children can verbalize where they hurt while others may only react by crying. Each child must be approached with these differences in mind. Any differences that fall out of the realm of what is considered normal growth and development should be noted by the nurse and other members of the health-care team.

For an infant or a nonverbal child, the nurse begins the health history with an interview of the parents, grandparents, foster parents, stepparents, nannies, older siblings,

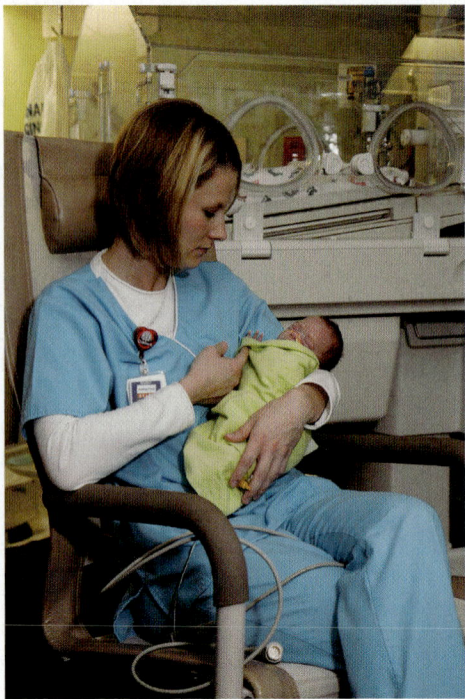

Figure 21-1 Pediatric nurse holding a child.

Growth and Development

Pediatric care can occur in a variety of settings including the hospital, clinic, school, or rehabilitation center. Regardless of location of service, measurement and assessment of pediatric growth and developmental milestones should be included in routine health screening and physical assessment. Growth and development occurs across varying settings and can be influenced by the environment. It is essential that the nurse understand ways to promote normal growth and development regardless of location. The nurse must have a vast knowledge about growth and development and ways to encourage healthy attainment of milestones (Ward & Hisley, 2009).

Children primarily learn through stimulation and play. Play helps children develop fine and gross motor skills, hand-eye coordination, communication skills, social skills, problem-solving skills, and memory development (Barrett, 2012). Nursing care should focus on providing toys and stimulation that are appropriately based on the developmental age of the child and the situation. Toys and stimulation that are appropriate for school may not be acceptable in the hospital. The nurse should have knowledge about what types of activities and toys are appropriate for varying situations. The nurse can encourage the family members to bring the child's favorite things from home to minimize stress and create a sense of safety for the child as he or she receives care in different settings. When hospitalization is required, health restoration is a priority, but consideration of growth and development must be included in the nursing plan of care. Collaboration with the child life specialist can be helpful to identify appropriate resources for the child, regardless of location of service.

Source: Barrett, L. (2012). Toys that are S.A.F.E. (Sturdy, Age Appropriate, Fun and Economical). *EParent Magazine,* (October, 2012). Retrieved from www.eparent.com; Ward, S., & Hisley, S. (2009). *Maternal-child nursing care: Optimizing outcomes for mothers, children & families.* Philadelphia, PA: F.A. Davis.

Where Research and Practice Meet:
Health Insurance Portability and Accountability Act

The nurse must remember to comply with the **Health Insurance Portability and Accountability Act** of 1996 (HIPAA) when assessing and caring for the pediatric patient. This privacy act ensures that the child's health information is protected while allowing the flow of health information needed to ensure high-quality health care (U.S. Department of Health and Human Services, 2012).

and adult guardians who accompany the child to the health-care setting. After introductions are made, it is important to clarify the identity of the person who has brought the child in for care.

Young children need to feel secure before engaging in conversation with the nurse. In this instance, the nurse should establish a rapport with the parent first. Once the child feels comfortable with the nurse present, the child may be more apt to contribute to the interview process. The child may be able to add important pieces of information needed for optimum care.

The older school-age child may elect to be interviewed without the parent in the room. This allows the child to speak freely of his concerns and to ask questions regarding his health. The nurse should speak with the parent separately to determine if the parent has specific concerns or issues that may need to be addressed during the visit.

With the adolescent, the nurse may ask the parent to leave the room during the discussion of issues related to social and sexual content. The adolescent needs to know that a discussion can take place without the parent's knowledge to allow for the provision of appropriate medical and nursing care that will ensure the safety of the child. Exceptions to maintaining confidentiality involve instances concerning abuse or a life-threatening situation.

 Nursing Insight—Family dynamics

Family dynamics are assessed by observing the behaviors between the child and his parent.
Questions to consider:

- During a health-care visit, does the parent or caregiver seem appropriately concerned about the problem?
- Does the parent or caregiver have the information that a responsible parent would know regarding the child's illness, past medical history, and immunizations? Is the parent or caregiver a reliable historian?
- Is the parent or caregiver providing comfort to the child if the child is frightened?
- Does the parent or caregiver appear angry about being in the office?
- Is the parent or caregiver aware of the needs of the child?
- Does the child look well cared for?

ASKING QUESTIONS

The interview is conducted in a comfortable room with available seating for the parent and with eye-level interaction with both the parent and the child. An unhurried environment

encourages the parent to ask questions appropriate to the health of the child. The nurse projects a genuine interest in and a desire to help the child and family. This lays the foundation for a positive therapeutic relationship.

Beginning with open-ended questions allows for concerns to be explored, as the nurse invites the child or parent to tell his story by asking, "How can I help you today?" or, for a problem-oriented visit, "What made you come in today?" (Hogan-Quigley, Palm, & Bickley, 2011). This type of question allows the parent to recount the history of the present condition, also known as the chief complaint. A focused or problem-oriented health history is then obtained.

When clarifying the child's history, the nurse may use the mnemonic **OLD CAT** (Hogan-Quigley et al., 2011) to ask the appropriate questions. For example, a child complaining of pain would be asked these questions:

Onset: "When did the pain start?"
Location: "Where is the pain?"
Duration: "How long does the pain last?"
Character: "Can you tell me on on a scale of 1 to 10 how bad it is?" Or, for a younger child, ask the parent, "How much pain do you think the child is experiencing?" or use a pain scale that is appropriate for the child's level of development.
Aggravating/Alleviating: "What has made the pain better or worse?"
Timing: "When does the pain start/stop?"

After the chief complaint is determined, the child's past medical history is reviewed. This includes past acute illnesses and history of chronic illnesses, immunization history, hospitalizations, emergency room visits, serious injuries, operations, and current medication usage. Inquiries are made as to the use of any over-the-counter medications, herbal preparations, or folk remedies and any history of allergic reactions to food, medications, and environmental allergens. Information regarding reactions experienced by the child to a reported allergen is noted on the patient's chart.

 Cultural Diversity: Use of Complementary and Alternative Medicine

During the pediatric assessment, the nurse must assess the use of complementary and alternative medicine (CAM). CAM is a broad term that defines a wide variety of practices that generally are not a part of Western medicine. Some of these practices include the use of herbal medicines, dietary supplements, acupuncture, massage, biofeedback, yoga, spiritual practices, and others. Refer to Table 21-1 to review commonly used herbal preparations.

According to the National Center for Complementary and Alternative Medicine (2011), more than one-third of adult Americans use some form of CAM. Kundu and colleagues (2011) conducted a study of the medical staff at a large metropolitan children's hospital about physician attitudes regarding the use of CAM. More than two-thirds of the medical staff was aware of their patients' use of CAM, and an equal number recommended CAM to their patients. Unfortunately, the positive attitude about CAM therapies did not translate into a collaborative effort between the pediatricians and the CAM providers. Only 4% of pediatricians reported that they communicated regularly

Table 21-1 Commonly Used Herbal Preparations

Herbal Medicine	Common Indications	Contraindications	Nursing Considerations
Aloe Vera	Oral: constipation Topical: minor skin irritations	Oral: intestinal obstruction, acute surgical abdomen, inflammatory bowel disease	Oral preparations may cause abdominal pain Oral preparations should not be given to children under 12 years of age
Bilberry	Diarrhea	Pregnancy Lactation	Increased risk of bleeding if used concomitantly with anticoagulant and antithrombotic medications May cause nausea
Cayenne Pepper	Analgesic Oral gargle: sore throat Topical: muscle spasms	Oral: stomach ulcers, irritable bowel syndrome Topical: cannot be applied to open wounds	Oral preparations should not be used in patients with gastrointestinal or renal disease Topical preparations may cause a burning sensation and redness of the skin
Chamomile	Pain associated with colic, teething, stomachaches	Do not use if allergic to daisies, marigolds, or ragweed	Be alert for a hypersensitivity reaction Should not be used concomitantly with anticoagulant use, particularly warfarin (Coumadin)
Echinacea	Common cold Fever Inflammation of the mouth and pharynx	Do not use in presence of tuberculosis, multiple sclerosis, HIV, or AIDS	The immune-stimulating effect of echinacea may interfere with the action of immunosuppressant medications
Fennel	Colic and stomach spasms Upper respiratory infections	None identified	May have a laxative effect
Feverfew	Migraines Rheumatic diseases	Pregnancy Lactation	Not to be used in children under the age of 2 years
Licorice	Oral: cough, gastritis Topical: eczema	Diabetes Hypertension Liver or renal disease	Safe for short-term use in children May cause hypokalemia, dysrhythmias, hypertension
Saint John's Wort	Mild depression Anxiety	History of photosensitivity	Common side effects include restlessness, fatigue, frequent urination, headache Multiple herb-drug interactions
Tea Tree Oil	Topical: skin infections	Not to be used on eczematous lesions	Allergic contact dermatitis is common
Valerian	Insomnia	Liver disease	Increased risk of bleeding if used concomitantly with anticoagulant and antithrombotic medications

Source: National Center for Complementary and Alternative Medicine, http://nccam.nih.gov

with their patients' CAM providers (Kundu, Tassone, Jimenez, Seidel, Valentine, & Pagel, 2011).

A culturally competent nurse takes the time to become familiar with the health practices and beliefs of the diverse cultures in the community in which the nurse practices. The nurse understands that "important components of culture are dynamic and always changing, are shared by other members of the same cultural group, are learned from birth via language, socialization, and acquisition, and that the culture adapts to the specific conditions of the group such as the environment, ethnicity, religion or spirituality, education, occupation, time orientation, socialization, health practices and beliefs, and prevalent health conditions" (Ward, 2013). The nurse must value and respect those practices and adapt the intake history to determine communication and decision-making practices within the family and account for **ethnocultural** (relating to a particular ethnic group) beliefs about health and illness. For an example of a transcultural nursing assessment tool, visit http://www.culturediversity.org/assmtform.htm (Transcultural Nursing, 2012).

 Cultural Diversity: Avoid Stereotyping

Stereotyping an individual or a family based on a specific racial or cultural background, or assuming that all members of a particular culture subscribe to the traditions, beliefs, and customs associated with that culture, must be avoided. Length of time in the country, level of education, level of acculturation, and economic status all affect the degree to which the culture shapes the parent's approach to health care (Purnell, 2009). The nurse must be aware of how the patient's culture may affect views on health care and inquire about this during the health history and entire assessment process.

The impact of the current illness is evaluated by inquiring about the child's daily activities, using the mnemonic **SODA** to ask the appropriate questions:

Sleep: "How has your child been sleeping?"
Output: "How many times per day do you _____?" (Use the expression the family has

adopted to convey urine/stool output.) Or, for the younger child ask, "How many wet diapers has he had today?"

Diet: "How much fluid has your child taken in today?" "Has the illness affected the child's appetite or diet?"

Activity: "Has the child's activity level changed since he has been ill?"

Interviews are commonly concluded by asking if the parents have any other concerns or problems they would like to discuss.

COMPREHENSIVE HEALTH HISTORY

When a child is seen for a well-child visit, a comprehensive health history is necessary. Components of a child's health history include family medical and social history, immunizations, past medical history, developmental milestones achieved, patterns of daily activities, and a review of systems.

Family Medical and Social History

The family medical and social history includes documenting the current household makeup and the age and health of each family member. Document the following:

- Ages and cause of death of any deceased parents, grandparents, and siblings
- Chronic illnesses experienced by family members
- Inherited diseases
- Parents' professions, religious affiliations or spiritual beliefs, and family activities
- For the older child, interviewed without the presence of the parent, the social history must also include information regarding grade level, friendships, drug or alcohol use, smoking, sexual activity, and safe sex practices

Past Medical History

A thorough birth history can provide valuable information about the health status of a younger child. The history of the pregnancy, labor and delivery, and the health of the baby at birth are documented, including the birth weight and APGAR scores, if available. In addition, any difficulties with feeding, breathing, jaundice, or other medical problems in the early neonatal period must be documented.

The past medical history in children includes documentation of all acute illnesses. Chronic illnesses and the medications that have been prescribed are listed as well as the use of any herbal products and home remedies. If the child's chart is available, all encounter forms are reviewed to determine the reason for the visits, resultant medical diagnoses, and outcomes of previous treatments.

Immunizations

Common childhood diseases the child may have had, as well as any immunizations received, are documented, and the chart is reviewed before the interview to determine if the immunizations are current. Maintaining current immunization status protects the child and family against preventable communicable diseases. The Centers for Disease Control and Prevention (CDC) reviews and updates the immunization schedule regularly, so it is important for the nurse to be aware of and follow the most current guidelines (CDC, 2012a). The CDC Web site provides the most current child immunization schedules: http://www.cdc.gov/vaccines/schedules/index.html.

Developmental Milestones

A solid foundation in growth and development is a necessity for the nurse working in a pediatric setting. The developmental assessment is essential to determine if a child's development is within the normal range, delayed, or the child is at risk. Developmental milestones can be assessed using the **Denver II Screening Test** in children from birth to 6 years of age. The Denver II assesses personal–social, fine motor–adaptive, gross motor, and language skills (Frankenburg, Dobbs, Archer, Shapiro, & Bresnick, 1992). The nurse also documents the child's behaviors during administration of the test, including compliance, interest in surroundings, fearfulness, and a subjective measure of the child's attention span. After the test has been administered, the parents may be asked if the child's performance was characteristic of his normal behaviors. Referral is needed when the child has "failed" the test with two or more delays, if there is no improvement in areas of concern 3 months after the initial screen, or if the child is determined to be "un-testable" at two consecutive screenings.

Administering the 125-item test requires training. Information on training sessions and testing materials can be obtained through the following link: http://www.denverii.com/DenverII.html.

Patterns of Daily Activities

SLEEP. The nurse must determine both the number of hours and the quality of sleep the child receives each night. Sleep requirements change as the child grows, and each child's sleep requirements are different. Newborns sleep about 16 or 17 hours a day, typically in stretches of 2 to 3 hours at a time. Babies are typically able to sleep through the night by age 6 months. Children also differ in their ability to sleep. Some can sleep anywhere under any conditions while others suffer sleepless nights if there is even the slightest change in their normal routine. Naps may be a part of a child's life up to the preschool years. Children may experience nightmares or night terrors that can disrupt sleep. Nightmares may reflect the struggles children experience during the day or the fears a child has regarding separation, impulses, or conflicts. Night terrors occur during the first few hours of sleep. Nightmares and night terrors can be frightening experiences for a child; a child can recount her nightmares. However, the child has no recollection of night terrors.

NUTRITION. The questions a nurse asks regarding nutrition are based on the child's age. If the infant is breastfed, information is gathered as to how often and for how long the child is fed at each feeding and how many wet diapers are changed in the course of one day. With sufficient breast milk intake, the infant will have six or more wet diapers and gain weight.

For the infant who is receiving formula, information is gathered as to the type of formula, the amount taken at each feeding, and the number of feedings per day. It is also important to note if and when juices or solid foods have been started and whether supplements or vitamins have been prescribed.

When assessing children and adolescents, a 24-hour recall elicits the food items eaten in a typical day and reflects sociocultural trends. In addition, the nurse must document food allergies for all children. Foods and caloric intake should be appropriate for age and developmental level

(Table 21-2). Analysis of the child's food intake is compared with the foods suggested on MyPlate.gov for children over the age of 2 years. The servings for children are based on age, gender, and activity. Table 21-3 displays the recommended servings for each food group based on age, gender, and an activity level of less than 30 minutes per day. For those who participate in more than 30 minutes of physical activity per day, the number of servings may need to increase, provided they do not exceed the recommended daily caloric intake (go to www.choosemyplate.gov/food-groups). The "plate" on this Web site provides a familiar visual representation of the amount of food from each food group one should consume at each meal. The recommendations are that fruits and vegetables should cover one-half of the plate, proteins fill slightly less than one-quarter of the plate, grains fill just over one-quarter of the plate, and the dairy is represented by a glass in this "place setting." The nurse must be familiar with this Web site to better educate children and families.

Macronutrients

Daily caloric intake must have a balance of the macronutrients—protein, carbohydrates, and fat. Together, these macronutrients provide for a healthy diet.

PROTEIN. Ten to 35% of daily caloric intake must come from protein sources such as dairy products, eggs, lean meat, seafood, poultry, beans and peas (e.g., pinto, lentils, lima, split pea, and white beans), soy products (e.g., soy beans, tofu, and veggie burgers), and nuts and seeds (e.g., almonds, peanuts, and sesame seeds). Protein intake each week should include 8 ounces of seafood because this is a good source of lean protein and omega-3 fatty acids. After the age of 2 years, whole milk should be switched to low-fat or skim milk.

CARBOHYDRATES. Carbohydrates account for 45% to 65% of the daily caloric intake. Carbohydrate sources include grains, fruits, and vegetables. Half of all grain servings per day should be whole grains like quinoa, oatmeal, and brown rice or pasta.

FAT. Contrary to popular belief, not all fat is bad fat. In fact, 20% to 35% of daily caloric intake should be from fat. Saturated fats, those that are solid at room temperature, are implicated in the development of heart disease. Animal fat (meat and milk products) is the main source of saturated fats. It becomes important to recommend skinless poultry, lean meat, and fat-free milk when preparing meals for children. Unsaturated fats are those that are liquid at room temperature, known as oils; olive oil, canola oil, and soybean oil provide healthy alternatives to saturated fats.

Table 21-2 Average Daily Caloric Requirements for Children

Age	Daily Caloric Requirements
0–1 month	100–110 kcal/kg per day
2–4 months	90–100 kcal/kg per day
5–60 months	70–90 kcal/kg per day
>5 years	1,500 kcal for first 20 kg + 25 kcal for each additional kg

Source: Hay, W. W. Jr., Levin, M., Sondheimer, J., & Deterding, R. (2010). *Current diagnosis & treatment: Pediatrics* (20th ed.). New York, NY: Lange Medical Books/McGraw-Hill.

Case Study The Child at Risk for Obesity

Tariq is a 14-year-old African American adolescent who is at the 80th percentile for weight with a BMI in the overweight category. He leads a relatively sedentary lifestyle and spends about 4 hours a day playing video games. The family history is significant for parents who are both overweight. Tariq's father is being treated for hyperlipidemia, and his mother was recently diagnosed with type 2 diabetes. A maternal grandmother also has type 2 diabetes. The parents bring Tariq to the clinic today because they recognize their son is at risk and are motivated to improve health outcomes for their child.

critical thinking questions

1. What are the risk factors that may contribute to developing future health problems?

2. As an overweight child, what health problems is he at risk for developing in the future?

3. What strategies can be implemented at this time to prevent obesity and its associated complications?

◆ See Suggested Answers to Case Studies on Davis*Plus*.

Table 21-3 Recommended Food Group Servings by Age

Food Group	Children 2–3 Years Old	Children 4–8 Years Old	Girls 9–13 Years Old	Girls 14–18 Years Old	Boys 9–13 Years Old	Boys 14–18 Years Old
Protein	2 oz	4 oz	5 oz	5 oz	5 oz	6.5 oz
Vegetables	1 cup	1.5 cups	2 cups	2.5 cups	2.5 cups	3 cups
Fruit	1 cup	1–1.5 cups	1.5 cups	1.5 cups	1.5 cups	2 cups
Grain (at least ½ of the grains should be whole grains)	1.5 oz whole grain 1.5 oz other grains	2.5 oz whole grain 2.5 oz other grains	3 oz whole grain 3 oz other grains	3 oz whole grain 3 oz other grains	3 oz whole grain 3 oz other grains	4 oz whole grain 4 oz other grains
Dairy	2 cups	2.5 cups	3 cups	3 cups	3 cups	3 cups
Fats	3 tsp	4 tsp	5 tsp	5 tsp	5 tsp	6 tsp

PLAY, ACTIVITIES, AND SCHOOL. Patterns of play and children's activities reflect the interests of the child, the family financial circumstances, work schedules of the parents, environmental safety, and the availability of after-school activities. Throughout infancy, learning takes place in the context of sensory stimulation. The parent can provide insight into whether there is sufficient stimulation in the immediate environment to help the child learn. For example, talking and singing adds auditory stimulation. Holding, cuddling, and consoling the infant provides the tactile sensory stimulation for developing a sense of trust and facilitates the bonding process.

As the child matures, continued supervision of the child's activities is needed to encourage social competence and healthy habits. Information is gathered about the daily routine of the child; the contact the child has with playmates, older siblings, and adults; and whether the child has an opportunity to develop gross and fine motor skills or has attended community programs such as Head Start. For school-age children, additional information is gathered regarding achievement with schoolwork, special education needs, extracurricular activities, and interaction with peers.

An understanding of the patterns of daily activities allows the nurse to make suggestions for a healthy lifestyle to the parent or child, alert the primary care provider of potential problems, and provide anticipatory guidance as appropriate to the situation.

Review of Systems

Much like the physical examination, the **review of systems** (a series of questions about each body system) is best conducted with a head-to-toe approach, starting with a general question regarding each body system. The review of systems includes the following areas:

- General: usual weight, change in weight, weakness, fatigue, fever, or allergies
- Skin: rashes, pruritus, turgor, changes in color, indications of injury, acne, changes in nails or hair
- Head, Eyes, Ears, Nose, Throat (HEENT): injury to head, headaches, dizziness; eye infections, itching or watering eyes, behaviors indicating change in visual acuity, use of glasses, date of last eye exam; ear infections, behaviors indicating change in hearing; nose bleeds, colds, hay fever, sinus infections; sore throats, tonsils, dentition, caries
- Neck: neck pain, enlarged lymph glands, neck range of motion
- Chest: respiratory infections, asthma, chronic cough, wheezing, shortness of breath, breast changes
- Cardiovascular: heart murmur, palpitations, date of last blood work
- Gastrointestinal: regurgitation, vomiting, changes in bowel habits, constipation, diarrhea, food intolerance, abdominal pain, changes in appetite or eating pattern
- Genitourinary: *General*—dysuria, urgency, odor to urine, date of last urinalysis, signs of puberty, urethral or vaginal discharge, presence of lesions, sexual habits, contraceptive use, and symptoms or history of sexually transmitted infections; *males*—changes in groin/scrotum/glans, presence of circumcision; *females*—**menarche** (the first menstrual period), date of last menstrual period, dysmenorrhea, and date of last Pap smear (if appropriate)
- Musculoskeletal: injuries, fractures, weakness, clumsiness, gait, muscle pains
- Neurological: seizures, tics, psychiatric diseases, anxiety, depression
- Endocrine: history or symptoms of thyroid disease or diabetes or diseases that affect normal growth

---

 Now Can You—**Discuss the health history for the child?**

1. State the major components of a comprehensive health history for the child?
2. Ask appropriate questions about the child's health?
3. Discuss important elements in the review of systems?

Health Assessment

When examining children, the approach to the physical assessment is based on the child's age, cognitive level, and degree of illness. Infants can be examined from head to toe without difficulty. Some children are fearful of any examiner and are uncooperative. Others seem to enjoy the experience as something new. As a guideline, an exam starts with the least invasive actions and concludes with the most distressful actions. For example, it is easier to examine the posterior lung fields with the caregiver holding the child on her lap early in the exam while leaving the examination of the ears and mouth for the end of the exam.

ANTHROPOMETRIC MEASUREMENTS

Before the physical assessment, vital signs and **anthropometric measurements** (growth measurements of length, weight, and head circumference) are taken and recorded. Growth charts from the National Center for Health Statistics (NCHS) were revised in 2000 to include body mass index-for-age (BMI-for-age) percentiles. These growth charts can be found at http://www.cdc.gov/growthcharts/charts.htm (CDC, 2012b).

Length

Length is measured in the infant while he is lying supine on a measuring tray or board. If a measuring board is not available, the nurse holds the head in midline while an assistant holds the hips and knees extended flat on a paper-covered table. Points are marked at the top of the head and the heels of the feet, the child is moved, and the distance between markings is measured. For the older child a **stadiometer** (a device used to measure a standing height) is used to obtain a standing height. The child removes his shoes and stands with his back to the stadiometer, with the back of the heels and shoulders touching the wall.

Weight

The weight of an infant is measured using an infant scale lined with a thin paper cover. After the scale setting is balanced, the infant's clothing is removed and the child is weighed in either a supine or sitting position. The nurse protects the child from an accidental fall by placing a hand over the infant without direct contact. Older children are weighed on a standing scale. The same scales should be used to measure height and weight at each visit.

Body Mass Index

Once weight and height are assessed, body mass index (BMI) can be calculated. The BMI is used to assess total body fat and nutritional status. In children, the BMI is represented as a percentile, allowing a comparison to other children of the same age and gender. BMI is assessed at least once a year at the annual well-child appointment.

 Diagnostic Tools Body Mass Index (BMI)

A BMI-for-age plotted below the 5th percentile indicates a child who is underweight; a BMI-for-age between the 5th and less than the 85th percentile is considered a healthy weight; children with a BMI-for-age between the 85th and less than the 95th percentile are considered overweight; and those with a BMI-for-age greater than 95% are considered obese.

 Assessment Tool Body Mass Index (BMI)

The BMI-for-age is calculated by dividing the weight in kilograms by the meter height squared. Because most health-care providers obtain height in centimeters, an alternative calculation is to divide the weight in kilograms by the centimeter height squared multiplied by 10,000. For example, the BMI for an 8-year-old boy who weighs 26 kg with a height of 135 cm is calculated as follows: 26 divided by 135^2 (18,225) × 10,000 = 14.26. A BMI of 14.26, plotted on the growth chart between the 10th and 25th percentile, is a healthy weight. The nurse can help the family calculate their child or teen's BMI by accessing the CDC Web site (http://apps.nccd.cdc.gov/dnpabmi) (CDC, 2012c).

Head Circumference

For children 3 years of age and younger, head circumference measurements are done at routine well-child visits. The head's largest circumference is measured by placing the tape over the lower forehead, above the pinna of the ears, and over the occipital prominence (Fig. 21-2). This measurement is recorded in centimeters and displayed as a percentile. As with weight and height, evidence of growth within the percentiles remains consistent over time, with normal values according to age and gender reflecting normal development. When there is a deviation, either below or above the percentile from the previous visit, it may signify a potential problem. The nurse informs the primary care provider of these findings.

Skinfold Thickness Measurements

A skinfold thickness measurement is not used in a routine assessment but taken when the health assessment indicates, such as when the child is obese. The skinfold thickness measurement denotes the degree of adipose tissue or body fat. In addition to calculating and plotting the BMI once yearly, as recommended by the American Academy of Pediatrics (AAP, 2003), skinfold thickness measurements can add to the objective assessment of obesity in children and adolescents who are at risk. The nurse might measure the degree of skinfold thickness in the triceps or abdominal areas. The average of two consecutive readings is used as the skinfold thickness measurement. The reliability of the skin fold measurement is entirely dependent on correct measurement technique.

VITAL SIGNS

Temperature

Vital signs consist of temperature, pulse, respirations, and blood pressure (Table 21-4). A variety of digital and tympanic thermometers are available. The route used for assessing temperature depends on the age and developmental level of the child. Newborn temperature is assessed via the axillary route. The tip of a digital thermometer is placed in the axilla with the arm held against the side of the body until the temperature registers. Rectal temperatures are not routinely measured. If a rectal temperature is desired, caution is taken not to insert the thermometer more than 1/2 inch. In older children, tympanic membrane or temporal temperatures are obtained (Fig. 21-3). Because temperatures register within

Table 21-4	Average Range for Pediatric Vital Signs			
Age Group	HR	RR	BP Systolic	BP Diastolic
Infant	80–150	25–55	65–100	45–65
Toddler	70–110	20–30	90–105	55–70
Preschooler	65–110	20–25	95–110	60–75
School-age	60–95	14–22	100–120	60–75
Adolescent	55–85	12–18	110–125	65–85

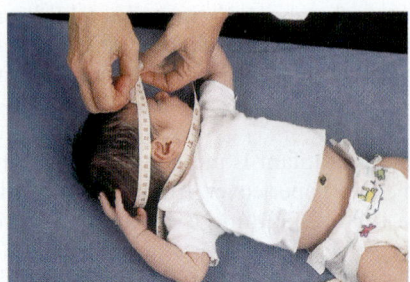

Figure 21-2 Measuring head circumference.

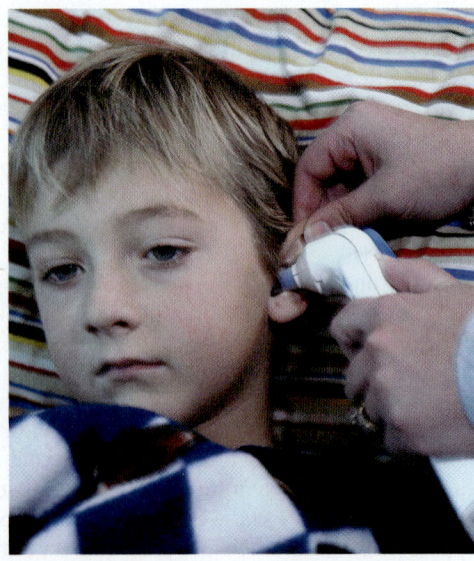

Figure 21-3 Taking tympanic temperature.

seconds, this route is a convenient one in pediatrics. The route used is charted when recording the child's temperature.

Pulse

Assessing the pulse in newborns and children requires concentration. The heart rate is variable and changes with illness. The apical pulse is counted for a full minute while the infant or child is quiet. With an uncooperative infant, the femoral arteries are palpated in the inguinal area, or the brachial arteries in the antecubital fossa.

Respirations

Respirations are to be counted for 1 full minute and can be assessed accurately only when the infant or child is not crying. A good time to count them is when a child is sleeping or resting quietly in a parent's arms. If possible, it is wise to start the vital sign assessment with respirations. There is a great deal of variability in the respiratory rate in children. Infants and young children are diaphragmatic breathers. The nurse can visually count the number of respirations by observing the abdomen as the child breathes.

Blood Pressure

Blood pressures are measured during well-child visits or routine physicals beginning when the child reaches 3 years of age. Readings are especially important for children with cardiac, pulmonary, or kidney disease; dehydration; or complaints of dizziness, regardless of age. For radial blood pressures to be accurate, selection of the cuff size is an important consideration. Appropriate cuff size is one in which the width of the bladder is approximately 40% and the length is approximately 80% of the circumference of the arm (Jarvis, 2012). Electronic blood pressure devices with varying cuff sizes are also available.

PHYSICAL ASSESSMENT

General Impression

As the nurse meets the child and the parents and engages in conversation with them, an impression begins to take form. This subjective feeling about the child encompasses many areas of assessment. As the nurse conducts the health history and performs the physical assessment, additional notions regarding the child and family develop. Not only is the uniqueness of the child portrayed, but a reflection of the child's family life becomes evident.

Take note of the behaviors of the child as he interacts with his parents. How does the child react to questions? What is the child's speech like? Is the child quiet, pleasant, talkative, uninterested, or angry? For the younger child, does the child listen to parents, interact in a meaningful way, or engage in age-appropriate behavior?

Hygiene and nutritional status are also examined. Is the child clean and appropriately dressed for the season? Body size, skin color, eyes, and the condition of the hair are observed for evidence of a good overall nutritional state.

Skin Assessment

The skin is assessed for color, turgor, and lesions. Skin color reflects ethnicity, diet, disease, and injury. Variations in tone are a result of genetic composition. Carotenemia, a benign yellowing of the skin caused by excessive carotene in the blood, may be present in the child with a diet high in yellow and orange vegetables, or yellowing of the skin and sclerae may indicate a dysfunction of the liver. Pallor may indicate anemia. Cyanosis may indicate a compromised cardiorespiratory state. Petechial lesions may be indicative of an infectious process or a blood disorder. Ecchymotic lesions may also indicate a blood disorder or be a tell-tale sign of past accidental or non-accidental injuries.

The nurse can assess the child's skin turgor for evidence of dehydration by grasping a small area of skin and pulling up. Once released, the skin should quickly return to its normal position. Skin that remains in the "tenting" position for several seconds indicates absence of skin turgor or presence of skin turgor with inadequate hydration.

If a rash is present or if jaundice is suspected, the nurse determines if the skin blanches, or turns pale. The nurse applies pressure to the skin with the thumbs about 1 to 2 inches apart. This presses the normal pink and darker colors out. In the presence of jaundice, there is a yellowish underlying color. Petechial lesions do not blanch, which may indicate a serious bacterial infection in an ill child. The primary health-care provider should be notified immediately.

The skin examination concludes with the inspection and documentation of the texture of the hair and the condition of the scalp, palms, and nails. Cradle cap is common in newborns and infants and is identified by thick, crusty scales over the scalp. The older child is monitored for lice or ticks.

Normal nails are pink and convex, with white edges extending over the end of the fingers. In children with cardiac disease, nails are examined for evidence of clubbing. Nail biting is a nervous habit that is evidenced by very short nails without the normal white edges.

The palms are examined for the normal flexion creases. Normally there are three creases. In a small section of the population, the two horizontal creases fuse to form a single horizontal palmar crease. This is a common finding in many genetic disorders, particularly Down syndrome. If this palmar crease is evident on only one hand, the child may have no genetic disorders.

✿ Cultural Diversity: Skin Assessment

Assessment of skin, hair, and nails in dark-skinned people requires knowledge of the integumentary differences in various cultures. **Melanin** is the pigment that gives color to skin and hair and protects against ultraviolet rays. For this reason, dark-skinned individuals have a lower incidence of skin cancer. Light-skinned individuals generally have a mild body odor and white sclera. Darker-skinned individuals tend to have a strong body odor and sclera that may be slightly yellow with small black marks. The hair of African Americans tends to be coarse, fragile, and dry, requiring daily care to maintain the health of the hair and scalp. In contrast, hair of Asians tends to be smooth and silky (Jarvis, 2012).

Head Assessment

The head is observed for symmetry and shape. Beyond the newborn period, head shape abnormalities in the infant may be caused by **craniosynostosis,** a premature fusing of one or more of the cranial sutures, or from gravitational influences caused by the infant's head being kept in the same position for an extended period of time. An odd head shape can develop because of the malleability of the skull bones. The supine sleep position has greatly reduced the incidence of sudden infant death syndrome. However, infants who are placed in the recommended supine position for sleep are at increased risk for **deformational posterior plagiocephaly**, or flattening, of the occiput.

The skull is palpated to evaluate fontanelles, sutures, contusions, or other swellings. Fontanelles are fibrous-membrane-covered areas where two or more skull bones converge. Although there are six fontanelles, the two most commonly evaluated are the posterior and anterior fontanelles. The posterior fontanelle closes within 1 to 3 months after birth, while the diamond-shaped anterior fontanelle remains open until 12 to 18 months of age.

The anterior fontanelle (AF) is the most significant fontanelle for evaluation (Fig. 21-4). A larger AF or one with a delayed closure may signify an infant with hypothyroidism, Down syndrome, **achondroplasia** (congenital dwarfism), or increased intracranial pressure. Assess the fontanelles when the infant is held in a sitting position. Depression of the AF may be indicative of dehydration; fullness of the AF is a potential sign of increased intracranial pressure.

The face is examined for general appearance and the comparison of features to those of the parents. Unusual features are noted, such as a **micrognathia** (shortened chin), low-set ears, flattened nasal bridge, enlarged or protruding tongue, **allergic shiners** (dark, under-eye rings) or a wide and flattened **philtrum** (the vertical groove from the bottom of the nose to the upper lip).

Neck Assessment

Lymph nodes of the head and neck are palpated systematically, starting at the preauricular area, proceeding to the postauricular area, and then to the occipital nodes (Fig. 21-5). Next, the tonsillar nodes at the angle of the mandible are examined, followed by the submandibular and submental nodes under the chin, the cervical chain of lymph nodes, and finally the supraclavicular area. Size, shape, mobility, and tenderness are documented. It is common for young children to have palpable, painless, movable nodes up to 1 cm in diameter. Pain upon palpation may be indicative of an upper airway infection. The trachea is palpated for midline placement and masses. A lateral deviation of the trachea may be caused by a mass or a collapsed lung. The thyroid gland is examined for enlargement, nodules, and goiters.

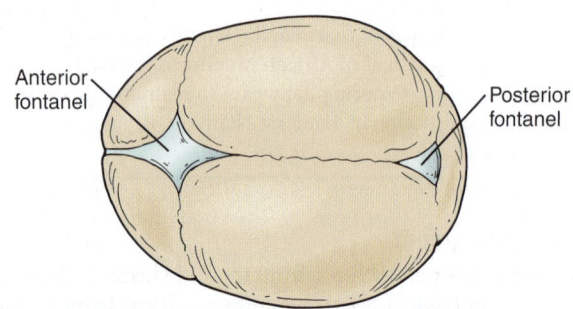

Figure 21-4 Anterior and posterior fontanelles.

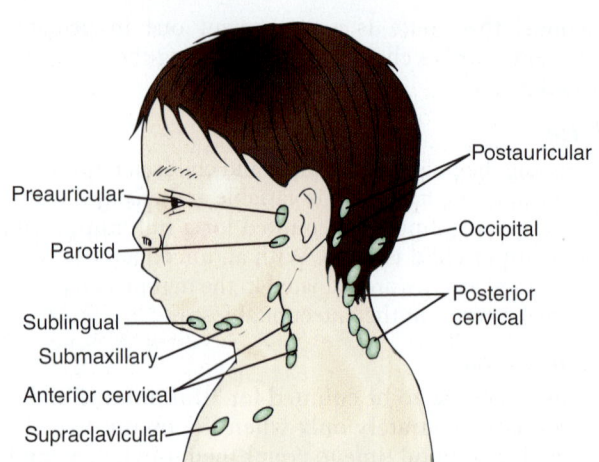

Figure 21-5 Lymph nodes of the head and neck.

Eye Assessment

Observation of the eyes includes assessment of symmetry, shape, and placement in relation to the nose. In addition, the nurse can assess for symmetry and size of the pupils and their response to light. The conjunctiva and lids are observed for conjunctivitis, styes, or **chalazions** (small discrete swellings of the upper lid that develop when a meibomian oil gland becomes blocked). The sclerae are inspected for color. The nurse notes erythema, swelling, or discharge from the eye. Documentation of the presence of discharge includes type (e.g., watery or purulent), color, amount, and associated symptoms. Treatment depends on the cause, which may be bacterial, viral, or an allergen.

 Assessment Tool Visual Acuity

Visual screening for children can begin at the age of 2 1/2 years. There are a variety of charts that will assist in the assessment of visual acuity. Visual acuity for each eye is assessed by occluding the contralateral eye with a plastic paddle. With all charts the objects, letters, and numbers decrease in size. The Allen chart requires the child to identify common objects; the "tumbling E" requires the child to identify the direction to which each E is facing; and the Snellen charts require the child to identify letters or numbers.

To ensure optimal eye health in children, testing for ocular alignment and visual acuity is essential (Hogan-Quigley et al., 2011). Assessment of visual acuity depends on the age of the child. Infants begin to use a steady gaze to regard faces or objects with interesting patterns. The nurse observes for and documents this finding during the physical exam. Any difference in visual acuity between one eye and the other is abnormal and requires a referral to a specialist. In addition, children are referred for further evaluation if they have a visual acuity reading of less than 20/50 or after failing a second screening.

TESTING FOR OCULAR ALIGNMENT. A common method for assessing ocular alignment is the Hirschberg corneal light reflex test, in which a light is shone directly into the child's eyes and note is taken of the position of the corneal light reflection in both eyes. The reflection should fall in the same location on the cornea of each eye. Displacement of the corneal light reflection in one eye is indicative of strabismus.

The second screening test is the cover–uncover test, in which the child is asked to focus on a distant object across the room. The nurse covers the first eye while watching the second eye for any movement. The cover is then removed from the first eye, which is observed for any movement. If no movement is detected, ocular alignment is intact. The examination is repeated on the opposite eye.

The red reflex is tested by viewing the pupil through an ophthalmoscope from a distance of 10 inches. If the pupil appears red, the finding is normal. A white retinal reflex may indicate cataracts, retinoblastoma, or chorioretinitis.

TESTING FOR COLOR BLINDNESS. Children should be screened at least once during the school-age years for the ability to discriminate between red, yellow, and green. A common method for detecting color blindness is the use of the Ishihara pseudochromatic charts. Each chart consists of a field of colored dots, each with a number in the center of the colored field: The inability to identify these numbers indicates color blindness.

Ear Assessment

The external ears are examined for size, shape, placement, pain, and presence of drainage from the ear canal. The pinna of the ear should be above the imaginary horizontal line drawn from the medial and lateral canthi toward the occiput. Low-set ears may indicate a congenital anomaly such as Down syndrome. To assess for pain, the nurse moves the pinna of the ear up and down. If the child complains of pain when pressure is applied to the tragus, the canal is examined for evidence of otitis externa. **Cerumen** (ear wax) may be seen on the external ear or in the external canal with an otoscope. Purulent drainage may indicate a foreign body in the external ear canal or a ruptured tympanic membrane. Any clear drainage noted from the ear, particularly after head trauma or with cranial infections, should be reported to the health-care provider immediately because this fluid may indicate a cerebrospinal fluid leak.

 Nursing Insight—*Use of a small cotton swab to clean the ear*

The nurse can instruct parents on the use of a small cotton swab to clean the ear. A small cotton swab should be used to clean only the external ear, and not the ear canal. When a small cotton swab is used in the ear canal, the cerumen is pushed back into the canal where it cannot be moved out by the mechanical action of the tiny ear hairs. Cerumen tends to dry, harden, and become difficult to remove over time. Impacted cerumen in the ear canal may lead to hearing deficits.

When an otoscope is used, the canal should be positioned for the optimal viewing of the tympanic membrane and canal. As a general rule, the pinna is pulled down and back for children younger than 3 years and up and back for older children. The child is positioned to prevent injury or discomfort. With the parent's help to gently restrain the child from moving, the otoscopic examination can take place with the child either sitting on the parent's lap or in the supine position.

The nurse understands that holding the otoscope upside down allows the nurse the use of one hand to help hold the child's head and the other to position the stem of the otoscope against the child's head for more stability. The tympanic membrane is examined for the presence of normal anatomical landmarks (Fig. 21-6).

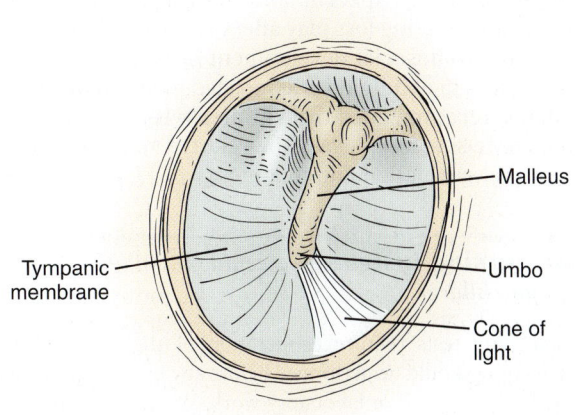

Figure 21-6 Tympanic membrane landmarks.

Malleus

Tympanic membrane

Umbo

Cone of light

Visual loss of these landmarks may be because of erythema, fullness behind the tympanic membrane, inflammation, purulent exudate, or fluid. Because of the anatomical structure of their ears, infants and young children are prone to developing otitis media. The eustachian tubes are shorter and more horizontally positioned, enabling viruses and bacteria to travel to the middle ear. Infants who are breastfed, do not attend day care, and are fed in an upright position have decreased rates of otitis media.

 Cultural Diversity: Otitis Media

Research has shown that otitis media is more prevalent for children of certain ethnicities. These ethnicities include Alaskans, American Indians, Hispanics, and Canadians based on less access to medical care and cultural belief about when to see a health-care provider (Ward, 2013).

HEARING SCREENING. In the older cooperative child, a tuning fork is used to assess bone and air conduction of sound. The Weber test involves striking the tines of the tuning fork and immediately placing the handle of the tuning fork midline on top of the child's head. The nurse asks the child in which ear he hears the sound best. If hearing is normal, sound is heard equally in both ears. Sound heard in one ear better than the other indicates a conductive hearing loss.

The **Rinne test** assesses air and bone conduction of sound. Bone conduction is tested by placing the handle of the vibrating tuning fork on the mastoid process behind the ear. The child informs the nurse when he no longer can hear the sound of the vibrating tuning fork and the nurse immediately moves the tines forward to within 1 to 2 inches of the auditory meatus. The child should hear the air-conducted sound of the vibrating tines twice as long as he heard the bone-conducted sound.

Tympanometry assesses the status of the middle ear. The nurse places a probe into the ear canal. The amount of sound that is reflected by the tympanic membrane is measured along with the pressure in the canal. The tympanogram delineates the movement of the eardrum as stiffness, floppiness, or normal eardrum movement.

Early detection of hearing loss is important to prevent delayed hearing, speech, and language development (Box 21-1). Hearing loss may affect both the academic success and psychosocial development of the child. Because hearing loss in childhood is associated with middle ear disease, it is recommended that children with positive results from office screening exams be referred to an audiologist for further evaluation and treatment.

 Nursing Insight—*Screening techniques for children*

Screening tests require cooperation of the child. Hearing screening should be performed before any invasive procedures such as injections or laboratory work. With testing, the nurse assesses for frequency (pitch) and the decibel level (loudness). Frequency is defined as the number of vibrations a sound creates per second. As the frequency increases, the pitch of the sound also increases. The frequency range is 250 to 6,000 hertz (Hz). For a normal finding, the child should hear at all frequencies at the 20-dB range.

Conditioned play audiometry is a common test for children older than 3 years. In this test, the child is asked to engage in a play-oriented activity, like placing a colorful block in a box each time a sound is heard. The child is subjected to sounds of different frequencies that a child with normal hearing could hear.

A conventional audiogram assesses hearing acuity by asking the child to raise her hand or press a button each time a sound is heard. The child must be able to understand the language spoken, be able to follow directions, pay attention, and wait to listen to the sounds.

 Optimizing Outcomes—**Hearing screening**

All children should be screened for hearing loss as needed. A hearing impairment may interfere with normal psychosocial development, communication among friends, and educational pursuits. Some children may be at greater risk for hearing loss because of overexposure to high levels of noise associated with yard work, listening to music at concerts and via earphones, and through chronic ear infections, ototoxic drugs, head injuries, including abuse, or diseases. Children with known risk factors for hearing loss should be monitored more closely and at more frequent intervals.

Nose/Sinus Assessment

The nasal mucosa is inspected for color and inflammation. Pale, boggy mucosa is a typical finding in a child with allergic rhinitis. The nasal mucosa appears erythematous with upper respiratory infections. Note any bleeding of the

---

Box 21-1 Risk Factors for Hearing Loss in Preschoolers

- Family history of childhood hearing loss
- Delayed hearing, speech, or language development
- Prior infections with meningitis, mumps, or otitis media
- Head trauma

---

mucosal lining because this can indicate injury. Purulent discharge from the nose may indicate a viral or bacterial condition. Purulent discharge occurring in one nostril is suggestive of a foreign object in the other nostril. The septum is inspected for the midline position. Maxillary sinuses are detected via x-ray exam by age 4, with other sinuses radiologically evident by age 6 (Hogan-Quigley et al., 2011). These areas are palpated for tenderness, using the thumbs of both hands and holding the child's head.

Throat/Mouth Assessment

The examination of the throat and mouth is saved for last in younger, less cooperative children. The nurse may ask the child to see "all of the tongue." Eliciting the sound "eeehh" flattens the tongue better than "aaahh," and visualization of the posterior pharynx is possible without the use of the tongue blade. The palate, uvula, tonsils, and mucous membranes are observed and assessed for color, exudate, and odor. The lips are observed for shape, symmetry, color, dryness, fissures at the corners of the mouth indicative of vitamin B_2 (riboflavin) deficiency, and clefts.

The teeth are inspected for number present, condition, color, alignment, and caries. Tooth eruptions occur at varying rates. Generally, when counting teeth on visual examination, the nurse can expect one tooth per month after 6 months of age until all 20 deciduous teeth are in place. The gingival tissue is inspected for color and condition. The gingival tissue is the same color as the surrounding mucous membranes and should not be hypertrophied or show evidence of bleeding.

 Cultural Diversity: Throat and Mouth Assessment

Melanin is the primary determinant of skin color in humans. The melanin in the skin is produced by melanocytes found in the basal layer of the epidermis. The melanocytes of different individuals are dependent on the genetic code. In some individuals and ethnic groups, the expression of the melanin-producing genes produces a greater or lesser concentration of skin melanin. The darker the skin, the more melanin is present. Patchy hyperpigmentation is a normal finding for dark-skinned individuals because of an increased level of melanin.

Chest Assessment

The nurse inspects the chest for size, shape, symmetry, respiratory effort, and breast development. In infants, the anteroposterior diameter is fairly equal to the lateral diameter. By 2 years of age, the lateral diameter is greater than the anteroposterior diameter. Equal anteroposterior and lateral diameter after the age of 2 years may indicate chronic lung disease. A chest that is larger on the left than on the right may indicate an enlarged heart or a collapsed right lung. **Pectus carinatum** (protrusion of the chest) and **pectus excavatum** (abnormal depression of the lower portion of the sternum) are abnormal chest shapes caused by sternal deviations.

 Nursing Insight—*Retractions*

With any increased work of breathing, retractions are observed. When the trachea or the smaller airways of the lungs experience air flow restriction, the pressure within the chest is reduced. As a result, the intercostal muscles are drawn inward in an attempt to assist in breathing. This drawing inward is visible as intercostal retractions. Retractions may also be seen in the substernal, subcostal, and suprasternal notch regions.

Normal breast development begins in girls between 10 and 14 years of age. Boys also undergo breast changes, and many show evidence of breast development. For the female, the breast development is documented using the Tanner Staging of Development of Secondary Sex Characteristics (Table 21-5). Breast assessment is important at every well-child visit for early detection of precocious puberty. Girls must be taught breast self-exam when breast tissue begins to develop.

Lung Assessment

Lung sounds are best auscultated with the child in a sitting position. The nurse instructs the child to take slow deep breaths through an open mouth. Using a stethoscope with an appropriately sized pediatric diaphragm, the nurse systematically auscultates the five lobes of the lungs, anteriorly and posteriorly, beginning with the apices and then moving side to side to compare bilateral lung sounds. In an infant, auscultation of lung sounds is best done early in the exam, while the child is quiet.

Direct observation of a child's breathing can help determine inadequate oxygenation status. For instance, a child with tachypnea (a rapid respiratory rate is 80 to 120 breaths/minute), shallow breathing, and use of accessory muscles means respiratory distress. Conversely, the child with slow breathing means the child does not have the energy for adequate oxygenation. Quiet breath sounds with an increased work of breathing means that air is not entering into the lung fields. An alteration in depth, **hyperpnea** (too deep), is associated with fever, and **hypopnea** (too shallow) is associated with central nervous system depression.

The child's posture can also indicate adequate or inadequate oxygenation. The child in respiratory distress sits in a tripod position sitting upright, leaning forward on outstretched arms with the jaw thrust forward. This particular position helps maximize opening up the airway and use of accessory muscles of respiration. Because a child with respiratory difficulties is often anxious, it is important to allow him to assume the position of comfort, which is usually the position that is easiest for the child to breathe.

BREATH SOUNDS. Normal breath sounds can be classified as bronchial, bronchovesicular, or vesicular. Adventitious sounds of these three classifications are described as crackles, wheezes, and rhonchi, respectively. Bronchial breath sounds are loud, high-pitched, and heard only over the trachea. The inspiratory and expiratory sounds are equal in length. Bronchovesicular breath sounds are of intermediate intensity and pitch, with equal inspiratory and expiratory phases. These sounds are best heard between the scapulae and over the mainstem bronchi. If bronchial or bronchovesicular sounds are heard elsewhere, it is indicative of an area of consolidation. Vesicular breath sounds are heard throughout the lung fields. These soft and low-pitched sounds have a longer inspiratory phase than an expiratory one. Decreased or absent breath sounds indicate a serious condition such as asthma, atelectasis, emphysema, pneumothorax, or acute respiratory distress syndrome (ARDS).

 Nursing Insight—*Lung assessment and breath sounds*

The nurse will more accurately assess the lungs by creating a quiet environment, placing the child in the best position for

Table 21-5 Tanner Staging of Development of Secondary Sex Characteristics					
Sex Characteristics	**Scoring**				
	1	2	3	4	5
Breast development in females	Slight to no elevation of papilla	Breast buds appear; areolar widening with slight elevation	Entire breast enlarged with no protrusion of the papilla or nipple	Enlargement of the entire breast with formation of secondary mound of areola and papilla	Mature breast with protrusion of nipple only. No protrusion of the papilla
Pubic hair development in females	None	Sparse, lightly pigmented, straight along border of labia	Darker and increasing amount on labia and pubis. Distribution in typical female inverted triangle	Coarse, thicker, curly. Increasing amount, less than adult	Adult female triangle with extension of hair onto medial thighs
Pubic hair and genital development in males	No pubic hair. Preadolescent genitalia	Scant, long, slightly pigmented pubic hair. Slight enlargement of scrotum and testes; scrotum reddens and becomes more textured	Pubic hair darker, starting to curl and extends across pubis. Scrotum and testes continue to enlarge. Penis becomes longer and slightly wider.	Pubic hair is coarse, curly, less quantity than adult. Scrotum is darker; penis increases in length and breadth. Glans is broader.	Adult distribution of pubic hair with extension to medial thighs; genitalia adult in size and shape

Source: Adapted from Tanner, J. M. (1962). *Growth at adolescence* (2nd ed.). Oxford: Blackwell Scientific.

auscultation, warming the diaphragm of the stethoscope before auscultation, placing the stethoscope on the child's bare skin, and comparing bilateral breath sounds.

focus on safety

Important respiratory signals

The nurse must recognize that normal breath sounds are equal bilaterally in intensity, rhythm, and pitch. The following respiratory signals may indicate that a respiratory condition causing distress is present in a child:

- Noisy breathing or snoring (air passing through a narrowed upper airway) may indicate nasal polyps, foreign body obstruction, choanal obstruction, hypertrophied adenoid tissue, or obesity.
- Grunting is caused by the glottis closing at the end of expiration and may suggest respiratory distress or pneumonia.
- Nasal flaring (intermittent outward movement of the nostrils) happens on inspiration and is a form of accessory muscle use found in a variety of conditions such as respiratory distress syndrome (Venes, 2013).
- Coughing (a forceful expiratory effort) is a normal process that clears the throat but can indicate an infection, asthma, lung disease, or sinusitis.
- **Stridor** (a high-pitched, harsh sound occurring during inspiration) results from air moving through a narrowed trachea and larynx and can indicate croup (Venes, 2013).
- Wheezing (a musical noise) results from air moving through mucus or fluids in a narrowed lower airway that is associated with asthma.
- Hoarseness is a rough quality in the child's voice and can mean that the airway is inflamed.
- Crackles is a fine, high-pitched sound heard on inspiration or expiration produced by air passing over retained airway secretions or the sudden opening of collapsed airways found in several respiratory conditions (Venes, 2013).
- Rhonchi are a low-pitched wheezing, snoring, or squeaking sound indicating a partial airway obstruction. Mucus or other secretions in the airway, bronchial hyperreactivity, or tumors that occlude respiratory passages can cause airway obstruction (Venes, 2013).
- Color changes in the skin (e.g., pallor, mottling, and cyanosis) are significant respiratory signals and usually indicate cardiac involvement.
- Chest pain is caused by alteration in chest structures, nonpulmonary involvement, or a variety of respiratory conditions.
- **Clubbing** (excessive growth of the soft tissues at the ends of the fingers or toes) is usually associated with chronic hypoxia and pulmonary disease.

Critical Nursing Action Adventitious Lung Sounds

A 3-year-old child is brought into the clinic with a chief complaint of recent coughing. The mother states that the child has no fever or cold symptoms, but began coughing several days ago. The nurse auscultates all lung fields and hears wheezing and localized rhonchi on the left side but normal vesicular sounds on the right side. The nurse must notify the health-care provider immediately for further evaluation and treatment.

Cardiac Assessment

The chest is inspected for symmetry and pulsations, and all peripheral pulses are palpated (Table 21-6). In slim children, pulsations from the heart may be visible. The nurse begins palpation with the carotid pulse, making note of any distended neck veins, and continues with the brachial and radial pulses. Capillary refill is assessed as well as changes in the fingernails (e.g., clubbing of the fingers) is noted. Peripheral edema and cyanosis are assessed during palpation of the femoral, popliteal, posterior tibial, and dorsalis pedis pulses.

Continued palpation of the chest can identify the presence of thrills, which are a consequence of blood flowing rapidly from high pressure to low pressure. The rough vibrating sensations are felt by placing the palm of the hand over the chest. Some ventricular septal defects result in thrills at the lower left sternal border. Pulmonary stenosis may cause a thrill at the upper left sternal border, whereas aortic stenosis is frequently palpable in the suprasternal notch.

Nursing Insight—*Point of maximal impulse (PMI)*

The point of maximal impulse (PMI), or area of most intense pulsation, and the point of apical impulse, or the impulse corresponding to the apex of the heart, are usually located in the same area of the chest. Generally, the apical impulse is found just lateral of the left midclavicular line (MCL) and fourth intercostal space (ICS) in children younger than 7 years. For children older than 7 years, it is found in the fifth ICS. The stethoscope is placed over this area for auscultation of the apical pulse.

Auscultation begins with the diaphragm of the stethoscope, and further evaluation of the heart sounds is done with the bell of the stethoscope (Fig. 21-7). To assess for the first heart sound (S_1—the "lub" sound), the nurse begins at the fourth or fifth *left* ICS at the MCL. The first heart sound reflects the closure of the mitral and tricuspid valves and signifies the beginning of ventricular contraction or systole. The second heart sound (S_2—the "dub" sound) reflects the closure of the pulmonary and aortic valves and signifies the beginning of atrial contraction or diastole. The nurse hears "lub dub."

During inspiration, the S_2 sound may be audible as a split sound because the pulmonary valve closes slightly

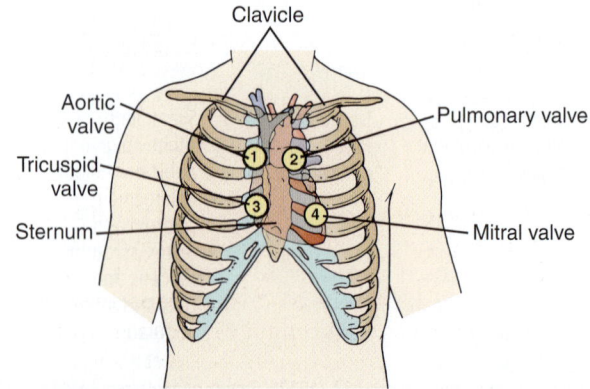

Figure 21-7 Four points of cardiac auscultation.

Table 21-6 Cardiac Assessment Techniques

Assessment Technique	What to Look For	Normal Findings	Abnormal Findings	Rationale
Inspection	Skin color, shape, and symmetry of chest, clubbing	Pink, symmetrical chest	Pallor, cyanosis, asymmetry of chest shape and movement, hyperdynamic precordium	Poor cardiac output; deoxygenated circulating blood, ventricular failure or hypertrophy, tachycardia
Palpation	Skin and body temperature, moisture, chest movement, point of maximal impulse (PMI)	Warm, dry, symmetrical movement, PMI at 4th or 5th ICS at midclavicular line	Cold extremities, dry flaky skin, diaphoresis; thrills or heaves	Poor circulation, heart failure, ventricular hypertrophy
Percussion	Heart shape and size	Normal size and shape for age and weight	Enlarged heart, axis deviation	Heart failure and hypertrophy
Auscultation	Murmurs, other sounds	No murmurs, innocent murmurs; quiet precordium	Murmurs, clicks, rubs, snaps	Structural defects, increased workload of heart and volume overload

Source: © Judith M. Marshall (2006).

later than the aortic valve. This physiological splitting is heard as a "lub-dub" and is within the context of normal. If splitting is also heard during expiration, this is suggestive of pulmonary valve pathology.

Two other heart sounds may be heard during the cardiac cycle. The S_3 and S_4 heart sounds are both heard in diastole. A physiological S_3 is heard frequently in children and young adults. It is heard best at the apex in a left lateral lying position by listening for the sound in early diastole right after the S_2. It is called a ventricular gallop and, because of the cadence of the rhythm, sounds like the word "Kentucky." Although an S_3 is most likely a finding not associated with heart disease, the finding should be documented and reported. S_4, heard in late diastole, is heard only in children who have congenital heart disease such as pulmonary hypertension and pulmonic stenosis. It is never a normal finding and must be reported to the primary health-care provider. The sound is sometimes compared with the word "Tennessee."

Murmurs are attributed to turbulent blood flow within the vessels. The nurse assesses for intensity, location, radiation, timing, and quality. Innocent murmurs are systolic, musical, or vibratory and of low intensity. The Still's murmur is the most common murmur and is located over the mid- or lower left sternal border. This murmur may be heard in well children, those with fever, after exercise, or in children with anemia when cardiac output is increased. A venous hum is a continuous soft, hollow sound that disappears when the child is supine. Diastolic murmurs usually indicate pathology.

Abdominal Assessment

The child should lie quietly in the supine position. The assessment begins with an inspection of the abdomen and its contour, which may be flat, round, protuberant, or scaphoid (shaped like a boat). Visible peristalsis may be noted in a thin child, and should be documented and reported. The umbilicus and inguinal areas are inspected for bulging, and note is made of any scars, rashes, lesions, or piercings.

The abdomen is divided into four quadrants: right upper quadrant (RUQ), left upper quadrant (LUQ), right lower quadrant (RLQ), and left lower quadrant (LLQ) (Fig. 21-8). The terms epigastric, umbilical, periumbilical, and suprapubic can also be used to describe symptoms and physical findings that are specific to these areas.

After inspection, the abdomen is auscultated in all four quadrants to assess for bowel motility. These high-pitched sounds occur every 5 to 10 seconds, so it is important for the nurse to allow enough time to adequately assess frequency and character of the bowel sounds. The absence of bowel sounds or high-pitched tinkles in the presence of abdominal distention and/or peritoneal signs suggests an acute abdominal condition. A child who is experiencing signs of a bowel obstruction has absent bowel sounds below the obstruction. The nurse must listen for up to 1 minute before determining the absence of bowel sounds in any one quadrant.

Palpation of the abdomen occurs last so as not to disrupt bowel sounds. Palpation is divided into light palpation and

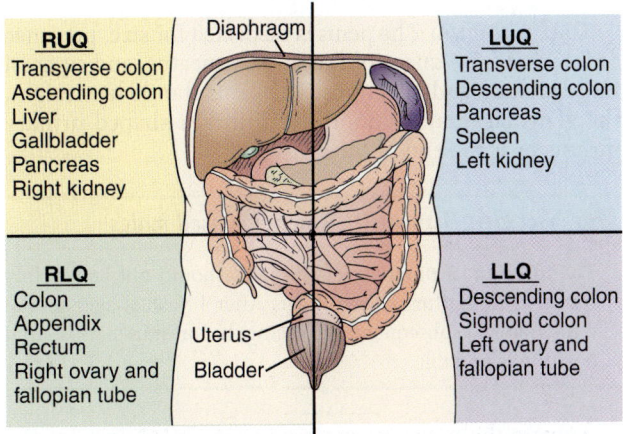

Figure 21-8 Abdomen divided into quadrants and organs in each quadrant.

deep palpation. Light palpation assists in identifying abdominal tenderness. Deep palpation is useful when assessing for the liver, kidneys, spleen, inguinal lymph nodes, and abnormal masses. If a mass is encountered, it is reported, noting its location, size, shape, consistency, and tenderness. Throughout the abdominal assessment, the nurse observes for changes in facial expression, guarding, and tensing of the abdominal muscles.

 Nursing Insight—*Palpation of the abdomen*

To minimize the sensation of tickling during palpation of the abdomen, the nurse may palpate through a layer of light clothing or place the child's hand on top of the nurse's hand while palpating. To relax the abdominal muscles, bend the child's knees until feet are flat on the exam table. Palpate any tender or painful areas last. The suprapubic area may feel tender if the child's bladder is full. Consider having the child empty the bladder before the abdominal assessment.

Genitourinary and Perineal Assessment

Both males and females are assessed for Tanner staging of hair growth, evidence of normal development for the age of the child, signs of sexual abuse, and precocious puberty.

FEMALE GENITALIA. The femoral nodes should be palpated. Enlarged nodes may indicate the presence of a sexually transmitted infection or something as simple as an inflamed hair follicle after shaving. The external genitalia of the female (the labia minora, labia majora, clitoris, vaginal opening, and urinary meatus) are examined for the presence of lesions, discharge, and irritation. The nurse must be able to visualize the vaginal and urethral openings. Occasionally the labia minora are fused because of adhesions, making this assessment difficult to impossible; this finding must be reported to the primary health-care provider for further evaluation and separation of the labia minora. A malodorous vaginal discharge may indicate the presence of a foreign body, especially in young children, or an infection. Vaginal exams in young children need to be completed by trained examiners. The American College of Obstetricians and Gynecologists (ACOG) (2011) recommends the first gynecological visit between the ages of 13 and 15 years and the first pelvic exam at age 21 years, sooner if the child is sexually active.

MALE GENITALIA. The penis is inspected for size, presence of foreskin, placement of the urinary meatus, and signs of inflammation and infections. The penis should be straight, the glans clean and smooth, and the slit-shaped urinary meatus near the end of the glans.

 Nursing Insight—*Uncircumcised males*

The foreskin of uncircumcised males should not be forcibly retracted until after 1 year of age. After 1 year of age, genital retraction and subsequently replacing the foreskin to its neutral position is possible.

Palpate the penis for masses and nodules. Inspect the scrotum for size, shape, symmetry, and presence of testicles. An enlarged scrotum should be transilluminated to assess for **hydrocele** (accumulation of serous fluid in the scrotum) versus a possible hernia. The nurse places a penlight under the scrotum; the scrotum will exhibit a red glow with a hydrocele but not with a hernia. The testicles are palpated for size and shape. Testicles are roughly the same size and smooth in contour. A testicle that is hard or in which a nodule is palpated must be reported to the primary health-care provider for further examination to rule out a tumor. The nurse must also report if one or both testicles have not descended. Males are instructed in testicular self-examination by the age of 14 years. Testicular cancer, while rare, is the most common cancer in males age 15 to 34 years (U.S. Preventative Services Task Force [USPTF], 2011).

ANAL EXAMINATION. The anus is not routinely examined in children unless indicated by abdominal, bowel, rectal, or stool abnormalities. If an anal examination is indicated, the child is placed in a side-lying position with the knees flexed. The area is examined for anal placement, lesions, trauma, irritation, fissures, bleeding, leakage of stool, and hemorrhoids as well as general cleanliness. Tone can be assessed by lightly touching the anus and observing for the anal reflex. If a digital exam is necessary, educate the child about the procedure in an age-appropriate manner, provide distraction during the procedure, and ask the child to "push down like he is trying to have a bowel movement," or other term used by child to indicate defecation, to help relax the anal sphincter.

Musculoskeletal Assessment

Much of the musculoskeletal exam can be done while observing the child enter and move about the exam room. The child is observed for range of motion, symmetry of movement, general alignment, and any deformities. Each joint is palpated for range of motion and the presence of any erythema or swelling.

The child's muscles are assessed for strength of movement. For upper extremity strength, the child is asked to hold both arms out to the sides and then out to the front. The child is asked to hold these positions as the nurse applies downward pressure to both arms. The symmetry of strength in both hands can be assessed by having the child squeeze the nurse's index fingers. The strength of the legs can be tested by asking the child who is lying supine to raise his legs while the nurse applies downward pressure on the legs. Screening for scoliosis is usually done between 9 and 15 years of age. A scoliometer can be used to assess for the condition as well as noting if the back appears straight and the hips are even.

Neurological Assessment

Mental status can be assessed by observing the infant interact with the parent, or by asking the older child to answer questions and listening for clear speech in the responses. This can be assessed in the course of a normal interview. Most of the assessment of motor functioning is done during the skeletal examination. In addition, the child can be asked to hop, skip, or jump to assess symmetry of movement. The nurse might suggest a game such as "hop on one foot." Sensory testing is done if there is a question regarding sensory functioning.

Cerebellar function is checked by observing the child's posture and gait or by using the finger-to-nose test. Young children perceive this test as a game and readily cooperate.

The Romberg test assesses cerebellar functioning; the child is assessed for the ability to stand without swaying while standing with eyes closed and arms outstretched.

The child is also assessed for persistence of primitive reflexes, which normally disappear during infancy. Babinski, Moro, palmar, plantar, and tonic neck reflexes are a few that are seen in the neonate but that disappear over time. Persistence of these reflexes may indicate cerebral dysfunction. Deep-tendon reflexes (DTRs) are elicited using the reflex hammer. DTRs are difficult to elicit in some children, and a distraction may be needed while testing reflexes.

Cranial nerve assessment is an integral part of the physical examination and may be completed throughout the exam or as a separate part of the exam (Table 21-7). For instance, the nurse can assess the muscles for facial expression during the interview. The nurse also examines the pharynx, tongue, and muscles of mastication during the examination of the mouth. The nurse understands that abnormal results of the cranial nerve exam may indicate a brain injury, infection, or compression of a particular nerve.

 Cultural Diversity: Physical Aspects of a Cultural Assessment

An important aspect of any physical assessment is sensitivity to cultural diversity. The nurse assesses each system based on the child's particular race and culture (Table 21-8).

 Now Can You—Discuss the importance of a health assessment for a child?

1. State the major components of a health assessment for the child?
2. Describe alterations in a health assessment for the child?
3. Discuss the physical aspects of a cultural assessment?

The Child in Pain

Whether hospitalized, in a clinic, or in the home, a child may experience pain related to an acute injury, medical or surgical condition, or disability. A child's pain may be either acute or chronic. All pain is not the same for all people. The skill of the nurse lies in helping the child to convey the kind and intensity of the pain he is experiencing and then determining the best way to manage pain (pharmacological and nonpharmacological).

 Nursing Insight—What is pain?

Pain is whatever the child says it is. What one person experiences as mild pain, another may experience as severe pain. With the use of pediatric pain scales, most children are able to communicate their level of pain very clearly. The important thing is for the nurse to listen to the child rather than prejudge what the child should feel.

UNDERSTANDING PAIN IN CHILDREN FROM A DEVELOPMENTAL PERSPECTIVE

How children perceive and express pain is a dynamic process. There are multiple factors to consider when assessing a child in pain, including age, developmental level, temperament, the type and severity of the pain, and environmental and psychological factors. Probably one of the most significant influences is the cognitive level of the child. For this reason, it is very important for the nurse to have a sound understanding of the cognitive development of children and those situations in which cognitive development may be delayed, altering how the nurse will assess for pain. Infants and children up to age 2 are in Piaget's *sensorimotor stage* of cognitive development. Although they

---

Table 21-7 Cranial Nerve Testing	
Cranial Nerve	**How to Test**
I. Olfactory	Ask the child to close both eyes and have the child identify smells. Rarely done during a routine examination.
II. Optic	Perform vision screen for test of visual acuity and color vision, test for peripheral vision, and examine the optic disc with the ophthalmoscope.
III. Oculomotor	Ask the child to follow an object through the six cardinal positions of gaze. Assess for pupillary response and drooping of upper lids.
IV. Trochlear	CN III, IV, and VI are tested together.
V. Trigeminal	Observe child chewing on a cracker. With eyes closed, gently stroke different areas of the face with a cotton ball to assess sensory function.
VI. Abducens	CN III, IV, and VI are tested together.
VII. Facial	Observe child's facial expressions during the interview and exam. May need to ask child to frown and then smile.
VIII. Acoustic	Cause a loud sound and assess if child turns to the sound.
IX. Glossopharyngeal	Stimulate gag reflex.
X. Vagus	Assess uvula in midline. Assess ability to swallow by asking child to do so.
XI. Accessory	As the nurse provides resistance, ask child to shrug shoulders and turn head side to side.
XII. Hypoglossal	Observe infant sucking on a bottle. Ask child to stick out the tongue. Listen for clarity of speech.

Table 21-8 Physical Aspects of a Cultural Assessment

General Appearance	Assessment	Conditions Associated With Certain Cultures
Skin	Melanin is responsible for the variation in skin colors and tones. It protects the skin from harmful ultraviolet rays. Darker-skinned children have lighter pigmentation on palms, lips, and nail beds.	Melanoma is higher among Caucasians than among African Americans and Hispanics.
Endocrine Sweat Glands	Caucasians and African Americans tend to have a stronger body odor while Asians and American Indians have a mild body odor.	There may be increased body image disturbance with increased body odor.
Hair	African American hair is typically thick, spiraled, thick and kinky, or can be straight.	African Americans' scalp has a tendency to be drier.
Eyes	In light-skinned individuals, the sclera is white. In darker-skinned individuals, the sclera can be slightly yellow with small black marks. (Ward & Hisley, 2009).	Epicanthal folds frequently occur in Asians and Caucasians
Ears	The eustachian tube is shorter and wilder, more horizontal, and the external auditory canal is shorter and has a slope opposite to an adult's ear in children of all races.	Otitis media is more common in Alaskans, American Indians, Hispanics, and Canadians.
Nose	Appearance of the nose is dependent on racial characteristics (e.g., broad or flat) but develops more fully during adolescence in all cultures.	Sinusitis is more prevalent in African Americans.
Mouth	Salivation begins at 3 months and 20 deciduous teeth erupt between 6 and 24 months in children of all races dependent on general state of health. All 20 teeth should be present by 2 1/2 years and are lost starting at 6 to 12 years of age. Patchy hyperpigmentation is normal and common in darker-skinned people.	Cleft lip and cleft palate are more common in Native Americans and Asians and less common in African Americans. African Americans have more tooth decay than other races. Non-White races have the poorest oral health habits.
Heart	In children of all cultures the heart's position in the chest is more horizontal, and the apex of the heart is located at the fourth intercostal space.	Heart disease and stroke are higher among African Americans. African Americans have a higher incidence of hypertension. African American children and adolescents have higher total cholesterol than children of other ethnicities.
Lungs	Respiratory development (size of thoracic cavity) continues throughout childhood and reaches full development by adolescence. Lung health among cultures depends on prenatal and postnatal exposure to environmental toxins. Occurrence of respiratory tract infections or asthma vary among cultures.	Tuberculosis and asthma are more prevalent among African Americans.
Genitourinary	Darkly pigmented people have darker nipples, areola, labia majora, and scrotum.	African American girls enter puberty and begin menstruating about 1 to 1 1/2 years earlier than Caucasian girls. The decision to circumcise boys is based on culture. In the United States a high percentage of males get circumcised. However, in other countries—Great Britain, Sweden, Australia, and Canada—circumcision is considered unnecessary.
Abdomen	In children of all cultures the abdominal wall is easier to palpate because it is less muscular.	Lactase is the digestive enzyme needed for absorption of lactose (milk sugar). The incidence of lactose intolerance is high in American Indians, Asians, and African Americans.
Musculoskeletal	Caucasian males are taller than African American and Asian males. Caucasian females are about the same height as African American females. Asian females are shorter than Caucasian and African American females.	Growth spurts mark time for significant growth. Height varies in each cultural group and is influenced by genetics and nutrition.
Neurological	In children of all cultures the neurological system is not fully developed at birth but develops as the child grows. Developmental milestones happen in an orderly sequence although the exact age at which they occur varies and is based on a multitude of factors.	No matter what the culture, a complete developmental assessment is necessary at routine well-child visits. Developmental delays need to be documented and reported.

Source: Ward (2013).

certainly experience pain, they do not understand it. Older infants and younger toddlers learn to anticipate painful events, both from repeated exposure to it (as in chronic illness) or from parental anxiety. As a toddler becomes verbal, she will use words such as "boo-boo" or "owie" to express pain. However, the toddler will not be able to describe it.

Children ages 2 to 7 years progress through *preoperational* cognitive development. Children ages 2 to 4 years are in the substage of preconceptual development. Ages 4 to 7 years progress through the substage of intuitive development. As a group, these children often believe they are experiencing pain as a form of punishment. They recognize the presence of pain but may not report it because they believe that the adults around them already know it exists. Children in this age range, especially those in the toddler and preschool years, can point to the area of pain but will be unable to describe it.

Piaget's stage of *concrete operational* development encompasses ages 7 to 11 years. In this stage, children begin to understand that injury and illness may be accompanied by pain, but they do not understand the cause. The older school-age child develops a greater understanding of the relationship between pain and illness, injury, and diagnostic procedures. These children also understand and use much more descriptive words to express their pain, such as pain that "comes and goes" or is cramping, burning, dull, or sharp. School-age children are beginning to differentiate between physical and psychological or emotional pain.

Formal operational thought, the final stage of Piaget's cognitive development theory, occurs between ages 11 and 18 years of age but may continue into early adulthood. The ability to think abstractly and use logic allows this age group to develop an advanced understanding of pain and its causes and to describe that pain in more detail. However, the need for control and the independence of adolescents is significantly impacted by the presence of pain. They may not admit to experiencing pain if they think they should "grin and bear it" like they perceive an adult might or if they believe the nurse thinks the pain should be tolerated.

PAIN ASSESSMENT AND MANAGEMENT

Ongoing assessment is essential for the child experiencing pain. Proper pain assessment requires identification of the type of pain the child is experiencing, the origins of either physiological or psychological pain, and the behavioral patterns associated with the pain. Pain assessment tools are invaluable for obtaining a child's perception and for the younger or disabled child as well as the parent's view of pain levels. There are several statistically reliable pain scales available for use with children of different ages and stages of cognitive development. The most commonly used pain scales are the numeric scale, the Wong Faces Scale, the FLACC, and CHEOPS pain scales (Fig. 21-9, Tables 21-9 and 21-10). Accurate pain assessment also requires an understanding of multiple factors, not the least of which is cognitive development, education of the child and family regarding the pain assessment tool being used, and consistency in application of the chosen tool.

The nurse should familiarize the child and family with an appropriate pain scale during hospitalization or a clinic visit, when the child is injured or ill, or for a medical procedure or surgery. The nurse understands that it is important to use the same pain scale according to age, developmental stage, and cognitive function level. In addition to the pain scales, the nurse asks about intensity, duration, and location of the pain; the effects of movement on the severity of pain; any aggravating and alleviating factors; and, if appropriate, previous interventions that alleviated the pain. It is useful to know what experiences the child has had with pain, including previous surgeries, illnesses, or congenital conditions. A child's ability to manage pain is sometimes related to the child's position in the family or his experience of illnesses in other close family members. Pain has many

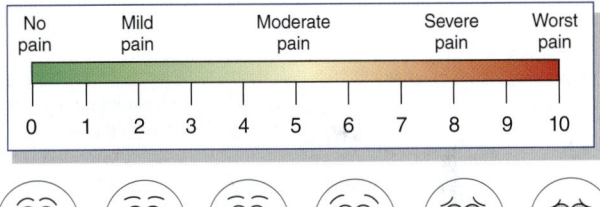

Figure 21-9 Pain scales. *A,* Numeric pain scale (about 12 years or older). *B,* Wong-Baker Faces pain scale (preschool through school-age).

Table 21-9	FLACC Pain Scale		
Categories	**Scoring**		
	0	1	2
Face	No particular expression or smile; disinterested	Occasional grimace or frown; withdrawn	Frequent to constant frown, clenched jaw, quivering chin
Legs	Normal position or relaxed	Uneasy, restless, tense	Kicking, or legs drawn up
Activity	Lying quietly, normal position, moves easily	Squirming, shifting back and forth, tense	Arched, rigid, or jerking
Cry	No cry (awake or asleep)	Moans or whimpers, occasional complaint	Crying steadily, screams or sobs, frequent complaints
Consolability	Content, relaxed	Reassured by occasional touching, hugging, or talking to; distractible	Difficult to console or comfort

Each of the 5 categories—(F) Face; (L) Legs; (A) Activity; (C) Cry; (C) Consolability—is scored from 0 to 2, which results in a total score between 0 and 10.

Table 21-10 CHEOPS Pain Scale

Children's Hospital Eastern Ontario Pain Scale (CHEOPS)
(Recommended for children 1–7 years old)—A score greater than 4 indicates pain

Item	Behavioral		Definition	Score
Cry	No cry	1	Child is not crying.	
	Moaning	2	Child is moaning or quietly vocalizing silent cry.	
	Crying	2	Child is crying, but the cry is gentle or whimpering.	
	Scream	3	Child is in a full-lunged cry; sobbing; may be scored with complaint or without complaint.	
Facial	Composed	1	Neutral facial expression.	
	Grimace	2	Score only if definite negative facial expression.	
	Smiling	0	Score only if definite positive facial expression.	
Child Verbal	None	1	Child not talking.	
	Other complaints	1	Child complains, but not about pain, e.g., "I want to see mommy" or "I am thirsty."	
	Pain complaints	2	Child complains about pain.	
	Both complaints	2	Child complains about pain and about other things, e.g., "It hurts; I want my mommy."	
	Positive	0	Child makes any positive statement or talks about others things without complaint.	
Torso	Neutral	1	Body (not limbs) is at rest; torso is inactive.	
	Shifting	2	Body is in motion in a shifting or serpentine fashion.	
	Tense	2	Body is arched or rigid.	
	Shivering	2	Body is shuddering or shaking involuntarily.	
	Upright	2	Child is in a vertical or upright position.	
	Restrained	2	Body is restrained.	
Touch	Not touching	1	Child is not touching or grabbing at wound.	
	Reach	2	Child is reaching for but not touching wound.	
	Touch	2	Child is gently touching wound or wound area.	
	Grab	2	Child is grabbing vigorously at wound.	
	Restrained	2	Child's arms are restrained.	
Legs	Neutral	1	Legs may be in any position but are relaxed; includes gentle swimming or separate-like movements.	
	Squirm/kicking	2	Definitive uneasy or restless movements in the legs and/or striking out with foot or feet.	
	Drawn up/tensed	2	Legs tensed and/or pulled up tightly to body and kept there.	
	Standing	2	Standing, crouching, or kneeling.	
	Restrained	2	Child's legs are being held down.	

descriptors: mild, moderate, severe, chronic, stabbing, burning, pricking, aching, throbbing, or dull. Pain is also expressed nonverbally with facial expressions, guarding, and muscle tension.

Mild pain is a slight discomfort. Its management may include minor analgesics along with comfort measures or distraction. However, engaging in a distraction does not mean that the child has no pain. It is simply a coping mechanism that diverts a child's attention from the pain for a finite period of time. Pharmacological intervention for mild pain starts with analgesics such as children's acetaminophen (Tylenol) or children's ibuprofen (Advil or Motrin) and is administered on a scheduled or as-needed basis.

Although moderate pain may also be relieved by using distraction, the child experiences much stronger unpleasant sensations. Using a child's vivid imagination is very effective in pain management, as long as it is used in conjunction with regularly timed analgesic administration, including milder opioids such as codeine in varying combinations of acetaminophen (Children's Tylenol).

Severe pain causes pallor, sweating, **piloerection** (elevation of the hair above the skin), dilated pupils, increased respiration and blood pressure, and muscle tension. However, if pain has been prolonged, the child's body may have become accustomed to it, in which case marked increases in vital signs may not be noted. Again, that does not mean that the child is not experiencing pain. When brief, intense pain subsides, the child's body may respond with a lower blood pressure or pulse rate.

Management of severe pain, often associated with surgical interventions, usually calls for strong analgesics like morphine sulfate (Astramorph). The maximum allowable dosage according to the child's weight in kilograms may be started in the recovery room and followed by regular dosing, within the allowable limit for the specific child, to ensure adequate pain coverage.

Acute pain occurs 24 to 48 hours after trauma or surgery. It is initially experienced as severe pain and gradually subsides over time. With orthopedic trauma, a short period of auto-anesthesia can occur that belies the extent of the injury. Because narcotics do not relieve all of the pain following surgery, they can be accompanied with some success by comfort measures, such as holding a hand or encouraging the child "to send his pain to you by squeezing your hand tightly."

Chronic pain in children is any pain lasting more than 3 months. It can result in fear of reinjury, anorexia, weight loss, changes in sleep patterns, guarded movements, a rigid facial expression, and an overall diminishment of the child's joy of living. Management of chronic pain involves careful observation of which pain relief measures work best for a particular child. Decreasing pain to acceptable levels allows the child to carry on with as many age-appropriate activities as possible given the circumstances of his illness or condition. Table 21-11 shows a comparison of acute and chronic pain.

Medication: Morphine Sulfate (Astramorph)

(**mor**-feen **sul**-fate)

Morphine sulfate (Astramorph) is an opioid analgesic. It is frequently used for children with severe or chronic pain. It can be given PO, IV, IM, epidurally, or via a patient-controlled analgesia pump (PCA).

Dosage Recommendations

PO, RECT (Adults and Children less than 50 kg) Usual starting dose for moderate to severe pain in opioid-naive patients—0.3 mg/kg q 3 to 4 hr initially

PO (Children greater than 1 mo) Prompt-release tablets and solution—0.2 to 0.5 mg/kg/dose q 4 to 6 hr as needed. Controlled-release tablet—0.3 to 0.6 mg/kg/dose q 12 hr

IM, IV, SQ (Adults and Children less than 50 kg) Usual starting dose for moderate to severe pain in opioid-naive patients—0.05 to 0.2 mg/kg q 3 to 4 hr, max: 15 mg/dose

IM, IV, SQ (Neonates) 0.05 mg/kg q 4 to 8 hr, max dose: 0.1 mg/kg. Use preservative-free formulation

IV, SQ (Children greater than 1 mo) Continuous infusion, postoperative pain—0.01 to 0.04 mg/kg/hr. Continuous infusion, sickle cell or cancer pain—0.02 to 2.6 mg/kg/hr

IV (Neonates) Continuous infusion—0.01 to 0.03 mg/kg/hr

Epidural (Children greater than 1 mo) 0.03 to 0.05 mg/kg, max dose: 0.1 mg/kg or 5 mg/24 hr. Use preservative-free

Source: Data from Vallerand, A. H., & Sanoski, C. A. (2014). *Davis's drug guide for nurses* (14th ed., pp. 880–884). Philadelphia, PA: F.A. Davis.

---

focus on safety

Naloxone (Narcan)

When giving morphine sulfate (Astramorph), be sure to have the opioid antagonist naloxone (Narcan) available if respiratory depression occurs. Narcan completely blocks the effects of opioids including central nervous system effects and respiratory depression. The dose for children is 5 to 10 mcg/kg (0.01 mg/kg).

Source: Data from Vallerand, A. H., & Sanoski, C. A. (2014). *Davis's drug guide for nurses* (14th ed., pp. 898–900). Philadelphia, PA: F.A. Davis.

Nursing Insight—Myths about pain management

- Children do not feel pain with the same intensity as adults.
- Children cannot tell where they hurt.
- Children will tell you if they are really having pain.
- Children become accustomed to pain.
- Narcotic analgesics are dangerous for children because they become addicted or go into respiratory distress.
- If children can be distracted, they are not in pain.
- If children say they are in pain, but do not look in pain, they do not need to be medicated.
- Being in pain for only a little while is not that bad.
- After children have undergone surgery, they should not be given analgesia until they can vocalize pain because they received enough anesthetic to "cover" their pain.
- The best way to give analgesics is intramuscularly.
- Children with neurological impairments do not feel pain as much as other children.
- Children, especially boys, should learn to tolerate pain; they will make better, stronger adults.

Children react to pain and its management in individual ways that also correspond to their developmental level (Table 21-12). Responses to analgesia, time, route, and dose are documented to enable nurses across all shifts to provide a continuum of care for the child.

Table 21-11 Characteristics of Acute and Chronic Pain

Acute Pain	Chronic Pain	Chronic Cancer Pain
Identifiable cause	Cause hard to find	Usually identifiable cause
Short duration	Lasts longer than 3 months	Duration varies
Sudden onset	Begins gradually and persists	Onset varies
Well defined	May or may not be well defined	May or may not be well defined
Limited	Unlimited	Unlimited
Decreases with healing	Persists beyond healing time	May persist beyond healing
Reversible	Exhausting and useless	Exhausting and useless
Signs and symptoms present	Signs and symptoms absent	Signs and symptoms absent
Anxiety	Depression and fatigue	Depression, fatigue, and anxiety

Table 21-12 Pain Management Strategies

Age (Guideline Only)	Concerns/Reactions	Distraction	Environment
Infant/Toddler (0–3 Years)	Separation anxiety Protest Despair Denial	Pacifier Swaddling Rocking Eye contact Music Picture books	Controlled lighting and noise Use treatment room
Preschool (3–6 Years)	Separation anxiety Concerns with body image Develops fantasies with illness and treatment Battle for control	Distraction kit Deep breathing Bubble blowing Counting Singing	Use treatment room Music Controlled lighting and noise
School Age (6–11 Years)	Has questions regarding body and illness Concerns of helplessness, passivity, and dependency Tend to be phobic and develop fears Anger	Deep breathing Hand squeezing Riddles/trivia Pretend games Talking Distraction kit	Use treatment room Music Controlled lighting and noise
Teens (12 and older)	Illness interferes with struggle for independence Illness is a major threat to developing self-image Very threatened by helplessness and loss of privacy Denial, withdrawal, anger, hostility, disappointment	Imagery Tablet Deep breathing Hand squeezing Talking Jokes Distraction kit	Use treatment room Music Controlled lighting and noise

focus on safety

Handoff communication

Handoff communication is an interactive process for relaying important patient information from one health-care team member to another (e.g., change of shift report between nurses) and allowing time for the person assuming care of a patient to ask questions. This communication typically occurs face-to-face at the bedside or in a taped format. Another type of handoff communication is partnership rounding, when nurses complete focused assessments and engage the patient in the conversation (Grant & Colello, 2009).

To improve patient safety and decrease medical errors caused by miscommunication, it is important to use a standardized format for handoff communication and to educate staff in its use. Handoff communication must be clear and concise to avoid unnecessary information obscuring the more important facts about the patient. One method for standardizing communication between health-care team members is to use the Shift Report Hand-off Guide (see *DavisPlus*). This form provides a situational method for communicating pertinent patient information and is widely used in many health-care systems (Institute for Healthcare Improvement, 2012) and can be modified for use between disciplines. The essential components are Situation, Background, Assessment, Recommendation, and Discharge Plan (SBAR). The Situation encompasses pertinent admission information and current issues; Background includes code status, current care (IVs/wounds/drains), pertinent lab and diagnostic test results, pertinent medications, recent interventions and their effectiveness, and focused physical assessment findings. Assessment relates to what the caring nurse believes is happening with the patient, any concerns the nurse may have, and issues with discharge planning. Recommendations refer to any follow-up needed in regard to current orders, care left undone or that which needs follow-up, and any pending treatments or procedures. Discharge Plan is a way to ensure the patient's needs continue to be met once they have returned home.

The Child With a Disability

Disabilities may be congenital or genetically based or develop from illness, injury, or disease progression (see Table 21-13). Regardless of the cause, families of children with disabilities are beset with emotional upset and confusion about the reality of not having the child they expected (i.e., one without a disability). In addition, the family is often distressed about the child's pain and her experiences with surgery, treatments, procedures, and repeated clinic appointments. The child is apt to have ongoing physical, occupational, or speech therapy, and parents often need to perform physically painful procedures at home to promote their child's development. Other ongoing treatments and procedures include respiratory therapy, gavage feedings, medication administration, using assistive devices, planning special diets, taking care of elimination needs, and implementing special techniques to maintain the musculoskeletal system. Understanding the child with a disability includes knowing about emotional, developmental, and physical concerns as well as comprehending caregiver fatigue and the concept of resiliency.

Parental Involvement	Preparation	Positions	Post-Procedure Comforting
Encourage parental presence, provide guidance and, if possible, comfort/cuddle baby during procedure	Prepare parent: offer explanations of what they will see and hear Develop a plan "who will do what"	Swaddle Cuddle	Soothe Swaddle Hold and rock Soft music Soothing voice
Encourage parental presence and provide guidance in encouraging participation during strategies	Medical play with relevant medical equipment and participation Pre-procedural teaching Reassurance of what child is to expect—focus on senses	Lap Parent or staff may support patient or have other close physical contact Present patient with choices	Praise and reward (stickers) Medical play Play Stories
Encourage parental presence and provide guidance Encourage parents to be part of the team	Simple medical terms to describe what will happen Allow appropriate play with medical equipment Explain reasons for various components of tests and allow appropriate participation by patient	Lap Parent may support patient or have other close physical contact Present patient with choices	Praise, reward (stickers) Play, medical play Stories Evaluate procedures and discuss suggestions for next time
Ask permission of patient for parental involvement Encourage parents to be part of the team	Clarify misconceptions and initiate discussions about the past experiences with procedures Allow appropriate participation by patient Pre-procedural teaching utilizing medical play	Present patient with choices Plan positioning with teen	Praise, reward (stickers) Play, medical play Stories, evaluate procedures and discuss suggestions for next time

Where Research and Practice Meet:
Handoff Communication

In a 15-year study by The Joint Commission (TJC) of **sentinel events** (unexpected events resulting in death or serious injury) occurring within health-care facilities, communication was identified as a major factor in medical errors, with handoff communication contributing to "an estimated 80% of serious preventable adverse events" (2010). For this reason, TJC identified a National Patient Safety Goal mandating health-care facilities to "improve the effectiveness of communication among caregivers" (The Joint Commission, 2010). Go to http://www.jointcommission.org/standards_information/npsgs.aspx for more information.

UNDERSTANDING THE CHILD WITH A DISABILITY

Emotional Concerns

Raising a child with a disability is distressing because of the disruption of the normal routine, the conveyance of continuous "bad news" or prognostics, the reconfirmation of future emotional and physical concerns, and the awareness of financial implications the diagnosis and treatment provoke. These financial concerns include medical care that is not covered by insurance or government-sponsored health-care programs as well as expenses incurred for child care or respite care. Often, a parent is required to stop working and become a full-time caregiver resulting in further economic distress. The nurse can help the family access community resources that can provide ongoing emotional support.

Across Care Settings: Insurance for children

The nurse can teach the family about how to obtain health insurance for their child. Health insurance provided to children through state and national programs is free or low-cost. The costs are different depending on the state and the family's income. When there are charges for health care, the charges are minimal. Children who have health insurance generally have better health throughout their childhood. Benefits of insurance for children include (1) receiving needed immunizations that prevent disease, (2) receiving treatment for acute as well as recurring illnesses, and (3) receiving preventative care to keep the child healthy.

It is important to note that in some cases children who are eligible for Medicaid cannot enroll in the state program because Medicaid provides comprehensive health benefits.

Developmental Concerns

Many congenital problems are repaired surgically either shortly after birth or once the child is physically developed and strong enough to withstand the rigors of surgery. Parents and the child need constant support from health-care personnel to sustain a loving environment for the child with a disability who may be undergoing the same growth

Table 21-13 Common Genetic Disorders

Genetic Disorder/Incidence	Common Assessment Findings
Cystic fibrosis/1:2,500 Caucasians	Infancy: Failure to thrive, frequent pneumonias Childhood: Chronic pulmonary disease, malnutrition
Down syndrome/1:800–1,000. 1:1,250 if mother is under age 25 years; 1:100 if mother is >40 years of age.	Flattened nasal bridge resulting in wide-set eyes; low set ears, Simian crease, developmental delays. Co-morbidities: diabetes, celiac disease, congenital heart defects
Sickle cell disease/1:500 African Americans	Anemia, pain, frequent infections
Klinefelter syndrome/1:600 males	Speech delay, possible learning disabilities, gynecomastia during puberty, smaller genitalia after puberty, infertility
Thalassemia/1:25,000 Mediterranean/Asian/African American descent	Anemia, pallor, facial deformity, hepatomegaly, splenomegaly, cardiomegaly, brittle bones
Neural tube defects/1:1,000	Learning disabilities, bowel and bladder dysfunction, paralysis of the lower extremities, latex allergy
Fragile X syndrome/1:1,500 males; 1:2,500 females	Mild to severe mental retardation; speech and language difficulties

and development changes as any other child of the same age. However, because of constant medical and surgical interventions, the child may demonstrate either signs of regression to more immature behaviors or surprising evidence of what some call a "maturity beyond their years." The latter has been observed in children with cancer who are faced with pain and/or body image disturbances, such as alopecia or extreme weight loss, and with their own mortality as they might understand it at their age.

Physical Concerns

The child with a disability undergoing surgery, especially at a younger age, may experience rapid fluid and electrolyte changes. These conditions may require intensive care procedures that are worrisome to parents and often painful for the children. Children with severe congenital heart problems face a lifetime of corrective procedures to augment initial surgeries or pharmacological therapies that consume time, energy, and finances. In addition, both parent and child need to learn physical self-care techniques, such as diabetes or anticoagulation monitoring. Often, abnormalities affect several body systems so that visits must be made to several different medical specialists who may require multiple pharmacotherapeutic regimens. Throughout all this, families must learn to care for the physical needs of the child.

 Nursing Insight—*Caring for the child with a disability*

- Maintain a respectful attitude toward the parent and the child.
- Listen carefully to the parent's concerns, realizing that parents often "know their child best."
- Assess the child's skills for coping with pain or fatigue.
- Evaluate how social and health-care agencies can assist parents and the child to manage the disability—financial, medical, and community services.
- Evaluate the need for respite care and reliable community resource providers.

Caregiver Fatigue

Caring for a child with a significant disability takes its toll on the entire family. Respite care agencies were developed in response to the needs of parents of extremely disabled children to give short-term relief from the 24-hour surveillance and care often required in cases of severe disability. As medical advancements have increased the life expectancy of disabled children, so too have the number of disabled children or premature births resulted in larger numbers of children and families requiring long-term medical care and social systems to support their needs.

Most disabilities in childhood result in multiple visits to clinics, hospitals, or rehabilitation centers, thus disrupting normal activity and sleep patterns. It requires much more energy for a disabled child to perform even the simplest task than it does for a healthy child. It has been estimated that a severely disabled child needs to perform a simple task, such as getting into "puppy position" or standing independently for 15 seconds, 10,000 more times than a physically healthy child to accomplish it. These children have extra requirements for stamina, calories, vitamins, minerals, and protein to accomplish normal daily activities, let alone learning developmentally appropriate mental skills. These children also need additional sleep but may have more trouble getting enough sleep if the demands of their care interfere with a normal sleep pattern. All of these factors contribute to caregiver fatigue.

Resiliency

Coping mechanisms give rise to resiliency in children and their families. Resiliency theory defines the protective factors in families, schools, and communities that exist in the lives of children. Four common attributes of resilient children include social competence, problem-solving skills, autonomy, and a sense of purpose and future. Nurses can help parents and children develop resiliency and positive self-esteem by fostering a mix of love and nurturing in the face of overwhelming stressors (Pizzolongo & Hunter, 2011). Emotional security and maturity provide the foundation for resiliency (Box 21-2).

Box 21-2 Ways to Promote Resiliency

- Express love and gratitude
- Foster competency and positive attitudes
- Nurture positive emotions
- Encourage helping others
- Teach peace-building skills
- Reinforce positive behaviors
- Reduce stress

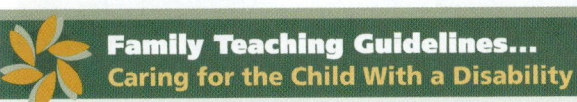

Family Teaching Guidelines...
Caring for the Child With a Disability

HOW TO: Care for the child with a disability

TOPIC: The nurse will improve the care of the family and a child with a disability

ESSENTIAL INFORMATION:

- Maintain a respectful attitude toward the parent and the child.
- Assess the child's communication strategies and incorporate them in the nursing plan of care.
- Listen carefully to the parent's concerns, realizing that parents often "know their child best."
- Evaluate how social and health-care agencies can assist parents and the child to manage the disability—financial, medical, and community services.
- Assess the child's skills for coping with pain or fatigue.
- Evaluate the need for respite care and reliable community resource providers.

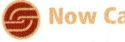 **Now Can You—**Describe the child in pain and understand the child with a disability?

1. Describe developmentally appropriate assessments of pain in children?
2. Discuss common medications used in the treatment of pain in children?
3. Understand the child with a disability?

Across Care Settings

There are several options for the delivery of nursing care in the hospital setting. Pediatric nursing care in the hospital for families is holistic, based on normal growth and development, emphasizing the optimization of preventative health and safety measures yielding positive health outcomes. Hospitalized nursing care is required when the child becomes ill, and the level of care is based on the available health-care resources and the amount of in-depth treatment that must be provided.

Hospital: When a child enters the hospital, it may be an entirely new experience where both the child and family are exposed to an unfamiliar medical environment. The hospital may be a specialty children's hospital located in a separate building especially designed for children or may be part of a general care hospital. Hospitals provide many health-care services, such as emergency care, specialized inpatient care, surgery, critical care, diagnostic tests and treatments, therapies, patient education, and other specialized services.

Children's Hospital: A specialty pediatric hospital that is specially designed and managed specifically for children that provides various health-care services, such as emergency care, specialized inpatient care, surgery, critical care, diagnostic tests and treatments, patient education, and other specialized services where physicians, nurses, child life specialists, other health-care providers, and employees are specially trained to work with children.

Day Hospital: A specialized hospital that serves children who require medical treatments such as blood transfusions, chemotherapy, steroid pulse therapy, IV hydration, IV antibiotic therapy, immunoglobulin therapy, or Remicade (infliximab) infusions.

Areas for Care in the Hospital

Twenty-Four-Hour Observation Unit: A short-stay hospitalization experience is also known as 24-hour observation. A 24-hour observation occurs when a child becomes suddenly ill and will most likely recover quickly. The child may need a shortened hospital stay for observation and specifically for treatments such as rehydration, aerosol treatment for acute asthma, or medication for an allergic reaction. At the conclusion of the 24-hour period, the child is reassessed and it is then determined whether continued hospitalization is needed or whether the child can be discharged home. The pediatric nurse provides acute nursing care and then quickly begins to prepare the child and family for discharge. As a part of discharge process, the nurse explains specific medical orders as well as when to notify the primary health-care provider with any questions, concerns, or change in condition.

Ambulatory Surgery Center: A surgical center is where children receive minimal surgical treatment, recover from the procedure, and are discharged soon after the surgery.

Children are more vulnerable to the stress of hospitalization because they do not have a full range of coping mechanisms such as highly developed problem-solving skills. The child and family are also introduced to an entirely new group of people and are exposed to uncomfortable or painful treatments and procedures, to other cultures and languages, and to many new and difficult stressors (Leininger, 1988). The pediatric nurse must provide skilled, safe, and competent care and be supportive in their adaptation to this unfamiliar and potentially frightening environment.

Fast Track Care: Children who have a minor illness such as an ear infection often go to an acute care facility, sometimes termed urgent care. This is a

Critical Nursing Action Caring for the Child at Home After Minor Surgery

Nurses teach parents how to care for their child at home after minor surgery. Care includes:

- Taking the child's axillary temperature
- Assessing the child's level of consciousness
- When to begin giving the child liquids
- When to offer liquids based on type of surgery, prescribed diet, and age
- When to offer solid food based on type of surgery, prescribed diet, and age
- What type of activity is expected or should be encouraged
- What are the actions and side effects of medications
- What are the signs and symptoms of infection
- What are signs of poor airway exchange
- How to use assistive devices and medical equipment and perform home treatments
- How to contact a nurse, pharmacist, health-care professional, or community agency
- When to call the doctor

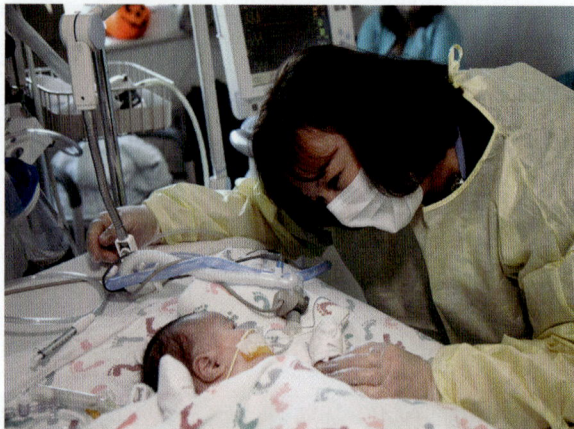

Figure 21-10 Child in critical care unit.

focus on safety

Critical illness

Common problems of critical illness are shock, acute respiratory failure, chronic respiratory failure, infection, sepsis, renal failure, neurological conditions, bleeding and clotting disorders, or multiorgan dysfunction. Nursing interventions for the illness are complex and ongoing. In this type of setting, the pediatric nurse usually cares for just one or two patients at a time to meet the multifaceted health-care and emotional support needs of the child and family.

standalone facility or a facility housed in a public business such as a grocery store or shopping mall. In a hospital or community setting, there is a "fast track" system where less urgent children are quickly assessed, treated by a physician, and then discharged home. Sometimes, after the child receives an initial assessment and treatment, she is admitted to a hospital depending on the diagnosis and subsequent treatment.

Emergency Department: Emergency care is provided in a hospital or health-care facility that provides quick treatment for children who have become suddenly ill or experienced a severe injury. Emergency departments (ED) are open 24 hours per day and 7 days per week. Children who arrive in the emergency department first receive a rapid screening or triage assessment to establish the nature and severity of their presenting illness. If the illness or injury is severe, the child is treated in an urgent manner, and all necessary procedures, treatments, and tests are performed immediately. The emergency department may have several areas of treatment, including a general and minor care area; a resuscitation room; or specialty areas for specific populations such as children, women, or persons requiring mental health care.

Critical Care Unit: When critical care of the child is required, the child is admitted to the critical care unit, usually through the emergency department or the operating room. A child who becomes very ill on a medical–surgical floor is transferred into a pediatric critical care unit. After delivery, a newborn who requires intensive care is transferred to a neonatal intensive care unit. Other types of critical care units where children might receive care include cardiac, surgical, or psychiatric critical care units. In any of these units, the child is extremely ill and receives specialized care, medication, IV fluid, and respiratory or ventilator support (Fig. 21-10).

Reasons for Accessing Medical Care

Each year, millions of children visit emergency departments for everything from primary care to severe, life-threatening injuries and illnesses.

Injuries to children between the ages of 1 and 14 years account for 33% of ED visits. These injuries are most often caused by falls and striking or being struck by another person or object (Forum on Child and Family Statistics, 2011). Head and neck injuries resulting from bicycle and motor vehicle accidents; concussions from contact sports; and strains, sprains, and fractures explain a large percentage of those visits. In adolescents aged 15 to 19, injuries because of more violent reasons (e.g., motor vehicle accidents, sports, and assaults) account for over half of all ED visits for injuries (Table 21-14).

Illnesses that include fever, cough, vomiting, and diarrhea are leading causes of visits to the ED. Additional reasons include upper respiratory infections, abdominal pain, and asthma. Many of these children are triaged to the urgent care or "treat and release" area of the ED and rarely need admission to the hospital. Of those half a million pediatric ED visits per year warranting admission, the most frequent reasons are infections of the respiratory system, urinary tract, and skin. The particular examples included in this chapter are epistaxis (nosebleed), poisoning caused by ingestion of medicine, and lead poisoning.

Epistaxis (nosebleed) is common in children. Most cases are clinically benign events; however, a serious nosebleed or a high-risk child experiencing a nosebleed may warrant accessing a care facility. The greatest concern occurs when family members or caretakers become upset at the sight of blood, which may appear excessive even from

Table 21-14 Injuries by Age Group

Age Group	Most Common Fatal Injury by Age Group	Most Common Nonfatal Injuries by Age Group
Infancy	Suffocation	Head injury, fractures, and sprains resulting from falls Motor vehicle accidents because of improperly installed car seats Burns caused by sunburn, stoves, cigarettes, bathwater, electrical outlets Choking on food or foreign bodies Suffocation caused by cords and strings
Toddler	Drowning	Head injury, fractures, and sprains resulting from falls Motor vehicle accidents Drowning Poisoning Burns caused by sunburn, stoves, cigarettes, bathwater, electrical outlets
Preschool	Drowning	Head injury, fractures, and sprains resulting from falls Motor vehicle accidents Burns caused by sunburn, stoves, cigarettes, bathwater, electrical outlets Poisonings Firearms
School-age	Motor vehicle accident	**Ages 5–9 years:** Head injury, fractures, and sprains resulting from falls Being struck by or against another person or object Animal bites Insect bites **Ages 10–12 years:** Head injury, fractures, and sprains resulting from falls Being struck by or against another person or object (sports injuries) Overexertion
Adolescents	Motor vehicle accident	Being struck by or against another person or object (sports injuries) Overexertion Motor vehicle accidents

Source: Centers for Disease Control and Prevention (CDC). (2012d). CDC childhood injury report. Retrieved from http://www.cdc.gov/safechild/Child_Injury_Data.html

a small nosebleed. Nosebleeds are related to the increased vascularity of nasal mucosa.

Critical Nursing Action Controlling Epistaxis (Nosebleed)

Don gloves and put the child in a sitting position, leaning forward. Apply direct pressure to the anterior nasal septum for 10 to 15 minutes. Remind the child to breathe through the mouth, so he does not become anxious. Applying ice to the nose area is beneficial. If a large amount of blood loss occurs, the nurse must monitor vital signs. In cases of severe nose bleeding that persists beyond 10 to 15 minutes, nasal packing may be required, as well as topical epinephrine. When an infection is present, antibiotics may be ordered. It is essential that the nurse keep the child and family quiet and calm by providing support and reassurance. It is important that families are able to demonstrate first aid measures necessary to control an occurrence of epistaxis.

Poisoning caused by ingestion of medicine contributes to 60,000 pediatric ED visits per year and accounts for another 500,000 calls to poison control centers (Morbidity and Mortality Weekly Report, 2012). Common medication ingestions include acetaminophen and iron. Caustic ingestions include hydrocarbons and corrosives (Table 21-15).

Acetaminophen (Tylenol), widely available in many brands and in many over-the-counter cold and flu medications, is one of the most common toxic ingestions worldwide (National Library of Medicine, 2011). Toxic ingestion requires proper care in a medical facility. Farrell Pediatrics (2014) describes the symptoms of acetaminophen overdose as they occur in four phases from the time of ingestion until 3 weeks post-ingestion.

Treatment of acetaminophen overdose is most successful if started within 8 hours of the ingestion with N-acetylcysteine (NAC) solution. NAC binds to the metabolite of acetaminophen, preventing its absorption and subsequent metabolism by the liver. This foul-smelling antidote is most often given orally and may be mixed with fruit juice to increase palatability. If the child cannot tolerate it orally, a nasogastric tube can be inserted. NAC is given every 4 hours for 20 to 72 hours, depending on the level of toxicity and the child's response to therapy.

The most common heavy metal ingestion is lead. Lead is found in contaminated soil, water that flows through old lead pipes or faucets, food stored in bowls glazed or painted with lead, toys, jewelry, and even in some folk remedies.

Cultural Diversity: Lead Exposure in Folk Medicines

Folk medicines used by Indian, Middle Eastern, West Asian, and Hispanic cultures may contain high levels of lead. During a health assessment interview, inquire as to the use of Greta, Azarcon (coral, Luiga, Maria Luisa, or Rueda), Ghasard, or Ba-baw-san.

Table 21-15 Common Toxic Ingestions

Ingestion of . . .	Leads to . . .
Acetaminophen—found in many over-the-counter medicines	Phase 1 (0–24 hr): Often asymptomatic. Nausea, vomiting Phase 2 (18–72 hrs): RUQ abdominal pain, poor appetite, tachycardia, hypotension Phase 3 (72–96 hr): Above symptoms. Liver dysfunction, jaundice, encephalopathy. Acute renal failure. Death from multisystem organ failure. Phase 4 (4 days to 3 weeks): Those who survive have complete recovery and resolution of organ failure.
Iron—vitamin or iron supplements	Vomiting Hematemesis Diarrhea − +/−bloody stools Abdominal pain Metabolic acidosis Coagulopathy Shock Coma
Lead—lead paint used before 1978 May be inhaled or ingested	Neuro: learning disabilities, motor deficits GI: abdominal pain, nausea, vomiting, constipation, anorexia Renal: tubular damage Heme: hemolysis, iron deficiency MS: muscle and joint pain Soft tissue: blue-black line in gum margins Endocrine: short stature
Hydrocarbons—distillates of petroleum: gasoline, kerosene, furniture polish, Freon	Gagging, choking, coughing, respiratory distress with aspiration of hydrocarbons Nausea, vomiting, lethargy, tremors
Corrosives—strong acids and alkaline products: batteries, ammonia, bleach, sodium hydroxide (drain cleaners)	Severe burning of the gastrointestinal tract leading to strictures Swelling/edema of oropharynx leading to respiratory obstruction Violent vomiting Hemoptysis Drooling Shock

Lead interferes with normal body function and is toxic to organs such as the heart, bones, intestines, kidneys, and reproductive system. It also interferes with nervous system development, which causes permanent learning and/or behavior disorders. Symptoms of lead poisoning include abdominal pain, confusion, headache, anemia, irritability, coma, and death.

The Centers for Disease Control standard for elevated blood lead level is 25 (mcg/dL) of the whole blood for adults. For children, the number is set lower at 5 (mcg/dL) of blood. Routine screening for lead poisoning occurs during the latter part of infancy during well-child care visits. To treat lead poisoning, the source of the lead is removed and chelation therapy is administered in the hospital.

 ***Across Care Settings:* Decreasing exposure to lead**

The incidence of lead poisoning has decreased with the removal of sources of lead in gasoline, lead paint, and water supplies. However, lead can still be found in tap water because most of the lead comes from the corrosion of older pipes that leach into the water supply after sitting in the pipes for several hours.

If mixing formula from powder or concentrate, advise parents to flush water from the system by running the tap for 1 to 2 minutes before using the water. Nurses can also promote decreased lead exposure in tap water by encouraging parents to contact the water authority to determine the lead content in the water. The EPA states that 15 parts per billion is acceptable.

Visit http://www.cdc.gov/nceh/lead for more information on the prevention of lead poisoning in children (CDC, 2012e).

If ingestion of lead occurs, the child may be seen in a clinic or hospitalized. The following is a nursing care plan for the child who has ingested lead.

Ways to Decrease the Stress of Hospitalization

When a child is hospitalized, the family undergoes stress. Family visitation and the family-centered care have dramatically helped children and families cope with the stress of a hospitalization. Despite the availability of parental rooming in, the parent may also be coping with other children at home or the need to work, which could lead to separation from the child, even though family visitation is encouraged. It is important to remember that the ill child depends on his parents as the primary source of coping and comfort. To help a child of any age adapt to the stress of hospitalization, the pediatric nurse can suggest rooming-in to the parents, where they stay in the room both during the day and through the night (see Table 21-16).

Nursing Care Plan The Child at Risk for Lead Poisoning

Nursing Diagnosis: Risk for poisoning related to environmental lead exposure

Measurable Short-Term Goal: Child's lead blood level will remain less than 5 mcg/dL.

Measurable Long-Term Goal: The child will not be exposed to lead in the home environment.

NOC Outcomes:

Safe Home Environment (1910)—Physical arrangements to minimize environmental factors that might cause physical harm or injury in the home

NIC Interventions:

Environmental Risk Protection (8880)
Home Maintenance Assistance (7180)
Parent Education: Childrearing Family (5566)

Nursing Interventions:

1. Assist caregivers to evaluate child's environmental risk for lead exposure (specify, e.g., if he or she lives or plays in housing built before 1978, has had a sibling or playmate diagnosed with lead poisoning, or ingests imported spices).

   RATIONALE: All children should be screened for lead poisoning at ages 1 and 2. The highest risk is from ingestion of lead-based paint, which was outlawed for use in homes in 1978 but other sources include imported Indian spices.

2. Assist family with identifying sources of lead in the child's environment: old lead-based paint, pottery not intended to hold food or liquid, imported spices, playing in dirt contaminated with old paint flakes (specify others as appropriate, e.g., hobbies).

   RATIONALE: The family may be unaware of lead sources in their environment.

3. Monitor child's blood lead levels as obtained (specify frequency).

   RATIONALE: The child may have no obvious symptoms, even with high lead levels.

4. Explain significance of child's blood lead level to family (specify if further screening or treatment is indicated).

   RATIONALE: Sharing information allows the family to participate in care decisions for the child.

5. Monitor for behavior changes and attainment of developmental milestones and explain expected characteristics for age to family.

   RATIONALE: Lead poisoning may cause behavior disorders or delayed development. The family is most likely to notice changes in behavior and can report on the child's developmental abilities.

6. Teach the family about the risks of lead poisoning for pregnant women and small children in terms the family can understand, including brain injury, developmental disabilities, kidney damage, and anemia.

   RATIONALE: This information can help protect others in the family or neighborhood.

7. Administer chelation therapy as ordered (specify: drug, dose, route, and times and additional interventions as appropriate, e.g., mixing EDTA with a local anesthetic).

   RATIONALE: (Specify action of the particular drug here: calcium disodium succinate [EDTA] and succimer or British antilewisite [BAL]).

8. Monitor lead levels and toxic side effects of chelation therapy (specify for drug, e.g., hematological, renal, and hepatic indicators).

   RATIONALE: Lead levels may increase at first as lead moves out of tissues into blood. (Specify toxic side effects of drug.)

9. Ensure adequate daily fluid intake and output during drug therapy (specify amount for child).

   RATIONALE: Chelating agents are excreted by the kidneys.

10. Provide verbal and written information to family on how to eliminate lead to make the home safe: professional cleaning, eliminate peeling paint, do not allow child to chew on painted surfaces, wipe down painted surfaces with a wet cloth, wet-mop floors rather than vacuuming, and do not store food in opened cans (specify others as indicated).

    RATIONALE: Vacuuming may spread lead dust around rather than remove it.

11. Teach parents to identify if pottery or ceramics in the home are intended to be used for food or liquids or are for ornamental use only.

    RATIONALE: The family may be unaware of the risk of lead leaching out of pottery designed for decoration only.

12. Instruct family to drink or mix infant formula with water from the cold tap only.

    RATIONALE: Lead from the pipes dissolves more easily in hot water than in cold.

13. Instruct family member to teach child not to eat paint chips or dirt and to wash his or her hands and face before eating or drinking.

    RATIONALE: Helps prevent ingestion of environmental lead.

(continued)

Nursing Care Plan The Child at Risk for Lead Poisoning (continued)

14. Notify appropriate agencies (specify, e.g., public health department) about child's environmental exposure and collaborate with other entities to improve environmental safety for all children.

    RATIONALE: Lead exposure is a community problem that should be addressed as a health issue.

15. Refer family for assistance from local lead abatement program (specify) or social service organizations as appropriate.

    RATIONALE: Poor families are often the victims of lead exposure in urban housing. The nurse acts as a patient advocate ensuring the environment is made safe for habitation.

Table 21-16 Erikson's Developmental Tasks and What May Happen During Hospitalization

Age	Developmental Task	What May Happen During Hospitalization	The Nurse Can
Infant	Trust vs. mistrust	Separation anxiety Stranger anxiety Disruption in normal routine	Encourage consistency among caregivers. Encourage the parents to stay with the infant. Encourage bonding. Allow the infant's home routine whenever possible. Comfort the infant; rock, hold, cuddle, swaddle. Encourage parents to bring familiar toys/blanket from home. Communicate with parents.
Toddler	Autonomy vs. shame and doubt	Regression Separation anxiety Negative behavior Increase in tantrums Fearfulness	Encourage consistency among caregivers. Encourage the parents to stay with the toddler. Allow the child's home routine whenever possible. Encourage parents to bring familiar toys/blanket from home. Communicate with parents. Allow the child to participate in care whenever possible. Use therapeutic play. Offer praise. Ensure a safe environment.
Preschool	Initiative vs. guilt	Play restrictions Fearfulness Thinks that hospitalization is a punishment	Encourage consistency among caregivers. Encourage the parents to stay with the preschool child. Allow the child's home routine whenever possible. Encourage parents to bring familiar toys from home. Communicate with parents. Allow the child to participate in care whenever possible. Use therapeutic play. Offer praise. Ensure a safe environment. Encourage use of the playroom and interaction with other children. Explain a procedure, treatment, and/or surgery in simple terms. Allow the child to ask questions. Encourage realistic choices whenever possible.
School Age	Industry vs. inferiority	Play restrictions Questions identity Increased need for attention Regression Fear of bodily mutilation	Encourage the parents to stay with the school-age child. Allow the child's home routine whenever possible. Encourage parents to bring familiar toys from home. Communicate with parents. Allow the child to participate in care whenever possible. Use therapeutic play. Offer praise. Ensure a safe environment. Encourage use of the playroom and interaction with other children. Explain a procedure, treatment, and/or surgery in simple terms. Allow the child to ask questions. Encourage realistic choices whenever possible. Encourage the child to verbalize feelings. Alleviate fears about changes in body image. Respect the child's privacy.

Table 21-16	Erikson's Developmental Tasks and What May Happen During Hospitalization (continued)		
Age	**Developmental Task**	**What May Happen During Hospitalization**	**The Nurse Can**
Adolescent	Identity vs. role confusion	Concerns about body image Separation from peers Loss of independence Decrease in socialization	Encourage visits or contact from peers. Explain a procedure, treatment, and/or surgery in understandable terms. Be honest. Allow the teen to ask questions. Encourage realistic choices whenever possible. Encourage the teen to verbalize feelings. Alleviate fears about changes in body image. Respect the teen's privacy. Encourage parent's involvement in care. Recognize the teen's tendency to reject authority.

The nurse can also use creativity in helping the child to gain control over the environment by encouraging the child to bring something from home to familiarize the room and make it personal. They might also encourage the child to draw a picture or design that can be hung up in the hospital room or give him a choice to watch a movie or select a game that he would like to play.

THERAPEUTIC PLAY

Therapeutic play, otherwise known as play therapy or medical play, has been shown to help to ease the stress of hospitalization and provide children with a means for dealing with their concerns and feelings.

 Nursing Insight—Therapeutic play

Therapeutic play is the use of play as therapy to help children who have had or will have a stressful experience. Therapeutic play may decrease the child's fear and anxiety. It may also help to correct misconceptions the child has about being in the hospital. There are two types of play techniques: directed and non-directed. Directed therapeutic play is guided by an adult who facilitates the play, including determination of the goals. In non-directed therapeutic play, the child is in control of the activity, although an adult may select the materials. Both types of play allow the child to demonstrate his or her emotions regarding the hospitalized experience.

Often, a child life therapist may be available to assist with therapeutic play and offer age-appropriate toys or distraction such as music or games. Therapeutic play also may help the child to cope with, and master, stressful experiences (Fig. 21-11). Pediatric nurses are encouraged to incorporate the use of therapeutic play in their everyday care of the child. By using play techniques and activities in all settings, including the emergency and outpatient departments, children benefit even if it means only that they are able to watch other children at play.

Therapeutic play can be used to prepare a child who requires an injection. The nurse or child life therapist encourages the child to play with equipment such as a needleless syringe filled with water, a doll, and an alcohol prep pad. After the injection, the nurse can then provide a bandage and a sticker for a reward. Another example is an

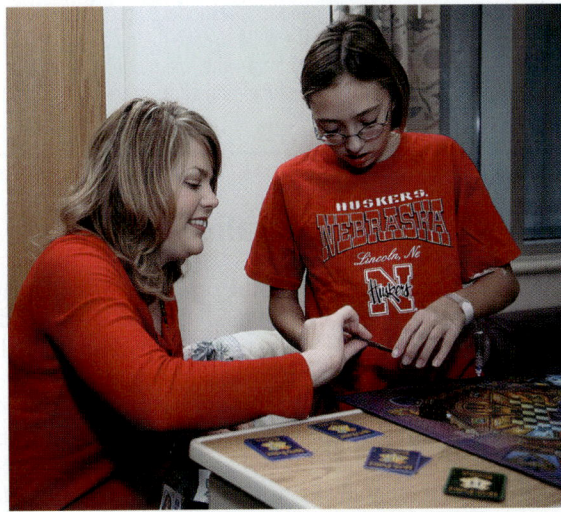

Figure 21-11 Child life specialist playing with child.

older child simulating the medical procedure (administering IV antibiotics), a therapeutic play technique that the nurse uses to discuss the process with the child, clarifying what is going to happen, and allowing him to release anxiety and decrease fears of the imminent situation.

GUIDED IMAGERY

Another way to help a child cope with the stress of hospitalization is the use of guided imagery. Guided imagery:

- Is a relaxation technique that aims to ease stress and to promote a sense of peace and harmony during a difficult time.
- Can be used by persons of all ages.
- Encompasses the power of the mind to help heal the body while maintaining a relaxed state including all of the body's senses (touch, smell, sound, sight, and vision) (Tusek, 2012).

ROLE MODELING

Role modeling is another way to decrease the stress of hospitalization and refers to a process by which the child learns certain behaviors by observing the behavior of others. Role modeling can help to decrease fears and anxieties as well as teach coping skills. Role models can be the people who are involved in the child's life, such as parents, grandparents, siblings, or teachers. Role models can also come from videotapes, movies, or even peers. Role models who are similar in age, sex, race, and attitudes are more likely to be imitated as well as models who have a caring demeanor (Watson, 2012). For example, a child might view a video about another child and her experience preparing for hospitalization and surgery. Viewing how the child in the video prepares for surgery may help the child who is facing surgery to find ways to cope with the anxiety and stress of the procedure.

Critical Nursing Action The Nurse Role Models for the Child

The pediatric nurse says "I am going to give you medicine that will help you get better." The nurse may need to role model by pretending to drink the medicine, encouraging the child to take the medicine. The child may be still somewhat hesitant after the role modeling but may eventually drink the medicine. The nurse then offers praise and allows the child to select a colorful sticker.

Parents With a Hospitalized Child

Parents with a hospitalized child often need to debrief and tell their story about the events that led to their child's hospitalization. Nursing assessment of parental needs, knowledge, concerns, expectations, and coping abilities is imperative to direct nursing actions that ease parental role stress. Parental stressors include sights and sounds of the hospital, changes in the child's behavior or appearance, changes in the parental role, unknown outcome, financial concerns, guilt or anger over the situation, and frustration about the function of the entire family (Fig. 21-12).

Seeking parental advice about the best way to approach their child, acknowledging parental need for involvement, and anticipating stressful events are integral to appropriately caring for the child in a family-centered manner. The communication between the pediatric nurse and family members must be genuine, and the plan of care must include resources available in the hospital as well as the community.

 Nursing Insight—Nursing interventions to help parents cope with the child's hospitalization

- Before admission, if possible, visit the hospital to see where the child will be staying.
- Encourage constant and open communication with the health-care team.
- Encourage visitation of parents, friends, and family members. The number of visitors may be limited depending on the child's condition.
- Perform ongoing assessment to ensure that the nurse fully understands any changes in the plan of care for the child.
- Observe for the need for crisis intervention, should the child's condition deteriorate or change.
- Encourage the parents to participate in the child's care, while being supportive of the child and family.

"What to say"—*Developing a plan of care*

Admission to the hospital is a critical period for both the child and parents. The nurse can ease the experience by including the parents in the plan of care. The nurse can request information from the parents about the child's personal routine as well as the child's perception of hospitalization.

- What are your child's daily routines related to eating, elimination, sleeping, bathing, and play?
- Who are the important people in your child's life?
- Does your child have a favorite toy or attachment object?
- Has your child had previous hospitalizations?
- What has your child been told about hospitalization?
- Does your child have any fears that the staff should know about?
- Have there been any recent changes or problems in your child's life?
- How does your child usually react to pain or when frightened?

The nurse must recognize the parent's concerns, including possible guilt, fear, or other anxieties about the child's hospitalization. The pediatric nurse plans care ensuring the promotion of trust by the child and parents through prompt attention to the child's needs. The nurse provides opportunities for the child and family to participate in care and by including parental preferences and home schedules so that care is provided in a familiar and consistent manner. The nurse can also provide positive reinforcement for the parents that may help alleviate some stress. Finally, the nurse ensures an ongoing evaluation of the plan of care is necessary to make needed adaptations and modifications.

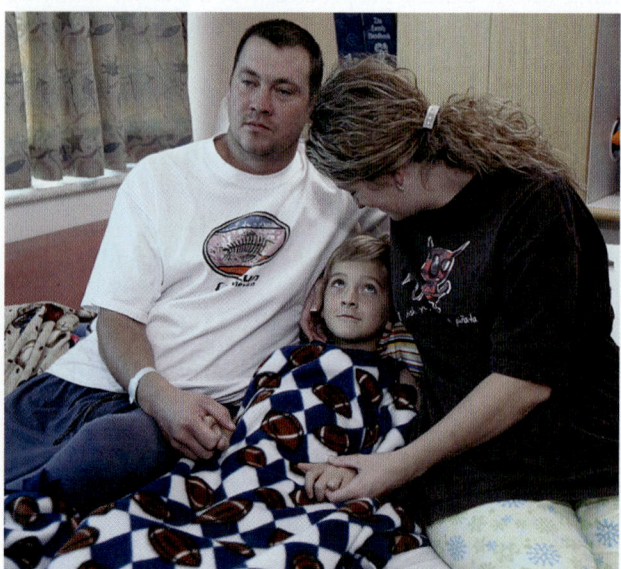

Figure 21-12 Parents at the bedside of a child in the hospital.

Nursing Insight—Effects of a hospitalized child on parents

Parenting an ill child can be stressful and demanding on both the child and the parent. During the period of illness, the child can begin to recover, become gradually sicker, or suddenly begin to exhibit behaviors that give the parents cause for great concern. Symptoms such as withdrawal, lack of activity, or irritability in performing basic functions may be a signal that the child's condition is worsening. During these times, continued parenting of a hospitalized child has many dimensions, such as interpreting the child's behaviors, teaching the child new skills or how to perform basic functions again, helping a child understand the words and language of health-care providers, and offering support during frightening experiences. Hospitalization has been demonstrated to be equally stressful for the parent as for the child. Parents may describe themselves as feeling incapable because of their loss of control over the situation and their inability to be able to protect their child. Some observed behaviors of parents include anxiety, denial and withdrawal, guilt, and fear (including concerns by the parents that they may have had a causal effect on their child's illness). There are ways that the nurse can help parents cope with the stressful situation during a child's hospitalization.

The pediatric nurse has a critical role in assisting parents in adapting to the child's hospitalization. The plan of care for the hospitalized child begins with the admission process when the pediatric nurse includes the parents in a conversation about important information about the child while at the same time offering support. The planning stage, with parental involvement, includes setting goals and objectives that are used to evaluate overall care. The plan of care also includes home routines, preferences, developmental needs, and identification of special needs.

Holistic Nursing Care for the Child

The child who requires general care in the health-care setting may be admitted for testing or treatment of an illness or disease. Holistic care measures include bathing, feeding, rest and safety measures, medication administration, infection control, and fever-reducing measures. Parents may wish to provide much of the care their child needs in regard to bathing and feeding. These measures are comforting to the child and parent and reduce anxiety in both. The nurse is responsible for these activities in addition to the child's safety. The nurse also provides emotional and spiritual support as needed.

 Nursing Care Plan The Hospitalized Child

Nursing Diagnosis: Anxiety related to unfamiliar environment and procedures

Measurable Short-Term Goal: The child will experience decreased feelings of apprehension and anxiety.

Measurable Long-Term Goal: The child will not experience avoidable anxiety during hospitalization.

NOC Outcomes:
  Anxiety Level (1211) Severity of manifested apprehension, tension, or uneasiness arising from an unidentifiable source
  Anxiety Self-Control (1402) Personal actions to eliminate or reduce feelings of apprehension, tension, or uneasiness arising from an unidentifiable source

NIC Interventions:
  Anxiety Reduction (5820)
  Security Enhancement (5380)
  Calming Technique (5880)

Nursing Interventions:

1. Approach the child and parent(s) in a calm and reassuring manner, providing teaching and anticipatory guidance as appropriate.
   RATIONALE: Feelings of anxiety or apprehension in the caregiver are easily transmitted to the patient and family. Knowledge reduces fear of the unknown.

2. Encourage the family to stay overnight, bring the child's favorite toys or security objects, and maintain routines as appropriate.
   RATIONALE: Familiarity enhances the child's feeling of safety in a strange environment.

3. Provide a pacifier for an infant or rock, hold, or comfort an older child as needed.
   RATIONALE: Comfort measures will vary by age, culture, and individual preference.

4. Perform any invasive or painful procedures in a place other than the patient's room. Allow a family member to be present during procedures if desired.
   RATIONALE: The patient's room should become and remain a safe place where the child is able to relax. Family presence is reassuring for the child.

5. Encourage the family, and the child, if age-appropriate, to participate in care activities such as bathing, feeding, medication administration, or help with dressing changes.
   RATIONALE: Reduces unnecessary anxiety from having a stranger perform tasks. An older child will feel less anxiety if allowed some control over how things are done.

Global Health Case Study Anna

Anna is the 13-year-old daughter of Mexican immigrants. Anna attends a local middle school and is capable of communicating in English. Her parents, Dolores and Benito, are migrant farm workers and understand very little English. They live in a community that is primarily Spanish speaking and adhere to their cultural practices. Because the family is in this country illegally, they are extremely fearful of entering the health-care system. For the last month, Anna has experienced bloody diarrhea and abdominal pain daily, resulting in a 10-lb weight loss. Dolores sought help from the **Curandero** (a man in the Mexican culture who practices folk medicine) in their community, but Anna is becoming weak and fatigued and is no longer able to attend school. The family reluctantly takes Anna to the hospital.

critical thinking questions

1. What resources would you enlist to help you establish a relationship with this family?

2. How would these resources impact the delivery of care?

◆ See Suggested Answers to Global Health Case Studies on Davis*Plus*.

BATHING

Family home practices and preferences for bathing are assessed on admission of the child. Bathing of infants can be accomplished at the bedside using a portable tub. For infants younger than 6 months or for those who have head lag, the nurse supports the head and neck with one hand while using the other hand to wash. If a tub bath is contraindicated, a bed bath can be given. Precautions are taken to control the water temperature so that it does not exceed 100°F (37.8°C) and to quickly cover areas of the body after washing. The parent may welcome the respite from caring for the child or may wish to continue bathing the child in the hospital. Toddlers and preschoolers may enjoy a bath in a larger tub. Although they can wash some body areas without supervision, most children need reminders or prompting to wash. Never leave a child alone while tub bathing. Older children may be able to shower and groom themselves with little assistance. Privacy is valued by the older child. A child who is feeling ill or who has tubes, drains, or dressings may be unable to ambulate to the bathroom for washing or to immerse herself in water. A sponge bath is appropriate in this case.

Shampooing hair during the bath may be part of daily care for children. Again, the nurse can assess family preferences and practices. Shampoo basins can be used at the bedside to wash hair. African American children or those with braiding or dreadlocks require special care. Braids are left in place for several weeks and care of the hair and scalp is individualized for each child. Parents may be asked for instructions in hair care.

The nurse can use bath time to observe parent–child interaction and to assess the child. Language skills and social skills can also be assessed during the bath. The skin is assessed for lesions, rashes, turgor, color, and circulatory integrity. Muscle tone is easily assessed along with adequate respiratory status. This can also be a time for the child to become acquainted with the nurse as a caring, supportive person.

Critical Nursing Action Key Actions in Caring for the Child Confined to Bed

The child confined to bed is at risk for skin breakdown. The nurse should do the following:

- Keep the skin clean and dry.
- Assess nutritional status for adequate protein.
- Use the draw sheet for position changes.
- Assess skin for irritated areas.
- Assess for pressure ulcers by looking for the "red flush" (the first sign of tissue compromise and ischemia).

FEEDING

Basic knowledge of nutritional requirements is essential when working with children. Formula-fed infants require no more than 24 to 32 ounces of iron-fortified formula daily. For infants who have a gastrointestinal disturbance, pulmonary failure, or are in congestive heart failure, it may be difficult to ingest the required amount of calories without tiring, and gavage (nasogastric or gastric) feedings may be necessary.

For the older child, assess preferences by taking a diet history and asking about routines at mealtimes. Children are often prescribed an "as tolerated" diet, and they are able to select foods that appeal to them. It is best to gently encourage the intake of wholesome and nutritious foods and snacks. Foods ingested are also important for their fluid content (e.g., gelatin and ice pops). Parents can be encouraged to bring in favorite foods from home. Cultural preferences may make a difference in whether or not a child eats while hospitalized.

Nursing Insight—*Encouraging adequate food and fluid intake*

- Offer small portions at frequent intervals.
- Host a "tea party" using medicine cups filled with the child's favorite drink.
- Make food into fun shapes (trace a smile face with a spread on a sandwich; use a cookie cutter to make different shapes for sandwiches).
- Offer incentives of more time doing a favored activity.
- Offer two choices ("Would you like to use a straw or a colored cup for your drink?"). This allows autonomy.

REST

Hospitalization disrupts a child's normal daily routine as well as his sleep pattern. The pediatric nurse can assess normal sleep patterns, including both nighttime hours of sleep and daytime naps. Most pediatric units allow parents to "sleep-in." This provides both the parent and child with comfort and creates an environment with decreased levels of unfamiliarity and anxiety. The nurse understands that children up to the age of 5 may take an afternoon nap. If the child's condition allows, uninterrupted naptimes should be included in the plan of care.

SAFETY MEASURES

Safety measures instituted on a pediatric unit are based on the developmental level of each child to protect him from harm. Safety measures include keeping toxic materials out of reach, identifying children with name bands, and knowing the whereabouts of children on the unit. The nurse must also provide a safe environment in the hospital room and in the transport of children from their room to other departments in the hospital.

The nurse uses two patient identifiers by checking the name band before any treatment or medication is administered. Name bands can be removed by the child easily, or they may inadvertently fall off, leaving the nurse with no means to verify a child's identity. If a child is found without a name band, the child's name must be verified and a new name band applied to an extremity. The nurse cannot depend on all children to correctly identify themselves. Younger children may answer to any name or may not answer at all. When a name band is not on a child's extremity, medications or treatments are administered only after a parent or nurse has identified the child and the name band has been replaced.

The nurse is responsible for keeping children safe on the pediatric unit and knowing the whereabouts of the child on the unit. Many pediatric units have alarms and restricted access at stairways, elevators, and the entrance to the unit. The nurse can review with the older child the places she is allowed to go and the activities she can engage in while a patient on the unit. Limits must be set and enforced. To prevent child abduction, pediatric personnel must be vigilant about visitors.

Provide a safe environment. In the child's room, safety features are used on high chairs and strollers, and beds are kept in the locked position with the height of the bed in the lowest position. Crib side rails are elevated when the child is in the bed. Bubble tops may be needed to prevent a child from climbing over the rails. Check the room for any small articles that may be left behind in a bed, such as syringe covers and alcohol wipes. All items must be removed from the bed because they present a choking hazard.

Safety concerns regarding the transport of children are based on their developmental level. Infants can be carried short distances in the room or on the unit. For longer transports to other areas of the hospital, bassinets, cribs, strollers, wheelchairs, or special vehicles are used (e.g., wagon with raised sides). The wagon can be painted in bright colors, and some have plastic bubble tops in the shape of small automobiles. Children enjoy this type of transport. It is important to check that restraint devices like a seat belt in a stroller are securely fastened and that the child is not left unattended during transport.

MEDICATION ADMINISTRATION

When administering medications to a child, the pediatric nurse needs to consider the developmental level of the child. Each age group responds differently to the medication administration process. Administering medications to an infant may require additional assistance to minimize movement, particularly with injections. The infant needs immediate cuddling and comfort after medication administration. A toddler may consider medications to be a punishment. Often a child will close his mouth tightly and refuse to take the medication. To minimize this, it might be useful to let the toddler administer medications to a doll or play with a needleless syringe if receiving oral liquid medications. To increase compliance of the toddler, it may be necessary for the nurse to allow a parent to administer the oral medications. Offer immediate praise after medication administration. The preschooler will want to take charge of the medication and, in some instances, this may be appropriate. Oral medications in a cup or syringe can be self-administered by the preschooler under direct and close supervision. The preschooler will benefit from some therapeutic play before medication administration. Offer simple explanations about the medications and why the child is receiving them. The school-age child is far more cooperative but still fears a loss of control and pain and will negotiate with almost every intervention. It is best to allow a school-age child as much control and choice as possible and to offer praise and rewards after medication administration. The school-age child will want to know what the medications are for and how they work. Offer age-appropriate explanations and allow time for questions. The adolescent is far more advanced in his thought processes, will be able to understand more detailed explanations, and will want a greater role in his health-care decisions. The nurse must be patient and allow time for more complex questions from the adolescent.

If the child takes medications at home, ask the parent how the child prefers to take the medications (e.g., whole with juice, crushed in applesauce, one at a time, etc.). If the child does not normally take medications at home but will be going home with routine medication, the nurse may need to help the parent decide on ways to administer the medications to the child.

Educating the child and parent about the medications being administered is important. Explanations about the purpose of the medication, why the child is taking it, dosing, frequency, and common side effects must be discussed at the fifth grade level for parents and at an age-appropriate level for the child. It is prudent to provide written information on all medications and may be necessary to create a chart of the daily medications, doses, and the times they are to be administered. Additional information to provide to the child and parents about any medications includes drug-drug interactions, duration of the medication therapy, what to do if a dose is missed or vomited, and how to store the medications. Assess the level of understanding of the parents and child prior to discharge. For any medication that requires psychomotor skills to administer, such as eye drops, gastrostomy tube administration, or subcutaneous injections, provide ample time for demonstration and return demonstration by the parents and child, if appropriate. Provide time for the parents to ask questions and express concerns they may have about the medications.

Nurses are well educated in the six rights of medication administration:

- Right patient
- Right medication
- Right dose
- Right route
- Right time
- Right documentation

In addition to these rights, two additional key aspects of medication administration have been identified and need to be followed:

- Right reason (the ordered medication is appropriate for the patient)

- Right response (did the administered medication have the desired effect)?

Despite the education of health-care professionals in the rights of safe administration of medications, medication errors in the health-care setting continue to be a leading cause of adverse medical events.

With advancing technology, there are many electronic systems available to help decrease the number of medication errors. Barcode Medication Administration (BCMA) technology allows for the scanning of a barcode on each medication and IV fluid. The scan verifies that the medication scanned is the medication that was ordered. In addition to verifying the right medication, BCMA technology verifies some of the aforementioned rights of administration—right dose, right time, and right route. In many institutions, the patient identification band is also barcoded and scanned with each medication pass to verify that the medications are being given to the right patient. BCMA does not replace the need for the nurse to follow the rights of administration. It is simply an electronic double-check of the first five rights of administration. The nurse must attend to all eight rights regardless of the presence of the BCMA system. Lynas (2010) reports that with the implementation of bar-coded medications, the medication error rate has been reduced by 70% to 80% in those institutions that use BCMA technology. While medication errors are still likely to occur in the best of circumstances, barcode medication administration provides the opportunity for improved outcomes in the safe delivery of medications (Fowler, Sohler & Zarillo, 2009) (Fig. 21-13).

INFECTION CONTROL MEASURES

Each year, health-care–associated infections affect 2 million people and account for 80,000 deaths from those infections. The majority of these infections are because of poor hand hygiene practices of health-care professionals. According to the Institute for Healthcare Improvement (IHI) (2011), compliance by health-care workers with mandated hand hygiene guidelines is less than 50%. To improve compliance and decrease health-care-associated infections, the IHI has published a "How-to" guide for health-care facilities with implementation and compliance guidelines for improving hand hygiene practices. The IHI publications "How-to Guide: Improving Hand Hygiene" and the "Hand Hygiene Monitoring Tool" can be found at http://www.ihi.org/knowledge/Pages/Tools/HandHygieneMonitoringTool.aspx. Best practices for hand hygiene are (IHI, 2011):

- Use of waterless, alcohol-based hand rubs is the preferred method for hand hygiene. These rubs are highly bactericidal and rapidly kill many of the viruses and fungi that cause health-care–associated infections. Rubs used in sufficient amounts to cover the hands and fingers are rubbed into the skin for a minimum of 15 seconds and until the hands are dry.
- Hand washing with water and soap in sufficient amounts to cover all surfaces of the hands and fingers with 15 seconds of rubbing that causes friction is to be done when hands are visibly soiled, after using the restroom, before eating, and after caring for patients with diarrhea. Single-use towels are used to dry the hands and turn off the faucet to avoid recontamination.
- Gloves are to be used properly in direct-care situations in which there is a high risk of exposure to bodily fluids. Gloves must be changed when moving from a contaminated area to a clean site on the same patient. Once gloves are removed, the health-care worker must perform hand hygiene immediately.

Transmission of infection requires three essential elements: an offending microorganism, a susceptible host, and a method of transmission to infect the host. The offending microorganism can be brought into the hospital setting with the ill child or can be part of the new environment. Main routes of transmission include contact, droplet, airborne, common vehicle, and vector borne. Fundamental isolation precautions include hand washing and gloving, the appropriate placement of a patient in isolation appropriate for disease process, and the use of barrier gear to protect the caregiver and prevent further transmission of infection.

The Healthcare Infection Control Practices Advisory Committee (HICPAC, 2011) lists two tiers of isolation precautions. The first tier is "standard precautions" that integrate the features of universal precautions designed to reduce the risk of transmission of blood-borne pathogens. The second tier is "transmission-based precautions" that are intended to prevent the transmission of pathogens from those with infectious diseases. Transmission-based precautions include airborne, droplet, and contact precautions (HICPAC, 2011). When caring for children in a hospitalized setting, the specific guidelines from the Centers for Disease Control and Prevention should be followed for procedures related to the type of precautions implemented for the patient (HICPAC, 2011).

The experience of isolation for a child can be perceived in negative ways. In the preschool years, when magical thinking is the predominant manner of processing information, the child may perceive the situation as a punishment for some previous thought or action. Once the precautions are in place and the child and family are coping with the restrictions, the child may need diversional activities. Child life specialists can assist in the selection of age-appropriate games and toys. Once a toy is

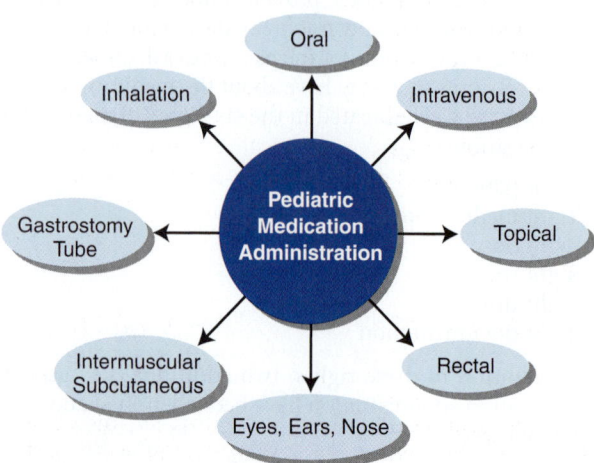

Figure 21-13 Routes of medication administration.

brought into a precaution room, it must be cleaned before other children can play with the toy. Visitors need not be restricted from the room, but they do need specific instructions on how to protect themselves and the patient. Isolation guidelines are placed on the door with step-by-step instructions on what is required prior to entering the room. Hand washing before and after leaving the room is essential.

FEVER-REDUCING MEASURES

Fever (a temperature greater than 100.4°F [38.0°C]) accompanies many childhood illnesses. A fever is a natural and beneficial response to the invasion of an offending organism and can help "kill" the virus or bacteria. If a child with a fever is very uncomfortable and irritable, his fever may be treated with antipyretics (e.g., acetaminophen and nonsteroidal anti-inflammatory drugs [NSAIDs]) or by using environmental measures. Antipyretics work to lower the set point at the thermoregulatory center in the hypothalamus.

focus on safety

Aspirin (salicylates)

Aspirin (salicylates) is not given because of the correlation between the use of aspirin and the development of Reye syndrome in children with viral infections.

Acetaminophen (Children's Tylenol) is available in suppository, liquid, and capsule form. It can be given every 4 to 6 hours with no more than five doses in a 24-hour period; there is little risk of hepatic toxicity. Ibuprofen (Children's Advil), a common NSAID, is given to children as a fever-reducing measure. This drug is given every 6 hours and may be an advantage when rest is crucial or when administering medications to the child is a challenging task. Dyspepsia and nausea are common side effects of ibuprofen. The medication, taken as a chewable tablet, caplet, or liquid, can be given with food or after meals if gastrointestinal (GI) upset occurs. The child should be monitored for GI bleeding. Dosing for ibuprofen is dependent on the temperature of the child.

Medication: Dosage Recommendations for Acetaminophen (Children's Tylenol)

(a-seet-a-**min**-oh-fen)

Age	Dosage
Neonates (0–4 weeks)	10–15 mg/kg/dose every 6–8 hours
Infants (1–12 months)	10–15 mg/kg/dose every 4–6 hours, as needed, not to exceed 5 doses in 24 hours
Children (1–12 years)	10–15 mg/kg/dose every 4–6 hours, as needed, not to exceed 5 doses in 24 hours
Children (>12 years)	325–650 mg every 4–6 hours, as needed, not to exceed 4 grams in 24 hours

Source: Vallerand, A. H., & Sanoski, C. A. (2014). *Davis's drug guide for nurses* (14th ed., pp. 112–113). Philadelphia, PA: F.A. Davis.

A fever less than 102.6°F (39.2°C) warrants a dose of 5 mg/kg of body weight. If a child's temperature is greater than 102.6°F (39.2°C), the dose is increased to 10 mg/kg of body weight. The efficacy of antipyretic medication is assessed by retaking the child's temperature 1 hour after administration.

Environmental measures are effective in reducing fevers in children. Cooling measures, such as reducing room temperature, applying cool compresses to the skin, and wearing a light layer of clothing, are effective alone or after the antipyretic is given.

A cooling blanket, which has coils through which a refrigerated solution circulates, may be necessary to control hyperthermia. The cooling blanket is placed on the bed, covered with a sheet, connected, and set to a temperature of 98.6°F (37°C). The temperature is decreased according to the child's response to cooling. Rectal temperature must be monitored every 15 minutes while the child is on the blanket, and the child must be assessed for shivering. Cooling blankets are only used in circumstances warranting an immediate drop of a very high fever.

EMOTIONAL AND SPIRITUAL SUPPORT

Parents may be in need of emotional and spiritual support when a child is hospitalized. It is important for the nurse to be "in the moment" with parents and other family members. Conveying a caring attitude and listening closely to what the parent is really saying is important in making a connection with them. The relationship that the nurse creates with parents and family members is basic to healing and is an expression of spirituality (Dossey, Keegan, Guzzetta, & Kolkmeier, 2009).

The nurse helps family members by listening to their concerns, clarifying any misconceptions, and helping the family develop coping strategies to decrease stress and optimize functioning. Coping resources include using both the strength from within and the support from resources in the community.

 Collaboration in Caring—*Spiritual care*

The parents and child may find comfort in talking with a priest, monk, chaplain, deacon, rabbi, imam, or other trusted person with religious ties. Spiritual care may come from a particular faith community that has shared beliefs and values. At times when parents ask, "why is this happening to my child?" it may be beneficial for the nurse to arrange a meeting with people from their faith community to discuss the parents' concerns and issues.

Preparing Children for Procedures

EXPLAINING PROCEDURES

As a child grows and develops cognitively, his understanding of his experiences changes as well as his response to the events. To an adolescent, a venipuncture may be an annoyance, but to a toddler, it may be a frightening experience that is stressful not only to the child but to the parent as well. Developmental characteristics dictate how to approach the child and what to say to the child. What the nurse conveys to the patient and the parents can diminish the anxiety and fearfulness associated with common procedures.

Critical Nursing Action Preparing an Infant for a Procedure

- Describe the procedure to the parents, explaining what will happen and how long it will take. Encourage the parent to stop you at any point if there is a question.
- Remind parents that infants often cry for reasons other than discomfort but be honest about any discomfort the infant may experience with the procedure.
- Identify what restraints may be used and give an explanation as to why they are needed.
- Allow parents to decide whether they would like to be present for the procedure. Parents may prefer to leave the room and return immediately following the procedure to comfort their child.

Critical Nursing Action Preparing a Toddler for a Procedure

- Describe the procedure to the parents, explaining what will happen and how long it will take.
- Use play to demonstrate the procedure to the toddler; encourage him to demonstrate or practice with a doll or teddy bear.
- Use simple, concrete language to describe the procedure and how it might feel to the toddler. Limit preparation to 5 to 10 minutes because of the short attention span of the toddler.
- Identify what restraints may be used and explain why they are needed.
- Allow parents to decide whether they would like to be present for the procedure. Parents may prefer to leave the room and return immediately after the procedure to comfort their child. Allow the parents to stroke their child or speak soothingly to their child if they remain in the room.

Critical Nursing Action Preparing a Preschooler for a Procedure

Explain the procedure in terminology the child can understand. Begin preparation immediately prior to the procedure so the child will not worry for hours or days. Use play to demonstrate the procedure to the child; encourage her to demonstrate or practice with a doll or teddy bear.

Set limits for the child so she is aware of expectations. For example, tell her she can yell and scream as much as she wants but must hold very still. Give legitimate choices to the child whenever possible. Allow parents to decide whether they would like to be present for the procedure. Parents may prefer to leave the room and return immediately after the procedure to comfort their child. Allow the parents to stroke their child or speak soothingly to their child if they remain in the room. Use distraction techniques such as deep breathing, singing, or squeezing a parent's or nurse's hand.

Critical Nursing Action Preparing a School-Age Child for a Procedure

Explain the procedure in terminology that the child can understand. Children in this stage of development have a good concept of time, so preparation can begin in advance of the procedure. For the younger school-age child, use play to demonstrate the procedure and if possible have the child demonstrate on and practice positioning with a doll or teddy bear. Allow the child to touch and explore equipment to be used in the procedure and involve the child in simple tasks during the procedure when possible. Set limits for the child so she is aware of expectations. For example, tell her she can yell and scream as much as she wants but must hold very still. Give legitimate choices to the child whenever possible. Allow parents and the child to decide together whether parents will be present for the procedure. Some school-age children may be modest about exposing body parts in front of family members. Allow the parents to stroke their child or speak soothingly to their child if they remain in the room. Teach the child techniques such as deep breathing, counting, reciting a silly rhyme, or anything else that might help distract and relax the child during the procedure.

Critical Nursing Action Preparing an Adolescent for a Procedure

Describe the procedure, explaining exactly what will happen and how long it will take.

Encourage the adolescent to stop you at any point if she has a question. Be honest. Describe potential risks and pain associated with the procedure, but don't dwell on it. Allow the adolescent to take as active a role as possible in the procedure. Practicing positioning or demonstrating the equipment prior to the procedure helps give the adolescent a sense of control. Provide a peer video of the procedure if possible. If possible, allow the adolescent to make decisions such as when the procedure should take place. Allow the adolescent the option of having a parent present. Offer tips for distraction such as deep breathing, relaxation, counting, or squeezing an object or parent's hand.

Critical Nursing Action Before, During, and After a Procedure

Before:
1. Think through the procedure in advance and anticipate problems.
2. Gather all equipment and check to make sure it functions properly.
3. Establish trust by getting to know the child first.
4. Through the use of play, allow the child to "perform" the procedure on her doll, teddy bear, or other appropriate surrogate.
5. Offer a coping strategy such as guided imagery or relaxation breathing.
6. Give the child realistic choices.
7. Be sure informed consent is signed.
8. Wash hands.
9. Let the child know that it is "OK" to cry.

During:
1. Whenever possible, schedule all treatments away from the child's bed or "safe area."
2. Expect the child to do well.

3. Talk to the child and ask how he is doing.
4. Keep the child informed as to the progress of the procedure.
5. Use distraction techniques such as pop-up picture books, bubbles, "shutting off the pain switch," or other techniques that have been practiced before the procedure.
6. When appropriate, give the child some control by allowing him to make some of the decisions.
7. Involve the parent to provide comfort to the child, if the parent is able. Sometimes a parent's presence at the procedure may not be beneficial for the child.

After:

1. Praise the child for completing the procedure.
2. Provide an opportunity for the child to verbalize feelings.
3. If the parents were not involved in the procedure, comment on a positive aspect involving the child during the procedure. "Jill was able to help out and keep still when she was asked to do so! She did a great job!"
4. Give a reward (e.g., stickers, small toy, or previously agreed-on reward negotiated with parents).
5. Document the child's response to the procedure and outcomes.

 Nursing Insight—*Distraction*

A distraction kit is a set of materials that help divert the child's attention to a more pleasant experience than the painful experience.

• Appropriate for any age
• Use before, during, and after procedure
• Can also suggest holding someone's hand really tight, say "ouch" really loud, count to 10 or count backwards, sing a song, or pretend to be somewhere else

 Nursing Insight—*The environment*

• Use designated treatment rooms when possible.
• Child's inpatient room should be kept as a "safe area" whenever possible.
• Optimal lighting for a procedure should be sufficiently bright and focused on safety but otherwise without glare.

 Nursing Insight—*Preparing the parent*

• Relieve parental anxiety so they can help prepare and reassure the child or youth.
• Provide an explanation of what they will see and hear.
• Use simple explanations that are developmentally appropriate to explain how, why, where, and when.

Source: Stollery Children's Hospital, Edmonton, Alberta, Canada.

❝What to say❞—*Using developmentally appropriate words*

For children with beginning language skills, use simple terms that are familiar to the child, such as "go potty," "owie," and "boo-boo." For the concrete thinker who takes what is said literally, do not use words that may frighten the child (e.g., "*dye* in your vein," "*shot* in the arm," "*cut* out the tonsils," and "*take* your temperature"). Instead, use "*special medicine* in your vein," "*special medicine* in your arm," "*make* your tonsils *better*," "*check* to see if your temperature *is working*." For all children, be honest and they will learn to trust you.

INFORMED CONSENT

Informed consent involves providing the patient with the necessary knowledge to make a decision regarding health care. Informed consent implies that the person understands the benefits and risks of treatment or the refusal of treatment. The person must also be legally able to give consent by virtue of his age. In most of the United States and Canadian provinces, the age of legal consent is 18. An exception is made for the adolescent younger than 18 who is married, a parent, self-supporting, or a member of the military (Peoples Law Library of Maryland, 2012). Informed consent can be obtained from these emancipated minors. In some jurisdictions, the age of consent varies for girls aged 14 years and older for contraception advice and gynecological procedures. For most children, the parent or legal guardian is the person who gives consent for their care.

Written informed consent is required before diagnostic procedures, medical treatments, or surgical procedures. It is also required prior to immunizations or any treatment with inherent risks.

 legal alert—**Obtain written consent before a procedure**

Informed consent must be obtained before a procedure is performed. It is the physician's responsibility to explain the procedure and the risks and benefits of treatment. Alternatives to the prescribed treatment also should be discussed. When signed by the emancipated minor or parent, an informed consent is a legal document denoting that the emancipated minor or parent understands the nature of the procedure, risks, and benefits. The nurse serves as a witness to the signature.

 Nursing Diagnoses Potential Nursing Diagnoses for the Child Undergoing Procedures or Surgery

• Anxiety related to the procedure
• Pain related to break in skin integrity

 Where Research and Practice Meet: Informed Consent

For children who are part of a research study, consent needs to be obtained. Assent seeks to obtain the child's agreement to participate in the study and assurance that he understands all the material presented to him regarding the study (Unguru, Sill, & Kamani, 2010). Depending on the age of the child, the material is presented in terms that the child can comprehend. Assent implies that sufficient education about the project, the process, and the consequences have been explained fully and that the child is sharing in the decision-making process.

- Knowledge deficit related to unfamiliarity of procedure
- Interrupted family process related to demand of surgery or procedure
- Risk for fluid volume deficit related to NPO status, nausea, vomiting, or bleeding

Common Procedures

IV LINES

In the hospital, children may require IV therapy for fluid maintenance or replacement, before diagnostic testing, blood product replacement, medication administration, or preoperatively. IV fluids may be administered through a peripheral line, a central venous access, or a peripherally inserted central catheter.

PERIPHERAL IV LINES

A peripheral line with a normal saline lock is used to keep the vein open for the possibility of future IV therapy, or for the child who requires intermittent medication administration. The tubing is capped at the end with an injection cap that allows for multiple punctures. Once the medication is disconnected from this tubing and the line flushed, the child can ambulate unencumbered by the IV pole and tubing. The hospital's protocol for flushing the peripheral intermittent infusion device is followed. The normal saline lock is secured to prevent accidental dislodgement. For the younger child who has a normal saline lock inserted in the dorsum of the hand, a cover with cling wrap may be necessary to prevent the child from manipulating or pulling out the normal saline lock (Fig. 21-14).

CENTRAL VENOUS ACCESS

Children with a condition necessitating long-term IV access are candidates for central venous access devices. The IV catheter is inserted into a large vein such as the vena cava, subclavian, jugular, or femoral vein. Broviac, Hickman, and Groshong catheters are used for access. These catheters are multilumen and accommodate more than one IV therapy. After insertion, a chest x-ray exam is done to confirm proper positioning of the catheter. With a central venous access device, the child is not subjected to multiple IV "sticks." It is easily accessed for medication and fluid administration as well as blood draws without the pain associated with further needle punctures.

PERIPHERALLY INSERTED CENTRAL CATHETER

The peripherally inserted central catheter line (PICC line) can be left in place for up to 4 months. It is inserted above the antecubital fossa into the median, cephalic, or basilic vein and threaded into the superior vena cava. PICC lines are most often used for long-term antibiotic and analgesic therapy (Fig. 21-15). These lines may also be threaded just to the head of the clavicle. This is considered a midline placement and is often used for antibiotic therapy. The hospital's protocol for PICC line flushing and dressing changes over the insertion site is followed.

VASCULAR ACCESS PORT

A vascular access port is another central venous access device that is implanted under the skin and is used for long-term fluid or medication administration. The Infuse-A-Port or Port-A-Cath is not visible and no dressing is required (Fig. 21-16). Although the child may be restricted from contact sports, he can swim or shower without restrictions. To access this device, the nurse palpates for placement, cleanses the area, and uses the Huber needle to puncture the port's central diaphragm.

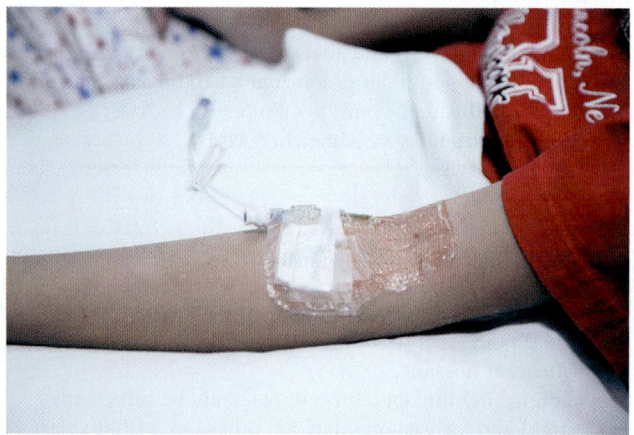

Figure 21-15 PICC line.

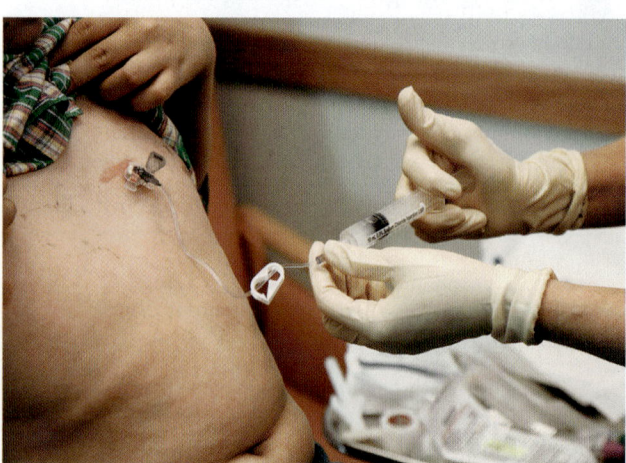

Figure 21-16 Infuse-A-Port.

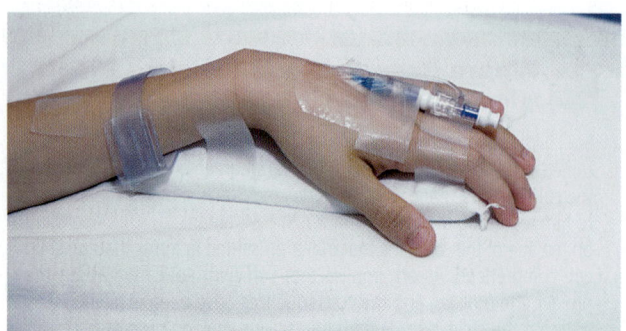

Figure 21-14 Normal saline lock.

focus on safety

Risk of infection

With any procedure in which the skin barrier is compromised, adhere to sterile techniques for dressing changes over IV sites and to monitor for signs and symptoms of infection (change in temperature, erythema, edema, or pain at IV site and tenderness on palpation).

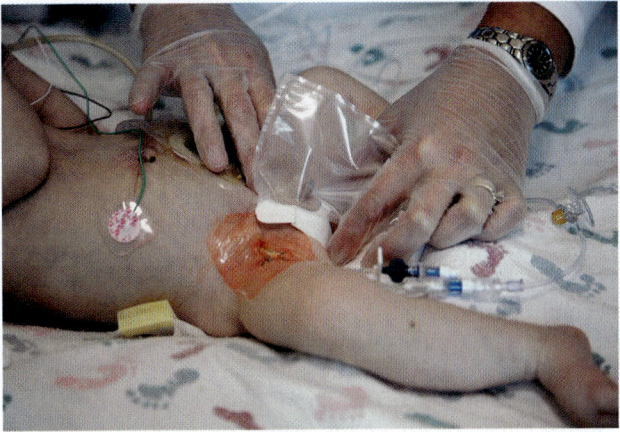

Figure 21-17 Urine collection bag.

MEASURING INTAKE AND OUTPUT

The pediatric nurse carefully assesses the intake and output in children, especially those with vomiting, diarrhea, fever, nasogastric suctioning, draining wounds, and burns; presurgical patients; and children with cardiac, renal, or respiratory illnesses. Table 21-17 describes calculation of daily maintenance fluid requirements. The nurse measures intake for the breastfed infant by recording "breastfed" (or by weighing the infant before and after the feeding and recording the increase in weight as ounces or milliliters consumed) on the intake sheet. For infants with congestive failure or a respiratory illness like bronchiolitis, the nurse also asks about the length of time the feeding took to complete. Expending too much energy in feeding may be deleterious to the child's health. **Gavage** (feeding a patient via a feeding tube passed through the nose into the stomach) feedings may be necessary for the child in congestive heart failure. IV fluids may be required for the child struggling to breathe with a dyspneic respiratory condition.

For the child who wears diapers, the diaper can be weighed before and after use to determine urinary output. Diapers are weighed on a gram scale, and output is determined by subtracting the weight of a dry diaper from the weight of a wet one. Each gram is equal to about 1 milliliter; therefore, the difference is the amount of urine output in milliliters. The method used to measure normal urinary output is 1 to 2 mL/kg per hour.

X-RAY EXAMS

Children require x-ray exams for diagnostic purposes. They are also essential when checking for the placement of a chest tube, central line, or a feeding tube. For the younger child needing an x-ray exam, the nurse may be asked to help position the child for an optimal view. A

lead apron is worn to protect against unnecessary exposure to radiation. Pregnant women should not assist because fetal tissue is especially sensitive to damage by x-rays.

SPECIMEN COLLECTION

Urine Sample Collection

To collect a urine sample, children may require either catheterization or a clean-catch specimen. A catheterized specimen is obtained using sterile technique. Bladder catheterization can be a traumatic experience for both the child and the parents. Distraction techniques can be helpful in decreasing anxiety and fear. A lubricant with 2% lidocaine is used to eliminate the discomfort of catheterization. If a clean-catch specimen is requested, the nurse places a urine collection bag around the perineal area after cleaning the perineum and surrounding skin (Fig. 21-17). The infant is diapered and the bag monitored for urinary output. The urine must be removed from the bag and sent to the lab within 30 minutes of voiding.

Stool Sample Collection

Stool samples are frequently obtained for ova and parasites (O&P), to determine the causative agent for a diarrheal condition, or to check for the presence of occult blood. If the child is toilet-trained, he can use the potty chair or the toilet with a collection hat under the seat. In a non-potty trained child, stool from the diaper is collected. Samples are transferred into a collection cup using tongue blades. O&P samples are sent to the lab as soon as possible. When lab services are not provided 24 hours a day, the sample should be refrigerated as soon as possible.

Blood Sample Collection

Having blood drawn can be a traumatic event. Preparation and support during the procedure alleviates some of the fear and pain associated with venipuncture. Trauma can be alleviated by using distraction techniques with the child prior to the venipuncture. Application of EMLA cream, a topical analgesic containing lidocaine and prilocaine, anesthetizes the skin before any painful procedure. The cream is applied to the site, covered with

Table 21-17	Calculation of Daily Maintenance Fluid Requirements
Child's Weight	**Daily Maintenance Fluid Requirement**
0–10 kg	100 mL/kilogram of body weight
11–20 kg	1,000 mL + 50 mL/kilogram for each kg >10
>20 kg	1,500 mL + 20 mL/kilogram for each kg >20

Example:
A child weighs 48 kg. For the first 20 kg the child needs 1,500 mL. For the next 28 kg, the child needs 20 mL/kg. So, 1,500 mL + (28 kg × 20 mL) = 1,500 mL + 560 mL = 2,060 mL/day

a transparent dressing for 1 hour, and removed prior to the venipuncture.

Throat Culture Collection

A rapid strep test or a throat culture can be used to diagnose group A streptococci as the cause of sore throat. If the rapid strep test is positive, an antibiotic is prescribed. If the rapid strep test is negative, a culture to grow the bacteria is done to confirm the results. A throat culture is more accurate than the rapid strep test, but it may take several days to obtain results. Most children do not tolerate throat cultures very well. For younger children it may be helpful to place the child on the parent's lap facing forward and have the parent place one arm across the child's chest and over his arms, and one hand on the child's forehead. The child is now sufficiently restrained to obtain a specimen safely. The nurse uses a tongue blade to push the tongue downward and swabs the posterior pharynx with two sterile cotton-tipped applicators (Fig. 21-18).

 focus on safety

Epiglottitis

One caveat exists regarding throat cultures. Throat examinations and cultures should not be performed on a child who has suddenly developed a high fever; is drooling; has severe sore throat, hoarseness, stridor; and sits in a tripod position. This history indicates the possibility of epiglottitis. Eliciting the gag reflex, as happens with a throat culture, in this child may cause the inflamed epiglottis to completely obstruct the airway.

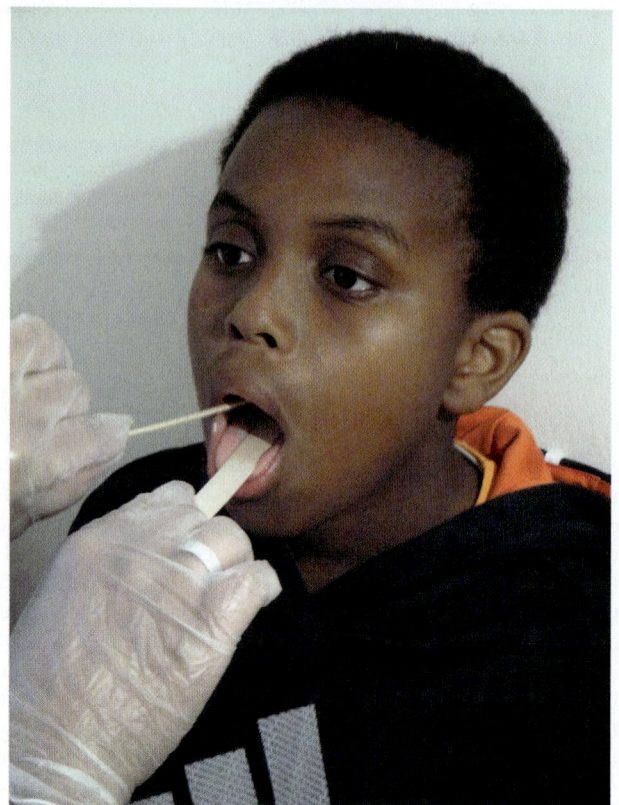

Figure 21-18 Throat culture.

Cerebrospinal Fluid Collection

A lumbar puncture (LP) is a necessary procedure to rule out sepsis or meningitis. It can also be scheduled as a procedure for children undergoing treatment for cancer. The nurse prepares the child for an LP by telling the family and the child the reason for the procedure and teaching distraction methods to the child. Practicing the position required for the procedure can be helpful with the older child. An hour before the LP, EMLA cream can be applied to the skin at the designated site. This makes the procedure less painful. With the lumbar puncture, a needle is inserted into the subarachnoid space at the level of L4 or L5 to withdraw cerebrospinal fluid (CSF) for analysis. An infant is seated upright with the head bent

forward. An older child must lie on his side with the head flexed, hips and knees flexed, and the back arched while being firmly held to make sure he does not move. CSF samples are sent for culture, glucose, red blood cells, and protein.

After the LP, vital signs are taken. The child is encouraged to lay flat for 1 hour and drink fluids. The child may complain of a headache or pain at the site of the LP. Frequent neurological assessment is performed to note changes in status. Complications such as nerve trauma, infection, bleeding, or pressure effects are rare.

Enteral Tube Feedings

When a child is unable to take adequate nutrition by mouth, an alternate feeding method is used to maintain and promote growth in the child. The type of feeding method selected depends on the child's medical condition. Children can be nourished through an oro- or nasogastric feeding tube or a gastrostomy tube. Feedings may be administered as a bolus or a continuous infusion. Bolus feedings are given at relatively the same rate as an oral feeding would normally be taken and are the preferred method to deliver formula in children who cannot tolerate oral feedings. Formula given as a continuous infusion is placed on a feeding pump and regulated to be administered over a predetermined number of hours. Continuous infusions are often preferred in children with serious cardiac defects to decrease the workload of the heart while providing enteral nutrition. To allow underweight infants or children to gain weight, a continuous feeding may be given during hours of sleep to boost calorie intake without interfering with a normal daily

Labs: Analysis of Cerebrospinal Fluid

	Pressure (mm Hg)	Protein (mg/dL)	RBCs	Glucose (mg/dL)	WBCs
Infant	<200	20–170	None	34–119	0–30
Child	<200	5–40	None	60–80	0–20

RBCs = Red blood cells, WBCs = White blood cells.
Source: Data from Van Leeuwen, A. M., Poelhuis-Leth, D., & Bladh, M. (2013). *Davis's comprehensive handbook of laboratory and diagnostic tests with nursing implications* (5th ed.). Philadelphia, PA: F.A. Davis.

feeding/eating schedule (see Procedure 21-1: Inserting an Oro- or Nasogastric Tube Procedure).

OROGASTRIC AND NASOGASTRIC FEEDING TUBES. For newborn infants requiring gavage feedings (a feeding done using a tube that is passed through the nares and into the stomach; the food is in liquid form, usually at room temperature), the orogastric route is preferred because newborns are obligate nose breathers. The tube is inserted and then removed at the end of the bolus feed. If the tube is to be left in place, the nasogastric route should be considered. Nasogastric tube feedings are preferred over total parenteral nutrition because they preserve the stomach's mucosa, allow the digestive process to continue, and are cost-effective.

 Nursing Insight—*Psychosocial needs of the infant receiving gavage feedings*

The time taken to administer a gavage feeding can be used in the same way as in a regular feeding. Place the infant comfortably in the mother's arms with the head elevated. Provide the

---

 Procedure 21-1 Inserting an Oro- or Nasogastric Tube

Purpose

To maintain optimum nutrition using a feeding tube that is passed through the mouth or nares and into the stomach

Equipment

- Oro- or nasogastric tube
- Tap water or a water-soluble lubricant
- Syringe
- pH indicator paper

Steps

1. Wash hands and don gloves.
2. Determine tube length required by measuring from the nose to the earlobe and to the midway point between the end of the xiphoid process and the umbilicus (Fig. 21-19).

   RATIONALE: *Proper measurement determines the distance that the catheter is inserted.*

3. Note the measurement by finding the manufacturer's black mark on the proximal end of the tube near the nares.
4. Lubricate the tube with tap water or a water-soluble lubricant. Follow manufacturer guidelines.

   RATIONALE: *Lubrication eases catheter insertion.*

5. Using the dominant hand, gently direct the tube toward the back of the throat or, if using the nose, toward the occiput.

6. Aspirate stomach contents.

   RATIONALE: *Indicates proper placement.*

7. Check for proper placement using the method following the institution's policy:

   a. Use pH indicator paper for assessment of gastric aspirate.

   b. Inject a small amount of air into the tube while auscultating over the stomach; the nurse should hear a "swoosh" as the air enters the stomach.

   c. Obtain an x-ray film to verify placement. This method is not practical for every feeding, but is often used after initial placement of the oro- or nasogastric feeding tube when used for continuous feeding.

   RATIONALE: *Indicates proper placement.*

 focus on safety

Risks with an oro- or nasogastric tube

There are some risks with an oro- or nasogastric tube. The liquid from the feeding or medication may enter the lungs and possibly cause pneumonia. The feeding tubes may also cause the child discomfort. The tube can also become plugged, causing pain, nausea, or vomiting.

Teach Parents

It is important for parents to understand the purpose of the feeding tube. Enteral tube feedings offer complete nutrition, but children often need additional water flushes to provide for maintenance fluid requirements. Parents must be able to recognize signs that the NG tube is not functioning properly or may be displaced. If the child is discharged home with the NG tube in place, parents need to know how to check placement, administer feedings, secure the NG tube to the child's face, and recognize signs of intolerance to feedings.

Documentation

6/18/10 1300 8f nasogastric tube inserted in left nostril without difficulty. Placement of the tube confirmed. Nasogastric tube secured.

— D. Naccarini, RN

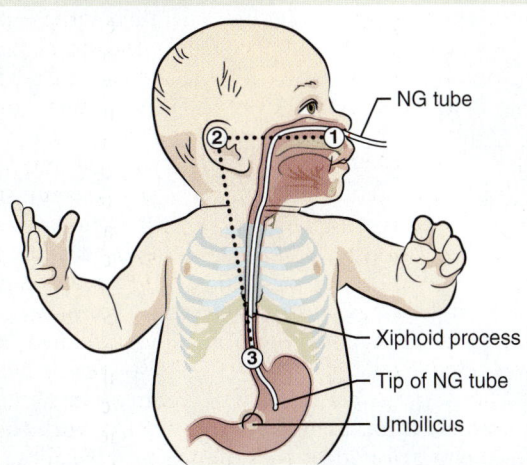

Figure 21-19 Nasogastric tube insertion measurement.

NG tube

Xiphoid process

Tip of NG tube

Umbilicus

infant with a pacifier to help simulate an actual feeding. Non-nutritive sucking has been shown to increase weight gain and decrease crying and to allow for the normal muscular development of the mouth and tongue.

Once placement of the tube is confirmed and the child is in position, the nurse administers a bolus feeding of room-temperature formula via gravity through an appropriately sized syringe attached to the feeding tube. The formula-filled syringe is held less than 12 inches above the infant. When the feeding is complete, the tubing is flushed with tap water to prevent clogging of the lumen, the syringe is removed, and the feeding port capped. To decrease the chance of regurgitation, the infant is burped after the bolus is infused. Follow hospital guidelines for nasogastric gavage feedings. The nurse must remember that the amount of water should be only the amount required to successfully flush the length of tubing; excess water may result in overfeeding.

GASTROSTOMY FEEDING TUBES. When a child requires enteral tube feedings over a longer period of time, such as those with oral feeding aversions or neurological dysfunction, a gastrostomy tube (GT) is an alternative to the nasogastric tube. A GT is inserted through the abdominal wall into the stomach. The GT is secured internally and externally with a variety of bumpers depending on the manufacturer of the GT. Some physicians also secure the GT in place with external sutures for the first 7 to 10 days postoperatively.

After the initial insertion, the GT is left open to gravity drainage for 12 to 24 hours and the wound site observed for signs of infection. Stoma care and assessment are important nursing interventions because of the potential for leakage of gastric secretions onto the periostomal skin. Guidelines for feeding the child through a gastrostomy tube are similar to nasogastric tube feedings. Figure 21-20 shows two of the many types of gastrostomy tubes available.

focus on safety

Gastrostomy tubes

A gastrostomy tube may move into the duodenum and cause an obstruction as it occludes the pyloric sphincter. Mark the tube with indelible ink to make it is easy to observe for migration. The nurse must report any vomiting, abdominal distention, or evidence of bile drainage as aspirate.

Ostomies

An ostomy is a surgical opening from either the small or large bowel to the surface of the abdomen to allow for fecal elimination (Fig. 21-21). An ostomy may be needed for a variety of reasons, including trauma, obstruction, disease, and infection. It may be needed on a temporary basis to allow the bowel sufficient time to heal or permanently when the child's condition does not allow for ostomy reversal.

For infants and toddlers, the parent assumes all responsibility for the care of the ostomy. The nurse assists the parents by clarifying misconceptions, addressing concerns about caring for the child with an ostomy, and providing teaching guidelines regarding ostomy care. It is necessary for the nurse to feel comfortable discussing difficult issues with the child. If the child is unable or unwilling to verbalize his feelings, the nurse may attempt to engage the child through the use of play or art by bringing crayons and paper to the child's room and giving the child time to process the current events in his life. The child may be able to express himself through art or play more readily than through words. A child life specialist may provide additional ways for the child to communicate his "stories" about how the ostomy is affecting his everyday life. Nurses must be aware of community resources and refer the parents and child to appropriate support groups. Through participation in support groups, the parents and child will be able to talk with others who face the same issues and have struggled with similar concerns.

Older children must be encouraged to become independent in the care of their ostomy. A school-aged child needs to learn all aspects of ostomy care, including removal

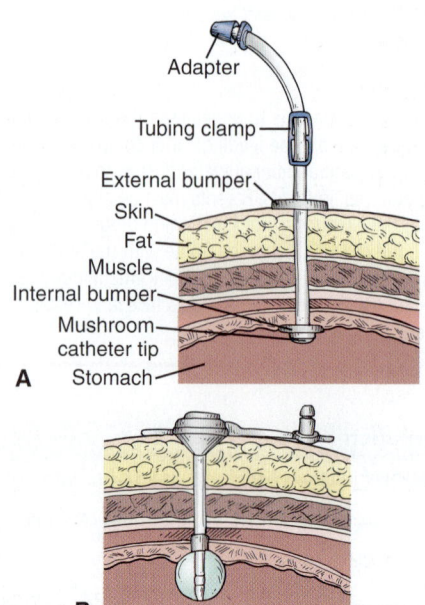

Figure 21-20 Gastrostomy tubes. *A,* PEG. *B,* Mic-Key.

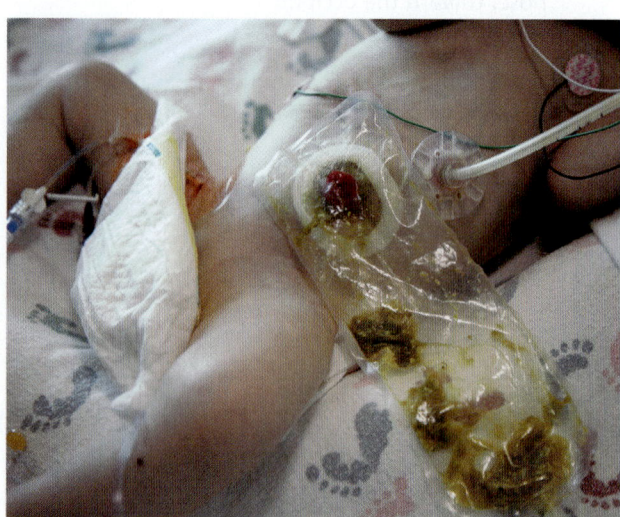

Figure 21-21 Child with an ostomy.

and reapplication of the ostomy appliance and periostomal skin care. The child must be aware of the signs and symptoms of potential complications to report to the school nurse or parents. Nurses and parents must be aware of the special needs of all adolescents (peer group and self-acceptance, sexuality, and depression) and how those needs may be further affected in the presence of an ostomy. When the child is in the school setting, there should be an arrangement made with the school nurse to allow for adequate time and privacy for maintenance of the ostomy and for storage of ostomy supplies.

RESTRAINING THE CHILD

Physical Restraint

Restraining a child may be a necessary intervention to ensure a child's safety during a procedure or to prevent injury to an operative site. Parents as well as the child need to be informed as to why a restraint is necessary. Once the restraint is applied, the child must be checked and documentation made as to the condition of the skin and circulation of the affected extremity. The extremity is checked every 15 minutes for 1 hour after initial application and then every 1 to 2 hours to ensure the child's safety. Follow hospital protocol.

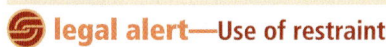 **legal alert**—Use of restraints

The Joint Commission has specific information about caring for the patient with restraint and seclusion. The nurse must assess:

- Signs of injury associated with the application of restraint or seclusion
- Nutrition/hydration
- Circulation and range of motion in the extremities
- Vital signs
- Hygiene and elimination
- Physical and psychological status and comfort
- Readiness for discontinuation of restraint or seclusion

For more information go to http://www.jointcommission.org/

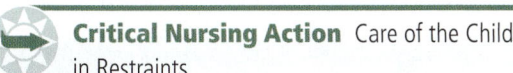 **Critical Nursing Action** Care of the Child in Restraints

1. Remove restraints every 2 hours to assess skin and provide range of motion to the affected extremity.
2. If appropriate, provide supervised time with restraints off to allow the child to engage in activities of daily living (e.g., toileting, feeding, reading a book, watching TV, etc.).
3. Encourage games and activities that promote growth and development.
4. Reapply restraints.
5. Document condition of skin, nursing care given with restraints off, and removal and reapplication of restraints.
6. Teach parents how to remove and reapply restraints.

Common types of restraints used for children are the elbow restraint and the papoose restraint. The elbow restraint prevents the child from flexing the elbow, therefore preventing the child's hands from reaching the head (Fig. 21-22). They prevent the child from pulling out an IV line in a scalp vein or other peripheral line. If the child is recovering from

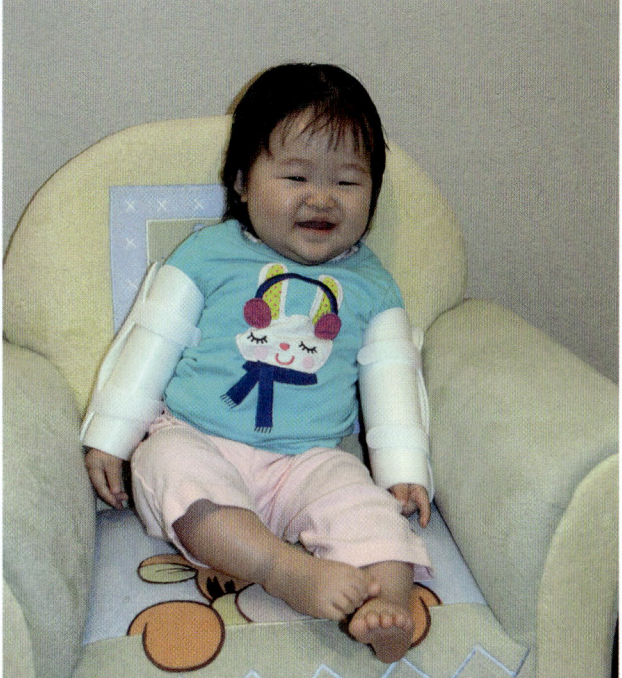

Figure 21-22 Elbow restraint.

cleft lip repair, the elbow restraint prevents the child from touching the incision area. Most children tolerate this type of restraint without problems related to skin integrity or circulatory compromise. Elbow restraints should be removed, one at a time, every hour to allow for exercise of the arm. The child must be supervised when the restraints are removed.

The papoose restraint is much like swaddling an infant. It is a total body restraint. The papoose restraint temporarily immobilizes an infant or small child for an examination or procedure that involves the head, neck, or throat (Fig. 21-23). This is ideal to keep the child safe during venipuncture, throat examination, insertion of a nasogastric tube, or administration of ophthalmic, otic, or oral medications.

Pharmacological Restraint

In addition to physical restraints, pharmacological restraints can be administered to children during diagnostic and therapeutic procedures. Sedation of children is administered to allow the safe completion of a procedure. Chloral hydrate (Aquachloral) is a nonbarbiturate sedative–hypnotic drug commonly used in children to produce sedation. The drug

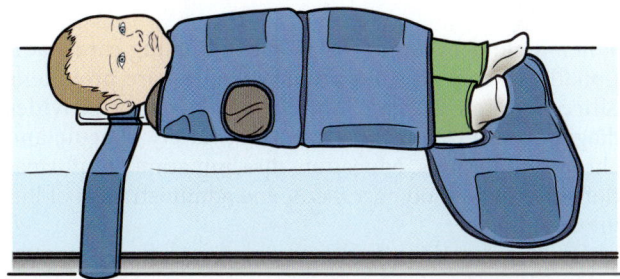

Figure 21-23 Place the baby on his back to sleep.

Medication: Chloral Hydrate (Aquachloral)

(klor-al **hye**-drate)

Points to Remember:

- As a sedative or antianxiolytic, administer 25 mg/kg per day PO divided every 6 to 8 hours up to 500 mg per single dose.
- As a sedative for dental and medical procedures, administer 50 to 75 mg/kg 30 to 60 minutes prior, may repeat if needed. Do not exceed 1 gram total for an infant or 2 grams total for a child.
- As a hypnotic, administer 50 mg/kg PO up to 1 g per single dose, max of 2 grams/day.
- Peak time is 1 hour.
- Assess level of consciousness at time of peak effect. Notify health-care provider if desired sedative effect not reached.
- Duration of action is 4 to 8 hours.
- Dilute chloral hydrate syrup in juice or water to decrease gastric irritation.
- Monitor for dizziness, confusion, excessive sedation, and paradoxical excitation.

Source: Vallerand, A. H., & Sanoski, C. A. (2014). *Davis's drug guide for nurses* (14th ed. pp. 312–314). Philadelphia, PA: F.A. Davis.

decreases anxiety and induces sleep without respiratory depression or suppression of the cough reflex.

 Nursing Diagnoses Potential Nursing Diagnoses for the Child Across Care Settings

Family Processes, altered related to health condition (specify), injury, violence
Growth and Development, altered related to trauma, hospitalization, congenital defects, prolonged pain, and separation from family
Fear related to unfamiliar environment, separation from family
Pain, chronic related to effects of condition (specify)
Poisoning, high risk for related to age-specific environmental hazards
Self-esteem, chronic low related to disfigurement, separation
Sleep Pattern Disturbance related to pain, fear
Social Isolation related to physical handicap, hospitalization, terminal illness

Community Settings

Children have special health-care needs for which families, nurses, and other health-care providers collaborate to create a family-centered plan of care. Today, children are apt to receive the majority of their health care in a community setting. Community settings are on the front line of prevention and early detection, and these settings may be located in neighborhood clinics, schools, shopping malls, or health-care centers.

PRIMARY HEALTH-CARE PROVIDER'S OFFICE OR CLINIC

When a child becomes ill, pediatric nursing care traditionally takes place in a primary health-care provider's office or clinic setting. This medical facility provides diagnosis and treatment related to a variety of acute and chronic conditions, education, dissemination of information, well childhood check-ups, and administration of immunizations.

Health information is also provided, and discussions are held with the family about how to take care of the child at home, providing well childhood check-ups, and administering scheduled immunizations. It is important that caregivers

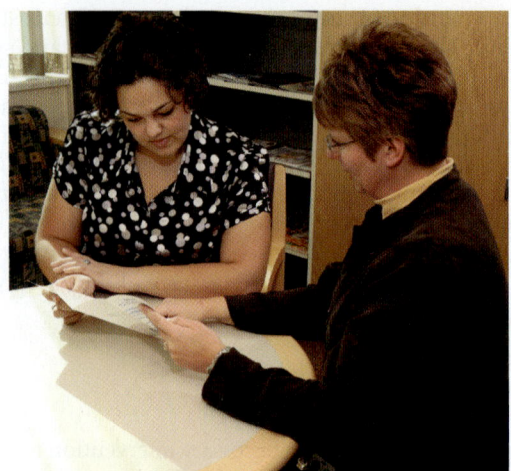

Figure 21-24 The nurse provides community resources to parents.

understand the importance of accessing a primary health-care provider to receive comprehensive care about their child's condition. The pediatric nurse in this setting can recommend additional community resources for the family (Fig. 21-24).

 focus on safety

Keeping children safe in the home

In the home, parents must think like a child thinks. Suggest that parents get down on the floor in their home to see what their child sees (e.g., electrical plugs and outlets, tablecloths ready to be pulled, and hot coffee mugs on the edge of the table). Be sure to store all chemicals and medications out of children's reach. In the hospital, toxic and nontoxic materials should be stored in a locked utility room, on the top shelf of a cabinet, or in another location where children do not have ready access. Utility rooms, kitchens, medication carts, treatment rooms, and supply rooms are locked, denying access to children. Play areas should be locked unless the child is accompanied by an adult.

 **Family Teaching Guidelines...**
Teaching Tips for Families

HOW TO: The nurse can tell the family to bring a list of questions or concerns to discuss when visiting the primary care physician's office.

ESSENTIAL INFORMATION:

- Bring a list of any allergies that the child has along with medications the child is currently taking.
- Be ready to share information as to how the child is growing and changing. Keep track of the child's developmental progress.
- Inquire about resources including community organizations that may provide assistance.
- Ask about how to receive care after normal business hours or emergency care.
- Request to meet the health team members who will be working with the child (a nurse, a referral coordinator, or a medical assistant).

focus on safety

Prevention is key to child safety

Infant Safety

- The home needs to have a smoke and carbon monoxide detector and fire extinguisher.
- The car seat is placed in a backward-facing position in the backseat of the vehicle.
- Crib safety: the distance between slats of railings less than 2 3/8 inches to prevent head entrapment or strangulation, no sharp edges, mattress snug, bumper pads are suggested.
- Furniture paint should be nontoxic and positioned to avoid cords, windows, curtains, blinds, outlets, and lamps.
- Bottles are warmed slowly in hot water, and the microwave is never used to warm a bottle.
- Keep hot liquids and foods away from the baby.
- Never attach pacifier with clip to infant's clothes or around neck.
- Keep one hand on infant when changing the infant's diaper.
- Never leave the baby alone on a high surface.
- Do not let infant sleep in a playpen.
- Never leave baby unattended in high chair, stroller, or swings. Walkers are not recommended.
- Make sure the infant's toys have no removable small parts that can present choking hazards.
- The bath water must be below 120°F. Test the water before the baby's bath. Keep one hand on infant at all times in bathtub.

Toddler Safety

- Prevent burns by keeping items like boiling pots, curling irons, and other hot items out of the toddler's reach. Turn pot handles in on stove.
- Prevent choking by maintaining an environment that is free of any small toys or objects that a toddler could swallow.
- Prevent poisoning by keeping all toxic chemicals locked in drawers or on the top shelves of cabinets.
- Prevent drowning by keeping toilet seat lids down and bathtubs drained completely when not in use. Never leave a child alone in any depth of water.

Pre-School Safety

- Teach the child about stranger danger.
- Fire safety includes teaching stop, drop, and roll and how to exit the home in case of a fire.
- Survey the playground for sharp objects and other unsafe objects.
- Teach the child to wear a helmet when riding bikes.
- Teach the parents about safe boundaries.

School Age

- Keep car doors locked.
- Use the buddy system when walking home from school.
- Teach crossing the street safely.
- Teach about safe touch.
- Keep toxic chemicals locked up and out of the child's reach.
- Keep the Poison Control Center number handy.
- Ride in backseat of car.
- Teach hand washing.

Adolescent

- Teach behaviors that contribute to unintentional injuries and violence including:

  Tobacco use
  Alcohol and other illicit drug use
  Sexual risk behaviors
  Unhealthy dietary behaviors
  Physical inactivity
  Lack of wearing seat belts
  Firearm safety

Across Care Settings: Clinics

In a community, there can be one general care clinic or many types of specialty clinics:

- **Allergy & Asthma Clinic:** A clinic for children that provides comprehensive services for diagnosis and treatment of allergy and asthmatic conditions
- **Audiological Clinic:** A clinic for children where they are assessed for auditory conditions, may receive newborn hearing screenings, obtain treatment for otitis media, or receive hearing aids
- **Cardiology Clinic:** A clinic for children that provides comprehensive services for diagnosis and treatment of congenital and acquired heart conditions
- **Dermatology Clinic:** A comprehensive clinic for the evaluation of children with conditions related to acute, chronic, or genetic integumentary conditions
- **Diabetes Clinic:** A consultation and management clinic for children who are diagnosed and are living with diabetes
- **Eating Disorders Clinic:** A consultation clinic employed by physicians, psychologists, dietitians, and social workers that is specifically designed for children with eating disorders, such as anorexia nervosa or bulimia
- **Endocrinology Clinic:** A clinic for children that provides comprehensive services for diagnosis and treatment of endocrine and metabolic conditions
- **Gastroenterology—Nutrition Clinic:** A clinic for children that provides comprehensive services for diagnosis and treatment of gastrointestinal, nutritional, and liver conditions
- **Genetic Clinic:** A clinic for children that provides comprehensive services for diagnosis and treatment of inborn errors of metabolism and biochemical genetic conditions along with genetic counseling of patients and prenatal testing
- **Immunology Clinic:** A clinic for children that provides comprehensive services for diagnosis and treatment of children with unusual infections, primary immune deficiencies, or complement deficiencies
- **Infectious Disease Clinic:** A clinic for children that provides comprehensive services for diagnosis and treatment of acute infections or chronic infections
- **Neurology Clinic:** A clinic for children with neurological conditions such as spina bifida, cerebral palsy, or autism who require comprehensive care and treatment
- **Oncology Clinic:** A clinic for children that provides comprehensive services for diagnosis and treatment of cancer
- **Ophthalmology Clinic:** A clinic for children that provides comprehensive services for diagnosis and treatment of ophthalmological conditions
- **Orthopedics:** A clinic for children that provides comprehensive services for diagnosis and treatment of acute and chronic musculoskeletal and bone conditions
- **Pulmonary/Cystic Fibrosis Clinic:** A clinic for children that provides comprehensive services for diagnosis and treatment for acute and chronic respiratory conditions

- **Rheumatology Clinic:** A clinic for children that provides comprehensive services for diagnosis and treatment of arthritis, lupus, and inflammatory conditions
- **Urology Clinic:** A clinic for children that provides comprehensive services for diagnosis and treatment of acute, chronic, and congenital genitourinary conditions

The pediatric patient may also receive health-care services in other community settings. These settings include:

Community Centers: A community-based center where the pediatric nurse provides health screening and education, emphasizing health promotion and disease prevention

Preventative Medicine Center: A community-based center that provides a comprehensive menu of pediatric testing, diagnosis, and treatment related to acute and chronic conditions

Home Health Care: Health-care services provided by nurses and other health-care professionals in the child's home

Medical Home: An ongoing source of health care providing primary care services that is both ongoing and comprehensive

 Nursing Insight—*Medical home*

A medical home provides comprehensive primary care services on an ongoing basis, in a manner that encourages a positive relationship with the child, family, and the health-care team. The child lives in the facility because of complex care needs. The concept of a medical home has gained attention, particularly in the care of children who have special medical needs, are homeless, or who do not have health insurance (Bachrach et al., 2011). The care is provided in a manner that is family-centered, coordinated, culturally sensitive, and accessible. Quality of life can be improved for all children, especially those with special needs, with the collaboration of families, insurers, employers, government, medical educators, and other components of the health-care system, through the care provided in a medical home.

 Critical Nursing Action Outcomes of a Medical Home and Coordinated Care

Children with special needs receive coordinated ongoing comprehensive care within a medical home based on these outcomes:

- Families of children with special health-care needs will have adequate private and/or public insurance to pay for the services needed.
- Children will be screened early and continuously for special health-care needs and will have increased wellness.
- Services for children with special health-care needs will be organized in a manner that fosters trust, considers the family's cultural and religious beliefs, and builds support for the child and family.
- Families of children with special needs will partner in decision making at all levels and will be satisfied with the services they receive.
- All youth with special needs will receive the services necessary to make appropriate transitions to adult health care, work, and independence.

Families will have increased satisfaction with their health care.
(American Academy of Pediatrics, 2008)

 Nursing Insight—*Benefits of a medical home*

- A child regularly sees the same primary care physician and staff.
- There is coordination of care for the child.
- There is an open exchange of information in an honest and respectful manner.
- There is support for finding resources and information related to all stages of growth and development and medical conditions.
- The family is connected to information and family support organizations.
- The medical home partnership promotes health and quality of life as the child grows and develops.

Mobile Health-Care Unit: A portable van that visits neighborhoods, schools, and other community locations where children can obtain screening, diagnosis, and treatment related to a variety of medical conditions, receive immunizations, and receive well childhood check-ups or basic care.

Rehabilitation Service: Services that can be provided in a community-based center or hospital where children can receive occupational, physical, audiology, and/or speech therapy.

School Setting: Schools offer basic nursing care for minor acute conditions, disease management, and teaching about health promotion and disease prevention, as well as play a role in advocacy, screening, and counseling services.

State Health Program: Each state works with its federal and local partners to help children remain healthy and safe. The programs and services help prevent illness and injury, promote healthy places to live and work, provide education to help people make good health decisions, and ensure that states are prepared for emergencies or natural disasters (National Center for Injury Prevention and Control, 2012).

The Department of Health and Human Services: The United States government's principal agency for protecting the health of all Americans and providing essential human services, especially for those who are least able to help themselves (U.S. Department of Health and Human Services Health Resources and Services Administration, Maternal and Child Health Bureau, 2012).

Specialty Camps: Specialty camps are a recreational, educational, and supportive resource where children can play, learn how to care for and cope with their condition, and meet other children who share the same medical condition (e.g., Asthma Camp, Arthritis Camp, Diabetes Camp, and Ventilator Assistive Camp). In specialty camps, activities are planned that help children alleviate stress, interact with their peers, achieve mastery over planned activities, and provide a diversion from the challenges of coping with their illness or condition.

Churches, Synagogues, Mosques: Faith community health centers integrate care of the spirit with care of physical body and mind. Nurses who practice in a faith-based health center provide spiritual comfort and counseling in keeping with the religious beliefs of the center. Faith communities offer a wide variety of health-related services, including health promotion education, disease prevention, immunizations, and referrals to appropriate resources.

Faith Community Nursing is recognized as a nursing specialty by the American Nurses Association (ANA). This specialty is governed by the individual state Nurse Practice Act, the ANA Scope and Standards for Registered Nurses, and the ANA Scope and Standards for Faith Community Nurses (International Parish Nurse Resource Center [IPNRC], 2012).

 Nursing Insight—Maternal and child health bureau

This U.S. Department of Health and Human Services Web site offers information about equal access for all to quality health care in a supportive, culturally competent, family and community setting (U.S. Department of Health and Human Services Health Resources and Services Administration, Maternal and Child Health Bureau, 2012).

After a child has received the needed health care, parents may wonder how to continue to care for their child and his or her special needs. Families must be given information about follow-up care especially related to rehabilitation. Follow-up care can help ensure that the child returns to normal functioning, learns to adapt to his or her condition, or reaches the highest, most realistic level of health.

CARE IN THE SCHOOL SETTING

Care in school settings is provided by nurses who specialize in the prevention of illness, help children with special health-care needs, and assist in the early identification of health concerns for children. The purpose of the National Association of School Nurses is to advance the delivery of professional school health services to promote optimal health and learning in students. School nursing is a specialty practice whose members help children maintain good health practices, along with academic success. The school nurse's role is to facilitate normal development, promote health and safety, and intervene with actual and potential health problems. The school nurse also provides case management services and collaborates with other professionals to maintain the family unit, instill self management skills, and promote self advocacy (National Association of School Nurses, 2012).

The school health nurse also plays a leadership role in the support of a coordinated school health initiative. There are eight potential areas in which the school health nurse may be involved:

- Provide the experience and resources in health education including developing health information and health programs.
- Provide activities and health information, including increasing the awareness and education of staff and faculty of the school, and keep accurate health records.
- Assess the health of students and provide access to health care.
- Counsel and advise staff in the early identification of psychological or social issues.

- Provide health education about nutrition, encourage healthy eating and snacking behaviors, and review and improve offerings of school menus.
- Work with students and physical education teachers to encourage physical activity including students who may have special health-care needs.
- Report and intervene when there are hazardous situations within the school, including crisis intervention.
- Provide leadership and collaborative partnerships with community agencies to meet the health-care needs of children and their families.

 Nursing Insight—School nurses are the link between health and education

- Provide education on health-related topics such as nutrition.
- Assist special needs children with their unique needs.
- Help families' access health care.
- Complete important screenings such as vision, hearing, and scoliosis.
- Offer counseling, primary health-care services, and emergency care.
- Ensure communicable disease control by tracking immunizations and tuberculin skin test.
- Work with teachers in the identification of children at high health risk.
- Supply information for community referral and follow-up.
- Serve as advocates for children through medical case management, child abuse recognition, and crisis intervention and triage.
- Assist in the creation of community-wide disaster plans.
- Use individualized care plans and individualized family service plans.

HEALTH SCREENINGS

Health screening is a way to test or examine children for the presence of a disease, illness, chronic condition, developmental delays, or mental health issue. Health screening plays an important role in the early diagnosis and management of selected illnesses or conditions and the initiation of treatment, which can then prolong and improve lives. Community settings often provide primary care along with health screening and surveillance. **Health surveillance** is the continuous observation related to tracking health conditions and risk behaviors. Nurses, physicians, and other health-care professionals gather ongoing information about disease incidence, demographics of an illness, and implementation of policies that may prevent further spread of diseases.

Children are screened for iron-deficient anemia during well-child care visits. Children with a positive family history for acquired cardiac disease or hypercholesterolemia may be screened for elevated cholesterol levels. High-risk children are screened for tuberculosis.

Iron-Deficiency Anemia Screening

The incidence of iron-deficiency anemia (IDA) has been steadily declining since the 1970s because, in part, of the use of iron-fortified formulas and the decrease in use of whole milk for infants. There are no data available for the prevalence of IDA in children 6 to 12 months of age. However, in children aged 1 to 3 years, iron deficiency remains common at 6.6% to 15%, with 0.9% to 4.4% developing IDA; this accounts for 40% of anemia in children (Baker, Greer, & The Committee on Nutrition, 2010). For this reason, the American Academy of Pediatrics (2013) recommends screening for IDA at 1 year of age by hemoglobin and hematocrit measurement.

Cholesterol Screening

While there are certainly populations of children at risk from hypercholesterolemia, such as children with a family history, recent studies suggest that cholesterol screening in childhood may help to identify those at risk and decrease the development of cardiovascular disease in adulthood (Ritchie, Murphy, Ice, Cottrell, Minor, Elliott, et al., 2010). In 2011, the American Academy of Pediatrics (AAP) made significant changes to their guidelines for cholesterol screening. Based on new recommendations of the National Heart, Lung and Blood Institute (2011), AAP guidelines now call for cholesterol screening at least once between the ages of 9 and 11 years and again between 17 and 21 years (AAP, 2011). A child with evidence of a high total cholesterol (greater than 200 mg/dL) is treated with a weight loss plan and dietary modifications. A weight loss plan is implemented after an assessment by a health-care provider of the dietary habits and activity level of the child and family. For weight loss to be successful, the family must participate together to bring about effective change in the overweight child. Dietary modifications include a decrease in foods with saturated fats (e.g., whole milk and fatty cuts of meat) and an increase in dietary fiber from fruits and vegetables. In some cases it may be necessary for a child to be placed on a lipid-lowering medication.

Tuberculosis Screening

Tuberculosis (TB) screening is recommended for children at high risk; those who are foreign-born; those who travel to or have household visitors from a country with a high prevalence of TB; and those in contact with people who are homeless, incarcerated, infected with HIV, or are IV drug users. Other risk factors include living with a household member who has an active case of TB, a chronic condition such as diabetes or renal failure, or who is immunocompromised. Tuberculin skin testing (TST) for latent TB infection is administered to children who have one or more risk factors associated with TB (CDC, 2010).

 Collaboration in Caring—_The nurse's role in health screening and surveillance_

The nurse has a key role in health screening and surveillance:

- Pay attention to voiced parental concerns.
- Ask questions about the child's growth and development.
- Observe the child's mental, physical, and spiritual state (not just a diagnosed condition).
- Note any risk factors that may be present.
- Document specific observations and findings.
- Provide community resources and make appropriate referrals.
- Track disease incidence and demographics of illnesses.
- Implement policies that may prevent further spread of diseases.
- Initiate follow-up care for any concerns and conditions.

Summary Points

- The nurse becomes acquainted with the norms of pediatric nursing practice in the context of caring for the child across care settings and understands that the nurse's practice must be individualized for the unique needs of the child.

- When examining infants, children, and adolescents, the approach to the assessment will be based on the child's age, developmental and cognitive level, and, when ill, the extent of the illness.

- A culturally competent nurse takes the time to become familiar with the health practices and beliefs of the diverse cultures in the community in which she practices.

- Much like the physical examination, the review of systems is best conducted with a head-to-toe approach, starting with a general question regarding each body system.

- Children react to pain and its management in ways that correspond to their developmental level. Accurate pain assessment depends on the consistent use of an assessment tool familiar to both the child and parent.

- Caring for the child with a disability takes a toll on the entire family. The pediatric nurse must be aware of all available resources within the community to assist the family in the care of the disabled child.

- Currently there are myriad options for the delivery of nursing care ranging from the traditional hospital inpatient environment to the broader community setting. Pediatric nursing care for families is holistic, based on normal growth and development, emphasizing the optimization of preventative health and safety measures yielding positive health outcomes.

- There are several ways to help children and families adapt to the stress of hospitalization. The pediatric nurse can suggest rooming-in to the parents, where they stay in the room both during the day and through the night.

- Holistic care measures include feeding, rest and safety, medication administration safety, infection control, and fever-reducing measures. The nurse also provides emotional and spiritual support as needed. The nurse is also responsible for these activities in addition to the child's safety.

- Explanations of procedures must be given at a developmentally appropriate level, avoiding words that may be unintentionally frightening.

- Community settings are on the front line of prevention and early detection, and these settings may be located in neighborhood clinics, schools, shopping malls, or health-care centers.

Review Questions

Multiple Choice

1. When preparing a 4-year-old child for a procedure, the pediatric nurse must be aware of the child's developmental status. Which nursing action demonstrates awareness of the child's developmental status?
A. Demonstrating the procedure on the child's teddy bear.
B. Providing a peer video of the procedure for the child to view.
C. Explaining the procedure to the child the day before the actual procedure occurs.
D. Discussing the procedure at length with the child.

2. The 10-year-old child is receiving preoperative teaching prior to a tonsillectomy. Which response by the nurse uses a developmentally appropriate explanation of the operation?
A. "Don't worry; the doctor will cut your tonsils out while you are asleep."
B. "The shot that you will receive in your arm will only help the pain a little bit."
C. "Don't worry about the operation; it is really not a big deal."
D. "The doctor will give you special sleeping medicine before she operates."

3. There are many myths regarding children and pain levels. Which statement regarding pain management in pediatrics is true?
A. Children cannot tell where they hurt.
B. The child who is neurologically impaired does not feel pain.
C. Children should not receive narcotics because they will become addicts.
D. The use of special pain scales allows children to better express their level of pain.

4. The pediatric nurse uses the head-to-toe approach when conducting a physical assessment on an infant. Which sequence represents correct technique?
A. Heart rate, urine output, respiratory rate, and presence of bowel sounds
B. Head circumference, lung sounds, presence of bowel sounds, urine output
C. Presence of eye drainage, abdominal pain, lung sounds, and urine output
D. Urine output, skin color, skin turgor, heart rate, and bowel sounds

5. During a well-baby visit, the pediatric nurse initiates teaching related to health promotion and prevention of illness. Which nursing statement is appropriate to include in the teaching session?
A. "Call the pediatrician if the baby has a temperature of 99°F (37.2°C)."
B. "If you smoke, be sure to blow the smoke away from the baby's face."
C. "Call the pediatrician if you notice a change in the baby's activity level or feedings."
D. "We want to watch the baby's weight gain, so feed the baby when she cries."

6. The nurse is caring for a toddler hospitalized after a motor vehicle accident. Based on Erikson's developmental model, which behavior would you anticipate can occur as a result of the hospitalization?
A. Regression to a previous behavior
B. The belief that they are being punished
C. Fear of bodily mutilation
D. Loss of independence

7. What is the nurse's responsibility in educating families about how to care for their child at home after minor surgery?
A. Taking the child's rectal temperature
B. Assessing their child's level of consciousness
C. Teaching about the signs and symptoms of infection
D. Teaching about the signs of poor air exchange

8. A parent in the pediatric clinic states that she has been giving her 1-year-old aspirin (ASA) for his fever. What response by the nurse is best?
A. Ensure the parent knows the normal dose of 10 mg/kg.
B. Teach the parent to only use 5 doses per day.
C. Instruct the parent not to use aspirin on a child.
D. Make sure the parent can take the child's temperature.

9. A child with special needs has moved into the community. Which health-care resource should the school nurse direct the child's family toward?
A. Medical home
B. Pediatric clinic
C. Home health care
D. Community center

10. A nurse is providing anticipatory guidance to the parents of an infant. The nurse explains that, for children of this age, the most common fatal injury is which of the following?
A. Drowning
B. Suffocation
C. Electrocution
D. Heavy metal poisoning

See Answers to End of Chapter Review Questions on Davis*Plus*.

REFERENCES

American Academy of Pediatrics (2003). Measurement of skin fold thickness in childhood. Retrieved from http://pediatrics.aappublications.org/content/42/3/538

American Academy of Pediatrics (AAP). (2005). Recommendations for Preventive Pediatric Health Care (RE9353). Retrieved from http://www.aappolicy.aappublications.org/sub-journals/pediatrics/html

American Academy of Pediatrics. (2008). Retrieved from http://pediatrics.aappublications.org/content/110/1/184.full

American Academy of Pediatrics (AAP). (2011). Physicians recommend all children, ages 9–11, be screened for cholesterol. Retrieved from www.aap.org/en-us/about-the-aap/aap-press-room/Pages/study-supports-universal-Cholesterol-Screening-of-Children.aspx

American College of Obstetricians and Gynecologists (ACOG). (2011). Your first gynecologic visit. Retrieved from http://www.acog.org/For_Patients/faq150.pdf?dmc=1&ts=20120328T1200494902

American Nurses Association (ANA). (2010). *Nursing: Scope and standards of practice*. Washington, DC: Nursesbooks.org

Bachrach, 2011 A., Isakson, E., Seith, D., & Brellochs, C. (2011). *Pediatric medical homes: Laying the foundation of a promising model of care.* National Center for Children in Poverty: Columbia University.

Baker, R., Greer, F. R., & The Committee on Nutrition. (2010). Diagnosis and prevention of iron deficiency and iron-deficiency anemia in infants and young children (0-3 years of age). *Pediatrics, 126*(5), 1040–1050. doi:10.1542/peds.2010-2576

Centers for Disease Control and Prevention (CDC). (2010). Latent tuberculosis infection: A guide for primary health care providers. Retrieved from http://www.cdc.gov/tb/publications/LTBI/diagnosis.htm

Centers for Disease Control and Prevention (CDC). (2012a). Recommended immunization schedule for persons aged 0 through 18 years. Retrieved from http://www.cdc.gov/vaccines/schedules/hcp/imz/child-adolescent.html

Centers for Disease Control and Prevention (CDC). (2012b). Individual growth charts. Retrieved from http://www.cdc.gov/growthcharts/charts.htm

Centers for Disease Control and Prevention (CDC). (2012c). BMI percentile calculator for child and teen. Retrieved from http://apps.nccd.cdc.gov/dnpabmi/

Centers for Disease Control and Prevention (CDC). (2012d). CDC childhood injury report. Retrieved from http://www.cdc.gov/safechild/Child_Injury_Data.html

Centers for Disease Control and Prevention (CDC). (2012e). National poison prevention week, 50th anniversary. *Morbidity and Mortality Weekly Report, 61*(2), 177. Retrieved from http://www.cdc.gov/mmwr/preview/mmwrhtml/mm6110a4.htm?s_cid=mm6110a4_w

Dossey, B. M., Keegan, L., Guzzetta, C. E., & Kolkmeier, L. G. (2009). *Holistic nursing: A handbook for practice* (5th ed.). Sudbury, MA: Jones & Bartlett.

Farrell Pediatrics. (2014). Retrieved from http://www.farrellpediatrics.com/acetaminophen-dosage/Farre

Forum on Child and Family Statistics. (2011). Child injury and mortality. Retrieved from http://www.childstats.gov

Fowler, S., Sohler, P., & Zarillo, D. F. (2009). Bar-code technology for medication administration: Medication errors and nurse satisfaction. *Medsurg Nurse, 18*(2), 103–109.

Frankenburg, W. K., Dobbs, J. B., Archer, P., Shapiro, H., & Bresnick, B. (1992). The Denver II: A major revision and restandardization of the Denver developmental screening test. *Pediatrics, 89*(1), 91–97.

Grant, B., & Colello, S. (2009). Engaging the patient in handoff communication at the bedside. *Nursing, 39*(10), 22–26.

Hay, W. W. Jr., Levin, M. Sondheimer, J., & Deterding, R. (2010). *Current diagnosis & treatment: Pediatrics* (20th ed.). New York, NY: Lange Medical Books/McGraw-Hill.

Healthcare Infection Control Practices Advisory Committee (HICPAC). (2011). Department of Health and Human Service, Centers for Disease Control and Prevention. Retrieved from http://www.cdc.gov/HAI/settings/outpatient/basics-infection-control-plan-2011

Hogan-Quigley, B., Palm, M. L., & Bickley, L. (2011). *Bates' nursing guide to physical examination and history taking.* Philadelphia, PA: Lippincott Williams & Wilkins.

Institute for Healthcare Improvement. (2011). How-to guide: Improving hand hygiene. Retrieved from http://www.ihi.org/knowledge/Pages/Tools/HowtoGuideImprovingHandHygiene.aspx

Institute for Healthcare Improvement. (2012). *SBAR Technique for Communication: A Situation al Briefing Model.* Retrieved from http://www.ihi.org/knowledge/Pages/Tools/SBARTechniqueforCommunication-ASituationalBriefingModel.aspx

International Parish Nurse Resource Center. (2012). Fundamentals of Parish Nursing. Retrieved from www.parishnurses.org/Fundamental-sofpn.aspx

Jarvis, C. (2012). *Physical Examination & Health Assessment.* Canada: Elsevier. The Joint Commission. (2010). Center for Transforming Healthcare's Hand-Off Communications Project. *Joint Commission Online.* Retrieved from http://www.centerfortransforminghealthcare.org/projects/detail.aspx?Project=1

Kundu, A., Tassone, R., Jimenez, N., Seidel, K., Valentine, J., & Pagel, P. S. (2011). Attitudes, patterns of recommendation, and communication of pediatric providers about complementary and alternative medicine in a large metropolitan children's hospital. *Clinical Pediatrics, 50*(2), 153–158.

Leininger, M. (1988). Leininger's theory of nursing: Cultural care diversity and universality. *Nursing Science Quarterly, 1*(4), 152–160.

Lynas, K. (2010). A step forward for medication safety: Stakeholders agree to a common standard for barcoding pharmaceuticals. *Canadian Pharmacists Journal, 143*(2), 62.

Morbidity Mortality Weekly and Report. (2012). Retrieved from http://www.cdc.gov/mmwr/

National Association of School Nurses. (2012). Retrieved from http://www.nasn.org/

National Center for Complementary and Alternative Medicine. (2011). What is complementary and alternative medicine? Retrieved from http://www.nccam.nih.gov/health/whatiscam

National Center for Injury Prevention and Control. (2012). Retrieved from http://www.cdc.gov/ncipc/cmprfact.htm

National Heart, Lung and Blood Institute. (2011). Expert panel on integrated guidelines for cardiovascular health and risk reduction in children and adolescents: Summary report. Retrieved from http://www.nhlbi.nih.gov/guidelines/cvd_ped

National Library of Medicine. (2011). Acetaminophen overdose. Retrieved from http://www.nlm.nih.gov/medlineplus/ency/article/002598.htm

Peoples Law Library of Maryland. (2012). Emancipation of a minor. Retrieved from http://www.peoples-law.org/children/emancipation/emancipationhome.htm

Pizzolongo, P. J., & Hunter, A. (2011). I am safe and secure: Promoting resilience in young children. *Young Children,* (March 2011), 67–69.

Purnell, L. D. (2009). *Guide to culturally competent health care* (2nd ed.). Philadelphia, PA: F.A. Davis.

Ritchie, S. K., Murphy, E. C., Ice, C., Cottrell, L. A., Minor, V., Elliott, E., & Neal, W. (2010). Universal versus targeted blood cholesterol screening among youth: The CARDIAC project. *Pediatrics, 126*(2), 260–265. doi:10.1542/peds.2009-2546

Stollery Children's Hospital, 8440-112 Street, Edmonton, Alberta, Canada.

Tanner, J. M. (1962). *Growth at adolescence* (2nd ed.). Oxford: Blackwell Scientific.

Transcultural Nursing. (2012). Transcultural nursing assessment tool. Retrieved from http://www.culturediversity.org/assmtform.htm

Tusek, D. (2012). What is guided imagery? Retrieved from http://www.guidedimageryinc.com/guided.html

Unguru, Y., Sill, A. M., & Kamani, N. (2010). The experiences of children enrolled in pediatric oncology research: Implications for assent. *Pediatrics, 125*(4), 876–883. doi:10.1542/peds.2008-3429

U.S. Department of Health and Human Services. (2012). Insure kids now! Retrieved from http://www.insurekidsnow.gov/questions.asp#why1

U.S. Department of Health and Human Services Health Resources and Services Administration, Maternal and Child Health Bureau. (2012). Retrieved from http://www.mchb.hrsa.gov

U.S. Preventative Services Task Force (USPTF). (2011). Screening for testicular cancer: Reaffirmation recommendation statement. *Annals of Internal Medicine, 154*, 483–486.

Vallerand, A. H., & Sanoski, C. A. (2014). *Davis's drug guide for nurses* (14th ed.). Philadelphia, PA: F.A. Davis.

Van Leeuwen, A. M., Poelhuis-Leth, D., & Bladh, M. (2013). *Davis's comprehensive handbook of laboratory and diagnostic tests with nursing implications* (5th ed.). Philadelphia, PA: F.A. Davis.

Venes, D. (Ed.). (2013). *Taber's cyclopedic medical dictionary* (22nd ed.). Philadelphia, PA: F.A. Davis.

Ward, S. (2013). *Pediatric nursing care: Best evidence-based practices.* Philadelphia, PA: F.A. Davis.

Ward, S., & Hisley, S. (2009). *Maternal-child nursing care: Optimizing outcomes for mothers, children & families.* Philadelphia, PA: F.A. Davis.

Watson, J. (2012). *Human caring science: A theory of nursing* (2nd ed.). Sudbury, MA: Jones & Bartlett Learning.

Wong, D. L., Hockenberry-Eaton, M., Wilson, D., Winkelstein, M. L., & Schwartz, P., (2009). *Wong's essentials of pediatric nursing* (8th ed.). St. Louis, MO: C.V. Mosby.

CONCEPT MAP

Health Assessment:
- Anthropometric measurements; vital signs; general impression
- Complete physical assessment based on child's race and culture
  - Skin: color; turgor; hair; nails
  - HEENT: shape/symmetry; fontanels; ocular alignment; visual acuity; color blindness; hearing screening; thyroid; lymph glands
  - Chest: shape/symmetry; respiratory effort; breast development
  - Lungs: adventitious sounds; stridor
  - Cardiac: pulses; heart sounds; murmurs; edema
  - Abdomen: contour, umbilicus; inguinal area; bowel sounds; organ palpation
  - GU/Perineal: genitalia; anus; Tanner staging/hair; signs of sexual abuse
  - Musculoskeletal: symmetry of movement; ROM; body alignment; strength
  - Neurological: mental status; motor/sensory functioning; persistence of primary reflexes

Across Care Settings:
- Teach family how to obtain insurance for child
- Promote decreasing exposure to lead in the community

Cultural Diversity:
- To establish therapeutic relationships, avoid stereotyping based on specific race/culture
- Lead is found in some folk medicines
- Be aware of all physical assessment findings that vary by culture

The Child in Pain:
Assessment: → age, developmental level; temperament; type/severity of pain; environmental/psychological factors; cognitive level
- Use pediatric-specific scales: numeric; FLACC; Wong faces; CHEOPS
- Descriptors: mild; moderate; severe; acute; chronic
Management: → pharmacologic, distraction, verbal comforting

Obtaining the Health History:
- Establish relationship with child/family
- Comply with HIPAA regulations
- ID culturally based health practices; use of CAM
- Ask open-ended questions: OLDCAT; SODA
  - Family/social/past medical history
  - Immunizations
  - Developmental level
  - Patterns of daily activities → sleep; nutrition; play; activity; schoolwork
  - Review of body systems

The Child With a Disability:
- Multiple potential causes
- Emotional, developmental, and physical concerns for child and family
- Financial concerns/burden
- May need multiple surgeries/ongoing care
- Family → at risk for caregiver fatigue
- Nursing: help parent/child develop resiliency

Where Research Meets Practice:
- Poor communication among caregivers is a major factor contributing to medical errors

Caring for the Child in the Hospital, the Community, and Across Care Settings

Focus on Safety:
- Use evidence-based handoff communication methods
- Recognize signals of impending respiratory conditions/distress
- To keep children safe in hospital/home: Prevention is key
- Use naloxone to reverse opioid toxicity
- No aspirin for child with Reye's syndrome
- No throat cultures for child with epiglottisis
- G-tubes can migrate; cause pyloric obstruction
- Critical illnesses → complex ongoing care, e.g., shock, sepsis, acute respiratory failure

Hospital-Based Care

Community Settings

Holistic Nursing Care:
- Bathing/shampooing
- Nutrition: feeding; diet hx/routines; home food
- Rest: parents sleeping-in; naps
- Safety: name bands; alarm unit exits; storing toxics; transportation issues
- Medication administration
- Infection control; child in isolation
- Fever reduction

Decreasing Stress of Hospitalization:
- Emotional support of parents → assess needs, knowledge, concerns; include them in plan of care; allow/encourage participation in care
- Therapeutic play
- Guided imagery
- Include home practices/preferences when appropriate

Hospital Procedures:
- Explanation based on developmental level
- Obtain informed consent → give parents information to decide
- Common procedures:
  - IV access; peripheral CVAD; PICC; ports
  - I&O: include breastfeeding; gavage; weighing diapers
  - X-ray exams
  - Enteral feedings: oro-/nasogastric; G-tube

Specimen Collection:
- Stool/urine: depends on potty training
- Blood: address fears and discomfort
- Throat cultures
- LP: positioning for and assessments

- Multidisciplinary approach using a family-centered plan of care
- PCP office/clinic
- Community centers
- Preventative medicine center
- Home health
- Medical home
- Rehab service
- State health programs
- Department of HHS
- Speciality camps
- Mobile health unit
- Faith-based centers
- Schools
- Clinics

What to Say:
- How to use Q-tips correctly
- Use developmentally appropriate words in speaking to child

Critical Nursing Action:
- Notify provider ASAP of adventitious breath sounds
- Teach home care to parents of child having minor surgery
- Techniques for controlling epistaxis
- Care to prevent skin breakdown in immobile child
- Nursing responsibilities pre- and post-procedures on children
- Prepare child for procedures using age-specific strategies to allay fears/anxiety
- Follow skin assessment, removal, and documentation policies when using restraints

Restraining a Child:
- Instruct parents
- Follow assessment and documentation policies and TJC standards
- Types: elbow, papoose, pharmacological

Now Can You:
- Complete a comprehensive health history/health assessment on a child across all care settings
- Discuss all components of holistic, safe, and evidence-based nursing care across the health-care continuum

Nursing Insight:
- Assess family dynamics
- Screening tests require child's cooperation
- Perception and expression of pain r/t multiple factors
- Pain is whatever the child says it is
- Use of therapeutic play decreases fear/anxiety
- Non-nutritive sucking beneficial during gavage
- Increase fluid intake → tea party, colored straws

Caring for the Child With a Psychosocial or Cognitive Condition

True joy, happiness and inner peace come from the giving of ourselves to others.

—Henri Nouwen

LEARNING TARGETS *At the completion of this chapter, the student will be able to:*

◆ Discuss vulnerability and resilience, culture, diversity, health disparities, and barriers to child and adolescent mental health.

◆ Examine the conditions related to various psychological and cognitive conditions.

◆ Explore the risk factors that contribute to various psychological and cognitive conditions.

◆ Prioritize developmentally appropriate and holistic nursing care for various psychological and cognitive conditions.

◆ Demonstrate awareness of issues impacting access and referral to appropriate community resources.

◆ Develop teaching plans and discharge criteria for parents whose children have various psychological and cognitive conditions.

PICO(T) Questions

The intent of evidence-based practice (EBP) is to provide nursing care that integrates the best available evidence. An initial step in EBP is to write a PICO(T) question that effectively guides the research. A PICO(T) question is an acronym that stands for population (P), intervention or issue (I), comparison of interest (C), outcome (O), and timeframe (T). Depending on the question, all or some of the question components are used in the research process. Use these

PICO(T) questions to spark your thinking as you read the chapter.

1. Do (P) children with learning disorders have a (O) higher incidence of (I) depression than (C) children without learning disorders?

2. Is there a (O) screening tool that most accurately identifies (P) children suffering with (I) anxiety disorders?

 Evidence-Based Practice

McMenamy, J., Sheldrick, R. C., & Perrin, E. C. (2011). Early intervention in pediatrics offices for emerging disruptive behavior in toddlers. *Journal of Pediatric Health Care, 25*(2), 77–86.

The purpose of this study was to explore parenting interventions used with families of preschool-aged children experiencing early attention-deficit/hyperactivity disorder (ADHD) and oppositional defiant disorder (ODD) symptoms. The incidence of ADHD and ODD is estimated to be from 3% to 18% of school-aged children. Studies have suggested that symptoms of these disorders may appear in early childhood. One study found that symptoms demonstrated in preschool-aged children will continue through

and are evident in 50% of adolescents. Research has suggested that future diagnoses of ADHD and ODD are often evident by externalizing symptoms during preschool-aged children and increases the risk for conduct disorders before the age of 10. Children with ADHD and ODD are also at a higher risk for disorders demonstrated by internalizing symptoms, such as anxiety and depression. Research also indicates that the parents of children with ADHD and ODD symptoms experience increased stress,

Evidence-Based Practice (continued)

which may lead to negative parenting approaches. Though use of stimulant medication is the first line treatment for school-aged children with ADHD, it is generally not prescribed for preschool-aged children making behavioral treatment the first choice. This type of intervention often includes parent education programs; one such program identified by the authors is "The Incredible Years Program" (IYP). In addition, early screening and counseling are mainstays in providing services for families of children experiencing ADHD and ODD.

Participants in this study included families from two different cities in Massachusetts. One city was located in central Massachusetts and considered small; Boston was the other city included in the study. Participants were selected by responding to screening questionnaires, which parents were asked to complete during scheduled well-child visits. The Infant Toddler Social-Emotional Assessment was used to screen potential participants. Five subscales of the tool were used: Aggression, Compliance, Hyperactivity/Impulsivity, Peer Aggression, and Attention Skills. Eligibility to participate in the study was determined by scoring at or above the 80th percentile on any of the five subscales. This questionnaire was also re-administered at the completion of the intervention and at a 6-month follow-up visit. At one site, 341 (55%) of 629 parents completed the questionnaire. Fifty-nine (17%) were found to have children who met the researchers' criteria for elevated ADHD/ODD symptoms. Of that cohort, 43 families were successfully contacted, and of that group 18 (42%) agreed to join the Parenting Resource and Education Project (PREP), which combined parent education and screening for the purpose of the research. Seven participants from this site had an annual income below $25,000. All mothers but one completed high school, and eight attended college. Thirteen of the children were Caucasian, one was Asian, and four were Hispanic. Eighty families were identified through the second site; 59 (74%) completed the questionnaire, and 17 (28%) met the criteria for inclusion; 10 were successfully contacted of which five enrolled in the PREP program. Four of the families in this group had an annual income below $25,000. Four of the children in this cohort were African American, and one was Caucasian. All of the mothers completed high school, and three completed college. The final total sample size combining both sites included the parents (caregivers) of 23 children.

Data were gathered through the use of multiple screening tools and questionnaires. All of the tools and questionnaires had documented reliability and validity and had been used in previous studies. The Achenbach Child Behavior Checklist is a 118-item tool that was used to assess behavior in three domains: total problems, externalizing, and internalizing. The LIFT Parenting Practices Interview is a 43-item questionnaire used to determine parent domains of discipline (i.e., harsh parenting, inconsistent discipline, appropriate discipline, and positive parenting strategies). The Parenting Stress Index is a 25-item tool used to assess the degree of perceived stress among parents related to parenting roles. The Parent Satisfactions Questionnaire (PSQ) was used to assess parents' satisfaction with the discussion of topics included during the intervention, (i.e., child behavior and development). The Likert-scale questionnaire included 40 items. The Pediatrician Satisfaction Questionnaire (PedSQ) is a 12-item Likert-scale tool used to assess the provider's satisfaction with screening procedures, the value of the information provided by the screening, schedule disruption, and impact of the procedures and parenting program sessions on time and effort.

The PREP intervention involved parent participation in a 10-week parenting education group, which met for 2 hours weekly in the pediatrician's office. The IYP curriculum was used and included strengthening parent skills through play, praise and reward, effective limit setting, and handling misbehavior. Sessions included video-taped vignettes, group discussion, and homework. Sessions were co-led by a doctoral student in clinical psychology and a nurse practitioner.

Mothers' satisfaction as assessed through the PSQ at the end of the project reported an overall satisfaction: 79% (n=15) reported being satisfied or greatly satisfied with the child's progress, 100% reported being satisfied or very satisfied with the program, and 100% noted that they would recommend the program to others. Ninety-four percent (n=18) considered the strategies recommended to change the child behavior as appropriate or very appropriate; 85% (n=16) reported feeling confident or very confident in their ability to manage behavior problems; 94% (n=18) reported that the program was helpful in managing personal and family problems. Mothers reported an improvement in child behavior in six of seven areas (i.e., compliance, attention, a decrease in internalizing behaviors, a decrease in externalizing behaviors, aggression, and activity level). The 6-month follow-up reported continued change with the exception of the attention skill, which dropped to below the significance level. Ten providers responded to the PedSQ. All reported little or no negative impact on their workload, office space, schedule, and time in relation to the project activities. Seven of 10 reported a moderate to significant change among the parents in each group. The researchers concluded that there was an overall improvement in parenting skills and a decrease in parenting stress among the participants as well as a decrease in aggression and an increase in compliant behaviors among the children of the participants. Both parents and providers reported a high level of satisfaction.

1. How is this information useful to clinical nursing practice?

2. Based on these findings, what are implications for further research?

See Suggested Responses for Evidence-Based Practice on Davis*Plus*.

Introduction

This chapter provides a review of the developmental aspects of various psychological and cognitive conditions. The discussion includes an examination of the various psychological and cognitive conditions and developmentally appropriate and holistic nursing care. Information about diagnostic and laboratory testing and medications is given. Teaching plans and discharge criteria for parents whose children have various psychological and cognitive conditions are incorporated.

 Nursing Insight—*Institute of Medicine Consensus Report*

The 2009 Institute of Medicine (IOM) Consensus Report identified mental illness and substance abuse disorders in children and adolescents as a costly concern, economically and psychosocially, not only for the individual and family, but for society as well (Institute of Medicine of the National Academies, 2009). The IOM reports that an increasing number of the psychiatric disorders that affect children and adolescents are preventable through mental health promotion (encouraging mentally healthy families and social environments) as well as prevention (measures that avoid the occurrence of mental illness). Because many of the psychiatric and behavioral disorders present in adulthood have their origins during childhood (*Healthy People 2020,* 2014; IOM, 2009), it makes even more sense to address them as early on as possible.

Understanding the normal neurological, cognitive, and emotional development of children is important in determining if they are functioning within their appropriate developmental level. For example, developmentally expected anxiety in infants and young children may suddenly arise as a fear of strangers or in response to separation from caregivers. This typically occurs between 7 to 12 months and peaks between 9 to 18 months but decreases for most children by age 2 1/2. Also, a child may have an inherent anxious temperament and may be inhibited when encountering new situations, people, or objects and may respond to these with fear and withdrawal. Likewise, nurses note that normal behaviors for young children (e.g., imaginary friends, concrete thinking, etc.) are interpreted differently when displayed in adults (as signs of schizophrenia). Awareness of language development is important in determining learning disabilities, developmental disabilities, or autism. It is important for the nurse to have a good history of developmental milestones, including language development, sensory perception, emotion regulation, motor skills, attention, and memory.

Vulnerability and Resilience

Vulnerability and resilience are important topics in the care of children. Vulnerability toward maladjustment or resilience in the face of adversity may be passed on from one generation to the next. It is important that the nurse working with children and their families understand this concept. Vulnerability is defined as those characteristics of a child that may predispose him to a disorder. A child's vulnerability is affected by a number of risk factors such as genetics, temperament, environment, and exposure to threats of mental health (Sroufe, 2009). Mental, emotional, or behavioral illness develops through the interplay of factors from each of these domains. Resilience, on the other hand, refers to the child's capacity to use adaptive and positive resources, internal and external, to cope with adversity. Like vulnerability, resilience is multifaceted and is influenced by genetics, temperament, environment, and timing.

Growth and Development

The child with a pervasive developmental disorder such as autism is characterized by developmental deficits in language and communication, social reciprocity, and patterns of interests and behaviors. Children diagnosed with autistic disorders have a greater percentage of delayed attainment of all developmental milestones. Children with cognitive conditions rely heavily on caregivers to get basic needs met. This can be associated with the child's inability to gain independence and self-sufficiency (Meilleur & Fombonne, 2009). Research has identified that regression of growth and development may occur in children with these cognitive disorders known as regressive autism. Losses of language and communication skills, and changes in social engagement and responsiveness, have been exhibited in children diagnosed with regressive autism. Causes of developmental losses are hypothesized but primarily unknown. Prior to developmental losses, children may display subtle changes in development such as abnormal head circumference. Increasing awareness and knowledge about regressive developmental disorders will allow for better identification of these children (Meilleur & Fombonne, 2009).

Nurses should become knowledgeable of various psychosocial and cognitive conditions and their effects on normal growth and development. Developmental disabilities are known to occur with children affected with fragile X syndrome, Down syndrome, fetal alcohol spectrum disorder, learning and cognitive disorders, and autism spectrum disorder (Ward & Hisley, 2009). Early identification of children affected with psychosocial and cognitive conditions is essential to prevent loss and or regression of growth and development. The nurse should assess for behavioral abnormalities and delays in achievement of developmental milestones. The nurse should promote attainment of growth and development while being attentive to known deficits. Special consideration should be taken to encourage attainment of motor and speech skills (Matson, Mahan, Kozlowski, & Shoemaker, 2010). The nurse should encourage the child's independence through exploration and decision making when appropriate. Collaboration with occupational, physical, and speech therapists should be considered based on the needs of the child. The nursing plan of care should be individualized to the child's specific abilities and needs. The nurse should teach parents the normal stages of growth and development and methods to promote achievement of milestones as well as prevention strategies for regression. The nurse should educate the family on ways to help the child develop independence based on his or her own personal abilities.

Sources: Matson, J., Mahan, S., Kozlowski, A., & Shoemaker, M. (2010). Developmental milestones in toddlers with autistic disorder, pervasive developmental disorder-not otherwise specified and atypical development. *Developmental Neurorehabilitation, 13*(4), 239–247.

Meilleur, A., & Fombonne, E. (2009). Regression of language and non-language skills in pervasive developmental disorders. *Journal of Intellectual Disability Research, 53*(2), 115–124.

Optimizing Outcomes—Understanding resilience in the face of vulnerability

It is important to keep in mind that not all offspring of parents with mental health issues go on to develop mental health-related problems themselves. Children of parents or caregivers with mental health issues who do not exhibit any maladjustment or symptoms of mental illness during childhood are known to be resilient children. The best outcome gained from understanding resilience and the factors that encourage resilience can be used to prevent illness and promote good mental health for all children. Mental health promotion efforts focus on the development and nurturance of the innate and learned resilience of children and their families to maintain high levels of mental health (IOM, 2009).

Culture, Diversity, and Health Disparities

Culture and diversity have a significant influence on children's and families' cognitive and psychosocial health. **Culture** is considered to be an external and acquired phenomenon. It is the complex set of beliefs and attributes passed on within a group. What is considered mental illness in one culture may not be in another. **Ethnicity** refers to groups of people who share similar cultural characteristics (i.e., common language, religion, food, and beliefs about health). **Race** is used to describe categories of people, mostly based on physical characteristics (e.g., skin color and shape of nose). **Diversity** refers to the fundamental differences between cultures. The nurse must be able to recognize the place of cultural values, beliefs, and customs for each family, as well as to respect the definitions brought forth from each diverse culture. With the ever-growing virtual world, the physical world has opened exponentially, creating numerous situations that will test the nurse's knowledge of and openness toward others.

Nursing Insight—Understanding mental health disparities in children

One issue that deserves attention from the nursing community involves health disparities. Health-care disparities or inequalities in racial and ethnic minorities are widespread compared with those in non-minorities (Coker, Rodriguez, & Flores, 2010). Children from lower-income families or those within the juvenile justice system suffer greater instances of mental illness and are less likely to receive timely diagnosis or treatment (Children's Defense Fund, 2010). Immigrant children also suffer from disparities in mental health-care delivery. For instance, the nurse must recognize that new immigrants may be concerned with learning the language and getting and keeping a job. These parents may focus only on their children's basic health-care needs (e.g., vaccines and treatment for ear infection) and may not at all attend to their children's cognitive and psychosocial health needs. It is important that the nurse do a thorough assessment of health-care needs, including cognitive and psychosocial well-being.

Given the magnitude of mental health disparities in children and adolescents, nurses at all levels of practice, along with other health-care providers, must become better prepared to implement strategies designed to reduce health-care disparities. Nurses are well positioned to take a leadership role in the movement toward abating and eliminating health-care disparities through awareness and advocacy.

Cultural Diversity: Promoting Understanding of Culture in Diverse Families

It is important that nurses gain an in-depth understanding regarding the culture of various people; acquire sensitivity and empathy in working with diverse families (e.g., give up preconceived notions or generalizations about particular ethnic or racial groups); and attain skills in relationship building with children, adolescents, and parents or caregivers of various ethnic and racial backgrounds. It is recommended that nurses working with children and families of diverse socioeconomic backgrounds take an approach of listening, providing as much positive feedback as possible for what families are doing well and keep resilience-promoting strategies in mind. Using anticipatory guidance, nurses working with children and their families may be most effective suggesting alternative ways of handling a specific cognitive or psychosocial-related concern. In this way, nurses can provide health and psychoeducation in a nonthreatening way to help families decide what works best for them.

Strategies outlined above for nurses to decrease health-care disparities also apply in working with families who may be poor, disenfranchised, and affected by substance abuse, family violence, and child maltreatment.

Barriers to Child and Adolescent Mental Health

There are a number of barriers to the diagnosis and treatment of children's cognitive and psychosocial health. A brief overview is provided here to help the nurse gain an understanding of the issues in order to intervene to minimize these barriers. Though there are increasing efforts to educate the public, the stigma of mental illness continues to be a major barrier to accessing mental health services for children and their families (Mukolo, Heflinger, & Wallston, 2010). The health-care community and the lay public have long been skeptical about whether young children, in particular, experience clinically significant mental health disorders, such as depression or anxiety. There is a prominent belief that childhood is a "sacred" happy time free of problems. Health-care providers have also had a role in perpetuating barriers by minimizing or dismissing parents' or caregivers' concerns. Parents may be told that the child is simply going through a stage that will pass, when there are indeed grounds for concern (e.g., early signs of autism spectrum disorder). It is important for the nurse to understand that this type of thinking may lead to several issues for children, adolescents, and their families such as (1) not getting screened on a timely basis for disordered behaviors and emotional difficulties can be attenuated or resolved if early intervention is sought in a timely fashion, (2) having a sense of shame for the family if a child or adolescent is eventually diagnosed with a mental health problem that might have been prevented or attenuated earlier, and (3) inability to receive adequate mental health or psychosocial treatment when indicated because of lack of resources (Hinshaw, 2006). One particular barrier that relates not only to mental health concerns, but to health in general, is that of health-care illiteracy. Even well-educated people may be "illiterate" when coping with mental illness and related health care.

Mental Illness In Children

Children and adolescents are not immune to mental and emotional illnesses. Mental illness in young people may be confusing and frightening for children and families. The disorders can be devastating, particularly if they are not detected and treated (National Institute of Mental Health [NIMH], 2009b).

ANXIETY

While children commonly experience transient anxieties at various developmental points, clinically significant anxiety must be recognized as a problem. It is important to distinguish between developmentally expected anxiety, anxious temperament, and symptoms of a disorder. The following diagnostic categories related to anxiety disorders have been identified in the *Diagnostic and Statistical Manual of Mental Disorders* (DSM-V): separation anxiety disorder, panic disorder, agoraphobia, specific phobia, social anxiety disorder, generalized anxiety disorder, substance-induced anxiety disorder, and posttraumatic stress disorder (American Psychiatric Association [APA], 2013).

Signs and Symptoms

Criteria common to all anxiety disorders in childhood are as follows (DC:0-3R):

- Anxiety that does not abate or gets worse over time (persistent)
- Anxiety that pervades more than one aspect of the child's life
- Significant distress or avoidance of feared situations
- Impaired functioning or development in response to the anxiety

Diagnosis

As with any emotional or psychiatric difficulty, a complete physical, psychosocial, and family history helps reveal genetic, biological, and familial contributors to anxiety. Differentiation between the categories of anxiety disorders is related to the type of fear exhibited by the child.

In **separation anxiety disorder**, children experience:

- Overwhelming fear of becoming separated from or losing a caregiver (Fig. 22-1).

Panic disorder usually begins in adolescence but may start earlier.

Symptoms of a panic attack might include:

- Palpitations
- Sweating
- Shaking
- Nausea
- Dizziness
- Fear of dying

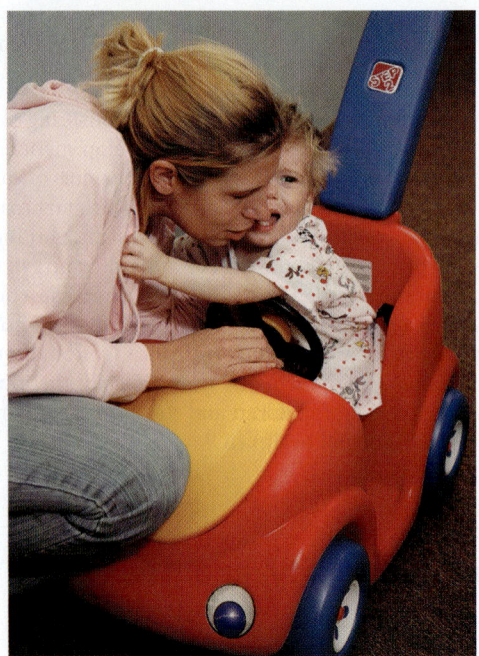

Figure 22-1 This child is displaying signs of separation anxiety.

- Tingling sensations
- Chills or hot flushes

Agoraphobia refers to the fear of and avoidance of certain places or situations (e.g., fear of leaving home) or being in open or crowded places. **Specific phobia** refers to unrelenting fear of certain objects or situations (e.g., spiders, storms, snakes, or water). These may be difficult to evaluate because at each developmental stage children and adolescents have various expected fears. Children with **social anxiety disorder** avoid social situations. In **generalized anxiety disorder**, children experience excessive worry about everything, including peer relationships, social acceptance, and pleasing others. **Posttraumatic stress disorder** occurs in response to a perceived or actual threat to one's life or safety. There is a clear precipitant, and a reaction is generally understandable. The response may persist for weeks, months, or years and is accompanied by panic symptoms.

Anxiety often presents in the form of somatic complaints like stomachaches and restlessness (American Academy of Child & Adolescent Psychiatry [AACAP], 2010a). The pediatric nurse can recognize anxiety problems when a child persistently presents with symptoms that do not have a recognizable physical cause.

Prevention

There are specific measures that a nurse may undertake to help prevent anxiety disorders from occurring or to lessen their impact on children. Simply paying attention to any signs of anxiety is the first step in recognizing clinically significant symptoms. Children and adolescents are more likely to respond to someone who takes the time to listen and care.

Current Western culture is filled with scary images, whether in the form of games, movies, television, or actual events in the news. It is important for the nurse to understand and to help parents think about how and when to protect children from the influx of information that might be overwhelming.

Collaborative Care

Nursing Care. There are several evidence-based therapies provided by qualified advanced practice clinicians. The pediatric nurse is aware of some of these therapies to assist parents in finding a referral. The Coping Cat Program is designed for children ages 7 to 13 with anxiety disorders, and the CAT Program is for adolescents (Podell, Mychailyszyn, Edmunds, Puleo, & Kendall, 2010). Both of these cognitive–behavioral programs are designed to help the child develop skills to cope with anxiety and provide techniques to decrease fears through systematic exposure to the feared object. These programs are intended to be used with children and adolescents who have social anxiety disorder, generalized anxiety disorder, and social phobia.

The FRIENDS program was designed for the parents as well as their children with anxiety disorders (Podell et al., 2010). It is similar to the Coping Cat in that it uses cognitive–behavioral techniques to help children and their families cope with anxiety. FRIENDS is an acronym that provides a relatively easy reminder for management of anxiety:

- Feeling worried?
- Relax and feel good.
- Inner thoughts.
- Explore plans.
- Nice work so reward yourself.
- Don't forget to practice.
- Stay calm, you know how to cope.

This program has proved to be useful in reducing the risk of development of anxiety disorders in children (Kösters, Chinapaw, Zwaanswijk, van der Wal, Utens, & Koot, 2012).

Education/Discharge Instructions

The nurse can provide health teaching for families related to healthy coping and communication.

Additional teaching interventions may involve teaching relaxation and deep breathing as well as problem-solving techniques.

Where Research and Practice Meet: The Effectiveness of the FRIENDS Program

Essau, Conradt, Sasagawa, and Ollendick (2012) conducted a large study designed to further test the effectiveness of the FRIENDS program for prevention and treatment of anxiety and depressive disorders in children and adolescents. They studied 638 children in the German school system. The children were divided randomly into an intervention group of 302 children and a control group of 336 children. Children in the intervention group participated in a 10-week course of the FRIENDS program, plus two additional booster sessions. Their parents participated voluntarily in four parent sessions. Children in the control group were given the opportunity to participate in the program 6 months after the study was conducted. Both groups received pretest and posttest measures as well as follow-up measures at 6 and 12 months. The researchers found that while there was little statistical difference between the two groups in the immediate posttest, there were significant positive differences for the intervention group at the 12-month follow-up. This was true for both anxiety and depressive symptoms. The intervention group were also less likely to avoid problem-solving than the control group.

It is important for the nurse to understand studies like this one. Knowing what is available to help children who may be susceptible to anxiety and depression will assist in both prevention and care of difficulties.

 Complementary Care: *Mindful Breathing*

Mindfulness means paying attention in the present moment. Paying attention to one's breathing may be a way of coping with anxiety. The teaching works best before an anxiety episode.

The nurse teaches slow breathing by telling the child to (Fig. 22-2):

- Consciously direct your attention to your breathing.
- Breathe in slowly, paying attention as the air enters nose and mouth and fills your lungs.
- Breathe out slowly, paying attention as the air leaves your body.
- Allow your mind to follow the breath in and out.
- Imagine yourself in a rubber raft riding the gentle waves of your breath.

POSTTRAUMATIC STRESS DISORDER

Posttraumatic stress disorder (PTSD) is an anxiety disorder that occurs in response to a real or perceived trauma or threat to one's life or safety. Children of all ages may be involved in traumatic situations related to human (e.g., abuse, violence, war, etc.) or environmental (e.g., natural disasters, automobile accidents, etc.) causes. While some may exhibit little or no negative immediate or long-term consequences of the trauma, or are easily comforted and can move on, others are vulnerable to PTSD.

Signs and Symptoms

After a trauma, a child or adolescent with PTSD exhibits symptoms within each of the following sets of reactions:

- Re-experiencing the trauma through flashbacks, nightmares, or physical sensations
- Avoiding reminders of anything or any place that triggers memories
- Physiological symptoms of anxious arousal (e.g., insomnia, startle response, or sense of panic) (APA, 2013).

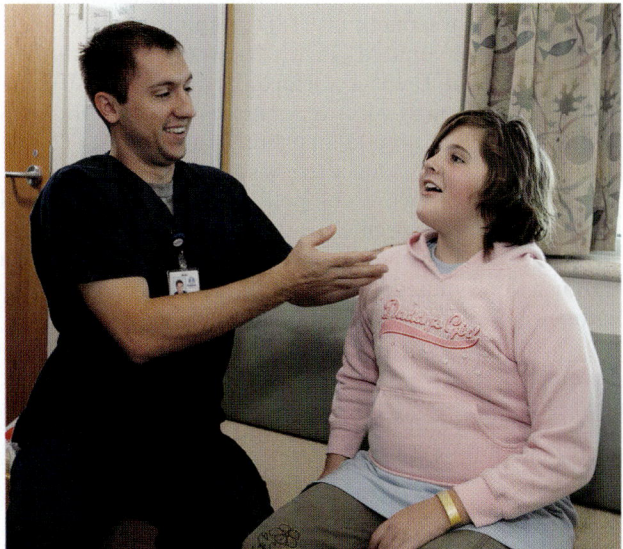

Figure 22-2 The nurse teaches the child how to reduce anxiety with slow breathing.

Diagnosis

Diagnosis is based on the exhibited symptoms within the sets of reactions. There are clear developmental differences across childhood and adolescence (Scheeringa, Zeanah, & Cohen, 2011)) that will need to be accounted for in making a definitive diagnosis.

Prevention

Preventing traumatic experiences from causing emotional and physical damage is an important aspect of this condition.
Possible preventive factors might include:

- Promoting resilience in at-risk families and children (prior to traumatic events)
- Promoting resilience in general (teaching safety measures for potential risk factors (e.g., environmental disasters, "stranger-danger," etc.)
- Early research on pharmacological measures to prevent PTSD has been promising.
- Creating and implementing programs that ensure safety

Collaborative Care

Nursing Care. Many children who endure posttraumatic distress may not be brought into a mental health-care facility for clinical intervention. Some seriously traumatized children enter treatment through the court system after having experienced abuse or serious loss within the family of origin. The nurse may come in contact with these children in primary care or in school or other settings.

In the community, the nurse is instrumental in educating parents about the symptoms and helping the family and child by making referrals for appropriate services. The nurse can reinforce the importance of providing a secure home base for the child, one that includes the family's or caregiver's willingness to be available to and comfort the child without judgment.

As with each of the anxiety disorders, being aware of the resources available for treatment of PTSD is important. Mental health professionals equipped to help the young person process and cope with the sequelae of trauma can provide various types of cognitive behavior therapy with or without medication intervention. Pharmacological intervention for treatment of PTSD in children and adolescents has been limited. In a review of extant studies, Strawn, Keeshin, DelBello, Geracioti, & Putnam (2010) reported that although selective seratonin reuptake inhibitors (SSRIs) are often used as first line treatment of PTSD in children and adolescents, there is scarce evidence supporting the practice. More compelling evidence was found about supporting specific treatment of symptoms as they arise (i.e., antiadrenergic agents for hyperarousal, alpha agonists for sympathetic symptoms, alpha-1 agonists or antipsychotics for intrusive thoughts, etc.).

 Medication: Selective Serotonin Reuptake Inhibitors (SSRIs)

Children may be prescribed SSRIs because these are the treatment of choice not only for depression, but also for the management of anxiety. They are useful in decreasing the avoidant behaviors and intrusive thoughts engendered by PTSD (Lubit, 2012).

Education/Discharge Instructions

The nurse can teach the family that psychotherapy and psychopharmacotherapy together may be most helpful for children suffering with PTSD. It is important to help parents and families understand the immediate and ongoing impact that a traumatic event may have in the young person's life.

Mood Disorders

Pediatric mood disorders may take the form of **major depression** (serious, time-limited depression), **dysthymic disorder** (longer-term, less-intense depression), or **bipolar disorder** (consisting of mood swings between depression and mania). These disorders are sometimes more difficult to diagnose in children and adolescents than in adults because of developmental phases and the lack of language and cognitive skills to describe symptoms and experiences.

DEPRESSION

Depression may be situational or related to environmental factors combined with genetic and biological factors.

Signs and Symptoms

Five key features must be present and persistent for most days during a period of 2 weeks for the diagnosis of a major depressive disorder in children and adolescents. This list of symptoms is compiled based on several diagnostic classification publications to reflect a developmentally sensitive criterion (APA, 2013).

- Persistent sad or irritable mood—reported feeling sad or empty or observed by others (e.g., appears tearful). This mood is different from the child's baseline emotional and behavioral state and is unrelated to events that may cause temporary distress or sadness (e.g., getting a time-out).
- Loss of interest in activities once enjoyed (**anhedonia**)—reported by child or observed by others.
- Significant change in appetite or body weight—difficulty sleeping or oversleeping.
- Fatigue or loss of energy.
- Feelings of worthlessness or excessive/inappropriate guilt.
- Decreased ability to think or concentrate or to make decisions; an example is a drop in grades and/or school performance.
- Recurrent thoughts of death or suicide with or without a suicide plan, and in younger children, consistent engagement in activities or play that involve themes of death and suicide.

Diagnosis

Diagnosis is based on the exhibited depressive symptoms.

Collaborative Care

Nursing Care. The most important aspect of helping a depressed child is to ensure safety. It is recommended that any nurse working with a child who is depressed understand how to deal with the potential suicide ideation or intent.

Because depression often goes unrecognized in children or adolescents, the nurse is instrumental in determining the presence of signs and symptoms. Pediatric and school nurses are in a position to observe changes in a child's behavior and demeanor as well as grades. Developing a trusting relationship with a child and asking about feelings or thoughts may provide evidence of underlying depression and provide the child with a first step in feeling better.

Education/Discharge Instructions

Nurses can talk with the parent(s) or caregiver(s) of a child about suspected depression and suggest referral to a counselor, pastor, chaplain, or spiritual director for evaluation and treatment.

BIPOLAR DISORDER

Bipolar disorder (BPD), also known as manic–depression, is a mood disorder that is evidenced by significant mood swings (from depression to mania) (APA, 2013).

Signs and Symptoms

Because BPD is a combination of major depression and mania, the nurse must be aware of symptoms associated with BPD. Both manic and depressive symptoms, as described by the National Institute of Mental Health (2009a) are listed:

Mania	Depression
Overly happy, irritable, silly, and elated	Persistent sad or irritable mood Worried, feeling empty
Overly inflated self-esteem; grandiosity Increased energy, feels jumpy or "wired"	Loss of interest in activities once enjoyed
Decreased need for sleep—able to go with very little or no sleep for days without tiring	Change in eating and sleeping habits Physical agitation or slowing Loss of energy
Increased talking—talks too much, too fast; changes topics too quickly; cannot be interrupted	Feelings of worthlessness or inappropriate guilt Difficulty concentrating
Distractibility—attention moves constantly from one thing to the next	Recurrent thoughts of death or suicide
Hyper-sexuality—increased sexual thoughts, feelings, or behaviors; use of explicit sexual language	
Increased goal-directed activity or physical agitation	
Disregard of risk—excessive involvement in risky behaviors or activities	
Impulsive behavior, such as spending sprees	

Source: National Institute of Mental Health, (2009a).

Nursing Care Plan The Depressed Child

Nursing Diagnosis: Ineffective individual coping or impaired adjustment related to depression

Measurable Short-Term Goal: Child will use positive talk to interrupt negative thinking about self.

Measurable Long-Term Goal: Child will demonstrate increased self-esteem by accepting positive feedback from others.

NOC Outcomes:
Active Listening (4920)
Self-Esteem (1205) Personal judgment of self-worth

NIC Interventions:
Self-Esteem Enhancement (5400)
Active Listening (4920)

Nursing Interventions:

1. Listen actively to child, displaying interest without judgment or responding too quickly.

   RATIONALE: Active listening shows attention to the message and respect for the child's thinking and perceptions.

2. Monitor and help the child to identify statements reflecting perceived self-worth.

   RATIONALE: Provides information about distorted or negative perceptions.

3. Assist the child to examine perceptions that are self-reflected in negative "self-talk" and turn these into positive statements of self-worth.

   RATIONALE: Allows replacement of negative self-evaluations with positive statements that enhance self-esteem.

4. Encourage the child to identify personal strengths and accept valid positive responses from others.

   RATIONALE: Helps the child develop positive self-esteem.

5. Assist child to set realistic goals to enhance self-esteem, providing appropriate praise or rewards for progress.

   RATIONALE: Positive reinforcement supports progress in meeting realistic personal goals.

Diagnosis

Diagnosis is based on a thorough history and physical as well as the identification of the significant mood swings (from depression to mania). Often family members or significant others can describe the behavior that may help lead to a diagnosis.

Prevention

The following therapeutic parenting and education strategies are helpful for the family.
　Preventive strategies include:

- Practice and teach relaxation techniques
- Use firm restraint holds to control rages
- Prioritize battles and let go of less important matters
- Reduce stress in the home
- Use good listening and communication skills
- Use music and sound, lighting, water, and massage to assist the child with waking, falling asleep, and relaxation
- Stress reduction at school
- Prepare for stressful situations by developing coping strategies beforehand
- Engage the child's creativity through activities that express and channel gifts and strengths
- Provide routines, structure, and freedom within limits (National Institute of Mental Health, 2009a)

Collaborative Care

Nursing Care. It is important for the nurse to recognize that if a child is in an acutely manic state, the child is struggling against internal feelings and is not just being a "bad child." Psychotherapy and medication are indicated.

Education/Discharge Instructions

Instructions that can be given to the family:

- Remove harmful objects from the home (or lock them in a safe place) that could be used to inflict harm to self or others during a rage, especially guns.
- Keep medications in a locked cabinet.
- Teach the family to watch for the child's response/reaction to medication(s).
- Instruct the family that it may take 2 to 3 weeks before the medications become effective.
- Instruct the family that if symptoms escalate and become uncontrollable they need to contact their healthcare professional.
- Instruct the family to visit the following Web site for more information about bipolar disorder: http://www.bpkids.org, a parent-led organization that provides supportive information for children, caregivers, and families. (National Institute of Mental Health, 2009a)

 Now Can You—Differentiate between depression and bipolar disorder?

1. Describe the signs and symptoms of depression and bipolar disorder?
2. Describe nursing care for the child with depression or bipolar disorder?

SUICIDE

Suicide represents a devastating consequence resulting from any number of psychiatric difficulties. This is a serious public health problem that affects children and adolescents. Suicide is the third leading cause of death for youth between the ages of 10 and 24. The top three methods used in suicides of children and adolescents include firearm (46%), suffocation (37%), and poisoning (8%). Many more children and adolescents survive suicide attempts than actually die from such attempts. A nationwide survey performed by the Centers for Disease Control and Prevention found that 15% of the youth in grades 9 to 12 in public and private schools in the United States reported seriously considering suicide, 11% reported creating a plan, and 7% reporting trying to take their own life in the preceding 12 months. Each year, approximately 149,000 youth between the ages of 10 and 24 receive medical care for self-inflicted injuries at emergency departments across the United States (CDC, 2009).

Signs and Symptoms

The nurse suspects suicide potential when faced with any of the following in the child or adolescent:

- Symptoms of depression or other mental illnesses
- Withdrawal from friendships
- Expression of hopelessness
- Isolative behavior
- Personality changes
- Decline in schoolwork
- Giving away personal possessions that were once prized
- Preoccupation with death in writing or playing
- Refers to dying or no longer being around
- Access to a method of suicide (e.g., medications or weapons)

Diagnosis

If the nurse is concerned that a child or adolescent might be suicidal, the nurse must ask the child about suicidal thoughts or behaviors. This information may help to save the child's life.

- "Have you thought about doing something to hurt yourself or take your life?"
- "Do you ever wish you were not alive?"
- "What would you do if you were to hurt yourself?"

Prevention

The school nurse is in a position to recognize children or adolescents who might be suicidal. The nurse must ask about suicide ideation. The nurse can discern: Does the child have a plan? Is that plan possible (i.e., is the means to self-harm accessible)? Has the child attempted suicide before? Foremost, if any of these factors are present, the nurse must refer the child (and family) to a mental health professional who can assess the level of risk. The child or adolescent may need immediate hospitalization to remain safe.

✳ **Nursing Insight**—*Primary and secondary prevention strategies*

- Identify school-based programs that target students who are at risk for dropping out of school and assist the child or adolescent to remain involved in school.
- Cognitive–behavioral techniques may be used with a suicidal child or adolescent by conducting exercises, activities, and discussions that assist them to connect their thoughts with their behaviors.

Collaborative Care

Nursing Care. The nurse is supportive of the child or adolescent and supportive of the medication regime. Pharmacological treatments include medications to treat the underlying psychiatric difficulty (Table 22-1).

focus on safety

Suicidal behavior related to antidepressant therapy

In 2004, the U.S. Food and Drug Administration issued a "black box" warning that SSRIs may increase the risk of suicide in children and adolescents. Studies have been conducted since that have weighed the benefits of using antidepressants versus the potential costs have not generated a great deal of clarity. Subsequent studies discussed by Goodman, Murphy, and Storch (2007) related that the increased incidence of suicide ideation and attempt was not universal, nor was it related only to those diagnosed with depression but also in children taking SSRIs for other disorders. The evidence is controversial because other studies have shown antidepressants to be very effective in decreasing the suicide risk by effectively dealing with the underlying causes. Several factors have been proposed to explain the occurrence of suicidal ideation in children treated with these medications: (1) The prescription may be an inadequate dose, and therefore the depression is not treated. (2) An energizing phenomenon, which describes a situation in which the depressive symptoms related to energy decrease before the mood symptoms, may occur, thus making it more possible for the depressed individual to have the energy to attempt suicide. (3) The emergence of an activation syndrome may be related to a toxic reaction to the medication. (4) Motor restlessness related to akathisia (motor restlessness that may appear as a side effect of antipsychotic medication) may occur. (5) A shift from depression to mania in a not-yet-diagnosed bipolar child may occur. (6) Idiosyncratic reactions (perhaps related to gene-drug reactions) may occur (Goodman et al., 2007).

Education/Discharge Instructions

Instruct the family to provide protective measures for the child: remove all potentially self or other harmful objects from the home such as guns or other weapons. Rid cupboards of poisons, lock medicines away, and provide close, constant supervision. Assist the family in identifying strengths and resources available (e.g., crisis or suicide hot lines, counseling, and inpatient treatment facilities).

SCHIZOPHRENIA

Schizophrenia is a serious chronic mental health disorder that is thought to be the result of abnormalities in neurodevelopmental processes that occur early (i.e., prenatal, infancy, and early childhood) as well as later (i.e., late childhood and adolescence) in life. The disorder typically begins in late adolescence or early adulthood, but it is possible for children as young as 5 or 6 to exhibit signs (Loth, 2012).

Signs and Symptoms

Schizophrenia has the following signs and symptoms:

- Hallucinations (hearing voices, seeing things, or experiencing strange sensations)
- Delusions (false beliefs, e.g., beliefs that the radio is sending special messages)
- Disorganized speech and behavior
- Decreased or "flattening" of affect (visible expression of mood), speech, and motivation (APA, 2013)

Table 22-1 Pharmacological Treatments for Psychological Difficulties

Category	Medications	Uses
Antianxiety	**Beta blockers**	Anxiety
	propanolol (Inderal)	
	Alpha blockers	
	clonidine (Catapres)	
Antidepressants	**Selective serotonin uptake inhibitors (SSRIs)**	Depression Anxiety OCD Elective mutism
	fluoxetine (Prozac) sertraline (Zoloft) paroxetine (Paxil) citalopram (Celexa) escitalopram (Lexapro) fluvoxamine (Luvox)	
	Tricyclics	Enuresis
	imipramine (Tofranil) clomipramine (Anafranil)	Autism
	Other	
	bupropion (Wellbutrin) venlafaxine	
Mood Stabilizer	lithium carbonate (Lithobid, Lithane, or Eskalith)	Bipolar disorder Mania ODD ADHD
Anticonvulsants	valproate (Depakote)	Bipolar disorder Mania
Antipsychotics	**Traditional**	Autism
	haloperidol (Haldol)	Psychosis
	Atypical	Tourette's syndrome
	risperidone (Risperdal)	Behavioral problems related to other psychiatric disorders (conduct disorder, ADHD, MR)
	olanzapine (Zyprexa) quetiapine (Seroquel) ziprasidone (Geodon) aripiprazole (Abilify)	
Stimulants	methylphenidate (Ritalin and Concerta) dextroamphetamine (Dexedrine and Adderall)	ADHD
Nonstimulants	atomoxetine (Strattera)	ADHD

Diagnosis

A diagnosis of schizophrenia is based on a mental health interview that includes a comprehensive developmental and family history.

Collaborative Care

Nursing Care. Early treatment for schizophrenia usually involves pharmacological agents (e.g., atypical antipsychotics), adolescent and family psychoeducation, and psychotherapy aimed at increasing level of functioning. To obtain the best outcome, the adolescent and family should always stay in treatment. Acute treatment for active psychosis (e.g., hallucinations, delusions, fearfulness, and acting out) consists of maintaining the safety of the child and others. It is frightening to lose sight of reality. Families of children with schizophrenia, like those with any chronic difficult illness, may need ongoing support. There are organizations that offer support and advocacy for families of the mentally ill. One such organization is the National Alliance on Mental Illness (NAMI; www.nami.org), which provides parents and families with important information.

Education/Discharge Instructions

Patient education involves reminding the child and family about the importance of taking the medications as well as informing them of the related side effects. Reinforce ongoing psychotherapy and support.

Psychosocial and Cognitive Disorders

REACTIVE ATTACHMENT DISORDER

Reactive attachment disorder (RAD) is a relatively rare condition characterized by significant difficulties in forming emotional attachments with others (AACAP, 2011a). Children with RAD have generally experienced early life trauma or loss, making it difficult for them to form meaningful and vital connections. Attachment difficulties can be recognized as early as infancy and definitely by the age of 5 (Lubit, 2012).

 Nursing Insight—*Understanding reactive attachment disorder*

Infants develop attachments during their earliest months and years of life. John Bowlby (1909–1990) studied the impact of maternal deprivation on childhood development. Mary Ainsworth (1913–1999) studied forms of attachment, identifying traits that described an infant's security in relationship to its mother. In establishing reliable attachments to their earliest caregivers, infants are afforded the framework for future trusting relationships. These attachments create situations within which the child can safely test out physical and emotional boundaries, as well as a context within which to develop the ability to regulate emotions.

Children who have not been afforded consistent and nurturing presence early in their lives become either anxiously attached or detached in relation to others. Infants and children diagnosed with attachment disorders have usually endured neglect and/or maltreatment or have experienced severe trauma. Vulnerable children are those within the foster care and international and domestic adoption system who have previously been abandoned or abused. These are the children who have most clearly experienced disrupted early attachment. Infants with mothers with significant postpartum depression or mental illness may not have had the opportunity to bond and attach healthily.

Signs and Symptoms

Signs and symptoms of RAD (APA, 2013) include:

- Marked disturbance in ability to relate socially, manifesting either:

- Emotional withdrawal or inhibition
  - Inability to seek or accept warmth from others
  - Inability to show or respond to affection
- Marked disinhibition
  - Indiscriminant willingness to seek comfort even from strangers
  - Excessive trust of strangers
- Infants with serious insecure attachment may exhibit severe feeding difficulties not related to a physiological cause

Diagnosis

The pediatric nurse can aid in the diagnostic process by parental report and observing how the child interacts around parents and strangers.

Prevention

As with many of the childhood and adolescent disorders that are related to early trauma, prevention lies in educating parents and caretakers and providing them with mental health services prior to becoming parents. Adoptive parents should be aware of the difficulties that may have been experienced by their children prior to adoption. While it is not always possible to avoid attachment difficulties, nurses can help parents and caregivers cope with the sequelae.

Collaborative Care

Nursing Care. Because attachment disorders in infants and children result from the lack of opportunity to experience a caring relationship, this opportunity is offered as a first step in treatment. Developing trust through meeting the child's basic needs or responding to cries or tantrums or listlessness with patience and consistency is exceptionally important. A child with RAD has no true concept about which basic needs will be met. RAD is a rare but serious condition. Families who present with a child with symptoms should be referred for psychotherapy (AACAP, 2011a).

Education/Discharge Instructions

Parents of children with RAD need a great deal of support. They should be educated about attachment and bonding and about how to deal with a child who has difficulty making interpersonal connections. These parents often benefit from involvement in a support group with other families of children with RAD.

ATTENTION-DEFICIT/HYPERACTIVITY DISORDER

Attention-deficit/hyperactivity disorder (ADHD) is familiar to parents, schoolteachers, and others who know the child. Images of the overactive, talkative child "bouncing off the walls" and always in trouble are likely portrayed. ADHD is one of the most publicized and prevalent psychiatric conditions of childhood. A child can have attention-deficit disorder with or without hyperactivity. The category of ADHD without hyperactivity typically has symptoms of distractibility. While ADHD without hyperactivity garners much less attention than ADHD with hyperactivity, it can cause just as much difficulty in the life of the child and the family.

The CDC has indicated that 9.5% of the children in the United States have been diagnosed with ADHD. That is a significant increase over the 3% to 7% reported in the DSM-IV-TR. Parent-reported ADHD increased at an even greater rate (22% increase) (CDC, 2011a). As with other psychiatric disorders, particularly autism spectrum disorders, it is yet unclear if the increase in numbers is a result of better case-finding, increased public awareness, or actual increase in the disorder.

Signs and Symptoms

Signs and symptoms of attention-deficit/hyperactivity disorder include:

- Inattention
  - Often fails to give close attention to details or makes careless mistakes in schoolwork, work, or other activities
  - Often has difficulty sustaining attention in tasks or play activities
  - Often does not seem to listen when spoken to directly
  - Often does not follow through on instructions and fails to finish schoolwork, chores, or duties in the workplace (not due to oppositional behavior or failure to understand instructions)
  - Often has difficulty organizing tasks and activities
  - Often avoids, dislikes, or is reluctant to engage in tasks that require sustained mental effort (such as schoolwork or homework)
  - Often loses things necessary for tasks or activities (e.g., toys, school assignments, pencils, books, or tools)
  - Is often easily distracted by extraneous stimuli
  - Is often forgetful in daily activities
- Six (or more) of the following symptoms of hyperactivity-impulsivity have persisted for at least 6 months to a degree that is maladaptive and inconsistent with developmental level:
  - Hyperactivity
    - Often fidgets with hands or feet or squirms in seat
    - Often leaves seat in classroom or in other situations in which remaining seated is expected
    - Often runs about or climbs excessively in situations in which it is inappropriate (in adolescents or adults, may be limited to subjective feelings of restlessness)
    - Is often "on the go" or often acts as if "driven by a motor"
    - Often talks excessively
  - Impulsivity
    - Often blurts out answers before questions have been completed
    - Often has difficulty awaiting turn
    - Often interrupts or intrudes on others (e.g., butts into conversations or games)

Although ADHD is most often diagnosed in early school-age children, symptoms can be seen in much younger children. Children with these symptoms often have difficulty with school performance as well as social and peer interaction. While poor school performance is usually the driving factor in seeking help for children with these symptoms, difficulty with peer groups and family relationships are just as evident. Many children with ADHD also have comorbid conditions such as depression, anxiety, oppositional defiant disorder, and learning disabilities.

Table 22-2 Characteristics of Attention-Deficit/Hyperactivity Disorder	
Developmentally inappropriate or maladaptive symptoms consisting of either inattentive symptoms (first column), hyperactive or impulsive symptoms (second column), or a combination (both columns).	
Inattention	**Hyperactivity or Impulsivity**
Distractibility	Excessive energy and activity
Inability to complete projects	Restlessness
Easily bored	Overactivity
Disorganized	Inability to sit still or stay in one place for long
Inattentiveness	Excessive talking
Avoidance of detailed tasks	Poor boundaries—interrupts or intrudes
Forgetfulness	Difficulty delaying

Diagnosis

Evaluations for ADHD are conducted by advanced practice nurses, physicians, and other health-care providers. For appropriate assessment of ADHD, the child must first meet the diagnostic criteria outlined in the DSM-IV-TR (APA, 2013) (Table 22-2).

When the criteria are met, the final diagnosis requires evidence of the child's behavior in a variety of settings, such as classroom, during homework, or playtime. Evidence is obtained by asking parents, teachers, and other caregivers to complete rating scales about behavior. Additional information needed includes the age at onset of symptoms, duration of symptoms, and degree of impaired functioning.

Collaborative Care

Nursing Care. ADHD is evaluated by using a variety of rating scales that asks the caregiver or teacher to rate the child's behavior (e.g., behavior occurs extremely often, often, sometimes, rarely, or never). A school nurse is trained to perform observations of the child while in class to assist in the information gathering. These scales in combination with a clinical family interview provide the examiner with valuable information to determine a diagnosis. A thorough clinical interview with the child is also important in determining the appropriate diagnosis and treatment.

The most effective treatment for ADHD is a combination of pharmacological and psychosocial interventions. Using both modalities allows for the control or abatement of symptomatic behavior by the medication while at the same time working on changing maladaptive behavior patterns through therapy with the child and family. When recommending psychosocial intervention, clinicians must keep in mind the developmental level of the child and family. Also, from a developmental psychopathology perspective, it is important to inform the family that early intervention works best and that the child and family may have periods of adaptive and maladaptive behavior.

Education/Discharge Instructions

The nurse can educate the family in behavioral techniques for helping the child focus and maintain appropriate

> ### Medication: ADHD
>
> Stimulants are the most commonly used medication for this condition. Ritalin and other forms of methylphenidate, amphetamine salts (Adderall), and atomoxetine (Strattera), a nonstimulant medication, are commonly used in this condition.
>
> Methylphenidate also is prescribed in a transdermal patch form for children 6 years and older.
>
> This patch was designed for children who were unable to swallow any tablets or capsules.

behaviors. Education about pharmacological interventions is also important.

When providing psychosocial care, the nurse recognizes that children often respond to therapeutic approaches that include behavioral therapy, rewards (sticker charts), and positive versus negative reinforcement (used as often as possible when child demonstrates acceptable behavior). School nurses are in a position of supporting teachers and other staff in the use of behavioral charts. Pediatric nurses in the community can offer support to parents and families in ongoing use of behavior modification.

Some families may resist medications. Other families may put all of their faith into medications, thus not following through with the entire treatment plan. It is important for the nurse to help the family make use of all of the treatment options available to them and to participate actively with their health provider(s) in developing a plan for their child.

OPPOSITIONAL DEFIANT DISORDER AND CONDUCT DISORDER

Antisocial behavior is at the core of disordered behavior that can often explode into clinical disorders most often known as oppositional defiant disorder (ODD) and conduct disorder (CD).

ODD and CD have multifactorial and complex etiologies. Studies have identified a number of biological and psychosocial factors that may be associated with the development of CD and ODD in children and adolescents.

Signs and Symptoms

ODD has these signs and symptoms:

- Frequent temper tantrums
- Excessive arguing with adults
- Often questioning rules
- Active defiance and refusal to comply with adult requests and rules
- Deliberate attempts to annoy or upset people
- Blaming others for his or her mistakes or misbehavior
- Often being touchy or easily annoyed by others
- Frequent anger and resentment
- Mean and hateful talking when upset
- Spiteful attitude and revenge seeking (AACAP, 2011b)

Conduct disorder has the following signs and symptoms:

- Breaking rules without obvious reason
- Cruel or aggressive behavior toward people or animals (e.g., bullying, fighting, using dangerous weapons, forcing sexual activity, and stealing)
- Failure to attend school (truancy beginning before age 13)
- Heavy drinking and/or heavy illicit drug use
- Intentionally setting fires
- Lying to get a favor or avoid things they have to do
- Vandalizing or destroying property (MedLine Plus, 2011).

Diagnosis

Diagnosis is accomplished using the behavioral criteria presented. It is important to note that many children who meet the criteria for ODD or CD often have comorbid mental health problems and may also function poorly in interpersonal relationships with peers and caregivers (AACAP, 2011b).

Prevention

Early assessment of these conditions is important, using multimethod and multi-informant approaches that include self-report scales, child interview, parent interview, physical assessment, observation of child–parent interaction, and thorough family assessment (e.g., history of exposure to violence in the family and community).

When working with children and adolescents who exhibit ODD or CD, it is important for the nurse to be aware and manage personal feelings that may be aroused by the patient and family. The nurse can educate the family about the family-based prevention and intervention programs.

Collaborative Care

Nursing Care. Children with ODD or CD may be prescribed medications from a number of categories such as stimulants for ADHD symptoms, antipsychotics for behavior regulation, mood stabilizers for regulation of high and low mood presentations, and antianxiety agents.

Nurses who work with families that have children with ODD or CD must be mindful of the stress that these disorders have on the whole family. It may be exhausting for parents to cope with the defiant behaviors. Siblings may be put at risk simply spending time with the misbehaved child. Respite care (short-term care) can give the family a "rest" from the child who has the disorder. Encouraging family members to learn coping skills and take care of personal needs as well as the child's may be useful in helping them to find balance in daily living.

Education/Discharge Instructions

Nursing care for these conditions also includes educating the family about medications. It is important that the child and family understand the action, potential side effects, and additional information about prescribed medications. In addition, the nurse should educate families about community resources available for respite and the importance of psychotherapy.

> ### Nursing Diagnoses Oppositional Defiant Disorder and Conduct Disorder
>
> - Ineffective coping related to personal vulnerability
> - Impaired social interaction related to hostile, negative, and defiant behavior
> - Chronic low self-esteem related to difficulties with positive social interactions
> - Compromised family functioning related to inadequate information and family disorganization

Tic Disorders

Tics are sudden, painless, non-rhythmic behaviors that are either motor (related to movement) or vocal and that appear out of context—for example, grimacing in class. They are fairly common in childhood; tics are generally temporary conditions that resolve on their own. For some children, however, the tics persist over time, becoming more complex and severe. These tics can impact a person's capability to function (Disorders.org, 2011).

Examples of simple motor tics:

- Eye blinking
- Facial grimacing

Examples of complex motor tics:

- Hand gestures
- Jumping

Examples of simple vocal tics:

- Throat clearing
- Grunting

Examples of complex vocal tics:

- Meaningless changes in volume and pitch of speech
- Echolalia (repeating last heard sounds or words) (APA, 2013)

TOURETTE'S SYNDROME

Tourette's syndrome (TS) is included in a spectrum of tic disorders, which includes transient and chronic tics. It is an inherited neuropsychiatric disorder with an onset in childhood. TS is characterized by multiple physical (motor) tics and at least one vocal (phonic) tic. There is usually a premonitory urge prior to the tic. The tics can be repressed temporarily.

Signs and Symptoms

Children with TS often exhibit symptoms of other disorders, similar to obsessive compulsive disorder (OCD), autism spectrum disorders, and attention-deficit/hyperactivity disorder (ADHD). Children with coexisting disorders are more likely to suffer depression, low self-esteem, negative peer acceptance, and poor school performance than those with tics alone.

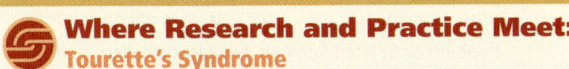

> **Where Research and Practice Meet:**
> **Tourette's Syndrome**
>
> Rivera-Navarro, Cubo, and Almazán (2009) studied the differences in perception regarding the communication and impact of a diagnosis of Tourette's syndrome (TS) on patients, as well as their relatives and physicians. All groups perceived different causes for the difficulty of the diagnosis of TS. However, the physicians and the relatives both noted that the symptoms of TS were often hidden behind family guilt. It was recommended as a result of this study that an effort should be made to improve the communication of such a diagnosis to family members to facilitate better understanding of this diagnosis (Rivera-Navarro, Cubo, & Almazán, 2009).

Some examples of TS behavior are the following:

- Eye blinking
- Neck jerking
- Abdominal tensing
- Touching
- Stomping
- Facial contortions
- Retracing steps

These symptoms can last from several hundred milliseconds to several seconds or longer.

These symptoms are irresistible and separated by periods of non-tic behavior (APA, 2013).

Diagnosis

> **Diagnostic Tools** Tourette's Syndrome
>
> The nurse can help the family recognize certain features of TS to assist in the diagnosis of the condition:
> - The child may have both multiple motor and one or more vocal tics present at some time but not necessarily concurrently.
> - The tics occur several times a day.
> - The tics occur almost every day or intermittently throughout a period of more than 1 year.
> - The onset of tics is before age 18 years.
> - The disturbance is not caused by the direct physiological effects of a substance or a general medical condition. (APA, 2013)

Collaborative Care

Nursing Care. The nurse working with a child with TS must recognize the impact the disorder has on the child's functioning and social relationships. The nurse can help family members and teachers understand that the child cannot control the tics. The child may become self-conscious and worried that he will blurt out words or utterances at inopportune times, so the nurse uses active listening. The child may also be shunned or laughed at by peers who do not understand the behavior; therefore, professional counseling may be needed.

Tic disorders do not often cause impairment of daily living. In fact, many of the manifestations are actually mild. Nursing interventions are predominantly geared toward helping the child and family cope with the disorder.

Education/Discharge Instructions

Parents need to be aware of the fact that TS and other tics can create stress for the child and that the child may experience low self-esteem. The nurse can help the parents watch for signs that the child is being bullied by peers or siblings. Instruct the family to watch for signs of coexisting disorders such as ADHD or OCD.

Maltreatment of Children

Child maltreatment includes abuse and neglect of a child less than 18 years of age by anyone who is in a caregiver or custodial role (e.g., a parent, foster caregiver, clergy, coach, or teacher). The most common forms of abuse are physical, sexual, emotional abuse, and neglect (CDC, 2012a). **Child physical abuse** may result in injury inflicted by beating, pushing, kicking, pinching, burning, or choking. **Physical abuse** includes traumatic brain injury, which manifests as symptoms related to head trauma as a result of forceful shaking of the infant or young child.

Child sexual abuse involves any sexually related act, usually between a child and an adult (related or not) that can include fondling, forced or assented oral sex or intercourse, sodomy, exposing children to adult sexual behavior (e.g., showing pornography to children), and exploiting through child pornography or prostitution.

Child emotional abuse includes any behavior, attitude, or failure to act that disrupts children's socio-emotional development and mental health. Some examples include shaming or humiliating (ascribing derogatory labels to the child, e.g., "you are worthless"), and intimidating (threatening and frightening).

Child neglect involves failure to provide emotional and physical care as well as opportunity for education. Neglect is most common but also the most difficult to identify.

Other types of abuse include **Munchausen-by-proxy syndrome** in which a person, usually the mother, deliberately makes the child sick. **Electronic sexual luring** is enticing children via computer or other electronic means.

 Nursing Insight—*Incidence of child maltreatment*

Statistics gathered routinely by the U.S. Department of Health and Human Services track the incidence of child maltreatment and give a breakdown of the incidence of the various types of maltreatment. Abuse is counted based on the number of times the child is found to be a victim. The federal fiscal year 2010 duplicate victim rate was 10.0 victims per 1,000 children in the population. The unique victim rate was 9.2 victims per 1,000 children in the population (http://www.acf.hhs.gov/programs/cb/pubs/cm10/cm10.pdf#page=31).

- More than five children die every day as a result of child abuse.
- Child abuse occurs at every socioeconomic level, across ethnic and cultural lines, within all religions, and at all levels of education (http://www.childhelp.org/pages/statistics).

Signs and Symptoms

The signs and symptoms of abuse are multifaceted (Table 22-3).

It is also important to note that posttraumatic stress disorder found in children or the adolescent can be maltreatment undetected or not caught early in the presentation of such symptoms.

Diagnosis

Diagnosis of physical, sexual, or emotional abuse or neglect may take time, and a thorough family history, physical examination, and developmental assessment are necessary for diagnosis. It may be necessary to x-ray various areas of the body in addition to obtaining serum chemistry lab tests to determine any infection, drug induction, or toxicity.

Table 22-3 Physical, Sexual, Emotional Abuse, Neglect, and Munchausen by Proxy

Type of Abuse	Tactics of Abuse	Possible Signs and Symptoms in the Child
Physical: Bodily injury caused by intentional or unintentional physical aggression	Beating, hitting, slapping, poisoning, kicking, pinching, biting, shoving, choking, pulling hair, burning Excessive corporal punishment	Suspicious bruises, welts, or burns Unexplained fractures or dislocations New and healing or healed lacerations or abrasions Wariness of adults or caregivers Fearful of going home Acting out with aggression
	Shaken baby syndrome	Retinal hemorrhages CNS injury
	Munchausen by proxy	Prolonged or recurrent illnesses or injuries that cannot be explained
Sexual: Sexual acts involving an adult and a child	Penetration, incest, rape, oral sex, sodomy, fondling Violations of bodily privacy Exposing children to adult sexuality	Inappropriate or precocious interest in or knowledge of sexuality Poor peer relationships Sudden changes in behavior (regressive, acting out, sexual behavior, enuresis, recurrent urinary tract infections, redness and swelling of genitalia)
	Commercial exploitation Sexual exploitation (prostitution or pornography)	Running away from home or substance abuse Rapidly declining school performance Suicide attempts
Emotional: Attitude, behavior, or failure to act that interferes with a child's mental health or social development	Intimidation, belittling, shaming, lack of affection and warmth, habitual blaming, ignoring or rejection, extreme punishment, exposure to violence, child exploitation, child abduction	Apathy, depression Hostility Difficulty concentrating
Neglect: Pattern of failing to meet basic needs	Physical, educational, emotional	Clothing unsuited to the weather Poor hygiene Hunger Lack of supervision

Prevention

focus on safety

Risk factors for maltreatment

If a nurse can identify risk factors related to the maltreatment, the harm to children may be prevented. Children who are at risk for maltreatment include:

- Children with disabilities
- Children of very young parents
- Children of young single mothers who live in poverty
- Parents who suffer from mental or chronic physical illness
- Parents who have:
  - extremely stringent ideas of discipline may use harsh punishment
  - excessive stress
  - marital conflict
- Parental substance abuse
- Intergenerational history of abuse

Collaborative Care

Nursing Care. The nurse is instrumental in the care of children who have experienced any type of abuse. There are primary and secondary preventive strategies that the nurse can use:

- Discuss with parents ways to discipline the child that do not involve physical or verbal aggression.
- Educate parents regarding birth control to decrease unintended pregnancies.
- Instruct mothers about the use of alcohol or drugs during pregnancy and the impact it has on the growing baby.
- Decrease the use of drugs or alcohol by new parents.
- Improve the availability of and access to health care across the spectrum of the family's life.
- Educate children and adolescents about the body and personal boundaries.
- Advocate for political initiatives to help avoid and ultimately stop child abuse.

Professionals who report child abuse are not revealed to the family in question unless the caller chooses to disclose this information. While all reports are taken seriously, not all reports result in the removal of the child from the home. Every report is investigated, but action may or not be taken depending on the assessment (Childhelp National Child Abuse Hotline, 2012). It is also important to note that the nurse is required to report any suspicion of child abuse or neglect.

Education/Discharge Instructions

- Provide parents with information regarding "normal" stages of growth and development.
- Provide family education about what to expect from parenthood.
- Instruct parents on how to cope with some of the difficult times related to raising a child.
- Help parents develop resources for support, such as babysitters, family members, and community resources.

legal alert—Report cases of child abuse

To report suspected child abuse, the nurse can call the local enforcement agency and/or follow the clinical setting's guidelines for reporting abuse. All U.S. states have mandatory reporting guidelines for professionally licensed healthcare workers/providers. It can be a difficult experience to report child abuse because of possible consequences to the child, family, and professional. It is important to remember that all allegations of child abuse must first be investigated before confirmed. After documented confirmation, the child will be placed in a safe environment free of abuse.

National Hotline in USA: 1-800-4-A-CHILD or 1-800-422-4453

For more information consult the link:

http://www.helpguide.org/mental/child_abuse_physical_emotional_sexual_neglect.htm#online

Substance Use and Abuse

Substance abuse refers to the repeated use of illicit substances (drugs or alcohol or inhalants) despite the negative consequences. **Substance dependence/addiction** refers to the physiological and/or emotional reliance on that substance with tolerance and withdrawal symptoms noted (APA, 2013).

Nursing Insight—*Substance use and abuse*

Children and adolescents may abuse any of the same substances abused by adults. The major factors determining which substances are used are availability and cost. Some of the more common substances of abuse for children and adolescents include alcohol, tobacco, marijuana, cocaine, ecstasy, methamphetamine, other forms of stimulants, prescription medications (e.g., the child's own prescription or medications stolen from a family member), and inhalants (e.g., glue, gasoline, and white-out).

Signs and Symptoms

The American Academy of Child & Adolescent Psychiatry (AACAP, 2010b) published a list online of some of the warning signs that a young person might be abusing alcohol or drugs:

- Physical: fatigue, repeated health complaints, red and glazed eyes, and a lasting cough
- Emotional: personality change, sudden mood changes, irritability, irresponsible behavior, low self-esteem, poor judgment, depression, and a general lack of interest
- Family: starting arguments, breaking rules, or withdrawing from the family
- School: decreased interest, negative attitude, drop in grades, many absences, truancy, and discipline problems
- Social problems: new friends who are less interested in standard home and school activities, problems with the law, and changes to less conventional styles of dress and music

Diagnosis

Diagnosis of substance use and abuse is based on the physical, emotional, and social factors exhibited by the child. A thorough family history is essential along with information about the child's physical and emotional health.

Prevention

Parents can help prevent substance abuse in their families. This does require an investment of time and energy into their children's and adolescent's lives. Parents can:

- Communicate their concerns about substance use
- Clearly state what the expectations are for behavior
- Get acquainted with the friends of the children and adolescents
- Have full knowledge of the location of the children
- Establish rules that are developmentally appropriate for the age of the child

Parents concerned about their children's mental health should seek treatment because untreated psychiatric disorders can increase the risk of substance abuse (AACAP, 2010b).

Collaborative Care

Nursing Care. Initial nursing care involves the use of screening tools to assess drug and alcohol use in children. The nurse is in an ideal position to identify adolescents at risk for substance abuse, especially if there is a strong family and genetic history of abuse. Two tools that can be used in the identification of substance abuse are the CRAFFT (Knight, Sherritt, Shrier, Harris, & Chang, 2002) and the CAGE (Ewing, 1984). Both of these tools use simple acronyms to assist in the evaluation of drinking or drug use (Table 22-4).

The CRAFFT is recommended by the American Academy of Pediatrics' Committee on Substance Abuse for use as a screening tool with adolescents. It consists of a series of six questions developed to screen adolescents for high risk alcohol and other drug use disorders simultaneously. It is a short, effective screening tool meant to assess whether a longer conversation about the context of use, frequency, and other risks and consequences of alcohol and other drug use is warranted.

Screening using the CRAFFT begins by asking the adolescent to "Please answer these next questions honestly"; telling him or her "Your answers will be kept confidential"; and then asking three opening questions.

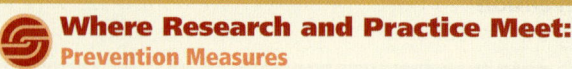

Where Research and Practice Meet:
Prevention Measures

Some preliminary work has been funded by Substance Abuse and Mental Health Services Administration, the National Institute of Mental Health, the National Institute on Drug Abuse, and the National Institute on Alcohol Abuse and Alcoholism with some initial recommendations for a multifaceted approach to address prevention of substance abuse in children and adolescents. Strategies have been developed to later be tested for effectiveness in various population groups. Universal prevention measures would be shared with the general public. Selected prevention measures have been created that target subgroups that have a significantly higher probability of developing a mental, emotional, or behavioral disorder (Institute of Medicine of the National Academies, 2009).

If the adolescent answers "No" to all three opening questions, the provider only needs to ask the adolescent the first question—the CAR question. If the adolescent answers "Yes" to any one or more of the three opening questions, the provider asks all six CRAFFT questions.

CRAFFT is a mnemonic acronym of first letters of key words in the six screening questions. The questions are asked exactly as written.

C Have you ever ridden in a CAR driven by someone (including yourself) who was "high" or had been using alcohol or drugs?

R Do you ever use alcohol or drugs to RELAX, feel better about yourself, or fit in?

A Do you ever use alcohol/drugs while you are by yourself, ALONE?

F Do you ever FORGET things you did while using alcohol or drugs?

F Does your family or FRIENDS ever tell you that you should cut down on your drinking or drug use?

T Have you gotten into TROUBLE while you were using alcohol or drugs?

Table 22-4 The CRAFFT and CAGE Tools Use Simple Acronyms to Assist in the Evaluation of Drinking or Drug Use

Evaluating the Child for Substance Abuse: Two common ways of evaluating for substance abuse are CRAFFT and CAGE.

CRAFFT	CAGE
Have you ever ridden in a **C**ar driven by someone (including yourself) who was high or had been using alcohol or drugs?	Have you ever felt like **C**utting down on your drinking?
Do you ever use alcohol or drugs to **R**elax, feel better about yourself, or fit in?	Have people made you **A**ngry by talking about your drinking?
Do you ever use alcohol or drugs while you are by yourself **A**lone?	Have you ever felt **G**uilty about your drinking?
Do you ever **F**orget things you did while using alcohol or drugs?	Do you ever need a drink first thing in the morning to have enough **E**nergy or to feel ready for the day?
Do your **F**amily or **F**riends ever tell you that you should cut down on your drinking or drug use?	
Have you ever gotten into **T**rouble while you were using alcohol or drugs?	
Scoring: 2 or more positive items indicate the need for further assessment.	Scoring: 2 or more positive answers = an alcohol problem. Note: this tool is used with individuals 16 and older
Source: Reprinted from Center for Adolescents Substance Abuse Research at Children's Hospital, Boston.	*Source:* Ewing, J. A. (1984). Detecting alcoholism: The CAGE questionnaire. Public Domain.

For more information, link to the following Web site http://www.ceasar-boston.org/CRAFFT/index.php

Education/Discharge Instructions

- Be alert to early signs of substance use (e.g., smelling alcohol or cigarette smoke)
- Observe for changes in mood or odd behavior when the adolescent returns home (AACAP, 2010c).

The nurse can help the child and family find community resources that may help conquer the substance abuse problem. The most promising appears to be a family-based, family-supported approach (Gifford, 2011).

Eating Disorders

Eating disorders that are mostly apparent in adolescence are classified into four categories that include **anorexia nervosa** (purging or withholding), **bulimia nervosa** (binging and purging), **binge eating disorder** (binging without purging), and eating disorder not otherwise specified (APA, 2013).

Eating disorders most often affect females, but adolescent males are also known to suffer from these illnesses.

focus on safety

Risk factors for development of an eating disorder

- Family genetics
- Rigidity, ritualism in home
- Stressful life event
- Hormonal and physiological changes associated with puberty
- "Picky" eater in childhood
- Participation in sports that focus on the pursuit of thinness (APA, 2013); (Assessment Technologies Institute, 2010)

Signs and Symptoms

- Inordinate concern and gross distortion of body image and body weight
- Preoccupation with food
- Hide behaviors related to food and caloric intake from others
- Depression
- Anxiety
- Family discord; conflict avoidance
- Weight loss up to 85% of ideal body weight
- Consuming caloric intake but then purging by vomiting
- Vigorous physical activity
- Amenorrhea
- Weakness
- Fatigue (APA, 2013; Townsend, 2012).

focus on safety

Anorexia nervosa

Anorexia nervosa can become a life-threatening problem or cause death because of severe weight loss that can result in electrolyte imbalance and hemodynamic instability.

Diagnosis

Diagnostic criteria for anorexia nervosa:

- Weight less than 85% of expected weight
- Distorted body image
- Absence of three consecutive menstrual cycles

Diagnostic criteria for bulimia nervosa:

- Lack of control over eating
- Recurrent inappropriate compensatory behavior to prevent weight gain, such as vomiting
- Cycle of binge eating and inappropriate compensatory behaviors occurring at least twice a week for 3 months (APA, 2013)

 Assessment Tool Eating Disorders

The nurse can also use astute assessment skills to help diagnose the child or adolescent suspected of an eating disorder. The nurse needs to determine:
- Perception of issue, shape, and weight
- Eating habits
- Mental status: cognitive distortions: "my life is over if I gain 5 pounds"
- Participation in rigorous physical regimen
- Vitals: blood pressure, pulse, and temperature will be low
- Lanugo
- Jaundice
- Cool extremities with poor skin turgor
- Dental erosion, if purging
- Peripheral edema
  (Assessment Technologies Institute, 2010)

Laboratory tests
Abnormal lab results associated with eating disorders:
- Hypokalemia
- Hyponatremia
- Anemia
- Leukopenia
- Increased liver enzyme levels
- Elevated bilirubin level
- Decreased levels of follicle-stimulating hormone
  (Assessment Technologies Institute, 2010; Van Leeuwen, Poelhuis-Leth, & Bladh, 2011)

Diagnostic tools
- Electrocardiogram changes such as prolongation of the QT interval, bradycardia, and ventricular tachycardia with a risk of sudden death also need to be evaluated. (Macías-Robles, Perez-Clemente, Maciá-Bobes, Alvarez-Rueda, & Pozo-Nuevo, 2009)

Prevention

The nurse is in the best position to identify early cases of eating disorders and refer for preventive individual and family treatment. The nurse has to keep in mind that the assessment needs to be conducted within a growth and developmental perspective and that intervention is considered within a family-based approach.

Collaborative Care

Nursing Care. Mental health nursing care measures are essential in the treatment of a child or adolescent diagnosed with an eating disorder. The nurse can employ these measures if the child is admitted to a mental health-care facility or teach the parents these care measures to use in the home environment. Such measures include:

- Provide a highly structured environment
- Involve patient in decision making and participation in the plan of care

- Assist patient in setting realistic weight goals
- Promote cognitive reframing: assist patient in changing the negative perception to a positive one
- Monitor patient's weight, vitals, intake and output, caloric intake, and exercise (Assessment Technologies Institute, 2010).

There are no drugs that are specifically for eating disorders; however, there are medications that treat the core symptoms of eating disorders. For example, selective serotonin reuptake inhibitors have been useful in reducing obsessive compulsive behaviors and craving for carbohydrates (Townsend, 2012).

Education/Discharge Instructions

When making referrals for treatment, it is important to consider the skill level of the treatment clinician, and often a team approach with expertise in this area of health and mental health works best. It is important to instruct families that treatment for eating disorders can take a long time and that family members will be involved in the recovery.

Obesity

Obesity in children and adolescents is widespread and is considered to be an important U.S. and international public health problem. The percentage of children aged 6 to 11 years in the United States who were obese increased from 7% in 1980 to nearly 20% in 2008. Similarly, the percentage of adolescents aged 12 to 19 years who were obese increased from 5% to 18% over the same period (CDC, 2012b).

Overweight is defined as having excess body weight for a particular height from fat, muscle, bone, water, or a combination of these factors. **Obesity** is defined as having excess body fat.

Overweight and obesity are the result of "caloric imbalance"—too few calories expended for the amount of calories consumed—and are affected by various genetic, behavioral, and environmental factors (CDC, 2011b).

The rates are rising in the countries that are more economically developed (Linnard-Palmer, 2010).

Childhood obesity is of epidemic proportions, and while obesity is not currently classified as an eating disorder, the psychological factors involved are significant (Fig. 22-3). Being overweight or obese deserves a multidisciplinary approach to correct the issues presented. Individuals with obesity present with many physiological problems that go along with obesity including hypertension, diabetes, shortness of breath, and increased risk for cardiovascular disease (Townsend, 2012). In addition to the physiological problems encountered, children who are overweight or obese may experience psychosocial difficulties because they may be teased or bullied by peers, leading to difficulties with self-esteem and social development.

🌼 *Nursing Insight*—*Obesity*

Today there is a movement in schools to prevent childhood obesity. In the last 30 years, the national incidence of childhood

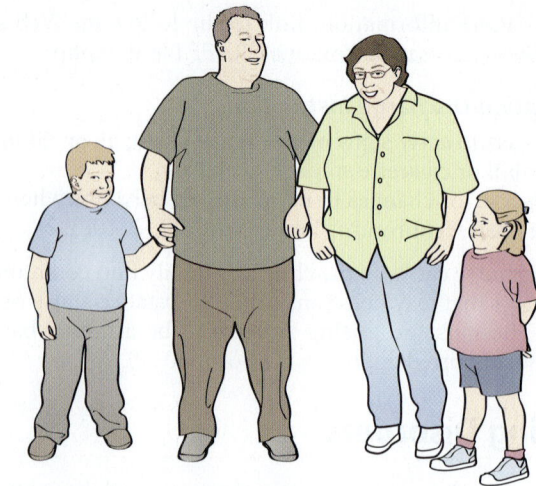

Figure 22-3 Childhood obesity is of epidemic proportions in the United States.

obesity among 12- to 19-year-olds has more than tripled. Today, more than a third of all teenagers across the United States are categorized as either overweight or obese. "It's especially alarming because the consequences of childhood obesity aren't felt today. They're felt 10, 20 years down the road" (Gersib, 2010, p. 1). Schools have made decisive efforts to address the obesity problem after a thorough assessment of their contribution to this issue:

- Cutbacks to physical education programs have reduced the opportunities for physical activity during the school day.
- Walking and biking to school is much less common than in generations past.
- Electronic sedentary behaviors (ESB), including television viewing, computer use (excluding use for homework), and gaming-system use, are on the rise.

During an average school day, students in Nebraska spend more than 3.5 hours engaging in ESB activities. In fact, 35% of students spend 5 or more hours each day in front of the television! In addition, 2009 statistics released by Lincoln Public Schools (LPS) reported that the rate of overweight and obese LPS fifth graders that receive free or reduced-cost meals in the bottom 50% of the income range is an alarming 12 points higher than the district-wide average. Almost 48% of these low-income students were determined to be either overweight or obese. It's clear there are socioeconomic factors at play in the childhood obesity issue as well. It is so important to get government, community leaders, and schools together to identify problems, develop solutions, and impact positive change on the community. One such program is *Teach a Kid to Fish*. This program instills healthy habits and develops a love of physical activity and the outdoors early in life. *Safe Routes Nebraska*, a federally funded program, supports building safer walking and biking routes to school. Schools, parent-teacher organizations, and other community groups can also access resources and information that can make it easier for children to become active during the time directly before and after school (Gersib, 2010).

Signs and Symptoms

Childhood obesity is determined by plotting the **body mass index (BMI)** percentile on a growth chart. The BMI = weight (in kg) divided by height (in meters) squared.

A BMI-for-age between the 5th and less than the 85th percentile is considered a healthy weight; children with a BMI-for-age between the 85th and less than the 95th percentile are considered overweight; and those with a BMI-for-age greater than or equal to 95% are considered obese. (Linnard-Palmer, 2010)

❝What to say❞—*About the child's weight problem*

When parents ask the nurse about a delay in their child's weight problem, the nurse can respond by asking relevant questions such as:

- Does your child have an elevated heart rate or increased blood pressure (even at rest)?
- Do you feel your child is overweight?
- Is your child breathless with minimal activity or movement?
- Does your child find it difficult to walk, run, or play for any extended period of time?
- Does your child (or do parents) report any bullying or teasing about being overweight?

Cultural Diversity: Disparities in Childhood Obesity

There are significant racial and ethnic disparities in obesity prevalence among U.S. children and adolescents. In 2007–2008, Hispanic boys aged 2 to 19 years were significantly more likely to be obese than non-Hispanic white boys, and non-Hispanic black girls were significantly more likely to be obese than non-Hispanic white girls (CDC, 2012b).

Certainly there are other factors that come into play such as poverty that impacts the ability to consume healthy foods. Social and cultural factors impact the perception in some cultures that obesity reflects wealth (Linnard-Palmer, 2010). Because food is expensive, many times children are told to "clean up their plates, finish all that is on their plate" even when the child is quite full already. Not wanting to disappoint their parents or caregivers, children will completely eat what is on their plates.

Diagnosis

Diagnosis of obesity is based on an excess of fat in proportion to lean body mass. The BMI correlates closely with total body fat, which is estimated using dual-energy x-ray absorptiometry scanning in children who are overweight and obese (Schwarz, 2012).

Prevention

Communities are the cornerstone for preventive interventions that increase the accessibility of fresh foods and physical activity, implement policies to reduce the marketing of unhealthy foods to children and adults, and help make informed and healthy nutritional choices easier, affordable, and accessible (Blumenthal, 2012; Plachta-Danielzik, Landsberg, Lange, Langnäse, & Müller, 2010; Swinburn, 2009).

For example, at the national level, several initiatives have been launched to address some of these issues. The Affordable Care Act 2010 has mandated inclusion of menu labeling in restaurants and on vending machines. The Healthy Hunger-Free Kids Act 2010 has set nutritional standards for foods served in schools and child care facilities. There are expanded efforts to promote breastfeeding in a number of Baby Friendly hospitals. Also, accommodations are being considered at the workplace for breastfeeding mothers. Furthermore, the Let's Move Campaign is mobilizing all sectors of society to get involved in reversing childhood obesity rates within a generation. As part of this initiative, the Child Care State Challenge is encouraging the adoption of voluntary standards for physical activity, limits on screen time, healthy beverages, and promoting the availability of healthy foods in child care settings (Blumenthal, 2012).

At the community level, new affordable housing neighborhoods like Greenbridge, Washington are being designed and built as models for creating an environment that promotes healthy diets and active lifestyles for their residents. In this predominantly immigrant community where more than 15 languages are spoken, more than 54% of adults are overweight or obese, and more than 85% of adolescents in grades 8, 10, and 12 do not meet the physical activity recommendations set by the federal government. A national program funded by the Robert Wood Johnson Foundation, Healthy Kids, and Healthy Communities promotes community-based solutions. This community has focused on shaping the environment to encourage healthy behaviors among families, with special attention to children who are at the highest risk. In addition to elementary schools, Head Start programs, and Boys and Girls Clubs, community gardens have been cultivated to grow fresh fruits and vegetables. Local parks and walking paths have also been built. Public health clinics are readily accessible in neighborhoods as well. Community centers also provide free exercise classes (Blumenthal, 2012). Motivated communities can make a difference and have an impact on our nation's children and adolescent obesity incidence and prevalence rates.

Collaborative Care

Nursing Care. Because obesity is such a pervasive problem in society today, nursing care measures are geared toward helping the child and family recognize the problem and help the child to return to a healthier state. Obesity is a sensitive subject to address with the child or adolescent and their parents. It will be important for the nurse to address the obesity as well as the child. It can be addressed purely from a physical perspective, that is, addressing the concerns of potential health risks in the future (e.g., diabetes, hypertension, and weight related disorders). Offer education and support because this condition needs to be approached from an emotional perspective as losing weight over time is doable. The change of lifestyle habits of the family become much easier to do when the entire family engages in new healthy habits together. This prevents the child or adolescent from feeling singled out. It is also important to come from a positive perspective, such as asking the family what has gone well before or what are the current healthy habits the family engages in. What does the family like to do? Families will stick with what is fun and what they like to do. What is the family willing to try? Set the goals with the family's input. With this "buy in" early on in the change process, the family will be motivated to act on the proposed and recommended changes.

Education/Discharge Instructions

- Inquire about the family's perception of food and weight.
- Conduct a comprehensive individual and family history (determine if there is a history of diabetes, dyslipidemia, or cardiovascular disease).
- Perform a thorough physical assessment.
- Teach the child and family about the value of a 24-hour recall, reflecting the dietary habits of the individual and family.
- Discuss an activity inventory of the individual and family to determine the amount of time spent in playing video games, watching TV, and other sedentary activities within a 24-hour period.
- Suggest fun-filled family activities such as walking, playing catch, and going to the zoo or park.
- Discuss the ordered laboratory tests (e.g., metabolic profile) with the family, both the purpose and results of such tests.
- Obtain a current height, weight, and BMI. Assess the past data.
- Inform the family that the Women Infants and Children programs provide healthy food selections.
- Educate new parents about healthful attitudes about food and feeding.

The nurse also communicates to the child and family that dieting is not suggested for children and adolescents. In fact, in the long run restrictive eating often contributes to continued overweight or to other eating problems. Nevertheless, focusing on healthy eating habits that can last throughout the lifetime is essential. It is important to empathize with the child who expresses dissatisfaction with his weight and provide education and guidance related to healthful eating and exercise.

? Global Health Case Study Hector Martinez

Hector Martinez is an 8-year-old boy who is in the third grade at a local elementary school. He lives at home with his parents and four other siblings ranging in age from 2 to 13 years of age. He weighs 150 pounds (68 kg) and is 4 foot 2 inches tall. The diet of the family consists of tortillas (cooked in saturated fat), beans, and rice at least twice a day. There are no fresh fruits or vegetables in the family's diet. The family mostly consumes high-fructose drinks such as soda. After school and on weekends, Hector sits at home and watches the television or plays video games. Once in a while he participates in after-school activities and is required to attend gym class once a week. The family's income and resources are limited with no access to health care.

critical thinking questions

1. Name two priority nursing diagnoses related to this situation.

2. Discuss the importance of family education and specific strategies that the nurse can use to teach the family to address Hector's weight problem.

◆ See Suggested Answers to Global Health Case Studies on DavisPlus.

Sleep Disorders

Adequate sleep is essential to good health. Sleep difficulties are relatively common in children and adolescents. It is estimated that between 20% and 25% of children and adolescents suffer from some type of sleep disturbance (Nutter, 2012). There are nearly 80 sleep disorders that affect children and adolescents (Sleep Education, 2012). These disorders cause varying degrees of symptoms and distress, but all are important to recognize and ameliorate. Sleep can be viewed as a part of normal growth and development because some sleep problems are considered normal and subside as the child grows. There is a reciprocal relationship between sleep disorders and other psychiatric disorders. In other words, many psychiatric disorders cause difficulties with sleep (e.g., depression, anxiety, ADHD, etc.), and conversely, a child whose sleep is impaired is more susceptible to stress-induced disorders (Bonuck & Grant, 2012). A good nursing assessment is essential in identifying sleep problems in children and in differentiating between physiological/psychological disorders versus developmental or behavioral issues (e.g., poor sleep hygiene, long daytime naps, caffeine consumption, etc.).

Signs and Symptoms

- Difficulty falling asleep at night
- Difficulty returning to sleep after waking up during the night
- Waking up frequently during the night
- Light sleep; not deep sleep
- Sleepiness and low energy during the day
- Daytime irritability
- Snoring or periods of sleep apnea

 Nursing Insight—*Common causes of sleep problems in children*

- Nightmares
- Sleep terrors
- Sleepwalking
- Episodes of insomnia
- Irregular sleep routine
- Caffeine intake
- Sleep apnea
- Restless leg syndrome

Diagnosis

A child who presents with sleep difficulties must receive a thorough physical examination to rule out physiological causes. It is important to assess sleep patterns as well as quality of sleep. Sleep disorders are considered based on a positive answer by the parent or caregiver to one or more of these questions:

- Is it hard for your child to fall asleep?
- Is it hard for your child to stay asleep through the night?
- Does your child wake up feeling tired?
- Is your child sleepy during the day?

Prevention

The nurse must listen carefully to the parents' concerns about the child's sleeping issues. It is important to discover this problem early and to understand the causes of sleep disturbances as well as to implement prevention and intervention strategies. Early identification and intervention are important in preventing significant emotional, developmental, and physical difficulties. The nurse educates parents about healthy sleep hygiene, management of respiratory disorders, pediatric depression, anxiety, and developmental and mental health diagnoses as a means of prevention of ongoing difficulties.

Collaborative Care

Nursing Care. The nurse can help the family by providing support while listening without passing judgment and providing information on healthy sleep habits. The American Academy of Sleep Medicine has developed a Web site for teachers (K–12) to help them better understand sleep in their students. The guidelines listed in Box 22-1 are also helpful for the nurse and the family.

Education/Discharge Instructions

Encourage the family to continue with follow-up care with the health-care provider and help them locate community resources such as a support group.

Case Study Sleeping Issues

Paul is 4 years old, and according to his mother, he has had sleeping difficulties since he was a baby. He voices many fears, makes demands, and sometimes has tantrums at bedtime. He says he is afraid of the dark even though he has a nightlight in his room. Paul complains of being hungry as soon as he lies down in bed. Unless his mother stays in the room with Paul until he falls asleep, he does not stop crying and often becomes upset for no apparent reason. Paul takes an afternoon nap until 5:00 p.m. Now that the family is expecting a new baby, they wish to have Paul's sleeping difficulties under control. He has a bedtime of 8:00 p.m., but he does not get to sleep until 11:00 p.m. or midnight unless he has not napped during the day.

critical thinking questions

1. Name the priority nursing diagnosis related to this situation.
2. Discuss the importance of parental education and specific sleep hygiene techniques that the nurse can teach.

◆ See Suggested Answers to Case Studies on Davis*Plus*.

 Now Can You—Discuss sleep disorders?

1. Explain how a nurse would assess a child who complains of a sleep disorder.
2. How can a sleep disorder be diagnosed?
3. Can you describe healthy sleep habits?

Developmental Disabilities

Developmental disability is a term that encompasses a number of serious disorders affecting the child's mental and/or physical developmental processes. The developmental disorders that will be discussed in this section are Down syndrome (DS), fragile X syndrome (FXS), and intellectual disabilities (formerly mental retardation). Each of these is evidenced by global delays in developmental

---

Box 22-1 Top 10 Healthy Sleep Habits for Children and Teens

1. Only use your bed for sleeping.
2. Avoid drinking caffeine in the afternoon and at night.
3. Avoid taking naps in the late afternoon or in the evening.
4. Avoid large meals right before bedtime.
5. Dim household lights at night and let in plenty of sunlight in the morning.
6. Create a healthy sleep environment in your bedroom with:
   a. Dim lighting
   b. A comfortable temperature
   c. Soothing sounds
   d. No TV or computer
7. Turn off all of these items at least 30 minutes before your bedtime:
   a. Computer
   b. TV
   c. Movies and videos
   d. Video games
   e. Cell phone or other popular technological devices
8. Develop a bedtime routine that helps you relax by:
   a. Eating a healthy snack or light dessert
   b. Brushing your teeth
   c. Taking a warm bath or shower
   d. Reading
   e. Listening to relaxing music
9. Go to bed at or near the same time every night, even on weekends.
10. Discuss any ongoing sleep problems with your parent or doctor.

Source: The American Academy of Sleep Medicine (2012).

---

functioning. There is wide variability in the classification of developmental disabilities. In addition to the three mentioned in this section, others include, but are not limited to, autism spectrum disorders, fetal alcohol syndrome disorders, and attention-deficit/hyperactivity disorder (ADHD) (CDC, 2011c). Each of these additional diagnoses will be discussed individually in this chapter. Developmental disabilities may co-occur with a variety of physical conditions such as seizures, sensory impairments, speech and language problems, and cerebral palsy. The incidence of developmental disabilities has increased significantly from 1997 to 2008 (Boyle, Boulet, Schieve, Cohen, Blumberg, Yeargen-Allsopp, et al., 2011; CDC, 2011c). Whether this is related to better screening and diagnosis, greater public awareness, or actual increased incidence is unclear (Boyle, et al., 2011). Continued screening is essential.

There are a number of conditions that may be responsible for these disorders. Genetic conditions that cause developmental disabilities, such as fragile X syndrome or Down syndrome, result when abnormal genes are inherited from parents or when there are errors in genetic combinations. Metabolic conditions such as phenylketonuria (PKU) can lead to developmental disabilities if not recognized and treated early. Pregnancy-related problems include alcohol ingestion or viral infection such as rubella. In addition, trauma or asphyxia during the birth process can lead to inadequate oxygen availability and may also cause developmental disabilities.

Prevention

Promoting good prenatal care will aid in preventing some of the developmental disabilities.

The nurse communicates to families that the most preventable forms of developmental disabilities are related to prenatal nutrition and abstinence from alcohol (CDC, 2012a). Genetic counseling may also be helpful, particularly in families where the parents are older or where there is history of fragile X syndrome.

Collaborative Care

Nursing Care. Nursing assessment of children with developmental disabilities includes information from the mother's prenatal history, birth history, and child's developmental progress. Each of these assessment categories provides the nurse and family with valuable information. The nurse understands that there is not one portrait of a developmentally disabled child and knows that each child with a disability has unique needs.

An important aspect of nursing care is ongoing communication with the family about the child's specific disability, treatment measures, and medications. Another focus of nursing care is helping the family build life skills for the child based on the degree of disability. The goal is for the child or adolescent to develop the greatest level of functioning and skills possible to maintain daily living. The nurse can encourage the family to use physical therapy, speech and language therapy, and special educational opportunities.

Education/Discharge Instructions

The nurse can teach the family about community resources such as the Special Olympics or schools for therapeutic horseback riding instruction. Group activities can build both motor and learning skills as well as provide socialization.

 ### Across Care Settings: Special education and related services

For eligible school-aged children (including preschoolers), special education and related services are available through the public school system. The schoolteacher, nurse, and parents work together to develop an Individualized Education Plan (IEP). This plan addresses the child's unique needs and provides the services to meet the needs of each child.

FRAGILE X SYNDROME

Fragile X syndrome (FXS) is the most common cause of developmental and intellectual disabilities in children (CDC, 2011d). It is a genetic disorder in which the protein necessary for normal brain development is not manufactured. It may be hard to discern infants who have Fragile X syndrome and infants with other disorders based on physical characteristics alone. Identification is based on awareness of the potential signs and symptoms as well as family genetic history. It is imperative that early identification of the disorder be made and that early intervention with the child and family begin so there is the best opportunity to maximize positive outcomes for the child and family. The nurse has an important role to help identify the disorder and then provide family education and

support and connect families with appropriate special education and health services.

Signs and Symptoms

Fragile X syndrome has the following signs and symptoms:

- Physical features: large head; elongated face; prominent ears, chin, and forehead
- Developmental delays: not reaching milestones in line with children in the same age group
- Learning disabilities: difficulty learning new skills; poor intellectual development
- Social/behavioral difficulties: poor communication, self-abuse, no eye contact, difficulty paying attention (CDC, 2011d)

Diagnosis

Diagnosis is made through DNA testing to find changes in the fragile X mental retardation (*FMR1*) gene. DNA testing is generally not done unless there is a known family history of the disorder or unless the physical symptoms are present.

Collaborative Care

Nursing Care. While there is no known cure for FXS, the nurse can help the family access and use early intervention services. Families need encouragement to take advantage of health care and social services available. They also need information about growth and development and anticipatory guidance to raise the child according to his or her developmental level.

Education/Discharge Instructions

The nurse can provide the family with information related to FXS and the potential sequelae. If medications are prescribed, particularly to deal with the behavioral symptoms, the nurse can provide valuable medication education and support.

DOWN SYNDROME

Down syndrome (DS) is the most common and readily identifiable chromosomal abnormality associated with developmental disabilities (National Dissemination Center for Children and Youth with Disabilities [NICHCY], 2010). New terminology identifies the child as having an intellectual disability. During cell development, the fetus receives 47 chromosomes instead of the normal 46. The extra chromosome changes the development of the body and the brain.

Signs and Symptoms

Common signs and symptoms of DS at birth include:

- Poor muscle tone
- Slanting eyes with folds of skin at the inner corners (epicanthal folds)
- Hyperflexibility
- Short, broad hands with a single crease across the palms of one or both hands
- Broad feet with increased space between the first and second toes
- Flat bridge of the nose
- Short, low-set ears
- Short neck with extra folds of skin
- Small head

- Small oral cavity and airway
- Short, high-pitched cries in infancy

Nursing Insight—*Down syndrome health-related issues*

In addition to distinct physical appearance, children with DS frequently have health-related issues:

- Heart defects
- Decreased immune function
- Gastrointestinal anomalies
- Visual and hearing difficulties
- Speech difficulties
- Hypothyroidism

Sleep apnea is also a problem noted in these children. Assessment of the child's sleep patterns is conducted asking the caregiver if the child snores and has pauses in breathing during sleep. If that is the case, then further evaluation is needed, and it begins with sleep studies that include electroencephalography.

Diagnosis

The diagnosis of DS is usually made from a chromosomal blood test shortly after birth. In addition, just as intelligence varies in the normal population, there is a wide variation in the DS population regarding cognitive abilities, behavior, and developmental progress.

Collaborative Care

Nursing Care. Nursing care of a child with DS is similar to that of any developmental disorder. The nurse must be sensitive to the needs of parents who have learned the newborn has the disorder. Helping parents cope and providing them with resources is an important nursing intervention.

Early intervention with children who have DS has become much more sophisticated. Early intervention serves to provide the best possible individualized care to children with DS so these individuals can make the most of personal capabilities. Nursing care is geared to the special physical, developmental, and emotional needs of each child. The nurse can coordinate programs designed to help children with DS. These programs offer speech therapy, cognitive and social skills, self-help skills, and occupational and physical therapies that may improve gross and fine motor development. The nurse is also in a good position to help families cope emotionally with living with a child with this disability.

Education/Discharge Instructions

The nurse can educate parents and families about the resources available for children with DS.

Collaboration in Caring—*Raising public awareness*

The nurse has a responsibility to raise public awareness and acceptance about children with DS. Children with DS can be included in mainstream educational curriculum and society. The parent, nurse, school personnel, and other individuals in the community can develop an IEP. The nurse can help the child with DS throughout the life span as the child grows into adulthood. Through improved public acceptance and increased community resources, more opportunities for persons with disabilities to live and work independently in the community are possible.

INTELLECTUAL DISABILITIES

In October, 2010, President Barack Obama signed *Rosa's Law,* changing the designation "mental retardation" to "intellectual disability" (National Dissemination Center for Children with Disabilities [NICHCY], 2011a). Intellectual disability may present across the spectrum, with minimal impairment at one end, to severe impairment at the other. There are a number of potential causes of intellectual disability. In addition to those mentioned earlier, PKU and the use of alcohol or drugs during pregnancy, other difficulties during pregnancy and birth (e.g., prematurity, low birth weight, lack of oxygenation, environmental toxins, illnesses, and malnutrition), or after birth (e.g., whooping cough, chickenpox, measles, *Haemophilus influenzae*, or exposure to environmental toxins) can contribute. Poverty may increase these risk factors.

Signs and Symptoms

Three criteria must be present for the diagnosis of intellectual disabilities to be made:

- An intelligence quotient (IQ) score significantly below average (i.e., below 70—average score is 100)
- Limitations in functions of daily life, such as communication, social situations, or school activities
- Onset before the age of 18 (APA, 2013).

There are four levels of developmental disabilities:

- Mild: IQ between 55 and 69; the person is generally able to live independently; by far the largest group of developmentally disabled children
- Moderate: IQ between 40 and 54; the person is able to function semi-independently
- Severe: IQ between 25 and 39; the person generally requires institutionalization or very close monitoring
- Profound: IQ below 25; the person requires total care

Diagnosis

Diagnosis of intellectual disabilities is based on determination of intellectual (i.e., IQ, reasoning, learning, and problem solving) and adaptive functioning (American Association on Intellectual and Developmental Disabilities [AAIDD], 2010). The diagnosis is also based on delays in reaching developmental milestones or inability to perform developmental tasks. The official diagnosis of intellectual disability is performed by a qualified health-care provider or a collaborative team of clinicians. These clinicians assess developmental progress at various stages of development and perform intelligence and achievement testing. With a confirmed diagnosis of developmental disabilities, the nurse can assess the level of functioning of the child and the family and determine their current level of need. The nurse can communicate to parents that using standardized tests can further suggest a diagnosis.

Prevention

Preventative measures that address education of parents prior to and during pregnancy may help prevent intellectual disabilities. As with all developmental disabilities, recognition of and amelioration of environmental and maternal health risk factors decreases the possibility of intellectual disability. In addition, promoting health and safety measures for the infant, toddler, and young child (e.g., nutrition, safety awareness, lead prevention, child safety seats, etc.) is essential.

Collaborative Care

Nursing Care. Nursing care of the children with developmental disabilities includes information gained from the mother such as prenatal history, birth history, and child's developmental progress. Each of these assessment categories provides the nurse and family with valuable information.

There is not one portrait of a developmentally disabled child. Some mildly disabled children may not appear "different." The nurse knows that each child with a type of disability has unique needs.

An important aspect of nursing care is ongoing communication with the family about the child's specific disability, treatment measures, and medications. The nurse communicates to families that the most preventable forms of developmental disabilities are related to prenatal nutrition and abstinence from alcohol. Tell families that genetic counseling that may also be helpful, particularly in families in which the parents are older or when there is history of FXS. Promoting good prenatal care, encouraging parents to have their children immunized, and enforcing safe practices when bike-riding or playing may help prevent developmental disabilities.

Education/Discharge Instructions

Another focus of nursing care is helping the family find educational resource tools that are directed toward building life skills for the child based on the degree of disability. The goal is for the child or adolescent to develop the greatest level of functioning and skills possible to maintain daily living. The nurse can encourage the family to use physical, speech, and language therapy. The nurse can teach the family about community resources such as the Special Olympics or schools for therapeutic horseback riding instruction. Group activities can build both motor and learning skills as well as provide socialization.

AUTISM SPECTRUM DISORDERS

Autism spectrum disorders (ASDs) can be first diagnosed in infancy or childhood. Symptoms typically appear by age three (CDC, 2011e). The DSM-V defines autism spectrum disorder as a continuum of disorders that involve limitations in social relatedness, verbal and nonverbal communication, and the range of interests and behaviors (APA, 2013).

Signs and Symptoms

ASDs have these signs and symptoms:

- Persistent qualitative impairment in social reciprocity (i.e., unable to engage in socially appropriate communication).
- Impaired communication (using no language, or using deviant speech with errors in tone, prosody, pitch, grammar, or pragmatics [taking turns]).
- Restrictive or repetitive behaviors, interests, or activities.

 Nursing Insight—*Autism spectrum disorders*

The reported number of children with ASDs has increased since the early 1990s. The estimated incidence in 2004 was 1 in 166 children. The most recent reporting by the CDC (2011e) indicated an increase in prevalence by 2008 to 1 in 88 children. Whether this reflects a true increase in prevalence or an increase in reporting continues to be a matter of speculation. The factors involved in understanding the potential increase in prevalence include that the true prevalence rates 10 or 20 years ago are difficult to ascertain retrospectively, changes in diagnostic criteria (e.g., the concept of autism is now viewed as a spectrum of disorders), a heightened public awareness of autism, and increased media coverage of affected children and families (CDC, 2011e).

Diagnosis

In 2003, a partnership between the American Pediatric Association and the Centers for Disease Control and Prevention created a program called First Signs (http://www.firstsigns.org/delays_disorders/other_disorders.htm).

This widely disseminated public awareness campaign was designed to increase pediatric primary care provider and parental awareness about the signs and symptoms of autism. Based on this awareness, a thorough developmental history is conducted that can lead to an early diagnosis. Recent speculation on a relationship between vaccinations and autism has been disproved (IOM, 2009).

 Critical Nursing Action Understanding Autism Spectrum Disorder

The CDC has developed an initiative entitled "Learn the Signs. Act Early" which has a three-pronged approach to improving detection and care of children with ASD and other developmental disorders (www.cdc.gov/milestones). The 3-tiered program focuses on health education, early screening and intervention, and research and evaluation. The CDC offers education related to helping parents understand and track early developmental milestones, encouraging them to act early if they have questions or concerns about their child's progress. The campaign partners with systems from state, territorial, and national efforts to broaden collaborative efforts to help parents and professionals. The research and evaluation component of the program strives to continually develop resources and tools for early identification and referral.

The CDC developed the following guidelines, employing the acronym Autism A.L.A.R.M. to highlight important information the nurse can use in helping families with autistic children.

Autism is prevalent

- 1 out of 6 children is diagnosed with a developmental disorder and/or behavioral problem.
- 1 in 88 children is diagnosed with an ASD. Developmental disorders have subtle signs and may be easily missed.

Listen to patients:

- Early signs of autism are often present before 18 months.
- Parents usually do have concerns that something is wrong.
- Parents generally do give accurate and quality information.
- When parents do not spontaneously raise concern, ask if they have any concerns.

Act early:

- Know the subtle differences between typical and atypical development.
- Learn to recognize red flags.
- Improve the quality of life for children and their families through early and appropriate intervention.

Refer:

- To the Web for sources related to early intervention of autism or a local school program.
- To an autism specialist, or team of specialists, immediately for a definitive diagnosis.
- To audiology to rule out a hearing impairment.
- To local community resources for help and family support.

Monitor:

- Schedule a follow-up appointment to discuss concerns more thoroughly.
- Look for other features known to be associated with autism.
- Educate parents and provide them with up-to-date information.
- Advocate for families with local early intervention programs, schools, respite care agencies, and insurance companies.
- Continue surveillance and watch for additional or late signs of autism and/or other developmental disorders.

Collaborative Care

Nursing Care. Nurses who work in primary care settings can provide care for children with autism. Awareness of the need for early intervention is important because of the substantial cortical plasticity (the ability of tissues to grow during early brain development). There are many successful nonmedical treatments for children with autism. One of the most important interventions involves early language development. Poor functional communication skills also contribute significantly to the problematic behaviors that some autistic children display (e.g., poor frustration tolerance and aggression toward self or others). Equally important are interventions that address social competence. The nurse can teach parents that social skills training and acquisition groups provide the child with an opportunity to learn and practice appropriate social relatedness (Kasari, Rotheram-Fuller, Locke, & Gulsrud, 2012).

The nurse can assist the child and family in coping with this disorder. Children with ASDs respond best to structure and predictability. Learning and social interactions is approached systematically and gradually, allowing the child to develop comfort with the concepts. As with the schizophrenic child, it is important to stay aware of the child's physical boundaries and reluctance to be touched by others.

Education/Discharge Instructions

Parents can be taught the A.L.A.R.M. acronym as a means of understanding ASD and its treatment.

FETAL ALCOHOL SPECTRUM DISORDER

The **teratogenic effects** (causing abnormal development of the embryo) of alcohol have long been recognized. Warnings against drinking while pregnant are carried on all alcoholic beverages. Still, fetal alcohol spectrum disorder (FASD) is a common disorder with a range of physical and neurodevelopmental problems that are known to be completely preventable. The CDC estimates the occurrence of FASD at 40,000 babies/year (CDC, 2012b). FASD results from maternal consumption of alcohol during pregnancy. Data show that alcohol intake at any time of pregnancy is harmful.

FASD describes a continuum of alcohol-related disorders that includes fetal alcohol syndrome (FAS), alcohol-related neurodevelopmental disorder (ARND), alcohol-related birth defects (ARBD), and fetal alcohol effects (FAE) (Substance Abuse and Mental Health Services Administration [SAMHSA], 2012).

Signs and Symptoms

Nurses working in the nursery or in the neonatal intensive care unit may be able to identify the physiological features of FASD. Other symptoms become apparent as the child's development progresses.

- **FAS:**
  - Abnormal facial features (i.e., epicanthal folds, flat mid-face, short nose, short eye openings, thin upper lip, underdeveloped jaw, and groove in upper lip)
  - Growth problems
  - Hyperactive behavior
  - Learning and attention difficulties
  - Poor motor skills
  - Developmental delays or disabilities
- **ARND:**
  - Intellectual disabilities
  - Behavioral problems
  - Learning problems
  - Poor attention
  - Poor judgment
  - Poor impulse control
- **ARBD:**
  - Physiological problems (heart, kidneys, orthopedic, and/or hearing)

Diagnosis

Early diagnosis is important, but often very difficult without definitive evidence of maternal alcohol ingestion. A diagnosis of FASD requires a comprehensive history, including information on maternal consumption of alcohol during pregnancy. Physical characteristics at birth can alert the nurse that the infant needs further testing for this syndrome.

Prevention

The nurse can communicate to families that FASD and ARND are 100% preventable, and as such, it is important to develop prevention programs to reduce the rates of these disorders. Nurses can provide information to families about the effects of alcohol on the fetus. School nurses especially can facilitate early education regarding alcohol consumption during pregnancy. Because there are no guidelines about safe consumption rates for pregnant women, the public must know that the safe amount is no alcohol intake during pregnancy. In addition, nurses can help to identify cases of FASD and help families seek appropriate services.

Collaborative Care

Nursing Care. While there is no cure for FASD, nurses must understand that early intervention and referral can help the child and family function optimally. Involving the child in early education such as the birth-to-three services as an infant and in special education as a preschooler can help her learn adaptive skills to use throughout life. Help parents or caregivers work with their child and learn about limitations and strengths of the child.

Education/Discharge Instructions

Women of childbearing age can be informed of the preventability of FAS through abstinence from alcohol ingestion during pregnancy. Parents with a child who has FAS must be taught how to cope with behaviors and given resources to help them deal with their limitations.

Learning Disabilities and Cognitive Impairment

The nurse understands that a child may manifest challenges in more than one specific learning area, including math, reading, and organizing skills. Early learning challenges are influenced by emotional and social competencies, auditory processing and language skills (e.g., memory and ability to retrieve), perceptual motor skills, motor planning (e.g., sequencing and visual memory), visual/spatial processing skills, and ability to modulate sensory information. The ability to learn involves many of these skills working together. Increased information about learning issues may help identify this condition early and initiate preventive interventions. Learning disabilities are very common. The U.S. Department of Education reported in 2010 that 1 out of 5 people in this country has a learning disability (NICHCY, 2011b).

There are several learning disabilities including, but not limited to:

- Reading Disorder (Dyslexia)—significantly impaired ability to read; words or letters may be "mixed up" or distorted, making it impossible to recognize what others see.
- Arithmetic Disorder (Dyscalculia)—significant inability to understand or recognize numbers or functions of numbers, or copy them correctly, or follow sequences.
- Writing Disorder (Dysgraphia)—difficulties forming letters or writing within a prescribed space.
- Language Disorder (delays in or lack of ability to understand or express verbal communication).
  (NIH, Eunice Kennedy Shriver National Institute of Child Health & Human Development, 2010)

Signs and Symptoms

Signs and symptoms of learning disabilities commonly seen in children include:

- Academic achievement significantly less than would be expected for her age, education, and level of intelligence
- Significant interference with academic performance or activities that require reading, math, or writing skills (APA, 2013)

The nurse understands that a multidimensional approach is used to assess early learning patterns. The recommended areas for assessment include functional, emotional, and developmental capacities, auditory processing and language, visuospatial capacities, and regulatory-sensory processing patterns.

Diagnosis

Diagnosis is made through comprehensive assessments involving interviews and observation. Definitive testing is recommended before a learning disorder or challenge is diagnosed.

Prevention

Early identification of learning challenges are conducted before a child is fully immersed in an academic environment so that early intervention can begin. Early identification and treatment gives the child the greatest potential for a good outcome.

Collaborative Care

Nursing Care. The nurse communicates to the family that the child's strengths are incorporated as part of assessment, early prevention, and intervention. The nurse can fully inform the parents about their child's rights and entitlements in the public school sector. Often, children who enter public education with a learning challenge or disability will have an Individualized Education Plan (IEP) that is revised every few months.

Education/Discharge Instructions

The nurse can teach the parents about how to capitalize on their child's strengths. School nurses are particularly useful in providing education and support to children and their families.

Elimination Disorders

ENCOPRESIS

The DSM-V describes **encopresis** as the passage of feces into inappropriate places and locations repeatedly such as on the wall, clothing, or furniture (APA, 2013). Encopresis is primary (in children who have not become consistently continent by age 5) or secondary (children who have been continent and then become incontinent for a period of time). The child may present with either constipation with fecal incontinence because of overflow of feces, or without constipation.

Signs and Symptoms

Common signs and symptoms of encopresis are:

- Constipation
- Pain and straining with defecation
- Anxiety about defecating in a specific place
- Anal fissure
- Fecal retention

Diagnosis

Diagnostic criteria for encopresis include:

- Placement of feces into inappropriate places occurring once a month for at least 3 months
- Occurs in child at least 4 years old or older (APA, 2013)

Collaborative Care

Nursing Care. It is important for the nurse to talk to the parents about the child's defecation patterns during a medical appointment. The nurse also understands that it is important to take a thorough history of bowel habits and

Where Research and Practice Meet:
Encopresis

Coehlo (2011) evaluated both the medical and family approach to the problem of encopresis in children. The results showed when both medical and behavioral strategies were used with children that greater success was observed. Some of the strategies that were recommended were nutritional changes, bowel training, use of oral stool softeners, and behavioral modifications. Family support and education was vital as progress was monitored and changes made in the treatment plan. A multidisciplinary team, including the child and parents, provide the best support for the most effective treatment plan. Even with the most effective treatment, children with encopresis generally take up to 6 months or longer to regain bowel control. Times of transition can interfere with the progress. Dedication and time will reap positive outcomes for both the child and the family. Achievement of this milestone can then be a family celebration. (Coehlo, 2011).

In nearly all published series, boys are much more commonly affected than girls. As much as 80% of affected children are boys.

---

toilet training. Monitoring the occurrence of constipation will give an indicator of the cause(s). It is also important to evaluate the child's dietary habits, focusing on the amount of fiber and liquids the child consumes.

Education/Discharge Instructions

Once defecation patterns have been established, the nurse can then make recommendations. A high-fiber diet can prevent constipation. The nurse can also talk to the parents to determine any life transitions that may be happening in the child's life such as moving, a new baby in the household, or loss of a caregiver.

It is important for the nurse to help the family understand healthy toilet training. Making defecation nonstressful and rewarding may help the child change the behavior. A child's potty is recommended to help the child position him- or herself to push stool out adequately. Because family stress and change can contribute to encopresis, referral of the family for counseling may be in order

Summary Points

- Vulnerability is defined as a pre-dispositional factor, or set of factors, that makes a disordered state possible. Resilience is a dynamic developmental process reflecting evidence of positive adaptation despite significant life adversity.

- There is research indicating that health-care disparities in racial and ethnic minorities are widespread compared with those in non-minorities, and barriers such as mistrust, fear, and discrimination stand in the way of optimal mental health outcomes in ethnically diverse families.

- Though there are increasing efforts to educate the public, the stigma of mental illness continues to be a major barrier to accessing mental health services for children and their families.

- Mental illness in children includes conditions such as anxiety, depression, posttraumatic stress disorder, suicide, bipolar disorder, schizophrenia, and autism spectrum disorder.

- The most effective treatment for attention-deficit/hyperactivity disorder is a combination of pharmacological and nonpharmacological interventions. Using both modalities allows for the control or abatement of symptomatic behavior.

- Child maltreatment is considered to be any action or failure to act by a person that endangers a child's physical or emotional health and development. A person is abusive if the person fails to nurture the child, physically injures the child, or relates sexually to the child.

- The nurse is in an ideal position to identify adolescents at risk for substance abuse, especially if there is a strong family and genetic history of abuse, referring for treatment as early as possible. Treatment might involve family psychoeducation regarding substance abuse.

- Anorexia nervosa can become a life-threatening problem or cause death because of severe weight loss that can result in electrolyte imbalance and hemodynamic instability.

- Communities are in a pivotal position to significantly impact the childhood and adolescent obesity issue.

- A number of factors can cause developmental disabilities: genetic conditions, such as Down syndrome or fragile X syndrome; metabolic conditions such as phenylketonuria; or pregnancy-related problems, including alcohol ingestion or viral infections such as rubella.

- The nurse recognizes that it is important to take a complete nursing history when assessing the child with elimination disorders.

Review Questions

Multiple Choice

1. In the emergency department, a 10-year-old child complains of dizziness, palpitations, sweating, and tingling sensations. The mother tells the nurse that recently her child has been talking about the fear of dying. The pediatric nurse analyzes these behaviors as signs and/or symptoms related to what condition?
   A. Attention-deficit/hyperactivity disorder
   B. Panic disorder
   C. Posttraumatic stress disorder
   D. Suicidal tendencies

2. The pediatric nurse working with at-risk children understands the term "resilience" to mean which of the following?
   A. Child's characteristics that predispose him or her to a disorder
   B. Ability of child to use resources to help cope with adversity
   C. Immune system functioning of the child to combat illness
   D. Child's belief that his life and his health are in his control

3. A nurse notes the diagnosis of "agoraphobia" on a child's chart. What does the nurse understand this to mean?
   A. Fear of the unknown
   B. Fear of small spaces
   C. Fear of leaving home
   D. Fear of death

4. A child has a diagnosis of dysthymic disorder. What assessment findings by the nurse are consistent with this condition?
A. Loss of interest in activities once enjoyed
B. Serious time-limited depression
C. Long-term, less intense depression
D. Inability to recognize feelings

5. The nurse working with children understands that in what time frame do symptoms of schizophrenia usually occur?
A. School age
B. Toddler
C. Early teens
D. Late teens and early adulthood

6. A child has the following behaviors: deliberately tries to annoy people, displays frequent anger and resentment, and blames others for all her problems. What disorder could this child have?
A. Oppositional defiant behavior
B. Conduct disorder
C. Schizophrenia
D. Attention-deficit/hyperactivity disorder

7. A nurse notes that a child has the diagnosis of echolalia on her chart. What assessment finding does the nurse expect with this condition?
A. The child will ask the nurse to repeat statements.
B. The child pretends to not hear what the nurse says.
C. The child repeats the last heard words or sounds.
D. The child says the same thing over and over again.

8. How many children does the nurse understand die of child abuse each day?
A. 1 to 2
B. greater than 5
C. 5 to 10
D. unknown

9. A nurse assesses a middle school child and finds a body mass index (BMI) in the 92nd percentile. What category does this place the child in?
A. Normal
B. Above normal
C. Overweight
D. Obese

10. The nurse working with children and adolescents knows that what percentage of this population suffers from sleep disorders?
A. 10% to 15%
B. 15% to 20%
C. 20% to 25%
D. 30% to 40%

See Answers to End of Chapter Review Questions on Davis*Plus.*

REFERENCES

American Academy of Child & Adolescent Psychiatry (AACAP). (2010a). Anxiety disorder resource center. Retrieved from http://www.aacap .org/cs/anxiety_disorder_resource_center/anxiety_disorder_faqs# anxietyfaq2

American Academy of Child & Adolescent Psychiatry (AACAP). (2010b). Substance abuse resource center. Retrieved from http://www.aacap .org/cs/substance_abuse_resource_center/substance_abuse_faqs# question5

American Academy of Child & Adolescent Psychiatry (AACAP). (2010c). Teens: Alcohol and other drugs. Retrieved from http://www.aacap .org/AACAP/Families_and_Youth/Facts_for_Families/Facts_for_ Families_Pages/Teens_Alcohol_And_Other_Drugs_03.aspx

American Academy of Child & Adolescent Psychiatry (AACAP). (2011a). Facts for families #85: Reactive attachment disorder. Retrieved from http://www.aacap.org

American Academy of Child & Adolescent Psychiatry (AACAP). (2011b). Facts for families # 72: Children with oppositional defiant disorder. Retrieved from http://www.aacap.org

American Association on Intellectual and Developmental Disabilities [AAIDD]. (2010). Retrieved from http://aaidd.org/

American Psychiatric Association (APA). (2013). *Diagnostic and statistical manual of mental disorders (DSM-V)* (5th ed.). Washington, DC: Author.

Assessment Technologies Institute. (2010). *RN mental health nursing,* (8th ed.). Content mastery series review module. Stilwell, KS: Assessment Technologies Institute.

Blumenthal, S. (2012). *Poverty and obesity: Breaking the link.* Retrieved from http://www.huffingtonpost.com/susan-blumenthal/poverty-obesity_ b_1417417.html?ncid=edlinkusaolp00000008

Bonuck, K., & Grant, R. (2012). Sleep problems and early developmental delay: Implications for early intervention. *Intellectual & Developmental Disabilities, 50*(1), 41–52.

Boyle, C. A., Boulet, S., Schieve, L. A., Cohen, R. A., Blumberg, S. J., Yeargen-Allsopp, M., & Kogan, M. D. (2011). Trends in the prevalence of developmental disabilities in US children, 1997–2008. *Pediatrics, 127,* 1034–1042 . Retrieved from http://pediatrics.aappublications.org/ content/early/2011/05/19/peds.2010-2989 doi:10.1542/peds.2010-2989

Bulechek, G. M., Butcher, H. K., & Dochterman, J. M., & Wagner, C. (2013). Nursing interventions classification (NIC) (6th ed.). St. Louis, MO: Elsevier Mosby.

Centers for Disease Control and Prevention (CDC). (2009). Suicide prevention Retrieved from http://www.cdc.gov/violenceprevention/ pub/youth_suicide.html

Centers for Disease Control and Prevention (CDC). (2011a). ADHD, Data & Statistics. Retrieved from http://www.cdc.gov/ncbddd/adhd/data .html

Centers for Disease Control and Prevention (CDC). (2011b). Basics about Childhood Obesity. Retrieved from http://www.cdc.gov/obesity/ childhood/basics.html

Centers for Disease Control and Prevention (CDC) (2011c). About Developmental Disabilities. Retrieved from http://www.cdc.gov/ncbddd/ developmentaldisabilities/index.html

Centers for Disease Control and Prevention (CDC). (2011d). Fragile X Syndrome Retrieved from http://www.cdc.gov/ncbddd/fxs/index.html

Centers for Disease Control and Prevention (CDC). (2011e). Autism Spectrum Disorders. Retrieved from http://www.cdc.gov/ncbddd/ autism/index.html

Centers for Disease Control and Prevention (CDC). (2012a). Child Maltreatment Prevention. Retrieved from http://www.cdc.gov/Violence Prevention/childmaltreatment/

Centers for Disease Control and Prevention (CDC). (2012b). Childhood Obesity Facts. Retrieved from http://www.cdc.gov/obesity/childhood/ data.html

Childhelp National Child Abuse Hotline. (2012). Misconceptions of reporting child abuse. Retrieved from http://www.childhelp.org/get_help

Children's Defense Fund. (2010). Mental Health Fact Sheet. Retrieved from http://www.childrensdefense.org/child-research-data-publications/ data/mental-health-factsheet.pdf

Children's Hospital Boston. (2009). The CRAFFT screening tool. CeASAR: The Center for Adolescent Substance Abuse Research. Retrieved from http://www.ceasar-boston.org/CRAFFT/index.php

Coehlo, D. P. (2011). Encopresis: A medical and family approach. *Pediatric Nursing, 37*(3), 107–112.

Coker, T. R., Rodriguez, M. A., & Flores, G. (2010, Jun). Family-centered care for US children with special health care needs: Who gets it and why? *Pediatrics, 125*(6), 1159–1167. Epub 2010, May 3. doi: 10.1542/peds.2009-1994

Disorders.org. (2011). *Tic disorders.* Retrieved from http://www.disorders .org/tic-disorders/

Essau, C. A., Conradt, J., Sasagawa, S., & Ollendick, T. H. (2012). Prevention of anxiety symptoms in children: Results from a universal school-based trial. *Science Direct, 43,* 450–464.

Eunice Kennedy Shriver National Institute of Child Health & Human Development (NIH) (2010). Retrieved from http://www.nichd.nih.gov/ Pages/index.aspx

Ewing, J. A. (1984). Detecting alcoholism: The CAGE questionnaire. *Journal of the American Medical Association, 252*(14), 1905–1907.

Gersib, M. (2010). From fat to fit: How Nebraska can free itself from childhood obesity. *Prairie Fire: The Progressive Voice of the Great Plains*. Retrieved from http://www.prairiefirenewspaper.com/2010/01/from-fat-to-fit

Gifford, S. (2011). Family Involvement is Important in Substance Abuse Treatment. *Psych Central*. Retrieved from http://psychcentral.com/lib/2011/family-involvement-is-important-in-substance-abuse-treatment/

Goodman, W. K., Murphy, T. K., & Storch, E. A. (2007). Risk of adverse behavioral effects with pediatric use of antidepressants [Electronic version]. *Psychopharmacology, 191*(87), 87–96.

Healthy People 2020. (2014). Retrieved from http://www.healthypeople.gov/

Hinshaw, S. (2006). The stigmatization of mental illness in children and parents: Developmental issues, family concerns, and research needs. *Journal of Child Psychology and Psychiatry, 46*(7), 714–734.

Institute of Medicine of the National Academies. (2009). Preventing Mental, Emotional, and Behavioral Disorders Among Young People: Progress and Possibilities Retrieved from http://www.iom.edu/Reports/2009/Preventing-Mental-Emotional-and-Behavioral-Disorders-Among-Young-People-Progress-and-Possibilities.aspx

Johnson, M., Bulechek, G., Butcher, H., McCloskey Dochterman, J., Maas, M., Moorhead, S., & Swanson, E. (2013). *NANDA, NOC, and NIC linkage: Nursing diagnoses, outcomes, & interventions* (2nd ed.). St. Louis, MO: Elsevier Mosby.

Kasari, C., Rotheram-Fuller, E., Locke, J., & Gulsrud, A. (2012). Making the connection: Randomized controlled trial of social skills at school for children with autism spectrum disorders. *Journal of Child Psychology& Psychiatry, 53*, 431–439. doi:10:11/j.1469-7610.2011.02493.x

Knight, J. R., Sherritt, L., Shrier, L. A., Harris, S. K., & Chang, G. (2002). Validity of the CRAFFT Substance Abuse Screening Test Among Adolescent Clinic Patients. *Archives of Pediatrics and Adolescent Medicine, 156*, 607–614.

Kösters, M. P., Chinapaw, M., Zwaanswijk, M., van der Wal, M. F., Utens, E., & Koot, H. M. (2012). Study design of 'FRIENDS for Life': Process & effect evaluation of an indicated school-based prevention programme for childhood anxiety & depression. *BMC. Public Health*, 12, 86. doi:10.1186/1471-2458/12/86/prepub

Linnard-Palmer, L. (2010). *Peds notes: Nurse's clinical pocket guide*. Philadelphia, PA: F.A. Davis Company.

Loth, A. K. (2012). Childhood-Onset Schizophrenia. *Medscape Reference*. Retrieved from http://emedicine.medscape.com/article/914840-overview

Lubit, R. (2012). Reactive Attachment Disorder. *Medscape Reference*. Retrieved from http://emedicine.medscape.com/article/915447-overview

Macías-Robles, M., Perez-Clemente, A., Maciá-Bobes, C., Alvarez-Rueda, M., & Pozo-Nuevo, S. (2009). Prolonged QT interval in a man with anorexia nervosa. *International Archives of Medicine, 2*(23). doi:10.1186/1755-7682-2-23

Medline Plus. (2011). Retrieved from http://www.nlm.nih.gov/medlineplus/

Moorhead, S., Johnson, M., Maas, M. L., & Swanson, E. (2013). Nursing outcomes classification (NOC) (5th ed.). St. Louis, MO: Elsevier Mosby.

Mukolo, A., Heflinger, C. A., & Wallston, K. A. (2010). The stigma of childhood mental disorders: A conceptual framework. *Journal of the American Academy of Child and Adolescent Psychiatry, 49*, 92–198.

National Dissemination Center for Children and Youth with Disabilities (NICHCY). (2010). Down Syndrome, NICHCY Disability Fact Sheet #4. Retrieved from http://www.nichcy.org/wp-content/uploads/docs/fs4.pdf

National Dissemination Center for Children and Youth with Disabilities (NICHCY). (2011a). Intellectual Disabilities, NICHCY Disability Fact Sheet #8. Retrieved from http://nichcy.org/wp-content/uploads/docs/fs8.pdf

National Dissemination Center for Children and Youth with Disabilities (NICHCY). (2011b). Learning Diabilies, NICHCY Disability Fact Sheet #7. Retrieved from http://www.nichcy.org/wp-content/uploads/docs/fs7.pdf

National Institute of Mental Health (NIMH). (2009a). What are symptoms of bipolar disorder? Retrieved from http://www.nimh.nih.gov/health/publications/bipolar-disorder/what-are-the-symptoms-of-bipolar-disorder.shtml

National Institute of Mental Health (NIMH). (2009b). *Treatment of Children with Mental Illness: Frequently asked questions about the treatment of mental illness in children*. Retrieved from http://www.nimh.nih.gov/health/publications/treatment-of-children-with-mental-illness-fact-sheet/index.shtml

Nutter, D. A. (2012). Pediatric Sleep Disorders. *Medscape Reference*. Retrieved from http://emedicine.medscape.com/article/916611-overview

Plachta-Danielzik, S., Landsberg, B., Lange, D., Langnäse, K., & Müller, M. (2010). 15 years of the Kiel Obesity Prevention Study (KOPS). Results and its importance for obesity prevention in children and adolescents *Bundesgesundheitsblatt Gesundheitsforschung Gesundheitsschutz, 53*(3), 707–715.

Podell, J. L., Mychailyszn, M., Edmunds, J., Puleo, C., & Kendall, P. C. (2010). The Coping Cat Program for anxious youth: The FEAR plan comes to life. *Science Direct, 17*, 132–141.

Rivera-Navarro, J., Cubo, E., & Almazán, J. (2009). The diagnosis of Tourette's syndrome: Communication and Impact, *Clinical child psychology and psychiatry, 14*(1); 13–23

Scheeringa, M. S., Zeanah, C. H., & Cohen, J. A. (2011). Review: PTSD in children and adolescents: Toward an empirically based algorithm. *Depression & Anxiety, 28*(9), 770–782. doi:10.1002/da.20736

Schwarz, S. (2012). Obesity in Children. Retrieved from http://emedicine.medscape.com/article/985333-overview

Sleep Education. (2012). Retrieved from http://www.sleepeducation.com/default.aspx

Sroufe, L. A. (2009). The concept of development in developmental psychology. *Child Developmental Perspective, 3*, 178–183. doi:10:1111/j.1750-8606.2009.00103.x

Strawn, J. R., Keeshin, B. R., DelBello, M. P., Geracioti, T. D. Jr., & Putnam, F. W. (2010). Psycho-pharmacological treatment of posttraumatic stress disorder in children and adolescents: A review. *Journal of Clinical Psychiatry, 71*(7), 932–941.

Substance Abuse and Mental Health Services Administration (SAMHSA). (2012). Major depression in children and adolescents. Retrieved from http://store.samhsa.gov/term/Depression

Swinburn, B. (2009). Obesity prevention in children and adolescents. *Child and Adolescent Psychiatric Clinics of North America, 18*(1), 209–223.

The American Academy of Sleep Medicine. (2012). Retrieved from www.sleepeducation.com

Townsend, M. (2012). *Psychiatric mental health nursing: Concepts of care in evidence-based practice* (7th ed.). Philadelphia, PA: F.A. Davis.

Van Leeuwen, A., Poelhuis-Leth, D., & Bladh, M. (2011). *Davis's comprehensive handbook of laboratory and diagnostic tests with nursing implications* (4th ed) Philadelphia, PA: F.A. Davis.

Ward, S., & Hisley, S. (2009). *Maternal-child nursing care: Optimizing outcomes for mothers, children & families*. Philadelphia, PA: F.A. Davis.

CONCEPT MAP

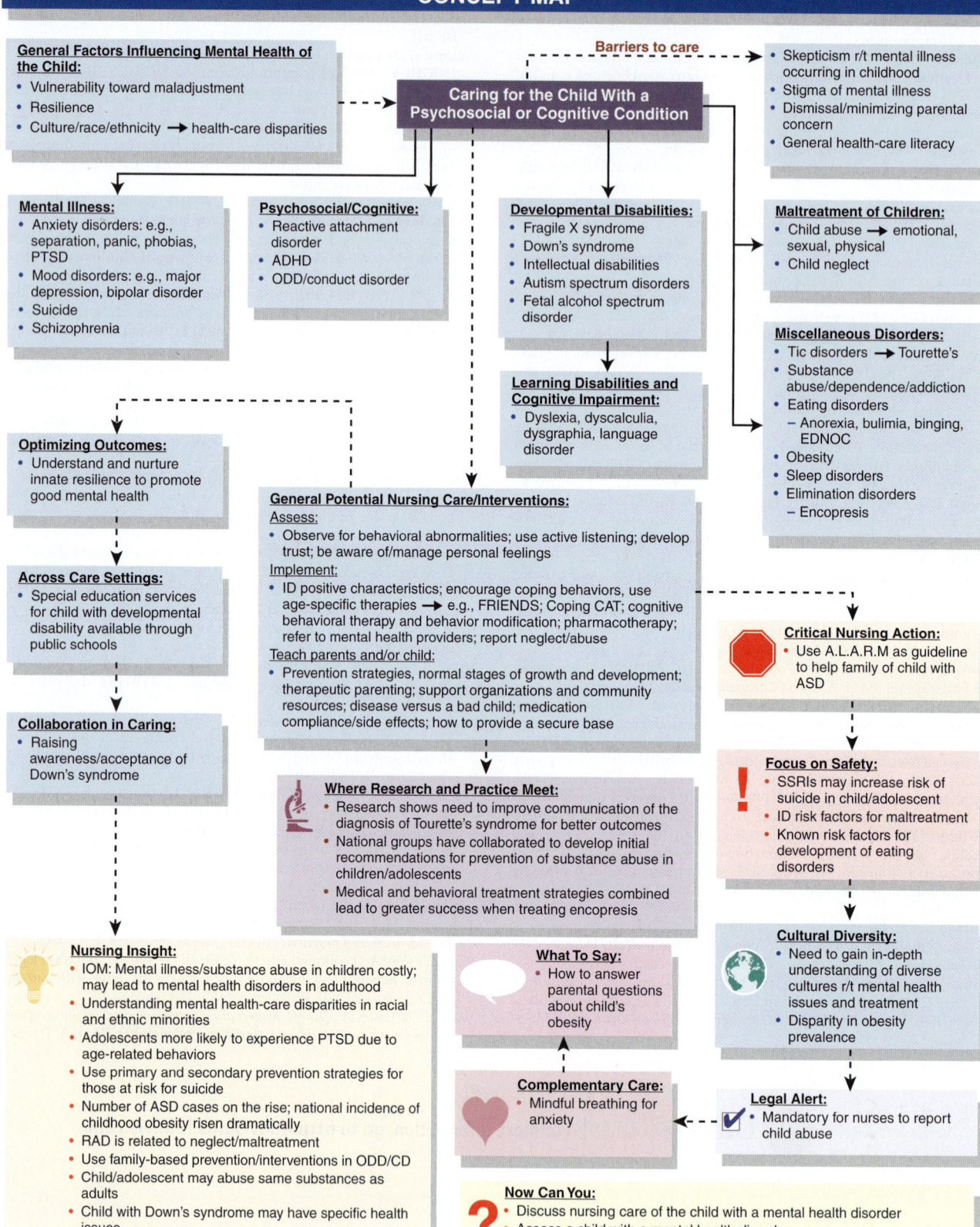

Barriers to care

Caring for the Child With a Psychosocial or Cognitive Condition

General Factors Influencing Mental Health of the Child:
• Vulnerability toward maladjustment
• Resilience
• Culture/race/ethnicity ➝ health-care disparities

- Skepticism r/t mental illness occurring in childhood
- Stigma of mental illness
- Dismissal/minimizing parental concern
- General health-care literacy

Mental Illness:
• Anxiety disorders: e.g., separation, panic, phobias, PTSD
• Mood disorders: e.g., major depression, bipolar disorder
• Suicide
• Schizophrenia

Psychosocial/Cognitive:
• Reactive attachment disorder
• ADHD
• ODD/conduct disorder

Developmental Disabilities:
• Fragile X syndrome
• Down's syndrome
• Intellectual disabilities
• Autism spectrum disorders
• Fetal alcohol spectrum disorder

Maltreatment of Children:
• Child abuse ➝ emotional, sexual, physical
• Child neglect

Miscellaneous Disorders:
• Tic disorders ➝ Tourette's
• Substance abuse/dependence/addiction
• Eating disorders
  – Anorexia, bulimia, binging, EDNOC
• Obesity
• Sleep disorders
• Elimination disorders
  – Encopresis

Learning Disabilities and Cognitive Impairment:
• Dyslexia, dyscalculia, dysgraphia, language disorder

Optimizing Outcomes:
• Understand and nurture innate resilience to promote good mental health

Across Care Settings:
• Special education services for child with developmental disability available through public schools

Collaboration in Caring:
• Raising awareness/acceptance of Down's syndrome

General Potential Nursing Care/Interventions:
Assess:
• Observe for behavioral abnormalities; use active listening; develop trust; be aware of/manage personal feelings
Implement:
• ID positive characteristics; encourage coping behaviors, use age-specific therapies ➝ e.g., FRIENDS; Coping CAT; cognitive behavioral therapy and behavior modification; pharmacotherapy; refer to mental health providers; report neglect/abuse
Teach parents and/or child:
• Prevention strategies, normal stages of growth and development; therapeutic parenting; support organizations and community resources; disease versus a bad child; medication compliance/side effects; how to provide a secure base

Critical Nursing Action:
• Use A.L.A.R.M as guideline to help family of child with ASD

Focus on Safety:
• SSRIs may increase risk of suicide in child/adolescent
• ID risk factors for maltreatment
• Known risk factors for development of eating disorders

Where Research and Practice Meet:
• Research shows need to improve communication of the diagnosis of Tourette's syndrome for better outcomes
• National groups have collaborated to develop initial recommendations for prevention of substance abuse in children/adolescents
• Medical and behavioral treatment strategies combined lead to greater success when treating encopresis

Nursing Insight:
• IOM: Mental illness/substance abuse in children costly; may lead to mental health disorders in adulthood
• Understanding mental health-care disparities in racial and ethnic minorities
• Adolescents more likely to experience PTSD due to age-related behaviors
• Use primary and secondary prevention strategies for those at risk for suicide
• Number of ASD cases on the rise; national incidence of childhood obesity risen dramatically
• RAD is related to neglect/maltreatment
• Use family-based prevention/interventions in ODD/CD
• Child/adolescent may abuse same substances as adults
• Child with Down's syndrome may have specific health issues
• Known common causes of sleep problems in children

What To Say:
• How to answer parental questions about child's obesity

Complementary Care:
• Mindful breathing for anxiety

Cultural Diversity:
• Need to gain in-depth understanding of diverse cultures r/t mental health issues and treatment
• Disparity in obesity prevalence

Legal Alert:
• Mandatory for nurses to report child abuse

Now Can You:
• Discuss nursing care of the child with a mental health disorder
• Assess a child with a mental health disorder
• Plan safe and effective care for a child with a mental health disorder

one
two
three
four
five
six
seven

Ongoing Care of the Child in the Hospital and in the Community

Caring for the Child With a Respiratory Condition

All things share the same breath—the beast, the tree, the man . . . the air shares its spirit with all the life it supports.

—Chief Seattle

LEARNING TARGETS *At the completion of this chapter, the student will be able to:*

◆ Describe the anatomy and physiology of the respiratory system.

◆ Examine common conditions of the respiratory system.

◆ Prioritize developmentally appropriate and holistic nursing care measures for common conditions of the respiratory system.

◆ Explore diagnostic, laboratory testing and medications for common conditions of the respiratory system.

◆ Develop teaching plans and discharge criteria for parents whose children have common respiratory conditions.

PICO(T) Questions

The intent of evidence-based practice (EBP) is to provide nursing care that integrates the best available evidence. An initial step in EBP is to write a PICO(T) question that effectively guides the research. A PICO(T) question is an acronym that stands for population (P), intervention or issue (I), comparison of interest (C), outcome (O), and timeframe (T). Depending on the question, all or some of the question components are used in the research process. Use these PICO(T) questions to spark your thinking as you read the chapter.

1. Do (I) overweight (P) adolescents with asthma (O) have more asthma attacks (C) than adolescents of average weight with asthma?

2. What is (O) the primary role of the nurse when working with the (P) parents of an infant with (I) cystic fibrosis (CF)?

Evidence-Based Practice

Danhauer, J. L., Johnson, C. E., & Caudle, A. T. (2011). Survey of K–3rd-grade teachers' knowledge of ear infections and willingness to participate in prevention programs. *Language, Speech & Hearing Services in Schools, 42,* 207–222.

The purpose of this study was to determine elementary school-teachers' experience with, knowledge of, and attitudes toward ear infection and their willingness to participate in prevention programs to prevent ear infections. The American Academy of Pediatrics (AAP) maintains that most children have at least one ear infection by the age of 3. Early diagnosis and management are recommended to avoid the complications of infection, namely speech, language, hearing, academic, and social development problems, which may ultimately impact children's ability to learn. Though some predisposing factors cannot be avoided, prevention includes avoidance of passive cigarette smoke, pacifier use, and bottle propping. Breastfeeding, frequent hand washing, and limiting participation in day care are also known to reduce the incidence of ear infections. In the United States, acute otitis media (AOM) is the most common reason for visits to a primary care provider and antibiotic prescriptions for children age 6 and

(continued)

Evidence-Based Practice (continued)

younger, costing $3 billion to $5 billion annually. Several studies have explored the use of complementary and alternative medicines (CAMs). In one study, regularly chewing gum was found to reduce the incidence of ear infections by 40%. Other studies have specified the use of xylitol, a naturally occurring sugar alcohol, as a prophylaxis for AOM based on the fact that chewing exercises the pharyngeal and eustachian tube structures. Xylitol is also used to prevent dental caries and its anti-adhesive properties prevent bacteria from attaching to the pharyngeal and eustachian tube structures. Two double-blind clinical trials supported the notion that AOM could be reduced by as much as 40% through the regular use of xylitol gum five times a day. Studies have indicated that children rated the taste of the gum as positive 86% of the time, which supports compliance. In most studies, teachers have generally expressed concern about the distraction caused by chewing gum in the classroom, as well as concerns regarding safety and school policies.

A request for participation was e-mailed to all 112 kindergarten through third-grade teachers in all 14 elementary schools in Santa Barbara, California. "Demographics for the schools included 77 African American/Black, 103 Asian American, 1,593 Caucasian/White, 29 Filipino, 3,807 Hispanic/Latino, and 6 Pacific Islander students, with a total enrolment of 5,791 students" (p. 209). Twenty-nine of the 112 teachers (26%) agreed to participate in the survey. The sample included participants from all but 5 schools. Participants included 28 females and 1 male: 17 were greater than 45 years of age, 8 were 36 to 45 years of age, and 4 were 25 to 35 years of age. The numbers of participants from the 9 schools ranged from 1 to 7 (mean of 3.3). Twenty-one of the teachers had more than 10 years of experience, 6 had between 5 and 10 years of experience, and 1 had less than 5 years of experience. Eight participants taught kindergarten, 8 taught first grade, 5 taught second grade, and 8 taught third grade. All of the participants were regular classroom teachers.

Data were gathered through the use of Survey Monkey. The survey contained 37 items and included questions about demographics, teacher preparation and continuing education, knowledge of and ability to recognize ear infections, knowledge and attitudes toward preventing infections, and willingness to participate in a prevention program. The researchers summarized the survey results as follows:

- Approximately half of the teachers can recognize signs of ear infections.
- Most teachers knew that ear infections could cause hearing loss and impact learning.
- Over half of the teachers didn't know that ear infections could be prevented.
- Approximately two-thirds of the teachers didn't know if their schools would allow participation in a prevention program.
- The majority of teachers would be willing to participate in a prevention program.
- None of the schools allowed gum chewing.
- Over half of the teachers indicated that they would be willing to allow gum chewing to prevent ear infections.
- Most teachers were interested in obtaining more information about ear infections and prevention.

The researchers concluded that teachers were interested in participating in a prevention program. The survey identified obstacles that would prevent the use of xylitol chewing gum. Obstacles included the fact that the gum would need to be used 5 times a day, which included 3 doses during the school period. Other concerns were in regard to choking and the time needed for facilitating and supervising the gum chewing. The researchers further noted that these results were most likely generalizable to other schools in other states, especially in regard to gum chewing policies.

1. How is this information useful to clinical nursing practice?
2. Based on these findings, what are implications for further research?

See Suggested Responses for Evidence-Based Practice on *DavisPlus*.

Introduction

This chapter provides a review of the anatomy and physiology and developmental aspects of the respiratory system. The discussion includes an examination of the various respiratory conditions including developmentally appropriate and holistic nursing care. Information is given about diagnostic and laboratory testing and medications. Teaching plans and discharge criteria for parents whose children have various respiratory conditions are incorporated.

Respiratory conditions are common causes of illness among children and can be acute, severe, or even life threatening. Children can experience chronic respiratory illnesses that affect growth and development and overall lifestyle. An astute awareness of common respiratory conditions helps the nurse provide holistic care to the child and family (Ward, 2013).

A & P review **The Respiratory System**

The respiratory system (Fig. 23-1) consists of the upper respiratory tract, which comprises the nose, nasal cavity, sinuses, pharynx, larynx, and trachea and the lower respiratory tract, which includes the lungs, bronchi, bronchioles, and alveoli. The anatomy and physiology of the respiratory system in children differs from that of the adult population. The most obvious difference between the anatomy and physiology is size.

Ventilation (breathing) involves taking in oxygen through the nose and mouth and then delivering it to the lungs. The nose has cilia (small hairlike projections) and mucus-producing cells that line the nostrils to prevent small particles from entering the nasal cavity. The mucus is a protective mechanism to trap foreign matter that enters the nasopharyngeal cavities.

The Respiratory System

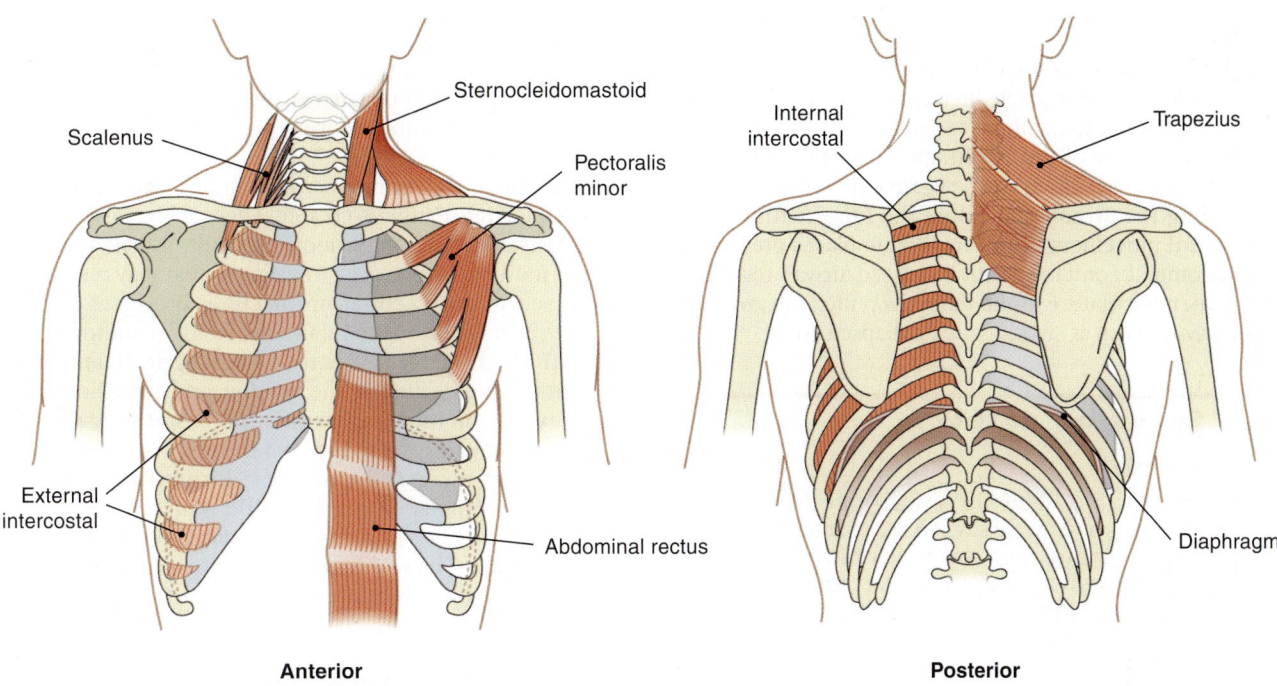

Figure 23-1 The respiratory system.

Growth and Development

The child with a respiratory condition can easily become overwhelmed and burdened with the disease process and extensive medical therapies. For example, cystic fibrosis is a multisystem respiratory disease that requires extensive medical management to minimize recurrent lung infections. Treatment for cystic fibrosis requires chest physical therapy, exercise regimens, and medications (Neufeld & Keith, 2012). Additionally, alterations in oxygenation and perfusion can impact the child's ability to participate in physical activity and play. Because of these factors, the child with a respiratory condition is vulnerable to alterations in regular growth and development. While treating and preventing respiratory complications, focus on promoting regular growth and development is essential.

Nursing care of the child with a respiratory condition should maintain a balance of disease symptom management and promotion of regular growth and development. This can be accomplished by providing developmentally appropriate toys that promote oxygenation and the stimulation needed for growth.

For example, bubbles and pinwheels are toys that promote deep breathing and lung expansion as well as the development of motor skills and fine motor movement. The nurse should understand the child's abilities and limitations and provide growth and developmental activities that are appropriate. Activity that supports airway maintenance and adequate oxygenation is essential. The child should be encouraged to participate in activities and allowed to rest as needed. The child with a respiratory condition such as cystic fibrosis and asthma require lifelong medical care and often need frequent hospitalization. Frequent hospital admissions can result in delays or regression of developmental milestones based on environmental changes and social isolation. The nurse should educate the family about strategies to prevent disease regression and hospital readmission to avoid this.

Source: Neufeld, K., & Keith, L. (2012) Special needs populations: Care of the patient with cystic fibrosis. *Association of PeriOperative Nurses Journal, 96*(5), 528–539.

The oxygen then passes from the pharynx to the larynx. To prevent any food or liquid from entering the larynx, the epiglottis closes over the opening of the larynx during swallowing. A cough reflex expels foreign bodies. From the larynx, air passes through the trachea, which branches into the left and right bronchi. The bronchi divide into smaller branches called bronchioles. The bronchioles end in a cluster of air sacs called the acinus.

Individual air sacs, called alveoli, exchange oxygen and carbon dioxide. Oxygen exchange with the bloodstream occurs in the capillaries. Oxygen attaches to the red blood cells and is transported to the rest of the body. Carbon dioxide diffuses from the bloodstream into the alveolus where it is transported out of the body during exhalation. ◆

Developmental Aspects of the Respiratory System

The airway of the newborn is narrow and more easily occluded than that of an adult. Newborns are obligatory nose breathers; they do not use their mouth for breathing. The cough of a newborn is usually nonproductive because they produce little respiratory mucus. Because they lack this cleansing function, they are more susceptible to respiratory infections. Newborns have a highly developed sense of smell, and the mucous membranes are highly vascular. The ethmoid and maxillary sinuses are present at birth, though the frontal and sphenoidal sinuses are not fully developed until the child is 6 to 8 years of age. The lymphoid tissues, or tonsils, are absent at birth and grow more rapidly in the child than any other tissue. By age 7, the tonsils present at adult size.

Children younger than the age of 6 are abdominal-breathers instead of thoracic-breathers. The intercostal muscles are too weak to facilitate respiration, causing the child to rely on the use of the diaphragm for inspiration. As the diaphragm moves downward, negative pressure is created, expanding the alveoli and filling the lungs with air. The downward movement of the diaphragm places pressure on the abdominal contents. With increased airway resistance, the weak musculature of the thorax is pulled inward, causing retractions, as if sucking on a collapsed straw.

focus on safety

Retractions

Retractions are a pulling in of the soft tissue of the chest wall with inspiration and occur when the accessory muscles are used for breathing. This is an abnormal finding and requires the nurse to conduct a more thorough respiratory assessment. In the chest, common sites for retractions include suprasternal, supraclavicular, intercostal, subcostal, and substernal areas.

The respiratory system of the toddler has expanded to hold a greater volume. The expanded distances between various structures of the respiratory tract decrease the risk of infections. The tonsils and adenoids of the toddler are increasing in size. The eustachian tubes remain short and horizontal during the toddler and preschool-age years, providing easier access for nasal bacteria to enter the ear.

The epiglottis of children age 8 and younger is longer and flaccid (floppy), making it more susceptible to swelling that can lead to airway occlusion. The epiglottis is small and does not close properly, and the larynx and the glottis are higher in the younger child's neck, which makes the child more prone to aspiration. The thyroid, cricoid, and tracheal cartilages are immature and are easily collapsible with flexion of the neck. There are fewer functional muscles in the neck, and the increased amount of soft tissue makes the younger child more susceptible to infection and edema.

The trachea in children is shorter and narrower in diameter than in adults. To compare, the trachea of a newborn is approximately 4 mm in diameter, about the diameter of a drinking straw (or as a general rule, the size of the infant's or child's little finger). By age 6, the diameter of the trachea is approximately 12 mm, while an adult's trachea is from 18 to 20 mm in diameter. A child's trachea bifurcates (separates into two branches) at the third thoracic vertebra, but an adult's trachea bifurcates at the sixth thoracic vertebra. In addition to the higher level of bifurcation, the angle of the right bronchus (one of the two large branches of the trachea) is much sharper in children. Because of the narrow lumen of the trachea, excess mucous production can easily produce an obstruction.

The right bronchus is shorter, wider, and more vertical than the left; therefore, inhaled foreign bodies more often lodge in the right bronchus. The bronchioles of the infant are little more than a thin layer of muscle and are elastic-lined with ciliated epithelium. Lung tissue is also immature at birth and continues to grow and develop until about the

age of 12. Children have less alveolar surface for gas exchange than adults. The surface area increases ninefold by the age of 12. The alveoli increase in number from 25 to 300 million during this time, along with increasing size and functionality. The maturity of the alveoli enhances ventilation and respiration, thereby promoting more effective gas exchange.

Because of the differences in a child's airway, the force needed for ventilation is greater. There is increased friction and resistance, making it more difficult to generate ventilation in the presence of airway edema that may result from hypersensitivity reactions or infectious processes.

The average full-term infant has 20 to 50 million alveoli at birth (Light, 2011a). There is a rapid growth and maturation of alveoli during the toddler and preschool ages. This expansion improves ventilation; respiratory rates decrease significantly from those of the newborn. The alveoli continue to increase in number during the school-age period, reaching approximately 300 million by 8 years of age (Light, 2011a). Lung development is complete by 5 to 6 years of age. The respiratory structures of the adolescent are of approximately adult size and capacity.

Critical Nursing Action Respiratory Rate

In assessing the respiratory rate of a child, the nurse understands that the rate and depth of respirations can be impacted by crying, physical activity, anxiety, anemia, acid-base disturbances, fever, central nervous system disturbances, and salicylate ingestion. The child's respiratory rate is assessed in correlation with other overall physical findings. When assessing the respiratory rate of the pediatric patient, the nurse counts for a full minute (Table 23-1).

Because the respiratory system is undergoing a process of development during childhood, the child is more prone to develop respiratory problems. In addition, the child does not have the immunity that adults have to many infectious agents. Therefore, respiratory infections occur more frequently in the pediatric population.

Because children are prone to respiratory illness, it is important for the nurse to know the normal values for arterial blood gases to deliver effective care (Table 23-2). Pediatric nurses must consider these factors when caring for pediatric patients.

Congenital Respiratory Conditions and Structural Anomalies

There are a variety of congenital respiratory conditions and structural anomalies in children. It is essential that the nurse have a good understanding of the diagnosed condition along with an understanding of signs and symptoms and prescribed care.

CHOANAL ATRESIA

Choanal atresia is a congenital malformation of the nose in which there is blockage of the posterior side of the nose. It occurs when fetal development of the posterior choanae fails to develop properly. Bony atresia occurs 90% of the time; membranous atresia occurs 10% of the time

Table 23-1 Average Respiratory Rates in Children

Preterm	Newborn	1 Year	3 Years	6 Years	10 Years	14 Years	18 Years
40–70	30–50	20–40	20–30	16–22	16–20	14–20	16–20

Source: Sawer, S. S. (2012). *Pediatric physical examination & health assessment* (p. 99). Sudbury, MA: Jones & Bartlett Learning.

Table 23-2 Arterial Blood Gas Values

Age Group	PCO_2	PO_2	HCO_3^-	pH	O_2 Saturation
Birth, cord, full term	31–66 mm Hg	60–70 mm Hg	17–24 mEq/L	7.32–7.49	40%–90%
2 months–2 years	26–41 mm Hg	80–95 mm Hg	16–23 mEq/L	7.34–7.46	95%–99%
Child	35–45 mm Hg	80–95 mm Hg	22–26 mEq/L	7.35–7.45	95%–99%
Adult	35–45 mm Hg	80–95 mm Hg	22–26 mEq/L	7.35–7.45	95%–99%

Source: Van Leeuwen, A. M., & Poelhuis-Leth, D. J. (2011). *Davis's comprehensive handbook of laboratory and diagnostic tests: With nursing implications* (4th ed.). Philadelphia, PA: F.A. Davis.

Medication: Medications Related to Respiratory Conditions

Therapeutic Category	Indication(s)	Action(s)
Antibiotics (oral, parenteral, inhalation)	Abscess, bacterial pneumonia, cystic fibrosis, empyema, pharyngitis, sinusitis, tonsillitis, tuberculosis. Inhaled antibiotics are used in cystic fibrosis.	Treats respiratory tract bacterial infections.
Antihistamines (oral)	Allergic rhinitis, asthma.	Counteracts the effects of histamine on a receptor site used to treat allergies, hypersensitive reactions, and colds.
Anticholinergics (inhalation)	Acute or chronic wheezing in asthma or chronic lung disease.	Produces bronchodilation (without systemic effects) and inhibits the muscles from tightening around the bronchi (large airways).
Antiviral agents (oral, parenteral)	Influenza virus types A and B.	Treats the flu symptoms. Antiviral agents do not destroy their target pathogen; instead they inhibit their development.
B_2, Agonists (oral, inhalation)	Asthma, chronic obstructive lung disease.	Acts as a smooth muscle relaxant resulting in bronchodilation.
Caffeine (oral)	Apnea.	Stimulates the respiratory center.
Corticosteroids (oral, parenteral, inhalation)	Asthma.	Acts as a potent anti-inflammatory agent.
Cough suppressants (oral)	Common cold, bronchitis, pneumonia, sinusitis.	Treats a cough (productive or dry). For a productive cough (with phlegm), the cough syrup contains an expectorant to help loosen mucus. For a dry cough the cough syrup contains suppressants (antitussives) in an attempt to suppress the urge to cough.
Decongestants (oral)	Common cold.	Reduces swelling and congestion.
Expectorants (oral)	Common cold, pneumonia.	Reduces viscosity of thick mucus secretions.
Leukotriene receptor antagonists (inhalation)	Asthma, bronchitis, constricted airways.	Inhibits leukotrienes that cause inflammation.
Mast-cell stabilizers (inhalation)	Asthma (maintenance).	Prevents or controls certain allergic disorders.
Recombinant human deoxyribonuclease I (rhDNase) (inhalation)	Cystic fibrosis.	Helps delay cystic fibrosis progression by improving lung function and reducing the risk for respiratory tract infections and thins and loosens mucus.
Racemic epinephrine (inhalation)	Croup, bronchiolitis.	Produces bronchodilation.
RSV vaccine (IM injection)	Respiratory syncytial virus.	Provides infection-fighting antibodies to help protect high-risk infants' vulnerable lungs.

Source: Ward (2013).

(Schroeder & McColley, 2011, p. 266). Most cases are unilateral, though both sides of the nose may be affected. A child with bilateral choanal atresia usually displays respiratory problems during development. The occurrence of choanal atresia ranges from 1:5,000 to 1:8,000 live births and is twice as common in females (Schroeder & McColley, 2011).

Signs and Symptoms

Unilateral choanal atresia may not be evident at birth because neonates may be able to breathe sufficiently through one side of their nose.

- Choanal atresia may be asymptomatic until signs of respiratory infection, nasal discharge, or persistent nasal obstruction occur.
- Children with bilateral choanal atresia may have difficulty with nasal breathing and make vigorous attempts to inspire and suck with their lips.
- Cyanosis may be evident.
- Because infants breathe through their mouths while crying, they may appear pink, yet turn blue when quiet.
- The infant may have difficulty eating because of difficulty breathing.
- The child may choke or regurgitate formula or breast milk while being fed because of difficulty coordinating chewing, breathing, and swallowing.
- Failure to gain weight may occur because of feeding difficulty.
- Choanal atresia is associated with other congenital anomalies. Fifty percent of the time, choanal atresia is seen as part of CHARGE syndrome (Schroeder & McColley, 2011). This includes:
  - Coloboma of the eye
  - Heart defects
  - Atresia (choanal)
  - Retarded growth and development
  - Genitourinary hypoplasia
  - Ear anomalies

Diagnosis

Diagnosis of choanal atresia is established by the inability to pass a firm catheter through each nostril 3 to 4 cm into the nasopharynx. The diagnosis is confirmed by computerized tomography (CT) scan with intranasal contrast that shows narrowing of the posterior side of the nose.

Prevention

Though this condition may not be prevented, good prenatal care provides an opportunity to promote optimal prenatal development.

Collaborative Care

Nursing Care. Nursing care for choanal atresia may involve the initial diagnosis of the defect by observation and assessment for the patency of the nose by failure to pass a nasal catheter. Overall nursing care depends on the type of defect and the extent of surgical correction. Immediate care of a child with choanal atresia includes airway maintenance and starting gavage feeding to prevent aspiration and poor nutrition. Care of the infant before surgery includes caregiver/parent education and maintenance of IV fluids while the child is kept on "nothing by mouth" status.

Surgical Care. Depending on the extent of the defect, the immediate concern may include resuscitation. An airway may be placed and, in some cases, intubation or tracheostomy is needed. If the infant is able to learn to mouth breathe, surgery can be delayed. Surgical correction involves the removal of the obstruction, which corrects the problem. The surgery may be done through the nose (transnasal) or through the mouth (transpalatal). Definitive repair may involve transnasal puncture and stenting or resection. Recurrent stenosis may occur, requiring dilation, reoperation, or both.

 focus on safety

Aspiration precautions

Because the child may have difficulty with feeding, aspiration precautions must be observed. The baby is fed in a semi-upright position with periods of rest to facilitate breathing. The nurse also instructs the caregiver to protect the child against respiratory infection by practicing good hand washing and avoiding densely populated public places, such as day cares, grocery stores, and malls.

Education/Discharge Instructions

Discharge instructions include wound care (keeping the wound clean and dry) and prevention of infection. The importance of adequate fluids and resumption of feeding is also stressed. Parents are taught how to keep the child's nostrils clean by gently cleansing the rim of the nostrils with a warm, soft cloth. A clean nasal area prevents dry mucus from accumulating in the child's nostrils, facilitating breathing. The nurse can encourage the parents to elect for early treatment, especially if the condition is bilateral.

ESOPHAGEAL ATRESIA (EA) AND TRACHEOESOPHAGEAL FISTULA (TEF)

EA is the failure of the esophagus to develop a continuous passage characterized by the presence of a blind pouch. The proximal and/or distal portions of the esophagus may or may not be connected to the trachea by a fistula (TEF). A TEF creates an abnormal communication between the trachea and the esophagus. Anomalies are caused by defective separation, incomplete fusion, or failure of the structure to hollow out. When a fistula is present, it is between the distal esophagus and the airway 85% of the time (Thilo & Rosenberg, 2011, p. 44). EA without a fistula occurs about 10% of the time (Sullivan & Kinane, 2011, pp. 283–287). TEF is often associated with other anomalies, which may involve the kidneys, heart, limbs, or spine. The defect occurs in approximately 1 in 3,000 live births and is commonly associated with **polyhydramnios** (the presence of excess amniotic fluid in the amniotic sac) that is related to the presence of a gastrointestinal (GI) obstruction (Bishop, 2011, p. 478).

 Nursing Insight—*Variations of esophageal atresia with or without tracheoesophageal fistula*

The nurse understands that there are different anatomical variations of EA with or without TEF:
- EA with distal TEF (85.8% of the cases)
- Isolated EA (7.8%)

- Isolated TEF (4.2%)
- EA with proximal TEF (0.8%)
- EA with double TEF (1.4%)

This anomaly occurs during fetal development when the tracheoesophageal groove fails to close, resulting in incomplete separation of the trachea and esophagus. The esophagus and trachea begin forming from the foregut in the 4- to 6-week-old embryo. The caudal part of the foregut forms a ventral diverticulum that develops into the trachea. The horizontal part of the trachea and esophagus fold and then join together to form the septum that divides the foregut into ventral larynx and trachea and the dorsal part of the long tube called the esophagus. During this process of formation, the posterior deviation of the tracheoesophageal septum leads to failure of closure between the trachea and esophagus (Fig. 23-2).

Signs and Symptoms

- Excessive drooling and secretions
- Frothing and bubbling at the mouth and nose
- Cyanosis
- Respiratory distress
- Choking with attempted feeding
- Inability to pass orogastric tube into the stomach

Clinical symptoms may intensify with feeding leading to regurgitation, choking, and aspiration.

In cases of isolated TEF, symptoms may occur later in life with the child having chronic respiratory problems and abdominal distension because of air building up in the stomach. Because EA and TEF have been associated with other congenital anomalies that occur in the musculoskeletal, GI, cardiac, and genitourinary systems, a thorough assessment by the nurse is necessary.

Diagnosis

If not diagnosed with prenatal sonogram, most neonates are diagnosed soon after birth or during infancy because TEF is a life-threatening condition. TEF is confirmed by

focus on safety

Checking the mother's obstetric history

When the nurse is caring for a newborn and observes the baby to be drooling excessively, and/or having persistent choking spells and color changes with feedings, it is important for the nurse to check the mother's obstetric history. If there is history of polyhydramnios, the nurse must report the observed symptoms to the baby's pediatrician immediately. These symptoms are highly suspicious of EA and TEF.

observing an early onset of respiratory distress accompanied by signs and symptoms described earlier, as well as possibly the inability to pass a nasogastric or orogastric tube. Confirmatory diagnosis is made through radiography. Barium should not be used because of the risk of aspiration, though a small amount of a dilute water-soluble agent can be used for contrast (Bishop, 2011, p. 478). Chest films are taken to determine the patency of the esophagus or the presence and level of the blind pouch.

 Nursing Diagnoses Esophageal Atresia With or Without Tracheoesophageal Fistula

- Ineffective airway clearance related to excessive secretions
- Altered nutrition: Less than body requirement related to inadequate ingestion of nutrients
- High risk for infection related to accumulation of secretion in the lungs
- Altered family processes related to frequent hospitalization/prolonged sickness
- Impaired family social interaction related to situational crisis
- High risk of aspiration related to excessive drooling and poor swallowing and inability to clear secretions

Prevention

Though this condition may not be prevented, good prenatal care provides an opportunity to promote optimal prenatal development.

Most Common Types of Esophageal Atresia and Tracheoesophageal Fistula

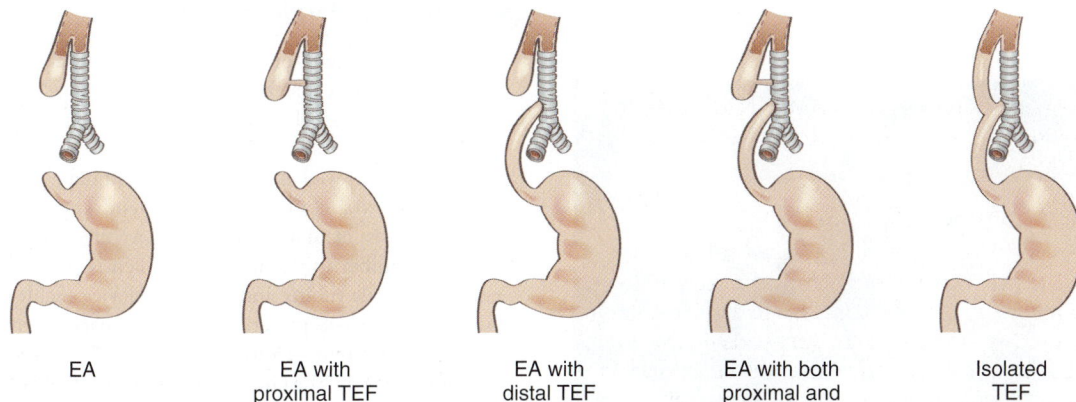

| EA | EA with proximal TEF | EA with distal TEF | EA with both proximal and distal TEF | Isolated TEF |

EA = Esophageal atresia
TEF = Tracheoesophageal fistula

Figure 23-2 Esophageal atresia and tracheoesophageal fistula.

Collaborative Care
Nursing Care.

Critical Nursing Action Nursing Assessment

When assessing a child diagnosed with EA or TEF, the nurse watches for subtle changes in the child's color, respiration, behavior, heart rate, and general health. Subtle changes often occur before technology is able to recognize these changes. It is essential to have emergency equipment ready at the bedside. It is also important to remember that the child has an uncanny ability to compensate. When the child is no longer able to compensate, the child "crashes" and then may then have a poor probability of recovery.

Immediately after birth, treatment is aimed at maintaining a patent airway and preventing aspiration of secretions. Although EA and TEF are surgical emergencies, discretion is used about performing immediate surgical corrections. Highly compromised neonates, such as those who are premature, those with concurrent congenital anomalies, and those who are in poor physical condition, should not be operated on immediately.

Surgical Care. After life-sustaining measures are given, surgical corrections may come in stages that may be palliative in nature (e.g., gastrostomy and drainage of esophageal pouch). The goal of surgery is to close the fistula and attach the two sections of the esophagus. Artificial ventilation may be required in the beginning, and the child can be weaned off the artificial ventilation as the condition improves. However, endotracheal (ET) intubation is often avoided because it may worsen abdominal distention because of the connection between the trachea and esophagus (Fig. 23-3).

Before surgical correction, the neonate is not given oral feedings, but IV (parenteral) fluids instead. The nurse positions the neonate at a 30- to 45-degree elevation of the head to protect the trachea from secretions, and the head is turned to the side to prevent aspiration and drain secretions. Suctioning is done regularly and at frequent intervals. A nasogastric or orogastric tube with continuous, low suctioning is likely to be placed by the health-care provider into the blind pouch and is monitored for patency. The tube should not be irrigated because this may

cause aspiration. Hydration and fluid and electrolyte balance are monitored. Often antibiotic therapy is started because aspiration pneumonia is inevitable.

focus on safety

Preoperative and postoperative suctioning

Preoperatively, any nasogastric or orogastric tube placement for suctioning must be done carefully and gently and progression stopped immediately if any resistance is met because this can lead to a perforation of esophageal tissue in an infant with an anomaly. Tube placement is usually done by the primary care provider. Postoperative oral or nasal suctioning of the infant with EA or TEF must also be done extremely carefully to avoid disruption of the repairs. Carefully measure the catheter and do not insert any further than the distance from the nares to the ear lobe.

Immediately after the surgical correction, nurses must monitor vital signs at regular intervals. The site requiring correction is usually in the thoracic cavity, so the nurse expects the baby to return with a chest tube and possibly still be intubated with an ET tube. Infants with chest tubes are carefully handled to avoid dislodging of the tube. Suctioning of the oropharyngeal area is kept to a minimum to avoid disruption of the surgical repair.

Postoperatively, the nurse performs vigilant assessments on all body systems to detect any complications or new problems. Because the child may have low blood counts and a decrease in fluid volume, the nurse must regulate plasma or blood transfusion and the IV infusions adequately. To maintain adequate nutrition, gavage feeding may be initiated by the second or third postoperative day. Gavage feedings are administered slowly while watching the child closely for any untoward manifestations, such as aspiration. The child requires prolonged hospitalization, so the family must be informed about the lengthy hospital stay and the myriad of ongoing treatments. After the child has recovered, he may be discharged to the care of the parents. Emphasize to the family the need for frequent follow-up visits to ensure that no complications or problems are present.

Nursing Insight—*Chest tubes*

Removal of air, fluid, or blood from the pleural, pericardial, or mediastinal spaces may be facilitated by the placement of chest tubes. The purpose of closed chest suction is to remove air and fluid from the thoracic cavity and to improve postoperative lung re-expansion, as well as to treat pneumothorax. The chest tube is connected to a closed drainage system. The closed drainage systems consist of an underwater seal, a collection chamber, and suction chamber in a single unit, which is subsequently connected to sterile tubing and a suction device (Schlosser, 2013). Suction is applied as prescribed by the primary care provider and typically ordered at –15 to –20 cm H_2O (Schlosser, 2013). To function properly, the chest drainage system needs to be placed a minimum of 1 foot (30 cm) below the level of the lungs.

Nursing considerations:
• Explain procedure to the child and parents.
• Note character, consistency, and amount of drainage in the collection chamber.

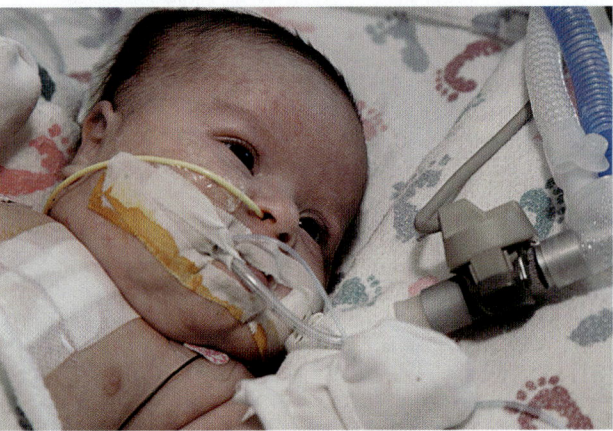

Figure 23-3 Child with an endotracheal tube.

- Note integrity of the tubing and chest tubes every 2 to 4 hours.
- Carefully coil the tubing and secure to the edge of the bed, avoiding pressure or kinks in the tubing.
- Mark drainage level according to the policy of your institution.
- Never clamp the tube when moving or transporting the child.
- Encourage coughing and deep breathing according to the policy of your institution.
- Check the rate and quality of respirations and auscultate the lungs according to the policy of your institution.
- Instruct the child and parents to report any breathing difficulty.
- Notify the primary care provider of changes in color, decreased oxygen saturation, rapid or shallow breathing, chest pain, or excessive bleeding.
- Check the chest tube dressing according to the policy of your institution.
- Do not routinely milk or strip the chest tubes because it can cause negative pressure, which may damage lung tissue (Schlosser, 2013).
- Document observations, routine care, dressing appearance, drainage, and functioning of the chest drainage system according to your institution's policy.

Education/Discharge Instructions

After corrective surgery, the majority of the infants lead normal lives. The potential for the complication of post-operative infection can be prevented by instructing the parents to keep the wound clean and dry. Instruct the parents on carefully observing the infant during feeding and to report any difficulty swallowing. Parents also need to be instructed on proper feeding and positioning to avoid aspiration. In addition, parents must be educated on signs of respiratory infection, as well as on the signs of a stricture, which may be demonstrated by refusal to eat and can require dilation. If complications do occur, they are challenging, especially during infancy. Prognosis depends on the presence or absence of other associated anomalies.

ACUTE RESPIRATORY DISTRESS SYNDROME (ARDS)

ARDS is a life-threatening condition that is characterized by increased pulmonary capillary permeability and pulmonary edema, which leads to hypoxemia, reduced lung compliance, and alveolar infiltrates. An acute underlying illness or injury predisposes to ARDS. A primary insult with sepsis, viral pneumonia, smoke inhalation, aspiration of gastric contents, hydrocarbon ingestion or aspiration, or near drowning may progress to ARDS (Albietz, Czaja, Dobyns, Grayck, & Mourani, 2011). Infection is the most common cause and is often associated with respiratory syncytial virus (RSV) in children. Indirect lung injury, such as that in the case of pancreatitis, shock, burns, trauma, drug overdoses, and blood transfusions may also precipitate an insult, which may lead to ARDS. The underlying disease or disorder influences the mortality rate. Mortality in adults can be as high as 90% with underlying liver disease and as low as 10% in children with RSV. The average mortality rate overall is 40% (Albietz et al., 2011). Multisystem organ failure is a frequent complication of ARDS, has a major impact on the prognosis, and is the leading cause of death in both adults and children.

As the disease progresses the alveolar-capillary membrane becomes more permeable. As exudate enters the alveolar spaces, the lung becomes less compliant and susceptible to pulmonary edema. This further leads to decreased surfactant production, which exacerbates alveolar instability. Swelling leads to atelectasis, and gas diffusion is impaired (Albietz et al., 2011; Thilo & Rosenberg, 2011). As a result, there is a decrease in oxygen entering the bloodstream, which may lead to multisystem organ damage.

Family Teaching Guidelines...
Care for the Child With Esophageal Atresia and/or Tracheoesophageal Fistula

TOPIC: Esophageal Atresia With or Without Tracheoesophageal Fistula

In many hospitals, the nurse takes responsibility in preparing parents for discharge and home management. There are several topics that the nurse must teach parents to care for the child who has a diagnosis of EA and/or TEF:

- In the case of tracheotomy, nurses must teach parents proper sterile technique of suctioning and how to handle the equipment appropriately.

- Verify that all emergency calling numbers are written down so emergency care could be provided in a serious situation.

- Ensure parents know how to identify respiratory distress.

- Confirm parents know feeding techniques for gastrostomy tube and how to handle tube plugging and dislodging.

- Instruct parents in performing CPR before the child goes home.

- Encourage parents to use different toys and games to promote stimulation during regular care (e.g., encourage mobilization or action play to help the child reach developmental milestones and divert the child's mind, which may help the child cope during the prolonged sickness). Mobilization can be as simple as holding or rocking, while action play can be games, toy figures, or crafts.

- Involve other siblings in adapting the young child with EA or TEF. It is essential that the family help the child with EA or TEF learn socialization and interaction with others.

- Ensure the family knows how to operate equipment and knows proper maintenance of the equipment used at home.

Signs and Symptoms

In previously healthy infants and children, respiratory distress and hypoxia can occur within 24–48 hours of the insult. The earliest phases may include the following (Albietz et al., 2011):

- Dyspnea
- Tachypnea
- Normal chest examination
- Mild hypoxemia
- Hypercapnia

Hypoxemia and respiratory distress worsen over the next several hours. Symptoms may include, but are not limited to, the following (Albietz et al., 2011):

- Cyanosis
- Tachycardia
- Irritability
- Dyspnea
- Coarse rales
- Radiological evidence of alveolar infiltrates, which is indicative of pulmonary edema. This is initially noted in the dependent lung.
- Pulmonary hypertension
- Moderate to severe hypoxemia

As ARDS progresses over the next 2 to 10 days, there is more evidence of diffuse alveolar infiltrates and decreased lung volume. Symptoms may include (Albietz et al., 2011):

- Tachypnea
- Tachycardia
- Signs of consolidation
- Diffuse rhonchi
- Sepsis syndrome
- Diffuse alveolar infiltrates

Pulmonary fibrosis and pneumonia occur as ARDS progresses beyond 10 days and may include the following (Albietz et al., 2011):

- Symptoms as above
- Recurrent sepsis
- Evidence of multisystem organ failure
- Recurrent pneumonia
- Progressive lung restriction
- Impaired tissue oxygenation

Diagnosis

Diagnosis of ARDS is based on four diagnostic criteria, which include the following (Albietz et al., 2011):

- An acute underlying illness or injury
- Bilateral lung infiltrates evidenced on chest radiography
- Absence of heart failure or left atrial hypertension
- Presence of severe hypoxemic respiratory failure

ARDS is usually diagnosed in a patient who is in the hospital from a critical illness such as shock, sepsis, or other trauma. Diagnostic tests may include:

- Arterial blood gases
- Chest x-ray
- Other blood tests that can find an infection that may be causing ARDS
- CT scan of the lung
- Electrocardiogram and echocardiogram to rule out cardiac causes

Prevention

The incidence of ARDS may be decreased through primary prevention of traumatic injuries by use of child car restraints, bicycle helmets, and protective sports gear. Some infectious illnesses primarily affecting the respiratory tract may be prevented through compliance with recommended immunizations and good hand washing hygiene. RSV passive immunization with immunoglobulins can inhibit more serious illness in vulnerable patients.

Collaborative Care

Nursing Care. Caring for children with ARDS requires advanced training and technical skills. Nursing care for children with ARDS also requires a vigilant nursing assessment and monitoring of vital signs. The nurse must accurately record and report significant changes in vital signs to the physician. Calories and fluids are provided intravenously; therefore, the nurse monitors exact intake and output. In addition, the child with ARDS requires supportive care. The child will be placed in intensive care, and both the respiratory and cardiovascular status will be monitored closely. Care includes positioning, pain and anxiety control, maintenance of nutrition, and infection control practices. Ventilator support may be required as the disease progresses and requires the nurse to be sensitive to the psychological support of both the child and family. Education should include an explanation of procedures and assisting the family to understand test results and evidence of disease progress.

Medical Care. Medical management is directed at improving oxygenation and ventilation and often includes use of mechanical ventilation with attention to positive end-expiratory pressure (PEEP). Medical management of ARDS includes several broad areas (Albietz et al., 2011; Cheifetz, 2011).

Monitoring includes continuous blood pressure measurements, central venous pressure monitoring, and ABS analysis to assess for adequate oxygenation, ventilation, fluid volume, and cardiac functioning. Daily chest radiography may also be ordered to monitor for the incidence of air leaks. Laboratory studies may be ordered to monitor renal, liver, and GI functioning as well as for infection surveillance. Fluids may be restricted to reduce intravascular volume because of the potential for pulmonary edema related to increased pulmonary capillary permeability.

Most people with ARDS will need mechanical ventilator assistance with a low tidal volume. Use of a high tidal volume can overdistend the lungs and can lead to lung inflammation and ventilator-associated lung injury. For milder symptoms, oxygen may be delivered using a properly fitting face mask. PEEP is considered an essential component of ventilation. Use of PEEP helps expand alveoli and increases lung volume.

Prone positioning has been demonstrated to improve postural drainage and ventilation of collapsed portions of the lungs. Use of inhaled nitric oxide, which causes pulmonary vasodilation increasing blood flow, has been found to improve oxygenation though research has not demonstrated an overall significant improvement in survival rates. Surfactant therapy has been studied as a potential treatment for ARDS though has not been consistently found to be beneficial in children. Use of extracorporeal membrane oxygenation (ECMO), which removes the blood from the body and then returns it, has also been used in adults, though according to Cheifetz (2011), there are limited data addressing its use in children. Though ECMO is a life-saving therapy, it is also considered invasive with a high risk of bleeding.

Education/Discharge Instructions

Parents need to be instructed that long-term care follow-up and monitoring of the pulmonary system will be needed. Albietz et al. (2011) noted that one study reported that 3 out of 10 children were still symptomatic with 7 of 10 experiencing severe hypoxemia at rest up to 4 years after discharge. Parents need to understand the importance of a smoke-free environment, providing proper nutrition, avoiding infections, and ensuring compliance with immunizations.

CYSTIC FIBROSIS

Cystic fibrosis (CF) is an inherited autosomal-recessive disorder that causes the production of thick mucus that blocks exocrine glands and affects several body systems, including respiratory, gastrointestinal, and reproductive systems. CF is the most common cause of chronic respiratory disease in children and is accompanied by multiple, severe respiratory infections. The increased mucus production in the airways causes obstruction and stasis of fluid, providing a rich habitat for bacterial growth. In addition, the pancreatic ducts are often blocked by mucus, prohibiting the secretions of pancreatic enzymes necessary for the metabolism of food nutrients. In later childhood, the reproductive system is affected because ovarian ducts and the vas deferens may be occluded, leading to infertility. There is also an increased loss of sodium, causing salt depletion in children with CF.

CF is more common in Caucasians and occurs in approximately 1 in 3,000 live births. The incidence in African Americans is 1 in 15,000 to 20,000; the incidence in Hispanics is 1 in 4,000 to 10,000 live births (John & Brady, 2012a, p. 735). CF is transmitted as an autosomal-recessive trait, which means that a child can receive a defective gene from either parent. When both parents carry the defective gene, there is a 75% chance that the child will inherit one CF gene from each parent and manifest the disease. There is a 50% chance that the child will inherit one defective gene and one normal gene from each parent and become a carrier of the disease. There is a 25% chance that the child will inherit only normal genes and be free of CF.

The CF genes have been found on chromosome 7, which encodes cystic fibrosis transmembrane conductor regulator (CFTR) protein. CFTR normally regulates the chloride channel and facilitates the activity of other chloride and sodium channels at the cell surface. Abnormal functions of CFTR cause a disruption of sodium ion transport across the exocrine and epithelial gland cells and make the cell walls impermeable to chloride ions. This causes an excess of sodium and chloride found in the sweat of children affected by CF. In addition, the loss of sodium and water from the airways increases the viscosity of the mucus and disrupts the ciliary mechanism (hairlike process) that is intended to clear the airways, predisposing the child to recurrent respiratory infections.

A similar transport defect occurs in the pancreatic and bile ducts. With inadequate excretion of pancreatic enzymes for food breakdown, children experience varying levels of protein and fat absorption. With reduced protein and fat absorption, there is weight loss and failure to thrive, requiring an affected child's diet to be high in protein and calories. Fat is excreted in the stool, resulting in abnormal bowel patterns, including steatorrhea, diarrhea, and abdominal pain.

The mucus gland produces thin, free-flowing secretions, but in CF it produces thick mucus that accumulates and obstructs the different organs. In newborns, thick secretions may plug the small intestine and lead to failure in passing meconium (the first feces of a newborn infant, which is greenish black, odorless, and tarry) (Venes, 2013). In the gastrointestinal system, thick secretions impair the digestive system and lead to malnutrition in childhood.

 Nursing Insight—*Meconium ileus*

Meconium ileus may be the initial presentation of CF in the neonate. This is demonstrated by a meconium stool that is described as thick and sticky and present in 15% of newborns with CF. Meconium ileus may cause an obstruction which requires surgical removal.

Signs and Symptoms

CF affects the different vital organs of the body, and children with the condition show a wide range of signs and symptoms. The severity of the symptoms varies from child to child. Because CF is a multisystem disease (failure of two or more organ systems), the symptoms are presented according to the body system affected:

- Gastrointestinal tract symptoms include:
  - Meconium ileus
  - Prolonged jaundice
  - Steatorrhea
  - Rectal prolapsed
- Respiratory symptoms include:
  - Crackles
  - Wheezes
  - Diminished breath sounds
  - Dry productive cough
  - Tachypnea, hypoxia, and cyanosis
- Integumentary symptoms include:
  - Salty-tasting tears and skin
- Secondary consequences include:
  - Dehydration
  - Malnutrition
  - Intestinal atresia
  - Idiopathic pancreatitis
  - Biliary cirrhosis
  - Cholestasis

- Emphysema and atelectasis
- Prolonged hypoxia
- Hemoptysis
- Bacterial pneumonia
- Diabetes
- Anemia
- Failure to thrive
- Osteoporosis
- Common characteristics include a child that is:
  - Thin and underweight (classified as less than or equal to 10th percentile for height and weight on a standardized growth chart)
  - Has a barrel chest
  - Has a protuberant abdomen and distention
  - Has wasted buttocks
  - Has thin extremities
  - Is listless and lethargic
  - Has delayed development of secondary sex characteristics and infertility
  - Has occlusion of the vas deferens in males
  - Has occlusion of the ovarian ducts in females

Diagnosis

The diagnosis of CF is based on the child's signs and symptoms, including a positive history of the disease in the family, absence of pancreatic enzymes, increase in the electrolyte concentration of sweat, and chronic pulmonary involvement. Chest x-ray films show patchy atelectasis and obstructive emphysema. A quantitative sweat chloride test is performed on sweat obtained by iontophoresis of pilocarpine. The results of the sweat chloride test are determined differently depending on the age of the child. A chloride concentration of greater than 60 mEq/L is diagnostic of CF. The normal values of sweat chloride test are usually less than 40 mEq/L. A concentration between 30 to 59 mmol/L for infants less than 6 months or from 40 to 59 mmol/L in older children is considered within an intermediate range (John & Brady, 2012a). Pancreatic dysfunction is also clinically apparent. Tests for direct documentation of enzyme secretion are invasive and are not routinely done for children. Pulmonary function tests are done in older children. These tests help to evaluate the progression of the disorder and provide direction for suitable treatment.

Prevention

There is no known prevention for this disease process. In families where there is a known case of CF, identification of carriers may assist the parents in family planning decisions.

 Across Care Settings: Promoting respiratory function

To ensure respiratory function, a multidisciplinary approach is taken. A physician, nurse, respiratory therapist, social worker, dietitian, and psychologist are the important professionals in the management of a child with CF.

Collaborative Care

Nursing Care. The goal of treatment is to ensure respiratory function, enhance nutrition, promote growth and development, and encourage independence in an individual child and family. The potential for the complications related to respiratory infection and malnutrition can be reduced or prevented by instructing the parents on proper nutrition, medication compliance, good hand washing, and avoiding contact with persons with respiratory infections.

Medical Care. Airway clearance and antibiotic use are the key treatment modalities for lung disease related to CF. Ensuring respiratory function in children entails controlling infection and improving aeration. These care measures are achieved via medicated aerosol therapy, chest physiotherapy (percussion and postural drainage), and antibiotic therapy (Fig. 23-4). Some children with CF may have a central venous access device for frequent antibiotic administration. Evidence-based medications routinely used in the treatment of CF include inhaled mucolytic agents, recombinant human DNAse (Pulmozyme), inhaled hypertonic saline, and medication for chronic Pseudomonas infections, which include inhaled tobramycin (TOBI) and oral azithromycin (Federico et al., 2011).

Most children with CF have a complete loss of pancreatic function and inadequate digestion of fats and protein; therefore, an important aspect of management is to replace the pancreatic enzymes. Enzyme replacement is administered with meals and snacks so the digestive enzymes are mixed with food in the duodenum. Enzyme replacement should not exceed 2,500 lipase units/kg per meal (Carter & Marshall, 2011). The nurse must explore the best way of administering oral capsules with the family and the child.

 Optimizing Outcomes—Nutrition

The best outcome for a child with CF is a well-balanced, high-protein, high-caloric diet. Pancreatic insufficiency results in malabsorption of fat-soluble vitamins (vitamins A, D, E, K). Daily vitamin supplementation is recommended. The nurse can also work closely with family to prevent infection as well as optimize nutrition and growth of a child.

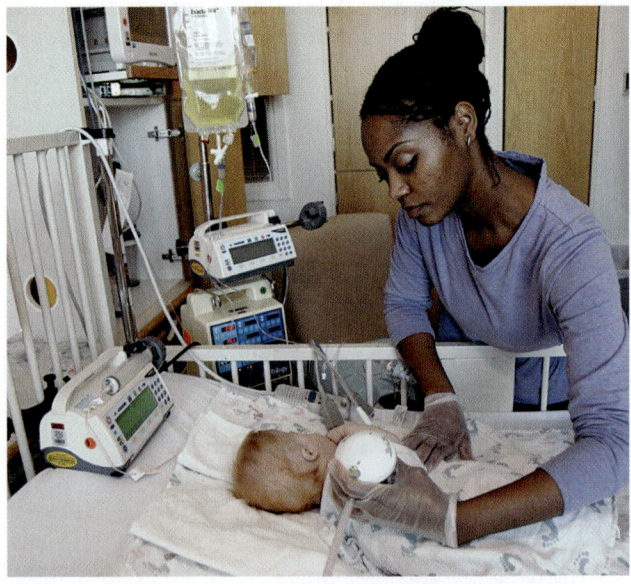

Figure 23-4 Chest physiotherapy is performed to loosen and remove lung secretions. Percussion and vibration are used over the affected areas of the lungs.

Education/Discharge Instructions

 Across Care Settings: Caring for the child with cystic fibrosis at home

It is essential that the nurse teach parents how to care for their child at home. After the diagnosed and acute phase of illness, the family is prepared for home management and assists in promoting child growth and development with limitations.

- Teach the family about the nature of the disease and prepare them to manage day-to-day minor complaints.
- Assist the family in arranging for the portable suction machine and about the proper suctioning technique at home.
- Instruct the family to do the respiratory therapy before a meal because chest physiotherapy may induce vomiting "of the thick tenacious mucus."
- Teach the family different techniques used for chest physiotherapy and postural drainage and coughing exercises based on their child's age. The child needs to be suctioned, followed by chest physiotherapy and inhalation to liquefy the thick secretions.
- Teach the family about preferred meal plans, high-caloric diet, and mixing pancreatic enzyme with meal.
- Instruct the family to monitor the child's weight to ensure proper growth patterns.
- Teach the family how to administer medications properly.
- Inform the family how to access community resources and how to contact their home health nurse.

 Nursing Care Plan The Child With Cystic Fibrosis

Nursing Diagnosis: Risk for infection due to impaired body defense system

Measurable Short-Term Goal: The child will remain free from symptoms of infection during hospitalization.

Measurable Long-Term Goal: The parents will implement measures to prevent infection.

NOC Outcomes:
Risk Control (1902) Personal actions to prevent, eliminate, or reduce modifiable health threats
Immune Status (0702) Natural and acquired appropriately targeted resistance to internal and external antigens

NIC Interventions:
Health Education (5510)
Infection Protection (6550)
Medication Management (2380)

Nursing Interventions:

1. Wash hands or use approved alcohol-based hand rubs, before and after providing care.

   RATIONALE: Appropriate hand hygiene helps prevent infection outbreaks, reduces transmission of antimicrobial-resistant organisms, and reduces overall infection rates.

2. Monitor temperature every 4 hours. Report a single temperature greater than 101.3°F (38.5°C) or three temperatures greater than 100°F (38°C) in 24 hours to the care provider.

   RATIONALE: Fever is often the first indication of infection.

3. Observe for and report additional signs of infection such as increased mucus production, persistent cough, tachypnea, difficulty breathing, or cyanosis.

   RATIONALE: Increased mucus production in the airways causes obstruction and stasis of fluid, providing a rich habitat for bacterial growth. Early detection of infection allows for prompt and appropriate intervention.

4. Monitor and report laboratory values as ordered, such as complete blood count with differential, serum protein, serum albumin, and cultures.

   RATIONALE: Laboratory values are correlated with the child's history and physical examination to provide a global view of the patient's immune function and nutritional status.

5. Encourage fluid intake and a high-calorie balanced diet, emphasizing proteins, fatty acids, and vitamins.

   RATIONALE: Nutrients benefiting the immune system include essential amino acids, linoleic acid, vitamin A, folic acid, vitamin B_6, vitamin B_{12}, vitamin C, vitamin E, Zn, Cu, Fe, and Se. Efficient immune function may be affected by deficiencies in one or more of these nutrients.

6. Instruct the child and parents on principles of medication management: prophylactic antibiotics, medicated aerosol therapy, chest physiotherapy (CPT), and deep breathing and cardiovascular exercise.

   RATIONALE: Instruction empowers the child and family to manage care. Medicated aerosol therapy, CPT, and deep breathing exercises help reduce atelectasis and risk for infection and promote healing.

7. Encourage use of community resources, such as the Cystic Fibrosis Foundation.

   RATIONALE: The use of community resources may help support the family to find ways to prevent infection and increase the possibility of a positive adjustment to the condition.

The nurse must help the parents understand that caring for a child with CF can be challenging. There are sufficient resources and help lines that can assist parents, and the nurse uses these resources to provide adequate health education to parents and older children.

Nursing Diagnoses Cystic Fibrosis

- Ineffective airway clearance related to thickened secretions
- Ineffective breathing patterns related to tracheobronchial obstructions
- Altered Nutrition: Less than body requirement related to inability to digest and/or loss of appetite
- Altered growth and development related to inadequate thickening of nutrients
- High risk for infection related to impaired body defense system
- Altered family processes related to frequent hospitalization/prolonged sickness

⑤ legal alert—Use ethical considerations when conducting research involving children

In conditions such as CF, it is important for the pediatric nurse to conduct research for the advancement of knowledge. It is also important for the nurse to protect the children when conducting research. Children are under the legal age limit, and research requires the consent of the parent or legal guardian. Children are especially vulnerable because of their immaturity and inability to decide for themselves.

When conducting research in the pediatric setting, be sure to:

- Obtain written consent from the parents or legal guardians.
- Obtain written assent from mature children (generally age 12–13 and older).
- Use the ethical principles of beneficence, non-malfeasance, autonomy, veracity, justice, fidelity, and professional integrity.
- Review the institutional protocols carefully, ensuring that the highest standards of research are addressed.
- Secure clearance from the Institutional Review Board at the institution.

Be sure to design the research so that:

- Children's rights are respected.
- Children are protected from harm and discomfort.
- Children's parents or legal guardians are provided the information necessary for them to give their informed consent.
- Children's rights to anonymity and confidentiality are ensured.

Source: Code of Federal Regulations Subpart A Sec. 46.102. (2009). *Basic HHS Policy for Protection of Human Research Subjects.* Office of Human Subjects Research. National Institute of Health: Bethesda, MD.

⑤ Now Can You—Describe congenital respiratory conditions and structural anomalies?

1. Prioritize developmentally appropriate and holistic nursing care for respiratory conditions?
2. Develop teaching plans and discharge criteria for parents whose children have respiratory conditions?

Upper Airway Disorders

RHINOSINUSITIS

Nursing Insight—*Sinuses*

Sinuses are hollow air spaces in the human body. In relation to the respiratory system, each sinus cavity has an opening into the nose for free exchange of air and mucus and is joined with the nasal passages by a continuous mucous membrane lining. The maxillary (behind the cheek) and ethmoid (between the eyes) sinuses are small but present at birth. The sphenoid sinuses, located behind the ethmoid sinuses, begin to develop in the first 2 years of life but are not fully visible on radiograph until about 6 years of age; they reach their permanent size by about age 12. The frontal sinuses are located between the lamina of the frontal bone and begin to develop around 7 years of age. The child's sinus cavities are not fully developed until 20 years of age, which makes the child vulnerable to sinus infection.

Rhinosinusitis was formerly referred to as sinusitis. The term rhinosinusitis more accurately acknowledges the fact that both the "nasal and sinus mucosa are involved in similar and concurrent inflammatory processes" (Yoon, Kelley, & Friedman, 2011, p. 470). Rhinosinusitis is caused by either viral or bacterial infections. The most common bacterial pathogens associated with rhinosinusitis are *S pneumonia, H influenza, M catarrhalis,* and β-hemolytic streptococci (Yoon et al., 2011).

Normally, mucus collects in the sinuses and drains into the nasal passages. When children have a cold or an allergy attack, the sinuses become inflamed and drainage is difficult. In addition, air is trapped within the already blocked sinus along with pus or other secretions. This inflammation and accumulation of secretions can lead to congestion and infection. There is usually accompanying facial pain, headache, and fever. Approximately 5% to10% of upper respiratory tract infections becomes complicated with the development of acute sinusitis. The main sites for sinusitis in children under 10 are the maxillary and ethmoid sinuses. For children over 10 the frontal sinuses are more commonly involved.

Rhinosinusitis may be either acute or chronic. Rhinosinusitis is considered chronic if it persists for more than 3 months. Allergies, nasal deformities, cystic fibrosis, nasal polyps, and HIV infection predispose children to chronic sinus infections.

Signs and Symptoms

The nurse observes for the following signs and symptoms in a child that is indicative of rhinosinusitis:

- A cold lasting more than 10 to 14 days, sometimes with low-grade fever
- Cough that is worse at night because of sinus drainage
- Fever
- Facial pain (may or may not be present)
- Eyelid edema (when the ethmoid sinuses are involved)
- Thick yellow-green nasal discharge
- Postnasal drip leading to sore throat, cough, bad breath, nausea, and vomiting
- Headaches (usually not before age 6)
- Maxillary or dental pain
- Decreased ability to smell (**hyposmia**)
- Ear pressure or fullness

- Irritability and fatigue
- Poor appetite

Diagnosis

When the child comes to the health-care facility, diagnosis of acute rhinosinusitis is determined by a physical examination and the presence of purulent nasal discharge, nasal obstruction, and facial pain, pressure, or fullness with symptoms from 10 to 30 days (John & Brady, 2012a). Sinus aspirate culture is the only accurate method of diagnosis but is not practical for routine use. Radiographic imaging studies are done in the presence of symptoms indicative of orbital, intracranial, or soft tissue abscess; if acute rhinosinusitis is unresponsive to 48 hours of antibiotics; or if the child has chronic unresponsive asthma or chronic and reoccurring rhinosinusitis.

 Nursing Insight—*Diagnosing rhinosinusitis*

Rhinosinusitis is difficult to diagnose in children because respiratory infections are more frequent during childhood.

Prevention

Prevention of rhinosinusitis includes instructing the parents on allergy management, measures to relieve nasal airway obstructions, and attention to persistent nasal discharge. Because viral rhinosinusitis is more commonly associated with day-care settings, smoking in the home, and the presence of siblings with respiratory infections, preventive measures also include attention to proper hand washing, tissue disposal, covering the nose and mouth while coughing, elimination of smoking in the home, and alternative child care options.

Collaborative Care

Nursing Care. The nurse's primary responsibilities in caring for the child with rhinosinusitis include assessment, medication administration, providing comfort measures, and providing instructions to the parents.

Medical Care. Medical management for uncomplicated bacterial rhinosinusitis includes a prescription of antibiotics. Amoxicillin (Amoxil) is generally considered the first line of treatment because it is safe and inexpensive (John & Brady, 2012a). Azithromycin (Zithromax), clarithromycin (Biaxin), erythromycin (Benzamycin), or trimethoprim/sulfamethoxazole (TMP-SMX) (Bactrim) are indicated in the presence of allergy to amoxicillin (Amoxil). Though there is no randomized controlled trial to support the use of topical decongestants, they are sometimes used with older children, though limited to 5 days to avoid rebound swelling (John & Brady, 2012a). Saline irrigation via a nasal spray or neti pot® may be helpful with acute or chronic rhinosinusitis to help thin secretions. Acetaminophen (Children's Tylenol) and ibuprofen (Children's Advil) may be used for pain relief. A cool-mist humidifier and oral fluids can relieve dry mucous membranes associated with mouth breathing.

Surgical Care. Surgery is necessary a small percentage of the time to remove a physical obstruction and drain the sinuses. The surgeon opens and widens the natural pathways of the sinuses by inserting an endoscope. The surgeon also may recommend adenoidectomy as part of the

treatment for sinusitis because infection in the adenoids can cause symptoms similar to sinusitis (American Academy of Otolaryngology, Head and Neck Surgery, 2011). The nurse's primary responsibility is to recover the child after surgery.

Education/Discharge Instructions

The nurse teaches the child and parents the importance of avoiding rhinosinusitis during a cold or allergy attack by promoting rest, liquids, and good nutrition. Instruct the parents on the use of saline nasal sprays, adequate oral fluids, and cool-mist humidifiers to help relieve sinus discomfort. Parents also need to be instructed on the importance of completing the full course of antibiotic therapy to treat the cause of the bacterial infection.

 Complementary Care: *Chiropractic Care and Chronic Rhinosinusitis*

Complementary care measures have been increasingly used for children. A good knowledge and understanding of these approaches helps the nurse provide information about these therapies. Chiropractors are one of the professional complementary care providers most often used for children and are licensed in all states. The professional fees are covered by third-party payers including Medicare and most leading insurance carriers. Chiropractors do not prescribe pharmaceuticals or perform surgery. Spinal manipulation is the principal therapeutic option. Spinal

---

Family Teaching Guidelines...
How to Avoid Rhinosinusitis (Sinusitis)

TOPIC: How to Keep the Child's Sinuses Clear

ESSENTIAL INFORMATION:

- Use an oral decongestant or a nasal spray decongestant when initial signs and symptoms appear. Gently have the child blow the nose, blocking one nostril while blowing through the other one. It is also important to remember that a nasal spray decongestant can cause rebound swelling after 3 days of usage.
- Ensure that the child drinks plenty of fluids to keep nasal discharges thin.
- Apply heat via warm compresses or heating pad (on low heat) over the inflamed area.
- Use a cool-mist humidifier in the same room or area occupied by the child.
- Avoiding air travel during the symptomatic period is recommended. In the event that there is a need for the child to fly, a nasal spray decongestant may be used before airplane takeoff to help prevent blockage of the sinuses and allowing mucus secretions to drain.
- Avoiding contact with known allergens is important.
- Using air conditioners to help ensure even room temperature is helpful.
- Using electrostatic filters attached to heating and air conditioning equipment to help remove allergens from the air is necessary.

Source: Academy of Otolaryngology, Head and Neck Surgery (2011).

manipulation is a form of manual therapy that involves the movement of a joint beyond its usual end range of motion but not past its anatomical range of motion. Chiropractors engage in health promotion and treatments of pediatric conditions such as otitis media, asthma, allergic rhinitis, sinusitis, infantile colic, and enuresis. An initial visit to the chiropractic clinic lasts for about 45 minutes; follow-up visits are generally 15 to 20 minutes. Adverse effects from chiropractic adjustments are rare. Families who use this complementary therapy rarely abandon their mainstream health-care provider or traditional medical practices.

Chiropractic treatment of rhinosinusitis is based on the theory that abnormal positioning of spinal bones interferes with healthy nerve impulses and that sinus drainage, nasal congestion, and headaches may be triggered by nerve impulses caused by misalignment of spinal bones.

"What to say"—*How to talk to parents about chiropractic therapy*

The nurse approaches the family with compassion and sincerity. Expressions of caring are conveyed in the following statements:

Nurses are in a position to be asked by parents about chiropractic therapy. When asked, the nurse provides parents with the basic knowledge in nontechnical terms. The nurse speaks in an open-minded, nonjudgmental fashion, avoiding terms such as "unproven" or "unconventional." The nurse also elicits values, beliefs, and influences that led the parents to opt for the complementary therapy. When possible, the nurse supports the parents' decisions and offers to obtain more information for the family.

NASOPHARYNGITIS

Nasopharyngitis, also referred to as the common cold or an upper respiratory infection (URI) is a viral infection of the respiratory tract that involves the nose and throat. It occurs throughout the year but the highest incidence occurs during the early fall until the late spring and lasts for about 7 days. Young children have an average of six to ten URIs per year but 10% to 15% of children have at least 12 infections per year. Thirty percent to 40% of URIs are caused by rhinoviruses; other causes include enteroviruses, respiratory syncytical viruses (RSV), influenza, and parainfluenza viruses (Yoon et al., 2011). Rhinovirus is more common in the early fall and late spring season, RSV primarily in the winter and spring, and the parainfluenza virus in autumn. Adenovirus and coronavirus produce epidemics during the winter and spring. The common cold spreads easily from one person to another. Viruses causing the ailment are spread by small and large particle aerosols.

Signs and Symptoms

- Gradual onset
- Rhinorrhea (clear and watery at first then becoming thicker and more purulent)
- Sore throat
- Difficulty swallowing (**dysphagia**)
- Mild cough
- Low-grade fever
- Red nasal membranes

- Mild conjunctival irritation or redness
- Anterior cervical lymphadenopathy
- Clear chest sounds
- Headache
- Malaise

Diagnosis

Diagnosis is based on the presenting symptoms. It is important to rule out other conditions that are possibly more harmful than the common cold. Routine laboratory examinations are not generally necessary in diagnosing a common cold. Pathogens associated with colds may be detected by culture, antigen detection, or serological methods. A specific etiological diagnosis is useful only when treatment with antiviral agents is being considered.

Prevention

The importance of good health as the major preventive measure for children not to catch cold is also stressed. Prevention means that children are given adequate nutrition, rest, and sleep. Good hand washing and care in avoiding touching eyes and nose can help prevent the spread of the URI. Instruct parents on the avoidance of secondhand smoke and crowded places during cold seasons. Instruct parents to avoid contact with persons known to have URI symptoms.

Collaborative Care

Nursing Care. Nursing care for the child with a viral URI is supportive and is directed toward parent education and symptomatic relief of pain, fever, and congestion. Symptomatic treatment includes fluids, antipyretics, and rest. Nasopharyngitis causes discomfort especially for the infant. The nurse elevates the head or crib, which helps with the child's drainage of secretions. Normal saline nose drops may help thin nasal secretions. Maintaining adequate fluid intake in the child is important because it prevents dehydration and keeps secretions thinned for easier expulsion. Fruit juices and gelatins may be offered to the child to increase fluid intake. The nurse communicates to the parents to avoid milk and milk products in excess because this makes secretions thick and sticky. It may be helpful if nurses offer these fluids in tiny colorful cups or glasses with straws so they are more attractive to the child. The nurse can also stress the importance of rest. Children are given play activities such as puzzle games, story books, crayons, and art materials to decrease boredom.

Medical Care. The use of antihistamines, decongestants, and cough medications is not recommended for children under 4 years of age and is used with caution in children younger than 6 years old (John & Brady, 2012a). If recommended by the primary care provider, antihistamines may be prescribed to help dry up nasal secretions. Parents are instructed to administer antihistamines with caution because they dry up the bronchial secretions, which in turn may make the cough worse. Antihistamines can also cause dizziness and drowsiness. Antibiotics are not recommended for a dry hacking cough. Most cough mixtures contain alcohol so the medication needs to be administered with caution.

Education/Discharge Instructions

Because the hands are the primary vehicle for transmission of the cold virus, the parents and child can be instructed on good hand washing, tissue disposal, and cleaning of toys, tables, and other items used by the child to prevent the spread of infection. The nurse advises the parents that disposable wipes and tissue papers used for secretions are disposed in sealed plastic bags.

Parents are instructed on the use of normal saline nasal drops or spray before feedings to reduce thick or crusted mucus. Suctioning the nares with a bulb syringe can assist in removing secretions. Parents are also instructed on how to prepare homemade saline nose drops by mixing 8 oz of distilled water, a half teaspoon of salt, and a quarter teaspoon of baking soda. This mixture can be kept up to 24 hours if refrigerated, though it should be brought to room temperature before use.

PHARYNGITIS

Pharyngitis is an inflammation of the mucosa of the pharynx that frequently results in sore throat. It occurs most commonly in winter and is spread by close contact. The incidence is high among children and declines in late adolescence and adulthood. Approximately 85% of sore throats are viral in nature, of which adenovirus is the most common (Yoon et al., 2011). Fifteen to 25% of the cases of pharyngitis are caused by group A beta-hemolytic streptococci (GABHS).

Pharyngitis can either be a short illness with no symptoms or could result in severe, life-threatening illness. In cases of the latter, the causative agent is group A beta-hemolytic streptococci, which may lead to acute rheumatic fever, scarlet fever, or acute glomerulonephritis. Colonization of the pharynx by GABHS may produce either asymptomatic or acute infection. The M protein is the major virulence factor of GABHS and facilitates resistance to phagocytosis by polymorphonuclear neutrophils. Type-specific immunity develops during infection and provides protective immunity to subsequent infection with that particular M serotype.

Signs and Symptoms

- Often an abrupt onset
- Fever
- Sore throat
- Difficulty swallowing
- Headache
- Abdominal pain
- Inflamed, red, and enlarged pharynx and tonsils, which are often covered with exudates
- Anterior cervical lymphadenopathy
- The presence of petechiae on the palate; a fine, red, sandpaper-like rash on the trunk or abdomen; and a strawberry tongue are common findings with a group A streptococcus infection

Viral pharyngitis is usually self-limiting with symptoms subsiding in 3 to 5 days unless superimposed by sinusitis or parapharyngeal or peritonsillar abscess.

Diagnosis

Throat culture remains a good way to diagnose streptococcal pharyngitis (Fig. 23-5). A false-positive culture can occur if other organisms are misidentified as GABHS, and children who are streptococcal carriers may have positive cultures. False-negative cultures are attributed to a variety

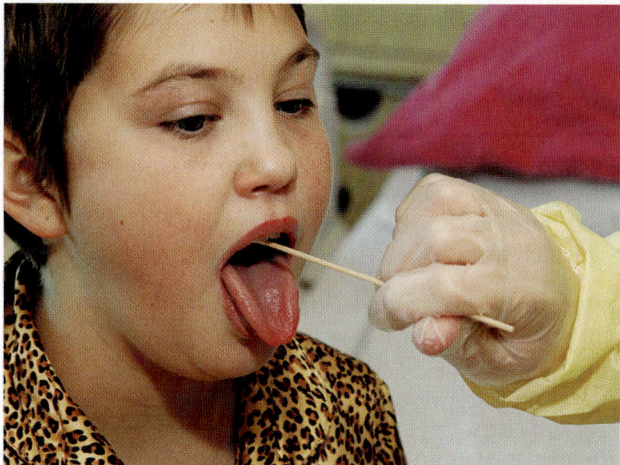

Figure 23-5 Use a long, sterile cotton swab to swab a culture from the back of the child's throat.

of causes, including an inadequate throat swab specimen and a patient's covert use of antibiotics (Smith, 2011). Diagnostic test kits with rapid identification of GABHS are available for use at the office or clinic settings. These rapid tests have high specificity. Therefore, a positive result generally does not need a throat culture confirmation. The throat culture does give information about susceptibility of the organism to specific antibiotics.

Prevention

Good hand washing, covering the nose and mouth when coughing, and care in avoiding touching eyes and nose can help prevent the spread of the pharyngitis. Instruct parents on the avoidance of secondhand smoke and crowded places during flu seasons. Instruct parents to avoid contact with persons known to have pharyngitis.

Collaborative Care

Nursing Care. Nursing care for the child with pharyngitis is generally supportive and is directed toward parent education with regard to ensuring fluid administration, prevention of dehydration, and providing symptomatic relief of pain and fever. The nurse instructs parents about administering oral penicillin and analgesics as prescribed. Emphasize bedrest, especially during the acute phase of the illness. A cold or warm compress to the neck is helpful to relieve pain. If the child is old enough, warm saline gargles and throat lozenges may be offered to the child to soothe the painful throat. A cool-mist humidifier may be used to help moisten nasal pharyngeal mucosa. Food and fluids are given as tolerated because swallowing is painful. Cool and bland liquids are less painful to swallow than hot and solid foods. The child should not be forced to eat if there is intense pain upon swallowing. Rather, foods that are high in nutrients and energy can be offered when the child can tolerate eating. Hand washing by the caregivers, including both nurses and parents, is done to prevent the spread of the infection.

Medical Care. Viral pharyngitis is generally treated with supportive care as needed, which includes pain and fever relief with acetaminophen or ibuprofen. Most untreated cases of streptococcal pharyngitis resolve in a few days.

The objective of antibiotic therapy is to hasten clinical recovery and prevent acute rheumatic fever. Antibiotics may be started immediately without culture. Oral penicillin is the prescribed treatment of choice. Oral penicillin is inexpensive and is given 2 or 3 times a day for 10 days. Oral amoxicillin (Amoxil) is suitable for children because it is available as chewy tablets or as a suspension. Oral erythromycin (Erythrocin) is indicated in children allergic to penicillin.

Education/Discharge Instructions

For children who are cared for at home, it is important that the nurse instruct the parents to give the full dose of the antibiotic prescribed even though the child shows signs of improvement. This is a very important aspect in the management of pharyngitis to prevent valvular damage of the heart. Instruct parents on methods used to provide pain and fever relief, such as administering acetaminophen (Children's Tylenol) or ibuprofen (Children's Advil) and use of a cool-mist humidifier. Discuss the importance of providing food and fluids as tolerated in the form of a cool and bland diet. Because organisms may be harbored on inanimate items, such as bathroom cups, toothbrushes, or orthodontic devices, parents are instructed to clean or discard the item as appropriate to prevent reinfection. Children may return to school once they are afebrile and have taken the antibiotics for at least 24 hours.

TONSILLITIS

Inflammation of the tonsils often occurs with pharyngitis, which may lead to the diagnosis of tonsillitis or tonsillopharyngitis. Tonsillitis is an inflammation of the tonsils, which are masses of lymphoid tissue located within the pharynx. Tonsils protect the respiratory and alimentary tracts from infection by inducing secretory immunity and regulating the production of secretory immunoglobulin. Tonsils normally enlarge progressively between 2 and 10 years of age and reduce progressively during preadolescence, which makes the tonsils of children larger than those of adults. Nearly all children in the United States experience at least one episode of tonsillitis. Viruses and group A beta-hemolytic streptococcus are the most common cause of infection in tonsillitis.

Signs and Symptoms

There are several types of tonsillitis: acute, recurrent, chronic, and peritonsillar abscess. The signs and symptoms differentiate the types of tonsillitis.

The presenting symptoms in acute tonsillitis include:

- Fever
- Chills
- Foul breath (halitosis)
- Dry throat
- Dysphagia (difficulty in swallowing)
- Referred otalgia (pain in the ears)
- Headache
- Malaise (fatigue)
- Muscular pains
- Enlarged cervical nodes
- Enlarged tonsils (tonsils that are observed to touch at the midline are called "kissing tonsils" or are 4+ in size)
- Airway obstruction may occur because of enlarged tonsils and lead to mouth breathing

Symptoms usually resolve in 3 to 4 days; however, some patients may remain symptomatic for up to 2 weeks, even during therapy. Recurrent tonsillitis presents with multiple episodes of the illness in a year.

Symptoms of chronic tonsillitis include:

- Foul breath (halitosis)
- Chronic sore throat
- Foreign body sensation
- A history of expelling foul tasting, smelly, cheesy lumps

Symptoms of peritonsillar abscess include:

- Severe throat pain
- Fever
- Drooling
- Foul breath (halitosis)
- Difficulty opening the mouth
- Changes in voice quality
- Partial deafness may occur as a result of the inflammatory process brought about by the infection

Diagnosis

Diagnosis is based on the presenting symptoms and inspection of the throat.

Prevention

Good hand washing, covering the nose and mouth when coughing, and care in avoiding touching eyes and nose can help prevent the spread of the organism that causes tonsillitis. Instruct parents to avoid secondhand smoke and crowded places during flu seasons. Also, instruct parents to avoid contact with persons known to have pharyngitis, which is often associated with the development of tonsillitis.

 Medication: Erythromycin

(eh-rith-roe-**mye**-sin)

Indications:
IV, PO: Infections caused by susceptible organisms including upper and lower respiratory tract infections and otitis media

Actions: Suppresses protein synthesis at the level of the 50S ribosome.

Therapeutic Effects: Bacteriostatic action against susceptible bacteria spectrum: streptococci, staphylococci, and gram-positive bacilli.

Contraindications and Precautions:
CONTRAINDICATED IN: Hypersensitivity

Adverse Reactions and Side Effects: CNS: Seizures, EENT: Ototoxicity, CV: QTC prolongation, ventricular arrhythmias, GI: Nausea, vomiting, abdominal pain, Derm: Rashes

Route and Dosage:
Children PO: 30 to 50 mg/kg in divided doses q 6 to 8 hr.
Neonates PO: 20 to 50 mg/kg per day divided q 6 to 12 hr.

Nursing Implications:
1. Inform parents of medication administration.
2. Prepare to administer around the clock.
3. Use calibrated measuring device for liquid preparations.
4. Do not crush or chew delayed-release capsules or tablets; swallow whole.

Source: Data from Vallerand, A. H., & Sanoski, C. A. (2014). *Davis's drug guide for nurses* (14th ed.). Philadelphia, PA: F.A. Davis.

Collaborative Care

Nursing Care. Nursing care of tonsillitis requires nursing care similar to that of pharyngitis. Cool-mist humidifiers help maintain hydration of the mucous membrane during periods of mouth breathing. Warm saline gargles, throat lozenges, and antipyretics may be ordered to reduce discomfort. A soft or liquid diet is preferred.

Medical Care. Medical management consists of antibiotics, antipyretics, and analgesics. Penicillin, erythromycin (Erythrocin), and amoxicillin (Amoxil) are the commonly prescribed antibiotics. Cephalosporins or clindamycin (Cleocin) are more effective for patients with chronic conditions.

Surgical Care. Tonsillectomy (surgical removal of the tonsils) is used for recurrent or chronic tonsillitis. There are no criteria for the number of infections before tonsillectomy is carried out (Smith, 2011). The American Academy of Otolaryngology and Head and Neck Surgery (2011) suggests the occurrence of three or more treated infections per year as sufficient to necessitate a surgical intervention. Surgery is performed 6 weeks after an acute infection has been resolved.

After the surgery, children are kept on their side to facilitate drainage of secretions. Providing comfort and reducing activities that may aggravate bleeding is a priority. Coughing, clearing the throat, and blowing the nose are to be avoided. Secretions and vomitus are checked for fresh blood. Because the throat is sore after surgery, the nurse can apply ice packs and an ice collar to provide relief. Food and fluids are offered when the child is alert: cool water, crushed ice, and flavored ice-pops are the initial foods to be given. However, red- or brown-colored fluids are not given so the nurse is able to distinguish the drainage, which might be fresh or old blood. As the child begins to tolerate food, items such as gelatin, cooked fruit, sherbet, soup, and mashed potatoes are offered. Foods to avoid include milk, ice cream, and pudding because they coat the mouth and throat and cause the child to clear the throat, which may cause bleeding.

Education/Discharge Instructions

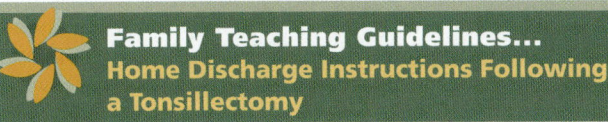

Family Teaching Guidelines...
Home Discharge Instructions Following a Tonsillectomy

TOPIC: The nurse can teach the parents to:

♦ Keep the child away from highly seasoned food and "sharp" foods (e.g., nacho chips) for a period of 2 weeks. The scab is most likely to be dislodged at 8 to 12 days.

♦ Have the child avoid gargling and vigorous tooth brushing.

♦ Instruct the child that he or she should not cough or clear the throat.

♦ Limit the child's activities that may result in bleeding.

focus on safety

Signs of bleeding after tonsillectomy

When the nurse is caring for a post-tonsillectomy child, if the child is continuously swallowing, it is indicative of bleeding. Additional signs to be observed are restlessness, increased pulse rate, and pallor (late symptom).

 Now Can You—Enhance communication?

1. Perform activities to increase the child's communication and interaction with the nurses during illness and hospitalization?
2. Describe ways to enhance the children's feelings of control over their care?

CROUP

Croup is a generic term encompassing a heterogeneous group of illnesses affecting the larynx, trachea, and bronchi. The lateral walls of the trachea below the level of the vocal cords are marked by swelling and erythema. Croup is described according to the main anatomical area affected. Epiglottitis, supraglottitis, laryngitis, laryngotracheobronchitis and bacterial tracheitis encompass the croup syndrome. Croup commonly affects children between 3 months and 5 years of age, most often at around 2 years of age. The incidence is higher in boys, and it is most frequent during the winter months. The incidence of epiglottitis has dramatically decreased since the introduction of the Hib vaccine in the late 1980s.

Viral agents, particularly the parainfluenza viruses (types 1, 2, and 3), and RSV are the most common cause of croup and account for the majority of cases (Smith, 2011). *Streptococcus pyogenes*, *S pneumoniae*, and *Staphylococcus aureus* are the common causes of epiglottitis while *Haemophilus influenzae*, *S aureus*, and *Corynebacterium diphtheriae* are involved in bacterial tracheitis.

Signs and Symptoms

The symptoms of croup can be explained in terms of the anatomical structure of children. The subglottic region of the larynx is held within the rigid ring of the cricoid cartilage. Symptoms are related to the extent of upper airway involvement and the infectious agent responsible for the croup. Croup can lead to obstruction because children have a narrow larynx, such that a decrease in airway diameter causes a decrease in airflow, leading to the symptoms of croup.

Acute laryngotracheitis
- Usually viral (parainfluenza, adenovirus, RSV)
- Peak age is 3 to 36 months
- Gradual, acute onset during the night
- URI symptom
- Seal-bark cough
- Mild to moderate dyspnea
- Symptoms worse at night
- Low-grade fever
- Respiratory rate less than 50

Spasmodic croup
- Usually viral
- Peak age is 3 to 36 months
- Generally no preceding illness, though may have coryza

- Sudden onset often at night
- Fever variable
- Barky cough
- Hoarseness

Epiglottitis
- Usually caused by *Haemophilus influenzae type B* (Hib)
- Peak age is 1 to 5 years
- Rapid onset
- Sore throat
- Dysphagia
- Anxiety related to inspiratory distress without significant stridor (John & Brady, 2012a)
- Drooling
- Muffled speech
- Toxic appearance
- Tripod positioning
- Marked distress
- High fever ranging from 101.8°F to 104°F (38.8°C to 40°C)

Laryngotracheobronchitis (LTB)
- Usually caused by *Staphylococcus aureus* (John & Brady, 2012a)
- Peak age is 3 to 36 months
- Acute onset
- Hoarseness
- Barky cough
- Inspiratory stridor
- Toxic appearance
- Purulent sputum
- Marked distress
- High fever 102.2°F (39°C)

Bacterial tracheitis
- Considered a bacterial complication of a viral disease
- Can lead to a life-threatening airway obstruction severe enough to cause respiratory arrest
- Preceded by upper respiratory tract infection
- Croupy cough
- Stridor unaffected by position
- Toxic appearing
- High fever
- Stridor
- Hoarseness
- Dyspnea
- Retractions and nasal flaring
- Thick purulent tracheal secretions

Laryngitis
- More common in older children
- Usually caused by a virus
- Hoarseness
- May have upper respiratory symptoms including coryza, sore throat, and nasal congestion
- Malaise
- Low-grade fever
- Headache
- Myalgia

ACUTE EPIGLOTTITIS

Acute epiglottitis or supraglottitis is a sudden, potentially lethal condition characterized by high fever, sore throat, dyspnea, and rapidly progressing respiratory obstruction.

Acute epiglottitis is considered a medical emergency and is considered a serious obstructive inflammatory condition that requires immediate attention.

 ### Nursing Insight—*Epiglottis*

A common scenario is that the child goes to bed asymptomatic and awakens with complaints of sore throat and pain or swelling accompanied by a febrile state. The classic sign of acute epiglottitis is when the child sits upright in a tripod position with the chin thrusted out (sniff position). The child's mouth is open with drooling, a protruding tongue, and dysphagia. The child is irritable and restless with a thick and muffled voice and frog-like croaking sound on inspiration. Suprasternal and substernal retractions may be visible. The nurse notes that the child breathes slowly, the throat is red and inflamed, and there is a distinctive large, cherry-red, edematous epiglottis.

 ### focus on safety

Hospitalization

Symptoms that warrant hospitalization are progressive stridor, severe stridor at rest, respiratory distress, hypoxia, cyanosis, and depressed mental status (confusion, altered levels of consciousness, etc.).

Diagnosis

Diagnosis of the croup syndrome is based on the signs and symptoms along with the history. Because of the severity of the respiratory distress, immediate treatment takes priority over testing. Soft tissue imaging of the neck and chest demonstrates the classic presentation of subglottic narrowing or the "**steeple sign**." When epiglottitis is suspected, blood cultures are ordered to identify the causative organism. A radiograph of the lateral neck may present with the "thumb sign," which describes the x-ray appearance of the epiglottis (John & Brady, 2012a). The diagnosis of a bacterial cause for croup, such as in the case of bacterial tracheitis and LTB, can be confirmed by an elevated white blood cell count, which includes leukocytosis with a left shift. Bacterial tracheitis can be differentiated from epiglottitis by a slower onset, the absence of the thumb sign, and classic symptoms presented in epiglottitis.

Prevention

Routine immunization with Hib provides primary prevention of epiglottitis. Good hand washing, proper tissue disposal, and covering the nose and mouth when coughing are effective methods of preventing spread of infection.

 ### focus on safety

Epiglottitis

If epiglottitis is suspected, DO NOT attempt to visualize the throat with a tongue blade because this may cause a laryngospasm leading to an immediate airway occlusion. If the health-care provider plans to do a direct laryngoscopy, the nurse prepares for tracheal intubation because of the potential for an airway occlusion. The insertion of an artificial airway may rapidly improve the child's respiratory status.

Collaborative Care

Nursing Care. The nursing care measures for the various causes of croup depend on the causative organism. The most important goal in the treatment of children with croup is maintaining the airway and providing adequate respiratory exchange. The nurse stays at the child's side to reduce child and parent anxiety, observes for worsening symptoms, and helps the child maintain a position that supports maximum airway and respiratory exchange. Key areas of nursing responsibility include maintaining the airway, providing rest and humidification, monitoring fluid balance, and administering medications as prescribed. Changes in condition are based on observations and assessment of the child's response to therapy, including careful observation of the child's response to his or her surroundings (changes in level of consciousness).

Medical Care. Commonly, mild cases of croup are treated with cool mist. A high-humidity, cool air vaporizer may be used at home in the child's room. In the hospital setting, oxygen hoods for infants and oxygen tents for toddlers are used. Cool mist is thought to moisten airway secretions to facilitate clearance, soothe inflamed mucosa, and provide comfort and reassurance to the child thereby lessening anxiety. Nebulized racemic epinephrine (Micronefrin or Vaponefrin) (0.25 to 0.5 mL in 3 mL of a normal saline solution) or *l*-epinephrine (5 mL of 1:1,000 solution) are equally effective to cause mucosal vasoconstriction and consequently decrease subglottic edema, thus relieving the symptoms (Vallerand & Sanoski, 2014). This treatment is indicated for those with moderate to severe stridor at rest or when stridor does not respond to cool mist. Observe the child after nebulization to assess the airway and side effects of the delivered medication.

Corticosteroids are also given to children to decrease the edema in the laryngeal mucosa through their anti-inflammatory action. IM dexamethasone (Decadron) and nebulized budesonide (Pulmicort) are widely used (Sharma & Conrad, 2011).

Antibiotic therapy is indicated for epiglottitis and bacterial tracheitis. Combinations of ampicillin and sulbactam (Unasyn) are the drugs most often prescribed. Antibiotics are not used in the management of viral croup.

Education/Discharge Instructions

Parents are instructed on the use of cool-mist humidification, as well as the potential to use a steamy bathroom to help modify respiratory symptoms. If the child has been hospitalized and discharged on medications, the parents also need instructions on the importance of compliance and the proper administration and dosage of medications. Parents are also instructed on symptoms of potential side effects of the medications and the symptoms of a worsening condition (e.g., specifically increased signs of respiratory distress, restlessness, and confusion).

❀✿ **Nursing Diagnoses** Upper Respiratory Disorders

- Risk for ineffective airway clearance related to excessive secretions, inflammation, or obstruction in the airway
- Risk for ineffective breathing pattern related to tracheobronchial inflammation or obstruction
- Risk for imbalanced nutrition: Less than body requirements related to discomfort with swallowing
- Anxiety related to perceived threat of hospitalization, or to invasive procedures or changes in health status of the child
- Risk for deficient fluid volume related to inadequate fluid intake or excessive losses through abdominal route
- Pain related to procedures or increased pressure in the middle ear (specific to otitis media)
- Disturbed sensory perception: Auditory related to inflammation and edema in the middle ear (specific to otitis media)
- Fatigue related to increased respiratory effort

OTITIS EXTERNA AND OTITIS MEDIA

Infectious ear disorders may be divided into otitis externa, which is an inflammation or irritation of the outer ear and ear canal; and otitis media, which is a suppurative infection of the middle ear cavity.

Otitis Externa

Although it is popularly called swimmer's ear, it can occur in situations that do not involve swimming. It usually affects older children and teens whose ears are exposed to persistent excessive moisture. It occurs more often in warm climates and during the summer. Otitis externa involves an inflammatory reaction of the external auditory canal, which may also include the pinna or tympanic membrane.

External otitis is commonly caused by *Pseudomonas aeruginosa*, especially in association with swimming in pools or lakes (Smith, 2011). Fungal infections with *Candida* and *Aspergillus* may also be the causative agents. Excessive wetness as in swimming or bathing, dryness of the air canal, lack of cerumen, presence of other skin pathology, digital trauma, and a foreign body make the skin of the ear canal vulnerable to infection. Otitis externa may develop in up to 20% of children with tympanostomy tubes and is associated with *Staphylococcus aureus*, *Streptococcus pneumoniae*, *Moraxella catarrhalis*, *Proteus*, *Klebsiella*, and occasional aerobes (Smith, 2011).

Signs and Symptoms

- Itching
- Pain, accentuated when the pinna or targus are moved and with chewing
- Feeling of pressure or fullness (may be either conductive or sensorineural)
- Occasionally hearing loss
- Rare **otorrhea**, which is defined as inflammation with purulent discharge
- Erythema and edema of the ear canal
- Cerumen may become whitish
- Absence of fever

Diagnosis

Examination of the ear and the occurrence of the presenting symptoms including a positive history confirm the diagnosis. On otoscopy (the use of the otoscope in examining the ear), the ear canal appears swollen and debris may be present. The patient may resist insertion of the otoscope because of pain. A culture may be done for bacteria or fungus when the otitis externa does not appear to be improving.

Prevention

Parents and children can prevent future episodes of otitis externa by keeping the external ear canal dry. Earplugs may be worn when swimming, though some sources discourage the use to prevent reinfection (Smith, 2011; Yoon et al., 2011). During bathing, shower caps or earplugs with petroleum jelly may be used. Strategies to promote ear canal dryness include drying the ear canals using a hair dryer on a low setting. Solutions that can promote drying the ear canal after swimming include a mixture of half rubbing alcohol and half vinegar, Burow solution, or diluted isopropyl alcohol. Two to three drops may be squirted into the ear, which would then be allowed to run out. Children are instructed to avoid scratching or cleaning the external ear canal.

Collaborative Care

Nursing Care. The goal of nursing care is to manage pain, treat the infection, and educate the family on strategies to prevent reinfection. Pain relief may be managed with the use of analgesics and warm compresses or a heating pad to the affected ear. Antibiotic or antifungal eardrops may be prescribed. The nurse educates parents on the proper dose and method of administering the drops as well as on strategies to prevent reinfection.

Medical Care. Antibiotic or antifungal eardrops are prescribed for a course of 7 to 10 days. Corticosteroids are also effective in treating most forms of external otitis. If the ear canal is swollen, a cotton wick is inserted into the ear canal so that the eardrops travel into the end of the canal. Analgesics are given to relieve pain.

Education/Discharge Instructions

Parents and child education include strategies included under prevention in addition to instructing the parents on the proper dose and method of administering the eardrops.

Otitis Media

Otitis media (OM) is an infection of the middle ear. It is one of the most prevalent conditions of early childhood. *Streptococcus pneumoniae, Haemophilus influenzae, Moraxella catarrhalis,* and *S pyogenes* group A streptococci are the most common causes of infection in otitis media (Petersen-Smith & McKenzie, 2012). Tobacco smoke, including passive or secondhand smoke, aggravates the otitis media by impairing mucociliary function with subsequent congestion of soft nasopharyngeal tissues.

 Nursing Insight—*The pathology of otitis media*

The pathology of otitis media is understood by reviewing the structure and functions of the eustachian tube in children. The eustachian tubes in children are shorter, wider, and more horizontal in infants than in adults. The eustachian tube carries out three functions:

- Protection of the middle ear from nasopharyngeal secretions
- Drainage of secretions produced in the middle ear
- Ventilation of the middle ear, which serves to equalize air pressure within the middle ear with atmospheric pressure in the external ear canal and to replenish oxygen that has been absorbed

Because of this structure of the eustachian tubes in children, drainage is often impaired, which results in retention of secretions and air in the middle ear. The horizontal position also facilitates the movement of pathogens up the eustachian tube from the pharynx into the middle ear. Edema resulting from upper respiratory infection, allergic rhinitis, or hypertrophic adenoids interferes with the functions of the eustachian tube.

The following factors lead to otitis media in children:

- The eustachian tubes are short, wide, and straight and lie in a horizontal plane.
- The cartilage lining is undeveloped, making the tubes more distensible. The normally abundant pharyngeal lymphoid tissue readily obstructs the eustachian tube openings in the nasopharynx.
- Immature humoral defense mechanisms increase the risk of infections.
- The lying-down positions of infants favor the pooling of fluid, such as formula, in the pharyngeal cavity.

The incidence is highest among children between 6 months and 2 years with 39% of infants experiencing their first case of acute otitis media by 9 months and 62% by 24 months of age (Petersen-Smith & McKenzie, 2012). By 6 years of age, 75% of children have had one or more episodes of otitis media. In addition to the physical discomfort and economic costs related to otitis media, there is evidence that children with recurrent otitis media are at risk for both hearing loss and speech delay.

Otitis media presents in several forms: acute otitis media (AOM), otitis media with effusion (OME), and chronic otitis media with effusion (COME). The term otitis media is a frequently used, general term and refers to an inflammation of the middle ear without reference to etiology or pathogenesis. More specifically, acute otitis media is inflammation of the middle ear space with the rapid onset of the signs and symptoms of acute infection, such as fever and ear pain. Otitis media with effusion occurs when there is fluid in the middle ear space without symptoms of acute infection. Some references note that OME is also referred to as chronic OM (Yoon et al., 2011). COME is a persistent middle ear infection with discharge through a tympanic membrane perforation. OME may occur independent of AOM or may be the result of a persistent, unresolved AOM lasting for more than 3 months (Smith, 2011). OME may occur after an ear infection has run its course and fluid remains trapped behind the eardrum. COME refers to a condition in which fluid remains in the middle ear for a long time even though there is no infection.

 Nursing Insight—*Breastfeeding and otitis media*

A direct link has been established between OM and infant feeding methods. Infants who have been breastfed have a lower incidence of OM than those who have been bottle fed. The number of episodes of OM decreases significantly with increased duration and exclusive breastfeeding. Breast milk contains immunoglobulin A (IgA), which offers protection against allergies and viruses. Because of the position of the infant during breastfeeding, there is less likelihood of reflux of milk in the ear, whereas bottle feeding increases the chances of milk getting into the ear.

Signs and Symptoms
- Acute otitis media
  - **Otalgia** (acute ear pain)
  - Irritability
  - Otorrhea
  - Fever, which may be as high as 104°F (40°C)
  - Poor feeding

- Rubbing or pulling at the affected ear
- Bulging tympanic membrane, air fluid level, or visualization of purulent material on otoscopic examination
- Postauricular and cervical lymph glands and lymph node enlargement
- Otitis media with effusion (OME) or chronic OM
  - Often asymmetric and afebrile
  - Intermittent complaints of ear pain
  - Feeling of fullness in the ear, popping or a feeling of "talking in a barrel" (Petersen-Smith & McKenzie, 2012)
  - Complaint of hearing loss
  - Dizziness or impaired balance
  - Chronic vomiting and failure to thrive may be related to chronic OME (Petersen-Smith & McKenzie, 2012)

Diagnosis

Diagnosis is based on signs and symptoms as well as an otoscopic examination. An otoscopic examination reveals that in AOM the intact membrane appears bright red and bulging with no visible landmarks or light reflex. The usual landmarks of the bony prominences from the long and short processes of the malleus are obscured by the outwardly bulging membrane. In OME, otoscopic examination reveals a slightly injected, dull gray membrane, obscured landmarks, and a visible fluid level or meniscus behind the eardrum if air is present above the fluid.

Prevention

To minimize the recurrence of otitis media, the parents are instructed to eliminate identified environmental allergens, feed infants in an upright position, avoid propping the bottle, and encourage medical follow-up to check for complications such as chronic hearing loss. There may also be an advantage to avoiding pacifiers (Vergison, Dagan, Arguedas, Bonhoeffer, Cohen, Dhooge, et al., 2010). Exclusive breastfeeding until at least 6 months of age is also considered protective (Petersen-Smith & McKenzie, 2012). Parents are also instructed to avoid excess exposure to individuals with upper respiratory infections and secondhand smoke. Xylitol syrup or xylitol containing gum has been suggested as potentially protective, though studies are currently under way to validate this effect (Klein & Pelton, 2011).

Collaborative Care

Nursing Care. The goal of nursing care is to manage pain, treat the infection, and educate the family on strategies to prevent reinfection. Pain relief may be managed with the use of analgesics and warm compresses or a heating pad to the affected ear. Antibiotic or antifungal eardrops may be prescribed. The nurse educates the parents on the proper dose and method of administering the drops as well as on strategies to prevent reinfection.

Medical Care. The guidelines published in 2004 by the American Academy of Pediatrics and the American Academy of Family Physicians remain the current recommendation for the diagnosis and management of AOM (American Academy of Pediatrics (AAP): American Academy of Family Physicians, 2004a; Petersen-Smith & McKenzie, 2012). Recommendations include controlling fever and pain with either acetaminophen (Children's Tylenol) or ibuprofen (Children's Advil). The cause of AOM has changed from primarily bacterial to primarily viral in recent years because of an increasing administration of vaccines that decrease the incidence of bacterial infections; withholding the use of antimicrobials is advised unless a bacterial cause is clearly evident. The first line of drug choice is amoxicillin (Amoxil) given for 10 days (Smith, 2011).

For resistant infections or severe illness with fever greater than 102.2°F (39°C), amoxicillin-clavulanate (Augmentin) may be used. Care may also include high doses of cefdinir (Omnicef) combined with tympanocentesis (drainage of fluid from the middle ear using a small-gauge needle to puncture the tympanic membrane) (Venes, 2013). Use of decongestants and antihistamines are not considered helpful. Ofloxacin (Floxin) or ciprofloxacin antimicrobial ototopical drops (Cipro) may be prescribed if the tympanic membrane is perforated, if the child has ear drainage, or if the child has patent pressure equalizing tubes (PET) in his or her ears.

Medical management of children with OME involves identifying risks for speech, developmental language, and learning problems and documenting each visit for the presence of effusion (AAP, 2004b). Children not considered to be at risk are watched for 3 months and referred to an otolaryngologist as symptoms indicate.

Surgical Care.

 Nursing Insight—*Patent pressure equalizing tubes*

Though once considered a common procedure for equalizing middle ear pressure, use of pressure equalizing tubes (PETs) for healthy children with persistent middle ear effusion is now under reconsideration (Petersen-Smith & McKenzie, 2012). Some sources indicate that insertion of PETs in children under age 3 with a history of persistent OME does not result in significant improvement or improved speech and language acquisition (John & Brady, 2012b). Current practices recommend waiting 6 months for bilateral effusion resolution and 9 months for unilateral effusion resolution before a decision is made to insert PETs.

Surgical insertion of pressure equalizing tubes remains a common treatment for persistent OME. The tubes are inserted into the tympanic membrane via a myringotomy and generally remain in place for several months subsequently falling out on their own. The procedure, which takes approximately 15 minutes, may be done in an outpatient setting. Parents are instructed on the administration of eardrops if prescribed postoperatively. The health-care provider may also recommend strategies to avoid having water enter the ear, though generalized water precautions are also controversial. Parents may be instructed to have the child wear earplugs while bathing or swimming. Placement of PETs promotes an increase in language acquisition through improved hearing.

Education/Discharge Instructions

Antibiotics are used judiciously in the management of otitis because of the increasing resistance of the pathogens. Health education from the nurse is important if a decision is made to treat the condition with an antimicrobial agent. The full course of the antimicrobial therapy must be strictly followed. The nurse tells the parents that if the child fails to respond to this initial antimicrobial management within 48 to 72 hours, another assessment must be done to confirm AOM and exclude other causes of illness or ineffective antibiotic response.

focus on safety

Rupture of the tympanic membrane

The rupture of the tympanic membrane brings immediate relief of pain, a gradual decrease in temperature, and the presence of a purulent discharge in the external auditory canal. Rupture of the tympanic membrane may lead to scarring and hearing loss.

 Now Can You—Recognize upper airway disorders and provide discharge education?

1. Identify the symptoms of the various upper airway respiratory conditions?
2. Prepare home care and management plans for children with tonsillitis, croup, epiglottitis, rhinosinusitis, and otitis media?

Lower Airway Disorders

BRONCHITIS

Bronchitis is a nonspecific bronchial condition in which there is inflammation of the bronchial tubes. It is unusual for children to be diagnosed with bronchitis alone; other associated upper and/or lower respiratory tract conditions are more likely to be involved because of the close proximity of the respiratory tract structures. Tracheobronchitis is a more common term used when the trachea is prominently involved.

Bronchitis may be acute or chronic. Acute bronchitis is commonly preceded by a viral upper respiratory tract infection and may last for 1 to 3 weeks. The incidence of acute bronchitis is highest during the winter months. Children are usually affected in their first 4 years of life. Chronic bronchitis lasts for months or years and is more common among adults, particularly smokers. The incidence of chronic bronchitis in children is also more often associated with cigarette smoking or the presence of secondhand smoke, as well as with the presence of another chronic condition, such as allergies, asthma, and cystic fibrosis.

Viruses are usually the causative organism. The tracheobronchial epithelium is invaded by the infectious agent, and this leads to activation of inflammatory cells and release of cytokines, giving way to the occurrence of symptoms. If the tracheobronchial epithelium becomes significantly damaged or hypersensitized, then a protracted cough may last for 1 to 3 weeks.

Signs and Symptoms

- Dry, hacking cough that becomes more productive and purulent over time and worsens at night
- Rhinorrhea occurring 3 to 4 days after onset of a cough
- Signs of nasopharyngeal infection and conjunctivitis
- Coarse breath sounds, rhonchi, and coarse, changing rales
- Low-grade or no fever
- Low substernal discomfort or burning in the chest
- Chronic bronchitis is characterized by the presence of a productive cough lasting more than 3 months

Diagnosis

Because a virus is usually the causative organism, bronchitis is diagnosed based on the child's symptoms. In children older than 6 years of age, *M pneumoniae* can be a common cause, and bronchitis can then be determined by the identification of this bacterium.

Prevention

Good hand washing, covering the nose and mouth when coughing, and care in avoiding touching eyes and nose can help prevent the spread of the organisms that cause bronchitis. Instruct parents on the avoidance of secondhand smoke, dust exposure, known allergens, air pollution, and crowded places during flu seasons. Instruct parents to avoid contact with persons known to have bronchitis.

Collaborative Care

Nursing Care. Nursing care is generally directed toward providing supportive care and the provision of adequate air exchange. To be able to provide oxygenation, the nurse must ensure that the airway is open and free of obstruction. The airway can be opened by administering prescribed bronchodilators. The nurse encourages the child to clear the airway from secretions by coughing. Use of a cool-mist humidifier at the bedside may help liquefy secretions, which promotes expectoration when coughing. Secretions are disposed of in sealed plastic bags. The nurse suggests to the parents that is not unusual for a young child to swallow secretions instead of coughing them out, which may cause the child to vomit these accumulated secretions during the night.

Medical Care. For acute bronchitis, care is primarily supportive. Symptom relief may include use of antipyretics, analgesics, and humidity. Cough suppressants are administered with caution because they interfere with clearance of secretions. The condition is self-limiting, and antibiotics, though often prescribed, do not hasten improvement in uncomplicated cases. The treatment for chronic bronchitis depends on the cause or underlying condition. The chronic cough associated with asthma or other underlying chronic conditions may be treated with bronchodilators, cromolyn sodium (Nasalcrom), corticosteroids, and anticholinergic agents (John & Brady, 2012a).

Education/Discharge Instructions

Home care may include instructing the parents on the use of a cool-mist humidifier, providing sufficient fluids and nutrition, and encouraging the child to expectorate secretions. Parents are instructed to avoid exposing the child to secondhand smoke, environmental pollutants, and known allergens.

BRONCHIOLITIS AND RESPIRATORY SYNCYTIAL VIRUS

Bronchiolitis is an inflammation of the bronchioles and small bronchi. It is also referred to as "infectious asthma, asthmatic bronchitis, wheezy bronchitis or virus induced asthma" (John & Brady, 2012a, p. 730). Bronchiolitis causes lower respiratory tract obstruction because of inflammation and edema, which may lead to bronchospasms. Bronchiolitis is usually caused by viral pathogens, such as respiratory syncytial virus (RSV), adenovirus, and parainfluenza virus (types 1, 2, and 3), among others. RSV accounts for the majority of cases of bronchiolitis, which peaks in the winter, generally beginning as early as September or October and continuing through April or May. Bronchiolitis is common among children age 2 years and younger. Nearly 80% of the cases of bronchiolitis occur in children younger than 1 year of age (John & Brady, 2012a). By the age of 2, nearly every child has been exposed to the virus.

Bronchiolitis is highly contagious and spreads by direct contact with respiratory secretions or from particles on contaminated objects. Bronchiolitis is easily spread from hand to eye, nose, and mucous membranes.

The peak period for a child to acquire RSV is December through March. RSV most often begins as an infection in the nasal epithelial cells. The RSV virus then replicates in the host cell. The host cell is destroyed, and virus particles are released to propagate the infection. The infection results in the destruction of the epithelial cells of the respiratory tract (Weinberger, 2011). Exposure to RSV triggers a humoral immune response. Primary RSV infection results in only a weak antibody response with IgM, IgG, and IgA produced (John & Brady, 2012a). This response is not enough to destroy the virus completely or to prevent upper respiratory tract replication of the virus. Consequently, an upper respiratory tract illness develops. High levels of neutralizing antibodies are required to prevent the progression of infection from the upper respiratory tract to the lower respiratory tract.

Signs and Symptoms

- Upper respiratory infection (URI) symptoms of cough, coryza, and rhinorrhea lasting 3 to 7 days
- Respiratory distress marked by noisy, raspy breathing and cyanosis
- Audible wheezing
- Retractions
- Rales and prolonged expiratory phase of respirations
- Tachypnea
- Low to moderate fever up to 102°F (38.9°C)
- Decreased appetite and poor feeding
- Pharyngitis
- Depending on the duration of symptoms and oral intake, dehydration may be manifested by poor tearing, dry mucous membranes, and poor skin turgor
- Thick mucus, exudate, and mucosal edema obstruct the smaller airways (bronchioles) leading to a reduction in expiration, air trapping, and hyperinflation of the alveoli
- The obstruction interferes with gas exchange, possibly leading to hypoxemia (decreased oxygen) and hypercapnia (increased carbon dioxide in the blood), which in turn leads to respiratory acidosis
- May be accompanied by otitis media and conjunctivitis
- May result in hospitalization

Diagnosis

Positive identification of RSV is accomplished by either of two methods: enzyme linked immunosorbent assay (ELISA) or rapid immunofluorescent antibody from direct or aspiration of nasal secretions or nasopharyngeal washings (John & Brady, 2012a; Smith, 2011). Chest x-ray films reveal hyperaeration, hyperinflation, atelectasis, areas of collapse, and flattened diaphragm indicating air trapping.

Arterial blood gases reveal decreased pH and a $PaCO_2$ greater than 45 mm Hg, indicating respiratory compromise and potential failure. Complete blood count shows increased white blood cells (WBC), which is indicative of infectious processes. Pulse oximetry provides evidence of decreasing oxygen saturation (Smith, 2011).

Prevention

Proper hand washing, reducing exposures to and transmission of RSV, and avoiding secondhand smoke are the best means of prevention. The monoclonal antibody palivizumab (Synagis) is given IM to high-risk infants and shown to be effective in reducing the complications of RSV, hospitalization, and associated morbidities as prophylaxis for high-risk infants (Federico et al., 2011).

Collaborative Care

Nursing Care. RSV is treated symptomatically through maintenance of hydration, fever control, oxygenation, and keeping the mucous membranes clear of mucus. Children may be managed at home. Hospitalization is recommended for children who have some other underlying illness or are in a debilitated state. In the hospital, nursing care includes head elevation of 30 to 40 degrees, oxygen saturation monitoring, and cool-mist therapy combined with oxygen administered by hood or tent in concentrations sufficient to alleviate dyspnea and hypoxia. The nurse administers IV fluids until the child shows signs of improvements.

Strict isolation is required for patients infected with RSV virus because it is easily spread from hand to eyes or nose and other mucous membranes. The nurse emphasizes hand washing and that contact precautions such as the use of gown, gloves, and masks are required (Fig. 23-6). Parents need to know that the first 24 to 72 hours is the critical time and in most cases there is complete recovery.

Medical Care. The clinical goal is to return the child to a normal respiratory status. Medical therapy is aimed at relief of respiratory distress, improvement in oxygenation, and alleviation of airway obstruction.

An antiviral agent such as RSV-IGIV or RespiGam has been used as a prophylactic to prevent RSV in high-risk children. This antiviral agent may be administered via endotracheal tube, hood, or tent. When an antiviral agent is administered, crystallization of the medication can occur in the nares, endotracheal tube, or eyes. An antiviral agent can be teratogenic (an environmental agent capable of producing a birth defect) to the fetus of a pregnant woman.

Additional medical management may include inhaled or oral corticosteroids, chest physiotherapy, and antibiotics. Antibiotics are not routinely used unless there is another associated bacterial infection (Weinberger, 2011).

Education/Discharge Instructions

Educate parents on the importance of watching for signs of worsening conditions, such as signs of respiratory distress and dehydration, and on when to seek care. Instruct parents on the use of cool-mist humidification, providing fluids, and fever control. Parents can be instructed to manage rhinitis through the use of saline drops and nasal suctioning. Guidelines for feeding an infant with signs of mild respiratory distress may include smaller, more frequent feedings, upright

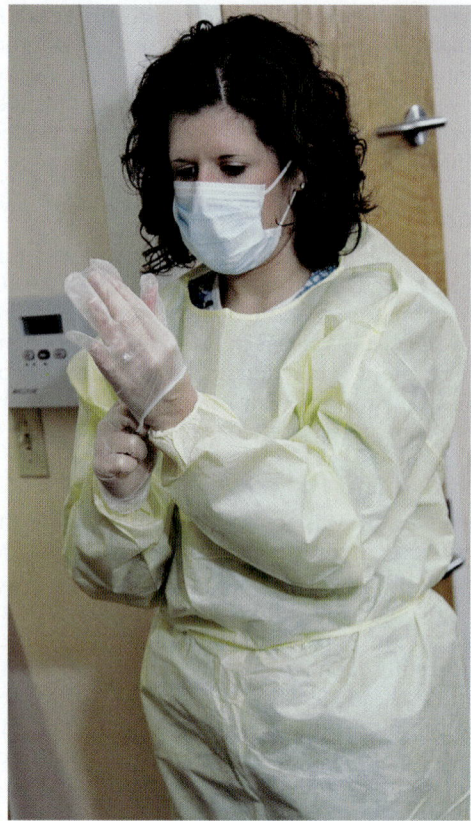

Figure 23-6 When a child has respiratory syncytial virus, contact precautions, such as the use of gowns, gloves, and masks, are required.

positioning, strategies to prevent vomiting, and observing for signs of respiratory distress during feeding.

PNEUMONIA

Pneumonia is a lower respiratory tract infection of the pulmonary parenchyma. It is more common in infancy and early childhood. It may occur as a primary infection or secondary to another illness or infection. Pneumonias are classified as lobar, bronchopneumonia, and interstitial. Lobar pneumonia involves lobes of the lungs. Bronchopneumonia begins with involvement of the terminal bronchioles that become clogged with mucopurulent exudate and forms consolidated patches in the lungs, while interstitial pneumonia is more or less confined to the alveolar walls (Smith, 2011).

The term "community-acquired pneumonia" is defined as pneumonia in a previously healthy individual, which was contracted outside the hospital setting. Hospital-acquired (nosocomial) pneumonia refers to pneumonia that is acquired in the hospital setting (Light, 2011).

Viral pneumonia, a more common form, involves RSV infection in infants and parainfluenza and adenoviruses in older children, whereas *Streptococcus pneumoniae* is the common pathogen causing bacterial pneumonia. Viral pneumonia accounts for 45% of pneumonia cases (Light, 2011). A viral infection can have a secondary bacterial infection 6 to 8 days after initial onset because of viral insult of protective mechanisms.

Aspiration pneumonia may occur as a result of aspiration of foreign material into the lower respiratory tract.

Lung inflammation, which may or may not be associated with consolidation, is referred to as pneumonitis (John & Brady, 2012a).

 Nursing Insight—*Typical or atypical pneumonia*

Pneumonia may also be typical or atypical. An atypical pneumonia indicates a lack of localization in the patterns of consolidation (John & Brady, 2012a). The most common causes of atypical pneumonia include *Mycoplasma pneumoniae* and *Chlamydophila pneumoniae* (Light, 2011).

Most often, pneumonia is a complication of a preexisting infection or a condition produced when a patient's defense mechanisms have been weakened and the causative agent multiplies and is spread through the lymphatic system, bloodstream, and sinuses. The severity is related to the virulence of the invading microorganism (Light, 2011).

Signs and Symptoms

The symptoms of pneumonia are variable depending on the site affected, cause, and age of the child. Common symptoms may include the following:

- URI symptoms (cough, coryza, rhinorrhea) lasting 3 to 7 days
- Onset
  - Viral: acute, gradual
  - Bacterial: acute, gradual
  - Mycoplasma and Chlamydia: slow
- Fever
  - Low to moderate, up to 102°F (38.9°C) with viral pneumonia
  - Acute onset of high fever with bacterial pneumonia greater than 102.2°F (greater than 39°C)
  - Mycoplasma and Chlamydia greater than 102.2°F (greater than 39°C)
- Clinical findings
  - Viral: cough, coryza, hoarseness, crackles, wheezing, stridor
  - Bacterial: cough, dyspnea, tachypnea, rales, decreased breath sounds, grunting, retractions, toxic appearance
  - Mycoplasma and Chlamydia: persistent productive cough (sputum may be rust colored or bloody), malaise, headache (John & Brady, 2012a)
- Additional symptoms, which vary with cause, location, and age of the child:
  - Chest pain
  - Retractions
  - Nasal flaring
  - Malaise
  - Decreased appetite
  - Rhonchi or fine crackles
  - Decreased breath sounds
  - Varying degrees of respiratory distress, which may include restlessness, pallor, cyanosis, grunting, and prolonged expiration
  - Abdominal distention
  - Palpable liver and spleen related to pressure from hyperinflated lungs (John & Brady, 2012a)

Diagnosis

Clinical features and chest x-ray exams aid in the diagnosis of pneumonia. It is not always possible to identify the causative agents based on x-ray exams alone. Clinical history, the child's age, and laboratory examinations help in identifying the causative agent. Radiographic examination shows diffuse or patchy infiltration with peribronchial distribution. A sputum culture may help determine the cause when bacterial pneumonia is suspected. The WBCs will be elevated and greater than 20,000/mm³ with predominant neutrophils in the case of bacterial pneumonia (John & Brady, 2012a). In the case of a critically ill or immunocompromised child, a blood culture may be indicated (Light, 2011). A septic workup to include blood, urine, and cerebral spinal fluid (CSF) cultures may also be done in infants under 2 months of age (John & Brady, 2012a).

 Diagnostic Tools Chest Radiograph

The chest radiograph aids in the diagnosis of pneumonia. Opacities, seen as white areas on the x-ray plate, represent consolidation and are typical in cases of pneumonias.

Prevention

Prevention of pneumonia includes immunization. The American Academy of Pediatrics (2012) recommends seasonal flu vaccine for all persons beginning at age 6 months and older. The Centers for Disease Control and Prevention (2012) recommends "pneumococcal conjugate vaccine (PCV13) for all children younger than 59 months old and for adults with certain risk factors. Children 24 months or older who are at high risk of pneumococcal disease should also receive the pneumococcal polysaccharide vaccine (PPSV23). High-risk children should also receive the pneumococcal vaccine.

Collaborative Care

Nursing Care. Nursing care is primarily directed toward providing supportive care and educating the family about the illness and management. Supportive care includes ensuring adequate hydration, which will help in thinning secretions. Oxygen administration via nasal cannula with cool mist, chest physiotherapy, and postural drainage are initiated for patients requiring hospitalization (Fig. 23-7).

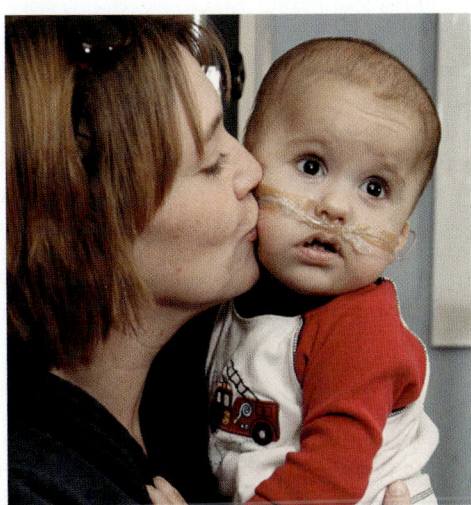

Figure 23-7 Oxygen administration via nasal cannula.

Labs: Sputum Culture and Sensitivity

To establish the causative organism and the most effective and appropriate antibiotic, culture and sensitivity tests of the sputum are performed. Coughed out sputum is difficult to obtain from children, especially those who are very young. A specimen may be obtained via a direct throat swab immediately after coughing. In some cases, a sterile catheter may be inserted directly into the trachea through the endotracheal tube or during direct laryngoscopy. During sleep, children usually swallow their sputum; therefore, an early morning fasting specimen obtained via gastric aspiration may also be obtained. The gastric content can be collected before breakfast by inserting the naso-oral tube into the stomach.

The nurse must place the specimen in the appropriate container and properly label it with the patient's name, the nature of the specimen, date and time collected, and the examination desired. Ideally, the specimen must be sent immediately to the laboratory. If this is not feasible, the specimen is kept in a refrigerator until it is taken to the laboratory. Results of the test may be reported in 2 or more days.

Supplemental oxygen may be necessary with children experiencing significant respiratory distress and who would be easily fatigued by activities. IV fluids help prevent dehydration. Elevating the head of the bed will promote improved air exchange of the lungs.

Nursing care measures such as changing the child's clothes and linen take place frequently to prevent chills. Positioning the child on the affected side naturally splints the chest and reduces pleural rubbing that causes discomfort. Assess the child's sputum for color, amount, and consistency. The sputum assessment must be recorded in the child's record.

To detect any change in condition, assess vital signs and breath sounds. Also assist the child and the parents in alleviating anxieties through continuous emotional support and reassurance.

Medical Care. Most cases of pneumonia can be treated at home with rest and fluids and symptomatic management with analgesics and antipyretics. Antibiotics are given for bacterial pneumonia and not for viral pneumonia. If antibiotics are given, the drugs may range from amoxicillin (Amoxil) to the third-generation cephalosporins, depending on the severity of the condition. Bronchodilators also might be used. Analgesics may reduce the pain associated with coughing.

Education/Discharge Instructions

Treatment of a child with pneumonia is supportive depending on the severity of the symptoms. Education includes instructing the parents on the importance of adhering to the prescribed antibiotic regimen. Parents of infants may need to be instructed to continue frequent, small feedings because the child may tire easily. Inform the parents that complete recovery from pneumonia may occur in about 2 weeks. Even if the child is feeling better after treatment, gradual return to normal activities like school and play are encouraged.

Nursing Diagnoses Lower Respiratory Disorders

- Risk for ineffective airway clearance related to excessive secretions in the airway, tracheobronchial inflammation, or obstruction
- Risk for ineffective breathing pattern related to tracheobronchial inflammation or obstruction

- Risk for impaired gas exchange related to ventilation perfusion imbalance
- Anxiety related to perceived threat of hospitalization, or to invasive procedures or changes in health status of the child
- Risk for deficient fluid volume related to inadequate fluid intake or excessive losses through abdominal route
- Fatigue related to increased respiratory effort

 Now Can You—**Recognize lower airway disorders and provide discharge education?**

1. Identify the symptoms of the various upper airway respiratory conditions?
2. Prepare home care and management plans for children with bronchiolitis, bronchitis, and pneumonia?

Infectious Conditions

PERTUSSIS

Pertussis, or whooping cough, is a highly contagious bacterial infection of the respiratory tract that causes paroxysmal cough. A "whooping" sound is produced as the child tries to take a breath. The disease is still a major cause of morbidity and mortality in children younger than 2 years. According to the Centers for Disease Control and Prevention (CDC), during 2012 outbreaks of pertussis were reported in a majority of states. An increased number of cases were reported in 49 states and the District of Columbia up through November 21, 2012, compared with the same time period in 2011. In 2010, 27,500 cases were reported. As of January 5, 2013, surveillance systems indicated that more than 41,000 cases were reported to the CDC during 2012, which included 18 pertussis-related deaths, the majority of which occurred among infants younger than 3 months of age. The incidence rate of pertussis among infants exceeds that of all other age groups. The second highest rates were among children 7 through 10 years old in addition to an increased rate among adolescents 13 and 14 years of age (CDC, 2013).

The causative organism is *Bordetella pertussis*, a gram-negative coccobacillus. The disease is spread via droplet infection and direct contact with discharges from respiratory mucous membranes of an infected child. Pertussis is highly contagious; approximately 80% to 90% of susceptible individuals exposed to the infection develop the disease.

In this condition, *B pertussis* attaches to and multiplies on the respiratory epithelium, starting in the nasopharynx and ending primarily in the bronchi and bronchioles (John & Brady, 2012a). A tracheal cytotoxin is produced that is responsible for the local epithelial damage that produces the respiratory symptom.

Signs and Symptoms

Pertussis is divided into three stages: catarrhal, paroxysmal, and convalescent stages. The classic cough of pertussis lasts from 6 to 10 weeks (John & Brady, 2012a). Each of the stages lasts for 2 to 4 weeks (Ogle & Anderson, 2011). The incubation period ranges from 6 to 21 days (John & Brady 2012a).

CATARRHAL STAGE
- Lasts 1 to 2 week
- Upper respiratory infection similar to common cold
- Mild cough, coryza, and sneezing
- Low-grade fever less than 101°F (38.3°C)

PAROXYSMAL STAGE
- Lasts 2 to 4 weeks
- Fever absent or minimal
- Persistent staccato, paroxysmal cough ending with an inspiratory whoop
- Cyanosis, sweating, prostration, and exhaustion from coughing (Ogle & Anderson, 2011)
- Coughing may be accompanied by a red face and protruding tongue
- Conjunctival hemorrhage and facial petechiae may occur related to the force of the cough
- Saliva, mucus, and tears may flow from nose, eyes, and mouth during cough
- Vomiting may accompany coughing

CONVALESCENT STAGE
- Lasts 3 weeks to 6 months
- Symptoms diminish over that period of time
- Coughing becomes less severe and paroxysms and whoops slowly disappear
- Cough may persist for months and is aggravated by physical stress and respiratory irritants

Diagnosis

It is not easy to diagnose pertussis because the initial symptoms are similar to those of other upper respiratory tract infections. The diagnosis of pertussis is based on a history of severe coughing, with or without a whoop, reddening of the face during coughing, and incomplete or absent pertussis vaccination.

When blood testing is performed, there is profound lymphocytosis, usually more than 70% of the total WBC count, which often increases to 20,000 to 40,000 or even 100,000 cells/mm². Chest radiography may show focal atelectasis and/or peribronchial cuffing.

The criterion standard for diagnosis of pertussis is isolation of *B pertussis* in a culture from a swab taken from nasopharyngeal secretions. Polymerase chain reaction (PCR) testing to detect DNA is also commonly done. The CDC recommends both culture and PRC tests if a child has a cough lasting longer than 3 weeks. Many health-care professionals now consider serological testing with enzyme linked immunosorbent assay (ELISA) to be the criterion testing standard (Ogle & Anderson, 2011).

Prevention

Primary preventive care occurs through vaccination against the disease with DTaP. The vaccine is a combination of diphtheria, pertussis, and tetanus toxoids. DTaP is recommended at 2, 4, 6, and between 15 and 18 months with a booster at 4 to 6 years. A booster is also recommended for adolescents between 11 and 12 years of age. The vaccine has an efficacy of 70% to 90% and may not prevent the illness entirely, but it has been shown to lessen disease severity and duration (Smith, 2011).

Collaborative Care

Nursing Care. The goals of nursing care include limiting the number of paroxysms; observing the severity of cough; and maximizing nutrition, hydration, rest, and recovery (Guinto-Ocampo, & McNeil, 2010). During hospitalization, the nurse can implement droplet precaution. Droplet precaution is an isolation technique that decreases transmission of organisms when an infected child coughs, sneezes, or spits (Venes, 2013). Droplet precautions are recommended for 5 days after the commencement of therapy or 3 weeks after the onset of paroxysmal cough if no antimicrobial therapy has been given. During hospitalization, the nurse must vigilantly monitor the child's vital signs and oxygen saturation. Nursing care also centers on the child's hydration and nutritional status. If the child is unable to drink, an IV infusion is given. The nurse accurately records coughing, feeding, vomiting, and weight changes.

Medical Care. Antibiotic therapy is given to eradicate the infection, reduce morbidity, and prevent complications. Erythromycin (Erythrocin) is the drug of choice for pertussis. It is given at 40 to 50 mg/kg per day (not to exceed 2 g) four times in a day for 14 days (Ogle & Anderson, 2011). Children allergic to erythromycin (Erythrocin) are given trimethoprim sulfamethoxazole (Bactrim) (Smith, 2011). Corticosteroids may be used to reduce the severity of the illness although it increases the risk of masking a superinfection.

Education/Discharge Instructions

The nurse also instructs the parents that no special diet is required for the child because the child is fed according to what is tolerated. The same is true for the child's activities. For as long as the child can tolerate, he or she can participate in regular activities and play. The prognosis for recovery is good for children who are well-managed. It is important for the nurse to emphasize the importance of follow-up checks.

 Nursing Insight—What if the family expresses concerns about having the child immunized with the pertussis vaccination?

In December 2005, the American Academy of Pediatrics approved recommendations from the Committee on Infectious Disease for universal vaccination of DTaP for adolescents at the 11- or 12-year visit to boost protection against pertussis.

PULMONARY TUBERCULOSIS

Tuberculosis (TB) is a chronic bacterial infection, usually of the lungs that is spread through the air. *Mycobacterium tuberculosis* is its most common causative agent. There was a declining rate of TB until the mid-1980s, when outbreaks drew new attention to TB. This outbreak was brought about by the increase in immunosuppressed individuals, particularly those with HIV, as well as an increase in drug-resistant strains.

Aside from *M tuberculosis*, *Mycobacterium bovis* may also affect children because the microorganism may be present in unpasteurized milk or milk products. Latent tuberculosis infection occurs after the inhalation of infective droplet nuclei of *M tuberculosis*. Conditions such as lowered body resistance, HIV infection, malnutrition, untreated upper respiratory tract infection, and other debilitating conditions increase the chance acquiring an active infection.

Transmission of tuberculosis is person-to-person through airborne droplet nuclei. It rarely occurs by direct contact with infected discharge or a contaminated fomite (any substance that adheres to and transmits infectious material) (Venes, 2013). Young children with tuberculosis rarely infect other children or adults because the tubercle bacilli are sparse in the endobronchial secretions of children and cough is often absent or lack the force necessary to suspend the infectious particles (John & Brady, 2012a; Smith, 2011).

When the organism enters the lungs, there is proliferation of epithelial cells that surrounds and encapsulates the multiplying bacilli as a way of warding it off. This process forms the typical tubercle. The extension of the primary lesion causes progressive tissue destruction as it spreads within the lungs. The tubercle bacilli are carried to most tissues of the body through the blood and lymphatic vessels. Tuberculosis that infects other body systems includes:

- Tuberculosis meningitis, which involves the brain and is demonstrated by symptoms of headache, nausea, vomiting, and other signs of increased intracranial pressure. This type of TB is fatal without treatment.
- Glandular tuberculosis extends into the lymph nodes. Symptoms include tenderness and immobility of the node. Treatment may include incision and drainage.
- Miliary tuberculosis involves invasion and erosion of the blood vessels of the lungs.
- Skeletal tuberculosis is associated with osteomyelitis and arthritis. (Ogle & Anderson, 2011; Smith, 2011)

Other forms of tuberculosis are abdominal or gastrointestinal (GI) tract tuberculosis, which occurs from swallowing infected material. It may involve associated tuberculosis peritonitis. Urogenital tuberculosis involves the kidneys. Once a person becomes infected with the organism, progression may occur in three different directions. The infection can heal, which occurs 90% of the time; the person may experience a primary infection that leads to an active case of TB; or a primary infection heals and the organism becomes dormant, which reactivates months to years later, generally in relation to something that causes stress or major life changes. This occurs in approximately 10% of individuals. Once infected with the organism, the person will have a positive tuberculin skin test regardless of whether an active case occurred.

Signs and Symptoms

Many children with TB may be asymptomatic and do not develop symptoms early in the infection. When symptomatic, children present with the same clinical manifestations as adult patients, which include:

- Low-grade fever
- Mild cough
- Night sweats
- Flu-like symptoms that resolve within a week may be observed
- Anorexia and weight loss may follow as the disease progresses

Diagnosis

The diagnosis of TB in children is challenging because children exhibit a variety of symptoms. Exact diagnosis of TB is based on the child's physical signs and symptoms, the history of exposure to TB, x-ray films that may show evidence of *M tuberculosis* infection, and laboratory cultures that may confirm the diagnosis. Early morning gastric contents from the stomach may be helpful in diagnosing TB. However, it takes about 4 weeks for the culture test to confirm the diagnosis because the bacillus grows slowly on a culture medium. Skin testing for TB is based on delayed hypersensitivity (Blosser, Brady, & Royal, 2012). The test does not become positive until 3 weeks to 3 months after the person has inhaled the organism. A positive TB skin test is indication for a radiographic evaluation, which may suggest, but not confirm, the diagnosis. The positive skin test does not indicate an active case, only that the person has become infected with the organism. Skin testing is also not always accurate; up to 40% of children with positive cultures have negative skin tests (Blosser et al., 2012). The accuracy may be impacted by the presence of HIV, malnutrition, viral illnesses, and poor injection technique or interpretation error. The diagnosis is confirmed by a positive culture of sputum or other body fluids, such as urine, gastric lavage, or spinal fluid.

 ### Cultural Diversity: Bacille Calmette-Guérin Vaccine

Bacille Calmette-Guérin (BCG) vaccine is a preparation of a dried, living, but attenuated culture of *Mycobacterium bovis*. It is used worldwide in areas with a high incidence of tuberculosis (TB) to provide passive TB immunity to infants and to protect adults who have an unavoidable risk of TB infection. In many foreign countries where BCG vaccination is widely used, the tuberculin skin test (TST) is not useful because patients vaccinated with BCG will have a positive skin test (Venes, 2013).

The BCG vaccine is not routinely given in the United States because researchers have shown that BCG vaccine has worked well in some situations, but poorly in others. The best use of BCG vaccination appears to be the prevention of life-threatening forms of tuberculosis in infants and young children.

Prevention

Prevention is directed toward avoiding contact with the organism. This includes screening populations at risk to identify and treat infected persons, which helps avoid secondary transmission from close contact. Health-care settings can avoid transmission through the use of appropriate physical ventilation of air around the infected case. Health-care facilities should have adequate ventilation with air exhausted to the outside via negative-pressure ventilation (Smith, 2011). In addition, health-care providers should have annual testing. BCG is the only available vaccine that is not routinely used in the United States. Studies demonstrate varying degrees of protection, ranging anywhere from no protective efficacy to 90% protection (Smith, 2011). Drinking pasteurized milk helps decrease transmission of *M bovis*.

Collaborative Care

Nursing Care. Nursing care is supportive and directed toward educating the parents to adhere to the medication regime. Supportive care also involves ensuring the patient has adequate rest, nutrition, and hydration, as well as aiding fever reduction and avoiding exposure to others. Most individuals receive care on an outpatient basis through clinics, schools, or a public health setting. However, in

cases of serious infection and involvement of other organs, children may need hospitalization. Children started with drug therapy are not contagious and require only standard precautions. Children with no cough and negative sputum smears may be cared for without isolation. Children with contagious infections must be placed in isolation.

During the child's hospitalization, the nurse must work closely with the family and the child to ensure that optimal care is provided. The nurse can explain the nature of disease and how children are at high risk of getting the infection. The nurse must emphasize good hand washing to reduce the chance of transmission from one person to another. Nurses can also teach children to cover their nose and mouth with tissue paper when sneezing and coughing. Proper disposal of the tissue paper in wastebaskets must also be emphasized.

During hospitalization, the nurse must assist the child in collecting different specimens for the diagnosis, which includes sputum for culture. Children are unable to cough properly, so sputum may be difficult to collect from the young child.

Medical Care. Treatment generally involves a 9-month regimen of isoniazid and rifampin (Smith, 2011). The drugs are administered daily for the first 1 to 2 months, then may be administered daily or twice weekly for the remaining time. The addition of pyrazinamide to the regimen given daily for the first 2 months may reduce the duration of therapy to 6 months (Smith, 2011). Adherence and compliance can be strengthened by directly observed therapy (Smith, 2011). Direct observation therapy (DOT) means that a health-care worker or other responsible, mutually agreed-on individual is present when medications are administered to the child. DOT has been recommended as treatment for children and adolescents with TB in the United States because it decreases the rate of relapse, treatment failures, and drug resistance.

Education/Discharge Instructions

The family of the child can be informed about the benefits of DOT. Nurses can discuss with the family about the methods for giving the medicines (e.g., tablets may need to be crushed well to facilitate its oral intake). The availability of liquid preparation in syrup form may be explored. The nurse can tell the family that they need to follow precautionary measures to prevent latent infection. The nurse emphasizes regular follow-up visits and regular intake of medications.

 ### Global Health Case Study Tuberculosis

Twelve-year-old Maria is brought to the urgent care clinic by her parents for a complaint of nonproductive cough, night sweats, fatigue, and weight loss for the past 4 weeks. Maria was recently adopted from an orphanage in a relatively poor Latin American country known for poor primary health prevention practices. Little is known of her immunization status or contact with infectious diseases. Maria has been in the United States for 6 weeks. Since that time, her parents have noted that she has lost 6 lb. The orphanage reported that little information was known about her birth parents except that she is of Latin American descent. She was born full term without complications, though the birth mother received minimal prenatal care. At birth Maria weighed 6 lb and measured 19 in. At the time of adoption the orphanage reported that Maria weighed 72 lb and was 57 in. in height. During a physical assessment, the nurse notes the following:

- T = 100.9°F
- P = 90
- R = 25
- BP = 107/67
- Weight = 66 lb (30 kg) (5th percentile on age appropriate growth chart)
- Height = 57 in (145 cm) (25th percentile on age appropriate growth chart)
- Skin is pale and dry
- Mucous membranes are dry
- Lungs: diminished breath sounds in the bases, crackles bilaterally
- Abdomen: scaphoid, active bowel sounds in all four quadrants
- Appears tired, though cooperative

critical thinking questions

1. Are these findings normal or pathological?
2. What actions should the nurse take?
3. What should be included in parent teaching?

◆ See Suggested Answers to Global Health Case Studies on *DavisPlus*.

INFLUENZA

Influenza, or flu, is a common infection of the respiratory system caused by viruses. Infants and children are most vulnerable to the influenza virus. It is estimated that children are 3 times more likely to become ill with influenza than adults are. The American Lung Association notes that in the United States influenza and its related complications result in an estimated 226,000 hospitalizations and anywhere from around 3,000 to 49,000 deaths annually; particularly older individuals and those with chronic medical conditions die from influenza in the United States (American Lung Association, 2013a). The disease rapidly spreads worldwide in seasonal epidemics. Influenza is most common during the winter months.

Labs: Tuberculin Skin Test

The TST is an exact indicator whether a child has been infected with the tubercle bacillus. The TST consists of injecting a measured amount of the intermediate strength of 5 tuberculin units of tuberculin purified protein derivative intradermally to form a small wheal in the forearm. In 48 to 72 hours, a positive reaction is marked by an area of red induration (an area of hardened tissue). Reactions are classified based on the diameter of the induration. A reaction greater than or equal to 15 mm is considered positive in children 4 years of age and older. A reaction of 10 mm in size are considered positive in children younger than 4 years of age and with high risk factors, such as underlying kidney disease, diabetes, or known contact with a health-care worker or other person with active TB. A reaction of 5 mm of induration is considered positive in immunocompromised patients (Blosser et al., 2012). A reaction of less than 2 mm, without blistering, is considered a negative TST. The American Academy of Pediatrics recommends that administration and interpretation of the TST be performed and read by trained health-care professionals (Fig. 23-8).

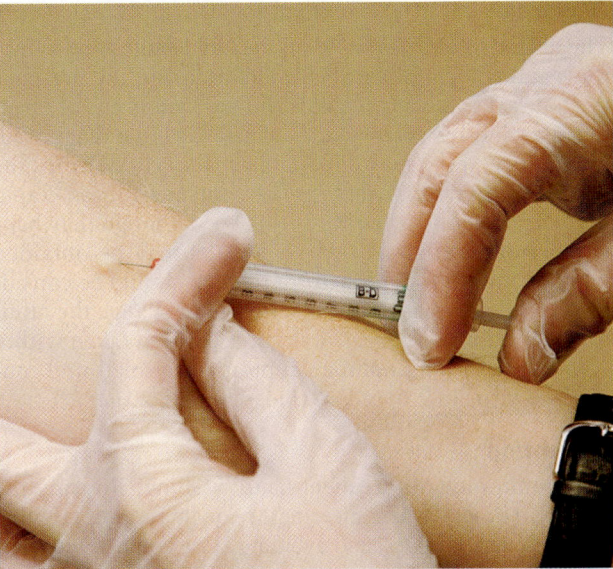

Figure 23-8 Nurse is performing a tuberculin skin test.

Three types of virus cause influenza. Influenza types A and B are the major influenza pathogens and cause epidemics. These viruses mutate and create different strains. Influenza type C causes mild symptoms and does not cause epidemics. Regular H1N1 and H3N2 are categorized under type A influenza and are included in the seasonal flu vaccine. Type B viruses are generally not found in humans, although they can cause illness with less severe symptoms. Type C viruses cause mild illness in humans and are not typically included in the seasonal flu vaccine (American Lung Association, 2013a). Influenza is spread through droplets when an infected person coughs, sneezes, or speaks. Indirectly, articles contaminated by nasopharyngeal secretions may spread the infection. Infected individuals shed the virus for 1 to 2 days before symptoms appear and may continue to shed the virus in increasing amounts for as long as 2 weeks (Blosser et al., 2012). Influenza causes a lytic (cellular destruction) infection of the respiratory epithelium with loss of ciliary function, decreased mucus production, and desquamation of the epithelial layer. These changes may permit secondary bacterial invasion directly from the epithelium or through the middle ear space.

Signs and Symptoms

- Abrupt onset of fever
- Facial flushing
- Chills
- Headache
- Myalgia
- Malaise
- Diarrhea, nausea, and vomiting
- Cough
- Coryza
- Dry or sore throat
- Photophobia, tearing, burning, and eye pain may occur
- Complications include severe viral pneumonia, encephalitis, and secondary bacterial infections such as otitis media, sinusitis, or pneumonia
- Flu symptoms in children are similar to that of adults, except that children have higher degrees of fever of up to 105.1°F (40.6°C)

Diagnosis

The diagnosis of flu is based on the child's signs and symptoms and epidemiological considerations. In the presence of a known epidemic, a child who has symptoms of fever, malaise, and respiratory illness may easily be diagnosed. Laboratory tests may also isolate the virus from the nasopharynx if done early in the course of illness. Rapid influenza diagnostic tests are available, although they have varying degrees of sensitivity. Results may be obtained within 15 minutes, but their routine use should be considered based on whether the results would change the clinical care. Nasopharyngeal swabs or aspiration taken within 72 hours of the onset of the symptoms can isolate and confirm the virus in 2 to 6 days (Blosser et al., 2012).

Prevention

Prevention includes frequent hand washing, covering the mouth and nose when sneezing or coughing, properly disposing of used tissues, and avoiding close contact with persons who may have become infected. Influenza vaccines are now widely used for prevention. There are two routes for the vaccines: IM and nasal spray. Vaccination is recommended annually to populations at risk because the flu virus is continuously changing. Current guidelines recommend that all children ages 6 months to 18 years be immunized with 2 doses being administered during the first year of immunization (AAP Updates Recommendations for Flu Vaccine, 2014). In addition, health-care providers should receive a yearly influenza vaccine to protect themselves and prevent spread to patients and their families.

Collaborative Care

Nursing Care. Because influenza is a self-limiting condition, nursing care is supportive. Depending on the severity of influenza, the child recovers within 1 to 2 weeks. The nurse must emphasize to the parents the importance of adequate rest and sleep. When the child has the flu, more fluids are offered. An electrolyte solution is recommended. The nurse can reiterate the importance of having an annual vaccination.

Medical Care. In uncomplicated cases, influenza is treated symptomatically because symptoms usually recede in 48 to 72 hours. Adequate rest and fluid intake are important components of the regimen. For fever and pain, acetaminophen (Children's Tylenol) or ibuprofen (Children's Advil) is given. Antiviral drugs such as oseltamivir (Tamiflu), amantadine (Symmetrel), and rimantadine (Flumadine) are currently used to manage influenza. These medications are usually given in the first 48 hours to decrease the severity and duration of the illness (Blosser et al., 2012). Antibiotics are given when there is evidence of a superimposed bacterial infection, like prolonged fever and deterioration of the condition.

 Medication: Oseltamivir (Tamiflu)

(o-sel-**tam**-i-vir)

Indications: Used for uncomplicated acute illness due to influenza infection in adults and children greater than 1 year of age that have had symptoms for greater than 2 days
   Prevention of influenza in patients greater than 1 year

Unlabeled Use: Treatment or prophylaxis for infection in infants less than 1 year and of patients symptomatic for 2 days with severe illness.

Actions: Inhibits the enzyme neuraminidase, which may alter virus particle aggregation and release.
THERAPEUTIC EFFECTS: Reduced duration of flu-related symptoms

Contraindications and Precautions:
CONTRAINDICATED IN: Hypersensitivity and children less than 1 year old

Adverse Reactions and Side Effects:
CNS: Insomnia, vertigo, seizures, abnormal behavior, agitation, confusion, delirium, hallucinations, nightmares **RESP:** bronchitis, **GI:** nausea, vomiting

Route and Dosage:
PO:
Children greater than 88 lb (40 kg): 75 mg twice daily for 5 days
Children 50.6 to 88 lb (23–40 kg): 60 mg twice daily
Children 33 to 50.6 lb (15–23 kg): 45 mg twice daily
Children less than 33 lb (15 kg) and less than 1 year: 30 mg twice daily

Nursing Implications:
1. Monitor influenza symptoms. Additional supportive treatment may be indicated to treat symptoms. Treatment should be started as soon as possible from the first sign of flu symptoms. Administer with food or milk to minimize GI irritation.
2. Drug should be used within 10 days of constitution.
3. Caution patients/parents that Tamiflu should not be shared with anyone even if they have the same symptoms.
4. Tamiflu is not a substitute for flu shots according to immunization guidelines.
5. Advise patient to consult health-care professional before taking any medications concurrently with Tamiflu.
6. Advise patients to report behavior changes.
7. Follow dosage as indicated by the health-care provider.

Source: From Vallerand, A. H., & Sanoski, C. A. (2014). *Davis's drug guide for nurses* (14th ed.). Philadelphia, PA: F.A. Davis.

Education/Discharge Instructions

Parents can be instructed to ensure adequate rest, hydration, and nutrition as well as provide fever control as necessary. Continued education includes a reminder of the importance of receiving the influenza vaccine as well as frequent hand washing, covering the mouth and nose when sneezing or coughing, properly disposing used tissues, and avoiding close contact with persons who may have become infected.

 ### Nursing Insight—Salicylates (aspirin)

The nurse can instruct the parents to avoid giving salicylates (aspirin) because of the possibility of Reye syndrome. Reye syndrome is an encephalitis-like illness following a viral infection. Reye syndrome is highly associated with the intake of salicylates (aspirin) during the course of the viral disease. The symptoms include nausea, vomiting, lethargy, and indifference; in severe cases, there may be irrational behavior, delirium, and rapid breathing. Warn parents to watch out for these symptoms, especially if aspirin has been given to the patient prior to consultation.

 Now Can You—Recognize infectious respiratory disorders?

1. Differentiate the causes and symptoms among the various infectious respiratory conditions?
2. Provide guidelines to parents and children regarding prevention of infectious respiratory conditions?

Pulmonary Noninfectious Irritation

FOREIGN BODY ASPIRATION

Foreign body (FB) aspiration refers to any solid or liquid substance that becomes caught in the respiratory tract and blocks air passage. Young children are at greater risk of aspirating foreign bodies because of curiosity and the habit of putting things in the mouth. Foreign body aspiration may occur at any age, but it is most common among toddlers. A total of 4,100 deaths from unintentional ingestion or inhalation of food or objects occurred in 2006 (Warshawsky, 2012). The incidence in children from ages 0 to 4 years was 0.5/100,000 population. The most frequently aspirated objects are organic food items such as peanuts, popcorn, hot dogs, or vegetable matter and fruit gel snacks. Non-food objects include balloons, coins, pen tops, and pins (Warshawsky, 2012).

In the child, the aspirated object may stay in the same place of obstruction or move with air. There is a possibility that if the child forcefully coughs, the object may be spit out. During the presence of the FB the bronchioles and bronchi may become larger during inspiration and smaller during expiration. Small objects may cause little damage, and large objects may occlude the whole airway passage, causing more severe symptoms. A sharp object not only blocks the airway but also may lead to severe trauma, and the child may have complications such as inflammation and abscess, atelectasis, and emphysema.

Signs and Symptoms

Signs and symptoms of FB aspiration vary with location (John & Brady, 2012a).

- Laryngeal FB
  - Rapid onset of hoarseness
  - Chronic, croupy cough
  - Aphonia (inability to speak)
  - Unilateral wheezing
  - Recurrent pneumonia
- Tracheal FB
  - History of brassy cough
  - Hoarseness
  - Dyspnea
  - Possible cyanosis
  - Homophonic wheeze (musical and having the same sound)
  - "Audible slap and palpable thud sound produced by the momentary expiratory effect of the FB at the subglottic level" (John & Brady, 2012a, p. 728)
- Bronchial FB
  - Most objects are aspirated into the right mainstem bronchus because it is at a less acute angle than the left mainstem bronchus
  - Initial findings similar to those seen in tracheal or laryngeal FB aspiration
  - Blood-streaked sputum
  - Metallic taste (if metallic object was aspirated)
  - May have few initial symptoms if the object did not cause obstruction and was nonirritating
  - Homophonic wheeze
  - Emphysema-like changes result in hyporesonance or hyperresonance
  - Diminished breath sounds
  - Crackles, rhonchi, and wheezes

The child's condition may worsen with the total obstruction and the child may become cyanotic or unconscious. Delay in removal of the FB may be fatal.

Diagnosis

The child's history and physical signs help in the diagnosis of FB aspiration. In children, an FB is suspected in the presence of acute or chronic pulmonary lesions. The nurse can communicate to the family that an x-ray exam with fluoroscopic examination can be helpful in locating the site of the aspirated object. Definitive diagnosis of FB aspiration is through bronchoscopic examination.

The nurse who is knowledgeable in assessing respiratory emergencies can make a difference in saving the child's life. The CUPS (critical, unstable, potentially unstable, and stable) assessment method may be a useful tool for the nurse because it includes actions that the nurse can take for each level of emergency.

Assessment Tool Pediatric Respiratory Emergencies

Assessment	Critical	Unstable	Potentially Unstable	Stable
Airway	Completely or severely obstructed	Partially obstructed, excessive secretions or blood	Open with secretions	Open
Breathing rate	May be slow, absent, or very fast with periods of slowing	Increased	Occasionally increased	Normal
Breathing effort	Absent or greatly increased with periods of weakness	Increased	Normal	Normal
Breath sounds	Grunting, faint, or absent	Wheezing or stridor, decreased breath sounds	Normal or slight wheezing	Normal
Skin color	Pale, mottled, or blue	Pink or pale	Pink	Pink
Inspection	Normal, decreased, or absent chest movement	Normal or decreased chest movement	Runny nose, red eyes, fever	Runny nose
Actions	Immediately open airway, suction, give high-concentration oxygen with assisted ventilation, and transport	Move at moderate pace; give high-concentration oxygen; prepare for transport; reassess frequently	Move at moderate pace; help into position of comfort; give high-concentration oxygen; prepare for transport	Begin focused history and physical exam

Source: Data from Rahm, N. S., Hansen, J. D., & Sanddal, N. D. (1997). *Critical trauma care by the basic EMT.* Bozeman, MT: Critical Illness and Trauma Foundation, Inc.

Prevention

Prevention of foreign body aspiration includes educating parents and caregivers. Parents are instructed to avoid giving nuts, uncooked carrots, or other foods that are broken into pieces to infants and children before the molars have erupted. In addition, balloons, marbles, coins, tiny toys, or toys with small pieces (e.g., button eyes or beads are not to be given to small children). Instruct parents to keep toxic substances out of the reach of young children. Force feeding is also to be avoided.

Collaborative Care

Nursing Care. In the hospital, the nurse must closely monitor the child's vital signs and assess the level of consciousness. The nurse can explain any procedures to the parents to help allay anxieties. Initially, the child may be placed on "nothing by mouth" status, and the family is encouraged to follow the medical regimen. The nurse can provide a cool-mist vaporizer and administer antibiotic therapy if deemed appropriate.

The nurse, especially in the community, plays a very important role in foreign body aspiration because the community nurse is involved in health care in the home setting where the accidents commonly occur. In the community setting, the nurse must be skillful in the Heimlich maneuver and can provide health education to parents regarding the procedure.

Medical Care. If a large object has been swallowed, it may be difficult for the child to remove the FB spontaneously by coughing. In this case, the child will need instrumental assistance to remove the obstruction. The nurse understands that delays in the treatment may lead to swelling in the obstructed site and inflammation may set in, hampering the removal of the object. The FB may also adhere to the lumen of the air passage.

Medical management involves the removal of FBs from the respiratory tract by direct laryngoscopy or bronchoscopy. The child is hospitalized during and after the procedure for observation of laryngeal edema and respiratory distress.

Education/Discharge Instructions

Parents can be taught about safety precautions to avoid FB aspiration. For instance, the nurse can communicate to the parents that toys must not have small detachable parts and food should be cut into small bits appropriate for the child's age.

 ### Collaboration in Caring—*The Heimlich maneuver*

The Heimlich maneuver is a life-saving way of removing the FB. In a choking child older than 1 year of age, abdominal thrusts are necessary. In a choking infant, back blows and chest compressions are performed. The community health nurse can encourage the parents to complete a cardiopulmonary resuscitation course (CPR) at the American Red Cross, the American Heart Association (AHA), or other community agencies that teach CPR.

Heimlich maneuver on a conscious child older than 1 year of age:

1. Standing behind the child wrap your arms around the child's waist. With the fist of one hand, place the thumb side against the child's abdomen, slightly above the umbilicus. Grasp the fist with the other hand.

2. Squeeze the child's abdomen using quick inward and upward thrusts.

The Heimlich Maneuver

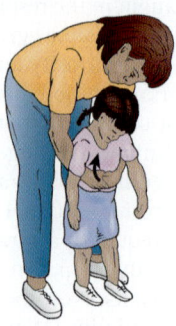

3. Continue the thrusts until the obstruction has been relieved or the child becomes unconscious.

4. Establish unresponsiveness by tapping and shouting "Are you alright?"

5. If the child is unresponsive and apneic or gasping, call for help or activate the emergency response system.

6. Begin CPR starting with 30 chest compressions.

7. Each time the airway is opened using a head-tilt, chin-lift, check for an object and if visible, remove it. Never perform a blind finger-sweep.

Heimlich maneuver on an infant:

1. Lay the infant on your arm or thigh with the infant's head face down.

2. Give five blows to the infant's back using the heel of your hand.

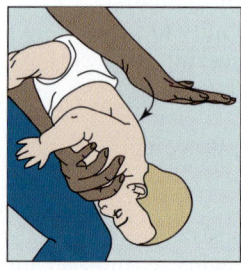

3. If the airway obstruction continues, turn the infant over with head down and give five chest thrusts using two fingers at a distance of 1 fingerbreadth below the nipple level in midline.

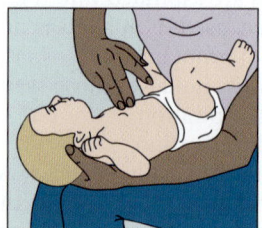

4. Do not perform abdominal thrusts on the infant because it can damage the infant's liver.

5. Check the infant's mouth for any obvious obstructions that can be removed.

6. Do not perform a blind finger-sweep to retrieve an object.

7. If necessary, repeat the sequence and ask for help to call 911.

8. If the infant becomes unconscious, begin CPR with chest compressions.

9. After 30 compressions, open the airway.

10. Before beginning rescue breathing, check the mouth for an FB. Remove if the object is visible—do not do a blind finger-sweep.

11. Attempt ventilation and follow with chest compressions until the object is removed.

12. Activate the emergency response system after 2 minutes if no response.
(AHA, 2010)

SMOKE INHALATION INJURY

Burns and fires are the third leading cause of death in the United States and the leading cause of death of children in the home (Lafferty, 2012). Small children are more vulnerable to smoke inhalation injuries because they are less likely to escape a confined space, have smaller airways, and higher respiratory rates that increase exposure to smoke (Serebrisky, 2012). Sixty percent to 80% of fire-related deaths in the United States are associated with smoke inhalation injury. Smoke is a mixture of gases and aerosolized particulate matter generated by combustion. Incomplete combustion produces noxious substances that, when inhaled, are toxic to humans.

Smoke inhalation may cause three types of injury: heat, chemical, and systemic. Smoke tends to be dry but with high temperature. Heat produces immediate injury to the mucosa, resulting in erythema, ulceration, and edema, thus compromising the upper airway. If significant edema ensues, symptoms related to obstruction such as dyspnea, stridor, and cyanosis occur. Chemical injury is related to the inhalation of substances generated during combustion. Irritant gases such as carbon dioxide combine with water in the lungs to form corrosive acids; aldehydes cause denaturation of proteins, cellular damage, and edema of pulmonary tissues (Lafferty, 2012).

Systemic injury occurs from gases formed during combustion that are nontoxic to the airways but may cause injury or death by interfering with oxygen utilization. Carbon monoxide (CO) and hydrogen cyanide are substances that can be formed when materials such as silk, nylon, polyurethane, and organic matter are burned. These substances are considered as asphyxiant and lead to neurological symptoms (Lafferty, 2012).

Signs and Symptoms

- Cough
- Bronchospasm
- Dyspnea and stridor
- Shortness of breath
- Hoarseness
- Eyes may be red and irritated by smoke
- Skin may range from pale to bluish, to cherry red
- Soot may be present in the nostrils or throat
- Upper airway passages may become swollen within 24 hours of the injury
- Headaches related to exposure to CO, which is present in all fires
- Nausea and vomiting related to CO exposure
- Chemical asphyxiants and low levels of oxygen may cause changes in the mental status
- Confusion, fainting, seizures, and coma are potential complications
- Burns in the face and neck may accentuate the symptoms
- Chemical injury may result in erythema, edema, and ulceration of the airways

Diagnosis

Diagnosis of smoke inhalation is based on the signs and symptoms of the injury, especially in survivors of the fire. However, the nurse understands that diagnosis of CO poisoning requires careful neurological examination and is based on compatible history and clinical findings. Basic diagnostic studies may include chest radiography, pulse oximetry, and laboratory work to include electrolytes, blood gases, complete blood count, blood urea nitrogen, and creatinine. A bronchoscopy may be done to assess the degree of damage done to the airways and to allow for suctioning of secretions and debris.

Prevention

The prevention of smoke inhalation injuries includes instillation of smoke and CO detectors in the home, planned and practiced escape routes, and visible access to police and fire department numbers in the event of an emergency. Children can also be involved in practicing escape routes and be instructed where to find police and fire emergency numbers.

Collaborative Care

Nursing Care. It is important for the nurse to remember that nursing care of children with smoke inhalation involves prioritizing life-sustaining systems of respiration and circulation. Nurses assist in emergency intubation and monitor the patients accordingly. Signs of CO poisoning are recorded and reported without delay.

Recovery for children with minor burns and smoke inhalation have good recovery rates, provided adequate nutrition is given when the patient is medically cleared to have oral intake. The nurse can offer foods that are attractively served so that the child is encouraged to eat. Favorite toys may be placed at the bedside so that the child is not bored and will maintain normal development. For infants, a child life specialist can offer stimulation and calming music. Nurses can encourage parents to participate in the care of the child.

Medical Care. Treatment is aimed at managing upper airway obstruction and possible CO poisoning. Urgent attention to the adequacy of airway, breathing, and circulation is obligatory. The immediate administration of 100% oxygen via a high-flow system is important to reverse tissue hypoxia. If the child is comatose, intubation is recommended to deliver the highest possible fraction of inspired oxygen (FIO_2) and to prevent CO_2 retention. After the initial stabilization, treatment of concomitant burn injury is initiated. Up to 50% of patients with an inhalation injury require initial intubation and its associated care. Ventilator assistance may be needed depending on the severity of the injury. Fluids are administered to maintain fluid and electrolyte balances. Because inhalation injuries may predispose the airway to infection, antibiotics may be ordered.

Education/Discharge Instructions

Parents are instructed to follow-up if they believe the child's condition is worsening after discharge. Signs of a worsening condition may include hoarse voice, difficulty breathing, prolonged coughing spells, and mental status changes (e.g., confusion). Instruct the parents to ensure the child avoids cigarette smoke because this may trigger shortness of breath and irritation of the injured respiratory tract. If inhalers and pain medications are prescribed, instruct the parents on dosing and administration of those medications.

PASSIVE SMOKING

Passive smoking is defined as a nonsmoker's inhalation of the smoke coming from the smoker. The smoke inhaled by nonsmokers is called environmental tobacco smoke (ETS). This is also referred to as secondhand smoke (SHS). There is conclusive evidence about the ill effects of smoking and ETS on health. The findings on passive smoking and disease have been the foundation of the push for smoke-free environments and for educating parents concerning the effects of their smoking on their children's health.

The nonsmoker breathes "sidestream smoke" from the burning tip of the cigarette and "mainstream smoke" that has been inhaled then exhaled by the smoker (American Cancer Society, 2012). Sidestream smoke has a higher concentration of cancer-causing agents than mainstream smoke (American Cancer Society, 2012). ETS contains more than 7,000 chemicals, 250 of those chemicals are potentially harmful, and 69 are known or suspected carcinogens (American Cancer Society, 2012). Inhalation of ETS may bring both short- and long-term effects. The short-term effects are manifested as irritation to the upper airways, while the long-term effects are related to the consequences of inhaling the chemicals in ETS such as nicotine and CO for prolonged periods of time.

It is estimated that more than 2.6 million children ages 12 to 17 are cigarette smokers (Burns & Dunn, 2012). In 2010, 19.3% of the adults in America were cigarette smokers, demonstrating a slight decrease from 20.9% in 2005 (CDC, 2011).

Health effects of SHS on children include ear infections, more frequent asthma attacks, respiratory infections, respiratory symptoms (coughing, sneezing, and shortness of breath), and increased risk for sudden infant death syndrome (SIDS). The CDC estimates that up to 150,000 to 300,000 new cases of bronchitis and pneumonia occur annually, and from 7,500 to 15,000 hospitalizations related to SHS exposure also occur annually in children aged 18 months or younger (CDC, 2012). **Third-hand smoke** is a term used to define exposure that a child gets from contact with surfaces that over time have absorbed smoke exposure through dust inhalation, dermal exposure, and ingestions (Sockrider & Farber, 2011). The burning of tobacco releases nicotine in the form of a vapor that can be adsorbed onto surfaces, such as walls, floors, carpeting, drapes, and furniture. Nicotine in this form can exist on these surfaces for days, weeks, and months. Babies and children are at greater risk of exposure to third-hand smoke because they function closer to these surfaces, especially the floor. They also tend to touch and put in their mouths different items from contaminated surfaces.

Signs and Symptoms

- Stuffy, runny nose
- Watery eyes
- Sneezing
- Bronchitis
- Wheezing
- Headache
- Nausea
- Pneumonia
- Asthma
- Allergies
- Otitis media
- Middle ear effusion
- Premature coronary artery disease
- Low birth weight
- SIDS
- Cognitive delay

Diagnosis

The diagnosis of conditions related to passive smoking is based on history and evidence of exposure to ETS. Exposure can be estimated by measuring the biomarker cotinine. This biomarker is sensitive to tobacco exposure that has occurred in the previous 4 days (Sockrider & Farber, 2011). The marker can be extracted from urine, saliva, blood, and other tissues. Measurements of several components of ETS have been made in homes, workplaces, and public places to characterize the contribution of smoking to indoor air pollution. Dangerous levels of ETS components usually come within those measures.

Prevention

Children can be protected from the effects of SHS by providing the following instructions to parents:

- Do not allow anyone to smoke inside the home
- Ensure that there is no smoking allowed in day-care settings
- Ensure that the child's school promotes a smoke-free environment, both inside and out
- Choose businesses that are smoke-free
- Do not allow persons to smoke while riding with children in a car

Collaborative Care

Nursing Care. The nurse plays an active role through health education, especially to parents. The nurse, through health education, must emphasize the negative effects of smoking, both for the smokers and the recipients of environment tobacco smoke. To support "stop smoking campaigns" means the nurse must be a good role model and give up any personal smoking habits.

Nurses must also support the call of the World Health Organization for the right of every child to grow up in an environment free of tobacco smoke. Efforts are made by the nurses to persuade parents, especially pregnant women, to give up smoking. This is one way of advocating for the rights of children.

Medical Care. Treatment for children is focused on the specific ailments that exposure to ETS has produced. One of the most important components to be addressed in passive smoking is its control. Strategies to control ETS are currently being undertaken by both the government and private sectors through education, regulation, legislation, and litigation.

Education/Discharge Instructions

"What to say"—Third-hand smoke

The nurse tells the parents that third-hand smoke refers to exposure that a child gets from contact with surfaces that over time have absorbed smoke. Children come in contact with third-hand smoke through dust inhalation, dermal exposure, and ingestions. The burning of tobacco releases nicotine in the form of a vapor that can be adsorbed onto surfaces, such as clothing, walls, floors, carpeting, drapes, and furniture. Nicotine in this form can exist on these surfaces for days, weeks, and months. Babies and children are at greater risk of exposure to third-hand smoke because they function closer to these surfaces, particularly the floor. They also tend to touch and mouth items from the contaminated surfaces. The best way to prevent exposure is to promote a totally smoke-free environment, not only in the home, but also in the car and in day-care settings (CDC, 2011).

 Now Can You—Recognize noninfectious respiratory conditions?

1. Differentiate the causes and symptoms among the various noninfectious respiratory conditions?
2. Provide safety guidelines to parents and children regarding prevention of noninfectious respiratory conditions?

Respiratory Conditions Related to Allergens

ALLERGIC RHINITIS

Allergic rhinitis is an inflammation of the nasal membranes predominantly in the child's nose and eyes. Airborne particles of dust, dander, or plant pollens in children who are allergic to these substances cause allergic rhinitis. It appears alone or in combination with a cold.

 Nursing Insight—How does inflammation of the nasal membranes occur?

Inflammation of the mucous membranes is characterized by a complex interaction of inflammatory mediators and is triggered by an immunoglobulin E (IgE)-mediated response to an extrinsic protein.

The mediators that are immediately released include histamine, tryptase, chymase, kinins, and heparin. The mast cells quickly synthesize other mediators including leukotrienes and prostaglandin D_2. These mediators then lead to the symptoms of rhinorrhea.

Next, mucous glands are stimulated, leading to an increase of secretions produced. Vasodilation then leads to congestion and pressure. Sensory nerves are also stimulated,

leading to sneezing and itching. This sequel happens in a matter of minutes and is called the early phase response.

In the next 4 to 8 hours there is a complex interplay of neutrophils, eosinophils, lymphocytes, and macrophages. This interplay brings about continued inflammation, termed as the late phase response. The phase may persist for days, and systemic effects range from fatigue to sleepiness to malaise to generalized weakness.

Signs and Symptoms

- Mouth breathing, snoring, and nasal speech
- Clear, thin, watery rhinorrhea
- Nasal congestion and inflammation
- Bogginess of the nasal mucous membranes—may appear pale to purplish
- Nasal crease—horizontal crease across the lower third of the nose (John & Brady, 2012b)
- Itching or rubbing nose referred to as an "allergic salute"
- Nasal stuffiness and postnasal drip
- Sneezing
- Congested cough or night cough
- Itching palate, pharynx, nose, or eyes
- Hoarseness and frequent attempts to clear the throat
- Redness of the conjunctiva, tearing, and edema of the lid and periorbital area
- Allergic shiners (dark periorbital swelling)
- Enlarged tonsils and adenoids
- Cobblestone appearance of pharynx and/or palpebral conjunctivae
- Fatigue
- School performance issues related to lack of sleep
- Dennie lines, Morgan fold, or atopic pleats—extra groove in lower eyelid (Venes, 2013)

Diagnosis

A thorough history and physical examination of the child confirm allergic rhinitis. A nasal smear is done to determine the number of eosinophils in the nasal secretions. A radioallergosorbent test is done to determine specific IgE antibodies. Skin testing is often done to identify the specific allergen.

Prevention

The key to preventing an allergic rhinitis is in learning to avoid known allergens. Strategies for controlling exposure include the following:

- Avoiding exposure to tobacco smoke
- To avoid dust mites, use pillow and mattress covers, wash bed linens weekly in 130°F (54.4°C) water, remove stuffed animals from the bedroom, replace bedroom curtains with blinds, remove carpet from bedroom, and wet mop solid surface floors weekly
- Remove pets from the home
- Repair water leaks, reduce indoor humidity to less than 50%
- Avoid outdoor activity when pollution, mold, and pollen levels are high

Collaborative Care

Nursing Care. Nursing care is primarily directed toward providing supportive care and educating the family about the illness and management. Supportive care includes ensuring rest, nutrition, and adequate hydration, which will help in thinning secretions.

Medical Care. Treatment for allergic rhinitis in the child involves pharmacological management. Pharmacological management includes short-acting antihistamines, longer acting histamines, nasal corticosteroid sprays, decongestants, and leukotriene inhibitors. There is evidence to prove that high-dose allergy shots are recommended if the allergen cannot be removed and if the child's symptoms are hard to control. This includes regular injections of the allergen given in increasing doses, which in turn help the body to adjust to the allergen.

Education/Discharge Instructions

Education includes giving instruction on environmental control strategies as noted under prevention. In addition, the nurse reviews the prescribed medications with the parents and patient, giving instructions for use in the case of inhalers or internasal sprays, as well as reviewing dosage, common side effects, and contradictions.

 Across Care Settings: Education

Education about environmental control measures involves both the avoidance of known allergens (substances to which the patient has IgE-mediated sensitivity) and the avoidance of nonspecific irritants and triggers. In the clinic setting, the nurse can explore possible allergens of the child with the parents to obtain important information that might determine the cause of the allergic rhinitis. Parents must understand the possible complications that allergic rhinitis may cause. These complications range from otitis media, eustachian tube dysfunction, and acute sinusitis to chronic sinusitis.

ASTHMA

Asthma is the most common chronic disease in childhood and is characterized by the triad symptoms of bronchial smooth muscle spasm, inflammation and edema of the bronchial mucosa, and production and retention of thick, tenacious, pulmonary secretions leading to airway obstruction. Asthma affects over 6.7 million people and nearly 1 in 11 children in the United States (Covar, Fleischer, & Boguniewicz, 2011). The mortality rate for asthma is 28 out of 1 million children annually (Covar et al., 2011). Prevalence and mortality rates are higher among minority and inner-city children. Risk factors include environmental factors, such as air pollutants, allergen exposure, exposure to tobacco smoke, and strong chemical odors. Other factors include low socioeconomic status and health-care disparities (Redjal, 2011). The term **status asthmaticus** is used to refer to persistent and intractable asthma in which the child does not respond to therapy and a medical emergency ensues.

 Cultural Diversity: Asthma

In the United States, the poor, especially of African American or Hispanic background, experience disproportionally high rates of both asthma prevalence and morbidity (John & Brady, 2012b; Rance, O'Laughlen, & Ting, 2011). There is great worldwide variability in prevalence, with industrialized areas having consistently high rates. African American children have a 60% higher prevalence of asthma in addition to 260% higher prevalence of emergency room visits. African American children also have a hospitalization rate of 250% higher than white children as well as a 500% higher mortality rate (Rance et al., 2011). The incidence of asthma in African American adolescent males is also reported to be as high as 27% (Rance et al., 2011). Factors associated with the higher rates include underutilization of the National Asthma Education and Prevention Program (NAEPP) guidelines (National Heart, Lung, and Blood Institute, 2007) and the underutilization of inhaled corticosteroids as a control therapy.

Genetic, environmental/extrinsic, and intrinsic factors predispose the child to develop asthma. Although allergens play an important role in asthma, 20% to 40% of children with asthma have no evidence of allergic disease. Among the extrinsic factors are allergens such as dust, pollen, animal hairs, chemical sprays, perfumes, baby powder, molds, and foods such as nuts, chocolates, oranges, and chicken. Conditions such as changes in weather, pollution, and smoke may also trigger an attack. Intrinsic factors include exercise, anxiety, strong emotions such as fear and laughter, and infections.

When any of the factors trigger an asthma attack, the response comes in 10 to 20 minutes. The allergen/antigen binds to the allergen-specific immunoglobulin E (IgE) surface, causing activation of resident airway mast cells and macrophages. Pro-inflammatory mediators, such as histamine and leukotrienes, are released. They provoke contraction of the airway's smooth muscles, increased mucus secretion, and vasodilation. Consequently, microvascular leakage and exudation of plasma into the airway walls cause them to become thickened and edematous with subsequent lumen constriction (Redjal, 2011).

Signs and Symptoms

- Recurrent wheezing
- Shortness of breath
- Nonproductive cough
- Chest tightness or pain
- Exercise intolerance
- Prolonged expiratory phase of respirations
- Tachypnea
- Retractions and nasal flaring
- History of allergies
- History of atopic dermatitis
- Nasal polyps
- History of nighttime cough
- Family history of atopy (asthma, allergic rhinitis, or atopic dermatitis)

Diagnosis

The asthma diagnosis for the child is based on clinical symptoms, history, physical examination, and to a lesser extent, laboratory tests. Diagnostic studies may include pulse oximetry to measure oxygen saturation, blood gases to determine carbon dioxide retention and hypoxemia, complete blood count, pulmonary function tests to assist in determining the degree of disease, peak expiratory flow rate, allergy testing, and chest radiography to evaluate

Labs: Blood Gases

Blood gases are used to evaluate respiratory and metabolic functioning through determining the acid-base balance of the blood by the measurement of oxygen and carbon dioxide. Blood gases may be obtained through arterial, venous, capillary, or cord blood. Normal values vary depending on the source. During normal metabolic processes, oxygen is used and carbon dioxide is produced. Various disease conditions impact the levels of each gas in different ways. Blood gas measurements provide information that may help the primary care provider manage metabolic or respiratory disorders. Arterial blood gases measure the amount of dissolved oxygen and carbon dioxide present in arterial blood and reveal the acid-base state and how well the oxygen is being carried to the body. Common measures obtained from blood gases include pH, which measures free H^+ (hydrogen) ion concentration in the circulating blood. The pH is regulated and the acid-base ratio maintained through the work of the lungs and kidneys. The pH is elevated (alkaline) in respiratory or metabolic alkalosis and decreased (acid) in the case of respiratory or metabolic acidosis. The amount of carbon dioxide in the blood is determined by the partial pressure of carbon dioxide (PCO_2) measurement. The PCO_2 is primarily controlled by the lungs. As the CO_2 level increases, the pH decreases. The lungs also help compensate for metabolic disturbances. HCO_3^- represents the bicarbonate ion. As the HCO_3^- level increases so also does the pH. The amount of oxygen dissolved in the blood is measured by the partial pressure of oxygen (PO_2) measurement. The amount of oxygen bound to hemoglobin is determined by oxygen saturation (O_2Sat).

hyperinflation and the potential for coexisting infection (John & Brady, 2012b).

 Nursing Insight—*Blood gases and asthma*

Airway diseases, such as asthma that causes respiratory structures to become less compliant, may lead to carbon dioxide retention and subsequent respiratory acidosis. Interference with breathing causes the CO_2 rate to increase and the pH to drop. Ongoing carbon dioxide retention can lead to chronic respiratory acidosis. Conditions that increase respiratory rates, such as hyperventilation, anxiety, pulmonary embolus, salicylate poisoning, and fever, lead to respiratory alkalosis, which is demonstrated by a loss of CO_2 and an increase in pH.

Prevention

Prevention is directed toward day-to-day management of asthma. This includes educating the parents and child on the importance of identifying environmental factors that trigger an attack; compliance with medication; and how to use and clean inhalers, spacer devices, or aerosol equipment as needed (John & Brady, 2012b). In addition, parents and children need to understand how to manage asthma in settings away from home, how to recognize when there is a need to seek additional assistance, and the importance of regular follow-up.

Collaborative Care

Nursing Care. Nursing care for children with asthma involves assisting with relief of symptoms and providing health education to patients and family. Asthma attacks are frightening and stressful both for the child and family; therefore, the nurse has a calm approach in its initial management. Administering quick-relief medications without delay is important. Essential nursing interventions include giving medications on time, liquefying secretions through adequate hydration, positioning the child properly (head of bed elevated 30 degrees) to provide comfort, and lung expansion. The side-lying and semi-prone positions are also recommended. It is vital that the nurse reports and records the child's respiratory assessment and responses to medications so that appropriate management may be initiated immediately. The nurse can also ensure that respiratory treatments happen in a timely manner and that ordering a prn (as needed) treatment may be necessary.

Medical Care. Treatment consists of early relief of symptoms through drug therapy and prevention of further attacks through allergen control, environmental manipulation, health education, and attainment of self-management skills. The goal is to enable the child to have as regular a life as possible by keeping the lung function within normal limits. The nurse provides adequate health education about the use of a peak flow meter to help the parents increase their capacity to care for the child.

Drug therapy depends on the level of severity of the disease. There are two approaches to this therapy: (1) the quick-relief or rescue medications and (2) the long-term control medications.

The U.S. Department of Health and Human Services (2007), the National Asthma Education and Prevention Program, expert panel give guidelines for the diagnosis and management of asthma via revised age-related classification schemes for asthma severity (Tables 23-3, 23-4, and 23-5).

Table 23-3 Criteria for Classification of Asthma Severity in Children 0–4 Years of Age

Severity	Day Symptoms	Night Awakenings	SABA Use*	Limit to Activity
Intermittent	≤2 days/week	None	None	≤2 times/week
Mild Persistent	3–6 days/week	1–2 times/month	>2 days/week	Minor
Mod. Persistent	Daily	3–4 times/month	Daily	Some
Severe Persistent	Several times/day	>1 time/week	Several times/day	Extremely

*Short-acting beta 2 agonists (SABA), such as albuterol, does not include prevention of exercise-induced bronchospasm (EIB).

Source: The U.S. Department of Health and Human Services (2007). National asthma education and prevention program. Expert panel report 3: Guidelines for the diagnosis and management of asthma.

Table 23-4 Criteria for Classification of Asthma Severity in Children 5–11 Years of Age

Severity	Day Symptoms	Night Awakenings	SABA Use*	Limit to Activity
Intermittent	≤2 days/week	≤2 times/month	≤2 days/week	None
Mild Persistent	≥2 days/week but not daily	3–4 times/month	≥2 days/week but not daily	Minor limitations
Mod. Persistent	Daily	≥1 times/week but not nightly	Daily	Some limitation
Severe Persistent	Throughout the day	Often nightly	Several times/day	Extremely limited

*Use of short-acting beta 2 agonists (SABA), such as albuterol, does not include prevention of exercise-induced bronchospasm (EIB).

Source: The U.S. Department of Health and Human Services (2007). National asthma education and prevention program. Expert panel report 3: Guidelines for the diagnosis and management of asthma.

Table 23-5 Criteria for Classification of Asthma Severity in Children >12 Years of Age

Severity	Day Symptoms	Night Awakenings	SABA Use*	Limit to Activity
Intermittent	≤2days/week	≤2 times /month	≤2 days/week	None
Mild Persistent	≥2 days/week but not daily	3–4 times/month	≥2 days/week but not daily	Minor limitations
Mod. Persistent	Daily	≥1 times/week but not nightly	Daily	Some limitation
Severe Persistent	Throughout the day	Often nightly	Several times/day	Extremely limited

*Use of short-acting beta 2 agonists (SABA), such as albuterol, does not include prevention of exercise-induced bronchospasm (EIB).

Source: The U.S. Department of Health and Human Services (2007). National asthma education and prevention program Expert panel report 3: Guidelines for the diagnosis and management of asthma.

The guidelines recommend daily anti-inflammatory agents to control the levels of persistent asthma, with increasing doses of medication as necessary. The use of low-dose control medications, such as inhaled steroids, cromolyn sodium (Intal), nedocromil (Tilade), or an anti-leukotriene agent such as a montelukast sodium (Singulair) tablet is recommended for children with mild, persistent asthma (Fig. 23-9). A higher dose of steroids with the addition of long-acting beta antagonists may be needed for moderate and severe persistent asthma. For quick relief of bronchospasm and for children with asthma, short-acting inhaled beta antagonists are recommended. For more detailed information of the guidelines visit http://www.nhlbi.nih.gov/guidelines/asthma/index.htm.

ASTHMA ACTION PLAN

The Asthma Action Plan (Fig. 23-10) is an educational communication tool used between the health-care provider and the patient, along with their family and caregivers, to properly manage asthma and respond to asthma episodes. The Asthma Action Plan is completed by the child's primary care provider. It includes the symptoms and management for each color zone including peak flow measurements appropriate for each color zone. Nurses can provide adequate instructions on how to use, interpret, and complete the form.

A peak flow meter (Fig. 23-11), which can be purchased over the counter, is an essential companion for the Asthma Action Plan for children older than 6 years. The peak flow meter is a portable handheld device that is used to measure the ability to push air out of the lungs. To determine the child's zone for children younger than 6 years, the symptoms alone are used. The "personal best" peak flow is determined when the child is symptom free. A peak flow meter package usually contains a form where peak flow

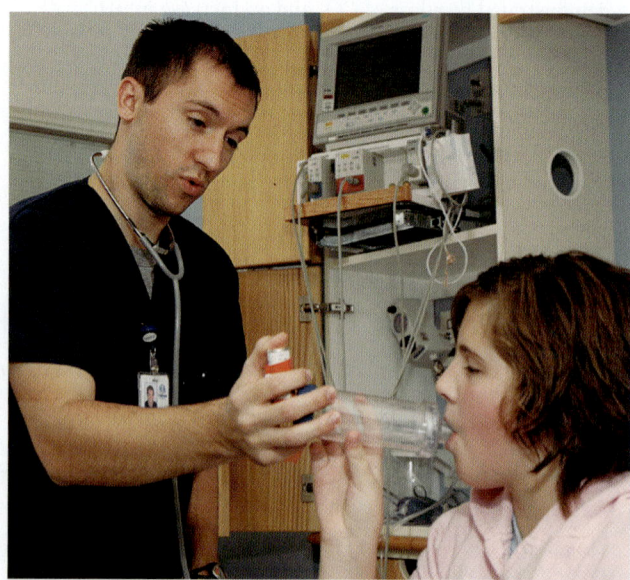

Figure 23-9 The respiratory therapist helps the child use a metered dose inhaler.

Asthma Action Plan

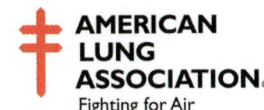

AMERICAN LUNG ASSOCIATION.
Fighting for Air

General Information:

- Name _____
- Emergency contact _____ Phone numbers _____
- Physician/healthcare provider _____ Phone numbers _____
- Physician signature _____ Date _____

Severity Classification
○ Intermittent　　○ Moderate Persistent
○ Mild Persistent　○ Severe Persistent

Triggers
○ Colds　　○ Smoke　○ Weather
○ Exercise　○ Dust　　○ Air Pollution
○ Animals　○ Food
○ Other _____

Exercise
1. Premedication (how much and when) _____
2. Exercise modifications _____
_____

Green Zone: Doing Well　　　　　**Peak Flow Meter Personal Best =**

Symptoms

Control Medications:

- ■ Breathing is good
- ■ No cough or wheeze
- ■ Can work and play
- ■ Sleeps well at night

Medicine	How Much to Take	When to Take It
_____	_____	_____
_____	_____	_____
_____	_____	_____

Peak Flow Meter

More than 80% of personal best or _____

Yellow Zone: Getting Worse　　　**Contact physician if using quick relief more than 2 times per week.**

Symptoms

Continue control medicines and add:

- ■ Some problems breathing
- ■ Cough, wheeze, or chest tight
- ■ Problems working or playing
- ■ Wake at night

Medicine	How Much to Take	When to Take It
_____	_____	_____
_____	_____	_____
_____	_____	_____

Peak Flow Meter

Between 50% and 80% of personal best or
_____ to _____

IF your symptoms (and peak flow, if used) return to Green Zone after one hour of the quick-relief treatment, THEN

- ○ Take quick-relief medication every 4 hours for 1 to 2 days.
- ○ Change your long-term control medicine by _____
- ○ Contact your physician for follow-up care.

IF your symptoms (and peak flow, if used) DO NOT return to Green Zone after one hour of the quick-relief treatment, THEN

- ○ Take quick-relief treatment again.
- ○ Change your long-term control medicine by _____
- ○ Call your physician/Healthcare provider within _____ hour(s) of modifying your medication routine.

Red Zone: Medical Alert　　　　**Ambulance/Emergency Phone Number:**

Symptoms

Continue control medicines and add:

- ■ Lots of problems breathing
- ■ Cannot work or play
- ■ Getting worse instead of better
- ■ Medicine is not helping

Medicine	How Much to Take	When to Take It
_____	_____	_____
_____	_____	_____
_____	_____	_____

Peak Flow Meter

Less than 50% of personal best or
_____ to _____

Go to the hospital or call for an ambulance if:

- ○ Still in the red zone after 15 minutes.
- ○ You have not been able to reach your physician/healthcare provider for help.
- ○ _____

Call an ambulance immediately if the following danger signs are present:

- ○ Trouble walking/talking due to shortness of breath.
- ○ Lips or fingernails are blue.

Figure 23-10 Asthma Action Plan. *Source:* Used with permission of American Lung Association, © 2012.

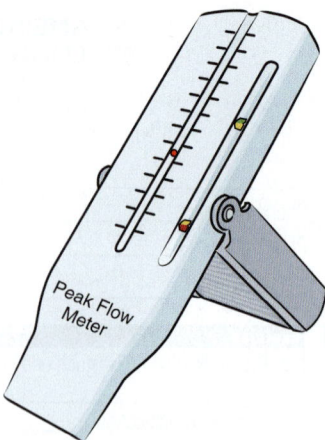

Figure 23-11 Peak flow meter.

readings are recorded regularly. A personal best normal may be obtained from measuring the patient's own peak flow rate. Therefore, it is important for the patient, parents, and the doctor to discuss what is considered "normal" (Procedure 23-1).

Education/Discharge Instructions

Asthma education is critical and is directed at addressing activities discussed in the section on prevention. The community nurse can offer health education to families that emphasizes correctly adhering to the treatment regimen, preventing infection, and avoiding asthma triggers. Nurses are in the best position to provide health education because they are in contact with the patients and the parents most of the time.

 Procedure 23-1 Using a Peak Flow Meter

The peak flow meter is a portable handheld device that is used to measure the child's ability to push air out of the lungs. The American Lung Association recommends the following steps in using the peak flow meter (American Lung Association, 2013b).

Purpose

The purpose of a peak flow meter is to keep track of the results and help the parents and child to learn about asthma. Keeping a daily record may also help determine if the child's asthma is getting worse.

Equipment

- Peak flow meter
- Peak flow record

Steps

1. Before each use, make sure the sliding marker or arrow on the peak flow meter is at the bottom of the numbered scale (zero or the lowest number on the scale).

   RATIONALE: *Initial calibration ensures an accurate reading.*

2. Instruct the child to stand up straight and to remove gum or any food from the mouth.

   RATIONALE: *Proper body alignment is essential for an accurate reading.*

3. Instruct the child to take a deep breath and to put the mouthpiece of the peak flow meter into the mouth. Close the lips tightly around the mouthpiece. Be sure to keep the tongue away from the mouthpiece.

   RATIONALE: *A tight seal is necessary for measuring an accurate reading.*

4. Instruct the child to take in one breath and to then blow out as hard and as quickly as possible. Blow a "fast hard blast" rather than "slowly blowing" until all of the air is emptied from the lungs.

RATIONALE: *A fast hard blast empties all the air from the lungs. This helps ensure an accurate measurement.*

5. Teach the parents that the force of the air coming out of the lungs causes the marker to move along the numbered scale. Record the number where the marker landed on a *peak flow record*.

   RATIONALE: *Teaching the parents about how to use and record the measurement of the peak flow meter increases their capacity to care for the child.*

6. Repeat the entire routine three times (if the routine is done correctly the numbers from all three tries are very close together).

   RATIONALE: *Repeating the entire routine three times helps ensure accurate data collection.*

7. Record the highest reading. Do not calculate an average.

   RATIONALE: *The highest reading provides the most accurate data.*

8. Measure the peak flow rate at the same time each day. A good time to measure the peak flow rate is between 7 and 9 a.m. and between 6 and 8 p.m. Note: It may be a good idea to measure the peak flow rate before or after using asthma medicine.

   RATIONALE: *A consistent time of day provides the best information about the child's ongoing lung function.*

9. Keep a chart of the peak flow rates on a *peak flow record*.

   RATIONALE: *Having written documentation of information about the lung function from day to day may help with early identification of problems.*

 focus on safety

Peak flow meter

A peak flow meter package usually contains a *peak flow record* where the peak flow readings are recorded regularly.

Procedure 23-1 Using a Peak Flow Meter (continued)

Teach Parents

Teach parents about the child's personal best. The "personal best" peak flow is determined when the child is symptom free. It is important for the child, parents, and doctor to discuss what is considered "normal." Remind parents of the need to discuss the readings with the physician.

Documentation

01/31/2013 0900 Peak flow meter used. Green zone, good control; 80% of personal best, no symptoms noted. Continues to take usual medication.

N. Kramer, RN-C. Kildare RN

 Where Research and Practice Meet:
Asthma Care for African American Children

The underutilization of the National Asthma Education and Prevention Program (NAEPP) guidelines and inhaled corticosteroids as controller therapy is well documented in the literature and one of the greatest obstacle to improving outcomes for children with asthma (Rance et al., 2011) The guidelines provide information and guidance about the most current disease management with the goals of improving quality of care and reducing disparity. The guidelines also provide criteria for classification of asthma severity according to age and symptoms, which support treatment plans. The nurse is instrumental in improving these outcomes and compliance through ensuring the guidelines are used consistently among all populations. The nurse is also in the position to use the guidelines in assessing severity of patient symptoms and in properly documenting and reporting to the primary care provider. Using the severity criteria guidelines can become a mainstay in acquiring the history and physical condition of all children with known or suspected asthma. The guidelines can also be used to provide education to parents and patients regarding management and compliance (National Heart, Lung, and Blood Institute, 2007).

 Nursing Insight—Spacers

The nurse understands that for children less than 5 years of age, a spacer or a valved holding chamber (VHC) is recommended and is attached to the metered-dose inhaler (MDI). A spacer may deliver the medication to the child's lungs better than an inhaler alone and may be easier for the child to use than an MDI alone. In addition, for ease of delivery, child-sized masks are available that fit the VHC. With this device there is more medication deposited in the lungs and less systemic side effects. After VHC use, the nurse can have the child follow with mouth washing and spitting to decrease swallowing medication and side effects including, in the case of inhaled corticosteroids, prevention of oral *candidiasis* (U.S. Department of Health and Human Services, 2007).

 Across Care Settings: **What to do in cases of an acute asthma attack**

An asthma attack may occur anytime and anywhere. It may happen in the home, at a school, in a mall, or in a park. To guide parents, teachers, and people who work in places where children go, the nurse can provide the following tips:

Teachers and school administrators can be familiar with the health history of the child. It is important to coordinate care and share information with the school health nurse. The nurse also knows the school district's rules and regulations regarding carrying asthma medications to school, including where the medications are to be kept and how to use the medications. In coordination with the child's physician and parents, the nurse can fill out an emergency asthma action plan, including the child's triggers. The nurse needs to post emergency phone numbers in case of an attack. In addition, the nurse must know the child's peak flow readings, the child's personal best, and when the child runs into trouble. The nurse can also educate the teachers and other personnel who come in contact with the child.

Parents must be sure to carry the child's quick-relief medications. It is helpful if the school-age child carries it, too, along with the instructions about how the medication is used.

Nurses can give information on environmental control and creating an allergen-free environment. In addition, through community health education, the nurse can emphasize that when a child exhibits difficulty breathing, wheezing, and coughing, it is important to be calm and reassure the child. It is important to find out if the child's medicine is available; if not, call 911.

Personnel in parks, malls, and play areas can be briefed about possible pediatric emergencies including management in an emergency situation.

 Now Can You—**Recognize respiratory conditions related to allergies?**

1. Differentiate the causes and symptoms among the various respiratory conditions caused by allergic responses?
2. Provide care guidelines to parents and children regarding prevention exacerbation of symptoms related to respiratory conditions caused by environmental factors?

Summary Points

◆ The differences between the adult and child respiratory system affect function and subsequent respiratory conditions.

◆ It is essential that the nurse has a good understanding of congenital respiratory conditions and structural anomalies in children, along with an understanding of signs and symptoms and prescribed treatment.

◆ Nurses must provide adequate emotional support to parents whose children have life-threatening respiratory conditions.

◆ The diagnosis, signs and symptoms, and nursing care measures are important in caring for children with respiratory conditions.

◆ Nursing care for children with infectious respiratory conditions includes close monitoring and correct treatment to prevent spread of infection.

◆ Nursing care for noninfectious respiratory conditions is aimed at managing the upper airway to prevent obstruction and further damage.

◆ During health teachings, nurses emphasize to parents an awareness of the ill-effects of the different forms of air pollutants, including environmental tobacco.

◆ The goal for children with asthma is to enable the child to have as normal of a life as possible by keeping the lung functioning within normal limits.

◆ The nurse can educate the family about the benefits of the child wearing a medical alert bracelet.

Review Questions

Multiple Choice

1. The pediatric nurse is aware that the child with cystic fibrosis has discharge planning needs. Which is important to communicate to the family during discharge teaching?
   A. Importance of a well-balanced, low-protein, high-calorie diet
   B. When and how to administer pancreatic enzymes
   C. Use of vitamin supplements is not needed with pancreatic enzymes
   D. Nature and course of the disease including self-limiting nature

2. A 2-year-old child is discharged from the outpatient surgical unit after having a tonsillectomy. What statement by the parent indicates to the nurse that discharge teaching has been effective?
   A. "I will administer cherry-flavored acetaminophen (Tylenol) for pain."
   B. "It is important to have my child gargle to prevent an infection."
   C. "I will bring my child to the emergency department if I see excessive swallowing."
   D. "I will offer my child ice cream to help soothe the pain in the throat."

3. The nurse is providing care to an infant being discharged after surgical correction of choanal atresia. Which topic is appropriate for the nurse to include in the discharge teaching for this infant?
   A. Gastrostomy feedings
   B. Direct observation therapy
   C. Nebulizer treatments
   D. Appropriate technique for cleaning nostrils

4. What information about pediatric respiratory anatomy and physiology is important for nursing care?
   A. Newborns are obligatory nose breathers.
   B. Sinuses are not developed until around age 10.
   C. Neonates are able to breathe from the diaphragm.
   D. Babies and children are not prone to aspiration.

5. The nurse is teaching home care to the parents of a child with chronic sinus infections. What information does the nurse provide?
   A. Have the child blow his nose vigorously before using decongestant spray.
   B. Steroids are usually required in children who have sinus infections.
   C. Ice packs over the inflamed sinuses will help with comfort and swelling.
   D. Using decongestant sprays for more than 3 days can cause rebound swelling.

6. An emergency department physician is preparing to directly visualize the larynx of a child suspected of having epiglottitis. What action by the nurse is most important?
   A. Allow the child to assume a position of comfort.
   B. Have an intubation tray at the bedside.
   C. Put on a face mask in addition to gloves.
   D. Have the parents sign an informed consent.

7. A child has otitis externa with a swollen ear canal. What intervention does the nurse teach the parents for instilling eardrops?
   A. Use a warm moist pack prior to the eardrops.
   B. Have the child lay flat for 20 minutes afterwards.
   C. Drip the medication onto the cotton ear wick.
   D. Chill the eardrops before administering them.

8. The nurse reads on a child's chart that she is having a tempanocentesis. For what medical condition is this warranted?
   A. Conductive hearing loss
   B. Otitis externa
   C. Infected eustachian tubes
   D. Otitis media

9. The nurse is caring for a 16-year-old admitted with suspected bacterial pneumonia. Which action by the nurse takes priority?
   A. Administer antibiotics as ordered.
   B. Obtain a sputum sample for culture.
   C. Start an IV for maintenance fluids.
   D. Give acetaminophen (Tylenol) for fever.

10. A child is brought to the emergency department, and the parents report frequent episodes of harsh coughing that causes the child's face to turn red. The parents also report the child's eyes are red, and she frequently coughs so hard she vomits. What question by the nurse is most important?
    A. Is anyone else in the family sick?
    B. Is she allergic to anything known?
    C. Has she had a high fever lately?
    D. Are her immunizations up to date?

See Answers to End of Chapter Review Questions on Davis*Plus*.

REFERENCES

AAP Updates Recommendations for Flu Vaccine. (2014). Retrieved from http://pediatrics.aappublications.org/content/early/2012/09/04/peds.2012-2308.full.pdf

Albietz, J. A., Czaja, A. S., Dobyns, E. L., Grayck, E. N., & Mourani, P. M. (2011). Critical care. In W. W. Hay, M. J. Levin, J. M. Sondheimer, & R. R. Deterding (Eds.), *Current diagnosis and treatment* (20th ed., pp. 358–361). New York, NY: McGraw-Hill.

American Academy of Family Physicians. (2005). Asthma Action Plan. Retrieved from http://www.nhlbi.nih.gov/files/docs/public/lung/asthma_actplan.pdf

American Academy of Otolaryngology, Head and Neck Surgery. (2011). Retrieved from http://entnet.org/

American Academy of Pediatrics (AAP). (2012). Policy statement: Recommended childhood and adolescent immunization schedules–United States. *Pediatrics, 129*(2), 385–386.

American Academy of Pediatrics (AAP): American Academy of Family Physicians. (2004a). Clinical practice guidelines: Diagnosis and management of acute otitis media. *Pediatrics, 113*(5), 1451–1465.

American Academy of Pediatrics (AAP): American Academy of Family Physicians. (2004b). Clinical practice guidelines: Otitis media with effusion. *Pediatrics, 113*(5), 1413–1429.

American Cancer Society. (2012). *Secondhand smoke.* Retrieved from http://www.cancer.org/cancer/cancercauses/tobaccocancer/second-hand-smoke

American Heart Association (AHA). (2010). Part 1: Executive summary: 2010 American Heart Association guidelines for cardiopulmonary resuscitation and emergency cardiovascular care. *Circulation, 122,* S640–S656. doi:10.1161/CIRCULATIONAHA.110.970889

American Lung Association. (2013a). Lung-disease influenza. Retrieved from http://www.lung.org/lung-disease/influenza

American Lung Association. (2013b). Measuring your peak flow. Retrieved from http://www.lung.org/lung-disease/asthma/living-with-asthma/take-control-of-your-asthma/measuring-your-peak-flow-rate.html

Bishop, W. P. (2011). The digestive system. In K. J. Marcdante, R. M. Kliegman, H. B. Jenson, & R. E. Behrman (Eds.), *Nelson's essentials of pediatrics* (6th ed., pp. 477–481). Philadelphia, PA: Elsevier.

Blosser, C. G., Brady, M. A., & Royal, R. B. (2012). Infectious diseases and immunizations. In C. E. Burns, A. M. Dunn, M. A. Brady, N. B. Starr, & C. G. Blosser (Eds.), *Pediatric primary care* (5th ed., p. 468). Philadelphia, PA: Elsevier.

Bulechek, G. M., Butcher, H. K., Dochterman, J. M., & Wagner, C. (2013). *Nursing interventions classification (NIC)* (6th ed.). St. Louis, MO: Elsevier Mosby.

Burns, C. E., & Dunn, A. M. (2012). Environmental health issues. In C. E. Burns, A. M. Dunn, M. A. Brady, N. B. Starr, & C. G. Blosser (Eds.), *Pediatric primary care* (5th ed., pp. 1074–1076). Philadelphia, PA: Elsevier.

Carter, E. R., & Marshall, S. G. (2011). The respiratory system. In K. J. Marcdante, R. M. Kliegman, H. B. Jenson, & R. E. Behrman (Eds.), *Nelson's essentials of pediatrics* (6th ed., pp. 499–524). Philadelphia, PA: Elsevier.

Centers for Disease Control and Prevention (CDC). (2011). *Morbidity and Mortality Weekly Report (MMWR), 60*(35), 1207–1212.

Centers for Disease Control and Prevention (CDC). (2012). *Secondhand smoke (SHS).* Retrieved from http://www.cdc.gov/tobacco/basic_information/secondhand_smoke/

Centers for Disease Control and Prevention (CDC). (2013). *Outbreaks.* Retrieved from http://www.cdc.gov/pertussis/outbreaks.html

Cheifetz, I. M. (2011). Pediatric acute respiratory distress syndrome. *Respiratory Care, 56*(10), 1589–1599.

Code of Federal Regulations Subpart A Sec. 46.102. (2009). *Basic HHS Policy for Protection of Human Research Subjects.* Office of Human Subjects Research. National Institute of Health: Bethesda, MD: http://www.hhs.gov/ohrp/humansubjects/guidance/45cfr46.html

Covar, R. A., Fleischer, D. M., & Boguniewicz, M. (2011). Allergic disorders. In W. W. Hay, M. J. Levin, J. M. Sondheimer, & R. R. Deterding (Eds.), *Current diagnosis and treatment* (20th ed., pp. 1054–1068). New York, NY: McGraw-Hill.

Federico, M. J., Kerby, G. S., Deterding, R. R., Baker, C. D., Balasubramaniam, V., Zemanick, E. T., et al. (2011). Respiratory tract & mediastinum. In W. W. Hay, M. J. Levin, J. M. Sondheimer, & R. R. Deterding (Eds.), *Current diagnosis and treatment* (20th ed., pp. 487–535). New York, NY: McGraw-Hill.

Guinto-Ocampo, H., & McNeil, B. K. (2010). Pertussis. eMedicine. Retrieved from http://emedicine.medscape.com/article/967268-overview

John, R. M., & Brady, M. A. (2012a). Respiratory Disorders. In C. E. Burns, A. M. Dunn, M. A. Brady, N. B. Starr, & C. G. Blosser (Eds.), *Pediatric primary care* (5th ed., pp. 708–738). Philadelphia, PA: Elsevier.

John, R. M., & Brady, M. A. (2012b). Atopic and rheumatic disorders. In C. E. Burns, A. M. Dunn, M. A. Brady, N. B. Starr, & C. G. Blosser (Eds.), *Pediatric primary care* (5th ed., pp. 497–516), Philadelphia, PA: Elsevier.

Johnson, M., Moorhead, S., Bulechek, G., Butcher, H., Maas, M., & Swanson, E. (2012). *NIC and NOC linkages to NANDA-L and clinical conditions* (3rd ed.). St. Louis, MO: Elsevier Mosby.

Klein, J. O., & Pelton, S. (2011). *Acute otitis media: Prevention of recurrence.* Retrieved from http://www.uptodate.com/contents/acute-otitis-media-in-children-prevention-of-recurrence

Lafferty, K. A. (2012). Smoke inhalation. Retrieved from http://emedicine.medscape.com/article/771194-overview

Light, M. J. (2011). Anatomy of the lung. In M. J. Light, C. J. Blaisdell, D. N. Homnick, M. S. Schechter, & M. M. Wienberger (Eds.), *Pediatric pulmonology* (pp. 1–14). Elk Grove Village, IL: American Academy of Pediatrics.

Moorhead, S., Johnson, M., Maas, M. L., & Swanson, E. (2013). *Nursing outcomes classification (NOC)* (5th ed.). St. Louis, MO: Elsevier Mosby.

National Heart, Lung, and Blood Institute (NHLBI): National Asthma Education and Prevention Program. (2007). Expert Panel Report 3: Guidelines for the diagnosis and management of asthma. Retrieved from http://www.nhlbi.nih.gov/guidelines/asthma/asthgdln.pdf

National Heart, Lung, and Blood Institute (NHLBI); National Institutes of Health; U.S. Department of Health and Human Services. (2007). Asthma Action Plan. Retrieved from http://www.nhlbi.nih.gov/health/public/lung/asthma/asthma_actplan.pdf

Ogle, J. W., & Anderson, M. S. (2011). Infections: Bacterial & spirochetal. In W. W. Hay, M. J. Levin, J. M. Sondheimer, & R. R. Deterding (Eds.), *Current diagnosis & treatment* (20th ed., pp. 1201–1203). New York, NY: McGraw Hill.

Petersen-Smith, A. M., & McKenzie, S. B. (2012). Ear disorders. In C. E. Burns, A. M. Dunn, M. A. Brady, N. B. Starr, & C. G. Blosser (Eds.), *Pediatric primary care* (5th ed., pp. 652–668). Philadelphia, PA: Elsevier.

Rahm, N. S., Hansen, J. D., & Sanddal, N. D. (1997). Critical trauma care by the basic EMT. Bozeman, MT: Critical Illness and Trauma Foundation, Inc.

Rance, K., O'Laughlen, M., & Ting, S. (2011). Improving asthma care for African American children by increasing national asthma guideline adherence. *Journal of Pediatric Health Care, 25*(4), 235–249.

Redjal, N. (2011). Wheezing and asthma. In C. D. Berkowitz (Ed.), *Berkowitz's pediatrics: A primary care approach* (4th ed., pp. 491–501). Elk Grove, IL: American Academy of Pediatrics.

Sawer, S. S. (2012). *Pediatric physical examination & health assessment* (p. 99). Sudbury, MA: Jones & Bartlett Learning.

Schlosser, P. A. (2013). Bioinstrumentation: Principles and techniques. In M. F. Hazinski (Ed.). *Nursing care of the critically ill child* (3rd ed., pp. 1005–1007). St. Louis, MO: Elsevier.

Schroeder, J. W., & McColley, S. (2011). Congenital abnormalities of the upper airway. In M. J. Light, C. J. Blaisdell, D. N. Homnick, M. S. Schechter, & M. M. Wienberger (Eds.), *Pediatric pulmonology* (p. 266). Elk Grove Village, IL: American Academy of Pediatrics.

Serebrisky, D. (2012). Smoke Inhalation injury. Retrieved from http://emedicine.medscape.com/article/1002413

Sharma, G. D., & Conrad, C. (2011). Croup, epiglottitis, and bacterial tracheitis. In M. J. Light, C. J. Blaisdell, D. N. Homnick, M. S. Schechter, & M. M. Wienberger (Eds.), *Pediatric pulmonology* (pp. 347–375). Elk Grove Village, IL: American Academy of Pediatrics.

Smith, S. (2011). Pharyngitis. In K. J. Marcdante, R. M. Kliegman, H. B. Jenson, & R. E. Behrman (Eds.), *Nelson essentials of pediatrics* (6th ed., pp. 386–388). Philadelphia, PA: Elsevier.

Sockrider, M., & Farber, H. J. (2011). Secondhand tobacco smoke exposure and active smoking in childhood and adolescence. In M. J. Light, C. J. Blaisdell, D. N. Homnick, M. S. Schechter, & M. M. Wienberger (Eds.), *Pediatric pulmonology* (pp. 391–421). Elk Grove Village, IL: American Academy of Pediatrics.

Sullivan, B., & Kinane, T. B. (2011). Congenital lung anomalies. In M. J. Light, C. J. Blaisdell, D. N. Homnick, M. S. Schechter, & M. M. Wienberger (Eds.), *Pediatric pulmonology* (pp. 278–307). Elk Grove Village, IL: American Academy of Pediatrics.

Thilo, E. H., & Rosenberg, A. A. (2011). The newborn infant. In W. W. Hay, M. J. Levin, J. M. Sondheimer, & R. R. Deterding (Eds.), *Current diagnosis & treatment* (20th ed., pp. 44–46). New York, NY: McGraw Hill.

U.S. Department of Health and Human Services. (2007). National asthma education and prevention program. Expert panel report 3: Guidelines for the diagnosis and management of asthma. Full report 2007. NIH Publication No. 07–4051. Bethesda, MD: NHLBI Health Information

Center. Retrieved from http://www.nhlbi.nih.gov/guidelines/asthma/asthgdln.htm

Vallerand, A. H., & Sanoski, C. A. (2014). *Davis's drug guide for nurses* (14th ed.). Philadelphia, PA: F.A. Davis.

Van Leeuwen, A. M., & Poelhuis-Leth, D. J. (2011). *Davis's comprehensive handbook of laboratory and diagnostic tests: With nursing implications* (4th ed.). Philadelphia, PA: F.A. Davis.

Venes, D. (2013). *Taber's cyclopedic medical dictionary* (22nd ed.). Philadelphia, PA: F.A. Davis Company.

Vergison, A., Dagan, R., Arguedas, A., Bonhoeffer, J., Cohen, R., Dhooge, I., et al. (2010). Otitis media and its consequences: Beyond the earache. *Lancet 10,* 195–203.

Ward, S. (2013). *Pediatric nursing care: Best evidence-based practices.* Philadelphia, PA: F.A. Davis.

Warshawsky, M. E. (2012). Foreign body aspiration. Retrieved from http://emedicine.medscape.com/article/298940

Weinberger, M. M. (2011). Bronchiolitis. In M. J. Light, C. J. Blaisdell, D. N. Homnick, M. S. Schechter, & M. M. Wienberger (Eds.), *Pediatric pulmonology* (pp. 377–390). Elk Grove Village, IL: American Academy of Pediatrics.

Yoon, P. J., Kelley, P. E., & Friedman, N. R. (2011). Ear, nose, & throat. In W. W. Hay, M. J. Levin, J. M. Sondeheimer, & R. R. Deterding (Eds.), *Current diagnosis & treatment* (20th ed., pp. 470–473). New York, NY: McGraw Hill.

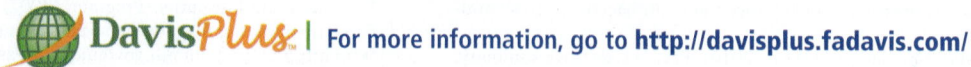

Davis*Plus* | For more information, go to **http://davisplus.fadavis.com/**

CONCEPT MAP

Diagnostics **Caring for the Child With a Respiratory Condition** Anatomical differences

Could Precipitate a Condition:
- Smaller nares
- Epiglottis: longer, higher, flaccid
- Trachea: shorter, narrower, higher bifurcation
- Increased friction and resistance→difficult ventilation
- Lung tissue immature at birth
- < 6 yrs: abdominal breather
- Less mature immune system

Oxygenation:
- Pulse oximetry
- Arterial blood gases

Function:
- Pulmonary function test
- Slow vital capacity
- Lung volume and capacity

Infectious Conditions:
- Pertussis/whooping cough
- Tuberculosis
- Influenza

Noninfectious Irritation:
- Foreign body aspiration
- Smoke inhalation injury
- Passive smoking-3rd hand smoke

Radiological:
- X-rays
- CT scan
- Fluoroscopy

Visualization:
- Laryngoscopy
- Bronchoscopy
- Thoracoscopy
- Endoscopy
- Otoscopy

Lab Studies:
- Lung tissue biopsy
- Blood cultures

Upper Airway Disorders:
- RHINO
- Sinusitis/nasopharyngitis/pharyngitis
- Tonsillitis
- Croup/croup syndrome
- Otitis media/externa

Lower Airway Disorders:
- Bronchitis
- Pneumonias
- SARS
- Bronchiolitis/RSV

Congenital Conditions/Structural Anomalies:
- Choanal atresia
- Esophageal atresia and TEF
- Diaphragmatic hernia
- ARDS
- Bronchopulmonary dysplasia
- Cystic fibrosis

Disorders Related to Allergens:
- Allergic rhinitis
- Asthma

Focus on Safety:
- Use aspiration precautions when feeding a child with a respiratory illness

General Potential Nursing Care:
- Assessment: airway patency; color; LOC; cardiac assessment; posture; respiratory rate; chest symmetry percussion/palpation; auscultation; sputum
- Promote adequate oxygenation: clean nasal area; suction; chest PT; vaporizer; oximetry/ABG results; CPAP/mechanical ventilation; stat rx for asthma
- Aspiration precautions; watch feeding position
- Monitor vital signs
- Maintain adequate nutrition and fluid balance
- Protect against infection; hand washing
- Infection processes: possible strict isolation; antibiotic therapy; prevent transmission
- Care of the postop child
- Promote normal development

Critical Nursing Actions:
- Correlate respiratory rate to overall physical findings/factors that impact it
- During a complete assessment, nursing instinct can ID subtle changes before technology
- Assess resp. status/prevention resp. infection in infant with BPD

Clinical Alert:
- Retractions indicate use of accessory muscles/respiratory difficulty
- Maternal polyhydramnios is associated with esophageal atresia
- Use care/accurate technique with postoperative suctioning/tube placement
- ARDS might necessitate use of assisted mechanical ventilation
- Continuous swallowing may indicate postoperative tonsillectomy bleeding
- Rupture tympanic membrane → decrease in pain, temp, purulent ear discharge → scarring and hearing loss
- Know symptoms of acute epiglollitis requiring hospitalization/use of tongue blade to assess can cause laryngospasm

Nursing Insight:
- There are different variations of esophageal atresia
- Understand the purpose of and nursing considerations for chest tubes
- Pneumonia can be typical or atypical
- Avoid use of salicylates for fever due to potential for Reye syndrome
- Otitis media occurs less in breastfed infants
- RSV-IGIV can prevent RSV
- 11- to 12-year-olds need pertussis booster
- Children < 5 need a space with their MDI

Complementary Care:
- Use of chiropractic care for asthma/rhinitis/sinusitis

Cultural Diversity:
- BCG vaccine used worldwide to prevent life-threatening form of TB
- There are higher asthma rates in poor African American/Hispanic children

Collaboration in Caring:
- Encourage parents to learn the Heimlich maneuver

Across Care Settings:
- Cystic fibrosis → multidisciplinary collaboration/extensive family teaching
- Teach how to avoid/control allergens
- Asthma → requires awareness by multiple community partners/collaborative treatment

Where Research And Practice Meet:
- Use of NAEPP guidelines and inhaled steroids can decrease the disparity in care of African American children with asthma

Now Can You:
- Discuss anatomical differences and respiratory assessment in the child
- ID signs/symptoms, care for the child with a congenital respiratory disorder
- Prepare home care and management plans

Caring for the Child With a Gastrointestinal Condition

 Stomach trouble in children can be a common complaint because of a variety of physical (eating too much) or psychological reasons (stress). In most cases a child's stomachache is not serious however; the pain is genuine and must be addressed. Common causes of stomachaches include constipation, milk allergy, urinary tract infections, strep throat, appendicitis, and emotional upset. The nurse teaches parents when to call the health-care provider. For instance, call when a baby with stomach pain draws her legs up toward the abdomen or when a young child has recurrent stomach distress and/or has trouble sleeping. Also, tell parents that sudden pain or pain that persists, change in bowel habits, vomiting, fever of 100.4°F (40°C), sore throat, or headache warrants a call to the health-care provider.

—American Academy of Pediatrics (AAP), 2014

LEARNING TARGETS *At the completion of this chapter, the student will be able to:*

- Describe the anatomy and physiology and developmental aspects of the gastrointestinal system.
- Examine common conditions of the gastrointestinal system.
- Prioritize developmentally appropriate and holistic nursing care for common conditions of the gastrointestinal system.
- Explore diagnostic, laboratory testing and medications for common conditions of the gastrointestinal system.
- Develop teaching plans and discharge criteria for parents whose children have common gastrointestinal conditions.

PICO(T) Questions

The intent of evidence-based practice (EBP) is to provide nursing care that integrates the best available evidence. An initial step in EBP is to write a PICO(T) question that effectively guides the research. A PICO(T) question is an acronym that stands for population (P), intervention or issue (I), comparison of interest (C), outcome (O), and timeframe (T). Depending on the question, all or some of the question components are used in the research process.

Use these PICO(T) questions to spark your thinking as you read the chapter.

1. Does (I) delaying the introduction of gluten in (P) infants' diet until at least 1 year of age (O) decrease the rate of celiac disease (C) compared with introducing gluten earlier?

2. Is there a (O) higher incidence of (I) Crohn's disease in (P) children who were bottle-fed (C) compared with those who were breastfed?

Evidence-Based Practice

Sharp, D. B., Santos, L. A., & Cruz, M. L. (2009). Fatty liver in adolescents on the U.S.-Mexico border. *Journal of the American Academy of Nurse Practitioners, 21,* 225–230.

The purpose of this study was to describe the physical and metabolic characteristics of children diagnosed with fatty liver disease and to determine the presence of nonalcoholic fatty liver disease (NAFLD). In recent years fatty liver disease has become the most common cause of liver disease in children and adolescents. Studies have found that children of Hispanic origin have a higher prevalence of fatty liver disease than other racial groups in the United States as well as a higher rate of overweight (21.8% versus 12.3% for white children). The prevalence of children with a body mass index (BMI) of greater than or equal to 95% has increased to 17% in recent years. The development of fatty liver disease is of concern because it may lead to chronic end-stage liver disease later in life. In addition, children with fatty liver disease are also more likely to have hypertension, hypertriglyceridemia, hypercholesterolemia, and type 2 diabetes. Data from national health surveys indicate that NAFLD is on the rise and estimates that 60% of adolescents with elevated liver alanine aminotransferase (ALT) are overweight. One percent of overweight adolescents have ALT levels more than twice the normal level, which may suggest the presence of advanced liver disease.

A retrospective chart review was performed to gather data from the pediatric population of a gastroenterology clinic in El Paso, Texas, which is considered a U.S.-Mexico border city. The population of El Paso is 583,419 of which 79% are of Hispanic or Mexican descent. Diagnosis of fatty liver disease was based on an elevated ALT as well as ultrasound evidence. Patients aged 8 to 18 years of age were identified from the chart review on which 32 met the criteria. Data were gathered to include demographic information as well as laboratory and clinical evidence. Clinical and laboratory evidence included ALT, aspartate aminotransferase (AST), triglycerides, high-density lipoprotein (HDL), low-density lipoprotein (LDL), total cholesterol, and fasting glucose and insulin levels. Height and weight information was used to calculate BMI. The researchers also determined the number of children and adolescents who fell under their criteria for "metabolic syndrome," which they defined as including the presence of three or more abnormalities (e.g., BMI greater than or equal to the 95th percentile for age and gender, triglycerides greater than or equal to 150 mg/dL, HDL less than or equal to 35 mg/dL, fasting blood sugar greater than or equal to

100 mg/dL, and ALT greater than or equal to 30 units/L). The researchers also determined the number of children and adolescents with AST greater than 35 units/L, cholesterol greater than 200 mg/dL, fasting insulin at greater than or equal to 20 microunits/mL, and LDL greater than or equal to 130 mg/dL.

The subjects included 24 males and 1 female and ranged in ages from 8 to 18 years of age: 4 (13%) were between 8 and 11 years and 21 (87%) were between 12 and 18 years of age. One potential subject was eliminated because of a history of chemotherapy treatment for cancer, which also can cause liver changes not related to NAFLD. Twenty-five subjects were of Mexican American descent, and all were overweight as defined by a BMI at the greater than or equal to the 95th percentile. Results were as follows:

- ALT levels
  - 13.8% had levels twice the normal
  - 27.5% had levels three times the normal
  - 48.3% had levels four times the normal
- 86% had elevated AST levels
- 45% had elevated triglycerides
- 26% had elevated total cholesterol
  - 53% had low HDL
  - 20% had elevated LDL
- 17% had elevated fasting blood sugar
- 82% had elevated fasting insulin levels

Fifteen patients had three or more of the risk factors, which the researchers used to define metabolic syndrome. Four subjects had four or more risk factors.

The researchers conclude that clinical and laboratory findings in this population were consistent with the diagnosis of NAFLD. They further concluded that their findings were consistent with previous studies, which found that fatty liver disease and NAFLD are more common in boys, increases with age, and that children of Hispanic and Mexican descent are more susceptible to NAFLD.

1. How is this information useful to clinical nursing practice?

2. Based on these findings, what are implications for further research?

See Suggested Responses for Evidence-Based Practice on Davis*Plus*.

Introduction

This chapter provides a review of the anatomy and physiology and developmental aspects of the gastrointestinal system. The discussion includes an examination of the various gastrointestinal tract conditions including developmentally appropriate and holistic nursing care. Information about diagnostic and laboratory testing and medications is explored. Teaching plans and discharge criteria for parents whose children have various gastrointestinal conditions are incorporated.

A & P review **The Gastrointestinal System**

The gastrointestinal (GI) system (Fig. 24-1) is responsible for ingestion, digestion, absorption, metabolism, and elimination of solid and liquid nutrients. Each organ in the system performs a specific function in this process. The GI system is divided into two basic portions, the upper and

Growth and Development

The child with a gastrointestinal condition such as celiac disease, Crohn's disease, gastroesophageal reflux, or short bowel syndrome is highly susceptible to alterations in physical growth and development. Conditions affecting the gastrointestinal tract can impair the body's ability to digest and absorb nutrients resulting in failure to thrive. Failure to thrive can pose detrimental consequences on a child's physical growth and development. Failure to thrive impairs the child's ability to gain weight, grow, and fight against infection. Failure to thrive also hinders the child's psychosocial, motor maturation and intellectual development. Because of the multiple ways in which growth and development are affected by failure to thrive, early identification and treatment is needed (Nutzenadel, 2011).

Nursing care for the child with a gastrointestinal condition should promote a balanced nutrition required for healthy growth and development. The proper

treatment of failure to thrive in childhood consists of treatment of the underlying illness combined with nutritional treatment that addresses the mechanism of the accompanying failure to thrive (Nutzenadel, 2011). The nurse should collaborate with the nutritionist to implement an appropriate oral, enteral, or parenteral diet needed to optimize caloric intake. The nurse should closely monitor the child's height, weight, BMI, and weight-to-length ratio observing for an upward trajectory on the growth chart. Nutritional support with a dietitian may be helpful to provide effective education about lifelong dietary changes needed to promote growth. The nurse should educate the family about the importance of compliance with the dietary changes to prevent complications of the disease process.

Source: Nutzenadel, W. (2011). Failure to thrive in childhood. *Duetsches Arzteblatt International, 108*(38), 642–649.

The Gastrointestinal System

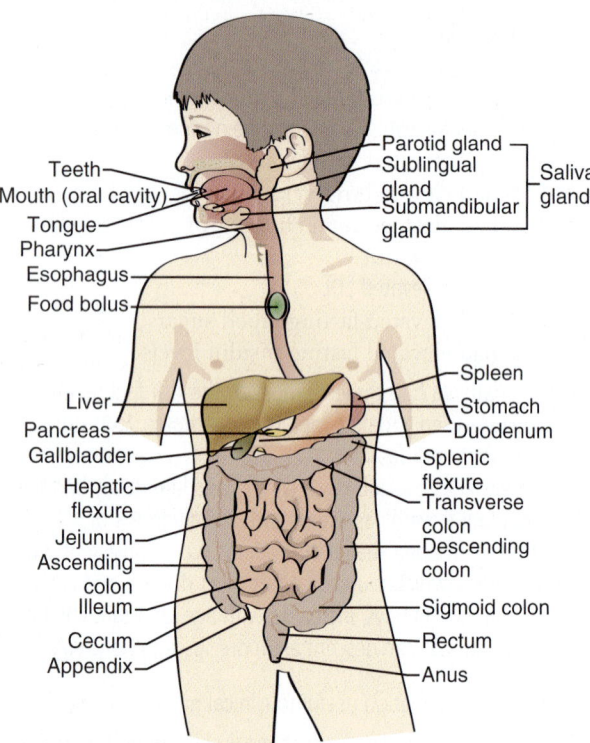

Figure 24-1 Gastrointestinal system.

the lower. The upper portion includes the mouth (teeth and gums), the esophagus, and the stomach. The lower portion consists of the small intestine, large intestine (colon), rectum, and anus. In addition, other organs are a significant part of the GI system: the liver, pancreas, and gallbladder.

The upper portion of the GI system is responsible for nutrient intake or ingestion: the mouth and esophagus. The tongue senses the taste and texture of food, which initiates salivation. The salivation that occurs in the mouth initiates the beginning of the digestive process. The saliva releases two enzymes: amylase and ptyalin. These enzymes begin the breakdown of complex starches into disaccharides. The esophagus transports food to the stomach by the process of peristalsis. In the stomach, food mixes with gastric fluids and is then propelled into the small intestine.

The lower portion of the GI system handles the remainder of the digestion, absorption, and metabolism processes with the assistance of the liver and pancreas. The small intestine does most of the work of absorption through a system of villi and folds, which increases the absorptive surface. The small intestine further convert disaccharides into monosaccharides. Hindrance of this process can lead to diarrhea. The small intestine is primarily responsible for absorption of carbohydrates, fats, proteins, minerals, and vitamins into the systemic circulation. The duodenum forms the first portion of the small intestine. Pancreatic and bile ducts empty in the upper portion of the duodenum. The duodenum is followed by the jejunum, where the majority of water, protein, carbohydrates, and vitamins are absorbed. Fat breakdown occurs mainly in the jejunum through the secretion of lipases by the pancreas. The lymphatic system then absorbs fats. Proteins are converted to amino acids by the pancreatic enzyme trypsin and are absorbed via the capillary walls of the villi and into the systematic circulation. The last and longest segment of the small intestine is the ileum, which absorbs bile salts, vitamins C and B_{12}, and chloride.

The large intestine takes care of elimination. The contents of the small intestine enters the cecum through the ileocecal valve, which is located in the right lower quadrant of the abdomen and forms the beginning of the large intestine. The appendix, which is described as a blind tube containing lymphoid tissue, is attached to the cecum. The ascending colon rises along the right anterior portion of the abdomen, followed by the transverse colon, which lies horizontally across the abdomen, and then forms the descending colon along the left lateral abdomen. The sigmoid colon follows the descending colon into the pelvic cavity. The sigmoid colon then connects to the rectum, where stool is stored until it is expelled through the anal canal and through the anus. Elimination culminates in the removal of solid waste products through defecation.

Accessory Structures

The liver is located below the right diaphragm and is the largest and heaviest organ in the body. The liver is a vascular organ composed of right and left hepatic lobes. The liver is responsible for metabolizing carbohydrates, fats, and proteins and also breaks down toxic substances such as drugs. In addition, the liver stores vitamins and iron and produces antibodies, bile, prothrombin, and fibrinogen for coagulation.

The gallbladder, which lies within the inferior surface of the liver, stores bile, which is produced by the liver. The bile is then secreted into the duodenum through the cystic duct and common bile duct, where it assists in the digestion of fats.

The pancreas can be found between the spleen and stomach in the left upper quadrant of the abdominal cavity. The pancreas produces pancreatic enzymes, which are excreted into the duodenum by way of the pancreatic duct. The pancreatic enzymes assist in the metabolism of proteins, fats, and carbohydrates. Insulin and glucagon are also produced by the pancreas and secreted directly into the bloodstream. ◆

Developmental Aspects of the Gastrointestinal System

The gastrointestinal system plays an essential role in a child's growth and development. Because the GI system is complex, the nurse must understand the ways in which each developmental stage contributes to the promotion of the health of the child. The infant has several physiological mechanisms in place to ensure the adequate intake of nutrients. The infant has a built-in safeguard to prevent choking while swallowing and sucking. The posterior portion of the tongue that separates the mouth and throat is raised against the soft palate while the infant sucks. This allows the infant to suck and breathe at same time. The infant also has a longer posterior soft palate, which assists her in swallowing milk. In addition, the passage from mouth to pharynx is smaller, which helps to control the amount of liquid that is taken in. The nurse can teach the parents that the infant's stomach usually empties in 2.5 to 3 hours, and this is the reason that the infant has frequent feedings. Digestion takes place in the intestines so it is important that the intestines function properly. In addition, the liver and pancreas do not mature until 6 months of age. The nurse therefore tells the parents that infants younger than 4 months of age do not require solid foods. Pancreatic lipase is essential for fat and protein metabolism but is not adequately secreted until age 1 year, which limits the body's ability to absorb fats, such as those present in cow's milk. This information reinforces the need to carefully introduce foods into the infant diet, limiting foods to those that are specially prepared for infant digestion.

 Nursing Insight—*Infant bowel sounds*

In the newborn, bowel sounds are audible within the first few hours of life. A newborn with a scaphoid abdomen or signs of respiratory distress is evaluated carefully for bowel sounds and/or decreased breath sounds in the chest, which may be evidence of congenital diaphragmatic hernia. A congenital diaphragmatic hernia is an opening between the chest and abdominal cavities through which abdominal organs may herniate into the chest cavity, compromising respiratory and cardiac structures.

 Nursing Insight—*Developmental aspects*

Breastfed infants tend to have "watery" stools. Formula-fed infants' stools are soft and sometimes "seedy." Infants do not absorb water as rapidly as older children. When **defecating** (evacuation of the bowels, feces), the infant may appear to be straining because of immature muscle coordination (Venes, 2013).

Infants' digestive system is immature but adequate, and growth is rapid. Infants gain 1.5 lb (680 g)/month, double their weight by 6 months, and triple it by 1 year. By 2 years, the child's salivary glands reach adult size. The average toddler gains 5 to 6 lb (2.3–2.7 kg) per year. The stomach capacity increases to about 500 mL, and the liver matures to become more efficient in vitamin storage, **glycogenesis** (the formation of glycogen from glucose [Venes, 2013]), and amino acid changes. The growth of the child's digestive system slows during the toddler years, which leads to a reduction in caloric needs from those of the infant period. The average toddler needs approximately 102 kcal/kg (46 kcal/lb) as opposed to 108 kcal/kg (50 kcal/lb) during infancy. Since the toddler characteristically has a decreased appetite and reduced metabolic rate, his appetite may be sporadic or appear finicky. Because of this sporadic behavior, the toddler may also go on food fads or "jags," preferring only one item and refusing other foods that she has preferred in the past.

The preschool-age child continues to have appetite fluctuations, with periods of overeating or refusal to eat. The preschool-age child gains about 4 to 5 lb (1.8–2.3 kg) per year. By age 4 to 5, the GI system is mature enough for the child to eat a full range of food, with stools becoming more like those of adults. School-age children gain about 4 to 6 pounds (1.8–2.7 kg) per year. When the child reaches the middle-school years, the GI tract has become relatively stable. The digestive systems of the middle-school child and adolescent are adult size and fully functional. Stools are usually passed once per day and are well formed. The liver and spleen enlarge during the adolescent growth spurt, though do not change in function.

 **Family Teaching Guidelines...**
Dealing With Food Fads or Jags With Young Children

TOPIC: The nurse will promote good nutrition in children

ESSENTIAL INFORMATION:

- Reassure the parents that food fads or jags are normal at this age and that the tendencies will pass.
- Stress that a little patience will keep both parents and child from further gastrointestinal upsets.
- Suggest that the parents not force the child to eat foods he is not interested in but to provide a variety of nutritious foods during meals and for between-meal snacks in the amount appropriate for the child's age.
- Inform the family about resources when they need additional help.
- Go to www.nal.usda.gov/fnic/, www.choosemyplate.gov/, and www.aap.org for more information on this topic.

Structural Gastrointestinal Disorders

INGUINAL HERNIA

Inguinal hernia is the most common type of hernia in children, accounting for 80% of all childhood hernias. An inguinal hernia arises from the failure of the processus vaginalis to atrophy and close during the eighth month of gestation. This provides a canal that allows for abdominal fluid or structure (bowel, ovary, or fallopian tube) to extend up to or through the inguinal ring into the scrotum or labia.

This type of hernia is eight to ten times more common in males with a 7% to 30% incidence among premature children (Gaylord & Petersen-Smith, 2012). An inguinal hernia is defined as the protrusion of bowel through the inguinal canal and is usually evident by a protrusion in the inguinal area and a bulging of the scrotal sac (Sundaram, Hoffenberg, Kramer, Sondheimer, & Furuta, 2011). In females, the hernia may involve a protrusion through the round ligament into the labia. Inguinal hernias in the pediatric population are generally considered indirect, meaning that the hernia passes through the internal abdominal ring, traverses the spermatic cord through the inguinal canal, and emerges at the external inguinal ring.

Signs and Symptoms

Inguinal hernias can have any of the following symptoms:

- Bulge on either side of pubic bone
- Burning, gurgling, or aching sensation at the bulge
- Pain or discomfort that increases while bending, coughing, or lifting
- Heavy or dragging sensation in groin
- Weakness or pressure in groin

Diagnosis

An inguinal hernia is identified by swelling in the inguinal area that extends toward or into the scrotum. Most inguinal hernias are observed by 6 months of age with more than 50% diagnosed before 1 year of age.

Prevention

Though this condition may not be prevented, good prenatal care provides an opportunity to promote optimal fetal development in utero.

Collaborative Care

Nursing Care. The majority of inguinal hernias are managed through surgical correction on an outpatient basis. The initial nursing care of the child hospitalized for the hernia repair involves parental education and preoperative preparation of the child.

Surgical Care. Elective surgical correction is the treatment of choice for the child. After surgery, the nurse can inform the parents that the child's vital signs are monitored frequently and that the child's position will be changed often to avoid undue stress on the surgical area.

Traditional postoperative measures such as assessing the child's vital signs and bowel sounds as well as maintaining fluid and electrolyte balance, monitoring pain, and ensuring return to normal bowel elimination are also done. Postoperative complications can be prevented by instructing the parents to keep the wound clean and dry and to change wet or soiled diapers as soon as possible for children who are not toilet trained.

 Nursing Insight—*Incarcerated hernia*

An incarcerated hernia is a portion of the intestine that cannot be returned to the abdominal cavity. The condition causes obstruction or pain and if left untreated can lead to strangulation (Venes, 2013). This condition requires prompt referral and correction to prevent the bowel from becoming strangulated and necrotic.

Education/Discharge Instructions

If the child has an inguinal hernia, the nurse can tell the parents that the surgery will repair the defect caused by the hernia. Recovery from an inguinal hernia is usually rapid, and the child will return home the same day as the surgery. Discharge instructions include informing the parents on wound care and the importance of keeping the surgical site clean and dry. The nurse also tells the parents the child can resume normal activity in 4 to 6 weeks and that he may be given a prescription for stool softeners to prevent straining during defecation (Venes, 2013).

UMBILICAL HERNIA

The nurse understands that umbilical hernia is the most common type of hernia in infants. An umbilical hernia is the protrusion of the intestine through the abdominal fascia, which is often identifiable during crying, defecation, or coughing (Fig. 24-2). An umbilical hernia occurs as a result of failure of the umbilical ring to close, which normally begins at the end of the first trimester. The incidence of umbilical hernias is estimated at 1 out of every 6 live births. Umbilical hernias are more common in premature and low-birth-weight infants and ten times more common in African American children. Umbilical hernias are also more common in children with Down syndrome and in children with hypothyroidism.

Signs and Symptoms

- The majority of umbilical hernias are asymptomatic.
- Umbilical hernias are more prominent when the infant is crying.

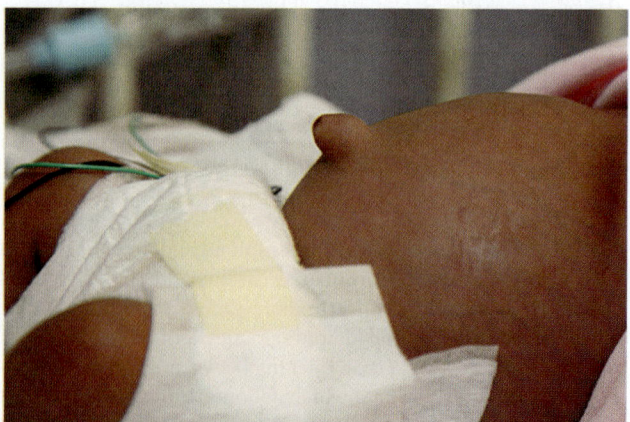

Figure 24-2 An umbilical hernia is the protrusion of the intestine through the abdominal fascia.

Diagnosis

Umbilical hernias can be identified as a soft midline swelling in the umbilical area, which can be reduced with pressure.

Prevention

Though this condition may not be prevented, good prenatal care provides an opportunity to promote optimal fetal development in utero.

Collaborative Care

Nursing Care. Most umbilical hernias resolve spontaneously by 3 to 5 years of age, though there is a decreased likelihood of spontaneous closure for a hernia larger than 1.5 cm in diameter or for one with a large, proboscis-like defect (elongated or extensible tubular process). The initial nursing care of the child hospitalized for the repair of an umbilical hernia involves parental education and preoperative preparation of the child. The majority of umbilical hernias are managed on an outpatient basis.

Surgical Care. Surgery is considered for a persistent hernia beyond the age of 5, an incarcerated hernia, or a hernia that enlarges dramatically. Vital signs are done frequently in the postoperative period. Postoperative care also includes keeping the wound clean and dry as well as managing the child's pain. A pressure dressing is generally applied for 48 hours postoperatively. The child may resume a normal diet and activity postoperatively. Postoperative complications of umbilical hernia repair are rare.

Education/Discharge Instructions

Prior to surgery the nurse instructs the parents about umbilical hernia and prognosis for the spontaneous resolution of the umbilical hernia. If surgery is required, parents are instructed to have the child avoid strenuous activities after surgical correction for 2 to 3 weeks and resume a normal diet as tolerated. Nursing care is similar to care of a child with an inguinal hernia.

ANORECTAL MALFORMATIONS

Anorectal malformations range from simple, such as an imperforate anus, to include other associated anomalies of not only the GI system but also the genitourinary (GU) system and pelvic organs. The incidence of anorectal malformation is approximately 1 in 4,000 to 5,000 births and is more common in males (Gaylord & Yetman, 2012). As one of the most common groups of congenital defects, these abnormalities are caused by abnormal or arrested development of the GI system. The location of the abnormality and actual organ systems involved is related to the week of gestation at which the development was disrupted. The etiology of anorectal malformations is unknown.

Signs and Symptoms

Rectal atresia (closure of the rectal passage) may initially present as a normal appearing anal opening but is later detected as an abnormal situation and is a complete obstruction that precludes the passage of stool. Immediate surgical intervention is mandatory for rectal atresia.

Rectal stenosis (constriction or narrowing of the rectal passage) includes vomiting, abdominal distention, and difficulty passing stool. Rectal stenosis may present with a ribbon-like or narrow stool, which is not always readily apparent at birth.

Absence of a rectal opening is referred to as an **imperforate anus.** An imperforate anus defect can be manifested in several forms, which include a fistula or connection from the distal rectum to the perineum or GU system. Passage of meconium through the vagina, urethra, or an opening under the scrotum is early evidence of an imperforate anus though the presence of a fistula may not be evident at birth. In the presence of an imperforate anus, as peristalsis increases, meconium is forced through the abnormal passage.

More extensive defects may present with evidence of a rectal connection to the vagina or urethra as the opening through which the stool passes.

Diagnosis

Diagnosis is made by physical examination and radiological imaging (x-ray), which indicates the level of the defect and location of fistula formation (Bishop, 2011; Shilyansky & Pitcher, 2010). The visualization of gas in the bladder or urethra during imaging also indicates the presence of a fistula connection between the bowel and associated structure (Bishop, 2011). Magnetic resonance imaging of the lumbosacral spinal cord is required for all children presenting with an imperforate anus to rule out the presence of a tethered spinal cord, which is common in children with this malformation (Bishop, 2011). An ultrasound (outlines the shape of tissues and organs) of the abdomen and pelvis, an IV pyelogram (provides information about the structure and function of the kidney, ureter, and bladder), and voiding cystogram (radiography of the bladder) are performed to evaluate associated defects of the urinary tract.

Prevention

Though this condition may not be prevented, good prenatal care provides an opportunity to promote optimal fetal development in utero.

Collaborative Care

Nursing Care. Overall nursing care depends on the type of defect and the extent of surgical correction. The child is kept NPO (nothing by mouth); therefore, the care of the infant before surgery includes parent education and maintenance of IV fluids. In addition to basic needs of the child undergoing surgery of the GI tract, pain control and the importance of infection control post-surgery must be stressed related to the location of the surgical incision and the potential for fecal or urinary contamination. The nurse also communicates to the family that, postoperatively for high anorectal malformations, a colostomy is placed and subsequent colostomy care is also required.

Surgical Care. Management of anorectal malformations may require extensive treatment, depending on the extent of the defect and associated organ involvement, including GI, urinary, and reproductive systems. Repeated manual dilation can be used to treat anal stenosis. The creation of a new anal opening may be used to correct anatomically lower anorectal defects.

A two-stage repair is generally necessary for anatomically higher anorectal defects. The first stage of anorectal repair involves resection and the creation of a temporary colostomy. The second stage involves "the closure of the colostomy and a pull through procedure in which the blind pouch of the rectum is anastomosed to the anus" (Shilyansky & Pitcher, 2010).

Common postoperative nursing measures are done such as monitoring frequent vital signs and intake and output, fluid maintenance, pain control, and offering developmental appropriate play. With the presence of a colostomy, the nurse stresses the importance of good skin care and infection control in the postoperative period. Nasogastric decompression is often required early in the postoperative period. Oral feedings are generally initiated with the reestablishment of peristalsis and once stooling has begun.

Education/Discharge Instructions

Discharge instructions include colostomy care, wound care, prevention of infection, and the procedure for anal dilation, if appropriate for the defect. The importance of adequate fluids is also stressed. The parent is instructed on the potential need for dietary fiber and the possible use of stool softeners or bulking agents. In addition, the parent is advised about the potential for delayed toilet training.

 Now Can You—Identify structural gastrointestinal disorders?

1. Identify structural GI disorders?
2. Identify signs and symptoms of structural GI disorders?
3. Identify nursing care for structural GI disorders?

Obstructive Gastrointestinal Disorders

HYPERTROPHIC PYLORIC STENOSIS

The etiology of hypertrophic pyloric stenosis (Fig. 24-3) is unknown. Suggested causal theories include a deficiency in inhibitory neuronal signals or molecular causes, such as a mechanism similar to that of Hirschsprung's disease (Sundaram et al., 2011). Ganglionic cell immaturity has also been suggested as a causative factor. Hypertrophic pyloric stenosis typically occurs in a healthy male infant.

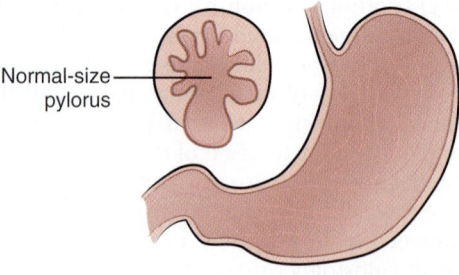

Hypertrophic Pyloric Stenosis

Normal-size pylorus

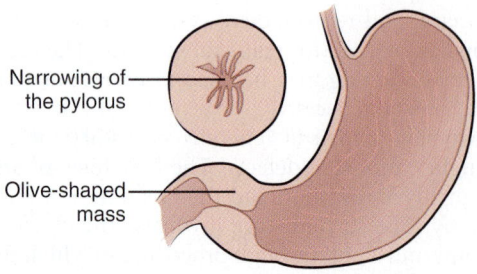

Narrowing of the pylorus

Olive-shaped mass

Figure 24-3 Hypertrophic pyloric stenosis.

 Cultural Diversity: Occurrence of Hypertrophic Pyloric Stenosis

Hypertrophic pyloric stenosis occurs in approximately 6 to 8 of 1,000 live births in the United States (Bishop, 2011). The incidence of pyloric stenosis is more common in the Caucasian population compared with 1.8 per 1,000 live births in the Hispanic population and 0.7 in the African American population. Males, especially firstborns, are affected two to four times more often than females are, and there may be a positive family history.

Signs and Symptoms

There is a pattern of normal feedings and new onset of non-bilious vomiting. The vomiting usually begins with episodes of regurgitation during the first few weeks of life (Gaylord & Yetman, 2012). Vomiting usually occurs immediately after a feeding and may become projectile in nature. The infant generally appears hungry immediately after vomiting and eagerly wants to feed again.

Other symptoms are as follows:

- Insatiable appetite
- Weight loss
- Dehydration
- Constipation
- Olive-shaped mass
- Visible reverse, or left to right, peristalsis may be observable in the left upper quadrant

 clinical alert

Vomiting

Projectile vomiting is the classic and most common symptom of hypertrophic pyloric stenosis.

Diagnosis

Diagnosis of hypertrophic pyloric stenosis can be made by palpating the pyloric mass. The mass is olive-shaped, moveable, firm, and best palpated from the left side and located above and to the right of the umbilicus in the mid-epigastrium (the superior central portion of the abdomen) beneath the liver edge (Bishop, 2011; Gaylord & Yetman, 2012). An abdominal x-ray film may show an enlarged stomach with diminished or absent gas in the intestine (Bishop, 2011). Examination of the pylorus on ultrasound shows elongation and thickening of the pylorus, which may be confirmed by a barium upper GI series. Confirmation by an upper GI series demonstrates a "string sign," which is caused by the barium passing through a narrowed pylorus (Bishop, 2011).

 Diagnostic Tools   Ultrasound

A diagnosis is often made after the history and physical examination. The diagnosis can be established 60% to 80% of the time by an experienced examiner. If the diagnosis of hypertrophic pyloric stenosis is inconclusive, an ultrasound can be used to demonstrate an elongated muscular mass surrounding a long pyloric canal. Ultrasound confirms the diagnosis of hypertrophic pyloric stenosis.

Prevention

Though this condition may not be prevented, good prenatal care provides an opportunity to promote optimal fetal development in utero.

Collaborative Care

Nursing Care. Initial care of the child with the diagnosis of pyloric stenosis includes a careful history and assessment of the child. The nurse needs to be alert to signs of dehydration, such as changes in skin turgor, appearance of the mucous membranes, depressed fontanelle, presence or absence of tears, urine output, and changes in vital signs as well as weight loss and evidence of discomfort.

Before surgery, the child is given nothing by mouth (NPO), and a nasogastric tube is inserted to provide gastric decompression. Surgery may be performed without delay in infants without dehydration and electrolyte imbalances. If dehydration is present, the dehydration imbalance is corrected with IV fluids and administration of appropriate electrolyte therapy.

Surgical Care. Treatment for hypertrophic pyloric stenosis is surgery called a **pyloromyotomy** (incision and suture of the pyloric sphincter). It is performed by laparoscopy (abdominal exploration) with an endoscope. The pyloric mass is split without cutting the mucosa and the incision is closed (Sundaram et al., 2011).

Postoperative care includes monitoring vital signs frequently. The nurse communicates to the family that it is common for the infant to experience some vomiting in the first 24 to 36 hours after surgery (Gaylord & Yetman, 2012). Fluid balance is maintained through administration of IV fluids and oral liquids as tolerated. Whether or not bowel sounds are present, feeding begins 6 hours after surgery. Pedialyte 15 mL is given every 2 hours for 2 consecutive feeds, if the baby tolerates this with no vomiting, then it is advanced to half-strength formula 15 mL every 2 hours for 2 consecutive feeds. If no vomiting, then advanced to 30 mL for 2 consecutive feeds, then 45 mL for 2 consecutive feeds and finally 60 mL for 2 consecutive feeds. If the baby vomits, then the baby stays at that level until 2 consecutive feeds are tolerated. It is important for the nurse to continue to monitor for signs of dehydration and for the infant's response to oral fluids. After surgery, the family members can be instructed on the importance of saving wet diapers that are weighed to measure output. Postoperative care also includes monitoring the surgical site for signs of infection, keeping the wound clean and dry, and providing pain relief. The potential for complication of postoperative infection can be prevented by instructing the parents to keep the wound clean and dry and to change wet or soiled diapers as soon as possible for children who are not toilet trained.

Education/Discharge Instructions

Discharge instructions include care of the incision and observation for signs of infection. The nurse must instruct the parent to observe the infant's response to feedings because some vomiting may still occur within the first 48 hours postoperatively. Vomiting beyond 48 hours must be reported to the child's health-care provider.

🌼 **Nursing Diagnoses** Hypertrophic Pyloric Stenosis

- Fluid Volume Deficit related to the effects of frequent vomiting
- Nutritional Imbalance: Less than Body Requirements related to vomiting and gradual reintroduction of feedings
- Pain related to surgical trauma
- Risk for Infection related to surgical incision
- Parent knowledge deficit related to postoperative care of the infant

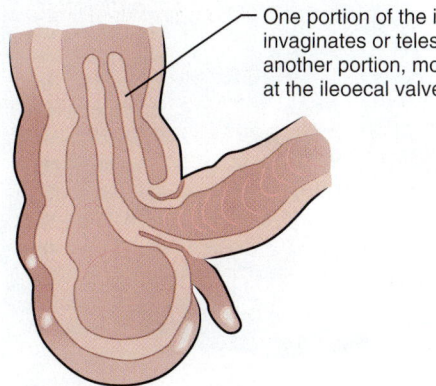

One portion of the intestine invaginates or telescopes into another portion, most commonly at the ileoecal valve.

Figure 24-4 Intussusception.

INTUSSUSCEPTION

Intussusception is a condition that occurs when one portion of the intestine that invaginates or telescopes into another portion, most commonly at the ileocecal valve (Venes, 2013) (Fig. 24-4). Most of the time, intussusception occurs in the first 2 years of life, but children can be susceptible until early school age (Sundaram et al., 2011). Intussusception is more common in males and is the most common cause of intestinal obstruction in children 5 months to 3 years of age (Starr, Blosser, Brady, Burns, Dunn, & Petersen-Smith 2012). Suggested predisposing factors to the development of intussusception include the presence of polyps, Meckel's diverticulum, Henoch–Schönlein purpura, constipation, lymphomas, lipomas, parasites, rotavirus, adenovirus, and the presence of foreign bodies. Intussusception may also occur as a complication of cystic fibrosis (Sundaram et al., 2011).

Signs and Symptoms

- Acute abdominal pain caused by the spasm of the telescoping bowel
- Pain frequently mimics the pain experienced by "colicky" infants
- Infants may pull their legs up toward the abdomen
- Pain is relieved once the abdomen relaxes
- Vomiting may or may not be present and it may or may not be projectile
- Fever
- Dehydration
- Abdominal distention
- Lethargy
- Grunting noises because of pain

---

 focus on safety

Abdominal pain in children

In children, abdominal pain can be referred from an extra-abdominal source such as pneumonia, a urinary tract infection, or testicular torsion or can be associated with a systemic disease. Abdominal pain is a common complaint in ill children and can be found in GI conditions as well as streptococcal pharyngitis, lower lobe pneumonia, sickle cell disease, cystic fibrosis, and other conditions. A child's abdominal pain experience is usually limited, and the child may be unable to accurately describe or pinpoint the location or sensation.

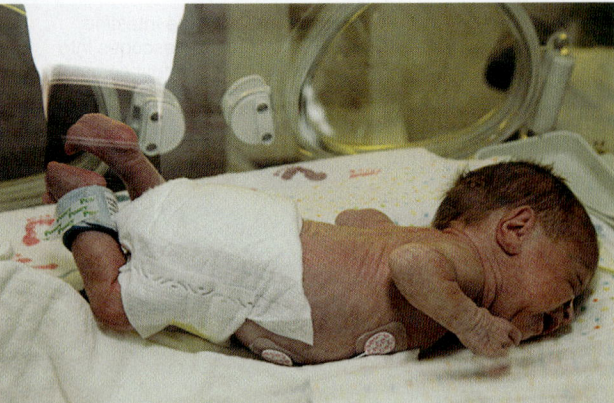

Figure 24-5 Infant with paroxysmal, episodic abdominal pain displays screaming and drawing up the legs.

 Assessment Tool Classic Symptomatic Triad for Intussusception

The classic symptomatic triad for intussusception includes:
- Paroxysmal, episodic abdominal pain with vomiting every 5 to 30 minutes
- Screaming and drawing up legs with periods of calm, sleeping, or lethargy between episodes (Fig. 24-5)
- Stool, possibly diarrheal in nature, with blood (Starr et al., 2012, p. 761).

Diagnosis

Diagnosis of intussusception is based on a history of the characteristic symptoms and the physical findings during examination. The presence of a "sausage-shaped" mass in the upper right quadrant (Dance's sign) during palpation of the abdomen is indicative of intussusception (Starr et al., 2012). Although the upper right quadrant is the most common site, the mass may be felt in other abdominal areas too. The abdomen is distended and tender on palpation, and bowel sounds may be either increased or decreased.

 Diagnostic Tools Intussusception

A flat-plate x-ray film of the child can appear normal early in the course of the disorder. However, an abdominal ultrasound confirms the diagnosis in the majority of cases (Bishop, 2011).

Prevention

Though this condition may not be prevented, good prenatal care provides an opportunity to promote optimal fetal development in utero.

Collaborative Care

Nursing Care. When the child has been diagnosed with intussusception, the nurse can provide information about the condition and reassurance to the parents. The nurse is responsible for monitoring the infant for signs of perforation, peritonitis (inflammation of the abdominal cavity), or shock in addition to evidence of increased pain. The nurse also monitors and records the child's stools. The spontaneous passing of a stool may indicate a resolution of the obstruction. Postoperative care is similar to that of the child surgery for pyloric stenosis.

 focus on safety

Signs of perforation and peritonitis

The child with perforation has acute pain, beginning over the perforated area and spreading over the abdomen. The abdomen may become rigid, and the child may experience nausea and vomiting, tachycardia, fevers, chills, sweats, confusion, and decreased urinary output (Venes, 2013). There is moderate or mild abdominal pain that worsens with movement. Fever, change in bowel habits, and malaise are also common. In addition, the child has nausea, loss of appetite, and fever or hypothermia. During the nursing assessment, the nurse notes that the abdomen is distended with decreased bowel sounds (Venes, 2013).

Medical Care. A barium or air enema is used to both diagnose and treat intussusception. In radiological reduction, the barium (contrast media) or air allows visualization of the telescoped bowel. The pressure applied by the enema may cause the telescoped bowel to return to its normal position, thus relieving the obstruction. Reduction rates are reported as high as 65% to 90% through the instillation of barium or air. If the treatment is managed through radiological reduction, the child is observed for passage of stool and barium or contrast material as indicated. The nurse monitors the child's vital signs and ongoing assessment of her overall condition. If radiological reduction is ineffective or if peritonitis, perforation, or shock is evident, prompt surgical correction is required (Sundaram et al., 2011).

Surgical Care. If the child is having surgery, preparation before surgery includes placing the child NPO, inserting a nasogastric tube, and initiating IV fluid therapy. The surgical procedure either repairs the bowel or removes any portion that has been permanently damaged.

Education/Discharge Instructions

Discharge instructions include care of the incision and observation for signs of infection. Parents can be taught about feeding, dehydration, and appropriate pain management strategies.

MALROTATION AND VOLVULUS

Abnormal rotation of the intestine around the superior mesenteric artery during fetal development may lead to malrotation of the intestine. Malrotation may be present in utero, appear during early infancy, or later on in childhood. Malrotation is the most serious type of intestinal obstruction because it may lead to intestinal necrosis, peritonitis, perforation, and death related to a complete twisting of the intestine around itself, or volvulus. The incidence of malrotation is approximately 1 in 500 live births.

Signs and Symptoms

Symptoms of malrotation or volvulus may occur at any age but are most common in the first month of life.

- A major symptom is intermittent bilious or green vomit

- Additional symptoms include abdominal distention, recurrent abdominal pain, lower GI bleeding, a palpable epigastric mass, dehydration, lethargy, and shock.
- The child's stools may be bloody, which suggests ischemia and possibly gangrene of the bowel.

focus on safety

Bowel infarction

Without surgical correction, ischemia can lead to infarction of the bowel, which is demonstrated by painful abdominal distension and shock. Older children show recurrent abdominal pain, intermittent vomiting, chronic diarrhea, and symptoms related to failure to thrive or **malabsorption** (inadequate absorption of nutrients from the intestinal tract) (Venes, 2013).

focus on safety

Shock

Signs of shock include tachycardia; tachypnea; hypotension; and cool, clammy, or cyanotic skin (Venes, 2013).

Diagnosis

Diagnosis is based on history, physical examination, and radiographic studies such as barium enema and upper GI series, which is the definitive procedure to diagnose the condition. This abnormal condition has a characteristic corkscrew, coiled, or bird's beak appearance.

Prevention

Though this condition may not be prevented, good prenatal care provides an opportunity to promote optimal fetal development in utero.

Collaborative Care

Nursing Care. Preoperative nursing care includes IV hydration to restore fluid and electrolyte balance, nasogastric suction, and administration of IV antibiotics.

Surgical Care. Timely repair of this condition is indicated to prevent potential complications. Surgical treatment for malrotation and volvulus includes resection of nonviable intestinal segments with anastomosis (surgical connection). Short bowel syndrome is a potential postoperative complication because extensive portions of the bowel are either reconstructed or removed. Postoperative care is comparable to that of an infant or child undergoing abdominal surgery.

Education/Discharge Instructions

Postoperative care and discharge instructions are similar to that of the child surgery for pyloric stenosis.

Nursing Care Plan   A Child Who Has Undergone Abdominal Surgery

Nursing Diagnosis: Imbalanced Nutrition: Less than body requirements related to inability to ingest nutrients by mouth

Measurable Short-Term Goal: The child will receive adequate fluid intake.

Measurable Long-Term Goal: The child will obtain adequate nutrients to meet metabolic needs and for optimal healing.

NOC Outcomes:
Nutritional Status (1004) Extent to which nutrients are ingested and absorbed to meet metabolic needs

NIC Interventions:
Nutrition Therapy (1120)
Diet Staging (1020)

Nursing Interventions:

1. Maintain NPO status as ordered by health-care provider.

   RATIONALE: To promote bowel rest and healing after the surgical procedure.

2. Auscultate for presence of bowel sounds every 4 hours for 24 hours and then every shift thereafter.

   RATIONALE: Adequate bowel motility is required before the reintroduction of oral fluids and foods.

3. Assist mother with pumping and storing breast milk if appropriate.

   RATIONALE: Pumping helps to maintain milk production. Breast milk contains maternal antibodies, which may aid gastrointestinal healing.

4. Maintain IV access and administer fluids and medications as prescribed. Monitor intake and output.

   RATIONALE: To provide short-term fluid, electrolyte, and caloric support (specify actions of medications) and maintain fluid balance.

5. Collaborate with the care provider to slowly reintroduce oral clear liquids and progress to small, frequent feedings as tolerated. (For infants, progress from glucose, water, or oral rehydration solution to half-strength formula or breast milk).

   RATIONALE: To determine tolerance of oral fluids and foods by introducing in small amounts.

Now Can You—Identify obstructive gastrointestinal disorders?

1. Identify obstructive GI disorders?
2. Identify signs and symptoms of obstructive GI disorders?
3. Identify nursing care for obstructive GI disorders?

Inflammatory Disorders

PEPTIC ULCER DISEASE

Peptic ulcer disease (PUD) refers to a variety of upper gastrointestinal tract disorders that result from gastric acid–related injury and cause inflammation and subsequent ulceration (Bishop, 2011). Duodenal ulcers are more common than gastric ulcers in children (Sundaram et al., 2011).

 Nursing Insight—*Gastric ulcer*

The most common cause of gastric ulcer is infection with the gram-negative organism *Helicobacter pylori* with an estimated 50% of the world population infected with this organism (Bishop, 2011; Uc & Pandrangi, 2010). Risk factors for acquiring *H pylori* include low socioeconomic status and poor sanitation. Transmission of *H pylori* is person-to-person or by contaminated water (Starr et al., 2012).

Secondary ulcers are more likely to be peptic in origin and may occur as a result of factors such as stress, medication, or underlying conditions. Risk factors for PUD in children include:
- *Helicobacter pylori* infection
- Drugs
  - Nonsteroidal anti-inflammatory drugs (NSAIDs)
  - Bisphosphonates
  - Potassium supplements
- Family history
- Stress
- Sepsis
- Head trauma
- Hypotension

(Bishop, 2011; Sundaram et al., 2011)

Signs and Symptoms

Children with PUD may present with a wide range of symptoms or the patient may be asymptomatic:

- Abdominal pain (epigastric, worsening after meals)
- Dyspepsia
- Nausea and vomiting
- Excessive belching, hiccupping, and regurgitation
- Nocturnal awakening
- Anorexia
- Poor feeding
- Weight loss
- Hematemesis
- Melena
- Iron deficiency anemia

Diagnosis

Upper GI endoscopy is considered the most accurate and definitive test for diagnosis of PUD. Upper GI barium radiography may further indicate the presence of ulcerated depression (Sundaram et al., 2011). Additional diagnostic studies may include laboratory studies to identify anemia, fluid and electrolyte deficiencies, dehydration, and sepsis. Specific testing for *H pylori* is controversial and is only done if there is endoscopic evidence of ulceration or suggested organic disease (Starr et al., 2012). Tests specific for the identification of *H pylori* include (1) a histological exam and culture of biopsies obtained from endoscopy, (2) urea breath test (sensitive in children older than 2 years, (3) serum IgG antibody titer for *H pylori*, and (4) measurement of *H pylori* antigens in stool specimens (Sundaram et al., 2011).

Prevention

The most common cause of PUD, *H pylori,* is associated with poor sanitation, contaminated water, and person-to-person contact. Appropriate prevention is directed at teaching proper hand washing and avoidance of potential sources of contaminated water. Child and parent health promotion and maintenance education is directed at instructing family members in strategies to avoid stress and instructing them on the complications related to the use of caffeine and NSAIDs.

Collaborative Care

Nursing Care. Nursing care for children with PUD centers on stabilization of the child, decreasing the gastric acid, and determining the cause of the inflammation that results in the ulceration. The child may be discharged when the condition stabilizes and oral feeding is tolerated.

Medical Care. PUD is treated with antibiotics (in the presence of *H pylori*), histamine agonists, and/or proton pump-inhibitors, which may be administered IV if bleeding is present. A nasogastric tube is placed for decompression of the stomach in the presence of severe gastric or esophageal hemorrhage. Antacids are generally unacceptable for use in children because of the volume needed to suppress and neutralize gastric acid. Histamine agonists and proton pump-inhibitors usually produce a response in 4 to 8 weeks (Sundaram et al., 2011).

Education/Discharge Instructions

Child and parent education needs to stress the importance of compliance with medication and dietary management, which includes avoiding certain foods identified by the child or family such as caffeinated soda, fatty foods, chocolate, and spicy foods. Avoiding eating late night snacks also helps. Bland diets have not been proven to promote healing. In addition, stress reduction is necessary to successfully treat PUD in children. Discharge instructions also include teaching the child and family about the

Labs: Urea Breath Test

The urea breath test requires the child to swallow a tablet or drink a solution containing urea, which is composed of nitrogen and carbon. The carbon dioxide exhaled is then measured and indicates the presence of *H pylori* in the stomach. Urease, which breaks down into ammonia and carbon dioxide, is an enzyme produced by *H pylori* (Uc & Pandrangi, 2010).

importance of avoiding substances that cause pain such as NSAIDs.

INFLAMMATORY BOWEL DISEASE

Inflammatory bowel disease (IBD) is a general term often used to refer to two major forms of chronic intestinal inflammatory conditions, Crohn's disease and ulcerative colitis, which have common epidemiology and clinical features. Both Crohn's disease and ulcerative colitis are characterized by extraintestinal and systemic features, yet they are distinct disorders as described in the following sections.

Crohn's Disease

Crohn's disease is a chronic inflammatory disease characterized by periods of exacerbations and remissions. Crohn's disease can affect any portion of the gastrointestinal (GI) tract. The bowel may present with a combination of non-sequential areas of pathology and disease-free sections of bowel. Crohn's disease rarely affects the oropharynx, esophagus, and stomach; the small bowel is affected 25% to 30% of the time; the colon and anus are affected 25% of the time; the ileocolonic region is affected up to 40% of the time; and diffuse disease occurs 5% of the time (Starr et al., 2012). Crohn's disease is characterized by skipped lesions or areas of inflammation anywhere in the upper or lower GI tract. Because of these "skip" areas, the appearance is often described as cobblestone (Starr et al., 2012). Affected areas are described as containing varying degrees of edema, erythema, ulceration, friability, and thickening of the bowel wall and mesentery. Common features of Crohn's disease include abscess formation, fistulas, and perianal disease (Cronin, 2011). The majority of Crohn's disease occurs in the terminal ileum, with resultant potential nutritional deficiencies (Starr et al., 2012).

The occurrence of Crohn's disease is 400 out of 100,000 and has increased during the past few decades. It is more common in Caucasians and affects males and females equally. The age at onset is between 10 and 20 years, and the condition occurs throughout the life span with peaks in the second, fourth, and sixth decades of life. Twenty-five percent to 40% of cases are diagnosed in childhood and adolescence, and the incidence in siblings is higher than that of the general population. Although the cause of Crohn's disease is unknown, it is thought that the susceptibility to Crohn's is most likely inherited and involves a genetically determined response that is immunologically mediated (Starr et al., 2012).

Signs and Symptoms

Children with Crohn's disease may have an acute or insidious onset.

- Abdominal pain
- Diarrhea
- Blood and mucus in the stool
- Urgency and **tenesmus**
- Sensation of incomplete emptying after defecation
- Anorexia
- Weight loss

Clinical presentation of Crohn's disease varies extensively depending on the area of the intestine that is involved and the severity of the inflammation (Bishop, 2011). If the disease is limited to the colon, symptoms are similar to those of ulcerative colitis. Upper GI tract involvement is manifested by vomiting and epigastric pain. Small bowel involvement is manifested by the following signs and symptoms:

- Cramp-like pain commonly located in the right lower quadrant
- Lower right quadrant tenderness and a feeling of fullness
- Postprandial pain
- Anemia
- Lethargy
- Perianal abnormalities, such as skin tags and fistulas
- Partial or complete bowel obstruction (Bishop, 2011)

Extraintestinal signs and symptoms may include, but are not limited to, the following:

- Fever
- Growth delay
- Delayed sexual development
- **Arthralgias** (joint pain)
- Arthritis in the large joints
- Stomatitis (inflammation of the mouth, lips, tongue, and mucous membranes)
- Aphthous ulcers
- **Uveitis** (inflammation of the eye)
- Conjunctivitis
- Renal stones
- **Erythema nodosum** (a tender, red, nodular rash on the shins) (Starr et al., 2012; Venes, 2013).

Diagnosis

Diagnosis is based on client history, physical findings, and laboratory results. Laboratory findings may include leukocytosis, microcytic anemia, low serum iron and total iron-binding capacity, low serum albumin, thrombocytosis, and elevated sedimentation rates and C-reactive protein. An upper GI series with small bowel follow-through or computed tomography (CT) scan is used to determine small bowel involvement. Endoscopy and colonoscopy are the most useful diagnostic methods and may demonstrate segmented lesions with thickened circular folds and a cobblestone appearance of the bowel wall with longitudinal ulcers and transverse fissures as well as a narrowed lumen, fistulas, and the string sign (Bishop, 2011; Cronin, 2011; Sundaram et al., 2011). Cross-sectional imaging and information about bowel wall thickening can be provided by CT scan; the extent of lumen disease can be provided by magnetic resonance imaging (MRI) (Cronin, 2011). Radiography is not considered diagnostic, though it can highlight areas of inflammation, narrowing, obstruction, and dilation (Cronin, 2011).

Prevention

Though the cause of Crohn's disease is unknown, it is thought that the disease is most likely inherited. Preventive activities are directed toward physical, social, and psychological health maintenance activities, which promote growth and development through proper nutrition, sleep/rest, physical activity, stress reduction, medication compliance, and lifestyle.

Collaborative Care

Nursing Care. Nursing care includes the administration of medication and nutritional management, emotional support, and community referral (Starr et al., 2012). The focus of care during periods of remission involves monitoring compliance. As symptoms resolve, the child may resist taking medications. The adolescent with Crohn's disease presents unique challenges in the treatment of her disease. Adolescents have a natural desire to be "normal" and to be like their peers. This may lead the adolescent to resist taking prescribed medications that cause obvious side effects, such as those experienced with prolonged use of steroids.

Medical Care. The goals of treatment include controlling the disease, including remission, preventing relapses, and maintaining normal nutrition, growth, and lifestyle (Starr et al., 2012). In children, the treatment for Crohn's is pharmacological, nutritional, surgical, and psychosocial (Starr et al., 2012). The choice of treatment depends on location and severity of the disease as well as complications. Several categories of pharmacological agents are used to treat Crohn's disease. Initially the focus is on reducing inflammation. Drugs known as 5-aminosalicylic acid, or 5-ASA are the most commonly used and include sulfasalazine (Azulfidine), balsalazide (Colazide and Colazal), or mesalamine (Asacol, Lialda, and Pentasa) products (Cronin, 2011; Sundaram et al., 2011).

Corticosteroids are effective for reduction of inflammation in moderate to severe disease and may be given orally, rectally, or IV for acute exacerbations. Metronidazole (Flagyl) and ciprofloxacin (Cipro) have demonstrated effectiveness in the treatment of perianal complications. Antibiotics such as ampicillin (Marcillin), gentamicin (Garamycin), clindamycin (Cleocin), and metronidazole (Flagyl) are effective during acute exacerbations (Starr et al., 2012).

Immunosuppressive medications are useful with corticosteroid-resistant disease (Starr et al., 2012). Immunomodulators, which change the way the immune system responds to inflammation, are also used to treat Crohn's disease. Immunomodulators are known as thiopurines or immunosuppressants. Immunosuppressants decrease the activity of the immune system. Immunosuppressants used to treat Crohn's disease may include azathioprine (Imuran and Azasan), 6-mercaptopurine (6MP and Purinethol), tacrolimus (Prograf), and methotrexate (MTX, Rheumatrex, and Mexate) (Cronin, 2011).

For children with Crohn's disease that does not respond to other treatments, a biological drug, infliximab (Remicade), is often prescribed (Sundaram et al., 2011). Infliximab is an antibody that attaches itself to the inflammation-promoting protein, tumor-necrosis factor-alpha (TNF-alpha). Other biologicals include an anti-TNF medication, which is used to treat other immune system disorders such as rheumatoid arthritis. Certolizumab (Cimzia) is another anti-TNF blocker approved recently for Crohn's disease.

Additional treatment may include (1) antibiotics, such as ampicillin, sulfonamides, cephalosporins, tetracycline, and metronidazole; (2) antidiarrheal agents; and (3) fluid replacement and nutritional supplements. Hospitalization, total parenteral nutrition, and gastric decompression may be required during severe episodes of the disease.

Surgical Care. Surgery for a child with Crohn's disease may be indicated if the child does not respond to medical treatment or in the case of bowel strictures, obstruction, perforation, toxic megacolon, intractable bleeding, or diarrhea. Surgical correction involves removal or resection of the diseased segment with resection or anastomosis (connection). The nurse communicates to the family that surgical repair does not cure Crohn's disease but removes an effected portion of the bowel (Cronin, 2011; Sundaram et al., 2011).

Education/Discharge Instructions

Teach the child and family about nutritional management, which may include the following:

- Frequent, small meals
- High-protein and high-carbohydrate diet
- Vitamin and iron supplement in the presence of lactose intolerance
- Restriction of irritating and poorly absorbed foods, such as fried food and carbonated drinks
- During inflammatory periods, decrease foods that stimulate peristalsis, such as high-fiber food because they promote water retention
- Nutritional supplements may be needed to maintain nutrition and normal growth

Provide child and family education regarding the disease process and medication management. Psychosocial referral may be necessary to assist the child and family in coping with the disease. The child and family may face issues related to school absences and tardiness, need for special bathroom privileges at school, and issues related to self-esteem because of small stature caused by steroid use, or the presence of an ostomy (Dunn, 2012).

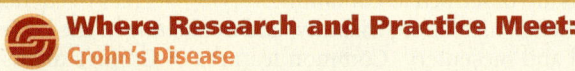

Where Research and Practice Meet: Crohn's Disease

Research exploring the use of an enteric-coated fish oil preparation in adults with Crohn's disease found that those who received the fish-oil preparation were less likely to have relapses than patients who received placebos. Fish oil has been found to not only have anti-inflammatory actions but also to increase the absorption of nutrients resulting in improved nutrition (Blosser, 2012; Wiese, Lashner, Lerner, DeMichele, & Seidner, 2011).

Medication: Steroid Side Effects

Cardiovascular: Edema, hypertension, congestive heart failure
Central nervous system: Vertigo, seizures, psychoses, headache
Dermatological: Acne, skin atrophy, impaired wound healing, petechiae, bruising
Endocrine and metabolic: Cushing's syndrome, growth suppression, glucose intolerance, and sodium and water retention
Gastrointestinal: Peptic ulcer, nausea, vomiting
Genitourinary: Menstrual irregularities
Neuromuscular and skeletal: Muscle weakness, osteoporosis, fractures
Ocular: Cataracts, elevated intraocular pressure, glaucoma

Source: Data from Vallerand, A. H., & Sanoski, C. (2014). *Davis's drug guide for nurses* (14th ed.). Philadelphia, PA: F.A. Davis.

Across Care Settings: Promoting growth

Nutritional therapy may be helpful in correcting malnutrition and promoting growth (Dunn, 2012; Sundaram et al., 2011). A well-balanced, high-protein diet is recommended for children whose symptoms do not prohibit oral intake. Fiber-containing foods, such as seeds, popcorn, and corn, may produce symptoms and obstructions in children with intestinal stricture though there is no evidence that avoiding specific foods influences severity of the disease in most children (Sundaram et al., 2011). A dietitian teaches the family how to provide for adequate nutrition to promote growth. High-calorie liquid supplements may be recommended as well as supplemental vitamins, especially the fat-soluble vitamins, and minerals.

Emotional support is another important nursing intervention for both the child and family in the management of this chronic condition. The nurse can communicate to the family that the child with Crohn's disease may experience depression, anxiety, and low self-esteem. Early detection of psychological problems requires referral, which often involves both the child and family.

⚙ Nursing Diagnoses The Child With Crohn's Disease

- Imbalanced Nutrition: Less than Body Requirements related to inability to ingest and absorb food and nutrients
- Risk for Fluid Volume Deficit related to excessive losses through diarrhea
- Pain related to inflammation and irritation of the bowel
- Potential for Delayed Growth and Development related to effects of physical illness and inability to maintain nutritional needs
- Anxiety related to threat to self-concept from change in health status

Ulcerative Colitis

Ulcerative colitis is an acute or chronic inflammation of the colon, which is characterized by recurring bloody diarrhea (Starr et al., 2012). Unlike Crohn's disease, ulcerative colitis involves a continuous segment of the colon and usually involves the epithelial lining of the bowel. The pathology of ulcerative colitis is described as a superficial, acute inflammation of mucosa with microscopic crypt abscess (Bishop, 2011).

The cause of ulcerative colitis is unknown. The probability of a genetically determined and an altered immunologically mediated response to the intestinal mucosa is likely (Starr et al., 2012). Infectious agents, autoimmune responses, and environmental factors play a role though no specific responsible agents have been identified (Bishop, 2011; Starr et al., 2012).

The incidence of ulcerative colitis is increasing, especially in industrialized countries, though it is relatively uncommon in tropical and underdeveloped countries (Starr et al., 2012). Ulcerative colitis is more common in the Jewish population. In addition, there is a higher risk in families who have a close relative with ulcerative colitis (Bishop, 2011). The overall incidence of ulcerative colitis in the United States is 10 to 20 cases per 100,000 (Starr et al., 2012). The peak onset occurs between ages 15 and 25, with approximately 20% of the cases occurring in children and adolescents younger than 20 years (Starr et al., 2012).

Signs and Symptoms

- Abdominal pain
- Bloody diarrhea
- Bowel elimination urgency
- Tenesmus (a painful spasmodic contraction of the anal sphincter leading to the sensation of constantly needing to empty the bowel)
- Left lower quadrant pain with cramping
- Pain that increases before defecation and passing flatus (Starr et al., 2012)
- Weight loss
- Delays in growth and sexual maturation

Other manifestations, though not present in all cases, may include the following:

- Arthritis/arthralgias of the large joints
- Oral ulcers
- **Primary sclerosing cholangitis** (chronic liver inflammation leading to scarring of hepatic ducts)
- Uveitis
- Skin lesions such as those found in pyoderma gangrenosum (a rare, ulcerating skin disease) and erythema nodosum (a tender, red, nodular rash) (Bishop, 2011; Starr et al., 2012).

Diagnosis

Diagnosis of ulcerative colitis in a child is based on history and physical findings. Radiological and endoscopic examinations are used to evaluate the characteristics and location of the lesions.

Prevention

As with Crohn's disease, the cause of ulcerative colitis is unknown. It is thought that the disease is most likely inherited. Preventive activities are directed toward physical, social, and psychological health maintenance activities, which promote growth and development through proper nutrition, sleep and rest, physical activity, stress reduction, medication compliance, and lifestyle.

Collaborative Care

Nursing Care. Similar to Crohn's disease, nursing care includes medication and nutritional management, emotional support, and community referrals (Starr et al., 2012). These can be found through the Crohn's & Colitis Foundation of America (www.ccfa.org) and other related organizations. There are also support mechanisms via Facebook and Twitter. However, social media safety must be stressed. In addition, a referral is made to an ophthalmologist to rule out ophthalmological manifestations of the disease. Psychosocial therapy may be indicated because depressive disorders are common (Starr et al., 2012).

Medical Care. Goals of the treatment of ulcerative colitis include disease control, inducing remission, preventing relapse, and achieving normal growth and lifestyle (Starr et al., 2012). Pharmacological, nutritional, surgical, and psychosocial management may be included in the plan of care. IV or oral steroids are used for moderate to severe ulcerative colitis, with dosages tapered when the child is in remission.

Immunomodulatory agents such as vitamins, minerals, and natural foods as well as azathioprine (Imuran) or 6-mercaptopurine (Purinethol) are used to wean the patient off of steroids (Bishop, 2011). Aminosalicylates relieve symptoms and inflammation in the intestines and help IBD go into remission (Bishop, 2011). Iron supplementation is given to correct anemia, and antispasmodics may be given before meals (Starr et al., 2012).

⚙ Labs: Laboratory Findings for Ulcerative Colitis

Laboratory findings for ulcerative colitis may include elevated sedimentation rate, microcytic anemia, and elevated white blood cell count with left shift, antineutrophil cytoplasmic antibodies present in 66% (Bishop, 2011).

Surgical Care. Ulcerative colitis is curable surgically with a total mucosal proctocolectomy with the ileal pouch–anal anastomosis as the most common restorative surgery. Failed medical therapy and persistent hemorrhage are the most common indications for surgical correction.

Education/Discharge Instructions

The nurse can communicate to the family that nutritional recommendations include use of a diet high in protein and carbohydrates with normal fat and decreased roughage. Vitamin and iron supplements are recommended.

 Now Can You—Distinguish between Crohn's disease and ulcerative colitis?

1. Discuss the differences between Crohn's disease and ulcerative colitis?
2. Discuss nursing care for Crohn's disease and ulcerative colitis?

FAILURE TO THRIVE

Failure to thrive (FTT) is not a diagnosis but a description of a condition that usually occurs in infancy and is characterized by failure of the infant to meet age-appropriate weight gain (Starr et al., 2012). It is known that FTT infants do not obtain or are unable to take in enough nutrition to adequately meet standard growth and weight expectations. Failure to thrive may be one of the earliest signs of several gastrointestinal disorders, such as ulcerative colitis; complications related to a gastrointestinal disorder, such as inflammatory bowel disease; or associated with disorders characterized by structural obstruction, such as pyloric stenosis. Additional major causes of FTT related to gastrointestinal disorders include gastroesophageal reflux, Crohn's disease, lactose intolerance, Hirschsprung's disease, hepatitis, pancreatic insufficiency, irritable bowel disease, and malabsorption diseases and milk intolerance. Starr et al. (2012) have identified the following criteria that may be used to define FTT:

- Weight less than 80% of median weight for length
- Weight for length less than 80% of ideal weight
- Weight for length less than the 10th percentile
- Body mass index for chronological age less than 5th percentile
- Weight for chronological age and sex less than 5th percentile or more than 2 standard deviations below the mean
- Length for chronological age and sex less than 5th percentile
- Weight deceleration crossing more than two major percentile lines on age- and population-appropriate growth chart
- Height, head circumference, and developmental skills may be affected
  (Starr et al., 2012, p. 773)

Three basic causes of FTT are inadequate caloric intake, inadequate caloric absorption, and excessive caloric expenditure (Starr et al., 2012). Certain situations from a psychosocial perspective are also related to the development of FTT. Families in vulnerable situations (e.g., poverty, young and/or single parent, and mentally ill or substance-abusing parents) or those in which child abuse or neglect exist are at risk for FTT. More than 80% of the cases are caused by nutritional deficiency without an underlying medical condition (Krebs, Primak, & Haemer, 2011; Stevens, Gentry, & Michener, 2008). Prevalence rates in the United States are estimated to be between 5% and 10% (Starr et al., 2012).

Signs and Symptoms

Assessment of the signs and symptoms of failure to thrive is accomplished by tracking the growth rate of the infant or child to determine if an actual lack of adequate progression exists. Physical examination and evaluation of the child's developmental status is also important because lack of sufficient nutrition on an ongoing basis will affect the child's cognitive and emotional development. Beyond that, it is important to develop an understanding of the underlying cause(s).

Historically, health-care providers distinguished FTT according to organic (medical conditions or illnesses that would affect the child's ability to take in or use nutrition) versus nonorganic (related to abuse, neglect, or attachment difficulties) classifications. In recent years, however, these distinctions have been less useful because many children with FTT exhibit symptoms of both causes (Krebs et al., 2011). A comprehensive approach toward the evaluation of FTT includes a thorough prenatal, birth, medical, social, developmental, and nutritional history; physical examination; and limited laboratory evaluation. Key signs and symptoms impact multiple body systems and include but are not limited to the following (Starr et al., 2012):

- Diarrhea, constipation, and vomiting
- Evidence of recurring infection
- Abdominal distention
- Loss of subcutaneous fat
- General wasting (with inflammatory disease, HIV, and cerebral palsy)
- Signs of dehydration
- Evidence of abuse or neglect
- Scaling skin (with zinc deficiency)
- Edema (with protein deficiency)
- Alopecia
- Spoon-shaped nails (with iron deficiency or GI disease)
- Labial fissures (with vitamin deficiency)
- Respiratory compromise (with cystic fibrosis and bronchopulmonary dysplasia)
- Lymphadenopathy, hepatosplenomegaly, masses, and distention (with inborn errors of metabolism and immunodeficiency)
- Inability to be comforted
- Preference or lack of preference for close, personal interaction or touch

Diagnosis

In addition to a thorough history, physical examination and nursing assessment diagnostic studies are included as well as a feeding history and a developmental assessment. Laboratory studies generally provide a low yield for diagnosing FTT in the absence of findings pointing toward an organic cause. Screening laboratories may include a chemistry panel, complete blood count, and iron panel.

Nursing Insight—*Failure to thrive*

During a nursing assessment the nurse can discern:
- How does the caretaker interact with the child?
- Are there signs of abuse or neglect?
- Does the caretaker understand appropriate feeding amounts and routines?
- Does the caretaker mistakenly believe that a healthy adult diet (e.g., lower fat) is also healthy for an infant?

Prevention

Primary prevention and health promotion activities include good pre- and postnatal care and education, which include instructing the new parents on what to expect and how to promote growth and development in the child, proper feeding and burping the child, informing the parents of the availability of community resources such as the Women, Infant and Children (WIC) program, and instructing the parents of the importance of their own personal self-care.

Collaborative Care

Nursing Care. A comprehensive history and physical examination are vital in identifying the source of the problem and developing a plan of care. The goal of care is on restoring and providing nutritional management, which may involve an interdisciplinary care team. In some cases of FTT, a specialized intervention by developmental pediatric or mental health-care providers is required. Nurses identify these cases and provide education regarding feeding practices and the importance of support for families. The nurse can also provide support and reassurance to new mothers who are struggling with FTT infants and young children. While nursing care must address the physiological needs of the child, it must also encompass the emotional needs. If the nurse suspects neglect or abuse, steps must be taken to notify the appropriate child protection agency.

 Nursing Diagnoses Failure to Thrive

- Imbalanced Nutrition: Less than body requirements related to inability to ingest or digest food or absorb nutrients because of biological or psychological factors
- Delayed Growth and Development related to inadequate caretaking, environmental and stimulation deficiencies, or physical/psychosocial conditions
- Risk for Impaired Parenting related to unmet social and emotional needs of parental caregivers, ineffective role modeling, insufficient knowledge or crisis

Education/Discharge Instructions

Nurses can provide education related to feeding practices and instructing the parents about the availability of community resources that may assist in providing emotional and social support as well as access to basic resources, such as food and clothing.

 Nursing Care Plan Imbalanced Nutrition

Nursing Diagnosis: Imbalanced Nutrition: Less Than Body Requirements related to inadequate nutrient intake

Measurable Short-Term Goal: Child will ingest adequate nutrients.

Measurable Long-Term Goal: Child will demonstrate appropriate growth for age on normal curve.

NOC Outcomes:
   Appetite (1014) Desire to eat when ill or receiving treatment
   Nutritional Status: Food and Fluid Intake (1008) Amount of food and fluid taken into the body over a 24-hour period

NIC Interventions:
   Nutritional Monitoring (1160)
   Nutrition Therapy (1120)
   Nutrition Management (1100)

Nursing Interventions:

1. Monitor weight daily on same scale and at same time during hospitalization and at every encounter in community-based care.

   RATIONALE: Assists in early identification and correction of nutritional deficiencies to prevent complications from malnutrition.

2. Provide favorite high-protein, high-calorie, nutritious foods and drinks in small frequent meals (specify for child).

   RATIONALE: Child is more likely to eat familiar foods, and small frequent meals may be better tolerated during illness.

3. Ensure that mealtime is pleasant and uninterrupted. Schedule treatment and procedures at times other than feeding time. Do not mix medications in food offered during mealtimes.

   RATIONALE: Child may refuse to eat essential foods if they have been associated with unpleasant activities, smells, or tastes.

4. Encourage additional nutritious, high-calorie snacks as tolerated by child (e.g., milkshakes and string cheese).

   RATIONALE: Supplemental nutrition may provide the additional calories and nutrients via the preferred oral route.

5. Initiate oro- or nasogastric nutrient supplementation as determined by the health-care provider.

   RATIONALE: The ill child may be unable to ingest adequate calories and nutrients orally.

APPENDICITIS

Appendicitis is an inflammation of the appendix, which is a small sac-like structure at the end of the cecum. Appendicitis is considered the most common condition requiring abdominal surgery in childhood (Bishop, 2011). In appendicitis the lumen of the appendix becomes obstructed with fecal matter, lymphoid tissue, tumor, parasite, foreign body, or inspissated (thickened) cystic fibrosis secretions, which cause the appendix to become distended and subject to ischemia and necrosis (Starr et al., 2012). The characteristic symptoms are caused by the inflammation around the infected appendix with approximately "a 36- to 72-hour maximum window from the onset of pain to the rupture of the gangrenous appendix" (Starr et al., 2012, p. 758). Rupture of the appendix usually occurs within 48 hours of onset of the symptoms (Bishop, 2011).

The incidence of appendicitis increases with age, with the average age of occurrence at between 6 and 10 years of age (Starr et al., 2012). The incidence is slightly higher in boys than in girls and more common in Caucasians (Starr et al., 2012). The risk of perforation is twice as likely for children younger than 5 years of age. Perforation occurs in approximately one-third of children before treatment is initiated (Starr et al., 2012).

Signs and Symptoms

The most reliable diagnosis of appendicitis is gained through an evaluation of the sequencing of the symptoms (Starr et al., 2012).

- One of the earliest symptoms is periumbilical pain (pain around the umbilicus). This pain often awakens the child peaking at 4-hour intervals. The periumbilical pain subsides and then is followed by the classic sign of right lower quadrant pain.

  Additional symptoms include:

- Vomiting generally follows periumbilical pain, unlike the vomiting associated with gastroenteritis, which precedes the pain
- Anorexia
- Stools described as low in volume and mucus-like, diarrhea is atypical
- Constipation
- High fever may be associated with perforation; otherwise the child may be afebrile or have a low fever

 focus on safety

Appendicitis

Perforation is suspected when abdominal pain is suddenly relieved without intervention. In that case the physician is notified immediately (Starr et al., 2012). The child needs immediate attention and transport to a nearby health-care facility.

Diagnosis

The child diagnosed with appendicitis experiences a progression of symptoms with no single test providing overall confirmation of the diagnosis. Laboratory findings may demonstrate an elevated white blood cell count. An elevated white blood cell count does not distinguish simple appendicitis from perforated appendicitis. Children with appendicitis may also have a normal white blood cell count. An abdominal radiograph may reveal fecal matter, or some other obstruction, although this rarely confirms the diagnosis. If there is uncertainty in young children, ultrasound and CT scan may help differentiate abdominal pain from other causes though the usefulness is variable (Bishop, 2011; Sundaram et al., 2011).

 Nursing Insight—*Appendicitis physical examination*

Symptom	Physical Signs
Rebound tenderness (Fig. 24-6)	Presence of involuntary guarding, rebound tenderness with pain over McBurney's point, which is located 1.5–2 inches in from the right anterior superior iliac crest on a line toward the umbilicus—best elicited on palpation.
Heel-drop jarring test	Stands on toes for 15 seconds, then drops on heels—inability to stand straight or climb stairs; winces when getting off examination table.
Psoas sign	Abdominal pain with right hip flexion against resistance
Obturator sign	Pain on passive internal rotation of the flexed right thigh
Rovsing's sign	Deep pressure in lower left abdominal quadrant elicits pain with a sudden release (Starr et al., 2012).

Prevention

Appendicitis is a surgical condition that cannot be prevented.

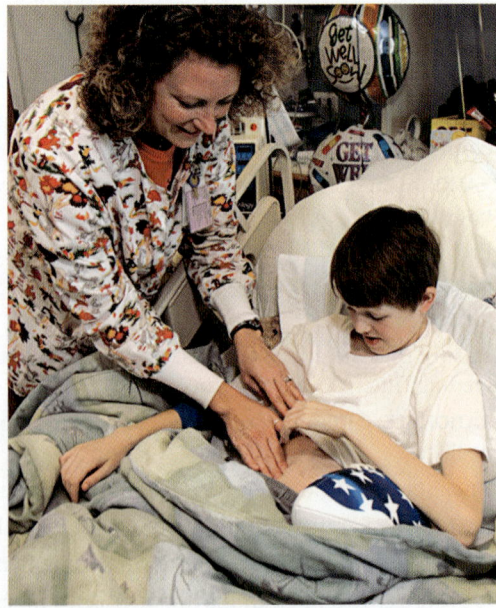

Figure 24-6 Appendicitis physical examination reveals rebound tenderness.

Collaborative Care

Nursing Care. Nursing care of the child with appendicitis who has undergone an appendectomy includes monitoring intake and output, wound care, and pain control. The child will be NPO for 24 hours or until peristalsis returns. Most children are discharged to home in 2 to 3 days. If the procedure is performed by laparoscope (abdominal exploration with an endoscope) (Venes, 2013), the child may remain in the hospital overnight or be discharged the day of surgery. If perforation occurred, drains may protrude from the incision or the wound and remain open to prevent infection and allow healing. In the case of a perforated appendix, IV antibiotics are given for 7 to 14 days. The child generally remains NPO with a nasogastric tube in place until bowel function returns.

Surgical Care. Treatment for children who have appendicitis is surgical, and an appendectomy is curative if performed before perforation. If perforation occurs, a course of postoperative antibiotics is needed (Bishop, 2011). The potential for the complication of postoperative infection can be prevented by instructing the parents to keep the wound clean and dry.

 ### Cultural Diversity: Empacho

Empacho is a Spanish word for indigestion, stomach pains, and cramps. A common belief in the Hispanic culture is that the symptoms are caused by a ball of undigested food on the stomach wall and often because of being forced to eat more than is needed and desired (Spector, 2012). The presence of the food ball causes vomiting, pain, diarrhea, and cramping. Treatment includes massaging and pinching the spine (Spector, 2012).

Education/Discharge Instructions

Discharge instructions include informing the parents on wound care and the importance of keeping the surgical site clean and dry and monitoring the site for signs of infection. The parents are instructed on pain management and the progression of activity over a 2-week period and the resumption of normal nutritional intake as directed by the health-care provider and as tolerated.

OMPHALITIS

Omphalitis is an infection of the umbilical stump. This occurs once the umbilicus is colonized with streptococci, staphylococci, or gram-negative organisms, which may cause a local infection (Thilo & Rosenberg, 2011).

Signs and Symptoms

- Redness and edema of the soft tissue around the umbilical stump
- Foul-smelling drainage

Diagnosis

Local and systemic cultures are obtained to confirm diagnosis (Thilo & Rosenberg, 2011).

Prevention

Prevention through good perinatal care and parent education about keeping the umbilical stump clean and dry is paramount to preventing the occurrence of omphalitis.

Collaborative Care

Nursing Care. Nursing care of omphalitis is aimed at prevention and education of the parent. The potential for infection can be minimized by keeping the cord clean and dry. Several methods may be used to provide cord care, which include use of an antimicrobial agent such as bacitracin (Baciguent) or use of triple dye (contains gentian violet, proflavine hemisulfate, and brilliant green) to paint the umbilical stump. Other experts suggest swabbing the umbilical stump with alcohol; cleansing it with soap and water; cleansing it with sterile water, a neutral pH cleanser, or povidone-iodine; or natural healing with no treatment.

Medical Care. IV broad-spectrum antibiotics, such as nafcillin (Unipen), vancomycin (Vancocin), or third-generation cephalosporins (Cefotaxime), are used to treat omphalitis (Thilo & Rosenberg, 2011).

Education/Discharge Instructions

Before discharge, the parent or caregiver needs to be instructed on the recommended method of cord care and the importance of placing the diaper below the level of the cord to avoid irritation. Parents are also instructed regarding the expected process for stump deterioration and symptoms of infection that is reported to the health-care provider. Cord separation generally takes place in 10 to 14 days.

MECKEL'S DIVERTICULUM

Meckel's diverticulum arises from a remnant of fetal development in the midgut, which normally is obliterated by the seventh to eighth week of gestation. Failure of this destructive process results in an omphalomesenteric problem (referring to the umbilicus and mesentery fistula or fibrous band) (Venes, 2013). The fibrous band, known as Meckel's diverticulum, connects the small intestine to the umbilicus. A Meckel's diverticulum averages 1 to 10 cm in length and is the most common congenital malformation of the GI tract. It occurs in 2% of the population and is usually present before 2 years of age. Meckel's diverticulum is twice as common in males as females (Hanna, 2011). Males are also three times more likely to experience complications than females (Sundaram et al., 2011). Hanna (2011) describes features of Meckel's diverticulum using a rule of 2's, that is, "2% of the population, located within 2 ft (60–100 cm) of the ileocecal valve, usually 2 in. (5 cm) long, and most (well over 50%) present before age 2 years" (Hanna, 2011, p. 75).

Signs and Symptoms

Symptoms of Meckel's diverticulum are recognized in childhood, with 65% in children younger than 5 years of age and the peak at 2 years of age. Manifestations include the following:

- Abdominal pain described as periumbilical or lower abdominal and similar to appendicitis or volvulus
- Pain may be vague and recurrent
- Painless rectal bleeding (more often found in the older child)
- Stools described as bright or dark red with mucus or of a "currant jelly" appearance
- Rectal bleeding accompanied by pain in infants
- Severe anemia and shock can occur in undiagnosed disease

Diagnosis

Diagnosis in the child is based on history, physical examination, and radiography, specifically a nuclear medicine scan. A radionuclide scintigraphy or Meckel scan detects the presence of gastric mucosa and has an overall diagnostic accuracy of 90%. A radionuclide or Meckel scan is an imaging study that uses injection and detection of radioactive isotopes to create images of body parts (Bishop, 2011). A Meckel scan is more effective in the identification of diverticulum, which may be difficult to visualize with plain films, CT, or barium studies. Abdominal radiographs and barium enema are not useful for diagnosis. The child is also screened for anemia.

Prevention

Though this condition may not be prevented, good prenatal care provides an opportunity to promote optimal fetal development in utero.

Collaborative Care

Nursing Care. Nursing care is similar to that of any child undergoing surgery as well as monitoring for shock, blood loss, and providing rest. Preoperative antibiotics may be ordered if diverticulitis (inflammation of the diverticulum [Venes, 2013]) has occurred. If obstruction has occurred, fluid and electrolyte imbalances are corrected before surgery. Postoperative care includes fluid replacement and gastric decompression and evacuation via nasogastric tube.

Surgical Care. Treatment for symptomatic Meckel's diverticulum involves surgical removal of the diverticulum or pouch to prevent hypovolemic shock from hemorrhage (Sundaram et al., 2011). Surgical repair is more common in children younger than 2 years of age, which accounts for 50% of those requiring surgery. Refer to the nursing care plan: A Child Who Has Undergone Abdominal Surgery. The potential for postoperative infection can be prevented by instructing the parents to keep the wound clean and dry and to change wet or soiled diapers as soon as possible for children who are not toilet trained.

Education/Discharge Instructions

Discharge instructions include teaching the parents about wound care and the importance of keeping the surgical site clean and dry as well as monitoring the site for signs of infection. The parents are instructed on pain management and the progression of activity over a 2-week period and the resumption of normal nutritional intake as directed by the health-care provider and as tolerated.

PANCREATITIS

Pancreatitis is an inflammation of the pancreas, particularly in the parenchyma. **Parenchyma** refers to the functional tissue of an organ as opposed to its supporting structure (Venes, 2013). Pancreatitis may be acute or chronic. Acute pancreatitis is considered reversible in contrast to chronic pancreatitis, which causes irreversible changes to the function and structure of the pancreas (Bai, Lowe, & Husain, 2011). Premature activation of digestive enzymes within the pancreas can lead to injury and subsequent pancreatitis (Bai et al., 2011). Triggers for pancreatitis in children differ from those of adults and in most cases are idiopathic. In children, common causes include drugs, hypertriglyceridemia, biliary microlithiasis, trauma, or viral infection. Less common causes include collagen vascular disorders and parasitic infestations (Bishop, 2011). A **microlith** is a tiny stone or calculus that is also associated with pancreatitis (Venes, 2013).

Chronic pancreatitis involves irreversible changes in the structure and function of the pancreas caused by recurrent or persistent attacks of pancreatitis and more common in hereditary pancreatitis and cystic fibrosis (Bai et al., 2011; Bishop, 2011). Reoccurring attacks of pancreatitis leads to scarring of the small and large pancreatic ducts, stone formation, duct stasis, and inflammation.

Signs and Symptoms

Clinical signs and symptoms of pancreatitis are nonspecific and vary with age:

- Abdominal pain (be sure to assess frequency of the pain) (Bai et al., 2011)
  - Epigastric location: steady, ache-like, and worse in recumbent position
  - Back pain
  - Radiation of pain to the back
  - Diffuse pain
  - Guarding pain
- Nausea and vomiting (the most common presenting symptom in children under 3 (Lowe, 2010)
- Abdominal distention
- **Grey Turner sign:** a discoloration or bruising and induration of skin on flank (Lowe, 2010)
- **Cullen's sign:** bluish discoloration of periumbilical region caused by a hemorrhage (Lowe, 2010)
- Low-grade fever
- Hunched-over or knee-to-chest position (Petersen-Smith & McKenzie, 2009)
- Dehydration or shock
- Jaundice
- Symptoms of diabetes mellitus and malabsorption—may develop late in the course of chronic pancreatitis (Lowe, 2010)

Diagnosis

Baseline laboratory studies include serum amylase and lipase levels as well as complete blood count, C-reactive protein, and phosphorus levels. Elevated serum amylase or lipase levels, which occur as a result of pancreatic injury, support the diagnosis of pancreatitis. As pancreatitis progresses, lipase levels remain elevated longer than amylase levels, making lipase a better choice for diagnostic testing. Amylase and lipase are measured at least daily along with a complete blood count, C-reactive protein, and phosphorus level. In addition, infants and toddlers are more likely to be diagnosed through serum lipase levels because they demonstrate fewer signs and symptoms (Park, Latif, Ahmad, Bultron, Orabi, Bhandari, et al., 2010).

Imaging studies are important for the diagnosis of pancreatitis because enzyme levels are not 100% sensitive or specific (Bai et al., 2011). Ultrasound is the diagnostic study of choice because it allows for the detection of edema, which is present in most cases. Ultrasound is preferred over a CT scan because it can detect gallstones as a cause of pancreatitis. CT is generally not recommended to evaluate initial presentation unless diagnosis is unclear. There are no current guidelines recommending the use of MRI (Bai et al, 2011).

Prevention

Prevention of pancreatitis includes maintaining a well-balanced, low-fat diet, controlling triglycerides, and educating the child and parents on the impact of drug and alcohol abuse on the pancreas.

Collaborative Care

Nursing Care. Nursing care for pancreatitis is supportive and includes management of fluid balance, nutritional support, and pain control. The child is placed on bowel rest (NPO) when pancreatitis is suspected. A nasogastric tube (NG) is placed to maintain stomach decompression. Vomiting necessitates the use of IV fluid replacement. Pre- and postoperative nursing care would be consistent with that provided for general abdominal surgery.

Medical Care. Some controversy exists regarding the use of opioid analgesics for pain relief, which is said to potentially cause spasms of the **sphincter of Oddi** (Bishop, 2011; Lowe, 2010). The sphincter of Oddi is located at the opening of the common bile duct into the duodenum (Venes, 2013). Lowe (2010) notes the use of morphine increases pressure on the sphincter and subsequently leads to further inflammation of the pancreas. This action is common to all narcotics, which are often recommended for the treatment of pain with pancreatitis. A broad-spectrum antibiotic may be considered if the child is febrile and has evidence of extensive pancreatic necrosis.

Surgical Care. Surgical management, though rare, may be indicated in patients whose pancreatitis is caused by severe abdominal trauma or major ductal abnormalities.

Education/Discharge Instructions

Chronic pancreatitis is rare in children. Care involves educating the patient and family about signs and symptoms that indicate a recurrence and complications.

GALLBLADDER DISEASE

Though gallbladder disease, or cholelithiasis, is relatively uncommon in childhood, gallstones may develop at any age and in utero. Cholelithiasis is the presence of stones in the gallbladder and is often associated with hyperlipidemia, obesity, pregnancy, use of birth control pills, infection, bile stasis, congenital anomalies, use of TPN, and family history (Punia, Garg, Bisht, Dalal, & Mohan, 2010). Children with cystic fibrosis, hemolytic disease, Crohn's disease, and Wilson's disease are at greater risk for gallstone formation. The chemical irritation that causes obstructed flow of bile from the gallbladder to the cystic ducts is called cholecystitis and is often associated with gallstones. Pancreatitis is the most common complication of gallstone disease in children (Sokol & Narkewicz, (2011).

Signs and Symptoms

- Right upper quadrant pain, often radiating substernally or to the right shoulder
- Pain episodes often occur after eating
- Pain episodes more common after ingestion of fatty or greasy foods
- Pain may be diurnal but is usually worse at night
- Sudden onset of severe, sharp right upper quadrant pain and localized tenderness is associated with biliary obstruction (Starr et al., 2012)
- Nausea and vomiting
- Jaundice
- Fever (with cholecystitis)
- Pear-shaped palpable mass in the right upper quadrant

Diagnosis

Common diagnostic and laboratory studies are generally normal unless calculi have lodged in the extrahepatic biliary system (Sokol & Narkewicz, 2011). The following are commonly ordered when evaluating for gallbladder disease.

- Liver function tests, bilirubin and C-reactive protein—may be elevated in the presence of ductal stones
- Amylase and Lipase—may be elevated if pancreatitis is also present
- CBC—may demonstrate leukocytosis when cholecystitis is present
- Plain abdominal x-ray—may reveal radiopaque stones
- Ultrasound—is the best imagining technique and will show stones, sludge, and anatomic alterations, such as dilation of the duct system
- CT Scan—provides information similar to that of the ultrasound though involves radiation

Prevention

Prevention of cholelithiasis includes maintaining a well-balanced, low-fat diet, controlling hyperlipidemia, weight control, and educating the child and parents on the impact of birth control pills on the gallbladder.

Collaborative Care

Nursing Care. Nursing care of the child admitted with symptomatic cholecystitis is supportive and includes management of fluid balance, nutritional support, and pain control. The child is placed on NPO status, and gastric decompression via NG tube is initiated. IV antibiotics may be ordered if fever is present.

Surgical Care. When cholelithiasis causes symptomatic cholecystitis, surgical removal of the gallbladder is necessary. Laparoscopic cholecystectomy is the treatment of choice for symptomatic cholelithiasis (Emami, Garrett, Anselmo, &

 Where Research and Practice Meet:
Controversy on the Use of Nutritional Support

The literature also reflects controversy on the use of nutritional support. According to Lowe (2010) "starvation has long been considered part of standard care in patients with acute pancreatitis" (p. 436). Recent research suggests that length of stay is reduced and clinical outcomes improve when feeding is started early (Bai et al. 2011; Lowe, 2010; Park et al., 2010). Though limited data are available on children, studies indicate that oral feeding is well tolerated in adults with mild acute pancreatitis and that feeding can be initiated early in the course of treatment (Bai et al., 2011; Lowe, 2010; Park et al., 2010). Low-fat diets are most often recommended. Nutritional support in cases of severe acute pancreatitis is provided via nasogastric and nasojejunal feedings, though studies suggest that oral feedings early in the course of treatment provide benefits with fewer complications than parenteral nutrition (Lowe, 2010). Total parenteral nutrition (TPN) is usually not recommended though may be used when enteral feeds are not well tolerated (Bai et al., 2011). Formula composition remains an institutional choice.

Nguyen, 2010; Sokol & Narkewicz, 2011). Use of lithotripsy or use of shock waves to break up the stones has not been approved for use in children (Sokol & Narkewicz, 2011). Postoperative care for the child undergoing a laparoscopic cholecystectomy is routine and brief because the length of stay is generally 1.6 days (Emami et al. 2010). Traditional GI postoperative nursing care measures are employed.

Education/Discharge Instructions

Discharge instructions include informing the parents on wound care and the importance of keeping the surgical site clean and dry as well as monitoring the site for signs of infection. The parents are instructed on pain management and the progression of activity over a 2-week period and the resumption of normal nutritional intake as directed by the health-care provider and as tolerated.

 ### Cultural Diversity: Genetic Predisposition for the Development of Gallstones

Native American Indians (especially Pima Indians) and persons of Hispanic origin have a genetic predisposition for the development of gallstones (Sokol & Narkewicz, 2011). Native Americans have the highest rates of gallstones in the United States. Mexican American men and women of all ages also have high rates of gallstones. Obesity and higher cholesterol levels are factors.

Functional Gastrointestinal Conditions

Characteristics of disorders described as functional include the presence of clusters of symptoms related to dysfunction in the gastrointestinal (GI) tract or in the "processing of information originating from the GI tract" (Yacob & DiLorenzo, 2009, p. 254). This definition stresses the importance of viewing functional disorders using a biopsychosocial model emphasizing not only physiological symptoms but also sociocultural and psychosocial influences (Yacob & DiLorenzo, 2009).

IRRITABLE BOWEL SYNDROME

Irritable bowel syndrome (IBS) is a common cause of recurrent abdominal pain in children. IBS affects males and females equally, with diagnosis usually during school age and adolescence. IBS is characterized by chronic pain and changes in bowel habits and affects the large intestine. Symptoms are linked to visceral hypersensitivity and altered motility (Ebach, 2011). The cause of IBS is thought to involve a combination of factors, including motor, autonomic, and psychological functions. A diagnosis of IBS is generally made by ruling out organic causes for the symptoms, such as other inflammatory diseases, lactose intolerance, and parasitic infections.

IBS is sometimes referred to as "nervous stomach" or spastic colon. IBS is classified as a functional GI disorder because the symptoms occur when the intestines, or bowels, function improperly. When the intestines are exposed to certain "triggers," they respond with muscle spasms instead of normal peristalsis. These muscle spasms result in one or more of the symptoms of IBS. Triggers that can cause the

symptoms of IBS to "flare" include eating large amounts of food at one time; eating spicy, high-fat, or gas-causing foods; or stress. Most children with IBS have various symptoms including variable stool patterns, alternating between constipation and diarrhea.

Signs and Symptoms

Children with IBS have abdominal pain beginning with a change in stool frequency or consistency (Bishop, 2011). IBS does not cause constant symptoms, and exacerbations can occur at any time. Other symptoms include flatus, bloating, constipation, diarrhea, or a combination of both constipation and diarrhea. Children with frequent bouts of IBS or those who suffer several symptoms simultaneously may experience headache, nausea, anorexia, and weight loss.

 Assessment Tool Irritable Bowel Syndrome

The Rome Criteria III provides a criteria guideline that is commonly used by physicians to diagnose IBS (Yacob & DiLorenzo, 2009). Using the Rome Criteria III, symptoms "include all the following occurring at least once per week for at least 2 months before diagnosis" (Starr et al., 2012, p. 764).
- Abdominal discomfort or pain "associated with two or more of the following at least 25% of the time" (Starr et al., 2012, p. 764)
  - Improved with defecation
  - Onset associated with a change in frequency of the stool
  - Onset associated with a change in form of the stool
- No evidence of inflammatory, anatomical, metabolic, or neoplastic disorder that would explain symptoms

  Additional symptoms of IBS may include:

- Pain described as dull or cramping
- Tenesmus
- Fever
- Weight loss
- Abnormal stool frequency (i.e., four or more per day or two or fewer per week)
- Abnormal stool form (i.e., lumpy and hard, loose and watery, or alternating between diarrhea and constipation)
- Straining, urgency, or feeling of incomplete bowel emptying
- Bloating or feeling distended
- Dyspepsia
- **Hematochezia** (stools containing red blood rather than tarry stool)
  (Venes, 2013)
  (Bishop, 2011; Starr et al., 2012)

Diagnosis

Since there is no specific test or procedure to diagnose IBS, the diagnosis is based on clinical signs and symptoms, history, and physical assessment. The history includes finding a family pattern of IBS and discovering the triggering events or psychosocial factors. A diagnosis of IBS is also made by ruling out other GI disorders (Andresen, Keller, Pehl, Schemann, Preiss, & Layer, 2011). Recommended laboratory studies to verify the diagnosis and rule out other conditions include CBC, erythrocyte sedimentation rate (ESR), c. reactive protein, urinalysis and optional serum electrolytes, thyroid-stimulating hormone, blood glucose/ HbA1c, and renal and liver function studies.

Prevention

Prevention and control of the symptoms of irritable bowel syndrome include maintaining a well-balanced, low-fat diet; avoiding caffeine, fatty and gas-causing foods, and cruciferous vegetables; and avoiding large meals.

Collaborative Care

Nursing Care. Nursing care of the child admitted with symptomatic irritable bowel syndrome is supportive and includes management of fluid balance, nutritional support, and pain control.

Medical Care. The goal of management is to modify the symptoms and identify strategies for dealing with factors that trigger the symptoms (Starr et al., 2012). Treatment for IBS may include a combination of pharmacological and nonpharmacological therapies (Sherman, 2010). Identifying foods that trigger symptoms is most important. Triggers may include caffeine, fatty food, large meals, gas-producing foods, lactose, and cruciferous vegetables (Starr et al., 2012). Food diaries are very useful in helping determine what foods must be avoided. In addition, eating more fiber and less fatty foods seems to help prevent intestinal muscle spasms. Having the child drink plenty of liquids, including water, can promote regular stool elimination patterns. Healthy toilet training and toileting patterns can control some symptoms. Promoting a healthy routine for regular bowel elimination can decrease the symptoms and the stress related to worry about bowel movements at school or at other inconvenient times. Encouraging the child to adapt positive strategies for managing stress can prevent exacerbations.

 Collaboration in Caring—*Care of the child*

Children need a balance of school, physical activity, socialization, and other age-appropriate activities. Children need to be taught to share feelings, concerns, and other typical growth and development issues with a parent or other interested caring adult. Though rarely used, amitriptyline (Elavil) or selective serotonin reuptake inhibitors for symptoms of depression may be prescribed in difficult or persistent cases (Sherman, 2010; Starr et al., 2012). Through collaboration in caring, children can receive the care they need.

If constipation becomes a chronic problem, stool softeners may be indicated for short-term use. Antispasmodics such as hyoscyamine (Levsin), atropine (Atropine-Care), scopolamine (Isopto), and phenobarbital (Donnatal), and propantheline bromide (Pro-Banthine) may be used in severe cases. Probiotics and/or peppermint oil may provide some relief from bloating and flatulence (Starr et al., 2012; Summer, Hommel, & Todd, 2011).

 focus on safety

Irritable bowel syndrome

Symptoms of IBS accompanied by fever, severe abdominal pain, and/or vomiting blood require immediate attention. Surgical evaluation and/or intervention may be necessary.

Education/Discharge Instructions

Family support and education are the primary goals in nursing care (Summers et al., 2011). The nurse can assist the parent and child in developing strategies that will decrease symptoms. Nutritional strategies include eating more slowly, avoiding carbonated drinks, and including fiber in the diet. The child also needs support and assistance in developing strategies to reduce environmental stressors.

❝What to say❞—*Irritable bowel syndrome*

The nurse communicates to the family that stress can trigger the symptoms of IBS in many children. When family circumstances present stressful situations, parents may need help in dealing with situations that can exacerbate the symptoms of IBS. Family counseling may be an option. At home, parents and children can be taught to keep a diary of stressful events and foods so they can determine the triggers that cause "flares" of IBS. Teachers must also be aware of the condition and may need to be involved in helping the child reduce or cope with the stress related to school. The school counselor can be a good resource for the child.

INFANTILE COLIC

The cause of infantile colic is unknown. Several factors have been implicated in the development of colic, including both physical and psychological factors such as allergy, cow's milk intolerance, over- or underfeeding, inadequate burping, cigarette smoke, maternal anxiety, and familial stress (Starr et al., 2012). A stressful pregnancy and birth experience have also been suggested as potential underlying factors in the development of colic. Organic causes account for less than 5% of colic (Gahagan, 2011). On average, infants cry 2 to 3 hours per day; the infant with colic cries more than 3 hours per day (Starr et al., 2012).

Signs and Symptoms

Colic is described as persistent, unexplained crying or fussing in infants younger than 3 months of age (Starr et al., 2012). In addition, the infant has:

- Episodes that usually occur at the same time each day
- Episodes that often occur during the late afternoon or evening
- Pulling-up both legs and arms into a flexed position
- Frequent demand of feeding though fussy while feeding
- Excessive gas
- Difficulty in being consoled

Diagnosis

In the past, the "rule of threes" has often been used to diagnose colic and was based on a report of the symptoms occurring for more than 3 weeks during which the crying episodes occurred for more than 3 days of the week with crying for more than 3 hours a day. This definition is helpful in the diagnosis but has been found to be limited in that is does not define what is meant by crying and the necessity of waiting until 3 weeks to diagnosis (Gahagan, 2011). The incidence of colic is estimated to be about one-third of all infants (Starr et al., 2012).

Prevention

Prevention and control of the symptoms of colic include educating the new parents on techniques for feeding and burping the infant and avoiding cigarette smoke in the child's environment. Parents also need educational guidance on maintaining their own physical and psychosocial needs and reducing stress.

Collaborative Care

Nursing Care. Nursing care of the child admitted with symptomatic colic is supportive and includes management of fluid balance, nutritional support, and comfort needs.

Medical Care. Management of colic begins with ruling out acute conditions that cause abdominal pain. The goal of treatment for infantile colic is to manage the situation until the symptoms resolve because no cure exists (Box 24-1). Though anticholinergics, barbiturates, motility enhancing agents, and antiflatulents have been prescribed, practitioners generally avoid using these drugs because of their limited success and the lack of scientific data to support their effectiveness (Goldson & Reynolds, 2011).

Education/Discharge Instructions

An important key to management of colic is parent education. Parents need to be educated about the developmental characteristics of crying, factors that may trigger colic, and techniques for soothing the infant. Calming techniques may include sucking, soothing vocalizations, swaddling, rocking, reduced environmental stimulation, promotion of regularity, and car rides. Parents also need their efforts reassured as well as informed that the baby is in good health.

Cultural Diversity: Mexico and Eastern Europe

Chamomile, vervain, licorice, fennel, anise, peppermint, gingerroot, dill, caraway seeds, and mint, which have antispasmodic properties, are found in herbal teas and are used as remedies for colic in Mexico, Eastern Europe, and other cultures (Gahagan, 2011).

Where Research and Practice Meet: Probiotics

Research suggests the immature infant immune system may struggle with bacterial imbalances in the GI tract, which may benefit from the use of probiotics (Blosser, 2012; Savino, Cordisco, Tarasco, Locatelli, Biola, Oggero, et al., 2011). Probiotics improve motility and reduce gas and cramping. Several studies have suggested the use of acupuncture for infantile colic though results were not conclusive (Landgren, Kvorning, & Hallstrom, 2011; Skjeie, Skonnord, Fetveit, & Brekke, 2011).

Box 24-1 Management Strategies for Infantile Colic

The following are nursing strategies for an infant with infantile colic:

- Support parents.
- Assure parents that the child is in good health.
- Reinforce parents' efforts to comfort the child.
- Instruct parents on strategies to calm infant, such as swaddling, decreasing environmental stimulation, and rocking.
- Assess feeding techniques and instruct as needed.
- Provide an opportunity for parents to express frustrations.

Source: Starr, N. B., Blosser, C. G., Brady, M. A., Burns, C. E., Dunn, A. M., & Petersen-Smith, A. M. (2012). Gastrointestinal disorders. In C. E. Burns, A. M. Dunn, M. A. Brady, N. B. Starr, & C. G. Blosser (Eds.), *Pediatric primary care* (5th ed., pp. 739–788). St. Louis, MO: Elsevier.

ACUTE DIARRHEA

Though the term gastroenteritis has been used to describe diarrhea in the past, the term is now considered by many health-care providers to be a misnomer because the cause of diarrhea does not involve the stomach (Starr et al., 2012). Acute diarrhea is defined as excessive loss of fluid and electrolytes in the stool with the disruption occurring in the intestinal tract. Stool loss is considered excessive when it is more than 10 g/kg per day in children less than 2 years of age; stooling is described as occurring four or more times in 24 hours in children older than 2 years (Starr et al., 2012). Acute diarrhea with or without vomiting has multiple causes, which may include infections in or outside the intestinal tract, diet, medications, or toxic substances and can be classified by etiology or physiological mechanism, which includes secretory or osmotic (Bishop, 2011).

Osmotic diarrhea occurs as a result of malabsorption or maldigestion in which water is pulled into the bowel. This type of diarrhea is caused by noninfectious conditions such as lactose deficiency, overfeeding, malabsorption syndromes, and excess ingestion of hypertonic juices (those with high levels of carbohydrates), such as some sports drinks, fruit juices, and soda (Bishop, 2011).

Secretory diarrhea occurs when there is an increase in the active secretion of fluid or electrolytes into the stool. The most common cause of this type of diarrhea is bacterial, chemical reaction, or inflammation such as occurs in inflammatory bowel disease (Bishop, 2011). One of the most common side effects of antibiotic use is antibiotic-associated diarrhea (Barakat, El-Kady, Mostafa, Ibrahim, & Ghazaly, 2011).

Infectious agents associated with diarrhea include bacteria (*Campylobacter jejuni, Clostridium difficile, Yersinia enterocolitica, Salmonella, Shigella,* and enterohemorrhagic *Escherichia coli*) and viruses (human rotavirus and adenovirus) (Starr et al., 2012) (Table 24-1).

Nursing Insight—*Acute diarrhea*

Approximately 500,000 office visits and 55,000 hospitalizations in the United States occur annually in children for acute diarrhea. Infectious diarrhea is a leading cause of death for children worldwide (Tablang & Katz, 2012). Acute diarrhea causes 10% of preventable deaths in the United States, including 300 deaths annually in children between the ages of 1 and 4 (Starr et al., 2012). The literature suggests that the cause of morbidity and mortality from this illness is related to poverty and poor access to care.

Signs and Symptoms

- Increased frequency and fluid content of the stools with or without associated symptoms
- Parents are asked about the presence of other signs and symptoms, such as vomiting, fever, and pain with special attention to the number of wet diapers within the previous 24-hour period
- Signs of systemic illness may also be evident

The nurse also explores the history, which includes:

- Food allergies
- Recent travel, especially to a foreign country or residing in an area with untreated water

Table 24-1   Rotavirus

Rotavirus	Incidence	Protecting Children	Dehydration Secondary to Gastroenteritis
Viral gastroenteritis causes approximately 80% of all cases of diarrhea in children younger than 1 year with rotavirus, accounting for 50% of the cases of acute diarrhea in children.	The incidence for rotavirus does not vary between industrialized and developing countries, nor has incidence been shown to decrease with increased sanitation in developing nations.	Surviving an episode of rotaviral gastroenteritis confers partial immunity.	Rotaviral gastroenteritis is a self-limiting disease.
Rotavirus is the most common cause of diarrhea illness among children worldwide and accounts for approximately one-third of hospitalizations of children in industrialized countries.	The incubation period for rotavirus is approximately 1–3 days. This is followed by a 3- to 8-day period of fever, vomiting, diarrhea, and abdominal pain.	Subsequent cases are possible but tend to be milder and less life-threatening.	Deaths from rotavirus are caused by dehydration.
It is estimated that by 5 years of age, nearly every child will have had at least one episode of rotavirus-induced illness.	The disease is self-limiting. However, the vomiting and diarrhea in rotavirus may be severe enough to require intervention to prevent dehydration.	In 1998, a rotavirus vaccine was introduced called RotaShield. The vaccine was shown to be 100% effective in prevention of rotavirus infection but was quickly withdrawn after it was demonstrated that the vaccine was associated with a slightly higher risk of intussusception in infants.	Because most children with a diarrhea-type illness are cared for in the home, it is critical that the nurse educate the families on early signs of dehydration requiring medical treatment.
Epidemiological studies conservatively estimate that rotavirus-caused gastroenteritis is responsible for 352,000–592,000 deaths annually in children younger than 5 years, with 82% of these deaths occurring in the poorest of countries.	A primary factor in survival of rotaviral-induced gastroenteritis is access to adequate medical care.	The recommended 2007 immunization schedule for 0–6 years of age now currently includes a recommendation for a three-dose series of rotavirus vaccine (Rota).	Specific indicators of dehydration in infants include: • Decreased number wet diapers • Sunken fontanelle and eyes • Listlessness • Cool, pale skin
The primary transmission of this virus is via the fecal–oral route; however, the virus is very hearty and stable on surfaces for long periods of time, increasing the risk for transmission through contaminated surfaces or food.	Worldwide, children have limited access to rehydration therapy.	The first dose is recommended to be administered between 6 and 12 weeks of age, with the initial dose not to be started later than age 12 weeks (Goldman, 2012).	Families are given specific instructions regarding oral intake goals during treatment for rotavirus and instructed to return for follow-up if a child is unable to meet the goals or the appearance of any of the above symptoms of dehydration.
In addition, the virus has been found in the respiratory tract of infected individuals, raising concern for transmission via infectious secretions.	Most often, therapy primarily consists of oral rehydration. In the case of rotavirus, vomiting may limit the usefulness of oral rehydration and in the absence of access to IV hydration, death occurs secondary to fluid and electrolyte imbalances.		

- Dietary consumption, with special attention to the consumption of poorly cooked food, poultry, shellfish, unpasteurized or under-pasteurized milk or juice, home canned food, fresh produce, and raw or under-cooked eggs
- Day-care attendance
- Family members with similar symptoms
- Medications
- **Pica**
- Recent changes in weight or growth patterns
- Response to rehydration

Diagnosis

A thorough history that includes recent travel, day-care or school illness contacts, family members with similar illnesses, ingestion of medications and toxic substances, and a dietary history is included in an interview to determine diagnosis. In addition, information regarding the number of stools, frequency, and quality is elicited and includes when the symptoms began.

The physical examination focuses attention to the abdomen and perineum in addition to state of alertness, changes in the growth pattern, and the hydration status of the child. Laboratory tests are selected based on the suspected etiology and the overall health and appearance of the child. No blood tests may be indicated for an essentially well-appearing child. For a child demonstrating symptoms of toxicity, stool for culture and sensitivity (C&S), serum electrolytes, and a complete blood count (CBC) with differential are suggested. Diarrhea with weight loss suggests the need for serum electrolytes and CBC with differential. Evidence of blood in the stool with or without a history of antibiotic use suggests a need to assess stool for C&S, CBC with differential, and serum electrolytes.

Prevention

Prevention of acute diarrhea includes proper hand washing, food handling, and care of soiled diapers and clothing. In addition, some episodes of acute diarrhea can be avoided by avoiding overfeeding the child and use of excess juice in the diet.

Collaborative Care

Nursing Care. Care of the child hospitalized for acute diarrhea includes monitoring fluid intake and output, observing for signs of dehydration (see Chapter 31), offering fluids as indicated, and monitoring IV infusions if ordered. The skin integrity of the perineal and buttock areas must be monitored for irritation related to frequent stooling, and good perineal skin care must be provided.

Medical Care. Most incidences of acute diarrhea are self-limiting. Management of viral and most bacterial causes is primarily supportive. Treatment of acute diarrhea is determined by extent of the illness and the cause, with attention to hydration and dietary needs as appropriate and with prevention as a priority (Starr et al., 2012). Initially the priority is to restore and maintain hydration. Oral rehydration is generally attempted before IV hydration is initiated and is again related to the acuity of the illness and its effect on the child. A recent trend in rehydration of the child who is not experiencing vomiting is to allow the child to drink what she desires, which may include formula or milk, although other authors may consider this controversial. Traditional treatment of children with mild to moderate dehydration (less than 10%) includes oral rehydration for 24 hours (Ebach, 2011). The rehydrating solutions generally recommended include low amounts of glucose and electrolytes. Fruit juices, soda, sports drinks, and powered drinks are generally not recommended by those employing traditional treatments. Returning to full-strength formula is recommended as quickly as possible. Breastfed infants are allowed to nurse even during the time they are receiving rehydration treatment and may be fed more frequently for shorter periods of time. A regular diet may be provided once the child is rehydrated and can tolerate food.

Solid food is generally started within the first 24 to 48 hours and starts with bland, soft foods. Care needs to be taken to avoid foods with a high fat content and simple sugars. Foods generally well tolerated include vegetables, fruits, yogurt, complex carbohydrates, and lean meat.

Depending on the cause of the diarrhea, pharmacological treatment in general is not ordered for young children. Although antidiarrheals are generally not recommended, they may be used with caution in older children if the diarrhea persists beyond the initial infection. Metronidazole (Flagyl) is considered a first-line therapy for treatment of *C difficile* colitis (Ebach, 2011; Studer, 2011). The use of *Lactobacillus* (gram-positive, anaerobic, non–spore-forming bacilli) has been found to shorten the duration of the illness if used early in the process (Hitzeman, & Romo, 2011; Starr et al., 2012; Studer, 2011).

IV fluids are essential with "impaired circulation and possible shock; weight less than (8.8 to 11 lb) 4 to 5 kg or a child younger than 3 months; intractable diarrhea, lethargy, anatomic anomalies; failure to gain weight or continued weight loss despite oral fluids" (Starr et al., 2012, p. 781).

 Complementary Care: *Diarrhea*

Products containing *Lactobacillus acidophilus*, such as yogurt, can be used to decrease the incidence of rotavirus diarrhea in infants 5 to 24 months of age (Blosser, 2012). *Lactobacillus* is a nonpathogenic bacterium that produces lactic acid from carbohydrates and is normally found in dairy products and in the feces of infants fed by bottle. The addition of *L acidophilus* to the diet changes the bacterial flora of the GI tract, hence treating the overgrowth of pathogenic or diarrhea-causing organisms in the GI tract.

Education/Discharge Instructions

Education on preventive measures is essential. The child and parents need to be instructed on good hand hygiene. The nurse must reinforce proper hand washing to include not only that which follows toileting or diaper changes but also before and after eating and in the preparation of foods. In addition, appropriate care of soiled clothing and diapers is essential.

Across Care Settings: Schools, day care, and community

The most effective treatment for gastroenteritis for children in schools, day care, and community is prevention through good hand washing. Hand washing with water and soap in sufficient amounts to cover all surfaces of the hands and fingers with 15 seconds of rubbing that causes friction is to be done when hands are visibly soiled, after using the restroom or diaper change, before eating, and after caring for children with any type of secretions. Single-use towels are used to dry the hands and turn off the faucet to avoid recontamination.

CHRONIC DIARRHEA

Chronic diarrhea is defined as three or more stools passed per day for 14 days or longer, though healthy infants may pass 5 to 8 stools per day (Ebach, 2011; Starr et al., 2012). Chronic diarrhea is usually associated with a chronic condition, such as inflammatory bowel disease; malabsorption syndromes; overfeeding; formula protein intolerance; lactose intolerance; food allergies; viral, bacterial, or parasitic agents; radiation therapy; or immunodeficiencies (Sundaram et al., 2011). Inadequate management of acute diarrhea can also lead to chronic diarrhea. Chronic nonspecific diarrhea, or toddler's diarrhea, is the most common cause of chronic loose stools in childhood. The child with toddler's diarrhea generally has a normal growth and weight gain. The cause of toddler's diarrhea may be from excessive intake of sweetened drinks or fruit juices or a diet low in fat or high in non-digestible carbohydrates (Ebach, 2011).

Signs and Symptoms

Chronic diarrhea has clinical manifestations that reflect the underlying pathology. The nurse obtains information about the history of the diarrhea, including frequency and appearance. Information regarding weight loss, medications, and presence of associated symptoms is determined. Special consideration needs to be taken to determine the dietary history with special attention to the amount of fruit juice ingested per day. The parents also are asked whether the child has had stool incontinence and what treatments have been attempted at home in addition to recent travel and school exposure.

- Abdominal distention or tenderness
- Hyperactive bowel sounds

- Signs of weight loss
- Dehydration
- Perineal irritation
- Presence of undigested food particles in the stools
- Blood in the stool

Diagnosis

Diagnostic assessment may include stool for C&S, ova and parasites, fecal pH, occult blood, fat stain, and Clinitest for reducing substances (Procedure 24-1). Sweat chloride and lactose tolerance tests may be ordered to rule out cystic fibrosis or lactose intolerance. In addition, a CBC with differential, ESR, serum electrolytes, albumin level, liver function, and a urinalysis with culture are used as nonspecific indicators of illness. If laxative abuse is suspected, a stool laxative screen may be ordered (Juckett & Trivedi, 2011).

Prevention

Prevention of chronic diarrhea is similar to that of acute diarrhea and includes proper hand washing, food handling,

---

Procedure 24-1 Collecting Stool for Culture and Sensitivity and Ova and Parasites

Purpose

Collecting stool for culture and sensitivity and ova and parasites is used to detect the presence of bacterial overgrowth, to confirm bacterial gastroenteritis, and to assess sensitivity of specific antimicrobials.

Equipment

- Gloves
- Patient identification label
- Sterile culture tube and cotton swab to collect specimen
- Biohazard container

Steps

1. Don gloves.

   RATIONALE: *Prevents the spread of bacteria.*

2. Using the sterile cotton swab collect (scrape) a fresh, warm specimen of stool from the diaper or stool receptacle and place it into the sterile culture tube or a specimen may be obtained by inserting a rectal swab into the rectum and rotating for 30 seconds.

   RATIONALE: *Proper specimen collection is essential for correct analyzation.*

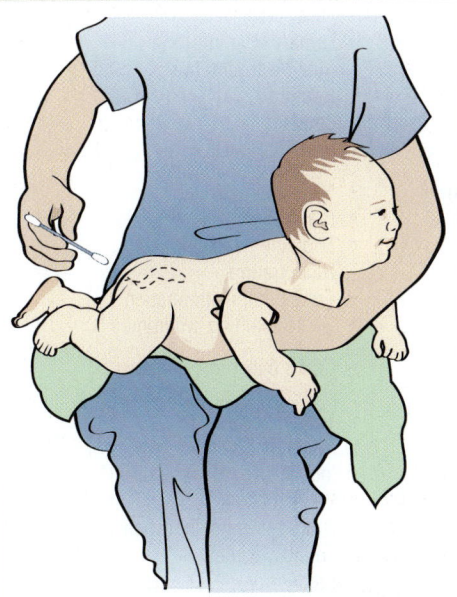

3. Label both the sterile culture tube and the biohazard bag with the patient's identification information.

   RATIONALE: *Accurate labeling is essential for correct patient identification.*

4. Place the sterile culture tube into the biohazard bag.

   RATIONALE: *To ensure that the properly identified specimen is safely transported to the laboratory.*

5. Deliver the fresh specimen of stool to the laboratory promptly after collection.

   RATIONALE: *Delays in transfer of the specimen may affect viability of the organism.*

 clinical alert

- Avoid external contamination of stool and deliver to laboratory promptly.
- Provide samples from several areas of the stool to ensure that organisms are isolated. Failure to do so may yield a false-negative result.
- Inform the lab of antimicrobial or antiamebic therapy within 10 days because it may yield false-negative results.
- Medications such as antacids, antibiotics, antidiarrheals, iron, and castor oil may interfere with analysis.

Teach Parents

Teach parents that a stool for culture and sensitivity is used to detect the presence of bacterial overgrowth, confirm bacterial gastroenteritis, and assess sensitivity of specific antimicrobials.

Teach parents that a stool for ova and parasites (O & P) is used to aid in diagnosis of parasites or their eggs.

Documentation
10/12/14 0900 Stool for culture and sensitivity, and ova and parasites collected from the diaper, labeled, placed in biohazard bag, and sent to laboratory via laboratory collection personnel.
N. Kramer, RN

Source: Van Leeuwen, & Poelhuis-Leth (2011).

and care of soiled diapers and clothing as well as avoiding over feeding the child and excess juice in the diet.

Collaborative Care

Nursing Care. The general nursing care of the child with chronic diarrhea is similar to that of acute diarrhea with special focus related to the underlying cause. As with acute diarrhea the child and parents need to be educated on primary prevention.

Medical Care. Management of chronic diarrhea involves treating the underlying cause. The treatment for toddler's diarrhea is a change or reduction in the child's intake of fruit juices.

Education/Discharge Instructions

Child and parent instructions are similar to those provided for acute diarrhea as they apply to the underlying cause.

 Global Health Case Study Chronic Diarrhea

Thirty-month-old Tammy is brought to the urgent care clinic by her parents for a complaint of diarrhea for the past 4 weeks. The stools are reported to occur between three and six times a day, are described as greasy, and are foul-smelling. Tammy's parents have also noted that she appears to have cramps, is bloated, passes an unusual amount of flatus, and lacks energy. Tammy was recently adopted from an orphanage in the relatively poor central Asian country of Kyrgyzstan, which is known for poor sanitation and water quality. Tammy has been in the United States for 6 weeks. Since that time her parents have noted that she has lost 2 lb. The orphanage reported that little information was known about her birth parents except that she is of Asian/Russian descent. She was born full term without complications, though the birth mother received minimal prenatal care. At birth Tammy weighed 6 lb and measured 19 in. At the time of adoption the orphanage reported that Tammy weighed 32 lb and was 37.5 in. in height. At the physical assessment the nurse notes the following:

- T = 98.6°F (37°C)
- P = 95
- R = 25
- BP = 107/67
- Weight = 30 lb (13.6 kg) (25th percentile on age-appropriate growth chart)
- Height = 37.5 in. (94 cm) (50th percentile on age-appropriate growth chart)
- Skin pale and dry
- Mucous membranes dry
- Abdomen distended with hyperactive bowel sounds
- Child appears tired though is cooperative

critical thinking questions

1. Are these findings normal or pathological?

2. What actions does the nurse take?

3. What is included in parent teaching?

◆ See Suggested Answers to Global Health Case Studies on Davis*Plus*.

VOMITING

Vomiting is the forceful expulsion of stomach contents. The type of emesis assists in identifying the cause. "Nonbilious vomit is generally caused by infection, metabolic,

neurologic, or psychological problems" (Starr et al., 2012, p. 742). **Bilious vomiting** (vomit containing bile) is more likely caused by an obstructive process. Bloody emesis is usually evidence of active bleeding in the GI tract, such as peptic ulcer disease or gastritis. The nurse communicates to the family that nausea and retching often accompany vomiting. Regurgitation in contrast is a more passive and effortless phenomenon. Table 24-2 lists the most common causes of vomiting related to origin.

Signs and Symptoms

Specific manifestations and diagnosis related to vomiting vary as greatly as the causes and origin of the illness. A thorough history and assessment must include a description of the onset, duration, quality and quantity, appearance, presence of undigested food, odor, and evidence of a precipitating event. The child's recent exposure to illness, injury, or stress, in addition to family history of a similar illness, needs to be determined. The parents or child are asked about the relation of the vomiting to the time of day, meals, or other activities. Associated symptoms, such as fever, diarrhea, ear pain, headache, and signs of increased intracranial pressure or urinary tract infection are also evaluated. Vomiting upon arising in the morning is often associated with neurological

Table 24-2	Common Causes of Vomiting
Origin	**Cause**
Upper GI	• Gastritis • Esophagitis • Pyloric stenosis • GERD
Small intestine	• Intestinal malrotation with volvulus
Colon	• Hirschsprung's disease • Intussusception • Fecal impaction
Liver or pancreas	• Hepatobiliary dysfunction
Infections	• Bacterial enteritis • Otitis media • Urinary tract infection • Viral gastroenteritis • Hepatitis • Sepsis • Chronic sinusitis
Neurological	• Hydrocephalus • Brain tumor • Migraine headache • Head trauma • Congenital malformation • Cyclic vomiting syndrome
Other	• Cow's milk protein allergy • Maternal drug exposure and withdrawal • Toxic ingestion • Appendicitis • Inborn error of metabolism • Pneumonia • Drug or alcohol ingestion • Eating disorders • Pregnancy • Diabetic ketoacidosis

involvement. The nurse also asks the parent or child about medications currently being taken to include over-the-counter, herbal, cultural, and homeopathic remedies (Starr et al., 2012). The nurse assesses the abdomen for the following:

- Distention
- Visible peristalsis
- Bowel sounds, depending on the cause of the vomiting, bowel sounds may be hyperactive or hypoactive
- Signs of dehydration
- Evidence of malnutrition

Diagnosis

In addition to a thorough history and physical examination, diagnostic studies may include urinalysis and culture, CBC, serum electrolytes, blood culture, liver function tests, and select abdominal imaging depending on suspected cause of the vomiting. Plain radiograph or ultrasonography of the abdomen may detect anatomical abnormalities. Endoscopy of the upper GI tract can be used if esophagitis is suspected. Further studies may include a toxicology screen, rapid strep test/throat culture, pregnancy test, or electroencephalogram depending on the suspected origin of the vomiting.

Prevention

If vomiting is related to improper feeding technique, prevention can be directed toward instructing the parents on proper formula preparation and positioning the infant during feeding.

Collaborative Care

Nursing Care. Nursing care is determined by cause and generally focuses on careful observation and support. Care is taken to carefully position the child who is vomiting to prevent aspiration. The nurse assesses for signs of dehydration and carefully monitors fluid intake and output. Oral hygiene may include rinsing the mouth or brushing the teeth after vomiting to dilute the hydrochloric acid that comes in contact with the teeth.

Medical Care. Management of vomiting is directed toward the treatment of the cause and prevention of complications. The degree of dehydration is determined and treated. For self-limiting causes of vomiting in childhood, the bowel is allowed to rest. Rehydration is generally initiated after 1 to 2 hours with nothing by mouth. Plain water, apple juice, soda, milk, and sports drinks are avoided. Depending on the child's age and size 0.5 to 2 oz of a rehydrating solution may be offered at 15-minute intervals. Breastfed infants may be nursed more frequently for shorter periods. Solids are avoided for 4 to 6 hours after which reintroduction is begun with bland solids, which may include complex carbohydrates, such as rice, wheat, cereals, yogurt, cooked vegetables, and lean meats. Fatty foods and those high in simple sugars are avoided.

When vomiting is of a limited duration and the cause is known, antiemetic drugs may be indicated. Adverse effects are rare with antiemetic use in children. Antiemetic medications that block chemoreceptor triggers include ondansetron (Zofran) or granisetron (Kytril) (Starr et al., 2012). The nurse understands that metoclopramide (Reglan) enhances peristalsis, and therefore gastric emptying. Phenothiazine (Phenergan) is used cautiously per rectum every 6 hours if vomiting is excessive, dehydration is imminent, and GI disease has been excluded.

Education/Discharge Instructions

If vomiting has been determined to be related to improper feeding technique, the caregiver needs instruction on food or formula preparation and a demonstration of correct positioning during and after feeding.

CYCLIC VOMITING SYNDROME

Cyclic vomiting syndrome (CVS) is a recurrent stereotypical spell of vomiting followed by periods of wellness (Sundaram et al., 2011). One-third of recurrent vomiting in children is caused by CVS, with a female-to-male ratio of 60:40. CVS is most commonly diagnosed between the ages of 3 and 7 (Starr et al., 2012). Starr et al. (2012) suggest that affected children "tend to have mothers and maternal grandmothers with a higher incidence of migraine headache, depression, anxiety, irritable bowel syndrome (IBS), and hypothyroidism" (Starr et al., 2012, p. 745). CVS is generally outgrown before or during the preteen years.

The typical child presents as well 90% of the time. However, during exacerbations significant costs are incurred and children miss an average of 24 days of school per year. Medical costs are related to IV rehydration, diagnostic studies, procedures, emergency room costs, and time taken off from work by the parent.

Signs and Symptoms

The following diagnostic criteria were defined by the North American Society for Pediatric Gastroenterology, Hepatology, and Nutrition (NASPGHAN) Consensus Statement on the Diagnosis and Management of Cyclic Vomiting Syndrome:

- At least 5 attacks over any interval, or a minimum of 3 attacks over a 6-month period
- Episodic attacks of intense nausea and vomiting lasting from 1 hour to 10 days and occurring at least 1 week apart
- Stereotypical in the individual patient
- Vomiting during attacks occurs at least 4 times/hour for at least 1 hour
- A return to baseline health between episodes
- Not attributed to another disorder
  (Li, Lefevre, Chelimsky, Boles, Nelson, Lewis, et al., 2008, p. 383)

The primary clinical manifestation is recurrent episodic vomiting, usually lasting 24 to 48 hours. The vomiting occurs at regular intervals, usually every 2 to 4 weeks. The condition may include a prodromal (initial or indicative of an approaching illness [Venes, 2013]) period during which the child may demonstrate signs of pallor, anorexia, nausea, abdominal pain, and lethargy. Once the episode resolves, a brief recovery period occurs during which the child returns to normal activities. Episodes generally occur in the middle of the night or early morning. Vomiting occurs on an average of six times per hour. Eighty-three percent of the time the emesis is described as bilious, with hematemesis (vomiting of blood) occurring approximately 32% of the time.

Associated GI symptoms include:

- Severe abdominal pain occurring 80% of the time
- Retching

- Anorexia
- Nausea
- Diarrhea

Systemic symptoms include:

- Headache
- Photophobia (light intolerance)
- Phonophobia (intolerance or fear of sound)
- Vertigo (sensation of moving in space or having objects move)

Infection, psychological stress, diet changes, or menstruation may be precipitating factors. A positive family history of migraine headaches may be present. On examination, the child may appear pale and listless, often lying in a position to decrease the pain, such as in a fetal position. Dehydration may be evident.

"What to say"—*Cyclic vomiting syndrome*

Essential questions the nurse asks to help determine the diagnosis include:

- Has the child had at least three episodes?
- Is the child completely asymptomatic between episodes?
- Are the episodes stereotypical?

Additional diagnostic red flags may include "severe headache, GI bleeding, unilateral abdominal pain, weight loss, failure to respond to any treatment, progressive worsening, abnormal neurological examination, triggering events, prolonged episodes requiring repeat hospitalizations, and a change in pattern or symptoms" (Starr et al., 2012).

Diagnosis

Diagnostic studies are used to rule out other conditions. Laboratory studies may include CBC with differential, electrolytes, glucose, liver function tests, metabolic screening (lactate, ammonia, amino acids, and porphobilinogen), urinalysis, urine culture, and urine organic acids. Imaging studies may include small bowel radiography, abdominal ultrasound, MRI or CT of the head or sinuses, and/or endoscopy.

Prevention

Prevention of cyclic vomiting includes balanced nutrition, maintaining a routine sleep/rest schedule, moderate exercise, avoiding food and environmental triggers, and stress management.

Collaborative Care

Nursing Care. Nursing care is supportive and includes management of fluid balance, nutritional support, and comfort needs.

Medical Care. Management is generally supportive care and includes fluid replacement, rest, and pharmacotherapy as needed. Careful monitoring and documentation of fluid intake and output during vomiting episodes are essential. Accurate assessment includes the type and appearance of the vomiting in addition to associated behavior. A calm stress-free environment is provided. Up to one-third of

children with cyclic vomiting suffer with migraines by age 9.5 years, and up to 50% are predicted to suffer migraines by age 15 years (Venkatasubramani & Li, 2010). A psychiatric evaluation may be indicated for cyclic vomiting because the symptoms can be associated with psychological stress.

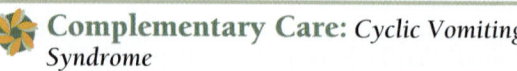

Complementary Care: *Cyclic Vomiting Syndrome*

Complementary therapy may include biofeedback, massage, and imagery (Slutsker, Konichezky, & Gothelf, 2010).

Education/Discharge Instructions

Family education includes considering lifestyle changes such as increasing exercise, maintaining well-balanced diet and good hydration, regular meal and sleep routines and schedules, and the recognition and avoidance of food and environmental and psychological triggers.

CONSTIPATION

Constipation is the difficult or infrequent passage of hard stool, which is often associated with straining, abdominal pain, or withholding behaviors. Frequency alone is not a good diagnostic criterion because children vary greatly in their stooling frequency. Phatak and Pashankar (2010) cite the NASPGHAN criteria for constipation as delay or difficulty in passing stools, for 2 or more weeks, and causing significant distress.

Constipation accounts for 3% of pediatric primary care clinic visits and 25% of pediatric gastroenterologist visits (Greenwald, 2010; Phatak & Pashankar, 2010). Studies estimate the prevalence of chronic constipation in North America to be between 2% to 27% of children and adults with a mean outpatient cost of $13,927 (Choung, Shah, Chitkara, Branda, Van Tilburg, Whitehead, et al., 2011). Constipation peaks between the ages of 2 and 4 and is more common in males than in females until adolescence, after which it is seen more frequently in females.

Constipation may occur secondary to an organic cause or in association with a systemic condition. Strictures and Hirschsprung's disease are included among organic causes. Systemic conditions that may be a factor in the development of constipation include hypothyroidism, hypercalcemia caused by hyperparathyroidism or vitamin D excess, and chronic lead poisoning. Drugs such as antacids, diuretics, iron supplements, opioids, antihistamines, and antiepileptics are also associated with constipation as a side effect. Children with spinal cord pathology may experience a loss of rectal tone and sensation.

Medication: Medications Used for Vomiting

A combination of medications is used for sedation and the relief of pain and nausea and vomiting. This may include a combination of diphenhydramine (Benadryl), lorazepam (Ativan), promethazine (Phenergan), ondansetron (Zofran), and ketorolac (Toradol) with ranitidine (Zantac). For severe abdominal pain, morphine may be added (Starr et al., 2012). Prophylactic medications for CVS include cyproheptadine (Periactin), sumatriptan (Imitrex), or amitriptyline (Elavil) (Starr et al., 2012).

Most constipation is considered idiopathic or functional with no clear underlying cause. Environmental and/or psychosocial factors such as travel, illness, dietary changes, and emotional factors may cause chronic constipation. Children may also experience constipation during toilet training, which is related to not wanting to take time from play or from overenthusiastic toilet training. Dilation and stretching of the rectum may come from repeated withholding. This leads to a decreased sensation or urge to pass stool. The most common cause of constipation in children is poor dietary intake of fiber and lack of exercise (Marchand, Di Lorenzo, & Jarczk, (2011).

Onset of constipation during infancy is generally associated with dietary causes. Constipation is less common in breastfed infants. Environmental changes and attention to controlling the passage of stool are more common causes of constipation in early childhood. Any feeling of discomfort during stooling may lead the child to deliberately withhold stool in the future.

In the school-age child, organic and environmental factors are considered. Fear of using school restrooms or embarrassment in asking the teacher is a common cause of constipation in early school-age children. Separation, change in routine, and change in eating and sleeping patterns may all contribute to the change seen in bowel habits. These children may try to "hold" their stool until a later time. When they do finally try to eliminate the stool, it may be very hard and painful. The longer the child holds the stool and delays elimination, the harder and larger the stool becomes and the more painful the process.

Signs and Symptoms

The major symptoms associated with constipation are poor appetite and straining with stools. Soiling is more common with the diagnosis of encopresis. Additional signs include:

- Stools are hard and blood may occasionally be seen in the outer surface of the stool
- Changes in stooling pattern (i.e., size, frequency, amount, and color)
- Pain with defecation
- Diarrhea leakage
- Tenderness in the area of the colon and small intestine
- Rectal fissures
- Withholding behaviors such as crossing legs, squatting, hiding in a corner, or dancing

Diagnosis

Diagnosis of constipation is based on the symptoms. An abdominal radiography and barium enema may be ordered for children who do not respond to treatment.

 focus on safety

Abdominal pain

Most children who are constipated usually have some abdominal pain caused by cramping. However, if the onset of constipation and severe abdominal pain is acute and/or accompanied by fever, vomiting, or other symptoms, the child must be evaluated for a bowel obstruction.

 Nursing Insight—Constipation

The majority of children have idiopathic or functional constipation. This classification is used when there is no identifiable reason or underlying cause for their constipation.

Prevention

Prevention of constipation can occur through good toileting habits and reinforcement of sitting on the toilet for defecation as well as maintaining a well-balanced diet and hydration and age-appropriate exercise.

Collaborative Care

Nursing Care. Care of the child with constipation begins with a careful assessment of bowel patterns, diet history, drug history, and environmental factors. The nurse asks the parent to describe the color, consistency, frequency, and characteristics of the stool.

Medical Care. The management of simple constipation can generally be accomplished by focusing on dietary intake and keeping the bowel relatively empty. Occasional constipation caused by dietary intake can be treated with adequate intake of water and other fluids, which assist in regulating elimination. A regular diet, rich in all nutrients coupled with an adequate amount of water and other fluids, is the best way to ensure normal bowel elimination patterns. Fresh fruit and vegetables add fiber and can relieve constipation (Maffei & Vicentini, 2011). Limiting dairy products such as cheese can also provide relief. However, many children can be "picky eaters" at times, preferring fast food or the same food for every meal. This type of eating can lead to disruptive bowel patterns including constipation. Occasionally, stool softeners may be needed to "train" the child and the bowels into a regular pattern of elimination. Giving the stool softener at bedtime allows it to work gently overnight to foster a morning elimination pattern. No medication is used on a long-term basis without a physician's prescription or health-care provider's guidance.

Chronic constipation may require strategies to restore a regular stooling pattern, hence shrinking the distended rectum to a normal size and promoting regular toileting practices. Therapy for chronic constipation may include bowel cleansing and maintenance therapy to prevent further stool retention. Initial treatment of chronic constipation includes removing hard, impacted stool, which may be accomplished through use of suppositories, enemas, and occasionally the use of polyethylene glycol electrolyte solution (GoLYTELY) administered orally or by nasogastric tube. A combination of mineral oil and enemas may be used for severe impaction for which suppositories are not effective. Rarely, surgical removal is needed.

Once the impaction is removed, maintenance therapy includes use of mineral oil, stool softeners, and laxatives. Stool softeners may not be effective for severe constipation. The safest laxatives are milk of magnesia and polyethylene glycol (MiraLax).

Bowel retraining includes developing good toileting habits and reinforcement of sitting on the toilet for defecation. A regular toileting time is established once or twice per day. The child sits on the toilet 5 to 10 minutes with positive behaviors reinforced.

Nursing Insight—*Enema*

An enema is given to remove stool and/or gas from the bowel. The health-care provider orders the enema and determines the next step(s) if the enema is unsuccessful. For an infant a catheter between 2.5 and 3.5 cm is used. For a child the catheter size is 5 to 7.5 cm. A common type of enema is a Fleet's® Enema. Prior to the procedure educate the parent and child (if appropriate) that the enema is inserted into the rectum, given slowly, and that there may be a feeling of abdominal distension.

The basic procedure includes the following important steps:
1. Use 2 patient identifiers to ensure the correct patient will receive the enema.
2. The tip of the enema is lubricated, but more water-soluble jelly can be applied as needed.
3. Apply a bed protector and ensure the child (depending on age) can readily reach a bedside commode chair, bathroom, or use a bedpan. The infant is diapered.
4. Gather hygiene supplies such as a basin, soap, water, towels, and washcloths.
5. Perform hand hygiene and don gloves.
6. Provide privacy.
7. Raise the bed to a comfortable working height.
8. Separate the buttocks and locate the anus.
9. Gently insert the tip of the enema into the child's rectum to the recommended depth with the tip directed toward the umbilicus.
10. After instilling the solution, gently remove the tip.
11. After an appropriate interval, transfer him to the bedside commode chair, bathroom, or bedpan.
12. Have the child expel the solution.
13. Clean the child's perianal area and help him resume a comfortable position in bed.
14. Measure the amount of returned solution and quality of the feces.
15. Dispose the used equipment and other items.
16. Remove gloves and perform hand hygiene.
17. Document the procedure in the child's records.

Optimizing Outcomes—Constipation

A 2½-year-old child has not passed a stool in 5 days. The parents report that the child has been eating and growing well and has no other symptoms of illness. They report that the last stool passed was firm and appeared to cause the child some discomfort. The parents also report no evidence of blood has been noted in the stool. In addition, the parents began toilet training the child approximately 3 weeks ago.

The best outcome for the family is to understand that the child is normal. The nurse can discuss toilet training readiness to include not only physical readiness but also mental and psychological readiness. In addition, the nurse can include instructions regarding the importance of water and high fiber in the diet and the avoidance of excessive refined carbohydrates.

Education/Discharge Instructions

Parent education is an important part of nursing care and includes instruction on dietary needs, toileting practices, and bowel cleansing as needed.

GASTROESOPHAGEAL REFLUX AND GASTROESOPHAGEAL REFLUX DISEASE

Gastroesophageal reflux (GER) is the return of gastric contents from the stomach through the lower esophageal sphincter into the esophagus. Classifications of reflux include physiological, also called functional, and pathological, often referred to as spitting up or regurgitation. Physiological reflux, or GER, is described as infrequent and episodic vomiting and is a common occurrence in many healthy infants. A decrease is seen as the esophagus elongates and matures. Starr et al. (2012) suggest that the occurrence of physiological GER is present in 73% of infants in the first month and is reduced to 50% by age 5 months. By 1 year less than 4% of infants continue to regurgitate.

Nursing Insight—*Functional GER*

Functional or physiological GER involves painless, effortless vomiting with no physical sequelae (Starr et al., 2012). Infants who spit up or regurgitate stomach content while maintaining normal nutrition meet the criteria for functional GER. Factors that impact the occurrence of functional GER include small stomach size, short esophagus, liquid diet, horizontal positioning, and frequent, large-volume feedings (Bishop, 2011).

Pathological reflux, or GERD, is frequent with associated physical dysfunction. The diagnosis of GERD is generally considered when reflux persists beyond 18 months of age and involves an increased frequency and duration of episodes (Bishop, 2011). GERD occurs in approximately 5% to 8% of all newborns and has been associated with apnea and other life-threatening events. GERD is often associated with esophagitis, failure to thrive, and aspiration pneumonia and is noted after there is a pathological and/or histological change because of reflux (Bishop, 2011). Children with GERD beyond 18 months are more likely to experience symptoms similar to an adult's.

The incidence of GER in healthy infants is approximately 40% to 50% as demonstrated by regurgitation followed by crying. The incidence of GER peaks at approximately 4 months of age, then steadily declines.

GERD is more common in premature infants and those born with neurological impairments. GERD can be identified in as many as 70% of low-birth-weight infants (1,700 g) with up to 85% of those infants becoming symptom free by 1 year of age (Starr et al., 2012). Reflux disease remains significant in 1% to 3% of older children.

The cause of GER is unknown and considered multifactorial. Neuromuscular immaturity of the lower esophagus, age, hormones, and intra-abdominal pressure are suggested as factors in the development of GERD. The following information will focus mainly on GER with some integration of information about GERD.

Signs and Symptoms

The most common symptoms of GER are vomiting and regurgitation that is nonbilious and includes undigested formula or food (Starr et al., 2012). Associated symptoms include the following:

- Irritability and fussiness
- Dysphagia or refusal to feed
- Choking

- Chronic cough
- Wheezing
- Apnea
- Weight loss
- Frequent respiratory infections
- Bloody vomit or hematemesis
- Hoarseness or sore throat
- Halitosis
- Chronic sinusitis and/or otitis media

Diagnosis

Diagnosis of GER is through history and physical examination. An upper GI series may be used to rule out anatomical abnormalities, but it does not provide information about the physiological function of the esophagus and is considered an unreliable diagnostic test for pathological GERD. Post-swallowing reflux can be observed through a barium swallow. A 24-hour intraesophageal pH monitoring study is essential in the diagnosis of GERD. If esophagitis, strictures, or Barrett's esophagus is suspected, an endoscopy with biopsy may be completed to confirm the diagnosis.

? Case Study Gastroesophageal Reflux

Two-month-old Ella was born via a normal spontaneous vaginal delivery. Her birth weight was 10 lb 2 oz (4.6 kg) and she was 22 in. (55.8 cm) long. Her parents are of Caucasian descent. Her mother's prenatal care was initiated during the third month of gestation, and the pregnancy was uncomplicated. Her mother states that Ella spits up four or five times per day. She reports that Ella has four or five soft yellowish-brown stools daily. Ella is breastfed, and her mother reports that Ella nurses every 3 to 5 hours. No solids have been initiated.

Ella is awake and resting quietly in her mother's arms. During the initial assessment, the nurse notes the following information: axillary temperature: 98.6°F (37°C); pulse, 106 beats per minute; respirations, 28 breaths per minute; weight is 13 lb 10 oz (6.2 kg); and length is 23.5 in. (59.7 cm). Ella appears pink, well nourished, and well hydrated. After the assessment, Ella began to fuss, at which time her mother offered her a bottle of Enfamil, which she takes eagerly. After completion of the bottle, Ella regurgitates a small amount of partially digested nonbilious liquid. Ella then closes her eyes and quietly falls asleep. The mother proceeds to tell the nurse that this is what normally occurs when Ella vomits.

critical thinking questions

1. Are these findings normal or pathological?

2. What actions does the nurse take?

3. What is included in parent teaching?

◆ See Suggested Answers to Case Studies on DavisPlus.

Prevention

Preventive activities can be directed toward instructing parents on proper formula preparation, feeding, and positioning the infant during and after feeding.

Collaborative Care

Nursing Care. Healthy, well-nourished infants need no treatment for physiological reflux. Common interventions include providing parent support and anticipatory guidance. The parents need to be reassured that there is no underlying disease.

Steps in managing reflux with no underlying structural problems may begin with evaluating and changing the volume of the feeding such as offering small amounts more often and burping frequently. Thickening of feedings with cereal, although controversial, can provide sufficient calories while reducing the volume. One teaspoon per ounce of dry infant cereal may be added to 1 to 2 ounces of formula. Care must be taken when adding cereal to formula because it increases the caloric density of the formula and decreases the amount of fluid intake. Intra-abdominal pressure increase can be avoided by positioning the infant in an upright position (generally no higher than a 45-degree angle) after feeding. Several studies have reported that a prone position decreases episodes of reflux. Since prone positioning has been associated with sudden infant death syndrome (SIDS), this position is only considered with extreme caution and when complications from GER exceed the risk of SIDS. In addition, right side-lying positioning facilitates gastric emptying.

Nursing care for either GER or GERD includes a thorough assessment of the infant's growth measurements and developmental patterns. Feeding patterns are evaluated, and the amount, type, and frequency of feedings are established with the pattern of regurgitation or emesis related to the feedings. In addition, information about positioning and burping after feedings are determined. A baseline respiratory status is important because of the risk of aspiration associated with GERD.

Medical Care. If the infant experiences complications, pharmacological therapy may be offered (Bishop, 2011). Proton-pump inhibitors, such as omeprazole (Prilosec), esomeprazole (Nexium), pantoprazole (Protonix), and lansoprazole (Prevacid), provide effective medical therapy for heartburn and esophagitis though are not recommended in the treatment of otherwise healthy infants (Baker, Tsou, Tung, Baker, Li, Wang, et al., 2010; Chen, Gao, Johnson, Niak, Troiani, Korvick, et al., 2012). H_2 inhibitors such as cimetidine (Tagamet) and ranitidine (Zantac) may also reduce heartburn though are considered less effective (Bishop, 2011). Prokinetic drugs, such as metoclopramide (Reglan), offer enhanced stomach emptying and increase lower esophageal sphincter control though the benefit is considered minimal (Bishop, 2011).

Surgical Care. Surgical treatment may be recommended for severe symptoms, such as those that are life threatening or unresponsive to nonsurgical interventions. The surgical intervention of choice for the treatment of GERD is a **Nissen fundoplication** (wrapping the gastric cardia with adjacent portions of the gastric fundus) (Venes, 2013). A feeding **jejunostomy** (a surgical creation of an opening into the jejunum) may be used for infants with severe neurological defects who cannot tolerate oral or gastric tube feedings (Bishop, 2011). Recent advances in surgical interventions for GERD have expanded the forms of fundoplication treatment options that provide fewer complications or need for repeat surgical intervention (Halbert, 2011; Rothenberg & Chin, 2010). The nurse provides post-operative surgical care.

Education/Discharge Instructions

Much of the initial nursing care focuses on educating the parents regarding dietary modifications, positioning, and pharmacological therapy if prescribed. The importance of frequent burping and suggested positions for burping is also discussed with the parents. Depending on the age of the child and the nature of the diet, education may also include information about dietary irritants (e.g., chocolate, caffeine products, citrus fruits, fruit drinks, and tomatoes). If treatment includes use of thickened feedings, the nurse demonstrates how to enlarge the hole in the nipple to better facilitate this type of feeding. Parents may also need to be reminded to avoid vigorous playing after feeding.

 Nursing Insight—*Gastroesophageal reflux*

Frequent use of an infant seat for positioning is avoided because it reduces truncal tone in infants and increases intra-abdominal pressure, which can promote reflux (Weill, 2008).

 Nursing Diagnoses The Child With Gastroesophageal Reflux

- Imbalanced Nutrition: Less than Body Requirements related to chronic vomiting or regurgitation
- Risk for Fluid Volume Deficit related to excessive losses through normal route
- Risk for Aspiration related to increased intragastric pressure with an incompetent cardiac sphincter
- Potential for Parental Knowledge Deficit related to lack of information concerning the child's care

HIRSCHSPRUNG'S DISEASE

Hirschsprung's's disease, also known as congenital aganglionic megacolon, is caused by a congenital absence of Meissner's and Auerbach's autonomic plexus in the bowel wall. This absence of ganglion cells results in lack of motility in the affected portion of the bowel (Sundaram et al., 2011). Hirschsprung's disease is usually limited to the distal colon. The absence of ganglion cells in the affected portion of the bowel results in lack of nervous system stimulation to that portion of the colon. This leads to abnormal or absence of peristalsis in the involved segment and an inability of the internal sphincter to relax. A complete or partial bowel obstruction may occur as a result of this inability of the smooth muscles to relax. This in turn leads to an accumulation of bowel contents in the involved segment of the bowel. The obstruction may extend proximally to involve varying portions of the colon (Fig. 24-7).

Hirschsprung

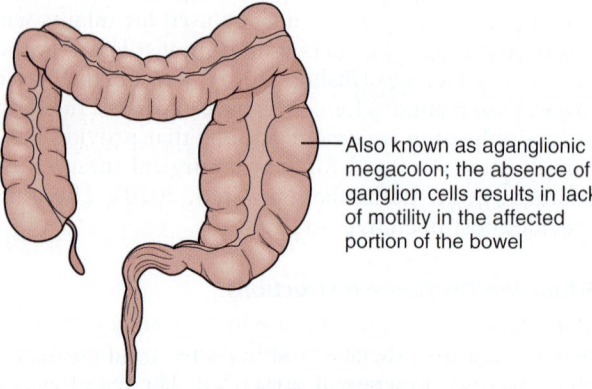

Also known as aganglionic megacolon; the absence of ganglion cells results in lack of motility in the affected portion of the bowel

Figure 24-7 Hirschsprung's disease.

The incidence of Hirschsprung's disease is 1 in 4,400 to 7,000 births (Mousa, 2010). It is the most common cause of neonatal obstruction of the colon and accounts for up to 33% of all neonatal obstructions (Gaylord & Yetman, 2012). The condition is familial, four times more common in males, and more common in children with trisomy 21 (Down syndrome) (Sundaram et al., 2011).

Signs and Symptoms

The history of the child with Hirschsprung's disease verifies the following signs and symptoms:

- Failure to pass meconium within the first 48 hours of life
- Failure to thrive
- Poor feeding
- Chronic constipation
- Down syndrome (Gaylord & Yetman, 2012)

Physical findings include:

- Vomiting
- Abdominal obstruction
- Failure to pass stools
- Diarrhea
- Flatus
- Explosive bowel movements

In older children, the initial symptom is chronic constipation (Mousa, 2010). The child's stools may be described as ribbon or pellet shaped and foul smelling.

 focus on safety

Enterocolitis

Enterocolitis (inflammation of the small intestine and colon) is the most ominous presentation of Hirschsprung's disease. Enterocolitis may present in an otherwise well infant with a history of constipation. The child with enterocolitis may present with an abrupt onset of foul-smelling diarrhea, abdominal distention, and fever. Rapid progression may indicate perforation of the bowel and sepsis. The major cause of death in Hirschsprung's disease is related to enterocolitis and sepsis, accounting for up to 30% of cases (Bishop, 2011; Mousa, 2010).

Diagnosis

Diagnosis in the newborn is suspected based on clinical presentation or intestinal obstruction and failure to pass meconium. Radiographic studies show evidence of a dilated loop of bowel. A barium enema often demonstrates the transition between the dilated proximal colon and the aganglionic distal segment, though this may not be evident until age 2 months or later (Sundaram et al., 2011). Absence of ganglion cells is determined by a biopsy. Rectal manometry and rectal suction biopsy are the easiest and most reliable indicators of Hirschsprung's disease (Sundaram et al., 2011). In anorectal manometry a balloon is distended in the rectum and measures the pressure of the internal anal sphincter. In normal patients, rectal distention initiates a reflex decline in internal sphincter pressure. In patients with Hirschsprung's disease, the pressure fails to drop or there is a rise in pressure with rectal distension.

Prevention

Because the condition is familial as well as associated with chromosomal disorders, prevention includes comprehensive prenatal care and counseling in families with a familial history of Hirschsprung's disease.

Collaborative Care

Nursing Care. Initial care of the child with Hirschsprung's disease involves preoperative assessment of the child's fluid and electrolyte status. The child is placed NPO (nothing by mouth), and a nasogastric (NG) tube is inserted. IV fluids and electrolytes are administered to prevent and/or correct imbalances. Accurate intake and output is maintained to include colostomy and nasogastric tube drainage.

Surgical Care. Correction of Hirschsprung's disease involves surgical resection of the affected bowel with or without a colostomy (Gaylord & Yetman, 2012; Sundaram et al., 2011). Surgical interventions generally include a temporary colostomy, with a subsequent ostomy takedown and reanastomosis at age 6 to 12 months. Other surgical options include excising the aganglionic segment and anastomosing the normal proximal bowel to the rectum 1 to 2 cm above the dentate line. Postoperative care includes routine post–abdominal surgical intervention such as physical assessment, NPO, pain management, wound care, and fluid maintenance. Patency of the NG tube is maintained along with monitoring for abdominal distention and assessing for return of bowel sounds.

Education/Discharge Instructions

The nurse instructs the parents how to care for the temporary colostomy. The instructions include care of the skin, appliance application, and referral to community resources. The parents also need to be instructed on the symptoms of complications, such as enterocolitis, leaks, and strictures at the site of anastomosis. Signs of leaks include abdominal distention and irritability. Constipation, vomiting, and diarrhea may indicate strictures. Signs of enterocolitis may include abdominal distention and pain in addition to fever, diarrhea, or shock-like symptoms (Sundaram et al., 2011).

 Now Can You—Discuss functional gastrointestinal conditions?

1. Discuss functional gastrointestinal conditions?
2. Discuss signs and symptoms of functional gastrointestinal conditions?
3. Discuss nursing care for functional gastrointestinal conditions?

Malabsorption Disorders

LACTOSE INTOLERANCE

Lactose intolerance is an inability to digest milk and some dairy products, which leads to symptoms of bloating, cramping, and diarrhea (Venes, 2013). This condition results from a deficiency in the enzyme lactase, which is necessary for the digestion of lactose in the small intestine where lactose is hydrolyzed into glucose and galactose. Hydrolysis is a chemical decomposition in which a substance is split into simpler compounds by taking up the elements of water (Venes, 2013).

Lactose intolerance can be categorized into at least four different types (Starr et al., 2012). Congenital lactase deficiency is an inborn error of metabolism, which becomes evident once the newborn consumes a lactose-containing product, such as human milk or formula products. This deficiency results from reduced or absence of lactase. Congenital lactase deficiency is rare and requires lifelong dietary restrictions.

Primary lactase deficiency, also referred to as late-onset lactase deficiency and lactase non-persistence, is the most common type of lactose intolerance (Starr et al., 2012). Primary lactase deficiency usually becomes evident after weaning and is more common in certain ethnic groups

---

 Cultural Diversity: Occurrence of Lactose Intolerance

Asian, Ashkenazi Jewish, American Indian, Hispanic, and African American populations experience a higher incidence of primary lactase deficiency in the United States population than do those of European American descent (Starr et al., 2012).

Secondary lactase deficiency, or lactose intolerance, occurs secondary to intestinal lumen injury. Damage to the intestine can decrease or destroy the enzyme lactase. The most common cause of secondary lactose intolerance is viral gastroenteritis (Ebach, 2011). Temporary or permanent lactose intolerance can be caused by disorders such as cystic fibrosis, celiac disease, and kwashiorkor (severe protein-deficiency form of malnutrition of children), as can various infectious processes such as giardiasis (infection with a flagellate protozoan), rotavirus (an RNA virus), or HIV. Secondary lactose intolerance can also be secondary to chemotherapy (Starr et al., 2012).

Developmental lactase deficiency can occur in infants born before 34 weeks of gestation and is related to the immaturity of the intestinal tract (Starr et al., 2012).

Signs and Symptoms

Lactose intolerance can have any of the following symptoms:

- Bloating
- Cramping
- Abdominal pain
- Flatulence
- Pain and diarrhea occur often within 30 minutes of the ingestion of lactose-containing products
- Recent history of viral gastroenteritis
- Signs in infants include vomiting, distention, abdominal pain after ingesting lactose-containing formula or the ingestion of cow's milk by the breastfeeding mother
- Severe watery diarrhea with stools positive for reducing substance may be evident in infants with congenital lactase deficiency.

Diagnosis

Lactose intolerance is diagnosed on the basis of the history and a decrease in symptoms with elimination of lactose products from the diet. Diagnosis is further confirmed with the reintroduction of lactose-containing foods and a flare of symptoms. The nurse can communicate to the family that "the breath hydrogen test is used to positively diagnose the condition." The breath hydrogen test measures hydrogen in the breath after a challenge with the ingestion of 50 grams of lactose (Venes, 2013).

Nursing Insight—*Diagnosing lactose intolerance in infants and toddlers*

An endoscopic visualization of the gastric mucosa and a digestive fluid sample may be needed with infants and toddlers because of the difficulty of performing the breath hydrogen test.

Prevention

Though some forms of lactose intolerance cannot be prevented, good prenatal care as well as strategies to avoid infection may prevent or reduce the incidence of the disease. Complications related to lactose intolerance may be reduced by educating parents on nutritional management.

Critical Nursing Action Lactose Intolerance

Dairy products are a major source of calcium, and vitamin D supplements are needed to prevent deficiency. Hard cheese, cottage cheese, or yogurt may be taken in place of milk.

Collaborative Care

Nursing Care. Care of the child and family dealing with lactose intolerance is primarily directed at diagnosis, support, and education.

Medical Care. Eliminating dairy products or the use of enzyme replacement may be used for the treatment of lactose intolerance. Reducing the amounts of dairy products instead of eliminating them is recommended by others. Soy-based formula can be substituted for formula or breast milk in infants. Most individuals can tolerate small amounts of lactose and are encouraged to include it in their diets. Milk products are better tolerated when taken at meal times. Enzyme tablets, such as Lactaid, Lactrase, and Dairy Ease, can be used to predigest the lactose in milk or supplement the child's own lactose. The enzyme tablets can be added to milk or sprinkled on dairy products.

clinical alert

Probiotics

Concern regarding the potential for decreased bone mineral density and osteoporosis in children and adolescents with lactose intolerance reinforces the recommendations for the ingestion of small amounts of dairy products with meals. **Probiotics** (food preparations containing microorganism) such as *Lactobacillus* can improve lactose intolerance when live cultures are fermented in dairy products. *Lactobacillus* is a nonpathogenic bacterium that produces lactic acid from carbohydrates and is normally found in milk, feces of infants fed by bottle, and adults. The active culture in yogurt provides a source of calcium for persons with lactose intolerance in addition to producing some of the lactose enzyme required for proper digestion.

Education/Discharge Instructions

Dietary education includes identification of the restrictions and alternative sources of dairy products, which can be included in the diet. Parents also need to be made aware of hidden sources of lactose such as its use as a bulk agent in certain medications. Parents are instructed to consult with pharmacists regarding the avoidance of lactose-containing medications. The parents also are directed to alternative sources of calcium, such as yogurt, that are appropriate for the child's diet.

CELIAC DISEASE

Celiac disease, also known as celiac sprue, gluten-induced enteropathy, and gluten-sensitive enteropathy, is a disorder in which the proximal small bowel mucosa is damaged as a result of dietary exposure to gluten and is second only to cystic fibrosis as a cause of malabsorption disease in children (Bishop, 2011). The disorder does not present until gluten products have been introduced into the diet, usually between 6 months and 2 years of age as table foods are introduced into the diet. Celiac disease is a permanent intolerance to gluten. Gluten consists of two protein components, glutenin and gliadin. The toxic protein component is thought to be that of gliadin (Hoffenberg & Flass, 2010). Gluten is found in wheat, rye, barley, and related grains. Rice does not contain toxic gluten and can be eaten freely, as can a special preparation of oats (Bishop, 2011).

The pathology shown with celiac disease reveals a diffuse lesion of the upper small intestinal mucosa. Short, flat villi, deepened crypts, and irregular vacuolated surface epithelial layer and crypt hyperplasia are seen via light microscopy (Strauch & Cotter, 2011). As the villi flatten out and atrophy, there is a decrease in the absorptive surface of the intestine. Malabsorption with a decreased fat absorption eventually impacts the absorption of proteins; carbohydrates; and the fat-soluble vitamins A, D, E, and K.

It is estimated that approximately 1 in 300 and up to 1% of the population in the United States has celiac disease, of which only a few are diagnosed (Strauch & Cotter, 2011). Women are three times more likely to be affected than men (Strauch & Cotter, 2011). The disease is also more common in persons of European decent and in those with type 1 diabetes, autoimmune thyroiditis, trisomy 21, Turner's syndrome, and IgA deficiency (Hoffenberg & Flass, 2010; Strauch & Cotter, 2011).

Cultural Diversity: *Occurrence of Celiac Disease*

Celiac disease primarily affects people of northern European descent. The average incidence of celiac disease in Europe is 1:1,000 live births with a range of 1:77 in Sweden to 1:198 in the Netherlands (Hoffenberg & Flass, 2010).

Signs and Symptoms

Early manifestations of celiac disease are nonspecific and include anorexia, irritability, weight loss, and listlessness. Classic presentation in the pediatric population begins around age 6 months to 2 years and is characterized by gastrointestinal manifestations as gluten products are introduced into the diet. Classic symptoms include the following:

- Diarrhea
- Abdominal distention and bloating
- Steatorrhea, which is described as bulky, greasy, foul-smelling, and putty-colored stool because of the large amount of undigested fat content
- Constipation
- Vomiting
- Abdominal pain
- Anorexia

Atypical symptoms include:

- Protuberant abdomen, loss of subcutaneous fat, hypotonia, anorexia, lethargy, and muscle wasting because of protein losses
- Anemia and bruising because of inadequate vitamin K absorption
- Growth retardation
- Osteoporosis
- Delayed puberty development
- Iron deficiency anemia
- Failure to thrive
- Abnormal liver function
- Dental enamel defects
- An atypical presentation of celiac disease may delay diagnosis until adult years because the extraintestinal manifestations overshadow the GI symptoms, which may be mild or entirely absent

Diagnosis

The combination of clinical symptoms and serological markers may suggest the diagnosis of celiac disease, though a small bowel biopsy is essential to confirm the diagnosis and is performed before gluten is eliminated from the diet (Hoffenberg & Flass, 2010). A positive biopsy reveals atrophy of the villi and deep crypts on the intestinal mucosa is the definitive test (Starr et al., 2010; Strauch & Cotter, 2011). Laboratory studies detect antigliadin and antiendomysial antibodies in addition to evidence of malabsorption and nutritional deficiencies. The nurse understands that the presence of antigliadin and antiendomysial antibodies and their disappearance when gluten is removed from the diet are important findings in the diagnosis.

Prevention

Though celiac disease cannot be prevented, symptoms may be reduced through careful dietary education and management to include understanding and reading labels as well as being directed to sources where gluten-free food may be obtained.

Collaborative Care

Nursing Care. Care of the child and family dealing with a gluten intolerance is primarily directed at diagnosis, support, and education.

Medical Care. The treatment of celiac disease is a gluten-free diet. Since gluten is found mainly in wheat and rye and to a smaller extent in barley and oat products, it is recommended that they be eliminated from the diet. Corn, rice, and millet are acceptable grains. Dietary consultation is helpful as well as referral to a celiac support group (Strauch & Cotter, 2011).

Education/Discharge Instructions

Tell parents that following a gluten-free diet can heal the damage to the intestine and prevents further damage. The child and parents need to be instructed on the hidden sources of gluten, which may be found in many processed foods, such as thickening agents, soups, and luncheon meats. Gluten is added to many foods as hydrolyzed vegetable protein. Supplemental calories, vitamins, and minerals are recommended during the acute phase. The nurse communicates to the parents that normal amounts of fat are suggested. Improvement is generally demonstrated within a week, though complete recovery and histological normality may require from 3 to 12 months (Strauch & Cotter, 2011). Teach the family about adverse symptoms when gluten is introduced to the diet, growth, and adherence to the gluten-free diet (GFD). Monitoring the child at intermittent intervals is essential. Periodic measurement of transglutaminase is recommended to determine dietary compliance or to reevaluate persistent symptoms after the initiation of the GFD. Intervals of a year or longer in the asymptomatic patient serve as a monitor of adherence to the GFD.

Optimizing Outcomes—Celiac disease

Celiac disease requires a lifelong commitment to diet control. Providing optimal outcomes for the child with celiac disease involves dietary guidance. For the best outcome, instruct the child and parents on the importance of carefully reading labels for hidden sources of gluten-based products. These can often be found in common foods, such as ice cream, hot dogs, luncheon meats, soups, and cookies.

Children with more severe mucosal damage have impaired digestion of disaccharides, especially in relation to lactose. This may also necessitate the need for temporary lactose restriction in the diet. General dietary needs include high calories and proteins with simple carbohydrates, such as fruits and vegetables. High-fiber foods, such as raw vegetables and fruits with skins, nuts, and raisins are avoided until bowel inflammation has been reduced. It is important to stress the lifelong need for diet control. Once the gluten-free diet has been introduced and symptoms are resolved, the child, and possibly the parents, may believe that the condition has been corrected.

legal alert—Obtain consent for genetic testing

In the case of genetic testing of children, the risks and benefits of testing are discussed with the child as appropriate for her level of development. Most testing requires only a blood sample with little physical risk, although there can be psychological risks to the child that include decreased self-worth, anxiety, and disruption of family bonds (Siegel, Alpert, & Goldstein, 2012). The best interest of the child is the primary consideration when genetic testing is ordered with counseling provided before the testing. When possible, both the parents and the child provide informed consent.

SHORT BOWEL SYNDROME

Short bowel syndrome (SBS) is a malabsorptive disorder that results from decreased mucosal surface area, which is usually caused by surgical resection of the small bowel. Factors such as dysmobility and overgrowth of bacteria can exacerbate the malabsorption. Volvulus, gastroschisis, necrotizing enterocolitis, and atresias are the most common causes of SBS in children. Crohn's disease is also a cause in older children. Trauma to the GI tract is a less common cause of SBS. The small intestine may be congenitally short in conditions in which bowel is lost in utero. Loss of a large portion of the bowel produces malabsorption and malnutrition. SBS results in compromised bowel function. Use of long-term parenteral nutrition has improved life expectancy, though long-term parenteral nutrition can cause complications that may lead to surgical intervention. For infants who experience a greater than 50% bowel resection or require IV nutrition for more than 2 months, the 5-year survival rate is estimated to be 73% (Sundaram et al., 2011). Liver failure and recurrent infection are the most common causes of mortality (Sundaram et al., 2011).

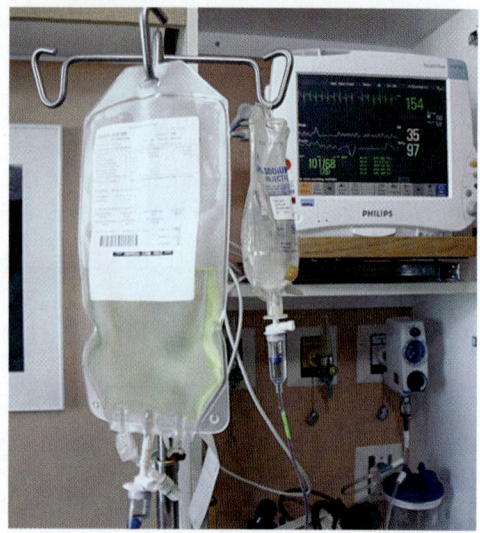

Figure 24-8 Total parenteral nutrition (TPN) is provided for the child who is unable to maintain adequate oral nutritional intake.

Signs and Symptoms

Malnutrition and diarrhea are the most common manifestations of SBS. Additional symptoms include:

- Steatorrhea
- Diarrhea caused by carbohydrate malabsorption
- Fatigue and lethargy
- Abdominal distention
- Foul-smelling stools
- Flatulence
- Weight loss
- Failure to thrive
- Potential for dehydration, acidosis, hyponatremia, and hypokalemia resulting from inadequacy of the short bowel to reabsorb fluid and electrolytes

Diagnosis

Diagnosis is confirmed by abdominal x-ray and ultrasound, endoscopy, colonoscopy, and CBC that reveals anemia. A stool sample may reveal presence of infection; blood; or unabsorbed sugar, fats, and protein.

Prevention

Preventive care is directed toward avoiding or reducing complications related to the disease process and treatment. This may include educating parents on appropriate hydration, nutrition, and medication compliance as well as care of the central line catheter.

Collaborative Care

Nursing Care. The focus of nursing care includes administration and monitoring of nutritional therapy. Care must be taken to avoid the complications of a central venous line (CVN) (a venous access device inserted into the vena cava to infuse fluids and medicines) and total parenteral nutrition (TPN) therapy (Venes, 2013) (Fig. 24-8). In addition, care focuses on maintaining adequate nutrition and preventing complications (Rahhal, 2010).

Administering enteral feeding is also an important part of nursing care. Enteral feeding tube care is also important

because care must be taken to observe for signs of dislodgement, infection, or occlusion. Feeding tolerance must also be included as part of nursing care. Input, output, specific gravity, and weights are assessed daily by the nurse. Stools are tested for occult blood, pH, and reducing substances in addition to monitoring for vomiting, changes in the appearance of the stools, and abdominal distention.

With prolonged hospitalization, the nurse needs to consider the child's emotional and developmental needs. Parents also need to be provided with psychosocial support and education to assist them in coping with the long-term effects of SBS. The plan of care includes attention to interventions to promote family adaptation.

Medical Care. The use of TPN via a central line is part of the initial treatment of SBS. The goal is to wean the child off IV nutrition progressing to enteral feedings via nasogastric or gastrostomy tube as soon as possible (Hennies, Dienhart, & Wessel, 2010; Rahhal, 2010).

Education/Discharge Instructions

The nurse communicates to the parents that the "main purpose of enteral nutrition is to stimulate the adaptive growth of the small intestine" (Rahhal, 2010). Oral feedings may be started as tolerated in order for the infant to learn to suck and swallow. Pacifiers are also encouraged for this purpose. TPN may be gradually decreased as enteral and oral feedings are increased.

Because children with SBS require long-term follow-up and care, parental education focuses on caring for the central line once the child is discharged. Additional instructions include assessing for hydration and managing medications. Teach parents about using a multidisciplinary approach that includes a gastroenterologist, nutritionist, pediatric surgeons, social worker, and speech and behavioral therapy (Rahhal, 2010). Home-care services provide the opportunity for children with SBS to receive carefully monitored care at home. The nurse may serve as a resource for connecting the family to the appropriate home-care agencies, nutritional support services, and supply sources.

Hepatic Disorders

BILIARY ATRESIA

Biliary atresia, or extrahepatic biliary atresia (EHBA), is an idiopathic, progressive, inflammatory process that may involve absence of some or all of the major intrahepatic and extrahepatic biliary ducts resulting in fibrosis and obstruction. Biliary atresia is the second most common liver disease diagnosed in infants with an incidence that ranges from 1 in 10,000 to 15,000 live births and is fatal within the first 2 years of life if not corrected (Schwarz, 2011). The incidence of biliary atresia in the United States is nearly twice as high in non-white infants compared with white infants (Leyva-Vega & Haber, 2010). Studies documenting incidence in certain populations vary though most often state that the ratio of male to female is relatively equal (Sokol & Narkewicz, 2011). The disease is more common in premature infants. The exact cause of biliary atresia is unknown. EHBA has two distinct presentations, postnatal and fetal, with differing mechanisms of development suggested. Infections and immune-related mechanisms are implicated in postnatal EHBS, which represents 65% to 90% of cases (Schwarz, 2011). In the fetal form, there is a congenital absence of patent biliary ducts.

Signs and Symptoms

The earliest clinical manifestation of EHBA and most outstanding feature is jaundice, which can be first observed in the sclera.

- Jaundice may also be evident at birth but usually is not apparent until 1 to 2 weeks of age (Bishop, 2011).
- Urine is dark and stains the infant's diaper.
- Stools are lighter than normal and often tan to white in color.
- The infant demonstrates poor weight gain and symptoms of failure to thrive resulting from poor fat metabolism.
- Pruritus (itching, burning, or tingling of the skin) and irritability are present, which are often evident by an infant who is difficult to comfort.
- Hepatomegaly (enlarged liver) is an early symptom and the liver is firm upon palpitation.
- Splenomegaly (enlargement of the spleen) occurs later (Sokol & Narkewicz, 2011).
- Ascites, bone fractures, and bleeding complications may occur later in life (Sokol & Narkewicz, 2011).

Diagnosis

Early diagnosis is the key to survival of the child with EHBA. Infants who have surgery within the first 60 days of life have an 80% chance of establishing bile flow, with the potential for successful correction. CBC, electrolytes, bilirubin, and liver enzymes are included in the diagnostic workup as well as a TORCH titer (lab test for presence of antibodies for Toxoplasmosis, Other infections, Rubella, Cytomegalovirus, and Herpes simplex) and sweat test (measures electrolytes excreted in a sweat test to rule out cystic fibrosis) to rule out other conditions with symptoms of jaundice and cholestasis. Biliary patency may be demonstrated by hepatobiliary scintigraphy (HIDA scan) but is not diagnostic (Sokol & Narkewicz, 2011). Endoscopic retrograde cholangiopancreatography can be performed in a very young infant and has 80% accuracy. Abdominal ultrasound is used to exclude anatomical abnormalities (Leyva-Vega & Haber, 2010). A percutaneous liver biopsy is used to confirm the diagnosis.

Prevention

Since the cause of biliary atresia is unknown, prevention of complications related to total parenteral nutrition (TPN), compliance with medication management, and education on strategies to promote growth and development is essential. A potential exists for some cases of biliary atresia to be related to postnatal infection and fetal development. Additional preventive activities include good prenatal care and postnatal infection control and parent education.

Collaborative Care

Nursing Care. The nurse educates the family about the disease process, plan of care, and the long-term nature of the condition.

Medical Care. Medical care is primarily supportive and focuses on providing nutritional support. Formula with medium-chain triglycerides and essential fatty acids is recommended as well as supplemental minerals including iron, zinc, and selenium and the fat-soluble vitamins A, D, E, and K. For the infant with moderate to severe failure to thrive, aggressive nutritional support in the form of continuous tube enteral tube feedings or TPN may be required. For advanced liver dysfunction, management is similar to that of the child with cirrhosis.

Surgical Care. Management also involves surgical resection to correct the obstruction and provide for the drainage of bile from the liver into the intestines. The Kasai's procedure, which is a hepatic portoenterostomy, may be performed to slow pathological changes that take place in the biliary duct (Bishop, 2011). Surgery is done as early as possible and preferably before 45 to 60 days of life (Sokol & Narkewicz, 2011). Cirrhosis, hepatic failure, and death occur by 18 to 24 months in the absence of surgical correction or transplant. In surgery done before 3 months of age, bile flow drainage is achieved approximately 60% to 80% of the time (Schwarz, 2011). A hepatic portoenterostomy involves resecting a section of the jejunum to the liver at the normal exit site of the hepatic duct to allow bile drainage into the small intestine. The jejunum may be looped to form a cutaneous double-barreled ostomy (Venes, 2013). Approximately one-third of infants regain normal liver function and become jaundice free after the Kasai's procedure. A middle third demonstrate liver damage and must be supported by medical and nutritional interventions, and the last third eventually require a liver transplant.

Nursing care immediately after a hepatic portoenterostomy is similar to that of the child following other major abdominal surgery. To help the child regain optimal health, providing nutritional support postoperatively involves special formulas, vitamins, and mineral supplements through parenteral and nasogastric tube feedings. For the infant with a double-barreled ostomy, bile is obtained from one site and re-fed into the other site after feeding.

Education/Discharge Instructions

The child's family needs to be instructed on and demonstrate skin and stoma care to be continued after discharge. The family also needs instruction on how to monitor and administer nutritional therapy. Side effects such as pruritus can be addressed through drug therapy and comfort measures. Postoperative risks and long-term complications are explained to include symptoms to observe for such as indications of GI bleeding, ascites (accumulation of fluid in the peritoneal cavity), and cholangitis. Psychosocial support is provided to the child and family to assist them in coping with the long-term nature of the condition, financial burden, uncertain prognosis, and potential waiting for transplant.

CIRRHOSIS

The development of cirrhosis and progressive liver failure characterizes chronic liver disease in childhood (Bishop, 2011). Cirrhosis is a pathological condition that occurs as an end stage to many liver and inflammatory conditions such as biliary atresia and chronic hepatitis leading to the development of diffuse hepatocyte injury, fibrosis, and formation of nodules, which eventually distort the vasculature of the liver leading to further complications such as portal hypertension (Sokol & Narkewicz, 2011). Though chronic liver disease is rare in children, it includes a wide range of disorders, such as malformations, genetic, drug-induced, vascular, infection, and autoimmune disease (Pariente & Franchi-Abella, 2010). Severe liver disease is also a complication of hemophilia and cystic fibrosis, which can lead to cirrhosis or irreversible damage. Chronic inflammation or disease causes scar tissue formation, which leads to impaired intrahepatic blood flow and ongoing necrosis resulting in further cirrhotic changes.

Signs and Symptoms

Manifestations of cirrhosis vary depending on the cause:

- General manifestations include jaundice, growth failure, muscle weakness, anorexia, nausea and vomiting, weight loss, swelling, and lethargy
- Impaired intrahepatic blood flow leads to anemia, abdominal pain, edema, ascites, and GI bleeding
- If the cirrhosis is secondary to a disorder of fat metabolism, such as obesity, hyperlipidemia, and insulin-resistant diabetes, steatorrhea may be observed (Bishop, 2011)
- Portal hypertension and ascites are common symptoms of cirrhosis in the child with biliary anomalies
- Splenomegaly is the most important sign of portal hypertension (Sokol & Narkewicz, 2011). Splenomegaly may be demonstrated by the presence of anemia, leukopenia, thrombocytopenia, and esophageal varices (Bishop, 2011). These conditions lead to easy bruising, epistaxis, and GI hemorrhage (Sokol & Narkewicz, 2011)
- Jaundice, dark urine, and pruritus are symptoms of biliary obstruction

Diagnosis

Diagnosis of cirrhosis is based on history, physical examination, laboratory values, and liver biopsy. Ascites, blood flow through the liver and spleen, and patency of the portal vein can be confirmed by Doppler ultrasonography, MRI or CT of the liver and spleen (Pariente & Franchi-Abella, 2010). Laboratory evaluation includes liver function tests, such as bilirubin, aminotransferase, ammonia, albumin, cholesterol, and prothrombin time. Liver biopsy may reveal evidence of nodules and fibrosis; endoscopy may reveal esophageal varices and bleeding.

Prevention

Preventive care is directed toward avoiding or reducing complications related to the disease process and treatment. This may include educating parents on appropriate hydration, nutrition, and medication compliance as well as care of the central line catheter if needed.

Collaborative Care

Nursing Care. Nursing care of the child with cirrhosis is similar to that of any child with a severe life-threatening disease. Interventions include monitoring for complications of malnutrition, hemorrhage, and hepatic failure in addition to providing comfort measures and emotional support for the child and family.

Medical Care. Goals of care management are similar to that of caring for a child with hepatitis and directed at preventing and treating complications because there is no successful treatment of cirrhosis. Malabsorption problems are treated with nutritional support, such as a low-fat, low-protein diet and supplemental fat-soluble vitamins. Fluid restrictions, diuretics, and low-sodium diet are used to treat ascites. Blood and blood products are administered for the treatment of bleeding complications, and hepatic encephalopathy is treated with a reduced-protein diet.

Surgical Care. The only definitive treatment for end-stage liver disease and cirrhosis is a liver transplant, which improves the prognosis for many children (Sokol & Narkewicz, 2011). A 90% 1-year survival rate has occurred as a result of a combination of surgical techniques and the use of immunosuppressive therapy. Emotional support is essential.

Education/Discharge Instructions

Parent education includes instruction on management of medication side effects and compliance with medication. Education on nutritional needs is important. The family may need referral for financial and/or psychological support as well as recommendations as to where available community resources can be located.

PORTAL HYPERTENSION

Portal hypertension is a common complication of cirrhosis. It is characterized by an "increase in portal vein pressure to more than 5 mm Hg greater than the inferior vena caval pressure" (Sokol & Narkewicz, 2011, p. 657). The increased pressure is caused by resistance to blood flow to and from the liver. The increased pressure causes collateral veins to form. Complications of portal hypertension include GI bleeding and esophageal varices (Sokol & Narkewicz, 2011). Non-cirrhotic causes of portal hypertension include, but are not limited to, acquired abnormalities of the portal and splenic veins, local trauma, peritonitis, pancreatitis, portal or splenic vein malformations, hypercoagulable states, tumor as a complication of bone marrow transplant or chemotherapy for acute leukemia, and congenital hepatic fibrosis (Sokol & Narkewicz, 2011).

Signs and Symptoms

Signs and symptoms of portal hypertension vary with the underlying cause and presentation (Table 24-3).

Diagnosis

Common diagnostic studies are similar to those used to diagnosis cirrhosis.

Prevention

Preventive care is directed toward avoiding or reducing complications related to the disease process and treatment. This may include educating parents on appropriate hydration, nutrition, and medication compliance as well as care of the central line catheter if needed.

Collaborative Care

Nursing Care. Nursing care of the child with portal hypertension is similar to that of any child with a severe life-threatening disease. Interventions include monitoring for complications of malnutrition, hemorrhage, and hepatic failure in addition to providing comfort measures and emotional support for the child and family.

Medical Care. Goals of care management are similar to that of caring for a child with hepatitis and directed at preventing and treating complications. Interventions include monitoring for complications of malnutrition, hemorrhage, and hepatic failure in addition to providing comfort measures and emotional support for the child and family. Bleeding must be controlled if varices are present and may include transfusion and use of vasopressor therapy.

Education/Discharge Instructions

Parent education includes instruction on compliance with medication and observation for and management of medication side effects. Families must be instructed on nutritional

---

Table 24-3 Signs and Symptoms of Portal Hypertension

Signs and symptoms of portal hypertension vary with the underlying cause and presentation.

Presentation	Cause	Signs & Symptoms	Comments
Prehepatic portal hypertention	• Acquired abnormalities of the portal and splenic veins • Portal or splenic vein malformations	• Splenomegaly in an otherwise well child • Recurrent episodes of abdominal distention resulting from ascites • Hematemesis and melena	In neonates there may be a history of omphalitis, sepsis, dehydration, or umbilical vein catheterization. History in older children may include trauma, peritonitis, hypercoagulable disease, or pancreatitis.
Suprahepatic vein occlusion or thrombosis (Budd-Chiari syndrome)	• No cause can be demonstrated in most children • In adults tumor, medication, and hypercoagulable states are common	• Abdominal pain • Tender hepatomegaly or acute onset • Abdominal enlargement caused by ascites • Jaundice • Vomiting • Hematemesis • Diarrhea • Less common: distended superficial veins on the back and anterior abdomen and dependent edema • Generally the signs and symptoms of cirrhosis	Hepatic obstruction may be secondary to tumor, abdominal trauma, hyperthermia, or sepsis. May occur following the repair of an omphalocele or gastroschisis. Oral contraceptive medications may cause hepatic vein thrombosis.
Intrahepatic portal hypertension • Cirrhosis • Veno-occlusive disease • Congenital hepatic fibrosis • Other	• Cirrhosis: see previous section • Veno-occlusive disease: most frequently occurs with bone marrow transplant. May develop after chemotherapy for acute leukemia. Additional causes include ingestion of pyrrolizidine alkaloids (bush tea or other herbal teas), or congenital immunodeficiency states. • Congenital hepatic fibrosis: rare autosomal recessive disorder. • Other: hepatoportal sclerosis, focal nodular regeneration of the liver and schistosomal hepatic fibrosis.		Congenital hepatic fibrosis is generally diagnosed by a liver biopsy. Autosomal recessive polycystic kidney disease is frequently associated with congenital hepatic fibrosis.

Source: Sokol & Narkewicz (2011).

needs. The family may need referral for financial and/or psychological support as well as recommendations as to where available community resources can be located.

 Nursing Insight—*Wilson's disease*

Wilson's disease is an autosomal recessive disease categorized as a chronic hepatic disorder characterized by the accumulation of toxic levels of copper in the liver as well as in the kidneys, brain, and cornea (Manolaki, Nikolopoulou, Daikos, Pangotakaki, Tzetis, Roma, et al., 2008). This disorder leads to injury of hepatic cells. The disease is caused by the mutation of a gene, which is involved in copper integration and transport though a protein (Emerick, 2010). The effect of the gene mutation is a reduced secretion of copper into the bile. This allows for copper accumulation in the hepatic cells.

Symptoms rarely present before age 3 and generally not until the second decade of life. Hepatic and hematological symptoms account for 40% to 60% of symptoms followed by neurological (30%) and psychiatric (10%) symptoms. Hepatic symptoms include jaundice, spider hemangiomas, portal hypertension, and hepatic failure. Treatment involves treatment with copper chelating agents, which is continued throughout life (Bishop, 2011).

NONALCOHOLIC FATTY LIVER DISEASE

The most common form of chronic liver disease in children today is nonalcoholic fatty liver disease (NAFLD), which is estimated to affect 10% of children in the United States (Croke & Sampson, 2012; Sokol & Narkewicz, 2011). The prevalence is related to obesity in the population with most cases occurring in overweight children and is more common in children with type 2 diabetes mellitus or hyperlipidemia (Sokol & Narkewicz, 2011). NAFLD is demonstrated by fatty changes in the hepatocytes and varying degrees of inflammation, swelling, and portal fibrosis (Bishop, 2011).

Signs and Symptoms

Children are often diagnosed during routine screening. NAFLD is insidious; most children are asymptomatic with abnormalities found upon a liver enzyme test or an abdominal ultrasound for an unrelated complaint (Croke & Sampson, 2012). Risk factors include obesity, insulin resistance, hypertension, and dyslipidemia. General complaints include the following:

- Fatigue
- Malaise
- Upper right quadrant discomfort or epigastric pain
- Central adiposity is present in 90% of children
- Hepatomegaly is a common finding (Croke & Sampson, 2012)

Approximately 30% of children diagnosed with NAFLD demonstrate **acanthosis nigricans**, which is indicative of insulin resistance (Sokol & Narkewicz, 2011). Acanthosis nigricans is defined as a chronic inflammatory skin disorder characterized by hyperpigmentation and hyperkeratosis (Venes, 2013).

Diagnosis

Laboratory studies may include elevation of aspartate aminotransferase/alanine transaminase (AST/ALT) ratio, increased prothrombin time, decreased albumin levels, and increased serum bilirubin (Croke & Sampson, 2012). Ultrasound is selected as the imaging study of first choice because of its lack of radiation exposure and cost compared with MRI or CT scan. A liver biopsy may be used to confirm the findings as well as differentiate NAFLD from alcoholic liver disease, though efforts are made to avoid invasive procedures in children who do not demonstrate evidence of excessive alcohol consumption or viral hepatitis (Croke & Sampson, 2012).

Prevention

The incidence of NAFLD can be reduced by decreasing the risk factors associated with obesity, type 2 diabetes mellitus, hypertension, and hyperlipidemia. Preventive activities may include nutritional counseling, weight reduction, increased activity, and medication compliance as appropriate to the cause.

Collaborative Care

Nursing Care. Care of the child and family dealing with NAFLD is primarily directed at early diagnosis, support, and education.

Medical Care. The goal of treatment is to prevent or reverse hepatic damage. Treatment includes diet and exercise. Management includes weight loss, control of hyperlipidemia and blood glucose levels, and behavioral intervention (Pozzato, Verduci, Scaglioni, Randaelli, Salvioni, & Rovere, et al., 2010). Nutritional counseling focuses on a low in saturated fat and high-fiber diet. Research suggests the benefit of nutritional behavioral interventions in reducing liver fat (Pozzato et al., 2010). Oral diabetic agents and/or insulin are used in diabetics to lower A1C levels to under 7.0% (Croke & Sampson, 2012). Studies have found some benefit from the use of vitamin E though strong evidence is lacking (Bishop, 2011; Croke & Sampson, 2012).

Education/Discharge Instructions

NAFLD is considered a family disease because of lifestyle factors. All family members need to be included in treatment and education, which includes nutritional counseling, increasing activity, and medication compliance.

HEPATITIS

Hepatitis may be acute or chronic and involves an inflammation of the liver. Hepatitis may be caused by viral, bacterial, fungal, or parasitic infections; and chemical or drug toxicity. Six distinct viruses have been identified as causing hepatitis: hepatitis A virus (HAV), hepatitis B virus (HBV), hepatitis C virus (HCV), in addition to hepatitis D virus (HDV), hepatitis E virus (HEV), and hepatitis G (HGV), which are not common (Smith, 2011). HAV, HEV, and HGV cause only acute infection. HBV and HCV cause chronic infections, whereas HDV has both acute and chronic forms. HAV and HEV are transmitted via the fecal–oral route, which is referred to as an enteral form of hepatitis. HBV, HCV, HDV, and HGV are transmitted via blood transfer or through intimate sexual contact, which is referred to as a parenteral form. Since the frequency of parenteral HCV transmission from infected blood products has been diminished by routine screening using anti-HCV antibody, the mother-to-infant transmission is now the primary mode of transmission in children, accounting for 60% of cases (Mohan, Gonzalez-Peralta, Fujisawa, Chang, Heller, Jara, et al., 2010). HCV infection may occur in utero or at the time of birth (Mohan et al., 2010). The risk of HCV from illicit IV drug use is 60% to 90% and 10% to 20% for those receiving chronic hemodialysis (Blosser, Brady, & Müller, 2012). Vaccines are available for the prevention of HAV and HBV. Although each type of hepatitis has unique characteristics, assessment findings and treatments have many similarities (Table 24-4).

Most cases of hepatitis in children are caused by HAV and are most common in ages 5 to 14 years (Smith, 2011). HAV is found in the stool of infected individuals and transferred by oral ingestion, which is easily spread in areas with poor sanitation. Poor hygiene is also an important factor in the spread of HAV. High-risk areas also include settings where there are a number of children and infants in a common area, such as day-care centers. Contact may occur directly through infected feces or indirectly through food and water contamination. Outbreaks have occurred in areas that have experienced sewage-contaminated water, infected food handlers with poor hygiene, and shellfish caught in water contaminated by sewage (Sokol & Narkewicz, 2011). The incubation period is 15 to 40 days (Sokol & Narkewicz, 2011).

HDV occurs only in patients with acute or chronic HBV infection, which causes it to be severe. The risk of HDV is reduced with hepatitis B vaccination. HDV is also more common in Mediterranean countries and among hemophiliacs and IV drug users (Blosser et al., 2012). HEV is more common in adults, uncommon in developed countries, and rare in the United States (Sokol & Narkewicz, 2011). High-epidemic areas include Southeast Asia; China; the Middle East; and parts of Africa, Mexico, and Central America (Sokol & Narkewicz, 2011). HEV produces a high incidence of mortality in pregnant women. The high-risk group for HGV includes transfusion recipients, IV drug users, and persons infected with HCV. Individuals infected with HGV are usually asymptomatic for liver involvement.

Signs and Symptoms

Characteristics for HAV, HBV, and HCV overlap considerably, are characteristic of the preicteric phase, and include the following:

- Headache
- Anorexia
- Malaise
- Abdominal pain
- Nausea and vomiting
- Dark urine precedes the jaundice phase (Sokol & Narkewicz, 2011). This phase lasts approximately 1 week and usually precedes the onset of clinically detectable disease (Smith, 2011).

The most common symptoms of the icteric phase include the following and may last several weeks:

- Jaundice
- Hepatomegaly
- Stools may appear clay-colored during this phase (Sokol & Narkewicz, 2011)
- Diarrhea is common in infants; constipation is more common in older children
- Poor weight gain

Prodromal symptoms (initial stages of the disease) often decline in children during the icteric phase (Smith, 2011). Young children are often asymptomatic or have a mild, nonspecific illness without icterus HAV, HBV, and HCV (Table 24-5).

Diagnosis

Diagnosis is based on history of exposure, symptoms, and serological testing for markers of hepatitis A, B, and C and liver function tests, specifically an elevation of ALT (an

---

Table 24-4 Hepatitis Viruses

	HAV	HBV	HCV	HDV	HEV
Type of virus	Enterovirus	Hepadnavirus	Flavivirus	Incomplete	Calicivirus
Transmission	Fecal–oral	Parenteral, sexual, vertical	Parenteral, sexual, vertical	Parenteral, sexual	Fecal–oral
Incubation period	15–40 days	45–160 days	30–150 days	20–90 days	14–65 days
Diagnostic tests	Anti-HAV IgM	HBsAg, anti-HBc IgM	Anti-HCV, PCR-RNA test	Anti-HDV	Anti-HEV IgM
Mortality rate	0.1%–0.2%	0.5%–2%	1%–2%	2%–20%	1%–2% (10%–20% in pregnant women)
Carrier state	No	Yes	Yes	Yes	No
Vaccine available	Yes	Yes	No	Yes (HBV)	No
Treatment	None	Interferon-α, (pegylated interferon in adults) nucleoside analogues (lamivudine, tenofovir, adefovir, entecavir)	Interferon-pegylated interferon plus ribavirin (Copegus, Rebetol)	Treatment for HBV	None

Source: Sokol, R. J., & Narkewicz, M. R. (2011). Liver and pancreas. In W. W. Hay, M. J. Levin, J. M. Sondheimer, & R. R. Deterding (Eds.), *Current diagnosis & treatment in pediatrics* (20th ed., pp. 631–673). New York, NY: Lange Medical Books/McGraw-Hill.

Table 24-5 Comparison of Hepatitis A (HAV), Hepatitis B (HBV), and Hepatitis C (HCV)

Clinical Features	HAV	HBV	HCV
Onset	Usually rapid, acute	More insidious	Usually insidious
Fever	Common and early	Less frequent	Less frequent
Anorexia	Common	Mild to moderate	Mild to moderate
Nausea and vomiting	Common	Sometimes present	Mild to moderate
Rash	Rare	Common	Sometimes present
Arthralgia	Rare	Common	Rare
Pruritus	Rare	Sometimes present	Sometimes present
Jaundice	Present	Present	Present

Source: Sokol, R. J., & Narkewicz, M. R. (2011). Liver and pancreas. In W. W. Hay, M. J. Levin, J. M. Sondheimer, & R. R. Deterding (Eds.), *Current diagnosis & treatment in pediatrics* (20th ed., pp. 631–673). New York, NY: Lange Medical Books/McGraw-Hill.

intracellular enzyme involved in amino acid and carbohydrate metabolism [Venes, 2013]), AST (an intracellular enzyme involved in amino acid and carbohydrate metabolism [Venes, 2013]), and serum total bilirubin. Liver biopsy may be required to establish the diagnosis and degree of disease, although it is rarely indicated in the diagnosis of HAV (Sokol & Narkewicz, 2011). The nurse understands that the presence of antigens or antibodies confirms and differentiates the diagnosis of HAV, HBV, and HCV. Serum immunological tests are not available to detect HAV, but there are two HAV antibody tests: anti-HAV IgG and immunoglobulin M (IgM). Anti-HAV is present at the onset and persists throughout life. A positive anti-HAV test indicates the presence of a current infection, immunity from a past infection, or immunization.

Prevention

Preventive measures include instructing the family on good hand washing (the single most effective preventive measure), food handling, careful disposal of excreta and stool or blood-contaminated objects, and safe sexual activity. Hepatitis A vaccine is recommended for routine immunization of all children beginning at age 12 months and for children who may be living in high-risk communities (Smith, 2011). Administer the second (final) dose 6 to 18 months after the first. Unvaccinated children, 24 months and older, who are at high risk should be vaccinated (American Academy of Pediatrics [AAP], 2012). Hepatitis B vaccine is recommended for routine immunization of all infants beginning at birth and for all children and adolescents through age 18 who have not been previously vaccinated (Smith, 2011).

Collaborative Care

Nursing Care. Nursing care is directed at maintaining comfort and providing adequate nutrition. The goal for management of viral hepatitis includes early detection, support, and monitoring of the disease, recognition of chronic liver disease, and prevention of spread of the disease.

Medical Care. Management of hepatitis is primarily supportive because there is no specific treatment (Smith, 2011). Management includes measures to provide rest to

the liver, hydration, adequate nutrition, and the prevention of complications. Severe dehydration, vomiting, a prolonged prothrombin time, or signs of encephalopathy are indications for hospitalization (Smith, 2011).

Immune globulin is given to children who have been exposed to a person with HAV within 2 weeks of exposure. Immune globulin is up to 90% effective when given during this time period (Blosser et al., 2012). The prognosis for children with HAV is usually good because most cases are mild and in most cases carrier states do not occur. Prevention of HBV infection after a one-time exposure such as a needlestick can be effectively prevented by the use of hepatitis B immune globulin (HBIG).

 Critical Nursing Action Prevention of Hepatitis A and Hepatitis B

Instruct the family on good hygienic practices:

- Wash hands after changing diapers and using the toilet.
- Wash hands before food preparation and eating.
- Carefully dispose of soiled diapers.
- Wash linen or clothing contaminated with stool separately in hot water.
- Clean contaminated household surfaces with bleach and water (1/4 cup of bleach to 1 gallon of water).
- Teach families about the importance of the HAV and HBV vaccinations..

Education/Discharge Instructions

Families need to be educated about preventive measures. Children with mild symptoms can be cared for at home, which necessitates the need to instruct the family regarding infection control, providing a well-balanced diet, and providing rest. Children with HAV are not considered infectious within a week after the onset of jaundice, and school attendance may be resumed. The family also needs to be instructed to avoid administering any medication to the child because normal doses of drugs may become dangerous because of the liver's inability to process them.

LIVER TRANSPLANTATION

Major indicators for liver transplantation in children include end-stage liver disease, acute fulminant hepatic failure, or complications from metabolic liver disorders (Sokol & Narkewicz, 2011). Advances in immunosuppression, improved surgical techniques and postoperative care, and better transplant candidate selection have increased the success of liver transplantation in children. Both cadaveric and living-related liver transplants are available for children in transplant centers. Transplant rejection is the most serious complication, and most children require immunosuppressive drugs for their lifetime (Sokol & Narkewicz, 2011). Repeated transplant occurs in approximately 10% of recipients. Survival rate of at least 2 to 5 years occurs in 80% to 90% of children (Sokol & Narkewicz, 2011). The incidence of liver transplant is approximately 600 children per year, one-third of which are infants with biliary atresia accounting for approximately 55% of transplantation (Turmelle & Sheperd, 2010). The second most common cause at 25% is liver-specific genetic/metabolic diseases such as cystic fibrosis, glycogen storage disease, familial cholestasis, and maple syrup urine disease (Turmelle & Sheperd, 2010). Acute liver failure, which includes Wilson's disease, acetaminophen toxicity, drug toxicities, and viral hepatitis account for approximately 10% of transplantation in children.

Prevention

Prevention can be directed toward reducing additional complications through monitoring for side effects and compliance with drug therapies.

Collaborative Care

Nursing Care. Nursing care of the child awaiting liver transplant is similar to that of any child with a severe life-threatening disease. Interventions include monitoring for complications and providing comfort measures and emotional support for the child and family. Postoperative nursing care includes monitoring for symptoms of rejection and infection. Observe for fever, increasing pain, redness, and swelling of the incisional site and changes in the liver function tests.

Surgical Care. Liver transplantation is the treatment option for acute liver failure and end-stage liver disease. It is the replacement of the diseased liver with a healthy liver allograft.

Education/Discharge Instructions

An important element of postoperative care includes child and family education. Families need to be assessed for their knowledge of the need for lifetime medication. The nurse must also be sensitive to the anxiety faced by families when the child is placed on a transplant waiting list. Family concerns may include issues related to transportation, finances, job loss, and lodging as well as care of other children in the family. A social worker is included on the interdisciplinary team to assist with the coordination of services and resources needed by the child and family.

Abdominal Trauma: Injuries

The leading cause of death in children and adolescents after the first year of life is caused by injuries. Injuries are responsible for more than 50% of all deaths in the 15- to 24-year age group (Lee & Marcdante, 2011). Motor vehicle injuries are the primary cause of accidental death in the United States with nearly 60% occurring with unrestrained children (Lee & Marcdante, 2011). Ten percent of serious trauma to children occurs as a result of abdominal and genitourinary injury, which includes contusion or laceration to liver, spleen, and kidneys (Lee & Marcdante, 2011) (Table 24-6). Nursing care measures include assessment, bedrest, pre- and postoperative care, administration of medications, NG tube and TPN, and education.

Table 24-6 Injuries Caused by Abdominal Trauma

Organ	Incidence and Description	Management
Abdomen	• Approximately 8% of pediatric trauma • Risk of blunt trauma injuries increased because of relative size and close proximity of organs • Penetrating trauma accounts for greater than 10% of pediatric abdominal trauma • Gunshot wounds involve multiple organs in 80% of the cases	• Serial examination is primary in decisions regarding surgical interventions • Surgical intervention may be required if persistent unstable vital signs along with aggressive fluid replacement • Laparoscopy may be indicated with peritoneal irritation and abdominal wall discoloration • CT is valuable for assessing intra-abdominal trauma
Spleen	• Most frequently injured abdominal organ in children • Positive Kehr's sign (pressure on the left upper quadrant eliciting left shoulder pain) related to diaphragmatic irritation from ruptured spleen • Spleen injury suspected with left upper quadrant abrasions or tenderness • Splenic injury may include capsular tear to a complete rupture	• CT scan can be used to grade splenic injury • Treatment of choice is nonoperative management • Surgery indicated for blood loss greater than 40 mL/kg or transfused blood in 24–36 hours or evidence of hemodynamic instability • With splenectomy, penicillin prophylaxis is recommended
Liver	• Accounts for 40% of all deaths associated with blunt abdominal trauma in children • Right lobe injuries are more common • Diagnosis based on Kehr's sign (pressure on the right upper quadrant eliciting right shoulder pain)	• Conservative management is recommended with ongoing monitoring of blood loss, hepatic function, and liver structure with serial CT scans or ultrasound • Operative management is reserved for life-threatening situation

(continued)

Table 24-6	Injuries Caused by Abdominal Trauma (continued)	
Organ	**Incidence and Description**	**Management**
Liver (continued)	• Severe hemorrhage is more common with liver injury than with other abdominal organs	
Pancreas and duodenum	• Less common in children than adults • Seen in bicycle handlebar injuries, motor vehicle crashes, and non-accidental trauma • Diagnosis difficult unless obvious injury to overlying structures • Diffuse abdominal tenderness, pain, and vomiting accompanied by elevation of amylase and lipase may be indicative of injury though often does not occur for several days after injury • Duodenal injuries include hematomas and perforation • Perforations are difficult to diagnose	• Management includes nasogastric suction and parenteral nutrition • Nonoperative management is appropriate for contusions • Surgical interventions may be required with distal transection • Perforation is not always obvious with a CT
Intestinal	• Injury occurs less often than with solid intra-abdominal organs • Risk varies with the amount of intestinal contents, that is, a full bowel is likely to shear more easily than an empty bowel • Lap belt or seat belt in a motor vehicle crash results in a sudden deceleration and increase in intraluminal pressure and can lead to perforation	• Presence of a contusion over the seat belt area and abdomen or back pain indicates a need to pursue the diagnosis of intestinal injury • Pneumoperitoneum in association with intestinal perforation occurs in about 20% of patients

Source: Lee, K. J., & Marcdante, K. J. (2011). The acutely ill or injured child. In K. J. Marcdante, R. M. Kliegman, H. B. Jenson, & R. E. Behrman (Eds.), *Nelson: Essentials of pediatrics* (6th ed., pp. 151–154). Philadelphia, PA: Elsevier.

focus on safety

Child restraints and protection

Injuries to hollow organs are increasing, partly related to the increasing number of improperly restrained children involved in motor vehicle accidents (Lee & Marcdante, 2011). Both parents and children need to be instructed on the proper use of seat belts, booster seats, and infant car seats as well as on the use of protective gear when riding bicycles, skateboards, or scooters.

Summary Points

◆ The gastrointestinal (GI) system of the child is immature compared with that of an adult, leading to variations in response to illnesses.

◆ Pyloric stenosis is characterized by projectile vomiting and a palpable olive-shaped mass in the epigastrium.

◆ One of the most common causes of intestinal obstruction in infancy is from intussusception.

◆ Anorectal malformations are usually evident at birth.

◆ The most common type of hernia in children is an umbilical hernia.

◆ Signs and symptoms of appendicitis include abdominal pain that begins in the periumbilical area and moves to the right lower quadrant, accompanied by a low-grade fever, nausea, and occasionally vomiting.

◆ Treatment focus for inflammatory bowel disease includes medication, nutrition, and often surgery.

◆ Nursing care of the child with celiac disease includes education about the gluten-free diet.

◆ The complications of peritonitis and perforation from appendicitis can be prevented by prompt recognition and diagnosis.

◆ Care of the child with gastroesophageal reflux (GER and GERD) can be managed by teaching the parents feeding and positioning methods to prevent or reduce reflux.

◆ Correction of Hirschsprung's disease involves surgical resection of the affected bowel with or without a colostomy.

◆ Malabsorption disorders include lactose intolerance, celiac disease, and short bowel syndrome.

◆ Progressive cirrhosis and death occur from untreated biliary atresia in most children by age 2.

◆ Cirrhosis is a pathological condition that occurs as an end stage to many liver and inflammatory conditions such as biliary atresia and chronic hepatitis.

◆ Hepatitis may be acute or chronic and involves an inflammation of the liver. Hepatitis may be caused by viral or bacterial infections, fungal or parasitic infections, or chemical and drug toxicity.

◆ Ten percent of serious trauma to children occurs as a result of abdominal and genitourinary injuries, which include contusion or laceration to liver, spleen, and kidneys.

Review Questions

Multiple Choice

1. A 6-week-old infant is admitted to the hospital with possible hypertrophic pyloric stenosis. Which symptom is most descriptive of pyloric stenosis in infants?
   A. Abdominal peristaltic waves passing from right to left
   B. Does not appear hungry without projectile vomiting
   C. Emesis usually occurs after a feeding and is projectile
   D. Decreased interest in feedings with weight loss

2. The pediatric nurse is monitoring a child for signs of bowel perforation. Which assessment finding supports the diagnosis of a bowel perforation?
   A. Acute pain over affected area
   B. Frequent bradycardia
   C. Increased urinary output
   D. An episode of bloody diarrhea

3. A neonate has the diagnosis of imperforate anus. Which definition of this diagnosis will the nurse provide to the neonate's parents?
   A. Complete obstruction preventing passage of stool
   B. Imperfect formation of the anus
   C. Partial occlusion of the anal opening
   D. Absence of a rectal opening

4. Which pediatric gastrointestinal disease is characterized by "skipped" areas of lesions?
   A. Crohn's disease
   B. Ulcerative colitis
   C. Hirschsprung's disease
   D. Malabsorption

5. A child has severe Crohn's disease that has not responded to any pharmacological therapies. Which classification of medication does the nurse anticipate being added to the medication regime?
   A. Corticosteroids
   B. Antibiotics
   C. Immunosuppressants
   D. Biological agents

6. Which nursing action is appropriate when assessing an obturator sign on pediatric patient?
   A. Perform deep palpation, letting up quickly
   B. Passively rotate flexed right thigh
   C. Percuss all four quadrants of the abdomen
   D. Flex the patient's neck sharply to the chest

7. What will the nurse assess with the pediatric patient to determine hematochezia?
   A. Blood in the vomit
   B. Blood in the stool
   C. Bile-colored vomit
   D. Straining with stool

8. A child with cyclical vomiting syndrome is seen in the clinic for another episode of vomiting. Which finding would indicate the need for further assessment by the nurse?
   A. Headache
   B. Photophobia
   C. Fever
   D. Vertigo

9. Which type of lactose intolerance is most prevalent in the pediatric population?
   A. Congenital lactase deficiency
   B. Primary lactase deficiency
   C. Secondary lactase deficiency
   D. Developmental lactose deficiency

10. The nurse is working with the family of a child diagnosed with nonalcoholic fatty liver disease. Which nursing action is the priority?
   A. Encouraging all family members to make healthy lifestyle changes
   B. Preparing the child and family for future liver transplantation
   C. Instructing parents to have genetic testing prior to future pregnancies
   D. Teaching the child and family about having a Kasai's procedure

See Answers to End of Chapter Review Questions on *DavisPlus*.

REFERENCES

American Academy of Pediatrics (AAP). (2012). *Recommended immunization schedule for prsons aged 0 through 6 years.* Retrieved from http://www2.aap.org/immunization/IZSchedule.html

American Academy of Pediatrics (AAP). (2014). Retrieved from http://www.aap.org/en-us/Pages/Default.aspx

Andresen, V., Keller, J., Pehl, C., Schemann, M., Preiss, J., & Layer, P. (2011). Irritable bowel syndrome-the main recommendations. *Deutsches Arzteblatt International, 108*(44), 751–760.

Bai, H. X., Lowe, M. E., & Husain, S. Z. (2011). What have we learned about acute pancreatitis in children? *Journal of Pediatric Gastroenterology and Nutrition, 52*(3), 262–270.

Baker, R., Tsou, V. M., Tung, J., Baker, S. S., Li, H., Wang, W., et al. (2010). Clinical results from a randomized, double-blind, dose-ranging study of pantoprazole in children aged 1 through 5 years with symptomatic histologic or erosive esophagitis. *Clinical Pediatrics 49*(9), 852–865.

Barakat, M., El-Kady, Z., Mostafa, M., Ibrahim, N., & Ghazaly, H. (2011). Antibiotic associated bloody diarrhea in infants: Clinical, endoscopic, and histopathologic profiles. *Journal of Pediatric Gastroenterology and Nutrition, 52*(1), 60–64.

Bishop, W. P. (2011). The digestive system. In K. J. Marcdante, R. M. Kliegman., H. B. Jensen, & R. E. Behrman (Eds.), *Nelson essential of pediatrics* (6th ed., pp. 463–498). St. Louis, MO: Elsevier.

Blosser, C. G. (2012). Complementary medicine. In C. E. Burns, A. M. Dunn, M. A., Brady, N. B. Starr, & C. G. Blosser, *Pediatric primary care* (5th ed., pp. 1085–1129). St. Louis, MO: Elsevier.

Blosser, C. G., Brady, M. A., & Müller, W. K. (2012). Infectious diseases and immunizations. In C. E. Burns, A. M. Dunn, M. A., Brady, N. B. Starr, & C. G. Blosser (Eds.), *Pediatric primary care* (5th ed., pp. 427–493). St. Louis, MO: Elsevier.

Bulechek, G. M., Butcher, H. K., Dochterman, J. M., & Wagner, C. (2013). Nursing interventions classification (NIC) (6th ed.). St. Louis, MO: Elsevier Mosby.

Chen, I., Gao, W., Johnson, A. P., Niak, A., Troiani, J., Korvick, J., et al. (2012). Proton pump inhibitor use in infants: FDA reviewer experience. *Journal of Pediatric Gastroenterology and Nutrition, 54*(1), 8–25.

Choung, R. S., Shah, N. D., Chitkara, D., Branda, M. E., Van Tilburg, M. A., Whitehead, W. E., et al. (2011). Direct medical costs of constipation from childhood to early adulthood: A population-based birth cohort study. *Journal of Pediatric Gastroenterology and Nutrition, 52*(1), 47–54.

Croke, B., & Sampson, D. (2012). Nonalcoholic fatty liver disease: Implications for clinical practice and health promotion. *The Journal for Nurse Practitioners, 8*(1), 45–50.

Cronin, E. (2011). Advances in the management of Crohn's disease. *Nurse prescribing, 9*(10), 499–506.

Dunn, A. M. (2012). Nutrition. In C. E. Burns, A. M. Dunn, M. A. Brady, N. B. Starr, & C. G. Blosser (Eds.), *Pediatric primary care* (5th ed.). Philadelphia, PA: Elsevier Saunders.

Ebach., D. R. (2011). Diarrhea. In W. P. Bishop (Ed.), *Pediatric practice gastroenterology* (pp. 41–54). New York, NY: McGraw-Hill.

Emami, C. N., Garrett, D., Anselmo, D., & Nguyen, N. X. (2010). Single-incision laparoscopic cholecystectomy in a pediatric population: A preliminary report. *The American Surgeon, 76*(10), 1047–1049.

Emerick, K. M. (2010). Wilson's disease. In W. P. Bishop (Ed.), *Pediatric practice gastroenterology* (pp. 356–366). New York, NY: McGraw-Hill.

Gahagan, S. (2011). Behavioral disorders. In K. J. Marcdante, R. M. Kliegman, H. B. Jensen, & R. E. Behrman (Eds.), *Nelson essential of pediatrics* (6th ed., pp. 45–61). St. Louis, MO: Elsevier.

Gaylord, N. M., & Petersen-Smith, A. M. (2012). Genitourinary disorders. In C. E. Burns, A. M. Dunn, M. A. Brady, N. B. Starr, & C. G. Blosser (Eds.), *Pediatric primary care* (5th ed., pp. 809–843) St. Louis, MO: Elsevier.

Gaylord, N. M., & Yetman, R. J. (2012). Perinatal conditions. In C. E. Burns, A. M. Dunn, M. A. Brady, N. B. Starr, & C. G. Blosser (Eds.), *Pediatric primary care* (5th ed., pp. 961–999). St. Louis, MO: Elsevier.

Goldman, R. (2012) Effectiveness of rotavirus vaccine in preventing severe acute gastroenteritis in children. *Can Family Physician. 58*(3): 270–271.

Goldson, E., & Reynolds, A. (2011). Child development and behavior. In W. W. Hay, M. J. Levin, J. M. Sondheimer, & R. R. Deterding (Eds.), *Current diagnosis & treatment in pediatrics* (20th ed., pp. 64–103). New York, NY: Lange Medical Books/McGraw-Hill.

Greenwald, B. J. (2010). Clinical practice guidelines for pediatric constipation. *Journal of the American Academy of Nurse Practitioners, 22*(7), 332–338.

Halbert, K. L. (2011). Nissen vs. toupet fundoplication in the treatment of gastroesophageal reflux disease. *Pediatric Nursing, 37*(4), 171–174.

Hanna, E. (2011). Gastrointestinal bleeding. In W. P. Bishop (Ed.), *Pediatric practice gastroenterology* (pp. 65–79). New York, NY: McGraw-Hill.

Hennies, G., Dienhart, M. C., & Wessel, J. (2010). Nutritional management in short bowel syndrome. *ICAN: Infant, Child, & Adolescent Nutrition, 2*(1), 26–31.

Hitzeman, N., & Romo, C. (2011). Probiotics for persistent diarrhea in children. *American Family Physician, 84*(1), 25–26.

Hoffenberg, E., & Flass, T. (2010). Celiac disease. In W. P. Bishop (Ed.), *Pediatric practice gastroenterology* (pp. 265–276). New York, NY: McGraw-Hill.

Johnson, M., Bulechek, G., Butcher, H., McCloskey Dochterman, J., Maas, M., Moorhead, S., & Swanson, E. (2012). *NANDA, NOC, and NIC linkage: Nursing diagnoses, outcomes, & interventions* (2nd ed.). St. Louis, MO: Elsevier Mosby.

Juckett, G., & Trivedi, R. (2011). Evaluation of chronic diarrhea. *American Family Physician, 84*(10), 1119–1126.

Krebs, N. F., Primak, L. E., & Haemer, M. (2011). Normal childhood nutrition & its disorders. In W. W. Hay, M. J. Levin, J. M. Sondheimer, & R. R. Deterding (Eds.), *Current diagnosis & treatment in pediatrics* (20th ed., pp. 273–299). New York, NY: Lange Medical Books/McGraw-Hill.

Landgren, K., Kvorning, N., & Hallstrom, I. (2011). Feeding, stooling and sleeping patterns in infants with colic – a randomized controlled trial of minimal acupuncture. *Complementary and Alternate Medicine, 11*(93), 1–9.

Lee, K. J., & Marcdante, K. J. (2011). The acutely ill or injured child. In K. J. Marcdante, R. M. Kliegman., H. B. Jensen, & R. E. Behrman (Eds.), *Nelson essential of pediatrics* (6th ed., pp. 141–145). St. Louis, MO: Elsevier.

Leyva-Vega, M., & Haber, B. A. (2010). Biliary atresia. In W. P. Bishop (Ed.), *Pediatric practice gastroenterology* (pp. 330–340). New York, NY: McGraw Hill.

Li, B. U. K., Lefevre, F., Chelimsky, G. G., Boles, R. G., Nelson, S. P., Lewis, D. W., et al. (2008). North American society for pediatric gastroenterology, hepatology, and nutrition consensus statement on the diagnosis and management of cyclic vomiting syndrome. *Journal of Pediatric Gastroenterology and Nutrition, 47*, 379–393.

Lowe, M. E. (2010). Acute and chronic pancreatitis. In W. P. Bishop (Ed.), *Pediatric practice gastroenterology* (pp. 429–440). New York, NY: McGraw Hill.

Maffei, H. V. L., & Vicentini, A. P. (2011). Prospective evaluation of dietary treatment in childhod constipation: High dietary fiber and wheat bran intake are associated with constipation amelioration. *Journal of Pediatric Gastroenterology and Nutrition, 52*(1), 55–59.

Manolaki, N., Nikolopoulou, A., Daikos, G. L., Pangotakaki, E., Tzetis, M., Roma, E., et al. (2008). Wilson disease in children: Analysis of 57 cases. *Journal of Pediatric Gastroenterology and Nutrition, 48*, 72–77.

Marchand, S., Di Lorenzo, C., & Jarczyk, K. S. (2011). Efficacy of fiber supplements in the management of constipation in young children. *ICAN: Infant, Child, & Adolescent Nutrition, 3*(1), 16–20.

Mohan, N., Gonzalez-Peralta, R. P., Fujisawa, T., Chang, M., Heller, S., Jara, P., et al. (2010). Chronic hepatitis C virus infection in children. *Journal of Pediatric Gastroenterology and Nutrition, 50*(2), 123–142.

Moorhead, S., Johnson, M., Maas, M. L., & Swanson, E. (2013). *Nursing outcomes classification (NOC)* (5th ed.). St. Louis, MO: Elsevier Mosby.

Mousa, H. (2010). Disorders of gastrointestinal motility. In W. P. Bishop (Ed.), *Pediatric practice gastroenterology* (pp. 277–294). New York, NY: McGraw Hill.

Pariente, D., & Franchi-Abella, S., (2010). Paediatric chronic liver disease: How to investigate and follow up? Role of imaging in the diagnosis of fibrosis. *Pediatric Radiology, 40*, 906–919.

Park, A. J., Latif, S. U., Ahmad, M. U., Bultron, G., Orabi, A. I., Bhandari. V., & Husain, S. Z. (2010). A comparison of presentation and management trends in acute pancreatitis between infants/toddlers and older children. *Journal of Pediatric Gastroenterology and Nutrition, 51*(2), 167–170.

Petersen-Smith, A. M., & McKenzie, S. B. (2009). Gastrointestinal disorders. In C. E. Burns, A. M. Dunn, M. A. Brady, N. B. Starr, & C. G. Blosser (Eds.), *Pediatric primary care* (4th ed., pp. 795–844). St. Louis, MO: Elsevier.

Phatak, U., & Pashankar., D. (2010). Retrieved from http://naspghan.org/

Pozzato, C., Verduci, E., Scaglioni, S., Randaelli, G., Salvioni, M., Rovere, A., et al. (2010). Liver fat change in obese children after a 1-year nutrition-behavior intervention. *Journal of Pediatric Gastroenterology and Nutrition, 51*(3), 331–335.

Punia, R. P. S., Garg, S., Bisht, B., Dalal, U., & Mohan, H. (2010). Clinicopathological spectrum of gallbladder disease in children. *Acta Paediatrica, 99*, 1561–1564.

Rahhal, R. M. (2010). Short bowel syndrome. In W. P. Bishop (Ed.), *Pediatric practice gastroenterology* (pp. 295–305). New York, NY: McGraw Hill.

Rothenberg, S. S., & Chin, A. (2010). Laparoscopic Collis-Nissen for recurrent severe reflux in pediatric patients with esophageal atresia and recurrent hiatal hernia. *Journal of Laparoendoscopic and Advanced Surgical Techniques, 20*(9), 787–790.

Savino, F., Cordisco, L., Tarasco, V., Locatelli, E., Biola, D. D., Oggero, R., & Matteuzzzi, D. (2011). Antagonistic effect of *Lactobacillus* strains against gas-producing coliforms isolated from colicky infants. *Microbiology, 11*(157), 1–7.

Schwarz, S. M. (2011). *Biliary atresia*. Retrieved from http://emedicine .medscape.com/article/927029-overview

Sherman, C. (2010). Latest review aims to simplify irritable bowel. *Clinical Advisor, 13*(2), 43–46.

Shilyansky, J., & Pitcher, G. (2010). Atresia, webs, and duplications. In W. P. Bishop (Ed.), *Pediatric practice gastroenterology* (pp. 219–232). New York, NY: McGraw Hill.

Siegel, B. S., Alpert, J. J., & Goldstein, R. (2012). The profession of pediatrics. In M. J. Marcdante, R. M. Kliegman, H. B. Jenson, & R. E. Behrman (Eds.), *Nelson essentials of pediatrics* (6th ed., pp. 1–11). Philadelphia, PA: Saunders.

Skjeie, H., Skonnord, T., Fetveit, A., & Brekke, M. (2011). A pilot study of ST36 acupuncture for infantile colic. *Acupuncture Medicine, 29*, 103–107.

Slutsker, B., Konichezky, A., & Gothelf, D. (2010). Breaking the cycle: Cognitive behavioral therapy and biofeedback training in a case of cyclic vomiting syndrome. *Psychology, Health & Medicine 15*(6), 625–631.

Smith, S. (2011). Infectious diseases. In M. J. Marcdante, R. M. Kliegman, H. B. Jenson, & R. E. Behrman (Eds.), *Nelson essentials of pediatrics* (6th ed., pp. 410–413). Philadelphia, PA: Saunders.

Sokol, R. J., & Narkewicz, M. R. (2011). Liver and pancreas. In W. W. Hay, M. J. Levin, J. M. Sondheimer, & R. R. Deterding (Eds.), *Current diagnosis & treatment in pediatrics* (20th ed., pp. 631–673). New York, NY: Lange Medical Books/McGraw-Hill.

Spector, R. E. (2012). *Cultural diversity in health and illness* (8th ed.). Upper Saddle River, NJ: Prentice-Hall.

Starr, N. B., Blosser, C. G., Brady, M. A., Burns, C. E., Dunn, A. M., & Petersen-Smith, A. M. (2012). Gastrointestinal disorders. In C. E. Burns, A. M. Dunn, M. A. Brady, N. B. Starr, & C. G. Blosser (Eds.), *Pediatric primary care* (5th ed., pp. 739–788). St. Louis, MO: Elsevier.

Stevens, M. G., Gentry, B. C., & Michener, M. D. (2008). What is the clinical workup for failure to thrive? *Journal of Family Practice, 57*(4), 264–266.

Strauch, K. A., & Cotter, V. T. (2011). Celiac disease: An overview and management for primary care nurse practitioners. *The Journal for Nurse Practitioners, 7*(7), 588–594.

Studer, K. M. (2011). Use of probiotics to prevent *Clostridium difficile*-associated diarrhea. *The American Journal for Nurse Practitioners, 15*(5/6), 8–12.

Summers, L., Hommel, K., & Todd, R. (2011). IBD in adolescents: Considerations for impact, development, and management. *Infant, Child, & Adolescent Nutrition, 3*(5), 268–273.

Sundaram, S., Hoffenberg, E., Kramer, R., Sondheimer, J. M., & Furuta, G. T. (2011). Gastrointestinal tract. In W. W. Hay, M. J. Levin, J. M. Sondheimer, & R. R. Deterding (Eds.), *Current diagnosis & treatment in pediatrics* (20th ed., pp. 595–630). New York, NY: Lange Medical Books/McGraw-Hill.

Tablang, M. V. F., & Katz, J. (2012). *Viral gastroenteritis*. Retrieved from http://www.emedicine.medscape.com/article/176515-overview

Thilo, E. H., & Rosenberg, A. A. (2011). The newborn infant. In W. W. Hay, M. J. Levin, J. M. Sondheimer, & R. R. Deterding (Eds.), *Current diagnosis & treatment in pediatrics* (20th ed., pp. 1–63). New York, NY: Lange Medical Books/McGraw-Hill.

Turmelle, Y., & Sheperd, R. W. (2010). Liver transplantation. In W. P. Bishop (Ed.), *Pediatric practice gastroenterology* (pp. 403–417). New York, NY: McGraw-Hill.

Uc, A., & Pandrangi, B. (2010). Gastritis and peptic ulcer disease. In W. P. Bishop (Ed.), *Pediatric practice gastroenterology* (pp. 190–200). New York, NY: McGraw-Hill.

Vallerand, A. H., & Sanoski, C. (2014). *Davis's drug guide for nurses* (14th ed.). Philadelphia, PA: F.A. Davis.

Van Leeuwen, A. M., & Poelhuis-Leth, D. J. (2011). *Davis's comprehensive handbook of laboratory and diagnostic tests with nursing implications* (3rd ed.). Philadelphia, PA: F.A. Davis.

Venes, D. (2013). *Taber's cyclopedic medical dictionary* (22nd ed.). Philadelphia, PA: F.A. Davis Company.

Venkatasubramani, N., & Li, B. U. K. (2010). Vomiting. In W. P. Bishop (Ed.), *Pediatric practice gastroenterology* (pp. 19–31). New York, NY: McGraw-Hill.

Weill, V. (2008). Gastroesophageal reflux in infancy. *Advance for Nurse Practitioners, 16*(1), 47–50.

Wiese, D. M., Lashner, B. A., Lerner, E., DeMichele, S. J., & Seidner, D. L. (2011). The effects of an oral supplement enriched with fish oil, prebiotics, and antioxidants on nutritional status in Crohn's disease. *Nutrition in Clinical Practice, 26*(4), 463–473.

Yacob, D., & DiLorenzo, C. (2009). Functional abdominal pain: All roads lead to Rome (criteria). *Pediatric Annals, 38*(5), 253–258.

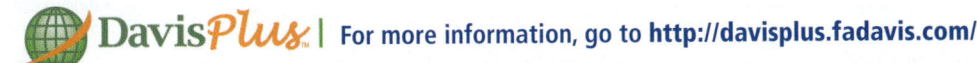

CONCEPT MAP

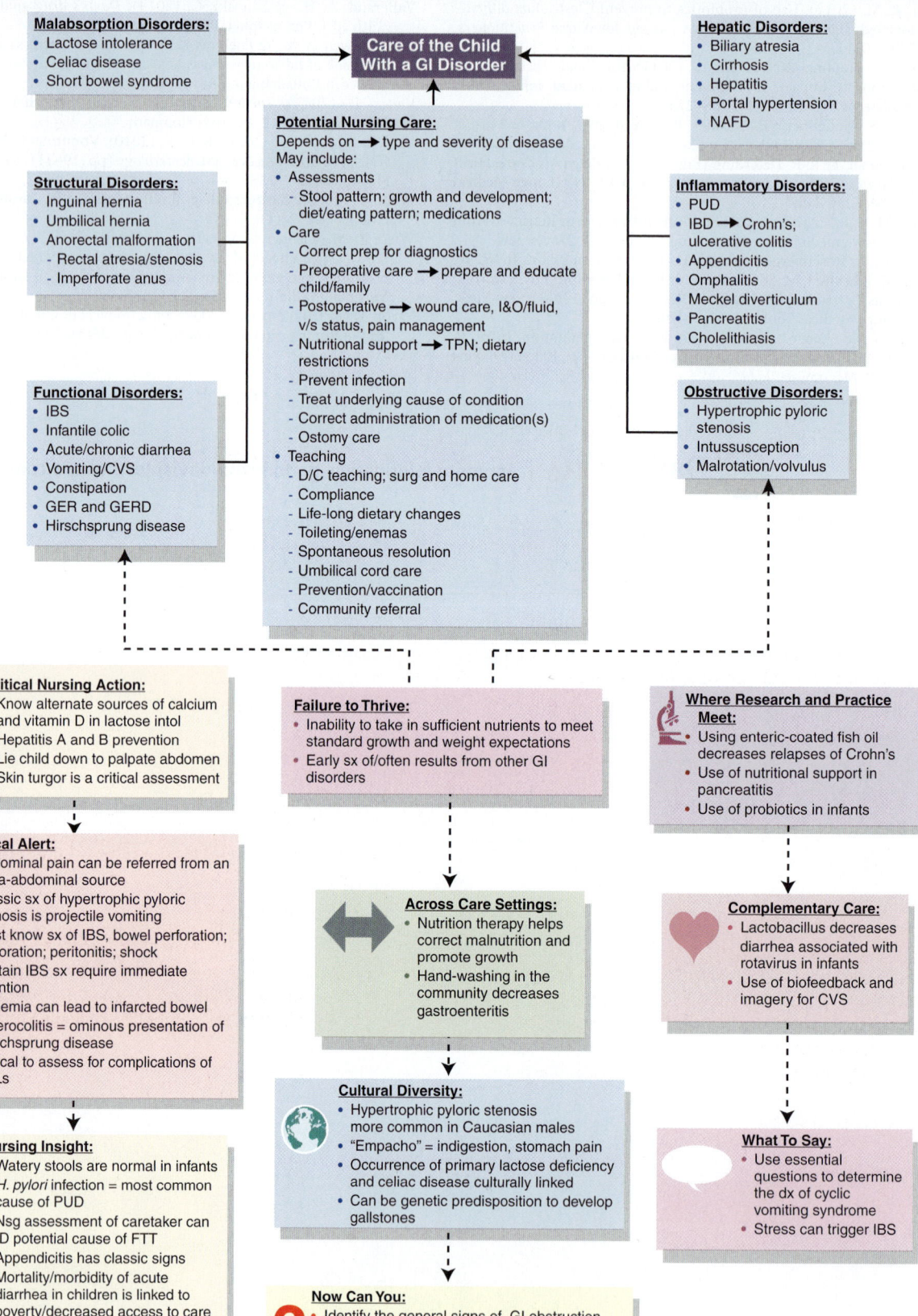

Malabsorption Disorders:
• Lactose intolerance
• Celiac disease
• Short bowel syndrome

Care of the Child With a GI Disorder

Hepatic Disorders:
• Biliary atresia
• Cirrhosis
• Hepatitis
• Portal hypertension
• NAFD

Structural Disorders:
• Inguinal hernia
• Umbilical hernia
• Anorectal malformation
  - Rectal atresia/stenosis
  - Imperforate anus

Potential Nursing Care:
Depends on → type and severity of disease
May include:
• Assessments
  - Stool pattern; growth and development; diet/eating pattern; medications
• Care
  - Correct prep for diagnostics
  - Preoperative care → prepare and educate child/family
  - Postoperative → wound care, I&O/fluid, v/s status, pain management
  - Nutritional support → TPN; dietary restrictions
  - Prevent infection
  - Treat underlying cause of condition
  - Correct administration of medication(s)
  - Ostomy care
• Teaching
  - D/C teaching; surg and home care
  - Compliance
  - Life-long dietary changes
  - Toileting/enemas
  - Spontaneous resolution
  - Umbilical cord care
  - Prevention/vaccination
  - Community referral

Inflammatory Disorders:
• PUD
• IBD → Crohn's; ulcerative colitis
• Appendicitis
• Omphalitis
• Meckel diverticulum
• Pancreatitis
• Cholelithiasis

Obstructive Disorders:
• Hypertrophic pyloric stenosis
• Intussusception
• Malrotation/volvulus

Functional Disorders:
• IBS
• Infantile colic
• Acute/chronic diarrhea
• Vomiting/CVS
• Constipation
• GER and GERD
• Hirschsprung disease

Critical Nursing Action:
• Know alternate sources of calcium and vitamin D in lactose intol
• Hepatitis A and B prevention
• Lie child down to palpate abdomen
• Skin turgor is a critical assessment

Failure to Thrive:
• Inability to take in sufficient nutrients to meet standard growth and weight expectations
• Early sx of/often results from other GI disorders

Where Research and Practice Meet:
• Using enteric-coated fish oil decreases relapses of Crohn's
• Use of nutritional support in pancreatitis
• Use of probiotics in infants

Clinical Alert:
• Abdominal pain can be referred from an extra-abdominal source
• Classic sx of hypertrophic pyloric stenosis is projectile vomiting
• Must know sx of IBS, bowel perforation; perforation; peritonitis; shock
• Certain IBS sx require immediate attention
• Ischemia can lead to infarcted bowel
• Enterocolitis = ominous presentation of Hirschsprung disease
• Critical to assess for complications of CVLs

Across Care Settings:
• Nutrition therapy helps correct malnutrition and promote growth
• Hand-washing in the community decreases gastroenteritis

Complementary Care:
• Lactobacillus decreases diarrhea associated with rotavirus in infants
• Use of biofeedback and imagery for CVS

Nursing Insight:
• Watery stools are normal in infants
• *H. pylori* infection = most common cause of PUD
• Nsg assessment of caretaker can ID potential cause of FTT
• Appendicitis has classic signs
• Mortality/morbidity of acute diarrhea in children is linked to poverty/decreased access to care
• Majority of children have idiopathic or functional constipation
• Avoid frequent infant seat use for infants with GERD

Cultural Diversity:
• Hypertrophic pyloric stenosis more common in Caucasian males
• "Empacho" = indigestion, stomach pain
• Occurrence of primary lactose deficiency and celiac disease culturally linked
• Can be genetic predisposition to develop gallstones

What To Say:
• Use essential questions to determine the dx of cyclic vomiting syndrome
• Stress can trigger IBS

Now Can You:
• Identify the general signs of GI obstruction
• Discuss various treatments for IBD
• Discuss the management of constipation
• Differentiate between regurgitation and GERD
• Differentiate between hepatitis A, B, and C

Caring for the Child With an Immunological or Infectious Condition

 "Infection prevention and control measures aim to ensure the protection of those who might be vulnerable to acquiring an infection both in the general community and while receiving care due to health problems, in a range of settings. The basic principle of infection prevention and control is hygiene"

—World Health Organization, 2014

LEARNING TARGETS *At the completion of this chapter, the student will be able to:*

- ◆ Describe the anatomy and physiology and developmental aspects of the immunological and infectious systems.
- ◆ Examine the common conditions of the immunological and infectious systems.
- ◆ Prioritize developmentally appropriate and holistic nursing care measures for common conditions of the immunological and infectious systems.
- ◆ Explore diagnostic and laboratory testing and medications for common conditions of the immunological and infectious systems.
- ◆ Develop teaching plans and discharge criteria for parents whose children have common immunological and infectious conditions.

PICO(T) Questions

The intent of evidence-based practice (EBP) is to provide nursing care that integrates the best available evidence. An initial step in EBP is to write a PICO(T) question that effectively guides the research. PICO(T) is an acronym that stands for population (P), intervention or issue (I), comparison of interest (C), outcome (O), and timeframe (T). Depending on the question, all or some of the question components are used in the research process. Use these

PICO(T) questions to spark your thinking as you read the chapter.

1. What are the (O) key considerations nurses should explain to (P) parents about (I) childhood immunizations?

2. What (I) nursing interventions are beneficial for school nurses working with (P) students who are HIV positive to assist students with (O) optimal functioning?

Evidence-Based Practice

Secor-Turner, M., Scal, P., Garwick, A., Horvath, K., & Wells, C. K. (2011). Living with juvenile arthritis: Adolescents' challenges and experiences. *Journal of Pediatric Health Care, 25*(5), 302–307.

The purpose of this study was to examine the challenges experienced by adolescents living with juvenile arthritis (JA). The prevalence of JA in persons under 18 years of age is approximately 113/100,000 and considered a common chronic condition of childhood. Children with JA experience joint pain and swelling, activity limitation, and have a higher incidence of depression. Limitations affect home, school, work, and social activities. National priorities have focused on the child to adult transition of care, though even with services in place, more than 50% of youths fail to receive comprehensive follow-up care. Unmet needs reported by youths with JA are often in educational, social, and emotional areas of experiences.

Participants in this study were recruited via e-mail and flyers. Contacts were made through client lists from a local chapter of the Arthritis Foundation and pediatric rheumatology clinics in Minnesota. Eligible participants included youths and young adults with JA between the ages of 14 and 29. A $25 gift card was provided to those who participated in the study. Those who agreed to participate in the study were divided into two groups (i.e., youths ages 14 to 21 and young adults ages 22 to 29). Five persons were in each group. The youth group included 3 females and 2 males, 4 of which were Caucasian. Their mean age was 16.2 years. The young adult group included 4 females and 1 male, of which 4 were Caucasian. Their mean age was 25.4 years.

Semi-structured interview questions were used to guide two focus groups (i.e., youth and young adult groups). One of the researchers was the moderator and note taker for each group with meetings lasting approximately 75 minutes each. Responses to the questions were transcribed verbatim, assigned coded categories, and eventually organized into five themes: health care, relationships, school, physical, and individual/personal. Two of the researchers were involved in the initial reading and coding of the transcripts. An independent third researcher with qualitative research experience resolved disagreements between the two initial coders.

Results were organized and reported under each of the five identified themes. For those in the youth groups, many of the health care–related challenges focused around medications and included cost, taking medications, and finding the medications that were effective. Concern was expressed over the need to battle insurance companies to get coverage for specific medications (e.g., etanercept [Enbrel]). Young adults reported that their biggest concerns were in managing health-care services, switching from a pediatric to adult rheumatologist, obtaining insurance, and family planning issues. These results are consistent with previous studies.

Relationship issues for youths focused on telling others about their disease and the lack of understanding by others. The young adult group noted that they had similar challenges with disclosure during their teen years. Young adults further noted concern with dating and feelings of isolation because they did not know other young adults with JA. Previous studies have identified social support as a key need for youths and young adults, and both desire health-care services to go beyond the medical aspects to include social and emotional needs.

School challenges were reported by the youth group to include involvement in sports, participating in gym class, doing schoolwork, and discussing JA with teachers. One participant noted that a teacher indicated that she needed to try harder and yelled at her, stating that she needed an attitude adjustment because she became tired during gym class. The young adult group noted that they had experienced similar challenges during their adolescence. Research notes that adolescents with JA are 17 times more likely to experience limitations in activities in a variety of settings.

Physical challenges for the youth group included managing pain and exercise. The young adult group noted the same concern, as well as a concern about the need to use assistive devices during their adolescence. Research notes that pain and decreased function has been associated with higher levels of depression.

The youth groups did not describe individual challenges, though the young adult group indicated concerns over feeling different than peers. They also noted that they missed out on activities because they often did not feel well.

The researchers concluded that variations between the two groups reflected developmental differences. Youths were more concerned with peer identification and less future oriented. Challenges were related to the present. Young adults were more concerned with the transition into adulthood, personal responsibility for their care, and forming relationships.

1. How is this information useful to clinical nursing practice?

2. Based on these findings, what are implications for further research?

See Suggested Responses for Evidence-Based Practice on Davis*Plus*.

Introduction

This chapter provides a review of the anatomy and physiology and developmental aspects of the immune system. The discussion includes an examination of the various infectious and immune conditions including developmentally appropriate and holistic nursing care. Information about diagnostic and laboratory testing and medications is given. Teaching plans and discharge criteria for parents whose children have various infectious and immune conditions are incorporated.

Growth and Development

The child with an infectious condition is usually isolated to control the spread of disease. Isolation from peers allows for limited exposure to play and social activities such as school. Limited interaction in social experiences can be detrimental to the child's growth and development. Nursing care for the child with an infectious condition focuses on treatment of the infectious disease process and maintenance of normal growth and developmental milestones. Because of the hyper-metabolic state that accompanies infection or illness, an adequate diet should be encouraged. The nurse should initiate a high-calorie diet to promote a healthy immune system. Proper hydration should be provided to reduce the risk of dehydration. The child should be given adequate rest periods as needed during recovery. Quiet activities can be initiated if the child has low levels of energy.

If the child is placed in isolation, the nurse should work with the child life therapist and the family members to provide appropriate toys and stimulation to the child. Social isolation limits the child's ability to develop and maintain interpersonal and verbal and nonverbal communication skills. Social interaction should be encouraged when appropriate. The nurse should provide education about prevention strategies and appropriate immunizations needed to reduce the rate of infection.

 Nursing Insight—*Public health concern*

Infectious and immune conditions represent a significant pediatric public health concern for the child, family, and the public. Prevention and control of infections and communicable diseases is a primary goal of national, state, and local health agencies, addressed largely through surveillance, public education, and immunization programs. Pediatric nurses are at the forefront of these efforts and are responsible for nursing care of children and families, as well as assisting families to become informed and educated so that they can take an active role in caring and advocating for their children.

A & P review An Important Line of Defense

The immune system protects the child from an attack of foreign intruders. The immune system is made up of cells, tissues, and organs that work in an organized manner to protect the body against invaders and infectious organisms (Fig. 25-1). At birth children have an intact, but often immature, immune system. Infants do carry maternal antibodies until approximately 6 months of age; however, they remain at a greater risk for infection than the general population. Germs, including bacteria and viruses, are foreign invaders, or *antigens*, which the immune system recognizes and responds to by producing proteins called *antibodies* to fight the antigens. Antibodies may be produced in the thousands but sometimes disappear after they have destroyed the antigens. Memory cells are cells that recall the original antigen and bring up the body's defenses if it invades the body again, and this level of protection is known as immunity (Centers for Disease Control and Prevention [CDC], 2013a).

The white blood cells (leukocytes) are part of the defense system. There are two basic types: phagocytes (neutrophils are the most common and fight bacteria) and lymphocytes (B lymphocytes and T lymphocytes), which seek out and destroy organisms that might cause disease. Leukocytes are produced or stored in the lymphoid organs: lymph nodes, bone marrow, thymus, spleen, and tonsils. The leukocytes circulate throughout the body via the blood. Antigens are foreign substances that invade the body. When an antigen is detected, several types of cells work together to recognize and respond to the invader. Mature B lymphocytes independently identify foreign antigens and differentiate into antibody-producing plasma cells (memory cells). Once the B lymphocytes have produced antibodies, these antibodies remember the invader so if the same antigen is presented to the immune system again, the antibodies can respond. Although antibodies can recognize an antigen, they are not capable of destroying it without the help of mature T cells that are antigen specific. Antibodies can also neutralize

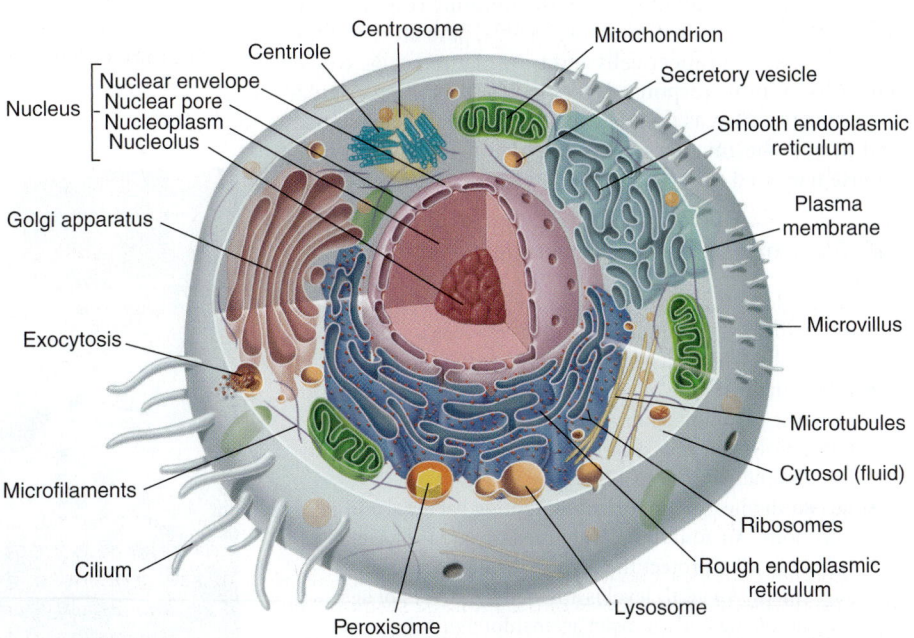

The Human Cell

Centrosome
Centriole
Mitochondrion
Secretory vesicle
Nuclear envelope
Nuclear pore
Nucleoplasm
Nucleolus
Nucleus
Smooth endoplasmic reticulum
Golgi apparatus
Plasma membrane
Microvillus
Exocytosis
Microtubules
Cytosol (fluid)
Microfilaments
Ribosomes
Cilium
Rough endoplasmic reticulum
Peroxisome
Lysosome

Figure 25-1 Typical cell.

toxins and activate a group of proteins that assist in killing bacteria, viruses, or infected cells.

The protection offered by the immune system is called immunity. There are three types of immunity: innate, adaptive, and passive. Innate (or natural) immunity is a general protection and includes the physical barriers of the body, like the skin and mucous membranes. The skin is the first line of defense in preventing diseases from entering the body. Adaptive (or active) immunity develops as children are exposed to diseases or immunized against diseases through vaccination. Passive immunity is acquired by the introduction of preformed antibodies into an unprotected individual, and it lasts for a short period of time. For example, passive immunity can occur from antibodies that pass from the mother to the fetus through the placenta or newborns that acquire immunity through breastfeeding.

The Body's Defense

The skin is the most important physical barrier and the body's first line of defense. It is the largest organ of the body and has several major functions:

- Protects the deeper tissues from injury
- Protects the body from foreign matter invasion
- Regulates temperature
- Aids in water retention
- Aids in synthesis of vitamin D
- Initiates the sensations of touch, pain, heat, and cold
- Mucous membranes provide a protective barrier against the entry of pathogens

Mechanical and chemical barriers also help protect the child. For instance, tears, urine, vaginal secretions, and semen have a role in primary defense against infection. The mechanical action of these fluids flowing out from the body carries with it unwanted intruders that may cause disease. An example of a chemical barrier is the acidic secretions of the stomach and digestive enzymes that serve to neutralize organisms taken into the body through the mouth. Chemical barriers in the gastrointestinal system can be maintained with good nutrition.

The body's second line of defense is the **immune response**. The overall purpose of the immune response is to defend the body against microorganisms, parasites, and foreign cells such as cancer cells and transplanted cells. Key to a normal immune response is the body's ability to recognize foreign substances as non-self and then to mobilize defenses and attack the invaders. A deficiency in the immune response may lead to serious illness in the pediatric patient. ◆

❋ Nursing Insight—*Immunoglobulins*

Immunoglobulins, also known as antibodies, are substances made by the body's immune system in response to diseases and other insults. The major types of immunoglobulins are:

- IgM is the first type of antibody made by the body in response to an infection. This antibody helps other immune system cells destroy foreign substances. An adult level is attained by 9 to 12 months of age.
- IgG antibodies are important in fighting bacterial and viral infections. An adult level is attained by 1 year of age.
- IgA antibodies protect the body's surface from foreign substances. An adult level is attained by 5 years of age.
- IgE causes the body to react against foreign substances such as fungus spores, animal dander, and pollen. An adult level is attained by early childhood.

❝What to say❞—*Children are more vulnerable to infections*

Parents ask why children are more vulnerable to infections. Not all situations are alike so it is important that the nurse tailor the response to the situation. Here is sample information the nurse can share with parents.

1. The skin has a thinner texture that is more susceptible to external irritants and a greater risk for the absorption of microorganisms because of the greater body surface area than adults.
2. Immunoglobulin A (IgA), secreted by the epithelial cells of the mucous membranes, does not reach adult levels until the child is 5 years of age, making children less resistant to organisms.
3. The endocrine glands that secrete sweat are not capable of mature function until 3 years of age, making children less able to regulate body temperature.

A way to help ensure a healthy immune system is to educate the family about the role of the immune system and the natural processes that help the body maintain resistance to disease. Nurses can support the child's immune system through nursing interventions such as meticulous skin care and measures that target the maintenance of important barriers (Fig. 25-2).

Congenital Immunodeficiency Disorders

Congenital immunodeficiency disorders of childhood include a number of rare disorders possibly associated with mutant genetic defects. These disorders, grouped as primary immunodeficiency disorders (PID), may result in lifelong impairment of immune system function. The impairment causes an increase in incidence, severity, and recurrence of infections.

There are four main groups of PID:

- Antibody deficiency, B lymphocyte defect
- Combined deficiency, T and B lymphocyte defect

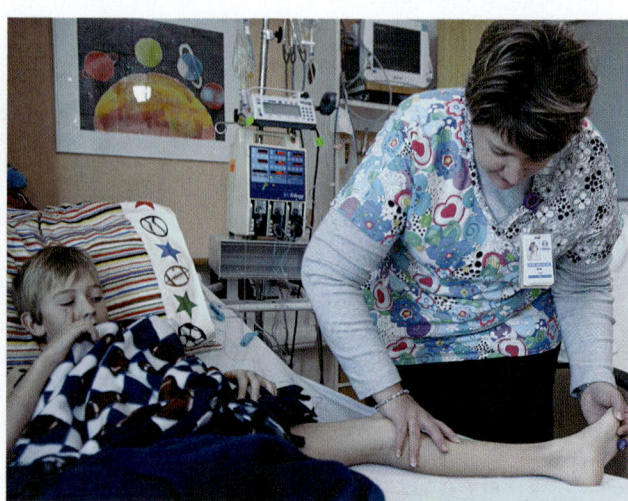

Figure 25-2 Assessing and maintaining skin care is an important role of the nurse.

- Phagocyte defect disorders (neutrophil or mononuclear cell disorders)
- Complement defect disorders (bacterial protein disorders)

ANTIBODY DEFICIENCY: B-CELL DISORDERS

In B-cell disorders, inadequate immunoglobulins are present. Maternal antibodies naturally protect newborns during the first few months of life; thus B-cell disorders do not become apparent until after 3 to 6 months of age, and some do not occur until later childhood or adulthood. In B-cell disorders, the child usually has recurrent infections, beginning with respiratory infections, sinus infections, and pneumonia. Some children have chronic gastrointestinal (GI) malabsorption syndromes and inflammatory bowel disease (e.g., Crohn's disease and ulcerative colitis) (Stewart, Johnston, & Liu, 2014).

COMBINED DEFICIENCY T- AND B-CELL DISORDERS

Diseases affecting B and T lymphocytes usually manifest before 6 months of age. Babies may have failure to thrive and suffer from severe infections, including septicemia and meningitis. Other features of this disorder cluster include recurrent candidiasis and prolonged diarrhea, both of which may cause severe diaper dermatitis. In these disorders, **opportunistic** infections caused by *Pneumocystis jiroveci* pneumonia and *Toxoplasma gondii* are seen (Stewart et al., 2014).

PHAGOCYTE DEFECT DISORDERS

These disorders also can occur very early in a child's life. They are manifested with dermatitis, impetigo, mouth ulcers, pneumonia, suppurative adenitis (infected lymph nodes), abscesses, and **osteomyelitis.** Wounds in children with this immune disorder do not heal properly.

COMPLEMENT DEFECT DISORDERS

This group of disorders can arrive at any age in childhood. Severe infections including meningitis, septicemia, and sinus or pulmonary infections are common. Associated autoimmune disorders may occur, including systemic lupus erythematosus, dermatomyositis, and scleroderma.

Signs and Symptoms

A good way of identifying if a child has primary immunodeficiency is by using Modell's 10 Warning Signs of Primary Immunodeficiency:

- 8 or more ear infections per year
- 2 or more serious sinus infections per year
- 2 or more months on antibiotics with little effect
- 2 or more pneumonias within 1 year
- Failure of infant to gain weight or grow normally
- Recurrent, deep skin or organ abscesses
- Persistent thrush in the mouth or on the skin after 1 year of age
- Need for IV antibiotics to clear infections
- 2 or more deep seated infections
- Family history of primary immunodeficiency (Stewart et al., 2014)

Diagnosis

Diagnosis of congenital immunodeficiency disorders is based on symptoms of congenital immunodeficiency disorders that begin in infancy. The actual diagnosis depends on the exact immune components involved. Laboratory testing should include a full blood count and immunoglobulin levels (especially IgA, IgG, and IgM). Additional tests will be ordered depending on the suspected disorder.

Prevention

Most primary or congenital immunodeficiency disorders are genetic and not preventable, but good prenatal care and education regarding care can decrease the associated clinical manifestations.

 Nursing Insight—Other common types of congenital immunodeficiency disorders

The onset of X-linked agammaglobulinemia occurs after 4 months of age, typically in males with low or absent IgM, IgG, and IgA antibodies and B lymphocytes. Treatment of these congenital immunodeficiency disorders is lifelong with the administration of intravenous immune globulin (IVIG) or (IV IgG [immunoglobulins]).

- **Autosomal recessive congenital agammaglobulinemia:** the onset is before 6 months, with both male and females affected. There are low B lymphocytes as well as low or absent immunoglobulins. IVIG treatment is lifelong.
- **Hypogammaglobulinemia:** selective IgA deficiency is the most common abnormality in this family, but there is no treatment specific to IgA except antibiotics or sometimes IVIG. It is possible to have acquired hypogammaglobulinemia from such disorders as nephrotic syndrome, and it is possible to have transient hypogammaglobulinemia and only antibiotics may be needed.
- **Severe combined immunodeficiency diseases (SCID):** includes T and B lymphocyte disorders, frequent prolonged diarrhea, and failure to thrive. Without treatment, children with SCID will usually die within the first years of life. Laboratory testing includes hypogammaglobulinemia and lymphopenia. Natural killer cells and B lymphocytes are often decreased. *Pneumocystis jiroveci* pneumonia with cough, dyspnea, and hypoxia is common as is persistent candida diaper dermatitis. Tonsils and lymph nodes may be absent. The main differential diagnosis is with pediatric HIV. There are several variants of SCID (Stewart et al., 2014).

Collaborative Care

Nursing Care. Nursing care for patients with congenital immunodeficiency disorders is complex, depending on the disorder. Many of these affected children are infants, and families are devastated by the diagnosis of these complex disorders.

The nurse obtains blood samples for laboratory tests based on the health-care provider's order. A complete blood count (CBC) with differential, immunoglobulin levels (IgA, IgG, IgM), T and B lymphocyte tests, and protein electrophoresis are drawn to determine types of immunoglobulin disorders. Additionally, pre- and post-immunization titers for routine immunizations (e.g., tetanus, diphtheria, mumps, and rubella) are drawn. These titers determine if the child has enough immunity to form a response to these immunizations. The nurse is instrumental in monitoring for frequency of infections, lack of response to antibiotic therapies, and the development of more severe infections, such as *Pneumocystis jiroveci* pneumonia. It is important to note that some live vaccinations may be contraindicated in immune disorders.

Education/Discharge Instructions

The nurse tells the family that continued monitoring of growth and development on standardized growth charts is done to assess for failure to thrive or weight loss patterns. Family support and education is essential to properly care for the child. Refer families to support groups and healthcare specialists.

 Nursing Insight—*Wiskott–Aldrich syndrome*

Wiskott-Aldrich syndrome is an example of an x-linked immunodeficiency syndrome occurring from genetic mutation but only occurring in males.

This disorder includes **thrombocytopenia** and eczema, so the symptoms include potential bloody diarrhea, cerebral hemorrhage, and later malignancies and autoimmune syndromes. Differential diagnosis includes leukemia and **idiopathic thrombocytopenic purpura (ITP)**. Survival later than adolescence is rare without treatment, which includes antibiotic prophylaxis with trimethoprim sulfamethoxazole (TMP-SMZ) (Bactrim or Septra) for *Pneumocystis jiroveci* pneumonia and IgG replacement therapy. Splenectomy is a possibility to decrease thrombocytopenia, and stem cell transplant can offer a cure (Stewart, et al., 2014).

Human Immunodeficiency Virus (HIV [AIDS])

HIV is the primary cause of AIDS in infants and children. The HIV virus selectively targets and destroys T helper cells (i.e., T4 or CD4), thereby destroying cellular immunity. The child is virtually unprotected against a number of opportunistic infections and bacterial, fungal, and viral diseases. Every system is potentially affected because the HIV virus integrates itself into the patient's genetic material (Fahrner & Romano, 2010) (Box 25-1).

However, the body's immune response may raise CD4 (helper T cell) levels for some time, creating a latent period that may last 10 years or more, before the child becomes sick. When CD4 levels drop, symptoms begin to appear and the change from HIV to AIDS begins. The Centers for Disease Control and Prevention (CDC) (2013b) indicate

that children who become infected with the HIV virus between 13 and 25 years old survive longer than people who become infected later in life. If a baby acquires HIV prenatally, the latency period may be brief and the child becomes ill quickly, developing AIDS in the first year of life, with a poor prognosis. Statistics show that from 1994 to 2006 mortality has decreased by 76% for HIV-infected children (Fahrner & Romano, 2010).

 Nursing Insight—*HIV in infants*

The following factors are associated with HIV in infants:

- Advanced maternal disease
- High maternal viral load
- Low maternal CD4+ count
- Prematurity
- In utero transmission
- High viral load in the first 2 months of life
- Lack of neutralizing antibodies
- Presence of p24 antigen
- AIDS-defining illnesses
- Early cytomegalovirus infection
- Early neurological disease
- Mycobacterium avium complex and anemia
- Failure to thrive
- Early-onset diarrhea

(Rivera, 2011)

Signs and Symptoms

Signs of HIV in children can include any of the following:

- Lymphadenopathy
- Hepatosplenomegaly and hepatitis
- Chronic diarrhea, with malabsorption
- Failure to thrive
- Oral thrush
- Skin infections
- Fevers
- Recurrent infections, including mucous membrane and skin infections
- Thrombocytopenia
- Developmental delay and loss of milestone achievements

Resulting conditions include:

- Cardiomyopathy
- Nephropathy

Diagnosis

Diagnostic testing for HIV infection in children is necessary whenever there is a suspicion that the child may have the virus. Diagnosis of HIV infection in children requires a multipronged approach using appropriate testing and clinical observation. In infants, the diagnosis can be complicated by the transmission of maternal antibodies. The CDC developed a separate classification system for pediatric HIV or AIDS in 1987 and then revised it in 1994 for children younger than 13 years. Because of passively acquired maternal antibodies in the first 18 months of life, there are separate criteria for this age group because this may confuse the infant's status with regard to HIV infection.

Box 25-1 Pancytopenia

Pancytopenia is an issue for children with HIV that may cause thrombocytopenia (low platelet count). Intravenous immune globulin (IVIG) is used to raise the platelet count. Another way to raise the platelet count is to use high-dose steroids. Sometimes WBC abnormalities also occur, including neutropenia, leukopenia, and lymphopenia. Epoetin alfa (Erythropoietin) is a newer medication that increases RBC and WBC production in such cases (Fahrner & Romano, 2010).

Labs: HIV Testing in Infancy

The HIV Nucleic Acid (RNA and DNA) Assay Test is the best diagnostic test, and the results are available within 1 week.

HIV blood cultures are a good diagnostic test. These cultures are expensive, and the results are available in 4 to 6 weeks.

The p24 antigen assay test measures the viral capsid (core) p24 protein in blood that is detectable during an acute infection. This test is most accurate at 6 months of age when maternal antibodies start to decline. Because these tests are not available in all sites, refer the family to a research center or the nearest pediatric HIV specialty center (Farhner & Romano, 2010).

For children age 13 and older, HIV antibody testing is the same as for adults, using the enzyme-linked immunosorbent assay (ELISA) test that identifies the presence of HIV antibodies. If the initial ELISA antibody test is positive, it merits repeating, and if the repeat test is still positive, it is necessary to add the Western blot test, which is a confirmatory indirect fluorescent antibody test.

Other tests that are now available have less accuracy. They include an oral fluid (not saliva) antibody test that needs a confirmatory Western blot, a urine test that needs a confirmatory Western blot, a rapid test that uses blood from a finger stick or oral fluid, and home testing kits. Only one kit, Home Access HIV Test System, using a finger prick, is approved by the Food and Drug Administration (National HIV and STD Testing Resources, CDC, 2012).

Prevention

The nurse should counsel pregnant women to follow the guidelines for mandatory HIV testing. This is the most significant way to decrease vertical transmission of HIV. Secondly, as the American Academy of Pediatrics Committee on Pediatric AIDS and Committee on Adolescence has noted, half of all new HIV infections in the United States are occurring among youths from ages 13 to 24 (Pediatric Clinical Practice Guidelines and Policies by the American Academy of Pediatrics, 2011). Therefore, nurses are instrumental in educating adolescents about HIV transmission, prevention, and testing. Use of condoms and safe sexual practices are also essential information for adolescents to hear.

Collaborative Care

Nursing Care. Caring for children with HIV or AIDS is a complex process that includes physical, psychological, and family care. The pediatric nurse assesses the family's support systems, coping mechanisms, and overall ability to care for the HIV-infected child. Social stigma is frequently associated with this diagnosis, and many families may feel isolated and face rejection. Because the diagnosis and treatment for HIV cause a family crisis, it is vital for the pediatric nurse to provide psychological support, monitor infection, manage pain, provide developmental care, monitor nutrition and immunizations, and focus on proper medication administration.

INFECTION. The primary concern for early and accurate identification of children with HIV infection is beginning treatment. The goals of treatment for children with HIV are to slow progression to AIDS, prevent further infections, promote normal growth and development, prevent complications including cancers, and prolong and improve quality of life.

If the mother is also infected with HIV, the nurse determines the best way to care for both patients. Priority nursing care focuses on decreasing the potential for opportunistic infection.

Nursing Insight—*Opportunistic infections*

HIV-infected children are at risk for infections that a child with normal immunity would not acquire and thus the term "opportunistic" is used to describe these infections. *Pneumocystis jiroveci* pneumonia is the most common opportunistic infection in children. The nurse must be ready to manage the infections that the child acquires. Often prompt and vigorous antimicrobial therapy for treatment of infections is needed. For this reason, according to current CDC (2013b) HIV and Resources Guidelines, all infants born to HIV-infected mothers are routinely started on a prophylactic antibiotic regimen for this organism. Trimethoprim sulfamethoxazole (TMP-SMZ) (Bactrim or Septra) is the agent of choice for this treatment. Intravenous immune globulin (IVIG) has also been used to prevent bacterial infections in young children. In addition, the nurse teaches the family signs and symptoms of infection and encourages them to limit the child's exposure to large crowds of people and to those with notable infections.

Candidiasis, a fungal infection, is the most common pathogen experienced by infected children, seen most easily with oral thrush and diaper dermatitis that are recurrent. Treatments include oral or topical nystatin (Mycostatin) and oral clotrimazole (Mycelex) troches. Other oral agents (e.g., ketaconazole [Nizoral] and fluconazole [Diflucan]) are used for resistant cases under special precautions.

Medication: Trimethoprim sulfamethoxazole (TMP-SMZ) (Bactrim or Septra)

(trye-**meth**-oh-prim/sul-fa-meth-**ox**-a-zole)

Indications: Prevention of *Pneumocystis jiroveci* pneumonia. Prevention of bacterial infections in an immunosuppressed child.

Actions: Combination inhibits the metabolism of folic acid in bacteria at two different points.

Therapeutic Effects: Bactericidal action against susceptible bacteria.

Contraindications and Precautions:
CONTRAINDICATED IN: Hypersensitivity to sulfonamides or trimethoprim, megaloblastic anemia secondary to folate deficiency, severe renal impairment, and children younger than 2 months of age.

Adverse Reactions and Side Effects: Hepatic necrosis, nausea, vomiting, diarrhea, toxic epidermal necrolysis, Stevens-Johnson syndrome, erythema multiforme, rashes, agranulocytosis, aplastic anemia, and phlebitis with IV insertion.

Nursing Implications:
1. Assess child for infection. Advise the family to notify the health-care provider for any signs of infection.
2. Assess for allergy to sulfonamides.
3. Monitor lab values periodically throughout therapy. May produce elevated serum bilirubin, creatinine, and alkaline phosphatase.

Source: Data from Vallerand, A. H., & Sanoski, C. A. (2014). *Davis's drug guide for nurses* (14th ed.), Philadelphia, PA: F.A. Davis.

The pediatric nurse addresses infection control information for day-care providers and school personnel about how to care for frequent diarrhea and to assess for candidiasis infections. These issues may create problems with diaper changes and keeping the genital areas free of a superinfection. Caretakers must use gloves properly and carefully, and body secretions must be properly disposed of in biohazardous waste containers. Universal precautions are enforced in all public areas and are especially important during participation in contact sports, during menstruation in girls, and for all sexually active teens.

PAIN MANAGEMENT. Pain management is a significant care concern for children with HIV. Pain in children can be multifactorial, resulting from inflammation, or from systemic manifestation of AIDS such as cardiomyopathy, drug toxicities, invasive secondary infections, and medical procedures used to monitor and treat the HIV infection. The majority of HIV-infected children report pain as a factor affecting their daily lives. Successful management of pain is based on the same principles of pain management found in other illnesses. Diligence in identification of pain, goals, and strategies to manage pain, implementation of nonpharmacological and pharmacological pain management strategies, and ongoing pain assessments are all-important in the plan of care. Pain control is a major factor in quality of life and hence a primary goal for the nurse.

 Complementary Care: *Nonpharmacological Adjuncts to Pain Management*

Pain management in children with HIV can be challenging. Proper pain management involves both pharmacological and nonpharmacological strategies. Nonpharmacological techniques are based on the child's own experiences and preferences. Some examples of nonpharmacological techniques include guided imagery, hypnosis, prayer, meditation, music, or aromatherapy. Nonpharmacological techniques such as *preparation, distraction,* and *relaxation* help with pain control for the child.

DEVELOPMENTAL CARE. Developmentally appropriate *preparation* before painful procedures has been shown to decrease the anticipation of pain, thus decreasing the pain experience. Child life specialists may assist the nurse to prepare the child for procedures. Preparation may include diagrams, pictures, handling equipment, meeting medical personnel, or visiting special rooms, such as recovery or the intensive care units.

Distraction can be useful, particularly for younger children. Techniques such as blowing bubbles, singing songs, blowing pinwheels, or reading a favorite book may turn their attention away from the procedure. Family members can be encouraged to participate in distraction by providing a favorite toy.

Relaxation can be effective in pain control and actually decreases pain in the child. Nurses can teach relaxation skills to parents early in the course of HIV. A deep sense of relaxation can be obtained through guided imagery or hypnosis. The nurse can encourage parents to use relaxation books that will help them direct the relaxation exercise with their child. Additional complementary and alternative therapies include massage, acupuncture, and vitamin and other dietary supplements.

 Across Care Settings: Head Start

Regarding education, Head Start, a federally funded preschool program, is mandated to enroll children with HIV in school. The Individuals with Disabilities Education Act (2004) guarantees all children with disabilities access to a free and appropriate education from birth through 21 years of age, and this includes children with HIV.

NUTRITION. Children who are HIV positive are adversely affected by malnutrition in the form of either weight loss or obesity, underscoring the need for continuous assessment and attention. Failure to thrive causes poor weight gain, often with weight lower than the 5th percentile. The child can experience chronic diarrhea, malabsorption-induced immunodeficiency, and adverse gastrointestinal (GI) effects of many HIV treatments. Causes of chronic diarrhea include Mycobacterium avium-intracellulare, Giardia, and Cryptosporidium. The nurse works closely with a nutritionist to develop a plan to manage the child's diet in interesting and vital ways.

Obesity is a common problem in children with HIV and a contributing factor to immune dysfunction. Obesity occurs as a result of side effects from some of the medications commonly used to treat HIV coupled with decreased physical activity. Early involvement of a nutritional expert to provide consultation with the family is beneficial. The nutritionist can address specific nutritional needs and provide education about healthy dietary choices. In addition, the nutritionist can perform a nutritional assessment that includes monitoring heights and weights, evaluating laboratory values, and screening for dietary difficulties.

Oral supplementation is recommended to proactively meet nutritional goals of underweight children with HIV. The overall goal of oral supplementation is prevention of malnutrition. In addition, aggressive oral care is emphasized to prevent oral lesions that may add to decreased intake. Another way to ensure adequate nutrition is the initiation of parenteral (tube) feedings. Parenteral feeding is used for the most severe cases in which all attempts at normal oral nutrition have failed. The inherent risks of invasive oral or nasal catheters can negatively affect the already immunocompromised child, making this a high-risk course of treatment. However, parenteral nutrition may correct the nutritional deficiencies and therefore is a consideration when other routes have failed.

IMMUNIZATIONS. Knowledge about immunizations for the child with HIV is important. B-cell dysfunction can influence how effective a vaccine is to an HIV-infected person. Most children with symptomatic HIV show a poor response to gaining immunity from vaccinations, and so it is suggested that they also receive **passive immunoprophylaxis** if exposed to a vaccine-preventable disease, such as measles or tetanus. In the past, HIV children did not receive live viral vaccines (e.g., MMR and varicella) because of the concern that they could actually develop these infections because of their immunosuppression. Now children can receive these vaccinations if their immunity is good, depending on their CD4 counts (T-cell counts). Also, if a child has received IVIG within the past 3 months, she receives vaccines at the midpoint between IVIG infusions because IVIG may decrease the response to vaccination.

Nursing Insight—*CDC recommendations for childhood vaccines*

Current CDC (2013c) recommendations for childhood vaccine administration for patients with HIV are as follows:
Contraindicated vaccines
- OPV (oral polio) vaccine
- Smallpox vaccination
- BCG (bacille Calmette-Guérin) vaccination
- Live attenuated influenza vaccine (LAIV) (intranasal flu vaccine)
- Yellow fever vaccine might have a contraindication or a precaution depending on the clinical parameters of the child's immune function
- Withhold MMR and varicella in severely immunocompromised persons
- HIV-infected infants without severe immunosuppression should routinely receive MMR vaccine as soon as possible upon reaching their first birthday (consideration should be given to administering the second dose of MMR vaccine as soon as 28 days after the first dose).
- MMR is recommended for all asymptomatic HIV-infected persons who do not have evidence of severe immunosuppression (CD4 levels less than 15%) (CDC, 2013c)

Specifically recommended vaccines for children with HIV or AIDS:
- Pneumococcal vaccination
- Consider Hib (if not administered in infancy)
- Meningococcal vaccination (CDC, 2013c)

Medical Care.

focus on safety

Administration of medication to children

The nurse can help the family understand the importance of antiretroviral therapy and teach parents the common side effects. Other considerations for antiretroviral therapy include actual administration of the medication to the child in a safe and effective manner, using the six rights of medication administration. It is important for the nurse to note that many antiretroviral medications are not well tolerated by children because of taste. In addition, the medication regimen can be quite complex, requiring the family to adhere to a complicated schedule of medication administration and monitoring. The nurse can assist the family with understanding the prescribed medicine routine by creating a written schedule of medications, common side effects, and when to call the physician (Tabor, 2009).

Intravenous immune globulin (IVIG) is used to boost the infected child's immune system, although practice shows it does not decrease the incidence of serious bacterial infections. There are only rare allergic reactions to IVIG and no drug interactions, and routine vaccinations are spaced out between IVIG dosing. Aerosolized or IV pentamidine (Dapsone) and atovaquone (Mepron) are medications that can be used for older children to prevent *Pneumocystis jiroveci* pneumonia (Fahrner & Romano, 2010).

Trimethoprim sulfamethoxazole (TMP-SMZ) (Bactrim or Septra) is used to prevent *Pneumocystis jiroveci* pneumonia as a prophylactic agent. However, there is a significant risk of neutropenia and thrombocytopenia with this drug, so the child's CBC must be closely monitored. There is also a significant Stevens-Johnson syndrome risk with the use of Trimethoprim sulfamethoxazole (TMP-SMZ) (Bactrim or Septra).

Selected medications are used for children and adolescents who are HIV or have AIDS (see Table 25-1).

Table 25-1 Selected Medications for Children Who Are HIV Positive or Have AIDS	
Medication	**Rationale**
An antibiotic used for prophylaxis and treatment of infection is trimethoprim sulfamethoxazole (TMP-SMZ) (Bactrim or Septra)	Trimethoprim sulfamethoxazole (TMP-SMZ) (Bactrim or Septra) is used in the prevention of *Pneumocystis jiroveci* pneumonia; major toxicities are thrombocytopenia and neutropenia
Antiretroviral drugs (HAART)	Nucleoside reverse transcriptase inhibitors (NRTI) include: Non-nucleoside reverse transcriptase inhibitors (NNRTI) Protease inhibitors (PI) Entry and fusion inhibitors (FI) Inegrase inhibitors (II) Chemokine receptor antagonists
zidovudine (AZT)	This is a type of nucleoside reverse transcriptase inhibitor
lamivudine (Epivir)	This is a type of nucleoside reverse transcriptase inhibitor
nevirapine (Viramune)	This is a type of non-nucleoside transcriptase inhibitor
nelfinavir (Viracept)	This is a type of protease inhibitor
enfuvirtide (Fuzeon)	This is a type of entry and fusion inhibitor
raltegravir (Isentress)	This is a type of integrase inhibitor

Nursing Insight—*Highly active antiretroviral therapy (HAART)*

Highly active antiretroviral therapy, or HAART, has become the cornerstone of medical treatment for HIV. Although these regimens keep changing as new drugs are created, currently, combining at least three drugs from two different classes is recommended. Unfortunately, many HAART drugs carry serious adverse effects. As of 2012, more than 20 antiretroviral drugs have been approved for pediatric use; greater than 15 of these have availability in pediatric formulation or capsule size. The current recommendation is to use a 3-drug NRTI regimen only when an NNRTI or a PI cannot be used as first-line treatment (Greenfield, 2012).

Education/Discharge Instructions

Symptomatic and supportive care of children with HIV or AIDS is similar to that for children with immunodeficiency conditions. Essential in the child's care are palliative and comfort care measures. Proper hygiene, comfortable clothing, good nutrition, play, rest, and social interaction are all important aspects of care for the child. The nurse ensures good communication between the family and health-care providers to facilitate a realistic ongoing treatment plan.

Adolescents present their own specific challenges when infected with HIV. Based on their desire to be independent, adhering to complicated treatment regimens may be a struggle. The nurse works closely with the adolescent to identify strategies for managing a complex medical illness with the need to be independent and socialize with peers. Often, referral to an adolescent support group is helpful for children in this age group.

It is critical to help the family access available resources including social services, financial aid, spiritual support, insurance coverage, and how to access community health clinics. Often, the acute care setting nurse who is intermittently involved in the child's care can initiate the coordination of ongoing care by contacting a case manager to guide the family through the complex health-care system. Although in the past, it was common for children with HIV to not be told their diagnoses, now many are living into adolescence and adulthood. There are guidelines for helping to tell children about their diagnosis through the American Academy of Pediatrics (AAP) (2013) and other national AIDS or HIV foundations, such as American Foundation for Children with AIDS (http://www.helpchildrenwithaids.org) and the Elizabeth Glaser Pediatric AIDS Foundation (http://www.pedaids.org).

Collaboration in Caring—*Collaboration between the family and others*

Care of the child with HIV or AIDS is complex and best managed through collaboration with the family and others (which may include a combination of nurses, physicians, pain specialists, a psychologist, nutritionist, social worker, child life specialist, and a schoolteacher). The family is encouraged to view the team members as a collaborative team of professionals and then see themselves as equal participants in their child's care.
Nurse: Provides coordination of team and acts as the bridge between the family and others, assists family and child to assume an active role in the care, identifies conditions requiring intervention, provides treatments or referrals as needed, and helps the family create a livable plan for their unique situation.
Physician: Provides and directs all medical care and monitors infections, complications, and growth and development.
Pharmacist: Provides the medication and acts as a resource to help the family understand drug actions, interactions, dosing parameters, and adverse side effects.
Pain specialist: Provides pharmacological and nonpharmacological management for acute and chronic pain.
Psychologist: Assists the child and family to identify positive coping strategies for living with HIV or AIDS.
Nutritionist: Provides early and ongoing support for nutritional needs.
Social worker: Provides support, community resources, and possible ways to manage finances.
Child life specialist: Provides support for normal development and coping strategies.
Schoolteacher: Assists family with a realistic educational plan through episodes of illness.

focus on safety

Stevens-Johnson syndrome

Stevens-Johnson syndrome, a potentially fatal syndrome, can be a side effect of trimethoprim sulfamethoxazole (TMP-SMZ) (Bactrim or Septra) or any type of sulfa. It can also be seen with other medications or viral illnesses. Stevens-Johnson syndrome begins with high fever, sore throat, cough, arthralgias, vomiting, and diarrhea. Next, erythematous macules begin to spread from head and neck down to the trunk. These may develop into hemorrhagic blisters and even involve the mucosa of the nose, mouth, and eyes. Associated disorders include gastrointestinal bleeding, renal problems, sepsis, pneumonitis, and ophthalmological issues. Children with Stevens-Johnson syndrome must be admitted rapidly to the pediatric intensive care unit for wound care, hydration, electrolyte issues, pain management, and nutritional assistance. IVIG is the treatment of choice for this sometimes fatal reaction (Burns, Dunn, Brady, Starr, & Blosser, 2013).

Medication adherence may be a problem with HIV-infected individuals of all ages. Nurses can educate themselves about the medications and adverse effects, to best support their patients. HIV medications are frequently changing and the CDC is an excellent source for current information (http://www.cdcnpin.org). For up-to-date information on pediatric dosing for HIV medications, see the following CDC Web site: http://www.cdc.gov/globalaids/docs/program-areas/pmtct/Peds%20Dosing%20Guide.pdf.

 Now Can You—Discuss human immunodeficiency virus (HIV)?

1. Discuss the developmentally appropriate and holistic nursing care for children with HIV or AIDS?
2. Explore diagnostic, laboratory testing and medications for children with HIV or AIDS?
3. Develop teaching plans and discharge criteria for parents whose children have HIV or AIDS?

Nursing Care Plan The Child With Immunosuppression

Nursing Diagnosis: Risk for Infection Related to Immunosuppression

Measurable Short-Term Goal: Child remains free from symptoms of infection.

Measurable Long-Term Goal: Child regains natural resistance to infection.

NOC Outcomes:
Immune Status (0702) Natural and acquired appropriately targeted resistance to internal and external antigens
Infection Severity (0703) Severity of signs and symptoms

NIC Interventions:
Infection Protection (6550)
Infection Control (6540)

Nursing Interventions:

1. Institute standard precautions and designated isolation precautions as appropriate.

   RATIONALE: Precautions protect the nurse, child, and family members from the transfer of microorganisms.

2. Demonstrate and instruct visitors to wash hands on entering or leaving the patient's room and to use protective equipment properly.

   RATIONALE: Hand washing and proper use of gloves, masks, or cover gowns eliminate major transmission routes for many organisms.

3. Monitor for systemic and localized signs of infection (specify frequency) when the child is hospitalized and at each interaction when providing community-based health care. Assess temperature, lung sounds, and condition of skin, as well as mucous membranes for pain, redness, and edema.

   RATIONALE: Fever or respiratory symptoms may be the only overt signs of infection in an immunosuppressed child. Systematic monitoring allows early recognition and treatment of infection.

4. Monitor laboratory values as obtained: absolute granulocyte count, white blood cell count, and differential results.

   RATIONALE: Changes in lab values alert the caregiver to developing infection. The immunosuppressed patient may not exhibit overt signs of an inflammatory response.

5. Promote a balanced diet of favorite foods, prepared and presented attractively. Allow only cooked fruits and vegetables if the child is neutropenic.

   RATIONALE: Deficient intake of protein; vitamins A, C, or E; iron; or zinc may have a detrimental effect on the immune system and place the child at increased risk for infection. Cooking fruits and vegetables helps to eliminate harmful organisms.

6. Encourage rest and sleep by providing a quiet environment and favorite toys or blankets (specify).

   RATIONALE: Sufficient rest and sleep help support the immune system.

7. Administer prophylactic or therapeutic antibiotics as prescribed (specify drug, dose, route, and time), following CDC and AAP recommendations.

   RATIONALE: Specify the action of prescribed medication.

Autoimmune Disorders

An **autoimmune disorder** is the immune response against one of the body's own tissues or cells. Autoimmunity results from the body's inability to distinguish self from non-self, wherein the immune system carries out immune responses against normal cells and tissues. The disorders can be organ specific or systemic, as in systemic lupus erythematosus, dermatomyositis, spondyloarthropathies, scleroderma, and hypermobility syndrome. Juvenile rheumatoid arthritis is discussed in the Evidence-Based Practice feature in this chapter and again, more at length, in Chapter 29.

 Nursing Insight—Other autoimmune disorders in childhood

Other autoimmune disorders, signs and symptoms, and nursing care measures are found in Table 25-2.

SYSTEMIC LUPUS ERYTHEMATOSUS

Systemic lupus erythematosus (SLE) is a multisystem chronic autoimmune disorder of the blood vessels and connective tissue. The basic pathophysiology of SLE includes autoantibodies that attach to the body proteins, creating antigen-antibody complexes. These antigen-antibody complexes are then deposited throughout the body, causing widespread tissue damage. The exact cause of SLE is unknown, although it is tied to genetic predisposition coupled with unidentified trigger(s) that cause the disease to activate. Suspected triggers include estrogen, infections, ultraviolet light, pregnancy, and certain drugs. The signs, symptoms, and course of disease are variable and dependent on the exact body systems that are affected, ranging from mild to life-threatening. SLE has unpredictable periods of exacerbation (flare-ups) and remissions (lessening in intensity or degree). SLE is most common in adolescent and young adult females, African Americans, and Hispanics.

Table 25-2 Autoimmune Disorders in Childhood

Autoimmune Disorder	Signs and Symptoms	Medical Management
Spondyloarthropathy: mostly found > age 10; +HLA B-27 test in 80%	Pain at tendon insertions—heel, tibial tubercle; low back pain; sacroiliitis	NSAIDs: ibuprofen (Advil) or naproxen (Naprosyn)
Enteropathic arthritis; includes Reiter's syndrome, celiac and inflammatory bowel disease (IBD)-associated arthritis	Uveitis, stomatitis (aphthous ulcers in mouth), hepatitis, erythema nodosum	NSAIDs: ibuprofen (Advil) or naproxen (Naprosyn) methotrexate (Rheumatrex) infliximab (Remicade)
Polyarteritis nodosa: vasculitis, caused by streptococcus, hepatitis B, parvovirus	Fever, painful nodules, purpura, myalgias/arthralgias, hypertension, proteinuria, hematuria, cardiac and CNS disease	Steroids (i.e., prednisone, prednisolone, or Medrol) methotrexate (Rheumatrex) azathioprine (Imuran) cyclophosphamide (Cytoxan)
Fibromyalgia: chronic pain syndrome	Fatigue, sleep disturbance, headache, musculoskeletal pain, trigger point pain, "fuzzy brain"	Low dose trazodone (Oleptro)

Source: Soep & Hollister (2009).

Signs and Symptoms

The symptoms are highly variable in both presentation and severity.

- Fever
- Malaise
- Chills
- Fatigue
- Weight loss

As the disease progresses, symptoms may include a characteristic malar photosensitive rash (butterfly rash on the face); arthritis; photosensitivity; serositis; proteinuria; immunological and hematological disorders such as hemolytic anemia, lymphocytopenia, thrombocytopenia, and vasculitis; and an abnormal antinuclear antibody (ANA).

Diagnosis

Diagnosis is based on laboratory tests that include a complete blood cell count with differential, metabolic chemistry panel, urinalysis, ANA, anti-DNA antibody, complement 3 (C3), complement 4 (C4), quantitative immunoglobulins, rapid plasma reagin, lupus anticoagulant, erythrocyte sedimentation rate, cardioreactive protein, and antiphospholipid antibodies. A negative ANA test excludes SLE diagnosis, while a positive ANA test does not definitively indicate SLE because more tests must be added to confirm the diagnosis (Burns et al., 2013).

Prevention

Prevention of exacerbations is the most important aspect for children with SLE. It is important for the family to understand the importance of rest and adequate nutrition to help maximize immune system function.

Collaborative Care

Nursing Care. Managing pain and inflammation, treating symptoms, and preventing complications are important nursing care measures. Excessive sunlight and stress can exacerbate the disease, so the nurse communicates this information to the child and family. SLE is a condition with varying signs and symptoms, and it requires continued careful assessment to ensure prompt recognition of an exacerbation. This disease often affects adolescents, so the facial rash, fatigue, and arthritic changes may put the child at risk for depression and altered body image.

 focus on safety

Systemic lupus erythematosus

This inflammatory autoimmune disease creates autoantibodies and affects multiple body systems. It involves B and T lymphocyte dysfunction, and the ANA is classically elevated in this disorder. SLE varies from mild to severe and life-threatening. Patients can experience central and peripheral nervous system symptoms including headaches, psychosis, seizures, and renal injury.

Medical Care. Treatment of pain and inflammation in mild SLE is generally accomplished with nonsteroidal anti-inflammatory medications (NSAIDs). Antimalarial medications are also used in mild SLE to control symptoms of arthritis, skin rashes, mouth ulcers, fever, and fatigue. Oral steroids are commonly used to control the disease (Procedure 25-1). Corticosteroids in forms such as prednisone, prednisolone, or Medrol are highly effective in reducing inflammation and symptoms, although they also have the serious side effect of immunosuppression. During an exacerbation period, corticosteroids may be initiated in high doses. After symptoms are under control, the dose is tapered down to the lowest therapeutic level. It is important to tell the parents that steroids must be tapered slowly when it is time to discontinue the medication.

The most potent type of medication used to treat severe SLE includes immunosuppressive agents. These medications are used when the disease has reached a serious state in which severe signs and symptoms are present. Immunosuppressive agents may also be prescribed if there is a need to avoid corticosteroids. The decision to use immunosuppressives requires serious consideration because of significant side effects, primarily related to general immunosuppression. Examples of immunosuppressive agents used in treatment of

Procedure 25-1 Oral Administration of Steroid Medication

Purpose

Steroid medication is used to treat a variety of conditions, including allergic and autoimmune disorders.

Equipment

- Gloves
- Patient identification label
- Oral medication
- Medication cup

Steps

1. Wash hands and don gloves.

RATIONALE: *Prevents the spread of bacteria.*

2. Check the child ID band and use two patient identifiers.

RATIONALE: *Prevents the accidental administration of medication to the wrong child. Also, it alerts the nurse to potential medication allergies that could imply an ordered medication should not be administered.*

3. Ensure the correct dosage and route of medication.

RATIONALE: *Steroid medication comes in liquid suspensions for younger children and in tablet form for older children. As a general rule, the suspensions are bitter in taste and may need to be followed by a sweet treat if allowable.*

4. Prepare the medication according to the child's developmental age.

RATIONALE: *Use a clean medication cup to administer steroid pills or suspension. The nurse may also mix the steroid suspension in a more palatable food, such as applesauce or pudding. If in suspension, make certain that the child receives the entire amount of the suspension in the food transport.*

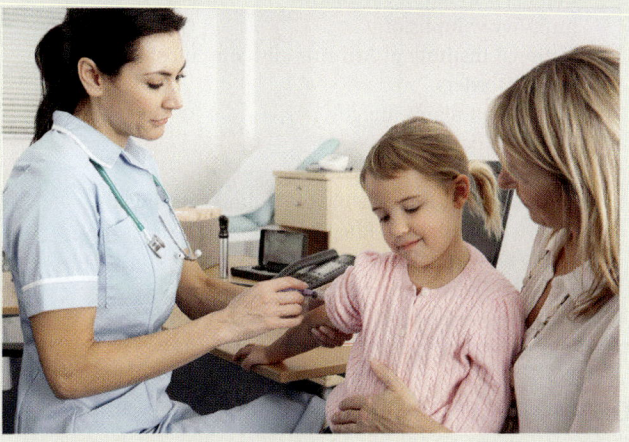

clinical alert

Steroids

Steroids must be tapered to avoid problems with the hypothalamic-pituitary-access (HPA). If steroids are given at a high dose for a long period, the body will interpret this as not needing to produce its own cortisol, which is dangerous. Steroid tapers or short bursts of steroid dosing (usually no more than 5 days) eliminate interference with the HPA and keep the body producing its own cortisol.

Teach Parents

Teach the parents that children on steroid medications may be irritable, very energetic, or have insomnia. It is essential to keep them away from infectious disease sources, especially while on steroids because their immunity may be altered.

Documentation
10/12/15 0900
M. Helming RN

SLE include azathioprine (Imuran), cyclophosphamide (Cytoxan), and methotrexate (Rheumatrex). Each medication has unique and serious risks such as bone marrow depression and hepatotoxicity. The nurse must reinforce information on the action of the medication as well as the side effects with the parents before administration of this medication.

Education/Discharge Instructions

Overall, children with SLE maintain good health, but the disease severity is variable. In addition to medication, parental education also focuses on palliative care and providing psychosocial support. It is important to tell parents to maintain good nutrition for the child. Although there is no specific diet for SLE, a balanced diet, low in salt (if the child becomes hypertensive or nephrotic), is encouraged. Rest and exercise include periods when the child is active during remissions and increases rest during exacerbation. Avoidance of sun exposure is stressed because of the

photosensitive rash that occurs with SLE. Use of sunscreen is important, and planning outdoor activities in the shade or staying indoors may be necessary. Because this condition may be difficult for the child and family to cope with and understand, encouraging the expression of feelings or joining a support group is encouraged. Parents should notify teachers, coaches, and others about their child's condition so they can help monitor the child and obtain necessary treatment if needed. It is also the nurse's responsibility to help the child and family identify possible triggers, such as sunlight and emotional stress and assist the family in finding ways to avoid them. Referral to support groups helps the child to adjust to life with SLE.

 Collaboration in Caring—*Systemic lupus erythematosus resources*

The nurse encourages an adolescent recently diagnosed with SLE to contact a local support group. In addition, several good resources are available online through the organizations located at the following Web sites:

- Lupus Foundation of America
  http://www.lupus.org/
- National Institute of Arthritis and Musculoskeletal and Skin Disorders
  http://www.niams.nih.gov
- SLE Foundation, Inc.
  http://www.lupusny.org/
- Association of Rheumatology Health Professionals, American College of Rheumatology
  http://www.rheumatology.org/
- Arthritis Foundation
  http://www.arthritis.org/

DERMATOMYOSITIS

Dermatomyositis is a relatively uncommon disorder found in children and adults. It is an autoimmune disorder characterized by muscle weakness and a distinctive rash. In children, the most common age range for onset is between 5 and 15 years of age.

Signs and Symptoms

- Proximal muscle weakness, especially in shoulders and pelvis
- **Heliotropic** violaceous (red-purple) rash around eyes and upper eyelids
- Possible malar rash similar to SLE, with edema of face and eyes
- Tenderness, stiffness of muscles, possible voice change, **dysphagia**

Diagnosis

Diagnosis is made clinically and requires the care of a rheumatologist. Clinical presentation is most important, but the following laboratory tests may be abnormal: liver function tests (elevated), white blood cell count (elevated), lymphocyte count (depressed), hematocrit (low), albumin (low), creatine kinase (elevated), and erythrocyte sedimentation test (elevated). Further testing includes electromyelogram testing, muscle biopsy, and magnetic resonance imaging of the quadriceps muscle (Volochayev, Csako, Wesley, Rider, & Miller, 2012).

Prevention

There is no known prevention for dermatomyositis. As an autoimmune disease, it may be associated with other autoimmune diseases, with interstitial lung disease, and with some cancers. Keeping the disease stable with medication and regular health care may prevent more serious sequelae and complications.

Collaborative Care

Nursing Care. This chronic autoimmune disorder can cause significant physical disabilities and possibly socially embarrassing facial and voice changes. Emotional care involves providing therapeutic listening for these children and support for coping mechanisms. Physical care involves monitoring these children for adverse effects of the potent medications used to treat this disorder, including long-term steroids and methotrexate (Rheumatrex).

Medical Care. Dermatomyositis is treated with long-term steroid administration. Steroids that are often used include methotrexate (Rheumatrex), cyclosporine (Sandimmune), hydroxychloroquine (Plaquenil), and intravenous immunoglobulin (IVIG) when needed (Soep & Hollister, 2009).

Education/Discharge Instructions

Parents are taught about medication management and potential side effects that can occur as a result of long-term steroid use.

SCLERODERMA

Scleroderma disorder has three identified types: the full disease, limited scleroderma, and localized scleroderma, in descending order of seriousness. Children who suffer from localized scleroderma have a better prognosis than children diagnosed with other types.

A common disorder occurring with scleroderma, and sometimes in other autoimmune diseases, is Raynaud's phenomenon, which can have its onset in children or adolescents. Raynaud's phenomenon is an intermittent, vasospastic disorder in which cold temperatures or stress put the child's fingers and/or toes into vasospasm, causing a color change to blue (cyanosis), then white (blanching), then red (as the blood flow returns). This disorder can be **idiopathic** or can be associated with a variety of rheumatological diseases, including scleroderma (Soep & Hollister, 2009).

Signs and Symptoms

Some common conditions related to scleroderma are:

- Raynaud's phenomenon
- Arthralgias
- Esophageal dysfunction (difficulty swallowing, gastroesophageal reflux)
- Potential renal, pulmonary, and cardiac dysfunction, including pulmonary hypertension
- Skin change can occur with localized scleroderma subtype, consisting of indurated, hypopigmented or hyperpigmented plaques called **morphea**, which can cause thickened skin, scar, atrophy, and contractures of underlying joints (Soep & Hollister, 2009).

Diagnosis

Diagnosis is based on the acronym, CREST syndrome (C = calcinosis (bony prominences), R = Raynaud's phenomenon, E = esophageal dysmotility (gastroesophageal reflux disease and motility issues), S = sclerodactyly (stiff skin over hands), and T = telangiectasia (tiny broken capillaries on skin). Numerous laboratory tests including ANA and anticentromere antibody are positive in scleroderma.

Prevention

This is an autoimmune disorder for which there is no known prevention. However, control of the disease and proper follow-up may help patients avoid or manage some of the most serious complications of the systemic type, such as pulmonary hypertension and gangrene of extremities.

Collaborative Care

Nursing Care. Nursing care for scleroderma involves physical support for the various symptoms and emotional support for the disabilities that can occur with some symptoms, such as pulmonary hypertension associated with marked dyspnea. Nurses can assist patients in understanding Raynaud's phenomenon by reducing stress, wearing mittens instead of gloves to keep the hands warm, using hand and foot warmers, and avoiding tobacco abuse, which further constricts arteries.

Care also includes monitoring laboratory testing for positive ANA titer; possible elevated erythrocyte sedimentation rate, testing for positive anticentromere antibody, and other rheumatological testing that differentiate this from other disorders. A dermatologist may follow localized morphea scleroderma, but rheumatologists follow limited and full scleroderma. Limited scleroderma has less risk for renal and cardiac issues but has more risk for pulmonary hypertension. The full form of scleroderma has been associated with severe renal disease, hardening of the skin, and early mortality. Radiological tests, such as esophageal motility tests and stress echocardiograms, may be needed to diagnosis this disorder.

Medical Care. Medications are variable depending on the associated disorders. There are some new medications such as iloprost (Ventavis) and sildenafil (Viagra) that have proven life-saving for pulmonary hypertension. Calcium channel blockers and topical nitroglycerin have been helpful in reducing the vasoconstriction of Raynaud's phenomenon.

Education/Discharge Instructions

Children with the more common localized or linear forms of scleroderma may have disfiguring white patches on the face, neck, and over the extremities. The extremities may have decreased mobility because of these hardened patches, so parents and children will need advice on sports participation and counseling on the possible disfigurement (www.scleroderma.org). The nurse will need to give information on topical medications, such as calcipotriene, or systemic medications, such as methotrexate (Trexall), and their potential adverse effects. In the rare case of juvenile systemic scleroderma, the nurse must work with the patient, family, and specialists involved in the care of potential end-organ diseases, such as cardiac, pulmonary, and renal disease.

 Complementary Care: *Biofeedback*

Biofeedback has been found helpful in controlling the vasospasm of Raynaud's phenomenon. Biofeedback is a technical process of monitoring the body's response to various stressors. Electrodes are attached to the skin, and they send signals to a monitor to represent heart rate, respiratory rate, blood pressure, skin temperature, sweating, and muscular function. A biofeedback therapist uses this information to help patients practice relaxation exercises to control these functions through breathing, relaxation techniques, and guided imagery. Vasospasm is a constriction of arterial blood vessels that can be modified through awareness of the process and halting it. In Raynaud's phenomenon, the vasospasm occurs both with exposure to cold and to stress.

HYPERMOBILITY SYNDROME

This disorder is also known as **ligamentous laxity**, and it may be seen in childhood. This disorder may be a component of what is commonly termed "double-jointedness."

Associated problems with this disorder include local or widespread pain, chronic fatigue, sleep problems, and early-age degenerative arthritis. Ehlers-Danlos syndrome and Marfan syndrome (elongated extremities and increased risk for aortic aneurysm) are two varieties of hypermobility syndromes. Potential accompanying disorders include irritable bowel syndrome, mitral valve prolapse, easy bruising, and anemia.

Signs and Symptoms

Hypermobility syndromes are indicated by these symptoms:

- Arthralgias
- Intermittent joint pain after exercise
- Occasional joint edema after exercise

Diagnosis

The child must meet five criteria: (1) hyperextension of knee, (2) palms can be on floor with knees extended, (3) hyperextension of elbow, (4) passive opposition of thumb to flexor surface of forearm, and (5) passive hyperextension of fingers so they are parallel with extensor surface of forearm. The Brighton Criteria and Beighton Scores are important diagnostic parameters for hypermobility syndromes.

Prevention

As an autoimmune disease, there is no known prevention at this time.

Collaborative Care

Nursing Care. Nursing care includes providing a graded conditioning program to support joints and prevent them from hyperextending (Soep & Hollister, 2009). Notify the child and family that recurrent sprains and strains of joints, ligaments, and tendons may take longer than usual to recover, and joint subluxation (partial dislocation) is more common. This may require limitations on sports and repeated orthopedic and physical therapy appointments. The nurse should inform the parents about the possibility of severe pain, poor balance, clumsiness, and early degenerative arthritis. Nurses should be aware that children with this disorder may need to see physical therapists, occupational therapists, rheumatology physicians, and orthopedists. Children may have associated needs for counseling and group support, as with the Hypermobility Syndromes Association (http://hypermobility.org).

Medical Care. Medical management consists of the proper knowledge about medication administration. The nurse teaches parents about common medications used for autoimmune diseases (Box 25-2).

Box 25-2 **Medications for Autoimmune Disorders**

NSAIDs: ibuprofen (Advil) or naproxen (Naprosyn)
Steroids (e.g., prednisone, prednisolone, Medrol)
methotrexate (Rheumatrex)
azathioprine (Imuran)
cyclophosphamide (Cytoxan)
infliximab (Remicade)
intravenous immune globulin (IVIG) (IgG [Immunoglobulins])
cyclosporine (Sandimmune)
hydroxychloroquin (Plaquenil)
pregabalin (Lyrica)

Education/Discharge Instructions

Parents must understand that proper medication administration is an important aspect of care for the child (see Box 25-2).

Allergic Reaction

ANAPHYLAXIS

Anaphylaxis is considered a medical emergency and the most severe allergic reaction possible. Both IgE- and non-IgE-mediated activities cause this life-threatening event, including the activation of mast cells, basophils, eosinophils, histamine, leukotriene, cytokines, T lymphocytes, and neutrophils, among other cells. Most importantly, this cascade of events activates the heart, lungs, and vasculature in a detrimental manner, including vasodilation, hypotension, and resultant shock. Histamine can cause coronary artery vasospasm and shorten diastole. Histamine stimulates bronchial smooth muscle contraction, causing bronchospasm. Increased vascular permeability causes laryngeal edema, closing the airway down. The body reacts violently to an antigen (foreign substance) that causes a hyperacute allergic response (Ferdman, 2012). Fatalities are caused by respiratory compromise and cardiovascular collapse, with respiratory failure being more common in pediatric mortality. Most reactions occur quickly after exposure, although food allergies can manifest from 25 minutes after exposure to several hours later. Insect stings and drug allergies cause the most rapid route to anaphylaxis, with an average of 5 to 20 minutes to onset (Ferdman, 2012).

 Nursing Insight—*Anaphylaxis-causing agent or event*

Identification of the anaphylaxis-causing agent or event is essential and often requires consultation with an allergist. Allergen immunotherapy given by an allergist may itself cause anaphylaxis, so it must be cautiously given and monitored. Most common causes of anaphylaxis are insect stings or bites (honeybee, bumblebee, wasp, yellow jacket, hornet, and fire ants). Other insects that have less potential for causing anaphylaxis are bedbugs, spiders, mosquitoes, or flies.

Vaccine reactions most commonly occur from the gelatin preservative in some vaccines. Egg-allergic children may react to egg-containing vaccines such as influenza and yellow fever. Reactions to preservatives, antibacterial agents, or components of the vaccine, including neomycin, can prompt anaphylaxis.

The most common medications that can cause anaphylaxis are the antibiotics from the penicillin family, followed by cephalosporin antibiotics, and then sulfonamides (e.g., with trimethoprim sulfamethoxazole (TMP-SMZ) (Bactrim or Septra), macrolides (e.g., erythromycin and clarithromycin), and quinolones (e.g., ciprofloxacin). In older children and teens, nonsteroidal anti-inflammatory drugs (NSAIDs) are the most common cause of a medication reaction. People allergic to NSAIDs may also be allergic to aspirin, although children rarely take aspirin.

Latex allergy, another allergic reaction, is less common, but exposure to latex in gloves, medical equipment, and other household equipment can cause anaphylaxis in children. Children who require multiple surgeries, who have congenital urological malformations, and who have myelomeningocele are notably more allergic to latex. Latex allergy can be less severe than anaphylaxis, resulting even in skin rashes and asthma (Ferdman, 2012).

Signs and Symptoms

Signs and symptoms of anaphylaxis develop suddenly and require prompt recognition and treatment:

- Wheezing
- Tachycardia
- Hypotension
- Cyanosis
- Alteration in level of consciousness
- Nasal congestion
- Angioedema (swelling around mouth and oropharynx)
- Facial edema
- Anxiety
- Hives and urticaria
- Nausea and vomiting
- Abdominal pain
- Laryngospasm
- A sense of impending doom
- Vascular collapse and cardiac arrest

 Nursing Insight—*Additional signs and symptoms of anaphylaxis*

Additional signs and symptoms that may occur with anaphylaxis include flushing, pruritus, rhinorrhea, sneezing, allergic conjunctivitis, and headache. Occasionally gastrointestinal (GI) symptoms such as abdominal cramping, nausea, vomiting, and diarrhea occur.

Diagnosis

Diagnosis of anaphylaxis is based on the child's history, skin prick allergy testing, and serum allergy testing, such as the radioallergosorbent test or ImmunoCAP test. Skin prick testing is contraindicated if the child is anaphylactic to a substance, as opposed to a lesser allergic reaction (Distler, 2010). It is important to differentiate true food allergies to those caused by cell-mediated food hypersensitivities (e.g., celiac disease, malabsorption syndromes, and food-induced colitis, which have more gastrointestinal symptoms). Also, it is important to differentiate between oral allergy syndrome, in which patients get tingling of the palate, tongue, lips, or oropharynx after ingesting certain foods, but they never get anaphylaxis. True anaphylactic food allergies can be life-threatening with respiratory or cardiac arrest, although some food allergies are only manifested by urticaria and pruritus.

Prevention

Prevention of anaphylactic reactions is an essential component of nursing care. Nurses should be vigilant about checking for allergies from patients, family members, the medical record, and allergy bracelets. Nurses should obtain excellent histories about allergic reactions and should document them carefully and prominently for all health-care team members to see. Some anaphylactic reactions occur upon first-time exposure, but others, including some bee stings, occur only on the second or subsequent exposures. If there is a family history of anaphylaxis, the nurse should counsel the patient and other health-care team members because the patient could well develop anaphylaxis also. Emergency medicines such as epinephrine and fast-acting antihistamine medications need to be available for immediate use. Patients with history of anaphylactic reactions should wear ID jewelry detailing the reactions, should carry wallet card identification of the anaphylactic reaction, and should carry life-saving medicine with them (or in the case of young children, the parents, school nurses, teachers, and other health-care team members should have access to emergency medications).

Collaborative Care

Nursing Care.

Critical Nursing Action Anaphylaxis

Immediate nursing care for anaphylaxis includes the following actions:

- Activate the emergency system
- Perform cardiopulmonary resuscitation
- Ensure adequate airway—endotracheal intubation or oxygen
- Administer epinephrine (Adrenalin)
- Place a tourniquet proximal to the site of injection or insect sting
- Keep the child lying flat, warm, and with feet slightly elevated
- Administer corticosteroids and antihistamines
- Determine the cause of the attack

For children who have experienced an anaphylactic reaction, the nurse must provide follow-up care to families to prevent recurrences. If the child has allergies that cannot be completely eliminated, a follow-up referral to an allergist for desensitization treatments or a self-administration epinephrine prescription, such as an EpiPen, is warranted. It is important that parents are taught to recognize early indicators of anaphylaxis and are confident in their ability to act quickly on this assessment.

focus on safety

EpiPen

The EpiPen Jr® autoinjector is used for children experiencing a life-threatening reaction. An injection of 0.15 mg of epinephrine (Adrenalin) is used for children between 33-66 lbs (15-30 kg), and an injection of 0.3 mg is used for children equal to or greater than 66 lbs (30 kg).

Parents must notify the school nurse, day-care providers, coaches, and other adult leaders who spend time with the child about the diagnosed allergy. Everyone working with the child must be taught how to use an EpiPen® or EpiPen Jr (epinephrine). EpiPens are usually kept in the school nurse's office. During sports activities, a second EpiPen may be given to the coach or the assistant. Along with documentation of the allergy, contact information, and the EpiPen that is on-hand, ready access to a phone for emergency medical assistance is a necessity (Ward, 2013).

Medical Care. Basic life support must be initiated with support of airway, breathing, and circulation. Administration of oxygen and initiation of an IV therapy with an isotonic crystalloid solution as soon as possible are standard treatment. Epinephrine (Adrenalin) injection is administered IM or IV to provide reversal of pulmonary bronchospasm and constriction of blood vessels, thereby improving respiratory status and blood pressure. Ongoing assessment for shock is necessary and can be treated via IV fluid bolus. Occasionally, antihistamines and corticosteroids may be added to further control symptoms after the initial stabilization. The majority of children respond positively to the treatment, with a full recovery (Ward, 2013).

Education/Discharge Instructions

In case of an allergic reaction, instruct the parent to administer the medication exactly as directed and call 911 immediately. Other education/discharge instructions include:

- Instruct the parents to teach the child to know his triggers
- Review correct administration technique for the EpiPen or EpiPen Jr (epinephrine)
- Teach the child to self-inject the epinephrine medication and what to do in case of an emergency
- Tell parents of children too young to self-inject and who are separated from them to discuss the allergy and how to use an autoinjector with another responsible adult

Collaboration in Caring—*Peanut allergies in school*

National data show that 4% of U.S. children have some type of food allergy. Children with food allergies more often suffer from other IgE-mediated issues (e.g., asthma, eczema, and allergic rhinitis) (Distler, 2010). Ninety percent of all food allergies are from peanuts, tree nuts, fish, shellfish, cow's milk, hen eggs, soy, and wheat. Many children outgrow these food allergies within the first decade of life, with the exception of a peanut allergy. Peanuts, tree nuts, and shellfish tend to be allergens that persist throughout life.

focus on safety

Creating a safe environment

The pediatric nurse plays a critical role in collaboration with the family and school personnel to create a safe environment for a child with peanut allergy to safely attend school. The nurse assists the family in establishing a coordinated plan including the following key components:

- Educate the school staff regarding peanut allergies. Include all staff who may be supervising this student and who may be in a position to recognize and intervene in an emergency.

Outline an emergency plan specific for the student to include:

- Specific instructions for staff in the event of a reaction
- Location of emergency medications
- Identification and elimination of exposure to the allergen
- Placement of emergency phone numbers in a designated area
- Establish a "peanut-free" zone in the cafeteria or a peanut-free table
- Send a letter to parents who may provide snacks to the child, such as parents of children in the same class, from a sports team, or a club, informing them of the presence of a child with a severe peanut allergy.

Medication: Diphenhydramine (Benadryl)

(dye-fen-**hye**-dra-meen)

Indications: Relief of allergic symptoms caused by histamine release, including anaphylaxis, allergic rhinitis, and allergic dermatoses. Relief of pruritus.

Actions: Antagonizes the effects of histamine at H_1-receptor sites. Significant CNS depressant and anticholinergic properties.

Therapeutic Effects: Decreased symptoms of histamine excess (sneezing, rhinorrhea, nasal and ocular pruritus, ocular tearing and redness, and urticaria).

Contraindications and Precautions:
CONTRAINDICATED IN: Hypersensitivity.

Adverse Reactions and Side Effects: Drowsiness, paradoxical excitation (more common in children), anorexia, and dry mouth.

Nursing Implications:
1. Provide child and family education regarding medication, caution not to exceed recommended dose.
2. Inform parents that medication may cause drowsiness or excitability in child.
3. Provide education regarding common side effect of dry mouth. Management strategies include frequent mouth care and oral rinses.

Source: Data from Vallerand, A. H., & Sanoski, C. A. (2014). *Davis's drug guide for nurses* (14th ed.), Philadelphia, PA: F.A. Davis.

 Now Can You—Care for the child with anaphylaxis?

1. Prioritize developmentally appropriate and holistic nursing care for children with anaphylaxis?
2. Develop teaching plans and discharge criteria for parents whose children have anaphylaxis?

Infectious Diseases of Childhood

The occurrence of infectious disease in children is the result of an interaction between several factors including the child, the environment, and the agent causing the illness.

There are two main models used to illustrate the interaction, the most common being the epidemiological triangle (Fig. 25-3). In the epidemiological triangle the host, environment, and agent make up the three sides of an equilateral triangle. The *host* is the organism from which a parasite obtains its nourishment, the *environment* is the surroundings or conditions that influence the organism, and the *agent* causes the actual effect (disease) (Venes, 2013). This model illustrates the codependence that these three factors have on one another and recognizes that a change in any one of the three factors will influence the risk or probability of a child contracting the disease.

Many factors such as age, gender, physical, and psychosocial factors all play a role in the susceptibility of the host to an infectious disease. The normal development of the child's immune system is also a major factor in many infectious diseases, especially during the early childhood years. The child has natural protection from maternal antibodies for up to the first 6 months of life; therefore, any sign of infection that occurs during this time is taken seriously and often an extensive medical work-up is initiated. Also, children under 6 months of age who show signs of infectious disease may be ill enough to be hospitalized because of some compromise in their maternal and natural immunity.

The final element in the triangle, the agent, contains specific information, including infectivity, pathogenicity, and virulence, that assists the nurse in developing the appropriate plan of care. **Infectivity** includes the mode of transmission, incubation period, and communicable period. The *mode of transmission* is how the pathogen actually gains access to the body. With this knowledge, the nurse can plan care to eliminate unnecessary portals of entry (e.g., multiple IV sites) and thoroughly inspect the skin for potential breaks that allow entrance of organisms. Knowledge about the *incubation period* (period of time when an organism invades the body and develops an onset of symptoms) and the *communicable period* (the time that the child is able to transmit the pathogen to others) allows the nurse to alert others that the child is infectious and to isolate the child for a certain period.

Pathogenicity is the percentage of those children exposed to the pathogen that will eventually develop the disease. This information is helpful to the nurse in the community when assessing citywide outbreaks. The nurse can notify schools, community centers, churches, shopping malls, and other public places that an outbreak exists and that it is best to avoid these areas, especially for high-risk children. *Virulence* is the severity of the health problems caused by the agent. The more virulent the disease the more necessary it is to curtail its spread. For example, in winter during an influenza outbreak, a number of schools close so they can be thoroughly cleaned and sanitized. Pathogenicity and virulence are often key considerations in development and implementation of public health programs.

The Chain of Infection model is also an important way to understand transmission of infection (Fig. 25-4). This model illustrates the exact steps that must occur for transmission and demonstrates possible ways to stop transmission of the disease.

The first link shows that pathogenic microorganisms, whether viruses, bacteria, or fungi, require a reservoir where the pathogen can grow. Reservoirs may be human hosts, animals, and the soil. With knowledge about the reservoir, the nurse can eliminate it to break the chain. A mosquito abatement program to control West Nile virus is an example of an attempt to alter the chain of infection via reservoir elimination. Public health immunization campaigns are examples of a way to decrease the reservoir for diseases.

The next two links in the chain involve the escape of the pathogen from the reservoir into the host. Knowledge

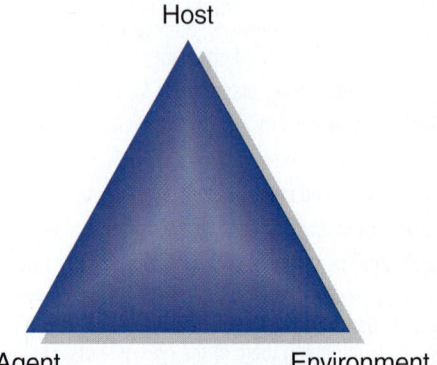

Figure 25-3 Epidemiological triangle.

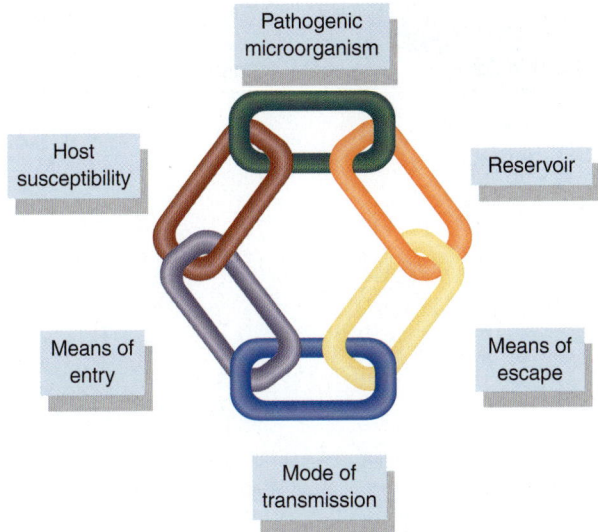

Figure 25-4 Chain of infection model.

about the routes of transmission (contact, droplet, airborne) enables the nurse to initiate appropriate isolation precautions. **Contact transmission** refers to infection that is contagious through skin, vomit, feces, urine, mucous membranes, and wounds. Droplet transmission implies a spread of organisms through close mucous membrane or respiratory secretions contact, as exemplified by rhinovirus that can cause the common cold and influenza. Airborne transmission refers to pathogens that may be suspended in the air and therefore spread over long distances. Examples of airborne transmission include measles, tuberculosis, and varicella (Virginia Department of Health, 2012).

The final link involves a susceptible host. Susceptibility of the host to infection is decreased mainly via good general health practices such as good hygiene, nutrition, overall good health, lack of immunity disorders, and a decrease in stress. A listing of infectious diseases and nursing care actions is shown in Table 25-3.

(Text continued on page 994)

Table 25-3 Communicable Diseases in Childhood

Disease	Signs and Symptoms	Nursing Care	Complications
Chickenpox (Viral) 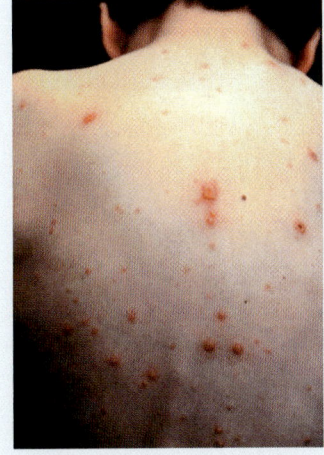 Causative Agent—Varicella-zoster virus, a herpes virus (VZV) Epidemiology—Highly contagious disease Peak Incidence—Late winter and spring Mode of Transmission—Airborne, spread through contact with respiratory droplets and contact with lesions Infection Control—The incubation period is from 10 to 21 days. Children are considered contagious 1–2 days before the eruption of lesions to the time when all lesions have crusted, or up to 7 days after appearance of the rash. The period of communicability may be prolonged in children who are immunocompromised. Airborne and contact precautions are needed for hospitalized children during the period of communicability. Varicella vaccination is increasingly used in childhood and adolescence,	Malaise, fever, possible URI, symptoms are followed by a rash. The rash is described as a "tear drop on a rose." It begins with a macule on a red base, then progresses to a clear vesicle, and later forms a crust. The lesions are severely pruritic, and eruptions may continue to occur for up to 5 days. Generally the rash first appears on the face and trunk but may spread anywhere on the body.	Nursing care is supportive with antipruritic lotions, baths, and antihistamines. Some children receive oral acyclovir (Zovirax), which is not curative but can slightly shorten the disease duration and intensity. IV acyclovir is used for immunocompromised child presenting with chickenpox. Must be used within 24 hours of onset to be effective. Varicella-zoster immune globulin (VZIG) may be given within 72 hours of exposure to immunocompromised children. VZIG provides only temporary immunity. Oral antihistamines, baking soda, oatmeal baths and lotions, such as Aveeno baths and calamine lotion are given to manage the itching.	Immunocompromised children have a high risk for complications (including those on steroids for treatment of asthma). The most common complications are bacterial superinfections with lesions, encephalitis, varicella, pneumonia, and immune thrombocytopenia purpura (ITP). Use of aspirin-containing medications has been linked with Reye's syndrome in children with Varicella-zoster (chickenpox).

(continued)

Table 25-3 Communicable Diseases in Childhood (continued)

Disease	Signs and Symptoms	Nursing Care	Complications
Chickenpox (Viral) (continued) so the incidence of varicella has decreased over time. However, it is unclear whether this vaccine provides lifelong immunity. Herpes zoster (shingles) is reactivated varicella that can occur especially in older and immunocompromised individuals; this is a result of the varicella virus remaining dormant in nerves after the disease.			
Diphtheria (Bacterial) 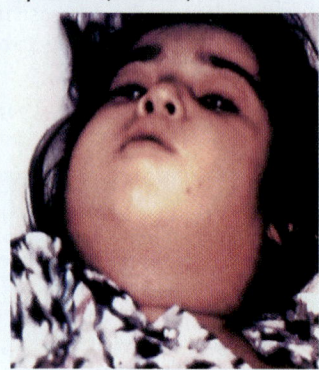 Causative Agent—*Corynebacterium diphtheriae* bacillus Epidemiology—This is a rare disease in United States; it can occur from raw milk and milk products. Peak Incidence—Occurs mostly in fall and winter in unimmunized or partially immunized persons. Mode of Transmission—Transmitted through respiratory droplets, contact with respiratory secretions, contact with skin lesions. Infection Control—The incubation period is 2–7 days (or may be longer) so if the disease is suspected, isolate the child. Droplet and contact precautions are used for hospitalized children. Immunization with recurrent boosters is the only effective means of control.	Signs and symptoms are mild in partially immunized or severe in unimmunized children. Low-grade fever, rhinorrhea, cough, sore throat, gray, adherent membrane in pharynx or trachea, possible skin ulcers, hoarseness, stridor, and pharyngitis are common. More severe signs and symptoms cause difficulty breathing because of narrowing of the upper airway.	Hospitalization is required with IV antitoxin (hyperimmune equine antiserum) and antibiotics (erythromycin or penicillin). All contacts are given prophylactic antibiotic treatment and immunization boosters.	Respiratory compromise is secondary to the endotoxin that is produced and a membrane that covers much of the upper airway. The membrane toxin can produce myocarditis, respiratory compromise, and peripheral and cranial neuropathies.
Infectious Mononucleosis (Viral) Causative Agent—Epstein-Barr virus (EBV) Epidemiology—Most persons become infected with EBV sometime during their life (usually adolescence or young adulthood). Peak Incidence—Ages 15–17 Mode of Transmission—This disease is transmitted via intimate contact with the saliva of an infected individual, but it is also infectious from blood. Infection Control—The incubation period is 30–50 days. Infected persons may shed virus intermittently and without symptoms throughout life.	Signs and symptoms include fever, severe exudative pharyngitis, and prominent cervical and often occipital lymphadenopathy lasting from 2–3 weeks. Fatigue and possible hepatosplenomegaly are also seen. A fine maculopapular rash may occur, especially if the patient is given amoxicillin (Amoxil) or ampicillin (Unasyn). In the lab, a positive monospot or heterophile test and atypical lymphocytes on a CBC/differential are classic.	Steroids are considered in the case of respiratory difficulty secondary to occlusive pharyngitis (but must be used cautiously). Bedrest and avoidance of strenuous activities, especially contact sports, is required (because of risk of splenic rupture).	Respiratory compromise is secondary to the airway swelling and exudative pharyngitis, aseptic meningitis, and encephalitis. Rarely, splenic rupture occurs. Possible mononucleosis hepatitis. Aseptic meningitis or encephalitis occurs. There is a possible occurrence of thrombocytopenia and agranulocytosis.

Table 25-3 Communicable Diseases in Childhood (continued)

Disease	Signs and Symptoms	Nursing Care	Complications
No isolation beyond standard precautions needed. There are other diseases, such as CMV, toxoplasmosis, and HIV that can cause a mono-like syndrome with similar symptoms.			
Rubella (virus)/German or 3-Day Measles Two forms: congenital and postnatal (after birth). Causative Agent—Rubeola virus Epidemiology—Up to 39 million cases worldwide each year Peak Incidence—In United States, mostly at age 6 months because infants are not vaccinated yet. Mode of Transmission—This disease is highly contagious. It is spread through placenta or nasopharyngeal secretions and fomites. Infection Control—Incubation period: 14–21 days.	Signs and symptoms include a prodrome of mild fever, sore throat, arthralgia, eye pain, GI upset. Lymphadenopathy follows and is noted for the occurrence of postauricular nodes. Other lymph nodes, such as cervical and occipital nodes, can become inflamed. The rash is a fine, light-pink, maculopapular rash on face then traveling to the chest and entire body.	Supportive care is given with antipyretics. Isolate the child from others while disease is active, usually for up to 1 week after rash starts.	The riskiest complications occur prenatally, in the first trimester to 16th week of pregnancy, and include mental retardation, deafness, eye disorders, cardiac defects, and stillbirth. Postnatal complications include arthritis, ITP, and encephalitis.
Haemophilus Influenzae Type b (Bacterial) Causative Agent—*Haemophilus influenzae type b* Epidemiology—Highly contagious disease Peak Incidence—Occurs most often in spring and summer with infants and children in day care. Mode of Transmission— Spreads via direct contact or inhalation of droplets from infected persons. Infection Control— The incubation period is unknown, and the disease is likely contagious for up to 3 days following onset of symptoms. The infectious agent may colonize in respiratory tract of an asymptomatic person. This disease is preventable with the vaccine.	Signs and symptoms begin as an upper respiratory infection. Bacteria subsequently pass into the blood and may be spread to sites throughout the body. Symptoms of infection are dependent on the site and may include sinusitis, otitis media, upper and lower airway infections, septic arthritis, and cellulitis. In infants this organism is a cause of sepsis.	Nursing care includes antibiotic administration. Prophylactic treatment with rifampin (Rifadin) is given to unimmunized people in the household.	Death may occur secondary to serious infections with *Haemophilus influenzae type b* if not treated.
Influenza (Viral) Causative Agent—The flu is caused by influenza viruses A, B, and C. A and B strains can cause epidemics, while C causes only mild illness in children. Subtypes including H1N1, H1N2, and H3N2 also exist. Recently, the virulent H1N1 strain caused deaths and severe disease, especially in young children, and it is now incorporated into the flu vaccine. Epidemiology—This disease is highly contagious. It occurs most often in spring and summer with infants and children in day care. Peak Incidence—This disease occurs more often in the winter months. Mode of Transmission—This disease	Signs and symptoms have a rapid onset of a high fever, myalgia, arthralgias, headache, sore throat, rhinitis, and nonproductive cough. Otitis media and nausea and vomiting are common in younger children with influenza.	Nursing care is supportive and includes antipyretics, bedrest, and keeping the child isolated until symptoms subside. Antiviral medications (zanamivir and oseltamivir especially) reserved for children with immunosuppression. These medications are started within 48 hours of symptom onset and are effective in decreasing duration and symptoms of flu.	Complications can include febrile seizures in young children. Secondary bacterial pneumonia and exacerbation of underlying chronic illness can be seen. Sepsis can happen in infants. Myocarditis and death can occur.

(continued)

Table 25-3 Communicable Diseases in Childhood (continued)

Disease	Signs and Symptoms	Nursing Care	Complications
Influenza (Viral) (continued) is transmitted via direct contact, droplets, and fomites contaminated with nasopharyngeal secretions. Infection Control—The incubation period is typically 1–4 days. Many types of flu are largely preventable or at least diminished with the injectable or intranasal vaccine. The exact vaccine is created each year based on predictions of flu types expected.			
Mumps (Parotitis) (Viral) 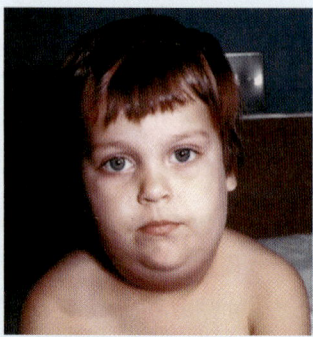 Causative Agent—Paramyxovirus Epidemiology—This disease is highly contagious. Peak Incidence—late winter to early spring, higher outbreaks among college-age persons if not vaccinated Mode of Transmission—The transmission of this disease spreads via droplets directly from an infected person (saliva and respiratory secretions). Virus may be airborne through infected droplets. Infection Control—The most contagious period is from 2 days before symptoms begin to 6 days after they end. Hospitalized children require droplet precautions.	Signs and symptoms are mild and systemic including malaise, low-grade fever, anorexia, ear pain and headache, and pain with chewing. As the disease advances, bilateral or unilateral parotid gland swelling appears; swelling generally peaks around the third day and lasts up to 6 days.	Nursing care is supportive and control of the signs and symptoms. Hydration and good nutrition are important care measures.	The main complication is orchitis in post-pubertal males. Sterility secondary to this complication is rare. Less common complications are oophoritis, pancreatitis, myocarditis, and deafness.
Pertussis (Bacterial) 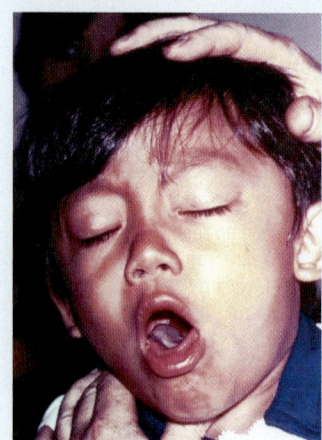 Causative Agent—*Bordetella pertussis* bacteria Epidemiology—This disease occurs in unimmunized or partially immunized persons, and outbreaks of pertussis	The initial signs and symptoms include a mild respiratory illness but with a cough that has a classic "whooping" sound, which is a high-pitched inspiratory sound. This persistent dry cough may last for months and includes coughing paroxysms and vomiting after coughing.	Nursing care includes the administration of antibiotics as ordered by the health-care provider. Infants younger than 6 months of age and those with severe disease are hospitalized for close observation of respiratory status. Nursing care also includes maintaining open airway and monitoring oxygen saturation.	Complications in infants, especially those younger than 6 months, include apnea, seizures, severe pneumonia, and pulmonary hypertension. In all children, bacterial pneumonia, seizures, encephalopathy, epistaxis, and even death can occur.

Table 25-3 Communicable Diseases in Childhood (continued)			
Disease	**Signs and Symptoms**	**Nursing Care**	**Complications**
more recently have led to recommendations for older children and adults to get re-vaccinated with booster doses of this vaccine. Adults and adolescents who are no longer immune provide a major reservoir for pertussis. It can also spread to incompletely immunized infants and children, with higher morbidity and mortality. Mode of Transmission—Transmission takes place through close contact with the infected person and aerosol droplet. Infection Control—The incubation period is 6–21 days. Hospitalized children should be placed on droplet precautions until the period of communicability has passed. Testing is possible through culture and PCR test.			
Pneumococcal Disease (Bacterial) Causative Agent—*Streptococcus pneumoniae*. Epidemiology—This disease is the leading cause of bacterial pneumonias in children except for newborns. Peak Incidence—Occurs in late winter and early spring when children spend more time in close quarters. Mode of Transmission—This disease spreads through contact with infected respiratory secretions. Infection Control—The incubation period is 1–3 days. There are 91 identified serotypes of pneumococcus, and three vaccines have been developed that address a number of serotypes. The vaccines are commonly given to young children and are offered to older children and teens who may not have received them, but who are at high risk of pneumococcal disease.	Signs and symptoms include upper respiratory infection, high fever, pleuritic chest pain, cough, chills, and dyspnea. Severe signs of respiratory distress are nasal flaring, grunting, retractions, rales, decreased breath sounds, tachypnea, wheezing, and stridor. The cough may be dry or productive and could include hemoptysis.	Nursing care includes the administration of penicillin (Bicillin), which is used for certain strains of pneumococcal disease. Other treatments for pneumonias include a wide range of antibiotics as determined by the health-care provider. Inpatient pediatric patients will have IV fluids and antibiotics. Viral pneumonias do not respond to antibiotics. Treat viral pneumonia with supportive care.	Complications can cause bacteremia in children, bronchiectasis, and airway compromise.
Poliomyelitis (Viral) 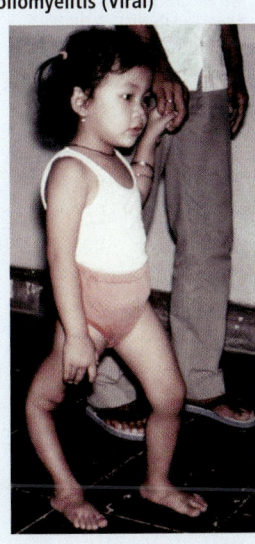	Signs and symptoms happen in the central nervous system with either non-paralytic or paralytic symptoms. Initially, children present with nonspecific symptoms such as low-grade fever and sore throat. The symptoms start mildly and then progress to transient pain and stiffness in the child's neck, back, and legs. Then symptoms may get severe, progressing to meningeal membranes. Signs of respiratory compromise may also occur. Paralytic polio is the most severe form and includes severe muscle pain followed	Nursing care is supportive. During the rehabilitation phase, physical therapy can maximize function.	Complications include permanent paralysis, respiratory arrest, and aseptic meningitis.

(continued)

Table 25-3 Communicable Diseases in Childhood (continued)

Disease	Signs and Symptoms	Nursing Care	Complications
Poliomyelitis (Viral) (continued) Causative Agent—Enterovirus Epidemiology—This disease is most common in infants and young children. Peak Incidence—In the United States, this has no peak incidence because of vaccination. Prior use of live vaccination did transmit some cases of polio, but only inactivated vaccine is now used. Mode of Transmission—This disease is transmitted via fecal–oral route primarily, but may also be transmitted through respiratory secretions. Infection Control—Standard and droplet precautions are used for hospitalized children to control the infection.	by paralysis in the legs but sometimes affecting other muscles, including those used in respiration.		
Roseola (Exanthem Subitum) (Viral) Causative Agent—Human herpes virus 6 or 7 Epidemiology—This disease occurs primarily in children. Occurs any time of the year. Peak Incidence—6–15 months of age Mode of Transmission—This disease is transmitted through oral, nasal, and conjunctival secretions. Infection Control - Incubation is 9–10 days. The most infectious period is during the febrile period before rash develops. Transmission of the disease is prevented through standard precautions and good hand washing.	Signs and symptoms may be asymptomatic or occur with just fever and no rash. Sudden high fever (usually 101°F (38.3°C) to higher than 103°F (39.4°C) and lasts 3–5 days. As fever begins to decrease, a discrete, red, maculopapular rash that fades when pressure is applied appears on the trunk. The rash then spreads to head and extremities and may last several days. Other signs and symptoms include URI, cervical lymphadenopathy, and lethargy.	Nursing care is supportive and includes fever-reducing measures. Monitor for febrile seizures.	Complications include a high fever.
Rubeola: Measles (Viral) 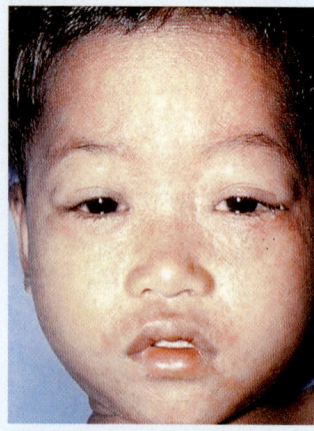 Causative Agent—Morbillivirus. Epidemiology—Occurs in outbreaks among unimmunized populations. Peak Incidence—Peaks in winter and spring. Mode of Transmission—The mode of transmission happens through the respiratory tract via droplets or direct contact with infectious secretions like blood or urine. This disease can also be transmitted via fomites. Infection Control—The incubation period is 8–12 days. Airborne and	Signs and symptoms include the prodromal phase lasting about 4–5 days and a moderate fever, cough, coryza, and conjunctivitis. Koplik's spots appear on the buccal mucosa 2 days before the onset of the rash (blue-white granules on erythematous base). The rash stage usually lasts about 3–4 days with a rise in fever up to 105°F (40.5°C). The rash first appears on forehead and behind the ears and then spreads to face, trunk, and upper and lower extremities. After 4–7 days rash begins to fade, and the temperature begins to drop. Other common symptoms can include anorexia, malaise, fatigue, and generalized lymphadenopathy.	Nursing care is supportive with antipyretics, bedrest, and increased fluids. Ensure the room is dark if photophobia occurs. Watch for complications and superinfections (otitis media and pneumonia).	Complications include pneumonia, otitis media, mastoiditis, encephalitis, and myocarditis. Younger children, medically fragile children, and children with underlying immunosuppression are at greater risk for complications.

Table 25-3 Communicable Diseases in Childhood (continued)

Disease	Signs and Symptoms	Nursing Care	Complications
contact precautions are recommended from 2 days before onset of symptoms until 5 days after appearance of the rash (about 14 days total). Measles is a reportable disease.			
Scarlet Fever (Bacterial) 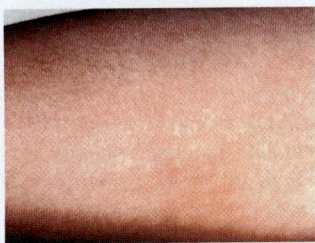 Causative Agent—Group A beta-hemolytic streptococci (GAS). Epidemiology—This disease is secondary to a pharyngeal infection with GAS. Peak Incidence—This disease is seen most frequently in late fall through spring. Mode of Transmission—This disease is spread through direct contact with infectious respiratory secretions. Infection Control—The incubation period is 2–5 days. Children with untreated infections remain contagious for weeks with the highest risk of transmission during the acute phase of the illness. Children should remain home from school until they have been on antibiotics for at least 24 hours and remain afebrile.	Signs and symptoms include acute onset with a fever, sore throat, rhinitis, headache, and tender cervical nodes. A sandpaper-like rash appears 12–48 hours after onset of symptoms. This rash is most prominent in creases and blanches to touch. In 3–4 days, the rash begins to fade, and the tips of toes and fingers begin to peel. On day 4 or 5 a bright red strawberry tongue develops.	Nursing care includes the administration of antibiotics, as determined by the health-care provider. Supportive nursing care is done for throat pain and fever.	Untreated strep infections may lead to retropharyngeal abscess, acute rheumatic fever, acute glomerulonephritis, toxic shock syndrome, bacteremia, and necrotizing fasciitis.
Tetanus (Bacterial) 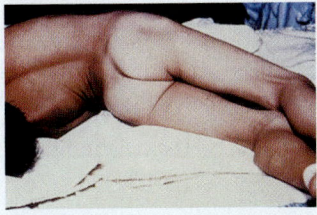 Causative Agent—*Clostridium tetani.* Epidemiology—Rare in United States. However, in other parts of the world neonatal tetanus is still a significant risk. Mode of Transmission—This disease occurs in humans through a cut or deep puncture wound that comes in contact with soil contaminated with the *Clostridium tetani* bacillus. Neonatal tetanus occurs in newborns delivered in unsanitary conditions. Infection Control—The incubation period for tetanus is 2–14 days. Prevention is immunization and postexposure prophylaxis.	Signs and symptoms of *Clostridium tetani* produce a neurotoxin that affects the muscles and nerves. Early signs are headache and restlessness followed by stiffness of the neck and jaw. The stiffness then progresses to painful spasms of the masticatory muscles accompanied by difficulty opening the mouth and dysphagia. Localized painful muscle spasm may begin to occur at the site of the wound. This disease eventually progresses up the trunk to the point of opisthotonos (a severe spasm of back muscles) causing the back to arch. As the neurotoxin spreads widely throughout the body, seizures are possible.	Nursing care includes the administration of tetanus immune globulin (TIG) to neutralize the neurotoxin. Antibiotics as determined by the health-care provider eliminate the bacillus from the body. Surgical debridement of the wound is done to control infection. An antispasmodic agent such as diazepam (Valium) is given to reduce spasms.	Complications include potential for spasms in all muscle groups. Laryngospasm and respiratory muscle spasms may compromise breathing and lead to death.

Nursing Insight—*Basic guidelines for infection control*

Infection Control Recommendation	Summary of Useful Practices
Cleaning and disinfection	Disinfect or sterilize surfaces, such as bed rails, computer keyboards, nightstands, phones, and toilets.
Cough etiquette/respiratory courtesy	Wear masks and/or cover mouth and nose when coughing or sneezing. Maintain a distance of 3 feet from others when you have a cold or flu.
Drug formulary restrictions	Limit prescribing privileges for antibiotics to designated specialists.
Hand hygiene	Use alcohol-based rubs when appropriate. Wash hands after contact with any blood, body fluids, or potentially contaminated items or patients.
Isolation procedures	Follow protocols for isolation of patients who are bleeding, coughing, giving off other excretions, secretions, or potentially hazardous body fluids. Segregate patients during outbreaks of infectious diseases. Separate immune-suppressed patients from others with potentially communicable diseases.
Laundry/linen and food service management	Gather patient clothing, eating utensils, gowns, sheets, and towels without contaminating other objects used in patient care. Wear a gown and gloves while collecting and washing laundry. Perform hand hygiene after laundry management procedures.
Personal protective equipment (PPE) use	Wear gloves, goggles, gowns, masks, and shoe covers while performing patient care procedures whenever exposure to blood, body fluids, aerosols, or splashes is possible. Dispose of PPEs in designated containers.
Resuscitation and invasive airway management	Avoid mouth-to-mouth contact with patients and wear PPE at all times, such as particulate respirators or masks. Disinfect or sterilize endoscopes, intubation equipment, nebulizers, face masks (e.g., for continuous positive airway pressure or supplemental oxygen), or other respiratory care devices.
Sharps (management of needles, wires, etc.)	Maintain sharps in open view to avoid accidental injuries. Never recap or manipulate needles used in patient care. Dispose of sharp objects in puncture-proof solid waste containers.
Source control	Supply/apply anti-infective rubs or soaps to patients to limit their colonization by disease-causing bacteria.
Standard precautions	Follow standard precautions during every patient encounter.

(Venes, D. (Ed.). (2013). *Taber's cyclopedic medical dictionary online* (22nd ed.). Philadelphia, PA: F.A. Davis.)

Infections

There are three types of infections: viral, fungal, and bacterial. Viruses (e.g., influenza, common cold viruses, and HIV) are microorganisms that are smaller than bacteria and do not grow without having a living cell as a host. The virus replicates itself in other living cells of people, animals, or plants. Fungal infections are pathological organisms including yeast and dermatophytes, such as tinea (e.g., athlete's foot and candida yeast infections). Fungal infections are most likely to occur in children with a compromised immune system (Venes, 2013). Bacterial infections are caused by single-celled living microorganisms and include such types as *Streptococcus*, *Staphylococcus*, and *Escherichia coli*. Bacteria can be found everywhere in the environment (see Chapter 23 for other common bacterial infections). It is important to understand the difference between viral, fungal, and bacterial infections so the proper medication is given. Limited antiviral antibiotics are available to treat some types of viral infections, antifungal agents are used to treat fungal infections, and antibacterial antibiotics treat bacterial infections.

 Nursing Insight—*Infections*

Human beings become colonized with certain bacteria shortly after birth. Some of these bacteria are actually beneficial and keep other pathogenic organisms that enter the body in check. Examples of healthy bacteria in human intestines include *Lactobacillus*, known as a probiotic if taken as a supplement. Infectious agents, whether bacteria, viruses, or fungi, can cause disease if there is a harmful proliferation of these pathogens that causes them to outweigh normal immunity and normal harmless bacteria (Blosser, Brady, & Royal, 2013).

Signs and Symptoms

Although each infectious condition has unique signs and symptoms, several symptoms are common in varying degrees among several illnesses. Common signs and symptoms of infection include:

- Fever
- Malaise
- Anorexia
- Pruritus (itching) from rashes

 Nursing Insight—*Pathophysiology of a fever*

The hypothalamus is the thermostat of the body. As blood circulates through the hypothalamus, it directs the various body organs to either conserve or dissipate the heat, (depending on the blood's temperature). If the body temperature is lower than normal, vasoconstriction, or shivering, is initiated to conserve heat, and chills occur to increase heat production. When a child has a fever (excess heat) the body's temperature, heart, and respiration rates increase. Vasodilation occurs, and the skin becomes flushed and warm to the touch. When the fever "breaks," the child may start to perspire, and the heart and respiration rates return to normal.

Diagnosis

Diagnosis of an infectious disease is confirmed by type of infection, signs and symptoms, and various diagnostic means.

 Diagnostic Tools Identification of an Infectious Disease

The following is a list of laboratory studies and diagnostic tests that are used to diagnose infection:
- Complete blood count (CBC) with differential
- Urinalysis
- Spinal fluid analysis
- Cultures from fluids, secretions, drainage (including blood, urine, sputum, nasal fluids, and wounds)
- Chest radiograph
- Computerized tomography (CT)

Prevention

 Across Care Settings: Caring for the child with an infectious disease

The majority of children with an infectious disease are cared for in the home or by a child care provider. Nursing care for the children and their families includes prevention of common illnesses along with their complications. Prevention of disease transmission within the family or community is essential. Key points to prevent transmission include:
- Good hand hygiene practices
- Covering the mouth and nose when coughing or sneezing
- Disposal or cleansing of articles contaminated with respiratory or gastric secretions such as tissues, blankets, and toys
- Use of antiseptic hand cleansers, such as alcohol-based hand gels
- Early identification of illness, with isolation from other children during infectious stages

Collaborative Care

Nursing Care. Building on the scientific foundation of immunology, the nurse provides specific care measures to promote immune function and to provide education to families.

Simple nursing actions, such as good skin care and optimal nutrition, help maintain the natural body barriers to disease and the natural immune response. The skin barrier is maintained by good hygiene measures such as hand washing and paying attention to any breaks or openings on the skin surface. Through good nutrition, the innate physical, chemical, and mechanical barriers are preserved, and the risk for infection is decreased. Adequate nutrition also promotes prompt healing and decreases the potential for skin breakdown. Maintaining barriers and the immune response is particularly important in children whose immune system is not yet fully mature and for children who are at risk for immunosuppression. Many children are more susceptible to disease in their early years until they develop greater immunity.

Nursing care for the child with an infectious disease also centers on accurate assessment, prevention of disease transmission, treating the signs and symptoms, teaching families about universal precautions, and preventing complications.

 Assessment Tool Key Components of Physical Assessment for the Child With an Infectious Disease

Vital Signs
- Temperature
- Heart rate
- Respiratory rate
- Blood pressure
- Pain

Respiratory Assessment
- Upper respiratory infection symptoms
- Breath sounds
- Work of breathing
- Pulse oximeter reading
- Skin/mucous membrane color
- Secretions; color, character, amount

Neurological Assessment
- Febrile seizures
- Early identification of neurological complications
- Level of consciousness

Gastrointestinal Assessment
- Fluid intake
- Presence of vomiting or diarrhea
- Level of hydration

Skin Assessment
- Presence of rash, pruritus, lesions

 focus on safety

CDC recommendations

Perform hand hygiene in ambulatory care settings:

A. Before touching a patient, even if gloves will be worn
B. Before exiting the patient's care area after touching the patient or the patient's immediate environment
C. After contact with blood, body fluids or excretions, or wound dressings
D. Prior to performing an aseptic task (e.g., placing an IV or preparing an injection)
E. If hands will be moving from a contaminated body site to a clean body site during patient care
F. After glove removal
G. Use soap and water when hands are visibly soiled (e.g., blood or body fluids), or after caring for patients with known or suspected infectious diarrhea (e.g., *Clostridium difficile* or norovirus). Otherwise, the preferred method of hand decontamination is with an alcohol-based hand rub.

Source: CDC (2013c).

The nurse assists families in managing the signs and symptoms. Fever is a common early symptom of bacterial and viral infections but not of most fungal infections. The nurse teaches parents about the use of acetaminophen (Children's Tylenol) or ibuprofen (Children's Advil) for treatment of fevers. It is essential that parents follow the directions on the medication label because there has been concern with overdosing children on antipyretic agents. Cool, moist compresses to the head and sponging or tepid baths can reduce the fever.

Malaise (weakness) tends to correlate with fevers, and providing a quiet, restful environment during the acute phase of illness may assist in the management of this symptom. If the child is anorexic, offering small amounts of fluids frequently helps keep the child hydrated. Sometimes a room-temperature, lemon-lime soft drink or ice-pop will taste good to the child. Also, offering small amounts of favorite foods, soft foods, or bland foods may help with the anorexia. If the anorexia becomes worrisome to parents, the nurse can encourage them to contact their health-care provider.

Pruritus is associated with many of the common infectious diseases and can be a source of distress for the child and a potential site for secondary infection because of skin breakdown. Parents may be advised to keep the child's fingernails short and place soft mittens on younger children to prevent scratching. Oatmeal or Aveeno® baths may provide some relief, as does Caladryl® lotion. Parents are advised to change bed linens frequently and avoid use of harsh soaps during the time of illness to avoid further irritation. Light clothing often helps keep perspiration and heat rashes to a minimum. An oral antihistamine such as diphenhydramine (Benadryl) may be useful in cases of severe pruritus.

Medical Care. Medical care for a patient with an infection will be specific for the actual pathogen that is present. Once the pathogen is diagnosed, the physician will order antibiotic therapy that is most appropriate for the patient and the disease process. The physician will also prescribe appropriate therapy to treat the symptoms associated with the disease process to keep the patient as comfortable as possible.

Education/Discharge Instructions

The nurse educates families and day-care providers about standard precautions. Emphasize hand washing, cleaning of toys and surfaces, and proper disposal of diapers. Educating the family about how to effectively control the itching is an important part of the nursing care plan. The pediatric nurse also provides education to families about the importance of excluding the child from school and other activities during the illness. Sound knowledge about the routes of transmission assists the nurse in developing a plan of care for the hospitalized child that includes environmental precautions that minimize the risk of transmission.

focus on safety

Reye's syndrome risk with use of aspirin

The administration of salicylates (aspirin) to children with acute viral illnesses, especially influenza and varicella (chickenpox), is linked to Reye's syndrome. This syndrome causes increased intracranial pressure and fat deposits in organs, causing children to become ill very quickly. It is critical that nurses teach parents about Reye's syndrome and provide education regarding use of aspirin-free medications for control of fever in children (National Reye's Syndrome Foundation, 2014).

 Optimizing Outcomes—Children with infectious diseases

The best outcome for the child with an infectious disease is the prevention and early identification of complications. The nurse pays careful attention to fluid deficit, upper respiratory tract infection, and neurological difficulties.

focus on safety

Complications

Although potential complications are specific to each illness, there are general symptoms that are associated with many of the infectious diseases. Children with infectious disease often are at risk for developing a fluid deficit caused by a combination of anorexia, nausea, vomiting, and sore throat. The nurse assists families in managing fluid deficit by offering the child small amounts of liquids frequently and offering favorite fluids to the child such as juice, soda, or water. Respiratory infections are also common. A cool steamer, decongestants, or gentle nasal suctioning with a bulb syringe may help diminish respiratory difficulty. Neurological symptoms include general lethargy (sluggishness or tiredness) that may progress to decreased responsiveness. Generalized irritability that progresses to inconsolable crying, seizures, or meningeal symptoms, including stiff neck and photophobia, may be present. Parents must be instructed to call the health-care provider if these neurological symptoms occur or the child is unresponsive.

 Critical Nursing Action Seeking Immediate Help

Respiratory symptoms are a major component of many of the common infectious illnesses of childhood. Respiratory symptoms of concern include increased work of breathing; inability to swallow, including drooling; muffled voice; or very rapid or slow respirations. The nurse instructs the family to seek help immediately if the child exhibits any of these signs of respiratory deterioration.

 Medication: Common Medications That Contain Salicylates (Aspirin)

Alka-Seltzer	Ecotrin
Anacin	Excedrin
Ascriptin	Kaopectate
Bayer Arthritis Pain	Pamprin
and Aspirin preparations	Pepto-Bismol
Bufferin	Sine-Off Sinus Medicaine
Doan's	St. Joseph Adult Aspirin
Dristan	Vanquish

Nursing Insight—*Sneeze and cough guidelines*

In response to the virulence of H1N1 especially, the CDC developed new cough and sneeze guidelines. Posters of this are available, and it is suggested that these guidelines be placed in prominent areas as reminders. The guidelines are as follows:
- Cover your mouth and nose with a tissue when you cough or sneeze.
- Put your used tissue in the wastebasket.
- If you don't have a tissue, cough or sneeze into your upper sleeve or elbow, not your hands.
- You may be asked to put on a face mask to protect others.
- Wash your hands often with soap and warm water for 20 seconds.
- If soap and water are not available, use an alcohol-based hand rub.
  (CDC, 2013d)

Viral Infections

There are more than 400 types of viruses, which are the smallest infectious agents known today. When a virus enters a cell, it can trigger a disease process immediately or remain dormant for many years. The virus can enter any organ of the body by attaching to the cell membrane and assembling the cells into a more mature form that is then capable of affecting other cells and taking over cellular function. Viruses are responsible for such diseases as fifth disease (erythema infectiosum), cytomegalovirus (CMV), herpes simplex virus, herpes zoster, and infectious mononucleosis.

FIFTH DISEASE (ERYTHEMA INFECTIOSUM)

This viral disease is common in childhood, and it is caused by human parvovirus B19. Most children do not get seriously ill with this virus, but children who are immunocompromised may become very ill. Pregnant women who acquire this disease from a child, if they have never developed antibodies to it, may unfortunately lose their babies because of hydrops fetalis (fetal death).

Signs and Symptoms

Fifth disease is known as the "slapped cheek" virus because it begins with a red rash on the face appearing as though the child's cheeks were slapped. The rash then spreads to the trunk and extremities, appearing more as a macular (flat) lacy-appearing erythematous exanthema (rash). Fever may occur and the rash, though usually gone in a week, can recur with heat exposure for up to 4 months.

Diagnosis

Diagnosis is made through clinical appearance of the signs and symptoms in most cases but can be accurately diagnosed with IgM Parvovirus B19 antibodies in the serum within 30 days of rash onset.

Prevention

Avoid exposure to other children with fifth disease. Maintain good hand washing techniques. Pregnant women must avoid all contact with fifth disease as it can fatally damage the fetus.

Collaborative Care

Nursing Care. Symptomatic relief, treatment of high fever, and warnings to keep children away from pregnant women are the main nursing care measures. The rash is not really uncomfortable. The nurse can help in early identification of this disease because of its classic appearance. If a pregnant woman has been exposed to this virus, she should see her obstetrics provider immediately (Richardson, 2013). Because the disease is spread by droplet through coughing and sneezing, droplet precautions should be instituted if a child is hospitalized. This usually implies the use of masks, gloves, eyewear, and keeping the child in a single room.

Medical Care. Use of acetaminophen (Children's Tylenol) or ibuprofen (Children's Advil) according to age-appropriate guidelines is useful for high fevers, sore throat, and headache that may accompany this disease.

Education/Discharge Instructions

The nurse should instruct the patient and family to maintain safe hygiene practices and use careful hand washing. The child should be kept away from potentially pregnant females. The rash can last at least a week, and it has been known to recur when the patient is exposed to heat. Do not use aspirin-containing products for these children because of the risk of Reye's syndrome.

CYTOMEGALOVIRUS INFECTIONS

Cytomegalovirus (CMV) is a member of the herpes family, which attaches to host cells to cause disease. CMV is transmitted via close contact with body fluids of an infected person. This virus may remain in a latent form within the child's body after the initial infection, and it can reactivate particularly with children who have immunodeficiency situations, as occurs in HIV and organ transplantation. The disease is not highly contagious, and transmission is easily prevented with good hand washing. Congenital CMV is possible and is usually associated with congenital defects such as vision or hearing damage. Children ages 1 to 3, teenagers, and pregnant women may have a high incidence of CMV infection. Young children in day care are a reservoir for this disease.

Signs and Symptoms

Some babies born with CMV are asymptomatic, while others experience hearing loss, a variety of neurological issues, and even intrauterine growth restriction. Older children may experience symptoms similar to infectious mononucleosis with fever, headache, rash, abdominal pain, and even hepatitis. CMV can also cause pneumonia and self-limited gastrointestinal symptoms. Children with immune disorders can become seriously ill from CMV, including fever and pneumonia. Retinitis, or inflammation of the retina, can cause blindness in CMV infection associated with AIDS. CMV hepatitis may also occur in transplanted livers.

Diagnosis

Urine, saliva, blood, and biopsy samples can be used for virus isolation to make a diagnosis. CMV pneumonia is suggested by radiograph and lung CT scan.

Prevention

CMV infection is a source of significant morbidity and mortality in immunocompromised children. Good hand washing is the best preventive measure. Disposable gloves should be worn when handling linen or underclothes soiled with feces or urine. CMV-negative blood should be provided to immunocompromised children.

Collaborative Care

Nursing Care. The most common symptom after resolution of the acute phase of the infection is fatigue, which may be present for as long as 18 months after the primary infection. Because CMV can be transmitted by direct contact, nursing care involves contact precautions and careful hand hygiene. The nurse notes if the patient has any signs of immune deficiency, which could have put him or her at risk of developing CMV infection. Inquire about frequent sore throats, respiratory infections, enlarged lymph nodes, and recurrent fevers, for example. The nurse should evaluate the patient for potential need for acetaminophen or ibuprofen for symptom control. The nurse should monitor the patient for vision changes, weight loss, anorexia, nausea, vomiting, shortness of breath, chest tightness, fever, and recurrent symptoms that can occur after the first signs of disease.

Medical Care. Ganciclovir (Cytovene), an antiviral agent, is primarily used in the treatment of life-threatening CMV in the immunocompromised population with CMV infection. Neutropenia, thrombocytopenia, and anemia are possible adverse effects of this drug.

Education/Discharge Instructions

The nurse educates the patients and family members about the risks of this disease and of the treatments. Teach the

---

 Medication: Ganciclovir (Cytovene)

(gan-**sye**-kloe-vir)

Indications:
Treatment of CMV retinitis in immunocompromised children.
Prevention of CMV infection in transplant children at risk.

Actions: CMV converts ganciclovir to its active form inside the host cell, where it inhibits viral DNA polymerase.

Therapeutic Effects: Antiviral effect directed against CMV-infected cells.

Contraindications and Precautions:
CONTRAINDICATED IN: HYPERSENSITIVITY TO GANCICLOVIR OR ACYCLOVIR.

Adverse Reactions and Side Effects:
Seizures, headache, malaise, drowsiness, ataxia,
GI bleeding, nausea, vomiting, increased liver enzymes
Neutropenia, thrombocytopenia, anemia
Hypotension, hypertension
Renal toxicity

Nursing Implications:
1. Pediatric dosing is not established.
2. Increased risk of bone marrow depression when used with antineoplastics or zidovudine.
3. Assess child during treatment of signs of infection, bleeding, or development of CMV retinitis.
4. Administer IV at slow rate, using in-line filter.
5. Advise child/family to notify health-care provider for any signs of bleeding.

Source: Data from Vallerand, A. H., & Sanoski, C. A. (2014). *Davis's drug guide for nurses* (14th ed.). Philadelphia, PA: F.A. Davis.

---

parent or caregiver to handle diapers or underclothing carefully, with good hand washing to prevent the spread of CMV. Universal precautions in acute and primary care settings will help to decrease the risk of spread to other children and women of childbearing age, where CMV infection can cause serious fetal harm. Pregnant employees in day-care centers and hospital nurseries should avoid caring for CMV patients. A patient with CMV will require optometry evaluations of the optic fundus if he or she has HIV/AIDS.

HERPES SIMPLEX VIRUS

The herpes simplex virus is extremely common, and it is estimated that many people are infected with it during childhood. There are 2 types: herpes simplex 1 and herpes simplex 2 (HSV-1 and HSV-2). Type 1 is primarily associated with mouth, lip, and facial lesions. Type 2 is primarily associated with genital lesions and neonatal cases through birth. The types can be mixed and each can be found in the other areas mentioned. Type 1 infections are more commonly known as "fever blisters" or "cold sores," and frequently they recur in the nasolabial area of the face with the presence of upper respiratory infections, fever, and exposure to stress or sunlight. Type 2 lesions originate with sexual activity. Herpes Type 1 is discussed here.

Signs and Symptoms

Small vesicles or erythematous form around the lips, base of nose, or in the genital area, in most cases. They may have a prodrome of pruritus or burning prior to developing, and most are painful when the vesicles break. These vesicles crust over as they are healing.

🌼 *Nursing Insight*—*Neonatal infections*

Babies can have skin, eye, and mouth lesions. The progression of disease in neonates is severe, causing risk for retinitis, encephalitis (brain inflammation), and microcephaly (small brain). The herpes simplex becomes disseminated (i.e., it invades the body).

Diagnosis

Diagnosis is obtained through culturing the fluid from the vesicles. It is possible to type the HSV as either 1 or 2. Spinal fluid, Pap smears, and Tzanck tests are other means to diagnose herpes simplex virus.

Prevention

Because herpes simplex is a contagious disease, observe careful hand washing techniques and universal precautions. In acute care settings, patients with herpes must not be exposed to immune-suppressed patients because of the risk of disseminated herpes infections. The virus can be transmitted by saliva and also by exposure to the mother's genitalia during childbirth. If a mother has a genital herpes outbreak around the time of delivery, the baby may be delivered by C-section.

Collaborative Care

Nursing Care. Careful hand washing and contact precautions (including avoiding kissing and touching) are necessary because HSV lesions can be infectious from saliva and from direct contact, especially with vesicular fluid, onto mucosal surfaces and through fissures in the skin. Teach parents to use separate towels and glasses for these children. For children with HSV-2, there may be concerns about inappropriate sexual exposures. For infants with neonatal disseminated HSV, the disease is very serious and is fatal for half of all neonates with untreated HSV that affects the central nervous system. Infants may suffer long-term neurological sequelae (Blosser et al., 2013). Nurses should use gloves when there are active herpes lesions in patients to avoid spreading infection to themselves or other patients.

Nurses should report any facial lesions that are tracking up the child's face, cheek, or nose close to the eye, because herpes in the eye can cause blindness if not treated immediately.

 Nursing Insight—*Herpetic Whitlow*

A disorder named "herpetic whitlow," or herpes infection on the fingers, was once common in nurses and dental workers whose hands were exposed to herpes viruses before the widespread use of gloves.

Medical Care. For children who have HSV-1 on the facial areas, the nurse may administer topical prescription antiviral medications, such as acyclovir (Zovirax) ointment or penciclovir (Denavir) ointment. These medications are not curative, but they lessen the duration and pain of HSV-2 genital lesions. Children, depending on their ages, may be also treated with IV, topical, or oral antiviral agents, usually acyclovir (Zovirax). Famciclovir (Famvir) and valacyclovir (Valtrex) are reserved for use in older adolescents and adults for acute episodes. For disseminated newborn infections, IV acyclovir (Zovirax) is the standard treatment, and long-term use of this medication is under investigation (Blosser et al., 2013).

Education/Discharge Instructions

Remind parents and patients that herpes simplex is most often a recurrent disease. While the first episode is generally the worst episode, herpes simplex can recur. In some patients, there is never a recurrence, but more commonly, the lesions will recur, and the frequency of recurrence may be associated with the patient's immune status and degree of stress. Education includes avoidance of sharing toothbrushes and lip cosmetics. Educate patients to avoid excessive sunlight because it can cause recurrences of herpes labialis, and for those patients who are sexually active, latex condoms should be recommended to prevent genital transmission of herpes. It is not known if herpes can be spread when there are no active skin lesions.

HERPES ZOSTER (SHINGLES)

The varicella-zoster virus (the same virus that causes varicella or chickenpox) causes herpes zoster. This virus is seen in older children and young adults. The first time the child is exposed to this virus, he or she contracts chickenpox. On a subsequent exposure, because of reactivation of the virus, herpes zoster occurs.

Signs and Symptoms

Initial signs and symptoms include cutaneous vesicular lesions that follow the nerve pattern on the face, trunk, and upper back area, usually affecting only one side of the body. The lesions resemble herpes simplex lesions, although they cluster in larger numbers normally and are more painful. The classic presentation is considered "dew drops on a red rose," implying a clear fluid vesicle on top of an erythematous base. There may be a prodrome of burning pain or pruritus before the lesions appear. It is important to note that the child may experience pain from the nerve involvement.

Diagnosis

Diagnosis of herpes zoster is based on patient history and physical examination findings. It is important to obtain any history of having chickenpox (varicella).

Prevention

Currently, the only prevention for herpes zoster is primary immunization with varicella vaccine. Once a patient has had varicella illness, the herpes virus remains dormant in nerve root endings and can resurface as herpes zoster at any point in life. However, immunosuppressed individuals, persons with other significant medical diseases, elders, and persons under stress are the most common people who experience herpes zoster.

Collaborative Care

Nursing Care. Patients with disseminated herpes zoster infections may be hospitalized. Otherwise, most patients can be taken care of in the home. Nursing care includes measures to decrease the itching and pain. Cool water compresses, cool baths, wet to dry Burrow's solution dressings three times in a day, and calamine lotion can relieve the itching or burning associated with herpes zoster. Acetaminophen (Children's Tylenol) may be given for pain. Do not administer aspirin products because of risk of Reye's syndrome. Acyclovir (Zovirax) is the treatment of choice for children with herpes zoster. There are separate dosages for over and under age 12, and acyclovir can be given by IV for fastest relief for disseminated herpes. It may be given orally, dependent on age, for recurrent episodes. The nurse must also observe the patients with disseminated zoster for meningitis, encephalitis, deafness, and uveitis of the eye.

Medical Care. Famciclovir (Famvir) or valacyclovir (Valtrex) are drugs administered to inhibit viral DNA synthesis, thus limiting the disease symptoms and duration, although no medications are curative. Acyclovir (Zovirax) is most commonly used for children.

Education/Discharge Instructions

Postherpetic neuralgia is common during, and subsequent to a herpes zoster outbreak. It is neurological pain that can have a burning sensation. Early use of antiviral medications such as acyclovir (Zovirax) will decrease the chance of postherpetic neuralgia. If pain continues, the patients need to report this to their health-care providers because there are some medications that can improve neuralgia.

Patients with herpes zoster should stay away from anyone who has not had varicella nor been immunized against varicella because there is risk of causing varicella in those individuals. Recurrence of herpes zoster necessitates a medical evaluation for underlying disease or immune suppression.

Nurses should educate patients to avoid directly touching the lesions or exposing another's skin and mucous membranes to the lesions.

Medication: ACYCLOVIR (Zovirax)

(ay-**sye**-kloe-veer)

Indications:
PO: Recurrent genital herpes infections. Localized cutaneous herpes zoster infections (shingles) and chickenpox (varicella).
IV: Severe initial episodes of genital herpes in non-immunosuppressed patients.
Mucosal or cutaneous herpes simplex infections or herpes zoster infections (shingles) in immunosuppressed patients. Herpes simplex encephalitis.
Topical
Cream: Recurrent herpes labialis (cold sores).
Topical
Ointment: Treatment of limited non–life-threatening herpes simplex infections in immunocompromised patients (systemic treatment is preferred).

Actions: Interferes with viral DNA synthesis.

Therapeutic Effects: Inhibition of viral replication, decreased viral shedding, and reduced time for healing of lesions.

Contraindications and Precautions:
Avoid in hypersensitivity to acyclovir or valacyclovir. Use cautiously in pre-existing, serious, neurological, hepatic, pulmonary, and fluid and electrolyte abnormalities. Renal impairment dose alteration if CCl less than 50 mL/minute.

Adverse Reactions/Side Effects:
CNS: seizures, dizziness, headache, hallucinations, trembling. GI: diarrhea, nausea, vomiting, liver enzymes, hyperbilirubinemia, abdominal pain, anorexia. GU: renal failure, crystalluria, hematuria, renal pain. Derm: Stevens-Johnson syndrome, acne, hives, rash, unusual sweating. Endo: changes in menstrual cycle. Hemat: thrombotic thrombocytopenic purpura/hemolytic uremic syndrome (high doses in immunosuppressed patients). Local: pain, phlebitis, local irritation. MS: joint pain. Misc: polydipsia.

Nursing Implications:
1. Assess lesions before and daily during therapy.
2. Monitor neurological status in patients with herpes encephalitis.
3. Lab Test Considerations: Monitor BUN, serum creatinine, and CCr before and during therapy. This may indicate renal failure.

Source: Data from Vallerand, A. H., & Sanoski, C. A. (2014). *Davis's drug guide for nurses* (14th ed.). Philadelphia, PA: F.A. Davis.

INFECTIOUS MONONUCLEOSIS

The Epstein-Barr virus is responsible for infectious mononucleosis, which is communicable during the active phase of the illness (7–10 days). Historically, infectious mononucleosis was first discovered as a disease that was transmitted through kissing. Although it can occur at any age, the disease is most commonly found in adolescents and young adults.

Signs and Symptoms

The cervical and often occipital lymph nodes become swollen, enlarged, and tender. Other symptoms are tonsillitis or pharyngitis with significant exudates, chills, fever (103.3°F [39.6°C]), headache, anorexia, and malaise. Also, during the initial disease phase, the spleen may become enlarged. Because rupture is possible, avoid palpating the spleen or placing any pressure over the area. Mononucleosis hepatitis is also possible in severe cases.

Diagnosis

The monospot test, or heterophile antibody test, was designed to detect the disease. A positive test result confirms the disease. If necessary, a blood test can be drawn to confirm the presence of Epstein-Barr virus. Sometimes the monospot test does not turn positive early in the disease. Therefore, it is useful to have a complete blood count and differential blood test because atypical lymphocytes and sometimes an increase in monocytes are seen on the differential cells early on in the condition.

Prevention

Because mononucleosis is considered most communicable by saliva, avoid kissing and close facial contact with patients with mononucleosis. This virus can also be spread by coughing, sneezing, and sharing of eating utensils. Adolescents who are not eating or sleeping properly, particularly in the late high school and college years, seem to have increased risk of infectious mononucleosis related to high stress and lowered immunity.

Collaborative Care

Nursing Care. Children can experience general fatigue or weakness for up to 6 weeks after the acute phase. Therefore, it is important that they continue to include rest periods and fluids during their normal daily routine. The nurse communicates to the caregivers that sharing drinking cups with family members and peers is not advisable, nor is close contact, such as kissing. Children and adolescents are typically removed from contact sports that could injure the liver or spleen for as long as the disease is active. Bedrest, maintaining hydration, decreasing fever, and isolation are required during the acute phase of the illness.

Education/Discharge Instructions

The nurse should educate the patient and family about the necessity of avoiding contact sports and roughhousing because of risk of rupture of the spleen. Patients with infectious mononucleosis are often eager to return to activities before their bodies are sufficiently healed, and it is possible to relapse with worsening symptoms. Use of acetaminophen should be avoided because of the greater risk of hepatotoxicity when the liver is enlarged. Alcohol should be avoided because of the risk of hepatomegaly.

Fungal Infections

Any disease introduced by a fungus is called a mycosis. Fungi are either unicellular (yeasts) or multicellular (molds) and larger than bacteria. Fungal diseases are categorized according to the particular body tissue they affect. Most infections in children are superficial subcutaneous infections of the skin, hair, nails, or mucous membranes associated with either overgrowth of fungi normally present or introduced through breaks in the skin. Superficial findings include slight itching, red or gray patches, dryness, and brittle hair. Transmission is by the inhalation of spores. There are four superficial fungal infections seen in children: tinea capitis, tinea pedis, tinea cruris, and tinea corporis (Table 25-4).

Table 25-4 Fungal Infections

Fungal Infection	Location	Treatment	Parent Information
Tinea Capitis (Ringworm)	Fungal infection that begins as an infection of a single hair follicle but spreads rapidly in a circular pattern and produces a 1-inch-diameter lesion. The circular pattern becomes filled with dirty-appearing scales, and the hairs involved break off. Alopecia (hair loss) can occur in patches, and pustular lesions (kerions) can also occur. This infection goes from the noninflammatory to the inflammatory stage over an 8-week period.	Oral griseofulvin (Fulvicin) is taken with fatty food to increase absorption. Selenium or ketoconazole shampoo is used to prevent transmission in the household. CBC, liver function tests (LFTs), and BUN/creatinine must be monitored when the child is taking griseofulvin (Fulvicin).	Adolescents are warned not to use alcohol because of tachycardia. Children do not need to be kept home from school. Family members must not share towels or combs. Linens and clothing should be laundered in hot water to decrease spread among family members. Hair regrowth takes up to 12 months.
Tinea Pedis (Athlete's Foot)	Fungal infection with skin lesions located between the toes and on the plantar surface of the foot. This condition may begin as fine scale and may macerate and become superinfected. It is intensely pruritic.	Liquid preparations of clotrimazole (Lotrimin) are used. tolnaftate (Tinactin) miconazole (Micatin)	Antiseptic foot baths. Wear cotton socks. Change shoes periodically. Use antifungal powders or spray in shoes. Do not let others share personal items such as footwear, towels, clothes, or sports equipment. Wear sandals or swim shoes in public showers and stockings or shoes in locker rooms.
Tinea Cruris (Jock Itch)	Fungal infection found on the inner aspects of thighs, groin, and scrotum; pink, pruritic rash with fine scale and sharp margins. More common in adolescent males, obese individuals, or with chafing.	Cream, liquid, or powder preparations of clotrimazole (Lotrimin) are used. tolnaftate (Tinactin) miconazole (Micatin)	Shower or bathe frequently. Dry scrotal area thoroughly when damp. Wear cotton underwear. Do not let others share personal items such as footwear, towels, clothes, or sports equipment.
Tinea Corporis (Epidermal layer of the skin)	Fungal infection of the epidermal layer of the skin that has a circular lesion with a clear center and scaly inflammation.	Topical clotrimazole (Lotrimin)	Do not let others share personal items such as footwear, towels, clothes, or sports equipment.

Source: Burns, C. E., Dunn, A. M., Brady, M. A., Starr, N. B., & Blosser, C. G. (2012). *Pediatric primary care* (5th ed.). Philadelphia, PA: Elsevier.

CANDIDA ALBICANS (ORAL THRUSH)

Most infants have natural yeast in their mouths called *Candida albicans*. Because of the immature immune system in infants, the yeast in their mouths can overgrow and lead to an infection called oral thrush. This fungal infection is quite common but can be exacerbated by the use of steroid inhalers or antibiotics. HIV patients are also at greater risk for thrush.

Signs and Symptoms

The main symptom is white plaques on the surface of the tongue and the buccal (cheek) membranes.

Diagnosis

C albicans is diagnosed via a microscopic examination of the plaques (Venes, 2013).

Prevention

The nurse educates parents about the prevention of oral thrush. If the infant is bottle-fed, oral thrush can be prevented by thoroughly cleaning the bottle nipples in hot water. If the infant is breastfed and the mother's nipples are sore and reddened, the nurse can encourage the mother to contact the health-care provider about possible use of an antifungal ointment on the nipples while the infant is also treated with nystatin (Mycostatin). Pacifiers are thoroughly cleaned in hot water.

Collaborative Care

Nursing Care. This fungal infection is painful, and the child may not eat well. Maintaining nutrition is a priority nursing care measure for the child. Small, frequent feedings and soft and bland foods during the infection for the older child may help ensure good nutrition. A soft toothbrush or gauze pad can be used to clean the mouth.

In babies with thrush, the baby's mouth should be rinsed out with water from a medicine cup after feedings. The baby's hands should be washed frequently with soap and water. Pacifiers and teething rings should be boiled for 5 to 7 minutes after each use during the course of infection. Toys that a child may chew on should be washed in hot, soapy water. Candidal diaper rash may occur especially if a baby has thrush because both are candidal overgrowths. If a baby is breastfeeding, the mother's nipples will need to be washed carefully, and if there are any cracks in the skin, there is risk of passing the candidal infection to the mother, especially into the breast ducts. Mothers with nipple thrush may need to be treated simultaneously with their infected babies.

Nurses need to administer the candidal medication with a dropper for infants and with instructions to swish and swallow the medications in the case of older children. (BabyCare Advice, 2013).

Medical Care. Nystatin (Mycostatin) is the medication that effectively treats thrush. It is administered with a gloved finger using a swab placed on the buccal membranes. The medication must be administered after feedings so it will remain in contact with the fungi rather than being washed away immediately during the feeding. Older children may be treated with *troches* (lozenges that dissolve by sucking on them), pastilles, or suspensions. Adolescents may be treated with fluconazole (Diflucan) orally for 7 to 14 days, depending on the severity (Sherman, 2009).

Education/Discharge Instructions

The nurse is aware that candidiasis can be a generalized infection, especially in newborns, causing a bright red diaper rash. It must be treated immediately to prevent it from becoming systemic. Parents are taught that changing diapers frequently, exposing the area to air, and applying nystatin (Mycostatin) ointment is important.

 Nursing Insight—*Urinary tract Candida*

Candida does not routinely cause urinary tract infections, but it is often asymptomatically present in the urine. It has the potential for causing cystitis or pyelonephritis. However, neonates or highly immunocompromised children may develop disseminated candidiasis from urinary tract candida, and treatment must be aggressive, as in other systemic fungal infection (Sherman, 2009).

 focus on safety

Systemic fungal infections

One systemic fungal infection, known as systemic mycosis, occurs primarily through inhalation of fungal spores. The specific fungal agent determines the course and severity of the infection. Systemic mycosis is not transmitted from person to person. Another type of systemic mycotic infection is aspergillosis, which is found in airborne dust particles, compost heaps, or air vents. The condition usually manifests in children who already have a weakened immune system. Aspergillosis usually affects open spaces in the body, such as cavities that have formed in the lungs from preexisting lung diseases. It is characterized by a slow-progression, chronic illness and spreads rapidly through the bloodstream to the brain and kidneys. This infection is very serious and difficult to treat. The main medical treatment for aspergillosis is the administration of IV amphotericin B (Amphocin) and supportive management for complications from either the active disease or subsequent treatment.

Also, invasive candidiasis, another systemic fungal infection, is now being seen mostly in hospitalized patients as the fourth most common cause of nosocomial bloodstream infection or sepsis in the United States (Sherman, 2009). It occurs most often in leukemic and cancer patients on chemotherapy or in dialysis patients. A newer class of antifungal agents that kill, rather than just inhibit, the growth of the bloodstream candida is called the **echinocandin** class; it works by attacking the cell walls and is best used if the organisms are resistant to fluconazole (Diflucan).

OTHER FUNGAL INFECTIONS

Tinea Capitis

Tinea capitis (see Table 25-4) is also known as ringworm for its distinctive round shape and capacity to spread on the skin, with central clearing of the rash. This type of fungal infection is common and is known as a dermatophyte. Tinea grow on the scalp (tinea capitis), hands (tinea manuum), feet (tinea pedis), groin (tinea cruris), and skin (tinea corporis). Children are most prone to tinea capitis. Tinea capitis can cause *alopecia* (localized balding) because of loss of hair. Medical management in children includes a topical over-the-counter antifungal agent. Difficult cases are eradicated with oral medications such as griseofulvin (Fulvicin).

Histoplasmosis

This fungal infection can occur when mold spores are inhaled and they convert to yeast in the lungs. High-risk areas of mold include cleaning or excavating in old homes or schools, cutting firewood, gardening, and exploring barns and caves. Signs and symptoms include weight loss, fever, fatigue, dry cough and substernal chest pain, acute respiratory distress syndrome, meningitis in infants, pericarditis, and arthritis symptoms. Medical management for histoplasmosis includes amphotericin B (Amphocin) and a pediatric infectious disease health-care practitioner needs to monitor these children for complications.

Coccidioidomycosis

This fungal infection can occur from inhaling spore-forming molds into the lungs from the soil. It is common, especially to the southwestern U.S. states, and it is asymptomatic or self-limiting without treatment in most patients. Signs and symptoms include fever, malaise, respiratory distress, rash of erythema nodosum or erythema multiforme, weight loss, arthralgia, headache, and confusion. If needed, medical management is done with azole type antifungal medications such as itraconazole (Sporanox).

Pneumocystis Jiroveci Pneumonia

This fungus typically causes pneumonia. There is a risk of this condition in pediatric patients who are HIV and among other immunocompromised children. Signs and symptoms include nonproductive cough, weight loss, fever, chills, dyspnea, respiratory failure, tachypnea, and crackles and rhonchi in lungs. Prophylaxis is commonly managed with trimethoprim sulfamethoxazole (TMP-SMZ) (Bactrim or Septra). Other agents used for severe cases include parenteral pentamidine (Nebupent), atovaquone (Mepron), dapsone (Dapsone), and clindamycin (Cleocin) plus primaquine (Phosphate Tablets). Sometimes short courses of steroid therapy are used. Immunocompromised patients who do not have HIV should also receive prophylaxis (O'Keefe, 2012).

Bacterial Infections

 Nursing Insight—*Other common bacterial infections*

Common bacteria cause disease in the pediatric population. *Streptococcus pneumoniae, or pneumococcus,* is an alpha-hemolytic, aerotolerant anaerobic member of the genus

Streptococcus. S pneumoniae is a major cause of pneumonia and also responsible for pediatric otitis media and sinusitis. *Haemophilus influenza* is a gram-negative, coccobacilli bacterium and responsible for numerous cases of pediatric otitis media as well as sinusitis. *Moraxella catarrhal* is of the species *catarrhalis* in the genus *Moraxella* and also a cause of pediatric otitis media and sinusitis. The group A β-hemolytic streptococcus (*Streptococcus pyogenes*, or GAS) is a form of β-hemolytic streptococcus bacteria. It is a gram-positive bacterium responsible for the classic "strep throat." It is also seen in a variety of other pediatric disorders. This bacterium is also responsible for rheumatic fever and rheumatic heart disease. *Neisseria meningitidis*, often referred to as *meningococcus*, is a serious pathogen in the development of bacterial meningitis, which is sometimes fatal. Sequelae of meningitis include neurological issues and hearing deficits. Children and adolescents with meningitis typically have high fever, extremely stiff neck (nuchal rigidity), vomiting, and headache, with the later development of a rash that is stellate, resembling stars. Rapid treatment for meningitis is required. Bacterial meningitis must be differentiated from viral meningitis, which is usually not as severe. See Chapter 23 for other common bacterial infections.

Medication: AMOXICILLIN (used for several types of childhood bacterial infections) Amoxil, DisperMox, Moxatag

(a-mox-i-*sill*-in)

Indications: Treatment of: skin and skin structure infections, otitis media, sinusitis, respiratory infections, and genitourinary infections. Endocarditis prophylaxis. Postexposure inhalational anthrax prophylaxis.

Actions: Binds to bacterial cell wall, causing cell death.

Therapeutic Effects: Binds to bacterial cell wall, causing cell death. Therapeutic effects: Bactericidal action; spectrum is broader than penicillins. Spectrum: Active against: Streptococci, pneumococci, enterococci, *Haemophilus influenzae, Escherichia coli, Proteus mirabilis, Neisseria meningitides, N gonorrhoeae,* shigella, *Chlamydia trachomatis,* salmonella, *Borrelia burgdorferi,* and *H pylori Helicobacter.*

Contraindications and Precautions:
CONTRAINDICATED IN: Hypersensitivity to penicillins (cross-sensitivity exists to cephalosporins and other beta-lactams); tablets for oral suspension (DisperMox) contain aspartame; avoid in patients with phenylketonuria.
Use cautiously in: severe renal insufficiency (pdose if CCr >30 mL/min); infectious mononucleosis, acute lymphocytic leukemia, or cytomegalovirus infection (risk of rash); OB, Lactation: Has been used safely.

Adverse Reactions and Side Effects: CNS: SEIZURES (high doses). GI: pseudomembranous colitis, diarrhea, nausea, vomiting, liver enzymes. Derm: rash, urticaria. Hemat: blood dyscrasias. Misc: liver reactions including ANAPHYLAXIS, SERUM SICKNESS, superinfection.

Interactions: Drug-Drug: Probenecid: renal excretion and blood levels of amoxicillin—therapy may be combined for this purpose. May alter effect of warfarin. May alter effectiveness of oral contraceptives. Allopurinol may increase the frequency of rash.

Nursing Implications:
1. Instruct patients to take medication around the clock and to finish the drug completely as directed, even if feeling better. Advise patients that sharing of this medication may be dangerous.
2. Pedi: Teach parents or caregivers to calculate and measure doses accurately. Reinforce importance of using measuring device supplied by pharmacy or with product, not household items.
3. Review use and preparation of tablets for oral suspension (DisperMox).

4. Advise patient to report the signs of superinfection (furry overgrowth on the tongue, vaginal itching or discharge, loose or foul-smelling stools) and allergy.
5. Instruct patient to notify health-care professional immediately if diarrhea, abdominal cramping, fever, or bloody stools occur and not to treat with antidiarrheals without consulting health-care professionals.

Source: Data from Vallerand, A. H., & Sanoski, C. A. (2014). *Davis's drug guide for nurses* (14th ed.). Philadelphia, PA: F.A. Davis.

Nursing Diagnoses The Child With an Infectious Disease

Hyperthermia related to disease process
Risk for fluid volume deficit related to decreased intake
Impaired skin integrity related to pruritus
Deficient knowledge related to disease process and self-care

Case Study Infant With Pertussis

A 3-month-old infant is admitted with a history of "cold" symptoms for the last 2 weeks. The parents report the symptoms of fever, malaise, and a hacking cough that seems much worse at night. The cough tends to come in clusters and has been increasing in intensity over the past 3 days. The parents have brought the infant into the emergency room because he is now vomiting during the coughing spells and then turns blue around his mouth. An initial diagnosis of pertussis is made.

critical thinking questions

1. The parents ask about transmission of pertussis for themselves and for the other children. How would the nurse best respond?

2. What preparations should the nurse take now to prevent the spread of this disease?

3. What actions should the nurse take during a coughing spell?

4. The family asks about the length of the illnesses. What is the nurse's response?

◆ See Suggested Answers to Case Studies on Davis*Plus*.

Animal-Borne Infectious Diseases

Animals serve as a reservoir for certain infectious diseases, including rabies, West Nile virus, and avian influenza. Nurses participate in prevention of these diseases through education for families about strategies that minimize exposure to infected animals, mosquitoes, and infected birds.

focus on safety

Animal safety

The nurse proactively talks to families and children about the risk of approaching unknown animals. Typically, rabies is not readily noticed through behavior of infected animals; for this reason children should be warned to be wary of unfamiliar animals.

RABIES

Rabies is an acute viral infection of the nervous system caused by Rhabdoviridae Lyssavirus. The primary agent for this virus is carnivorous wild animals. Transmission of this disease occurs through direct contact with the brain tissue or the saliva from infected animals. The typical incubation period for rabies is 3 to 8 weeks but may extend for several months. Transmission is primarily through saliva from a bite from the infected animal, although contamination of mucous membranes, including the eyes, mouth, and nose, and aerosol transmission have occurred. When a potentially risky animal bite occurs, the animal is captured, if possible, and tested for rabies while isolated. Death may occur within days of the onset of symptoms of rabies. Treatment must be initiated as soon as possible after exposure and before the onset of symptoms.

Signs and Symptoms

Signs and symptoms are related to the infection of the central nervous system, which causes fulminant brain disease and death.

Early symptoms include:

- Nonspecific conditions, such as headache, fever, and general weakness

Later symptoms include:

- Anxiety
- Insomnia
- Confusion
- Paralysis
- Hallucinations
- Agitation
- Hypersalivation
- Difficulty swallowing
  (CDC, 2013c)

The respiratory tract is then affected, leading to spasms that cause severe impairment of respiratory function, including respiratory arrest.

Diagnosis

Diagnostic tests are performed on samples of saliva, serum, spinal fluid, and skin biopsies of hair follicles at the nape of the neck for rabies antigen. Human saliva can also be tested for the virus by polymerase chain reaction, and serum and spinal fluid may be tested for antibodies to rabies virus (CDC, 2013c).

Prevention

Rabies prevention is twofold; all domestic animals that can receive rabies vaccinations should receive them at the appropriate ages and intervals. All people, and children in particular, should be taught to stay away from wild animals that may carry rabies. Reporting of unusual animal behaviors, including mouth frothing, unprovoked attacks, and being around in daylight if normally nocturnal, should occur. The local animal control officer can be contacted to check any suspicious animal sightings. If an animal has bitten a child or adult, the animal is usually destroyed, or if caught, quarantined and checked for rabies signs. Some animals are sacrificed to detect for the presence of rabies.

Collaborative Care

Nursing Care. The nurse cleanses the wound and administers human rabies immune globulin (HRIG) and the rabies vaccine series. The nurse must instruct the patient and family regarding follow-up and provide support to the family as needed.

Medical Care. Exposure treatment for rabies includes wound cleansing with a virucidal agent, administration of HRIG, and administration of a rabies vaccine series. The rabies postexposure vaccinations consist of 4 doses of rabies vaccine given on the day of the exposure. These vaccines are then administered again on days 3, 7, and 14. These vaccines are highly effective if given rapidly after exposure to rabies (CDC, 2013c).

Education/Discharge Instructions

focus on safety

Postexposure treatment for rabies

Because of the traumatic nature of treatment postexposure, seriousness of rabies, and poor prognosis, exercising caution with unknown animals is essential. Most exposures to rabies occur through bites of wild animals, which allow contaminated saliva to enter the bite wound. If an animal has injured a child, the parents must contact their health-care provider immediately.

CAT SCRATCH DISEASE

This infection is common in the pediatric age group where children are playing with and holding kittens or cats. The bacterium *Bartonella henselae* is the source of infection through a cat scratch or bite in which cat saliva penetrates the human skin.

Signs and Symptoms

Within 3 to 10 days, a papule or vesicle (blister) develops at the site, followed by regional lymphadenopathy (lymph node enlargement), and the enlarged lymph nodes can last for months. Because many children are scratched or bitten in the hands and forearms, the most common nodes involved are the epitrochlear nodes (near elbow) and axillary nodes (under arms) which drain the hands and arms but also the neck or groin. Sometimes only one node is inflamed and the child may have a fever.

Diagnosis

Diagnosis is based on signs and symptoms and sometimes diagnostic testing with lymph node biopsy. Laboratory testing can be done in suspected cases of cat scratch disease. The tests include an enzyme-linked immunosorbent assay to detect serum antibodies. This test is not always accurate, and it can take at least 2 weeks and up to 8 weeks to develop a positive titer (Nervi, 2013).

Prevention

Children are taught to avoid rough play with cats, and any scratches or bites should be cleansed with antiseptic solutions immediately (Richardson, 2013). There is some evidence that flea-infested cats are at higher risk for transmitted cat scratch disease, so flea prevention should be instituted.

Collaborative Care

Nursing Care. The nurse treats the wounds and assesses the lymph nodes. Because there are more serious sequelae possible, including hepatosplenomegaly (liver and spleen enlargement) and encephalopathy, the nurse must observe the patient carefully for fever, headache, neck stiffness, and abdominal pain especially. It is important to note that immunocompromised patients may become much more ill with this disorder.

Medical Care. Antibiotics such as azithromycin (Zithromax) and erythromycin may be ordered to decrease the risk of a bacterial infection. Additional medications that can be used for older children include doxycycline, and for those over age 18, quinolones such as Cipro can be used.

Education/Discharge Instruction

Nurses can teach patients and families about proper administration of medication and about preventive care to avoid another episode of cat scratch disease.

WEST NILE VIRUS

West Nile virus causes an infection that is spread by mosquitoes that become infected when they bite infected birds, and standing, stagnant water is a risk factor for the breeding of these mosquitoes (Burns et al., 2013). The incubation period for West Nile virus is from 2 to 14 days, and the risk is highest to immunosuppressed children and adults. In rare cases, the virus can lead to encephalitis, meningitis, myocarditis, and hepatitis.

Signs and Symptoms

Nonspecific symptoms can be mild, including:

- Fever
- Weakness
- Headache
- Myalgia
- Anorexia
- Nausea
- Vomiting

Diagnosis

Diagnosis of West Nile virus is confirmed by specific IgM antibody in serum or in cerebrospinal fluid. Serial cultures are needed to watch changes during acute and convalescent samples (Burns et al., 2013).

Prevention

West Nile virus is most associated with mosquito-borne illness, so during the seasons (often late summer and early autumn) when it is most risky, children may not be allowed outdoors for recess or for after-school activities. It is also advisable for parents not to keep any sources of free-standing water in their yards because they are breeding grounds for mosquitoes.

Collaborative Care

Nursing Care. Nurses must educate people on the risks of West Nile virus, preventive care, and observation for worsening symptoms (Burns et al., 2013).

Medical Care. Treatment is supportive based on the signs and symptoms. Most patients who are infected with West Nile virus recover without incident. Less commonly, nearly 1 in 150 people infected with West Nile virus may develop severe symptoms including headache, high fever, neck stiffness, disorientation, tremor, seizures, muscle weakness, paralysis, numbness, vision loss, and coma. These severe symptoms may last several weeks and require hospitalization, IV fluids, and respiratory and neurological support (CDC, 2013f). Severe sequelae include meningitis and encephalitis, with the risk of permanent neurological defects. Infants born from women who were infected during pregnancy need to be evaluated for congenital defects.

Education/Discharge Instructions

Responding to parental concerns, nurses can help them plan strategies for minimizing exposure to mosquito bites. Of particular concern is also minimizing possible side effects related to systemic absorption of insect repellents. Although diethyltoluamide (DEET)-containing insect repellents are most effective as preventative agents, they can be neurotoxic; there are numerous organic and nontoxic natural insect repellents available that some parents prefer to use for children. Advise parents to keep their children dressed with long-sleeved shirts and pants during the peak season, and also mosquito nets can be used for baby carriers.

 Nursing Insight—*Use of insect repellents*

Concerned about exposure to insect bites and the possibility of infectious disease transmitted through this route, parents at times apply insect repellents such as DEET directly on their children. "Insect repellents containing DEET (*N, N*-diethyl-*m*-toluamide, also known as *N, N*-diethyl-3-methylbenzamide) with a concentration of 10% appear to be as safe as products with a concentration of 30% when used according to the directions on the product labels." The American Academy of Pediatrics recommends that repellents with DEET are not to be used on infants younger than 2 months old (AAP, 2013). The nurse provides education about the application of insect repellents. The insect repellent must be applied to the child's clothing. Applying the insect repellent to the clothing decreases the chance of systemic absorption (through the skin) of a potentially harmful substance. DEET has been known to cause neurotoxicity, especially in children, if absorbed through the skin. There are organic and safer insect repellents available, but none have the efficacy of DEET.

INFLUENZA PANDEMICS

Influenza pandemics are recurring events. In the past century influenza pandemics occurred in 1918, 1957, and 1968. Humans can become sick when infected with viruses from animal sources, such as avian influenza virus (subtypes H5N1 and H9N2) and swine influenza virus (subtypes H1N1 and H3N2). The avian influenza, known commonly as bird flu, refers to an influenza virus that occurs naturally in birds worldwide. Although occurring chiefly in infected poultry, certain subtypes of the virus may mutate and transfer to humans. Because this strain of virus has not been previously circulated in the human population, the potential for an influenza pandemic is present. More than 600 cases of avian flu have been identified since 2003, notably in Asia, Europe, the Near East, and Africa.

This flu can be highly fatal, but it is thought to be very rarely transmitted from human to human (CDC, 2013d). The swine flu has been previously rare in human beings but presents similarly to typical flu. It is most often seen in people who work with pigs, and notable risks for children include petting zoos, fairs, and raising pigs for show or clubs (CDC, 2013d). Because of a genetic mutation going from swine to people, this disease developed rapidly in 2009 and is also called "variant flu." In 2009, a variety of swine flu, known as H1N1 became a worldwide pandemic. In the 2012 to 2013 influenza reporting time, even though H1N1 is now included in the routine flu vaccination, 138 children died of flu (all types) (CDC, 2013d). Severe pneumonia and acute respiratory distress are also possible.

Avian Influenza: Signs and Symptoms

- Cough
- Sore throat
- Fever
- Myalgia

    Other signs and symptoms include:

- Nausea
- Diarrhea
- Vomiting
- Abdominal pain
- Altered mental status
- Seizures leading to death

Avian Influenza: Diagnosis

Diagnosis includes "a viral swab from the throat or nose of the ill person early in the disease. This swab is sent out to a lab for culture or molecular testing. Also, lower respiratory tract specimens can be analyzed for critically ill patients. Serum tests for antibody levels done at two different times may suggest avian flu" (CDC, 2013d).

Swine Influenza (H1N1 Variant): Signs and Symptoms

- Fever and chills
- Fatigue and malaise
- Arthralgias and myalgias
- Sore throat
- Cough
- Rhinorrhea
- Possible diarrhea
- Possible vomiting

    In children, other conditions may arise:

- Neurological symptoms: seizures and mental status changes
- Reye's syndrome risk if aspirin taken with flu
- Death

Swine Influenza (H1N1 Variant): Diagnosis

Rapid flu tests are available, but sometimes the results are not accurate. A flu swab should be taken from a nasopharyngeal test. Accuracy depends on the test quality, the sample collection method, and how much virus the person may be shedding at the time of the test. Sometimes diagnosis is made solely based on clinical symptoms, especially during the time of flu epidemics.

Prevention of Pandemic Flu

A campaign to prevent pandemic flu involves careful hand washing, use of alcohol-based hand sanitizers, and covering the mouth when coughing or sneezing. Strong immunization campaigns to vaccinate all people eligible for vaccination are the most important aspect of prevention. Public education, with which nurses are often involved, is essential in dispelling myths about flu vaccination and educating the public on how to prevent flu. Testing for flu is an important part of understanding and tracking the epidemiology of influenza. Continued research is needed to find more effective influenza vaccines.

Collaborative Care

Nursing Care. Nurses should not administer aspirin to any patients with influenza, especially under age 21, because of the risk of Reye's syndrome. Acetaminophen is generally safe to use for fever control, headache, and arthralgias associated with influenza. Encourage intake of liquids and foods as tolerated. Warm liquids may be soothing for sore throats. Children with influenza should not be in day care or school until they are fully over the disease to prevent contagiousness.

Nurses must observe for risk of serious sequelae, especially in children. These include neurological and respiratory issues because there is a potential for rapid decline and death in children.

Medical Care. Treatment of flu includes supportive and symptomatic care, including aggressive treatment of complications such as pneumonia. Two influenza medications may also be used: oseltamivir (Tamiflu) and zanamivir (Relenza). These are neuraminidase inhibitors that are active against both influenza A and B types.

Education/Discharge Instructions

Educate the public about the risks of influenza, no matter which type. Also, nurses can inform the public about the highest risk populations, who should definitely be vaccinated against influenza each year or monitored carefully if they have contraindications to the vaccine:

- Children younger than 5, but especially younger than 2 years of age
- Pregnant women
- Adults over 65
- American Indians and Alaskan natives
- Children and adults with chronic medical conditions such as asthma, chronic lung disease, neurological disorders, sickle cell anemia and other blood disorders, renal and hepatic disorders, metabolic diseases, cardiac diseases, and immune-deficient disorders
- Children and teens younger than 19 years of age on long-term aspirin therapy (because of Reye's syndrome)
- People on long-term steroid therapy (CDC, 2013c)

    Provide medication instructions:

- Zanamivir (Relenza) is approved for use in patients age 5 and older.
- Oseltamivir (Tamiflu) is approved for patients age 2 weeks and older.

- Older influenza medications, amantadine and rimantadine, are not considered highly effective and may not cover H1N1 flu variants.
- Oseltamivir (Tamiflu) and zanamivir (Relenza) are indicated for use if the virus has been active for less than 48 hours. They will not cure the flu, but they may lessen its severity by slowing the spread of the virus.

These medications may also be used preventively for people over age 1 and who have been exposed to the flu.

- Oseltamivir (Tamiflu) is given in suspension or capsule forms, usually twice a day for 5 days. Common side effects include nausea, vomiting, GI upset, and diarrhea.
- Zanamivir (Relenza) is given in an inhaled form within 48 hours of flu symptom onset, especially from age 7 and up. It also can be used preventively for patients age 5 and older if exposed to flu. It is inhaled twice a day for 5 days. For prevention, it is inhaled once daily for 10 days. Patients with asthma and other respiratory conditions usually have a contraindication to the use of Relenza.

Tamiflu resistance is being noted in about 2% of the global cases of H1N1 variant flu in 2013.

 Global Health Case Study Pandemic Flu

Chang is a 10-year-old boy living in mainland China. His father keeps flocks of poultry in their yard, and one of Chang's tasks is feeding the poultry and cleaning up their excrement. Chang develops a dry cough and fever of 101°F (38.3°C). He is nauseated with loss of appetite and has mild diarrhea. His father is beginning to develop the same symptoms. There is no local hospital, and the only physicians and nurses are located in the hospital three villages away. There is also word that several of Chang's neighbors are becoming ill with similar symptoms.

critical thinking questions

1. What is the definition of a pandemic?
2. Why are there no vaccines for pandemics?
3. What is the main treatment for avian influenza?
4. What are the main symptoms of avian influenza?
5. What are the high-risk complications of avian flu?

◆ See Suggested Answers to Global Health Case Studies on *DavisPlus*.

Immunizations

There is a direct correlation between infant immunization rates and the rates of diseases that have become preventable by immunization. Diseases such as polio and smallpox have been essentially eradicated in the United States (Stevenson, 2009). Although polio immunization is still given, smallpox immunization is no longer required. In other parts of the developing world, however, some of these diseases are still present. The cornerstone of infectious disease prevention in pediatrics is an immunization program in which the child receives the necessary vaccines. Vaccines are produced by using weakened or killed microbes, inactivated toxins, or subunits of disease-causing microbes. The goal of an immunization program is to bring about active immunity to guard

 Family Teaching Guidelines...
Preparing for an Influenza Pandemic

HOW TO: Actions taken by individuals and communities help to decrease the impact of an influenza pandemic. Nurses can work with families to provide them the information needed to prepare adequately.

ESSENTIAL INFORMATION: When working with families, the nurse can:

1. Discuss the differences between seasonal flu and pandemic flu.
2. Describe actions being taken by the health-care community to monitor and prepare for the pandemic and encourage families to take an active role.
3. Assist families to establish their own plan for care in the event of a pandemic including:
   ◆ Store a 2-week supply of food and water for the family.
   ◆ Maintain a supply of needed medications.
   ◆ Maintain a supply of over-the-counter medications needed to treat symptoms of flu.
   ◆ Establish a plan for family members living alone.
4. Encourage families to become involved with community groups to help prepare and plan for the pandemic.
5. Reinforce basic infection control techniques to limit spread of influenza.
6. Provide families with links to CDC resources with preparation checklists. Encourage them to use the checklists to assist in preparation.

against the onset of a specific antigen. The immune system response occurs through an exposure to a naturally occurring antigen or artificially through a vaccine-mediated exposure.

 Nursing Insight—Vaccine

The general requirements for development and implementation of a vaccine are:
- There must be a risk of the disease for the individual or population.
- The risk of the vaccine itself must be minimal and outweighed by the risk of the disease.
- The vaccine must be given at a time when it is effective.
- The immunization itself must be effective in promoting an immune response.

National Institutes of Health MedlinePlus (2013)

An understanding about the different types of vaccines can assist the nurse in planning care that maximizes the effectiveness of vaccine and anticipates possible complications that can occur. Traditional vaccines include *inactivated vaccines*, *live attenuated vaccines* (weakened), *and toxoids*. Inactivated vaccines are produced when the disease-causing microbe is killed but is still capable of inducing the human body to produce antibodies (e.g., inactivated poliovirus vaccine). They are very safe and require little special handling. These types of vaccines stimulate a relatively weak immune response. For this reason, repeated boosters are required.

The *live virus (attenuated) vaccine* is made by using a disease-causing organism that is not killed but is grown under special conditions designed to decrease virulence (e.g., measles vaccine). Vaccines made with live organisms require special care, such as refrigeration. Live vaccines have the potential for mutation, allowing the organism to revert to a more virulent form. Because of the increased risk of mutation, live vaccines are not recommended for children (or adults who have close proximity to the child) with compromised immune systems.

A *toxoid vaccine* is used in an inactivated form and is effective in producing an immune response geared toward a toxin-producing organism. The toxoid has been treated with either heat or a chemical to weaken its toxic effect but retains its antigenicity (e.g., tetanus toxoid).

More recent vaccine development has produced subunit vaccines, polysaccharide vaccines, conjugate vaccines, and recombinant vaccines. *Subunit vaccines* use only a portion of the virus or bacterium to produce the desired immunological response without the undesirable effects that occur with some of the other surface antigens (e.g., *Bordetella pertussis* vaccine included in the acellular DPT). The subunit vaccine produces immunity to *B pertussis* with less risk so it may be more safely given to infants and young children. Some bacteria possess a polysaccharide outer capsule that protects them from recognition and phagocytosis by the immune system. Organisms with this coating include *Haemophilus influenzae type b* (Hib), *Streptococcus pneumoniae*, and *Neisseria meningitides*, each of which may produce a very serious case of pneumonia or meningitis in infants or young children.

Polysaccharide vaccines (Pneumovax), made from portions of the polysaccharides making up the protective capsule of these organisms, have long been available and are effective in producing immunity in children older than 2 years of age. At exposure the polysaccharide capsule does not elicit a T-cell response; the duration of immunity is variable and not lifelong. In addition, these antigenic components are not recognized by the immune system of children younger than 2 years of age, and it is children in this age group who are at highest risk for serious pulmonary or neurological infection resulting from these bacteria.

The development of *conjugate vaccines* has provided an option for protecting infants and young children. The conjugate vaccine links a recognizable antigen with the "hidden" bacterial antigen, thereby enabling the immature immune system to identify the bacteria as non-self and respond. In this way, the infant's T cells may identify the otherwise unrecognizable antigen, providing both an improved primary response and conferring immunological memory. An example of a conjugate vaccine used in children younger than 2 years of age is the Hib vaccine. Before the advent of this vaccination, pediatric meningitis resulting from Hib infection was a common cause of morbidity in infants.

Production of the *recombinant vaccine* uses genetic engineering to insert the genes for production of the antigens desired into a low-virulent vector. The vector then can be used to easily produce quantities of the antigen for further purification into a subunit vaccine. The only recombinant vaccine currently used is hepatitis B virus (HBV). The HBV surface antigen is injected into yeast cells that produce quantities of the antigen for use in vaccination against hepatitis B.

Prevention

 Across Care Settings: The Advisory Committee on Immunization Practices

The Advisory Committee on Immunization Practices develops and revises the immunization guidelines each year. There are four primary health-care provider immunization schedules:

- Ages birth to 6 years
- Ages 7 to 18 years
- Combined ages birth to 18 years
- Catch-up schedule ages 4 months to 18 years

Collaborative Care

Nursing Care. The primary nursing goal related to vaccinations for children is to ensure up-to-date immunizations for all children based on their particular health status. The pediatric nurse has several roles in the area of immunization. Addressing family concerns regarding immunizations is an important role of the nurse. The nurse also plays a key role in organizing and carrying out vaccination programs and distributing accurate and timely information regarding childhood immunizations. The nurse reminds parents when the next immunizations are due. In addition, the nurse must use the current immunization schedule and recognize that the complicated schedule may pose some challenges for parents. The CDC makes parent-friendly versions of the immunization schedules and publishes them in Spanish. All schedules are downloadable for free at http://www.cdc.gov/vaccines/schedules/index.html.

Specific immunization schedules are as follows:

- Immunization schedule for children ages 0 to 6: http://www.cdc.gov/vaccines/schedules/downloads/child/0-6yrs-schedule-pr.pdf
- Immunization schedule for children and teens ages 7 to 18: http://www.cdc.gov/vaccines/schedules/downloads/child/7-18yrs-schedule-pr.pdf
- Immunization Schedule for Catch-Up Immunizations ages 4 months through 18 years: http://www.cdc.gov/vaccines/schedules/downloads/child/catchup-schedule-pr.pdf

Information about vaccinations is readily available via the worldwide Web, which has both benefits and disadvantages. Through the Web, parents are bombarded with information regarding the types and safety of immunizations. The nurse's role is to stay abreast of current information and discuss the parents' concerns. Contacting and immunizing high-risk unimmunized children, such as children who are homeless, immigrants, refugees, home schooled, frequently mobile, or who have a chronic or life-threatening illnesses, is also an important nursing function. The nurse is actively involved in statewide reporting of adverse effects of the vaccine.

Nursing Insight—*The role of the nurse*

A nurse working in a pediatric or family practice clinic is aware of the extensive program that the CDC has available called CDC's Vaccines for Children (VFC). This program allows eligible children (often uninsured or underinsured) to receive free vaccinations. Statistics for 2010 revealed that approximately 82 million VFC vaccine doses were administered free to 40 million children at a U.S. government cost of $3.6 billion. Providers in this program agreed to meet certain vaccine requirements such as monitoring vaccine expiration dates and storing vaccines at the required temperature ranges (CDC, 2013b).

legal alert—Vaccine Information Statements (VIS)

The nurse also ensures that the parent has a vaccine information sheet that records the immunizations. The CDC publishes Vaccine Information Statements (VIS) forms. The pediatric nurse or health-care provider is responsible to give parents or guardians the form prior to the child's immunizations. The National Childhood Vaccine Injury Act of 1986 requires by law that all vaccine recipients or parents/guardians of children receiving vaccines be given these one-page (two-sided) information sheets created by the CDC that discuss the risks and benefits of certain vaccinations. The legal mandate, as stated in the National Childhood Vaccine Injury Act, is that providers must:

- *Give the appropriate VIS to the recipient or to the recipient's parent or legal representative with each dose of vaccine.*
- Give the VIS prior to administration of the vaccine.
- Give the VIS each time the vaccine is given (not just with the first dose) and record certain information in the patient's permanent medical record.
(CDC, 2013b)

Over the years, there have been an increasing number of immunizations that have been marketed, especially for children. Newborn infants are now receiving a hepatitis B vaccine, but many of the other vaccines are started at 2 months of age. Many are given in a primary series to develop the child's immunity in his or her early years, and then some, but not all, are followed with booster doses later in childhood, adolescence, and adulthood. The pediatric nurse is familiar with pediatric immunizations and each year's updated immunization schedule. See Table 25-5 for detailed information about vaccination.

Table 25-5 Vaccines		
Vaccine Type	**Vaccine Brand Name(s)**	**Average Ages Given (see CDC annual charts for specifics because this changes)**
Hepatitis A Hepatitis B	1. Hepatitis A: VAQTA; Havrix 2. Hepatitis B: Engerix B; Recombivax HB 3. Hepatitis A & B combination:Twinrix	1. Ages >12 months for both 2. Approved for all ages 3. Ages >18 years
Diphtheria Tetanus Pertussis	1. Diphtheria, Tetanus Toxoid, and Acellular Pertussis DTaP: DAPTACEL; Infanrix; Tripedia. 2. Diphtheria, Tetanus Toxoid, and Acellular Pertussis (DTaP) + Hepatitis B + Inactivated Polio: Pediarix 3. DTap + Inactivated Polio: KINRIX 4. Tetanus Toxoid, Reduced Diphtheria, and Acellular Pertussis: Adacel 5. Tetanus Toxoid, Reduced Diphtheria, and Acellular Pertussis: Boostrix 6. There are other varieties for adults with just diphtheria and tetanus or tetanus alone.	1. Tripedia: ages 6 weeks to 7 years; Infanrix: ages 6 weeks to 7 years; DAPTACEL: ages 6 weeks to 6 years 2. Ages 6 weeks to 6 years 3. Ages 4 to 6 as fifth dose of DTaP and fourth dose of IPV 4. Booster for ages 11–64 5. Booster for ages 10 and older
Measles (rubeola) Mumps Rubella (German measles) Varicella	1. Measles alone: Attenuvax 2. Measles, Mumps + Rubella: MMR II 3. Measles, Mumps, Rubella + Varicella: ProQuad 4. Mumps alone: Mumpsvax 5. Rubella alone: Meruvax II 6. Varicelle alone: Varivax	1. Ages 12 months and older 2. Ages 12 months and older 3. Ages 12 months to 12 years 4. Ages 12 months and older 5. Ages 12 months and older 6. Ages 12 months and older, with optional second dose
Haemophilus influenzae type b (Hib)	1. Haemophilus B: ActHIB 2. Haemophilus B: Hiberix 3. Haemophilus B: PedvaxHIB 4. Haemophilus B + Hepatitis B: Comvax	1. Ages 2–18 months 2. Ages 15 months to 4 years 3. Ages 2–71 months 4. Ages 6 weeks to 15 months
Pneumococcus	1. Pneumococcal Polyvalent: Pneumovax 23 2. Pneumococcal 7 Valent: Prevnar 3. Pneumococcal 13 Valent: Prevnar 13	1. For >50 years or >age 2 with increased risk for pneumococcal disease 2. Ages 2, 4, 6 and 12–15 months 3. Ages 6 weeks to 5 years for otitis media prevention; Ages 6 weeks to 17 years for invasive disease prevention >age 50 for pneumonia/invasive disease prevention

(continued)

Table 25-5 Vaccines (continued)

Vaccine Type	Vaccine Brand Name(s)	Average Ages Given (see CDC annual charts for specifics because this changes)
Polio Inactivated (Live oral polio no longer used in United States)	1. Inactivated polio: IPOL	1. As young as 6 weeks
Gardasil or Cervarix for HPV (optional)	Quadrivalent HPV: Gardasil Bivalent HPV: Cervarix	1. Approved ages 9–26 years in boys and girls 2. Approved ages 9–25 in girls
Meningitis (usually required before college or dormitory housing)	1. Menveo 2. Menactra 3. Menomune *All 3 varieties cover slightly different subtypes	1. Ages 2–55 years 2. Ages 9 months to 55 years 3. Ages 2 years and up
Influenza (optional)	1. Influenza Trivalent A + B injection: Fluzone, Fluviron, Fluarix and others 2. Influenza Quadrivalent A + B: Fluarix Quadrivalent 3. Live intranasal Trivalent A+B: FluMist 4. Live intranasal Quadrivalent A + B: FluMist Quadrivalent	1. Fluzone is approved age 2 years and up; Fluviron is approved for age 4 years and up 2. Approved for 3 years and up 3. and 4. FluMist is approved for ages 2–49 years
Rotavirus vaccines	1. Rotarix: 2 oral doses 2. RotaTeq: 3-dose series	1. Approved for 6–24 weeks 2. Approved for 6–32 weeks

Source: Food and Drug Administration Biologics/Vaccines/Approved Products (FDA), 2013. Retrieved from http://www.fda.gov/BiologicsBloodVaccines/Vaccines/ApprovedProducts/UCM093833

The primary immunizations of childhood for boys and girls are:

- Hepatitis A and B
- Diphtheria
- Tetanus
- Pertussis
- Measles (rubeola)
- Mumps
- Rubella (German measles)
- *Haemophilus influenzae type B*
- *Pneumococcus*
- Polio
- Gardasil or Cervarix (optional)
- Meningitis (usually required before college or dormitory housing)
- Influenza (optional)

 Nursing Insight—*Pertussis vaccine*

The nurse is aware of the resurgence of pertussis because of a lapse in re-vaccination practices. In 2009, there were over 16,000 documented cases of pertussis, of which 12 were fatal. Most of the infected individuals were adolescents and adults who had the capability of infecting infants (Rutecki, 2012). A new version of adult pertussis vaccine has been created (Tdap) to be given with tetanus and diphtheria updates. This vaccine is acellular, or weakened, because many children experienced significant adverse effects from full pertussis vaccine in the past.

 Nursing Insight—*Influenza vaccine*

The influenza vaccine, which used to be recommended only for adults and high-risk children, is now recommended universally from ages 6 months to 18 years in the pediatric group. Influenza-related complications in children ages 24 months and younger are just as dangerous as they are for those people age 65 and older. With the advent of H1N1 influenza strain in 2009, when it was declared a pandemic by the World Health Organization, the H1N1 vaccine is now included with the annual flu vaccine, which is a combination of three strains that are predicted to be the most virulent that year. In 2009 when H1N1 was first discovered, there were numerous fatalities with H1N1 and high morbidity was noted in children and young adults. Because of its great risks, H1N1 is now always covered in the annual flu vaccine. In the past, persons with egg allergies could never have an influenza vaccine, but now there are some new guidelines for potential administration of the vaccine in some people with mild egg allergies, under very specific conditions and under physician oversight for risk of anaphylactic reaction (National Institutes of Health, 2003).

 Nursing Insight—*Vaccine combinations*

In addition, there are numerous companies creating a variety of combined immunizations to decrease the number of injections at a given time. The benefit of combined vaccines is reduction in number of injections overall and improved vaccination timeliness and coverage. However, there is one main disadvantage to combination vaccinations, which is increased risk of adverse reactions (Koslap-Petraco, 2010). For example:

- The MMR and Varicella vaccines are available in a combination product, MMRV, with the brand name of ProQuad.
- Kinrix is the brand name of the combination of DTap-IPV.
- Pentacel contains DTap, IPV, and Hib.

The nurse is diligent in maintaining current knowledge about the medication's action and potential side effects and any contraindications to immunizations. In addition, the nurse is skilled in the actual administration of the vaccine. Setting up immunization clinics and long-term tracking of children who have and have not received immunizations is important as well as accurate documentation and follow-up care. The nurse who works in the infectious disease area must cultivate specific channels for keeping up to date. The nurse uses current information to discuss the immunization plan and concerns with the family prior to immunization.

Education/Discharge Instructions

 Nursing Insight—*Parental concerns*

Addressing parental concerns about the safety of vaccination is a major role of the pediatric nurse. Over the past 25 years, the number of childhood vaccines given has actually more than doubled. Children may now receive approximately 24 vaccines during the first 2 years of life (Stevenson, 2009). Many parents are concerned their child's immunity cannot withstand so many vaccinations so close together. Some parents believe it is better for children to actually experience the disease and gain natural immunity, but this is untrue and potentially dangerous.

 Where Research and Practice Meet:
Thimerosal

Information on vaccinations from the media can be confusing to parents and guardians because there are many Web sites that are actually anti-vaccine sites. In 1999, a concern arose about giving vaccinations with thimerosal (a mercury-related preservative once found in many vaccines) to young children. This was based on a flawed 1998 research study that suggested the rise in autism and other neurological disorders was associated with the thimerosal in vaccinations. No research since that time has found any causal relationships (Stevenson, 2009). This caused many parents to refuse MMR vaccine for their children, but the study has now been discredited and removed from the literature (Koslap-Petraco, 2010). Therefore, the nurse needs to assure parents that there is no link between MMR vaccine and autism; no further studies have shown any issue. Genetic links to autism are being explored instead (Autism Today, 2012).

 Family Teaching Guidelines...
Education About Immunizations

HOW TO: Increasing immunization administration and compliance requires that the nurse work with the family to address the administration of the vaccine as well as their educational concerns.

ESSENTIAL INFORMATION: When working with families the nurse can:

- Discuss the actual administration and potential side effects of the vaccine with the parents.
- Develop programs and materials that educate parents about immunizations.

- Identify opportunities for administering immunizations by providing immunization clinics in nontraditional settings such as churches, synagogues, mosques, community centers, or shopping malls.
- Provide opportunities and encourage parents to communicate their concerns about immunizations.
- Encourage parents to investigate immunizations using reputable Web sites and other resources.
- Assist the parents in understanding how to keep track of immunizations and when the next immunizations are due.
- Assist parents in investigating funding resources for immunizations (this is a possible barrier to immunization for many families).

 Critical Nursing Action Identifying Contraindications to Immunizations

Only one universal contraindication exists:

- Previous severe allergic reaction (anaphylaxis) to the vaccine or its component of vaccine.

Individual vaccines may have additional contraindications and precautions. Safe administration of vaccines requires the nurse to screen for contraindications and precautions prior to administration. Refer to the CDC table of contraindications and precautions for most common vaccinations at http://www.immunize.org/catg.d/p3072a.pdf.

 focus on safety

Adverse effects of immunizations

Local effects are mild and occur most frequently (soreness, redness, and pain at the site of injection). These effects can be managed through local application of heat or ice to the site. Systemic effects are less frequent and include fever and mild irritability. These are managed with acetaminophen (Children's Tylenol) administration before immunization, continuing every 4 hours as needed for 24 hours. An allergic reaction is rare but serious. The pediatric nurse and parents should watch for signs of an allergic response and seek medical assistance immediately should their child exhibit any of the following symptoms: high fever; altered mental status, including excessive irritability, lethargy, non-responsiveness, or seizures; increased work to breathe; hoarseness or wheezing when breathing; hives; or pale or cool skin.

The immunizations are administered according to manufacturers' recommendations. During the immunization process, the nurse takes the time to address the unique concerns of each family. The parent's role after immunization is to understand and treat side effects. It is important for the nurse to communicate to parents when to call the health-care provider. Once parental concerns have been addressed, the child can be released from the clinic when there are no signs of adverse reaction.

 Now Can You—Safely give immunizations?

1. Identify the different types of vaccines?
2. Discuss prevention and nursing care measures related to vaccines?
3. Identify education and discharge instructions for family education regarding immunizations?

Resistant Organisms

In recent years, there has been a steady increase in the incidence of infections with antibiotic-resistant organisms in the United States and in many countries around the world. Several factors have been associated with the genesis and spread of these organisms. On a global scale, bacterial resistance, as a result of misuse, is an escalating problem in many countries providing an ever-increasing reservoir for resistant organisms to thrive.

 ### Cultural Diversity: Global Antibiotic Use

Some countries sell general antibiotics over the counter, allowing the public to purchase them indiscriminately, increasing the likelihood of inappropriate and incomplete use of them. Conditions for the development of antibiotic-resistant organisms include overcrowded living conditions and lack of potable water and basic sanitation. With global travel, the increase in community-acquired, antibiotic-resistant organisms in the world has accelerated. Giving antibiotics for viral infections; using stronger, newer antibiotics when not necessary; and not completing antibiotic courses all contribute to antimicrobial resistance. Antibiotic-resistant organisms can be transmitted directly from an infected or colonized person (as in nasal colonization), from a health-care worker, or from fomites: inanimate objects such as durable medical equipment, stethoscopes, name badges, and jewelry worn by health-care workers (Pong, 2012). Health-care providers and others can carry methicillin-resistant Staphylococcus aureus (MRSA) in the nares and on the skin, without becoming ill, but this can pass MRSA on to more susceptible individuals. Patients on ventilators often are colonized with resistant bacteria. It is vital for the nurse to recognize the risk factors for antibiotic resistance: being hospitalized, having prior antibiotic therapy, and living in a chronic health-care facility (Pong, 2012).

Signs and Symptoms

When infected, patients exhibit the same types of symptoms as with drug-susceptible organisms, but the organisms have more resistance to standard antibiotic therapies.

Diagnosis

MRSA is diagnosed through laboratory culture and clinical appearance. MRSA has both a hospital strain and a community-acquired strain, and these bacteria are genetically altered, being more resistant to standard antibiotics. These strains, as well as drug-resistant *Streptococcus pneumoniae,* are the most common resistant organisms seen in pediatric patients. Vancomycin-resistant enterococci is another common type of resistant organism, found mostly in acute care settings. In most cases, a purulent lesion that is suspicious for being MRSA contaminated should be incised, drained, and cultured for full diagnosis and appropriate treatment.

Prevention

Careful hand washing is considered the most important preventive activity for preventing resistant organism disease. Alcohol-based hand sanitizers and foam cleaners are used throughout health-care facilities. Careful

infection-control surveillance by acute and chronic care facilities includes implementing isolation procedures, taking appropriate cultures, and close monitoring (Pong, 2012). Within the community, nurses can promote public awareness and infection control measures in addition to teaching the public to finish antibiotic treatments and use antibiotics appropriately. Not finishing the full prescribed course of the antibiotic can lead to increasing resistance.

Collaborative Care

Nursing Care. Nurses are the bridge between the actual infection and public health awareness. The CDC (2013e) has implemented core strategies to reduce the spread of MRSA (see Table 25-6).

Communicable and immunological treatments include measures taken to care for a child with MRSA:

- Isolate the child by assigning the patient to a private room.
- Use standard precautions throughout the hospital stay.
- Wash hands with a chlorhexidine-soap solution.
- Don disposable, non-sterile gloves when coming in contact with body fluids or wounds.
- Wear a protective gown when entering the patient's room.
- Wear a filtered mask if the child has a productive cough or if handling respiratory secretion.
- Caps and overshoes are not required.
- Change protective garments between patients.
- Close the patient's door.
- Keep all equipment such as thermometers, stethoscopes, and sphygmomanometers in the patient's room and disinfect or destroy after use.
- Place laundry in water-soluble bags and use designated waste bags.
- Use labeled biohazard bags for contaminated waste or specimens that are collected and need to be sent to the laboratory.
- Special precaution for food trays and dishes and utensils is not needed.
- Avoid transfer to other areas if possible. However, if transport is necessary, use standard precautions.
- Document pertinent data.
- Notify the environmental services department to thoroughly clean the room after discharge. (Ward, 2013)

 ### Nursing Insight—*Probiotics*

Probiotics are foods or dietary supplements containing living microorganisms. These bacteria change the intestinal flora, improving growth or activity of certain bacteria. A classic example is the use of yogurt, which contains Lactobacilli, natural probiotics, to prevent candida infection that is often a result of antibiotic use because the antibiotics kill organisms that keep the natural fungi in balance. Today it is possible to purchase probiotic pills to prevent disease. One such probiotic is *Lactobacillus acidophilus,* which can be found naturally in some forms of yogurt but is also available commercially in supplements. Probiotics have been used to treat acute viral gastroenteritis, prevent antibiotic-associated gastroenteritis, and prevent necrotizing enterocolitis in low-birth-weight infants (Starr,

Table 25-6 Core Strategies to Reduce the Spread of MRSA

Assess hand-hygiene practices	Ensure easy access to soap and water/alcohol-based hand gels • Education for health-care personnel and patients • Observation of practices, particularly around high-risk procedures (before and after contact with colonized or infected patients) • Feedback – "Just in time" feedback if failure to perform hand hygiene observed
Implement contact precautions	Use of gown and gloves for patient care, don equipment prior to room entry • Remove gown and gloves prior to room exit • Assign a single room (preferred) or cohort placement for MRSA-colonized/infected patients • Use of dedicated nonessential items may help decrease transmission because of contact with these fomites (e.g., blood pressure cuffs, stethoscopes, and IV poles and pumps)
Recognize previously colonized patients	Patients can be colonized with MRSA for months • There is no single "best" strategy for discontinuation of isolation precautions for MRSA patients • Recognizing previously colonized or infected patients who have not met criteria for discontinuing isolation allows them to be subject to interventions in a timely fashion
Rapid reporting of MRSA lab results	Facilities should have a mechanism for rapidly communicating positive MRSA results from laboratory to clinical area • Allows for rapid institution of interventions on newly identified MRSA patients
Providing MRSA education for health-care providers	To improve adherence to hand hygiene • To improve adherence to interventions (e.g., contact precautions) • Encourage behavioral change through a better understanding of the problem

Source: CDC (2013e).

Blosser, Brady, Burns, Dunn, & Petersen-Smith, 2012). It is believed that, once in the colon, the probiotics act to reinforce the mucosal barrier through reducing gut permeability and enhancing local immune response, such as IgA release.

Education/Discharge Instructions

"What to say"—*Home care instructions*

The nurse provides home care instructions to the parents of a 2-year-old child presenting with symptoms of a viral illness. The parents tell the nurse they are unhappy with the health-care provider's decision not to prescribe antibiotics. Not all situations are alike; the nurse can tailor interaction to the situation.

• Tell me more. What has been your past experience with treating similar illnesses?

• What are your concerns with this illness? What do you believe will happen if antibiotics are prescribed to treat your child at this time?

• What are your plans to care for your child? Under what circumstances will you contact your health-care provider to discuss a change in treatment plan?

Summary Points

♦ There are many infectious disorders and immune diseases that especially impact the pediatric population.

♦ The immune system acts as the body's primary defense system and includes concepts such as active and passive immunity, immunoglobulins, and immune response.

♦ Congenital immunodeficiency disorders have four main groups of disorders associated with mutant genetic abnormalities. These children face lifelong compromise in their immune response, leading to increased risk of infectious disease.

♦ HIV is the primary cause of AIDS in infants and children. This disease spectrum causes increased risk of life-threatening opportunistic infections from bacteria, virus, and fungi especially.

♦ Autoimmune disorders involve the body creating an immune response against its own tissues or cells.

♦ Anaphylaxis is the most severe type of allergic reaction, often causing hypotension, shock, and possibly cardiorespiratory arrest.

♦ Infectious diseases are common in children, in part because of the growth of the immune system.

♦ Diseases generally fall into three categories: viral, bacterial, and fungal.

♦ Pandemic infections, including avian influenza and swine flu, have impacted on the health of people of all ages, but children are particularly at risk for serious and sometimes fatal outcomes.

♦ Animal-borne infectious disease remains a significant risk for the pediatric population.

♦ The cornerstone of infectious disease prevention in pediatrics is an immunization program in which children receive necessary vaccines.

◆ Excessive global use of antibiotics has led to increased antibiotic resistance and the appearance of resistant organisms such as MRSA.

Review Questions

Multiple Choice

1. The nursing faculty explains to a group of students about the body's immune response. What action by the immune response is most important for its functioning?
   A. Creating and maintaining immunoglobulins
   B. Inducing a febrile response to an invading organism
   C. Producing a mechanical barrier against infection
   D. Recognizing non-self material and reacting to it

2. A child with a congenital immunodeficiency is scheduled for a routine vaccination. What instruction is most important for the nurse to provide the parent before they leave the clinic?
   A. "If your child has a little temperature give acetaminophen (Tylenol)."
   B. "Keep your child away from other children for the next few days."
   C. "Let's schedule your return visit to have blood drawn for a titer."
   D. "Put ice on the injection site 4 times a day for 15 minutes."

3. A 1-year-old child who is HIV positive has a recurrent diaper infection. Which medication does the nurse anticipate teaching the parents about?
   A. Amoxicillin (Amoxil)
   B. Clotrimazole (Mycelex)
   C. Fluconazole (Diflucan)
   D. Nystatin (Mycostatin)

4. The pediatric intensive care unit nurse receives a report from the emergency department about a 10-year-old child being admitted with Stevens-Johnson syndrome. Which medication does the nurse prepare to administer to this child?
   A. Acyclovir (Zovirax)
   B. Fluconazole (Diflucan)
   C. Intravenous immune globulin (IVIG)
   D. TMP-SMZ (Bactrim)

5. The nurse is teaching a teen and family about systemic lupus erythematosus. Which information about this disease is correct?
   A. Excessive fatigue makes symptoms worse.
   B. High-dose steroids will make you drowsy.
   C. Pain control usually requires narcotics.
   D. Sunlight will help get rid of the facial rash.

6. The nurse reads on a child's medical record that he has a heliotropic violaceous rash around his eyes. Which disease process does the nurse suspect?
   A. Dermatomyositis
   B. Rheumatoid arthritis
   C. Scleroderma
   D. Systemic lupus erythematosus

7. A parent rushes her child to the emergency pediatric clinic after she picks up her baby from day care and sees a bright red spot on his cheek that looks as if he was slapped by a caregiver. Which information does the nurse anticipate providing to the mother?
   A. Keep your child away from any pregnant women while he is sick.
   B. The rash will probably spread to the trunk, arms, and legs.
   C. Warm baths with oatmeal will decrease the pain from the rash.
   D. You can treat your child's fever with salicylates (baby aspirin).

8. The clinic nurse is evaluating a teen who reports extreme fatigue and a sore throat. On physical exam, the nurse notes swollen, tender occipital lymph nodes and an enlarged area on abdominal palpation. Which diagnostic testing does the nurse anticipate being ordered as the priority?
   A. Complete blood count
   B. Monospot test
   C. Rheumatoid factors
   D. Titer for Epstein-Barr virus

9. A nurse is providing community education on preventing mosquito-borne diseases in children. Which instruction is most appropriate for the nurse to provide?
   A. Avoid spraying repellent directly onto your child's skin.
   B. DEET-containing repellent can be sprayed on the clothes.
   C. Dress your baby warmly even on hot days when going outside.
   D. Keep babies less than 1 year of age inside at all times.

10. The family practice nurse is teaching a student about different types of vaccines. Which information about vaccines is correct?
    A. Attenuated vaccines are used only in adults.
    B. Inactivated vaccines prevent disease reactivation.
    C. Live virus vaccines need occasional boosters.
    D. Toxoid vaccines contain highly potent viruses.

See Answers to End of Chapter Review Questions on *DavisPlus*.

REFERENCES

American Academy of Pediatrics (AAP). (2013). Retrieved from www.AAP.org

Autism Today. (2012). Retrieved from http://www.autismtoday.com/articles/Genetic_Factors_in_Autism.htm

Avian Influenza. (2013). Retrieved from http://www.cdc.gov/flu/avianflu/avian-in-humans.htm

BabyCare Advice. (2013). Retrieved from http://www.babycareadvice.com/babycare/general_help/article.php?id=50

Blosser, C. G., Brady, M. A., & Royal, R. B. (2013). Infections, diseases, and immunizations. In C. E. Burns, A. M. Dunn, M. A. Brady, N. B. Starr, & C. G. Blosser (Eds.). *Pediatric primary care* (5th ed.). Philadelphia, PA: Elsevier Saunders.

Bulechek, G. M., Butcher, H. K., Dochterman, J. M., & Wagner. (2013). *Nursing interventions classification (NIC)* (6th ed.). St. Louis, MO: Elsevier Mosby.

Burns, C. E., Dunn, A. M., Brady, M. A., Starr, N. B., & Blosser, C. G. (Eds.). (2013). *Pediatric primary care* (5th ed.). Philadelphia, PA: Elsevier Saunders.

Centers for Disease Control and Prevention (CDC). (2013a). Retrieved from http://www.cdc.gov/vaccines/vac-gen/howvpd.htm#why

Centers for Disease Control and Prevention (CDC). (2013b). Retrieved from http://www.cdc.gov/hiv/resources/guidelines/

Centers for Disease Control and Prevention (CDC). (2013c). Retrieved from http://www.cdc.gov/vaccines/pubs/vis/vis-facts.htm

Centers for Disease Control and Prevention (CDC). (2013d). Retrieved from http://www.pandemicflu.gov/plan/checklists.html

Centers for Disease Control and Prevention (CDC). (2013e). Retrieved from http://www.cdc.gov/HAI/pdfs/toolkits/MRSA_toolkit_white_020910_v2.pdf

Centers for Disease Control and Prevention (CDC). (2013f). Retrieved from http://www.cdc.gov/ncidod/dvbid/westnile/wnv_factsheet.htm

Distler, J. W. (2010). Food allergy in children. *Advance for NPs and PAs, 1*(2), 27–30.

Fahrner, R., & Romano, S. (2010). HIV infection and AIDS. In P. J. Allen, J. A. Vessey, & N. A. Schapiro (Eds.). *Primary care of the child with a chronic condition* (5th ed.). St. Louis, MO: Elsevier Mosby.

Ferdman, R. M. (2012). Anaphylaxis. In K. Reuter-Rice & B. Bolick (Eds.). *Pediatric acute care: A guide for interprofessional practice*. Burlington, MA: Jones & Bartlett Learning.

Food and Drug Administration Biologics/Vaccines/Approved Products. (2013). Retrieved from http://www.fda.gov/BiologicsBloodVaccines/Vaccines/ApprovedProducts/UCM093833

Greenfield, R. A. (2012). Pediatric HIV infection. Retrieved from http://emedicine.medscape.com/article/965086-overview

Johnson, M., Moorhead, S., Bulechek, G., Butcher, H., Maas, M., & Swanson, E. (2012). *NIC and NOC linkages to NANDA-L and clinical conditions* (3rd ed.). St. Louis, MO: Elsevier Mosby.

Koslap-Petraco, M. (2010). Child and adolescent immunization: Current issues and updates. *Advance for Nurse Practitioners, 18*(8), 8–12.

Moorhead, S., Johnson, M., Maas, M. L., & Swanson, E. (2013). *Nursing outcomes classification (NOC)* (5th ed.). St. Louis, MO: Elsevier Mosby.

National HIV and STD Testing Resources, CDC. (2012). Retrieved from http://www.HIV test.org/faq.aspx#pregnancy

National Institutes of Health. (2003). Understanding vaccines: What they are and how they work. Retrieved from http://niaid.nih.gov/NIH publication No. 03-4219

National Institutes of Health MedlinePlus (2013). Oseltamivir. http://www.nlm.nih.gov/medlineplus/druginfo/meds/a699040.html

National Reye's Syndrome Foundation. (2014). Retrieved from http://reyessyndrome.org/

O'Keefe, C. (2012). Fungal infections. In K. Reuter-Rice & B. Bolick (Eds.). *Pediatric acute care: A guide for interprofessional practice*. Burlington, MA: Jones & Bartlett Learning.

Pediatric Clinical Practice Guidelines and Policies by the American Academy of Pediatrics. (2011). Retrieved from http://pediatrics.aappublications.org/site/aappolicy/index.xhtml

Pong, A. (2012). Resistant organisms. In K. Reuter-Rice and B. Bolick (Eds.). *Pediatric acute care: A guide for interprofessional practice*. Burlington, MA: Jones & Bartlett Learning.

Richardson, B. (2013). *Pediatric primary care: Practice guidelines for nurses* (2nd ed.). Burlington, MA: Jones & Bartlett Learning.

Rivera, D. M. (2011). Pediatric HIV infection. Emedicine. Retrieved from http://emedicine.medscape.com/article/965086-overview

Rutecki, G. W. (2012). Pertussis: No longer "Whooping" but still a serious public health problem. *Consultant, 52*(4), 259.

Sherman, C. (2009). Candidiasis: New agents for invasive infections. *The Clinical Advisor,* 20–23.

Soep, J. B. & Hollister, J. R. (2009). Rheumatic diseases (Chapter 27). In W. W. Hay, M. J. Levin, J. M. Sondheimer, & R. R. Deterding (Eds.). *Current diagnosis and treatment: Pediatrics* (19th ed.). New York, NY: McGraw Hill.

Starr, N. B., Blosser, C. G., Brady, M. S., Burns, C. E., Dunn, A. M. & Petersen-Smith, A. M. (2013). Gastrointestinal disorders. In C. E. Burns, A. M. Dunn, M. A. Brady, N. B. Starr, & C. G. Blosser (Eds.). *Pediatric primary care* (5th ed.). Philadelphia, PA: Elsevier Saunders.

Stevenson, A. M. (2009). Factors influencing immunization rates. *The Clinical Advisor,* November, 19.

Stewart, L. J., Johnston, R. B., & Liu, A. H. (2014). Immunodeficiency. Chapter 31. In W. W. Hay, M. J. Levin, J. M. Sondheimer, & R. R. Deterding (Eds.). *Current diagnosis and treatment: Pediatrics* (19th ed.). New York, NY: McGraw Hill.

Vallerand, A. H., & Sanoski, C. A. (2014). *Davis's drug guide for nurses* (14th ed.). Philadelphia, PA: F.A. Davis.

Venes, D. J. (2013). *Taber's cyclopedic medical dictionary* (22nd ed.). Philadelphia, PA: F.A. Davis. Virginia Department of Health. (2012). Standard precautions and transmission-based precautions. Retrieved from http://www.vdh.virginia.gov/epidemiology/surveillance/hai/StandardPrecautions.htm

Virginia Department of Health. (2012). Standard precautions and transmission-based precautions. Retrieved from http://www.vdh.virginia.gov/epidemiology/surveillance/hai/StandardPrecautions.htm

Volochayev, R., Csako, G., Wesley, R., Rider, L. G., & Miller, F. W. (2012). Polymyositis and dermatomyositis and differences among clinical and demographic groups. *Open Rheumatology Journal, 6*(2012 June), 54–63. doi:10.2174/1874312901206010054

Ward, S. (2013). Pediatric nursing care: Best evidence-based practices. Philadelphia, PA: F.A. Davis.

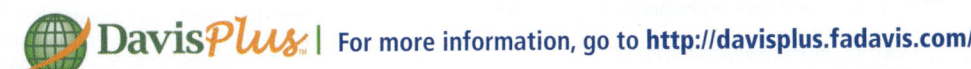

DavisPlus | For more information, go to **http://davisplus.fadavis.com/**

CONCEPT MAP

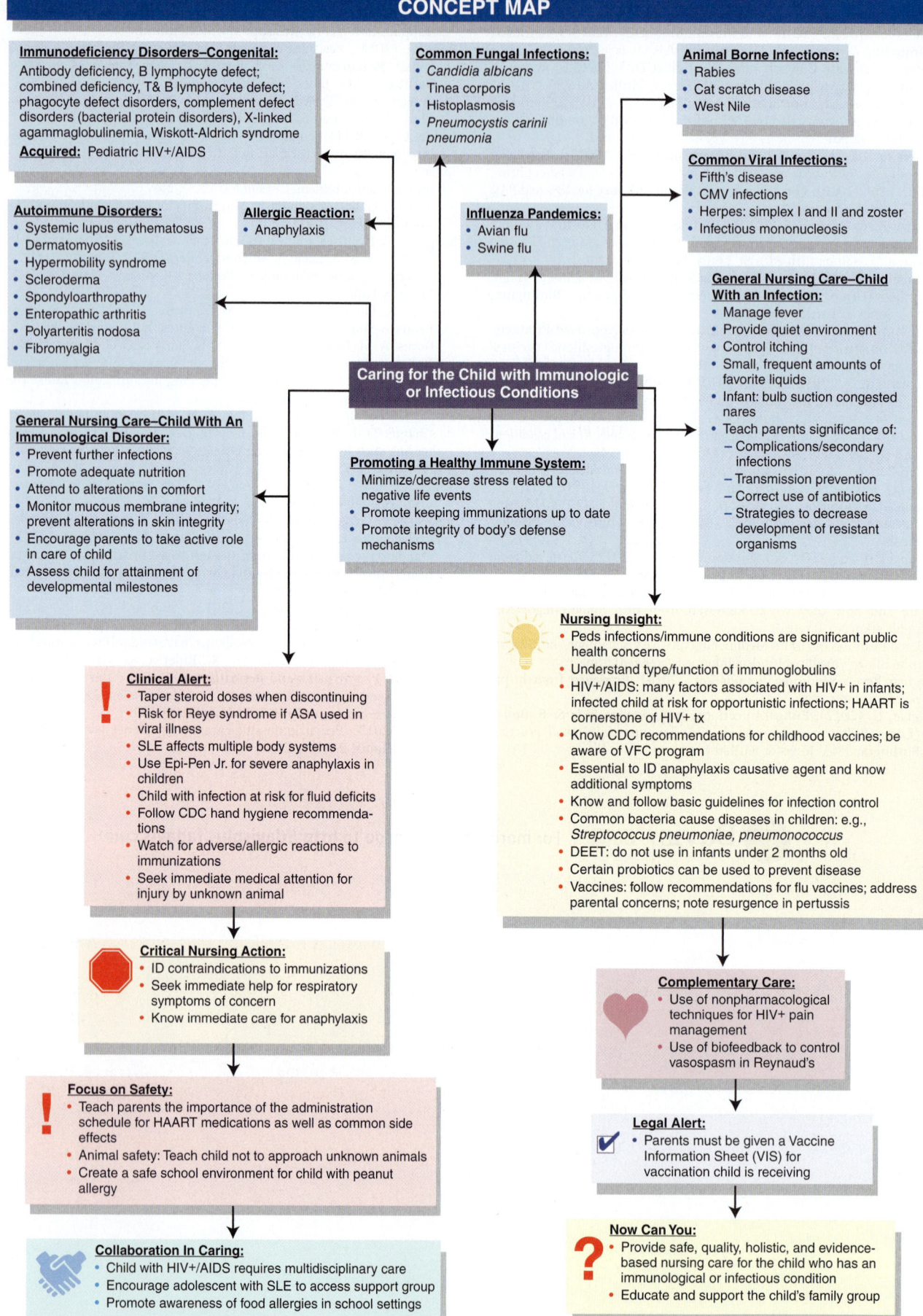

Immunodeficiency Disorders–Congenital:
Antibody deficiency, B lymphocyte defect; combined deficiency, T& B lymphocyte defect; phagocyte defect disorders, complement defect disorders (bacterial protein disorders), X-linked agammaglobulinemia, Wiskott-Aldrich syndrome
Acquired: Pediatric HIV+/AIDS

Common Fungal Infections:
• *Candidia albicans*
• Tinea corporis
• Histoplasmosis
• *Pneumocystis carinii pneumonia*

Animal Borne Infections:
• Rabies
• Cat scratch disease
• West Nile

Common Viral Infections:
• Fifth's disease
• CMV infections
• Herpes: simplex I and II and zoster
• Infectious mononucleosis

Autoimmune Disorders:
• Systemic lupus erythematosus
• Dermatomyositis
• Hypermobility syndrome
• Scleroderma
• Spondyloarthropathy
• Enteropathic arthritis
• Polyarteritis nodosa
• Fibromyalgia

Allergic Reaction:
• Anaphylaxis

Influenza Pandemics:
• Avian flu
• Swine flu

General Nursing Care–Child With an Infection:
• Manage fever
• Provide quiet environment
• Control itching
• Small, frequent amounts of favorite liquids
• Infant: bulb suction congested nares
• Teach parents significance of:
 – Complications/secondary infections
 – Transmission prevention
 – Correct use of antibiotics
 – Strategies to decrease development of resistant organisms

Caring for the Child with Immunologic or Infectious Conditions

General Nursing Care–Child With An Immunological Disorder:
• Prevent further infections
• Promote adequate nutrition
• Attend to alterations in comfort
• Monitor mucous membrane integrity; prevent alterations in skin integrity
• Encourage parents to take active role in care of child
• Assess child for attainment of developmental milestones

Promoting a Healthy Immune System:
• Minimize/decrease stress related to negative life events
• Promote keeping immunizations up to date
• Promote integrity of body's defense mechanisms

Nursing Insight:
• Peds infections/immune conditions are significant public health concerns
• Understand type/function of immunoglobulins
• HIV+/AIDS: many factors associated with HIV+ in infants; infected child at risk for opportunistic infections; HAART is cornerstone of HIV+ tx
• Know CDC recommendations for childhood vaccines; be aware of VFC program
• Essential to ID anaphylaxis causative agent and know additional symptoms
• Know and follow basic guidelines for infection control
• Common bacteria cause diseases in children: e.g., *Streptococcus pneumoniae, pneumonococcus*
• DEET: do not use in infants under 2 months old
• Certain probiotics can be used to prevent disease
• Vaccines: follow recommendations for flu vaccines; address parental concerns; note resurgence in pertussis

Clinical Alert:
!
• Taper steroid doses when discontinuing
• Risk for Reye syndrome if ASA used in viral illness
• SLE affects multiple body systems
• Use Epi-Pen Jr. for severe anaphylaxis in children
• Child with infection at risk for fluid deficits
• Follow CDC hand hygiene recommendations
• Watch for adverse/allergic reactions to immunizations
• Seek immediate medical attention for injury by unknown animal

Critical Nursing Action:
• ID contraindications to immunizations
• Seek immediate help for respiratory symptoms of concern
• Know immediate care for anaphylaxis

Complementary Care:
• Use of nonpharmacological techniques for HIV+ pain management
• Use of biofeedback to control vasospasm in Reynaud's

Focus on Safety:
!
• Teach parents the importance of the administration schedule for HAART medications as well as common side effects
• Animal safety: Teach child not to approach unknown animals
• Create a safe school environment for child with peanut allergy

Legal Alert:
☑
• Parents must be given a Vaccine Information Sheet (VIS) for vaccination child is receiving

Collaboration In Caring:
• Child with HIV+/AIDS requires multidisciplinary care
• Encourage adolescent with SLE to access support group
• Promote awareness of food allergies in school settings

Now Can You:
?
• Provide safe, quality, holistic, and evidence-based nursing care for the child who has an immunological or infectious condition
• Educate and support the child's family group

Caring for the Child With a Cardiovascular Condition

 I dedicate this chapter to the children with cardiac disease who I have cared for over the last 25 years in the PICU, Cardiology, and Cardiovascular surgery. There are many children who have had immediate and lasting results from treatment (those I rarely see in follow-up), and then there are those I see chronically, year after year, perhaps since infancy, who have grown to college age. These children have the strength to survive and to live day to day with the constant reminder of their illness. They live with tachycardia, cyanosis, shortness of breath, and poor growth patterns and low exercise tolerance. Year after year, month after month, or even week after week these children return for blood tests, electrocardiograms, echocardiograms, and invasive procedures such as cardiac catheterizations and multiple surgeries, rarely complaining and often striving to live the best life they can. They give me strength.

—Judy Marshall RN, NP

LEARNING TARGETS *At the completion of this chapter, the student will be able to:*

- Describe the anatomy and physiology and developmental aspects of the cardiac system.
- Discuss congenital heart disease (heart defects) and its effect on children.
- Examine the conditions related to cardiac diseases.
- Prioritize developmentally appropriate and holistic nursing care for cardiac conditions.
- Explore diagnostic and laboratory testing including the importance of interventional cardiac catheterization procedures and medications for cardiac conditions.
- Develop teaching plans and discharge criteria for parents whose children have cardiac conditions.

PICO(T) Questions

The intent of evidence-based practice (EBP) is to provide nursing care that integrates the best available evidence. An initial step in EBP is to write a PICO(T) question that effectively guides the research. A PICO(T) question is an acronym that stands for population (P), intervention or issue (I), comparison of interest (C), outcome (O), and timeframe (T). Depending on the question, all or some of the question components are used in the research process. Use these PICO(T) questions to spark your thinking as you read the chapter.

1. What are the (O) most important (I) teaching points nurses should explain to (P) parents of children who are taking beta blockers for heart failure?

2. What are the (O) most important (I) evidence-based nursing interventions when caring for (P) infants in the first week following surgery to repair congenital heart defects?

Evidence-Based Practice

Evans, W. N., Acherman, R. J., Castillo, W. J., & Restrepo, H. (2011). The changing occurrences of tetralogy of Fallot and simple transposition of the great arteries in southern Nevada. *Cardiology in the Young, 21,* 281–285.

The purpose of this study was to examine the prevalence of tetralogy of Fallot and simple transposition of the great arteries in Hispanic and non-Hispanic children of one western state. Tetralogy of Fallot and transposition of the great arteries are among the most easily recognized and most common cyanotic cardiac malformations. Research has determined that the incidence of tetralogy of Fallot is approximately 30 to 40 infants/100,000 live births, and the incidence of simple transposition of the great arteries is about 20 to 30 infants/100,000 live births. Racial and temporal differences have been studied by others. Temporal and racial differences were reported between African American and Caucasian in one southeastern state though it was concluded that the variations were related to improved detection.

A database of congenital cardiac defects covering a 30-year period was used to determine changes in racial and temporal incidences. This database included all live and terminated pregnancies occurring in the largest populated county in southern Nevada. The Hispanic population of this county has increased from 5% in 1980 to 28% in a 30-year period. The racial distribution of the non-Hispanic population of that county has remained consistent at 85% Caucasian, 10% African American, and 5% Asian. For the purpose of analysis, the data were subdivided or grouped into six 5-year periods. Data were further divided into Hispanic and non-Hispanic groups though there were no further subdivisions for other racial groups. Data were analyzed using chi-square, linear regression, and *t*-tests; the p-value was set at a ≤0.05 significance level. The analysis identified 249 children born with tetralogy of Fallot and 78 born with simple transposition of the great arteries. Those identified as having tetralogy of Fallot included 152 males (61%) and 97 females (39%); 63 (25%) were identified as Hispanic and 186 (75%) non-Hispanic. Those of Hispanic origin included 33 (52%) females and 30 (48%) males. There were 64 females (34%) and 122 (66%) males of non-Hispanic descent. The researchers determined that the difference between the male and female ratios and between the Hispanic and non-Hispanic patients was statistically significant (p=0.01). Among the 249 patients with tetralogy of Fallot, 22 (9%) were identified as having Down syndrome though there was not a significant difference between Hispanic and non-Hispanic patients in this category.

Of the 78 patients with simple transposition of the great arteries, 50 (64%) were male and 28 (36%) were female. Twenty-eight (36%) were Hispanic and 50 (64%) non-Hispanic. Of the 28 Hispanic patients, 19 (68%) were male and 9 (32%) were female. Of the non-Hispanic population, 31 were male (62%) and 19 (38%) were female. The researchers determined that there was no significant difference between male and female ratios nor between Hispanic and non-Hispanic populations. Down syndrome was not identified in any of these patients.

The researchers noted the following trends:

- The incidence of simple transposition in the non-Hispanic population was 20/100,000 live births in the 1980s.
- The incidence of simple transposition in the non-Hispanic population was 9/100,000 live births in the 2000s.
- The incidence of simple transposition in the Hispanic population was 20/100,000 live births in the 1980s.
- The incidence of simple transposition in the Hispanic population was 30/100,000 live births in the 2000s.
- The incidence of tetralogy of Fallot in the non-Hispanic population was 40/100,000 live births in the 1980s.
- The incidence of tetralogy of Fallot in the non-Hispanic population was 50/100,000 live births in the 2000s.
- The incidence of tetralogy of Fallot in the Hispanic population was 30/100,000 live births in the 1980s.
- The incidence of tetralogy of Fallot in the Hispanic population was 80/100,000 live births in the 2000s.

The researchers concluded that data analysis demonstrated a significant upward trend in the incidence of tetralogy of Fallot in the Hispanic population. Non-Hispanic upward trends were determined as not significant. The researchers further noted that their findings were in contrast to most studies (i.e., this study found a significantly higher increase in the incidence of Hispanic females versus males born with tetralogy of Fallot though the reverse was found to be significant for the non-Hispanic population). Though there was a slight upward trend in the incidence of simple transposition of the great arteries among the Hispanic population, it was not determined to be significant. The incidence of simple transposition demonstrated a downward trend in the non-Hispanic population and was determined to be slightly short of statistical significance (p=0.052). The researchers further indicated that the results of this study suggested interaction between genetics and the environment.

1. How is this information useful to clinical nursing practice?

2. Based on these findings, what are implications for further research?

See Suggested Responses for Evidence-Based Practice on Davis*Plus.*

Introduction

This chapter provides a review of the anatomy and physiology and developmental aspects of the cardiac system. The discussion includes an examination of the various cardiac diseases including developmentally appropriate and holistic nursing care. Information about diagnostic and laboratory testing and medications is given. Teaching plans and discharge criteria for parents whose children have various cardiac conditions are incorporated. Children with cardiac problems are a complex population of patients. The heart is integral to all other bodily systems. While a child can survive on one kidney or one lung, heart disease is not self-limited and affects most other bodily systems. Cardiac diseases are often associated with other syndromes (Table 26-1).

A & P review *Understanding the Heart*

Anatomy

A child's heart contracts 60 to 180 times per minute depending on his or her age. The heart never stops beating although it decelerates during rest and sleep and accelerates during excitement, exercise, or illness.

Chambers

The heart consists of four chambers, two of which act as reservoirs (atria) and two as pumping chambers (ventricles) to direct the blood flow of the heart (Fig. 26-1).

The right atrium is a reservoir, or collecting chamber, for the peripheral venous return. The right atrium receives deoxygenated blood from the entire body (except lungs) through the superior and inferior vena cava

Table 26-1 Syndromes Associated With Cardiac Disease		
Syndrome/Disease/ Chromosomal Aberrations	**Cardiac Defect/Condition**	**Other Physical Findings**
Down Syndrome	AV canal, VSD	Down's facies, developmental delay
Noonan Syndrome	Pulmonic valve stenosis, LVH	Elfin facies, pectus deformity, joint laxity, undescended testes, spine abnormalities, hypotonia, seizures
Williams' Syndrome	Supravalvular aortic stenosis, PA stenosis	Williams' facies: include a small upturned nose, long philtrum (upper lip length), wide mouth, full lips, small chin, and puffiness around the eyes. Hypercalcemia, dental abnormalities, renal problems, sensitive hearing, hypotonia, joint laxity, overly friendly personality
DiGeorge or Velocardiofacial Chromosome	Interrupted aortic arch, truncus arteriosus, VSD, PDA, TOF	Decreased immune response, low-set ears, palate problems, hypoparathyroidism, hypocalcemia
Duchenne's Muscular Dystrophy	Cardiomyopathy	Generalized weakness and muscle wasting first affecting the muscles of the hips, pelvic area, thighs, and shoulders. Calves are often enlarged.
Marfan Syndrome	Aortic aneurysm, aortic and/or mitral regurgitation	Arms disproportionately long, tall and thin with laxity of joints, dislocation of lenses, spinal problems, stretch marks, hernia, pectus abnormalities, restrictive lung disease
Trisomy 18	VSD, PDA, PS	Multiple joint contractures, spina bifida, hearing loss, radial aplasia (underdevelopment or missing radial bone of forearm), cleft lip, birth defects of the eye
Trisomy 13	VSD, PDA, dextrocardia	Omphalocele, holoprosencephaly (an anatomical defect of the brain involving failure of the forebrain to divide properly), kidney defects, skin defects of the scalp
CHARGE	TOF, truncus arteriosus, vascular ring, interrupted aortic arch	*C*oloboma of the eye, *H*eart defects, *A*tresia of the choanae, *R*etardation of growth and development, *G*enital abnormalities, and *E*ar abnormalities and deafness.
Fetal Alcohol Syndrome	VSD, PDA, ASD, TOF	Growth deficiencies, skeletal deformities, facial abnormalities, organ deformities: genital malformations, kidney and urinary defects, central nervous system handicaps
VATER (VACTERLS)	VSD and others	*V*ertebral anomalies, vascular anomalies, *A*nal atresia, *C*ardiac anomalies, *T*racheo–esophageal (T–E) fistula, *E*sophageal atresia, *R*enal anomalies, radial dysplasia, *L*imb anomalies, *S*ingle umbilical artery
Turner's Syndrome	CoA, ASD, AS	Kidney problems, high blood pressure, overweight, hearing difficulties, diabetes, cataracts, and thyroid problems, lack of sexual development, a "webbed" neck, a low hairline at the back of the neck, drooping of the eyelids, dysmorphic, low-set ears, abnormal bone development, multiple moles

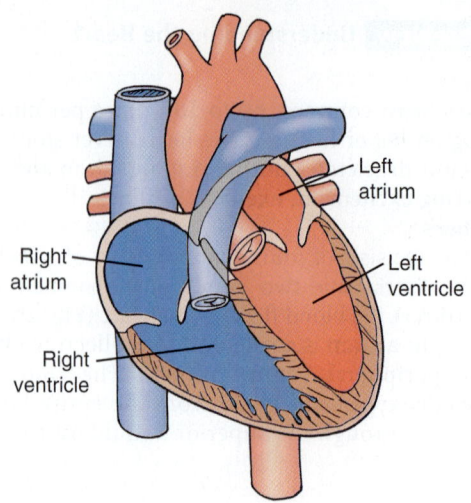

Figure 26-1 Chambers of the heart.

and coronary sinus with an approximate oxygen saturation of 70%.

The left atrium receives fully oxygenated blood from the lungs through the pulmonary veins, with an approximate oxygen saturation of 100% (Venes 2013). The ventricles are the remaining two chambers in the heart. From the atria, blood empties into the ventricles through atrioventricular valves. The right ventricle has smaller muscle mass with **trabeculated** surfaces. The right ventricle receives blood from the right atrium and pumps it into the lungs via the pulmonary artery. The left ventricle typically is thicker with a smooth interior. The left ventricle receives blood from the left atrium and pumps it into the systemic circulation via the aorta (Venes, 2013).

Valves

There are four valves in the heart. Two are atrioventricular (AV) valves connecting the atria and ventricles (Fig. 26-2). The tricuspid valve connects the right atrium to the right ventricle and is so named because it consists of three cusps or "doors" that *open* to allow blood flow into the adjoining chamber and then *close* to prevent backflow. The mitral valve, called a bicuspid valve for its two cusps, connects the left atrium to the left ventricle. The aortic and pulmonary

valves are both tricuspid and are called semilunar valves because each cusp looks like a half-moon. The pulmonary valve is located at the junction of the right ventricle and pulmonary artery. It prevents regurgitation of blood from the pulmonary artery to the right ventricle. The aortic valve, located at the junction of the left ventricle and the ascending aorta, prevents **regurgitation** into the left ventricle (Venes, 2013).

Vessels

Aside from the chambers and the valves in the heart, there are major vessels that lead to and from the heart. The venae cavae carry the blood from body tissues to the right atrium. The superior vena cava enters from above the heart and carries blood from the head, arms, and upper body. The inferior vena cava enters from below the heart and carries blood from the legs, abdominal organs, and lower part of the body. The pulmonary artery is the only named artery in the body that carries deoxygenated blood. It is called an artery because it carries blood away from the heart, but because it arises from the right ventricle, it carries deoxygenated blood. It carries this blood to the pulmonary capillary bed, where it interfaces with the alveoli in the lungs and "picks up" oxygen. From the lungs, the blood returns to the heart through the pulmonary veins into the left atrium (the only veins that carry oxygenated blood). The blood leaves the left ventricle through the aortic valve, through the aorta, and out to the body (Fig. 26-3).

Normal Flow

It is important to understand the flow of blood through the cardiovascular system because an interruption in any one of the vessels, valves, or chambers causes a disruption in the cardiac output. Figure 26-4 shows a schematic representation of normal blood flow through the heart.

Physiology

The simplest way to understand the physiology of the heart is to comprehend that the purpose of the heart is to pump blood. This vital pumping function provides a means to carry oxygen via the hemoglobin to the tissues. Without oxygen delivery, cells die and ultimately body systems fail. The heart must maintain a cardiac output at all times.

Cardiac output is the amount of blood discharged from the left or right ventricle per minute (Venes, 2013). Cardiac output is the product of stroke volume (SV) and heart rate (HR) (CO = SV + HR).

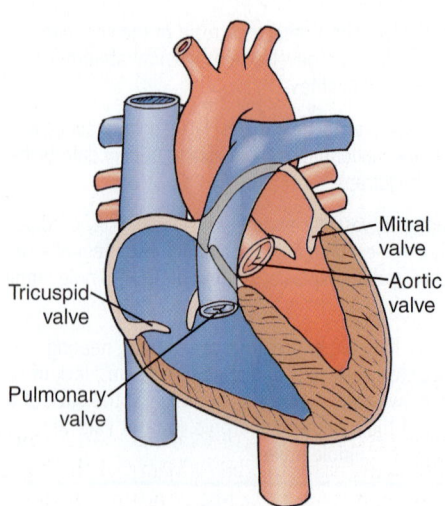

Figure 26-2 Valves of the heart.

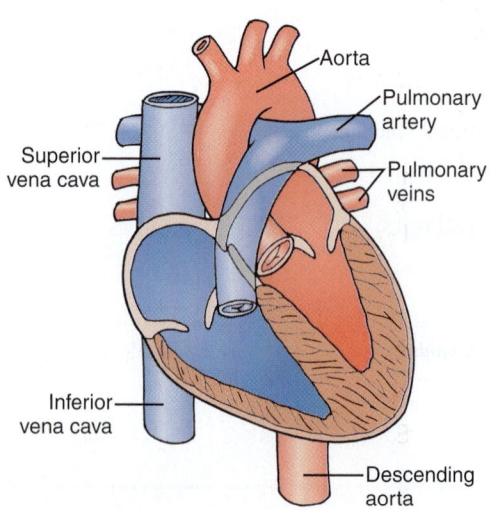

Figure 26-3 Vessels of the heart.

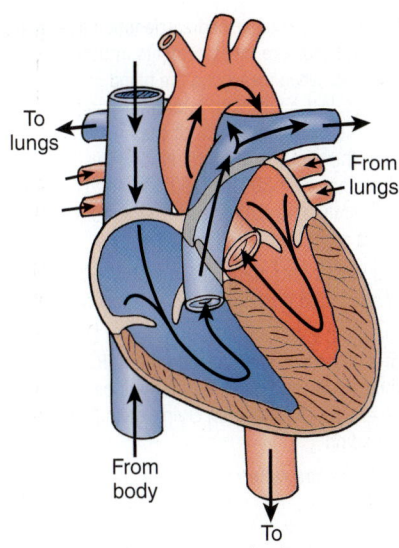

Figure 26-4 Normal blood flow.

Stroke volume is the amount of blood ejected by the left ventricle with each heartbeat (Venes, 2013). Stroke volume is the product of preload, afterload, and contractility (inotropy) (SV = Preload × Afterload × Contractility).

An altered cardiac output limits the blood's ability to provide oxygen to the tissues. Because heart rate and the size of the heart vary with the size of the child, the volume of cardiac output will vary accordingly. A variety of methods measure cardiac output with varying degrees of accuracy. The Fick equation is the most accurate way to measure cardiac output (Fig. 26-5).

Preload, Afterload, and Contractility

The concepts of preload, afterload, and contractility are integral to the understanding of heart disease and congestive heart failure and the treatment of these conditions. Most cardiac medications will affect one or all of these properties of the cardiac cycle.

Preload is equivalent to the venous blood return to the atria from the body and end diastolic volume of the heart. Afterload is the aortic impedance or the wall stress.

Contractility is the force exerted at ejection taking into account the end diastolic volume and the wall stress. ◆

Prevention of Heart Disease in Children

Some congenital heart defects and heart disease in children can be prevented with good prenatal care, vitamins, and low viral exposure. However, most often congenital

$$\text{Pulmonary flow } (Q_p) = \frac{V_{O_2}}{C_{PV} - C_{PA}}$$

$$\text{Systemic flow } (Q_s) = \frac{V_{O_2}}{C_{AO} - C_{MV}}$$

Figure 26-5 Fick equation.

heart defects are attributed to genetic causes, and gene therapy may be developed in the future to prevent the development of cardiac defects. However, often there is no known reason why children develop cardiac defects, and therefore it is difficult to prevent. Women planning on getting pregnant should maintain optimal health. Smoking, excessive alcohol consumption, and illicit drug use should all be avoided. The woman should get good sleep and eat a healthy diet. Exercise is always important. Women who are obese, smoke, or have diabetes have an increased risk of delivering a child with a cardiac defect. In addition, all women of childbearing years, whether or not they are planning a pregnancy, should take folic acid supplements (400 mcg/day) at least 1 month prior to conception. It is well documented that folic acid administration given prior to conception and during pregnancy will prevent or reduce the chance of neural tube defects. This is also true of some cardiac defects. Currently existing diseases such as diabetes, thyroid, mental illness, or sexually transmitted diseases should be well controlled prior to conception. Some medications to treat these diseases may be teratogenic (causing birth defects), and these drugs must be weaned or stopped under the guidance of a physician or nurse practitioner.

Caring for the Child With a Cardiovascular Condition

Growth and Development

Promoting growth and development for the child with a cardiovascular condition involves a variety of interventions. The child with a cardiovascular condition requires adequate sleep, nutrition, and rest to maintain optimal health and wellness. The child with a cardiovascular condition may require more rest than the healthy child because of activity intolerance and fatigue from the underlying cardiac condition. To optimize regular growth and development, activities should be tailored to the child's energy level. During low levels of energy, frequent naps and quiet play may be warranted. Crying can be stressful on the child and quickly use up reserved energy. The nurse should provide education to the family about being attentive to the child's cry to conserve energy. Supplemental oxygen may be indicated to alleviate shortness of breath with activity, promote rest, and reduce stress.

Frequent hospitalization or surgery may be required to correct cardiac defects and manage disease regression. The nurse should frequently assess the child for delays in growth and development because of chronic hospitalization. The nurse should educate the family about promoting healthy nutritional intake, prevention of infection and complications of the disease process, and lifestyle changes required to prevent disease regression and comorbidities. The nurse should encourage the family to create a sense of normalcy for the child. The nurse and the family should understand that because of limitations with activity and chronic hospitalization, the child may experience delays or lags in growth and development. The nurse should encourage the healthy attainment and maturation of the child with activities and stimulation that are appropriate.

Source: Ward & Hisley (2009).

Congestive Heart Failure

Many congenital and acquired cardiac conditions result in congestive heart failure (CHF). Much of the basic nursing care of a patient with a cardiac condition is dependent on the degree of the CHF.

Cardiac failure occurs when the heart can no longer fully accomplish its intended purpose. CHF, or simply, heart failure, is characterized by the inability of the cardiac muscle to perform its proper function of moving blood forward. Blood is "congested" in a backward direction. The heart's pumping action is lost so the blood backs up into other areas of the body such as the lungs or the liver. This backward congestion of fluid eventually fills into the periphery. Congenital heart disease (CHD), dysrhythmias, or other cardiac diseases such as cardiomyopathy or Kawasaki's disease can lead to CHF.

Signs and Symptoms

The signs and symptoms of CHF vary with age and whether the fluid is more congested on the right or left side. Infants present with:

- Poor feeding
- Poor growth
- Irritability
- Shortness of breath or excessive sweating
- In advanced stages, an enlarged liver or edema develops

Older children show:

- Poor growth
- Shortness of breath and exercise intolerance

Peripheral edema in children does not present in the same way as in adults. Ascites rarely occurs in children except in the most dramatic cases and more often in teenagers.

Babies and toddlers exhibit:

- Puffy eyelids
- Swelling of hands and feet
- Bulging fontanelle

Diagnosis

Diagnosis includes patient history and physical examination findings including vital signs (blood pressure and pulses may be diminished), weight gain, or changes in breath sounds. Diagnostic measures include **B-type natriuretic peptide**, chest x-ray exam, exercise test, echocardiogram, magnetic resonance imaging, and cardiac catheterization.

Collaborative Care

Nursing Care. Nursing care measures include keeping the child comfortable. Fluid collections in the brain, periphery, and abdomen make the child irritable. Often, a patient in CHF is restless because of an altered breathing pattern related to fluid in the abdomen and in the pulmonary bed. Therefore, implement oxygenation nursing interventions to ensure appropriate oxygenation levels. Nursing care for the child with congestive heart failure includes good skin care.

Careful monitoring and follow-up care is necessary in CHF. Because of the risk of dehydration, fluid restriction is not often used in children.

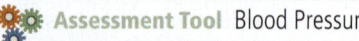 **Assessment Tool** Blood Pressure

Though one of the most important assessment tools for the pediatric cardiac patient, accurate blood pressure monitoring may be the most difficult to achieve. The American Heart Association (AHA, 2014a; Gómez-Marín,

Prineas, & Råstam, 1992) published a scientific paper outlining the proper technique of blood pressure measurements in both children and adults. In summary, remember when measuring the blood pressure on a child:

- Cuff size: select a cuff with a bladder width (measured top to bottom) that is at least 40% of the arm circumference midway between the shoulder and the elbow. This typically will allow cuff length coverage of 80% to 100% of the circumference of the arm. Too small of a cuff gives false high measurements, and too large of a cuff gives false lows.
- Manual versus automatic: often when child has tachycardia, the automatic blood pressure cuff will not pick up the rapid pulse.
- Environment: a child may be frightened by the potential discomfort of a blood pressure measurement. Remember to approach the child slowly and explain what will be done. Even with these measures, the child is often crying giving an inaccurate (often too high) reading.
- A blood pressure, when taken on a child, is always performed on a bare arm.

Medical Care. CHF is treated with medications because of the congenital defects.

 Critical Nursing Action Medications

Positive inotropes such as digoxin (Lanoxin), or even the stronger dopamine drugs, are used when poor contractility is the cause of CHF. If increased preload is the cause, then diuretics such as furosemide (Lasix) or hydrochlorothiazide (Aquazide) may be used. Vasodilators such as captopril (Capoten) or enalapril (Vasotec) are prescribed if increased afterload is the causative factor. Often all three are used in conjunction.

Surgical Care. Surgical repair for CHF is based on correcting the defect as outlined in Table 26-4: Surgical Repairs of Cardiac Defects.

Education/Discharge Instructions

Discharge instructions include monitoring vital signs, how to recognize signs and symptoms, and uses and side effects of medication. Teach parents that a good exercise plan may help to make the heart muscle stronger and help to prevent the CHF. Even moderate walking is beneficial. However, a vicious cycle may occur because the child may not feel well enough to exercise or even walk, leading to worsening of the symptoms. When the parent understands the signs and symptoms, medication can be given before the child reaches a critical state.

Congenital Heart Disease

Congenital heart disease is a defect in the heart, great vessels, or a noted disease pattern after birth. Congenital heart defects occur in approximately 4 to 8 per every 1,000 live births (Ubeda Tikkanen, Rodriguez Oyaga, Arroyo Riaño, Maroto Álvaro, & Rhodes, 2012). There are various ways by which the nurse can recognize a congenital heart defect, including recognizing the shunting pattern and recognizing cyanotic versus acyanotic congenital heart defects (Table 26-2).

Signs and Symptoms

Most signs and symptoms are related to the oxygenation status of the defect. Overall signs and symptoms are also related to the contractility state or if the patient is in heart failure. Congenital heart defects are sometimes classified as

Table 26-2 Classification of Cardiac Defects

Class	Name	Prevalence (% of all defects)	Types or Forms	Associated Defects
L–R Shunt	Atrial–septal defect	5–10 (50–100)	Secundum or primum or sinus venosus	PAPVR or mitral valve prolapse
	Ventricular septal defect	20–25 (200–250)	Perimembranous, muscular, multiple	PDA, CoA, AV prolapse
	Patent ductus arteriosus	5–10 (50–100)	Large shunt or small	
	AV canal	0.02 (0.20)	Complete or partial; balanced or unbalanced	AV regurgitation. 30% of cases occur with Down syndrome
	Partial anomalous pulmonary venous return	<1 (10)	TAPVR	ASD
Obstructive Lesions	Pulmonary stenosis	5–8 (50–80)	Valvular, subvalvular, supravalvular (PA)	VSD, Noonan syndrome
	Aortic stenosis	0.05 (0.50)	Valvular, subvalvular, supravalvular	Bicuspid aortic valve, Williams' syndrome, IHSS
	Coarctation of the aorta	5–10 (50–100)	Preductal, postductal, ascending aorta, descending aorta	Bicuspid AV, aortic hypoplasia, VSD, PDA, abnormal MV
	Interrupted aortic arch	0.01 (0.10)	Type of coarctation, types A, B, C	PDA, VSD, bicuspid AV, MV deformity, truncus arteriosus, subaortic stenosis
Cyanotic Defects	Transposition of the great arteries	0.05 (0.50)	D type, L-type,	ASD, VSD, PDA, PS
	Tetralogy of Fallot	0.10 (1.00)	PS or PA or absent PV with PS	May be cyanotic or acyanotic if PS is mild
	Total anomalous pulmonary venous return	0.01 (0.10)	Supracardiac, cardiac draining into RA, cardiac draining into the coronary sinus, infracardiac; obstructive	ASD or PFO
	Tricuspid atresia	1–2 (10–20)		ASD, VSD, PDA, CoA, TGA
	Pulmonary atresia	<1 (10)	Variable RV sizes	ASD, PFO or PDA
	Epstein's anomaly	<1 (10)	Variable degrees of displacement	WPW, RA hypertrophy, ASD
	Truncus arteriosus	<1 (10)	Types I–IV showing various placements of PA arising from the aorta	Large VSD, right aortic arch, DiGeorge syndrome
	Single ventricle	<1 (10)	DILV or RV	ASD, PS, PA, CoA, VSD, asplenia, polysplenia, TGV
	Double outlet right ventricle	<1 (10)	Types are by the position of the VSD: subaortic VSD, subpulmonary VSD, remote VSD, subaortic VSD with PS, doubly committed VSD	VSD, PS
	Splenic syndromes	<1 (10)	Asplenia and polysplenia	Various redundant cardiac structures or absence of structures

The numbers in the parentheses indicate the number of infants born with defects out of 100,000 live births.
Source: © Judith M. Marshall (2014).

cyanotic versus acyanotic; many, but not all, cardiac defects involve mixing of blood. If the deoxygenated or venous blood from the right side of the heart is forced into the left side of the heart (called right to left shunting), as in cyanotic defects, the overall oxygen saturation of the blood will drop. The range may vary from normal (96%–100%) to as low as 70%. In acyanotic defects the oxygenated blood shunts from the left to the right. This type of mixing will not affect the overall oxygenation status.

In the presence of normal hemoglobin, a decrease in the oxygen saturation to 85% will cause an outward sign of cyanosis (bluish coloration) that appears around the lips, nose, and mouth of babies and toddlers and in the nailbeds of older children. If the decreased oxygen state is chronic, the child eventually will develop clubbing of the fingernails. The longer and lower the oxygen saturation, the more evident the clubbing. One physiological explanation for this change is that the capillaries enlarge (dilate) to accommodate the low saturation in an attempt to deliver more blood to the periphery (Schwartz & Richards, 2012).

Another long-term effect of low oxygenation is polycythemia. Polycythemia is the increase in the red blood cell production in response to the low oxygen output. The patient has hemoglobin levels greater than 15 g/dL. The condition also causes thickening of the blood and predisposes the child to thrombi and stroke. Low oxygenation and thickened blood will often cause the heart muscle to work harder in an effort to circulate more oxygen. This leads to muscular hypertrophy and eventually to pump failure.

Diagnosis

The diagnosis of a heart murmur usually starts with a referral after a murmur is detected. Sometimes other symptoms are present, such as shortness of breath or high blood pressure in children. Diagnostic screening of suspected congenital defects includes a chest x-ray exam and electrocardiogram (ECG). Most are confirmed by echocardiography or cardiac catheterization. The echocardiogram gives information such as location and size of the defect and can give indirect measurement of pressure. A cardiac catheterization will give direct measurements of the pressure in the chambers and vessels and gradients (difference of pressure) across the valves. A magnetic resonance angiogram or computed tomography angiogram provide additional information for specific defects.

Collaborative Care

Nursing Care. Nursing care for the patient with CHD is similar for all of the various types of lesions. To avoid repetition, nursing care will be discussed here and specific nursing care topics will be outlined in each case. Nursing care entails monitoring and maintaining the child's oxygen and nutritional status. Educate the family about the importance of rest periods and managing the child's fatigue. Emotional care is also essential for the child and the family as well because this condition will most likely involve many types of surgeries and many hospitalizations. Provide emotional support by listening and supplying the family with resources for understanding the disease and the prognosis and treatment plan. When the family is interested, help them fulfill their spiritual needs. Even if not religious, a family may request a spiritual person to be present in the room.

Medical Care. Medical management usually focuses on treating the CHF that may develop because of the specific defect and includes preload-reducing agents such as furosemide (Lasix), positive inotropes such as digoxin (Lanoxin), and contractile function agents such as carvedilol (Coreg) (Table 26-3).

Surgical Care. For congenital heart defects, provide care to the child related to post-surgical concerns.

Surgical repair of congenital heart defects is outlined in each heart condition and is found in Table 26-4.

Preoperative care for the child undergoing cardiac surgery is similar to care of other surgical patients. A thorough history and physical is essential to identify recent changes in the past medical history. Each institution will develop a preop checklist. The nurse can also provide and support the education given to the family regarding the type of surgery and the process of the surgery (e.g., surgery time, recovery times, and expectations).

Postoperative care of the child who has had reparative cardiac surgery is complex and almost always includes an admission to the intensive care unit. See Critical Nursing Action: Postoperative Management.

Exercise and stress reduction are two nonpharmacological approaches to congenital heart defects. Although the only method to "cure" a defect is through surgery, complementary or alternative methods may help the patient to live a higher quality of life.

Table 26-3 Commonly Used Cardiac Medications

Drug Class	Name of Drug
Class I - Na+ Channel Blockers – 1A	quinidine procainamide disopyramide phosphate
Class I – Na+ Channel Blockers – 1B	lidocaine mexiletine
Class I – Na+ Channel Blockers – 1C	propafenone flecainide
Class II – Beta-Adrenergic Blockers	propranolol atenolol metoprolol sotolol
Class III – Prolongs Repolarization	amiodarone
Class IV – Calcium Channel Blockers	verapamil diltiazem
Miscellaneous	digoxin – cardiac glycoside adenosine – endogenous nucleoside
Drugs Used in Pump Failure – Vasoconstrictors	epinephrine levarterenol (norepinephrine)
Drugs Used in Pump Failure – Positive Inotropes	dopamine dobutamine milrinone
Drugs for Bradycardia	isoproterenol
Epinephrine (see above)	atropine
Diuretics	furosemide chlorothiazide bumetanide
Drugs for Hypertension – Calcium Channel Blockers	amlodipine
Drugs for Hypertension – Ace Inhibitors	captopril enalapril lisinopril
Angiotensin Receptor Blockers	losartan
Antithrombotic Agents	warfarin (Coumadin) clopidogrel aspirin heparin enoxaparin (Lovenox)
Hypercholesterolemia Drugs	pravastatin cholestyramine nicotinic acid

Source: Vallerand, A. H., & Sanoski, C. A. (2014). *Davis's drug guide for nurses* (14th ed.). Philadelphia, PA: F.A. Davis.

focus on safety

The patient with CHD

Safety measures when caring for a patient with CHD include placing the child on a pulse oximeter, even if it seems the child does not have an immediate oxygenation problem. The same holds true with a cardiac monitor. These children are at high risk for deoxygenation and dysrhythmic episodes.

Education/Discharge Instructions

Discharge instructions and parent education include monitoring vital signs and how to recognize signs and symptoms of cardiac failure. The parent will be given ranges of vital signs appropriate for the child's age and circumstance. For example, some patients may have a lower or higher than expected range for their age because of the type of cardiac disease. Parents should learn cardiopulmonary resuscitation.

If the child is discharged to home with oxygen, the parents will also have a pulse oximeter in the home. The parent will be taught to observe for subtle signs of CHF such as shortness of breath, decreased appetite, irritability, swelling, and weight gain. Discharge instructions include medication use, effects, and side effects. The nurse ensures that the parent is receiving education about medications that is appropriate for their learning style and comprehension level. Each medication should be reviewed for specifics.

Postoperative teaching points will answer the family's questions about diet, exercise, activity, and return to school. A proper diet for a cardiac patient includes balanced, healthy food choices for good bone healing and avoidance of junk food and empty calories. Fluid restriction is not encountered as often as in the adult population but may be used for patients in severe congestive heart failure or older children. Infants and younger children can dehydrate much easier; therefore, this practice is avoided in this age range.

Postoperative care also includes care of the surgical wound. In general, the area is to be kept clean and dry, and often the Steri-Strips are left in place until they fall off. The parents are taught how to watch for wound healing and signs of infection, such as redness at the site or fever.

Typically, when a sternal approach is used the bone must be allowed to heal for 6 weeks. This means an infant or baby must be cradled when picked up or carried (i.e., avoid lifting the child from under the arms), and older children should not use backpacks. Exercise guidelines are specific for each condition and based on protection of the surgical site and bone healing time. For older children, no contact sports are allowed in the first 6 weeks to 6 months after surgery until the bone is healed. Occasionally, a child may be fitted with a protective vest to prevent injury to the chest when returning to sports. The nurse teaches parents that a good exercise plan might help to make the heart muscle stronger and help to prevent CHF. Parents are also taught that the child with a cardiac condition may be incapable of doing certain strenuous exercises and may need to modify or avoid physical activity. There may be a fine line between encouraging the child to engage in physical activity for the benefits and inhibiting the child from doing physical exercise for fear of getting sicker. The nurse helps the parents balance the decision for the types and amounts of exercise. Generally, the child may return to school when the bone is healed.

The nurse provides parents with community-based resources to set up home-bound schooling. Discharge education also includes support systems for children who also have other conditions such as Down syndrome.

Segmental Classification of Congenital Heart Defects

In the United States, cardiac defects occur in 8 to 12 per 1,000 (1%) live births (Park, 2009). There are several approaches to classifying heart lesions. Table 26-2 outlines the segmental approach, which is organized by the type of defective physical structure. This segmental approach classifies the defect in relation to the septum (pl. septae) (chamber walls), vessels and valves, conal–truncal defects, and combination defects (Mavroudis, Backer, & Idriss, 2013).

The traditional way of classifying heart defects is not always exact because the shunting and flow may change over the natural course of the disease process.

LEFT-TO-RIGHT SHUNT LESIONS

Atrial Septal Defect

Atrial septal defect (ASD) is a simple defect of the atria. During fetal development, the septal wall forms between the fourth and eighth weeks of life when two septae, the primum and secundum, stretch across the center of the common atrium (Fig. 26-6). Eventually, these septae overlap (but not completely) and form a small opening called the foramen ovale. The foramen ovale is a necessary structure during fetal life but should close within hours after birth. Sometimes the foramen ovale may persist until 1 year of life. An ASD results when the two septae fail to overlap properly. There are two variations of the defect that differ in the location of the defect on the septal wall: primum ASD (high on the septal wall) and secundum ASD (low on the wall).

Signs and Symptoms

Possible symptoms of ASD include:

- Possible murmur
  - Blowing to harsh systolic murmur heard best at 2nd intercostal space left sternal border
  - May radiate to apex or back
- Possible right ventricle (RV) heave or a thrill (abnormal tremor accompanying a vascular or cardiac murmur felt on palpation) (Venes, 2013)
- Possible right atrial enlargement caused by fluid overload from left-to-right shunting through the opening in the atrial wall
- Possible right ventricular enlargement, which is the source of the RV heave
- Right axis deviation (evidence of ventricular enlargement) on an ECG recording
- A fixed, split, second heart sound
- Hepatomegaly as a result of this fluid overload
- Signs and symptoms of cardiac failure (these signs gradually worsen with time unless the defect is repaired)
  - Shortness of breath
  - Respiratory distress

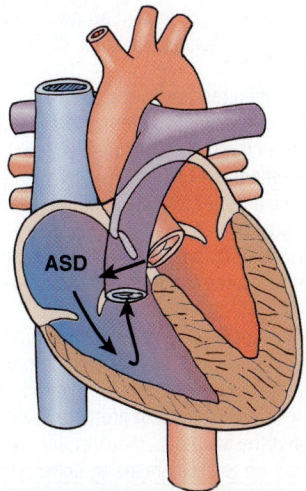

Figure 26-6 Atrial septal defect.

- Periorbital edema
- Failure to thrive
- Increased respiratory infections may be noted
- Risk for stroke because of the tendency of blood pooling leading to increased risk of thrombus formation

Diagnosis

The ASD is confirmed by echocardiography or cardiac catheterization. A chest x-ray exam and ECG support the diagnosis.

Collaborative Care

Nursing Care. Nursing care focuses on postoperative management of the child. If a closure device is used, the nurse is aware of the signs and symptoms of complications of the device, such as bleeding, tamponade, or migration of the device. Signs and symptoms such as chest pain, palpitations, sudden hypotension, and dehydration or anemia warrant further investigation.

Surgical Care. Without treatment, certain types of ASDs may close spontaneously in the first year of life, and the child typically shows no outward signs of a malformation. The ASD, if not closed spontaneously, can be closed with a surgical procedure or interventional cardiology in which a closure device is inserted.

Critical Nursing Action Postoperative Management

Provide immediate postoperative care in the intensive care unit:

- Record the vital signs frequently until the child is stable.
- Monitor fluid status. Accurately measure the intake and output of all fluids.
  - Maintain vascular access systems via:
    - A peripheral IV is used to administer fluid and medications.
    - A central venous pressure line is inserted in a large vessel in the neck or groin and is used to measure central venous pressure in the right atrium.
    - Intracardiac catheters are inserted in the right atrium, left atrium, and pulmonary artery and are used to measure the pressures inside the cardiac chambers that provide essential information about cardiac output, blood volume, pulmonary pressures, ventricular function, and drug therapy response.
  - Maintain chest tubes that remove secretions and re-expand the lungs. Check drainage for quantity and color.
- Assess for complications such as cardiac, neurological, pulmonary, renal, or hematological changes, infection, or delayed growth and development.
  - Assess and maintain respiratory status.
    - Respiratory assessment is performed frequently, and oxygen is delivered via mechanical ventilation.
    - Suction secretions.
  - Monitor blood lab values for postoperative bleeding and post-pump electrolyte imbalances.
- Assess for signs and symptoms of infection. Manage pain via comfort measures and the administration of medication.
- Provide emotional support and information about home care.
  - Consider the child's level of development to provide developmentally appropriate care.
  - Ensure rest, which is essential to promote healing and decrease the workload of the heart.
  - Group nursing care to avoid imposing unnecessary fatigue and weakness.

focus on safety

Complications

- Renal failure is considered when the output is less than 1 mL/kg per hour along with an elevation in serum creatinine and blood urea nitrogen.
- Postoperative hemorrhage is considered when there is excessive chest tube drainage greater than 5 to 10 mL/kg in 1 hour or more than 3 mL/kg per hour in 3 consecutive hours.

Education/Discharge Instructions

See Education/Discharge Instructions for Cardiovascular Conditions in Children.

Ventricular Septal Defect

A ventricular septal defect (VSD) is the most common congenital heart defect. Fortunately, it is one of the mildest. A VSD forms in much the same way as an ASD. In fetal development, at the approximate gestational age of 4 to 8 weeks, the wall is formed when a superior and inferior limb (like a divider) of tissue come together to create a wall between the two chambers (Fig. 26-7). A defect in the formation of this wall can be a single opening, or the wall may be fraught with multiple defects, sometimes referred to as a Swiss cheese VSD.

The defect may be located anywhere on the ventricular septal wall. Usually, those in the muscular septum close spontaneously. If left alone, individuals can live a long, normal life. In the worst cases, the child suffers from right ventricular overload from left-to-right (acyanotic) shunting of blood caused by the high-pressure gradient from the left to the right side. Generally, a VSD is repaired surgically. However, in the future, the use of a transcatheter closer device may be more common.

Signs and Symptoms

Mostly asymptomatic

- Large VSD with a significant left-to-right shunt: signs of right ventricular failure
  - Shortness of breath
  - Feeding difficulties

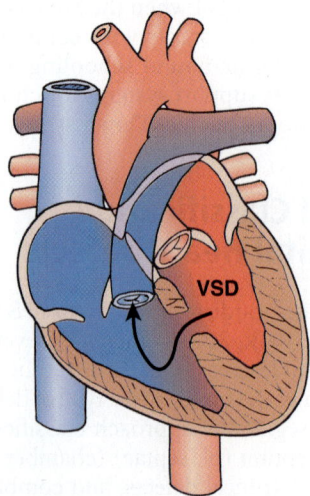

Figure 26-7 Ventricular septal defect.

- Poor growth
- Easy fatigability
- Recurrent pulmonary infections
- Murmur
  - A harsh murmur along with a thrill at the lower left sternal border
  - Pansystolic

Diagnosis

Diagnosis is based on an audible heart murmur along with other signs and symptoms. Additional tests, such as a chest radiograph and ECG, support the diagnosis. An echocardiogram, cardiac catheterization, and/or cardiac magnetic resonance imaging (MRI) confirm the diagnosis.

Collaborative Care

Nursing Care. Nursing care focuses on postoperative management of the child.

Medical Care. Care of the child with VSD is similar to that of the child with ASD.

Education/Discharge Instructions

See Education/Discharge Instructions for Cardiovascular Conditions in Children.

Patent Ductus Arteriosus

A patent ductus arteriosus (PDA) is the simplest form of vessel defect (Fig. 26-8). Remember that the ductus arteriosus is a normal structure during fetal life. In utero, the pulmonary resistance is high because the lungs are filled with fluid rather than air. The blood is oxygenated through the placenta by the umbilical vein. Instead of the blood flowing from the pulmonary artery (PA) to the lungs, the ductus is a "pop-off" valve for the large volume of fluid. As the blood flow follows the "path of least resistance," the blood moves through the ductus, into the aorta, and out to the body tissues. Directly after birth and the baby's first breaths, the pulmonary resistance drops and the blood flows from the PA into the lungs. Because there is decreased flow through the PDA, the duct starts to close. Changes in prostaglandin level assist the closure as well. In 8% to 10% of the population, the PDA remains open (Park, 2009). It can take as long as 1 year for the PDA to close completely.

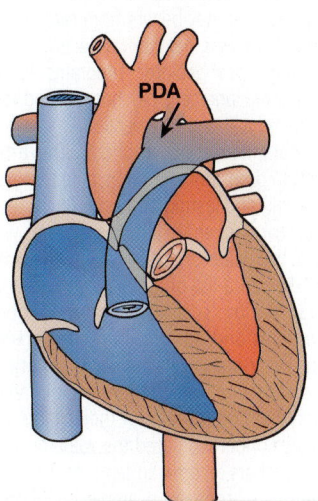

Figure 26-8 Patent ductus arteriosus.

The pediatric cardiologist monitors the asymptomatic child up to 1 year for spontaneous closure of the PDA.

If a large PDA is not closed, severe long-term sequelae may ensue. At birth, the pulmonary resistance is higher than the left-sided pressures. As this gradient reverses, the left-sided pressure forces blood toward the right side through the PDA. Eventually, the fluid congests the right side of the heart and the pulmonary bed. The right ventricle hypertrophies as it attempts to mobilize fluid forward. The defect occurs alone or in combination with coarctation of the aorta.

Signs and Symptoms

Symptoms of PDA can include:

- The PDA murmur is distinctive in sound and location
  - Best heard at the left subclavicular margin
  - Described as machine-like, to and fro, or continuous
- Frequent colds
- Susceptibility to respiratory syncytial virus
- Fatigue
- Poor feeding
- Poor growth pattern
- Blood pressure reveals a wide pulse pressure

Diagnosis

The presence of the characteristic machine-like murmur under the left clavicle, along with symptoms of heart failure, leads to the diagnosis of PDA. A chest radiograph shows an enlarged heart and evidence of an excessive blood flow to the lungs. An echocardiogram confirms the diagnosis, demonstrating the size of the ductus arteriosus and enlargement of heart chambers because of the extra blood flow.

Collaborative Care

Nursing Care. Nursing care focuses on post-surgical measures, such as wound care, monitoring vital signs, and ensuring adequate hydration and nutrition. If this is closed with a transcatheter closure device, monitor for signs of migration. If the device dislodges, the child will suddenly have a wide pulse pressure. At that point, the cardiac interventionist is notified for further actions.

Medical Care. A PDA may be closed surgically or with a transcatheter device. The PDA may also be closed using the medication indomethacin (Indocin).

> ### 🌼 *Nursing Insight*—*Subacute bacterial endocarditis prophylaxis*
>
> If the child has a high risk for bacterial endocarditis, the physician provider will prescribe antibiotics before dental work and surgery. The child may require this for only 6 months after the defect is repaired. Be aware of the published American Heart Association (AHA) guidelines. In 2007, the AHA made sweeping changes to the guidelines for prophylaxis needed for patients with known cardiac disease. The guideline changes were made because:
> - Infectious endocarditis (IE) is much more likely to occur from frequent exposure such as teeth brushing, chewing, or toothpicks than from a one-time occurrence of a tooth extraction or gastrointestinal/genitourinary procedure.
> - Risk-benefit ratio: Prophylaxis will prevent only a very small number of IE, and the risk of antibiotic resistance is high.
> - Good oral hygiene is more effective than a onetime dose of antibiotics.

Education/Discharge Instructions

See Education/Discharge Instructions for Cardiovascular Conditions in Children.

Atrioventricular Canal Defect

An atrioventricular canal defect (AVC) is also known as complete AVC or endocardial cushion defect (ECD). This defect is somewhat of a combination of an ASD and VSD. However, it is much more than that because it involves the valves. In its simplest definition, an AVC is a large hole in the center of the heart. Embryologically, the endocardial cushion fails to form properly. There are openings on the atrial wall and the ventricular wall, and the tricuspid and mitral valves come together to form one large valve (Fig. 26-9). These defects are often seen in children with Down syndrome (Pettersen, 2013). This defect must be repaired surgically if the child is to live a normal life span. Although the blood is mixed through this large open space, the shunt is left to right and the child is not cyanotic. There are many variations of this defect including partial ECD.

Signs and Symptoms

Signs and symptoms of cardiac failure will gradually worsen with time unless the defect is repaired:

- Shortness of breath
- Respiratory distress
- Periorbital edema
- Failure to thrive
- Increased respiratory infections
- Distended liver may be noted

Diagnosis

A complete physical examination, including auscultation of the heart and lungs, helps in the diagnosis. A heart murmur is verified. Additional tests such as chest x-ray and ECG support the diagnosis. Tests such as an echocardiogram, cardiac catheterization, and/or cardiac MRI confirm the diagnosis.

Collaborative Care

Nursing Care. Nursing care focuses on postoperative management of the child. Postoperative education also includes support systems for children who also have concomitant Down syndrome.

Medical Care. Care of the child with AVC is more complex than that of the child with ASD and or VSD. Prior to surgery, nursing care is geared toward optimizing the cardiac output and ensuring adequate weight gain.

 Nursing Insight—*Care of the child with congenital heart defects*

The hospital nurse most often cares for a child with a congenital heart defect when the child is admitted for surgery. Occasionally, a child with a defect may be admitted for reasons not related to the heart. The child is always monitored for signs of congestive heart failure (CHF) and measures taken to prevent fatigue, fluid overload, or infections. If a school nurse has a student with a congenital heart defect, the cardiologist or cardiology nurse practitioner submits letters to the school that outline the plan of care and any physical or activity restrictions. Anyone caring for a child who is taking cardiac medications must understand the effects, side effects, and proper dosing.

 Where Research and Practice Meet:
Exercise Testing and Training in Children With Congenital Heart Disease

Doctors from Children's Hospital of Boston conducted a review of literature regarding cardiac rehabilitation programs for patients under the age of 18. Articles were published between January 1981 and November 2010. A total of 16 clinical studies were reviewed. The researchers were concerned that although cardiac rehabilitation programs are widely accepted and shown to improve outcomes for patients with acquired cardiac disease, very few programs exist for the pediatric population of patients with CHD. Therefore, the researchers postulated that children with cardiac defects might benefit from cardiac rehabilitation programs. In this review of the literature, the researchers used the OXFORD classification for evidence-based medicine (Centre for Evidence-Based Medicine [CEBM], 2013). The youngest patient in this study was 4 years old. The number of patients per each study was anywhere from 1 to 103 and were in programs lasting from 2 weeks to 10 months. In summary, the researchers felt that, of the cardiac rehabilitation programs studied, there was not consistency in the types of programs or outcomes measurements. The programs varied in their level of intensity, frequency, and duration of exercises. The studies also did not take into account that the children with cardiac disease may have other comorbidities of the pulmonary, musculoskeletal, or neurological system that may benefit from cardiac rehabilitation programs. The review also showed that many aspects often seen in adult programs were missing from pediatric programs such as nutritional counseling, risk-factor management, psychosocial and vocational training, and most important, educational intervention.

The overall recommendations found in the articles were that cardiac rehabilitation programs should be at least 12 weeks in length, 2 to 3 times per week, and lasting at least 40 minutes. One important discovery was that cardiac rehabilitation programs were dramatically underutilized, and the value of such programs was not appreciated. The researchers outlined a list of factors that potentially contributed to the under-appreciation, such as a limited number of specialists or specialized facilities and poor insurance coverage. Other factors included provider- or patient-related factors. Patient factors were expense, logistics of getting to facility or having time to get to facility, or parental anxiety born out of fear for their child's ability to exercise safely. Providers also underestimated the value or availability of such programs. The researchers recommended that changes be made at all levels of the health-care arena, for example, in policies, protocols, and awareness initiatives (Ubeda Tikkanen et al., 2012).

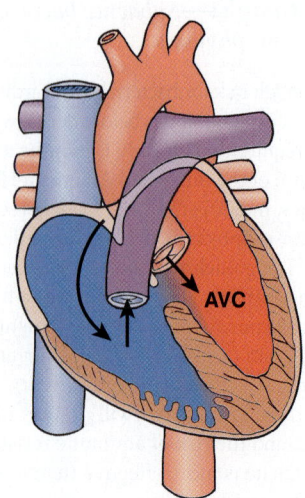

Figure 26-9 Atrioventricular canal defect.

Education/Discharge Instructions

See Education/Discharge Instructions for Cardiovascular Conditions in Children.

OBSTRUCTIVE LESIONS

Pulmonic Stenosis

Pulmonic stenosis, or pulmonic valve stenosis, is a malformation of the pulmonary artery or pulmonic valve. The narrowing of the valve causes an increased workload on the right ventricle (Fig. 26-10), which in turn leads to CHF with symptoms such as hepatomegaly. This condition is frequently associated with Noonan syndrome and is part of the combination condition called tetralogy of Fallot.

 Nursing Insight—*An insufficient valve*

Valves may be congenitally malformed or become physically altered because of disease. If the valve does not close properly, there may be leakage called regurgitation or insufficiency when the valve is stiff or stenotic. When the valve is insufficient, the ventricle must pump with greater force to push blood through a stiff or "sticky" door. Because of the backflow of blood, the ventricle pumps with a greater force of contraction because there is more volume and thus more stretch (Starling's law). This constant increased force eventually tires the cardiac muscle. The nurse is aware of the signs and symptoms of CHF.

Signs and Symptoms

A heart murmur is the most common sign of pulmonic stenosis.

- Grade II to IV out of VI systolic murmur, may have ejection click

During periods of increased blood pressure, such as with excitement, exercise, crying, or fever, the child may experience dyspnea (breathlessness) or in the most severe cases, brief moments of cyanosis when the blood flow does not reach the pulmonary bed.

Diagnosis

The diagnosis is confirmed by the presence of a heart murmur, by electrocardiogram (ECG), and by echocardiogram.

Cardiac catheterization measures the degree of pulmonary stenosis. An ECG will show right ventricular hypertrophy.

Collaborative Care

Nursing Care. Care measures help the patient to reduce stressful situations that may cause high blood pressure.

Surgical Care. Depending on the gradient (difference in the pressure measurements between chambers or across the defect), the cardiologist may choose to observe the child closely over time before recommending an intervention. Surgical interventions include balloon angioplasty or valvuloplasty (a procedure that reopens narrowed blood vessels and restores forward blood flow) or open-heart surgery. Because this valve is in an area of low flow and low pressure, these children often do well with one intervention but are monitored periodically for restenosis.

Education/Discharge Instructions

See Education/Discharge Instructions for Cardiovascular Conditions in Children.

Aortic Stenosis

Aortic stenosis, or aortic valve **stenosis** (AS or AVS), is a malformation and narrowing in the aorta or around the aortic valve (Fig. 26-11). A narrowing in this area causes an increased workload on the left ventricle that eventually leads to **hypertrophy** (increase in size) and heart failure. This condition may also be acquired after birth. Variations of this defect are supra- and subvalvar stenosis and have an association with bicuspid aortic valve.

Signs and Symptoms

Aortic stenosis can be indicated by several symptoms:

- A murmur may be audible
  - During the systolic phase of the cardiac cycle.
  - A click may be heard, and a thrill may be noted.
- The child may have chest pain or fatigue and syncope on exertion.
- Critical AS causes heart failure in neonates.

Diagnosis

Diagnosis is based on the clinical findings and echocardiogram with a chest x-ray exam and ECG supporting the

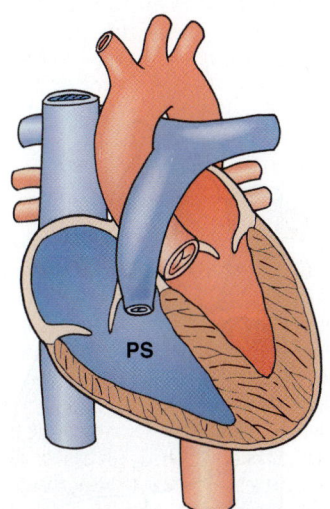

Figure 26-10 Pulmonary stenosis.

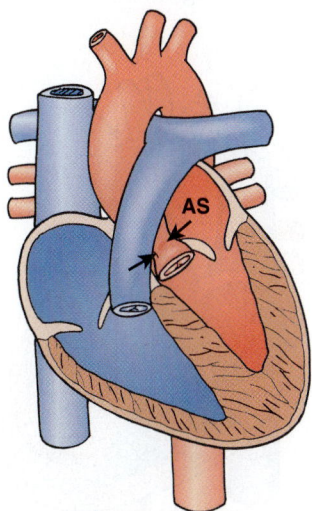

Figure 26-11 Aortic stenosis.

diagnosis. An ECG may show left ventricular hypertrophy. Cardiac catheterization is the definitive test, also measuring the exact gradient.

Collaborative Care

Nursing Care. Nursing care is based on medical and/or postoperative management. In critical situations with very narrow valves, preload and afterload reduction medication is indicated. Because this valve is in a high-flow, high-pressure area, it is more critical to correct.

Surgical Care. A balloon angioplasty or valvuloplasty is performed to open the narrow area with a balloon. Another treatment mode is surgical intervention to repair or replace the valve. Aortic stenosis requires lifelong monitoring.

Education/Discharge Instructions

See Education/Discharge Instructions for Cardiovascular Conditions in Children.

Coarctation of the Aorta

Coarctation of the aorta (CoA) is a narrowing or stricture of the descending aorta distal to the carotid arteries. The coarctation is classified by its location: preductal, ductal, or postductal (Fig. 26-12). Normally, blood pressure (BP) in the legs should be higher or equal to that in the arms. When a BP in the lower extremities measures greater than 10 mm Hg less than that in the upper extremities, the practitioner suspects a CoA (Park, 2009). Occasionally, the BP in the right arm is higher than in the left. This usually occurs with a preductal coarctation in which the blood flow to the left arm is supplied by the flow of blood through the ductus, which is a lower pressure system. For this reason, if only one upper extremity is used as comparison with the lower extremities, it should be the right arm. If a child is hypertensive, CoA is suspected.

Signs and Symptoms

Symptoms of CoA can be:

- Murmur
  - Not always present
  - Systolic ejection murmur heard at upper right sternal border and left sternal border
  - Cycle radiates to left axilla and left intrascapular area of the back
- The child may show signs of CHF

- The child may have pain in the legs or cyanotic lower extremities

Diagnosis

The classic diagnostic feature of this defect is a high gradient, which is the difference in the pressure measurements between the arms and legs.

Collaborative Care

Nursing Care. Nursing care focuses on postoperative management of the child. The child is followed by the health-care provider for evidence of restenosis. The nurse assists in this monitoring by proper evaluation of the upper and lower blood pressures. Post-surgically, the child may have severe rebound hypertension. The ventricles have become very accustomed to pushing hard against the narrowed area in the aorta. When this area is opened up, the heart muscle still wants to contract strongly against the gradient. If there is nothing to push against, there is still an abnormally high blood pressure. This is controlled by antihypertensive agents for 6 months to a year after surgery and may be required through life.

Medical Care. Pharmacological treatment includes afterload-reducing agents, which control the blood pressure. Two such agents are captopril (Capoten) or enalapril (Vasotec).

Surgical Care. Surgery is always indicated for this condition. Invasive treatment for older infants and adolescents involves a balloon angioplasty and stent placement.

Education/Discharge Instructions

See Education/Discharge Instructions for Cardiovascular Conditions in Children.

CYANOTIC CONGENITAL HEART DEFECTS

Tricuspid Atresia

Tricuspid atresia (TA) is caused by an error in the formation of the tricuspid valve. As a single defect, this condition is incompatible with life because no blood from the right atrium reaches the right ventricle and thus the right ventricular outflow tract leading to the PA and the lungs. For this reason, most children born with TA also have comorbidity with a septal defect such as ASD or VSD as well as a PDA. The deoxygenated blood must reach the pulmonary bed to sustain life (Fig. 26-13).

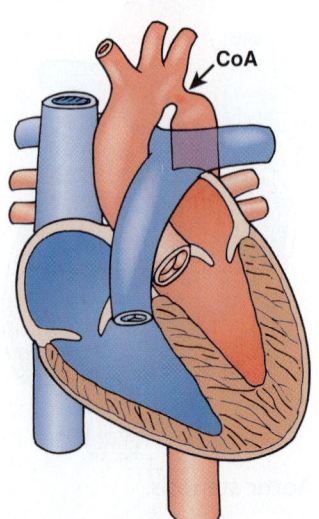

Figure 26-12 Coarctation of the aorta.

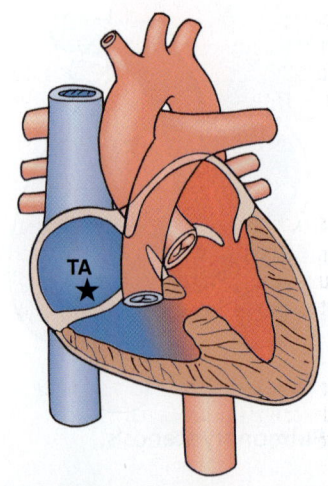

Figure 26-13 Tricuspid atresia.

Signs and Symptoms

The initial signs are dramatic; as the PDA starts to close in the hours after birth, the child becomes severely

- Cyanotic
- Tachycardic
- Dyspneic

A heart murmur is generally present at the left sternal border that is pansystolic.

Diagnosis

Tricuspid atresia may be discovered during a routine prenatal ultrasound imaging or at birth based on the signs and symptoms. Diagnostic testing includes ECG, echocardiogram, chest radiograph, and cardiac catheterization.

Collaborative Care

Nursing Care. Nursing care focuses on postoperative management of the child. Prostaglandins keep the PDA from closing, allowing blood flow from the right side of the heart to reach the lungs. Use of this medication can sustain an open PDA for a short time, but more definitive treatment with a balloon septostomy or a shunt surgery will eventually be done.

Surgical Care. Tricuspid atresia requires emergency intervention. Initially, the neonate is given PGE$_1$ to keep the PDA from closing. In addition, if there is no ASD or patent foramen ovale (PFO), an emergent balloon atrial septostomy is performed to ensure survival. The next step is to perform a systemic-pulmonary shunt if the pulmonary blood flow is deficient or a PA band if the pulmonary blood flow is excessive. Eventually a Glenn procedure may be done, and Fontan procedure is the definitive surgery.

 Nursing Insight—Pulmonary atresia

Pulmonary atresia is a fatal defect if not corrected or **palliated** (treated to reduce effect) early in life. Pulmonary atresia is absence of the pulmonary valve, pulmonary artery, or both (Fig. 26-14).

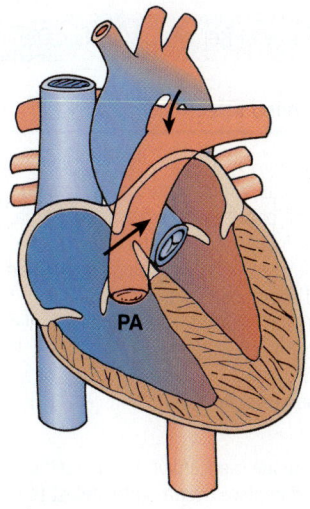

Figure 26-14 Pulmonary atresia.

The child must have an ASD or PFO (the opening present in utero and at birth that closes spontaneously) and/or a PDA to survive. A PDA will allow blood to flow into the lungs for oxygenation.

If the pulmonary valve and/or pulmonary artery are not present, the cardiac team performs emergency procedures to save the child's life. Initially, prostaglandin (PGE$_1$) is infused to maintain patency (free flow) of the PDA. A balloon atrial septostomy (formation of an opening in a septum) is then performed to create an ASD (Venes, 2013). This procedure allows the flow of blood from the right side to the left. Primary surgical repair includes a shunt (diversion) or a conduit (channel). Later, a Fontan procedure (a procedure used to repair complex single ventricle–type congenital heart defects) may be needed. See Table 26-4.

Education/Discharge Instructions

See Education/Discharge Instructions for Cardiovascular Conditions in Children.

Table 26-4 Surgical Repairs of Cardiac Defects

Repair and Intended Effect	Defects	Potential Long-Term Implications and Sequelae
Palliative Repairs		
PA banding: • A restrictive band is placed around the main pulmonary artery to decrease uncontrolled pulmonary blood flow and prevent the development of pulmonary hypertension and eventual right heart failure.	VSD, single ventricle, tricuspid atresia	Eventual decreased O$_2$ saturations with growth and aging, right ventricular hypertrophy, if the band becomes too tight with growth of the child. Excessive flow to left pulmonary artery and left pulmonary HTN r/t stenosis of the right pulmonary artery, related to possible migration and encroachment on the right PA. Possible revision of banding.
Blalock-Taussig shunt (modified): • A Gore-Tex graft conduit is placed between the right or left subclavian artery and the ipsilateral pulmonary artery to provide controlled pulmonary blood flow.	Cyanotic heart defects such as HLHS, TOF, pulmonary atresia, tricuspid atresia	Mild pulmonary artery distortion at site of anastomosis, inability of shunt size to increase with growth and aging, thrombus formation on graft site, potential coronary ischemia r/t pulmonary "steal" of blood flow during diastole.
• Sano shunt • A Gore-Tex graft conduit is placed between the single ventricle and the pulmonary artery to provide controlled pulmonary blood flow.	Cyanotic heart defects such as HLHS, pulmonary atresia, tricuspid atresia, single ventricle defects	Mild pulmonary artery distortion at site of anastomosis, thrombus formation on graft site, inability of shunt size to increase with growth and aging.

(continued)

Table 26-4 Surgical Repairs of Cardiac Defects (continued)

Repair and Intended Effect	Defects	Potential Long-Term Implications and Sequelae
• Atrial septectomy • A communication is surgically created by tearing a hole or incision between the left and right atria. This encourages mixing of blood flow at the atrial level and encourages pulmonary blood flow. More invasive than ballooning of septum as seen in Rashkind procedure. Considered to be a palliative procedure prior to complete repair.	Single ventricle physiology with intact atrial septum, un-repaired TGA.	Eventual development of heart failure if further palliation or repair is not sought.

Definitive (or Complete) Repairs

Patch closures • Native cardiac tissue (pericardium) or a prosthetic patch is sutured in place over a septal defect to effectively close the communication between the atria or ventricles.	ASD, VSD, AV canal	Incomplete closure of defect, dysrhythmia, potential for patch dehiscence, AV block (VSD closures)
• Ductal ligation • A tie or clip is placed around the patent ductus arteriosus and tightened to prevent excessive pulmonary blood flow from the aorta.	PDA	Incomplete closure of ductus and associated residual pulmonary shunting, mobilization of device.
• COA repair • Narrowing in the proximal, distal, or arch of the aorta is reduced or eliminated via surgical resection of stenosed area, patch placement to increase aortic diameter, subclavian flap aortoplasty or bypass grafting.	Coarctation of aorta	Restenosis or recoarctation of affected portion of aorta, transient spinal ischemia and associated paraplegia, paradoxical hypertension, possible need for re-repair or angioplasty
Valvuloplasty • A malformed, damaged, or stenotic valve is surgically revised to correct the associated malfunction.	Destructive endocarditis, valvular stenosis	Incomplete or unsuccessful revision of affected valve; thromboemboli formation, additional valvular damage and possible need for valve replacement.
• Artificial valve replacement • A faulty or damaged native valve is replaced with a valve made of either human or animal tissue or a mechanical valve.	Endocarditis, failed Ross, valvular stenosis	Need for a lifetime of replacement prosthetic valve procedures, need for long-term oral anticoagulation, thromboemboli formation, aortic or pulmonary insufficiency.
Ross procedure • A damaged or dysfunctional aortic valve is removed and replaced with the patient's pulmonic valve, which is then replaced with a donor homograft valve.	Destructive endocarditis, valvular aortic stenosis	Aortic/pulmonary valve stenosis, gross valvular dysfunction, aortic or pulmonary insufficiency, potential for a lifetime of possible prosthetic valve replacements, risk for heart block.
Konno procedure* • A faulty aortic valve is replaced with a prosthetic valve while the narrowed aortic root is enlarged via patch placement to increase systemic blood flow.	Any left-ventricular outflow tract obstruction such as aortic valve hypoplasia, subaortic stenosis	Potential failure of aortic valve graft and persistent aortic stenosis, thromboemboli formation on grafted valves, potential need for lifelong oral anticoagulation, potential for development of heart block, aortic insufficiency.
Damus-Kaye-Stansel procedure • Prosthetic conduits are placed between the proximal main pulmonary artery and the aorta and between the right ventricle and the distal pulmonary artery. Existing VSD is closed and the existing aortic valve may be closed or left unclosed. This procedure attempts to reroute in appropriate pulmonary and systemic blood flow	TGA with VSD; Double outlet right ventricle (DORV) with VSD.	Aortic insufficiency, thromboemboli formation in cases of complete aortic valve closure, need for periodic surgical conduit replacements, coronary ischemia.
Rastelli • The main pulmonary artery is divided from its incorrect origin on the LV and is reattached to the RV using a prosthetic conduit. A tunnel is then created between the existent VSD and aorta, effectively rerouting blood from the LV to systemic outflow.	DORV, TGA + VSD + subaortic stenosis/pulmonic stenosis truncus arteriosus type I.	Conduit obstruction and resultant heart failure, dysrhythmia, thromboemboli formation, failure of prosthetic conduits to allow increased flow with growth and aging, implicit need for eventual RV-PA conduit replacements.
Arterial switch (ASO) • The great arteries (main pulmonary artery and aorta) are divided from the LV and RV respectively	TGA	Dysrhythmia, coronary artery obstruction, LV ischemia and dysfunction, aortic insufficiency, supravalvular pulmonic

Table 26-4 Surgical Repairs of Cardiac Defects (continued)

Repair and Intended Effect	Defects	Potential Long-Term Implications and Sequelae
and reattached to their appropriate locations on the RV (MPA) and LV (aorta). The coronary arteries are also divided from the MPA and transplanted to the neo-aorta.		stenosis, branch pulmonary artery stenosis.
Staged Repairs		
Modified Norwood • The main pulmonary artery is divided from the branch pulmonary arteries and patched to the hypoplastic aortic arch, creating a hybrid systemic arterial outflow from the RV. An atrial septectomy is created via catheterization or surgical incision to allow for left to right shunting, so that oxygenated pulmonary venous blood is directed toward systemic outflow. A systemic–pulmonary shunt (Sano or Blalock-Taussig) is created to allow pulmonary arterial blood flow because the creation of single ventricle physiology only has a direct connection to systemic outflow. This stage creates a single ventricle that is responsible for pulmonary and systemic circulation.	Stage 1 repair for HLHS	Coronary ischemia caused by diastolic "steal" of aortopulmonary shunt if BT shunt is used, pulmonary artery distortion, cyanosis, aortic outflow obstruction, tricuspid insufficiency, potential stenosis of systemic-pulmonary shunt, failure to thrive, feeding difficulties, dysrhythmia.
Glenn • The systemic–pulmonary shunt (BT or Sano) is taken down or ligated with clips. The SVC is connected to the branch pulmonary arteries. The existent ASD is enlarged if necessary to allow for continued left-to-right shunting of oxygenated blood into the systemic outflow. This stage attempts to reduce the workload of the heart so that the single ventricle is only pumping to the systemic circulation.	Stage 2 repair for HLHS, tricuspid atresia	Elevated upper body venous pressures related to increased PVR, hypoxemia, upper body swelling, headache, dysrhythmia, stenosis at area of SVC-PA anastomosis, development of aortopulmonary collateral vessels.
Fontan • The procedure attempts to establish separate pulmonary and systemic circulations by attaching the IVC directly to the RPA-SVC anastomosis with a Gore-Tex extracardiac conduit. This allows for passive flow of systemic venous return directly to the pulmonary arteries and completely bypasses the RA. The existent single ventricle continues to receive pulmonary arterial flow and pump to the systemic circulation via the neo-aorta constructed in Stage 1 repair. Other Fontan techniques route caval flow through a conduit partly routed through the RA, which may lead to complications. Newer techniques bypass the RA completely. Occasionally, fenestrations, or holes, are created between the IVC-RPA conduit and the RA to allow for a "pop-off" of extra fluid, which is thought to prevent some postoperative complications.	Stage 3 repair for HLHS, tricuspid atresia	Obstruction of conduit leading to systemic venous pooling, thromboemboli formation, dysrhythmia, systemic venous hypertension, protein-losing enteropathy, right heart failure leading to hepatosplenomegaly.
Infrequent Repairs		
Blalock-Taussig shunt (Classic) • The right or left subclavian artery is divided from the aorta and attached to the ipsilateral (same side) pulmonary artery to provide controlled pulmonary blood flow.	Cyanotic heart defects such as HLHS, TOF, pulmonary atresia, tricuspid atresia	Mild pulmonary artery distortion at site of anastomosis, resultant ischemia to hand or arm on ipsilateral side of anastomosis with associated limb length discrepancy and perfusion, potential coronary ischemia related to pulmonary "steal" of blood flow during diastole.
Waterston-Cooley shunt • A connection is created between the ascending aorta and the right pulmonary artery to increase pulmonary blood flow; now considered obsolete as a result of development of superior shunts. This procedure is RARELY performed today.	Cyanotic heart defects	Right pulmonary artery distortion at site of anastomosis, inadequate pulmonary blood flow and persistent cyanosis, excessive pulmonary blood flow and development of pulmonary hypertension, right pulmonary artery stenosis and possible need for major reconstructive surgery.

(continued)

Table 26-4 Surgical Repairs of Cardiac Defects (continued)

Repair and Intended Effect	Defects	Potential Long-Term Implications and Sequelae
Potts shunt • A connection is created between the descending aorta to the left pulmonary artery to increase pulmonary blood flow; now considered obsolete as a result of development of superior shunts. This procedure is RARELY performed today.	Cyanotic heart defects	Left pulmonary artery distortion at site of anastomosis, inadequate pulmonary blood flow and persistent cyanosis, excessive pulmonary blood flow and development of pulmonary hypertension, difficulty of shunt take-down.
Senning • Conduits or baffles made from pericardium or synthetic material are placed between the RA and the LV pulmonic outflow and between the LA and the RV aortic outflow. These conduits allow appropriate pulmonary and systemic circulation without switching placement of the great arteries.	TGA	Atrial dysrhythmias, baffle obstructions or leaks, right heart failure related to use of right ventricle as systemic pump. Tricuspid or mitral insufficiency, thromboemboli.
Mustard • Conduits or tunnels are created between the RA and the LV pulmonic outflow and between the LA and the RV aortic outflow using atrial tissue. These conduits allow appropriate pulmonary and systemic circulation without switching placement of the great arteries.	TGA	Atrial dysrhythmias, conduit obstructions or leaks, right heart failure related to use of right ventricle as systemic pump. Tricuspid or mitral insufficiency, thromboemboli.

* Ross-Konno procedure combines replacement of aortic valve with native pulmonary valve and aortic root enlargement.
Source: © Judith M. Marshall (Data from Mavroudis, Backer, & Idriss, 2013).

 focus on safety

Survival of the child

With any congenital defect, as long as there is mixing of oxygenated and deoxygenated blood, the child survives. A more definitive surgery, such as a Fontan procedure, is performed at a later date to correct the condition.

 Nursing Insight—*Epstein's malformation*

Epstein's malformation occurs when the tricuspid valve is displaced into the right ventricle (Fig. 26-15). Typically, in this condition, an ASD is present. The ventricle and the atria may become hypertrophied and this condition is often associated with supraventricular dysrhythmias, particularly Wolff-Parkinson-White syndrome. With Epstein's malformation, the child may live normally or require treatment. Surgical intervention is the treatment of choice.

Epsteins

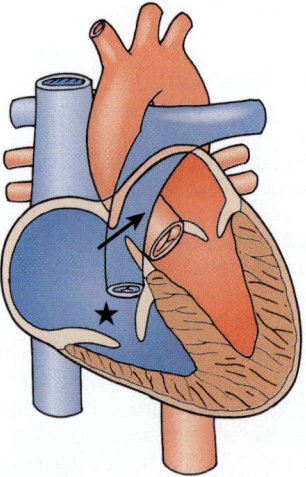

Figure 26-15 Epstein's malformation.

Total Anomalous Pulmonary Venous Return

Total anomalous pulmonary venous return (TAPVR) is a condition in which the pulmonary blood flow returns to the heart through the right atrium rather than the left (Fig. 26-16). The child usually has an ASD, allowing the blood to flow back to the left ventricle and out to the body tissues. As a consequence of the ASD, mixing of venous blood with arterial blood may occur, causing a cyanotic condition. One problem for a child with TAPVR is that a high volume of blood returns to the right side of the heart, causing right-sided hypertrophy and enlargement. If an ASD is not present, the health-care provider will create one with a balloon septostomy. A variation of this condition is partial anomalous pulmonary venous return (PAPVR), in

which two of the veins return blood to the left side and two of the veins return blood to the right side. Other variations are simply in routing of the blood flow back to the heart.

Signs and Symptoms

TAPVR can be indicated by several symptoms:

• Murmur
  • Systolic ejection murmur heard best in pulmonic area that radiates throughout lung field
• Cyanosis
• Respiratory distress
• Lethargy
• Poor and rapid breathing

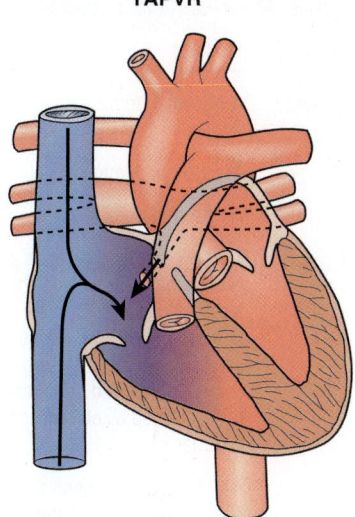

Figure 26-16 Total anomalous pulmonary venous return.

- Poor feeding
- Frequent respiratory infections
- Signs of heart failure

Diagnosis

Diagnosis is based on signs and symptoms and diagnostic testing including ECG, echocardiogram, chest x-ray exam, and cardiac catheterization.

Collaborative Care

Nursing Care. Nursing care focuses on postoperative management of the child.

Surgical Care. The treatment for TAPVR is complete surgical repair (see Table 26-4). Post-surgery, the child can live a full, normal life and is followed by the health-care provider routinely (every 1 to 2 years) for any reoccurring stenosis.

Education/Discharge Instructions

See Education/Discharge Instructions for Cardiovascular Conditions in Children.

CONAL–TRUNCAL DEFECTS

Conal–truncal defects develop during the formation of the trunk dissection. Embryologically, the pulmonary artery and the aorta begin as a large "trunk." The ventricles then fold over, the atria rise into position, and the great vessels form when the trunk twists around and forms a septum, dividing the vessel into two walls. Transposition of the great vessels and truncus arteriosus occur in children when there is a disruption in this process.

Transposition of the Great Arteries or Vessels

Transposition of the great arteries or vessels (TGA or TGV) occurs in utero when the signals cross, and instead of twisting, there is simply a septation and the aorta arises from the right side of the heart and the pulmonary artery arises from the left (Fig. 26-17).

Signs and Symptoms

Symptoms appear at birth or soon afterwards and include:

- Cyanosis
- Shortness of breath

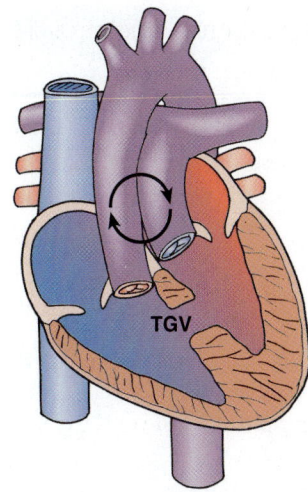

Figure 26-17 Transposition of the great vessels.

- Poor feeding
- Eventual clubbing of the fingers and toes
- Murmur not always present

Diagnosis

Diagnosis is based on signs, and diagnostic testing includes pulse oximetry, ECG, echocardiogram, chest x-ray exam, and cardiac catheterization. If an echocardiogram is done before birth, it is called a fetal echocardiogram.

Collaborative Care

Nursing Care. Nursing care focuses on postoperative management of the child. The child's condition is followed up by a health-care provider throughout life to monitor for signs of stenosis around the anastomosis sites.

Surgical Care. The severity of the signs and symptoms direct the timing of treatment. TGA in all cases must be surgically corrected, typically with an arterial switch operation (ASO). This surgery is considered a definitive repair, and the prognosis is good.

Education/Discharge Instructions

See Education/Discharge Instructions for Cardiovascular Conditions in Children.

 Nursing Insight—*Diagnosis of cardiac defects and disease through genetics*

As early as 1795, and possibly before, scientists theorized that physical attributes were transmitted genetically. The early work of Maupertuis, Darwin, and Mendel laid the groundwork for genetic theories. DNA was discovered in 1869. Watson and Crick determined that DNA was a double-strand helix in the 1950s. By the year 2000, the scientists with the Human Genome Project mapped the human genes. Only a short 12 years later, many diseases can be traced directly to a deletion or defect of a particular gene. Genes responsible for many cardiac diseases and defects are outlined on the National Institutes of Health Web site Genetics Home Reference (National Library of Medicine, 2014) (Table 26-5). One example of how this information can be used in the treatment of cardiac disease is in the case of channelopathies (NYU Cardiac and Vascular Institute, 2013). Channelopathies are defects of the electrolyte channels in cardiac muscle that leads

Table 26-5 Genetic Testing Used for Cardiac Defects, Cardiomyopathy, and Syndromes Associated With Cardiac Problems

Gene (and Purpose)	Condition	Cardiac Effect	Pattern
PKP2	Arrhythmogenic right ventricular cardiomyopathy (ARVC)	Dysrhythmia, cardiomyopathy	Autosomal dominant
ELN (elastin)	Supravalvular aortic stenosis (SVAS)	Valvar	Autosomal dominant
TNNI3 (troponin I)	Familial restrictive cardiomyopathy	Cardiomyopathy	Autosomal dominant
22q11.2 deletion	DiGeorge syndrome, velocardiofacial syndrome, Shprintzen syndrome, and conotruncal anomaly face syndrome	Multiple defects of heart (conotruncal), face, immune system	The deletion may occur as a random event during the formation of reproductive cells or in early fetal development. Those with the deletion can pass to their offspring and only one copy of an altered gene is necessary, so it is classified as an autosomal dominant disorder.
RYR2 and *CASQ2*	Catecholaminergic polymorphic ventricular tachycardia (CPVT)	Dysrhythmia	*RYR2* gene: autosomal dominant *CASQ2* gene: autosomal recessive
FBN1 (fibrillin-1)	Marfan	Valvular (aortic) Other defects of eyes, spine, laxity in ligaments	Autosomal dominant
IDS (I2S enzyme)	Mucopolysaccharidosis type II (MPS II)	Heart valve abnormalities can cause the heart to become enlarged (ventricular hypertrophy)	X-linked recessive pattern
PTPN11, SOS1, RAF1, *KRAS, NRAS,* and *BRAF* (tissue formation) **Most common bolded**	Noonan syndrome	Pulmonary valve stenosis, hypertrophic cardiomyopathy, multiple other system defects	Autosomal dominant
DMD	Duchenne's and Becker's muscular dystrophy	Cardiomyopathy and other muscular disorders	X-linked recessive
KCNE1 and *KCNQ1* (potassium channel)	Jervell and Lange-Nielsen syndrome	LQT Syndrome, profound hearing loss	Autosomal recessive pattern

Source: National Library of Medicine, (2014).

to dysrhythmia disturbances and sudden death. Testing for the specific gene *KCNE1* allows health-care providers to determine if a patient has a higher potential for lethal dysrhythmias and thus justifies specific treatment modalities for these patients (Kontula, Swan, Marjamaa, & Lahtinen, 2011).

Truncus Arteriosus

Truncus arteriosus is a complicated cyanotic lesion with a poor prognosis if not treated surgically. In truncus arteriosus, the trunk has neither twisted nor formed a septum. There are multiple variations of the condition, classed I to IV, but the general physiology is that the aorta and pulmonary arteries (PAs) are combined, with full mixing of blood (Fig. 26-18). Sometimes the PAs arise from the aorta, either ascending or descending.

Signs and Symptoms

Symptoms of truncus arteriosus include:

- Cyanosis
- Congestive heart failure
- Low cardiac output
- Systolic ejection murmur with possible thrill at left sternal border

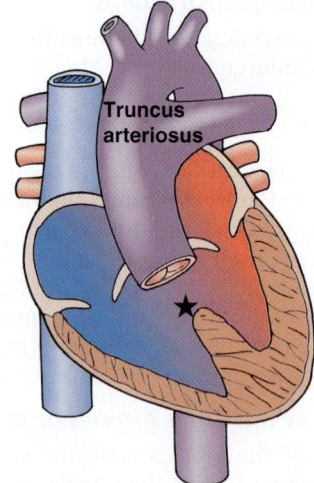

Figure 26-18 Truncus arteriosus.

Diagnosis

Diagnosis is based on signs and diagnostic testing that include pulse oximetry, ECG, echocardiogram, chest radiograph, and cardiac catheterization.

Collaborative Care

Nursing Care. Nursing care focuses on postoperative management of the child.

Surgical Care. This condition requires palliative and complete surgical repair (see Table 26-4). Treatment for children includes aggressive medical regimen with inotropic medications along with preload and afterload reduction.

Education/Discharge Instructions

See Education/Discharge Instructions for Cardiovascular Conditions in Children.

Tetralogy of Fallot

Tetralogy of Fallot (TOF) is a combination defect. *Tetra* is from the Latin root "four" and Fallot is the name of the physician who defined it as a syndrome or common grouping. There are always four associated conditions: VSD, overriding aorta, hypertrophic RV, and pulmonary stenosis or atresia. With advanced technology and early screening, this condition is diagnosed at an early age. As recently as the 1980s, TOF was undetected for many years, and in developing countries remains so even today.

Signs and Symptoms

TOF can be indicated by the following symptoms:

- Tachypnea
- Dyspnea on exertion
- Growth failure
- Cyanosis after ductus arteriosus closes
- Loud systolic ejection murmur that is described as harsh and radiating
- Right ventricular hypertrophy (Fig. 26-19) caused by a stenotic vessel and high pulmonary vascular resistance (PVR)

focus on safety

Tetralogy of Fallot

The hallmark sign of TOF is cyanosis with crying or playing, which is relieved by squatting or drawing up the legs. These episodes (called "TET" spells) are cyanotic events exacerbated by excitement and crying, then relieved by a decrease in pulmonary vascular resistance.

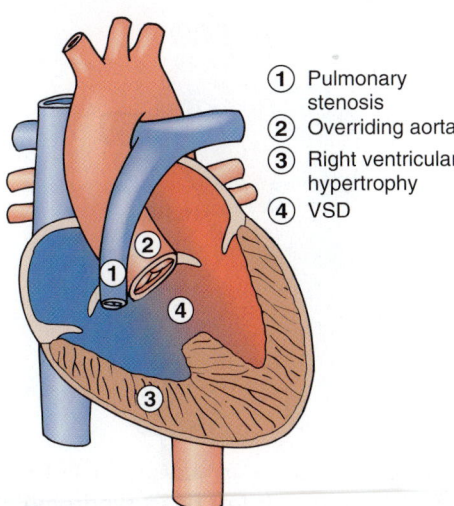

1. Pulmonary stenosis
2. Overriding aorta
3. Right ventricular hypertrophy
4. VSD

Figure 26-19 Tetralogy of Fallot.

Diagnosis

Diagnosis of TOF is based on signs and symptoms such as cyanosis, breathing difficulties, fainting, fatigue and weakness, slow growth, or developmental delay. Tests, including ECG, echocardiogram, chest x-ray exam, and cardiac catheterization support and confirm the diagnosis.

Collaborative Care

Nursing Care. Pre-surgical care involves preventing or minimizing symptoms associated with the defect.

Surgical Care. See Table 26-4 for definitive surgical treatment.

Education/Discharge Instructions

See Education/Discharge Instructions for Cardiovascular Conditions in Children.

 Nursing Insight—*Auscultation of heart murmurs*

Most heart sounds are made through the opening and closing of valves or blood flow through an abnormal opening. The typical points for auscultating heart sounds are shown in Figure 26-20. When listening for each valve, the auscultation landmarks are not located above the valve itself but in the direction of the flow of blood. Therefore, the aortic and pulmonic valves are best heard above the valve and the tricuspid and mitral sounds are best heard below the valve (Tables 26-6 and 26-7).

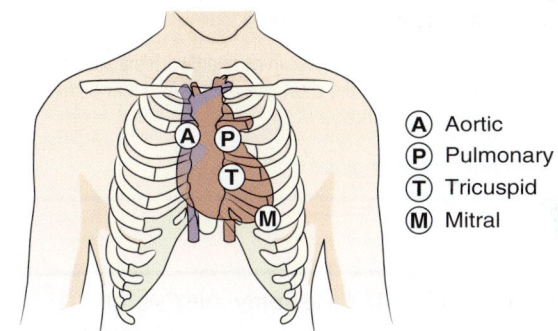

(A) Aortic
(P) Pulmonary
(T) Tricuspid
(M) Mitral

Figure 26-20 Auscultation points.

Table 26-6	Heart Murmurs	
Location of Sound	**Associated Defect or Conditions**	**Phase**
Aortic	Ao valve stenosis	Systolic
	Supravalvular aortic stenosis	
	Subvalvular aortic stenosis	
	Aortic regurgitation	Diastolic
Pulmonic	Pulmonary valve stenosis	Systolic
	ASD	
	PA stenosis	
	Ao stenosis	
	Coarctation of the aorta	
	PDA	
	PAPVR	
	TAPVR	
	Pulmonary ejection murmur	
	Pulmonary flow murmur	
	Pulmonary insufficiency	Diastolic

(continued)

Table 26-6 Heart Murmurs (continued)

Location of Sound	Associated Defect or Conditions	Phase
Mitral	Mitral regurgitation Aortic stenosis MV Prolapse Vibratory innocent murmur HOCM	Systolic
	Mitral stenosis	Diastolic
Tricuspid	VSD Tricuspid regurgitation TOF Vibratory innocent murmur HOCM	Systolic
	Tricuspid stenosis	Diastolic

Table 26-7 Classification of Murmurs

Grade	Description
1	Soft murmur, heard under quiet conditions usually by an expert
2	Quiet murmur, heard even if it is noisy
3	Moderately loud murmur, easily heard
4*	Loud murmur associated with a thrill
5	Very loud murmur heard with the edge of the stethoscope tilted against the chest plus a thrill
6	Very loud murmur that can be heard with the stethoscope 5–10 mm from the chest plus a thrill. Also may be heard without a stethoscope.

*Diastolic murmurs are only graded to 4.

? Global Health Case Study Alex's Story

This case study is based on a true story. Alex was a 27-year-old male from Mongolia. He came to the United States on a student/work visa. He was required to have a physical exam to work at a local department store, so was advised to go to a doctor of nursing practice (DNP) clinic to get a routine physical and pay cash because he did not have health insurance. At first glance, the DNP noted that Alex was cyanotic and had clubbing of the fingernails. Because of a language barrier, Alex was not able to tell the DNP that he was born with tetralogy of Fallot, which was never repaired because he had no access to surgical care in his country. The DNP knows that it is difficult to determine the incidence of congenital heart defects in developing nations because of poor data collection. In addition, it is difficult to compare these statistics to those from developed nations because those children born with CHD in developed nations will survive because of technology and medical advances and access to care, while those born in developing nations usually die before their first year. The DNP was surprised to learn that he had lived this long with this type of cyanotic defect. The DNP accessed the necessary resources for Alex to be admitted to a local children's hospital immediately. Within 6 months of the procedure, Alex had normal oxygen saturation measurements, his heart rate normalized, but his fingernails remained clubbed. Alex was able to stay in the United States to begin his education in computer programming.

critical thinking questions

1. Besides assessing vital signs, what other diagnostic tool could the DNP use to assess his oxygenation status?

2. What other definitive testing might be done next to diagnose Alex's condition?

3. The DNP knows that this type of defect requires what type of treatment?

4. Why was Alex, at 27 years old, seen at a children's hospital?

◆ See Suggested Answers to Global Health Case Studies on Davis*Plus*.

Complex Single Ventricle–Type Defects

Complex single ventricle defects are cyanotic conditions with full mixing of oxygenated and deoxygenated blood. The main concern is that there is only one physiological pumping chamber or ventricle. A VSD may be present. In these conditions, **palliative** procedures allow the child to grow until a definitive repair may be performed. Hypoplastic left heart syndrome is a condition in this category.

 Nursing Insight—*Hypoplastic left heart syndrome*

Hypoplastic left heart syndrome is a life-threatening defect that must be treated shortly after birth to sustain life. The ventricle is extremely small or hypoplastic and unable to maintain an adequate cardiac output. The right ventricle must act quickly as the primary pumping mechanism of the cardiac system (Fig. 26-21). This is possible only if there is a left-to-right connection. If there is no ASD, an artificial shunt or pathway must be created shortly after birth (see Nursing Insight: Pulmonary Atresia). Prostaglandin (PGE_1) is given to keep the PDA open. A Norwood procedure is the first stage in the process along with a Blalock-Taussig (BT) shunt. Eventually, a Glenn procedure provides more blood flow and, ultimately, a Fontan procedure is performed. If these surgeries are not suitable, the only other option for treatment is a cardiac transplantation. Rarely,

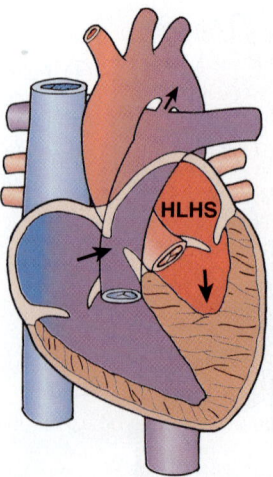

Figure 26-21 Hypoplastic left heart syndrome.

in the most severe cases, palliative or end of life care measures are discussed with the family. Advocate for the family to access these resources.

3. Prioritize developmentally appropriate and holistic nursing interventions for a child with congenital heart disease?

4. Explore diagnostic and laboratory testing including medications for a child with congenital heart disease?

"What to say"—*Children with cardiac defects*

Often families of children with cardiac defects are given a poor prognosis. Children with hypoplastic left heart syndrome (HLHS) have a bleak future. The nurse can help the family simply by allowing time to express their feelings of sadness and possibly anger. Other caring actions include facilitating meetings with other supportive services, such as pastoral care or social workers to assist the family through the grieving process.

Nursing Insight—*Remembering the names of cardiac defects*

One way to remember cyanotic defects is to know that all defects starting with a "T" are cyanotic defects. There is no special reason; it is just a convenient way to remember which defects may be cyanotic.

Nursing Diagnoses: Congenital Heart Defects

• Decreased cardiac output related to structural factors of congenital heart defect and ineffective contraction of the cardiac muscle
• Ineffective breathing pattern related to pulmonary congestion and decreased cardiac output
• Activity intolerance related to decreased cardiac output

Now Can You—**Understand the congenital heart disease?**

1. Discuss the anatomy and physiology of the heart?
2. Identify signs and symptoms in a child with congenital heart disease?

? Case Study Infant With a Heart Murmur

Abby, a 1-month-old infant, is seen in the community clinic for a heart murmur first noted at birth. The clinic nurse obtains a history from the mother about the infant's weight gain, feeding patterns, and behavior. The mother reports that the baby has "gained some weight, tires when feeding, and sleeps most of the time." The nurse then performs a nursing assessment and hears an aortic murmur. This type of murmur is detected as an abnormal, soft blowing sound heard during the systolic phase of the cardiac cycle. The murmur may be a sign of aortic valvular disease such as aortic stenosis.

critical thinking questions

1. What suggestions can the nurse give Abby's mother about feeding the baby?

2. Discuss important aspects about oral medication administration.

◆ See Suggested Answers to Case Studies on Davis*Plus*.

Cardiac Diseases

Children with cardiac diseases are at risk for alterations in growth and development, nutrition, psychosocial functioning, and schooling. Other risks include infection, acquiring other diseases, and even cardiopulmonary arrest. Sometimes these children have significantly altered lifestyles and undergo constant medical treatment.

SUBACUTE BACTERIAL ENDOCARDITIS

Subacute bacterial endocarditis (SBE), also known as infective endocarditis, occurs subsequent to a bacterial infection or introduction of an infective agent into the child's bloodstream. SBE is commonly seen in patients with an unrepaired congenital heart defect or valve disease, but can also occur in normal hearts. The infection may be caused by an invasive procedure such as surgery, urological procedures, or most often, dental cleaning. The bacterium in the bloodstream adheres to a rough area in the heart such as a stenotic valve or an area of turbulent flow. The bacterium colonizes and causes tissue destruction.

Signs and Symptoms

SBE can have vague symptoms:

• Low-grade fever
• Malaise
• Loss of appetite
• Muscle aches

Acute illness can also indicate SBE:

• High fever
• Chills
• Sweating
• Stiff joints
• Back pain

If SBE is a prolonged untreated illness:

• Symptoms of heart failure (Venes, 2013).

Diagnosis

A thorough medical history and a physical exam are essential to diagnosis. The history includes symptoms, questions about a heart murmur or valve replacement, surgery, any recent risk factors for a bacterial or fungal infection (e.g., dental procedures or catheter for dialysis), recent fever, chills, or flu-like symptoms lasting more than 2 weeks. A physical exam may reveal eye hemorrhage petechiae, fluid in the lungs, or signs of a stroke. Blood cultures to identify bacteria or fungi in the bloodstream may detect endocarditis.

Prevention

Prevention of SBE starts with the understanding of the causative factors of SBE. Parents of children with the risk factors of contracting SBE should be proactive in obtaining the prophylaxis if deemed necessary.

Collaborative Care

Nursing Care. Teach the family about the importance of preventative measures if their child is at risk for SBE. When caring for a child with SBE, monitor vital signs including temperature to assess for evidence of infection. A parent may be worried about the prognosis of having SBE. The child may fully recover or may be required to have a valve replacement if the valve is damaged by the infective process. Be supportive of the parents' emotional and spiritual needs in this situation by providing education about what the future might hold.

 focus on safety

Dental care

Because the bacteria responsible for infective endocarditis enters the bloodstream often through the gums, safety concerns for SBE are related to prevention based on the American Heart Association (AHA) guidelines that state good dental care is essential. Care is taken to prevent any subsequent infections.

Medical Care. SBE is treated with antibiotics, but the most effective approach is prevention. The guidelines for administration and dosage of prophylactic antibiotics are determined by the American Dental Association (ADA) and the AHA. Guidelines for when to prescribe prophylaxis treatment were updated in April 2007:

- Patients with prosthetic cardiac valve
- Patients who previously had endocarditis
- Patients with congenital heart disease in the following categories only:
  - Unrepaired cyanotic congenital heart disease, including those with palliative shunts and conduits
  - Completely repaired congenital heart disease with prosthetic material or device, whether placed by surgery or catheter intervention, during the first 6 months after the procedure
  - Repaired congenital heart disease with residual defects at the site or adjacent to the site of a prosthetic patch or prosthetic device (that inhibit endothelialization)
  - Cardiac transplantation recipients with cardiac valvular disease or in the first 6 months post-transplant

If valve destruction occurs, the valve may need to be repaired or replaced.

Education/Discharge Instructions

The parents of a child with subacute bacterial endocarditis should be counseled regarding how to prevent future infections and how to recognize when an infection may occur. Any febrile illness should be reported to the provider as soon as possible. If the child sustained any valvular damage, follow-up visits should be made at regular intervals, for example, every 2 to 3 months initially and eventually moving to every 6 months or a year.

KAWASAKI'S DISEASE

Kawasaki's disease, also known as mucocutaneous lymph node syndrome, is a multisystem disease affecting the cardiovascular system. The cause is unknown, but a defective immune response to an infectious process is thought to be responsible. Kawasaki's disease is not congenital or contagious. During the acute phase, diffuse vasculitis leads to long-term cardiovascular problems in 1 out of every 5 patients affected. One long-term sequela of Kawasaki's disease is aneurysm formation in arterial vessels (all aneurysms are concerning, but most worrisome are those of the coronary arteries). Other sequelae are myocarditis or rhythm disturbances.

Signs and Symptoms

Signs and symptoms of Kawasaki's disease are the result of vasculitis affecting all organ systems. Together with persistent fever (5 days or more spiking to 104°F [40°C]), if the patient has four of the five signs listed below, a Kawasaki's diagnosis can be made:

- Skin rash
- Cervical lymphadenopathy, typically unilateral, greater than 1.5 mm in diameter
- Edema and erythema of hands and feet with eventual peeling of skin
- Irritation and inflammation of the mouth with "strawberry tongue," erythema, and cracking lips
- Conjunctivitis without exudate

Diagnosis

There is no specific test to detect Kawasaki's disease. Children with a fever along with other signs and symptoms in the presence of vessel aneurysm are diagnosed with Kawasaki's disease. A complete blood count, erythrocyte sedimentation rate (ESR), electrocardiogram, and echocardiogram are done help to confirm diagnosis. Occasionally, cardiac catheterization is indicated to diagnose aneurysm formation. Other inflammatory diseases, such as Rocky Mountain spotted fever, scarlet fever, or toxoplasmosis, need to be ruled out.

Prevention

Because the cause is unknown, it is difficult to discuss prevention. As with any other type of disease, a proper, balanced diet, hydration, and healthy living will aid the child in the healing process.

Collaborative Care

Nursing Care. Physical care of a patient with Kawasaki's disease centers on supportive treatment of the symptoms and on giving the prescribed medications. Emotional and spiritual care may be necessary if the child suffers the sequelae of aneurisms and the family is facing a lifetime of treatment and monitoring. Preoperative care and postoperative care will be required only if the child undergoes surgery for aneurism repair.

"What to say"—*Communicating to the family*

Communicate to the family that the initial episode and the immediacy of the treatment that was delivered determine the frequency of follow-up visits to the health-care provider. After the initial event, children receive a medication called dobutamine (Dobutrex) or an exercise stress test to assess the vascular response to exercise. Coronary bypass surgery is rarely needed, and a very small number of children with Kawasaki's disease–related complications require a cardiac transplantation.

Medical Care. Care of the child with Kawasaki's disease begins with the administration of IV immunoglobulin (IVIG) and aspirin (ASA), which are used primarily for their anti-inflammatory effects. Other treatments such as steroids, plasma exchange, or cytotoxic agents may be used if this initial therapy is ineffective (AHA, 2014b).

 focus on safety

Anticoagulant medication precautions

Instruct the family about precautions if the child is taking anticoagulant medications. The child is monitored closely because of the risk of infection, bleeding, and bruising.

Education/Discharge Instructions

The parents should be aware that follow-up visits are essential. If the child is on anticoagulant therapy, appropriate blood testing and monitoring should be adhered to. The child may have activity restrictions if there are aneurisms involved.

 focus on safety

Thrombus formation

Teach parents that children with aneurysm formation as a result of Kawasaki's disease require long-term follow-up for continued assessment related to other vascular changes such as stenosis or tortuosity (twisting) (AHA, 2014b; Park, 2009). Tell parents in the event of thrombus (blood clot) formation, the treatment is the same as for any patient who is at risk for a myocardial infarction. Thrombotic agents, such as streptokinase (Streptase), urokinase (Abbokinase), and alteplase (Activase), are used with some success in thrombus formation. Long-term use of anticoagulants such as warfarin (Coumadin) or clopidogrel (Plavix) may also be used to prevent thrombus formation in the engorged or aneurysmal vessels.

 Across Care Settings: **American Heart Association**

The American Heart Association (www.heart.org) has complete up-to-date information about diagnosis and treatment of Kawasaki's disease (AHA, 2014b).

CARDIOMYOPATHY

Cardiomyopathy (CM) is a condition in which the cardiac muscle becomes dilated, hypertrophied, stiff, or inflamed. There are various classifications and causes, but the end result is the same. The cardiac muscle no longer functions adequately, and treatment must ensue to sustain life.

 Nursing Insight—*Three classes of cardiomyopathy*

Dilated (DCM) or congestive cardiomyopathy is the most common form and is caused by weakened contractions leading to dilation of all four chambers of the heart. The weakened contractions are caused by myocardial damage as a result of toxic agents. Dilated cardiomyopathy is caused by myocardial damage from chemotherapy, microbes, bacteria, viruses, immunological defects, or nutritional disorders.

Hypertrophic cardiomyopathy (HCM) is usually a familial disorder. It is a condition in which the ventricle is hypertrophied, swollen, or thickened in the absence of other cardiac conditions. The pumping mechanism of the ventricle is usually hyperdynamic, and the filling is hindered because of thickening of the ventricle.

Restrictive cardiomyopathy (RCM) is the least occurring type of cardiomyopathy and is characterized by unusually noncompliant ventricular walls that fail to relax. The size of the ventricle is normal, but the atria are enlarged because of the impaired diastolic filling caused by stiffness in the ventricle (Park, 2009).

Signs and Symptoms

The child with CM has a variety of vague symptoms such as:

- Weakness
- Excessive tiredness
- Shortness of breath
- Exercise intolerance
- Heart palpitations
- Chest pain
- Poor feeding
- Slow weight gain
- Syncope (fainting)
- Light-headedness

Diagnosis

Diagnosis includes a complete physical examination that may reveal a murmur, gallop, and venous congestion as demonstrated by hepatomegaly or distended neck veins. An electrocardiogram may show right- or left-sided enlargement and possible Q waves. Tachycardia, cardiac rhythm disturbances, or ventricular ectopy is often seen. An echocardiogram provides the exact diagnosis. A family history of cardiomyopathy or sudden death of unknown causes in a family member may also alert the practitioner to seek a definitive diagnosis for CM.

Prevention

CM often cannot be prevented because the causes are familial or genetic in many cases. For CM caused by infections, it is important that families know that any infection in a child should be treated seriously and acted on as soon as possible under the direction of a physician or nurse practitioner.

Collaborative Care

Nursing Care. Nursing care measures include alleviating the symptoms with prescribed medications and monitoring for worsening signs. After the diagnosis, the child with CM is closely monitored for further complications, preferably through a recognized cardiomyopathy program. Communicate to the family that frequent echocardiograms are warranted to assess the size and function of the ventricular wall and to note improvement or deterioration of the condition. The family must also understand that the child is placed on activity restrictions to prevent overstimulation of the heart muscle (Park, 2009).

Medical Care. Medical management includes a medication regimen that is aimed at improving function of the cardiac muscle. Angiotensin-converting enzyme (ACE) inhibitors or angiotensin receptor blockers have positive inotropic properties influencing the force of muscular contractility (Venes, 2013) and must be continued until the muscle becomes stronger; the need for these medications may be lifelong. Other medical treatment includes beta-blocker therapy and nutritional supplementation, particularly with carnitine (Carnitor or l-carnitine). Diuretic and inotropic therapy is also recommended, except in the case of hypertrophic CM.

Surgical Care. Cardiac transplant is the focus of surgical management.

Medication: Carvedilol

(kar-**ve**-dil-ole)

Beta (β)-Adrenoreceptor blocker, -adrenergic

Indications: Carvedilol is indicated for the treatment of mild to severe heart failure of ischemic or cardiomyopathic origin.

Actions: Beta blockers slow tachycardia and vasodilation; carvedilol decreases peripheral vascular resistance, decreases renal vascular resistance, reduces plasma renin levels, and increases atrial natriuretic peptide levels.

Therapeutic Effects: Increases stroke volume, decreases blood pressure and improves renal flow, decreases heart rate.

Contraindications and Precautions: Monitor for possible deterioration of congestive heart failure (CHF), liver injury, bronchospastic disease, and thyrotoxicosis.

Adverse Reactions and Side Effects: Chest pain, dizziness, hyperglycemia, bradycardia, nausea.

Route and Dosage:
Oral: 0.07 mg/kg per dose
Maximum dose: 0.5 mg/kg
Once or twice daily dosing
  Reduce dose for bradycardia less than 55 beats per minute

Nursing Implications:
1. Initiate with low dose and titrate up as tolerated.
2. Monitor blood pressure for 1 hour after initial dosing.
3. Monitor blood pressure, pulse, and ECG frequently.
4. Take with food.

Source: Vallerand, A. H., & Sanoski, C. A. (2014). *Davis's drug guide for nurses* (14th ed). Philadelphia, PA: F.A. Davis.

Education/Discharge Instructions

The education for patients with cardiomyopathy is similar to those with congestive heart failure. The parents must adhere to the medication and follow-up regimen. Discharge instructions and parent education include monitoring vital signs and how to recognize signs and symptoms of cardiac failure. The parent will be given ranges of vital signs appropriate for the child's age and circumstance. For example, some patients may have a lower or higher than expected range for their age because of the type of cardiac disease. Occasionally, the parent should learn cardiopulmonary resuscitation (CPR) and how to measure basic vital signs such as heart rate, respiratory rate, and blood pressure. If the child is discharged to home with oxygen, the parents will also have a pulse oximeter in the home. The parent will be taught to observe for subtle signs of CHF such as shortness of breath, decreased appetite, irritability, swelling, and weight gain.

Discharge instructions include medication use, effects, and side effects. The nurse will ensure that the patient is receiving education appropriate for his or her learning style and comprehension level. Each medication should be reviewed for specifics.

The parents should be instructed about diet, exercise, activity, and returning to school. A proper diet for a cardiac patient includes balanced, healthy food choices for good bone healing and avoidance of junk food and empty calories. Fluid restriction is not encountered as often as in the adult population but may be used for the patient in severe congestive heart failure or the older child. As discussed earlier, infants and younger children can dehydrate much easier; therefore, this practice is avoided in this age range. Exercise guidelines are based on tolerance levels for each individual patient.

 Nursing Insight—*Rheumatic fever*

Rheumatic fever (RF) is a group-A hemolytic streptococcal infection affecting multiple body systems such as the heart, the joints, subcutaneous tissue, and, at times, the nervous system. Typically arising as an acute pharyngitis, it occurs most often in children aged 5 to 15 years. Two to 3 weeks after the initial infection, the organism invades the bloodstream and deposits on the valves of the heart (vegetation) causing permanent damage. The aortic and mitral valves are most frequently involved. The mitral damage may result in mitral stenosis or mitral regurgitation. Aortic regurgitation also results from rheumatic fever (AHA, 2014b; Parrillo, 2012). The signs and symptoms of RF coupled with a history of strep pharyngitis lead to the diagnosis. Typically 5 major criteria (called Jones criteria) are present to give a diagnosis of rheumatic fever:

- Arthritis (predominantly involving the large joints and is migratory [moves from joint to joint])
- Carditis and valvulitis
- Sydenham's chorea (jerky purposeless movements of hand, changes in handwriting, emotional outbursts)
- Erythema marginatum (a circular red rash) with clearly demarcated raised edges seen most often on the trunk

- Subcutaneous nodules (palpable nodules in the subcutaneous tissue)
  There are 4 minor criteria:
- Arthralgia
- Fever
- Elevated ESR or C-reactive protein
- Prolonged PR interval

Prevention of rheumatic fever is aimed at treating the initial strep infection early. Once a child has had RF, prompt recognition of a new infection will prevent a second RF attack and reduce the chances of progression of severity of heart disease. Heart failure management is an important nursing care measure. Medical treatment for rheumatic fever is antibiotic administration and use of anti-inflammatory medications, specifically aspirin.

Education and discharge instructions include telling parents that children who have had rheumatic fever may require a valve replacement during their lives. A valve replaced in infancy or childhood must be replaced every 5 years to accommodate the child's growth. Valves replaced during adolescence can last up to 10 years.

Additional Cardiac Conditions

CARDIAC TRAUMA

Blunt cardiac trauma (BCI) is uncommon and can result from a variety of injuries, such as a motor vehicle crash or sports activity. Seat belt use has reduced the incidence of BCI, but even a child wearing a seat belt or other protective equipment in a car can sustain cardiac trauma. Cardiac trauma can be seen in child abuse cases. Cardiac trauma will occur in less than 5% of children with thoracic trauma. The chest wall of a child has more compliance than adults, and rib and sternal fractures will be seen less often. This may cause an underdiagnosis of trauma. Many cases may self resolve. Damage to the heart muscle occurs as the result of a direct blow to the thorax overlying the heart (e.g., a baseball or steering wheel). Electrocution (injury from electricity) can also cause damage to the cardiac muscle. In cardiac trauma, the particular damage to the heart can be a ventricular rupture, a great vessel tear, damage to the pericardial sac or coronary arteries, septal or valvular injuries, cardiac tamponade, myocardial infarction, comorbidities or sternal fracture, or dysrhythmias. Commotio cordis is a type of trauma caused by a small dense object colliding with the chest at a rapid velocity as is the case with a baseball or hockey puck. This may produce a lethal dysrhythmia if this occurs during the relative refractory period (most vulnerable) of the cardiac cycle.

Signs and Symptoms

The signs and symptoms are related to the type of cardiac trauma sustained and include:

- Bruising
- Pain, mild to severe (probably related mostly to surface musculoskeletal pain)
- Pulsus paradoxus or pulse deficit
- Muffled heart sounds or murmur
- Dysrhythmia
- Shortness of breath
- Hypotension
- Severe cardiac shock

Diagnosis

The diagnosis is made based on a thorough history including the type of trauma, force of trauma, associated injuries and symptoms, and loss of consciousness. The diagnosis of the extent of cardiac trauma is made with electrocardiogram (ECG); echocardiogram; cardiac enzymes, specifically troponin I; and chest x-ray exam. All of these tests will indicate cardiac muscle damage. A computed tomography or multigated acquisition scan may be helpful in determining other injuries, but does not correlate to outcome. Other labs include a complete blood count to detect anemia from hemorrhage.

 Nursing Insight—*FAST (Focused Assessment With Sonography in Trauma)*

The FAST test is a bedside ultrasound that may be used to detect hemopericardium.

Prevention

Prevention of cardiac trauma also goes hand in hand with safety. Provide safety instructions about sports, crashes, and seat belt use to parents for wherever the child lives, goes to school, and plays.

Collaborative Care

Nursing Care. Nursing care is based on the extent and exact type of the injury. Initial nursing care includes bedrest. Activity restrictions are enforced until the cardiac muscle heals. In addition, antiarrhythmics, inotropic agents, and pericardiocentesis (aspiration of fluid from the pericardial sac) may be required. A cardiac rehabilitation program is recommended.

Medical Care. Medical management focuses on monitoring and giving medications to prevent or alleviate congestive heart failure or dysrhythmias.

Education/Discharge Instructions

Education focuses on recognition of complications and preventing further injury. The child may be fitted with a special vest to prevent further contusion. The patient will have exercise restrictions for 2 to 4 weeks or more depending on the extent of the damage. The child may be on extensive bedrest until the cardiac muscle heals.

 focus on safety

Sports gear

Children should wear appropriate safety gear when playing sports and be properly restrained when riding in a motor vehicle.

Nursing Insight—Cardiac tumors

Cardiac tumors are rare in children and are almost exclusively rhabdomyomas (Park, 2009). Other tumors are teratomas, fibromas, and myxomas. Most cardiac tumors are benign but significant because they occupy space and may restrict the normal filling of the heart and flow of blood. Surgical removal is the treatment of choice for cardiac tumors. At times, it is surgically unsafe to remove the tumor, and a cardiac transplant is needed. A long-term consequence of cardiac tumors includes scar tissue formation, which in turn may lead to dysrhythmias. If the child with cardiac tumor develops dysrhythmias, the nurse should perform cardiac monitoring procedures and call the health-care provider for an ECG interpretation.

Nursing Insight—Hypercholesterolemia–hyperlipidemia

The etiology for hypercholesterolemia–hyperlipidemia in children is classified as primary or secondary. A primary cause is hereditary predisposition (Park, 2009), and children may develop atherosclerotic lesions as early as infancy. Hypercholesterolemia is more often a result of secondary causes. Secondary causes are exogenous (originating outside an organ), endocrine, or

Table 26-8	Cholesterol Levels in Children		
	Desirable	**Borderline**	**Associated With Higher Risk**
Total cholesterol	<170	170–199	200 or more
LDL cholesterol	<110	110–129	130 or more

Source: American Heart Association, 2014, July 17.

metabolic disorders; liver diseases; renal diseases; or other miscellaneous reasons such as anorexia nervosa or collagen diseases. Children with cardiac transplant have a high incidence of hyperlipidemia because of the immunosuppressant drug cyclosporine-A (Neoral). In addition, children with cardiac transplant form **atherosclerotic** lesions at a very rapid rate and risk facing coronary artery bypass graft, or worse, a second transplant surgery. Communicate to the family that treatment of hyperlipidemia for children with a transplanted heart is more aggressive than for the general population. If the patient has a received a heart transplant, ensure routine lipid panels are performed.

HYPERTENSION

High blood pressure, or hypertension (HTN), is an elevated blood pressure and is uncommon in children, though the incidence is rising along with childhood obesity. The American Heart Association has current recommendations for blood pressure assessment in children (Urbina, Alpert, Flynn, Hayman, Harshfield, Jacobson, et al., 2008)

Signs and Symptoms

HTN can manifest in a variety of symptoms.

- Signs and symptoms depend on the underlying causes.
- Elevated blood pressure is a key sign.
- A young child may be irritable.
- An older child may complain of:
  - Changes in vision
  - Dizziness
  - Headaches

Diagnosis

Taking a detailed medical and thorough family history is important in the diagnosis of HTN. A child is hypertensive if the blood pressure is above the 95th percentile for age, height, and gender. As a screening tool, consider any reading greater than 20 mm Hg above normal blood pressure for the child's age. A teenager's blood pressure is considered high based on adult values for treatment purposes and follows the same guidelines as adults. The extent of further testing is based on the degree of blood pressure elevation. High blood pressure or HTN may indicate a coarctation of the aorta, kidney disease, left ventricular hypertrophy, or early-onset familial hypertension. Some cardiology centers conduct HTN follow-up for families with a strong history.

Prevention

HTN in children is usually related to an underlying physical cause such as kidney disease or coarctation of the aorta. Prevention is reliant on monitoring to prevent HTN in these settings, but often HTN is the first symptom.

Family Teaching Guidelines...
Hypercholesterolemia–Hyperlipidemia

TOPIC: The nurse will educate the family about hypercholesterolemia–hyperlipidemia.

ESSENTIAL INFORMATION:

- There are two types of primary hypercholesterolemia–hyperlipidemia: familial hypercholesterolemia and familial combined hyperlipidemia. The standards for childhood cholesterol levels are different from those for adults (Table 26-8).
- Although the standard levels are different, the treatment goals are similar to those for adults and include diet modification, exercise, and medication. A recommended balanced nutrition is one that provides less than 10% of total calories from saturated fatty acids, 30% or less of total calories from fat, and less than 300 mg of cholesterol each day. Help the family decrease the fat and cholesterol intake to 7% of fatty acids, 25% or less of total calories from fat, and less than 200 mg of cholesterol per day.
- Pharmacological treatment is recommended for children older than 8 years of age whose low-density lipoprotein (LDL) cholesterol is high.
- Recommendations for screening children after age 2 and no later than 10 years older are:
  - At least one parent with high cholesterol
  - A family history of early heart disease such as a male parent or grandparent with congenital heart disease (CHD) before age 55 or a female parent or grandparent with CHD before age 65
  - Family history of diabetes, hypertension, or obesity
  - Child with obesity (greater than 85th percentile)
  - Immunosuppressant drug use (AHA, 2014b)

Collaborative Care

Nursing Care. Nursing care for the child with HTN is based on education about the condition, diet, exercise, lifestyle modification, and medication. The nurse is aware that vital signs will include more frequent blood pressure measurements. The nurse uses proper technique of blood pressure measurements and cuff size in children of all ages.

Medical Care. Medications for high blood pressure or HTN include beta blockers and ACE inhibitors.

focus on safety

Managing hypertension

Safety is related to managing HTN to prevent worse problems such as stroke or circulation problems.

Education/Discharge Instructions

Education includes teaching parents to administer antihypertensive medications on time and not skip doses to prevent rebound effect. Education about the condition, diet, exercise, lifestyle modification, and medication should begin as soon as the diagnosis is confirmed.

Cultural Diversity: Hypertension

Based on familial predisposition, HTN has a higher incidence among African American children than in other ethnic groups. Nursing care for this group of children includes educating the child and family about the condition, promoting a reasonable sodium intake, and teaching the family how to reduce the saturated fat and cholesterol in their diet.

PULMONARY ARTERIAL HYPERTENSION

Pulmonary arterial hypertension (PAH) is a condition of high blood pressure in the lungs. It may result from cardiac defects or may be idiopathic (without recognizable cause). It is often associated with cor pulmonale and is a severe disease resulting in death if not treated. Normally, the desired pulmonary blood pressure is low, allowing blood to flow easily from the right side of the heart. The pressure in the right side of the heart is lower than in the left (the left reflecting the systemic blood pressure). If the pressure in the lungs is high, as with PAH, the right ventricle must pump harder to force the blood to the lungs. Over time, this wears on the ventricle and causes right ventricular hypertrophy. Eventually, the heart fails and congestive symptoms develop.

Signs and Symptoms

Pulmonary hypertension often has multiple symptoms:

- Shortness of breath (dyspnea), especially during exercise
- Chest pain
- Weakness
- Fatigue
- Dizziness
- Leg swelling
- Fainting episodes

Diagnosis

In the early stages of the disease, a physical exam may be normal because diagnosis of PAH may take several months. However, as the condition progresses, a physical exam shows a heart murmur, enlargement of the neck veins, liver and spleen enlargement, leg swelling, parasternal heave, ascites, and clubbing.

Diagnostic tests such a pulmonary arteriogram, echocardiogram, chest radiograph, cardiac catheterization, and pulmonary function tests may help confirm the diagnosis.

Prevention

Prevention is related to getting early and consistent care of cardiac defects. Sometimes this condition is not preventable.

Collaborative Care

Nursing Care. The patient's prognosis is often poor, and he or she will face a lifetime of medications. Focus on providing education and support for the family. Focus care on reducing respiratory sequelae by providing for frequent rest periods and monitoring the respiratory status carefully through vital signs and pulse oximetry. Provide oxygen and adjust according to need. The nurse will provide essential medications.

Medical Care. Treatment for pulmonary arterial hypertension includes oxygen, which relaxes the arteries of the lungs; medications used specifically for pulmonary hypertension (see Nursing Insight); calcium channel blockers that relax the blood vessels; and diuretics that decrease the volume in the vessels. However, these treatments may have an untoward effect of lowering the overall blood pressure.

Nursing Insight—*Medications used for pulmonary hypertension*

- Phosophodiesterase—type 5 (PDE-5) inhibitor. PDE-5 is found in the pulmonary vascular smooth muscle and degrades cyclic guanosine monophosphate (cGMP). When this chemical is inhibited, cGMP levels increase and causes smooth muscle relaxation. This eventually decreases the pulmonary arterial pressure.
  - **Sildenafil (Revatio, Viagra)**—most commonly used. Reconstituted at a concentration of 2.5 mg/mL. Best ordered as "sildenafil" or "Revatio" rather than "Viagra" for insurance purposes.
  - **Tadalafil (Adcirca, Cialis)**
- Endothelin receptor antagonist, which relaxes pulmonary arterial vasculature:
  - **Bosentan (Tracleer)**—liver function tests (LFTs must be done monthly) so you may receive faxed LFT results. Bosentan is teratogenic category X so pregnant women and women of childbearing age should not handle the medication (main concern is in the dust). Medication dissolves in water, should not be crushed.
- Direct dilator of pulmonary arterial vascular beds:
  - **Inhaled treprostinil (Tyvaso)**
  - **Treprostinil (Remodulin—IV or Subcutaneous)**—half-life is 3 to 4 hours. Is started in the hospital and then given as subcutaneous continuous infusion at home.
- Prostacyclin, a direct-acting pulmonary vasodilator:
  - **Epoprostenol (Flolan)**—The half-life is 2 to 3 minutes and is given IV. Children can be on this medication at

home if they have a peripherally inserted central catheter line. This medication can never be stopped, for any length of time. Parents are instructed on what to do if the infusion becomes interrupted.

Education/Discharge Instructions

Teaching points include discussion about diet, exercise, and medication. The diet may be higher in calories to accommodate for the energy expenditure of this pulmonary-related disease. The child may have very low exercise tolerance and will have limited abilities to exercise. That does not mean the patient should not exercise at all but may have to enroll in a specialized cardiac rehab program.

NEURALLY MEDIATED SYNCOPE

Neurally mediated syncope (NMS), also called vasovagal syncope, is a condition caused by an exaggerated response to a normal bodily function. In normal function, the **baroreceptors** in the carotid artery regulate blood pressure during certain situations. When the body is stressed during extreme heat, pain, fright, or prolonged standing, the initial response is a release of epinephrine, stimulating the sympathetic nervous system. A classic presentation is when a child faints when a parent is brushing his or her hair. This stimulation in turn raises the blood pressure. The baroreceptors send messages to control the blood pressure. In neurally mediated syncope, the baroreceptor response is exaggerated, causing the blood pressure and the heart rate to drop rapidly and significantly.

Signs and Symptoms

Symptoms of NMS include:

- Temporary loss of consciousness (a fainting spell)
- Seizure (rare)

Diagnosis

A thorough history and other tests rule out other diagnoses, such as seizures or Long QT syndrome. The definitive diagnosis of neurally mediated syncope is made via the tilt test but can be made on history alone.

 Diagnostic Tools Tilt Test

NMS is diagnosed with a tilt table test. Assist the child by placing him or her in a supine position on a table equipped with a foot board. The table may be tilted to an upright position anywhere between 45 and 90 degrees. After a short time, the table is tilted to a full 90-degree angle so that the child stands upright. This maneuver may or may not reproduce the fainting or symptoms. If the tilt test is positive, the nurse will see a remarkable drop in blood pressure or heart rate, and the child will experience syncope or presyncope (dizziness or light-headedness). If the child does not exhibit any symptoms, such as syncope or light-headedness, the table is laid flat again and isoproterenol (Isuprel) is administered to stimulate a fast heart rate. This chemical mimics the fight or flight (fear, pain, or anxiety) response that may occur before episodes of syncope. The table is then tilted again to elicit a syncopal response or a drop in the blood pressure. If there is no response or change in vital signs, the test is considered negative and other causative factors are evaluated. If parents want to learn more about this test, they can go to the Mayo Clinic Web site (www.mayoclinic.org) (Mayo Clinic Staff, 2012).

Prevention

Prevention includes maintaining good hydration and preventing situations that may lead to syncope.

Collaborative Care

Nursing Care. Monitor for frequency, severity, and precipitating factors of syncope. Nursing care for NMS may be as simple as increasing the child's sodium and water intake.

 focus on safety

Communication

It is important to communicate to the family that NMS is concerning based on the potential for injury if the child loses consciousness. If a teen with syncope is of driving age, in some states the teen must be syncope-free for 6 months before driving again.

Medical Care. An adrenocorticosteroid such as fludrocortisone (Florinef) may be given to retain fluid. The next level of medical treatment is a beta blocker, which regulates the exaggerated response.

Education/Discharge Instructions

The family and the patient should be encouraged to learn to recognize those activities that put them at greatest risk for a syncopal event. The child should maintain adequate hydration, especially in the summer heat. The patient is instructed not to stand in one place for a long time and bend the knees or sit down if a syncopal event is imminent.

LONG QT SYNDROME

Long QT syndrome (LQTS) is an electrophysiological condition predisposing the child to fatal dysrhythmias such as ventricular tachycardia, torsade de pointes, and ventricular fibrillation (Fig. 26-22). LQTS is a familial disorder, and if one child is affected, all siblings and parents are tested for the disorder. There are a variety of known factors and genetic chromosomal markers in a person with LQTS. LQTS is among a group of channelopathies (defects of the ion channels on the cardiac cell membrane). Currently, genetic researchers are studying this phenomenon in hopes of a better treatment or developing a cure. A prolonged QT interval can also be acquired from medications and various toxins (http://archive-org.com/org/a/azcert.org/2012-12-20_1013917_7/Drug_Lists/). The child and family are most

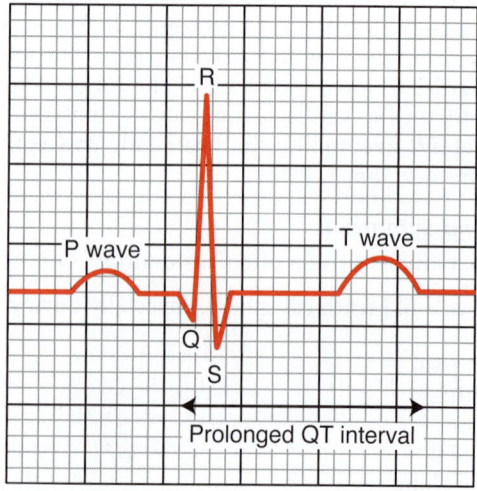

Figure 26-22 Prolonged QT.

likely unaware that they have this problem. Because sudden death is one of the symptoms, the child's first episode may be the last.

Signs and Symptoms

Symptoms of LQTS can include:

- History of fainting triggered by intense emotions, vigorous physical activity, swimming, auditory stimuli (such as a school bell), and upon awakening
- Palpitations
- Seizure
- Sudden death

Diagnosis

An ECG is performed in all children with seizures of sudden onset, fainting, or near drowning episodes. The child may be asymptomatic and may present at routine exam with a prolonged QT on ECG.

Prevention

Prevention of the dysrhythmias caused by LQTS is accomplished by taking prescribed medications.

Collaborative Care

Nursing Care.

focus on safety

Teenagers

Teenagers with LQTS can undergo risk stratification to determine the risk for dysrhythmias and the need for medication. If the risk for dysrhythmias is high, the teen should not be allowed to drive until dysrhythmias are under control for 6 months.

Medical Care. The primary treatment is medication. The most frequently used medications are beta blockers. Treatment also includes pacemaker-defibrillator (insertion) or left cardiac sympathetic denervation. It is important that the nurse communicates to the family that the most common cause of treatment failure is noncompliance with medication.

Education/Discharge Instructions

 Across Care Settings: **Schools**

If a school nurse has a student with LQTS or any other cardiac concern, care is taken that school staff is trained in proper cardiopulmonary resuscitation techniques and an automated external defibrillator placed in the school. Advocate for the child to propose an alternative solution to the ringing of the school bell because the loud bell can be a stimulus to an arrhythmic event.

RHYTHM DISTURBANCES

Rhythm disturbances are an alteration in the normal electrical flow within the heart. Figure 26-23 shows the normal electrical conduction pattern identified as PQRST. Any alteration in this pattern will alter the normal flow, filling, and emptying of the heart. This alteration in flow affects the cardiac output.

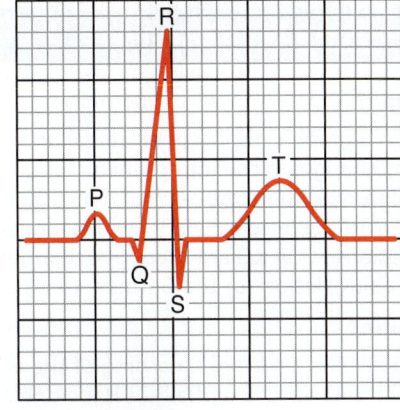

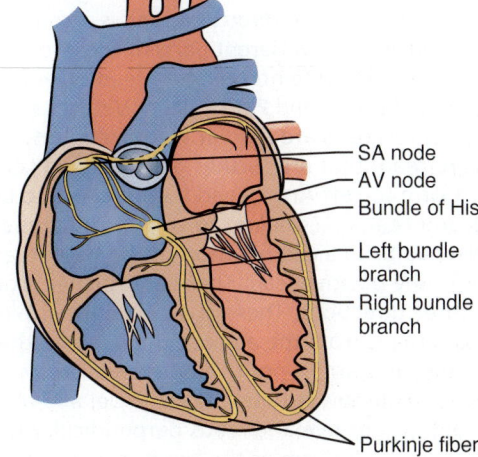

Figure 26-23 PQRST electrophysiology.

Signs and Symptoms

Dysrhythmias can be indicated by:

- Palpitations
- Shortness of breath
- Congestive heart failure (CHF) symptoms
- Syncope
- Dizziness

Diagnosis

Diagnosis is based on a rhythm interpretation of the ECG (Procedure 26-1). The concern with all dysrhythmias is the effect on cardiac output. All rhythm disturbances can be grouped into three categories: too fast, too slow, or absent. Lethal rhythms are those producing little or no cardiac output and unless corrected will lead to cardiac death.

Tachycardia is the name for a fast heart rate. It describes any condition in which the heart beats faster than the standard pediatric heart rate values and includes sinus tachycardia, supraventricular tachycardia, atrial tachycardia, atrial flutter, atrial fibrillation, junctional tachycardia, and ventricular tachycardia. If the heart rate is too fast, the diastolic phase shortens in relation to the length of the full cardiac cycle. The ventricle is not allowed enough filling time; the stroke volume is less, therefore decreasing the cardiac output. The lethal rhythms in this category are torsade de pointes and ventricular fibrillation.

Bradycardia is the name for a slow heart rate. This is any condition in which the heart beats slower than the

Procedure 26-1 Obtaining a 12-Lead Electrocardiogram (ECG)

Purpose

An ECG is a graphic display of electrical activity produced by changes in the intracellular charge of the cardiac muscles. The components of an ECG are marked with the letters PQRST (see Fig. 26-23). The abbreviations ECG/EKG are used interchangeably. (The K is the abbreviation for the German *kardio* [cardiac].)

Equipment

A 12-lead ECG is a surface recording of the electrical activity of the heart. Essentially, it is looking at the heart from different angles, by measuring the flow of current from different directions. This is accomplished by putting leads on different parts of the body and the chest. There are three groupings of leads: Limb Leads, Augmented Leads, and Precordial or Vector Leads.

The Limb Leads are bipolar leads (requiring two leads to read) that are further grouped into Lead I (Right Arm to Left Arm), Lead II (Right Arm to Left Leg), and Lead III (Left Arm to Left Leg). Augmented Leads read from a combination of the two other leads to the positive lead. These are further grouped into three directions. These are aVR: right arm is positive and reads from the apex of the heart to the apex, aVL: left arm is positive and reads across the right ventricle toward the left ventricle, and aVF: foot (left) is positive and reads perpendicular from the top to the bottom of the heart in a cephalocaudal direction. Precordial leads are also known as V-Leads or chest leads. These leads are unipolar and measure the electrical activity in the transverse plane or a cross section of the heart.

Steps: Setting Up the Machine

1. First, set up the ECG machine.

RATIONALE: *It is best to have the machine ready to go before placing the electrodes on the child because it may be difficult to obtain an artifact-free recording from an agitated child.*

Steps: Prior to Attaching the Leads

1. Put in demographic data

RATIONALE: *To ensure that accurate data are recorded, the correct spelling of the child's name, date of birth, and the medical record number is important. These items are all crucial components of proper identification of the patient. From a legal standpoint, it will prevent errors in diagnosis and treatment plans.*

2. Change leads view

RATIONALE: *The recording machines are typically set up as a 12-lead ECG, with a continuous Lead II rhythm strip, as opposed to a 3-lead rhythm strip. Make sure the machine is on the correct recording mode.*

3. Gain

RATIONALE: *The gain is 10 mm/mV for pediatrics, and every subsequent recording should be the same. Do not compare two different 12-lead ECG recordings done at different gains.*

4. Speed

RATIONALE: *The standard default speed should be set at 25 mm/second. The recorder can be set for different speeds depending on the purpose of the recording.*

Steps: Lead Placement

1. Skin preparation

RATIONALE: *Clean the chest lead placement area with alcohol or usual skin prep, if necessary. If the patients have chest hair, as in adolescent boys, shave the electrode areas.*

2. Limb lead placement

RATIONALE: *Proper lead placement includes:*

a. *White – Right Arm or Shoulder*

b. *Black – Left Arm or Shoulder*

c. *Red - Left Leg or Abdomen*

d. *Green – Right Leg or Abdomen*

3. Vector lead placement

RATIONALE: *Proper lead placement includes:*

a. *V1 - 4th intercostal space, just to the right of the sternum*

b. *V2 - 4th intercostal space, just to the left of the sternum*

c. *V4 - On the midclavicular line and 5th intercostal space*

d. *V6 - On the midaxillary line, horizontal with V4*

e. *V5 - Between V6 and V4*

f. *V3 - Between V4 and V2*

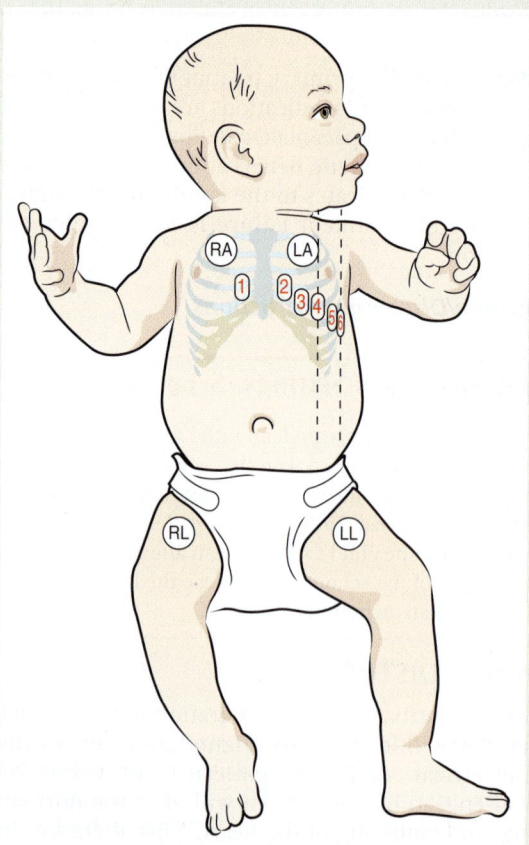

Electrocardiogram (ECG).

Procedure 26-1 Obtaining a 12-Lead Electrocardiogram (ECG) (continued)

Steps: Recording

RATIONALE: *To ensure an accurate recording:*

1. 12-Lead Recording
   a. Make sure there is little to no movement.
2. Press the button for a Rhythm Strip.

Steps: Troubleshooting

RATIONALE: *When no signal or a poor signal is observed, the following is considered:*

1. Have the cables been correctly connected?
2. Is the equipment functioning correctly?
3. Could external electrical equipment interference be a problem?
4. Was skin preparation adequate?
5. Could the electrodes suffer from:
   a) The gel drying out?
   b) Poor adhesion?

Teach Parents

Teach parents the reasons the procedure is being performed on the child.

Documentation

The baby had a 5-beat run of ventricular tachycardia, and the provider ordered a 12-Lead ECG. The underlying rhythm was sinus. The procedure was completed according to protocol and the technician downloaded the data to the computer system so the cardiologist may analyze. There was no further evidence of ventricular tachycardia throughout the procedure or afterward.

J. Marshall, RN

standard pediatric heart rate values. This type of dysrhythmia most commonly includes sinus bradycardia and junctional and idioventricular rhythms. In a bradycardic child, the cardiac output is affected because the heart rate is slow. Initially, the body tries to compensate by increasing the contractile force, thus increasing the stroke volume. Eventually, this will plateau or the cardiac muscle may not be strong enough to compensate as in CHF or cardiomyopathy. The lethal rhythms in this category are asystole and agonal rhythms.

Blocks are disruptions in the flow of electrical current throughout the heart. They include bundle branch block (BBB) and first-, second-, and third-degree blocks. First- and second-degree type I blocks and BBB may cause no interference in the cardiac output, whereas second- and third-degree blocks are more severe and require intervention to maintain adequate circulation. The latter rhythms will be lethal if not corrected.

Prevention

Prevention of the dysrhythmias caused by rhythm disturbances is accomplished by taking prescribed medications. The family should be instructed to avoid activities that will promote the rhythm disturbance such as dehydration, increased exercise, or Valsalva maneuvers.

Collaborative Care

Nursing Care.

 Collaboration in Caring—*Nurses caring for children with heart dysrhythmias*

The nurse working in a cardiac area with children who experience dysrhythmias and require cardiac telemetry can acquire specific knowledge about the ECG and learn about basic dysrhythmia interpretation. When caring for children on a cardiac floor or in the intensive care unit, nurses can acquire more advanced information through a course on 12-lead ECGs. Working with the clinical

education department to provide training in Pediatric Advanced Life Support and a pediatric emergency course is essential.

 Optimizing Outcomes—Rhythm disturbances

Determine the baseline rhythm and recognize changes that will facilitate the best outcome for a child with a dysrhythmia. Know ramifications of these changes. Important critical thinking questions the nurse can ask about rhythm disturbances are:

- Is the rhythm potentially fatal?
- Will it alter the cardiac output?

 Nursing Insight—*Pulseless electrical activity*

Pulseless electrical activity (PEA), formerly known as electromechanical dissociation, is a condition in which the observer will see an electrical rhythm on the cardiac monitor, but there is no cardiac output and therefore no pulse. Pathologically, there is no communication between the electrical and mechanical components of the heart. The nurse should remember to treat the patient, not the rhythm. If this situation is noted, the nurse should obtain a blood pressure and pulse rate and then consider the underlying causes (Chameides & Ralston, 2011). The underlying causes of PEA are as follows (often referred to as the Hs and Ts):

- Hypovolemia
- Hypoxia
- Hydrogen ion (acidosis)
- Hypo-/Hyperkalemia
- Hypoglycemia
- Hypothermia
- Toxins
- Tamponade
- Tension pneumothorax
- Thrombosis (heart or lung)
- Trauma

Discovering and correcting the underlying causes will correct the PEA.

Nursing Insight—*Sinus dysrhythmias*

A normal irregular rhythm in which the rhythm varies with respiration is called sinus dysrhythmia. Sinus dysrhythmia has no adverse effect on the cardiac output.

- The heart rate increases with inspiration. (Remember: "*Inspiration*" and "*Increase*" both start with an "I").
- The heart rate decreases with expiration.

What if the child presents to the pediatrician's office with "an irregular rhythm"? A simple, inexpensive, and noninvasive ECG will determine the etiology of irregular rhythms. If the heart rate speeds up when asking the child to take a breath and slows down when asked to exhale and hold it out, the diagnosis can be made.

Invasive Tests

CARDIAC CATHETERIZATION

Cardiac catheterization is an invasive test performed for a number of reasons. The purpose of the cardiac catheterization is to determine the pressures within the child's heart vessels and to provide a radiographic picture of the anatomy by measuring the size and shape of vessels, valves, and ventricles. A cardiac catheterization is necessary to perform a myocardial biopsy. Corrective procedures, called interventional catheterizations, may be performed in the cardiac catheterization lab.

 ### Diagnostic Tools Cardiac Catheterization

The cardiac catheterization procedure takes place in a cardiac catheterization lab where the child is sedated or anesthetized. First, an introducing sheath is placed in a major vessel such as the femoral vein or artery. Next, a long hollow tube or catheter is threaded through this sheath and into the heart. The physician uses real-time radiographic study (fluoroscopy) to monitor the movement of the catheter and to prevent perforation. During a cardiac catheterization, pressure is measured in the ventricles and the vessels. The normal pressure of the left ventricle correlates with the normal blood pressure for age. The normal pressures in the right ventricle and right and left atria are similar to those of an adult patient. Elevated pressures can indicate a variety of illnesses and will usually support or refute the suspicions of the diagnostician. For example, high pressure in the right ventricle may indicate a ventricular septal defect with left-to-right shunting, pulmonary artery stenosis, or pulmonary hypertension. Radiopaque dye is injected through the catheter, and the flow of the dye is observed on fluoroscopy. The "shape" of the dye is the shape of the inside of the heart, giving a picture of the anatomy of the ventricle, valves, vessels, and any defects that may be present.

The overall risks for the child undergoing a cardiac catheterization are minimal. Because this is an invasive procedure, know the risks of bleeding, infection, thrombus, dysrhythmia, perforation, stroke, or even death.

 ### focus on safety

Post-catheterization

Post-catheterization, monitor the child's pressure dressing in the groin as well as the heart rate, respirations, and blood pressure (Box 26-1).

ANGIOGRAPHY

Angiography helps to assess the structure and function of the ventricles, vessels, and valves. It is also useful to determine

---

Box 26-1 Typical Post-Cardiac Catheterization Medical Orders

Admit to post-surgical observation unit.

VS every 15 minutes 4 times, then every 1 hour 4 times, then every 2 hours 2 times, then every 4 hours for 24 hours.

Check pulses with vital signs, especially on affected extremity.

Check pressure dressing along with vital signs for evidence of bleeding.

Keep O₂ saturation above _____.

Call house officer or resident on call for heart rate (age-related), blood pressure (age-related) _____ (age and baseline dependent), and temperature ≥101.1°F (38.4°C).

Call the hospitalist for complaints of abdominal pain or no urine output.

Give acetaminophen (Children's Tylenol) for pain.

Give antiemetic per health-care provider orders for nausea.

Keep flat in bed for 6 hours.

Check pressure dressing with vital signs for bleeding.

Call the hospitalist for complaints of abdominal pain or no urine output.

Increase diet as tolerated.

---

size and location of septal defects. After placement of the catheter in the heart, radiopaque contrast medium is injected into the chambers and vessels of the heart. If there is a defect, the contrast highlights septal openings, narrow vessels, and extra vessels. An angiogram provides important information to the physicians to direct the medical and surgical treatment.

BIOPSY

Biopsy of the myocardium is performed routinely for children who have had a cardiac transplant or to determine the cause of myocarditis or cardiomyopathy. Children with cardiac transplant undergo routine biopsies to assess for rejection. Several small pieces of myocardial tissue are removed and then analyzed by a laboratory specialist for cellular changes. The sample may also contain microbial organisms responsible for the cellular changes seen in cardiomyopathy.

CLOSURE DEVICES

It is possible to close simple congenital intracardiac communications or shunts in the cardiac catheterization laboratory rather than with major surgery. Atrial septal defects and an opening called a patent foramen ovale (PFO) are closed with transseptal closure devices. The cardiologist places these transseptal closure devices across the septum, through the defect, and deploys the device to form a seal around the opening. In the case of a patent ductus arteriosus (PDA) closure, a plug type device is used.

By approximately 6 weeks after the closure device is placed, the child's own tissue grows over the device, creating a seal through endothelialization (growth of new tissue), and by 6 months a permanent seal forms. Yearly follow-up visits to the cardiologist are recommended along with an ECG, an echocardiogram, and possibly a chest radiograph. The provider will explain the risk of embolization of the device. Embolization occurs when the device becomes dislodged from its intended location, migrating to the atria, pulmonary artery, ventricle, or aorta. Monitor for signs or symptoms of embolization and provide support with education.

OPENING DEVICES

Angioplasty or Valvuloplasty

Narrow vessels or valves may be opened or dilated with a balloon angioplasty or valvuloplasty as an initial treatment, or a stent may be placed in a vessel as a long-term treatment (Fig. 26-24). This treatment is performed during a cardiac catheterization procedure. A special catheter with a balloon is passed into the heart and into the narrow vessel. The balloon is then inflated, causing the stenotic area to expand. Sometimes the stenosis recoils days, months, or years after the balloon procedure. The procedure may then be repeated, but this time, a stent (a wire mesh tube) is placed over the balloon. The balloon is again inflated and the stent is left in place. This repair is permanent and requires surgical extraction if removal is necessary.

Balloon Atrial Septostomy

Balloon atrial septostomy is an emergent palliative procedure necessary to keep the child alive when the heart has no means of blood flow to the pulmonary system or body such as in tricuspid atresia or hypoplastic left heart. A catheter with a balloon is passed into the right atrium, pushed across the septum or through a PFO, and an entry way to the left atrium is created. The balloon is inflated and then pulled forcefully across to the right atrium, creating an opening large enough to accommodate blood flow. Infusion of prostaglandin is a palliative treatment prior to the septostomy to keep the PDA open and allow blood flow to the pulmonary bed or to the body.

Collaborative Care

Nursing Care. Be aware of specific aspects of caring for a child in the post-cardiac catheterization period. After cardiac catheterization, the child has a pressure dressing placed in the groin area at the insertion site. If an internal jugular vein is used, a small bandage covers the site on the neck.

Monitor the heart rate, respirations, and blood pressure and make sure to note that it is in the same measured range as pre-catheterization. If tachycardia is identified post-catheterization, pain or dehydration is considered to be the underlying cause. Acetaminophen (Children's Tylenol) is given for the pain. If the child is dehydrated, administer fluid boluses per health-care provider's order. Signs of infection are rare in the first few hours post-catheterization.

Children with cardiac disease may be cyanotic so it important to obtain a baseline oxygen saturation and monitor the child with that number in mind. Some children with heart disease normally have a value as low as 85%. Confirm the range of normal oximeter readings with the health-care provider.

The child may be placed on cardiac telemetry if dysrhythmias were induced during the catheterization. Normally, if the child has a non-electrophysiological diagnosis, any dysrhythmias seen during the procedure disappear when the catheters are removed, but subsequent monitoring may be required.

There are specific growth and development issues to consider post-catheterization. After a cardiac catheterization, a child is required to lie flat for up to 6 hours depending on the insertion site of the catheter. The supine position minimizes the risk of bleeding through the insertion site. A younger child may need to be restrained with leg immobilization devices to keep the leg straight. Older children or adolescents are usually cooperative, unless they are developmentally delayed. Administer sedation if necessary to keep the child still, but this may delay the discharge and holds certain risks. Generally, an infant or child does well if the mother is allowed to stay at the bedside or hold the child. Allowing the infant to feed is also calming.

Communicate to the family that after a cardiac catheterization, the child will continue the same medications as before. If any devices such as closure devices or stents remain in the body, the child will take a baby aspirin for 6 months after the procedure. The aspirin prevents clot formation while endothelialization occurs around the artificial device. Subacute bacterial endocarditis prophylaxis precautions are followed by the health-care provider for 6 months for device placement patients. Tell the family that after 6 months of placement of the device, no special precautions are needed.

 clinical alert

Blood pressure post-interventional catheterization

The child's blood pressure should remain within normal limits **post-interventional catheterization.** One specific measurement to watch is the pulse pressure, which is the difference between the systolic and diastolic blood pressure. A normal pulse pressure range is 40 mm Hg. Children with PDA have a wide pulse pressure (greater than 40 mm Hg). After the closure of a PDA, the pulse pressure should be within normal range. A sudden widening of the pulse pressure post-procedure may indicate a dislodged or embolized device. This event requires urgent measures by the physician or resident in-house, who must be contacted immediately. Embolization of the device can cause stroke, thromboembolic events, or death.

Communicate to the family that the child's growth must be considered before placing a stent. Some stents are expandable and must be re-dilated at a later date to accommodate for the growth of the child. If it is known that a child must have a more definitive surgery, a stent may be placed, knowing that it will be extracted at a later date. Risks include vascular tear or embolization of the device. Absorbable stents are in the experimental phase.

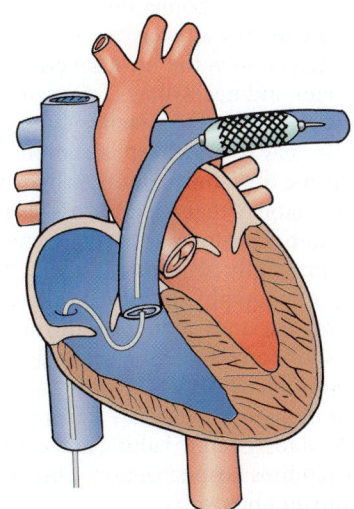

Figure 26-24 Balloon angioplasty with stent.

Surgical Interventions

Surgical repair may be palliative repair or complete anatomical repair. Palliative repair is usually considered when the child is very young and the complete anatomical repair is too complex for him or her to tolerate. The surgeons perform a temporary, palliative repair to allow the child time to grow and develop to a point when the more definitive procedure may be tolerated. The child may be cyanotic after a palliative repair but less cyanotic than if the surgery were delayed. These children are followed closely by the cardiologist until the time when a complete repair may be done. A complete repair is considered a cure or definitive treatment. However, as the child grows or hemodynamic requirements change, a complete repair may have to be revised.

PACEMAKERS

Pacemakers are used to treat cardiac conditions such as heart block or severe bradycardia, sick sinus syndrome, lethal dysrhythmias, and some junctional or idioventricular rhythms. Pacemaker therapy may be internal or external, temporary or permanent; external pacing is always temporary. The surgeon may elect to place temporary pacing wires if the child has complications of heart block during surgery or if the surgical area is near or on the conduction tissue.

Collaborative Care

Nursing Care. Communicate to parents that permanent pacemakers may be placed in the abdomen in younger children and in the subclavicular area in older children. Consideration is taken for children who are athletic because the pacemaker generator must be protected.

Pacemaker generators must be replaced every 5 to 10 years. When a pacemaker is placed in an infant, a replacement may be necessary 15 times in his or her lifetime. Currently the American Heart Association and American College of Cardiology do not recommend pacemaker placement for neurally mediated syncope.

Nursing care of the pacemaker postoperative patient is the same as for any surgical procedure, including watching for signs of infection and ensuring the incision remains intact. Communicate to the family that follow-up care requires routine pacemaker testing as recommended by the pacemaker center placing the device. Essential information for the family is to understand that after initial follow-up procedures, evaluation of the pacemaker is usually performed every 6 months to 1 year but can be as often as every 3 months.

CARDIAC TRANSPLANTATION

Cardiac transplantation requires complex multidisciplinary management and is used as a treatment for severe, life-threatening cardiac conditions. Transplantation is performed only under the most grave of circumstances, in situations in which the child would otherwise die.

A progressive heart transplantation program includes a cardiomyopathy treatment program to prevent the need for transplantation. The transplantation team attempts to correct the condition early on and to prevent the child's condition from progressing to the point of no return. It is certainly more desirable to perform a transplant long before the child is gravely ill, but it is also difficult to justify the need for transplantation to a family whose child is playful and seems "normal" to them. Although survival rates continue to improve, there are limitations.

Although transplantation saves lives and greatly improves the quality of life, it is often said that transplantation is exchanging one disease for another. Living with a

focus on safety

Complications of cardiac transplantation

The four main complications of cardiac transplantation are:

- Rejection
- Infection
- Post-transplant lymphoproliferative disorder
- Transplant coronary artery disease

transplanted heart is considered a chronic condition, but it is manageable. The child and his or her family must follow a strict regimen of medication, diagnostic tests, blood tests, and clinic follow-up.

 Across Care Settings: **The transplantation team**

The cardiac transplantation team consists of nurse practitioners, physicians, surgeons, nurses, social workers, medical psychologists, religious leaders, school nurses, and school officials. Most importantly, the child, his or her parents, and extended family are involved in the caretaking decisions. The child and family must be hyper-compliant with the regimen to prevent rejection of the cardiac muscle.

Collaborative Care

Nursing Care. The priority nursing intervention is to help the family understand the importance of medication compliance. There is no room for a less than rigorous approach when administering the medications. This is a difficult endeavor, but the positive aspect is that the child will live. The medication regimen includes as many as three antirejection medications (immunosuppressants), antihypertensive drugs, electrolyte supplements, diuretics, anticoagulants, and antihyperlipidemics. These medications must be given every day. The immunosuppressant drugs prevent the body's immune system from rejecting the transplanted heart muscle and must be given within a 1-hour window every 12 hours.

Another important nursing intervention is communicating to the family about the frequent follow-up visits to the clinic, which will help ensure close monitoring by the cardiac transplantation team. Sometimes the child will come to the hospital as frequently as every week for follow-up care.

Myocardial rejection is the most severe consequence of cardiac transplant and necessitates frequent follow-up and biopsies. Rejection can lead to systemic failure, and depending on the grade, may require hospitalization. Following the transplant, educate the family about cardiac catheterization with myocardial biopsy that is performed as often as every 2 weeks in the initial postoperative phase and during times of rejection. The family also must understand that every year, coronary angiography with cardiac catheterization is performed on regular intervals depending on the transplant center to assess for coronary atherosclerosis, a side effect of the immunosuppressant drugs. Myocardial rejection is the most severe consequence of cardiac transplant. Myocardial rejection can lead to systemic failure, and depending on the grade, usually requires hospitalization. This necessitates frequent follow-up and biopsies.

Children who have received a transplanted heart are subject to many emotional and psychological issues. Because it is difficult to live one's life with any heart defect or other chronic defects, imagine a life of a child locked into this intensive medical regimen. Children who received their transplant as infants or toddlers may be more adjusted psychologically (because it is the only life they know) but may suffer more developmental delays. These children may have suffered brain anoxia or are delayed because of frequent hospitalizations. Most children do well, attending school and continuing on to college. Psychosocial adjustment depends on the coping skills and support systems of the child and the family. In addition, physical growth can be stunted because of frequent prednisone dosing. Alterations in growth and development also have an emotional impact on the child's life.

Nursing Care for the Child With a Cardiac Condition in the Hospital

The nursing plan of care for the child in the pediatric intensive care unit (PICU) with a cardiac condition consists of assessment, outcomes, intervention, and evaluation.

Caring for post-cardiac surgical patients generally requires admission to a PICU for recovery. PICU admission requires specific care by highly trained nurses. The child typically stays in the PICU for approximately 2 to 3 days for simple repairs and 5 to 10 days for more complicated repairs. The child is then transferred to a cardiac step-down or cardiac care unit. If the child has other body system failures or does not respond well to the surgery, very lengthy postoperative PICU admissions may ensue. The PICU stay is also influenced by the child's condition before surgery or any perioperative complications. The patient in the PICU is intubated, has chest tubes, a nasogastric tube, and Foley catheter. There are also multiple peripheral and central IV lines and temporary pacer wires. Post-surgical patients have a large dressing on the surgical site (mid-sternum or lateral). When this dressing is removed, there are usually Steri-Strips or Dermabond(tm) on the skin.

Nursing care for the child in the PICU integrates important concepts such as assessment, nutrition, hygiene, activity, and psychosocial care. Emphasis for care also includes taking vital signs, maintaining growth and development, administering medications, performing lab tests, and interpreting an ECG.

 Critical Nursing Action Postoperative Vital Signs

The routine for vital signs (VS) in the PICU is much more rigorous than on a general or telemetry floor. Typically, recovery of cardiac surgical patients takes place in the PICU rather than in the post-anesthesia unit. These patients may be very sick and require close monitoring and a one-on-one patient assignment. The VS are taken every 15 minutes for the first few hours, then every 30 minutes, and then every hour until the child is stable. Adjust the frequency depending on the stability of the patient. All changes in VS, no matter how subtle, are documented and reported to the health-care provider.

Growth and development is a consideration for any hospital admission. Often PICU patient's post-cardiac surgery are heavily sedated or chemically paralyzed to maintain stability. When caring for a sick child, it is important to consider the child's level of development. Soft music can be played for any child, and older children are given explanations about any touching or procedures that will occur even if they cannot respond. Encourage the parents to talk to the child, as well. It has been documented that after sedated or chemically paralyzed patients are brought to consciousness, the child can tell their caretakers about events and conversations heard throughout the day. Never assume that your patient cannot hear what is said.

 legal alert—Administer medication properly

It is crucial to understand the desired and undesired effects of the child's medication. Before giving any medication, check the proper dosage and route. At times, pediatric medications are given in very small amounts, and an error in decimal placement can mean a fatal overdose or other detrimental effects. The nurse applies current knowledge about the 6 rights of medication administration and accurately documents the medication and child's tolerance of the medication (Ward, 2013). When the patient is on a cardiac monitor, be sure to observe for both subtle and obvious changes. Postoperative dysrhythmias may be caused by electrolyte disturbances or trauma caused by surgery.

Nursing Insight—_Laboratory values_

Laboratory values are unstable, and close monitoring is necessary. Electrolyte measurement, particularly potassium, is perhaps the most critical lab test in the initial postoperative period because the cardiac bypass machine hemolyzes the cells, thus creating a high concentration of extracellular potassium. Hemoglobin and hematocrit tests check for possible bleeding, and coagulation factors can be affected by pump time. The child will probably be on a ventilator, and arterial blood gases must be assessed frequently to determine the concentration of the gases, like carbon dioxide and oxygen.

TRANSFERRING THE STABLE CHILD TO A SURGICAL OR MEDICAL UNIT

Commonly, a pediatric patient with a newly diagnosed cardiac condition is treated in a tertiary care center for more specialized treatment. When the post-surgical child becomes more stable, she or he is transferred to the surgical or cardiac floor. The nurse on this type of unit is trained in caring for cardiac patients, and the unit is equipped with telemetry monitoring. The stable child requires less frequent vital signs monitoring every 4 hours.

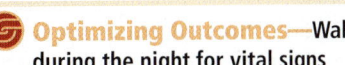 **Optimizing Outcomes—Waking the child during the night for vital signs**

The best outcome for a child with a cardiac condition is proper healing along with adequate growth and development. Studies show that sleep is necessary for proper healing and that a full sleep cycle allows certain hormones (cortisol and growth hormone) and chemicals necessary for healing and growth (Copstead-Kirkhorn & Banasik, 2013). Be sure to assess if the child needs to be awakened during the night for vital signs or can be allowed uninterrupted sleep. Many necessary vital signs can be taken directly from the monitor while observation of respirations, color, and comfort can be assessed without touching the child.

Medications given to patients on the medical/surgical unit usually do not require constant monitoring or adjusting. Some children are admitted to a medical/surgical unit for the sole purpose of starting a new medication and monitoring its effects. It is also important to draw blood for laboratory analysis to track certain conditions that may affect the cardiac system, such as anemia or coagulopathies.

Nursing Care Plan The Child With a Cardiac Condition

Nursing Diagnosis: Cardiac Output, Decreased related to alterations in preload, afterload and inotropic function of the heart

Measurable Short-Term Goal: The child will maintain heart rate, respirations, and blood pressure within acceptable limits (specify).

Measurable Long-Term Goal: The child will tolerate daily activity without signs of cardiac decompensation.

NOC Outcomes:
Cardiac Pump Effectiveness (0400) Adequacy of blood volume ejected from the left ventricle to support systemic perfusion pressure.
Vital Signs (0802) Extent to which temperature, pulse, respiration, and blood pressure are within normal range.

NIC Interventions:
Cardiac Care (4040)
Fluid/Electrolyte Management (2080)
Medication Administration (2300)
Vital Signs Monitoring (6680)

Nursing Interventions:

1. Assess vital signs: blood pressure, respirations, lung sounds, and apical and peripheral heart rate for a full minute (specify frequency). Monitor temperature every 4 hours.

   RATIONALE: Changes in cardiac output will be reflected in changes in blood pressure, respiratory status, and heart rate. Fever and infectious processes increase cardiac workload.

2. Provide continuous cardio-respiratory monitoring and evaluation of oxygen saturation levels as ordered.

   RATIONALE: Continuous cardiac monitoring provides objective data about cardiac functioning. Oxygen saturation above 95% indicates adequate respiratory status.

3. Weigh the child daily at the same time, on the same scale, and dressed in the same manner. Evaluate for edema.

   RATIONALE: Congestive heart failure results in fluid accumulation reflected by weight gain and edema. Decreased weight may indicate therapeutic effects of treatment.

4. Administer supplemental humidified oxygen as ordered.

   RATIONALE: Adequate oxygenation enhances tissue perfusion and decreases tachypnea and metabolic demands. Humidification moistens secretions to keep the airway clear.

5. Administer cardiac, diuretic, and other medications as ordered by caregiver (specify drug, dose, route, and times).

   RATIONALE: (Specify the action of the particular drug related to cardiac output.)

6. Promote adequate rest and uninterrupted sleep by clustering nursing care. Collaborate with parents to reduce stress for child.

   RATIONALE: Rest and stress management reduce the work of the heart.

7. Position the child upright at a 30- or 60-degree angle (semi-Fowler's position).

   RATIONALE: Elevating the head of the bed enhances lung expansion, decreases venous return to the heart, redistributes blood to dependent areas, and relieves pressure on the diaphragm.

8. Monitor fluid and electrolytes as obtained. Maintain fluid restrictions if ordered (specify).

   RATIONALE: Excess fluid volume increases the work of the heart, while electrolyte alterations interfere with the electrophysiology and function of the cardiac muscle.

9. Provide ongoing education and support to the family. Encourage verbalization of concerns, feelings, and questions.

   RATIONALE: Adequate knowledge and emotional support lessens the family's and child's anxiety levels.

Nursing Care for the Child With a Cardiac Condition in the Community

Caring for the child with a cardiac condition in a community-based clinic includes:

- Monitor heart rate, blood pressure, respiratory rate, and oxygen saturation. Compare the vital sign values to the vital signs from previous visits.
- Review medications and changes noted by the caregiver. Verify medications and provide teaching about the medication. Ensure that the family has enough refills and is receiving the proper dosage. Occasionally

medications are adjusted during a phone triage visit. Proper documentation is also essential. Medications are frequently altered at clinic visits related to growth of the child. Adjustments may also need to be made because of medical insurance requirements and financial cost to the family.

Typically the school nurse does not perform lab tests in the school setting. Laboratory tests are performed in conjunction with the clinic visit. Tests are ordered depending on the previous lab values and the medications taken. In addition, there will be no electrocardiogram equipment in the school, although if the child has a Holter monitor or event recorder in place, the school nurse is responsible for reapplying electrodes or helping the child complete a diary.

The school nurse is familiar with the location and use of the defibrillation equipment placed in the school.

Nursing Insight—*Warfarin (Coumadin)*

Many children require warfarin (Coumadin) to prevent thrombus. The prothrombin time (PT) and international normalized ratio (INR) are checked on a routine basis. Shortly after initiation of warfarin (Coumadin), the PT/INR is checked frequently until stabilized. After stabilization, the follow-up is usually every 1 to 3 months. Communicate to the family that the response to warfarin (Coumadin) is affected by diet. The present recommendations are to adjust the warfarin (Coumadin) dosage rather than the diet. Also note if any changes have been made to the warfarin (Coumadin) dosage.

Across Care Settings: Monitoring the child at home

If a Holter monitor or event recorder is ordered for home use, they are applied in the clinic setting. Parents may also be given other recording devices for home use, such as an apnea monitor or pulse oximeter. Parents are advised not to become too preoccupied with these devices and learn to rely on their own instincts or assessment skills. The child may return to the clinic where an echocardiogram is performed to assess for changes in the chamber size or valve disease. Electrocardiogram (ECG) monitoring includes a 12-lead ECG that provides a snapshot view of potential or existing dysrhythmias and estimated chamber size or strain on the heart muscle. Explain to the parents that this test often takes 1 hour.

Across Care Settings: Returning to school

Inevitably, the child will return to school. Frequently, the school nurse or other school officials will be called on to provide care for this child. At the minimum, schools should have an automatic external defibrillator device installed. Personnel having direct contact with the child should complete a cardiopulmonary resuscitation (CPR) course. Often, it is the school nurse who first identifies a cardiac problem, hears a murmur on a routine visit to the office, or the child has a syncopal or palpitation episode. A child with long QT syndrome may have a first event while participating in school activities such as physical education, swimming, or even when the school bell is sounded, so the school nurse must be prepared to respond immediately.

The school nurse also has other responsibilities. Typically, vital signs in the school setting will coincide with administration of medication or an untoward event. If there is an event, the school nurse is responsible for stabilization until emergency medical service arrives on the scene. Children may be taking medication frequently during the day, which necessitates administration by the school nurse who understands the actions, interactions, and side effects of medications.

Across Care Settings: The homebound child

The homebound child or one who visits the cardiac clinic often requires specific nursing care. Often, his parents or other

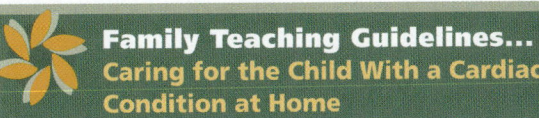

Family Teaching Guidelines...
Caring for the Child With a Cardiac Condition at Home

TOPIC: Teaching the child and family about the cardiac condition is essential to help ensure proper growth and development. Important information includes cardiopulmonary resuscitation, vital signs, medications, the disease entity, and resources.

ESSENTIAL INFORMATION:

VITAL SIGNS: Parents may still wake up during the night to take the child's vital signs, as is done in the hospital setting. There is rarely a need for a full-time nurse for cardiac reasons alone, but a home health nurse may evaluate the child at intervals to see if help at home is needed.

MEDICATION: Often, children with cardiac disease require lifelong medication administration. Some require medication only until the surgery is completed and within the initial postoperative period. As in the case with the cardiac transplant child, the family must receive essential information related to the timing and the routine of medication administration. In other cases, the cardiac drugs may be given safely with basic instructions. Teach the family that one of the most important aspects of medication administration is proper dosing. Many of the medications are given in a liquid form. The medication dosing is done in milliliters (mL) or cubic centimeters (cc) and not teaspoons (tsp) or other household measures, and the parent is given a measuring device for administering these medications accurately.

DISEASE ENTITY: It is important to educate the family about the disease entity itself. Because there are many resources in print and on the Internet, it is important to ensure that the child and family are receiving and reading the most up-to-date and accurate information possible. An informed family and child will be less anxious and perhaps more compliant. Educating families also builds a relationship necessary for a team approach in treating the cardiac disease.

primary caregivers extend care into the home or community. One philosophy of family-centered care is that the parent or primary caretaker always knows the child best, and the nurse relies on the parents' judgment if they call with concerns.

focus on safety

Cardiopulmonary resuscitation

CPR training provided by a certified CPR instructor or fire department personnel is essential because many cardiac diseases predispose to dysrhythmias.

The following are resources for families and children:

American Heart Association: www.heart.org

Cardiomyopathy Association: www.cardiomyopathy.org

Children's Heart Society: www.childrensheart.org

Congenital Heart Information Network: www.tchin.org

Heart Rhythm Society: www.hrsonline.org

Heart Transplant: www.cota.org, www.a-s-t.org, www.ishlt.org

Kawasaki's Disease: www.kdfoundation.org

Complementary Care: *Caring for Children with Cardiac Conditions*

There are non-pharmaceutical, nonsurgical, and nonelectrical adjuvant therapies for cardiac defects and disease. There are no alternative cures for these diseases, but some activities will keep the symptoms to a minimum.

Diet: Balanced nutrition helps maintain a healthy weight and allows for nutrients, which will boost the immune system. Reducing fat intake will help to lower cholesterol and reduce the chance of additional strain on the heart caused by atherosclerotic disease (AHA, 2014c).

Exercise: In a child with a cardiac disease or defects, certain exercises can be detrimental. Each patient has an individualized exercise plan tailored for his or her cardiac disease.

Good Sleep Patterns: Children, especially teenagers, should start to develop a healthy sleeping pattern. Sleep allows for cortisol and growth hormone release, which is essential for cellular repair. It also helps with stress reduction and allows for proper lifestyle functioning and learning throughout the day.

Stress Reduction: Maintaining a stress-free or low-stress lifestyle helps to keep the blood pressure within normal range.

Alcohol, Drugs, Smoking: Teenagers are counseled to avoid alcohol, illicit drugs, and smoking cigarettes or marijuana because all of these will have detrimental effects on the circulation and oxygen-carrying capacity.

Homeopathic or Nutritional Supplements: The general population may believe that if something is "natural," then it will be good for you, but that is not always the case. These supplements are always reviewed with the health-care providers—physician, pharmacist, and/or doctor of nursing practice—because supplements can interact with medications or cause tachycardia or bradycardia. Most of these supplements are not regulated by the Food and Drug Administration, and there is no quality or quantity control on the ingredients or consistency.

Other Complementary or Alternative Therapies: Complementary or alternative therapies such as therapeutic touch, meditation, cupping, acupuncture, or prayer may be employed by the family. These types of therapies can be psychologically beneficial to the family and the child.

Summary Points

- The main concern with children with cardiac disease is that they have an alteration in cardiac output affecting all cellular function.

- Congenital heart disease describes a congenital defect in the heart, valves, or great vessels. Congenital heart defects occur in about 1% of all pregnancies and in 1 in 170 live births.

- Disease includes problems with the structure, function, and electrical conduction within the heart.

- Children with cardiac diseases are at risk for alterations in health such as growth and development, nutrition, psychosocial implications, and schooling, as well as being at an increased risk for infection, acquiring other diseases, and even cardiopulmonary arrest. Sometimes these children have significantly altered lifestyles and undergo constant medical treatment. The nurse must have a good understanding of common cardiac diseases in children and be able to provide essential nursing care measures.

- The nurse provides nursing care to the child who has undergone procedural treatments with closure devices or surgery.

- The nursing plan of care for the child with a cardiac condition consists of assessment, outcomes, intervention, and evaluation.

- Post-cardiac surgical patients generally require admission to a pediatric intensive care unit (PICU) for recovery. PICU admission requires specific care by highly trained nurses.

- When the post-surgical child becomes more stable, he or she is then transferred to the surgical or cardiac floor.

- The parents or other primary caregivers extend care into the home or community.

- Teaching the child and family about the cardiac condition is essential to help ensure proper growth and development. Essential information includes cardiopulmonary resuscitation, vital signs, medications, the disease entity, and resources.

Review Questions

Multiple Choice

1. Which heart valve prevents regurgitation of blood from the pulmonary artery into the right ventricle?
   A. Aortic
   B. Mitral
   C. Pulmonary
   D. Tricuspid

2. A nurse suspects an infant of having advanced heart failure. Which clinical manifestation of heart failure did the nurse assess to reach this conclusion?
   A. Enlarged liver
   B. Feeding problems
   C. Poor growth
   D. Sweating excessively

3. A nurse is teaching parents of a child who has an atrial septal defect (ASD) about possible treatment options. Which treatment option does the nurse include in the teaching session?
   A. Heart transplant
   B. Spontaneous closure
   C. Surgical repair
   D. Use of a closure device

4. Which hormone is partly responsible for ensuring that the ductus arteriosus closes normally?
   A. Estrogen
   B. Human growth hormone
   C. Progestin
   D. Prostaglandin

5. A child has aortic stenosis. What manifestation does the nurse assess for?
   A. Aortic aneurysm
   B. Left ventricular failure
   C. Right ventricular atrophy
   D. Tricuspid regurgitation

6. A nurse is caring for a child hospitalized with possible channelopathy. What nursing action is most important for this child?
   A. Continuous cardiac monitoring
   B. Frequent blood pressures
   C. Total bedrest until corrected
   D. Treatment of hypertension

7. The parents of a child diagnosed with Kawasaki's disease ask the nurse to explain the disease and symptoms. Which response by the nurse is the most appropriate?
   A. Bacterial infection after an invasive procedure
   B. Chronic viral infection of unknown origin
   C. Genetic defect causing vessel abnormalities
   D. Vasculitis affecting all organs of the body

8. A child has restrictive cardiomyopathy. What information given to parents by the nurse is correct?
   A. Caused by toxic agents
   B. Least common form
   C. Most common form
   D. Often a familial disorder

9. A child with cardiomyopathy is prescribed a beta blocker. Which drug does the nurse teach the parents about?
   A. Carvedilol (Coreg)
   B. Flecainide (Tambocor)
   C. Quinidine (Quinaglute)
   D. Verapamil (Calan)

10. A child has been diagnosed with long QT syndrome. The nurse counsels the family to have genetic testing. Which family members does the nurse encourage to be tested?
   A. All female siblings
   B. All male siblings
   C. Parents only
   D. Parents and all siblings

See Answers to End of Chapter Review Questions on Davis*Plus*.

REFERENCES

American Heart Association (AHA). (2014a). Recommendations for blood pressure measurement in humans and experimental animals. doi:10.1161/_01.HYP.0000150859.47929.8e

American Heart Association (AHA). (2014b). Kawasaki disease. Retrieved from http://www.heart.org/HEARTORG/Conditions/More/CardiovascularConditionsofChildhood/Kawasaki-Disease_UCM_308777_Article.jsp

American Heart Association (AHA). (2014c). Healthy diet goals. Retrieved from http://www.heart.org/HEARTORG/GettingHealthy/NutritionCenter/HealthyDietGoals/Healthy-Diet-Goals_UCM_310436_SubHomePage.jsp

American Heart Association (AHA). (2014, July 17). What your cholesterol levels mean. Retrieved from http://www.heart.org/HEARTORG/Conditions/Cholesterol/AboutCholesterol/What-Your-Cholesterol-Levels-Mean_UCM_305562_Article.jsp

Bulechek, G. M., Butcher, H. K., Dochterman, J. M., & Wagner, C. (2013). *Nursing interventions classification (NIC)* (6th ed.). St. Louis, MO: Elsevier Mosby.

Centre for Evidence-Based Medicine (CEBM). (2013). EBM Tools: Finding the Evidence: Levels of Evidence 1; Levels of Evidence 2. Retrieved from http://www.cebm.net/?o=1025

Chameides, L., & Ralston, M. (2011). *Pediatric advanced life support.* Dallas, TX: American Heart Association.

Copstead-Kirkhorn, L. E., & Banasik, J. L. (2013). *Pathophysiology* (5th ed.). St. Louis, MO: Elsevier.

Gómez-Marín, O., Prineas, R. J., & Råstam, L. (1992) Cuff bladder width and blood pressure management in children and adolescents. *J Hypertens, 10*(10):1235–1241.

Johnson, M., Moorhead, S., Bulechek, G., Butcher, H., Maas, M., & Swanson, E. (2012). *NIC and NOC linkages to NANDA-L and clinical conditions* (3rd ed.) St. Louis, MO: Elsevier Mosby.

Kontula, K., Swan, H., Marjamaa, A., & Lahtinen, A. M. (2011). KCNE1 D85N polymorphism—a sex-specific modifier in type 1 long QT syndrome? *BMC Med Genet, 12*(11). doi:10.1186/1471-2350-12-11

Mavroudis, C., Backer, C. L., & Idriss, R. F. (2013). *Pediatric cardiac surgery* (4th ed.). Oxford, UK: Wiley-Blackwell.

Mayo Clinic Staff. (2012). Tilt table test. Retrieved from http://www.mayoclinic.org/tests-procedures/tilt-table-test/basics/definition/prc-20019879

Moorhead, S., Johnson, M., Maas, M. L., & Swanson, E. (2013). *Nursing outcomes classification (NOC)* (5th ed.). St. Louis, MO: Elsevier Mosby.

National Library of Medicine (US). Genetics Home Reference [Internet]. Bethesda (MD): The Library; 2014 Jul 28. Heart and circulation; [reviewed 2014 May; cited 2014 Jul 31]. Available from http://ghr.nlm.nih.gov/conditionCategory/heart-and-circulation

NYU Cardiac & Vascular Institute. (2013). New Guidelines for Cardiovascular Genetic Testing. Retrieved from http://cvi.med.nyu.edu/news/press-releases/new-guidelines-cardiovascular-genetic-testing

Park, M. (2009). *The pediatric cardiology handbook: Mobile medicine series* (4th ed.). Philadelphia, PA: Elsevier Mosby.

Parrillo, S. J. (2012). Rheumatic Fever in Emergency Medicine. Retrieved from http://emedicine.medscape.com/article/808945-overview

Pettersen, M. D. (2013). Pediatric Complete Atrioventricular Septal Defects. Retrieved from http://emedicine.medscape.com/article/893914-overview

Schwartz, R. A., & Richards, G. M. (2012). Clubbing of the Nails. Retrieved from http://emedicine.medscape.com/article/1105946-overview

Ubeda Tikkanen, A., Rodriguez Oyaga, A., Arroyo Riaño, O., Maroto Álvaro, E., & Rhodes, J. (2012). Paediatric cardiac rehabilitation in congenital heart disease: A systematic review. *Cardiology in the Young, 22,* 241–250. doi:10.1017/S1047951111002010

Urbina, E., Alpert, B., Flynn, J., Hayman, L., Harshfield, G. A., Jacobson, M., et al. (2008). Ambulatory blood pressure monitoring in children and adolescents: Recommendations for standard assessment: A scientific statement from the American Heart Association Atherosclerosis, Hypertension, and Obesity in Youth Committee of the Council on Cardiovascular Disease in the Young and the Council for High Blood Pressure Research. *Hypertension, 52,* 433–451. doi:10.1161/HYPERTENSIONAHA.108.190329

Vallerand, A. H., & Sanoski, C. A. (2014). *Davis's drug guide for nurses* (14th ed.). Philadelphia, PA: F.A. Davis.

Venes, D. (2013). *Taber's cyclopedic medical dictionary* (22th ed.). Philadelphia, PA: F.A. Davis.

Ward, S. (2013). *Pediatric nursing care: Best evidence-based practice.* Philadelphia, PA: F.A. Davis.

Ward, S., & Hisley, S. (2009). *Maternal-child nursing care: Optimizing outcomes for mothers, children & families.* Philadelphia, PA: F.A. Davis.

CONCEPT MAP

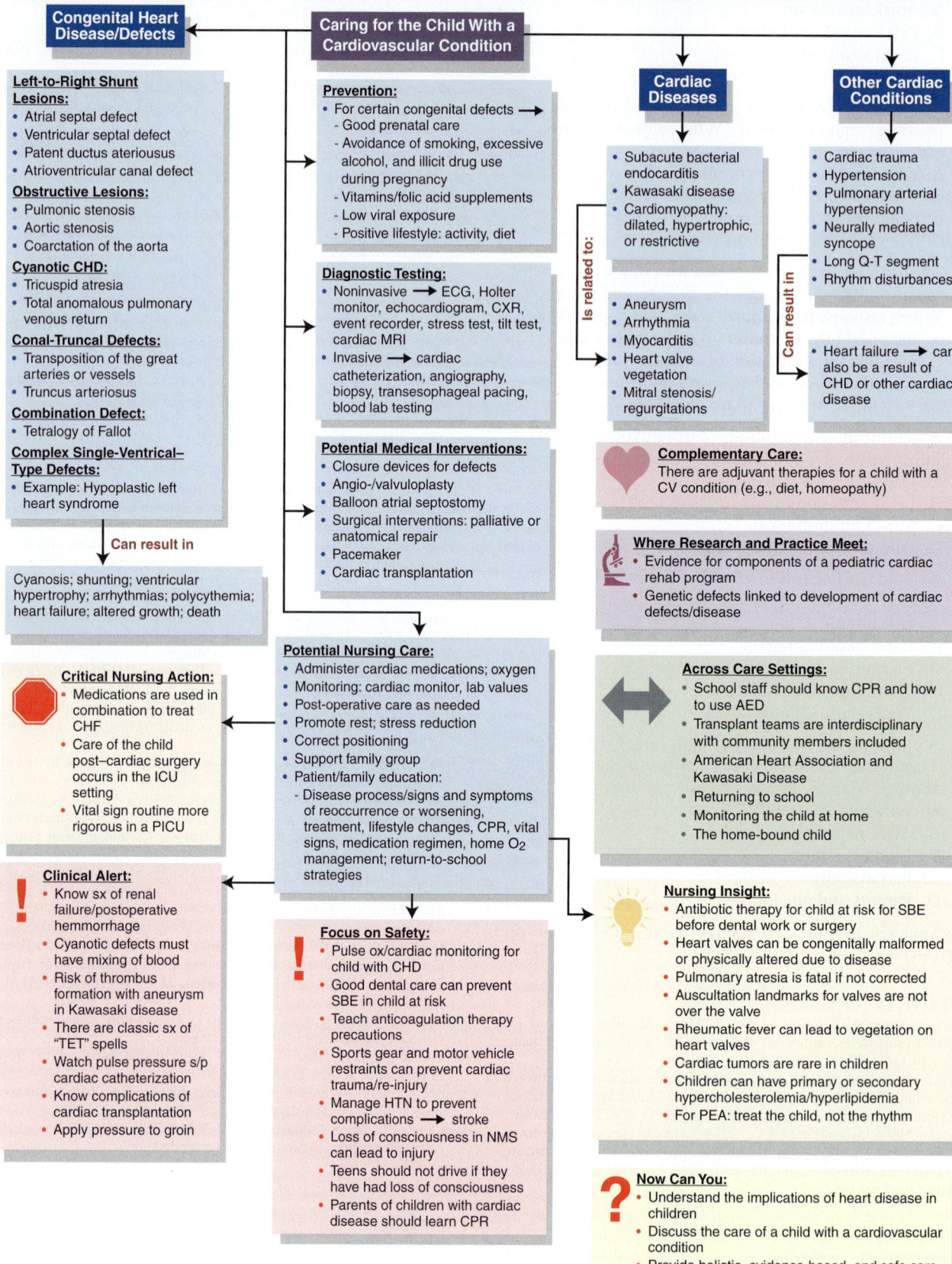

Congenital Heart Disease/Defects

Left-to-Right Shunt Lesions:
• Atrial septal defect
• Ventricular septal defect
• Patent ductus ateriousus
• Atrioventricular canal defect

Obstructive Lesions:
• Pulmonic stenosis
• Aortic stenosis
• Coarctation of the aorta

Cyanotic CHD:
• Tricuspid atresia
• Total anomalous pulmonary venous return

Conal-Truncal Defects:
• Transposition of the great arteries or vessels
• Truncus arteriosus

Combination Defect:
• Tetralogy of Fallot

Complex Single-Ventrical– Type Defects:
• Example: Hypoplastic left heart syndrome

Can result in

Cyanosis; shunting; ventricular hypertrophy; arrhythmias; polycythemia; heart failure; altered growth; death

Caring for the Child With a Cardiovascular Condition

Prevention:
• For certain congenital defects ➔
  - Good prenatal care
  - Avoidance of smoking, excessive alcohol, and illicit drug use during pregnancy
  - Vitamins/folic acid supplements
  - Low viral exposure
  - Positive lifestyle: activity, diet

Diagnostic Testing:
• Noninvasive ➔ ECG, Holter monitor, echocardiogram, CXR, event recorder, stress test, tilt test, cardiac MRI
• Invasive ➔ cardiac catheterization, angiography, biopsy, transesophageal pacing, blood lab testing

Potential Medical Interventions:
• Closure devices for defects
• Angio-/valvuloplasty
• Balloon atrial septostomy
• Surgical interventions: palliative or anatomical repair
• Pacemaker
• Cardiac transplantation

Cardiac Diseases

• Subacute bacterial endocarditis
• Kawasaki disease
• Cardiomyopathy: dilated, hypertrophic, or restrictive

Is related to:

• Aneurysm
• Arrhythmia
• Myocarditis
• Heart valve vegetation
• Mitral stenosis/ regurgitations

Other Cardiac Conditions

• Cardiac trauma
• Hypertension
• Pulmonary arterial hypertension
• Neurally mediated syncope
• Long Q-T segment
• Rhythm disturbances

Can result in

• Heart failure ➔ can also be a result of CHD or other cardiac disease

Complementary Care:
There are adjuvant therapies for a child with a CV condition (e.g., diet, homeopathy)

Where Research and Practice Meet:
• Evidence for components of a pediatric cardiac rehab program
• Genetic defects linked to development of cardiac defects/disease

Potential Nursing Care:
• Administer cardiac medications; oxygen
• Monitoring: cardiac monitor, lab values
• Post-operative care as needed
• Promote rest; stress reduction
• Correct positioning
• Support family group
• Patient/family education:
  - Disease process/signs and symptoms of reoccurrence or worsening, treatment, lifestyle changes, CPR, vital signs, medication regimen, home O_2 management; return-to-school strategies

Across Care Settings:
• School staff should know CPR and how to use AED
• Transplant teams are interdisciplinary with community members included
• American Heart Association and Kawasaki Disease
• Returning to school
• Monitoring the child at home
• The home-bound child

Critical Nursing Action:
• Medications are used in combination to treat CHF
• Care of the child post–cardiac surgery occurs in the ICU setting
• Vital sign routine more rigorous in a PICU

Clinical Alert:
• Know sx of renal failure/postoperative hemmorrhage
• Cyanotic defects must have mixing of blood
• Risk of thrombus formation with aneurysm in Kawasaki disease
• There are classic sx of "TET" spells
• Watch pulse pressure s/p cardiac catheterization
• Know complications of cardiac transplantation
• Apply pressure to groin

Focus on Safety:
• Pulse ox/cardiac monitoring for child with CHD
• Good dental care can prevent SBE in child at risk
• Teach anticoagulation therapy precautions
• Sports gear and motor vehicle restraints can prevent cardiac trauma/re-injury
• Manage HTN to prevent complications ➔ stroke
• Loss of consciousness in NMS can lead to injury
• Teens should not drive if they have had loss of consciousness
• Parents of children with cardiac disease should learn CPR

Nursing Insight:
• Antibiotic therapy for child at risk for SBE before dental work or surgery
• Heart valves can be congenitally malformed or physically altered due to disease
• Pulmonary atresia is fatal if not corrected
• Auscultation landmarks for valves are not over the valve
• Rheumatic fever can lead to vegetation on heart valves
• Cardiac tumors are rare in children
• Children can have primary or secondary hypercholesterolemia/hyperlipidemia
• For PEA: treat the child, not the rhythm

Now Can You:
• Understand the implications of heart disease in children
• Discuss the care of a child with a cardiovascular condition
• Provide holistic, evidence-based, and safe care for the child with a CV condition

Caring for the Child With an Endocrinological or Metabolic Condition

"**E**ven when all is known, the care of a man is not yet complete, because eating alone will not keep a man well; he must also take exercise. For food and exercise, while possessing opposite qualities, yet work together to produce health."

—Hippocrates

LEARNING TARGETS *At the completion of this chapter, the student will be able to:*

◆ Describe the anatomy and physiology and developmental aspects of the endocrine system.

◆ Examine the common conditions of the endocrine system.

◆ Prioritize developmentally appropriate and holistic nursing care measures for common conditions of the endocrine system.

◆ Explore diagnostic testing, laboratory testing, and medications for common conditions of the endocrine system.

◆ Develop teaching plans and discharge criteria for parents whose children have common endocrine conditions.

PICO(T) Questions

The intent of evidence-based practice (EBP) is to provide nursing care that integrates the best available evidence. An initial step in EBP is to write a PICO(T) question that effectively guides the research. A PICO(T) question is an acronym that stands for population (P), intervention or issue (I), comparison of interest (C), outcome (O), and timeframe (T). Depending on the question, all or some of the question components are used in the research process. Use these

PICO(T) questions to spark your thinking as you read the chapter.

1. What are (O) the evidence-based practices that nurses should teach (P) adolescents with diabetes who are going to be (I) using an insulin pump?

2. On average, do (P) 8-year-old children with type 1 diabetes demonstrate (O) the same level of accuracy (I) in measuring their blood glucose levels (C) compared with their parents?

 Evidence-Based Practice

Smaldone, A., & Ritholz, M. D. (2011). Perceptions of parenting children with type 1 diabetes diagnosed in early childhood. *Journal of Pediatric Health Care, 25*(2), 87–95.

The purpose of this study was to examine the perceptions of parents regarding their psychosocial adaptation in providing long-term care for children diagnosed with type 1 diabetes (T1DM) by age 5 or younger. Research has noted that the incidence of T1DM is on the rise with the greatest increase in young children. Though T1DM is more commonly diagnosed during puberty, approximately 15% to 20% of new cases are now diagnosed in children

5 years of age or under. The literature notes that diagnosing T1DM is more difficult in young children because they may not present with the classic symptoms, which can lead to a more serious presentation (e.g., diabetic ketoacidosis [DKA]). Early, non-classic symptoms in children may include enuresis and constipation. T1DM presents further challenges for parents in that children are limited in their language and cognitive ability to communicate

(continued)

symptoms and are often picky eaters. Studies have indicated that the incidence of depression in mothers of newly diagnosed diabetic children is approximately 30% and related to ongoing concerns about management and adapting to the daily demands of the disease.

Participants in this study were recruited from a diabetes day camp for children and by word of mouth. Criteria for inclusion were that the parents had 1 or more children diagnosed with T1DM by the age of 5. Either one or both parents of the same child were allowed to participate, though couples were interviewed separately. Participants received $50 for their participation. The participants included 14 parents (i.e., 3 mothers, 3 fathers, and 4 couples). These 14 parents represented 11 children diagnosed by age 5 or younger (mean = 3.2 years or age at the time of diagnosis). At the time of diagnoses, 36% of the children were in DKA. One parent was Hispanic, and 13 were identified as non-Hispanic white. The mean age of the parents at the time of the study was 41.7 years of age. One hundred percent of the parents were married and living with their partner. Ten were college graduates, and the other 4 had some college education. All of the fathers in the study worked full-time, 2 of the mothers worked full-time, 2 worked part-time, and 3 were not employed outside the home. Of the 11 children represented by the parents in the study, 7 were female and 10 were hospitalized at the time of diagnosis. The current mean age of the children was 11.1; the mean duration of their diabetes at the time of the study was 8.0 years. One mother had 2 children with T1DM, and another mother had herself been a diabetic for 25 years. Ten of the children had transitioned from injections to use of an insulin pump.

Data were collected through interviews using open-ended questions. Interviews were completed by the researchers, took place at the participant's home, were audio recorded, and transcribed. Transcripts were coded independently by each researcher. Two of the parents in the study were also asked to review the findings for accuracy in interpretation. Three major themes were identified: (1) diagnostic experiences: frustrations, fears, and doubts; (2) adapting to diabetes; and (3) negotiating developmental transitions. In regards to "diagnostic experiences," parents expressed concern over not being taken seriously. Some noted that they felt abandoned, unsupported, and a lack of empathy from the primary care provider. Parents also expressed reluctance to leave the hospital and hesitancy about their own ability to manage the care of their child.

In relation to the theme of "adapting to diabetes," parents felt overwhelmed and self-doubt. Several parents noted that sharing the care responsibility with the other parent, and sometimes another family member (e.g., a grandparent) eased the adjustment process. Parents noted that the use of informal feedback and verification of impressions with the other parent regarding symptoms and decisions regarding daily care increased comfort and ability to adapt. The majority of mothers noted that participation in a support group helped them learn from the experience of others and lessened the feeling of isolation. Most of the fathers did not find the support group helpful.

In relation to the theme of "negotiating developmental transitions," parents noted anxiety over some of the firsts in their child's life (e.g., going to school, staying with a relative other than the parents, and staying overnight at a friend's house). Parents acknowledged the need for their children to have normal childhood experiences but most of the time noted that they sometimes felt a lack of understanding from relatives, other parents, and school personnel. However, one mother noted that the school nurse took time to attend training with the family on the use of the insulin pump. Concerns were also expressed about the child's future ability to be independent and leave home. Parents who were able to collaborate with the health-care team regarding treatment decisions perceived that the care was more effective.

The researchers conclude that parents' perception of diagnoses and treatment effectiveness can improve with increased collaboration and communication with the parents during those experiences. Providers need to be aware of the parents' feelings of isolation and concern with mastery of the disease and care needed. This is ongoing and occurs through anticipatory guidance during every contact with the family and child.

1. How is this information useful to clinical nursing practice?

2. Based on these findings, what are implications for further research?

See Suggested Responses for Evidence-Based Practice on Davis*Plus*.

Introduction

This chapter provides a review of the anatomy and physiology and developmental aspects of the endocrine system. The discussion includes an examination of common endocrine conditions including developmentally appropriate and holistic nursing care. Information about diagnostic and laboratory testing and medications is given. Teaching plans and discharge criteria for parents whose children have common endocrine conditions are incorporated.

The endocrine system is composed of multiple organs throughout the body. These organs secrete hormones that regulate various bodily functions. Hormones are proteins consisting of amino acid chains or steroids derived from fatty (cholesterol-derived) substances. Hormones act as "messengers," moving from system to system coordinating the functions of many parts of the body. In the care of children, it is important to remember that the endocrine system controls growth and development as well as energy use and energy stores; it also controls levels of sugar, salt, and fluids in the bloodstream. Hormones regulate a child's response to stress or physical trauma and play a vital role in sexual development.

Growth and Development

The child with an endocrinological condition may experience variations in normal growth and development, particularly with physical growth. Growth changes are closely associated with deficiencies in the pituitary hormone and can result in delayed skeletal growth or short stature, associated with hypopituitary deficiencies, or accelerated growth, associated with pituitary hyperfunction. The nurse must recognize the cause of the alterations in growth as complications of the endocrinological condition and not necessarily associated with disturbances in growth and development. Nursing care should include assessment and measurement of normal growth patterns including height, weight, head circumference, and body mass index. The nurse should also assess for the presence of abnormal physical characteristics for age and body build. Proper administration of medications is required to correct disturbances in hormone levels and should be closely regulated by the nurse. The nurse should educate the child and the family about medical treatment and target goals for growth and development.

The child with an endocrinological condition may experience emotional distress because of alterations in hormone levels, bullying from peers, and low self-esteem. Nursing care should include assessment of the child's emotional well-being and acceptance of the disease process. The nurse should assess for emotional distress of the child and make referrals to psychological counseling when indicated.

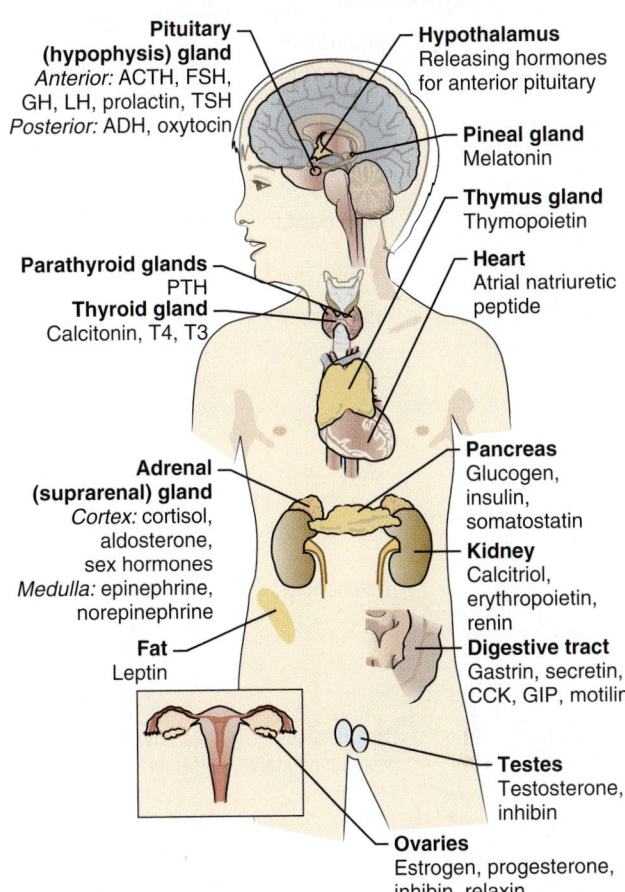

The Endocrine System

Figure 27-1 Anatomy and physiology of the endocrine system.

A & P review The Endocrine System

The glands that make up the endocrine system include the hypothalamus, pituitary gland, thyroid, parathyroids, adrenal glands, pineal body, and reproductive glands (ovaries and testes) (Fig. 27-1). The hypothalamus is located in the center of the brain and is the main control center of the body. Its function is to communicate the messages of the central autonomic nervous system to the organs and glands of the endocrine system, thus maintaining homeostasis throughout the body.

The pituitary gland is connected to the hypothalamus by a stem-like structure. It has two parts: the anterior and the posterior pituitary. It is said that the pituitary gland is the "master" because of its effect on growth and the functions of other glands in the body. The thyroid gland is located in the front of the neck just below the larynx. The two lobes of the thyroid are connected by an isthmus, which is a small band of tissue. The thyroid produces two hormones called thyroxin (T_4) and triiodothyronine (T_3).

There are four parathyroid glands, two embedded on the posterior side of each lobe of the thyroid gland. The parathyroid glands produce parathyroid hormone (PTH) and are responsible for calcium regulation. The adrenal glands are located on the top of each kidney. Each gland has an outer (cortex) portion and an inner (medulla) portion. The hypothalamus controls the adrenal glands by directing the anterior pituitary to release adrenocorticotropic hormone (ACTH) releasing hormone. The adrenal cortex and the medulla produce different hormones. The pancreas is located in the abdomen, just behind the stomach near the duodenum. It functions as both an endocrine (without ducts) gland by secreting hormones and also as an exocrine (with ducts) gland. As an endocrine gland, it secretes both insulin and glucagon, which are carried to the cells through the bloodstream. These two pancreatic hormones have antagonistic effects on metabolism. The pancreas also functions as an exocrine gland, producing and secreting digestive enzymes directly into the small intestine through ducts.

The gonads, namely the ovaries in females and the testes in males, produce several steroidal sex hormones. Generally, these sex hormones produce and regulate changes in the male and female body at puberty.

Table 27-1 discusses the hormones secreted by the endocrine system and related physiology. Some of these endocrine glands secrete more than one hormone, and some hormones function in more than one way. Endocrine physiology is based on the function of each hormone and an intricate feedback regulation. Feedback is the process by which an organ or tissue either reacts positively or negatively based on the response or action of the target cells or the circulating hormone. Stress, temperature, and nutritional status can influence feedback regulation. Figures 27-2 and 27-3 show examples of positive and negative feedback (Ward, 2013). ◆

Pathophysiological Conditions of the Endocrine System

Conditions of the endocrine system are a result of either an over- or underproduction of the hormones or stimulating hormone. Endocrine diseases are also caused by the hyper- or hypo-response of the target organ or cell. A critical nursing assessment is essential to competent nursing care (Table 27-2).

Table 27-1 Hormone Table

Hormone	Produced by or Stored in	Function and Action (Physiology)	Target Organ or Cell	Other Feedback Loop Regulation Factors
Growth hormone–releasing hormone (GHRH)	Hypothalamus	Causes release of GH from somatotrophs in the anterior pituitary	Anterior pituitary	GHRH and somatostatin have antagonistic effects on the production and release of GH
Somatostatin	Hypothalamus	Inhibits GH and TSH	Anterior pituitary	GHRH and somatostatin have antagonistic effects on the production and release of GH
Thyrotropin-releasing hormone (TRH)	Hypothalamus	Stimulates production and release of TSH	Anterior pituitary	Thyroid hormone levels Dopamine can stimulate or inhibit release Inhibition of serotonin GABA Somatostatin CRH
Corticotropin-releasing hormone (CRH)	Hypothalamus	Stimulates production and release of ACTH	Anterior pituitary	Stress ACTH levels
Gonadotropin-releasing hormone (GnRH)	Hypothalamus	Causes release of FSH and LH	Anterior pituitary	FSH LH Testosterone Estrogen Progesterone
Antidiuretic hormone	Hypothalamus/posterior pituitary	Acts directly on target cells increasing membrane permeability to water	Renal collecting ducts and distal tubules	Regulated by osmotic pressure of plasma (osmolality) Osmoreceptors in hypothalamus mediate the response Set point influencing stimulation: Concentrated body fluids = release of ADH = increased reabsorption of water Dilute body fluids = inhibition of ADH = decreased reabsorption of water
Oxytocin	Hypothalamus/posterior pituitary	Effects not as important in children Stimulates milk ejection Stimulates smooth muscle contraction of the uterus at birth Assists in maternal attachment Found in seminal fluid	Uterus, breasts	Progesterone levels Stimulation of nipples Stimulation of cervix by fetus
Growth hormone	Anterior pituitary	Causes growth of ALL body tissues that are capable of responding to it Promotes mitosis and cellular growth Affects metabolic processes by increasing the rate of protein synthesis, thus decreasing protein catabolism, slowing carbohydrate use, and increasing mobilization of fats Increases use of fats for energy Increases linear growth acting on the growth plates of long bones Secretion (pulsatile and circadian) greatest during sleep (stages 3 and 4) and adolescence and least during old age Stimulates production of insulin-like growth factor-1 (IGF-1) somatomedin	All cells in body, liver, IGF-1	Hypothalamus: GHRH Somatostatin Sleep Exercise Physical activity Trauma Stress

Table 27-1 Hormone Table (continued)

Hormone	Produced by or Stored in	Function and Action (Physiology)	Target Organ or Cell	Other Feedback Loop Regulation Factors
Thyroid-stimulating hormone (TSH)	Anterior pituitary	Stimulates the thyroid to produce and secrete thyroid hormone	Thyroid	TRH Dopamine Somatostatin Thyroid hormones
Adrenocorticotropic hormone (ACTH)	Anterior pituitary	Stimulates production of glucocorticoids	Adrenal glands	Glucocorticoids
Prolactin	Anterior pituitary	Stimulates breast growth Stimulates milk production	Breasts	May be related to immune response Estrogen Dopamine
Luteinizing hormone (LH)	Anterior pituitary	Stimulates ovulation	Testes, ovaries,	Pulsatory regulation of GnRH when levels of sex hormones are adequate
Follicle-stimulating hormone (FSH)	Anterior pituitary	Stimulates maturation of ovarian follicle and sperm production	Testes, ovaries	Pulsatory regulation of GnRH when levels of sex hormones are adequate
Thyroxine (T_4) Triiodothyronine (T_3)	Thyroid gland	Influences metabolic rate Needs iodine for production	Affects cells in body in metabolism, growth, development; specific systems: cardiac, neurological, reproductive	Hypothalamus: pituitary-thyroid feedback system TSH released by anterior pituitary TRH produced by the hypothalamus
Parathyroid hormone (PTH)	Parathyroid glands	Helps maintain homeostasis through regulation of calcium PTH Acts on bones and renal tubules increasing serum calcium levels In bone, increases osteoclastic activity releasing calcium from bone into the extracellular fluid In kidneys, increases calcium reabsorption (decreasing urine calcium levels) Stimulates activation of vitamin D (increasing intestinal calcium absorption)	Bones, kidneys, intestines	Serum calcium levels Reciprocal with PTH levels PTH and calcitonin are antagonistic
Calcitonin	Parathyroid glands	Increases bone formation by osteoblasts Inhibits bone breakdown by osteoclasts Decreases serum calcium levels Promotes conservation of hard bone	Bone, kidneys	Concentration of ionized calcium
Insulin	Islets of Langerhans (beta cells of pancreas)	Facilitates diffusion of glucose into the cells Increases uptake and decreases release of amino acids, thus inducing protein synthesis Has role in lipid formation Stimulates secretion of somatomedin	All cells	Glucose levels in blood (hyperglycemia or hypoglycemia)
Glucagon	Islets of Langerhans (alpha cells of pancreas)	Increases blood glucose Stimulates breakdown of glycogen Stimulates gluconeogenesis Stimulates lipolysis	Liver	Glucose levels in blood (hypoglycemia or hyperglycemia) Elevated amino acids in blood that lead to gluconeogenesis Exercise

(continued)

Table 27-1	Hormone Table (continued)			
Hormone	**Produced by or Stored in**	**Function and Action (Physiology)**	**Target Organ or Cell**	**Other Feedback Loop Regulation Factors**
Cortisol—glucocorticoids	Adrenal cortex	Primarily affect glucose metabolism Influence use of fats and proteins Anti-insulin: raise blood sugar Decrease glucose uptake by fat and muscle cells Increase glucose synthesis Gluconeogenesis: production of energy (glucose) from amino acids (protein) Protein catabolism releasing muscle stores of proteins – provides amino acids Lipid catabolism Increase cholesterol Immune and inflammation functions Fetal lung maturation and surfactant production Cognitive functions	All cells, liver	Hypothalamic secretion of CRH Pituitary secretion of ACTH Physiological and psychological stress Renin-angiotensin system (mineral)
Aldosterone—Mineralocorticoids	Adrenal cortex	Maintain normal salt and water balance, sodium retention, and potassium excretion	Distal tubule of the kidney	Extracellular potassium ion concentration Angiotensin II
Sex steroids—androgens	Adrenal cortex	Have minor role in development of secondary sex characteristics Are main source of androgens in girls and women	Secondary sex organs, seminal vesicles, brain, bone, breasts	Estrogens Thyroid hormone Pregnancy Estrogen-containing preparations Androgens Synthetic progestins (norethindrone, norgestrel, desogestrel, norgestimate) Glucocorticoids Growth hormone Insulin Obesity Acromegaly Hypothyroidism Hyperinsulinemia
Epinephrine and norepinephrine	Adrenal medulla	Increase heart rate Increase contractile force of heart Dilate bronchioles Increase metabolism Lipolysis Decrease gastric motility Decrease motor function (not essential) Vasoconstrict (norepinephrine)	Heart, blood vessels, lungs, all cells	Regulated by the sympathetic nervous system Exercise Bleeding Low blood sugar Stress

GABA, gamma-aminobutyric acid.
Source: Ward (2013).

"What to say"—*Offering support*

An endocrine condition can be frightening to both children and parents. It is important to allow the parents and child to express the signs and symptoms in their own language. The parent can interject a more-detailed answer for the child or you may ask the parent more-detailed questions based on the child's statement. Use these questions to assess the situation:

1. When did you first notice your child's illness?

2. What are specific signs and symptoms you have noticed?

3. Has your child experienced changes in growth or appearance?

4. Has the illness disrupted the child's and family's usual routines?

5. Has a complete health history and physical examination been completed?

6. What kind of medical testing has been done so far?

7. Are you or the child frightened by the illness?

8. What kind of support system do you have in place? (Ward, 2013)

Positive Feedback Loop

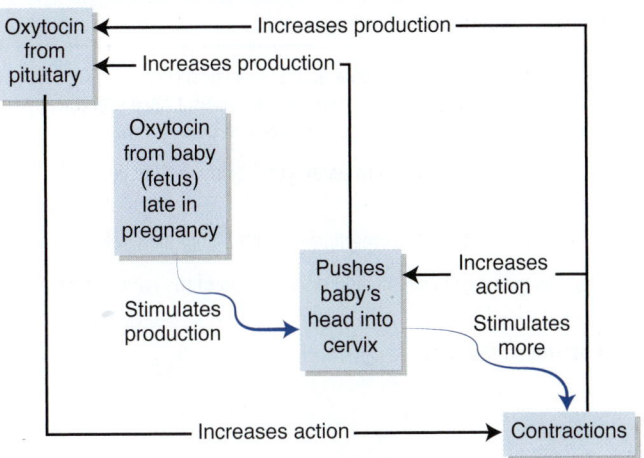

Figure 27-2 Positive feedback loop.

Negative Feedback Loop

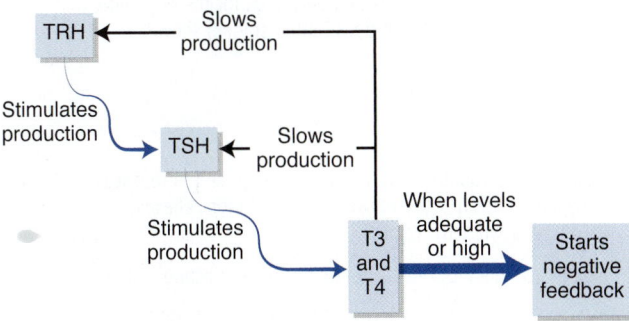

Figure 27-3 Negative feedback loop.

 Nursing Insight—*Ways to offer support to families and children with endocrine conditions*

- Listen attentively
- Be present in the moment, giving your full attention to the child and family
- Provide accurate and ongoing information
- Clarify questions
- Help families find and use community resources
- Assist parents with scheduling follow-up appointments
- Help families to find reliable online resources
- Discuss health promotion measures such as diet and exercise (Ward, 2013)

CONDITIONS OF THE ANTERIOR PITUITARY

The anterior pituitary gland is responsible for the production of many hormones that influence and regulate growth, metabolic activity, and sexual development. Conditions of the anterior pituitary result in either an over- or underproduction of the hormones or stimulate hormones. These conditions will cause growth hormone deficiency, gigantism, or precocious puberty.

Pituitary Hypofunction

Pituitary hypofunction, or hypopituitary, causes growth hormone deficiency (GHD), an endocrine condition caused by a decreased production of growth hormone (GH). Children with this condition present with short stature (below the 5th percentile) and demonstrate delayed skeletal growth. GHD is also referred to as pituitary dwarfism, acquired growth hormone deficiency, isolated growth hormone deficiency, congenital growth hormone deficiency, and panhypopituitarism

Table 27-2 Critical Nursing Assessment of the Endocrine System		
Body System	**Symptoms**	**Physical Examination Findings**
General assessment	Recent weight gain or loss, fatigue, malaise, weakness, fevers, intolerance to heat or cold, increased sweating, or night sweats	Obesity, thinness, and dehydration
Skin, nails, and hair	Changes in skin pigment; excessive dryness or moisture, itching; recent hair loss or change in the texture of the hair on head or body; changes in nail shape or brittleness of nails	Pigment differences in the skin; skin excessively warm, moist skin, diaphoretic, or smooth In hyperthyroidism, rough, dry, and flaky skin In hypothyroidism, dull, coarse, and brittle hair In hirsutism, abnormal or absent genital hair in puberty; pitted, grooved, or brittle nails
Head	Headache, dizziness, or vertigo	Frontal lobe bulging or bossing In hyperparathyroidism, flat fontanelle
Eyes	Redness, dryness, bulging, and visual disturbances	Exophthalmos, redness, visual impairment, lid lag, and periorbital edema
Ears	No history of findings directly related to the endocrine system	No physical findings directly related to the endocrine system
Nose	Stuffy nose	No physical findings directly related to the endocrine system
Mouth and throat	Mouth sores do not heal; difficulty with swallowing; hoarseness or voice change	Enlarged tongue, fine tremors of the tongue, and fruity breath odor
Neck	Swelling in the neck or goiter and pain	Thyroid enlargement; unilateral or bilateral and tracheal displacement; "buffalo hump" Difficulty in assessing the thyroid in an infant because of the short neck

(continued)

Table 27-2 Critical Nursing Assessment of the Endocrine System (continued)

Body System	Symptoms	Physical Examination Findings
Breast	Breast development either early or late	Early breast development before age 8 yr, delayed breast development, neonatal breast development (from transplacental estrogen; normal finding), or gynecomastia in boys
Respiratory, thorax, lungs	No history of findings directly related to the endocrine system	Skeletal deformities related to parathyroid gland dysfunction
Cardiovascular	Palpitations, tachycardia, and high blood pressure	Tachycardia, bradycardia, hypertension with a bounding pulse
Peripheral vascular	Coldness, numbness, tingling, and discoloration of the hands and feet	Cool, delayed capillary refill, and discoloration of the hands or feet
Gastrointestinal	Decreased or increased appetite, increased thirst, nausea, vomiting, abdominal pain, diarrhea, and weight gain or loss not related to food intake or deliberate dieting	A full, round abdomen
Urinary	Frequency, nocturia, polyuria; kidney stones; and pain in the flank, groin, or suprapubic region or low back	No physical findings directly related to the endocrine system
Genitalia	Testicular pain or lumps, undescended testicles; unusual menstrual history (When did menarche start [at what age]? What was the date of last menstrual period and what was the duration? Has there been any amenorrhea? Has a gynecological examination been performed?)	Are ambiguous genitalia present? Are the genitalia swollen, or is the scrotum asymmetric? Is the penis large for the boy's age (precocious puberty). What does Tanner staging show?
Neurological	Tremor, tic, coordination problems, numbness or tingling, memory disorder, nervousness, mood change, psychosis, or seizures	Peripheral neuropathy, hyperactivity of deep tendon reflexes In hyperthyroidism, hypoactivity of deep tendon reflexes In SIADH, asymmetric pupils
Hematological	No history of findings directly related to the endocrine system	No physical findings directly related to the endocrine system
Endocrine	History of endocrine disorders and/or need for or current use of hormone replacement therapy	Abnormal examination of the testes, ovaries, or thyroid gland
Musculoskeletal	Broken bones noted from unusual circumstances; joint pain or stiffness; muscle pain or cramps; weakness; and gait problems	Skeletal deformities related to parathyroid gland dysfunction, spasms, current or recent fractures in various stages of healing, limited range of motion, and spine and back deformities

SIADH, syndrome of inappropriate antidiuretic hormone.

Source: Ward (2013).

(Kemp, 2013). The incidence of GHD has been reported to be about 1 out of every 3,500 children (Kemp, 2012; U.S. National Library of Medicine, National Institutes of Health, 2012). It is unclear whether the incidence between boys and girls differs although males may be referred more often than females for short stature because it is believed that small females are more accepted in our society.

The cause of hypopituitarism is often unknown and idiopathic in nature. Advances in genetic mapping have allowed identification of at least three genetic mutations as causative factors of GHD (U.S. National Library of Medicine, National Institutes of Health, 2012). In addition, there are many other causes both congenital and acquired, including trauma, CNS infections, and tumors in the region of the hypothalamus or pituitary as well as secondary causes such as cranial irradiation and transient causes such as psychosocial deprivation (Trip-Hoving, Van Alfen-Vander Velden, & Otten, 2009; Whittemore, Smaldone, & Steiner, 2013).

 Nursing Insight—*Etiology*

- CNS tumor, including craniopharyngioma–47%
- CNS malformation–15%
- Septo-optic dysplasia–14%
- Leukemia–9%
- CNS radiation–9%
- CNS trauma–3%
- Histiocytosis–2%
- CNS infection–1%
  (Kemp, 2012)

Signs and Symptoms

Usually, in the neonatal period, infants with GHD are of normal birth weight and length. The delayed or absent growth begins to be assessed in the first 2 years of life. Delayed growth of less than 2 inches (4 to 5 centimeters) in a year is to be evaluated further. Assessment must be done carefully and consistently at each visit to the pediatrician. The rate of growth can be measured using the metric system to increase the preciseness of the measurement. If a child's height or weight plateaus (i.e., stays the same), further evaluation is warranted.

Other signs and symptoms of growth hormone deficiency include:

- Delayed closure of the anterior fontanelle
- Delayed dental eruption
- Greater weight-to-height ratio
- Increased abdominal (truncal) fat
- Decreased muscle mass
- Poor development of bridge of nose giving a pixie-like appearance
- Protrusion of the frontal skull bones
- Delayed puberty, including a high-pitch voice and a small penis or testes in boys
- Hypoglycemia

It is important to alert the health-care provider about episodes of frequent or recurrent hypoglycemia, prolonged jaundice, or micropenis in the neonatal period because these may indicate the possibility of congenital hypopituitarism (Whittemore et al., 2013).

 Critical Nursing Action Proper Growth Assessment

It is imperative that the nurse plot the child's height and weight accurately at each outpatient visit on the appropriate growth chart (Fig. 27-4). If the child is of short stature (below the 5th percentile) and is not chartable on the usual chart or has a syndrome known for short stature, the nurse accesses the Centers for Disease Control and Prevention (CDC) (2009) "Clinical Growth Charts" Web site (http://www.cdc.gov/growthcharts/clinical_charts.htm) for the most appropriate chart. It is important to use the same growth chart at each visit. Weigh the patient the same way each time; for example, an infant is completely undressed (including diaper), and a young child is dressed in underwear only. Standardized techniques for measuring height are used in the clinical setting.

Diagnosis

A diagnostic work-up begins with a review of all previous growth charts to determine the rate of growth. Special attention is given to children in less than the 5th percentile or to any child whose growth has ceased, which is evidenced by

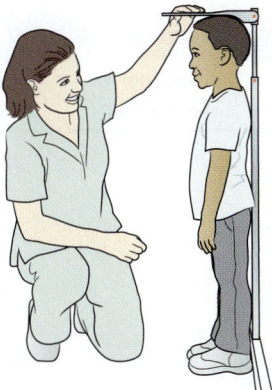

Figure 27-4 The nurse is measuring the child's height to ensure growth and development are on target.

a flat line or plateau on the growth chart. Bone age determination by radiograph of the wrist, knee, or hand is usually less than the child's chronological age, thus indicating a delayed skeletal maturation. Magnetic resonance imaging (MRI) of the brain is performed to rule out a brain tumor. Table 27-3 outlines specific laboratory tests for endocrine conditions to confirm the diagnosis. Other pituitary function tests, which stimulate or suppress growth hormone (GH) release, are performed. The GH stimulants are typically insulin or arginine. The suppression test is done after giving glucose. Other stimulants include arginine, levodopa (L-dopa), clonidine, and glucagon (Kemp, 2012). When peak GH levels are less than 10 nanograms per liter (ng/L) after stimulation, the diagnosis is confirmed.

Prevention

GHD is not preventable in most cases. Preventive measures in caring for the child with GHD are through education with the goals of controlling stress, preventing and monitoring for signs of GHD insufficiency, and promoting age-appropriate development. The child's growth is monitored with each checkup. Parents need to be cognizant of the potential for emotional stress caused by small stature. Parents also need to be instructed on ensuring that the child is in compliance with hormone replacement therapy as well as potential side effects of the treatment.

Collaborative Care

Nursing Care. Assist the child in reaching the goals of treatment, which are that the child achieves a normal

(Text continued on page 1073)

Table 27-3 Common Laboratory Tests for Endocrine Conditions

Hormone Produced	Function/ Description	Common Tests of Endocrine Function	Purpose of Test	Significance of Results as Related to the Endocrine System
Adrenal Glands				
• Aldosterone	• Salt, water balance	Aldosterone levels (normal values vary by age)	• Evaluate hypertension of unknown cause • Suspected hyperaldosteronism • Suspected hypoaldosteronism	Increased Levels • Adenomas • Bilateral hyperplasia of aldosterone-secreting cells • Secondary to conditions caused by increased renin levels (e.g., diuretic or laxative abuse) • Cirrhosis

(continued)

Table 27-3 Common Laboratory Tests for Endocrine Conditions (continued)

Hormone Produced	Function/ Description	Common Tests of Endocrine Function	Purpose of Test	Significance of Results as Related to the Endocrine System
Adrenal Glands				
• Aldosterone (continued)				Decreased Levels • Addison's disease • Hypoaldosteronism • Diabetes • Excess secretion of deoxycorticosterone • Turner's syndrome
• Cortisol	• Stress reaction	Cortisol and Challenge Tests • ACTH stimulation, rapid test • CRH stimulation • Dexamethasone suppression • Metyrapone stimulation	• Determine adrenal hyperfunction (e.g., Cushing's disease) • Determine adrenal hypofunction (e.g., Addison's disease)	Increased Levels • Adrenal adenoma • Cushing's syndrome • Hyperglycemia • Stress Decreased Levels • Addison's disease • Hypopituitarism • Adrenogenital syndrome
• DHEA-S	• Body hair development at puberty	DHEA-S levels (normal values vary by age and gender)	• Evaluate for androgen excess, including congenital adrenal hyperplasia and adrenal tumor • Evaluated for female infertility, amenorrhea, hirsutism	Increased Levels • Cushing's disease • Hirsutism • Polycystic ovary • Anovulation • Ectopic ACTH-producing tumors • Hyperprolactinemia • Virilizing adrenal tumors Decreased Levels • Addison's disease • Adrenal insufficiency • Pregnancy • Psychosis related to adrenal insufficiency
• Epinephrine and norepinephrine	• Blood pressure regulation, stress reaction, heart rate	Catecholamines: blood and urine levels (levels vary by age)	• Assists in diagnoses of some tumors and pheochromocytoma • Used to evaluate acute hypertensive episodes	Increased Levels • Diabetic acidosis • Hypothyroidism • Some tumors and pheochromocytoma • Strenuous exercise Decreased Levels • Autonomic nervous system dysfunction • Orthostatic hypotension
Hypothalamus				
• Growth hormone-releasing hormone (GHRH)	• Stimulates growth hormone production by the pituitary	Growth hormone stimulation and suppression tests (normal values vary by age and gender)	Assists in diagnoses of • Acromegaly • Dwarfism • Growth retardation in children • Gigantism in children • Used to monitor treatment of growth retardation	Increased Levels • Acromegaly • Anorexia nervosa • Cirrhosis • Uncontrolled diabetes • Gigantism (pituitary) • Hyperpituitarism • Stress • Ectopic GH secretion from neoplasms Decreased Levels • Adrenocortical hyperfunction • Dwarfism (pituitary) • Hypopituitarism

Table 27-3 Common Laboratory Tests for Endocrine Conditions (continued)

Hormone Produced	Function/ Description	Common Tests of Endocrine Function	Purpose of Test	Significance of Results as Related to the Endocrine System
• Thyrotropin-releasing hormone (TRH)	• Stimulates TSH production in the pituitary	Thyrotropin (TSH) levels	Assists in diagnosis of • Congenital hypothyroidism • Hypothyroidism or hyperthyroidism • Pituitary or hypothalamic dysfunction	Increased Levels • Congenital hypothyroidism in neonate • Ectopic TSH-producing tumors • Primary hypothyroidism • Secondary hyperthyroidism related to pituitary hyperactivity • Thyroid hormone resistance • Thyroiditis Decreased Levels • Graves' disease • Primary hyperthyroidism • Secondary hypothyroidism • Excessive thyroid hormone replacement
• Corticotropin-releasing hormone (CRH)	• Stimulates ACTH production by the pituitary	Refer to Cortisol and Challenge Tests under the adrenal glands	Refer to Cortisol and Challenge Tests	Refer to Cortisol and Challenge Tests
• Gonadotropin-releasing hormone (GnRH)	• Stimulates LF and FSH production by the pituitary	Human chorionic gonadotropin levels (levels vary by week of gestation)	• Assists in diagnosing HCG-producing tumors • Confirms pregnancy • Assists in diagnosing ectopic pregnancy or threatened or incomplete abortion • Assists in determining whether hormone levels are adequate to maintain pregnancy • May help detect neural tube defects prenatally	Increased Levels • Ectopic HCG-producing tumor • Erythroblastosis fetalis • Multiple gestation pregnancy • Pregnancy Decreased Levels • Ectopic pregnancy • Incomplete abortion • Intrauterine fetal demise • Spontaneous abortion • Threatened abortion
• Prolactin inhibitory hormone (PIH, Dopamine)	• Inhibits prolactin production	Prolactin levels (levels vary by age and gender)	• Assists in diagnoses of the primary hypothyroidism • Evaluation of postpartum lactation failure	Increased Levels • Increased adrenal insufficiency (secondary to hypopituitarism) • Anorexia nervosa • Breastfeeding • Hypothalamic and pituitary disorders • Primary hypothyroidism • Insulin-induced hypoglycemia • Pituitary tumor • Polycystic ovary • Pregnancy Decreased Levels • Severe hemorrhage after obstetric delivery that causes pituitary infarction (Sheehan's syndrome)
• Arginine vasopressin (AVP), also called antidiuretic hormone (ADH), produced by the hypothalamus, stored and secreted by the pituitary	• Water balance	Antidiuretic hormone level	• Assists in the diagnosis of malignancy associated with syndrome of inappropriate ADH secretion • Differentiates between neurogenic and nephrogenic diabetes insipidus • Detects CNS trauma or disease that may be demonstrated by impaired ADH secretions	Increased Levels • Pain, stress, or exercise • Nephrogenic diabetes insipidus • Disorders involving the central nervous system, thyroid gland, and adrenal gland • SIADH Decreased Levels • Nephrotic syndrome • Pituitary diabetes insipidus

(continued)

Table 27-3 Common Laboratory Tests for Endocrine Conditions (continued)

Hormone Produced	Function/ Description	Common Tests of Endocrine Function	Purpose of Test	Significance of Results as Related to the Endocrine System
Ovaries				
• Estrogen	• Female sexual characteristics	Estradiol levels (levels vary with age and gender)	• Assists in diagnosing adrenal and estrogen-producing tumors	Increased Levels • Adrenal and estrogen-producing tumors • Feminization in children • Gynecomastia • Hyperthyroidism Decreased Levels • Primary and secondary hypogonadism • Turner's syndrome
• Progesterone	• Female sexual characteristics	Progesterone levels (levels vary with age, gender, and pregnancy stage)	• Evaluates for risk of early or spontaneous abortion • Identifies for risk of ectopic pregnancy	Increased Levels • Congenital adrenal hyperplasia • Ovarian tumors Decreased Levels • Galactorrhea-amenorrhea syndrome • Primary or secondary hypogonadism • Threatened abortion
Pancreas				
• Glucagon	• Glucose regulation	Fasting and post-prandial glucose (blood sugar) (levels vary with age in infants and young children) Glucagon levels (levels vary with age)	• Assists in the diagnosis of glucagon deficiency and suspected renal failure	Increased Levels • Acromegaly • Acute stress • Cushing's syndrome • Diabetes • Glucagonoma • Pancreatic adenoma • Pancreatitis • Pheochromocytoma • Renal disease • Shock and trauma • Strenuous exercise • Thyrotoxicosis • Vitamin B_1 deficiency Decreased Levels • Addison's disease • Galactosemia • Glucagon deficiency • Hereditary fructose intolerance • Hypopituitarism • Hypothyroidism • Malabsorption syndrome • Maple syrup urine disease • Poisoning resulting in severe liver disease • Starvation
Parathyroid Glands				
• Parathyroid hormone (PTH)	• Regulates blood calcium	Parathyroid levels (levels vary with age)	• Assists in diagnoses of causes of primary and secondary hyperparathyroidism	Increased Levels • Primary or secondary hyperparathyroidism Decreased Levels • DiGeorge syndrome • Hyperthyroidism • Nonparathyroid hypercalcemia • Secondary hypoparathyroidism

Table 27-3 Common Laboratory Tests for Endocrine Conditions (continued)

Hormone Produced	Function/ Description	Common Tests of Endocrine Function	Purpose of Test	Significance of Results as Related to the Endocrine System
Pituitary Gland				
• Prolactin	• Milk production	Refer to Prolactin levels under the hypothalamus	• A blood test that measures the level of the hormone in the body	• In women, a prolactin test is ordered if she displays symptoms of prolactinoma, a benign tumor on the pituitary gland or if she is having infertility problems, irregular menstrual periods or to rule out problems with the pituitary gland or hypothalamus • In men a prolactin test is ordered if he displays the symptoms of prolactinoma or to investigate testicular or erectile dysfunction or to rule out problems with the pituitary gland or hypothalamus
• Growth hormone (GH)	• Stimulates childhood growth, cell production, helps maintain muscle and bone mass in adults	Refer to Growth Hormone under the hypothalamus	• Measures the amount of human growth in the blood	• Too much growth hormone during childhood can cause a child to grow more than normal and too little growth hormone can cause a child to grow less than normal
• ACTH	• Stimulates cortisol production by the adrenal glands	Refer to Cortisol, challenge tests, and DHEA-S under adrenal glands	• Measures the level of adrenocorticotropic hormone (ACTH) in the blood	• A higher than normal level of ACTH may indicate the adrenal glands are not producing enough cortisol as in Addison's disease or Cushing's disease. A lower than normal level of ACTH may indicate the pituitary gland is not producing enough cortisol as in hypopituitarism
• TSH	• Stimulates thyroid hormone production	Thyroid-stimulating hormone levels (levels vary with age)	• Assists in the diagnoses of hypothyroidism, hyperthyroidism, and pituitary dysfunction	Increased Levels • Congenital hypothyroidism • Primary hypothyroidism • Thyroiditis • Secondary hyperthyroidism related to hyperactive pituitary Decreased Levels • Graves' disease • Primary hyperthyroidism • Secondary hypothyroidism
• LH, FSH	• Regulation of testosterone and estrogen, fertility	Luteinizing hormone levels (levels vary with age and gender as well as menstrual phase in women)	• Assists in differentiating between primary and secondary causes of gonadal failure • Used to evaluate precocious puberty, both male and female infertility, and response to therapy used to induce ovulation	Increased Levels • Gonadal failure • Primary gonadal dysfunction • Anorchia Decreased Levels • Anorexia nervosa • Malnutrition • Pituitary or hypothalamic dysfunction • Severe stress
		Follicle-stimulating hormone levels (levels vary with age, gender, and menstrual phase)	• Assists in differentiating between primary and secondary causes of gonadal failure (i.e., pituitary or hypothalamic) • Used in fertility testing	Increased Levels • Gonadal failure • Gonadotropin-secreting pituitary tumors • Klinefelter's syndromes • Orchitis • Precocious puberty • Primary hypogonadism • Turner's syndrome

(continued)

Table 27-3 Common Laboratory Tests for Endocrine Conditions (continued)

Hormone Produced	Function/ Description	Common Tests of Endocrine Function	Purpose of Test	Significance of Results as Related to the Endocrine System
Pituitary Gland				
• LH, FSH (continued)			• Evaluates early sexual development and maturation failure • Assists in diagnosing menstrual disturbances and gynecomastia	Decreased Levels • Anorexia nervosa • Anterior pituitary hypofunction • Hypothalamic disorders • Polycystic ovary disease • Sickle cell anemia • Pregnancy
Testes				
• Testosterone	• Male sexual characteristics	Testosterone levels (levels vary by age and gender)	• Assists in diagnosing hypergonadism, precocious puberty, and male infertility • Differentiates between primary and secondary hypogonadism	Increased Levels • Adrenal hyperplasia • Adrenocortical and gonadal tumors • Hyperthyroidism • Idiopathic sexual precocity • Polycystic ovaries Decreased Levels • Anovulation • Cryptorchidism • Delayed puberty • Down syndrome • Klinefelter's syndrome • Primary and secondary hypopituitarism • Malnutrition
Thyroid Gland				
• T_4 (thyroxine)	• Helps regulate the rate of metabolism	Total and free thyroxine levels (T_4) (levels vary with age and gender)	• Assesses for signs of hypothyroidism or hyperthyroidism • Monitors response to therapy for hypothyroidism or hyperthyroidism	Increased Levels • Hyperthyroidism • Hypothyroidism treated with T_4 • Thyrotoxicosis caused by Graves' disease • Obesity • Excess intake of iodine • Acute psychiatric illness • Hepatitis Decreased Levels • Hypothyroidism • Strenuous exercise • Late stage pregnancy
• T_3 (triiodothyronine)	• Helps regulate the rate of metabolism	Total and free triiodothyronine levels (T_3) (levels vary with age and pregnancy status)	• Assists in diagnosing T_3 toxicosis and assessing for TSH and T_4	Increased Levels • Hyperthyroidism • Iodine deficiency • Pregnancy • T_3 toxicosis • Treated hyperthyroidism Decreased Levels • Hypothyroidism • Malnutrition • Late stage pregnancy
• Calcitonin	• Helps regulate bone status, blood calcium	Calcitonin and Calcitonin Stimulation Tests (levels vary by gender)	• Assists in diagnosing hyperparathyroidism and thyroid cancer • Used to monitor serum calcium levels	Increased Levels • Hypercalcemia • Thyroid cancer • Chronic renal failure • Pancreatitis • Pernicious anemia • Pheochromocytoma • Thyroiditis Decreased Levels n.a.

Sources: Endocrine Syndromes (2011); Van Leeuwen, Poelhuis-Leth, & Bladh (2011).

growth rate and eventually reaches a normal adult height. Another important aspect of nursing care includes patient and family teaching about the condition and its treatment and providing as much support as possible. Parents need to be taught about GH replacement therapy, its preparation, and administration of the subcutaneous injections. Just as with other daily subcutaneous injections, rotating sites, potential side effects, and actions to take if necessary must be taught to the parents. Parents are prompted to think of ideas that would decrease the child's stress regarding the daily injections. Help the patient and family plan and understand individual patient goals and the progress made toward achievement. Typically the most important goal is improved growth and psychological acceptance of body image. Help the family to monitor the status of these vital outcomes.

clinical alert

Accurate growth measurements

When a child is diagnosed with GHD, careful and consistent growth measurements are essential as well as plotting the measurements on the appropriate growth chart. The nurse may require training in how to properly weigh or measure the child. The CDC Web page (http://www.cdc.gov) has information about body mass index for children and teens outlining proper technique for home measurements, which may also be useful in the clinical environment (CDC, 2011).

focus on safety

Daily weights to ensure accurate medication doses

When the child is hospitalized, daily weights may be performed for the purposes of recalculating medication dosages. A conscientious nurse may notice if the dose ordered is now inaccurate based on the most current weight. Often in today's high-tech environment, the electronic medical record may alert the nurse or the pharmacist if the dosage is inappropriate. Weighing in kilograms is often more accurate because many medications are dosed in kilograms for the pediatric population.

Medical Care. Medical management includes the administration of human recombinant GH (replacement therapy with daily subcutaneous injections). Recombinant human GH is a safe treatment for children with idiopathic short stature, but it is not without its adverse reactions. Be aware of all possible side effects of replacement GH, including increased intracranial pressure (ICP), gynecomastia, arthralgia, and edema. Children who complain of a headache must be carefully monitored because this may be the only sign of ICP. Managing these side effects may require a temporary reduction or cessation of the GH dose. This therapy can decrease a child's sensitivity to insulin, causing hyperglycemia. Other side effects of human growth hormone medications are outlined in Table 27-4.

Education/Discharge Instructions

Children with GHD can be small framed and of short stature. It is important to stress to the family to treat the child for his or her age, not size. Frequently, teachers or other adults treat a child with GHD differently than a child of the same age and normal size. Children with GHD are

Table 27-4	Side Effects of Human Growth Hormone Medications
System	**Adverse Reactions**
Cardiovascular	• Mild edema of the hands and feet • Hypertension
Central Nervous System	• Headache • Intracranial hypertension • Insomnia • Fever, malaise, and dizziness with the use of somatropin (Zorbtive)
Dermatological	• Rash • Increased growth of preexisting nevi • Local lipoatrophy or lipodystrophy with subcutaneous administration • Exacerbation of psoriasis with use of somatropin (Saizen)
Endocrine and Metabolic	• Hyperglycemia • Hypothyroidism • Insulin resistance
Gastrointestinal	• Pancreatitis • Flatulence, vomiting, nausea, abdominal pain, gastritis, gastroenteritis, pharyngitis with the use of somatropin (Zorbtive)
Hematological	• Slight risk of developing leukemia
Local	• Pain at injection site
Neuromuscular and Skeletal	• Arthralgia • Carpal tunnel syndrome • Pain in the hip and back • Scoliosis • Myalgia • Weakness
Otic	• Otitis media
Renal	• Glycosuria
Respiratory	• Rhinitis
Miscellaneous	• Flu-like symptoms • Hypersensitivity reactions

Sources: Taketomo et al. (2012); Vallerand & Sanoski (2014).

encouraged to play sports of all types if they are able to compete because size does not always determine ability. They are encouraged to dress age-appropriately. Supporting the family to help the child attain a positive self-image is of the utmost importance. The nurse helps the child realize that self-determination and confidence, not height, achieve goals. Classmates can sometimes be insensitive to the child's feelings and can even tease the untreated short child. Adolescence, because of the focus on body image, can be an especially difficult time. It is best to begin treatment as early as possible before the psychological effects of short stature may have a lasting impact.

Encourage parents to take the child with GHD to the dentist regularly because the GH treatments cause the child's teeth to be softer and much more susceptible to cavities.

Also provide parents with appropriate supportive resources. Specific foundations have Web sites that allow families to network with other families undergoing the same treatment. Some reliable resources include the Human Growth Foundation and the Magic Foundation (http://www.magicfoundation.org/www), which includes online videos that address this topic. Even though these videos are for adults, they may help the family to explain the disease to the child. The University of Kansas Medical Center Genetics Education Center has a Web site (http://www.kumc.edu/gec/) with a wealth of knowledge regarding genetic diseases including those that affect stature. These Web sites may offer solutions to financial support because the GH treatments can be expensive, and even with insurance the family may have high co-pays. The drug companies that provide GH replacement products have assistance programs for families who cannot pay for the treatments (Human Growth Foundation, 2012; The Magic Foundation, 2013; University of Kansas Medical Center Genetics Education Center, 2012).

"What to say"—*Helping children express themselves*

Children can be apprehensive about daily injections of any kind. It is important for the nurse to be as honest as possible regarding the GH treatments. For example, a nurse does not tell a child that an injection will not hurt. The nurse can help the child express her or his feelings by asking the following questions:

- "How do you feel?"
- "What do you tell your friends about your condition and the GH medication?"
- "How have you changed since the GH treatments began?"
- "What advice do you have for other children beginning GH treatment?"

Collaboration in Caring—*A team approach*

The nurse can make referrals for psychological counseling for the child or family if warranted. Even when the nurse is not certain about the child's psyche, a referral can be made and the decision left to the specialist.

Pituitary Hyperfunction

Pituitary hyperfunction, or precocious puberty (early or premature), is a condition that occurs with overactivity of the pituitary gland. Generally, puberty occurs between 8 and 13 years of age in girls and between 9½ and 14 in boys. In girls, precocious puberty begins when any of the following secondary sexual characteristics develop before 8 years of age: breasts, armpit or pubic hair, mature external genitalia, and the first menstruation. In boys, precocious puberty begins when any of the following secondary sexual characteristics occur before 9 years of age: mature external genitalia; growth of body hair, including facial, underarm, abdominal, chest, and pubic hair; increase in size of and mass of muscles; deepening of the voice; and change in the shape of the face and skeleton.

Most often, precocious puberty is idiopathic in girls. The incidence is about 5 times higher in girls than in boys

(Kaplowitz, 2013). Precocious puberty is caused by central nervous system (CNS) abnormalities, or lesions such as a benign hypothalamic tumor; other types of brain tumor; or brain injury. Other known causes include post-infections (encephalitis or meningitis); congenital adrenal hyperplasia; tumors of the ovary, adrenal gland or testicle; exogenous sources; or androgens.

Signs and Symptoms

Similar characteristics of precocious puberty appear in boys and girls as well as ones specific to each sex. In boys, the following signs and symptoms may be seen:

- Facial hair
- Penile growth
- Increased masculinity
- Testicular enlargement
- Voice changes

In girls these characteristic signs and symptoms are likely:

- Breast development
- Onset of menarche
- Ovary enlargement
- Cysts on ovaries

Commonly seen in both boys and girls are the following:

- Axillary hair
- Pubic hair
- Body odor
- Acne
- Emotional lability
- Mood swings
- Growth spurts in height
- Advanced bone age equals increased skeletal growth, which in turn equals increased height initially. If untreated, epiphyseal plates (growth plates) close early and growth stops.

Diagnosis

Blood tests to diagnose this condition include measurement of luteinizing hormone (LH), follicle-stimulating hormone (FSH), testosterone, or estradiol. Testing to stimulate the release of gonadotropins confirms the diagnosis. In addition, radiological studies are used to calculate the child's bone age. Because of the high incidence of CNS involvement, skull computed tomography (CT) and/or MRI is usually indicated.

The nursing assessment includes a complete history and assessment of the child's pubertal status. This includes a Tanner staging of sexual maturation documenting breast, genital, pubic hair, and testicular development. Growth charts demonstrate the exact age of the linear growth spike. The history also includes exposure to hormones, CNS infection or trauma, and the family history of the age at puberty onset.

Prevention

Pituitary hyperfunction cannot be prevented. Some of the risk factors for precocious puberty, such as sex and race, can't be avoided; although, risk factors can be reduced by ensuring that the child avoids external sources of estrogen and testosterone such as can be found in prescription medications for adults or dietary supplements containing

focus on safety

Exogenous hormones

Many commercially purchased female products contain estrogen. Facial creams, hair products, and other "beauty" aids can contain hormones or placenta extracts. Some shampoos specifically marketed to African Americans have been found to contain hormones. Children can readily absorb enough of these exogenous hormones to present with precocious puberty.

The nurse must alert parents of the dangers of hidden toxins in everyday products that can harm their children. They must also be cognizant of "endocrine disruptors," which are found on the National Institute of Environmental Health Sciences (NIEHS) Web site (http://www.niehs.nih.gov/).

estrogen or testosterone. Medication compliance, stress reduction, and maintaining a normal weight are also preventive activities.

Collaborative Care

Nursing Care. The nurse assists in providing treatment for precocious puberty. Help monitor the success of the treatment by using the correct growth charts and facilitating blood levels of gonadotropins and sex steroids. When treatments are stopped, puberty promptly begins. Consistent, accurate record keeping of the child's growth rate must be documented because while on treatment, the child's growth rate declines. Continue to assess and document the progression or regression of the child's secondary sex characteristics. Nursing care also focuses on the accuracy of medication delivery. Provide accurate information to both the child and the family about medication preparation, action, and administration techniques.

Medical Care. Treatment for CNS tumors may involve resection or radiation of the lesion. Pharmaceutical treatment includes gonadotropin-releasing hormone (GnRH) agonists, which, in the past, were given via subcutaneous injection daily or as a depot injection once every 3 to 4 weeks. More recently, a 3-month formulation has shown great promise. Histrelin or Supprelin LA is a permanent implant device that automatically releases the inhibitor subcutaneously over the course of the year. The child is monitored by an endocrinologist and returns each year for a new implant until he or she reaches an age when puberty will normally occur. These treatments suppress the release of gonadotropins by acting on the pituitary gland (Kaplowitz, 2013; Taketomo, Hodding, & Kraus, 2012). Treatments cause a decrease in growth rate and a stabilization or regression in development of secondary sexual characteristics; size of the breasts, ovaries, uterus, and testes as well as erection frequency all decrease.

Education/Discharge Instructions

It is important to approach the child in a manner appropriate to his or her level of emotional and cognitive development. Information provided to both the child and family includes the physical changes that the child is experiencing as well as on the child's disturbed body image. Help is given to the child and family about manner of dress. Loosely fitting clothing may help to conceal the abruptly changing body image. The nurse can also make referrals to a therapist.

Depending on the age of the child, he or she can be included in the teaching as much as appropriate. Providing information about normal development during puberty helps the caregivers and the child understand the physical and emotional changes that occur with the early onset of puberty. Most importantly, the nurse guides the family toward evidence-based methods and away from fads and crazes.

 Optimizing Outcomes—**Financial resources**

Helping the parents identify financial resources for assistance if necessary ensures the best outcomes of the care and treatments given. GnRH analog depot treatments are very costly and can range from $700 to $1,000 per injection. These treatments are usually covered by the insurance companies, but some require the injection to be given in the health-care provider's office. For those with limited insurance resources, some pharmaceutical companies provide assistance and give treatments at limited or no cost.

 Across Care Settings: **Referrals**

Precocious puberty has an effect on the child and family both psychologically and psychosocially. It is important for the primary care pediatrician to make referrals to an endocrinologist and psychologist as soon as possible. Especially in very young children, early referrals can help to prevent serious psychological trauma and help the child begin to adjust to his or her changing body. Communication among members of the entire team is essential for ongoing collaboration and the best possible outcomes.

Gigantism and Acromegaly

Although both gigantism and acromegaly have the same cause, they are different in assessment and management. Acromegaly occurs in adulthood when the long bones of the legs and arms have stopped growing (Understanding Acromegaly, n.d.). As an adult disease, it will not be discussed further in this chapter.

In children, before closure of the bone growth plates, the condition is known as gigantism. Gigantism is caused by large amounts of GH resulting in excessive growth of the long bones in a child. Gigantism is a rare disease that affects about 3 to 6 out of every million people in the United States. Gigantism is caused by the uncontrolled hypersecretion of GH by the pituitary. In most cases, the cause of this excessive production of GH is a noncancerous tumor on the pituitary. Rarely, gigantism may be associated with other diseases such as multiple endocrine neoplasms, McCune Albright syndrome, neurofibromatosis, or Carney complex (Diaz-Thomas, 2012).

Children affected by gigantism can grow to extraordinary heights and are usually greater than 2 standard deviations above expected height. It also affects the child's muscle and organ growth, making the child look very large for his or her age. It may be noted as early as the sixth to ninth month of life. Gigantism involves changes in the way the body functions and can delay puberty. Over time, these changes can cause complications (such as cardiomegaly or tumors) that can be life threatening (Diaz-Thomas, 2012). Diabetes has been reported. Early diagnosis and treatment can prevent irreversible changes that may ultimately lead to a premature death. Mortality rates can be two to four times higher in these patients because of the strain this excessive growth has on the vital organs, such as the heart (Diaz-Thomas, 2012).

 Nursing Insight—Understanding acromegaly/ gigantism

To understand the causes and treatment of acromegaly/ gigantism, the nurse understands the three important hormones that circulate throughout the body to regulate many of the body's most basic activities:

- Growth hormone (GH)
  - The pituitary releases GH in short spurts throughout the day and night, resulting in constantly varying GH levels.
  - When a person has gigantism, abnormally high levels of GH are released by the pituitary. Too much GH causes changes in physical characteristics and other aspects of the body.
- Insulin-like growth factor (IGF-1)
  - IGF-1 levels rise whenever GH levels rise, but IGF-1 is released more evenly than GH, and IGF-1 levels remain higher longer.
- Somatostatin
  - Somatostatin controls the amount of GH in the body.
  - This knowledge has led to the development of treatments for gigantism.
  - Somatostatin analogs last much longer than natural somatostatin providing better control over excessive GH levels.

Signs and Symptoms

The signs and symptoms of gigantism may include the following:

- Rapid growth during childhood combined with obesity
- Swelling of soft tissue
- Skin tags
- Muscle weakness
- Fatigue
- Skin changes (thickening, oiliness, acne, and hirsutism)
- Coarsening of facial features, including forehead, nose, lips, tongue, and jaw.

Besides the changes in appearance, gigantism produces body function changes like the following:

- Arthralgia (arthritis-like joint pain)
- Delayed onset of puberty
- Amenorrhea or irregular menstruation in girls
- Excessive perspiration (hyperhidrosis) (Diaz-Thomas, 2012)

Diagnosis

The best way to diagnose acromegaly is to measure serum GH levels after an overnight fast and then again after giving a glucose drink (oral glucose tolerance test). A glucose ingestion of 75 grams would lower a healthy person's GH level to less than 1 ng/mL. In a child with gigantism and an overproduction of GH, this reduction would not be seen.

As a response to increases in GH, insulin-like growth factor (IGF-1), produced in the liver, also increases. IGF-1 levels are much more stable over time than GH; therefore, it provides a more reliable test than GH levels.

Because more than 90% of children with gigantism suffer from benign tumors of the pituitary gland (an adenoma), other tests such as head scans by MRI or by CT look specifically for pituitary growths or tumors. These tumors are usually the source of the excessive GH secretion.

Prevention

Because gigantism cannot be prevented, care involves early diagnosis and treatment, which can prevent irreversible changes that can ultimately lead to a premature death. Progressive, untreated disease can cause serious complications, such as hypertension, cardiomyopathy, and subsequent cardiovascular disease, osteoarthritis, diabetes mellitus, polyps of the colon, sleep apnea, carpal tunnel syndrome, hypopituitarism, uterine fibroid tumors, spinal cord compression, and vision loss. The focus of care is aimed at preventing the numerous complications of this condition. The nurse must remember that lifelong monitoring and evaluation are vital to maintain optimal health. This is a very rare disorder, with few clinical examples in pediatrics. Multi-team efforts can help to extend and normalize life as much as possible. The earliest interventions can help prevent many serious complications that can lead to a premature death.

Collaborative Care

Nursing Care. Provide supportive, assistive care toward achieving the goal of the treatment plan. An accurate assessment is one of the most important aspects of clinical care. Using the correct growth chart and meticulously documenting height and weight will allow the nurse to track changes at each outpatient visit. When a child is affected by gigantism, the patterns of abnormal growth are quite recognizable. Rather than just unusual tallness, there is a characteristic body build consisting of heavy thick bones, especially jaw, and unusually large hands and feet. The nurse is cognizant of types and normal ranges of laboratory values. In addition to assessment, understand the uses and side effects of the medication that the child receives. Medication regimens, including how to administer subcutaneous injections, and the importance of regular health-care provider visits are part of family education.

Medical Care. Medication is the treatment of choice if surgery cannot be performed or if the surgeon cannot completely remove the tumor. Somatostatin analogs or dopamine agonists are effective in reducing the release of GH secretion. The dopamine agonists are often used as an adjunct to somatostatin analogs such as octreotide. Somatostatin analogs are given with a pump or long-acting depot injections. A newer preparation of GH-receptor antagonists have shown promise in the adult population but have not been studied in children (Diaz-Thomas, 2012; Eugster, 2011).

Surgical Care. If there is a tumor, surgical removal is warranted. It has been found that surgery is the curative treatment of choice in 80% of the cases. Postsurgical care after pituitary tumor excision requires precise critical neurosurgical care. Neurological and vital signs are taken frequently. Depending on the surgical site (sometimes it is removed through the nasal passage), care also includes observations and documentation of dressing, wound, and drainage. The first dressing change is often done by the surgeon or advanced practice nurse. Each hospital will have a distinct protocol or health-care provider's order set regarding the appropriate postoperative care.

Radiation is not recommended in children because of the complications and side effects to other bodily functions. Gamma knife radiation can pinpoint the beam of radiation to a specific spot but affects other growth hormone functions. If used at all in children, it is used with caution (Diaz-Thomas, 2012; Eugster, 2011).

Education/Discharge Instructions

Follow-up home care may be needed in some cases depending on the status of the child's health and the resources available to the family. In the first few weeks of treatment, the family will benefit if a home-health nurse reinforces the discharge teaching and gives them a sense of confidence regarding the medication delivery and care of the child.

CONDITIONS OF THE POSTERIOR PITUITARY

Diabetes Insipidus

Antidiuretic hormone (ADH) acts on the kidneys to conserve water by controlling the kidneys' urine output. ADH is secreted by the hypothalamus and stored in the posterior pituitary gland before it is released into the bloodstream. When sufficient ADH is secreted, the amount of urine output is decreased to avoid dehydration. Diabetes insipidus (DI) is a hypofunction of the posterior pituitary gland and is classified in two ways: by either a deficient production of ADH or lack of response to ADH. *Neurogenic* (central DI) occurs when the production or secretion of ADH is insufficient because of damage to the pituitary gland or hypothalamus. *Nephrogenic* DI is the lack of the kidney's appropriate response to normal levels of ADH. In children, this is most often a genetic cause that is discovered early in life (Bichet, 2011; Srivatsa, Majzoub, & Kappy, 2010). When a child has diabetes insipidus, there is insufficient ADH resulting in excessive production of extremely dilute urine, causing the child to be excessively thirsty.

 Nursing Insight—*The classes of diabetes insipidus have differing etiologies*

Central diabetes insipidus (or neurogenic) is caused by damage directly to the pituitary gland, such as head injury, neurosurgery, a genetic disorder, and other diseases. *Nephrogenic* diabetes insipidus is related to a problem in the kidney caused by drugs or chronic disorders, such as kidney failure, sickle cell disease, or polycystic kidney disease. Generally occurring *suddenly*, diabetes insipidus can be a result of either medical or surgical conditions:

Surgical (most common causes):

- Damage caused by neurosurgery (i.e., hypothalamus or pituitary gland)
- Brain injury or tumor excisions

Medical (most common causes):

- Hypothalamus malfunction (insufficient ADH production)
- Pituitary gland malfunction (ADH is not released into the bloodstream)
- Vascular abnormalities or cerebral vascular accident, or "stroke"
- Infection
- Encephalitis—brain inflammation
- Meningitis—inflammation of meninges
- Sarcoidosis—inflammation of the lymph nodes and other tissues throughout the body
- Tuberculosis—infectious disease
- Family heredity—genetic defect (Greenbaum, 2011; Srivatsa et al., 2010)

Signs and Symptoms

Diabetes insipidus causes an excessive production of extremely dilute urine leading to excessive thirst. Symptoms in the infant include the following (Zeitler, Travers, Nadeau, Barker, Kelsey, & Kappy, 2011):

- Poor feeding
- Failure to thrive
- Fussiness
- Frequent saturated diapers
- Vomiting
- Constipation

Symptoms in the older child and teen may include:

- Irritability
- Excessive thirst (polydipsia)
- Excessive urine production (polyuria)
- Craving for cold water
- Enuresis (nocturnal bed wetting)
- Nocturia

Children of all ages may experience:

- Vomiting
- Constipation
- Fevers
- Dry skin
- Weight loss (Ward, 2013)

Diagnosis

After a complete history, physical examination, and daily log of fluid and dietary intake and output patterns (polyuria greater than 2 L/m²), the first morning urine is usually collected after an overnight fast and subsequently

 clinical alert

Dehydration

Dehydration can be seen in all cases, causing the infant or child to be irritable with many other manifestations, including dry mucous membranes, decreased skin turgor, decreased tears when crying, sunken fontanelle, and tachycardia. If dehydration is severe, the child's pulse may be "thready" and very rapid. Hypotension may also be present and could lead to hypovolemic shock. If dehydration occurs, it is important to administer IV fluids.

focus on safety

Ways to prevent IV infiltration

Inserting an IV in children can be challenging. The IV insertion sites are small and delicate. In addition, during an insertion, a child may wiggle or thrash around, making the procedure difficult. The vessel walls can become easily damaged. Ways to prevent IV infiltration include:

- Use clear tape to secure the IV site.
- Use an armboard to secure the site.
- Avoid using butterfly needles for infusions.
- Assess the site and surrounding tissue hourly.
- Avoid opaque restrictive dressing wrapped around the site.
- Use a vein viewer or a transilluminator when inserting an IV.
- Tape the IV insertions area securely enough to stabilize the site without causing constriction.

tested for urine specific gravity. The serum is also tested for osmolarity and sodium. Hyperdilute urine (specific gravity of 1.005 or less) with elevated serum osmolarity (greater than 290 Osmol/kg) and serum sodium (as high as 170 mEq/L) confirms the diagnosis. Diagnosis can be difficult in infants because they naturally excrete dilute urine. A 24-hour urine collection determines total daily urine output (Zeitler et al., 2011).

Diagnostic Tools   Diagnosis of Diabetes Insipidus

The definitive diagnosis of diabetes insipidus can be made with a water deprivation test. This test will also discern the type of DI (i.e., neurogenic or nephrogenic). This test requires close supervision of the patient's vital signs, weight, and lab tests (i.e., urine and serum osmolality as well as serum sodium as often as every hour). The usual protocol for monitoring is every 2 hours for the first 4 hours, and then hourly. During this test, the child may become febrile and develop hypotension. The test starts after breakfast and the first void. After body weight, serum osmolality, and sodium are measured, the child is deprived of fluid until dehydration occurs. The child is weighed according to protocol, which may be as often as every 2 hours, allowing no more than 2% to 5% loss of body weight (Bichet, 2011; Miller, Libber, & Plotnick, 2009). Each time the child voids, the urine is measured for volume, osmolality, and specific gravity. The serum sodium and osmolality are obtained after the first 4 hours and then every 2 hours following. The test can be stopped if the specific gravity is 1.020 or higher, urine osmolality is greater than 600 mOsmol/kg, serum osmolality is greater than 300 mOsmol/kg, serum sodium is greater than 145 mEq/L, body weight loss is greater than 5%, the child shows signs of volume depletion, or there are time constraints. The infant younger than 6 months is not deprived of water more than 6 hours, a child between 6 to 24 months is not deprived longer than 8 hours, and the child older than 24 months is not deprived more than 12 hours. Upon termination, the weight, vital signs, plasma sodium, plasma and urine osmolality, and urine specific gravity are obtained. A specimen is also sent for levels of plasma ADH, which is increased after dehydration tests in patients with hereditary nephrogenic DI.

This test is not done on newborns or young infants. The alternate test is to give desmopressin and measure the urine osmolality at baseline and every 30 minutes for 2 hours. If there is no increase in the urine osmolality (at least 100 mOsmol/L above baseline) the infant may have hereditary nephrogenic DI. Subsequent DNA testing for mutation will confirm the diagnosis (Bichet, 2011; Miller et al., 2009).

Prevention

Prevention of DI may not always be possible. In many cases, the condition is present at birth (congenital). DI may also be caused by head trauma, neurosurgery, or infection. Medication

compliance and access to water are needed to prevent dehydration. Children and families also need to plan ahead by carrying water with them and by keeping a supply of medication available everywhere (e.g., school or travel). A medical alert bracelet or medical alert card is also encouraged.

Collaborative Care

Nursing Care. It is important for the nurse to remember that a diet low in solutes helps this condition. Generally, infants are given breast milk because it is naturally low in solutes. Protein content in diets should be about 6% of an infant's diet and only 8% of a young child's caloric intake. This should be enough to allow normal growth but not cause a solute excess.

Closely monitor the child for subtle signs of impending dehydration or fluid imbalance by closely monitoring urine output and fluid intake. This is best done through daily weights. This nursing task is performed using standard conditions (e.g., same scale, infant completely undressed including diaper, and young child in underwear with socks only). Output measurements must also be exact and include weighing diapers in grams for infants. All urine is caught in a container or urinal to enable precise measurement in milliliters. Any diapers containing stool are identified. Each institution may have a unique protocol on measuring mixed stool and urine diapers. Accurate documentation is essential to professional communication.

Caring for a child during the water deprivation test can be difficult. The child becomes very irritable because of thirst, and it may be difficult for the child to understand why he or she cannot drink. It will take patience on the part of the parents and nursing staff as the child becomes more and more irritable. The nurse and parents can alternate holding and comforting the child as well as using distraction methods.

This condition demands close monitoring of the fluid and electrolyte balance to prevent complications (Miller et al., 2009). Family involvement is the key to successful home management. Common gastrointestinal illnesses that either increase fluid needs or decrease intake must be identified, and the nurse must alert parents to the seriousness of these conditions that can lead to life-threatening fluid and electrolyte imbalances.

clinical alert

Hypernatremic dehydration

Poor skin turgor or tenting of abdominal skin is not always seen. When the child has hypernatremic dehydration, skin turgor is not decreased despite the state of dehydration (Srivatsa et al., 2010). Hypernatremia places the child at an increased risk for seizures. If left untreated, diabetes insipidus can cause a child to have brain damage and impaired mental function such as retardation or attention-deficit/hyperactive disorder (ADHD), short attention span, or restlessness (Srivatsa et al., 2010).

Medical Care. The health-care provider will differentiate between central (neurogenic) and nephrogenic diabetes insipidus before decisions are made regarding treatments and nursing care. For central diabetes insipidus, when polyuria is persistent, intranasal, parenteral, or oral doses of desmopressin (DDAVP) are the treatments of choice.

The diuretic hydrochlorothiazide (Microzide) is given in combination with chlorpropamide (a sulfonylurea compound) to decrease urine volume by up to 75%. Accurate administration of medications is a key factor when providing nursing care. The intranasal form of desmopressin (DDAVP) may be difficult to give. Special care is taken to give the medication accurately and to teach the parents proper administration.

Nephrogenic diabetes insipidus is not treated with DDAVP because of the pathology of the receptor sites, thus making the kidney unresponsive. In this setting, thiazide diuretics, a potassium-sparing diuretic, such as amiloride (Midamor), and a nonsteroidal prostaglandin, such as indomethacin (Indocin) or aspirin, are all useful treatments.

Education/Discharge Instructions

Patient and parent teaching, as with most conditions, is important. Early discovery and care of the child with diabetes insipidus is important. This condition demands close monitoring of the fluid and electrolyte balance to prevent complications (Miller et al., 2009). Family involvement is the key to successful home management. Helping the family by beginning a log of accurate intake, output, and daily weight while the child is still hospitalized can be the greatest asset and can optimize outcomes for this very challenging care situation. Parents must be taught to replace fluids in the very young child or infant because these patients cannot be relied on to accurately express thirst nor can these patients obtain a drink on their own.

 Collaboration in Caring—*Collaboration with parents*

Collaboration with the parents helps to manage the child's care at home. It is important to also keep the health-care provider alerted to episodes of dehydration. Early recognition of the disease, in addition to the ability to recognize excessive fluid losses and then replace these losses, is the key to long-term survival. A dietitian and pediatric endocrinologist will work closely with the health-care provider and the family to care for this child.

Syndrome of Inappropriate Antidiuretic Hormone

Syndrome of inappropriate antidiuretic hormone (SIADH) is caused when excessive levels of ADH are produced and is rare in children. ADH normally causes the kidneys to conserve water. This syndrome causes water retention and electrolyte imbalance—specifically decreased serum sodium. This is counterintuitive because despite a decrease

in osmolality and electrolytes, the body is still producing excessive ADH, causing more water reabsorption, thus leading to even more dilution and decrease in osmolality. Eventually, this results in water intoxication. The hypersecretion can be from overproduction in the hypothalamus or oversecretion from the posterior pituitary (Greenbaum, 2011; John & Day, 2012).

SIADH occurs most frequently in children with neonatal hypoxia, CNS infections, or intrathoracic disease in association with certain drugs (e.g., chlorpropamide, vincristine, imipramine, and phenothiazines) and can occur in postoperative patients (Srivatsa et al., 2010). Among premature neonates, the syndrome most often accompanies brain injury and is closely associated with intracranial hemorrhage. It can also be caused by hypoxia and positive pressure ventilation. In other cases, some medications (diuretics) and chemotherapy may produce ADH. Other causes may include the following: meningitis, encephalitis, brain tumors, psychosis, head trauma, Guillain-Barré syndrome, damage to the hypothalamus or pituitary gland during surgery, lung diseases, and positive pressure ventilation.

Signs and Symptoms

Children experience and express symptoms differently. Symptoms of SIADH may include:

- Nausea and vomiting
- Seizures
- Headache
- Muscle cramps
- Weakness
- Personality changes such as irritability, combativeness, confusion, drowsiness, hallucinations, stupor, and coma (John & Day, 2012),

Other signs and symptoms may include:

- Increased blood pressure
- Weight gain with no externally visible edema
- Decreased urine output despite a high specific gravity
- Fluid and electrolyte imbalance

As the electrolyte (especially sodium) levels decrease, the child becomes lethargic and confused. Often, if the child is old enough, complaints of a headache are also common. Eventually, altered levels of consciousness followed by seizures and coma can be seen.

Diagnosis

SIADH is diagnosed through laboratory testing.

 Diagnostic Tools Serum Levels

Laboratory serum levels are monitored and a diagnosis is confirmed when the following values are found (Srivatsa et al., 2010):
- High urine osmolality (greater than 1,200 Osmol/kg)
- High urine specific gravity (greater than 1.030)
- Urine sodium continues to reflect the intake of sodium despite low serum sodium
- Low serum osmolality (less than 275 mOsmol/kg)
- Low serum sodium (less than 135 mEq/L)
- Decreased blood urea nitrogen (less than 10 mg/dL)
- Decreased hematocrit
- Serum bicarbonate remains steady
- Serum potassium is usually normal

 Medication: Accurate Administration of Intranasal Medication Doses

Intranasal desmopressin (DDAVP) can be administered through a rhinal tube. Ensure the child blows his or her nose before the medication is given. Positioning the child on the side while the medication is given enhances the absorption of the medication. Children's Hospitals and Clinics of Minnesota, Family Services and Resources (2011) provide a well-written resource for medication administration.

Prevention

Because there is no clear underlying cause for SIADH, prevention includes attention to safety related to head trauma, good prenatal care, and avoidance of infectious diseases. Careful attention and recognition of symptoms, which may be experienced by the child with head trauma or infectious diseases, and referral or notification of the primary care provider can lead to quicker initiation and response to treatment.

Collaborative Care

Nursing Care. Fluid restriction is the most difficult aspect of nursing care. This restriction can be challenging to maintain, especially if the child is old enough to reach the sink or water fountain. Fluid intake by all routes must be recorded as intake. The nurse must meticulously monitor and record all intake and output. Sometimes, the placement of a Foley catheter is necessary or weighing soiled diapers in grams is needed to ensure accurate measurements of output. The nurse must remember to obtain the weight of a clean diaper so that it can be subtracted from that of the soiled diaper weight before recording the output. The child's family members must also be made aware of fluid restrictions and the need for careful monitoring and recording of intake and output.

Certain medications are given with meals to prevent any unnecessary fluid intake. If the child is thirsty, he or she can be offered hard candy to suck, providing the child's medical condition does not contraindicate the sugar. To prevent water reabsorption in the intestines, tap water and saline enemas are avoided. Irrigate all oral tubes with normal saline rather than with water to prevent pulling of sodium thus creating an even greater electrolyte imbalance. Oral mucous membranes can be kept moist by providing frequent mouth care. Avoid alcohol-based mouthwashes because these dry out the mucous membranes. The nurse must also monitor the child's nutritional status. A diet high in sodium and protein is encouraged because this increases urine excretion.

Neurological assessments are also imperative. Assessing level of consciousness, headache (if child can verbalize), and seizure activity can be indications of severe electrolyte imbalance. Seizure precautions must be set up and implemented at the bedside.

Finally, the nurse evaluates the child for fluid retention. When fluid retention is suspected, monitoring of input and output (I&O), baseline weight, and daily weight is essential. The nurse evaluates patients for edema in dependent areas and assesses the child's lungs to detect overhydration and monitor skin turgor carefully. Each of these assessments

focus on safety

Hyponatremia

It is critical to remember that the hyponatremia (low serum sodium of less than 125 mEq/L) may cause seizures in the child with SIADH. Keeping the serum sodium level near normal is the goal of treatment. The pediatric nurse must be thorough and accurately track intake, output, and daily weights of the child. Along with the primary health-care provider, an endocrinologist, often a nephrologist, a neurologist, and possibly a pediatric intensive care specialist may need to be consulted if the child manifests severe clinical, neurological symptoms.

must be clearly communicated to subsequent health-care provider and the nurse who will assume care for the child.

Medical Care. Medical management includes treating the underlying cause or disorder in addition to correcting the fluid and electrolyte imbalance. Fluid restriction is the cornerstone of care for a child with SIADH. Fluids are generally reduced to two-thirds of maintenance levels (Zeitler et al., 2011). Hypertonic sodium chloride solution is given if severe hyponatremia and severe neurological disease are present. Corticosteroids are given only when adrenal insufficiency is present. Vasopressin is effective in altering permeability of the renal collecting ducts, which allows for the reabsorption of water (Vallerand & Sanoski, 2014). Oral urea therapy has also been found to be an effective and safe treatment in children (Srivatsa et al., 2010).

Education/Discharge Instructions

Educating parents about the importance of fluid balance is a significant aspect of teaching the care of a child with SIADH. The family must also be taught that a daily weight of the child is the most important indicator of fluid balance. Maintaining fluid balance and avoiding excessive fluid intake is also emphasized. Be sure to include hidden sources of water in foods to optimize the outcomes of this child's care. Family members are taught to measure the urine output accurately, using whatever is appropriate for the child (e.g., diaper weights, urinal use, or toilet "hats"). In addition to teaching all of the care aspects for the child with SIADH, include basic information about SIADH and its causes, signs, and symptoms.

 Now Can You—Describe conditions of the anterior and posterior pituitary?

1. Describe conditions of the anterior pituitary?
2. Discuss nursing care for conditions of the anterior pituitary?
3. Describe conditions of the posterior pituitary?
4. Discuss nursing care for conditions of the posterior pituitary?

CONDITIONS OF THE THYROID

Hypothyroidism

Hypothyroidism is defined as thyroid insufficiency. In hypothyroidism, the thyroid gland is underactive and secretes too little thyroid hormone for the body to function normally. If left untreated, hypothyroidism can lead to a goiter. The thyroid gland secretes thyroid hormones, which control the speed of metabolism. Brain development, as well as the normal growth of the child, depends on normal levels of thyroid hormone. Hypothyroidism was once referred to as cretinism and was thought to be a major cause of severe mental retardation, but this view is not held today. Infants can be born with congenital hypothyroidism; acquired hypothyroidism can develop in children of any age. Congenital hypothyroidism affects about one in every 4,000 newborns in North America and is usually caused by dysgenesis or disorders of embryogenesis (Jospe, 2011). In older children and young adults, hypothyroidism can also cause diverse symptoms including slowed heart rate, chronic tiredness, and inability to tolerate cold. The child may feel physically tired and mentally fatigued, thus learning may be impaired.

Disorders of intrathyroid metabolism or goitrous congenital hypothyroidism are uncommon and are demonstrated by low levels of thyroxine and triiodothyronine and high levels of FSH, with consequent goiter formation (Jospe, 2011). The incidence of this type of disorder is one in 30,000 live births (Jospe, 2011).

Hashimoto's thyroiditis is the most common cause of acquired hypothyroidism in children and is also known as autoimmune or lymphocytic thyroiditis (Jospe, 2011). Hashimoto's thyroiditis is 25% to 35% more common among family members, in girls with the incidence peaking during adolescents, and the most common cause of goiter (Jospe, 2011; Zeitler et al., 2011). Other causes of acquired hypothyroidism include thyroidectomy, subacute thyroiditis, cranial or spinal radiation, or exposure to goitrogenic drugs such as lithium, iodine, thioamides, or resorcinol (Whittemore, Smaldone, & Steiner, 2013).

Signs and Symptoms

Hypothyroidism has varying levels of manifestations from subtle (in infancy) to overt (as the child matures).

In an infant, the signs and symptoms include:

- Prolonged newborn jaundice
- Poor feeding
- Constipation
- Cool, mottled skin
- Hypotonia
- Increased sleepiness
- Decreased crying
- Larger fontanelles
- Umbilical hernia
- Large, thick tongue

As the child begins to grow and mature, manifestation of hypothyroidism may include:

- Short stature for age
- Delayed dentition
- Delays in major developmental milestones
- Weight gain
- Hypotonia
- Puffy facial features
- Severe mental retardation
- Protruding abdomen
- Umbilical hernia
- Thick, dry, scaly, pale or mottled skin
- Sparse, coarse, dry or brittle hair

Symptoms in the older child are more overt and much like those found in the adult. These symptoms include:

- Bradycardia
- Fatigue
- Hypothermia
- Hoarse voice
- Dry, flaky skin
- Puffiness in the face (especially around the eyes)
- Impaired memory and difficulty in thinking (appears as a learning disability)
- Drowsiness, even after sleeping through the night
- Delayed or arrested puberty
- Heavy or irregular menstrual periods (in girls at the age of puberty)
- Constipation

Diagnosis

Congenital hypothyroidism is usually detected during the routine newborn screening. Every state in the United States requires routine neonatal screening by the measurement of thyroid-stimulating hormone (TSH) values in the cord blood or through a heel stick (Jospe, 2011). Positive newborn screening results are confirmed by a serum sample. Abnormally low levels of thyroxine (T_4) and high TSH confirm the findings (Zeitler et al., 2011, p. 955). Further diagnosis may include a scan of the thyroid gland to establish the cause of congenital hypothyroidism though it is not necessary because it does not impact the treatment (Zeitler et al., 2011).

Prevention

It is essential that the nurse is aware that congenital hypothyroidism is an important cause of mental retardation. Complications are preventable with the earliest identification and subsequent treatment. Educating parents regarding the signs and symptoms helps to identify the condition early so treatment can be started as soon as possible. It is important to inform families who have infants with this condition that lifetime treatment does prevent mental retardation. Newborn lab results must be assessed, and follow-up for any abnormal results is mandatory. The most common cause of hypothyroidism in the United States is Hashimoto's thyroiditis, which cannot be prevented. Although hypothyroidism is not preventable, intellectual disabilities and delayed growth and development may be reduced or prevented through prompt recognition and treatment.

Collaborative Care

Nursing Care. Nursing care is based on the child's response to the illness. The main focus of care is to educate the family on the importance of compliance with the medication regimen, periodic monitoring of thyroid function, and on establishing a normal pattern of growth without complications.

Medical Care. The focus of medical management is treatment with thyroid hormone replacement therapy. Children with hypothyroidism are treated with levothyroxine sodium (Synthroid). Doses are determined based on age and weight. Iodine supplementation is also appropriate in some cases. The easiest supplements are given in the diet. The goal of treatment is normal hormone levels within the infant's first 4 weeks of life. Frequent visits to the health-care provider for follow-up blood tests and adjustments of the dose are necessary. Once the child's hormone levels are properly adjusted, return outpatient visits are needed every 2 to 3 months for the first 3 years of life. Thyroid hormone treatment may be needed for life; treatment is simple, inexpensive, and easily monitored.

 Nursing Insight—*Formula*

Soy-based formula may cause a decrease in the absorption of levothyroxine (Synthroid). Switching an infant from a milk-based formula to a soy-based formula may increase the dose of thyroid hormone needed to maintain a euthyroid status (having a normally functioning thyroid gland) (Bhatia, Greer, & the Committee on Nutrition, 2008).

Education/Discharge Instructions

Educating the parents about the disorder and on the treatment plan is the main focus of teaching. Parents need to be instructed on methods that can be used to administer the medication as well as about adverse effects. Parents are taught proper administration of the medication. The pills can be crushed in a spoon, dissolved with a small amount of water or other liquid immediately before administration, and administered to the child with a syringe, dropper, or nipple (Taketomo et al., 2012).

Parents need to be informed that careful and regular monitoring of the child's growth, weight gain, and developmental milestone progression helps to validate that the dosing and medication administration are sufficiently accurate to achieve positive results. Laboratory blood tests of T_4 and TSH every 4 to 6 months during the first year of life and every 2 to 4 months afterward also keep close track of the child's hormone levels. Parents are encouraged to seek early evaluation and intervention to any problems that become readily recognizable. Educating the parents completely at the very beginning regarding the diagnosis, its signs and symptoms, care, treatment, and outcomes of care ensures that they know what to watch for and are aware of the most effective care possible. For children whose condition is not rapidly diagnosed or treated, the return of normal thyroid function may take a long time. The child may exhibit dramatic changes in behavior. Continued care by the health-care provider, the endocrinologist, and a psychotherapist may be necessary.

Graves' Disease

Graves' disease (hyperthyroidism), which is considered an autoimmune disorder, is the most common cause of hyperthyroidism in children (Huang, 2010; Whittemore et al., 2013). The incidence of hyperthyroidism in children ranges from 1 to 8 per 100,000. Graves' disease is most common in young to middle-aged women with a male/female ratio of 1:6. Hyperthyroidism also tends to run in families. Incidence increases with age, reaching a peak during adolescence. It is rare in children younger than 5 years of age (Huang, 2010). Though the terms hyperthyroidism and thyrotoxicosis are often used interchangeably, they are not synonymous. "Thyrotoxicosis is a general term that refers to any condition that elevates circulating thyroid hormones while hyperthyroidism refers only to the subset of thyrotoxic disorders that are due to increased function of the thyroid gland itself" (Huang, 2010, p. 119). Thyrotoxicosis may be caused by thyroid gland dysfunction, as in the case of hyperthyroidism, or may result from excessive stimulation of normal thyroid tissue such as in Graves' disease and TSH-secreting pituitary adenomas (Huang, 2010).

Signs and Symptoms

Excessive thyroid hormone affects all organ systems of the body. Symptoms of Graves' disease are identical to those of hyperthyroidism, with the addition of three other symptoms. Although these symptoms present somewhat differently in each child, they include:

- Goiter (enlarged thyroid gland that may cause a bulge in the neck and dysphagia)
- Raised, thickened skin over the shins, back of feet, back, hands, or face
- Swollen, reddened eyes that bulge (exophthalmos)

Other signs and symptoms can include:

- Tachycardia with palpitations
- High blood pressure
- Moist skin
- Increased perspiration
- Shakiness and tremor
- Hyperreflexia
- Audible thyroid bruit
- Nervousness
- Confusion
- Emotional lability
- Poor concentration and decreased school performance
- Hyper-defecation
- Increased appetite accompanied by weight loss
- Difficulty sleeping
- Constant stare
- Sensitivity of eyes to light
- Changes in menstrual periods

Diagnosis

As with other thyroid conditions, blood levels of thyroid hormones confirm the diagnosis. These hormones are elevated. TSH levels are decreased because the high levels of T_3 and T_4 inhibit the anterior pituitary's production of TSH (Whittemore et al., 2013).

Prevention

Because Graves' disease is an autoimmune condition, the best prevention is careful observation to better facilitate diagnosis and management. The nurse must be aware of the fact that infants born to women with a current or past history of Graves' disease may present with neonatal Graves' disease (Whittemore et al., 2013). In addition, research suggests a genetic predisposition to Graves' disease (Ploski, Szymanski, & Bednarczuk, 2011). Careful attention and recognition of symptoms and referral or notification of the primary health-care provider can lead to quicker initiation and response to treatment. In addition, complications and exacerbation of symptoms may be prevented by educating the parents and child on the proper use of medication and on proper diet and rest.

Collaborative Care

Nursing Care. Physical assessment is first and foremost in the care of the child with Graves' disease. The astute nurse may identify these children when they are referred for evaluation of symptoms of ADHD. A complete history including school performance, easy distractibility, and sleep pattern disturbances will aid in the ongoing care of the child. Once the child is diagnosed, the parents and child are taught the importance of following the prescribed treatment regimens. The nurse knows that treatment for hyperthyroidism is individualized for each patient. Ultimately, the goal of treatment is to

---

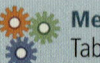 **Medication:** Accurate Administration of Hormone Tablets

Hormone tablets (or any pills) are not mixed in a full bottle of formula. It is best to avoid ruining the taste of the infant's sole source of nutrition. Second, placing the medication in a full bottle will require the baby to drink the entire bottle to obtain the entire dose. Leaving even a small amount of formula on the bottom of the bottle could mean that the child may be under-dosed. Most drug references state that hormone tablets mix very unevenly in solution, and it is difficult for them to stay in suspension. It is best to crush and mix it in a small amount of fluid immediately before administration. The solution is then drawn up into an oral syringe and given before the feeding.

restore the thyroid gland functioning in which the production of thyroid hormone is at normal levels.

It is essential for the nurse to recognize the signs and symptoms of both hyperthyroidism and hypothyroidism. A sudden release of thyroid hormones can result in a thyroid storm, which can lead to heart failure and shock. A sudden onset of restlessness, fever, diaphoresis, and tachycardia is reported immediately because this may indicate a thyroid storm. The only indication for care in the hospital as an inpatient is if the child with hyperthyroidism experiences a thyroid storm.

 focus on safety

Thyroid storm

A thyroid storm is a rare and potentially fatal complication of hyperthyroidism. It typically occurs in patients who experience a precipitating event such as surgery, infection, or trauma. A thyroid storm must be recognized and treated on signs and symptoms alone because laboratory confirmation often cannot be obtained in a timely manner. Patients typically appear markedly *hypermetabolic* with high fevers, tachycardia, nausea and vomiting, tremulousness, agitation, and psychosis if untreated. Patients may also become stuporous or comatose with hypotension.

Medical Care. Medical management is directed at decreasing thyroid hormone levels and includes treatment with antithyroid medication, radioactive iodine therapy, and subtotal thyroidectomy.

Treatment may include (Gurgul & Sowinski, 2011; Zeitler et al., 2011):

- Antithyroid medications (PTU-propylthiouracil or MTZ-methimazole) to help lower the level of thyroid hormones by blocking the synthesis of T_3 and T_4. Pharmacotherapy has been used effectively but has side effects (Table 27-5). Severe effects can be fatal.
- Radioactive iodine therapy (in the form of a pill or liquid), which damages thyroid cells (destruction can take 6 to 18 weeks) to decrease the production of thyroid hormones.
- Surgery to remove the overactive nodule of the thyroid (subtotal thyroidectomy).
- Beta-blocking agents (Inderal) to block the action of thyroid hormone on the body (these drugs do not change the levels of thyroid hormone in the blood but make the patient feel better by relieving tachycardia, restlessness, and tremors).

Table 27-5 Side Effects of Antithyroid Medications

Mild Effects	Severe Effects (can be fatal)
Skin rash	Agranulocytosis (sore throat, high fever)
Mild leukopenia	Lupus-like syndrome
Loss of taste	Hepatitis
Arthralgia	Hepatic failure
Loss/abnormal hair pigmentation	Glomerulonephritis

Surgical Care. The surgical option is used as a last resort when other treatments have not resulted in permanent remission or when the parents cannot comply with the medication regimen. Surgery may be recommended for the child experiencing adverse effects from antithyroid medication or if they have experienced a relapse after 2 years of treatment (Chiapponi, Stocker, Mussack, Gallwas, Hallfeldt, & Ladurner, 2011). This requires a sensitive approach to the family and entails a thorough discussion between the primary health-care provider and family. Some providers believe that total thyroidectomy is the preferred, definitive treatment for patients with Graves' disease (Chiapponi et al. 2011; Peroni, Angiolini, Vigone, Mari, Chiumello, Beretta et al., 2012).

Education/Discharge Instructions

Children with Graves' disease are treated on an outpatient basis for the most part. The parents need to know the significance of continuing the medication regimen even after the symptoms of hyperthyroidism have resolved. Parents must also be taught to watch for medication side effects. The importance of routine blood tests must also be emphasized as well as following through with all return visits to the health-care provider. If referrals are made, the importance of keeping these appointments must also be stressed.

Even though the child is being treated for hyperthyroidism, the signs and symptoms of hypothyroidism must also be taught to the family so that if treatments become toxic they would know what symptoms to observe in the child. Emergency numbers and referrals must be provided to the family in the event that any severe reactions occur.

The importance of a low-stress, low-pressure environment is also reinforced because increased tension could exacerbate the symptoms. The child may also exhibit sudden bursts of emotion such as crying, excitement, or irritability. The family is taught to expect these feelings and that the ill child is not able to control them. The importance of discussing feelings with the child is stressed to minimize these outbursts. Parents are instructed to notify the child's school nurse and teacher about these feelings. The school nurse may need to be involved in the medication regimen during school operational hours. In this case, a note from the child's health-care provider is required. The teachers must also be alerted to the child's illness and the potential lack of focus in class. It may even be necessary to have the child tutored so that the child is able to catch up to the lessons.

CONDITIONS OF THE PARATHYROID

Hypoparathyroidism

Hypoparathyroidism is a rare condition in which there is inadequate production of parathyroid hormone (PTH). It can also occur when the PTH that is produced cannot be used by the body or the kidneys and bones cannot respond to the production of PTH. This deficiency of PTH decreases the calcium level in the blood and increases the phosphate levels (Zeitler et al., 2011).

Hypoparathyroidism may be either inherited or acquired. It can result from a variety of causes:

- Underdeveloped parathyroid glands at birth (inherited)
- Medical treatment (radiation to thyroid gland, drug treatment, thyroid or parathyroid surgery) (acquired)
- An underlying medical condition such as cancer, neck trauma, Wilson's disease (high level of copper in

tissues), an excess of iron in tissues, and low levels of magnesium (acquired)

- Idiopathic (i.e., the parathyroid suddenly stops functioning for no known reason)
- Associated with other conditions (e.g., DiGeorge syndrome)

 Nursing Insight—DiGeorge syndrome

DiGeorge syndrome is an example of a defect in parathyroid gland development. DiGeorge syndrome is composed of hypoparathyroidism, T-cell abnormalities, and cardiac anomalies (Kelly & Levine, 2010).

Signs and Symptoms

The following signs and symptoms often appear in children with hypoparathyroidism:

- Poor tooth development
- Vomiting
- Headaches
- Mental deficiency
- Seizures
- Uncontrollable, painful spasms of the face, hands, arms, and feet
- Irritability
- Muscle rigidity
- Abdominal distention
- Apnea causing irregular cyanosis

Diagnosis

A thorough history and physical is completed. Care is taken to assess for the presence of muscle spasms, twitches, or a history of seizure activity. History or presence of vomiting with abdominal distention is noted as well as episodes of apnea with or without cyanosis. Blood work, including calcium (low), phosphate (high), magnesium (low), and low PTH, confirms the diagnosis (Jospe, 2011). Bone or soft tissue abnormalities (increased bone density) are evaluated with radiographs and CT scans (Zeitler et al., 2011). A 12-lead electrocardiogram (ECG) may reveal a prolonged QT interval.

Prevention

There is no action that can be taken to prevent either hereditary or sustained acquired hypoparathyroidism. With vitamin D therapy and supplemental calcium, most people will have minimal symptoms. Complications can be prevented or reduced by instructing the parents and child on the importance of reporting symptoms such as tingling or burning sensation in fingers, toes, or lips and muscle twitching or cramping as well as medication compliance and follow-up.

Collaborative Care

Nursing Care. Hypocalcemia, which produces the symptoms of hypoparathyroidism, such as seizures, tetany, and laryngospasms, requires IV calcium. The nurse must continuously monitor the child with telemetry for cardiac arrhythmias and blood pressure for life-threatening hypotension. Seizure precautions are maintained until calcium levels approach a normal level. Once serum calcium levels are greater than 7.5 mg/dL the IV calcium can be stopped.

 Critical Nursing Action Calcium Administration

It is important for the pediatric nurse to scrupulously check the IV site for accurate placement because infiltration of the IV calcium supplements causes extravasation and sloughing of the tissue around the site. IV calcium supplements must be properly calculated, diluted, and administered strictly according to the hospital's standards of care and protocols. Oral calcium and vitamin D are administered as soon as possible. Monitor the success of the oral forms of calcium and vitamin D for at least 24 hours after IV calcium is stopped because "rebound" hypocalcemia can occur. The nurse must be alert for subtle changes in the child's status.

 Nursing Insight—Assessing for hyperreflexia of muscles

Assess for hyperreflexia (increased action of the reflexes) by tapping on the facial nerve. If there is a spasm of the facial muscles, this is a positive Chvostek sign (facial muscle spasm) and confirms the fact that the child has muscle pain, cramps, and probably twitches. These muscle manifestations may progress to numbness and tingling of the hands and feet as well as stiffness. Remember infants and small children cannot express these manifestations and therefore just cry to communicate pain.

Medical Care. The goal of medical management is to maintain the calcium in a low-normal range while avoiding hyperphosphatemia. In the acute phase of hypoparathyroidism, calcium is administered IV; diuretics may be prescribed in that circumstance as well to prevent over-excretion of calcium in the urine and to reduce the amount of calcium and vitamin D needed. The active form of vitamin D, 25-dihydroxyvitamin D, is preferred in the treatment of hypoparathyroidism (Zeitler et al., 2011). Urinary calcium secretion is monitored to avoid the risk of renal parenchyma calcification. Long-term medical care includes medication administration of calcium and vitamin D multiple times a day as well as regular checks of serum and urine electrolytes. The child is monitored for the development of long-term complications (e.g., cataracts and soft tissue calcification) as well as nephrolithiasis, which can impact renal function.

Education/Discharge Instructions

Teaching the families about the disease, its signs and symptoms, and the importance of lifelong treatment optimizes the outcomes of the child's care. A lifelong regimen of dietary or supplemental calcium and vitamin D is usually required to restore calcium and mineral balance. If phosphorus levels are extremely elevated, a diet may be given that excludes high-phosphorus foods such as eggs and dairy products.

Hyperparathyroidism

Hyperparathyroidism is rare in children. Primary hyperparathyroidism is more common in females and in adolescents. It is caused by overactive parathyroid glands that produce high levels of PTH, which results in increased levels of serum calcium (Kelly & Levine, 2010). The excess calcium leads to osteoporosis and osteomalacia (both bone-weakening diseases). High levels of PTH cause the bones to demineralize, which increases the serum calcium levels. PTH also acts on the kidney to conserve calcium and excrete phosphate. Another result of the increased serum calcium is the development of kidney stones (Kelly & Levine, 2010). Kidney stones form because of the high levels of calcium excreted into the urine by the kidneys. Primary hyperparathyroidism may develop as a result of one of the following conditions (Kelly & Levine, 2010):

- Single or multiple benign tumors in the parathyroid glands
- Parathyroid hyperplasia (excessive growth of normal parathyroid cells)
- Parathyroid malignancies (rare)
- Certain endocrine disorders, such as type I and II multiple endocrine neoplasia syndromes

Signs and Symptoms

At least 50% of patients with primary hyperparathyroidism have no symptoms, and approximately 1% of cases go undiagnosed. When symptoms do occur, they are generally attributed to persistently high levels of calcium. Symptoms include:

- Bone and joint pain
- Bone loss leading to osteoporosis with possible bone fractures
- Muscle weakness
- Abdominal discomfort because of pancreatitis
- Heartburn
- Nausea and vomiting
- Constipation
- Lack of appetite
- Peptic ulcers
- Kidney stones
- Excessive thirst
- Excessive urination
- Depression
- Anxiety
- Memory loss
- Excessive drowsiness or fatigue

Diagnosis

Although this diagnosis is frequently delayed in children, it is usually detected when the child becomes symptomatic. Children with symptoms of renal colic or nephrolithiasis are evaluated for hyperparathyroidism. Evaluation of elevated blood calcium and PTH levels is diagnostic in children (Kelly & Levine, 2010). If radiographs are performed, the child's bones may show signs of rickets (Zeitler et al., 2011) (Fig. 27-5).

Prevention

There is no known prevention for primary hyperparathyroidism, but early recognition of the symptoms may promote compliance with treatment and reduce overall complications. People who are at risk for this condition can avoid dehydration. Risk factors generally refer to adults and include being older, female, obese, and having depression, though inherited endocrine problems can also lead to hyperparathyroidism.

Collaborative Care

Nursing Care. Nursing care consists of medical and surgical management. Nursing care focuses on fluid management and consistent monitoring of the child's intake, output, and electrolyte balance.

Medical Care. Because hyperparathyroidism is demonstrated by hypercalcemia, initial treatment focuses on reducing osteoclastic bone reabsorption (Kelly & Levine, 2010). Initial management may include the use

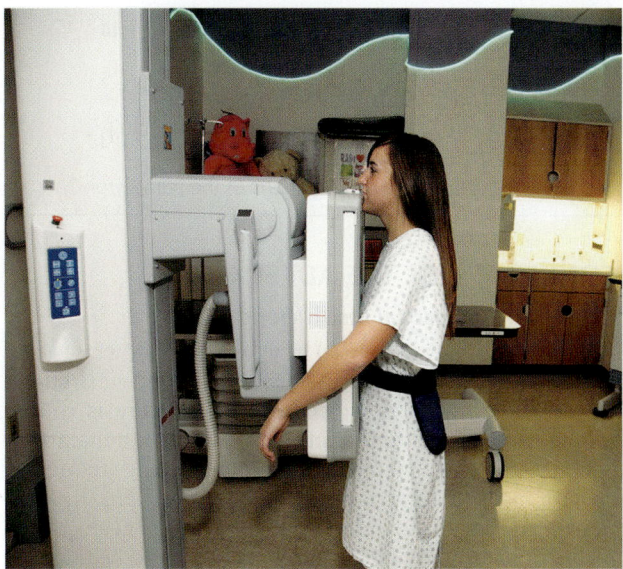

Figure 27-5 A radiograph taken to diagnose rickets.

of medications, such as oral phosphate, pamidronate, calcitonin, or etidronate disodium to treat hypercalcemia associated with hyperparathyroidism (Kelly & Levine, 2010). Administration of IV fluids and diuretics may assist with the increased excretion of calcium in children not in renal failure (Zeitler et al., 2011). A diet low in calcium may also be ordered.

Surgical Care. Parathyroidectomy is effective and restores the normal blood calcium levels. This surgery has few complications and is the treatment of choice in children with primary hyperparathyroidism (Kelly & Levine, 2010). Unfortunately, if diagnosis is late, this surgical procedure cannot reverse the late effects of hyperparathyroidism on other organs such as the kidneys.

Preoperative care includes increasing the child's intake and careful monitoring of I&O. The nurse also monitors IV fluids and dietary restrictions. Urine is strained when renal calculi are suspected. Monitor the child for safety in the presence of muscular weakness. Postoperative care of the child after removal of the parathyroid glands is focused on airway management and frequent assessments for respiratory distress or airway obstruction because of edema at the surgical site. As with all surgical procedures, continual monitoring for signs of infection and hematoma is done.

Education/Discharge Instructions

The child and family are taught to consistently observe for signs and symptoms of hypocalcemia. Learning to administer calcium supplements is invaluable because this treatment may be needed for life. Family members are taught to realize that frequent blood draws may be necessary initially to monitor calcium and phosphorus levels. The nurse can explain to the family that eventually the lab work can be done less frequently, but it needs be stressed that these blood tests are an important part of the continued health care of the child. The primary health-care provider may recommend that the child take particular nutritional supplements because a child with primary hyperparathyroidism may develop deficiencies. Vitamins C and K as well as manganese are necessary for normal bone formation.

Now Can You—Describe conditions of the thyroid and parathyroid?

1. Describe conditions of the thyroid?
2. Discuss nursing care for conditions of the thyroid?
3. Describe conditions of the parathyroid?
4. Discuss nursing care for conditions of the parathyroid?

CONDITIONS OF THE ADRENALS

Acute Adrenocortical Insufficiency

Adrenal crisis may be caused by any of the following: rapid withdrawal from steroid therapy, sepsis, surgical stress, bleeding into the adrenal glands, pituitary necrosis, or thyroid hormone replacement in someone with adrenal insufficiency. The following factors increase the chance of developing adrenal crisis: septic shock, adrenal insufficiency, and use of steroid medications (Zeitler et al., 2011). If the child has any of these risk factors, the health-care provider must be notified.

Nursing Insight—_An adrenal crisis is a life-threatening condition_

Adrenal crisis is a life-threatening condition in which the anterior pituitary gland does not make enough adrenocorticotropic hormone (ACTH). ACTH is responsible for regulating the adrenal gland (a gland atop each kidney that makes hormones that regulate bodily functions). Adrenal crisis is a medical emergency, and children with adrenal crisis require _immediate_ treatment (Whittemore et al., 2013). Parents need to seek emergency medical care at once if they suspect an adrenal crisis.

Critical Nursing Action Steroid Administration

Steroid administration is never stopped abruptly. Steroids must be slowly weaned according to the health-care provider's orders. An abrupt withdrawal can cause an adrenal crisis (Zeitler et al., 2011).

Signs and Symptoms

The child in adrenal crisis may exhibit any of these symptoms. Yet, it is important for the nurse to remember that these symptoms may also be caused by other, less serious health conditions. However, it is vital to report any of the following signs and symptoms to the health-care provider:

- Weakness
- Ongoing fatigue
- Nausea
- Vomiting
- Loss of appetite
- Weight loss
- Low blood pressure
- Abdominal pain
- Fever
- Confusion or coma
- Diarrhea
- Cyanosis
- Dehydration

Diagnosis

Tests to diagnose adrenal crisis may include chest radiograph, CT scan of the abdomen, and blood tests that detect ACTH and electrolyte levels, red blood cells, and other autoimmune or endocrine disorders (Whittemore et al., 2013).

Prevention

Prevention of adrenal crisis involves ongoing assessment of the ill or hospitalized child with a history of congenital adrenal hyperplasia. Parents are educated to recognize symptoms that indicate the beginning of an acute adrenal crisis as well as the need for "stress" doses of hydrocortisone when their child has a febrile illness, surgery, or trauma (Whittemore et al., 2013). If the child is hospitalized, the nurse must notify the health-care provider if adrenal crisis is suspected.

Collaborative Care

Nursing Care. Be cognizant of the fact that this crisis can be fatal and may quickly appear. The nurse must ensure continuous assessment; recognition of the signs and symptoms is essential. It may be necessary to take the child's vital signs every 15 minutes, always carefully watching for the most subtle signs of the onset of shock. Subtle signs of shock may include a slight cooling of the hands and feet along with a decrease in skin color. For instance, the infant's periphery goes from pink to extreme pallor. The nurse must monitor IV fluid rates and remain in constant communication with the health-care provider so that responses to the treatments are known and counteracted if necessary.

Medication administration is also a significant part of nursing care. Medications are given as prescribed by the health-care provider. Once the child has stabilized, clear, oral fluids can be initiated slowly. It would defeat the purpose if, in the child's eagerness to drink, he or she began to vomit again. For this reason, encourage the child to drink slowly. If the child refuses to drink, other forms of liquid such as ice pops, frozen ice, gelatin, or broth may give the child incentive to take fluids orally. In this situation, parents are often in a state of confusion and shock because the treatments and changes in their child's condition occur rapidly. Keep the parents informed by providing frequent updates on the child's condition as well as an explanation of the treatments. To decrease the parents' fear, noting slight improvements in the child's status helps them remain positive. Because neurological symptoms can be so devastating, remind the parents that these are only temporary and that paralysis can be reversed once the child is stabilized.

Recognize that fluid shifts may also occur quickly, so lab values must be reviewed often. Cortisone and sodium chloride treatments are often given rapidly to rectify ominous situations. A consequence of this rapid treatment is an abnormally low potassium level, such that the child may be at risk for flaccid paralysis or seizures. Continue ongoing observation and frequent assessment of the child.

Medical Care. Initially, steroid IV hydrocortisone (A-Hydrocort) and antibiotic drugs are needed to treat an adrenal crisis. If the child is vomiting or unconscious, the nurse gives these medications by injection or IV. Because of fluid loss, the child is given IV fluids to reverse dehydration, electrolyte imbalances, and hypovolemia (Zeitler et al., 2011). If the child is in severe crisis and has a decreased blood pressure, vasopressor may be used to raise the child's blood pressure quickly by vasoconstriction. When these conditions are corrected and

Labs: Potassium Depletion

Because treatments for adrenal crisis cause potassium depletion, it is crucial to keep a close watch on the child's lab values. Be mindful of the warning signs of hyperkalemia and hypokalemia (apnea, cardiac arrhythmias, paralysis, poor muscle control, and weakness).

the child is stable, cortisone medications and sodium chloride may be given orally. Sodium balance is maintained by replacing aldosterone with synthetic steroids that aid in sodium retention (Zeitler et al., 2011).

Education/Discharge Instructions

Discharge preparation is started as soon after the crisis as possible. Keep in mind the readiness of the parents to learn. Be sure that the parents are ready to listen and learn about the care of the child at home. In some cases, it may be necessary to wait until the parents feel secure about the fact that their child will be going home under their care. Parents and the child need to be taught as appropriate that medication will be required throughout the child's life. Parents may also benefit by being taught how to give hydrocortisone IM, which may be needed if the child vomits. Explain the need for careful monitoring of the child in the presence of illness, stress, or surgery because this may require the necessity of contacting the health-care provider for an adjustment in dose. Parents need to know that some teens do not take prescribed medication doses because of the side effects. The nurse can reassure parents that this may happen and to call the primary pediatrician if it does. Provide parents with information about obtaining a medical ID bracelet or necklace for the child.

Cultural Diversity: Shock in Dark-Complexioned Children

When assessing for shock in children with a dark complexion, remember to look at the palms of the hands, soles of the feet, and lips to ascertain color changes; pale or bluish skin tone is common.

CHRONIC ADRENOCORTICAL INSUFFICIENCY

Chronic adrenocortical insufficiency, or Addison's disease, is the result of an underactive adrenal gland. An underactive adrenal gland produces insufficient amounts of cortisol and aldosterone.

Nursing Insight—*Cortisol and aldosterone*

Cortisol is a steroid hormone that helps to control the body's metabolism of fats, proteins, and carbohydrates; suppresses inflammatory reactions in the body; and affects immune system functions. Aldosterone is a steroid hormone that controls sodium and potassium in the blood.

The onset of this disease may occur at any age. Most of the time, the cause of the disease is unknown. The majority of Addison's disease cases are caused by the actual destruction of the adrenal glands through cancer, infection, an autoimmune process, or other diseases (Donohoue, 2010). Other causes may include the following:

- Use of corticosteroids as a treatment (such as prednisone) may cause a slowdown in production of natural

corticosteroids by the adrenal glands and mimic Addison's disease (Whittemore et al., 2013).
- Certain medications used to treat fungal infections may block production of corticosteroids in the adrenal glands, causing signs and symptoms similar to those of Addison's disease.
- Rarely, Addison's disease is inherited as an X-linked, recessive trait; the gene responsible for the condition is located on the X chromosome and passed down from a healthy female carrier to her sons, who are affected. In this form, symptoms typically begin in childhood or adolescence.

Failure to produce adequate levels of cortisol can occur for different reasons. Corticosteroids play an important role in helping the body fight infection and promote health during physical stress. The problem may be caused by a disorder of the adrenal glands themselves or by inadequate secretion of ACTH by the pituitary gland (Donohoue, 2010). The lack of adrenal hormones may cause:

- Elevated levels of potassium
- Extreme sensitivity to the hormone insulin, which is normally present in the bloodstream, and may lead to low blood sugar levels
- Increased risk during stressful periods, such as surgery, infection, or injury

Primary Adrenal Insufficiency

Most cases of primary adrenal insufficiency are caused by the gradual destruction of the adrenal cortex, the outer layer of the adrenal glands, by the body's own immune system. About 70% of reported cases of Addison's disease are caused by autoimmune disorders, in which the immune system makes antibodies that attack the body's own tissues or organs and slowly destroy them (Donohoue, 2010). Adrenal insufficiency occurs when at least 90% of the adrenal cortex has been destroyed. As a result, often both glucocorticoid (cortisol) and mineralocorticoid (aldosterone) hormones are lacking (Triantafyllou, Mavrides, Katzos, Printza, & Papachristou, 2010). Sometimes only the adrenal gland is affected, as in idiopathic adrenal insufficiency. In other cases, additional endocrine glands are also affected, as in the polyendocrine deficiency syndrome.

Polyendocrine Deficiency Syndrome

The polyendocrine deficiency syndrome is classified into two separate forms:

- Type I occurs in children, and adrenal insufficiency may be accompanied by underactive parathyroid glands, slow sexual development, pernicious anemia, chronic *Candida* infections, chronic active hepatitis, and hair loss (Venes, 2013).
- Type II, often called *Schmidt's syndrome*, usually affects young adults. Features of type II may include an underactive thyroid gland, slow sexual development, diabetes, and loss of pigment on areas of the skin (vitiligo) (Venes, 2013).

Scientists believe that the polyendocrine deficiency syndrome is inherited because frequently more than one family member tends to have one or more endocrine deficiencies.

Signs and Symptoms

It is important to note that mild symptoms of Addison's disease may manifest only when the child is under physical stress. The most common symptoms of Addison's disease may be seen individually or in any combination. Each child experiences symptoms very differently. Classic signs of Addison's disease include hyperpigmentation, hyponatremia, poor vascular tone, hypoglycemia, ketonemia, and hyperkalemia (Thabet, Bozarth, & Barboi, 2012). The nurse needs to regularly observe for any of the following symptoms (Donohoue, 2010):

- Weakness
- Fatigue
- Dizziness
- Rapid pulse
- Dark skin that is first noted on hands and face
- Black freckles
- Bluish-black discoloration around the nipples, mouth, rectum, scrotum, or vagina
- Weight loss
- Dehydration
- Loss of appetite
- Intense salt craving
- Muscle aches
- Nausea
- Vomiting
- Diarrhea
- Cold intolerance

If left untreated, Addison's disease can lead to severe abdominal pain, extreme weakness, low blood pressure, kidney failure, and shock, especially when the child experiences physical stress. Although the symptoms of Addison's disease may resemble other problems or medical conditions, it is best for the nurse to encourage the parents to consult the child's health-care provider to confirm the diagnosis.

The symptoms progress slowly and are usually ignored until a stressful event such as an illness or an accident causes the child's condition to worsen (Donohoue, 2010). This is called an Addisonian crisis, or acute adrenal insufficiency. In most cases, symptoms are severe enough that patients seek medical treatment before a crisis occurs. However, in a few children, symptoms first become readily apparent during an Addisonian crisis.

focus on safety

Symptoms of an Addisonian crisis

Symptoms of an Addisonian crisis include sudden penetrating pain in the lower back, abdomen, or legs; severe vomiting and diarrhea; dehydration; low blood pressure; and a loss of consciousness. If left untreated, a child with Addison's disease in crisis can die (National Institutes of Health (NIH) Publication No. 14–3054, 2014).

Diagnosis

Aside from the clinical symptoms and the signs found on physical examination, including low blood pressure, a diagnosis of Addison's disease is usually confirmed by laboratory tests. Typically, a patient has low blood sodium, high potassium, and low blood sugar. The initial test for adrenal insufficiency is the measurement of serum cortisol levels. The serum cortisol level is drawn in the morning between 6:00 a.m. and 8:00 a.m. The levels are the highest at this time because of circadian rhythm. Cortisol levels greater than 20 mg/dL are considered normal, whereas levels less than 3 mg/dL are diagnostic of Addison's disease (Whittemore et al., 2013). Levels lower than this must be considered within the clinical context.

Prevention

Preventive measures in caring for the child with Addison's disease are through education with the goals of controlling stress, preventing and monitoring for an Addison's crisis, and maintaining growth and development. Parents need to be cognizant of stress in the environment, which may include febrile illnesses, surgery, injury, and emotional stress. Stress increases the body's demand for cortisol. Parents also need to be instructed on ensuring that the child is in compliance with hormone replacement therapy. In addition, parents can be instructed on the administration of IM hydrocortisone in the case of vomiting. If the child becomes ill, injured, or needs surgery, the health-care provider is notified regarding the potential need for dosage adjustment.

Collaborative Care

Nursing Care. Nursing care of the hospitalized child in adrenal crisis is similar to that of the child with congenital adrenal insufficiency. When a child is hospitalized in an adrenal crisis, the focus of nursing care is on fluid and electrolyte replacement. Closely monitor for signs of hypovolemic shock. The nurse understands that peripheral circulation must be checked often. Frequently, hourly assessments help the nurse detect subtle changes that can be the earliest indicators of potential imbalances not yet detected by laboratory tests.

Medical Care. Addison's disease is treatable with oral forms of the missing hormones. Cortisol (Solu-Cortef) is available in tablet form, and it is given 2 to 3 times a day. This medication helps maintain the child's blood glucose levels (NIH Publication No. 14–3054, 2014).

If the patient has an illness accompanied by vomiting, an IM injection of cortisol (Solu-Cortef) must be given at home. Then the patient must be taken to an emergency room for further treatment. All patients or their parents must have a dose of Cortisol (Solu-Cortef) available at home and be instructed on the proper technique to administer it during a crisis.

Education/Discharge Instructions

Parents need to be aware of the diligent commitment that is necessary to giving the child medications routinely and regularly. They must plan medication delivery into their day so that it is never forgotten. The morning rush to school, the bus, or carpool may not be the best time to plan the cortisol replacements. Parents must also know that the drug cannot be stopped suddenly and that if the child is unable to ingest it because of vomiting, the injectable hydrocortisone must be given IM. Teaching IM injections is also necessary. Another important aspect of parent teaching involves providing information on the side effects of the drug as well as on the signs and symptoms of adrenal crisis. A home free of stress is the best environment for a child with Addison's disease because the body needs increased cortical hormones during times of stress and this child's body is unable to produce the hormone. During times of emotional stress or physical stress, the parents may have to give additional hormone replacements. Because dehydration and stressful situations are the likely triggers of a crisis, instructing parents to keep the child well-hydrated in situations such as extreme heat, exercise, or influenza is warranted. These conditions are discussed before discharge so that the parents feel in control when at home.

One of the best recommendations to make to parents when caring for a child with Addison's disease is to purchase a medical alert bracelet or tag for the child to wear. This would ensure that the treatment of a child in crisis would not be delayed. It is also important to teach the family and the child about electrolyte loss (especially sodium) during vigorous exercise or on extremely hot days when the child would perspire. Eating more salty food and drinking more water in the hot weather helps the child maintain a mineral balance in his or her body, which will ward off a crisis.

 Optimizing Outcomes—**Hormone treatment**

The best outcome of care for the child is optimized with adequate hormonal treatment. Hormone treatment helps maintain a normal growth pattern. Even though a child with Addison's disease rarely grows beyond the fifth percentile, development during puberty is normal (Vallerand & Sanoski, 2014).

 focus on safety

Cortisone insufficiency

When caring for this child, whether in the hospital or clinic, the pediatric nurse must be aware of the signs and symptoms observed before an adrenal crisis: headache, dizziness, and nausea or vomiting (stomachache) or "wobbly knees." By the time the child exhibits extreme weakness and mental confusion, the adrenal crisis is imminent. Parents also need ongoing support to manage the care and the medications of a child with Addison's disease. This is often very frightening for parents. A well-thought-through plan can help the parents be ready for any emergency.

 Collaboration in Caring—*The child with Addison's disease*

Along with the primary care provider, the endocrinologist is an important member of the team. Including the parents as members of this team will ensure that they will feel in better control of potential crisis situations. As the child matures and becomes a teenager, it is essential to include him or her as well so that the child is educated and understands the consequences of skipping doses of medication or of stress. The child also needs to be competent to administer emergency, injectable doses of the cortisone.

Cushing's Syndrome

Cushing's syndrome is a rare disorder that seldom is seen in persons younger than 20 years of age. It is hormonal in nature and presents when a person has been exposed to increased levels of cortisone for an extended period of time. When diagnosed in young children it is often caused by an adrenal tumor or prolonged steroid therapy. About 10 to 15 million new cases are diagnosed annually. It is estimated that only 10% of all individuals affected in a year are children (NIH Publication No. 08–3007, 2012). Although the true etiology of Cushing's syndrome is not clear, it can be because of several causes including the oversecretion of the pituitary, causing an excessive amount of serum ACTH and

of the adrenal gland, causing an overload of glucocorticoids, usually tumor related (Zeitler et al., 2011). Long-term administration or large doses of corticosteroids are also known to cause a child to present with Cushing's syndrome. If a child's adrenal glands are insensitive to normal levels of cortisone, then levels can become dramatically abnormal (Donohoue, 2010; Kumah-Crystal & Lomenick, 2011).

Signs and Symptoms

The signs and symptoms of Cushing's syndrome develop gradually, so insidiously, in fact, that it may be years before the child shows clearly visible signs of Cushing's syndrome. Often children are hypokalemic, causing alkalosis because of potassium excretion and hypercalcemia caused by excessive amounts of urinary calcium.

Common signs and symptoms of Cushing's syndrome include:

- Weight gain
- Pendulous abdomen
- Fatigue
- Muscle wasting
- Weakness
- Thin extremities
- Round "moon" face
- Facial flushing
- Fatty pad between shoulders (buffalo hump)
- Pink or purple stretch marks (striae) on abdominal skin, thighs, breasts, and arms
- The child's skin is also thin and fragile with little subcutaneous tissue causing easy bruising and slow healing

The child may exhibit the following:

- Depression
- Anxiety
- Irritability
- Euphoria
- Frank psychoses
- Irregular or absent menstrual periods in females
- Erectile dysfunction in males

 Nursing Insight—*Signs and symptoms of Cushing's syndrome*

Hyperglycemia may eventually lead to latent or overt diabetes, high blood pressure, or arteriosclerosis. Because of the excess production of androgens, signs and symptoms related to secondary sexual characteristics can also be seen.

Diagnosis

Children who are being evaluated for Cushing's syndrome must be seen by a pediatric endocrinologist because test result adjustments must be considered before the diagnosis is confirmed. Levels of cortisone are recorded so that escalating levels are clearly seen.

A 24-hour urine collection is a valuable tool to determine if the child's urine is clear of free cortisol. Because 24-hour urine collections can be very difficult to obtain in an infant and child, the test may need to be duplicated to obtain reliable results. It is important to remember that to correctly interpret the results of the 24-hour urinary free cortisol (UFC), the results must be "corrected" for the child's body surface area (Zeitler et al., 2011). Because cortisone is released by the child's body in response to stress, several other conditions could cause high UFC levels, for example, physical stress, such as overexertion or obesity, and emotional stress such as depression.

Cortisol levels can also be measured in a child's saliva by taking both a midnight and morning sample. Levels are usually at the lowest point at midnight and the highest in the morning (Moloney & Dowling, 2012; Zeitler et al., 2011). This normal pattern is lost in children with Cushing's syndrome and the midnight levels are not significantly different from the morning levels.

Diagnosis is based on the results of not only urine and saliva screening but also on serum blood levels, including fasting blood glucose and electrolyte levels as well as a bone scan for osteoporosis and a radiograph of the skull for an enlarged sella turcica. An MRI of the pituitary as well as a CT scan of the child's adrenal glands may also be performed (Zeitler et al., 2011). The medical history of the child may also hold the key to the diagnosis. A complete physical exam, including a review of growth charts, may indicate that there is a decline in linear growth with a simultaneous dramatic increase in weight (Baş, Çetinkaya, & Aycan, 2012; Kumah-Crystal & Lomenick, 2011). Testing does not stop with confirmation of a diagnosis. Additional results need to be investigated to determine the cause of the syndrome.

Prevention

Preventive measures in caring for the child with Cushing's syndrome are through education with the goals of controlling stress, preventing and monitoring for signs of adrenal insufficiency, and maintaining growth and development. Parents need to be cognizant of stress in the environment, which may include febrile illnesses, surgery, injury, and emotional stress. Stress increases the body's demand for cortisol. Parents also need to be instructed on ensuring that the child is in compliance with hormone replacement therapy. In addition, parents can be instructed on the administration of IM hydrocortisone in case of vomiting. If the child becomes ill, injured, or needs surgery, the health-care provider is notified about the potential need for dosage adjustment.

Collaborative Care

Nursing Care. Nursing care depends on the cause and the treatment of the illness. If the child has a surgical intervention, nursing care involves preoperative assessments and fluid hydration as well as postoperative assessments, pain control, and medication regimens. When a child's adrenal glands have been removed, cortisol replacement is necessary. This medication is best given early in the morning or every other day to decrease the side effects. This regimen closely mimics the body's normal diurnal pattern of cortisone secretion. The nurse needs to teach the child and family about the disease, its cause, and subsequent treatments. If a surgical intervention is indicated, thorough preoperative and postoperative teaching must be done. Often the operating room is a very frightening place for children. Many hospitals perform this teaching well before the procedure and have children tour and touch equipment when they are in a relaxed state of mind, which enables the day of the procedure to go much more smoothly.

Medical Care. Management varies depending on the cause with the goal of resolving hormone balance and reversing the symptoms of Cushing's syndrome. If the cause of Cushing's syndrome is long-term steroid therapy, treatment is directed at reducing the dose to the lowest possible therapeutic level needed to treat the underlying condition

(Ba et al., 2012). Treatments may include pharmaceuticals that inhibit the production of cortisol. Surgical excision is the treatment of choice for pituitary or adrenal gland tumors. If surgery is not possible, radiation therapy is used.

Surgical Care. Tumors in either the pituitary or in the adrenal glands require surgical excision. Referrals to a neurosurgeon are necessary (Jospe, 2011).

Education/Discharge Instructions

Teaching parents how to give the medication, including the injectable form for an emergency situation, helps gain the confidence necessary to manage a child recovering from Cushing's syndrome. It is important to inform the parents that the "Cushing-like" appearance will decrease as the child recovers. Finally, it is very important to alert the parents to watch for signs of adrenal insufficiency. If corticosteroid treatments are stopped, the child will exhibit signs of adrenal insufficiency. Encourage the family to have the child wear medical alert identification at all times.

Congenital Adrenal Hyperplasia

Children born with congenital adrenal hyperplasia (CAH) lack the ability to produce cortisol. The condition begins early during the fetal gestational period, and the infant is born with the disease. With this deficiency, or lack of cortisol, the negative feedback system fails, causing an excessive amount of corticosteroid-releasing hormone to be secreted from the hypothalamus as well as ACTH from the anterior pituitary (Zeitler et al., 2011). Overproduction of ACTH in turn causes the adrenal glands to become hyperplastic, causing an excessive amount of androgens to be secreted.

The most common cause of CAH is a result of a deficiency of 21-hydroxylase (an enzyme, steroid) which is seen in about 1 out of every 15,000 live births (Moloney & Dowling, 2012; Zeitler et al., 2011). This deficiency leads to two major problems: deficient production of both cortisol and aldosterone and shunting of steroid precursors that form androgens (Whittemore et al., 2013). The abnormal production of androgens causes an abnormal development of sexual organs in male infants and virilization in females. It results in the masculinization of females, which makes the sex of the baby unclear because of ambiguous genitalia (*pseudohermaphroditism*) or more male-like features.

Signs and Symptoms

Generally, the male infant has no physical differences until later in childhood when the early development of pubic hair, penile enlargement, or both are accompanied by accelerated linear growth and advancement of skeletal maturation (von Oettingen, Pou, Levitsky, & Misra, 2012). At birth, a female may have malformed external genitalia. The clitoris is enlarged, and there may be a fusion of the labial folds; this can give the female a male appearance externally. Internally, the uterus, fallopian tubes, and ovaries are normal (Whittemore et al., 2013; Zeitler et al., 2011).

Symptoms of cortisol deficiency include:

- Failure to thrive
- Weight loss
- Weakness
- Nausea and vomiting
- Poor appetite
- Hypoglycemia
- Cool, clammy skin
- Dizziness
- Confusion

Symptoms of aldosterone deficiency include:

- Vomiting
- Poor feeding
- Lethargy
- Dehydration
- Skin hyperpigmentation
- Fatigue

Diagnosis

Despite the fact that prenatal screening is used to diagnose CAH as early as possible, false positives indicate that the health-care provider needs to be cognizant of the clinical signs and symptoms postnatally; milder cases may be missed by the newborn screening programs (Whittemore et al., 2013). Elevated serum levels of 17-hydroxyprogesterone (17-OHP) may indicate the disease (Whittemore et al., 2013). It is important to note that these levels are highest in preterm infants. The levels decrease as infants mature, except in an infant with CAH, in whom the levels continue to escalate. Although considered a "social emergency," care must be taken to determine the actual diagnosis of the child with ambiguous genitalia. Chromosomes can be studied microscopically to determine the child's gender.

Prevention

Preventive measures in caring for the child with congenital adrenal insufficiency are through education with the goals of controlling stress, preventing and monitoring for signs of adrenal insufficiency, and maintaining growth and development. Parents need to be cognizant of stress in the environment, which may include febrile illnesses, surgery, injury, and emotional stress. Stress increases the body's demand for cortisol. Parents also need to be instructed on ensuring that the child is in compliance with hormone replacement therapy. In addition, parents can be instructed on the administration of IM hydrocortisone in the case of vomiting. If the child becomes ill, injured, or needs surgery, the health-care provider is notified about the potential need for dosage adjustment.

Collaborative Care

Nursing Care. Nursing care is similar to that of the child with Addison's disease. Health-care professionals must maintain a positive atmosphere from the moment the baby is born. In the delivery room, a positive emotional tone has a lasting effect on the parents' understanding of this disease. Care is directed at preventing and monitoring for acute adrenal crisis and educating the parents about the importance of medication compliance.

Medical Care. Nearly all children diagnosed with CAH are treated with replacement of glucocorticoids. By alleviating the deficiency of cortisol, the negative feedback loop suppresses ACTH secretion and thus prevents adrenal stimulation. The mineralocorticoid fludrocortisone (Florinef) or hydrocortisone (A-Hydrocort) is also given. Neither of these drugs has significant side effects at replacement doses (Whittemore et al., 2013). Side effects are seen only when doses exceed those necessary for replacement. If the levels are above normal, the child can acquire acne, an elevated blood pressure, or even growth retardation. Because all females with CAH are fertile, surgical repair can be performed once the replacement of hormones has begun (Jospe, 2011). Usually it is done before the girl's first birthday, and if necessary, may be further corrected before menarche.

Education/Discharge Instructions

Because these medications need to be given throughout the child's life, parents need to be instructed to give the medication regularly. Often, making the administration part of the family's routine will ensure that the medication is not forgotten. The alternative route to the oral medication, namely the IM medication, must also be taught in the event that the child has an illness in which oral doses are contraindicated. Emergency procedures, including IM injection of hydrocortisone, must be taught to the parents. It is essential for the family to know that if the medication cannot be given at all, the child must be taken to the emergency department of the closest hospital for treatment. It is always good advice to recommend that the child wear a medical alert bracelet.

"What to say"—*Congenital adrenal hyperplasia*

It is important to address congenital adrenal hyperplasia (CAH) and the decision about whether to wait to perform surgical correction until the child can participate in the discussions (Lee, Witchel, Rogol, & Houk, 2010). Questions to consider include:

- Because the surgery is usually cosmetic in nature, what harm would there be to wait?
- What are the consequences of early surgical repair?
- Will the nerve endings to the female's clitoris be damaged?
- What impact will the early surgery have on the child's sexuality in later life and on the sexual identity of the child?

Obviously, the decision is very complex and requires careful thought. The nurse can also examine personal thoughts about what makes up a child's sexuality.

Much parental teaching is needed not only regarding the medication and its various route and administration methods but also about this chronic illness and its treatment, as well as pre- and postoperative teaching if genital reconstruction is done. Emotional support of the parents is also essential for this lengthy process.

Family education, including for the siblings and grandparents, must be provided, and the nurse can best help the

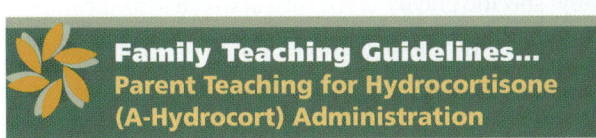

Family Teaching Guidelines...
Parent Teaching for Hydrocortisone (A-Hydrocort) Administration

ESSENTIAL INFORMATION:

- Medication must be used as prescribed.
- Parents must know to always have the injectable hydrocortisone available at home, school, and wherever the child travels.
- An emergency kit is kept on hand at all times with a cortisol supply to administer to the child during acute illness, vomiting, diarrhea, or during stressful circumstances. When oral doses cannot be tolerated, the injectable dose should be readily available (Moloney & Dowling, 2012).
- Administer the medication *on time* because this follows the child's body's normal cortisol release patterns.

parents address these family members. Referring to the infant as a "beautiful baby" will help the parents accept the baby as early as possible.

As with any lifelong illness, it is important for the parents to acknowledge the importance of regular check-ups. The primary pediatrician and the endocrinologist, pharmacist, dietitian, and nurse can work together to support the entire family to reach their maximum potential.

🦠⚙️ Nursing Diagnoses Congenital Adrenal Hyperplasia

- Risk for deficit fluid volume related to the excess salt excretion of the kidneys and the failure of the negative feedback system
- Risk for disproportionate growth related to initial accelerated growth and early fusion of the epiphyseal plates of the long bone
- Risk for impaired parenting related to the fact that the sex of the child may be uncertain until the karyotype result is determined
- Caregiver role strain related to a chronic, life-threatening illness that can cause strain on the entire family

---

Hyperaldosteronism

Hyperaldosteronism produces excessive secretion of aldosterone, which may be caused by an adrenal tumor or syndrome that is a result of an enzyme deficiency. Similar to other endocrine disorders, hyperaldosteronism becomes symptomatic with excessive sodium levels and deficient potassium levels as well as fluid retention (Zeitler et al., 2011).

Signs and Symptoms

The following are associated with excess cortisol (Whittemore et al., 2013):

- Weight gain
- Growth failure
- Osteopenia
- Delayed puberty
- Acne
- Purple striae
- Hirsutism
- Compulsive behavior

The following findings are associated with fluid retention:

- Hypervolemia
- Headache
- Hypertension
- Nocturnal enuresis
- Low specific gravity

The following findings are associated with hypokalemia:

- Muscle weakness
- Paresthesia
- Episodic paralysis and tetany
- Polydipsia
- Polyuria

Diagnosis

When a young child presents with hypertension, the health-care provider must rule out adrenal tumors. In addition to

---

🦠⚙️ Labs: Hyperaldosteronism

Lab results indicate decreased potassium level, increased aldosterone level, and decreased renin activity. Urinalysis reveals an elevated aldosterone level. A CT scan of the child's abdomen reveals an adrenal mass, and an ECG shows abnormalities that can occur with low potassium levels.

---

the hypertension, the child presents with hypokalemia and polyuria; if these conditions fail to respond to ADH administration, the clinical diagnosis of hyperaldosteronism is suspected. Diagnostic findings may include elevated plasma and urinary aldosterone and an abnormal glucose tolerance test (Zeitler et al., 2011). Imaging by the use of MRI or CT may assist with diagnosis when a tumor is suspected (Donohoue, 2010).

Prevention

Preventive measures in caring for the child with hyperaldosteronism are through education with the goals of preventing and monitoring for the adequacy of blood pressure control and treatment of hypokalemia as well as maintaining growth and development. Parents also need to be instructed on ensuring that the child is in compliance with hormone replacement therapy. Genetic counseling is provided when familial hyperaldosteronism is identified.

Collaborative Care

Nursing Care. Nursing care and treatment are similar to those for chronic adrenocortical insufficiency. Initially, the potassium depletion is replaced, and the diuretic spironolactone (Aldactone) causes diuresis and thus blocks the aldosterone effects by preserving potassium and promoting sodium and water excretion.

Any child admitted with hypertension is observed closely for the signs and symptoms of hyponatremia and hyperkalemia. Excessive thirst, bed wetting, or unexplained weakness raises suspicions in the nurse that the child has a serious illness. When vital sign assessments do reveal hypertension, it is important to notify the health-care provider immediately and to continue frequent vital signs until a provider performs a thorough physical. Once the diagnosis is confirmed, the nursing care focuses on preoperative care and teaching. The treatment plan must be followed, but more importantly, it must be taught to the family because the child will often need medication that must be adjusted for growth for the duration of the condition.

Postoperative care focuses on the child's immediate status and care on continual assessments of fluid balance, incision site, and adherence to the medication regimen. If diuretics are ordered, it is best to administer them as early in the day as possible to avoid bed wetting at night. Because the potassium supplements can be difficult to swallow, mixing them with strong flavored juice helps make the medication more palatable.

Medical Care. Treatment of hyperaldosteronism depends on the cause. Medical management may include use of glucocorticoids such as spironolactone. Surgical removal is recommended in the presence of a tumor (Zeitler et al., 2011). Long-term follow-up depends on the cause of hyperaldosteronism and may include blood pressure control and treatment of hypokalemia (Chrousos, 2012).

Surgical Care. In the presence of a tumor, surgical excision of the affected adrenal gland or tumor is recommended. Once the gland or tumor is excised, it is common for the child to experience hypoaldosteronism postoperatively. Hyperkalemia is also seen in this period because of the potassium replacements. Children may need mineralocorticoid supplementation for several months after the removal of the adrenal gland or tumor. Although postoperatively the blood pressure declines, it may not be sustained and may also need to be controlled with a sodium restriction diet, or antihypertensive medications.

Education/Discharge Instructions

The medication regimens are the focus of parent teaching (e.g., give diuretics early in the day). Alerting the parents to subtle signs of electrolyte imbalances is the best weapon against serious consequences. Parents should know the signs and symptoms of hypo- and hyperkalemia. The parents can also meet with a dietitian to discuss high-potassium foods that can be included in the child's diet. Being open and available to answer questions or to help the parents in any way is the best support that can be given to the family.

PHEOCHROMOCYTOMA

Pheochromocytoma is a condition caused by an adrenal gland tumor. Unlike other tumors, it may not be physically connected to the adrenal gland. In this case, it is called *extra-adrenal*. The tumor intermittently releases excessive catecholamines (i.e., epinephrine and norepinephrine) leading to episodic hypertension (Takeda, Hara, Kawaguchi, Nishiyama, & Takahasi, 2010). The peak incidence of pheochromocytoma is between the third and fifth decades of life with approximately 10% occurring in childhood. The occurrence of pheochromocytoma in the United States is rare with about 800 new cases diagnosed per year, of which the majority are benign and only 10% are malignant (Stöppler, 2010a).

Signs and Symptoms

Signs and symptoms of pheochromocytoma include the following:

- Hypertension is the most common symptom, which may be episodic
- Tachycardia
- Arrhythmias
- Palpitations
- Tachycardia
- Anxiety
- Headache
- Dizziness
- Blurred vision
- Poor weight gain
- Growth failure
- Nausea
- Vomiting
- Abdominal pain
- Pale, clammy skin
- Profuse sweating
- Cool extremities
- Polydipsia
- Polyuria

Pheochromocytoma may also mimic the signs and symptoms of diseases such as hyperthyroidism or diabetes mellitus.

Diagnosis

Thorough assessments begin with a complete medical history and physical examination. The classic diagnostic symptoms of pheochromocytoma include headache, sweating, and heart palpitations (Stöppler, 2010a). Additional studies to diagnosis pheochromocytoma may include blood chemistry and urinalysis to measure hormone levels, CT scan to locate tumor, and an MRI scan to create an image of the functioning adrenal gland (Donohoue, 2010; Zeitler et al., 2011).

Prevention

Preventive measures in caring for the child with pheochromocytoma are through education with the goals of controlling stress, monitoring for signs of hypertension, and maintaining growth and development. Parents also need to be instructed on ensuring that the child is in compliance with medication therapy and follow-up monitoring.

Collaborative Care

Nursing Care.

 Critical Nursing Action Pheochromocytoma

The child with pheochromocytoma can potentially be very ill. Remember to perform assessments frequently. Because the adrenal tumor may sometimes be visible abdominally, it is critical to remember *not* to touch or manipulate it in any way. Palpation can cause a further release of catecholamines increasing the likelihood of a severe hypertensive crisis that could cause potentially harmful tachyarrhythmias.

Nursing care includes caring for the child undergoing surgery to remove the tumor. As with any of these disorders, it is imperative that the nurse be alert during assessments for the most subtle signs of the impending disorder. Hypertension or hypertensive attacks are sometimes the first sign that must be acted on quickly by the nurse. Be sure to thoroughly document history of the symptoms and precipitating factors.

Frequent assessment of vital signs is essential preoperatively. The preoperative nurse notes any hypertensive states or signs of congestive heart failure. Blood glucose levels are also taken at least daily. Prompt reporting of any hyperglycemic readings is important.

Postoperatively, the nurse continues close observation and assesses for signs and symptoms of shock that could be caused from the removal of excess catecholamines. The hospital environment should be calm, just as it is preoperatively. Undue physical or emotional stress is avoided for the child's best possible recovery. Because normal visiting hours can cause stress, parents are allowed to room in and stay with the child anytime, day or night. This measure helps to alleviate the stress that leaving the child can cause. Distractive play is encouraged as long as it does not exceed the child's energy level.

Medical Care.
Tumor removal causes an excessive release of catecholamines, leading to severe hypertension and tachyarrhythmias. Other complications, including hypovolemic shock and catecholamine withdrawal, can cause a dramatic shift in blood pressure leading to hypotension. To avoid these challenging and life-threatening surgical complications, preoperative treatment with medication to inhibit the effects of the catecholamines is begun 1 to 3 weeks before surgery. The drug used most often is an adrenergic-blocking agent such as phenoxybenzamine (Dibenzyline) (Donohoue, 2010). This medication is long-acting, can be given by mouth every 12 hours, and is suitable for long-term use. This blocking agent may be combined with other adrenergic-blocking agents to increase the efficacy of the treatment. Treatment is continued to keep blood pressure within a normal range and to decrease or eliminate hypertensive attacks that include facial flushing, headaches, tachycardia, nausea and vomiting, and hyperglycemia.

Surgical Care.
Treatment of pheochromocytoma is through surgical removal. If the tumor is bilateral, both adrenal glands must be removed and the child placed on lifelong treatment

with mineralocorticoids and glucocorticoids. Tumor recurrence must be monitored through follow-up of blood pressure and catecholamine concentrations (Donohoue, 2010).

Education/Discharge Instructions

Parent teaching about the diagnosis focuses on the signs and symptoms of the condition. Careful observation of the precipitating factors that cause stress can be helpful to keep the child's metabolic needs at a minimum. Anxiety can cause stress, exaggerate the symptoms, and increase metabolism, which causes more catecholamines to be secreted and stimulates a severe hypertensive crisis with possible tachyarrhythmias as well. The parents need to know that touching or palpating the mass can further harm the child in the same manner as stress.

 Now can you—Describe conditions of the adrenals?

1. Describe conditions of the adrenals?
2. Discuss nursing care for conditions of the adrenals?

Metabolic Conditions

Metabolic conditions of the pancreas most often involve the destruction of the **islets of Langerhans** (contain insulin-producing beta cells), which causes a failure to produce and secrete enough insulin to digest the carbohydrates, proteins, and fats eaten by the child. Diabetes is one of the leading causes of chronic illness in the United States. Data from the 2014 National Diabetes Statistics Report indicate that approximately 208,000 people younger than 20 years of age have been diagnosed with either type 1 or type 2 diabetes, which accounts for 0.25% of all children in this age range (American Diabetes Association (ADA), 2011; CDC, 2014a). As American society unknowingly increases carbohydrate intake, the incidence of diabetes is on the rise. It is important to note that previously diabetes was classified as child (type 1—insulin dependent) or adult (type 2—non-insulin dependent) depending on the time of onset and insulin dependency. Today classification is much more complex because either type can affect a person of any age and can be either insulin dependent or non–insulin dependent.

- Type 1 diabetes mellitus: caused by cell destruction resulting in definite insulin dependency
- Type 2 diabetes mellitus: caused by insulin resistance in which the body fails to recognize and use insulin properly

TYPE 1 DIABETES MELLITUS

Type 1 diabetes mellitus is an autoimmune disease that arises when a child with a particular genetic makeup is exposed to any precipitating event, such as infection—particularly viral—or other environmental factors such as diet. This is the most common form of diabetes in persons younger than 40 years of age. Elevated blood glucose levels in excess of 200 mg/dL and elevated hemoglobin HbA_{1c} greater than 7.0% are indicative of type 1 diabetes mellitus (Ward, 2013). Because high glucose levels and ketoacidosis are critical situations, a child initially diagnosed with type 1 diabetes may be hospitalized to control the blood glucose level and determine what type, dose, and frequency of insulin works best for the child. Diet and other essential care measures are also initiated.

Signs and Symptoms

Classic and common symptoms of type 1 diabetes include:

- Polyuria
- Polydipsia
- Weight loss
- Muscle wasting
- Polyphagia
- Nocturia
- Tachycardia
- Blurred vision
- Fatigue
- Vaginal moniliasis

The following symptoms may be present as ketoacid accumulates (Whittemore et al., 2013):

- Abdominal pain
- Nausea and vomiting
- Fruity-smelling breath
- Weakness
- Mental confusion
- Coma
- Slow, labored breathing
- Flushed cheeks and face

focus on safety

Hypoglycemia or hyperglycemia

Teach parents to evaluate the child for the signs and symptoms of either hypoglycemia or hyperglycemia. In understandable terms, explain these signs and symptoms to the parents so they can watch for them at home.

Diagnosis

Primarily, elevated postprandial or random blood glucose levels (usually in excess of 200 mg/dL) and elevated hemoglobin levels (HbA_{1c}) (equal to or greater than 7.0%) are indicative of diabetes mellitus (Whittemore et al., 2013). A fasting blood sugar may be equal to or greater than 126 mg/dL (Whittemore et al., 2013). Urine glucose and ketones may also be increased. The child generally presents with the complaint of the usual triad of symptoms (polyuria, polydipsia, and polyphagia). Per health-care provider order, repeat fasting blood glucoses because at least 2 random elevated blood glucose studies help make the final determination of the diagnosis.

Prevention

Type 1 diabetes is not preventable, though people with type 1 diabetes can help prevent or delay the development of complications by keeping their blood sugar within a target range. Prevention includes adherence to dietary expectations and regular checkups, which include monitoring for changes in blood pressure and cholesterol. Additional preventive measures include the avoidance of smoking and compliance with immunizations as well as with the annual flu shot and pneumococcal vaccine. In the case of adolescents or children old enough to administer their own insulin, parents need to ensure that the child is compliant and following the medication regimen.

Collaborative Care

Nursing Care. Nursing care is individualized based on the needs of the child and family; therefore, the child care is organized around monitoring, stabilization, and education.

focus on safety

Nursing care related to developmental issues

The Infant and Toddler
- Management is up to caregiver(s)
- Consistency in intake is important, particularly carbohydrates
- Food can become a battleground between the caregiver(s) and child
- Carbohydrate consistency rather than a specific food group offers more flexibility than a structured meal plan
- Diluted insulin may be required for some infants
- Establish rituals and routines
- Find a specific place to perform blood tests and keep the supplies
- A toddler will feel more in control if able to predict and participate in activities
- Signs and symptoms of hypoglycemia may be mistaken for the toddler's temper tantrum

The Preschooler
- Characteristics of this age are increased motor maturity, friends, and magical thinking
- They understand simple explanations, which can allay fears
- Stress that the diabetes is not caused by being bad
- Play therapy using dolls and equipment will help them express feelings
- Need meal and snack supervision
- May be able to identify physiological feelings associated with hypoglycemia
- High-energy activities make them susceptible to hypoglycemia
- Caregiver(s) needs to be prepared with carbohydrates as well as emergency medicines

AGE-APPROPRIATE DIABETES TASKS
- Chooses and cleans finger for puncture
- Helps by holding still for injection
- Identifies a word or phrase to describe feeling of hypoglycemia
- Helps by choosing foods

The School-Age Child
- Incorporate the diabetes into a busy school day
- Care needs to be unobtrusive to avoid singling out the child
- Encourage the family to communicate with school personnel
- A school nurse needs to supervise blood glucose monitoring and insulin injections and educate others to recognize and treat hypoglycemia

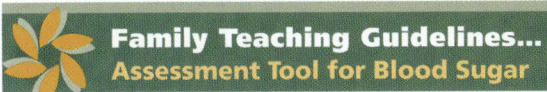

Family Teaching Guidelines...
Assessment Tool for Blood Sugar

ESSENTIAL INFORMATION:

Hypoglycemia (Low Blood Sugar)
- Cold, pale skin (cold sweat)
- Light-headedness
- Shakiness or hand tremors
- Sudden hunger (crave salt or sweet)
- Emotional outbursts (personality changes)
- Drowsiness or extremely tired
- Pounding heartbeat or palpitations
- Nervousness or dizziness
- Anxiety or irritability
- Sweating
- Headache, mental confusion, difficulty concentrating
- Numbness or tingling of lips or mouth
- Poor coordination or staggering, unable to walk
- Slurred or slow speech
- Dilated, enlarged pupils
- Fainting (needs emergency treatment immediately)

Hyperglycemia (High Blood Sugar)
- Loss of appetite, nausea or vomiting
- Increased thirst, even if consuming a large amount of liquids
- Weakness, stomach pains or aches
- Heavy, labored breathing
- Fatigue, tired, often sleepy
- Large amounts of sugar in urine
- Ketones in urine
- Frequent urination
- Blurred or double vision

- Caregiver(s) and the school nurse must plan ahead for field trips, school parties, and athletic events (e.g., send snacks, emergency medicine, and phone numbers)

AGE-APPROPRIATE DIABETES TASKS

- Performs finger puncture and blood glucose test
- Chooses injection site according to rotation schedule
- Pushes plunger on insulin syringe after the needle is inserted by parent or gives own injection
- Performs ketone testing
- Recognizes the need to eat on time to avoid hypoglycemia
- Knows treatment for hypoglycemia

The Adolescent

- Peer group acceptance and body image are important issues
- Risk-taking behaviors are common
- Challenging authority is common
- Missed injections, omitted tests, irregular meals, and dietary splurges are common
- Late adolescence is marked by future orientation and fewer peer group demands
- Shift from caregiver(s) responsibility to the adolescent taking responsibility for her or his condition
- Identify what is important to the adolescent (e.g., appearance, athletic ability, endurance, or weight)

AGE-APPROPRIATE DIABETES TASKS

- Records blood glucose values in diary
- Performs insulin injection
- Draws up and injects insulin
- Looks for patterns in blood glucose values
- Recognizes when to test for ketones
- Initiates treatment for ketones (fluids)
- Chooses correct foods for meals and snack
- Adds extra snack for increased activity
- Can choose appropriate foods at school and social gatherings (Ward, 2013)

Medical Care. The goals of medical management include optimal glycemic control, normal growth and development, minimizing complications, education, and attainment of emotional adjustment to diabetes. The treatment regimen includes monitoring blood sugar for hypoglycemia, hyperglycemia (see Table 27-6), and HbA_{1c} and establishing control through nutrition and meal planning, insulin therapy, exercise, prevention of complications, and education.

Blood Glucose and Ketone Monitoring. The ADA has recommended that the health-care provider weigh the benefits of lowering the child's blood glucose levels against the unique risk of hypoglycemia. Children with type 1 diabetes may lack the capacity to recognize and respond to hypoglycemic symptoms so blood sugar is monitored frequently. Hypoglycemic unawareness is a unique challenge for all pediatric health-care professionals and parents. Home glucose monitoring occurs 3 to 6 times per day (Fig. 27-6). With home testing, glucose control is more exact than in the past. The importance of home monitoring is a vital aspect of care. Parents can be reassured that the glucose monitor is generally covered under most insurance plans.

Urine testing for ketones is performed at least every 3 hours during a child's illness. Ketones also must be checked whenever blood glucose readings exceed 240 mg/dL or when the child experiences unexplained weight loss even if he or she is well. Ketones in the urine are indicative of insulin deficiency.

Insulin. Many factors influence the child's insulin requirements. Insulin needs are affected by the child's nutritional intake and physical energy expended as well as the child's emotional and stress level that accompany normal activities like growth spurts, puberty, and illness. Despite these variables that make insulin regulation extremely difficult, it is the foundation of treatment for a child with type 1 diabetes.

Many types of insulin are available today (Table 27-7). Generally, the type of insulin used for each individual patient is based on the child's blood glucose levels and the child's lifestyle (Whittemore, 2013). Combinations of short, intermediate, and long-acting insulin (premixed) are given

---

Table 27-6 Hypoglycemia and Hyperglycemia

Clinical Condition	Manifestations	Critical Nursing Actions
Hypoglycemia		
Too much insulin for amount of food eaten	Rapid onset Irritable Nervous	• Give 15 grams of carbohydrates (1/2 glass orange juice)
Injected insulin into muscle	Shaky feeling, tremors	• Recheck blood glucose in 15 minutes
Too much activity for insulin dose	Difficult to concentrate Difficult to speak	• If blood glucose is >70 mg/dL give another 15 grams of carbohydrates
Too much time between meals	Behavior change Confused Repeats over and over	• Recheck again in another 15 minutes
Too few carbohydrates eaten	Unconscious Seizure	• If unconscious, give IM glucagon
Illness or stress	Tachycardia Shallow breathing Pale, sweaty Hungry Headache Dizzy	

Table 27-6 Hypoglycemia and Hyperglycemia (continued)

Clinical Condition	Manifestations	Critical Nursing Actions
	Blurry or double vision Photophobic Numbness of mouth or lips	
Hyperglycemia		
Too little insulin for the food eaten	Gradual onset Lethargic Sleepy	• Give additional insulin at usual injection time
Illness or stress	Slow response Confused	• Use sliding scale doses for specific level of blood glucose
Too many carbohydrates eaten	Breathes deeply and rapidly Skin flushed and dry	• Increase fluids
Meals too close together	Mucous membranes dry	• If ketones are elevated, give an extra insulin injection
Too many snacks	Thirsty, hungry, dehydrated	
Insulin given just under skin	Weak, tired, headache	
Too little activity	Abdomen hurts Nausea and vomiting Blurry vision Shock	

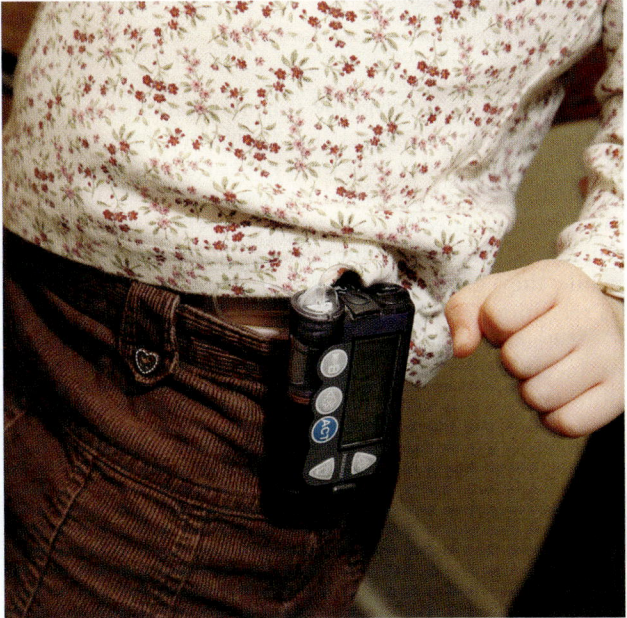

Figure 27-6 Wearing an insulin pump is a good way for children to regulate glucose levels.

subcutaneously throughout the day in an attempt to simulate the body's natural release of the hormone (Table 27-8).

• Humalog/NovoLog insulin is a short-acting insulin. It is clear and usually taken immediately before meals. This regular insulin works so quickly that it can even be taken after meals. It is usually used for children who are picky eaters or toddlers who do not always eat the same amount of food and thus can take the insulin right after they eat.

• Regular insulin is a rapid-acting insulin, which is also clear and begins to act quickly; it merely takes slightly longer to reach its peak than Humalog or NovoLog.

• NPH insulin is an intermediate insulin. It is cloudy and absorbs more slowly. It is made with a protein, enabling its slow release. Even though the peak and the duration can vary from child to child, generally when this insulin is taken in the morning it does not take effect until the afternoon.

• Ultralente insulin peaks somewhat more slowly than the previous NPH. It can be given at dinner, and its effects can help maintain a normal blood glucose level until morning.

• Lantus insulin is long-acting. It is a clear insulin that lasts 24 hours with steady levels, giving it nearly no

Table 27-7 Insulin

Insulin Name	Insulin Type	Onset	Peak Effect	Duration
Humalog/NovoLog	Rapid-acting	10–15 minutes	55 minutes	4 hours
Regular	Short-acting	30 minutes	95 minutes	6–9 hours
NPH	Intermediate-acting	2–4 hours	6–8 hours	12–15 hours
Ultralente	Intermediate-acting	4–6 hours	8–20 hours	24–36 hours
Lantus	Long-acting	1–2 hours	2–22 hours	24 hours

Sources: Chase & Eisenbarth (2011); Jospe (2011).

Table 27-8 Premix Insulin

Insulin Name	Insulin Type	Onset	Peak Effect	Duration
Lente	Premixed	1–2 hours	3–14 hours	18–20 hours
70/30 NPH/Regular	Premixed	30 minutes	Variable	12–18 hours
75/25 NPH/Humalog	Premixed	10–15 minutes	1–8 hours	12–15 hours

Source: Chase & Eisenbarth (2011).

peaking action. It is like NPH in that it is consistent and predictable in its action but can vary within the same child in the time it takes to peak from one day to the next. Lantus, like all types of insulin, is given subcutaneously, but because it cannot be mixed with any other insulin, it must be given as a separate injection.

- Lente, NPH/Regular, and NPH/Humalog are premixed insulin combinations that give the child the benefit of more than one type of insulin with a single injection. The premixed varieties are usually used by families who do not want to have to draw from several bottles.

 Critical Nursing Action Examples of Medical Orders for Insulin Administration

- Apidra Insulin 100 units/mL – give 1 unit(s) for every 12 grams of carbohydrates eaten
- Apidra Insulin 100 units/mL – give 1 unit(s) for every 50 mg/dL BS over 150

(BS 300 minus 150 = 150/50 = 3 units)
- Lantus Insulin 100 units/mL – give 5 units now
- Lantus Insulin 100 units/mL – give 5 units at bedtime

Lantus insulin (dosage determined by health-care provider) given daily at the same time once. In the case of an infant or toddler, the insulin is given after the meal based on the carbohydrate intake (Ward, 2013).

 focus on safety

Sick day rules
- Always give the prescribed insulin.
- Conduct glucose testing every 4 hours.
- Conduct ketone testing with each voiding.
- Give calorie-containing liquids in place of solid foods.
- Follow the usual meal plan (hospitalize the child if he or she cannot retain fluids and food).
- Encourage rest and sleep.
- Notify the health-care provider with concerns.

(Ward, 2013)

Insulin must be given by subcutaneous injection. Parents are taught to expect that their child may need 1 to 4 injections per day and that, generally, the more injections, the greater the blood glucose control. Children can be fearful of injections. Parents need time, patience, and encouragement. Give support to parents and caregivers while they give an injection to boost their confidence (Procedure 27-1).

With some children and adolescents, insulin pump use is increasing because the delivery of insulin is steady throughout the day, which most closely resembles the body's natural response. Recent research has shown that

 Procedure 27-1 Teaching Parents How to Inject Insulin

Purpose

To teach parents how to inject insulin

Equipment
- Insulin bottle from refrigerator (remove up to 1 hour before injection to allow it to warm to room temperature)
- Appropriate syringe (U-30, U-50, or U-100)
- Alcohol wipes
- Container for the dirty, used syringe

Steps

1. Check the expiration date on the insulin bottle.

   RATIONALE: *Ensures that the insulin has not expired.*

2. Wash hands.

   RATIONALE: *Prevents the spread of bacteria.*

3. Clean rubber stopper on insulin bottle with alcohol wipe.

   RATIONALE: *Promotes asepsis.*

4. Remove syringe cap and pull air into the syringe. Line up the end of the black plunger to the exact amount of the insulin dose needed.

   RATIONALE: *Ensures accurate dosage of insulin to be drawn up.*

5. Put the syringe needle through the bottle rubber top and push syringe plunger so that all the air goes from the syringe into the bottle.

Procedure 27-1 Teaching Parents How to Inject Insulin (continued)

6. Turn the insulin bottle upside down and pull the syringe plunger so that the insulin enters the syringe until the top of the black plunger exactly lines up with the dose of insulin to be given.

7. Remove every air bubble, always checking that the dose is exact.

RATIONALE: *Exact dosing is essential in managing the child's condition.*

8. Choose (or let the child choose) the site of the injection.

RATIONALE: *Allowing the child to participate may help him or her feel more in control of the condition.*

9. Clean the injection site with an alcohol swab.

RATIONALE: *Alcohol will decrease the presence of microorganisms.*

10. Pinch up the skin slightly and gently, with the syringe at a 90-degree angle (perpendicular) to the skin, with a dart-like motion, insert the needle into the skin, release the skin.

RATIONALE: *Ensures proper medication administration.*

11. Slowly inject the dose of insulin.

12. Discard the used syringe in a hard, rigid container with a tight-fitting lid.

Teach Parents

If the child expresses that the injection is painful, the following measures can be taken to decrease the pain:

- Inject room temperature insulin.
- Clear even the tiniest air bubbles from the syringe.
- Let the alcohol dry completely before injection.
- Tell the child to relax muscles in area of injection (the more tense the muscles during injection, the more painful the procedure).
- Use syringe-like dart to pierce skin quickly.
- Do not change the needle direction during insertion or withdrawal.
- Never reuse syringes.
- Rotate sites with each injection (giving the insulin in the *same* place twice in 1 day can cause

unnecessary discomfort for the child and undue stress on the tissue).

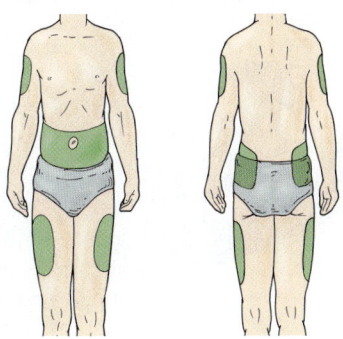

- Document exactly where each injection was given to avoid the same place more than once a day.
- Create and keep a Diabetes Management Notebook with the plan and a place to record daily blood sugar values as well as doses of insulin administered including injection site.

For example:

Date	Blood Glucose A.M.	Blood Glucose P.M.	Insulin Dose Given and Time	Injection Site	Given by
8/9/15	144		4 units regular at 0700	Right mid-arm	Mom
8/9/15	144		4 units regular 4 units NPH 1230	Left mid-thigh	Dad

Documentation

Mother gave 4 units of Regular at 0700 in right mid-arm in the morning, noted by N. Kramer, RN
Father gave 4 units of Regular and 4 units NPH at 1230 in left mid-thigh in the afternoon, noted by
N. Kramer RN

---

with proper training and follow-up, insulin pump therapy provides a lasting and effective treatment modality (Jospe, 2011; Whittemore et al., 2013). Because pumps can be easily mistaken for a cell phone, pager, or iPod, communication with schoolteachers regarding the use and occasional beep is essential (Fig. 27-7).

Caregiver knowledge is associated with better glucose control/outcomes in young children with diabetes (Hassan & Heptulla, 2010). Education is the main route by which a family achieves the best glucose control for the child with type 1 diabetes. The better the blood glucose is controlled, the less frequent the child experiences

complications. Education must focus on insulin types, use, administration, and schedule; meal planning, including the balance of carbohydrates, proteins, and fats; physical exercise; blood glucose monitoring; and extremity care.

Children with diabetes could use alternative therapies to help manage blood glucose levels and to prevent any of the complications associated with the condition:

- Lifestyle changes, particularly diet and exercise
- Medications, namely insulin for individuals with type 1 diabetes

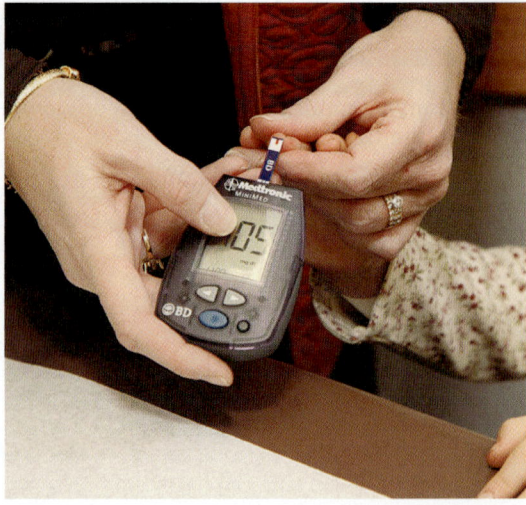

Figure 27-7 Home monitoring requires parents to perform glucose checks on the child with diabetes.

 Medication: Insulin Dosage and Frequency

Although the dosage of insulin is based on the individual needs of the child or adolescent, the precise dose needed for each individual child cannot be predicted. For children, common maintenance doses of insulin range from 0.5 to 1.0 unit per kilogram per day in divided doses (Taketomo et al., 2012).

For adolescents, common maintenance doses of insulin depend on weight and increased need for insulin during a growth spurt. An adolescent may require less than 1.2 units/kg/day during a growth spurt. A non-obese adolescent may require 0.4 to 0.6 units/kg/day, and an obese adolescent may require 0.8 to 1.2 units/kg/day (Taketomo et al., 2012). If 2 doses of insulin are the goal of treatment, then usually 60% to 75% of the insulin is given before breakfast with the remainder given with the dinner meal.

- Stress reduction and relaxation techniques
- Acupuncture for pain from nerve damage

Stressful life events can worsen diabetes in several ways. For example, stress stimulates the nervous and endocrine systems in ways that increase blood glucose levels and disrupt healthy behaviors (e.g., eating habits). Stress management is an integral part of the treatment of diabetes. Studies have shown that diabetics who participate in biofeedback sessions are more likely to reach normal blood glucose levels. Although other studies have produced results that contradict this, researchers and clinicians generally agree that long-term stress is likely to worsen diabetes and that biofeedback, tai chi, yoga, and other forms of relaxation may help motivate people with diabetes to change their habits to manage their condition.

Nursing Insight—*Education for families*

- Teach children and families how to count carbohydrates.
- Teach children and families about exercise in relation to insulin dosage and diet. Exercise plays an important role when regulating glucose levels. Blood glucose levels are decreased during periods of exercise. Children require less insulin. Children with type 1 diabetes who exercise must monitor their blood glucose levels carefully. Monitoring of the glucose levels must occur before, during, and after

exercise. Vigilant monitoring may prevent a hypoglycemic reaction. It is also important for children with diabetes to balance their carbohydrate intake and exercise to maintain normal blood glucose levels. The nurse can help children and families learn about a meal plan that takes into account age, size, weight, exercise level, medications, and other psychosocial and medical issues in relation to their exercise pattern.

- Teach children and families about blood glucose and ketone monitoring. Monitor blood glucose levels 3 to 6 times per day. Monitor urine ketones whenever blood glucose readings exceed 240 mg/dL, when children experiences unexplained weight loss, or if the child is ill.
- Teach children and families about the management of this chronic illness. The focus of follow-up care is helping children reduce symptoms and prevent or prolong the appearance of long-term complications. Standard follow-up care is determined on an as-needed basis, and children are seen by a health-care provider at least every 3 months for glucose and symptom monitoring.
- Teach children and families about diabetic ketoacidosis (DKA). DKA is a combination of hyperglycemia, ketosis, and acidosis resulting from severely deficient insulin in either type 1 or type 2 diabetes. Children are hospitalized so be sure to provide support to the family during this crisis. (Ward, 2013)

Family Teaching Guidelines...
Dealing With a Hypoglycemic Crisis

HOW TO: Recognize the signs of hypoglycemia (child is pale, sweaty, dizzy, "shaky" [tremors], confused, irritable, numb on lips or mouth and can have an altered mental status)

ESSENTIAL INFORMATION:

- Check blood glucose level
- If blood glucose is below 70 mg/dL, rapidly give one of the following sources of carbohydrates (about 10 to 15 grams each), the right amount to treat hypoglycemia:
  - 1/2 to 3/4 cup of orange or grape juice (a juice box is good when one is away from home)
  - 2 glucose tablets or 2 doses of glucose gel
  - 2 to 4 pieces of hard candy
  - 5 gumdrops
  - 1 to 2 tablespoons of honey
  - 1 small box of raisins
  - 6 oz regular (not diet) soda (about half a can)
  - 2 tablespoons of cake icing
- Recheck blood glucose in 15 minutes; if reading is still below 70 mg/dL, then give another glass of juice
- Recheck blood glucose again after another 15 minutes
- When blood glucose returns to at least 80 mg/dL, a more substantial snack (non-concentrated sugar) may be given (e.g., cheese and crackers, bread and peanut butter, etc.) if the next meal is more than 30 minutes away or if a physical activity or exercise is planned
- If the child is unconscious, glucagon is given either subcutaneously or IM (ADA, 2013)

***Across Care Settings*: A team approach**

The care of a child with type 1 diabetes is very complex. A team approach with the family at the core of the team is paramount. Based on age, the child is included in the plan and the care as much as possible (whenever appropriate). The most effective team consists of several members across the specialties within the hospital including primary pediatrician, pediatric endocrinologist, diabetes nutritionist and nurse educator, exercise physiologist, and mental health professionals for psychological support as needed. Lines of communication must be kept open to best serve the family and the child. It is also vital to include other significant adults (living in the home) into the diabetic child's plan of care.

The glucose balance of a child with type 1 diabetes is daunting (Table 27-9). Because glucose control highly depends on monitoring and regulating the child's diet, exercise, and insulin dose and administration, the significant people in the child's daily life must know the plan. That is, the child's teachers, coach, school nurse, counselor, principal, or assistant and even the "lunch mom" must know the appropriate parts of the plan to help actualize it. A child is not to be left unsupported at any time. Whatever the child is involved in away from the home, the responsible adults must know the appropriate care of the diabetic child.

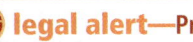 **legal alert—Protection from discrimination**

Students with diabetes are protected from discrimination by federal and some state laws, which establish legal responsibilities for the school. Children with disabilities are protected under the following federal laws: Section 504 of the federal civil rights law, the Individuals with Disabilities Education Act, and the Americans with Disabilities Act. Under the law, children with diabetes and/or other disabilities have the right to free public education appropriate to their needs. The parents or guardians have the legal right to have their child assessed; to request a meeting with the school regarding the child's Individualized Education Plan, which identifies specific services needed; and to be notified of and approve any changes in the plan (American Diabetes Association, n.d.).

Education/Discharge Instructions

Parents and children need to be instructed on the five major components of management and care: insulin types, diet and nutrition, exercise, stress management, and blood

---

 Nursing Care Plan The Child With Type 1 Diabetes

Nursing Diagnosis: Imbalanced Nutrition: Less than Body Requirements related to inability to metabolize carbohydrates

Measurable Short-Term Goal: The child will exhibit blood glucose levels between (specify range for age).

Measurable Long-Term Goal: The child will not experience hypoglycemia or diabetic ketoacidosis.

NOC Outcomes:
Nutritional Status: Biochemical Measures (1005)
  Body fluid components and chemical indices of
  nutritional status
Nutritional Status: Food and Fluid Intake (1008)
  Amount of food and fluid taken into the body
  over a 24-hour period

NIC Interventions:
Hyperglycemia Management (2120)
Hypoglycemia Management (2130)
Teaching: Prescribed Diet (5614)

Nursing Interventions:

1. Identify when the child and family are ready and motivated to learn all aspects of diabetic care.

   RATIONALE: Children and families need time to accept this chronic illness and will not be able to learn until they are ready for new information.

2. Teach child and family about the relationship between nutrition, insulin production and effect, exercise, and the specific treatment regimen prescribed for the child.

   RATIONALE: Understanding the underlying condition will help the child and family manage daily decisions regarding diabetes care.

3. Explain clearly the signs and symptoms of hypoglycemia, hyperglycemia, and diabetic ketoacidosis with appropriate treatment options.

   RATIONALE: Children are highly susceptible to hypoglycemia and cannot always verbalize exactly how they feel.

4. Teach and provide multiple opportunities for supervised practice of blood glucose testing and insulin preparation and administration.

   RATIONALE: Children and families learn best with multiple demonstrations and return demonstrations. Various scenarios will enhance their problem-solving and critical thinking skills.

5. Include the parents and child in the development of the diabetic management plan including blood glucose testing, diet, and exercise.

   RATIONALE: Plans that include the input from the child and the family are more likely to be successful.

Table 27-9 Plasma Blood Glucose and A₁c Goals

Age Group (Years)	Plasma Blood Glucose Goal Range (mg/dL)		Hemoglobin A₁c %	Rationale
	MORNING BEFORE MEALS	BEDTIME/ OVERNIGHT		
Toddlers and preschoolers (0–6 years)	100–180	110–200	>8.5%	High risk/vulnerability to hypoglycemia
School age (6–12 years)	90–180	100–180	>8%	Risk of hypoglycemia and low risk of complications prior to puberty
Adolescents and young adults (13–19 years)	90–130	90–150	>7.5%	Risk for severe hypoglycemia Developmental and psychological issues Lower goal >7.0% is reasonable if it can be achieved without excessive hypoglycemia

Sources: American Diabetic Association (2013); Ward (2013).

glucose and ketone monitoring. Long-term treatments focus on reducing symptoms and preventing complications. Each of these therapies is a vital part of effective metabolic control. Although children and adolescents can be taught to perform the components, family management has proven to afford the diabetic child an improved glycemic control (American Diabetes Association, 2013). Parents and children need to be instructed on how to inject insulin, monitor blood glucose, prevent hypoglycemia, and manage dietary requirements.

focus on safety

Management of diabetes

Attention to safety in the care of the diabetic child doesn't end when the child arrives at school or participates in extracurricular school activities. The child whose health depends on insulin requires 24-hour management. Families may feel concern regarding the safety of their child in relation to good diabetes management. All school members who have a responsibility to the diabetic child need to receive proper training. This may include the school nurse and classroom teachers but also coaches and staff. They need to understand the child's needs, how to identify emergencies, and who to contact when concerns arise (American Diabetes Association, 2011).

Nursing Diagnoses The Child With Type 1 Diabetes

- Risk for injury related to hypoglycemia or hyperglycemia
- Knowledge deficit related to management of type 1 diabetes
- Interrupted family processes related to management of the chronic illness
- Disturbed body image related to management of type 1 diabetes

TYPE 2 DIABETES MELLITUS

Unlike type 1 diabetes mellitus, type 2 diabetes mellitus is caused by the body's resistance to recognize and use insulin rather than a deficient production of insulin as in type 1. For years, type 2 diabetes was labeled as "adult-onset," but in the past several decades there has been an alarming increase in type 2 diabetes in young people. Insulin resistance occurs when the individual cells do not recognize the insulin molecule and resist its influence. The cell membrane does not allow the insulin to initiate the normal enzymatic

reactions that cause metabolism. The glucose cannot be used by the cells, the cells begin to be "starved," and the blood glucose levels slowly but steadily rise.

It is estimated that over one-third of all people with type 2 diabetes are undiagnosed. Though the incidence of type 2 diabetes is rare in children under 10, the increase of type 2 diabetes in the adolescent population has been dramatic over the past decade (ADA, 2013; CDC, 2014b). Three thousand six hundred (3,600) children were newly diagnosed with type 2 diabetes annually between 2002 and 2005. The annual rate of new cases for children younger than age 10 was 0.4/100,000 and 8.5/100,000 for children older than age 10. Rates were also higher among minority populations.

Cultural Diversity: High-Risk Populations

Populations at higher risk include African American, Hispanic/Latina Americans, Native American Indians, and Asian/Pacific Islander Americans (NIH, 2013). In addition to racial risk factors, those associated with the increased incidence include obesity; sedentary lifestyles; high-caloric, lipid-rich diet; and family history. In the Native American Indian population, 76% of new cases among 10- to 19-year-olds are considered to be type 2 diabetes. The incidence in Pima Indians is 51 per 1,000 cases (Whittemore et al., 2013).

Where Research and Practice Meet:
Bionic Pancreas

Boston University is currently testing a "bionic pancreas" in children between the ages of 12 and 20 years. The bionic pancreas is described as a "wearable device that combines continuous glucose monitor and two insulin pumps controlled by a computer program running on an iPhone to automatically give small doses of insulin or glucagon every 5 minutes as needed" (Children With Diabetes, 2013). Participants will attend a 2-week summer camp. Participants have a history of using an insulin pump for at least 3 months. While at camp, participants will be involved in normal camp activities and have the usual camp diet. Participants will wear a continuous glucose monitor. During 1 week, participants will be controlled by the "bionic pancreas." During the alternate week, the participants will have their own insulin pumps.

Signs and Symptoms

Children with type 2 diabetes often have no symptoms, and their condition is detected only when a routine exam reveals high blood glucose levels or complications appear. Occasionally, a child with type 2 diabetes may experience some of the following symptoms, which tend to appear gradually over time:

- Numbness or burning sensation of the feet, ankles, and legs
- Blurred or poor vision
- Impotence
- Fatigue
- Poor wound healing
- Obesity
- Unexplained weight loss
- Headache
- Symptoms of sleep apnea

In some cases, symptoms may mimic type 1 diabetes and appear more abruptly. These symptoms include:

- Polyuria
- Polydipsia
- Nocturnal enuresis or nocturia
- Yeast infections
- Whole body itching

Diagnosis

In the 2013 American Diabetes Association (ADA) position statement, specific criteria were established for type 2 diabetes testing in children:

- Overweight defined as a body mass index (BMI) greater than 85th percentile for age and sex, weight greater than 85th percentile for height, or weight greater than 120% of ideal weight for height
- Plus *two* of the following risk factors:
- Family history of type 2 diabetes in a first- or second-degree relative
- Race/ethnicity (Native American, African American, Latino, Asian American, Pacific Islander)
- Signs of insulin resistance or a condition associated with insulin resistance such as acanthosis nigricans (black-brown velvety skin condition on the back of the neck, axillae, or arms caused by too much insulin in the blood), hypertension, dyslipidemia, polycystic ovary syndrome, or small-for-gestational-age birth)
- Maternal history of diabetes or gestational diabetes mellitus

Blood glucose testing begins at about age 10 years or at the onset of puberty if younger. The frequency of this testing is about every 3 years. The preferred test is the fasting blood glucose level (ADA, 2013). Diagnosis is confirmed with fasting blood glucose results equal to or greater than 126 mg/dL or 2 random blood glucose readings equal to or greater than 200 mg/dL (Whittemore et al., 2013).

Prevention

Type 2 diabetes can be delayed or prevented through a healthy lifestyle. The risk of developing diabetes and complications related to it can be reduced through diet, physical activity, and maintaining a healthy weight. A large prevention study looked at persons with a high risk for diabetes and demonstrated that the development of type 2 diabetes was reduced by 58% during a 3-year period through weight loss, increased activity, and lifestyle changes (NIH Publication No. 09–5099, 2013). Increased awareness of the escalating type 2 diabetes crisis in the pediatric population can give the nurse the necessary tools to begin to fight this problem. Nurses, no matter what their care setting or work environment, teach the public about the value of weight control, active lifestyles, and role model a healthy example for teachers, families, and most importantly, children.

Collaborative Care

Nursing Care. Care of the child with type 2 diabetes may occur in a variety of settings and varies related to the developmental age of the child and the family's response to the diagnosis. Education is the main focus of care and will need to involve those who provide care to or interact with the child, such as parents, teachers, and day-care providers. Managing diet, exercise, lifestyle, and medication compliance as well as preventing complications are the focus of child and family education. The child and parents are provided with information about the disease, prognosis, self-care, the importance of follow-up, monitoring, and treatment needs. Refer to type 1 diabetes for more detail regarding nursing care as appropriate for the child's needs.

Consistent monitoring for complications of diabetes is a critical component of the care of a diabetic child. The nurse must be alert to the signs and symptoms of complications. The signs of acute complications include hypoglycemia, weight loss, and diabetic ketoacidosis. Long-term complications involve the degradation of vital body systems, including cardiopathy, nephropathy, neuropathy, and retinopathy. Many complications can have devastating effects, including growth failure, delayed puberty, menstrual disturbances, emotional disturbances, cataracts, impaired cognitive function, hyperlipidemia, and breakdown or buildup of subcutaneous tissue at injection sites.

Communicate not only with the primary health-care provider but with the endocrinologist, the nutritionist, the diabetic nurse educator, the pharmacist, the social worker, the school nurse, and the home health nurse, so that everyone is knowledgeable about the individual needs of each particular child and his or her family.

Medical Care. The management of type 2 diabetes can vary depending on the severity of the disease. With normal or near normal HbA$_{1c}$ levels, nutritional teaching, such as decreasing calories, and behavioral changes, especially increasing activity, are pivotal to successful therapy. Teaching lifestyle modification must include the entire family to ensure compliance. The ADA (2013) recommends increasing physical activity with the goal of engaging in moderate activity such as walking. Dietary recommendations include limiting the intake of sugar-sweetened drinks, reducing intake of fat and calories, and increasing dietary fiber (ADA, 2013).

With a mildly elevated HbA$_{1c}$ level (5.7%–6.4%) an oral hypoglycemic agent such as metformin (Actoplus Met) may be given (ADA, 2013). The medication, in combination with lifestyle modification, usually successfully lowers the blood glucose level. With severe presentation (greater than 9.0%), treatment is similar to that of type 1 diabetes. Insulin is given either IV or subcutaneously until the child is stabilized. Oral hypoglycemic agents can be given, particularly if the child has lost weight (Chase & Eisenbarth, 2011).

Complementary Care: *Resources*

Multiple complementary care Web sites and resources suggest the use of omega-3 fatty acid as a source of complementary care for persons with type 2 diabetes although a systematic review of the literature did not find any major harm or benefit (Wu, Micha, Imamura, Pan, Biggs, Ajaz, et al., 2012). Though some variation exists regarding the potential benefit of using omega-3 fatty acids as complementary care in the treatment of type 2 diabetes, sources note that because people with diabetes often have high triglyceride and low HDL, the use of eating foods or taking fish oil supplements may provide a benefit without affecting blood sugar (National Center for Complementary and Alternative Medicine, 2009).

Education/Discharge Instructions

Teaching the child, parents, teachers, counselors, coaches, and clergy is the primary focus of nursing care. Healthy eating habits and increasing activity in a sedentary lifestyle are very difficult. All of this must be done without compromising normal growth and development while improving the quality of life.

Provide diabetes education for the entire household (Table 27-10). For instance, if a grandmother resides in the patient's home, but was not included in the teaching, she may unknowingly sabotage the efforts to change eating habits and lifestyle. The nurse must be cognizant of any

---

Table 27-10 Teaching Parents, the Child, and the Adolescent About Diabetes

Parent Outcomes:
- Manage the child's diabetic condition
- Set realistic goals for the child and entire family
- Acquire confidence about providing diabetic care

Child and Adolescent Outcomes:
- Learn to manage diabetic care
- Learn to set realistic goals at and away from home
- Acquire confidence about self-care

Topic	The Nurse Will Teach the Parent(s) About the:	The Child Can:	The Adolescent Can:
The Diabetic Condition	• Type of diabetes • Treatment plan based on age and growth and development benefits of healthy lifestyle	• Give a simple explanation of the disease • Begin to learn diabetic self-care	• Give a more complete explanation of the disease • Perform diabetic self-care
Nutrition	• Importance of breastfeeding and dietary needs during growth and development • The principles of carbohydrate and medications in relation to daily lifestyle • The principles of carbohydrate exchange	• Begin to learn how to make appropriate food choices • Begin to learn the guidelines for meal and snack planning • Begin to understand social eating habits • Begin to learn about the principles of carbohydrate and medications in relation to daily lifestyle • Begin to understand carbohydrate exchange	• Make appropriate food choices • Know guidelines for meal and snack planning • Understand social eating habits • Apply the principles of carbohydrate and medications in relation to daily lifestyle • Apply the principles of carbohydrate exchange
Activities	• Way activity and glucose levels interact • Way younger children have high energy levels that affect blood glucose levels • Way habits such as walking and sports can promote better health	• Begin to understand sedentary activities such as television or computer gaming should be limited • Begin to understand that playing active games or engaging in activities such as walking and sports promote better health	• Limit television or computer gaming • Engage in active games or activities such walking and sports promote better health
Medications	• Way insulin acts and its adverse reactions • Way insulin is dosed • Way to administer insulin • Way insulin is stored • Way to create a medication schedule to fit the family's lifestyle	• Begin to understand the need for frequent supervision related to diet and insulin • Begin to understand how to plan diet and medication around lifestyle • Begin to understand the need for additional carbohydrates or insulin depending on the glycemic state	• Supervise self related to diet and insulin • Plan diet and medication around lifestyle • Recognize the need for additional carbohydrates or insulin depending on the glycemic state
Hypoglycemia and Hyperglycemia	• Signs and symptoms of hypoglycemia and hyperglycemia and how to respond to the situation	• Begin to understand the signs and symptoms of hypoglycemia and hyperglycemia and learn how to respond to the situation	• Understand and respond to the signs and symptoms of hypoglycemia and hyperglycemia

Table 27-10 Teaching Parents, the Child, and the Adolescent About Diabetes (continued)

Topic	The Nurse Will Teach the Parent(s) About the:	The Child Can:	The Adolescent Can:
Medical Emergency	• Cause and response to diabetic ketoacidosis	• Learn about the cause and response to diabetic ketoacidosis	• Understand and respond to diabetic ketoacidosis
Chronicity	• The risk of long-term, uncontrolled diabetes such as the effect on neurological and vascular systems	• Begin to understand the risk of long-term, uncontrolled diabetes such as the effects on neurological and vascular systems	• Understand and respond to the risk of long-term, uncontrolled diabetes and the effects on neurological and vascular systems
Psychosocial Adjustment	• Way to give responsibility to the child for the condition as it relates to developmental maturity • Way to teach others how to manage the diabetic condition • Way to incorporate diabetic care into the family's lifestyle with minimal stress • Way to find parental relief periodically so parents can "get away"	• Learn to manage the diabetic condition based on lifestyle and personal preferences such as peer relationships and daily activities at and away from home • Learn about the importance of weight control • Learn to incorporate healthy habits into everyday lifestyle	• Manage the diabetic condition based on lifestyle and personal preferences such as dating, sex and alcohol, and tobacco and drug use • Understand how peer pressure affects the management of diabetes • Manage weight control • Incorporate healthy habits into everyday lifestyle • Understand how puberty and hormonal changes affect the diabetic condition

Sources: Adapted from Atkinson, A., & Radjenovic, D. (2007). Meeting quality standards for self-management education in pediatric type 2 diabetes. *Diabetes Spectrum, 20*(1), 40–46; Ward, 2013.

factors that may make compliance difficult and talk to the parents and the child about home routines, especially those around mealtime and activities.

 Nursing Insight—*Education for families*

• Teach about diet management (decreasing caloric intake)
• Encourage behavioral changes: increasing activity
• Encourage lifestyle modification; include the entire family to promote compliance
• Discuss oral hypoglycemic agents
• Monitor for complications
  (Ward, 2013)

 Global Health Case Study Type 2 Diabetes

Twelve-year-old Angelina is brought to the urgent care clinic by her parents for a complaint of being tired and having a headache. She is also complaining of vaginal itching and an odorless thick white drainage. Angelina and her family recently emigrated from El Salvador. While doing a physical assessment, you notice the presence of acanthosis nigricans on the back of her neck and on her arms. Angelina also appears to be overweight. Family history includes a father and paternal grandmother with type 2 diabetes. Angelina's history indicates that menarche began at age 11.6, or approximately 8 months ago. Menstrual periods are regular, and she denies sexual activity, smoking, or drug use. A brief nutritional history indicates a diet low in fruits and vegetables and high in flour tortillas, white rice, and processed foods. Traditional foods, including tortillas, rice, and beans, are usually prepared using lard. Meals are eaten with the extended family, with a large meal at noon and a lighter meal in the evening. On physical assessment, the nurse notes the following:

• T = 98.6°F (37.0°C)
• P = 88
• R = 20
• BP = 136/84
• Weight = 122 lb (55 kg) (90th percentile on age-appropriate growth chart)
• Height = 59 in. (150 cm) (50th percentile on age-appropriate growth chart)
• BMI = 88th percentile for age, gender
• Skin pale and dry
• Mucous membranes moist and pink
• Lungs – clear breath sounds
• Abdomen – symmetrical and rounded, active bowel sounds in all four quadrants
• Appears tired, though is cooperative

critical thinking questions

1. Are these findings normal or pathological?
2. What actions should the nurse take?
3. What should be included in parent teaching?
◆ See Suggested Answers to Global Health Case Studies on *DavisPlus*.

Source: Kemp, C. (2005). Mexican & Mexican-Americans: Health Beliefs & Practices.

DIABETIC KETOACIDOSIS

Diabetic ketoacidosis (DKA) is the presenting complaint in nearly one-fourth of all newly diagnosed pediatric patients with type 1 diabetes mellitus (Dowling, 2013). It is a complex combination of hyperglycemia, ketosis, and acidosis resulting from severely deficient insulin in either type 1 or type 2 diabetes (although it is extremely rare in type 2 diabetes). The abnormal metabolism of carbohydrates, protein, and fat that leads to very high glucose levels causes DKA. It is important to know that DKA is the leading cause of death in children with type 1 diabetes.

In many cases, ketoacidosis is a common occurrence with young children who have difficulty verbalizing the classic signs and symptoms.

Signs and Symptoms

It is important to note that in the toddler age group, the classic manifestations of DKA are often absent. In addition, the signs and symptoms may be difficult for the child to verbalize. Many times the child is not known to be diabetic because the onset can often be insidious, but if it is known, a complete history, especially noting the compliance with insulin regimens and the name of the endocrinologist, is essential. Signs and symptoms of DKA include the following:

- Fatigue
- Malaise
- Nausea and vomiting
- Abdominal pain
- Polydipsia
- Polyuria
- Polyphagia
- Weight loss
- Fever

Other signs and symptoms include:

- Altered mental status (the child may be alert or in a coma)
- Tachycardia
- Tachypnea
- Hyperventilation (Kussmaul's respiration)
- Normal or low blood pressure
- Increased capillary refill time
- Poor perfusion
- Lethargy
- Weakness
- Acetone (fruity) odor of breath, which indicates metabolic acidosis

Diagnosis

Diagnosis is confirmed with a blood glucose of greater than 250 mg/dL, ketonuria, or ketonemia with a serum bicarbonate level of less than 18 mEq/L. The pH of the blood is less than 7.34 (Westerberg, 2013). The pH will indicate the degree of the acidosis (Chase & Eisenbarth, 2011).

focus on safety

Diabetic ketoacidosis

DKA is caused by insulin deficiency (Westerberg, 2013). Infection is the most frequent factor associated with the development of DKA, particularly in known diabetics. Aggressive evaluation for infection is always necessary. Antibiotic therapy should be strongly considered until the culture results are known. The following patient-related issues can also be considered:

- Patient has poor compliance with existing insulin regimens
- Patient exhibits underlying endocrine changes of adolescence

- Thelarche—before puberty, just at the beginning of rapid growth
- Adrenarche—activity of the adrenal cortex intensifies and hormones increase (at about 8 years of age)
- Menarche—the first menstruation usually occurs between 9 and 17 years of age
- The caregiver's lack of competence
- Insulin pump failure may occur
- Insulin noncompliance
- Prescription or illicit drug use
- New-onset diabetes

Prevention

Diabetic ketoacidosis can be prevented by close monitoring and control of blood sugars, especially in the presence of infection, other serious illnesses, trauma, or stress (Stöppler, 2010b). In addition, DKA may be prevented by taking extra insulin or other antidiabetic medication as prescribed by the health-care provider. The health-care provider is contacted to assist the family and child in seeking prompt attention as needed.

Collaborative Care

Nursing Care. Care of the patient with DKA is based on four essential physiological principles (Chase & Eisenbarth, 2011):

- Restore fluid volume
- Return child to a glucose utilization state by inhibiting lipolysis
- Replace the child's body electrolytes
- Correct acidosis and restore acid-base balance

Children in DKA are unstable. Fluids and electrolytes can shift rapidly, and the acid-base balance can fluctuate. Because of this instability, the nurse needs to carefully assess signs and symptoms and be prepared to revise treatment protocols as prescribed by the provider. The nurse can expect to rapidly change IV solutions and the need to adjust the plan before one therapy is completed. The outcome of care is to restore hemodynamic and acid-base balance slowly, reducing the acidosis and restoring the child to a normal stabilized state.

The diabetic child in DKA is usually in the intensive care unit. The pediatric intensive care unit nurse must assess the child rapidly, frequently, and thoroughly. The focus of nursing care is to replenish the intravascular volume. Fluid status can be determined by the child's weight, skin turgor, pulse rate, level of consciousness, and blood pressure. As fluid and electrolyte deficits are carefully replaced, the child slowly returns to an acid-base balance status. Ongoing maintenance fluids are then given.

Nursing assessment of acidosis can be ascertained by the presence of Kussmaul's respiration, flushed cheeks, acetone (fruity) breath, and complaints of back and abdominal pain. The bedside nurse is responsible for observing and documenting the child's response to each of the interventions. This requires a skilled nurse who understands and is comfortable with the care of a child in DKA.

With a child in DKA who is possibly comatose and is in the intensive care unit, stress levels of the parents and caregivers are increased. The nurse must stay calm and think clearly. Assessments may need to be made every 15 minutes. One aspect of assessment that is essential to know is the sound of Kussmaul's respiration. **Kussmaul's respiration** is very deep and laborious. In an attempt to correct the metabolic acidosis, the respiratory system works hard to "blow off" excess carbon dioxide. When a child breathes this way, some say it sounds like a locomotive.

With the diabetic child in the intensive care unit, there are many members of the health-care team working together in collaboration to prevent future episodes. In some cases, it was unknown that the child had diabetes, and the DKA is the first time the parents realize that their child is ill. Keeping lines of communication open between parents and health-care providers and realizing that the plan is ever-evolving keeps everyone focused on the best possible outcomes for each child.

Medical Care. Blood glucose is monitored every hour with the blood glucose goal results at approximately 100 to 180 mg/dL. When the child's blood glucose returns to a value below 200 mg/dL, 5% dextrose may be added back to the maintenance IV (Westerberg, 2013). Some health-care providers prefer a 2-bag system hanging at the bedside, one IV bag with and one without glucose. Given through a Y-port, the nurse is able to infuse either one fluid or the other or both if the child needs them.

Serum potassium levels must also need to be checked every 2 to 4 hours (Westerberg, 2013). Initially, DKA causes the child to be hyperkalemic. Acidosis, dehydration, and decreased insulin levels cause an increase in extracellular concentration, though potassium is depleted in the child with DKA. As the dehydration and acidosis improve, and insulin and glucose are given, the child becomes hypokalemic. When the child's urinary output is adequate, potassium may be added to the IV fluids. With normal potassium levels, the child in DKA may need potassium. With abnormally low potassium levels, the ill child may need as much as 20 to 40 mEq/L (Jospe, 2011). Placing the child on telemetry and obtaining an electrocardiogram may be needed to monitor for lethal arrhythmias.

Insulin infusions are begun at 0.1 unit/kg per hour. As the hyperglycemia and acidosis are corrected, the insulin rate is decreased (Jospe, 2011). The insulin infusion is continued until the pH and the acidosis are corrected.

The child's electrolytes are carefully monitored, and the acid-base balance is checked and documented every 2 to 4 hours. As the DKA is resolved, usually in 24 to 48 hours, and the child tolerates oral fluids, the insulin administration is switched to a subcutaneous regimen.

Education/Discharge Instructions

Education is directed at preventing DKA. Families must be taught to check and recheck blood glucose levels or urine ketone levels any time the child is sick (vomiting) or if a blood glucose result is greater than 240 mg/dL. Ideally, the parents are taught and become comfortable with the child's management plan before discharge. Meals and insulin administration are planned to give the child the most normal blood glucose level on average (HbA_{1c}). Parents need to know that long-term complications occur when blood glucose is abnormally high and that keeping the blood glucose at as normal a level as possible is the best protection their child can receive.

 Case Study Child With Type 1 Diabetes

It is the middle of December and this young family is busy with holiday preparations. The children only have a week left of school before the holiday break, and Johnny, the first-grader, has had a "runny nose." It is craft day and the children are excited. The 3-year-old sister begins to cry. She is flushed, seems feverish, and will not drink her favorite juice. The mother calls the clinic and states, "My daughter has vomited twice and is a newly diagnosed type 1 diabetic. I cannot get her to drink, what should I do? I think she may have the flu."

critical thinking questions

1. What is important to relay to the mother?

2. How can the mother convince the child to drink fluids?

3. What should the mother do for the fever?

4. Should the mother call 911 or take the child to the emergency department?

◆ See Suggested Answers to Case Studies on Davis*Plus*.

Now Can You—Discuss diabetes mellitus?

1. Examine the difference between type 1 diabetes mellitus and type 2 diabetes mellitus?
2. Discuss the nursing care for the child with type 1 diabetes?
3. Discuss the nursing care for the child with type 2 diabetes?
4. Discuss the nursing care for the child with diabetic ketoacidosis (DKA)?

Summary Points

◆ The endocrine system controls a child's growth and development.

◆ Hormones regulate a child's response to stress and physical trauma.

◆ Diabetes insipidus is a hypofunction of the posterior pituitary gland, which can be caused by either a deficient production of antidiuretic hormone or lack of response to antidiuretic hormone.

◆ Dehydration is a severe problem, causing the infant or child to be irritable with many other manifestations, including dry mucous membranes, decreased skin turgor (tenting of abdominal skin in infant), decreased tears when crying, sunken fontanelle, and tachycardia. The nurse must act quickly to avoid serious consequences of hypotension and shock.

◆ The pediatric nurse must be thorough and accurately track intake, output, and daily weights of the child because hyponatremia (low serum sodium less than 125 mEq/L) may cause seizures in the child with syndrome of inappropriate antidiuretic hormone.

◆ It is essential that the nurse is aware that congenital hypothyroidism is an important cause of mental retardation. Complications are preventable with the earliest identification and subsequent treatment.

◆ Adrenal crisis is a life-threatening condition in which the anterior pituitary gland does not make enough adrenocorticotropic hormone. Adrenal crisis is a medical emergency, and children with adrenal crisis require *immediate* treatment.

◆ With proper administration, pharmaceutical treatments can be successfully used with many endocrine disorders. The nurse must ensure that the medications are given accurately and that parents are taught techniques correctly.

◆ Educate parents regarding the signs and symptoms of endocrine conditions for the condition to be recognized early and treated as soon as possible.

◆ Insufficient amounts of cortisol and aldosterone cause Addison's disease.

◆ Diabetes is one of the leading causes of chronic illness in the United States.

◆ Type 2 diabetes is caused by the body's inability to recognize and use insulin rather than a deficient production of insulin as in type 1 diabetes and has become an epidemic in the pediatric population.

◆ Diabetic ketoacidosis is the presenting complaint in nearly one-fourth of all newly diagnosed pediatric patients with type 1 diabetes mellitus.

Review Questions

Multiple Choice

1. The pediatric nurse understands that which endocrine gland is responsible for calcium metabolism?
   A. Adrenal
   B. Hypothalamus
   C. Parathyroid
   D. Thyroid

2. A nurse is assessing a child who is in the 3rd percentile for growth. When arranging laboratory and other assessments, the nurse places priority on which endocrine gland?
   A. Adrenal
   B. Hypothalamus
   C. Pituitary
   D. Thyroid

3. The mother of a 7-year-old girl brings her daughter to the pediatrician's office for an annual examination. On assessment, the pediatric nurse notes signs or symptoms that may suggest a diagnosis of precocious puberty. Which assessment finding is inconsistent with the nurse's knowledge of this condition?
   A. Breast development
   B. Brittle hair
   C. Menstruation
   D. Some pubic hair

4. A child presents in the pediatric clinic where the parent reports that his facial features appear "coarser" than before and new onset of hyperhidrosis. Which diagnostic test does the nurse prepare the patient and parent for?
   A. 24-hour urinalysis
   B. Anti-insulin antibody
   C. Oral glucose tolerance test
   D. Serum hormone assay

5. A child has been diagnosed with a pituitary tumor. What medical management does the nurse prepare the child and family for?
   A. Chemotherapy
   B. Radiation treatments
   C. Steroid infusions
   D. Surgical removal

6. A child with diabetes insipidus is being monitored for fluid balance. Which assessment is the most accurate way to determine fluid balance?
   A. Daily weight
   B. Hemodynamic monitoring
   C. Intake and output
   D. Urine osmolality

7. The pediatric nurse monitoring electrolytes understands that at what level does hyponatremia pose the threat of causing seizures?
   A. Less than 150 mEq/L
   B. Less than 145 mEq/L
   C. Less than 130 mEq/L
   D. Less than 125 mEq/L

8. The pediatric nurse is providing care to a pediatric patient with primary adrenal insufficiency. Which item in the patient's history is the most likely cause of this condition?
   A. Autoimmune destruction
   B. Genetic abnormality
   C. Infectious process
   D. Steroid therapy

9. A nurse is reviewing laboratory findings in a child suspected of having Addison's disease. Which finding would be consistent with this condition?
   A. Albumen 4.0 g/dL
   B. Cortisol 2 mg/dL
   C. Potassium 4.4 mEq/L
   D. Sodium 139 mEq/L

10. A parent brings a child to the clinic and reports the child has episodes of sweating, headaches, and heart palpitations. Which medication does the nurse provide education to the parents on?
    A. Desmopressin (DDAVP)
    B. Methylprednisolone (Solu-Medrol)
    C. Phenoxybenzamine (Dibenzyline)
    D. Spironolactone (Aldactone)

See Answers to End of Chapter Review Questions on DavisPlus.

REFERENCES

American Diabetes Association (ADA). (n.d.). Living with diabetes: Legal protection. Retrieved from http://www.diabetes.org/living-with-diabetes/

American Diabetes Association (ADA). (2008). Nutrition recommendations and interventions for diabetes. *Diabetes Care*, Suppl 1, 61–78.

American Diabetes Association (ADA). (2011). Safe at school. Retrieved from http://www.diabetes.org/living-with-diabetes/parents-and-kids/diabetes-care-at-school/

American Diabetes Association (ADA). (2013). Standards of medical care in diabetes—2013. *Diabetes Care, 36,* Suppl 1, 11–66.

Atkinson, A., & Radjenovic, D. (2007). Meeting the quality standards for self-management education in pediatric type 2 diabetes. *Diabetes Spectrum, 20*(1), 40–46.

Baş, V. N., Çetinkaya, S., & Aycan, Z. (2012). Iatrogenic Cushing syndrome due to nasal steroid drops. *European Journal of Pediatrics, 171,* 735–736.

Bhatia, J., Greer, F., & the Committee on Nutrition. (2008, May 1). Use of soy protein-based formulas in infant feeding. *Pediatrics, 121*(5), 1062–1068. doi:10.1542/peds.2008-0564

Bichet, D. G. (2011, September). Treatment of nephrogenic diabetes insipidus (R. Sterns, Ed.). http://www.vivo.colostate.edu/hbooks/pathphys/endocrine/index.html

Bulechek, G. M., Butcher, H. K., Dochterman, J. M., & Wagner, C. (2013). *Nursing interventions classification (NIC)* (6th ed.). St. Louis, MO: Elsevier Mosby.

Centers of Disease Control and Prevention (CDC). (2009). Clinical growth charts. Retrieved from http://www.cdc.gov/growthcharts/clinical_charts.htm

Centers for Disease Control and Prevention (CDC). (2011). *About BMI for children and teens.* Retrieved from http://www.cdc.gov/

Centers for Disease Control and Prevention (CDC). (2014a). *National diabetes statistics report: Estimates of diabetes and its burden on the United States, 2014.* Atlanta, GA: U.S. Department of Health and Human Services. Retrieved from http://www.cdc.gov/diabetes/pubs/statsreport14/national-diabetes-report-web.pdf

Centers for Disease Control and Prevention (CDC). (2014b). *SEARCH for diabetes in youth.* Retrieved from https://www.searchfordiabetes.org/public/dsphome.cfm

Chase, H. P., & Eisenbarth, G. S. (2011). Diabetes mellitus. In W. W. Hay, M. J. Levin, J. M. Sondheimer, & R. R. Deterding (Eds.), *Current diagnosis & treatment,* New York, NY: Lange Medical Books/McGraw-Hill.

Chiapponi, C., Stocker, U., Mussack, T., Gallwas, J., Hallfeldt, K., & Ladurner, R. (2011). The surgical treatment of Graves' disease in children and adolescents. *World Journal of Surgery, 35,* 2428–2431. doi:10.1007/s00268-011-1238-9

Children's Hospitals and Clinics of Minnesota. (2011). *Family services and resources.* Retrieved from http://www.childrensmn.org/patientfamily/family-services-a-resources/education-materials-a-z#PFSDocListD

Children With Diabetes. (2013). *Bionic pancreas summer camp.* Retrieved from http://www.childrenwithdiabetes.com/studies/BionicPancreas2013Camp.htm

Chrousos, G. (2012). Hyperaldosteronism treatment & management. *Medscape: Drugs, diseases & procedures.* Retrieved from http://emedicine.medscape.com/article/920713-treatment

Diaz-Thomas, A. (2012). *Gigantism and acromegaly.* Retrieved from http://emedicine.medscape.com/article/925446-overview

Donohoue, P. A. (2010). Adrenal disorders. In M. S. Kappy, D. B. Allen, and M. E. Geffner (Eds.), *Pediatric practice endocrinology* (pp. 131–190), New York, NY: McGraw Hill Medical.

Dowling, L. (2013). The 4 'T's – aiding prompt diagnosis of type 1 diabetes in children. *Practice Nurse, 43*(2), 18–21.

Endocrine Syndromes. (2011, April 25). *Lab Tests Online.* Retrieved from http://labtestsonline.org/understanding/conditions/endocrine

Eugster, E. A. (2011, September). Pituitary gigantism (M. Geffner, Ed.). Retrieved from http://www.uptodate.com

Greenbaum, L. A. (2011). Fluid and electrolytes. In K. J. Marcdante, R. M. Kliegman, H. B. Jenson, & R. E. Behrman (Eds.), *Nelson's essentials of pediatrics* (6th ed., pp. 625–669). Philadelphia, PA: Elsevier.

Gurgul, E., & Sowinski, J. (2011). Primary hyperthyroidism-diagnosis and treatment: Indications and contraindications for radioiodine therapy. *Nuclear Medicine Review 2011, 14*(1), 29–32.

Hassan, K., & Heptulla, R. A. (2010). Glycemic control in pediatric type 1 diabetes: Goal of caregiver literacy. *Pediatrics, 125*(5), e1104–e1108. doi:10.1542/peds.2009-1486

Huang, S. A. (2010). Graves disease. In M. S. Kappy, D. B., Allen, & M. E. Geffner (Eds.), *Pediatric practice endocrinology* (pp. 94–102). New York: McGraw Hill Medical.

Human Growth Foundation. (2012). Retrieved from http://www.hgfound.org/

John, C. A., & Day, M. W. (2012). Central neurogenic diabetes insipidus, syndrome of inappropriate secretion of antidiuretic hormone, and cerebral salt-wasting syndrome in traumatic brain injury. *American Association of Critical-Care Nurses, 32*(2), 653–656. doi:http://doi.org/10.4037/ccn2012904

Johnson, M., Moorhead, S., Bulechek, G., Butcher, H., Maas, M., & Swanson, E. (2011). *NOC and NIC linkages to NANDA-I and clinical conditions* (3rd ed.). St. Louis, MO: Elsevier Mosby.

Jospe, N. (2011). Endocrinology. In K. J. Marcdante, R. M. Kliegman, H. B. Jenson, & R. E. Behrman (Eds.), *Nelson's essentials of pediatrics* (6th ed., pp. 625–669). Philadelphia, PA: Elsevier.

Kaplowitz, P. B. (2013). *Precocious puberty.* Retrieved from http://emedicine.medscape.com/article/924002-overview#a0199

Kelly, A., & Levine, M. A. (2010). Disorders of bone and mineral metabolism. In M. S. Kappy, D. B., Allen, and M. E. Geffner (Eds.), *Pediatric*

practice endocrinology (pp. 191–256). New York, NY: McGraw Hill Medical.

Kemp, C. (2005). Mexican & Mexican-Americans: Health Beliefs & Practices. Retrieved from https://bearspace.baylor.edu/Charles_Kemp/www/hispanic_health.htm

Kemp, S. (2012). Pediatric growth hormone deficiency. Retrieved from http://emedicine.medscape.com/article/923688-overview#showall

Kemp, S. (2013). Hypogonadism. Retrieved from http://emedicine.medscape.com/article/922038-overview

Khardori, R. (2013). Type I diabetes mellitus. Retrieved from http://emedicine.medscape.com/article/117739-overview#showall

Kumah-Crystal, Y., & Lomenick, J. P. (2011). Growth failure due to inhaled corticosteroid therapy. *Clinical Pediatrics, 50*(2), 159–161.

Lee, P. A., Witchel, S. F., Rogol, A. D., & Houk, C. P. (2010). Disorders of sex development. In M. S. Kappy, D. B., Allen, & M. E. Geffner (Eds.), *Pediatric practice endocrinology,* (300–320). New York, NY: McGraw-Hill.

The Magic Foundation. (2013). Retrieved from http://www.magicfoundation.org/

Miller, R. S., Libber, S. M., & Plotnick, L. P. (2009). Polyuria. *Textbook of pediatrics care.* Elk Grove, IL: American Academy of Pediatrics.

Moloney, S., & Dowling, M. (2012). Early intervention and management of adrenal insufficiency in children. *Nursing Children & Young People, 24*(7), 25–28.

Moorhead, S., Johnson, M., Maas, M. L., & Swanson, E. (2013). *Nursing outcomes classification (NOC)* (5th ed.). St. Louis, MO: Elsevier Mosby.

National Center for Complementary and Alternative Medicine. (2009). Diabetes and CAM: A focus on dietary supplements. Retrieved from http://nccam.nih.gov/health/diabetes/CAM-and-diabetes.htm

National Institute of Environmental Health Sciences. (n.d.). Endocrine disruptors. Retrieved from http://www.niehs.nih.gov/health/topics/agents/endocrine/

National Institutes of Health (NIH) Publication No. 08–3007. (2012, April). Cushing's syndrome. Retrieved from http://www.endocrine.niddk.nih.gov/pubs/cushings/cushings.aspx

National Institutes of Health (NIH) Publication No. 09–5099. (2013). Diabetes prevention program (DPP). Retrieved from http://diabetes.niddk.nih.gov/dm/pubs/preventionprogram/

National Institutes of Health (NIH) Publication No. 14–3054. (2014, Jan). Adrenal insufficiency and Addison's disease. Retrieved from http://www.endocrine.niddk.nih.gov/pubs/addison/addison.aspx

Peroni E., Angiolini, M. R., Vigone M. C., Mari, G., Chiumello, G., Beretta, E., & Weber, G. (2012). Surgical management of pediatric Graves' disease: An effective definitive treatment. *Pediatric Surgery International, 28*(6), 609–614. doi:10.1007/s00383-012-3095-5

Ploski, R., Szymanski, K., & Bednarczuk, T. (2011). The genetic basis of Graves' disease. *Current Genomics, 12*(8), 542–563.

Srivatsa, A., Majzoub, J. A., & Kappy, M. S. (2010). Posterior pituitary and disorders of water metabolism. In M. S. Kappy, D. B., Allen, & M. E. Geffner (Eds.), *Pediatric practice endocrinology* (pp. 94–102). New York, NY: McGraw Hill Medical.

Stöppler, M. C. (2010a). *Pheochromocytoma.* Retrieved from http://www.medicinenet.com/phenochromocytoma/article.htm

Stöppler, M. C. (2010b). *Diabetic ketoacidosis.* Retrieved from http://www.emedicinehealth.com/diabetic_ketoacidosis/page9_em.htm

Takeda, K., Hara, N., Kawaguchi, M., Nishiyama, T., & Takahasi, K. (2010). Parathyroid hormone-related peptide-producing non-familial pheochromocytoma in a child. *International Journal of Urology, 17,* 673–676.

Taketomo, C. K., Hodding, J. H., & Kraus, D. M. (2012). *Pediatric & neonatal dosage handbook: A comprehensive resource for all clinicians treating pediatric and neonatal patients* (19th ed.). Hudson, OH: Lexi-Comp.

Thabet, F. I., Bozarth, X. L., & Barboi, A. C. (2012). Myopathy as the initial presentation of Addison's disease. *Journal of Pediatric Neurology, 10,* 309–312. doi:10.3233/JPN-120580

Triantafyllou, P., Mavrides, P., Katzos, G., Printza, N., & Papachristou, F. (2010). A girl with progressive fatigue and hyponatremia: Answer. *Pediatric Nephrology, 25,* 2271–2273. doi:10.1007/s00467-009-1404-6

Trip-Hoving, M., Van Alfen-Van der Velden, J. A., & Otten, B. J. (2009). Psychosocial deprivation as a cause of growth retardation in children. National Center for Biotechnology Information. Retrieved from http://www.ncbi.nlm.nih.gov/pubmed/19900333

Understanding Acromegaly. (n.d.). Acromeagaly info: Novartis. Retrieved from http://www.acromegalyinfo.com/info/understanding/home.jsp

University of Kansas Medical Center Genetics Education Center. (2012). Dwarfism/Short Stature. Retrieved from http://www.kumc.edu/gec/support/dwarfism.html

U.S. National Library of Medicine, National Institutes of Health. (2012). Growth hormone deficiency–children. Retrieved from http://www .nlm.nih.gov/medlineplus/ency/article/001176.htm

Vallerand, A. H., & Sanoski, C. A. (2014). *Davis's drug guide for nurses* (14th ed.). Philadelphia, PA: F.A. Davis.

Van Leeuwen, A. M., Poelhuis-Leth, D. J., & Bladh, M. L. (2011). Davis's Comprehensive Handbook of Laboratory and Diagnostic Tests (Version 14.0.4) [Computer software]. Philadelphia, PA: F.A. Davis Company.

Venes, D. (2013). *Taber's cyclopedic medical dictionary* (22nd ed.). Philadelphia, PA: F.A. Davis Company.

von Oettingen, J., Pou, J. S., Levitsky, L. L., & Misra, M. (2012). Clinical presentation of children with premature adrenarche. *Clinical Pediatrics, 51*(12), 1140–1149.

Ward, S. (2013). *Pediatric nursing care: Best evidence-based practices.* Philadelphia, PA: F.A. Davis.

Westerberg, D. P. (2013). Diabetic ketoacidosis: Evaluation and treatment. *American Family Physician, 87*(5), 337–346.

Whittemore, B. J., Smaldone, A., & Steiner, R. D. (2013). Endocrine and metabolic disorders. In C. E. Burs, A. M. Dunn, M. A. Brady, N. B. Starr, & C. G. Blosser (Eds.), *Pediatric primary care* (5th ed., pp. 529–556). Philadelphia, PA: Elsevier.

Wu, J. H., Micha, R., Imamura, F., Pan, A., Biggs, M. L., Ajaz, O., et al. (2012). Omega-3 fatty acids and incident type 2 diabetes: A systematic review and meta-analysis. *British Journal of Nutrition, 107,* Suppl 2: S214–S227. doi:10:1017/S0007114512001602

Zeitler, P. S., Travers, S. H., Nadeau, K., Barker, J., Kelsey, M. M., & Kappy, M. S. (2011). Endocrine disorders. In W. W. Hay, M. J. Levin, J. M. Sondheimer, & R. R. Deterding (Eds.),*Current diagnosis and treatment: Pediatrics* (20th ed.). New York, NY: McGraw Hill.

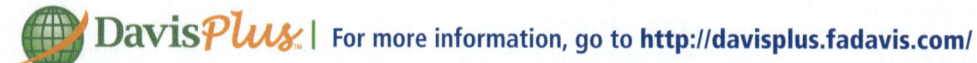

DavisPlus | For more information, go to **http://davisplus.fadavis.com/**

CONCEPT MAP

Caring for the Child With an Endocrinologic or Metabolic Condition

Organs:
- Hypothalamus
- Pituitary gland
- Thyroid and parathyroid
- Adrenal gland
- Pancreas
- Pineal body
- Ovary or testes

Hormones:
- ADH
- Growth hormone
- TSH; PTH
- ACTH-releasing
- Aldosterone
- Insulin

General Potential Nursing Care:
Assessments: thorough nursing history; school performance; sleep patterns; growth measurements, including skeletal; presence of abnormal physical characteristics for age and body build; vital signs; heart rate/rhythm/perfusion; urine output; daily weight, I&O; fluid/electrolyte balance; neurological assessment
Interventions: approach child using correct emotional and cognitive developmental level; address body image issues; manage stress; encourage exercise/activity/adjust diet; provide emergency treatments for acute conditions; care of the post-surgical child; care of the child with chronic illness; includes collaborative and interdisciplinary care
Teaching: about condition itself; treatments; resources/foundations; administration of, compliance with and side effects of medications; treatments for home care (i.e., wts, I&O); follow-up appoinments; S & S of complications

Adrenal Conditions:
- Adrenocortical insufficiency
  - Acute: life threatening < ACTH
  - Chronic: Addison's disease
  - Cushing's syndrome
- CAH: congenital adrenal hyperplasia
- Hyperaldosteronism
- Pheochromocytoma
  - Adrenal tumor

Metabolic Conditions—Pancreatic:
- Type I diabetes
  - Autoimmune
- Type II diabetes
  - → With all, failure to produce sufficient insulin
  - → DKA: prevalent in Type I

Thyroid Conditions:
- Hypothyroidism: untreated = goiter
- Hyperthyroidism: Graves disease

Parathyroid Conditions:
- Hypoparathyroidism: inherited or acquired
- Hyperparathyroidism: leads to osteoporosis; osteomalacia

Pituitary Conditions
Anterior →
- Hypopituitary: GHD
- Hyperfunctioning pituitary
  - Precocious puberty: sex characteristics < age 8–9
  - Acromegaly/gigantism: abnormal/overgrowth hands/feet/facial features

Posterior →
- Diabetes insipidus: < ADH production, gross water loss
- SIADH: > ADH, gross water retention

Clinical Alert:
!
- Exogenous hormones in OTC feminine products
- Accurate growth assessment necessary for child with GHD
- Dehydration can lead to hypovolemic shock
- Tenting not always seen in hypernatremic dehydration r/t SIADH
- Hyponatremia can precipitate seizures
- A thyroid storm is potentially fatal
- Know signs/symptoms of impending adrenal crisis; untreated Addisonian crisis can be fatal
- Hyperglycemia increases susceptibility to infection; infections major fx associated with DKA
- Teach parents signs/symptoms of hyper-/hypoglycemia

Critical Nursing Action:
- Accurate assessment of ht/wt (growth assessment)
- Daily weights necessary to calculate accurate medication doses in children
- Assess IV site for Ca⁺ infusion
- Never stop steroid therapy suddenly
- Never touch/manipulate visible adrenal tumor (pheochromocytoma)
- Nursing care for child with DM Type I r/t developmental issues
- Know correct insulin orders r/t type

Optimizing Outcomes:
- Help parents to access financial resources for CnRH tx.
- Use hormones to treat Addison's disease

Cultural Diversity:
- Assess palms/lips for color for changes in dark complected child
- Certain ethnic groups are at higher risk for developing Type II DM

Nursing Insight:
- There are many ways to offer families/children support (e.g., listening, providing info)
- GH, IGF-I, somatostatin are involved in acromegaly
- Classes of diabetes insipidus have different etiologies
- Soy-based formula may decrease absorption of levothyroxine
- DiGeorge syndrome = defect in development of parathyroid gland
- Know how to assess hyperreflexia
- An adrenal crisis is life-threatening
- 10–15% of those with DM are children < 18 with Type I
- Dietary plan in Type I DM crucial to proper blood glucose maintenance

Where Research and Practice Meet:
- Type I diabetes is not purely genetic; environmental factors
- Use of bionic pancreas

What to Say:
- Help child express anxiety about daily injections (meds to rx endocrine condition)
- Discussion r/t surgical correction of CAH should include child

Across Care Settings:
- Team approach for DM Type I treatment

Legal Alert:
☑
- Children with DM are protected from discrimination r/t receiving free public education

Collaboration in Caring:
- Psychological counseling is part of the team approach
- Endocrinologist important team member

Now Can You:
?
- Describe conditions of the anterior/posterior pituitary
- Explain nursing care for conditions of the thyroid
- Discuss diabetes mellitus Type I and II and associated nursing care

Focus on Safety:
!
- Know sick day rules for diet/meds in Type I DM
- Teach all school members care of the child with DM

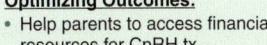

chapter

28

Caring for the Child With a Neurological or Sensory Condition

 Men ought to know that from the brain, and from the brain only, arise our pleasures, joy, laughter and jests, as well as our sorrows, pains, grief, and tears.
—Hippocrates (about 400 B.C.)

LEARNING TARGETS *At the completion of this chapter, the student will be able to:*

- ◆ Describe the anatomy and physiology and developmental aspects of the neurological system.
- ◆ Examine common conditions of the neurological system.
- ◆ Prioritize developmentally appropriate and holistic nursing care for common conditions of the neurological system.
- ◆ Explore diagnostic testing, laboratory testing, and medications for common conditions of the neurological system.
- ◆ Develop teaching plans and discharge criteria for parents whose children have common neurological conditions.

PICO(T) Questions

The intent of evidence-based practice (EBP) is to provide nursing care that integrates the best available evidence. An initial step in EBP is to write a PICO(T) question that effectively guides the research. A PICO(T) question is an acronym that stands for population (P), intervention or issue (I), comparison of interest (C), outcome (O), and timeframe (T). Depending on the question, all or some of the question components are used in the research process. Use these

PICO(T) questions to spark your thinking as you read the chapter.

1. What are (O) evidence-based practices for (P) nurses caring for an infant suspected of suffering from (I) abusive head trauma?

2. What are (I) beneficial strategies that nurses can teach (P) parents of children with spina bifida to (O) optimize bowel function?

 Evidence-Based Practice

Brustrom, J., Thibadeau, J., John, L., Liesmann, J., & Rose, S. (2012). Care coordination in the spina bifida clinic setting: Current practice and future directions. *Journal of Pediatric Health Care, 26*(1), 16–26.

The purpose of this study was to describe the goals for, and the process used, in care coordination. In addition the study examined the perceived effectiveness and barriers in care coordination as determined by clinical care coordinators and families of children with spina bifida. Care coordination for the person with spina bifida involves multidisciplinary support and occurs over the lifetime of the person. Multiple specialties are involved in comprehensive, life span coordination of care for the individual

with spina bifida, which include but are not limited to orthopedic, neurology, urology, gastroenterology, developmental pediatrics, and nursing as well as coordination of social, occupational therapy, nutritional, financial, and educational services. Previous literature describes care coordination as a "process of organizing services in such a way that they can be used easily by people with spina bifida and their families, with the ultimate goal being to, first, teach the family, and later the young adult with spina

Evidence-Based Practice (continued)

bifida to independently navigate medical, educational, and financial systems necessary to ensure as much self-sufficiency as possible" (p. 17). Care coordination is generally understood as a service provided by one member of the patient care team who coordinates services provided by a multidisciplinary team. Care coordinators also facilitate future appointments and referrals and ensure treatment plans are agreed on and communicated to the family. Previous research notes that effective care coordination can provide better communication, improved connection with community resources and support, better understanding of care goals, improved family relationships with providers, reduced caregiver strain, fewer trips to the clinic, fewer complications, and fewer hospitalizations.

Participants in this study included clinic staff from seven spina bifida clinics in the United States. Focus groups were also held with parents/caregivers whose children were under the care of each of those clinics. Currently there are 121 spina bifida clinics in the United States. Potential participants for this study were selected from 63 clinics that responded to a previous survey done by the Spina Bifida Association (SBA). Responses to the SBA survey were grouped and stratified according to size, location, number of active patients younger than 21, and level of care coordination services provided. These were further grouped into four regions of the United States. Eight clinics agreed to participate though one subsequently dropped out related to staffing changes. Caregivers included in the focus groups were recommended to the researchers by clinic staff.

Of the 7 clinics selected, 2 were from the eastern part of the United States, 2 from the Midwest, 2 from the south, and 1 from the Pacific region. The mean population served by the clinics was 310.7 and ranged from 150 to 600 clients. Seventy-five percent (75%) of the population served were Caucasian, though half of one clinic's population was Hispanic. Six of the clinics served clients whose ages ranged from birth to mid-twenties; one clinic served clients whose ages ranged into the thirties. Clients were served at no-charge in 2 clinics with 50% or more of the clients at the other 5 clinics insured by Medicaid. Clients served were from predominately low to middle socioeconomic backgrounds. All but 1 clinic averaged 10 to 15 clients per day with the other clinic averaging 20 to 30 per day. Forty-three clinic staff and 38 caregivers participated in the study. Staff members included 9 clinic directors and 11 nurse/clinic coordinators (categorized as one because of job responsibilities). Other types of staff represented in the total were medical specialists, therapists, social workers, and business managers. The average staff tenure was 10.5 years and ranged from 6 months to 30 years. The average number of years the caregivers attended the clinics was 8 years and ranged from 1 to 18 years. All caregiver participants except one were the birth or adoptive mothers of children with spina bifida. The one outlier was a father. The age ranges for the children of the caregivers was 2 to 21 years of age and averaged 9 years. Most participants lived from 1 to 2 hours' drive away from the clinic.

Data were gathered through the use of semi-structured interviews with clinical staff; focus groups were used to obtain information from the caregivers. Research activities at each of the clinic sites included 5 to 9 staff interviews and 1 caregiver focus group. Individual interviews with staff ranged from 20 to 60 minutes. Focus groups averaged 3 to 7 participants and lasted form 1½ to 2 hours. Focus group participants received $40 cash or $20 gas cards, depending on the clinic policy, as an incentive to participate. Staff participation was voluntary and without monetary incentive. A focus group facilitator guide and a staff interview guide were developed for the project. The guides included questions related to the purpose of the project. Data from the interviews and focus groups were transcribed and coded by two independent analysts. Coded data were entered into an analysis program, which helped generate themes.

Results were organized under the following themes: goals of care coordination, care coordination processes and procedures, perceived effectiveness of care coordination, and care coordination barriers and facilitators. The goals of care coordination can be summarized as follows: (1) considering each child and family holistically and meeting their overall needs, (2) coordinating multiple services to be provided during one visit, and (3) assisting children in gaining increased independence and reaching their full potential. Recommendations obtained from the theme of care coordination included improving communication among families, scheduling appointments on one day, and those appointments that needed to be at a better time to meet family needs. Providing families with more information and access to community resources, improving communication among the clinic care team with more involvement in the care conference, and improving communication between the clinic care team and the family was also noted. Barriers mentioned by both staff and caregivers included insufficient staffing, clinic day logistics (too long of a day and too many providers trying to see patients at one time), lack of community resources or ability to communicate their availability, lack of team meetings and communication among team members, lack of sufficient insurance coverage and reimbursement, and families' hesitancy to communicate needs to staff. Facilitators identified by both staff and caregivers included dedicated staff and use of a single staff to coordinate care, all specialists available on the same day, linking families to resources, providing opportunities for families to interact with each other, team meetings to facilitate communication, teamwork, and providing resources for transportation. Most of the staff and caregivers noted that services were effective and beneficial. Caregivers stated that they were generally happy with the care provided, though they made recommendations for changes as noted under barriers and facilitators. Staff believed that the services they provided increased access for families and helped reduce burdens. Care coordinator staff members considered their role as a liaison between families and providers.

The researchers conclude that though care coordination can be complicated and time consuming, both staff and caregivers/families agree that it results in benefits to the clients and family members and may reduce the burden to families. The results of the study suggested the importance of adequate staffing and teamwork, as well as family involvement in the plan of care.

1. How is this information useful to clinical nursing practice?

2. Based on these findings, what are implications for further research?

See Suggested Responses for Evidence-Based Practice on Davis*Plus*.

Introduction

This chapter provides a review of the anatomy and physiology of the nervous system followed by a discussion of factors that influence alterations in consciousness. An examination of the various neurological conditions with developmentally appropriate and holistic nursing care is included. This chapter also provides a review of the alterations related to non-traumatic neurological conditions and sensory and language disorders. Information about diagnostic and laboratory testing and medications is given. Teaching plans and discharge criteria for parents whose children have various neurological conditions are incorporated.

Neurological conditions can happen at any time of growth and development and may lead to poor long-term developmental outcomes for the child. Competent neurological assessment and recognition of neurological conditions are done by highly skilled nurses so the child can meet his or her most realistic potential.

A & P review The Nervous System

The nervous system is made up of the central nervous system (CNS), which consists of the brain and spinal cord and the peripheral nervous system (PNS) (Fig. 28-1). The PNS consists of the cranial nerves, the spinal nerves, and peripheral nerves. The PNS is subdivided into the sensory-somatic

The Nervous System

☐ **Central Nervous System**
  Brain
  Spinal cord
☐ **Peripheral Nervous System**
  Cranial nerves
  Spinal nerves

Intercostal nerve
Radial nerve
Cauda equina
Median nerve
Ulnar nerve
Sciatic nerve
Femoral nerve
Digital nerve
Common peroneal nerve
Deep peroneal nerve
Tibial nerve
Superficial peroneal nerve
Saphenous nerve

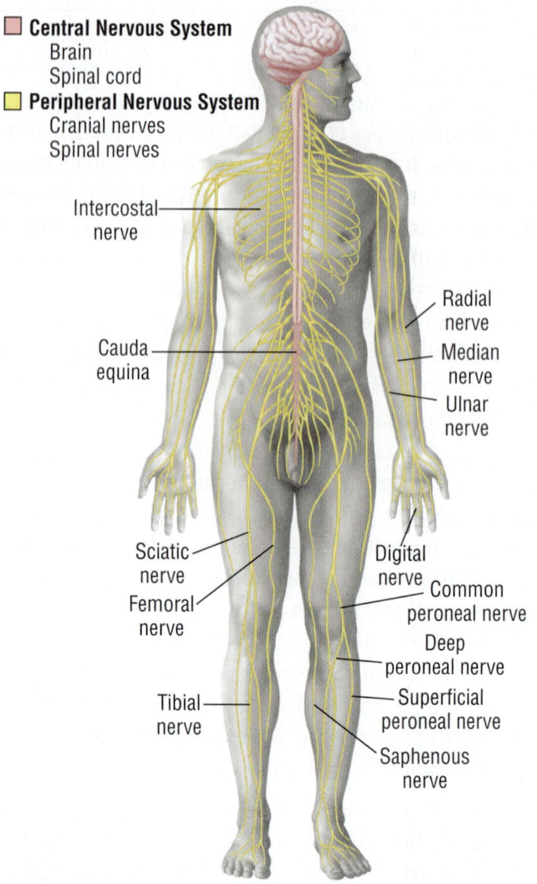

Figure 28-1 Anatomy and physiology of the neurological system.

Growth and Development

The child with a neurological condition such as cerebral palsy is at greater risk for limited intellectual development than typically developing children because of impaired physical mobility and altered sensory and perceptual changes. Intellectual capacity impacts daily-life functioning; verbal, memory, and literacy skills; functional mobility; self-care; and social functioning (Smits, Ketelaar, Gorter, Schie, Becher, Lindeman, et al, 2011). With limited intellectual capacity, the child is highly likely to have decreased growth and development.

Nursing care of the child with a neurological condition should focus on maximizing the child's intellectual, cognitive, and motor abilities through comprehensive rehabilitation services. The nurse understands that impaired physical mobility is associated with decreased muscle control and strength. Physical therapy is required to assess and treat motor dysfunctions. The nurse should implement range of motion exercises and position the child to promote tendon stretching to encourage mobility, increase circulation, and prevent contractures. The nurse understands that activities of daily living and play promote motor growth and development. The nurse should encourage the child to use fine and gross motor skills while completing these tasks such as eating with a utensil and getting dressed. The nurse should allow time for the child to complete the task. The nurse should position toys that encourage rolling and reaching. Education about keeping physical therapy appointments and wearing proper brace wear and adaptive equipment is important.

The nurse understands that sensory and perceptual changes are caused by cerebral damage. The nurse should provide assistance with accepting or learning alternative methods for living with diminished vision or hearing. The child can benefit from varied forms of sensory and perceptual input. Technologies such as tablet devices and personal computers have provided new ways for children with sensory changes to communicate and interact. The nurse should encourage the use of these adaptive devices to enhance sensory input. The nurse should educate the family about maximizing the usage of the child's intact senses when possible.

Smits, D., Ketelaar, M., Gorter, J., Schie, P., Becher, G., Lindeman, E., et al. (2011). Development of non-verbal intellectual capacity in school-age children with cerebral palsy. *Journal of Intellectual Disability Research, 55*(6), 550–562. doi:10.1111/j.1365-2788.2011.01409.x. Epub 2011 Mar 25.

---

nervous system and the autonomic nervous system. The brain is a network of nerve cells called neurons, which consist of axons and dendrites. Axons take information away from the cell body, and dendrites bring information to the cell body. Brain tissue may be white or gray. White matter consists of axons that are coated with myelin, which allow nerve impulses to travel rapidly, and gray matter is made of neuronal cell bodies and surrounds the cerebral hemispheres, thus forming the cerebral cortex. Areas of gray matter are also found deep in the brain and include the basal ganglia (affect movement), the hypothalamus (maintains homeostasis and regulates blood pressure, heart rate, and temperature), and the thalamus (processes sensory impulses and sends them to the cerebral cortex). Another important structure of the nervous system is the spinal cord.

The spinal cord is a mass of nerve tissue encased in a vertebral column, and the cord contains sensory and motor pathways. The spinal cord does not extend the length of the vertebral canal. A disruption in the pathway from the brain to the PNS and spinal cord results in altered neurological function (Bickley & Szilagyi, 2013). ◆

Altered Level of Consciousness

Consciousness comprises two components: arousal and thought content. Arousal or level of consciousness (LOC) is awareness of the environment by which the child is alert and responsive to environmental stimuli.

LOC is controlled by the reticular activating system and the cerebral hemispheres of the brain. A child may experience various levels of consciousness depending on the neurological condition. An alteration in content of thought may be caused by internal or external factors including structural, metabolic, and psychogenic. Structural factors are abnormalities of the anatomy of the brain. Metabolic factors include infections, trauma, congenital anomalies, vascular anomalies, and toxins (McCance & Huether, 2010). Psychogenic factors are influenced by psychological disturbances within a child.

Altered LOC is a significant indicator of neurological dysfunction. The most common cause of altered LOC in children is infection of the brain and meninges (American Academy of Pediatrics [AAP], 2010). When determining the etiology of an altered state of consciousness, organic and functional causes are evaluated. Abnormal responses and nursing actions to assess the state of consciousness are identified in Table 28-1.

Unconsciousness is a state in which a child's cerebral function is depressed. Unconsciousness ranges from a stupor (aroused only with vigorous or unpleasant stimulation) to a coma (state of unconsciousness when the child cannot be aroused even by painful stimuli) (Venes, 2013).

The unconscious child requires astute and continuous monitoring. The nurse carefully monitors vital signs, LOC, reflexes, and pupil reaction. In addition, the nurse carefully and meticulously documents the objective data obtained to determine any deterioration that may alter therapy. The cause of the patient's unconscious state guides the nursing care and medical management. Also a nurse should assess the child for any seizure activity that may occur as a result of cerebral ischemia and edema. A **persistent vegetative**

state is a complete unawareness of the environment accompanied by sleep-wake cycles.

INCREASED INTRACRANIAL PRESSURE

Whether the pathological process is structural or metabolic, increased intracranial pressure (ICP) can lead to secondary (preventable) brain injury. Therefore, prompt diagnosis and aggressive treatment of increased ICP is essential to limiting secondary brain injury in children with a neurological insult (Pitfield, Carroll, & Kissoon, 2012). A delicate balance exists between the volume of the intracranial vault and the contents including the brain, blood, and **cerebrospinal fluid (CSF)**. The CSF is the fluid of the brain and spinal cord that supplies nutrients and removes waste products and also serves as a watery cushion that absorbs shock to the central nervous system (CNS) (Venes, 2013). The **intracranial pressure** is the pressure of the CSF in the subarachnoid space between the skull and the brain. The cranium and vertebral body form a rigid container, and if any of its contents increase, an increase in ICP occurs. As brain volume expands, some compensation is possible as CSF and blood move into the spinal canal and extracranial vasculature. The normal ICP is 0 to 10 mm Hg. Once the ICP reaches approximately 20 mm Hg, small increases in blood volume can result in extreme elevations in ICP (Piña-Garza, 2013) (Fig. 28-2).

focus on safety

Monro-Kellie hypothesis

The pressure-volume relationship among the blood, ICP, volume of CSF, brain tissue, and cerebral perfusion pressure is known as the Monro-Kellie hypothesis or Monro-Kellie doctrine. The hypothesis states that if one of the components increases, the other components must compress. The body tries to compensate by an increase in CSF absorption, a decrease in CSF production, a reduction in blood volume, or a decrease in brain mass. When compression is exhausted, the ICP rises. As a result of increased ICP, blood flow and oxygen delivery may be compromised. When blood flow and oxygen decrease, secondary brain injury occurs (Mokri, 2001; Scanlon & Sanders, 2010).

 Nursing Insight—*Increased intracranial pressure*

Increased ICP can have devastating and long-term consequences for the child and family. Infants and children whose fontanelles have not closed are able to compensate for increased ICP for a short time. The child's fontanelles bulge, and cranial sutures may spread apart to accommodate the increased volume.

 Nursing Insight—*Cerebral perfusion pressure*

The difference between the mean arterial pressure within the cerebral vessels and ICP is termed **cerebral perfusion pressure (CPP)**. The CPP is calculated by subtracting the ICP from the mean arterial pressure (MAP): (CPP = MAP – ICP).

One of the primary dangers of increased ICP is that decreasing cerebral perfusion can cause ischemia. As the ICP nears the level of the mean systemic pressure, it is more difficult for blood to enter the intracranial space. The body's natural response to a decrease in CPP is to increase blood pressure and dilate the blood vessels in the brain. The vasodilation results

Table 28-1	States of Consciousness Technique and Patient Response	
State	**Technique**	**Response**
Alertness	Speak in a normal tone of voice	An alert patient answers appropriately while opening his eyes and responding fully.
Lethargy	Speak in a loud voice	A lethargic patient opens his eyes but appears drowsy; answers questions appropriately but falls asleep easily.
Obtundation	Shake gently to arouse	An obtunded patient opens his eyes and looks at the stimuli; appears slightly confused; alertness and interest in surroundings are decreased.
Stupor	Use a painful stimuli	A stuporous patient only responds to painful stimuli; verbal responses are absent or slow; responsiveness to a painful stimuli ceases.
Coma	Apply repeated painful stimuli	A comatose patient does not respond to internal or external stimuli; he remains in an un-arousal state with eyes closed.

Source: Bickley & Szilagyi (2013).

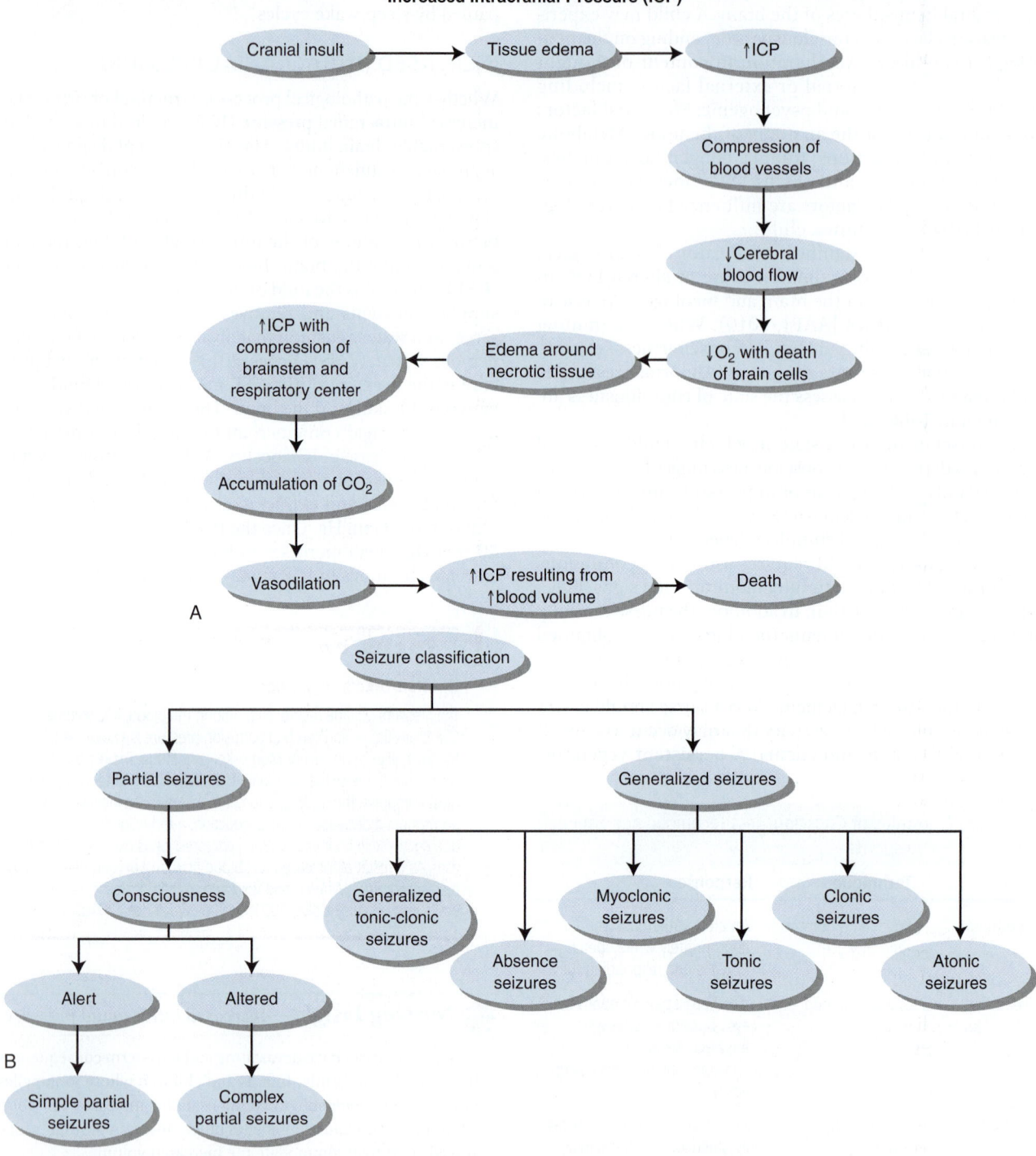

Figure 28-2 Algorithm for increased intracranial pressure.

in increased cerebral blood volume that increases ICP and lowers CPP further. This vicious cycle results in widespread reduction in cerebral blood flow and perfusion leading to ischemia and brain infarction. CPP is maintained at greater than 50 to 70 mm Hg with increased ICP because a lower level may result in secondary hypoxic–ischemic injury (Kochaneck, Carney, Adelson, Ashwal, Bell, Bratton, et al., 2012). An increase in blood pressure may also make intracranial hemorrhages bleed more quickly, which increases ICP (Scanlon & Sanders, 2010). If brainstem compression is involved, the respiratory center is affected and respiratory depression and arrest may occur.

Signs and Symptoms

The clinical features of ICP vary according to the child's age and the rate at which the pressure increases. The signs and symptoms of a child with increased ICP are related to cerebral edema and ischemia and may include the following (Table 28-2):

Early Signs in Children:

- Change in LOC
- Irritability
- Lethargy
- Headache
- Nausea and emesis

Table 28-2 Signs and Symptoms of Increased Intracranial Pressure in Infants

Early Signs and Symptoms	Late Signs and Symptoms
Headache	Further decrease in LOC
Emesis	Bulging fontanelles (infant)
Change in LOC	Decreasing spontaneous movements
Decrease in GCS score	Posturing
Irritability	Papilledema
Sunsetting eyes	Pupil dilation with decreased or no response to light
Decreased eye contact (infant)	Increased blood pressure
Pupil dysfunction	Irregular respirations
Cranial nerve dysfunction	Cushing's triad (late, ominous sign)
Seizures	See Table 28-3–Types of Seizures and Signs and Symptoms

- Diplopia and blurred vision
- Seizures

 Nursing Insight—*Cushing's triad*

A child with significantly increased intracranial pressure may exhibit Cushing's triad. Symptoms of Cushing's triad are hypertension (with widening pulse pressure), bradycardia, and an irregular respiratory pattern. Cushing's triad is a late sign and usually indicative of impending herniation (the displacement of the brain through the foramen magnum) (Venes, 2013).

Diagnosis

The diagnosis of increased ICP is based on signs and symptoms exhibited by the child and diagnostic test results. **Papilledema** (a mass of blown-out blood vessels located around the optic nerve) is an important sign of increased ICP. This finding can be observed when the nurse assesses the child's eyes with an ophthalmoscope.

 Diagnostic Tool Determining Increased Intracranial Pressure

Magnetic resonance imaging (MRI) or computed tomography (CT) is used to determine the etiology and severity of increased ICP. As a rule, CT contrast is avoided in the presence of intracranial bleeding. The child's ICP can also be monitored by inserting an intracranial catheter.

Prevention

Safety and injury prevention, educational strategies, and anticipatory guidance on safety issues are essential to decrease many preventable injuries in children (Brain Injury Association of America 2012; Centers for Disease Control and Prevention [CDC], 2012a).

Collaborative Care

Nursing Care. Closely monitor the pediatric patient with increased ICP because changes in the neurological status can occur very quickly and may have life-threatening

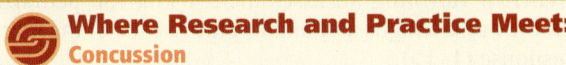 **Where Research and Practice Meet:**
Concussion

A research study conducted by Zuckerman, Lee, Odom, Solomon, Forbes, and Sills (2012) found that in sport-related concussions, athletes 13 to 16 years old take longer to return to their neurocognitive and symptom baselines than athletes 18 to 22 years old. The Concussion in Sport Group (CIS) recommends greater caution regarding return to play with children and adolescents. Proper assessment and management of concussions in children are crucial to prevent long-term sequelae.

consequences. The nurse's initial assessment provides a baseline by which the child's progress is evaluated. The goals of the child's care are to provide general supportive care and prevent secondary injury.

When caring for the child with an altered state of consciousness, carefully monitor the child's neurological status by assessing LOC with the use of a pediatric Glasgow Coma Scale (GCS). The pediatric GCS consists of three components of assessment: eye opening, motor, and auditory/visual responses (Fig. 28-3).

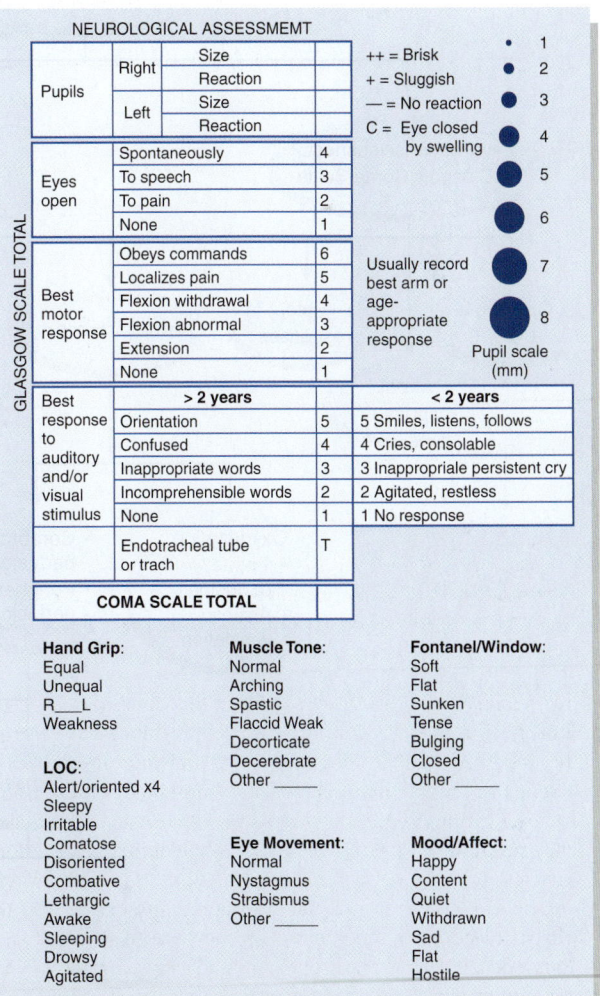

Figure 28-3 The pediatric Glasgow Coma Scale.

When performing an assessment using the pediatric GCS, the nurse assigns a numeric value to each of the levels of response (1–15).

- Score of 9–15 (unaltered state of consciousness)
- Score of 8–4 (state of coma)
- Score of 3 or below (deep coma)

Coma scale scores may fluctuate if a change in neurological state occurs, including cerebral ischemia; the administration of medications, including paralytics and sedatives; and a regaining of consciousness.

The nurse carefully monitors, measures, and documents vital signs, LOC, reflexes, and pupil reaction as prescribed by the health-care provider or as dictated by facility policy. The frequency of vital sign measurement is dependent on the etiology, neurological status, and cerebral involvement. Any change in vital signs needs to be evaluated because the child's condition can deteriorate rapidly. The child's vital signs may need to be assessed every 15 minutes or more often if the neurological state or physical state is unstable. If the child's condition is stable, vital signs are measured every 2 hours (Fig. 28-4).

Cerebral infections can cause elevated temperatures so the child's temperature must be measured every 2 to 4 hours. Antipyretics such as acetaminophen (Children's Tylenol) or ibuprofen (Children's Advil) are administered by the nurse to lower the child's temperature. Cooling the environment, applying a hypothermic blanket, or providing a tepid bath is also used to decrease body temperature.

The head of the bed can be elevated 15 to 30 degrees and the child's head maintained in a midline position to prevent jugular compression and facilitate venous drainage. Perform passive range-of-motion exercises at least every 2 hours to prevent development of contractures.

A priority for any child with an alteration in consciousness is obtaining and maintaining a patent airway. Inadequate oxygenation or excess carbon dioxide causes cerebral blood vessels to dilate, resulting in an increase in ICP. The child is intubated if the Glasgow Coma Score is less than 8 (Kochaneck et al., 2012). In addition, if the child is intubated, monitor the ventilator equipment. It is important to maintain normal ventilation in children. Sometimes positive end expiratory pressure is necessary to maintain oxygenation saturations above 95%.

The nurse meticulously monitors respiratory status including respiratory rate and rhythm, use of accessory muscles, apnea, breath sounds, and level of oxygenation. A child in a light coma still may be able to cough and swallow and maintain adequate respiratory function. A child in a deep coma may be unable to swallow or adequately handle

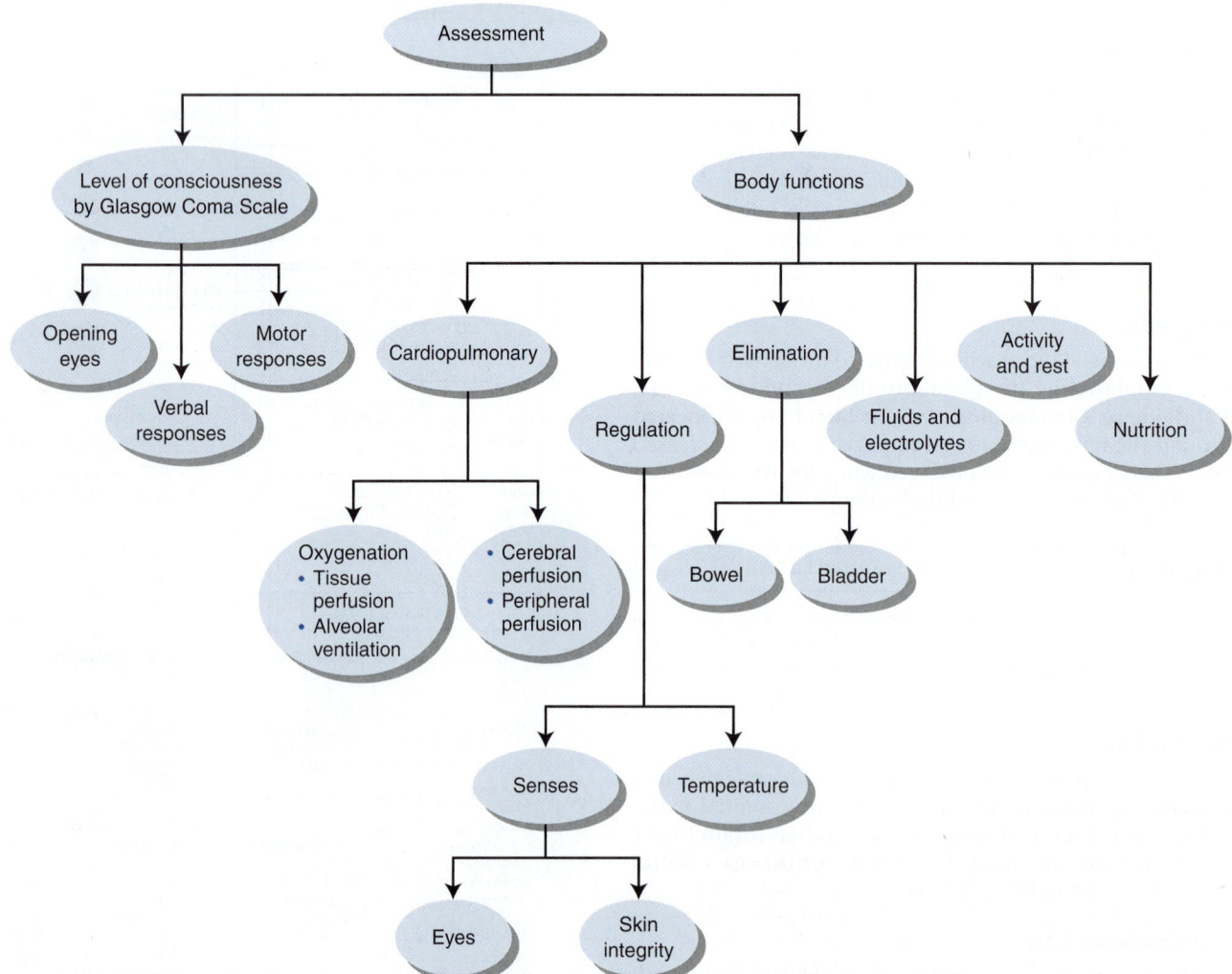

Figure 28-4 Caring for the unconscious child.

oral secretions. It is important to note that the gag reflex of an unconscious child may be impaired. The airway must be suctioned to remove secretions that may obstruct the airway or that may be aspirated. Be careful when suctioning the child's airway because ICP may increase.

If the child's condition deteriorates, hyperventilation, with a bag valve mask (e.g., Ambu Resuscitator®), may be performed until the ICP decreases. Hyperventilation is aimed at keeping a low level of serum PCO_2 so that cerebral blood flow decreases and reduces cerebral blood volume, thereby reducing ICP. Prolonged hyperventilation is avoided because it may cause hypotension as a result of decreased venous return (Kochaneck et al., 2012). Mild hyperventilation may be prescribed by some health-care providers. If the child is not intubated, supplemental oxygenation will be necessary. If possible, the child should be positioned on the side to decrease possible airway obstruction.

A child who cannot maintain respiratory function needs to be mechanically ventilated. The child may need ventilator assistance for only a short time or may be dependent on the ventilator indefinitely. When caring for a mechanically ventilated child, monitor the arterial blood gases. Administer medications to sedate or relax the child to prevent injury related to manipulation of the endotracheal tube or accidental extubation.

The unconscious child who is intubated for an extended period of time requires a tracheostomy. The nurse performs tracheostomy care for these patients. The nurse changes the child's position at least every 2 hours and performs chest physiotherapy to prevent respiratory complications of atelectasis and pneumonia.

Critical Nursing Action Assessing for Hypothermia

When using a hypothermic blanket, monitor the patient's temperature continuously to prevent **hypothermia** (a body temperature below 95°F [35°C]). Hypothermia causes shivering and increased ICP.

Complementary Care: *The Benefits of Massage Therapy*

When caring for any child, the nurse can incorporate therapeutic massage. The child may benefit from the many positive results of massage (e.g., decreased blood pressure, increased circulation, increased skin tone, and improved peristalsis). Benefits of massage may also include decreased anxiety, decreased skin breakdown, and decreased constipation.

Focus on Safety

Care measures

Two care measures are important for patient safety: (1) never place the patient's head lower than the body; this position significantly increases the patient's ICP, and (2) administer IV fluid cautiously because hypertonic IV solutions have an osmotic effect. Normal saline, lactated Ringer's solution, and albumin are primarily used. Hypotonic IV fluids (a combination of dextrose [5% or 10%] and sodium chloride [0.22% or 0.3%]) are avoided because they cross the blood–brain barrier resulting in increased cerebral edema and ICP.

If a child has increased ICP and has inadequate circulation, fluid administration takes priority over concern about cerebral edema. Fluid restriction is contraindicated in children who are poorly perfused with brain pathology or are hypovolemic (have an insufficient amount of fluid in the circulatory system) because hypovolemia results in decreased cerebral perfusion. The nurse closely monitors fluid balance by accurately measuring and recording intake and output.

The child with increased ICP is predisposed to seizures. Monitor seizures for such factors as frequency, severity, and type of seizure. The nurse places the child under seizure precautions, which includes padded side rails or bed rails, oxygen and suction equipment readily available, IV access, and anticonvulsant medications at the bedside according to physician prescription.

Medical Care. The nurse administers antiseizure medications such as phenytoin (Dilantin) as prescribed by the health-care provider. This medication controls seizures but may cause gingival hyperplasia, which is a long-term effect. The nurse observes for swelling and bleeding of the child's gums and provides good dental hygiene. Parents must be taught about the necessity of performing proper hygiene when their child is taking this medication. Also, medications must be administered to decrease cerebral edema based on the health-care provider's order. A drug frequently prescribed is mannitol (Osmitrol).

Medication: Mannitol (Osmitrol)

(man-i-tol)

Classifications: Osmotic diuretic, diagnostic agent

Indications: Reduction of intracranial pressure and treatment of cerebral edema

Actions: Increases the osmolality of the glomerular filtrate, preventing the reabsorption of water and resulting in a loss of sodium chloride and water

Contraindications: Use cautiously with hypersensitivity, anuria, and active intracranial bleeding

Incompatibilities: Do not add to blood products

Adverse Reactions and Side Effects: CNS: Confusion, headache; **ENTT:** blurred vision; **CV:** chest pain, pulmonary edema, tachycardia; **GI:** nausea, thirst, vomiting; **GU:** renal failure, urinary retention, dehydration, hyperkalemia, hypernatremia, hypokalemia, hyponatremia; **LOCAL:** phlebitis at the IV site

Route and Dosage: Reduction of intracranial/intraocular pressure: 1 to 2 g/kg as a 15% to 20% solution over 30 to 60 minutes.

Nursing Implications:
1. Do not administer electrolyte-free mannitol with blood products. If blood is administered, add at least 20 mEq of NaCl to each liter of mannitol.
2. Confer with physician regarding placement of an indwelling Foley catheter (except when used to decrease intraocular pressure).
3. Administer by IV infusion undiluted.

Evaluation/Desired Outcomes:
1. Urine output of at least 30 to 50 mL/hr or an increase in urine output in accordance with patient parameters set by physician
2. Reduction in intracranial pressure
3. Reduction in intraocular pressure
4. Excretion of certain toxic substances

Source: Vallerand, A. H. & Sanoski, C. A. (2014). *Davis's drug guide for nurses* (14th ed.). Philadelphia, PA: F.A. Davis.

Barbiturates may also be administered to reduce ICP. Barbiturates cause the blood vessels in the brain to constrict, but the blood vessels in the rest of the body to dilate. Carefully monitor volume status and blood pressure. The use of steroids with increased ICP is controversial. Corticosteroids have no effect on cytotoxic brain edema resulting from metabolic, infectious, or hypoxic–ischemic disorders (Alderson & Roberts, 2009). The child with increased ICP may require analgesia and sedation. The child who is hospitalized for increased ICP is usually in an intensive care unit or in an area where he is closely monitored. Overstimulation from the child's environment, in addition to fear and pain, may increase the ICP.

Pain and agitation is treated aggressively if increased ICP is present. Nursing actions that may increase ICP include endotracheal suctioning, bathing, and positioning. If the child's ICP becomes dangerously high, the child is sedated and, if necessary, paralyzed. Narcotics such as morphine (Astramorph) or fentanyl (Sublimaze) and benzodiazepines such as lorazepam (Ativan) are titrated to the desired effect.

Optimizing Outcomes—Intracranial pressure monitoring

A pressure line is inserted to accurately monitor ICP. Several types of monitoring devices are available, including intracranial bolts, intraventricular catheters, and intraparenchymal fiberoptic catheters. Intracranial pressure monitoring is indicated for the child who has a GCS score <8, who exhibits signs of increasing ICP, who is post major neurosurgical procedures, or who has a high probability of having increased ICP. The best outcome for ICP monitoring is to maintain cerebral perfusion pressure between 50 and 70 mm Hg, for an ICP <20 mm, and monitor for occurrences such as herniation or bleeding.

Surgical Care. A **craniotomy** (an incision through the cranium) is recommended only when all other measures have been unsuccessful. A complication of a craniotomy is herniation of the brain through the defect, leading to further edema and an increase in ICP (Brain Trauma Foundation, 2012). After a craniotomy, assess the child for signs and symptoms of infection and increased ICP postoperatively. The nursing care measures discussed above also apply to postoperative care of the child.

Education/Discharge Instructions

Provide education that incorporates knowledge of head injury and postprocedural care for the child as well as prevention measures, medications, referrals, and potential complications.

Nursing Diagnoses The Child With Increased Intracranial Pressure

- Impaired mobility related to altered neurological functioning
- Impaired gas exchange related to increased intracranial pressure
- Risk for impaired skin integrity related to decreased mobility and incontinence
- Risk for infection related to invasive hospital procedures
- Risk for aspiration related to enteral feeding
- Risk for altered bowel elimination related to decreased peristalsis

SEIZURE DISORDERS AND EPILEPSY

A **seizure** is an electrical disturbance within the brain, resulting in changes of motor function, sensation, or cognitive ability. Seizure activity is classified according to the area of the brain experiencing the abnormal electrical activity and the neuromuscular sensory and psychogenic alteration from the electrical conduction disturbance. The incidence and onset of seizure disorders varies by age and underlying physical or pathological condition. Seizures may be genetically linked in susceptible children, or the etiology may be unknown. Seizures can result from a traumatic brain injury, an infection in the central nervous system, toxic ingestion, endocrine dysfunction, atrial–venous malformation, or an anoxic episode. Neonates may develop seizures because of intrapartum or postpartum anoxic episodes, maternal ingestions or exposure to teratogens, and prenatal infections. Hypoglycemia and congenital malformations can also cause neonatal seizures in the first month of life.

An estimated 2.2 million Americans have epilepsy, with approximately 150,000 new cases diagnosed in the United States each year. Approximately 1 in 26 people will develop epilepsy at some point in their lives, and the onset of epilepsy is highest in children and older adults (Institute of Medicine of the National Academies, 2012).

Nursing Insight—*Febrile seizures*

Febrile seizures are the most common form of first-time seizure in childhood and are usually seen in children younger than 3 years of age. Children may experience a febrile seizure between the ages of 6 months to 5 years, but the most common occurrence is in the first 1 to 2 years of life. The exact etiology of febrile seizures has not been clearly identified. There may be a family history of seizure activity or febrile seizures. A simple febrile seizure is a brief (less than 15 minutes), generalized episode that occurs only once during a 24-hour period in a febrile child without any evidence of metabolic imbalance, history of prior febrile seizure, or intracranial infection. A complex febrile seizure lasts longer than 15 minutes and recurs within 24 hours. Antipyretics and anticonvulsant therapy may be administered, but this treatment is controversial in prophylaxis therapy and prescribed more frequently in complex febrile seizures. There is a slightly increased incidence of epilepsy in children with febrile seizures over the general population, especially if other types of seizures or abnormal CNS development are present in the child or the family (Hampers & Spina, 2011; Robertson & Shilkofski, 2012; Steering Committee on Quality Improvement and Management, Subcommittee on Febrile Seizures, American Academy of Pediatrics, 2008).

Signs and Symptoms

Seizures are classified as generalized or partial (focal) (Table 28-3).

Diagnosis

Seizures are diagnosed clinically with the use of neurological testing. Neurological testing procedures are used to determine the etiological epileptic focal center in the brain causing the abnormal electrical activity. In-depth testing of

Table 28-3 Types of Seizures and Signs and Symptoms

Type of Seizures	Brain Location/Cause	Signs and Symptoms
Partial (Focal)	Localized to one area	One area is affected: hands, lips, wrist, arms, or face. Impaired loss of consciousness at onset.
Partial complex (psychomotor)	Temporal lobe	Loss of consciousness and loss of awareness or surrounding. Changes in behavior (lip smacking, picking, inappropriate mannerisms, confusion) follow the seizure.
Partial simple		Lasts 5 minutes, child only remembers the aura. Automatisms are noted. No loss of consciousness or awareness. Motor signs are isolated to one area of the body and then spread to the rest of the body. May experience senses such as buzzing sounds, tingling, flashing lights, anxiety, fear, or anger.
Generalized		
Tonic-clonic	Genetic predisposition or brain injury secondary to anoxia	Partial simple and complex seizures evolve to generalized seizures. Aura is experienced followed by loss of consciousness and tone. Patient falls to the floor with tonic-clonic muscle contractions. Patient is postictal and confused after the seizure is over. Loss of urine may occur.
Atonic: loss of muscle tone, drop attacks. Absence (petit mal)		Sudden drop to the floor caused by loss of motor muscle tone. Seen in children 2 to 4 years of age. No loss of consciousness but experiences loss of awareness. Nonconvulsive. Periods of staring or minor movements lasting seconds. May occur several times a day, interferes with learning and schoolwork.
Tonic		Stiffening of the body that is sustained, involving all four extremities.
Myoclonic	Metabolic etiology	Single or multiple jerks or flexion of limbs.
Clonic		Intermittent rhythmic jerking, 1–3 per second, may start in one body location and move or migrate to another location.
Myoclonic and akinetic		Complete or total lack of movement.

the neurological system helps to classify the type of seizure and determine appropriate anticonvulsant therapy. The neurological exam to diagnose seizures consists of a cranial nerve assessment, deep tendon reflex, sensory and motor response, level of consciousness, and hearing and pupil checks. A CT scan or an MRI is performed to look for CNS malformation, lesions, neoplasms, hemorrhage, trauma, foreign body, or edema. An angiography is done to assess for arteriovenous malformations that may be hereditary. New-onset seizures may suggest malignant neoplasms and warrant emergent neuroimaging.

Electroencephalogram (EEG) is the accepted standard test for diagnosing a seizure disorder. The EEG evaluates the electrical activity of the brain while the brain is in a sleepy or drowsy state and also when stimulated (Fig. 28-5). Loud noises, bright lights, and rapid flashing images are presented during the procedure, and the resulting electrical brain wave response is graphed. This information is useful to the neurologist in diagnosing the type of seizure activity, especially if the history and exam do not support a clear diagnosis. Video EEG can also be done if the EEG is inconclusive or if the child experiences sleep and waking onset seizures. Positron emission tomography is performed if brain structures require outlining or mapping before a surgical procedure, but is not routinely indicated for seizure evaluations. **Pseudoseizures**, or false seizures, are evaluated as neurological episodes until determined to be psychological or not pathological in nature and etiology.

Prevention

In nearly two-thirds of the cases of epilepsy, a specific underlying etiology is not found (CDC, 2012b). Preventable events such as traumatic and/or anoxic brain injuries, brain infections, or stroke are causes of epilepsy.

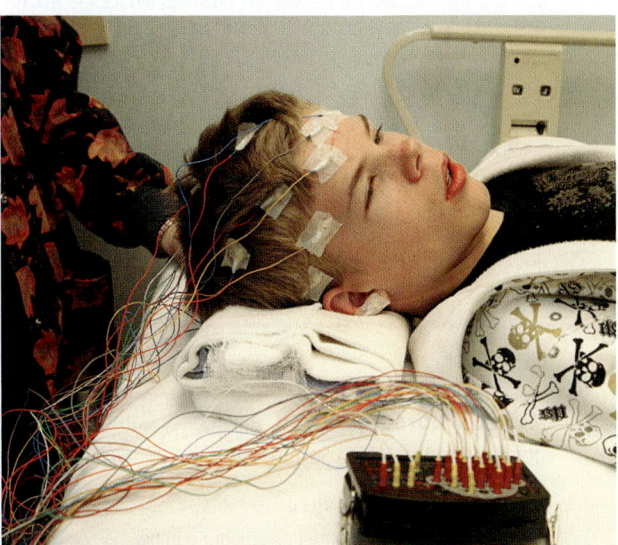

Figure 28-5 The EEG evaluates the electrical activity of the brain while the brain is in a sleepy or drowsy state and when stimulated.

Collaborative Care

Nursing Care. The nurse completes a detailed history of the seizure event, an in-depth review of the child's prenatal and postnatal history, and review of systems. The event history must include antecedent events that may have precipitated the seizure such as dehydration, video-gaming, exercise, or any ingestion of substances that may cause seizures. Information regarding the type of activity during the seizure, any loss of consciousness, loss of urine, noises made, cyanosis, and history of present illness is also retrieved from the persons who witnessed the event. Because of the genetic predisposition of some types of seizures, a family history and type of seizure activity must be obtained. The neurological exam is completed by the physician or a neurological specialist.

Seizure management is a collaborative effort among the nurse, the medical team, the primary care provider, and the family. Specific nursing care for a child with seizures is determined by the type of seizure. If the etiological agent for the seizure is pathological in origin, seizures are managed medically until the cause can be resolved. If the cause is a brain tumor, the mass is excised. If the cause is endocrine dysfunction, it is resolved. If infection is present, appropriate antibiotic therapy is initiated. If the cause of the seizure is unknown and a structural abnormality is not present, the child is placed on an anticonvulsant therapy specific for the type of seizures being experienced.

focus on safety

Seizure precautions

- Maintain airway patency; ensure nothing is placed in the child's mouth during a seizure. A loose tooth may be aspirated or knocked out. Suctioning may be necessary after the seizure is over.

- Monitor oxygenation saturation; the child's color should remain pink. The pulse oximeter should read 95% or greater and the heart rate is normal or slightly raised.

- Administer IV medications. When administering IV medications during a seizure, give the medication slowly to reduce the risk of side effects such as respiratory or circulatory failure.

- Raise and pad the side rails when the child is in a bed or the crib; the child needs to be protected from injury (Fig. 28-6).

- Teach parents about the importance of having the child wear a medical alert bracelet. The child who has seizures is advised to wear a medical identification bracelet at all times.

- Also provide emotional support to the child and family. Allow the child and family to express their feelings, offer a support group, and remind the family to treat the child as normally as possible.

Critical Nursing Action Emergency Care for the Child Having a Seizure

1. In the community setting call 911.
2. In a hospital, use the designated emergency number.
3. Maintain a patent airway. If the airway is occluded, open the airway with a jaw thrust maneuver. Administer oxygen if needed and available. Do not put anything in the mouth. If the situation

warrants emergency medical care, qualified health-care personnel can insert an appropriate-sized oral airway.
4. Loosen restrictive clothing to ensure adequate circulation to essential body organs.
5. Administer medications such as diazepam (Valium), lorazepam (Ativan), or fosphenytoin (Cerebyx) as ordered by the physician. These medications are not administered to a neonate because they are toxic as a result of immature liver function.
6. Monitor respiratory status and circulatory status throughout the seizure.
7. Position the child in a lateral position to prevent **aspiration** (entry of secretions into tracheobronchial passages) (Fig. 28-7).
8. Inform the child that he or she has just had a seizure. Tell the family that the child may still be confused and disoriented for a short time.
9. Stay with the child. Support is essential because a seizure is frightening to both the child and family.
10. Document all important details about the seizure, the care provided, and the condition of the child after the seizure and give notification to the physician.

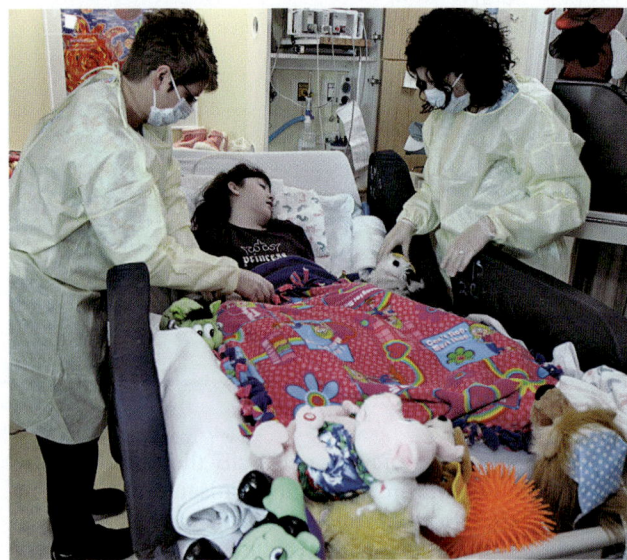

Figure 28-6 An important nursing care measure is padding the side rails.

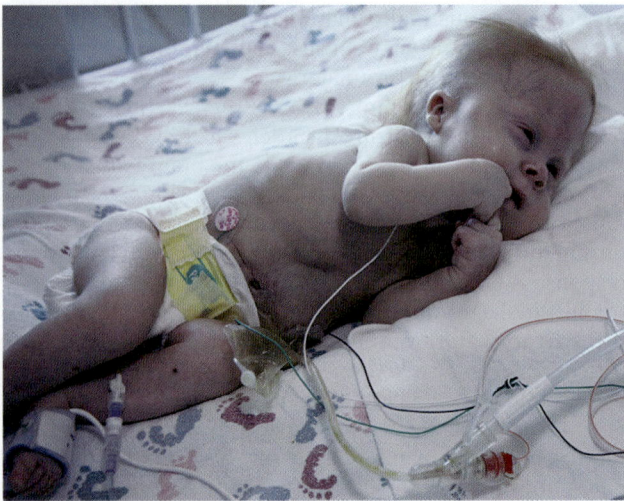

Figure 28-7 When the seizure is over, place the child in the recovery position on the left lateral recumbent position.

Airway management and client safety are priority nursing interventions for the child experiencing a seizure. The child who has experienced a seizure needs continuous monitoring of respiratory status because seizure medications can cause a decreased level of consciousness, apnea, and hypotension. Additionally, after the postictal phase, the child may need to be reoriented.

The hospitalized child receives continuous cardiac, respiratory, and oxygen monitoring. Centrally located monitoring on the nursing unit for ease of observation in case of seizure activity is necessary. Baseline seizure activity for some children may be several seizures a day without compromise. The child must be continually monitored while an inpatient. All caregivers of children with seizures must be instructed in CPR.

Medical Care. Antiepileptic drug (AED) therapy is the main treatment for seizure management in children with epilepsy. Many medications are available and have varying therapeutic effects on the brain (Table 28-4). Monotherapy (one drug) is the desired goal of epilepsy treatment. However, polytherapy (more than one drug) may be initiated when a child has intractable epilepsy or seizure control is improved with the synergistic effects of two antiepileptic medications.

Many anticonvulsant medications can become toxic when taken on a daily basis. Baseline liver function, renal function, and hematological values are assessed before initiation of pharmacotherapy and retained for future reference. Anticonvulsant drug serum levels are also monitored to maintain therapeutic levels. Children may outgrow a certain dosage and begin having seizures because of lowered serum levels. Drug serum levels are assessed every 3 to 6 months.

 Nursing Insight—*Epilepsy*

In refractory cases of epilepsy, other supplemented treatments such as vagus nerve stimulation or the ketogenic diet (high-fat, adequate-protein, low-carbohydrate) may be implemented.

Surgical Care. Epilepsy surgery is most commonly performed when a seizure focus is located in a single area of the brain.

Education/Discharge Instructions

Medication information such as type of medication, dose, route, and frequency of dosing must be explained to the parents. The regimen must also be adhered to in the day-care setting. The child is not left alone until the seizures have been controlled and he or she is seizure-free for several months. Adolescents may drive (depending on state laws) and participate in sports as long as therapeutic serum anticonvulsant drug levels are within normal range and the adolescent is seizure-free for at least 6 months.

School nurses and teachers are informed about the child's seizure condition and follow institutional procedures if the child experiences a seizure in school or day care. The Epilepsy Foundation (2012) encourages school nurses to have an updated and individualized seizure action plan in place for all children with a history of seizures. Medical alert identification bracelets are worn by younger children and may be worn by older children and adolescents (Robertson & Shilkofski, 2012; Vendrame & Loddenkemper, 2012).

Table 28-4 Commonly Prescribed Antiepileptic Drugs (AEDs)				
Type of Seizure	**Medication**	**Dose Range**	**Adverse Reactions**	**Nursing Care**
Partial Complex (Psychomotor)	carbamazepine (Tegretol)	10–30 mg/kg per day in divided doses. Increase until best response is achieved.	Drowsiness, nausea, liver changes, increased appetite.	Give with food but not with milk.
	valproic acid (Depakene)	0.1 mg–0.2 mg/kg/day in two or three divided doses per day.	Confusion, ataxia, nystagmus, nausea, gingival hyperplasia, bleeding disorders.	Always give with food and monitor serum drug levels. Teach parents about oral hygiene and wearing a medical alert tag. Teach parents to watch for adverse effects indicating toxicity.
	phenytoin (Dilantin)	5 mg/kg per day in two to three divided doses.	May cause dizziness, drowsiness, or physical incoordination. Avoid abrupt discontinuation of use. Daily multivitamin is recommended while on this medication.	Always give with food and monitor serum drug levels. Teach parents about oral hygiene and wearing a medical alert tag. Teach parents to watch for adverse effects indicating toxicity. Give with water, juice, or milk.
	phenobarbital (Luminal)	Infants 5–6 mg/kg per day in one or two divided doses.		

(continued)

Table 28-4 Commonly Prescribed Antiepileptic Drugs (AEDs) (continued)

Type of Seizure	Medication	Dose Range	Adverse Reactions	Nursing Care
Partial Complex (Psychomotor)–cont.	fosphenytoin (Cerebyx)	Children 1–6 years, 6–8 mg/kg per day in one or two divided doses. Loading dose of 10–20 mg/kg. Then 4–6 mg/kg per day.		
Generalized Tonic-Clonic	valproic acid (Depakene) and carbamazepine (Tegretol). phenytoin (Dilantin). phenobarbital	May be an inexpensive medication.	Monitor for sleepiness, hyperactivity, drowsiness, and school performance changes.	
	Ketogenic diet high in fat and low in protein and carbohydrates.	Causes a high level of ketones, which decreases myoclonic or tonic-clonic seizure activity.	Nausea, vomiting, headache, drowsiness, dizziness.	This diet is hard to maintain for a long period of time because of the lack of food variety and difficulty of food preparation and parental involvement.
Absence (Petit Mal)	ethosuximide (Zarontin) or valproic acid	3–8 mg/kg per day		Avoid antacids.
Partial Simple	topiramate (Topamax)	1–3 mg/kg per day	Weight loss, dizziness, diarrhea, cognitive dysfunction.	Avoid antidepressants and antacids.

 Now Can You—Discuss seizures and related nursing care?

1. Identify the difference between generalized and focal seizure?
2. Identify the medications for the different types of seizures?
3. Identify developmentally appropriate and holistic nursing care for a child with a seizure disorder or epilepsy?

Inflammatory Neurological Conditions

MENINGITIS

Meningitis is an inflammation of the structures in the central nervous system (CNS) caused by an infectious process. The meninges are composed of three membranes that cover the brain and protect it from injury and infection: the dura mater, arachnoid mater, and pia mater. These structures house arterioles, venules, and cerebrospinal fluid that protects, bathes, and provides chemical functional support for the brain and its contents. Meningitis is either septic or aseptic. Septic or pyogenic meningitis is caused by a bacterial pathogen such as *Streptococcus pneumoniae*, *Neisseria meningitidis*, *Escherichia coli*, or *Haemophilus influenzae* type B. Aseptic meningitis is caused by a known or unknown viral agent typically presenting at peak seasonal viral illness intervals in the fall and winter.

Meningitis can develop at any time during childhood. During the neonatal period, meningitis results from a pathogen transmitted during the labor and delivery process or while in utero. The most common types of neonatal meningococcal infections are caused by herpes simplex, group B beta-hemolytic *Streptococcus*, and *E coli*. In older infants and children, a peak incidence of *S pneumoniae* is noted in the winter months. In summer months, bacterial

organisms such as *N meningitidis* and nonbacterial agents such as rhinoviruses and adenoviruses are more prevalent. *Haemophilus influenzae* type B, once a deadly pathogen, has almost been eradicated now with scheduled routine childhood immunizations (CDC, 2012c).

Bacterial meningitis is the result of bacterial dissemination from a nasopharyngeal or a hematological inoculation. The pathogen migrates into the cerebrospinal fluid and imbeds in the subarachnoid space. The body reacts to the infiltration with a severe inflammatory response and white blood cell proliferation. Systemic septicemia, surgical procedures involving the CNS, a penetrating wound, otitis media, sinusitis, cellulitis of the scalp or facial structure, dental caries, pharyngitis, and orthopedic diseases and procedures are also antecedent events leading to bacterial meningitis.

Nursing Insight—*Viral or aseptic meningitis*

The etiological pathogen in viral, or aseptic, meningitis is a viral agent. The most common pathogens are herpes and adenovirus; in most cases the etiological agent is unknown. Some cases are the result of partially treated bacterial meningitis (Kleigman, Stanton, St. Geme, Schor, & Behrman, 2011). Clinically the child with viral meningitis presents with the same vague or subtle symptoms; however, the child does not become toxic or as acutely ill as the patient with bacterial meningitis. Diagnosis is based on CSF analysis, CSF Gram stain, and culture. Results are typically negative unless a viral agent is identified. If left unrecognized and untreated, meningitis may progress rapidly to a critical state depending on the age of the patient and the etiological pathogen. Younger infants and children succumb rapidly to meningitis, and children with meningococcemia, *H influenzae* type B, and *E coli* become toxic and deteriorate quickly if untreated.

Labs: Cerebrospinal Fluid Analysis

A lumbar puncture is performed to collect cerebrospinal fluid (CSF). Normal CSF is clear and colorless. In infections, CSF pressure may be increased, and it may appear cloudy. Increases in CSF protein and decreases in glucose are commonly seen in bacterial meningitis.

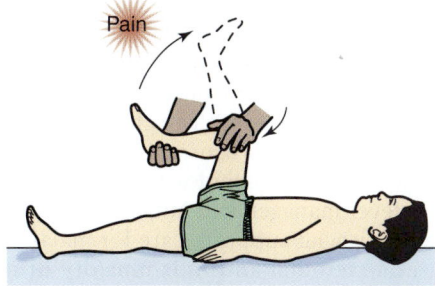

A. Kernig's sign

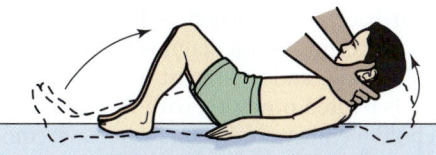

B. Brudzinski's sign

Figure 28-8 Classic findings on examination for a child suspected of meningitis include *A*, a positive Kernig's or *B*, Brudzinski's sign.

Signs and Symptoms

A child with meningitis may initially appear to be mildly ill with general vague or subtle signs and symptoms such as:

- Fever
- Headache
- Stiff neck
- Lethargy and/or irritability
- Nausea and/or vomiting

Diagnosis

Conduct a review of the current illness with specific information obtained regarding duration of symptoms, ill contacts in the family or school settings, seizures, loss of sleep or weight, anorexia, emesis, behavioral changes, and immunization status. A complete blood count (CBC) reveals an elevated white blood cell count and any clotting deficiencies. A disseminated intravascular coagulation panel is collected to rule out a coagulation disorder when the child presents with petechial hemorrhage, shock, and meningococcemia. Blood cultures are obtained to identify the potential hematological origin. A lumbar puncture is also performed for CSF analysis including chemistry and cell counts as well as culture and Gram stain for bacterial or viral diagnosis. Meningitis is diagnosed based on the results of the lumbar puncture.

Assessment Tool Kernig's or Brudzinski's Sign

Classic findings on examination for a child suspected of meningitis include a positive Kernig's or Brudzinski's sign (Kleigman, et al., 2011). These exams indicate meningeal irritation resulting in hyperreactive reflexes. The test for Kernig's sign (Fig. 28-8*A*) is conducted with the child lying supine with the hips flexed. As the nurse straightens the leg, the child either cries out or resists the leg extension. If the child experiences pain behind the knee as the knee is fully extended, this is an abnormal finding. Bilateral increased resistance and pain on extension of the knee is a positive Kernig's sign and may indicate meningeal irritation.

Brudzinski's sign (Fig. 28-8*B*) is conducted with the child lying flat. The nurse attempts to raise the head toward the child's chest and place the chin on the chest. If there is pain or resistance, the child immediately flexes the hip and knee. If the child exhibits flexion of the hips and knees when the nurse performs the maneuver, meningeal inflammation may be present (Bickley & Szilagyi, 2013).

Prevention

The pneumococcal conjugate vaccine is a routine childhood immunization that is effective at preventing pneumococcal meningitis. Additional recommendations for the meningococcal vaccination include children age 2 and older with immunodeficiency and those under 21 who have not been vaccinated.

Collaborative Care

Nursing Care. Essential nursing care includes assessing neurological status at least every 2 to 4 hours. The child's level of consciousness and the use of a pediatric Glasgow Coma Scale, pupil response, and overall activity provide clues to the child's neurological status (e.g., increase in intracranial

pressure [ICP] or response to antibiotic and fluid therapy). In small infants, ICP can be subjectively monitored by palpating the anterior fontanelle while the patient is lying supine. If the fontanelle is tense and bulging, this may suggest increased ICP, particularly when combined with photophobia, irritability, a high-pitched cry, anorexia, and emesis. Infants with open fontanelles and an enlarging head circumference during or post meningitis infection may indicate hydrocephalus and must be monitored. The child with an increasing head size and symptoms of increased ICP requires radiological evaluation such as a CT scan or MRI (Fig. 28-9). To prevent additional increased ICP, the child's room is kept quiet, dim, and without loud or noxious visual, auditory, or olfactory stimuli.

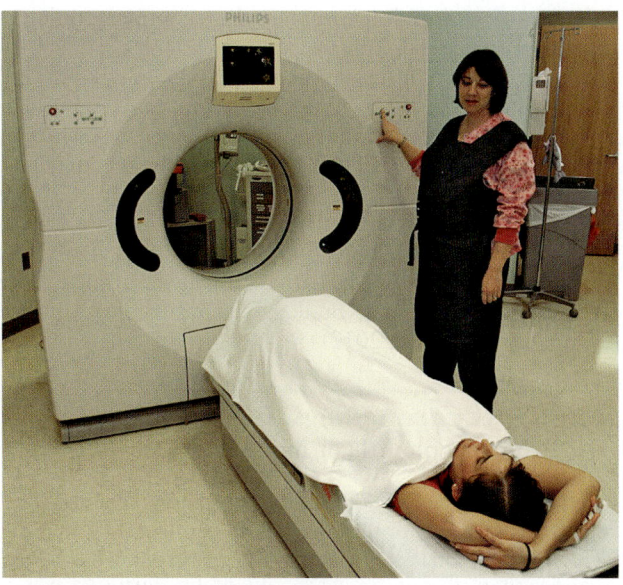

Figure 28-9 The child with an increasing head size and symptoms of increased ICP requires radiological evaluation, such as a CT scan.

Medical Care. The onset of seizure activity associated with meningitis is managed medically, and seizure precautions are maintained at all times. The child with meningitis may develop new-onset seizures and is treated with anticonvulsant therapy. The child is also kept NPO (nothing by mouth) until nausea and vomiting has been resolved. Comfort care includes a dim room, antipyretic therapy for fever management, nutrition as tolerated, and emotional and social support. Care for malaise includes massage, non-steroidal anti-inflammatory drugs, warm baths, and rest.

Treatment for meningitis varies depending on whether it is viral or bacterial in origin. A lumbar puncture with CNS analysis confirms the diagnosis. Viral meningitis is often self-limiting, and treatment is supportive. Bacterial meningitis is treated promptly with IV antibiotics.

Household members and others who have come in close contact with someone diagnosed with meningococcal meningitis are advised to take antibiotics to prevent becoming infected.

Surgical Care. Surgery is usually delayed in a child with acute brain infection unless ICP and cerebral edema is compromising outcomes. Factors predisposing an individual for the development of nosocomial meningitis are reviewed and care taken to minimize the development of meningitis after craniotomy.

Education/Discharge Instructions

Infections of the CNS can be a cause of distress to the family. Educate the family and the child about the disease, preventing injury, and early detection of complications. Also explain that long-term parenteral access is maintained with a peripherally inserted central catheter, and IV antibiotics can be continued at home with the assistance of a home health nurse.

ENCEPHALITIS

Encephalitis is usually viral in origin and occurs with an acute febrile illness that is characterized by cerebral edema and infection of surrounding meninges. Less common etiologies are fungal, bacterial, and parasitic infections, exposure to toxins or drugs, and cancer. The most common types of viral encephalitis are caused by arthropod-borne viruses (mosquito-borne) and the herpes simplex type I. Systemic viral illnesses such as rabies, mononucleosis, and poliomyelitis may also result in encephalitis. Depending on the source of the encephalitis and the severity of the illness, signs and symptoms of the virus develop within hours to weeks after exposure. Encephalitis caused by bacteria usually results in a more serious illness (Steiner, Budka, Chaudhuri, Koskiniemi, Sainio, Salonen, et al., 2010).

 Across Care Settings: Complications from encephalitis or meningitis

The complications resulting from encephalitis or meningitis may include motor or cognitive deficits, seizure disorders, hearing or vision loss, memory loss, and paralysis. If a child has permanent or lingering problems, the treatment plan for them is multidisciplinary. This multidisciplinary approach optimizes the child's recovery and maximizes skills necessary for life.

Signs and Symptoms

The signs and symptoms experienced by children vary from mild to life-threatening. The severity of the illness depends on the child's age, immune system stability, underlying cause, and duration of illness.

- Confusion
- Headache
- High fever
- Photophobia
- Lethargy
- Nuchal rigidity
- Seizures
- Coma

Diagnosis

The diagnosis of encephalitis mimics signs and symptoms of other neurological disorders. When obtaining a history and physical, ask the parent about exposure to possible sources of encephalitis (McCance & Huether, 2010). Assess the child's skin for any lesions that might be vector bites. Ask the child and family about possible exposure to mosquitoes, bats, or other sources of encephalitis. The family needs to be questioned about outdoor play, camping trips, unvaccinated pets, wild animals, medication, and recent illnesses. MRI or CT is used to determine any cerebral edema, shifts within the brain, or focal lesions. The healthcare provider may also order cerebral fluid analysis, an electroencephalogram, and lab work. Brain biopsy is the test for a definitive diagnosis (Steiner et al., 2010).

Prevention

To help prevent viral encephalitis, educate parents and others in the community on prevention methods and early detection and intervention.

 Across Care Settings: Community education about DEET

Educate parents and others in the community about DEET as a way to help prevent viral encephalitis. Insect repellents containing DEET (N, N-diethyl-*m*-toluamide, also known as N, N-diethyl-3-methylbenzamide) should be used according to the directions on the product labels. The American Academy of Pediatrics recommends that repellents with DEET are not to be used on infants younger than 2 months old (AAP, 2012a).

Collaborative Care

Nursing Care. Be astute when caring for a child with encephalitis because of the rapid neurological changes that may occur with the illness. Provide care and support for the child and the family during the acute and convalescent phases of the disease process. During the acute phase of the disease, administer IV fluids, medications, and nutrition (Table 28-5). Seizure precautions must be initiated because of cerebral edema and increased ICP. To decrease ICP, perform interventions such as ongoing neurological assessments, ensuring the child is afebrile and seizure free, maintaining hemodynamic stability, and positioning the child to avoid neck-vein compression. Also carefully monitor the child's fluid and electrolyte balance and watch for syndrome of inappropriate antidiuretic hormone (SIADH) (Steiner, et al., 2010).

Table 28-5 Neurological or Non-Traumatic Condition Medications

Drug	Action	Dosage Recommendations	Laboratory Monitoring	Main Side Effects
baclofen (Lioresal)	Reduction of skeletal spasms associated with upper motor neuron lesions	PO 2–7 y.o.: 10–15 mg/d divided q8h, may increase by 5–15 mg/d divided q8h; ≥8 y.o.: 10–15 mg/d divided q8h, may increase by 5–15 mg/d q3d (max 60 mg/d); also available for intrathecal pump administration	Monitor periodic serum glucose and liver function tests	Transient drowsiness; abrupt discontinuation of intrathecal administration may result in high fever, altered mental status, exaggerated rebound spasticity, and muscle rigidity
carbamazepine (Tegretol)	Partial, generalized tonic-clonic, and mixed seizures	PO <6 y.o.: 10–20 mg/kg/d, gradually increase, max 35 mg/kg/d in 3–4 divided doses; 6–12 y.o.: 100 mg bid, gradually increase to 400–800 mg/d in 3–4 divided doses (max 1 g/d)	Serum therapeutic range: 5–12 mcg/mL Monitor CBC, serum electrolytes, liver function test	Allergic rashes; nausea; diplopia; blurry vision; drowsiness; aplastic anemia; leukopenia (transient); agranulocytosis
lamotrigine (Lamictal)	Partial seizures, Lennox-Gastaut syndrome, adjunct therapy for tonic-clonic, absence, myoclonic seizures	*If given with valproic acid*: PO 2–16 y.o.: 0.2 mg/kg/d × 2 wk, then 0.5mg/kg/d × 2 wk, then 1 mg/kg/d (max 5 mg/kg or 250 mg/d) *If given with any anticonvulsant other than valproic acid*: PO 2–16 y.o.: 1 mg/kg bid × 2 wk, then 2.5 mg/kg bid × 2 wk, then 5 mg/kg bid (max 15 mg/kg/d or 400 mg/d)	None	Dizziness; ataxia; somnolence; headache; nausea; diplopia; blurred vision; rhinitis; Stevens-Johnson syndrome
levetiracetam (Keppra)	Partial seizures as adjunct with other AEDs	PO 4–16 y.o.: 20 mg/kg/d in 2 divided doses, may increase by 20 mg/kg every 2 wks up to 60 mg/kg/d	Monitor periodic CBC, liver function test	Asthenia; headache; somnolence; behavioral changes
mannitol (Osmitrol)	Reduction of intracranial pressure and cerebral edema	1–2 g/kg as a 15%–20% solution over 30–60 min	Closely monitor serum and urine electrolytes and kidney function	Fluid and electrolyte imbalance; hyponatremia
oxacarbazepine (Trileptal)	Partial seizures as monotherapy or adjunct to other AEDs	PO 4–16 y.o.: 8–10 mg/kg/d divided bid (max 600 mg/d) gradual increase to target dose (divided bid) based on weight: 20–29 kg 900 mg/d; 29.1–39 kg 1,200 mg/d; >39 kg 1,800 mg/d	Monitor periodic sodium, T_4 level	Somnolence; ataxia; headache; dizziness; nausea
phenobarbital (Phenobarbital)	Generalized tonic-clonic, partial seizures, and status epilepticus	Child: PO/IV 3–8 mg/kg Neonate: PO/IV 3–4 mg/kg/d (max 5 mg/kg/d) Status epilepticus – Child: IV 15–18 mg/kg in single or divided doses (max 20 mg/kg) Neonate: IV 15–20 mg/kg in single or divided doses	Serum therapeutic range: 15–40 mcg/mL	CNS depression; somnolence; irritability; cognitive impairment; rash; agranulocytosis; respiratory depression
phenytoin (Dilantin)	Generalized tonic-clonic and some partial seizures	PO/IV, 15–20 mg/kg loading dose, then 5 mg/kg in 2–3 divided doses	Serum therapeutic range of 10–20 mcg/mL Monitor periodic CBC and CMP	Drowsiness; rashes; nystagmus; hirsutism; folate deficiency; gingival hyperplasia; agranulocytosis; aplastic anemia
topiramate (Topamax)	Partial seizures used as adjunct	PO 2–16 y.o.: 1–3 mg/kg at hs × 1 wk, then increase by 1–3 mg/kg/d in 2 divided doses every 1–2 wks to a target range of 5–8 mg/kg/d	Monitor periodic CBC	Fatigue; speech problems; somnolence; dizziness; ataxia; psychomotor slowing; confusion; nystagmus; difficulty concentrating; memory difficulties
valproic acid (Depakene) divalproex sodium (Depakote)	Absence, mixed, myoclonic, complex partial seizures	PO/IV 15 mg/kg/d in divided doses when total daily dose >250 mg, increase at 1 wk intervals by 5–10 mg/kg/d (max 60 mg/kg/d)	Serum therapeutic range 50–100 mcg/mL Monitor periodic CBC with platelet count, CMP	Sedation; drowsiness; nausea; vomiting; prolonged bleeding time; pancreatitis; bone marrow depression

Sources: Vallerand & Sanoski (2014); Ward (2013).

Nursing Care Plan The Child With Meningitis

Nursing Diagnosis: Decreased Intracranial Adaptive Capacity related to inflammatory process secondary to microbial invasion of the central nervous system

Measurable Short-Term Goal: The child will not experience complications from increased intracranial pressure (ICP).

NOC Outcomes:
Neurological Status (0909) Ability of the peripheral and central nervous system to receive, process, and respond to internal and external stimuli
Tissue Perfusion: Cerebral (0406) Adequacy of blood flow through the cerebral vasculature to maintain brain function

NIC Interventions:
Intravenous Therapy (4200)
Neurological Monitoring (2620)
Cerebral Edema Management (2540)
Seizure Precautions (2690)

Nursing Interventions:

1. Implement universal precautions. Initiate airborne or droplet isolation for first 24 hours of antibiotic administration for bacterial meningitis (specify). Instruct family in correct isolation procedures.

   RATIONALE: Universal precautions help prevent transmission of infection. Respiratory isolation prevents droplet transmission of bacteria to family and caregivers until the prescribed antibiotic has been implemented for 24 hours.

2. Initiate and maintain IV access (specify fluids and rate) as ordered. Monitor hourly intake and output, notifying the caregiver if urine output is less than 0.5 to 1 mL/kg per hour.

   RATIONALE: IV access is required for optimal medication administration; fluids promote adequate hydration; decreased output may signal impending SIADH.

3. Administer prescribed IV antibiotic, antiviral, steroid, and antipyretic medications as prescribed (specify drug, dose, route, and times).

   RATIONALE: Antimicrobial medications should be administered as soon as possible. Drugs that are specific for the cultured microorganism will be most effective in combating infection. Steroids reduce cerebral edema, decreasing meningeal irritation to help prevent complications such as hearing loss, hydrocephalus, and learning disorders.

4. Monitor vital signs every 1 to 4 hours (specify, depending on severity of symptoms). Place on cardiac monitor as indicated (specify).

   RATIONALE: Changes in vital signs such as tachycardia, tachypnea, and hypertension with widening pulse pressure signal increasing ICP and possible septicemia.

5. Monitor neurological status and symptoms closely; compare with baseline for child and notify caregiver of significant changes.

   RATIONALE: Decreased consciousness and changes in reflexes may signal increasing ICP.

6. Maintain the child in a quiet darkened environment with padded side rails up when in bed. Teach family about seizure precautions.

   RATIONALE: Promotes comfort by reducing noise, light, and activity. Padded side rails may help prevent injury in the event of seizure activity. Empowers family to participate in care.

Medical Care. Treatment for encephalitis is determined by the etiology. Viral encephalitis is treated with an antiviral medication such as acyclovir (Zovirax) (McCance & Huether, 2010). Encephalitis of a bacterial origin is treated with a narrow-spectrum antibiotic. Other medications that may be prescribed are antipyretics, anticonvulsants, analgesics, and anti-inflammatory agents (Steiner et al., 2010).

Surgical Care. Maintaining effective cerebral perfusion and decreasing ICP is the goal of treatment. However, surgical decompression may be necessary for sustained increased ICP and cerebral edema.

Education/Discharge Instructions

Parents are given instructions about discharge referrals and signs of infection or changes in level of consciousness. Health instruction for this condition involves primary prevention strategies to prevent another occurrence as well as monitoring for any potential seizure activity.

Global Health Case Study Environmental Hazards

A nurse is teaching nonmedical volunteers who will be traveling to Malawi about environmental hazards they might be exposed to while in this foreign country. To better prepare volunteers for their trip, identify major causes of illness and death in the country.

critical thinking questions

1. What are three environmental hazards you would expect to find in this community?

2. As the nurse conducted a community health assessment and reviewed the epidemiological triad model, he noted that

malaria is prioritized as a major focus for nursing intervention for the population of Malawi and for people traveling to the country. What types of individuals are more susceptible to malarial infection?

3. What precautions can the nurse teach parents and volunteers to help prevent transmission of malaria through insect bites?

4. What resources would the nurse recommend for the travelers to access and review before leaving on their trip?

◆ See Suggested Answers to Global Health Case Studies on Davis*Plus*.

REYE'S SYNDROME

Reye's syndrome is a rare illness that progresses quickly and does not have a favorable outcome. Reye's syndrome is primarily associated with the administration of acetylsalicylic acid (aspirin) during viral illnesses and affects children between the ages of 4 and 14 years of age. A decline in the incidence of Reye's syndrome has been evident in the recent past, primarily because of the decreased administration of acetylsalicylic acid and parental education about the disease.

Reye's syndrome affects all organs of a child's body but causes the most damage to the brain and liver. The brain is affected by an increase in ICP, and other organs are affected by an accumulation of fat. The disorder is considered to be a two-phase illness because it usually occurs in conjunction with a viral infection, especially varicella (chickenpox) or influenza (flu). The child usually develops symptoms several days after a viral illness (Kleigman et al., 2011).

Signs and Symptoms

The signs and symptoms of the illness are a result of hyperammonemia, hypoglycemia, and an increase in short-chain fatty acids found in the serum after the liver becomes involved. Symptoms of Reye's syndrome include:

- Restlessness
- Vomiting
- Drowsiness
- Seizures
- Loss of consciousness

There are several stages of Reye's syndrome. The child may progress through all of the stages or stop at any stage if treatment is effective (McCance & Huether, 2010).

 Nursing Insight—*The stages of Reye's syndrome*

Stage   I: Lethargy, vomiting, drowsiness, liver dysfunction
Stage II: Disorientation, combativeness, aggressiveness, delirium, hyperactive reflexes, hyperventilation, shallow breathing, stupor, liver dysfunction
Stage III: Obtundation, coma, decorticate posturing, hyperventilation
Stage IV: Deepening coma, large and fixed pupils, decerebrate posturing, loss of ocular reflexes, liver dysfunction
Stage V: Loss of deep tendon reflexes, seizures, flaccidity, respiratory arrest, usually no liver function

Diagnosis

Because a number of inherited metabolic diseases present with many of the same symptoms as Reye's syndrome, these illnesses need to be excluded before a diagnosis of Reye's syndrome can be made. When obtaining a history and physical, ask about recent viral illnesses and the use of any medications containing acetylsalicylic acid. Perform a complete neurological assessment. A definitive diagnosis of this syndrome is established with a liver biopsy obtained during the illness or at autopsy. Other diagnostic tests that are ordered are serum tests including liver enzymes, blood glucose, ammonia level, coagulation studies, and others to exclude metabolic inherited disorders. The child may have a lumbar puncture to rule out infections, including meningitis and encephalitis (Kleigman et al., 2011).

Prevention

Medications containing aspirin are not given for the treatment of any viral illness in childhood. Many over-the-counter medications contain salicylates (aspirin) so it is important to instruct parents to read the medication label carefully and consult with the pharmacist or healthcare provider if they are uncertain of the contents of the medication.

Collaborative Care

Nursing Care. Be sure to perform a neurological assessment because of the high incidence of increased ICP and brain injury. The child's level of consciousness, seizure activity, and reflex function are assessed to determine the stage of the illness. If the child is experiencing respiratory difficulty, monitor the oxygen saturation concentration with the use of pulse oximetry. Supplemental oxygen is administered via nasal cannula. If the child's condition worsens, the child may need intubation and mechanical ventilation. The health-care provider may insert an arterial line to monitor blood pressure and obtain arterial blood gases. Remember to assess the insertion site for complications of infection and leaking. The nurse initiates seizure precautions if the child demonstrates signs of increased ICP. Invasive procedures are performed, and the child is handled carefully because of the risk of bleeding as a result of liver involvement. Emotional support is provided to the child and parents.

Medical Care. To reduce the risk of increased ICP, carefully administer IV fluids. The IV fluids may include glucose to correct hypoglycemia and potassium, chloride, and sodium to correct electrolyte imbalances. Corticosteroids are prescribed to decrease cerebral edema and inflammation, and insulin may be administered to increase glucose metabolism. Diuretics may be prescribed to enhance fluid elimination, resulting in decreased ICP.

Education/Discharge Instructions

There is an excellent chance of recovery when Reye's syndrome is diagnosed early and treated promptly. Health instruction for this condition involves teaching parents to avoid administering aspirin or aspirin-containing medications as well as reviewing medication labels carefully.

"What to say"—*Can I give my child aspirin?*

For many years, childhood illnesses and discomforts were managed with the administration of aspirin (acetylsalicylic acid) because it is a component found in many over-the-counter medications to relieve fever, muscle aches, and nausea (Table 28-6) (National Reye's Syndrome Foundation, 2012). If a parent asks, "Can I give my child aspirin?" the nurse responds, "No product containing acetylsalicylic acid is given to any person younger than 19 years of age experiencing a viral illness because of the risk of Reye's syndrome. It is important for you to always check the medication label or ask the pharmacist if the medication contains aspirin."

GUILLAIN-BARRÉ SYNDROME

Guillain-Barré Syndrome (GBS) is a rare, self-limiting, and potentially debilitating disease in which the body's immune system produces antibodies against its own nerves, resulting in muscle weakness or paralysis. Loss of function can range from fatigue and lethargy to complete paralysis of the lower limbs extending upward, affecting upper motor and sensory neuron pathways.

School-age children are most susceptible, and more males than females are affected. The exact cause of GBS is unknown. The syndrome may follow an antecedent gastrointestinal or respiratory illness. Commonly occurring etiological pathogens are *Mycoplasma pneumonia*, the Epstein–Barr virus, cytomegalovirus, *Varicella*, and *Campylobacter jejuni*. Inflammatory mediators penetrate the Schwann cells in the nerve axons, causing demyelination (removal of the myelin sheath of nerve tissue) and denuding (loss of nerve covering) of the neuronal pathways, resulting in decreased conduction of sensory and motor peripheral and spinal pathways. Areas of nerve involvement are assessed and monitored as nerve function and sensation is blocked or slowed. Some cases of GBS have been linked to several vaccines, such as meningococcal, influenza, swine vaccine, and rabies vaccine, but the evidence is weak and anecdotal (DiFazio & Kao, 2012; Israeli, Agmon-Levin, Blank, Chapman, & Shoenfeld, 2012).

Table 28-6 Medications Containing Acetylsalicylic Acid

Nonprescription Products	Prescription Products
Alka-Seltzer	Darvon
Excedrin	Norgesic
Pepto-Bismol	Robaxisal
Anacin	Talwin
Kaopectate	Butalbital
BC	Percodan
Pamprin	Roxiprin
	Lortab
	propoxyphene
	Soma

Signs and Symptoms

Signs and symptoms of GBS usually progress quickly and the muscle weakness begins in the legs and spreads to the arms (ascending paralysis):

- Muscle weakness
- Numbness
- Paresthesias
- Paralysis
- Areflexia in arms and legs
- Hypotension
- Respiratory distress

Diagnosis

Diagnosis of GBS is based on clinical and laboratory procedures. Elevated CSF protein levels in the absence of infection support the clinical diagnosis. Sensory and motor nerve conduction studies, such as electromyography, define the subtype classification and degree of inflammatory involvement; results will demonstrate blocked impulses or conduction slowing along the peripheral motor and sensory nerve endings (Pluta, Lynm, & Golub, 2011).

Prevention

Exactly what triggers GBS is unknown, but it is thought to follow a preceding viral or bacterial infection. Vaccinations against the flu also have been documented as precipitating factors. Outcomes improve if the disorder is diagnosed and treated early.

Collaborative Care

Nursing Care. Vigilant clinical monitoring related to the progression of motor, sensory, and functional losses and the degree of respiratory compromise are the priority nursing assessments. As GBS progresses, monitor pulse oximetry, respiratory function, ease of breathing, and lung sounds for potential atelectasis leading to pneumonia. Respiratory support is provided with intermittent positive pressure breathing, cough assist, and incentive spirometry. Frequent repositioning is also required every 2 hours. To maintain urinary output, it may be necessary to use an indwelling urinary catheter or intermittent clean catheterization. Parenteral or enteral nutrition is maintained if the child is unable to meet nutritional intake needs or is experiencing dysphagia.

Be sure to assess the pain level in the child. GBS is painful and requires opioid analgesia that is administered on a scheduled basis to treat the severe neuralgia. Children with GBS may underreport the pain associated with the neuritis and expect the nurse to understand their discomfort, so be sure to proactively manage the pain in GBS.

Immobilization can lead to muscular contracture and loss of function after the inflammation has subsided. Passive range-of-motion exercises, frequent position changes, and hand and foot orthotics or splints may be used temporarily to preserve function and prevent contractures. Skin integrity over bony prominences or pressure areas must be monitored and managed aggressively with padding, close inspection, and frequent repositioning. Age-appropriate developmental activities are provided daily as the child is able. Offer visual and auditory stimulation frequently to meet the child's cognitive, social, and emotional needs. School work, crafts, and books provide respite from the boredom and may prevent behavioral and emotional disorders related to the debilitation and limitations of the disease.

Medical Care. Supportive measures are the hallmark of care for patients with GBS. Plasma exchange and IV immunoglobulin therapies shorten the disease duration, support the recovery phase, and reduce the duration of disability (El-Bayoumi, El-Refaey, Abdelkader, El-Assmy, Alwakeel, & El-Tahan, 2011; Hughes, Swan, & vanDoorn, 2012). Corticosteroids are initiated to slow the inflammatory response.

Education/Discharge Instructions

Family education is extremely important because the rate of recovery may be prolonged depending on the degree of disease involvement. Counseling on expectations upon discharge is critical to promote positive patient outcomes.

 Nursing Diagnoses Guillain-Barré Syndrome

- Ineffective breathing patterns related to ascending loss of nerve function
- High risk for alteration in airway clearance related to muscle weakness and/or paralysis
- Alterations in comfort related to neuralgia
- Social isolation related to debilitation and limitations imposed by the child's disease
- Powerlessness related to loss of function and sensation

JUVENILE MYASTHENIA GRAVIS

Juvenile myasthenia gravis (MG) is an autoimmune disease in which antibodies are directed against the postsynaptic membrane of the neuromuscular junction, resulting in muscle weakness. It is relatively uncommon in childhood and has many clinical features similar to that seen in adults. Juvenile MG causes weakness of skeletal muscles and can lead to a variety of symptoms. The muscles most frequently affected are those used for eye movement, chewing, swallowing, and breathing (Finnis & Jayawant, 2011).

Signs and Symptoms

Common symptoms of MG in children are:

- Ptosis
- Diplopia
- Difficulty swallowing, chewing, and speaking
- Weakness or paralysis of skeletal muscles

Diagnosis

The diagnosis of juvenile MG is based on the clinical symptoms and the course of characteristic progressive weakness. Diagnosis is confirmed by electrophysiology and nerve conduction studies. Antibodies to acetylcholine receptor antibodies may also be detected in the serum. An edrophonium (Tensilon) test may corroborate the diagnosis. When Tensilon (edrophonium chloride), a short-acting anticholinesterase, is administered IV, there is marked improvement of the muscle weakness.

Prevention

Prevention is difficult because the exact cause of juvenile MG is unknown. However, there is a link with tumors of the thymus gland, and CT scan of the chest is performed to rule out thymoma (Finnis & Jayawant, 2011).

Collaborative Care

Nursing Care. Monitor for the major complications of MG, which involve the airway. Clinical monitoring related to the progression of fatigue, motor function, and respiratory compromise is the nurse's priority. The muscle weakness and fatigue typically worsen during the day or at times of stress. It is important to identify factors that may cause exacerbations or "flare-ups." Emphasize the importance of rest. Additionally, nursing interventions focus on monitoring respiratory function and status, nutritional needs, and preventing complications.

Medical Care. Acetylcholinesterase inhibitors (neostigmine or pyridostigmine) are used to treat the symptoms and to prevent exacerbations. Plasmaphoresis or IV immunoglobulins are other effective treatments for acute illness. Medication dosing is arranged so that peak action is during mealtime. Because the medication is given during mealtime, carefully observe the child to monitor for aspiration and eating difficulties. The child and parents are taught the importance of strict administration of medications and potential side effects, which include nausea, vomiting, diarrhea, abdominal cramps, and increased salivation (Vallerand & Sanoski, 2014).

---

 focus on safety

Distinguishing cholinergic crisis from myasthenic crisis

Be able to distinguish **cholinergic crisis** (pronounced muscular weakness and respiratory paralysis caused by excessive acetylcholine found in patients with myasthenia gravis as a result of overmedication with anticholinesterase drugs) from myasthenic crisis. A serious complication of MG is muscle weakness and respiratory failure. Myasthenic crisis is often caused by undermedication, perhaps because of a skipped dose of medication, but could also be precipitated by an illness or infection (Finnis & Jayawant, 2011; Lewis, 2010).

Surgical Care. Because of the presumed role of the thymus in the pathogenesis of MG, thymectomy is usually performed if a thyoma is present. After surgery typical postoperative care is provided that focuses on thorough assessment, addressing pain control, maintaining hydration, and giving comfort care measures.

Education/Discharge Instructions

Provide education that includes health instruction related to the course of the disease. Family members are taught to recognize symptoms that may indicate an exacerbation, such as increased muscle weakness. Additional instructions for strict adherence to the anticholinesterase medication dosing schedule should be included.

BOTULISM

Botulism is a rare but serious infection resulting from ingesting spores of the bacteria *Clostridium botulinum* from contaminated food products (honey) or soil. There are several forms of botulism: food-borne, infant, and wound. Infant botulism may range from mild to severe and often occurs in babies younger than 6 months.

Signs and Symptoms

Symptoms may range from mild constipation to impaired neurological function and respiratory failure. (CDC, 2012d; Kleigman et al., 2011).

- Afebrile
- Constipation
- Weakened cry
- Weakness (drooping eyelids)
- Descending paralysis

Diagnosis

Diagnosis is often made based on history, clinical symptoms, and physical examination. A stool sample can confirm diagnosis. Electromyography is used to help confirm the diagnosis.

Prevention

The American Academy of Pediatrics (2012b) recommends that honey is not given to a child younger than 12 months of age.

Collaborative Care

Nursing Care. Nursing interventions are focused on promoting recovery and reducing risk of respiratory complications. Treatment is supportive in mild cases. Supportive treatment includes airway management and strategies to reduce the risk of health-care-associated infection. Most children fully recover without any complications. However, recovery may be prolonged after a severe illness (AAP, 2012b; CDC, 2012d).

Medical Care. Administration of a human botulinum immunoglobulin may be indicated in more severe cases to decrease the sequelae. Botulism immune globulin is a sterilized solution made from human plasma. It contains antibodies capable of neutralizing neurotoxins type A and B (Vallerand & Sanoski, 2014).

Education/Discharge Instructions

Health instruction for this condition includes preventative education. If the child received immunoglobulin, parents are cautioned to avoid live vaccinations for approximately 5 months after administration.

Developmental Neurological Conditions

SPINA BIFIDA

Neural tube defects (NTDs) are a group of birth defects in which malformations of the brain and spinal cord occur and the structures lack protection of soft tissue and bone. NTDs develop when the neural tube fails to close during fetal development. Usually, the nerves below the defect are impaired, although some sparing of nerves with subsequent partial functioning may occur (CDC, 2012e).

Spina bifida is the most frequently occurring and permanently disabling birth defect in the United States. No two people affected by this disorder are alike. It accounts for approximately two-thirds of all NTDs. Spina bifida is derived from the Latin words meaning "cloven backbone." It is a congenital spinal deformity occurring early during gestation (18 to 28 days). The etiology of the disorder can be multifaceted, including environmental and genetic risks. Environmental predisposing factors include exposure to prolonged hyperthermia, poor nutrition, diabetes mellitus, and the consumption of seizure medications during early pregnancy. There is a localized defect of the vertebral arch and no spinal cord or meningeal involvement. A dimple or tuft of hair may be seen on the infant's back (March of Dimes, 2013).

If the child has a **meningocele**, a protruding sac is located on the cervical, thoracic, or lumbar spine at the level of the defect and a thin layer of muscle and skin usually covers the lesion. Meninges (membranes) protrude through the defect in the spine, but no involvement of neural elements is present. Neurological functioning is usually not affected.

A **myelomeningocele** is the most severe form of spina bifida and is evident on delivery. The meninges protrude through the defect, and the meninges contain spinal cord elements. It appears as a very pronounced skin defect, usually covered by a transparent membrane and may even have neural tissue attached to the inner surface. The higher the defect is located on the spine, the greater the loss of spinal cord function because usually no neurological function is found below the defect. The bony prominences of the unfused neural arches can be felt at the defect's lateral border. When the child is born, the membrane covering the defect may be intact or may leak cerebrospinal fluid (CSF). If the membrane is not intact, the risk for infection and neuronal damage is increased. Until the defect is surgically closed, CSF may accumulate, which results in further dilation and enlargement of the sac, and further neuronal damage may occur. The involvement of the spinal cord has greater implications for the function of the child during childhood.

Signs and Symptoms

The signs and symptoms demonstrated by children with spina bifida vary depending on the level of the lesion and the type of defect. Spina bifida occulta is the least severe form, and signs and symptoms include:

- Visualization of meningocele or myelomeningocele
- Weakness
- Paralysis
- Sensory loss

The signs and symptoms of severe spina bifida include:

- Visualization of the myelomeningocele
- Neurological deficits
- Hip and joint deformities
- Impaired bowel and bladder function

Diagnosis

After 12 to 14 weeks of pregnancy, prenatal diagnosis can be made if the defect is visible through ultrasound examination. During pregnancy, maternal serum testing of alpha-fetoprotein is performed to determine the presence of an NTD. An elevated alpha-fetoprotein level may indicate an NTD because open neural defects leak this substance into surrounding amniotic fluid, and a small portion is absorbed into the mother's blood. On delivery, the defect is usually visible, and a diagnosis is made. The defect is examined to determine the type and severity of the defect, and contents of the sac are assessed for meninges, CSF, and spinal cord. An MRI or a CT scan identifies the neurological structures contained in the sac.

Prevention

Spina bifida may be prevented by controlling environmental factors that increase the risk of a woman having a child with the disorder. It is imperative the pregnant women receive education on these risk factors. Women who are pregnant should decrease exposure to hyperthermia (e.g., saunas and hot tubs). A pregnant patient with diabetes mellitus must be closely monitored. The patient must understand the importance of maintaining blood glucose levels within a normal range by adherence to an appropriate diet, exercise regimen, and medication therapy. Some antiseizure medications may result in spina bifida. A woman receiving these medications needs to notify the physician immediately if she becomes pregnant so the medication therapy can be altered. Every woman of childbearing age is advised to ingest 400 mcg of folic acid per day to prevent neural tube birth defects. Good nutrition is also an important preventative measure, and sources of folic acid include green leafy vegetables, liver, legumes, orange juice, fortified breakfast cereals, and multivitamins (Everette, 2011).

Collaborative Care

Nursing Care. Upon delivery, the nurse assesses the defect for the type of contents in the sac and measures the defect. A priority nursing concern is prevention of injury and infection of the sac. The sac must be assessed for indications of infection including redness, purulent drainage, bleeding, and necrosis. If the sac ruptures and leaks CSF, the patient is at risk of developing meningitis.

 Critical Nursing Action Preventing Injury of the Sac

After birth, as quickly as possible and using sterile techniques, cover the defect with a sterile non-adhesive dressing moistened with sterile saline to maintain moisture and prevent drying. The dressing is changed every 2 to 4 hours as prescribed and when soiled. Place the newborn in a prone position and do not place a diaper over the defect to prevent pressure on the sac, rupture, and infection of the sac.

Evaluate the orthopedic function of the newborn. A low thoracic lesion may cause total flaccid paralysis of the lower body. A small sacral lesion may cause only patchy areas of decreased sensation in the feet. Movement or lack of movement of the extremities is assessed and documented. The child may have contractures of the hips, knees, and ankles, and the hips may be dislocated. Prevent joint contractures or further joint contractures by performing passive range-of-motion exercises but do not perform range-of-motion exercises with the hips because hip displacement is common. Clubfeet is a common orthopedic complication of spina bifida because the fetus cannot move the lower extremities in utero. As the child gets older, locomotion is facilitated with the use of braces, wheelchairs, and walkers.

The bladder and bowel function of children with spina bifida may be affected to varying degrees. During the neonatal period, assess the voiding and defecation patterns of the newborn. The newborn who constantly dribbles urine may have a neurogenic bladder and may experience urinary retention and overflow with a risk of urinary tract infections. A newborn who voids at spaced intervals may be able to achieve some level of urinary continence later in life because there is some innervation of the bladder.

 Critical Nursing Action Do Not Obtain a Rectal Temperature

Do not obtain a rectal temperature of a child with spina bifida because rectal irritation and rectal prolapse may occur.

Constipation and impaction are common complaints associated with spina bifida. The child's diet needs to include fiber and fluid. If constipation occurs, stool softeners and laxatives are administered. A child with spina bifida may not be able to feel the urge to defecate, and bowel incontinence may result. The child may need to wear diapers, and as he or she gets older, psychosocial disturbances including depression, embarrassment, and shame may be experienced. If adequate innervation of the bowel exists, bowel training is attempted.

Medical Care. Treatment is dependent on the form of spina bifida. Children with the mildest form, spina bifida occulta, often do not need treatment. The initial goals of treatment include reducing neurological deficits and preventing complications (Thompson & Segal, 2010).

A child with more pronounced spina bifida is at risk for neurological complications, including meningitis, because of the possibility of infection of the CSF and meninges and the possibility of hydrocephalus because an obstruction to CSF absorption may occur. Approximately 70% to 90% of children with myelomeningocele develop hydrocephalus (Spina Bifida Association, 2013). Early signs of infection include irritability, elevated temperature, and lethargy. IV antibiotics are administered to prevent infection preoperatively and postoperatively. Anticholinergics may also be administered to improve urinary continence while antispasmodics may be given to control bladder spasms. The patient who is in a wheelchair for the majority of the day is prone to skin breakdown of the coccyx because of pressure. Areas where orthopedic devices apply pressure need to be padded well and assessed frequently (Brustrom, Thibadeau, John, Liesmann & Rose, 2012; Liptak & El Samra, 2010).

Surgical Care. A **laminectomy** (the excision of a vertebral posterior arch, usually to remove a lesion or herniated disk) and closure of the defect is performed as soon after birth as possible to preserve the neurological function present, prevent infection or rupture, improve the appearance, and allow for easier handling of the baby (Venes, 2013).

Preserving skin integrity is an important nursing responsibility. Preoperatively, ensure no pressure is placed on the vulnerable defect. Postoperatively, the surgical incision is protected by not applying pressure on the area. Perineal irritation and skin breakdown may occur if incontinence is a problem. Check the perineum for stool and urine and change the diaper as needed. The infant's vital signs and neurological function are monitored closely to identify changes that may indicate infection. Perform dressing changes using sterile technique and assess the surgical site for redness, purulent drainage, and odor. The site must also be assessed for CSF leakage.

Because hydrocephalus may develop after surgical repair, measure the infant's head circumference as prescribed. Assess the fontanelles for bulging and cranial sutures for separation. The infant is maintained in a position that does not place pressure on the surgical site. Provide postoperative pain management because when the infant cries, intracranial pressure (ICP) increases. Pain management must be administered carefully so neurological impairment does not occur.

 focus on safety

Latex allergy

Children with spina bifida demonstrate sensitivity to latex. The proposed theory is that these individuals become sensitized after repeated exposure to latex early in life. Nurses caring for children with spina bifida provide a latex-free environment. Referrals can be made so families can obtain information regarding a latex allergy. Helpful organizations include the Spina Bifida Association of America and the American Latex Allergy Association.

Education/Discharge Instructions

Parents are given instructions for post-procedural care and instructed to report signs of infection or worsening neurological deficits. Health instruction includes education on common medical problems that occur with spina bifida as well as interdisciplinary follow-up for these conditions, which include mobility, skin care, and bowel and bladder function. Referral to community resources and support groups may be beneficial in helping parents adjust to living with a chronic illness.

HYDROCEPHALUS

The term hydrocephalus is derived from the Greek, *hydor* (water) and *kephale* (head). CSF is formed and secreted by the choroid plexus (the ventricle's highly vascular lining). Newborns produce approximately 25 mL of CSF per day, and children produce between 25 and 500 mL per day (Greenberg, 2010). After it is secreted, the CSF circulates through the intracranial vault and the spinal cord. In hydrocephalus, there is an increase of CSF production, impedance to CSF absorption, or an obstruction of flow. As the fluid volume increases in the ventricles, pressure increases within the intracranial vault. Many functions are served by the CSF, including buffering of the brain, helping maintain normal chemical balances, and assisting in the maintenance of the important blood–brain barrier.

Congenital anomalies, including Chiari I and II malformations, Dandy-Walker syndrome, and aqueductal stenosis, are the most common causes of hydrocephaly during the neonatal and early infancy periods. Acquired hydrocephaly occurs after birth and in infancy, usually resulting from intraventricular hemorrhage as a result of prematurity (Greenberg, 2010). Other causes of acquired hydrocephaly include tumors, head injury, bleeding, and infections.

There are two categories of hydrocephalus. Communicating hydrocephalus occurs when there is full communication between the subarachnoid space and ventricles. The causes of communicating hydrocephalus are defective absorption of CSF (most often), overproduction of CSF (rarely), and venous drainage insufficiency (occasionally). Non-communicating hydrocephalus occurs when CSF flow

within the ventricular system or the ventricular outlets to the arachnoid space is prevented. Non-communicating hydrocephalus occurs when there is obstruction of the flow of CSF (extraventricular or intraventricular) and includes tumors, anatomical malformations, or cerebral edema. Most cases of hydrocephalus are obstructive (McAllister, 2012).

 ### Cultural Diversity: Head Circumference and Infants of Asian Heritage

The standard head circumference chart used today was developed in Denver, Colorado, in the 1960s and was based on Caucasian American samples. This assessment tool does not allow for any difference in standards with reference to ethnicity. Infants of Asian heritage generally have smaller head circumferences in comparison to Caucasian infants. When Asian infants are measured using the current tool, the measurement obtained may indicate the infant is small for gestational age (SGA). However, this may not be true. The infant may be considered to be at risk for medical diseases and complications based on data that may not be accurate. When using the current tool to obtain a head circumference measurement of an Asian infant, recognize that the data obtained may not be accurate with regard to ethnicity. Determine if the infant exhibits other physical findings associated with SGA.

Signs and Symptoms

The signs and symptoms of hydrocephalus vary based on the child's age and the cause and rate of hydrocephalus development (Fig. 28-10). The child may demonstrate signs and symptoms of increased ICP if the disorder is severe enough:

- MacEwen's sign (tapping on the skull near the junction of the frontal, temporal, and parietal bones yields an unusually resonant sound)
- Difficulty holding the head upright
- Prominent forehead
- Head enlargement
  (McCance & Huether, 2010)

Diagnosis

Congenital hydrocephalus can be diagnosed with ultrasound during a prenatal examination or be discovered during

Signs and Symptoms of Hydrocephalus

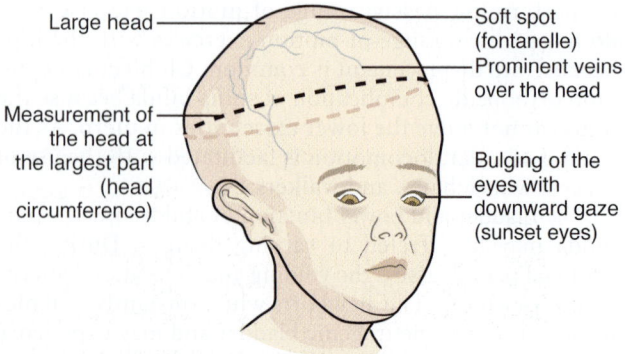

Figure 28-10 Signs and symptoms of hydrocephalus.

infancy or even early childhood. Hydrocephalus is discovered by observing the signs and symptoms exhibited by the patient, such as increasing head circumference inconsistent with normal growth.

 Diagnostic Tools Hydrocephalus

The primary means of diagnosis is through imaging studies (e.g., CT, MRI, and ultrasound), which usually reveal enlargement of ventricles. A cisternogram (radiographic evaluation) is used to evaluate CSF flow dynamics in the child's brain and spinal cord. During the procedure, dye is injected into the subarachnoid area around the brain. Once the dye has circulated through the CSF path, a series of pictures is taken. The procedure is performed to reveal CSF concentration, leakage, obstruction, and pressure.

A lumbar puncture is used to examine CSF and measure pressure. The health-care provider performs transillumination to show abnormalities of the various areas of the child's head. Thinning or separation of the bones of the skull is identified with radiographs of the skull. An ultrasound of the brain possibly may show ventricular dilation, hydrocephalus, or intraventricular bleeding.

Prevention

To reduce the risk of hydrocephalus, pregnant females are encouraged to obtain early prenatal care and follow-up for early detection. If the child has a ventriculoperitoneal shunt, preventing and promptly treating infections is essential.

Collaborative Care

Nursing Care. Carefully examine the child to identify the presence of any immediate life-threatening symptoms. These symptoms exhibited by the child may be indicative of increased ICP or infection. Perform nursing actions related to increased ICP and the proposed course of treatment. The child's head circumference is obtained (Procedure 28-1) and documented to identify any major changes that need to be evaluated.

Medical Care. Medical treatment is not effective in long-term treatment of chronic hydrocephalus.

Acetazolamide (Diamox) and furosemide (Lasix) medications affect CSF dynamics by decreasing CSF secretion. Isosorbide (Dilatrate or ISMO) increases CSF reabsorption although its effectiveness is questionable.

 Assessment Tool Head Circumference Measurement

Birth to 3 months Note the average head size at birth is 33–38 cm (12–14 inches)	Head circumference increases 2 cm/month (0.75 inch)
4–6 months Note the average head size at 6 months is 43 cm (17 inches)	Head circumference increases 1 cm/month (0.4 inch)
6 months to a year Note the average head size at 1 year is 46 cm (18 inches)	Head circumference increases 0.5 cm/month (0.2 inch)

By 1 year of age the child's head size has increased by 33%.

Source: Normal Growth of Young Children-*Pediatrics*-About.com, 2012.

Surgical Care. A procedure performed to relieve increased ICP is called endoscopic third ventriculostomy. An endoscope is introduced and used to visualize the floor of the ventricle, and a fenestration is made that allows the CSF to flow around the obstruction (Greenberg, 2010).

Procedure 28-1 Measuring Head Circumference

Purpose

Measuring head circumference is an important component of evaluation of a child's growth as well as his or her health status.

Equipment

- Flexible, non-stretchable tape measure
- Child's chart

Steps

1. Obtain a flexible, non-stretchable tape measure (preferably one in which one end inserts into the other end).

2. Allow the parent to hold the child in his or her arms or lap.

   RATIONALE: *Parents holding the child may help decrease the child's anxiety.*

3. Remove braids, barrettes, or other hair decorations.

   RATIONALE: *The hair must lie flat to obtain an accurate measurement of head circumference.*

4. Place the tape measure over the most prominent part of the occiput (back of the head) and just above the supraorbital ridges (above the eyebrows).

   RATIONALE: *The landmarks ensure accurate measurement.*

5. Pull the tape measure snugly to compress the hair and underlying tissues.

   RATIONALE: *Ensures accurate measurement.*

6. Read the measurement to the nearest 0.1 cm or 1/8 inch.

7. Document the measurement on the chart.

Clinical Alert If an abnormal circumference is found based on the child's age, reposition the tape and measure the head circumference again. The new measurement should agree with the first measurement within 0.2 cm or 1/4 inch.

Teach Parents

To help ensure an accurate head circumference measurement, teach the parents how to hold the child firmly while offering verbal comfort and encouragement.

Documentation

9/10/10 1200 Head Circumference 43 cm (17 inches)

– T. Martin, RN

The main surgery for hydrocephalus is the placement of a ventriculoperitoneal shunt (Fig. 28-11). A ventricular shunt means a catheter is placed in the lateral ventricle where a one-way valve is set at a desired pressure to drain the CSF. Then, a distal catheter that terminates in the peritoneal cavity or alternate drainage site is placed. The peritoneal cavity is the preferred site for placement of the distal catheter because of easy accessibility and decreased risk of complications.

focus on safety

Alternate shunt placements

Sites for shunt drainage placement, other than the peritoneal cavity, are the right atrium of the heart and the pleural space of the lungs. The alternate sites pose the risks of pleural effusion, emboli, pneumothorax, respiratory distress, and endocarditis.

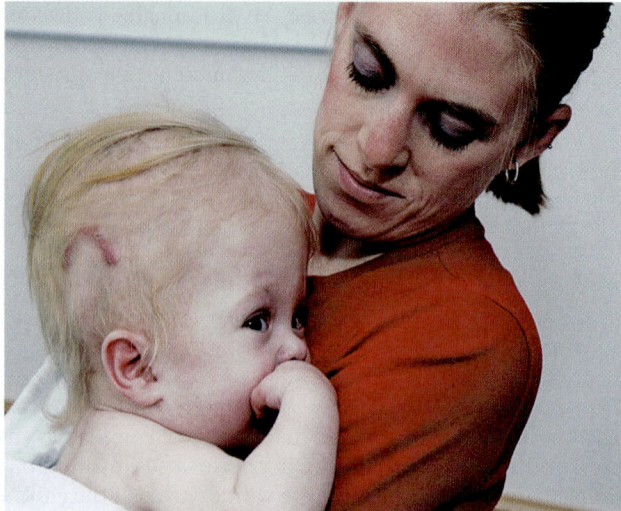

Figure 28-11 A child may have a shunt placed to drain excessive intracranial CSF.

Preoperatively ensure support of the child's head. The child requires frequent position changes of the head because hydrocephalus causes the skin of the scalp to thin, and prolonged pressure may result in impaired skin integrity. Prior to the shunt surgery, do not use scalp veins for IV therapy because the IV may be located near the surgical site.

The child who is to receive a ventricular shunt receives a preoperative IV antibiotic to help prevent development of infection. During the preoperative period, medications including acetazolamide (Diamox) and furosemide (Lasix) may be prescribed to decrease the production of CSF. These medications are sometimes used to postpone the need for shunt insertion.

focus on safety

Complications of a ventriculoperitoneal shunt

The placement of a ventriculoperitoneal shunt can present complications such as hemorrhage, subdural hematoma, CSF leakage, bradycardia, and injury to structures located in the area of surgery. The child is monitored because the fenestration may close or narrow resulting in enlarged ventricles and increased ICP. The child may also be at risk for meningitis and encephalitis postoperatively because the shunt is placed in the ventricles of the brain and any introduction of infectious agents causes a potentially life-threatening illness. Infective complications occur in approximately 5% to 10% of shunt operations. Most shunt infections occur within the first 3 months after the surgical procedure and are more frequent in children younger than 6 months of age (Sgouros, 2011).

In the postoperative period, neurological assessment is paramount. Irritability, lethargy, or other alterations in neurological function may be indicative of meningitis or increased ICP. Assess and document the child's vital signs and neurological assessments every 15 minutes or as prescribed by the surgeon. The child's head circumference is measured daily, and the fontanelles are assessed for bulging and the sutures examined for separation. Because of the possibility of a shunt malfunction, an ophthalmologist examines the child's eyes to detect pressure on the optic nerve, which, if not treated promptly, causes irreversible damage. Safety precautions are implemented

because pain and fever may cause the child to become disoriented.

When positioning the child, elevate the head no higher than 30 degrees to prevent ventricular decompression and place the child on the nonoperative side to prevent pressure on the shunt. If increased CSF occurs, the physician may prescribe for the child to be elevated higher than 30 degrees. The shunt may be manually purged but only in extreme cases because of the risk of a subdural hematoma.

When assessing the abdomen, auscultate for hypoactive or absent bowel sounds to identify a paralytic ileus. Obtain an abdominal circumference measurement to assess for distention. To promote accuracy, put a mark on the abdomen so the tape measure is placed in the same spot every time. If peritonitis develops, the child may complain of diffuse abdominal pain and tenderness along with nausea and vomiting.

When taking vital signs, pay particular attention to an elevated temperature and rapid pulse rate. Peritonitis results in leukocytosis (an increase in white blood cells); therefore, lab results are closely monitored. Observe for signs of hypovolemia and shock resulting from loss of electrolytes and fluids into the abdominal cavity and assess for rebound tenderness and muscle rigidity.

Postoperatively, the child receives IV antibiotics and is monitored for infection. Observe for redness along the shunt tract in addition to palpating for warmth to assess for infection. Other signs of shunt infection are fever, irritability, lethargy, abdominal discomfort, and apnea (Greenberg, 2010). The most common organisms that cause CSF infections in infants and children are *Staphylococcus aureus* and *Staphylococcus epidermidis*. Adolescents are more likely to experience an infection resulting from *Propionibacter acne*, which is a slow-growing infection of the CSF.

focus on safety

Shunt infection

Common signs and symptoms demonstrated by a child with a shunt infection include decreased level of consciousness, irritability, increased ICP, seizures, poor feeding, and an alteration in vital signs.

Education/Discharge Instructions

Communicate to the parents that a child with hydrocephalus needs continuous monitoring and assessment because hydrocephalus is a lifelong disorder. Educate parents so they can recognize complications of hydrocephalus, including increased ICP and shunt malfunction (e.g., kinking and plugging within the ventricle from tissue or exudate or obstruction at the distal end from thrombosis or displacement of the tubing because of growth). Shunt infection can happen at any time but most often occurs 1 to 3 months after placement. Instruct parents to assess for common signs and symptoms (e.g., nausea and vomiting, headache, change in customary behavior, lethargy, unresponsiveness, or elevated temperature). Explain that the child will not be able to participate in contact sports because of the possibility of shunt damage. The importance of safe transport and positioning (a reclining car seat) is also emphasized.

CEREBRAL PALSY

Cerebral palsy (CP), the most common permanent physical disability of childhood, is characterized by physical impairment and mild to severe physical and mental dysfunction. The United Cerebral Palsy Foundation (2012) estimates that approximately 764,000 adults and children in the United States have at least one symptom of CP. CP is a nonprogressive neurological disorder that results from brain injury occurring before cerebral development is complete. Because brain development continues for the first 2 years of life, the disorder can be a result of brain injury occurring not only during the prenatal period but also during the perinatal and postnatal periods. Prenatal risk factors include asphyxia, infections (e.g., rubella, cytomegalovirus, and toxoplasmosis), intracranial hemorrhage, blood incompatibility, and trauma. The perinatal risk factors for CP are low birth weight, birth at less than 32 weeks of gestation, and intracranial hemorrhage. Postnatal risk factors include viral encephalitis, bacterial meningitis, falls, child abuse, and motor vehicle crashes.

The amount of disability varies because some children with CP may only have minimal disability and can lead relatively normal lives while others require extensive assistance. There are four types of CP. Spastic CP is the most common type. A child with spastic CP has stiff muscles because of increased muscle tone, and the muscles are predisposed to contracture. Children with this type of CP have poor control of posture, coordinated movement, and balance. Spastic CP is often classified according to the limbs affected (i.e., diplegia, hemiplegia, quadriplegia, monoplegia, and triplegia). Children with spastic diplegia (both legs are involved) have difficulty walking because of tight muscles in the hips and legs and may have scissoring (legs turn inward and cross at the knees) (National Institute of Neurological Disorders and Stroke, 2012; CDC, 2012f).

Children with ataxic cerebral palsy have difficulties with balance and depth perception. They walk with an unsteady gait, demonstrate poor coordination, and often have fine motor control problems. Athetoid CP or dyskinetic CP is characterized by uncontrolled involuntary writhing movement of extremities. In severe cases, the facial muscles may be affected, and drooling, speech difficulties, and grimacing may occur. In mixed CP, a child has two or more types of CP. Some of the common symptoms of mixed CP are difficulty or inability to walk, speech difficulty, swallowing

problems, breathing difficulties, bowel or bladder incontinence, seizures, vision problems, learning disabilities, hearing deficits, attention or behavioral problems, and impaired senses (National Institute of Neurological Disorders and Stroke, 2012) (Fig. 28-12).

Signs and Symptoms

The signs and symptoms vary depending on the area of the brain involved and the extent of damage.

- Muscle rigidity
- Muscle spasticity
- Poor control of posture
- Ataxia

Diagnosis

Diagnosis of CP is primarily based on clinical symptoms demonstrated by the child and a history of delay in reaching developmental milestones. The child may exhibit various muscular **hypotonia** (low muscular tension) or **hypertonia** (high muscular tension). A child with CP may demonstrate hand preference by 6 months of age instead of 12 months. An important sign of CP is persistence of some primitive infant reflexes (i.e., Moro and crossed extensor reflexes) because these reflexes normally disappear between 6 months and 12 months of age. CT, MRI, and cerebral ultrasound are tests used to diagnose alterations in brain integrity that is often present with CP.

Prevention

While the exact cause of cerebral palsy is unknown, there are risk factors that may increase the risk of having a child

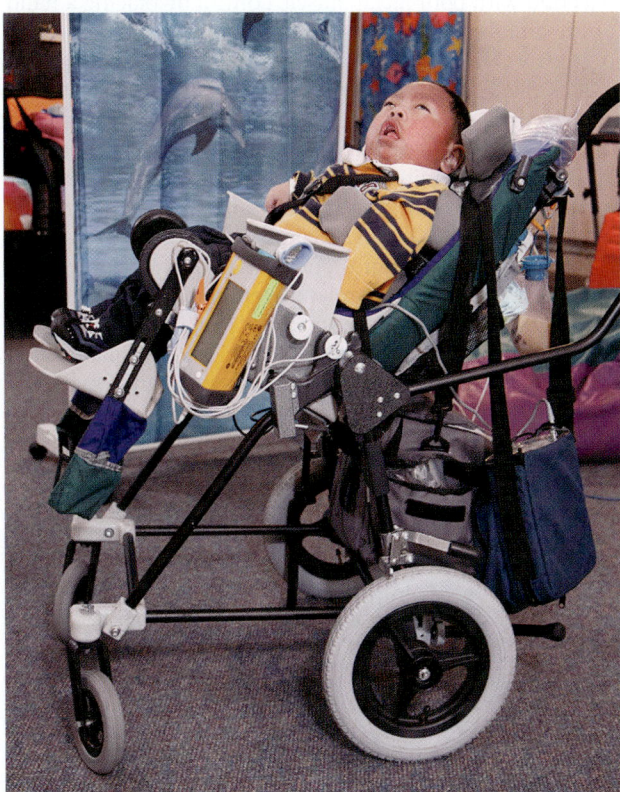

Figure 28-12 The child with cerebral palsy has physical impairment and has mild to severe physical and mental dysfunction.

with cerebral palsy. The nurse provides education about various risk factors, including infection during pregnancy, premature birth, and injury and stresses the important of routine prenatal counseling and visits.

Collaborative Care

Nursing Care. The child with CP has some degree of muscular dysfunction. Splints and braces may be necessary to facilitate muscle control and improve body functioning. Assistive devices are necessary to allow the child to perform these tasks, including large-handled brushes and toothbrushes. Encourage the child to perform self-care tasks. Clothing should be easy to manipulate. To reduce muscle spasms and prevent fatigue, allow frequent rest periods.

Children with CP may or may not demonstrate intellectual deficits. The degree of deficit depends on the severity of brain injury. Children with CP need intellectual stimulation. If possible, the child with CP is enrolled in school to foster relationships, self-esteem, and normalcy. Participating in activity programs helps incorporate play into exercise. Toys are chosen based on cognitive, not chronological, age. The environment needs to be safe because the child may not comprehend the concept of danger.

A child with CP may experience feeding problems because of impaired muscle control and strength. If the child can feed independently, he or she is encouraged to do so. Utensils with large handles may be used for easier manipulation. The child must be fed in an upright position and not hurried while eating because of the danger of aspiration. Assistance is provided by standing behind the child and guiding the hand to the mouth. Stabilize the mandible in a child with poor facial muscle control by placing a hand on the child's mandible.

Medical Care. Administer medications that reduce muscle spasms. Skeletal muscle relaxants may be used for short-term control with older children and adolescents. Dantrolene (Dantrium) is administered to decrease spasticity, but the child must be monitored for hepatic impairment. The use of baclofen (Lioresal) has proven to be an effective muscle relaxant. Baclofen (Lioresal) can be administered intrathecally via an implanted infusion pump to provide continuous and controlled relief. Neurolytic agent nerve blocks provide a temporary decrease in spasticity for localized applications. Paralysis of specific muscles can be achieved by the injection of botulinum (Botox), but the long-term effects have not been determined. Antianxiety medications such as diazepam (Valium) may be administered to older children and adolescents to reduce excessive motion and tension. Children with CP are at increased risk for seizures. Medications, including phenobarbital (Luminal) and phenytoin (Dilantin), may be administered to control seizures (American Academy of Neurology and Child Neurology Society, 2013).

Surgical Care. The child who does not respond to conservative management may need surgical intervention. Surgical procedures provide joint stability and balanced muscle power and may include tendon lengthening, release of spastic wrist flexor muscles, and correction of spastic hip adduction. Selective dorsal rhizotomy (severing of dorsal sensory fibers that have an abnormal response resulting in spasticity) may be performed to improve the child's ability to sit, stand, and walk.

Education/Discharge Instructions

Provide education that incorporates knowledge of expected growth and development as well as early detection of deterioration and signs and symptoms of infection. The health-care needs of a child with CP are complex and will require a multidisciplinary approach to improve health and functional outcomes.

Case Study Infant Amy Moore

Infant Amy Moore, 9 months old, has been referred to a neurologist by a pediatrician for evaluation. The neurologist questions the infant's mother about her pregnancy, the birth, and Amy's physical and psychosocial development. The mother states Amy is her first child, and she had a complicated pregnancy. She was diagnosed with cytomegalovirus at 26 weeks of gestation and pregnancy-induced hypertension at 28 weeks. She delivered Amy at 32 weeks because of rapid progression of the hypertension. At birth, Amy weighed 2 pounds and 9 ounces, and her Apgar scores at birth were 3 and 6. Based on her initial assessment, Amy was transferred to the neonatal intensive care unit (NICU) and remained there for 65 days. Amy was mechanically ventilated for 26 days and received enteral feedings. While in the NICU, Amy had a small intraventricular hemorrhage. Amy weighed 4 pounds and 10 ounces when discharged. The mother states that she is concerned about Amy's physical and psychosocial development. Physical assessment findings are as follows: poor eye contact, anterior fontanelle soft spot, slight drooling of oral secretions, mild head lag, few facial expressions, hypotonic extremity muscles, and right-handedness noted.

critical thinking questions

1. What risk factors predisposed Amy to CP?

2. What physical assessment findings demonstrated by Amy are indicative of CP?

◆ See Suggested Answers to Case Studies on Davis*Plus*.

Neurological Injuries

DROWNING OR SUBMERSION INJURIES

Drowning or submersion injuries (SI) involving children are usually preventable, yet more than 1,500 children in the United States die every year from submersion injuries. Drowning ranks fifth among the leading causes of unintentional injury death in the United States. Males are approximately four times more likely to experience an SI than females. Children younger than 3 years of age and adolescents 15 to 19 years of age are at the highest risk. Submersion injuries in a child may have various causes (e.g., accidental, trauma, seizure, and abuse) (CDC, 2012g; Encyclopedia of Children's Health, 2012).

Drowning or SI are a major cause of death and disability in children. Children are at risk for these injuries because of the inability to swim, fatigue, inadequate muscle strength, and lack of knowledge of water safety. A child who has an SI may have only short-term complications or may have long-term, life-altering disabilities. Early and aggressive medical treatment is paramount in the care of the child, and the child's prognosis depends on the treatment provided.

A submersion injury occurs when a child who is submerged in water tries to breathe and aspirates water (wet drowning) or has a laryngospasm without aspiration (dry drowning). The most significant contributing factors to morbidity and mortality are hypoxemia with decreasing oxygen delivery to vital tissues. Central nervous system (CNS) damage may occur during the incident (primary injury) or may result from ongoing pulmonary injury, injury caused by reperfusion, or multi-organ dysfunction (secondary injury). Early resuscitation is associated with an improved prognosis.

Signs and Symptoms

The signs and symptoms of drowning vary depending on age, how long the child was submerged, and the temperature of the water (Encyclopedia of Children's Health, 2012). Common symptoms include:

- Confusion or coma
- Hypothermia
- Dysrhythmias
- Tachypnea
- Tachycardia
- Hypoxia
- Seizures

 Nursing Insight—*Drowning affects many organ systems*

Neurological
- Alterations in level of consciousness
- Cerebral edema and/or anoxia

Respiratory
- Respiratory distress (cyanosis, hypoxia, and/or wheezing)

Circulatory
- Hypovolemia
- Hypothermia

Cardiac
- Ventricular dysrhythmias

Diagnosis

Diagnosis consists of assessing many systems. Arterial blood gas analysis detecting for carboxyhemoglobin and methemoglobinemia, continuous pulse oximetry, and chest radiography all help assess the respiratory system. Computed tomography (CT) and cervical spine imaging are used to evaluate the neurological system. The cardiovascular system is evaluated with echocardiography and electrocardiography. Laboratory tests usually include complete blood count, blood coagulation studies, liver enzymes, renal function tests (blood urea nitrogen and creatinine), serum electrolytes, and serum glucose (CDC, 2012g; Shepherd, 2011; Topjian, Berg, Bierens, Branche, Clark, Friberg, et al., 2012).

 Assessment Tool Orlowski Scale

Clinicians use the Orlowski scale to predict the likelihood of neurologically intact survival. Each item is assigned one point. If a child has a score of 2 or less, there is a 90% likelihood of a complete recovery. If a child has a score of 3 or more, there is a 5% chance of survival (Mickalide & Carr, 2012; Shepherd, 2011).
- Three years of age or older
- Submersion time greater than 5 minutes
- No resuscitation efforts for more than 10 minutes after rescue
- Comatose on admission to the emergency room
- Arterial pH less than 7.10

Prevention

Prevention strategies are multifaceted and include behavioral change, use of safety devices (e.g., pool fencing and swimming lessons), and improvement of legislation that promotes injury prevention programs. The main factors that affect drowning risk are lack of swimming ability, unsupervised water access, lack of close supervision while swimming, failure to wear life jackets, alcohol use, and seizure disorders (CDC, 2012g). Anticipatory guidance that includes home safety education and interventions may reduce injury rates.

Collaborative Care

Nursing Care. When caring for a patient admitted because of drowning, a priority nursing responsibility is assessing and maintaining the airway. If respiratory or cardiac arrest occurs, life support measures are implemented. Suctioning is performed to remove debris, secretions, or emesis that may obstruct the airway (Mickalide & Carr, 2012g). Insert a nasogastric tube to remove gastric contents and relieve abdominal distention to reduce the risk of vomiting and aspiration. Oxygenation is a primary concern. A non-rebreather mask is used if the child is not intubated. Oxygen saturation and respiratory status must be closely monitored in case respiratory deterioration occurs (Shepherd, 2011). The child who is in respiratory compromise (hypoxic or apneic) or is unconscious needs immediate intubation.

Medical Care. Evaluate the child for symptoms that indicate other injuries including head or spinal trauma. Antibiotics are administered as a precautionary measure.

 Assessment Tool Pediatric Early Warning Score

The Pediatric Early Warning Score (Fig. 28-13) is an assessment tool used for many neurological conditions and identifies pediatric deterioration as well as determines activation of the rapid response team up to 11 hours prior to a code event (Akre, Finkelstein, Erickson, Liu, Vanderbilt & Billman, 2010). During this critical time period, alert the health-care provider and the rapid response team of any needed changes in the child's plan of care such as more frequent assessments or additional medical consultation (Robson, Cooper, Medicus, Quintero, & Zuniga, 2012).

 Focus on Safety

Cricoid pressure

To avoid vomiting during intubation, apply cricoid pressure or empty the stomach contents with a nasogastric tube (Topjian et al., 2012; Trethewy, Burrows, Clausen, & Doherty, 2012).

Education/Discharge Instructions

Neurological injury with long-term sequelae secondary to hypoxic brain injury remains a major problem in the management of children with submersion injuries. Provide education and support to assist the family in caring for a child with neurological impairment. The child may need rehabilitation and long-term follow-up.

TRAUMATIC BRAIN INJURY

Traumatic brain injury (TBI) occurs when a jolt or blow to the head disrupts the normal function of the brain. The effects of a TBI may be as mild as a brief loss of consciousness

Royal Alexandra Hospital for Sick Children, Brighton-Paediatric Early Warning Score

	0	1	2	3	Score
Behavior	Playing/appropriate	Sleeping	Irritable	Lethargic/confused Reduced response to pain	
Cardiovascular	Pink or capillary refill 1–2 seconds	Pale or capillary refill 3 seconds	Grey or capillary refill 4 seconds. Tachycardia of 20 above normal rate	Grey and mottled or capillary refill 5 seconds or above. Tachycardia of 30 above normal rate or brachycardia	
Respiratory	Within normal parameters, no recession or tracheal tug	> 10 above normal parameters, using accessory muscles, 30+% FiO₂ or 4+ liters/min	> 20 above normal parameters recessing, tracheal tug, 40+% FiO₂ or 6+ liters/min	5 below normal parameters with sternal recession, tracheal tug, or grunting. 50% FiO₂ or 8+ liters/min	
Score 2 extra for 1/4 hourly nebulizers or persistent vomiting following surgery.					

Figure 28-13 Pediatric Early Warning Score (PEWS) is an early warning scoring system that uses markers to judge severity of the child's condition and may improve the overall management of the acutely ill child. *Source:* Adapted from Monaghan, A. (2005). Detecting and managing deterioration in children. *Paediatric Nursing, 17*(1), 32.

or as severe as a vegetative state or death. Each year in the United States, approximately 1.7 million people experience a TBI; 50,000 die (2,685 are children), and as many as 5.3 million persons are currently living with a long-term disability. Each year, many children from 0 to 14 years of age experience varying degrees of brain injury. Approximately 470,000 children are seen in emergency departments for accidents involving a head injury and 37,000 of those evaluated are hospitalized (Brain Injury Association of America, 2012; CDC, 2012a; Faul, Xu, Wald, & Coronado, 2010). The primary causes of pediatric TBIs are motor vehicle crashes, bicycle accidents, sports trauma, violence, and falls. Any child with a TBI must be evaluated for child abuse (Fig. 28-14).

A TBI can be classified as penetrating (e.g., bullet entering the brain) or blunt injury (e.g., fall from a tree). A TBI is further classified as primary or secondary. Primary injury occurs directly from the trauma, and secondary injury is a result of complications (e.g., cerebral ischemia and hemorrhage). Children are predisposed to head injury because their heads are larger in relation to their body size, they have a more unsteady gait, and they have thinner, softer cerebral tissue. Direct brain injury occurs when the skull vault is penetrated. A skull fracture may or may not be present. Indirect brain injury results when structural deformation occurs. Rotational acceleration and deceleration forces are usually present in motor vehicle crashes, and they produce tearing and shearing injuries of the brain (CDC, 2012a).

Signs and Symptoms

Symptoms of traumatic brain injury can include:

- Scalp laceration
- Alteration in level of consciousness
- Seizures

Diagnosis

A CT or magnetic resonance imaging (MRI) identifies intracranial bleeding, compression of cerebral tissue, the presence of penetrating foreign objects, and skull fractures. An electroencephalogram is prescribed to determine if the child has brain activity abnormalities. Intracranial pressure (ICP) monitoring, cerebral blood flow, and cerebral perfusion pressure are measured if increased ICP is present. Cerebral oxygenation is monitored with the use of jugular venous bulb saturation and concentration or near infrared spectroscopy (Kim & Gean, 2011).

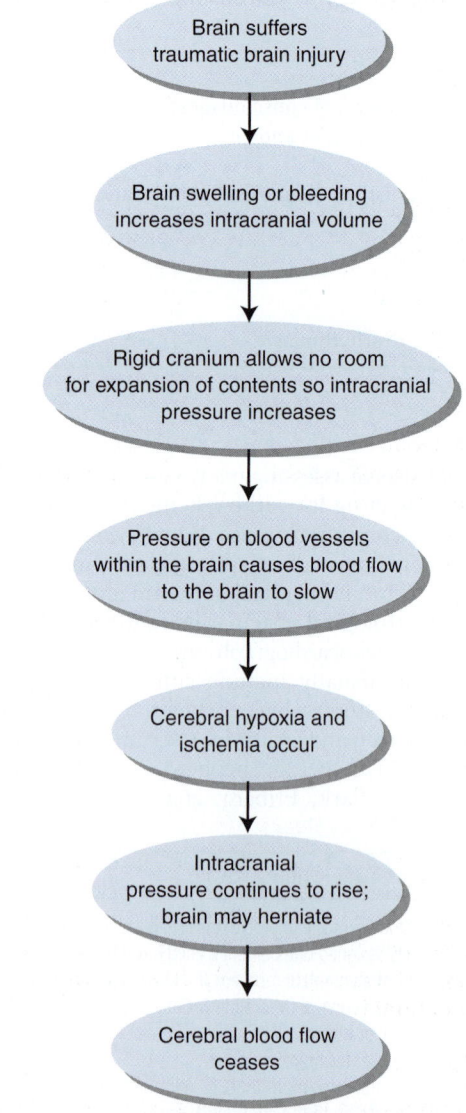

Brain suffers traumatic brain injury

↓

Brain swelling or bleeding increases intracranial volume

↓

Rigid cranium allows no room for expansion of contents so intracranial pressure increases

↓

Pressure on blood vessels within the brain causes blood flow to the brain to slow

↓

Cerebral hypoxia and ischemia occur

↓

Intracranial pressure continues to rise; brain may herniate

↓

Cerebral blood flow ceases

Figure 28-14 Traumatic brain injury.

Prevention

The health-care team can incorporate injury prevention education and anticipatory guidance into encounters with the child and family. Community-based primary prevention educational initiatives increase awareness and can reduce the risk of exposure. Effective preventive measures (e.g., helmets, seat belts and car seats, effective sporting equipment, and home safety inspection) can reduce the risk of TBI.

Collaborative Care

Nursing Care. The child with a TBI needs immediate care to prevent life-threatening complications or death. Airway patency is a priority. Deliver supplemental oxygen via a bag-valve-mask device, per order, until the airway is established. Assessment of the child's neurological status is imperative. Use the pediatric Glasgow Coma Scale to evaluate neurological status. The child's pupil size and reactivity are assessed, and a difference or change is reported. Reflexes are assessed to determine brainstem involvement, and if the brainstem is injured, the child's prognosis is poor. Palpate the skull to identify any fractures or depressions. Signs of a basal skull fracture include leakage of cerebrospinal fluid from the ears or nose, hemotympanum (blood in the middle ear), mastoid ecchymosis (Battle's sign), and periorbital ecchymosis (raccoon eyes) (Caton-Richards, 2010; Kochanek, Carney, Adelson, Ashwal, Bell, Bratton, et al., 2012). Assess the patient for increased ICP and ensure appropriate measures are implemented.

Medical Care. Under the direction of medical orders, the child may need to be intubated and mechanically ventilated if a patent airway is not possible because of injury to the neck or pharynx, if level of consciousness is depressed, or if the neurological state is expected to deteriorate.

The attending health-care provider may recommend that the nurse insert two large-bore IV needles and administer isotonic fluid to maintain adequate circulation. IV fluids are warmed if hypothermia is a concern. If the child does not respond to fluid boluses or blood loss is greater than 30% of the child's total blood volume, blood products are administered (Heyser, 2012).

 Critical Nursing Action Basal Skull Fracture

Do not insert a nasogastric tube if a basal skull fracture is suspected because the tube may enter the brain through the fracture. Insert an orogastric tube if needed instead.

Education/Discharge Instructions

TBI is a leading cause of disability. Discharge education will be specific to the degree of brain injury. A multidisciplinary team will guide rehabilitation. Parents are given emotional support and resources to prepare them for challenges they may encounter taking care of a child who has suffered a brain injury.

ABUSIVE HEAD TRAUMA

Abusive head trauma (formally referred to as shaken baby syndrome) is a non-accidental injury caused by picking up an infant or child by the shoulders or upper torso and shaking him or her (Centers for Disease Control and Prevention, National Center for Injury Prevention and Control, 2014). Abusive head trauma results from major rotational forces and angular deceleration encountered when an infant is shaken forcefully. The injury may be intentional or unintentional. Most victims of shaken baby syndrome are younger than 6 months of age, and the source of the abuse is usually the father or a male acquaintance of the mother. The prognosis for an infant depends on the severity of the injury and response to medical therapy. Complications a child may experience are neuromotor impairment, visual impairment, and developmental delays (Herman, Makoroff, & Corneli, 2011; Liley, Stephens, Kaltner, Larkins, Franklin, Tsey, et al., 2012).

Signs and Symptoms

Symptoms of severe cases of abusive head trauma include:

- Seizure activity
- Apnea
- Bulging or full fontanelles
- Coma
- Hemorrhage (retinal or intracerebral)
- Bradycardia
- Complete cardiovascular collapse

Symptoms of less severe cases of abusive head trauma include:

- Vomiting
- Hypothermia
- Poor feeding
- Failure to thrive
- Increased sleeping
- Lethargy
- Irritability
- Difficult to arouse

Diagnosis

To diagnosis abusive head trauma, a CT scan or MRI is used to determine if a subdural or subarachnoid hemorrhage is present. An ocular fundoscopic exam is used to assess for retinal hemorrhage, a classic sign of abusive head trauma.

 Nursing Insight—*Abusive head trauma*

Recognizing abusive head trauma can be challenging. The hallmark of abusive head trauma is an absence of external trauma to the head, face, and neck of an infant along with massive intracranial or intraocular bleeding. Inconsistencies between health history and physical examination are further investigated.

Prevention

Identifying risk factors and increasing awareness of potential stressors parents and other caregivers may experience while caring for an infant are important measures in preventing this type of injury. Teaching parental skills related to coping with a crying infant is also a crucial preventative measure (Barr, 2012; Barr, Rivara, Barr, Cummings, Taylor, Lengua, et al., 2009).

Collaborative Care

Nursing Care. Nursing care of abusive head trauma involves initiation and maintenance of respiratory and cardiovascular support, if necessary. Upon admission, assess for increased ICP and visible injuries. Gathering a health history and critical information about the abusive event is essential.

The child may have long-term impairment. Long-term impairment requires ongoing therapy that may consist of total care of self-care deficits, gastrostomy tube feedings, a tracheostomy, and pressure ulcer prevention. Additionally, prevention of complications such as infection, contractures, or decreased muscle tone for children in a vegetative state is important. The long-term outcome for a child with abusive head trauma may be uncertain. The child may have minimal deficits or complications or he or she may experience severe and life-altering complications. The child's prognosis is affected by many variables, including the degree of cerebral involvement, areas of the brain affected, severity of intracranial hemorrhaging, and medical management provided.

Medical Care. Initial care measures include maintaining oxygenation, inserting a nasogastric or orogastric tube, assessing for seizure activity and implementing seizure precautions, and maintaining adequate fluid and nutritional intake. Documenting the data is also important.

 legal alert—Legal and ethical responsibility

Nurses are legally and ethically required to report any incidences of probable abuse to the appropriate child welfare and law enforcement agencies. It is recommended that health-care facilities have relevant policy and procedural guidelines in place for a child admitted with abusive head trauma. Accurate documentation in the medical record is of great importance because the record may be used in court.

Education/Discharge Instructions

The nurse must honestly address parental concerns and questions and provide information about agencies that can provide assistance and support them. The parents need to realize the child may never return to the prior level of cognitive and physical functioning. Discharge instructions regarding home management and monitoring, indications to see the health-care provider, and follow-up appointments are given to the caregiver. Of the infants who survive, long-term neurological complications may include cognitive and behavioral disturbances, motor and visual deficits, and seizures; therefore, the family must be provided with community resources.

SPINAL CORD INJURY

The incidence of spinal cord injury (SCI) is based on pediatric demographics, gender, and age of the child. SCIs are seen more in the summer with bike riding, swimming and diving activities, football playing, and motor vehicle collisions. Spinal cord injuries have been associated with traumatic births and child abuse in children younger than 1 year of age. SCIs are also associated with fighting with guns and knives and other forms of violence (Parent, Mac-Thiong, Roy-Beaudry, Sosa, & Labelle, 2011).

SCI involves injury to the spinal cord in any or all of the following regions: cervical, thoracic, lumbar, or sacral. SCIs are caused by direct or indirect force causing a contusion or bruising, compression, hemorrhage, or significant vascular damage resulting in paresthesia (loss of sensation) or paralysis (loss of function) below the level of injury.

There are four types of SCIs: (1) cord resection, when the spinal cord is completely severed; (2) cord laceration, caused by a blunt instrument such as a knife; (3) cord contusion, caused by swelling and edema; and (4) cord injury, in which there is no necrosis or obvious injury.

There are three phases of SCI injury: acute, secondary, and chronic. The acute phase begins at the immediate time of injury and lasts through a few days later and is characterized by damage to the tissues resulting in cell necrosis. Immediately after the insult, there is hemorrhage and edema combined with electrolyte and fluid shifts. The cord then experiences a spinal shock that lasts for 24 hours. The secondary phase occurs at the time of injury and continues over several weeks. The child's neurological status at this phase determines recovery outcomes. The chronic phase is marked with scarring and progression or regression of function. Understand that complete resection of the spinal cord results in complete loss of motor function and sensation below the area of injury. Regardless of the mechanism of injury, the result is either temporary or permanent loss or alteration of autonomic, motor, and sensory function (Gepp & Nadal, 2012; Helgeson, Gendelberg, Sidhu, Anderson, & Vaccaro, 2011).

Nursing Insight—*Spinal cord injury without radiographic abnormality*

Spinal cord injury without radiographic abnormality (SCIWORA) is a closed spinal cord injury resulting in stretching of the spinal cord without bony involvement or radiographic abnormalities. SCIWORA occurs in more than 50% to 70% of spinal cord injuries in children. SCIWORA usually occurs in children younger than 8 years of age because they are at risk for high cervical injuries because of their disproportionately larger head in relation to their body. As the child grows, the spinal cord becomes less elastic but is covered by strengthened bony prominences; this added protection accounts for better resistance to injury as the child ages. The long-term outcome for children with SCIWORA is related to the etiology of the injury and the degree of functional loss (Schottler, Vogel, & Sturm, 2012; Vogel, Betz, & Mulcahey, 2011).

Signs and Symptoms

Signs and symptoms vary depending on the level of the injury. Immediately following the injury, there is temporary loss of spinal reflex activity below the level of the injury causing a disruption of sympathetic nervous system function. This results in vasodilation, hypotension and bradycardia. This is referred to as spinal shock and subsides with the return of the reflexes. The severity of the symptoms depends on whether the entire cord is injured (complete) or only partially injured (incomplete).

Injuries at any level can cause:

- Increased muscle tone (spasticity)
- Loss of normal bowel and bladder control (may include constipation, incontinence, or bladder spasms)
- Numbness
- Sensory changes
- Pain
- Weakness or paralysis

Diagnosis

The International Standards for Neurological and Functional Classification of Spinal Cord Injury identify two levels of spinal cord loss and function. Tetraplegia, currently replacing the term quadriplegia, is caused by an SCI at the cervical level that involves all four extremities. Paraplegia is the result of thoracic, lumbar, or sacral injury loss of function and sensation in the lower extremities (Kirshblum, Burns, Biering-Sorensen, Donovan, Graves, Jha, et al., 2011).

The clinical diagnosis of SCI and SCIWORA is made both clinically and radiologically. Loss of motor function, sensation, and anal tone clinically define the level of injury and degree of involvement. A radiological examination with spine series, CT scan, or MRI identifies the type of injury, the presence of hemorrhage or inflammation, and the degree of bony involvement, if any (Easter, Barkin, Rosen, & Ban, 2011).

Prevention

Public awareness efforts targeting both children and parents are essential in primary prevention strategies. Many spinal cord injuries can be prevented by implementing safe injury control practices. Providing education about the leading causes of spinal cord injury and ways to prevent them may influence changes in behavior to adopt these measures to prevent injuries (CDC, 2012a; Shriners Hospitals for Children, 2012).

Focus on Safety

Autonomic dysreflexia

Autonomic dysreflexia is a stress syndrome caused by massive amounts of stimuli overloading the autonomic system, which results in hyperactive sympathetic stimulation. This leads to a myriad of symptoms such as extreme anxiety, headache, visual and auditory sensation changes, nausea, seizures, hypertension, peripheral vascular dilation or flushing, and bradycardia. This situation is an emergent condition requiring immediate management of hypertension, cardiac, and neurological complications.

Collaborative Care

Nursing Care. The priorities of spinal cord injury care are attention to airway management, breathing or ventilatory support, circulation support, disability identification, and exposure of known and unknown physical limitations. Immediate cervical (c-spine) immobilization is maintained continuously. Treat an SCI with full-body immobilization and maintain with lumbar–thoracic–sacral orthotics, which are rigid body casts that maintain neuromuscular alignment until the injury is resolved.

Provide emotional and social support because the child with a spinal cord injury and his or her family have unique collective and individual needs. The younger child does not understand the loss of function immediately and is more concerned with parental presence and fear issues. The older child understands the loss of function and sensation and is more cooperative and eager to return to normal living as much as possible. Encourage older children and adolescents to participate in their own care as much as possible. All daily activities such as bathing, dressing, eating, grooming, and bowel and bladder contents elimination are performed by the older child as he or she is able.

The adolescent presents a unique developmental challenge. The realization about the loss of friends, athletic participation, and social disruption may place the teen at risk for depression, withdrawal, isolation, and suicide. Look for these changes and recommend antidepressant medication to promote optimal function and return to a healthy emotional status. The child with SCI requires lifelong care and support. This places a financial, mental, physical, and emotional strain on the family. Recognize caregiver role strain and offer or encourage respite care for the caregivers as needed.

Medical Care. If a child has a high cervical injury or if an open airway cannot be maintained, a temporary or permanent tracheostomy is necessary for the child to breathe. Mechanical ventilation may be a lifelong need for patients with a high C4 injury. Cardiovascular and circulatory support is maintained with adequate fluid resuscitation, inotropic medications, and blood products to maintain circulation, cardiac output, and renal function during the immediate posttraumatic event.

Also monitor appropriate daily fluid intake and output measurements and ensure adequate daily fluid requirement needs are met. Enteral feedings may be needed until the child is able to chew and swallow without threat of aspiration. A child with altered oral pharyngeal motility or dysphagia may require an oral pharyngeal motility study before oral feedings.

The child with an SCI may be placed in skeletal traction or a halo device for immobilization and alignment of the spine. Methylprednisolone (Medrol) may be used after the initial injury to reduce spinal cord inflammation (Easter et al., 2011). Pain management is also a priority. Early respiratory physiology is initiated to minimize complications.

A child immobilized by an SCI may have slowed peristaltic function and may require medications such as metoclopramide (Reglan), laxatives, or stool softeners to prevent constipation, gastric overdistention, and fecal impaction. Bowel training may be a chronic issue for most children with SCI. Stool bulking with high-fiber foods may promote stool formation. Lower intestinal evacuation may be necessary with enemas, suppositories, and colonic irrigations (Vogel, Betz, & Mulcahey, 2012; White & Thumbikat, 2012).

Surgical Care. Generally there are two back surgery approaches: open back surgery and minimally invasive spine surgery. In SCI, an open back approach is used. The goal of this surgery, following an SCI, is to stabilize the bony elements of the spine and relieve pressure on the spinal cord.

Collaboration in Caring—*Spinal cord injury*

Nursing care of the child with an SCI is an interdisciplinary approach. Multidisciplinary teams manage the aspects of care together to promote continuity and coordination of care. The child works together with the family; medical team; physical, speech, occupational, and respiratory therapists; and social workers to coordinate the services needed for individualized care, focusing on achieving patient outcomes and optimizing resources.

Education/Discharge Instructions

SCI patients will require extensive rehabilitation to achieve a maximum level of functioning. In preparation for discharge home, educational resources and information on resources and preventing secondary complications will be beneficial to help the patient, family, and caregivers manage the lifelong, complex care needs of the child.

Nursing Diagnoses Spinal Cord Injury

- Impaired urinary elimination related to neuromuscular alteration
- Constipation related to sensory and motor impairment
- Ineffective individual coping related to traumatic spinal cord injury and potential loss of function
- Impaired physical mobility related to neuromuscular functional loss
- Risk for injury related to loss of sensation and motor function
- Risk for impaired skin integrity related to loss of sensation
- Situational alteration in self-esteem related to change in lifestyle

Nontraumatic Neurological Conditions

HEADACHES

Headaches are common during childhood and become more common and more frequent during adolescence. Headaches are classified as primary or secondary and further classified into subtypes according to the International Classification of Headache Disorders (ICHD-II) (International Headache Society, 2013). The ICHD-II is a useful tool in classifying acute and chronic headaches in school-age children and adolescents but lacks sensitivity in diagnosing benign headaches in preschool and younger children (Roser, Bonfert, Ebinger, Blankenburg, Ertl-Wagner, & Heinen, 2013). The ICHD-II classifies major groups of headache disorders and provides diagnostic criteria to assist in improving the diagnosis, treatment and care of a child with headaches.

Triggers of primary headaches have been identified as lack of sleep, stress, exercise, hunger, loud noise or persistently loud noises, weather changes, and hormonal changes caused by menstrual cycles in females. Secondary headaches are associated with an organic disorder such as trauma, vascular changes, infectious processes, substance use, brain neoplasms, or psychogenic issues. A detailed health history and neurological examination is essential because more than 98% of children with brain tumors have objective assessment findings (Lewis, 2010). Headaches are further classified into subtypes based on descriptive symptoms and frequency of disturbances.

Tension Headache

Tension headaches are common among school-age children and are associated with stress.

Signs and Symptoms

A tension headache is located in the back of the head at the base of the skull and can include:

- A dull, moderate pain
- Pain may radiate bilaterally, just above the neck and shoulders
- Affected sleep for children with these headaches
- Loss of vision, nausea, photophobia, and auditory sensitivity are *not* associated with tension headaches.

Migraine Headache

Migraine headaches are another type of headache and can be present in the preschool or school-aged child. Most often, there is a family history of migraines.

Signs and Symptoms

Signs and symptoms of migraine headaches include:

- Radiating pain located on one side of the head with a throbbing or pulsating quality.
- Preceding aura accompanied by nausea, vomiting, diaphoresis, pallor, photophobia, and auditory sensitivity. (Aura may be sensed by a noxious smell, bright lights, or a change in vision.)
- Not easily remedied with rest alone and typically require prophylactic and acute management.

Nursing Insight—*Other signs and symptoms of migraine headaches*

A range of other signs and symptoms can help in the diagnosis of migraine headaches. A classic finding in the health history is that when the child has a headache, he or she wishes to lie in a dark, quiet room with a cold towel placed over the face. Other signs and symptoms include:
- Throbbing and/or pulsing pain, usually unilateral
- Nausea
- Vomiting
- Photosensitivity
- Sound sensitivity
- Blurred vision
- Abdominal pain (also called abdominal migraine)

Cluster Headaches

Cluster headaches are a series of headaches over a period of weeks or months that vary in intensity and can be very debilitating.

Signs and Symptoms

Signs and symptoms of cluster headaches include:

- Unilateral pain, behind one eye, resulting ptosis (drooping), pupil constriction, erythema, and edema of the affected eye
- Rhinorrhea with clear drainage in the absence of an upper respiratory illness (Hershey, 2012; Lewis, 2010).

Diagnosis

Headache diagnoses are based on clinical symptoms according to the ICHD-II criteria. Diagnosis is based on inclusion and exclusion of clinical criteria. Clinical diagnosis is difficult with a young child because of cognitive and communication barriers. A history of headache signs is difficult to piece together because the symptoms may mimic those of other minor pediatric illnesses. Neuroimaging studies are warranted with sudden severe onset of headaches, history of trauma, family history of brain neoplasms or vascular malformations, change in neurological function, signs of increased intracranial pressure or visual disturbances, new seizure onset, unexplained ataxia, or alterations in level of consciousness.

Diagnostic assessment begins with a full neurological examination, history of present illness, family headache history, review of symptoms, and headache history including patterns, antecedent events, and symptom management. Decisions for diagnostic neuroimaging, lumbar puncture, or electroencephalogram testing are based on patient data obtained at the time of the neurological evaluation. Routine neuroimaging is not indicated in the presence of a normal neurological exam (Blume, 2012; Hershey, 2012; Ozge, Termine, Antonaci, Natriashvili, Guidetti, & Wober-Bingol, 2011).

Prevention

Child and family education can target ways to prevent headaches. Migraine prophylaxis includes identification and management of headache triggers and medications such as topiramate (Topamax), sumatriptan (Imitrex), ergotamine (Cafergot), nonsteroidal anti-inflammatory drugs, antiemetics, and sedative analgesics.

Collaborative Care

Nursing Care. Combined pharmacological and nonpharmacological therapies along with child and family education can successfully manage the child with primary headaches. Nonpharmacological therapies include lifestyle modification and psychotherapeutic measures. Educate the family on recognition of headache aura, prophylaxis strategies, and management intervention, including medication, relaxation strategies, and environmental modifications (e.g., noise reduction and dim or dark room). Evaluate the effectiveness of the medication and monitor for adverse reactions. Treatment also involves rest and stress-reduction strategies such as soothing baths, music, guided imagery, or massage therapy.

Medical Care. Acute episodes are treated with acetaminophen (Children's Tylenol) and ibuprofen (Children's Advil). Other pharmacological prophylactic medication such as beta blockers, calcium channel blockers, antidepressants, and anticonvulsants or a combination of these can also help the child cope with primary headaches. IM or intranasal dihydroergotamine is used for moderate to severe migraines in adolescents (Hershey, 2012; Ozge et al., 2011; Robertson & Shilkofski, 2012). Pharmacology therapy is individualized to the child's needs.

 Nursing Insight—Headaches and surgery

> Surgical treatment is usually not indicated for headaches. Treatments targeting deactivation of trigger points and occipital nerve stimulation are of growing interest and research (Evans, 2013).

Education/Discharge Instructions

Health education for this condition includes ensuring medications are taken as prescribed. Keeping a record of headaches is helpful to observe improvements and evaluate for contributing factors.

Sensory Conditions

EYE DISORDERS

Children may experience a myriad of common eye disorders. The parent may notice an abrupt change or changes in vision function. Children are not acutely aware of changes in vision or eye disturbances and may not voice complaints of vision difficulty unless there is an injury. Common childhood eye disorders are classified as refractive disorders, astigmatism, amblyopia, strabismus, or organic diseases (Chou, Dana, & Bougatsos, 2011) (Table 28-7).

Nursing Insight—Vision

> Vision occurs when light reflects from an object and passes through the cornea, aqueous humor, pupil, lenses, and vitreous humor and is finally absorbed by the retina. The retina is composed of rods and cones that are used in night, color, daylight, and eye movement functions. The rods and cones communicate electrical energy to the retina, which then sends an impulse to the optic nerve that is relayed to the visual cortex of the brain. The majority of the blood vessels radiate from the optic nerve and the retina. The fovea centralis, which is located in the center of the macula about 2.5 disc diameters from the optic nerve, is responsible for color perception.

Refractive Disorders

The most common category of vision disorders in children is refractive errors (Wojciechowski, 2011). Light refraction is the bending of light as it passes through a lens. As light passes through an opening in the pupil, the lens directs the light to the retina to initiate vision. In very young infants, the light rays fall behind the retina because of the shallowness of the eye.

HYPEROPIA. Most children are hyperopic (farsighted). The severity of hyperopia diminishes as the child ages. Risk factors for refractive error include retinopathy of prematurity and family history of high refractive error.

Signs and Symptoms

Signs and symptoms of hyperopia include:

- Unclear vision at close range
- Clearer vision at a far range
- Trouble focusing on projects requiring close range vision, prompting loss of interest (in young children)

Diagnosis

If a child reports headaches, dizziness, or eye strain after doing schoolwork, hyperopia is suspected and a referral is made for complete vision assessment. Hyperopia usually diminishes by age 5, but in some cases may still persist.

Prevention

Parents play a key role regarding early diagnosis and prevention. If parents notice visual disturbances in the child

Table 28-7 Common Acute Eye Disorders

Eye Disorder	Cause/Organism	Signs and Symptoms	Treatment
Conjunctivitis	An inflammation of the conjunctiva caused by bacterial, viral, or allergic agents.	Excessive tearing, erythema, and edema with clear, watery discharge, yellow or green drainage, and eyelid crusting. Bacterial and viral agents are difficult to discriminate clinically without a culture. Viral usually seen in children older than 6 years of age with a clear watery drainage. Allergic: cobblestoning and pallor of the conjunctiva, pruritus, watery clear drainage.	Apply warm soaks to remove crusting, use good hand hygiene and apply cool compresses to edematous eyes. Antibiotic ointment or solutions are used for bacterial infections. Family education includes good hand hygiene before and after touching the eye, non-sharing of personal items such as pillowcases and washcloths, and careful disposal of used tissues and wipes. Older children who wear contact lenses or use cosmetics must discard used materials and begin use of new materials after the infection has resolved. School attendance is permissible after the discomfort and drainage has subsided, usually after 24 hours of treatment. If symptoms are not improved in 24 to 48 hours the family seeks additional follow-up medical care. Conjunctivitis associated with herpes may be treated with oral or parenteral antiviral agents. Herpetic ophthalmicus is one of the leading causes of vision loss in children. Allergic conjunctivitis is treated with allergen avoidance and antihistamines.
Neonatal Conjunctivitis–Ophthalmia Neonatorum	Chemical irritation caused by maternal sexually transmitted diseases acquired at birth. *Chlamydia, gonorrhea, herpes.*	Purulent drainage either white or yellowish.	Prophylactic antibiotic ointment is used in all neonates. Lack of treatment can cause eye damage.
Stye	A localized inflammatory swelling of one or more of the glands of the eyelid. They are mildly tender and may discharge some purulent fluid (Venes, 2013).	Painful, erythematous lesion on the lid margin. Slight edema, some lymph node tenderness or induration.	Apply warm, moist compresses with an antibiotic ointment. Good hand hygiene is necessary.
Chalazion	Granuloma of the meibomian gland on the eyelid. Cause unknown.	Hard, small nodule on either eyelid may be painful.	Applying warm moist compresses and massage, with antibiotic ointment, may resolve the condition spontaneously. Surgical removal or steroid injections may be used to reduce size and symptoms such as ptosis.
Blepharitis Marginalis	Staphylococcal infection of the lid margin.	Erythematous eyelid margin with crusted eye drainage.	Apply an antibiotic ointment to the lower affected eyelid. Apply warm, moist compresses to remove crusting drainage.
Keratitis	Inflammation and infection of the corneal layers caused by bacterial, viral, fungal, or foreign body infiltration.	Very painful, excessive tearing, photophobia, and erythema.	An ophthalmologist must examine the cornea to monitor or treat potential scarring and prevent loss of vision.
Periorbital Cellulitis	Inflammation of the subcutaneous tissues and skin about the eye may be bacterial or viral.	Edema, pain, erythema in the skin and orbital folds of the affected eye.	Use IV antibiotic therapy for 7 days.
Blocked Tear Duct	Obstruction of the nasolacrimal tear duct causing inflammation or cystitis.	Tearing, yellow drainage, crusting, small bump in the inner canthus of the affected eye. Usually unilateral, may be painful.	Apply warm compresses and gently massage the lacrimal sac with the forefinger, milking any exudates toward the nose. This condition may require probing of the duct by an ophthalmologist if no improvement is noted in 6 months.

Sources: American Association for Pediatric Ophthalmology and Strabismus (2012); Burns, Dunn, Brady, Start, & Blosser (2013).

such as unclear vision at a close range or difficulty focusing on projects, it is important to take the child to a health-care provider for further assessment.

Collaborative Care

The main care for these children is wearing glasses with corrective convex lenses. The lenses focus the light rays on the retina to correct the refractive disorder. Routine follow-up examinations are important.

Education/Discharge Instructions

Tell parents that refractive errors are treated with corrective lenses. Parents should also know refractive surgery may be performed in children to prevent amblyopia (American Association for Pediatric Ophthalmology and Strabismus, 2012).

MYOPIA. Some children develop myopia (nearsightedness) during their school years, particularly if there is a familial history of myopia. About 30% of school-aged children and adolescents in the United States have myopia (Vitale, Sperduto, & Ferris, 2009). In myopia, light rays do not reach the retina, which causes blurred vision at a far range and clear vision at a close range. This condition continues to progress in severity until puberty when progression plateaus (American Association for Pediatric Ophthalmology and Strabismus, 2012; Wojciechowski, 2011). An important risk factor for the development of simple myopia is a family history of myopia.

Signs and Symptoms

Signs and symptoms of myopia include:

- Squinting
- Complaints of difficulty seeing objects that are far away
- Inability to see the blackboard, television, or street signs but able to clearly read a book or a computer screen at close range

Diagnosis

Vision screening begins about 3 years of age or earlier if there are risk factors of visual impairment (U.S. Preventative Task Force, 2011).

Prevention

To prevent permanent visual impairment, early detection through screenings is essential.

Preventative measures also include parental education about the warning signs of vision problems.

Collaborative Care

Myopia or blurred distance vision and reduced distance visual acuity can be improved with appropriate minus-power lenses.

Laser assisted surgery keratomileusis (LASIK) is available for the adolescents if desired. The age for LASIK surgery is controversial. If the procedure is performed before full eye growth maturity has been reached, additional surgery may be needed (U.S. Food and Drug Administration, 2012).

Education/Discharge Instructions

Parental education includes the importance of follow-up care and options available for correction of myopia. Schedule follow-up appointments for the child and stress the importance of keeping these appointments. Also, provide community resources to families about where to purchase corrective lenses. If the family cannot afford corrective lenses, contact a case manager who can help the family.

ASTIGMATISM. Astigmatism is an irregular curvature or uneven contour of the eye resulting in impaired light refraction. The cause is unknown. Astigmatism may be present at birth or acquired. Light rays are unevenly distributed in the eyes, causing blurred vision at all distances. This condition is associated with birth hyperopia and myopia.

Signs and Symptoms

Signs and symptoms of astigmatism include:

- Blurred vision at all distances, even with corrective lenses

Diagnosis

If a child complains of headaches, blurry vision, or dizziness after doing close work or difficulty reading, he or she is referred to an ophthalmologist for exact diagnosis. Diagnosis is confirmed with history and thorough ophthalmological examination.

Prevention

Prevention and early detection of astigmatism through school and community screenings are recommended to decrease preventable childhood visual impairment (Agency for Health Care Research and Quality, 2014).

Collaborative Care

Correction of astigmatism includes corrective lenses and routine follow-up examinations to monitor for amblyopia.

Education/Discharge Instructions

Parents are given education on the importance of follow-up care and treatment options available for correction of astigmatism. They are also instructed to promote eye protection and report any changes in visual acuity to the health-care provider, which may include the pediatrician and/or ophthalmologist.

 Nursing Insight—*Amblyopia*

Amblyopia ("lazy eye") is one of the most common monocular eye disorders in children leading to loss of vision. Strabismus and anisometropia are the most prevalent forms of amblyopia in children. **Strabismus**, or a cross-eyed appearance, results in malalignment of the eyes (see later discussion). **Anisometropia** is a condition in which the refractive power of the eyes is unequal (Venes, 2013). If the refractive errors are significantly different in one eye, the child becomes dependent on the eye that is more easily focused, leading to an irreversible loss of vision potential. Vision screening is strongly recommended by the American Academy of Pediatrics (2014) over the course of childhood to detect amblyopia early enough to allow successful treatment. Because many affected children are asymptomatic, early detection of abnormal visual function requires effective screening throughout early childhood. Amblyopia may be resolved if it is detected at an early age. It is recommended that preschoolers be screened for visual acuity using the Snellen E chart. Treatment is initiated during the preschool years if possible. The success of amblyopic therapy diminishes after age 6 (Olitsky, Hug, Plummer, & Stass-Isern, 2011; U.S. Preventative Services Task Force, 2011).

The goal of amblyopia treatment is to improve visual acuity of the weaker eye and prevent permanent loss of vision or visual impairment. Occlusion therapy, or patching of the normal eye, is done to restore strength and function to the lazy eye (Fig. 28-15). Duration of occlusion therapy is widely debated. No clear evidence exists for length of occlusion theory (Li & Shotton, 2009; Stewart, Moseley, & Fielder, 2011). Child and parental compliance with occlusion therapy is complicated and stressful for the entire family. Children are too young to appreciate the significance of the therapy and attempt to remove or hide the patches. Compliance is better if patching is disguised behind eyeglasses or if patching time is shortened. Amblyopia is also treated with corrective lenses for up to 6 months or until improvement plateaus, then eye muscle repair surgery may be indicated (Olitsky et al., 2011). If amblyopia it is not treated, permanent loss of vision may occur.

 Optimizing Outcomes—Early vision screening

Early screening for all children at risk for amblyopia and aggressive, prompt treatment will result in the best outcome and prevention of visual impairment.

Strabismus

Strabismus is a condition of non-parallelism in the different fields of gaze causing visual lines to cross even when focused on the same object. Weakened or misaligned extraocular muscles pull the eyes in different directions resulting in a cross-eyed appearance. The child attempts to compensate for this unequal vision by preferentially choosing to use one eye and not the other eye. When the child focuses on an object, one eye wanders off of the focused object while the other eye looks straight ahead. The child then experiences two separate images instead of one and develops a stronger eye.

Strabismus occurs in 2% to 7% of children, affecting males and females equally, and has an inherited pattern in about half of the cases. Pseudostrabismus is an appearance of crossed eyes but is a result of physical attributes such as prominent epicanthal folds and a flattened nasal bridge. Children outgrow this condition over time. True strabismus

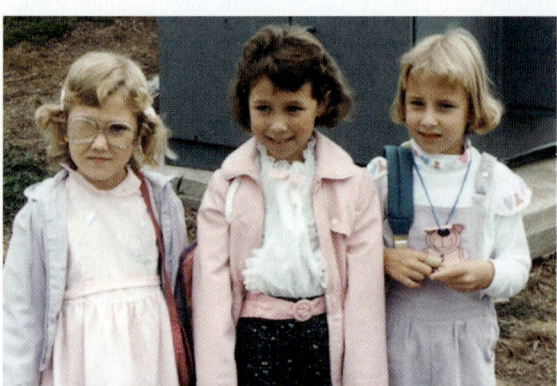

Figure 28-15 Occlusion therapy or patching of the normal eye is done to restore strength and function to the lazy eye.

does not change without intervention and can lead to amblyopia and loss of vision (Stewart, Moseley, & Fielder, 2011). Any other disease that causes vision loss may also cause strabismus.

Signs and Symptoms

Signs and symptoms of strabismus include:

- Persistent squinting
- Head tilting
- Clumsiness
- Decreased visual acuity

Intermittent strabismus is seen in normal children younger than 3 years of age when the child is tired, ill, or with a sudden change in light or distance.

Diagnosis

Childhood screening is begun as early as 3 to 6 months of age. The corneal light reflex test and the cover test are performed to detect strabismus, but the cover test is the most reliable. The cover test is more sensitive in that eye movement is noted in response to covering and uncovering the child's eye while focusing on an object. This test requires the child's cooperation. The cover test is performed by having the child focus on a toy or favorite object and covering one eye. If the uncovered eye moves, that eye was not fixated on the object and strabismus is suspected. Three forms of strabismus describe the eye deviation noted on an exam:

- Esotropia: eye turns toward the midline of the face or nose
- Exotropia: eye turns away from the midline of the face
- Hypertropia: eye turns toward the forehead or a downward turning

 Assessment Tool Hirschberg Asymmetrical Corneal Light Reflex Test

The Hirschberg asymmetrical corneal light reflex test is performed by holding a penlight or flashlight in front of the child's face. The light reflection is noted on the cornea in both eyes. Symmetrical placement on both eyes at the same time and in the same location on each eye designates negative corneal light reflex exam results and indicates normal muscle alignment. Positive asymmetrical corneal light reflex test results occur when the light falls slightly medially to the center of the pupil on the iris. The presence of an asymmetrical corneal light reflex is a positive exam and is suggestive of strabismus. A cover test is then performed.

Prevention

Early identification and recognition of all children suspected for strabismus is critical to prevent vision loss. To prevent visual loss, a family history of strabismus is done. Parents need to understand that farsightedness may be a contributing factor suggestive of strabismus.

Collaborative Care

Nursing Care. Treatment of strabismus involves ocular patching of the stronger eye to force the weaker eye to work independently and "exercise" to strengthen extraocular muscles. Occlusion therapy is conducted under the care of a pediatric ophthalmologist. Patching is most successful if implemented before age 3 to 4 years. Glasses are also prescribed for the child.

Medical Care. Botulinum toxin A (Oculinum) (Botox) may also be used for treatment of strabismus in children. Botox can be used in conjunction with, or as an alternative to, surgery. The toxin is injected into the extraocular muscle, causing misalignment and produces a temporary muscle shortening resulting in a parallelism of vision. The Botox effects last for up to 3 months, and repeat injections may be performed. Potential complications include retrobulbar hemorrhage, ocular needle penetration, and ptosis.

Surgical Care. If conservative therapy is not effective, eye muscle repair surgery may be needed (Olitsky et al., 2011).

Education/Discharge Instructions

Provide families and children with referral sources, support groups, information, and schooling. School-based screening programs are essential for early detection, identification, and initiation of treatment of strabismus-related eye disorders. The school nurse may also be involved when treatment is needed during school hours.

 Nursing Insight—*Color blindness*

Color blindness is an X-linked recessive inheritable color vision deficiency that causes loss of accurate color perception. Males are more affected (8%) than females (less than 0.5%). Color blindness may be selective, partial, or complete (all colors). Complete color blindness is rare and results in perception of only shades of gray. Color blindness is a deficiency of photosensitive pigments (red, green, blue, or yellow) located in the cones of the retina. Color blindness is untreatable, nonprogressive, and non-debilitating (Adams, Verdon, & Spivey, 2009).

Color blindness is detected using colored charts called the Ishihara Test plates (Fig. 28-16). Each chart is composed of colored dots with a number located in the center of the plate in a different color, usually yellow, red, green, or brown. The child is asked to identify the number or the shape in the center of the chart. A child without a color vision deficiency sees the object clearly. A child with color blindness sees only the plate of dots without an image, or the image is blurred and indistinct.

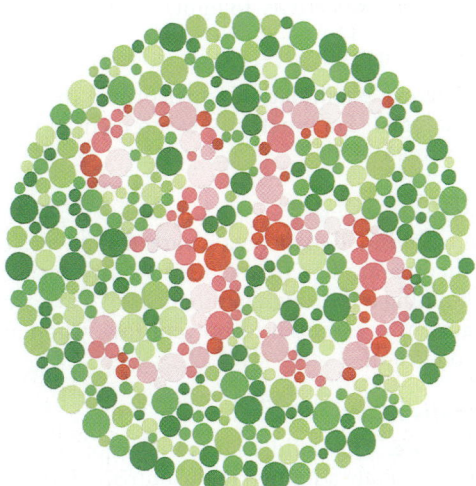

Figure 28-16 Color blindness is detected using colored charts called Ishihara Test plates.

Children can learn to compensate for their color deficiency with support from family members, teachers, and friends. Some alterations in daily function may be affected, but they can be compensated for with minor behavioral alterations. For instance, at a traffic signal the child will need to learn to identify the signal by order rather than by color. Assistance with clothing selection may be necessary as well as labeling the clothes. Provide reassurance to parents that color blindness does not lead to loss of vision.

Nystagmus

Nystagmus is a rapid, irregular, involuntary eye movement caused by a disorder of the central nervous system that may be congenital or acquired. There are many types of nystagmus.

Congenital nystagmus is usually mild and non-progressive and persists into adulthood. Brain injuries are the most common cause of acquired nystagmus. Any child who develops nystagmus early in life is evaluated for an underlying central nervous system cause. Prognosis is based on the etiological cause (American Association for Pediatric Ophthalmology and Strabismus, 2012).

Signs and Symptoms

Signs and symptoms of nystagmus include:

- Eyes that rotate in a lateral direction, clockwise or counterclockwise direction, up and down, or any combination of these movements.
- Repetitive and involuntary eye movement that may be managed by gaze redirection.

Diagnosis

If an identifiable cause is not clear, neuroimaging, such as an MRI, is warranted to rule out the possibility of a neoplasm.

Prevention

Preventative measures include providing information to families that nystagmus can be inherited or may develop after an accident or illness and is often a symptom of an underlying eye or medical problem (American Optometric Association, 2012). If low vision is suspected, parents must seek medical advice from a health-care provider to prevent further visual loss.

Collaborative Care

Nursing Care. Acquired nystagmus treatments are based on the existing etiology and may include pharmacological, optical, and surgical approaches (Thurtell & Leigh, 2012). Significant refractive error is corrected with glasses or contact lenses.

Surgical Care. Extraocular surgery may correct some forms of congenital nystagmus. Goals of surgery include increasing visual acuity, alleviating an abnormal head position, or decreasing the amplitude of nystagmus (American Association for Pediatric Ophthalmology and Strabismus, 2012).

Education/Discharge Instructions

Before discharge, parents will receive instructions about home care, medications, and recognizing signs of complications.

Cataracts

A cataract is a clouding or a haziness of the corneal lens. Significant irreversible vision disorders are caused by cataracts. Cataracts can be located unilaterally in one eye or bilaterally in both eyes. Cataracts can be acquired or congenital, resulting in partial or complete occlusion, or both. Acquired cataracts can be caused by maternal infection acquired during pregnancy, trauma to the eye, radiation, or systemic diseases. Some cataracts are a result of family inheritance patterns. Congenital cataracts are present in neonates with syndrome anomalies or mothers with TORCH (toxoplasmosis, rubella, cytomegalovirus, herpes simplex or HIV) infection during pregnancy. Congenital cataracts can be autosomal dominant in genetically linked families. However, X-linked and recessive genetic situations have been reported (Olitsky et al., 2011).

Signs and Symptoms

During an eye exam with an ophthalmoscope, a cataract is usually visualized by the examiner. Signs and symptoms of cataracts include:

- Abnormal or absent red reflex
- Excessive tearing and extraocular movements
- Strabismus
- Abnormal cover test
- Photophobia
- Decreased visual acuity

Diagnosis

A pediatric ophthalmologist performs a complete eye examination. Diagnosis is made when the lens appears cloudy or there is a white or dulled red reflex.

Prevention

Early detection and diagnosis of a congenital cataract prevents loss of visual acuity. Prevention also includes a referral to a pediatric ophthalmologist when low vision is suspected.

Collaborative Care

Nursing Care. In cataract care, a change in eyeglasses and or more lighting may be all that is required for better vision. The child who is undergoing a cataract removal is usually admitted to the outpatient surgery unit. Prior to the procedure, nursing care includes preparing the child and family for surgery, administering any medications, and providing health education regarding recovery and limitations of activity. Preoperative visual status baseline is also obtained.

Surgical Care. In most cases, a laser procedure is performed to remove the cataract. Because the eye is still growing, a permanent lens is not placed until eye growth has reached maturity. When the eye has reached full development, the child can return to surgery where a small incision is made in the eye to place a permanent lens. The child can wear a standard corrective contact lens until a permanent lens can be placed.

Postoperative nursing care for the child includes monitoring nausea, emesis, pain, hemorrhage, and signs of infection. Keep the child free from wrenching, coughing, crying, and active play that can cause increased intraocular pressure (IOP). Postoperative eye drops also include a steroid preparation to reduce inflammation and prevent adhesions. Mydriatic eye drops prevent adhesions of the pupils, and topical antimicrobial eye solutions prevent infection. Postoperative education for the family and child includes signs and symptoms of infection, hemorrhage, increased IOP, and activity restrictions until cleared by the health-care provider.

Education/Discharge Instructions

Follow-up care of the child is based on loss of visual acuity. Some children need glasses for correction of refraction errors. Other children may need an antiglaucoma medication to prevent IOP development. If amblyopia is evident, the non-surgical eye is patched to force the operative eye to "exercise," which strengthens the extraocular muscles (Hager, Schirra, Kohnen, Seitz, & Kasmann-Kellner, 2012).

Glaucoma

Glaucoma is an increase of the IOP in the eye caused by an obstruction or impaired outflow of aqueous humor (clear fluid), which leads to retinal damage and eventual necrosis of the optic nerve. Optic nerve cupping is seen with ophthalmoscope examination. The eye enlarges because of increased IOP, causing a thinned, cloudy-appearing cornea. The sclera may appear bluish. Glaucoma can be congenital or acquired. Some cases of pediatric glaucoma are caused by eye trauma or from surgical procedures. Congenital or infantile glaucoma is a rare condition presenting with corneal opacification (or clouding), corneal enlargement, and eye pain. Another rare type of congenital glaucoma is when the iridocorneal (the junction of the iris and the cornea) angle of the eye at the canal of Schlemm causes an obstruction of outflow of aqueous humor from the eye. This condition appears in the first year of life and, if left untreated, results in blindness (American Association for Pediatric Ophthalmology and Strabismus, 2012).

Signs and Symptoms

Signs of infantile glaucoma include a triad of symptoms:

- Buphthalmos (enlarged eye globe)
- Epiphora (excessive tearing)
- Photophobia (sensitivity to light)

Diagnosis

A complete eye examination is performed by a pediatric ophthalmologist. **Tonometry** (measurement of tension) is used to evaluate IOP.

Prevention

Although childhood glaucoma is rare, some types of pediatric glaucoma are hereditary. Preventative measures include obtaining a thorough family history. Early detection and treatment is essential to prevent low vision and preserve good vision.

Collaborative Care

Nursing Care. The child who is undergoing surgery for glaucoma is usually admitted to the outpatient surgery unit and then may be transferred to the pediatric floor. Prior to the procedure, nursing care includes preparing the child and family for surgery, administering any medications, and providing health education regarding recovery and limitations of activity. Preoperative visual status baseline is also obtained.

Surgical Care. Early surgical intervention is done to remove obstructions and allow the flow of aqueous humor into the canal of Schlemm. Provide preoperative, family-centered care and education about the condition. Prior to the procedure, the child is premedicated with a topical anesthetic to obtain a reliable eye pressure measurement. Also, before surgery, prevent IOP increase by maintaining a quiet, calm environment with dim lighting. Anti-glaucoma medications provide temporary relief of IOP. Postoperatively analgesia is given for pain as well as using anxiety reduction strategies such as distraction, massage, music, and parental presence. Favorite toys, pacifiers, and blankets are used to comfort the child.

Education/Discharge Instructions

Prior to discharge, teach the parents about eye dressings, medications, signs and symptoms of infection and increased IOP, activity limitations, and follow-up care.

Retinoblastoma

Retinoblastoma is a malignant tumor of the retina seen in children, usually before the age of 5. It is a rare condition, accounting for fewer than 3% of the cases of childhood cancers. This tumor can spread to the optic nerve and invade the brain, lymph nodes, facial bones, and bone marrow (Pichi, Lembo, DeLuca, Hadjistilianou, & Nucci, 2013).

Signs and Symptoms

In retinoblastoma a whitish or yellow color of the pupil called leukocoria or cat's eye reflex is noted instead of the usual red reflex (Venes, 2013). Late signs and symptoms of retinoblastoma include:

- Visual acuity disturbances
- Pain
- Inflammation
- Hyphema (blood in the anterior chamber of the eye) (Venes, 2013)

Diagnosis

Diagnosis is made when either the absence or abnormality of the red reflex is noted during examination of the fundus of the eye using direct ophthalmoscopy. An MRI confirms diagnosis and staging of the tumor.

Prevention

Genetic counseling can help families understand the risk of retinoblastoma. This information is important if there is a prior family history of retinoblastoma.

Collaborative Care

Nursing Care. Nursing care is supportive and includes preoperative/postoperative education regarding the treatment plan, expected side effects, and ongoing health-care needs of the child. The plan of care is individualized for each child. Priority nursing interventions include preparing the family for postoperative appearance and/or visual changes, pain control, and psychosocial support.

Medical Care. Treatment is often multifactorial and primarily depends on the size and location of the tumor, age of the child, and the degree of metastatic disease. Management of the disease is based on unilateral or bilateral presentation and degree of cancer infiltration. If the eye is saved and vision is still present but altered by the tumor, other therapies such as radiation are used to shrink the tumor. Systemic chemotherapy is used to treat metastases. Once the tumor invades other organs, the success of treatment is diminished. Chemotherapy drugs include etoposide (VP-16, VePesid), carboplatin (Paraplatin, Paraplatin AQ), vincristine (Oncovorin, Vincasar PFS), and cyclophosphamide (Cytoxan, Neosar, Procytox) (Zage & Herzog, 2011).

Surgical Care. Because this tumor is a rapidly progressing cancer, aggressive treatment including laser, radiation or cryotherapy (use of ice compresses), or enucleation (removal of the eye) is necessary for increased survival. Health instruction includes postprocedure care for the child and potential recognition of complications such as bleeding or infection.

Education/Discharge Instructions

The child will be followed routinely to screen for recurrence of disease. Family members of any child with a retinoblastoma are advised to have regular eye examinations (Korones, 2009).

 Nursing Insight—*Eye injuries*

Foreign bodies

When a child has a foreign body penetrating the eye, careful history of the injury and assessment dictate immediate action. An intraocular penetration injury or laceration (tear) to the cornea or eye globe requires an immediate transport to the local emergency room. An eye shield is used to prevent further trauma, and all bleeding must be controlled before transport.

In foreign body penetration, vision loss is prevented by prompt medical treatment. The triage nurse must be able to recognize an emergent situation from a non-emergent injury. If a foreign body is visualized in the conjunctival sac, a physician can carefully remove the object using a cotton-tipped applicator or warmed normal saline irrigation. Glass particles are removed carefully using a cotton-tipped applicator. Sand, gravel, and dirt are flushed with warm normal saline. Foreign bodies need to be removed meticulously to avoid a corneal abrasion.

Corneal abrasion

Corneal abrasion is a nonpenetrating injury to the cornea. Common objects that cause an abrasion include contact lens, human fingers, animal nails, sticks, flying objects, pens, pencils, and glass. Corneal abrasions are painful. Treatment is necessary if purulent eye drainage is present. Medications include topical antibiotic solutions or ointments if infection is suspected. Analgesics may be administered for pain. An eye patch is placed to prevent the child from rubbing or scratching the eye causing further irritation and potential self-inoculation of bacteria. An ophthalmologist reexamines the child in 1 to 2 days.

Chemical burns

In the emergency room, chemical burns to the eye are treated with rapid eye flushing for 15 to 30 minutes followed by pH analysis of the chemical agent. Eye patching and referral to an emergency room or an ophthalmologist is essential to evaluate for further treatment.

Critical Nursing Action Chemical Burns

Nursing care of the patient with a chemical burn requires prompt assessment. The nurse assesses the injury and monitors the patient for signs of infection, hemorrhage, and increased IOP. Provide emotional and social support for the child and family. Stress the importance of follow-up care that involves evaluation of the cornea for scarring and IOP testing to determine postinflammatory response. Instruct the family that patching and eye medication may be required at home. School and normal activities are allowed after physician consultation.

HEARING DISORDERS

Hearing Loss

Hearing loss is one of the most common disabilities in the United States. Early detection and intervention are essential to maximize outcomes. Hearing loss can be caused by several factors:

- Genetic causes
- Non-genetic causes (meningitis or maternal TORCH infections during pregnancy, in particular cytomegalovirus)
- Idiopathic or unknown causes

Fluid accumulation in the middle ear from allergies or colds can be a contributing factor for hearing impairment in children. Seventy-five percent of children experience at least one ear infection before the age of 3. Hearing loss affects approximately 17 children in 1,000 under 18 years of age. Two to three children per 1,000 are born with hearing abnormalities. Of these children, 90% are born to parents who can hear (AAP, 2012c; National Institute on Deafness and Other Communication Disorders, 2012).

Hearing loss may also be caused by conduction abnormalities associated with structural anomalies of the inner and outer ear or sensory neural hearing loss caused by central nervous dysfunction. Central nervous system dysfunction includes damage to the cerebral cortex, brainstem, or cranial nerve VIII. Hearing loss is also seen with severe neurological insult from trauma, anoxia, infections, or malformations.

A hearing disorder can involve a combination of both conductive and sensory-neural abnormalities. Sensory-neural hearing loss is a common sequela of bacterial meningitis, affecting approximately 10% of these children. Rapid identification and prompt treatment can prevent post-meningitis hearing loss (Pace & Pollard, 2012). Hearing loss is quantified in terms of severity and degree of functional disability and may be unilateral or bilateral (Table 28-8).

Signs and Symptoms

Common signs and symptoms of hearing loss include:

- Child lacks the startle reflex
- Child does not turn toward source of sound
- Child does not follow verbal directions or respond when called by name
- Child has delayed speech or speech that is difficult to understand
- Child has difficulty with articulation

Table 28-8 Classification of Hearing Loss

Level of Hearing Loss	Range	Description
Normal	0 dB–15 dB	No impairment – able to hear all speech sounds
Slight	16 dB–25 dB	Vowel sounds are heard clearly, may miss some consonant sounds
Mild	26 dB–40 dB	Hears some speech
Moderate	41 dB–55 dB	No speech heard
Moderate/severe	56 dB–70 dB	No speech heard
Severe	71 dB–90 dB	No speech heard and no other sounds heard
Profound loss	91 dB or more	No speech and no other sounds heard

Source: American Speech-Language-Hearing Association (2012).

 Nursing Insight—Risk factors

Critical risk factors for hearing loss in neonates also include extracorporeal membrane oxygenation, systemically administered ototoxic medications, phototherapy, and severe hypoxic ischemic encephalopathy post-resuscitation or asphyxia.

Diagnosis

Hearing loss is determined by otoscopic examination and audiological testing. A routine otoscopic examination is performed by a health-care provider to evaluate the presence of a middle ear effusion or otitis media (Fig. 28-17). Part of the otoscopic examination also involves the use of the pneumoscope to assess for tympanic membrane mobility.

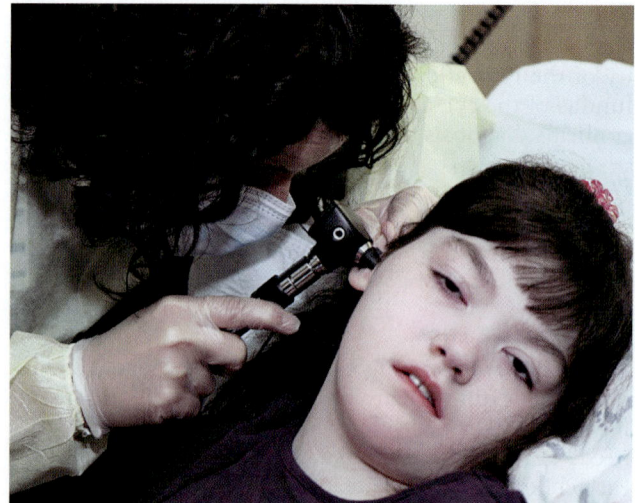

Figure 28-17 A routine otoscopic examination of the child is performed by a health-care provider to evaluate the presence of middle ear infection or otitis media.

If the hearing loss continues to be suspected, a **tympanogram** (radiographic examination of the eustachian tubes and middle ear after introduction of a contrast medium) may be completed (Venes, 2013). The tympanogram evaluates the tympanic membrane (TM) compliance to air pressure. An ear-tight probe containing a small speaker, microphone, and air pump is placed into the external auditory canal. The probe then determines the flexibility of the TM in response to positive and negative pressure levels. The normal result is a mountain peak plotted on a graph depicting the positive and negative pressure levels. A flat or absent mountain peak suggests a conductive hearing loss caused by obstruction.

Diagnostic Tools Audiological Testing

Audiological testing may include one or several procedures:

The otoacoustic emissions test or an auditory brainstem evoked response (ABER) performed by a licensed, certified audiologist further defines the degree of hearing loss. This is a very reliable test that measures acoustic responses produced by the inner ear and cochlear function. A small probe is placed in the outer ear canal and senses sounds that are reflected or echoed back out of the ear. This bounced back sound is the otoacoustic emission that may spontaneously occur or be evoked.

The automated ABER records electrical activity in response to auditory stimuli received from electrodes placed on the scalp. The electrical impulse reflects cochlear, auditory brainstem, and cranial nerve VIII vibration pathways. The ABER places a series of clicking sounds through earphones placed over the infant's or child's ears. The sounds are then converted to waveforms and detected as electrical activity by the scalp sensors. The strength of the stimulus level is in the normal voice and hearing range of 35 to 50 dB. The ABER is useful for screening newborns with congenital hearing loss or postneonatal intensive care therapies such as mechanical ventilation.

Audiography can be performed in children older than 3 years of age who are able to cooperate and follow directions. This test requires the child to raise his hand in response to normal hearing tones. The screening is performed under the supervision of a clinically competent audiologist, speech pathologist, or appropriately supervised personnel (American Speech-Language-Hearing Association, 2012).

Prevention

Early detection and intervention for children with hearing loss has been recommended by the Joint Committee on Infant Hearing (2007) and the Centers for Disease Control and Prevention (2012h). A universal infant hearing screening before 1 month of age is recommended. Newborn readiness for discharge includes a hearing screening evaluation. If newborn hearing loss is suspected, a more extensive audiological evaluation is recommended by 3 months of age. Adolescents are encouraged to turn down radios, stereos, and personal music devices such as iPods, MP3 players, and cell phones to prevent hearing loss.

Collaborative Care

Nursing Care. Simple conduction loss caused by cerumen (earwax) impaction can be treated with over-the-counter preparations, water irrigations, and foreign body removal. Nurses provide emotional, educational, and collaborative support for the child with a hearing loss and his or her family. Sign language services may be required as well as visual aids that support nonverbal communication and lip reading. The family needs to investigate home safety measures that protect the hearing-impaired child from inadvertent injury.

Supervision may be required at all times. Other assistive communication techniques include lip reading, finger spelling, and cuing. The family can use cued speech, a visual communication system that uses hand and mouth shapes along with gestures to cue a sound or a consonant. This serves as a supplement to lip reading and sign language.

Medical Care. Medical management of hearing loss begins by 6 months of age (Joint Committee on Infant Hearing, 2012). Appropriate treatment for hearing loss is based on underlying pathological conditions, presence of organic diseases, severity of the hearing loss, degree of frequency loss, and any CNS abnormalities. Ear infections are treated with appropriate antimicrobial therapy with close follow-up to monitor for the hearing loss or language delays as well as to monitor response to therapy.

Surgical Care. Children who have chronic ear infections may have surgery to restore inner ear function with myringotomy tubes placed in the tympanic membrane for effusion drainage and pressure equilibrium. Stapedectomy (excision of the stapes to improve the hearing) and tympanoplasty (restores function to the sound-transmitting mechanism of the middle ear) have been shown to be effective in restoring the hearing for conduction disorders. Severe to profound hearing loss is treated using cochlear implants that provide sound awareness and support speech development. Cochlear implants carry a risk of meningitis.

Education/Discharge Instructions

To relieve anxiety, parents will need preparation of what to expect with a child undergoing general anesthesia and instructions on caring for a child with tympanostomy tubes for preventing complications.

Nursing Insight—*Amplification aids*

Amplification aids (hearing aids) are small microphones that amplify sounds. Amplification devices are fitted to infants as young as 4 weeks old. Most children with mild to moderate hearing loss require some form of amplification. The amplification frequency and ranges are predetermined. The amplification device is placed in the child's ear, turned on, and then the volume of amplification is adjusted to the child's comfort level. In preverbal children, nonverbal cues of irritability such as crying, restlessness, or agitation may signal the need to adjust the volume. Care and maintenance of the hearing aid involve keeping the unit clean and dry with a dry cloth, avoiding water immersion, and replacing batteries frequently. Background noise can be distracting to infants wearing a hearing aid. Hearing aids can be removed while sleeping. High-pitched sounds called acoustic feedback can also be disrupting. This sound may not be realized by the hearing-impaired child but can be easily remedied by turning the volume down on the hearing aid, removing the aid, and inspecting the ear for cerumen impaction, cleaning the device, or ensuring proper installation in the external ear canal.

legal alert—Follow rules set forth in the Individuals With Disabilities Education Act

Children identified with a hearing loss begin school at an early age to prevent early developmental delays in speech and language development. All levels of education should have hearing conservation and loss prevention curricula.

The school nurse can play a pivotal role in initiating and monitoring these programs. Early intervention services are implemented in the family using a multitiered approach. The Individuals with Disabilities Education Act of 2004 (http://idea.ed.gov/) (2004) ensures that children older than 3 years of age receive assistive services throughout the school years up to age 21.The hearing-impaired child needs support services in school and elsewhere to communicate and learn. Early recognition, prevention, treatment, and support services combined with healthy family and individual coping ensures optimal growth and development for the child with a hearing disorder. Hearing-impaired children can have the same cognitive ability as children who have no hearing loss. Hearing loss accounts for most language delays seen in children.

 Nursing Insight—Communicating with the hearing-impaired child

- Recognize behavioral cues suggestive of hearing loss.
- Obtain the child's attention before speaking.
- Face the child when talking.
- Position yourself at the child's eye level.
- Talk slowly and loudly.
- Modify the environment; unnecessary noises are reduced.
- Offer emotional support: A child with a hearing loss may face a potential stigma associated with the communication difficulty.

Language Disorders

Communication is a process of complex interaction involving the exchange of information, feelings, ideas, and interactions. Verbal speech together with a language framework provides the basic component of communication. Nonverbal gestures, tones, and body movements provide as much if not more communication than words. Language development is the process of giving and receiving of information as well as processing and organizing meaning to exchange information, thoughts, and feelings. The ability to understand what is said is receptive language. The ability to clearly speak to others is expressive language. Speech impairment is an inability to make voice sounds or produce quality sounds; children may experience any combination of hearing, speech, and/or language disorders.

Children understand more than they can express at a very early age because language is learned last. The majority of a child's speech should be clearly understood by 3 to 4 years of age. Most communication skills are learned by age 5. Approximately 5% of all children have a language disorder.

 Nursing Insight—A language quick reference tool

The child's language should be understood:
- 50% of the time by age 2 years
- 75% by age 3 years
- 100% by age 4 years
- Sentences should be as long as their age

Signs and Symptoms

Children with a receptive language disorder may have:

- Difficulty understanding what others are saying
- Problems following directions that are verbally given to them
- Difficulty organizing their thoughts

Children with an expressive language disorder have difficulty using language to express their thoughts or needs and may exhibit:

- Difficulty forming sentences
- Trouble finding the correct words when speaking
- A decreased vocabulary when compared with other children of the same age
  (National Institute on Deafness and Other Communication Disorders, 2012)

Diagnosis

Diagnosis determines that the communication skills are considered delayed and the child is not meeting predictable developmental sequencing for their age.

Prevention

Prevention centers on early detection and intervention for young children with a language disorder. Early discovery of hearing loss can prevent other forms of delay in child development such as social or emotional development.

Collaborative Care

Nursing Care. The nurse is in a key position to recognize speech and language developmental delays. Knowledge about development milestones assists the nurse in recognizing children who are at risk or experiencing a difficulty. The overall nursing goal of early recognition is to prevent communication, language, and literacy delays that significantly impact the child at an early age, potentially for life.

 **Family Teaching Guidelines...**
Language Disorder

HOW TO: Tell the family that a language disorder is a child's impaired ability to understand or use words correctly, to express one's self, to follow directions, to understand words, or any combination of these conditions.

ESSENTIAL INFORMATION:

- Help the child learn how to say speech sounds correctly.
- Help the child improve language comprehension such as increasing vocabulary.
- Help the child with conversational and storytelling skills.
- Help the child and family understand the disorders may impact the child's educational and social interactions.

Advise the family about how to find a speech pathologist in the community; schools, rehabilitation, community and private clinics, and home services may be utilized to meet the child's needs (American Speech-Language-Hearing Association, 2012).

Education/Discharge Instructions

The emphasis of parent teaching is to provide therapy support and encourage the child. Nurses may provide education and supportive community resources for parents to help enhance the child's communication skills, develop goals for effective therapy at home, and help with transition to school.

 Nursing Diagnoses Language Disorders

- Social isolation related to inability to communicate, decreased level of consciousness, and/or hospitalization
- Impaired verbal communication related to articulation difficulties or environmental deprivation
- Parental knowledge deficit related to lack of understanding of normal language development

Summary Points

- ◆ Increased intracranial pressure (ICP) can have devastating and long-term consequences for the child.

- ◆ A seizure is an electrical disturbance within the brain, resulting in changes of motor function, sensation, or cognitive ability.

- ◆ Encephalitis is usually viral in origin and occurs with an acute febrile illness characterized by cerebral edema and infection of surrounding meninges. Signs and symptoms of encephalitis include disorientation, confusion, headache, high fever, photophobia, lethargy, aphasia, hallucinations, seizures, nuchal rigidity, and coma.

- ◆ Guillain-Barré syndrome (GBS) is a rare self-limiting disease characterized by clinical manifestations of ascending muscle weakness and/or paralysis.

- ◆ There are two categories of hydrocephalus. Communicating hydrocephalus occurs when there is full communication between the subarachnoid space and ventricles. Non-communicating hydrocephalus occurs when CSF flow within the ventricular system or the ventricular outlets to the arachnoid space is prevented. Most cases of hydrocephalus are obstructive.

- ◆ Cerebral palsy is a non-progressive neurological disorder that results from brain injury occurring before cerebral development is complete.

- ◆ Drowning or submersion injuries (SIs) are a major cause of death and disability in children.

- ◆ The priorities of trauma care for a child with a spinal cord injury are initiated with primary attention to airway management, breathing and/or ventilatory support, circulation support, disability identification, and exposure of known and unknown physical limitations.

- ◆ Headaches are common during childhood and become more common and more frequent during adolescence. Headaches are classified as primary or secondary and further classified into subtypes according to the International Classification of Headache Disorders (ICHD-II).

- ◆ Children may experience a myriad of common eye disorders, which may present as an abrupt change or changes in vision function.

- ◆ Hearing loss is one of the most common disabilities in the United States. Early detection and intervention are essential to maximize. Early detection and intervention for young children with a language disorder prevents many forms of delay in child development.

Review Questions

Multiple Choice

1. A pediatric nurse is offering a health prevention lecture in the community. Which topic is appropriate to include in this lecture?
   A. The use of DEET-containing products is contraindicated in school-aged children.
   B. Avoiding areas infested with mosquitoes can be helpful in preventing encephalitis.
   C. The incidence of Reye's syndrome has increased because of the use of acetaminophen (Tylenol).
   D. The varicella vaccine is not to be given to children with arthritis or Kawasaki's disease.

2. A 3-year-old with a history of hydrocephalus has recently undergone a ventriculo-peritoneal shunt insertion. Which postoperative intervention is the most appropriate?
   A. Assessing for signs of infection and for neurological function
   B. Maintaining the head of the bed at a 90-degree angle
   C. Encouraging the patient to lie on the operative side
   D. Encouraging the patient to lie supine for the first 24 hours

3. The pediatric nurse is admitting a child with a history of seizure activity. What will the nurse ensure is at the bedside to implement seizure precautions?
   A. A ventilator
   B. Suction equipment
   C. Intubation equipment
   D. Soft restraints

4. A child is admitted to the intensive care unit following a motor vehicle crash. The student nurse uses the Glasgow Coma Scale to evaluate the child's neurological status. When using this tool, for which assessment does the registered nurse intervene?
   A. Verbal response
   B. Orientation
   C. Eye opening
   D. Motor response

5. A child has a hearing loss following several ear infections. Which area of assessment is a priority for this child?
   A. Language problems
   B. Balance problems
   C. Head size out of the norm
   D. Metabolic disorders

6. A child is brought to the emergency department with a chemical burn to the eye. Which action by the nurse takes priority?
   A. Attaching the child to the cardiac monitor
   B. Determining the composition of the chemical
   C. Assessing how this injury could have occurred
   D. Flushing the eye with saline or water for 15 minutes

7. An infant has been fitted with amplification devices for a hearing loss. What will the nurse include in the teaching plan for this infant?
   A. Wash the devices with cool water and pat dry weekly.
   B. Irritability can indicate the devices are turned up too loud.
   C. The child will eventually need surgery to correct the hearing loss.
   D. Very few children need amplification devices for mild hearing loss.

8. A nurse is assessing growth and development in a 4-year-old child. Which sentence indicates the child is probably speaking appropriately for her age?
   A. "I hungry."
   B. "No! No nap!"
   C. "Play ball with me."
   D. "I want to go to the park."

9. A child is being assessed with the Ishihara Test plates. The nurse understands that this tests what part of neurological function?
   A. Expressive speech
   B. Color blindness
   C. Ocular nerve function
   D. Coordination

10. A child's medical record states he has an altered level of consciousness. What is the priority problem for the nurse to assess for this child?
   A. Trauma
   B. Abusive head trauma
   C. Infection of the brain or meninges
   D. Brainstem abnormality

See Answers to End of Chapter Review Questions on Davis*Plus*.

REFERENCES

Adams, A. J., Verdon, W. A., & Spivey, B. E. (2009). Color vision. In W. Tasman, & E. A. Jaeger (Eds.), *Duane's foundations of clinical ophthalmology* (15th ed., Chapter 19). Philadelphia, PA: Lippincott Williams & Wilkins.

Agency for Health care Research and Quality. (2014). U.S. Preventative Services Task Force). Retrieved from http://www.ahrq.gov/professionals/clinicians-providers/guidelines-recommendations/uspstf/index.html

Akre, M., Finkelstein, M., Erickson, M., Liu, M., Vanderbilt, L., & Billman, G. (2010). Sensitivity of the Pediatric Early Warning Score to identify patient deterioration. *Pediatrics, 125*(4), e763–e769.

Alderson, P., & Roberts, I. (2009). Corticosteroids for acute traumatic brain injury. *Cochrane Database of Systemic Reviews, 25*, Issue 1. Art. No.: CD000196. doi:10.1002/14651858.CD000196.pub2

American Academy of Neurology and Child Neurology Society. (2013). Practice Parameter: Pharmacologic treatment of spasticity in children and adolescents with cerebral palsy (an evidence-based review). Report of the Quality Standards Subcommittee of the American Academy of Neurology and the Practice Committee of the Child Neurology Society. Retrieved from http://www.neurology.org/content/74/4/336.full.pdf

American Academy of Pediatrics (AAP). (2010). Altered mental status. *Pediatric Care Online*. Retrieved from https://www.pediatriccareonline.org/pco/ub/view/Point-of-Care-Quick-Reference/397246/0/altered_mental status_

American Academy of Pediatrics (AAP). (2012a). Insect repellents. Retrieved from http://www.healthychildren.org/english/safety-prevention/at-play/pages/Insect-Repellents.aspx

American Academy of Pediatrics (AAP). (2012b). Botulism. Retrieved from http://www.healthychildren.org/English/health-issues/conditions/infections/Pages/Botulism.aspx

American Academy of Pediatrics (AAP). (2012c). Healthy Children.org: Health issues: Hearing loss. Retrieved from http://www.healthychildren.org/English/health-issues/conditions/developmental-disabilities/Pages/Hearing-Loss.aspx

American Academy of Pediatrics. (2014). Instrument-based pediatric vision screening policy statement. Retrieved from http:/www.aap.org/

American Association for Pediatric Ophthalmology and Strabismus. (2012). Retrieved from http://www.aapos.org/

American Optometric Association. (2012). Nystagmus. Retrieved from http://www.aoa.org/x9763.xml

American Speech-Language-Hearing Association. (2012). Types of hearing loss. Retrieved from www.asha.org/

Barr, R. G. (2012). Preventing abusive head trauma resulting from a failure of normal interaction between infants and their caregivers. *Proceedings of the National Academy of Sciences of the United States of America, 16*(109 Suppl 2), 17294–17301. doi:10.1073/pnas.1121267109

Barr, R. G., Rivara, F. P., Barr, M., Cummings, P., Taylor, J., Lengua, L. J., & Meredith-Benitz, E. (2009). Effectiveness of educational materials designed to change knowledge and behaviors regarding crying and shaken-baby syndrome in mothers of newborns: A randomized, controlled trial. *Pediatrics, 123*(3), 972–980. doi:10.1542/peds.2008-0908

Bickley, L., & Szilagyi, P. (2013). *Bates' guide to physical examination and history taking* (11th ed.). Philadelphia, PA: Lippincott Williams & Wilkins.

Blume, H. K. (2012). Pediatric headache: A review. *Pediatric Reviews, 33*(12), 562–576. doi:10.1542/pir.33-12-562

Brain Injury Association of America. (2012). Retrieved from http://www.biausa.org/

Brain Trauma Foundation. (2012). Decompressive craniectomy for the treatment of intracranial hypertension. *Pediatric Critical Care Medicine, 13*, S53–S60.

Brustrom, J., Thibadeau, J., John, L., Liesmann, J. & Rose, S. (2012). Care coordination in the spina bifida clinic setting: Current practice and future directions. *Journal of Pediatric Health Care, 26*, 16–26.

Bulechek, G. M., Butcher, H. K., Dochterman, J. M., & Wagner, C. (2013). *Nursing interventions classification (NIC)* (6th ed.). St. Louis, MO: Elsevier Mosby.

Burns, C. E., Dunn A. M, Brady, M. A., Starr, N. B., & Blosser, C. G. (2013). *Pediatric Primary Care* (5th ed.). Philadelphia, PA: Elsevier Saunders.

Caton-Richards, M. (2010). Assessing the neurological status of patients with head injuries. *Emergency Nurse, 17*, 28–31.

Centers for Disease Control and Prevention (CDC). (2012a). Injury prevention & control: Traumatic brain injury. Retrieved from http://www.cdc.gov/TraumaticBrainInjury/statistics.html

Centers for Disease Control and Prevention (CDC). (2012b). Epilepsy. Retrieved from http://www.cdc.gov/epilepsy/

Centers for Disease Control and Prevention (CDC). (2012c). Meningococcal disease. Retrieved from http://www.cdc.gov/meningococcal/

Centers for Disease Control and Prevention (CDC). (2012d). Botulism. Retrieved from http://www.cdc.gov/nczved/divisions/dfbmd/diseases/botulism/

Centers for Disease Control and Prevention (CDC). (2012e). Spina Bifida. Retrieved from http://www.cdc.gov/ncbddd/spinabifida/

Centers for Disease Control and Prevention (CDC). (2012f). Cerebral Palsy. Retrieved from http://www.cdc.gov/ncbddd/cp/index.html

Centers for Disease Control and Prevention (CDC). (2012g). Unintentional drowning: Get the facts. Retrieved from http://www.cdc.gov/homeandrecreationalsafety/water-safety/waterinjuries-factsheet.html

Centers for Disease Control and Prevention (CDC). (2012h). Hearing loss in children. Retrieved from http://www.cdc.gov/ncbddd/hearingloss/

Centers for Disease Control and Prevention, National Center for Injury Prevention and Control. (2014). Injury Center: Violence prevention. Retrieved from http://www.cdc.gov/ViolencePrevention/pub/PediatricHeadTrauma.html

Chou, R., Dana, T., & Bougatsos, C. (2011). Screening for visual jmpairment in children ages 1–5: Systematic review to update the 2004 U.S. Preventive Services Task Force Recommendation. Rockville (MD): Agency for Healthcare Research and Quality. Report No.: 11-05151-EF-1.

DiFazio, M. P., & Kao, A. (2012). Pediatric Guillain-Barre syndrome. Retrieved from http://emedicine.medscape.com/article/1180594-overview

Easter, J. S., Barkin, R., Rosen, C. L., & Ban, K. (2011). Cervical spine injuries in children, part II: Management and special considerations, *Journal of Emergency Medicine, 41*, 252–256.

El-Bayoumi, M. A., El-Refaey, A. M., Abdelkader, A. M. El-Assmy, M. M., Alwakeel, A. A., & El-Tahan, H. M. (2011). Comparison of intravenous immunoglobulin and plasma exchange in treatment of mechanically ventilated children with Guillain Barre syndrome: A randomized study. *Critical Care, 15*(4), R164. doi:10.1186/cc10305

Encyclopedia of Children's Health. (2012). Near-drowning. Retrieved from http://www.healthofchildren.com/N-O/Near-Drowning.html

The Epilepsy Foundation. (2012). Retrieved from http://www.epilepsy.com/

Evans, R. W. (2013). A rationale approach to the management of chronic migraine. *Headache, 53*(1): 168–176. doi:10.1111head.12014

Everette, M. (2011). A review of the folate intake of childbearing aged women. *Currernt Nutrition & Food Service, 7*, 82–91.

Faul, M., Xu, L., Wald, M. M., & Coronado, V. G. (2010). *Traumatic brain injury in the United States: Emergency department visits, hospitalizations, and deaths 2002–2006.* Atlanta, GA: Centers for Disease Control and Prevention, National Center for Injury Prevention and Control.

Finnis, M. F., & Jayawant, S. (2011). Juvenile myasthenia gravis: A paediatric perspective. *Autoimmune Diseases,* volume 2011, Article ID 404101. doi:10.4061/2011/404101

Gepp, D., & Nadal, L. G. (2012). Spinal cord trauma in children under 10 years of age: Clinical characteristics and prevention. *Child's Nervous System, 28*(11): 1919–1924.

Greenberg, M. S. (2010). *Handbook of neurosurgery* (7th ed.). New York, NY: Thieme Medical Publishers.

Hager, T., Schirra, F., Kohnen, T., Seitz, B., & Kasmann-Kellner, B. (2012). Treatment of cataracts in childhood I: Clinical picture and surgical approach. *Ophthalmologe, 109*(12): 1233–1245.

Hampers, L. C., & Spina, L. A. (2011). Evaluation and management of pediatric febrile seizures in the emergency department. *Emergency Medicine Clinics of North America, 29*, 83–93.

Helgeson, M. D., Gendelberg, D., Sidhu, G. S., Anderson, G., & Vaccaro, A. R. (2011). Management of cervical spine trauma: Can a prognostic classification of injury determine clinical outcomes. *Orthopedic Clinics of North America, 43*, 89–96.

Herman, B. E., Makoroff, K. L., & Corneli, H. M. (2011). Abusive head trauma. *Pediatric Emergency Care, 27*(1), 65–69. doi:10.1097/PEC.0b013e31820349db

Hershey, A. D. (2012). Pediatric headache: Update on recent research. *Headache, 52*, 327–332. doi:10.1111/j.1526-4610.2011.02085

Heyser, G. (2012). Triaging pediatric head injury. *Advance for Nurses.* Retrieved from http://nursing.advanceweb.com/Features/Articles/Triaging-Pediatric-Head-Injury.aspx

Hughes, R. A., Swan, A. V., & vanDoorn, P. A. (2012). Intravenous immunoglobulin for Guillain-Barre syndrome. *Cochrane Database of Systemic Reviews, 11*(7), Cd002063. doi:10.1002/14651858.CD002063.pub5

Individuals With Disabilities Education Act. (2004). 20 U.S.C. § 1400.

Institute of Medicine of the National Academies. (2012, March). *Epilepsy Across the Spectrum: Promoting Health and Understanding.* National Academy of Sciences.

International Headache Society. (2013). IHS Classification ICHD-II. Retrieved from http://ihs-classification.org/en/

Israeli, E., Agmon-Levin, N., Blank, M., Chapman, J., & Shoenfeld, Y. (2012). Guillain-Barre syndrome. A classical autoimmune disease triggered by infection or vaccination. *Clinical Reviews in Allergy and Immunology, 42*, 121–130.

Johnson, M., Moorhead, S., Bulechek, G., Butcher, H., Maas, M., & Swanson, E. (2012). *NIC and NOC linkages to NANDA-L and clinical conditions* (3rd ed.). St. Louis, MO: Elsevier Mosby.

Joint Committee on Infant Hearing Year 2012 position statement: Principles and guidelines for early detection and intervention program. *Pediatrics, 106*(4), 795–817.

Kim, J. J., & Gean, A. D. (2011). Imaging for the diagnosis and management of traumatic brain injury. *Neurotherapeutics,8*, 839–853. doi:10.1007/S13311-010-0003-3

Kirshblum, S. C., Burns, S. P., Biering-Sorensen, F., Donovan, W., Graves, D. E., Jha, A., et al. (2011). International standards for neurological classification of spinal cord injury. *Journal of Spinal Cord Medicine, 34*(6), 535–546.

Kleigman, R. M., Stanton, B. M. D., St. Geme, J., Schor, N. F., & Behrman, R. E. (2011). *Nelson textbook of pediatrics* (19th ed.). Philadelphia, PA: W.B. Saunders.

Kochaneck, P. M., Carney, N., Adelson, P. D., Ashwal, S., Bell, M. J., Bratton, S., et al. (2012). Guidelines for the acute medical management of severe traumatic brain injury in infants, children, and adolescents (2nd ed.). *Pediatric Critical Care Medicine, 13*, S1–S82.

Korones, D. (2009). Retinoblastoma. The Merck Manual Home Health Handbook. Retrieved from http://merckmanuals.com/home/childrens_health_issues/childhood_cancers/retinoblastoma.html

Lewis, D. W. (2010). Headaches in children and adolescents. *Pediatric Annals, 39*, 388–390. doi:10.3928/00904481-20100623.02

Li, T., & Shotton, K. (2009). Conventional occlusion versus pharmacologic penalization for amblyopia. *Cochrane Database of Systemic Reviews,* Issue 4. Art. No.: CD006460. doi:10.1002/14651858.CD006460.pub2

Liley, W., Stephens, A., Kaltner, M., Larkins, S., Franklin, R. C., Tsey, K., et al. (2012). Infant abusive head trauma – Incidence, outcomes and awareness. *Australian Family Physician, 41*(10), 823–826.

Liptak, G. S., & El Samra, A. (2010). Optimizing health care for children with spina bifida. *Developmental Disabilities Research Review, 16*, 66–75.

March of Dimes. (2013). Spina bifida. Retrieved from http://www.marchofdimes.com/

McAllister, J. P. (2012). Pathophysiology of congenital and neonatal hydrocephalus. *Seminars in Fetal & Neonatal Medicine, 17*(5), 285–294.

McCance L., & Huether, E. (2010). *Pathophysiology: The biologic basis for disease in adults and children* (6th ed.). Maryland Heights, MO: Elsevier Mosby.

Mickalide, A., & Carr, K. (2012). Safe kids worldwide: Preventing unintentional childhood injuries across the globe. *Pediatric Clinics of North America, 59*, 1367–1380.

Mokri, B. (2001). The Monro–Kellie hypothesis: Applications in CSF volume depletion. *Neurology, 56*, 1746–1748. doi:10.1212/WNL.56.12.1746

Monaghan, A. (2005). Detecting and managing deterioration in children. *Paediatric Nursing, 17*(1), 32.

Moorhead, S., Johnson, M., Maas, M. L., & Swanson, E. (2013). *Nursing outcomes classification (NOC)* (5th ed.). St. Louis, MO: Elsevier Mosby.

NANDA International (2012). *Nursing diagnoses: Definitions and classifications 2012–2014.* NJ: Blackwell Publishing Ltd.

National Institute of Neurological Disorders and Stroke. (2012). Cerebral palsy. Retrieved from http://www.ninds.nih.gov/disorders/cerebral_palsy/cerebral_palsy.htm

National Institute on Deafness and Other Communication Disorders. (2012). Statistics about hearing, balance, ear infections, and deafness. Retrieved from www.nidcd.nih.gov/health/statistics/hearing.asa

National Reye's Syndrome Foundation. (2012). Retrieved from http://www.reyessyndrome.org

Normal Growth of Young Children - Pediatrics - About.com, 2012. Retrieved from http://pediatrics.about.com/cs/weeklyquestion/a/032002_ask.htm

Olitsky S. E., Hug D., Plummer L. S., & Stass-Isern M. (2011). Disorders of eye movement and alignment. In R. M. Kliegman, R. E. Behrman, H. B. Jenson, & B. F. Stanton (Eds.), *Nelson textbook of pediatrics* (19th ed., Chapter 615). Philadelphia: Elsevier Saunders.

Ozge, A., Termine, C., Antonaci, F., Natriashvili, S., Guidetti, V., & Wober-Bingol, C. (2011). Overview of diagnosis and management of paediatric headache. *Journal of Headache Pain, 12*(1), 13–23.

Pace, D., & Pollard, A. J. (2012). Meningococcal disease: Clinical presentation and sequelae. *Vaccine, 30,* (Suppl 2), B3–B9. doi:10.1016.j.vaccine.2011.12.062

Parent, S., Mac-Thiong, J. M., Roy-Beaudry, M, Sosa, J. F., & Labelle, H. (2011). Spinal cord injury in the pediatric population: A systematic review of the literature. *Journal of Neurotrauma, 28*(28)8, 1515–1524.

Pichi, F., Lembo, A., DeLuca, M., Hadjistilianou, T., & Nucci, P. (2013). Bilateral retinoblastoma: Clinical presentation, management and treatment. *International Ophthalmology.* doi:10.1007/s10792-012-9703-5

Piña-Garza, J. E. (2013). *Fenichel's clinical pediatric neurology: A signs and symptoms approach* (7th ed.). Philadelphia, PA: Elsevier Saunders.

Pitfield, A. F., Carroll, A. B., & Kissoon, N. (2012). Emergency management of increased intracranial pressure. *Pediatric Emergency Care, 28*, 200–207.

Pluta, R. M., Lynm, C., & Golub, R. M. (2011). Guillain-Barre syndrome. *Journal of the American Medical Association, 305,* 319. doi:10.1001/jama.305.3.319

Robertson, J., & Shilkofski, N. (2012). *The Harriet Lane handbook* (19th ed.). Philadelphia, PA: Elsevier Mosby.

Robson, M. A., Cooper, C. L., Medicus, L. A., Quintero, M. J., & Zuniga, S. A. (2012). Comparison of three acute care pediatric early warning scoring tools. *Journal of Pediatric Nursing, 28*(6), e33–e41. doi:10.1016/j.pedn.2012.12.002. Epub 2012 Dec 28.

Roser, T., Bonfert, M., Ebinger, F., Blankenburg, M., Ertl-Wagner, B., & Heinen, F. (2013). Primary versus secondary headache in children: A frequent diagnostic challenge in clinical routine. *Neuropediatrics, 185*(1), 55–59. doi:10.1055/s-0032-1325399

Scanlon, V. C., & Sanders, T. (2010). *Essentials of anatomy and physiology* (6th ed.). Philadelphia, PA: F.A. Davis Company.

Schottler, J., Vogel, L. C., & Sturm, P. (2012). Spinal cord injury in young children: A review of children injured at 5 years of age and younger. *Developmental Medicine and Child Neurology, 54*(12), 1138–1143.

Sgouros, S. (2011). Spina bifida, hydrocephalus and shunts. Retrieved from http://emedicine.medscape.com/article/937979-overview

Shepherd, S. M. (2011). Drowning. Retrieved from http://emedicine.medscape.com/article/772753-overview

Shriners Hospitals for Children. (2012). Spinal cord injury awareness. Retrieved from http://www.shrinershospitalsforchildren.org/Education/SCIAwareness.aspx

Spina Bifida Association. (2013). About Spina Bifida. Retrieved from http://www.spinabifidaassociation.org/site/c.evKRI7OXIoJ8H/b.8029551/k.99AA/Learn_about_SB.htm

Steering Committee on Quality Improvement and Management, Subcommittee on Febrile Seizures, American Academy of Pediatrics. (2008, June). Febrile seizures: Clinical practice guideline for the long-term management of the child with simple febrile seizures. *Pediatrics, 121*(6), 1281–1286. doi:10.1542/peds.2008-0939

Steiner, I., Budka, H., Chaudhuri, A., Koskiniemi, M., Sainio, K., Salonen, O., & Kennedy, P. G. (2010). Viral encephalitis: A review of diagnostic methods and guidelines for management. *European Journal of Neurology, 17*(8), 999–e57. doi:10.1111/j.1468-1331.2010.02970.x

Stewart, C. E., Moseley, M. J., & Fielder, A. R. (2011). Amblyopia therapy: An update. *Strabismus, 19*, 91–98.

Thompson, J. D., & Segal, L. S. (2010). Orthopedic management of spina bifida. *Developmental Disabilities Research Reviews, 16*, 96–103.

Thurtell, M. J., & Leigh, R. J. (2012). Treatment of nystagmus. *Current Treatment Options in Neurology, 14*, 60–72.

Topjian, A. A., Berg, R. A., Bierens, J. J., Branche, C. M., Clark, R. S., Friberg, H., et al. (2012). Brain resuscitation in the drowning victim. *Neurocritical Care, 17*(3), 441–467. doi:10.1007/s12028-012-9747-4

Trethewy, C. E., Burrows, J. M., Clausen, D., & Doherty, S. R. (2012). Effectiveness of cricoid pressure in preventing gastric aspiration during rapid sequence intubation in the emergency department: study protocol for a randomised controlled trial. *Trials, 16*(13), 17. doi:10.1186/1745-6215-13-17

United Cerebral Palsy Foundation. (2012). Cerebral Palsy Source. Retrieved from http://www.cerebralpalsysource.com/About_CP/facts_cp/index.html

U.S. Food and Drug Administration. (2012). LASIK. Retrieved from http://www.fda.gov/MedicalDevices/ProductsandMedicalProcedures/SurgeryandLifeSupport/LASIK/default.htm

U.S. Preventative Services Task Force. (2011). Vision screening for children 1 to 5 years of age: U.S. Preventative services task force recommendation statement. *Pediatrics, 127*, 340–346.

Vallerand, A. H., & Sanoski C. A. (2014). *Davis's drug guide for nurses* (14th ed.). Philadelphia, PA: F.A. Davis.

Van Leeuwen, A. M., Poelhuis-Leth, D. J., & Bladh, M. L. (2011). *Davis's comprehensive handbook of laboratory and diagnostic tests*. Philadelphia, PA: F.A. Davis.

Vendrame, M., & Loddenkemper, T. (2012). Approach to seizures, epilepsies, and epilepsy syndromes. *Sleep Medicine Clinics, 7*(1), 59–73. doi:10.1016/j.jsmc.2012.01.006

Venes, D. (2013). *Taber's cyclopedic medical dictionary* (22nd ed.). Philadelphia, PA: F.A. Davis Company.

Vitale, S., Sperduto, R. D., & Ferris, F. L. (2009). Increased prevalence of myopia in the United States between 1971–1972 and 1999–2004. *Archives of Ophthalmology, 127*, 1632–1639.

Vogel, L, C., Betz, R. R., & Mulcahey, M. J. (2012). Spinal cord injury in children and adolescents. *Handbook of Clinical Neurology, 109*, 131–148.

Ward, S. (2013). *Pediatric nursing care: Best evidence-based practices*. Philadelphia, PA: F.A. Davis.

White, J. P., & Thumbikat, P. (2012). Acute spinal cord injury. *Surgery, 30*(7), 326–332.

Wojciechowski, R. (2011). Nature and nuture: The complex genetics of myopia and refractive error. *Clinical Genetics, 79*(4), 301–320.

Zage, P. E., & Herzog, C. E. (2011). Retinoblastoma. In R. M. Kliegman, R. E. Behrman, H. B. Jenson, & B. F. Stanton (Eds.). *Nelson textbook of pediatrics* (19th ed., Chapter 496). Philadelphia, PA: Elsevier Saunders.

Zuckerman, S. L., Lee, Y. M., Odom, M. J., Solomon, G. S., Forbes, J. A., & Sills, A. K. (2012). Recovery from sports-related concussion: Days to return to neurocognitive baseline in adolescents versus young adults. *Surgical Neurology International, 3*, 130. doi:10.4103/2152-7806.102945

CONCEPT MAP

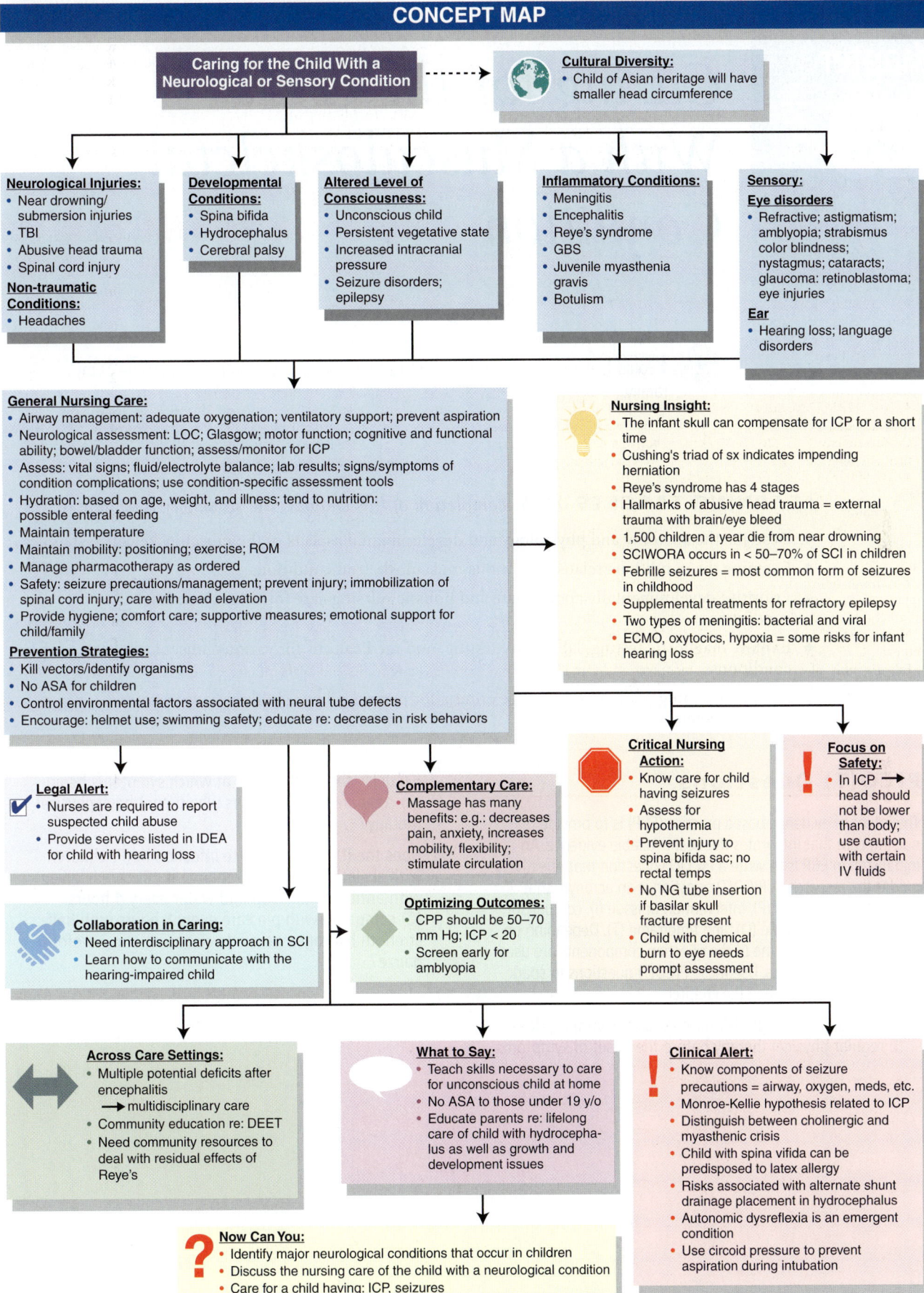

Caring for the Child With a Neurological or Sensory Condition

Cultural Diversity:
• Child of Asian heritage will have smaller head circumference

Neurological Injuries:
• Near drowning/submersion injuries
• TBI
• Abusive head trauma
• Spinal cord injury
Non-traumatic Conditions:
• Headaches

Developmental Conditions:
• Spina bifida
• Hydrocephalus
• Cerebral palsy

Altered Level of Consciousness:
• Unconscious child
• Persistent vegetative state
• Increased intracranial pressure
• Seizure disorders; epilepsy

Inflammatory Conditions:
• Meningitis
• Encephalitis
• Reye's syndrome
• GBS
• Juvenile myasthenia gravis
• Botulism

Sensory:
Eye disorders
• Refractive; astigmatism; amblyopia; strabismus color blindness; nystagmus; cataracts; glaucoma: retinoblastoma; eye injuries
Ear
• Hearing loss; language disorders

General Nursing Care:
• Airway management: adequate oxygenation; ventilatory support; prevent aspiration
• Neurological assessment: LOC; Glasgow; motor function; cognitive and functional ability; bowel/bladder function; assess/monitor for ICP
• Assess: vital signs; fluid/electrolyte balance; lab results; signs/symptoms of condition complications; use condition-specific assessment tools
• Hydration: based on age, weight, and illness; tend to nutrition: possible enteral feeding
• Maintain temperature
• Maintain mobility: positioning; exercise; ROM
• Manage pharmacotherapy as ordered
• Safety: seizure precautions/management; prevent injury; immobilization of spinal cord injury; care with head elevation
• Provide hygiene; comfort care; supportive measures; emotional support for child/family
Prevention Strategies:
• Kill vectors/identify organisms
• No ASA for children
• Control environmental factors associated with neural tube defects
• Encourage: helmet use; swimming safety; educate re: decrease in risk behaviors

Nursing Insight:
• The infant skull can compensate for ICP for a short time
• Cushing's triad of sx indicates impending herniation
• Reye's syndrome has 4 stages
• Hallmarks of abusive head trauma = external trauma with brain/eye bleed
• 1,500 children a year die from near drowning
• SCIWORA occurs in < 50–70% of SCI in children
• Febrile seizures = most common form of seizures in childhood
• Supplemental treatments for refractory epilepsy
• Two types of meningitis: bacterial and viral
• ECMO, oxytocics, hypoxia = some risks for infant hearing loss

Critical Nursing Action:
• Know care for child having seizures
• Assess for hypothermia
• Prevent injury to spina bifida sac; no rectal temps
• No NG tube insertion if basilar skull fracture present
• Child with chemical burn to eye needs prompt assessment

Focus on Safety:
• In ICP → head should not be lower than body; use caution with certain IV fluids

Legal Alert:
• Nurses are required to report suspected child abuse
• Provide services listed in IDEA for child with hearing loss

Complementary Care:
• Massage has many benefits: e.g.: decreases pain, anxiety, increases mobility, flexibility; stimulate circulation

Collaboration in Caring:
• Need interdisciplinary approach in SCI
• Learn how to communicate with the hearing-impaired child

Optimizing Outcomes:
• CPP should be 50–70 mm Hg; ICP < 20
• Screen early for amblyopia

Across Care Settings:
• Multiple potential deficits after encephalitis → multidisciplinary care
• Community education re: DEET
• Need community resources to deal with residual effects of Reye's

What to Say:
• Teach skills necessary to care for unconscious child at home
• No ASA to those under 19 y/o
• Educate parents re: lifelong care of child with hydrocephalus as well as growth and development issues

Clinical Alert:
• Know components of seizure precautions = airway, oxygen, meds, etc.
• Monroe-Kellie hypothesis related to ICP
• Distinguish between cholinergic and myasthenic crisis
• Child with spina vifida can be predisposed to latex allergy
• Risks associated with alternate shunt drainage placement in hydrocephalus
• Autonomic dysreflexia is an emergent condition
• Use circoid pressure to prevent aspiration during intubation

Now Can You:
• Identify major neurological conditions that occur in children
• Discuss the nursing care of the child with a neurological condition
• Care for a child having: ICP, seizures

Caring for the Child With a Musculoskeletal Condition

 I could feel it in my bones, how I missed the heat of my country and the love of my family.

—Tony Perez (2012)

LEARNING TARGETS *At the completion of this chapter, the student will be able to:*

- ◆ Describe the anatomy and physiology and developmental aspects of the musculoskeletal system.
- ◆ Examine the conditions related to various musculoskeletal conditions.
- ◆ Prioritize developmentally appropriate and holistic nursing care for musculoskeletal conditions.
- ◆ Explore diagnostic testing, laboratory testing, and medications for various musculoskeletal conditions.
- ◆ Develop teaching plans and discharge criteria for parents whose children have various musculoskeletal conditions.

PICO(T) Questions

The intent of evidence-based practice (EBP) is to provide nursing care that integrates the best available evidence. An initial step in EBP is to write a PICO(T) question that effectively guides the research. A PICO(T) question is an acronym that stands for population (P), intervention or issue (I), comparison of interest (C), outcome (O), and timeframe (T). Depending on the question, all or some of the question components are used in the research process. Use these PICO(T) questions to spark your thinking as you read the chapter.

1. In (P) toddlers at high risk for muscular dystrophy, does (I) regular physical therapy before the onset of symptoms (O) delay the average age at which symptoms begin (C) compared with toddlers who do not have physical therapy?

2. Does the (I) rate of pin site infection in (P) children with skeletal traction (O) change if pin care is given with antibacterial soap and water every 4 hours (C) compared with pin care every 8 hours with half-strength hydrogen peroxide cleansing and Xeroform gauze?

Evidence-Based Practice

Flynn, J. M., Garner, M. R., Jones, K. J., D'Italia, J., Davidson, R. S., Ganley, T. J., et al. (2011). The treatment of low-energy femoral shaft fractures: A prospective study comparing the "walking spica" with the traditional spica cast. *Journal of Bone and Joint Surgery, 93*(23), 2196–2202.

The purpose of this study was to compare the use of the "walking spica" with the traditional spica cast management and patient outcomes. Previous research has noted that the use of a single-leg "walking spica hip" cast has been shown to be safe and effective for use in children with femoral shaft fractures.

The researchers performed a prospective study comparing the outcomes from a walking spica cast to the outcomes of a traditional spica cast in the management of a low-impact femoral shaft fracture in young children (aged 1 to 6 years). The study included 45 children ages 1 to 6 treated for low-energy femoral shaft fractures during a 3-year period. Six physicians agreed to participate in this study at the Children's Hospital of Philadelphia. The walking spica cast was described as a single-leg cast with a 45-degree angle of hip flexion and a 45-degree of knee flexion with the cast ending at the ankle.

Criteria for inclusion in the study were as follows:

- Children 1 to 6 years of age
- Diagnosis of low-energy femoral shaft fracture (diagnosis made by the treating physician)
- Fracture location classified as proximal, middle, or distal diaphysis

Exclusion criteria were as follows:

- High-energy fracture (e.g., MVA, fall from a significant height, or shortening of the bone by more than 2 cm)
- Open fracture
- Extension of the fracture into the metaphysis or physis
- Pathological fracture
- Concomitant fracture in another bone on the same side or the other femur
- Concomitant head injury
- Existing skeletal disorder
- Suspected child abuse
- Developmental delay

Forty-five children met the criteria at the time of admission. The type of cast used was determined by the physician who was assigned to the care of the child. Three surgeons used the traditional 1½ spica casts, and three surgeons used the walking spica hip cast. The casts were applied under anesthesia in the operating room during the reduction of the fracture. Follow-up examinations were made at 1 week, 2 weeks, 3 weeks, and between 5 to 8 weeks after the fracture reduction. The cast was usually removed at 6 weeks. The family was asked to complete two outcome questionnaires (i.e., a validated Impact on Family Scale and a 10-item yes or no questionnaire developed by the researchers and administered when the cast was removed). In addition, the inpatient record and radiograph studies were also reviewed.

Of the 45 children included in the study, 19 (42%) were treated with the walking spica cast, and 26 (58%) with the traditional 1½ spica cast. Both groups were similar in age, mean time between injury and treatment, mean length of hospitalization, distribution of fracture types, and fracture locations. It was noted that 16 (45%) of the children suffered the fracture as the result of a fall from a standing height. None of the patients were treated with traction prior to casting. Initial time to callus formation was 2.4 weeks for those treated with the traditional spica cast and 2.3 weeks for those treated with the walking spica cast. The mean time for fracture union was 6.3 weeks for both groups. Seventeen of the 19 patients treated with a walking spica cast were able to crawl while in the cast, which took an average of 2.3 weeks to develop this ability. Twelve of the 17 were also able to walk in the cast with a mean time of 3.3 weeks to develop this ability. None of the patients in the traditional spica cast was able to crawl, stand, or walk before removal of the cast.

The Impact on Family Scale revealed that children who were treated with the walking spica had a significantly lower burden on the family compared with children who were treated with the traditional spica cast (p=0.04). Findings from the questionnaire developed by the researchers included the following: 11 of the children treated with a traditional spica cast needed ambulance transport for follow-up appointments, mean cost of $505 per trip with $5 per mile, which was paid for by the insurance company. No child with a walking spica cast needed an ambulance for transport (p=0.001).

The researchers concluded that the results of this study supported previous study findings that a single-leg walking cast is effective for management of low-impact femoral shaft fractures in young children. There were two significant findings to support the use of the walking spica cast over the traditional spica cast. They were the burden on the family and the fact that an ambulance was not needed.

1. How is this information useful to clinical nursing practice?

2. Based on these findings, what are implications for further research?

See Suggested Responses for Evidence-Based Practice on Davis*Plus*.

INTRODUCTION

This chapter provides a review of the anatomy and physiology and developmental aspects of the musculoskeletal system. The discussion includes an examination of the various musculoskeletal tract conditions including developmentally appropriate and holistic nursing care. Information about diagnostic and laboratory testing and medications is given. Teaching plans and discharge criteria for parents whose children have various musculoskeletal conditions are incorporated.

Growth and Development

Conditions such as muscular dystrophy, clubfoot, osteogenesis imperfecta, spinal disorders, and orthopedic injuries can cause prolonged periods of immobilization. In addition to disease process, immobility may occur from treatments and therapies such as casts, traction, pins, and distraction devices (Ward & Hisley, 2009). The child with a musculoskeletal condition is affected with difficulties in mobility that can result in delays or abnormalities in achievement of developmental milestones in motor function and movement.

Nursing care of the child with a musculoskeletal condition should include regular assessment of growth and developmental milestones as well as impairments, physical restrictions, and limitations of musculoskeletal injuries affecting normal growth and development. Nursing interventions geared toward the patient's individual ability is important to maximize growth and development potential particularly during periods of immobility. Nursing interventions should include active and passive range of motion and treatment strategies geared toward preventing complications of the disease process or treatments of it. The nurse should educate the family about appropriate child self-care techniques to help foster coping with activity restrictions. It is also important that the nurse educate the family about ways to prevent exacerbations of chronic conditions to reduce the incidence of decline or delay in growth and development (Ward & Hisley, 2009).

The nurse should encourage physical and occupational therapy to assist with improvement in motor function and movement. Research has shown that a family-centered therapy approach is important for significant improvement in therapy responses. Family-centered therapy includes the involvement of the parents and family members in the identification of the child's impairments and developmental milestones as well as the development of an appropriate intervention plan. Significant improvements in outcomes have been identified when parents are actively involved with such therapies (Baker, Haines, Yost, DiClaudio, Braun, & Holt, 2012).

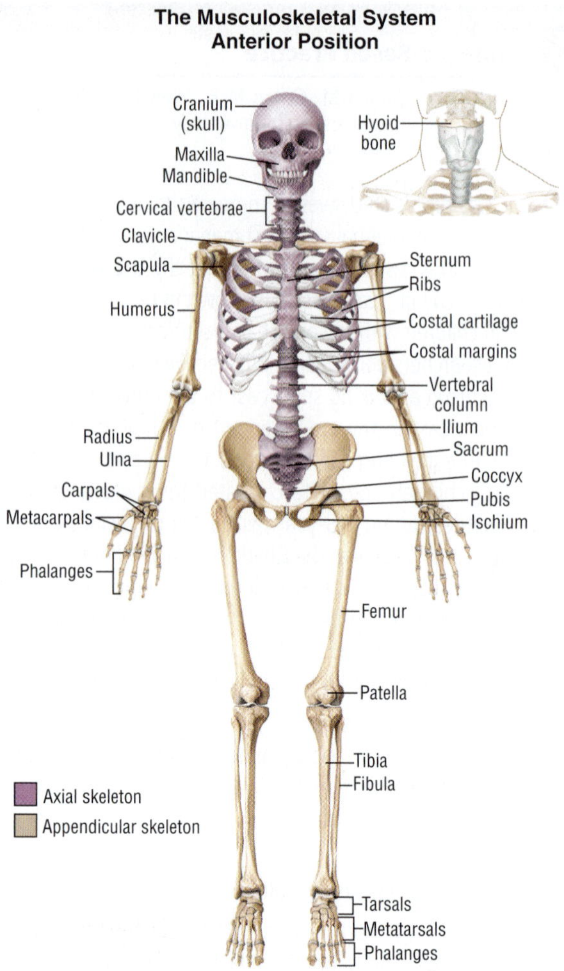

Figure 29-1a Skeletal system anterior view.

A & P review Understanding the Musculoskeletal System

Movement is made possible by the musculoskeletal system, which consists of the bones, joints, ligaments and tendons, and muscles (Figs. 29-1A and 29-1B). These structures provide protection for the vital organs inside the body. Children are more likely to suffer from conditions of the musculoskeletal system because their musculoskeletal system is still growing. On the positive side, because the bones are still growing in a child, a fracture heals much faster than in an adult. Conversely, if the fracture penetrates the growth plate in a child, growth of that bone is interrupted. Some conditions involving the musculoskeletal system may have only a slight effect on the child's ability to mobilize and be short-term. Other conditions may have a significant effect and be debilitating and long term.

Bones

Bones are classified by their size and shape. Long bones are found in the extremities, including the fingers and toes. Most childhood disorders are located in the long bones. Short bones are located in the ankle and wrist. Flat bones are located in the skull, scapulae, ribs, sternum, and clavicle. Irregular bones are the vertebrae, pelvis, and facial bones. Long bones consist of the epiphysis (rounded, end portion), the diaphysis (long, central portion), and the metaphysis (thin portion between the epiphysis and the diaphysis). Long bones grow in length at the epiphyseal plate (cartilage segment) when the cartilage segment cells grow away from the shaft of the bone. The cartilage cells are replaced by bone. The diaphysis of the long bones is covered by periosteum (an outer, sensitive layer). The width of the bone is increased by pressing against the periosteum. Some disorders, such as osteomyelitis, cause damage to the periosteum and can interrupt bone growth.

Bones need nutrients to grow. Calcium is a main component of bones and is required for bone formation, resorption (bone breakdown), and remodeling (new bone replacing old bone). Calcitonin, parathyroid hormone, vitamin D, other minerals, and enzymes all play a role in the processes of resorption and remodeling. The central part of a long bone contains the marrow. Red marrow produces red and white blood cells and platelets. Yellow marrow produces fat cells. Bones have an excellent blood supply, which enable the production of blood components for the body. Bone cells die, and the necessary production of blood components is interrupted if there is no blood supply to the long bones.

Joints

A joint is where two or more bones have contact with one another and allow for movement. Joints are classified as structural and functional, providing mechanical support. Fibrous joints are held together by a thin layer of strong

**The Musculoskeletal System
Posterior Position**

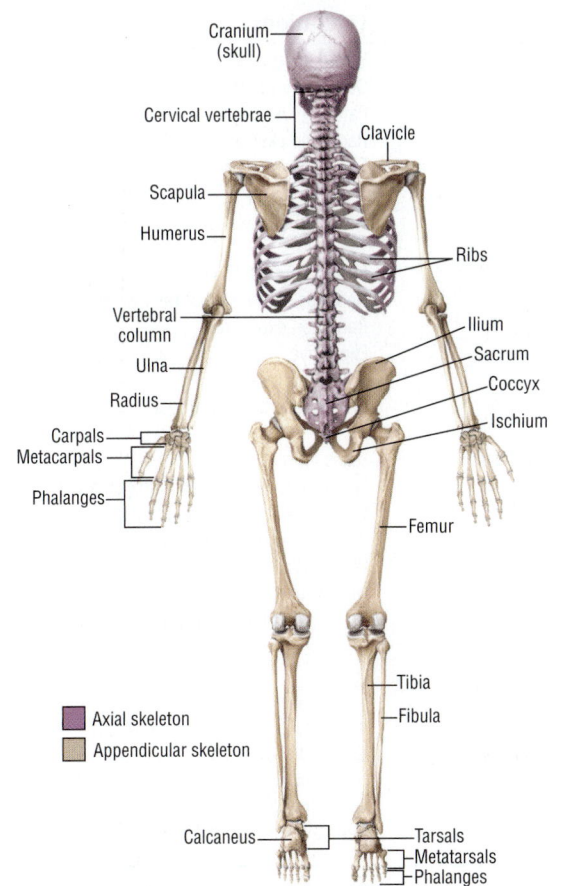

Figure 29-1b Skeletal system posterior view.

connective tissue and have no movement between the bones, such as in skull sutures. Cartilaginous joints attach bones by cartilage. These joints allow for little movement, for example, the ribs or spine. Synovial joints allow for more movement than the cartilaginous joints. Cavities between bones in synovial joints are filled with synovial fluid, which lubricates and protects the bones. Examples of synovial joints are found in the wrist, elbow, hip, and knee. Synovial joints can be subdivided into the following categories based on the type of movement.

A hinge joint occurs where the convex surface of one bone fits into the concave surface of another bone, making movement possible as found in the knee or elbow. A gliding joint allows for gliding movements between flat surfaces as one surface slides over another surface as found between the tarsal bones. Pivot joints allow for rotation around an axis such as the end of the radius rotating around the ulna as the palm of a hand is turned outward or inward. Compound joints are made up of several joints between a number of different bones and allow for a variety of movements such as the set of joints that move the skull on the vertebral column. A ball-and-socket joint allows for radial movement; examples are the joints in the hips and shoulders.

Ligaments and Tendons

Ligaments are fibrous bands of connective tissue linking two or more bones or cartilages together. They provide stability to a joint during both movement and rest. The blood supply to ligaments is very small, and they lack elasticity. Therefore, an injury to a ligament can take a long time to heal. Tendons are also fibrous connective tissue that attaches muscles to bones and other parts. There is also very little blood supply to the tendons, and an injury to a tendon can also involve a lengthy recovery.

Muscles

Muscles consist of striated muscles and smooth muscles. Skeletal muscle is a type of striated muscle that attaches to tendons. Skeletal muscles are used to create movement through contraction by applying force to bones and joints. These muscles can contract voluntarily (by somatic nerve stimulation) or can contract involuntarily through reflexes. Smooth muscle is a type of muscle found in the walls of all the hollow organs of the body (except the heart). Smooth muscles are involuntary muscles and are under the control of the autonomic nervous system. For example, smooth muscles regulate the flow of blood in the arteries, move food through the gastrointestinal tract, and expel urine from the bladder. ◆

Nurses play an important role in assisting the parents to find methods to help the child maintain normal growth and development and adapt to or overcome musculoskeletal system impairment. Casts, skin traction, skeletal traction, and distraction devices are ways to immobilize an extremity. The nurse evaluates the child through physical assessment (Box 29-1). Laboratory studies and diagnostic tests can help establish the cause and nature of the musculoskeletal injury or condition. The results of these tests are then used to help develop an appropriate plan of nursing care.

Children are by nature active, and their musculoskeletal system plays a major role in their growth and development. When their ability to interact with the environment is impaired, possibly through a musculoskeletal system disorder, they are at risk for impaired growth and development. Alterations in the musculoskeletal system may be related to a congenital defect such as muscular dystrophy, clubfoot, or osteogenesis imperfecta. Other alterations may be related to an acquired defect such as Legg-Calvé-Perthes disease, slipped femoral capital epiphysis, fractures, soft tissue or sports injuries, Osgood-Schlatter disease, osteomyelitis, juvenile arthritis, scoliosis, tetanus, or osteoporosis.

Casts, skin traction, skeletal traction, and distraction devices are ways to immobilize an extremity. The nurse evaluates the child through physical assessment. Laboratory studies and diagnostic tests can help establish the cause and nature of the musculoskeletal injury or condition (Box 29-2). The results of these tests are then used to help the nurse develop an appropriate plan of care.

While the child is hospitalized, coordinate a care conference to help plan discharge and home care. Preparing the family for discharge is essential to ongoing care of the child because there may be a need for a long-term cast or continued immobility. The family needs to learn about making adaptations in the home environment to ensure a safe environment and allow the child as much movement as possible. The family also needs psychosocial support to assist them in coping with the child's ongoing musculoskeletal condition. Help the family and the child achieve the best possible psychosocial outcome by arranging for home nursing care, physical and/or

Box 29-1 Diagnostic Tools Orthopedic Imaging Tests

Diagnostic Imaging Test	Benefits	Limitations
Radiograph	Easily available Visualizes fractures well No sedation needed Inexpensive	Two-dimensional Does not visualize soft tissue such as cartilage Patient must be positioned properly Radiation exposure
Fluoroscopy	Guides many orthopedic procedures Can be used with contrast Real-time radiography Inexpensive	Radiation exposure
Arthrography	Provides visualization of joints Three-dimensional view	Risk of reaction to contrast Depends on the skill of the radiographer Radiation exposure
Computed tomography (CT scan)	Cross-sectional view of anatomy Clearer than radiographs Software programs can show reconstruction Can use contrast media	Expensive May require sedation Risk of reaction to contrast
Bone scan (nuclear medicine)	Excellent at finding changes in bone as a result of infection, trauma, or tumor	Takes 4 hours Not always available on emergency basis Cannot distinguish benign from malignant tumors Radiation exposure to entire body IV access required
Ultrasound	Easily available No radiation No sedation needed Good for visualizing soft tissue masses and cysts Painless Inexpensive	Limited use Depends on the skill of the radiographer
Magnetic resonance imaging (MRI)	Visualizes hard and soft tissue and bone marrow No radiation	Not readily available No metal can be present in the vicinity Sedation may be needed Need experienced radiologist to read MRI

Box 29-2 Labs: Blood and Body Fluid Analysis for the Child With Alterations in Musculoskeletal Conditions

Diagnostic Test	Function of the Test	Indications	Normal Values
Complete blood count (CBC)	Blood sample evaluates many aspects.	Low platelets indicate a bleeding disorder. A high WBC count indicates a bacterial infection or septic arthritis.	Platelets: 150,000–400,000/μL WBC: 4500–10,000/μL

CBC differential	Breaks down WBC into various types (five total).
	Numbers indicate a percentage of total WBC.
	Indicates the type of infection.
		A high monocyte count indicates a long-term infectious process.
		Lymphocytes indicate an increase in viral illness.
		Eosinophils indicate an allergic or parasitic condition.
		Basophils indicate a chronic inflammatory condition.
		Neutrophils (polys)
		  Bands are immature neutrophils.
		  Segs are mature neutrophils.
		  (Left-shift describes an increase in the band neutrophils.)
		Suggests a severe bacterial infection such as sepsis.
			0% for bands and 31%–57% for segs
			Presence of bands is highly indicative of a bacterial infection

C-Reactive protein (CRP)	Measures a protein in blood that is released when an infection is present.	A normal level is 0–1.0 mg/dL or less than 10 mg/L.	Over 10 mg/L indicates an infection is present
Calcium and phosphate	Measures the amount of these minerals.	Low levels may indicate rickets.	Calcium: 8.5–11 mg Phosphorus: 3.0–4.5 mg/dL
Rheumatoid factor (Rh factor)	Measures the body's autoimmune response to an antigen.	If positive, may indicate juvenile arthritis. Not all children with juvenile arthritis have a positive Rh factor.	Negative
Erythrocyte sedimentation rate (ESR)	Measures the speed at which RBCs settle out in solution.	Elevated indicates septic arthritis. May also indicate infection.	0–10 mm/hr
Blood cultures	Measures whether microorganisms grow out in the lab.	Can identify an organism causing infection. Forty percent of children with septic arthritis have a positive blood culture.	No growth
Bone biopsies	Diagnose tumor or infection of the bone.	Osteomyelitis Bone tumor	Normal bone cells
Fluid aspiration from joints	Diagnose an infection of the joint or drain fluid from joint to relieve pressure.	Drainage is purulent. Culture of fluid is positive.	Clear fluid No growth from culture

occupational therapy, and ways to obtain durable medical equipment.

 Collaboration in Caring—*Care of a child with a musculoskeletal disorder*

Care of a child with a musculoskeletal disorder involves collaboration with the interdisciplinary team members, each having a specific role. Coordinate ongoing care and ensure the child's holistic needs are met. Teaching parents about the serial casting process, directing the family to a respite care center, and telling them how to provide home care is an essential nursing role. The physical therapist is usually one of the first members of the health-care team who initially assists the child out of bed after a procedure, such as orthopedic surgery or cast application. Assisting the child with gross motor movement, passive range-of-motion exercises, and arranging for ambulation aids and wheelchairs is done by the physical therapist. The occupational therapist works with the child's fine motor development and makes splints and orthotics that fit the child. The child life therapist is instrumental in helping with diversion activities to keep the child calm during painful procedures such as blood draws. A proper diet aids the healing process during which instructional sessions are conducted by a nutritionist. To help the transition home, the social worker communicates with the family about coping techniques and community resources to use with the child at home after discharge.

Common Musculoskeletal Conditions Found in Children

CLUBFOOT

Clubfoot is a common foot deformity diagnosed in newborns. Recent advances in genetics have identified that clubfoot is a genetic disorder. In fact, a recent study showed that there was a higher incidence of clubfoot in identical twins than with fraternal twins (Dobbs & Gurnett, 2011). There is also a possibility that the position of the fetus in utero influences the formation of clubfoot. There are four main classes of clubfoot determined by the cause and the response to treatment:

- Postural—benign form, usually resolves with stretches and casting
- Idiopathic—true congenital clubfoot with varied severity
- Neurogenic—usually with spina bifida
- Syndromic—associated with other anomalies and leads to rigid feet
(Carroll, 2012, p. 1)

Signs and Symptoms

In clubfoot, the foot:

- Is plantar flexed
- Has an inverted heel
- Has an adducted forefoot
- Is rigid and cannot be manipulated into a neutral position

Diagnosis

Diagnosis of clubfoot is made by visualization during the newborn nursing assessment.

Prevention

Because this is a genetic disorder, there are no preventive measures that can be taken.

Collaborative Care

Nursing Care. Treatment is begun as soon as possible after birth. Clubfoot can be treated with serial casting (replacing plaster casts) on the affected extremity(s) at specified intervals to permit progressively greater ranges of joint motion so that the maximum range needed for function may be restored. While casted, the affected extremity is manipulated into a more normal position, and a cast is applied to hold this position. In the beginning, the cast is changed frequently and eventually reduced to a less frequent basis until overcorrection of the position is achieved.

Nursing care for a child undergoing nonsurgical management of clubfoot also includes passive range of motion (ROM) and care of the cast application after manipulation. Because manipulation of the affected extremity with serial casting can cause discomfort while the muscles and ligaments are being stretched, pain medication is indicated. Neurovascular assessments (including assessing for swelling) must be done every 1 to 2 hours for the first 24 to 48 hours after cast application and every 4 hours thereafter until a new cast is placed. After application, the cast is left open to air to aid in the drying process, and the extremity is elevated.

 Nursing Insight—*Overcorrection*

Overcorrection is the goal for serial casting because the ligaments and muscles are shortened, and when the casts are finally removed, there is a tendency for these muscles and ligaments to pull the foot back into the clubfoot position. Overcorrection enables this pull to level off at a normal position. Communicate to the family that exercises, splints, special shoes, or casts may be prescribed on a long-term basis.

Medical Care. Medical management for clubfoot has evolved over the past 100 years. Dr. Hugh Owen Thomas used a forceful correction of the foot. Dennis J. W. Brown, MD (Australian surgeon), also used forceful correction then followed by his famous splint (Figs. 29-2A and 29-2B). Ignacio V. Ponseti, MD, of the University of Iowa, developed a technique in the 1940s in which he abducted and dorsiflexed the foot. Currently, after the manipulation of the foot, a cast is applied. The cast is then molded around the heel while the forefoot is abducted. The knee is flexed to 90 degrees. As early as the following day or anytime

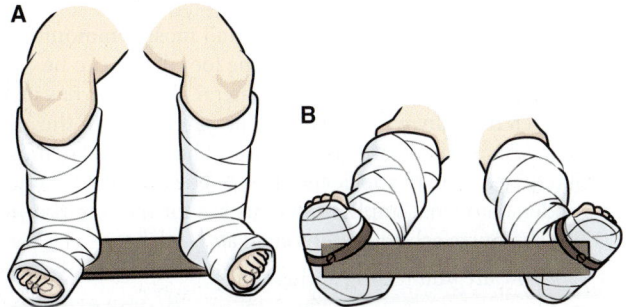

Figure 29-2a and b Browne splint.

thereafter, the casts are removed and then the foot is re-manipulated further into the abducted position. It takes up to seven different manipulations and castings to achieve the maximum position. The Browne splint is used after the final cast has been removed (Figs. 29-2*A* and 29-2*B*). These splints are worn for 23 hours per day until the child is about 3 years of age.

 Nursing Insight—*The Copenhagen technique*

Another method used to correct clubfoot is the Copenhagen technique that involves flexing and manipulating the foot, muscle stimulation, and applying a plaster cast. It is performed daily from birth until normalcy is achieved at about 6 weeks of age. After surgery, bandaging is used instead of splints until the child is walking. The foot is checked routinely until bone maturity is achieved in adolescence. Observe for swelling in the ankle and foot. The key to preventing swelling is to elevate the ankle and foot. Assess for drainage from the cast and for signs of infection, including purulent drainage, fever, and chills. Be aware that pain management is important postoperatively. Pain medication is initially administered IV with morphine sulfate (Astramorph). When the child can tolerate fluids and food, he or she can be switched to oral pain medication.

Surgical Care. Severe cases of clubfoot may require surgery when the infant is 9 to 12 months of age. An orthopedic surgeon lengthens the tendons to help ease the foot into a more normal position using a **tenotomy** (the operation of cutting and repositioning a tendon) of the Achilles tendon for lengthening. A tendon transfer can also be performed to prevent foot inversion and adduction of the metatarsus.

Surgical procedures also involve soft tissue releases, bone fusions, and joint releases. A standardized 4-step surgical procedure is done on children with clubfoot; first is a plantar release; second is a **Z-plasty** (incision made in the form of a Z, in which the points are transposed into the opposite spot) of the Achilles tendon; third is a Z-plasty of the tibialis posterior tendon; and fourth is an open reduction of the **talonavicular** (pertaining to the talus and navicular bones) joint with placement of **Kirschner wires** (K-wires) (steel wire placed through a long bone to apply traction to the bone) (Carroll, 2012).

However, some problems with surgical management are identified as overcorrection, recurrence, and pain. Each foot has a slightly different pathology, so management needs to be tailored to the individual child (Carroll, 2012).

❝What to say❞—*Talipes equinovarus (clubfoot)*

The most severe form of clubfoot and most commonly known is Talipes equinovarus. The foot defect can be unilateral (more common) or bilateral. A mother has just delivered a baby with clubfoot. The parents are in the delivery room and are visibly upset. The parents are most likely in a state of shock and denial. The family does not understand what implications this has for their newborn.

The nurse asks questions such as:

1. "How are you feeling at this time?"
2. "After you rest we can talk more about the baby's condition."

 Where Research and Practice Meet:
Idiopathic Clubfeet

Utrilla-Rodriguez, Martinez-Cañavete, and Casares (2012) studied 82 patients with idiopathic (pertaining to illnesses whose cause is either uncertain or as yet undetermined) clubfeet and had received treatment using a modified Copenhagen technique. In this study, all patients were less than 2 months old when enrolled. A physician and a physical therapist evaluated the infants at the time of enrollment. The foot deformities were rated according to the Harrold and Walker scale, which uses 3 grades to classify the deformity. Grade 1 is characterized by the ability to manipulate the feet into normal position. Grade II is when the clubfoot is persistent with manipulation and is less than or equal to 20 degrees. Grade III is when the clubfoot is persistent with manipulation and is greater than 20 degrees. Treatment sessions occurred 5 days per week for 30 minutes per foot, and a corrective splint is worn over the weekend. Minimum follow-up was 3 years. The objectives were to reposition affected joints, maintain reduction of the deformity, rebalance the muscles in the feet, and position the bones to the anatomically correct position. Stretching and manipulation began starting with the correction of adduction (movement of a limb toward the median plane of the body), then the cavus, the hindfoot varus (posterior part of the foot), and lastly the equinus. These manipulations were performed by experienced pediatric physical therapists. Manipulations of the bones were performed, and stimulation of the muscles was done by using a toothbrush, rubbing it to the hypotonic muscles to the lateral and anterior-lateral area of the foot. The authors noted that there is a lack of published data regarding the use of the toothbrush being able to produce a response of the muscle, but the authors' experience has observed a muscle response as a perineal muscle contraction. After the bone manipulation and stimulation, cotton bandages and two strips of plaster were applied to maintain the proper foot position. An additional cotton bandage was used to cover the plaster strips. Neurovascular assessments were done to ensure adequate circulation to the extremity. This procedure was done daily for about 6 weeks. At that point, maximum abduction had been achieved. A maintenance splint was then applied that maintained the foot in the correct position. It used elastic straps and plastic as well as metal bracing materials to maintain the foot in an abducted, dorsiflexed position with outward rotation of the foot and the knee in a 90-degree flexed position. The parents were also taught to do the exercises five times per day. When the child reached 7 or 8 months of age, the infant was gradually released from this splint and put in pre-walking shoes that have an inverted internal border. Physical therapy was initiated and gradually increased so that ROM was preserved. When the child began to walk, a shoe with good support, a tongue, and laces replaced the pre-walking boots.

Correction criteria were used to evaluate the results with these patients; development of dorsiflexion and plantar flexion of the foot and heel in normal position with the foot in correct alignment were the criteria that were used. After 3 years of follow-up, 54% of the children did not need any surgical procedures and met all of the correction criteria. Two percent of the children needed a tenotomy of the Achilles tendon, and 44% needed a posterior release.

3. "What do you know about clubfoot and the treatment?"
4. "Can I stay with you to offer support while you hold the baby?"

Education/Discharge Instructions

In either case, serial casting or surgery, instruct the family to keep the cast clean. The young child needs to be diapered in such a way that the cast is outside the edges of the diaper. Double diapering and changing the diaper

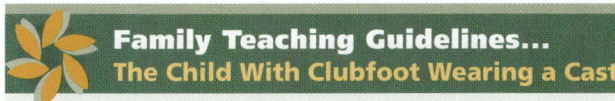

Family Teaching Guidelines...
The Child With Clubfoot Wearing a Cast

HOW TO:

Teach the parents how to care for their child with a clubfoot who is wearing a cast. Instruct the parents to:

◆ Give the child emotional support and reassurance that he can return to his normal activities soon after the cast is removed.

◆ Maintain the child's normal development by playing, reading, and spending time with the child.

◆ Keep the cast and surrounding area clean and dry and reposition him every 2 hours.

◆ Elevate the affected extremity and use good hygiene to prevent skin breakdown.

◆ Notify the health-care provider if the child has a fever, signs and symptoms of infection, or unrelieved pain.

◆ Take the child to the health-care professional if the cast is damaged (soft, loose, or cracked) or cast syndrome is suspected.

ESSENTIAL INFORMATION:

◆ Follow-up care is essential.

◆ Inform the parents that there may be a potential for reoccurrence of the clubfoot.

◆ Teach the parents about the importance of monitoring cast complications.

frequently are also methods to keep the cast clean. The older child may have to change underwear frequently. It is not feasible to bathe the child in a tub of water with bilateral long leg casts with an abduction bar so a sponge bath is given. Provide the family with emotional support. Distraction techniques and age-appropriate toys can help the child to handle the long recovery process.

It is also important to stress that the child needs to continue with growth and developmental milestones. The infant or child can be placed on a blanket on the floor and explore his or her surroundings while supervised. Adjustments can be made so that the infant or child can continue to develop gross motor, fine motor, cognitive, and language milestones.

 Nursing diagnoses A Child With Clubfoot

- Impaired Physical Mobility related to external devices (casts) secondary to serial casting for Clubfoot
- Impaired Parenting related to growth and development lag secondary to serial casting for Clubfoot
- Risk for Impaired Skin Integrity related to external devices (casts) secondary to serial casting for Clubfoot
- Knowledge Deficit related to management and home care of a child who has been casted for management of Clubfoot

LEGG-CALVÉ-PERTHES DISEASE

Legg-Calvé-Perthes disease (LCPD) has an insidious onset and is accepted as a disorder of growth. LCPD is considered a multifactorial condition caused by genetic and environmental factors, which may be a precursor to the disease (Kim, 2011). The disease starts with an interrupted blood supply to the femoral head.

Catterall (1971) (in Wenger & Pandya, 2011) developed a classification system to determine the severity of the disease. The four different groups define the radiographic appearance during the greatest bone loss.

- Catterall I & II are when less than 50% of the femoral head is involved, whereas
- Catterall III & IV have greater than 50% of the femoral head involved and a potentially poor prognosis (Wenger & Pandya, 2011).

Medical treatments using physical therapy and bracing are used as well as surgical containment procedures, which are both successful methods for treatment (Wenger & Pandya, 2011). It can take 18 months to 4 years for this condition to resolve.

 Where Research and Practice Meet:
Incidence of LCPD

A systematic review of racial and geographic factors in the incidence of LCPD was performed by Perry, Machin, Pope, Bruce, Dangerfield, Platt, et al. (2012). The studies that were reviewed had been performed between 1969 and 2009. Race was the single most important factor in determining risk for this disease. In South Africa, blacks had the least incidence whereas Caucasians had the greatest incidence. Mixed race children had moderate risk. There was also a strong correlation between latitude and incidence. For every 10-degree increase of latitude, the incidence of LCPD increased. LCPD was 8.8% greater in Caucasian regions than in East Asian regions. Incidence in South Asia was 2.9 times greater than East Asian regions.

Where Research and Practice Meet:
Prognostic Factors

A systematic review of prognosis and prognostic factors was undertaken by Cheng, Lam, and Ng (2011). The findings indicated that 60% to 80% of children with LCPD had excellent results on follow-up. This follow-up continued for 40 years. Children who were diagnosed with the disease between 5 and 7 years of age had a significantly better outcome than children who were diagnosed with the disease after 8 or 9 years of age. The age at the time of healing is a more important prognosticator than the age at onset of the disease. LCPD occurs 4 times more frequently in boys than girls, but girls have a poorer prognosis.

There are 4 stages of LCPD:

- Aseptic necrosis (flattening of the femoral head)—is the precipitating factor, it lasts several weeks and presents with synovitis and a decrease in ossification in the nucleus of the femoral head secondary to ischemia
- Revascularization—can occur rapidly through **recanalization** (reestablishment of an opening through a vessel that had been previously occluded) of the existing blood vessels within a few weeks, or it can last 6 to 12 months when new blood vessels are formed; increased joint space, increased cartilage thickness, decrease in size and density of femoral head
- New bone formation—lasts 1 to 2 years, collapse and **superolateral** (above and to the side) displaced head, avascular bone is reabsorbed
- Regenerative phase—reconstitution of femoral head with remodeling and final healing
  (Joseph, 2011)

Signs and Symptoms

In LCPD, the child complains of:

- Hip or knee soreness or stiffness
- Pain that increases with activity and decreases with rest
- A painful limp
- Quadriceps muscle atrophy
- Joint dysfunction
- Limited ROM

Diagnosis

A radiograph establishes the initial diagnosis LCPD. The definitive diagnosis is made by magnetic resonance imaging (MRI) and radiographic studies, which show osteonecrosis.

Prevention

There are no preventive measures that can be taken.

Collaborative Care

Nursing Care. Obtaining a history is important in assessing the child with possible LCPD. This history will uncover how long the child has been limping and the severity of the pain. The child describes the pain as increasing in intensity with activity and decreasing with rest. The nurse's assessment of ROM will help determine limitations on abduction and internal hip rotation. An assessment of the thigh and buttock area will reveal a wasting of the muscles. A shortening of the extremity on the affected side indicates that the femoral head has collapsed. The goal of nursing care is to keep the femoral head in the acetabulum, and this is done during an initial period of non–weight bearing when a brace is generally used.

When the child is receiving conservative hospitalized care, assess the skin for breakdown. Preparing the child and family for a radiographic exam and MRI is done. If the child is being treated with a brace, collaboration with the **orthotics team** (a team of experts who teach others how to use orthopedic appliances) is required. The child is maintained on bedrest to reduce the inflammation and restore motion. Pain management is included in the nursing plan of care.

Medical Care. Early medical treatments focused on periods of hospitalization and complete non–weight bearing. Later on, medical management involves increased non–weight bearing and using a brace that is worn for 2 to 4 years. Another type of medical management involves the child remaining in a Montreal abduction plaster cast for a year or more. This type of cast allows weight bearing with the femoral head and is determined to be not harmful in the healing process. One problem with this cast is that multiple clinic visits and hospitalizations for repeat casting, followed by the need to regain hip and knee motion are needed. The Toronto brace can replace casting allowing for full knee flexion while maintaining hip placement. Less frequently, traction or a spica cast is used.

Surgical Care. Surgical osteotomies (cutting through a bone) are performed to reposition the femoral head to maintain optimal position for healing. A femoral or Salter **osteotomy** is performed for LCPD. After surgery a spica hip cast is required, so implement the usual postoperative care measures in addition to the care of a child in a cast. Pain relief is achieved with the administration of nonsteroidal anti-inflammatory drugs (NSAIDs) such as ibuprofen (Children's Advil).

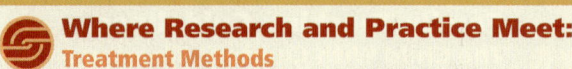

Where Research and Practice Meet: Treatment Methods

A study performed by Herring (2011) examined whether one of three nonoperative methods or two surgical methods produced a significantly better outcome in the management of LCPD. The three nonoperative methods were bracing, no treatment, and ROM exercises. The surgical procedures were femoral osteotomy and Salter osteotomy. Results showed there were no significant differences between the nonsurgical treatments and also no significant differences between the surgical groups. In addition, there was no significant difference between the nonsurgical and the surgical methods for treatment if the child was less than 8 years of age at onset. If the child was older than 8 years, the surgical treatment was significantly more effective in certain types of LCPD.

Education/Discharge Instructions

Ongoing management after discharge from the hospital consists of conservative therapy for 1 to 3 years. Communicate to the family that initially the child will need to avoid weight-bearing activities and that mobility restrictions are maintained. While the child has mobility restrictions, ROM is implemented. Because it is difficult for a child to remain on bedrest, emotional support and diversional activities are essential. It is also important to teach the family about home care. Discuss the importance of adaptive play. After the physician has communicated that the condition has resolved, the child can return to normal activity in about 3 to 4 months.

 Across Care Settings: Visiting nurse

After diagnosis in the health-care practitioner's office, the child with LCPD is to be cared for at home by a visiting nurse and physical therapist. The visiting nurse can:

- Assess the family support systems while the child and family are in their own environment.
- Ensure that the family is able to provide the care needed.
- Ensure compliance with the use of the conservative devices.
- Ensure the non–weight bearing status of the child.
- Assess the knowledge of the parents and child about ongoing care.
- Encourage the use of creative quiet activities and hobbies.
- Arrange for physical therapy for ROM exercises and to ensure that the child is safe while walking with a non–weight bearing device.
- Ask the family about follow-up care with the physician.

 Nursing Diagnoses A Child With Legg-Calvé-Perthes Disease

- Risk for Injury related to altered mobility secondary to Legg-Calvé-Perthes Disease treatment
- Impaired Physical Mobility related to external devices secondary to Legg-Calvé-Perthes Disease treatment
- Risk for Impaired Skin Integrity related to external devices secondary to Legg-Calvé-Perthes Disease treatment
- Body Image Disturbance related to immobility secondary to Legg-Calvé-Perthes disease
- Knowledge Deficit related to management and home care for a child with Legg-Calvé-Perthes disease

SLIPPED CAPITAL FEMORAL EPIPHYSIS

Slipped capital femoral epiphysis (SCFE) affects 10.8 per 100,000 children (Kuzyk, Kim, & Millis, 2011, p. 667). A higher proportion of children with SCFE are obese. The cause is unknown, but there is a genetic component and it may be related to endocrine abnormalities. When this condition occurs, the capital femoral epiphysis (top of the femur) slips through the epiphysis (growth plate) in a posterior direction. Conditions associated with SCFE are hypothyroidism, renal osteodystrophy, and post–radiation therapy.

Signs and Symptoms

SCFE symptoms appear gradually. Acute slip symptoms are present for less than 3 weeks. Chronic slip symptoms are present for more than 3 weeks.

- Pain in the groin or referred pain to the thigh or knee is the child's primary presenting complaint. This occurs because the child is externally rotating the leg to relieve pressure on the hip joint. The parent usually notices that the child is limping and favoring that extremity.
- During examination, the child complains of pain during internal rotation of the hip.
- The hip does not fully rotate internally, and abduction is limited.
- The affected leg may be shorter if the child has a moderate or severe slip.

Diagnosis

Radiographic studies are used to diagnose SCFE. Typically, the frog-leg lateral view will show a mild step-off of the anterior femoral epiphysis with its corresponding metaphysis in a posteroinferior direction (Wu, & Pollock, 2011, p. 1095).

 Assessment Tool Slipped Capital Femoral Epiphysis

SCFE is classified by stage and severity:

Stage
- Preslip—The child complains of weakness in the leg, pain in knee or hip when standing or walking for long periods of time. Acute slip—The child falls and then reports hip pain.
- Chronic slip—The femoral head gradually slips off the femoral neck and then remodels for the incorrect position.
- Acute-on-chronic—Slow progressive slip that then becomes more displaced when the child falls.

Severity
- Grade I: Preslip—There is a widening of the physis without any displacement of the epiphysis.
- Grade II: Minimal slip—There is a one-third displacement of the femoral head from the femoral neck.
- Grade III: Moderate slip—There is more than one-third but less than one-half displacement of the femoral head from the femoral neck.
- Grade IV: Severe slip—There is more than one-half displacement of the femoral head from the femoral neck.

Prevention

There are no preventive measures that can be taken because the cause is idiopathic.

Collaborative Care

Nursing Care. Once a child has been diagnosed with SCFE, no weight bearing is permitted. Assist the family in adjusting to the sudden hospitalization, non–weight bearing status of the child and the impending surgery. The goal of nursing care is to prevent further slippage. No ROM is attempted if the child has an acute slip because it may cause further damage. Communicate to the family that the hip cannot be reduced manually because that will cause further damage to the femoral head. Bedrest with the child in traction decreases **synovitis** (inflammation of a synovial membrane) in the hip. If the child has an acute slip, split Russell's traction may be instituted for a few days before surgery.

Medical Care. When a child has been diagnosed with SCFE in one hip, the other hip is also assessed to ensure that there are not any subtle or early changes of SCFE in the contralateral hip (Wu & Pollock, 2011).

Surgical Care. Surgery (pinning) is the intervention of choice for a child with mild to moderate SCFE. The pinning consists of a percutaneous insertion of a large screw or pin into the femoral head to hold it in place. There is a small incision, and the child stays in the hospital for less than 24 hours. After 1 week, the child may bear full weight and the pin is removed at a later date.

With severe SCFE, an osteotomy is required, which consists of a breaking and resetting of the bone. This prevents further slippage and restores hip motion to normal. It is a much more extensive surgery, requiring a longer hospitalization and prolonged immobilization.

After surgery, postoperative pain management is managed with IV narcotics and changed to oral narcotics once the child is tolerating liquids and solid food. Also monitor the neurovascular status frequently and collaborate with physical therapy to teach the child crutch walking. The physical therapy initiates ambulation with crutches. After that, continue ambulation with the child who is using crutches.

Education/Discharge Instructions

The child is discharged when pain is controlled with oral narcotics and the child can ambulate safely with crutches. It is helpful to arrange for a visiting nurse to ensure that the child can ambulate safely with crutches at home. If the child still needs assistance with ambulation at home, a physical therapist can visit the home and reinforce teaching.

FRACTURES

Fractures occur when a bone undergoes more stress than it can absorb. Skeletal fractures account for 10% to 15% of all childhood injuries. The most common causes of fractures are falls and motor vehicle and bicycle crashes. There are differences between a fracture in a child and a fracture in an adult. A child's bone heals faster because of a higher metabolic rate and because the epiphyseal plate (growth plate) is still open. However, any damage to the epiphyseal plate can result in a limb length discrepancy, joint incongruity, and a progressive angular deformity of the limb.

Fractures are characterized as closed or open. A **closed reduction** has no break in the skin. The health-care practitioner aligns the fractured ends by manually manipulating the extremity or traction under conscious sedation or general anesthesia. The goal is to reduce the fracture as soon as possible. With an open fracture the bone has penetrated through the skin. An **open reduction** requires surgery when the fracture cannot be reduced by closed methods or when torn muscles or ligaments need to be repaired. It is designated type I, II, or III based on the degree, severity of soft tissue damage, size of the wound, and amount of contamination. The potential for infection is greatest with an open fracture.

✳ Nursing Insight—*Fractures*

Fractures are associated with development. During birth, one type of fracture that occurs is when an infant has a fracture of the collarbone. Otherwise, fractures in infancy are rare because the infant has limited mobility. During the first 2 years of life, fractures can be commonly caused by mobility injuries or as the result of physical maltreatment. Stress fractures have become prevalent in adolescent girls doing high-impact activities like gymnastics, cheerleading, and low vitamin D levels.

Signs and Symptoms

Classification of fractures involves identifying the locations and description of the fracture. The location is where the fracture occurs along the shaft of the bone. The signs and symptoms of fractures are described in terms of the amount of injury.

❝What to say❞—*Severity of the fracture*

Communicate to the family that the severity of the fracture depends on the amount of force placed on the bone and the strength of the bone, the size of the bone, and the direction of the force. Once a bone is fractured, an inflammatory response occurs. **Osteoblasts** (bone-forming cells) activate within 24 hours to begin making new bone. A callus forms during the first few weeks. Complete callus formation and establishment of compact bone takes 4 to 12 weeks. **Remodeling** (rounding off angles and filling in hollows) continues for up to 1 year. In children, the ends of the bone do not need to be perfectly aligned because the bone has an enhanced ability to remodel.

Diagnosis

A fracture is suspected by presenting symptoms, trauma history, and physical examination of the child. Radiograph exam is the primary method to diagnose fractures. When a radiograph is performed, at least two views are taken (anteroposterior and lateral). The joints above and below the suspected fracture must be included in the radiographic evaluation. Computed tomography (CT) scans, MRI, fluoroscopy, and myelograms are also used to diagnose fractures (Box 29-3).

⚙ Assessment Tool   Classification of Fractures by Location

Epiphyseal
Type I
   Separation of epiphysis
   May be mistaken for a sprain
   Does not usually affect growth

Box 29-3 **Performing the Neurovascular Assessment**

- Pain—Does the child complain of pain in the affected limb? Is it relieved by narcotic medication? Does it become worse when fingers or toes are flexed? If yes, notify physician immediately (compartment syndrome).

- Sensation—Can the child feel touch on the extremity? Is two-point discrimination decreased? If yes, notify the physician immediately (compartment syndrome).

- Motion—Can the child move fingers or toes? Lack of movement may indicate nerve damage.

- Temperature—Does the affected limb feel warm? Does it feel cool? A cool extremity may change to feeling warm if a blanket is placed over it and the extremity is elevated. If the extremity is still cool after these interventions, there is poor circulation.

- Capillary refill time (CRT)—Apply brief pressure to the nail bed and note how quickly pink color returns to the nail bed. CRT of less than 3 seconds is the norm. If CRT is greater than 3 seconds, circulation is poor.

- Color—Note the color of the affected limb. Compare it to the color of the unaffected limb. Pink is the norm. If the color is paler than in the unaffected limb, circulation is poor.

- Pulses—Check pulses distal to the injury or cast. If the pulse is difficult to locate, assess with a Doppler. If the cast covers the foot or hand, it may not be possible to check the pulse, but the other neurovascular assessment can be implemented.

Type II
   Fracture separation of the epiphysis
   Circulation remains intact
   Does not usually affect growth
Type III
   Fracture through the epiphysis into the joint
   Does not usually affect growth if reduced properly
Type IV
   Fracture through epiphysis into the joint and the metaphysis
   Open reduction and internal fixation necessary
Type V (rare occurrence)
   Crush injury to epiphyseal plate
   Results in premature closure of the epiphyseal plate
   Growth arrest occurs
Diaphysis
Proximal
Midshaft
Distal

Prevention

Fractures can be prevented by teaching parents to buckle-up children. Using protective gear for contact sports may help prevent fractures. Preventing falls in young children is also an important preventative measure. Teaching children safety while biking and walking as well as the use of a seat belt in cars has a preventative effect.

Collaborative Care

Nursing Care. Obtain a history from the child and family describing how the injury occurred. In cases in which maltreatment is involved, it is helpful to ask the child how the injury occurred in the absence of the caregiver. Depending on the type and location of the fracture, children generally heal without complications.

Nursing care involves preventing complications such as limping, decreased ROM, and nerve deficits. Other complications that can occur with fractures are shock, fat emboli, deep vein thrombosis, pulmonary embolism, and infection. Late complications that can occur are mal-union, nonunion, refracture, joint stiffness, reflex sympathetic dystrophy, loss of reduction, posttraumatic arthritis, delayed union, and pseudoarthritis.

Medical Care. Specific, closed reduction, medical management depends on the type and location of the fracture. If the bones are not displaced, no reduction of the fracture is needed. If the bones are displaced, a reduction of the fracture is needed, in which the ends of the bone are placed close together or aligned. In either case, the bone must be immobilized.

After closed reduction, perform frequent checks to assess for pain, numbness, or tingling. Nursing actions that can help to prevent complications and restore function are frequent neurovascular assessments, notifying the health-care provider of any changes, elevating the affected extremity above the level of the heart, and applying cold packs (15-minute intervals) for the first 24 hours after the injury.

Surgical Care. Open reduction includes internal fixation that is used to stabilize the bone ends until healed. Internal fixation is achieved with percutaneous pins or with screws, plates, or rods. For example, an intramedullary fixation rod can be placed in the shaft of the femur. After the bone has healed, the hardware can be removed.

Immediately after the open reduction, the affected bone must be immobilized to maintain the position of the fracture, prevent rotation and shearing of the fracture, and permit active muscle contraction. Immobilization is achieved with splints, braces, casts, external fixators, or traction. Immobilization relieves pain and allows for ease of movement of the unaffected areas of the body. It is important to mobilize the child as quickly as possible to avoid hazards of immobility.

Open fractures present additional concerns. The potential for infection from contamination is great. Antibiotics must be administered in the emergency department and continued for at least 3 days after the injury. Surgery for wound cleansing, debridement, and stabilization of the fracture needs to be performed urgently. If the wound is small, the surgeon may surgically close the wound. Most often, the wound is left open and draining until the infection is eradicated. The child may have to return to surgery later for more debridement or closure of the wound.

After surgery (open reduction), if the child has any open wounds or pins from traction or a distraction device, assess the wound(s) and perform pin care every 8 hours to prevent infection. For any type of fracture, it is critical to assess and manage pain. IV opioids are administered for the first 24 hours. Once the child is tolerating liquids and a regular diet, pain medication is switched to the oral route. Acetaminophen (Children's Tylenol) with codeine or oxycodone (Percocet) is the preferred narcotic. It is important to differentiate between pain and muscle spasms with a child who has had a fractured femur. Muscle spasms are extremely painful. Diazepam (Valium) is the best choice for an antispasmodic medication. Muscle spasms generally subside after the first week. A child in a spica hip cast eats small, frequent meals to avoid abdominal distention. The child also increases fluids and fiber in the diet to prevent constipation. The child and family may experience anxiety related to the unplanned hospital admission and possible surgery. Provide emotional support to the child and the family.

clinical alert

Compartment syndrome

The classic sign of compartment syndrome (related to casting) is an unrelenting pain that is unrelieved by narcotics. This is one of the 5 Ps that are described later in this chapter. The priority intervention for compartment syndrome is prevention. Prevention is achieved by elevating the extremity to prevent excessive swelling and performing frequent neurovascular checks. When compartment syndrome occurs, notify the health-care provider immediately.

Critical Nursing Action Caring for a Child With a Fracture in a Cast

- Elevate the extremity with the cast on pillows for at least the first 24 hours (Fig. 29-3).
- Avoid indenting the cast.
- Assess the extremity for swelling and discoloration.
- Observe the extremity for sensation and movement.
- Notify a health-care professional immediately if abnormalities are noted.
- Follow activity restrictions.
- Do not allow the affected limb to hang down for any length of time.
- Prevent the child from putting anything inside the cast.
- Keep a clear path for ambulation.
- Ensure the child uses crutches appropriately.
- Encourage rest.
- Encourage good nutrition to promote healing (Table 29-1).
- Encourage quiet activities.
- Ensure child moves joints above and below cast.

Collaboration in Caring—*Caring for a child with a fracture*

- A child life specialist can initiate play to help reduce the anxiety of a child with a fracture. He or she can assist the child with working through fears and frustrations with medical play, art therapy, and distraction.

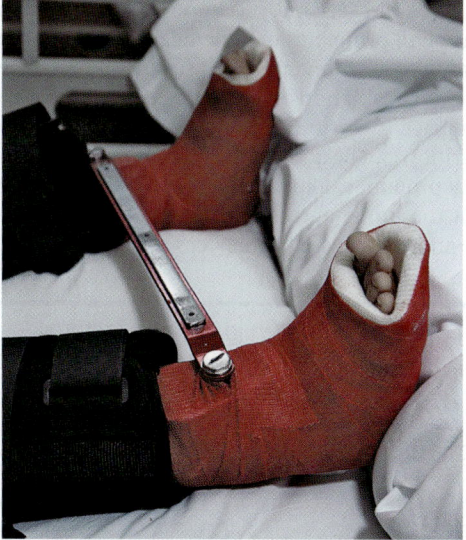

Figure 29-3 A cast is applied to the affected extremity to keep it immobile while healing.

Table 29-1 Daily Nutritional Requirements for Musculoskeletal Health

Nutrient	Toddler	Preschool	School Age	Teen Girl	Teen Boy
Protein	13 g	19 g	34 g	46 g	52 g
Sources and amounts: meat, poultry, and fish (7 g per oz), eggs (6 g), dried beans and peas (8 g per ½ cup), tofu (4 g per ½ cup), milk (8 g per cup), yogurt (11 g per cup), American cheese (6 g per oz)					
Iron	7 mg	10 mg	8 mg	15 mg	11 mg
Sources and amounts: liver (6.7 mg per oz), ground chuck (1 mg per oz), iron-fortified cereal (6 mg per ¼ cup), lentils (1 mg per ½ cup), kidney beans (2.6 mg per ½ cup)					
Calcium	500 mg	800 mg	1,300 mg	1,300 mg	1,300 mg
Sources and amounts: milk (290 mg per cup), yogurt (207 mg per ½ cup), cheddar cheese (204 mg per oz), ice cream (85 mg per ½ cup), spinach (120 mg per ½ cup)					
Vitamin D	200 units	200 units	200 units	200 units	200 units
Sources and amounts: synthesized from skin exposure to ultraviolet light; added to some foods and supplements; salmon (149 units per oz), canned tuna (50 units per oz)					
Vitamin C	15 mg	25 mg	45 mg	65 mg	75 mg
Sources and amounts: orange (70 mg per medium raw), orange juice (63–97 mg per ¾ cup), green pepper (60 mg per ½ cup raw), strawberries (49 mg per ½ cup), kiwi (70 mg each), broccoli (39 mg per ½ cup raw)					

Sources: Data from American Heart Association (AHA) (2013); Institute of Medicine (IOM) (2011).

- Social services personnel may also be available to assist the family on admission to the emergency department and can continue to support the family during the child's hospitalization. At discharge, they can arrange for transportation and identify helpful community resources.
- A schoolteacher or tutor can assist a child who is hospitalized for an extended period of time.
- A physical therapist will ensure that the child is safe while walking with crutches and provide passive and active ROM exercises to the other extremities. Once the cast is removed, the physical therapist will institute exercises to increase muscle strength in the affected extremity.

Education/Discharge Instructions

Discharge teaching helps parents feel more comfortable caring for their child at home. It is important to review the management plan, principles of bone healing, how to perform a neurovascular assessment, and cast care. Parents need to be taught about adaptations to the home environment that need to be in place to ensure the child's safety. Teach the family that nutrition can be addressed by providing a well-balanced diet with protein, calcium, and iron. The physical therapist can visit the home and help the family learn methods for transfer and use of assistive devices at home.

? Case Study The Child With a Fracture Who Has Complications

A 12-year-old child was admitted with a femur fracture. He has a morphine sulfate (Astramorph) patient-controlled analgesia (PCA) that has a dose that is safe and effective. The leg is elevated on two pillows, and ice packs are in place. The nurse performs a neurovascular assessment with the first morning vital signs. During the following hour, the child complains that on the numerical pain scale, the pain is 10 out of 10. The nurse checks the history recorded on the PCA pump and determines the requested number of doses. The neurovascular assessment reveals that the pulse is absent and the extremity is cool and pale. The capillary refill time is greater than 3 seconds (Fig. 29-4) (Box 29-4).

critical thinking questions

1. What is occurring with this child?
2. What does the nurse do first?
3. If this is determined to be compartment syndrome, what will occur?
4. How can the nurse help the child and family during this emergency situation?

◆ See Suggested Answers to Case Studies on Davis*Plus*.

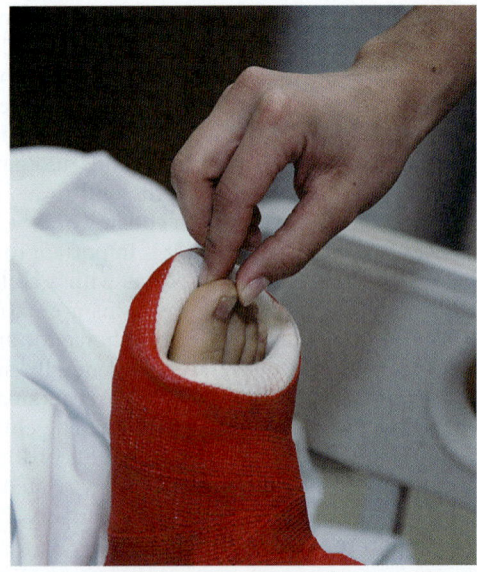

Figure 29-4 The nurse assesses capillary refill time.

Box 29-4 Assessment Tool Classification by Type of Break

TRANSVERSE
Line crosses the shaft at a 90-degree angle

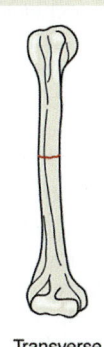

Transverse

SPIRAL
A diagonal line coils around the bone
Caused by a twisting force

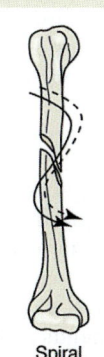

Spiral

OBLIQUE
A diagonal line across the bone

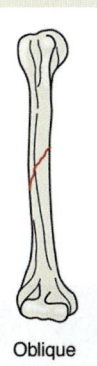

Oblique

GREENSTICK
Bone is bent but not broken
More common in children

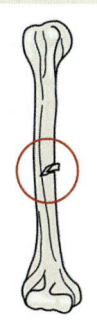

Greenstick

COMMINUTED
Three or more fracture fragments

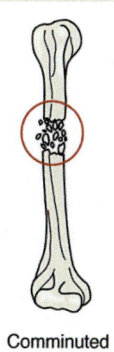

Comminuted

COMPRESSION
Bone becomes wider and more flat
Usually seen in the spine

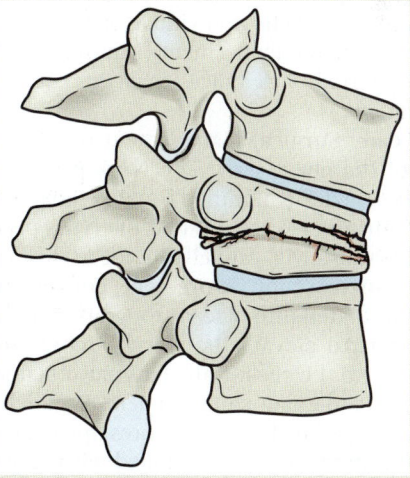

PECTUS EXCAVATUM

Pectus excavatum is a congenital condition consisting of a posterior depression of the sternum and affecting the adjacent costal cartilages. It is the most common congenital deformity of the chest, but the cause is not clearly understood. Infants and young children rarely complain of symptoms that would affect their ability to participate in activities. However, older children and adolescents develop cardiorespiratory symptoms during physical exercise.

Signs and Symptoms

Signs and symptoms of pectus excavatum can include:

- Sunken chest wall at the sternum
- Fatigue
- Shortness of breath
- Chest pain
- Tachycardia

Some children only present with the sunken chest wall as a symptom.

Diagnosis

A chest radiograph, pulmonary function test, CT scan of the chest, stress test, laboratory studies such as chromosome or enzyme studies, electrocardiogram, and an echocardiogram are used to make the diagnosis.

Prevention

Because it is a congenital deformity, there are no known preventive measures.

Collaborative Care

Nursing Care. Nursing care is supported with physical therapy. Mild or moderate cases are treated with an exercise and posture program with follow-up every 6 to 12 months. A posture program teaches individuals about proper posture and body alignment enhancement (National Posture Institute, 2014). Fitted back braces may be required for the pediatric patient.

Surgical Care. Surgical management involves a reconstruction of the chest wall. The Nuss procedure or an open repair called the modified Ravitch technique is typically used for severe cases. When the Nuss procedure is performed, a substernal tunnel anterior to the heart is created using thoracoscopy. A pre-bent, convex steel bar is inserted and rotated into place through the thoracoscope. Its function is to elevate the sternal depression and is fixed securely to the chest wall. This bar remains in place for 2 to 3 years to ensure a permanent remodeling of the sternum. The open technique requires open chest surgery in which the sternum is repositioned with an osteotomy and the costal cartilage is reformed as well. A wire or a strut is placed under the sternum to keep it in place (Frantz, 2011).

Postoperative care of the orthopedic pediatric patient includes assessment of vital signs, pain, monitoring of surgical site, return of bowel sounds, and postoperative voiding. Postoperatively, advance the diet as tolerated according to age. Administer pain medications and use diversional activities as a useful method for nonpharmacological pain relief.

 Nursing Insight—*Preventing pneumonia*

Respiratory care includes assessment and methods to increase lung expansion to prevent pneumonia. An incentive spirometer is used for the school-age and adolescent child (Fig. 29-5). Younger children are not able to understand how to use the incentive spirometer but use creative measures to encourage expansion of the lungs (e.g., blowing a pinwheel, bubbles, a musical instrument, or a small folded paper triangle across the bedside table).

Education/Discharge Instructions

Discharge teaching includes how to care for the child after discharge such as assessing for signs and symptoms of infection that would require the parent to notify the health-care provider. Discuss when the child should return to the health-care provider for follow-up.

POLYDACTYLY/SYNDACTYLY

Polydactyly is defined as a condition in which the child has more than the normal number of fingers or toes. Syndactyly is defined as the fusion of one or more fingers or toes. This condition could be a result of a congenital disorder or a result of a severe burn injury where scarring fused the two phalanges together.

Signs and Symptoms

In polydactyly, there are six or more fingers or toes on the hand or foot. It can occur on one or both hands and/or one or both feet. In syndactyly, two or more phalanges of the fingers or toes are fused together. The fused bones appear as one digit with an extra-wide nail and finger or toe. It can occur on one or both hands and/or one or both feet. It can occur as a result of a congenital deformity or as a result of a burn injury where the bones of the fingers or toes have fused together.

Diagnosis

Diagnosis is made by visualization of the digits.

Prevention

Prevention of polydactyly is not achievable because it is a congenital defect. However, if it occurred as a result of

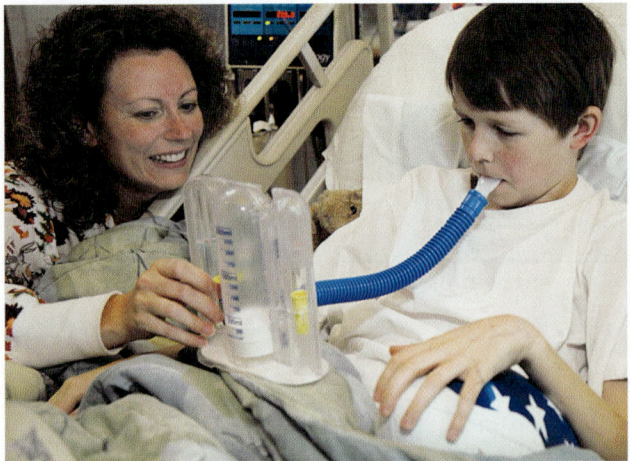

Figure 29-5 Blowing into incentive spirometer helps expand the lungs and prevent pneumonia.

a burn injury, preventing the burn injury would prevent the defect.

Collaborative Care

Nursing Care. Offer parents support until a decision is made about corrective surgery. If the decision is made to not repair the defect with surgery, the child will live with the defect. The child is adaptable and may adjust to the deformity without difficulty, or ongoing support may need to be continued through counseling.

Surgical Care. Treatment is to surgically remove the extra finger or toe. The procedure is performed by a hand surgeon (with reconstructive surgery background) or an orthopedic surgeon (Venes, 2013). The surgery for syndactyly is more complex than surgery for polydactyly. The skin, muscles, nerves, tendons, ligaments, blood vessels, and the bones must be separated. Sometimes the bones are shorter, so the surgeon will perform an osteotomy and place a distractor. The distractor consists of pins that are placed in the two bone fragments. A wire is passed through connections at the end of each of the pins. Once the callus has started to form, the health-care provider turns the device so that the two bone fragments are distracted from each other. Usually a quarter of a turn with an Allen wrench is done twice per week. After about 6 weeks, the desired length has been achieved and the device and wires can be removed under anesthesia. Skin grafts are placed at the time of the initial surgery to close the wound where there is a shortage of skin. Standard postoperative care is provided with special attention to the surgical area and graft site if applicable.

Education/Discharge Instructions

Discharge teaching helps parents feel more comfortable caring for their child at home. It is important to review the management plan, principles of bone healing, how to perform a neurovascular assessment, and how to care for the Kirschner wires (K-wires) using pin care techniques.

DISLOCATED RADIAL HEAD

Dislocated radial head is a form of dislocation. The head of the radius slips and becomes dislocated as a result of an injury. As with all other dislocations, it is a complete separation of the bone from the articular surfaces of the joint. Subluxation is only a partial displacement of the joint. The most frequent sites of dislocation or subluxation are the thumb, elbow, shoulder, wrist, finger, knee, and hip. If the dislocation is a result of trauma, damage to blood vessels, nerves, ligaments, and soft tissue surrounding the joint can occur. Neurovascular compromise can occur to the extremity distal to the injury. There is a genetic predisposition to dislocation such as a child with **Marfan's syndrome** (a hereditary degenerative disorder of connective tissue, bones, muscles, and ligaments).

Signs and Symptoms

Signs and symptoms of dislocated radial head include:

- Severe pain
- Inability to move the affected limb
- Abnormal contour of the joint
- Bruising at the joint

Diagnosis

Diagnosis is made by a radiograph of the affected area.

Prevention

Prevention can occur by avoidance of the injury that would cause the dislocated radial head.

Collaborative Care

Nursing Care. It is important to obtain an accurate history regarding the details of the injury from the child and the caregiver. Time of injury as well as the description, angle of force, and the child's immediate sensations will aid in the management of the injury. It is also important to obtain information about any previous dislocation or subluxation injuries.

Medical Care. In a mild case, the affected area is stabilized in a splint for 10 to 14 days. After that, intense active ROM is used to regain full use of the extremity.

Surgical Care. Surgery consists of an open reduction and internal fixation to stabilize the fracture or dislocation. Bone grafting from the iliac crest may be necessary to connect the head fragment to the radial shaft. Monitor the neurovascular status frequently after the injury and after the reduction or intervention. Ensure that the child maintains proper positioning of the extremity (Sommers & Brunner, 2011).

Education/Discharge Instructions

Review the management plan, principles of bone healing, how to perform a neurovascular assessment, and care of the suture line.

SOFT TISSUE INJURIES

Soft tissue injuries (sprains and strains) are unusual in young children. These injuries are more often seen in the adolescent age group. The growth plate of the epiphysis is weaker than the ligaments in younger children because of the new bone formation and is prone to fracture rather than sprains or strains. With puberty, skeletal growth declines, and the growth plates begin to close. The growth plates become less susceptible to injury, and the ligaments and tendons become more susceptible to injury. The ankle is the most frequently sprained or strained joint. The prognosis is good for first- and second-degree sprains. Severe sprains (third-degree) have an increased risk of recurrent injury, persistent instability, and traumatic arthritis.

Signs and Symptoms

Sprain and strain share some signs and symptoms, but it is important to differentiate the two. Signs and symptoms of sprain include:

- Pain
- Swelling
- Bruising
- Instability
- Loss of the ability to move and use the joint

Signs and symptoms of strain include:

- Pain
- Limited motion
- Muscle spasms
- Muscle weakness

- Swelling
- Cramping
- Inflammation

Diagnosis

A history is obtained from the child and the parents. The history and a physical exam reveal important information about the injury, swelling, and local hemorrhage at the injury site. The child's most painful area is examined last. An x-ray exam is performed if there is an obvious fracture or misalignment.

 Assessment Tool Sprains Are Classified According to Severity

First Degree
Mild; ligament is stretched and the affected joint is stable
Minimal pain, swelling, ecchymosis
Full ROM and weight bearing

Second Degree
Moderate; ligament is partially torn and joint laxity is present
Moderate pain, swelling, ecchymosis
Motion is slightly limited and painful
Mild joint laxity with tenderness over the joint
Inability to bear weight

Third Degree
Severe; ligament is completely torn and joint is unstable
Significant swelling and severe ecchymosis occurs within the first 30 minutes
Severe pain over the joint makes examination difficult
Cannot bear weight or otherwise use the extremity

Prevention

Because a sprain is the result of an accident, preventing the accident would prevent the initial injury. Pre- and post-workout stretching will help to keep joints pliable. After healing the initial injury, prevention of a reinjury is the most effective. Using a number of techniques such as the prophylactic use of an ankle brace and physical therapy for stretching and strengthening exercises will strengthen the joint.

Collaborative Care

Nursing Care. Immediately after the initial injury, it is most important to use the RICE acronym (Fig. 29-6):

R—Rest; resting the injured extremity prevents further injury and allows the ligament to heal

I—Ice; ice for the first 48 hours, keep ice packs in place for 15-minute intervals to decrease swelling

C—Compression; apply an Ace wrap or some other method to apply pressure to the affected joint to help reduce swelling

E—Elevation and early motion of the affected joint; elevation reduces swelling and early motion of the affected joint helps keep the full ROM

Medical Care. Immobilization of the joint is recommended based on the severity of the injury. Mild sprains are immobilized with external support with an elastic bandage, brace, or ankle lacer. Moderate sprains require a posterior splint or cast for 2 to 3 weeks in conjunction with crutches. Severe sprains require conservative or surgical management with a cast for 4 to 6 weeks and no weight-bearing activities. Early motion after the injury, with gentle stretching and a strengthening program, speeds recovery.

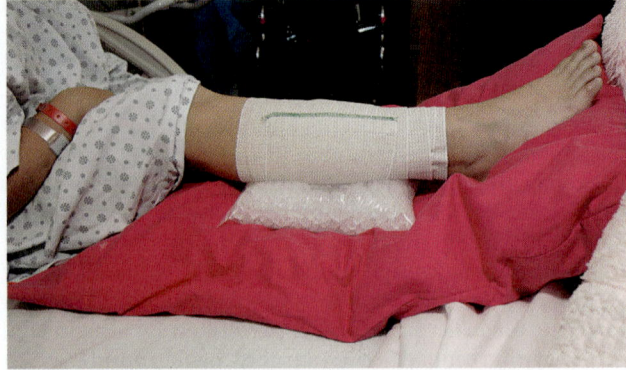

Figure 29-6 The nurse uses the "RICE" acronym.

Collaboration with the physical therapist is necessary in caring for the child with a soft tissue injury. The physical therapist teaches the patient quadriceps and hamstring exercises, an ROM program for ankle injuries, and crutch walking. To prevent nerve damage, the physical therapist ensures that the patient bears weight on his or her hands, not the axillae.

Education/Discharge Instructions

The nurse has an important role in teaching home care for the child with a soft tissue injury. Teach the proper technique for wrapping the affected joint and ensure that it is followed. Communicate to the caregiver that it is important to start wrapping the area distally and work up to the proximal area beyond the level of the injury. The child needs a physical activity restrictions school note for the physical education teacher and coach. If the child has a mild sprain, sports activities can be resumed in 2 to 3 weeks. If the child has a moderate sprain, the child can participate in partial weight-bearing activities using crutches and return to full weight-bearing and sports activities gradually. If the child has a severe sprain, sports activities can be resumed in approximately 4 to 8 weeks.

SPORTS INJURIES

One-half of boys and one-quarter of girls ages 8 to 16 participate in competitive sports. Sports injuries occur as a result of these competitive sports in three-quarters of all middle and high schools in the United States. Subsequently, the increase in popularity of competitive sports, recreational sports, and cheerleading has significantly increased the number of overuse injuries, sprains, strains, and dislocations. The causes of these injuries may be a result of inadequate health physicals, hazardous practice and play areas, training and practice errors, improper safety equipment, improper nutrition, overtiredness, and a limited awareness or concern for the possible risk factors. Sports injury may involve fractures, sprains, and strains as well as knee and elbow injuries.

A child who participates in sports in which the legs are being used, such as skiing, soccer, football, or track, is at risk for a knee injury such as a tear in the anterior cruciate ligament (ACL). The injury occurs when the ACL is stretched or torn during a sudden twisting motion when the feet stay planted one way and the knee turns the opposite way.

A child who participates in sports in which the arms are being used, such as baseball, basketball, or tennis, is at risk for an elbow injury. This injury is commonly known as "Little Leaguer's elbow." This sport injury involves a repetitive forward motion of the arm, and the child is not able to extend the elbow fully. This is because of injury to the muscle consisting of tiny tears and contractures.

Signs and Symptoms

A ruptured or torn ACL causes:

- Instability and pain in the knee

  In an elbow injury, signs and symptoms are:

- Pain and tenderness
- Loss of full extension of the elbow (24 to 48 hours after the injury)

Diagnosis

Diagnosis of a sports injury is based on an x-ray exam followed by an MRI.

Prevention

Because sports injuries are the result of an accident, preventing the accident while participating in a particular sport would prevent the injury. Pre- and post-workout stretching will help to keep joints, muscles, tendons, and ligaments pliable.

Collaborative Care

Nursing Care. Management for a knee injury depends on whether the injury is mild or severe and whether there was a twisting action involved in the injury. A mild injury is treated with rest and ice. A topical anesthetic is applied locally to minimize pain, and oral pain medication can be given. After 24 hours, heat is applied, which aids in healing.

Medical Care. If the injury is more severe and the knee joint fills with fluid, a physician will aspirate the excess synovial fluid. A cast may need to be applied to completely immobilize the joint. It takes the same length of time for a severe ligament injury to heal as a bone; therefore, the cast remains in place for about 8 weeks.

If the injury involved a severe twisting motion, the kneecap may be dislocated (slips around to the posterior side of the knee). The knee appears deformed and a healthcare provider slides the kneecap back into place immediately. The child is placed in a leg immobilizer for about a week. If this type of injury occurs frequently, surgery on the ligaments is necessary. Quadriceps exercises, which consist of straight leg–raising exercises, help prevent a kneecap dislocation from occurring again.

For an elbow injury, exercises to strengthen the flexor muscles help prevent further injury. Children need extra protection against injury to the epiphyseal plates until they have fused (between the ages of 14 and 17 years of age). To prevent elbow injuries, children who participate in ball sports need time to warm up. Pitching breaking balls and curve balls is discouraged. Pitching is also limited to six innings per week with a 3-day rest period between games. Management of the "Little Leaguer's elbow" consists of applying ice for 15 minutes three times per day. Administering an anti-inflammatory agent may help the child be comfortable. Cortisone injections into the

joint can also be helpful, but only a limited number can be used. Management for a more severe case consists of rest and immobilization of the elbow until pain, tenderness, and limited movement disappear. Permanent damage to the epiphyseal line and an elbow deformity can be the result of this injury.

Surgical Care. An arthroscopy is performed to examine the joint and repair torn ligaments or cartilage with an arthroscope. This method is a minimally invasive surgical procedure on a joint. Small incisions are made so the joint is not opened up fully. The recovery time is significantly reduced because this type of procedure lessens trauma to the connective tissue. Scarring is also reduced because of the small incisions.

Education/Discharge Instructions

Review the management plan, principles of healing, how to perform a neurovascular assessment, and care of the suture line. If a joint is immobilized, instruct the patient and family on how to care for the patient with the immobilizer and any special instructions on the use of the immobilizer. Maintaining the extremity in an elevated position is also an important instruction.

OSGOOD-SCHLATTER DISEASE

Osgood-Schlatter disease is a common cause of knee pain (Fig. 29-7). It is a problem of overuse in active older school-age children or adolescents. It is more prevalent in boys and occurs in boys between the ages of 12 and 15 years and in girls between the ages of 10 and 12 years (Weiler, Ingram, & Wolman, 2011).

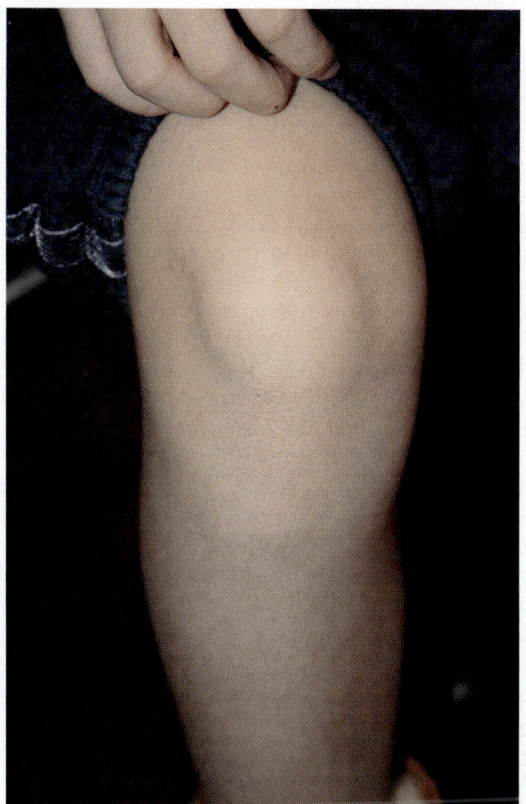

Figure 29-7 Osgood-Schlatter "bump."

It is an irritation of the patellar ligament at the tibial tuberosity. It is caused by a repetitive injury resulting in inflammation and small avulsions (tearing away) of the bone. The cycle continues with new bone forming each time the injury and the body attempts to heal (Weiler et al., Ingram, & Wolman, 2011). Osgood-Schlatter disease does not result in long-term complications, and the prognosis is good. Sports activity does not have to be eliminated but must be reduced enough to control the pain. When pain is tolerable a gradual increase in exercise may occur but must be titrated to a level that is tolerable for the child. Occasionally, in severe cases, pain in the knees during running or jumping can continue to occur for many years later.

Signs and Symptoms

Signs and symptoms of Osgood-Schlatter disease include:

- Pain below the kneecap that is aggravated by activity and relieved by rest
- The child experiences pain when asked to squat or extend the knee against resistance
- Symptoms resolve around the time skeletal growth ceases (about puberty)

Diagnosis

A radiograph of the knee is performed to rule out a tumor. History and the presenting symptoms assist in making this diagnosis.

Prevention

This occurs in the "right child" (usually a genetic pattern) at the "right age" (usually pre-adolescence and just before a big growth spurt) doing the "right activity" (usually involves running or jumping). Because it is genetic in origin and strikes pre-adolescents, it is not possible to prevent the disease. However, early recognition can help minimize the severity of the disease.

Collaborative Care

Nursing Care. Pain management is an important nursing action for a child with Osgood-Schlatter disease. The pain medication of choice is an NSAID. The knee is iced after exercising. An elastic wrap or neoprene sleeve over the knee during activity also helps to relieve the pain.

Medical Care. After radiographic study is performed, conservative management is continued such as rest and ice to the knee. Nierenberg, Falah, Keren, and Eidelman (2012) developed an algorithm for treating Osgood-Schlatter disease. Initially, tibial tuberosity pain is treated with conservative medical therapy.

Surgical Care. Generally these children can be treated effectively without surgery. However, when pain continues over the tibial tubercle, a painful ossicle has formed. The surgery is performed after the child has reached bone maturity to avoid damage to the epiphyseal plate (Weiler et al., 2011). A radiograph shows the ossicle and an **apophysis** (an offshoot or projection especially from a bone) is performed, which consists of the excision and trimming of the apophysis.

Education/Discharge Instructions

Teach the family about activity limitations. Provide support by helping the child cope with the restrictions on activities and social interactions. The nurse collaborates with the physical therapist to teach the child exercises to strengthen the upper body. The physical therapist also teaches the child to perform lower extremity isometrics. These exercises help the child maintain strength while the injured knee heals. Once the symptoms improve, the child returns to normal activities.

TORTICOLLIS

Torticollis ("twisted neck") is characterized by a stiff neck causing a lateral flexion contracture of the cervical spine musculature. It can be congenital or acquired. Congenital torticollis is a fibrosis of the sternocleidomastoid muscle that rotates the newborn's head to the opposite side, becoming evident during the first 2 weeks after birth. Babies may develop positional plagiocephaly (asymmetrical head shape) or frontal bulging. Spinal misalignment can lead to other orthopedic problems. Spasmodic torticollis has recurrent and transient spasms. Delayed development can occur because the child is unable to turn its head to see, hear, and touch.

Signs and Symptoms

Signs and symptoms of torticollis include:

- Twisted neck
- Spasmodic torticollis has recurrent and transient spasms

Diagnosis

Diagnosis is made beginning with assessing the development of the infant. Next an examination is performed with special attention to the neurological and eye assessments. Radiographs and an MRI scan of the spinal cord and brainstem will usually be performed if there are developmental delays noted or there is no known cause of the torticollis.

Prevention

There are no preventive measures for congenital torticollis.

Collaborative Care

Nursing Care. Nursing care is supportive to physical therapy. Provide support through teaching and ensuring that the parents understand the treatment measures and prescribed exercises.

Medical Care. The main medical management is physical therapy. Treatment with botulinum toxin (Botox) also has been effective in inhibiting the spasms of the muscle (Venes, 2013).

Surgical Care. Surgery has been effective by dividing the sternocleidomastoid muscle (Venes, 2013). Nursing care for the child undergoing surgery is to provide the typical pre- and postoperative care, including monitoring of vital signs, care of the suture line, and assessing for the return of bowel sounds and postoperative voiding. Advance the diet to the appropriate food choices for the child's age. Administer pain medication and use diversional activities for nonpharmacological pain control.

Education/Discharge Instructions

Inform the family that physical therapists perform interventions to strengthen muscles, correct imbalances, increase cervical spine ROM, and increase posture. Active stretching, positioning strategies, functional play, and neurodevelopmental interventions are used to treat this disorder (Mayer, 2012).

OSTEOMYELITIS

Osteomyelitis is an infection of the bone and the tissues around the bone and needs immediate treatment. It occurs most commonly in healthy children. It can cause massive destruction of bone, sepsis, and possibly death. Osteomyelitis often involves the long bones in the lower extremities in children, but it can involve any other bone in the body.

Although many bacteria can cause osteomyelitis, the most common bacteria is *Staphylococcus aureus*. Bacteria lodge and multiply in the middle of the bone where circulation is sluggish. The infection spreads to the ends of the bones and can destroy the epiphyseal plate in children. The inflammatory process produces pus, edema, and vascular congestion in the area of infection (Fig. 29-8A–C). Pressure in the bone increases and eventually cuts off the blood supply, causing necrosis. The body attempts to lay down new bone over the necrotic bone. The prognosis is good if the osteomyelitis is treated promptly with IV antibiotics. However, when the infection weakens the bones, pathological fractures can develop.

 Nursing Insight—*Osteomyelitis*

The following can cause acute osteomyelitis:
- An open fracture
- Penetration of the skin by a contaminated object
- A septic joint
- An infected wound
- Bacterial infection from somewhere else in body, like dental caries
- Blunt trauma

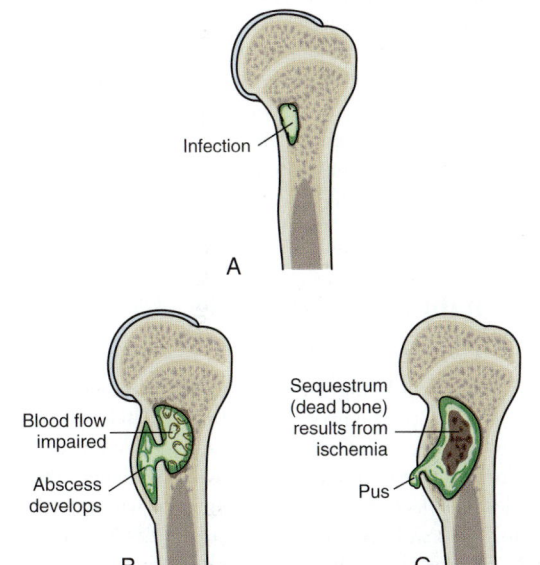

Figure 29-8 Sequence of osteomyelitis development. *A*, Infection begins. *B*, Blood flow is blocked in the arc of infection, and an abscess with pus forms. *C*, Bone dies within the infection site, and pus continues to form.

Signs and Symptoms

Signs and symptoms of osteomyelitis include:
- Pain in the affected bone
- Fever
- Irritability
- Guarding the affected limb
- Localized tenderness, redness, warmth, and pain on palpation
- Occasionally, soft tissue swelling around the area

Diagnosis

Osteomyelitis is suspected when the child presents with the signs and symptoms. The child's history may reveal a fall or bumping of the affected extremity. History also reveals a recent infection such as a cold or otitis media. Radiographic exam and a bone scan confirm the diagnosis. Blood cultures help determine the causative bacteria.

Prevention

Osteomyelitis can be prevented by ensuring that a wound that may be deep enough to allow bacteria to come in contact with a bone or joint is treated with sufficient antibiotics so that it does not spread to the bone or joint.

Collaborative Care

Nursing Care. The main nursing care for osteomyelitis is to administer a course of broad-spectrum antibiotics. Antibiotics are begun after blood cultures are drawn. The exact antibiotic prescribed will depend on the causative bacteria. The child is hospitalized while on antibiotic therapy. It is important to evaluate the child's response to the antibiotic therapy about 2 or 3 days after the initial dose. If the child demonstrates a good response to the IV antibiotic therapy, more blood cultures are drawn, IV antibiotics are stopped, and the child continues therapy on oral antibiotics for 4 to 8 weeks at home.

Medical Care. If the child demonstrates poor response to the IV antibiotic therapy, antibiotic therapy is continued for a much longer period. Monitor laboratory values such as the erythrocyte sedimentation rate (ESR). This lab study is a good indication of whether the infection is resolving. As the infection resolves, the ESR decreases to normal. Palliative measures such as rest, oral pain medication, good

Where Research and Practice Meet:
Staphylococcus Aureus (SA) Osteomyelitis

A study done by Belthur, Birchansky, Verdugo, Mason, Hulten, Kaplan, et al. (2012) evaluated the risk factors for pathological factors in children with *Staphylococcus aureus* (SA) osteomyelitis. They compared 17 children who were treated for a pathological fracture as a result of SA osteomyelitis with a group of 49 children who had SA osteomyelitis without any pathological fractures. Most of the children with pathological fractures had methicillin-resistant Staphylococcus aureus while only 2 had methicillin-sensitive Staphylococcus aureus. They also discovered that children with the fractures had a more complex infection and inflammatory response; the fractures may have been in response to the infection and inflammatory response.

nutrition, and diversional activities can also help the child tolerate the lengthy hospitalization.

Surgical Care. Surgical management for osteomyelitis usually requires surgery for debridement and temporary stabilization of the bone with a **Kirschner wire** (**K-wire**), which is a steel wire placed through a long bone to apply traction to the bone, with an antibiotic implanted in the bone cement. Further surgery is performed to reconstruct the bone using a distractor and an external fixator (Baumbach, Hobolm, & Wozasek, 2011).

Postoperative nursing care includes monitoring vital signs, pain, effect of pain medication, surgical wound, pin care if necessary, return of bowel sounds, and postoperative voiding as well as advancing diet to appropriate diet for age. Using distraction techniques are good nonpharmacological pain relief techniques. This child receives IV antibiotics. Insertion of a peripherally inserted central catheter (PICC) line is usually needed. This will allow the child to be discharged home with a visiting nurse and home infusion therapy service. Collaborate with the case manager to coordinate these services. If the child is not full–weight bearing, then physical therapy will also be involved to ensure that the child is able to safely ambulate with crutches or a pediatric walker.

Education/Discharge Instructions

The nurse has an important role in teaching home care for the child with osteomyelitis. The child may be discharged on a regimen of home IV antibiotics. Teach parents about the importance of antibiotic compliance because this requires a sustained commitment from the family. Antibiotics that can be scheduled every 8 to 12 hours may have a better compliance rate than more frequently scheduled antibiotics. The child may return to school if the antibiotics are on a 12-hour schedule. A home school teacher or tutor is needed if the antibiotics are scheduled more frequently.

 Nursing Insight—*Chronic osteomyelitis*

Chronic osteomyelitis is uncommon and occurs when bone tissue dies as a result of the lost blood supply. The frequency of chronic osteomyelitis has diminished because of an increased awareness of the need for prompt, aggressive treatment. The management for chronic osteomyelitis is prolonged, painful, and frustrating for the child and family. Pain control is an important nursing action for the child with chronic osteomyelitis. It is important to make the child as comfortable as possible. For the first few days of hospitalization, the affected limb is placed in a splint. Oral analgesics, including acetaminophen (Children's Tylenol), ibuprofen (Children's Motrin), or narcotic analgesics such as acetaminophen with codeine (Percocet) can be used to manage pain. The IV site is monitored for infiltration because the antibiotics used to treat osteomyelitis are caustic to the veins. A PICC or tunneled central line is placed if IV therapy continues for more than 2 to 3 days. Diversional activities are employed while the child is in the hospital and at home, while activity is limited.

 Now Can You—**Discuss various musculoskeletal conditions?**

1. Describe the signs and symptoms of various musculoskeletal conditions?
2. Describe the holistic nursing care measures for a child with various musculoskeletal conditions?

JUVENILE ARTHRITIS

Juvenile arthritis is an autoimmune inflammatory process with unknown origin but is thought to be triggered by an infection. Peak onset occurs in two different age groups (between 1 and 3 years of age and between 8 and 12 years of age). Females are affected twice as frequently as males. Symptoms can range from very mild to very severe. Juvenile arthritis is not a childhood version of rheumatoid arthritis. The prognosis of juvenile arthritis is considered good. Success related to how the child and family cope with the condition is based on how well the child meets developmental milestones. If juvenile arthritis occurs in a younger child, growth retardation is more likely to occur.

The child with juvenile arthritis has a pattern of remissions and exacerbations. The prognosis for children with juvenile arthritis is that 60% to 70% will have remissions. Approximately 45% will still have active disease 10 years after diagnosis, which results in disability in adulthood. Three different types are described in Table 29-2.

 Nursing Insight—*Human leukocyte antigens (HLAs)*

Human leukocyte antigens (**HLAs**) (any of the multiple antigens on all nucleated cells in the body that identify the cells as "self") play a role in juvenile arthritis. There is chronic inflammation of the synovial membrane with effusion and destruction of the articular cartilage. Immune complexes in the blood and synovial tissue initiate the inflammatory response by activating the plasma protein complement. Excessive fluid is produced that is watery, thin, and lacks mucin. The synovium swells, and thickened villi and nodules protrude into the joint cavity. A restriction in the joint capsule and ligaments leads to a decreased joint movement and tendonitis. **Ankylosis** (adhesions causing immobility in the joint) also develops between joint surfaces, which can further limit joint mobility.

 Collaboration in Caring—*Adolescents living with juvenile arthritis*

The adolescent living with juvenile arthritis faces many challenges. Because juvenile arthritis is a lifelong illness, Secor-Turner, Scal, Garwick, Horvath, and Wells (2011) performed research to determine what challenges these adolescents face. They used focus groups with adolescents (14–21 years of age) and young adults (22–29 years of age). The results of the study identified five areas that presented challenges to adolescents. These challenges are identified as:

- Health care
- Relationships

Table 29-2 Types of Juvenile Arthritis

	Polyarticular	Oligoarthritis	Systemic Onset
Number of Joints Involved	Five or more	Four or fewer	Any number
Joints Affected	Usually small joints of fingers and hands Weight-bearing joints Same joint on both sides	Usually large joints, knees, ankle, elbow Usually particular joint on one side of body	Any joint
Sex Affected	Girls more than boys	Girls more than boys (most common type)	Boys and girls equally
Body Temperature	Low-grade fever	Low-grade fever	High spiking fever lasting for weeks or months
Other Symptoms	Stiffness and minimal joint swelling Rheumatoid nodules on elbow or other body area receiving pressure from chairs, shoes Rheumatoid factor in 20% of cases ANA titer is possible Elevated WBC, complement, and erythrocyte sedimentation rate	Iridocyclitis (eye inflammation) Painless joint swelling with little redness ANA titer (possible) HLA antigen (possible in boys)	Macular rash on chest, thighs Inflammation of heart and lungs Anemia Enlarged lymph nodes, liver, and spleen Rarely rheumatoid factor and ANA titer Elevated WBC

- School
- Physical
- Individual

Health-care challenges relate to the management of the medications on a daily basis. The issues included taking the medications, finding medications that were effective, cost of the medications, and concerns about understanding insurance particularly with regard to coverage for the medications. This also progressed as the adolescent or young adult became able to become independent in managing their arthritis and health care.

Relationship challenges focused on disclosing the disease and people not understanding what the adolescent was going through with the disease. They expressed the inability to explain the disease process. The young adults faced similar issues: when to tell, or not.

School challenges had to do with playing sports, participating in physical education classes, getting schoolwork done on time, and talking to their teachers about their arthritis. Young adults faced similar challenges. Pain and exercising were the major factors affecting physical challenges in both age groups. Also noted was that chronic pain had an effect on mental health as well as the physical health.

Adolescents did not identify individual challenges, but young adults described the feeling of being different from their peers and having to miss activities that their peers were doing. Conclusions from this study identify the need to create transitional programs that will assist these adolescents to cope with the challenges that they are facing and be able to become more independent as a young adult. Nurses can assist these adolescents by referring them to the Arthritis Foundation and making referrals for home care needs. The school nurse is a part of the team to assist the adolescent in meeting these challenges. The school nurse can assist the adolescent in dealing with physical limitations and with strategizing how to inform teachers of the adolescent's limitations.

Signs and Symptoms

Signs and symptoms of juvenile arthritis include:

- Joints that are swollen, tender, and warm to touch
- Joints that are stiff and have loss of motion, especially in the morning
- Limited ROM

Systemic signs and symptoms include:

- Malaise
- Fatigue
- Lethargy
- Late afternoon fever with a temperature spike up to 105.1°F (40.6°C)

Diagnosis

There is no actual test for juvenile arthritis; therefore, diagnosing juvenile arthritis is difficult. The diagnosis is made by excluding other conditions that may cause similar symptoms or other possible causes such as viral infections. Any child with joint swelling or pain that has lasted longer than 6 weeks is assessed for possible juvenile arthritis. The child protects the affected joint and may even refuse to walk if the joint is a weight-bearing joint. The child may also have a rash.

The white blood count (WBC) and ESR are important laboratory values to monitor. The character, frequency, and severity of systemic and **articular** (joint capsule) manifestations are critical factors in diagnosing juvenile arthritis. Radiographs or bone scans to detect changes in bones and joints are used in diagnosis.

Prevention

Because the onset of the disease is not clearly understood, there are no known preventive measures that can be taken.

Collaborative Care

Nursing Care. Nursing care is supportive and includes pain management. If the child is hospitalized, monitor the child's vital signs, pain and effectiveness of pain medication, and response to any therapies. Using distraction techniques is also an effective nonpharmacological pain relief measure. Encouraging the child to maintain and continue development is an important nursing role. Collaboration with Child Life Services is a key nursing intervention.

Optimizing Outcomes—Prevent injury and long-term disability

The best outcomes for the child with juvenile arthritis are to prevent injury and long-term disability.

Medical Care. Medications are a key factor in the management of the child with juvenile arthritis (Box 29-5).

Medical management is supportive. Application of heat and passive and active ROM exercises will help to keep the child with juvenile arthritis as active as possible. Physical therapy will play an important role in the care of these children.

Surgical Care. Surgery is generally not indicated for children with juvenile arthritis. When surgery is indicated it is usually for a joint replacement surgery. Postoperative nursing interventions include monitoring vital signs, caring for the suture line, and assessing for the return of bowel sounds and postoperative voiding. Monitor fluid status as well as advance the diet as appropriate for the child's age. Administer pain medication and use diversional activities for nonpharmacological pain control.

Education/Discharge Instructions

Juvenile arthritis requires teaching the child and family about the disease and proper care. Teach caregivers how to assess the child's joints for warmth, tenderness, pain, and limitations in ROM. The family must be alert for increasing irritability, guarding, and refusal to bear weight and take action by encouraging rest. Help parents learn proper positioning of the inflamed joints and the appropriate application of heat or cold. A physical therapist can design an exercise program with isometric exercises and passive ROM. Part of home care also includes the need for a diet high in fiber,

---

Box 29-5 Medications for Juvenile Arthritis

- NSAIDs (nonsteroidal anti-inflammatory drugs). Only a few NSAIDs have been approved for use with juvenile arthritis. The approved NSAIDs are:
  - ibuprofen (Children's Advil): Safe dose range 30–50 mg/kg/day in 3–4 divided doses per day with a maximum dose of 2.4 g/day for children 6 months to 12 years. Safe dose range 400–800 mg 3–4 times daily with a maximum dose of 3,600 mg/day for children older than 12 years.
  - naproxen (Aleve): Safe dose range is 10–15 mg/kg/dose every 12 hours with a maximum dose of 1,000 mg/day in children over 2 years of age. Safe dose range of 250–500 mg twice daily with a maximum of 1.5 g/day for adults.
  - tolmetin (Tolectin): Safe dose range is 20 mg/kg/day in 3–4 divided doses initially, followed by a maintenance dose of 15–30 mg/kg/day in 3–4 divided doses. Safe dose range is 400 mg three times per day initially, followed by a maintenance dose of 600–1,800 mg/day in 3–4 divided doses with a maximum dose of 2,000 mg/day.
  - choline magnesium trisalicylate (Trilisate): Safe dose range is 30–60 mg/kg/day in 3–4 divided doses for children. Safe dose range is 3 g/day at bedtime or in 2–3 divided doses.
  - indomethacin (Indocin): Safe dose range is 1–2 mg/kg/day in 2–4 divided doses with a maximum of 4 mg/kg/day in children greater than 2 years. Safe dose range is 25–50 mg 2–4 times daily in adults.
  - diclofenac (Cataflam): Safe dose range is 50 mg 3–4 times daily for adults
- If an NSAID is selected, it is usually chosen based on dosing schedule, patient preference, or medication taste because there is a lack of agreement on the best NSAID for patients with juvenile arthritis.
- Disease-modifying antirheumatic drugs (DMARDs) are agents that prevent or relieve rheumatism. Some of the more commonly used DMARDs are:
  - methotrexate (Rheumatrex): Safe dose range is 10 mg/m^2 once weekly, initially and may be increased to 20–30 mg/m^2 in children. Safe dose range is 7.5 mg weekly, maximum dose of 20 mg/week and is decreased when a response occurs. It is effective in polyarticular JA and has been used for the past 10 years. The most common side effect of methotrexate (Rheumatrex) is gastrointestinal symptoms.
  - cyclophosphamide (Cytoxan): Safe dose for PO induction is 2–8 mg/kg/day in divided doses for 6 days or longer. Maintenance of 2–5 mg/kg twice weekly in children. Safe dose for PO is 1–5 mg/kg/day for adults.
  - sulfasalazine (Azulfidine): Safe dose range is 30–50 mg/kg/day in 2 divided doses. Initiate therapy at 1/4–1/3 of planned maintenance dose

and increase every 7 days until maintenance dose is reached. Not to exceed 2 g/day in children 6 years or older. Safe dose is 500 mg–1 g/day for 1 week then increase by 500 mg/day every week up to 2 g/day in 2 divided doses. If no benefit, then increase to 3 g/day in 2 divided doses for adults.
  - infliximab (Remicade): Safe dose range is 3 mg/kg followed by 3 mg/kg 2 and 6 weeks after initial dose and then every 8 weeks. May be adjusted up to 10 mg/kg if partial response in adults. May be used with methotrexate (Rheumatrex).
- New drugs potentially available for use with juvenile arthritis are:
  - leflunomide (Arava) is an immunosuppressant. Loading dose is 100 mg daily for 3 days. Maintenance dosing is 20 mg/day. If intolerance occurs it may be decreased to 10 mg day. The side effects of these drugs are diarrhea, elevated liver enzymes, alopecia, and rash. They have been approved for use in adult patients with adult RA but have not yet been approved for use with children. There is a teratogenic potential that would be of concern with children, particularly adolescent girls.
  - etanercept (Enbrel). Safe dose in children 4–17 years is via SC injection and is 0.8 mg/kg/week up to 50 mg as a single injection if the child weighs more than 63 kg. If the child weighs between 31 and 62 kg, and then 0.8 mg/kg/week in two injections either the same day or separated by 3–4 days. If the child weighs less than 31 kg, then 0.8 mg/kg/week as a single injection. Safe dose in adults is via SC injection and is 50 mg once weekly. It has been found to reduce the signs and symptoms of moderately severe to severe polyarticular juvenile arthritis. It is a potent inhibitor of tumor necrosis factor, which is a key proinflammatory cytokine found in the synovial tissue of patients with juvenile arthritis.
  - prednisone (Deltasone): Safe dose range is 0.1–2 mg/kg/day in 1–4 divided doses in children. Safe dose range is 5–60 mg/day as a single or divided dose in adults.
- Other corticosteroids are potent and administered at the lowest possible dose and for the shortest possible period of time. Side effects such as Cushing's syndrome, osteoporosis, increased risk of infection, glucose intolerance, cataracts, and growth retardation can occur.

Source: Vallerand, A. H., & Sanoski, C. A. (2014). *Davis's drug guide for nurses* (14th ed.). Philadelphia, PA: F.A. Davis.

protein, calcium, and adequate fluid intake. Develop a plan of care that aids parents in providing age-appropriate activities and reinforces independent activities. After an exacerbation, the child needs to be encouraged to resume pre-exacerbation activities. It is best to involve the child in the decision-making process as much as possible. Psychosocial adjustment of the child is assessed by school performance and peer activities. Attending professional counseling sessions or support groups can be encouraged.

 Nursing Diagnoses A Child With Juvenile Arthritis

- Chronic pain related to joint inflammation secondary to Juvenile Arthritis
- Impaired physical mobility related to joint discomfort and stiffness secondary to Juvenile Arthritis
- Altered family processes related to a situational crisis (child with a chronic illness) secondary to Juvenile Arthritis

TRANSIENT SYNOVITIS OF THE HIP

Transient synovitis of the hip is similar to septic arthritis of the hip. The mean age of the child at diagnosis is 5.7 years.

Signs and Symptoms

Signs and symptoms of transient synovitis of the hip include:

- Fever
- Painful hip (one side only)
- Limp

Diagnosis

Sultan and Hughes (2010) developed and tested an algorithm to differentiate the two diagnoses of transient synovitis of the hip and septic arthritis of the hip. The use of the algorithm prevents the unnecessary invasive ultrasound guided aspiration of the synovial fluid of the joint. Septic arthritis of the hip is diagnosed by a positive aspirate culture from the affected joint or when the cultures are negative. If the cultures are positive, then the diagnosis is confirmed as septic arthritis of the hip; if the cultures are negative, then the diagnosis of transient synovitis of the hip is confirmed.

Prevention

Transient synovitis of the hip is a form of arthritis in which the cause is unknown. Therefore, there are no preventive procedures.

Collaborative Care

Nursing Care. Because transient synovitis resolves spontaneously in about 7 to 10 days, nursing care is supportive. Family education about the condition is important.

Medical Care. Medical management includes limiting activity so the child is more comfortable. However, there is no danger of untoward effects if the child maintains normal activity. NSAIDs can be prescribed to reduce pain.

Education/Discharge Instructions

It is important to inform the parents and child that the synovitis resolves spontaneously. In addition, long-term complications are not usually seen. The child will need to take the prescribed NSAIDs for comfort. Instructions on the dose, frequency, route, and potential side effects of the medication are given to the parents prior to discharge. The parents are also instructed to call the health-care provider if the child experiences unexplained pain or a

limp with or without a fever. In addition, the health-care practitioner can be contacted if the pain lasts longer than 10 days, gets worse, or the child suffers a high fever.

MUSCULAR DYSTROPHIES

Muscular dystrophies (MDs) are a group of muscle disorders that cause the gradual wasting of symmetrical groups of skeletal muscle. It is the most common group of muscle disorders in childhood. All MDs are a result of a genetic defect that causes the degeneration of muscle fibers. Most MDs are identified in early childhood. Thirty percent of the time, MD is caused by a spontaneous mutation, and 65% of MD cases are sex-linked recessive disorders. MDs are divided into three types: pseudohypertrophic muscular dystrophy (Duchenne's muscular dystrophy), congenital myotonic dystrophy, and facioscapulohumeral muscular dystrophy.

Duchenne's is the most common type of MD. Duchenne's muscular dystrophy is a sex-linked recessive disease, so it generally only affects males. Duchenne's muscular dystrophy affects 1 in 3,600 males. Females are usually carriers. In a case such as a female child with Turner's syndrome, in which the child receives only one X chromosome from the mother, the female child could have Duchenne's muscular dystrophy.

Congenital myotonic dystrophy is an autosomal dominant inherited disease. The disease process begins while the fetus is in utero. The infant usually dies before 1 year of age because of the inability to maintain respiratory function. Facioscapulohumeral muscular dystrophy is an autosomal dominant trait carried on chromosome 4. Symptoms progress slowly, making a normal life span possible.

Signs and Symptoms

MD is a disease where there is progressive symmetrical muscle wasting and weakness without loss of sensation. In Duchenne's muscular dystrophy, the child develops the following signs and symptoms:

- Symptoms first appear after the child is able to walk, usually about 3 to 7 years of age
- A waddling, wide-based gait
- Calf muscles that become weak and hypertrophied
- The leg, pelvis, arm, shoulder, and cardiac muscles are weak and hypertrophied (Poliachik, Friedman, Carter, Parnell, & Shaw, 2012)

With congenital myotonic dystrophy, the signs and symptoms include:

- Severe muscle weakness at birth
- Respiratory muscle degeneration leading to inadequate respiration

Signs and symptoms of facioscapulohumeral muscular dystrophy include:

- Occurs after the child is 10 years old
- Facial weakness: the child becomes unable to wrinkle the forehead and cannot whistle

 Assessment Tool Gowers' Maneuver

A child with muscular dystrophy uses the Gowers' maneuver to rise from the floor. The Gowers' maneuver is when the child must move to a kneeling position with hands also on the floor to stabilize. Then the child, while keeping hands on the floor, rises to feet. The child comes to a standing position by using the hands to walk up the legs until in a standing position.

Diagnosis

Children with a positive family history are at risk for Duchenne's muscular dystrophy. These children are monitored for clinical symptoms that do not usually appear until preschool years. Serum creatinine kinase (CK) levels are monitored. CK levels are elevated in the early stages of the disease. As muscle bulk decreases, the CK levels also decrease. Definitive diagnosis is made by **muscle biopsy** (the removal of muscle tissue for microscopic examination and chemical analysis) and **electromyelogram** (a graphic record of resting and voluntary muscle activity as a result of electrical stimulation) (Venes, 2013). Diagnosis of congenital myotonic dystrophy is based on serum enzyme analysis and muscle biopsy. Muscle biopsy and serum enzyme analysis are used for diagnosing facioscapulohumeral muscular dystrophy.

Prevention

MDs are genetic; prevention is not possible once conception has occurred. Genetic testing should be done when the parents state they have already had a child with MD or MD has occurred in a close relative.

Collaborative Care

Nursing Care. Nursing care for MD is aimed at maintaining independent living for the child as long as possible. Help foster the patient's independence and self-care. It is important to teach the child how to achieve an optimal level of functioning, making adaptations so he or she can participate in self-care measures. Encouraging the child to be involved in activities that will maintain independence is important. For example, swimming is a good activity to achieve independence because when the child is in the water, exercises can be done without the child feeling the weight of his or her body.

These children rarely live beyond 20 years of age. Because death is usually a result of respiratory complications, the key is to prevent respiratory infections. Monitoring the respiratory status is critical. Any respiratory infection must to be treated quickly and aggressively with antibiotics, postural drainage, and chest physiotherapy (CPT).

Also be sure to monitor the child's skin. As the child's mobility decreases, the skin can deteriorate quickly. It may be necessary to arrange for a special bed with an air cushion that can assist the caregiver in turning the child frequently.

Transferring the child in and out of bed and into a chair may eventually need to be performed with a Hoyer lift. Toileting can become an issue when the child is no longer able to ambulate and is required to wear diapers. Safety factors are essential in the care of the child with MD.

Nutrition is another nursing care focus. Monitor the child's weight gain. A diet that is low in calories and high in protein helps prevent obesity. A high-fiber diet and adequate fluid intake help prevent constipation.

Assessment of the child's mobility is an important nursing action to help the child maintain ambulation for as long as possible. Active and passive ROM are also performed. Splinting and bracing may be recommended by the physician to prevent contractures.

Medical Care. Antibiotics are ordered to treat respiratory infections and ensuring that the child has as few respiratory infections as possible. The flu shot is highly recommended for these children. Coordination of care with physical therapy, occupational therapy, respiratory therapy, and durable medical equipment is essential in the medical management for these children.

Surgical Care. Surgery is not usually required to treat children with MD; however, these children may also suffer from scoliosis or dislocated hips. When this occurs, surgery to repair the scoliosis or to treat the hip dislocation is warranted, and standard postoperative care is provided.

Education/Discharge Instructions

Teach the family to provide meticulous skin care. It is important for the child to begin a regimen of stool softeners and laxatives to help prevent constipation. Recognize that the child and family need emotional support. Encourage the child and family to participate in support groups or spiritual care. The Muscular Dystrophy Association is an excellent resource for these families and children (http://www.mda.org/). Parents are referred for genetic counseling. With MD, the parents must watch their child pass away gradually.

Collaboration in Caring—*A child with muscular dystrophy*

Coordination of the child's health care requires collaboration with:

- Families
- Physicians
- Physical therapists
- Nutritionists
- Social workers
- Medical equipment companies
- Faith communities
- Visiting nurses

Assess the family's ability to cope with their child's chronic illness and poor prognosis and provide the necessary support and community resources to the family. Help the family find proper community and online resources because the child will eventually need an electric wheelchair, Hoyer lift, and modifications to the home environment.

Complementary Care: *Muscular Dystrophy*

Children who suffer from MD often turn to alternative or complementary therapies because there is no cure. Qigong is now accepted as an innovative exercise program for children with MD and may lower the rate of decline in general health.

Nursing Diagnoses A Child With Muscular Dystrophy

- Impaired Physical Mobility related to chronic degenerative disease process secondary to Muscular Dystrophy
- Self-care Deficits; Bathing/Hygiene, Dressing, and Grooming related to chronic degenerative disease process secondary to Muscular Dystrophy
- Risk for Injury related to decreasing mobility secondary to chronic degenerative disease process secondary to Muscular Dystrophy
- Fatigue related to increased energy expenditure secondary to Muscular Dystrophy
- Altered Grieving related to chronic and terminal illness secondary to Muscular Dystrophy

- Altered Family Processes related to chronic and terminal illness secondary to Muscular Dystrophy
- Impaired Gas Exchange related to diminishing muscle function secondary to Muscular Dystrophy
- Altered Nutrition related to chronic and debilitating disease process secondary to Muscular Dystrophy

SCOLIOSIS

Scoliosis is a non-painful lateral curvature of the spine and is the most common spinal deformity in children. The spine either curves laterally in only one direction (C curve) or in two opposite directions (S curve). There is a lateral deviation and rotation of each vertebra, which accentuates the deformity. Idiopathic scoliosis is common in female children and in families in which another member has been affected by scoliosis. Idiopathic scoliosis is the predominant form, and there is no recognizable cause. Unequal leg lengths, such as untreated developmental dysplasia of the hip (DDH), can cause scoliosis. Congenital scoliosis is related to vertebral anomalies. It can also be associated with other congenital anomalies, such as myelomeningocele (spina bifida), osteogenesis imperfecta, or MD. Paralytic scoliosis occurs in association with neuromuscular diseases such as cerebral palsy, paraplegia, and quadriplegia.

Signs and Symptoms

Signs and symptoms of scoliosis include:

- Unequal shoulder heights
- Scapula prominences
- Rib prominences
- Chest asymmetry
- Leg length discrepancy
- Skin has hairy patches, nevi, café au lait spots, lipomas, and dimples

Diagnosis

Diagnosis is confirmed by radiography. The physician looks at the **Cobb's angle** (a measure of the curvature of the spine in degrees). The number of degrees helps the physician decide what type of management is necessary. A curve of the spine that is 10 to 15 degrees is considered mild, and the child will be assessed for scoliosis at regular checkups until pubertal maturation and growth are complete. A curve between 15 and 40 degrees (mild) will generally suggest a back brace. A curve of more than 40 degrees (severe) revealed by x-ray exam requires management, and the child is referred to an orthopedic surgeon.

Prevention

Idiopathic scoliosis has no known cause, so prevention is not possible.

Collaborative Care

Nursing Care. Scoliosis screening is a critical nursing action. The child is evaluated for scoliosis screening at each health-care maintenance visit until the child reaches bone maturity (Larson, 2011). The evaluation begins with a general inspection of the back in the standing and sitting position. Asymmetries are noted. Differences in shoulder height are measured from the floor to the **acromioclavicular joints** (the joint between the acromion and the acromial end of the clavicle) bilaterally. Head alignment is also evaluated. The head should be in the midline and align perfectly over

the sacrum. The spine should be seen during flexion, extension, and side-bending motions. Tanner's stage and age of menarche in girls is also noted. Assessing rib heights in both the thoracic and lumbar regions is done. The spine is palpated for deviations not easily seen. Both iliac crests are palpated simultaneously to determine if there is an uneven pelvis. Watch for limping during ambulation. Assess for a high arch, which may indicate a tethered spinal cord. If scoliosis is suspected, a neurological exam needs to be performed by evaluating motor, sensory, and reflex functions of both upper and lower extremities. Assess for the abdominal reflex and the anal wink reflex also. Severe scoliosis can lead to respiratory compromise because the lung under the shortened side of the body will not be able to fully expand. Severe scoliosis can also have a negative effect on the hips and knees (Fig. 29-9).

Medical Care. Bracing and exercise are the usual medical treatments for mild cases of scoliosis. Bracing stops the progression of scoliosis. The molded brace is worn 23 hours per day. The patient may only remove the brace to shower. The adolescent wears a special T-shirt under the brace to prevent skin irritation. Communicate to the child and family that compliance with bracing improves the outcome for this condition. The major problem with bracing is body image. Many adolescents do not want to wear the brace at school or while they are with their friends. Also tell the family that the best way to increase compliance is to include the adolescent in decisions. Exercises recommended by a physical therapist help the muscles in the back gain strength.

✿ Complementary Care: *Exercise and Bracing*

Thompson (2011) revealed that outcomes from exercises alone and chiropractic therapy are rarely therapeutic in managing scoliosis. Transcutaneous electrical stimulation has also proved ineffective. Exercises are of benefit when used in conjunction with bracing to maintain and strengthen the muscles of the back and abdomen.

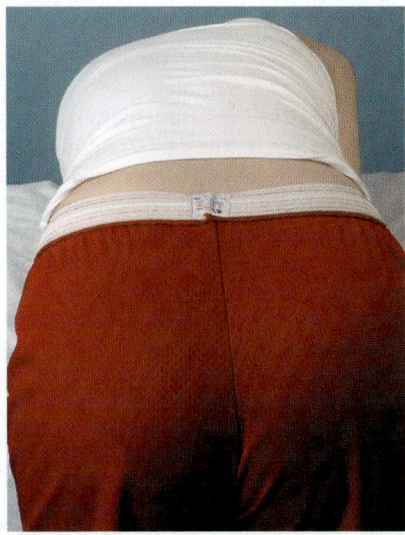

Figure 29-9 The child is asked to bend at the waist with arms hanging loosely. This is called the Adam's position or the bend-over test. Scoliosis is obvious in this adolescent.

Nursing Care Plan The Child With a Musculoskeletal Disorder

Nursing Diagnosis: Mobility: Physical, Impaired related to physical disability or mechanical restrictions.

Measurable Short-Term Goal: The child will engage in activities appropriate within current physical limitations.

Measurable Long-Term Goal: The child will regain maximum mobility.

NOC Outcomes:

Mobility (0208) Ability to move purposefully in own environment independently with or without assistive device

Transfer Performance (0210) Ability to change body location independently with or without assistive device

NIC Interventions:

Activity Therapy (4310)
Environmental Management (6480)
Self-Care Assistance: Transfer (1806)

Nursing Interventions:

1. Monitor the child for complications of immobility (specify, e.g., peripheral pulses, capillary refill, skin integrity, muscle weakness).

   RATIONALE: Provides prevention or early recognition of complications to decrease their severity.

2. Allow the child to make as many realistic choices as possible and encourage independence in activities of daily living.

   RATIONALE: Empowers the child by allowing him to exercise as much control as possible over self and the environment.

3. Select appropriate transport for the child and promote as much mobility as possible (specify, such as a wheelchair, crutches, stretcher, go-cart, or stroller).

   RATIONALE: Mobility promotes normality and helps prevent feelings of isolation.

4. Encourage the child to go to the playroom if possible or arrange for the child life specialist therapist to visit the child.

   RATIONALE: Increases child's mobility and decreases isolation. The child life specialist promotes normal growth and development.

5. If the child is immobile for a long period of time, plan periodic rearrangement and redecoration of the room with input from the child as appropriate.

   RATIONALE: Change breaks up the monotony of the immobilization and provides an opportunity for engagement and creativity.

Surgical Care. The health-care provider may suggest that surgery be delayed as long as possible because the fusion of the vertebrae will stop spinal growth. However, a spinal fusion is necessary when pulmonary function becomes compromised, sitting or walking becomes difficult because of poor balance, pain, curves are noted as severe by x-ray exam, and for cosmetic reasons. Instrumentation (an application of metal screws, bolts, or wires to straighten the spine) is usually performed with the spinal fusion. The instrumentation holds the vertebrae in place until the fusion has healed.

When surgery is scheduled, the nurse helps the child and parents understand what may happen before and after the procedure. Prior to surgery, a tour of the intensive care unit (ICU) can help alleviate the child's anxiety. It is also important to stress that after surgery the child will have an indwelling urinary catheter in place. Teach ROM exercises before surgery.

In the postoperative phase, the child remains in the ICU overnight. Assess vital signs and neurological status every 1 to 2 hours after surgery. Once the child is stable, she is transferred to the inpatient area where vital signs and neurological assessments continue to be performed every 4 hours. Monitoring fluid balance and renal function is important because the kidneys are hypoperfused during surgery. The child may also have had blood transfusions.

The child may also have a chest tube in place. The chest tube will be hooked up to suction at first and then placed on water seal. When drainage has ceased, the chest tube is removed. Radiography is usually performed the day after chest tube removal to ensure that no pneumothorax is developing. Incentive spirometry, CPT, and coughing and deep breathing exercises are used to prevent atelectasis and pneumonia. Also assess for signs and symptoms of infection every 4 hours, such as fevers, chills, redness and pain at the incision site, and drainage from the incision site.

Assess circulation in the child's lower extremities, the incision, the bowel sounds in all four quadrants, and the softness of the abdomen each time vital signs are assessed. Any changes in the neurovascular status and signs of redness, swelling, drainage, or dehiscence (separation of the suture line) must be reported to the physician.

Pain from a spinal fusion surgery can be severe. Various methods are used to control pain in the postoperative patient. Continuous infusion of an opioid can be used for nonverbal patients. PCA is effective and commonly used for those patients who are able. In some cases, an epidural with bupivacaine (Marcaine) anesthetic alone or combined with an opioid such as morphine sulfate (Astramorph) or hydromorphone (Dilaudid) is used with success (Fig. 29-10). Pain management is usually switched to the oral route by

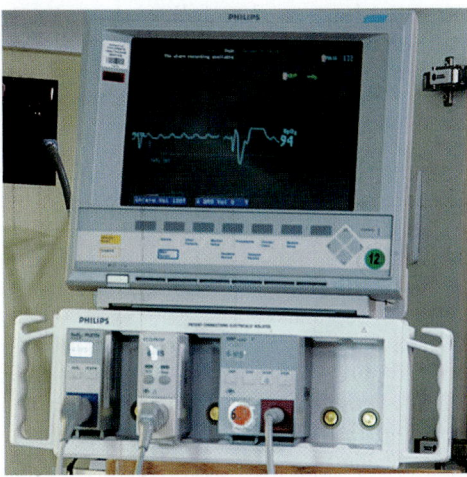

Figure 29-10 While the child is receiving narcotics, the nurse monitors oxygen saturation.

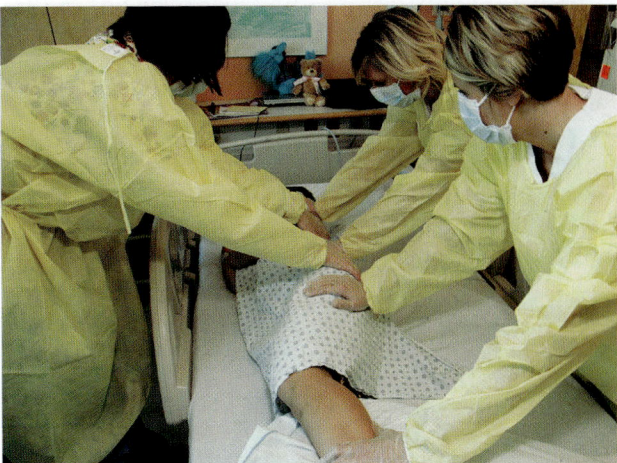

Figure 29-11 The patient must be turned using the logrolling technique.

postoperative day 3. The oral analgesic of choice is acetaminophen (Tylenol) with codeine. Acetaminophen (Children's Tylenol) with codeine can be administered to children who are too young for oxycodone (Percocet) and is available in a liquid form, if needed. For older children, oxycodone (Percocet) can be used as the oral drug of choice.

The surgeon may require the patient to wear an orthotic brace. Collaboration with the orthotist is necessary to ensure that the brace fits properly. Check for pressure points under the brace for the first couple of days after implementation of the brace. ROM exercises are also performed to keep the uninvolved extremities from becoming weak.

Ambulation is permitted (usually about 5 days postoperatively). Early mobilization is important in the care of the child who has had a spinal fusion to prevent atelectasis, pneumonia, pulmonary emboli, phlebitis, and skin breakdown. Perform passive ROM to all extremities. To turn the patient, use the logrolling technique.

 Critical Nursing Action Logrolling

Positioning of the patient is also an important nursing action. The patient must be turned using the logrolling technique. Logrolling involves two or more nurses turning the patient in complete unison. The head, shoulders, hips, and legs are turned as one unit, thereby keeping the back in a straight line as the patient is turned (Fig. 29-11).

A nutritionist helps prevent constipation by suggesting adding fiber and fluids to the diet. Foods high in iron, folate, and vitamin C are added to the patient's diet. Psychosocial aspects of care for this child include nursing actions that maintain or build his or her self-esteem. Because some musculoskeletal conditions have visible deformities, address body image concerns and anxiety. Certain situations may create an inability for the child to interact physically or socially or may cause the child to feel alienated from the peer group. Other psychosocial concerns related to the family are daily living routines and family functions, continued care of other siblings, and financial burdens. Compliance with the treatment regimen is important to ensure the best outcome for the child.

Collaboration with physical therapy is necessary to assist with ambulation training in addition to ROM exercises. The physical therapist also teaches strengthening and isometrics exercises. The wheelchair may need to be adjusted if the child is wheelchair-bound. The orthotist fabricates the orthotic brace and makes any necessary adjustments.

Education/Discharge Instructions

The nurse arranges for home care. Important information that is included in a discharge-teaching plan is:

- A caregiver must be home with the child at all times until the health-care provider determines if it is safe to leave the child unattended (based on age and recovery)
- The child will need durable medical equipment for the home environment, such as an elevated toilet seat and shower chair
- A hospital bed may also be needed in some circumstances
- Activity restrictions such as:
  - No twisting or bending
  - No lifting of heavy objects
  - No contact or high-impact sports for 2 years
- The child may return to school about 4 to 6 weeks after surgery
- Teach parents to be alert for unfavorable signs such as:
  - Pain
  - Infection
  - Difficulty breathing
- Teaching the family about the brace care including the signs and symptoms of skin breakdown
- Instruct the caregiver that the patient's head is not raised more than 30 degrees without the jacket brace
- Provide the family with information about community resources that are available
- Arrange for counseling for the adolescent, particularly if there is non-compliance with wearing the brace
- Encourage the adolescent to be as active as possible in their care based on health-care provider's orders
- Stress to the parents that it is important to keep follow-up appointments

Global Health Case Study Idiopathic Scoliosis

A 17-year-old girl, Gerseld, has a history of severe idiopathic scoliosis. She was brought to the United States for treatment because her ability to walk long distances has diminished in the past 2 years. Gerseld was brought here by missionaries who were able to pay for her to come but not any family members. There is a host family who Gerseld can stay with while she is recuperating. Gerseld is otherwise healthy.

Gerseld has just arrived from the postanesthesia care unit (PACU) after a posterior spinal fusion with instrumentation. She had a blood loss of 1,200 mL and received packed red blood cells and 450 mL of cell saver in the operating room. She also received 2 L of lactated Ringer's solution in the PACU. Gerseld has a central line for IV access. Her vital signs are heart rate, 90 to 110 beats/min; blood pressure, 105/58; and temperature 97.2°F (36.2°C). Her face, hands, and feet are edematous. Her urine output is less than 1 mL/hr via Foley catheter. Urine appears dark yellow. Gerseld denies discomfort and appears relaxed.

critical thinking questions

1. What assessment data place Gerseld at risk for complications?

2. Taking into consideration the characteristics of the adolescent stage of growth and development, what can the nurse do to optimize Gerseld's plan of care?

3. Taking cultural and spiritual care into consideration, what can the nurse do to ensure that Gerseld receives care that is culturally competent and addresses her spiritual needs?

4. What does the nurse need to tell the host family about discharge planning for the home care instructions?

◆ See Suggested Answers to Global Health Case Studies on *DavisPlus*.

KYPHOSIS

Kyphosis is a non-painful spinal curvature in the sagittal plane. It is commonly described as "hunchback." Slight kyphosis is found in the normal spine. Families usually seek treatment when the kyphosis becomes noticeable. In children, kyphosis is caused by a congenital or acquired condition. Some congenital causes of kyphosis are ankylosing spondylitis, metabolic disorders, osteogenesis imperfecta, spina bifida, Paget's disease, and Scheuermann's disease, which causes juvenile or adolescent kyphosis because there are wedge-shaped vertebrae in the thoracic region. In acquired kyphosis, the child can voluntarily bend the spine to correct the curvature. In addition, there is no underlying evidence of structural changes seen with acquired kyphosis. Kyphosis is potentially serious because of the risk of progressive deformity.

Signs and Symptoms

Signs and symptoms of kyphosis include:

- Uneven shoulder height in the child
- Complaints of pain in the thoracic region

Diagnosis

Kyphosis is most commonly diagnosed in early adolescence during routine back screening for scoliosis. If kyphosis is suspected, a complete examination includes a complete orthopedic and neurological exam. Radiographs confirm the diagnosis and are used to follow progression of the disease. If the curve exceeds 50 degrees, it is considered abnormal (kyphotic).

Prevention

There are no preventive measures that can be taken because the cause is idiopathic.

Collaborative Care

Nursing Care. Nursing care is similar to the nursing care of the child with scoliosis.

Medical Care. Nonsurgical management is recommended for acquired kyphosis when the curve is between 50 and 70 degrees. It is possible to treat the child with continued observation and thoracic hyperextension exercises, or a brace may be needed.

Surgical Care. Surgical management is recommended when the curve is greater than 70 degrees. Anterior–posterior spinal fusion is the surgery of choice. The child with congenital kyphosis does not respond well to bracing, so surgery is necessary. The nursing care for the child with a surgical repair for kyphosis is the same as for the child with scoliosis, and standard postoperative measures are provided.

Education/Discharge Instructions

Education and discharge instructions are similar to the education/discharge instructions for scoliosis.

LORDOSIS

Lordosis is a spinal curvature in the sagittal plane (Fig. 29-12). It is seen in conjunction with flexion contractures of the hip, scoliosis, obesity, DDH, and SCFE. Slight lordosis is present in the normal spine and is not considered a major deformity.

Signs and Symptoms

Lordosis is commonly described as "swayback," an excessive backward cavity of the spine.

Diagnosis

The parents may first notice that the child's clothing is not fitting properly. This may precipitate a visit to the primary care provider. If lordosis is suspected, the full

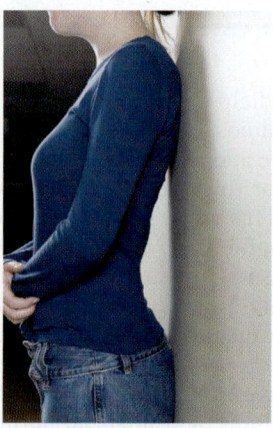

Figure 29-12 Slight lordosis is present in the normal spine and is not considered a major deformity.

diagnostic exam includes a full orthopedic and neurological examination. Radiographs confirm the diagnosis and are used for follow-up progression of the disease. MRI, CT scans, and nuclear scans can also be used to determine a more detailed view of the spine in the back.

Prevention

The cause is unknown but has been thought to be associated with poor posture and a congenital predisposition to the development of lordosis. Prevention involves reducing the predisposing factors such as obesity, MD, DDH, or neuromuscular disorders.

Collaborative Care

Nursing Care. Reducing the predisposing factors can also be temporarily achieved with postural exercises and support garments. Teaching is an important nursing function. As with scoliosis, teaching is necessary regarding the use and care of the back brace. Exercises along with the use of a back brace are also important.

Medical Care. Medical management incorporates observation. As with scoliosis, once the spinal abnormality has been identified, the health-care practitioner monitors the curvature. Physical therapy is instituted to provide exercise programs to maximize physical function. If the curvature is stable and less than 30 degrees, observation is the treatment of choice. If the curvature is greater than 30 degrees and is worsening, bracing is instituted. As with scoliosis, compliance with the bracing protocol is imperative in achieving the best possible outcome.

Surgical Care. As with scoliosis, surgery is indicated in the most severe cases of lordosis. Surgery is similar to the surgery to correct scoliosis. Bracing after surgery is also generally required.

Education/Discharge Instructions

Because the surgery is similar to scoliosis surgery, nursing care and education/discharge teaching are basically the same as for patients recovering from scoliosis surgery.

TETANUS

Tetanus (lockjaw) is a preventable, acute, and potentially fatal disease. Tetanus occurs when an exotoxin, which is produced by an anaerobic, gram-positive bacillus (*Clostridium tetani*) forms spores. The spores are found in soil, dust, and human gastrointestinal tracts. These spores enter the body through wounds such as burns; stabs; minor, unnoticed breaks in the skin; and the umbilical cord of a newborn.

 Cultural Diversity: Tetanus

Spores entering through the umbilical cord of the newborn are seen more often in developing countries, where women are not immunized against tetanus, contaminated instruments are used to cut the umbilical cord, or poultices are made from cow dung or fermented milk and used for cord care. The greatest incidence of tetanus is during warmer months when people are outdoors more frequently.

Prevention of tetanus is the best defense. For the organism to grow in the human, four requirements must be fulfilled: a presence of tetanus spores, an injury to the tissues, wound conditions that enable multiplication of the spores, and a susceptible host. When the natural defense mechanisms fail, the organism proliferates and forms exotoxins known as tetanospasmin. Tetanospasmin affects the central nervous system through the neuron axons and the vascular system.

Signs and Symptoms

Symptoms of tetanus can develop between 5 and 15 days after the initial wound:

- Progressive stiffness and tenderness of the muscles in the neck and jaw
- **Trismus** (difficulty opening the mouth)
- **Risus sardonicus** (a peculiar grin) is also present because of facial muscle spasms

As the disease progresses, there is more involvement of the muscles in the body:

- **Opisthotonos** (rigid and severe arching of the back, with the head thrown backwards) posturing occurs
- Board-like rigidity of the abdomen and limb muscles
- Difficulty swallowing
- Hypersensitive to stimuli such as a slight noise, bright lights, and gentle touch (these stimuli trigger paroxysmal muscular contractions lasting from seconds to minutes)

 Nursing Insight—Disease progression

As the disease progresses further, the contractions recur with increasing frequency until they are almost continuous. Laryngospasm and tetany of the respiratory muscles develop. As a result, secretions accumulate, atelectasis and pneumonia develop, and finally respiratory arrest occurs. During all of these phases of symptomatology, the child remains alert. Pain and distress can be determined through the child becoming tachycardic, sweating, and having an anxious expression. Generally, the child remains afebrile. If a fever occurs, it is only a mild fever.

Diagnosis

Diagnosis is based on patient history and physical examination findings.

Prevention

Prophylactic therapy is administered after trauma. Tetanus antitoxin is no longer available in the United States. An unprotected or inadequately immunized child who has sustained an injury that is prone to tetanus needs to be given tetanus immune globulin. Tetanus toxoid (tetanus toxin modified so that its toxicity is reduced, while retaining its capacity to promote active immunity) is administered (Venes, 2013). The child continues to receive the complete immunization for tetanus at the correct intervals. Tetanus is rare in countries with an excellent immunization program. However, in developing countries where children are not routinely immunized, tetanus has a higher mortality rate. Recovery from an infection from tetanus does not guarantee natural immunity, so the tetanus immunization series should begin.

Collaborative Care

Nursing Care. In the case of a tetanus infection, communicate to the family that the administration of antibiotics will be prescribed to control the proliferation of exotoxin. Antibiotics of choice are penicillin G (Pfizerpen) or erythromycin (Erythrocin). Tetracycline (Sumycin) is used in older children whose dentition is complete.

If prophylaxis is not used, management in the acute phase of the disease is through aggressive support given in the ICU. The child is closely monitored and given respiratory support in a quiet environment. Fluids and electrolytes as well as caloric intake are monitored closely. Initiate nasogastric (NG) enteral feedings for the child. In the case of severe laryngospasm, total parenteral nutrition or enteral feedings through a gastrostomy tube may need to be initiated. Recurrent laryngospasm may necessitate endotracheal intubation and mechanical ventilation.

One key to providing nursing care for the child with tetanus is to control or eliminate stimulation from light, sound, and touch. Avoid unnecessary handling and sudden or loud noises and perform frequent neurological and vital sign assessments. Assess oxygen saturation and arterial blood gases regularly. Emergency equipment must be placed close to the child's bed. Oropharyngeal suctioning is done when there is an accumulation of secretions. Assess for excessive central nervous system depression and for muscle spasms. The child must be maintained on total parenteral nutrition or enteral feeds through an NG tube or gastrostomy tube.

Collaborate with the respiratory therapist and physician to ensure that the child receives adequate respiratory support and that seizures are kept under control. Also collaborate with the pharmacist regarding the administration of the medications to eradicate the exotoxin from the child. Nursing care is clustered so that the child has a chance to rest and recover from the stress of the intervention.

Medical Care. Medication administration is an important nursing action to keep the child as comfortable as possible. If a neuromuscular blocking agent is being used, pay close attention to the effects of those agents (Box 29-6).

Nursing Insight—*Neuromuscular blocking agent*

Important ideas to remember when caring for a child treated with a neuromuscular blocking agent are the following:
* The child has total paralysis, including respiratory function.
* The child is not able to communicate.
* The child is anxious.
* The child is aware of all surrounding activity.
* The child is terrified.

Collaboration in Caring—*Providing holistic care*

* Anticipate the child's needs.
* Explain all procedures.
* Never leave the child alone.
* Reduce anxiety in the child by using a calm, reassuring manner.
* Support and understand the child's fear.
* Encourage the parents to stay with the child.
* Medicate the child with an anxiolytic (antianxiety agent).
* Assess hydration and nutrition.

Box 29-6   Medication: Pharmaceuticals Used for Tetanus

Medications are used to alleviate the muscle spasms and seizures.

* Diazepam (Valium) (dose of 0.1–0.2 mg/kg IV every 4–6 hours) is the drug of choice to control seizures. It is a benzodiazepine, anxiolytic, and an anticonvulsant (Okoromah & Lesi, 2009).
* Dantrolene sodium (Dantrium) is a skeletal muscle relaxant and can be effective. Caution is used when administering to a child with cardiac or pulmonary impairment. Unnecessary exposure to light is avoided. This medication is allowed to extravasate into the surrounding tissue. Discontinue if benefits are not evident in 45 days (Acara & Tschudy, 2012).
* Neuromuscular blocking agents are used when the child is suffering severe unresponsive tetanus. These two are non-depolarizing neuromuscular blocking agents.
* Vecuronium bromide (Norcuron) is an intermediate-acting neuromuscular blocking agent. Initial dose is 0.08–0.1 mg/kg IV with maintenance doses of 0.01–0.15 mg/kg every 30–60 minutes, as needed. It may cause arrhythmias, rash, and bronchospasm. It is used with caution in patients with renal or hepatic failure and neuromuscular disease. Infants from 7 weeks to 1 year of age are more sensitive to the medication and may have a longer recovery period. Children from 1–10 years of age may need higher and more frequent doses. Neostigmine (Prostigmin), pyridostigmine (Mestinon), and edrophonium (Enlon) are antidotes. Onset is 1–3 minutes. Duration is 30–90 minutes.

Source: Vallerand, A. H., & Sanoski, C. A. (2014). *Davis's drug guide for nurses* (14th ed.). Philadelphia, PA: F.A. Davis.

Education/Discharge Instructions

If the child survives the acute illness, then the recovery is usually complete. Discharge teaching includes:

* Teach the family that tetanus is preventable
* Inform the family of the benefits of immunization and the immunization schedule
* Teach the family that convalescence may be prolonged
* Tell the family that multidisciplinary rehabilitation and home nursing may be required

---

 Now Can You—Discuss tetanus?

1. Describe the prophylaxis management for a child at risk of tetanus?
2. Describe the symptoms of tetanus?
3. Describe the critical nursing actions needed to care for a child with tetanus?
4. Describe the medications and the important facts regarding the medications for a child with tetanus?

OSTEOGENESIS IMPERFECTA

Osteogenesis imperfecta (OI), or brittle bone disease, is the most common genetic disorder of the bone. OI is a group of autosomal dominant diseases characterized by excessive fragility of the bones causing a high rate of fracture. It occurs equally in all races and is equally prevalent between males and females. It is a biochemical defect that causes a decrease in the synthesis of collagen. It affects all connective tissue in the body. Children may become disabled as a result of the severe deformities.

Any undue stress on the bone causes a fracture (e.g., changing the infant's diaper can cause a femur fracture). The fracture heals within the normal period, but the bone lacks the normal strength. Bone deformities such as bowing and growth pattern disturbances occur. Some newborns die of complications caused by the extreme fragility of the bones. When caring for an infant who presents with a fracture, it is important to rule out OI as well as child abuse.

Signs and Symptoms

Signs and symptoms of OI include:

- Lax joints
- Small, weak muscles

Diagnosis

Diagnosis is based on the severity of clinical symptoms and the level of disability. There are five major types of OI that are based on severity and the mode of genetic transmission.

A unique feature of this disease is that there is very little bruising or swelling, only tenderness at the fracture site. Laboratory studies are not useful in the diagnosis of OI. Radiographic studies show multiple normal callus formations at new fracture sites, evidence of previous fractures, and skeletal deformities. In addition, radiographs will reveal generalized osteopenia, which is an insufficiency of bone. A collagen biopsy will confirm the diagnosis.

Prevention

There are no known preventative measures as this condition is genetic.

Collaborative Care

Nursing Care. An important intervention is to teach the parents of an infant just diagnosed with OI to watch for signs of a fracture. Communicate that the signs of fracture include irritability, fever, and refusal to eat. Tell parents of an older child that signs to watch for are pain, swelling, and possible deformity at the site.

Body composition is a risk factor for increased bone fractures in these children. These children typically have a decreased amount of calcium and vitamin D intake. Individualized nutritional support is recommended to help increase the intake and absorption of calcium and vitamin D (Chagas, Roque, Peters, Lazaretti-Castro, & Martini, 2011). Patients who are treated with olpadronate (a bone-resorption inhibitor) therapy show a greater increase in spinal bone mineral content and bone mineral density.

Medical Care. Bisphosphonates such as pamidronate (Aredia), alendronate (Fosamax) and zoledronic acid (Reclast) have been studied for use with children with OI. Studies continue using these medications. Bisphosphonate (Reclast) is an inhibitor of osteoclastic bone resorption and is used in management for moderate to severe forms of OI. The best regimen and the long-term outcomes of bisphosphonate (Reclast) therapy are unknown. Management with bisphosphonate (Reclast) is an adjunct therapy for children with OI and is used in conjunction with physical therapy, rehabilitation, and orthopedic care. Other therapies that are being researched are using growth hormone, increased vitamin D intake, maintaining physical activity, and a potential for gene therapy.

Surgical Care. Surgical management includes an operation to reduce fractures, correct spinal deformities, and straighten long bones. Intramedullary rodding of the femur is not a perfect solution but can provide stability to a deformed bone.

A solid intramedullary rod is easier to insert but does not grow with the child and needs to be replaced every 2 to 4 years. A telescoping intramedullary rod is more complicated to insert but can be adjusted as the child grows.

If the child is going for surgery to reduce and immobilize a fracture, ensure that the child is adequately hydrated with IV fluids. Postoperative care involves frequent vital sign and neurovascular assessments. Pain management is also an important critical nursing action. IV narcotics are administered as indicated. If the child is old enough to use a PCA, it is used to keep pain control at a more constant, therapeutic level. When the child is able to tolerate solid food, pain medication is changed to an oral narcotic such as acetaminophen (Children's Tylenol) with codeine. Children with OI have excessive fluid loss through their skin, so they have a much greater need for hydration. Assess hydration status with every vital sign assessment.

Education/Discharge Instructions

Communicate to parents that the child's development may be delayed because of increased dependence on parents and decreased social interactions. Play and physical therapy are used with these children; the family can play with the child. The physical therapist directs ROM and muscle-strengthening exercises. The physical therapist also helps the child regain mobility after surgery or a fracture and ensures that the child can use the ambulatory devices safely. If deformities are present, ambulatory devices such as a walker or wheelchair may be necessary.

Encourage parents to receive genetic counseling. Causing a fracture is the biggest fear of these parents. Focus information toward the specific type of OI. Specific instructions about how to hold their infant, change the infant's diaper, and position their infant to reduce the possibility of fracture are reviewed to help parents feel comfortable caring for their infant. The goal is to achieve a balance between protecting the child from fractures and allowing the child to live as normal a life as possible.

OSTEOPOROSIS

Osteoporosis is a condition that has been known to develop in postmenopausal women. The bones lose density and calcium and become brittle. Osteopenia, or low bone mass between 1 and 2.5 standard deviations below the norm, precedes osteoporosis. Children can develop osteoporosis related to imbalanced nutrition or some pathological conditions.

Premature, very-low-birth-weight infants often suffer from osteopenia of prematurity because bone mass is acquired in the last weeks of gestation. These infants may have an inability to ingest sufficient nutrients because of their prematurity or other health problems related to their prematurity. Activity is often less in premature infants so there is a decreased amount of mechanical loading on their bones.

Older children may acquire osteoporosis as a result of decreased mechanical loading. Children who have a health condition that results in decreased ambulation or minimal pressure on the long bones are at risk for osteoporosis. Children with any of the following diseases are at risk for osteoporosis: spina bifida, cerebral palsy, juvenile arthritis, OI, diabetes, growth hormone deficiency, and Turner's syndrome. Immobilization can also lead to osteoporosis, so children who are immobilized in traction or children who are wearing a cast are at risk.

Many adolescents do not ingest the necessary requirements of calcium and vitamin D, which puts them at risk for osteoporosis later in life. Some lifestyle choices also put adolescents at risk for osteoporosis (e.g., smoking, using alcohol, drinking excessive amounts of soda, and keeping their weight very low).

Signs and Symptoms

The precursor to osteoporosis is osteopenia. Osteopenia is when the bone mineral density (BMD) is lower than normal but not low enough to be osteoporosis. A child with osteopenia is at greater risk to develop osteoporosis. In osteopenia, the bones become thinner and existing bone cells are reabsorbed faster than new bone can be made. Mineral, heaviness, and structure of the bones are lost thereby making them at greater risk for fracture. Eating disorders or problems with metabolism prevent the body from absorbing and using vitamins and minerals that would prevent osteopenia. Chemotherapy and steroids can also increase the likelihood of osteopenia developing. Exposure to radiation is yet another treatment that can lead to osteopenia. Other assessment data that would increase the risk of developing osteopenia are:

- Family history of osteoporosis
- Being thin
- Being Caucasian or Asian
- Limited physical activity
- Smoking
- Drinking cola drinks regularly
- Drinking excessive amounts of alcohol (adolescents)

All of these factors that can lead to osteopenia will eventually lead to osteoporosis because osteopenia is a precursor to osteoporosis. There are actually no signs and symptoms of osteopenia. There is no observable pain or change as the bone becomes thinner. The risk of a fracture increases as the bone becomes less dense.

Osteoporosis is a disease that strikes silently. Signs or symptoms may not become apparent for years. In many cases, osteoporosis is first diagnosed when a bone is fractured. Sometimes symptoms appear:

- Pain
- Height loss
- Compression fracture(s) of the back

Diagnosis

The diagnosis of osteoporosis in children includes a dual energy x-ray absorptiometry (DXA) or bone mineral densitometry. A t-score (total score) is a score that is compared with the peak bone mineral density of a healthy 30-year old adult. A t-score of 0 means that the patient's BMD is equal to that of this 30-year old adult with a peak BMD. The difference is measured in standard deviations (SDs). SDs below 0 are indicated by negative numbers. The lower the SD means the greater the risk for fracture. A t-score (or total score) less than 2.5 SDs from the mean indicates osteoporosis.

In children, the diagnosis is a more complex process. DXA scans can be performed, but t-scores are not reported. A z-score is a BMD that has been compared with an individual who is matched to the child. A BMD z-score using the standardized bone density and taking age, gender, bone age, height, and weight are needed to determine if osteoporosis is present. The diagnostic criteria for children

include a DXA scan with a BMD z-score of less than 2.0 SDs in addition to a history of fractures from a minimum of a standing height (Kirouac, 2011).

Diagnosis includes CBC, ESR, urinalysis, chemistry panel, arthritis panel, serum protein electrophoresis, and x-ray of the involved bones. It becomes apparent when an infant or child suffers a fracture, and the x-ray exam confirms this diagnosis.

Prevention

Nurses play a significant role in preventing osteoporosis in children. Education with children, parents, and the community at-large are the target audience (Kirouac, 2011). The intake of calcium and vitamin D are crucial for preventing osteopenia and for reaching peak bone mass in school-age and adolescent girls. Calcium is ingested through drinking milk and eating leafy green vegetables. Vitamin D allows for the proper absorption of calcium and is ingested through eating fatty fish, fish oils, and milk and cereal. Vitamin D can also be created in the body by having short exposure to sunlight on a daily basis.

Collaborative Care

Nursing Care. Nursing care includes encouraging dietary intake of calcium and vitamin D, physical activity to promote bone strength, and psychosocial care. Calcium intake is an essential nutrient in bone growth and strength. When dietary intake of calcium does not reach recommended levels, the child cannot reach the genetically predetermined peak bone mass.

Physical activity is a major factor in skeletal development and bone mass. The maximum effect of physical activity on bone takes place in the young child before the epiphyseal plates close.

 Nursing Insight—*Psychosocial adjustment*

Psychosocial adjustment for children with osteoporosis can be an issue. A study by Michielsen, Van Wijk, and Ketelaar (2010) evaluated the quality of life in children with congenital limb deficiency. Their psychosocial functioning is comparable to their peers. Children who have suffered a limb deficiency as a result of trauma have to deal with the loss of the limb. If the child is an adolescent, the child must deal with the loss as well as their altered self-image.

Medical Care. Many treatments are not for use with children. They are used in postmenopausal women and men over age 70. There are more limited treatment modalities available for children such as nutrition and exercise. Good nutrition includes a diet high in calcium and vitamin D, while exercise includes strength and resistance training, which strengthen bones. Bisphosphonates, a class of drugs that prevents the loss of bone mass, are used in extreme cases. They decrease the activity of the cells that cause bone loss while increasing bone density and reducing the risk of fracture. Pamidronate (Aredia) has been used with limited experience in children. Alendronate (Fosamax) and zoledronic acid (Reclast) have no data available for use in children.

Education/Discharge Instructions

Education includes information about calcium, vitamin D, nutrition, and exercise. If the child has had long-term corticosteroid therapy or chemotherapy, the child is at risk for osteopenia and osteoporosis, so parents must be informed and encouraged to see the health-care provider.

Cultural Diversity: Caring for a Hispanic Child

Families of Hispanic background believe in *mal ojo* or "the evil eye." They believe that the *mal ojo* causes an illness that affects children and occurs when someone with special powers looks at or admires a child but does not touch the child. For this reason, it is very important for a nurse to touch the child when making an admiring statement about him. The parents may call a *curandera* or *curandero* to treat the child through touch and prayer. They may have the child wear special amulets or charms to protect him from the *mal ojo*. Hispanic families believe that the saints help their sick child recover. They may place holy pictures of saints on or near their child. It is very important to respect this practice and not replace the pictures, amulets, or charms on or near the child in the absence of the parents.

Immobilizing Devices

Casts, boots, splinting devices, skin traction, skeletal traction, and distraction devices are several different methods to immobilize an extremity. Each of these methods is effective in treating musculoskeletal conditions in the child. There are benefits and risks associated with each of these methods. Specific nursing interventions need to be initiated with each of these immobilization devices (Fig. 29-13).

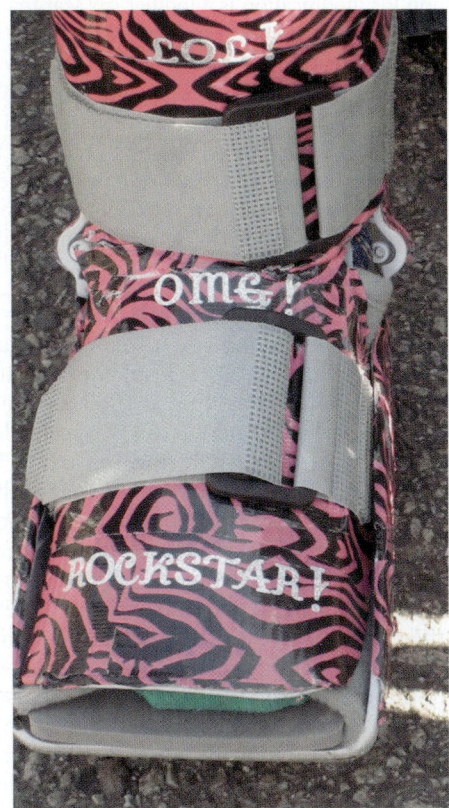

Figure 29-13 Decorated boot.

CASTS

Casts are a solid mold applied for immobilization purposes for fractures, dislocations, and other injuries. Casts are made of either a synthetic material such as fiberglass or plaster of Paris. Fiberglass is preferred because it is lighter in weight and dries within 30 minutes. Plaster of Paris casts take about 10 to 72 hours to dry.

There are four categories of casts: upper extremity, lower extremity, spinal or cervical, and total body (Fig. 29-14). An upper extremity or lower extremity cast provides absolute immobility of the affected extremity (Fig. 29-15). A complex or extensive fracture may require a rigid spinal or

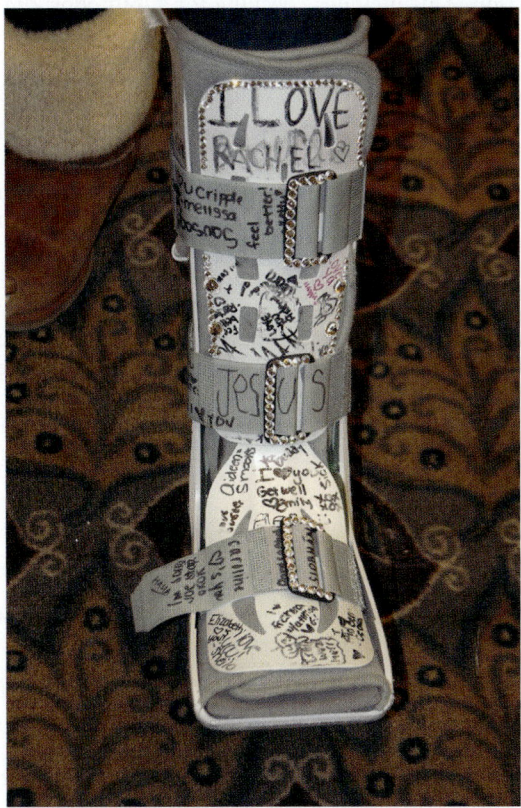

Figure 29-14 Types of casts.

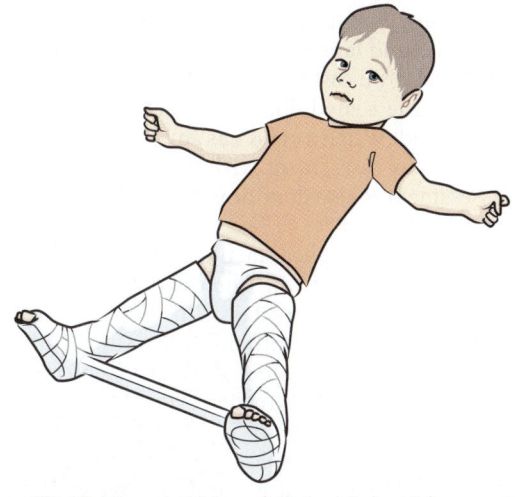

Figure 29-15 The child in a bilateral short leg cast with an abduction bar.

cervical cast for a long period of time. A total body cast such as a spica hip cast (also called a spica cast) immobilizes the hips and thighs so that bones or tendons can heal properly after hip surgery. A bilateral long leg cast with an abduction bar (crossbar connects the cast together at ankle level) is also used for significant immobilization. Both the spica hip and bilateral long leg cast with an abduction bar encases both legs to the toes.

When a child is placed in a total body cast with abduction bar, it is easier for parents to manage care than when a child is in a spica hip cast with no bar. Teach parents that the cast needs to be changed periodically. The two most common reasons to change a cast are when it becomes soiled or wet. Also, incision sites under a cast need to be assessed for infection. This includes checking for a foul odor, drainage from inside the cast, or staining through the cast.

Cast Complications

The major complication is **compartment syndrome**. Compartment syndrome develops when pressure within a closed fascial compartment is raised when inflammation occurs in the tissue that is surrounded by the fascia. This causes a decrease in blood flow and perfusion to the muscle that is surrounded by the fascia. Intracompartmental pressure increases, and blood flow to the tissue distal to the affected compartment can stop, thereby causing ischemia and eventually necrosis. There are two assessments that can be performed. The first is the neurovascular assessment (Box 29-3). The second is to assess for the 5 Ps:

- Pain unrelieved by narcotics
- Pallor
- Pulselessness
- Paresthesia
- **Poikilothermia** (a body temperature that varies with the temperature of its surroundings)

Application of ice and elevation can help to alleviate the risk of compartment syndrome. Any child at risk for compartment syndrome has the extremity elevated and ice applied. Administration of narcotic pain medication after pain assessment can also be implemented.

Collaborative Care

Nursing Care. Nursing care of the child in a cast begins with the child and family. For example, allow a preschoolage child to apply a cast to a doll. Then, give the child time to play with the casted doll before actually applying the cast to the child. When a child has any type of cast, perform a neurovascular assessment with vital signs. A neurovascular assessment is also done any time neurovascular compromise is suspected.

After the cast is applied, facilitate drying of the cast by leaving the cast open to air. The cast has a hollow sound when it is dry. Children treated with a fiberglass spica hip cast are placed in the bed with pillows to support the lower extremities. During the course of the drying phase and ongoing cast care, the child is turned every 2 hours. Frequent turning helps to facilitate drying and prevents cast syndrome if the child is in a spica hip cast. At times, the cast is bivalved meaning that it is cut down one or both sides with scissors to allow for expansion. The bivalved procedure is done to alleviate pressure, monitor for infection, or

to help maintain proper hygiene. After the cast is bivalved, the affected extremity is elevated when the child is in bed, in a chair, or in a wheelchair.

Nursing Insight—*Cast drying*

It is never acceptable to use a hair dryer to facilitate drying. The heat from the hair dryer can cause a burn injury under the cast. Instruct the family that careful handling of the cast is an important intervention that prevents dents in the cast. Dents can cause pressure points on the tissue under the cast and ultimately result in a pressure sore.

Elevation of the affected extremity helps with the child's pain control and prevents damage caused by pressure. If the child has a single-extremity cast, a waterproof plastic sleeve can be used to protect the cast and provide a seal during bathing. It is also important to explain to parents of a child in a cast that the child needs to be held. Help parents adjust to holding their child with a cast.

Hygiene is a major concern for a child in any type of cast but especially a spica hip cast or bilateral long leg casts with an abduction bar. Understand that protecting the proximal edges of the long leg casts and the perineal area of the spica hip cast from soiling is a key hygienic intervention that is achieved by petaling or bivalving the cast.

Nursing Insight—*Modifications for a child in a spica hip cast*

Modifications need to be made for a child in a spica hip cast. The spica hip cast prevents the child from sitting normally; therefore, parents need a way to help their child adapt. One suggestion for modification is a toddler car seat that does not have sides. Toddler car seats are designed to help the small child with a spica hip cast to sit fairly normally. They also have a 5-point restraint system. Another suggestion is allowing a child to sit in a wagon with side rails. Feeding a child in a spica hip cast can also be a challenge. Placing the child in the prone position on the floor is a good modification and makes it easier for the child to feed themselves. Allowing the child to have supervised time while prone on a blanket helps the child to maintain developmental milestones.

Bathing the child with a cast is also an important nursing intervention. If the child has a small extremity cast, a typical bath can be taken as long as the cast is protected from water (Figs. 29-16*A* and 29-16*B*). A large plastic bag can be placed over the cast during the bath. The best method is to purchase a plastic cast cover at a pharmacy. They come in pediatric sizes for long and short arm or leg casts. The hole is small but expands to allow the casted extremity to be inserted, and then it contracts to prevent water from entering. The child also keeps the extremity outside the edge of the tub while bathing or showering; however, it is the least effective of the three methods discussed. If the child is in a bilateral long-leg cast with an abduction bar or a spica hip cast, teach the parent how to bathe the child by giving a sponge bath. In addition, frequent diaper changes help prevent complications such as skin breakdown and infection. Good perineal care is essential for children of all ages.

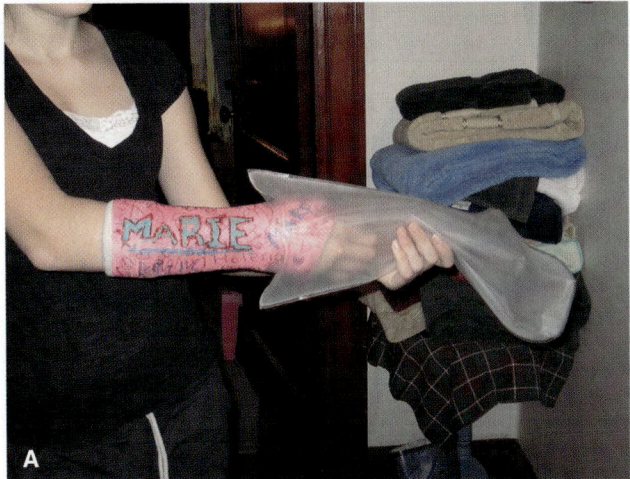

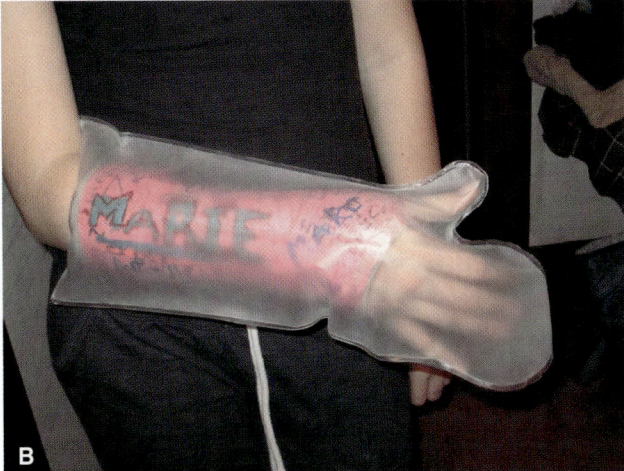

Figures 29-16a and b Cast cover for showering.

The child is prone to constipation because of inactivity while immobilized in a cast. Teach the family about the importance of good fluid intake, a diet high in fiber, and calling the health-care professional about laxatives or stool softeners if needed.

Sometimes the child experiences some itching under the cast. Itching can be prevented by keeping the skin in good condition by turning the child every 2 hours and keeping the cast clean and dry. It is important to tell parents that some children try to push items under the cast to scratch the area. Teach the parents and the child that absolutely nothing is placed in the cast. If the itching is severe, instruct the parent to call the health-care provider about medication.

Cast care also includes taking care of the cast when it is being removed. Explain to the child that the sound of the cast saw is loud and can be frightening. It is difficult for the child to believe that the saw will not cut his or her skin. Reassure the child that she will not be injured with the cast removal. When the cast is removed, the child's skin is dry and flaky and the muscles are weak and possibly stiff. It is important to consider the child's emotions about the cast because the child may have grown used to it and think of it as a part of him.

Cast syndrome is a complication that can occur when a child has been placed in a spica cast. This syndrome occurs when a portion of the duodenum is compressed between the superior mesenteric artery and the aorta, causing vomiting, abdominal distention, and bowel obstruction.

Critical Nursing Action Cast Syndrome

Cast syndrome can be prevented by three nursing interventions:

- Frequent repositioning
- Fluids and increased fiber in the child's diet
- Cutting a "belly hole" or a window in the cast to allow for abdominal expansion

PRINCIPLES OF TRACTION

Recognize that the main principle of traction is to reduce dislocations and immobilize fractures in the child. During the application of traction, one body part is pulled in one direction (traction) against a counterpull in the opposite direction (countertraction). The traction and the countertraction are the actual weights and pulleys. There are two main types of traction: skin traction and skeletal traction.

Skin Traction

Skin traction is used for an extremity with a type of strapping material applied to the limb. Skin traction is used for short periods of time. Bryant's traction is one type of skin

Procedure 29-1 Petaling or Bivalving a Cast

Purpose

The purpose of petaling a cast is to promote good hygiene by protecting the perineal area of the spica hip casts from soiling.

Equipment

- 1-inch waterproof adhesive tape
- Plastic bag to place adhesive tape on
- Scissors

Steps

1. Use scissors to cut 1-inch-wide strips of waterproof adhesive tape. The length of the

waterproof adhesive tape is approximately 1½ to 2 inches long.

RATIONALE: *Waterproof adhesive tape helps provide a protective barrier for the skin.*

2. The edge on one end of both pieces of the waterproof adhesive tape must be rounded.

RATIONALE: *Rounded edges keep the waterproof adhesive tape edges from rolling.*

3. Apply the first strip of waterproof adhesive tape to any edge of the cast that is likely to become soiled by urine or stool.

(continued)

Procedure 29-1 Petaling or Bivalving a Cast (continued)

4. Tuck the straight (unrounded) end inside the cast.

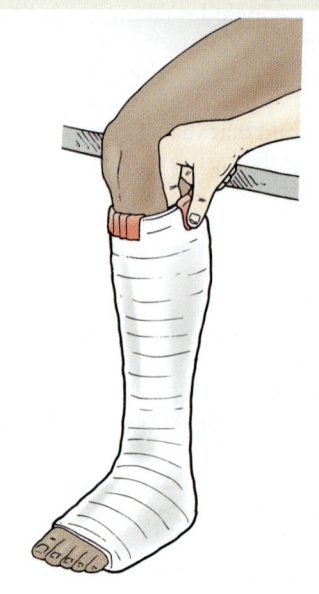

5. With your forefinger, gently ensure that the inside end of the tape is flat and not sticking to the child's skin.

6. Repeat the procedure, overlapping each additional strip, until all rough edges are completely covered.

Clinical Alert It is a good idea to petal the edges of the cast that are likely to be soiled by urine and feces on the first postoperative day and preferably before the Foley catheter is removed.

Teach Parents

Teach the parents that diapering needs to be modified. To achieve this, a small diaper or peri-pad is placed in the perineal area with all edges of the cast outside this small diaper. Then a larger diaper is placed outside the smaller diaper and taped in the normal fashion. Ensure that the perineal edges of the cast remain outside the diaper.

Documentation

1/9/10 0900 Upper edge of cast soiled and moist. Cast petaling performed. Waterproof adhesive tape to the upper edge of the cast. After petaling, the cast is noted to be clean and dry. No adverse reactions noted.

—M. O'Connor, MS, RN

---

traction and is used to treat developmental dysplasia of the hip, shortened limb, and femur fractures in children younger than 2 to 3 years of age. The child must weigh less than 26.4 lb (12 kg) to use Bryant's traction. In Bryant's traction, the child lies supine with thighs flexed and the hips slightly off the bed. Moleskin straps are applied to the child's calves, and the pull is in only one direction. The nurse understands that the child's body is the countertraction. In modified Bryant's traction, the hips remain on the bed, but the legs are abducted.

Russell's traction is another type of skin traction that is used when the child weighs more than 26.4 lb (12 kg). It is most often used to stabilize femur fractures until a callus forms. With this type of traction, the child lies supine with hip flexed and abducted. There are two lines of pull in Russell's traction, and the hips need to remain in alignment (Fig. 29-17). The child has a trapeze secured on a crossbar above the bed to assist with repositioning and maintaining upper body strength. In this type of traction a sling is placed under the knee. The placement of the sling is assessed frequently. Countertraction is increased with the foot of the bed elevated and the head of the bed flat.

Collaborative Care

Nursing Care. Nursing care for the child in skin traction requires a neuromuscular assessment to the affected extremity every 4 hours. Watch for web space numbness in fingers and toes. Web space numbness may indicate compartment syndrome. For any child in traction, it is necessary to assess circulation, sensation, pain, pallor, cyanosis, movement, and decreased pulse every 2 to 4 hours.

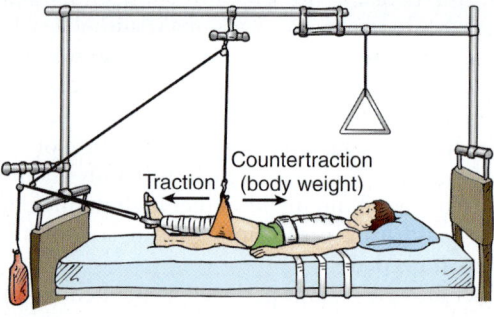

Figure 29-17 The child in Russell's traction (with trapeze).

Ensure that the traction weights are checked and hanging free and that the child is in alignment with the traction. Skin traction needs to be removed and reapplied every 4 hours.

Perform skin care every 4 hours. The skin under the straps needs to be inspected and treated with rubbing alcohol to remove the body oils, which might cause the straps to slip. Pay close attention to the bony prominences that can break down easily. Do not massage bony prominences and ensure protective foam is in place. If the child has Ace wraps, protect the Ace wraps from urine and stool. Have two sets of Ace wraps for the child, keep one set washed and be ready to use the spare ACE wrap in case the first ACE wrap becomes soiled. While the child is in traction, initiate diversional activities to keep the child occupied while in traction (e.g., movie videos, board and video games, puzzles, blocks, and other toys that are easy for the child to handle).

Skeletal Traction

Skeletal traction is used when more pulling force is needed than can be withstood by skin traction. Since the advent of newer orthopedic devices that achieve similar outcomes as skeletal traction and allow the child to be cared for at home rather than in the hospital, skeletal traction is used much less frequently. However, skeletal traction is still used when the weight of the traction needs to be more than 5 lb.

In children, skeletal traction is used for long periods of time until the bone is ready for casting or **open reduction** (surgery to place the bones in their proper position). Many children needing skeletal traction have sustained multiple injuries. In skeletal traction, a pin is placed through the bone distal to the fracture. It is extremely important to note that with skeletal traction, the weights cannot be removed. There are three common forms of skeletal traction: Crutchfield tongs, 90/90 femoral traction, and Dunlop traction.

CRUTCHFIELD TONGS. Crutchfield tongs are used in the management of cervical and thoracic fractures. The tongs are placed into the child's skull (Fig. 29-18). The pull is along the axis of the spine. The traction usually hangs off the head of the bed. The countertraction is the body. The tongs need to be assessed every 8 hours and as needed for placement and looseness. Use logrolling to turn the child in Crutchfield tongs. When this type of traction is used, pin care (gently cleansing the wound with saline-moistened gauze and applying antibiotic ointment with a cotton-tipped applicator if prescribed by the physician) needs to be done every shift. Neurovascular signs need to be assessed every 4 hours (more often if needed) because of the pressure on the spinal cord. Other important nursing care measures include pain control, meeting nutrition and elimination needs, providing proper hygiene, maintaining developmental milestones, giving emotional support, and allowing for spiritual care. The family can be encouraged to express feelings of worry, helplessness, and frustration.

90/90 FEMORAL TRACTION. The 90/90 femoral traction is most commonly used to treat femur fractures and complicated femur fractures. A pin is placed in the femur, distal to the fracture. Weights are attached to a sling that supports the calf and also to the pin that causes the traction (Fig. 29-19). The body is the countertraction. Femoral traction is more effective in children older than 6 years of age. Often femoral traction is used for the first 2 to 3 weeks after a femur fracture until enough of a callus forms. After a callus forms, a spica hip cast is applied. Perform pin care every shift or according to the hospital policy. Also be sure to meet the holistic health needs of the child and family.

Maintaining the child in this type of alignment can be challenging. Sometimes there is a need for restraints to keep the child in proper alignment. If restraints are needed,

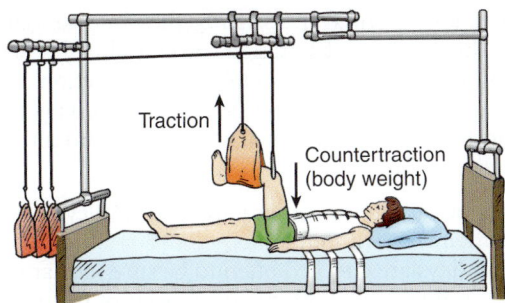

Figure 29-19 The 90/90 femoral traction is most commonly used to treat femur fractures and complicated femur fractures.

hospital policy needs to be strictly followed and obtain an order from the health-care provider. Generally, a hospital restraint policy states that the restraints need to be removed every 2 hours for 10 minutes while the child is awake and every 4 hours for 10 minutes while the child sleeps. The restraint order also needs to be renewed by the physician every 24 hours. A better solution than restraints is constant supervision by parents, family members, friends, and hospital staff. Often a hospital will have a volunteer program or a child life specialist who can help with diversion activities.

DUNLOP TRACTION. Dunlop traction is used in the management of a supracondylar fracture of the humerus. In this type of traction, a pin is placed in the humerus, distal to the fracture. Weights are attached to the forearm and to the pin that causes the traction. The body is the countertraction (Fig. 29-20).

Volkmann's ischemia can occur with children in Dunlop traction. The child complains of numbness, tingling, and a decreased sensation in the fingers. An important nursing intervention is to ask the child to wiggle the fingers to help relieve the discomfort.

Collaborative Care

Nursing Care. Assessment is the key nursing care measure for a child in skeletal traction. Neurovascular status must be assessed carefully every 1 to 2 hours for the first 48 hours and then every 4 hours after that if there is no compromise in circulation. Know the symptoms of compartment syndrome and report them to the physician immediately.

Be sure to understand the principles of traction and the reason why the traction has been applied. Maintaining the alignment of the traction with the child can be a challenge. By nature, children are unable to remain still in bed for extended periods of time. Realign the child in the bed often. Emphasis is on ensuring that the shoulder, hip, and leg are in a straight line with the lines of traction. Diversional

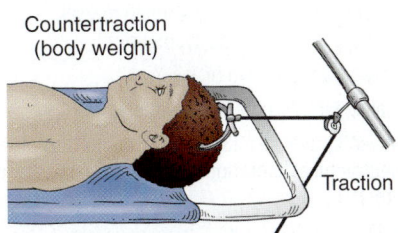

Figure 29-18 Crutchfield tongs are used in the management of cervical and thoracic fractures.

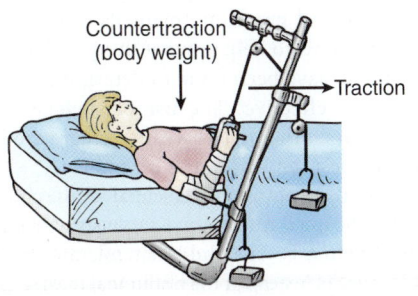

Figure 29-20 Dunlop traction is used in the management of a supracondylar fracture of the humerus.

activities are essential in assisting the child to maintain proper alignment. Collaboration with the child life specialist also helps the child. Maintaining the traction also involves assessing the desired line of pull with the relationship between the distal part and the proximal part. The nurse ensures that:

- The ropes are in the center part of the pulley, taut, and are intact, without knots.
- The pulleys are checked often to be sure they are in their original place and that the wheels of the pulley move freely.
- The amount of the weights is correct and that they are hanging freely.
- The bed is positioned with the head or the foot of the bed elevated as ordered so that the correct amount of pull is achieved with the traction and countertraction.
- The skeletal traction is not removed. If a child needs to be moved or if the traction needs to be adjusted, contact the health-care provider.

To prevent skin breakdown, place the child on an alternating-pressure mattress or a foam mattress overlay. A nursing assessment of the child's body is done to look for redness or breakdowns, especially on bony prominences receiving the greatest pressure. Wash and dry the child's skin daily or more frequently if needed. Change the child's position every 2 hours to relieve pressure. Assess pin sites every 8 hours for signs and symptoms of infection to prevent osteomyelitis.

Managing the child's pain is essential so use pharmacological and nonpharmacological care measures. Also use good judgment about the administration of pain medication by not waiting too long to administer pain medication and being alert for any adverse side effects. Effective pain control methods include epidural with bupivacaine (Marcaine) and a narcotic such as morphine sulfate (Astramorph) or hydromorphone (Dilaudid), patient-controlled analgesia with morphine sulfate (Astramorph), or hydromorphone (Dilaudid). Antispasmodics such as diazepam (Valium) will give relief to the child with muscle spasms. Also ask the parents to participate in pain assessment and pain management by offering comfort measures. Diversional activity also might help manage pain. Be sure to involve the child life specialist in this aspect of care. Work collaboratively with the physical therapist to perform passive and active range-of-motion exercises to prevent weakness in uninvolved extremities. If pain is under control, the child may be able to perform minimal activities of daily living while on bedrest.

 ### Nursing Insight—*Pin care*

Pin site infection has been a problem for nursing practice. Hospital policy and procedure manuals each have a specific procedure to follow to help prevent this problem. A few multicenter studies have been done to determine which method is in fact most effective. The use of skeletal traction has declined greatly in the past 15 years so there are few studies regarding the best method to use for pin care.

Maintaining good nutrition is essential for the child in skeletal traction. The hospital nutritionist can visit with the family to discuss healthy meals. The child may tolerate six small meals and healthy snacks instead of the traditional meal schedule. Offer the child healthy drinks and snacks. A sticker reward chart is an effective measure to encourage good nutrition and reward healthy food choices. The child also needs to be assessed for regular elimination to ensure he or she does not become constipated or acquire a urinary tract infection. Also, be alert to the child in skeletal traction because serious complications can occur. **Osteomyelitis** (inflammation of bone and marrow, usually caused by infection) is a major, serious complication. Prevent complications such as pneumonia, circulatory compromise, ischemia, and problems of disuse with uninvolved extremities. Any circumferential dressing has a potential to cause impaired circulation so dressings are assessed for tightness. Any restrictive bandages or devices are also assessed to ensure that they are neither too tight nor too loose. Prepare the family for discharge and offer psychosocial support.

 ### Nursing Insight—*Distraction devices*

Distraction devices are usually used to lengthen a bone. The surgeon performs an **osteotomy** (cuts through a bone) and places the distraction device. A distraction device can be placed in any long bone such as the femur and mandible, as well as in bones in the hand and the foot. Nursing care of the child with a distraction device is much the same as for the child in skeletal traction.

 ### Now Can You—Discuss nursing care for musculoskeletal conditions?

1. Discuss the nursing care for a child with a cast?
2. Describe the principles of traction?
3. Describe the nursing care for skin and skeletal traction?

! focus on safety

Falls

Children in general are at great risk for falls while hospitalized. The Pediatric Fall Risk Tool is used to determine the fall risk. It is performed during the initial assessment and then reassessed when there is a change in the child's status. The Pediatric Fall Risk Tool assesses:

- History of falls within the past 3 months (Score 0 = No or 3 = Yes)
- Physical alterations (Score 0 = No or 3 = Yes) to any of the list below:
  - Surgery within admission
  - Underlying medical condition of seizures
  - History of vertigo or syncope
  - Guillain-Barré syndrome
  - Multiple sclerosis
  - Alteration in visual acuity
- Functional Status: altered mobility (Score 0 = None, 1 = Weak, 2 = Impaired or age-specific, learning to walk, 3 = Crutches, walker, brace, or orthostatic hypotension)
- Equipment (Score 0 = No or 3 = Yes)
  - IV, saline lock, IV pole, Foley catheter
- Cognitive/Psychosocial (Score 0 = oriented to own ability, 2 = Neurological limitations because of illness or behavioral concerns)
  - Impaired mental status

- Developmental delay
- Behavioral concerns
- Depression
- Oppositional deficit behavior
- Medications that alter equilibrium (Score 0 = No, 3 = Yes)
  - Anticonvulsants
  - Narcotics
  - Antipsychotics
  - Sedatives
  - Chemotherapy
  - Hypotensive medications

When this score is determined, it will reveal a number between 0 and 17. If the score is between 0 and 7, the child is at low risk for falls, if it is greater than or equal to a score of 8, then the child is at high risk for falls.

Ensure that the bed is the correct size, in the lowest position with the wheels locked. Side rails need to be up when the child is in the bed or crib. Clothes need to fit, and the child needs to wear skid-proof footwear. All IV tubes, drains, and catheters need to be secured. Ensure that spills and clutter are cleaned up. Teach the patient and family regarding these safety measures. If the child is in the high-risk category, all of the low-risk interventions need to be implemented as well as the following interventions. Hourly rounds to check on the child and attend to their needs are important. The child does not get out of bed without assistance. Evaluate whether patient care sitters may be necessary. All unnecessary equipment and furniture is removed from the room. Determine the need for physical therapist or occupational therapist consults or the need for a psychiatric or social worker for any behavioral issues. Also request the assistance of the child life therapist for play activities. A special wristband on the child and a sign on the door can flag others that the child is at risk for a fall.

Summary Points

- Growth and development of the musculoskeletal system play a major role in the normal growth and development of the child.

- Nurses play an important role in assisting the parents to find methods to help the child maintain normal growth and development as well as adapting or overcoming musculoskeletal system impairment.

- Care of a child with a musculoskeletal disorder involves collaboration with the interdisciplinary team members, each having a specific role.

- When caring for a child with a musculoskeletal condition, a neurovascular status must be assessed carefully and every 1 to 2 hours for the first 48 hours. A thorough neurovascular status consists of pain, sensation, motion, temperature, capillary refill time, color, and pulses.

- Clubfoot is a term used to describe a foot deformity diagnosed in newborn infants. The most severe form of this condition resembles a "club" and is called talipes equinovarus. It requires long-term follow-up because there is a residual lifelong atrophy of the calf muscle.

- Nursing care for a child undergoing nonsurgical management of clubfoot includes passive range of motion and care of the cast application after manipulation.

- There are four stages of Legg-Calvé-Perthes disease (LCPD): aseptic necrosis, revascularization, new bone formation, and the regenerative phase. It is a self-limiting disease, and it can take from 18 months to 4 years for the child to emerge from it. The child needs to participate in non–weight-bearing activities during the course of the disease.

- Nursing care of the child with slipped capital femoral epiphysis (SCFE) includes bedrest, assisting the family in adjusting to the sudden hospitalization, non–weight-bearing status of the child, and the impending surgery. After surgery, monitor the neurovascular status frequently and manage pain.

- Nursing diagnoses for a child with a fracture include risk for injury related to external devices, impaired physical mobility related to external devices, and risk for impaired skin integrity related to external devices.

- In pectus excavatum, surgery is performed to elevate the sternal depression and secure it to the chest wall. A bar remains in place for 2 to 3 years to ensure a permanent remodeling of the sternum.

- The surgery for syndactyly is more complex than surgery for polydactyly. The skin, muscles, nerves, tendons, ligaments, blood vessels, and bones must be separated. Sometimes the bones are shorter so the surgeon will perform an osteotomy and place a distractor. The distractor consists of pins that have been placed in the two bone fragments.

- Dislocated radial head is a form of dislocation. The head of the radius slips and becomes dislocated as a result of an injury.

- Soft tissue injuries are sprains and strains and are unusual in young children. Sprains and strains are often seen in the adolescent age group.

- The increase in popularity of competitive sports, recreational sports, and cheerleading has significantly increased the number of overuse injuries, sprains, strains, and dislocations.

- The major signs and symptom of Osgood-Schlatter disease include pain below the kneecap that is aggravated by activity and relieved by rest and pain when asked to squat or extend the knee against resistance.

- Congenital torticollis becomes evident during the first 2 weeks after birth. Delayed development can occur because the child is unable to turn her head to see, hear, or touch.

- All types of osteomyelitis require immediate treatment.

- The child with juvenile arthritis will have joints that are swollen, tender, and warm to touch and limited range of motion (ROM). The joints will have a loss of motion and will be stiff, especially in the morning. Intermittent joint pain that lasts longer than 6 weeks is suspected for juvenile arthritis.

- Treatment of transient synovitis of the hip includes limiting activity so the child is more comfortable. However, there is no danger of untoward effects if the child maintains normal activity. Nonsteroidal anti-inflammatory medications (NSAIDs) can be prescribed to reduce pain.

♦ In Duchenne's muscular dystrophy, the symptoms first appear after the child is able to walk, usually about 3 to 7 years of age. The child develops a waddling, wide-based gait and uses the Gowers' maneuver to rise from the floor.

♦ Positioning of the child after surgery for scoliosis is an important nursing action. The child must be turned using the logrolling technique.

♦ Early mobilization is important in the care of the child who has had a spinal fusion. Early mobilization prevents atelectasis, pneumonia, pulmonary emboli, phlebitis, and skin breakdown.

♦ Kyphosis is a non-painful spinal curvature of the spine and is commonly described as "hunchback."

♦ Lordosis is commonly described as "swayback," an excessive backward cavity of the spine.

♦ Prevention of tetanus is the best defense; tetanus prophylaxis through immunization is the key to preventing this condition.

♦ Reliable prenatal diagnosis about osteogenesis imperfecta (OI) is not currently available. Diagnosis is based on the severity of clinical symptoms and the level of disability.

♦ Research shows that an intake of calcium in school-age and adolescent girls plays an important role in preventing the development of osteoporosis.

♦ Casts, boots, splints, skin traction, skeletal traction, and distraction devices are effective methods in treating musculoskeletal conditions in the child.

♦ Complications can occur when a child is immobilized in a cast. The major complication that can occur is compartment syndrome, which is caused by an accumulation of fluid in the fascia.

♦ Symptoms of compartment syndrome include pain, pallor, pulselessness, paresthesia, and paralysis.

♦ A nursing assessment of a child in a cast includes the 5 Ps: pain unrelieved by narcotics, pulse present at the distal site, pallor, paresthesia, and paralysis.

♦ Recognize that the main principle of traction is to reduce dislocations and immobilize fractures in the child.

♦ Distraction devices are usually used to lengthen a bone; the surgeon cuts through a bone and places the distraction device.

Review Questions

Multiple Choice

1. The pediatric nurse is caring for a 5-year-old child in traction related to a broken femur. Which action by the nurse takes priority?
   A. Assess neurovascular status every 4 hours.
   B. Provide diversional activities for the child.
   C. Educate parents on the principles of traction.
   D. Provide high-protein, high-fiber menu items.

2. The nurse consults the child life specialist to help plan care for a child who is immobilized and is increasingly anxious. Which is the priority intervention for this child?
   A. Allowing the school to provide a tutor
   B. Providing diversional activities
   C. Consulting a social worker
   D. Administering pain medication

3. The nurse is preparing a 7-year-old child to have a cast removed from his leg. Which statement would be most appropriate to prepare the child for the procedure?
   A. "As soon as the cast comes off, you can get up and move around."
   B. "The sound of the cast saw is very loud and may be a little scary."
   C. "You must sit very still so we don't accidentally hurt your leg."
   D. "Don't worry; you will be asleep during the cast removal."

4. A nurse reads the diagnosis of neurogenic clubfoot on an infant's chart. Which other diagnosis does the nurse expect to find when reviewing the medical record?
   A. Osteogenesis imperfecta
   B. Spina bifida
   C. Muscular dystrophy
   D. No associated diagnosis

5. The pediatric nurse is aware that which is the precipitating cause of Legg-Calvé-Perthes disease?
   A. Genetic abnormality
   B. Interruption in blood flow
   C. Birth trauma
   D. Dietary deficiency

6. The pediatric nurse understands that which classification of fracture has the most potential to affect growth?
   A. Type III
   B. Type V
   C. Closed
   D. Open

7. Which explanation by the pediatric nurse is most appropriate for a child with ankylosis?
   A. ROM restrictions in the vertebrae
   B. Adhesions causing joint immobility
   C. Curvature of the cervical spine
   D. Bowed legs caused by low calcium

8. A nurse visiting a day care notices a boy trying to get up off the floor by kneeling, rising to his feet while keeping his hands on the floor, then walking his hands up his legs until he is standing. Which assessment finding does this nurse document?
   A. Positional instability
   B. Gowers' maneuver
   C. Kernig's sign
   D. Grey Turner's sign

9. The nurse is providing care to a child diagnosed with lordosis. Which common term might the parents have heard to describe this condition?
   A. Hunchback
   B. Swayback
   C. Spinal curvature
   D. Flat feet

10. A nurse admitting a child to the intensive care unit is told the child has risus sardonicus. Which disease process does the nurse suspect the child has?
   A. Scoliosis
   B. Osteogenesis imperfecta
   C. Duchenne's muscular dystrophy
   D. Tetanus

See Answers to End of Chapter Review Questions on Davis*Plus*.

REFERENCES

Acara, K., & Tschudy, M. (2012). *Harriet Lane handbook: A manual for pediatric house officers* (17th ed.). St. Louis, MO: Mosby.

American Heart Association (AHA). (2013). Retrieved from http://www.heart.org/HEARTORG/

Baker, T., Haines, S., Yost, J., DiClaudio, S., Braun, C., & Holt, S. (2012). The role of family-centered therapy when used with physical or occupational therapy in children with congenital or acquired disorders. *Physical Therapy Reviews, 17*(1) 29–36.

Baumbach, S. F., Hobohm, L., & Wozasek, G. E. (2011). A treatment strategy for complex cases of osteomyelitis in children and its applicability on three exemplary cases. *Journal of Pediatric Orthopedics, 20*(6), 432–435. doi:10.1097/BPB.0b013e3283458846

Belthur, M. V., Birchansky, S. B., Verdugo, A. A., Mason, Jr., E. O., Hulten, K. G., Kaplan, S. L., et al. (2012). Pathologic fractures in children with acute Staphylococcus aureus osteomyelitis. *Journal of Bone and Joint Surgery, 94-A*(1), 34–42. doi:10.2106/JBJSJ.01915

Bulechek, G. M., Butcher, H. K., Dochterman, J. M., & Wagner, C. (2013). *Nursing interventions classification (NIC)* (6th ed.). St. Louis, MO: Elsevier Mosby.

Carroll, N. C. (2012). Clubfoot in the twentieth century: Where we were and where we may be going in the twenty-first century. *Journal of Pediatric Orthopedics, Part B, 21*(1), 1–6. doi:10.1097/BPB.0b013e32834a99f2

Chagas, C. E. A., Roque, J. P., Peters, B. S. E., Lazaretti-Castro, M., & Martini, L. A. (2011). Do patients with osteogenesis imperfecta need individualized nutritional support? *Nutrition, 28*, 138–142. doi:10.1016/j.nut.2011.04.003

Cheng, J. C., Lam, T. P., & Ng, B. K. (2011). Prognosis and prognostic factors of Legg-Calve-Perthes disease. *Journal of Pediatric Orthopedics, 31*(2), S147–S151.

Dobbs, M. B., & Gurnett, C. A. (2011). Genetics of clubfoot. *Journal of Pediatric Orthopedics, Part B, 21*(1), 7–9. doi:10.1097/BPB.0b013e328349927c

Flynn, J. M., Garner, M. R., Jones, K. J., D'Italia, J., Davidson, R. S., & Ganley, T. J. (2011). The treatment of low-energy femoral shaft fractures: A prospective study comparing the "walking spica" with the traditional spica cast. *Journal of Bone and Joint Surgery, 93-A* (23), 2196–2202. doi:10.2106/JBJSJ.01165

Frantz, F. W. (2011). Indications and guidelines for pectus excavatum repair. *Current Opinions in Pediatrics, 23*, 486–491. doi:10.1097/MOP.0b013e32834881c4

Herring, J. A. (2011). Legg-Calvé-Perthes disease at 100: A review of evidence-based treatment. *Journal of Pediatric Orthopedics, 31*(2), S137–S140.

Institute of Medicine (IOM). (2011). Retrieved from http://www.iom.edu/

Johnson, M., Moorhead, S., Bulechek, G., Butcher, H., Maas, M., & Swanson, E. (2012). *NIC and NOC linkages to NANDA-L and clinical conditions* (3rd ed.) St. Louis, MO: Elsevier Mosby.

Joseph, B. (2011). Natural history of early onset and late-onset Legg-Calve-Perthes disease. *Journal of Pediatric Orthopedics, 31*(2), S152–S155.

Kim, H. K. W. (2011). Legg-Calve-Perthes disease: Etiology, pathogenesis, and biology. *Journal of Pediatric Orthopedics, 31*(2), S141–S146.

Kirouac, N. (2011). Osteoporosis in children: Implications for nursing. *Journal of the Pediatric Endocrinology Nursing Society*, 271–274. doi:10.1016/j.pedn.2011.02.—2

Kuzyk, P. R., Kim, Y., & Millis, M. B. (2011). Surgical management of healed slipped capital femoral epiphysis. *Journal of American Academy of Orthopedic Surgeons, 19*(11), 667–677.

Larson, N. (2011). Early onset scoliosis: What the primary care provider needs to know and implications for practice. *Journal of the American Academy of Nurse Practitioners, 23*, 392–403. doi:10.1111/j.1745-7599.2011.00634.x

Mayer, R. (2012). PTs stress a stretching and positioning program designed to specifically meet the child's needs. *Advance for Physical Therapy & Rehab Medicine*, Retrieved from http://physical-therapy.advanceweb.com/Editorial/Content/PrintFriendly.aspx?CC=248128

Michielsen, A., Van Wijk, I., & Ketelaar, M. (2010). Participation and quality of life in children and adolescents with congenital limb deficiencies: A narrative review. *Prosthetics and Orthotics International, 34*(4), 351–361. doi:10.3109/03093646.2010.495371

Moorhead, S., Johnson, M., Maas, M. L., & Swanson, E. (2013). *Nursing outcomes classification (NOC)* (5th ed.). St. Louis, MO: Elsevier Mosby.

National Posture Institute. (2014). Public posture programs. Retrieved from http://www.npionline.org/programs/public/index.html

Nierenberg, G., Falah, M., Keren, Y., & Eidelman, M. (2012). Surgical treatment of residual Osgood-Schlatter disease in young adults: Role of the mobile osseous fragment. Ortho Supersite. doi:10.3928/01477447-20110124-07. Retrieved from http://www.orthosupersite.com/print.aspx?rid=80661

Okoromah, C. A. N., & Lesi, A. F. E. (2009). Diazepam for treating for tetanus (review). *The Cochrane Collaboration published in the Cochrane Library 2009, Issue 1.*

Perez, T. (2012). BrainyQuote.com. Retrieved from BrainyQuote.com Web site: http://www.brainyquote.com/quotes/quotes/t/tonyperez197438.html

Perry, D. C., Machin, D. M. G., Pope, D., Bruce, C. E., Dangerfield, P., Platt, M. J., et al. (2012). Racial and geographic factors in the incidence of Legg-Calve-Perthes' disease: A systematic review. *American Journal of Epidemiology, 175*(3), 159–166. doi:10.1093/aje/kwr293

Poliachik, S. L., Friedman, S. D., Carter, G. T., Parnell, S. E., & Shaw, D. W. (2012). Skeletal muscle edema in muscular dystrophy: Clinical and diagnostic implications. *Physical Medicine Rehabilitation Clinics of North America, 23*(1), 107–122. doi:10.1016/j.pmr.2011.11.016

Secor-Turner, M., Scal, P., Garwick, A., Horvath, K., & Wells, C. K. (2011). Living with juvenile arthritis: Adolescents' challenges and experiences. *Journal of Pediatric Health Care, 25*(5), 302–307. doi:10.1016/jpedhc.2010.06.004

Sommers, M. S., & Brunner, L. S. (2011). *Diseases and disorders: A nursing therapeutics manual (RnDisease4™)* (based on 4th edition). F.A. Davis Company. Powered by Skyscape. Version: 14.0.3/2011.5.26.

Sultan, J., & Hughes, P. J. (2010). Septic arthritis or transient synovitis of the hip in children. *Journal of Bone & Joint surgery (Br), 92-B*, 1289–1293.

Thompson, G. H. (2011). The spine. In R. M. Kliegman, B. M. D. Stanton, J. St. Geme, N. F. Schor, & R. E. Behrman. *Nelson textbook of pediatrics* (19th ed.). Philadelphia, PA: Saunders.

Utrilla-Rodriguez, E. M., Martinez-Cañavete, M. J. G., & Casares, J. A. C. (2012). Conservative treatment of clubfoot using modified Copenhagen method. *Pediatric Physical Therapy, 24*, 51–56. doi:10.1097/PEP.0b013e31823dcd25

Vallerand, A. H., & Sanoski, C. A. (2014). *Davis's drug guide for nurses* (14th ed.). Philadelphia, PA: F.A. Davis.

Venes, D. (Ed.). (2013). *Taber's cyclopedic medical dictionary* (22nd ed.). Philadelphia, PA: F.A. Davis.

Ward, S., & Hisley, S. (2009). *Maternal-child nursing care: Optimizing outcomes for mothers, children & families.* Philadelphia, PA: F.A. Davis.

Weiler, R., Ingram, M., & Wolman, R. (2011). Osgood-Schlatter disease. *British Medical Journal, 343*:d4534. 1–2. doi:10.1136/bmj.d4534

Wenger, D. R., & Pandya, N. K. (2011). A brief history of Legg-Calvé-Perthes disease. *Journal of Pediatric Orthopedics, 31*(2), S130–S136.

Wu, G. S., & Pollock, A. N. (2011). Slipped capital femoral epiphysis. *Pediatric Emergency Care, 27*(11), 1095–1096.

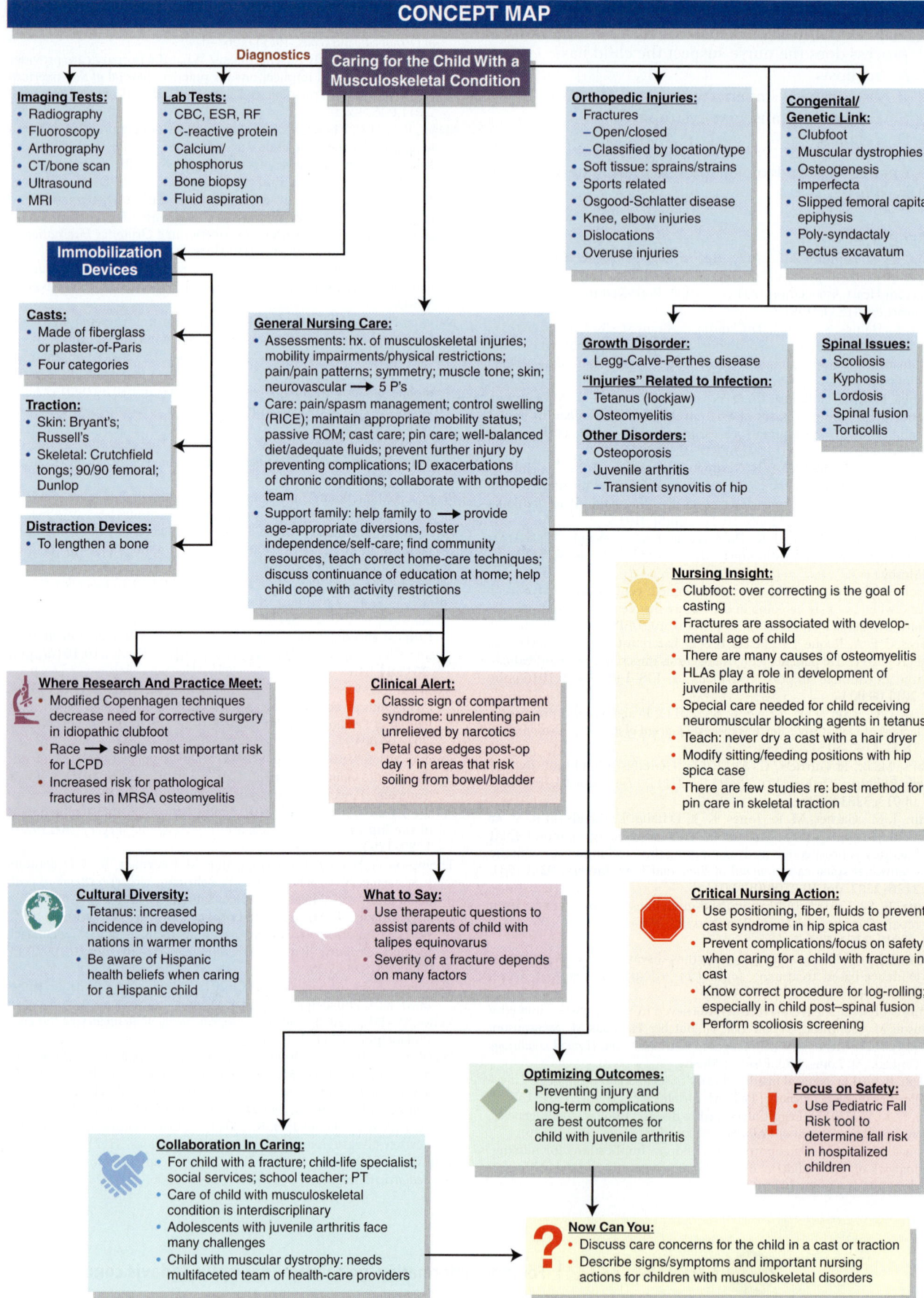

CONCEPT MAP

Diagnostics

Caring for the Child With a Musculoskeletal Condition

Imaging Tests:
- Radiography
- Fluoroscopy
- Arthrography
- CT/bone scan
- Ultrasound
- MRI

Lab Tests:
- CBC, ESR, RF
- C-reactive protein
- Calcium/phosphorus
- Bone biopsy
- Fluid aspiration

Orthopedic Injuries:
- Fractures
  - Open/closed
  - Classified by location/type
- Soft tissue: sprains/strains
- Sports related
- Osgood-Schlatter disease
- Knee, elbow injuries
- Dislocations
- Overuse injuries

Congenital/Genetic Link:
- Clubfoot
- Muscular dystrophies
- Osteogenesis imperfecta
- Slipped femoral capital epiphysis
- Poly-syndactaly
- Pectus excavatum

Immobilization Devices

Casts:
- Made of fiberglass or plaster-of-Paris
- Four categories

Traction:
- Skin: Bryant's; Russell's
- Skeletal: Crutchfield tongs; 90/90 femoral; Dunlop

Distraction Devices:
- To lengthen a bone

General Nursing Care:
- Assessments: hx. of musculoskeletal injuries; mobility impairments/physical restrictions; pain/pain patterns; symmetry; muscle tone; skin; neurovascular ⟶ 5 P's
- Care: pain/spasm management; control swelling (RICE); maintain appropriate mobility status; passive ROM; cast care; pin care; well-balanced diet/adequate fluids; prevent further injury by preventing complications; ID exacerbations of chronic conditions; collaborate with orthopedic team
- Support family: help family to ⟶ provide age-appropriate diversions, foster independence/self-care; find community resources, teach correct home-care techniques; discuss continuance of education at home; help child cope with activity restrictions

Growth Disorder:
- Legg-Calve-Perthes disease

"Injuries" Related to Infection:
- Tetanus (lockjaw)
- Osteomyelitis

Other Disorders:
- Osteoporosis
- Juvenile arthritis
  - Transient synovitis of hip

Spinal Issues:
- Scoliosis
- Kyphosis
- Lordosis
- Spinal fusion
- Torticollis

Nursing Insight:
- Clubfoot: over correcting is the goal of casting
- Fractures are associated with developmental age of child
- There are many causes of osteomyelitis
- HLAs play a role in development of juvenile arthritis
- Special care needed for child receiving neuromuscular blocking agents in tetanus
- Teach: never dry a cast with a hair dryer
- Modify sitting/feeding positions with hip spica case
- There are few studies re: best method for pin care in skeletal traction

Where Research And Practice Meet:
- Modified Copenhagen techniques decrease need for corrective surgery in idiopathic clubfoot
- Race ⟶ single most important risk for LCPD
- Increased risk for pathological fractures in MRSA osteomyelitis

Clinical Alert:
- Classic sign of compartment syndrome: unrelenting pain unrelieved by narcotics
- Petal case edges post-op day 1 in areas that risk soiling from bowel/bladder

Cultural Diversity:
- Tetanus: increased incidence in developing nations in warmer months
- Be aware of Hispanic health beliefs when caring for a Hispanic child

What to Say:
- Use therapeutic questions to assist parents of child with talipes equinovarus
- Severity of a fracture depends on many factors

Critical Nursing Action:
- Use positioning, fiber, fluids to prevent cast syndrome in hip spica cast
- Prevent complications/focus on safety when caring for a child with fracture in cast
- Know correct procedure for log-rolling; especially in child post–spinal fusion
- Perform scoliosis screening

Optimizing Outcomes:
- Preventing injury and long-term complications are best outcomes for child with juvenile arthritis

Focus on Safety:
- Use Pediatric Fall Risk tool to determine fall risk in hospitalized children

Collaboration In Caring:
- For child with a fracture; child-life specialist; social services; school teacher; PT
- Care of child with musculoskeletal condition is interdisciplinary
- Adolescents with juvenile arthritis face many challenges
- Child with muscular dystrophy: needs multifaceted team of health-care providers

Now Can You:
- Discuss care concerns for the child in a cast or traction
- Describe signs/symptoms and important nursing actions for children with musculoskeletal disorders

Caring for the Child With an Integumentary Condition

 In almost all diseases, the function of the skin is, more or less, disordered; and in many most important diseases, nature relieves herself almost entirely by the skin. This is particularly the case with children. However, the excretion, which comes from the skin, is left, unless removed by washing or by the clothes. Every nurse keeps this fact constantly in mind: if the nurse allows the sick to remain unwashed, or their clothing to remain on them after being saturated with perspiration or other excretion, the nurse is interfering injuriously with the natural processes of health just as effectually as if the nurse were to give the patient a dose of slow poison by the mouth. Poisoning by the skin is no less certain than poisoning by the mouth—only it is slower in its operation.

—Florence Nightingale

LEARNING TARGETS *At the completion of this chapter, the student will be able to:*

◆ Describe the anatomy and physiology and normal function of the skin.

◆ Examine the conditions related to various skin conditions.

◆ Prioritize developmentally appropriate and holistic nursing care for various skin and burn conditions.

◆ Explore diagnostic and laboratory testing and medications for various skin and burn conditions.

◆ Develop teaching plans and discharge criteria for parents whose children have various skin and burn conditions.

PICO(T) Questions

The intent of evidence-based practice (EBP) is to provide nursing care that integrates the best available evidence. An initial step in EBP is to write a PICO(T) question that effectively guides the research. A PICO(T) question is an acronym that stands for population (P), intervention or issue (I), comparison of interest (C), outcome (O), and timeframe (T). Depending on the question, all or some of the question components are used in the research process. Use these PICO(T) questions to spark your thinking as you read the chapter.

1. Is (I) severe acne (O) more common in (P) teenage girls than (C) teenage boys?

2. Does (I) application of aloe vera gel (O) speed healing of non-blistered sunburned skin in (P) children under age 6?

Evidence-Based Practice

McCullough, A. C., Seifried, M., Zhoa, X., Hasse, J., Kabat, W., Yogev, R., et al. (2011). Higher incidence of perineal community acquired MRSA infections among toddlers. *BMC Pediatrics, 11*(96), 1–6. doi:10.1186/1471-2431-11-96

The purpose of this study was to examine incidence of perineal community acquired methicillin-resistant Staphylococcus aureus (CAMRSA) infections among toddlers. Though MRSA is one of the most common pathogens found in hospitalized patients, its incidence is increasing among children in the community setting. According to the Centers for Disease Control and Prevention (CDC) CAMRSA has some unique molecular features that distinguish it from health-care acquired MRSA. Research indicates that the incidence of MRSA infections among children increased sixfold between 2002 and 2007. Previous research has also noted an increased incidence of perineal MRSA associate with children in day-care settings.

A retrospective, descriptive chart review was used to gather data. This study was completed in a children's hospital located in Toledo, Ohio, and included the charts of all pediatric patients under the age of 18 who received care during a 7-month period and who had a positive culture for MRSA. Data were reviewed and compared for social and demographic information as well as for a history of skin and soft tissue infection (SSTI) and antimicrobial susceptibilities. Patient charts were also examined for incidence of systemic cardiovascular, gastrointestinal, respiratory, and nervous system diseases, type of care, (i.e., outpatient, inpatient, or emergency care), and site of infection.

Data were analyzed using a Fisher's exact test with a p-value of less than 0.05 considered as statistically significant. Fisher's exact test is used to determine if there are nonrandom associations between two categorical nominal variables. It is commonly used when sample sizes are small. Sixty-three patients with MRSA infections were identified of which 58 (92%) met the CDC clinical criteria for CAMRSA infections. It was noted that all of the patients in this cohort had SSTIs. Twenty-five (43%) of the children were ages 0 to 3, 19 (33%) were ages 4 to 12, and 14 (24%) were ages 13 to 18. Thirty-six (62%) patients were female. Thirty-four (62%) were African American, 16 (29%) were Caucasian, and 5 (9%) categorized as other. The researchers also noted that 74% of the CAMRSA patients were considered from lower socioeconomic groups compared with 51% of the hospitals' total pediatric population admitted

for all causes. Twenty-four (41%) of the children had SSTI and 19 (33%) did not have a preexisting condition. Preexisting conditions were identified as follows:

- Respiratory disease—22 (38%)
- Gastrointestinal—9 (16%)
- Cardiovascular—3 (5%)
- Nervous system—1 (2%)

In children ages 0 to 3, the incidence of perineal SSTI was 76% (n=19) though accounted for only 11% (n=2) of children ages 4 to 12. None of the children ages 13 to 18 had a perineal SSTI. Extremity infections were more common in the older age groups with 13 (69%) each in both the 4 to 12 and 13 to 18 age groups. Only 3 (12%) were identified in the 0 to 3 age group. The researchers noted that there was a significant association between site of infection and age group.

The sites of infection were as follows:

- Face—4 (7%)
- Lower extremity—18 (31%)
- Perineal—21 (36%)
- Trunk—4 (7%)
- Upper extremity—11 (19%)

The researchers conclude that the findings from their study are consistent with the national trend of a sixfold increase in MRSA among children with the majority being CAMRSA. They further note that there is a significant association between age and site of infection with perineal infections more common in children ages 0 to 3. They suggested that the increased rate of colonization with CAMRSA in this group could be association with the use of diapers or dermabrasion caused by vigorous wiping of the area during diaper changes.

---

1. How is this information useful to clinical nursing practice?

2. Based on these findings, what are implications for further research?

See Suggested Responses for Evidence-Based Practice on Davis*Plus*.

Introduction

This chapter provides an overview of skin conditions that are common during infancy, childhood, and adolescence. The discussion includes an examination of the various skin conditions including developmentally appropriate and holistic nursing care. Information about diagnostic and laboratory testing and medications is given. Teaching plans and discharge criteria for parents whose children have various skin conditions are incorporated.

Growth and Development

The child with an integumentary condition may experience increased emotional insecurity because of decreased self-esteem and disturbances in self-image related to alterations in appearance from acne, scars, or burns. The nurse caring for the child with an integumentary condition should focus on promoting a positive self-esteem. The nurse understands that learning and mastering tasks can increase confidence. The nurse should encourage the child to participate in activities that promote learning, self-confidence, and acceptance. Activities and stimulation should be individualized to each child's developmental age and situation. The nurse should assess for signs of avoidance and social isolation. The nurse should encourage the child to interact with others normally to encourage social and cognitive development.

It is important that the nurse cares for the integumentary condition and also attends to the child's self-image. The nurse should provide an environment of openness that fosters a sense of well-being to the child. The nurse should provide education to the child about the disease process and treatment expectations in a nonjudgmental manner that fosters open communication and trust. The nurse should encourage parental involvement to better ease the child's discomfort and acceptance of the disease process.

A & P review   The Skin

The skin is the largest organ in the body; its main purpose is to protect the deeper tissues from injury and from foreign matter invasion. The skin also protects the body from exposure to a variety of environmental, pest, tactile, and chemical irritants on a daily basis that can disrupt the effectiveness of the skin as a protective barrier. Other functions of the skin include synthesis of vitamin D from ultraviolet light, aiding in water retention, and ridding the body of toxins. The skin also helps regulate temperature and initiates the sensations of touch, pain, heat, and cold in the body.

The skin has three layers: the epidermis, the dermis, and the subcutaneous fatty layer (Fig. 30-1). These three layers act to provide the body with a barrier against external invaders. Each layer of the skin contains specific properties. The epidermis is the outlet for the sweat glands, and the hair follicles protrude through this layer. The dermis contains the nerves, muscles, connective tissue, sebaceous and sweat glands, blood vessels, and lymph channels. The subcutaneous

fatty layer separates the skin from the underlying tissue as well. While all the accessory structures of the skin—the hair, nails, sebaceous glands, exocrine glands, and apocrine glands—are present at birth, most are immature and cannot function to their full potential until middle childhood.

While most skin conditions are common across the age span, children are often at a higher risk for certain skin conditions based on their large body surface area and still maturing immune system (Table 30-1). The Association of Women's Health, Obstetric and Neonatal Nurses (AWHONN) Neonatal Skin Condition Score (NSCS) is a good assessment tool for newborns (Table 30-2). ◆

✺ *Nursing Insight*—*Infant skin and temperature*

An infant's skin is thin and contains very little subcutaneous fat. For this reason, temperature regulation becomes an important issue because the infant tends to lose heat rapidly. Take care not to leave an infant uncovered and exposed for a prolonged time. Because of their immature neurological system and large body surface area, infants have more difficulty in regulating their body temperature.

Skin Lesions

A skin lesion is a circumscribed area of altered tissue (Venes, 2013). When assessing the skin for a lesion, it is important to note the size, shape, color, and texture. The two main types of lesions are primary and secondary. Primary lesions include macules, papules, patches, nodules, tumors, vesicles, pustules, bullae, and wheals. Macules,

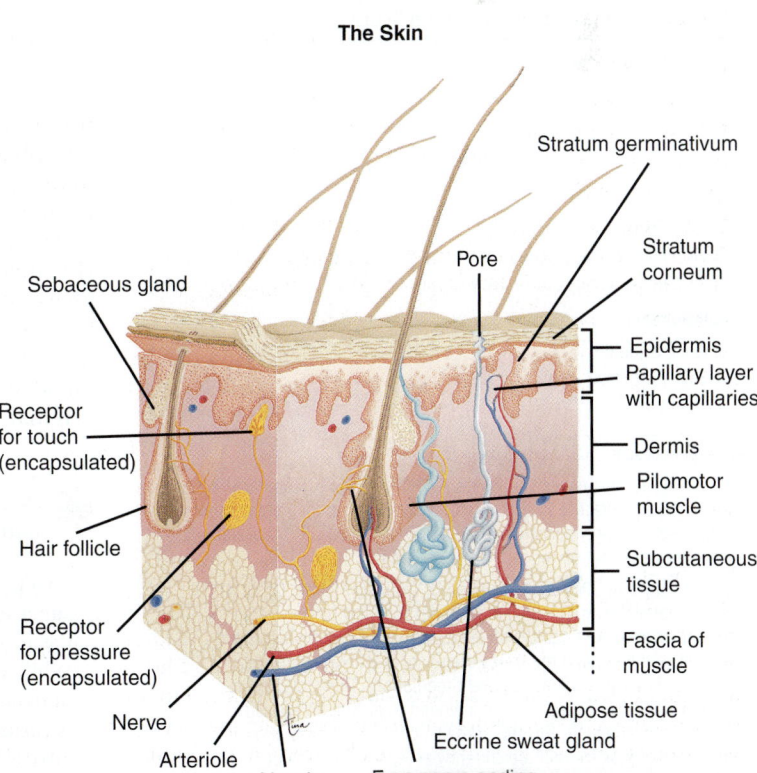

The Skin

Stratum germinativum

Pore

Stratum corneum

Sebaceous gland

Epidermis

Papillary layer with capillaries

Receptor for touch (encapsulated)

Dermis

Pilomotor muscle

Hair follicle

Subcutaneous tissue

Receptor for pressure (encapsulated)

Fascia of muscle

Adipose tissue

Nerve

Eccrine sweat gland

Arteriole

Free nerve ending

Venule

Figure 30-1 The skin has three layers: the epidermis, the dermis, and the subcutaneous fatty layer.

Table 30-1 Integumentary Changes as Children Grow

Newborn	Child	Adolescent
Skin is thin.	Skin thickens with age.	Skin reaches adult thickness.
Friction can cause blistering easily.	Friction and shear are not as destructive to the child's skin, but skin is still developing the bond between epidermis and dermis.	The epidermis and dermis are bound together and firm.
Eccrine sweat glands are functional.	Eccrine sweat glands are functional.	Eccrine sweat glands are fully functional, and testosterone increases sweating in the male.
Apocrine sweat glands are not functional.	Apocrine sweat glands grow larger preparing for pubescence.	Apocrine sweat glands are mature at puberty.
Color is lighter than normal for race and ethnicity. Newborns and infants should avoid direct exposure to the sun.	Color is normal for race and ethnicity. Skin is easily sunburned, especially in fair-haired, fair-skinned children.	Color is normal for race and ethnicity, functional at adult levels. Melanin is normal and provides some UV protection; however, protection from direct sun is still important.

papules, and nodules are found in children and adolescents with acne. Vesicles and pustules are seen in the child with chickenpox and impetigo. Wheals are often seen in the child with an allergic reaction. Secondary lesions are those that happen as a result of changes from the primary lesions. They include crusts, scales, lichenification, scars, keloids, fissures, erosions, and ulcers (Table 30-3).

Notably visible lichenification, or the thickening of the skin with hyperpigmentation, is often found on children who have atopic dermatitis. Ulcers may be associated with cancer. Scars are the result of a wound. Keloids, seen mainly in persons of color, result from hypertrophy of the scar tissue that extends beyond the wound edges (Venes, 2013).

Wounds and Wound Healing

Typical wounds found in the child are a result of cuts, scrapes, and burns and can be secondary to surgical intervention. When an injury has occurred, skin healing has three phases, and these often overlap. The first stage, inflammation, reflects the skin's initial healing response and lasts about 2 to 5 days. This is a preparatory stage for repair. Under normal circumstances, the wound seals itself with blood coagulation, followed by vasodilation that allows the leukocytes to ingest the bacteria and debris at the site of the injury (Fishman, 2006). In the second phase, proliferation, the blood flow is reestablished to the site, and natural debridement occurs. In this phase, lasting 2 days to 3 weeks, the wound contracts and a fine layer of epithelial cells cover the site of new collagen (Fishman, 2006). Finally, during remodeling, the third phase, collagen production occurs that allows for scar formation. This phase, lasting 3 weeks to 2 years, allows the collagen to increase the tensile strength of the newly mended tissue. Scar strength is only 80% as strong as the original tissue (Fishman, 2006) (Fig. 30-2).

Table 30-2 AWHONN Neonatal Skin Condition Score Tool

AWHONN Neonatal Skin Condition Score (NSCS)

Dryness

1 = Normal, no sign of dry skin
2 = Dry skin, visible scaling
3 = Very dry skin, cracking or fissures

Erythema

1 = No evidence of erythema
2 = Visible erythema, <50% body surface
3 = Visible erythema, ≥50% body surface

Breakdown

1 = None evident
2 = Small, localized areas
3 = Extensive

Note: perfect score = 3, worst score = 9.

This scoring system, developed for the AWHONN/NANN Neonatal Skin Care Research-Based Practice Project (RBP4) was adapted from a visual scoring system used in a previous study (Lane and Drost, 1993). This tool can facilitate assessment of neonatal skin condition.

Source: Copyright 2007 by Association of Women's Health, Obstetric and Neonatal Nurses. This skin assessment tool may be duplicated for use in the clinical setting. It is understood that institutions may have different resources, and the states or provinces where the institutions are located may promulgate different regulations. This tool does not define a standard of care, nor is it intended to dictate an exclusive course of management. This tool presents general methods and techniques of practice that are currently accepted and used by recognized authorities.

 Nursing Insight—*Superficial wound management*

As a pediatric nurse, it is important to note that in the area of superficial wound management, wounds are often closed with tissue adhesives (e.g., DERMABOND®) that work like glue. While the adhesive is effective in wound closure, the cosmetic outcome is not statistically different from suturing (Coulthard, Esposito, Worthington, van der Elst, van Waes, & Darcey, 2010). Tending to wounds in this way has decreased both child and parent anxiety.

Table 30-3 Common Skin Lesions and Associated Conditions

Lesion Name	Description	Associated Condition (Example)
Primary Lesions		
Macules	Flat, circumscribed area that has color change: <1 cm in diameter	Freckles, flat moles, petechiae, measles, scarlet fever
Papules	Raised, circumscribed area: 1 cm diameter	Warts, moles, lichen planus, scabies
Patches	Macule that is flat and nonpalpable, irregular shape: 1 cm diameter	Port-wine stains, café-au-lait spots, capillary hemangiomas
Nodules	Raised, firm, circumscribed (deeper than a papule), 1–2 cm diameter	Lipomas, erythema nodosum
Tumors	Raised and solid; may be clear, deep in the dermis, 2 cm in diameter	Lipomas, hemangiomas, neoplasms, benign tumors
Vesicles	Raised, circumscribed, superficial, filled with serous fluid, 1 cm in diameter	Varicella, herpes zoster (shingles)

(continued)

Table 30-3 Common Skin Lesions and Associated Conditions (continued)

Lesion Name	Description	Associated Condition (Example)
Pustules	Raised, superficial, like vesicle, but fluid is purulent	Impetigo, acne
Bullae	Vesicle 1 cm in diameter	Blister
Wheals	Raised, irregular shape, cutaneous swelling, solid; diameter is variable (usually transient)	Urticaria, insect bites, allergic reaction
Secondary Lesions Crusts	Dried body fluid on the skin surface: serum, pus, or blood	Disease where the skin weeps: eczema, impetigo, seborrhea

Table 30-3 Common Skin Lesions and Associated Conditions (continued)

Lesion Name	Description	Associated Condition (Example)
Scales	Raised cluster of keratinized cells, irregular, diameter is variable, can be thick or thin, dry or oily	Seborrheic dermatitis, dry skin, skin flaking after allergic reaction
Lichenification	Rough, thickened epidermal area often in the flexor surface of extremity	Chronic dermatitis
Scars	Fibrous tissue, thin or thick, coloration may be lighter or darker than surrounding skin	Healing wound of any etiology
Keloids	Fibrous tissue (scar) of irregular shape, raised and grown beyond the boundary of the original wound	Postoperative wound healing (more common in persons of color)
Fissures	Linear crack in the epidermis may be deeper; moist or dry	Athlete's foot; cracks at the corner of the mouth or anus

(continued)

Table 30-3 Common Skin Lesions and Associated Conditions (continued)

Lesion Name	Description	Associated Condition (Example)
Erosions	Depressed, moist, loss of part of the epidermis	After rupture of vesicle or bulla (e.g., varicella)
Ulcers	Concave, moist, loss of epidermis and dermis	Ulceration: stasis, decubitus

Nursing Care Plan   The Child With Eczema

Nursing Diagnosis: Impaired Skin Integrity related to inflammatory processes

Measurable Short-Term Goal: The child will regain skin integrity.

Measurable Long-Term Goal: The child will not experience secondary infection.

NOC Outcomes:
Tissue Integrity: Skin and Mucous Membranes (1101) Structural intactness and normal physiological function of skin and mucous membranes.
Allergic Response: Localized (0705) Severity of localized hypersensitive immune response to a specific environmental (exogenous) antigen.

NIC Interventions:
Infection Protection (6550)
Skin Care: Topical Treatments (3584)
Pruritus Management (3550)

Nursing Interventions:

1. Review family history for allergies or eczema.

   RATIONALE: Assists with diagnosis of lesions because infantile eczema is often associated with familial tendencies.

2. Assess child's skin lesions for location, size, color, type, drainage, signs of secondary infection, and any precipitating factors the family can identify.

   RATIONALE: Provides baseline data from which to evaluate improvement or worsening of the condition. Intense itching and scratching may disrupt skin integrity further and lead to secondary infections.

3. Administer cool compresses or medications as ordered to relieve itching and treat secondary infection (specify drug, dose, route, and times).

   RATIONALE: Cold helps reduce irritation. Antihistamines and/or topical steroids may be prescribed to reduce inflammation and pruritus, and antibiotics may be required for secondary infection.

4. Teach the family to promote skin hydration by bathing child in a lukewarm bath without harsh soaps and to apply emollient lotions liberally to damp skin.

   RATIONALE: Hot water and harsh soaps may exacerbate the skin irritation. Emollient lotions help trap moisture next to the skin to reduce irritation and itching.

Nursing Care Plan The Child With Eczema (continued)

5. Teach the family to dress child in light, soft, nonirritating clothing and to keep the child's fingernails short, smooth, and clean.

   RATIONALE: Overheating and irritating fabrics may increase pruritus and inflammation. Nail care may help prevent secondary infection from itching.

6. Assist the family to identify and remove potential irritants from the child's environment, including harsh detergents, perfumes, rough fabrics, and animal dander.

   RATIONALE: A nonirritating environment helps decrease the likelihood of flare-ups of the condition.

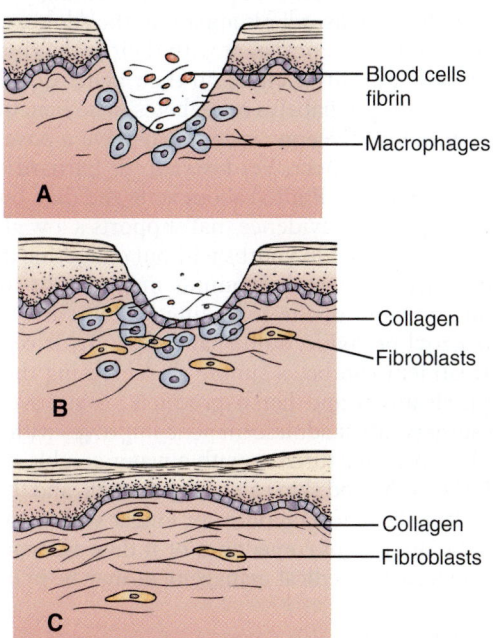

Figure 30-2 Three phases of wound healing. *A,* Inflammation. *B,* Proliferation. *C,* Remodeling.

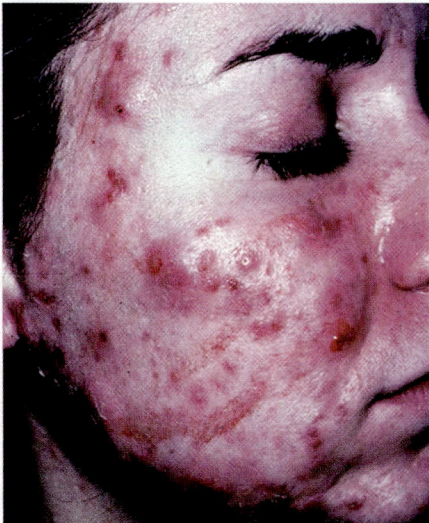

Figure 30-3 Acne generally begins in the teen years.

Skin Infections

A number of invaders can affect the skin, and these can be bacterial, viral, or fungal in nature. While most of the skin conditions resulting from these invaders respond quickly to treatment, others require an extended time for healing. The specific pathogens that are responsible for the infection, as well as the treatment and sequela of the infection, affect the healing response. Three specific pathogens are identified as the most frequent causes of bacterial skin infections: *Staphylococcus aureus, Streptococcus,* and *Pseudomonas.* Viral infections can be caused by any number of viruses, but those encountered the most often include a member of the poxvirus group, herpes simplex I or II, and the human papillomavirus. Fungal infections are also caused by a wide variety of pathogens, the most common being *Candida albicans.*

BACTERIAL INFECTIONS

Acne

Acne vulgaris is the most common bacterial skin disorder treated by physicians in adolescents (Fig. 30-3). Although acne generally begins in the teen years, it can begin earlier in some children. The onset of adrenal androgenic hormones in the prepubertal child is the primary reason for the occurrence of acne.

 Nursing Insight—*Acne during adolescence*

With the increase in the androgenic hormones during adolescence, there is an increase in the size of the sebaceous glands, and consequently, more sebum secreted. With the increase in sebum secretion, the follicle (a small secretory sac) enlarges, placing the person at risk for a keratin plug. These plugs result in the presence of a closed comedo that is called a "whitehead." At times, the comedo becomes inflamed and creates enough pressure to rupture. If a follicle is dilated enough to reach the skin surface, a comedo may form what is often called a "blackhead." Hyperpigmentation (increase in color) in the area of insult will remain for weeks to months. If the area is aggravated by mechanical means, such as scratching, squeezing, or harsh chemical cleansers, a scar may form. When inflammation deepens into the dermis, there is a potential for scarring as well as walling off of infection in cysts. Often, adolescents who have excessive sebum have more acne present because sebum is a growth medium for *Propionibacterium acnes* (*P acnes*) (Alexis & Lamb, 2009).

Signs and Symptoms

Signs and symptoms of acne can be mild, moderate, or severe and progress in the following pattern:

- Increased sebum production
- Follicular hyperkeratinization
- *Propionibacterium acnes (P acnes)* within the follicle
- Inflammation with papules, pustules, or nodules

Signs and symptoms of mild acne include open **comedones**, closed comedones, and no inflammatory lesions. An open comedo, which has a black head, has an open follicular orifice with oxidized lipids, keratinocytes, and melanocytes. A closed comedo, which has a white head and pustule, has a closed follicular orifice with sebum and keratinous substances.

Moderate acne will have a mix of noninflammatory comedones and inflammatory pustules and papules, while severe acne will have an increased number of inflammatory papules, pustules, and nodules with evidence of scarring (Courtenay, 2011). Severe acne is a significant progression of the signs and symptoms listed.

Diagnosis

A thorough skin assessment is the method of diagnosis for acne along with a complete history. For an assessment, the nurse can prepare the teen by making sure his or her face, scalp, chest, and back are exposed and cleansed of all makeup and powders. Laboratory tests are ordered when an underlying endocrine disorder is suspected.

❝What to say❞—*Assessing acne in an adolescent*

Adolescents may suffer a psychological burden related to their acne. The nurse must realize that it is important to elicit information from the adolescent about his or her feelings and relationships and if acne is affecting these relationships. If necessary, the nurse can refer the adolescent for further support and intervention.

When assessing acne in an adolescent, the nurse asks specific questions that guide the acne treatment regimen:

"When did your acne begin?"

"What types of cleansing products, makeup, or moisturizers and hair care products are you currently using?"

"What medications are you taking, including over-the-counter and natural products?"

"Have you noticed certain foods, activities, or environmental factors that affect your acne?"

"Do you notice a change in your acne related to your menses?"

"What other dermatological problems have you had recently or in the past?"

"Does anyone tease you in person, in writing, on the Internet, or via text or phone conversations about your acne?"

"Can you tell me how you feel about having acne?"

Prevention

Acne can be prevented in some adolescents with care in skin cleansing, decreasing rubbing, and picking of the existing comedones. Avoiding oil-based cleansing and moisturizing products in the areas where acne breakouts are occurring, for example, the forehead and nose, which is often referred to as the "T zone," may be beneficial as well. Oil-based makeup and other occlusive cover-ups are not helpful in resolving acne breakouts and may worsen them.

Stress and diet are controversial in regard to acne. In a large randomized controlled study, milk intake was found to exacerbate acne in some adolescents (Melnik, 2012). With this in mind, a dietary consult may benefit the adolescent in choosing appropriate dairy foods that will satisfy their body's need for calcium. Stress does not alone increase sebum production but has been shown to increase acne because of the corticotropin-releasing hormone that rises during the stress response. Stress may, therefore, make acne worse in some adolescents at particularly taxing times.

If an endocrine disorder is apparent, the adolescent may find dietary changes consistent with their endocrine disorder may have a positive effect on their acne. Consider an adolescent with prediabetes or diabetes, who benefits from a diet with a low glycemic index, may have a positive decrease in acne (Spencer, Ferdowsian, & Barnard, 2009). Information remains limited about acne and diet, but there is a growing body of evidence that supports a low glycemic index diet helps even in youths without endocrine disorder (Melnik, 2012). Over-the-counter medications for acne have one or more of the following ingredients: salicylic acid, benzoyl peroxide, sulfur, and alpha hydroxyl acids. Acne treatment can be as simple as decreasing the use of abrasive cleansers and harsh products or as involved as minor surgery. Most adolescent acne improves with cleansing and proper moisturizing with a water-soluble moisturizer. However, if good skin care is not enough, and they have suffered from acne for 3 months or longer without a reduction in the number of comedones or if they are worsening, a more aggressive medical management may be in order.

Collaborative Care

Nursing Care. It is important to teach the adolescent about proper treatment of the acne. Prior to any type of acne care, pretreatment includes assisting the adolescent in cleansing the area of treatment, gently. Be sure to assess the acne area including the face, chest, and back in good light. Posttreatment measures include gently cleansing or using a cool cloth to soothe the immediate inflammatory effects of tissue disruption and provide comfort.

Nursing care also includes teaching the adolescent about medications used in the treatment of acne including antimicrobials (topical or oral antibiotics), retinoid, and/or hormonal therapy.

Medical Care. Medical treatment for acne includes pharmacological treatments including antimicrobials, retinoids, and hormonal therapy. Antimicrobials include erythromycin (Ery-Tab) (topical or oral), clindamycin (Cleocin) (topical or oral), tetracycline (Sumycin) (oral), minocycline (Minocin) (oral), and doxycycline (Vibramycin) (oral). Retinoids include tretinoin (Retin A) (topical), tazarotene (Tazorac) (topical), and isotretinoin (Accutane) (oral).

If young women are experiencing hyperandrogenic states, the treatment is relative to the etiology of the disease process. For instance, in polycystic ovary syndrome (PCOS), metformin (Fortamet) is the primary treatment to manage insulin resistance. If the androgen hormones are elevated without the diagnosis of PCOS, spironolactone

(Aldactone) may be used as an oral agent to decrease the hormone production. Some young women without hyper-androgenic states, but who experience menstrual cycle acne breakouts, may benefit from low-dose oral birth control pills.

Light-based adjunctive therapies may also be employed. Light therapies include broad-spectrum, continuous-wave, visible light sources (e.g., blue light or red light). It is believed that the light produces free radicals that kill the acne-causing bacteria on the skin:

- For mild to moderate acne
- In clinic biweekly treatment

Laser sources including the potassium titanyl phosphate laser, pulsed dye laser, and infrared laser are used. Laser treatment is used for treatment and scar reduction and does one of these things: reduced comedones by oxidizing the acne-causing bacteria; and at more intense levels, will burn the sebaceous sac; and/or burn the follicular sac. Be aware that there is a risk of thermal burn (Aziz-Jalalie, Tabaie, & Djavid, 2012).

Education/Discharge Instructions

Teaching and reinforcing proper skin care and medication management is essential for the adolescent with acne. Acne treatment tends to be very drying and must not be covered with moisturizers or makeup. Teaching the teen how to use the medication at bedtime may increase adherence to the treatment regimen. Medication for acne is found in Table 30-4.

 Cultural Diversity: Culturally Diverse Adolescents

For culturally diverse adolescents the health-care provider must carefully choose topical treatments that are not excessively drying. If retinoids are used, for instance, a cream preparation is preferred. Post-inflammatory hyperpigmentation is a greater problem in culturally diverse adolescents and significantly more noticeable during acne treatment and post-acne than in the Caucasian population (Alexis & Lamb, 2009).

 Critical Nursing Action Cleansing the Adolescent's Face

The nurse uses these steps when cleansing the adolescent's face:

1. Use a warm moist cloth with antibacterial soap to soak away some of the crusting and then gently wipe away as much crusting as possible before applying the antibiotic topical ointment.
2. Apply the prescribed antibiotic topical ointment with a cotton swab or the finger of a gloved hand.
3. Apply a water-soluble moisturizer.
4. Encourage good hand washing techniques before and after the cleansing.
- **Note:** If the teen is cooperative, allow him or her as much autonomy in cleansing and treating the area as possible, while teaching-coaching them through the process.

 Nursing Insight—*Tetracycline (Sumycin), minocycline (Minocin), and doxycycline (Vibramycin)*

Tetracycline (Sumycin), minocycline (Minocin), and doxycycline (Vibramycin) can all cause photosensitivity with prolonged exposure to sunlight or tanning beds. Patients must be instructed regarding this risk along with education to avoid pregnancy while taking any of these medications because they can cause permanent discoloration of the offspring's teeth if exposed in utero during the second half of pregnancy or in children younger than 8 years.

 legal alert—Isotretinoin (Accutane)

Isotretinoin (Accutane) has been shown to cause severe birth defects. Therefore, women must not take this medication if there is any chance of becoming pregnant. Be sure to discuss this with all adolescents. Pregnancy tests must be performed before treatment with this medication, monthly during treatment, and 1 month after the cessation of treatment. Women considering this treatment must use two forms of birth control. Visit iPLEDGE: Committed to Pregnancy Prevention program at http://www.ipledgeprogram.com/ to view the information appropriate for patients undergoing isotretinoin (Accutane) treatment. Other side effects include hypercholesteremia, drying of the mucous membranes, decreased night vision, headaches, depression, and liver damage.

Give adolescents strict instructions not to share this medication with peers and to report any change in mood. Suicidal tendencies have been linked to isotretinoin (Accutane) therapy. If a teen is under the legal age limit, the parents or guardians must read, complete, and sign a designated form that proves they have been informed about the risks associated with isotretinoin (Accutane). The iPLEDGE Program is designed to ensure safe administration, prescription, and consumption of this medication. There are exact guidelines that must be followed when filling the prescription. The physician informs parents or guardians about the specific rules and regulations associated with this medication (iPLEDGE, 2005).

 Nursing Insight—*Liver enzymes*

Liver enzymes must be drawn once a month to ensure that liver damage is not occurring from the isotretinoin (Accutane). Medication refills are not authorized unless the individual submits to the pregnancy testing guidelines and has blood testing of the liver enzymes. Teens are particularly difficult to manage because they often feel invincible and because they are not as likely to be compliant with this treatment unless a direct effect is seen quickly in their acne improvement.

Impetigo Contagiosa

Impetigo contagiosa is a bacterial infection of the skin often found on and around the mouth and nose of the child or elsewhere on the face (Fig. 30-4). It may also appear on the hands, neck, trunk, buttocks, or extremities. Infants and children less than 5 years old are at greatest risk to have impetigo. It is generally caused by *Staphylococcus aureus*. On

Table 30-4 Medications for Acne

Name	Indications	Actions	Therapeutic Effect
erythromycin (E-Mycin)	Treatment of acne	Inhibits protein synthesis of bacterial ribosome	Anti-infective
clindamycin (Cleocin)	Treatment of skin infections: acne	Inhibits protein synthesis of bacterial ribosome	Anti-infective
tetracycline (Sumycin)	Treatment of various infections: acne	Inhibits protein synthesis of bacterial ribosome	Anti-infective
tretinoin (Retin-A)	Acne, acute promyelocytic leukemia, wrinkles	By stimulating the transcription process, it increases epidermal cell mitosis and epidermal cell turnover	Anti-acne, antineoplastic, retinoid
adapalene (Differin)	Acne, chloasma, keratosis	Thought to normalize epithelial cells	Retinoid-like effect
tazarotene (Tazorac)	Acne, psoriasis, wrinkles	Studies suggest: inhibits growth of human keratocyte	Retinoid
minocycline (Minocin)	Treatment of various infections: acne	inhibits growth of human keratocyte	Anti-infective
doxycycline (Vibramycin)	Treatment of various infections: acne Treatment of anthrax	Inhibits protein synthesis of bacterial ribosome	Anti-infective
isotretinoin (Accutane)	Acne	Reduces sebaceous gland size and inhibits sebaceous gland activity	Anti-acne, retinoid

Source: Data from Vallerand, A. H., & Sanoski, C. A. (2014). *Davis's drug guide for nurses* (14th ed.). Philadelphia, PA: F.A. Davis.

Contraindications and Precautions	Adverse Reactions and Side Effects	Route and Dosage	Nursing Implications
Hypersensitivity, known alcohol intolerance	Nausea/vomiting, rashes	Topical and systemic	Assess child for infection. Obtain specimen for culture and sensitivity before dosing. Assess for improvement in the child's condition.
Hypersensitivity, previous pseudomembranous colitis, severe liver impairment	Diarrhea, rashes, pseudomembranous colitis	Topical and systemic	Assess child for infection. Obtain specimen for culture and sensitivity before dosing. Monitor bowel elimination. Assess for improvement in the child's condition.
Hypersensitivity, known alcohol intolerance, pregnancy, lactation	Nausea/vomiting, diarrhea, photosensitivity	Systemic	Assess patient for infection. Obtain specimen for culture and sensitivity before dosing. Monitor liver and kidney functions. Assess for improvement in the child's condition.
Hypersensitivity	Oral: Dysrhythmia Topical: Erythema, scaling, dryness, itching, photosensitivity	Systemic and topical Oral: capsule, liquid filled: 10 mg Topical cream: 0.02%, 0.025%, 0.05%, 0.1% Topical gel/jelly: 0.01%, 0.025%, 0.04%, 0.1% Topical solution: 0.05% Usually used once per day before bed	Assess patient for sensitivity. Assess for superinfection. Assess for improvement in the child's condition.
Hypersensitivity	Erythema, scaling, dryness, itching, photosensitivity	Topical gel: 0.1% Solution 0.1% Usually used once per day before bed	Assess patient for sensitivity. Assess for superinfection. Assess for improvement in the child's condition.
Hypersensitivity, pregnancy	Topical: erythema, scaling, dryness, itching, photosensitivity	Safety not established in children <12 years old Topical cream: 0.05%, 0.1% Topical gel/jelly: 0.05%, 0.1%	Assess patient for sensitivity. Assess for superinfection. Assess for improvement in the child's condition.
Hypersensitivity, known alcohol intolerance, pregnancy, lactation	Nausea/vomiting, diarrhea, photosensitivity	Systemic	Assess patient for infection. Obtain specimen for culture and sensitivity before dosing. Observe for change in skin pigmentation. Monitor liver and kidney functions. Assess for improvement in the child's condition.
Hypersensitivity, known alcohol intolerance, pregnancy, lactation	Nausea/vomiting, diarrhea, photosensitivity	Systemic	Assess patient for infection. Obtain specimen for culture and sensitivity before dosing. Monitor liver and kidney functions. Assess for improvement in the child's condition.
Hypersensitivity, pregnancy	Dermatologic: cheilitis, dry skin, itching. Endocrine metabolic: serum triglycerides raised Hepatic: hepatotoxicity Psychiatric: aggressive behavior, depression, violent behavior	Systemic Safety and effectiveness in children <12 years not established 1 mg/kg/day ORALLY in 2 divided doses	Obtain a pregnancy test, two tests at baseline, followed by tests monthly during therapy, at the completion of therapy, and 1 month after the discontinuation of therapy. Assess for depression, psychosis, suicidal ideation, or aggressive behavior. Monitor hepatic function by obtaining a lipid panel; weekly or biweekly intervals. Register for iPLEDGE Program: www.ipledgeprogram.com Assess for improvement in the child's condition.

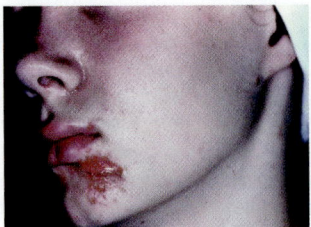

Figure 30-4 Impetigo is a highly contagious bacterial infection.

rare occasions, other bacteria may be responsible for the skin infection, including methicillin-resistant Staphylococcus aureus (MRSA) (Kim, Lee, Lee, Lee, & Yoon, 2012).

The lesions begin as a vesicle or pustule surrounded by edema (swelling) and erythema (redness). Later these lesions erupt, leaving honey-colored exudate. This exudate becomes crusty in appearance and sticky to the touch. The child may experience pruritus (itching) that is not usually painful. Over time, impetigo clears leaving no residual scarring in the absence of scratching or picking.

Signs and Symptoms

Signs and symptoms of impetigo include:

- Vesicles, pustules
  - Upon rupture, lesion with honey-colored exudates; exudate dries into a crusty, sticky residue
- Mild edema
- Erythema
- Pruritic

Diagnosis

Impetigo is diagnosed through assessment. Rarely does the diagnosis require laboratory testing by culture. A diagnostic culture is needed if the health-care provider is unsure of the exact diagnosis and is investigating a differential diagnosis such as contact dermatitis or herpes virus.

Prevention

Impetigo is very contagious and passed by touch from the infected child to others. Good hand washing and keeping a child at home for 24 hours after the induction of the antibiotic will decrease the spread of impetigo in the child's environment.

Collaborative Care

Nursing Care. The nurse informs the family that some providers may allow for spontaneous resolution by encouraging strict hygiene measures if the child is home and not requiring day-care or school involvement.

Medical Care. Medical treatment for impetigo is pharmacologically based. Topical antibiotics such as mupirocin (Bactroban) may be used if the skin lesions are limited. Oral antibiotics are given for widespread infections and may include amoxicillin/clavulanate (Augmentin), dicloxacillin, or erythromycin (E.S.S.) (Box 30-1).

💬 **What to say**—*Teaching about impetigo*

When the nurse is caring for the child with impetigo, it is important to teach the child and caregiver:

"Do not be embarrassed; this occurs quite commonly."

"It is very important to wash your hands."

"Try not to scratch the lesions."

"Change pillowcases nightly until the lesions are no longer oozing or flaking."

Box 30-1 **Common Medications Used for Impetigo**

- mupirocin (Bactroban) (topical)
- dicloxacillin (Dycill) (oral)
- cephalexin (Keflex) (oral)
- clindamycin (Cleocin) (oral)

Methicillin-Resistant Staphylococcus aureus (MRSA)

MRSA is a contagious bacterium that is resistant to treatment from beta-lactam antibiotics such as methicillin also called meticillin, amoxicillin (Amoxil), penicillin G (Bicillin L-A) and oxacillin (Bactocill). Hospital acquired MRSA may result in more systemic infections, but community acquired MRSA is usually limited to the skin and soft tissue.

Nursing Insight—*Methicillin-resistant Staphylococcus aureus (MRSA)*

Originally, MRSA was seen only as a hospital acquired infection, but the emergence of community acquired MRSA in the 1990s was a product of the new USA300 strain of staph (Landrum, Neumann, Cook, Chukwuma, Ellis, Hospenthal, et al., 2012). The rates for MRSA rose throughout the 1990s and reached a peak in the mid-2000s. The rates have slowly declined every year since 2006, but MRSA continues to be an infection seen within the community and hospital setting. Those at highest risk of infection are children in day-care settings, children and adolescents in athletics, and those who frequent athletic facilities despite the fact that the gymnasiums and other fomites are not likely to be the reason for the transmission. Rather, it is the proximity of children with others that increases their risks (Markely, Edmond, Major, Bearman, & Stevens, 2012).

Signs and Symptoms

Signs and symptoms of MRSA include vesicles, pustules, **furuncles**, and **carbuncles.** Upon rupture, the exudate is white to yellow. Then a small central opening develops with varnish-colored exudate. As the skin heals, the crusts are brown and dry like most scabs. Other signs and symptoms include:

- Mild edema
- Erythema
- Tender to painful depending on the location and level of induration and infection

MRSA infections are often found in areas covered by hair such as the axilla, nape of the neck, and groin but can occur anywhere on the body where a scratch or scrape has disrupted the integrity of the skin. The lesions begin as a papule or pustule surrounded by edema (swelling) and erythema (redness), a common sign of inflammation. Some lesions will develop into carbuncles (commonly termed boils) with a deeper pocket of infection and more discomfort. MRSA often presents as a singular lesion but can be seen in clusters with no discernible pattern.

The most common presentation in a mild case of MRSA skin infection is the child brought to the provider's office with complaint of "spider bite." If the lesion has erupted or been scratched open, the lesion will look much like other skin and soft tissue infections including impetigo and varicella (chickenpox), with an open center and thin crusting over the surface. A thorough history, and as needed, a culture of the lesion, will aid in diagnosis.

Diagnosis

MRSA is diagnosed through clinical assessment. However, a culture is warranted if the lesion is one of many, a recurrent lesion, or if the child has impaired immunity as well as any child recently released from the hospital.

Prevention

MRSA is contagious and is passed skin to skin as well as from inanimate surfaces to the skin. Personal prevention can be achieved by good hand washing. Children are taught good hand and personal hygienic practices. Athletes can shower immediately after events and avoid sharing any personal items, like razors and towels; uniforms are cleaned after every event. Furthermore, the parent or caregiver can keep any wound clean and covered especially when they are in contact with other people. An over-the-counter antibacterial cream or ointment may be needed.

Schools, day cares, and athletic facilities can cleanse the environment regularly with a good bactericidal spray or wash. Hospitals have specific cleansing routines after dismissal of patients from a room or suite. Terminal (final) cleaning of the room is well defined by the Centers for Disease Control and Prevention. Hospital cleaning professionals are trained how to completely clean a room from top to bottom with attention to all areas where the patient may have had any contact (CDC, 2008). In the home setting, regular unscented bleach is very effective in killing bacteria and viruses on hard surfaces.

 Nursing Insight—*Bleach solution*

A bleach solution can be easily prepared by mixing 1 tablespoon of bleach for every 1 quart of water. A bucket and cloth or spray bottle can be used. Always make sure that you mix this solution in a well-ventilated area. Bleach water solution loses its antibacterial effects within 24 hours, so it needs to be made on the day it is to be used.

Collaborative Care

Nursing Care. Careful hand washing and the use of universal precautions are essential when caring for every child who has acquired MRSA, especially in the spread of this infection. A diet high in protein promotes wound healing, and consuming a variety of foods is an important factor in maintaining overall good health. A skin culture may be warranted by which the type of pathogen is determined that helps ensure proper diagnosis.

Medical Care. The first line of treatment for MRSA is the administration of an oral antibiotic and a topical cream or ointment:

- vancomycin (Vancocin) (IV)
- clindamycin (Cleocin) (IV/IM/PO), dicloxacillin (PO)
- mupirocin (Bactroban (topical)

❝What to say❞—*Teaching about MRSA*

When the nurse is caring for the child with MRSA, it is important to teach the child and caregiver:

"This is a common skin infection."

"It is very important to wash your hands."

"Try not to scratch the lesions."

"Keep the area covered until it scabs over."

"Use the medication as prescribed for the entire duration prescribed."

Cellulitis

Cellulitis is a spreading bacterial infection that enters via existent openings in the skin caused by dermatological conditions or trauma that then spreads into the interstitial space. The most common bacteria causing cellulitis are *Streptococcus pyogenes* and *Staphylococcus aureus* (Venes, 2013), particularly *S pyogenes*. The most frequent location of cellulitis is the face and extremities, particularly the lower legs, but cellulitis can occur anywhere on the body (Venes, 2013). The method of injury will impact the cellulitis treatment. For instance, a cellulitis that results post–dog bite is treated differently than a cellulitis that results from an insect bite. The clinician will often reference the *Sanford Guide to Antimicrobial Therapy* (Gilbert, Moellering, Eliopoulos, Chambers, & Saag, 2011) in such instances (Box 30-2).

Signs and Symptoms

Signs and symptoms of cellulitis include skin that is:

- Red to purplish red
- Swollen or indurated
- Warm or hot to touch
- Tender or painful to touch

The child may be feverish, and it is likely that he or she will experience discomfort on palpation of the indurated area. Often the child experiences malaise, fever, and chills. **Lymphadenitis** (inflammation of the lymph nodes) may or may not be present in the region.

Diagnosis

A complete history and physical is the usual method of diagnosis. Lab tests, radiological testing, or surgical biopsy is used only in the presence of severe infection. Complete blood counts and blood cultures are ordered to rule out **septicemia** (infection of the blood) if symptoms warrant.

> **Box 30-2 Common Medications to Treat Cellulitis**
> **Penicillin G (Bicillin L-A) IM**
>
> - amoxicillin (Amoxil) PO
> - ceftriaxone (Rocephin) IM
> - cephalexin (Keflex) (PO)
> - clindamycin (Cleocin) IV
> - If MRSA is considered (exudates present)
>   - sulfa (Bactrim) (PO)
>   - doxycycline (Vibramycin) (PO)

Prevention

To help prevent cellulitis, tell the caregiver about these simple care measures when the child has a skin wound:

- Wash the child's wound daily with soap and water.
- Apply an over-the-counter antibiotic cream or ointment.
- Watch for signs of infection such as redness, pain, and drainage.

Collaborative Care

Nursing Care. Depending on the location of the cellulitis and the total surface area of the induration as well as the age of the child, the medical management may differ. Most cases of cellulitis are handled in the outpatient arena. Cellulitis that manifests on the face and neck, genitals, or over a joint are more worrisome and may cause systemic infection. Orbital cellulitis is fairly common in children and may lead to hospitalization for IV antibiotics.

If a child has a severe case of cellulitis, hospitalization and IV antibiotics may be necessary. In addition, steroids to decrease inflammation such as prednisolone (Pediapred) may be ordered but are not routine. Another nursing intervention for symptom control is the administration of an anti-inflammatory medication such as ibuprofen (Children's Advil) or acetaminophen (Children's Tylenol).

Medical Care. Medications are important in the management of cellulitis, and these medications are often used:

- penicillin G (Bicillin) IM
- amoxicillin (Amoxil)
- ceftriaxone (Rocephin)
- cephalexin (Keflex)
- clindamycin (Cleocin)

If MRSA is considered (based on history or suspect abscess), these medications are used:

- vancomycin (Vancocin) (IV)
- clindamycin (Cleocin) (IV/IM/PO)
- dicloxacillin (PO)

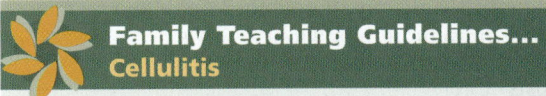

Family Teaching Guidelines...
Cellulitis

TOPIC: How to teach parents important information about how to care for their child with cellulitis:

1. Administer all antibiotics as prescribed. Stress to the caregiver not to stop the antibiotics when the skin appears to have improved. The caregiver must realize that failure to finish the antibiotics may result in recurrence of the infection.
2. Use warm, moist packs to relieve discomfort as needed. If cool, moist packs relieve discomfort, this is acceptable.
3. Use analgesics such as ibuprofen (Children's Advil) or acetaminophen (Children's Tylenol) if necessary for comfort. If the skin infection is in a limb, elevate the limb to provide comfort and decrease swelling.

ESSENTIAL INFORMATION:

Contact the health-care practitioner if the redness or edema appears to be worsening, if the child's pain is increasing, or if the temperature remains above 101.5°F (38.6°C) 48 hours after the beginning of antibiotic administration.

Medication: Penicillin G Benzathine (Bicillin L-A)

(pen-i-**sill**-in, gee, ben-za-theen)

Pregnancy Category: B

Indications: Treatment of a wide variety of infections: pharyngeal/tonsil/skin as well as prophylaxis for rheumatic fever.

Actions: Binds to bacterial cell wall, resulting in cell death.

Therapeutic Effects: Bacteriostatic action against susceptible bacteria spectrum: Streptococci, Staphylococci, and some gram-negative organisms

Contraindications and Precautions:
CONTRAINDICATED IN: Hypersensitivity

Adverse Reactions and Side Effects:
Pain at injection site
Gastrointestinal: Diarrhea, epigastric distress, nausea/vomiting
Endocrine: Rash
Respiratory: Anaphylaxis

Nursing Implications:
1. Assess for history of hypersensitivity.
2. Observe patient for signs of anaphylaxis for a minimum of 15 minutes after injection.
3. Reconstitute with D5W or 0.9% NaCl.
4. Administer deeply in a well-developed muscle mass.

Source: Data from Vallerand, A. H., & Sanoski, C. A. (2014). *Davis's drug guide for nurses* (14th ed.). Philadelphia, PA: F.A. Davis.

focus on safety

Group A streptococcus

Group A streptococcus can cause necrotizing fasciitis (flesh-eating bacteria). Be alert to the following clinical manifestations of necrotizing fasciitis: severe pain, bruising, crepitus, or bullae filled with bluish/purple-colored fluid over the induration (an area of hardened tissue) (Venes, 2013).

Optimizing Outcomes—Family adherence

The best outcome for a child with cellulitis who is receiving an antibiotic is for the family to be adherent and administer the entire medication as prescribed. If the family has a history of nonadherence to a medical plan, or if the child cannot take the medication as prescribed, the nurse must notify the health-care practitioner immediately. The health-care provider may then choose to order a single dose of IM penicillin G (Bicillin L-A) or a 3-day regimen of ceftriaxone (Rocephin) instead of the oral medication. Using a topical anesthetic such as EMLA (lidocaine/prilocaine) at the injection site at least an hour before the injection helps decrease the pain.

Nursing Diagnoses Cellulitis

- Impaired skin integrity related to inflammatory process damaging skin
- Pain related to inflammatory changes in tissues from infection
- Ineffective tissue perfusion: peripheral related to edema

VIRAL INFECTIONS

Molluscum Contagiosum

Molluscum contagiosum is a skin infection caused by a poxvirus. This condition is a self-limiting viral disease common in children lasting from 6 to 18 months. Transmission is through direct contact with contaminated objects or by sexual contact. Transmission of the virus is significantly easier when the skin is wet.

Signs and Symptoms

Signs and symptoms of molluscum contagiosum include small flesh- or pink-colored papules (pearl-like), that are no larger than 2 to 6 mm in diameter. The central depression of the papule may have an exudative plug. Groups of papules range from a few to several hundred. In children, the papules are found predominately on the trunk and face; in adolescents, they are on the inner thighs, genitals, and pubic areas. Papules are never seen on the palms or soles in any age group.

Diagnosis

The condition is diagnosed by assessing the skin for lesion typology. A family history may reveal that the virus has recently affected other family members. Adolescents may share a history of sexual contact with an infected partner thus predisposing them to this skin condition.

Prevention

A child who has molluscum contagiosum should use the bathtub alone, rather than have communal bathing with siblings. The tub is disinfected after a bath, and the child's towels are not shared. There are no special covering of the lesions for normal activities of daily living because the child and his family may already have or have had the viral infection.

Collaborative Care

Nursing Care. The nurse communicates to the family that no specific diagnostic testing or intervention is required for mild cases because they resolve on their own. If medications are prescribed, proper instruction in medication name, dose, interval, and potential adverse effects are discussed.

Medical Care. Generally, molluscum contagiosum will self-resolve. In more severe cases, medical treatment may require the daily use of topical tretinoin (Retin A) to irritate the skin and in turn stimulate the immune system to respond to this viral condition. If this is unsuccessful, the health-care provider may choose **curettage** (cutting away), or **cryrotherapy** (freezing each lesion with liquid nitrogen). Complications from these treatments may include scarring. A secondary infection would require treatment with topical or oral antibiotics.

 Nursing Insight—*Molluscum contagiosum*

Use of aggressive, potentially scarring treatment is reserved for children who are experiencing significant emotional upset because of the presence of the molluscum contagiosum. Trading the small but often multiple lesions for scars is not advantageous to child or family. A child psychologist or psychiatrist is a part of the child's health-care team to help with psychosocial aspects of this condition.

Education/Discharge Instructions

The nurse instructs the family in good hand hygiene, to redirect the child from picking at the lesion to prevent autoinnoculation, and if treated to allow any scabbing to fall off naturally.

 Complementary Care: *Molluscum Contagiosum*

Topical agents that promote healing are frequently used for rashes: Cow udder balm (bag balm), green tea extract, vitamin E preparations, aloe vera, milk, calamine, and colloidal oatmeal can be helpful natural agents used in this skin condition.

Human Papillomavirus

Human papillomavirus infections (warts) are common among children. The human papillomavirus causes warts by invading the epithelial cells in the skin. The wart is transmitted by direct skin-to-skin or mucous membrane contact and from hard surface areas such as plantar warts from gymnasium floors. The usual incubation period is 2 to 6 months, but in some cases there is a latency period. Three types of warts occur in children: common warts (verruca vulgaris), plantar warts (verruca plantaris), and flat warts (verruca plana).

Signs and Symptoms

Common warts can appear anywhere on the body and appear:

- Rough (cauliflower-looking appearance)
- Raised or flat
- Flesh-colored

At times, there will be a central black dot. They may appear alone or in clusters. (Fig. 30-5)

Plantar warts are found on the soles of the feet on weight-bearing surfaces. They are difficult to differentiate from corns and calluses but usually have a small dark dot near the center secondary to **thrombosed** vessels. Plantar warts cause foot pain if they grow large and can be surgically removed if painful and not responding to other treatments. Flat warts generally occur on the face or legs and are sometimes flesh-colored and rarely rough. They are usually not painful, nor do they itch unless other skin irritation is present.

Diagnosis

Diagnosis is based on presenting signs, symptoms, and visual inspection. Often the family makes a diagnosis at home and treats the wart with over-the-counter medications before seeking medical advice. Health-care provider advice is usually sought after a long period of failed resolution, or an increase in the number or size of the warts.

Prevention

Primary prevention of warts can begin with avoiding exposure to the virus that is shedding from others. Good hand washing is imperative. Avoid touching the warts of others because the wart virus may transfer to another person's skin.

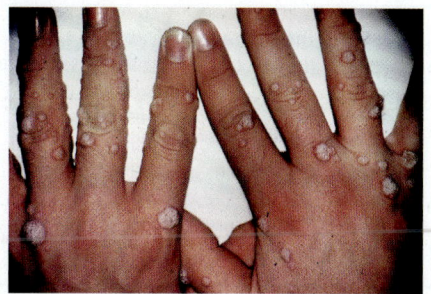

Figure 30-5 Warts are a cutaneous elevation of the skin.

Using slippers or sandals in public areas may decrease the incidence of plantar warts. Secondary prevention or a decrease in personal wart proliferation can be achieved by covering the child's warts and not touching or scratching the warts.

Collaborative Care

Nursing Care. The nurse communicates to the caregiver that most of the time no intervention is needed for warts because 75% of warts resolve on their own within 2 years. Several medications, both over-the-counter and prescription, are available for wart treatment (Table 30-5).

If cryotherapy (liquid nitrogen) is needed, the nurse will prepare the patient by describing the procedure to the parent and the child, tailoring the information to the child's developmental age. Pain may occur during and immediately after cryotherapy. Use of age-appropriate distraction techniques and motivational reward for holding still will be beneficial to most children. After the procedure is done the nurse applies occlusive dressings if needed.

Medical Care. If over-the-counter treatments are not working, parents typically seek medical care for the child. Medical management of warts includes the following: Flat warts are treated with cryotherapy (liquid nitrogen) or topical application of 5-fluorouracil (Efudex), imiquimod (Aldara), or tretinoin (Retin-A). Raised warts are treated with cryotherapy and often a follow-up regimen of salicylic acid or imiquimod (Aldara). If warts are on the face, imiquimod (Aldara) is gentler and less likely to scar than using cryotherapy or salicylic acid. Plantar warts and very large or deep warts may require curettage.

Education/Discharge Instructions

Important aspects of education for parents with children who have warts include:

- Reminding the patient and family that these are viral in nature, and to be careful to reduce spreading

- Encouraging the child to discuss concerns and fears about appearance
- Re-teaching medication adherence before the child leaves the office
- If the child had curettage or cryotherapy, teach wound management and signs and symptoms of infection; continued or increased pain is a warning sign and would warrant a call to the health-care practitioner
- Healing after cryotherapy takes 4 to 7 days. If prescribed, encouraged the patient or parent to begin salicylic acid after 1 week's time

 Complementary Care: *Tape and Adhesives*

There is some evidence that application of duct tape and other adhesive to a wart one night a week for 6 weeks is effective in wart resolution. This is likely because of occlusion of the wart and irritation of the surface creating an immune response that kills the virus. This avant-garde technique may work when aggressive salicylic acid or liquid nitrogen is not chosen by the patient and/or the family (Bruggink, Gussekloo, & Berger, 2010).

Herpes Simplex Virus 1

Herpes simplex virus 1 (HSV-1) is the common cold sore (Fig. 30-6). HSV-1 can cause painful blisters on mucosal surfaces of the skin, and the most common location for HSV-1 is on the face, usually on the lips and in or near the mouth and nose. HSV-1 can also affect the sclera or the eyelid (Venes, 2013). It can accompany fever, stress, extremely dry lips, or extensive sun exposure, and it can occur soon after such prodromal incidents.

Signs and Symptoms

The infection, HSV-1, is evident by watery blisters in the skin or mucous membranes of the mouth or lips. After the

Table 30-5 Human Papillomavirus (Warts)			
Type of Wart	**Common Wart (verruca vulgaris)**	**Flat Wart (verruca plana)**	**Plantar Wart (verruca plantaris)**
Treatment and Description	Topical: keratolytic acids (OTC)	Topical tretinoin cream (prescription)	Topical keratolytic acids
	This topical treatment is applied by dropper or cotton swab. Place the thick liquid directly on the top of the wart taking care to keep this highly acidic fluid off the surrounding skin. The wart will peel away in layers as the acid kills the superficial layers one at a time.	This topical treatment is applied by using a gloved hand or finger in a thin coating.	This topical treatment is applied by dropper or cotton swab. Place the thick liquid directly on the top of the wart taking care to keep this highly acidic fluid off the surrounding skin. The wart will peel away in layers as the acid kills the superficial layers one at a time.
	Liquid Nitrogen Cryosurgery		**Liquid Nitrogen Cryosurgery**
	The application of liquid nitrogen to the wart by the practitioner is a common method that often expedites the wart's demise. The practitioner will direct a narrow flow of the liquid nitrogen to the wart directly, causing it to freeze and therefore killing the warty tissue. This is mildly painful but efficient.		(with paring and topical chemodestruction to enhance its effectiveness) The application of liquid nitrogen to the wart by the practitioner is a common method that often expedites the wart's demise. The practitioner will direct a narrow flow of the liquid nitrogen to the wart directly, causing it to freeze and therefore killing the warty tissue. This is mildly painful but efficient.

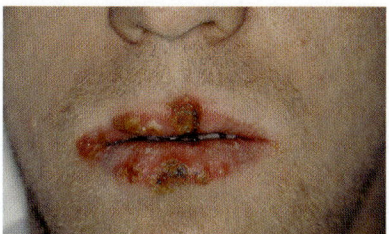

Figure 30-6 Herpes simplex virus 1. Cold sore.

virus has been introduced into the body, it establishes a latent infection. There is usually tenderness, burning, tingling, or itching before the sore actually appears based on a variety of stimuli such as a febrile illness, emotional stress or ultraviolet light exposure. The sore usually begins as a red rash progressing on to blisters (vesicles) that open up, leaving a painful ulceration. These ulcerations are virulent and highly contagious as evidenced by the increasing prevalence of HSV-positive persons as they age (Van Wagoner, & Hook, 2012). The lesions will resolve without intervention in 7 to 18 days depending on the depth of the lesion and the presence of continuing illness or stress.

Diagnosis

When the child and family arrive at the clinic, the nurse communicates to them that no specific diagnostic testing is required and that visualization of the lesion is often the only procedure required to diagnose the condition. A family history may reveal that the virus has recently affected other family members. If a differential diagnosis is needed, the health-care provider may perform a viral culture of an open area to determine if the lesions are the herpes virus or a different virus such as the varicella virus (chickenpox), which is similar in appearance.

Prevention

The nurse instructs the family to avoid contact with persons who have active herpetic lesions. Families avoid sharing of utensils and drinking items, especially when someone is ill or has an active lesion. In the school environment, avoidance of the mouth on the water fountain and shared sports bottles is very helpful in avoiding HSV-1. Using a good lip balm with sunscreen when out of doors is recommended.

Collaborative Care

Nursing Care. Rarely are topical treatments helpful in speeding the healing process but over-the-counter topical preparations such as docosanol (Abreva) can be used by children older than 12 years for local relief of symptoms and may limit the length of the outbreak (Usatine & Tinatigan, 2010).

Medical Care. For children over the age of 2 who have **gingival** herpetic lesions and are not drinking well, the clinician may choose to use a topical treatment of "Magic Mouthwash," a preparation with multiple recipes but commonly made of equal parts liquid diphenhydramine (Benadryl Allergy®), aluminum hydroxide/magnesium hydroxide (Mylanta), and viscous lidocaine in equal parts. This wash can be swished and spit in an older child or carefully applied with a cotton-tip applicator in a younger child.

Even though there are no treatments that can cure this viral infection, there are medications that decrease the length

of the outbreak and/or increase the intervals between outbreaks. Acyclovir (Zovirax) is a prescribed oral medication that can be prescribed for a child older than the age of 2 for their first outbreak or for outbreak suppression. Dosing for acyclovir (Zovirax) is 15 mg/kg/day divided into 5 doses for a 7-day course (Usatine & Tinatigan, 2010). Topical acyclovir (Zovirax) is also available in a 5% cream or ointment to be applied to lesions 5 times per day for 4 days.

Education/Discharge Instructions

Hand washing and keeping eating utensils, washcloths, and hand towels segregated after use are vital to control the spread of HSV-1 to other people.

Often, the child is not the only family member suffering from recurrent HSV-1. Each family member who has active viral lesions must follow all instructions as previously discussed. Parents can take care to not kiss their children on the face when they have an active HSV-1 lesion on their lip because the virus could easily be wiped by the child into their eyes, nose, or oral mucous membranes.

 Across Care Settings: Supporting the child during treatment

- The community nurse has an important role in supporting the child and family during herpes simplex virus 1 (HSV-1) treatment. Tell the child and family the origin, signs, and symptoms of the virus in age-appropriate language.
- Create an environment of trust; allowing the child to keep a parent close may help the child cope better with the clinic visit.
- Monitor pain response throughout the visit to determine if the parent will need information about adequate pain control such as acetaminophen (Children's Tylenol).

FUNGAL INFECTIONS

Cutaneous Candidiasis

Candida albicans is the most common of the *Candida* fungi (yeast). It lives naturally in the gut and oral mucosa but is not a threat to intact skin. *Candida* overgrowth can occur

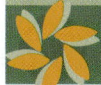 **Family Teaching Guidelines...**
Herpes Simplex Virus (HSV-1)

TOPIC: The nurse will promote ways of decreasing transmission of HSV-1 and preventing subsequent outbreaks.

ESSENTIAL INFORMATION: Teach the child to keep his or her hands away from the face.

- Teach the child good hand washing techniques. To wash the proper amount of time, young children can be taught to sing the alphabet song while rubbing their hands together.
- Decrease stressful situations.
- Avoid prolonged sun exposure.
- Moisturize the lips and use a moisturizing sunscreen on the lips during the summer months.

in newborns who acquire this fungal infection during the birth process from the vaginal canal of an infected mother. Children who have an immune disorder are at risk for developing oral (thrush) or diaper area candidiasis. Children who use corticosteroid inhalers for allergy and asthma prophylaxis and treatment may develop oral candidiasis as well. Rinsing the mouth after each inhaler dose decreases the likelihood of developing oral candidiasis.

Signs and Symptoms

Candidiasis has the following signs and symptoms:

- Oral, including mucous membranes, tongue, buccal (cheek) area, or gingival (gums): Whitish-gray plaques that cannot be removed
- Skin: fine, red or pink raised papules on the skin with a scalloped border
  - "Satellite lesions" are typical: stray papules present near the border of the moist rash area

In candidiasis, the rash feels pruritic and/or tender.

Diagnosis

A thorough history of the mother and the child's existing conditions and a current visualization of the lesions helps diagnose this condition. Recent use of an antibiotic, diabetes, or an immune deficiency disorder are risk factors for candidal infections. If there is a need for a differential diagnosis, a fungal culture can be obtained.

Prevention

Cleaning infants' baby bottle nipples with soap and water and allowing them to thoroughly dry decreases the chance of candidiasis from unclean utensils. Keeping the infant's diaper area as dry as possible and using moisture barriers on clean, dry skin of the diaper area will also decrease the chance of candida overgrowth. Children who rinse their mouth after inhaled corticosteroid use will reduce their chance of oral candidiasis.

Collaborative Care

Nursing Care. With a gloved hand, the nurse uses a swab to apply the medication to the insides of both cheeks. Remember to use a separate swab for each cheek, applied with a gloved finger in a thin layer on the infected area 2 or 3 times per day. Remember, skin is clean and thoroughly dry before application of antifungals.

Medical Care. Oral candidiasis is treated with kinesthetic nystatin (Mycostatin) orally after each feeding or 2 or 3 times per day. Topical treatment for skin infections includes nystatin (Mycostatin), clotrimazole (Lotrimin), miconazole (Monistat), or ketoconazole (Nizoral) ointment.

 Complementary Care: *Diaper Rash Creams*

Different areas of the United States, as well as other countries, make and market diaper rash creams for barrier protection against candida and other diaper rashes. Some have very catchy names like "Bum Boosa Bamboo Diaper Rash Ointment" or "Boudreaux's Butt Paste." Parents may choose trendy or expensive preparations, but some of the easiest to acquire and least expensive are the simpler preparations with petrolatum jelly or zinc oxide (e.g., Vaseline® or Desitin®) (Wondergem, 2010).

 Nursing Insight—Assessing oral thrush: Is it formula or breast milk on the infant's tongue?

Sometimes after an infant drinks formula or breastfeeds, a white film is noted on the tongue. To differentiate the formula or breast milk from oral thrush, the nurse can use a tongue blade to gently scrape the white film. If the nurse can remove the film, it is formula or breast milk. If the nurse cannot remove the film, it is thrush. (Procedure 30-1)

Education/Discharge Instructions

In relation to obtaining a fungal culture, remind the parent(s) that a drop of blood after a feeding may occur because of the mother's nipple rubbing against the area where the culture was obtained. This is not cause for concern and will stop within 24 hours. Serious bleeding that does not stop with gentle pressure would be unusual and would require emergency action. The final culture is not available for 48 to 72 hours; preliminary culture results may be available sooner, and parents are given permission to call for results after this time.

Tinea Capitis, Tinea Corporis, Tinea Cruris, and Tinea Pedis

Tinea capitis, tinea corporis, tinea cruris, and tinea pedis (dermatophytoses) are fungal infections that affect the skin, scalp, or nails (Fig. 30-8). Children of all ages are affected. It may be spread from person to person or from animal (especially cats) to person. These infections may also be spread by contact with inanimate objects such as clothing, furniture, or bed linen of another infected person. Some children may be colonized but remain asymptomatic.

These common fungal infections are as follows:

Tinea capitis—involves the scalp, is characterized by scaly, pruritic patches, can be associated with breakage of the hair, usually seen in prepubertal children between the ages of 1 and 10 years

Tinea corporis—involves the skin of the body, is characterized by a round to oval lesion with maculopapular border with central clearing often with scaling, except the scalp, groin, hands, and feet; seen in children and adolescents; sometimes referred to by the common term ringworm even though no "worm" is involved

Tinea cruris—known as "jock itch"; characterized by red, scaly skin that involves the inner thighs, inguinal creases, or perineal area (rare before adolescence)

Tinea pedis—known as "athlete's foot"; characterized by red, scaly, pruritic skin that may develop weeping and involves the kinesthetic webbed areas of the toes and feet, seen in children and adolescents

Signs and Symptoms

Other signs and symptoms of these infections include:

- Pruritic rash with round, scaly, pink to red lesions, often with central clearing, creating a circular lesion
- On the head, hair loss may occur in the area of the rash

Procedure 30-1 Obtaining a Fungal Culture

Purpose

The purpose of obtaining a fungal culture is to test for the presence of fungi, and if found, identify the type (Fig. 30-7).

Equipment

- Gloves
- Tongue blade
- Sterile cotton swab
- Sterile test tube

Steps

1. Explain the procedure to the child in age-appropriate terms.

   RATIONALE: *A simplified explanation may help decrease anxiety.*

2. Gather all supplies.

   RATIONALE: *To ensure proper supplies are available prior to the procedure.*

3. Depress the tongue with a tongue blade.

   RATIONALE: *Using a tongue blade keeps the child's mouth open and the tongue out of the way.*

4. Aseptically place a sterile cotton swab against a plaque. Vigorously rub the plaque with the cotton swab.

   RATIONALE: *Twirling the swab exposes all sides of the swab to the plaque.*

5. After swabbing, place the swab into a covered, sterile test tube provided by the laboratory and place in a biohazard bag.

   RATIONALE: *Maintains universal precautions.*

6. Have the specimen transported to the lab within 15 to 30 minutes.

   RATIONALE: *Timely delivery will help ensure accuracy of test results.*

Clinical Alert The nurse must remember that attempting to remove the oral thrush can cause the lining of the oral mucosa to bleed.

Note

The specimen must have a label with the child's name, identification numbers, date/time of collection, and the nurse's name or initials.

Caution: Monitor the child's mucosa for bleeding.

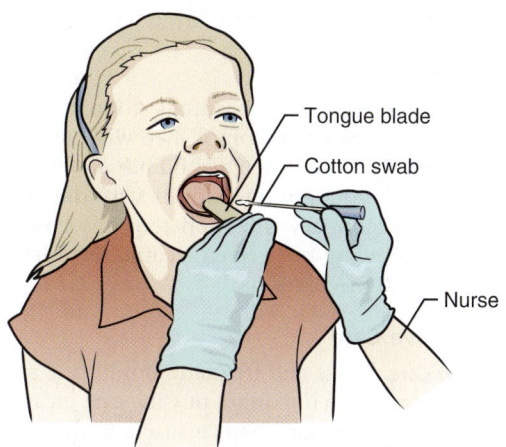

| Tongue blade
| Cotton swab
| Nurse

Documentation

9/25/15 1500 An oral culture was obtained. Child tolerated the collection without difficulty; no pain or bleeding noted.

—C. Kildare, APRN, FNP

Figure 30-7 Obtaining a fungal culture.

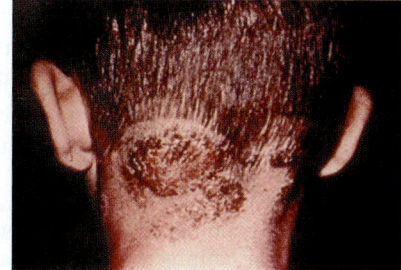

Figure 30-8 Ringworm is a fungal infection that affects the skin, hair, or nails.

Diagnosis

The diagnosis of tinea is made by visual inspection using a Wood's lamp that discloses yellowish gold fluorescent coloration. A potassium hydroxide preparation of scrapings is also diagnostic, demonstrating groups of thick-walled spores and myriad short thick angular hyphae resembling spaghetti (Petros, 2010).

Prevention

Have family pets checked at the veterinarian if they experience areas of fur loss, excessive itching, or self-grooming. Encourage good hand washing. Have children and adolescents in sports activities bathe as soon as they are home from practice or games to remove fungal spores that may be the skin. Do not share **fomites** (objects that can carry infection) like bath and hand towels, combs and brushes, hats, helmets, and intimate apparel.

Collaborative Care

Nursing Care. The nurse must stress that everyone in the family needs to be treated and that it is essential not to share hair brushes or bath towels. Specifically, with tinea capitis the affected area of hair growth may take 6 to 12 months to grow or it may not grow back at all. The nurse can provide emotional support and suggest hairstyles to help conceal tinea capitis.

Medical Care. Treatment for tinea infections includes antifungal medications.

- griseofulvin (Fulvicin or Grisactin) oral
- fluconazole (Diflucan) oral or topical shampoo
- miconazole (Monistat) buccal tablet or topical,
- terbinafine (Lamisil) oral or topical

For most types of tinea infections, treatment with antifungal drugs in the form of skin creams, lotions, or ointments is adequate. If the infection is widespread or affects the hair or nails, griseofulvin (Fulvicin or Grisactin) in tablet form is prescribed for the child. The medication must be taken for at least 6 weeks to be effective. Absorption of the medication is enhanced if it is given with a high-fat meal. Other drugs such as miconazole (Monistat), fluconazole (Diflucan), and terbinafine, an antifungal shampoo, are often recommended. Terbinafine (Lamisil) has been approved for children over 4 years of age, and fluconazole shampoo is approved for children over 12 days of age (Petros, 2010).

Education/Discharge Instructions

The child is checked periodically throughout treatment to be sure a proper response is noted. The nurse must stress the importance of completing the recommended treatment even after the lesions appear to be cleared. For treatment of tinea pedis, education should include wearing lightweight *dry* socks, well-ventilated shoes, and adequate cleaning of shower areas to prevent spread of the infection.

 Now Can You—Discuss bacterial, viral, and fungal skin infections?

1. Name one skin condition in each category (bacterial, viral, and fungal) and its signs and symptoms, diagnosis, and prevention?
2. Discuss the holistic nursing interventions for the named conditions?
3. Discuss education/discharge instructions for the named conditions?

Hypersensitive Skin Reactions

DERMATITIS

Dermatitis is an inflammatory rash marked by itching and redness that occurs as a result of numerous conditions. There are three common classifications of dermatitis in children: **atopic**, contact, and **seborrheic**.

Atopic Dermatitis

Atopic dermatitis is a chronic skin condition with three distinct phases (acute, subacute, and chronic) with no known etiology. In the infant, the rash usually presents on the head, face, and lateral arms and legs. In the older child,

---

Labs: Liver Enzymes

When griseofulvin (Grifulvin V) is used, baseline liver enzymes are evaluated and are rechecked every 6 weeks. Alternate treatment is warranted if tests are abnormal.

---

the rash presents in the folds of the arms and legs and occasionally on the eyelids and neck.

This condition is found in children with allergies and in children whose family has a history of allergies, asthma, and rhinitis. Approximately 50% of persons with atopic dermatitis present in the first year of life and an additional 30% in the years between ages 1 and 5. Although the etiology may be genetic, the child may also have immunological impairment. It is also possible for the etiology to be environmental in nature (e.g., pollution, indoor allergens such as cigarette smoke, or infections).

Signs and Symptoms

The child with atopic dermatitis has a red, raised rash that is both pruritic and painful with red papules that may have a serous exudate (clear fluid) during the acute phase. The rash is dry and easily cracks and excoriates in the subacute phase. If the disease progresses and the rash become chronic, the skin thickens, lichenification may be present, and the papules can become fibrotic.

Diagnosis

A complete family history and visual assessment of the child reveals the common signs of this condition. Blood tests reveal an increase in circulating IgE antibodies.

Prevention

The priority preventative measure is stopping a secondary infection, which can be accomplished with good skin care and close monitoring. When a child has atopic dermatitis, prevention of secondary infection is very important. Prevention of a secondary infection requires good hygiene processes, following prescribed treatment protocols, and maintaining skin hydration.

Collaborative Care

Nursing Care. Close and frequent monitoring and assessment of the rash is an important nursing care measure. Some children should use non-soap cleansers to decrease drying and subsequent secondary infection, examples include Johnson and Johnson Gentle Cleansing Wash®, Cetaphil®, Neutrogena Extra Gentle Cleanser®, and Neutrogena Ultra Gentle daily cleanser® for the adolescent needing a daily face wash. Warm, not hot, bathing water will decrease irritation. Encourage the adolescent to keep the water a bit cooler, avoid excessive scrubbing with exfoliating scrubs and cloths, and pat dry. Moisturizing immediately after bathing with emollients, such as Cetaphil Moisturizing Cream® or Eucerin®, locks in moisture and decreases dry, flaky, or itchy skin (National Eczema Organization, 2012).

Education/Discharge Instructions

Nurses need to reinforce gentle cleansing and the use of tepid to slightly warm water for bathing as well as the appropriate emollients. Encourage patients to practice itch-scratch avoidance and to keep fingernails trimmed short with no sharp edges. Teach parents the signs and symptoms of secondary infection including a fever remaining above 101.5°F (38.6°C) or evidence of red, painful, pus-filled lesions.

Contact Dermatitis

Contact dermatitis can occur if an allergen or skin irritant is encountered (Venes, 2013). In children, the irritant agents that cause this type of skin sensitivity are often soaps or detergents with fragrances or dyes. For infants, the diaper area is especially prone and could be the result of diaper perfumes, cloth diaper detergents, or diaper wipes (Fig. 30-9) (Jacob, Herro, Guide, Cunningham & Connelly, 2012). Diaper dermatitis is one form of irritant contact dermatitis and can be caused by prolonged exposure to urine and feces. Diaper dermatitis is characterized by an erythematous, confluent maculopapular rash that is prominent on convex surfaces and in the folds. Children playing out of doors may encounter varying plant life that can cause contact dermatitis, like poisonous oaks, ivies, or sumacs. As children get older and begin to wear jewelry and watches, contact dermatitis may be present from specific types of metals, commonly nickel, but any metal can be a source of allergen (Usatine & Riojas, 2010).

Signs and Symptoms

Signs and symptoms of contact dermatitis include the following:

- Irritated, inflamed, and pruritic rash within 48 hours of contact with the offending agent
- Vesicles and bullae that may be present in the area
- Urticaria (hives) when there is contact with an allergen
- Vesicles that may weep serous fluid

Diagnosis

A complete history of contacts both in and out of doors for a child appearing in the community health clinic helps determine the diagnosis. If a differential diagnosis is required because there are atypical lesions, a biopsy may be performed. Vesicular lesions that present in children may also include varicella and impetigo. These etiologies are ruled out before a diagnosis of contact dermatitis is considered.

 Nursing Insight—*Patch testing*

If the offending agent is not easily determined, an allergist may be an appropriate referral to determine if allergic contact dermatitis is the diagnosis. One method of determining an allergy is by completing patch testing. The allergist prepares the proper concentration of allergens in a paraffin base and places this on the child's skin, usually the back, holding it in place with hypoallergenic tape. The patch is left in place for varying times based on the type of allergy being assessed (48 hours of wear is standard). After the time has passed, the skin is assessed for reaction that is measured by redness and edema (Figure 30-10).

Prevention

Children going into heavily weedy or wooden areas can wear long sleeves, long pants, and socks to prevent contact with poisonous plants. Strict avoidance of known allergens in the home, including soaps and fragrances, will decrease the incidence of allergic contact dermatitis. Prevention of irritant contact dermatitis is avoidance of known substances that have resulted in rash and, for infants, frequent changing of diapers.

Collaborative Care

Nursing Care. If the nurse notices that there are weepy lesions, a drying agent like an over-the-counter product such as Domeboro® powder (active ingredient, aluminum sulfate) may bring relief. For pruritic relief, cool baths are effective. For a longer effect, a low dose of over-the-counter hydrocortisone (Cortisone-10) cream can be applied with a gloved finger. Oral steroids such as prednisolone (Orapred) are used only if more than 10% of the child's body surface area is involved. If discomfort from agents such as poison ivy or oak is the concern, a topical anesthetic such as Dermoplast® may bring relief.

Nursing care of diaper dermatitis is aimed at allowing the area to heal in an environment of minimal moisture. This can be accomplished by frequent diaper changes, allowing the area to "air" dry, and the use of barrier ointments that include white petrolatum or zinc oxide.

Medical Care. Over-the-counter topical medications are used for comfort, and if necessary, the provider may order an antipruritic by mouth like hydroxyzine (Atarax). If greater than 10% of the child's body is involved, prescribing an oral steroid is common. Prednisolone (Orapred) dosed at 0.14 mg to 2 mg/kg/day in once daily or divided dosing is prescribed.

 Complementary Care: *Topical Agents*

Topical agents that promote healing are frequently used for dry skin rashes: cow udder balm (bag balm), green tea extract or red

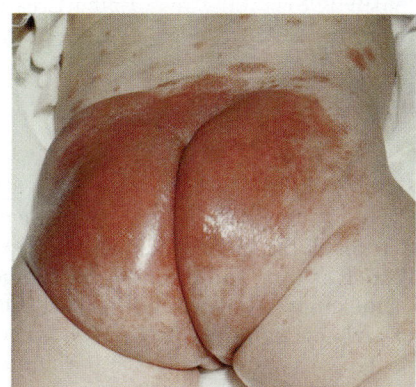

Figure 30-9 Contact dermatitis can occur if an allergen or skin irritant is encountered.

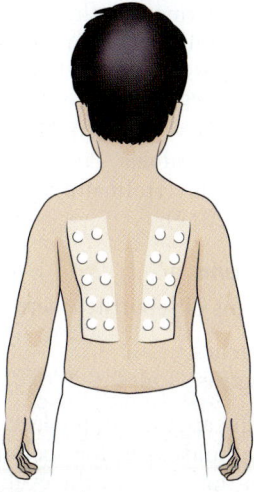

Figure 30-10 Patch testing.

tea (steeped and cooled), vitamin E preparations, aloe vera, milk, calamine, and colloidal oatmeal. Adding baking soda to the bath or a few drops of chamomile, lavender, or calendula oil can reduce itching and promote moisture retention in the skin.

Education/Discharge Instructions

Nurses teach preventative methods when children and adolescents present with this diagnosis. Medication management, when prescribed, is reinforced. If the child is suffering from severe pruritus, they may require a sedative for sleeping purposes. Sleep aid medications considered safe and effective for children include diphenhydramine (Benadryl Allergy [over-the-counter for children over 2 years of age]) and hydroxyzine (Atarax [prescribed]). If an oral steroid such as prednisolone (Pediapred) is ordered for the inflammation, remind parents that the child must complete the dose in the exact way it was prescribed, particularly if a tapering prescription is needed. The nurse must also teach parents that prednisolone (Pediapred) must be taken with food and may cause excessive wakefulness in a child.

 ### Collaboration in Caring—*A severe allergic reaction*

The parents must notify the school nurse, day-care providers, coaches, and other adult leaders who spend time with the child about the diagnosed allergy. Everyone working with the child must be taught how to use an EpiPen® or EpiPen Jr.® (epinephrine). EpiPens are usually kept in the school nurse's office. During sports activities, a second EpiPen may be given to the coach or the assistant. Along with documentation of the allergy, contact information, and the EpiPen that is on-hand, ready access to a phone for emergency medical assistance is a necessity.

 ### Nursing Diagnoses Contact Dermatitis

- Impaired Skin Integrity related to allergic reaction
- Acute Discomfort related to inflammation of the skin
- Alteration in Sleep Pattern related to pruritus

Seborrheic Dermatitis

Chronic seborrheic dermatitis affects 2% to 5% of the population. Although it can affect young children, the peak incidence occurs in persons aged 18 and older. There are many theories about the etiology of seborrheic dermatitis. This condition may have a genetic predisposition. In immunosuppressed individuals, *Pityrosporum ovale* may be the offending fungus (Hofmann-Wellenhof, Pellacani, Halvehy, & Soyer, 2012).

Signs and Symptoms

Signs and symptoms of seborrheic dermatitis include:

- Red to pink patches
- Loose yellow, greasy scales

The rash usually appears on the face, the cheek bones, and the nasolabial folds as well as behind the ears. It can also be found on the scalp, in the eyebrows, and on the upper chest and upper back.

Diagnosis

The child who is diagnosed with seborrheic dermatitis has the defined rash. The nurse understands that the particular look of the rash differentiates it between other conditions such as lupus, rosacea, and atopic or contact dermatitis.

Prevention

If a child has had seborrheic dermatitis in the past, and it clears, it can be prevented by preemptive treatment. Daily or at least three times a week, an anti-seborrheic shampoo can be used to cleanse the area of skin that is prone to breakout.

Collaborative Care

Nursing Care. The nurse is aware that antifungal therapy is used if the etiology is *P ovale*. If the condition is not fungal in nature, topical corticosteroids may be used intermittently. It is important for the nurse to remember that low-dose corticosteroid topical applications are to be used on the face and other thinner skin surfaces. For the hair, antiseborrheic shampoos that contain one of the following active ingredients can be used: coal tar (T/Gel® Therapeutic Shampoo Stubborn Itch), ketoconazole (Nizoral®), selenium sulfide (Selsun Blue®), or zinc pyrithione (Denorex®).

Medical Care. Medical treatment for seborrheic dermatitis includes antifungal therapies and topical corticosteroids, if indicated, for inflammation.

Education/Discharge Instructions

The nurse communicates to the child and family it is more efficacious if the child or adolescent rotates the types of shampoos. Some of the shampoos are marketed as "anti-dandruff" shampoos.

CUTANEOUS SKIN REACTIONS

Cutaneous skin reactions are a manifestation of an allergic response. The offending allergen can be introduced into the system in a variety of ways such as ingestion, inhalation, or coming into direct contact.

Signs and Symptoms

There are four basic types of skin reactions in an allergic response:

- **Exanthema** (eruption)
- **Urticarial** (itching)
- **Blistering** (swelling)
- **Pustular** (a small elevated skin lesion filled with white blood cells)
  (Venes, 2013)

Diagnosis

Visual assessment along with a complete history may help the nurse determine the cause. The nurse can find out specific details such as time and place of onset, ingested prescription medications, over-the-counter medications, bug bites, use of herbal or cultural remedies, and their relationship to the cutaneous eruptions. It is important to note that medication reactions can occur with the first dose of medication or even with a medication that the child has taken for months or years.

Prevention

Prevention includes telling parents to report any medications the child is taking to assess for potential cross reactivity. Alert the health-care practitioner to all allergies. Also, it is important for parents to keep all allergy-producing foods and airborne irritants out of the child's room, home, and school or care center and alert friends and family to the allergy.

Collaborative Care

Nursing Care. It is paramount that the nurse looks beyond the outer surface of the skin and assesses for the root of the problem that may be a life-threatening condition associated with a systemic allergic response. An allergic reaction can be mild or a severe immediate hypersensitivity to an excessive release of chemical mediators affecting the entire body from medications, insects, foods, immunizations, diagnostic contrast media, or the administration of blood products. During the assessment phase, the nurse must examine the face for swelling, especially around the lips, and including the tongue. It is essential that the nurse check the throat, using a light, but avoid using a tongue blade. Use of a tongue blade may stimulate more oral or pharyngeal swelling. Check nasal passages for edema (swelling) and erythema (redness) to ensure a patent airway. Airway compromise is a medical emergency.

The nurse must recognize the key assessments in a systemic allergic response. Any edema or laryngospasms in the airway have the potential to cause blockage. If airway obstruction is noted, the emergency medical system must be initiated, and circulation, airway, and breathing are begun. The nurse must assess for cyanosis and listen for audible sounds of upper airway respiratory distress such as wheezing or stridor. Assessing the vital signs, specifically, hypotension, which may lead to vascular collapse and cardiac arrest and is a critical indication that the allergic response may be systemic. A nonjudgmental approach helps the nurse obtain the essential information that is necessary to determine which agent is the cause of the reaction.

Medical Care. Treatment measures include administering epinephrine (Adrenalin), keeping the child lying flat and warm with the feet slightly elevated, and administering oxygen if available. Immediate transport to an emergency medical facility is essential.

 focus on safety

EpiPen®

The EpiPen Jr.® autoinjector is used for children experiencing a life-threatening reaction. An injection of 0.15 mg of epinephrine (Adrenalin) is used for children up to 33 lb (15 kg), and an injection of 0.3 mg is used for older children and adults. If a severe allergic reaction occurs, the medication is administered by IM injection immediately (Rhoads, 2009). Be sure to check the expiration date on the EpiPen® or EpiPen Jr.®

Education/Discharge Instructions

The nurse communicates to the child and family that is important to know the offending allergen and that it can be introduced into the system through ingestion, inhalation, or coming into direct contact. Reinforcing the signs and symptoms of the allergic response as well as emergency treatment is essential information for the child and family.

Infestations

PEDICULOSIS CAPITIS

Pediculosis capitis, head lice, is a common childhood condition that can be passed among friends and family. Approximately 6 to 12 million school-aged children are infested yearly. There are three kinds of lice: scalp (pediculosis capitis), body (pediculosis corporis), and pubic area (pediculosis pubis). The lice pierce the skin and suck blood. The bites can cause severe itching and can predispose the child to a secondary infection.

 Cultural Diversity: Pediculosis

African Americans have the lowest incidence of head lice. Hair type is likely the reason why the common head louse cannot hold the hair follicle, stay on the head, and subsequently lay eggs (CDC, 2010a).

Signs and Symptoms

Signs and symptoms of pediculosis include:

- Live lice
  - Tend to live near the nape of the neck and behind the ears
- Louse eggs (nits)
  - Can be found anywhere along the shaft of the hair; the older the nits are, the more distal
  - Pearlescent teardrop in shape, initially laid at the base of the hair shaft
  - Fluoresce blue under a Wood's lamp

 focus on safety

Nits on the eyelashes

Nits on the eyelashes of a child are sometimes a sign of sexual abuse. The nurse must report any suspicious findings.

Diagnosis

For lice, the clinical presentation and identification of the louse and/or its eggs is important. Persistent itching of the head is the classic sign.

Prevention

To prevent lice, all children must avoid the use of one another's combs, barrettes, hats, and headbands. Children who are involved in sports may pick up lice in batting helmets and other protective headgear that is shared. These fomites can easily carry lice from child to child.

In the home or the school or day-care setting, children with active lice need treatment as well as their environment. All associated persons affected by lice are also treated.

Collaborative Care

Nursing Care. The nurse educates the family about over-the-counter lice treatments that may be helpful in the care of lice. The nurse can explain to the child and family that anyone can get lice if in close proximity to others who happen to have it. Lice are common in school-age children, and there is no need for embarrassment. Guide the parents to resolution through treatment.

Medical Care. Over-the-counter lice treatments may be helpful. Types of pediculicide treatments include pyrethroids such as permethrin (Nix) and malathion (Ovide) and antiparasitics, including benzyl alcohol (Ulesfia), lindane (Kwell), spinosad (Natroba), and ivermectin (Stromectol). Ivermectin is used orally in hard to manage cases of head lice (Chosidow, Giraudeau, Cottrell, Izri, Hofmann, Mann, et al., 2010). Malathion (Ovide) is recommended for children over the age of 2, and benzyl alcohol is not recommended for children under 6 months of age. Permethrin (Nix) is not recommended for infants under 2 months of age, and spinosad does not have proven safety in children less than 4 years of age.

When the child is over the age of 2, the best, first-line pharmacological shampoo with the fewest incidence of resistance is malathion (Ovide). Both malathion (Ovide) and benzyl alcohol outperform permethrin (Nix) (CDC, 2010a).

"What to say"—*Pediculosis*

When parents inquire about lice, the nurse:

- Asks family members if there is a recent history of another family member with infestation
- Asks the school nurse or day-care provider if there is lice infestation in that setting
- Communicates that a "nit check" of each individual will help the family members determine who needs treatment
- Reminds family members and friends that because they may acquire lice from the affected child, they can take the same treatment actions (The National Pediculosis Association, Inc., 2011)

Education/Discharge Instructions

The nurse instructs the family to wash the hair according to the product's instructions. If a child is unable to tolerate these shampoos, former remedies including the use of asphyxiants like petrolatum and food oils (e.g., olive oil) can be used. Once the shampoo is rinsed from the hair, remove nits by backcombing with a fine-tooth comb while the hair is still wet (nits are easier to remove when the hair is damp).

The nurse stresses to the caregiver to implement housecleaning (e.g., dust, vacuum, and scrub); wash clothing and bedding; and wipe off hats, helmets, and toys. If a soft or cloth toy like a stuffed animal is not washable, it must be bagged in a sealed plastic bag and away from family members' rooms for 14 days. Launder all bed linens in hot water. Pillows are washed if possible, or thrown away if used by the child to avoid reinfestation. Anti-lice sprays can be used for furniture and other environmental objects that are not disposable, but the most important cleaning is vacuuming. Hair care items can be boiled (hot water above 140°F) or soaked in anti-lice shampoo and never shared (The National Pediculosis Association, Inc., 2011).

The nurse instructs the family member to remove nits from eyelashes by applying petrolatum jelly to the eyelashes twice a day for 8 days. The family member can

Family Teaching Guidelines...
Pediculosis

TOPIC: The nurse will discuss how to prevent the spread of pediculosis

ESSENTIAL INFORMATION:

- Assess for lice using good lighting and examining the child's head to identify both live lice (very small and brown or black) and nits.
- Separate sections of the hair, paying particularly attention to the area behind the ears and the nape of the neck.
- Teach the family member that this dandruff-like appearance cannot be easily removed by combing because of the sticky adherence of the nit.

check the school's anti-lice policy; children must remain home from school until lice-free. The child may be required to be checked by the school nurse or day-care provider before returning. Tell the family member that the child is rechecked for infestation in 7 to 10 days, sooner if the child is itching incessantly or the itching is interfering with sleep.

Complementary Care: *Wet-Combing the Hair*

Wet-combing the hair that is moistened with water and food oil, (e.g., olive oil) is very effective and safe in small children and may preclude the need for a medicated shampoo. Parents can use a nit comb to carefully comb the hair in its entirety while removing live lice and nits and disposing of them in a sealed plastic bag.

focus on safety

Neurotoxicity

Lindane (Kwell) shampoo is an insecticide and can cause neurotoxicity, seizures, and death. There is an FDA Black Box warning that this shampoo is only to be used as a second-line treatment and retreatment is avoided, and the American Academy of Pediatrics no longer recommends it as a pediculicide (Federal Drug Administration [FDA], 2009). Care is employed with families to make sure that only affected adults will use the product, not children.

SCABIES

Scabies results from a mite infestation with *Sarcoptes scabiei*. Children with a weakened immune system are at increased risk. Scabies is transmitted by close personal contact with an infected person and is more common in persons who live in crowded conditions or share a bed.

The scabies mite cannot survive for more than 3 days away from the skin. Scabies is a common condition found worldwide that does not discriminate based on race or social class.

Mite infestation is highly transferable, and while children of all ages are affected, it is most commonly seen in children younger than 2 years of age.

Signs and Symptoms

Signs and symptoms of mite infestation include:

- Pruritic (worse at night), linear rash under the skin that may appear as a burrow
- Intermittent red or pink papules of inflammation

Scabies is commonly found:

- On the hands and webs of the fingers
- Along the waistband
- In the armpits and groin

 Nursing Insight—Mite infestation

In this condition, the female arachnid mite burrows into the outer layer of the epidermis and lays her eggs, leaving a trail of debris and feces (scybala). The larvae hatch in approximately 2 to 5 days and proceed to the surface of the skin. This cycle repeats every 7 to 14 days. The original mite dies in the burrow after 4 to 5 weeks. The scabies rash is red streaked and appears linear from the burrowing. The mites, eggs, and their excrement can cause intense itching, especially at night. There are also signs of papules that are a result of inflammation secondary to infestation.

Diagnosis

In assessing for scabies, it is essential to check all pruritic areas for the primary burrows and secondary inflammatory papules (raised, circumscribed lesions) (CDC, 2010b). A skin scraping may be viewed under the microscope for evidence of the mite, eggs, or feces. As an alternate assessment tool, the nurse can use clear adhesive tape (wrapping or packing tape), apply to the area of the linear rash, press firmly, and then lift away. Place the adhesive tape on a slide and evaluate under microscopy. The mites and eggs are easily identifiable under the microscope (Walter, Heukelbach, Fengler, Worth, Hengge, & Feldmeier, 2011). This technique is especially gentle for a child who would not tolerate skin scraping as well. If scabies are not identifiable by visual inspection, microscopic examination is completed.

Prevention

Do not share a bed, clothing, or intimate touch with a person who has scabies. Children should avoid sleeping in the same bed as a parent or sibling with scabies. Even if only one member of the family has scabies, the entire family is treated.

Collaborative Care

Nursing Care. The nurse teaches the family how to use the medication after a bath and what to look for if there is minor skin irritation. Further, the nurse reminds the family that all members having exposure need to be treated at the same time to decrease the likelihood of re-infestation.

The nurse suggests to the parents that a dishwasher with no other contents works well for cleaning washable toys and hair items. Treating all clothing, bedding, towels, and cloth toys by washing them in hot water and then placing them in the dryer is necessary to kill all scabies.

Medical Care. Permethrin 5% cream (Elimite) is approved for infants over 2 months of age.

 focus on safety

Permethrin 5% (Elimite)

Avoid permethrin 5% cream or lotion (Elimite) in persons with known allergy to chrysanthemums. No serious side effects have been noted with permethrin 5% cream or lotion (Elimite), but some children will experience mild burning sensation upon application; a few others may experience redness or itching. Identifying these potential mild effects will help the caregiver determine that there is an allergic reaction to the cream or lotion.

Education/Discharge Instructions

First, a warm soap and water bath is given, and then permethrin 5% cream or lotion (Elimite) is applied and left on for 8 to 14 hours. The cream or lotion is applied from the neck to the toes avoiding mucous membranes and the genitals. Children under 2 years of age can have the cream applied to their scalp and temples and covered with a cap. Overnight treatment is easiest. Treatment is repeated in 1 week. All persons in close contact with the child are treated concurrently (Currie & McCarthy, 2010). For severe cases, ivermectin (Stromectol) may be used orally, and the family is instructed to return to their health-care provider for follow-up and treatment. The rash and the itching may take up to 2 to 3 weeks to resolve because of the ongoing presence of the irritants of the mite until the stratum corneum has replaced itself.

 Nursing Diagnoses Lice and Mite Infestation

- Altered Comfort related to pruritus secondary to infestation
- Potential Altered Health Maintenance related to nonadherence of cleaning regimen
- Potential for Social Isolation related to isolation from peers during treatment
- Pain related to secondary infection
- Risk for Infection related to impaired skin integrity, primary infestation, secondary pruritus

Bites and Stings

INSECTS

The most common insect bite comes from the mosquito. Spider and tick bites are also prevalent among children. The stings experienced most frequently are from bees, wasps, and hornets, and in some parts of the United States, scorpions. Other insects are also likely to bite, such as some types of flies, fleas, and fire ants.

Signs and Symptoms

Mosquito bite:

- Red, edematous papule
- Pruritic
- Burning pain

Spider bite (e.g., widows, false black widows, and brown recluse):

- Red, edematous papule, wheal, or pustule, often solitary
- Pruritic

- Pain: mild to severe
- Local necrosis and systemic symptoms (rare)

 Tick bite:

- Small reddish area that may or may not be raised
- Sometimes pruritic
- Tick may still be attached
- Systemic symptoms associated with related diseases, including Rocky Mountain spotted fever and Lyme disease (Table 30-6)

 Bee, wasp, or hornet sting:

- Red, edematous papule
- Pain at the time of the sting
- If the reaction is systemic:
  - Generalized urticaria (hives)
  - Flushing
  - Angioedema with wheezing (rare)

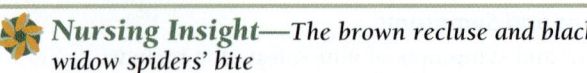

Nursing Insight—*The brown recluse and black widow spiders' bite*

The bite of the brown recluse spider begins with itching, pain, and erythema. The venomous sting advances into a purple lesion that signals the beginning of necrosis. The site becomes red with blisters, has a white ring, and is surrounded by irregular erythematous.

The black widow spider's bite leaves a stinging sensation at the time of the bite along with two fang bite marks, edema, petechiae, and erythema. The neurotoxin is usually self-limiting, but can result in a more severe anaphylactic reaction. A systemic reaction from the neurotoxic venom can occur in 1 to 3 hours, with symptoms peaking in 3 hours and then diminishing in 72 hours. A systemic reaction includes muscle rigidity of the abdomen and torso, muscle cramps near the bite, malaise, sweating, dizziness, restlessness, insomnia, nausea and vomiting, hypertension, arrhythmias, and **oliguria** (low urine output).

Table 30-6 Insect Bites

Bite	Local Reaction	Treatment for Local Reactions
Mosquitoes and Fleas Systemic reaction is possible: allergic reaction; wheezing, urticaria, laryngeal edema, shock	Red papules Itching, sometimes burning Local swelling (from foreign proteins) Minimal pain	Cleanse Cold compresses to the site Antihistamines, oral or topical
Bees, Wasps, and Hornets Systemic reaction is possible: urticaria, flushing, angioedema, pruritus, wheezing	Redness and swelling (from venomous enzymes) Mild pain	Remove stinger quickly by scraping, not pinching Cleanse Cold compresses to the site Elevate the extremity Antihistamines A dash of meat tenderizer with a drop of water on the sting, massaged in for approximately 5 minutes will decrease pain
Fire Ants Systemic and anaphylactic reaction is possible.	Redness, swelling, and induration (from neurotoxin, creates a histamine response) Red, itchy wheal that turns into a cloudy vesicle within 24 hours	Cleanse Cold compresses Antihistamines, oral or topical Elevate extremity
Ticks Systemic allergic reaction is possible. Lyme disease is possible: bull's-eye rash with erythema migrans, followed by fatigue, malaise, and joint pain	Tick is usually found with head burrowed into the skin The tick must be removed Area is generally reddened, and occasionally itchy	Remove tick Cleanse Cold compresses Monitor for rash over the next month
Brown Recluse Spider Systemic reaction is possible in 12–72 hours: fever, chills, malaise, arthralgia, nausea, and vomiting Intravascular hemolysis resulting in anemia	Red swollen "bull's-eye" wound that turns purplish with an outer area of white induration Skin necrosis occurs (the venom is proteolytic and cytotoxic)	Cleanse Apply ice to the site Apply topical antibiotic cream or lotion Seek emergency assistance
Black Widow Spider Systemic reaction possible in 1–3 hours, diminishing within 72 hours: muscle rigidity, malaise, sweating, nausea and vomiting, hypertension, arrhythmia, oliguria, restlessness, insomnia	Painful Redness and swelling Fang marks Petechiae branching out from site Stinging sensation	Cleanse Ice Antihistamine, orally Hydrocortisone topically Seek emergency assistance to manage any neurotoxic symptoms

Source: CDC (2011c).

Diagnosis

Diagnosis of insect bites and stings are based on the child's history and physical findings.

Prevention

To protect against insect bites and stings, the nurse can stress that children and adolescents adhere to the following directives when out of doors: wear light-colored clothing with minimal patterns, wear minimal perfumes or colognes, and cover the skin whenever possible to decrease the chance of insect bites and stings. Mosquitoes bite more in the dusk and darkness; protecting the child with bug repellent at this time will decrease the incidence of bites. Do not play in areas of dead foliage where spiders like to nest. Children should not play in live, blooming foliage to avoid bee stings. Playing in wooded areas is ok, but doing a thorough tick inspection upon reentering the home is absolutely necessary (CDC, 2011c).

Collaborative Care

Nursing Care. All bites are cleansed gently with soap and water and patted dry. Monitor bites for signs and symptoms of infection from the **vector** (e.g., insect or arachnid) and from secondary infection caused by scratching the bite site.

Specific care measures for mosquito bites and therefore mosquito-borne illnesses are the use of bug repellent sprays applied sparingly to the child's clothing to help decrease bites and therefore lower the risk for contracting West Nile virus, a significant mosquito-borne illness in the United States today. The CDC (2012c) is now recommending two new repellents that do not contain N-diethyl-m-toluamide (DEET), a common ingredient in most bug repellents. The two new repellents are oil of lemon eucalyptus or PMD (Repel) and picaridin (KBR 3023) (Cutter Advanced Insect Repellent), easily found in local stores that carry brand name bug repellent sprays (CDC, 2012c).

Education/Discharge Instructions

The first step is to remove all ticks immediately and properly. The nurse must remember to tell parents to remove a tick, grasping it firmly with fine-point tweezers where the mouth part is attached. Pulling gently is important to avoid squeezing of the tick's body (to avoid leaving any tick parts in the child) until it releases. The nurse explains to the parents to save the intact tick in a sealable bag in the freezer with the date of the bite recorded (in case the tick needs to be tested for disease). Stingers from bees, wasps, and hornets are removed immediately; they will come out in one piece with a singular tug or scrape. When the stinger is injected, the venom is already in the skin; however, the stinger can cause more irritation and pain and possibly a deep "foreign body" reaction if not removed immediately. After removal of any vector, cleanse the area with soap and water and pat dry.

 focus on safety

A severe reaction to a bite

A child who has had a severe reaction to a bee or wasp sting wears a medical alert bracelet or necklace and carries an EpiPen® (epinephrine) or EpiPen Jr.® School nurses, coaches, and other adults who provide care or guidance for these children should have access to the EpiPen®.

 focus on safety

Products with oil of lemon eucalyptus

When using insect repellents on children, spray or apply to the adult's hands first and then gently apply to the head, neck, and face avoiding the eyes, ears, nostrils, and mouth. Using this same method, apply to all exposed skin. Apply the repellent to the outside of clothing, not under clothing. Do not use products with oil of lemon eucalyptus on children under the age of 3 (CDC, 2012a). Other products, including KBR 3023 (Cutter) is acceptable for children 2 months and older. Remember, insect repellents are pesticides and cannot be applied to the skin of children for long periods of time. After an event out of doors, children can bathe and have their clothes placed in the washing machine.

 Now Can You—Identify the types of insect bites?

1. Identify the local symptoms of insect bites and stings?
2. Identify which spider bite may produce an anaphylactic reaction?
3. Discuss specific prevention measures for insect bites and stings?

ANIMAL BITES

Dog bites account for the majority of animal bites to children. In fact, in the United States, approximately 800,000 dog bites are reported each year, and 50% of them involve children. Boys are bitten more often than girls, and children between the ages of 5 and 9 are most at risk (National Center for Injury Prevention and Control, 2008). Often the child knows the animal and may have been bitten because of improper behavior such as interfering with feeding, playing, or taunting. Common locations for dog bites are the head and neck in children under 5 and extremities in older children. Upper extremities and face are common locations for cat bites.

Signs and Symptoms

DOG BITES. Children younger than 5 years are more likely to be bitten in the head and neck, while older children are more likely to be bitten on the extremities. Signs and symptoms for dog bites include:

- Scratches and abrasions
- Deep lacerations or punctures
- Crushing tissue and bone injury, including nerve/tissue/muscular/bone involvement

CAT BITES. Cats are more likely to bite a child's upper extremities and face. Signs and symptoms for cat bites include:

- Scratches and abrasions
- Puncture-like bites
- Complications, such as cat scratch disease, osteomyelitis, and septic arthritis (Baddour, 2011)

Diagnosis

Diagnosis of animal bites is based on patient history and physical findings. To diagnose a more severe problem, a radiographic evaluation may be required.

Prevention

Children under the age of 5 should be supervised when interacting with an animal (CDC, 2009). These young children may inadvertently upset the animal and subsequently be unable to protect themselves. Although the highest crude rate of bites occurs in children ages 5 to 9, these children are not always within an adult's sight when interacting with animals. Therefore, children must learn basic safety approaches to dogs and cats in their environment, including holding still and allowing a new animal to look at and smell the child's hand. Children who verbalize fear of dogs and cats can be exposed to them in very controlled environments if the parent desires. Spaying or neutering animals can help reduce aggressive behavior. National Dog Bite Prevention Week is the third full week in May annually (American Veterinary Medical Association, [AVMA], 2012).

"What to say"—*Animal bite prevention*

The nurse can teach the following safety tips to children and parents when encountering dogs or other unfamiliar animals:

- Never leave a child alone with an animal.
- Never put your face close to an animal.
- Avoid dogs and animals that are not familiar.
- Seek permission to touch or pet an animal.
- Avoid any contact with wild animals.
- Do not run away from aggressive animals. Lie down in a ball, protecting the face, and remain quiet.
- Never overexcite or tease an animal.
- Play with animals only when an adult is present.
- Report any strange behavior from an animal, even if it is a familiar animal.
- Do not disturb animals that are eating, sleeping, or nursing their young.

Collaborative Care

Nursing Care. The nurse must take an accurate history about the incident and gather information about the exact injury, circumstances surrounding the attack, and location of the animal if known. The animal bite requires a good cleaning with soap and water and thorough rinsing. The nurse can then cover the wound with a topical antibiotic and clean dry dressing that helps to protect it from infection. Small wounds can be closed with adhesive strips, and larger wounds may need suturing. Wounds over the joints must be further elevated and immobilized.

If the wound was a crushing injury from a larger or stronger animal, an evaluation in the practitioner's office or an emergency department is required to rule out damage to deeper structures. A tetanus booster is required if the child has not had one in the last 5 years (Schueler, Beckett, & Gettings, 2010). After wound treatment, antibiotics are considered for bites. Only 5% of dog bites will become infected, but approximately 80% of cat bites will become infected (Gilbert et al., 2011).

focus on safety

Rabid animal

It is essential the nurse find out if the animal is rabid. Human rabies immune globulin or human diploid cell rabies vaccine should be given to all children who have been bitten by an unknown wild or domestic animal that is positive for rabies or bitten by an animal in which rabies cannot be excluded (World Health Organization [WHO], 2011). Unknown dogs or other mostly domesticated animals may not require rabies prophylaxis. The local health department has information regarding best practice based on reported rabies cases in their area.

Medical Care. Antibiotics are given for dog bites in the child who has a compromised immunity, when the bite was over hand joints or involving the face, severe crushing injuries, or when the child presented for care distant from the time of original injury. First-line antibiotics are amoxicillin/clavulanate (Augmentin) followed by clindamycin (Cleocin). Cat bites are also treated with an antibiotic. First-line medication is amoxicillin/clavulanate (Augmentin), followed by cefuroxime (Ceftin) or doxycycline (Vibramycin) (Gilbert et al., 2011).

focus on safety

Animal bite

Animal bites are a reportable injury. Contact the local health department to obtain the appropriate paperwork. The nurse will need to know the type of animal, owner of animal if known, date and time of the bite, where the bite was treated, and what the treatment entailed (e.g., sutures or tetanus vaccination) as well as contact information for the child or guardian.

HUMAN BITES

Human bites can be quite common and usually occur in toddlers and young children. Human bites carry a higher risk for infection than do animal bites. Further, human bites may carry blood-borne diseases such as hepatitis B or C and HIV. Specifically, children with bites on the hand are at risk for osteomyelitis and septic arthritis.

Signs and Symptoms

Signs and symptoms of human bites include:

- Teeth marks without penetration
- Cutting or piercing of the skin
- Bruising, swelling, or tenderness
- Erythema, pain, or fever

Hand bites are at risk for osteomyelitis and septic arthritis, and all open skin bites are prone to infection.

Diagnosis

Diagnosis of a human bite is based on patient history and physical findings.

Prevention

Monitoring young children in tandem play is important to protect them from injuring each other or themselves.

Children who cannot express their feelings with words are more likely to strike out or bite. Parenting techniques such as time out, behavior modification, and positive reinforcement for good behavior may prevent future biting, but a swift intervention at the time of a bite will help a child of any age understand that the behavior is undesirable.

Collaborative Care

Nursing Care. The nurse must take an accurate history about the incident and gather information about the exact injury. After the bite, if the skin is broken, the nurse communicates to the family that both the biter and the bitten are at risk for blood-borne diseases. Both children need to be tested according to blood-borne pathogen exposure precautions.

The nurse irrigates the wound with Ringer's solution or with soapy water. Vigorously scrubbing the wound is not recommended. After irrigation, a topical antibiotic is gently applied to the area. The wound is then dressed, and the extremity is elevated. The area must be monitored daily for infection. If any infection is noted, the primary health-care practitioner must be notified. The child's immunization record needs to be evaluated by the nurse for status of tetanus coverage. The child can be cared for at home, alerting the parents to signs and symptoms of infection and proper wound care.

Medical Care. Amoxicillin/clavulanate (Augmentin) is the first-line antibiotic in the treatment of a human bite. If there is a penicillin allergy, a combination of clindamycin and ciprofloxacin (Cipro) or TMP-SMX (sulfamethoxazole/trimethoprim) (Bactrim) is warranted (Gilbert et al., 2011).

Education/Discharge Instructions

The nurse teaches the parent how to clean and dress the wound and monitor for potential infection: redness, swelling, streaking, and fever. Instructions on oral antibiotics are reinforced, if prescribed. Parents are reminded when to return to the health-care provider for a follow-up appointment

Diseases From Bites

LYME DISEASE

Lyme disease was named for the town of Lyme, Connecticut, in 1975 when there was a cluster of children with new onset juvenile rheumatoid arthritis that had previously suffered tick bites. Lyme disease is a tick-borne infection with multiple system involvement. It is an inflammatory response to the spirochete *Borrelia burgdorferi* and is the most common vector-borne disease in the United States. In 2010, there were 42 states affected, and yet 80% of the Lyme disease cases occurred in the Northeastern, Mid-Atlantic, and North Central states (CDC, 2012a).

✿ *Nursing Insight*—*Exposure to Lyme disease*

Exposure to Lyme disease can occur in any outdoor setting where ticks are endemic. The tick bite is often found on the head and neck, back, arms, and legs. Animals such as dogs and cats can also have the disease. Lyme disease occurs year round, with the highest incidence of infection in the summer. Children between 5 and 14 years of age are at highest risk because of outdoor

activities. Infection does not induce immunity. It takes 48 hours after contact with a human to introduce the spirochete into the feeding site where the tick has buried its head. Any rash that appears before 48 hours is an allergic reaction or infection, not Lyme disease. The infection is not contagious from person to person.

Signs and Symptoms

Lyme disease presents in three stages:

Early localized disease (3–30 days after bite)

- Red macule at the bite site
- Bulls-eye rash with a central macule and surrounding clear area, then an expanding rash (5–50 cm in circumference) (Venes, 2013)
- Possible systemic symptoms
  - Fatigue, headache, arthralgia (joint pain), neck pain, fever, and myalgia (muscle pain) (listed in order of prevalence)

Early disseminated disease (2 weeks after bite until chronic symptoms develop)

- Expands as a red, roundish, flat, non-pruritic, and non-vesicular (erythema migrans) rash; this is the most common manifestation of this stage
- Fatigue, headache, arthralgia (joint pain), and fever become more common
- Possible cranial nerve palsy, especially facial nerve palsy (bilateral facial nerve palsy is pathognomonic for Lyme [characteristic for specific disease])
- Meningitis (1% of affected children)
- Carditis (less than 1% of affected children)
- 90% will have positive serological conversion in this stage

Late disease (weeks to months after the initial bite)

- Arthritis, lasting up to many years but not considered chronic
  - Singular joint at a time, migrates from joint to joint, typically larger joints and primarily the knee(s)
  - Swollen and tender, rarely erythematous
  - Can bear weight but is uncomfortable (Shapiro, 2012)

Diagnosis

Diagnosis is determined by physical and history; incidence of tick bite may or may not be reported. Labs can confirm Lyme disease. Lab testing is not appropriate in the child who presents with erythema migrans and lives in or has just visited an area where Lyme disease is endemic. That child should be treated presumptively for Lyme disease.

⚙ Labs: Immunoassay

Lab testing is performed to determine if Lyme disease is present. The enzyme-linked immunosorbent assay (ELISA) is performed with follow-up of positive results with the Western blot for confirmation (Vermeulen, Verbakel, Notermans, Reimerink, & Peeters, 2010). The ELISA method may provide a false-positive result because of cross-reactive antibodies to other spirochetal infections. Seroconversion takes at least 6 weeks in Lyme disease, so the child is treated symptomatically while waiting for lab confirmation. The child will have specific IgM antibodies that will appear first at 3 to 4 weeks, peak at 6 to 8 weeks, and then decline. The IgG antibodies appear at 6 to 8 weeks.

Prevention

Avoiding play in wooded areas or using precautions in such environments will decrease the incidence of Lyme disease. Children can dress in long sleeves and long pants when in wooded areas; DEET spray is used when age-appropriate. At the end of the day of play (preferably within 2 hours), a shower or bath can be taken, followed by a tick check from scalp to toes. Clothing and other worn items are put in the clothes washer to avoid live ticks from roaming into the home. Pets can be combed and have tick collars or skin treatments as an added protection.

Collaborative Care

Nursing Care. During the history and physical, the nurse asks the family member if there has been an occurrence of a tick bite.

Medical Care. A 2-week course of oral antibiotics is given if infection is suspected. Amoxicillin (Amoxil) or cefuroxime (Ceftin) are the most often used antibiotics in children 8 years of age or younger. Doxycycline (Vibramycin) or tetracycline (Sumycin) is given to children older than the age of 8 years (Gilbert et al., 2011). If recurrent arthritis, central nervous system complications, or carditis occurs, treatment lasts for 4 weeks with IV ceftriaxone (Rocephin), cefotaxime (Claforan), or penicillin G (Bicillin L-A). With early detection and treatment, the prognosis is good; however, relapse can occur (Gilbert et al., 2011).

Education/Discharge Instructions

Teaching methods of tick bite prevention is invaluable. If the child is treated for Lyme disease whether presumptively or because of positive lab tests, the nurse reinforces the proper use of antibiotics, including compliance. Furthermore, the nurse reminds the family of follow-up appointments with the health-care provider.

ROCKY MOUNTAIN SPOTTED FEVER

Rocky Mountain spotted fever (RMSF) is a multisystem disease that can be mild, moderate, or severe. The onset can be either gradual or sudden. The greatest risk of mortality is to the child under the age of 4 or who presents late in the illness or without the characteristic rash (CDC, 2011b). Some ticks, the American dog tick and the Rocky Mountain wood tick, harbor the organism *Rickettsia rickettsii* that can be transmitted to the human host after a tick bite.

 Nursing Insight—*Rocky Mountain Spotted Fever*

Rocky Mountain Spotted Fever (RMSF) is one of the spotted fever rickettsioses with the highest incidence in the contiguous states of North Carolina, Oklahoma, Arkansas, Tennessee, and Missouri (CDC, 2011b). The peak season is June and July; however, that season is delayed in the state of Arizona to August and September (CDC, 2011b). The death rate overall for RMSF is 23% if untreated and less than 5% if treatment ensues early in the disease process (CDC, 2011b). The peak pediatric age for RMSF is 5 to 9 years of age; however, the majority of those affected are in their fifth decade. Those most at risk are males, Native Americans, and persons living in wooded areas (CDC, 2011b). The incubation period lasts 2 to 14 days after the bite of an infected tick; however, the majority of persons will be symptomatic on days 5 to 7.

Signs and Symptoms

Signs and symptoms of RMSF include:

- At onset, fever, headache (severe), malaise, myalgias (muscle pain), arthralgia (joint pain), and nausea with or without vomiting
- Severe abdominal pain that mimics appendicitis pain (greater than 60% of children)
- Edema
- Rash
  - Develops between days 3 and 5 of the disease (10% to 20% of patients will not have a rash)
  - Begins on the wrists and ankles and spreads centrally and out to the palms and soles
  - Macular/papular but may become petechial
  - No urticaria (hives)
  - Non-pruritic
  - Difficult to visualize in darker-skinned individuals (Sexton, 2011)

Diagnosis

Diagnosis of RMSF is based on the classic triad of presenting symptoms, which include rash, fever, and history of a tick bite. Often symptoms are vague and particularly difficult to diagnose if the child or parents do not recall a tick bite. The nurse asks questions about the child's history: outdoor play, playing with animals, history of a singular macule/papule that may have been the original tick bite site. A nonspecific rash with fever and a poor history will lead to laboratory testing.

Prevention

Instruct children to avoid playing in wooded areas. Using precautions in such environments will decrease the incidence of this condition; children can dress in long sleeves and long pants when in wooded areas. DEET spray is used when age-appropriate. At the end of the day of play (preferably within 2 hours) a shower or bath is taken, followed by a tick check from scalp to toes. Clothing and other worn items are placed in the clothes washer before placing in the dirty clothes to avoid live ticks from roaming into the home. Pets are combed and have tick prevention collars or treatments for added protection.

Collaborative Care

Nursing Care. The nurse communicates to the family that treatment is begun based on clinical symptoms and epidemiology. Teaching about the medication regimen will

 Labs: Complete Blood Count and Comprehensive Metabolic Panel

The nurse can expect a positive immunofluorescence assay (IFA) and elevations in white blood cell (WBC) count, thrombocytopenia (low platelets), and hyponatremia (a decreased concentration of sodium in the blood). This sodium imbalance is responsible for the edema seen in children. There may also be elevated liver enzymes (CDC, 2011b). The child's WBCs will likely remain low in the early stage and rise to slightly abnormal in later stages.

WBCs: 5,000 to 10,000/mm³. Later stage: 10,000 to 12,000/mm³
Platelets: 150,000 to 400,000/mm³. Thrombocytopenia less than 150,000/mm³
Na: 136 to 145 mEq/L. Hyponatremia 136 mEq/L
Bilirubin (total): 0.3 to 1.0 mg/dL. Hyperbilirubinemia 1.0 mg/dL

assist the family in adherence. Teaching about the typical course of the illness and expectations for return to wellness and full functioning will alleviate child and family fears (CDC, 2011b).

Medical Care. The first-line drug treatment for children over 45 kg is doxycycline (Vibramycin) dosed twice a day at 2.2 mg/kg/dose twice daily, up to 100 mg twice daily (Vallerand & Sanoski, 2014).

Chloramphenicol sodium succinate dosed at 50 mg/kg/day in 4 divided doses is indicated for smaller children and pregnant women (Vallerand & Sanoski, 2014). Supportive therapy for other symptoms resulting from RMSF may include antipyretics, anti-inflammatory medication, and IV fluids.

Education/Discharge Instructions

Time for recovery must be allowed after RMSF. Usually a child can return to school but time for rest must be allowed during and after the school day. The family may need to work with the school system to allow for limited hours in the school and work assigned for at home. Sports and other activities can be resumed as the child resumes normal activity levels. Monitoring the child's stamina even more closely is warranted if he or she was very ill and/or had prolonged hospitalization.

CAT SCRATCH DISEASE

Cat scratch disease (CSD) is a self-limiting illness lasting 6 to 12 weeks that begins with a scratch or bite from a cat (CDC, 2011a). Approximately 40% of domestic cats are reservoirs for the bacillus *Rochalimaea henselae*, which causes the disease response in humans (CDC, 2011a).

Signs and Symptoms

Signs and symptoms of CSD include:

- Tender **lymphadenopathy** (swollen lymph nodes) of the head, neck, and/or upper limbs
- General malaise and low-grade fever
- Headache
- Papule at site of original bite or scratch

Symptoms manifest 3 to 10 days after injury and take between 6 and 12 weeks to resolve (Nervi, Ressner, Drayton, & Kapila, 2011).

Diagnosis

A history of a cat scratch and the physical findings are used to diagnose CSD. If there is concern about a differential diagnosis, laboratory studies may be ordered.

Prevention

To prevent CSD parents can discourage rough play with cats and kittens. If a cat bite or scratch does occur, wash the wounds immediately in warm soapy water. Do not let the cat or child lick open wounds. Keep wounds covered if the child cannot protect the cuts from the animal.

Collaborative Care

Nursing Care. Communication to the family includes prevention techniques and the antibiotic regimen that has been prescribed. Other treatments and care are not typically indicated, but good hand hygiene and wound management is indicated.

Education/Discharge Instructions

Encourage the parents to monitor the scratch site for changes that might be indicative of worsening infection. Checking for increased redness, swelling, pain, and fever (temperature greater than 101.5°F [38.6°C]) warrants a return to the health-care provider.

Burns

The skin is an important organ system; the epidermal layer protects the body from infection, regulates body temperature, prevents fluid losses, helps with sensory function, manufactures vitamin D, and plays a role in body image determination. The dermal layer provides elasticity and durability to the skin. A burn injury interrupts each of these normal processes. Some children are at higher risk for burns because of their environment, their behavior, and their age. Burns are a result of either thermal, radiation, chemical, or electrical insult (Box 30-3).

CHILD DEVELOPMENT AND BURN INJURIES

Because, children develop in a predictable time frame, they are at risk for certain types of burn injuries at certain ages and developmental stages.

> *Infant growth* involves increasing gross motor and fine motor development. The infant is able to do things one day that he or she could not have done the day before. In addition, the infant is becoming mobile, which increases the risk for danger. Typically burn injuries seen in infants are:
> - A scald from reaching for items, like coffee, tea, or hot oil from deep fat fryers

---

Labs: Cat Scratch Disease

The health-care provider orders an IFA and ELISA for *R henselae* that has a sensitivity of 95% and specificity of 77% (Nervi et al. 2011). Rarely, a lymph node biopsy is warranted for confirmation of disease and to rule out cancers of the lymphatic system.

Box 30-3 Pediatric Burns Etiology and Incidence

- 450,000 Americans received treatment for burn injuries in 2008.
- 3,500 Americans died as a result of a burn injury in 2010.
- 3,000 of these deaths were a result of a residential fire.
- 75% of these deaths occur at the scene of the injury or during transport.
- 45,000 Americans were hospitalized with a burn injury in 2010, with about 55% receiving treatment in specialized burn centers. This percentage has steadily increased in recent years with growing recognition of the specialized care that these patients require.
- 94.8% of burn patients admitted to a burn center survive. 70% of burn victims are male with 30% female. 63% are Caucasian, 17% African American, 14% Hispanic, and 6% of other ethnicities (American Burn Association [ABA], 2011).
- "Scald burns from hot liquids account for 80% of all thermal injuries in children" (Green, 2010, p. 45).

- A scald from being placed in a bathtub, basin, or pan of water that was hotter than 120°F (48.9°C) (National Fire Protection Association [NFPA], 2011).
- A radiation burn from touching hot objects like a wood stove
- An electrical cord burn to the mouth from chewing on electrical cord that was plugged into the wall
- A flame and/or inhalation burn from a house fire

Toddler growth involves separating from the parents and finding independence. The infant freely explores the environment and observes parental behavior, copying it without knowing dangerous consequences. Typical burn injuries seen in toddlers are:

- A scald burn from pulling down hot items from tall surfaces
- A scald burn from attempting to turn on the bathtub faucet
- A flame burn from attempting to ignite a match or lighter
- A flame and/or an inhalation burn from a house fire
- A radiation burn from touching hot appliances like curling irons
- An electrical cord burn to the mouth from chewing an electrical cord that was plugged into the wall

"What to say"—*Communicating with the mother of a toddler*

The nurse is caring for Betsy, a toddler, who has a 40% scald burn that happened when her mother was cooking dinner. The toddler reached up and grabbed the handle of a boiling pot of water off the stove that subsequently spilled on her body. The toddler has deep partial-thickness and full-thickness burns to her scalp, face, neck, shoulder, arm, hand, chest, back, and feet. Betsy has dressings covering all of her wounds, which are beginning to swell. She is intubated and breathing on a ventilator. Today, when the mother enters her room, she immediately starts sobbing. What will the nurse say to the mother?

The nurse is open, honest, caring, and compassionate. Because the nurse does not know what Betsy's mother's first concern is today, good listening skills are of the utmost importance. Using therapeutic communication with open-ended questions is helpful when trying to communicate with the mother. The mother might say she is afraid that her child will die or might be fearful of how her child looks now and in the future. Once the mother opens up to the nurse, her questions and fears can be addressed. If the mother's main fear is if the child will survive, it is comforting for the mother to know that the nurse is with the child for the entire shift and that the child will be monitored frequently. If the mother's concern is about how her child looks now, the nurse can explain that the swelling that occurs during the first 48 hours is common and the nurse monitors frequently. It is also important to explain to the mother that the child's swelling will diminish after the first 48 hours. If the mother's fear is about the eventual scarring, then the nurse talks about the care of burns and possible reconstructive surgery in the future. In addition, referring the mother to a parent's burn support group is beneficial. Participation in a burn support group may help the mother discuss fears and concerns with other mothers and parents who have been in a similar situation.

Preschool child growth involves increased mobility and independence. The preschooler becomes inventive and uses magical thinking in daily activities. Typically burn injuries in preschoolers are:

- A scald burn may happen when running into the kitchen and getting in the way while a parent is cooking
- A radiation burn from touching hot appliances like a stove burner
- An electrical burn from playing with an electrical cord that had a frayed wire
- A radiation burn from touching hot appliances like a clothing iron
- A flame burn from trying to ignite a lighter or a match
- A flame and/or an inhalation burn from a house fire

School-age children's and adolescents' growth involve more freedom and access to adult items. These youth may use their independence to cook, light candles, and investigate situations without thinking about the danger. Typically burn injuries in school-aged children and adolescents are:

- A scald burn from cooking in the microwave, stove, or oven
- A flame burn from trying to ignite a lighter or a match
- A chemical burn from experimentation with chemical agents
- An electrical burn from climbing trees where electrical power lines of 14,000 volts or more are passing through the tree

---

⊗ focus on safety

Burn prevention

The nurse is instrumental in helping to prevent burn injuries in children of all ages. Prevention of burn injuries is included when discussing anticipatory guidance during the well-child visit. School nurses can teach burn prevention as part of health education during the National Burn Awareness Week (CDC, 2012b) in February and during the National Fire Prevention Week in October (NFPA, 2011).

Education for parents includes a discussion about smoke detectors that are installed in every sleeping room, outside each separate sleeping area, and on every level of the home, including the basement. For the best protection, the alarms should be interconnected, using wireless, battery-operated smoke detectors. Batteries on smoke detectors are checked on a monthly basis by pushing the test button, and batteries are changed at least once per year (NFPA, 2011). Water heaters are set no higher than 120°F (48.9°C) and should deliver shower or bath water at no higher than 100°F (37.8°C). Pot handles on the stove are turned in so they cannot be knocked or grabbed by curious children, and appliance cords are kept away from the edges of counters. Hot foods and liquids are also kept away from the edges of the table or countertops. Cigarettes, lighters, matches, and lit candles are kept out of reach of small children. For other burn prevention ideas, refer to the CDC, the American Burn Association (ABA), or the NFPA.

Across Care Settings: Burn centers

Burn centers treat both adults and children. Patients with burn injuries are referred to a verified burn center based on criteria for transfer from the American Burn Association (ABA, 2011) including the following:

- Partial-thickness burns of greater than 10% of the total body surface area
- Burns that involve the face, hands, feet, genitalia, perineum, or major joints
- Third-degree burns in any age group
- Electrical burns, including lightning injury
- Chemical burns
- Inhalation injury
- Burn injury in patients with preexisting medical disorders that could complicate management, prolong recovery, or affect mortality
- Any patients with burns and concomitant trauma (such as fractures) in which the burn injury poses the greatest risk of morbidity or mortality. In such cases, if the trauma poses the greater immediate risk, the patient's condition may be stabilized initially in a trauma center before transfer to a burn center. Physician judgment will be necessary in such situations and should be in concert with the regional medical control plan and triage protocols.
- Burned children in hospitals without qualified personnel or equipment for the care of children
- Burn injury in patients who will require special social, emotional, or rehabilitative intervention

BURN SEVERITY

Three factors—type of burn, depth of burn, and size and extent of the burn—determine the burn severity.

TYPE OF BURN

There are four major types of burn injury: **thermal, radiation, chemical,** and **electrical.** The classifications are described below.

- **Thermal burns** are the most common type of burn in childhood and occur as a result of contact with a flame, flash, or scald.
  - **Flame burns** occur from the ignition of combustible materials and contact with fire, fireworks, candles, and campfires.
  - **Flash burns** are caused by explosions, especially with combustible fuels like gasoline, kerosene, charcoal lighter, and fireworks or hairspray.
  - **Scald burns** occur when hot liquid is spilled on a child (e.g., oil, grease, coffee, hot tea, or soup) or from hot tap water in sinks and bathtubs or from steam.
  - **Contact burns** are caused by exposure to a hot object like an oven, hot iron, radiator, hot light bulb, or other heating device.
- **Radiation burns** occur when the skin of the child comes in contact with radiofrequency or ionizing agents. The most common radiation burn injury is sunburn. However, cancer patients undergoing radiation therapy can also suffer a radiation burn. Another form of radiation burn is exposure to radioactive material as with the nuclear plant meltdown.
- **Chemical burns** occur when the skin comes in contact with a chemical agent that is corrosive to the skin. Acids like sulfuric acid and muriatic acid are caustic to the skin. Alkaline agents like lye, lime, ammonia, and household cleaning agents are also caustic to the skin and cause injury.
- **Electrical burns** occur when electricity passes through or around the body as it seeks the fastest path of least resistance to the ground. Household current of 110 volts can cause a full-thickness burn injury to the corner of the mouth. Electrical lines that carry electricity throughout towns and cities typically carry 14,800 volts. High-tension wires can carry as much as 150,000 volts. Lightning can have between 10 and 100 million volts.

Nursing Insight—*Neck burn*

Best practice for prevention of neck burn scars state that a delay in splinting may result in earlier and more frequent surgeries for reconstruction (Healey & Katsu, 2010). During the recovery phase, hyperextension of the neck is required until the wound is healed. Positioning of the child with a neck burn begins during the resuscitative phase when the child is placed in the bed without a pillow (Healey & Katsu, 2010). To achieve neck extension, a foam roll or pillow is placed under the shoulders, a double-mattress where the head is extended over the top mattress, or wedges under the shoulders are placed.

DEPTH OF BURN

Depth of burn injury is another factor that is assessed (Fig. 30-11). Depth of injury used to be classified by degree (first, second, third, and fourth). These terms are no longer used in burn care. Burn depth is classified as:

- **Superficial Thickness:** presents with erythema (reddened) and pain for 2 to 3 days (e.g., a sunburn). These burns involve an intact epidermis without blisters. Because the skin is essentially intact, all functions of the skin remain intact. Several days following the burn injury, the outer layer of the epidermis sloughs off (peels). This depth of burn usually heals within 4 days without any scarring (Green, 2010).
- **Superficial Partial Thickness:** presents with erythema and blister formation. The blisters may burst and weep. It generally has a moist appearance to it. It bleeds easily and is very painful. The heat of the burn injury has damaged the epidermis and the outer portion of the dermis. Most of the time, these burns heal spontaneously within 3 weeks. Scarring will occur in these types of burns and take longer than 2 weeks to heal (Green, 2010).
- **Deep Partial Thickness:** presents with a white or pale color to the injured tissue. There are generally huge blisters, which burst, and the pale dermis is visible. This type of burn is extremely painful. If it does not become infected, it will heal within 3 to 9 weeks. Scarring will occur with this type of burn because it will take longer than 2 weeks to heal. Sometimes excision and grafting are performed to aid the healing process and diminish the severity of scarring (Green, 2010).
- **Full Thickness:** destroys the epidermis and dermis, and eschar is visible. A deep full-thickness burn may also damage the nerves, bones, and muscles.

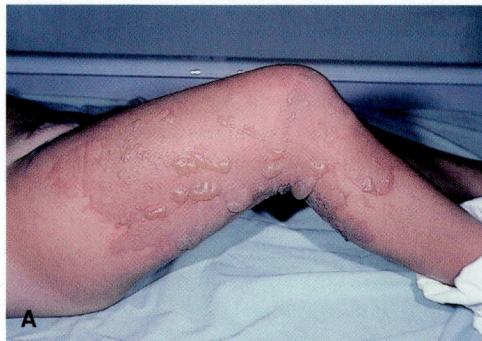
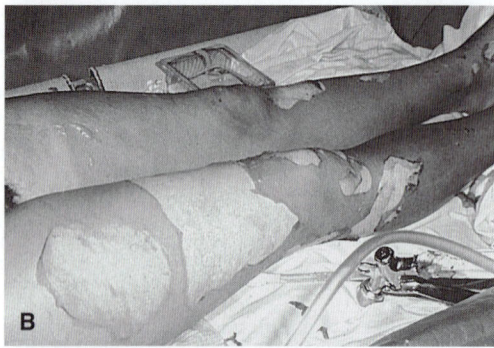
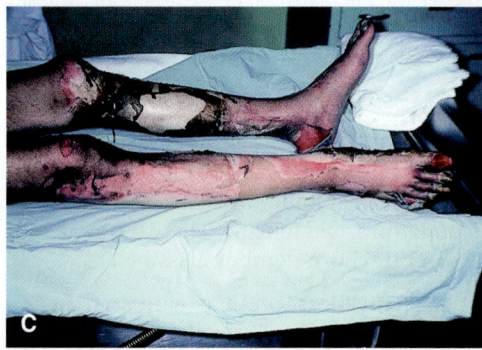

Figure 30-11 Classification of burns. *A*, Partial thickness (superficial). *B*, Partial thickness (deep). *C*, Full thickness.

SIZE OR EXTENT OF A BURN

The third factor that is used to determine the severity of a burn is the size or extent of the burn. The size of the burn is determined using a chart that calculates the **Total Burn Surface Area** (**TBSA**) (percentage of body surface area that has been affected by a burn injury). The **Rule of Nines** (Figure 30-12*A*) chart is used for adolescents. It uses one set of numbers for calculating the percentage for each body part. It is not recommended in infants and growing children. The **Lund and Browder Chart** (Figure 30-12*B*) is used in pediatric burn care. It allows for the estimation of TBSA, size and percent of burn injury that takes growth and development into account (Saffle & the Evidence-Based Guidelines Group, American Burn Association [ABA], 2001). A study by Sheridan et al. (1995) determined that the palm of a human hand is 0.5% of body surface area (Saffle & the Evidence-Based Guidelines Group, ABA, 2001) (Figure 30-12*C*).

PHASES OF A BURN

A burn also has three phases; the *first phase* is the **Burn Shock/Resuscitative Phase**. This phase is during the first

24 to 48 hours of the injury (Saffle & the Evidence-Based Guidelines Group, ABA, 2001). This phase is characterized by shock. The *second phase* of the burn injury is the **Recovery or Wound Healing Phase**. The major goal is to close the wound as quickly as possible. There is about a 2-week time period to remove the burned tissue and heal the wounds before infection becomes a problem. The *third phase* of the burn injury is the **Rehabilitation Phase**. The goals of this phase are to prevent scar contractures of the healed skin or skin grafts, aid scar maturation, and enable the child to reenter his or her social environment. The rehabilitation plan is initiated on admission and based on initial and ongoing assessments including:

- Depth of the burn and potential for prolonged healing of more than 10 days
- Location of the burn, anterior versus posterior
- Circumferential burn

Burn Care

A physician (burn surgeon, pediatrician, and reconstructive plastic surgeon), nurse or nurse practitioner, case manager, physical therapist, occupational therapist, social worker, psychologist or psychiatrist, and child life therapist all have significant roles in helping children heal the burn wounds. A child who has suffered a burn injury of greater than 30% needs specialized nursing care in an intensive care unit. Children with minor burns are cared for in a clinic or outpatient setting.

 Collaboration in Caring—*A team approach*

The care of a burned child requires interactions with the interprofessional team. During hospitalization, the nurse provides essential nursing care and acts as the advocate for the child and family. The nurse also coordinates care of other health-care professionals such as a physical therapist who helps the child maintain or regain physical function. An occupational therapist helps the child adapt to activities of daily living and also makes splints for treatment. A dietitian plans appropriate nutrition for immediate and long-term nutritional needs. As the child becomes more able to return to activities including school, the case manager, social worker or nurse, helps bridge any information gap between agencies. Long-term therapy, with rehospitalization and scar revisions, is another reason for an integrative team approach in which health-care professionals provide optimal care for the entire family.

Optimizing Outcomes—Best outcomes of burn care

The best outcome for a burned child is to include holistic nursing interventions from the following categories:

- Burn assessment
- Fluid resuscitation
- Prevention of infection
- Prevention of sepsis
- Prevention of pneumonia
- Pain management
- Maintaining circulation

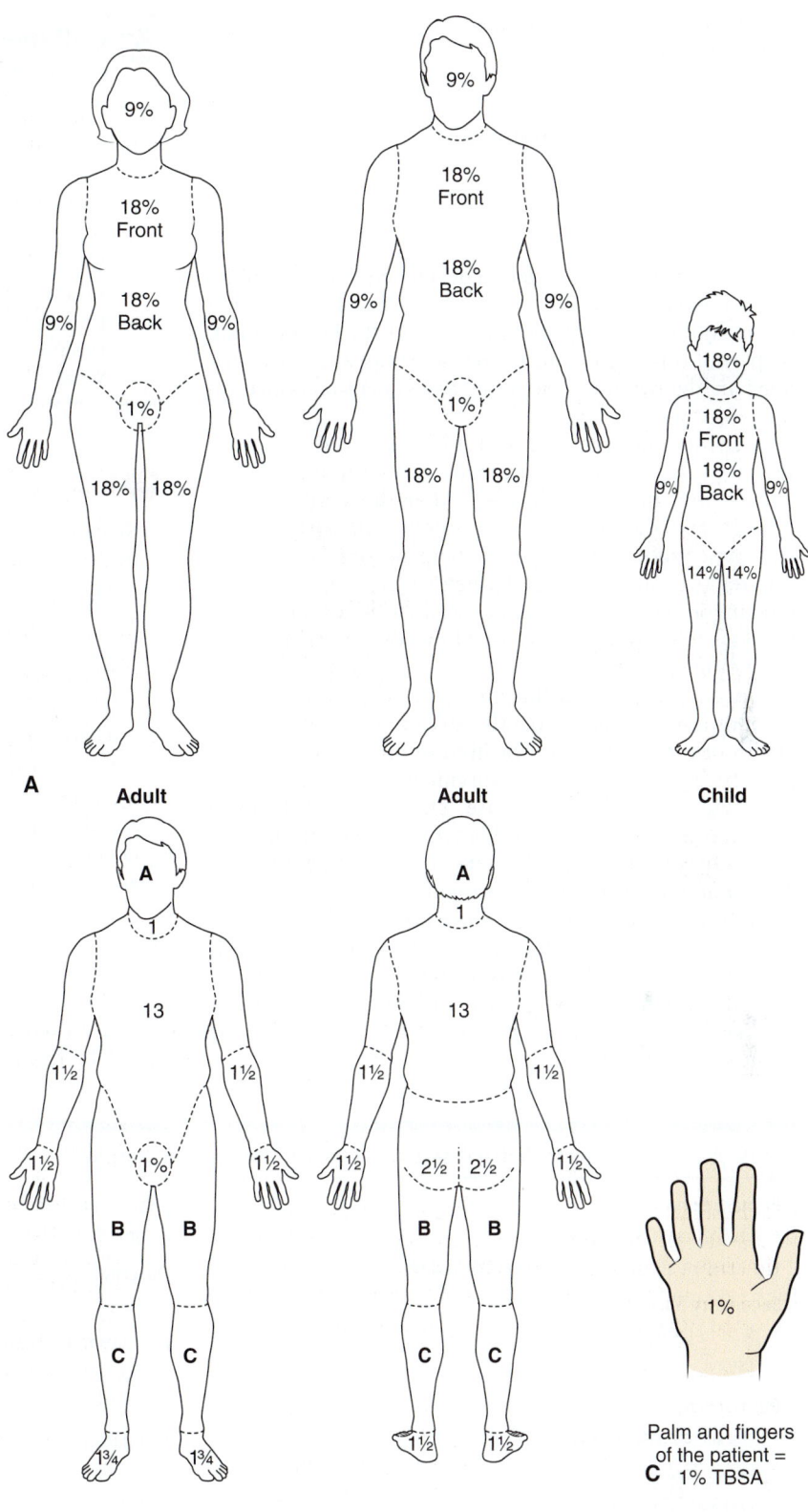

Figure 30-12 *A,* Rule of nines. *B,* Lund and Browder chart. *C,* Hand method.

	Age					
Area	**0**	**1**	**5**	**10**	**15**	**Adult**
A	9.50	8.50	6.50	5.50	4.50	3.50
B	2.75	3.25	4.00	4.50	4.50	4.75
C	2.50	2.50	2.75	3.00	2.50	3.50

- Promotion of good nutrition
- Pruritus management
- Psychological issues
- The rehabilitation phase
- Education/discharge instructions

BURN ASSESSMENT

The American Burn Association developed Practice Guidelines for Burn Care in 2001. This comprehensive document reviewed the literature about the care of the burn patient. As part of this document, the participating authors developed an algorithm for the initial assessment of a burn injury (Box 30-4).

Assessment of the burn history is vital. The initial assessment includes emergency care related to circulation, airway, and breathing (CABs). After the CABs are addressed and the child is being safely transported to an emergency room, the nurse or emergency medical technician removes all clothing and jewelry to decrease continued burning at any site. The child needs to be covered with blankets to keep warm because of the loss of heat through the wounds.

Once the child is in the emergency department, burn wounds are assessed for depth, surface area, and severity. Depth of the wounds is measured in millimeters or centimeters. Circumference measurements are also necessary to provide a full clinical picture. The surface of the burn wound is assessed for color, blanching, desiccation (dryness), turgor/elasticity, blisters, or sloughed blisters. TBSA and all other skin assessments are taken into consideration to help classify the burn. For some burn assessments, wounds are photographed with a camera that has a measurement-graphing lens. If the burn injuries are severe and encompass large areas of TBSA, some burn or emergency departments use video charting to record the clinical assessment.

 Collaboration in Caring—*Gathering important information*

The emergency health-care professionals will ask these questions to gather important information about the burn injury:

- "What caused the burn?"
- "When did this burn occur?"
- "Who was present or witnessed the injury?"
- "What first aid was given?"
- "How did the burn feel when it first occurred?"
- "How does the burn feel now?"
- "Has the child had any accidents or injuries before?"
- "What other medical history does this child have?"

 legal alert—Possible abuse or neglect

Remember to assess the burn injury for the possibility of neglect or physical abuse. Be alert for the following:

- The burn injury does not fit the story of what occurred.
- The developmental stage of the child does not fit the burn injury.
- The parent or guardian tells different versions of the injury to different members of the health-care team.
- There was a delay in seeking treatment.

It is extremely important to document the nursing assessment and the parents' account of the burn. Use quotations and document who made the statement. It is important to document the date and time of the injury as well as the date and time of the initial access to the health-care facility.

FLUID RESUSCITATION

Children with about 10% of TBSA burn will likely require IV fluid resuscitation. Children who suffer burns

---

Box 30-4 **Algorithm for Initial Assessment of a Burn Injury in the Hospital**

Primary Survey
- Airway, breathing, circulation
- Intubation, ventilation, vascular access, fluid resuscitation

Secondary Survey
- Head-to-toe examination
- History

Burn Specific
- Stop the burning process

Estimate Size of Burn
- Lund & Browder Chat
- Palm = 0.5% TBSA

Estimate Depth of Burn
- Examination of wounds
- Estimation of full thickness, deep partial thickness, superficial partial thickness

Begin Fluid Resuscitation
- Calculate total volume of fluids
- Administer per the protocol that was used

Determine Presence of Inhalation Injury
- Intubate if inflation injury is present

Determine Presence of Circumferential Burn
- Escharotomy to be performed, if present

Evaluation of Anatonie Area
- Face, hands, genitalia
- Provide treatment

Evaluation for Special Injuries
- Electrical, abrasive, drugs, cold, chemical
- Provide treatment

Determine Whether Injury Is Abusive or Neglectful
- Notify proper authorities

Treat Wounds
- Surgical debridement & dressing changes
- Hydrotherapy & dressing changes

Source: Adapted from Gibran (2006) in the American Burn Association Practice Guidelines for Burn Care published in the *Journal of Burn Care & Research.*

greater than 15% TBSA are at risk for developing hypovolemic and cellular shock. Children require more fluid per kilogram than adults and average 5.8 mL/kg/% burn of fluid resuscitation. The Parkland formula recommends 4 mL/kg/% burn/day and is acceptable for burn injury of 14% TBSA and less (Box 30-5). Whether the Parkland formula or the increased fluid formula of 5.8 mL/kg/% TBSA, the formula is administered in the same way. The first 50% of the formula is administered at the time of the burn in the first 8 hours. The remaining 50% is administered over the next 16 hours. In all cases, the formula that is used is a guideline. The child's urine output determines how well he or she is tolerating resuscitation; 0.5 to 1 mL/kg/hr of urine output is the goal during the resuscitative phase (Blumetti, Hunt, Arnoldo, Parks, & Purdue, 2008).

PREVENTION OF INFECTION

Prevention of infection for a child with a burn is critical in achieving wound closure. Burn wound infections originate from the patient because of the bacteria that is already found on the patient's body or as a nosocomial infection transmitted by others. Burn wound infections can be a serious complication that increases morbidity and mortality in the burned child. In fact, "75% of burn mortality is a result of infection, rather than burn shock or hypovolemia" (Rafla & Tredget, 2011, p. 6). Factors that have an influence in the morbidity and mortality of a child with a burn wound infection or sepsis are major burn injuries (typically greater than 30% TBSA), a significant full-thickness injury, prolonged open wounds, and delayed initial burn care (Rafla & Tredget, 2011).

Dressing change to wounds is performed once or twice daily. Maintaining aseptic technique during the dressing changes is essential. With patients who have burn injuries greater than 80%, two nurses perform the dressing change. Dressing changes to the face of an intubated child always requires two nurses. During the dressing change, if there is a break in sterile technique, the nurse informs the other nurse of the break and re-gloves to maintain asepsis. If there are signs of infection, the frequency of the dressing changes or the topical agent are adjusted by the health-care provider. When the dressing change is complete, the physical therapist performs range of motion exercises and applies splints. Wound cultures are also done once or twice per week to monitor for infection as well as monitor the type of bacteria that may be growing on the skin.

 Nursing Insight—*Infection control surveillance*

Infection control surveillance has led to systematic collection of data to monitor infection rates, trend data, and evaluate the current treatment methods. Infection control protocols include surveillance cultures from the patient, cohort patient care teams, strict enforcement of patient and health-care professional hygiene, hand sanitizer units, patient isolation, and monitoring antibiotic use as well as the antibiotic resistance/susceptibility patterns (Rafla & Tredget, 2011).

Prevention of wound infection requires assessment of the wound with each dressing change, looking for changes in wound color, character, odor, and amount of wound drainage. Factors that help prevent morbidity and mortality are early wound closure, topical antibiotics, prophylactic antibiotics, and advances in infection control (Rafla & Tredget, 2011). Strict aseptic technique is essential during a dressing change. A débriding dressing is chosen if necrotic tissue is seen during the dressing change. A protective, moist dressing is preferable if the wound is clean. Treatment of a wound infection may involve changing the topical agent or the frequency of the dressing changes. Different topical agents with benefits and risks and different wound closure techniques are listed in Box 30-6 and Box 30-7.

Nursing Insight—*Early burn excision and grafting*

A method for removal of burned tissue is to use **Early Burn Excision and Grafting** (a method of burn wound treatment that involves surgical excision and grafting with a split-thickness skin graft) (Greenwood, Kavanagh, & Mackie, 2010). Protocols have been developed at burn centers regarding excision and grafting of burns. The excision of the burn and application of a **split-thickness skin graft** (STSG) (surgically made skin graft that includes the epidermis and part of the dermis) are done under anesthesia in the operating room. The area of treatment is surgically debrided and the skin graft is harvested from an unburned area of the child's body. The STSG is prepared and then put into place over the wound to be treated. It is held in place with dissolvable sutures. The primary dressing is left untouched for about 7 days. Then, the primary dressing is removed and assessment made as to the **Graft Take** (percentage of the STSG that has healed and the wound is closed). If excision and grafting is not needed, topical antibiotics are used to protect the damaged skin from infection.

Box 30-5 **The Parkland Formula**

4 mL of IVF × weight in kg × %TBSA
   Give ½ of the total IVF volume over the 1st 8 hours.
   Give the second ½ at an even rate over the next 16 hours.
   Example: A child weighing 110 lb (50 kg) with a 20% TBSA burn requires:
   4 mL × 50 kg × 20% TBSA 4,000 mL
   1st 8 hours IVF 2,000/8 hours 250 mL/hr
   next 16 hours IVF 2,000/16 hours 125 mL/hr

Source: Kliegman, R. M., Stanton, B. M. D., St. Geme, J., Schor, N., Behrman, R. E. (2008). *Nelson's textbook of pediatrics* (19th ed.). Philadelphia, PA; Elsevier.

 Where Research and Practice Meet:
Burn Dressing

One of the newer dressing materials, Aquacel- Ag, was compared with petrolatum gauze in partial-thickness burns in a pediatric burn center. The results of this study demonstrated that Aquacel- Ag was safe and effective for the treatment of partial-thickness burns (Saba, Tsai, & Glat, 2009).

Box 30-6 Topical Agents to Treat Burns

Topical Agent	Benefits	Risks or Cautions
Silver Nitrate (0.5% AgNO$_3$	• Introduced in 1965 • Causes electrolyte abnormalities • Can be used on new split-thickness skin grafts without damaging the graft	• Induced electrolyte abnormalities • Staining of unburned skin and nails • Does not penetrate eschar • Cannot be used on the face • Applied as a wet dressing • Dressings must be dampened with AgNO$_3$ every 2 hours (Fuller, 2009)

Silver Sulfadiazine (AgSD)	• Introduced in 1968
	• Penetrates eschar more than AgNO$_3$
	• Does not cause electrolyte abnormalities
	• Can use on facial burns
		• Will destroy new split-thickness skin grafts
		• Contraindicated with
		  • Allergy to Sulfa
		  • G6PD
		  • Methemoglobinemia
		  • Formation of immune complexes
		• Adheres to exudate from partial-thickness burns to form a pseudoeschar, so must be cleansed during dressing changes (Fuller, 2009)

Sulfamylon (mafenide acetate)	• Will penetrate eschar the most • Used on burns to the ear to protect the cartilage	• Can be painful with application • Will destroy new split-thickness skin grafts
Acticoat™	• Antimicrobial, nanocrystallizing film of pure silver • Nonadherent • Nonabrasive • Sustained release of ionic silver • Effective against more than 150 pathogens • Can be used on split-thickness skin grafts, débrided burns, and donor sites • Held in place with sterile water-soaked gauze or dry gauze	• Cannot use sterile normal saline because it will cause precipitation of the salt out of the dressing • Cannot use with any topical antimicrobials (Ülkür, Oncul, Karagoz, Yeniz, & Celikoz, 2005)

Box 30-7 Skin Replacement Therapies

Type of Skin Replacement	Name of Product	Benefits	Risks
Temporary	Biobrane™	• Semipermeable temporary skin substitute • Nylon fabric with outer silicone film that is saturated with porcine collagen • Small holes that allow for drainage of exudates • Allows permeability for topical antibiotics • Indicated for partial-thickness burns • Can be used on excised wound beds with or without meshed autografts • Can be used on donor sites	• Can result in adherence to the wound and possibly needing debridement to remove (Shores, Gabriel & Gupta, 2007)

Temporary	Allografts	• Donated cadaver skin
		• Stored in a skin bank
		• Used as a temporary graft until autografting is possible
		• Contains epidermis and dermis
		• Aids in revascularization
			• Potential of disease transmission
			  • Now tested for HIV and Hepatitis B
			  • No tests for Hepatitis C
			• Difficulty in storing
			• Difficulty in obtaining (Shores et al., 2007)

Temporary	Transcyte (Dermagraft-TC)	• Human fibroblast-derived made of silicone • Has a polymer membrane and neonatal human fibroblast cells • Provides a transparent epidermis • Secretes human dermal collagen, matrix proteins, and growth factors	(Smith and Nephew Acticoat™ Antimicrobial Barrier Dressing Silcryst, 2014).

Box 30-7 Skin Replacement Therapies (continued)

Type of Skin Replacement	Name of Product	Benefits	Risks
Temporary	Xenograft	• Can be used on superficial partial-thickness and deep partial-thickness wounds • Can be used as a temporary barrier before grafting • Non-human, pig skin • Used on full-thickness injuries as a temporary covering • Can be used in partial-thickness burns • Available since 1965	• Potential for disease transmission • Doesn't always re-vascularize the wound (Shores et al., 2007)

Temporary to Permanent	Integra™	• Dermal matrix replacement
		• Two layers
		  • Collagen-glycosaminoglycan that biodegrades
		  • Thin silicone outer layer that acts as a barrier
		  • Allows for a neodermis to grow through the matrix
		  • Helps to cover large areas prior to donor site being available
		  • Aids in the collagen redevelopment and produces less severe scarring
			• Requires a second procedure to apply a thin split-thickness skin graft or application of cultured epithelial cells
			(Shores et al., 2007)

Permanent	Epicel®— Cultured epithelial autografts	• Cultured autologous keratinocyte product • Used for deep partial-thickness and full-thickness burns • Grown from a tiny skin biopsy taken from that patient • Co-cultivation with irradiated murine (mouse) cells	• Contraindicated for patients with amikacin, vancomycin, and bovine product sensitivities • Takes up to 4 weeks to grow the cultures • Only replaces the epidermal layer, so strength and durability of the skin that the dermis provides is lacking (Genzyme Biosurgery, 2014)

Permanent	Autografting	• **Split-Thickness Autografts (STSG)**
		  • Contain epidermis and upper layers of dermis of child's own skin
		  • Usually used for initial wound closure
		  • Donor sites will regenerate and can be used multiple times
		  • Graft can be stretched from 1:2 through 1:6 using a mesh machine
		
		• **Full-Thickness Skin Grafts (FTSG)**
		  • Contain epidermis and all of dermis
		  • Usually used in reconstructive phase
			• Permanent skin replacement that provides dermal and epidermal layers
			• Risk of graft loss because of infection
			• Scarring will occur, but if meshed, the mesh pattern will be visible within the scar
			• Initially cannot feel "soft touch"
			• Requires moisturization
			• Requires a second donor site of a split-thickness skin graft to cover the full-thickness donor site
			• Great risk of graft failure secondary to infection
			(Shores et al., 2007)

PREVENTION OF SEPSIS

To prevent sepsis (an infection in the blood), an IV catheter is placed through unburned skin, and an occlusive dressing is placed over the catheter. In a child with a major burn injury, this may not be possible. In those cases, the catheter is placed through burned tissue, and frequent catheter changes are required. For a major burn, a nonocclusive povidone-iodine dressing is changed every 2 to 4 hours. If the infection is invasive, surgical excision and IV antibiotics may be required (Rafla & Tredget, 2011).

PREVENTION OF PNEUMONIA

Children who have suffered a significant inhalation injury are prone to pneumonia. Pneumonia is treated quickly with traditional methods such as systemic antibiotics, vigorous chest physiotherapy, deep breathing, coughing, suctioning, and frequent turning. A newer method to prevent and treat pneumonia includes the use of high-frequency ventilation. Permissive hypercapnia has also been used with success (Rafla & Tredgett, 2011). Severely burned children are intubated and ventilated. Respiratory status is monitored hourly, and coordination with respiratory therapy is essential because ventilator changes may need to be adjusted frequently. Frequent assessment of the child's respiratory status and hourly vital signs are performed.

PAIN MANAGEMENT

A central line may be inserted upon admission for pain control. Pain is a significant issue in the care of the child with a burn because wound debridement hurts. The nurse administers IV pain medication 20 to 30 minutes before a dressing change using IV narcotics such as morphine

focus on safety

Proper equipment needed

When a child is intubated, it is important to ensure that emergency intubation equipment is nearby. Resuscitation bag appropriate for the size of the child and suction equipment must be assembled at the bedside and ready to be used in case of an emergency. Several of the correct size of suction catheters should also be at the bedside. An endotracheal tube of the same size and one that is one size smaller are placed near the head of the bed, and the tube size needs to be documented in the medical record. When an intubated child is being transported, a resuscitation bag and suction equipment, including catheters and a cardiorespiratory monitor, must accompany the child.

sulfate (MS-Contin). Non-narcotic pain control methods are also important. Diversional activities such as music, television, and visualization have also been helpful methods that assist with pain control. Involving child life services during the dressing change can be beneficial. Children as young as 3 years of age can participate in the dressing change by having them remove the dressing with supervision from the nurse or child life therapist. By participating in the dressing change, the child is given control over this painful procedure and therefore may be able to handle the dressing change better.

Complementary Care: *Distraction*

The nurse uses distraction as a good technique when changing the dressings for a child with burns. The type of distraction used is based on age and developmental stage (e.g., singing, counting, watching television, focusing on pictures, talking about familiar events or places, playing games, or blowing pinwheels or bubbles). If the child is anxious or has severe pain, medication may be required before and during distraction. The nurse must remember to praise the child when the dressing change is complete, with the focus on all of the positive behaviors that the child displayed.

MAINTAINING CIRCULATION

Nursing interventions for burn care ensures that circulation to the injured extremity is assessed and maintained. Decompression of circulation pressure on the tissue includes a

Where Research and Practice Meet:
Multi Modal Distraction

Miller, Rodger, Kipping, and Kimble (2011) conducted a study about children with burns who were treated in an outpatient department. The researchers compared Standard Distraction (SD) techniques to Multi Modal Distraction (MMD) techniques. The children in the SD group received standard pre-procedure care and had access to the toys in the waiting room. These children were administered non-narcotic medication to assist them with pain control. The children in the MMD group were introduced to a customized handheld MMD device that was interactive with the child through movement, touch screen, and multisensory feedback. The content on the device contained subject matter that helped the child prepare for a procedure as well as divisional technologies that the child could access during the procedure. The results of this study showed that the MMD group had a significant (p<0.001) reduction in pain intensity during a procedure.

fasciotomy and assessment of the muscle compartments. Compartment pressures are measured; pressures greater than 30 mm Hg in the tissue or pressures that are greater than 10 to 20 mm Hg of the diastolic pressure indicate increased compartment pressure and require emergency surgery. In many cases, muscle damage is so severe that the extremity cannot be saved resulting in amputation of the extremity. Entry and exit sites are the most common sites for severe circulation impairment and eventual amputation. Traditional pre- and postoperative nursing care measures are employed.

Nursing Insight—*Eschar and escharotomy*

Eschar has a waxy, white, gray, black, bright red, dry, and leathery appearance. There is a lack of pain while the eschar is intact and a prolonged capillary refill time. If the capillary refill time is impaired or the injury is **circumferential** (perimeter of the wound), an **escharotomy** (a surgical incision through the necrotic skin) is performed within the first 24 to 48 hours. This surgery allows the eschar to expand and allows the underlying blood vessels, nerves, ligaments, tendons, and bones to receive oxygenation (Green, 2010). A skin graft is also performed; a full- or split-thickness grafting depends on wound condition, location, thickness, size, and aesthetic concerns.

Nursing Insight—*Fasciotomy*

A deep full-thickness burn that is circumferential may require a **fasciotomy** (a surgical incision through the fascia) performed within the first 24 to 48 hours after the burn (Venes, 2013). This surgery allows the underlying blood vessels, nerves, ligaments, tendons, and bones to receive oxygenation. In severe burns, an **amputation** (removal of a limb or body part, as a result of the burn injury and a lack of adequate circulation to the extremity or body part) may be performed (Green, 2010; Venes, 2013).

PROMOTION OF GOOD NUTRITION

Promotion of good nutrition is another major issue during burn recovery because a balanced diet is necessary for wound healing. Patients are weighed at least 2 times per week. According to Graves, Saffle, & Cochran (2009), the majority of burn centers in the United States provide a high-calorie, high-protein diet for those patients tolerating an oral diet. Patients not tolerating an oral diet receive total parenteral and enteral nutrition. Advancement to enteral feedings and eventually oral feedings happen as the child recovers and can tolerate the diet. As soon as the patient is able, he or she is encouraged to sit in a chair, get out of bed, and walk, which may stimulate her appetite.

Nursing Insight—*Curling's ulcer*

Burn patients are at risk for **Curling's ulcer** (a form of peptic ulcer that sometimes occurs following the stress of a severe burn). H_2 antagonists (ranitidine [Zantac]) or proton pump inhibitors (pantoprazole [Protonix], omeprazole [Prilosec], and lansoprazole [Prevacid]) are administered to help prevent this ulcer.

activities of daily living and sleep. The pruritus of a burn injury arises in the skin because of inflammation, dryness, or the burn damage (Goutos, Dziewulski, & Richardson, 2009). Therapeutic strategies that act on the peripheral aspects of pruritus include a cooling of the burn scar, antihistamines, topical doxepin (Sinequan), local anesthetics, laser treatment, compression garments, and ondansetron (Zofran). The application of cooling agents such as showering or bathing and topical emollients are used as a temporary relief in many burns. Antihistamine medications have been instrumental in the relief of pruritus (Box 30-8).

Topical doxepin (Sinequan) is a tricyclic medication with potent histamine receptor-blocking abilities. "It has been found to be 50 times more potent than hydroxyzine (Vistaril) and 800 more times potent than diphenhydramine (Benadryl)" (Goutos et al., 2009, p. 224). Local anesthetics such as lidocaine are used to diminish nerve impulses by blocking sodium channels on neuronal cell membranes. Colloidal oatmeal has been shown to reduce pruritus because it forms an occlusive barrier on the skin and maintains optimal levels of hydration in the skin. Compression garments have been used for scar maturation for many years. Compression therapy can also be an effective treatment for burn pruritus. The mechanism of this is not clear, but it may be associated with a reduction in inflammatory cells and a decrease in histamine release.

 Nursing Insight—Urinary output

Urine output is monitored hourly, looking for 0.5 to 1 mL/kg/hr during the resuscitative phase. Urine output is expected to increase to 1 to 2 mL/kg/hr during the second 48 to 72 hours after the burn injury. After that, urine output of 1 mL/kg/hr is the goal. Foley catheter care must be performed according to hospital policy and procedure.

 Nursing Insight—Laser treatment

Laser treatment was performed in one study that involved pediatric patients and adult patients. The length of pruritus was improved in patients (by 1 month) and remained improved in these patients again at 6 and 12 months (Goutos et al., 2009, p. 225).

PRURITUS MANAGEMENT

Pruritus management is a common issue in the rehabilitative phase of injury. It is debilitating and can interfere with

Psychological Issues

Psychological issues play a major role in all phases of burn injury. However, psychological issues are greater for the child in the rehabilitative phase of the burn injury. Burn

---

Box 30-8 Antihistamine Medications for Pruritus

Medication	Mechanism of Action and Side Effects
chlorpheniramine (Chlor-Trimeton)	• Used for relief of allergic symptoms from histamine release • Antagonizes effects of histamine at H_2-receptor sites • Does not inactivate histamine • Causes drowsiness, dizziness, and sometimes excitation in pediatric patients • Administer 4 mg every 4–6 hours every 8–12 hours, but not to exceed 24 mg/day in children over 12 years of age • Administer 2 mg 3–4 times daily, but not to exceed 12 mg/day in children aged 6–12 years • Oral doses should be taken with food or milk to decrease GI irritation • Chewable tablets should not be swallowed whole and should be chewed well before swallowing
diphenhydramine (Benadryl)	• Used for relief of allergic symptoms caused by histamine release • Antagonizes effects of histamine at H_1-receptor sites • Does not inactivate histamine • Causes drowsiness, dizziness, headache, and paradoxical excitation in pediatric patients • Administer 25–50 mg every 4–6 hours but not to exceed 300 mg/day in patients >12 years of age • Administer 12.5–25 mg every 4–6 hours but not to exceed 150 mg/day in children aged 6–12 years • Administer 6.25–12.5 mg every 4–6 hours but not to exceed 37.5 mg/day in children aged 2–6 years

Box 30-8 Antihistamine Medications for Pruritus (continued)

Medication	Mechanism of Action and Side Effects
diphenhydramine (Benadryl) (continued)	• Oral doses should be taken with food or milk to minimize GI irritation • Capsule may be emptied and the contents taken with water or food • Oral disintegrating tablets and strips should be left in package until use. Do not push tablet through the blister. Place tablet on the tongue. Tablet will dissolve and be swallowed with saliva. No liquid is necessary
hydroxyzine (Atarax)	• Acts as an antipruritic • Blocks histamine$_1$-receptors • Causes drowsiness, agitation, dizziness, headache, wheezing, dry mouth, constipation, nausea, urinary retention, and flushing • Administer 2 mg/kg/day every 6–8 hours • Do not confuse hydroxyzine (Atarax) with lorazepam (Ativan) • Tablets may be crushed; capsules may be opened and administered with food or fluids • Suspension must be shaken well before administration
cyproheptadine (Periactin)	• Used for relief of chronic urticaria • Antagonizes the effects of histamine at H$_1$-receptor sites • Does not inactivate histamine • Causes drowsiness, excitation in children, blurred vision, palpitations, dry mouth, constipation, photosensitivity, rashes, and weight gain • Administer 4 mg every 8 hours or 4–20 mg/day in 3 divided doses in children >14 years of age • Administer 2–4 mg every 8–12 hours but not to exceed 16 mg/day in children 6–14 years • Administer 2 mg every 8–12 hours but not to exceed 12 mg/day in children 2–6 years • Do not confuse cyproheptadine with cyclobenzaprine • Administer with food, water, or milk to minimize GI upset
cetirizine (Zyrtec)	• Used for relief of chronic urticaria • Antagonizes the effects of histamine at H$_1$-receptor sites • Does not inactivate histamine • Dizziness, drowsiness (significant with doses >10 mg/day), fatigue, pharyngitis, and dry mouth • Administer 5–10 mg divided once or twice daily for children 6 years of age and older • Administer 2.5 mg once daily initially, may increase to 5 mg once daily or 2.5 mg every 12 hours in children 2–5 years • Administer 2.5 mg once daily, may increase to 2.5 mg every 12 hours in children 1–2 years • Administer 2.5 mg once daily in children 6–12 months • Do not confuse with Zantac (ranitidine) • Administer without regard to food
loratadine (Alavert, Claritin)	• Used for management of chronic idiopathic urticaria and hives • Blocks peripheral effects of histamine released during allergic reactions • Causes confusion, drowsiness (rare instances), paradoxical excitation, blurred vision, dry mouth, GI upset, photosensitivity, rash, and weight gain • Administer 10 mg once daily for children 6 years and older • Administer 5 mg once daily for children 2–5 years • For rapid-disintegrating tablets, place on tongue, may be taken with or without water
cimetidine (Tagamet)	• Unlabeled use for management of urticaria • Inhibits action of histamine at the H$_2$-receptor sites • Causes confusion, dizziness, drowsiness, hallucinations, headache, arrhythmias, constipation, neutropenia, and thrombocytopenia

Source: Vallerand & Sanoski (2014).

scars are visual, and children respond to peoples' reactions about their appearance once they have been discharged from the burn center.

THE REHABILITATION PHASE

During the rehabilitation phase, positioning and splinting the affected joint at regular intervals are important to wound healing. In conjunction with proper positioning and splinting, active range of motion will be restarted when the wounds heal, allowing for return of functional mobility. It is vital that

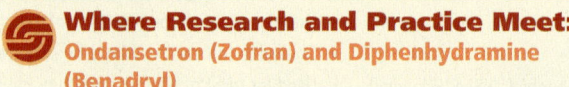

Where Research and Practice Meet:
Ondansetron (Zofran) and Diphenhydramine (Benadryl)

The effectiveness of ondansetron (Zofran) was compared with diphenhydramine (Benadryl) for treatment of pruritus in healing burn wounds in a single research study. Ondansetron (Zofran) was found to be significantly more effective ($p<0.05$) than diphenhydramine (Benadryl). The study raises the possibility that serotonin may play a role in preventing pruritus (Goutos et al., 2009).

once the child has entered the rehabilitation phase, more aggressive techniques for scar reduction may be used because the graft is stronger and more mature. Regular massage is necessary to aid in breaking up the scar formation. Daily stretches and exercises will aid in regaining and maintaining full range of motion. Pressure garments are applied and worn for 23.5 hours a day for 1 to 2 years (they are removed for ½ hour during bath time). Frequent follow-up at a burn clinic is necessary to make adjustments and assess adherence with the treatment plan (Healey & Katsu, 2010).

 Across Care Settings: **The rehabilitation phase**

During the rehabilitation phase, the child may be transferred to a rehabilitation center where he or she continues to receive intensive physical and occupational therapy. After discharge to home, physical and occupational therapy is continued. The child may need continued psychological treatments. If the child is enrolled in school or day care, communication must occur with the schoolteacher or day-care provider about the child's ongoing needs.

 Nursing Insight—*Reconstruction*

Reconstruction begins within weeks, months, or even years following the injury. Typically scar maturation occurs within 12 to 18 months after the injury so the reconstruction begins after scar maturation. As the scars mature, the scar becomes

 Where Research and Practice Meet:
Prevalent Psychiatric Disorders in Adolescents

Adjustment for adolescents presents a different set of circumstances and is based on level of maturity and willingness to participate in ongoing therapy and involvement in community resources. A study done by Thomas, Blakeney, Holzer, & Meyer (2009) investigated how prevalent psychiatric disorders were among adolescent long-term burn survivors. In the study, 50 youths were characterized by their parent or guardian as "troubled." The most common psychiatric disorders found in this study were:

- Anxiety (36%)
- Substance abuse (18%)
- Disruptive behavior disorders (14%)

The results of this study were then compared with previous reports about psychiatric disorders in adolescents and found that the incidence of psychiatric disorders was lower than in previous studies. However, in the comparison assessment, it was noted that there were higher rates of substance abuse and a shift in the type of behavior disorders. There were fewer reports of anxiety disorders, particularly posttraumatic stress disorders (Thomas et al., 2009).

In addition to the psychological effects on the burned child, the parents and siblings also suffer. The parents can suffer from feelings of anxiety about whether the child will live, the severity of the scars, guilt feelings that they could have prevented the injury, and grief over the loss of their normal child and possible loss of their child's life. Parent support groups in the burn unit and community are essential in helping parents cope with these issues. Siblings may also have psychological effects from the burn injury. They see that the burned child receives much attention and sometimes feel pushed aside. Siblings may be sad, confused, or angry that their sister or brother has been injured and may require personal counseling and use of ongoing community resources.

suppler, and the need for the surgery may diminish. Timing of the reconstructive procedures is determined by several factors that are based on the child's physical and psychological status. The child has to be emotionally prepared for the procedures and the possibility of missing school and social events. The child may suffer from anxiety related to surgical procedures or the hospitalization and require counseling. The child and parents also need to have realistic expectations about the benefits and risks of the procedure. It is extremely important to involve the child in the decision-making process about reconstructive surgery. Allowing the child to be part of the decision-making process means that the child "has bought in" to the conversation and understands the later commitment for the recovery requirements that are needed after the procedure is done (Klein, 2011).

Education/Discharge Instructions

Discharge planning includes a decision as to whether the child can be cared for at home or be admitted to a rehabilitation facility. A visiting nurse, physical therapist, and/or occupational therapist are involved in the child's home care. Parents are taught how to care for the wounds, perform the physical therapy, perform skin care and massage, and apply pressure garments and splints. The nurse tells the family about importance and compliance of follow-up appointments.

The entire family is impacted by a burned child. The central themes in families, according to Lehna (2010), are normalization and adjustment. The nurse tells the family that normalization is found in play, school, work, and family relations with siblings. The process of adjustment is varied and gradual and happens at school and in other social settings.

 Collaboration in Caring—*Reentry into society*

In an effort to assist with reentry into society, school reentry programs have been developed. The social worker, nurse, physical or occupational therapist, and child life therapist visit the child's school and assist the child with social skills and provide information to school staff and other parents. The health-care team can prepare a presentation for the child's classmates to help them understand the impact of a burn on their peer. They discuss what the child has been through and how their classmates can help their peer be accepted at school. Burned children have reported that this measure has helped them adapt and feel comfortable in school.

Burn camps have also been developed and invite children who have suffered burn injury to learn new coping skills while participating in fun activities. Therapists and nurses are employed at the camp to provide counseling and care for these children. Burned children have expressed that they feel safe in this setting. In addition, when the children return to a burn follow-up clinic, they may feel more accepted for who they are and find the clinic is a refuge from the stares that they encounter in public.

Injuries Associated With Burns

INJURIES ASSOCIATED WITH THE INHALATION OF TOXIC GASES

Burns of the airway occur as a result of heat from flames and inhalation of toxic gases. The inhaled poisons cause the lungs to fill with fluids causing sudden acute pulmonary edema.

Signs and Symptoms

- Singed eyebrows
- Singed nasal hairs
- Stridor
- Hoarseness
- **Carbonaceous sputum** (soot in sputum)
- Burns around the mouth and nose
- Edematous lips
- Black nasal or oral secretions
- Facial burns
- Hypoxemia
- History of:
  - Standing while clothes burned
  - Being in an enclosed space during the fire
  - Inhaling toxic gasses during the fire (Green, 2010, p. 46)

Diagnosis

Diagnosis is based on the history, physical assessment, and the signs and symptoms of sudden acute pulmonary edema (shortness of breath, dyspnea that worsens when lying down, a feeling of suffocating, wheezing, gasping for breath, anxiety, restlessness, and cough).

Collaborative Care

Nursing Care. The priority intervention for inhalation injury is administering oxygen and early intubation and ventilation. If early intubation is not possible, then an emergency tracheostomy is performed. Aggressive suctioning of the carbonaceous particles is also a main objective. Suctioning helps prevent the development of pneumonia. The nurse assesses for the deterioration of respiratory function and implements interventions to minimize the development of pneumonia. Frequent turning, chest physiotherapy, and suctioning are the most frequent nursing interventions. The nurse collaborates with the respiratory therapist, physicians, and other health-care providers to ensure optimal outcomes.

INJURIES ASSOCIATED WITH CHEMICAL BURNS

Chemical burns differ from thermal burns in that the burn tissue destruction continues until the chemical agent is removed.

Signs and Symptoms

Signs and symptoms of a chemical burn mimic skin and eye conditions. Depending on the chemical, specific signs are noted.

Diagnosis

Diagnosis is based on the history, physical assessment, and signs and symptoms that the particular chemical created on the affected body area.

focus on safety

Respiratory arrest

Respiratory arrest can occur as a result of the effect of the chemical on the central nervous system. Activate the emergency medical system and initiate cardiopulmonary resuscitation.

Collaborative Care

Nursing Care. The priority nursing care measure is removing the chemical agent by dilution or brushing it off. A chemical burn is never neutralized with another chemical. Neutralization causes a release of heat, which can increase the initial injury. Chemical burns as a result of contact with gasoline typically present as a partial-thickness burn with erythema. Resuscitation for children with these types of burns is similar to resuscitation for thermal burns and does not require grafting. However, children with chemical burns may acquire renal failure because of the nephrotoxic effect of the chemical that was absorbed by the body. The Parkland formula with lactated Ringers solution is used with the goal to maintain urine output of 0.5 to 1 mL/kg/hr.

Chemical burns as a result of phenol are mostly partial thickness. Phenol acts as a local anesthetic, so extensive damage can occur before the child feels the pain from the burn. Removal of this substance is done by spraying water on the burn surface; dabbing is contraindicated. Then the burn surface is wiped quickly with polyethylene glycol. These actions will virtually eliminate toxic symptoms and diminish the severity of the burn. The kidneys can also be affected from a chemical burn because there may be damage to the renal tubules and a precipitation of hemoglobin in the glomeruli. Neurologically, these children may have hyperreflexia and convulsions. Blood pressure is initially increased and then it decreases so the nurse initiates the proper measures to treat variance in blood pressure.

INJURIES ASSOCIATED WITH ELECTRICAL BURNS

Electrical burns fall into two categories: low-voltage injuries and high-voltage injuries. Low-voltage injuries typically occur in young children who are putting items like electrical cords in their mouth. When they bite through the protective covering, they come in contact with 110 volts or possibly 220 volts.

Signs and Symptoms

Low-voltage burns cause a full-thickness injury to the lip or the fingertip.

Diagnosis

Diagnosis is based on the history, physical assessment, and signs and symptoms that the particular voltage created on the affected body area.

Collaborative Care

Nursing Care. Low-voltage electrical burn injuries may be treated on an outpatient basis. The recovery phase of a low-voltage burn injury to the mouth is not much of an issue. However, the scar that forms presents with reconstruction challenges. Mouth splints have been used to stretch the scar and prevent the contracture at the corner of the mouth. However, this technique only stretches the scar, but does not deal with the problem of the portion of the circumoral area that has healed by contracture. A surgical method can be tried in which a full-thickness tongue flap is surgically attached to the excised scar. After 10 days, the flap is separated and the two sites are sutured closed. Two small **z-plasty** (a versatile plastic surgery technique that is used to improve the functional and cosmetic appearance of scars) revisions are performed within the next year. The surgery results allow the circumoral mucosa to appear normal, and the scar may be barely noticeable (Thorne, Chung, Gosain, Gurtner, Mehrara, Rubin, et al., 2014).

 Nursing Insight—High-voltage electrical burns

High-voltage burns are more dangerous in children than low-voltage burns, and survival is based on the type of current and other associated injuries. Children who have suffered a high-voltage burn injury and have no ECG changes, no history of loss of consciousness, or have a small percentage of total burn surface area can be treated in an emergency room and then cared for on an outpatient basis. However, more critically ill children who have suffered a high-voltage electrical burn and have upper extremity burn injuries, progressive neurological dysfunction of the burned extremity, vascular compromise, increased compartment pressure, or systemic clinical deterioration from suspected **myonecrosis** (death or necrosis of muscle tissue) are admitted to the hospital or burn center and require cardiac monitoring that includes watching creatine kinase levels that indicate muscle injury and troponin levels that indicate the heart muscle has been damaged (Arnoldo et al., 2010).

Nursing Care for Minor Burns

Minor burns are usually treated in a clinic or outpatient setting. An interprofessional team collaborates in providing care to these patients. In a clinic or outpatient setting, the nurse uses the concept of the six "Cs" to manage minor burns:

- Clothing: Remove any clothing that is hot or has been in contact with the offending chemical, if it is a new burn.
- Cooling: Burns need to be cooled immediately with cool (54°F) (12.2°C) saline-soaked gauze or any available clean cloth soaked in cool water, if it is a new burn. Caution: Do not use ice!
- Cleaning: Wash wound with mild soap and rinse well with water with each dressing change.
- Chemoprophylaxis: Bacitracin (AK-tracin) may be used topically to prevent infection. Other types of anti-infective agents are used in moderate and major burns. A tetanus booster (Td) is also administered if not administered within the previous 5 years.

 Where Research and Practice Meet:
Low-Voltage or High-Voltage Electrical Burns

A systematic review of the literature conducted by Arnoldo, Klein, and Gibran (2010) revealed that cardiac abnormalities could occur after either low-voltage or high-voltage burns. Nonspecific ST-T changes and atrial fibrillation were the most common cardiac abnormalities. The review of literature found that any child who suffered a low-voltage electrical burn and (1) had a history of a loss of consciousness, (2) had electrocardiogram (ECG) abnormalities, (3) had a burn that put he or she at risk for hemorrhage, or (4) had the need for circulation monitoring should be admitted to a health-care facility. The researchers also found ECG monitoring should be done on children who suffered an electrical burn.

 Global Health Case Study A Burned Child

Lapid (2008) described a case study of a Bedouin child who was brought in to an emergency room with infected burn wounds on the dorsum of both hands. The parents were reluctant to divulge exactly how the burn injury occurred. Eventually, they stated that the girl had been treated 5 days earlier by a traditional healer to cure her headaches. The "treatment" consisted of the traditional healer dripping a blue liquid on the dorsum of both hands in the shape of a spiral. The parents refused to identify the traditional healer but brought in a bag containing the substance that was used. The bag contained small blue crystals, which the healer had mixed with egg whites. The treatment was painful for the child. After 5 days, the child became febrile with signs of infection of pain, warmth, swelling, and redness around the burn. The parents decided it was time to seek treatment at the emergency room.

critical thinking questions

1. What evidence from the case study might lead the nurse to believe this injury was a result of abuse or neglect?
2. What cultural information might be helpful to the nurse?
3. What is the role of the nurse in this situation?
4. What treatment measure is done to stop the burning process?
5. Do traditional healers from other cultures treat burn injuries?

◆ See Suggested Answers to Global Health Case Studies on *DavisPlus*.

- Covering: Cover the burn with gauze to prevent infection, to decrease pain, and to absorb drainage. A moist wound heals much better than an open wound.
- Comfort: Give acetaminophen (Children's Tylenol) or ibuprofen (Children's Advil) to decrease the pain. Premedication for dressing changes is done 45 minutes before the dressing change to achieve maximum benefit from the pain medication. Pain medications are scheduled regularly to decrease pain in the child who has sleep, play, or mood alterations (Morgan, Bledsoe, & Barker, 2000).

 Cultural Diversity: Home Remedies

The nurse must learn about the culture of the family and their ways for treating burns. For instance, home remedies may have been used before the child is brought in to the emergency room. For example, an Asian child may have had toothpaste applied to a fresh burn and subsequently there was a delay in seeking treatment, or the Amish people may have treated a burn with B&W ointment and applied dressings from scalded burdock leaves.

 Now Can You—Discuss Burns?

1. Describe child development and burn injuries?
2. Discuss the type, depth, and size and extent of the burn?
3. Prioritize developmentally appropriate and holistic nursing care for burn conditions?

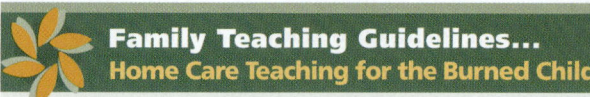

Family Teaching Guidelines...
Home Care Teaching for the Burned Child

TOPIC: The nurse will teach the family how to care for the burned child.

ESSENTIAL INFORMATION: When the child is discharged home, the parents will assume care of the burned child, so the nurse instructs parents on these measures:

◆ Bathing
◆ Skin care measures
◆ Massages with a non-perfumed moisturizer
◆ Wound dressing changes
◆ Knowledge about the signs and symptoms of infection
◆ Information about when to call the doctor or nurse practitioner
◆ Application of pressure garments
◆ Application of splints
◆ Importance of physical therapy
◆ Importance of occupational therapy
◆ Nutritional diet that contains high protein and calories
◆ Frequent follow-up appointments
◆ Attendance at a parent support group
◆ Attendance at a victim support group (if necessary)
◆ Participation in a school reentry program

Hypothermia

Hypothermia is secondary to cold air exposure, wet clothes, and immersion in water. Hypothermia is also present in victims of burns, when large amounts of skin are no longer present, or the child no longer has the capacity to hold heat. Mild hypothermia is a condition in which the child's core body temperature falls below 93.2°F (34°C). Hypothermia is a life-threatening emergency. The body loses heat in one of five ways: radiation, conduction, convection, evaporation, and respiration (Table 30-7).

Different developmental stages predispose the child to different types of exposure. Infants and young children are at higher risk because of their immature thermoregulatory system, thinner skin, and lack of subcutaneous fat. Older children are at high risk for hypothermia because they may lack the cognitive ability to evaluate risky situations. Adolescents are at risk for hypothermia because of risk-taking behaviors such as participating in outdoor activities without proper clothing and potentially the ingestion of alcohol or other illicit drugs. In children of any age, a trauma, brain disorder, or severe sepsis can also cause hypothermia because these conditions interfere with the thermoregulation system.

Signs and Symptoms

Signs and symptoms of hypothermia are dependent on its stage:

• Stage one: temperature between 93.2°F and 96.8°F (34°C–36°C)
• Shivering and piloerection (goose flesh)
• Vasoconstriction
• Increased metabolism
• Shallow breathing, fatigue, nausea, and visual disturbances

Table 30-7	Types of Heat Loss
Radiation	Heat loss from the head and areas with less subcutaneous fat and thin skin (e.g., prematurity of the newborn) This is the most rapid method of heat loss and accounts for at least 50% of heat loss
Conduction	The transfer of heat away from the body by direct contact with a cooler surface (e.g., wet clothing or immersion)
Convection	The transfer of heat away from the body by the movement of air over the skin surface (e.g., wind and drafts)
Evaporation	The transfer of heat away from the body (e.g., skin moisture turned to vapor as it is dried by the movement of air)
Respiration	Expiration of heat from the lungs (e.g., cold and windy weather)

• Poor fine motor coordination
• Local reaction: burning and numbness of extremities, pallor (pale/blue-gray) to erythema (redness)
• Stage two: temperature between 86°F and 93°F (30°C–34°C)
    • Violent shivering, pallor, and distal cyanosis
    • Poor gross motor coordination; stumbling
    • Confused but awake and alert
    • Local reaction: insensate (no feeling) and skin may blister from frostbite

Mild to moderate frostbite can resolve in rewarming with little to no sequelae (pathological conditions)

• Stage three: temperature less than 86°F (less than 30°C)
    • Stops shivering
    • Reduced consciousness moving to stupor
        • Paradoxical behavior (unusual); undressing
        • Metabolism slows to 1/2 of normal
    • Bradycardia and tachyarrhythmias
    • Respirations slow
    • Central nervous system stops
    • Multiple organ failure
        • Death
          (Corneli & Bolte, 2012)
          (See Table 30-8)

focus on safety

Other etiologies of hypothermia

The nurse must understand that metabolic or neurological etiologies may be the cause of hypothermia in children. The cause of hypothermia is investigated when no environmental explanation for hypothermia exists.

Nursing Insight—Hypothermia

Hypothermia is also associated with near drowning. When the child's body is immersed in water, heat is lost quickly. During a near drowning, the body tries to maintain core body temperature at the expense of losing heat in the extremities. Shivering is the body's way to re-warm the blood. Increased muscle tone and increased metabolism also occur.

Table 30-8 Hypothermia		
Classification	**Body Temperature**	**Clinical Symptoms**
Mild	93.2°F–96.8°F (34°C–36°C) (Venes, 2013)	Shivering Rapid heart rate Rapid respiratory rate Vasoconstriction Increased urine output As temperature decreases child becomes apathetic rather than excited, lethargic, and has impaired judgment
Moderate	86°F–93°F (30°C–34°C) (Venes, 2013)	Decreased heart rate Decreased respiratory rate Hypotension Loss of consciousness Decreased pupillary response
Severe	<86°F (30°C) (Venes, 2013)	Apnea Asystole Coma It may not be possible to readily differentiate between severe hypothermia and death

Diagnosis

A diagnosis of hypothermia in children is based on body temperature and relevant behaviors. If there is no etiology of prolonged exposure to the cold, the child will need differential diagnostics to determine if the etiology is neurological or metabolic.

Prevention

Monitoring children closely so they do not leave the house in inclement weather without adequate protection is essential information to pass along to parents. Teaching children to avoid walking on frozen lakes and ponds unless they are sure they are adequately frozen is very important. Emphasize to parents the need to protect the child from all bodies of water, especially in the cooler temperatures, to avoid both the incidence of accidental drowning and immersion hypothermia. Appropriate cold weather clothing is vital to keeping warm. Covering the head will help the child stay warm; covering the ears, hands, and feet helps reduce the chance of frostbite. Warm socks under waterproof footwear as well as mittens work well for children who are out of doors for short periods of time in the cold weather.

focus on safety

Wet clothing

Wet clothes increase the risk of hypothermia. The nurse or parents must remove wet clothing as soon as possible and replace with dry clothing.

Collaborative Care

Nursing Care. The nurse initiates emergency medical care by calling the emergency response team and by conducting a complete assessment of airway, breathing, and circulation.

Cardiopulmonary resuscitation is initiated if the child's condition warrants. The nurse must record core body temperature. Rectal temperatures are most accurate and are used during the rewarming process. However, if peritoneal lavage with warm fluids is used, the rectal temperature may not be reliable, and a central venous monitor will be more accurate.

Important nursing care measures include removing all cold and wet clothing, wrapping the child in warmed blankets, and administering warmed oxygen and warmed IV fluids to promote cardiac output. Vital signs and urine output are also monitored during the rewarming process. Electrocardiograms are used to give essential information about the heart, both rate and rhythm. The nurse must remember that ventricular or atrial dysrhythmias are possible in hypothermia. After these critical measures are implemented, the nurse raises the child's body temperature by using a forced air warming system (e.g., the Bair Hugger®). This type of system uses convection to heat the trunk area first (Allen, Salyer, Dubick, Holcomb, & Blackbourne, 2010).

Case Study Hypothermia

Eight-year-old Sam and his friends are planning to ice fish on a small farm pond about 100 yards from his backyard. Sam and his friends are cutting a small hole in the ice about 10 feet from the shore of the pond when a cracking sound sends Sam's friends running to shore. Sam has always been braver, and he continues his work to open an ice hole. In a little while, Sam's friends return to see his progress. As his friends watch from shore, they see Sam fall into the water near the edge of the pond. Sam's friends run to the house to tell Sam's mother. Sam's mother calls 911, then runs down to the pond and pulls him out. Her cold limp son lies on the ground while she waits for the emergency medical team to arrive. While she waits, she remembers that it is best to remove any wet clothing and begins to frantically undress Sam. She then covers him in the blankets that the friends have brought down to the pond. When the medical team arrives, they find him not breathing and unresponsive. Sam has no signs of respirations or heartbeat, and his body temperature is very cold. The team begins circulation, airway, and breathing, and Sam is transported to the local emergency room.

critical thinking questions

1. What are the priority nursing actions that you will perform when Sam enters your emergency department?

2. Sam's heart monitor shows asystole, and his rectal temperature is 71.6°F (22°C). What is the status of Sam's condition?

3. Is external rewarming the most effective method of rewarming after severe hypothermia?

◆ See Suggested Answers to Case Studies on Davis*Plus.*

Nursing Insight—*Peripheral IV infiltration*

Peripheral IV infiltration occurs when non-vesicant medications leak into the tissue instead of going into the accessed vein. Infiltration happens if the catheter is inserted improperly, the catheter becomes dislodged, or the IV catheter is not properly secured. Signs and symptoms of peripheral IV infiltration include swelling, pain at the insertion site, coolness of the skin, leakage at the insertion site, erythema, blistering, or lack of blood return. An essential nursing function is peripheral IV assessment every 4 hours or more often if needed.

Frostbite

Frostbite in children is an injury that results from prolonged exposure (more than an hour) to severe cold and usually affects the outer extremities (ears, cheeks, nose, hands, and feet). Crystal formations occur in the tissue and blood cells, which result in dehydration of the cells and ischemic damage.

Signs and Symptoms

Signs and symptoms of frostbite depend on severity:

- Mild to moderate
  - Reddened, cool to touch skin
  - Tingling or numbness
  - Mild swelling
  - Pain upon rewarming
- Severe
  - Pale, waxy, cool skin; feels "wooden"
  - Numbness, insensate (no feeling) that may not improve immediately with rewarming
  - Blisters
  - Extensive swelling
  - Blackened, necrotic (dead or dying) tissue; damage may extend down through the skin to the muscle and bone if severe or prolonged exposure
  (Torpy, 2011)

Diagnosis

Frostbite can be identified by the hard, pale, and cold quality of skin that has been exposed to the cold. The extent of the injury is determined upon rewarming.

Prevention

Monitoring children closely so they do not leave the house in inclement weather without adequate protection is essential information to pass along to parents. Appropriate cold weather clothing is vital to keeping warm. Covering the head will help the child stay warm; covering the ears, hands, and feet help reduce the chance of frostbite. Warm socks under waterproof footwear as well as mittens work well for children who are out of doors for short periods of time in the cold weather.

Collaborative Care

Nursing Care. Treatment for frostbite is much like core hypothermia treatment. Place the child in a warm area, remove all wet and cold clothing, and replace with warm nonrestrictive clothing. Remove watches and rings if present. Add warm blankets around the child and use the Bair Hugger® if available.

Do not rub, massage, or soak the frostbitten area (Torpy, 2011). Massage causes the crystals that have formed in the capillaries to break through causing damage in the area. After rewarming is complete, the affected extremity is wrapped in a soft cloth or gauze, and the child can be encouraged to rest. If no subsequent problems arise, the child can remove the soft cloth and return to indoor activities. If parents suspect continued problems, the health-care practitioner is notified.

✿⚙ Nursing Diagnoses Frostbite

- Impaired Skin Integrity related to freezing of the skin
- Ineffective Thermoregulation related to extended exposure to a cold environment
- Pain related to decreased circulation from prolonged exposure to cold

Pressure Ulcers

Pressure ulcers are the result of compression on one or more areas of the body for an extended period. This subsequently injures both the capillary bed and the soft tissues, allowing for decreased perfusion and subsequent breakdown. Because of this compression, the skin cells are deprived of nutrients and needed oxygen. Metabolic waste products then accumulate, causing the injury. Any delay in intervention may cause a deep sore to form.

Pressure ulcers occur in children with decreased mobility. Premature infants, infants who have motor delays and cannot easily move their head or extremities, and children with paralysis or other forms of limited mobility are at risk. Children who use mobility devices (e.g., crutches, walkers, and wheelchairs) are at risk for developing pressure ulcers in the weight-bearing tissue used while navigating with these devices. Children and adolescents in casts or body braces are also at risk if the apparatus is ill fitting or if the areas of pressure are not properly padded. Infants, children, and adolescents who are malnourished or have infections or anemia are at higher risk for ulceration. Children who are bed bound for any period of time, such as children with low cardiac output, are also at risk for ulceration. Children with decreased sensation to pressure or pain may also be at risk of developing skin breakdown and pressure ulcers. Friction and shear from caregivers moving the immobile child is yet another way to injure the skin and decrease local perfusion.

Signs and Symptoms

Signs and symptoms of pressure ulcers are dependent on the stage of the ulcer:

- Stage one
  - Intact skin
  - Not able to blanch, redness, usually over a bony prominence
  - May feel softer, warmer, or cooler than surrounding tissue
- Stage two
  - Partial-thickness loss of the dermis
  - Shallow, open ulcer
  - Pink wound bed, no sloughing
  - May be a blister instead of open ulcer
    - Does not include tape burn, skin tears, or dermatitis
- Stage three
  - Full-thickness loss of the dermis
  - Subcutaneous fat may be visible
  - Sloughing may be present
  - Possible tunneling
- Stage four
  - Full-thickness loss of the dermis
  - Exposed bone, tendon, or muscle (beyond the fatty layer)
  - Sloughing or eschar (necrotic, dead tissue) may be in the wound bed
  - Frequent tunneling

Stage three and four descriptions are anatomically dependent. Areas with little subcutaneous fat (e.g., bridge of nose, ear, back of head, and malleolus) may be quite shallow.

It is possible that some ulcers cannot be staged. This can happen when a full-thickness loss has occurred and the wound bed is covered with slough, either yellow, green, gray, or black. This type of wound will need debridement before staging can be performed (National Pressure Ulcer Panel, 2010).

The four stages of ulcer formation can assist the nurse in thorough skin assessment (Fig. 30-13). The earliest sign of skin damage is a reddened area on the skin that does not disappear within 30 minutes of removing the cause of the pressure or irritant. The skin can appear to have an abrasion and look raw or rubbed. Further damage extends through the dermis forming the ulcer.

 Cultural Diversity: Pressure Ulcers

In children with dark-pigmented skin, the area can look red or purple upon blanching.

Diagnosis

Diagnosis is based on a good nursing assessment using reliable tools. The Braden scale (http://www.bradenscale .com) is used to assess pressure ulcer risk every shift. The major components assessed in the scale are sensory perception, skin moisture, physical activity, mobility ability, nutrition, and friction and shear (Braden & Bergstrom, 1988). In the child who is postoperative, the Braden scale is less predictive, but a better tool is not yet available (Chen, Liu, & He, 2012) A standardized assessment tool such as the Neonatal Skin Condition Score for neonates may also be used as an assessment tool for at-risk neonates (Lund & Osborn, 2004). This tool is found on the Association of Women's Health, Obstetric and Neonatal Nurses (AWHONN) Web site: Search "neonatal skin condition score."

Prevention

Prevention of pressure ulcers is essential and begins by routinely moving and shifting the weight of the child off bony prominences on a regular basis. Movement must occur at least every 2 hours for the child who is confined to bed. A child in a sitting position (e.g., in a wheelchair) shifts her weight every 15 minutes, independently or with assistance. If the child wears braces, the skin is inspected for redness or irritation at least once a day. If any redness is noted, the nurse must not reapply the brace and must notify the health-care practitioner immediately.

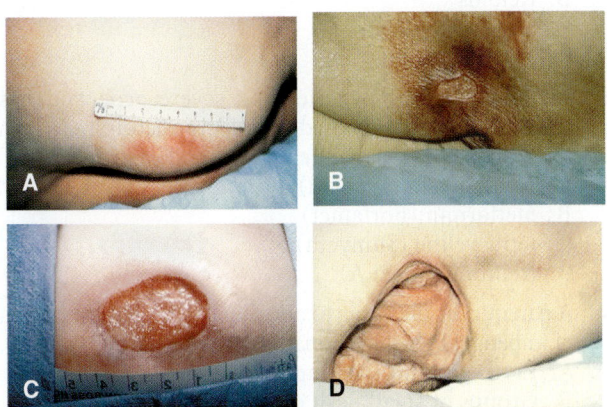

Figure 30-13 Stages of pressure ulcer. *A,* Stage 1. *B,* Stage 2. *C,* Stage 3. *D,* Stage 4.

Collaborative Care

Nursing Care. The nurse addresses the exact condition affecting the skin before a pressure sore actually develops. The nurse proactively addresses anemia. A diet high in iron may help prevent pressure ulcers. Keep bed clothing straight and wrinkle-free to decrease areas of pressure. Air, water, or gel mattresses and pads decrease pressure areas. The nurse keeps the child's skin both clean and dry. A variety of topical treatments are available (Table 30-9).

Careful inspection of a child's skin at least three times a day is essential. The nurse must note the color of the affected area, signs of infection, character of the skin lesion, wound edges, drainage, measure the diameter, and determine the depth of the pressure ulcer. Repositioning the child at least every 2 hours to relieve pressure on bony prominences as well as readjustment of tubes and other devices to protect the skin is necessary to prevent sores.

Stage one and two pressure ulcers are cleansed and allowed to dry. The nurse must also keep the child off the affected area as much as possible. With time and protective management, the wound resolves. Stage three ulcers may heal spontaneously as well. Some hydrophilic gels or hydrocolloid dressings may be used. In stage 4 ulcers, surgical debridement and closure may be needed.

Summary Points

- Children are often at a higher risk for certain skin conditions based on their large body surface area and still maturing immune system.

- A skin lesion is a circumscribed area of altered tissue. When assessing the skin for a lesion, it is important to note the size, shape, color, and texture.

- Typical wounds found in the child are a result of cuts, scrapes, and burns and can be secondary to surgical intervention.

- A number of invaders can affect the skin, and these can be bacterial, viral, or fungal in nature. While most of the skin conditions resulting from these invaders respond quickly to treatment, others require an extended time for healing.

- Methicillin-resistant Staphylococcus aureus (MRSA) is a contagious bacterium that is resistant to treatment from beta-lactam antibiotics.

- Contact, atopic, and seborrheic dermatitis is an inflammatory rash on the skin marked by itching and redness that occurs because of numerous conditions.

- Cutaneous skin reactions are a manifestation of an allergic response. The offending allergen can be introduced into the system in a variety of ways such as ingestion, inhalation, or coming into direct contact.

- Infestations in children include pediculosis and scabies mites.

- The most common insect bite comes from the mosquito. Spider and tick bites are also prevalent among children. The stings experienced most frequently are from bees, wasps, and hornets. Animal and human bites as well as diseases from these bites are common.

- Children are at risk for certain types of burn injuries at certain ages and developmental stages.

Table 30-9 Topical Treatments

Classification	Names	Precautions
Anesthetics	benzocaine (Americaine) lidocaine and prilocaine (EMLA)	Allergy Do not use over wounds Do not use over large areas: avoid the eyes
Antibacterial	bacitracin and polymyxin B (AK-Poly-Bac) neomycin (Myciguent) mupirocin (Bactroban)	Allergy Existing infection (for prevention of infection) Antibiotic resistance Use for only minor cuts/scrapes/burns
Antifungal	clotrimazole (Lotrimin) ketoconazole (Nizoral) miconazole (Aloe Vesta) nystatin (Mycostatin)	Cautious use in nail and scalp infections
Anti-itch	diphenhydramine (Benadryl)	Allergy Photosensitivity
Emollients	White petrolatum jelly Mineral oil Lanolin Glycerin	Allergy Choose fragrance-free products
Steroids	Varying strengths Strongest group I: betamethasone (Diprolene) Group II: dexamethasone (Decadron) Group III: triamcinolone 0.5% (Kenalog) Group IV: fluocinolone (Lidex) Group V: hydrocortisone 0.2% (A-Hydrocort) Group VI: desonide (Tridesilon) Group VII: hydrocortisone 1% (A-Hydrocort)	Allergy Repeated use in the same area of the skin will cause thinning of the skin and may inhibit the skin's ability to fight infection The lowest strength on the thin skin of the face and genitalia is used Avoid the eye area: places the patient at risk for glaucoma or cataract formation

Source: Vallerand, A. H., & Sanoski, C. A. (2014). *Davis's drug guide for nurses* (14th ed.). Philadelphia, PA: F.A. Davis.

- Three factors: type of burn, depth of burn, and size and extent of burn determine the severity.

- The best outcomes for a burned child include holistic nursing interventions from the following categories: burn assessment and fluid resuscitation and prevention of infection, sepsis, and pneumonia. Pain management, maintaining circulation, promotion of good nutrition, pruritus management, psychosocial issues, the rehabilitation phase, and education/discharge instructions are also important care measures.

- Injuries associated with burns include inhalation of toxic gases and injuries from chemical burns and electrical burns.

- Minor burns are usually treated in a clinic or outpatient setting. An interprofessional team collaborates in providing care to these patients.

- Hypothermia is a life-threatening emergency, and the body loses heat in one of five ways: radiation, conduction, convection, evaporation, and respiration.

- Frostbite in children is an injury that results from prolonged exposure (more than an hour) to severe cold and usually affects the outer extremities (ears, cheeks, nose, hands, and feet).

- Pressure ulcers are the result of compression on one or more areas of the body for an extended period; this subsequently injures both the capillary bed and the soft tissues, allowing for decreased perfusion and subsequent breakdown.

Review Questions

Multiple Choice

1. The nursing instructor is explaining the layers of skin to students. Which layer is inconsistent with knowledge of this topic?
   A. Dermis
   B. Epidermis
   C. Intradermis
   D. Subcutaneous fatty layer

2. When assessing for primary skin lesions on children, what does the nurse specifically look for?
   A. Crusts
   B. Keloids
   C. Scales
   D. Wheals

3. An adolescent is experiencing severe acne and has recently been diagnosed with prediabetes. Which medication does the nurse educate the adolescent about?
   A. clindamycin (Cleocin)
   B. metformin (Fortamet)
   C. tetracycline (Sumycin)
   D. trenitoin (Retin A)

4. A parent calls the clinic to ask about signs and symptoms of impetigo. Which information does the nurse provide?
   A. Erythema and swelling of the fingers
   B. Groups of small flesh colored or pink papules
   C. Painful, watery blisters often near the nose
   D. Pustules that have honey-colored exudate

5. A teen is prescribed griseofulvin (Grifulvin V). What teaching does the nurse provide the child and parents?
   A. Apply this medication only at night.
   B. Avoid sun exposure and tanning beds.
   C. Have liver enzymes checked every 6 weeks.
   D. Use two forms of birth control if you have sex.

6. A child has lice. The parent wants to know what to do with the child's stuffed animals. Which response by the nurse is most appropriate?
   A. Seal in a plastic bag in the garage for 2 weeks.
   B. Spray with an anti-lice fumigating product.
   C. Throw them away; they cannot be cleaned.
   D. Wash in hottest water possible and line dry.

7. A mother reports seeing "burrows" on her child's hands. Which medication does the nurse teach the mother about?
   A. lindane (Kuell)
   B. malathion (Ovide)
   C. permethrin 5% (Elimite)
   D. spinosad (Natroba)

8. The emergency department nurse knows that which type of bite has the highest risk of infection?
   A. Cat
   B. Dog
   C. Human
   D. Squirrel

9. The nurse provides anticipatory guidance to parents telling them the maximum water temperature for bathing children is which temperature?
   A. 100°F (37.8°C)
   B. 110°F (43.3°C)
   C. 120°F (48.9°C)
   D. 140°F (60°C)

10. The nurse working with children knows that which burn is the most common type of burn in the pediatric population?
   A. Contact
   B. Flame
   C. Scald
   D. Thermal

See Answers to End of Chapter Review Questions on DavisPlus.

REFERENCES

Alexis, A. F., & Lamb, A. (2009, January–February). Concomitant therapy for acne in patients with skin of color: A case-based approach. *Dermatology Nursing, 21*(1).

Allen, P. B., Salyer, S. W., Dubick, M. A., Holcomb, J. B., & Blackbourne, L. H. (2010, July). Preventing hypothermia: Comparison of current devices used by the US Army in an in vitro warmed fluid model. *Journal of Trauma, 69*(Suppl 1), S154–S156.

American Burn Association. (2011). Burn incidence and treatment in the United States: 2011 fact sheet. Retrieved from http://www.ameriburn.org/resources_factsheet.php

American Veterinary Medical Association (AVMA). (2012). National dog bite week. Retrieved from http://www.avma.org

Arnoldo, B., Klein, M., & Gibran, N. (2010). Practice guidelines for the management of electrical injuries. *Journal of Burn Care and Research, 27*(4), 439–447. doi:10.1097/01.BCR.0000226250.26567.4C

Association of Women's Health, Obstetric and Neonatal Nurses (AWHONN). (2007). Neonatal skin condition score. Retrieved from http://www.awhonn.org/awhonn/content.do?name=03_JournalsPubsResearch%2F3G4_NeonatalSkinCare.htm

Aziz-Jalali, M. H., Tabaie, S. M., & Djavid, G. E. (2012, March–April). Comparison of red and infrared low-level laser therapy in the treatment of acne vulgaris. *Indian Journal of Dermatology, 57*(2), 128–130.

Baddour, L. M. (2011). Soft tissue infection due to dog and cat bites. In Up to Date. Retrieved from http://www.uptodate.com/contents/soft-tissue-infections-due-to-dog-and-cat-bites?source=search_result&search=cat+bites&selectedTitle=1~20

Blumetti, J., Hunt, J. L., Arnoldo, B. D., Parks, J. K., & Purdue, G. F. (2008). The Parkland formula under fire: Is the criticism justified? *Journal of Burn Care & Research, 29*(1), 180–186. doi:10.1097/BCR.0b013e31815f5a62

Braden, B., & Bergstrom, N. (1988). The Braden scale for predicting pressure sore risk. Copyright 1988 by Barbara Braden and Nancy Bergstrom. All rights reserved. Retrieved from http://www.bradenscale.com

Bruggink, S., Gussekloo, J., & Berger M. Y. (2010). Cryotherapy with liquid nitrogen versus topical salicylic acid application for cutaneous warts in primary care: Randomized controlled trial. *CMAJ, 182*(15), 1624–1630.

Bulechek, G. M., Butcher, H. K., Dochterman, J. M., & Wagner, C. (2013). *Nursing interventions classification (NIC)* (6th ed.). St. Louis, MO: Elsevier Mosby.

Centers for Disease Control and Prevention (CDC). (2008). Guideline for disinfection and sanitization and sterilization in health care facilities, 2008. Retrieved from http://www.cdc.gov/hicpac/pdf/guidelines/Disinfection_Nov_2008.pdf

Centers for Disease Control and Prevention (CDC). (2009, May 14). Dog bite. Retrieved from http://www.cdc.gov/HomeandRecreationalSafety/Dog-Bites/biteprevention.html

Centers for Disease Control and Prevention (CDC). (2010a, November 2). Head lice. Retrieved from http://www.cdc.gov/parasites/lice/head/epi.html

Centers for Disease Control and Prevention (CDC). (2010b, November 2). Scabies. Retrieved from http://www.cdc.gov

Centers for Disease Control and Prevention (CDC). (2011a). Cat scratch disease. Retrieved from http://www.cdc.gov/healthypets/index.html

Centers for Disease Control and Prevention (CDC). (2011b). Rocky Mountain spotted fever. Retrieved from http://www.cdc.gov/rmsf/

Centers for Disease Control and Prevention (CDC). (2011c, November 15). Preventing tick bites. Retrieved from http://www.cdc.gov/lyme/prev/on_people.html

Centers for Disease Control and Prevention (CDC). (2012a). Lyme disease. Retrieved from http://www.cdc.gov/Lyme/

Centers for Disease Control and Prevention (CDC). (2012b, February). National Burn Awareness Week. Retrieved from http://www.cdc.gov/tobacco/calendar/feb/matopmal_burn-awareness/index.htm

Centers for Disease Control and Prevention (CDC). (2012c, August 27). West Nile virus: Insect repellent use and safety. Retrieved http://www.cdc.gov/ncidod/dvbid/westnile/qa/insect_repellent.htm

Chen, H., Liu, P., & He, W. (2012, February). The Braden scale cannot be used alone for assessing pressure ulcer risk in surgical patients: A meta-analysis. *Wound Management, 58*(2), 34–36, 38–40.

Chosidow, O., Giraudeau, B., Cottrell, J., Izri, A., Hofmann, R., Mann, S. G., et al. (2010). Oral ivermectin versus malathion lotion for difficult-to-treat head lice. *New England Journal of Medicine, 362*(10), 896.

Corneli, H. M., & Bolte, R. G. (2012, September 18). Clinical manifestations of hypothermia in children. In Up to Date. Retrieved from http://www.uptodate.com/contents/clinical-manifestations-of-hypothermia-in-children

Coulthard P., Esposito, M., Worthington, H. V., van der Elst, M., van Waes, O. J. F., & Darcey, J. (2010). Tissue adhesives for closure of surgical incisions. *Cochrane Database of Systematic Reviews,* (5).

Courtenay, L. A. (2011). A practical approach to the treatment of acne vulgaris. *Nursing Standard, 25*(19), 55–64.

Currie, B. J., & McCarthy, J. S. (2010). Permethrin and ivermectin for scabies. *New England Journal of Medicine, 362*(8), 717.

Davison, P. G., Loiselle, F. B., & Nickerson, D. (2010). Survey on current hydrotherapy use among North American burn centers. *Journal of Burn Care and Research, 31*(3), 393–399. doi:10.1097/BCR.0b013e3181db5215

Federal Drug Administration (FDA). (2009, June). Lindane shampoo and lindane lotion. Retrieved from http://www.fda.gov/Drugs/DrugSafety/PostmarketDrugSafetyInformationforPatientsandProviders/ucm110452.htm

Fishman, T. D. (2006). Wound care information network. Retrieved from http://www.medicaledu.com/phases.htm

Fuller, F. W. (2009). The side effects of silver sulfadiazine. *Journal of Burn Care & Research, 30*(3), 464–470. doi:10.1097/BCR.0b013e3181a28c9b

Genzyme Biosurgery. (2014). Epicel: Cultured epidermal autografts. Retrieved from http://www.accessdata.fda.gov/scripts/cdrh/cfdocs/cftopic/pma/pma.cfm?num=H990002

Gibran, N. (2006). Practice guidelines for burn care. Committee on Organization and Delivery of Burn Care, American Burn Association. *Journal of Burn Care and Research.* doi:10.1097/01.BCR.0000226084.26680.56

Gilbert, D. N., Moellering, R. C., Eliopoulos, G. M., Chambers, H. F., & Saag, M. S., (Eds.). (2011). *The Sanford guide to antimicrobial therapy 2011.* Sperryville, VA: Antimicrobial Therapy, Inc.

Goutos, I., Dziewulski, P., & Richardson, P. M. (2009). Pruritus in burns: Review article. *Journal of Burn Care and Research, 30*(2), 221–228. doi:10.1097/BCR,0b013e31898a2fa

Graves, C., Saffle, J., & Cochran, A. (2009). Actual burn nutrition care practices: An update. *Journal of Burn Care and Research, 30*(1), 77–82. doi:10.1097/BCR.0b013e318921f0d

Green, T. E. (2010). Pediatric burns: Initial response, lasting effects. *Nursing, 40*(8), 42–49. doi:10.1097/01/NURSE.0000383896.57848.7a

Greenwood, J. E., Kavanagh, S., & Mackie, I. P. (2010). Revisiting protocols for burn injury management. *International Journal of Care Pathways, 14*(3), 88–95. doi:10.1258/jicp.2010.010013

Healey, T., & Katsu, A. (2010). Positioning and splinting of neck burns. *Joanna Briggs Institute*. Retrieved from http://joannabriggs.org/

Hofmann-Wellenhof, R., Pellacani, G., Halvehy, J., & Soyer, H. P. (Eds.). (2012). *Reflectance confocal microscopy for skin diseases*. Berlin, Germany: Springer-Verlag.

iPLEDGE. (2005). iPLEDGE: Committed to pregnancy prevention. Retrieved from https://www.ipledgeprogram.com/

Jacob, S. E., Herro, E. M., Guide, S., Cunningham, B., & Connelly, E. A. (2012). Allergic contact dermatitis to Pampers(tm) Drymax [Electronic Version]. *Pediatric Dermatology*. doi:10.1111/j.1525-1470.2011.01588.x

Johnson, M., Bulechek, G., Butcher, H., McCloskey Dochterman, J., Maas, M., Moorehead, S., & Swanson, E. (2012). *NANDA, NOC, and NIC linkage: Nursing diagnoses, outcomes, & interventions* (2nd ed.). St. Louis, MO: Elsevier Mosby.

Kim, W. J., Lee, K. R., Lee, S. E., Lee, H. J., & Yoon, M. S. (2012). Isolation of the causative microorganism and antimicrobial susceptibility. *Korean Journal of Dermatology, 50*(9), 788–794.

Klein, M. B. (2011). Burn reconstruction. *Physical Medicine and Rehabilitation Clinics of North America, 22,* 311–325. doi: 10.1016/j.pmr.2011.01.002

Landrum, M. L., Neumann, C., Cook, C., Chukwuma, U., Ellis, M. W., Hospenthal, D. R., et al. (2012). Epidemiology of Staphylococcus aureus blood and skin and soft tissue infections in the US military health system, 2005-2010, *Jama 308*(1), 50–51.

Lapid, O. (2008). Copper sulphate burns to the hands, a complication of traditional medicine. *Journal of Burn Care and Research, 29*(3), 544–547. doi:10.1097/BCR.0b013e318171183

Lehna, C. (2010). Sibling experiences after a major childhood burn injury. *Pediatric Nursing, 36*(5), 245–252.

Lund, D., & Osborne, J. (2004). Validity and reliability of the neonatal skin condition score. *Journal of Obstetric, Gynecological and Neonatal Nursing, 33*(3), 320–327.

Markely, J. D., Edmond, M. B., Major, Y., Bearman, G., & Stevens, M. P. (2012). Are gym surfaces reservoirs for Staphylococcus aureus? A point prevalence survey. *American Journal of Infection Control, 40*(10), 1008–1009.

Melnik, B. C. (2012). Diet in acne: Further evidence for the role of nutrient signaling in acne pathogenesis. *Acne Derm Venereol, 92,* 228–231.

Miller, K., Rodger, S., Kipping, B., & Kimble, R. M. (2011). A novel technology approach to pain management in children with burns: A prospective randomized controlled trial. *Burns, 37*(3), 395–405. doi:10.1016/j.burns.2010.12.008

Moorhead, S., Johnson, M., Maas, M. L., & Swanson, E. (2013). *Nursing outcomes classification (NOC)* (5th ed.). St. Louis, MO: Elsevier Mosby.

Morgan, E. D., Bledsoe, S. C., & Barker, J. (2000). Ambulatory management of burns [Electronic Version]. *American Family Physician, 62*(9), 2015–2026.

National Eczema Organization. (2012). All about atopic dermatitis. Retrieved from http://nationaleczema.org/

National Fire Protection Association. (2011). Educational Messages Advisory Committee. Retrieved from http://www.nfpa.org/itemdetail .asp?categoryid=1068&itemid=25474&ur...0public%20educators/ educational%messages%advisory%20committee

The National Pediculosis Association, Inc. (2011). Retrieved from http:// www.headlice.org/

National Pressure Ulcer Panel. (2010). National pressure ulcer stages/ categories. Retrieved from http://www.npuap.org/resources/educational- and-clinical-resources/npuap-pressure-ulcer-stagescategories/

Nervi, S. J., Ressner, R. A., Drayton, J. A., & Kapila, R. (2011, November 21). Cat scratch disease. Retrieved from http://emedicine.medscape.com/ article/214100-overview#a0104

Petros, H. (2010). What's your assessment? *Dermatology Nursing, Clinical Year in Review.* 46–65.

Rafla, K., & Tredget, E. E. (2011). Infection control in the burn unit. *Burns, 37,* 5–15. doi:10.1016/j.burns.2009.06.198

Rhoads, J. (2009). Managing bites and stings. *The Nurse Practitioner, 34*(8), 37–43.

Saba, S. C., Tsai, R., & Glat, P. (2009). Clinical evaluation comparing the efficacy of Aquacel- Ag Hydrofiber- dressing versus petrolatum gauze with antibiotic ointment in partial-thickness burns in a pediatric burn center. *Journal of Burn Care and Research, 30*(3), 380–385. doi:10.1097/BCR.0b013e3181a2898f

Saffle, J., & the Evidence-Based Guidelines Group, American Burn Association. (2001). Practice guidelines for burn care. *Official Publication of the American Burn Association. Journal of Burn Care & Rehabilitation.* Retrieved from http://www.ameriburn.org/PracticeGuidelines2001.pdf

Schueler, S. J., Beckett, J. H., & Gettings, S. (2010, November 8). Dog bites: Tetanus. http://www.freemd.com/dog-bites/treatment-tetanus.htm

Sexton, D. (2011, March 16). Clinical manifestations and diagnosis of Rocky Mountain spotted fever. In Up to Date. Retrieved from http://www.uptodate.com/contents/clinical-manifestations-and- diagnosis-of-rocky-mountain-spotted-fever?source=search_result& search=rmsf&selectedTitle=1~43

Shapiro, E. D. (2012, October). Lyme disease: Clinical manifestations in children. In Up to Date. Retrieved from http://www.uptodate.com/ contents/lyme-disease-clinical-manifestations-in-children?source= search_result&search=lyme&selectedTitle=5~150

Sheridan, R. L., Petras, L., Basha, G., Salvo, P., Cifrino, C., Hinson, M., et al. (1995, Nov–Dec). Planimetry study of the percent of body surface represented by the hand and palm: Sizing irregular burns is more accurately done with the palm. *Journal of Burn Care & Rehabilitation, 16*(6), 605–606.

Shores, J. T., Gabriel, A., & Gupta, S. (2007). Skin substitutes and alternatives: A review. *Advances in Skin and Wound Care, 20*(9), 493–508. Retrieved from http://www.nursingcenter.com/prodev/cearticleprint .asp?CE_ID=742183

Smith & Nephew Acticoat™ Antimicrobial Barrier Dressing Silcryst. (2014). Acticoat antimicrobial dressing. Retrieved from http://www .acticoat.com

Spencer, E. H., Ferdowsian, H. R., & Barnard, N. D. (2009). Diet and acne: A review of the evidence. *International Journal of Dermatology, 48*(4), 339.

Thomas, C. R., Blakeney, P., Holzer, C. E., & Meyer, III, W. J. (2009). Psychiatric disorders in long-term adjustment of at-risk adolescent burn survivors. *Journal of Burn Care and Research, 30*(3), 458–463. doi:10.1097/BCR.0b013e3181a28c36

Thorne, C., Chung, K., Gosain, A., Gurtner, G., Mehrara, B., Rubin, J., et al. (2014). *Grabb and Smith's plastic surgery* (7th ed.). Minneapolis, MN: Wolters Kluwer.

Torpy, J. M. (2011). Frostbite. *JAMA, 306*(23), 2633. doi:10.1001/ jama.2011.1799

Ülkür, E., Oncul, O., Karagoz, H., Yeniz, E., & Celikoz, B. (2005). Comparison of silver-coated dressing (acticoat), chlorhexidine acetate 0.5% (Bactigrass), and fusidic acid 2% (Fucidin) for topical antibacterial effect in methicillin-resistant Staphylococci-contaminated wounds [Electronic Version]. *Burns, 31*(7), 874–877.

Usatine, R. P., & Riojas, M. (2010). Diagnosis and management of contact dermatitis. *American Family Physician, 82,* 249–255.

Usatine, R. P., & Tinitigan, R. (2010). Nongenital herpes simplex virus. *American Family Physician, 82*(9), 1075–1082.

Vallerand, A. H., & Sanoski, C. A. (2014). *Davis's drug guide for nurses* (14th ed.). Philadelphia, PA: F.A. Davis.

Van Leeuwen, A. M., Poelhuis-Leth, D. J., & Bladh, M. L. (2011). *Davis's comprehensive handbook of laboratory and diagnostic tests*. Philadelphia, PA: F.A. Davis.

Van Wagoner, N. J., & Hook III, E. W. (2012). Herpes diagnostic tests and their use. *Current Infectious Disease Report, 14,* 175–184.

Venes, D. (Ed.). (2013). *Taber's cyclopedic medical dictionary* (22nd ed.). Philadelphia, PA: F.A. Davis.

Vermeulen, M. J., Verbakel, H., Notermans, D. W., Reimerink, J. H., & Peeters, M. F. (2010, March). Evaluation of sensitivity, specificity and cross-reactivity in Bartonella henselae serology. *Journal of Medical Microbiology, 59,* 743–745.

Walter, B., Heukelbach, J., Fengler, G., Worth, C., Hengge, U., & Feldmeier, H. (2011). Comparison of dermoscopy, skin scraping, and the adhesive tape test for the diagnosis of scabies in a resource-poor setting. *Archives of Dermatology, 147*(4), 468.

Wondergem, F. (2010, July/August). Napkin dermatitis and its treatment. *Journal of Community Nursing, 24*(4), 21–26.

World Health Organization (WHO). (2011, September). Rabies: Fact sheet. Retrieved from http://www.who.int/mediacentre/factsheets/fs099/en/

CONCEPT MAP

Caring of the Child With an Integumentary Condition

Nursing:
- Assess bite area
- Assess for systemic reaction → necrosis, anaphylaxis
- Tread local symptoms
- Cover area
- Prevent complications: cellulitis, tetanus, other infections
- Teach: repellants, approach to animals

Bites/Stings:
- Insect
- Animal
- Human

- Lyme disease
- Rocky Mtn. Spotted Fever
- Cat scratch disease
- Rabies

Infestations:
- Head lice
- Scabies

Nursing:
- ID risk factors → quarters, socioeconomic status
- Total body assessment
- Complete treatment of:
  – Family
  – Environment
  – Community
- Non-judgemental attitude key

Hypersensitvity Skin Reactions:
Dermatitis:
- Atopic
- Contact
- Seborrheic
Cutaneous:
- Exanthema
- Urticarial
- Blistering
- Pustular

Other:
- Hypothermia
- Frostbite
- Pressure ulcers

Nursing Insight:
- Use proper terms for skin conditions
- Infants lose heat rapidly due to having little subcutaneous fat
- Adolescents with excess sebum experience more acne
- Be aware of acne meds that cause photosensitivity; assess liver enzymes every month when on Accutane
- Not all children having molluscum contagiosum receive aggressive treatment due to potential scarring
- Must differentiate between oral thrush and residual breast milk
- Use of patch test can determine an allergy
- Spider bites can result in anaphylaxis
- Lyme disease results from tick bite → prevalent in high-tick areas
- Fasciotomy may be needed in treatment of circumferential burn
- Monitor hourly urine output during burn treatment
- Hypothermia is associated with near drowning

Burns:
- Severity of burns determined by →

Type:
- Thermal
- Radiation
- Chemical
- Electrical

Depth (i.e., Thickness):
- Superficial
- Superficial partial
- Deep partial
- Full

Size/Extent:
- Using TBSA
- Using Lund and Browder chart

Skin Lesions:
- Primary:
  – Macules, papules, tumors, pustules, wheals, bullae
  – Secondary → due to changes in primary
  – Crusts, scars, scales, fissures, keloids, ulcers

Skin Infections:
- Bacterial
  – Acne, impetigo, MRSA, cellulitis
- Viral
  – Molluscum contagiosum, HPV, HSV-1
- Fungal
  – Cutaneous candidiasis, tinea capitus/corporis/cruris/pedis

Nursing:
- ID allergen/irritant
- Use drying agent/cool baths
- Topical/oral meds
- Maintain skin integrity
- Assist with self-image issues

Clinical Alert:
- Strep-A can cause necrotizing fascitis
- There is an Epi-Pen Jr. for children having allergic responses
- Nits on eyelashes may be a sign of child sexual abuse
- Post–animal bite: essential to determine if animal is rabid; animal bites are reportable injuries
- Wear Medic-Alert if child has had a severe insect bite reaction
- Respiratory arrest can occur after a chemical burn
- Have emergency equipment nearby if child is intubated
- Core body temp below 95°F (35°C) = life-threatening emergency
- Wet clothing can potentiate hypothermia

Burn Phases:
- Burn shock/resuscitation
- Recovery/wound healing
- Rehabilitation

Nursing:
- Identify lesion/organism
- Maintain clean, intact skin
- Monitor exudate
- Use good hand washing
- Control itching
- Thoroughly cleanse environmental transmission items
- Prevent spread/self-innoculation
- Treat sequelor
- Teach about mouth rinse for inhaled steroids
- Instruct re: need for frequent diaper changes

Nursing—Moderate to Major Burns:
- Emergent: CAB
- Assess burn → characteristics/category
- Fluid resuscitation → Parkland formula
- Prevent infection sepsis, pneumonia
- Maintain circulation to injured extremity
- Promote adequate nutrition
- Pain management: IV opioids
- Wound care: debridement, escharotomy, cleansing
- Grafting

Focus on Safety:
- Qwell shampoo can cause neurotoxicity
- Permetherin cream not for use in those with chrysanthemum allergy
- Insect repellent with oil of lemon eucalyptus should not be used in children under 3 yrs old
- Use anticipatory guidance when teaching about burn prevention

Family Teaching Guidelines:
- Caring for child with cellulitis
- Decreasing transmission/preventing outbreaks of HSV-1
- How to assess for/prevent spread of head lice

What to Say:
- Assessing acne in adolescents
- Teach child and caregiver about impetigo
- How to prevent animal bites
- Gathering important information about a burn injury

Complementary Care:
- Duct tape for wart resolution
- Topical agents for rashes: bag balm, aloe vera, vitamin E preps, diaper rash creams
- Distraction: good technique during burn dressing changes

Collaboration in Caring:
- For child with severe allergy: teach all in the community use of Epi-Pen
- A team approach needed to care for the severely burned child

Legal Alert:
- Accutane acne treatment can cause birth defects; inform child-bearing women
- Assess child with burn injuries for possibility of neglect/abuse

Cultural Diversity:
- Treatment for acne should be specific to skin type of culture
- African Americans have a lower incidence of head lice
- Be aware of culturally specific burn treatments
- In pigmented skin, pressure ulcers can blanche red/purple

Across Care Settings:
- Burn centers treat both adults and children
- Community support needed for child during treatment for HSV-1

Now Can You:
- Name at least four conditions affecting the skin and state priority interventions for each
- Identify the components of holistic, evidence-based, patient-centered nursing care for the child with an integumentary condition

Caring for the Child With a Genitourinary Condition

 "He who has health, has hope and he who has hope, has everything."

—Arabian Proverb

LEARNING TARGETS *At the completion of this chapter, the student will be able to:*

- ◆ Describe the anatomy and physiology of the genitourinary system.
- ◆ Examine common conditions of the genitourinary system.
- ◆ Prioritize developmentally appropriate and holistic nursing care measures for common conditions of the genitourinary system.
- ◆ Explore diagnostic testing, laboratory testing, and medications for common conditions of the genitourinary system.
- ◆ Develop teaching plans and discharge criteria for parents whose children have common genitourinary conditions.

PICO(T) Questions

The intent of evidence-based practice (EBP) is to provide nursing care that integrates the best available evidence. An initial step in EBP is to write a PICO(T) question that effectively guides the research. A PICO(T) question is an acronym that stands for population (P), intervention or issue (I), comparison of interest (C), outcome (O), and timeframe (T). Depending on the question, all or some of the question components are used

in the research process. Use these PICO(T) questions to spark your thinking as you read the chapter.

1. Is there a (O) higher incidence of (I) enuresis in (P) children where one or both parents also had enuresis?

2. Does (I) the use of moist cleansing wipes after urination (O) lower the rate of urinary tract infections (P) in adolescent girls (C) compared with the use of toilet paper?

 Evidence-Based Practice

Zelikovsky, N., Dobson, T., & Norman, J. (2011). Medication beliefs and perceived barriers in adolescent renal transplant patients and their parents. *Pediatric Nephrology, 26,* 951–959. doi:1007/s00467-011-1805-1

The purpose of this study was to examine the beliefs of adolescents who have undergone kidney transplants and their parents regarding medication and perceived barriers related to taking medications. Kidney transplant is a cost-effective way to eliminate dialysis and provide the best opportunities for healthy growth and development in children who have experienced end-stage renal disease. This also reduces family conflict, improves academic functioning, and improves health-related quality of life, though it requires a lifetime of compliance to a daily medication regimen of immunosuppressant therapy. The authors noted a limited availability of research

that explores the beliefs of adolescents who have experienced transplantation for chronic disease. Research regarding the perception of adult mediation challenges note that benefits generally outweigh barriers; chronically ill patients express concerns about negative side effects and the long-term impact of medication use. The authors also stated that one study exploring the belief of pediatric transplant patients noted patients understood that their health depended on following the medication regimen. Previous studies have expressed the concern of parents regarding the side effects of long-term medication use. Regardless of the type of chronic illness,

Evidence-Based Practice (continued)

common concerns include cognitive factors (forgetting, difficulty with a complex regimen, and time management) and lifestyle changes (interference with activities, being away from home, and routine changes) as well as concern with psychosocial factors and family issues (i.e., conflict, lack of support, peer pressure, and behavioral issues).

Participants in this study were recruited from a pediatric kidney transplant program in one northeastern state. Potential candidates were selected from a transplant list. Criteria for participation included being between the ages of 13 and 20, having a functioning kidney transplant, and taking immunosuppressant medications. Patients who did not speak English proficiently and those with a cognitive delay were excluded. Those who met the criteria were contacted during regular clinic appointments to determine willingness to participate. Those agreeing to participate completed a demographic questionnaire, which included questions about age, race/ethnicity, parent education, family income, family size, and number of children living at home. Data were collected regarding patient and parent perception of mediation barriers through the use of two tools, both of which had proven reliability and validity. The Adolescent Medication Barriers Scale (AMBS)/Parent Mediation Barriers Scale (PMBS) were used to determine perceived barriers. The surveys included 17 and 16 items respectively and were rated using a Likert scale. A 10-item Beliefs about Medications Questionnaire (BMQ) was also administered. The focus of this questionnaire included exploring the necessity for taking the medication and concerns about side effects.

Forty adolescents and their parents were included in the study. The mean age of the participants was 16.5 years, ranged from 13 to 20, and included 20 males and 20 females. The race/ethnicity of the participants included Caucasians 67.5%, African Americans 17.5%, Hispanics 7.5%, Asians 2.5%, American Indians 2.5%, and Biracial 2.5%. The mean income of the families was $61,000 and ranged from $11,000 to $191,000. Four or fewer family members were found in 62.5% of the participants, and 37.5% had 5 to 8 members. This was further delineated by the number of children in the families (i.e., 72.5% had 2 or fewer children, and 27.5% had 3 to 6 children). A minimum of a high school education or GED was found in 27.5% of the mothers, 32.5% had some additional training or college courses, 20% had obtained a college degree, and 20% had a graduate or professional degree. Of the fathers, 5.1% had not graduated from high school, 38.5% had completed high school or had a GED, 23.1% had partial additional training or college courses, 17.9% had a college degree, and 15.4% had a graduate or professional degree.

Data were analyzed using a one-way analysis of variance (ANOVA) and t-tests. Beliefs about medications and barriers were examined in relation to various demographics (i.e., patient age, parent education, income, and family size). The biggest concerns expressed by younger adolescents (ages 13–16) were in relation to forgetting to take mediation, scheduling the medication, and the potential impairments or side effects from taking the medication. No significant differences were noted in the parents' perception of barriers and beliefs about medications in relation to the age of their child, ethnicity, gender, or parental education. Though results were not statistically significant, the researchers note that the rating of perceived barriers increased in relation to a larger family size as evident by more concern with adolescent frustrations (e.g., not wanting to have others see him or her take medications, mediations getting in the way of activities, changes in appearance, and tired of taking medications) and the need for parents to remind the adolescent to take his or her medication. Significance was noted between parents' income levels, their need to remind the adolescent to take the medications, and adolescents' concern with medication harmfulness. The researchers noted that families in low (less than $30,000) and high (greater than or equal to $100,000) income brackets expressed more concern than those in a middle ($31,000–99,000) income bracket. Adolescents also expressed greater concern than parents over issues such as swallowing as well as taste and number of medications needed. Parents expressed more concern over the need to take medication to maintain health than did the adolescents.

The researchers conclude that younger adolescents had a greater number of concerns over taking medication than did older adolescents. Concerns included forgetfulness, organization, and scheduling. The researchers suggested that this may be related to the fact that parents are more likely involved in managing the child's regimen at this age, hence leading to more adolescent dependency and less confidence as well as the possibility that less information is retained by children during the clinic visits. They further noted that the significance of income level may be related to the availability of resources and necessity to work with the lower income families and with the possibility of both parents working in high-demanding jobs and having less time at home with the higher income level families.

1. How is this information useful to clinical nursing practice?

2. Based on these findings, what are implications for further research?

See Suggested Responses for Evidence-Based Practice on Davis*Plus*.

Introduction

This chapter provides a short review of the anatomy and physiology of the genitourinary system, as well as fluid and electrolyte balance, followed by a discussion of a variety of renal and reproductive problems. The discussion includes an examination of the various genitourinary conditions, including developmentally appropriate and holistic nursing care. Information about diagnostic and laboratory testing and medications is given. Teaching plans and discharge criteria for parents whose children have various genitourinary conditions are incorporated. Genitourinary conditions vary from hereditary anomalies to infectious diseases and sometimes traumatic injuries. These types of conditions occur in both genders throughout childhood, ranging from the newborn period through adolescence. Nurses must have the requisite knowledge about the genitourinary system and knowledge about the factors that affect its functions, which then help them provide safe and competent nursing care.

CARING FOR THE CHILD WITH A GENITOURINARY CONDITION

A & P review The Kidneys

The kidney is divided into an outer cortex and inner medulla (Fig. 31-1). The outer cortex is composed of the glomeruli and convoluted tubules of the nephron and blood vessels. The medulla is composed of the renal pyramid. Urine leaves the papilla of a pyramid to collect in a minor calyx. The minor calyces come together to make the major calyces and then the renal pelvis.

Each kidney is surrounded by adipose tissue to protect it from trauma, although kidneys can be injured by blows to the abdomen and such trauma as often occurs in motor vehicle accidents. Kidneys receive their blood supply through a single renal artery that comes from each side of the aorta, one to each kidney. The renal artery subdivides into five segmental arteries that feed each kidney. Each segmental artery further subdivides into multiple branches several times; the smallest of these are the afferent arterioles, which feed the glomeruli.

The glomerulus is a tuft of capillaries in a thin-walled capsule termed Bowman's capsule. While blood flows into the glomerulus through the afferent arteriole, it leaves through the efferent arteriole. Fluid and blood particles are filtered through capillary membranes into a fluid-filled space in Bowman's capsule. The filtered blood is termed the filtrate.

The tubular components of the nephron are divided into four parts. The first part is a coiled portion termed the proximal convoluted tubule, and this drains Bowman's capsule. The second part is a thin loop termed the loop of Henle, while the third part is the distal convoluted tubule. The fourth and final part is the collecting tubule, which joins several tubules together to collect filtrate. About 85% of the nephrons are cortical nephrons, so termed because they are on the superficial portion of the cortex. The remaining 15% of the nephrons penetrate deeper into the medulla and are involved with urine concentration.

Functions of the kidney include removal of waste products, filtering the blood, maintaining fluid and electrolyte

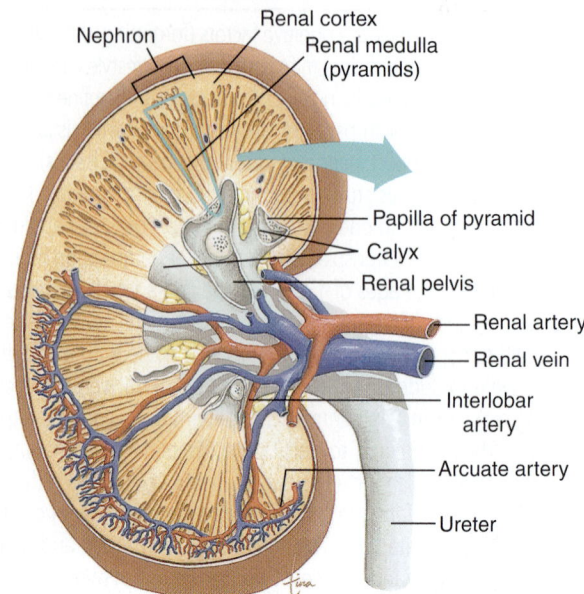

The Kidney

Figure 31-1 Anatomy of the kidney.

balance (e.g., sodium, potassium, calcium and phosphorus), maintaining acid-base balance, and releasing hormones:

- Renin: blood pressure regulation
- Calcitriol: Vitamin D activation for healthy bones
- Erythropoietin: red blood cell production

Monitoring kidney function includes:

- Glomerular filtration rate (GFR)
  - Amount of blood filtered by the glomeruli
  - 125 mL/minute
- Creatinine clearance (reflects GFR)
  - 85 to 135 mL/min
- Creatinine
  - 0.5 to 1.5 mg/dL
- BUN
  - 10 to 30 mg/dL
- Urine specific gravity
- UA (no protein, blood) ◆

Fluid and Electrolyte Balance

Children are at a greater risk for fluid and electrolyte imbalance than adults because they have a proportionately greater amount of body water, require more fluid intake, and subsequently excrete more fluid. Fluid balance implies that the liquid in the body is regulated in such a way as to maintain homeostasis (a state of equilibrium). The body's intake and output of fluid in a 24-hour period is approximately the same. A fluid deficit occurs when fluids are lost by diaphoresis, vomiting, diarrhea, or hemorrhage. A fluid overload occurs from conditions that create impaired fluid excretion, such as kidney disease or congestive heart failure. Fluid overload also can occur because of excessive administration of IV fluids (Venes, 2013). Fluid balance is measured by daily discrepancies in body weight and by monitoring fluid intake and output.

Growth and Development

The child with a genitourinary condition may experience alterations in mastery of growth and developmental milestones such as potty training. Conditions such as hypospadias, ambiguous genitalia, and renal and bladder disorders predispose the child to alterations in elimination. Disturbances in elimination or surgical repair of the genitourinary system can have a negative impact on growth and development. The nurse should provide education to the family and the child about surgical repair and other treatments as appropriate to avoid disturbances in growth and development. If the child is having alterations with elimination because of the genitourinary condition, the nurse should encourage coping and acceptance of the disease process. Problems with the "private parts" can be embarrassing and emotional for the child. The nurse should provide appropriate psychosocial and emotional support to the parents and the child. The nurse should explore for feelings of guilt or blame and refer to a counselor if needed.

Source: Ward S., & Hisley, S. (2009). *Maternal-child nursing care: Optimizing outcomes for mothers, children & families.* Philadelphia, PA: F.A. Davis.

Nursing Insight—*Fluid measurements in ounces and millimeter equivalents*

Ounces	Milliliters
0.25	7.5
0.50	15
1.0	30
2.0	60
3.0	90
4.0	120
5.0	150
6.0	180
7.0	210
8.0	240
9.0	270
10.0	300
11.0	330
12.0	360
13.0	390
14.0	420
15.0	450

(Ward, 2013)

focus on safety

Calculation of daily maintenance fluid requirements for intake and output

To determine fluid maintenance for intake use:

Body surface area for children greater than 22 lb (10 kg): 1,500 to 2,000 mL/m2 per day.

OR

Child's Weight	Daily Maintenance Fluid Requirement
0–10 kg (0–22 lb)	100 mL/kg of body weight
11–20 kg (24.2–44 lb)	1,000 mL + 50 mL/kg for each kg >10
>20 kg (>44 lb)	1,500 mL + 20 mL/kg for each kg >20

To determine fluid maintenance for output use:

Infant 2 to 3 L/kg per hour

Toddler/Preschooler 2 mL/kg per hour

School age 1 to 2 mL/kg per hour

Adolescent 0.5 to 1 mL/kg per hour

(Ward, 2013)

Nursing Insight—*Risk for fluid and electrolyte imbalance*

Children are at a greater risk than adults for fluid and electrolyte imbalance because children have:

- A greater body surface area
- A higher percentage of total body water (the volume of total body water decreases with increasing age)
- A greater potential for fluid loss via the gastrointestinal tract and skin

- An increased incidence of fever, upper respiratory infections, and gastroenteritis
- A greater metabolic rate
- Immature kidneys that are inefficient at excreting waste products
- Kidneys that have a decreased ability to concentrate urine
- Increased risk for developing hypernatremia based on their inability to verbalize thirst

The body is continually losing water in urine and stool and by evaporation from the skin and lungs. If the child is not taking in enough fluids to make up for the amount lost, he or she can become dehydrated. Dehydration occurs when the amount of fluids leaving the body is greater than the amount of fluids being taken into the body.

TYPES OF DEHYDRATION

Depending on the cause of the fluid loss, a child will lose water and electrolytes.

Dehydration is classified as isotonic, hypotonic, or hypertonic.

Isotonic dehydration occurs when electrolyte and water deficits are present in balanced proportions (sodium and water are lost in equal amounts). Serum sodium remains in normal limits (130–150 mEq/L). This is the most common type of dehydration. Hypovolemic shock is the greatest concern.

Hypotonic dehydration occurs when the electrolyte deficit exceeds the water deficit. Serum sodium concentration is less than 130 mEq/L. Physical signs are more severe with smaller fluid losses.

Hypertonic dehydration is the most dangerous type and occurs when water loss is in excess of electrolyte loss. Sodium serum concentration is greater than 150 mEq/L. Seizures are likely to occur.

Assessment is a priority nursing action when caring for the child with a fluid and/or electrolyte imbalance. The astute nurse must recognize fluid deficit and excess as well as electrolyte imbalance and then provide the proper care. Sometimes emergent care is required when IV replacement of fluids and electrolytes is essential.

Nursing Insight—*Fluid deficit and excess*

Fluid deficit (to determine normal values use calculation of daily maintenance fluid requirements)

Causes	Signs and Symptoms	Nursing Care Measures
Diminished fluid intake	Dry skin	Determine underlying cause
Diaphoresis	Dry mucous membranes	Replace fluids
Vomiting Diarrhea	Poor skin turgor Thirst Scaphoid abdomen	Replace electrolytes Oral hydration
Nasogastric suction	Poor perfusion	IV hydration

Fever	Decreased urinary output	Measure intake and output
Hemorrhage	Weight loss	Monitor vital signs
General fluid deficit	Fatigue	Monitor laboratory values (electrolytes)
	Tachycardia	
	Tachypnea	Nursing care measures listed
	Decreased blood pressure	
	High urine specific gravity	
	High hematocrit	

Fluid excess (to determine normal values use calculation of daily maintenance fluid requirements)

Causes	Signs and Symptoms	Nursing Care Measures
Excessive oral intake	Pulmonary edema (crackles)	Determine underlying cause
Hypotonic fluid overload	Weight gain (fluid retention)	Decrease fluid intake
Kidney disease	Lethargy	Administer diuretics
All causes	Decreased level of consciousness	Monitor vital signs
	Slow, bounding pulse	Monitor laboratory values (electrolytes)
	Low urine specific gravity	Nursing care measures listed
	Decreased hematocrit	

Pathophysiology of Dehydration

In the early phases of dehydration, fluids with some electrolytes are lost from the extracellular fluid. If the fluid loss continues, loss of the intracellular fluid can occur. Hypovolemic shock occurs when there is an insufficient amount of fluid in the circulatory system, and subsequent death can result (Fig. 31-2).

The main electrolytes are sodium (the primary electrolyte of the extracellular fluid) and potassium (the primary electrolyte of the intracellular fluid). These electrolytes keep the body in balance by maintaining muscle contraction, heart rhythm, and brain function. Normal values for sodium are 130 to 150 mEq/L, and potassium values are 3.5 to 5.5 mEq/L. An imbalance in one or both of these electrolytes can cause illness in children. Calcium imbalance can also pose problems for children. The normal value for calcium is 8.8 to 10.8 mEq/L.

 Nursing Insight—*Electrolyte imbalance*

Sodium (Na⁺) deficit (hyponatremia; serum sodium concentration <130 mEq/L)

Causes	Signs and Symptoms	Nursing Care Measures
Decreased sodium intake	Dehydration	Determine underlying cause
Excessive sweating	Nausea	Determine underlying cause

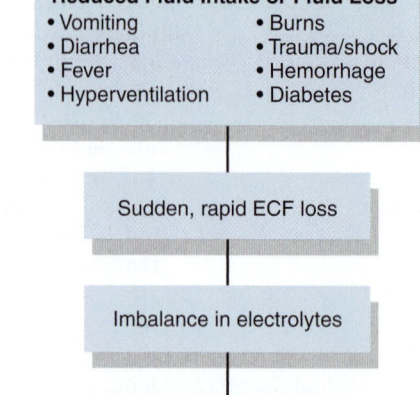

Pathophysiology of Dehydration

Reduced Fluid Intake or Fluid Loss
- Vomiting
- Diarrhea
- Fever
- Hyperventilation
- Burns
- Trauma/shock
- Hemorrhage
- Diabetes

Sudden, rapid ECF loss

Imbalance in electrolytes

Loss of ICF

Cellular dysfunction

Hypovolemic shock

Death

Figure 31-2 Pathophysiology of dehydration.

Fever	Weakness	Administer IV fluids with the appropriate amount of sodium added
Malnutrition	Lethargy	Monitor laboratory values (electrolytes)
Vomiting	Abdominal cramping	Determine underlying cause
Diarrhea	Dizziness	Determine underlying cause
Nasogastric suction	Weak pulse	Measure output and calculate fluid requirements
Diabetic ketoacidosis	Decreased blood pressure	Contact health-care provider for specific orders
Kidney disease	Hematuria, tea or red-colored urine	Contact health-care provider for specific orders

Sodium (Na⁺) excess (hypernatremia; serum sodium concentration ≥145 mEq/L)

Causes	Signs and Symptoms	Nursing Care Measures
Excessive salt intake	Oliguria	Determine underlying cause

Fever	Nausea	Monitor neurological status
High insensible water loss	Vomiting	Monitor laboratory values (electrolytes)
Diabetes insipidus	Muscle twitching	Administer desmopressin (DDAVP) per health-care provider order
Hyperglycemia	Lethargy	Contact health-care provider for specific orders
Kidney disease	Vomiting Encephalopathy Overload of fluid in the lungs	Contact health-care provider for specific orders

Potassium (K⁺) deficit (hypokalemia; serum potassium concentration ≤3.5 mEq/L)

Causes	Signs and Symptoms	Nursing Care Measures
Diuresis	Muscle weakness	Determine underlying cause
Starvation	Muscle cramping and stiffness	Monitor vital signs
IV fluid without potassium added	Hypotension	Offer high-potassium foods
Diarrhea	Hyporeflexia	Administer oral potassium supplements (assess for adequate output before administration)
Vomiting	Cardiac arrhythmias (tachycardia or bradycardia)	Administer IV potassium based on health-care provider's order
Nasogastric suction	Fatigue	Obtain electrocardiogram (ECG) (for IV potassium bolus)
Administration of diuretics or corticosteroids	Drowsiness	Monitor laboratory values (electrolytes)
Burns that are healing		Evaluate acid-base status
Metabolic alkalosis	Apnea Cyanosis Nausea Vomiting Diarrhea	Contact health-care provider for specific orders

Potassium (K⁺) excess (hyperkalemia; serum potassium concentration ≥5.5 mEq/L)

Causes	Signs and Symptoms	Nursing Care Measures
Increased intake of potassium	Muscle twitching	Determine underlying cause

Severe dehydration	Muscle weakness	Monitor vital signs
	Flaccid paralysis	Obtain ECG
Rapid administration of IV potassium chloride	Hyperreflexia	Administer IV fluids as ordered
Potassium-sparing diuretics	Oliguria	Administer IV insulin to facilitate potassium moving into cells (if ordered)
Burns	Apnea (respiratory arrest)	Monitor laboratory values (electrolytes)
Kidney disease (failure)	Bradycardia	Evaluate acid-base status
Adrenal insufficiency (Addison's disease)	Ventricular fibrillation (cardiac arrest)	Begin cardiopulmonary resuscitation
Metabolic acidosis	Rapid breathing Confusion Lethargy Severe metabolic acidosis that can lead to shock or death	Contact health-care provider for specific orders

Calcium (Ca²⁺) deficit (hypocalcemia; serum calcium concentration <8.8 mEq/L)

Causes	Signs and Symptoms	Nursing Care Measures
Inadequate dietary intake	Tetany	Determine underlying cause
Vitamin D deficiency	Convulsions	Administer oral calcium supplement as prescribed
Feeding cow's milk to infants	Neuromuscular irritability	Administer IV calcium slowly and monitor IV site for irritation
Adrenal insufficiency	Tiredness Weakness Dizziness Nausea Vomiting Diarrhea Loss of appetite Stomachache Joint aches and pains	Monitor laboratory values (electrolytes)

Calcium (Ca²⁺) excess (hypercalcemia; serum calcium concentration >10.8 mEq/L)

Causes	Signs and Symptoms	Nursing Care Measures
Excessive vitamin D intake	Weakness	Determine underlying cause
Acidosis	Fatigue	Obtain ECG

Immobilization (prolonged periods of time)	Constipation	Monitor laboratory values (electrolytes)
Increased bone catabolism	Anorexia	Contact health-care provider for specific orders
Hyperthyroidism	Nausea	Contact health-care provider for specific orders
Kidney disease	Vomiting Thirst Bradycardia (cardiac arrest)	Contact health-care provider for specific orders

Nursing care for fluid and electrolyte imbalances centers on recognizing the underlying causes of dehydration and electrolyte imbalance and then replacing water loss and electrolytes. Another nursing care measure is education. Explain to parents the signs and symptoms of dehydration and the importance of offering clear liquids.

 Critical Nursing Action Fluid and Electrolyte Imbalance Nursing Interventions

Nursing interventions for fluid and electrolyte imbalance include:

- Obtain daily weights (same scale, same time, and wearing the same clothing) (infants are weighed naked and often older children are weighed only in their underwear).
- Measure intake and output (weigh diapers to assess output).
- Assess hydration status, which includes assessing for presence of tears, skin turgor, anterior fontanelle (up to 18 months), sticky mucous membranes, sunken eyeballs, urine and stool output, weight loss, tachycardia, tachypnea, decreased blood pressure, temperature, and thirst.
- Obtain laboratory tests including specific gravity, hematocrit, blood urea nitrogen, creatinine, Na+, K+, and Ca++.
- Assess the type of acid-base disturbance (metabolic acidosis, metabolic alkalosis, or respiratory acidosis).
- Administer oral clear liquids as ordered (1–2 oz every hour).
- Start an IV for fluid and electrolyte replacement as ordered by the health-care provider.
- Before administering IV potassium (K+), ensure the child has voided (to prevent tubular necrosis).
- Cleanse perineal area and apply protective topical ointment.

Encourage the parents to be involved in the care of child.

- Educate the parents about signs and symptoms of dehydration, rehydration, and when to call the health-care provider.
- Encourage parents to be compliant with follow-up appointment(s).

 Critical Nursing Action Assessing Peripheral IV Infiltration

Peripheral IV infiltration occurs when the IV catheter moves out of the vein and the administered fluid then enters the surrounding tissue. Assessing the peripheral IV site every 4 hours is a critical nursing action. Use the Pediatric Peripheral IV Infiltration scale to watch for peripheral IV infiltration:

Grade 0
- No symptoms
- Flushes with ease

Grade 1
- Localized swelling (1%–10%)
- Flushes with difficulty
- Pain at the site

Grade 2
- Slight swelling at the site (up to ¼ of the extremity above or below site, or 25%–50% of the extremity above or below site)
- Presence of redness
- Pain at the site

Grade 3
- Moderate swelling at the site (¼ to ½ of the extremity above or below site, or 25%–50% of the extremity above or below site)
- Pain at the site
- Skin cool to touch
- Blanching
- Diminished pulse below site

Grade 4
- Severe swelling at the site (more than ½ of the extremity above or below site, or more than 50% of the extremity above or below site)
- Infiltration of blood products, irritants, and/or vesicants (any amount of swelling)
- Skin cool to touch
- Skin breakdown/necrosis
- Blistering
- Diminished or absent pulse
- Pain at site
- Capillary refill greater than 4 seconds

Sources: Pop, S. (2012); Children's Hospital; Medical Center Dallas, Dallas, TX.

If peripheral IV infiltration occurs, stop the infusion immediately. Helpful nursing measures are elevating the extremity, applying warm packs, and using a compression dressing. For more advanced infiltrations, Bacitracin (Baciguent) is applied topically, and the site is covered with a dressing. Call the health-care provider for medical orders in severe situations. Reassess the site frequently and accurately document the site as well as nursing care measures.

Common Disorders of the Urinary System

In addition to a physical assessment and history, a urinalysis provides data for assessment of common disorders of the urinary system. Table 31-1 presents normal urinalysis data.

URINARY TRACT INFECTIONS

An acquired infection of the urinary system caused by a bacterium, virus, or fungus is referred to as a **urinary tract infection** (UTI). Most often, UTIs are ascending and start distally, at the urethral area, causing urethritis or cystitis. If they start in the upper tract, they cause ureteritis and pyelitis, or pyelonephritis (Kliegman, Stanton, St. Geme, Schorr, & Behrman, 2011). The probability of an ascending UTI depends on the virulence of the organism and the status of health and immunity of the child (McInerny, Adam, Campbell, Kamat, Kelleher, & Hoekelman, 2009). The most common organism noted with UTI is *Escherichia coli* (Burns, Dunn, Brady, Starr, & Blosser, 2009; Feld & Mattoo, 2010).

Gender, age, race, renal tissue, poor hygiene, constipation, nutritional status, and adaptive and resistant qualities of the causative agents as well as structural abnormalities,

Table 31-1 Normal Urinalysis	
Urinalysis	**Normal Values**
Appearance	Clear
Color	Amber yellow
Odor	Aromatic
pH	4.6–8.0 (average 6.0)
Osmolarity	50–1,400 mOsm/L
Protein	None or up to 8 mg/dL 50–80 mg/24 hr (at rest) <250 mg/24 hr (exercise)
Specific gravity	Adult: 1.005–1.030 (usually 1.010–1.025) Elderly: values decrease with age Newborn: 1.001–1.020
Leukocyte esterase	Negative
Nitrites	Negative
Ketones	Negative
Crystals	Negative
Casts	None present
Glucose	Brand new specimen: negative 24-hour specimen: 50–300 mg/day or 0.3–1.7 mmol/day (SI units)
White blood cells (WBCs)	<5/hpf
WBC casts	Negative
Red blood cells (RBCs)	<5/hpf
RBC casts	None

catheterization, urinary tract instrumentation, and sexual activity all contribute to the incidence and etiology of this disease (Burns et al., 2009). Constipation results in incomplete bladder emptying, resulting in residual urine in the bladder, which reduces the innate defense of the child.

Newborns, particularly if born prematurely, or infants with a low birth weight have a higher incidence of UTIs. In girls, UTIs peak during infancy and during toilet training, and uncircumcised boys have a greater risk of contracting UTIs (Kliegman et al., 2011).

 Nursing Insight—*Risk factor for UTIs*

The most significant risk factor for UTI is the presence of a urinary tract abnormality that causes urinary stasis, obstruction, reflux, or dysfunctional voiding, as in vesicoureteral reflux (VUR) (Axton & Fugate, 2008). **Pyelonephritis** (an infection in the renal pelvis) also contributes to UTI and causes renal scarring with repeated infections. Alterations that interfere with elimination (such as constipation) create a risk for UTIs. Conditions associated with chronic perineal irritation such as poor hygiene, nylon or spandex undergarments, masturbation,

pinworms, diaper rash, sexual activity, sexual abuse, prolonged baths, or bubble baths can cause UTI (Tschudy & Arcara, 2012). Other important associations to consider in UTIs include difficulty with toilet-training, neurogenic bladder, and/or a history of abnormal voiding patterns (Tschudy & Arcara, 2012; Kliegman et al., 2011).

Nursing Insight—*Facts about UTIs*

Facts about UTIs include:
- The higher the infection in the urinary system, the more likelihood of pyelonephritis as opposed to lower (cystitis) (Tschudy & Arcara, 2012).
- Within the first 2 years of life, infections that progress into the renal parenchyma frequently cause scarring, resulting in hypertension and sometimes leading to chronic renal failure (inability of the kidneys to function adequately) (Kliegman et al., 2011).
- There is a high occurrence of UTIs in the newborn period, followed closely by ages 1 to 3 months with the most frequent pathogen as *E coli.* (Burns et al., 2009).
- Group B streptococcal and other blood-borne pathogens are related to newborn UTIs.
- *Enterococcus* and *Pseudomonas* occur more frequently when the child has recurrence of UTI, anatomy that is abnormal, or neurogenic bladder (Tschudy & Arcara, 2012, p. 480).
- Children who are hospitalized or have catheterizations frequently have UTIs, most commonly caused by enterococcus and *Pseudomonas* (Tschudy & Arcara, 2012, p. 480).
- Decrease in the use of indwelling catheters has decreased UTIs.
- When a child has an indwelling catheter, replacement of a new catheter prior to antibiotic therapy reduces frequency of relapse of UTIs (Lerma & Nissenson 2012, p. 343).

Signs and Symptoms

Unique developmental related signs and symptoms accompany UTIs. In the neonate, signs and symptoms include:

- Failure to thrive
- Jaundice
- Hypothermia
- Vomiting or diarrhea
- Cyanosis
- Abdominal distention
- Lethargy
- Sepsis

In the infant, signs and symptoms include:

- Poor feeding
- Fever (especially related to pyelonephritis)
- Vomiting or diarrhea
- Malodor
- Dribbling urine
- Abdominal pain/colic irritability
- Malaise
- Poor weight gain
  (Burns et al., 2009, p. 872)

In the toddler and preschooler, signs and symptoms include:

- Abdominal pain
- Vomiting or diarrhea
- Flank pain
- Fever (especially related to pyelonephritis)
- Malodor
- Altered voiding pattern
- Diaper rash
- Enuresis
- Malaise
  (Gaylord & Starr, 2009, p. 872)

In school-age and adolescent children, signs and symptoms include:

- Enuresis
- Malodor
- Classic dysuria with frequency, urgency, and discomfort
- Fever/chills (especially related to pyelonephritis)
- Abdominal pain
- Flank pain
- Malaise
- Vomiting or diarrhea
  (Burns et al. 2009, p. 872)

Malodor is often noticed by parents with children 1 to 3 years of age with a UTI. However, the malodor in this case is not correlated strongly with a diagnosis of UTI (Gauther, Gouin, Phan, & Gravel, 2012). The ammonia odor of urine is attributed to normal flora breaking down urea.

 ### Nursing Insight—*UTIs in adolescents*

Adolescents can hide the true nature for seeking health care. With the adolescent, it is important in the review of systems to check for the classic symptoms of UTI within the context of the genitourinary system. Symptoms may include "dysuria, urgency, frequency, discharge, and bleeding" (Tschudy & Arcara, 2012).

Diagnosis

An accurate diagnosis determines the treatment and is based on the urine culture and sensitivities (Tschudy & Arcara, 2012). Diagnosis of a UTI includes obtaining a urinary culture that confirms the pathogen and the exact type of bacteria present in the urine. Suprapubic aspiration (SPA) or catheterization with 50,000/mL bacterial growth can also indicate a UTI (McInerny et al., 2009, p. 2610). In infants and children ages 2 to 24 months, researchers found SPA more invasive and painful and the results similar to, but not as effective as, urinary catheterization (Finnell, Carroll, Downs, & the Subcommittee on Urinary Tract Infection, 2011). When a child is intensely ill, however, a catheterization or SPA is the choice in all age groups to detect UTIs (McInerny et al., 2009).

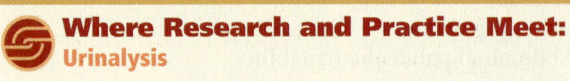 **Where Research and Practice Meet:**
Urinalysis

A urinalysis that is normal does not rule out the presence of a UTI. Therefore, a culture and sensitivity is done if there is any possibility of

a UTI (McInerny et al., 2009). A complete blood count with differential, a test for blood urea nitrogen (BUN), creatinine, and a C-reactive protein is done for the child less than 1 year of age who appears sick or whose symptoms and signs suggest pyelonephritis (Burns et al., 2009, p. 873). In an infant less than 1 year of age who has a fever without a focus or possible sepsis, blood cultures are done (Burns et al., 2009, p. 873). To localize the actual infection, imaging studies are delayed for 3 to 6 weeks after an infection for follow-up. If, however, obstruction is suspected, imaging studies are done immediately.

 ### Diagnostic Tools Determining Problems With the Urinary Tract

There is variance from institutions, and it is best to view the American Academy of Pediatrics Web site for the best possible recommendations for UTIs (Tschudy & Arcara, 2012).

- The AAP recommends that children less than 2 years of age with a first occurrence of UTI should have ultrasonography in the acute phase and cystography or renal cortical scan (McInerny et al., 2009, p. 2612). The renal ultrasound depicts the ureters but does not discern if there is an infection.
- A voiding cystourethrogram (VCUG) depicts urethral and bladder anatomy and is appropriate usually 2 to 6 weeks following an infection (McInerny et al., 2009). Some researchers believe a VCUG should be done after the first febrile UTI. Health-care providers should remember that children who are from a disadvantaged background and who may not have a consistent primary health-care provider may have already had a UTI or febrile infection that was not followed up on (Wan, Skoog, Hulbert, Casale, Greenfield, Cheng, et al., 2012). An IV pyelogram assists with identifying the size, shape, and position of the urinary system as well as elimination function by noting length of time for passage of contrast material through the kidneys.
- Nuclear cystography visualizes the bladder and is good for detecting VUR.
- Nuclear cortical scanning detects tubular damage and scarring.
- A nitrite test is used to assess if urinary gram-negative bacteria (particularly *E coli, Klebsiella,* and *Proteus*) are present.

Prevention

Table 31-2 outlines urinary tract infection risk factors. UTI parents need to teach children to void frequently, wash hands after elimination, wear loose-fitting clothes, and teach girls to wipe from front to back. Cotton underwear for both genders is preferable because it decreases moisture by allowing more aeration than nylon underwear. Finally, constipation, if it is an issue, needs to be prevented. Parents can talk with their health-care provider about best treatment and practices to prevent constipation (National Kidney and Urologic Diseases Information Clearinghouse [NKUDIC], 2011). Tell parents it is also important for the child to drink plenty of water for his or her age to prevent dehydration and enhance the immune system's infection-fighting abilities.

Collaborative Care

Nursing Care. The goals of nursing care are to collaborate with the patient, family, and other health-care providers along the continuum of care needed to diagnose and treat UTIs. With every diagnostic test and medication ordered, the nurse provides developmentally appropriate education for the entire family.

Obtain a history that identifies risk factors, signs and symptoms, medications, and nutritional and fluid intake

Table 31-2 Urinary Tract Infection Risk Factors

- Lack of circumcision in male infants
- Male infants in the first 6 to 8 postnatal months
- Lack of breastfeeding in first 6 postnatal months
- Constipation
- Dysfunctional voiding pattern
- Recent history of antibiotics
- Urinary tract infection in the past 6 months
- Indwelling catheters or intermittent catheterization
- Family history of recurrent urinary tract infection
- Recent sexual intercourse
- Use of a diaphragm for birth control or spermicidal agents

Source: Adapted from Feld & Mattoo (2010).

and output parameters. A nursing assessment is done of the external genitalia, noting irritation, pinworms, sexual abuse, or trauma (Kliegman et al., 2011). Also, for girls, inspect the perineal area for redness, edema, discharge, labial adhesions, and vaginitis. In males that are not circumcised, "dribbling, threadlike stream, and urethral ballooning" is assessed (Burns et al., 2009, p. 872). Note

any dimpling in sacral area (Burns et al., 2009). Other assessments include vital signs, growth and development, pain, tenderness, a mass in the flank area, or fecal impaction (Gaylord & Starr, 2009, p. 871). Notice odors associated with the urine and record intake and output.

Typically, patients who require IV fluids or IV antibiotics, neonates, and infants identified as high-risk are admitted to the hospital. All infants younger than 1 month with suspected UTI, even if not febrile, are admitted. There may be other reasons for admission based on the healthcare provider and/or family's collaborative decision (Tschudy & Arcara, 2012).

Medical Care. Parenteral and oral antibiotics are used to treat UTIs, and a urine culture must be obtained prior to starting the therapy (Wan et al., 2012). The AAP recommends parenteral antibiotics for children with toxic symptoms, dehydration, vomiting, or noncompliance. IV antibiotics are usually given for 14 days to toxic children or those with pyelonephritis. Oral antibiotics for 2 to 4 days for uncomplicated cases are thought by some sources to be as effective as 7 to 10 days of oral treatment (Tschudy & Arcara, 2012, p. 481). Table 31-3 lists the most common urinary tract anti-infective agents, side effects, and related nursing interventions.

Table 31-3 Common Urinary Tract Anti-Infective Agents, Side Effects, and Related Nursing Interventions

Anti-Infective	Side Effects	Nursing Intervention
cefotaxime (Claforan)	Mild diarrhea, mild abdominal cramping	Monitor fluid intake.
ampicillin (Principen)	Nausea, vomiting, diarrhea, rash	Hold medication and notify health-care provider if rash or diarrhea develops. With prolonged therapy monitor renal, hepatic, and hematology lab work.
gentamicin (Gentamicin Pediatric)	Serious side effects are ototoxicity and nephrotoxicity.	Monitor urinalysis. Know that the therapeutic peak is 5–10 mcg/mL and the trough is 2 mcg/mL. The family needs to notify the health-care provider if balance, hearing, urinary, or vision problems occur even after drug is completed.
ceftriaxone (Rocephin)	Serious side effects are antibiotic-associated colitis manifested as severe abdominal pain, tenderness, fever, and diarrhea that is severe and watery.	Assess bowel pattern or pain. Monitor intake and output.
cefixime (Suprax)	Serious side effects are Stevens-Johnson syndrome, nephrotoxicity, blood dyscrasias, and superinfections.	Monitor BUN and serum creatinine. Monitor intake and output. Teach parents how to recognize signs of superinfection (e.g., furry tongue, perineal itching). Tell parents to give this medication with yogurt/buttermilk to decrease superinfections by maintaining intestinal flora.
cephalexin (Keflex)	Serious side effects are antibiotic-associated colitis, superinfections, nephrotoxicity with preexisting renal disease, angioedema, bronchospasm, and anaphylaxis especially if allergies to penicillin or cephalosporins.	Monitor intake and output for nephrotoxicity. Assess bowel activity and stool consistency and increasing gastrointestinal effects. Take this medication with food or milk if mild gastrointestinal upset occurs. Assess mucous membranes and tongue for white patches.
sulfamethoxazole-trimethoprim (Bactrim)	Serious side effects are fatalities secondary to Stevens-Johnson syndrome, toxic epidermal necrolysis, fulminant hepatic necrosis and other blood dyscrasias such as agranulocytosis and aplastic anemia.	This medication is contraindicated in children younger than 2 months of age; kernicterus may result if used with newborns. Monitor intake and output. Assess skin for pallor, purpura, and rash or overt signs of bleeding or swelling.

(continued)

Table 31-3 Common Urinary Tract Anti-Infective Agents, Side Effects, and Related Nursing Interventions (continued)

Anti-Infective	Side Effects	Nursing Intervention
sulfamethoxazole-trimethoprim (Bactrim) (continued)		Monitor hematology, liver and renal function lab results. The family needs to report new symptoms (e.g., bruising, fever, sore throat, or other skin reactions).
nitrofurantoin (Macrobid)	Serious side effects are Stevens-Johnson syndrome, liver toxicity, peripheral neuropathy, and impairment of pulmonary function.	Monitor for peripheral neuropathy (e.g., numbness and/or tingling of extremities). Monitor for liver toxicity signs and symptoms. Monitor respiratory system and chest pain, cough, or difficulty with respirations.
ciprofloxacin (Cipro)	This medication has several IV incompatibilities so be sure to check with the pharmacist. Serious side effects are superinfection, nephrotoxicity, cardiac arrest, cerebral thrombosis, and arthropathy that may occur in children younger than 18 years.	Monitor intake and output. Ensure that fluid intake maintained. Use caution regarding sun exposure affecting eyes and skin. If the child wears contact lenses, remove them if taking ophthalmic solution or ointment.

 Nursing Insight—*Broad-spectrum antibiotics*

Emphasize the importance and rationale for taking all antibiotics for the entire designated time, along with adequate intake of fluids. For children on low-dose antibiotics prophylactically, medication taken at night allows the drug more time to eliminate the infection in the bladder.

Education/Discharge Instructions

Teach the family signs of infection depending on the age of the child including the importance of hand washing, which is the most important measure for reducing infection (Axton & Fugate, 2008). Assist parents in understanding the relationship of fecal soiling and constipation as an increased cause of infection. Constipation prevention

or intervention includes collaboration with the health-care provider regarding increased dietary and fluid intake as well as administering stool softeners and laxatives and teaching the child to establish normal bowel habits (Feld & Mattoo, 2010). If appropriate, reinforce the risk factors related to contracting UTIs (Feld & Mattoo, 2010, p. 454).

VESICOURETERAL REFLUX

Normally, urine should flow downward from the kidneys through the ureters into the bladder and urethra. In vesicoureteral reflux (VUR), the urine backflows from the bladder to the ureters and sometimes back to the kidneys. The disorder occurs at the vesicoureteral junction, which normally creates a one-way valve for the urine to enter the bladder without being refluxed back into the ureters or

---

Nursing Care Plan The Child With a UTI

Nursing Diagnosis: Impaired Urinary Elimination related to tissue inflammation

Measurable Short-Term Goal: The child will be able to void adequate amounts of clear urine without burning, frequency, or urgency.

Measurable Long-Term Goal: The child will not experience renal complications.

NOC Outcome:
Urinary Elimination (0503) Collection and discharge of urine

NIC Interventions:
Medication Administration (2300)
Pain Management (1400)
Specimen Management (7820)

Nursing Interventions:

1. Assess history of urinary tract problems, family dynamics, and understanding of urinary elimination and hygiene.

   RATIONALE: Recurrent UTIs may indicate lack of knowledge about urinary hygiene or may be an indication of sexual abuse.

2. Collaborate with the care provider regarding the collection of a urine specimen for culture and sensitivity and follow-up culture, if ordered, after antibiotic administration is completed.

   RATIONALE: A urine culture will help determine the causative organism and the antibiotic that will be most effective against the organism. Follow-up testing will determine if the causative organism has been eliminated by the antibiotic.

Nursing Care Plan The Child With a UTI (continued)

3. Instruct family to administer medications as prescribed, including antipyretics, analgesics, and the full course of antibiotics (specify drugs, doses, routes, and times).

   RATIONALE: An antipyretic reduces fever associated with a UTI. Urinary tract analgesics provide symptomatic relief from burning pain, frequency, and urgency. Antibiotics must be maintained at a consistent blood level for a prescribed number of days to eliminate the causative organism.

4. Assist the caregiver to plan for optimal nutrition and fluid intake that is individualized for the child (specify for age).

   RATIONALE: Good nutrition and adequate hydration is required for healthy immune response and optimal renal function.

5. Teach the child and/or family about good genital hygiene practices: wiping from front to back and washing hands before and after elimination.

   RATIONALE: Prevents fecal–urinary contamination and the spread of infection.

6. Provide the child and family with education about prevention of urinary tract infections, including obtaining adequate fluids, voiding frequently, recognizing UTI signs and symptoms, and the necessity of completing the full course of antibiotics.

   RATIONALE: Provides knowledge for child and family and empowers them to prevent recurrent infections.

---

kidneys. VUR is found as a common cause of children with UTI, and it is most frequently diagnosed between ages 2 and 3. VUR is more common in girls, is familial, and is more common in Caucasians. It is a cause of UTI in infants and children and is more commonly diagnosed after the first or second UTI episode.

Primary Vesicoureteral Reflux

A child may be born with a valvular defect at the ureter and bladder junction because of insufficient fetal growth of the ureter. The resultant valvular defect allows urine to back-flow from the bladder to the ureters. As a child grows and the ureters lengthen, this type of VUR may resolve spontaneously (NKUDIC, 2011).

Secondary Vesicoureteral Reflux

In secondary VUR, there may be an obstruction from an abnormal tissue fold within the urethra, which causes urine to flow backwards to the ureters. It is more often bilateral in this case (NKUDIC, 2011). When urine refluxes backwards into the kidneys, it can cause **hydronephrosis** (distension of the kidney) and risk for pyelonephritis (kidney infection, as opposed to bladder infection).

Gradations of VUR are provided in the International Reflux Grading System, with a range from Grade I to Grade V (Fig. 31-3). These gradations were created based on the appearance of the renal pelvis and calyces on VCUG (radiography of the bladder and urethra by use of a radiopaque contrast medium).

Signs and Symptoms

The most common presentation for VUR is recurrent UTI. Flank pain, abdominal pain, and enuresis may coexist, although developmentally, toddlers are seldom capable of describing these symptoms. The major risk of VUR is the development of acute pyelonephritis because of the backflow of urine toward the kidney. Even one episode of febrile acute pyelonephritis can cause renal damage in children (Burns et al., 2009).

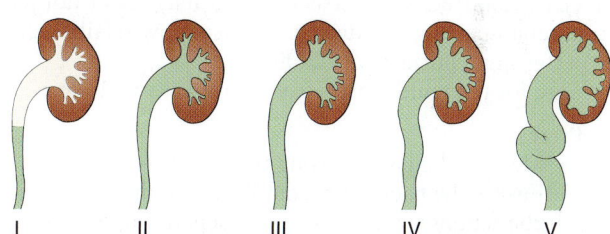

Figure 31-3 Gradations of VUR are found in the International Reflux Grading System ranging from Grade I to Grade V.

These children also have these signs and symptoms:

- Fever
- Nausea and vomiting
- UTI symptoms

 Nursing Insight—*Children younger than 2 years old*

The risks of persistent VUR, especially in children younger than 2 years old, are significant because it is the most common cause of UTI and renal scarring. Children with UTI who are younger than 2 years of age may more easily develop sepsis and become gravely ill. The American Urologic Association recommends continuous antibiotics for children less than age 1 who have had febrile UTIs or VUR Grades III to V. Infants with high-grade reflux do not tend to resolve as spontaneously as those with low-grade reflux.

Diagnosis

Diagnosis of VUR is most consistently based on the VCUG radiograph which identifies the bladder, urethra, and ureters during micturition. Radiographic contrast material is observed as it refluxes back into the ureters and kidneys from the bladder. Renal ultrasound, nuclear scan, or IV pyelography (IVP) are ancillary tests that also may be ordered.

 Diagnostic Tools VCUG Results According to the International Reflux Classification

- Grade I: Urine backs up into the ureter only
- Grade II: Urine backs up into the ureter, renal pelvis, and collecting system without dilation
- Grade III: Reflux into the collecting system with mild dilation, slight ureteral tortuosity, and no or slight blunting of the fornices
- Grade IV: Moderate dilation of the renal pelvis and calyces with complete obliteration of the sharp angle of the fornices (McCarthy, 2011)

Prevention

VUR may be genetic and physiological. Prevention centers on preventing UTI and pyelonephritis when children have VUR.

Collaborative Care

Nursing Care. Nursing care for nonsurgical VUR includes vigilance in preventing and treating UTIs, especially because there is significant risk for the more dangerous pyelonephritis. Renal scarring and damage are also hazards of VUR. Children with persistent VUR may suffer not just from renal scarring and disease but also growth failure and hypertension (Burns et al., 2009).

Care for the child who is having a VCUG includes:

Pretest
- Identify the patient using two identifiers.
- Ensure the patient has complied with dietary restrictions.
- Obtain a history and nursing physical assessment, including vital signs and lab work.
- Remove all external metallic objects.
- Obtain a list of current medications. Determine allergies, including a reaction to iodinated contrast medium and assess substance abuse issues.
- Instruct the patient to void or apply a clean diaper.
- Ensure the test is performed before an upper gastrointestinal study or barium swallow.
- Record the last day of an adolescent's menstrual period to determine the possibility of pregnancy.
- Have the legal guardian sign an informed consent.
- Review the procedure with the patient (age appropriate) and family and address questions and/or concerns.

During the test
- The procedure takes approximately 30 to 60 minutes.
- A Foley catheter is inserted.
- The catheter is filled with iodinated contrast medium to eliminate air pockets and is inserted until the balloon reaches the meatus.
- When ¾ of the iodinated contrast medium has been injected, a radiographic exposure is made while the remainder of the iodinated contrast medium is injected.
- When the patient is able to void, the catheter is removed and the patient urinates while images of the bladder and urethra are recorded.
- Have emergency equipment ready.
- Observe standard precautions.

- Place the patient on the examination table in a supine or lithotomy position.
- Collaborate with the x-ray technician to ensure a radiograph film is taken of the kidney, ureter, and bladder to ensure that barium or stool does not obscure visualization of the urinary system.
- Monitor the patient's vital signs and for complications (e.g., allergic reaction to the iodinated contrast medium, anaphylaxis, and bronchospasm).

Post-test
- Tell parents that the examination report will be sent to the health-care provider who will discuss the results.
- Instruct the parents to resume the child's usual diet and medications as directed by the health-care provider.
- Monitor vital signs and neurological status per institutional protocol.
- Notify the health-care provider if the patient has elevated temperature or abnormal vital signs.
- Monitor for a reaction to the iodinated contrast medium such as rash, urticaria, tachycardia, hyperpnea, hypertension, palpitations, nausea, or vomiting.
- Instruct the parents to report symptoms such as fast heart rate, difficulty breathing, skin rash, itching, chest pain, persistent right shoulder pain, or abdominal pain immediately to the nurse or health-care provider.
- Maintain adequate hydration based on kilograms of weight.
- Recognize parent's anxiety related to delayed test results.
- Reinforce any information given by the health-care provider related to further testing and follow-up appointments.
- Answer any further questions or concerns. (Van Leeuwen, Poelhuis-Leth, & Bladh, 2011, pp. 586–588)

Optimizing Outcomes—Children With VUR and UTI

A thorough nursing assessment promotes the best outcome for a child with VUR and UTI. Because infants and small children cannot express urinary discomfort easily, nurses can observe for discomfort during voiding or straining to void, dribbling of urine, and starting and stopping of the stream. Fever of unknown origin and irritability may be suspicious for UTI in nonverbal children especially. Nurses must take extreme care to obtain a reliable clean-catch urine specimen through assisting older children in the collection of the sample and through proper handling of a bagged specimen in younger children.

Medical Care. The treatment plan varies based on the grade of the actual reflux. In Grades I and II, the mildest types of reflux, the VUR may resolve spontaneously as the child grows up (in 85% of the cases), and grade III VUR may resolve spontaneously in only 50% of children (Burns et al., 2009). In children with more severe grades of reflux, such as Grades IV and V, surgical intervention may be required, and the child needs to be seen by a pediatric urologist and pediatric nephrologist.

Many children who are managed medically take prophylactic long-term antibiotics in addition to anticholinergic agents, such as oxybutynin chloride (Ditropan), to reduce bladder pressure. Also refer to Table 31-3 for common side effects of urinary tract anti-infective agents and related nursing interventions.

Surgical Care. Surgical management ranges from abdominal surgery to less invasive endoscopic surgery. Candidates for surgery include children with recurrent breakthrough pyelonephritis, renal inflammation, fever, and reflux that haven't improved within 1 year of diagnosis. Several surgical approaches are available, usually involving the ureter, but a new outpatient surgical technique using Deflux is used. Deflux is composed of complex sugars that form a gel that is inserted into the ureter to stop urine from refluxing back into the ureters (NKUDIC, 2011). Nurses caring for the postsurgical patient must be vigilant in monitoring intake and output as well as maintaining the patient's pain control.

Education/Discharge Instructions

Nurses play a vital role in educating the parents and family members about signs and symptoms of UTI and the importance of medication in this chronic disorder. It is the pyelonephritis secondary to VUR that causes renal scarring and damage, so early identification and treatment of UTIs is important.

UNEXPLAINED PROTEINURIA

This commonly asymptomatic disorder tends to occur after age 8 and is associated with upright activities during the daytime hours. Routine office urinalysis may discover proteinuria (loss of proteins, such as albumin or globulins, in the urine). Proteinuria ranges from simple and reversible etiologies to complex, life-threatening causes. More benign etiologies of proteinuria include orthostatic (from supine to seated or standing) or postural (affected by posture) proteinuria.

 focus on safety

Other causes of proteinuria

Other causes of proteinuria include protein in the urine that occurs after fever or hardy exercise. When the patient's temperature subsides or the patient has not exercised heavily for 48 hours, the proteinuria subsides as well. In this case, it is wise to obtain a urine sample potentially associated with exercise and compare it to one produced after 48 hours without heavy exercise (Helming, 2009).

 Where Research and Practice Meet:
Prophylactic Antibiotics

Many children with VUR are treated with prophylactic antibiotics, such as a daily low dose of an antibiotic. Children on medication are followed by urine culture periodically (every 2 or 3 months). Prophylactic antibiotics are often recommended until the child has been free of infection for a long time. However, other researchers disagree and say it may not be necessary for children with VUR to take urinary antibiotic prophylaxis for VUR because it may lead to antibiotic resistance and may not be necessary in many cases for long-term treatment (Alconcher, Meneguzzi, Buschiazzo, & Piaggio, 2009).

 Nursing Insight—*Pathological etiologies for proteinuria*

More grave, pathological etiologies for proteinuria include glomerulonephritis, polycystic kidney disease, renal trauma, chronic pyelonephritis, acute tubular necrosis, obstructive uropathy, Henoch-Schönlein purpura, and congestive heart failure. Pregnancy and certain medications can cause proteinuria as well. Associated signs and symptoms for more pathological proteinuria include the potential presence of hematuria, edema (including periorbital edema), hypertension, fatigue, impaired growth and failure to thrive, dysuria (painful urination), frequency, oliguria (diminished urine), and costovertebral angle (CVA) tenderness or flank pain (Helming, 2009).

Signs and Symptoms

The dipstick must show 1+ (30 mg/dL) or higher level of proteinuria to be considered significant. False-positive readings for proteinuria are possible with highly concentrated urine, with specific gravity greater than 1.015, and in this case, the proteinuria must be 2+ or higher to be considered significant. Proteinuria may also be noted in infected urine, often along with leukocytes, hematuria, and positive nitrates (Helming, 2009).

 focus on safety

Potential signs of renal disease

Note potential signs of renal disease:
- Periorbital (around the eye orbit) edema
- Peripheral edema
- CVA tenderness
- Bladder distension
- Renal masses

(Glass, 2011)

Diagnosis

Proteinuria is found on dipstick in about 10% of all children ages 8 to 15. The child needs to void at bedtime and not again until the morning the specimen is obtained. Obtain serial first-voided (the first urine of the morning) specimens for urinalysis at least 3 times over a 2-week span if orthostatic proteinuria is suspected. It is advisable to send urine for culture and sensitivity to rule out a UTI. Any urinalysis containing proteinuria, especially higher than 1+, along with possible hematuria, white blood cells, casts, crystals, and bacteria, is more suspicious for urological or renal disease. Additional renal serum tests that should be ordered include BUN and creatinine. A 12- or 24-hour urine test for creatinine (a chemical waste product of muscle metabolism) and protein may suggest pathology.

Further diagnostic testing may include renal ultrasound, VCUG, and testing for antistreptolysin titer (ASO) to rule out post-streptococcal glomerulonephritis. Referral to a urologist or nephrologist is necessary when proteinuria is persistent, of a high level, or is associated with other urinary abnormalities.

Prevention

Proteinuria can sometimes be prevented by avoiding extreme exercise and minimizing fever occurrences.

Collaborative Care

Nursing Care. In the clinic setting, the nurse instructs the parent or child on how to obtain a first-voided morning specimen to test for orthostatic or postural proteinuria. Make certain the parent understands whether the specimen is to be returned to the clinic or to a laboratory. Nurses can perform an accurate urine dipstick test by obtaining proper quantities of urine to dip the sticks into and then by waiting the appropriate amount of time to test each specimen (Fig. 31-4).

In the clinic, the nurse also assesses weight, blood pressure, pulse, and growth, which may be impaired with renal disease. Additionally, the nurse performs an abdominal examination to assess for renal masses and extended bladder.

Education/Discharge Instructions

If the child requires further testing in the inpatient or outpatient settings, the nurse is instrumental in educating parents about what each test entails. Sometimes it is possible to obtain educational handouts geared for the lay public to help patients understand what urinary disorders mean and how various urological tests are performed. In this case, the nurse's role is largely that of an educator. Nurses also make certain that patients receive the proper follow-up after proteinuria is discovered. This may infer return visits to the clinic and the establishment of appointments with a pediatric urologist or nephrologist.

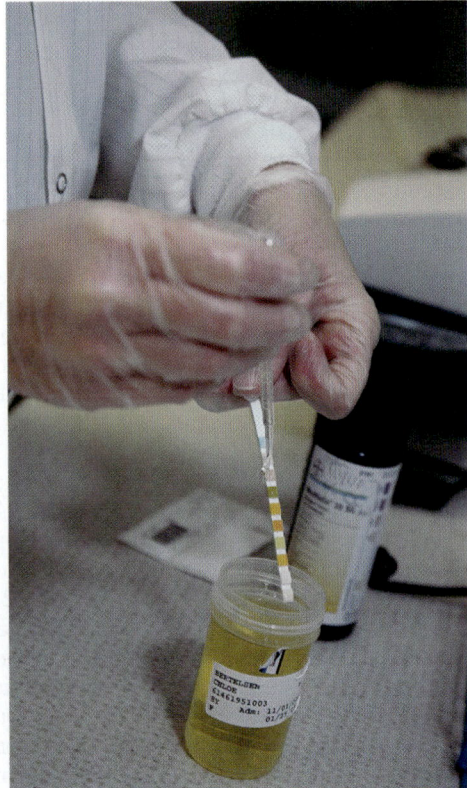

Figure 31-4 Nurses can perform an accurate dipstick test.

HEMATURIA

Asymptomatic gross (visible) and microscopic hematuria is considered somewhat common in children. Although rare, microscopic hematuria can be the first sign of renal disease. The most common etiologies for microscopic hematuria are UTI, post-streptococcal glomerulonephritis, hypercalciuria (with or without renal calculi), and structural abnormalities (e.g., single kidney) (Helming, 2009). It is especially important for children with gross hematuria to undergo a significant urological work-up.

Conversely, gross hematuria in children is more serious, indicating a possibility of IgA nephropathy, hypercalciuria with or without calculi, post-streptococcal glomerulonephritis, renal trauma, coagulopathy (a disorder of blood coagulation), hydronephrosis, epididymitis (inflammation of the epididymis, usually associated with a sexually transmitted infection), and tumor. UTI may cause microscopic or gross (macroscopic) hematuria. It is also important to note that strenuous exercise may induce hematuria as well as certain viral and bacterial illnesses. Occasionally, external irritation may cause hematuria (e.g., from bubble baths, soaps, and scratching) (Helming, 2009).

Signs and Symptoms

The main sign of hematuria is blood in the urine; it can be either microscopic (only seen on dipstick or laboratory analysis) or macroscopic (visible to the eye).

Diagnosis

The color of the urine may be significant; tea-colored or brownish urine often signifies a urological disorder. Pink or red urine with or without blood clots, but without protein, usually originates in the lower urinary tract. If higher than 1+ hematuria is present on dipstick, then it is necessary to obtain a microscopic urinalysis to check for red blood cells (RBCs). Pseudohematuria is a condition that shows a false-positive dipstick but no RBCs on microscopic lab examination.

Urinalysis that reveals hematuria along with casts and proteinuria is highly suspicious for renal disease. UTI may show hematuria along with mild proteinuria but without casts. Significant proteinuria and presence of casts often signifies the risk of more severe renal disease. Urine culture is suggested to rule out UTI in cases of hematuria, and a complete blood and platelet count are needed early. Further diagnostic work-up may first include renal ultrasound, and if necessary, IVP (a dye study that cannot be done if the child is allergic to the IVP dye or shellfish), cystoscopy (scope into bladder), and VCUG. Referral to a pediatric urologist or nephrologist is necessary in cases of hematuria suggesting the potential for renal disease (Burns et al., 2009).

> ### ✿ *Nursing Insight*—*Hematuria*
>
> In children, the major cause of asymptomatic and atraumatic (no trauma) hematuria is renal disease, while in adults, the major cause of hematuria is malignancy. The patient's age is significant in the evaluation of hematuria, and knowing whether it is microscopic versus gross hematuria makes a significant difference in the diagnostic work-up. The use of radiological studies and cystoscopy are variable in children, whereas adult guidelines are more specific. It is suggested that follow-up of

hematuria in children is necessary even after a negative work-up. This implies that children should have laboratory urinalysis periodically even if they have had negative work-ups for renal disease (Tu & Shortliffe, 2010).

Prevention

The types of hematuria that may be preventable are associated with UTIs, and to some extent, with renal calculi. Use the same techniques that prevent UTIs. Renal calculi, which occur in children, may sometimes be prevented by decreasing intake of certain foods, depending on the type of renal stone identified.

Collaborative Care

Nursing Care. Based on development, if the child cannot voluntarily provide a urine specimen, be sure to use the appropriate bagging technique to obtain the specimen. A clean-catch specimen may be needed. Obtain a urine specimen by collecting urine from a bag that fits over the perineum in females or over the penis in males (see Procedure 31-1). The skin must be dry for the bags to adhere, and it is ideal to cleanse the perineum in girls or penis in boys before placing the plastic collecting bag. The bag must be removed as soon as the child voids to avoid fecal contamination. Transfer the urine to a sterile collection container using universal precautions and send it to the laboratory immediately. The nurse is also responsible for accurately testing the urine with a dipstick, ensuring that there is an adequate sample, and allowing the proper time limits for testing.

Education/Discharge Instructions

Depending on the cause of the hematuria, the nurse is called on to educate the child and parent about necessary laboratory and procedural tests, in addition to giving an understandable explanation of the cause of the hematuria. In the case of UTI, the nurse educates the family in the proper techniques of collecting a urine specimen.

GLOMERULONEPHRITIS

Glomerular disease (glomerulonephritis) can be a result of primary kidney disease or secondary multisystem diseases that cause damage to the glomerulus. Both primary and secondary diseases are accompanied with histological evidence that captures the glomerular damage and resultant clinical manifestations and needed treatment. Glomerulonephritis, or nephritis, as it is also known, can be divided into (1) acute, (2) intermittent, or (3) chronic types. Further, nephritis is also classified according to primary and secondary types. Primary glomerulonephritis occurs when the glomerulus is the structure that is impaired in some way. Secondary glomerulonephritis implies that renal issues are secondary to systemic disease. Such diseases include Henoch-Schönlein purpura, systemic lupus erythematosus, and drug hypersensitivity reactions (Burns et al., 2009). Figure 31-5 shows glomerular filtration and tubular reabsorption.

Acute Glomerulonephritis

Inflammation of the glomeruli (tubules of the kidney) is called glomerulonephritis. Interference with the glomeruli filtering waste products from the blood gives rise to acute

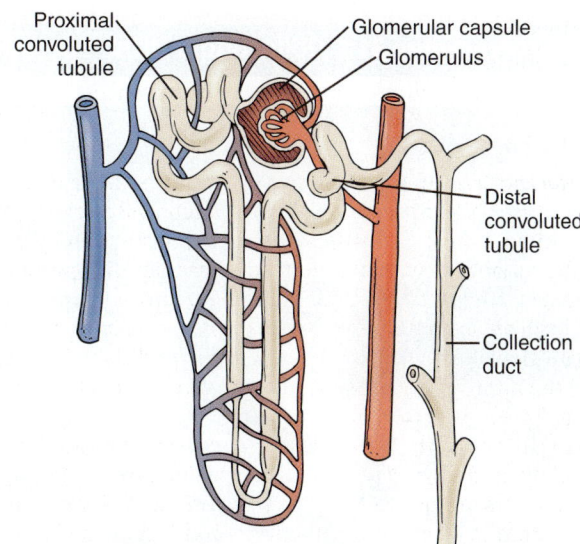

Figure 31-5 The nephron showing glomerular filtration and tubular reabsorption.

and chronic clinical manifestations. If the inflammation follows the course of an infection, it is called post-infectious glomerulonephritis. If it can be directly attributed to the streptococcus organisms, it is called post-streptococcal glomerulonephritis.

> ### Nursing Insight—*Post-streptococcal glomerulonephritis*
>
> Although it is not common, it is possible for children to develop an acute glomerulonephritis within 2 weeks following an acute Group A beta-hemolytic streptococcal infection, even if it was successfully treated with antibiotics. Antigen-antibody complexes with the streptococcal bacteria form and are then deposited in the glomeruli, causing damage. Infections that were missed or not cultured may cause patients to develop this sequelae. Consider not only Group A beta-hemolytic streptococcal pharyngitis but also other potential sources of this bacteria, such as impetigo.

Signs and Symptoms

Signs and symptoms of glomerulonephritis include:

- Gross hematuria, either tea- or red-colored urine
- Edema, which may be seen in the periorbital region (around the eye orbits)
- The child may develop hypertension and headache
- Severe disease causes ascites because of fluid shifting

Diagnosis

If the child has not had a diagnosed streptococcal infection in the previous 2 weeks, it is possible that the health-care provider will order a serum ASO titer that will indicate exposure to the bacteria. Serum complement (C3) is another blood test that may be positive. Urine microscopic hematuria may still be noted up to 1 year after this disease resolves. Laboratory tests such as BUN and creatinine are used to assess renal function. If children do not fully recover, they may develop nephrotic syndrome and require a renal biopsy.

Procedure 31-1 Collecting a Urine Specimen (Fig. 31-6)

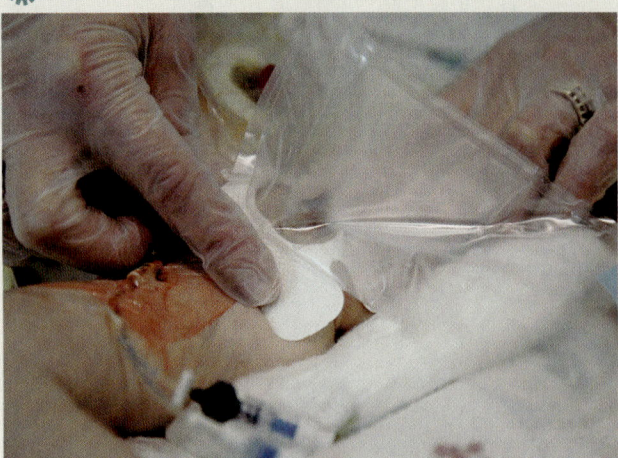

Figure 31-6 The nurse collects specimens in a bag that fits over the perineum in females or over the penis in males.

Purpose

The purpose of collecting a urine specimen is to screen for early signs of disease.

Equipment

- Packaged urine culture set (usually contains three antiseptic towelettes and a sterile urine collection plastic container)

Steps

1. Wipe (or have the child wipe) the labia or penis with the three provided iodine or antiseptic solution towelettes. In occasional situations, it is considered appropriate to use just soap and water to wash these areas. The customary procedure is to wipe the areas 3 times. In males, wipe the urethral tip 3 times in a circular fashion, once with each wipe. In a female, holding the labia open to expose the urethra, wipe the right side top to bottom and discard the wipe. Then repeat this on the left side, discarding the wipe. Wipe top to bottom over the central area where the urethral meatus is and discard that wipe.

   RATIONALE: *Cleansing removes normal flora that may contaminate a urine culture and make it impossible to tell which organisms are pathogens.*

2. Ask the child to begin to urinate into the toilet, bedpan, or urinal, and then stop urinating.

   RATIONALE: *This action flushes away urine in the distal urethra, which may be contaminated with normal flora from the skin.*

3. Position the sterile urine container so that it catches the "mid-stream" urine, which needs to be about 3 to 4 ounces of urine.

4. Remove the container and cap it, taking care not to contaminate the inner container with your gloved hands.

   RATIONALE: *Removing the container keeps the specimen sterile.*

5. Allow the child to finish voiding into the toilet, bedpan, or urinal.

Clinical Alert Do not keep a urine culture at room temperature any longer than 10 minutes. If the specimen cannot be sent to the laboratory immediately, it is necessary to refrigerate it in a plastic specimen bag to prevent the overgrowth of organisms that interfere with the interpretation of the culture and sensitivity to specific antibiotics. The specimen is plated on a nutrient medium, and bacteria that are present are allowed to grow and then are counted. Usually, different antibiotic discs are placed on the inoculated medium to show which ones decrease the colony counts (sensitivity).

Teach Parents

Parents may be responsible for collecting urine cultures from their children at home or in the medical office, so they must be instructed on the sterile techniques of handling the specimen. If the specimen is collected at home, it may need to be refrigerated before bringing it to the laboratory.

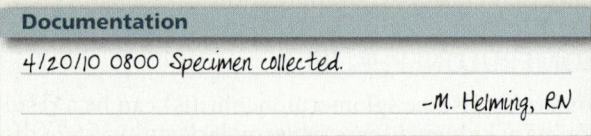

Documentation
4/20/10 0800 Specimen collected.
—M. Helming, RN

Note: Time and date of the urine collection must appear on the label and in the chart. The label should also contain the patient's name and other identifying information, such as identification number.

Prevention

Preventative measures focus on preventing infections with the streptococcus organisms. Teach families standard prevention measures such as hand washing, cleaning the perineal area, and keeping the child home when he or she is ill or shows signs of acute infection.

Collaborative Care

Nursing Care. Nurses support family members through this frightening and uncommon disorder.

Assess the child's pharynx and upper respiratory tract for signs of acute infection and obtain a streptococcal culture. In addition to a rapid-streptococcal test, send a full streptococcal

culture swab to the laboratory for a confirmatory exam. Monitor children for hypertension and urinary output.

Children who develop significant oliguria, gross hematuria, and hypertension are hospitalized because of the risk of associated acute renal failure. The child's renal status is carefully monitored to make certain there is no severe renal dysfunction. Dietary restrictions such as sodium, potassium, and fluid intake are necessary. In most cases, the disorder begins to resolve within 2 or 3 weeks.

Medical Care. Children with glomerulonephritis may be ill enough to be hospitalized. The etiology of glomerulonephritis must be determined, and infectious sources such as streptococcus are treated with appropriate antibiotics.

Children with post-streptococcal glomerulonephritis require antibiotic therapy if an infection is still found. Fluid imbalances require monitoring of fluid intake and output as well as possible treatment with diuretic medications and antihypertensive drugs. Children with severe glomerulonephritis may require peritoneal dialysis or hemodialysis. Corticosteroids may be useful to manage the acute process.

Education/Discharge Instructions

Patients who are developmentally old enough to understand as well as family members can be educated to get prompt medical care for cases of impetigo and streptococcal pharyngitis, which can lessen the risk of acute glomerulonephritis. However, sometimes glomerulonephritis can occur even though the infection is treated, up to several weeks later. Advise patients and families to take the antibiotic treatments until fully completed to avoid resistant organism development and recurrence of infection.

 Case Study Post-Streptococcal Glomerulonephritis

Sara is a 4-year-old girl who is taken to the pediatric emergency department with edematous eyelids and swollen abdomen. Sara's mother reports that along with her daughter's swollen eyelids, her daughter has a decreased appetite and has been very fatigued for the past several days. Sara's vital signs are normal except for her blood pressure, which is 140/90. The systems review and physical exam are negative except for lesions on her ankles and a "doughy" or "dense" feeling to her abdomen, which is slightly firm to touch. The ankle lesions are circular and crusted with sticky yellow drainage, which Sara scratches during the exam. Sara's mother reports that her daughter is allergic to amoxicillin (Amoxil) and develops a rash.

critical thinking questions

1. What does the nurse suspect is the cause of Sara's signs and symptoms?

2. What other questions does the nurse ask Sara's mother?

3. What other laboratory tests are anticipated?

4. What are two other laboratory tests that would confirm a diagnosis of post-streptococcal glomerulonephritis?

5. What type of diet will be ordered for Sara?

6. What antibiotic could be given to Sara because she is allergic to amoxicillin?

7. What patient teaching would the nurse provide to the mother before Sara goes home?

◆ See Suggested Answers to Case Studies on Davis*Plus*.

Chronic Glomerulonephritis

Chronic glomerulonephritis involves several glomerular diseases that, unlike acute post-streptococcal glomerulonephritis, do not have a tendency toward spontaneous recovery. Advanced pathological damage to the glomeruli silently occurs. Damage to the glomerular membrane causes permeability and electrical charge changes that permit passage rather than filtering of protein molecules. Proteinuria and hematuria finally surface with a urinalysis obtained during a clinic visit. Renal failure can be an outcome depending on the degree of damage done to the glomerular

membrane. Types of chronic glomerulonephritis include IgA nephropathy, hereditary nephritis, benign recurrent nephritis, and membranoproliferative nephritis.

IgA nephropathy is more common in males of European or Asian descent. It is also known as Berger's disease. A virus or heavy exercise may precede the presence of microscopic hematuria that lasts only about 72 hours. Usually, there is no hypertension, no edema, and the prognosis is good. If proteinuria persists or the serum creatinine level elevates, there is a risk of it progressing to chronic renal insufficiency.

Hereditary nephritis can be caused by many disorders, but Alport's syndrome is the most prominent. It is more common in males and presents before age 15 as an X-linked genetic disorder. It presents with microhematuria (on dipstick or urinalysis) and sometimes macrohematuria (gross, visible hematuria) and proteinuria. Associated disorders are deafness and ocular disease which, if accompanied by hypertension, can signal a risk for progression to end-stage renal disease.

Benign recurrent nephritis is also called "thin basement membrane disease"; it is an inherited disorder as well. An upper respiratory infection may bring on episodes of micro- and macro-hematuria plus proteinuria. Most renal laboratory values are otherwise normal. This disease is mild unless it is associated with deafness or ocular disease, which can imply a risk of renal failure.

Membranoproliferative glomerulonephritis is sometimes referred to as "chronic nephritis." Kidney biopsy helps to distinguish this from other types. It can occur after acute nephritis and can be associated with anorexia, malaise, and intermittent vomiting. The renal function deteriorates so that prognosis is guarded in this case. Some cases respond to steroid treatment (Burns et al., 2009).

Signs and Symptoms

Signs and symptoms of acute glomerulonephritis include:

- Decrease in the urine output
- High blood pressure
- Headaches
- Periorbital edema
- Increased abdominal girth
- Swelling of the labia or scrotum
- Hematuria, microscopic or macroscopic
- Proteinuria
- Abnormal BUN and creatinine

Diagnosis

Diagnosing chronic glomerulonephritis includes the use of diagnostic laboratory tests similar to that of acute or chronic renal failure: urinalysis, blood chemistry, BUN, serum creatinine, and pH.

Prevention

Primary prevention involves decreasing the incidence of acute glomerulonephritis by appropriate and early streptococcal pharyngitis and impetigo treatment. Then, careful medical and nursing care of acute glomerulonephritis will help to decrease the incidence of chronic glomerulonephritis.

Collaborative Care

Nursing Care. The patient is monitored vigilantly for nephrotic syndrome, chronic renal failure, end-stage renal disease, chronic or malignant hypertension, heart failure, pulmonary edema, chronic or recurrent UTIs, and infection. The nurse monitors weight, abdominal girth, electrolytes (e.g., hyperkalemia with potential electrocardiogram changes) as well as acidosis and inadequate renal perfusion. If renal failure eventually occurs, the patient and family are prepared for the possibility of dialysis and renal transplant.

Nursing care also depends on the degree of renal insufficiency or failure. The overall management principles for treating chronic glomerulonephritis are related to treating the etiology of primary disease or secondary disease that affects the glomerulus, preventing immune responses (or limiting them), and correcting problems of edema, hyperkalemia, or hyperlipidemia, if present. Dietary management may include restriction of salt and fluid along with instituting low-potassium foods. Careful monitoring of urine output, along with weight and abdominal girth, is necessary.

Trusting, supportive, developmentally appropriate relationships are established through the caring interventions of the nurse and other health-care providers. Long-term follow-up, possible renal biopsies every 2 to 5 years, and vigilant observations for possible renal failure become part of the patient's and family's everyday life.

Medical Care. The use of plasma exchange may be instituted in severe cases to decrease the amount of circulating immunoglobulins that are damaging the kidney. When hypertension is present, it is generally related to fluid overload, and loop diuretics such as furosemide (Lasix) may be given to reduce the circulating intravascular fluid volume.

Education/Discharge Instructions

Chronic glomerulonephritis is a serious disease that may manifest in hypertension, nephrotic syndrome, and renal failure, so children are vigilantly monitored for electrolyte and fluid imbalances as well as for deteriorating renal function. Proper diet may require instruction from a dietitian. Educate families on the delicate balance of fluid and salt in this disease as well as on the potential complications that can occur if the disease is not properly managed. Children may require emotional support and counseling to live with this chronic condition because their energy levels may be severely decreased. Tell parents that activity levels may be restricted at certain points of development.

HEMOLYTIC UREMIC SYNDROME

Hemolytic uremic syndrome (HUS) is the most common cause of acute renal failure (ARF) in children. HUS is most commonly associated with children ingesting beef contaminated with E coli, although other organisms, such as shigella, coxsackievirus, adenovirus, salmonella, ECHO virus, pneumococci, and rickettsia have been implicated. This potentially lethal outcome is most commonly seen in young children between 6 months and 3 years of age, but can occur in all age groups (Hay, Levin, Sondheimer, & Deterdin, 2009).

focus on safety

E coli O157:H7

Undercooked ground beef has been one of the primary sources of *E coli* O157:H7 that can cause HUS. Meat should be cooked until it reaches a temperature of 160°F (71.1°C) and is no longer pink. *E coli* outbreaks have occurred in fast-food and other restaurants and have been found in unpasteurized cider, milk, juice, alfalfa sprouts, strawberries, and most recently, raw spinach.

It is believed that an endotoxin is produced from the dangerous bacteria in the gastrointestinal tract and results in inflammation causing capillary wall destruction. This occurs also within the glomerular arterioles, and as the endothelium of the glomerulus becomes more edematous, platelets aggregate at the site of injury. A clot then forms that impedes renal circulation. This stimulates increased rennin production, which results in hypertension. These platelets are damaged, and this results in thrombocytopenia or a drop in the platelet count to less than 100,000/μL for a period of 1 to 2 weeks. The overall effect damages the glomerular blood vessels, resulting in a lesser glomerular filtration rate, lowered urine output, acute renal failure, and hypertension. The clotting and inflammatory process may also affect the respiratory system and any other body system.

focus on safety

At-risk populations

Young children and older adults are at-risk populations for developing HUS from *E coli* O157:H7, so it is prudent to investigate whether any person with diarrheal illness has eaten contaminated food. Stool culture tests for *E coli* O157:H7 are available at most clinics and are ordered by a health-care provider if there is a suspicion of contaminated food.

Signs and Symptoms

Classically, HUS includes a triad of symptoms: thrombocytopenia, anemia, and ARF. Other signs and symptoms include:

- Gastroenteritis (inflammation of the intestines as a result of infection) with abdominal pain, vomiting, and bloody diarrhea
- Potential upper respiratory infection
- Hematuria
- Proteinuria
- Pallor
- Lethargy
- Irritability
- Decreasing urine output
- Hepatosplenomegaly
- Dehydration
- Possible seizures
- Consciousness alteration
- Anemia with high reticulocyte count
- Thrombocytopenia

Diagnosis

HUS can endure from several days to 3 weeks. Diagnosis of HUS includes critical analysis of laboratory results. About 15% of children can progress to end-stage renal disease (Hay et al., 2009). In HUS, laboratory abnormalities show an elevation in BUN and creatinine levels. **Hyperkalemia** (elevated potassium level) also may occur because of decreased urinary excretion. Serum glucose levels may drop because of increased metabolic needs but may also rise if the pancreas is affected, and some children require insulin. Other affected electrolytes include calcium, which decreases, and phosphorus, which rises. The platelet count drops to below 140,000, which is called **thrombocytopenia** (Van Leeuwen et al., 2011, p. 421). The reticulocyte count rises, which refers to immature RBCs being produced from the bone marrow as a response to the hemolytic anemia to try to improve oxygenation (Van Leeuwen et al., 2011, p. 1149).

Prevention

Teach parents and other caregivers to make certain that ground beef is fully cooked to 160°F (71.1°C). Avoidance of fecal contamination on fruits and vegetables, using proper cleaning, and if possible, using pasteurized products such as pasteurized apple cider is important.

Collaborative Care

Nursing Care. The child suffering from HUS is ill enough to be in intensive care and require dialysis. Monitor the child's level of consciousness, signs of increased intracranial pressure, congestive heart failure, bleeding, and hypertension. Fluid intake and output is measured every 4 hours and up to every hour if the child is critically ill. Daily weights are essential, and the nurse needs to assess electrolyte balances (sodium, potassium, chloride, and bicarbonate) as well as arterial blood gas measurements. The BUN and creatinine are important to measure to determine if renal status is worsening, and the child may be at risk of needing dialysis. The lungs should be assessed for signs of congestive heart failure such as rales. Assess for peripheral and periorbital edema because these are indicators of worsening renal and cardiac status.

Monitor the child's vital signs frequently for hypertension and tachycardia. It is recommended that children with HUS have electrocardiographic monitoring to assess for possible changes such as widened QRS complexes, heart block, and peaked T waves caused by hyperkalemia.

 Assessment Tool Hemolytic Uremic Syndrome (HUS)

Be observant for the risks related to HUS:
- Signs of bleeding associated with thrombocytopenia, petechiae, epistaxis (nosebleed), prolonged bleeding at venipuncture sites, and ecchymosis
- Signs of increased intracranial pressure, including change in level of consciousness and risk of seizure
- Abdominal symptoms are the primary presenting complaints for children and occur in the form of diffuse abdominal pain, intussusception (telescoping of the bowel), nausea and vomiting, diarrhea, and fever. These abdominal symptoms may present up to 1 week after exposure to the *E coli* O157:H7 toxin.

Medical Care. Antibiotics are contraindicated in treating HUS because they may worsen the situation.

Education/Discharge Instructions

Teach patients and families to properly cook all ground beef products to an internal temperature of 160°F (71.1°C). Ensure a restaurant also properly cooks the meat at the noted temperature. It is recommended that people should order ground beef that is well-done and no longer pink or red in color. Educate patients and families about epidemic outbreaks that have occurred with a variety of produce types, including apple cider and spinach. Produce should be carefully selected and washed, although this may still not entirely eliminate the risk of infection.

legal alert—Hemolytic uremic syndrome

Children who have been exposed to undercooked beef or other products containing *E coli* O157:H7 may seek legal remedies for their suffering. Severe illness, possibly chronic renal problems, and death have been outcomes of pediatric HUS. Restaurants and food producers who are responsible for contaminated products have legal liability for personal injury. Some years ago, many outbreaks of HUS forced the fast-food industry to cook all beef sufficiently so that no redness persisted and the internal temperature of the thickest portion of the beef reaches 160°F (71.1°C).

HENOCH-SCHÖNLEIN PURPURA

Henoch-Schönlein purpura (HSP) includes a range of mild to severe glomerulonephritis and renal insufficiency. This disease is classified as a **vasculitis** (inflammation of blood vessels) because there is a component of inflammation in the arteries. HSP typically follows an upper respiratory tract infection during the ages from 6 months old to adulthood (Burns et al., 2009). Unfortunately, up to 20% of children with HSP can progress to end-stage renal failure.

Signs and Symptoms

Signs and symptoms of HSP include:

- Hematuria
- Hypertension
- Bloody diarrhea
- Crampy abdominal pain
- Rash with palpable purpura (raised purpura), features found especially on the lower extremities and buttocks
- Joint pain and swelling
- Scrotal swelling in males

Diagnosis

Diagnosis is not difficult if the classic symptoms of rash, gastrointestinal complaints or hematuria, and arthritis are present. The diagnosis of HSP depends on clinical findings and history. There is not a specific laboratory test for the disorder, although an elevated serum IgA level, elevated sedimentation rate, elevated platelet count, and elevated white blood cell count may be present. Urinalysis may show hematuria. A stool guaiac test (a test for unseen blood in stool) may be positive.

Prevention

The best way to prevent HSP is to thwart upper respiratory tract infections and seek medical care if this kind of infection occurs.

Collaborative Care

Nursing Care. Although most children recover spontaneously from HSP, some children can relapse and some can recover very slowly, continuing to show hematuria up to 2 years later. Children with HSP are at risk of complications of intussusception (telescoping of the bowel), intestinal hemorrhage, intestinal perforation, and central nervous system and severe renal complications. Monitor children with HSP for signs of bleeding, pallor, vital sign alterations, abdominal pain, oliguria, and urine abnormalities.

Medical Care. Corticosteroids are used in treatment of HSP, although they may not be sufficient (Hays et al., 2009). Corticosteroids assist with the abdominal and joint pain as well as the edema but do nothing to assist the renal compromise. Some children may require immunosuppressant medications and even a renal transplant.

Education/Discharge Instructions

Assure families that most cases of HSP tend to last up to 1 month and then resolve without severe sequelae. However, some children get a rash intermittently for up to 1 year, and some children can have a recurrence of HSP. If nephritis occurs, there may be hypertension and renal insufficiency. Parents are told to observe for signs and symptoms of the disease and to have the child monitored periodically by health-care providers, especially by a pediatric nephrologist or urologist (Burns et al., 2009).

NEPHROTIC SYNDROME

Nephrotic syndrome is a disorder of the renal system in which excessive protein is excreted into the urine. Associated problems include hyperlipidemia (excessively high lipids), hypoalbuminemia (low blood albumin), and edema although these may not be present in all cases at all times. It appears that the glomerular membrane may become more permeable, thus allowing more protein to be excreted. It may result from allergic, infectious, vascular, malignant, autoimmune, or idiopathic (unknown) reasons. It occurs 15 times more often in children than adults, with peak incidence from ages 2 to 6 years of age (Burns et al., 2009).

Signs and Symptoms

Signs and symptoms of nephrotic syndrome include:

- Edema, especially periorbital and dependent (e.g., feet and ankles)
- Decreased urine production
- Possible ascites with respiratory compromise because of enlarged abdomen
- Hypertension
- Anorexia
- Diarrhea
- Vomiting
- Growth failure and muscle wasting if prolonged illness

Diagnosis

Urinalysis may show protein levels of 2+ or greater, hyaline or granular casts, microhematuria, and high specific gravity. Cholesterol levels may be elevated, and serum albumin levels may be low. A kidney biopsy may be required.

Prevention

Based on the cause of nephritic syndrome, prevention can be promoted through regular visits to a health-care provider.

Collaborative Care

Nursing Care. Hospitalization may be needed if the disease is severe. Fluid and electrolyte balance, weight, and degree of edema are monitored. Be aware of the disease manifestations and the need for possible kidney biopsy.

Medical Care. Diuretics and albumin replacement may be used early on in the disease. Salt may be restricted. The primary medication used is prednisone, given in higher doses

initially to induce remission and then tapered down to handle the inflammation, potentially over several months (Burns et al., 2009).

Education/Discharge Instructions

Teach parents how to monitor for protein levels using a dipstick in the urine at home. Routine immunizations are given only during remission because the child may be on steroids, which may decrease response to immunizations.

Case Study Preschooler With Nephrotic Syndrome

Grant, a 4-year-old, has been in preschool but was sent home because of an upper respiratory infection and slight fever. In several days, he returned to normal. However, 2 weeks later his mother noticed that his eyelids were puffy, and that he had gained 2 pounds since having his cold. His ankles were slightly swollen, and his abdomen seemed distended. She took him to the health-care provider who assessed the dipstick results for urine, which was 2+ proteins. Grant was also pale, tired, and slightly irritable. His mother said his appetite had decreased since his respiratory infection. He was admitted to the local pediatric hospital where he was diagnosed with nephrotic syndrome.

critical thinking questions

1. Discuss important aspects of a health history and physical assessment.
2. What are common nursing care measures for Grant?
3. What other questions does the nurse ask?
4. What laboratory tests will be ordered by the health-care provider?
5. What procedure would confirm nephrotic syndrome?
6. What medications might be ordered by the health-care provider?
7. Discuss important discharge instructions.

◆ See Suggested Answers to Case Studies on Davis*Plus*.

 Now Can You—**Discuss common disorders of the urinary system?**

1. Explain why the early diagnosis of UTIs is critical?
2. Examine acute and chronic glomerulonephritis and related nursing care measures?
3. Describe gradations of VUR?
4. Discuss HUS and nephrotic syndrome as well as related nursing care measures?

Structural Defects of the Urinary System

Although theoretically the urinary tract system is composed of two ureters, one bladder, and one urethra that appears independent of the kidneys, the two systems are intertwined. Abnormalities with the urinary tract system ultimately affect the other systems. The abnormalities may be anatomical, infectious, cellular, inflammatory, functional, or maturational.

Bladder exstrophy is a urinary tract system structural abnormality that can damage the kidney. Another example is a kidney disease, **hydronephrosis**, an accumulation of urine in the renal pelvis that results from an obstruction. These structural defects also compromise kidney function, resulting in hypertension, metabolic acidosis, inability to concentrate urine, urinary stasis and infection, and chronic renal failure.

Other structural defects of the urinary system are referred to as obstructive uropathy, which are structural or functional abnormalities that also result in retrograde flow of urine back into the renal pelvis. The most common of these obstructive uropathies is ureteropelvic junction obstruction (an obstruction or stenosis of the ureteropelvic valve between the renal pelvis and ureters). The outcome of untreated obstructive uropathy is chronic renal failure caused by damage to the renal parenchyma from hydronephrosis.

 ### Nursing Insight—*Hydronephrosis*

The term hydronephrosis means swollen upper urinary tract. It is not always from obstruction, but it can restrict urinary outflow, which can lead to renal deterioration. Hydronephrosis is acute or chronic, and it can occur antenatally (before birth) or postnatally. In children, hydroureter implies a ureter that is dilated. Hydronephrosis is often associated with vesicoureteral reflux VUR (Lusaya, 2011). Hydronephrosis can be found antenatally during an ultrasound. It is associated with a higher incidence of VUR (Mathew, Abdelsalam, Saslow, Amendolia, Nakhla, Kemble, et al., 2009). In children, especially in newborns, the physical examination is abnormal when hydronephrosis is present. An abdominal mass can be an enlarged kidney from hydronephrosis. A palpable bladder, especially in a boy, may mean hydronephrosis in the urethral area. A child with external ear abnormalities or low-set ears (below an imaginary line drawn from the eye to the side of the head) may have congenital kidney problems. Also, a single umbilical artery may be associated with congenital anomalies (abnormalities) of the kidney and urinary tract (Lusaya, 2011). If a child has hydronephrosis, it is important to determine the underlying cause to discover how best to treat this condition.

EXSTROPHY OF THE BLADDER

Exstrophy of the bladder is a congenital defect in which the abdominal and anterior bladder walls do not fuse during fetal development. This results in the anterior surface of the bladder being open on the abdominal wall. Exstrophy comes from the Greek meaning "turn inside out." The tissue that usually covers the bladder also does not form correctly, and it is separated so the bladder is fully exposed. The defect has a variety of degrees of severity. There are a number of associated congenital anomalies or other structural alterations (e.g., epispadias, cryptorchidism, chordee (downward penis), anus malposition, rectal prolapse, and widely split symphysis pubis (Association for the Bladder Exstrophy Community, 2012).

Signs and Symptoms

The visualization that the bladder is open on the abdominal wall is the main determinant of this condition.

Diagnosis

Ultrasound is the tool used to diagnose exstrophy of the bladder.

Prevention

Prevention is promoted through good prenatal care and prenatal nutrition. Early detection of exstrophy of the bladder in utero can assist the family to deliver at a neonatal intensive care unit that is capable of proper care measures needed for the infant's overall health and to promote a good health outcome.

Collaborative Care

Nursing Care. Nursing care measures for exstrophy of the bladder focus on physical assessment, vital signs monitoring, fluid and electrolyte balance, infection prevention, nutrition maintenance, psychological care, and pre- and postsurgical care. After birth and until surgery, the open area is kept clean because urine on the skin can cause irritation and possibly introduce infection. Diapers are applied to fit loosely and changed frequently. The exposed bladder is covered with Vaseline gauze per health-care provider's orders.

Surgical Care. Surgery is necessary within the first 24 to 48 hours of the infant's life in this rare disorder. The surgical procedure puts the bladder back into the abdomen, the separated pelvic bones are brought together, and the abdominal skin is closed. The bladder may need to be augmented to improve its size, and urinary diversion is sometimes required. If there are associated abnormalities, these may need surgery at a later time (Association for the Bladder Exstrophy Community, 2012). Standard postoperative nursing care measures are performed, which include vital sign monitoring, ongoing physical assessment, pain control and comfort measures, administration of IV fluids and electrolytes, maintaining nothing by mouth status until dietary orders are given, skin care, intake and output monitoring, surgical site assessment, and psychosocial and developmental assessment of the child. Remember to hold and cuddle the child when orders have been written to increase activity as tolerated.

Education/Discharge Instructions

The nurse teaches the family to provide care for their infant including incisional care postoperatively. If the infant is discharged prior to reconstructive surgery, parents will need to be instructed to change diapers frequently and to cover the defect with plastic wrap to decrease the risk of infection and ulceration. The nurse must teach the family the signs and symptoms of urinary tract infections and when to seek care. The nurse must educate and support the family in regard to what are realistic long-term outcomes of both functional and cosmetic results depending on the exact components of the infant's genitourinary defects.

 ### Across Care Settings: Exstrophy of the bladder

The nurse prepares day-care providers and school nurses to care for infants and children with exstrophy of the bladder. Education for care providers involves proper diapering, hygiene maintenance, education about the congenital anomaly, and other associated anomalies, if applicable. Later on, preparation for psychosexual problems that may arise as the child reaches adolescence may be needed.

Renal Trauma

In the emergency department, the nurse is prepared for all situations, and genitourinary (GU) system traumas account for approximately 10% of all injuries. A GU system trauma includes the scrotum, penis, urethra, ureters, bladder, and kidneys. For those patients with trauma to the abdomen, there are about 10% to 15% GU injuries that are concurrent.

Kidney trauma is present in about 8% to 10% of abdominal trauma situations. History of injury relates to blunt and penetrating abdominal injury. Blunt trauma examples are injuries from sports, violence, motor vehicle injuries, and falls from high places. Kidney injury occurs more often from blunt trauma. Blunt abdominal trauma often is not the only damage that occurs because there may be multisystem injuries, but kidneys are known for rupturing from blunt trauma. Penetrating trauma examples are often caused by animal bites, gunshot wounds, or stabbings. Death with renal trauma is secondary to hemorrhage or multisystem damage. Children must be observed for covert symptoms of hemorrhage because they can compensate and not show hypovolemia until in great distress. Also, it is important to recognize that children's kidneys are more anterior and mobile (greater amount of space in the abdomen) as well as greater in size compared with the child's body and often are less protected by adipose tissue (Blair, 2011).

Signs and Symptoms

With critical injuries involving renal trauma, children show the following signs and symptoms:

- Grey-Turner's sign (ecchymosis localized in the flank area and flank tenderness)
- Palpable mass
- Hematuria
  (Blair, 2011)

 Nursing Insight—*Hematuria*

Hematuria is most often considered the cardinal marker of renal injury but not seen that often. The presence of any degree of hematuria is regarded as a potential indication of underlying renal injury or anomaly. Hematuria out of proportion to the mechanisms of injury should suggest a congenital anomaly or neoplasm.

Diagnosis

Understanding the actual injury mechanisms assists in diagnosing the extent of the renal injury. Diagnosis of renal trauma is confirmed by history and clinical findings as well as diagnostic studies that may include focused abdominal sonography for trauma, computerized tomography, and diagnostic peritoneal lavage (Blair, 2011).

Prevention

Prevention of morbidity and mortality is gained through proper emergency care in situations including car accidents and athletic injuries.

Collaborative Care

Nursing Care. Because renal trauma is a critical injury, advanced trauma life-support guidelines are followed. The goal of nursing care is prevention of renal morbidity and mortality. Kidney injuries are assessed with grades I through V. Blunt trauma, such as bruising without any urinary extravasation (grades I, II, and III), is treated conservatively. Treatment includes bedrest, analgesia, and prophylactic antibiotics. Grades IV and V renal trauma require referral to the urologist (Table 31-4).

Nursing care measures center on recognizing a renal injury and the potential urgency. The nurse gathers a detailed history of the problem. Sometimes a lengthy admission process is not possible because of the impending surgery. Performing a nursing assessment including vital signs, growth and development, nutritional and immunization status, and a thorough physical examination is essential. The nurse gains crucial information such as the precipitating event, allergies, medications, general state of health, and previous hospitalizations or surgeries. Also, the nurse gathers information including possible previous renal disease, increased blood pressure, or the presence of only one kidney, which presents its own special needs (Blair, 2011).

Table 31-4 Grades I–V Kidney Injuries	
Grade	**Extent of Kidney Injury**
Grade I	Renal contusion with microscopic hematuria: urological studies normal Subscapular hematoma, not expanding with no parenchymal laceration
Grade II	Perirenal hematoma, not expanding, confined to renal retroperitoneum Laceration less than 1 cm parenchymal depth of renal cortex without urinary extravasation
Grade III	Laceration greater than 1 cm parenchymal depth of renal cortex without collecting system rupture or urinary extravasation
Grade IV	Laceration through the cortex, medulla, and collecting system Main renal artery or vein injury with contained hemorrhage
Grade V	Laceration resulting in a completely shattered kidney Avulsion of the renal hilum, devascularization of the kidney

Note: Advance one grade for bilateral injury up to grade III.

Source: Adapted from Blair. (2011). Overview of genitourinary trauma. *Urologic Nursing, 31*(3), 142. (Blair is quoting from Moore, E. E., Shackford, S. R., Pachter, H. I., McAninch, J. W., Browner, S. B., Chamption, Y. H. R., et al. (1989) Organ injury scaling: Spleen, liver, and kidney. *The Journal of Trauma, 29*(12), 1664–1668.

Surgical Care. Surgery may be required if abdominal exploration is needed. Prepare both the child and family for the surgery and immediate postoperative care. Essential abbreviated information is communicated because the family may not understand the full situation. Serious injury to the urinary system often requires astute observation in the critical care unit. Nursing care is tailored to the identified problems in order of importance, and the nurse must develop a care plan that deals with the multifaceted problems.

After surgery the child is placed on bedrest for initial observation and remains on bedrest for 3 days after internal bleeding has subsided. Monitoring vital signs; urinary, respiratory, cardiac, and gastrointestinal status; and the surgical incision is essential. Priority actions also include monitoring intake and output, measuring weight and abdominal girth, administering IV fluids, and managing pain. Report signs of inadequate renal perfusion (hypotension) and acidosis and observe for edema, oliguria, or anuria.

Collaborative care that includes psychological support is also important (Blair, 2011). Psychosocial care of the family includes encouraging the parents to remain at the bedside, relaying appropriate developmental information, and minimizing stressors experienced by the child. Remind the family to avoid discussions at the bedside that may upset the child. Respect and support the family's decisions about medical care but advocate through the proper channels for the child if the best interest of the child is in question. Notify a hospital chaplain for spiritual care if the family desires.

Education/Discharge Instructions

Inform the family to follow health-care provider instructions and keep clinic appointments. Educate the family on potential complications that may occur years later such as hypertension or proteinuria. The American Academy of Pediatrics, American Academy of Family Physicians, and the Medical Society of Sports Medicine recommend avoiding heavy contact sports or collisions.

Renal Failure

ACUTE KIDNEY INJURY

Acute renal failure in children is now referenced as acute kidney injury (AKI), resulting in a treatable condition manifesting as an increase in nitrogenous waste products and lack of homeostasis regulation by the kidney (Blayney, 2013). In AKI there is a rapid downward spiral of renal filtration function accompanied by an increase in serum creatinine concentration or increase in blood urea nitrogen concentration. Therefore, AKI is a life-threatening syndrome in which there is a sudden decreased capacity of the kidneys to eliminate waste products, resulting in an inability to maintain fluid and electrolyte or acid-base balance (Sreedharan & Avnder, 2011). Acute kidney injury has a significant morbidity and mortality for critically ill pediatric patients, especially if children have suffered a multisystem organ failure (Walters, Porter, & Brophy, 2009).

 Nursing Insight—*Biomarkers*

Acute kidney injury biomarkers include neutrophil gelatinase-associated lipocalin, interleukin-18, and kidney injury molecule 1 (Blayney, 2013; Sreedharan & Avner, 2011).

Regardless of age, AKI is divided into pre-renal, intrarenal (intrinsic), and post-renal (obstruction) categories (Blayney, 2013). Table 31-5 outlines the common diseases under each category. The pre-renal injury, with sudden reduction of circulation to the kidneys, is most often a result of dehydration in children, such as shock, acute gastrointestinal losses, or congestive heart failure as well as increased vascular resistance of the kidneys (McInerny et al., 2009). Pre-renal AKI stems from significantly reduced cardiac output because of a depletion of volume or hypotension with resultant compensatory severe vasoconstriction. The nephrons are usually intact structurally and functionally with the **fractional excretion of sodium** (FENa), which tests the kidney's ability to concentrate urine and retain

Table 31-5 Common Causes of Acute Kidney Injury		
Pre-Renal	**Intrinsic Renal**	**Post-Renal**
Dehydration	Glomerulonephritis	Posterior urethral valves
Hemorrhage	Postinfectious/Poststreptococcal	Ureteropelvic junction obstruction
Sepsis	Lupus erythematosus	Ureterovesicular junction obstruction
Hypoalbuminemia (severe)	Henoch-Schönlein purpura	Ureterocele
Cardiac failure	Membranoproliferative Anti-glomerular basement membrane Hemolytic uremic syndrome Acute tubular necrosis Cortical necrosis Renal vein thrombosis Rhabdomyolysis Acute interstitial cystitis Tumor infiltration Tumor lysis syndrome	Tumor Urolithiasis Hemorrhagic cystitis Neurogenic bladder

sodium, usually less than 1% sodium with little or no sediment in the urine (Perrin & MacLeod, 2013).

Intrarenal structure, also known as intrinsic structure, reflects the kidney's response to continued injurious effects to the kidney from untreated pre-renal status resulting in structural as well as functional harm of the nephrons. An FENa greater than 1% with presence of sediment and casts in the urinalysis is evident. Intrarenal AKI can result from pyelonephritis, especially in infants, resulting in tissue damage (Beetz, 2012; Jetton & Askenazi, 2012; Quigley, 2012). Renal tissue damage can also occur from aminoglycosides, antibiotics, or poisoning from chemicals including "carbon tetrachloride, diethylene glycol, heavy metals" (McInerny et al., 2009, p. 2798). Additional reasons include nephrotoxic substances (e.g., nephrotoxic drugs, ischemia, or inflammatory responses releasing mediators that do further damage to the basement membrane and renal tubular epithelial cells).

Post-renal causes result from obstruction in the urinary system's ability to pass urine (Workeneh & Batuman, 2012). Positive renal outcomes, including normal renal filtration, usually occur with correction of the obstruction unless there is severe obstruction of the urinary tract system or kidney dysplasia (Kliegman et al., 2011; Perrin & MacLeod, 2013).

 Nursing Insight—*Understanding acute kidney injury*

Congenital heart disease surgery, sepsis, and nephrotoxic medications are also common causes of AKI (McInerny et al., 2009). Understanding the cause helps reverse post–renal failure.

focus on safety

Seizures

Seizures may occur secondary to the fluid and electrolyte imbalances or because of "hypocalcemia, hypertensive encephalopathy, uremia, and water intoxication" (McInerny et al., 2009, p. 2799).

 Nursing Insight—*Adolescents with acute kidney injury*

The new description for adolescents with AKI is "an abrupt reduction in kidney function defined as an absolute increase in creatinine of 0.3 mg/dL, or a percentage increase of more than 50% or a reduction in urine output (documented oliguria of 0.5 mL/kg/hr for more than 6 hours" (Perrin & MacLeod, 2013, p. 401).

 Nursing Insight—*The RIFLE classification*

AKI now utilizes the RIFLE classification, which is particularly useful in improving the understanding of outcomes (Workeneh & Batuman, 2012). Based on work done in 2004 from the Acute Dialysis Quality Initiative, new valid criteria is referred to as RIFLE and used for standardization of AKI (Workeneh & Batuman, 2012). RIFLE was later modified and validated for pediatric purposes (pediatric modified RIFLE or pRIFLE)

(Table 31-6). The acronym uses the estimated creatinine clearance and urine output to discern the **R** (Risk of renal dysfunction), **I** (Injury to the kidney), **F** (Failure of), or **L** (Loss of kidney function), and **E** (End-stage kidney disease) damage of the AKI (Walters et al., 2009; Workeneh & Batuman, 2012).

 Nursing Insight—*Fluid and electrolyte balance*

Hypotonic fluids used in excess can cause hyponatremia and anemia, which affects the central nervous and cardiac systems (McInerny et al., 2009). If there is an overload of potassium (hyperkalemia) or inadequate ability of the kidneys to excrete potassium, life-threatening hyperkalemia may cause cellular damage and increased neuromuscular excitability and possibly lead to cardiac arrhythmias (McInerny et al., 2009). With AKI, hydrogen ion excretion and bicarbonate reabsorption by the kidneys are insufficient. The resultant acidosis promotes further hyperkalemia resulting from the movement of intracellular potassium into the extracellular space as the body attempts to accommodate the higher hydrogen ion concentration. Respiratory compensation for an underlying metabolic acidosis may cause low carbon dioxide pressure resulting from tachypnea or Kussmaul's respiration. Failure of renal phosphate excretion with AKI can lead to hyperphosphatemia and inversely, hypocalcemia. Tremors and seizures may then occur (McInerny et al., 2009).

 ### Where Research and Practice Meet: pRIFLE

A retrospective study analyzing 390 children who underwent cardiac surgery utilized the serum creatinine criteria pRIFLE and showed that those who had no increase in serum creatinine postoperative days 1 and 2 were negatively predicted to incur AKI (Table 31-6). If there was a rise in serum creatinine on the first postoperative day, AKI was predicted to occur within 48 hours (area under the curve=0.65). Because AKI is not uncommon after pediatric heart surgery, monitoring the serum creatinine level would be proactive in providing quality patient care.

Table 31-6	Pediatric-Modified RIFLE (pRIFLE)	
Criteria	**Estimated CCI**	**Urine Output**
Risk	eCCI decrease by 25%	<0.5 mL/kg/hr for 8 hr
Injury	eCCI decrease by 50%	<0.5 mL/kg/ for 16 hr
Failure	eCCI decrease by 75% or eCCI <35 mlk/min/1.73 meter squared	<0.3 mL/kg/hr for 24 hr or anuric for 12 hr
Loss	Persistent failure > 4 weeks	
End-stage	End-stage renal disease (persistent failure >3 months)	

eCCI, estimated creatinine clearance; pRIFLE, pediatric risk, injury, failure, loss, and end-stage renal disease
Source: Kliegman et al. (2011).

Signs and Symptoms

Lab reports of electrolytes and serum osmolality with covert non-oliguric symptoms resulting in elevation of serum creatinine or changes in electrolytes are important to monitor (McInerny et al., 2009) (Table 31-7).

A thorough physical exam to uncover problems of pre-renal, intrinsic renal, or post-renal manifestations is critical. Pre-renal causes are associated with hypovolemia signs and are evidenced by:

- Tachycardia
- Dry mucous membranes
- Poor peripheral perfusion
  (Kliegman et al., 2011, p. 1819)

Other signs and symptoms of hypovolemia include:

- Poor skin turgor
- Flat jugular veins
- Weight loss
  (Perrin & MacLeod, 2013, p. 402)

Signs and symptoms relative to extracellular fluid indications from decreased renal circulation from vasodilation or cardiovascular disease include:

- Edema
- Ascites
- Weight gain
- Increased central venous pressure and pulmonary artery wedge pressure
  (Perrin & MacLeod, 2013, p. 402)

Intrarenal or intrinsic AKI is evidenced by:

- Peripheral edema
- Rales

- Cardiac gallop
- Potential presence of a rash and arthritis, suggesting systemic lupus erythematosus or Henoch-Schönlein purpura
  (Kliegman et al., 2011, p. 1819)

Post-renal findings include:

- Palpable flank masses might indicate "renal vein thrombosis, tumors, cystic disease, or urinary tract obstruction"
  (Kliegman et al., 2011, p. 1819)

 Nursing Insight—*Anuria*

Children with AKI in general do not have "complete **anuria** unless a catastrophic renovascular event or urinary obstruction has occurred" (McInerny et al., 2009, p. 2799). With **oliguria** or some degree of anuria, the effects of retention of fluid in spaces can manifest as "edema, water intoxication, vascular overload with congestive heart failure, pulmonary edema, hypertension, or any combination" (McInerny et al., 2009, p. 2799). The prognosis of AKI depends on the underlying condition precipitating the decline in function (Kliegman et al., 2011, p. 1822).

Diagnosis

Determining if the cause of the acute kidney injury is pre-renal, intrarenal, or post-renal requires a very careful history, analysis of symptoms, and physical examination. A previous medical history helps to determine any previous infections such as acute glomerulonephritis or neurogenic bladder. Genetic problems, such as a horseshoe-shaped kidney or only one kidney, can be uncovered.

Table 31-7 Signs and Symptoms of Electrolyte Imbalances in Acute Kidney Injury

Electrolyte Imbalance	Clinical Manifestations	Clinical Treatment
Hyperkalemia (>6.0 mEq/L) Results from inability to adequately excrete potassium derived from diet and catabolized cells. In metabolic acidosis, there is also movement of potassium from intracellular fluid to extracellular fluid.	Peaked T waves, widening of QRS on ECG Dysrhythmias: ventricular dysrhythmias, heart block, ventricular fibrillation, cardiac arrest Diarrhea Muscle weakness	Eliminate all intake of potassium (dietary, parenteral, or TPN) Eliminate administration of alkalinizing agents such as Kayexalate orally or in a retention enema when K+ is >7.0 mEq/L Other drugs may be ordered by physician including calcium gluconate 10% solution, sodium bicarbonate, and regular insulin when K+ is >7.0 mEq/L Administer dialysis if other methods to reduce the potassium level are ineffective
Hyponatremia In the acute oliguric phase, hyponatremia is related to the accumulation of fluid in excess of solute.	Change in level of consciousness Muscle cramps Anorexia Abdominal reflexes, depressed deep tendon reflexes Cheyne-Stokes respirations Seizures	Electrolyte replacement, sodium bicarbonate Dialysis to correct severe electrolyte disturbance
Hypocalcemia Phosphate retention (hyperphosphatemia) depresses the serum calcium concentration. Calcium is deposited in injured cells. Hyperkalemia and metabolic acidosis may mask the common clinical manifestations of severe hypocalcemia.	Muscle tingling Changes in muscle tone Seizures Muscle cramps and twitching Positive Chvostek's sign (contraction of facial muscles after tapping facial nerve just anterior to parotid gland)	Calcium gluconate Low phosphorus diet Phosphate binders (e.g., Tums tablets, calcium acetate, and sevelamer hydrochloride [Renagel]) and aluminum-based binders not used to prevent possible aluminum toxicity. Calcium IV not given (except for tetany to prevent calcium salt deposition into tissues) Dialysis to correct severe electrolyte disturbance

A through nursing physical assessment undergirds selection of lab work that provides underlying clues to diagnosis. Common laboratory data routinely obtained are a urinalysis, blood chemistry, blood urea nitrogen, serum creatinine, and pH.

AKI can also be diagnosed by finding toxins in the blood. Toxins are found if there has been exposure to heavy metals or organic solvents, which can cause acute tubular necrosis. Other epidemiological nephrotoxic agents include treatment with aminoglycosides, amphotericin B, contrast, or chemotherapeutic agents (Lerma & Nissenson, 2012).

 Nursing Insight—Decline in kidney function

An undiagnosed decline in kidney function may be a chronic kidney disease heralded by "urinary abnormalities, fatigue, pallor, slowed linear growth, poor school performance, and anorexia extending over a period" (McInerny et al., 2009, p. 2799).

 Diagnostic Tools Renal Biopsy

Renal biopsy is useful and ordered by the health-care provider if the cause of the AKI cannot be ascertained. However, contraindications to percutaneous renal biopsy include sepsis, uncontrolled high blood pressure, infection, hemorrhagic diathesis, parenchymal malignancy, or infection. After the biopsy, bleeding is the most frequent problem but is rarely a critical issue that would require operative strategies. The bleeding is usually controlled by the person's own hemodynamic processes. In conjunction with a biopsy, renal ultrasound has advantages, such as pinpointing obstructive uropathy and helping identify fluid collecting in perirenal spaces, which assists in differentiating cysts and masses that are solid and can illustrate the actual flow of blood with use of the Doppler.

 Nursing Insight—Renal tubular function and fractional excretions of sodium and urea

To identify tubular function, understanding fractional excretions of sodium (FENa) and urea are useful, particularly with AKI patients who have oliguria. To calculate the FENa, the urine sodium excretion is divided by the filtered sodium load.

A FENa less than 1% may indicate that the client has developed acute tubular necrosis. A FENa greater than 1% may be seen in clients who are taking diuretics, suffering with pre-renal azotemia, or who may have chronic kidney disease (CKD) (Lerma & Nissenson, 2012).

Prevention

Nurses need to identify patients at risk for AKI and intervene as soon as possible (Yaklin, 2011). Prevention includes monitoring for preexisting medical conditions and preventing them if possible. Also, avoiding hypoxia through close observation of drugs with nephrotoxicity is important (Murphy & Byrne, 2010).

Collaborative Care

Nursing Care. Analyzing whether AKI is pre-renal, intrarenal, or post-renal through assessment of the associated symptoms and physical findings is crucial in diagnosing,

---

Labs: **Complete Blood Count and Urinalysis**

A complete blood count (CBC) helps identify evidence of renal anemia and gives information regarding the platelets and red and white blood cells that would provide clues of infection and types of anemia (Tables 31-8 and 31-9). If the values are outside normal ranges, then more lab investigation is important (e.g., understanding if erythropoietin therapy is needed or if there are other causes such as infection, hyperparathyroidism, or deficiencies in vitamins such as B_{12} and folic acid) (Lerma & Nissenson, 2012; Thomas, 2008).

It is also important for the nurse to review urinalysis, serum blood urea nitrogen, serum creatinine, creatinine clearance, BUN-to-creatinine ratio, and biomarkers (Perrin & MacLeod, 2013, p. 403).

Table 31-8 Common Urinalysis Findings of Acute Kidney Injury

Urinalysis Findings	Interpretation
Urinary Sediment	Intrinsic kidney failure
Color	"Dirty" brown: intrinsic renal failure Reddish brown: acute glomerulonephritis Bilious tinge: mixed hepatic and renal failure
Proteinuria	Glomerulonephritis Interstitial nephritis Toxic and infectious causes
Casts	Red blood cell (RBC) casts Glomerulonephritis or vasculitis White blood cell (WBC) casts Interstitial nephritis Granular casts: glomerulonephritis Uric acid crystals: tumor lysis syndrome Calcium oxalate crystals: ethylene glycols
Ingestion	acetaminophen (Tylenol) crystals: acetaminophen (Tylenol)

---

treating, and caring for the sequelae of AKI. The sequelae are different depending on the patient's health status.

The nursing responsibilities for care of the patient with AKI are multiple and require significant patience with a child who has a changing level of consciousness and irritability. It is important to monitor laboratory results and identify hemodilution from overload of fluids with a reading of "decreased hemoglobin, hematocrit and serum sodium" (Perrin & MacLeod, 2013, p. 406).

Nursing care also involves increasing renal perfusion and preventing fluid, electrolyte, and acid-base imbalances. If the acid-base, fluid, and electrolyte status remains unimproved, then renal replacement therapy (RRT) is considered. The RRT of hemodialysis, peritoneal dialysis, hemofiltration, and renal transplant are discussed further on in this chapter.

Good communication with parents and their children, with use of therapeutic communication measures, helps reduce anxiety from uncertainty. Compassionate and collaborative care helps promote quality of life for children, even when facing death (Crozier & Hancock, 2012).

Table 31-9 Laboratory Differential Diagnosis of Acute Kidney Injury

	Pre-Renal		Intrarenal		
	CHILD	NEONATE	CHILD	NEONATE	POST-RENAL
Urine Na+ (mEq/L)	<20	<20–30	>40	>40	Variable, may be >40
FENa* (%) Should not be obtained after a diuretic is given—renders the test inaccurate	<1	<2–5	>2	>2.5	Variable, may be >2
Urine osmolality (mOsm/L)	>500	>300–500	>300	>300	Variable, may be <300
Serum BUN-to-creatinine ratio	>20	≥10	>10	>10	Variable, may be >20
Urinalysis	Normal		RBCs WBCs Casts Proteinuria		Variable to normal Possible crystals
Comments	History: diarrhea, vomiting, hemorrhage, diuretics Physical: volume depletion		History: hypotension, anoxia, exposure to nephrotoxins Physical: hypertension, edema		History: poor urine stream and output Physical: flank mass, distended bladder

*FENa, fractional excretion of sodium (%) = [(urine sodium/plasma sodium) + (urine creatinine/plasma creatinine)]/100; RBCs, red blood cells; WBCs, white blood cells

 legal alert—Be sure to record an accurate weight measurement

An inaccurate weight recorded in the patient electronic record can cause life-threatening harm for the patient. It is critical that when delegating to non-licensed health-care providers, such as nursing assistants, the nurse carefully monitors that the weight measures are being done properly and that the body mass index is plotted. Be sure to obtain accurate weight on the same scale, at the same time of day, and with the patient wearing the same clothing (infants are weighed naked and older children often only have on their underwear). The weights are ordered once a day, before feedings, and every 12 hours for critically ill children. Given that the patients may be on steroids, diuretics, or experiencing side-effects of nausea, vomiting, and diarrhea from antibiotics, the weight is very important, as is an accurate record of intake and output (Thomas, 2008).

 focus on safety

Fluid requirements

Children who have certain fluid requirements prescribed to increase urinary output may inadvertently experience **iatrogenic fluid overload** (damage caused by treatment). It is critical to be meticulous when monitoring a child with replacement fluids to prevent iatrogenic fluid overload. The nurse also detects fluid overload by monitoring weight daily and recording intake and output.

 Collaboration in Caring—*The dietitian*

Monitoring nutritional intake is important to help the health-care provider make treatment decisions.

Collaboration with a dietitian is important. It is estimated that around 40% of patients with AKI are reported as malnourished, with protein malnutrition a contributing factor to mortality. Often, children suffering anorexic appetites secondary to AKI are particularly difficult to assist with food selection. The child's favorite foods may be forbidden, so working as a team with the nutritionist, family, and child can be life-saving. It is also important to remember that some parents see the success of their role based in part on how their child eats their meals. The anorexia, therefore, is a substantial cause for worry by parents (Thomas, 2008).

Medical Care. It is critical to monitor the peak and the trough of medications that are nephrotoxic, with trough 1 hour before administration and peak level drawn immediately after medication is given. The nurse maintains aseptic technique when drawing medication blood levels to prevent infection in a child who is already at risk for infection from renal injury (Perrin & MacLeod, 2013).

 Nursing Insight—*Complications*

Collaboration with the health-care team is critical to ensure AKI complications are reduced or prevented, depending on whether the etiology is pre-renal, intrarenal, or post-renal. Early recognition with a good nursing assessment assists with a medical diagnosis. Appropriate nursing intervention aids in preventing AKI progression to parenchymal damage and increasing renal failure (Tables 31-10 and 31-11). The complications of AKI are variable, depending on the underlying etiology.

Table 31-10 Complications of Acute Kidney Injury

Metabolic	Cardiovascular	Gastrointestinal	Neurological	Hematological	Infection	Other
Hyperkalemia	Pulmonary edema	Nausea	Neuromuscular	Anemia	Pneumonia	Hiccups
Metabolic acidosis	Arrhythmias	Vomiting	irritability	Bleeding	Septicemia	Increased
Hyponatremia	Pericarditis	Malnutrition	Asterixis (flapping		Urinary tract	parathyroid
Hypocalcemia	Pericardial	Gastrointestinal	tremor)		infection	hormone
Hyperphosphatemia	effusion	hemorrhage	Seizures			Low total
Hypermagnesemia	Pulmonary		Mental status			triiodothyronine
Hyperuricemia	embolism		change			Low thyroxine
	Hypertension					Normal free
	Myocardial					thyroxine
	infarction					

Table 31-11 Medications Used to Treat Complications of Acute Kidney Injury

Medication	Action/Indication	Nursing Implications
Hyperkalemia • Kayexalate • calcium gluconate 10% • albuterol	Exchanges sodium for potassium Counteracts potassium-induced increased myocardial irritability Shifts potassium to the cells	May require up to 4 hours to take effect. Monitor for ECG changes. IV infiltration may result in tissue necrosis. Give by inhalation.
Metabolic Acidosis • sodium bicarbonate or sodium citrate	Helps correct metabolic acidosis by exchanging hydrogen for potassium	Do not mix with calcium. Complications include fluid overload, hypertension, and tetany.
Hypocalcemia • calcium gluconate 10%	Used in the presence of tetany; provides ionized calcium to restore nervous tissue function to control serum phosphorus	Administer slowly to prevent bradycardia. Monitor for ECG changes.
Malignant Hypertension (B/P >95% for age) • sodium nitroprusside, nitroglycerin	Relaxes smooth muscle in peripheral arterioles	Administer by continuous IV infusion; fall in blood pressure is seen within 10–20 min.

Education/Discharge Instructions

The long-term outcome for AKI relates to the etiology. Referral to a nephrologist as well as renal replacement therapy (RRT) sometimes will prevent further complications arising from AKI (Perrin & MacLeod, 2013).

The family of a child with acute kidney injury is cared for holistically; close physical observations of nutrition, intake and output, and vital signs are necessary to prevent future chronic renal failure. Additionally, counseling for emotional support is necessary (Bunchman, 2012). Also, tell the family about the importance of working with the dietitian (Yaklin, 2011). The AAP Pediatric Nutritional Handbook (2009) provides extensive age-appropriate nutritional counseling that relates to the renal disorder, and collaborating with a dietitian is of paramount importance (American Academy of Pediatrics (AAP, 2009a).

For children and their families who face end-of-life circumstances, palliative care and hospice may be helpful. The World Health Organization (WHO) definition of palliative care is "an approach that improves the quality of life of patients and their families facing the problems associated with life-threatening illness. The prevention and relief of suffering by means of early identification and impeccable assessment and treatment of pain and other problems (physical, psychosocial, and spiritual) is essential (Crozier & Hancock, 2012, p. 199).

 Nursing Diagnoses Acute Kidney Injury

- Ineffective tissue perfusion; renal related to hypovolemia and reduced arterial blood flow
- Excess fluid volume related to renal failure
- Imbalanced nutrition, less than body requirements related to altered metabolic requirements
- Risk for infection related to malnutrition, intubation, and indwelling catheters, drains, or IVs
  (Perrin & MacLeod, 2013, p. 411)

CHRONIC KIDNEY DISEASE

The term chronic kidney disease (CKD) has replaced the previous term of chronic renal failure or chronic renal

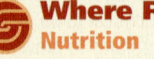 **Where Research and Practice Meet:**
Nutrition

Evidence-based indicators for adequate nourishment are used for home care and include the following age-appropriate information:
- Maintenance of body weight (with no evidence of excessive fluid intake or output)
- Maintenance of the albumin level at 3.5 to 4.0 g/dL
- Maintenance of the total protein level at 6 to 8 g/dL
- Normalizing serum electrolytes
  (Perrin & MacLeod, 2013)

insufficiency but excludes those children less than 2 years of age whose quick response to treatment cannot be estimated alone by the glomerular filtration rate (Table 31-12). For those children older than 2 years of age, the glomerular filtration rate may progressively deteriorate through 4 separate stages, and the rate varies from patient to patient.

 Nursing Insight—*A developmental perspective of CKD*

Developmentally, the etiology of CKD in children is age-related and dependent on the organs that are affected. For children younger than 2 years old, obstructive uropathy or renal hypodysplasia is the common underlying problem. For children between 2 and 5 years of age, neonatal vascular accidents, renal hypodysplasia, and obstructive uropathy are factors. For older children and adolescents, glomerulonephritis, lupus nephritis, or reflux nephropathy are the underlying etiologies. Genetic considerations include polycystic kidney disease, congenital nephritic syndrome, and sickle cell disease. For some, the course of the disease may eventually be fatal unless RRT and dialysis are initiated and sometimes followed by kidney transplantation (Daugirdas, 2011; Lerma & Nissenson, 2012).

Children with renal disease beginning in infancy and those with a congenital etiology are at risk for growth failure and for progression to end-stage renal disease (**ESRD**). Genetic counseling is promoted in family planning in these situations. It is also important for early detection of CKD for the following reasons:

• Timely surgical intervention, so early in-utero surgery can occur
• Knowledge that each disorder requires different treatments and has varying prognoses
• Information about genetic counseling because early diagnosis and treatment for siblings can be initiated if a hereditary or metabolic disease is discovered
• Attention to the timing and donor selection for renal transplantation
(Klein, 2010, p. 608)

 Nursing Insight—*CKD complications*

Each stage of CKD has its own complications. Healy (2011) observes, including stage 1, CKD has an overall complication rate of "70% hypertension, 37% anemia, 17% metabolic bone disease, and 12% growth failure" (p. 1749). Chronic kidney disease also differs in children compared with adults (whose major causes are diabetes and obesity). Prevention of long-term potential complications is integrated into the nursing plan of care.

 Nursing Insight—*Recommendation from the National Kidney Foundation*

The National Kidney Foundation (2013) recommends that patients and families with a background of diabetes, hypertension, or renal disease follow their glomerular filtration rate with their health-care provider to ensure early intervention to slow the process. Reduction of the glomerular filtration results in fluid, electrolyte, and acid-base imbalances, causing damage and abnormalities in all organ systems.

 Cultural Diversity: Kidney Failure

The following information underscores the importance of being aware and preventing health-care disparities. African Americans constitute about 32% of all patients treated for CKD in the United States. Also, anyone with high blood pressure, diabetes, or a family history of kidney disease is at risk for CKD and should have an evaluation via a kidney function test. The Centers for Disease Control and Prevention (2013) note that CKD is the ninth leading cause of death in the United States. Lerma and Nissenson (2012) identify the following points about renal diseases in African Americans:

1. The incidence and prevalence of renal diseases are highest among African Americans.
2. Renal disease among African Americans is characterized by an earlier onset and a more rapid progression to end-stage renal disease.
3. High blood pressure and diabetes account for more than two-thirds of the new cases of end-stage renal disease.
4. Renal disease progression can be effectively prevented and/or attenuated by appropriate blood pressure and blood sugar control.
(p. 482)

Signs and Symptoms

Table 31-13 outlines the pathophysiology that underlies the signs and symptoms of CKD. The most common pathophysiological findings at the time of diagnosis are related to (1) fluid and electrolyte/acid-base abnormalities, (2) metabolic abnormalities, (3) hormone alteration, (4) uremia, and (5) growth restriction (Klein, 2010, p. 608).

Table 31-12	Four Stages of Chronic Kidney Disease According to Glomerular Filtration Rate (GFR)	
Percentage of Reduction of GFR	**Stage of Renal Failure**	**Glomerular Filtration Rate as Applied to Children Age 2 and Older***
35%–55% of normal	1. Reduced renal reserve	≥90
25%–35% of normal	2. Renal insufficiency	60–89
20%–25% of normal	3. Renal failure	30–59
Less than 20% of normal	4. End-stage renal disease (ESRD)	15–29*

*If GFR <15, dialysis is needed

Table 31-13 Pathophysiology of Chronic Kidney Disease

Signs and Symptom	Mechanism
Accumulation of nitrogenous waste products	Decrease in glomerular filtration rate
Acidosis	Decreased ammonia synthesis Impaired bicarbonate reabsorption Decreased net acid excretion
Sodium retention	Excessive renin production Oliguria
Sodium wasting	Solute dieresis Tubular damage
Urinary concentrating defect	Solute dieresis Tubular damage
Hyperkalemia	Decrease in glomerular filtration rate Metabolic acidosis Excessive potassium intake Hyporeninemic hypoaldosteronism
Renal osteodystrophy	Impaired renal production of 1, 25-dihydroxycholecalciferol Hyperphosphatemia Hypocalcemia Secondary hyperparathyroidism
Growth retardation	Inadequate caloric intake Renal osteodystrophy Metabolic acidosis Anemia Growth hormone resistance
Anemia	Decreased erythropoietin production Iron deficiency Folate deficiency Vitamin B_{12} deficiency Decreased erythrocyte survival
Bleeding tendency	Defective platelet function
Infection	Defective granulocyte function Impaired cellular immune functions Indwelling dialysis catheters
Neurological symptoms (fatigue, poor concentration, headache, drowsiness, memory loss, seizures, peripheral neuropathy)	Uremic factors Aluminum toxicity Hypertension
Gastrointestinal symptoms (feeding intolerance, abdominal pain)	Gastroesophageal reflux Decreased gastrointestinal motility
Hypertension	Volume overload Excessive renin production
Hyperlipidemia	Decreased plasma lipoprotein lipase activity
Pericarditis, cardiomyopathy	Uremic factor(s) Hypertension Fluid overload
Glucose intolerance	Tissue insulin resistance

Source: Used with permission from Sreedharan, R., & Avner, E. (2011). In R. M. Kliegman, B. M. D. Stanton, St. J. W. Geme, N. F. Schor, & R. E. Behrman, *Nelson's textbook of pediatrics* (19th ed., p. 1823). Philadelphia, PA: Elsevier Saunders.

Additional conditions that are diagnosed secondary to severe uremia include congestive heart failure, pericarditis, uremic pleuritis, encephalopathy, and gastrointestinal bleeding (Klein, 2010).

Actual signs and symptoms of CKD are:

- Failure to thrive or anorexia
- Nausea
- Vomiting
- Loss of appetite
- Lethargy
- Headaches
- High blood pressure
- Reduced urine output
- Polyuria and polydipsia
- Bed wetting
  (Thomas, 2008, p. 297)

"What to say"—*Gathering information from the parents*

The nurse asks the parents if the child has any of the following symptoms:

- Malaise
- Poor appetite
- Vomiting
- Bone pain
- Headache
- Polyuria

The nurse also asks the parents if the child has had any of the following signs and symptoms in the past:

- Perinatal complications
- Oligohydramnios
- Recurrent urinary tract infections
- Enuresis

In addition, the nurse asks the parent:

- "Is there any family history of renal disease?"
- "Is there any family history of hearing impairment?"

Diagnosis

Physical examination findings of CKD have correlations with underlying pathophysiological mechanisms with all major body systems including skeletal, cardiopulmonary, neurological, endocrine and reproductive, hematological, gastrointestinal, integumentary, immunological, HEENT, and the abdomen (Table 31-14).

Common urinalysis findings associated with CKD include a urinary sediment; color ranging from dirty brown, reddish brown, to bilious tinge; proteinuria; and casts (Lerma & Nissenson, 2012; McCance, Huether, Brashers, & Rote, 2010; Thomas, 2008).

Labs: CKD Laboratory Findings

Laboratory findings are reflected in elevated blood urea nitrogen and serum creatinine along with hyperkalemia, hyponatremia, acidosis, hypocalcemia, hypophosphatemia, and elevated uric acid. A CBC is essential along with serum cholesterol and triglyceride levels, which are often increased.

Table 31-14 Physical Examination Findings Correlated With Underlying Pathophysiological Mechanisms for Chronic Kidney Disease

Organ System	Physical Findings	Correlation With Pathophysiological Mechanisms
Skeletal	Osteitis fibrosa (bone inflammation with fibrous degeneration) Bone demineralization (principally subperiosteal loss of cortical bone in the fibers, lateral ends of the clavicles, and lamina dura of the teeth) Spontaneous fractures, bone pain; osteomalacia (rickets or rachitic changes) with end-stage renal failure Edema Absent patella	Bone resorption associated with hyperparathyroidism, vitamin D deficiency, and demineralization Lowered calcium and raised phosphate levels
Cardiopulmonary	Hypertension, pericarditis with fever, chest pain, pericardial friction rub, pulmonary edema, Kussmaul's respiration Flow murmur Gallop Rub	Extracellular volume expansion as cause of hypertension Hypersecretion of renin also associated with hypertension Fluid overload associated with pulmonary edema and acidosis leading to Kussmaul's respiration
Neurological	Encephalopathy (fatigue, loss of attention, difficulty problem solving) Peripheral neuropathy (pain and burning in the legs and feet, loss of vibration sense and deep tendon reflexes) Loss of motor coordination, twitching, fasciculations, stupor, and coma with advanced uremia Hypotonia Irritability	Uremic toxins associated with end-stage renal disease
Endocrine and Reproductive	Retarded growth in children (short stature) Osteomalacia High incidence of goiter Sexual dysfunction: menorrhagia, amenorrhea, infertility, and decreased libido in women; decreased testosterone levels, infertility, and decreased libido in men	Decreased growth hormone Elevated parathyroid hormone Decreased thyroid hormone Elevated hormones: luteinizing hormone (LH), follicle-stimulating hormone, prolactin, and LH-releasing hormone; decreased testosterone, estrogen, and progesterone
Hematological	Anemia, usually normochromic, normocytic; platelet disorders with prolonged bleeding times (increase in bleeding gums)	Reduced erythropoietin secretion associated with loss of renal mass, leading to reduced red cell production in the bone marrow; uremic toxins associated with shortened red cell survival
Gastrointestinal	Anorexia, nausea, vomiting Mouth ulcers, stomatitis, bad breath (uremic fetor), hiccups, peptic ulcers, gastrointestinal bleeding, and pancreatitis associated with end-stage renal failure	Retention of urea, metabolic acids, and other metabolic waste products, including methylguanidine
Integumentary	Abnormal pigmentation and pruritus	Retention of urochrome, contributing to sallow, yellow color High plasma calcium levels associated with pruritus
Immunological	Increased risk of infection that can cause death; decreased response to vaccination	Suppression of cell-mediated immunity Reduction in number and function of lymphocytes Diminished phagocytosis
HEENT	Retinal changes Preauricular pits Hearing deficit	Uremic toxins
Abdomen	Palpable kidneys Suprapubic mass	

Diagnosis is also based on fluid, electrolyte, and acid-base abnormalities including identifying potassium (usually high), degree of fluid volume overload, and sodium imbalance. Diagnosis of metabolic abnormalities is made through calcium and phosphate serum elevations and increased parathyroid hormone (PTH), which promotes phosphate and calcium excretion. Assessment of active vitamin D is necessary because there is a vitamin D deficiency, which reduces the absorption of calcium in the gut and causes skeletal problems secondary to PTH.

CKD diagnostic tests that are frequently ordered by the health-care provider to assess for the fluid, electrolyte, and acid-base abnormalities; metabolic abnormalities; hormone alterations; uremia; and growth restriction include chest radiographs, bone films, renal ultrasounds, and electrocardiograms if the child is hyperkalemic (Klein, 2010).

Prevention

Malnutrition of the pregnant woman has correlation with renal disease for herself as well as for the unborn child. Hence, good prenatal care is of the utmost importance. After birth, it is also important to plot the child's growth on a standardized growth chart because growth delays alert a health-care provider to potential renal problems.

With the emphasis now on prevention and early assessment to spot CKD, prognosis has improved (Daugirdas, 2011). Future experience with biomarkers such as interleukin-18, neutrophil gelatinase-associated lipocalin, and kidney injury molecule 1 may allow for prevention by determining earlier if kidney disease is present. Intervening quickly can prevent further renal damage (Perrin & MacLeod, 2013).

Collaborative Care

Nursing Care. A through nursing assessment includes correlating the pathophysiology with the affected organ systems. The goals of nursing care for a patient with CKD are mutually established by the health-care provider and family. Collaboration with the health-care team is essential so that the quality of the child's life is extended as long as possible as the renal capacity diminishes affecting all organ systems.

It is important to provide the best possible nutrition. Nutrition has the greatest impact on renal recovery (AAP, 2009a). Given the many changes that occur with CKD, normal nutrition is challenged. Collaborate with a

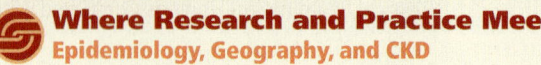

Where Research and Practice Meet:
Epidemiology, Geography, and CKD

McClellan, Plantinga and McClellan (2012) conducted a study on epidemiology, geography, and CKD. The purpose of the study was to correlate renal epidemiology of CKD with the environmental and geographical variations. Environmental characteristics such as temperature and elevation, as well as geographical variations of natural disasters were studied. Findings showed that the place of residency can be a risk factor related to the occurrence and progression of CKD.

dietitian who helps with meal planning to counteract growth restriction.

Pastoral care may be needed because this chronic disease takes its toll on the entire family as ESRD occurs. Also, the nurse can discuss renal transplant with the family.

Medical Care. Once the diagnosis is made from a well-taken history and laboratory results are completed, medications are ordered (Table 31-15).

Nursing Diagnoses CKD

- Fluid volume excess related to fluid retention and decreased kidney function
- Risk for infection related to depression of immunological defenses, invasive procedures or devices, and changes in dietary intake or malnutrition

Table 31-15 Medications Commonly Used for Children With Chronic Kidney Disease

Medication	Action or Indication	Nursing Considerations
Vitamin and mineral supplement (Nephrocaps)	Add vitamins and minerals missing from heavily restricted diet	Only prescribed vitamins should be used; over-the-counter brands may contain elements that are harmful.
Phosphate-binding agents: calcium carbonate (Tums), calcium acetate (PhosLo), or sevelamer hydrochloride (Renagel)	Reduce absorption of phosphorus from the intestines	Ensure that phosphate-binding agent is aluminum-free.
calcitriol (Rocaltrol)	Replace the calcitriol that kidneys are no longer producing to keep calcium balance normal	Monitor serum calcium level. Ensure that calcium supplement is provided.
epoetin alfa (Epogen, Procrit)	Stimulates bone marrow to produce red blood cells, treats anemia caused by CRF	Given by IV or subcutaneous injection. Monitor blood pressure because hypertension is an adverse effect. Monitor hematocrit and serum ferritin level according to facility guidelines.
Iron supplementation	Treat iron deficiency when epoetin alfa (Epogen) is prescribed	May be administered orally or IV during hemodialysis.
Growth hormone (GH)	Used to stimulate growth in children with CRF	Record accurate height measurements at regular intervals.
Antihypertensive agents: Angiotensin-converting enzyme (ACE) inhibitor (enalapril, lisinopril) Loop diuretics	Used with proteinuric kidney disease because it slows the progression to ESRD Used when volume overload is present	Monitor renal function and electrolyte balance.

- Risk for imbalanced nutrition, less than body requirements related to the inability to ingest or digest adequate nutrients (Doenges, Moorhouse, & Murr, 2013, p. 1070)

Renal Replacement Therapy

Renal replacement therapy (RRT) is the treatment option for end-stage renal disease (ESRD) and is also used for acute kidney injury (AKI). For the child with chronic kidney disease CKD, discussion with the family often starts when the child is in Stage 4 of the disease. RRT for children is a momentous decision for the family while they await a possible donor kidney. The transplant team collaborates with the family to orient them to the transplant process, which includes a facility tour as well as meeting other families who have had a similar journey and whose children are now stable.

Commonly accepted criteria to begin RRT in children include:

- Volume overload with evidence of pulmonary edema or hypertension
- Hyperkalemia greater than 6.5 mEq/L despite conservative measures (greater than 6.0 mEq/L if hypercatabolic)
- Metabolic acidosis with pH less than 7.2 or HCO_3^- less than 10
- Blood urea nitrogen (BUN) greater than 150 (lower if rising rapidly)
- Neurological symptoms secondary to uremia or electrolyte imbalance
- Calcium and phosphorus imbalance (e.g., hypokalemia with tetany or seizures in the presence of a high serum phosphate level)
- Dialyzable toxin or poison (e.g., lactate, ammonia, alcohol, barbiturates, ethylene glycol, isopropanol, methanol, salicylates, or theophylline) (Tschudy & Arcara, 2012, p. 495)
- Other important criteria are "uremic induced mental changes, or neuropathy or pericarditis" (Perrin & MacLeod, 2013, p. 413).

Table 31-16 gives the relative and absolute indicators for RRT.

Table 31-16 Relative and Absolute Indicators for Renal Replacement Therapy
Relative Indicators
• Age of child
• GRF 10%
• Primary renal disease and comorbid conditions
• Failure to thrive
• Developmental delay
• Inability to function at school
• Inadequate electrolyte and metabolic control
• Poor nutritional status
Absolute Indicators
• Pulmonary edema
• Uncontrollable hypertension
• Pericarditis
• Uremic encephalopathy
• Refractory nausea and emesis
Source: Box 32-2 in Klein, 2010, p. 810.

Nursing Insight—Three methods of RRT

There are three methods of RRT:
1. **Hemofiltration**, also known as continuous renal replacement therapy (CRRT)
2. Peritoneal dialysis (PD)
3. Hemodialysis (HD)
(Perrin & MacLeod, 2013)

HEMOFILTRATION

In the pediatric setting, hemofiltration, or CRRT, is a broad category that results in removing water by filtration through an extracorporeal system. Continuous arteriovenous hemofiltration (CAVH) is a CRRT subcategory treatment frequently used to remove solutes through "diffusion, convection, or both" (Blayney, 2013, p. 774). CAVH facilitates kidney function through an **extracorporeal** (outside the body) continuously running circuit occurring at a slow rate. The circuit is connected to an arterial and venous catheter with "passage of arterial blood through the filter [which] results in the formation of an ultrafiltrate of plasma that consists of water and non-protein bound solutes. The filtered blood is then returned to the patient through the venous catheter" (Blayney, 2013, p. 774). It is similar to hemodialysis, but is continuous, and because it is slower, it is stabilizing for patients who have more organ dysfunction, such as patients with shock or bone marrow transplants. It is also effective for neonates or small infants who are less likely to tolerate hemodialysis. CAVH, in some settings, has been replaced by continuous venovenous hemofiltration that is more precise ultrafiltration (Blayney, 2013).

Signs and Symptoms

Signs and symptoms of complications related to hemofiltration or CRRT include:

- Hypotension
- Electrolyte imbalances
- Coagulation abnormalities
- Bleeding
- Sepsis
(Perrin & MacLeod, 2013, p. 418)

Diagnosis

Careful understanding of the diagnoses that created the need for hemofiltration or CRRT is important.

Prevention

Careful intervention by the nurse helps to prevent possible hypothermia. Specifically, hypothermia in small infants can be reduced through blood warmers. However, the nurse can also use other external warming devices such as "radiant warmers, body warmer, heating mattresses, and solution heaters" (Blayney, 2013, p. 777).

Collaborative Care

Nursing Care. Prior to hemofiltration or CRRT, the goals of care include stabilizing fluid balance and assessing BUN, creatinine, glucose, and partial thromboplastin time (PTT) before initiating the procedure. Once hemofiltration, or

CRRT, commences, vital signs are monitored along with fluid balance every 30 minutes. The ultrafiltration rate is assessed every hour with replacement fluid set by the nephrologist. The patency of all the circuits is carefully checked, including looking for clots. Analysis of PTT and clotting studies are monitored every 1 to 3 hours (Perrin & MacLeod, 2013, p. 417).

Education/Discharge Instructions

Teach parents to monitor for complications related to CAVH, which include "fluid and electrolyte imbalances, bleeding/thromboembolic events such as anemia that results from excessive clot formation in the filters and hypovolemia if excessive volumes of ultrafiltrate is removed" (Blayney, 2013, pp. 775–776). Regardless of type of RRT, nutritional needs are important, and involvement of a dietitian is ideal (Thomas, 2008).

HEMODIALYSIS OR PERITONEAL DIALYSIS

The choice of dialysis, **hemodialysis** (HD) or **peritoneal dialysis** (PD), is dependent on the medical diagnosis, age, and symptoms that indicate the timing of starting RRT. Dialysis may be done through the peritoneal wall (PD) or through cleansing the blood by using a dialysis machine (HD). It is important to note that while dialysis is usually reserved for children in ESRD as a result of chronic renal failure, it may also be needed in acute renal failure if BUN and creatinine levels elevate (Sreedharan & Avner, 2011).

Peritoneal Dialysis

The process of PD uses the peritoneal membrane (abdominal lining) to filter blood and purify it. Using a dialysis solution composed of dextrose sugar and other minerals in water, it is inserted into the child's abdomen through an abdominal catheter. Through an osmotic process, the dialysis solution draws toxins, excess water, and waste chemicals from the blood into the dialysis solution. From there, it is drained through an abdominal tube out of the abdomen. The amount of time the dialysis solution is in the abdomen is termed the dwell time, and the entire process of filling and emptying the abdomen is termed an exchange. Table 31-17 outlines the advantages and disadvantages of peritoneal dialysis in children with ESRD.

There are two essential types of peritoneal dialysis: continuous ambulatory peritoneal dialysis (CAPD) (offers the greatest freedom) and continuous cycling peritoneal dialysis (CCPD). With CAPD the patient or parent will fill the abdomen with the dialysate with a dwell time set by the health-care provider. CCPD can be used as intermittent peritoneal dialysis or intermittent peritoneal dialysis given at night (Snyder, 2013). CCPD uses a machine termed "a cycler" to provide numerous exchanges during a child's sleep time. In the morning, the child has one exchange with a dwell time that lasts for the whole day, with a potential of adding a mid-afternoon treatment. In contrast, CAPD does not require a cycler machine. Instead, the dialysis solution is run from a plastic bag through the catheter, and it remains in the abdomen for several hours with a sealed catheter. After this dwell time has passed, the patient's dialysis solution with the waste products must be drained into a special disposal

Table 31-17	Advantages and Disadvantages of Peritoneal Dialysis in Children With End-Stage Renal Disease

Advantages

- Ability to perform dialysis treatment at home
- Easier than hemodialysis, especially in infants
- Ability to live a greater distance from medical center
- Freedom to attend school and after-school activities
- Less restrictive diet
- Less expensive than hemodialysis
- Promotes independence (adolescents)

Disadvantages

- Catheter malfunction
- Catheter-related infections (peritonitis and at the site)
- Impaired appetite (because of full peritoneal cavity)
- Negative body image
- Caregiver burnout

Source: Sreedharan & Avner (2011), Table 529-7, p. 1826.

bag, and then another cycle of dialysis solution is begun. The duration and prescribed amount of dialysate are individualized. Having nocturnal intermittent dialysis enables daytime activities. Peritoneal dialysis, unlike hemodialysis, must be performed daily (Sreedharan & Avner, 2011).

 Nursing Insight—PD and adolescents

Adolescents may lack adherence to the PD protocol. Also, based on their age, body image, and self-esteem, they may be affected by the appearance of an external catheter (Klein, 2010). It is important to suggest professional counseling to help adolescents adapt to PD.

Signs and Symptoms

Signs and symptoms of PD complications include:

- Potential peritonitis
- Catheter dysfunction and obstruction
- Pain
- Pulmonary complications
- Fluid and electrolyte imbalance (Blayney, 2013, pp. 768–769)

There are not many contraindications to a patient having PD, except "neonates with omphalocele, diaphragmatic hernia, or gastroschisis" (Blayney, 2013, p. 761). If a patient has had abdominal surgery, but minimal abdominal adhesions and no draining wounds, PD is still possible. If there are urinary diversions such as polycystic kidneys, colostomy, gastrostomy, or prune-belly syndrome, PD is still used. PD can be useful if a patient experiences rejection from a renal transplant. As long as the "allograft has been placed in the extraperitoneal space," PD can be used for this diagnosis also (Blayney, 2013, p. 761).

Diagnosis

Prior to PD, acute kidney injury or chronic kidney disease is diagnosed.

Prevention

The nurse who assesses the patient carefully regarding intake and output, lab work, and vital signs and ascertains that these findings are within normal limits helps reduce complications by determining if it is safe to start the PD. Also, once the cycle is completed, the nurse who discerns carefully that the dialysate return is "clear enough to read newspaper print through it" or quickly reports if it is cloudy, helps prevent peritonitis or PD complications (Perrin & MacLeod, 2013, p. 419).

Collaborative Care

Nursing Care. Nursing care is directed at preventing or identifying peritoneal dialysis complications. The riskiest problem with peritoneal dialysis is the chance of peritonitis, an infection of the abdominal peritoneum. This is extremely serious and requires urgent antibiotic therapy, hospitalization, and follow-up with the child's nephrologist (Blayney, 2013). To prevent infection, monitor the abdominal catheter sites for signs of infection or malfunctioning equipment and make certain that the returning dialysate solution remains clear if in the hospital setting. Usually, *Staphylococcus aureus* is the source of peritoneal infection, and cephalosporins and vancomycin hydrochloride (vancomycin hydrochloride injection) are frequently used for treatment. Yet today, because of vancomycin-resistant bacteria, vancomycin hydrochloride injection is not used as frequently.

focus on safety

Watch for complications

Clinical issues with PD include "hernia development, leaking, catheter exit site or tunnel infection, catheter migration, cuff extrusion and catheter outflow obstruction by the omentum or other intra-abdominal structures" (Klein, 2010, p. 611).

Monitor for pain during PD because it may be present even though the patient may not complain. If the pain is caused by inflow of the dialysis infusion, decrease the rate or infuse smaller volumes of the dialysate. Pain can also occur from the catheter being in a pocket instead of the peritoneal area, and distention can occur. This may indicate a need for the nurse to insert a new catheter. Pain also can occur once the cavity of the abdomen is emptied completely, so arranging for a small amount of residual fluid by decreasing the outflow time to less than 5 to 10 minutes reduces this pain (Blayney, 2013).

When the cycle is completed, disconnect the tubing aseptically, cap the access, and uses a sterile dressing to cover the site. The patient is then placed on a scale and weighed to judge the adequacy of fluid removal and to assess if kidney function has improved (Perrin & MacLeod, 2013).

Medical Care. Adherence to the required medication and fluid regimen are necessary along with dialysis treatment for optimal patient outcomes (Snyder, 2013). The nurse also discusses the family's understanding of the common medications that children take in association with having dialysis. Examples include Nephrocaps, phosphate-binding

agents, calcitriol, epoetin alfa (Epogen), iron supplements, vitamin D analog to accomplish low calcium levels, human growth hormone for growth failure, antihypertensives, and stool softeners (Snyder, 2013).

Education/Discharge Instructions

Assist parents and older children in learning about PD and preventing complications. Parents can learn how to monitor for infection if the PD is given at home. If the dialysate return is cloudy, it indicates a potential infection or problem and parents must notify the health-care provider immediately (Klein, 2010; Thomas, 2008).

School nurses and the school environment need to understand about the PD, the common medications, and the times the patient will be absent from school as a result of having PD.

Collaboration in Caring—*Peritoneal dialysis*

The nurse, family, and child work together with the health-care provider with regard to the PD and to determine when a new catheter needs to be inserted. The family also works closely with the dietician to learn about a renal diet that promotes health. The family has a working relationship with the surgeon who placed the catheter, and that surgeon is available when it is removed. When the catheter is removed, sterile technique is used and the tip of the catheter is sent into the lab for a culture, according to institutional policy (Blayney, 2013).

Nursing Diagnoses Peritoneal Dialysis

- Acute pain related to instillation of dialysate, temperature of dialysate
- Risk for infection, peritoneal related to invasive procedure, presence of catheter, dialysate
- Risk for fluid volume excess related to retention of dialysate
- Risk for ineffective coping related to disability requiring change in lifestyle
- Chronic sorrow related to chronic disability

Hemodialysis

To prevent accumulation of unwanted fluid and toxins, hemodialysis (HD) removes unwanted products by extracorporeal circulation through a dialyzer (Fig. 31-7). In adolescents and children in the United States with ESRD, HD is preferred. Extra water, extra salt, and toxic waste products are removed while the blood pressure and electrolytes, such as potassium, calcium, sodium, and bicarbonate, are kept in balance (Goldstein, 2011). Ideally, dialysis is not started in an emergency because in this situation vascular access is temporary. It is important to avoid using the cephalic vein, subclavian catheter, or starting the access in the nondominant vessels of the arm because it is best to have these veins available for future access (Goldstein, 2011).

Permanent and temporary vascular access means are available. Permanent vascular access is offered through an **arteriovenous (AV) fistula**, AV graft, and dual lumen catheters with Dacron cuffs (Klein, 2010, p. 612). Access through the permanent port ideally occurs after a waiting period of 2 to 6 weeks, which allows the AV fistula to

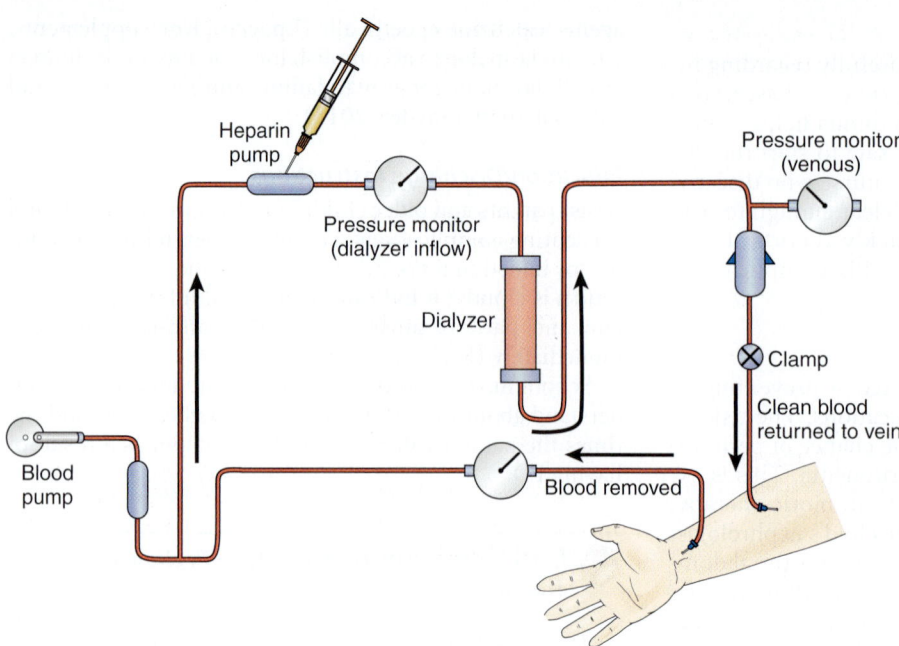

Figure 31-7 The hemodialysis process.

become stronger. For young children with reduced blood flow to extremities, a temporary access is created using an indwelling central venous catheter. This catheter can be placed in the femoral or internal jugular veins for short dialysis periods. HD for children should occur at a pediatric center for dialysis (Sreedharan & Avner, 2011).

The preferred type of vascular access is the AV fistula (Goldstein, 2011). In the AV fistula type, a surgeon connects an artery directly to a vein, commonly in the forearm and around the wrist. Waiting a few months before using the AV fistula allows maturing and healing of the arterial-venous vessels. This process allows more blood flow into the vein, so it grows stronger and larger. Eventually, the vein can support repeated HD connections. A bruit is a noise heard on auscultation that can best be detected over an AV fistula to make certain it is patent. The bruit is heard best at the incision. Also, a thrill can be palpated. Palpating and listening for the bruits is important to discern if thrombosis or stenosis has occurred as a complication (Thomas, 2008).

The AV graft is reserved for children with small veins that do not properly form a fistula over time. It requires a synthetic tube such as polytetrafluoroethylene to be implanted under the skin of the forearm. In comparison to the AV fistula, AV grafts have a higher pressure within the arterial venous connection, making them less compliant (Thomas, 2008).

Many children must be hemodialyzed 3 times a week at an outpatient dialysis center. It is possible to arrange for home HD if families meet the criteria of having running water and a parent and/or caretaker who is able to understand how to do HD (Thomas, 2008). Because each treatment lasts 3 to 4 hours, it is disruptive to the child's time, although it is possible for the child to read, write, complete homework, play video games, and watch television during this process. HD can be done in the hospital or in the home setting and is administered at night, over a longer duration, which assists in removing waste with fewer potential adverse effects such as hypotension (Snyder, 2013).

> ### Nursing Insight—*Hemodialysis and teenagers*
>
> Teenagers are usually started on HD rather than PD. Sometimes a preemptive transplant is done rather than to require the patient to experience dialysis (Lerma & Nissenson, 2012; Klein, 2010).

Signs and Symptoms

Criteria related to HD depend on the presence of the following signs and symptoms:

- Glomerular filtration rate (GFR) less than 15 mL/min per 1.73 meters squared
- Intractable complications of AKI
- Higher GFR (Blayney, 2013, p. 769)

At the onset of HD, a child may experience several side effects related to quick alterations in the body's chemical and water balance. These side effects include:

- Hypotension (low blood pressure)
- Weakness, dizziness, and nausea from the hypotension
- Muscle cramps secondary to electrolyte imbalances (Snyder, 2013)

Diagnosis

The underlying choice to use HD is determined by the health-care provider in partnership with the family. Based on diagnosis, it is important to relate the necessity of HD and what level of renal failure has occurred.

Prevention

For the patient who must monitor his or her own potassium nutritionally, it is important to know and avoid foods high in potassium, such as bananas, nuts, broccoli, dried fruits, oranges, cantaloupe, and tomatoes.

To prevent complications of HD, complete a thorough nursing assessment prior to starting HD. Common complications include:

- Hypotension and hypovolemia
- Fluid shifts and disequilibrium
- Hypervolemia
- Bleeding
- Anemia
- Infection
- Febrile reactions
(Blayney, 2013, pp.771–772)

Collaborative Care

Nursing Care. Administering HD to a child is a highly specialized form of nursing that requires additional training. The child best suited for HD has someone who can assist with the PD process at home, or they should live close to a dialysis center.

It is imperative to keep the AV fistula, AV graft, or venous catheter clean and safe. First, the access site must be kept clean and used only for HD (e.g., no drawing blood from the site). To keep the access site safe, tell the child that he or she cannot wear jewelry near the site, cannot have a blood pressure taken on the affected arm, and cannot bruise the site.

Fluid and dietary restrictions are necessary between dialysis sessions. HD has the benefit of rapidly improving the uremic child, somewhat normalizing growth rates, skeletal maturation, and sexual development, which may all be impaired in ESRD (Thomas, 2008).

Critical Nursing Action Arteriovenous Fistulas

Provide the following health promotion teaching to a child and family related to the care of a newly acquired AV fistula for HD treatment:

- Wash the access site with soap and warm water each day, and always before dialysis.
- Instruct the child to not scratch the area or to remove scabs.
- Check the access site daily for signs of infection, including warmth and redness.
- Check that there is blood flow in the access device daily. There should be a vibration (called a thrill) over the access. If this is absent or changes, a health-care provider at the dialysis center should be notified immediately.
- Take care to avoid traumatizing the arm where the access site is located; do not wear tight clothes, jewelry, carry heavy items, or sleep on the access site arm.
- Remind health-care providers not to take blood or measure blood pressure on the access site arm.
- Rotate needle on the access site. Use gentle pressure to stop bleeding when the needle is removed. If bleeding occurs later, apply gentle pressure; call a health-care provider if bleeding does not stop within 30 minutes or if bleeding is excessive.

Education/Discharge Instructions

HD can take place in the home, the clinical setting, or a dialysis center. Regardless of setting, collaborate with the family, health-care team, and case manager to plan for home care. Ensure support through multidisciplinary meetings that include the social worker, dietician, financial counselor, physicians, and primary nurse (Blayney, 2013). The child on HD often misses school and social activities,

leading to isolation and emotional problems, so counseling may be necessary.

Nursing Diagnoses Hemodialysis

- Excess fluid volume related to renal disease with minimal urine output
- Noncompliance with dietary restrictions related to denial of chronic illness
- Ineffective Health Maintenance related to deficient knowledge regarding hemodialysis procedure, restrictions, blood access care
- Powerlessness related to treatment regimen
- Risk for infection related to exposure to blood products or risk of developing hepatitis B

Kidney Transplant

Children with progressive renal disease leading toward end-stage renal disease (ESRD) are referred for a kidney transplant evaluation.

Nursing Insight—*Causes of ESRD*

- Polycystic kidney disease
- Inherited disease in which the kidneys overgrow with cysts that destroy good nephrons
- Tubular disorders: renal tubular acidosis, Fanconi's syndrome
- Urinary tract abnormalities: reflux nephropathy, posterior ureteral valves, neurogenic bladder
- Obstructive disorders: renal calculi, retroperitoneal fibrosis, prostatic hypertrophy
- Autoimmune disorders: Goodpasture's disease, Wegener's disease, systemic lupus erythematosus, IgA nephropathy
- Primary glomerular disorders with nephrotic syndrome
- Renal vasculitis diseases: polyarteritis nodosa, Henoch-Schönlein purpura
- Rare causes: hemolytic-uremic syndrome, thrombotic thrombocytopenic purpura, nephrotoxic agents, renal cell carcinoma, renal aplasia, scleroderma, amyloidosis, tubulointer.stitial nephritis

The child and his or her family are evaluated to help provide the best transplant outcome. Children with ESRD become transplant candidates if there may be better quality of life for the child and if the child can withstand the significant surgical risks of transplantation. The child must not be significantly immunocompromised prior to transplant. If the results of the evaluation are positive, then the child is placed on the national waiting list. The United Network for Organ Sharing (UNOS) has data identifying all patients who are waiting for a transplant and maintains a computer network to link all organ donation centers and transplant centers.

Children who receive renal transplants receive them either from unrelated donors who have died or from living donors. The living donors may be relatives who have ideal tissue matches, close friends, or parents. Over 50% of children who have a transplant receive from a living donor. Some children receive a preemptive transplant, which implies that the child has received a donated kidney before starting dialysis. This process has less chance of rejection (destruction of transplanted material at the cellular level) of the new kidney and longer life for the transplanted kidney. A high percentage of children receiving renal allografts have good outcomes (Healy, 2011).

Optimizing Outcomes—Kidney transplant

It is necessary to help the child remain as healthy as possible until a kidney transplant is available. The optimal outcome is long-term good health for the child.

focus on safety

Three requirements needed to receive a kidney transplant

- Compatible blood-type (ABO)
- Knowledge of a tissue match
  - "HLA" human leukocyte antigen
- Compatible cross match
  - Panel reactive antibody (PRA) or cytotoxic antibody level a significant factor
  - 0% to 100% PRA level: greater than 25% PRA will get more powerful immunosuppressive after transplant

Signs and Symptoms

Signs and symptoms of ESRD include:

- Swelling and edema
- Anemia
- Weakness and fatigue
- Shortness of breath
- Changes in urination
- Rash or itchy, dry skin
- Elevated blood urea nitrogen (BUN) and creatinine
- Uremia, buildup of waste
- Altered electrolytes
- Hypertension
- Tachycardia
- Tachypnea

Prevention

To prevent rejection, children who receive renal transplants are on long-term immunosuppressive and steroid medications. Medications include such drugs as FK506, Prograf, cyclosporine, and steroids. Blood levels are monitored for medication adjustment of dosage as needed. These drugs increase the child's risk for infection and can cause Cushing's syndrome by affecting glucocorticoids. Steroids can also raise serum glucose level, giving the potential for development of diabetes mellitus. In addition, steroids affect bone mineralization and strength, which can cause impairments in a growing child. Growth hormone has been used to counteract this problem (Healy, 2011).

Collaborative Care

Nursing Care. Any transplant recipient needs a thorough nursing assessment related to possible infection, imbalance of fluid and electrolytes, and rejection. Children who receive transplants remain on protein-restricted diets to avoid overloading the kidneys and help the child maintain proper

nutrition. Be sure to assess growth and development and provide developmentally appropriate activities. Collaborate with social workers, child life therapists, pastoral care, psychiatrists, counselors, financial assistance experts, educators, and other health-care providers to ensure the best outcome for the child.

Critical Nursing Action Kidney Transplant Evaluation

- A 2- to 3-day inpatient evaluation is done prior to the transplant
- A complete history and physical is obtained
- A psychosocial assessment is done
- A financial counselor is notified
- Certain laboratory tests are performed
  - Cross match, HLA/PRA markers, ABO, tissue typing
  - CBC, PT/PTT, INR, CMP
  - Hepatitis B, C, CMV, EBV, HSV, VZV, HIV, VDRL
  - Hemoglobin A1C
  - PPD
- Certain diagnostic tests are preformed:
  - CXR, EKG, 2-D echo, abdomen CT, abdomen US and vascular studies
  - Cardiology stress test and/or cardiac catheterization
  - Urological system evaluation
  - Pulmonary function tests
  - Comorbidity clearance and consulting

The United Network for Organ Sharing's definition of responsibilities for nurses and transplant coordinators is delineated by phase (Brennan & McEnhill, 2011). Hence, the nursing care interventions that follow are outlined by phase and are related to medical and surgical management and include education and discharge instructions.

Candidate Phase: The patient is waiting to be put on the transplant list.
- Reinforce treatment options provided to patient/family and complete medical history of child and parents.
- Encourage good nutritional support prior to and after transplant in collaboration with dietitian.
- Conduct a comprehensive physical assessment of child.
- Coordinate multiple diagnostic studies to be completed and ensure that any problems are corrected prior to listing the child as transplant candidate.
- Ensure that a living donor is healthy and compatibility is ensured through HLA matching.
- Conduct a psychosocial assessment of parent and child to ensure compliance.
- Assess that histocompatibility testing is done.
- Organize care and schedule tests needed prior to transplant.
- Answer questions and reinforce lifestyle commitments and changes that are required.
- Administer standard immunizations a minimum of 6 weeks prior to transplantation.
- Measure viral titers prior to transplantation to ensure vaccination adequacy.
  (Blayney, 2013; Williams, Bonin, Emory, Tate, Thompson, & Wood, 2011, p. 494)

Renal Transplant Phase: The actual transplant, pre- and postoperative

- Provide education about medications and treatments.
- Monitor bleeding, infection, or indications that the kidney is functioning abnormally; also monitor closely for increased blood pressure.
- Monitor respiratory and cardiac functions with immediate detection and referral to transplant team if any abnormalities are found.
- Monitor fluid status for either hypovolemia or hypervolemia.
- Monitor hourly intake urine and output.
- Monitor serum electrolytes and liver enzymes.
- Monitor vital signs and central venous pressure.
- Monitor for oliguria.
- Administer IV fluids.
- Administer diuretics.
- Administer dialysis or continuous venovenous hemofiltration (if needed).
- Monitor for wound infection.
- Monitor laboratory studies.

Assess for Surgical Complications

- Monitor findings from diagnostic tests.
- Monitor for **lymphoceles** (an abnormal collection of lymphatic fluid because of leakage from severed lymphatics surrounding the iliac vessels or the renal hilum of the donor kidney).
- Monitor for thrombosis of the renal artery or renal vein.
- Monitor for renal artery stenosis.

Assess for Urological Complications

- Monitor for obstruction.
- Monitor for urine leakage.

Assess for Medical Complications

- Monitor for adverse effects from immunosuppressive agents.
- Monitor for signs and symptoms of infection.
- Administer medication for urinary tract infection (UTI), pain, fever, nausea, and myalgias.

Medical Care. Table 31-18 provides common immunosuppression medications following a renal transplant.

Education/Discharge Instructions

Education and discharge instructions would take place during the **recipient phase** or post-surgery. Prepare the patient and family for discharge and homecare including medications, lab work, and follow-up care. The patient and family require integrated collaboration for physical, immunological, and psychosocial support. The goal is to help the child have a "normal" life though lifelong implications of transplant. Help parents and the child understand signs of possible rejection and/or infection. In addition, explain what follow-up care is necessary (Hatch & Greenstein, 2011; Williams et al., 2011).

 Critical Nursing Action   Signs and Symptoms of Kidney Transplant Rejection

Signs of kidney transplant rejection in children include hypertension, decreased urinary output, fever, weight gain, tenderness over donated kidney, edema, graft site pain, and increasing BUN and creatinine levels (Thomas, 2008).

Educate parents about:

- Follow-up care
- Immunizations
- Immunosuppressive therapy
- Dietary compliance and avoiding undercooked food
- Activities and play
- Medications
- Schooling
- Wearing masks in crowded public places and not being in contact with ill people
- Good oral care and dental visits
- Adolescents transitioning to self-management

 Nursing Insight—*Resources for patients and families*

- http://www.kidney.org—National Kidney Foundation
- https://www.aakp.org—American Association of Kidney Patients
- http://www.victoryjunction.org—Victory Junction Camp
- Local transplant centers

Table 31-18 Common Immunosuppression Medications Following a Renal Transplant		
Medication	**Action**	**Common Side Effects**
tacrolimus (Prograf)	Inhibits T-Cell activation	• GI upset (nausea, vomiting, diarrhea) • Hair loss • High blood glucose • Infection
mycophenolate (CellCept)	Inhibits T-Cell and B-cell proliferation	• GI upset • Infection • Leukopenia
Steroids (prednisone, prednisolone, methylprednisolone)	Suppresses migration of WBCs	• Depression • Mood swings • Slowed growth • Changes in appetite • Weight gain • Acne

(continued)

Table 31-18 Common Immunosuppression Medications Following a Renal Transplant (continued)

Medication	Action	Common Side Effects
cyclosporine (Gengraf, Neoral, Sandimmune)	Inhibits T-Cell signaling and T-Cell activation	• GI upset • Headaches • Elevated blood pressure • Hair growth • Hyperkalemia • Infection
azathioprine (Imuran)	Inhibits WBC production	• GI upset • Infection

Source: Williams, J., Bonin, S., Emory, B., Tate, A., Thompson, G., & Wood, S. (2011). The pediatric renal transplant process (p. 497). Retrieved from www.homehealthcarenurseonline.com

---

Where Research and Practice Meet:
Quality of Life

Quality of life is affected by advanced renal pathology, whether considering adults who had renal problems in childhood or children with chronic kidney disease (CKD). In comparison with healthy children, those children having mild to moderate CKD had lower "physical, school, emotional, and social domain scores" (Gerson, Wentz, Abraham, Mendley, Hooper, Butler, et al., 2010, p. e349). From this cross-sectional research of children aged 2 to 16, it is apparent that earlier intervention is needed for school-related difficulties as well as improving growth. Data analysis indicated that even children with early kidney disease can have quality of life difficulties. Collaboration with schools and obtaining school-based home services can potentially prevent some negative quality of life issues (Gerson et al., 2010).

Functional Disorders of the Urinary Tract

DYSFUNCTIONAL ELIMINATION SYNDROME

Dysfunctional elimination syndrome (DES), also called voiding dysfunction, is an abnormal but common pediatric elimination pattern associated with bladder and bowel withholding and incontinence. DES refers to the inability to efficiently empty the bladder, and this may be associated with urinary tract infection (UTI), constipation, incontinence, and other issues (Desantis, Leonard, Preston, Barrowman, & Guerra, 2011).

 Nursing Insight—*Functional voiding disorders*

There are numerous types of functional voiding disorders. **Urge incontinence** is the most frequently seen type of voiding dysfunction. Urodynamic studies show bladder storage problems and persistent bladder contractions that cause urgency and excess voiding withholding such as crouching, leg crossing, squatting, or dancing.

Lazy bladder syndrome occurs when children delay voiding and the detrusor muscle of the bladder weakens while the bladder itself enlarges. This causes incomplete voiding, minimal urge to void, and voiding infrequently, associated with increased bladder capacity (Canadian Urological Association, 2012).

Giggle incontinence is the leakage of urine when children are laughing, and there may be some bladder instability. Anticholinergic drugs can assist with this as well as the attention-deficit/hyperactivity (ADHD) drug methylphenidate (Ritalin).

Bladder-sphincter dyssynergia refers to a bladder disorder with elevated bladder pressure but a decrease in urine flow, leaving residual urine. The child may return quickly to the restroom after just leaving it.

Vaginal voiding is associated with dribbling after voiding caused by some urine flowing into the vaginal vault. This urine then dribbles out with standing or activity. This problem may be remedied by weight loss in overweight girls and having the girl sit backwards or straddle a toilet seat so urine is directed downward.

Signs and Symptoms

Signs and symptoms of DES include:

- Frequency in voiding
- Urinary incontinence
- Urgency
- UTI
- Occasional constipation

Diagnosis

Diagnosis is determined by signs and symptoms and physical examination including examining the back for sacral hairy tufts and gluteal asymmetry that may be associated with neurogenic bladder issues such as spina bifida. The rectum and colon are examined for evidence of constipation. The genitalia are also examined for physical abnormalities.

Diagnostic tests include a voiding cystourethrogram, flat plate of the abdomen to assess for constipation, uroflowmetry to assess voiding flow and velocity, and the addition of electromyography to assess the pelvic floor musculature.

Prevention

Prevention focuses on avoiding complications such as urinary incontinence, vesicoureteral reflux, hydronephrosis, and pyelonephritis.

Collaborative Care

Nursing Care. Nurses assist in helping children with voiding dysfunction by identifying issues, asking the child at various times of day if he or she has voided.

Monitoring stool elimination is also essential because some children with DES have constipation issues. The muscles used to control stooling are the same as the bladder control muscles, and this can interfere with voiding. Assess for any emotional or social problems resulting from a child's embarrassment or shame associated with voiding dysfunction. Promote adequate hydration by ensuring that the child is hydrated by drinking 8 ounces of water with each meal to maintain dilute and less acidic urine. Encourage the child to void every 2 hours. Voiding charts and diaries may assist in behavioral tracking and recording of successes.

Help the child maintain a normal bowel regimen, with or without the use of enemas and stool softeners, such as polyethylene glycol (MiraLax) or lactulose syrup. The child needs to sit on the toilet for 1 minute for each year of age after eating to let the gastrocolic reflex relax to induce bowel elimination. Girls with an inflamed perineum from leaking urine may be soothed with baking soda sitz baths and use of barrier creams.

 ### Complementary Care: *Using Biofeedback for DES*

Biofeedback training assists the child with gaining control over the bladder muscles and relaxing the external sphincter. The child wears an electromyogram (EMG) patch near the perineum or abdomen to assist with biofeedback training. Biofeedback assists the child to coordinate pelvic floor muscle relaxation with bladder contraction, even using a video game format. The child learns to relax these muscles to gain EMG tracings that promote normal voiding (Desantis et al., 2011).

Medical Care. If a child suffers from recurrent urinary tract infection (UTI), she may need antibiotic treatment and prophylaxis. Trimethoprim-sulfamethoxazole (Bactrim or Septra) and nitrofurantoin (Macrodantin) are the most common antibiotics used to treat prophylaxis of UTI. Anticholinergic drugs can help giggle incontinence.

Education/Discharge Instructions

Assist the family with obtaining psychological counseling for the patient, which is vital. Associated psychological and educational problems include learning disabilities, ADHD,

low motivation, sensory problems, and family issues. Parents and other family members may need assistance in dealing with these issues.

 ### Collaboration in Caring—*The American Academy of Pediatrics*

The American Academy of Pediatrics (2009b) recommends the following toilet training tips:

- **Decide which words to use.** Choose the words your family will use to describe body parts, urine, and bowel movements. Remember that other people will hear these words too, so pick words that will not offend, confuse, or embarrass anyone. Avoid negative words like "dirty," "naughty," or "stinky." They can make your child feel ashamed and embarrassed. Talk about bowel movements and urination in a simple, matter-of-fact manner.
- **Pick a potty chair.** A potty chair is easier for a small child to use because there is no problem getting onto it and a child's feet can reach the floor. Special books or toys for "potty time" may help make this more enjoyable for your child.
- **Know the signs.** Before having a bowel movement, your child may grunt or make other straining noises, squat, or stop playing for a moment. When pushing, his face may turn red. Explain to your child that these signs mean that a bowel movement is about to come. Your child may wait until after the fact to tell you about a wet diaper or a bowel movement. This is actually a good sign that your child is starting to recognize these body functions. Praise your child for telling you, and suggest that "next time" he let you know in advance. Keep in mind that it often takes longer for a child to recognize the need to urinate than the need to move bowels.
- **Make trips to the potty routine.** When your child seems ready to urinate or have a bowel movement, go to the potty. It may also be helpful to make trips to the potty a regular part of your child's daily routine, such as first thing in the morning, after meals, or before naps.
- **Try training pants.** Once your child starts using the potty with some success, training pants can be used. This moment will be special. Your child will feel proud. (AAP, 2009b).

Family Teaching Guidelines...
Toilet Training

TOPIC: Tips for Toilet Training

Normally, toilet training, which begins in the toddler to preschool years, is complete by about age 4. Training occurs first for nocturnal bowel control and second, for daytime bowel control. Then the child may be prepared for daytime bladder control, and lastly, nocturnal bladder control. The child is not ready for toilet training until he or she can voluntarily control the bladder sphincter, which requires physiological, psychological, and social development (Burns et al., 2009). Discourage the parents from forcing a child to toilet train before he or she shows signs of readiness.

Signs that the child is ready for toileting include:

- Showing an interest in toileting: about 24 months of age
- Telling parents or caretakers of the need to use the toilet: occurs on average at 26 months in girls and 29 months in boys
- The ability to stay dry for at least 2 hours: occurs at average 26 months for girls and 29 months for boys
- The ability to stay dry for the entire day: occurs at average 32 months for girls and 35 months old for boys (Burns et al., 2009)

There are many resources available to guide parents and caretakers on toilet training, such as children's books, parental guides, day-care provider guides, behavior charts, special potty chairs, and games.

ENURESIS

One of the most distressing childhood issues is **enuresis** (bedwetting). The definition of enuresis is the "involuntary discharge of urine" (*Taber's Online Medical Dictionary*, 2011).

Nursing Insight—*Dysfunctional voiding syndrome and enuresis*

There is a distinction between dysfunctional voiding and enuresis. In enuresis, the child voids normally and fully, but not at the socially acceptable time. In voiding dysfunction or DES, there is an abnormal emptying or storage in the bladder.

Nursing Insight—*Other issues associated with enuresis*

Enuresis may carry a genetic etiology. If one or both parents have suffered from enuresis, there is a higher likelihood their offspring may suffer, too. Chromosomal studies show a genetic predisposition for enuresis. Fifty percent of children with enuresis have one parent who suffered from it. Developmental delays in other areas, such as speech, motor, and growth, may accompany enuresis issues (Burns et al., 2009).

There are different types of enuresis: primary nocturnal enuresis (PNE) and primary and secondary enuresis. PNE is bedwetting during the night. Primary enuresis occurs when children have never been able to gain urinary control. Secondary enuresis refers to the presence of enuresis after a child has achieved dryness for 6 to 12 months. A small percentage of primary enuresis has a pathophysiological cause, but the majority of cases are functional, caused by something that is not pathophysiological. Besides genetics and developmental delay, some children with enuresis are thought to have small bladder capacity; difficulty with arousing during the night to void; low levels of antidiuretic hormone (ADH), which keeps people from voiding at night; stress; and other family disruptions such as a new baby at home, school phobias, or parental divorce.

Cultural Diversity: *Enuresis*

Toileting patterns and expectations vary among different cultural and ethnic groups. Enuresis may be considered more problematic for some cultures than for others, and expectations of bladder and bowel control vary among parents, teachers, health-care professionals, and day-care providers as well.

Signs and Symptoms

Signs and symptoms of enuresis include:

- Patterns of urinary urgency, crossed legs, jiggling behaviors, holding of genitals
- Foul-smelling urine odor
- Behavior problems, developmental delays, or possible ADHD
- Encopresis (involuntary loss of stool after normal time of control)
- Diabetes mellitus (polyuria, polydipsia, polyphagia, weight gain or loss)
- Obstructive sleep apnea
- Psychological stress
- Signs of sexual abuse

Diagnosis

Diagnosis is based on patient history and physical examination to rule out other medical conditions as the cause of enuresis.

Prevention

Enuresis is sometimes genetic, making prevention associated with awareness of familial incidence. In other cases, enuresis may be related to a variety of conditions, some of which can be prevented by medications or counseling.

Collaborative Care

Nursing Care. It is important to determine if this is primary or secondary enuresis. Enuresis is not considered abnormal until it is outside the range of 5 to 6 years of age. Nurses need to counsel parents on this fact and make them aware of developmental norms for toileting.

Complementary Care: *Enuresis*

- 4 to 6 sessions of hypnotherapy can train a child to awaken when his or her bladder feels full.
- Bed alarms are very popular with a higher success rate than medications; a bell or buzzer is triggered when the child begins to void. Eventually, the child usually learns to wake, but it may take up to 12 weeks of treatment (Burns et al., 2009).
- Not every child with enuresis is suffering psychological problems, but there is an increased incidence of psychological issues in secondary enuresis, including parental divorce, school trauma, hospitalization, and sexual abuse. Acupressure or massage therapy can be useful in some cases of psychological-induced enuresis.
- Citrus foods, carbonated or caffeinated drinks, red dyes, and artificially colored candy may contribute to enuresis. Elimination trials can be advised by nurses.
- Motivational therapy uses rewards, such as a star chart, where the child receives a star for dry nights or days. Children are taught to become more sensitive to body cues for voiding. Rewards can be associated with achieving a certain number of dry nights.

Medical Care. In extreme cases of enuresis, the child may be given medication to control the bladder. Many children are embarrassed by this problem, and school functions, camp, and sleepovers become problematic. Some parents use medication only as needed for these special occasions. The most commonly prescribed medication to treat enuresis is desmopressin (DDAVP), a synthetic analogue of ADH. This medication, administered orally, acts to lower nocturnal urinary production. DDAVP is available in

0.2 mg tablets given in dosages of 0.2 mg to 0.6 mg per night. It is not to be used under age 6, and there is still a risk of hyponatremia (low sodium), which can be dangerous, even causing seizures. A prior form of DDAVP, the nasal form, has been withdrawn from the market because of high risk of hyponatremia and seizures. Children who are hypertensive or who have risk of fluid or electrolyte imbalance (e.g., children with cystic fibrosis) should not use DDAVP oral tablets (Burns et al., 2009).

Medication: Imipramine (Tofranil)

(im-**ip**-pra-mean)

Indications: Depression, enuresis, bulimia, attention deficit disorder in children, obsessive-compulsive disorder, panic disorder

Actions: Tricyclic antidepressant known to increase the effect of norepinephrine and serotonin in the body. It also possesses anticholinergic side effects.

Contraindications and Precautions:
- Cardiovascular disease
- Seizure disorder
- Children younger than age 6
- Concomitant use of MAO inhibitors, such as Nardil and Parnate; cannot take Tofranil within 2 weeks of taking an MAO inhibitor drug
- Recent myocardial infarction

Adverse Reactions and Side Effects:
- Nervousness, anxiety, emotional instability
- Fainting, convulsions
- Constipation, nausea, vomiting
- Fatigue, sleep disorders
- Dry mouth
- Gynecomastia
- Confusion, hallucinations
- High or low blood pressure
- Tremor, numbness

Route and Dosage: Pediatric: short-term only, not for children younger than age 6

Dosing: Dosing is 0.9 to 1/5 mg/kg/day. Initially 10 to 25 mg tab daily 1 hour before bedtime. The dose can be increased by 25 mg/day to a maximum of 50 mg/day for children 6 to 12 years or a maximum of 75 mg/day for children older than 12 years.

Nursing Implications:
1. Risk of potential suicidal ideation during initiation of upward titration of this medication, especially in children and adolescents.
2. Toxic and possibly fatal drug interactions can occur with concomitant use of MAO inhibitors (e.g., Nardil, Parnate), SSRI drugs (e.g., Prozac, Paxil), and clonidine (antihypertensive drug also used for ADHD).
3. Blood pressure and heart rate should be assessed before treatment, and an initial electrocardiogram (ECG) should be taken. Serial ECGs may be needed with dose adjustments to monitor for prolonged PR and QT intervals and flattened T waves.
4. Nurses must assess patients for mood alterations, hallucinations, confusion, and laboratory abnormalities (leukocytes, blood glucose, and renal and hepatic status).
5. There is a significant risk of agitation, arrhythmias, hallucinations, fever, dyspnea, seizures, and vomiting in acute overdose. Treatment consists of gastric lavage, use of charcoal, and a stimulant cathartic. Additional supportive measures are heart monitoring, respiratory status monitoring, and possibly use of antiarrhythmic and anticonvulsant agents.

Source: Vallerand & Sanoski (2014).

Medication: Oxybutynin Chloride

Oxybutynin chloride is used for immediate release or extended release. This anticholinergic drug is used to defer incontinence. It is not used for children under 5 years of age. It is effective for daytime enuresis. The dose is 5 mg orally once daily. If needed, the health-care provider increases the dose as tolerated in 5 mg increments up to a maximum of 20 mg per day. Side effects include mouth dryness, urinary retention, and constipation (Vallerand & Sanoski, 2014).

Education/Discharge Instructions

Teaching includes explaining to the parents that sometimes enuresis is a result of the developmental stage of the child, or the child is a deep sleeper who does not feel the urge to void. In some cases, this may improve as the child grows, but it should be monitored. Avoidance of fluids close to bedtime, avoidance of diuretic beverages or substances (e.g., coffee, tea, chocolate, and colas), and use of reward charts are other techniques useful to parents. Many commercial items are available to assist parents. These include mattress pads with alarms, watches with reminders to void, books on staying dry, and absorbent underwear.

Other complementary care modalities have been developed to assist in the management of enuresis. Nurses should familiarize themselves with these to instruct parents and children with this problem. One behavioral treatment that has proven very useful involves conditioning through the use of a battery-operated bedwetting alarm, a device that wakens the child if the bedding becomes wet.

? Global Health Case Study Enuresis

Ahmed is a 10-year-old boy whose mother complains he has new onset diurnal enuresis. Ahmed and his family are refugees from a war-torn area of the Middle East. He is being evaluated by a DNP working for a medical mission hospital in the area. His mother reports he has had nightmares and frequent crying episodes since they moved into the refugee camp. Ahmed's physical examination includes the following data: Ahmed's weight is in the 10th percentile, and his height is in the 50th percentile. He is Tanner Stage I. He has a macular pink rash on his antecubital fossa and popliteal areas. He also has complaints of mild suprabupic pain to palpation, without rebound or guarding. He has no flank pain. The remainder of his exam is normal. His laboratory analysis reveals the urine dipstick shows 1+ proteinuria without hematuria or nitrites.

critical thinking questions

1. What questions does the nurse need to ask Ahmed?

2. What questions does the nurse need to ask Ahmed's mother?

3. What laboratory test(s) should the DNP anticipate will be needed if they are available at the medical mission hospital?

4. With the mild suprapubic pain and proteinuria, what is the next test that should be ordered?

5. What is the most likely medication Ahmed may be given if there is risk for UTI?

After Ahmed's medical visit, his urine culture is sent to the local lab and is found negative for infection. However, the protein level remains elevated. A few days later Ahmed's suprapubic pain has gone away, but his mother is worried because he is still having enuresis accidents several times during the day and at night. The DNP decides to check Ahmed for orthostatic proteinuria.

1. How do you instruct Ahmed's mother to collect this sample?

2. Given the circumstances, it is unlikely that Ahmed will be prescribed any medication for enuresis. What creative ideas might the nurse devise to explain the enuresis and to help his mother deal with the problem?

3. Do you think Ahmed's environment, genetics, and psychosocial situation have anything to do with the enuresis?

◆ See Suggested Answers to Global Health Case Studies on Davis*Plus*.

Now Can You—Discuss functional disorders of the urinary tract?

1. Name several different types of functional voiding disorders?
2. Describe nursing care for children who experience DES and enuresis?
3. Explain toilet training guidelines and tips for children?

Reproductive Disorders Affecting Girls

VULVOVAGINITIS

There are various etiologies of **vulvovaginitis** (inflammation of the vulva and vagina) in prepubertal girls. Candidiasis, a yeast organism, is the most common source of this disorder. Vulvitis (vulvar inflammation) may be isolated or occur with vaginitis, which is vaginal inflammation. The prepubertal girl is sensitive to lack of estrogen, lack of protective hair, and lack of labial fat pads as well as the influence of poor hygiene and proximity of the anus to the vulva. Clothing, soaps, and other chemicals may be irritating to vulvar skin. Tight jeans, ballet leotards, nylon tights, underwear, and bathing suits may all contribute to maceration and vulvar infection, especially if the weather is warm and there is associated sweating. It is common for young girls to void with their legs together, which increases the risk of urine refluxing into the vagina. Candidiasis is often associated with bubble baths in young girls, and this may also lead to urinary tract infection (UTI).

Nonspecific vulvovaginitis, without a clear etiology, is found in 25% to 75% of all cases in prepubertal girls. Fecal organisms have been found and so may be a cause of vulvovaginitis in some cases because of poor hygiene and possibly wiping back to front, spreading anal organisms. Candida, bacteroides, and some other streptococcal species have also been noted. Gram-negative *Escherichia coli* organisms have been cultured from girls with vulvovaginitis, and these may be fecal in origin. Normal flora including lactobacilli, diphtheroids, and *Staphylococcus epidermidis* have been noted on vaginal cultures of vulvovaginitis.

If infections that are sexually transmitted such as those caused by *Neisseria gonorrhea*, *Chlamydia trachomatis*, *Trichomonas*, herpes simplex, and human papillomavirus are found, there is high suspicion of sexual contact, either voluntary or because of sexual assault (Helming, 2009).

Signs and Symptoms

Signs and Symptoms
- Vulvar itching
- Discharge can vary from glutinous gray-white to purulent, blood-tinged, foul-smelling and brown, green, or thick white curds

Diagnosis

Diagnosis is based on patient history, clinical findings, and pH testing of vaginal secretions. Pseudohyphae (branching yeast organisms) may be found on microscopy where the pH is less than 4.5. Also, under the microscope, clue cells (large epithelial cells with bacteria) may indicate bacterial vaginosis, and trichomonads may indicate trichomonads infections. Other organisms may be found on Pap smears in adolescents (Candida or trichomonads) (Van Leeuwen et al., 2011).

Prevention

Instruct the parents and children to avoid predisposing factors for vaginitis. Use of antibiotics is sometimes associated with Candida vaginitis.

Collaborative Care

Nursing Care. Instruct young girls to wipe from the front to the back after voiding to avoid contaminating the perineum with stool. Educate patients in complementary care measures.

 Complementary Care: *Vaginal Candidiasis*

Complementary care for vaginal candidiasis includes:

1. Wearing cotton underwear to allow better ventilation
2. Avoiding wearing wet clothing, such as bathing suits, for long periods
3. Avoiding bubble baths as well as perfumes or powder near the vaginal area
4. In menstruating females, avoiding use of scented sanitary pads or tampons
5. Avoiding excessive sugars and simple carbohydrates in the diet
6. Eating yogurt because the natural lactobacilli maintain normal bacterial balance

---

Medical Care. Medical management of vaginal candidiasis in prepubertal girls is best accomplished with over-the-counter antifungal remedies such as miconazole (Monistat) and clotrimazole (Gyne-Lotrimin) creams applied topically, avoiding internal insertion until the adolescent years.

 Nursing Insight—Recurrent vaginal candidiasis

Recurrent vaginal candidiasis can be a sign of diabetes mellitus or other immune-suppressive illness.

---

 focus on safety

Vaginal foreign bodies

Insertion of a foreign object, normally by the young girl herself, usually from ages 2 to 9, has been noted to cause vaginal bleeding and/or odoriferous and blood-stained vaginal discharge. The problem normally is remedied through removal and a simple Betadine irrigation (Helming, 2009). Sexual abuse must be ruled out first. It may be necessary for the nurse to obtain social services and counseling services to investigate possible sexual abuse.

Education/Discharge Instructions

Suggest tub baths with clear, warm water 1 to 2 times daily for 10 to 15 minutes, followed by washing with a bland soap such as unscented Dove™, Basis™, Aveeno™, or Neutrogena™. The soap isn't applied to the vulvar area, and the vulva should never be scrubbed. Avoid shampooing the hair in the bathtub, so the vulva is not exposed to shampoo chemicals. Showering is sometimes a better option for personal hygiene.

After bathing, instruct the patient to gently pat dry the vulvar area. Sleeper pajamas are not recommended because of their occlusive nature. Underwear should be all cotton for greater ventilation. Underwear should be washed in mild, unscented detergent without bleach.

Some health-care providers recommend a small amount of A + D ointment™, Vaseline™, or Desitin™ ointment to be applied to protect the vulvar skin. Loose-fitting clothing is ideal, especially in warm weather.

LABIAL ADHESIONS

Labial adhesions are most common in girls from 3 months to 6 years old. This disorder is defined as the fusion of the labia minora because of inflammation, infection, trauma, and estrogen deficit.

Signs and Symptoms

- A thin film that develops over the labia, from the posterior aspect to the anterior aspect
- The vaginal introitus and urethral meatus are not visible
- Dysuria
- Urinary incontinence
  (Helming, 2009)

 focus on safety

Child maltreatment

Any scarring that is not midline or is severe and dense should raise the suspicion of child sexual abuse or trauma.

Diagnosis

Diagnosis is based on signs and symptoms and common associated problems such as dysuria and incontinence if urine is trapped or dribbling after voiding in toilet-trained girls.

> **Medication:** Antifungal Agents
>
> Miconazole (Monistat-Derm), Nystatin (Mycostatin), and clotrimazole (Mycelex) are antifungal agents used topically in the vaginal area. Based on the health-care provider order, one of these medications is applied topically to the external vagina once or twice daily in children. It can be applied also through a vaginal applicator in adolescents.

Prevention

Monitor for complications of UTI caused by obstruction of urine flow.

Collaborative Care

Nursing Care. Conduct a thorough nursing assessment of the newborn and infant during health-care visits. Be sure to report abnormal findings to the health-care provider. Assess for dysuria and incontinence. Ask the parent about signs and symptoms of UTIs.

Medical Care. Treatment with hormone cream such as Premarin cream 0.625 mg bid for 10 to 14 days is the standard treatment.

Surgical Care. Surgery for lysis of adhesions may be performed as determined by the health-care provider.

Education/Discharge Instructions

Communicate to the family that the condition may have spontaneous resolution over time or with treatment.

AMENORRHEA

Amenorrhea refers to the absence of menses. **Primary amenorrhea** occurs by age 14 if there has been no growth or development of secondary sexual characteristics (e.g., pubic hair, axillary hair, and breasts). Primary amenorrhea also is defined as no menses by age 16 if there are secondary sexual characteristics already. **Secondary amenorrhea** means that the girl or woman has had menses already, but there is no menses for 6 months if she has had normal periods or for the length of time equivalent to three cycle intervals if she has had irregular cycling. There are several possible causes: congenital abnormalities or absence of the uterus, fallopian tubes, or ovaries; deficiency of gonadotropin-releasing hormone from the pituitary; chromosomal disorders such as Turner's syndrome; lactation; menopause (premature or normal); hypothyroidism or hyperthyroidism; chemotherapy; polycystic ovarian syndrome (PCOS); diabetes mellitus; stress; excessive exercise, weight loss, anorexia, or bulimia; and pregnancy. Pregnancy must always be considered as a cause of secondary amenorrhea, even if the patient denies sexual contact (Arthur, 2011). In addition, certain medications can cause amenorrhea, including birth control pills and medroxyprogesterone acetate (Depo Provera), which is given as a contraceptive injection.

Signs and Symptoms

Primary amenorrhea
- Delayed puberty
- The Tanner stages of sexual characteristic development show delay

Secondary amenorrhea
- Signs and symptoms of pregnancy
- Mastalgia (breast tenderness) or breast enlargement
- Nausea and vomiting
- Urinary frequency
- Enlarged uterus
- Chadwick's sign

Nursing Insight—*Other underlying conditions*

- Hypothyroidism as evidenced by fatigue, hoarseness, constipation, and an enlarged thyroid gland
- Hyperthyroidism as evidenced by oily skin and hair, diaphoresis, tachycardia, diarrhea, and a goiter (enlarged thyroid gland)
- PCOS as evidenced by hirsutism (excessive facial and body hair) and obesity
- Corpus luteum cysts that cause intermittent pain in the lower abdominal quadrant
- Other cysts that can grow and rupture, causing significant lower abdominal quadrant pain as well as peritoneal signs of rebound, guarding, and rigidity

Diagnosis

In the absence of menses, a number of laboratory tests and other diagnostic tests are often necessary in the diagnostic evaluation of amenorrhea.

 Diagnostic Tools Determining Reason for Amenorrhea

- Genetic testing may be required to determine disorders such as Turner's syndrome.
- Pelvic ultrasound or transvaginal (ultrasound wand in the vaginal canal) is used to test for pregnancy, ovarian cysts, and other gynecological abnormalities. Patients normally are required to drink four 8-ounce glasses of water 1 hour before a pelvic ultrasound to elevate the bladder to view the pelvic organs.

Prevention

It is important to educate adolescent girls and boys about how pregnancy occurs and various birth control methods.

Collaborative Care

Nursing Care. Evaluate the patient with amenorrhea for signs and symptoms of pregnancy including weight gain, unprotected coitus, fatigue, nausea and vomiting, and mastalgia. A urinary human chorionic gonadotropin (HCG) test is given, and the patient is informed that it may turn positive within days after a missed menses. In cases of possibly false negative urine pregnancy tests, it is necessary to administer the serum HCG test to determine pregnancy status. If a parent is present with a girl who may be pregnant, the nurse should attempt to have the parent wait outside to speak confidentially to the adolescent girl by suggesting that at this age it is common to interview young women alone. Invite the parent or guardian back at the conclusion of the discussion. This sometimes allows the opportunity for a young woman to discuss the possibility of pregnancy or her concerns about contraception and sexually transmitted diseases.

Education/Discharge Instructions

Assist the patient in constructing a calendar depicting her abnormal menstrual pattern. Young girls often need to be educated about variations in menstrual cycles and why it is essential that they keep track of their cycle days, intervals, and duration. Girls who have eating disorders such as anorexia nervosa or bulimia may incur secondary amenorrhea because of weight loss and associated alterations in estrogen. When body fat significantly decreases, amenorrhea or oligomenorrhea (infrequent menses) may occur. Young girls who exercise heavily (e.g., gymnasts or distance runners) may develop menstrual disorders as well as young girls with eating disorders. In the circumstance of adolescent females, those with primary amenorrhea may have family members who have experienced the same issue.

 Nursing Insight—*Imperforate hymen*

In cases of imperforate hymen (without opening), a surgical intervention is required. In amenorrheic patients, if laboratory testing is normal, a trial of medroxyprogesterone acetate (Depo Provera), 5 or 10 mg daily for 5 or 10 days in 1 month is given in an attempt to elicit the menses by causing a progesterone withdrawal bleed. Some patients are placed on oral contraceptive agents to regulate the menses.

Reproductive Disorders Affecting Boys

VARICOCELE

Varicoceles are defined as abnormal dilations in the testicular veins, normally unilateral and affecting the left testicle. Most varicoceles arise after age 9, and 16% of adolescents and 20% of adult males have varicoceles. The etiology of this disorder remains unknown, but it is now considered the most common cause of male infertility that is correctable (Helming, 2009).

Signs and Symptoms

Signs and symptoms of a varicocele include:

- "Bag of worms" appearance
- Thickened spermatic cord
- Distended veins while standing
- Decrease in varicocele when laying supine
- Testes often smaller
- Pain or heaviness in scrotum

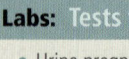 **Labs:** Tests for Amenorrhea

- Urine pregnancy test (urinary human chorionic gonadotropin [HCG]) are available over-the-counter and at clinics.
- Serum pregnancy tests show positive pregnancy results and approximate duration of the pregnancy. These tests are considered more accurate than urine pregnancy tests and identify pregnancy earlier.
- Thyroid stimulating hormone is a general test for hypothyroidism and hyperthyroidism. This test may be accompanied by a free thyroxine test to specify the disorder more clearly.
- Prolactin level is a test that shows hyperprolactinemia, which may be seen with hypothyroidism or with a benign pituitary adenoma. Prolactin is a hormone produced in the pituitary gland and is associated with breastfeeding.
- Follicle-stimulating hormone test which may be low in PCOS.
- Luteinizing hormone test that may be elevated in PCOS.
- Testosterone test that shows levels that may be high in PCOS, in addition to dehydroepiandrosterone levels.

(Van Leeuwen et al., 2011)

Diagnosis

Doppler ultrasonography helps to definitively determine the presence of varicocele. Semen analysis may also be done in older males.

Prevention

Prevention is important to prevent later infertility. The nurse recommends that the patient see the urologist about potential surgical treatment.

Collaborative Care

Nursing Care. Because this condition affects the genital area, emotional support is needed for the patient and family of males contemplating surgical procedures. For the older child, testicular self-exam is taught. Athletic supporters may help with the heaviness sensation.

Surgical Care. Surgical ligation (binding or tying) of the spermatic veins is the curative approach to preserve fertility. Nursing care centers on caring for the postsurgical patient. Standard postoperative measures are implemented through overall assessment and assessment of the surgical area, vital signs, bleeding, pain, respiratory status, intake and output, level of consciousness, nausea and vomiting, and fluid and electrolyte balance.

Education/Discharge Instructions

Immediate home care includes low-level activities and rest. Teach parents signs and symptoms of infection and how to assess for pain. Loose-fitting diapers are recommended. Prevent the child from using riding toys during play. Instruct the parents to call the health-care provider with concerns or questions.

CRYPTORCHIDISM

Cryptorchidism is defined as absent, undescended, or ectopic testicles. This is the most common male congenital anomaly, noted in 2% to 4% of all newborns males. It may result from hormonal, anatomical, or chromosomal variations. Prematurity increases the risk of cryptorchidism. Intersex conditions such as congenital adrenal hyperplasia may be associated. In 80% of the cases, the testicles are palpable but undescended, and the scrotal sac is empty as well as potentially flat or small. This condition must be distinguished from retractile testes, which are descended testicles that rise up into the groin area but can be pushed down into the scrotum. Retractile testes are very common in young males. The remaining 20% of cases are nonpalpable testes, which may actually be in the abdomen or inguinal area or may not be present at all (Helming, 2009).

The major risk associated with cryptorchidism is testicular cancer, which remains a lifetime risk even if the child has surgical repair. There is also risk of decreased fertility, testicular torsion, and increased trauma. If the testis does not descend permanently by age 6 months, surgical intervention is needed. All patients with a history of cryptorchidism must be vigilant with testicular self-exam and have annual testicular exams by a health-care provider.

Signs and Symptoms

Signs and symptoms of cryptorchidism include the following:

- A retractile testis has descended but retracts with exam and physical stimulation.

- An ectopic testis is outside the normal pathway (e.g., in the groin, abdominal wall, or perineum).
- After 1 year of age, it is uncommon for the testes to spontaneously descend.
- In 85% of affected males, the undescended testicle is unilateral and on the right (Helming, 2009).

Diagnosis

Diagnosis is based on patient history, physical examination findings, and imaging tests.

Prevention

Be aware that the risk of infertility may be decreased with surgical treatment although the risk of testicular cancer remains high throughout life.

Collaborative Care

Nursing Care. Gentle compression of the inguinal canals should reveal a palpable nodule in undescended testicles (Fig. 31-8). Counsel the parents of the child about the surgery and the benefits of surgery for infertility. Be prepared to counsel parents about the emotional upset of increased lifelong risk of testicular cancer.

Surgical Care. The child will receive general anesthesia and sometimes a caudal block prior to surgery (Shields & Tanner, 2010). The surgical repair is called an orchiopexy and is usually done between ages 6 months to 12 months. This surgery is minimally invasive and may involve a laparoscope that is used to locate and pull down the undescended testicle into the scrotal sac, anchoring it there.

Education/Discharge Instructions

Similar education/discharge instructions apply to the patient who has undergone an orchiopexy as do patients with varicocele. Tell parents that despite orchiopexy surgery, boys with this condition have a risk of infertility throughout life as well as a testicular cancer (Hudson, Balic, Nation, & Southwell, 2010).

✿ **Nursing Insight**—*Hydrocele*

A hydrocele is a collection of fluid in the scrotal sac, related to a patent processus vaginalis, which is the channel that gives fluid the ability to move from abdomen to groin. Peritoneal abdominal fluid can pass into this patent canal, enlarging the scrotal sack. This canal is patent in the majority of all newborns

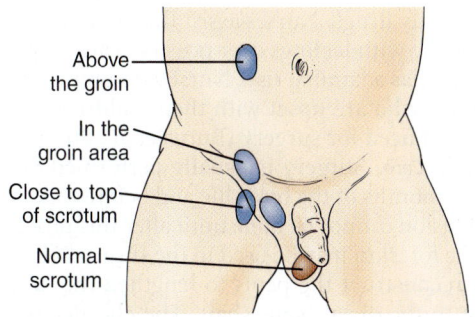

Figure 31-8 An undescended testis is palpable in various areas and needs to be surgically corrected.

at birth, and in the first month of life, the incidence decreases and again decreases by the age of 18 to 24 months. While this condition can rarely occur in females, primarily in intersex conditions, it is common enough in males that it must be repaired if it has not resolved by 1 year. If a hernia is found with it, earlier surgical repair is necessary.

HYPOSPADIAS AND EPISPADIAS

Hypospadias and epispadias are possibly genetic congenital conditions that imply an abnormal positioning of the urethral meatus in boys. In **hypospadias**, the meatus is inferior to its usual position. In **epispadias**, the meatus is superior to its usual position, and a surgical correction with possible penile urethral lengthening may be necessary. Hypospadias may cause chordee, which is a bending of the penis that may later present problems with intercourse. Young males with hypospadias may not be able to urinate standing, and there may be associated cryptorchidism. Patients need to be referred early to pediatric urologists for surgical repair (Helming, 2009).

Signs and Symptoms

Signs and symptoms of hypospadias include:

- Opening of the urethra below the tip on the bottom side of the penis
- Incomplete foreskin
- Curvature of the penis during erection
- Abnormal position of the scrotum in relation to the penis

Signs and symptoms of epispadias are:

- Opening of the urethra above the tip of the penis
- Curvature of the penis
- Urinary incontinence

Diagnosis

Diagnosis is based on patient history, physical examination findings, radiography, and ultrasound.

Prevention

Nurses must be aware of potential voiding dysfunction and chordee issues.

Collaborative Care

Nursing Care. The etiology of hypospadias is uncertain, but there has been an increased incidence in the 1990s associated with low-birth-weight babies and babies born to mothers who had undergone in vitro fertilization or had taken fertility drugs. Nurses assist the mothers and fathers with dealing with feelings over possibly causing this disorder. It also has a familial risk. Nurses are prepared to counsel parents who are upset with their children's congenital defects and need for surgery (Burns et al., 2009).

Surgical Care. Surgery is usually performed during the second 6 months of the boy's life and before toilet training. Circumcision cannot be done until after this procedure because the foreskin may be used in the surgical repair. Techniques reconstruct the penis to lengthen the urethra and bring it to the distal penis shaft. The chordee is straightened, and often foreskin is used as a graft, so children born with hypospadias cannot be circumcised.

The child may have a urethral stent or Foley catheter in place to allow urine drainage because of potential obstruction of voiding from surgical edema. A compression dressing termed a penile wrap may be used. The nurse observes for swelling (some is expected), hematoma, and any purulent discharge, fever, or erythema indicating possible infection. Instruct the caregiver to have the child soak in warm water for 20 minutes before the surgical follow-up appointment to loosen the dressing. Potential surgical complications may include urethral fistula (an opening that allows urine to leak to the surface), stenosis, return of the meatus to its original site postsurgically, and strictures at the site of the anastomosis.

Education/Discharge Instructions

Teach parents to watch for evidence of urinary tract infection (e.g., fever; cloudy, foul urine; and hematuria). These pediatric patients also often suffer acute pain related to bladder spasm, incisional pain, and pain related to infection. Oxybutynin chloride (Ditropan) is an anticholinergic medicine that may relieve bladder spasm. Adverse effects of Ditropan include dry mouth and flushed face.

 Nursing Insight—*Gynecomastia*

Sixty percent of males may have temporary **gynecomastia** (breast enlargement) during puberty, especially between the ages of 12 and 14 years old. This often coincides with one side of the scrotum growing faster than the other. Gynecomastia may be one of four types:

- Type I is considered benign and self-limited. It occurs during Tanner stages II and III, and most cases are unilateral. The problem may persist for 2 years. It may be associated with an imbalance in testosterone and estrogen levels or increased prolactin hormone. A 1 cm to 3 cm round, mobile mass may be palpated under the areola (Helming, 2009).
- Type II is painful gynecomastia without any associated disease.
- Type III is gynecomastia that results from obesity.
- Type IV is related to hypertrophy of the pectoral muscles.

"What to say"—*Gynecomastia*

- Teach the patient and parents that gynecomastia is usually a temporary condition.
- If obesity is an issue, collaborate with the patient and family members to establish an age-appropriate dietary plan. Referral to a dietitian may be useful.
- Explain to the family and patient that it may be necessary to have certain blood tests to eliminate any risk of pathological causes of the gynecomastia.
- Discuss ways the child can respond to hurtful comments from other children.
- Discuss with parents that an enlarging mass or a mass that persists more than 2 years requires a diagnostic work-up to consider the differential diagnoses of breast tumor, Klinefelter's syndrome (decreased facial hair, eunuch body, normal or borderline to low IQ, and micro-orchidism), drug-induced gynecomastia, and thyroid disease.

TESTICULAR TORSION

Testicular torsion is considered an emergency, and surgical intervention must occur within a 4- to 8-hour time frame from the onset of symptoms or the patient risks the need for orchiectomy (testes resection). Loss of one testis through **orchiectomy** has been documented to decrease sperm counts and reduce fertility. This emergency condition is most common in growing males between the ages of 10 and 19. It is possible to have intermittent torsion which may resolve itself but can develop into a full emergency (Helming, 2009).

During the neonatal period, testicular torsion can occur because the processus vaginalis about the spermatic cord and testis can twist, causing partial or complete vascular compromise. In ages above the neonatal period, the etiology of testicular torsion is distinct; the testicle normally is attached to the tunica vaginalis, but periodically, the testicle is not attached and it hangs free to twist around the spermatic cord. This can cause torsion with painful ischemia and loss of the testis. Testicular torsion is the cause of 16% to 27% of all cases of acute scrotal pain, and thus it must be ruled out in all cases (Helming, 2009).

Signs and Symptoms

Neonates:
- Scrotum appears dusky colored
- Solid mass is palpated
- Scrotal edema prevents transillumination (inspecting the testis by passing a light through the scrotum)
- Minimal or no pain from testicular motion

Older males:
- Severe and persistent pain that may begin gradually
- Trauma and physical exertion may promote the development of torsion
- Pain may be severe enough to awaken patients at night and prevent ambulation
- Fever, anorexia, nausea, and vomiting

 Nursing Insight—*Testicular torsion*

Other essential clinical signs include:
- The torsed testicle may be lying horizontally or appear higher in the scrotal sac than the opposite testicle.
- Although most commonly the situation is unilateral, it may be bilateral.
- Scrotal edema is usually present within 12 hours.
- Especially in the neonate, the testicle may feel quite hard.
- One way to differentiate the diagnosis of testicular torsion is to attempt to elicit the cremasteric reflex, which is normally absent on the torsion side.
- Prehn's sign, which is relief of pain from elevating the testicle, is also usually absent in torsion.

Diagnosis

Diagnosis is based on patient history, physical examination findings, and Doppler ultrasonography.

 Assessment Tool Doppler Ultrasonography

Doppler ultrasonography is the preferred diagnostic test, and it is ordered immediately if torsion is suspected. In testicular torsion, the testicle may be enlarged and may reveal decreased or absent blood flow. The Doppler test can also differentiate between ischemia and inflammation, such as that seen in orchitis (inflammation of a testis) and epididymitis (inflammation of the epididymis) often associated with gonorrhea. In the case of possible false-negative results on Doppler ultrasound, a technetium scintigraphy test shows definitive testicular torsion. Urinalysis is normal in most of the cases of testicular torsion (Glass, 2011).

Prevention

Be aware of the signs and symptoms of testicular torsion to seek emergency care for the patient immediately.

Collaborative Care

Nursing Care. Offer support to the patient and family about this emergency situation because it may be frightening. Prior to surgery, complete a through nursing assessment and history. Be sure to ask about allergies. Obtain medical orders including pain medication. Vital signs are necessary, and the patient is NPO. A surgery consent form must be signed by the parents or guardian and witnessed by the nurse. Keep the patient calm by using distraction techniques.

Surgical Care. Manual detorsion (surgery for torsion of a testicle) by the urologist is done with sedation and local anesthesia to provide immediate mitigation of pain. Surgery is performed within 4 to 8 hours, and an **orchiectomy** may be required if the testicle becomes necrotic and cannot be salvaged. However, if the surgeon is able to save or detorse the testicle, it will be sutured into the scrotum so that it is no longer able to twist. The other testicle is also stabilized in this same way to prevent recurrence of the torsion. This latter procedure is called orchiopexy. A synthetic testicle can be put in place at a later date, if the testicle is removed (Nursing Articles, 2010).

Postoperative orders include assessment, physical dressing observation, vital signs, pain management, fluids as tolerated, tracking intake and output, and emotional support. The patient is discharged when he is stable.

Education/Discharge Instructions

Teach the parents about the importance of assessing the surgical site, signs and symptoms of infection, hydration, loose-fitting clothing, and follow-up appointments.

PHIMOSIS

This condition refers to a situation in which the foreskin is so tight that it cannot be retracted over the glans penis. It can be acquired from infection or inflammation underneath the foreskin, or it can be congenital. There are two types of phimosis. Primary or physiological phimosis occurs in the first 6 years of life when the glans has not totally separated from the epithelium. Secondary or pathological phimosis occurs when the foreskin cannot be retracted although it was previously retracted.

Signs and Symptoms

Signs and symptoms of phimosis include:
- Possible infection or inflammation of the penis
- Presence of paraphimosis
- Dysuria
- Pain
- Abnormal, intermittent urine stream

- Inability to retract foreskin
- Pinpoint opening of foreskin

Collaborative Care

Nursing Care. Nursing care centers on promoting gentle cleansing of the penis and gentle stretching of the foreskin but only to the point of resistance. Counsel parents that a tight foreskin in uncircumcised males is normal and most often resolves by the age of 6. Circumcision is then suggested unless symptoms do not resolve.

Medical Care. In this condition, the health-care provider may suggest the use of low-dose topical steroid cream to promote successful retraction.

Surgical Care. Circumcision may be indicated for an unresolved condition, infection, or urinary obstruction. Postoperative orders include assessment, pain management, fluids as tolerated, and discharge when the patient is stable.

Education/Discharge Instructions

If the child has had surgery, teach the parents about the importance of assessing the surgical site, signs and symptoms of infection, hydration, loose-fitting clothing, and follow-up appointments.

PARAPHIMOSIS

Paraphimosis is a condition in which the foreskin is retracted and it cannot be reduced (returned) to its normal position. It is more common in adolescents and can occur after masturbation, forceful retraction, or sexual abuse.

Signs and Symptoms

Signs and symptoms of paraphimosis include:

- Bluish discoloration of glans and foreskin
- Edema of glans and foreskin
- Risk of necrosis of penis

Prevention

Tell the older child to avoid forceful retraction of the foreskin.

Collaborative Care

Nursing Care. Nursing care centers on promoting gentle cleansing of the penis and gentle stretching of the foreskin but only to the point of resistance. An application of an ice pack for a short period of time may decrease foreskin and glans swelling. The family may need to consult a urologist to reduce the foreskin. If surgery is needed, prior to the procedure complete a through nursing assessment and history. Be sure to ask about allergies. Obtain medical orders including pain medication. Vital signs are necessary, and the patient is NPO. A surgery consent form must be signed by the parents or guardian and witnessed by the nurse. Keep the patient calm by using distraction techniques.

Surgical Care. In severe cases, this is a surgical emergency in which a surgical release of the constricting band of tissue must be done to prevent necrosis of the glans. Postoperative orders include assessment, vital signs, pain management, fluids as tolerated, tracking intake and output, and emotional support. The patient is discharged when he is stable.

Education/Discharge Instructions

If the child has had surgery, teach the parents about the importance of assessing the surgical site, signs and symptoms of infection, hydration, loose-fitting clothing, and follow-up appointments.

Reproductive Disorders Affecting Both Girls and Boys

AMBIGUOUS GENITALIA

Approximately 1 out of 2,000 newborns are born in the United States with ambiguous genitalia, which cannot be properly identified as either male or female genitalia. In males, it is more typical to have underdeveloped genitalia, and in females, overdeveloped genitalia are more common (Fig. 31-9). The etiology may be related to fetal or maternal hormonal imbalances. The new terminology is **disorders of sex development**. One example is congenital adrenal hyperplasia, in which excess male hormones are produced in a female fetus. Another example occurs when a male fetus has testicles that do not develop properly, do not make enough testosterone, or the child cannot use the testosterone properly (Achermann, Eugster, & Shulman, 2011).

Signs and Symptoms

Signs and symptoms may represent any number of possibilities, including these examples:

- An enlarged clitoris that resembles a small penis
- Fusion of the labia that resembles a scrotum
- The penis may not form or is very small
- The urethral meatus is at base, not tip, of penis

Diagnosis

Diagnosis includes a family history of congenital adrenal cortical hyperplasia, amenorrhea, and infertility in aunts or maternal history of prostaglandin, androgen, or danazol (Danocrine, a synthetic androgen used for endometriosis) use. Diagnosis is also based on the fact that the infant has both ovaries and testes. The external genitalia may vary from fully masculine to nearly fully feminine.

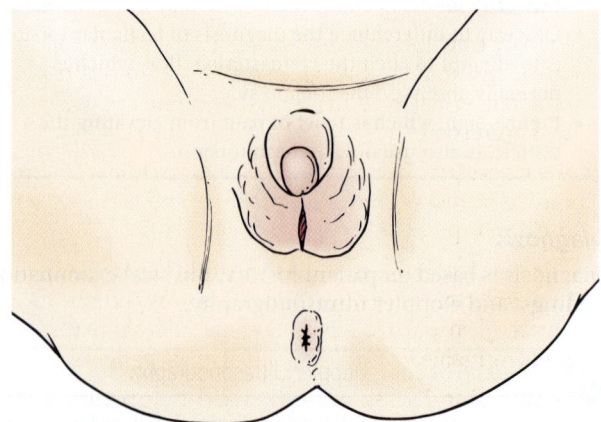

Figure 31-9 Ambiguous genitalia.

Prevention

Some of these disorders are genetic defects, and there may be no prevention. It is important for pregnant mothers to avoid any teratogenic medications that might cause birth defects.

Collaborative Care

Nursing Care. Care of the newborn follows standard care measures. Additional nursing care measures involve a great deal of support for the family members. The nurse assists the patient's family by suggesting endocrinology and genetic referrals.

Medical Care. Some patients with ambiguous genitalia become surgical candidates and need to see the urologist as well as a plastic surgeon. Sex assignment may be needed in some cases but is determined at a later date when laboratory test results are available (Achermann et al., 2011).

Education/Discharge Instructions

Help the family find proper support and community resources such as support groups, faith communities, and public health nurses. The family may need assistance with normal newborn care as well as emotional support. If the institution employs nurse case managers, ensure a relationship is established prior to hospital discharge.

 Now Can You—Discuss reproductive disorders in girls and boys?

1. Explain family teaching measures for vulvovaginitis?
2. Describe causes of secondary amenorrhea?
3. Examine care measures for hypospadias and epispadias?
4. Discuss ambiguous genitalia?

Summary Points

◆ It is essential for pediatric nurses to understand the pathophysiology of the renal system, renal disorders, acute kidney injury, and chronic kidney disease.

◆ Assessment of the genitourinary system is a priority nursing action when caring for the child with a fluid and/or electrolyte imbalance. The astute nurse recognizes fluid deficit and excess as well as electrolyte imbalance and then provides the proper care.

◆ Urinary tract infection is a very common infection in infants, children, and adolescents. In infants and young children, it may be difficult to determine the usual signs and symptoms of UTI.

◆ Vesicoureteral reflux (VUR) is a backflow of urine caused by anatomical abnormalities, and there is risk for the development of acute pyelonephritis.

◆ The most common etiologies for gross hematuria include hypercalciuria with or without stones, hypertension, and glomerulonephritis. Asymptomatic microhematuria has no identifiable cause in the majority of patients.

◆ Glomerular disease can be caused by primary kidney disease or secondary multisystem diseases that cause damage to the glomerulus.

◆ Hemolytic uremic syndrome (HUS) is considered the most common cause of acute renal failure (ARF) in children. Hemolytic uremic syndrome (HUS) is most commonly associated with children ingesting beef contaminated with *Escherichia coli* O157:H7.

◆ Abnormalities of the urinary tract system ultimately affect the kidneys. The abnormalities may be anatomical, infectious, cellular, inflammatory, functional, or maturational.

◆ The most common causes of renal trauma are motor vehicle accidents.

◆ Collaboration with the health-care team is critical so that acute kidney injury complications are reduced or prevented depending on whether the etiology is prerenal, intrarenal, or post-renal.

◆ The goals of nursing care for a patient with chronic renal disease are mutually established with the patient and family. Collaboration with the health-care team is essential so that the quality of life can be extended as long as possible because the renal capacity diminishes and affects all organ systems.

◆ The pRIFLE classification system helps to standardize acute kidney injury in the pediatric population.

◆ Renal replacement therapy (RRT) has three modalities: CCRT, peritoneal dialysis, and hemodialysis and each of these modalities has advantages and disadvantages.

◆ Nutrition is one of the most important interventions for positive outcomes in renal disease.

◆ Children in need of a renal transplant are placed on a waiting list and are registered with the United Network for Organ Sharing (UNOS), which keeps a computer network to link all organ donation centers and transplant centers.

◆ Enuresis can be primary or secondary. Culture influences how enuresis is evaluated and treated. Nurses can be very helpful in providing education for non-medicinal therapies for enuresis, including integrative therapies.

◆ Assess dysfunctional elimination syndrome (DES) in children by identifying issues, asking the child when he or she has voided, and asking the child if it is possible to hold back voiding if no bathrooms are available. Potential emotional and social problems may result related to shame and embarrassment.

◆ Genital and reproductive disorders in girls include amenorrhea, labial adhesions, Candida vulvovaginitis, nonspecific vulvovaginitis, and ambiguous genitalia.

◆ Genital and reproductive disorders in boys include varicocele, hypospadias, epispadias, hydrocele, testicular torsion, cryptorchidism, gynecomastia, and ambiguous genitalia.

Review Questions

Multiple Choice

1. A nurse is reviewing the laboratory values for a child with a genitourinary condition. Which lab value would require the nurse to intervene as the priority?
  A. Blood urea nitrogen (BUN): 32 mg/dL
  B. Creatinine: 3.6 mg/dL
  C. Creatinine clearance: 135 mg/minute
  D. Urinalysis: trace blood

2. A nurse is explaining to a group of students that pediatric patients are at greater risk for fluid and electrolyte imbalances than adults. Which is the best explanation for this condition?
   A. Higher percentage of total body water
   B. Hypernatremia caused by frequent drinking
   C. Kidneys with high concentrating abilities
   D. Smaller body surface area as compared with adults

3. A teenager participates in outdoor summer sports. The coach finds the teen sitting under a tree obviously dehydrated and with severe muscle weakness. For what electrolyte imbalance should the nurse assess as the priority?
   A. Hypercalcemia
   B. Hyperkalemia
   C. Hypomagnesemia
   D. Hyponatremia

4. A school-aged child is brought to the clinic by a parent who reports enuresis and malodorous urine. A routine urinalysis is normal. Which action by the nurse is best?
   A. Assess the child for toileting practices.
   B. Encourage the child to drink extra water.
   C. Facilitate a voiding cystourethrogram.
   D. Send urine for a culture and sensitivity.

5. A nurse is teaching a community parent group about various childhood genitourinary diseases. Which prevention method does the nurse teach the parents related to hemolytic uremic syndrome?
   A. Cook ground beef to an internal temperature of at least 160°F (71.1°C).
   B. Encourage your child to drink plenty of water throughout the day.
   C. Monitor your child's urinary output and report a decrease immediately.
   D. Seek rapid medical care if your child develops an upper respiratory illness.

6. The nurse assesses a child for Grey-Turner's sign. What technique is most appropriate for the nurse to use?
   A. Auscultates for renal bruits over the flanks
   B. Inspects for bruising over the flank area
   C. Palpates for an obvious abdominal mass
   D. Percusses for tympany over the kidney area

7. The nurse caring for a child with chronic kidney disease understands that which is the most common complication from this disorder?
   A. Anemia
   B. Bone disease
   C. Growth failure
   D. Hypertension

8. A nurse is assessing children at risk for chronic kidney disease. Which laboratory finding is most consistent with this condition?
   A. Calcium: 9.2 mg/dL
   B. pH: 7.16
   C. Potassium: 4.2 mg/dL
   D. Sodium: 140 mg/dL

9. A child is receiving peritoneal dialysis. Which potential complication does the nurse place greatest emphasis on preventing?
   A. Infection
   B. Migrating catheter
   C. Pain
   D. Urinary tract infection

10. A nurse is teaching a parent group about potty training. Which information does the nurse provide?
   A. A girl will be able to stay dry all day long by about 20 months.
   B. Choose a potty chair that is a little too big so the child feels grown up.
   C. If the child tells you after the fact about a wet diaper, he is not ready to train.
   D. Your child may show interest in toileting at around 2 years of age.

See Answers to End of Chapter Review Questions on Davis*Plus*.

REFERENCES

Achermann, J. C., Eugster, E. A., & Shulman, D. I. (2011). Ambiguous genitalia. *The Journal of Clinical Endocrinology and Metabolism, 96*(3), 33A–34A. Retrieved from http://jcem.endojournals.org/content/96/3/33A.full.pdf+html

Alconcher, L. F., Meneguzzi, M. B, Buschiazzo, R., & Piaggio, L. A. (2009). Could prophylactic antibiotics be stopped in patients with history of vesicoureteral reflux? *Journal of Pediatric Urology, 5*(5), 383–388.

American Academy of Pediatrics. (2009a). *Pediatric nutrition handbook* (6th ed.). Elm Grove Village, IL: AAP.

American Academy of Pediatrics. (2009b). Toilet training. Retrieved from http://www2.aap.org/publiced/BR_ToiletTrain.htm

Arthur, R. (2011). Gynecological guidelines. In J. Cash and C. Glass (Eds.), *Family practice guidelines* (2nd ed.). New York, NY: Springer.

Association for the Bladder Exstrophy Community. (2012). Retrieved from http://www.bladderexstrophy.com

Axton, S., & Fugate, T. (2008). *Pediatric nursing care plans for the hospitalized child* (3rd ed.). Upper Saddle River, NJ: Pearson Education, Inc.

Beetz, R. (2012). Evaluation and management of urinary tract infections in the neonate. *Current Opinions in Pediatrics, 24*(2), 205–211.

Blair, M. (2011). Overview of genitourinary trauma. *Urologic Nursing, 31*(3), 139–145.

Blayney, F. (2013). Renal disorders. In M. Hazinski, *Nursing Care of the Critically Ill Child* (3rd ed.). St. Louis, MO: Elsevier Mosby.

Brennan, J., & McEnhill, M. (2011). Use of nurse practitioners in pediatric kidney transplant: A model for providing comprehensive care to children and families. *Progress in Transplantation, 21*(4), 306–311.

Bunchman, T. E. (2012, March). Kids and kidney disease not child's play. *Nephrology Times, 5*(3), 2. doi:10.1097/01.NEP.0000413834.04316.f3

Burns, C. E., Dunn, A. M., Brady, M. A., Starr, N. B., & Blosser, C. G. (2009). *Pediatric primary care*. St. Louis, MO: Saunders Elsevier.

Canadian Urological Association. (2012). Dysfunctional elimination in children. Retrieved from http://www.uroinfo.ca

Centers for Disease Control and Prevention (CDC). (2013). Retrieved from http://www.cdc.gov/diabetes/projects/kidney/htm

Crozier, F., & Hancock, L. (2012). Pediatric palliative care: Beyond the end of life. *Pediatric Nursing, 38*(4), 198–203.

Daugirdas, J. (2011). *Handbook of chronic kidney disease management*. Philadelphia, PA: Lippincott Williams & Wilkins.

Desantis, D. J., Leonard, M. P., Preston, M. A., Barrowman, N. J., & Guerra, L. A. (2011). Effectiveness of biofeedback for dysfunctional elimination syndrome. In Pediatrics: A systematic review. *Journal of Pediatric Urology, 7*(3), 342–348. http://dx.doi.org.libraryproxy.quinnipiac.edu/10.1016/j.jpurol.2011.02.019

Doenges, M., Moorhouse, A., & Murr, C. (2013). *Nursing diagnosis manual* (4th ed.). Philadelphia, PA: F.A. Davis.

Feld, L., & Mattoo, T. (2010). Urinary tract infections and vesicoureteral reflux in infants and children. *Pediatrics in Review, 31,* 451–463. doi:10.1542/pir.31-11-451

Finnell, S., Carroll, A., Downs, S., & the Subcommittee on Urinary Tract Infection (2011). Diagnosis and management of an initial UTI in febrile infants and young children. *Pediatrics - Official Journal of the American Academy of Pediatrics.* doi:10.1542/peds.2011-1332

Gauther, M., Gouin, S., Phan V., & Gravel, J. (2012). Association of malodorous urine with urinary tract infection in children aged 1 to 36 months. *Pediatrics, 129*(5), 885–890. doi:10.1542/peds.2011–2856. Epub 2012 Apr 2.

Gaylord, N. M., & Starr, N. B. (2009). Chapter 34, Genitourinary disorders. In C. E. Burns, A. M. Dann, M. A. Brady, N. B. Starr, & C. G. Blosser, *Pediatric primary care* (4th ed.). Philadelphia, PA: Elsevier Saunders.

Gerson, A., Wentz, A., Abraham, A., Mendley, S., Hooper, S., Butler, R., et al. (2010). Health-related quality of life of children with mild to moderate chronic kidney disease. *Pediatrics - Official Journal of the American Academy of Pediatrics.* doi:10.1542/peds.2009–0085

Glass, C. (2011). Genitourinary conditions. In J. Cash & C. Glass (Eds.), *Family practice review* (2nd ed., 251–286). New York, NY: Springer.

Goldstein, S. (2011). Chronic dialysis. In A. Rudolph, G. Listiz, L. First, & A. Geshen, *Rudolph's pediatrics* (22nd ed.). Philadelphia, PA: McGraw-Hill.

Hatch, D., & Greenstein, S. (2011). Pediatric kidney transplantation treatment and management. Retrieved from http://emedicine.medscape.com/article/1012654-treatment#aw2aab6b4b4

Hay, W. W., Levin, M. J., Sondheimer, J. M., & Deterdin, R. R. (2009). *Current diagnosis and treatment in pediatrics* (19th ed.). New York, NY: McGraw-Hill.

Healy, P. (2011). Transplantation. In A. Rudolph, G. Listiz, L. First, & A. Geshen *Rudolph's pediatrics* (22nd ed.). Philadelphia, PA: McGraw-Hill.

Helming, M. (2009). Genitourinary disorders in children: A review of less common presentations. *Advance for Nurse Practitioners, 17*(3), 24–29.

Hudson, J. M., Balic, A., Nation, T., & Southwell, B. (2010). Cryptorchidism. *Seminars in Pediatric Surgery, 19*(3), 215–224.

Jetton, J. G., & Askenazi, D. J. (2012). Update on acute kidney injury in the neonate. *Current Opinion in Pediatrics, 24*(2), 191–196.

Klein, M. S. (2010). Chapter 32, Kidney disease, chronic. In P. J. Allen, J. A. Vessey, & N. A. Schapiro, *Primary care of the child with a chronic condition.* St. Louis, MO: Elsevier Mosby.

Kliegman, R. M., Stanton, B. M. D., St. Geme, J. W., Schor, N. F., & Behrman, R. E. (2011). *Nelson's textbook of pediatrics* (19th ed.). Philadelphia, PA: Elsevier Saunders.

Lerma, E., & Nissenson, A. (2012). *Nephrology secrets* (3rd ed.). Philadelphia, PA: Elsevier Mosby.

Lusaya, D. (2011). Hydronephrosis and Hydroureter. Retrieved from http://emedicine.medscape.com/article/436259-overview

Mathew, S., Abdelsalam, E , Saslow, J., Amendolia, B., Nakhla, T., Kemble, N., et al. (2009). Mild postnatal hydronephrosis is not associated with increased vesicoureteral reflux. *The Internet Journal of Pediatrics and Neonatology, 11*(1), 12.

McCance, K., Huether, S., Brashers, V., & Rote, N. (2010). *Pathophysiology: The biological basis for disease in adults and children.* Maryland Heights, MO: Elsevier Mosby.

McCarthy, K. (2011). Vesicoureteral reflux imaging. Retrieved from http://emedicine.medscape.com/article/414836-overview#a19

McClellan, A. C., Plantinga, L., & McClellan, W. (2012). Epidemiology, geography and chronic kidney disease. *Current Opinion in Pediatrics, 21*(3), 323–328.

McInerny, T., Adam, H., Campbell, D., Kamat, D., Kelleher, K., & Hoekelman, R. (2009). *American academy of pediatrics textbook of pediatric care.* Elk Grove Village, IL: American Academy of Pediatrics.

Murphy, F., & Byrne, G. (2010). The role of the nurse in the management of acute kidney injury. *British Journal of Nursing, 19*(3), 146–152.

National Kidney Foundation. (2013). Retrieved from https://www.kidney.org

National Kidney and Urologic Diseases Information Clearinghouse (NKUDIC) (2011). Retrieved from http://kidney.niddk.nih.gov/

Nursing Articles. (2010). Testicular torsion. Retrived from http://studynursing.blogspot.com/2010/12/torsion-of-testicular torsion.html

Perrin, K., & MacLeod, C. (2013). *Understanding the essentials of critical care nursing* (2nd ed.). Indianapolis, IN: Pearson.

Pop, S. (2012). A pediatric peripheral intravenous infiltration assessment tool. *Infusion Nurses Society, 4*(1), 243–248.

Quigley, R. (2012). Developmental changes in renal function. *Current Opinion in Pediatrics, 24*(2), 184–190.

Shields, L., & Tanner, A. (2010). Surgical procedures on children. In L. Shields, *Perioperative care of the child* (pp. 77–78). London: Wiley Blackwell.

Snyder, R. (2013). *What you must know about dialysis: The secrets to surviving and thriving on dialysis.* Garden City Park, NY: Square One Publishers.

Sreedharan, R., & Avner, E. (2011). Chronic kidney disease. In R. M. Kliegman, B. M. D. Stanton, St. J. W. Geme, N. F. Schor, & R. E. Behrman, *Nelson's textbook of pediatrics* (19th ed., p. 1822). Philadelphia, PA: Elsevier Saunders.

Taber's Online Medical Dictionary. (2013). Retrieved from http://www.tabers.com/tabersonline/ub/view/Tabers/144109/40/urine

Thomas, N. (2008). *Renal nursing* (3rd ed.). St. Louis, MO: Bailliere Tindall/Elsevier.

Tschudy, M., & Arcara, K. (2012). *The Harriet Lane handbook* (19th ed.). Philadelphia, PA: Elsevier Mosby.

Tu, W. H., & Shortliffe, L. D. (2010). Evaluation of asymptomatic, atraumatic hematuria in children and adults. *Nature Review Urology, 7,* 189–194. Published online 9 March 2010. doi:10.1038/nrurol.2010.27

Vallerand, A. H., & Sanoski, C. A. (2014). *Davis's drug guide for nurses* (14th ed.). Philadelphia, PA: F.A. Davis.

Van Leeuwen, A. M., Poelhuis-Leth, D. J., & Bladh, M. L. (2011). *Davis's comprehensive handbook of laboratory and diagnostic tests.* Philadelphia, PA: F.A. Davis.

Venes, D. J. (2013). *Taber's cyclopedic medical dictionary* (22nd ed.). Philadelphia, PA: F.A. Davis.

Walters, P, Porter, C., & Brophy, P. (2009). Dialysis and pediatric acute kidney injury: Choice of renal support modality. *Pediatric Nephrology, (24)*1, 37–48. doi:10.1007/s00467-008-0826-x

Wan, J., Skoog, S., Hulbert, W., Casale, A., Greenfield, S., Cheng, E., et al. (2012). Section on urology response to new guidelines for the diagnosis and management of UTI. *Pediatrics - Official Journal of the American Academy of Pediatrics.* doi:10.1542/peds.2011–3615

Ward, S. (2013). *Pediatric nursing care: Best evidence-based practices.* Philadelphia, PA: F.A. Davis.

Williams, J., Bonin, S., Emory, B., Tate, A., Thompson, G., & Wood, S. (2011). The pediatric renal transplant process. Retrieved from www.homehealthcarenurseonline.com

Workeneh, B., & Batuman, V. (2012). Acute kidney injury. *Medscape Reference Drugs, Diseases, and Procedures.* Retrieved from http://emedicine.medscape.com/article/243492-overview

Yaklin, K. (2011). Acute kidney injury: An overview of pathophysiology and treatments. *Nephrology Nursing Journal, 36*(1), 13–18.

CONCEPT MAP

Caring for the Child With a Genitourinary Condition

Reproductive Disorders—Boys:
- Varicocele; cryptorchidism; hydrocele; hypo-/hyperspadas; gynecomastia; testicular torsion; phimosis; paraphimosis; ambiguous genitalia

Reproductive Disorders—Girls:
- Vulvovaginitis; vaginal foreign body; labial adhesions; amenorrhea; ambiguous genitalia

Fluid/Electrolyte Balance:
- Fluid volume excess/deficit and electrolyte imbalances in children have a variety of causes
- Children at greater risk for F/E imbalances
- Measured by daily discrepancies in body weight; monitoring I&O

Structural Disorders:
- Abnormality in urinary tract system; can affect kidney function
- Bladder exstrophy
- Hydronephrosis
- Ureteropelvic junction obstruction

Renal Failure:
Acute Kidney Injury
- Sudden decrease in renal function; life-threatening syndrome; significant morbidity/mortality for critically ill children
- RIFLE classification system improves outcomes
- Signs/symptoms correlate to cause: Pre-, intra-, and postrenal
- Key ⟶ ID child at risk and prevent

Chronic Kidney Disease:
- Irreversible deterioration of kidney function
- Etiology varies by age (e.g., neonatal vascular accidents, adolescent glomerulonephritis, polycystic kidney disease)
- Progresses through four stages

Urinary System Disorders:
- UTI
  - *E. coli* most common organism
- Vesicoureteral reflux
  - Backflow of urine to ureters/kidney
  - Treatment plan varies according to age
- Unexplained proteinuria
  - 30 mg/dL or higher; simple to life-threatening causes
- Hematuria
  - Gross or microscopic; can indicate serious issues
- Glomerular disease
  - Can be primary or secondary
- ➤ Glomerulonephritis: acute/chronic/postsecondary
  - Glomerular damage affecting function
- ➤ Hemolytic uremic syndrome
  - Cascade of events; affects filtration; involves clotting and inflammation; affects other systems; most common cause of ARF in children
- ➤ Henoch-Schonlein purpura
  - Type of vasculitis; follows URIs
- ➤ Nephrotic syndrome
  - Excessive protein excretion in urine

Functional Disorders:
- Dysfunctional elimination syndrome; bladder/bowel withholding/incontinence
- Enuresis: involuntary discharge of urine

Renal/GU Trauma:
- Related to blunt/penetrating abdominal injury
- Can affect: scrotum, penis, urethra, ureters, bladder, kidney

Renal Replacement Therapy—ESRD:
- Hemofiltration/CRRT
- Peritoneal dialysis (PD)
  - Peritoneal membrane acts as filter
- Hemodialysis
  - Mechanical filtration/dialyzer
  - Vascular access ⟶ A/V fistula or graft

Cultural Diversity:
- Toileting patterns vary by culture
- African Americans constitute 32% of all persons treated for kidney failure

Kidney Transplant:
- Cadaver or living donor
- Phases: candidate, renal transplant, recipient
- Long-term pharmacotherapy posttransplant
- Potential for organ rejection ongoing

Critical Nursing Action:
- Care of the child with F/E imbalance
- Correct teaching r/t new AV fistula
- Completion of a pre–kidney transplant evaluation within correct time frame
- Know the symptoms of organ rejection

Legal Alert:
- ☑ Legal consequences when *E. coli* O157.H7 infections result in severe injury
- Inaccurate weight can cause life-threatening harm to critically ill child

What to Say:
- Health info/hx to obtain r/t suspected CRF
- Teach about gynecomastia

Clinical Alert:
- ! Calculate daily maintenance fluid requirements using child's BSA or weight in kilograms
- Fever/hardy exercise can cause proteinuria
- Look for symptom of renal disease with proteinuria
- Young children/older adults at risk for HUS r/t *E. coli* infection
- Iatrogenic fluid overload can be caused by fluid tx. to raise urine output
- Seizures can occur secondary to F/E imbalances
- Observe for complications of peritoneal dialysis
- r/o sexual abuse first for child showing sx. of vaginal foreign body

Nursing Insight:
- Urinary tract abnormalities causing stasis/obstruction = most significant risk for UTI
- Proteinuria can have a more grave etiology
- Hydronephrosis: swollen upper urinary tract
- Hematuria is a cardinal marker of renal injury
- NGAL, IL-15, KIM-I = biomarkers for AKI
- Use of RIFLE classification in AKI can improve outcomes
- FEna is a diagnostic index of tubular function
- Collaboration is critical to reduce/prevent AKI complications
- CKD etiology is age-related and dependent on organs affected; each stage of CKD has its own complications
- ESRD has many etiologies imbalances
- Referral to National Kidney Foundation can help families cope with renal failure in a child
- Adolescents may not adhere to PD protocols
- Enuresis may carry a genetic link
- Recurrent vaginal candidiasis can be a symptom of DM
- Amenorrhea can be r/t underlying causes
- 60% of males have temporary gynecomastia during puberty

Complementary Care:
- Use of biofeedback for DES
- For enuresis: hypnotherapy, acupressure, massage
- Strategies for managing vaginal candidiasis

Where Research and Practice Meet:
- A normal urinalysis does not mean UTI is not present
- There are pros and cons to prophylactic antibiotic use for VUR
- pRIFLE creatinine criteria predictive for AKI in children post–cardiac surgery

Now Can You:
- ? Name common disorders of the renal/urinary systems; discuss reproductive disorders for girls and boys
- Provide evidence-based, safe, and holistic care for the child with a genitourinary disorder

Across Care Settings:

- Day-care/school nurses need teaching regarding care of the child with bladder exostrophy
- Child post–kidney transplant needs multidisciplinary care in the community

Focus on Safety:
- ! Undercooked beef is primary source of *E. coli* causing HUS
- There are three requirements needed to receive a kidney transplant

Caring for the Child With a Hematological Condition

 A Nurse's Wish

To be a nurse requires dedication,
With years of study and preparation.
I pray for guidance and humbly ask,
That I will do well with this chosen task.
When illness strikes or pain demands,
And a life is placed within my hands,
Give me compassion, knowledge and skill
To do the things that comfort and heal.
Suffering makes patients' fear grow worse.

And they seek reassurance from their nurse.
Help me see things from their point of view.
And always to know what is best to do.
May I have a part, in some small way?
In restoring good health to a child today!
Let my work be all that I want it to be,
I ask the great healer to work through me.

—Author Unknown

LEARNING TARGETS *At the completion of this chapter, the student will be able to:*

- Describe the anatomy and physiology and developmental aspects of the hematological system.
- Examine common conditions of the hematological system.
- Prioritize developmentally appropriate and holistic nursing care measures for common conditions of the hematological system.
- Explore diagnostic, and laboratory testing and medications for common conditions of the hematological system.
- Develop teaching plans and discharge criteria for parents whose children have common hematological conditions.

PICO(T) Questions

The intent of evidence-based practice (EBP) is to provide nursing care that integrates the best available evidence. An initial step in EBP is to write a PICO(T) question that effectively guides the research. PICO(T) is an acronym that stands for population (P), intervention or issue (I), comparison of interest (C), outcome (O), and timeframe (T). Depending on the question, all or some of the question components are used in the research process. Use these

PICO(T) questions to spark your thinking as you read the chapter.

1. Do (P) children with acute idiopathic thrombocytopenia purpura (ITP) whose condition resolves without treatment have (O) a lower rate of (I) recurrence compared with (C) children with acute ITP who receive treatment?

2. What (I) nonpharmacological pain management strategies do (P) patients with sickle cell disease state are (O) most effective for moderate pain?

Evidence-Based Practice

Dale, J. C., Cochran, C. J., Roy, L., Jernigan, E., & Buchanan, G. R. (2011). Health-related quality of life in children and adolescent with sickle cell disease. *Journal of Pediatric Health Care, 25*(4), 208–215.

The purpose of this study was to examine the quality of life of children and adolescents with sickle cell disease (SCD). The incidence of SCD is 1 in 500 African Americans and 1 in 1,000 to 1,400 Hispanic Americans. Acute complications for SCD include acute chest syndrome, stroke, splenic sequestration, infection, aplastic crisis, priapism, acute pain, and vaso-occlusive crisis. Chronic complications include delayed growth and development, avascular necrosis of femoral head, pulmonary hypertension, renal disease, and gallstones. Both acute and chronic complications can impact the child's health-related quality of life (HRQOL) because of hospitalizations, activity limitation, and school absences. Some studies have found that HRQOL can be improved and pain reduced through use of hydroxy-urea, stem cell transplant, or physical therapy. Health is defined by the World Health Organization as the absence of disease and infirmity and the presence physical, mental, and social well-being. Quality of life includes physical and psychosocial health and impacts a person's beliefs and perceptions. In comparison to healthy children, research has noted a negative response to HRQOL among children with chronic diseases. These studies also note that parent perceptions of child HRQOL has been found to be rated worse overall than that of the child. Participants in this study were selected from a convenience sample of patients who were involved in a sickle cell program at a children's medical center in Dallas, Texas. Potential participants included children between 8 and 18 years of age diagnosed with either sickle cell anemia (95.2%) or sickle β zero thalassemia (4.8%). Additional participation criteria included ability to read, write, or verbalize information in either English or Spanish. Those excluded were patients who had previously experienced a stroke, participated in a chronic transfusion program, or were experiencing acute complications at the time of the clinic visit during which participants were selected. Potential participants included 234 patients who were being followed by the clinic at the time enrollment took place. Of that total, 124 agreed to participate, 6 declined, and an additional 104 were not approached. The study included one parent or proxy for each child in the sample. The mean age of the participants was 13; the mean school level of the participants was seventh grade; all but one participant were African American. Fifty-two percent were male. Demographic data noted that the children in this cohort missed an average of 3 days of school, were too ill to play, and needed an average of 3 days of care during the previous month. During the past year 50% of the children required hospitalization and 74% were seen in the emergency department. Half of the mothers and 66% of the fathers were educated at the high school level or lower. Seventy-eight percent of the parent respondents were the mother, 12.1% were

the father, 4.0% were grandmothers, and 5.7% were identified as guardians. Twenty percent of the parents noted that the child's illness interfered with their job, and 27% said it interfered with their ability to concentrate). A group of 10,241 healthy participants and their families with similar demographics who were newly enrolled in a state health insurance program also completed the survey and were used as a comparison group.

Data were gathered through the use of the PedsQL 4.0 survey, which is a multidimensional self-report instrument that includes 23 items and is rated on a Likert scale. This survey measures opinions or attitudes about problems related to physical, emotional, social, and educational functioning. The parent survey uses identical questions and asks the parent's perception of the child's functioning in each area. This survey has previously been proven to be reliable and valid for both well and chronically ill children. The survey was also available in the Spanish language for Spanish-speaking participants. An information form was used to obtain the demographic data. Data were analyzed using t-tests and ANOVA. Analysis of survey results found that there was a significant difference between the responses of the healthy children and the children with SCD as well as a significant difference between the children with SCD and their parents' perceptions of the child's HCQOL. Only 1 correlation was significant among the responses of the children, which was a weak reverse correlation between the number of hospitalizations and reduced school functioning scores. There were 4 significant correlations among the parents related to the number of hospitalizations (i.e., overall HRQOL and educational, emotional, and psychosocial health). A significant correlation was also noted between emergency department visits and emotional health. Overall, children with SCD described their HRQOL significantly better than their parents did.

The researchers conclude that their findings were similar to those noted in previous research of children with other chronic conditions in that children with SCD and their parents perceived their overall HRQOL to be lower than that of healthy children. Previous studies also noted parent ratings of HRQOL significantly lower than the ratings of the children in those studies.

1. How is this information useful to clinical nursing practice?
2. Based on these findings, what are implications for further research?

See Suggested Responses for Evidence-Based Practice on Davis*Plus*.

Introduction

This chapter provides a review of the anatomy and physiology and developmental aspects of the hematological conditions. The discussion includes an examination of the various hematological conditions including developmentally appropriate and holistic nursing care. Information is given about diagnostic and laboratory testing and medications. Teaching plans and discharge criteria for parents whose children have various hematological conditions are incorporated. In addition, blood transfusion therapy, bone marrow transplant, apheresis, and thrombosis are reviewed.

A hematological disorder in a child can have various causes including injury, nutritional deficit, genetic disorder, infection, congenital problem, or any number of blood-related conditions. A thorough history and physical examination are essential in the diagnosis and care of the child with a hematological disorder because the condition can be insidious in nature. To understand the disorders affecting children that involve the hematological system, it is imperative to comprehend the normal function of the blood and formed elements.

CARING FOR THE CHILD WITH A HEMATOLOGICAL CONDITION

A & P review Hematological System

The hematological system is a complex, yet fascinating system. The blood is composed of two parts: the fluid portion called plasma and the cellular portion. The solutes in the plasma include albumin, electrolytes, proteins, clotting factors, fibrinogen, globulins, and circulating antibodies. The cellular portion consists of the formed elements (red blood cells [RBCs], white blood cells [WBCs], and platelets).

The primary function of the RBCs (erythrocytes) is to transport hemoglobin that carries oxygen from the lungs to the tissues. The life span of a normal RBC is approximately 120 days. Leukocytes (WBCs) are mobile units of the body's protective system. Most leukocytes migrate to areas of serious inflammation and provide a rapid defense against any foreign agent. WBCs are also important in immune system mediation. The life span of a leukocyte is specific to the cell type.

Megakaryocytes are cells that give rise to platelets. Platelets are small fragments of megakaryocytes. Platelets are the smallest of all formed blood elements and are not really cells because they do not possess a cellular structure. The primary function of platelets is hemostasis and vascular repair after injury to a vessel wall. Platelets aggregate to form a plug. Their life span is approximately 7 to 10 days. Almost one-third of all circulatory platelets can normally be found in the spleen. In normal circumstances, platelets are removed by the liver and spleen in 10 days if not utilized in a clotting (Fig. 32-1). ◆

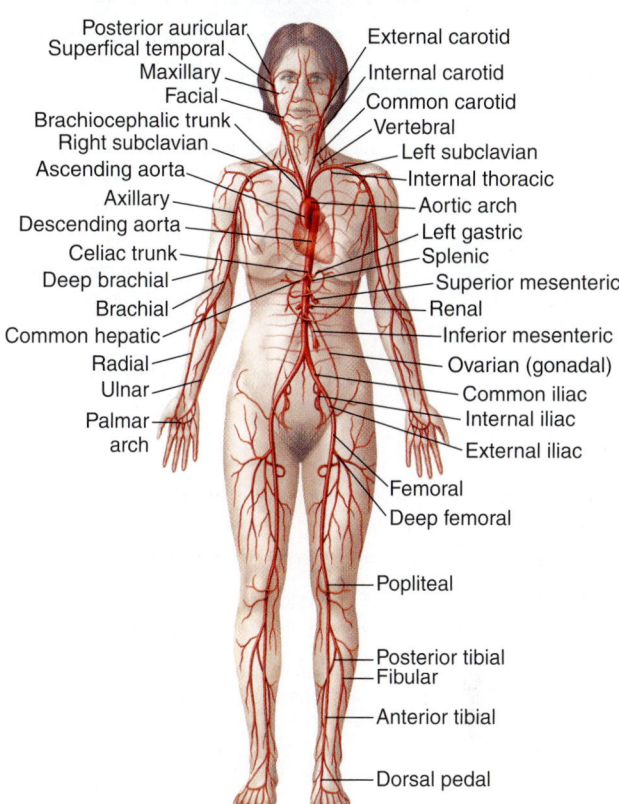

Hematological System

Figure 32–1 A & P of the circulatory system.

Common Hematological Conditions

Several common hematological conditions can occur in children. Some of these are acute in nature and with proper care can be easily managed. Others can be life-threatening or cause a chronic illness that can permanently impact the lifestyle of the child and his or her family. It is essential that the nurse understand the necessary assessment, nursing care measures, medications, laboratory tests, and important teaching aspects associated with these conditions (Tables 32-1, 32-2, and 32-3).

ANEMIA

One of the most common hematological conditions of infancy and childhood is anemia (a decrease in the number of red blood cells [RBCs]). The reduction in circulating RBCs decreases the oxygen-carrying capacity of the blood. For the majority of patients, anemia is not a disease but rather a symptom of other diseases.

> ✳ *Nursing Insight*—*Causes of anemia*
>
> - Decreased production of RBCs, such as in bone marrow failure and myelodysplastic syndromes
> - Increased destruction of RBCs, such as in sickle cell anemia or hereditary spherocytosis
> - Acute or chronic blood loss
>   It is important to identify the cause of anemia so that the treatment plan can be tailored to the child's specific needs.

Growth and Development

Iron-deficiency anemia and other hematological conditions can greatly impact the child's ability for normal growth and development. Iron deficiency leads to increased fatigue and poor concentration required for social interaction and cognitive stimulation. Research shows that this lack of social interaction is linked to poor motor development and cognitive impairment in children (O'Sullivan, 2013). Attention to growth and development must be a factor in the nursing plan of care to avoid delays.

The nurse understands that the child with a hematological condition such as iron deficiency may experience greater amounts of fatigue than a healthy child. It is important to provide activities that are developmentally stimulating and that conserve energy. Nutritional therapy can help to replace electrolytes and calories that are required for healthy activity. The nurse should educate the family about the proper dietary modifications and vitamin supplements appropriate for the child. Education about health promotion is essential to avoid reoccurrences of the disease process.

Source: O'Sullivan, S. (2013). Iron deficiency: The developing child at risk. *World of Irish Nursing, 21*(2) 41–42.

Table 32-1 Assessment of the Child With a Hematological Disease

System	Review of Symptoms (Symptoms: Subjective, Historical, or Current)	Physical Exam (Signs: Objective, Current)
• General	• Fatigue, malaise, weakness, lethargy, exercise intolerance, history of bleeding disorder, transfusions or need for medications to control clotting, exposure to toxins. Fever, chills, and infections if WBCs are deficient	• Ruddy face, hands, and feet; sweating; severe and sudden pain in bones, joints, back pain, and chills with G6PPD
• Skin, Nails, Hair	• Jaundice, pallor, rubor stated by patient or family (may not be evident on exam), history of bruising or petechiae	• Jaundice, pallor, or rubor noted by the provider on exam. Spooning of nails is indicative of iron-deficiency anemia. Multiple bruises and different stages of healing, pruritus (caused by mast cell activation), petechiae, superficial ecchymoses, purpura, and unusually heavy menstrual flow
• Head	• Headache, dizziness, or vertigo	• Abnormal facial bone structure (thalassemia)
• Eyes	• Visual disturbances (polycythemia)	• Pale outer canthus, scleral icterus (jaundice), retinal hemorrhage
• Ears	• No specific problems with hematology	• No specific problems with hematology
• Nose	• History of epistaxis	• Epistaxis, gingival bleeding, bullous hemorrhage on the buccal mucosa
• Mouth and Throat	• Pale mucous membranes, increased bleeding of gums with or without brushing	• Pale mucous membranes, easy bleeding of gums, red painful tongue, smooth glossy tongue (atrophic glossitis), mouth erosions
• Neck	• No specific problems with hematology	• No specific problems with hematology
• Breast	• No specific problems with hematology	• No specific problems with hematology
• Respiratory/Thorax Lungs	• Exertional dyspnea, coughing up blood (hemoptysis), tachypnea	• No specific problems with hematology
• Cardiovascular	• Palpitations, history of central vein thrombosis, nocturia, glossitis	• Transient heart murmur, cardiomegaly, iron overload on T2 MRI exam, tachycardia, pedal edema
• Peripheral Vascular	• Coldness, numbness, pain in legs (DVT)	• Cool, delayed cap refill, full bounding pulse, unilateral swelling of calf (DVT), brown discoloration of skin (venous stasis)
• Gastrointestinal	• GI distress (polycythemia), GI disorders that may cause poor absorption of iron or vitamins, blood in stool, pica, glossitis, dysphagia, weight loss, malabsorption, and diarrhea with steatorrhea, gallstones (sickle cell)	• Positive guaiac testing, hepatomegaly, atrophic gastritis, and splenomegaly, black tarry stools in newborn
• Urinary	• Blood in urine	• Reduced GFR and uremia in cases of anemia of renal failure
• Genitalia	• Increased bleeding with menses	• No specific problems with hematology
• Neurologic	• Coordination problems, headaches, irritability, light-headedness, restless leg syndrome, impaired psychomotor or mental development, may contribute to ADHD and decreased cognitive function in adolescents. Paranoid ideation, dementia, hallucinations, and distorted senses, paresthesias to spastic ataxia, somnolence, memory impairment	• Intracranial hemorrhage
• Hematologic	• History of hematological disorders, need for or current use of iron or other supplements, family history of bleeding disorder	• Noticeable bleeding anywhere on exam, unexplained hemorrhage or bleeding from IV sites after trauma or sepsis
• Endocrine	• No specific problems with hematology	• No specific problems with hematology
• Musculoskeletal	• Pain in joints and bones. Delayed growth pattern	• Abnormal skeletal structure

Source: Ward (2013).

Table 32-2 Medications

Medication/ Supplement Name	Dosage/Route/Timing	Action	Comments
• Aspirin (Bayer Aspirin, Bufferin)	• ½–1 baby aspirin/day or QOD	• Antiplatelet	• Effects can last as long as 1 week
• Coagulation factors	• Dosing is variable according to disease and coagulation studies	• Used as a replacement in coagulopathies when the factor deficiency is known and replaceable	• Usually replaced in IV infusion therapy unit
• warfarin (Coumadin, Jantoven, Warfilone)	• Dosing is individualized 1–10 mg/day in adjusted or variable doses	• **Anticoagulants** • Given in conditions with high risk for thrombi (thrombocytosis, Factor V Leiden, or polycythemias)	• Oral dosing
• desmopressin (DDAVP)	• Dosing sub Q – 0.3 mcg/kg 30 minutes prior to procedure	• **Hormones** • Used for von Willebrand's disease, helps to promote replacement of vWF	• Monitor serum sodium
• desferrioxamine (Desferal)	• 50 mg/kg/dose every 6 hours or 90 mg/kg/ dose every 8 hours, not to exceed 1 g/dose or 6 g/day	• **Antidotes** • Given with thalassemia and other diseases requiring hy- pertransfusions as an iron chelation agent	• Given IM, IV, or subcutaneous
• erythropoietin (Epogen, EPO, Erythropoietin, Procrit)	• Dosing is individualized. 25–300 units/kg 3–7 times per week.	• **Antianemics** • Given for anemias of all types especially for anemia of renal disease	• Given subcutaneously or IV
• heparin (Calcilean, Calciparine, Hepalean, Heparin Leo, Hep-Lock, Hep-Lock U/P)	• Dosing individualized and adjusted with a PTT between 60 and 85 seconds. Loading dose 75 units/kg for 10 minutes then reduce to 28 units/kg/hr maintenance	• **Anticoagulants** • Given in conditions with high risk for thrombi (thrombocytosis, Factor V Leiden, or polycythemias)	• Patient is hospitalized. Care- fully determine appropriate concentration because there are different formulations
• hydoxyurea (Droxia, Hydrea, Mylocel)	• 15 mg/kg/day daily	• **Antineoplastics** • Given for sickle cell anemia to increase concentration of hemoglobin F, which has protective properties against hemoglobin S	• Increase dose by 5 mg/kg/day every 12 weeks to a maximum dose of 35 mg/kg/day. Reduce dosage alternating with erythropoietin
• enoxaparin (Lovenox)	• Dosing (prophylaxis) 0.75 mg/kg/dose every 12 hours for infants • Children: 0.5 mg/kg/dose every 12 hours • Treatment: Infants: 1.5 mg/kg/dose every 12 hours • Children: 1 mg/kg/dose every 12 hours	• Given in conditions with high risk for thrombi (thrombocytosis, Factor V Leiden, or polycythemias)	• Can be given as outpatient, and family is instructed to give subcutaneously. Transition from heparin dosing to Lovenox—draw antifactor Xa 4 hours after dosing

Source: Ward (2013).

Table 32-3   PT, PTT, INR, Platelet Aggregate Testing

Platelets	• Number of platelets will determine efficacy of clotting
PT	• Extrinsic pathway • Vitamin K deficiency • Used to assess Coumadin dosing
INR	• Extrinsic pathway • Provides uniformity in testing for Coumadin dosing • May be therapeutically high
aPTT	• Intrinsic pathway • Shows if patient is adequately heparinized • Vitamin K deficiency
Platelet aggregation	• Aspirin use • Not usually tested but may determine appropriate Plavix dosing

Signs and Symptoms

Anemia may be insidious, and the child may be asymptomatic because of compensatory mechanisms. The child with mild anemia may be asymptomatic and not diagnosed until blood work is obtained. Initial signs of anemia vary but may include:

• Fatigue
• Shortness of breath
• Headache
• Difficulty concentrating
• Dizziness
• Pale skin

The child with moderate to severe anemia will have overt signs and symptoms:

• Irritability
• Fatigue
• Delayed motor development
• Tachycardia
• Shortness of breath
• Decreased activity level
• Pale skin
• Listlessness
• Systolic heart murmur
• Hepatomegaly, congestive heart failure (Nathan, Orkin, Ginsburg, & Look, 2009)

focus on safety

Screening guidelines

According to the 2010 clinical report by the American Academy of Pediatrics, hemoglobin and hematocrit are evaluated once during infancy (between 9 and 12 months of age) and again during early childhood (between 1 and 5 years of age). Additional preventive screening includes checking children in late childhood (between 5 and 12 years of age) and again in adolescence (between 14 and 20 years of age). The benefit of ongoing screening can identify children who may need treatment to prevent anemia (Baker, Greer, & The Committee on Nutrition, 2010).

Diagnosis

For the child diagnosed with anemia, a thorough history and physical examination are essential to establish a possible etiology. Complete blood count (CBC) and reticulocyte count are obtained to evaluate the hemoglobin and hematocrit. Anemia exists when the hemoglobin content is less than required to meet the oxygen demands of the body.

 Nursing Insight—Hemoglobin, hematocrit, and CBC

Hemoglobin is the iron-containing pigment of the RBC that carries oxygen from the lungs to the tissues. The hemoglobin level is measured as the amount of hemoglobin per deciliter of whole blood. The average hemoglobin in the blood varies based on the age and gender of the individual.

Normal hemoglobin (Hgb) (g/dL) lab values for children are:
Newborn: 12.7–18.6 g/dL
2 Months: 9.0–14.0 g/dL
2 Years: 10.5–12.7 g/dL
6–12 Years: 11.2–14.8 g/dL
12–18 Years: 10.7–15.7 g/dL

Hematocrit is the percent of whole blood that is composed of RBCs. The hematocrit measures both the number and size of the RBCs and is approximately three times greater than the hemoglobin value. The hematocrit indirectly measures the hemoglobin. The average hematocrit value in children lies between 35% and 45% (Van Leeuwen, Poelhuis-Leth & Bladh, 2011).

A child's CBC measures the formed elements in the blood, including RBCs, white blood cells (WBCs), and platelets, providing valuable information with regard to illnesses and disease processes that may be occurring. In addition to the quantitative analysis, the blood cells of the CBC can also be evaluated for shape, size, and color.

Prevention

Anemia caused by clinical conditions such as sickle cell disease, hereditary spherocytosis, and disorders of the red blood

Labs: Blood Values According to Age

Be knowledgeable about the age-specific laboratory value norms for the child. Based on the child's age, there may be variations in expected ranges (Tables 32-4, 32-5, and 32-6). Generic adult values should not be translated for pediatric patients.

 Labs: Complete Blood Count, Reticulocyte, and Peripheral Smear Lab Values for Children

When evaluating the presence of anemia, initial laboratory tests include CBC and a reticulocyte count. The CBC includes hemoglobin, hematocrit, RBC indices, platelet count, WBC count with a differential, and a peripheral smear to examine the morphology of the RBCs. For the patient with suspected anemia, the peripheral blood smear is imperative to confirm the appropriate diagnosis (Goldman & Schafer, 2012). The peripheral blood smear consists of a glass slide coated on one side with a thin layer of blood. The slide is stained with a dye and reviewed under a microscope to identify the red cell characteristics to confirm a diagnosis (Speller-Brown, Eimicke, & Martin, 2011).

Table 32-4   Laboratory Blood Values According to Age

Age/Blood Component	Newborn	2 Months	2 Years	6–12 Years	12–18 Years	Comments
Red blood cells (RBCs)	4.1–5.74	2.7–4.9	3.9–5.03	4.93–5.3	3.7–5.5	Measure of bone marrow function
Hemoglobin (Hgb) (g/dL)	12.7–18.6	9.0–14.0	10.5–12.7	11.2–14.8	10.7–15.7	Amount of hemoglobin/dL of whole blood
Hematocrit (Hct) (%)	37.4–56.1	28.0–42.0	31.7–37.7	34.0–43.9	33.0–46.2	Percentage of packed RBC to whole blood, approximately 3 times the Hgb content
White blood cells (WBCs)	6.8–14.3	5.0–19.5	5.3–11.5	4.5–10.1	4.4–10.2	Differential count is more important than the total number of WBCs
Platelets ($\times 10^3$/mm^3 [mcL])	164–586	164–586	206–459	189–403	175–345	Platelets contribute to blood clotting

Table 32-5   Normal White Blood Cell Differential Count According to Age

Age/White Blood Cell Component	Function	Newborn	2 Months	2 Years	6–12 Years	12–18 Years
Neutrophils (%)	Phagocytosis	19–49	15–35	13–33	32–54	34–64
Eosinophils (%)	Allergic reactions	0–4	0–3	0–3	0–3	0–3
Basophils (%)	Inflammatory reactions	0–1	0–1	0	0–1	0–1
Lymphocytes (%) (B cells and T cells)	Humoral immunity (B cell) and cellular immunity (T cell)	38–46	42–72	46–76	27–57	25–45
Monocytes (%) (macrophages)	Phagocytosis and antigen processing	0–9	0–6	0–5	0–5	0–5

Table 32-6   Red Cell Laboratory Values for Children

Test	Reference Range	Comments
Mean corpuscular volume (MCV)	79–95 µm^3	Average size of a single RBC, expressed as cubic microns (µm^3)
Mean corpuscular hemoglobin (MCH)	25–33 pg/cell	Average weight of the Hgb within a RBC, expressed in picograms (pg)
Mean cell hemoglobin concentration (MCHC)	31%–37% Hgb [g]/dL RBC	Average concentration of Hgb in each RBC
Reticulocyte count	0.5%–1.5%	Measure of the production of mature RBCs by the bone marrow
Peripheral smear	Size, shape, and structure of the RBCs as well as an estimate of the amount of Hgb in the RBCs	Can indicate variations in size and shape of RBCs, microcytic, macrocytic, or normocytic

Source: Hillman, Ault, Leporrier, & Rinder (2011).

cell often do not respond to traditional preventive measures. Anemia caused by iron deficiency and poor nutrition may be prevented by following screening guidelines and encouraging a well-balanced diet. Additionally, preventing exposure to lead-containing items such as paint, gasoline, and other household hazards may prevent the development of anemia.

Collaborative Care

Nursing Care. Nursing care for a child with anemia varies based on the etiology. The nurse would be responsible for administering and monitoring blood transfusions and other pharmacological treatments prescribed.

 ### Nursing Insight—*Evaluating a CBC*

Blood Elements	Increase	Decrease
RBC (Hgb/Hct)	Polycythemia	Anemia
WBC	Leukocytosis	Leukopenia
Platelets	Thrombocytosis	Thrombocytopenia

Medical Care. Treatment for anemia varies based on the etiology. To effectively replenish the RBCs, the underlying cause must be identified. For children with mild anemia, the nurse provides supportive care through diet or vitamin supplement. Children with moderate to severe anemia may need an RBC transfusion to restore blood volume. For specific types of anemia such as decreased production of RBCs, hematopoietic growth factors may prove beneficial in decreasing the need for blood transfusions.

Education/Discharge Instructions

Important home care instructions from the nurse are necessary for children with anemia to prevent complications that may occur. The teaching required for a child with a chronic illness is more extensive than for the child who has an acute self-limiting episode of anemia. The family must be made aware of the clinical signs and symptoms that may indicate anemia. The nurse teaches the family that alterations in daily activities may be necessary such as quiet play, allowing for periods of rest, and a diet high in iron. The caretaker must be able to identify signs and symptoms of anemia in the home setting such as pallor, fatigue, dizziness, and lethargy. Additional teaching must be completed on how to administer iron supplements if necessary for the child's treatment plan. The child with anemia may also need to have laboratory tests and medical exams periodically to evaluate the status of the anemia.

IRON-DEFICIENCY ANEMIA

The most prevalent nutritional disorder worldwide is iron-deficiency anemia. According to the World Health Organization (2013), approximately 30% of the population is affected with iron-deficiency anemia. Iron-deficiency anemia is defined as a microcytic, hypochromic anemia caused by an inadequate supply of iron (Goldman & Schafer, 2012). Iron is essential for the production of hemoglobin. When iron stores are inadequate, the production of hemoglobin is diminished. As a result of the decrease in hemoglobin, there is a decreased oxygen-carrying capacity of the blood. Iron-deficiency anemia is more common in infants. Premature infants are at a high risk because of their decreased fetal iron supply.

 ### Where Research and Practice Meet:
Iron-Deficiency Anemia in Infants and Children

In the United States, the incidence of iron-deficiency anemia in infants and children has decreased over the last several decades. Many children affected by this type of anemia live well below poverty level and have some type of racial or ethnic disparities. As of summer 2013, the most recent data by Brotanek and colleagues (2007) revealed that Hispanic toddlers are more likely than Caucasian and black toddlers to have iron-deficiency anemia as a result of the risk factors of being overweight. In addition to racial and ethnic risk factors, the age of the child is also significant; infancy, early childhood (specifically age 1 to 3 years), and adolescence are stages in which the risk factors are increased because of depletion of maternal stores, diet, and rapid growth. Since the 1960s, there has been a steady decline in the prevalence of iron-deficiency anemia related to the increased usage of iron-fortified foods, formulas, and the utilization of the Women, Infants, and Children Program (Turgeon, 2012).

Factors associated with the development of iron-deficiency anemia in infants and children often include:

- Stopping breastfeeding too early
- Giving formula that is non-iron-fortified
- Prolonging bottle-feeding
- Drinking more than 2 cups of cow's milk a day (Children 12 months and older)

 ### *Across Care Settings:* Women, Infants, and Children (WIC) program

Since the implementation of the Women, Infants, and Children (WIC) program, the incidence of iron-deficiency anemia has decreased. According to Oliveira, Frazão, and Smallwood (2010), WIC provides funds for infant formula to approximately 60% of all formula purchased in the United States. The target populations for WIC participants who need supplemental nutrition include:

- Pregnant women (through pregnancy and up to 6 weeks after birth or after pregnancy ends)
- Breastfeeding women (up to infant's first birthday)
- Non-breastfeeding postpartum women (up to 6 months after the birth of an infant or after pregnancy ends)
- Infants (up to the first birthday) and children up to their fifth birthday

---

It is important for the nurse to recognize the presence of iron-deficiency anemia (Box 32-1). Because it has been associated with abnormal infant behavior, growth, and development, it needs to be corrected. Toddlers have picky food preferences that are often low in iron. Adolescents are also vulnerable to iron-deficiency anemia because of rapid growth and sometimes poor eating habits. The pathophysiology of iron-deficiency anemia can be related to various factors such as a decreased supply of iron, impaired absorption of iron, increased demand for iron, or blood loss.

Signs and Symptoms

The signs and symptoms of iron-deficiency anemia vary with the severity of the disorder. If a child has a mild

Box 32-1   Common Causes of Iron-Deficiency Anemia

DECREASED IRON SUPPLY

Inadequate iron supply at birth

Nutrition

- Deficient iron intake
- Excessive milk
- Limited solid foods
- Poor eating habits, vegetarian diet, increased fast foods

INCREASED IRON DEMANDS

Growth

- Low birth weight, twins or multiple births
- Prematurity/infants
- Adolescents
- Pregnancy
- Cyanotic congenital heart diseases (e.g., tetralogy of Fallot)

BLOOD LOSS

Acute

Chronic

Parasite infection

GI tract (the most common site)

INABILITY TO FORM HEMOGLOBIN

Lack of vitamin B_{12} (e.g. pernicious anemia)

Folic acid deficiency

IMPAIRED ABSORPTION

Presence of iron inhibitors

- – Phytates, phosphates, or oxalates
- – Gastric alkalinity
- Malabsorption syndrome (e.g. celiac disease, severe prolonged diarrhea, post-gastrectomy, inflammatory bowel disease)

iron-deficiency anemia, he or she may be asymptomatic. This deficiency may not be apparent until laboratory tests are performed (decreased hemoglobin/hematocrit). For children with moderate to severe iron-deficiency anemia, signs and symptoms include:

- Irritability
- Fatigue
- Delayed motor development
- Tachycardia
- Shortness of breath
- Decreased activity level
- Pale skin
- Conjunctival pallor
- Listlessness
- Systolic heart murmur
- Hepatomegaly

 ### Nursing Insight—*Pica*

Pica, the eating of items of non-nutritive value such as starch, clay, ice, or paper (Nathan et al., 2009) may also be associated with iron-deficiency anemia. Iron deficiency, alone or with anemia, may result in impairment of cognitive skills that may not be reversible.

Diagnosis

Diagnosis of iron-deficiency anemia is based on patient history and physical examination findings. Laboratory tests that are frequently performed include those that quantify or describe hemoglobin, iron concentration, and morphological changes in the RBC.

Prevention

Collaborative Care

Nursing Care. Stress to parents that prevention is the key to avoiding iron-deficiency anemia. Parents can ensure that their children eat iron-rich foods such as beans, meat, fortified cereals, eggs, and green leafy vegetables. If oral iron supplements are prescribed, the nurse will teach parents how to properly administer them to the child.

Medical Care. Early identification and recognition of iron-deficiency anemia is essential. Many instances of iron-deficiency anemia can be avoided with the appropriate food selections. The dietitian provides nutritional counseling and assists with obtaining recommended iron-fortified formula and cereal.

Oral iron supplements may be prescribed if dietary treatment is not successful. The recommended dosage of elemental iron is 3 mg/kg per day based on body weight in 1 to 2 divided doses. The severity of the anemia dictates the monitoring frequency of laboratory testing and follow-up with the health-care provider. Several days after initiating iron replacement therapy, the reticulocyte count will rise, which is an indicator of RBC production. Children who are compliant with oral iron replacement therapy usually have a clinical response to the iron supplement therapy within 1 to 2 weeks. The health-care provider communicates to the parents the importance of compliance with iron administration and of follow-up visits to monitor hemoglobin, hematocrit, and reticulocyte count (Speller-Brown et al., 2011).

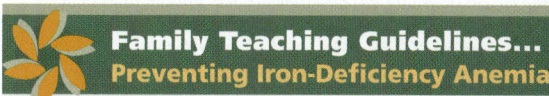

Family Teaching Guidelines...
Preventing Iron-Deficiency Anemia

TOPIC: Tell parents to prevent iron-deficient anemia:

- "Feed your infant breast milk or commercial infant formula recommended for the first 12 months of life."
- "Are you aware of community resources such as WIC to provide assistance with formula and iron-fortified foods?"
- "Be sure to use iron-fortified cereal from 6 to 12 months of age."
- "Do not feed your infant cow's milk before 12 months of age because it does not contain iron and essential nutrients. After 12 months of age, limit the amount of cow's milk to 18 to 24 ounces per day."
- "Offering solids before giving the bottle helps prevent iron deficiency."
- "Tell adolescents on a vegetarian diet or weight reduction diet to understand proper dietary alternatives. Red meats, beans, whole grains, nuts, and iron-fortified cereals are good sources of iron."

Education/Discharge Instructions

 Critical Nursing Action Education About Oral Iron

Educating parents on the proper administration of oral iron is a vital nursing responsibility. The iron supplement needs to be taken between meals because absorption is improved in an acidic environment. Administering this medication with a glass of orange juice may also enhance absorption. Iron supplements should not be taken with tea or dairy products because they may adversely affect the absorption process. Inform parents that liquid iron preparations may stain teeth so it is important to administer the medication with a dropper or drink it through a straw. Encourage the child to rinse his or her mouth after taking this liquid medication.

- Inform parents that iron can be constipating and it is necessary to increase the fiber and water intake to prevent this possible complication.
- Inform parents that possible side effects of iron therapy include gastric upset, nausea, vomiting, and constipation. Black, tarry stools are a common finding and are normal for children taking iron supplements.
- Inform parents to keep no more than a 1-month supply in the home and to store it out of reach of small children because ingestion of excessive quantities may be toxic or even fatal (Speller-Brown et al., 2011).

 focus on safety

An overweight child diagnosed with iron-deficiency anemia

The clinic nurse is vigilant for overweight infants who may have iron-deficiency anemia. While most infants diagnosed with iron-deficiency anemia are underweight, do not be misled. Infants who are overweight may also have this disorder. Many of these infants are overweight because of excessive milk ingestion, known as "milk baby." These infants are chunky, pale, and have a "porcelain-like" appearance. Other clinical features of these "milk babies" include poor muscle development and they are susceptible to infections. It is essential to obtain a comprehensive nutritional history from the parents.

 Global Health Case Study Iron-Deficiency Anemia

Jean is a 9-month-old immigrant from Haiti to the United States who is visiting a health-care provider at the Head Start clinic. During the initial history, his 18-year-old mother reports that she just immigrated to the United States and has never brought her child to a health-care provider. She has limited resources including transportation; she is living with extended family members in crowded living quarters. The nursing assessment reveals the infant has pallor to the hands, feet, and lips and is lethargic. The mother reports that Jean "drinks lots of milk," and states, "I give him milk whenever he cries." She also informs you that she has been feeding him the milk "all the kids drink in the household." She has tried some baby food but has no money to purchase it regularly." After a blood draw, the nurse notes that his laboratory results are hemoglobin 8.8 and hematocrit 26.3. Jean's vital signs include an axillary temperature of 97.6°F (36.4°C), a heart rate of 166 beats per minute,

respiratory rate of 32 breaths per minute, and blood pressure of 92/45.

critical thinking questions

1. From a nursing perspective what is your primary concern?

2. What community resource can you suggest to Jean's mother?

◆ See Suggested Answers to Global Health Case Studies on Davis*Plus*.

SICKLE CELL DISEASE

One of the most common genetic hematological conditions present in children is sickle cell disease (SCD). This disorder is transmitted via an autosomal recessive pattern of inheritance. Both parents of the child must have the sickle cell gene for the child to have SCD. The primary defect in this type of genetic disease is that the globin chain in normal hemoglobin A (HbA) is partially or completely replaced by hemoglobin S (HbS). HbS has a substitution of the amino acid valine for glutamine, which is more sensitive to the changes in the oxygen concentration in the blood. When a patient has a large amount of HbS and a decrease in oxygen levels, these abnormal hemoglobins clump together within the cell and change the shape from donut-like to a sickled shape (Hillman, Ault, Leporrier, & Rinder, 2011). The two most significant pathophysiological features of this disease include tissue ischemia as a result of the occlusions and the inherited fragility of the sickled cells (Fig. 32-2). Once RBCs sickle, they are more fragile and easily destroyed. The surfaces of these sickled cells are also sticky and adhere to the blood vessel walls. The shape of the sickled cell does not promote good oxygenation or movement throughout the circulatory system, hence clinical symptomatology results. If the RBCs cannot circulate through the vascular system and there are occlusions, hypoxemia may result that could lead to ischemia, infarcts, and possible tissue death (Turgeon, 2012). The average life span of a sickled RBC is approximately 8 to 21 days (Nathan et al., 2009). As a result of the shortened life span of the RBCs, children with SCD have an increased amount of hemolysis as evidenced by their chronic anemia.

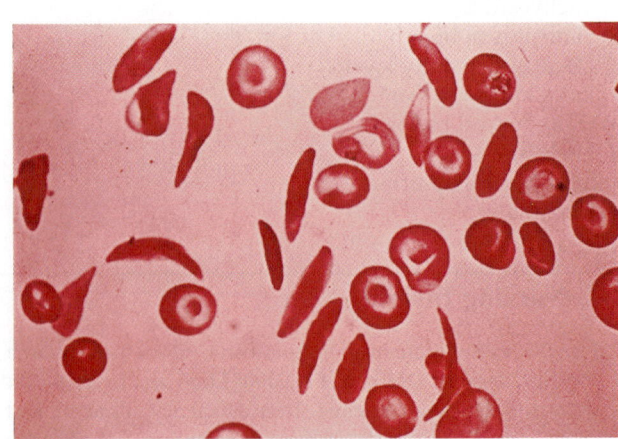

Figure 32–2 In sickle cell disease, the shape of the cell changes from a donut shape to a sickled shape.

Nursing Insight—*Complications*

Complications related to occlusion of blood vessels include splenic sequestration, functional asplenia, avascular necrosis of the femoral head, leg ulcers, hand-foot syndrome (dactylitis), and chronic organ damage. Additional complications secondary to hemolysis include anemia, cholelithiasis (gallstones), jaundice, and retarded growth and sexual maturation. The most severe complications are the occurrence of acute chest syndrome, priapism (painful and continuous erection of the penis), splenic sequestration (separation), and a cerebrovascular accident (CVA). These conditions are medical emergencies and treatment must be obtained immediately to prevent permanent disability or a life-threatening event (Hillman et al., 2011).

 Nursing Insight—*Inheritance*

Consistent with the genetic pattern of inheritance, hemoglobin genes come from both parents. If one parent has SCD and the other parent does not, the child has only the sickle cell trait. If one parent has SCD and the other has sickle cell trait, there is a 50% probability (1 out of 2) that the child will have either the SCD or the sickle cell trait. When both parents have sickle cell trait, they have a 25% probability (1 out of 4) of having a child with SCD or who will become a carrier of the disease (Fig. 32-3).

 Cultural Diversity: Sickle Cell Disease

Approximately 8% of the African American population in the United States is a carrier of sickle cell trait (Speller-Brown et al., 2011). Children affected by this condition are usually of African American or Mediterranean descent. Although rare, this genetic disorder may be seen in other populations such as those of Caribbean, South and Central American, Arab, and East Indian ancestry (Turgeon, 2012).

Patients with sickle cell trait have the heterozygous form of the disease. They usually are asymptomatic because they possess one sickle and one normal gene. The child with the trait may be affected only in certain situations such as high altitudes, periods of extreme stress such as dehydration, and females later in life during pregnancy. Children with SCD have the homozygous form of the disorder, indicating that both genes are abnormal (Turgeon, 2012).

Signs and Symptoms

Because SCD is a blood disorder, all organs of the body may be affected. The symptom that is most evident in a child with sickle cell anemia is the result of the vaso-occlusion of the blood vessels from the sickled red blood cells and hemolysis, which causes pain. The pain can be found anywhere in the body. Infants less than 6 months of age are often asymptomatic. According to Speller-Brown and colleagues (2011), other symptoms seen in children with SCD are:

- Weakness
- Pallor
- Fatigue
- Tissue hypoxia
- Jaundice as a result of RBC hemolysis

  Resulting conditions include:

- Chronic hemolytic anemia
- Increased susceptibility to infections
- Hand-foot syndrome (dactylitis)
- Enuresis and nocturia
- Stroke
- Avascular necrosis of the shoulder or hip
- Acute chest syndrome (severe pneumonia)
- Priapism
- Cholelithiasis
- Leg ulcers
- Delayed physical growth and sexual maturation

Diagnosis

Accurate assessment and diagnosis are essential for appropriate treatment. In utero, chorionic villus biopsy is done on the fetus when both parents are aware they carry the sickle cell trait. This testing allows infants to be identified early to elicit the appropriate diagnosis and prophylactic. Newborn screening is a standard in all 50 states. However, recognize that all parents may not be aware of their newborn screening results. In addition, children born outside the United States may not have received any screening tests at birth.

The newborn screening serves as only a screening tool and not a definitive diagnosis. Toddlers and preschool children who visit the health-care provider with nonspecific symptoms and are anemic undergo a thorough history and physical. If the etiology of the anemia is undetermined, a screening for SCD is indicated.

Diagnostic tests often used to diagnose SCD or the trait include thin-layer isoelectric focusing (IEF), high performance

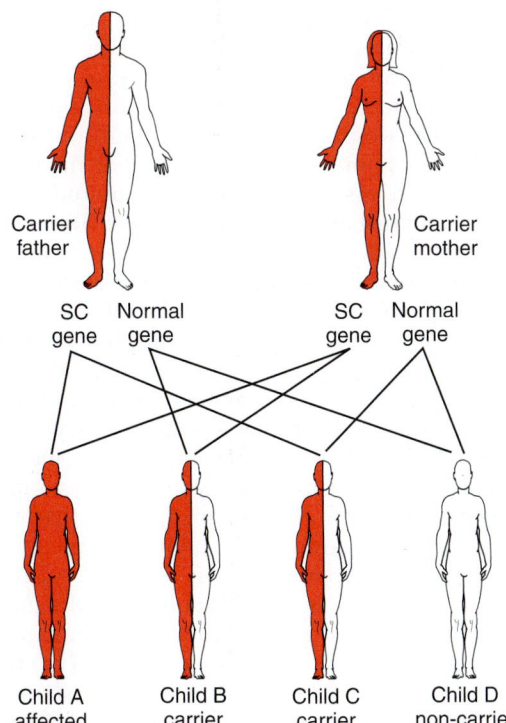

Carrier father   Carrier mother

SC gene   Normal gene   SC gene   Normal gene

Child A affected   Child B carrier   Child C carrier   Child D non-carrier

Figure 32–3 Pattern of inheritance of sickle cell disease.

liquid chromatography (HPLC), and hemoglobin electrophoresis (Turgeon, 2012). The hemoglobin electrophoresis assay separates the various types of hemoglobin and quantifies the percentage of various hemoglobins present. Laboratory tests including a CBC and reticulocyte count are also necessary. Expected laboratory findings for SCD are decreased hemoglobin and hematocrit and an elevated reticulocyte count.

Diagnostic Tools Further Testing for Infants Suspected of Having Sickle Cell Disease

When SCD is suspected, infants will require further testing, such as an IEF, HPLC, or a hemoglobin electrophoresis. A hemoglobin electrophoresis is a more specific blood test that identifies SCD versus sickle cell trait in a child (Turgeon, 2012).

Prevention

Sickle cell disease is a genetically transmitted disease that may affect every organ of the body. Raising awareness is paramount in preventing the transmission of this chronic, lifelong disease. Genetic counseling and follow-up of genetic screening at birth may assist parents in being aware of susceptibility and proper care of a child with SCD. Family members who are carriers of the sickle cell trait should take necessary precautions when planning pregnancies and participating in high-risk behaviors such as becoming dehydrated with excessive physical activity, high altitudes, and/or the need for anesthetics or surgical procedures.

Collaborative Care

Nursing Care. The nurse provides supportive and specific care based on the type of crisis present. Nursing care focuses on rest, hydration, pain control, and adequate oxygenation.

When providing nursing care to patients with sickle cell crisis, attempts are made to coordinate nursing care to allow adequate rest periods and to minimize unnecessary interruptions. Nursing care includes administering and monitoring adequate hydration (oral or IV).

Another essential nursing care measure is monitoring respiratory status and oxygenation of sickle cell patients. The child with sickle cell crisis may be at risk for an acute pulmonary event that may be a result of the disease itself or the use of opiates. A complete respiratory assessment includes signs and symptoms of respiratory distress, including auscultation of lung sounds to detect decreased and abnormal breath sounds, respiratory effort and quality, continuous monitoring of oxygen saturations, color and perfusion, and any necessary laboratory or radiographic studies. If abnormal findings are present, the nurse immediately informs the health-care provider so treatment can begin. For example, if the patient's oxygen saturation is consistently less than 90% on room air, supplemental oxygen is indicated. Pneumonia and pulmonary infarcts occur more often in this patient population.

Assessment Tool Pain Assessment

Pain assessment is documented for all patients. The use of a standardized pain assessment tool provides more accurate assessment data. A developmentally appropriate pain assessment tool also must be used for all patients in health-care settings. Pain assessment tools are used to assess the pain on admission, reassess pain, and determine treatment effectiveness. The Joint Commission's National Patient Safety Goals recommends pain assessment as the fifth vital sign.

A complete nursing history is obtained to determine what pain measures have worked for the child in the past. Pain control can be pharmacological or nonpharmacological. A combination of both is preferred.

Nursing Insight—*Bone marrow transplant*

A treatment modality to cure sickle cell patients with numerous complications is a bone marrow transplant. However, this treatment is not without risks, and most patients are not able to find a compatible donor match.

Complementary Care: *Nonpharmacological Pain Interventions*

In addition to administering medications for pain control, the use of nonpharmacological interventions has proven to be beneficial for many patients experiencing painful episodes from a sickle cell crisis. This may include distraction, guided imagery, relaxation techniques, music therapy, comfort care, cutaneous stimulation, and play therapy. If available, a child life specialist or other interdisciplinary team member can be consulted to assist in providing nonpharmacological interventions.

Medical Care. Treatment for SCD is the early identification and treatment of hypoxic episodes. Hydration is essential. The fluid requirement recommendations are 1.5 times above the child's normal calculated requirements. Adequate hydration promotes dilution and diminishes the possibility of hypoxic episodes. In addition to hydration, pain management is essential to adequately treat a painful vaso-occlusive crisis.

At home, the initial management consists of oral pain medication consisting of acetaminophen (Children's Tylenol), ibuprofen (Children's Advil), or acetaminophen with codeine (Children's Tylenol-Codeine) for mild to moderate pain. If the child continues to have pain, hospitalization may be required. For the hospitalized child with vaso-occlusive crisis, opioids such as immediate and sustained release morphine (Duramorph), oxycodone (OxyContin), hydromorphone (Dilaudid), or methadone (Methadose) may be administered around the clock. Morphine (Duramorph) is often considered the drug of choice. It may be administered by patient-controlled analgesia (PCA) (Hillman et al., 2011). Meperidine (Demerol) is sometimes avoided because of the possible central nervous system toxicity (Speller-Brown et al., 2011). PCA is an appropriate method of pain management for children who are able to manage their own pain relief. Another medication that may be used for painful crises and does not have the common side effects of the opiate drugs is ketorolac (Toradol). Ketorolac (Toradol) is a parenteral anti-inflammatory drug that has been found to be effective in reducing pain associated with a vaso-occlusive crisis. The recommended duration of ketorolac (Toradol) should not exceed 5 days because of the increased risk of gastritis and gastrointestinal bleeding.

Medication: Toradol (Ketorolac)

(tor-ah-dal) (Kee-**toe**-role-ak)

Indications: Short-term (less than 5 days) management of moderate to severe pain, including postoperative pain

Actions: Inhibits prostaglandin synthesis by decreasing activity of the enzyme cyclooxygenase, which results in a decrease of prostaglandin precursors

Therapeutic Effects: Pain relief

Route and Dosage:
Manufacturer's recommendations:
Single dose treatment
IM: 1 mg/kg as a single dose
Maximum dose: 30 mg
IV: 0.5 mg/kg as a single dose
Maximum dose: 15 mg
Multiple-dose treatment:
IM OR IV: 0.5 mg/kg every 6 hours. Do not exceed 5 days of treatment.
Oral dose:
Initial dose: 20 mg
Maintenance dose: 10 mg every 4 to 6 hours
Maximum dose: 40 mg/day
(Dosage information retrieved from http//www.drugs.com, 2013)

Contraindications and Precautions:
CONTRAINDICATED IN: Hypersensitivity to Toradol, acetylsalicylic acid (Children's Aspirin), or other nonsteroidal anti-inflammatory drugs (NSAIDs); patients with peptic ulcer disease or anyone with bleeding tendencies

Adverse Reactions and Side Effects: Dizziness, headache, rash, diarrhea, gastrointestinal (GI) pain, bleeding, prolonged bleeding times, anaphylaxis, hypersensitivity reactions

Nursing Implications:
1. Instruct the patient and parents on medication administration.
2. Do not exceed 5 days of total use.
3. May cause drowsiness and impair ability to perform activities requiring mental alertness.

Source: Vallerand & Sanoski (2014).

focus on safety

Hypertransfusion therapy

Children who have experienced numerous hospitalizations, CVA, or acute chest syndromes may be candidates for hypertransfusion therapy. These patients receive blood transfusions every 3 to 4 weeks to increase their amount of hemoglobin A. This treatment regimen is not without potential risks, which may include the transmission of various infectious diseases, an acute transfusion reaction, or iron overload from multiple blood transfusions. When blood transfusions are administered, often the quantity of the iron contained in the blood transfusion is greater than the body's ability to excrete, resulting in an iron overload. Iron overload occurs frequently because each unit of blood provides approximately 200 to 250 mg of elemental iron (Bryant & Norville, 2011). Sickle cell patients receiving hypertransfusion regimens are also advised to receive chelation therapy to prevent organ damage from iron accumulation. Treatment with chelation therapy for iron overload must be considered when a serum ferritin level is greater than 1,000 mcg/L (Hillman et al., 2011). Several chelating agents are available for prevention and treatment of iron overload.

focus on safety

When a child is asplenic

A child with a temperature greater than 101.5°F (38.6°C) requires immediate medical attention because most children with SCD are "functionally asplenic." When a child is asplenic, he or she does not have the ability to filter certain encapsulated bacteria. This allows the bacteria to multiply within the bloodstream, causing a low-grade bacterial infection or serious sepsis. Children with SCD generally are asplenic by the age of 3 to 5 years. The major cause of death in children with SCD who are less than 5 years old is overwhelming infection because of *Streptococcus pneumoniae, Haemophilus influenzae* type b, and *Neisseria meningitidis* (Nathan et al., 2009). If a child with SCD has a fever, immediate treatment involves blood cultures and the implementation of parenteral broad-spectrum antibiotics. Children with SCD often receive prophylactic oral penicillin at home to prevent overwhelming sepsis. The nurse knows that this critical information is necessary for parents to ensure the child receives the pneumococcal and *H influenzae* type b vaccine and other routine vaccinations.

Education/Discharge Instructions

Across Care Settings: Education about SCD

Children and families affected by SCD must learn to cope with a lifelong chronic illness. Families must be knowledgeable of the signs and symptoms of sickle cell crisis so they can report them to their primary health-care provider. The community-based nurse can educate the family about the goals of ongoing care including the prevention of complications associated with infections, hypoxemia, and vaso-occlusive crisis. Ensure that parents understand that strenuous activities may precipitate dehydration resulting in hypoxia; these activities should be avoided. Parents should also be knowledgeable about possible complications such as management of pain and fever, splenic sequestration, priapism, acute chest syndrome, and stroke. All of these complications could result in permanent disability or death.

Teach parents how to avoid a sickle cell crisis by providing rest and adequate hydration. Patients with SCD are on prophylactic penicillin to prevent overwhelming sepsis and supplemental folic acid to assist with red blood cell production. Adherence to these medications is critical in preventing complications associated with this disease. In addition to scheduled medications, all required immunizations should be administered per AAP guidelines. Parents must be aware that preventable illnesses have the potential to be life threatening for a patient who is asplenic.

In the event a patient experiences a mild sickle cell crisis at home, instruct him or her to stop what he or she is doing, rest, drink fluids, and take the prescribed pain medication. If improvement is not observed, notify the physician and anticipate the need for the patient to see a health-care provider or to go to the nearest emergency facility for additional treatment.

Nursing Diagnoses Sickle Cell Disease

- Knowledge deficit related to home care related to the disease process
- Pain related to tissue hypoxia secondary to vaso-occlusive crisis

- Alteration in tissue perfusion related to anemia
- Activity intolerance related to anemia
- Risk for injury related to anemia
- Altered family process related to hospitalization
- Ineffective coping related to chronic illness
- Fluid volume deficit related to decreased fluid intake and the kidney's ability to concentrate urine
- Risk for infection related to limited splenic filtering abilities

 Case Study Sickle Cell Disease

Michael is a 12-year-old boy with a history of SCD. He also has a history of numerous admissions to the hospital for pain crisis and has been on hypertransfusion therapy for approximately 3 years. Today, in the emergency department, Michael complains of pain in his chest (on visual numeric scale 8 out of 10 reported) and fever. Objective findings on the physical assessment include bilateral breath sounds with rhonchi and an audible moist cough, sclera noted to be slightly jaundiced, and all other findings within normal limits. His oxygen saturation is 87% on room air. Michael's vital signs are the following: heart rate, 121 beats per minute; respiratory rate, 28 breaths per minute; temperature, 101.5°F (38.6°C) orally; and blood pressure on the left upper extremity, 139/96. Complete blood count with WBC = 25, Hgb = 6.8, Hct = 20.2, and platelet count is normal. The reticulocyte count = 6.8%.

critical thinking questions

1. In addition to respiratory status, what are the other concerns?

2. What are important nursing interventions?

3. What information will the nurse teach the parents?

◆ See Suggested Answers to Case Studies on Davis*Plus*.

THALASSEMIA

The word "thalassemia" originates from the Greek word "thalassa" meaning "the sea" because the first cases identified were in children of Mediterranean descent. Thalassemia is an inherited autosomal recessive condition that results in a deficiency of the alpha or beta globin protein needed for the production of hemoglobin. Beta-thalassemia is the most common inherited genetic disorder in the world (Turgeon, 2012). There are three forms of beta-thalassemia:

- Thalassemia minor (or thalassemia trait) is asymptomatic or with mild microcytic anemia.
- Thalassemia intermedia is similar in signs and symptoms similar to splenomegaly (enlarged spleen) with severe anemia.
- Thalassemia major is the most severe form, also known as Cooley's anemia.
  (Hillman et al., 2011)

In addition to beta-thalassemia, there is alpha-thalassemia, which occurs when the alpha-chain is affected. These patients are sometimes mistakenly diagnosed with iron-deficiency anemia. The severity of alpha-thalassemia is based on the number of alpha genes affected. If the patient has 1 or 2 missing alpha genes, he or she is most likely asymptomatic or has a mild anemia. A patient missing 3 alpha genes is classified as having Hgb H disease, which is characterized by an excess of beta-chains, resulting from minimal production of

alpha-chains in the bone marrow and development of hemoglobin H as a result (Turgeon, 2012).

Signs and Symptoms

Children with beta-thalassemia who are symptomatic have:

- An enlarged liver and spleen
- Mild jaundice
- Growth retardation
- Moderate to severe anemia
- Increased risk of infections secondary to splenomegaly or splenectomy

 Nursing Insight—*Red blood cells*

Children with beta-thalassemia experience diminished erythropoiesis (less production of RBCs), in which the body attempts to increase RBC production to compensate for the anemia (Turgeon, 2012). When the hemoglobin level declines and severe anemia is present, bones that normally do not produce RBCs take on this function. As a result, there may be bony deformities such as frontal bossing or maxillary prominence from the excess cell production. These children also have an increased susceptibility to infection secondary to their nonfunctioning spleen.

Diagnosis

A thorough history and physical examination are necessary for diagnosis. Frequently performed laboratory tests include those that quantify or describe hemoglobin such as a CBC with red cell indices. Laboratory studies often reveal decreased hemoglobin and hematocrit, hypochromia, microcytosis, low mean corpuscular volume (MCV), and increased reticulocyte count (Turgeon, 2012).

Prevention

Thalassemia is a chronic, lifelong illness that requires adherence with all special aspects of care to ensure optimal quality of life. Most patients with beta-thalassemia will require blood transfusion therapy for life or a bone marrow transplant, which is curative. Patients receiving chronic transfusion therapy may experience iron overload requiring chelation therapy to prevent additional complications, such as multiorgan failure. Thalassemia is transmitted genetically, therefore genetic counseling is strongly recommended to prevent disease transmission.

Collaborative Care

Nursing Care. Children with beta-thalassemia are dependent on transfusions to maintain their hemoglobin to improve the quality of their life. The blood transfusions prevent extramedullary hematopoiesis, promote growth

Labs: Hemoglobin Electrophoresis

Hemoglobin electrophoresis can distinguish the type and severity of the thalassemia. Electrophoresis separates hemoglobin variants based on molecular charge. Hemoglobin is then described in order of relative abundance, detecting normal or abnormal cells (Van Leeuwen et al., 2011). Based on the results of the hemoglobin electrophoresis, a referral to a hematologist may be warranted for further evaluation.

and development, and reduce infections. The goal of nursing care for children with beta-thalassemia major (Cooley's anemia) is to prevent hypoxia by providing blood transfusion therapy usually every 3 to 4 weeks for the child's lifetime (Hillman et al., 2011).

Children with beta-thalassemia may experience numerous complications related to their disease and/or to the treatment of their disease. As a result of chronic transfusion therapy, these children are at high risk for developing hemosiderosis. Hemosiderosis is the accumulation of iron in the organs of the body.

Children with beta-thalassemia (Cooley's anemia) may be cured of their disorder with a bone marrow transplant (Hillman et al., 2011). Finding a suitable match may pose a challenge because of the limited donors available. Younger children often fare significantly better than older children who are treated with bone marrow transplant, primarily because their organs have not sustained substantial damage from the chronic transfusion therapy that may have caused iron overload.

focus on safety

Accumulation of iron (hemosiderosis)

As a result of the chronic blood transfusion therapy, in which each unit contains approximately 200 mg of iron, iron may accumulate in the body. The body does not have a mechanism to remove the iron. Excess iron is stored in the tissues and organs (hemosiderosis). Hemosiderosis must be treated to prevent toxic levels of iron in the body and possible death. Iron may be removed from the body by using drugs called chelating agents that bind with the iron and allow for excretion through the urine and stool. Chelating agents include deferasirox (Exjade) and deferoxamine B (Desferal). The patient's clinical condition often determines which chelating agent will produce the best outcome. Other factors that influence chelating selection include the route of administration, cost, and severity of iron overload.(Hillman et al., 2011). Several chelating agents are available for prevention and treatment of iron overload.

Comparison of Exjade and Desferal	deferoxamine B (Desferal)	deferasirox (Exjade)
Route of administration	Parenteral, usually subcutaneously or IV	Oral
Plasma half-life	Short (minutes), requires constant delivery	Long (8–16 hr) Remains in plasma for 24 hours
Therapeutic index	High at moderate doses	High in iron-overloaded patients
Annual cost ($)	10,000–25,000	24,000–58,000

Deferoxamine B (Desferal) is rapidly excreted in the urine. It must be administered IV or subcutaneously over a period of 8 to 10 hours, usually at bedtime, at least 5 days a week. Most parents can be taught how to insert the butterfly catheter and administer the drug via an infusion pump at home without difficulties. The treatment process with deferoxamine B (Desferal) may become burdensome and expensive, and the issue of adherence is quite often a concern for health-care professionals. Routine monitoring of iron levels is indicated for patients on chelation therapy to evaluate compliance and effectiveness of treatment. Patients at risk for hemosiderosis are evaluated for long-term complications. Complications that may occur are a result of iron deposits that may damage vital organs causing hearing loss, diabetes, organ failure, and ultimately, death.

Education/Discharge Instructions

Patients with this chronic hematological disorder require supportive care and teaching by the nurse. The nurse addresses the importance of blood transfusion therapy and chelation to ensure adherence with the treatment regimen to promote quality of life. Teach the family the appropriate technique for administration of the chelation therapy. Other teaching aspects include meticulous hand washing because these children are often asplenic, which increases their susceptibility to infection. Be sure to alert parents to seek medical attention if the child develops a temperature of 101.5°F (38.6°C). If the child has a fever, inform the parents that antibiotic prophylaxis may be indicated. Also, instruct the family on the importance of genetic counseling and referrals to community resources for support.

HEREDITARY SPHEROCYTOSIS

Hereditary spherocytosis (HS) is a hemolytic anemia acquired via autosomal-dominant inheritance and is caused by an abnormal RBC membrane. In most cases, there is a defect of the red cell skeletal protein called spectrin, or it may also include the proteins involved in the attachment of the spectrin to the membrane (Hillman et al., 2011). The severity of the disease is directly contingent on the amount of the spectrin deficiency.

The cellular defect results in an abnormal RBC membrane. The malformed cell membrane has a smaller surface area in relation to a normal RBC and an alteration in the actual shape of the cell from donut-like to that of a spherocyte. The new shape makes it difficult for the RBCs to circulate through the body, particularly to the spleen, which leads to sequestered cells and early destruction (Turgeon, 2012). HS does not involve an abnormality of the hemoglobin. Rather it is an inherited disorder that actually transforms the configuration of the red cell membrane (Turgeon, 2012).

Signs and Symptoms

Signs and symptoms of HS include:

- Hyperbilirubinemia
- Jaundice
- Anemia
- Splenomegaly or splenectomy

Some children acquire this condition later in life with anemia, jaundice, splenomegaly, or with an aplastic crisis often linked to a viral infection. The anemia may range from mild to severe based on the extent of compensation by the body.

Diagnosis

The diagnostic work-up for HS includes a thorough history and physical examination. A CBC is collected, and laboratory tests often reveal a low hemoglobin level between 7 and 10 g/dL and a negative Coombs test. The peripheral smear reveals small, dense, spherical red cells. The MCV is usually normal, and there is increased red cell osmotic fragility, which is a measure of the lysis of spherocytes.

Prevention

HS is a genetically transmitted condition; therefore, the primary strategy for prevention is genetic counseling to decrease the possible transmission of this blood disorder. Some children with moderate to severe HS may require a splenectomy. Nurses must educate patients and families about the role of the spleen in preventing infections and how those with HS may be more susceptible to various infections. Patients should adhere to prophylactic antibiotics and immunization schedules to prevent overwhelming infections. In addition, meticulous hand washing and following the principles of preventing infections must be included as part of the patient's plan of care.

Collaborative Care

Nursing Care. Children with HS generally are not hospitalized unless they experience a severe crisis requiring a blood transfusion and supportive care. Prior to administering a blood product, most institutions require that informed consent be obtained. Give parents oral or written information on the risks and benefits, possible adverse reactions, and the overall information about the transfusion process. Be sure to follow the institution's policies and procedures when administering blood to ensure patient safety. Blood counts, including a CBC, are obtained post-transfusion to determine if treatment was effective and to provide additional supportive care if indicated.

Medical Care. Children with severe hemolysis may require folic acid supplementation (Speller-Brown et al., 2011). Folic acid supplementation is recommended to stimulate the production of red blood cells and protein synthesis. During severe crisis, hospitalization may be required for supportive care and blood product transfusions.

Critical Nursing Action Pneumococcal and Haemophilus Influenzae Type b (Hib) Vaccine

Children with hereditary spherocytosis (HS) should receive the pneumococcal and *Haemophilus influenzae* type b (Hib) vaccine before the splenectomy to prevent life-threatening bacterial infections. Children can also be given prophylactic penicillin to prevent fatal infections.

Surgical Care. Children who have less than 80% of normal spectrin content are candidates for a splenectomy. The splenectomy eliminates the anemia and is reserved for children with moderate to severe cases of HS. After a splenectomy, the spherocytosis of the RBCs continues, although the cells no longer become sequestered in the spleen. The red cell survival improves to near normal. Postoperative care includes the following:

- Monitoring vital signs as per institution policy for postoperative care until the child's condition is stable
- Administering IV fluids, pain medications, and antibiotics if ordered
- Assessing the surgical site for the signs and symptoms of bleeding or infection
- Monitoring intake and output

Education/Discharge Instructions

Patients with hereditary spherocytosis must be educated on supportive care measures and include teaching parents of children with severe hemolysis of HS about the folic acid supplementation regimen. Educate parents to pay careful attention to infection control principles for a child who has

undergone a splenectomy; all patients who have had a splenectomy must have antibiotic prophylaxis and receive appropriate immunizations. Promote meticulous hand washing by all who are in contact with these patients because they have increased susceptibility to infection. Instruct parents on the proper method for taking a temperature. Inform parents to seek medical attention immediately if the child develops a temperature of 101.5°F (38.6°C). Remind parents that routine visits to their health-care provider must be scheduled to evaluate blood counts and the need for immunizations. Provide support to the child and family to help them cope with this lifelong illness. Encourage the family to use community resources for psychosocial support.

HEMOPHILIA

The most common group of hereditary bleeding disorders, hemophilia is caused by a deficiency or absence of factor VIII (hemophilia A) or factory IX (hemophilia B) and plasma proteins required for normal blood clotting. This group of bleeding disorders is inherited sex-linked recessive. The mother is the carrier of the X-linked deficiency, and the sons are those affected with the disorder (Munn & Valdiviez, 2011).

In children with hemophilia, the coagulation process cannot be completed, so bleeding is prolonged. A common misconception is that bleeding is faster in these patients, but this is not the case. The prolonged bleeding is what causes the clinical manifestations to be evident. The child with a greater degree of factor deficiency experiences more bleeding episodes than the child with mild deficiency. Hemophilia A is classified as mild, moderate, or severe based on the degree of deficiency present.

 Cultural Diversity: The Royal Disease

Hemophilia has been present for centuries throughout the world. Often, members of the royal English family married into royalty of other countries. Hemophilia has been referred to as "the royal disease." The marriage of England's Queen Victoria and Prince Albert hallmarked the beginning of hemophilia in the British royal line. Queen Victoria, who had nine children, was a carrier of the hemophilia gene. As a result, hemophilia was transmitted to most of the royal houses of Europe (Stevens, 1999). A specific example of the royal disease is the case of the Czar and Czarina of Russia, Nicholas II and his wife, Alexandra. As a granddaughter of Queen Victoria of England, Alexandra was a carrier of the same genetic mutation that afflicted several of the major European royal houses and passed the disease to her only son, Alexei. Because the family was killed by the Bolsheviks in 1918, it is not known whether any of the couple's four daughters (Olga, Tatiana, Maria, and Anastasia) inherited the gene as carriers as their mother had before them.

Signs and Symptoms

Often a child with hemophilia is diagnosed after presenting with bleeding or there is a known family history of bleeding disorders. Common presenting signs and symptoms include the following:

- Bruising
- Excessive bleeding (circumcision, tooth loss)

- Oozing after a circumcision
- Intracranial hemorrhage in the neonate as a result of childbirth
- Soft tissue bleeding
- Swelling or stiffness of joints, especially the knees
- Decreased range of motion of extremities
- Painful joints
  (Munn & Valdiviez, 2011)

Most children are free of symptoms until they crawl or walk. In infancy, a bleeding disorder may be discovered at the time of circumcision. In older children, excessive bleeding may occur with a tooth extraction or tooth loss. For the child with hemophilia who experiences frequent bleeds in the joints, there may be long-term consequences including mobility limitations, bony changes, and crippling deformities.

 Nursing Insight—*Seeking medical attention*

Children with bleeding disorders often experience hemarthrosis (a bloody effusion within a joint) and soft tissue bleeding (Munn & Valdiviez, 2011). Children who have hemarthrosis often seek medical attention after a minor injury in which there is swelling, or pain in the affected joint.

Diagnosis

For the child who experiences moderate to severe bleeding from minor procedures or bleeding into large joints, diagnostic testing is warranted. Common diagnostic tests may include a prothrombin time (PT) and a partial thromboplastin time (PTT) (Table 32-7). The most important test is the direct assay of plasma factor activity level for hemophilia A and B (Hillman et al., 2011). Based on the type of factor deficiency and the percentage of factor level in the plasma, the diagnosis and the type and the classification of hemophilia are confirmed.

Prevention

Hemophilia is a genetically transmitted condition; therefore, the primary strategy for prevention is genetic counseling to decrease the possible transmission of this blood disorder. Patients with hemophilia require education on how to determine if a bleed is present and methods to treat and prevent further episodes. Strategies to prevent bleeding episodes are essential. Patient must be instructed to avoid aspirin and aspirin-containing products, IM injections, and avoidance of activities that may cause injuries. Safety precautions at home must be reinforced to the family. Patients are taught to use safety equipment such as helmets, car seats, and seat belts to protect the child. In addition, avoidance of common household items such as bunk beds, ladders, and play toys such as skateboards, trampolines, and other high-risk items. Patients that require factor supplementation are instructed on how to properly administer factor products at home safely to prevent injury.

Collaborative Care

Nursing Care.

 Collaboration in Caring—*An interdisciplinary approach*

A collaborative interdisciplinary approach is essential in the care of children with hemophilia. The school nurse and others such as coaches, day-care providers, or team leaders who interface with the child must be aware of the condition and taught about emergency care if needed. Parents must be notified by whoever is working with the child so proper care can be sought.

The nurse initiates prompt treatment of bleeding episodes. The identification of the deficient factor is imperative to administer the proper replacement factors. The number one nursing priority for all patients with bleeding disorders is always patient safety, prevention of additional complications, and promoting wellness and quality of life.

 focus on safety

Hemophilia

The majority of patients with hemophilia can be safely managed at home by informed and educated family members. Depending on the severity of the bleed, such as a bleed into a joint, a head injury, or internal trauma, patients may require close observation and inpatient hospitalization.

Medical Care. Recombinant factor products are the main treatment of hemophilia patients (Munn & Valdiviez, 2011). These manufactured clotting factors are genetically engineered, thus reducing the transmission of various infectious diseases. After years of receiving replacement factor products, some children may develop inhibitors to the specific coagulation proteins. The development of inhibitors poses a unique treatment challenge to manage these patients. Changes or additions to the treatment regimen may be necessary to provide adequate replacement factors.

Table 32-7 Laboratory Tests to Diagnosis Bleeding Disorders		
Test	**Range**	**Significance**
Prothrombin time (PT)	10–14 sec	Measures the extrinsic pathway for bleeding, requires fibrinogen, prothrombin, and factors V, VII, and X. Prolonged times may indicate deficiencies of vitamin K liver factors, malabsorption, and liver disease.
Partial thromboplastin time (PTT)	22–35 sec	Measures the intrinsic pathway for bleeding, requires factors V, VIII, IX, X, XI, and XII and fibrinogen and prothrombin. Prolonged times may indicate a bleeding disorder.

Note: The above reference ranges are taken from a manufacturer or a single institution; check specific institutional guidelines.

Education/Discharge Instructions

For children with severe hemophilia, prophylactic doses of recombinant factor products may be administered in the home setting by caretakers to prevent bleeding episodes. The nurse instructs family members how to administer these factor products by IV access. Older, mature children may assume the responsibility of self-administering factor products at home after instruction has been completed. One of the most important steps toward independence for adolescents with hemophilia is learning how to self-administer medications. Proper administration of factor products at home improves the quality of life, decreases hospitalizations, reduces missed days in school, and prevents long-term complications for children with this chronic illness.

Administration of replacement factor products:

1. Prepare the setting: gather supplies, wash hands, and have environment ready for medication administration
2. Medication preparation: mix the factor concentrate with sterile water per instructions
3. Set up: draw contents of the reconstituted drug into a syringe to be ready to administer IV
4. Prepare child for treatment to be given
5. IV access: insert a butterfly needle into a vein so you can infuse factor medication
6. Injection: infuse the factor concentrate to treat bleeding episode or to administer as prescribed for preventive measures
7. Dispose of sharps and syringe in appropriate containers

 Nursing Diagnoses Bleeding Disorders

- Risk for injury related to bleeding tendencies
- Pain related to bleeding episodes in joints and muscles
- Knowledge deficit related to home care
- Potential for impaired physical mobility related to bleeding in the joints and muscles

VON WILLEBRAND'S DISEASE

One of the most common inherited bleeding disorders is von Willebrand's disease (vWD) (Munn & Valdiviez, 2011), which was first described in 1926 by Eric von Willebrand (Turgeon, 2012). This disorder is transmitted via an autosomal dominant pattern of inheritance, affecting males and females equally. This disease is characterized by a deficiency of von Willebrand factor (vWF) and has variable clinical manifestations. It plays an important role in the early phase of hemostasis by enhancing platelet aggregation and adhesion. The vWF assists in forming the "platelet plug" to

---

 Family Teaching Guidelines...
The Child With Hemophilia

HOW TO: Teach the Family How to Care for the Child With Hemophilia

Because there is no known cure for hemophilia, the interdisciplinary health-care team members, including physicians, nurses, rehabilitative services, social workers, child life specialists, and school personnel, are instrumental in teaching the family about how to care for their child with hemophilia.

Recommendations for families are to seek health care at a facility with a comprehensive hemophilia care center. If the treatment regimen is followed, these children can live long and productive lives. It is essential that the health-care team members teach the family about the prevention of bleeding to avoid complications. If a bleeding episode occurs, the family is instructed on the proper interventions to take. In the instance that the child has a soft tissue injury or bleeding into a joint, before seeking medical attention the family initiates supportive measures (i.e., application of pressure to bleeding site, ice, elevation, and rest) (Munn & Valdiviez, 2011). Other family teaching tips include:

- Instruct families on the signs and symptoms that require prompt medical attention. Most importantly, any trauma to the head or a change in the level of consciousness is a medical emergency.
- Teach families about the factor replacement products, including how to obtain the product. Often parents are instructed on how to administer prophylactic doses of factor replacement at home.

- Ensure families are aware that safety is of utmost importance. Injury prevention is reviewed at all stages of development because risk factors change based on the child's development and age. Contact sports are highly discouraged. The child is fitted for a safety helmet to prevent head injury when bike riding.
- Explore with families any home environmental factors that may pose a safety risk (e.g., mobility issues, bunk beds, and stairs).
- Inform families that, for children who have experienced bleeding into the joints, physical therapy may be necessary to preserve and maintain functional status. The physical therapist is a key member in the collaboration with the family to provide comprehensive care.
- Ensure children wear a medical alert bracelet in the event that a medical emergency occurs outside the home when his or her caretaker or parent is not present.
- Review with families the purpose of genetic counseling and why it is recommended (Munn & Valdiviez, 2011).
- Collaborate with other health-care professionals such as a nurse case manager or social worker who can assist with insurance issues, help obtain medications and supplies, locate rehabilitation services, coordinate home nursing care, and assist with other concerns. The social worker is also available for emotional and psychosocial support.
- Relay that resources are available at comprehensive hemophilia centers and also online by the National Hemophilia Foundation at www.hemophilia.org.

the damaged endothelium and also acts as a carrier protein for coagulation factor VIII (Hillman et al., 2011).

Signs and Symptoms

When there is a deficiency of vWF, signs and symptoms of prolonged bleeding times may include:

- Epistaxis
- Menorrhagia
- Bleeding from the oral cavity
- Easy bruising
- Excessive bleeding following minor surgery or dental extraction

Diagnosis

Often children are diagnosed with vWD when excessive bleeding is present with a simple tooth loss or a minor procedure such as circumcision. A comprehensive family history is essential. The family history reveals similar bleeding manifestations in other family members because vWD is an inherited bleeding disorder. A complete physical examination is essential to detect clinical abnormalities for bleeding tendencies such as multiple sites of bruising. For a child who is experiencing moderate to severe bleeding, a thorough diagnostic evaluation is warranted. The nurse obtains blood samples for PT, PTT, fibrinogen, thrombin time, platelet function assay, CBC, vWF, and vWF antigen.

Prevention

vWD is a genetically transmitted blood disorder; therefore, the primary strategy for prevention is genetic counseling to reduce the transmission of the disease. The teaching priority for patients with vWD is directed on controlling and preventing bleeding episodes. Patients are instructed on how to administer desmopressin (DDAVP), which is administered at home intranasally. Tell the family to contact the health-care provider if the patient has symptoms of an upper respiratory infection such as a runny nose or congestion; this may decrease the effectiveness of the intranasal DDAVP. Teaching about DDAVP also includes a reduction in fluid intake to prevent overhydration and possible hyponatremia. DDAVP therapy is most effective for patients with mild bleeding episodes. Teach parents to alert the health-care provider if bleeding episodes are not controlled or the patient has complaints of headaches.

Collaborative Care

Nursing Care. For the child identified with an inherited bleeding disorder such as hemophilia or vWD, the health-care provider recommends a medical alert bracelet be worn to alert health-care personnel and others about the child's condition.

Medical Care. Treatment for this disorder includes the administration of DDAVP, a synthetic analog of the antidiuretic hormone vasopressin. This hormone increases the plasma vWF and factor VIII after the administration by releasing vWF from its endothelial cell storage to produce an immediate increase in the plasma levels. This medication improves platelet function and shortens the bleeding time. This treatment method may be effective in correcting the bleeding defect of vWD. In addition to the primary function of DDAVP, there may be secondary stabilization of additional factor VIII. Other treatment modalities of

vWD include the IV administration of Humate-P and/or the administration of cryoprecipitate or fresh frozen plasma (Hillman et al., 2011).

Education/Discharge Instructions

Nursing care includes instructing parents about common sites of bleeding such as the nose, gums, and internal bleeding. Even the smallest nosebleed (Fig. 32-4) can be upsetting to a child and parent. Education can also be focused on controlling the bleeding by applying pressure, applying ice, and seeking medical attention. Educate adolescent females on what constitutes excessively heavy menses. The nurse's teaching also includes tips to avoid an embarrassing moment during periods of heavy menstrual flow, such as wearing two maxi pads and not wearing light-colored pants or skirts. Small children can be instructed to avoid nose picking, vigorous nose blowing, and strenuous activity that may cause a nosebleed. Teach children to sneeze with their mouth open and gently blow the nose if needed. Avoid the use of acetylsalicylic acid (Children's Aspirin) or NSAIDs, which may promote bleeding episodes. Children prone to epistaxis can use cool mist humidification as a preventive measure. Gentle flossing and usage of a soft bristle toothbrush is encouraged.

IMMUNE THROMBOCYTOPENIA

Immune Thrombocytopenia (ITP) is the most frequently occurring thrombocytopenia of childhood. The cause of this hemorrhagic disorder is unknown, although it may be an autoimmune response to a disease-related antigen (Munn & Valdiviez, 2011). The characteristic features include **thrombocytopenia** (an abnormal decrease in the number of blood platelets) and **purpura** (discoloration caused by a hemorrhage beneath the skin).

ITP is a disorder of increased platelet destruction caused by antiplatelet antibodies. These antiplatelet antibodies attach to the child's own platelets, and the body's immune system eliminates the platelets, erroneously identifying them as bacteria. The antibodies responsible for this response are glycoprotein anti-IIb and IIIa and are identified in children diagnosed with ITP (Munn & Valdiviez, 2011). ITP is classified by duration; lasting a few months to a year

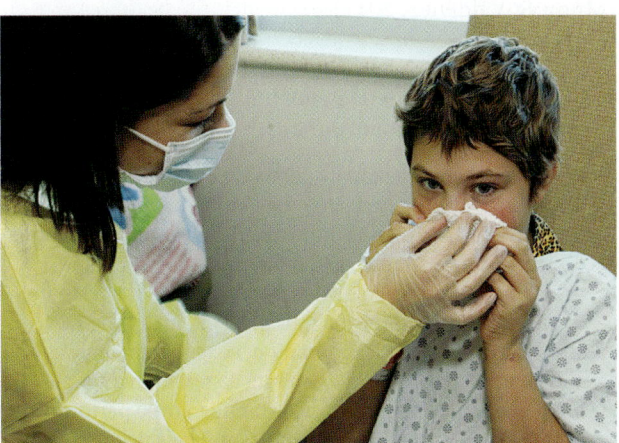

Figure 32–4 When a nosebleed occurs, the nurse can provide simple first aid measures that may assist in stopping the bleeding.

or chronic, lasting longer than a year. The more common type of ITP is often of shorter duration.

Newly diagnosed ITP is characterized by a normal platelet count within 6 months of diagnosis with no evidence of relapse. Approximately two-thirds of children diagnosed with acute ITP achieve complete remission (Turgeon, 2012).

 Nursing Insight—*Chronic immune thrombocytopenia*

Chronic ITP is most common in adults. However, a small percentage of children have this chronic condition. Chronic ITP is defined as the persistence of thrombocytopenia (usually less than 150,000) that lasts longer than 12 months (Turgeon, 2012). In some chronic ITP cases, there seems to be a strong correlation with the development of systemic erythematosus lupus (Turgeon, 2012).

Signs and Symptoms

The clinical presentation of ITP is generally a previously healthy child who may have had a recent viral infection and the following symptoms:

- Petechiae
- Bruising
- Mucocutaneous bleeding
- Epistaxis
- Menorrhagia
- Internal bleeding such as intracranial hemorrhage (rare occurrence)

Diagnosis

A thorough history and physical examination are essential. Most of these patients appear healthy, with the exception of bruising and bleeding. ITP is a diagnosis made by exclusion because there are no tests that confirm the diagnosis (Munn & Valdiviez, 2011).

Newly diagnosed ITP is often benign, self-limiting, and often occurs in children younger than 10 years of age after an upper respiratory infection; after childhood diseases such as measles, rubella, mumps, and chickenpox; and it may also occur after an infection with parvovirus B19 (Munn & Valdiviez, 2011).

"What to say"—*Diagnosing idiopathic (immune) thrombocytopenia purpura*

Communicate to the family about how ITP is diagnosed. It is essential that the nurse tell the family that there are no definitive tests to establish the diagnosis. Explain that other disorders such as lupus, leukemia, and lymphoma must be ruled out (Munn & Valdiviez, 2011). Numerous tests are required to confirm the diagnosis of ITP, including CBC and peripheral smear examination, coagulation analysis, and possible bone marrow aspirate if steroid therapy is implemented. A bone marrow aspirate may be performed to rule out an underlying malignancy. The CBC often shows isolated and usually severe thrombocytopenia, usually a platelet count of less than 20,000 (normal platelet count is 150,000 to 400,000). The peripheral smear is often

normal with the exception of thrombocytopenia with normal-size to large platelets (Munn & Valdiviez, 2011).

 Nursing Insight—*Accurately diagnosing ITP*

Often the child who appears in the emergency department with ITP may be erroneously identified as a child who is an abuse victim. ITP and child abuse may be easily confused. An accurate history and physical and evaluation of CBC will assist the health-care team in determining the actual cause of the observed bruising or bleeding.

Collaborative Care

Nursing Care. The majority of patients with acute ITP may have spontaneous resolution of the disorder with no treatment (Turgeon, 2012). The treatment for ITP among pediatric hematologists is not consistent, although recommendations from the American Society of Hematology have been established. General guidelines recommend that children who have a platelet count greater than 20,000 and are asymptomatic do not require treatment, and platelet counts are monitored. Small toddlers and active children with bruising and petechiae with platelet counts less than 20,000 are treated aggressively to avoid the most serious complication of a life-threatening intracranial bleed. Unless severe life-threatening bleeding is present, transfusion of platelets is not recommended to treat acute ITP because the antibodies attach to the infused platelets and destroy the new platelets in a similar fashion as the destruction of the patient's own platelets.

Medical Care. Treatment strategies for thrombocytopenia may include steroid administration, intravenous immune gamma globulin (IVIG) administration, or anti-D antibody (WinRho® SDF) administration. Children with exceptionally low platelet counts and acute bleeding require inpatient hospitalization with close observation because of the potential of a rare complication of a cerebrovascular bleed. These children may also receive a 2- to 3-day course of IVIG intravenously. The mechanism of action of IVIG is to prevent antibody attachment to the platelets, thereby preventing platelet destruction in the spleen. A vast majority of patients who receive IVIG experience a substantial rise in platelet count within 48 hours. Inpatient care may include bedrest, monitoring of vital signs and adverse reactions during the administration of IVIG, and daily blood counts.

 clinical alert

The administration of IV anti-D antibody

The newest treatment modality for acute ITP patients with an Rh(D)-positive blood type is the administration of IV anti-D antibody. The mechanism of action of anti-D antibody is to bind to the RBCs, which are selectively destroyed in the spleen instead of platelets. The anti-D antibody coats the Rh(D)-positive RBCs with antibody, only for Rh(D)-positive patients. The anti-D-coated cells saturate the capacity of the spleen receptors, and the platelets are spared. A common side effect of anti-D antibody is a transient hemolytic anemia that often resolves as the IgG disperses. It is important that the nurse communicate to the family the other possible side effects of anti-D antibody (e.g., fever, chills, or headache after infusion). A paramount nursing action is close observation and monitoring of the child's vital signs.

Surgical Care. In selected children for whom medical treatment has failed and there have been acute life-threatening bleeding episodes, a treatment modality may include a splenectomy. These patients must be older than 5 years of age and have low platelet counts that impact their activities of daily living (Munn & Valdiviez, 2011). However, advancements in medical treatment for ITP have diminished the need for the major surgical procedure of a splenectomy. Postoperative nursing care measures include:

- Monitoring vital signs as per institution policy for postoperative care until the child's condition is stabilized
- Administering IV fluids, pain medications, and antibiotics if ordered
- Assessing the surgical site for the signs and symptoms of bleeding or infection
- Monitoring intake and output

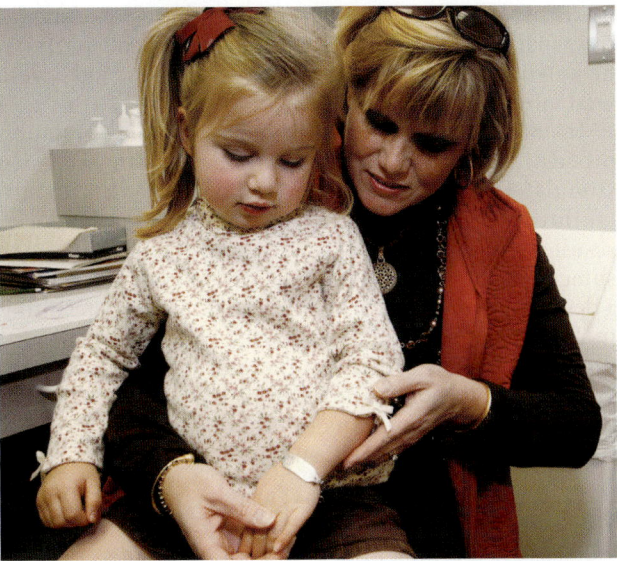

Figure 32–5 Any child who has immune thrombocytopenia purpura (ITP) should wear a medical alert bracelet.

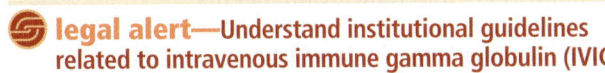 **legal alert—Understand institutional guidelines related to intravenous immune gamma globulin (IVIG)**

IVIG is a blood product and may require informed consent based on institutional guidelines. This plasma-based product is derived from multiple donors and has the potential to transmit infectious diseases. During the administration of this blood, frequent vital signs are monitored to observe for possible adverse reactions, such as fever, chills, hypotension, nausea, and headache. Safe administration of IVIG must include product-specific information for administration guidelines such as administration rates (Munn & Valdiviez, 2011).

 focus on safety

Intracranial bleeding

Ensure that caretakers are knowledgeable about identifying the most serious complication of ITP—an intracranial bleed. Parents must report any changes in level of consciousness or behavior, severe headaches, vision changes, ataxia, slurred speech, complaints of weakness or numbness, and severe vomiting not associated with nausea.

Education/Discharge Instructions

Teach the family that the most important information related to this condition is the child's safety. Advise parents to restrict activities such as contact sports and high-risk activities such as bicycle riding, roller skating, and riding motor scooters. Parents must be instructed on how to manage a bleeding episode in the home. Most common sites of bleeding would be minor cuts, scrapes, and nosebleeds. Instruct parents to apply pressure to the injury site. If the bleeding is from the nose, the nurse can instruct the caretaker to have the child lean down and forward, pinch the bridge of the nose, and if possible, apply ice. For severe bleeding that does not stop with manual pressure, the caregiver must seek medical attention. Other important teaching strategies include avoiding the use of acetylsalicylic acid (Children's Aspirin) or other aspirin-containing products, injections, the use of straight-edge razors, the use of tampons, or inserting a thermometer or suppository into the rectum. Instruct caregivers to report signs or symptoms of bleeding immediately and to provide a safe environment to prevent trauma such as using a nail file as opposed to clippers for nail grooming. It is essential that the nurse recommends to parents of a child with chronic ITP that a medical alert bracelet be worn (Fig. 32-5).

 Case Study Immune Thrombocytopenia

Kelly is a 4-year-old child who has just had a respiratory infection last week. When she woke up this morning to go to day care, she had bruises and petechiae. She did not have a fever. The parents immediately phoned the pediatrician and were told to bring the child to the emergency department. Her physical examination was unremarkable except for her bruising, petechiae and a platelet count of 6,000. All of Kelly's other labs were within normal limits. She was admitted to the hematology oncology unit.

critical thinking questions

1. What is the goal of Kelly's treatment?
2. What would you expect Kelly's treatment to consist of?

◆ See Suggested Answers to Case Studies on DavisPlus.

DISSEMINATED INTRAVASCULAR COAGULATION

Disseminated intravascular coagulation (DIC) is a hematological illness that is secondary to an underlying disease (Hillman et al., 2011). Some disease states in which children may develop DIC include sepsis (usually gram-negative bacteria), hypoxemia, major trauma with severe tissue injury, malignancy, thrombotic thrombocytopenic purpura, hemolytic uremic syndrome, extensive burns, and severe viral infections (Hillman et al., 2011).

In children with DIC, there is an abnormal coagulation process. This process is characterized by an excessive stimulation of normal coagulation that results in microthrombi. These microthrombi are released, and as a result more coagulation factors and platelets are consumed and produced. When the process occurs, there is a destruction of platelets and coagulation factors resulting in hemorrhaging and thrombosis. When this clinical diagnosis of DIC is evident, there is accompanying decreased platelet count, increased prothrombin, decreased fibrinogen, and a buildup of fibrin degradation products that may develop into DIC and tissue ischemia.

Signs and Symptoms

- Excessive bleeding from orifices or from other locations because of minor procedures
- Hematomas
- Petechiae or purpura
- Hypotension

A resulting condition includes:

- Progression to multiorgan failure caused by infarctions and ischemia

Diagnosis

There is no single test that confirms the diagnosis of DIC. The diagnosis is based on the combination of the child's clinical condition and laboratory tests pertinent to coagulopathies (Hillman et al., 2011). Children with DIC often demonstrate suspicious findings that include thrombocytopenia, prolonged PT, prolonged PTT, decreased fibrinogen, and increased D-dimer.

Prevention

DIC is often a complication of other disease processes; therefore, the most important aspect of prevention is to identify the underlying cause and treat appropriately. Important nursing responsibilities include early identification of risk factors that predispose patients to develop DIC, recognizing clinical signs and symptoms of DIC, and communicating findings with the health-care provider for prompt interventions.

Collaborative Care

Nursing Care. When caring for a child with DIC, the nurse's primary intervention is to assess the child and provide supportive care for the symptomatology. Monitor for signs of hemorrhage, bleeding (Procedure 32-1), petechiae, cutaneous oozing, dyspnea, lethargy, pallor, increased heart rate, decreased blood pressure, headache, dizziness, muscle weakness, and restlessness. Monitor for internal bleeding by checking both the urine and stool for occult blood. If the child is bleeding, it is important not to disturb clots, use pressure, apply ice to control bleeding, and measure blood loss. The nurse also obtains necessary laboratory tests and administers supportive treatments such as blood and factor products per physician's orders (Burke & Salani, 2013).

> **"What to say"**—*Disseminated intravascular coagulation*
>
> When a child is critically ill and has the diagnosis of DIC, parents are informed of the plan of care and course of treatment. In the intensive care unit, the nurse orients families to the unit procedures, equipment, and treatments. The possibility of excessive bleeding from multiple sites may occur and could be upsetting to family members. The nurse communicates to families about the occurrence of excessive bleeding to help decrease anxiety. Identifying areas of knowledge deficits and ensuring consistent caregivers during this time of crisis are important nursing interventions. Provide families with honest answers in clear and concise terms.

Medical Care. Children with DIC are critically ill and may require management in the intensive care unit. The administration of blood and factor products is often necessary. Prognosis for DIC has improved significantly over the last two decades because of advances in supportive care such as improved antibiotics, antifibrinolytic therapy, and improvement in transfusion therapy.

Education/Discharge Instructions

Because DIC is not a primary disease, parents should understand the importance of treating infections and the triggers that were identified to cause this coagulation disorder. Preventing complications of the primary illness will play a key role in preventing the development of DIC.

APLASTIC ANEMIA

Aplastic anemia is a rare illness but one of the most serious hematological conditions that generally afflicts adolescents and young adults. This condition, characterized by **pancytopenia** (a reduction in all cellular elements of the blood, white blood cells, platelets, and red blood cells), is caused by bone marrow hematopoiesis failure (Hillman et al., 2011). The clinical course may be acute and may progress to severe bone marrow suppression with the possibility of rapid deterioration leading to death. The condition could also have an insidious onset and chronic course (Turgeon, 2012). Classification can range from moderate aplastic anemia to very severe aplastic anemia.

 Nursing Insight—*Pancytopenia*

Pancytopenia is a common finding in aplastic anemia. In pancytopenia all formed elements of the blood are depressed at the same time. A patient with pancytopenia has neutropenia, decreased white blood cell count, anemia, decreased hemoglobin count, and thrombocytopenia.

Aplastic anemia is heredity (a congenital disorder) or an acquired illness. Hereditary aplastic anemia (a congenital disorder) is relatively rare, but it can occur with diseases such as Fanconi's anemia. Fanconi's anemia is inherited as an autosomal recessive trait. Fanconi's anemia accounts for 25% to 30% of all cases of childhood aplastic anemia

(Turgeon, 2012). Children with congenital aplastic anemia have chromosomal breakages and structural abnormalities that increase the incidence of various malignancies such as leukemia.

The majority of aplastic anemia cases are considered to be acquired and the specific cause is never determined (Box 32-2). Other forms of aplastic anemia are considered secondary to etiological agents that are usually associated with various environmental factors and physical conditions.

Signs and Symptoms

The presenting signs and symptoms of a child with aplastic anemia vary by severity of bone marrow suppression:

- Pancytopenia
- Bleeding
- Bruising
- Fatigue
- Pallor
- Dizziness

 Nursing Insight—*Signs and symptoms of aplastic anemia*

The child's symptoms are related to the degree of pancytopenia. Anemia, pallor, dizziness, and fatigue may be present because of a decreased RBC count. Increased bleeding and bruising, petechiae, and epistaxis may be attributed to a low platelet count. Increased susceptibility to infections and oral ulcerations that do not respond well to antibiotics are related to a low WBC count. The most common presenting symptom is bleeding, usually from the nose, mouth, and gastrointestinal tract. The nurse is aware that the child with aplastic anemia characteristically does not have the clinical finding of hepatosplenomegaly or lymphadenopathy. The child with this clinical finding is usually diagnosed with leukemia.

Diagnosis

To confirm the diagnosis of aplastic anemia and to rule out other hematopoietic diseases, a bone marrow aspirate and biopsy is performed. The results of the bone marrow aspiration generally reveal a fatty marrow with few developing blood cells. Children who are suspected to have aplastic anemia require a thorough history and physical and laboratory tests, including a CBC with differential. The findings of the CBC usually are consistent with all cell lines depressed.

Box 32-2 Causative Factors of Acquired Aplastic Anemia

- High-dose radiation
- Autoimmune disorders
- Pregnancy
- Infectious processes
  - Hepatitis
  - Epstein-Barr virus
  - HIV
  - Cytomegalovirus (CMV) infection
  - Infectious mononucleosis
- Nonpharmacological agents
  - Benzene
  - Lindane (insecticide)
  - Kerosene
  - Heavy metals
- Pharmacological agents
  - Chemotherapy
  - Chloramphenicol
  - Selected antiepileptics (carbamazepine)
  - Sulfonamides
  - Penicillamine
  - Nonsteroidal anti-inflammatory drugs (NSAIDs)
  - Antithyroid drugs
  - Psychotropics (e.g., clozapine)
  - Certain cardiovascular drugs
  - Penicillamine
  - Antithyroid drugs
  - Certain cardiovascular drugs

 Procedure 32-1 Obtaining a Fecal Occult Blood Test Sample

A fecal occult blood test is performed to detect hidden (occult) blood in the stool (Fig. 32-6).

Equipment

- Hematest supplies
- Gloves
- Sterile tongue blade
- Chemical reagent

Steps

1. Wash hands and don gloves.

   RATIONALE: *Prevents the spread of bacteria.*

2. Verify the identity of the patient using two patient identifiers.

   RATIONALE: *Accurate patient identification is necessary in the delivery of safe care.*

3. Check the manufacturer's instructions for specific Hematest supplies.

   RATIONALE: *Following the correct instructions ensures proper administration of the test as well as accurate results.*

4. Keep the Hematest supplies at room temperature.

   RATIONALE: *Extreme temperatures may damage the Hematest supplies.*

5. Use a sterile tongue blade to remove a sample of stool from the diaper.

   RATIONALE: *A sterile tongue blade helps to prevent contamination of the collected specimen.*

6. Place a smear of stool on both windows of the Hematest card as indicated in the instructions.

(continued)

Procedure 32-1 Obtaining a Fecal Occult Blood Test Sample (continued)

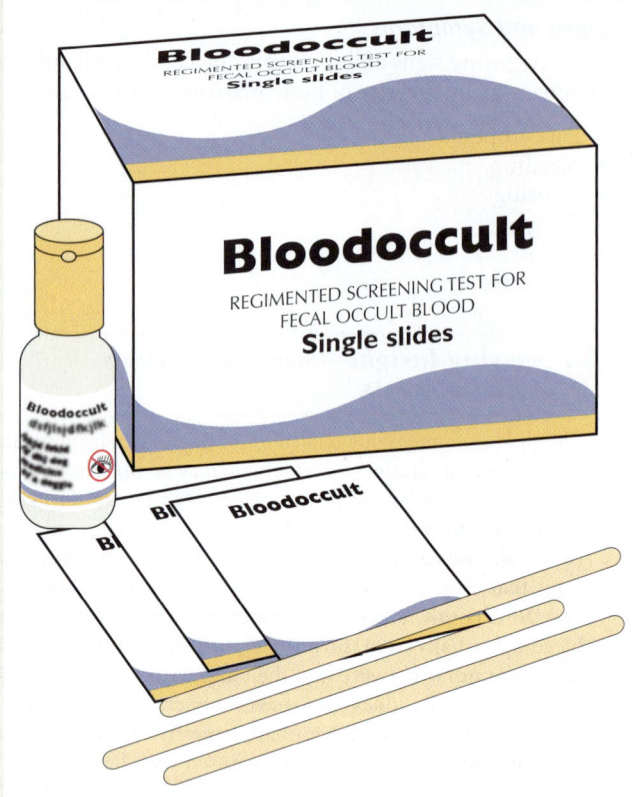

Figure 32–6 Obtaining a fecal occult blood test sample.

RATIONALE: *Collecting an adequate amount of stool is necessary to complete the test.*

7. Cover the windows with the paper flaps and wait the correct amount of time before reading the results.

RATIONALE: *It is important to follow the manufacturer's instructions.*

8. Apply the recommended drops of developing solution to the Hematest card.

RATIONALE: *It is important to follow the manufacturer's instructions for an accurate reading.*

9. Read the back flap of the sample card within the recommended time of application of developing solution.

RATIONALE: *Reading the card within the recommended time is essential to performing the test accurately.*

10. The Hematest card changes color to indicate the test results.

RATIONALE: *A change in color may indicate occult blood in the stool.*

Clinical Alert When the nurse records results, it is important to notify the health-care provider of any abnormal findings. In addition, the nurse checks the expiration date on the developing solution.

Teach Parents

It is important to teach the parents the rationale for the test.

Documentation

2/19/2015 at 1300 Stool Hematest negative

D. Salani, RN

Prevention

For patients with inherited aplastic anemia, genetic counseling is recommended to prevent transmission. For patients who have acquired aplastic anemia, if the causative is identified, exposure to or use of the product (such as a medication) is avoided.

Collaborative Care

Nursing Care. Nursing care for children with aplastic anemia varies based on the severity of illness and determination of causative factors. If the causative factor of the aplastic anemia has been identified, immediate removal of the agent is necessary. Some patients may respond to medical treatment and support. In these cases, a hematopoietic stem cell transplant may not be warranted. If there is no identified cause of the severe aplastic anemia and a suitable stem cell donor is identified, the treatment of choice is a hematopoietic stem cell transplant (HSCT). For best outcomes and long-term survival, every effort must be made to proceed to transplant as soon as possible. Following the stem cell transplant, nursing care consists of supportive care, immunosuppressive therapy, or the administration of hematopoietic growth factors. All patients diagnosed with aplastic anemia are extremely susceptible to infectious agents. These patients may not exhibit the "classic signs of infection."

 Critical Nursing Action Supportive Care

For all patients with aplastic anemia, and especially those who are preparing for HSCT, the nursing care plan often consists of supportive care including transfusions of RBCs and platelets. Transfusions are used cautiously to prevent development of antibodies (alloimmunization) and possible graft versus host disease if this patient proceeds on to transplant. Antibiotics are often given to treat infections but are generally not recommended prophylactically.

Critical Nursing Action Pancytopenia

This special population of pediatric hematology patients requires diligent nursing assessments secondary to their pancytopenia. These children may experience numerous complications from neutropenia, anemia, or thrombocytopenia. When caring for children who are neutropenic, the nurse does not traditionally see the hallmark signs of infections such as redness, swelling, and pus because these patients do not have the neutrophils to provoke such a response. The nursing care plan is used to monitor the subjective responses of the child.

Medical Care. Drug therapy is often the first line of therapy while searching for a potential bone marrow donor. The two most common immunosuppressive drugs used in treating aplastic anemia include antithymocyte globulin (ATG) and high-dose cyclosporine (Neoral, Gengraf). ATG is a horse or rabbit serum containing polyclonal antibodies against human T cells, and cyclosporine is also a T cell–suppressing agent. Immunosuppressive therapies work with the child's immune system. The mechanism of action is to stimulate the bone marrow to produce cells or to reduce the patient's immune response, thereby allowing the bone marrow to work. Combined ATG and cyclosporine is the gold standard for first-line immunosuppressive therapy. There is usually a 75% to 85% response rate (Turgeon, 2012).

Another treatment modality includes the administration of hematopoietic growth factors. These growth factors are copies of substances that occur naturally in the body and attempt to stimulate the bone. Sometimes combinations of these growth factors are used to treat aplastic anemia.

 focus on safety

Antithymocyte globulin (ATG)

Children with aplastic anemia who receive ATG require specific nursing care related to the administration of this medication. Although rare, a severe anaphylactic reaction may occur (e.g., hypotension, tachycardia, shortness of breath, or chest pain). Because there is a potential risk for anaphylaxis, an ATG test dose is often administered to determine if there is a potential for an adverse reaction to this medication. The child may have no adverse reaction to the test dose but still may have a reaction to ATG. If the child has been identified as being "allergic" to ATG, administration of this medication can still take place after a desensitization process or administration of premedications such as antihistamine and steroids.

Education/Discharge Instructions

Because of variations in severity of aplastic anemia, the nurse's teaching plan correlates with the child's clinical condition. Provide reassurance and support to families, including basic explanations of the disease process and recommended treatment plan. It is important for the nurse to review the child's prescribed drugs and discuss possible adverse reactions. Children can continue a normal lifestyle with some restrictions. The nurse communicates to the

---

 Nursing Care Plan The Child With Aplastic Anemia

Nursing Diagnosis: Risk for Infection related to decreased white blood cell count

Measurable Short-Term Goal: Patient will be afebrile within 24 hours of initiation of antibiotic therapy.

Measurable Long-Term Goal: Patient will have a decrease in the incidence of infections.

NOC Outcome:
Immune Status (0702) Natural and acquired appropriately targeted resistance to internal and external antigens

NIC Interventions:
Infection Protection (6550)
Medication Administration (2300)

Nursing Interventions:

1. Monitor child's temperature, blood pressure, pulse, and respirations (specify frequency).

   RATIONALE: To identify fever, tachycardia, tachypnea, hypotension, or other possible signs of sepsis and allow early intervention.

2. Perform hand washing or use antimicrobial hand gels/foams before and after caring for the patient. Teach family to use hand hygiene.

   RATIONALE: Hand washing reduces the spread of infection.

3. Administer antibiotics and acetaminophen per care provider's orders (specify drug, dose, route, and times).

   RATIONALE: (State the action of the antibiotic and acetaminophen here.) Aspirin and NSAIDs are usually not used because they may increase bleeding.

4. Maintain protective isolation per institution guidelines (specify).

   RATIONALE: Individualized isolation precautions avoid contact with infectious agents.

5. Provide or assist family member to provide meticulous oral and skin hygiene.

   RATIONALE: Reduces the portals of entry for infections.

6. Instruct family and visitors that no fresh fruits, vegetables, flowers, or plants are allowed in the child's room.

   RATIONALE: Some fresh fruits, vegetables, flowers, and plants may harbor bacteria or viruses.

family that monitoring the child's CBC is imperative, so changes in condition from mild to moderate aplastic anemia are noted. Children and their families must be aware of signs and symptoms of pancytopenia. Patients with moderate to severe aplastic anemia are encouraged to schedule regular rest periods, avoid contacts with crowds, and avoid sources of infections (e.g., sick contacts, soil, standing water). Injury prevention may include using a soft toothbrush for oral hygiene, ensuring a safe play environment, and avoiding the use of tampons for adolescent girls. Stress the importance of meticulous oral hygiene and diligent hand washing. For additional education materials and resources for family teaching, refer families to the Aplastic Anemia and MDS International Foundation at www.aamds.org.

NEUTROPENIA

Neutropenia occurs when an absolute neutrophil count is less than 1,000/mcL in infants younger than 1 year of age and 1,500/mcL for those older than 1 year of age.

 Nursing Insight—Absolute neutrophil count (ANC)

The ANC is the total number of white blood cells multiplied by the percentage of neutrophils (segs and bands).

The National Cancer Institute neutropenia grading system classifies slight neutropenia as grade 1 with ANC of less than 2,000, minimal neutropenia as grade 2 with ANC of less than 1,500, and moderate neutropenia as grade 3 with ANC less than 1,000. The most severe neutropenia is grade 4 with an ANC of less than 500. When caring for children with neutropenia, the nursing plan of care is based on the severity of neutropenia present.

Neutropenia is further classified as an acquired or congenital illness. Acquired neutropenia is more common than the congenital form. Viral infections (e.g., HIV, Epstein-Barr virus, hepatitis A and B, and respiratory syncytial virus) are often a common cause of acquired neutropenia (Turgeon, 2012). Acquired neutropenia is often referred to as secondary neutropenia because it occurs as a result of an illness or of treatment of an illness (e.g., chemotherapy, radiation therapy, immunosuppressive agents, specific medications, and malignancies). It can also result as part of the normal aging process.

Congenital neutropenia (also known as primary neutropenia) is usually caused by a genetic abnormality that results in profound neutropenia. Some examples include severe combined immunodeficiency syndrome, Wiskott-Aldrich syndrome, and Kostmann's syndrome. Often these congenital neutropenia disorders are associated with the future development of more serious illnesses such as myelodysplastic syndromes or acute myelogenous leukemia.

Signs and Symptoms

Signs and symptoms of neutropenia include:

- Fever
- Lymphadenopathy
- Organomegaly
- Pallor
- Bruising
- Petechiae

 clinical alert

Infection

Observe the child for any underlying infection, especially the mouth, skin, ears, and perianal area. A fever may be the only clinical sign that an infection is present. Often the child with neutropenia may not have the classic signs of an underlying infection, so the nurse must pay close attention to the subtle signs that may be present. The reason these children do not display the classic signs and symptoms is that they do not possess the cells (i.e., neutrophils) to evoke such a response, such as redness, swelling, or pus.

Diagnosis

The child diagnosed with neutropenia requires a meticulous history and physical examination. The child's height and weight are plotted on the growth chart to evaluate for any underlying genetic illness or deviations from the norm. The child's laboratory work-up is based on the findings from the history and physical. In most cases a CBC with differential and a peripheral smear will be performed. An important area to focus on is the ANC as opposed to the total WBC count. If the child has other clinical findings such as anemia, thrombocytopenia, or high MCV with normal B_{12}, a bone marrow aspirate may be indicated. The bone marrow aspirate is helpful in ascertaining the cause and treatment regimen for the neutropenia. Usually the child with congenital neutropenia has a normal cellularity with absence of mature neutrophils in the bone marrow sample. If a bone marrow aspirate cannot be obtained, a bone marrow biopsy may be required. Additional diagnostic tests may include cytogenetics (identification of chromosomes), including flow cytometry (laser device in a specialized laboratory is used for the counting and measuring of cells).

Prevention

For patients with congenital neutropenia who are considering pregnancy, genetic counseling is recommended. For patients with neutropenia as a result of an illness such as a blood cancer, prevention is focused on treating the underlying disease and close monitoring of blood counts. Patients receiving immunosuppressive therapy should be aware of when the nadir (time of lowest blood counts) occurs related to treatment, and neutropenic precautions are observed.

Collaborative Care

Nursing Care. In children with congenital neutropenia, the nursing plan of care is based on the degree of neutropenia and physical findings. In patients with acquired neutropenia, the etiology must be evaluated. One of the most important aspects of nursing care for neutropenic patients includes monitoring for infections by checking for fever, evaluating absolute neutrophil count, and performing physical exams. In the event an infection is suspected, treatment of a documented infection in the neutropenic patient is dependent on the organism that is isolated. Empiric therapy, usually with a broad-spectrum antibiotic, is usually implemented during the period of time in which culture results are pending. Once culture results are obtained, antibiotic therapy is evaluated for sensitivities and adjusted accordingly.

Medical Care. Treatment may range from supportive measures to the administration of colony-stimulating factors, and in most severe cases to bone marrow transplant if necessary.

The administration of granulocyte colony-stimulating factor such as GCSF (Neupogen) stimulates the bone marrow to produce more neutrophils.

Instruct parents of a child who has had an exposure to chickenpox (i.e., any type of varicella illness) to immediately contact a health-care provider. Administering the varicella-zoster vaccine may be helpful to the neutropenic child who might be exposed to an outbreak of chickenpox.

 Nursing Insight—*Hematopoietic growth factors*

Granulocyte colony-stimulating factors (GCSF) are powerful regulators of blood cell proliferation that stimulate the bone marrow to produce granulocytes and stem cells releasing them into the bloodstream. Growth factors are given to prevent profound neutropenia and decrease susceptibility to life-threatening infections. In the home setting, this medication is given by subcutaneous injection once daily by the child's caregiver. Possible side effects include fever, bone pain, headache, and local reaction at the injection site.

Education/Discharge Instructions

The child who has neutropenia, whether it is congenital or acquired, needs specific teaching on management. Families are instructed on when and how to appropriately wash their hands. Hands are washed with soap and water for at least 10 to 15 seconds using a circular motion. Friction (rubbing) is the most important aspect of hand washing because it assists in removing germs from the hands.

Teach parents how to appropriately check the child's temperature. Remind them to never check a temperature rectally because this route may cause a tear in the rectal mucosa, promoting an entrance for bacteria. Parents need to seek medical attention if the child develops a temperature of 101.5°F (38.6°C). Instruct caregivers to keep the neutropenic child away from anyone who is sick or has recently received live vaccines.

Teaching the family about meticulous oral hygiene is also important. To prevent bacteria in the mouth, the child can use a soft toothbrush and rinse well after brushing. Good skin care is essential to prevent infections or breaks in the skin.

 Critical Nursing Action The Neutropenic Child

Families and children with neutropenia are taught the following measures to reduce the incidence of infection:

- Know when routine visits are scheduled.
- Know the signs and symptoms of infections, such as fever (greater than 101.5°F [38.6°C]).
- Know that acetylsalicylic acid (aspirin) or NSAIDs are not given to children with low counts.
- Avoid large crowds or anyone who may be sick with a cold, flu, etc.
- Keep the child's body clean by bathing every day and brush teeth after meals and before bedtime.
- Avoid hot tubs.
- Always be sure to wash the child's hands before eating or touching his or her face, eyes, nose, and mouth.
- Avoid constipation and straining to have a bowel movement by drinking 2 quarts of fluids each day, such as water, and use a stool softener.

- Avoid putting anything in the child's rectum, including thermometers and suppositories.
- Avoid exposure to fresh flowers or live plants.
- Avoid exposure to stool droppings from pets and cleaning bird cages or cat litter boxes.
- Do not share bath towels or drinking glasses with others, including family members.
- Avoid eating the following items:
  - Raw milk or milk products or any milk product that has not been pasteurized, including cheese and yogurt made from unpasteurized milk
  - Raw or uncooked meat, fish, chicken, eggs, or tofu
  - Foods that contain mold (e.g., blue cheese)
  - Raw honey (honey that has not been pasteurized)
  - Uncooked fresh fruit or vegetables that are not well cleaned
  - Outdated foods or foods left at room temperature for more than 2 hours
- Tell adolescents not to use tampons, vaginal suppositories, or douche.
- Tell adolescents to avoid manicures, pedicures, acrylic nails, or nail tips.
- Tell adolescents to use an electric shaver instead of a disposable blade razor.

 Now Can You—Discuss common hematological conditions in children?

1. Identify signs and symptoms of common hematological conditions?
2. Examine preventative measures for common hematological conditions?
3. Discuss education/discharge criteria for common hematological conditions?

Blood Transfusion Therapy

Because of recent advances in health care and more children living with chronic illnesses, blood transfusion therapy may be required as part of the nursing care plan. Illnesses such as hematological, oncological, and other chronic conditions often necessitate the use of blood products. Nurses must be knowledgeable about blood transfusion products and specific indications for each blood product (Table 32-8). Administration of blood may vary based on institution policy and procedures and the actual product being administered.

BLOOD PRODUCT ADMINISTRATION

Most blood transfusions are delivered in the hospital. The first responsibility of the nurse who is administering a blood transfusion to a child is to review the plan of care with the family and explain in detail the indications and process of a blood transfusion. The ordering health-care provider must obtain signed consent from the parent or guardian to administer blood to the child.

 legal alert—Obtain transfusion consent

Transfusion consent is obtained before the administration of any blood product; check institutional guidelines.

Table 32-8 Transfusion Products

Transfusion Product	Indications	Critical Nursing Actions
Red Blood Cells	Hemoglobin <8 grams on a stable patient with a chronic anemia. Hypovolemia caused by acute blood loss. Evidence of impending heart failure secondary to severe anemia. Patients on hypertransfusion regimen for SCD and history of: • Cerebrovascular accident • Splenic sequestration • Acute chest syndrome • Recurrent priapism • Preoperative preparation for surgery with general anesthesia • Hypoxia Children requiring increased oxygen-carrying capacity (i.e., complex congenital heart, intracardiac shunting, severe pulmonary disease—ARDS): • Shock states (decrease B.P., increased peripheral vasoconstriction pallor, cyanosis, diaphoretic, clamminess, mottled skin, increased oxygen requirement, decreased urinary output) • Cardiac failure • Respiratory failure requiring significant ventilatory support • Postoperative anemia	Observe for clinical signs and symptoms of anemia: • Fatigue • Syncope • Pallor • Tachycardia • Diaphoretic • Shortness of breath • Inability to perform activities of daily living Don appropriate personal protective equipment (PPE) for all blood product transfusions. Monitor vital signs per hospital policy and procedure. Monitor hemoglobin and hematocrit. During blood product infusions, observe for adverse reactions. Blood can be stored only in a designated blood refrigerator. Generally 10–15 mL/kg of packed red blood cells are transfused (Khilnani, 2005).
Autologous Blood (self-donated blood product)	For general scheduled surgical procedures in which there are clinical indications that a blood transfusion may be necessary during the intraoperative or postoperative period, the patient may elect to self-donate. Check with blood bank facilities for time criteria for this type of donation. For general surgical procedures, the recommended hemoglobin is 10 grams or greater and for orthopedic surgery the recommendation is hemoglobin of 11.5 or greater.	Verify with parents that self-donation has occurred. Patient identification and administration process is the same as for all other blood products.
Whole Blood or Packed Red Blood Cells (PRBC) Reconstituted With Fresh Frozen Plasma (FFP)	Hypovolemia caused by acute blood loss non-responsive to crystalloids • Hct <35% • Hypovolemia caused by acute massive blood loss (i.e., major trauma) • History of blood loss at delivery or large amount of blood drawn for lab studies (10% blood volume) • Cardiac patients Hct <40% (e.g., structural heart disease, cyanosis, or congestive heart failure) • Drop in Hgb to below 10 grams intraoperatively • Exchange transfusion	Same nursing actions applicable to red blood cell infusions. In major trauma situations, patient may be transfused with O negative blood, the universal donor. Use blood warmer and rapid infuser if available.
Platelets	Platelet count <20,000 Active bleeding with symptoms of DIC or other significant coagulopathies Platelet count <50,000 with planned invasive procedure (i.e., surgical procedure, central line insertion, does not include drawing blood, IM injection, or IV catheter insertion) Prevention or treatment of bleeding caused by thrombocytopenia (secondary to chemotherapy, radiation, or bone marrow failure) Treatment of patients with severe thrombocytopenia secondary to increased platelet destruction or immune thrombocytopenia associated with complication of severe trauma Massive transfusion with platelet dilution	Know normal platelet count (150,000 to 400,000). Obtain CBC. Assess bruising, petechiae, and bleeding.
Fresh Frozen Plasma (FFP)	Replacement for deficiency of factors II, V, VII, IX, X, XII; protein C or protein S Bleeding, invasive procedure, or surgery with documented plasma clotting protein deficiency (e.g., liver failure, DIC, or septic shock) Prolonged PT and/or PTT without bleeding Significant intraoperative bleeding (>10% blood volume/hr) in excess of normally anticipated blood loss that is at high risk of clotting-factor deficiency Massive transfusion Therapeutic plasma exchanges Warfarin anticoagulant overdose	Notify blood bank to thaw FFP; product must be used within 6 hours of thawing. Don appropriate PPE for all blood product transfusions. Monitor vital signs per hospital policy and procedure. Monitor coagulation studies. During FFP infusions, observe for adverse reactions.

Table 32-8 Transfusion Products (continued)

Transfusion Product	Indications	Critical Nursing Actions
Cryoprecipitate (CRYO)	Fibrinogen levels below 150 mg/dL with active bleeding Bleeding or prophylaxis in von Willebrand's disease or in factor VIII (hemophilia A) deficiency unresponsive to or unsuitable for DDAVP or factor VII concentrates Replacement therapy, bleeding or invasive procedure in patients with factor XIII deficiency Patients with active intraoperative hemorrhage in excess of normally anticipated blood loss who are at risk of clotting factor deficiency	Assess for signs and symptoms of bleeding. Don appropriate PPE for all blood product transfusions. Monitor vital signs per hospital policy and procedure. Monitor coagulation studies. During cryoprecipitate infusions, observe for adverse reactions.
Granulocytes (white blood cell transfusion)	Bacterial or fungal sepsis (proven or strongly suspected) unresponsive to antimicrobial therapy Infection (proven or strongly suspected) unresponsive to antimicrobial therapy	Type and crossmatch required for all WBC transfusions. Pre-medications may be ordered, such as antihistamines or acetaminophen.
Factor VII	Treatment of factor VII deficiency Treatment of factor VIII inhibitors Treatment of factor IX inhibitors Idiopathic uncontrolled bleeding	Assess for signs and symptoms of bleeding. Don appropriate PPE for all blood products, even recombinant. Monitor coagulation studies. If undiluted, dilute vial with indicated amount of sterile water and administer IV as per manufacturer's guidelines.
Factor VIII Concentrate	Hemophilia A (factor VIII deficiency) Patients with factor VIII inhibitors Patients with von Willebrand's disease	Assess for signs and symptoms of bleeding. Don appropriate PPE for all blood products. Monitor coagulation studies. Check product to see if refrigeration necessary. Record expiration date and lot number of product.
Factor IX Concentrate (prothrombin complex)	Treatment of hemophilia B Hemophilia A with factor VIII inhibitors Patients with congenital deficiency of prothrombin, factor VII, and factor X	Assess for signs and symptoms of bleeding. Don appropriate PPE for all blood products. Monitor coagulation studies. Record expiration date and lot number of product.
Intravenous Immunoglobulin (IVIG)	Congenital or acquired antibody deficiency Immunological disorders such as idiopathic thrombocytopenia (ITP), Kawasaki's disease Post-transplant patients used prophylactically, newborns with severe bacterial infections	Don appropriate PPE for all IVIG infusions. Monitor vital signs per hospital policy and procedure. Start infusion slowly and increase rate/titrate per physician orders. During IVIG infusion, observe for adverse reactions such as fever, chills, and headache. Product is obtained from pharmacy. Record expiration date and lot number of product.

Transfusion consent must include the description of the procedure for transfusion, risks and benefits, treatment alternatives, and appropriate signatures including those of the health-care provider, the patient if 18 years or older, the parent or other legal representative, and witness (American Association of Blood Banks [AABB], 2011). Provide the opportunity for the family to ask questions. The family has the right to revoke consent. After the consent process is complete, obtain the required blood samples from the patient. For example, if a child requires a packed red blood cell transfusion, a type and crossmatch is indicated to determine the ABO and Rh(D) factor and to reserve the donated red blood cells for this specific child.

 focus on safety

Blood transfusion safety measure

During the collection of a blood sample for crossmatch, a blood bracelet with the specific identifying numbers is placed on the child's extremity, and the nurse uses two patient identifiers. This safety measure is to ensure that the child receives the correct blood product crossmatched specifically for his or her blood type to prevent a fatality.

Optimizing Outcomes—Type and screen and type and crossmatch

The best outcome exists for the child when the nurse understands the difference between the type and screen and type and crossmatch.

Type and Screen
- Obtain a type and screen in anticipation that a child may need a blood transfusion
- Use the proper ABO group and Rh(D) type

Type and Crossmatch
- Obtain a type and crossmatch if almost certain the child will require blood.
- Use the proper ABO/Rh(D)-compatible donor red cells.
- Know that the type and crossmatch is good for 72 hours (AABB, 2011).

Blood is administered to the child after verifying that the correct blood product is available and that the child's clinical condition is stable (i.e., vital signs within parameters to safely administer blood). The nurse completes the pre-assessment process for blood administration. The nurse is aware that there are several clinical conditions that may delay the administration of a blood product:

- Fever greater than 101°F (38.3°C)
- Lack of IV access
- Child is unable to be closely monitored by nursing staff
- Complex medication regimen with drugs with potential for anaphylaxis

 Nursing Insight—*Understanding blood type*

When the clinical criterion is met, the nurse proceeds and obtains the correct product to be infused from the institution's blood bank or pharmacy. Understand that blood type is essential information for the nurse (Box 32-3).

 focus on safety

The administration process for blood products

Understand the administration process for blood products:

Pre-transfusion
- Do not call for the blood product until it is needed.
- Obtain a set of pre-transfusion vital signs to ensure patient is clinically stable.
- Verify the health-care provider's orders, including the appropriate product and volume to be infused. Check with institution policies and procedures. The transfusion must be started within 30 minutes after the blood has left the blood bank.
- The maximum time for the infusion is 4 hours. Transfusion needs to start immediately because of the risk of bacterial contamination and cell lysis. Most blood banks do not accept blood back after 30 minutes.
- Follow institutional policy for obtaining, verifying, and transporting blood products obtained from the blood bank.
- Complete appropriate forms and ensure accurate patient identification.
- Indicate product type and check for any special orders such as cytomegalovirus safe or irradiated.

Box 32-3 Understanding Blood Types		
Blood Type	**Can Give to:**	**Can Take From:**
A+	A+	A+, A–, O–
A–	A+, A–	A–, O–
B+	B+	B+, B–, O+, O–
B–	B+, B–	B–, O–
AB+	AB+	All types
AB–	AB–	A–, B–, AB–, O–
O+	A+, B+, AB+, O+	O+, O–
O–	All types	O–

- Always check to see if any premedications were ordered before administration.
- Use personal protective equipment. Be sure to wear goggles and gloves.
- All blood products must be checked at the patient's bedside by two appropriate health-care providers and using two patient identifiers as per the institution's policy.

Remember the two patient identifiers must match the number on the blood product and the wrist band.

Initiation of the Transfusion
- Obtain baseline vital signs.
- Start the infusion slowly for the first 15 minutes.
- Designate a nurse to remain with the patient for the first 15 minutes of transfusion in the event of an adverse reaction.

During the Transfusion
- Do not infuse any other solutions simultaneously with blood through the same IV line. The only exception to this is normal saline (AABB, 2011).
- Never add any medications to blood.
- Monitor vital signs per the institution's policy and procedures.
- All identification information that is attached to the blood product must remain attached until the transfusion is completed.
- Monitor for signs and symptoms of adverse reactions *(see adverse reactions)*.

Post-transfusion
- Save the transfusion bag for at least 1 hour after the transfusion has ended.
- The blood slip must be completely filled out with the institution's required information.
- As per the AABB guidelines, information to be included in the child's medical record must include the transfusion order, the type of blood product, the donor unit number, date and time of transfusion, pre– and post–vital signs, the volume infused, required signatures, and if applicable any transfusion adverse events (AABB, 2011).
- Place the chart copy and blood bank copy of the blood slip in an appropriate area to be kept on file as per policy and procedure.

 Cultural Diversity: Sensitivity to Cultural and Religious Beliefs

The nurse is aware of cultural and religious beliefs to provide the most culturally competent care to patients and their families. In most cases, the nurse is the primary health-care provider at the bedside and may experience some personal conflict when providing the necessary medical care. The nurse must be knowledgeable about various belief systems that impact care and be aware of the resources that are available to assist in these situations.

 Cultural Diversity: Jehovah Witness

People of the Jehovah's Witnesses faith are adamantly opposed to receiving blood and blood products. This belief is based on the literal interpretation of the Bible that states that to be transfused with blood is equivalent to eating it and therefore prohibited by scripture as cited in Leviticus 17:10-14; Acts 15:19, 20, 28, 29 and Genesis 9:3, 4. Jehovah's Witnesses believe that blood transfusions, even life-saving ones, are forbidden by scripture. Additionally, if blood is removed from the body, it cannot be re-infused (e.g., cell saver technology that could be used in the operating room). Self-donation is also prohibited based on this premise. Members of this faith would "abstain from blood" even if death is imminent.

When caring for a child from a Jehovah's Witnesses family, there may be an ethical and medical dilemma to provide quality medical care. The health-care team can explore all alternative methods of treatment to respect the family's beliefs. In some circumstances when the child's life is severely threatened, the courts may be called on. A court order may be required to proceed with the necessary medical treatment. The involvement of the court system relinquishes the family from making the decision for their child to have a blood transfusion. This transfer of responsibility may diminish the disgrace that the family might experience from other members of this religious group when this medical treatment is necessary to save the child's life (Linnard-Palmar & Kools, 2004).

Prevention

Safe administration of blood products must be observed for all transfusions, even in an emergency situation. Initially, verification of health-care provider's orders and awareness of the indication for the blood transfusion are necessary. Always use the two patient identifiers per institution guidelines. The use of a second witness and "double check" at the bedside is an additional safety measure to ensure safe administration of blood.

 Nursing Insight—Preventing transfusion reactions

To prevent transfusion reactions, the nurse:
- Always uses two patient identifiers
- Knows about blood product administration
- Knows about the types of transfusion reactions

TRANSFUSION REACTIONS

Most transfusion reactions occur during the initiation of a transfusion, but a reaction can occur at any time during this process (AABB, 2011). These reactions can vary from a mild reaction, such as mild fever, to the most severe complication of death. Children who have received multiple transfusions are at higher risk for developing a transfusion reaction (Bryant & Norville, 2011).

 legal alert—Transfusion reaction procedure and documentation

The nurse is aware of the appropriate procedure and documentation required for transfusion reactions when an adverse reaction occurs. The nurse checks specific institutional policies and procedures about transfusion reactions. Documentation includes completing a blood transfusion reaction form and submitting an incident report.

 Critical Nursing Action Blood Administration

Strict observance to the institutional policy regarding the administration of blood products is essential. The accuracy of patient verification with two patient identifiers is a critical nursing action that can help prevent a transfusion reaction.

Febrile Reaction

The most common blood transfusion reaction is a non-hemolytic **febrile reaction** in which the child develops a fever greater than 2°F (1.1°C) from the baseline temperature. These reactions generally occur on initiation of the transfusion but have been known to occur up to 12 hours post-transfusion.

Signs and Symptoms

Signs and symptoms that may be present during a transfusion reaction include fever and chills, which then may progress to more serious complications such as tachycardia, tachypnea, and hypotension.

Collaborative Care

Nursing Care. An important nursing care measure includes monitoring the child's temperature to recognize febrile reactions early and prevent progression. If the child is having a febrile response, the nurse stops the transfusion, monitors vital signs, and notifies the health-care provider.

Medical Care. With the increased use of leukocyte-depleted blood products, this type of reaction has diminished. Premedication with acetaminophen (Children's Tylenol) sometimes can prevent this type of adverse reaction.

Allergic Reaction

Another type of non-hemolytic reaction is an allergic reaction. This reaction occurs during a transfusion in which the child has had a previous exposure to a particular allergen in the blood product. The exposure to this allergen stimulates an antibody response, and an allergic transfusion reaction is then evident. An allergic reaction may occur on the second or subsequent transfusions.

Signs and Symptoms.

Signs and symptoms include rash, hives, pruritus, swelling of the lips, wheezing, and anxiety.

Collaborative Care

Nursing Care. If the nurse suspects an allergic reaction, stop the transfusion, monitor vital signs, and notify the health-care provider.

Medical Care. In most cases, the administration of an antihistamine such as diphenhydramine (Benadryl) resolves an allergic response. A histamine blocker such as ranitidine (Zantac) may be administered to aid in symptom relief. In severe allergic reactions, the child may require the administration of steroids such as hydrocortisone (Solu-Cortef) and possibly adrenaline (Epinephrine). For future transfusions for this child, prophylaxis care may be required with diphenhydramine (Benadryl) and hydrocortisone (Solu-Cortef).

Bacterial Contamination

Bacterial contamination is a rare non-hemolytic reaction that generally occurs during the initiation of the infusion. The actual contamination of the blood product can occur anywhere during the process of collection, storage, and administration. Guidelines from the AABB (2011) require strict adherence to the completion of all transfusions in 4 hours or less to prevent this from happening. There are strict guidelines for blood collection centers on screening of potential donors, collection, and storage of blood products.

Signs and Symptoms

Signs and symptoms that may occur during a transfusion of blood that is contaminated are shaking chills, fever, vomiting, diffuse erythema, and the onset of hypotension that may progress to shock. In severe cases hemoglobinuria, actual renal failure, and disseminated intravascular coagulation may develop.

Collaborative Care

Nursing Care. If any of the signs and symptoms are identified, the nurse stops the transfusion, monitors vital signs, starts a normal saline infusion, notifies the health-care provider, and prepares for emergency care (support oxygenation and ventilation, antibiotics, and vasopressors may be ordered). Additionally, nursing responsibilities include obtaining blood samples for culture and sensitivity and sending the blood product with tubing to the blood bank also to be cultured.

Circulatory Overload

Circulatory overload is a rare occurrence in children. This reaction occurs when the infusion is given too rapidly or an excessive quantity of blood is given.

Signs and Symptoms

Signs and symptoms include dry cough, dyspnea, rales, distended neck veins, hypertension or hypotension, bradycardia, tachycardia, clammy skin, and cyanosis of the extremities.

Collaborative Care

Nursing Care. The nurse understands the importance of accurate verification of health-care provider orders, double-checks the volume to be infused, and uses an IV pump. The nurse is aware of children who are on fluid restriction and the accuracy of intake and output. If any of the signs and symptoms are identified, the nurse stops the transfusion, monitors vital signs, places the child upright with feet in a dependent position to increase venous resistance, notifies the health-care provider, and prepares for emergency care (support oxygenation and ventilation as well as diuretics may be ordered).

Acute Hemolytic Transfusion Reaction

Acute hemolytic transfusion reaction is rare, but it is the most severe type of reaction. It occurs when the donor

RBCs and the recipient plasma are incompatible, and there is an ABO mismatch. Acute hemolytic transfusion reactions occur upon initiation after exposure to a small amount of blood (Hillman et al., 2011).

Signs and Symptoms

Symptoms include fever, shaking chills, pain at the IV site, tightness of the chest, difficulties breathing, impending sense of doom, pallor, jaundice, nausea or vomiting, red or black urine, flank pain, and progressive signs of shock such as tachycardia and hypotension.

Collaborative Care

Nursing Care. If any of the signs and symptoms are identified, the nurse stops the transfusion, monitors vital signs, starts a normal saline infusion, verifies patient identification, notifies the health-care provider, and prepares for emergency care (support oxygenation and ventilation, antihistamines, fluids, diuretics, and vasopressors may be ordered). Other nursing responsibilities include obtaining blood and urine samples and sending them to the laboratory to analyze for the presence of hemoglobin, which indicates intravascular hemolysis. Insert a urinary catheter to monitor the child's output more accurately.

focus on safety

Transfusion-related acute lung injury

Transfusion-related acute lung injury (TRALI) is a major cause of transfusion-related morbidity and mortality. This complication occurs when there is an antigen-antibody reaction. This is not characterized as the typical allergic reaction. The causes of TRALI reactions are the antibodies that are found in the donated blood. These are antibodies to human leukocytes. The donor antibodies are infused to the patient and begin to attach to the patient's white blood cells and form microaggregates. These microaggregates often end up in the lungs, which may result in a vascular permeability, pulmonary edema, and life-threatening events (Bryant & Norville, 2011).

The child who is experiencing TRALI may develop respiratory distress such as shortness of breath, hypoxia, hypotension, fever, and abnormal breath sounds. The reaction typically occurs within 1 to 2 hours after the transfusion has started and full-blown acute respiratory distress may occur within 6 hours. For mild cases of TRALI, supportive care is indicated. Based on the severity of symptoms, respiratory support with a ventilator may be indicated. If this complication is suspected, it is reportable to the FDA (Bryant & Norville, 2011).

Education/Discharge Instructions

 Nursing Insight—*Teaching parents*

Children receiving blood transfusions require thorough teaching by the nurse to ease anxiety. The first transfusion of a blood product may be frightening for the child. If available, the use of a child life therapist to provide developmentally appropriate medical play could assist the child in understanding this required treatment. Teach parents to be aware of the signs and symptoms of an adverse reaction and to report any possible reaction signs and symptoms to the nurse immediately. Teaching by the nurse is tailored specifically to the type of blood product being administered.

Now Can You— Explain Blood Transfusion Therapy?

1. Discuss blood transfusion therapy?
2. Identify transfusion reactions?
3. Discuss education/discharge criteria for children receiving blood transfusion therapy?

Bone Marrow Transplantation

Hematopoietic stem cell transplant (HSCT) is the treatment for some types of oncological illnesses and hematological diseases. There are several types of hematological diseases in which HSCT may be a treatment option. For instance, a child newly diagnosed with severe aplastic anemia who has a human leukocyte antigen–matched (HLA-matched) sibling donor may proceed immediately to transplant as curative treatment. Children with other hematological disorders who have severe sequelae, including sickle cell disease with multiple complications such as cerebrovascular accidents and acute chest syndrome, may also be candidates to undergo an HSCT. Children who require chronic transfusion therapy may have the indications for HSCT such as beta-thalassemia and Diamond-Blackfan anemia. Some genetic and autoimmune diseases are now being treated with HSCT.

In these conditions, a large volume of actual bone marrow is harvested and bone marrow transplantation (BMT) is performed. The preparative BMT regimen consists of the administration of "near lethal" doses of chemotherapy and/or radiation to ablate the diseased bone marrow. This preparative regimen results in severe myelosuppression and places the child at grave risk for infection.

After the preparative regimen, the bone marrow is surgically obtained and then infused through a central line. Day "0" of the transplant process is the day that the patient receives the infusion of the stem cells. Following the infusion of the stem cells, waiting begins for engraftment (when the donated cells start to grow and make new blood cells). This treatment is not without potential risks, including death. This type of therapy may have lifelong consequences for the patient and his or her family, such as chronic immunosuppression, multiorgan failure, graft rejection, graft versus host disease, and long-term late effects.

Nursing Insight—*Hematopoietic stem cell transplants (HSCT)*

There are three types of HSCT:
   In an **autologous transplant**, the ill child is his or her own donor of stem cells. These donor stem cells are obtained by harvesting the child's cells through peripheral access or directly from the bone marrow cavity. This method is not used in hematological diseases because hematological illnesses originate in the bone marrow.
   In an **allogeneic transplant**, the recipient's HLAs are matched to a compatible donor, usually a sibling. The sibling must be tested by a thorough genetic investigation to determine if he or she is a carrier of the same hematological illness as the patient or is a compatible match before the transplant can occur. In other cases, the allogeneic donor is an unrelated

donor but is someone who has been identified from the National Marrow Donor Program. Umbilical cord blood stem cell transplant is another allogeneic type of transplant. These rich stem cells are obtained from the childbirth process immediately after delivery of the infant. The ability to obtain stem cells in this manner is a viable alternative that recently became available.
   In a **syngeneic transplant**, the donor of the bone marrow is an identical sibling.

Nursing Insight—*Hematological diseases cured by HSCT*

Indications for HSCT are:
   Severe aplastic anemia
   Beta-thalassemia
   Sickle cell disease
   Fanconi's anemia
   Kostmann's disease
   Diamond-Blackfan anemia

The child with a hematological illness who receives an HSCT must be prepared to live with potential complications. The majority of these children receive the HSCT from an unrelated donor. This carries a greater risk of long-term complications such as acute and chronic graft versus host disease. Other complications that may occur can be a result of the preparative regimen from the chemotherapy or radiation. Additional complications may result from infections, immunosuppression, organ dysfunction, and psychosocial impact.

Apheresis

Some children with hematological diseases may require apheresis as part of their treatment plan. The name of the apheresis procedure is identified according to a specific blood component that is extracted. This process usually takes place in the hospital setting with specially trained staff. In most institutions, children must be greater than 11 lb (5 kg).

The process of apheresis is the selective removal of a specific blood component from a donor or child while re-transfusing the remaining components. The ultimate goal in using apheresis therapy is to deplete or collect a circulating cell or substance. Blood is removed from the child, pumped through a special cell separator in the apheresis machine that removes the specific desired component by centrifugal force, and then is returned to the patient. The mechanics of the apheresis machine are comparable to those of a dialysis machine and require two large-bore lines, one line to draw from and another to return the blood.

Nursing Insight—*Apheresis*

There are three types of apheresis.
   Plasmapheresis
   Plasmapheresis is removal of plasma containing harmful components such as circulating complexes, antibodies

(IgM, IgG), cholesterol, and toxins. Plasma alone is depleted from the child's blood and replaced by donor plasma or a plasma substitute that is re-infused along with the child's own red blood cells (RBCs), white blood cells (WBCs), and platelets. Critically ill patients who have conditions such as thrombotic thrombocytopenic purpura, meningococcemia, toxic ingestion, hemolytic uremic syndrome, Guillain–Barré syndrome, and systemic lupus erythematosus may require a plasmapheresis.

Erythrocytapheresis (Red Cell Exchange)

In erythrocytapheresis (red cell exchange), RBCs are removed from the patient's blood and replaced by leukocyte-depleted donor red blood cells that are re-infused to the patient along with the patient's own plasma, WBCs, and platelets. Sickle cell anemia with acute chest syndrome, cerebrovascular accident, or severe priapism may require red cell exchange.

Leukapheresis (Stem Cell Collection or Leukodepletion)

The purpose of stem cell collection is to harvest an adequate amount of stem cells/mononuclear cells as noted by a countable marker on the white cell called a CD34 antigen. Based on the disease or reason for collecting, there may be multiple sessions to collect sufficient targeted cells. These mononuclear cells (monocytes) are involved in the body's immune responses. The collected stem cells are processed by the blood service and are cryopreserved in liquid nitrogen for future use. These stem cells are re-infused at a later specific date after the preparative regimen has ablated the bone marrow. Patients with solid tumors are the usual candidates to have their own stem cells removed, treated, and re-infused. Another procedure that may be used to remove excess white blood cells is leukodepletion. Leukodepletion is primarily used for patients with high WBC counts such as patients newly diagnosed with acute or chronic leukemia or at risk for acute tumor lysis syndrome. Complications may develop during the apheresis process (Table 32-9).

Thrombosis

A possible hematological complication for patients with chronic illness includes the development of a thrombosis (blood clot). A thrombosis is an abnormal formation of blood constituents within the vascular system. Thrombi can be caused by a variety of factors, such as prolonged immobility, disease states, major surgery or trauma, hypercoagulability, venous access devices, obesity, medications, and hereditary factors. Additional complications of thrombi include stroke, deep vein thrombosis, and pulmonary emboli. Certain disease states promote a higher incidence of thrombi, such as sickle cell anemia, malignancies, and diseases of coagulation.

Table 32-9 Complications of Apheresis	
Complication	**Critical Nursing Actions**
Hypocalcemia	Obtain ionized calcium levels before treatment. Correct all abnormal levels before initiating treatment. For apheresis lasting longer than 1 hour, ionized calcium level is monitored every hour until the end of the procedure. Consider calcium drip if needed: • Calcium chloride: 20–25 mg/kg per dose used for acute hypocalcemia • Calcium gluconate: 100–500 mg/kg/day (Retrieved from www.drugs.com)
Hypotension	Hypotension may occur with onset of treatment. Be sure to have fluid readily available at the bedside. Patients receiving inotropic support may need an increase in the rate of administration.
Risk for Bleeding	Prothrombin time (PT), partial thromboplastin time (PTT), fibrinogen level, platelet count, Hct, and activated clotting time (ACT) are measured before and after apheresis. ACT is measured at the bedside at regular intervals, and citrate and/or heparin doses adjusted accordingly. Platelets or other blood products such as clotting factors may be required during the procedure.
Hypothermia	Hypothermia may result from the blood being circulated in the extracorporeal circuit outside the body. • Use blood warmer on pheresis machine. • Monitor frequent temperatures to avoid hypothermia. • Assess patient for other signs of hypothermia such as bradycardia and shivering. • Keep child warm with blankets and/or external warmer. • Increase ambient room temperature.
Transfusion Reaction	Use leukodepleted blood. Monitor for transfusion reactions from the replacement products. Follow the transfusion reaction protocol if this occurs. Consider administration of an antihistamine for patients receiving multiple treatments.
Infection	Maintain strict sterile technique with all IV lines.
Air Embolism	Monitor tubing and connection sites. Check that all are secured properly.
Thrombus	Obtain platelet count before catheter placement and be aware when possible transfusion of platelets is necessary. Flush vigorously with adequate volumes of normal saline as per institutional policy.

Signs and Symptoms

A blood clot in the lungs causes a sudden pain in the side of the chest, shortness of breath, light-headedness, or increased heart rate. If blood appears in the urine, there may be a blood clot in the kidneys. In the skin, small hemorrhagic spots may appear. If there is a blood clot in a large artery of an extremity (arm or leg), an obstruction occurs and the extremity becomes cold, pale, blue, and the pulse disappears below the obstructed site (Venes, 2013).

Diagnosis

Diagnosis of thrombosis is based on a nursing assessment of the lungs, urine, and skin or red, swollen, or tender extremity. A venogram (an x-ray test that shows the blood flow through the veins) is used as well as a Doppler ultrasound exam of a limb. A D-dimer blood test is also drawn.

Prevention

Preventing thrombus formation starts with early ambulation and use of assistive devices such as intermittent pneumatic compression or the usage of anti-embolism stockings. Hospitalized patients with potential risk factors are identified early, and preventive care is implemented. Patients who have thrombus formation are managed medically and observed for possible complications.

Collaborative Care

Nursing Care. Nursing care for children with hematological diseases includes a thorough assessment of the child's risk factors for developing a thrombus. When caring for a child at risk for thrombosis, a prophylactic plan of care is individualized for each child's condition, and interventions are reviewed daily for effectiveness. Nursing assessment also includes a thorough skin assessment under the stocking and compression device to evaluate for redness or skin breakdown. Implementing early ambulation when appropriate is an additional preventive measure.

The most serious complication associated with thrombi is the possibility of developing pulmonary emboli (sudden blockage in the lungs) that can result in a life-threatening event. Deep venous thrombosis occurs less often in children than in adults, but when it does, it has the same potential for pulmonary embolization and death. Institutions have implemented formal protocols to identify children at risk for thrombolytic events and implement preventive measures.

Medical Care. All children on prolonged bedrest and those at high risk have prophylaxis care, which may include compression stockings, intermittent pneumatic compression devices, and passive range of motion. Compression stockings and intermittent pneumatic compression devices are usually used on the lower extremities. These assistive devices may promote increased venous flow and decreased venous pooling and stasis. These devices can be discontinued when the patient is ambulatory. Some children may benefit from the administration of low molecular weight heparin therapy (Rummell, 2013).

Education/Discharge Instructions

Discharge teaching includes avoiding activities such as prolonged sitting and bedrest, which may precipitate clot formation. Other teaching includes smoking cessation and avoiding drugs that cause blood clots (such as birth control pills). Teaching families also includes telling them that when traveling for extended periods of time (airplane or car travel) to move from the seat if safely permitted to take a short walk. The use of anti-embolism stockings is encouraged for daily use if risk factors are high for clot formation.

Summary Points

◆ Blood is composed of two parts, the fluid portion called plasma and the cellular portion. The solutes include albumin, electrolytes, proteins, clotting factors, fibrinogen, globulins, and circulating antibodies. The cellular portion consists of the formed elements: red blood cells, white blood cells, and platelets.

◆ Several common hematological conditions occur in children. Some of these conditions can be acute in nature and with proper care can be easily managed. However, others can be life-threatening or cause a chronic illness that can permanently impact the lifestyle of the child and his or her family.

◆ The nurse can stress to the parents that the primary goal with regard to iron-deficiency anemia is prevention. Nursing care consists of nutritional counseling, assistance with obtaining recommended iron-fortified formula or cereal, and the administration of oral iron supplements.

◆ Children and families affected by sickle cell disease must learn to cope with this lifelong chronic illness. The community-based nurse can educate the family about the goals of ongoing care, including the prevention of complications associated with infections, hypoxemia, and vaso-occlusive crisis.

◆ Because there is no known cure for hemophilia, the interdisciplinary health-care team members including physicians, nurses, rehabilitative services, social workers, child life specialists, and school personnel are instrumental in teaching the family about how to care for their child with hemophilia.

◆ Aplastic anemia is rare but one of the most serious hematological conditions that generally afflicts adolescents and young adults. This clinical syndrome is characterized by pancytopenia (a reduction in all cellular elements of the blood) caused by bone marrow hematopoiesis failure.

◆ Neutropenia can be congenital or acquired. All patients will need specific teaching on home management, including infection prevention measures such as the importance of hand washing.

◆ The first responsibility of the nurse who is administering a blood transfusion to a child is to review the plan of care with the family, explain in detail the indications and process of a blood transfusion, and then obtain blood consent from the appropriate individual.

◆ During every transfusion the importance of strict observance to the institutional policy regarding the administration of blood products cannot be stressed enough. In addition, the accuracy of patient verification is a critical nursing action that prevents this type of acute hemolytic transfusion reaction.

◆ Some children with hematological diseases may require apheresis as part of their treatment plan. The process of apheresis is the selective removal of a specific blood component from a donor or child while re-transfusing the remaining components.

◆ A possible hematological complication for patients with chronic illness includes the development of a thrombosis. A thrombosis is an abnormal formation of blood constituents within the vascular system.

Review Questions

Multiple Choice

1. A nurse is reviewing the lab values for a toddler. The child's hemoglobin is 7.7 g/dL. How would the nurse characterize the child's results?
   A. Normal
   B. Slightly anemic
   C. Moderately anemic
   D. Polycythemia

2. A student nurse is teaching the mother of an infant ways to prevent iron-deficiency anemia. Which instruction causes the registered nurse to intervene and correct the teaching?
   A. "Give your child whole milk instead of low-fat milk."
   B. "Be sure to feed your child iron-fortified cereals."
   C. "Offer solid foods first, then give your child a bottle."
   D. "WIC can provide you with iron-fortified infant formula."

3. A nurse is reviewing a chart on a child who has sickle cell disease and notes the diagnosis "dactylitis." What does the nurse understand about this condition?
   A. Prolonged painful erection
   B. Atypical pneumonia
   C. Avascular necrosis of the hip
   D. Hand-foot syndrome

4. The pediatric nurse is aware that which disease process is the most commonly inherited genetic disease worldwide?
   A. Sickle cell anemia
   B. Beta-thalassemia
   C. Cooley's anemia
   D. Hemosiderosis

5. A child's lab values show red blood cells that are small, dense, and round with a hemoglobin value of 8.5 g/dL. Based on these laboratory findings, which disease process does the nurse suspect?
   A. Hemosiderosis
   B. Cooley's anemia
   C. Hereditary spherocytosis
   D. Hemophilia

6. A school-aged child is diagnosed with hemarthrosis after tripping and falling. Which diagnostic testing is the priority for this child?
   A. Hemoglobin and hematocrit
   B. Bilateral knee radiographs
   C. Partial thromboplastin time
   D. Plasma factor activity

7. When teaching the parents of a child diagnosed with von Willebrand's disease, which information is most appropriate for the nurse to provide?
   A. Boys are affected twice as often as girls.
   B. Only female children will be affected.
   C. Boys and girls are affected equally often.
   D. This disease is not inherited and occurs randomly.

8. A child is diagnosed with chronic immune thrombocytopenia. Which diagnostic platelet count supports this diagnosis?
   A. Below 5,000
   B. Below 10,000
   C. Below 50,000
   D. Below 150,000

9. A pediatric intensive care nurse is providing care to a patient with disseminated intravascular coagulation. Which treatment option is most appropriate for this patient?
   A. Treat the underlying condition
   B. Administer massive blood transfusions
   C. Therapeutic hypothermia
   D. Routine vitamin K administration

10. A child is admitted with neutropenia. Which nursing action takes priority?
    A. Place the child on contact isolation.
    B. Maintain strict handwashing.
    C. Disinfect belongings brought from home.
    D. Do not allow visitors in the child's room.

See Answers to End of Chapter Review Questions on DavisPlus.

REFERENCES

American Association of Blood Banks (AABB). *Standards for blood banks and transfusion services* (27th ed.). (2011). AABB Press: Bethesda, MD.

Baker, R., Greer, F., & The Committee on Nutrition. (2010). Clinical report: Diagnosis and prevention of iron deficiency and iron-deficiency anemia in infants and young children (0–3 years of age). *Pediatrics, 126*(5), 1040–1050.

Brotanek, J., Gosz, J., Weitzman, M., & Flores, G. (2007). Iron deficiency in early childhood in the United States: Risk factor and racial/ethnic disparities. *Pediatrics, 120*, 568–575.

Bryant, R., & Norville, R. (2011). Management of blood component deficiencies. In C. Baggott, D. Fochtman, G. V. Foley, & K. P. Kelly (Eds.), *Nursing care of children and adolescents with cancer and blood disorders* (4th edition, pp. 583–611). Glenview, IL: Association of Pediatric Hematology/Oncology Nurses.

Burke, M., & Salani, D. (2013). Hematology and oncologic emergencies requiring critical care. In *Hazinski nursing care of the critically ill child* (pp. 825–850). St. Louis, MO: Elsevier.

Dale, J. C., Cochran, C. J., Roy, L., Jernigan, E., & Buchanan, G. R. (2011). Health-related quality of life in children and adolescents with sickle cell disease. *Journal of Pediatric Health Care, 25*(4), 208–215.

Goldman, L., & Schafer, A. (2012). *Goldman's Cecil medicine* (24th ed.). Philadelphia, PA: Elsevier.

Hillman, R. S., Ault, K. A., Leporrier, M., & Rinder, H. M. (2011). *Hematology in clinical practice* (5th ed.). New York, NY: McGraw-Hill.

Linnard-Palmar, L., & Kools, S. (2004). Parents' refusal of medical treatment based on religious and/or cultural beliefs: The law, ethical principles and clinical implications. *Journal of Pediatric Nursing, 19*(5), 351–356.

Munn, J., & Valdiviez, L. (2011). Bleeding disorders and thromboses. In C. Baggott, D. Fochtman, G. Foley, & K. Patterson (Eds.), *Nursing care of children and adolescents with cancer and blood disorders* (4th ed., 818–876). Glenview, IL: Association of Pediatric Hematology Oncology Nurses.

Nathan, D. G., Orkin, S. H., Ginsburg, D., & Look, A. T. (2009). *Nathan and Oski's hematology of infancy and childhood* (7th ed.). Philadelphia, PA: W.B. Saunders.

Oliveira, V., Frazão, E., & Smallwood, D. (2010). Rising infant formula costs to the WIC program: Recent trends in rebates and wholesale prices. Retrieved from www.ers.usda.gov/Publications/ERR93/ERR93.pdf

Rummell, M. (2013). Cardiovascular disorders. In *Hazinski nursing care of the critically ill child* (pp. 181–482). St. Louis, MO: Elsevier.

Speller-Brown, B., Eimicke, T., & Martin, B. (2011). Management of red blood cell disorders. In C. Baggott, D. Fochtman, G. V. Foley, & K. P. Kelly (Eds.), *Nursing care of children and adolescents with cancer and blood disorders* (4th edition, pp. 766–817). Glenview, IL: Association of Pediatric Hematology/Oncology Nurses.

Stevens, R. (1999). The history of haemophilia in the royal families of Europe. *British Journal of Haematology, 105*(1), 25–32.

Turgeon, M. L. (2012). *Clinical hematology: Theory and procedures* (5th ed.). Philadelphia, PA: Lippincott Williams & Wilkins.

Vallerand, A. H., & Sanoski, C. A. (2014). *Davis's drug guide for nurses* (14th ed.). Philadelphia, PA: F.A. Davis.

Van Leeuwen, A. M., Poelhuis-Leth, D. J., & Bladh, M. L. (2011). *Davis's comprehensive handbook of laboratory and diagnostic tests*. Philadelphia, PA: F.A. Davis.

Venes, D. (Ed.). (2013). *Taber's cyclopedic medical dictionary* (22nd ed.). Philadelphia, PA: F.A. Davis.

Ward, S. (2013). *Pediatric nursing care: Best evidence-based practices*. Philadelphia, PA: F.A. Davis.

Women, Infants, and Children. (2014). Retrieved from http://www.fns.usda.gov/wic/women-infants-and-children-wic

World Health Organization. (2013). Micronutrient deficiencies. Iron Deficiency anaemia. Retrieved from http://www.who.int/nutrition/topics/ida/en/index.html

DavisPlus | For more information, go to **http://davisplus.fadavis.com/**

CONCEPT MAP

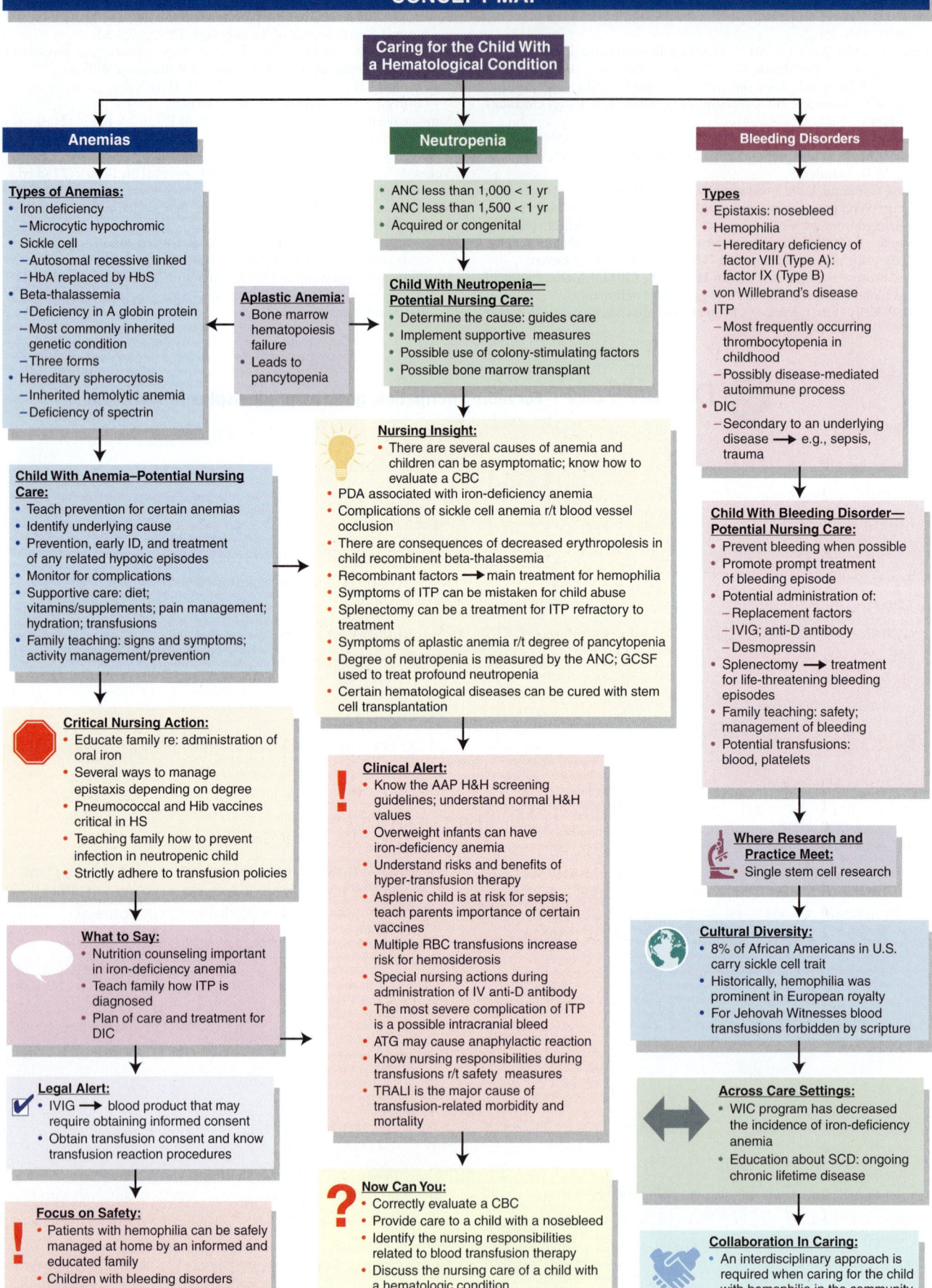

Caring for the Child With a Hematological Condition

Anemias

Types of Anemias:
- Iron deficiency
  - Microcytic hypochromic
- Sickle cell
  - Autosomal recessive linked
  - HbA replaced by HbS
- Beta-thalassemia
  - Deficiency in A globin protein
  - Most commonly inherited genetic condition
  - Three forms
- Hereditary spherocytosis
  - Inherited hemolytic anemia
  - Deficiency of spectrin

Child With Anemia–Potential Nursing Care:
- Teach prevention for certain anemias
- Identify underlying cause
- Prevention, early ID, and treatment of any related hypoxic episodes
- Monitor for complications
- Supportive care: diet; vitamins/supplements; pain management; hydration; transfusions
- Family teaching: signs and symptoms; activity management/prevention

Critical Nursing Action:
- Educate family re: administration of oral iron
- Several ways to manage epistaxis depending on degree
- Pneumococcal and Hib vaccines critical in HS
- Teaching family how to prevent infection in neutropenic child
- Strictly adhere to transfusion policies

What to Say:
- Nutrition counseling important in iron-deficiency anemia
- Teach family how ITP is diagnosed
- Plan of care and treatment for DIC

Legal Alert:
- IVIG ➞ blood product that may require obtaining informed consent
- Obtain transfusion consent and know transfusion reaction procedures

Focus on Safety:
- Patients with hemophilia can be safely managed at home by an informed and educated family
- Children with bleeding disorders should wear a Medical Alert bracelet

Neutropenia

- ANC less than 1,000 < 1 yr
- ANC less than 1,500 < 1 yr
- Acquired or congenital

Aplastic Anemia:
- Bone marrow hematopoiesis failure
- Leads to pancytopenia

Child With Neutropenia— Potential Nursing Care:
- Determine the cause: guides care
- Implement supportive measures
- Possible use of colony-stimulating factors
- Possible bone marrow transplant

Nursing Insight:
- There are several causes of anemia and children can be asymptomatic; know how to evaluate a CBC
- PDA associated with iron-deficiency anemia
- Complications of sickle cell anemia r/t blood vessel occlusion
- There are consequences of decreased erythropolesis in child recombinent beta-thalassemia
- Recombinant factors ➞ main treatment for hemophilia
- Symptoms of ITP can be mistaken for child abuse
- Splenectomy can be a treatment for ITP refractory to treatment
- Symptoms of aplastic anemia r/t degree of pancytopenia
- Degree of neutropenia is measured by the ANC; GCSF used to treat profound neutropenia
- Certain hematological diseases can be cured with stem cell transplantation

Clinical Alert:
- Know the AAP H&H screening guidelines; understand normal H&H values
- Overweight infants can have iron-deficiency anemia
- Understand risks and benefits of hyper-transfusion therapy
- Asplenic child is at risk for sepsis; teach parents importance of certain vaccines
- Multiple RBC transfusions increase risk for hemosiderosis
- Special nursing actions during administration of IV anti-D antibody
- The most severe complication of ITP is a possible intracranial bleed
- ATG may cause anaphylactic reaction
- Know nursing responsibilities during transfusions r/t safety measures
- TRALI is the major cause of transfusion-related morbidity and mortality

Now Can You:
- Correctly evaluate a CBC
- Provide care to a child with a nosebleed
- Identify the nursing responsibilities related to blood transfusion therapy
- Discuss the nursing care of a child with a hematologic condition

Bleeding Disorders

Types
- Epistaxis: nosebleed
- Hemophilia
  - Hereditary deficiency of factor VIII (Type A): factor IX (Type B)
- von Willebrand's disease
- ITP
  - Most frequently occurring thrombocytopenia in childhood
  - Possibly disease-mediated autoimmune process
- DIC
  - Secondary to an underlying disease ➞ e.g., sepsis, trauma

Child With Bleeding Disorder— Potential Nursing Care:
- Prevent bleeding when possible
- Promote prompt treatment of bleeding episode
- Potential administration of:
  - Replacement factors
  - IVIG; anti-D antibody
  - Desmopressin
- Splenectomy ➞ treatment for life-threatening bleeding episodes
- Family teaching: safety; management of bleeding
- Potential transfusions: blood, platelets

Where Research and Practice Meet:
- Single stem cell research

Cultural Diversity:
- 8% of African Americans in U.S. carry sickle cell trait
- Historically, hemophilia was prominent in European royalty
- For Jehovah Witnesses blood transfusions forbidden by scripture

Across Care Settings:
- WIC program has decreased the incidence of iron-deficiency anemia
- Education about SCD: ongoing chronic lifetime disease

Collaboration In Caring:
- An interdisciplinary approach is required when caring for the child with hemophilia in the community

Caring for the Child With Cancer

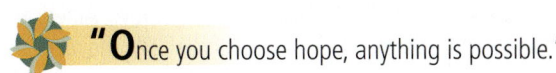

> "**O**nce you choose hope, anything is possible."

—Christopher Reeve

LEARNING TARGETS *At the completion of this chapter, the student will be able to:*

◆ Describe the anatomy and physiology related to the pattern of tumor progression.

◆ Examine common childhood cancers.

◆ Prioritize developmentally appropriate and holistic nursing care for common childhood cancers.

◆ Explore diagnostic and laboratory testing, and medications for common childhood cancers.

◆ Explore the negative and long-term effects of chemotherapy for children with common childhood cancers.

◆ Examine the medical emergencies that occur in children with common childhood cancers.

◆ Develop teaching plans and discharge criteria, including the psychological impact for parents whose children have common cancers.

PICO(T) Question

The intent of evidence-based practice (EBP) is to provide nursing care that integrates the best available evidence. An initial step in EBP is to write a PICO(T) question that effectively guides the research. A PICO(T) question is an acronym that stands for population (P), intervention or issue (I), comparison of interest (C), outcome (O), and timeframe (T). Depending on the question, all or some of the question components are used in the research process. Use these

PICO(T) questions to spark your thinking as you read the chapter.

1. Is there (O) a difference in the (I) rate of recurrence of non-Hodgkin's lymphoma in (P) children age 10 or younger (C) compared with children over age 10?

2. What (I) nursing interventions are shown to be (O) most beneficial in assisting (P) parents at the time they first learn of their child being diagnosed with cancer?

 Evidence-Based Practice

Martin, S., Calabrese, S. K., Wolters, P. L., Walter, K. A., Warren, K., & Hazra, R. (2012). Family functioning and coping styles in families of children with cancer and HIV disease. *Clinical Pediatrics, 51*(1), 58–64.

The purpose of this study was to compare family functioning and coping styles among children with cancer or HIV disease and their families. It is well known that serious illness in a child can have a profound impact on family functioning and coping. Serious illnesses impact family lifestyle, finances, and social relationships. According to the authors, the unique experiences of families of children with serious diseases are poorly understood. Previous research notes a lack of agreement on the findings. Some studies have noted that families do not experience long-term impairment, while others report significant negative effects on families. One study noted that a significant portion of participants met the criteria for psychiatric disorders or clinically significant dysfunction. Coping strategies may be implemented by families in response to stress caused by serious illness in a child. The strategies have

(continued)

Evidence-Based Practice (continued)

been categorized as active or passive. Active coping is goal-oriented, uses problem-solving techniques, and has been linked to positive psychological outcomes. Passive coping is associated with psychological dysfunction and may involve denial or disengagement. The authors note that, based on previous research, the perception of family coping remains unclear, hence a need for further research.

Participants in this study included the families or caregivers of 44 children with cancer and 65 children with vertically acquired HIV. Criteria for inclusion included children between the ages of 0 and 18 years of age who had been diagnosed at least 6 months prior. This study was done as part of a larger study conducted at the National Cancer Institute (NCI). Participants for the larger study were referred by medical providers from across the country. Data were collected during routine outpatient visits. With the exception of 18-year-old patients, the family or primary caregiver provided the responses. Responses were gathered through the use of questionnaires. These included the family assessment device (FAD), which contains a 12-item global functioning scale (GFS). This tool uses a 4-point Likert-type scale with responses ranging from "strongly agree" to "strongly disagree." The tool was designed to assess overall health and pathology in the family. The family crisis oriented personal evaluation scale (F-COPES) is a 29-item tool that uses a 5-point Likert-type scale with responses ranging from "strongly agree" to "strongly disagree." This tool measures coping strategies used to react to difficult circumstances. This tool includes 5 subscales: "Acquiring Social Support (actively seeking support from others; 9 items), Reframing (redefining stressful events to improve their manageability; 8 items), Seeking Spiritual Support (using involvement in an organized religion; 4 items), Mobilizing Family Support (ascertaining community resources and assistance from others; 4 items), and Passive Appraisal (minimizing reactivity to stressors; 4 items)" (p. 59). Reliability and validity for both instruments have been well established. A demographic questionnaire was also used to obtain data regarding race, gender, caregiver education, family composition, and caregiver relationship to the child.

Data were analyzed using analysis of variance to assess relationship of illness to family functioning and coping. *T*-tests were used to examine the differences between social support items. Pearson correlations were used to assess the relationships between functioning and coping strategies. The mean age of the patients in the cancer group was 10.9 years and ranged from 2 to 18. The mean number of years since their diagnosis was 3.5 years. Cancer diagnoses included 20% leukemia and 80% nervous system tumors. Sixty-one percent of the children had undergone radiation, 59% had used standard chemotherapy regimens, and 59% had experienced surgical resection. Eighty-two percent of those completing the questionnaires were mothers, and the mean education level of the caregiver was 14.6 years, with a range from 6 to 19 years. The mean age of the patients in the

HIV group was 11.2 and ranged from 3 to 18. The mean number of years since diagnosis was 9.8 years. The majority of children (86%) were on highly active antiretroviral therapy. The majority of respondents were mothers (75%), and the mean education level of the respondents answering the questionnaire, with the range of education being from 8 years of schooling to 19 years of schooling, was 13.7 years. Ninety-six percent of the caregivers for the children with cancer were a biological parent as opposed to 43% of the HIV children. Twenty-three percent of the family composition of the cancer patients were from a single-parent home compared with 38% of the HIV patients. The race designations of the cancer patients were as follows: Caucasian 64%, African American 23%, Hispanic 7%, Native American 0%, Asian/Pacific Islander 4%, and multiracial 2%. The race designations of the HIV patients were as follows: Caucasian 42%, African American 43%, Hispanic 11%, Native American 3%, Asian/Pacific Islander 0%, and multiracial 2%. Gender designations are as follows: Cancer patients included 57% males, and HIV patients included 54% males.

Twenty percent of the families in both the cancer and HIV groups scored at the unhealthy range of global functioning (GFS), which was not considered significantly different between groups. The researchers reported that families with children who had cancer scored significantly higher than the families with children who had HIV on the "Acquiring Social Support" subscale of the F-COPES scale. Further analysis found that families of children with HIV sought support among family members versus non-family members, which was more common in the families of children with cancer. The researchers also noted that lower GFS scores (indicating better functioning) among families with children who had cancer were noted to have higher F-COPES "Reframing" scores, which indicated more frequent use of reframing as a tool for coping. Among families with children who had HIV, lower GFS scores were correlated with higher F-COPES "Passive Appraisal" scores, which indicated minimizing reactivity to stress.

The researchers conclude that the majority of caregivers reported healthy family functioning with no between-group differences. In relation to coping, families of children with cancer relied more on social support than did families of children with HIV, though both groups also relied on family members for assistance with coping. The researchers further concluded that coping strategies and implications for family functioning vary depending on the condition and that active coping and reframing can improve functioning among families of children with cancer.

1. How is this information useful to clinical nursing practice?

2. Based on these findings, what are implications for further research?

See Suggested Responses for Evidence-Based Practice on Davis*Plus*.

Introduction

This chapter describes the anatomy and physiology related to the pattern of tumor progression in children with cancer. The discussion includes an examination of the common childhood cancers, including developmentally appropriate and holistic nursing care. Information is given about diagnostic and laboratory testing and medications. Teaching plans and discharge criteria are incorporated, including the psychological impact for parents whose children have common childhood cancers.

Cancer is a group of diseases in which there is out-of-control growth and spread of abnormal cells (**anaplasia**). Anaplastic cells resist normal growth controls. This abnormal cellular growth is also known as a neoplasm and is caused by one or a combination of three factors: (1) external or environmental stimuli, (2) viruses that can alter the immune system and let the cancer grow, and (3) chromosomal and gene abnormalities.

CARING FOR THE CHILD WITH CANCER

A & P review **Pattern of Tumor Progression**

A tumor originates as a single, transformed cell somewhere in the body. That cell must undergo a long process of growth and development before it can form a tumor. The cell also undergoes countless divisions to form a mass that may be made up of a billion cells at the time of diagnosis. Tumor cells have very stringent constraints placed on them as they grow. Each of the newly created cells must have a steady supply of nutrients to keep growing. While the tumor may not be directly next to a capillary, it may be close enough so that oxygen and nutrients can diffuse through tissue to tumor cells. If the tumor receives a continuous supply of nutrients and blood, it grows and invades surrounding tissue. Once a tumor grows past its critical phase, it induces growth of new blood vessels into the tumor mass. It can then grow much more rapidly and

produce a clinically detectable tumor. If a tumor does not receive adequate blood supply and nutrients, it can die. A tumor lacking a sufficient blood supply can also remain dormant for years and not grow beyond a certain size (Fig. 33-1). ◆

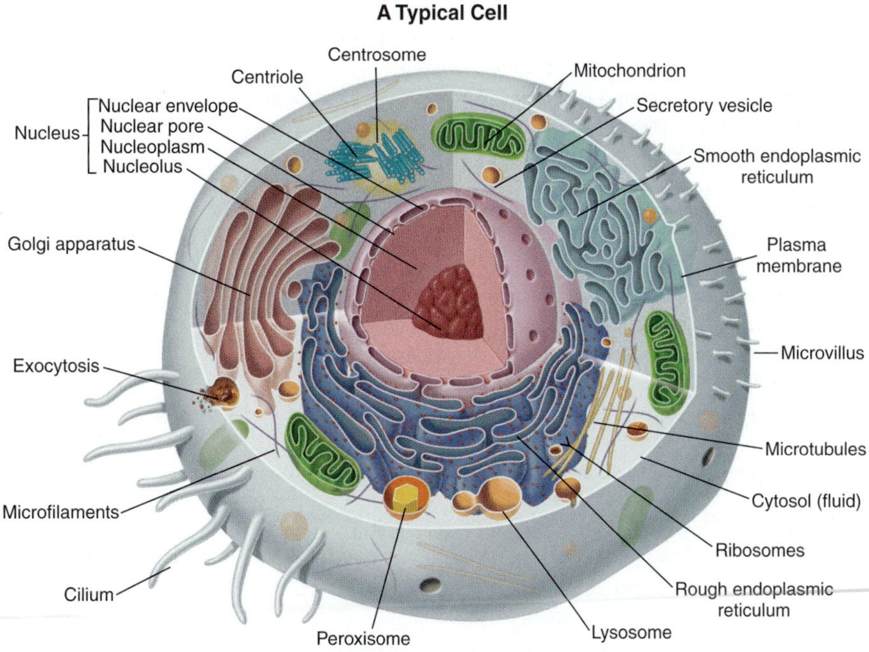

Growth and Development

The child with cancer experiences alterations or lags in growth and development because of altered nutrition, fatigue, pain, social isolation, and complications from the disease process requiring frequent hospital admissions. Nursing care for the child with cancer includes a variety of interventions geared toward minimizing the effects of the disease process on the child's growth and development.

Good nutrition is essential for the growing child to maintain normal growth and development. The child with cancer may experience altered nutrition, less than body requirements, because of the inability to ingest enough calories to meet the demands of the body and the disease process. The nurse should encourage the child to eat small, frequent, high-calorie meals to meet the body's increased metabolic needs. The nurse should promote good oral hygiene to prevent complications of pharmacological therapies. Enteral and parenteral nutrition should be implemented when needed. A nutritionist should be used to identify appropriate resources for the child.

Normal activity supports self-esteem and self-knowledge, so the nurse should encourage activity and play while allowing for adequate periods of rest because the child with cancer may fatigue easily. Quiet activities should be encouraged when the child has low levels of energy. The nurse should frequently assess the child's pain and implement appropriate pain relief measures to encourage activity and play.

Peer contact and schoolwork promote cognitive and social growth and development, so the nurse should encourage the child to attend school, or see peers when unable to attend school, to avoid social isolation. The nurse should work closely with schoolteachers and child life workers to identify schoolwork needs and support reentry to school when appropriate.

Source: Ward S., & Hisley, S. (2009). *Maternal-child nursing care: Optimizing outcomes for mothers, children & families.* Philadelphia, PA: F.A. Davis.

A Typical Cell

Labels: Centrosome, Centriole, Mitochondrion, Nuclear envelope, Nuclear pore, Nucleoplasm, Nucleolus (Nucleus), Secretory vesicle, Smooth endoplasmic reticulum, Golgi apparatus, Plasma membrane, Microvillus, Exocytosis, Microtubules, Cytosol (fluid), Microfilaments, Ribosomes, Rough endoplasmic reticulum, Cilium, Peroxisome, Lysosome

Figure 33-1 Typical cell.

Nursing Insight—*Cell division*

Normal cells divide in an orderly fashion through the four phases of cell division. Normal cells have a control mechanism that stops division when it is complete. Cancer cells have no control mechanism and keep dividing and replicating unchecked without stopping.

Nursing Insight—*Understanding cancer*

An oncogene is a gene found in a virus that has the ability to encourage a cell to become malignant (Venes, 2013). A tumor is a mass of abnormally growing cells that is either benign (not cancerous), with slow and limited noninvasive growth, or malignant (cancerous), a progressively virulent growth. Cancerous growths are divided further into solid tumors (e.g., a brain tumor) and systemic cancers, such as leukemia. Cancer is second only to accidents as the leading cause of death among children. It is important for the nurse to understand the terms associated with cancer (Box 33-1).

Nursing Insight—*Staging*

Staging describes the severity of the patient's cancer. It is the process of classifying tumors in relation to the degree of differentiation, possibility of responding to therapy, and prognosis (Venes, 2013).

> Stage 0 indicates early cancer that is present only in the layer of cells in which it began.
> Stage I, Stage II, and Stage III indicate more extensive disease, greater tumor size, and/or spread of the cancer to nearby lymph nodes or adjacent organs.
> Stage IV indicates that the cancer has spread to another organ(s).

Box 33-1 Terms Associated With the Cancer Patient

Roadmap—protocol or treatment plan that is "mapped out" to guide staff and families through the treatment course.

Protocol—complete explanation of a treatment plan, includes background, drug dosages and timing, and protocol requirements such as tests and laboratory specimens.

Clinical trials—medical research studies conducted with volunteers. Each study is designed to answer scientific questions and to find new ways to treat cancer.

Remission—the partial or complete disappearance of signs and symptoms of disease. This does not mean "cancer free." There could still be cancer cells that are undetectable in the body. Treatment will continue during this time.

Extravasation—leaking of vesicants that can cause tissue damage surrounding the IV or central line insertion site; blistering, blanching, or excoriation may lead to ulceration and deep skin sloughing.

Induction—chemotherapy given to achieve remission.

Consolidation—chemotherapy given after induction to control microscopic disease.

Maintenance—chemotherapy given on a long-term basis to maintain remission.

Palliative care—treatment given to relieve rather than cure symptoms caused by cancer. Supportive care services are usually involved. The patient may still receive chemotherapy or radiation.

Nursing Insight—*Differences between childhood and adult cancers*

Anatomically and physiologically, cancers in children differ greatly from the types of cancer occurring in adults. In children, many common malignancies arise from primitive embryonic tissue in which there is a strong environmental link related to the development of cancer.

Across Care Settings: **Common guidelines**

Common guidelines for childhood cancer survivors are:
- Childhood cancer survivors should have their height measured regularly.
- Pre-pubertal girls should be closely monitored for signs of early onset puberty.
- Patients who have evidence of impaired fertility should be referred to a specialist for ongoing assessment.
- Neck, spine, or brain radiotherapy may warrant ongoing thyroid function observation.
- Follow-up appointments are important.
- Give patients written summaries about their diagnosis, treatment, and possible late treatment side effects.
- A multidisciplinary team approach is important in the ongoing care of the patient.

Nursing Insight—*New therapies for cancer treatment*

The use of gene therapy is complex and in the early stages of usage for cancer patients. Gene therapy is used to understand and treat the genetic mutations that cause disease. *Immunotherapy,* the concept of boosting immune cells to destroy cancer cells, has been a goal of cancer treatment for many years. Limited success has been achieved with immunotherapy because cancer cells tend to evolve, mutating to evade immune detection.

Oncolytic agents are a growing area of gene therapy in which genetically engineered and altered viruses are used to target and destroy cancer cells while remaining innocuous to the rest of the body. *Gene transfer* is the insertion or transfer of a foreign gene into the cancer cell or surrounding tissue. Genes with a number of different functions have been proposed for this type of therapy. This area is vast and shows great possibilities for the future treatment of cancer.

Where Research and Practice Meet: **Long-Term Survival**

Childhood cancer survivors rates are improving. However, possible treatment effects discovered later in life may include problems with the cardiovascular, pulmonary, and/or endocrine systems or include possible renal issues and secondary tumors as well as cognitive, educational, neuropsychological, and/or social manifestations.

Now Can You—Discuss cancer in children?

1. Describe the pattern of tumor progression?
2. Differentiate between childhood and adult cancers?
3. Discuss new therapies for cancer treatment?

Common Childhood Cancers

PREVENTION OF COMMON CHILDHOOD CANCER

While prevention is not always possible with pediatric cancer, early detection is key in having a better prognosis and positive outcome. Today, health-care providers order x-rays and computed tomography (CT) scans more sparingly than in the past because limiting children's exposure to radiation may prevent future risks of developing cancer. The cause of cancer is still unknown, but genetics, environmental factors, and viruses may play a part in the development of childhood cancer. The typical warning signs of cancer may or may not apply to the type of cancers children acquire. However, a basic understanding of early warning signs is important. The American Cancer Society uses the word C-A-U-T-I-O-N to help recognize the seven early signs of cancer:

Change in bowel or bladder habits
A sore that does not heal
Unusual bleeding or discharge
Thickening or lump in the breast, testicles, or elsewhere
Indigestion or difficulty swallowing
Obvious change in the size, color, shape, or thickness of a wart, mole, or mouth sore
Nagging cough or hoarseness

Other symptoms may also indicate the existence of some types of cancer:

- Persistent headaches
- Unexplained loss of weight or loss of appetite
- Chronic pain in bones or any other areas of the body
- Persistent fatigue, nausea, or vomiting
- Persistent low-grade fever, either constant or intermittent
- Repeated infection

LEUKEMIA

The term leukemia refers to the cancers of the blood-forming cells or hematopoiesis. There are two types of blood-forming cells: myeloid and lymphoid. Myeloid cells (Fig. 33-2) differentiate and form into red blood cells, monocytes, granulocytes, and platelets. Lymphoid cells differentiate and form into B cells and T cells. In leukemia, normal hematopoiesis (production and development of blood cells) is altered. Immature blood cells multiply at the expense of normal blood cells. These immature blood cells also have a growth advantage over normal cellular elements because of their increased rate of proliferation (cell growth), a decreased rate of spontaneous apoptosis (cell death), or both (Kliegman, Stanton, St. Geme, Schor, & Behrman, 2011). The immature cells are known as blast cells. Normal bone marrow elements are replaced by large amounts of these immature lymphocytes (blast cells), which causes a "crowding out" of normal red blood cells (RBCs), platelets, and white blood cells (WBCs), resulting in **pancytopenia** (an abnormally low level of all

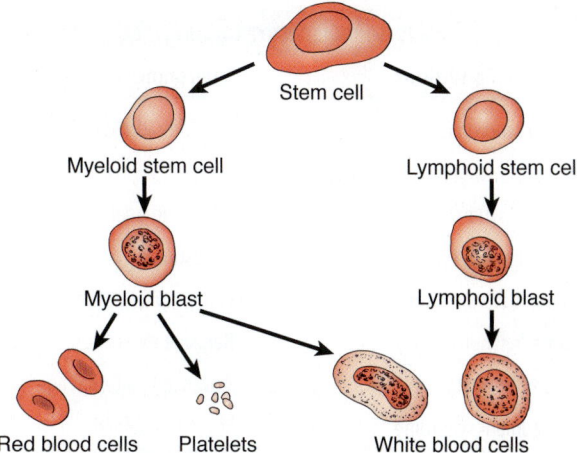

Figure 33-2 Myeloid cells differentiate and form into red blood cells, monocytes, granulocytes, and platelets.

blood cells produced by the bone marrow, including a low level of RBCs, WBCs, and platelets). Leukemia can develop at any point during the stages of normal lymphoid or myeloid differentiation in the bone marrow and can spread to the blood, lymph nodes, spleen, liver, central nervous system, or other organs in the body.

Classification of leukemia is based on the predominant cell line affected and the level of cellular differentiation. The terms myeloid and lymphoid denote the cell line involved. Both myeloid and lymphoid cell lines can proliferate into acute or chronic forms of leukemia. The three major classifications of childhood leukemia are acute lymphocytic leukemia, acute myelogenous leukemia, and chronic lymphocytic leukemia. Acute leukemia is a rapidly progressing disease that affects mostly immature, undifferentiated cells that are not able to perform their normal functions. Acute myelogenous leukemia affects all three types of blood cells, but the cells maintain some of their normal function, and chronic lymphocytic leukemia is a less rapidly progressing disease allowing for the production of mature, more differentiated cells. Chronic lymphocytic leukemia is rarely reported in children. Another type of leukemia, juvenile myelomonocytic leukemia, is rare and affects only 1% to 2% of children. It mostly affects children less than 4 years of age and is very difficult to treat. A disease related to leukemia is myelodysplastic leukemia (MDS). In MDS, the child's bone marrow does not produce enough WBCs, RBCs, and platelets. MDS ranges from mild to severe (Seattle Children's Hospital, 2013).

Acute Lymphocytic Leukemia

Acute lymphocytic leukemia (ALL) is the most common type of cancer in children. ALL accounts for 75% to 80% of all childhood leukemias and for approximately one-third of all childhood cancers. Approximately 2,800 children are diagnosed with ALL in the United States annually (Kliegman et al., 2011). The peak incidence is between 2 and 5 years of age. During infancy, boys are more likely than girls to develop ALL. The leukemic cells are usually acquired versus inherited. However, there is an increased risk among children with certain genetic disorders, such as Down syndrome. A variety of factors have been implicated that might predispose children to developing leukemia (Table 33-1).

Table 33-1 Factors Predisposing to Childhood Leukemia	
Genetic Conditions	**Environmental Factors**
Down syndrome	Ionizing radiation
Fanconi's syndrome	Drugs
Bloom's syndrome	Alkylating agents
Shwachman's syndrome	Nitrosourea
Klinefelter's syndrome	Epipodophyllotoxin
Turner's syndrome	Benzene exposure
Neurofibromatosis	Advanced maternal age
Li-Fraumeni syndrome	Severe combined immune deficiency

A current 5-year survival rate for ALL is 94% (St. Jude Children's Research Hospital, 2013).

Signs and Symptoms

The presenting symptoms of ALL vary widely, depending on the degree of infiltration of the bone marrow and other organs by leukemic cells. Most cases have an acute onset, while in other cases symptoms appear slowly.

- Fever occurs in approximately 50% of the cases
- Fatigue and lethargy
- ALL patients have anemia and are therefore pale
- Anorexia
- In more than one-third of children with ALL, especially the younger ones, bone or joint pain is present
- Parents may notice a limp or the child may refuse to walk

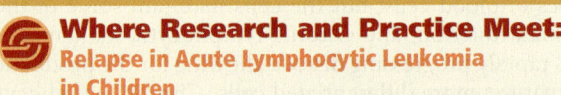

Where Research and Practice Meet:
Relapse in Acute Lymphocytic Leukemia in Children

Despite the improved treatment results for ALL, 20% to 30% of the children may have a relapse followed by a possible poor outcome. After the disease reoccurrence, the event-free survival is 25% to 40% and less than 20% for early relapse. This research examined 40 children (22 boys) with ALL who had their first relapse between 2004 and 2010. These children were consecutive relapse patients treated at 5 university hospitals in Finland. Of the 40 patients with relapses, 23 occurred while still on therapy, and 17 relapses happened while off therapy.

This pilot study used an ALL relapse protocol with well-known drugs and drug combinations using a concept of response-guided design. Relapse response was also measured in a logarithmic design. The primary end points were achievement of M1 marrow status and second remission. The remission induction rate was 90% with 10% induction mortality.

On the basis of this pilot study by Saarinen-Pihkala, Parto, Riikonen, Lahteenmaki, Bakassy, Glomstein, et al. (2011), the conclusion was made that an ALL marrow relapse non-responsive to steroids, vincristine, asparaginase, and anthracyclines was uncommon as was relapse non-responsive to alkylating agents. However, it was determined that classic drugs and well-known drugs can still be used during induction of ALL marrow relapse. It is hoped that this pilot data will be helpful for study groups planning new ALL relapse therapy strategies.

- Less common symptoms include headache, vomiting, difficulty in breathing, and low urine output. Bleeding under the skin, in the mouth, or sometimes in the eyes may be present. Petechiae can also be noted. Abdominal distention caused by an enlarged spleen, as well as enlarged lymph nodes are present in more than half of the patients. Hepatomegaly may also be present.

Diagnosis

A complete blood count and other blood tests are done to evaluate the WBC count, platelets, and liver and kidney function. A bone marrow aspirate is required to make the diagnosis of ALL. A finding of more than 25% abnormal lymphoblast cells (Fig. 33-3) in the bone marrow is diagnostic. Other samples in the bone marrow are sent for further testing and show chromosomal changes and better identify the specifics of the leukemia. The child's WBC count and age at diagnosis are the most important prognostic signs in ALL. The best prognosis is associated with a WBC count less than 5,000/mm^3 and an age of 2 to 9 years. The worst prognosis is associated with an initial WBC count of 50,000/mm^3 and an age older than 10 years. Infants younger than 1 year of age at the time of diagnosis also have a very poor prognosis.

Infants and patients with specific chromosomal abnormalities have a higher risk of relapse despite intensive therapy (Kliegman et al., 2011). Lumbar puncture is performed to assess for the presence of central nervous system (CNS) disease and staging of leukemia (Fig. 33-4). A chest radiograph is obtained to detect a mediastinal mass. Laboratory findings show liver or kidney involvement.

Diagnostic Tools Lumbar Puncture (LP)

LP, also known as a "spinal tap," is the introduction of a needle into the subarachnoid space of the lumbar spinal cord. The needle is inserted with a stylet into the interspace between the third and fourth lumbar vertebrae under strict sterile technique (Fig. 33-4). This test is usually done to remove a sample of cerebrospinal fluid (CSF) to test it for infection. For cancer patients, this procedure is also used to introduce chemotherapeutic agents into the CSF space. This is known as giving chemotherapy **intrathecally** (through the theca of the spinal cord into the subarachnoid space). Because some medications cannot cross the blood–brain barrier easily, physicians have obtained better results by introducing chemotherapeutic agents into the CSF space to kill cancer cells so they cannot "hide" behind the blood–brain barrier.

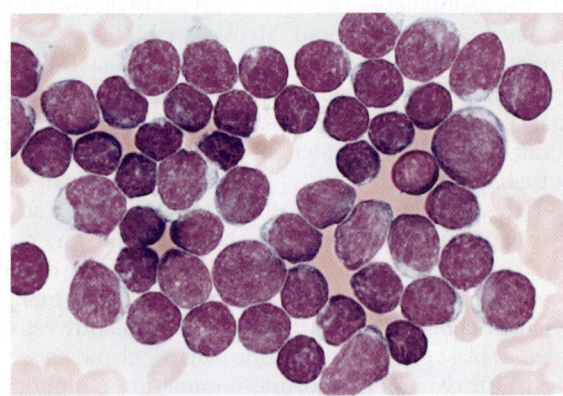

Figure 33-3 Dark-stained lymphoblast cells seen in acute lymphocytic leukemia (ALL), the most common type of childhood leukemia.

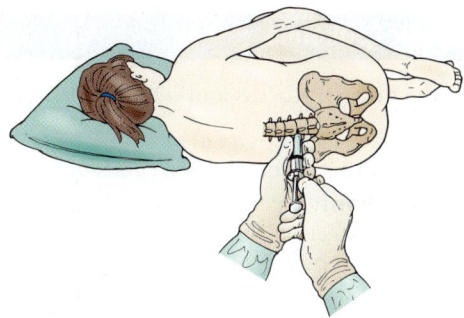

Figure 33-4 Lumbar puncture.

Collaborative Care

 Nursing Care. Without effective therapy and nursing care, ALL is fatal. Leukemia is treated with chemotherapy and includes three phases: remission-induction, consolidation, and maintenance. In the remission-induction phase, the tumor burden is reduced to an undetectable level. Ninety-five percent of children with ALL achieve remission during induction, which usually lasts 4 weeks. Once remission is achieved, most children relapse within a few months if treatment is stopped.

Complementary Care: *Visualization and Distraction*

The child may experience anticipatory anxiety before a procedure. The use of visualization and distraction can be helpful in these situations. When using visualization, be creative. Help the child imagine a trip to his or her favorite place. Have the child close his or her eyes while the nurse plays tour guide. Ask the child questions about the favorite place and encourage the child to be part of the story or trip. The nurse also uses distraction depending on the child's developmental level. Blowing bubbles, performing a magical light show, or simply reading a story can distract the child from the procedure.

Medical Care. Chemotherapy agents used for remission-induction are vincristine (Oncovorin), L-asparaginase (Elspar), and prednisone (Deltasone) or dexamethasone (Decadron). Children who have a worse prognosis are also given an anthracycline drug (chemotherapy drug that is known to affect and damage the heart, such as doxorubicin [Adriamycin]). Children with ALL also receive CNS prophylaxis. The prophylactic chemotherapy agent is injected intrathecally into the CSF space during an LP. Once the child is stable, the chemotherapy can be given in an outpatient setting.

The goal of the second phase, consolidation, is to destroy any residual leukemic cells. This phase starts immediately after remission is achieved and lasts about 6 months. Chemotherapy in this phase is frequently administered in high doses. Children are not usually hospitalized for this phase unless a complication arises. This phase may also require radiation.

The third phase, maintenance, controls the leukemia. It can last for 2 to 3 years after diagnosis. Today, remission can be induced in 95% of children.

The most common type of childhood cancer is acute lymphocytic leukemia (ALL). Within ALL there are a number of disease variations, one of which is called Philadelphia Chromosome Positive ALL (Ph+ ALL). Until recently, the preferred treatment for Ph+ ALL was to perform a stem cell transplant after the patient received 3 to 6 months of chemotherapy treatment. Even with this aggressive treatment, the cure rates were less than 50% and some of the children cured with stem cell transplant experienced serious long-term effects. Now new researched performed by Children's Oncology Group doctors has shown that treating children with Ph+ ALL using chemotherapy combined with a new drug called imatinib (Gleevec) can double cure rates. Based on these findings, stem cell transplants no longer are automatically considered to be the best way to treat children with Ph+ ALL (Children's Oncology Group, 2012).

Nursing Insight—*Bone marrow transplant*

Bone marrow transplant is the treatment option for children who have a second remission after relapse. This treatment involves giving the child high doses of chemotherapy and/or radiation to eradicate disease or cancer and then rescuing the patient with a source of stem cells that allows for recovery of healthy bone marrow.

There are two basic types of bone marrow transplants: autologous and allogeneic. In an autologous transplant, the patient's own peripheral blood or bone marrow is given back. An allogeneic transplant can be from a matched sibling, a relative, or an unrelated donor accessed through the National Marrow Donor Program.

Nursing Insight—*Biological therapy*

Biological therapy consists of high doses of hormones or other proteins that are normally made by the human body. Pharmaceutical companies can make these substances. These substances are made to prevent or treat damage to other systems of the body that may be caused by other leukemia treatments (Children's Hospital of Philadelphia (CHOP), 2013).

Education/Discharge Instructions

Parents are made aware of the importance of these children avoiding falls and "being careful" during play. Tell parents to monitor for signs of red dots called **petechiae** that are described as small (1 to 2 mm), red or purple spots on the body caused by broken capillaries that do not blanch or fade when pressed by the finger. With a low WBC count, tell parents to keep the child away from people who are ill and avoid crowded places, such as shopping malls.

Acute Myelogenous Leukemia

Acute myelogenous leukemia (AML) is the second most common type of leukemia seen in children. The principal defect in AML appears to be an arrest in the differentiation pathway of myeloid progenitors or precursors rather than abnormal growth kinetics. The molecular mechanism that leads to a block in differentiation is mostly unknown. AML can affect

---

Nursing Care Plan   The Child With Acute Lymphocytic Leukemia

Nursing Diagnoses: Risk for infection related to neutropenia from the disease process and treatment regimen

Measurable Short-Term Goal: The child will be afebrile.

Measurable Long-Term Goal: The child will not experience an infection during a neutropenic episode.

NOC Outcome:

Immune Status (0702) Natural and acquired appropriately targeted resistance to internal and external antigens

Risk Control: Infectious Process (1924) Personal actions to understand, prevent, eliminate, or reduce the threat of acquiring an infection

NIC Interventions:

Infection Protection (6550)
Surveillance (6650)

Nursing Interventions:

1. Monitor vital signs (specify frequency). Report a temperature 101.2°F (38.5°C) in a 24-hour period or 100.4°F (38.0°C) three times in a 24-hour period, or decrease in blood pressure to the physician.

   RATIONALE: Increased temperature, heart rate, and respiratory rate are signs of infection. A drop in blood pressure may be a late sign of septic shock.

2. Assess the child for areas of potential infection, such as mucosal ulcerations, breaks in the skin, and signs of localized signs of infection such as pain, redness, or swelling (specify frequency).

   RATIONALE: The skin and mucous membranes are the first line of defense against infection and openings in this protective barrier could be a portal for microbial entry. The child with neutropenia has diminished defense against infection, and sepsis may develop quickly.

3. Monitor laboratory values as obtained and report abnormal values to the physician.

   RATIONALE: Neutropenia from the disease process and chemotherapy increase the risk for infection. An elevated WBC count indicates an infectious process.

4. Wash hands thoroughly before and after providing care and teach the child and family when and how to wash their hands. Implement isolation precautions as ordered (specify).

   RATIONALE: Good hand hygiene is an effective and simple way to prevent transmission of infective microorganisms. Isolation precautions help protect the child from microorganisms in the hospital environment.

5. Instruct the family and visitors that no flowers, plants, fresh fruits, or vegetables should be brought into the child's room.

   RATIONALE: Promotes a safe environment for the child. Fresh plants and foods may carry infectious microorganisms that could be dangerous for the neutropenic child.

6. Flag the child's chart and alert all caregivers that the child must not use a drinking straw, have a rectal temperature taken, or receive rectal suppositories.

   RATIONALE: Protects the fragile mucous membranes of the mouth and rectum from mechanical injury, which could provide a portal for infection.

7. Administer antibiotic and antifungal medications as ordered and in a timely fashion (specify drug, dose, route, and times) and monitor for expected and adverse effects (specify).

   RATIONALE: Antibiotic therapy may be started in a child with a fever and who is neutropenic with an absolute neutrophil count of less than 500.

---

all three types of blood cells (Fig. 33-5). Accordingly, a standard classification system called the French–American–British system is used to differentiate AML into eight main types.

In the United States, AML constitutes 11% of the cases of childhood leukemia, with approximately 380 children diagnosed annually (Kliegman et al., 2011). AML is equally distributed among ethnic groups. Males and females are affected equally. Unlike ALL, the incidence of AML is constant from birth to 10 years of age, with a slight peak in adolescence. However, a neonate is more likely to have AML than ALL.

Signs and Symptoms

Children with AML may present with vague symptoms resembling the flu. Because blast cells replace the normal

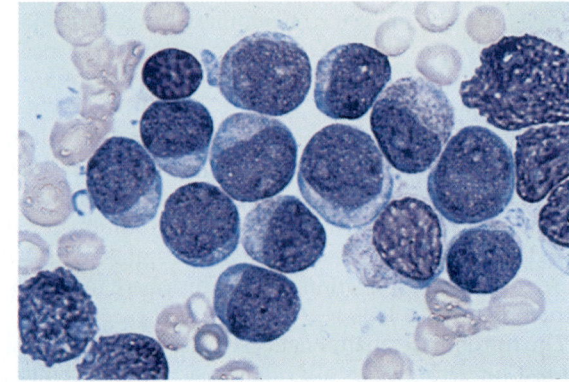

Figure 33-5 Acute myelogenous leukemia cells (AML).

blood cells in the bone marrow, children with AML often present with abnormal blood counts. A decreased number of RBCs may result in anemia that may lead to decreased oxygen delivery to the blood cells and tissue. Pallor, fatigue, headache, or dizziness may result.

- As a result of a decreased number of platelets, thrombocytopenia, petechiae, easy bruising, nosebleeds, or bleeding gums may be present.
- Fever and infection may be present as a result of decreased WBCs. Bone pain and arthralgias are less common complaints in childhood.
- Massive hepatosplenomegaly is uncommon except in infants with AML.
- Patients with AML present with signs and symptoms that infrequently occur with ALL, including subcutaneous nodules or "blueberry muffin" lesions, infiltration of the gingiva, signs and laboratory findings of disseminated intravascular coagulation, and discrete masses known as chloromas or granulocytic sarcomas that may occur in the absence of apparent bone marrow involvement (Kliegman et al., 2011).

Diagnosis

A bone marrow aspiration and analysis is required for a diagnosis of AML. The biopsy typically reveals a hypercellular marrow consisting of a pattern of cells with features that permit a subclassification of disease (Kliegman et al., 2011). The diagnosis is typically made when there are more than 25% malignant myeloid blast cells.

Collaborative Care

Nursing Care. Once diagnosis is made, treatment begins promptly, especially to control any copresenting symptomatology.

 Nursing Insight—*Therapies*

Treatment has improved significantly since the first effective therapies were introduced in the 1970s. The 5-year survival rate has increased from less than 5% in 1970 to 43% today as a result of treatment intensification, the incorporation of hematopoietic stem cell transplant into primary therapy, and enhanced supportive care (St. Jude Children's Research Hospital, 2013). Aggressive **multiagent chemotherapy** (using more than one type of chemotherapy, also called combination therapy) is successful in inducing remission in about 80% of patients. Up to 10% of patients die of either infection or bleeding before a remission can be achieved (Kliegman et al., 2011). More individualized therapies and better supportive care has pushed the survival rate of AML 3 years after diagnosis to 71% reported by St. Jude Children's Research Hospital (2013). Matched-sibling bone marrow or stem cell transplantation after remission has been shown to achieve long-term disease-free survival in 60% to 70% of patients (Kliegman et al., 2011).

Medical Care. Induction treatment includes the combination of cytarabine (Ara-C) and daunorubicin (Daunomycin). Other commonly used pediatric induction therapy regimens use cytarabine (Ara-C) and anthracyclines in combination with other agents such as etoposide (VP-16) and/or thioguanine (6-TG).

Education/Discharge Instructions

Parents of children who are discharged after receiving chemotherapy should be alert to signs and symptoms of infection, such as fever and fatigue, and should monitor for bruising if blood counts are low. The children usually receive a specific number of days of treatment and are not discharged until their blood count levels are safe and at a level determined to be an adequate return to baseline values.

Now Can You—**Discuss leukemia?**

1. Describe the main types of leukemia?
2. Describe the signs and symptoms of acute lymphocytic leukemia?
3. Describe three phases of acute lymphocytic leukemia chemotherapy treatment (remission-induction, consolidation, and maintenance)?
4. Discuss the purpose of a lumbar puncture?

Chronic Myelogenous Leukemia

Chronic myelogenous leukemia (CML) is a clonal disorder of the hematopoietic tissue (formation of blood cells) that accounts for 2% to 3% of all cases of childhood leukemia. About 99% of the cases are characterized by a specific translocation known as the Philadelphia chromosome. This disease has been associated with exposure to ionizing radiation, but very few children have a history of such exposure.

Signs and Symptoms

The presenting signs and symptoms of CML are nonspecific but include:

- Fever
- Fatigue
- Weight loss
- Anorexia
  (Kliegman et al., 2011)

CML is also characterized clinically by an initial chronic phase in which the malignant clone (cancerous alteration) produces an elevated leukocyte (WBC) count with increased numbers of immature granulocytes. In addition to leukocytosis, the blood counts may reveal mild anemia and thrombocytosis (increased number of platelets) (Kliegman et al., 2011). The spleen is often greatly enlarged, resulting in pain in the left upper quadrant of the abdomen.

The chronic phase typically ends 3 to 4 years after onset when the CML moves into an accelerated or "blast crisis" phase. At this point, the blood counts rise dramatically and cannot be controlled with drugs. Additional manifestations may occur, including hyperuricemia and neurological symptoms, which are related to increased blood viscosity with decreased CNS perfusion (Kliegman et al., 2011).

Diagnosis

A diagnosis is suggested by increased numbers of myeloid cells with differentiation to mature forms in the peripheral blood smear and bone marrow. Cytogenetic studies yield the presence of the characteristic Philadelphia chromosome (Kliegman et al., 2011).

Collaborative Care

Nursing Care. The optimum therapy is allogenic bone marrow or stem cell transplantation from a matched sibling, which is curative in up to 80% of children (Kliegman et al., 2011). Therefore, the main nursing care revolves around post bone marrow or transplant interventions.

Medical Care. Treatment of the signs and symptoms in the chronic phase can be controlled with hydroxyurea (Droxia, Hydrea), which gradually returns the leukocyte count to normal. This treatment is not definitive and does not eliminate the abnormal clone or prevent the progression of the disease. Therapy with interferon-a can produce a hematological remission in up to 70% of patients and cytogenetic remission in about 20% of patients (Kliegman et al., 2011). Combination chemotherapy is based on health-care provider order and has been successful in the treatment of these children.

Education/Discharge Instructions

Similar to ALL, parents are made aware of the importance of these children avoiding falls and "being careful" during play. Tell parents to monitor for petechiae on the skin that do not blanch or fade when you press your finger on them. With a low WBC count, the parents should keep the child away from people who are sick and avoid crowded places, like shopping malls.

SOLID TUMORS

Solid tumors in children differ significantly from those in adults. There are some solid tumors that children acquire that never develop in adults or if they do, are quite rare, such as neuroblastoma, Wilms' tumor, rhabdosarcoma, and osteosarcoma. The most common types of solid tumors found in children are discussed here. Solid tumors are named for the type of cells of which they are composed:

- Sarcoma is a cancer arising from connective or supporting tissues (e.g., bone or muscle).
- Carcinoma is cancer arising from the body's glandular cells and epithelial cells.
- Lymphomas are cancers of the lymphoid organs, such as the lymph nodes, spleen, and thymus, that produce and store infection-fighting cells.
- These cells also occur in almost all tissues of the body; therefore, lymphomas may develop in a wide variety of organs.

Brain Tumors

Tumors of the brain or of the CNS are the second most common cancer in children after leukemia. Brain tumors in children differ greatly from those seen in adults. Virtually all childhood brain tumors are primary tumors, meaning that they originate in the brain. In contrast, with adults, brain tumors are primarily metastatic, originating from another site and then spreading to the brain.

Brain tumors are divided into two types: supratentorial and infratentorial. Supratentorial tumors occur in the anterior two-thirds of the brain above the tentorium (dura matter located between the cerebrum and cerebellum, supporting the occipital lobes), primarily in the cerebrum. Infratentorial tumors are located in the posterior third of the brain, primarily in the cerebellum and brainstem and below the tentorium. The mortality rate among children and adolescents with brain tumors approaches 45% (Kliegman et al., 2011).

 Nursing Insight—*Glial tumors*

Glial cells are the major supportive and structural cells of the CNS because they form a framework supporting and nourishing nerve

cells. The most common type of primary brain tumors in children are glial tumors. An example of this tumor comprises the primitive neuroectodermal tumors, which arise almost exclusively in children. This tumor often resembles the early and undeveloped cells in an embryo and may be referred to as embryonal tumors. The most common site for this tumor is in the cerebellum.

 Nursing Insight—*Age-related differences in primary location of the tumor*

There are age-related differences in primary location of the tumor:

- Within the first year of life, supratentorial tumors predominate and include, most commonly, choroid plexus complex tumors and teratomas.
- From 1 to 10 years of age, infratentorial tumors predominate because of the high incidence of juvenile pilocytic astrocytoma (tumor of the brain or spinal cord composed of astrocytes) and medulloblastoma (an infiltrating malignant tumor of the roof of the fourth ventricle and cerebellum) (Venes, 2013).
- After 10 years of age, supratentorial tumors predominate (Kliegman et al., 2011).

Signs and Symptoms

Clinical manifestations of patients with brain tumors depend on the tumor location, tumor type, and the age of the child.

- Classic signs and symptoms are related to the tumor causing obstruction of CSF drainage paths, leading to increased intracranial pressure (ICP).
- Because their cranial sutures are open, infants may exhibit lethargy, irritability, and macrocephaly. They may also have a raised or tense fontanelle.
- Projectile vomiting is often seen in the morning with little warning, or a headache may be noted.

In young children, the diagnosis of a brain tumor may be delayed because the symptoms are often similar to those of a typical gastrointestinal illness (Kliegman et al., 2011). Subtle changes in personality, mentation, and/or speech may precede the classic signs and symptoms of brain tumors. Brainstem tumors are associated with cranial nerve abnormalities such as hemiparesis—a weakness on one side of the body—or a spastic gait. Older children may fall or stumble.

Diagnosis

Any child who displays signs of increased intracranial pressure (ICP) or other neurological signs, such as ataxia, visual disturbances (if able to ascertain), or hemiparesis, need to be referred for a complete neurological exam. The diagnostic work-up may include magnetic resonance imaging (MRI) or a CT scan. CT takes less time (5 to 10 minutes) and may be more appropriate if the child is able to lie still without sedation. An endocrine work-up may be required for tumors that occur in the pituitary area.

Collaborative Care

Nursing Care. First, the tumor is staged. Tumor tissue is needed for the pathologist to determine the histological diagnosis so that proper treatment can be determined.

Nursing Insight—*Performing the neurological exam*

The main focus of a physical assessment of a child with a brain tumor is the neurological exam. A patient's baseline assessment is important to detect any subtle changes. This exam includes vital signs; pupil size, equality, and response to light; level of consciousness (LOC); strength and equality of grip of hands; and movement of the legs. Head circumference and the assessment of the anterior fontanelle are extremely important in assessing an infant's ICP. Parents may first notice behavioral changes. The nurse performs frequent neurological exams to determine early changes in a child's condition. Detecting subtle changes in the neurological exam can be of great value in managing a child's condition and eventual prognosis. It is important for the nurse to remember that the neurological exam can change rapidly. Timely responses to neurological changes are of vital importance for the child with a brain tumor.

Good communication with the care delivery team is vital. Parents and the child need good emotional support and accurate information. Nurses are the pivotal coordinators of the care in this difficult situation. The nurse demonstrates a positive attitude and is reassuring to parents during difficult treatments to build a trusting relationship with the family.

"What to say"—*When a child is diagnosed with a brain tumor*

A 4-year-old child has just been diagnosed with a brain tumor. The pediatric nurse knows that the family is most likely in a state of shock. The family or the child does not understand the exact nature or future implications of a brain tumor. While caring for the child, the nurse treats him or her as normally as possible. It is acceptable to communicate with the child and family while the child plays. It is also important that the nurse support the parents or caregivers and allows them time to "absorb" the diagnosis.

What would the pediatric nurse say to the family?

- "It is important for you to verbalize and express your feelings."

- "You may find it helpful to talk with others who have had the same experience as you. I have contact information for a support group. Would you like me to make a call for you?"

- "I know this is a very difficult time for you. Let's take this one day at a time and make your child's daily routine as normal as possible."

Other nursing care measures include continued neurological assessments, airway and fluid maintenance, prevention of infection, pain management, adequate nutrition, and promotion of normal growth and development.

Medical Care. Treatment may include surgical resection, radiation therapy, chemotherapy, and or a combination of these, though in the last decade, chemotherapy has emerged as the standard care in the treatment of certain pediatric brain tumors, especially for children younger than 3 years of age. Several rounds of high-dose chemotherapy with stem cell rescue are now being offered for metastatic medulloblastoma, as well as for some other incurable brain tumors. The current 5-year survival rate for medulloblastoma is 85% (St. Jude Children's Research Hospital, 2013).

The goal of radiation therapy is to destroy the tumor while sparing normal brain tissue in the developing brain. Early use of radiation is done sparingly because of the desire to preserve intellectual growth and decrease the possibility of growth impairment. When radiation is used, the dose is usually high and the toxicity (poison level) can be severe. Radiation therapy to large areas of the brain can sometimes cause changes in brain function (Venes, 2013).

Surgical Care. After resection, postoperative care includes monitoring vital signs, performing an ongoing neurological assessment, administering IV steroids such as dexamethasone (Decadron) to prevent edema within the brain, assessing the surgical site, and helping the child to regain self-care skills and maintain age-appropriate development. Anticonvulsants are indicated for the child with a supratentorial tumor because seizures are possible. Two of the most common anticonvulsant drugs used in the pediatric population are fosphenytoin (Cerebyx) and phenytoin (Dilantin). The nurse should ensure the child's comfort and alleviate pain as well as offer support to the family.

focus on safety

Surgical resection

The extent of surgical resection (cutting out) of the tumor correlates with the prognosis. Radical resections are particularly important in children younger than 2 years of age because cranial radiation can be deferred in these patients. Because many of the brain tumors infiltrate into surrounding normal brain tissue, complete resection is not often possible.

Education/Discharge Instructions

It is important that parents are taught to monitor for headaches, blurred vision, pressure, confusion, or an altered LOC when taking their child home. Also teach parents to monitor for fever and check the incision site for signs of infection.

Neuroblastoma

Neuroblastoma is the third most common pediatric cancer after leukemia and brain tumors (Kliegman et al., 2011). Neuroblastoma is a tumor of nerve tissue that develops in infants and children. It develops from the tissues that form the sympathetic nervous system. The nervous system controls body functions like heart rate and blood pressure, digestion, and levels of certain hormones. Most commonly it develops in the abdomen within the tissues of the adrenal gland, but it may also be found in other areas like the brain, pelvis, mediastinum, and sympathetic ganglia. It can spread to the lymph nodes, liver, bones, and bone marrow (CHOP, 2011).

Neuroblastoma accounts for about 8% of all childhood cancers (Kliegman et al., 2011). Neuroblastoma is the most common diagnosed neoplasm in infants. The median age at diagnosis is 2 years. Ninety percent of all cases are diagnosed in children younger than 5 years. It can occasionally be seen in teenagers and young adults (CHOP, 2011). The incidence is slightly higher in boys than in girls, and in Caucasian, non-Hispanic children. In the United States there are about 800 new cases of neuroblastoma diagnosed per year (CHOP, 2011).

Signs and Symptoms

Children with neuroblastoma present with a wide variety of initial symptoms depending on the primary site of the tumor.

- Most commonly, the tumor is detected by palpation. On palpation the nurse notes that neuroblastoma crosses the midline. The tumor is noted as a hard, painless mass in the neck or abdomen.
- Masses of the thorax can be seen on radiographs and are usually an incidental finding on a film done to rule out pneumonia.
- If large enough, the tumor can produce edema of the lower extremities related to vascular compression.

Unfortunately, at the time of diagnosis, 75% of patients with neuroblastoma have a tumor that has already spread, or metastasized, to another site. Nearly one-half of the patients have widespread metastasis to the bone that causes bone pain. The bones of the skull and orbit are also frequently affected, so swelling and bruising around the eyes are common. The current 5-year survival rate for neuroblastoma is 75% (St. Jude Children's Research Hospital, 2013).

Diagnosis

Imaging studies, such as MRI and CT scan, may indicate the presence of a mass. A clear diagnosis of neuroblastoma can be made only by biopsy. Bone marrow aspiration may also be performed. Laboratory studies may be ordered because 95% of neuroblastomas secrete catecholamines. These are secreted in the urine, so vanillylmandelic acid and homovanillic acid tests are used to measure the level of catecholamines or catecholamine metabolites (breakdown products) in the urine.

 Nursing Insight—*Neuroblastoma*

Neuroblastoma is staged into low, average, and high-risk groups and into I through IV classification using the International Neuroblastoma Staging System (American Cancer Society, 2013a). The prognosis is determined by the age of the child, the stage of the tumor, and the histology of the tumor. The prognosis for children who have abdominal masses is poorer than for those with cervical, mediastinal, or pelvic tumors.

Collaborative Care

Nursing Care. During the treatment phase, a complete nursing assessment is vital to ensure that the child does not have an infection and his or her condition remains stable. Place emphasis on the child's comfort and alleviating pain. Supporting the child and the family during the diagnosis and treatment phase is most important. Encourage both the child and caregivers to share their feelings about the disease process and related treatments. Providing accurate information and education for the family is also important.

Medical Care. Treatment for neuroblastoma is determined by the stage of the disease and the age of the child. Initially, surgical resection is performed and followed by chemotherapy. In advanced stages of the disease, a complete surgical resection is sometimes not possible, and chemotherapy is initiated. Neuroblastoma is radiosensitive, but radiation alone is not curative. Radiation is used for tumor control in conjunction with chemotherapy and autologous or allogeneic bone marrow transplant.

Education/Discharge Instructions

Parents are taught to monitor the incision site for signs of infection and to watch the child for fever. It is best to keep children away from large crowds and ill people during the treatment phase. Teach parents about comfort measures, too.

Wilms' Tumor

Wilms' tumor (nephroblastoma) is a tumor that originates in one kidney or both kidneys (Kliegman et al., 2011). It is named after the German doctor, Max Wilms, who first described it in 1899. The actual cause of Wilms' tumor is unknown. Ninety percent of all kidney tumors are Wilms' tumors, and it is the fourth most common cancer in children. The average age at diagnosis is between 2 and 5 years (Kliegman et al., 2011). The disease occasionally affects older children, and girls and boys are equally affected. About 9 out of 10 children with Wilms' tumor are cured. A great deal of progress has been made in treating this disease with surgery, radiation, and chemotherapy (American Cancer Society, 2013b). The present 5-year survival rate is 90% (St. Jude Children's Research Hospital, 2013).

 Nursing Insight—*Genetics*

The majority of Wilms' tumor cases are sporadic, although 1% to 2% of patients have a family history. One Wilms' tumor gene has been located at 11p13, but only 20% of all Wilms' tumors carry that mutation (Kliegman et al., 2011).

Signs and Symptoms

The tumor is usually discovered on a routine physical exam or is felt or seen by a family member during bathing or routine care. Unlike neuroblastoma, the mass frequently presents on one side and seldom crosses the midline.

- Children with Wilms' tumor present with an abdominal mass that is usually painless.
- Hematuria, hypertension, and pain occur infrequently.
- Other symptoms may be aniridia (absence of the iris, the colored part of the eye), hemihypertrophy (an increased size of one-half of the body), or urinary defects such as cryptorchidism and hypospadias.

Diagnosis

A child presenting with an abdominal mass needs a timely diagnostic work-up. The nurse explains to the parents that ongoing laboratory and diagnostic testing include urine and electrolyte analysis and a complete blood count, and a renal or abdominal ultrasound, CT scan, or MRI of the abdomen are done. If metastasis is suspected, a chest x-ray exam is ordered.

Collaborative Care

Nursing Care. Nursing care for Wilms' tumor consists of a thorough health and history and nursing assessment. Foods high in calories and protein are important. If a child is unable to eat or meet basic caloric requirements for growth and development, dietary supplements, allowing the child food choices, and ensuring that food textures can facilitate eating might help. Enteral or parental feeding may be provided if necessary.

Critical Nursing Action Palpation of the Abdomen in a Child With Wilms' Tumor

Once a child has been diagnosed with Wilms' tumor, never palpate the abdomen or allow anyone else to do so. Palpating this kind of encapsulated tumor can cause it to rupture or lead to further metastasis. Be sure to place a warning sign on the child's hospital room door that says "No abdominal palpation."

Medical Care. Medical treatment includes both chemotherapy and post-radiation care. The most common chemotherapy drugs used for Wilms' tumor are actinomycin D, (Dactinomycin), and vincristine (Oncovorin). For tumors in more advanced stages, those with unfavorable histology, or those that recur after treatment, the following drugs are used: doxorubicin (Adriamycin), cyclophosphamide (Cytoxan), etoposide, irinotecan, and/or carboplatin (American Cancer Society, 2013b).

Surgical Care. A surgical removal of the mass, which usually involves taking the entire kidney, and biopsy are performed. After surgical resection for a Wilms' tumor, postoperative care is similar to care for children undergoing other abdominal surgeries. A critical postoperative assessment of the remaining kidney is necessary to ensure its function. Typical postoperative care measures are done. To track kidney function, closely monitor urine output for amount, color, clarity, presence of clots, pain, and laboratory values.

 Case Study Wilms' Tumor

A mother brings her 3-year-old to the pediatrician's office. She states that while giving her daughter a bath, she noticed a "lump" on her abdomen. The mother also says the child shows no abnormal behavior. She is sleeping and playing normally. However, the mother does state she is a picky eater but assumes that is normal for a preschooler. The mother is concerned about a "hernia or something." On physical examination by the pediatrician, a small mass in the abdominal cavity is discovered. The pediatrician sends the child for an abdominal CT scan. The CT confirms there is a mass on the left kidney. It is classified as a stage II Wilms' tumor.

critical thinking questions

1. What is the course of treatment for this child?

2. What information does the parent need to know about nutrition?

♦ See Suggested Answers to Case Studies on DavisPlus.

Education/Discharge Instructions

Teach parents to monitor the incision site for signs of infection as well as the child for a fever. Parents need to be aware of the child's nutritional intake and bowel movements. Stress the importance of follow-up appointments and clinic visits.

Rhabdomyosarcoma

Rhabdomyosarcoma is the most common pediatric soft-tissue sarcoma and accounts for 5% to 8% of all childhood

cancers (Kliegman et al., 2011). It arises from mesenchymal cells that are normally committed to skeletal muscle formation but can also arise from smooth muscle cells. There are two main types of rhabdomyosarcoma: embryonal rhabdomyosarcoma and alveolar rhabdomyosarcoma, along with some less common types (American Cancer Society, 2013c). These tumors occur at virtually any anatomical site but are most often found in the head and neck, genitourinary tract, extremities, and trunk. Rhabdomyosarcoma occurs with an increased frequency of patients with neurofibromatosis (Kliegman et al., 2011). Overall, two-thirds of children diagnosed with rhabdomyosarcoma will become long-term survivors. A current 5-year survival rate for rhabdomyosarcoma is 65% (St. Jude Children's Research Hospital, 2013). Children with distant metastatic disease at diagnosis have a poor prognosis, with only 30% surviving 5 years. It is most common in children less than 10 years of age but can occur in teens and adults. It is slightly more common in boys than girls (American Cancer Society, 2013c).

 Nursing Insight—*Rhabdomyosarcoma subtypes*

The embryonal type (resembling an embryo) accounts for about 60% of all cases, the most common type, and has an intermediate prognosis. The botryoid type resembles a "bunch of grapes" and accounts for 6% of cases. It is most often found in the vagina, uterus, bladder, nasopharynx, and middle ear. The alveolar type accounts for about 15% of cases. The tumor cells in this type tend to grow in cores that often have cleft-like spaces resembling alveoli. Alveolar tumors occur most often in the trunk and extremities and carry the poorest prognosis. The pleomorphic type (having many shapes) is quite rare in childhood (1% of cases). About 20% of rhabdomyosarcomas are considered to be undifferentiated (an alteration in cell character toward a malignant state) sarcomas (Venes, 2013).

 Where Research and Practice Meet: **Rhabdomyosarcoma**

Chromosomal translocations and genetic amplification events are being examined in relation to rhabdomyosarcoma (RMS) by the Children's Oncology Group. RMS has two major histological subtypes: embryonal rhabdomyosarcoma (EMS) and alveolar rhabdomyosarcoma (AMS). AMS tumors differ from EMS tumors by frequent occurrence in extremities and a worse prognosis, which is associated with early metastasis. At the genetic level, chromosomal translocations occur in tumors of the AMS subtype and appear as important events in RMS pathogenesis. Genome-wide screens also indicate frequent occurrences of gene amplification events in AMS tumors. Because gene amplification is an important mechanism for increasing oncogene copy number and expression, the overexpressed proteins are postulated to collaborate with the fusion oncoprotein generated by each translocation during oncogenesis. Each of these amplifications is associated with specific gene fusion subtypes and different clinical outcomes. The genes involved in frequent chromosomal translocations are *PAX3*, *PAX7*, and *FOXO1*. Researchers found that fusion gene amplification *PAX7-FOXO1* fusion status were each associated with a significantly improved outcome and perhaps a very good prognostic indicator (Duan, Smith, Gustafson, Zhang, Dunlevy, Gastier-Foster, et al., (2012).

Signs and Symptoms

Signs and symptoms of rhabdomyosarcoma depend on the location of the primary tumor and metastasis.

- In the head and neck, orbital or eyelid tumors may cause proptosis (a downward displacement of the eyeball) and may impair vision (Venes, 2013).
- Tumors in the nasopharynx may cause sinus obstruction or result in continual sinus drainage.
- If the tumor erodes through the bone to the brain, signs and symptoms of increased ICP (e.g., headache, vomiting, etc.) may be present.
- In the genitourinary tract, the bladder and prostate are the most common sites, and hematuria or urinary obstruction may result.
- Extremity sarcomas are seen as the affected area begins to swell. Erythema and tenderness may occur.
- Other sites can be any skeletal or smooth muscle and the intrathoracic, retroperitoneal, perineal, and perianal regions.

Diagnosis

Definitive diagnosis is established by biopsy. Investigating a lesion may help with diagnosis. Paratesticular lesions may be ignored for a long time by adolescents (Kliegman et al., 2011). A lesion in an extremity may be mistaken for a hematoma or hemangioma. Physical examination also includes attention to the lymph nodes. Radiographic studies include x-ray exams, CT scan, and MRI.

Collaborative Care

Nursing Care. Nursing care is based on which treatment options are prescribed (Kliegman et al., 2011). If surgical resection is done, monitoring of the surgical site is vital. If chemotherapy is the treatment, standard nursing care of the patient receiving chemotherapy is indicated.

Medical Care. Medical care is based on the primary tumor and disease stage (Kliegman et al., 2011). Patients with complete surgical resected tumors have the best prognosis. Unfortunately, most rhabdomyosarcomas are not completely resectable. Chemotherapy is the standard treatment.

Education/Discharge Instructions

Parents are taught about the importance of monitoring the surgical site and watching the child for a fever. Stress the importance of follow-up care and clinic visits. As with any child with cancer, remind parents to keep the child away from crowded areas and ill people. The child can resume normal activity depending on the treatment protocol and how they feel. Parents can be taught about quiet activities that integrate normal developmental socialization.

Retinoblastoma

Retinoblastoma is a malignant tumor that arises from the retina at the back of the eye during fetal life or early childhood. A retinoblastoma can grow rapidly or slowly. It may produce multiple tumors that can affect one or both eyes. It is sometimes recognized at birth. It affects mainly very young children. Retinoblastoma can often be seen by looking at a young person's eyes or by observing a photograph taken of the individual.

There is no racial or gender predominance, but there is a familial predisposition in about one-third of patients. Overall, 60% of cases are unilateral and nonhereditary. Bilateral involvement is found in 42% of those presenting when younger than 1 year of age and is even less common at older ages. Close to 95% of retinoblastomas are cured (Kliegman et al., 2011) (St. Jude Children's Research Hospital, 2013).

Signs and Symptoms

Usually retinoblastoma is detected by the caregiver, who notices a whitish glow in the pupil known as **leukocoria** (cat's eye reflex). This is seen instead of the red eye reflex typically seen in photographs and is the most common manifestation. Other signs include:

- Strabismus, red painful eyes, and blindness (late sign)

  Other, less common evidence of the tumor is:

- Visual impairment
- Abnormal appearance of the eye that consists of a change in color of the iris, pupils of unequal size, or increased pressure inside the eye

Diagnosis

Retinoblastoma is usually diagnosed via an examination under anesthesia using an ophthalmoscope. Orbital ultrasound and CT or MRI may be used to evaluate the extent of intraocular disease and extraocular spread.

Collaborative Care

Nursing Care. An important nursing care measure before surgery includes showing parents a photograph of another child who has had this type of surgery. Parents can then understand that the child's facial appearance will be nearly normal. It is also important to inform parents that after surgery the eyelid is usually closed, and their child will be wearing a patch over the operative eye. It is important to keep the operative site clean and dry. Postoperative medical orders may include eye socket irrigation and the application of an antibiotic ointment. Traditional postoperative measures such as airway and fluid maintenance, vital signs, pain management, and nutrition are also important.

 Nursing Insight*—*Additional treatment measures

Cryotherapy (freezing of the tumor) and photocoagulation (laser light treatment of the tumor) are used to treat small primary tumors.

Medical Care. Treatment for this tumor depends on the size and location of the tumor (or tumors), with the primary goal of being cured and a secondary goal of preserving vision. Primary enucleation (removal of the eye) is usually preformed if there is no potential for useful vision (Kliegman et al., 2011).

Education/Discharge Instructions

The child is usually discharged in 3 to 4 days after the surgery. The nurse teaches parents about care of the eye socket by showing them gentle irrigation of the area (with the prescribed solution) and then applying a thin coating of the prescribed antibiotic ointment. Eye gauze pads are applied until the wound has completely healed. Enforce good hand washing for the entire family. After about 3 weeks, the child is fitted for a prosthetic eye, and the child's facial appearance appears close to normal. Through the entire process, the nurse offers support to the child and family and encourages follow-up care.

BONE TUMORS

Malignant bone tumors account for approximately 5% of all childhood cancers. The two most common bone tumors are osteogenic sarcoma and Ewing's sarcoma (Kliegman et al., 2011).

Osteosarcoma

Osteogenic sarcoma, or osteosarcoma, is a bone tumor that usually occurs in the metaphysis (the growing portion of a bone) (Fig. 33-6). The long bones are more frequently affected than the flat bones such as the pelvis or skull. The leg is the most common site, with the femur (upper leg) being the most commonly affected bone, followed by the tibia (lower leg) and the humerus (upper arm). The high-risk period of developing osteosarcoma is during adolescent growth spurts. Often a traumatic event leads to the discovery of osteosarcoma as a secondary finding. Osteosarcoma can also occur as a complication of treatment for another tumor, especially at a site of prior radiation for a tumor such as retinoblastoma. These secondary radiation-associated osteosarcomas can occur 7 to 15 years after successful treatment of the primary tumor.

 Nursing Insight—*Osteosarcoma*

The cause of osteosarcoma is unknown. Certain genetic or acquired conditions may predispose children to the development of osteosarcoma. Children with hereditary retinoblastoma have a significantly increased risk of developing osteosarcoma (Kliegman et al., 2011). The annual incidence of osteosarcoma in the United States is 5.6 cases per million children younger than 15 years of age (Kliegman et al., 2011). There is a slightly lower incidence in African American children. Boys are usually more often affected than girls.

 Nursing Insight—*Osteosarcoma prognosis*

Presently, using modern therapy, the 5-year, event-free survival rate is 65% to 70% with an overall survival rate of 70% to 80%

(Ueki, Maeda, Seikimizu, Tsukushi, Nishida, & Horibe, 2013). St. Jude Children's Research Hospital (2013) reports a 5-year survival rate of 70%. Patients with nonmetastatic extremity osteosarcoma are cured with current multiagent treatment protocols 75% of the time. Patients with pelvic tumors do not have as good a prognosis as those with extremity tumors. From 20% to 30% of patients who have limited numbers of pulmonary metastases can also be cured with aggressive chemotherapy and resection of lung nodules. Patients with bone metastasis and those with widespread lung metastasis have an extremely poor prognosis (Kliegman et al., 2011).

Signs and Symptoms

Pain and swelling are the most common presenting symptoms. The pain increases with activity and weight bearing and may cause the child to limp. It is common for a child to have a dull, aching pain for several months before diagnosis.

Palpation at the site of the disease often reveals tenderness, swelling, warmth, and erythema.

Diagnosis

An x-ray film may include a sunburst pattern of the affected bone. An accompanying chest x-ray exam is performed to check for metastasis. A MRI of the entire bone is performed to evaluate the extent of the tumor. A nuclear medicine scan or bone scan may also be done to determine the extent of involvement in the bone (Kliegman et al., 2011). Nuclear tracer isotopes, such as technetium-99m or thallium-201, which are radioactive materials, show an increased uptake of radioactive material in the areas of the primary tumor as well as any area of metastasis. The most common site of distant metastatic spread of osteosarcoma is to the lung.

Certain laboratory tests, such as elevated blood serum levels of serum alkaline phosphatase or lactic acid dehydrogenase, can help make the diagnosis of osteosarcoma. Although the diagnosis of osteosarcoma may be strongly suspected after diagnostic studies, only a biopsy with microscopic examination provides final confirmation of osteosarcoma.

Collaborative Care

Nursing Care. For the child with osteosarcoma, monitoring and treating pain is important. Use age-appropriated pain scales to assess pain. To decrease the child's pain, use both pharmacological and nonpharmacological measures. Promote function and mobility and monitor the surgical site for redness, warmth, and signs of infection.

Medical Care. Children with osteosarcoma receive chemotherapy first to shrink the size of the tumor. Then the primary treatment goal is total eradication of the tumor.

Surgical Care. After chemotherapy, surgical resection of the affected bone is performed (Kliegman et al., 2011). Nursing care for the child postoperatively includes monitoring vital signs, performing ongoing nursing assessments, providing adequate pain control, and monitoring for signs and symptoms of infection. Emotional support of the child and family after surgical resection is another key aspect to help the child accept an altered body image.

 Nursing Insight—*Limb-sparing surgery or amputation*

Amputation was the surgical treatment used almost exclusively in the past. Today a limb-saving procedure is available.

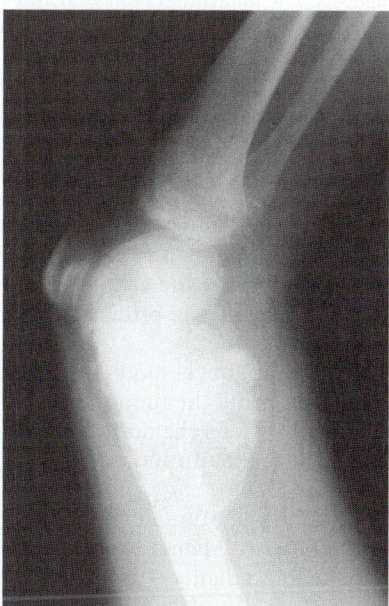

Figure 33-6 Osteosarcoma.

Limb-sparing surgery uses cadaver bone grafted into place to replace the section of bone that is resected with the tumor (or where the affected part of the bone is removed) and then replaced with a metal prosthesis. In the most severe cases, total limb amputation must be used. Various types of amputation can be done, including removal of the joint (disarticulation) or across-the-bone (transosseous) amputation. The decision as to which type is chosen must take into consideration the patient's lifestyle.

Education/Discharge Instructions

Tell parents it is important to monitor mobility function and pain when surgical resection has been performed. The overall goal is to prevent further amputation. While the child and family may want to preserve the limb, sometimes amputation with later prosthesis is a better choice when function of the limb is impaired or pain becomes uncontrollable. The child can resume normal activity depending on the treatment protocol and how he or she feels. Parents can be taught about quiet activities that integrate normal developmental socialization.

Ewing's Sarcoma

Ewing's sarcoma involves the bone as well as soft tissue. It tends to appear in the middle of bones, most often the femur, pelvis, ribs, upper arms, and thigh (Fig. 33-7). Ewing's sarcoma is a highly malignant bone tumor with a histological appearance that is different from that of osteosarcoma. There are two different types of tumors. The first type, Ewing's sarcoma family of tumors, refers to a group of small, round cell, undifferentiated tumors thought to be of neural crest origin that generally carry the same chromosomal translocation. The second type is called peripheral primitive neuroectodermal tumor. Both of these tumor types can arise in long bone or in soft tissue (Kliegman et al., 2011).

It is more often seen in young males than in females. Ewing's sarcoma commonly affects patients between 10 and 20 years of age. Annually between 300 and 400 cases are diagnosed in the United States each year. It is extremely rare among African American children and in Asian Americans (Kliegman et al., 2011).

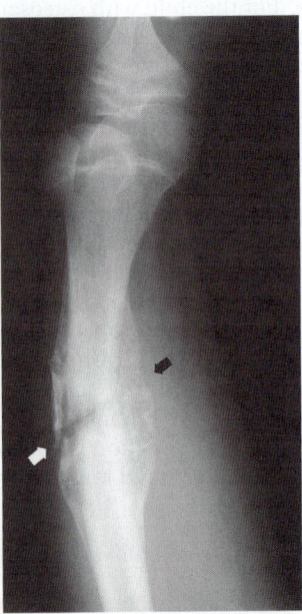

Figure 33-7 Ewing's sarcoma.

Nursing Insight—Prognosis

Patients with small, nonmetastatic, distally located extremity tumors have the best prognosis, with up to 85% having a 5-year survival rate when treated with chemotherapy, surgery, and/or radiation (Memorial Sloan Kettering Cancer Center, 2013). St. Jude Children's Research Hospital (2013) reports a 5-year survival rate of 65%. For the best prognosis, long-term follow-up is needed related to the chance of developing secondary malignancies. Late relapses, even 10 years after initial diagnosis, have been reported (Kliegman et al., 2011).

Signs and Symptoms

Clinical symptoms of Ewing's sarcoma are similar to those of osteosarcoma:

- Pain and swelling at the site of the tumor are the usual presenting symptoms (Memorial Sloan Kettering Cancer Center, 2013).
- The bone pain or swelling may be attributed to a sports injury, and caregivers may delay seeking care (Kliegman et al., 2011).
- When the tumor is present in the chest wall (Askin's tumor), the child may present with respiratory distress.
- The child with paraspinal or vertebrospinal tumors may present with symptoms of spinal cord compression.
- There may be systemic manifestations such as fever or weight loss.

Diagnosis

Diagnosis of Ewing's sarcoma is made via biopsy of the bone lesion. A complete staging procedure must be performed. A CT scan, MRI, or radionuclide bone scan is helpful in determining the primary site. Location of the primary tumor is important, especially with pelvic and sacral lesions, because those tumors are not able to be removed.

Nursing Insight—Metastasis

Ten to thirty percent of patients have metastatic disease at the time of diagnosis. The lung, other bones, and the bone marrow are the most common sites of metastasis. Widespread metastasis to other bones and the bone marrow may have a poor prognosis (Kliegman et al., 2011).

Collaborative Care

Nursing Care. Nursing care measures include assessment of unusual swelling and dilated surface blood vessels. Notice that the child may walk with a limp or have weakness on the affected side. Palpate the area and note any firm or non-tender enlargements. The primary nursing diagnosis is impaired mobility.

Medical Care. Multiagent chemotherapy is important because it can rapidly shrink the tumor and prevent new tumors from forming. Various chemotherapy treatment plans are used dependent on institution and established healthcare provider protocol.

Depending on the site of tumor involvement, radiation therapy may also be used (Memorial Sloan Kettering Cancer Center, 2013). When radiation treatment is performed, it is associated with the risk of radiation-induced secondary tumors, especially osteosarcoma, as well as failure of bone growth in skeletally immature patients.

Surgical Care. Surgical resection is preferred if possible. Postoperative care includes monitoring for signs and symptoms of infection, such as fever, redness, and warmth at the surgical site. Monitor drainage from the surgical site.

Education/Discharge Instructions

Discharge instructions include educating the parents about the signs and symptoms of infection such as fever, redness, and warmth at the surgical site. The child can resume normal activity depending on the treatment protocol and how he or she feels. Parents can be taught about quiet activities that integrate normal developmental socialization.

LYMPHOMAS

Lymphoma refers to a group of varied cancers that develop in the WBCs in the lymphatic system. Lymphatic tissue is present throughout the entire body and is a group of organs and tissues that are part of the immune system and also help to form new blood cells. These include the lymph nodes, small organs composed of lymphoid tissue at various parts of the body that are connected by lymphatic vessels; the spleen; the bone marrow; and the thymus gland just below the neck that produces one type of lymphocyte called the T cell. A lymphoma is a malignancy that arises from the lymphatic system.

Hodgkin's Disease

Hodgkin's disease (HD) consists of two types of lymphomas in children: Hodgkin's lymphoma (HL) and non-Hodgkin's lymphoma (NHL). Hodgkin's disease was first described in 1832 by the English physician Thomas Hodgkin. The major difference between the two types is that HL tends to involve the lymph nodes (those near the surface of the body), and NHL is frequently a disease of the tissues, especially the bowel, particularly in the region adjacent to the appendix, and in the upper midsection of the chest. In the United States, HD accounts for about 5% of childhood malignancies. Hodgkin's disease is rare in children younger than 5 years of age. There are three main age groups affected by Hodgkin's disease:

- Childhood form (younger than 14 years of age)
- Young adult form (15 to 34 years of age)
- Older adult form (55 to 74 years of age)

There is a male predominance in patients younger than 10 years of age, with an equal gender distribution in adolescence. People with a preexisting immunodeficiency, either congenital or acquired, have an increased risk of developing HD. The role of the Epstein–Barr virus is being studied in relation to HD. The Reed-Sternberg cell, a large cell with multiple or multilobulated nuclei, is considered the hallmark of HD, although similar cells are seen in mononucleosis (Kliegman et al., 2011). Currently the 5-year survival rate of children with HD is 95% (St. Jude Children's Research Hospital, 2013).

Hodgkin's Lymphoma
Signs and Symptoms

The onset of HL is not commonly acute in nature. The child may have symptoms for a long time before telling anyone or seeking care. A few patients may have no other presenting symptoms early in the disease other than swollen lymph nodes.

The disease is usually localized when patients present at the time of diagnosis:

- Painless, firm, cervical, or supraclavicular lymphadenopathy is the most common presenting sign.
- Inguinal or axillary sites are uncommon areas of presentation of lymphadenopathy. These lymph nodes are different than those associated with infection in that they are hard and not painful because they are filled with cancer cells.
- An anterior mediastinal mass is often present and can rapidly disappear with therapy.
- Systemic symptoms considered important in staging are unexplained fever, fever that comes and goes, weight loss, or drenching night sweats.
- Less common symptoms are lethargy, anorexia, and itching all over the body that cannot be explained (Kliegman et al., 2011).

Also less common are coughing, chest pain, and breathing problems if there are swollen lymph nodes in the chest. Excessive sweating, pain, or a feeling of fullness related to a swollen spleen or liver and skin blushing or flushing are other less common symptoms (National Institutes of Health (NIH), 2012).

Diagnosis

The only way to confirm HL is with a biopsy or removal of the enlarged lymph node. After biopsy confirms HL, several tests and scans are performed to determine the extent of spread: chest x-ray exam, CT scan, lymphangiogram to show abnormal nodes, MRI, bone scan, bone marrow biopsy, and blood tests.

Collaborative Care

Nursing Care. Nursing care for HL focuses on a thorough nursing assessment that includes monitoring the patient for fever and for painless lymph nodes in the neck, groin, or armpit area. Coughing or difficulty breathing and possible chest pain is noted as well as fatigue that does not go away. Pain, swelling, or a feeling of fullness in the abdomen is assessed. It is also important for the nurse to manage pain, provide comfort measures, and provide support to the child and the family. Obtain lab tests as ordered and prepare the child for imaging studies. Teaching the family about chemotherapy is necessary, if this is the prescribed treatment regimen.

Medical Care. Treatment for HL may include chemotherapy and radiation therapy, depending on the clinical stage at the time of diagnosis (Fig. 33-8). Diagnostic studies prescribed to monitor a child with HL may include a chest x-ray, CT scan, and MRI of the chest, abdomen, and pelvis. Pharmacological interventions are often prescribed to manage the patient's pain.

Education/Discharge Instructions

With a low WBC count, tell parents to keep the child away from people who are ill and avoid crowded places such as shopping malls. Teach the parents about comfort measures for the child. Stress the importance of follow-up appointments and clinic visits. The child can resume normal activity depending on the treatment protocol and how he or she feels. Parents can be taught about quiet activities that integrate normal developmental socialization.

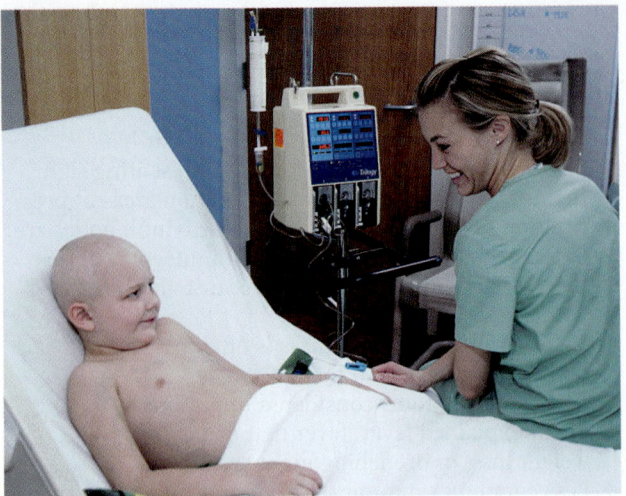

Figure 33-8 A child receiving chemotherapy.

Non-Hodgkin's Lymphoma

Malignant lymphoma is a cancer of lymphoid tissue or lymphatic system. NHL is different from HL in that there is no single focal origin (the malignant cells are rarely localized). NHL has a rapid onset and presents with widespread involvement. NHL results from malignant clonal proliferation of lymphocytes of T or B or indeterminate cell origin. There are four different types of NHL depending on how the cells look under the microscope:

- B-cell non-Hodgkin's lymphoma (Burkitt's and Burkitt's-like lymphoma) and Burkitt's leukemia
- Diffuse large B-cell lymphoma
- Lymphoblastic lymphoma (a malignancy of T cells)
- Anaplastic large cell lymphoma

There are two other types of lymphoma that occur in children: lymphoproliferative disease associated with a weakened immune system and rare non-Hodgkin's lymphomas that are more common in adults than children (National Cancer Institute, 2012).

Among children younger than 15 years of age, 60% of lymphomas are NHL. NHL is seen from infancy through adolescence, with a peak between the ages of 7 and 11. Boys are affected more than girls. The cause is unknown, although viral, genetic, immunological, and environmental factors have been implicated. Current 5-year survival rate for children with NHL is 80% (St. Jude Children's Research Hospital, 2013).

Signs and Symptoms

The presenting symptom of NHL is usually pain or swelling dependent on the initial site of involvement and the extent of disease spread. The most frequent sites of involvement are the abdomen, chest, and the head or neck region.

These lymphomas grow rapidly, and most children present with advanced-stage disease. Spread into the CNS may result in weakness of the facial muscles. Spread to the bone marrow may be associated with pale skin or bruising.

Diagnosis

Prompt tissue diagnosis and staging is important because of the rapid growth of lymphomas. Elevated levels of serum lactic dehydrogenase (greater than 500 units/L) correlate with tumor mass and are useful in deciding on therapy intensity. Other laboratory findings vary with the site or organs

involved. A CT scan or MRI of the chest or abdomen, or both, may assist in determining disease extent.

Collaborative Care

Nursing Care. Nursing care focuses on a thorough nursing assessment that includes monitoring the child for fever and for painless lymph nodes in the neck, groin, or armpit area. Assess for coughing, difficulty breathing, and possible chest pain. Fatigue that does not go away is also noted. Pain, swelling, or a feeling of fullness in the abdomen can occur. It is important for the nurse to provide pain management, comfort measures, and support to the child and the family. Obtain lab tests as ordered and prepare the patient for imaging studies such as a chest x-ray, CT scan, or MRI of the chest, abdomen, and pelvis.

Medical Care. Aggressive, multiagent chemotherapy is started as soon as possible once the diagnosis is made and tumor staging is complete. Intrathecal chemotherapy is given for CNS prophylaxis.

 focus on safety

Discarding chemotherapy drugs

When handling equipment or material that has contained chemotherapy drugs, discard it in a designated container that is properly labeled (Fig. 33-9). Chemotherapy drugs are considered hazardous waste material.

Education/Discharge Instructions

Discharge instructions and education for NHL includes monitoring the child for pain, infection, fever, and enlarged lymph nodes. Tell parents to watch for difficulty breathing. Teach parents about comfort measures. Stress the importance of follow-up appointments and clinic visits.

LIVER CANCER

In the United States, primary malignant liver tumors are the 10th most frequent pediatric malignancy (St. Jude Children's

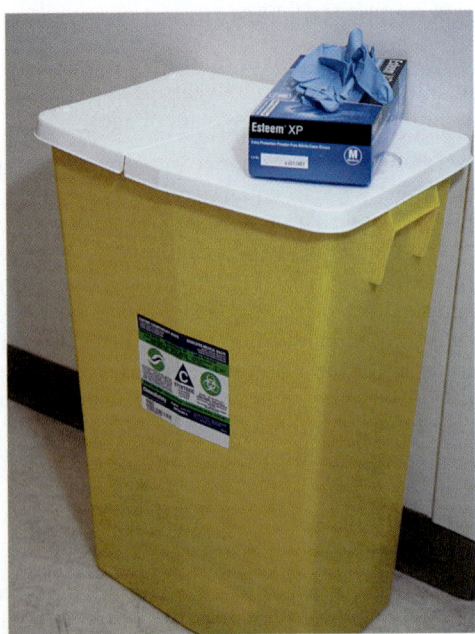

Figure 33-9 Chemotherapy waste receptacle.

Research Hospital, 2013). However, many other kinds of cancers can spread or metastasize to the liver. The two primary types of liver cancer are hepatoblastoma and hepatocellular carcinoma.

Signs and Symptoms

It is not uncommon for these symptoms to be present for months before a diagnosis is made.

- The first sign of liver cancer is a mass in the abdomen discovered by a family member or physician during a routine exam. It is usually located in the upper right side of the abdomen.
- Other symptoms the child might experience are a vague feeling of abdominal fullness, pain, vomiting, diarrhea, fever, abnormal weight loss, jaundice (yellow appearance of skin or sclera), or general itching.
- Occasionally, the liver may produce hormones that cause platelets to increase and the child has a very high platelet count.

Diagnosis

X-ray, ultrasound, CT scan, and MRI are used to diagnose liver cancer. These tests enable the physician to determine the severity and metastasis. The most common areas of metastasis are to other parts of the liver, the lungs, lymph nodes in the abdomen, and rarely, to the brain or bones. Biopsy of the liver cells confirms the diagnosis.

Collaborative Care

Nursing Care. See Holistic Nursing Care of the Child With Cancer.

 Nursing Insight—*Alpha-fetoprotein (AFP)*

Both hepatoblastoma and hepatocellular carcinoma produce a protein called alpha-fetoprotein (AFP), which can be detected in the blood via a simple blood test. If AFP levels fall, it indicates that treatment is working. If AFP levels rise, the tumor is not responding.

Medical Care. Chemotherapy is used first to shrink the size of the tumor. The best chance of curing liver cancer is surgical removal of the tumor. More than three-fourths of the liver can be removed without any problems because the liver can regenerate, or regrow. Hepatoblastoma responds well to chemotherapy, but hepatocellular carcinoma does not respond well to any known chemotherapy.

Education/Discharge Instructions

Instruct parents that it is important to follow up with all laboratory tests as ordered by the health-care provider. Parents must monitor the child for pain and discomfort and can call the health-care provider for medications as well as be taught nonpharmacological comfort measures. Stress the importance of follow-up appointments and clinic visits.

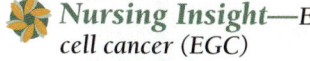 **Nursing Insight**—*Extragonadal germ cell cancer (EGC)*

Extragonadal germ cell cancers (EGCs) are tumors that originate in the sperm-forming cells in the testicles (male gonads)

or egg-producing cells in the ovary (female gonads). This type of cancer is located on the midline from the pineal gland to the coccyx. EGCs can be either benign or malignant. Most of the benign tumors occur in children. Surgical treatment can result in high rates of long-term survival and cure. Undescended testes are associated with an increased risk of testicular cancer (Kliegman et al., 2011).

Holistic Nursing Care of the Child With Cancer

Tailored holistic nursing care of the child with cancer is important to the child's survival and overall well-being. After diagnosis and staging and during the ongoing treatment, a thorough nursing assessment is crucial to maintain realistic optimal health and prevent complications. The nurse assesses for signs and symptoms of infection and bleeding. Additionally, the nurse monitors skin integrity (including mucous membranes), heart, kidney, bowel, lungs, musculoskeletal, and sensory function. Assessing the child's nutritional and pain status and evaluating the child's ability to meet normal growth and developmental milestones are also important.

There are several areas of nursing care for the child with cancer: maintaining nutrition, preventing infection, administering chemotherapy, addressing radiation side effects, understanding the use of surgery, managing pain, offering psychosocial support, managing negative and long-term effects of cancer treatments, and preventing medical emergencies. Understanding the psychological impact of pediatric cancer is also an important element of nursing care.

NUTRITION

Good nutrition is essential for the child with cancer to promote realistic optimal health and to maintain normal growth and development (Fig. 33-10). For the child with cancer, the demands of the illness and subsequent treatment can cause certain challenges. For example, children with cancer have elevated nutritional needs because of the disease itself and the effects of the treatment. At the same

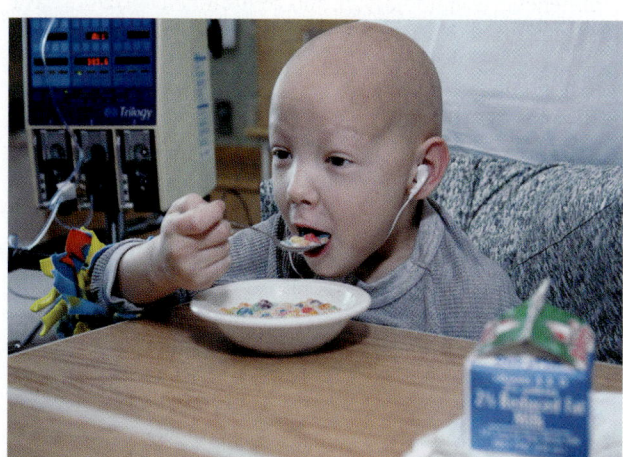

Figure 33-10 Good nutrition is essential for the growing child to maintain normal growth and development.

time, all children already have higher nutritional needs compared with adults for their normal growth and development (Bauer, Jurgens, & Fruhwald, 2011).

Parents frequently have anxiety about proper nutrition because the child can respond differently to treatment(s) and the desire and ability to eat and drink often change. Some children are able to eat enough food to have strength and energy to enjoy a normal level of activity; others are not. Poor nutrition can lead to tiredness or irritability, greater susceptibility to infections, and reduction of growth and developmental patterns.

The side effects of cancer therapy (nausea and vomiting, mouth sores, diarrhea, or constipation) can also make achieving adequate nutrition a challenge. Chemotherapy and radiation may interfere with the ability to chew and swallow. The child's sense of taste may change and his or her appetite may be poor.

A healthy immune system is a critical foundation of treatment. The immune system needs good nutrition for proper functioning. Proper immune function is possible only if the child obtains enough fluid intake and a high-calorie, well-balanced diet emphasizing proteins, fatty acids, vitamins, and minerals. The nurse offers suggestions to maintain good nutrition (Box 33-2). Encourage a diet that includes foods from all four food groups.

The nurse tries simple care measures first, such as offering small, frequent feedings, allowing the child food choices, choosing food textures that are appealing, and providing the child adequate time to eat. If the patient is unable to maintain good nutritional status, the nurse considers enteral tube feedings. If the gastrointestinal tract is not functioning well, total parenteral nutrition (TPN) via the IV route may be the only option. Communicate to the child and his or her parents that tube feedings or TPN may be temporary and that he or she may be able to eat independently again.

 Collaboration in Caring—*The role of a dietitian*

Consultation with the dietitian is essential to achieve the child's best nutritional outcome. If a child is unable to eat or meet basic caloric requirements for growth and development, the dietitian can recommend protein shakes and nutritional supplements. The dietitian teaches the child and family what foods would be best tolerated for certain conditions, like oral ulcerations or difficulty in swallowing.

INFECTION

A priority nursing action is preventing infection. It is essential that the nurse monitor for systemic and localized signs of infection every 2 to 4 hours (take the child's temperature every 4 hours). Report a single temperature greater than 101.2°F (38.5°C) in a 24-hour period or 100.4°F (38.0°C) 3 times in a 24-hour period.

The nurse provides meticulous skin care and maintains good hand washing. Instruct visitors to wash hands on entering and leaving the patient's room. Universal precautions and designated isolation precautions are instituted. Monitor and report laboratory values as ordered, such as absolute granulocyte count, white blood cell (WBC) count, complete blood count with differential, serum protein, serum albumin, and cultures. Encourage rest and sleep by providing a quiet environment.

It is important to teach the child and parents about the principles of prophylactic antibiotics and about the signs

---

Box 33-2 Suggestions for Nutrition

NAUSEA/VOMITING
- Offer plain, bland foods, such as cereal, canned or fresh fruit, rice, pasta, toast, mashed potatoes, soup, crackers, or plain meat.
- Avoid spicy, heavy, or fatty foods.
- If food smells bother the child, choose cold or room-temperature foods; use a cup with a lid.
- Do not offer solid food and liquid at the same time because this can induce nausea by making the child feel too full; give liquids 30 to 60 minutes after solid food.

DIARRHEA
- Offer plenty of liquids.
- Try bananas, rice, applesauce, toast, or tea.
- Decrease the fiber in the diet.

CONSTIPATION
- Provide extra liquids; offer beverages that contain caffeine, like coffee, tea, and cola.
- Increase fiber in the diet.
- Encourage the child to increase activity level.

POOR APPETITE
- Offer small amounts of food 4 or more times a day.
- Offer liquids between meals.
- Make every bite count by offering "power-packed foods."
- Start with small portions and gradually increase them.
- Allow the child to have foods and beverages that he or she especially likes.

SORE THROAT AND MOUTH
- Offer soft foods such as pudding, Jell-O®, macaroni and cheese, applesauce, bananas, ice cream, Italian ice, and popsicles.
- Avoid acidic foods like oranges and tomatoes, spicy foods, or foods that require a lot of chewing.
- Encourage good oral hygiene.

HEARTBURN OR REFLUX
- Do not give the child high-fat, spicy foods, caffeine, citrus juices, cinnamon, peppermint, or pepper.
- Keep the child upright for at least 1 hour after eating.

DIFFICULTY CHEWING OR SWALLOWING/DRY MOUTH
- Give the child soft, moist foods.
- Encourage sips of liquids while eating.
- Avoid hard foods that require a lot of chewing.
- Cut the food into small pieces.
- Use extra butter, sauces, or gravies.
- Offer hard candy to suck on.

BELCHING, INTESTINAL GAS, OR CRAMPS
- Avoid gas-forming foods such as cabbage, broccoli, cauliflower, cucumbers, beans, and carbonated beverages.
- Encourage the child to eat or drink slowly.
- Do not allow the child to chew gum.

and symptoms of infection to promote the best possible health for the child.

CHEMOTHERAPY

Chemotherapy is the primary treatment modality for many pediatric cancers. The nurse administers chemotherapy using a variety of drugs to destroy or kill cancer cells. The goal of chemotherapy is to reduce the primary size of the tumor by destroying cancer cells and to prevent those cells from spreading, or metastasizing.

Chemotherapy destroys these rapidly dividing and mutating cancer cells by interfering with cell division (Table 33-2). A variety of venous access devices are available to administer chemotherapy (Table 33-3).

Table 33-2 Chemotherapeutic Agents and Common Cancer Drugs

Agent	Indications	Route	Side Effects
asparaginase (Elspar, Kidrolase) Classification: Antineoplastic Pharmacological action: Enzyme	Acute lymphocytic leukemia (ALL)	IM and IV	Seizures, hyperglycemia Nausea and vomiting, rashes, coagulation abnormalities, hepatotoxic, pancreatitis, anaphylaxis (have emergency medications available)
bleomycin (Blenoxane) Classification: Antineoplastic Pharmacological: Antitumor antibiotics	Hodgkin's disease (HD), osteosarcoma, testicular embryonal cell carcinoma	IM, IV, and SQ	Pulmonary fibrosis Pneumonitis, hypotension, nausea and vomiting, anorexia, hyperpigmentation, rashes. Anaphylaxis: fever, chills
carboplatin (Paraplatin, Paraplatin AQ) Classification: Antineoplastic Pharmacological: Alkylating agent	Brain tumors, soft tissue sarcoma, osteosarcoma, retinoblastoma, neuroblastoma	IV	Ototoxicity, nausea and vomiting, constipation, diarrhea, stomatitis, renal and liver toxicity, hypocalcemia, hypokalemia, hyponatremia, hypomagnesemia, anaphylactic-like reactions
Corticosteroid (Dexamethasone, Decadron, Hydrocortisone, Prednisone) Classification: Corticosteroid Pharmacological: Systemic corticosteroids, anti-inflammatory	ALL, non-Hodgkin's lymphoma (NHL), HD, cerebral edema	PO, IV, and IT	Immunosuppression Weight gain, hypertension, anorexia, nausea and vomiting, acne, delayed wound healing, hirsutism, petechiae, osteoporosis, growth delay Cushingoid appearance
cyclophosphamide (Cytoxan, Neosar, Procytox) Classification: Antineoplastic, immunosuppressant Pharmacological: Alkylating agent	NHL, HD, ALL, neuroblastoma, Wilms' tumor, bone and soft tissue sarcoma, retinoblastoma	PO and IV	Myelosuppression Nausea, vomiting, anorexia, diarrhea, pulmonary and myocardial fibrosis, hemorrhagic cystitis, leukopenia, hematuria, alopecia, sterility, SIADH, may cause second neoplasm
daunorubicin (Daunomycin, Cerubidine) Classification: Antineoplastic Pharmacological: Anthracyclines	ALL, AML, osteosarcoma, soft tissue sarcoma	IV	Blistering, myelosuppression. Cardiotoxic: arrhythmias, acute cardiac myopathy-delayed, nausea and vomiting, stomatitis, potentiation of radiation, alopecia, rash, hyperpigmentation of nails
doxorubicin (Adriamycin, Adria, DOX, Rubex) Classification: Antineoplastic Pharmacological: Anthracyclines	ALL, AML, Osteosarcoma, soft tissue sarcoma, neuroblastoma	IV	Blistering, nausea and vomiting, stomatitis, esophagitis, diarrhea, red urine, anemia, hypersensitivity reaction, sterility. Cardiotoxic: arrhythmias, acute cardiomyopathy—delayed, potentiation of radiation, hyperpigmentation of nails, seizures, hypertension, edema, cough, shortness of breath, rash, thrombotic events
epoetin/erythropoietin (Epogen, EPO, Procrit) Classification: Biological response modifier Pharmacological: Hormone	Anemia	IV and SQ	Pulmonary edema, CHF, MI, hypotension, nausea and vomiting, anaphylaxis
etoposide (VP-16, VePesid) Classification: Antineoplastic Pharmacological: Podophyllotoxin derivative	AML, ALL, NHL, HD, bone and soft tissue sarcoma, Wilms' tumor, brain tumor, neuroblastoma, retinoblastoma	IV	Excessive leukocytosis, pain, and redness at subcutaneous site

(continued)

Table 33-2 Chemotherapeutic Agents and Common Cancer Drugs (continued)

Agent	Indications	Route	Side Effects

filgrastim (GCSF—granulocyte colony-stimulating factor) (Neupogen)
 	
Classification: Colony-
   stimulating factor
Pharmacological:
   Hematopoietic
   progenitor mobilizer
	Recovery drug for neutropenia	IV and SQ	Medullary bone pain

fluorouracil (5-FU, Adrucil) Classification: Antineoplastic Pharmacological: Antimetabolite	Brain tumors, germ cell tumors, osteosarcoma, soft tissue sarcoma, NHL, ALL	IV	Myelosuppression, nausea and vomiting (mild), mucositis (severe), hyperpigmentation of nails, nail loss, dermatitis, phototoxicity, myelosuppression, nausea and vomiting, diarrhea, neurotoxicity (encephalopathy, hallucinations), hepatotoxicity, hemorrhagic cystitis, alopecia, sterility, may cause second neoplasm
ifosfamide (Ifex) Classification: Antineoplastic Pharmacological: Alkylating agent	Stops methotrexate from harming the cells when given in high doses	IV	Allergic reactions: rash, urticaria, wheezing

leucovorin (Citrovorum factor, folinic acid, Wellcovorin)
 	
Classification: Antidote (for
   methotrexate), vitamins
Pharmacological: Folic acid
   analog
	Recovery drug to prevent hemorrhagic cystitis from ifosfamide and cyclophosphamide	IV and PO	Dose dependent on methotrexate level
			Given 24 hours after first methotrexate level has begun

mesna (Mesnex, Uromitexan) Classification: Antidote Pharmacological: Ifosfamide detoxifying agent	Prevention of ifosfamide-induced hemorrhagic cystitis	IV, PO, IM, and IT	Dizziness, drowsiness, headache, anorexia, diarrhea, nausea and vomiting, unpleasant taste, flushing, flu-like symptoms

methotrexate (MTX, Amethopterin)
 	
Classification:
   Antineoplastic
Immunosuppressant
Pharmacological:
   Antimetabolite
	ALL, osteosarcoma, NHL	IV	Myelosuppression, nausea and vomiting, stomatitis, alopecia, hepatotoxicity, neurotoxicity, photosensitivity, rash, pulmonary fibrosis, aplastic anemia

ondansetron (Zofran) Classification: Antiemetic Pharmacological: 5-HT$_3$ antagonist	Prevention of nausea and vomiting associated with chemotherapy	IV and PO	Headache, diarrhea, constipation, dry mouth, extrapyramidal reactions
PEG-L-asparaginase (pegaspargase) (Oncaspar) Classification: Antineoplastic Pharmacological: Enzymes	ALL, HD	IM and IV	Seizures, pancreatitis, lip edema, headache, nausea and vomiting, diarrhea, DIC, hemolytic anemia, pancytopenia, chills, night sweats
vincristine (Oncovorin, Vincasar PFS) Classification: Antineoplastic Pharmacological: Vinca alkaloids	Wilms' tumor, Ewing's sarcoma, brain tumor	IV	Altered LOC, blistering, peripheral neuropathy, alopecia, constipation, SIADH, seizure, nausea and vomiting

Note: IV, intravenous; IM, intramuscular; SQ, subcutaneous; PO, by mouth; IT, intrathecal.

Source: Vallerand & Sanoski (2014).

Table 33-3 Venous Access Devices

Name	Description	Advantage	Nursing Care
Central implanted ports, such as Infuse-A-Port, Mediport, Port-A-Cath, or Norport	A saucer-shaped plastic device with a self-sealing injection port that can be accessed from the top or side. Requires placement in operating room.	Decreased risk of infection. Placed under the skin, reducing the chance of becoming dislodged or pulled out. Limited noticeability (small bump under the skin). Patency is maintained by administering heparin after access. Little maintenance or care; child can participate in regular activities.	Cleanse skin with warm water and soap prior to use. Administer topical anesthetic such as EMLA (lidocaine and prilocaine) before accessing the port. Use a Huber needle to access the port. Observe child during medication administration for dislodgment of needle. When treatment is complete, the port must be surgically removed.
Central Groshong catheter	A silicone, flexible and clear catheter; at the proximal end, there is a closed-tip two-way valve. Requires placement in operating room.	Easy for self-administered medications and fluids. No heparin required. No clamping needed because of two-way valve. Minimal backflow. Decreases possibility of air embolism.	Weekly irrigation with normal saline. Parents can learn catheter care (site must be kept clean and dry). Teaching points include: (1) strenuous activity and water sports are restricted and (2) overall safety because the catheter protrudes from body and may be pulled out. Offer support based on body image disturbance.
Central tunneled catheter such as Broviac or Hickman	An open-ended silicone, flexible, radiopaque catheter. Requires placement in operating room.	Easy for self-administered medications and fluids. Decreases risk of infection.	Daily heparin flushes. Parents can learn catheter care (site must be kept clean and dry). When not in use, must be clamped. Teaching points include: (1) strenuous activity and water sports are restricted and (2) general safety precautions because the catheter protrudes from body and may be pulled out.
Peripherally inserted central catheters	Catheter made of Silastic or polyurethane material. Single or double lumen available. Inserted into antecubital fossa passing through the cephalic or basilic vein entering the superior vena cava.	Does not require placement in operating room. Pediatric nurse practitioners can insert the line using a small-lumen needle. Decreases risk of infection.	Flushed with saline using 5- to 10-mL syringe. Not suitable for rapid fluid replacement (small-lumen needle). Sometimes can be difficult to remove because of resistance.

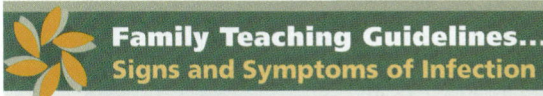

Family Teaching Guidelines...
Signs and Symptoms of Infection

HOW TO: Teach the Family How to Recognize Signs and Symptoms of Infection

The family needs to understand that any of these signs and symptoms, or a combination of them, must be reported to the physician immediately:

- Fever
- Decrease in temperature
- Runny nose (or other respiratory illness)
- Sore throat
- Childhood disease such as chickenpox
- Lethargy
- Pale or ashen color
- Chills
- Diaphoresis
- Poor appetite
- Poor fluid intake
- Nausea, vomiting, or diarrhea
- Decreased urination
- Foul smelling urine or pain or burning upon urination

ESSENTIAL INFORMATION:

The rectal mucosa is very vascular and an area of potential injury or a source of infection. Never take a rectal temperature or administer any rectal suppository or an enema.

RADIATION

Radiation therapy uses ionizing radiation to break apart the bonds within a cell, damaging it, and causing it to die. This treatment has evolved over the years with respect to children. Today, with the use of computed tomography (CT) and magnetic resonance imaging scans, it is possible to more precisely deliver radiation therapy to very specific, targeted areas. External beam radiation accounts for the majority of radiation treatments in children. The amount of radiation used is determined by the patient's age, tumor site, tumor size, tumor radiosensitivity, coexisting disease, and the use of other treatment modalities. The lowest effective dose of radiation is calculated and then delivered over a 3- to 6-week period. Treatment lasts just a few minutes. It is important for the child to remain still during treatment. Sometimes it may be necessary to sedate the child (Kliegman et al., 2011). Radiation is used with some hesitancy in children younger than 3 years of age because it can cause severe damage to healthy cells and restrict growth and fertility in the future. Nursing care includes measures that address the side effects of radiation.

clinical alert

Radiation side effects

- Nausea
- Alopecia
- Fatigue and malaise
- Low WBC
- Skin desquamation
- Mucous membrane inflammation and irritation

SURGERY

The child may have cancer-related medical conditions before surgery; therefore, the nurse understands that care measures are tailored to the child's pre- and postoperative nursing diagnoses. Before the development of chemotherapy and radiation, surgery was the principal treatment of children with solid tumors. Now surgery is used as an adjunct to both chemotherapy and radiation. Tumors are usually treated with chemotherapy and radiation first to reduce the size before surgical resection. The use of surgery varies widely depending on the child's diagnosis. Surgery is also an important role in the diagnosis of a tumor via biopsy. The biopsy sample may be obtained through a fine-needle aspiration or an open biopsy procedure.

 Nursing Insight—*Insertion of central venous catheters*

The insertion of central venous catheters is one of the most frequent surgical procedures performed (Fig. 33-11). These long-term central venous access devices make it safer to administer chemotherapy and total parenteral nutrition and are also used in administering antibiotics and obtaining blood specimens. Some of the catheters typically inserted in children include a Broviac or a Port-A-Cath.

 Nursing Diagnoses Children With Cancer

- Ineffective airway clearance related to excessive secretions
- Risk of injury (bleeding) related to thrombocytopenia
- Risk for fluid volume deficit related to vomiting and decreased oral intake
- Risk for infection related to neutropenia
- Pain related to diagnosis, disease process, and treatment
- Fatigue related to anemia
- Impaired oral mucosa related to oral ulcerations from cancer treatment
- Imbalanced nutrition: less than body requirements related to loss of appetite, nausea, vomiting, and mucositis

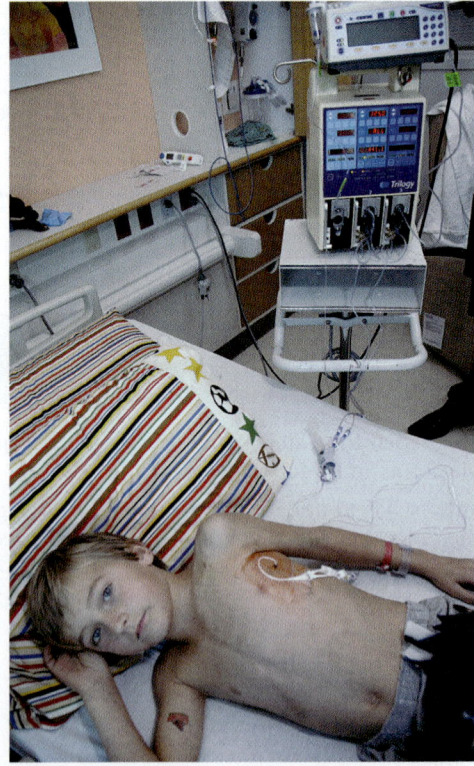

Figure 33-11 The insertion of a central venous catheter helps in administering chemotherapy and is one of the most frequent surgical procedures performed on children with cancer.

 Where Research and Practice Meet:
Exploring the Risk of Developing Cancer After CT Scans in Children

There are potential side effects of ionizing radiation exposure, particularly that of radiation from CT scans. According to a special report published in *Radiology 2011*, the incidence of using CT scans has increased more than 10% over the last 25 years. In one report published in 2012, children and adults who were scanned multiple times by CT scan were found to have a small risk in the development of leukemia and brain tumors in the decade after their first scan. This study examined more than 175,000 children and young adults led by researchers at the National Cancer Institute and the Institute of Health and Society at Newcastle University in the United Kingdom. Investigators estimated that for every 10,000 CT scans of the head performed in children aged 10 or younger, 1 case of leukemia and 1 case of a brain tumor would occur in the decade after the first CT beyond what would have been expected had no CT scans been done (Printz, 2013).

- Caregiver role strain related to disease process and frequent hospitalizations
- Ineffective coping related to cancer diagnosis
- Altered family process related to hospitalization

PAIN CONTROL

Controlling the child's pain is an essential nursing intervention. Pain associated with cancer can be acute or chronic. Four common types of pain found in children with cancer are tumor-related pain, impingement of tumor on nervous tissue, treatment-related pain, and post–lumbar puncture headaches. Postoperative pain is also a concern after tumor resection, biopsy, amputation, or central line placement. The most effective pain management strategies reported by children with cancer are use of effective pain medications combined with adequate rest and sleep, massage, heat, distraction, and social support.

Assessing Pain

It is imperative to use the appropriate pain assessment tool. The FLACC score for infants and young children, the Faces scale, and the numbers scale are used when children are asked to rate their pain (see Chapter 21 for pain assessment tools used in the care of children).

Pain Medications

- To manage the pain of cancer, the health-care provider may start with ordering acetaminophen (Children's Tylenol) and progress to a nonsteroidal anti-inflammatory such as naproxen or ibuprofen (Advil or Motrin) for children older than 6 months of age. Nonsteroidal anti-inflammatory agents are contraindicated in children with renal insufficiency or low platelet count.
- If these pain medications are insufficient, opioids are used and are administered orally, IV, IM, or can be delivered by a patient-controlled anesthesia device. Some are even available in a transcutaneous patch. Opioids for moderate pain are codeine (codeine sulfate or Tylenol with codeine). The opioid drug of choice is morphine (Duramorph) because of its extensive clinical usage and current published data. It is globally available and has controlled-release varieties. Doses are titrated for maximal effectiveness. Fentanyl (Duragesic) is a quick-acting opioid narcotic available in a transdermal patch. Hydromorphone hydrochloride (Dilaudid) is another opioid that is used to control pain. Methadone hydrochloride (Methadone) is being explored as a drug for use in the pediatric population and may offer an alternative to opioids.
- Procedural pain may require the additional use of benzodiazepines for sedation in addition to the pain medication. This class of drugs has a fast-acting sedative effect that offers a "dissociative effect" in which the child experiences an out-of-body-like experience that is effective for minor procedural sedation. Propofol (Diprivan) is an anesthetic agent used to reduce children's anxiety. It can be administered in intermittent bolus doses to provide adequate sedation during painful procedures such as a lumbar puncture.

 focus on safety

Ketamine hydrochloride (Ketamine HCl) and propofol (Diprivan)

Ketamine hydrochloride (Ketamine HCl) and propofol (Diprivan) are only to be given by a medical doctor with proper training in the use of anesthetic agents. It is given in a controlled environment with adequate resuscitation equipment available if needed. Nurses do not give either of these two agents.

 Nursing Insight—*Topical anesthetics*

Use topical anesthetics, such as EMLA (Astra Zeneca) cream, when possible for procedure-related pain. EMLA is a lidocaine/prilocaine 1:1 mixture. The nurse applies a thin coating of ointment to the projected insertion site(s) and covers the site(s) with a clear plastic occlusive dressing (such as Tegederm®). It is important to keep the cream on for at least 1 hour (sometimes longer) prior to the procedure.

PSYCHOSOCIAL SUPPORT

Psychosocial support is essential in providing holistic nursing care. Encourage 24-hour stay with parents and other family members or friends. Involve a child life specialist who can use therapeutic play or encourage arts and crafts. Video games, computers, handheld devices, or other technological equipment can be helpful when offering psychosocial support. Encourage visits to the playroom (if appropriate for the child's condition) while the child is in the hospital. Being present or simply listening can be powerful in the care of children with cancer. The nurse can also provide the family with community resources, reliable Internet sources, or information about support groups.

 Cultural Diversity: Communication and Language Challenges

Language, and the ability to understand it, is an important aspect of health literacy and is vital in a family's ability to use health information. Chinese and south Asian parents were interviewed over a 6-month period post–cancer diagnosis. Sixty-two percent of these parents had no difficulty communicating with providers. However 26% of parents struggled with English, and 12% of parents could not communicate with providers at all (Gulati, Watt, Shaw, Sung, Poureslami, Klaassen et al., 2012). Language as a

 Where Research and Practice Meet: **Propofol-Remifentanil and Propofol-Fentanyl**

In a study by Ince et al. (2013), researchers compared propofol-remifentanil and propofol-fentanyl for sedation during short hemato-oncological invasive procedures in children. Researchers found that for short hemato-oncological interventions, the propofol-remifentanil combination was also effective and suitable for early recovery outside the operating room for children older than 2 years in combination with propofol (Diprivan) and midazolam injection (Versed).

barrier to adequate health care continues to be problematic for non-English children and families in the United States. Language lines via the phone are now available in most health-care institutions, and if not, an appropriate interpreter must be provided. The results of this study indicated that parents and children must be able to understand their child's diagnosis, treatment, and outcomes.

 ### *Nursing Insight—Taking care of children with cancer*

The pediatric nurse knows that children with cancer want to be loved and treated like other children. Be sure to encourage these children to play and be involved in self-care activities as their condition allows. Encourage them to talk about their dreams, feelings, and fears. It is a privilege for the nurse to share in the lives of these brave children.

Negative Effects of Chemotherapy

Chemotherapy has several associated negative effects. The nurse must recognize and provide proper nursing care to promote the best health for the child during his or her treatment.

 ### focus on safety

Ataxia

Children with ataxia may have difficulty walking and are at risk for falling. Ataxia can be a result of the therapy or disease process. It may also be a result of certain medications. Be sure to evaluate the child's ability to walk safely. Evaluate the child's fall risk using the Humpty Dumpty Scale (Fig. 33-12) or other tools devised to assess the child's fall risk. Some children may need to use walkers or simply the assistance of an adult to walk. It is important to involve physical therapy to optimize the child's strength.

 Critical Nursing Action Recognizing Negative Effects of Chemotherapy

Chemotherapy is toxic to the body bcause it kills not only cancer cells but healthy cells as well. It is important that, as soon as chemotherapy is administered, the nurse ensures that the child is also well hydrated so that the chemotherapeutic agent (or toxin) is flushed out of the system. A way to ensure proper hydration is to measure the specific gravity of the urine. The urine specific gravity should be 1.012 or below. If it rises above this, IV fluid boluses are required.

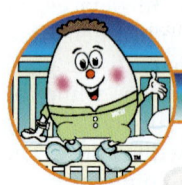

The Miami Children's Hospital Humpty Dumpty Falls™ Scale and Prevention Program

Preventing falls, enhancing safety.

Patient Safety is a top priority for hospitals nationwide. Pediatric safety prevention is a focal point of the educational endeavors at Miami Children's Hospital (MCH). Over the course of the past year, our facility has taken the lead in developing a tool to prevent pediatric falls and thereby enhance safety. This fall prevention program has been implemented, tested and proven to be an effective tool in the prevention of unintentional injury due to falls.

Miami Children's Hospital is pleased to inform you that its highly effective and acclaimed, Humpty Dumpty Falls™ Scale and Prevention Program is now available as a training module. Included in the kit are:

Falls Scale
- Humpty Dumpty Scale™ (inpatient/outpatient, Emergency Department)

Educational Tools
Materials may be customized for each facility.
- Patient falls safety protocol (inpatient/outpatient, Emergency Department)
- Falls Prevention-"We want you to know"
- PowerPoint Presentation

Signage
- Laminated sign for bed (inpatient)
- Stickers (inpatient, Emergency Department)
- Badges (outpatient)

References
- A two-hour training session (teleconference or onsite)
  * There is an additional cost for onsite instruction

Cost
- $399

Your facility may become a participant in the research studies.

This comprehensive packet will soon be available. If you would like to obtain more information, please contact: Maria Lina "Bing" Wood, ARNP, MSN, Director, Pediatric Intensive Care and ECLS Services at 305-669-6457 or via email at Bing.wood@mch.com

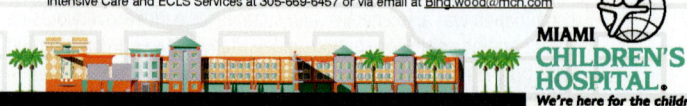

MIAMI CHILDREN'S HOSPITAL.
We're here for the children

MCH-HC06/06-O

Figure 33-12 Humpty Dumpty Scale.

NAUSEA AND VOMITING

Nausea and vomiting is a major negative effect of chemotherapy, and the nurse understands that the nausea may persist for weeks. Acute nausea begins 2 to 3 hours after chemotherapy starts, peaks at 4 to 10 hours, and lasts for 12 to 24 hours. Delayed nausea begins 1 to 5 days after chemotherapy, peaks 48 to 72 hours, and is less severe than acute nausea. Anticipatory nausea is psychological, and the nurse understands that it is important to medicate the child if he or she complains about nausea.

It is also important for the nurse to be knowledgeable about medications (antiemetics) that can prevent or lessen nausea and vomiting in children (Fig. 33-13).

Medication: Ondansetron (Zofran)

(on-**dan**-se-tron)

Classification: Antiemetic

Indications: Prevention of nausea and vomiting associated with chemotherapy or radiation therapy

Action: Blocks the effects of serotonin receptor sites

Contraindications: Hypersensitivity

Adverse Reactions and Side Effects: CNS: headache, dizziness, drowsiness, fatigue, weakness. **GI:** constipation, diarrhea, abdominal pain, dry mouth, increased liver enzymes. **Neuro:** extrapyramidal reactions

Route and Dosage:
PO (ADULTS AND CHILDREN GREATER THAN 11 YR)
Prevention of chemotherapy-induced nausea and vomiting: 8 mg 30 min prior to chemotherapy and repeated 8 hr later
PO (CHILDREN 4 TO 11 YR)
Prevention of chemotherapy-induced nausea and vomiting: 4 mg 30 min prior to chemotherapy and repeated 4 and 8 hr later
IV (CHILDREN 6 MO TO 18 YR)
Prevention of chemotherapy-induced nausea and vomiting: 0.15 mg/kg 15 to 30 min prior to chemotherapy and repeated 4 and 8 hr later

Nursing Implications:
Assess patient for nausea, vomiting, abdominal distension and bowel sounds prior to and following administration.

Source: Vallerand & Sanoski (2014).

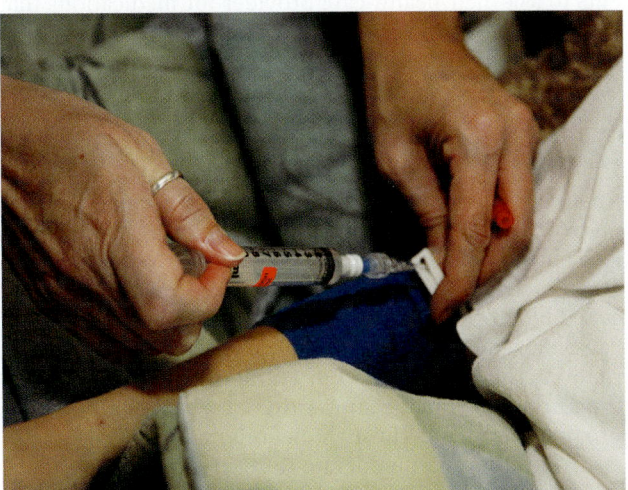

Figure 33-13 It is important for the nurse to be knowledgeable of medications (antiemetics) that can prevent or lessen nausea and vomiting in children receiving chemotherapy.

ALOPECIA

Hair loss (alopecia) is another negative effect associated with cancer treatment (Fig. 33-14). Not all children undergoing chemotherapy lose their hair. When it does occur, it may be devastating to the child and the family. Providing a wig or a hat and helping the child present a positive body image and peer acceptance are crucial. There are agencies (e.g., http://www.locksoflove.org/) that assist with providing the child with a wig.

❝What to say❞—*A child asks will my hair grow back?*

Many children who start chemotherapy have many questions, especially wanting to know "if my hair falls out, will it grow back?" Children worry about their appearance to an extent that depends on their age. The nurse explains that the hair will probably start to fall out 10 days to 2 weeks after chemotherapy begins and that it may fall out in sections. The nurse can assure the child that once the chemotherapy has been completed, his or her hair will grow back. Try to make this experience as positive as possible by emphasizing there are wigs available as well as head wraps and "cool" hats and caps to cover the child's head. Encourage the child to speak with others his or her age who have been through this experience. It is important for the nurse to emphasize the fact that just because his or her hair falls out, it does not change the person the child is inside. The child is the same person, who just looks a little different for a little while. The nurse can make this a special event by arranging for a first "cool hat" purchase before the child leaves the hospital.

Nursing Insight—*Looking different*

In a social sharing platform on Facebook®, Jane Bingham and Becky Sypin urged Mattel® to create "Bald and Beautiful Barbie"

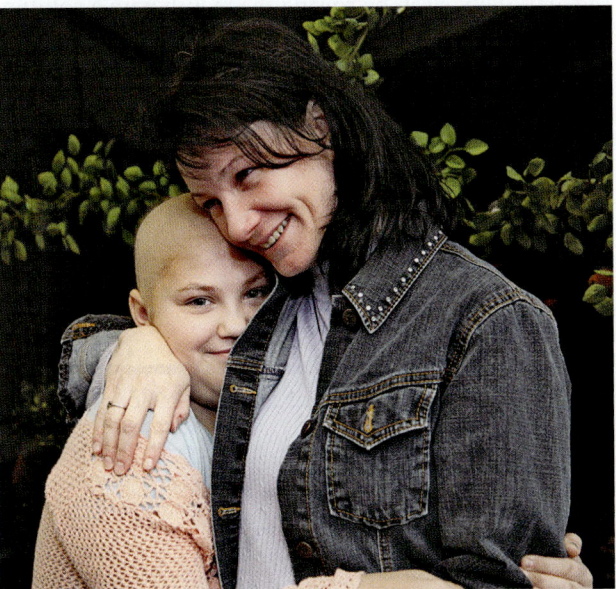

Figure 33-14 Alopecia is a negative effect associated with cancer treatment that can cause the child to feel self-conscious.

to comfort girls with cancer. Bingham, a survivor of non-Hodgkin's lymphoma joined her friend Becky Sypin, whose 12-year-old daughter lost all her hair after chemotherapy, and launched a campaign on Facebook® that quickly gained thousands of followers. Sypin approached Mattel® who initially declined but then agreed to distribute the doll exclusively to children's hospitals and other hospitals treating children with cancer in the United States and Canada. According to ABC-News.com, the doll will include "hats, scarves, and other fashion accessories to provide girls with a traditional fashion play experience. The wigs and hair coverings can be completely removed. These dolls are not available in retail stores, but through donation they are beneficial for girls who can play with them (Russo, 2012).

EXTRAVASATION

Chemotherapeutic drugs must be handled carefully to avoid **extravasation,** which is leaking of vesicants (Box 33-3) that can cause tissue damage surrounding the IV or central line insertion site; blistering, blanching, or excoriation may lead to ulceration and deep skin sloughing. In rare cases, vesicants can cause cellulitis that turns into a more severe infection. It is important to handle chemotherapy agents safely (Box 33-4). The nurse infusing these agents is specially trained and certified in the administration of chemotherapy agents. Flushing the line properly and ensuring a good blood flow can help prevent extravasation.

MUCOSITIS

Mucositis is a diffuse inflammation of the mucosa of the mouth, a change in the integrity of the mucous membranes characterized by soreness, redness, and swelling. Lesions on the mucous membranes allow bacteria to attach themselves to the affected areas and are a source of localized and systemic infection. Mucositis is caused by chemotherapy and radiation to the head and neck. It is essential to keep the oral cavity clean by rinsing the mouth with a solution

---

Box 33-3 **Agents Known to Cause Extravasation**
TPN and other hyperosmolar fluids Dilantin Chemotherapeutic agents (e.g., doxorubicin, daunorubicin, mitomycin C, vincristine, vinblastine, VP-16, and dacarbazine)

Box 33-4 **Safe Handling of Chemotherapeutic Agents**
• Use disposable gloves and gowns when handling or preparing chemotherapy medications to prevent contact with medication. • Use aseptic technique when administering medications. • Prepare drugs in a well ventilated room. • Dispose of all medications, contaminated needles, syringes, IV tubing, gloves, and gowns in an appropriate leakproof, puncture-resistant container.
Source: Alcoser & Rodgers (2003). *Journal of Pediatric Nursing, 18*(2), 103–112.

(e.g., chlorhexidine oral (Peridex), sodium bicarbonate swish and spit, Nystatin swish and swallow, a "magic mouthwash" consisting of milk of magnesia and Carafate, or others (variable by institution).

 Assessment Tool   Oral Assessment

It is important to inspect the oral cavity for problems related to cancer treatment:
- **Voice or cry** (normal, deep, or raspy-harsh)
- **Ability to swallow** (normal, pain, difficult to swallow)
- **Lips** (smooth, pink, moist, dry, cracked, ulcers, or bleeding)
- **Tongue** (midline, pink, moist, reddened, patches, film, blisters, or swollen)
- **Saliva** (normal, excessive, thick or strands, absent or decreased)
- **Mucous membranes** (pink, moist, red, coated, patches, ulcers, bleeding)
- **Gingiva** (pink, firm, edema with or without redness, bleeding)
- **Teeth** (clean, plaque, debris, condition)

DIARRHEA AND CONSTIPATION

Diarrhea may occur with chemotherapy. Assess the rectal mucosa to prevent infection. Gently cleaning the skin around the anus with a soft cloth and warm water is important. Applying a barrier cream (such as Desitin®) and allowing the irritated skin to be exposed to open air as much as possible may be necessary. Have the child drink plenty of clear fluids (based on 24-hour intake) and eat small amounts of soft, bland, low-fiber foods such as bananas, rice, noodles, white bread, or skinned chicken. Avoiding greasy, fatty, spicy, or fried foods as well as raw vegetables and fruits, and whole-grain breads (cereals, nuts, and popcorn) can help. It is also important to discourage gas-forming foods (beans, cabbage, and carbonated beverages) and limiting beverages with caffeine. Communicate to parents that they can contact the health-care provider about an over-the-counter medication for diarrhea such as loperamide (Imodium) or a prescription medication like diphenoxylate (Lomotil).

If the child becomes constipated, suggest foods high in fiber (fruits and vegetables) and drink plenty of fluid, such as water and juices. Normal activity and playing, if approved by the health-care provider, can help. Instruct parents to ask their health-care provider for medications that will help with the constipation. The health-care provider may prescribe medications such as docusate sodium (Colace) or bisacodyl (Dulcolax).

ANEMIA

Anemia can also be acquired during chemotherapy. Bone marrow suppression, nutritional deficiencies, and blood loss may all lead to anemia below 8 g/dL. While the cancerous cells are being killed, sometimes healthy cells such as red blood cells (RBCs) are also killed.

Some signs of anemia are severe fatigue, headache, irritability, or tachycardia. For children with mild anemia, the nurse can provide supportive care guidelines for improving the anemia through diet or vitamin supplementation. Children with moderate to severe anemia may need an RBC transfusion to restore blood volume. For anemia as a result of concomitantly administered chemotherapy, administer hematopoietic growth factors such as epoetin alpha (Epogen) that may prove beneficial in decreasing the need for blood transfusions.

THROMBOCYTOPENIA

Like RBCs, platelets can also be destroyed. Platelets are important for the clotting of the blood. Thrombocytopenia is a decreased number of platelets (less than 100,000 mcL). Thrombocytopenia develops as a result of increased destruction, decreased production, or loss of platelets. A platelet transfusion may be given if platelet counts drop to less than 50,000 mcL, if the patient has spontaneous bleeding, or if an invasive procedure is scheduled (Kliegman et al., 2011).

NEUTROPENIA

Neutropenic children have few white blood cells (WBCs) and often do not show signs of infection, such as swelling, redness, or drainage. The only sign may be fever. A fever in an oncology patient is 101.2°F (38.5°C) in a 24-hour period or 100.4°F (38.0°C) three times in a 24-hour period. Take only axillary or oral temperature.

A severe neutropenic patient has an absolute neutrophil count (ANC) less than 500/mm³. An ANC greater than or equal to 500 to 1,000/mm³ is considered moderately neutropenic, and an ANC greater than or equal to 1,000 to <1,500/mm³ is considered mildly neutropenic. When a child undergoing chemotherapy develops a fever, it is considered an emergency.

 Diagnostic Tools Calculating the Absolute Neutrophil Count (ANC)

Formula: (WBC × 10) × (Bands + Neutrophils)
Example: WBC = 8.8, Neutrophils = 82, Bands = 5
ANC = (8.8 × 10) × (82 + 5)
ANC = (88) × (87)
ANC = 7,656

Two sets of blood cultures are required for the neutropenic patient before the start of antibiotics. Antibiotics, determined by the health-care provider, such as ceftazidime (Fortaz), ampicillin (Unasyn), gentamycin (Garamycin), or Vancomycin Hydrochloride (Vancomycin Hydrochloride Injection) that treat both gram-positive and gram-negative bacteria, are started as soon as possible, no later than 1 hour after admission. More specific antibiotics are administered once culture and sensitivities are identified from the blood cultures. Monitor vital signs closely when administering antibiotics because of the release of endotoxin that may occur. Left unchecked, this condition may lead to septic shock. Filgrastim (Neupogen) is an injection also used in a neutropenic patient to increase the production of neutrophils. Neutrophils are important in maintaining the body's ability to fight infection.

 Optimizing Outcomes—**Neutropenic patient admitted to a pediatric unit**

To ensure the best outcome, a 2-year-old neutropenic oncology patient admitted to the inpatient pediatric unit should be placed in a private room. If a private room is not available, assigning the child to a room with someone noninfectious, such as a child with a fractured femur, is acceptable.

LONG-TERM EFFECTS OF CANCER TREATMENTS

Now that children with cancer are surviving longer, researchers are just beginning to understand the long-term effects of cancer treatments. Children undergoing cancer treatments are assessed for acute effects at the time but also need follow-up care in adulthood to assess for potential long-term effects. A long-term survivor of any cancer is considered a child who has been in remission for 5 years or who has been off cancer therapy for 2 years.

For example, high-tone hearing loss may be a side effect of cisplatin (Platinol). Other chemotherapeutic agents can cause loss of speech, impairment in depth perception, and increased response time, which can be a problem for the adolescent who wishes to drive. Lung problems can be caused by scarring of lung tissue or a reduction in lung elasticity during breathing. Shortness of breath and a reduced capacity to exercise can significantly impact the child. Kidney problems include bleeding, damage to the tubules that affects electrolyte exchange and salt balance, and protein wasting. Musculoskeletal defects involving the bones or soft tissue and teeth have been reported. Functional and/or mobility deficits may persist if an amputation was performed. Hormonal abnormalities that are often treatable may also exist. Cancer treatment can sometimes produce sterility. Hearing, skin problems, and cardiac dysfunction are some of the late side effects that children are left to deal with later in life.

Children who had radiation to the brain may show growth retardation, cognitive impairment, and/or learning disabilities. Damage to the hypothalamus may cause an irreversible disorder called diabetes insipidus. A type of nerve damage called peripheral neuropathy can lead to decreased reflexes and weakness. The thyroid gland is also sensitive to radiation and may pose problems later in life.

Medical Emergencies

Because of an altered state of health, a child with cancer is prone to various conditions that may constitute a medical emergency including accidents, infections, allergic reactions, or common childhood diseases. If one or more of these conditions is negatively affecting the child, the pediatric nurse must act quickly and notify the physician or oncologist caring for the child to prevent a life-threatening condition or further complications.

HEMORRHAGIC CYSTITIS

When caring for an oncology patient who is undergoing chemotherapy, using certain chemotherapy agents, such as cyclophosphamide (Cytoxan) or ifosfamide (Ifex), can cause hemorrhagic cystitis (bloody or painful urination). Radiation may also cause hemorrhagic cystitis.

Signs and Symptoms

Signs and symptoms in this condition can range from mild dysuria (painful urination) with urinary frequency to severe hemorrhage that is significant enough to damage the epithelial lining of the bladder. Patients also have leukocytes, erythrocytes, and clots in the urine.

Diagnosis

Diagnosis is based on the noted signs and symptoms.

Prevention

The best way to treat hemorrhagic cystitis is to prevent it with adequate hydration before and during the administration of chemotherapy.

Collaborative Care

Nursing Care. Be sure to test the urine for blood, pH, and specific gravity. The specific gravity should be 1.012 or below. If it is not, a bolus of IV fluid is required (Procedure 33-1). If the urine is positive for blood, send an immediate urinalysis sample to the lab and notify the physician immediately. Monitoring of intake and output is vital as well as a daily blood urea nitrogen (BUN) and creatinine. Mesna (Mesnex, Uromitexan) is a drug given to prevent hemorrhagic cystitis by helping to protect the lining of the bladder.

TUMOR LYSIS SYNDROME

Tumor lysis syndrome is a life-threatening condition that may develop in children with cancer. Tumors with high

---

 Procedure 33-1 Checking Urine Specific Gravity (Fig. 33-15)

Purpose

The purpose of checking the specific gravity of urine is to measure the concentration of the particles in the urine (Box 33-5).

Equipment

- Refractometer
- 3- or 5-mL syringe (needleless)

Steps

1. Have the child urinate into a urine collection receptacle.

   RATIONALE: *Collecting the urine in a nonsterile container is necessary to conduct the specific gravity test.*

2. Using a 3- or 5-mL syringe, draw up 0.5 mL of urine into the syringe.

3. Place the syringe into a universal precaution container.

   RATIONALE: *Promotes a safe environment.*

4. Take the urine specimen to the testing area.

RATIONALE: *A specific testing area promotes a safe environment.*

5. Open the refractometer.

6. Place 1 drop of urine in the center of the square opening.

7. Close the lid.

8. Look through the focused eyepiece to see the horizontal line clearly.

   RATIONALE: *Ensures accurate measurement of specific gravity.*

9. Note where the blue horizontal line crosses the markings (see picture below).

   RATIONALE: *The blue horizontal line that crosses the markings is the specific gravity reading.*

Clinical Alert If the institution does not have a refractometer, it is acceptable to use a urine dipstick, with the realization that this is not as detailed. The specific gravity markings on a urine dipstick are in increments of 0.005. On a refractometer, the markings are in increments of 0.001.

Teach Parents

The nurse can teach the parents about the purpose of a specific gravity measurement.

Box 33-5 Checking Urine Specific Gravity

SPECIFIC GRAVITY

- Check urine specific gravity for patients receiving Cytoxan, ifosfamide, cisplatin, high-dose carboplatin, or high-dose methotrexate.
- Specific gravity must be 1.012 or below before the start of chemotherapy and then for at least 24 hours after its completion.
- If at any time the specific gravity rises above 1.012, the patient should receive a fluid bolus (extra fluid). DO NOT turn off the main IV. The bolus is in addition to the main IV fluids.
- If giving more than two or three fluid boluses, notify the oncologist on call.

URINE pH

- Monitor when the patient is receiving methotrexate.
- Urine pH must be higher than 7.0 before starting methotrexate and must be maintained at that level until the methotrexate serum blood level is <0.1 mg/dL.
- Before receiving high-dose methotrexate, patients are hydrated with IV fluids of D5¼ with 40 mEq/L of $NaHCO_3$. The $NaHCO_3$ is needed to keep the urine alkalinized.

Documentation

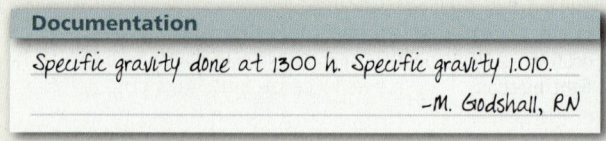

Specific gravity done at 1300 h. Specific gravity 1.010.

—M. Godshall, RN

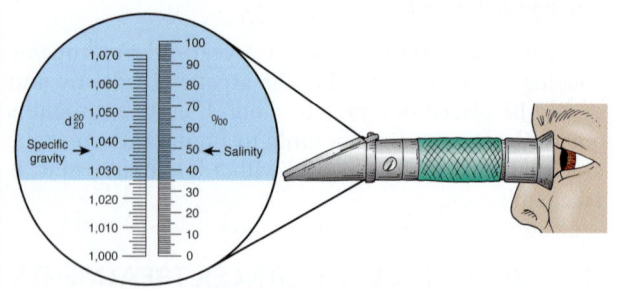

Figure 33-15 Urine specific gravity.

growth rates, large volume, or those that are widely disseminated as in Burkitt's lymphoma, lymphoblastic lymphoma, T-cell, and acute lymphocytic leukemia are associated with this disorder. Tumor lysis syndrome may result from cell death related to a chemotherapy agent or the malignancy itself.

Signs and Symptoms

Children develop lethargy, nausea and vomiting, oliguria, flank pain, pruritus, tetany, and altered level of consciousness. Renal failure can also occur.

Diagnosis

After the cell dies, there is a rapid (12 to 72 hours after treatment starts) release of intracellular contents (metabolites) that leads to hyperuricemia, hypocalcemia, hyperphosphatemia, and hyperkalemia. An astute nursing assessment and immediate laboratory results can help diagnose this condition.

Prevention

It is important to keep the urine alkalinized and maintain a low-phosphate diet.

Collaborative Care

Nursing Care. Administration of allopurinol (Aloprim) to reduce uric acid formation and promote excretion of by-products of purine metabolism is essential. Maintaining adequate hydration is also paramount. Monitoring electrolytes such as calcium, magnesium, phosphorus, and potassium as well as kidney function with measurements such as BUN and creatinine is very important. Sometimes dialysis or exchange transfusions are necessary to decrease the metabolic consequence that causes an even more severe effect on the child.

SEPTIC SHOCK

The patient who is neutropenic and has a fever is at great risk for septic shock. Septic shock happens in a child who is undergoing or has just finished chemotherapy and/or radiation. The level of the white blood cells (WBCs) that fight infection and invading organisms is extremely low (neutropenia).

Signs and Symptoms

Signs can include confusion, fever, increased respirations (tachypnea), decreased urinary output, and cold, clammy skin. The patient becomes pale, and the heart rate increases in an attempt to compensate, and then suddenly the patient's blood pressure plummets (late sign). Laboratory studies reveal acidosis and sometimes renal failure (Venes, 2013).

 Nursing Insight—*Hypotension*

Pediatric patients compensate for shock by increasing the heart rate. When that is no longer effective, the blood pressure falls rapidly.

Diagnosis

Vigilant monitoring of signs and symptoms by the nurse who is giving antibiotics to a neutropenic patient is crucial in diagnosing this condition.

 focus on safety

Septic shock

It is important to remember that this septic shock response can occur immediately or up to 48 to 72 hours later.

Prevention

When the child is admitted to the hospital with a fever, he or she is given an antibiotic regimen to cover both gram-positive and gram-negative bacteria within a 1-hour window of the patient arriving on the inpatient unit. As the antibiotic destroys the cell wall of the bacteria, endotoxin is released from the cell wall. This endotoxin starts a cascade and overwhelms the compromised body's ability to deal with the endotoxin.

Collaborative Care

Nursing Care. An ongoing nursing assessment is essential because, by the time the blood pressure drops, the situation is critical.

 Critical Nursing Action Nursing Care for Septic Shock

For a child who is neutropenic, admitted for a fever, and on antibiotics, the nurse must take vital signs every 10 to 15 minutes during the antibiotic administration to recognize signs of septic shock. Recognizing the other signs is also crucial. Remember that a drop in blood pressure is a late sign. Be ready to administer large amounts (1-L bags) of an isotonic fluid such as normal saline (20 mL/kg) rapidly to prevent circulatory collapse and possibly death. Be sure to check peripheral pulses and capillary refill to monitor perfusion (whether the blood is reaching the extremities). In an emergency, remember the cardiopulmonary resuscitation (CABs) and other emergent care measures:

Circulation
Airway
Breathing
Fluid resuscitation

Evaluation of etiology (complete blood count, electrolytes, disseminated intravascular coagulation panel, blood cultures, and liver and renal functions)

Blood products
Antibiotics
Vasopressors

 focus on safety

Other emergencies

• Superior vena cava syndrome—obstruction or thrombus in the superior vena cava

• Superior mediastinum syndrome—tracheal compression

• Pericardial effusion—fluid in the pericardial cavity, between the visceral and the parietal pericardium, and may produce symptoms of cardiac tamponade such as difficulty in breathing (Venes, 2013)

• Pleural effusion—fluid in the thoracic cavity between the visceral and parietal pleura, which may be seen on a chest radiograph if the fluid exceeds 300 mL (Venes, 2013)

- Abdominal emergencies—esophagitis, gastric hemorrhage, perirectal abscess, hemorrhagic pancreatitis, massive acute hepatomegaly, bowel obstruction
- Neurological conditions—stroke, seizure, spinal cord compression
- Shock—hypovolemic, cardiogenic, distributive
- Hyperleukocytosis—WBC count greater than 100,000/mm³

The Psychological Impact of Pediatric Cancer

The psychological impact that cancer has on the entire family is enormous. The feelings of shock, denial, confusion, and fear strike everyone. Families may feel someone or something is to blame for their child's illness. Adding to the stress is the feeling of having absolutely no control over any part of the situation. Feelings of any kind during this situation are normal because everyone reacts differently.

Sometimes one of the best sources of support for the parents is other parents who have gone through the experience of their child having cancer. It is important to encourage families to develop support systems whether they are family, friends, or other people who may be able to help in some way.

Many parents maintain a bedside vigil, which is understandable because they want to be there for their child. Because this can be very wearing and tiring (Fig. 33-16), the nurse can communicate to the parents that it is important that they get adequate rest and nutrition to avoid becoming sick themselves.

Depending on the child's age and level of understanding, it is important for the parents and health-care team to be honest with the child. A multidisciplinary approach is necessary, and the goal of the team is to communicate enough information so that the child can make sense of the situation without becoming overwhelmed. Information must be tailored to each child's developmental stage. The nurse must keep the lines of communication open.

Families may ask questions such as, Why did this happen? Why does my child suffer? What did I do wrong? These are normal feelings for families when a child is diagnosed with cancer. It is important to offer spiritual support when the child and family are ready. The child may feel a sense of spirituality through the nurse. The nurse can ask the hospital chaplain or Faith Community Nurse to visit on a regular basis, use prayer or meditation if requested, or read from a spiritual or inspirational text. Be sure to allow the child and family quiet time during the day to be alone and meditate if they choose.

Help the child and family express his or her feelings. Being present and giving reassurance that he or she is not being punished is important. Through the nurse's care, the child will know that he or she is loved. Many parents tell the nurse how they were touched deeply knowing that the nurse really cared for their child (Fig. 33–17).

 "What to say"—*To siblings of an ill child*

While children with cancer are undergoing many stressful events, a pediatric nurse does not forget about the sibling(s) of the children with cancer. Visiting a sick sibling is stressful for both the ill child and the sibling. The nurse can help make the sibling's day special by telling them a story or giving them a sticker or a coloring book and crayons. Encourage the ill child to color a picture for his or her sibling and hang it in the room. A sincere demeanor and common pleasantries, such as saying hello or calling the sibling by name, can make the visit special and less stressful.

? Global Health Case Study Family Dilemma

An 18-year-old adolescent named Lear is dying from liver cancer and is admitted to the pediatric unit. His parents are from Germany and speak limited English. Lear has learned the language quickly from attending school since arriving in the country 2 years ago. The nurse caring for this family notices that they do not want to talk about the fact that Lear is dying. The father tries to keep Lear's spirits up with conversation of their former country. The mother appears to be in denial and will not accept the possibility that Lear is dying. Lear is receiving antibiotic therapy and continued chemotherapy, which at this point is palliative. One day, when you are caring for Lear, he says to you that he is tired of being in pain and just wants to die. He says, "I know I am dying, but my family refuses to accept it." He is a mature young man, and you listen as he tells you of the dreams he had about going to college since arriving in America. He tells you that he wants you to speak to his oncologist and ask her to stop the chemotherapy treatment. Lear is 18 and legally an adult but wants the nurse to advocate for him because he is the only one in his family who is realistic about his future and disease progression.

critical thinking question

1. As Lear's nurse, how would you help him and his family so that he can experience a peaceful death?

◆ See Suggested Answers to Global Health Case Studies on *DavisPlus*.

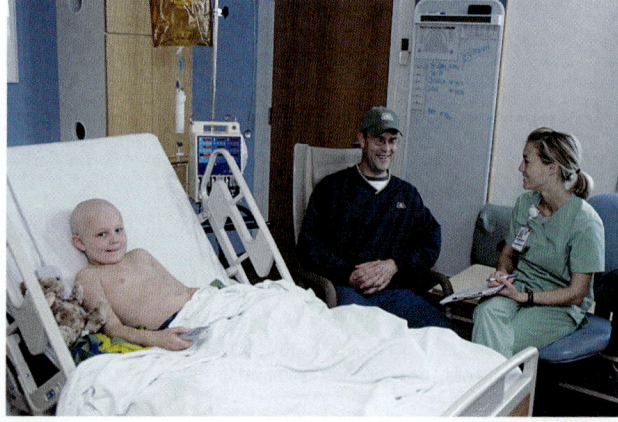

Figure 33-16 Many parents maintain a bedside vigil to support their child during treatment for cancer.

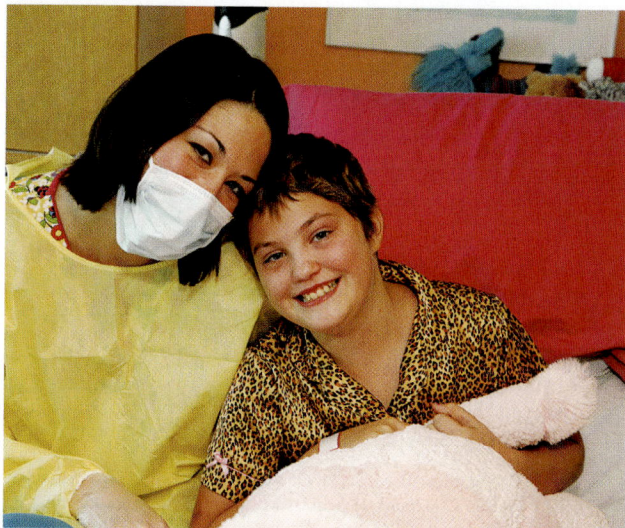

Figure 33-17 Through the nurse's care the child will know that he or she is loved.

Summary Points

- Cancer is a group of diseases in which there is out-of-control growth and spread of abnormal cells known as anaplasia (loss of the normal pattern of growth of cells).

- In children many common malignancies arise from primitive embryonic tissue in which there has been a strong environmental link related to the development of cancer.

- Acute leukemia is a rapidly progressing disease that affects mostly immature, undifferentiated cells. Chronic leukemia is a less rapidly progressing disease allowing for the production of mature, more differentiated cells.

- The most common types of solid tumors in children include brain tumors, neuroblastoma, rhabdosarcoma, retinoblastoma, and nephroblastoma (Wilms' tumor).

- The two most common bone tumors are osteogenic sarcoma and Ewing's sarcoma.

- Lymphoma is a malignancy that arises from the lymphatic system. Two types of lymphomas are seen in children: Hodgkin's disease (HD) and non-Hodgkin's lymphoma (NHL).

- Liver and extragonadal germ cell cancer are other types of cancer seen in children.

- Nursing care for a child with cancer includes maintaining nutrition, preventing infection, administering chemotherapy, addressing radiation side effects, understanding the use of surgery and related nursing diagnoses, controlling pain, offering psychosocial support, managing negative and long-term effects of cancer treatments, and preventing medical emergencies.

- Understanding the psychological impact of pediatric cancer is also an important element of care.

Review Questions

Multiple Choice

1. A 3-year-old child is admitted with a low neutrophil count 10 days after chemotherapy for acute lymphocytic leukemia. Which roommate selection would be the most appropriate for this child?
   A. 3-year-old with bronchiolitis
   B. 5-year-old with a fractured femur
   C. 4-year-old with a streptococcal infection
   D. 3-year-old with a history of diarrhea

2. The pediatric nurse provides teaching to the parents of a 6-year-old who is being discharged after chemotherapy. Which instruction by the nurse is the most appropriate?
   A. "Do not allow your child to play with any other children for a few days."
   B. "Be sure to encourage your child to brush his teeth vigorously every day."
   C. "If your child feels warm, be sure to take her temperature rectally."
   D. "Bring your child to the emergency department for fever of 101.2°F (38.4°C)."

3. A nurse reads a discussion of anaplasia in a child's progress notes. What does the nurse understand this term to mean?
   A. Lack of cell growth
   B. Out of control growth
   C. Slow deformed growth
   D. Benign growth

4. The nurse explains to parents of a child undergoing an oncological work-up that the exact cause of most cancers is unknown, but some factors are known to be involved. Which of the following is inconsistent with this understanding?
   A. Viruses
   B. Genetics
   C. Environmental exposures
   D. Bacterial infections

5. The parents of a 5-year-old child with acute lymphocytic leukemia are told their child is in remission and they want to stop chemotherapy. Which response by the nurse is the most appropriate?
   A. "Yes, we usually stop chemotherapy as soon as remission is achieved."
   B. "There is no scientific evidence that favors continuing or stopping treatment."
   C. "If treatment is discontinued, most children have a relapse within a short time."
   D. "Of course, the decision about treatments is entirely up to you as parents."

6. A child is admitted for an allogeneic bone marrow transplant. The nurse is aware that the donor marrow is coming from which source?
   A. A cadaver
   B. The child
   C. A sibling
   D. Lab created

7. A child has returned to the pediatric intensive care unit following a brain tumor resection. Which nursing assessment takes priority?
   A. Intracranial pressure
   B. Skin integrity
   C. Pain and discomfort
   D. Mobility

8. A child is noted to have leukocoria. Which diagnostic test does the nurse facilitate based on this assessment?
   A. Lumbar puncture
   B. Ophthalmic exam
   C. Abdominal ultrasound
   D. Muscle biopsy

9. The nurse reads in a child's chart that laboratory studies were positive for Reed-Sternberg cells. Which disease process does the nurse associate with this finding?
   A. Acute lymphocytic leukemia
   B. Rhabdomyosarcoma
   C. Glial cell brain tumor
   D. Hodgkin's disease

10. A child is hospitalized with Ewing's sarcoma. Which assessment finding is consistent with this diagnosis?
   A. Shortness of breath
   B. Bone pain and swelling
   C. Bloody diarrhea
   D. Ataxia and falls

See Answers to End of Chapter Review Questions on *DavisPlus*.

REFERENCES

Alcoser, P. W., & Rodgers, C. (2003). Treatment strategies in childhood cancer. *J Pediatric Nurs., 18*(2), 103-12.

American Cancer Society. (2013a). How is neuroblastoma staged? Retrieved from http://www.cancer.org/cancer/neuroblastoma/detailedguide/neuroblastoma-staging

American Cancer Society. (2013b). Wilms' tumor. Retrieved from http://www.cancer.org/cancer/wilmstumor/detailedguide/wilms-tumor-treating-general-info

American Cancer Society. (2013c). Rhabdomyosarcoma. Retrieved from http://www.cancer.org/cancer/rhabdomyosarcoma/detailedguide/rhabdomyosarcoma-what-is-rhabdomyosarcoma

Bauer, J., Jurgens, H., & Fruhwald, M. (2011). Important aspects of nutrition in children with cancer. *Advances in Nutrition, 2,* 67–77.

Children's Hospital of Philadelphia (CHOP). (2011). Neuroblastoma treatment and diagnosis in children. Retrieved from http://www.chop.edu/service/oncology/cancers-explained/neuroblastoma-diagnosis-and-treatment.html

Children's Hospital of Philadelphia (CHOP). (2013). Pediatric leukemias: Diagnosis and treatment. Retrieved from http://www.chop.edu/service/oncology/cancers-explained/leukemia-diagnosis-and-treatment.html

Children's Oncology Group. (2012). *Philadelphia Chromosome Positive ALL.* Retrieved from http://www.childrensoncologygroup.org/index.php/patients-and-families

Duan, F., Smith, L., Gustafson, D., Zhang, C., Dunlevy, M., Gastier-Foster, J., et al. (2012). Genomic and clinical analysis of fusion gene amplification in rhabdomyosarcoma: A report from the Children's Oncology Group. *Genes, Chromosomes & Cancer, 51*(7), 662–674.

Gulati, S., Watt, L., Shaw, N., Sung, L, Poureslami, I., Klaassen, R., et al. (2012). Communication and language challenges experienced by Chinese and South Asian immigrant parents of children with cancer in Canada: Implications for health services delivery. *Pediatric Blood Cancer, 58,* 572–578.

Kliegman, R. M., Stanton, B. M. D., St. Geme, J., Schor, N., & Behrman, R. E. (2011). *Nelson's textbook of pediatrics* (19th ed.). Philadelphia, PA: Elsevier Saunders.

Memorial Sloan Kettering Cancer Center. (2013). Pediatric cancer care: Ewing's sarcoma. Retrieved from http://www.mskcc.org/pediatrics/childhood/ewing-sarcoma

National Institutes of Health (NIH). (2012). Hodgkin's lymphoma. Retrieved from http://www.ncbi.nlm.nih.gov/pubmedhealth/PMH0001606/

Printz, C. (2013). Computerized tomography and cancer risk: The latest findings. *Cancer, 119*(4), 701–702.

Russo, M. (2012). Bald Barbie shows kids with cancer it is all right to look different. *The Cultureist.com.* Retrieved from http://www.thecultureist.com/2012/04/19/bald-barbie-promises-to-show-kids-with-cancer-its-ok-to-look-different/

Saarinen-Pihkala, U. M., Parto, K., Riikonen, P., Lahteenmaki, P. M., Bekassy, A. N., Glomstein, A., et al. (2012). RALLE Pilot: Response-guided therapy for marrow relapse in acute lymphoblastic leukemia in children. *Journal of Pediatric Hematology/Oncology, 34*(4), 263–270.

Seattle Children's Hospital. (2013). Cancer and tumors: Types of leukemia. Retrieved from http://www.seattlechildrens.org/medical-conditions/cancers-tumors/leukemia-types/

St. Jude Children's Research Hospital. (2013). Five-year cancer survival rates: 1962 vs. present. Retrieved from http://www.stjude.org/stjude/v/index.jsp?vgnextoid=5b25e64c5b470110VgnVCM1000001e0215acRCRD

Ueki, H., Maeda, N., Seikimizu, M., Tsukushi, S., Nishida, Y., & Horibe, K. (2013). Osteosarcoma after bone marrow transplantation. *Journal of Pediatric Hematology Oncology, 35*(2), 134–138.

Vallerand, A. H., & Sanoski, C. A. (2014). *Davis's drug guide for nurses* (14th ed.). Philadelphia, PA: F.A. Davis.

Venes, D. (Ed.). (2013). *Taber's cyclopedic medical dictionary* (22nd ed.). Philadelphia, PA: F.A. Davis.

WebMD.com. (2013). Retrieved from http://www.webmd.com/cancer/understanding-cancer-symptoms

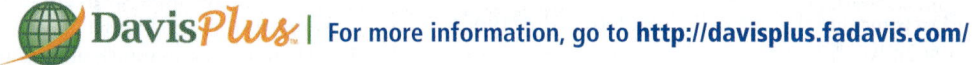

CONCEPT MAP

Caring for the Child With Cancer

Influences: Certain Viruses; Genetics → **Cancer** → **Anaplasia/neoplasm:** → **Malignant** → **Metastasis**

Benign

Types of Cancers in Children:
Leukemias:
- Acute lymphocytic leukemia
- Acute myelogenous leukemia
- Chronic myelogenous leukemia
- Juvenile chronic myelogenous

Solid Tumors:
- Brain tumors
  - Glial → astrocytomas; ependyomas
  - Primitive neuroectodermal tumor
- Neuroblastoma (Wilms' tumor)
- Nephroblastoma
- Rhabdosarcoma; retinoblastoma

Bone Tumors:
- Osteosarcoma; Ewing's sarcoma

Lymphomas:
- Hodgkin's/non-Hodgkin's

Liver Cancer
Extragonadal Germ Cell

Where Research and Practice Meet:
- EBV link to nasopharyngeal cancer
- Children who survive cancer often have TX-related late effects

Treatment Options

Collaboration in Caring:
- Nutritionist consult

Radiation Therapy:
- Use of lowest therapeutic dose over 3- to 6-wk period

Surgery:
- To diagnose cancer through biopsy; as adjuvant to chemo and radiation; resection of tumor; insert central venous catheter

HSCT—Bone Marrow Transplant:
- High-dose chemotherapy followed by stem cell rescue
- Autologous or allogeneic transplants

Gene Therapy:
- Developing slowly; to correct genetic defects

Chemotherapy:
- Primary treatment; use of drugs to kill cancer cells by interrupting cell division; toxic to some noncancerous cell lines

Holistic Nursing Care:
- Thorough physical assessment for side effects of all treatments
- Nutritional support
- Psychological support
- Pain management
- Immune support
- Prevent infection
- Administer chemo
- Prevent medical emergencies

Specific Nursing Care— Child Receiving Chemotherapy:
- Nausea/vomiting: anticipate timing; give antiemetics
- Alopecia: provide wig/wig info
- Extravasation: know drugs, know facility policy
- Mucositis: mouth care; appropriate products; close inspection; oral assessment tools
- Diarrhea/constipation: NO enemas if neutropenic; increased liquids; skin care to rectal area
- Anemia: assessment; transfusion
- Neutropenia: defined by absolute neutrophil count; protect from infection; neutropenic precautions
- Thrombocytopenia: pay attention to bleeding
- Pain control

Nursing Care—Oncologic/ Medical Emergencies:
- Hemorrhagic cystitis: urine for specific gravity/blood; IV fluid bolus; monitor I&O, BUN, and creatinine
- Tumor lysis syndrome: hydration; allopurinol; exchange transfusions
- Septic shock: intense monitoring and assessment of vital signs; triple antibiotic therapy; fluid resuscitation; possible ICU

What to Say:
- Have positive attitude; help family maintain normalcy
- Allow time to absorb dx
- Encourage verbalization; provide reassurance/ support group
- Include ill child in discussions
- Encourage sibling participation

Nursing Insight:
- Division of cancer cells is uncontrolled
- It is vital to perform a focused neuro exam on a child with a brain tumor
- Gene therapy for cancer is complex
- Bone marrow transplant is a treatment option in some cancers
- Many childhood malignancies arise from embryonic tissue
- How a cancer is staged describes its severity
- Oncogenes encourage malignancy
- Cryotherapy and photocoagulation can treat small tumors
- Use topical anesthetics for procedure-related pain

Critical Nursing Action:
- Never palpate abdomen of child with Wilms' tumor
- Hydration critical during chemotherapy administration
- Recognizing septic shock

Clinical Alert:
- Extent of bran tumor correlates with prognosis
- Chemotherapy is biohazardous waste
- Specific gravity by dipstick is not as accurate as by refractometer
- Septic shock response can be delayed
- Be aware of other oncological emergencies
- Know the side effects of radiation tx.

Family Teaching Guidelines:
- Recognizing signs of infection

Complementary Care:
- Visualization using scenarios meaningful to children
- Distraction

Cultural Diversity:
- Hispanic patients and pain control issues; cultural health beliefs

Now Can You:
- List/describe the cancerous growths that affect children versus adults
- Discuss various treatment modalities used in cancer treatment

Focus on Safety:
- Nurses may not administer the drugs ketamine or propofol
- Assess for treatment or disease-related ataxia → increases fall risk

chapter 34

Caring for the Child With a Chronic Condition or the Dying Child

 "Life is a treasure. People should enjoy it, even if digging to it, or through it, it is a challenge"

—Mattie Stepanek

LEARNING TARGETS *At the completion of this chapter, the student will be able to:*

- ◆ Describe chronic conditions and the dying process.
- ◆ Prioritize developmentally appropriate and holistic nursing care for various chronic conditions and children who are dying.
- ◆ Explore grief and caring for the professional caregiver.
- ◆ Develop teaching plans and discharge criteria for parents whose children have various chronic conditions and who are dying.

PICO(T) Questions

The intent of evidence-based practice (EBP) is to provide nursing care that integrates the best available evidence. An initial step in EBP is to write a PICO(T) question that effectively guides the research. A PICO(T) question is an acronym that stands for population (P), intervention or issue (I), comparison of interest (C), outcome (O), and timeframe (T). Depending on the question, all or some of the question components are used in the research process. Use these PICO(T) questions to spark your thinking as you read the chapter.

1. Do (P) siblings of children with chronic conditions demonstrate (O) a higher incidence of (I) behavioral issues than (C) sibling of children without chronic conditions?

2. What (I) nursing interventions are beneficial in (O) helping relieve caregiver burden in (P) parents of children with chronic conditions?

 Evidence-Based Practice

Alam, R., Barrera, M., D'Agostino, N., Nicholas, D. B., & Schneiderman, G. (2012). Bereavement experiences of mothers and fathers over time after the death of a child due to cancer. *Death Studies, 36,* 1–22.

The purpose of this study was to examine the gender differences and adjustments to the bereavement experiences of parents over time after the death of a child to cancer. Studies have found that the death of a child is associated with more intense grieving than that of a spouse. Depression, anxiety, and somatic complaints have been associated with chronic grief. Research indicates that the factors that impact grieving may include parent gender as a result of gender socialization and expectations experienced as the person develops into adulthood. Mothers are generally socialized to be the caregiver and nurturer, though with an increase in mothers working outside the home, some concern has been expressed over the mother's ability to maintain the roles. Fathers, on the other hand, have been socialized to be the provider. Other research has noted that fathers and mothers respond and demonstrate grieving in a different manner, though most have been shown to demonstrate some resolution by 18 months after the child's death. Successful adaption involves integrating the bereavement experience into daily life and subsequently coming to terms with the loss.

Evidence-Based Practice (continued)

Participants in this study were selected from eligible bereaved families whose child had been treated in a hematology and oncology unit of a large children's hospital. Twenty of 29 potential families agreed to participate. The participants included 18 mothers and 13 fathers. The mean age of the mothers was 40.8 and ranged from 27 to 50 years of age. The mean age of the fathers was 46.6 and ranged from 32 to 65 years of age. Of the 31 participants, 18 of the parents (13 mothers and 5 fathers) agreed to be interviewed twice providing data to compare grieving reactions at 6 months and 18 months after the child's death. Ninety percent of the parents were married or had a partner living in the home. Seventy-four percent of the participants were Caucasian. Other race/ethnicities were not identified in the information reported in the published article. Sixty-five percent of the parents were college graduates. The primary caregiver role was provided by the mother 98% of the time. The ages of the deceased children at the time of death ranged from 8 months to 20.7 years with a mean of 9.2. The length of the illnesses ranged from 4 days to 14.7 years. Leukemia (30%) and central nervous system conditions (35%) were the most common diagnoses. Twenty-six (87%) parents had surviving children. The majority (97%) of the homes involved dual-income families before the birth of children, and in all but one case the mother was the primary caregiver. Sixty-seven percent of the fathers kept working full time whereas the majority (61%) of mothers reduced or quit work to care for the ill child. After the child's death, 78% of the mothers continued to spend their time caring for surviving children. By 18 months post-death, all but one father and only 31% of the mothers had returned to work.

Data were analyzed using semi-structured interviews of which all but two took place in the parents' home. For the purpose of this study, data from interviews at 6 and 18 months were analyzed; parents were also interviewed at 12 months though the researchers found little variation between those interview results and the 6-month interview results. Length of the interviews ranged from 44 to 184 minutes with a mean of 87.7 minutes. Six open-ended questions were used addressing "(a) the child's illness, treatment, end of life, and death; (b) changes in daily routines, work, and relationship with friends and family following the death; (c) parents' current health; (d) changes in how parents relate to the deceased child; (e) spirituality and meaning regarding the illness and death of their child; and (f) coping strategies" (p. 5).

Results of the interviews were transcribed and analyzed for themes through the use of qualitative research software. The analysis codes were derived and evaluated by the researchers for agreement. The mothers focused on maintaining the connection with the deceased child. Over the 18-month period, fathers shifted their focus from their job to working on household projects and building a legacy to the deceased child.

In regard to the relationship with surviving children, fathers noted not being as involved as the mothers, and some reported struggling to connect with the children. Mothers on the other hand recognized the positive impact of having surviving children to care for as well as helping the children deal with their own grief. Spousal

relationships varied over time from continued improvement to ongoing struggles. At 18 months, improved relationships were attributed to professional help where struggles were attributed to ongoing differences in ability to communicate. In relation to extended family involvement, parents noted support was received at the 6 months period though indicated a significant reduction in communication with extended family by 18 months.

The researchers conclude that there were more gender differences among the first four themes. The main changes over time involved those related to employment attitudes, grief expression, coping, and relationships with extended family. Fathers were more work focused; mothers expressed more intense grief reactions, which lessened over time as well as were able to be more child-focused. Mothers continued to provide nurturing relationships with bereaved siblings. A range of spouse relationships were experienced among parents over time. Mothers were more likely to maintain a relationship with extended family. The researchers note that differences in parental bereavement over time may not be related only to gender socialization but also to the role the parent played in providing care to the dying child and the bond that was developed at that time.

1. How is this information useful to clinical nursing practice?
2. Based on these findings, what are implications for further research?

The following themes were identified: "(a) employment attitudes and practices, (b) grief expression, (c) coping with grief and bereavement, (d) relationships with surviving children, (e) communication with spouse, and (f) relationship with other family members" (p. 6).

In relation to employment practices, the 18-month interview responses noted that parental employment practices continued the pattern indicated at the 6-month interview. Fathers continued to provide for the family though changed priorities and attitudes toward employment in that most did not express the same enjoyment for their work as they did prior to the illness and death of their child. They focused on finding a way to build a legacy for their deceased child. The majority of mothers wanted to remain at home and focus on providing care and nurturing for the surviving children.

In regard to grief expression, analysis noted that by 18 months a stable gender difference existed. Grief was more openly expressed by the fathers whereas the intensity of pain lessened for mothers over time, hence, gaining more control over their expressions. The researchers also noted that fathers seemed to gain more confidence in their ability to express grief. In relation to the theme of coping with grief and bereavement, mothers focused more on home-related (child and family) strategies whereas fathers focused more on work. Over time most mothers continued to focus on providing care for the surviving children as well as speaking more to others about the grief.

See Suggested Responses for Evidence-Based Practice on Davis*Plus*.

Introduction

A **chronic condition** is a health situation that persists over time, usually longer than 3 months, or one in which recovery progresses slowly. A chronic condition is a physical, psychological, or cognitive impairment that places limitations on the child's daily activities and requires ongoing care. The condition may require that the child and family rely on assistance from other caregivers in the hospital or community settings in carrying out the activities of daily living. A chronic condition can be a congenital defect or a problem that occurs during fetal development. At birth, a chronic condition can arise from sepsis, prematurity, or intraventricular hemorrhage. It can also develop from a genetic predisposition. The chronic condition can be acquired sometime during the child's life as a result of an illness, accident, or injury.

 Nursing Insight—*Examples of chronic conditions*

Brain: Cerebral palsy, a seizure disorder, or post–infant meningitis sequela

Heart: Congenital heart disease, defects, or acquired heart disease

Lungs: Cystic fibrosis, bronchopulmonary dysplasia, asthma, airway stenosis, tracheal malacia, or restrictive lung diseases

Neuromuscular or skeletal: Muscular dystrophy, skeletal malformations, spinal muscular atrophy, mitochondrial disease, central congenital hypoventilation syndrome, spinal cord injury, or post–severe brain injury

Abdominal: Kidneys (renal failure), acquired or chronic liver dysfunction (biliary atresia, cirrhosis), or intestine (short bowel syndrome)

Skin: Eczema, dermatitis, or conditions such as Lyme disease that can cause chronic arthritis

Psychological: Depression, bipolar disorder, autism spectrum disorders, attention deficit disorder, attention-deficit/hyperactivity disorder

Cognitive: Down syndrome, developmental or learning disabilities

Conditions such as diabetes, cancer, and HIV are considered chronic. The condition may also have been acquired through an acute medical condition such as an infection or from a trauma such as near drowning, motor vehicle crash, traumatic brain injury, or abusive head trauma. Whatever the reason for the chronic condition, it becomes a lifelong situation for the child and family. The impact and adaptation to the condition depend on its severity, the age at which the insult occurred, the overall effect on the growth and developmental aspects, and the child's and family's responses to the condition.

The child with the chronic condition may require the use of adaptive devices (e.g., wheelchairs, walkers, braces, and crutches) that help to overcome environmental barriers (Schmitke & Scholmann, 2010) (Fig. 34-1). The nurse must remember that, when caring for the child with a chronic condition, the child may feel different than his peers.

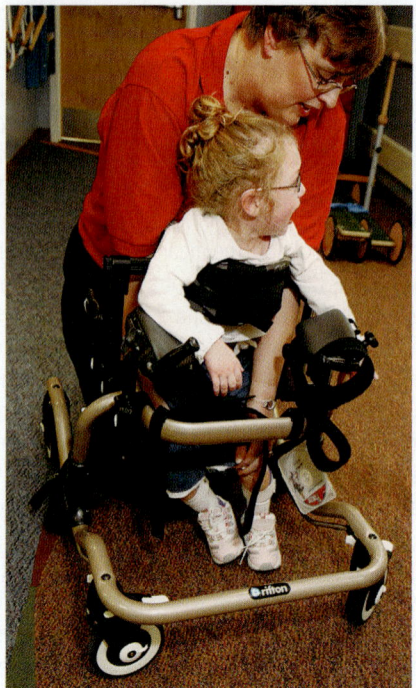

Figure 34-1 Some children who have a chronic condition require an adaptive device to help with mobility.

 Nursing Insight—*Other terms associated with a chronic condition*

Other terms used include children with activity limitations, restrictions to participation, impaired ability, or children who are physically challenged.

Disability is similar to a chronic condition in that it also refers to the limitations that prevent or interfere with a child's ability to perform daily activities.

Developmental disability refers to a group of conditions caused by an impairment in physical, learning, language, or behavior areas (Centers for Disease Control and Prevention [CDC], 2013).

Handicap is the inability to carry out tasks or access certain aspects of the environment because of one or more impairments.

CARING FOR THE CHILD WITH A CHRONIC CONDITION OR THE DYING CHILD

Growth and Development

The child with a chronic condition is faced with many challenges of daily life. The child with a chronic condition is more likely to experience frequent doctor and hospital visits, may feel different than other children, and may have limited activity because of the nature of the chronic condition or adaptive devices needed. Because of the challenges of living with a chronic condition, the child is predisposed to developmental delay and general growth failure (Ward & Hisley, 2009).

The nurse caring for the child with a chronic condition must foster healthy growth and development. The nurse understands that independence is a vital component of natural growth and development. The nurse should encourage the parents to not allow the child to become dependent on them for activities of daily living. The child should be allowed to make choices and participate in self-care activities to increase independence and a sense of control. The nurse should educate the child and family about healthy coping mechanisms such as listening, gaining knowledge about the disease process, and emphasizing the child's strengths. Keeping the child involved with peers is important to foster bonds and social interaction. Friends can help foster a sense of belonging and act as a means for coping.

Source: Ward S., & Hisley, S. (2009). Maternal-child nursing care: Optimizing outcomes for mothers, children & families. Philadelphia, PA: F.A. Davis.

A Chronic Condition and Its Relationship to Technology

In the United States today, the increase in chronic conditions may be partially attributed to technological life-saving and life-sustaining measures or technological devices that can now diagnose and treat diseases that previously were either undiagnosed or untreatable. For instance, the use of a refined diagnostic tool such as a 4D ultrasound has enabled health-care providers to find developmental problems while the infant is still in the mother's womb. Once the condition is diagnosed, health-care professionals can begin to develop a plan of care. The child who is born prematurely benefits from medical technology, such as a ventilator, that enables the infant to live. While technology has many benefits and has enabled some children to live, it can also cause them to be dependent on technology for survival. **Technology dependent** means the child is reliant on some type of medical device to compensate for the loss of normal use of a vital body function.

 Nursing Insight—*The Technology Related Assistance for Individuals With Disabilities Act*

In 1988 congress passed the Technology Related Assistance for Individuals with Disabilities Act (P.L. 103-218). This act was reauthorized in 1994, and in 1998 Congress enacted the Assistive Technology Act (P.L. 105-394), commonly known as the "Tech Act." The Tech Act program is administered by the National Institute on Disability and Rehabilitation Research, Office of Special Education and Rehabilitative Services of the U.S. Department of Education. Its main goal is to examine barriers for children and adults who need to access and obtain assistive technology. Assistive technology can enable individuals to participate in and contribute more fully to activities of their family, school, and community. Assistive technology devices are used to increase, maintain, or improve functional capabilities of individuals with disabilities. This includes ventilators for technology-dependent individuals.

Today, funding authorized by the Tech Act supports three programs, (1) assistive technology, state grant programs in 56 states and territories; (2) the Protection and Advocacy for Assistive Technology program in 56 states and territories; and (3) four national technical assistance programs. Thirty-two of the state assistive technology programs operate federal/state partnership alternative financing programs as described in President Bush's New Freedom Initiative. The Tech Act programs have been a major force in helping children and adults

with disabilities live more productively and independently (Consortium for Citizens with Disabilities, 2012).

A complete listing of state projects and links to state Web sites can be found on the Rehabilitation Engineering and Assistive Technology Society of North America Web site.

 Nursing Insight—*Understanding technology-dependent children*

Technology-dependent children are grouped according to the type of equipment required. According to a United States Congress report, the groups are designated from the most complex equipment to the least complex equipment required:

- Group 1—Children who require a ventilator
- Group 2—Children who require devices for total parenteral nutrition
- Group 3—Children who have a daily dependence on some other device for respiratory or nutritional support (e.g., tracheostomy, oxygen support, and tube feeding)
- Group 4—Children who require an apnea monitor, peritoneal dialysis or hemodialysis, or other devices such as catheters and colostomy bags
- Infants and children who fall into groups 1 and 3 are further defined as needing high-technology care; medically fragile (U.S. Congress of Technology Assessment, 1987)

Impact of a Chronic Condition

A chronic condition affects the family and child differently depending on the age at diagnosis. It can create a threat of the unknown, loss of control, and can have long-term effects yet to be discovered. Depending on the degree of illness, frequent hospitalizations or clinic visits may be needed. Frequent visits to the hospital or clinic visits can create stress because normal home routines

 Where Research and Practice Meet: **Does Home Nursing Coverage Affect the Sleep and Daytime Functioning of Parents of Ventilator-Assisted Children?**

Meltzer, Boroughs, & Downes (2010) examined the relationship between home-care nursing support, sleep, and daytime functioning of families of ventilator-assisted children. Thirty-six primary caregivers were surveyed in this descriptive study. It was discovered that daytime nursing coverage was not related to caregiver sleep or daytime functioning, but caregivers with less nighttime nursing coverage had significantly shorter sleep onset latency than caregivers with some night nursing (16–48 hours/week). Caregivers with regular night nursing (greater than 48 hours/week) had a total sleep time of almost 1 hour more than caregivers without regular night nursing (less than 48 hours/week). Caregivers with clinically significant signs of depression and sleepiness received significantly fewer hours of night nursing per week than caregivers without significant symptoms of depression and sleepiness. Home nursing support, in particular night nursing, is important for the health and well-being of family caregivers of ventilator-assisted children.

Where Research and Practice Meet:
Risk Factors for Morbidity and Mortality in Pediatric Home Mechanical Ventilation

In a study conducted by Reiter, Pernath, Pagel, Hiedi, Hoffman, Shoen, et al. (2011), risk factors were examined for morbidity and mortality in pediatric home mechanical ventilation. The researchers observed 54 patients; 26 of these patients had neuromuscular disease. In 16 patients, mechanical ventilation was initiated at less than 1 year of age. A total of 45 children were ventilated via tracheostomy and 9 by nasal mask. This study reviewed 68 of the severe emergencies that lead to 4 deaths. Respiratory causes were found in 48 of the cases (including 15 tracheostomy-related and 3 ventilator failures). Only age was correlated with incidence of emergencies, not underlying diagnosis or mode of ventilation. This study may help confirm young children may be more difficult and technically demanding to ventilate because of higher physiological vulnerability and less respiratory reserve. Information in this study contradicts earlier studies that show higher mortality probably linked to less optimal ventilator or monitoring technology as compared with more modern technology.

are disrupted and more demands are placed on the caregivers, who now must balance time between the sick child in the hospital and other responsibilities such as caring for other children as well as maintaining employment. An overwhelming lack of control can cause stress and may lead some parents to become controlling, overpowering, overprotective, and unable to function in a healthy manner. The family experiences social, financial, physical, and psychological strain as a result of the chronically ill child. The child also has to learn to cope with the condition including related medical experiences and unfamiliar people and places. The child can feel overwhelmed and unable to deal with the situation depending on age, coping mechanisms, and situation.

The nurse assists the family in developing an ongoing plan of care to meet the child's physical, emotional, and spiritual needs. Ongoing supportive resources help the family develop positive coping mechanisms. These resources might be in the form of connecting the family to other families that have a child with a similar condition, suggesting the family attend a formal support group, or involving a social worker who continues to determine what other avenues are available. Individual and family counseling also assist with the feelings of ongoing uncertainty and fear about the future.

IMPACT OF A CHRONIC CONDITION ON THE INFANT

In infancy, the developmental task is to achieve an emotional attachment or a bond with the primary caregiver. An infant with a prolonged hospital stay in the neonatal intensive care unit, where they require extensive medical care, impacts the natural formation of the parent-child bonding process. Additionally, painful procedures, alteration in feeding patterns such as the administration of formula or breast milk through a feeding tube, and altered sleep-wake patterns can impact the infant's long-term overall condition. Many hospitalized experiences can have a long-term impact on the infant by disrupting normal growth and developmental milestones.

Collaborative Care

Nursing Care. Priority nursing interventions for the infant or child with a chronic condition include rocking, holding, comforting, and using a soothing voice. It is also important to provide visual and auditory stimulation when one-on-one interaction is not possible. Brightly colored mobiles, calming music, and low lighting are also helpful in providing stimulation. It is important to group nursing care measures to minimize interruptions of nap and sleep time because rest is important in the recovery and healing process. The crib or patient's room is maintained as a safe place where no invasive procedures are performed. Drawing blood, starting IVs, and other invasive procedures are done in a designated treatment room. Anesthetic or analgesics are provided to minimize any pain and discomfort. The nurse encourages parents to hold the infant whenever possible, regardless of the amount of medical equipment attached to the infant (Fig. 34-2). Siblings can visit and participate in simple caretaking measures or create pictures to display in the room to help them feel a part of the care of the chronically ill child.

Case Study An Infant With a Chronic Condition

Shelly, a mother at 23 weeks' gestation with twins, developed HELLP syndrome (a condition characterized by *h*emolysis, *e*levated *l*iver enzymes, and *l*ow *p*latelets—a serious complication of preeclampsia) and went into premature labor. The birth was further complicated when the first baby died from a heart defect and the second baby experienced significant medical conditions. The living infant was placed on a ventilator and subsequently developed the chronic lung condition called bronchopulmonary dysplasia. After 3 months in the neonatal intensive care unit, the infant was transferred to a rehabilitation facility closer to home. As the days turned into months, the infant developed other conditions such as sepsis, pneumonia, and had one episode of cardiopulmonary arrest. With the decline in health, nurses at the rehabilitation faculty felt that the nursing care was no longer helpful and the child should be allowed to die. As time progressed, the infant's condition continued to deteriorate, and during this time the infant received extreme care measures that included oscillatory ventilation, numerous medications and other painfully invasive procedures. The parents voiced that everything possible should still be done for the infant. Later, the infant died at the rehabilitation facility at the age of 14 months.

critical thinking questions

1. The infant had several chronic conditions. How can the care given to the infant be viewed by the nurse?

2. What are extreme care measures?

3. Does the nurse suffer?

4. What if the nurse's beliefs about care differ from those beliefs of the institution?

◆ See Suggested Answers to Case Studies on DavisPlus.

IMPACT OF A CHRONIC CONDITION ON THE TODDLER

The toddler's main developmental task is initiating autonomy or self-control. When the child has a chronic condition, accomplishing this task is in jeopardy. The most frightening aspects of illness and hospitalization for the

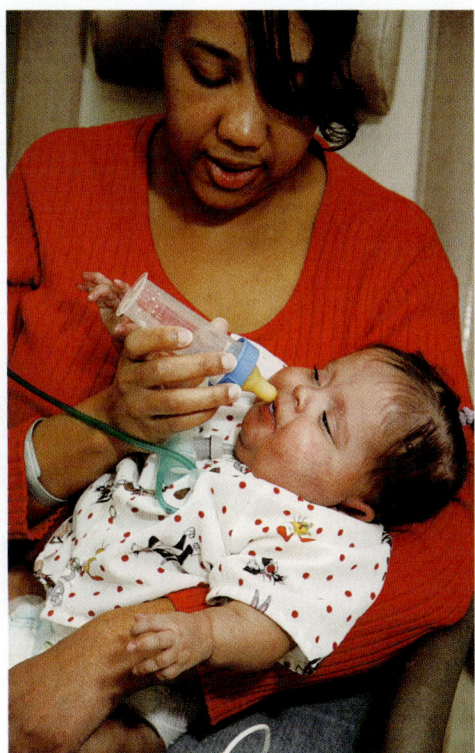

Figure 34-2 It is important for parents to hold and care for their chronically ill child.

toddler are pain, anxiety, and separation from parents. The toddler is also sensitive to bodily harm.

The child's chronic condition can hinder speech, gross motor development, and fine motor development; therefore, appropriate speech, physical, and/or occupational therapy is provided. Frequent or repeated hospitalizations cause the toddler stress. The toddler has a tremendous capacity to withstand the stress, provided that the relationship (attachment) to the parents or caregiver is maintained. The nurse encourages parents to stay with the child by giving the parents 24-hour unlimited visitation and proper sleeping accommodations. If a parent is unable to stay with the toddler, encourage him or her to designate another family member, such as a grandparent. This measure provides both safety and security to the toddler. The most common coping method employed by the chronically ill toddler is regression. Tell the family that regression can be expected, and it subsides, in time, after returning home.

 Nursing Insight—*Regression*

Regression is an abnormal return to an earlier reaction, characterized by emotions or behaviors that are inappropriate for the current age and may include the loss of recently acquired skills (Venes, 2013). Regression can be both physical and emotional. For example, physical regression occurs when a toddler refuses to continue bowel or bladder training. Regression can be considered emotional when a child refuses to talk, withdraws, or becomes easily irritated.

Collaborative Care

Nursing Care. Priority nursing interventions for the toddler with a chronic condition include maintaining the bond between the parents and child, promoting realistic developmental skills, and not reacting negatively to regression. Praise the child for all attempts at self-care. The nurse also gives parents instructions about realistic methods of discipline. Parents may be reluctant to enforce rules for the chronically ill child based on feelings and concerns about the child's condition. In turn, the child may react emotionally (naughtily) to inconsistent discipline patterns. Without consistent limitations, the toddler may feel insecure and unable to complete developmental tasks essential to the promotion of autonomy.

Pain management for the toddler includes administering medication and providing other traditional nursing comfort measures such as clean sheets, good hygiene measures, oral care, and skin care. Because the toddler needs a set routine, the nurse encourages parents to maintain the child's normal home schedule as much as possible. The nurse allows the child to express feelings through play, artwork, and activities. Have the nurse communicate with the toddler through a toy. For example, put a bandage on a stuffed doll before putting one on the toddler to help allay feelings of fear.

IMPACT OF A CHRONIC CONDITION ON THE PRESCHOOLER

The main developmental task of a preschooler is to create a sense of initiative. A painful treatment, isolation, separation from a parent, or loss of autonomy or mobility can be associated with chronic illness, and the preschooler is likely to interpret this experience as punishment for real or imagined wrongdoing. It is important to reassure the preschooler that this is not the case and that he or she is not being punished. Establishing a trusting relationship by explaining procedures honestly before they occur is essential. The preschooler with a chronic condition may react aggressively to the impact of illness by throwing toys, biting, hitting, and other aggressive ways that may be shocking to the parent. The preschooler may also regress, withdraw from others, wet the bed, have difficulty sleeping, or refuse to cooperate. Reassure the parents that this reaction is expected and temporary. The child also may have nightmares that symbolize fears so encourage the child to verbalize dreams and feelings if he or she wakes up crying. Young children accept the meanings of words literally. If death is associated with "going to sleep," the child may fear going to sleep.

Collaborative Care

Nursing Care. Priority nursing interventions include providing the preschooler with the opportunity to express fears and frustrations. At this age, storytelling and reading books about the illness may help the child to understand what is happening. The preschooler can express concerns through play. The nurse can ask the child life specialist for assistance with methods of play that will help the child express and communicate feelings. The nurse shares with the parents that the preschooler's sense of security is derived from schedules and rules. Parents are encouraged to maintain as normal a home schedule as possible and enforce consistent and realistic limits. The nurse teaches the parents that the child needs constant reassurance that nothing he or she has done has caused the illness. Honesty is important when explaining and preparing for procedures. The preschooler has a limited concept of time, so general terms like after lunch, after your nap, or at bedtime when describing time is best understood by the preschooler.

IMPACT OF A CHRONIC CONDITION ON THE SCHOOL-AGE CHILD

During the school-age period, the child's main developmental task is to achieve a certain degree of autonomy and independence and strive to develop a sense of industry. The school-age child takes pride in the ability to assume some new responsibility. Peer relationships become extremely important at this age. Separation from the peer group is often a difficult consequence of a chronic condition. The school-age child who experiences interrupted independence coupled with little peer interaction may show anger by refusing to comply with treatments. The school-age child can listen attentively but sometimes does not completely comprehend all of the information. He may be reluctant to ask questions or admit that he does not know the answer. It is easy for the child to misinterpret medical information. Remember that the school-age child has an increased awareness about the significance of illness but may not understand the lifelong consequences of the chronic condition.

Collaborative Care

Nursing Care. Priority nursing interventions for the school-age child include pain assessment and management. The nurse can use the FLACC pain scale (see Table 21-9), the numeric pain scale, or the Wong-Baker FACES pain scale (see Fig. 21-9). The child needs to be reassured that his or her personal behavior has not caused the illness. The nurse answers questions about treatment, procedures, and medications honestly and at a level the school-age child can understand. Play can be used as an outlet or a temporary escape from the illness or as another way of communication about the illness. Include peers or friends as appropriate during care or play activities. The nurse teaches parents how to help the child attain realistic independence by allowing him or her to play and/or socialize with friends, attend school, choose activities, and enjoy private time. The school-age child is aware of nonverbal cues and often understands more information than parents and caregivers realize. For this reason, it is important to encourage the child to maintain open and honest dialog with family and caregivers.

 Collaboration in Caring—*Child life specialist*

Whenever a child is diagnosed with a chronic condition, it is important to involve the Child Life Specialist. Because the child with a chronic condition often spends significant amounts of time in the hospital, the days can be long and boring. The Child Life Specialist is an expert in child development and therapeutic play. He assists with diversion activities during procedures, arranges for therapeutic play, or simply lets the child take time to play (Fig. 34-3).

IMPACT OF A CHRONIC CONDITION ON THE ADOLESCENT

Adolescence is a time of increasing independence, autonomy, and vulnerability. It is a time to ask, "Who am I?" and a time when self-esteem is closely related with peer

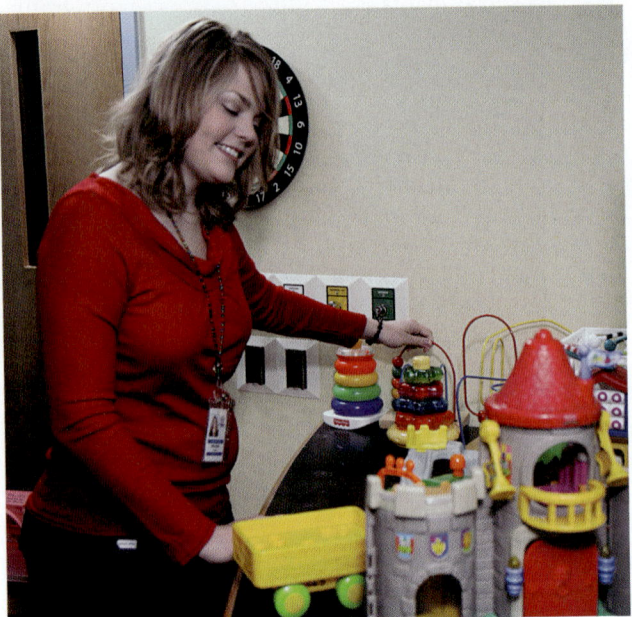

Figure 34-3 The child life specialist is called on to work with a child who has been diagnosed with a chronic condition.

acceptance. To complicate matters, during a chronic illness the adolescent may be placed on a pediatric unit or on an adult floor. Neither situation seems to be the right fit for the adolescent. Previously independent, the adolescent is now faced with a chronic condition and may be required to accept help from others. Dependence on caregivers and family for physical care, coupled with a lack of privacy, can disturb the adolescent's sense of autonomy and ability to make decisions. Based on this loss of independence, the adolescent may exhibit maladaptive coping behaviors such as hostility, anger, aggression, and sometimes noncompliance or refusal of treatment. Sometimes when presented with frequent medications, tests, appointments, and other procedures, the adolescent is easily overwhelmed and shows regression in behavior. Besides worrying about the condition, self-esteem, and identity, the adolescent may also show concern about the burdens and strains the family may now face. It is imperative to establish an open line of communication with the adolescent.

Collaborative Care

Nursing Care. Priority nursing interventions for the adolescent with a chronic condition include providing solitary time to help the adolescent regain control and have personal space. It is important to give the adolescent realistic choices to enhance control when possible. Realistic choices include when to bathe, sleep, eat, and visit with friends. The adolescent can be included in medical-related matters when possible. Peers can be a strong source of support for the adolescent, so peer interaction is important. The adolescent can be encouraged to expand networks of social support through peer groups and community programs when possible. A support group may help normalize the adolescent's crisis and give a new source of strength and hope. Maintaining contact with peers via social media is also important. Support groups are also available online.

IMPACT OF A CHRONIC CONDITION ON THE SIBLING

A chronic condition also has an effect on siblings. The siblings are affected in several ways such as experiencing decreased self-esteem, receiving less support from parents, exhibiting mood swings, lacking an understanding about the condition, and displaying a negative attitude toward the ill sibling's condition The sibling has feelings of jealousy, embarrassment, resentment, loneliness, and isolation. Siblings tend to feel isolated, act out in anger, feel guilty, lack understanding about the situation and display negative feelings and behaviors toward the ill child. If siblings are close in age, the chronic condition means the loss of a playmate. A young child, who has a vivid imagination, may believe he or she caused the condition or may fear that he or she might acquire the same condition as the sibling.

Collaborative Care

Nursing Care. Priority nursing interventions for the sibling is to promote family-centered care. Instruct parents to maintain familiar home routines as much as possible for the sibling. In addition, the nurse helps the parents include the sibling in simple care measures. Remind the parents that providing information about the ill child may decrease stress reactions in the sibling. Encourage sibling visitation and share age-appropriate information. If the sibling is too young, while important physician-family meetings are held, encourage them to draw a picture to hang up in the patient room. This activity occupies the siblings' time and helps them feel like they have done something to show how much they love their sister.

 Optimizing Outcomes—**The sibling**

How does the nurse handle "acting out" in the sibling? To achieve the best outcome give the sibling time to regain control and express feelings. To convey genuine understanding the nurse might say, "You seem very angry today (reflection). It is all right to be angry about your sister's condition and about the situation (validating the sibling's feelings). It must be difficult for you to have your sister in the hospital (empathizing and understanding)." The nurse can then help the sibling find a positive outlet for the anger such as art therapy (channeling). The nurse can encourage the sibling to tell an adult when the anger returns (providing an outlet).

The Child Living With a Chronic Condition

The percentage of U.S. children and adolescents with a chronic health condition increased from 1.8% in 1960's to more than 25% in 2007 (Halfon & Newacheck, 2010).

Asthma is the leading chronic condition in the United States, affecting about 6 million children. Other chronic conditions are sickle cell disease (SDS), bronchopulmonary dysplasia (BPD), congenital heart disease (CHD), cystic fibrosis (CF), type 1 and type 2 diabetes mellitus, epilepsy,

and chronic renal failure. Hemophilia, migraine, heart disease and the ever-growing problem of obesity are now included in the list of common chronic conditions. With the advancing technology and demand for critical care, it is estimated that by 2020 more than 600,000 patients per year will need extended critical care support (Choi, Donahoe, Zullo & Hoffman, 2011).

 Nursing Insight—*Children living with chronic conditions*

Children living with a chronic condition experience one or more of the following:
- Limitation(s) in motility appropriate for age and development
- Disfigurement, deformity or scarring
- Dependence on technology
- Dependence on assistive devices
- Dependence on medication
- Dependence on a special diet
- Ongoing need for medical care, appointments, treatments
- Ongoing need for special services
- Altered body image
- Dependence on others for basic daily needs
- Not being able to be or feel "normal"
- Missed days at school
- Not being able to participate in sports, social or extracurricular activities
- Missing out on school functions (i.e. dances, football games, etc)
- Lack of peer group or social support networks

Pediatric clinical samples and epidemiological data shows that 15% to 30% of chronically ill children are at risk for developing emotional and behavioral problems (Hysing, Davis, Nicholas, Wake & Lo, 2009).

 Nursing Insight—*Caregiver burden*

A child living with a chronic condition requires day-to-day care and can become a source of stress for parents and other caregivers. **Caregiver burden** is described as consistent stress, pressure, and anxiety in providing day-to-day care of a child with a chronic illness or disability while trying to maintain other family functions and demands. While caring for a loved one can bring personal fulfillment and satisfaction it can be associated with physical, psychological, and pose financial burdens for the caregivers. One of the greatest risks for caregivers is becoming ill themselves. Caregivers have high rates of insomnia, depression, don't eat well, are unable to exercise, take personal time, or seek preventative health care. One in five caregivers describes their health as fair or poor (Collins & Swartz, 2011). Financial burden becomes an issue as many caregivers must adjust their work schedules, take leaves of absences, or reduce work hours as a result of increased care responsibilities. More than 40% of caregivers have an annual household income below $50,000 (Collins & Swartz, 2011). Continuous health care is expensive. Other costs related to housing, lifestyle modifications, special equipment, and special services for the child are also expensive. Some of these costs may not be reimbursed by private health-care insurance plans.

Collaborative Care

Nursing Care. The nurse must communicate to the family that overwhelming feelings can be discussed with a health-care professional and that respite care is available.

Across Care Settings: Respite care

Respite care is short-term care offered to families living with a child who has a chronic condition. The main goal of respite care is to provide relief for family members of the burden and stress of sustained care by giving them a break in the daily challenges of caring for these children. Parents can also use respite care in situations in which someone besides them, such as home care nurses, can accompany the child to a doctor's appointment. The availability of respite care varies in every community and is not always paid for by private insurance. Sometimes state agencies or national programs can reimburse the family for respite care.

Global Health Case Study The Frequently Hospitalized Child

Samir is a 7-year-old boy from Sudan and has recently been admitted to the inpatient unit at the local children's hospital with a diagnosis of cerebral palsy, apnea, and seizure disorder. He has been admitted to the hospital numerous times since entering the US. Based on cultural expectations, soon after he was admitted, Samir's mother leaves the hospital and goes home to tend to another child who is 2 years old. When Samir is at home, the mother has difficulty getting anyone to watch him because of his apnea spells that can happen several times a day. The father refuses to stay alone with Samir for fear that "something might happen to Samir when he is alone with him." Some of the nurses on the unit talk despairingly about the mother because they think that the mother does not care about Samir, as evidenced by "dropping him off and leaving him alone." A few of the nurses fail to understand the complexity of the situation as well as the cultural implications. One nurse notices that the mother visits Samir every day at lunchtime, staying at his bedside for about 1 hour.

critical thinking questions

1. As a nurse leader, what can be said to the staff nurses when making judgments about the mother?

2. What kind of support systems does Samir's mother have in place at home? What can be done to increase support in the home?

3. Do you think this mother is suffering from "caregiver burden" and may be in need of respite care?

♦ See Suggested Answers to Global Healtth Case Studies on DavisPlus.

Emotional Responses to a Chronic Condition

When a child is diagnosed with a chronic condition the dynamics of the entire family is disrupted and emotional responses follow. Initially, the emotional response is shock and chaos. Family members continue to experience several feelings that include anger, fear, disbelief, anxiety and confusion. Emotional reactions differ depending on the specific diagnosis and whether there is a chance for the child to be cured. The parental reaction to the diagnosis of asthma will be different than the reaction to a diagnosis of cancer in their child. If a child has been ill for a long period, some parents may express relief at finally having an answer to the child's illness.

Potts and Mandleco (2011) found that children who do not focus on the positive aspects of the condition blame themselves and others as well as display negativity and irritability. Grieving parents may blame themselves or the other parent for not having been able to prevent the condition, especially if the condition is a congenital defect. In addition, parents may not be able to bond with the child. Sometimes, as a defense mechanism, a parent may be fearful of bonding with the child in case the child dies.

Collaborative Care

Nursing Care. The priority nursing intervention for the family's emotional responses to a chronic condition is communication, support, and understanding. The nurse communicates to the family that the child can continue to experience life as other children do, perhaps in moderation. Important information is communicated about the necessary treatment, procedures, medicine, and visits to the hospital or clinic. The nurse supports the family to help them normalize daily activities such as going to school and playing with friends. The nurse listens carefully to understand the family's concerns. Understanding is also important as parents of a child diagnosed with a chronic condition have been found to exhibit an initial grief reaction similar to that experienced with bereavement. They report episodes of recurrent sorrow, particularly at times of important transitions in the child's life that remind them that the child is not the same as other healthy children. The period of episodic grieving interspersed with periods of denial is called **chronic sorrow**. This lifelong sadness suggests these parents never reach closure about what has happened (Bowes, Lowes, Warner & Gregory, 2009). Discuss the importance of the parent's continued involvement in the care of the child through these recurrent sorrowful periods. Parents also need information about community resources.

"What to say"—*Talking about the chronic condition*

When talking about the child's chronic condition with the family, the nurse must be sure to use the child's name and personalize the discussion. It is important that the nurse avoid labeling the child by, for example, saying "CF kids." Instead, the nurse says, "Timmy will need ongoing care for his cystic fibrosis." This kind of communication places the emphasis on the child and not on the condition. It is also important to listen to the family so that home routines can be continued during hospitalization.

Caring for a Child With a Chronic Condition

The nurse assesses the language and nonverbal cues being used by the child and family. The nurse also determines the locus of control and where the decision–making process lies (with the parents exclusively or if it involves a larger social unit of the family). Consider the relevance of religious beliefs and spiritual practices, particularly about death, the existence of an afterlife, and the belief in miracles. Evaluate whether expressions of pain and related aspects are allowable in the culture or looked at as signs of weakness. Assessing how hope for future recovery is negotiated within the family is also important.

ESTABLISHING A THERAPEUTIC RELATIONSHIP

The nurse understands the importance of establishing a therapeutic relationship with the child and his or her family who are living with a chronic condition. This therapeutic relationship is vital when providing family-centered care because the family has a tremendous amount of responsibility in the care of the child. For the nurse to build a successful therapeutic relationship with the family, the nurse must first establish trust.

Critical Nursing Action Establishing Trust With the Family

The nurse takes the following actions when establishing trust:

- Consider the needs of the entire family; do not forget the siblings.
- Familiarize yourself with the child's condition and know about the disease process.
- Be open and honest.
- Show the family that the burden of care is understood. Burden of care includes the combination of physical, psychological, social, and financial burdens the family may face.
- Take time to listen to the child and to the caregiver.
- Include parents in the plan of care. Some parents like to participate in the child's care while the child is hospitalized. It is also important to maintain home rituals as much as possible while the child is hospitalized.
- Treat each child as an individual. It is essential that the nurse not label the child according to the disease process.
- Allow the child to make decisions about the care when possible. Decision making is especially important for the adolescent.
- Maintain confidentiality.
- Do not prematurely judge the parents. Some parents cannot stay with the child in the hospital based on personal needs and responsibilities.
- Arrange for continuity of nursing care.
- Assess the family's support systems and resources.

EDUCATION

Helping the family understand laws about educational services is important. The Individuals with Disabilities Education Act (IDEA) is the nation's federal special education law that ensures public schools provide for the educational needs of students with disabilities. IDEA requires that schools provide special education services to eligible students as outlined in a student's individualized education program (IEP). IDEA also provides specific requirements to guarantee a free appropriate public education for students with disabilities in the least restrictive environment. These are the protected rights of every eligible child in all 50 states and U.S. territories (National Center for Learning Disabilities, 2012).

Growth and Development

The child with a chronic condition may experience negative physical growth (growth failure) and developmental aspects. **General growth failure** means that the child grows more slowly and that the height and weight are in a lower percentile on the growth charts than for children of the same age. It may result from the condition itself or from related treatments and medications. Conditions such as cystic fibrosis or end-stage renal disease may significantly alter the growth process.

The pathophysiology of the condition may also affect the child's growth. For example, if the child has a severe hypoxia problem, the tissues may simply not receive the needed oxygen required to promote normal growth. Treatment measures associated with chemotherapeutic agents may hinder growth or damage usual organ functioning.

The child with altered growth may be delayed developmentally. The child may achieve developmental milestones much later than do peers or not at all. The nurse must be aware that the parents may positively or negatively affect the child's development. For instance, a parent, teacher, or guardian who is fearful of consequences of a child's condition may unduly restrict a child's opportunity for interaction and subsequently hinder development (e.g., parents of a child with autism do not allow him to play with peers). Conversely, some parents can embrace the child's condition and help the child attain the most realistic potential. The child's personality, temperament, and motivation may help or hinder developmental attainment.

An important nursing care measure related to growth is carefully plotting their growth using charts from the National Center for Health Statistics (NCHS) http://www.cdc.gov/nchs/about/major/nhanes/growthcharts/charts.htm. When a child is unable to take adequate nutrition by mouth, an alternate feeding method is used to maintain and promote growth in the child. The type of feeding method selected depends on the child's medical condition.

The nurse can encourage parents to maintain realistic developmental milestones. Helping the child interact with children of his or her own age (when possible) and creating a social network consisting of family, friends, and others in the community can help maintain development. Finding appropriate social activities also positively affects the child's development.

 legal alert—Observe federal laws providing educational services for children

Education for All Handicapped Children Amendments, PL 99-457 of 1986 expanded the scope of PL 94-142 to establish early intervention programs for infants and toddlers with disabilities. Free and appropriate public education (FAPE) includes an Individualized Family Service Plan for each family with infant and toddlers with disabilities.

In 1990, an amendment *(PL101-476)* was added to the Education for All Handicapped Children Act (EHA) by adding components that included renaming the EHA as *Individuals with Disabilities Education Act (IDEA)*. The amendment also replaced the phrase "handicapped child" with "child with a disability." This amendment provided transition services for a child by age 16 and extended eligibility to children with autism and traumatic brain injury. This act also defined Assistive Technology Devices and Services for children with disabilities. Additionally, it extended the Least Restrictive Environment clause.

Individuals with Disabilities Education Act (IDEA), *PL 105-17* of 1997 ensures that all children with disabilities have "access to the general curriculum" and that educators consider assistive technology (AT) devices and services on the IEPs of all students. Use of school-purchased devices (ATs) in a child's home or other setting is required if the child needs access to those devices to receive FAPE. Every child with a disability must have a written IEP, and parents have the right to question placement decisions and due process when settling differences. This also includes orientation and mobility services to the list of related services for children who are blind or who have visual impairments as well as for other children who may also need instruction when traveling around their school or to and from school.

The *Rehabilitation Act, PL 93-112* of 1973, prohibits discrimination against people with a disability. Section 504 specifies that each student who has a disability be entitled to accommodations needed to attend school and participate as fully as possible in school activities.

The *Education for All Handicapped Children Act, PL 94-142* of 1975, mandated that all children, even those with handicaps, be provided with public education and related services.

CULTURAL ISSUES

Understanding cultural diversity of the child who has a chronic condition is paramount. Culturally diverse considerations emphasize cultural sensitivity in both the hospital and community settings.

 Cultural Diversity: Dealing With a Chronic Condition

When working with a family dealing with a chronic condition, assess how the members express grief. Some families feel that grief is a private matter and tend to suppress feelings until they are alone. Other families outwardly express sorrow by crying or moaning. It is important to recognize how those beliefs and culture influence the family's reactions to grief and death.

The Dying Child

Dying is the total cessation of life. Death is difficult to comprehend and might be considered mysterious, ambiguous, or confusing for the child and family. The dying process is unique, and the exact time or date of death is unpredictable. When the child enters the dying process, the body begins to shut down physically as well as emotionally and spiritually. This failure might happen slowly or rapidly depending on the circumstance.

 Critical Nursing Action　Do Not Resuscitate

The **Do Not Resuscitate (DNR)** request means withholding life-sustaining treatment and requires that no attempt be made to revive a child who has clinically died. Withholding life-sustaining medical treatment includes decisions to withhold, withdraw, or limit medical treatment. Some medical ethicists feel that there is no difference between withholding and withdrawing treatment if the treatment is no longer beneficial to the child.

When making recommendations to withhold, withdraw, or limit medical treatment, the benefits of treatment must be weighed against the burden of continuing treatment for the child. A DNR order means that no lifesaving measures will be initiated in the event of cardiac or respiratory arrest. This decision also can mean removing medical equipment such as a ventilator or monitor, dialysis machine, feeding tube used for artificial nutrition, and IV fluids for hydration. Aggressive treatments such as chemotherapy or radiation therapy are also terminated.

The child and family participating in the process of withdrawal of life-sustaining therapy need consistency among health-care providers and the delivery of consistent messages. All members of the interdisciplinary team need to communicate effectively with each other so that families receive ongoing and reliable information.

PERCEPTIONS OF DEATH

Perceptions of death vary across the age continuum. The nurse prioritizes nursing actions and assists the child according to the appropriate developmental level to help make the transition to death fearless, peaceful, and painless. The causes of death among children ages birth to 19 vary; deaths in infants include prematurity, congenital defects, and infections. Death in toddlers and preschool commonly are the result of accidents and injuries. The most frequent causes of death in school-age children are cancers and unintentional injuries. The leading causes of death in adolescents are accidents, homicide, suicide, and cancer.

Understanding of death is related to the level of cognitive development. The infant's perception of death is based on the degree of discomfort and the reactions of the parent and others in the environment. The nurse can ensure that the infant's basic physiological needs are met, and she is able to build trust with caregivers. The nurse provides comfort through rocking, touch, non-nutritive sucking, and making sure familiar people and transitional or security objects (toys) are present (Hutton, Levetown, & Frager, 2010).

Toddlers have a more developed perception of death and can sense by the way that the parents react that something is wrong. The toddler is unable to distinguish fact from fantasy, which inhibits a true comprehension of death. Death for the toddler may mean separation from parents or disruption in routine. They see death as reversible. The dying toddler responds to the possibility of death with fear and sadness. It is important for the nurse to encourage parents to stay with the child by giving 24-hour unlimited visitation and ensuring their needs are met and comfort is maintained.

The preschool child seems to comprehend death more than can be verbalized. The preschooler is able to see the body changing and can understand that something is wrong. Fear of death may be present as early as 3 years of age, and nurses can discuss death simply and honestly in response to the child's questions. It is important for the nurse to keep answers short. The nurse remembers that the preschooler is a magical thinker and may view illness or injury as punishment for bad behavior. Reinforce that their condition is not caused by bad behavior. Because preschoolers are concrete thinkers, death should not be described as "going to sleep." A child of this age takes this response literally and fears going to sleep, so the nurse must never equate sleep with death. Provide concrete information about the state of being dead (e.g., a dead person no longer breathes or eats) (Hutton et al., 2010).

The school-age child often has a realistic understanding about the seriousness of the condition, but the understanding of death is not precise until he or she can understand the concept of time. Kübler-Ross (1983) found that after the age of 8 or 9 children understand the permanence of death. The school-age child is aware of nonverbal cues and often understands more of what is overheard than parents and nurses realize. Attempts to shield the school-age child from death can be perceived as distrust. The nurse must include children of this age in discussions about their care, condition, treatment or non-treatment, prognosis, and death. The school-aged child may request graphic details about death (e.g., burial and decomposition). The nurse evaluates for fears of abandonment, destruction, or body mutilation. It is important to foster the child's sense of mastery and sense of control (Hutton et al., 2010).

The adolescent has the capacity to understand death at the adult level but has difficulty accepting it as reality and often thinks that death can be defied. The adolescent thinks that the body is invincible, hence some of the risk-taking behaviors among this group. Adolescence is a difficult time to deal with death because establishing identity and independence is important. The adolescent has a fear of becoming dependent on parents. The nurse can help the family realize that even though the cognitive ability to understand death is present, the emotional maturity to face death is absent. The nurse and family include the adolescent in decision making. The adolescent might wish to write a final poem or message as well as say good-bye to friends. It is important to allow the adolescent to talk about feelings and disappointments about goals and experiences never to be attained. They may want to speak about unrealized plans (e.g., going to college, getting married, etc.).

BEFORE THE CHILD DIES

Before the child dies, the nurse completes the institution's checklist to ensure that all of the necessary institutional policies and procedures are followed. The nurse can contact the bereavement team before the death so they are ready to offer support when the death occurs. The nurse can also create a file that includes community resources that the family may need after the death to receive ongoing support.

A ledger may be created as a follow-up for acknowledging important times in the child's life (e.g., on the child's birthday or another special day). Later, the nurse can send a "thinking of you" card to let the family know that the child is still remembered on these occasions. The nurse can also make note of the child's death date to make a follow-up phone call that can allow parents to ask unanswered questions or express feelings.

Signs and Symptoms of Impending Death

The nurse recognizes physical signs of impending death. Knowing the normal physical processes may help the family through the experience.

 Assessment Tool Recognition of Physical Signs of Impending Death

- Loss of sensation
- Loss of the body's ability to maintain thermoregulation: skin may feel cool

- Skin color will be pale to eventually cyanotic (blue in color)
- Loss of bowel and bladder function
- Loss of awareness, consciousness, and slurring of speech
- Alteration in respiratory status
- **Cheyne-Stokes respirations** (a waxing and waning of respiration in the depth of breathing with regular periods of apnea)
- Noisy chest or respirations with the accumulation of fluid in the lungs or in the posterior pharynx
- Decreased, weak, or slow pulse rate
- Drop in blood pressure
- Confusion, delirium, or disorientation
- Weakness, fatigue
- Changes in pain perception
- Restlessness and agitation
- Alertness or alternation in sleep
- Decreased oral intake
- Seizures
  (End of Life Nursing Education Consortium [ELNEC], 2012)

Collaborative Care

Nursing Care. Once medical treatment is halted and the family has determined that death is inevitable, the focus of nursing care is about allowing the child to die. The nurse can shift from the curative technological approach to providing care that enables the child to move toward death by accessing his or her own inner resources. To help the child have a peaceful death, comfort measures are essential to help create a positive outcome at the time of the child's death as well as later on for the family. The nurse is aware of family needs and communicates genuine feelings of kindness and sympathy to the family.

 Critical Nursing Action Nursing Supportive Behaviors in End-of-Life Care

- Allow the parent to hold the child while life support is being discontinued
- Provide a peaceful dignified scene at the bedside
- Teach the family that the child can still hear you
- Encourage the family to talk to the child
- Use the team approach (Fig. 34-4)
- Encourage the family to ask questions
- Validate the family's caretaking decisions
- Provide continuity of care
- If the family is able, have them help care for the child

 Nursing Insight—*Presence*

The nurse responds sympathetically to the family at the time of the child's death. The death of a child is a sorrowful time for the family. One primary intervention for the nurse is to be present. Presence includes a receptive, nonverbal posture that signals to the family that the nurse is willing to sit quietly and listen. Being present may reduce the family's feelings of isolation. It is important to remember that the family may not need the nurse to say profound words. They may simply want the nurse's support and willingness to remain in the room.

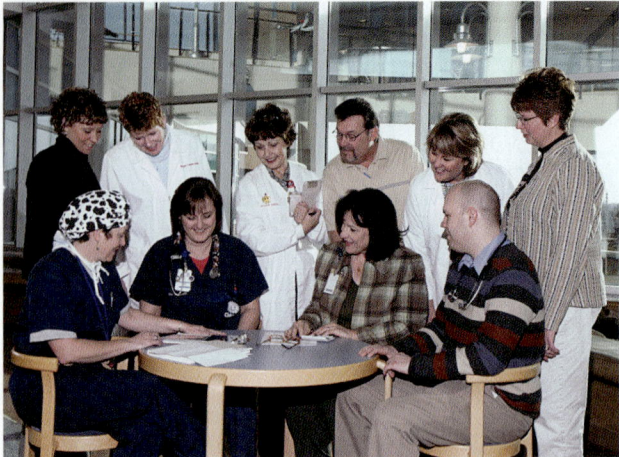

Figure 34-4 The health-care team is of tremendous support to parents and family of a chronically ill or dying child.

The nurse can perform the following nursing actions to support the dying process:

- Promote good communication with the health-care team
- Manage pain and discomfort
- Create a peaceful and comfortable environment
- Assist the child to die with dignity
- Cease unnecessary treatments
- Allow the family to express their end-of-life care wishes

Relationships are extremely important during the dying process, and physical contact is a major source of comfort to both the child and family. A simple touch from the nurse's hand, gently stroking the child's head, or the placement of a favorite toy next to the child shows the family that the nurse truly cares about the child. When a nurse offers touch, the family members may lean in toward the nurse and respond positively. The nurse must also be sensitive to a family who is not comfortable with being touched and may respond with stiffening or drawing back. In this situation, the nurse can quietly remove the hand and perhaps take a step back. The nurse must also have the insight to realize that this is not the time to share personal stories about loss. It is important for the nurse to keep the focus on the family.

It is important that the nurse give the family choices about what is possible during the dying process. The nurse can ask the family members if holding the child is desired. If death is imminent, the nurse must be sure to tell the family that death could occur while holding the child. Sometimes parents request to get into the bed with the child. This behavior is acceptable during the death of a child.

The nurse assesses the situation and creates a peaceful environment. Sometimes it is appropriate for the nurse to give the family short periods to be alone with the child, or the family may want a health-care professional in the room at all times. When the nurse presents these choices, if the family does not respond, ask the family again a few moments later because sometimes the family member cannot absorb everything that is occurring.

PALLIATIVE CARE, HOSPICE CARE, AND END-OF-LIFE CARE

Care of the dying child includes holistic nursing interventions that address the physical, emotional, and spiritual aspects of the child and family. Care of the dying child is addressed in three ways: palliative care, hospice care, and end-of-life care. These three ways are similar yet different from one another.

Palliative Care

With technological advances, nurses and other health-care professionals are faced with decisions as to when to stop treatment once it is initiated. **Palliative care** is a term that has drawn much attention in health care today.

 Nursing Insight—*Palliative care*

Palliative care is a philosophy of care that is defined as care that seeks to prevent, relieve, reduce, or soothe the symptoms produced by serious medical conditions or their treatment and to maintain a patient's quality of life. The World Health Organization defines palliative care as "Palliative care for children is the active total care of the child's mind, body, and spirit, and also involves giving support to the family" (ELNEC, 2012). The terms supportive care and palliative care may be used interchangeably.

Palliative care provides support and care for people, including children, facing life-threatening illnesses. The care is focused on enhancing the quality of life remaining by integrating physical, psychological, social, and spiritual care as defined by the child and family. An interdisciplinary team is aware of the child's needs and uses an approach and interventions that affirm life and neither hasten nor postpone death. Palliative care measures can coexist with curative measures. One goal of palliative care is to advocate for the needs of the child and family so that they can continue to live their lives with dignity and allow the child to die in a manner that is meaningful. Applications of palliative care interventions will vary with the setting and availability within that setting (ELNEC, 2012). Medical insurance payments or reimbursements now support this quality of care in some states (ELNEC, 2012).

 Where Research and Practice Meet:
Perceived Barriers

Perceived barriers to pediatric end-of-life care differ from adults because children may have more uncertainties with prognosis and discrepancies in treatment goals between staff members and family members, followed by barriers to communication. Improving staff education in communication skills and care of children in palliative care may improve this dilemma. It was found that uncertain prognosis (55%), family not being ready to acknowledge an incurable condition (51%), language barriers (47%), and time constraints were identified as the situations that caused the most uncertainty (Davies, Sehring, Partridge, Cooper, Hughes, Philip, et al., 2008).

Complementary Care: *Complementary and Alternative Medicine*

Complementary and alternative medicine (CAM) therapy includes popular care measures. It is defined by the National Institutes of Health (2012) as "a group of diverse medical and health care systems, practices, and products that are generally not considered part of conventional medicine." It is grouped into three groups such as natural products that include a variety of herbal medicines and vitamins, minerals, and natural products; mind and body medicine that includes meditation, acupuncture, and yoga; and manipulative and body practices such as spinal manipulation and multiple massage methods. In 2007, the National Health Interview Survey found that 17.7% of adults had used a non-vitamin, non-mineral approach like echinacea and fish oil. The same survey found that 12.7% of people had used deep breathing practices. Also found was that 8.6% of adults and 2.8% of children had used chiropractic or osteopathic medicine, and 8.3% of adults and 1% of children had used massage. These types of care measures may be beneficial for the dying child.

Advantages of CAM:

- Easy to understand
- Familiar methods
- Many are noninvasive
- Many have fewer side effects compared with medical treatments
- Help improve the overall quality of life
- Help maintain current state of health
- More holistic and in balance with nature (Suzuki, 2004).

Disadvantages of CAM:

- Some treatments are complex
- They have not undergone adequate testing of effectiveness
- Many herbal preparations and remedies lack Food and Drug Administration approval
- Many not covered by third-party reimbursement

 Nursing Insight—*What makes CAM controversial?*

One of the main controversies in the use of CAM is that many of the therapies have not been tested through research. CAM therapies have not been proven effective 100% of the time. Some health-care providers find that it is through pure belief that these measures work, similar to a placebo effect and that people who are drawn to CAM are desperate and "will try anything." In addition, some health-care providers are concerned that some patients may refuse traditional medicine based on belief in CAM.

Hospice Care

In 1967, Dr. Cicely Saunders established the first hospice, St. Christopher's Hospice in London. Hospice care is a form of health care that provides palliative (comfort) care across a variety of settings, based on the philosophy that dying is part of the normal life cycle. Hospice promotes the concept of "living until you die."

Hospice care uses a variety of services (medical equipment, diagnostic procedures, and therapeutic interventions) provided by a multidisciplinary group of health-care providers

consisting of physicians, nurses, and other personnel such as chaplains, health aides, and bereavement counselors.

 Critical Nursing Action A Hospice Approach to Nursing Care

The focus of care is on improving the quality of remaining life—that is, on palliative, not curative, measures. Additionally, it:

- Endorses family-centered care
- Meets the child's physical, emotional, social, and spiritual needs
- Promotes effective symptom control and pain management
- Includes the interdisciplinary team
- Supports the family decision for home or hospital care
- Offers coordinated care

Once hospice care is initiated, the nurse can help the family determine the best place for the child to spend the final days. Most children prefer to die at home surrounded by family. The concept of children's home hospice care is a growing alternative to inpatient hospital care for the dying child. Holistic care measures can be implemented easily in the home. The child who is cared for in the home receives nursing care that includes visits, treatments, medications, supplies, and equipment offered by the home care agency. At home, the child is exposed to normal daily activities and surrounded by family members as death draws near. When the child is at home, he or she may be able to continue to play with other children and "feel normal" for as long as possible.

The nurse understands that remaining in the home environment may not always be possible. Assuming care for a dying child can be an overwhelming duty. Some parents simply have too much grief to care for the dying child and other children along with household responsibilities. Hospice care also provides respite care that allows family members to "take a break" or "time off" to reenergize before returning to the role of primary caregiver. In addition to the actual care of the dying child, hospice care also offers professional support after the death of the child.

CHILDREN'S HOSPICE INTERNATIONAL. Children's Hospice International (2012) says it is important to give clear answers to children who are dying. Evasive answers may confuse the child. The nurse must remember that the child may be at a developmental level at which he or she may take conversations literally. When the nurse is talking to the child, it is important to remember:

- Do not tell the child that death is sleeping peacefully. The child may fear going to sleep.
- Do not tell the child abstract concepts like, "It is God's will" or "you are such a good boy that God wants you to be with him." He or she may start to misbehave so as not to die.
- Approach the child with compassion, honesty, support, and love.

(Adapted from Children's Hospice International, 2012)

End-of-Life Care

After it has been determined that the end of life is near (about 6 months) for the child, care measures can be initiated to help the child die peacefully and without pain.

End-of-life care recognizes that each child and family has unique needs at this time. **End-of-life care** must be accessible to the child and the family in their desired setting (the home, inpatient hospice, or intensive care unit). End-of-life nursing care is meant to provide the best quality of life possible for the child and family. It is a holistic approach to care that includes physical, emotional, social, and spiritual interventions. Quality of life can be enhanced by offering support to the bereaving child and family, relieving distressing symptoms, and providing respite.

The home is usually the preferred site and can provide a peaceful, supportive, and spiritual environment according to what the child and family desire. Encourage the family to include familiar items in the care of the child such as a favorite blanket, toy, picture, or other items of importance to the child. During the dying process, changes in care measures can be adjusted as needed, but drastic changes during the final stage should be avoided (ELNEC, 2012).

HOLISTIC CARE FOR THE DYING CHILD

End-of-life nursing care measures include managing discomfort and pain in the dying child. This can be difficult because pain is a subjective experience. Some children can clearly describe the pain while others cannot. Dying children who are nonverbal have the most difficulty in conveying pain (Table 34-1). The nurse can communicate to the family the necessity of pain management.

clinical alert

Principles of pain medication administration for the dying child

- Give pain medications orally for as long as possible.
- Alternate routes for pain medication administration include IV, subcutaneous, transcutaneous, transmucosal, rectal, nasal, epidural, and intrathecal. The enteral route (or through a gastrostomy tube) is the preferred route for children in the dying process.
- Consider using an appropriate adjuvant (a drug added to a prescription to hasten or increase the action of a principal ingredient in the medication).
- Adjuvants offer analgesia in certain situations and include anticonvulsants, antidepressants, or muscle relaxants (Box 34-1).

Box 34-1 Medications

Common medications for dying child are:

Narcotic	morphine (Duramorph)
	fentanyl sublingual tablets (Abstral)
	hydromorphone hydrochloride (Dilaudid)
	acetaminophen and codeine (Tylenol, Codeine)
Sedative	midazolam HCl syrup (Midazolam Hydrochloride Syrup)
	lorazepam (Ativan)
	diazepam tablets (Valium)
Anti-inflammatory	ibuprofen (Motrin)
	ketorolac (Toradol)
Antiemetic	ondansetron (Zofran)
	promethazine (Phenergan)
	metoclopramide (Reglan)
	prochlorperazine (Compazine)

Questions and concerns raised about the end of life are discussed with the nurse as they arise. When a child is dying, parents tend to want to protect him or her from death by avoiding the subject or not talking about death. Some parents feel that if they discuss death with the child, the child may lose hope. The nurse helps the family understand that the child may want to talk about death. The nurse communicates to the family that the child may not want to be left alone. The child may be more afraid of being abandoned. The nurse can also inform the family about other resources such as hospice nurses, child life specialists, chaplains or spiritual leaders, home care agencies, social workers, and support groups.

 Across Care Settings: **National Cancer Institute and the American Cancer Society Web sites**

The National Cancer Institute (NCI) has resources available by calling the Cancer Information Service toll-free at 1-800-4-CANCER (1-800-422-6237) or TTY (for deaf and hard of hearing callers): 1-800-332-8615. The NCI's Web site is located at http://www.cancer.gov. The American Cancer Society's Web site is http://www.cancer.org/.

Table 34-1 Holistic Care for the Dying Child

Comfort Measures	Emotional Support	Spiritual Interventions	Complementary Care
Manage pain Promote hygiene Provide oral care Use fresh linen and clothing Reposition Provide diet as tolerated	Active listening Show empathy Use distraction Encourage positive coping Encourage verbalization of feelings	Offer presence Use meditation Provide music Encourage prayer Suggest spiritual symbols	Use art therapy Discuss energy-based therapy (healing touch, therapeutic touch, Reiki) Promote relaxation Use guided imagery
Suggest physical therapy Suggest occupational therapy Help the family create new rituals when the old rituals no longer work because of the progression of the disease	Suggest psychotherapy Discuss support groups Discuss topics about grief, loss, isolation, fear, guilt, and relationships Discuss concerns about life after the child's death that relate to family, friends, and others	Read from spiritual text or poetry Allow for sacrament Contact the family's religious or spiritual community Discuss God/Higher Power or Spiritual Source	Discuss acupuncture Discuss aromatherapy Discuss reasonable activity

The National Cancer Institute fact sheets include the following:

- The NCI fact sheet about hospice care includes contact information for hospice organizations.
- The NCI Advance Directives fact sheet discusses a patient's rights regarding medical treatment.
- The NCI fact sheet on Home Care for Cancer Patients provides information and resources related to home care services.
- The NCI booklet Advanced Cancer: Living Each Day provides support to cancer patients, families, and friends.

The American Cancer Society offers information on:

- Learning about cancer
- Staying healthy
- Finding support and treatment
- Research
- Getting involved

 Cultural Diversity: Cultural Practices

The nurse is knowledgeable of cultural practices of the child and family. It is important for the nurse to include the right support person to facilitate the cultural care of the dying child. By including cultural rituals or customs, nursing care can ease the death process for the child and family. Special ceremonies or rites may be requested by the family and be accommodated whenever possible. Other cultural care measures may include use of spiritual texts and symbols, prayer or meditation, chanting, offering music, lighting a candle, listening in silence, being present in the moment, or including other methods of care as deemed appropriate by the culture. Always ask, do not assume you know what the family wants or needs.

 Nursing Diagnoses The Dying Child

- Pain related to frequent invasive procedures
- Alteration in Family Process related to frequent hospitalization
- Anxiety related to separation from caregivers
- Alteration in Nutrition: Less than Body Requirements related to decreased appetite from disease process
- Anticipatory Grieving by family related to prognosis of disease process and imminent death of child
- Social Isolation related to frequent hospitalizations
- Depression related to the potential for death
- Fear related to the child's understanding of the disease process and the unknown
- Altered Coping Mechanism related to parental anxiety and stress from imminent death of the child
- Knowledge Deficit related to the disease process, unknown outcome, and possible experimental treatment

AFTER THE CHILD DIES

After the child has died, the nurse talks to the family about the child's appearance and description of the death. The nurse describes the child's dress, hairstyle, if the child's eyes are open or closed, any noticeable injuries, positioning of the child, and what occurred at the moment of death. It is essential that the nurse give the family the choice of seeing the child alone or having the nurse accompany them into the room. If the family chooses to be alone, the nurse stays close by in case the family has questions or needs.

 Critical Nursing Action Handling the Child's Belongings

When handling the belongings of a child who has died, the nurse treats them gently and with respect. The nurse gives the belongings to the family in a special container or package, not simply placing them in a plastic bag because this action may appear insensitive. The nurse remembers that these items are the final possessions of the child, and the family will cherish them.

 Collaboration in Caring—*A father's story*

One father tells about a personal moment after the death of a child. The father said that as he held his adolescent daughter as she was dying, he felt her heart stop beating next to his chest. This was the actual moment when the daughter's heart took its last beat. The father treasures this moment. The nurse caring for the child was privileged to hear this father's story and collaborate with him in caring for his child during her death. The compassionate nurse is honored to be present for these moments in time, holding dear, and striving to make the tragedy of the death of a child special, positive, and memorable for the family.

 legal alert—**The death certificate**

A death certificate is an official government document that is issued to the nearest relatives of a dying person stating the fact, date, and cause of death. It relieves the family of the deceased from official, social, and legal obligations and enables the settlement of inheritance. The death certificate also authorizes the family to collect insurance and other benefits.

Grieving

From the moment a family has been informed about the child's fatal condition, the family's life changes direction and grieving begins (Fig. 34-5).

 Nursing Insight—*Grief*

Grief begins at the moment of diagnosis and fluctuates with remissions and exacerbations of the condition. It escalates at the time of death (though it may be mixed with feelings of relief and guilt) and continues at varying levels for years afterwards. Everyone grieves differently. Bereaved parents often experience renewed and intense grief on occasions that would have been significant benchmarks in the life of the deceased child such as birthdays, holidays, anticipated graduation from high school, and more (Hutton et al., 2010).

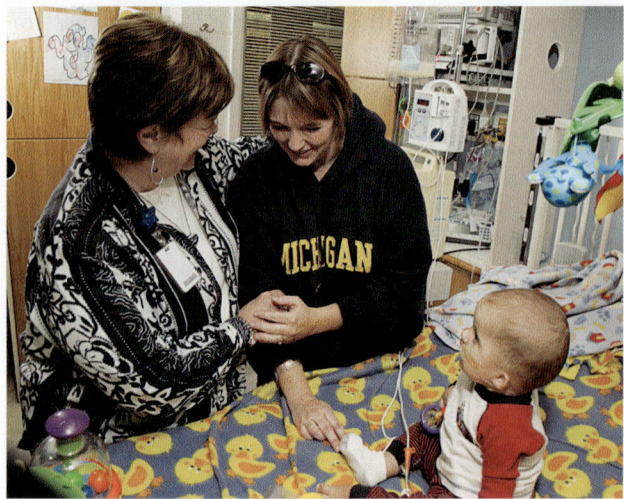

Figure 34-5 The hospital chaplain or another religious figure can offer spiritual support to the child and his or her family.

Signs and Symptoms

Grief can be an emotional response as well as a physical response to death. Somatic grief response can be described as:

- Feelings of tightness in the throat or chest, sighing
- Weakness or shortness of breath
- Preoccupation with the image of the deceased (e.g., hearing or seeing the person who died)
- Inability to focus on anything other than the loved one who died
- Emotionally distancing self from others
- Feelings of guilt
- Feeling responsible for the loved one's death
- Searching for what could have been done differently, thinking in terms of "if I only had done . . ."
- Hostile reactions that include feelings and expressions of anger
- Inability to complete daily tasks

Collaborative Care

Nursing Care. A holistic nursing plan of care is essential when caring for the grieving family.

The nurse offers ongoing emotional support to help the family understand the situation.

> 66**What to say**99—*After the death of a child*
>
> After the child's death, the family might ask the nurse questions such as, What did I do to deserve this? Did I do something wrong? Am I being punished? The nurse listens empathetically to the family and encourages them to "take it one day and sometimes one moment at a time." Help the family understand that there may be "good days" and that inevitably there will be "bad days." The nurse can give the family hope that over time the emotional pain may dissipate and that they can better understand the experience of their child's death.

GRIEF THEORIES

It is important for the nurse to understand the grieving process from well-known theories to provide proper care and support.

Kübler-Ross's Stages of Grief

Elisabeth Kübler-Ross (1983) described five stages of grieving.

DENIAL AND ISOLATION. This stage includes feelings of numbness, disbelief, and shock. Denial is a way of protecting the family and child from the emotional pain that may be too severe to handle all at once. The numbness helps the family and child by creating emotional distance from the pain, thereby allowing continuation of daily responsibilities. The nurse acknowledges feelings of numbness and reminds the family to slow down, "take it easy," pay attention to safety measures, and retain healthy habits.

ANGER. Anger can be one of the most difficult stages. At this point, the family and child have developed awareness about the reality of the diagnosis. The feelings of anger, fear, and guilt can be an overwhelming but a normal response to the impending death. Both the family and child may become angry with God or Higher Power or experience a spiritual crisis. The nurse gives spiritual care by sitting at the bedside or calling on a hospital chaplain or the family's personal clergy or spiritual leader to provide support. The nurse uses prayer, meditation, reading from a spiritual text, or just being present with the family. The nurse also encourages the family to find a positive outlet for the emotions. Positive outlets can include talking with other family members or friends, nurses, and families at the hospital or expressing feelings in a support group. Physical exercise is another positive way to release anger. Family members are encouraged to write their feelings down in a journal or draw to express emotions. The nurse helps the child to express anger through therapeutic play or art therapy.

BARGAINING. It is common for the family members to ask, "What did I do to make this happen?" It is normal for the family to try to bargain with either self or with God in hopes that the child's life will be spared. The family may express guilt at times for disciplining the child on occasion. The family may also feel punishment for personal life circumstances. Specifically, a mother might wonder if she caused the illness or injury during pregnancy. During this stage, it is natural for the family to make vows of personal improvement if the child is cured. It is important for the nurse to talk to the family about bargaining and reinforce that the child's illness is not anyone's fault.

DEPRESSION. When the illness can no longer be denied or bargained away, the family and child may begin to feel a profound sadness. The nurse understands that sadness or depression is to be expected. There are some warning signs that the nurse must be aware of that indicate extra help is needed during this period of depression (e.g., insomnia or excessive sleeping, nightmares, weight gain or weight loss, loss of concentration that interferes with the ability to function normally, overwhelming anger, and constant fear or worry about the physical wellness of other family members). If the nurse assesses that any of these signs are present, it is imperative to talk to the hospital social worker, physician, or a professional counselor to obtain help.

ACCEPTANCE. Accepting a child's illness and possible death means that the family or child has made an emotional adjustment to the illness. Although the family and child may still feel as if they are on an emotional roller coaster, the difficulties will become more predictable and manageable. At this phase, many family members find strength and joy in everyday living. Family members begin looking for meaning and a reason about why this happened to the child and what impact this experience may have on the future. The nurse remains present with the family and continues to offer support and encouragement. The nurse provides community resources for the family to help them continue in the grieving process.

Miles and Perry's Stages of Grief

Miles and Perry (1985), two other well-known grief theorists, identify three phases of parental grief.

PHASE 1. Phase 1 is a state of numbness and shock. The parents may seem to be in a trance and display no emotion. Some parents may try to comfort others, yet show no emotion themselves.

PHASE 2. Phase 2 is a period of intense grief. The parents may cry. Some parents express grief loudly with outbursts, while others cry quietly. Other parents display inappropriate silliness or euphoria. It is a mistake for the nurse to judge a parent as unaffected or uncaring because of the type of emotional reactions at the time of death.

PHASE 3. Phase 3 is a period of reorganization. Initially the parents are in a state of emotional shock and forget important information. Later parents can remember verbatim the information that was given at the time of the child's death.

Epperson's Theory of Grieving

It is important for the nurse to remember that no two families go through the grieving process at the same time or at the same pace. A family who experiences a sudden or catastrophic loss appears to go through a slightly altered grief process. Epperson's theory about catastrophic grief may be helpful in the emergency department setting. With the absolute loss of a child already evident, bargaining is absent and depression is replaced with remorse. According to Moroni-Leash (1994), Epperson's theory of the grieving process includes six phases.

HIGH ANXIETY. High anxiety is described as a time of great stress, with many physical manifestations of emotional upheaval. A nursing assessment of the family member finds agitation, rapid respiration and increased heart rate, irritability, muscular tension, and fainting along with digestive or bowel changes that may result in nausea and diarrhea. It is important to refer the family member to a health-care provider.

DENIAL. Denial is a protective emotional reaction to postpone the realization of the loss until sufficient psychological preparation has been made. This phase must not be hurried, and a period of acute denial is normal. However, the denial should not persist beyond the viewing of the child's body and after the family has departed the hospital. If denial continues, the nurse needs to refer the family member to a health-care provider or a professional counselor.

ANGER. Anger is a common emotional response and can be directed inwardly, toward another family member, or toward others. Usually the anger is a diffuse kind that lashes out at society or life in general, with the feeling that the loss was somehow "allowed" to occur. Many times, the anger may be an attempt to affix blame. The anger is usually brief. During an assessment, if the nurse sees that the anger persists, a complex underlying cause such as fear needs to be addressed further by a mental health specialist.

REMORSE. Remorse includes feelings of both guilt and sorrow. The family regrets that the accident or illness occurred and feels responsible that it could not be prevented. The nurse understands that this is the "if only . . ." stage. Nursing care includes giving the family repeated reassurance that personal actions were reasonable. In situations of true culpability, the responsible family member needs intensive support and counseling to come to terms with personal liability.

GRIEF. Grief is an intense period of overwhelming sadness. The duration and intensity of the grief depend on factors such as the medical condition of the child, existing support systems, and culpability in the disease or injury scenario. The nurse provides emotional support and genuine caring during this phase.

RECONCILIATION. Reconciliation is described as the final phase to be experienced and may be an end point to the acute family crisis. The nurse can tell the family that reconciliation is a time when the family begins to adapt to the existing circumstances and begins to move on with life.

 Cultural Diversity: The Hispanic Culture and Grief

Hispanics (Latinos) are persons of Mexican, Cuban, Puerto Rican, Central or South American, or other Spanish origins. As a result of this diversity, grieving behaviors surrounding the death of a child might take different forms. One example is a Hispanic family who is of the Catholic faith and who has a close extended family network within the social structure. Based on their culture and way of grieving, their infant child who has died is viewed as an angel who has returned to heaven. This belief brings comfort to the parents and the extended family, particularly the grandparents, and allows them to move on through the grieving process. To honor the deceased child, pictures are displayed in the home as a tribute, keeping the memory alive. There is a specified grieving time called *luto*. When this family is in *luto*, few celebratory activities take place, and usually no parties are attended and music is not played in the home. Outward expressions of happiness are discouraged for usually a year. In some instances, the relatives may wear black clothing to signify that they remember the loved one. If these traditions are not observed, there may be criticism from others. Any criticism is of the utmost concern to the family.

COPING PATTERNS

Grief reactions can differ. Certain behaviors by the family directly after a notification of illness or impending death tend to be magnifications of their predominant stress-coping behaviors in times of duress. In times of stress, the child and parents may revert backwards to familiar ways of coping. It is important to note that if there is too much damage to a familiar lifestyle or family structure, the child or parents may become unable to cope.

Collaborative Care

Nursing Care. The nurse recognizes the exhibited coping patterns, discovering ways to support the family directly or indirectly. The nurse listens, sits silently, refers the family to a pastoral care person, offers spiritual care such as prayer, or encourages journal writing or reading from a spiritual text. If the nurse notices that the behavior is destructive to self or others, it is necessary to call in a physician or a professional counselor. The nurse does not alter the coping pattern completely because alteration could strip the child and family completely of protective buffers and leave them exposed to more pain than is bearable.

Pathological Grief

On occasion, personal support systems do not adequately allow the individual to cope, and the family members may experience dysfunction or pathological grief. Intense grief feelings or a dysfunctional personality may easily bring on **pathological grief** (deviation from a healthy or normal grief) such as violence, addictions, or poor decision making.

Subtle signs are warning signs and may not necessarily indicate a severe problem. It is the intensity and duration of these behaviors that are the deciding factors indicating the need for professional help.

- Absence of grief such as showing little or no emotion
- Persistent blame or guilt
- Anxiety
- Aggressive and destructive outbursts
- Depression and suicidal thoughts or actions
- Unwillingness to speak about the deceased
- Expressing only positive or only negative feelings about the deceased
- Prolonged dysfunction in school
- Always assuming a caregiver role

 Nursing Care Plan The Grieving Family

Nursing Diagnosis: Grieving related to poor medical prognosis for child

Measurable Short-Term Goal: Family will explore their beliefs and feelings about the medical prognosis.

Measurable Long-Term Goal: Family will begin the grieving process, using resources and positive coping mechanisms.

NOC Outcomes:
Family Coping (2600) Family actions to manage stressors that tax family reserves
Grief Resolution (1304) Adjustment to actual or impending loss
Psychosocial Adjustment: Life Change (1305) Adaptive psychosocial response of an individual to a significant life change

NIC Interventions:
Anticipatory Guidance (5210)
Coping Enhancement (5230)
Family Integrity Promotion (7100)
Grief Work Facilitation (5290)

Nursing Interventions:

1. Develop a trusting relationship with child and family by spending time with them, using active listening techniques, and providing consistency in assignment of nurses to care for the child.

   RATIONALE: Enhances family comfort and enables the family to build trust with the nursing staff.

2. Assess the family's understanding, beliefs, and feelings about the child's prognosis.

   RATIONALE: Assists the family to organize and verbalize their concerns while allowing for correction of misunderstandings.

3. Provide ongoing information about the child's condition and what to expect next. Allow time for questions and reassurance.

   RATIONALE: Allows the family to understand what is happening and to prepare themselves for the next stage in a supportive environment.

4. Provide the child and family with a quiet space and protect their private time together from unnecessary interruptions.

   RATIONALE: Ensures privacy for the family to freely experience and show feelings without worrying about strangers and interruptions.

5. Encourage the family to participate in the child's care as much as possible, if desired.

   RATIONALE: Care provided by a familiar person may ease the child's anxiety and allows the family to demonstrate their love for the child.

6. Assist family to identify coping mechanisms and refer the family and child for spiritual care and/or professional support as needed (specify, e.g., pastoral care, family spiritual advisor, social services, grief counseling, or grief support groups).

   RATIONALE: Support systems can offer the family and child a constant source of support during the dying process and after the death of the child.

- Stealing or other illegal acts
- Signs of addictive behavior (e.g., drugs, food, or certain activities)

Pathological grief may manifest as suicidal ideation and can occur when an individual is notified about the death of a child. The individual may feel intense hopelessness, helplessness, and loss of love. It is very important that the nurse recognize these feelings and listen carefully to the individual who may be expressing suicidal ideas. The nurse immediately obtains professional psychiatric help for the individual.

The sudden loss of a child may be perceived like an emotional assault and an assertion of vulnerability. Therefore, sometimes an individual becomes violent when experiencing this significant loss in control. When the behavior of the individual escalates beyond the realm of verbal interchange, pathology is present. If the nurse notices that a family member displays a violent reaction, steps are taken to explain to other family members that they must avoid any confrontation with the individual. The nurse calls for the security guard to quietly remove the person to a private area away from others. It is essential that the nurse not be placed in a situation of personal risk. If the violent individual threatens the nurse or others, it is important to obtain help quickly and activate the facility's security personnel.

Homicidal ideation must never be ignored. Homicidal threats can occur when a child dies because of negligence (whether real or perceived, such as drunken driving or intentional violence). Sometimes after a cooling-down period, the individual regains a calm demeanor and the potential for violence may diminish. Most often, the violent individual is able to regain self-control and stabilize him- or herself. If this is not the case, the nurse calls for the security guard or the local police to deal with the individual.

Grief that is influenced by drugs and alcohol dramatically alters the individual's ability to work through the grieving process. Illegal narcotic or alcoholic substances cause emotional responses to be exaggerated and uncontrolled. The ability of family members to unite in support of each other can be greatly reduced in this situation. An important nursing management strategy is to call in other family members, friends, or professional counselors to provide immediate help and extended support for the individual under the influence of drugs or alcohol.

Extreme denial is another abnormal response to grief. Most often grief reaches its peak within 3 or 4 months after the bereavement. However, when this does not happen, psychosomatic, psychoneurotic, and psychotic reactions can occur with increased frequency. If an individual is unable to start accepting what has happened beyond the viewing of the child's body or extends grieving into months after the child's death, the nurse needs to be aware of a pathological denial response. The nurse helps the family member find an appropriate community resource or support group.

Saying Good-Bye

At the time of death, the parents of a dying child can be in extreme grief, and saying good-bye to the child is an important process.

Collaborative Care

Nursing Care. Facilitating saying good-bye is important, and the process is not rushed. It is paramount that, throughout the saying good-bye process, the nurse calls the child by name, which helps parents and family members feel that the nurse genuinely cares for the child. Allow family members adequate time to be alone with the child after death.

"What to say"—*Proper communication*

It is important to avoid platitudes such as "time heals all wounds," "you wouldn't want him to live like that," "you're lucky; it could have been much worse," or "you can always have another child." These phrases minimize the loss and have little comforting effect. They may be upsetting to the family and make them feel that somehow this child's life has limited value. It is better to say nothing if you do not know what to say. Some appropriate responses are:

"I'm sorry."

"This must be terribly hard for you."

"Is there anyone I can call for you?"

"Would you like me to stay with you for a while?"

During the good-bye, the nurse keeps the child covered up and as warm as possible. The parents may want to assist in the immediate postmortem care as a way of saying good-bye. Parents can give the child their last bath, comb the hair, wash the face, or dress the child in a clean set of clothing. Allowing parents to hold the child one more time as the final good-bye is said is an act of compassion. Extended family members, friends, and others may come to say good-bye as well. The nurse encourages parents and other visitors to talk about memories of the child. Crying is common for the parents, family, friends, and the nurse. If the nurse cannot keep personal emotional control, another nurse offers relief.

The nurse's role after the child's death is to be supportive and allow the family to dictate the "good-bye" timeline. If an extended time frame is needed to say good-bye, the nurse contacts pastoral care services to coordinate a private viewing time in the chapel. After the good-bye, it is important that the nurse ensure that the parents and others have departed from the hospital before transporting the child to the morgue.

Now Can You—Discuss the dying child?

1. Discuss the holistic nursing care for the dying child?
2. List the nursing diagnoses related to the dying child?
3. Assist the child and family through the grieving process?
4. Recognize pathological grief?

 Nursing Insight—*Supporting the family at the end of life*

The nurse
- Provides continuity of care
- Allows the parent to hold the child while life support is being discontinued

- Provides a peaceful dignified experience
- Teaches the family that the dying child, "can still hear you" and "it is all right to talk to the dying child"
- Uses the team approach with other health-care providers
- Allows family members adequate time to be alone with the child after death
- Allows time after death for additional questions and concerns
- Validates that everything possible was done for the child
- Encourages the family to care for the child after death if they are able (e.g., bathe and dress the body)

THE SIBLING SAYS GOOD-BYE

The sibling relationship is sometimes one of the most consistent and ongoing relationships for a child. It can involve many feelings and experiences, including disharmony. In a sibling relationship, the child may experience love, caring, sharing, comforting, playing, jealousy, envy, fighting, and blaming. To the child, the sibling is not only a brother or sister but also many times a playmate, friend, or support system. The child and sibling have learned and grown with each other, and now the relationship is lost. A visit from the sibling(s) is important.

When a child dies, the surviving sibling may be mistakenly overlooked. Sometimes overlooking another child is unintentional as the focus is placed on the child who died or on the parents. Sometimes there is a perception that the sibling will "be all right." The child may have been sent away to a grandparent or neighbor while the brother or sister was dying in the hospital. Sending the sibling away must not be viewed as negative behavior by the parent because the parent may be too overcome with personal emotions to care properly for the other child. When a child dies, the surviving sibling loses not only a brother or sister but sometimes also the grieving parents because they may be unable to attend to his or her needs. It is also important to remember that the sibling may experience guilt feelings, thinking he or she may have done "something" to make the child sick or has done something wrong and is now being punished. It is best to include the sibling in the dying and grief process.

Grief is individual, and children often alternate between expressing their grief or ignoring the situation. Some children play immediately after a death, even if the death is a sibling. Parents need to be informed that children use play as a coping mechanism, which doesn't minimize their grief. Some children may be uncomfortable seeing their parent's distress and may want to leave, while other children may want to stay and provide comfort to their parents. Keeping routines to enhance safety and comfort is essential for the sibling. Unacknowledged grief of a sibling may result in acting-out behaviors. Parents can still set limits and enforce usual discipline parameters. A sibling's schoolwork may deteriorate so it is important to let the child's teachers know about the situation. School counselors may help if they are comfortable talking about death with children (Hutton et al., 2010).

Collaborative Care

Nursing Care. The nurse encourages the family to include the sibling when saying good-bye. After the child has died, give the sibling a chance to say good bye, leave a personal item, or be alone with his or her sibling if desired. Allow the sibling to express personal wants and needs.

Critical Nursing Action The Sibling

The nurse's role in relation to the sibling consists of a variety of holistic nursing interventions:

- Listen and help the sibling express his or her feelings.
- Show the family how to acknowledge the sibling's presence during this difficult time (initiate a simple conversation, turn on cartoons, offer a drink or snack, or show the sibling how to touch the dying child).
- Explain the situation to the sibling and relate appropriate information in terms understandable for the sibling's age.
- Allow visitation during appropriate times.
- Help the sibling understand that he or she is not responsible for the sibling's death.
- Contact a child life specialist who can assist the sibling with art therapy.
- Encourage simple ways to be involved in the care such as making a final gift for the sibling to keep at the bedside.
- Remind the family that the sibling is also experiencing a loss.

RELATED ASPECTS OF CARE

Remembrance Packet

After the death of a child, ongoing nursing care includes creating a remembrance packet to give to the family. When creating this memory packet, the nurse gains permission from the parents to include personal aspects. If a camera is available, the nurse can take pictures of the child. Taking pictures can be especially important in the death of an infant if parents have not yet taken pictures. Sometimes the nurse may want to make a plaster impression of the child's hand or footprints. A lock of hair from the back of the child's head can be included in the remembrance packet. The nurse suggests to the parents that baptismal certificates, school papers, awards, or candles can also be incorporated into the remembrance packet. After the child's death, the nurse can mail a sympathy card to the parents that may also become a part of the remembrance packet.

Family Teaching Guidelines...
The Sibling Says Good-Bye

HOW TO: Teach the Family to Help the Sibling Say Good-Bye:

- Teach the family that it is important that the sibling be included in the grieving process and have the opportunity to say good-bye.
- Instruct families to allow the sibling to have short visits when possible.
- During visitation, encourage the family to have another support person with the sibling such as a friend or grandparent.
- Tell the family that the sibling can write letters or draw pictures for the child as a way of saying good-bye.

ESSENTIAL INFORMATION:

Kübler-Ross (1983) says that the child who has been included in the death and mourning process with the family is able to let go in a healthy way.

Sometimes the gathered items for the remembrance packet are refused by the parents. If permission is granted, place them in an envelope or box. Some parents are in such a state of shock they cannot accept the items but may ask for them at a later date.

Organ Tissue Donation

A discussion soon after death about organ tissue donation, in many states, is required by law. Organ tissue donation may be a sensitive issue for the nurse and family. The bereavement team knows when it is appropriate to approach the family. The **bereavement team** is a group of trained professionals who know how to approach the topic of organ tissue donation while maintaining dignity and respect for the deceased child. In some circumstances, the family may approach the nurse about organ tissue donation. Sometimes, the physician provides information about organ tissue donation.

Certain criteria must be met for the child to be an organ or tissue donor. Depending on the type of illness, criteria may not be met for organ tissue donation. Be aware of common questions that the family may ask about organ tissue donation to help the family make an informed decision. Sometimes after the organ tissue donation, the family of the child gains comfort in knowing that the death of the child enabled another child to live.

Funerals

The nurse may be asked by families to attend the funeral of the child. The presence of the nurse at the funeral is meaningful to the child's family and may bring the family comfort and convey a sense of caring for the deceased child. Attending the funeral is a personal decision for the nurse. While attending the funeral, the service may be difficult and bring up emotions for the nurse or it may assist the nurse in the grieving process and promote closure. Attending the service may be a meaningful way for the nurse to express feelings for the child and the family. If the nurse cannot attend the funeral, sending a card is a sign of caring about the child and family.

Caring for the Professional Caregiver

Caring for the dying child and family can be one of the greatest challenges presented to the nurse. A nurse caring for the dying child can experience personal emotions. One emotion is attachment, and it can vary from close contact with the child and family to distancing him- or herself from the situation. The nurse may also feel a sense of helplessness about not being able to alter the outcome of death, especially in an acute death situation. In caring for a child with a chronic condition, the nurse may have had more time to prepare for the child's death. Either way, the death of a child may not be easy for the nurse.

Caring for the child who is dying requires specialized knowledge and skill, sustaining an ongoing and special relationship with families, and at times advocacy. In addition, caring for a seriously ill or dying child requires compassion, sympathy, and empathy. This type of care can require enormous physical, emotional, and spiritual energy. Often the nurse is able to do this effortlessly. However, it is important to realize that the nurse can become depleted based on constant demands from the dying child and family. When the demands of care exceed personal energy, the nurse's personal energy may be threatened. This may be referred to as parallel suffering (ELNEC, 2012).

 ### Nursing Insight—*Burnout, compassion fatigue syndrome, and moral distress*

Burnout, compassion fatigue syndrome, and moral distress are important concepts.

- **Burnout** is a state of physical, emotional, and mental exhaustion caused by long-term involvement in emotionally demanding situations. It emerges gradually and is a result of emotional exhaustion and job stress.
- **Compassion fatigue syndrome** is characterized by a sense of helplessness, confusion, and isolation from supporters and can have a more rapid onset and resolution than burnout.
- **Moral distress** occurs when the nurse is unable to translate personal moral choices into action. The nurse acts in a manner contrary to personal or professional values which undermines integrity. During moral distress, the nurse experiences feelings of frustration, anger, and anxiety.

It is important for the nurse to pay attention to personal needs and recognize that certain actions can help relieve burnout, compassion fatigue syndrome, and moral distress. Sharing grief with the child's family after death can help both the nurse and family deal with feelings about the loss of the child. Most institutions have grief counselors and support services available to the nurse. Debriefing sessions with professional grief counselors after the child's death have proven to be helpful. Journal writing or art therapy is an avenue many nurses explore. Ask for personal support as well as to be supportive to other nurses. Consider organized support sessions after the death of a child. These post-clinical debriefings may be helpful for the nurse to talk with the physician or professional counselor for reassurance that a change in the nursing care would not have changed the outcome.

Another aspect is personal suffering that happens when the nurse feels little control over the practice environment. Even though caring for the dying child and family is a privilege that offers personal rewards, the nurse must recognize that personal suffering is possible. A good way to address the nurse's suffering is to attend a forum specifically for discussion, reflection, and shared understandings about suffering. During the forum, the nurse can express personal feelings, frustrations, and disappointments. The nurse can also use strategies in the work setting such as journal writing, art therapy, quiet time, a walk, prayer, or meditation that acknowledges and allows the nurse to process the grief and loss. Accept compassion and care from others. Self-care practices away from the workplace such as exercise, leisure activities with friends and family, and solitary time for reflection and renewal have great value. The nurse needs to refresh his or her spirit. It is important for the nurse to create healthy boundaries, setting proper limits for compassion and self-sacrifice with the child and his or her family as well as oneself.

Nursing Insight—*Paying attention to personal needs*

The nurse can pay attention to personal needs by asking:
- How do I feel?
- Am I comfortable caring for a child who is dying?
- Can I cope with the needs of the family as well?
- Am I becoming overwhelmed or attached when caring for this child and family?

If the nurse feels uncomfortable with any of these questions, it is time for reflection and self-care. The nurse understands that these feelings are normal and are a part of the human experience. It is important to know when the situation becomes too great to bear. It is difficult to help the patient and the family if the nurse is not coping. Remember there are employee assistance programs or forums at most institutions to assist the nurse with coping.

Summary Points

- A chronic condition is a health situation that persists over time, usually longer than 3 months, or one in which recovery progresses slowly.

- The increase in chronic conditions may be partially attributed to technological life-saving and life-sustaining measures or technological devices that can now diagnose and treat diseases that previously were either undiagnosed or untreatable.

- Technology-dependent children are grouped according to the type of equipment required.

- A chronic condition affects the family and child differently depending on the age at diagnosis.

- A child living with a chronic condition requires day-to-day care and can become a source of stress for parents and other caregivers.

- The nurse understands the importance of establishing a therapeutic relationship with the child and family who are living with a chronic condition.

- The child with a chronic condition may experience negative physical growth (growth failure) and developmental aspects.

- When the child enters the dying process, the body begins to shut down physically as well as emotionally and spiritually. This failure might happen slowly or rapidly depending on the circumstance.

- Perceptions of death vary across the age continuum. The nurse prioritizes nursing actions and assists the child according to the appropriate developmental level to help make the transition to death fearless, peaceful, and painless.

- The nurse recognizes physical signs of impending death. Knowing the normal physical processes may help the family through the experience.

- Once medical treatment is halted and the family has determined that death is inevitable, the focus of nursing care is about allowing the child to die. The nurse can shift from the curative technological approach to providing care that enables the child to move toward death by accessing his or her own inner resources.

- Grief begins at the moment of diagnosis and fluctuates with remissions and exacerbations of the condition.

- The nurse encourages the family to include the sibling when saying good-bye. After the child has died, give the sibling a chance to say good-bye, leave a personal item, or be alone with the sibling if desired.

- It is important to realize that the nurse can become depleted based on constant demands from the dying child and family. When the demands of care exceed personal energy, the nurse's personal energy may be threatened.

Review Questions

Multiple Choice

1. The pediatric nurse enters the room of an infant newly diagnosed with cerebral palsy and finds the mother tearful, looking over the infant's crib. The nurse places her hand on the mother's shoulder and the mother cries, "I wish my son were normal!" Which response by the nurse is most appropriate?
A. "I know what you mean. This is very difficult."
B. "Sit down and let's talk about how you're feeling."
C. "I am here to help you. I will come back later."
D. "Where is your husband? Can he help you now?"

2. The pediatric nurse working in an acute inpatient unit understands that a Do Not Resuscitate (DNR) order includes which measure?
A. Administering radiation therapy in an attempt to eradicate the disease
B. Administering antibiotic therapy as scheduled by the physician
C. Administering no lifesaving measures in the event of a respiratory arrest
D. Administering feeding via an oral-gastric tube for artificial nutrition

3. A 4-year-old's sibling has died. Even though she was told her sibling is dead, the child keeps asking when she will come back. The pediatric nurse knows this is an example of which item?
A. State of denial
B. Memory loss caused by stress
C. Developmental approach to death
D. Severe psychopathology

4. A 5-year-old's mother died. Now when anyone mentions her name, the child runs from the room screaming "Mommy, where are you? Why won't you come back?" Otherwise the child refuses to talk about his mother at all. Which intervention would be effective in helping this child explore his grief?
A. Talking to him about his feelings at bedtime
B. Encouraging him to write down his feelings
C. Telling him that his mother has gone away on a trip
D. Using creative activities such as drawing or play therapy

5. A child requires a ventilator and a feeding tube to live. Under the grouping proposed by a Congressional report on technologically dependent children, which category does this child fit into?
   A. Group 1
   B. Group 2
   C. Group 3
   D. Group 4

6. Which category best illustrates the consistent stress, pressure, and anxiety caused by caring for a chronically ill child?
   A. Moral distress
   B. Caregiver burden
   C. Role confusion
   D. Role strain

7. A family with a chronically ill child responds to changes in the child's condition with alternating periods of grief and denial. When documenting the behavior, which description is most appropriate?
   A. Maladaptive grief
   B. Caregiver role strain
   C. Chronic sorrow
   D. Impaired coping

8. A child with a chronic illness is way behind on the growth charts for height and weight as compared with peers of the same age. Which diagnosis does the nurse anticipate seeing when reviewing the medical record?
   A. Failure to thrive
   B. General growth failure
   C. Malnutrition
   D. Delayed development

9. Which federal law is most applicable to children who require special education?
   A. Education for All Handicapped Children Amendments
   B. The Rehabilitation Act
   C. Free and Appropriate Education Act
   D. Individuals with Disabilities Education Act

10. In working with terminally ill children, the nurse knows that in which age group are perceptions of death intertwined with fantasy?
   A. Toddler
   B. School-aged
   C. Preschool
   D. Adolescent

See Answers to End of Chapter Review Questions on *DavisPlus.*

REFERENCES

Bowes, S., Lowes, L., Warner, J., & Gregory, J. (2009). Chronic sorrow in parents of children with type 1 diabetes. *Journal of Advanced Nursing,* 65(5), 992–1000.

Bulechek, G. M., Butcher, H. K., Dochterman, J. M., & Wagner, C. (2013). *Nursing interventions classification (NIC)* (6th ed.). St. Louis, MO: Elsevier Mosby.

Centers for Disease Control and Prevention. (2013). Retrieved from http://www.cdc.gov/ncbddd/developmentaldisabilities/index.html

Children's Hospice International. (2012). Retrieved from http://www.chionline.org/resources

Choi, J., Donahoe, M., Zullo, T., & Hoffman, L. (2011). Caregivers of the chronically critically ill after discharge from the intensive care unit: Six months experience. *American Journal of Critical Care, 20*(1), 12–21.

Collins, L., & Swartz, K. (2011). Caregiver care. *American family Physician, (11)*, 1309–1317.

Consortium for Citizens with Disabilities. (2012). Retrieved from http://www.c-c-d.org/

Davies, B., Sehring, S., Partridge, J., Cooper, B., Hughes, A., Philip, J., et al. (2008). Barriers to palliative care for children: Perceptions of pediatric health care providers. *Pediatric, 121*(2), 282–288.

ELNEC: End of Life Nursing Education Consortium: Pediatric palliative care (August 23–24, 2012), Washington, DC.

Halfon, N., & Newacheck, P. (2010). Evolving notions of chronic childhood illness. *Journal of the American Medical Association, 303*(7), 665–666.

Hutton, N., Levetown, M., & Frager, G. (2010). *The hospice and palliative medicine approach to caring for pediatric patients* (3rd ed.). Glenview, IL: American Academy of Hospice & Palliative Medicine.

Hysing, M., Davis, E., Elgin, C., Wake, M., & Lo, S. K. (2009). The impact of childhood conditions and concurrent morbidities on child health and well-being. *Child Care Health Development, 3*(4), 418–429.

Kübler-Ross, E. (1983). *On children and death.* New York, NY: Macmillan.

Meltzer, L., Boroughs, D., & Downes, J. (2010). The relationship between home nursing coverage, sleep, and daytime functioning in parents of ventilator-assisted children. *Journal of Pediatric Nursing, 25*(4), 250–257.

Miles, M., & Perry, K. (1985). In M. C. Slota (Ed.), *Core curriculum for critical care nurses* (pp. 28–29). Philadelphia, PA: W.B. Saunders.

Moroni-Leash, R. (1994). *Death notification: A practical guide to the process.* Hinesburg, VT: Upper Access.

National Institutes of Health. (2012). What is complementary medicine. Retrieved from http://nccam.nih.gov/health/whatiscam

Potts, N., & Mandleco, B. (2011). *Pediatric nursing: Caring for children and their families* (3rd ed.). Clifton Park, NY: Delmar.

Reiter, K., Pernath, N., Pagel, P., Hiedi, S., Hoffman, F., Shoen, C., et al. (2011). Risk factors for morbidity and mortality in pediatric home mechanical ventilation. *Clinical Pediatrics, 50*(3), 237–241.

Schmitke, J., & Scholmann, P. (2010). Chronic conditions. In N. Potts & B. Mandleco, *Pediatric nursing: Care for children and their families* (pp. 493–515). Clifton Park, NY: Delmar.

Suzuki, N. (2004). Complementary and alternative medicine: A Japanese perspective. *Evidenced-based Complementary and Alternative Care, 1*(2), 113–118.

Technology Related Assistance for Individuals with Disabilities Act (2004–2007). Retrieved from http://www.napcse.org/FAQ-LAW.php

U.S. Congress of Technology Assessment. (1987). Retrieved from http://ota.fas.org/

Venes, D. (2013). *Taber's cyclopedic medical dictionary* (22nd ed.). Philadelphia, PA: F.A. Davis Company.

CONCEPT MAP

Nursing Insight:
- Know examples of and terms r/t chronic conditions
- Understand impact of chronic conditions on family/concept of caregiver burden
- Grief reactions vary over time
- Chronically ill children can regress
- Be aware of 1998 "Tech Act"
- Use "presence" at time of death
- Understand burnout, compassion fatigue, and moral distress in nurses

- Frequent hospitalization
- Chronic burden of care
- Threat of unknown
- Social, financial, psychological strain
- Stress/increased demands/role strain
- Interruption of normal routine
- Loss of control/powerlessness
- Balancing care with other responsibilities
- Need for ongoing supportive resources

Legal Alert:
- Be aware of laws re: provision of educational services
- Death certificate → official government document

Where Research and Practice Meet:
- Home night-nursing support improves health/well-being of families
- Perceived barriers to end-of-life care r/t uncertainties

Collaboration in Caring:
- Child life specialist

Complementary Care:
- Acupuncture; herbs; relaxation; prayers

Infant:
- Separation: disrupts bonding
- Alteration in growth and development

Toddler:
- Interruption of development: autonomy/self-control
- Hinders fine/gross motor skills
- Anxiety

Preschool Child:
- Interrupts initiative
- Perceives treatment as punishment
- Aggression; withdrawal; regression

School-Aged Child:
- Interrupts industry; peer interactions; independence
- Anger; refusal to comply with treatment

Adolescent:
- Loss of peer interaction negative self-esteem/sexual identity
- Loss of autonomy/control
- Maladaptive coping; worry about family

Sibling:
- Decreased self-esteem; less parental support; mood swings
- Loneliness/isolation

Nursing—Infant:
- Hold; rock; comfort; soothing voice
- Encourage parent–child bonding/holding
- Visual/auditory stimulation

Nursing—Toddler:
- Parent–child bond; promote realistic developmental skills
- Teach realistic methods of discipline
- Maintain normal schedule

Nursing—Preschool Child:
- Allow expression of fears/frustration
- Storytelling/books/dramatic play
- Normal schedule = security
- Use honesty; explain all procedures

Nursing—School-Aged Child:
- Clarify child's understanding of information
- Reassure: behavior doesn't cause illness
- Play can be an outlet
- Allow choices when possible
- Assess/manage pain

Nursing—Adolescent:
- Base care on "stage" of adolescence
- Allow choices to enhance control
- Peer/social support/use of social media

Nursing—Sibling:
- Promote family-centered care
- Maintain familiar routines
- Include sibling in simple aspects of care
- Provide information about ill child

Impact on family → **Chronic Condition**
Impact on child → **Caring for the Child With a Chronic Condition or the Dying Child**

Emotional Responses:
- Will differ depending on illness/prognosis
- Disrupted family dynamics
- Shock, fear, anger, disbelief anxiety, confusion, fear of bonding, chronic sorrow

Nursing Interventions:
- Understanding, communication, support
- Topics
  – Continue regular daily activities: incorporate disease into routine; help child to live life
- Treatments; procedures; meds
- Handling self-blame/chronic sorrow
- Participation in child's care

Other Important Aspects of Care
- Establish a therapeutic relationship
- Determine locus of control
- Relevence of religious practices
- Assess for alterations/delays in growth and development
- Promote/advocate for child's right to education
- Integrate cultural sensitivity

General Nursing Interventions: Dying Child
- Recognizes sx of impending death
- Therapeutic communication: relay sympathy, kindness
- Demonstrate caring: touch, placing toys
- Give family realistic choices in the process
- Provide information re: actual death of child
- Facilitate "saying good-bye"; no time limit; include sibling(s)
- Provide ongoing care for family after child's death
- Provide community resources

Grief
- Nursing care based on theory:
  – Kübler-Ross
  – Miles and Perry; Epperson
- Accept families in whatever stage of grief they are in
- Help families to retain healthy habits/find positive outlet for emotions
- Reinforce: illness is no one's fault
- Recognize coping patterns used and support family
- Identify pathological grief:
  – Suicidal/homicidal ideation
  – Addictive behaviors
  – Extreme denial
- Collaborate with licensed professionals
- Provide community resources

Palliative Care:
- Supportive/care for life-threatening illness
- Focus is on quality of life; alleviating/controlling distressing symptoms
- Medical model/hospital care
- Also addresses emotional/spiritual needs
- Can include curative therapies

Hospice Care:
- Comprehensive, multidisciplinary, holistic care
- Family-centered care
- Respite care/follow-up bereavement care for family
- Home hospice fosters "normality"

End-of-Life-Care:
- Facilitate discussions about death
- Continue palliative care: control pain
- Take proactive approach to impending death
- Create remembrance packet for family
- Provide care for the caregiver

Critical Nursing Actions:
- Establish trust with family, help siblings cope
- Hospice care focus → quality not cure
- Use supportive nursing behaviors during end-of-life care
- Understand all aspect of DNR
- Treat belongings of deceased child with respect

Optimizing Outcomes:
- Handle acting out in siblings with use of reflection/validation/channeling/ and providing an outlet

What To Say:
- Use child's name in discussions about disease
- Listen empathetically to family questions
- Avoid using platitudes at time of death

Across Care Settings:
- Use of respite care
- NCI and ACS have resources for families

Cultural Diversity:
- Culturally appropriate spiritual care and care of the dying child
- Special needs of the Latino culture related to grief
- Expressions of grief vary by culture

Now Can You:
- Define chronic conditions
- List three nursing diagnoses related to the dying process
- Differentiate between hospice and palliative care
- Assist the child and family throughout the grieving process

Caring for the Critically Ill Child

"The Pediatric Critical Care Nurse: A unique soul who passes thru your life for a minute but impacts it for an eternity."

—Author unknown

LEARNING TARGETS *At the completion of this chapter, the student will be able to:*

- Describe the anatomy and physiology and developmental aspects related to the critically ill child.
- Examine common conditions related to the critically ill child.
- Prioritize developmentally appropriate and holistic nursing care related to the critically ill child.
- Explore diagnostic and laboratory testing and medications related to the critically ill child.
- Develop teaching plans and discharge criteria for parents related to the critically ill child.

PICO(T) Questions

The intent of evidence-based practice (EBP) is to provide nursing care that integrates the best available evidence. An initial step in EBP is to write a PICO(T) question that effectively guides the research. PICO(T) is an acronym that stands for population (P), intervention or issue (I), comparison of interest (C), outcome (O), and timeframe (T). Depending on the question, all or some of the question components are used in the research process. Use these PICO(T)

questions to spark your thinking as you read the chapter.

1. What are the (I) evidence-based interventions that nurses can implement (O) to prevent ventilator-associated pneumonia in (P) critically ill children who are being mechanically ventilated?

2. Is the (I) use of continuous positive airway pressure (CPAP) (O) equally effective in (P) children under 5 years of age compared with (C) children over 5 years of age?

Evidence-Based Practice

Jones, B. L., Parker-Raley, J., Maxson, T., & Brown, C. (2011). Understanding health care professionals' views of family presence during pediatric resuscitation. *American Journal of Critical Care, 20*(3), 199–207.

The purpose of this study was to examine contrasting positions of health-care professionals regarding family presence during the resuscitation of a child. Family presence is described as the presence of a family member in a location that provides visual or physical contact with the child during an invasive procedure and includes resuscitation. Very often, it is the decision of the health-care professional as to whether family members may be present during resuscitation efforts directed toward their child. In the past, health-care professionals have expressed concerns, such as the

possibility that the experience may be too traumatic for the family, and that it may present a potential liability for health-care professionals and the institution. The concept of family-centered care recognizes the fact that better care, safety, satisfaction, and high quality outcomes result from family involvement. This belief recognizes the importance of the role of the family on the well-being of the patient and supports mutual collaboration with the members of the health-care team. This belief also includes family involvement in decision making. In 2002, the *Pediatric Advanced*

(continued)

Evidence-Based Practice (continued)

Life Support manual was revised to recommend supporting the option for family presence during resuscitation, though many professionals still do not allow family presence.

Previous research findings vary. The authors noted that one study suggested that if given a choice, 83% of parents would prefer remaining close to their child during resuscitation. Previous studies express the following professional concerns: the potential of family members to disrupt or interrupt treatment, the potential for family to become too emotionally vulnerable to deal with being present, and the possibility of the family not understanding the purpose of resuscitation and invasive procedures. Concerns expressed by staff also include legal vulnerability, increased stress, and need for prolonged resuscitation efforts related to family presence. Research has also suggested possible benefits for families (e.g., parent support, reassurance, healthier bereavement, and perception of participation in their child's care). The presence of family can provide emotional support for the child, translation of information, and a family spokesperson. Professionals in favor of family presence indicate that family presence provides families with more reassurance and confidence in the care provided. Professionals also mentioned that benefits to staff include more of a bonding with the family and suggests that family presence provides an opportunity to develop more rapport, which reinforces the strength of communication about the patient's prognosis.

This study included two phases of data collection, which utilized a mixed-method design (i.e., quantitative and qualitative). In the first phase, 137 health-care professionals were asked to complete a 23-item questionnaire addressing their views on family presence and their perception of the assumed views of those opposing this belief. Participants included physicians, nurses, and med students at one children's medical center in Austin, Texas. The 137 participants included 41 physicians, 87 nurses, and 9 medical students. Forty-two were men and 95 were women; 110 of the participants were Caucasian, 11 Hispanic, 5 Asian, 2 African American, 1 Native American, and 8 chose not to reveal ethnicity. The phase 1 questionnaire was designed to identify whether professionals were in favor of or opposed to family presence during resuscitation. The participants were also asked to identify their perception of professionals, whom they assumed had an opposing view. The survey provided the participants with a scenario and asked whether they agreed or disagreed with the physician's decision to allow family presence during resuscitation. The second part of the survey included 22 items rated on a 7-point, Likert-type scale with 1 being "extremely sympathetic" and 7 being "extremely unsympathetic." Questions were directed at determining the participants' viewpoints and their estimation of their opponents' views regarding sympathy

for families and professionals. The questions also included statements assessing concerns for risks linked to family presence and were rated on a scale in which 1 stood for "extremely concerned or risky" and 7 meant "extremely unconcerned or unrisky." The results of phase 1 noted that 95 participants were in favor of family presence and 42 were opposed. At the completion of phase 1, participants were asked if they were willing to participate in an interview about their beliefs. In phase 2, twelve respondents from phase 1 agreed to participate and were interviewed about the effects of family presence on patients' families and health-care professionals. Participants in phase 2 included 5 male physicians, 6 female physicians, and 1 female nurse. Interviews averaged 15 to 30 minutes and were audio recorded and transcribed. Eight participants supported family presence, and 4 disagreed with family presence during resuscitation.

Results indicated that 95 health-care professionals supported family presence in response to the scenario provided on the phase 1 survey, and 42 did not support it. Based on factor analysis, the researchers noted that professionals who supported family presence perceived that their counterparts who did not believe in family presence lacked sympathy for the family. Professionals who opposed family presence perceived that those who agree with family presence lacked sympathy for the trauma team. Health professionals from both sides expressed concerns for legal issues. Those in favor of family presence perceived that their opponents were excessively concerned with legal issues. Those who were opposed to family presence perceived that their opponents believed family presence provided a degree of legal protection avoiding false accusations. Those who opposed family presence underestimate their opponents' concerns for potential risks. Professionals on both sides of the question indicated that they have a high level of concern for professionals during resuscitation, though both underestimated their opponents concern for professionals. Both sides indicated that they believed they were more concerned for health-care professionals than their opponents.

The researchers concluded that the findings from this study add to a deeper understanding and clarification of previous studies regarding the advantages and disadvantages of family presence during pediatric resuscitation.

1. How is this information useful to clinical nursing practice?

2. Based on these findings, what are implications for further research?

See Suggested Responses for Evidence-Based Practice on *Davis Plus*.

Introduction

This chapter includes an examination of the critically ill child, including developmentally appropriate and holistic nursing care. Information is given about diagnostic and laboratory testing and medications. Teaching plans and discharge criteria are incorporated for parents whose children

are critically ill. The critically ill child is defined as a patient who is seriously injured or gravely ill and is at risk for potential or actual life-threatening health problems. The child requires closer monitoring and observation than is typically received on a general care unit. The critically ill child is highly vulnerable, unstable, and complex and therefore requires intensive and vigilant nursing care.

Critically ill children can present with a variety of medical conditions. Conditions requiring closer surveillance in a critical care area can include one or more of the following: recent major surgery, advanced analgesic techniques, organ system failure requiring technological support, and respiratory failure requiring advanced respiratory support.

Common problems of the critically ill child include gas exchange, perfusion, and fluid balance. These problems present the greatest challenges, including increased risk of morbidity and mortality. This chapter presents an extensive overview of the common problems and issues facing the critically ill child and nursing care.

CARING FOR THE CRITICALLY ILL CHILD

> ### Growth and Development
>
> The critically ill child is highly susceptible to delays or lags in growth and development because of prolonged hospitalization, stress from the critical care environment, and restricted activity. While caring for the critically ill child, the nurse understands that attention to promotion of regular growth and development is important to decrease the incidence of delays. The critical care environment can be stressful to the child because of changes in environment and daily routine. Sleep-wake cycles are interrupted by lights, sounds, procedures, and nursing cares. Faster recovery time is possible when the child feels at ease in the critical care environment. The nurse must encourage a non-stressful, soothing environment by minimizing unnecessary noise and decreasing stressful stimuli. The nurse must be cognizant of excessive noise, light, and sounds from conversation and medical equipment. Promoting comfort and rest is important to support healing for the critically ill child. The nurse should provide appropriate comfort measures to the child such as pain relief, repositioning, decreased physical restraint when possible, a day-night schedule, parental interaction, having personal items brought from home, and continuing home routines when possible. All measures are important to ensure a sense of security for the child.
>
> Play is important for development. While in the critical care environment, play may have to be passive. Appropriate passive activities that provide developmental stimulation include colorful mobiles, music, talking story books, and the child's favorite television shows. When the child is recovering, more active means of play can be initiated. The nurse should assess the individual developmental needs of the child and provide activities and stimulation that are unique to each situation. The nurse should provide education to the family about appropriate developmental activities. Assistance from a child life therapist, physical therapist, and occupational therapist can aid in providing appropriate therapies and activities that meet the developmental and medical needs of the critically ill child.
>
> Source: Ward S., & Hisley, S. (2009). *Maternal-child nursing care: Optimizing outcomes for mothers, children & families*. Philadelphia, PA: F.A. Davis.

Impact of a Critical Condition

Admittance to the critical care unit can be a traumatic and stressful experience for the critically ill child and his or her family. Regardless of developmental age, the critically ill child faces many issues related to the critical care environment. In addition to medical illness, the critical care environment introduces psychological stress caused by sleep disruptions, pain, and communication barriers. When caring for the critically ill child, the nurse appreciates the extremely vulnerable nature of the child and focuses interventions on promoting health and preserving development.

Critically ill children are often exposed to stress-inducing events and experiences. Because of the extreme nature of a critical illness, intensive medical treatment and interventions may be necessary. Invasive procedures are frequently necessary for the management of critical illnesses. These traumatic events and procedures can cause increased pain, fear, confusion, and anxiety for the child.

Another source of stress experienced by the critically ill child results from **sensory overload**. Sensory overload is a condition in which sensory stimuli are received at a rate and intensity beyond the level that the patient can accommodate (Jones & Fix, 2009). Sensory overload occurs from repeated stimulation to the visual, auditory, kinesthetic, gustatory, tactile, and olfactory senses. In the critical care environment, sensory overload occurs from constant light and noise from advanced medical technology and invasive monitoring devices. Sensory overload is also experienced from repeated stimulation from medical, personal, and nursing care that results in sleep interruptions. Sleep interruptions and sleep deprivation can occur because of physical and pharmacological barriers. Physical barriers include the presence of invasive lines and tubes and activity restrictions, which can cause anxiety, discomfort, and pain. Medications such as sedatives, opiates, and benzodiazepines can alter the sleep pattern in the critically ill child. Sensory overload causes increased amounts of physical and emotional stress on the critically ill child. Sensory overload has been associated with symptoms such as lethargy, behavioral changes, disorientation, panic, withdrawal, hallucinations, fear, and anxiety (Jones & Fix, 2009). Over time, these constant stressors have been shown to impair a child's ability to adapt and cope.

In addition to sensory overload, the critically ill child often experiences communication barriers caused by advanced medical equipment, invasive monitoring devices, and pharmacological barriers. Impaired communication can be devastating to the child and can lead to psychoemotional distress, including depression, anxiety, fear, anger, frustration, panic, sleep disorders, decreased self-esteem, and loss of control (Khalaila, Zbidat, Anwar, Bayya, Linton, & Syiri, 2011). Stress-inducing factors can greatly impact the overall health, well-being, and coping mechanisms of the critically ill child.

Collaborative Care

Nursing Care. Decreasing the stress experienced by the critically ill child is an integral part of nursing care in the critical care unit. To decrease the stress of an unfamiliar environment, encourage the family to bring the child's favorite articles from home. Personal items can evoke a sense of safety and security for the child. When invasive procedures are required, prepare the child to minimize stress associated with these procedures. The nurse provides developmentally appropriate explanations of procedures to the child. This may involve the use of a child life specialist who can assist with providing distraction methods and techniques that are developmentally appropriate. Distraction methods and coping mechanisms are identified prior to the procedure. The nurse involves the family and parents with procedures whenever possible. The family members and parents can aid with distraction and coping methods that will decrease the sense of fear and stress experienced by the critically ill child. Adequate pain management through pharmacological intervention is necessary to decrease the child's pain or discomfort during and after the procedure. The nurse advocates for optimal analgesia and sedation to decrease stressful experiences associated with painful procedures (Khalaila et al., 2011).

It is important to minimize the critically ill child's exposure to sensory overload and stimulation. Nursing care focuses on **clustering cares**. Clustering nursing cares is the most effective way to manage sensory overload experienced by the child. Clustering nursing cares involves minimizing interruptions in sleep and providing minimal amounts of stimulation. This involves grouping nursing interventions to allow for longer periods of rest in-between nursing cares. Clustering nursing care also aids in the maximization of sleep and rest, which can decrease anxiety and stress and increase coping mechanisms of the critically ill child (Jones & Fix, 2009).

Adequate sleep and rest is a priority for the critically ill child. Minimizing noise levels in the critical care environment is an important aspect of nursing care. Lower noise levels create a calmer environment that decreases stimulation of the child and promotes rest. Another way to promote sufficient sleep and rest is by providing an appropriate day and night schedule or routine. Be sure to organize major care events during normal daytime hours, allow for periods of quiet time with minimal noise and stimulation, close and open curtains as appropriate, minimize equipment noise and alarm levels, dim lights during the evening, and help to keep regular bedtime schedules and routines. Such nursing interventions can decrease sensory overload and minimize sleep deprivation associated with the intensive care environment.

Maximizing communication is important to reduce stress and anxiety experienced by the critically ill child. Be aware of, and sensitive to, communication difficulties of the child. The use of developmentally appropriate communication tools, such as alphabet boards and word or picture charts, can maximize communication with the critically ill child (Khalaila et al., 2011). Encourage the family members to interact with the child through speech and touch when appropriate. Supportive interpersonal interaction with family members can be therapeutic for the critically ill child who is unable to speak and may ameliorate stress and trauma experienced by some family members during admission to the critical care area (Broyles, Tate, & Happ, 2012).

Impact of the Critically Ill Child on the Family

The critical care environment can also be traumatic and stressful for the family of the child. Parents of critically ill children experience stress from a sense of the unknown due the child's critical medical condition, a loss of parental role, loss of normal family functions, foreignness of medical terms and equipment, and traumatic events experienced in the critical care environment. Parents and family members can directly witness traumatic events and procedures or be exposed to others experiencing traumatic events (Zimmerman & Bauersachs, 2012). Parents may also exhibit stress from financial concerns, isolation from other family members, limited visitation with their child, and the fear of losing their child. Parents can exhibit signs and symptoms of stress such as anxiety, depression, and fear that dramatically impact the family process (McAdam & Puntillo, 2009).

Collaborative Care

Nursing Care. Nursing interventions focused on the family are important aspects of care for the critically ill child. Family-centered nursing care is the best way to alleviate stress and anxiety that is experienced by the family members. **Family-centered care** is a philosophy of care that acknowledges that the family has the greatest influence over a child's health and well-being (Mundy, 2010). Incorporating a family-centered approach provides a positive effect on the overall well-being of the family. Nursing care focuses on maximizing parental involvement. The family is included in child care activities and decision-making processes as appropriate. These interventions promote individualized and holistic family-centered care.

Nursing interventions that focus on the family include strategies to reduce anxiety and distress, which are experienced by the parents and family members. Develop a trusting therapeutic and supportive relationship with the family through compassion and respect. Such interaction has been linked to an increase in satisfaction and a reduction in family members' symptoms (McAdam & Puntillo, 2009). Other nursing interventions that increase family-centered care include consideration of the physical and emotional needs of the parents and family members, providing appropriate communication about the critically ill child's medical condition, medical care and progress, and the identification of support systems and needs (Zimmerman, & Bauersachs, 2012). It is essential for the nurse to assess, identify, and understand the family's needs to improve family-centered care. Identifying the needs of parents enhances nursing communication and allows the nurse to incorporate the family's needs into the

---

Where Research and Practice Meet:
Minimizing Noise Levels in the Intensive Care Unit

Excessive noise in the intensive care unit can be detrimental to the critically ill child's recovery. Noise from unwanted sounds can increase negative effects such as slower healing and recovery process, sleep disturbances, cardiovascular stimulation, increased gastric secretion, pituitary and adrenal gland stimulation, and suppression of the immune response to infection. Staff conversation, telephones, televisions, and sound and alarms from invasive medical devices seem to be the most problematic noise experienced by patients and family members in the intensive care environment. Research shows that as many as 57% of intensive care unit patient arousals and awakenings are caused by noise (Lawson, Thompson, Saunders, Saiz, Richardson, Brown, et al., 2010). The World Health Organization recommends that noise levels inside the patient room should not exceed 30 dBA; yet, research has shown that noise levels range from 50 to 75 dBA (Xie, Kang, & Mills, 2009). Nursing staff in the intensive care environment must be conscious of noise levels and modify behaviors to reduce noise exposure to the patient. Noise reduction behaviors that are easy to incorporate into everyday nursing care include changing phones and pagers to vibrate mode when possible, avoiding loud conversation, limiting bedside conversation with colleagues, decreasing alarm sounds on medical devices, and establishing quiet times on each shift for at least an hour.

plan of care (Mundy, 2010). These holistic nursing interventions dramatically decrease the stress and anxiety experienced by the family members of a critically ill child.

Critical Nursing Action Promoting Family-Centered Care

Mundy (2010) suggests that the most important needs of the family during admission to the critical care environment are as follows:

- Frequent and timely communication about important changes in the child's medical condition and specific facts concerning the child's medical care, progress, and outcomes
- Having questions answered honestly
- Assurance that the best possible care is being given to the critically ill child
- Feeling that the health-care providers care about the critically ill child
- Feeling that the child is being handled gently by the health-care providers
- Feeling that there is hope
- The ability to see the child frequently and assist in the child's physical care

Important Aspects of Care for the Critically Ill Child

GROWTH AND DEVELOPMENT

The critically ill child may experience growth and development delays and/or regress to previous stages of development. Growth and development can be affected by life-saving medical treatments and interventions such as the prolonged use of sedative and paralytic medications and mechanical ventilation. Children requiring these medical interventions often are bed-bound and have restricted activity. These physical limitations present barriers to achieving developmental milestones. The critically ill child can experience delays in speech development because of the prolonged use of medical devices like endotracheal tubes and gastric feeding tubes. Growth and development may also be affected by the length of stay in the critical care unit. A longer hospital stay can increase the child's risk for experiencing growth and developmental delays.

Collaborative Care

Nursing Care. Excellent developmental care is important for children of all developmental ages who are admitted to the critical care unit. The nurse implements developmentally appropriate activities to stimulate the child's growth and development when appropriate. Consider utilizing a child life specialist to help incorporate developmentally appropriate activities and toys for the critically ill child. Physical and occupational therapists can assist with range of motion and therapeutic play activities that assist with the achievement of growth and development milestones.

NUTRITION

Nutrition is important for metabolism, growth, and repair. Because of the nature of acute illness, the critically ill child experiences increased metabolic requirements (Marshall, Cahill, Gramlich, MacDonald, & Heyland, 2012). Prolonged or continual stress depletes glycogen stores and creates a hypermetabolic state (Jones & Fix, 2009). Critically ill children can present with underlying protein energy malnutrition, which makes them particularly vulnerable to further nutritional depletion (Meyer, Harrison, Sargent, Ramnarayan, Habibi, & Labadarios, 2009). Observational research has shown that patients who receive less nutrition are more likely to experience adverse events, such as increased infectious complications and higher mortality (Meyer et al., 2009). Malnutrition is also linked to poor wound-healing and decreased skin integrity. Optimal nutrition is a necessity for the critically ill child because of their increased risk for malnutrition.

Collaborative Care

Nursing Care. The nurse recognizes that achieving and maintaining optimal nutrition is an essential therapeutic strategy for improving outcomes of the critically ill child. Prioritize nutritional therapy and implement goals into the plan of care that focus on achieving optimal nutritional care. The nurse ensures that nutritional targets are met by monitoring the intake and output and daily weight of the critically ill child. Lab values such as glucose levels, serum electrolytes, albumin, and protein levels are monitored regularly (Jones & Fix, 2009). It is also important that the nurse identifies patients with nutritional risk and assesses the adequacy of access for nutritional therapy. Consider a variety of nutritional methods including enteral and parenteral therapy. When administering nutritional feedings, monitor for potential complications and evaluate the effectiveness of nutritional feedings (Marshall et al., 2012).

PAIN

Pain management is important to promote healing and comfort for the critically ill child. Analgesics and sedative medications are commonly used for pain management and sedation. The consequences of poor pain management and inadequate sedation can be devastating. It is important to properly assess and manage the critically ill child's pain and sedation needs.

Collaborative Care

Nursing Care. A thorough pain assessment of the critically ill child includes both verbal and nonverbal assessments of pain. Be sure to assess for the physiological responses to pain including tachycardia, diaphoresis, sleep disturbances, hypertension, tachypnea, and nausea. Also monitor body and limb movements, facial expressions, posturing, and muscle tension for signs and symptoms of pain. Provide appropriate therapeutic interventions to relieve pain, including the use of pharmacological and nonpharmacological therapies.

focus on safety

Pharmacological intervention

When the critically ill child is receiving pharmacological intervention from analgesics or sedatives over an extended period of time, assess for signs and symptoms of physiological withdrawal. Signs and symptoms of analgesic or sedative withdrawal include nausea, vomiting, diarrhea, cramps, muscle aches, tachypnea, tachycardia, hypertension, delirium, tremors, seizures, agitation, and increased sensitivity to pain (Jones & Fix, 2009).

SKIN INTEGRITY

Maintaining skin integrity is an integral part of nursing care in any hospital setting for patients of all developmental ages. Maintaining skin integrity in the critical care environment can be difficult because of highly invasive medical interventions, equipment, treatments, and therapies. Hemodynamic instability, immobility, and compromised nutrition also increase risk for skin breakdown in the child. In addition to pressure ulcers, the child can experience diaper rash, skin tears, and IV extravasations. Skin breakdown increases the stress and pain experienced by the child and may increase the risk of infections or other complications. Treatment of skin breakdown adds financial burden to the hospital. Maintaining skin integrity is essential for the critically ill child because of the higher risk of mortality that is associated with the development of skin breakdown (Schindler, Mikhailov, Kuhn, Christopher, Conway, Ridling, et al., 2011).

Collaborative Care

Nursing Care. Exemplary skin care is an important outcome measure established by the American Nurses Association (Schindler et al., 2011). Recognize the importance of maintaining skin integrity in the critically ill child. Holistic nursing interventions to decrease skin breakdown include frequent turning and repositioning, the use of gel pads and pressure-reducing devices, repositioning of medical devices, decreasing friction and shear, and minimizing prolonged periods of head elevation in ventilated patients (Aust, 2011). Keeping the skin clean and dry, promoting mobility and movement when possible, and providing nutritional support are other important factors that promote skin integrity in the critically ill child. Special consideration is given to the medically sedated and or paralyzed child so that skin integrity is maintained.

CULTURAL OR SPIRITUAL ISSUES

Considerations about cultural and spiritual needs are important aspects of caring for the critically ill child and his or her family. Because of the extremely stressful nature of the critical care unit, cultural and spiritual issues may occur. Spiritual needs are often intensified in situations of crisis, such as coping with a critical illness and the unknown outcome of the disease process. Providing sensitive nursing care that addresses cultural and spiritual concerns is an important aspect to family-centered nursing care in the critical care environment.

Collaborative Care

Nursing Care. Nursing care focuses on assessing an individual family's social, cultural, and spiritual needs. Provide therapeutic communication and work to develop a trusting relationship. Developing a trusting relationship with open communication facilitates culturally competent and family-centered nursing care. Recognition of cultural and spiritual needs of the patient and family members is essential in providing culturally and spiritually competent nursing care. The nurse considers collaboration with medical translators, pastoral care workers, and chaplains to help facilitate cultural and spiritual needs.

 Cultural Diversity: Providing Culturally Competent Care

 Case Study Critically Ill Child

Charlotte, a 2-year-old child, developed fulminant hepatic failure (acute liver failure characterized by the rapid onset of hepatic encephalopathy and coagulopathy in patients with no known underlying liver disease). After being admitted to the pediatric critical care unit, the critical care nurse obtains a full medical history from Charlotte's parents, Jessica and Edward. Jessica explains that Charlotte has an unremarkable medical history, has no allergies, and takes no medications. Edward immediately informs the nurse that he and his family are active Jehovah's Witnesses. Edward explains to the nurse that their religious beliefs include abstaining from blood and that Charlotte is not to receive any blood transfusions. After completing an assessment of Charlotte, the nurse notes that Charlotte's skin and sclera appear jaundiced, and her capillary refill is 4 seconds. Her abdomen is swollen, and the liver is enlarged. The critical care nurse notes petechiae on Charlotte's chest and thorax. Charlotte's laboratory work reveals a hemoglobin level of 7.0 g/dL, a critically low value. After reviewing Charlotte's assessment data with the physician, a blood transfusion and preparations for a liver transplant are ordered.

critical thinking questions

1. How can the nurse provide culturally sensitive nursing care to Charlotte and her family?

2. How can the nurse take care of Charlotte's medical needs without compromising the beliefs of the family?

 legal alert—Life-threatening situation

If Charlotte's life is threatened, the health-care providers may give a blood transfusion. Section 24 of the *Human Tissue Act 1982* enacts that a medical practitioner who gives a child a blood transfusion against the expressed wishes of the parent is not committing a criminal offense. The blood transfusion must be treatment for a condition the child has, and without the transfusion the child is likely to die (Office of the Public Advocate Guardianship & Administration Act 1986, s42A).

3. What if the nurse's beliefs about medical treatment differ from the family members?

◆ See Suggested Answers to Case Studies on Davis*Plus*.

Common Problems of the Critically Ill Child

GAS EXCHANGE

Problems with gas exchange in children are a medical emergency and require immediate attention from the nurse. Problems with gas exchange may be caused by numerous conditions that affect oxygenation, ventilation, or both.

Nursing Care Plan Care of the Critically Ill Child

Nursing Diagnosis: Spiritual Distress, Risk for related to critical illness

Measurable Short-Term Goal: Family will have their spiritual needs met

Measurable Long-Term Goal: Family will maintain meaning and purpose in life

NOC Outcomes:

Spiritual Health (2001) Connectedness with self, others, higher power, all life, nature, and the universe that transcends and empowers the self

Comfort Status: Psychospiritual (2011) Psychospiritual ease related to self-concept, emotional well-being, source of inspiration, and meaning and purpose of one's life

NIC Interventions:

Spiritual Support (5420)

Coping Enhancement (5230)

Nursing Interventions:

1. Establish a therapeutic relationship with child and family with consistently assigned empathetic nurses.

   RATIONALE: To promote understanding and support child and family coping.

2. Reduce noise and excess stimulation while encouraging family presence with child.

   RATIONALE: Reduces stress for the child and family in the unfamiliar intensive care environment.

3. Respectfully explore family's cultural and spiritual expectations and needs based on the child's critical condition.

   RATIONALE: Provides information to meet the particular needs of the family during a time of stress.

4. Provide access to family and spiritual advisors, ensuring privacy or consultation as requested.

   RATIONALE: Provides a source of comfort and support to family.

5. Ensure that desired spiritual articles are available (specify, e.g., desired medals attached safely to gown) and shown appropriate respect.

   RATIONALE: Shows respect for the spiritual needs of the family.

6. Assist family to meet their needs with dignity by adjusting the constraints of the intensive care environment as possible. If impossible, explain clearly why this is so.

   RATIONALE: Common intensive care processes may be based on custom and may be altered if they do not interfere with the child's well-being.

Conditions that lead to the development of respiratory distress in children require advanced medical interventions and intensive nursing care and are often managed in the critical care unit. Understanding how to assess, monitor, and provide appropriate interventions to maximize gas exchange are a priority for the critical care nurse.

RESPIRATORY MANAGEMENT OF THE CRITICALLY ILL CHILD

Oxygen Monitoring and Assessment

When a child presents with respiratory distress, monitoring the respiratory status is critical. There are several techniques used to monitor the respiratory status in the critically ill child. Basic assessment of the respiratory system includes auscultation of the lung fields and assessing for respiratory distress including nasal flaring, cyanosis, retractions, and grunting. In the critical care unit, basic assessment is combined with more invasive techniques of respiratory assessment. Common methods for measuring gas exchange include monitoring of pulse oximetry, arterial and venous blood gas values, end-tidal carbon dioxide levels, transcutaneous carbon dioxide levels, and mixed venous oxygen saturation. In the critically ill child, both invasive and noninvasive monitoring techniques are used.

Noninvasive respiratory assessment techniques include pulse oximetry and transcutaneous carbon dioxide monitoring (Figs. 35-1A and 35-1B). Pulse oximetry uses a skin probe with an attached infrared light that measures transcutaneous oxygen saturation. Continuous pulse oximetry is used for children with gas exchange problems. Transcutaneous carbon dioxide monitoring is another noninvasive method used to assess gas exchange in the pediatric population. It involves the use of a skin electrode that measures carbon dioxide levels. Transcutaneous carbon dioxide monitoring may be indicated in addition to pulse oximetry in events of severe respiratory distress.

⚙ Diagnostic Tools Invasive Respiratory Assessment

Invasive respiratory assessment of the critically ill child includes arterial and venous blood gas sampling, end-tidal carbon dioxide monitoring, and mixed venous oxygen saturation monitoring. Arterial and venous blood gas values can be obtained through collection of arterial or venous blood, either through venipuncture or from an existing invasive line, such as an arterial line. Mixed venous oxygen saturation values (S_vO2) can be obtained through a pulmonary artery catheter and are a diagnostic indicator of oxygen demand and consumption by the body's tissues. S_vO2 monitoring in children may be indicated in events of severe and prolonged respiratory distress for invasive diagnostic monitoring. End-tidal carbon dioxide monitoring is an indirect

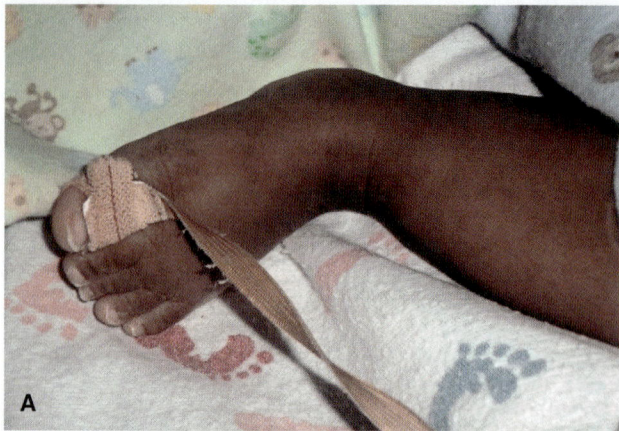

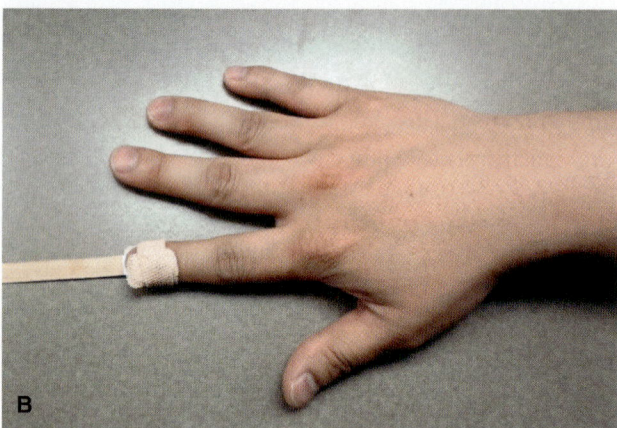

Figures 35-1a and b The pulse oximeter can be placed around the finger, toe, or foot whereas a transcutaneous carbon dioxide monitor is placed on the forearm, chest, or abdomen.

measurement of the production of carbon dioxide by the lungs and arterial carbon dioxide levels, measured from an existing endotracheal tube (Rasera, Gewehr, Domingues, & Junior, 2011).

 Nursing Insight—*Promoting skin integrity*

Because both pulse oximetry and transcutaneous monitoring use an external probe, precautions are taken to protect the skin of the critically ill child. The constant use of infrared light on the skin increases the risk for the development of skin breakdown. Frequently move the probe site and inspect the surrounding skin for redness and breakdown. Evidence shows that frequent movement of the skin probe is necessary to prevent thermal injury to the skin (Restrepo, Hirst, Wittnebel, & Wettstein, 2012). The pulse oximeter may be rotated from alternating sites including the toes, fingers, and around the foot. The transcutaneous carbon dioxide probe may be rotated on varying sites of the forearm, chest, and abdomen.

Methods of Administering Oxygen

The critically ill child with alterations in gas exchange often requires supplemental oxygen delivery. Supplemental oxygen can be supplied using various methods. Oxygen delivery methods may be invasive or noninvasive depending on the child's oxygen needs and ability to ventilate. Noninvasive methods of oxygen delivery will generally be attempted first unless more invasive therapy is indicated. Table 35-1 reviews noninvasive and invasive oxygen delivery methods.

 Case Study The Critically Ill Child With Acute Respiratory Failure

Henry, an 18-month-old child, is admitted to the pediatric critical care unit with a diagnosis of respiratory distress syndrome (RDS), following a viral illness. Upon assessment, Henry is lethargic, restless, and demonstrating nasal flaring and intercostal retractions. His oxygen saturation is 81% while receiving 100% oxygen via face mask. Arterial blood gas results reveal a pH of 7.29, CO_2 of 61, and HCO_3 of 20. Henry's parents are very upset and tell the nurse they don't understand how this could happen.

critical thinking questions

1. What should the nurse anticipate for Henry's treatment? What are the priority nursing interventions at this time?

2. What additional therapies and nursing interventions can the nurse initiate to maximize comfort and gas exchange in RDS?

3. How can the nurse explain what is happening and what to expect as a result of respiratory distress syndrome to Henry's parents?

4. Discuss ongoing priority assessments for Henry.

◆ See Suggested Answers to Case Studies on Davis*Plus*.

Intubation

Intubation is required for the critically ill child with respiratory failure. Intubation is an invasive procedure used when a child cannot maintain adequate oxygenation and/or ventilation. The intubation procedure may occur in a controlled situation, as a preventative measure, or emergently in the case of acute respiratory failure. Intubation requires insertion of an artificial airway (endotracheal, tracheal, or laryngeal tube) and ventilator support from a mechanical ventilator with supplemental oxygen administration.

The intubation procedure requires special equipment to maximize patient safety during the procedure. Standard equipment used for intubation includes a laryngoscope, endotracheal tube (ETT), monitoring equipment, a bag valve mask with oxygen source, suction device, and a tongue blade (Figs. 35-2*A* and 35-2*B*). ETT tubes come in various sizes and widths. The size of the tube is selected based on the age and weight of the child (Fig. 35-3). Sedation medications and analgesics are required during the intubation procedure to reduce pain, reduce the oxygen demand of the body, and reduce movement of the child to facilitate efficient and rapid intubation. Once the child is appropriately sedated, the health-care provider uses the laryngoscope to visualize the trachea of the child. The endotracheal tube is then inserted into the trachea and secured to the child's face. After the ETT is inserted, its correct position is verified with a chest x-ray, and then it is connected to the mechanical ventilator to facilitate gas exchange and ventilation.

Table 35-1 Methods/Modes of Oxygen Administration

Modes of Administering Oxygen	Indications	Invasive/Noninvasive
Nasal Cannula	Delivers low-flow oxygen, 24%–44% through nasal prongs at 1–6 L/min.	First-line option Noninvasive
Venturi Mask	Mixes oxygen with room air, creating high-flow enriched oxygen of a settable concentration. It provides an accurate and constant F_{IO_2}. Typical F_{IO_2} delivery settings are 24%, 28%, 31%, 35%, and 40% oxygen. The Venturi mask is often employed when the clinician has a concern about CO_2 retention.	First-line option Noninvasive
Oxygen Tent	Used for delivery of 28%–50% oxygen in an open system tent that is made of rigid plastic.	First-line option Noninvasive
Face Mask	The volume of the face mask is 100–300 mL. It delivers an F_{IO_2} of 40%–60% at 5–10 L/min. The face mask is indicated in patients with nasal irritation or epistaxis. It is also useful for patients who are strictly mouth breathers.	Second-line option Noninvasive
Non-Rebreathing Face Mask	Indicated when an F_{IO_2} >40% is required. It may deliver F_{IO_2} up to 90% at high-flow settings. Oxygen flows into the reservoir at 8–10 L/min.	Second-line option Noninvasive
High-Flow Nasal Canula	Delivers a high-flow oxygen through nasal prongs at 6–15 L/min.	Second-line option Noninvasive
Nasal BiPAP	Delivers bilevel positive airway pressure through a nasal mask.	Invasive
Facial CPAP	Delivers continuous positive airway pressure through a facial mask.	Invasive
Tracheostomy	Indicated for airway management and mechanical ventilation. Used for long-term mechanical ventilation and chronic ventilatory issues.	Invasive
Endotracheal tube	Used as short-term airway management and mechanical ventilation for management of conditions that require sedative, paralytic, or aggressive pharmacological pain management.	Invasive

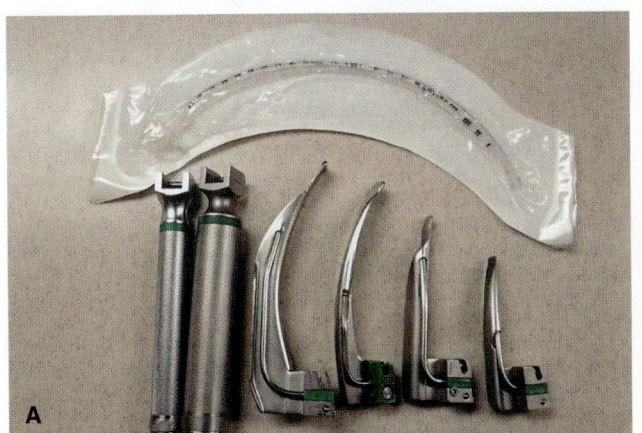 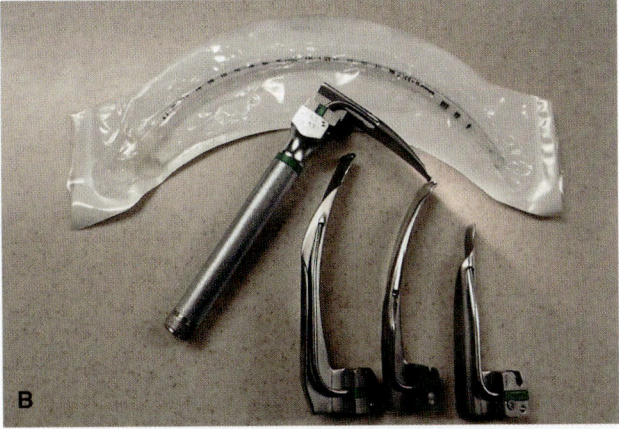

Figures 35-2a and b A laryngoscope and an endotracheal tube are important equipment required for intubation.

"What to say"—Emergent intubation

An emergent intubation may be a stressful procedure for both children and their caregivers. If a child has to be intubated emergently, the cause and onset of respiratory distress or arrest may have been unanticipated. Often, caregivers may be in shock or distraught initially, and even though they have questions, they may not be able to verbalize them appropriately. The role of the nurse includes supporting and educating the family members and identifying resources for them during this difficult time. Because the procedure and equipment for mechanical ventilation are invasive, it is important to emphasize interventions to reduce pain and discomfort to the child. Often, sedation is required with mechanical ventilation because it minimizes the child's responsiveness to stimulation. Educating the caregivers about the normal and anticipated responses may reduce anxiety and distress experienced regarding mechanical ventilation.

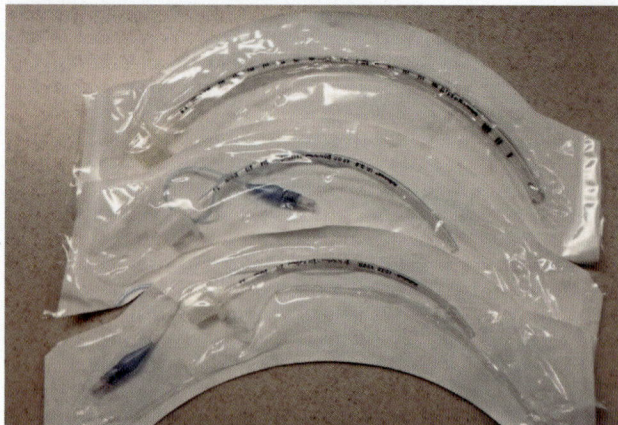

Figure 35-3 Endotracheal tubes range in sizes to accommodate children of different ages and weights. Endotracheal tube sizing formula = Internal diameter (mm) = 16 + age (y)/4, or use nares or little finger of patient.

Nursing Insight—*The nurse's role during intubation*

During the intubation procedure, the nurse is responsible for monitoring and supporting the critically ill child. Before the procedure, ensure that intubation equipment is prepared and functioning. Proper monitoring equipment, a suctioning device, and a bag valve mask with an appropriately sized mask and oxygen source are necessary to protect the patient's airway and to monitor the respiratory and cardiac status during the intubation procedure. The nurse prepares sedatives and analgesics needed. During the procedure, the nurse closely monitors the child and assists the health-care provider with the intubation procedure.

RAPID SEQUENCE INTUBATION. Intubation may occur in a nonemergent situation before a child undergoes sedation or to prevent anticipated complications in a high-risk

 Procedure 35-1 Closed-System Suctioning of the Endotracheal Tube

Purpose

The presence of an ETT impairs the cough reflex and may increase mucous production. The ETT is suctioned periodically to remove pulmonary secretions to promote bronchial hygiene and maintain patency of the artificial airway (Walsh, Hood, & Merritt, 2011). The frequency of the suctioning is determined by the caregiver based on the patient's condition. Closed-system suctioning is the most commonly used method for routine suctioning of the ETT. Closed-system suctioning involves the attachment of a sterile, closed, in-line suction catheter to the ventilator circuit, which allows passage of a suction catheter through the artificial airway without disconnecting the patient from the ventilator (AARC Clinical Practice Guidelines, 2010). The benefits of closed-system suctioning include continued delivery of oxygen, supportive positive pressure, lower risk of nosocomial infection, and reduced staff exposure (Walsh, Hood, & Merritt, 2011).

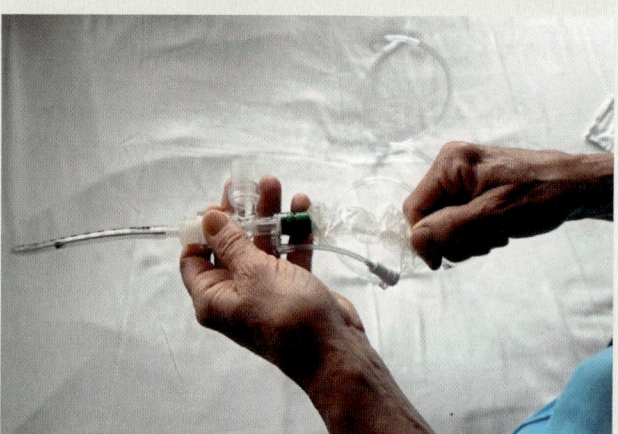

Closed system.

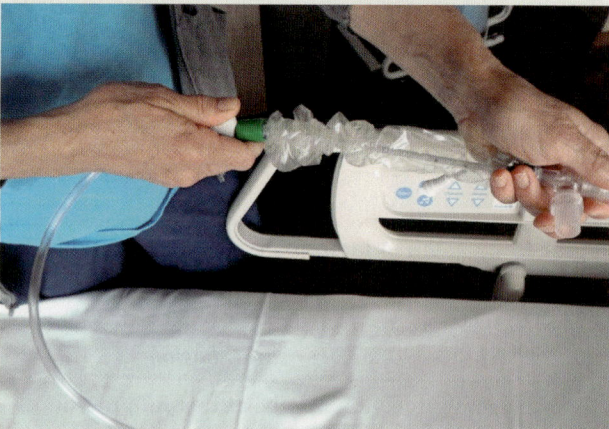

Suctioning the critically ill child.

Equipment

- Gloves
- Suction source (wall or portable) with canister setup
- Sterile saline, single use vial

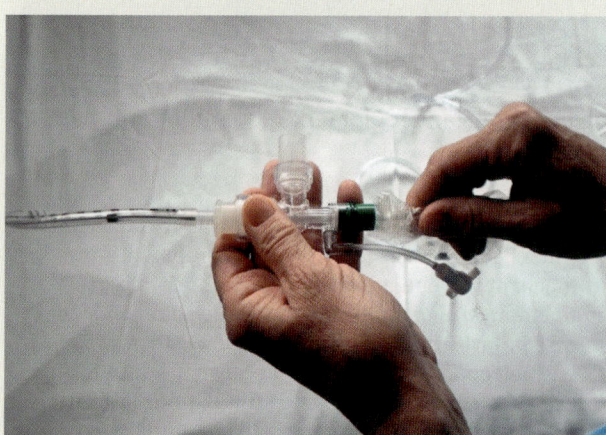

Attachment of a sterile, closed in-line suction catheter to the ventilator circuit.

Procedure 35-1 Closed-System Suctioning of the Endotracheal Tube (continued)

Steps

1. Wash hands and don gloves.

   RATIONALE: *Prevents the spread of bacteria.*

2. Auscultate the patient's lung sounds.

   RATIONALE: *It is necessary to assess the patient's lung sounds to identify need for suction and obtain a baseline assessment prior to suctioning.*

3. Hyperoxygenate the patient prior to suctioning as needed with 100% oxygen for 30 to 60 seconds. You can adjust the oxygen to give less than 100% oxygen when indicated.

   RATIONALE: *Hyperoxygenation increases oxygen available to the tissues during suctioning.*

4. Note the suction depth of the catheter. The tip of the closed, in-line catheter is advanced just past the end of the ETT.

   RATIONALE: *The tip of the catheter should not pass too far beyond the ETT to limit irritation and injury of the tracheal mucosa and carina.*

5. Check the suction device to ensure that there is appropriate suction pressure for the patient.

   RATIONALE: *Suction pressure for the pediatric population should range from 110 to 130 mm Hg and less than 100 mm Hg for the neonatal population.*

6. Consider the use of sterile normal saline lavage.

   RATIONALE: *Sterile normal saline lavage is not indicated for all patients on a routine basis. Sterile normal saline lavage may be useful for patients with a secretion retention problem or thick secretions. Saline instillation may dislodge bacteria and potentially distribute it to the lungs, which can lead to an increased risk of ventilator-associated pneumonia. If sterile saline lavage is indicated:*

   a. *Connect sterile normal saline vial to fluid instillation port*

   b. *Instill 1 to 2 mL of sterile saline if needed*

   c. *Allow ventilator to cycle several times to distribute sterile normal saline*

7. Quickly slide the catheter down the plastic sheath down the ETT until the desired length appears in the window. Avoid passing the catheter too far and irritating the carina.

8. Apply suction by squeezing on the suction control mechanism while withdrawing the catheter. The entire procedure should take 10 to 15 seconds.

9. Note the amount and characteristics of the aspirated secretions.

   RATIONALE: *It is necessary to monitor secretions removed from the ETT to identify complications or other lung injuries.*

10. Squeeze sterile normal saline while applying suction to rinse the inner lumen of the catheter.

    RATIONALE: *If the catheter is not cleaned between suctioning, adequate suction may not develop during the next suction pass and bacterial growth may occur inside the catheter.*

11. Auscultate the patient's lung sounds after suctioning. If the lung sounds remain coarse, the procedure may be repeated.

    RATIONALE: *Monitor effectiveness of suctioning.*

12. Remove gloves.

13. Perform hand hygiene.

    RATIONALE: *Prevents the spread of bacteria.*

14. Document findings in the patient's medical record.

Documentation

5/27/16 1000 In-line suctioning of the endotracheal tube completed. Secretion description: amount – large, color – white, consistency – thick. Patient tolerance: good.

                        CFrost, RN.

(AARC Clinical Practice Guidelines, 2010; Walsh, Hood, & Merritt, 2011).

---

patient. Intubation may also occur emergently in the development of acute respiratory distress or failure. Rapid sequence intubation (RSI) is a technique performed to gain control of the airway in the shortest amount of time. RSI is accomplished by sedating and paralyzing the patient to allow for easier intubation and the ablation of the gag reflex to prevent aspiration. The use of atropine (Atropine) may be indicated to prevent bradycardia. During RSI, the nurse administers an IV anesthetic followed by a rapidly acting dose of a neuromuscular blocking agent (Box 35-1). The combination of the two drugs adequately prepares the patient for immediate, direct laryngoscopy and intubation (Sagarin, Chiang, Sakles, Barton, Wolfe, Vissors, et al., 2002).

Collaboration in Caring—*Rapid sequence intubation*

When emergent intubation is necessary for the critically ill child, priority nursing interventions include communication and collaboration with health-care professionals in other disciplines. Additional health-care team members who are notified and present during the emergent intubation procedure include the primary health-care provider and respiratory team members. All health-care team members play a vital role in ensuring successful intubation for the maintenance of oxygenation and ventilation.

Box 35-1 Commonly Used Medications for the Intubated Child

Medication	Classification	Indication	Adverse Effects	Dosing and Antidotes	Nursing Implications
midazolam (Versed)	Benzodiazepine	Sedation or conscious sedation, anxiolysis, amnesia, status epilepticus, short-acting CNS depressant, after successful intubation used for airway control	Apnea, laryngospasm, respiratory depression, cardiac arrest, hypotension, cardiac arrhythmias, memory impairment in 90% of patients	Loading dose: 0.05–0.2 mg/kg IV Continuous infusion: 0.4–6 mcg/kg/min Reversal agent: flumazenil (Romazicon)	Monitor respiratory rate, BP, heart rate, oxygen saturation; pulse oximeter must be in place, maintain patent airway and adequate ventilation. Use with caution in patients with congestive heart failure, renal impairment, pulmonary disease, and hepatic dysfunction.
propofol (Diprivan)	Sedative, hypnotic	Induction of anesthesia, continuous anesthesia of mechanically ventilated patients	Apnea, bradycardia, hypotension	2–3 mg/kg IV push Continuous infusion: Initial rate of 25–50 mcg/kg/min Titrate based on patient response to a maximum: 150 mcg/kg/min	Monitor blood pressure, respiratory rate, heart rate, O$_2$ saturation, maintain patent airway and adequate ventilation, monitor serum lipids with use greater than 24 hr, monitor zinc and potassium levels. Short-acting, no analgesic properties; monitor depth of sedation.
ketamine (Ketalar)	Nonbarbiturate anesthetic/analgesic	Used as an anesthetic or as a sedative for short surgical procedures or dressing changes in adults and children. Used alone or in conjunction with other general anesthetics.	Respiratory depression, hypertension, tachycardia, tonic–clonic movements, vivid dreams, hallucinations, anorexia, nausea, vomiting	Sedation/Analgesia: Initial dose: 0.2–1 mg/kg/dose IV Continuous infusion: 5–20 mcg/kg/min	Monitor respiratory rate, BP, heart rate, oxygen saturation; pulse oximeter must be in place, maintain patent airway and adequate ventilation.
pentobarbital sodium (Nembutal)	Barbiturate	Sedative, hypnotic, and anticonvulsant Used to provide sedation and relieve anxiety and in high doses to induce coma in the management of cerebral ischemia and increased intracranial pressure	Respiratory depression, apnea, laryngospasm, bronchospasm or hypotension, nausea, vomiting	Children 6–18 months: 1–3 mg/kg. Max: 100 mg IV Children >18 months: 2 mg/kg. Additional 1–2 mg/kg every 5–10 min. Max: 5 mg/kg, rarely 6 mg/kg or 200 mg No known antidote	Monitor respiratory rate, BP, heart rate, oxygen saturation; pulse oximeter must be in place, maintain patent airway and adequate ventilation, monitor CNS and cardiovascular status.
lorazepam (Ativan)	Benzodiazepine	Sedation, antianxiety, anxiolysis, amnesia, status epilepticus	Rhythmic myoclonic jerking, paradoxical excitation, apnea, cardiac arrest, lethargy, confusion, depression, respiratory depression	0.02–0.05 mg/kg/dose IV push **Anxiety/Sedation associated with mechanical ventilation:** 0.02 mg/kg/dose–0.1 mg/kg/dose q 4 hr IV **Status epilepticus:** 0.l mg/kg/dose over 2–5 min; do not exceed 4 mg/dose; second dose = 0.05 mg/kg in 10–15 min IV Reversal agent: flumazenil (Romazicon)	Monitor respiratory rate, BP, heart rate, oxygen saturation; pulse oximeter must be in place, maintain patent airway and adequate ventilation.
fentanyl citrate (Sublimaze)	Opiate analgesic	Analgesia, generalized and regional anesthesia, sedation	Apnea, laryngospasm, cardiac arrhythmias, hypotension, bradycardia, chest wall rigidity,	Neonates: bolus 0.5–3 mcg/kg/dose Continuous infusion: 0.5–2 mcg/kg/hr IV	Monitor respiratory rate, BP, heart rate, oxygen saturation; pulse oximeter must

Box 35-1 **Commonly Used Medications for the Intubated Child** (continued)

Medication	Classification	Indication	Adverse Effects	Dosing and Antidotes	Nursing Implications
			respiratory depression, CNS depression	Children 1–12 years: bolus 1–2 mcg/kg/dose Continuous infusion: 1–5 mcg/kg/hr IV Children >12 yr old: bolus 0.5–1 mcg/kg/dose IV Reversal agent: naloxone (Narcan)	be in place, maintain patent airway and adequate ventilation.
methadone (Dolophine)	Opiate analgesic	Relief of moderate to severe pain	Shortness of breath, respiratory depression, headache, CNS depression, nausea, vomiting	0.1 mg/kg/dose every 4 hr × 2–3 doses, then every 6–12 hr as needed Maximum of 10 mg/dose PO Reversal agent: naloxone (Narcan)	Monitor telemetry, pain relief, respiratory and mental status and blood pressure.
hydromorphone (Dilaudid)	Opiate analgesic	Relief of moderate to severe pain	Confusion, sedation, hypotension, constipation, respiratory depression	0.015 mg/kg every 3–4 hr IV Reversal agent: naloxone (Narcan)	Monitor telemetry, pain relief, respiratory and mental status, and blood pressure.
morphine sulfate	Opiate analgesic	Relief of moderate to severe pain, supplement to anesthesia	Respiratory depression, hypotension, dizziness, cardiac arrest, shock	Initial: 0.05 mg/kg/dose IV every 2–4 hr Usual dosage range 0.1–0.2 mg/kg/dose IV every 2–4 hr Maximum dose: 15 mg/single dose. Reversal agent: naloxone (Narcan)	Monitor telemetry, pain relief, respiratory and mental status, and blood pressure.
cisatracurium besilate (Nimbex)	Neuromuscular blocking agent	Facilitates tracheal intubation by paralyzing skeletal muscle, skeletal muscle relaxant during mechanical ventilation, adjunct to general anesthesia	Bradycardia, hypotension, bronchospasm	Intubation dose: 0.1 mg/kg/dose IV Intermittent dose: 0.03 mg/kg/dose as needed to maintain neuromuscular blockade Continuous infusion: 1–4 mcg/kg/min Reversal Agent: neostigmine	Monitor respiratory rate, BP, heart rate, oxygen saturation; pulse oximeter must be in place, maintain patent airway and adequate ventilation. Has no effect on consciousness or pain threshold, must be used with adequate sedation.
vecuronium bromide (Norcuron)	Neuromuscular blocking agent	Facilitates tracheal intubation by paralyzing skeletal muscle, skeletal muscle relaxant during mechanical ventilation, adjunct to general anesthesia	Headache, dizziness, anxiety, weakness, palpitations, tremor, tachycardia, bronchospasm	0.1 mg/kg/dose IV. Repeat every hour as needed. May be administered as a continuous infusion at 1.5–2.5 mcg/kg/min IV Reversal agents: neostigmine, edrophonium, or pyridostigmine with atropine	Monitor respiratory rate, BP, heart rate, oxygen saturation; pulse oximeter must be in place, maintain patent airway and adequate ventilation. Has no effect on pain threshold, must be used with adequate sedation.
succinylcholine chloride (Anectine)	Neuromuscular blocking agent	Facilitates tracheal intubation by paralyzing skeletal muscle, skeletal muscle relaxant during mechanical ventilation, adjunct to general anesthesia Onset of flaccid paralysis is rapid (<1 min) after administration	Apnea, cardiac arrhythmias, increased intraocular pressure	1–2 mg/kg IV	Monitor respiratory rate, BP, heart rate, oxygen saturation; pulse oximeter must be in place, maintain patent airway and adequate ventilation, monitor effects with train of four. Has no effect on pain threshold, must be used with adequate sedation.

(continued)

Box 35-1 Commonly Used Medications for the Intubated Child (continued)

Medication	Classification	Indication	Adverse Effects	Dosing and Antidotes	Nursing Implications
succinylcholine chloride (Anectine) (continued)					Hyperkalemia Fasciculations Malignant hyperthermia Bradycardia
rocuronium (Zemuron)	Neuromuscular blocking agent	Facilitates tracheal intubation by paralyzing skeletal muscle, skeletal muscle relaxant during mechanical ventilation, adjunct to general anesthesia	Headache, dizziness, anxiety, weakness, palpitations, tremor, tachycardia, bronchospasm	0.6–1.2 mg/kg IV	Monitor respiratory rate, BP, heart rate, oxygen saturation; pulse oximeter must be in place, maintain patent airway and adequate ventilation.
etomidate (Amidate)	Anticholinergic	Induction agent that provides for cardiovascular stability	Nausea, seizure-like movements, adrenal suppression	0.1–0.3 mg/kg IV	Monitor respiratory rate, BP, heart rate.
atropine sulfate	Anticholinergic	Induction agent that provides for cardiovascular stability, treatment of symptomatic bradycardia	Tachycardia, palpitations, confusion, hypotension	0.01–0.05 mg/kg/dose IV	Monitor respiratory rate, BP, heart rate.

Source: Vallerand & Sanoski (2014).

COMPLICATIONS OF INTUBATION. Complications may occur during the initiation and maintenance of intubation. Insertion of the ETT requires passage of the tube through the vocal cords with the distal tip resting above the carina. Anatomical differences in the left and right bronchi often results in the passage of the tube into the right main stem bronchus. This results in ventilation of the right lung only and requires repositioning of the tube. Aspiration may also occur with intubation. Insertion of the ETT may trigger the gag reflex, and vomiting may occur. This increases the risk of vomitus being aspirated into the lungs and may result in aspiration pneumonia.

 focus on safety

Preventing aspiration

To prevent aspiration, suction equipment is available at the bedside. Insertion of a gastric tube is indicated to decompress and empty gastric contents.

Mechanical Ventilation

Goals of mechanical ventilation include optimizing pulmonary gas exchange, maximizing oxygen availability, relieving respiratory distress, and managing pulmonary mechanics. Mechanical ventilation may also be indicated in the critically ill child for non-pulmonary issues, such as when sedation is indicated for an invasive procedure or surgery. Mechanical ventilation includes the delivery of supplemental oxygen and management of respiratory functions. Various modes of mechanical ventilation are used to manage respiratory distress. Review Table 35-2 for different modes of mechanical ventilation. Management of mechanical ventilation requires vigilance and recognition of possible complications during therapy.

 Nursing Diagnoses The Critically Ill Child Receiving Mechanical Ventilation

- Impaired gas exchange related to acute respiratory failure
- Ineffective breathing pattern related to acute respiratory failure
- Ineffective airway clearance related to inability to clear secretions from endotracheal tube
- Pain (acute) related to invasive devices and monitoring equipment
- Disturbance in sensory perception related to sedatives, analgesics, and paralytics
- Risk for infection related to the presence of an artificial airway
- Risk for aspiration related to the presence of an artificial airway

Collaborative Care

Nursing Care. Nursing care for the mechanically ventilated child is extensive. In addition to providing basic nursing cares, nursing care of the mechanically ventilated child includes monitoring the ETT and the ventilator equipment, drawing and monitoring venous and arterial blood gases as indicated, and preventing complications associated with mechanical ventilation. The nurse is diligent to ensure proper function of the mechanical ventilator and equipment to achieve an appropriate therapeutic response.

 focus on safety

Managing the ETT

Managing the ETT is a priority of care for the mechanically ventilated child. Essentials of care include maintaining correct tube placement, preventing unplanned extubation, and maintaining tube patency. ETT placement may be measured with a daily chest x-ray. The location of the ETT is noted and monitored frequently by the nurse. Incorrect tube placement or tube dislodgement may result in decreased oxygenation and ventilation. If symptoms of respiratory distress occur post-intubation, the nurse immediately verifies correct tube placement and intervenes if necessary (Dalton, 2011).

Table 35-2 Modes of Mechanical Ventilation

Mode	Type: Negative Pressure or Positive Pressure Ventilation	Principles	Indications
BiPAP (**Bilevel Positive Airway Pressure**)	Positive pressure	Maintains positive pressure during inspiration and expiration.	Expiratory and inspiratory support for patients unable to protect their own airway. Reduces risk of respiratory muscle fatigue.
CPAP (**Continuous Positive Airway Pressure**)	Positive pressure	Maintains positive end expiratory pressure during spontaneous breathing cycle. Increases amount of air in lungs at end expiration.	Expiratory support. Reduces risk of respiratory muscle fatigue.
SIMV (**Synchronized Intermittent Mandatory Ventilation**)	Positive pressure A form of pressure support ventilation	Administers mandatory ventilator breaths at a preset level of positive airway pressure. Augments spontaneous tidal volume or inspiratory effort. Synchronizes with breathing pattern.	Respiratory failure requiring mechanical ventilation.
PRVC (**Pressure Regulated Volume Control**)	Controlled mode that combines pressure- and volume-controlled ventilation	A preset tidal volume is delivered at a set rate with the lowest possible pressure.	
HFOV (**High-Frequency Oscillatory Ventilation**)	Positive pressure	Delivers 60–100 breaths/min. Low tidal volumes. High pressures.	Failure of conventional mechanical ventilation, ARDS, and RDS.
ECMO (**Extracorporal Membrane Oxygenation**)		Modified form of heart and lung bypass. Bypasses cardiopulmonary system.	Failure of conventional mechanical ventilation, ARDS, and RDS. Severe cardiac and pulmonary damage or failure.

Sources: Jones & Fix (2009). Critical Care Notes; Cheifetez (2011).

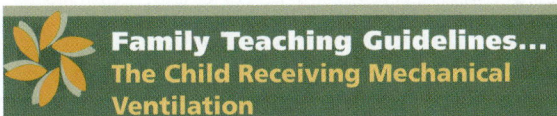

Family Teaching Guidelines...
The Child Receiving Mechanical Ventilation

TOPIC: Educating the Family About Mechanical Ventilation

ESSENTIAL INFORMATION:

♦ Teach the family about the purpose of mechanical ventilation and the goals of the therapy for the critically ill child.

♦ Explain how the ventilator and equipment functions to support the respiratory status of the critically ill child.

♦ Discuss strategies for measuring ventilator effectiveness including blood gas analysis, respiratory assessment, pulse oximetry reading, and end-tidal carbon dioxide monitoring.

♦ Give details about treatment strategies used to maximize the comfort level of the child receiving mechanical ventilation, including repositioning and the use of sedatives and analgesics.

♦ Encourage the family to interact with the critically ill child who is receiving mechanical ventilation during visitations. Explain that the family members can touch and talk to the child when appropriate.

♦ Consistently work with the health-care provider to keep the family updated about the condition of the child. Assist the family to understand what the goals and expectations of therapy are at all times.

Correct tube placement is maintained by proper securement of the ETT to the child's face. There are several techniques for securing the ETT. Policies and products used for securement vary. Based on the size of the child's face and the age of the child, a prefabricated securement device may be indicated. If the critically ill child's face is too small for a prefabricated securement device, the ETT is secured with cloth tape (Figs. 35-4*A* and 35-4*B*). Ensure that the tube is secured to prevent complications and frequently assess stability of the ETT; resecure the device when necessary. Moisture decreases the effectiveness of the securement device making the ETT vulnerable to position changes. The oral cavity is cleaned and suctioned frequently to decrease the amount of saliva on the securement device (Dalton, 2011).

Unplanned extubation may occur because of failure to secure the ETT and ventilator tubing, patient transfer, or self-extubation by the child. Unplanned extubation is an emergency because it compromises the child's respiratory status. Unplanned extubation often results in emergent reintubation and may increase the incidence of tissue trauma and hypoxia. To prevent unplanned extubation, assess placement and security of the ETT and ventilator tubing, monitor tubes during transfer, and assess the child's ability to remove the ETT. If there is risk of self-extubation, sedation medications and/or limb restraints may be initiated while the ETT is in place.

When ETT patency is compromised, gas exchange can be impaired. Tube patency is maintained by the use of suctioning devices. Suctioning is required because the tip of

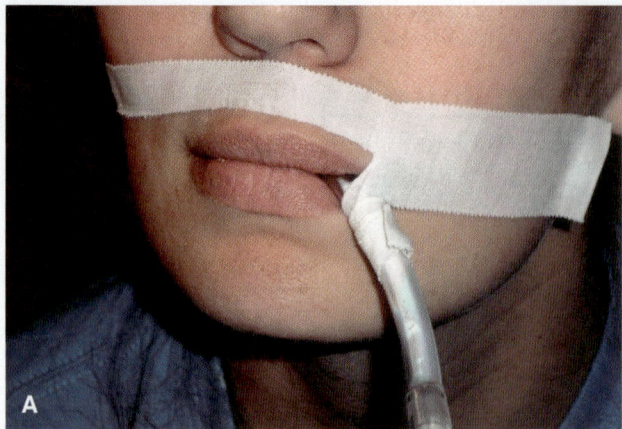

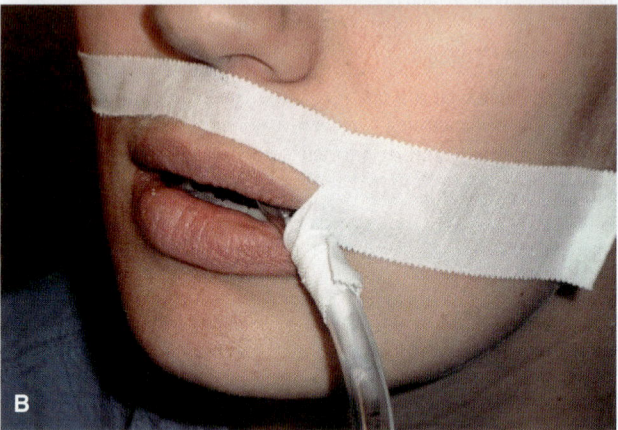

Figures 35-4a and b The endotracheal tube must be secured properly to the child's face to prevent dislodgement.

the ETT halts the mucociliary transport system. Additionally, in critically ill children a cough is often too weak to move secretions from the bronchi to the tip of the ETT (Ridling, Martin, & Bratton, 2003). The nurse ensures that proper suctioning equipment is available and functioning. Auscultate the lung sounds for evidence of secretions and suction the ETT when indicated to prevent aspiration or obstruction of the ETT from pulmonary secretions. Humidification and proper hydration can help to facilitate the mobilization of secretions (Dalton, 2011).

Consistent monitoring of the ventilator settings and alarms is necessary for the management of mechanical ventilators. Collaborate with the respiratory therapist to ensure proper functioning of the mechanical ventilator at all times. The nurse is responsible for assessing and evaluating ventilator alarms. Ventilator alarms must never be ignored or turned off. Ventilator alarms are frequently triggered by a problem with the patient or the equipment. Patient causes of ventilator alarms include biting of the endotracheal tube, obstruction from secretions, coughing or gagging, asynchronous breathing with the ventilator breaths, or episodes of apnea. Mechanical causes of ventilator alarms include kinking of the ventilator tubing, a leak in the endotracheal tube cuff, excess water in the ventilator tubing, a leak or disconnect in the ventilator system, an air leak from the presence of a chest tube, a malfunctioning oxygen system, or loss of power from the ventilator (Jones & Fix, 2009). Ventilator alarms require immediate attention and intervention. When

a ventilator alarm sounds, the nurse first checks the child then the ventilator for causes of the alarm. Auscultate breath sounds, suction the ETT when needed, assess for disconnects in the system, check the ventilator tubing, and remove excess water from the ventilator tubing. If the cause of the alarm cannot be found immediately, or the cause cannot be readily resolved and the patient's respiratory status is compromised, remove the patient from the ventilator and manually ventilate using a bag valve mask while alerting the respiratory therapist (Jones & Fix, 2009).

 Assessment Tool Troubleshooting Ventilator Alarms

The DOPE mnemonic is a useful assessment tool for ventilator alarm troubleshooting. The nurse caring for the ventilated child uses the **DOPE** mnemonic to assess for the source of the alarm. Assess for a **D**ISPLACED ETT, **O**BSERVE for an obstruction in the ETT, auscultate the lung fields to assess for a **P**NEUMOTHORAX, and finally, assess for **E**QUIPMENT failure.

Drawing blood gases is an essential nursing intervention used to monitor the effectiveness of mechanical ventilation. In most institutions, ventilator weaning is decided by the patient's blood gas values. The nurse is responsible for providing blood samples from invasive lines, either venous or arterial, for blood gas interpretation. Timely blood sampling is important for accurate blood gas analysis. Collaborate efficiently with the respiratory therapist and the laboratory for timely blood gas sampling and analysis.

 focus on safety

Frequent lab draws

With frequent lab draws, it is important to remember to use the minimum amount of blood required for an accurate blood gas sample to limit the amount of blood removed from the critically ill child.

Sedation and pain control are crucial for the mechanically ventilated child. The nurse is responsible for administering sedatives and analgesics to the child receiving mechanical ventilation to ensure adequate comfort and pain control as well as appropriate functioning of the ventilator. Frequently assess pain and sedation levels of the critically ill child receiving mechanical ventilation. Early identification of inadequate sedation is important to ensure that maximum comfort levels are met.

 Assessment Tool Assessing Sedation in the Mechanically Ventilated Child

Diligent nursing assessment of sedation and agitation is important to ensure positive outcomes in the ventilated child. Under-sedation can lead to inadvertent self-extubation, line removal, and other negative physiological issues. Over-sedation may affect the length of stay in the intensive care unit because of prolonged ventilation, increasing the risk of health care–acquired infections and cardiovascular compromise. The use of a valid tool to assess sedation and agitation is vital for the pediatric population. It improves interdisciplinary communication by reducing conflict related to differences in sedation assessment and improves patient outcomes by reducing the risk of over- or under-sedation (Lyden, Kramlich, Groves, & Bagwell, 2012).

The Richmond Agitation Sedation Score (RASS) is a commonly used tool that assists with sedation and agitation assessment. Using this scale, pediatric sedation and agitation are assessed according to the subjective judgment of the individual practitioner (Lyden et al., 2012). The RASS tool has three components of assessment: (1) observation, (2) response to verbal stimulation, and (3) response to physical stimulation. The use of the RASS tool is essential in the identification of inadequate sedation for the mechanically ventilated child. The nurse uses the tool to quickly identify sedation needs. Observe for agitation and response to verbal and physical stimulation in the critically ill child and collaborate with the health-care provider to identify target RASS levels and appropriate interventions based on the assessment score. Negative scores are associated with sedation, while positive scores are associated with agitation. Interventions are determined based on the desired RASS score.

Richmond Agitation Sedation Score		
RASS Score	**RASS Description**	
+4 Combative	Combative, violent, immediate danger to staff	
+3 Very agitated	Pulls or removes tube(s), catheter(s); aggressive	
+2 Agitated	Frequent non-purposeful movement, fights ventilator	
+1 Restless	Anxious, but movements not aggressive or vigorous	
0	Alert and calm	
−1 Drowsy	Not fully alert, but has sustained awakening (eye opening/eye contact) to voice (>10 seconds)	Voice stimulation
−2 Light sedation	Briefly awakens with eye contact to voice (<10 seconds)	Voice stimulation
−3 Moderate sedation	Movement or eye opening to voice (but no eye contact)	Voice stimulation
−4 Deep sedation	No response to voice, but movement or eye opening to physical stimulation	Physical stimulation
−5 Unarousable	No response to voice or physical stimulation	Physical stimulation

Source: Lyden, C., Kramlich, D., Groves, R., & Bagwell, S. (2012). Phase I: The development and content analysis of the Pediatric Sedation Agitation Scale. *Pediatric Nursing, 38(5),* 278–284.

There are many complications associated with mechanical ventilation. Nursing care focuses on reducing the risk of developing ventilator-associated infections and pneumonias and maintaining skin integrity. An ETT provides a direct pathway to the lungs for bacteria to enter. Patients receiving mechanical ventilation have decreased salivary secretion, and oral cavity hygiene worsens, resulting in bacteria overgrowth (Pedreira, Kusahara, Brunow de Carvalho, Nunez, & Peterlini, 2009). Bacterial overgrowth can lead to nosocomial infections, such as ventilator-associated pneumonia. To prevent the development of ventilator-associated pneumonia, diligent oral care is provided. Oral care includes assessment and frequent cleaning of the oral pharynx to facilitate the removal of plaque, bacteria, and debris. Minimizing bacteria in the oral pharynx will decrease the risk and incidence of nosocomial infections associated with the use of the mechanical ventilator (Pedreira et al., 2009).

Maintaining skin integrity in the mechanically ventilated child is a priority for the nurse. The mechanically

ventilated child is highly vulnerable to skin breakdown caused by the constant pressure of the artificial airway, increased immobility because of the use of sedatives and analgesia, and the inability to remove oral secretions. The ETT should remain in a semi-elevated position off the child's face and be repositioned frequently so that pressure does not build under the tube and cause skin breakdown. The ETT can be positioned with the holding device attached to the ventilator or elevated with a washcloth. The ETT is repositioned when possible to minimize skin breakdown around the mouth. The nurse considers repositioning the ETT when the securement device is changed. Frequent oral care is necessary to remove secretions and bacteria from the oral pharynx to prevent skin breakdown. Mouth moisturizer can be used to moisten the mouth and lips to prevent drying and cracking of the oral mucosa.

Frequent repositioning of the mechanically ventilated child is important to maintain skin integrity. Use caution when repositioning the child so that the ETT does not become dislodged or repositioned. The mechanically ventilated child is repositioned every 2 hours to relieve pressure points and maintain skin integrity. Pressure-reducing devices can be used for the back of the head, heels, and coccyx as needed. Prone positioning is occasionally warranted for the mechanically ventilated child (Schindler et al., 2011). Positioning in the prone position or reverse Trendelenburg may decrease work of breathing and allow for easier mobilization of secretions. Use care to ensure that pressure points are relieved with minor position changes at a minimum of every 2 hours when prone positioning is indicated (Aust, 2011).

Medical Care. Sedation and pain control are often necessary medical interventions for the mechanically ventilated child. Sedation is needed to facilitate sleep and rest, promote respiratory recovery, optimize gas exchange and consumption, enable the ventilator to support respiratory functions, and prevent ETT dislodgement. Sedation decreases the need for neuromuscular blocking agents and decreases ventilator time (Jones & Fix, 2009). Pain control is needed to reduce painful stimulation, relieve pain and discomfort associated with the presence of the artificial airway, and increase synchronization of breathing pattern with the mechanical ventilator. Sedation and pain control can be given through a variety of methods including intermittent or as-needed doses or as a continuous infusion. Regardless of the route of administration, adequate sedation and pain control are essential medical interventions for the mechanically ventilated child and should not be overlooked by the health-care provider or nurse.

Various drugs are combined to achieve desired levels of sedation and pain control for the mechanically ventilated child. Common classes of medications used for sedation and pain control include neuromuscular blocking agents, sedatives, and narcotics. Occasionally, neuromuscular blockade is necessary to promote respiratory recovery with full mechanical ventilator support. Neuromuscular blocking agents are used to reduce the oxygen demands of the body by reducing muscle movements and ease the facilitation of mechanical ventilation. Review Box 35-1 for commonly used sedative and analgesic medications for the mechanically ventilated child.

Complementary Care: *Adjuvant Therapies for Mechanical Ventilation*

There are many adjuvant medical therapies that can be used to augment mechanical ventilation for the critically ill child. Adjuvant medical therapies can help to facilitate oxygenation and ventilation and decrease airway inflammation. In some cases, respiratory distress is not relieved by the mechanical ventilator alone. In these cases, adjuvant medical therapies may be considered in addition to mechanical ventilation. See Table 35-3 to review adjuvant therapies used for the critically ill child with respiratory distress or failure.

MECHANICAL VENTILATOR WEANING. Mechanical ventilator weaning is an individualized process for the critically ill child. Weaning is based on several factors including blood gas results, pulse oximetry, end-tidal carbon dioxide values, lung compliance, and the clinical presentation of the child. Support from the ventilator is weaned to maintain normal blood gas results. The ventilator rate, tidal volume, and pressure support may be weaned to maintain blood gas

values within normal limits. Weaning of the ventilator should not occur if respiratory distress is present in the critically ill child, regardless of normal blood gas interpretation (Lillie & Jackson, 2010).

The respiratory status of the child is closely monitored during mechanical ventilator weaning. The child is observed for increased work of breathing and other signs of respiratory distress. Other important assessments include the level of fatigue and discomfort experienced by the child, vital signs, hemodynamics, oxygen and carbon dioxide levels, and blood gas values. If irregularities or abnormal assessment findings are noted, the weaning process may be adjusted.

EXTUBATION

Extubation is a unique process for the critically ill child. In contrast to the adult population, there is no evidence that supports weaning trials for extubation in the pediatric population. Extubation is based on many factors including the disease process, sedation and level of consciousness, fluid status and lung compliance. Each factor must be

Table 35-3 Adjuvant Medical Therapies for Mechanical Ventilation			
Therapy	**Indication**	**Principles**	**Nursing Considerations**
Nitric Oxide	Treatment of hypoxic respiratory failure associated with evidence of pulmonary hypertension	A low molecular weight compound that rapidly diffuses across the alveolar–capillary membrane into the smooth muscle of pulmonary vessels acting as a vasodilator by providing increased blood flow through the lungs and pulmonary artery dilation, reducing pulmonary artery pressure and right-to-left shunting.	Monitor for nitric oxide toxicity by evaluating the methemoglobin levels. Rebound pulmonary hypertension is a possible problem when stopping NO and must be weaned slowly. Closely monitor for respiratory distress, oxygen saturation, and vital signs.
Heliox	Treatment of acute and obstructive respiratory failure	A low-density molecule that easily penetrates the pulmonary vasculature. This results in improved gas exchange, lower airway resistance, and a reduction in work of breathing.	Wean heliox slowly and closely monitor for respiratory distress, oxygen saturation, and vital signs.
Bronchodilators	Treatment of restrictive airway disease, airway narrowing, and airway swelling	Medication that relaxes smooth muscles or airways and causes dilation of bronchi and bronchioles, which reduces resistance in the respiratory tract and improves airflow to the alveoli of the lungs.	Monitor for side effects of treatment including tachycardia, irregular heartbeat, nausea and vomiting, diarrhea, headache, and jittery or nervous feeling. Closely monitor for respiratory distress, oxygen saturation, and vital signs.
Corticosteroids	Treatment of airway inflammation	Medications that reduce the production of inflammatory chemicals to minimize tissue damage. Corticosteroids reduce airway inflammation and improve ventilation and gas exchange.	Monitor for side effects of steroid use including increased blood sugar, poor wound healing, hypertension, and mood swings.
Mucolytics	Used as an adjunct to standard pulmonary toileting and treatment of acute respiratory failure	Medication that reduces disulfide bonds in mucoproteins found in mucus to help loosen secretions for easier removal.	Closely monitor for respiratory distress, oxygen saturation, and vital signs.
CPT (Chest Physiotherapy)	Used as an adjunct to standard pulmonary toileting	External mechanical maneuvers, such as chest percussion and vibration, to augment mobilization and clearance of airway secretions.	Ensure that adequate pain relief and sedation are used to prevent pain associated with CPT therapy. Closely monitor for respiratory distress, oxygen saturation, and vital signs.

Source: Cheifetez (2011).

evaluated before extubation is considered. Extubation is most desirable when normal blood gas values have been reached, the ventilator settings are minimal, and the child presents with good lung compliance with the absence of respiratory distress.

For extubation to occur, the medical or surgical processes that suppressed the respiratory drive must be resolved. Medication infusions used for sedation that suppress the respiratory drive such as fentanyl (Abstral), midazolam (Versed), and propofol (Diprivan) must be stopped so that the respiratory drive is not compromised post-extubation. The child must be awake and able to support breathing with good lung compliance. Fluid status is considered prior to extubation. A child with fluid overload is highly vulnerable to respiratory distress and is therefore not a good candidate for extubation.

Good lung compliance in the critically ill child is measured by the ventilator settings and the clinical presentation. Ideally, a low ventilator respiratory rate is necessary for extubation. Depending on the age of the child, a ventilator respiratory rate of 6 to 10 is considered ideal for extubation. The lower the ventilator rate is before extubation, the more likely the child is able to support spontaneous ventilation after extubation. The peak inspiratory pressure should range from 16 to 25 cm H_2O before extubation. Lower peak inspiratory pressures indicate better lung compliance in the critically ill child. The tidal volume support from the ventilator must also be weaned before extubation. Full tidal volume support from the ventilator for children ranges from 6 to 8 mL/kg. Evidence shows that normal, unsupported tidal volumes for children range from 4 to 6 mL/kg. If the child can maintain spontaneous tidal volumes of 4 to 6 mL/kg, unsupported by a ventilator breath, he or she is a good candidate for extubation. Oxygen requirements are another consideration when determining when extubation is appropriate. Typically, a child will be more successful post-extubation with a lower pre-extubation oxygen need. Oxygen requirements less than 40% are ideal for extubation. A chest x-ray may be useful to identify areas of lung consolidation and evaluate how the fluid status is affecting the lungs. A chest x-ray alone is not a eliable indicator of readiness for extubation. Although a chest x-ray may be useful for detecting lung compliance issues, it may not match the clinical picture of the child and therefore is not a reliable indicator of readiness for extubation (Lillie & Jackson, 2010).

Once extubation criteria are met, the child can be extubated. Prior to extubation, all medical equipment is prepared. An appropriately sized bag valve mask and suction equipment should be readily available and functioning. Most critically ill children require supplemental oxygen post-extubation. A regular nasal cannula or a high-flow nasal cannula is commonly needed post-extubation and should be readily available. A high-flow nasal cannula is used for children with lung compliance issues, longer lengths of time on the ventilator, smaller physical size, and higher pressure support requirements received on the ventilator.

Once the medical supplies and personnel are ready, the critically ill child is prepared for extubation. Use developmentally appropriate language when educating the child about the extubation process. Extubation of the child is typically done with a respiratory therapist, a nurse, and a health-care provider at the bedside. The head of the bed is raised to 30 degrees to facilitate good lung expansion. The respiratory therapist and nurse work together to remove the ETT-securing device, deflate the cuff, and remove the ETT. The child is instructed to cough as the tube comes out. As the ETT is being removed, the child's mouth is suctioned simultaneously to remove secretions. Once the ETT is removed, supplemental oxygen is applied as needed.

Collaborative Care

Nursing Care. Complications can occur post-extubation because of the critically ill child's compromised respiratory state. Constant monitoring of the respiratory, cardiac, neurological, and fluid statuses are necessary interventions to promote positive outcomes in the extubated child. Closely monitor the oxygen saturations and vital signs while observing for signs and symptoms of respiratory distress. Supplemental oxygen is administered as needed to keep the oxygen saturation above 92%. Blood gases may be performed at intervals post-extubation to monitor gas exchange and assess for underlying acid-base imbalances.

 Across Care Settings: Transferring to a long-term care facility

In the critical care setting, providing excellent nursing care for the mechanically ventilated child is challenging. The nurse focuses on providing appropriate interventions to maximize outcomes related to the respiratory status and also provides care to support all body systems and care for the child holistically. Vigilance and assessment by the nurse are necessary for prevention and recognition of complications. This same type of care must be provided if it is determined that the child will be transferred to a long-term care facility after stabilization.

 Optimizing Outcomes—The extubated child

Optimizing outcomes for the extubated child requires vigilant nursing assessment and initiation of interventions to prevent complications. The nurse promotes the facilitation of gas exchange through positioning and adequate pulmonary hygiene. The extubated child is placed in an upright position to facilitate ventilation and gas exchange. Performing pulmonary hygiene is a priority for the child post-extubation. Coughing, deep breathing, and nasal/tracheal suctioning of the airway may be necessary to prevent atelectasis and increase mobilization of secretions.

 Now Can You—Care for the mechanically ventilated child?

1 Prioritize developmentally appropriate and holistic nursing care related to the critically ill child?
2. Explore diagnostic and laboratory testing and medications related to the critically ill child?
3. Develop teaching plans and discharge criteria for parents related to the critically ill child?

PERFUSION

Inadequate blood flow to the body's vital organs leads to critical illness and life-threatening complications. **Perfusion** refers to the delivery of oxygen and nutrient-rich blood to the tissues of the body. Adequate perfusion is necessary to support cellular metabolism and organ function. Inadequate perfusion, or **hypoperfusion**, may lead to organ dysfunction and failure. Treatment of illnesses that compromise perfusion in children often requires specialized management in the critical care unit. Common disease processes that increase the risk of perfusion abnormalities in children include cardiac disease, compromised immunity, endocrine disorders, gastrointestinal disease, genitourinary disease, liver disease, neurological disease, and renal disease. Any disease process or medical interventions that increase the risk of infection may put a child at risk for inadequate perfusion from sepsis. Management of perfusion abnormalities requires intensive assessment, monitoring, and intervention to prevent and treat complications. The goal in treating the child with inadequate perfusion includes restoring perfusion and supporting organ systems to preserve organ function and homeostasis. Treatment of perfusion abnormalities will be determined by the underlying cause, clinical presentation, and response to therapies. In this section we discuss perfusion abnormalities, including management of specialized monitoring devices and extensive nursing care for the critically ill child with perfusion abnormalities.

HYPOPERFUSION

Hypoperfusion may result from different physiological processes in the critically ill child. Disease processes that result in hypovolemia or vasodilation are the most common underlying causes of inadequate perfusion. Hypovolemia may be absolute as seen in conditions resulting in excessive fluid loss such as hemorrhage, severe vomiting, or diarrhea. Inadequate perfusion as a result of hypovolemia may also be classified as relative as a result of fluid third spacing. Perfusion abnormalities pertaining to relative hypovolemia are common in children with severe liver disease and malnutrition because lack of albumin production by the liver leads to sequestration of intravascular fluids clinically manifested by ascites and peripheral edema. Hypoperfusion also occurs secondary to disease processes that result in vasodilation. Vasodilation causes the blood pressure and mean arterial pressure to decrease, resulting in decreased arterial tone and blood flow to the vital organs. Certain disease processes, such as septic shock, result in both hypovolemia and vasodilation. Cardiac conditions may also lead to hypoperfusion in the critically ill child. In disease processes with cardiac conditions, organ failure may occur if the heart fails to adequately pump blood or afterload is severely increased.

Inadequate perfusion may occur primarily, leading to critical illness, or secondarily as the result of a preexisting disease process with predisposing risk factors. Inadequate perfusion can be detrimental to the critically ill child and requires early recognition and nursing intervention. Inadequate perfusion can lead to vascular compromise, tissue necrosis, and organ failure. It is the responsibility of the nurse to assess and recognize clinical manifestations of hypoperfusion and intervene appropriately.

Inadequate perfusion leads to the disruption of cellular processes, dysfunction of tissues, and ultimately failure of the vital organ systems. All organ systems are at risk for inadequate perfusion in the critically ill child. Organ hypoperfusion may occur through various processes. When a child is critically ill, the body activates the sympathetic nervous system in response to stress. Activation of the sympathetic nervous system increases blood flow to vital organs, such as the brain, lungs, and heart, leaving other organ systems such as the renal system, gastrointestinal system, and peripheral tissues at risk for inadequate perfusion. The renal system may be the first organ system to manifest dysfunction related to hypoperfusion. Renal hypoperfusion is clinically evident by decreased urine production and urinary output of less than 1 mL/kg/hr. Depending on the age of the critically ill child, when mean arterial pressure falls below 45 to 50 mm Hg, signs and symptoms of hypoperfusion may be evident.

Signs and symptoms of hypoperfusion may vary depending on the severity and duration of illness, disease progression, and compensatory ability of the child. Signs and symptoms of hypoperfusion may be generalized or more specific depending on organ system involvement. Generalized clinical manifestations of hypoperfusion in the critically ill child include decreased urinary output, decreased peripheral and pedal pulses, tachycardia, mental status changes and lethargy, delayed capillary refill, and pallor.

 clinical alert

Hypotension

Hypotension is considered a late sign of hypoperfusion in children and is considered ominous because there may be permanent damage to the affected organs.

FLUID BALANCE

To maintain adequate perfusion and homeostasis, fluid balance must be achieved and maintained. Many clinical conditions that result in critical illness also lead to fluid imbalances, which may include fluid volume deficit and/or fluid volume excess. Fluid imbalances may occur as a primary issue or as secondary to another underlying disease process, further compromising the critically ill child. Fluid volume deficit may contribute to absolute hypovolemia, compromising perfusion to the vital organs. Fluid loss may occur primarily through loss of blood or other bodily fluids or secondary to insensible losses, through processes such as respiration and from evaporation through the skin. Fluid volume excess may contribute to respiratory compromise, impairing ventilation and gas exchange. Fluid volume excess and fluid deficit may occur simultaneously, resulting in imbalances when the child is volume depleted within the vascular space, but fluid is present in excess amounts in the interstitial compartment, as in liver disease and sepsis. Maintaining optimum fluid balance presents a challenge for pediatric critical care providers. Fluid volume imbalances can potentially alter the function of organ systems and increase morbidity and mortality.

Nursing Diagnoses The Critically Ill Child With Altered Perfusion

- Fluid volume deficit/excess related to disease process: sepsis, shock, multiple dysfunction syndrome
- Decreased cardiac output related to disease process: sepsis, shock, multiple dysfunction syndrome
- Ineffective tissue perfusion (cardiopulmonary, gastrointestinal, renal, cerebral, peripheral) related to decreased cardiac output
- Risk for altered body temperature/hypothermia related to ineffective tissue perfusion and decreased cardiac output
- Risk for altered patterns of urinary elimination related to decreased perfusion to the kidneys and multiple dysfunction syndrome

Hemodynamic Management of the Critically Ill Child

HEMODYNAMIC MONITORING AND ASSESSMENT

Hemodynamic monitoring and assessment are indicated for measurement of cardiac, renal, and neurological function and as a guide for medication administration. Common conditions that alter perfusion and may require advanced hemodynamic monitoring include sepsis, shock, heart failure, cardiac dysrhythmias, traumatic brain injuries, renal failure, organ transplant, and extensive surgical cases. These conditions predispose the child to inadequate organ and tissue perfusion and require vigilant monitoring of hemodynamic status. Conditions that lead to the development of inadequate perfusion in children require advanced medical intervention and intensive nursing care. Understanding how to recognize the signs of inadequate perfusion and provide appropriate interventions to maximize tissue perfusion are a priority for the nurse (Hudson, 2013).

Hemodynamic monitoring assesses the primary factors that affect perfusion. This type of monitoring allows for assessment of vascular tone, organ function, and volume within the vascular system. Abnormalities in any of these factors may lead to inadequate perfusion and organ dysfunction. Treatment includes identifying and correcting the underlying causes of inadequate perfusion and supporting the body systems to maintain and optimize organ function.

Basic, noninvasive hemodynamic assessment includes measurement of systolic, diastolic, and mean arterial blood pressure. Fluid status and peripheral perfusion are other components of hemodynamic assessment of the critically ill child. Fluid status is monitored by the consistent measurement of intake and output including strict urine output, skin turgor, and evidence of edema. Peripheral perfusion is monitored by measurement of bilateral pulses, capillary refill, and core and skin temperature. The level of consciousness and mental status may also be monitored to assess cerebral perfusion. Advanced hemodynamic assessment for the child with inadequate perfusion includes invasive measurement of blood pressure, preload, afterload, cardiac output, central venous pressure, intracranial pressure, cerebral perfusion pressure, and oxygen consumption by the body's tissues. In the critically ill child with inadequate perfusion, both invasive and noninvasive monitoring techniques may be used.

The critically ill child with altered perfusion often requires additional monitoring of cardiac output and fluid status. This can be accomplished with more invasive monitoring techniques. A urinary catheter is commonly used for more accurate measurement of urine output. Other invasive hemodynamic monitoring techniques require venous or arterial access through invasive devices. Invasive devices that may be indicated for advanced hemodynamic monitoring include arterial lines, central venous catheters, pulmonary artery catheters, and intracranial pressure monitors (Fig. 35-5). See Table 35-4 to review commonly used invasive hemodynamic monitoring devices.

Insertion sites vary for each invasive hemodynamic monitoring device. Arterial catheters may be inserted into the radial, brachial, femoral, or dorsal pedis artery (Scales, 2010). Central venous catheters and pulmonary artery catheters may be inserted into the femoral, internal jugular, subclavian, transhepatic, or translumbar vein. Intracranial pressure monitors are inserted through the skull into the ventricle of the brain. The use of invasive hemodynamic monitoring devices requires specialized equipment and nursing care; therefore, invasive hemodynamic monitoring is most often instituted in the critical care environment.

INSERTION OF AN INVASIVE HEMODYNAMIC MONITORING DEVICE

Insertion of an invasive hemodynamic monitoring device is indicated for the critically ill child with inadequate perfusion. Insertion may occur in a controlled setting in the operating room for planned procedures and surgeries or emergently at the bedside as more advanced hemodynamic monitoring is indicated (Scales, 2010). The insertion requires special equipment. There are several commercially used kits for most invasive hemodynamic monitoring devices. The appropriate kit is selected based on type of hemodynamic monitoring indicated, insertion site access, and health-care provider preference. Other equipment needed includes sterile gloves, sterile gauze, sterile towels

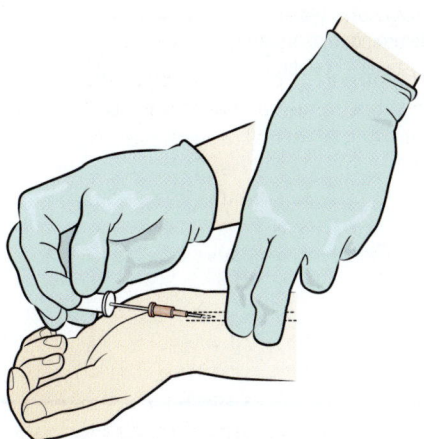

Figure 35-5 The arterial catheter is commonly used for invasive hemodynamic monitoring of the blood pressure. The arterial catheter is connected to pressure tubing that is leveled with the transducer for invasive monitoring of the blood pressure.

Table 35-4 Invasive Hemodynamic Monitoring

Hemodynamic Measurement	Measurment/ Calculation	Normal Range	Assessment	Clinical Indication
Cardiac Output (CO)	Stroke volume × heart rate	4–8 L/min	Reflects function of heart's ability to pump Organ perfusion	Low values: • Heart failure • Hypovolemia • Increased systemic vascular resistance High values: • Shock
Central Venous Pressure (CVP) or Right Atrial Pressure (RAP)	Measures volume of blood in right ventricle at the end of diastole	3–8 mm Hg	Measures right ventricular preload	Low values: • Hypovolemia • Increased pulmonary vascular resistance • Sepsis • Shock High values: • Right heart failure • Fluid overload
Pulmonary Artery Pressure (PAP)	Blood pressure in pulmonary artery	Systolic: 15–30 mm Hg Diastolic: 4–12 mm Hg	Measures right ventricular afterload Reflects pulmonary vascular resistance Reflects left ventricle compliance	Low values: • Hypovolemia • Valvular disease High values: • ARDS • Heart failure • Hypoxia • Sepsis • Shock • Right-to-left shunting • Pulmonary emboli
Pulmonary Artery Occlusion Pressure (PAOP) or Pulmonary Artery Wedge Pressure (PAWP)	Measures volume of blood in left ventricle at the end of diastole	2–15 mm Hg	Reflects volume of blood being ejected for systemic circulation Reflects pumping ability of the left ventricle	Low values: • Hypovolemia • Pulmonary emboli High values: • Cardiomyopathy • Fluid overload • Left heart failure
Mixed Venous Oxygen Saturation (S_VO2)	Percentage of oxygenated blood returning to heart after systemic circulation	60%–80%	Delivery and consumption of oxygen to tissue	Low values: • Acidosis • Decreased availability of oxygen • Hyperthermia • Insufficient hemoglobin • Poor perfusion • Seizures High values: • Burns • Liver failure • Renal failure • Sepsis • Shock

Source: Hudson (2013).

and drapes, cleaning solution such as chlorhexidine or Betadine, scalpel, suture, an appropriately sized catheter, sterile dressing, sterile scissors, pressure transducer kit, connection tubing, pressure tubing, pressure bag, and monitoring cable. Sedation medications and analgesics may

be indicated for the procedure. Occasionally 1% lidocaine solution is used at the insertion site.

The child is positioned so that the insertion site is readily assessable to the health-care provider. Once the child is appropriately medicated with anesthesia and analgesia, a sterile field is created by using sterile towels and drapes. The health-care provider locates the insertion site and uses a transducer needle to insert the catheter. Ultrasound guidance may be used to assist with insertion site location. A guide wire may be inserted to maintain placement while the catheter is prepared. Using the guide wire, the catheter is then advanced and sutured into place. The insertion site is then cleaned and covered with a sterile dressing. The catheter is immediately connected to the monitoring device for accurate invasive hemodynamic assessment (Hudson, 2013) (Fig. 35-6).

❝What to say❞—*Inadequate perfusion*

Interventions to care for the child with inadequate perfusion may often be overwhelming for the caregivers. Frequently, multiple interventions are required to restore adequate perfusion and maintain optimal organ function. Insertion of invasive lines, hemodynamic monitoring, and initiating interventions in response to clinical findings often occur emergently. When invasive procedures occur, they may trigger questions and concerns from the caregivers. The role of the nurse is to reinforce the purpose of these interventions and offer support as needed. The nurse constantly assesses the parents' needs as well as the needs of the child, utilizing additional resources to provide support as needed.

 Nursing Insight—The nurse's role during the insertion of an invasive hemodynamic monitoring device

During the insertion of an invasive hemodynamic monitoring device, the nurse is responsible for monitoring and supporting the critically ill child as well as assisting the health-care provider.

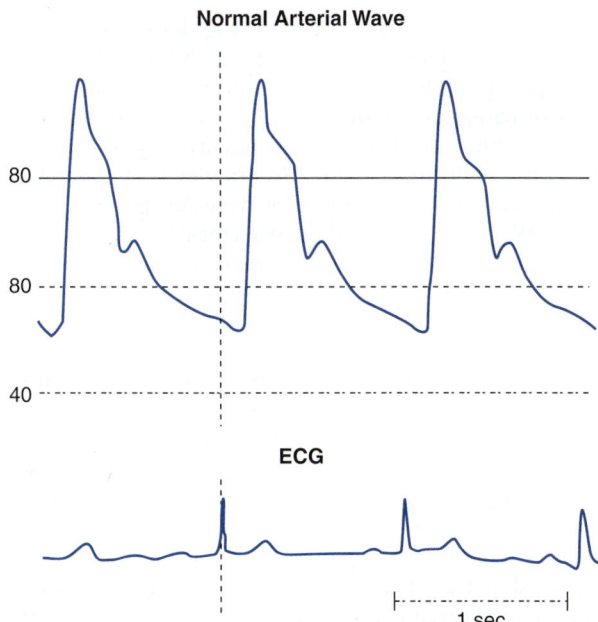

Figure 35-6 Monitoring waveforms provided by an invasive hemodynamic monitoring device is crucial for the critical care nurse.

Before the procedure, the nurse ensures that all equipment is prepared and functioning. This may require preparation of tubing for immediate connection and setup of invasive monitoring equipment. Sedatives and analgesics are prepared as needed. During the procedure, closely monitor the child's vital signs and assist the health-care provider as needed. After the procedure is complete, immediately connect the invasive hemodynamic monitoring device to the appropriate monitor and begin invasive hemodynamic assessment (Hudson, 2013).

COMPLICATIONS OF INVASIVE HEMODYNAMIC MONITORING DEVICES

Invasive hemodynamic monitoring poses many risks to the critically ill child. The presence of an invasive device adds to the risk for complications such as cardiac arrhythmias, arterial spasms, poor venous return, ischemia, hematomas, vessel perforation, infection, hemorrhage, air embolism, and thromboembolism. Complications of invasive device insertion include pneumothorax, or collapsed lung, and bleeding. Caution is maintained to prevent these complications from occurring.

Invasive hemodynamic monitoring devices can interrupt blood flow around the catheter through the arteries and veins. This increases the risk of ischemia and poor venous return distal to the insertion site. Any invasive device increases the risk of infection, which can be life threatening. Embolism is another risk factor in the use of invasive devices. Emboli may occur in the form of air entering an unsecured connection site or upon insertion or removal of the device. Emboli may also form at the insertion site or in the line and travel through the vascular system.

Invasive hemodynamic monitoring devices may be inserted into venous and arterial sites, increasing the risk of bleeding. Bleeding may occur slowly at the insertion site or rapidly if a disconnection occurs. If the invasive hemodynamic monitoring device becomes suddenly dislodged, hemorrhage may occur. Bleeding may also occur internally from perforation of the vessel and is often more insidious than an external hemorrhage. These complications can be devastating to the child. Recognize the signs and symptoms of each complication and intervene when needed.

Collaborative Care

Nursing Care. Hemodynamic assessment is a vital part of care for the critically ill child. Thorough hemodynamic assessment can assist with early detection and diagnosis of critical illness and aid with evaluation of the effectiveness of life-saving treatments and therapies. Complete a thorough hemodynamic assessment of the child. Hemodynamic assessment includes the measurement and monitoring of blood pressure, pulse, capillary refill, fluid status, mental status, temperature, and urine output (Hudson, 2013). These noninvasive assessments are crucial for early identification of hemodynamic instability in the critically ill child. Hemodynamic ranges differ for each age group. It is essential that the critical care nurse understand hemodynamic ranges for each age group, how to identify fluctuations from normal ranges, and when to intervene.

The presence of invasive hemodynamic monitoring devices allows for monitoring of hemodynamic parameters, which directly reflect cardiac function and fluid status. The specific type of monitoring that can be done depends on the type of invasive device present. Arterial lines allow for measurement of systolic, diastolic, and mean arterial pressures as well as sampling of arterial blood. Arterial lines may be indicated for monitoring conditions such as cardiac decompensation, neurological conditions, and shock. Central venous catheters allow for measurement of central venous pressure (CVP), also known as right atrial pressure. This type of monitoring is common in cardiac or shock conditions that result in hemodynamic instability and also in conditions in which strict fluid monitoring and fluid resuscitation are indicated. A pulmonary artery (PA) catheter (Swan-Ganz) is a specialized catheter specifically designed for hemodynamic monitoring. A PA catheter allows for monitoring of cardiac output (CO), CVP, pulmonary artery pressure (PAP), pulmonary artery wedge pressure (PAWP), and mixed venous oxygen saturation (S_VO2). A PA catheter is indicated in conditions with severe cardiac decompensation, hemodynamic instability, severe respiratory distress, and shock conditions (Hudson, 2013).

🦠 **Assessment Tool** The Pediatric Early Warning System

The nurse considers using the pediatric early warning system (PEWS) when the child's hemodynamic status is in question. The PEWS is a tool used for the early identification of children that are clinically decompensating. The PEWS tool helps the nurse to analyze the mental status and behavior, cardiovascular and respiratory status of the child, and determine when emergency intervention is needed. Children with invasive hemodynamic monitoring may need emergency medical intervention. The use of the PEWS tool can help the nurse identify when treatment is warranted.

The nurse caring for the critically ill child with altered perfusion may need to manage episodes of hypotension or hypertension. The nurse is responsible for the administration of fluid resuscitation and vasoactive medications needed to treat hypotension and hypertension. The nurse is responsible for the titration of vasoactive medications based on the hemodynamic assessment of the child. A thorough assessment is completed before any adjustments in vasoactive medication dosing are made. The nurse takes care not to titrate too quickly or too slowly and works to maintain appropriate hemodynamic parameters.

Critical Nursing Action Titrating Vasoactive Medications

During the administration of vasoactive agents, the nurse must closely monitor the critically ill child's hemodynamic status and response to treatments. Closely monitor the critically ill child with altered perfusion for significant vital sign changes, arrhythmias, decreased cardiac output, or decreased urinary output during titration of vasoactive medications. The nurse works closely with the health-care provider to determine hemodynamic goals for pulse, blood pressure, and medication dose titration or discontinuation parameters. Titration of vasoactive medications should not be too abrupt or too slow. The nurse should refer to the health-care provider's orders. The nurse adjusts vasoactive agents as needed to maintain appropriate blood pressure. Recognize that the peripheral blood flow is diminished with the administration of vasoactive medications. The peripheral pulses are monitored frequently, and the health-care provider is notified if the extremities become cold or mottled.

Monitoring the critically ill child with invasive hemodynamic monitoring devices requires increased assessment and vigilance to prevent complications. The nurse is responsible for catheter setup and functioning, catheter site care, and data interpretation. The nurse must understand how to properly level and zero catheter transducers, monitor waveforms, and interpret data provided by invasive hemodynamic monitoring devices. Data interpretation may be compromised if the device is not cared for properly. The nurse is properly educated about each type of invasive hemodynamic monitoring device and understands how to operate equipment to ensure proper functioning and accurate data interpretation (Hudson, 2013).

Invasive hemodynamic monitoring device setup varies for each catheter used. The nurse is responsible for assembling needed equipment; gathering tubing, cables, and transducers; and communicating with the medical and pharmaceutical team to ensure that fluids and equipment are readily available. To ensure consistency and accuracy of monitoring devices, the transducer must be calibrated regularly and placed in a consistent site. For arterial catheters and central venous pressure monitors, the transducer is calibrated at the phlebostatic axis. The phlebostatic axis represents the position of the atria and therefore reflects central blood pressure (Woodrow, 2009). The phlebostatic axis is located at the intersection of the fourth intercostal space and midaxillary line. Transducers are leveled against the phlebostatic axis at all times because transducers that are leveled higher or lower than the phlebostatic axis will produce inaccurate data and may result in inappropriate or unnecessary interventions. Monitor the level of the transducer and adjust the device as needed to maintain correct placement. The transducer may need to be adjusted to reflect patient position changes. **Zeroing** is the method of calibrating the monitoring system. Zeroing of all invasive hemodynamic monitoring devices must be done at least once a shift to ensure accurate data measurement (Woodrow, 2009).

Invasive hemodynamic monitoring devices greatly increase hemodynamic monitoring capabilities. The nurse must appropriately monitor and interpret data and waveforms provided by the device. An unmonitored waveform places the critically ill child at risk of harm. Closely monitor data and waveforms provided by the device and carefully monitor the consistency of the waveform provided by the device (Woodrow, 2009). If the waveform is inconsistent or dampened, the nurse assesses the patient, checks the equipment and connections, checks the level of the transducer, and considers recalibration of the device. Dampening refers to waveforms that consistently remain close to baseline. Waveforms that are dampened are considered inaccurate, and further assessment of the patient and equipment is warranted. Whenever invasive hemodynamic monitoring values are questionable, the nurse assesses for all possible causes of inaccuracy.

The positioning of invasive hemodynamic monitoring devices is important to maintain consistency and accuracy of hemodynamic measurements. The positioning of the catheter is also important to ensure accuracy of the measurements. For radial arterial catheters, the use of an arm board increases the accuracy of the measurement. The wrist may be hyperextended with an arm board to maintain correct position. Closely monitor the skin around the arm board for redness and skin breakdown. The arm board may be frequently repositioned to prevent skin breakdown.

Sampling from most invasive hemodynamic monitoring devices is a common practice. Depending on the device, venous or arterial blood can be drawn and used for blood gas analysis and comprehensive laboratory testing. Review and understand the procedure for correct sampling from each type of invasive hemodynamic monitoring device. Once a sample has been taken from the device, the nurse ensures that the device has been flushed properly to maintain accuracy of monitored data. Care is taken to avoid sampling errors. Errors of sampling or interpretation can cause or contribute to increased morbidity and mortality of the critically ill child.

Most invasive hemodynamic monitoring devices are not used for medication administration. The devices must be clearly labeled to avoid accidental medication infusion. Medications that are infused into an invasive hemodynamic monitoring system may cause complications and increase morbidity in the critically ill child. Prior to medication administration, assess the infusion port to ensure that it is an appropriate site for infusion.

clinical alert

Avoid medication administration into the arterial catheter

Arterial catheters are not to be used for medication administration. Drugs flowing under arterial pressure into smaller arteries and capillaries can cause necrosis and tissue damage (Woodrow, 2009). The arterial catheter must be clearly labeled to avoid infusion errors. Prior to medication administration, the nurse closely assesses the infusion port to ensure that it is not part of the arterial catheter system.

An invasive hemodynamic monitoring device is a site for potential thrombus formation, which may later release emboli that can occlude vessels and cause ischemia. To reduce the risk of thrombosis formation from a device, the patency must be maintained. Flush the catheter with 0.9% normal saline to ensure patency. To reduce the risk of thrombosis from an arterial catheter, the patency is maintained using a solution running slowly through the transducer at a rate of 3 mL/hr with the use of a pressure bag inflated to 300 mm Hg (Woodrow, 2009). This rate may be decreased to a minimum of 1 mL/hr depending on the fluid status of the child. Monitor the pressure bag and ensure that it remains inflated to 300 mm Hg to ensure adequate fluid flow through the arterial catheter and catheter patency.

Removal of most invasive hemodynamic monitoring devices is a nursing responsibility. Prior to removal, record any data needed, disconnect the monitoring cable, and prepare for device removal. Removal of invasive hemodynamic monitoring devices is performed sterilely. The nurse should start by removing the dressing and sutures to expose the device. Take proper care to apply pressure to the device insertion site during removal of the device. After removal of an invasive device, the nurse should be especially cautious of bleeding. Pressure is applied for at least 5 minutes to stop arterial bleeding. Pressure for up to 20 minutes may be indicated for femoral sites. A pressure

Where Research and Practice Meet:
Central Line-Associated Bloodstream Infections

Complications of invasive hemodynamic monitoring devices pose great risk to the critically ill child. While the placement of a central line can be a life-saving intervention for the critically ill child, it also poses great risk for the development of nosocomial bloodstream infections. Central line-associated bloodstream infections (CLABSIs) are a significant source of morbidity and mortality for the critically ill child (Hatler, Buckwald, Salas-Allison, & Murphy-Taylor, 2009). Research findings demonstrated that certain nursing practice guidelines helped decrease incidence of CLABSIs in pediatric patients. These guidelines include skin antisepsis, sterility when working with line insertion site or dressing, hand hygiene, daily assessment of necessity of line, discontinuation of line at earliest opportunity, and facility protocol adherence when caring for lines on a daily basis (Miller-Hoover & Small, 2009).

dressing may be applied if indicated (Woodrow, 2009). Closely monitor the insertion site periodically and assess for bleeding and bruising as well as color, warmth, sensation, movement, pulse, and capillary refill distal to the insertion site.

Invasive hemodynamic monitoring devices may impair blood flow and perfusion. Altered perfusion to distal limbs leads to ischemia and tissue damage or necrosis. Frequent vascular assessment of the distal limbs is essential for the detection and prevention of tissue ischemia. Observe the distal skin for color, warmth, sensation, movement, pulse, and capillary refill (Woodrow, 2009). If impaired perfusion is suspected, the nurse immediately notifies the health-care provider. Prompt discontinuation of the device is completed to prevent neurovascular impairment and loss of limb when invasive monitoring is no longer warranted.

An invasive hemodynamic monitoring device also increases the risk of bleeding and hemorrhage. When internal bleeding from a vessel occurs into the surrounding tissues, a hematoma may form. Hemorrhage may occur because of oozing blood from the insertion site and from accidental disconnection of tubing from the catheter device. Arterial catheters carry a higher risk of bleeding than other centrally inserted catheters (Woodrow, 2009). The invasive hemodynamic monitoring device should be visible at all times when possible. Frequently monitor the insertion site to assess condition and monitor for blood loss. The connections of the device must remain secure. Monitor connection sites and tubing to ensure secure connections at all times.

Global Health Case Study The Critically Ill Child With Altered Perfusion

Anna, a recent refugee, is a 6-year-old who was brought in to the emergency department by her mother with complaints of worsening fever, lethargy, and abdominal pain for the past 48 hours. Anna has not had proper medical care in her homeland and has a history of congenital heart disease with renal and genitourinary system involvement. She has a history of chronic urinary tract infections and finished a course of antibiotics for an infection 6 weeks ago. Her mother states that Anna has not been eating well and has become increasingly lethargic over the last 2 days. She has had a fever for the last 24 hours with a maximum temperature of 103.4°F (39.7°C). Anna's mother brought her in because she has not voided in the last 8 hours and is refusing to eat or drink anything. Laboratory tests reveal protein and elevated white and red blood cells in Anna's urine. Her white blood cell count is also elevated. Anna is admitted to a medical-surgical unit for management of a urinary tract infection and dehydration.

Anna receives a dose of IV antibiotics and is started on maintenance IV fluids to correct dehydration. The nurse notes that Anna is lethargic, has weak pulses, and has poor capillary refill in her lower extremities. A urinary catheter has been inserted, and Anna's urinary output over the last 2 hours has been 10 mL/hr. Her vital signs reveal a heart rate of 128 bpm and a temperature of 102.0°F (38.9°C).

Four hours later, the nurse assesses Anna and discovers that she is unresponsive. She is cold and clammy, has absent pedal pulses, and is taking short, shallow breaths. Assessment of vital signs reveals decreased heart rate and blood pressure. Total urinary output over the last 4 hours is 15 mL. The nurse performs a severe sepsis screening on Anna with positive results. Anna is transferred to the intensive care unit for management of severe sepsis and shock.

critical thinking questions

1. What predisposing factors did Anna have for the development of septic shock?

2. What is the pathophysiological process that leads to hypoperfusion in sepsis?

3. What clinical manifestations did Anna have related to hypoperfusion? What were the early signs? What late signs did she have?

4. What types of treatment and therapies do you anticipate the physician ordering to treat Anna?

5. What is the goal of her treatment?

◆ See Suggested Answers to Global Health Case Studies on Davis*Plus*.

"What to say"—*The critically ill child with altered perfusion*

The nurse is instrumental in communicating with the family about the child's condition. Here are important topics to teach the family.

- Teach the family about hemodynamic assessment techniques including invasive and noninvasive monitoring devices.

- Discuss the purpose of monitoring, the expected findings based on clinical condition, and the plan of care based on clinical findings.

- Prior to nursing intervention, explain to the family the purpose of medical management techniques of the critically ill child with altered perfusion, including the use of vasoactive medications, fluid boluses, and blood product administration.

- Consistently work with the health-care provider to keep the family updated about the condition of the critically ill child. Assist the family to understand what the goals and expectations of therapy are at all times.

Providing excellent care for the child with altered perfusion may be very challenging for the nurse. The responsibility to recognize and restore adequate perfusion to reestablish and maintain vital organ function is a primary intervention for the nurse. Vigilance and assessment by the nurse are necessary for prevention and recognition of complications.

 Now Can You—**Care for the critically ill child with altered perfusion?**

1. Provide nursing care to a child with the insertion of invasive lines, hemodynamic monitoring, and interventions associated with altered perfusion?

2. Provide nursing care to a child with altered perfusion?

? **Case Study** The Critically Ill Child With Multiple Organ Dysfunction Syndrome

Zoey, a 20-month-old child with a history of gastroschisis, was originally admitted to the pediatric critical care unit for a life-saving intestinal transplant. Immediately following transplant, Zoey developed Klebsiella pneumonia and required mechanical ventilation for respiratory support. Despite multiple antibiotic therapies, Zoey's condition deteriorated. Following an episode of sepsis with multi-drug resistant enterococcus, Zoey's kidney function declined and she developed renal insufficiency. Because of several days of oliguria, increased blood urea nitrogen and creatinine, and electrolyte disturbances, Zoey was treated with continuous renal replacement therapy. Zoey's condition worsened over time. Her respiratory status continued to decline. Because of severe respiratory acidosis, Zoey was transitioned to high-frequency ventilation. Zoey developed recurrent sepsis with gram-positive and gram-negative infections. She experienced severe hypotension, hypothermia, and whole body ischemia. Vasoactive medications were initiated to treat the hypotension and whole body ischemia. A warming unit was applied to treat her hypothermia. Because of the severe state of her illness and the high mortality rate of multiple organ dysfunction syndrome, extracorporeal membrane oxygenation therapy was initiated.

critical thinking questions

1. Describe the treatment approach for multiple organ dysfunction syndrome.

2. What supportive therapies can be initiated in this case?

3. Zoey's parents have difficulty understanding why she is not getting better with all the help of the machines. As the nurse, how would you address the parents' questions and concerns?

◆ See Suggested Answers to Case Studies on Davis*Plus*.

Medical Care. Medical management of the critically ill child with altered perfusion includes constant regulation of blood pressure and fluid status to prevent inadequate perfusion. Treatment of inadequate perfusion consists of fluid resuscitation using IV crystalloid or colloid solutions. The choice of solution depends on the clinical presentation, comorbidities, and underlying condition of the child. When fluid replacement is not successful in restoring adequate perfusion, vasoactive medications may be administered.

Fluid resuscitation is indicated for the critically ill child with hypoperfusion and low blood volume. Fluid resuscitation is accomplished by using an isotonic crystalloid or colloid solution. Crystalloid solutions, such as 0.9% normal saline or lactated Ringer's solution, are typically used for fluid resuscitation. Treatment volumes range from 10 to 20 mL/kg depending on the severity of hypoperfusion, age, weight, vital signs, and fluid status of the child.

Colloid solutions may be administered to the critically ill child with hypoperfusion when crystalloid solutions alone are inadequate. Colloid solutions increase blood volume and effectively restore blood pressure. Colloid solutions, such as whole blood and plasma, are given when hypoperfusion presents with anemia or blood loss. Human serum albumin is another type of colloid solution that may be indicated for the child with hypoperfusion from fluid volume deficit. Human serum albumin expands the vascular volume and draws fluid into the cells to restore colloidal osmotic pressure. Treatment volume with colloid solutions vary for each child based on age, weight, fluid status, and severity of anemia. Like crystalloid solutions, transfusion volumes for colloid solutions range from 10 to 20 mL/kg. The critically ill child with severe hypoperfusion will likely receive a transfusion of 20 mL/kg or more if indicated.

When fluid resuscitation alone is not successful in restoring perfusion, vasoactive medications may be initiated. Vasoactive medications result in increased cardiac output, vasoconstriction, and increased blood flow to the vital organs. Vasoactive medications used in combination with fluid resuscitation are very effective in restoring adequate perfusion. Most vasoactive medications are infused IV through a continuous drip. Vasoactive medications can be titrated to the desired effect. Multiple vasoactive medications can be used simultaneously if indicated. See Box 35-2 to review commonly used vasoactive medications in the critically ill child with altered perfusion.

Optimizing Outcomes—Early recognition of cardiac arrest

When caring for the child with altered perfusion, the goal of nursing care is to provide stabilization and maximize perfusion to the vital organs. When cardiac function is severely compromised and the child is hemodynamically unstable, the risk of cardiac arrest increases. When cardiac arrest occurs, the heart fails to pump, and perfusion to vital organs ceases. Without perfusion and oxygenation, vital organs such as the brain may suffer irreversible injury

---

Box 35-2 Vasoactive Medications

Medication	Classification	Indication	Dosing	Adverse Effects
dopamine (Intropin)	Inotrope, vasopressors	Adjunct to standard measures to improve blood pressure, cardiac output, urine output in treatment of shock unresponsive to fluid replacement, vasoconstriction	0.5–3 mcg/kg/min – stimulate dopaminergic receptors, producing renal vasodilation. 3–20 mcg/kg/min – stimulate dopaminergic and beta-1 adrenergic receptors, producing cardiac stimulation and renal vasodilation	Tachycardia, vasoconstriction, cardiac conduction abnormalities, decreased urine output
epinephrine (Adrenalin)	Antiasthmatics, bronchodilators, vasopressors	Management of reversible airway disease caused by asthma or COPD, severe allergic reactions, cardiac arrest, upper airway obstruction and croup, maintenance of heart rate and blood pressure, vasoconstriction	0.05–0.2 mcg/kg/min 0.01 mg/kg	Hypertension, arrhythmias, vasoconstriction, tachycardia, urinary retention
norepinephrine (Levophed)	Vasopressor	Produces vasoconstriction and myocardial stimulation, which may be required after adequate fluid replacement in the treatment of severe hypotension and shock, vasoconstriction	0.1–1 mcg/kg/min	Hypertension, arrhythmias, vasoconstriction, tachycardia, organ ischemia, gangrene of extremities
vasopressin (Pitressin)	Hormones, antidiuretic hormone	Management of pulseless VT/VF unresponsive to initial shocks, asystole, or pulseless electrical activity and management of vasodilatory shock, vasoconstriction	0.0005–0.01 units/kg/min	Vasoconstriction, arrhythmias, bronchoconstriction, cutaneous necrosis
phenylephrine (Neo-Synephrine)	Vasopressor	Treatment of hypotension and vascular failure in shock, supraventricular tachycardia, and as a vasoconstrictor in regional analgesia	0.1–0.5 mcg/kg/min	Headache, tachycardia, decreased cardiac output, metabolic acidosis, decreased urine output

(continued)

Box 35-2 Vasoactive Medications (continued)

Medication	Classification	Indication	Dosing	Adverse Effects
isoproterenol (Isuprel)	Antiasthmatic, beta$_1$- and beta$_2$-adrenergic agonist, bronchodilator, and sympathomimetic	Treatment of decreased cardiac output, AV block, bradyarrhythmias, vasoconstrictive shock, and asthma or COPD	0.05–2 mcg/kg/min	Chest pain, palpitations, tachycardia, ventricular arrhythmias, profound hypotension, bronchial irritation
dobutamine (Dobutrex)	Inotrope	Management of heart failure caused by depressed contractility from organic heart disease or surgical procedures, vasodilation	2.5–15 mcg/kg/min	Hypertension, ectopic heartbeats, tachycardia, angina
milrinone (Primacor)	Inotrope	Short-term treatment of CHF unresponsive to conventional therapy with digoxin, diuretics, and vasodilators, vasodilation	0.25–0.75 mcg/kg/min	Arrhythmias, hypotension, abnormal liver function tests
nitroprusside (Nipride)	Antihypertensive, vasodilator	Management of hypertensive crisis, vasodilation	0.3–10 mcg/kg/min	Hypotension, palpitations, hypoxia

Source: Vallerand & Sanoski (2014).

or damage. Early recognition and treatment of cardiac arrest with basic life support and pediatric advanced life support according to the American Heart Association guidelines increase survival rate and outcomes for children.

Maintenance of normothermia plays a critical role in preventing complications in the child with hypoperfusion. A forced air warming unit may be initiated to prevent or treat hypothermia. A warming unit distributes warm, temperature-controlled air across the body. The warming unit increases the temperature of the peripheral tissues, which allows warmer blood to circulate to the body's core, preventing or treating hypothermia.

Invasive medical management of perfusion and fluid balance issues for the critically ill child includes hemodialysis and extracorporal membrane oxygenation (ECMO). Hemodialysis and ECMO may be indicated when other means of providing adequate perfusion and fluid balance have failed. These highly sophisticated forms of technology improve perfusion and fluid issues by managing the roles of affected body systems to allow the organs to rest and recover from injury. Hemodialysis is indicated for the child with acute or chronic renal failure or with inadequate renal perfusion. Hemodialysis replaces the role of the kidneys and works to filter and remove waste and extra fluid from the blood. ECMO is indicated for the child with cardiac dysfunction and/or severe respiratory failure when conventional or high-frequency ventilation methods have failed. ECMO is a modified form of cardiopulmonary bypass that can provide temporary support of the pulmonary and/or cardiac circulation (Dalton, 2011). Through ECMO, the blood is oxygenated and circulated, diminishing the workload of the heart and lungs. Both hemodialysis and ECMO are used for the critically ill child of all ages and disease processes.

TRANSITIONING FROM INTENSIVE CARE

Transitioning from intensive care occurs when the critical illness has improved or is resolved and invasive monitoring is no longer indicated. Length of stay in the intensive care unit varies depending on severity of illness and response to treatment. The critically ill child may be transitioned to a progressive care status or unit prior to full transition to a general care floor. Progressive care provides care to patients whose needs are not critical enough for intensive care but too complex for the general care floor. Most institutions transition from intensive to progressive care. When the child has recovered enough, a general care floor is typically indicated before the transition home.

Parents of the critically ill child may be apprehensive to transition to the general care floor. The transition can be stressful because of location change, new care providers and policies, and lack of close monitoring. Parents can be actively involved in the care of the child including discussion about transition from intensive care to the general care floor. The nurse assists the family in coping with the transition to the general care floor and concentrates on supporting the child's recovery. Transition to the general care floor should be viewed in a positive light as a step toward transitioning home.

Although medicine and nursing care is at the forefront in advancement in medical treatment and technology, it is not always enough to save the critically ill child. Occasionally, the child is gravely ill, and medical treatment and technology only sustain life. Such illnesses include multi-organ system failure and brain death. In these circumstances, withdrawal of medical support may be indicated. Withdrawal of medical support includes the termination of medical treatments and therapies that are sustaining life. Once the decision to withdraw treatment has been made, support from the mechanical ventilator and medication infusions may be discontinued, and other means of supporting the body systems may be stopped to allow a natural death to occur. When withdrawal of care is indicated, the nurse must compassionately support the family members with the transition.

Summary Points

◆ The critically ill child is defined as a patient who is seriously injured or gravely ill and is at risk for potential or actual life-threatening health problems.

◆ The critical care environment is stressful to the critically ill child and the family members because of sensory overload, change in family processes, and the unknown of the critical care environment.

◆ Growth and development, nutrition, skin integrity, pain control, and cultural/spiritual issues are important aspects to recognize when caring for the critically ill child.

◆ Problems with gas exchange in children may be caused by numerous conditions that affect oxygenation, ventilation, or both and represent a medical emergency that requires immediate attention from the nurse.

◆ Many modes of oxygen administration can be used for the critically ill child with respiratory distress. Intubation is required for the critically ill child with respiratory failure requiring mechanical ventilation.

◆ The critically ill child receiving mechanical ventilation requires diligent nursing care to maintain safety and respiratory function.

◆ Inadequate blood flow caused by altered perfusion to the body's vital organs leads to critical illness and life-threatening complications in the critically ill child.

◆ Invasive hemodynamic monitoring devices are common for the critically ill child with altered perfusion and require specialized nursing care.

◆ Medical and nursing management of the critically ill child with altered perfusion includes the use of fluid resuscitation, vasoactive medications, hemodialysis, and extracorporeal membrane oxygenation.

Review Questions

Multiple Choice

1. A 10-year-old child was admitted with sepsis and acute renal failure. Today the health-care provider informs the parents that the child now has multisystem failure and brain death. The provider asks about withdrawing life support. Which intervention by the nurse is most appropriate?
   A. Leave the room to allow the parents to grieve for their child alone
   B. Answer any questions the family has before leaving them alone
   C. Tell the family that they will grieve but eventually will be alright
   D. Quietly remove the child from life-supporting equipment

2. Which intervention by the nurse is most appropriate to prevent sensory overload in the critically ill child?
   A. Leave the TV on all the time for comfort
   B. Create "quiet time" without interruptions
   C. Leave lights on so the child will not be scared
   D. Keep the child highly sedated to allow sleep

3. The nurse working in a pediatric intensive care unit that operates under the philosophy of family-centered care would place the highest priority on which intervention?
   A. Allowing unrestricted visiting by anyone in the family
   B. Having a parent or grandparent stay in the hospital at all times
   C. Involving the parents as much as possible in their child's care
   D. Teaching the family to provide most nursing care for the child

4. A nurse is caring for a patient with continuous pulse oximetry. Which important safety measure does the nurse incorporate into this child's care?
   A. Move the oximeter probe daily
   B. Assess distal pulses every 4 hours
   C. Remove condensation each shift
   D. Turn the child every 2 hours

5. The nurse is planning to suction a patient who is intubated and being mechanically ventilated. After auscultating lung sounds, which action does the nurse take next?
   A. Rinse the catheter with normal saline
   B. Perform sterile normal saline lavage
   C. Hyperoxygenate the patient
   D. Perform hand hygiene

6. The nurse assesses a child for hypoperfusion. What assessment finding is a late sign of hypoperfusion?
   A. Tachycardia
   B. Mental status change
   C. Decreased urine output
   D. Hypotension

7. A child has an arterial line in place. Which nursing action is the priority?
   A. Check all connections to ensure they are secure
   B. Flush the system two times per shift with saline
   C. Give neuromuscular blocking agents on time
   D. Institute protective isolation while the line is present

8. A child with hypoperfusion needs an infusion of a crystalloid solution. Which solution should the nurse choose based on this child's needs?
   A. 5% dextrose in water
   B. Whole blood
   C. Albumin
   D. Normal saline

9. A 5-year-old child has a radial arterial line in place. The nurse assesses the child's fingertips to be cool and pale. Based on these assessment findings, which intervention is the most appropriate?
   A. Reposition the arterial line
   B. Loosen the tape on the arterial line
   C. Document the findings in the chart
   D. Notify the health-care provider

10. A child is moving from the pediatric intensive unit to the regular pediatric floor. The parents seem upset. Which response by the nurse is the most appropriate?

A. "Aren't you happy your child is getting better?"

B. "I'd like to know more about what concerns you."

C. "This is great because it means he'll go home soon!"

D. "Don't worry; the staff on this unit is wonderful."

See Answers to End of Chapter Review Questions on *DavisPlus*.

REFERENCES

AARC Clinical Practice Guidelines. (2010). Endotracheal suctioning of mechanically ventilated patients with artificial airways. *Respiratory Care, 55*(6), 758–764.

Aust, M. (2011). Pressure ulcer prevention. *The American Journal of Critical Care, 20*(5), 376.

Broyles, L., Tate, J., & Happ, M. (2012). Use of augmentative and alternative communication strategies by family members in the intensive care unit. *American Journal of Critical Care, 21*(2), 21–32.

Cheifetez, I. (2011). Management of acute lung injury. *Respiratory Care, 56*(9), 1258–1272.

Dalton, H. (2011). Extracorporeal life support: Moving at the speed of light. *Respiratory Care, 56*(9), 1445–1456. doi:10.4187/respcare.01369

Hatler, C., Buckwald, L., Salas-Allison, Z., & Murphy-Taylor, C. (2009). Evaluating central venous catheter care in a pediatric intensive care unit. *American Journal of Critical Care, 18*(6), 514–520.

Hudson, K. (2013). Hemodynamic monitoring. Retrieved from http://dynamicnursingeducation.com/class.php?class_id=49&pid=18

Jones, J., & Fix, B. (2009). *Critical care notes: Clinical pocket guide.* F.A. Davis Company.

Khalaila, R., Zbidat, W., Anwar, K., Bayya, A., Linton, D., & Syiri, S. (2011). Communication difficulties and psychoemotional distress in patients receiving mechanical ventilation. *American Journal of Critical Care, 20*(6), 470–479.

Lawson, N., Thompson, K., Saunders, G., Saiz, J., Richardson, J., Brown, D., et al. (2010). Sound intensity and noise evaluation in a critical care unit. *American Journal of Critical Care, Nov 19*(6), 88–98.

Lillie, B., & Jackson, M. (2010). Pediatric invasive mechanical ventilation. *Journal for Respiratory Care Practitioners, 23*(2), 14–16.

Lyden, C., Kramlich, D., Groves, R., & Bagwell, S. (2012). Phase I: The development and content analysis of the Pediatric Sedation Agitation Scale. *Pediatric Nursing, 38*(5), 278–284.

Marshall, A., Cahill, N., Gramlich, L., MacDonald, G., & Heyland, D. (2012). Optimizing nutrition in intensive care units: Empowering critical care nurses to be effective agents of change. *American Journal of Critical Care, 21*(3), 186–194.

McAdam, J., & Puntillo, K. (2009). Symptoms experienced by family members of patients in intensive care units. *American Journal of Critical Care, 18*(3), 200–209.

Meyer, R., Harrison, S., Sargent, S., Ramnarayan, P., Habibi, P., & Labadarios, D. (2009). The impact of enteral feeding protocols on nutritional support in critically ill children. *The Journal of Human Nutrition and Dietetics, 22*(5), 428–436.

Miller-Hoover, S., & Small, L., (2009). Research evidence review and appraisal: Pediatric central venous catheter care bundling. *Pediatric Nursing, 35*(3), 191–201.

Mundy, C. (2010). Assessment of family needs in neonatal intensive care units. *American Journal of Critical Care, 19*(2), 156–163.

Pedreira, M., Kusahara, D., Brunow de Carvalho, W., Nunez, S., & Peterlini, M. (2009). Oral care interventions and oropharyngeal colonization in children receiving mechanical ventilation. *The American Journal of Critical Care, 18*(4), 319–328.

Rasera, C. C., Gewehr, P. M., Domingues, A. M., & Junior, F. F. (2011). Measurement of end-tidal carbon dioxide in spontaneously breathing children after cardiac surgery. *American Journal of Critical Care, Sept 20*(5), 388–394.

Restrepo, R. D., Hirst, K. R., Wittnebel, L., & Wettstein, R. (2012). AARC clinical practice guideline: Transcutaneous monitoring of carbon dioxide and oxygen: 2012. *Respiratory Care, Nov 57*(11), 1955–1962.

Ridling, D. A., Martin, L. D., & Bratton, S. L. (2003). Endotracheal suctioning with or without instillation of isotonic sodium chloride solution in critically ill children. *Journal of Critical Care, 12*(3), 212–219.

Sagarin, M. J., Chiang, V., Sakles, J. C., Barton, E. D., Wolfe, R. E., Vissors, R. J., et al. (2002). Rapid sequence intubation for pediatric emergency airway management. *Pediatric Emergency Care, 18*(6), 417–423.

Scales, K. (2010). Arterial catheters: Indications, insertion, and use in critical care. *British Journal of Nursing, 19*(19), S16–S21.

Schindler, C., Mikhailov, T. A., Kuhn, E. M., Christopher, J., Conway, P., Ridling, D., et al. (2011). Protecting fragile skin: Nursing interventions to decrease development of pressure ulcers in pediatric intensive care. *The American Journal of Critical Care, 20*(1), 26–34.

Vallerand, A. H., & Sanoski, C. A. (2014). *Davis's drug guide for nurses* (14th ed.). Philadelphia, PA: F.A. Davis.

Walsh, B., Hood, K., & Merritt, G. (2011). Pediatric airway maintenance and clearance in the acute care setting: How to stay out of trouble. *Journal of Respiratory Care, 56*(9), 1424–1444.

Woodrow, P. (2009). Arterial catheters: Promoting safe clinical practice. *Nursing Standard, 24*(4), 35–40.

Xie, H., Kang, J., & Mills, G. H. (2009). Clinical review: The impact of noise on patients' sleep and the effectiveness of noise reduction strategies in intensive care units. *Critical Care, 13*(2), 208.

Zimmerman, K., & Bauersachs, C. (2012). Empowering NICU parents. *International Journal of Childbirth Education, 27*(1), 50–53.

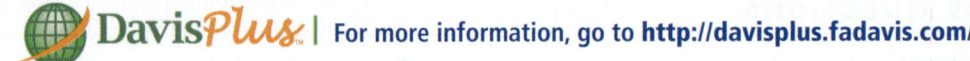

DavisPlus | For more information, go to http://davisplus.fadavis.com/

CONCEPT MAP

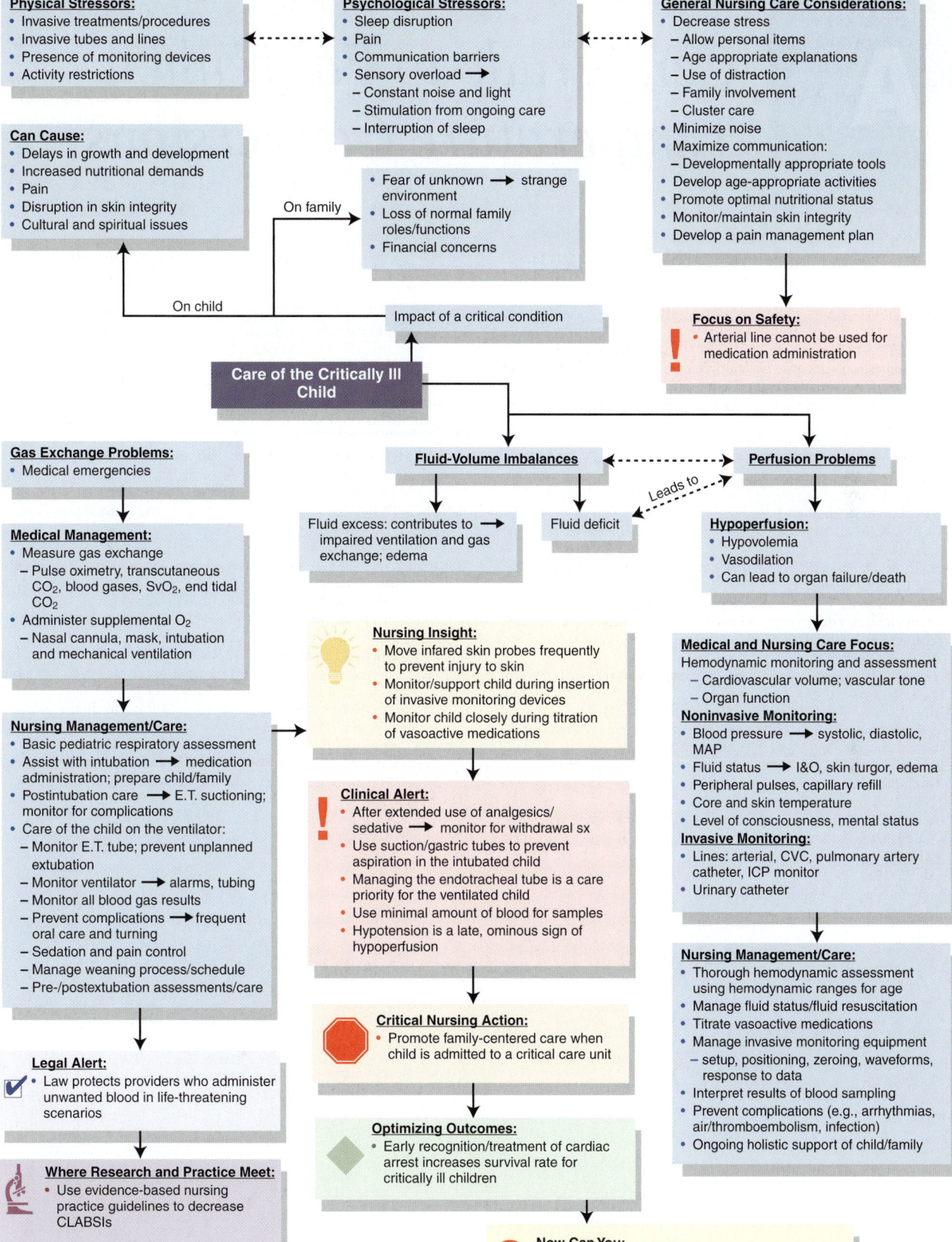

Physical Stressors:
- Invasive treatments/procedures
- Invasive tubes and lines
- Presence of monitoring devices
- Activity restrictions

Psychological Stressors:
- Sleep disruption
- Pain
- Communication barriers
- Sensory overload →
  - Constant noise and light
  - Stimulation from ongoing care
  - Interruption of sleep

General Nursing Care Considerations:
- Decrease stress
  - Allow personal items
  - Age appropriate explanations
  - Use of distraction
  - Family involvement
  - Cluster care
- Minimize noise
- Maximize communication:
  - Developmentally appropriate tools
- Develop age-appropriate activities
- Promote optimal nutritional status
- Monitor/maintain skin integrity
- Develop a pain management plan

Can Cause:
- Delays in growth and development
- Increased nutritional demands
- Pain
- Disruption in skin integrity
- Cultural and spiritual issues

On family
- Fear of unknown → strange environment
- Loss of normal family roles/functions
- Financial concerns

On child

Impact of a critical condition

Care of the Critically Ill Child

Focus on Safety:
! • Arterial line cannot be used for medication administration

Gas Exchange Problems:
- Medical emergencies

Fluid-Volume Imbalances

Perfusion Problems

Leads to

Medical Management:
- Measure gas exchange
  - Pulse oximetry, transcutaneous CO_2, blood gases, SvO_2, end tidal CO_2
- Administer supplemental O_2
  - Nasal cannula, mask, intubation and mechanical ventilation

Fluid excess: contributes to → impaired ventilation and gas exchange; edema

Fluid deficit

Hypoperfusion:
- Hypovolemia
- Vasodilation
- Can lead to organ failure/death

Nursing Insight:
- Move infared skin probes frequently to prevent injury to skin
- Monitor/support child during insertion of invasive monitoring devices
- Monitor child closely during titration of vasoactive medications

Medical and Nursing Care Focus:
Hemodynamic monitoring and assessment
  - Cardiovascular volume; vascular tone
  - Organ function

Noninvasive Monitoring:
- Blood pressure → systolic, diastolic, MAP
- Fluid status → I&O, skin turgor, edema
- Peripheral pulses, capillary refill
- Core and skin temperature
- Level of consciousness, mental status

Invasive Monitoring:
- Lines: arterial, CVC, pulmonary artery catheter, ICP monitor
- Urinary catheter

Nursing Management/Care:
- Basic pediatric respiratory assessment
- Assist with intubation → medication administration; prepare child/family
- Postintubation care → E.T. suctioning; monitor for complications
- Care of the child on the ventilator:
  - Monitor E.T. tube; prevent unplanned extubation
  - Monitor ventilator → alarms, tubing
  - Monitor all blood gas results
  - Prevent complications → frequent oral care and turning
  - Sedation and pain control
  - Manage weaning process/schedule
  - Pre-/postextubation assessments/care

Clinical Alert:
! • After extended use of analgesics/sedative → monitor for withdrawal sx
- Use suction/gastric tubes to prevent aspiration in the intubated child
- Managing the endotracheal tube is a care priority for the ventilated child
- Use minimal amount of blood for samples
- Hypotension is a late, ominous sign of hypoperfusion

Nursing Management/Care:
- Thorough hemodynamic assessment using hemodynamic ranges for age
- Manage fluid status/fluid resuscitation
- Titrate vasoactive medications
- Manage invasive monitoring equipment
  - setup, positioning, zeroing, waveforms, response to data
- Interpret results of blood sampling
- Prevent complications (e.g., arrhythmias, air/thromboembolism, infection)
- Ongoing holistic support of child/family

Critical Nursing Action:
- Promote family-centered care when child is admitted to a critical care unit

Legal Alert:
☑ • Law protects providers who administer unwanted blood in life-threatening scenarios

Optimizing Outcomes:
◆ • Early recognition/treatment of cardiac arrest increases survival rate for critically ill children

Where Research and Practice Meet:
- Use evidence-based nursing practice guidelines to decrease CLABSIs

Now Can You:
? • Provide safe, quality, evidence-based, and holistic care for the critically ill child and family

appendix A

Centigrade to Fahrenheit Temperature Conversions

Conversion Formulas	
°F = (°C × 9/5) + 32, or (°C × 1.8) + 32	
°C = (°F – 32) × 5/9, or (°F – 32) × 0.55	
°C	**°F**
35.0	95.0
35.2	95.4
35.4	95.7
35.6	96.1
35.8	96.4
36.0	96.8
36.2	97.2
36.4	97.5
36.6	97.9
36.8	98.2
37.0	98.6
37.2	99.0
37.4	99.3
37.6	99.7
37.8	100.0
38.0	100.4
38.2	100.8
38.4	101.1
38.6	101.5
38.8	101.8
39.0	102.2
39.2	102.6
39.4	102.9
39.6	103.3
39.8	103.6
40.0	104.0
40.2	104.4
40.4	104.7
40.6	105.1
40.8	105.4

Expected Temperatures in Children

Age	Fahrenheit (°F)	Centigrade (°C)
2 months	99.4	37.5
4 months	99.5	37.5
1 years	99.7	37.7
2 years	99.0	37.2
4 years	98.6	37.0
6 years	98.3	36.8
8 years	98.1	36.7
10 years	98.0	36.7
12 years	97.8	36.6

Photo and Illustration Credits

NURSING CARE PLANS

NIC and NOC information. Bulechek et al. (2009) *Nursing interventions clinical skills*, (5th ed.). St. Louis, MO: Elsevier; Moorhead et al. (2009). *Nursing outcomes classification*, (4th ed.). St. Louis, MO: Elsevier.

CHAPTER 2

Figure 2-1 Courtesy of Public Health Practice, St. Cloud, MN.

CHAPTER 3

Figure 3-1 Courtesy of Family Ties Project, Washington, DC. Life Planning for Families Affected by HIV/AIDS.

CHAPTER 4

Figure 4-1 Centers for Disease Control and Prevention, 2014.

Figure 4-2 Centers for Disease Control and Prevention, 2014.

Figure 4-3 United States Department of Agriculture, www.ChooseMyPlate.gov

Figure 4-4 Dillon, P. (2007). *Nursing health assessment: A critical thinking, case studies approach* (2nd ed., p. 612). Philadelphia, PA: F.A. Davis.

Figure 4-5 Dillon, P. (2007). *Nursing health assessment: A critical thinking, case studies approach* (2nd ed., p. 631). Philadelphia, PA: F.A. Davis.

Figure 4-6 Dillon, P. (2007). *Nursing health assessment: A critical thinking, case studies approach* (2nd ed., p. 634). Philadelphia, PA: F.A. Davis.

Figure 4-7 Dillon, P. (2007). *Nursing health assessment: A critical thinking, case studies approach* (2nd ed., p. 635). Philadelphia, PA: F.A. Davis.

Figure 4-8 Dillon, P. (2007). *Nursing health assessment: A critical thinking, case studies approach* (2nd ed., p. 640). Philadelphia, PA: F.A. Davis.

Figure 4-9 Dillon, P. (2007). *Nursing health assessment: A critical thinking, case studies approach* (2nd ed., p. 641). Philadelphia, PA: F.A. Davis.

Figure 4-10 Dillon, P. (2007). *Nursing health assessment: A critical thinking, case studies approach* (2nd ed., p. 641). Philadelphia, PA: F.A. Davis.

Figure 4-11 Dillon, P. (2007). *Nursing health assessment: A critical thinking, case studies approach* (2nd ed., p. 642). Philadelphia, PA: F.A. Davis.

Figure 4-12 Dillon, P. (2007). *Nursing health assessment: A critical thinking, case studies approach* (2nd ed., p. 642). Philadelphia, PA: F.A. Davis.

Figure 4-13 Dillon, P. (2007). *Nursing health assessment: A critical thinking, case studies approach* (2nd ed., p. 642). Philadelphia, PA: F.A. Davis.

Figure 4-14 The Nemours Foundation. (2012). *How to perform a testicular self-examination*. Retrieved from http://www.kidshealth.org/teen/sexual_health/guys/tse.html

Breast Self-Examination, Step 6. Venes, D. (2013). *Taber's cyclopedic medical dictionary* (22nd ed., p. 332). Philadelphia, PA: F.A. Davis.

CHAPTER 5

Figure 5-1 Dillon, P. (2007). *Nursing health assessment: A critical thinking, case studies approach* (2nd ed., p. 612). Philadelphia, PA: F.A. Davis.

Figure 5-2 Dillon, P. (2007). *Nursing health assessment: A critical thinking, case studies approach* (2nd ed., p. 612). Philadelphia, PA: F.A. Davis.

Figure 5-3 Dillon, P. (2007). *Nursing health assessment: A critical thinking, case studies approach* (2nd ed., p. 613). Philadelphia, PA: F.A. Davis.

Figure 5-4 Scanlon, V., & Sanders, T. (2015). *Essentials of anatomy and physiology* (7th ed., p. 502). Philadelphia, PA: F.A. Davis.

Figure 5-6 Scanlon, V., & Sanders, T. (2015). *Essentials of anatomy and physiology* (7th ed., p. 508). Philadelphia, PA: F.A. Davis.

Figure 5-7 Scanlon, V., & Sanders, T. (2015). *Essentials of anatomy and physiology* (7th ed., p. 509). Philadelphia, PA: F.A. Davis.

Figure 5-13 Scanlon, V., & Sanders, T. (2015). *Essentials of anatomy and physiology* (7th ed., p. 512). Philadelphia, PA: F.A. Davis.

Figure 5-14 Dillon, P. (2007). *Nursing health assessment: A critical thinking, case studies approach* (2nd ed., p. 613). Philadelphia, PA: F.A. Davis.

Figure 5-16 Dillon, P. (2007). *Nursing health assessment: A critical thinking, case studies approach* (2nd ed., p. 617). Philadelphia, PA: F.A. Davis.

Figure 5-19 Scanlon, V., & Sanders, T. (2015). *Essentials of anatomy and physiology* (7th ed., p. 503). Philadelphia, PA: F.A. Davis.

Figure 5-20 Scanlon, V., & Sanders, T. (2015). *Essentials of anatomy and physiology* (7th ed., p. 504). Philadelphia, PA: F.A. Davis.

Figure 5-21 Scanlon, V., & Sanders, T. (2015). *Essentials of anatomy and physiology* (7th ed., p. 501). Philadelphia, PA: F.A. Davis.

CHAPTER 6

Figure 6-2 Hatcher, R. A., et al. (2005). *A pocket guide to managing contraception.* Tiger, GA: Bridging the Gap Foundation.

CHAPTER 7

Figure 7-1 Courtesy of National Human Genome Research Institute, Bethesda, MD.

Figure 7-2 Scanlon, V., & Sanders, T. (2015). *Essentials of anatomy and physiology* (7th ed., p. 535). Philadelphia, PA: F.A. Davis.

Figure 7-3 Scanlon, V., & Sanders, T. (2015). *Essentials of anatomy and physiology* (7th ed., p. 522). Philadelphia, PA: F.A. Davis.

Figure 7-5 Scanlon, V., & Sanders, T. (2015). *Essentials of anatomy and physiology* (7th ed., p. 536). Philadelphia, PA: F.A. Davis.

Figure 7-7 Scanlon, V., & Sanders, T. (2015). *Essentials of anatomy and physiology* (7th ed., p. 539). Philadelphia, PA: F.A. Davis.

Figure 7-8 Scanlon, V., & Sanders, T. (2015). *Essentials of anatomy and physiology* (7th ed., p. 523). Philadelphia, PA: F.A. Davis.

Figure 7-9 Scanlon, V., & Sanders, T. (2015). *Essentials of anatomy and physiology* (7th ed., p. 531). Philadelphia, PA: F.A. Davis.

Figure 7-10 Scanlon, V., & Sanders, T. (2015). *Essentials of anatomy and physiology* (7th ed., p. 525). Philadelphia, PA: F.A. Davis.

Figure 7-12 Polan, E. U., & Taylor, D. R. (2007). *Journey across the life span: Human development and health promotion* (3rd ed., p. 77). Philadelphia, PA: F.A. Davis.

Figure 7-13 Polan, E. U., & Taylor, D. R. (2007). *Journey across the life span: Human development and health promotion* (3rd ed., p. 77). Philadelphia, PA: F.A. Davis.

Figure 7-14 Courtesy of National Human Genome Research Institute, National Institutes of Health, Bethesda, MD.

Figure 7-15 Courtesy of National Human Genome Research Institute, National Institutes of Health, Bethesda, MD.

Figure 7-16 Courtesy of National Human Genome Research Institute, National Institutes of Health, Bethesda, MD.

Figure 7-18 Venes, D. (2005). *Taber's cyclopedic medical dictionary* (20th ed., p. 1165). Philadelphia, PA: F.A. Davis.

CHAPTER 8

Figure 8-4 Dillon, P. (2007). *Nursing health assessment: A critical thinking, case studies approach* (2nd ed., p. 840). Philadelphia, PA: F.A. Davis.

Figure 8-6 Chapman, L., & Durham, R. (2009). *Maternal-newborn nursing: The critical components of nursing care* (1st ed., p. 49). Philadelphia, PA: F.A. Davis.

Figure 8-7 Venes, D. (2009). *Taber's cyclopedic medical dictionary* (21st ed., p. 432). Philadelphia, PA: F.A. Davis.

Figure 8-8 Chapman, L., & Durham, R. (2009). *Maternal-newborn nursing: The critical components of nursing care* (1st ed., p. 49). Philadelphia, PA: F.A. Davis.

Figure 8-9 Dillon, P. (2007). *Nursing health assessment: A critical thinking, case studies approach* (2nd ed., p. 834). Philadelphia, PA: F.A. Davis.

Figure 8-12 Dillon, P. (2007). *Nursing health assessment: A critical thinking, case studies approach* (2nd ed., p. 834). Philadelphia, PA: F.A. Davis.

Figure 8-15 Chapman, L., & Durham, R. (2009). *Maternal-newborn nursing: The critical components of nursing care* (1st ed., p. 69). Philadelphia, PA: F.A. Davis.

Figure 8-16 Chapman, L., & Durham, R. (2009). *Maternal-newborn nursing: The critical components of nursing care* (1st ed., p. 62). Philadelphia, PA: F.A. Davis.

CHAPTER 9

Figure 9-4 Dillon, P. (2007). *Nursing health assessment: A critical thinking, case studies approach* (2nd ed., p. 833). Philadelphia, PA: F.A. Davis.

Figure 9-5 Dillon, P. (2007). *Nursing health assessment: A critical thinking, case studies approach* (2nd ed., p. 836). Philadelphia, PA: F.A. Davis.

Figure 9-6 Dillon, P. (2007). *Nursing health assessment: A critical thinking, case studies approach* (2nd ed., p. 836). Philadelphia, PA: F.A. Davis.

Figure 9-7 Dillon, P. (2007). *Nursing health assessment: A critical thinking, case studies approach* (2nd ed., p. 837). Philadelphia, PA: F.A. Davis.

Figure 9-8 Dillon, P. (2007). *Nursing health assessment: A critical thinking, case studies approach* (2nd ed., p. 837). Philadelphia, PA: F.A. Davis.

Figure 9-9 Dillon, P. (2007). *Nursing health assessment: A critical thinking, case studies approach* (2nd ed., p. 837). Philadelphia, PA: F.A. Davis.

Figure 9-10*AB* Dillon, P. (2007). *Nursing health assessment: A critical thinking, case studies approach* (2nd ed., p. 631). Philadelphia, PA: F.A. Davis.

Figure 9-11*A–D* Dillon, P. (2007). *Nursing health assessment: A critical thinking, case studies approach* (2nd ed., p. 635). Philadelphia, PA: F.A. Davis.

Figure 9-12*AB* Dillon, P. (2007). *Nursing health assessment: A critical thinking, case studies approach* (2nd ed., p. 840). Philadelphia, PA: F.A. Davis.

Figure 9-13*AB* Dillon, P. (2007). *Nursing health assessment: A critical thinking, case studies approach* (2nd ed., p. 641). Philadelphia, PA: F.A. Davis

Procedure 9-2 Performing Leopold Maneuvers 1–4 Venes, D. (2009). *Taber's cyclopedic medical dictionary* (21st ed., p. 1319). Philadelphia, PA: F.A. Davis.

CHAPTER 10

Figure 10-2 Copyright 2001, The Dr. Spock Company.

Figure 10-8 Chapman, L., & Durham, R. (2009). *Maternal-newborn nursing: The critical components of nursing care* (1st ed., p. 90). Philadelphia, PA: F.A. Davis.

Figure 10-9 Courtesy of Indiana Perinatal Network.

CHAPTER 11

Figure 11-1 Venes, D. (2005). *Taber's cyclopedic medical dictionary* (20th ed., p. 1757). Philadelphia, PA: F.A. Davis.

Figure 11-3 Wedding, M. S., & Toenjes, S. A. (1998). *Medical laboratory procedures* (2nd ed., p. 57). Philadelphia, PA: F.A. Davis.

Figure 11-4 Chapman, L., & Durham, R. (2009). *Maternal-newborn nursing: The critical components of nursing care* (1st ed., p. 107). Philadelphia, PA: F.A. Davis.

Figure 11-5 Holloway, B., Moredich, C., & Aduddell, K. (2006). *OB peds women's health notes: Nurse's clinical pocket guide* (p. 43). Philadelphia, PA: F.A. Davis.

Figure 11-6 Holloway, B., Moredich, C., & Aduddell, K. (2006). *OB peds women's health notes: Nurse's clinical pocket guide* (p. 45). Philadelphia, PA: F.A. Davis.

Figure 11-8 Gilbert, E. S., & Harmon, J. S. (2003). *Manual of high risk pregnancy and delivery* (3rd ed., p. 562). St. Louis, MO: Mosby.

Figure 11-9 Chapman, L., & Durham, R. (2009). *Maternal-newborn nursing: The critical components of nursing care* (1st ed., p. 105). Philadelphia, PA: F.A. Davis.

Figure 11-10 Chapman, L., & Durham, R. (2009). *Maternal-newborn nursing: The critical components of nursing care* (1st ed., p. 115). Philadelphia, PA: F.A. Davis.

Figure 11-11 Dillon, P. (2007). *Nursing health assessment: A critical thinking, case studies approach* (2nd ed., p. 785). Philadelphia, PA: F.A. Davis.

Figure 11-12 Scanlon, V., & Sanders, T. (2007). *Essentials of anatomy and physiology* (5th ed., p. 491). Philadelphia, PA: F.A. Davis.

Figure 11-13 Scanlon, V., & Sanders, T. (2007). *Essentials of anatomy and physiology* (5th ed., p. 59). Philadelphia, PA: F.A. Davis.

Figure 11-15 Chapman, L., & Durham, R. (2009). *Maternal-newborn nursing: The critical components of nursing care* (1st ed., p. 110). Philadelphia, PA: F.A. Davis.

Figure 11-16 Chapman, L., & Durham, R. (2009). *Maternal-newborn nursing: The critical components of nursing care* (1st ed., p. 94). Philadelphia, PA: F.A. Davis.

Figure 11-17 Chapman, L., & Durham, R. (2009). *Maternal-newborn nursing: The critical components of nursing care* (1st ed., p. 94). Philadelphia, PA: F.A. Davis.

Figure 11-19 Chapman, L., & Durham, R. (2009). *Maternal-newborn nursing: The critical components of nursing care* (1st ed., p. 92). Philadelphia, PA: F.A. Davis.

Figure 11-20 Chapman, L., & Durham, R. (2009). *Maternal-newborn nursing: The critical components of nursing care* (1st ed., p. 96). Philadelphia, PA: F.A. Davis.

Figure 11-21 Chapman, L., & Durham, R. (2009). *Maternal-newborn nursing: The critical components of nursing care* (1st ed., p. 96). Philadelphia, PA: F.A. Davis.

CHAPTER 12

Figure 12-1 Holloway, B., Moredich, C., & Aduddell, K. (2006). *OB peds women's health notes: Nurse's clinical pocket guide* (p. 63). Philadelphia, PA: F.A. Davis.

Figure 12-7D Chapman, L., & Durham, R. (2009). *Maternal-newborn nursing: The critical components of nursing care* (1st ed., p. 202). Philadelphia, PA: F.A. Davis.

Figure 12-9 Holloway, B., Moredich, C., & Aduddell, K. (2006). *OB peds women's health notes: Nurse's clinical pocket guide* (p. 53). Philadelphia, PA: F.A. Davis.

Figure 12-11 Chapman, L., & Durham, R. (2009). *Maternal-newborn nursing: The critical components of nursing care* (1st ed., p. 155). Philadelphia, PA: F.A. Davis.

Figure 12-12 Chapman, L., & Durham, R. (2009). *Maternal-newborn nursing: The critical components of nursing care* (1st ed., p. 157). Philadelphia, PA: F.A. Davis.

Figure 12-15 Chapman, L., & Durham, R. (2009). *Maternal-newborn nursing: The critical components of nursing care* (1st ed., p. 149). Philadelphia, PA: F.A. Davis.

Figure 12-16 Chapman, L., & Durham, R. (2009). *Maternal-newborn nursing: The critical components of nursing care* (1st ed., p. 149). Philadelphia, PA: F.A. Davis.

Figure 12-17 Dillon, P. (2007). *Nursing health assessment: A critical thinking, case studies approach* (2nd ed., p. 837). Philadelphia, PA: F.A. Davis.

Figure 12-18 Holloway, B., Moredich, C., & Aduddell, K. (2006). *OB peds women's health notes: Nurse's clinical pocket guide* (1st ed., p. 55.) Philadelphia, PA: F.A. Davis.

Figure 12-19 Holloway, B., Moredich, C., & Aduddell, K. (2006). *OB peds women's health notes: Nurse's clinical pocket guide* (1st ed., p. 56). Philadelphia, PA: F.A. Davis.

Figure 12-20 Holloway, B., Moredich, C., & Aduddell, K. (2006). *OB peds women's health notes: Nurse's clinical pocket guide* (1st ed., p. 57). Philadelphia, PA: F.A. Davis.

Figure 12-21 Chapman, L., & Durham, R. (2009). *Maternal-newborn nursing: The critical components of nursing care* (1st ed., p. 186). Philadelphia, PA: F.A. Davis.

Figure 12-22 Chapman, L., & Durham, R. (2009). *Maternal-newborn nursing: The critical components of nursing care* (1st ed., p. 187). Philadelphia, PA: F.A. Davis.

Figure 12-23 Chapman, L., & Durham, R. (2009). *Maternal-newborn nursing: The critical components of nursing care* (1st ed., p. 193). Philadelphia, PA: F.A. Davis.

Figure 12-24 Chapman, L., & Durham, R. (2009). *Maternal-newborn nursing: The critical components of nursing care* (1st ed., p. 186). Philadelphia, PA: F.A. Davis.

Figure 12-25 Chapman, L., & Durham, R. (2009). *Maternal-newborn nursing: The critical components of nursing care* (1st ed., p. 186). Philadelphia, PA: F.A. Davis.

Figure 12-26 Chapman, L., & Durham, R. (2009). *Maternal-newborn nursing: The critical components of nursing care* (1st ed., p. 186). Philadelphia, PA: F.A. Davis.

Figure 12-27 Chapman, L., & Durham, R. (2009). *Maternal-newborn nursing: The critical components of nursing care* (1st ed., p. 186). Philadelphia, PA: F.A. Davis.

Figure 12-29 Chapman, L., & Durham, R. (2009). *Maternal-newborn nursing: The critical components of nursing care* (1st ed., p. 189). Philadelphia, PA: F.A. Davis.

Figure 12-32 Chapman, L., & Durham, R. (2009). *Maternal-newborn nursing: The critical components of nursing care* (1st ed., p. 191). Philadelphia, PA: F.A. Davis.

Figure 12-33 Chapman, L., & Durham, R. (2009). *Maternal-newborn nursing: The critical components of nursing care* (1st ed., p. 192). Philadelphia, PA: F.A. Davis.

Figure 12-34 Chapman, L., & Durham, R. (2009). *Maternal-newborn nursing: The critical components of nursing care* (1st ed., p. 182). Philadelphia, PA: F.A. Davis.

Figure 12-35 Chapman, L., & Durham, R. (2009). *Maternal-newborn nursing: The critical components of nursing care* (1st ed., p. 194). Philadelphia, PA: F.A. Davis.

Figure 12-37 Chapman, L., & Durham, R. (2009). *Maternal-newborn nursing: The critical components of nursing care* (1st ed., p. 162). Philadelphia, PA: F.A. Davis.

Figure 12-42 Chapman, L., & Durham, R. (2009). *Maternal-newborn nursing: The critical components of nursing care* (1st ed., p. 163). Philadelphia, PA: F.A. Davis.

Figure 12-45 Chapman, L., & Durham, R. (2009). *Maternal-newborn nursing: The critical components of nursing care* (1st ed., p. 164). Philadelphia, PA: F.A. Davis.

CHAPTER 13

Figure 13-5 Chapman, L., & Durham, R. (2009). *Maternal-newborn nursing: The critical components of nursing care* (1st ed., p. 167). Philadelphia, PA: F.A. Davis.

CHAPTER 14

Figure 14-1A–C Chapman, L., & Durham, R. (2009). *Maternal-newborn nursing: The critical components of nursing care* (1st ed., p. 198). Philadelphia, PA: F.A. Davis.

Figure 14-2 Chapman, L., & Durham, R. (2009). *Maternal-newborn nursing: The critical components of nursing care* (1st ed., p. 199). Philadelphia, PA: F.A. Davis.

Figure 14-3 Chapman, L., & Durham, R. (2009). *Maternal-newborn nursing: The critical components of nursing care* (1st ed., p. 208). Philadelphia, PA: F.A. Davis.

Figure 14-4 Chapman, L., & Durham, R. (2009). *Maternal-newborn nursing: The critical components of nursing care* (1st ed., p. 205). Philadelphia, PA: F.A. Davis.

Figure 14-6 Chapman, L., & Durham, R. (2009). *Maternal-newborn nursing: The critical components of nursing care* (1st ed., p. 209). Philadelphia, PA: F.A. Davis.

Figure 14-16 Chapman, L., & Durham, R. (2009). *Maternal-newborn nursing: The critical components of nursing care* (1st ed., p. 211). Philadelphia, PA: F.A. Davis.

Figure 14-17 Chapman, L., & Durham, R. (2009). *Maternal-newborn nursing: The critical components of nursing care* (1st ed., p. 223). Philadelphia, PA: F.A. Davis.

Figure 14-18 Chapman, L., & Durham, R. (2009). *Maternal-newborn nursing: The critical components of nursing care* (1st ed., p. 226). Philadelphia, PA: F.A. Davis.

Figure 14-19 Chapman, L., & Durham, R. (2009). *Maternal-newborn nursing: The critical components of nursing care* (1st ed., p. 213). Philadelphia, PA: F.A. Davis.

CHAPTER 15

Figure 15-1 Chapman, L., & Durham, R. (2009). *Maternal-newborn nursing: The critical components of nursing care* (1st ed., p. 252). Philadelphia, PA: F.A. Davis.

Figure 15-2 Scanlon, V., & Sanders, T. (2007). *Essentials of anatomy and physiology* (5th ed., p. 467). Philadelphia: F.A. Davis.

Figure 15-3 Holloway, B., Moredich, C., & Aduddell, K. (2006). *OB peds women's health notes: Nurse's clinical pocket guide* (p. 83). Philadelphia, PA: F.A. Davis.

Figure 15-4 Chapman, L., & Durham, R. (2009). *Maternal-newborn nursing: The critical components of nursing care* (1st ed., p. 234). Philadelphia, PA: F.A. Davis.

Figure 15-5 Dillon, P. (2007). *Nursing health assessment: A critical thinking, case studies approach* (2nd ed., p. 844). Philadelphia, PA: F.A. Davis.

Figure 15-7 Chapman, L., & Durham, R. (2009). *Maternal-newborn nursing: The critical components of nursing care* (1st ed., p. 240). Philadelphia, PA: F.A. Davis.

Figure 15-12 Courtesy of Medela Corporation, McHenry, IL.

Figure 15-13 Courtesy of Medela Corporation, McHenry, IL.

Figure 15-14 Chapman, L., & Durham, R. (2009). *Maternal-newborn nursing: The critical components of nursing care* (1st ed., p. 316). Philadelphia, PA: F.A. Davis.

Figure 15-15 Courtesy of Medela Corporation, McHenry, IL.

Figure 15-16 Chapman, L., & Durham, R. (2009). *Maternal-newborn nursing: The critical components of nursing care* (1st ed., p. 321). Philadelphia, PA: F.A. Davis.

Figure 15-18 Chapman, L., & Durham, R. (2009). *Maternal-newborn nursing: The critical components of nursing care* (1st ed., p. 257). Philadelphia, PA: F.A. Davis.

Figure 15-19 Chapman, L., & Durham, R. (2009). *Maternal-newborn nursing: The critical components of nursing care* (1st ed., p. 258). Philadelphia, PA: F.A. Davis.

Figure 15-20 Chapman, L., & Durham, R. (2009). *Maternal-newborn nursing: The critical components of nursing care* (1st ed., p. 258). Philadelphia, PA: F.A. Davis.

Figure 15-22 Chapman, L., & Durham, R. (2009). *Maternal-newborn nursing: The critical components of nursing care* (1st ed., p. 261). Philadelphia, PA: F.A. Davis.

CHAPTER 16

Figure in Procedure 16-1. Holloway, B., Moredich, C., & Aduddell, K. (2006). *OB peds women's health notes: Nurse's clinical pocket guide* (1st ed., p. 83). Philadelphia, PA: F.A. Davis.

CHAPTER 17

Figure 17-5 Chapman, L., & Durham, R. (2009). *Maternal-newborn nursing: The critical components of nursing care* (1st ed., p. 341). Philadelphia, PA: F.A. Davis.

Figure 17-9 Chapman, L., & Durham, R. (2009). *Maternal-newborn nursing: The critical components of nursing care* (1st ed., p. 348). Philadelphia, PA: F.A. Davis.

Figure 17-11 Chapman, L., & Durham, R. (2009). *Maternal-newborn nursing: The critical components of nursing care* (1st ed., p. 338). Philadelphia, PA: F.A. Davis.

Figure 17-12 Chapman, L., & Durham, R. (2009). *Maternal-newborn nursing: The critical components of nursing care* (1st ed., p. 351). Philadelphia, PA: F.A. Davis.

CHAPTER 18

Figure 18-1 Chapman, L., & Durham, R. (2009). *Maternal-newborn nursing: The critical components of nursing care* (1st ed., p. 323). Philadelphia, PA: F.A. Davis.

Figure 18-2 Chapman, L., & Durham, R. (2009). *Maternal-newborn nursing: The critical components of nursing care* (1st ed., p. 306). Philadelphia, PA: F.A. Davis.

Figure 18-4 Chapman, L., & Durham, R. (2009). *Maternal-newborn nursing: The critical components of nursing care* (1st ed., p. 326). Philadelphia, PA: F.A. Davis.

Figure 18-5 Chapman, L., & Durham, R. (2009). *Maternal-newborn nursing: The critical components of nursing care* (1st ed., p. 296). Philadelphia, PA: F.A. Davis.

Figure 18-6 Chapman, L., & Durham, R. (2009). *Maternal-newborn nursing: The critical components of nursing care* (1st ed., p. 294). Philadelphia, PA: F.A. Davis.

Figure 18-7 Chapman, L., & Durham, R. (2009). *Maternal-newborn nursing: The critical components of nursing care* (1st ed., p. 287). Philadelphia, PA: F.A. Davis.

Figure 18-8 Dillon, P. (2007). *Nursing health assessment: A critical thinking, case studies approach* (2nd ed., p. 857). Philadelphia, PA: F.A. Davis.

Figure 18-9 Dillon, P. (2007). *Nursing health assessment: A critical thinking, case studies approach* (2nd ed., p. 856). Philadelphia, PA: F.A. Davis.

Figure 18-10 Dillon, P. (2007). *Nursing health assessment: A critical thinking, case studies approach* (2nd ed., p. 856). Philadelphia, PA: F.A. Davis.

Figure 18-11 Dillon, P. (2007). *Nursing health assessment: A critical thinking, case studies approach* (2nd ed., p. 857). Philadelphia, PA: F.A. Davis.

Figure 18-12 Courtesy of Mead Johnson Nutritionals.

Figure 18-13 Courtesy of Mead Johnson Nutritionals.

Figure 18-14 Chapman, L., & Durham, R. (2009). *Maternal-newborn nursing: The critical components of nursing care* (1st ed., p. 295). Philadelphia, PA: F.A. Davis.

Figure 18-15 Chapman, L., & Durham, R. (2009). *Maternal-newborn nursing: The critical components of nursing care* (1st ed., p. 295). Philadelphia, PA: F.A. Davis.

Figure 18-16 Chapman, L., & Durham, R. (2009). *Maternal-newborn nursing: The critical components of nursing care* (1st ed., p. 295). Philadelphia, PA: F.A. Davis.

Figure 18-18 Dillon, P. (2007). *Nursing health assessment: A critical thinking, case studies approach* (2nd ed., p. 859). Philadelphia, PA: F.A. Davis.

Figure 18-19 Dillon, P. (2007). *Nursing health assessment: A critical thinking, case studies approach* (2nd ed., p. 861). Philadelphia, PA: F.A. Davis.

Figure 18-20 Dillon, P. (2007). *Nursing health assessment: A critical thinking, case studies approach* (2nd ed., p. 860). Philadelphia, PA: F.A. Davis.

Figure 18-21 Dillon, P. (2007). *Nursing health assessment: A critical thinking, case studies approach* (2nd ed., p. 860). Philadelphia, PA: F.A. Davis.

Figure 18-23 Dillon, P. (2007). *Nursing health assessment: A critical thinking, case studies approach* (2nd ed., p. 861) Philadelphia, PA: F.A. Davis.

Figure 18-24 Dillon, P. (2007). *Nursing health assessment: A critical thinking, case studies approach* (2nd ed., p. 862). Philadelphia, PA: F.A. Davis.

Figure 18-25 Chapman, L., & Durham, R. (2009). *Maternal-newborn nursing: The critical components of nursing care* (1st ed., p. 290). Philadelphia, PA: F.A. Davis.

Figure 18-26 Chapman, L., & Durham, R. (2009). *Maternal-newborn nursing: The critical components of nursing care* (1st ed., p. 306). Philadelphia, PA: F.A. Davis.

Figure 18-27 Dillon, P. (2007). *Nursing health assessment: A critical thinking, case studies approach* (2nd ed., p. 863). Philadelphia, PA: F.A. Davis.

Figure 18-28 Dillon, P. (2007). *Nursing health assessment: A critical thinking, case studies approach* (2nd ed., p. 864). Philadelphia, PA: F.A. Davis.

Figure 18-29 Dillon, P. (2007). *Nursing health assessment: A critical thinking, case studies approach* (2nd ed., p. 864). Philadelphia, PA: F.A. Davis.

Figure 18-30 Chapman, L., & Durham, R. (2009). *Maternal-newborn nursing: The critical components of nursing care* (1st ed., p. 292). Philadelphia, PA: F.A. Davis.

Figure 18-31 Dillon, P. (2007). *Nursing health assessment: A critical thinking, case studies approach* (2nd ed., p. 864). Philadelphia, PA: F.A. Davis.

Figure 18-32 Dillon, P. (2007). *Nursing health assessment: A critical thinking, case studies approach* (2nd ed., p. 865). Philadelphia, PA: F.A. Davis.

Figure 18-33 Chapman, L., & Durham, R. (2009). *Maternal-newborn nursing: The critical components of nursing care* (1st ed., p. 292). Philadelphia, PA: F.A. Davis.

Figure 18-34 Dillon, P. (2007). *Nursing health assessment: A critical thinking, case studies approach* (2nd ed., p. 873). Philadelphia, PA: F.A. Davis.

Figure 18-35 Dillon, P. (2007). *Nursing health assessment: A critical thinking, case studies approach* (2nd ed., p. 866). Philadelphia, PA: F.A. Davis.

Figure 18-37 Chapman, L., & Durham, R. (2009). *Maternal-newborn nursing: The critical components of nursing care* (1st ed., p. 323). Philadelphia, PA: F.A. Davis.

Figure 18-38 Chapman, L., & Durham, R. (2009). *Maternal-newborn nursing: The critical components of nursing care* (1st ed., p. 328). Philadelphia, PA: F.A. Davis.

Figure 18-39 Chapman, L., & Durham, R. (2009). *Maternal-newborn nursing: The critical components of nursing care* (1st ed., p. 324). Philadelphia, PA: F.A. Davis.

Procedure 18-3, first photo Dillon, P. (2007). *Nursing health assessment: A critical thinking, case studies approach* (2nd ed., p. 866). Philadelphia, PA: F.A. Davis.

Procedure 18-3, second photo Dillon, P. (2007). *Nursing health assessment: A critical thinking, case studies approach* (2nd ed., p. 866). Philadelphia, PA: F.A. Davis.

Procedure 18-3, third photo Dillon, P. (2007). *Nursing health assessment: A critical thinking, case studies approach* (2nd ed., p. 866). Philadelphia, PA: F.A. Davis.

Table 18-2 Palmar grasp Dillon, P. (2007). *Nursing health assessment: A critical thinking, case studies approach* (2nd ed., p. 866). Philadelphia, PA: F.A. Davis.

Table 18-2 Toe or plantar grasp. Dillon, P. (2007). *Nursing health assessment: A critical thinking, case studies approach* (2nd ed., p. 866). Philadelphia, PA: F.A. Davis.

Table 18-2 Rooting or sucking reflex. Dillon, P. (2007). *Nursing health assessment: A critical thinking, case studies approach* (2nd ed., p. 871). Philadelphia, PA: F.A. Davis.

Table 18-2 Extrusion reflex. Dillon, P. (2007). *Nursing health assessment: A critical thinking, case studies approach* (2nd ed., p. 871). Philadelphia, PA: F.A. Davis.

Table 18-2 Stepping reflex. Dillon, P. (2007). *Nursing health assessment: A critical thinking, case studies approach* (2nd ed., p. 870). Philadelphia, PA: F.A. Davis.

Table 18-2 Tonic neck or flexing reflex. Dillon, P. (2007). *Nursing health assessment: A critical thinking, case studies approach* (2nd ed., p. 868). Philadelphia, PA: F.A. Davis.

Table 18-2 Glabellar reflex. Dillon, P. (2007). *Nursing health assessment: A critical thinking, case studies approach* (2nd ed., p. 872). Philadelphia, PA: F.A. Davis.

Table 18-2 Babinski reflex. Dillon, P. (2007). *Nursing health assessment: A critical thinking, case studies approach* (2nd ed., p. 869). Philadelphia, PA: F.A. Davis.

Table 18-2 Moro reflex. Dillon, P. (2007). *Nursing health assessment: A critical thinking, case studies approach* (2nd ed., p. 868). Philadelphia, PA: F.A. Davis.

Table 18-2 Magnet reflex. Dillon, P. (2007). *Nursing health assessment: A critical thinking, case studies approach* (2nd ed., p. 873). Philadelphia, PA: F.A. Davis.

Table 18-2 Galant reflex or trunk incurvation reflex. Dillon, P. (2007). *Nursing health assessment: A critical thinking, case studies approach* (2nd ed., p. 873). Philadelphia, PA: F.A. Davis.

Table 18-2 Crawling reflex. Dillon, P. (2007). *Nursing health assessment: A critical thinking, case studies approach* (2nd ed., p. 872). Philadelphia, PA: F.A. Davis.

Table 18-2 Crossed extension. Dillon, P. (2007). *Nursing health assessment: A critical thinking, case studies approach* (2nd ed., p. 872). Philadelphia, PA: F.A. Davis.

CHAPTER 19

Figure 19-2 Courtesy of McLeod Regional Medical Center, Florence, SC.

Figure 19-3 Courtesy of St. Luke's University, Bethlehem, PA.

Figure 19-5 Courtesy of McLeod Regional Medical Center, Florence, SC.

Figure 19-6 Courtesy of McLeod Regional Medical Center Florence, SC.

Figure 19-7 Stevens, B., Johnston, C., Petryshen, P., & Taddio, A. (1996). Premature infant pain profile: Development and initial validation. *Clinical Journal of Pain, 12*(1), 13–22.

Figure 19-8 Courtesy of St. Luke's Hospital, Bethlehem, PA.

Figure 19-9 Courtesy of St. Luke's Hospital, Bethlehem, PA.

Figure 19-10 Courtesy of William A. Silverman, MD.

Figure 19-11 Courtesy of McLeod Regional Medical Center, Florence, SC.

Figure 19-12 Courtesy of St. Luke's Hospital, Bethlehem, PA.

Figure 19-13 Courtesy of St. Luke's Hospital, Bethlehem, PA.

Figure 19-15 Courtesy of St. Luke's Hospital, Bethlehem, PA.

Figure 19-18 Courtesy of McLeod Regional Medical Center, Florence, SC.

CHAPTER 21

Figure 21-2 Dillon, P. (2007). *Nursing health assessment: A critical thinking, case studies approach* (2nd ed., p. 856). Philadelphia, PA: F.A. Davis.

Figure 21-9 *Wong's essentials of pediatric nursing* (6th ed). St. Louis, MO: Mosby. Copyright by Mosby, Inc.

Figure 21-23 Chapman, L., & Durham, R. (2013). *Maternal-newborn nursing: The critical components of nursing care* (2nd ed., p. 433). Philadelphia, PA: F.A. Davis.

CHAPTER 23

Figure 23-1 Dillon, P. (2007). *Nursing health assessment: A critical thinking, case studies approach* (2nd ed., p. 394). Philadelphia, PA: F.A. Davis.

Figure 23-10 *Asthma Action Plan* used with permission. © 2012 American Lung Association, www.lung.org

Collaboration in Caring: Heimlich maneuver, back blows. Hopkins, T., & Myers, E. (2007). *Medical surgical notes* (2nd ed., p. 168). Philadelphia, PA: F.A. Davis.

Collaboration in Caring: Heimlich maneuver, chest thrusts. Hopkins, T., & Myers, E. (2007). *Medical surgical notes* (2nd ed., p. 168). Philadelphia, PA: F.A. Davis.

CHAPTER 24

Figure 24-1 Jones, S. (2009). *Pocket anatomy and physiology* (1st ed., p. 184). Philadelphia, PA: F.A. Davis.

Heimlich maneuver, back blows. Hopkins, T., & Myers, E. (2007). *Medical surgical notes* (2nd ed., p. 168). Philadelphia, PA: F.A. Davis.

Heimlich maneuver, chest thrusts. Hopkins, T., & Myers, E. (2007). *Medical surgical notes* (2nd ed., p. 168). Philadelphia, PA: F.A. Davis.

CHAPTER 25

Figure 25-1 Jones, S. (2009). *Pocket anatomy and physiology* (1st ed., p. 12). Philadelphia, PA: F.A. Davis.

Table 25-3 Chickenpox. Courtesy of the Centers for Disease Control and Prevention.

Table 25-3 Diphtheria. Courtesy of the Centers for Disease Control and Prevention.

Table 25-3 Mumps. Courtesy of the Centers for Disease Control and Prevention.

Table 25-3 Pertussis. Courtesy of the Centers for Disease Control and Prevention.

Table 25-3 Poliomyelitis. Courtesy of the Centers for Disease Control and Prevention.

Table 25-3 Rubeola: Measles. Courtesy of the Centers for Disease Control and Prevention.

Table 25-3 Scarlet fever. Courtesy of the Centers for Disease Control and Prevention.

Table 25-3 Tetanus. Courtesy of the Centers for Disease Control and Prevention.

CHAPTER 27

Figure 27-1 Jones, S. (2009). *Pocket anatomy and physiology* (1st ed., p. 231). Philadelphia, PA: F.A. Davis. Originally from Gilroy, A. M., MacPherson, B. R., Ross, L. M., Schuenke, M., Schulte, E., & Schumacher, U. (2009). *Atlas of anatomy*. New York, NY: Thieme.

Figure 27-2 Ward, S., (2014). *Pediatric nursing care: Best evidence-based practices* (1st ed., p. 347). Philadelphia, PA: F.A. Davis.

Figure 27-3 Ward, S., (2014). *Pediatric nursing care: Best evidence-based practices* (1st ed., p. 347). Philadelphia, PA: F.A. Davis.

CHAPTER 28

Figure 28-1 Jones, S. (2009). *Pocket anatomy and physiology* (1st ed., p. 231). Philadelphia, PA: F.A. Davis. Originally from Gilroy, A. M., MacPherson, B. R., Ross, L. M., Schuenke, M., Schulte, E., & Schumacher, U. (2009). *Atlas of anatomy*. New York, NY: Thieme.

Figure 28-2 Piña-Garza, J. E., (2013) *Fenichel's clinical pediatric neurology: A signs and symptoms approach* (7th ed., p. 94). Philadelphia, PA: Elsevier Saunders.

Figure 28-3 Teasdale, G., & Jennett, B. (1974). Assessment of coma and impaired consciousness. A practical scale. *The Lancet, 2*(7872), 81–84.

Figure 28-4 Wong, J., Wong, S., & Dempster, J. K. (1984). Care of the unconscious patient: A problem-oriented approach. *American Association of Neuroscience Nurses, 16*, 145.

Figure 28-8*AB* Williams, L. S., & Hopper, P. D. (2011). *Understanding medical surgical nursing* (4th ed., p. 1134). Philadelphia, PA: F.A. Davis.

Figure 28-13 Ward, S., (2014). *Pediatric nursing care: Best evidence-based practices* (1st ed., p. 546). Philadelphia, PA: F.A. Davis.

Figure 28-16 Scanlon, V., & Sanders, T. (2007). *Essentials of anatomy and physiology* (5th ed., p. 209). Philadelphia, PA: F.A. Davis.

CHAPTER 29

Figure 29-1*A* Jones, S. (2009). *Pocket anatomy and physiology* (1st ed., p. 24). Philadelphia, PA: F.A. Davis. Originally from Gilroy, A. M., MacPherson, B. R., Ross, L. M., Schuenke, M., Schulte, E., & Schumacher, U. (2009). *Atlas of anatomy*. New York, NY: Thieme.

Figure 29-1B Jones, S. (2009). *Pocket anatomy and physiology* (1st ed., p. 25). Philadelphia, PA: F.A. Davis. Originally from Gilroy, A. M., MacPherson, B. R., Ross, L. M., Schuenke, M., Schulte, E., & Schumacher, U. (2009). *Atlas of anatomy.* New York, NY: Thieme.

CHAPTER 30

Figure 30-1 Scanlon, V., & Sanders, T. (2007). *Essentials of anatomy and physiology* (5th ed., p. 91). Philadelphia, PA: F.A. Davis.

Figure 30-3 Goldsmith, L. A., Lazarus, G. S., & Tharp, M. D. (1997). *Adult and pediatric dermatology* (p. 351). Philadelphia, PA: F.A. Davis.

Figure 30-4 Williams, L. S., & Hopper, P. D. (2007). *Understanding medical surgical nursing* (3rd ed., p. 1226). Philadelphia, PA: F.A. Davis.

Figure 30-5 Williams, L. S., & Hopper, P. D. (2007). *Understanding medical surgical nursing* (3rd ed., p. 1237). Philadelphia, PA: F.A. Davis.

Figure 30-6 Dillon, P. (2007). *Nursing health assessment: A critical thinking, case studies approach* (2nd ed., p. 297). Philadelphia, PA: F.A. Davis.

Figure 30-8 Dillon, P. (2007). *Nursing health assessment: A critical thinking, case studies approach* (2nd ed., p. 241). Philadelphia, PA: F.A. Davis.

Figure 30-9 Dillon, P. (2007). *Nursing health assessment: A critical thinking, case studies approach* (2nd ed., p. 246). Philadelphia, PA: F.A. Davis.

Figure 30-11A Trofino, R. B. (1991). *Nursing care of the burn-injured patient*, plate 1, Philadelphia, PA: F.A. Davis.

Figure 30-11B Trofino, R. B. (1991). *Nursing care of the burn-injured patient*, plate 2, Philadelphia, PA: F.A. Davis.

Figure 30-11C Trofino, R. B. (1991). *Nursing care of the burn-injured patient*, plate 3, Philadelphia, PA: F.A. Davis.

Figure 30-13A–D Dillon, P. (2007). *Nursing health assessment: A critical thinking, case studies approach* (2nd ed., p. 237). Philadelphia, PA: F.A. Davis.

CHAPTER 31

Figure 31-1 Scanlon, V., & Sanders, T. (2015). *Essentials of anatomy and physiology* (7th ed., p. 464). Philadelphia, PA: F.A. Davis.

CHAPTER 32

Figure 32-1 Jones, S. (2009). *Pocket anatomy and physiology* (1st ed., p. 197). Philadelphia, PA: F.A. Davis. Originally from Gilroy, A. M., MacPherson, B. R., Ross, L. M., Schuenke, M., Schulte, E., & Schumacher, U. (2009). *Atlas of anatomy.* New York, NY: Thieme.

Figure 32-2 Harmening, D. L. (2009). *Clinical hematology and fundamentals of hemostasis* (5th ed., p. 211). Philadelphia, PA: F.A. Davis. From Bell, A., Hematology. In *Listen, look and learn.* Health Education Resources, Inc., Bethesda, MD.

CHAPTER 33

Figure 33-1 Jones, S. (2009). *Pocket anatomy and physiology* (1st ed., p. 12). Philadelphia, PA: F.A. Davis.

Figure 33-3 Harmening, D. L. (1997). *Clinical hematology and fundamentals of hemostasis* (3rd ed., p. 176). Philadelphia, PA: F.A. Davis.

Figure 33-5 Harmening, D. L. (1997). *Clinical hematology and fundamentals of hemostasis* (3rd ed., p. 176). Philadelphia, PA: F.A. Davis.

Figure 33-6 McKinnis, L. N. (2005). *Fundamentals of musculoskeletal imaging* (2nd ed., p. 56). Philadelphia, PA: F.A. Davis.

Figure 33-7 McKinnis, L. N. (2005). *Fundamentals of musculoskeletal imaging* (2nd ed., p. 76). Philadelphia, PA: F.A. Davis.

Figure 33-12 Miami Children's Hospital, Miami, FL.

CHAPTER 34

Figure 34-2 Harmening, D. L. (1997). *Clinical hematology and fundamentals of hemostasis* (3rd ed., p. 176). Philadelphia, PA: F.A. Davis.

Figure 34-3 Harmening, D. L. (1997). *Clinical hematology and fundamentals of hemostasis* (3rd ed., p. 176). Philadelphia, PA: F.A. Davis.

Figure 34-5 McKinnis, L. N. (2005). *Fundamentals of musculoskeletal imaging* (2nd ed., p. 56). Philadelphia, PA: F.A. Davis.

Figure 34-6 McKinnis, L. N. (2005). *Fundamentals of musculoskeletal imaging* (2nd ed., p. 76). Philadelphia, PA: F.A. Davis.

CHAPTER 35

Figure 35-1AB University of Nebraska Medical Center.
Figure 35-2AB University of Nebraska Medical Center.
Figure 35-3 University of Nebraska Medical Center.
Figure 35-4AB University of Nebraska Medical Center.
Figure 35-6 Lewis, S., Dirksen, S., Heitkemper, M., Bucher, L., & Camera, I. (2011). *Medical-surgical nursing: Assessment and management of clinical problems* (7th ed., p. 1687). Maryland Heights, MO: Elsevier Mosby.

Figure 35-7 Lewis, S., Dirksen, S., Heitkemper, M., Bucher, L., & Camera, I. (2011). *Medical-surgical nursing: Assessment and management of clinical problems* (7th ed., p. 1689). Maryland Heights, MO: Elsevier Mosby.

The Richmond Agitation Sedation Score. Ely, E. W., Gautam, S., May, L., Truman, B., Francis, J., Margolin, R., et al. (2001). A comparison of different sedation scales in the ICU and validation of the Richmond Agitation Sedation Scale (RASS) [abstract]. *American Journal of Respiratory and Critical Care Medicine, 163,* A954.

Index

Note: The letter b indicates a boxed feature on the page. The letter f indicates a figure. The letter t indicates a table.

A

A & B spells, 731
A & P (anatomy and physiology) review
  breasts, lactation and, 558–560f
  endocrine system, 1061f, 1062t–1064t, 1065f
  epidural space, 494, 495f
  fetal circulation, 199–200f, 709
  fetal skull, 415, 417f
  gastrointestinal system, 921–922f
  heart, 1019f–1021, 1020f
  hematological system, 1315f
  immune system, 971f–972
  integumentary system, 1205f
  kidneys, 1260f
  menstrual cycle, 143f, 144f
  musculoskeletal system, 1162f–1163f
  nervous system, 1114f
  neurological system, 709
  newborn at risk, 708–709f
  oogenesis, 135f
  pregnancy hormones, 223f
  primary germ layer, formation of, 196f, 197f, 199f, 201
  respiratory function, newborn, 708–709
  respiratory function, normal, 639–640
  respiratory system, 874–875f
  spermatogenesis, 150f, 151
  tumor progression, 1353f
Abarelis, 180t
Abdomen
  abdominal pain in children, 927
  acute abdomen in the neonate, 686
  cesarean birth procedure and care, 539f–542, 540f, 541f
  children, assessment of, 801f–802
  circumference measures, neonates, 673f
  congenital diaphragmatic hernia, 923
  cultural diversity, 804t
  gastroschisis and omphalocele, 744f–745
  inguinal hernia, 924
  Leopold maneuvers, 270–272
  maternal postpartum adaptations, 570–571f
  neonatal assessment, 684–686, 685f
  pain in, 321, 949
  premature newborn assessment, 729t
  prenatal physical examination, 270
  quadrants of, 801f
  scaphoid abdomen, 717
  trauma, injuries from, 963t–964t
Abdominal aorta, neonatal circulation, 643f
Abdominal muscles, postpartum exercises, 595f
Abdominal rectus, 570–571f, 875f
Abdominal tuberculosis, 901–903f
Abducens nerve, 803t
Abduction, safety measures, 555f–556
Ablation, 117
Abortion, 176–178, 201
Abortion, spontaneous. See Miscarriage
Abortus, 340
Abraham's Balm, 183
Abruptio placentae, 322, 345bf–346b, 527t, 528, 530–531
Absolute neutrophil count (ANC), 1338, 1379
Abstinence, 164
Abuse
  abusive head trauma, 1141–1142
  adolescents, safety guidance for, 99–100
  child abuse, overview, 853–855, 854t
  evidence-based practices, 30
  family, effect on, 74
  postpartum care for victims of, 631t–632
  SATELLITE Sexual Violence Assessment, 254

signs of, 274
trends in, 36, 42
Access to care
  advocacy about, 20
  children's health insurance, 809
  disparities in, 34–35
  health trends, 38
  health-care settings, 9–10
  language and cultural barriers, 12
  medical homes, 49
  medication costs, 1075
  mental health care, 843–844
  neighborhood deprivation, 717
  postpartum care, 632–633
  prenatal care, 248
  primary care settings, overview of, 832–835
  reasons for accessing care, 812–814
  rural and nonrural care, 787
  vulnerable populations, 41–44
Accessory nerve, 803t
Accessory nipples, 682
Accidents, 36, 97–98b, 399. See also Injuries; Trauma
Acculturation, 76
Accutane, 316, 1213
ACE wrap, 1196
Acesulfame potassium, 301
Acetaminophen, 813–814t, 823
ACHES, oral contraceptive pill symptoms, 169
Achilles tendon, clubfoot correction, 1166
Achondroplasia. See Dwarfism
Acidemia, 445
Acidosis, 445, 670, 724t, 1105–1107
Acme, uterine contractions, 413, 414f
Acne, 676, 1208t, 1211f–1213, 1214t–1215t
Acoustic nerve, 803t
Acoustic stimulation, 396
Acquired growth hormone deficiency, 1065–1067f, 1073t–1074
Acrocyanosis, 463t, 642, 665, 666b, 670f–671, 675
Acromegaly, 1075–1077
Acromion process, 421f–422
Active acquired immunity, 656
Active phase, labor, 431–433f, 432t
Active transport, 198
Activity. See also Exercise
  neonatal physiologic transition, 657–659
  postpartum care, 572
Actonel, 119
Acupressure and acupuncture, 302, 484–485
Acute abdomen, 686
Acute epiglottitis, 892–893
Acute glomerulonephritis, 889
Acute hemolytic transfusion reaction, 1344
Acute intracranial hemorrhage (ICH), 736b–737
Acute kidney injury (AKI), 1281–1286t, 1282t, 1283t, 1284t, 1285t
Acute lymphocytic leukemia (ALL), 1355f–1358, 1356ft, 1357f
Acute myelogenous leukemia, 1355f, 1357–1359, 1358f
Acute pyelonephritis, 364–365
Acute respiratory distress syndrome (ARDS), 799–800, 881–883
Acyclovir, 1000
Adam's position, 1185f
Adaptive devices, 1388f
Adaptive immunity, 972
Addiction, 61, 73–74, 390–391, 855–857, 856t
Addisonian crisis, 1088
Addison's disease, 1087–1089

Adenocarcinoma, 108–109
Adenovirus, 888–890, 898–900
Adhesions, tissue, 538
Adhesives, warts and, 1220
Adipose tissue, 141f–142, 794, 1205f
Adjuvant therapies, breast cancer, 114
Admissions data, labor, 427
Adnexa, 134
Adolescents. See also Children, health assessment
  acne, 1211f–1213, 1214t–1215t
  adolescent mothers and infant bonding, 590–591
  blood tests, normal values, 1318, 1319t
  breast development, 141f–142
  childhood obesity and, 31f–32
  chronic conditions, impact of, 1392–1393
  common injuries, 812–813t
  daily fluid requirement, 1261
  dental care, 96–97
  depo-provera, bone health and, 172–173
  developmental milestones, 780–783b, 781t, 782f
  developmental tasks of, 94b
  diet and nutrition, 93–96, 95f
  fatty liver, 921
  gynecological examination, 101–105f, 103t, 104f
  health promotion and screening, 82, 83t–84t, 85b
  health trends, 37
  hospitalization, stress of, 817t
  immunizations, 92, 93f–94f
  informed consent and, 782
  intimate partner violence and, 401
  juvenile arthritis, 1180–1181
  menstrual disorders, 105–106
  mental health care, access to, 843–844
  nutrition guidance, 1172t
  oral contraceptives and, 169
  pain management, 808t–809t
  play and, 92t
  pregnancy
    complications of, 398
    developmental tasks, 239, 281
    entry into care, 281–282
    expectant fathers, 283–284
    nursing care of, 282–283
    postpartum care, 597
    risks for and prevention of, 278–281, 279t, 280b
  procedures, preparation for, 824
  puberty, 144–145t, 146f
  renal transplants, 1258–1259
  reproductive health care, legal issues, 160
  safety issues, guidance for, 97–100, 98b, 833
  sexuality, guidance on, 92, 167
  sickle cell disease, 1314
  skin cancer, 100–101
  skin development, 1206t
  sleep and rest, 97, 860–861b
  smoking tobacco, 281
  violence against, 30
  vital signs, 794ft–795
Adoption, maternal support, 597–598
Adrenal crisis, 1086–1087
Adrenal glands
  adrenal crisis, 1086–1087
  adrenocortical insufficiency, chronic, 1087–1092
  congenital adrenal hyperplasia, 687, 1090–1092
  Cushing's syndrome, 1089–1090
  endocrine conditions, laboratory tests, 1067t, 1068t